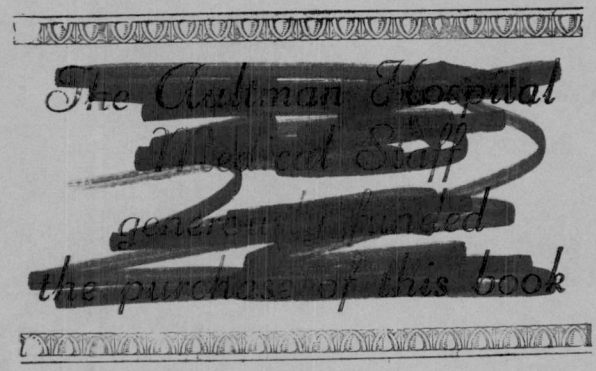

Miller's Anesthesia

SIXTH EDITION

Volume **1**

Miller's Anesthesia

SIXTH EDITION

Volume
1

Edited by

Ronald D. Miller, M.D.

Professor and Chair, Department of Anesthesia and Perioperative Care
Professor of Cellular and Molecular Pharmacology
University of California, San Francisco
School of Medicine
San Francisco, California

Atlas of Regional Anesthesia Procedures illustrated by

Gwenn Afton-Bird, M.S.

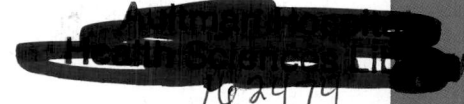

ELSEVIER
CHURCHILL
LIVINGSTONE

ELSEVIER
CHURCHILL
LIVINGSTONE

The Curtis Center
170 S Independence Mall W 300E
Philadelphia, Pennsylvania 19106

MILLER'S ANESTHESIA

ISBN 0-443-06618-3 (set)
9997629035 (Vol. 1)
9997629043 (Vol. 2)
Indian Edition ISBN 0-8089-2338-2 (set)
9996006611 (Vol. 1)
9996006670 (Vol. 2)
e-dition ISBN 0-443-06656-6

Distributed in the United Kingdom by Churchill Livingstone, Robert Stevenson House, 1-3 Baxter's Place, Leith Walk, Edinburgh EH1 3AF, Scotland, and by associated companies, branches, and representatives throughout the world.

Library of Congress Cataloging-in-Publication Data
Anesthesia / [edited by] Ronald D. Miller ; atlas of regional anesthesia procedures
   illustrated by Gwenn Afton-Bird.–6th ed.
      p. ; cm.
   Includes bibliographical references and index.
   ISBN 0-443-06618-3 (set)
   1. Anesthesia–Atlases. I. Miller, Ronald D.
   [DNLM: 1. Anesthesia. 2. Anesthesiology–methods. 3. Anesthetics–therapeutic use.
WO 200 A573 2005]
RD81.A54 2005
617.9'6–dc22

2003055832

Publisher: Natasha Andjelkovic
Senior Developmental Editor: Ann Ruzycka Anderson
Publishing Services Manager: Tina Rebane
Project Managers: Jodi Kaye and Mary Anne Folcher
Design Manager: Steven Stave

Printed in The United States of America

Last digit is the print number: 9   8   7   6   5   4   3   2   1

Contributors

J. Jeff Andrews, M.D.
Professor and Vice Chair for Education, Department of Anesthesiology, University of Alabama School of Medicine, University of Alabama at Birmingham, Birmingham, Alabama

Michael K. Ang-Lee, M.D.
Staff Anesthesiologist, Western Washington Medical Group, Providence Everett Medical Center, Everett, Washington

William P. Arnold III, M.D.
Associate Professor of Anesthesiology, University of Virginia School of Medicine, Charlottesville, Virginia

Solomon Aronson, M.D.
Glencoe, Illinois

David J. Baker, D.M.
Department of Anesthesiology and Critical Care, SAMU de Paris, Hôspital Necker-Enfants Malades, Paris, France

James Baker, M.D.
Assistant Clinical Professor, Department of Anesthesiology and Perioperative Care, University of California, San Francisco, San Francisco, California

Steven J. Barker, M.D.
Professor and Head, Department of Anesthesiology, University of Arizona College of Medicine, Tucson, Arizona

Perry S. Bechtle, D.O.
Professor, Department of Anesthesiology, Mayo Clinic College of Medicine, Rochester, Minnesota; Consultant in Anesthesia, Mayo Clinic, Jacksonville, Florida

James D. Beckman, M.D.
Assistant Clinical Professor, Department of Anesthesiology, Weill Medical College of Cornell University; Attending Anesthesiologist, Hospital for Special Surgery, New York, New York

Jonathan L. Benumof, M.D.
Professor, Department of Anesthesiology, University of California, San Diego, School of Medicine, San Diego, California

Charles B. Berde, M.D., Ph.D.
Professor, Department of Anesthesia (Pediatrics), Harvard Medical School; Chief, Division of Pain Medicine, Department of Anesthesiology, Perioperative and Pain Medicine, Children's Hospital, Boston, Massachusetts

Sean M. Berenholtz, M.D.
Assistant Professor, Department of Anesthesiology and Critical Care Medicine, Johns Hopkins University School of Medicine, Baltimore, Maryland

David J. Birnbach, M.D.
Professor, Department of Anesthesiology and Obstetrics and Gynecology; Associate Director, Institute for Women, University of Miami School of Medicine; Chief, Women's Anesthesia, Jackson Memorial Medical Center, Miami, Florida

Susan Black, M.D.
Professor, Department of Anesthesiology, University of Alabama School of Medicine, University of Alabama at Birmingham, Birmingham, Alabama

Russell C. Brockwell, M.D.
Associate Professor, Department of Anesthesiology, University of Alabama at Birmingham, School of Medicine; Chief of Anesthesiology, Department of Veterans Affairs, Birmingham Veterans Affairs Medical Center, Birmingham, Alabama

David L. Brown, M.D.
Professor and Head, Department of Anesthesia, University of Iowa Carver College of Medicine, Iowa City, Iowa

Ingrid M. Browne, M.D.
Visiting Assistant Professor, University of Miami School of Medicine, Miami, Florida

Michael K. Cahalan, M.D.
Professor and Chair, Department of Anesthesiology, University of Utah School of Medicine, Salt Lake City, Utah

Enrico M. Camporesi, M.D.
Professor and Chairman, Department of Anesthesiology, State University of New York Upstate Medical University; Attending Anesthesiologist and Director, Hyperbaric Treatment Unit, University Hospital; Attending Anesthesiologist, Veterans Affairs Medical Center; Consultant, Crouse Hospital, Syracuse, New York; Attending Anesthesiologist, Specialty Surgery Center, Liverpool, New York

Charles J. Coté, M.D.
Professor, Departments of Anesthesiology and Pediatrics, Northwestern University Feinberg School of Medicine; Vice Chairman, Director of Research, Department of Pediatric Anesthesiology, Children's Memorial Hospital, Chicago, Illinois

Roy F. Cucchiara, M.D.
Professor, Department of Anesthesiology, Mayo Clinic College of Medicine, Rochester, Minnesota; Consultant and Professor, Mayo Clinic, Jacksonville, Florida

Bernard J. Dalens, M.D.
Associate Professor, Department of Anesthesia, Laval University, Quebec City; Anesthesiologist, Center Hospitalier Universitaire de Quebec, Sainte Foy, Quebec, Canada

Brian M. Daniel, R.R.T.
Adult Clinical Team Leader, Department of Respiratory Care, University of California, San Francisco, San Francisco, California

Clifford S. Deutschman, M.S., M.D.
Professor, Departments of Anesthesia and Surgery, University of Pennsylvania; Director, Fellowship in Critical Care; Director, Fellowship in Anesthesia/ Critical Care Research; and Attending Physician, Surgical Critical Care Service, Hospital of the University of Pennsylvania, Philadelphia, Pennsylvania

Sudhir Diwan, M.D., M.S.
Director, Quad-Institutional Pain Fellowship, Department of Anesthesiology, Weill Medical College of Cornell University, New York, New York

John V. Donlon, Jr., M.D.
Staff Anesthesiologist, North Shore Cataract and Laser Center, Stoneham, Massachusetts

D. John Doyle, M.D., Ph.D.
Staff Anesthesiologist, Department of General Anesthesiology, Cleveland Clinic Foundation, Cleveland, Ohio

John C. Drummond, M.D.
Professor and Chair, Department of Anesthesiology, University of California, San Diego, School of Medicine, San Diego, California

Richard P. Dutton, M.D., M.B.A.
Associate Professor, Department of Anesthesiology, University of Maryland School of Medicine; Director of Trauma Anesthesiology, R. Adams Cowley Shock Trauma Center, University of Maryland Medical System, Baltimore, Maryland

Edmond I. Eger II, M.D.
Professor, Department of Anesthesia and Perioperative Care, University of California, San Francisco, San Francisco, California

Neil E. Farber, M.D., Ph.D.
Associate Professor, Departments of Anesthesiology, Pediatrics, Pharmacology, and Toxicology, Medical College of Wisconsin; Director, Pediatric Anesthesia Research, Children's Hospital of Wisconsin, Milwaukee, Wisconsin

Ronald J. Faust, M.D.
Professor, Department of Anesthesiology, Mayo Clinic College of Medicine; Consultant in Anesthesiology, Mayo Clinic, Rochester, Minnesota

Thomas W. Feeley, M.D.
Helen Shafer Fly Distinguished Professor of Anesthesiology and Head, Division of Anesthesiology and Critical Care, University of Texas M.D. Anderson Cancer Center, Houston, Texas

Marc Allan Feldman, M.D., M.H.S.
Head, Section of Anesthesia, Cole Eye Institute, The Cleveland Clinic Foundation, Cleveland, Ohio

Lee A. Fleisher, M.D.
Robert Dunning Dripps Professor and Chair of Anesthesia, Professor of Medicine, University of Pennsylvania School of Medicine, Philadelphia, Pennsylvania

Alejandro Recart Freire, M.D.
Staff Anesthesiologist, Padre Hurtado General Hospital, Santiago de Chile, Chile

Kazuhiko Fukuda, M.D.
Department of Anesthesia, Kyoto University Hospital, Kyoto, Japan

David M. Gaba, M.D.
Associate Dean for Immersive and Simulation-Based Learning and Professor of Anesthesia, Stanford University School of Medicine; Director, Patient Simulation Center of Innovation, VA Palo Alto Health Care System, Palo Alto, California

Thomas J. Gal, M.D.
Professor, Department of Anesthesiology, University of Virginia; Attending Anesthesiologist, University of Virginia Health Systems, Charlottesville, Virginia

Simon Gelman, M.D., Ph.D.
Professor and Chairman Emeritus, Department of Anesthesiology, Brigham and Women's Hospital, Harvard Medical School, Boston, Massachusetts

Peter S. A. Glass, M.B., Ch.B.
Professor and Chairman, Department of Anesthesiology, State University of New York at Stony Brook; Anesthesiologist-in-Chief, University Hospital at State University of New York at Stony Brook, Stony Brook, New York

David Glick, M.D., M.B.A.
Assistant Professor, Department of Anesthesia and Critical Care, University of Chicago; Medical Director, Postanesthesia Care Unit, University of Chicago Hospitals, Chicago, Illinois

Lawrence T. Goodnough, M.D.
Professor of Medicine and Pathology and Immunology, Department of Pathology, Washington University School of Medicine; Director of the Blood Bank, Barnes-Jewish Hospital, St. Louis, Missouri

Mark T. Grabovac, M.D.
Assistant Clinical Professor, Department of Anesthesiology and Critical Care Medicine, University of California, San Francisco, San Francisco, California

William J. Greeley, M.D., M.B.A.
Professor of Anesthesia and Pediatrics, University of Pennsylvania School of Medicine; Chair and Anesthesiologist-in-Chief, Department of Anesthesiology and Critical Care Medicine, The Children's Hospital of Philadelphia, Philadelphia, Pennsylvania

George A. Gregory, M.D.
Professor Emeritus, Department of Anesthesiology and Pediatrics, University of California, San Francisco, School of Medicine, San Francisco, California

Gerald A. Gronert, B.S., M.D.
Professor Emeritus, Department of Anesthesiology, University of California, Davis, School of Medicine, Davis, California

Michael A. Gropper, M.D., Ph.D.
Professor, Departments of Anesthesia and Physiology, University of California, San Francisco; Director, Critical Care Medicine, University of California, San Francisco, San Francisco, California

Raymond Hernandez, B.A., R.R.T.
Department of Respiratory Care, University of California, San Francisco, San Francisco, California

Zaharia Hillel, M.D.
Professor, Department of Anesthesiology, Columbia University College of Physicians and Surgeons; Director, Cardiac Anesthesia, St. Luke's–Roosevelt Hospital Center, New York, New York

Terese T. Horlocker, M.D.
Professor, Department of Anesthesiology, Mayo Clinic College of Medicine, Rochester, Minnesota

Eileen Connolly Inda, B.A., M.D.
Attending Anesthesiologist, Boys Town National Research Hospital, Omaha, Nebraska

Roger A. Johns, M.D.
Professor, Department of Anesthesiology and Critical Care Medicine, The Johns Hopkins University School of Medicine; Consultant, The Johns Hopkins Hospital, Baltimore, Maryland

Jean L. Joris, M.D., Ph.D.
Professor Department of Anesthesia and Intensive Care Medicine, University of Liège; Head, Department of Anesthesia and Intensive Care Medicine, Centre Hospitalier Universitaire de Liege, Liege, Belgium

Alan D. Kaye, M.D., Ph.D.
Professor and Chairman and Program Director, Department of Anesthesiology, and Professor, Department of Pharmacology, Texas Tech University Health Sciences Center, Lubbock, Texas

Judy R. Kersten, M.D.
Professor, Departments of Anesthesiology, Pharmacology, and Toxicology, Medical College of Wisconsin, Milwaukee, Wisconsin

Kevin K. Kim, M.D.
Department of Anesthesia and Perioperative Care, University of California, San Francisco, San Francisco, California

James Kindscher, M.D.
Professor and Vice Chair, Department of Anesthesiology, Kansas University School of Medicine; Medical Director, Operating Rooms, Kansas University Medical Center, Kansas City, Kansas

Donald D. Koblin, M.D., Ph.D.
Professor, Department of Anesthesia and Perioperative Care, University of California, San Francisco, School of Medicine; Staff Anesthesiologist, Veterans Affairs Medical Center, San Francisco, California

W. Daniel Kovarik, M.D.
Clinical Associate Professor, Department of Anesthesiology, University of Vermont School of Medicine, Burlington, Vermont; Director of Pediatric Anesthesiology, Maine Medical Center, Portland, Maine

Ian J. Kucera, Pharm.D., M.D.
Assistant Professor of Anesthesiology, Texas Tech University Health Sciences Center, Lubbock, Texas

Merlin D. Larson, M.D.
Clinical Professor, Department of Anesthesia and
Perioperative Care, and Clinical Professor, Moffitt-Long
Hospitals, University of California, San Francisco,
San Francisco, California

Cynthia A. Lien, M.D.
Professor of Clinical Anesthesiology, Weill Medical
College of Cornell University; Attending
Anesthesiologist, New York Presbyterian Hospital,
New York, New York

Lawrence Litt, M.D., Ph.D.
Professor, Department of Anesthesia and Perioperative
Care, University of California, San Francisco;
Attending Anesthesiologist, University of California,
San Francisco Affiliated Hospitals, San Francisco,
California

Linda L. Liu, M.D.
Associate Professor of Clinical Anesthesia, Department
of Anesthesia and Perioperative Care, University
of California, San Francisco, School of Medicine,
San Francisco, California

David A. Lubarsky, M.D., M.B.A.
Emanuel M. Papper Professor and Chair, Department
of Anesthesiology, Perioperative Medicine and Pain
Management, University of Miami School of
Medicine, and Professor, Department of
Management, University of Miami School of
Business; Chief of Staff, Jackson Health System,
Miami, Florida

Alex Macario, M.D., M.B.A.
Associate Professor of Anesthesiology and Health
Research and Policy, Stanford University School of
Medicine; Director, Fellowship in Management of
Perioperative Services, Department of Anesthesia,
Stanford University Medical Center, Stanford,
California

Michael E. Mahla, M.D.
Professor, Departments of Anesthesiology and
Neurosurgery, University of Florida College of
Medicine; Anesthesiology Residency Program
Director, Shands Hospital at the University of Florida,
Gainesville, Florida

Vinod Malhotra, M.D.
Department of Anesthesiology, New York Presbyterian
Hospital–Weill Cornell Medical Center, New York,
New York

Jonathan B. Mark, M.D.
Professor and Vice Chairman, Department of
Anesthesiology, Duke University School of
Medicine; Chief, Anesthesiology Service,
Veterans Affairs Medical Center, Durham,
North Carolina

Jackie L. Martin, Jr., M.D.
Associate Professor, Division of Cardiac Anesthesiology,
Department of Anesthesiology and Critical Care
Medicine, Johns Hopkins University School of
Medicine, Baltimore, Maryland

J. A. Jeevendra Martyn, M.D.
Professor, Department of Anesthesiology, Harvard
Medical School; Anesthetist and Director, Clinical
and Biochemical Pharmacology Laboratory,
Massachusetts General Hospital; Anesthetist-in-Chief,
Shriners Hospital for Children, Boston, Massachusetts

Maureen McCunn, M.D.
Assistant Professor, Department of Anesthesiology and
Critical Care, University of Maryland School of Medicine;
Medical Director of Neurotrauma Critical Care and
Physician Director of Continuous Renal Replacement
Therapies, R. Adams Cowley Shock Trauma Center,
University of Maryland Medical System, Baltimore,
Maryland

Matthew D. McEvoy, M.D.
Resident, Department of Anesthesiology, Medical
University of South Carolina College of Medicine,
Charleston, South Carolina

Brian P. McGlinch, M.D.
Assistant Professor of Anesthesiology, Mayo Clinic
College of Medicine, Rochester, Minnesota

Berend Mets, M.B., Ch.B., Ph.D.
Eric A. Walker Professor and Chair, Department of
Anesthesiology, Pennsylvania State University College
of Medicine, Milton S. Hershey Medical Center,
Hershey, Pennsylvania

Ronald D. Miller, M.D.
Professor and Chair, Department of Anesthesia and
Perioperative Care, Professor of Cellular and Molecular
Pharmacology, University of California, San Francisco,
School of Medicine, San Francisco, California

Jørgen Viby Mogensen, M.D.
Professor, Department of Anaesthesia, Copenhagen
University Hospital, Rigshospitalet, Copenhagen,
Denmark

Terri G. Monk, M.D.
Professor, Department of Anesthesiology, Duke
University School of Medicine; Anesthesiologist,
Duke University Medical Center and Veterans Affairs
Medical Center, Durham, North Carolina

Richard E. Moon, B.Sc., M.D., C.M., M.Sc.
Professor of Anesthesiology, Associate Professor of
Medicine, Departments of Anesthesiology and
Medicine, and Attending Anesthesiologist and
Pulmonologist, and Medical Director, Center for
Hyperbaric Medicine and Environmental Physiology,
Duke University Medical Center, Durham,
North Carolina

Kenjiro Mori, M.D.
Department of Anesthesia, Takamatsu Red Cross
  Hospital, Takamatsu, Japan

Jonathan Moss, M.D., Ph.D.
Professor of the College, The University of Chicago,
  Pritzker School of Medicine; Professor and Vice
  Chairman for Research, Department of Anesthesia
  and Critical Care, The University of Chicago
  Hospitals, Chicago, Illinois

Sheila M. Muldoon, M.D.
Professor, Department of Anesthesiology, Uniformed
  Services University of the Health Sciences, Bethesda,
  Maryland

Phillip S. Mushlin, M.D., Ph.D.
Vice Chairman, Faculty Development and Education,
  and Anesthesiologist, Brigham and Women's
  Hospital, Department of Anesthesiology,
  Perioperative and Pain Medicine, Boston,
  Massachusetts

Mohamed Naguib, M.B., B.Ch., M.Sc., M.D.
Professor of Anesthesia, University of Iowa; Professor,
  University of Iowa Health Care, Roy J. and Lucille A.
  Carver College of Medicine, Iowa City, Iowa

Shinichi Nakao, M.D.
Department of Anesthesiology, Kansai Medical
  University, Osaka, Japan

Patrick J. Neligan, M.A., M.B., B.Ch.
Assistant Professor, Department of Anesthesia,
  University of Pennsylvania; Attending Physician,
  Surgical Critical Care Service, Hospital of the
  University of Pennsylvania, Philadelphia,
  Pennsylvania

Dorre Nicholau, M.D., Ph.D.
Clinical Professor, Department of Anesthesia and
  Perioperative Care, University of California,
  San Francisco, San Francisco, California

Susan C. Nicolson, M.D.
Professor of Anesthesia, University of Pennsylvania,
  Director, School of Medicine; Director, Division of
  Cardiothoracic Anesthesia, and Attending
  Anesthesiologist, Department of Anesthesiology and
  Critical Care Medicine, The Children's Hospital of
  Philadelphia, Philadelphia, Pennsylvania

Claus U. Niemann, M.D.
Assistant Professor in Residence, Department of
  Anesthesia and Perioperative Care, University
  of California, San Francisco, School of Medicine,
  San Francisco, California

Ervant V. Nishanian, M.D., Ph.D.
Assistant Professor and Director of Cardiothoracic
  Anesthesiology, Columbia University College of
  Physicians and Surgeons, New York, New York

Edward J. Norris, M.D., M.B.A.
Associate Professor, Department of Anesthesiology and
  Critical Care Medicine, The Johns Hopkins Medical
  Institutions; Director, Vascular and Endovascular
  Anesthesia, The Johns Hopkins Hospital, Baltimore,
  Maryland

Daniel Nyhan, B.Sc., M.B., M.D.
Professor, Department of Anesthesia, The Johns Hopkins
  University School of Medicine; Chief, Cardiac
  Anesthesia, The Johns Hopkins Hospital, Baltimore,
  Maryland

Christopher J. O'Connor, M.D.
Associate Professor of Anesthesiology, Rush Medical
  College; Director, Cardiothoracic Anesthesia, Rush
  University Medical Center, Chicago, Illinois

Fredrick K. Orkin, M.D., M.B.A., M.Sc.
Professor of Anesthesiology and Health Evaluation
  Sciences, Department of Anesthesiology,
  Pennsylvania State University College of
  Medicine; Anesthesiologist, Milton S. Hershey
  Medical Center, Hershey, Pennsylvania

Paul S. Pagel, M.D., Ph.D.
Director, Cardiac Anesthesia, and Professor,
  Department of Anesthesiology, Medical College
  of Wisconsin; Professor of Biomedical Engineering,
  Marquette University, Milwaukee, Wisconsin

Piyush M. Patel, M.D.
Professor, Department of Anesthesia, University of
  California, San Diego; Staff Anesthesiologist, Veterans
  Affairs Medical Center, San Diego, California

Ronald Pauldine, M.D.
Assistant Professor, Department of Anesthesia and
  Critical Care Medicine, Johns Hopkins University
  School of Medicine; Staff, John Hopkins Bayview
  Medical Center, Baltimore, Maryland

Isaac N. Pessah, Ph.D.
Professor, Department of Molecular Biosciences;
  Director, Center for Children's Environmental Health
  and Disease Prevention, University of California,
  Davis, Davis, California

Peter J. Pronovost, M.D., Ph.D.
Associate Professor, Departments of Anesthesiology and
  Critical Care Medicine and Surgery, Johns Hopkins
  University School of Medicine, School of Public
  Health, and School of Nursing; Medical Director,
  Center for Innovations in Quality Patient Care,
  Johns Hopkins Medical Institutions, Baltimore,
  Maryland

Thomas E. Quinn, M.D.
Clinical Fellow, Department of Critical Care Medicine,
  University of California, San Francisco, San Francisco,
  California

Marcus Rall, M.D.
Director, Center for Patient Safety and Simulation
TuPASS, Department of Anesthesiology and Intensive
Care Medicine, University of Tuebingen Medical
School and University Hospital, Tuebingen, Germany

Ira J. Rampil, M.S., M.D.
Professor of Anesthesiology and Neurological Surgery
and Director of Clinical Research, State University of
New York at Stony Brook, Stony Brook, New York

J. G. Reves, M.D.
Vice President for Medical Affairs and Dean, Medical
University of South Carolina School of Medicine,
Charleston, South Carolina

Michael F. Roizen, M.D.
Professor, Departments of Anesthesiology and Medicine,
State University of New York Upstate Medical University;
President, CNY Biotechnology Corporation, Syracuse,
New York

Stanley H. Rosenbaum, M.D.
Professor of Anesthesiology, Internal Medicine, and
Surgery and Vice Chairman for Academic Affairs,
Department of Anesthesiology, Yale University School
of Medicine, New Haven, Connecticut

Steven Roth, M.D.
Associate Professor of Anesthesia and Critical Care and
Chief, Department of Neuroanesthesia, University
of Chicago, Chicago, Illinois

David M. Rothenberg, M.D.
Professor, Department of Anesthesiology, and Associate
Dean, Rush Medical College; Medical Director,
Surgical Intensive Care Unit, Rush University Medical
Center, Chicago, Illinois

John C. Rowlingson, M.D.
Professor of Anesthesiology and Director of Pain
Medicine Service, Department of Anesthesiology,
University of Virginia School of Medicine,
Charlottesville, Virginia

Marc A. Rozner, M.D., Ph.D.
Associate Professor, Departments of Anesthesiology
and Cardiology, University of Texas M.D. Anderson
Cancer Center; Adjunct Assistant Professor,
Department of Integrative Biology and
Pharmacology, University of Texas-Houston
Health Science Center; Associate Anesthesiologist,
University of Texas M.D. Anderson Cancer Center,
Houston, Texas

John J. Savarese, M.D.
Joseph F. Artusio, Jr. Professor and Chairman,
Department of Anesthesiology, Weill Medical College
of Cornell University; Anesthesiologist-in-Chief,
Department of Anesthesia, New York Presbyterian
Hospital, New York, New York

Alan J. Schwartz, M.D., M.Ed.
Clinical Professor of Anesthesia, University of
Pennsylvania School of Medicine; Director of
Education and Program Director, Pediatric
Anesthesiology Residency, Department of
Anesthesiology and Critical Care Medicine, The
Children's Hospital of Philadelphia, Philadelphia,
Pennsylvania

Johanna Schwarzenberger, M.D.
Assistant Professor of Anesthesiology, Division of
Pediatric Anesthesiology, Columbia University College
of Physicians and Surgeons, New York, New York

Debra A. Schwinn, B.S., M.D.
James B. Duke Professor of Anesthesiology, Professor
of Pharmacology and Cancer Biology, Professor of
Surgery, Vice Chairman for Research, and Director of
Molecular Pharmacology Laboratory and Perioperative
Genomics, Department of Anesthesiology, Duke
University Medical Center, Durham, North Carolina

Daniel I. Sessler, M.D.
Professor of Anesthesiology and Pharmacology,
Vice Dean for Research, Associate Vice President for
Health Affairs, Director of Outcomes Research
Institute, and Lolita and Samuel Weakley
Distinguished University Chair, University of
Louisville, Louisville, Kentucky

Steven L. Shafer, M.D.
Professor, Department of Anesthesia, Stanford
University School of Medicine, Stanford, California;
Adjunct Professor of Biopharmaceutical Science,
University of California, San Francisco, San Francisco,
California; Staff Anesthesiologist, VA Palo Alto Health
Care System, Palo Alto, California

Nigel E. Sharrock, M.B., Ch.B.
Assistant Clinical Professor of Anesthesia, Weill Medical
College of Cornell University; Attending
Anesthesiologist, Department of Anesthesiology,
Hospital for Special Surgery, New York, New York

Koh Shingu, M.D.
Professor and Chair, Department of Anesthesiology,
Kansai Medical University, Moriguchi, Osaka, Japan

Frederick E. Sieber, M.D.
Associate Professor, Department of Anesthesia and
Critical Care Medicine, Johns Hopkins University
School of Medicine; Chair, Department of Anesthesia,
Johns Hopkins Bayview Medical Center, Baltimore,
Maryland

Robert N. Sladen, M.B., Ch.B.
Professor of Anesthesiology and Vice Chair, Department
of Anesthesiology, Columbia University College of
Physicians and Surgeons; Director, Cardiothoracic
and Surgical Intensive Care Units, Columbia
Presbyterian Medical Center of the New York
Presbyterian Hospital, New York, New York

Thomas F. Slaughter, M.D.
Professor and Director of Cardiothoracic Anesthesia,
Virginia Commonwealth University Reanimation
Engineering Shock Center, Virginia Commonwealth
University, Richmond, Virginia

Donald R. Stanski, M.D.
Professor, Department of Anesthesia, Stanford
University School of Medicine, Stanford, California

John K. Stene, M.D., Ph.D.
Professor, Department of Anesthesiology, Pennsylvania
State University College of Medicine; Co-Director,
Surgical Intensive Care Unit, Pennsylvania State
University Milton S. Hershey Medical Center,
Hershey, Pennsylvania

Paul E. Stensrud, M.D.
Pediatric Cardiac Anesthesiologist, Department
of Anesthesiology, Mayo Clinic, Rochester,
Minnesota

James M. Steven, M.D., S.M.
Associate Professor of Anesthesia, University of
Pennsylvania School of Medicine; Chief Medical
Officer, Attending Anesthesiologist, and Associate
Anesthesiologist-in-Chief, Department of
Anesthesiology and Critical Care Medicine, The
Children's Hospital of Philadelphia, Philadelphia,
Pennsylvania

Gary R. Strichartz, Ph.D.
Professor of Anesthesia (Pharmacology), Harvard
Medical School; Vice Chair for Research, Department
of Anesthesiology, Perioperative and Pain Medicine,
Brigham and Women's Hospital, Boston,
Massachusetts

Vijayendra Sudheendra, M.D.
Department of Cardiothoracic Anesthesia and Critical
Care Medicine, Cleveland Clinic Foundation,
Cleveland, Ohio

Lena S. Sun, M.D.
Associate Professor of Anesthesiology and Pediatrics,
Columbia University College of Physicians and
Surgeons; Chief, Pediatric Anesthesiology, Children's
Hospital of New York, New York, New York

James F. Szocik, M.D.
Clinical Associate Professor, Department of
Anesthesiology, University of Michigan, Ann Arbor,
Michigan

Timothy J. Tautz, M.D.
Assistant Professor and Director, Malignant
Hyperthermia Diagnostic Laboratory, Department
of Anesthesiology and Pain Medicine, University
of California, Davis, School of Medicine, Davis,
California

Stephen J. Thomas, M.D.
Topkins–Van Poznak Distinguished Professor of
Anesthesiology, Department of Anesthesiology, Weill
Medical College of Cornell University; Vice Chair,
Department of Anesthesiology, Weill Cornell Medical
Center–New York Presbyterian Hospital, New York,
New York

Daniel M. Thys, M.D.
Professor of Anesthesiology, Columbia University
College of Physicians and Surgeons; Chairman,
St. Luke's-Roosevelt Hospital Center, New York,
New York

Kevin K. Tremper, M.D.
Professor and Chair, Department of Anesthesiology,
University of Michigan, Ann Arbor, Michigan

Robert D. Truog, M.D.
Professor of Anesthesia (Pediatrics) and Professor of
Medical Ethics, Harvard Medical School; Division
Chief, Critical Care Medicine, Children's Hospital,
Boston, Massachusetts

Kenneth J. Tuman, M.D.
Professor of Anesthesiology, Rush Medical College;
Vice Chair, Department of Anesthesiology, Rush
University Medical Center, Chicago, Illinois

Thomas C. Vary, Ph.D.
Professor, Department of Cellular and Molecular
Physiology, Pennsylvania State University College
of Medicine, Hershey, Pennsylvania

Daniel P. Vezina, M.D., M.Sc.
Assistant Professor and Director of the Perioperative
Echocardiography Service, Department of
Anesthesiology, Department of Internal Medicine,
Division of Cardiology, University of Utah School
of Medicine; Director of Cardiology,
Echocardiography Laboratory, Veterans
Administration Hospital, Salt Lake City, Utah

David B. Waisel, M.D.
Assistant Professor, Department of Anesthesia, Harvard
Medical School; Director, Pediatric Anesthesia
Fellowship Program, Children's Hospital, Boston,
Massachusetts

David C. Warltier, M.D., Ph.D.
Senior Vice Chairman, Department of Anesthesiology;
Professor of Anesthesiology, Pharmacology, and
Toxicology, Medical College of Wisconsin; Professor
of Biomedical Engineering, Marquette University,
Milwaukee, Wisconsin

Denise J. Wedel, M.D.
Professor, Department of Anesthesiology, Mayo Clinic
College of Medicine, Rochester, Minnesota

Paul F. White, Ph.D., M.D.
Professor and Holder of the Margaret Milam McDermott Distinguished Chair in Anesthesiology, Department of Anesthesiology and Pain Management, University of Texas Southwestern Medical Center at Dallas, Dallas, Texas

Roger D. White, M.D.
Professor of Anesthesiology, Mayo Clinic College of Medicine; Consultant in Anesthesia and Internal Medicine, Mayo Clinic, Rochester, Minnesota

William C. Wilson, M.D.
Associate Clinical Professor, Department of Anesthesiology, University of California, San Diego, San Diego, California

Christopher L. Wu, M.D.
Associate Professor of Anesthesiology, The Johns Hopkins University School of Medicine; Staff, The Johns Hopkins Hospital, Baltimore, Maryland

C. Spencer Yost, M.D.
Professor, Department of Anesthesia and Perioperative Care, University of California, San Francisco, School of Medicine; Attending Physician, Moffitt-Long Hospital, University of California, San Francisco, San Francisco, California

Chun-Su Yuan, M.D., Ph.D.
Professor, Department of Anesthesia and Critical Care, The Pritzker School of Medicine, The University of Chicago, Chicago, Illinois

Contributors to the Companion Video CD-ROM

Michael K. Cahalan, M.D.
Professor and Chair, Department of Anesthesiology, University of Utah School of Medicine, Salt Lake City, Utah

Lydia Cassorla, M.D.
Clinical Professor, Department of Anesthesia and Perioperative Care, University of California, San Francisco, San Francisco, California

Adam B. Collins, M.D.
Assistant Clinical Professor, Department of Anesthesia and Perioperative Care, University of California, San Francisco, San Francisco, California

Andrew T. Gray, M.D., Ph.D.
Associate Professor, Department of Anesthesia and Perioperative Care, University of California, San Francisco, San Francisco, California

Joan Howley, M.D.
Associate Clinical Professor, Department of Anesthesia and Perioperative Care, University of California, San Francisco, San Francisco, California

Jeffrey Katz, M.D.
Professor, Department of Anesthesia and Perioperative Care, University of California, San Francisco, San Francisco, California

Errol Lobo, M.D.
Associate Professor, Department of Anesthesia and Perioperative Care, University of California, San Francisco, San Francisco, California

Manuel Pardo, Jr., M.D.
Sol Shnider Endowed Chair for Anesthesia Education and Associate Professor of Clinical Anesthesia, Department of Anesthesia and Perioperative Care, University of California, San Francisco, San Francisco, California

Donald Taylor, M.D.
Assistant Professor, Department of Anesthesia and Perioperative Care, University of California, San Francisco, San Francisco, California

Maurice S. Zwass, M.D.
Professor of Clinical Anesthesia, Departments of Pediatrics and Anesthesiology, University of California, San Francisco; Associate Director of the Pediatric Intensive Care Unit, UCSF Children's Hospital, San Francisco, California

Preface to the Sixth Edition

The Fifth Edition of *Anesthesia* is widely recognized as the most complete and thorough analysis and presentation in the specialty of anesthesiology. As with past editions, all contributing authors were instructed to revise their chapters in a manner that ensured a contemporary treatment of the subject matter. The Sixth Edition was designed to retain all of the strengths of the Fifth Edition, in addition to responding to the new and challenging aspects of our specialty. To help us with that analysis, Dr. Lee A. Fleisher, the Chair of Anesthesia at the University of Pennsylvania, Dr. Roger A. Johns, Professor of Anesthesia at Johns Hopkins University, and Drs. Jeanine P. Wiener-Kronish and William L. Young, both Vice Chairs of Anesthesia at the University of California-San Francisco were added to the team of consulting editors.

We decided to add new chapters on implantable cardiac pulse generators; civil, chemical, and biologic warfare; anesthesia for robotic surgery; perioperative blindness; complementary and alternative therapies finding information on the Internet; and human performance in patient safety. These chapters represent major issues that have affected not only anesthesiology but medicine in general. All of the remaining chapters are fully revised and updated, including new author teams on many chapters, which facilitates the offering of contemporary information in a thorough and clinically relevant manner.

A CD-ROM with video segments was first introduced in the Fifth Edition. The intent was to provide a verbal and visual description of some of the more technically demanding procedures described in the text. That concept proved to be quite successful, and we are again including a video CD-ROM in this new edition. The new videos include segments on patient positioning; code blue simulation; Fastrach intubation; thoracic epidural, ultrasound-guided nerve blocks; ultrasound-guided peripheral venous access; and needle cricothyrotomy. The video segments are referenced in the text by a video icon in the margins. We hope that the expanded video feature facilitates and improves the mastering of the many technical aspects of our specialty.

A new feature of this work is the **e-dition**™ website, which will be started this year. This website provides regular weekly updates from experts in the field, so that *Anesthesia* can stay current year after year. Full text, illustrations, and videos are provided and are fully searchable. You can download illustrations to PowerPoint to enhance your presentations and lectures. References are linked to Medline or directly to full-text articles where available, which will expand your search capabilities. Other added-value features include drug information from the Mosby Drug Consult, sample test questions, and important anesthesiology-related web links.

We wish to acknowledge the long-term participation of Roy F. Cucchiara, Edward D. Miller Jr., J. Gerald Reves, and Michael F. Roizen, who all served as consulting editors on the previous edition. We are grateful for the tireless help of Dosia Matthews, who handled all communication with contributors and the publisher and facilitated the traffic of manuscripts and page proofs. We also wish to acknowledge the support of dedicated staff at Elsevier — Publisher Natasha Andjelkovic, Senior Developmental Editor Ann Ruzycka Anderson, Project Managers Jodi Kaye and Mary Anne Folcher, Publishing Services Manager Tina Rebane, Multimedia Producer Bruce Robison, Design Manager Steven Stave, and Marketing Manager Emily McGrath-Christie.

RONALD D. MILLER, M.D.
*Chairman, Department of Anesthesia and Perioperative Care
University of California-San Francisco
San Francisco, California*

Table of Contents

VOLUME 1

SECTION I: INTRODUCTION

Chapter 1
History of Anesthetic Practice   3
Merlin D. Larson

SECTION II: SCIENTIFIC PRINCIPLES

Chapter 2
Scope of Modern Anesthetic Practice   55
Stephen J. Thomas and Frederick K. Orkin

Chapter 3
**Basic Principles of Pharmacology Related
   to Anesthesia**   67
Steven L. Shafer and Debra A. Schwinn

Inhaled Anesthetics

Chapter 4
Mechanisms of Action   105
Donald D. Koblin

Chapter 5
Uptake and Distribution   131
Edmond I. Eger II

Chapter 6
Pulmonary Pharmacology   155
Neil E. Farber, Paul S. Pagel, and David C. Warltier

Chapter 7
Cardiovascular Pharmacology   191
*Paul S. Pagel, Judy R. Kersten, Neil E. Farber, and
   David C. Warltier*

Chapter 8
**Metabolism and Toxicity of Inhaled
   Anesthetics**   231
Jackie L. Martin, Jr.

Chapter 9
Inhaled Anesthetic Delivery Systems   273
Russell C. Brockwell and J. Jeff Andrews

Intravenous Anesthetics

Chapter 10
Intravenous Nonopioid Anesthetics   317
*J. G. Reves, Peter S. A. Glass, David A. Lubarsky, and
   Matthew D. McEvoy*

Chapter 11
Intravenous Opioid Anesthetics   379
Kazuhiko Fukuda

Chapter 12
Intravenous Drug Delivery Systems   439
Peter S. A. Glass, Steven L. Shafer, and J. G. Reves

Other Drugs Commonly Used in Anesthesia

Chapter 13
**Pharmacology of Muscle Relaxants and Their
   Antagonists**   481
Mohamed Naguib and Cynthia A. Lien

Chapter 14
Local Anesthetics   573
Gary R. Strichartz and Charles B. Berde

Chapter 15
Complementary and Alternative Therapies   605
Michael K. Ang-Lee, Chun-Su Yuan, and Jonathan Moss

Chapter 16
The Autonomic Nervous System   617
Jonathan Moss and David Glick

Physiology and Anesthesia

Chapter 17
**Respiratory Physiology and Respiratory Function
   During Anesthesia**   679
William C. Wilson and Jonathan L. Benumof

Chapter 18
Cardiac Physiology   723
Lena S. Sun and Johanna Schwarzenberger

Chapter 19
Hepatic Physiology and Pathophysiology   743
Phillip S. Mushlin and Simon Gelman

Chapter 20
Renal Physiology   777
Robert N. Sladen

Chapter 21
**Cerebral Physiology and the Effects of Anesthetics
   and Techniques**   813
Piyush M. Patel and John C. Drummond

Chapter 22
Neuromuscular Physiology and Pharmacology   859
J. A. Jeevendra Martyn

Chapter 23
Statistical Methods in Anesthesia   881
Stanley H. Rosenbaum

SECTION III: ANESTHESIA MANAGEMENT

Preoperative Preparation

Chapter 24
Risk of Anesthesia   893
Lee A. Fleisher

Chapter 25
Preoperative Evaluation   927
Michael F. Roizen

Chapter 26
Pulmonary Function Testing   999
Thomas J. Gal

Chapter 27
Anesthetic Implications of Concurrent Diseases   1017
Michael F. Roizen and Lee A. Fleisher

Chapter 28
Patient Positioning   1151
Ronald J. Faust, Roy F. Cucchiara, and Perry S. Bechtle

Chapter 29
Malignant Hyperthermia   1169
Gerald A. Gronert, Issac N. Pessah, Sheila M. Muldoon, and Timothy J. Tautz

Monitoring

Chapter 30
Fundamental Principles of Monitoring Instrumentation   1191
James F. Szocik, Steven J. Barker, and Kevin K. Tremper

Chapter 31
Measuring Depth of Anesthesia   1227
Donald R. Stanski and Steven L. Shafer

Chapter 32
Cardiovascular Monitoring   1265
Jonathan B. Mark and Thomas F. Slaughter

Chapter 33
Transesophageal Echocardiography   1363
Daniel P. Vezina and Michael K. Cahalan

Color Plates

Chapter 34
Electrocardiography   1389
Zaharia Hillel and Daniel M. Thys

Chapter 35
Implantable Cardiac Pulse Generators, Pacemakers, and Cardioverter-Defibrillators   1415
Marc A. Rozner

Chapter 36
Respiratory Monitoring   1437
Richard E. Moon and Enrico M. Camporesi

Chapter 37
Renal Function Monitoring   1483
Solomon Aronson

Chapter 38
Neurologic Monitoring   1511
Michael E. Mahla, Susan Black, and Roy F. Cucchiara

Chapter 39
Neuromuscular Monitoring   1551
Jørgen Viby Mogensen

Chapter 40
Temperature Monitoring   1571
Daniel I. Sessler

Chapter 41
Perioperative Acid-Base Balance   1599
Patrick J. Neligan and Clifford S. Deutschman

VOLUME 2

Anesthesia Techniques

Chapter 42
Airway Management   1617
Thomas J. Gal

Chapter 43
Spinal, Epidural, and Caudal Anesthesia   1653
David L. Brown

Chapter 44
Nerve Blocks   1685
Denise J. Wedel and Terese T. Horlocker

Color plates

Chapter 45
Regional Anesthesia in Children   1719
Bernard J. Dalens

Perioperative Fluid Therapy

Chapter 46
Fluid and Electrolyte Physiology   1763
Alan D. Kaye and Ian J. Kucera

Chapter 47
Transfusion Therapy   1799
Ronald D. Miller

Chapter 48
Autologous Transfusion   1831
Lawrence T. Goodnough and Terri G. Monk

SECTION IV: SUBSPECIALTY MANAGEMENT

Chapter 49
Anesthesia for Thoracic Surgery   1847
William C. Wilson and Jonathan L. Benumof

Chapter 50
Anesthesia for Cardiac Surgery Procedures   1941
Daniel Nyhan and Roger A. Johns

Chapter 51
Anesthesia for Pediatric Cardiac Surgery   2005
William J. Greeley, James M. Steven, and Susan C. Nicolson

Chapter 52
Anesthesia for Vascular Surgery   2051
Edward J. Norris

Chapter 53
Neurosurgical Anesthesia   2127
John C. Drummond and Piyush M. Patel

Chapter 54
Anesthesia and the Renal and Genitourinary
    Systems   2175
Vinod Malhotra, Vijayendra Sudheendra, and Sudhir Diwan

Chapter 55
Anesthesia and the Hepatobiliary System   2209
Christopher J. O'Connor, David M. Rothenberg,
    and Kenneth J. Tuman

Chapter 56
Organ Transplantation   2231
James Baker, C. Spencer Yost, and Claus U. Niemann

Chapter 57
Anesthesia for Laparoscopic Surgery   2285
Jean L. Joris

Chapter 58
Anesthesia for Obstetrics   2307
David J. Birnbach and Ingrid M. Browne

Chapter 59
Resuscitation of the Newborn   2345
George A. Gregory

Chapter 60
Pediatric Anesthesia   2367
Charles J. Coté

Chapter 61
Anesthesia for Orthopedic Surgery   2409
Nigel E. Sharrock, James D. Beckman, Eileen Connolly Inda,
    and John J. Savarese

Chapter 62
Anesthesia for the Elderly   2435
Frederick E. Sieber and Ronald Pauldine

Chapter 63
Anesthesia for Trauma   2451
Richard P. Dutton and Maureen McCunn

Chapter 64
Chemical and Biological Warfare Agents: The Role
    of the Anesthesiologist   2497
David J. Baker

Chapter 65
Anesthesia for Eye, Ear, Nose, and
    Throat Surgery   2527
John V. Donlon, Jr., D. John Doyle, and Marc Allan Feldman

Chapter 66
Anesthesia for Robotic Surgery   2557
Ervant V. Nishanian and Berend Mets

Chapter 67
Anesthesia for Laser Surgery   2573
Ira J. Rampil

Chapter 68
Ambulatory Outpatient Anesthesia   2589
Paul F. White and Alejandro Recart Freire

Chapter 69
Anesthesia at Remote Locations   2637
Paul E. Stensrud

Chapter 70
Clinical Care in Altered Environments: At High and
    Low Pressure and in Space   2665
Richard E. Moon and Enrico M. Camporesi

Chapter 71
The Postanesthesia Care Unit   2703
Thomas W. Feeley and Alex Macario

Chapter 72
Acute Postoperative Pain   2729
Christopher L. Wu

Chapter 73
Chronic Pain   2763
John C. Rowlingson

SECTION V: CRITICAL CARE MEDICINE

Chapter 74
Overview of Anesthesiology and Critical
    Care Medicine   2787
Linda L. Liu and Michael A. Gropper

Chapter 75
Respiratory Care   2811
Mark T. Grabovac, Kevin K. Kim, Thomas E. Quinn, Raymond
    Hernandez, and Brian M. Daniel

Chapter 76
Pediatric and Neonatal Intensive Care   2831
W. Daniel Kovarik

Chapter 77
Nutritional Aspects   2887
John K. Stene and Thomas C. Vary

Chapter 78
Cardiopulmonary Resuscitation: Basic and
    Advanced Life Support   2923
Brian P. McGlinch and Roger D. White

Chapter 79
Brain Death   2955
Kenjiro Mori, Koh Shingu, and Shinichi Nakao

SECTION VI: ANCILLARY RESPONSIBILITIES AND PROBLEMS

Chapter 80
Medical Information on the Internet   2973
Ira J. Rampil

Chapter 81
Quality Improvement   2979
Peter J. Pronovost and Sean M. Berenholtz

Chapter 82
Perioperative Blindness   2991
Steven Roth

Chapter 83
Human Performance and Patient Safety   3021
Marcus Rall and David M. Gaba

Chapter **84**
Patient Simulators   3073
Marcus Rall and David M. Gaba

Chapter **85**
Teaching Anesthesia   3105
Alan J. Schwartz

Chapter **86**
Operating Room Management   3119
James Kindscher

Chapter **87**
**Electrical Safety in the Operating
    Room**   3139
Lawrence Litt

Chapter **88**
**Environmental Safety Including Chemical
    Dependence**   3151
William P. Arnold III and Dorre Nicholau

Chapter **89**
**Ethical and Legal Aspects of Anesthesia
    Care**   3175
David B. Waisel and Robert D. Truog

Appendix
Système International   3199

INDEX   i

COMPANION VIDEO CD-ROM

Video **1**
Patient Positioning in Anesthesia
Lydia Cassorla

Video **2**
Code Blue Simulation
Manuel Pardo and Adam B. Collins

Video **3**
Fastrach Intubation
Donald Taylor

Video **4**
Thoracic Epidural Placement
Errol Lobo

Video **5**
Ultrasound-Guided Nerve Block
Adam B. Collins and Andrew T. Gray

Video **6**
Ultrasound-Guided Peripheral Venous Access
Adam B. Collins and Andrew T. Gray

Video **7**
Needle Cricothyrotomy
Adam B. Collins

Video **8**
**Pulmonary Catheter and Transesophageal
    Echocardiography**
Michael K. Cahalan

Video **9**
**Strategies for Successful Placement of Double-
    Lumen Endobronchial Tubes and Bronchial
    Blockers for Lung Separation**
Jeffrey Katz

Video **10**
Demonstration of the Anesthesia Machine
Joan Howley

Video **11**
Caudal Block in Pediatrics
Maurice S. Zwass

Miller's Anesthesia

SIXTH EDITION

Volume 1

Introduction

1 History of Anesthetic Practice

Merlin D. Larson

Cardiopulmonary Physiology 4
Respiration 4
Intravascular Pressures 6

**Autonomic Nervous System and
Neurohumoral Transmission 8**

**Historical Development of Theories
of Pain 9**

Surgical Procedures before 1846 10

**Introduction of General
Anesthesia 12**
Background 12
Gas Inhalation 12
Beginning of Inhaled Anesthesia 13
Aftermath 15
Priority for Discovery 16

**Development of Inhalation
Agents 16**
Chloroform 16
Nitrous Oxide 17
Unsatisfactory Inhaled Anesthetics 17
Fluorinated Anesthetics 18

Needles and Syringes 19

Intravenous Fluid Therapy 20
Crystalloids 20
Blood Transfusions 21

**Introduction of Regional
Anesthesia 22**
Early Attempts at Local Anesthesia 22
Cocaine 22
Regional Blocks 23

**Neuraxial Block and Acute
Pain Service 24**
Spinal Analgesia 25
Epidural Analgesia 27

Intravenous Anesthetics 28

Muscle Relaxants 30
Initial Contact with Arrow Poison 30
Mechanism of Action 30
Introduction into Clinical Medicine 30

Anesthesia Apparatus 33
Early Delivery Systems 33
Compressed Gases and Reducing Valves 33
Carbon Dioxide Absorption 34
Controlled Vaporizers 34
Ventilators in the Intensive Care Unit 35

Stress-Free Anesthesia 35

**Airway Management and
Resuscitation 36**
Masks and Airways 36
Tracheal Tubes 37
Laryngoscopes 39
Alternatives to the Laryngoscope 39
Resuscitation 39

**Anesthetic Accidents and
Complications—Preventive
Measures 40**

Biographical Sketches 42
Virginia Apgar 42
Arthur E. Guedel 43
John Snow 44

The first anesthetics were given to ameliorate the pain associated with dental extractions and minor surgery. As the complementary fields of surgery and anesthesiology matured together, new skills were required of the anesthesiologist, including expertise in resuscitation, fluid replacement, airway management, oxygen transport, operative stress reduction, and postoperative pain control.

Today, personnel from the anesthesiology department are scattered in several locations throughout the hospital, from the ambulatory care center to the intensive care unit. Organizing the background of these various activities into a coherent historical document is therefore complicated by the diverse roles that anesthesiologists play in the modern hospital.

One approach to the history of anesthesiology is to relate in detail the events surrounding the 1846 public demonstration of ether anesthesia by William T. G. Morton (1819-1868).[1-4] This event represents the starting point from which anesthesiology emerged as a specialty. Although the ether demonstration was dramatic and enacted by interesting personalities, it was just the opening act of the pain control story. Since 1846, there has been enormous progress and change in the specialty of medicine that has become known as anesthesiology, and these changes often have occurred in small, incremental steps that are hardly noteworthy on their own. Most operations in the modern operating room could not have been performed before the great progress in anesthetic practice that took place in the years between 1925 and 1960, but historians often overlook these advances, because they were introduced without the drama and spectacle of previous developments.

In addition to the advancements of the 20th century, it is necessary to look prior to mid-19th century to appreciate the groundwork laid by those curious individuals who sought a scientific understanding of cardiopulmonary physiology and pain. These fundamental discoveries provide the physiologic foundation for safe anesthetic practice. A brief survey of these developments is provided in the opening sections of the following narrative. Dentists, priests, musicians, pediatricians, engineers, ophthalmologists, neurophysiologists, pharmacologists, urologists, otolaryngologists, surgeons, ministers, dilettantes, philosophers, physiologists, missionaries, chemists, South American Indians, and anesthesiologists all had a role in shaping the practice of contemporary anesthesiology, one of the most fascinating stories in the history of medicine.

I have attempted to describe and reference the origins of ideas relating to modern anesthetic practice, but the issue of priority is vague on some topics and may be open to question by other historians of specific subjects. I have attempted to verify information from several sources, including original manuscripts whenever possible. Notably lacking are early references to anesthetic methods in Asia, because these texts and manuscripts are difficult to obtain. The historical developments of the subspecialties are not documented, but that information can be obtained from specialized textbooks. Perhaps Sir William Osler (1849-1919) expressed the difficulties of the medical historian best when he related the *History of British Medicine* in an address to the British Medical Association in 1897.[5]

> To trace successfully the evolution of any one of the learned professions would require the hand of a master—of one who, like Darwin, combined a capacity for patient observation with philosophic vision. In the case of medicine, the difficulties are enormously increased by the extraordinary development, which has taken place during the 19th century. The rate of progress has been too rapid for us to appreciate, and we stand bewildered and as it were, in a state of intellectual giddiness, when we attempt to obtain a broad, comprehensive view of the subject.

CARDIOPULMONARY PHYSIOLOGY

Respiration

Although volatile and gaseous anesthetics have changed over the past 150 years, there are two gases that will always be a part of anesthetic practice. How oxygen and carbon dioxide are consumed and produced and how they interact with the body has been the subject of intense research over the past 400 years. The ability to manipulate the pressure of these gases in the tissues has contributed much to the success of intensive care medicine. Because of the importance that carbon dioxide and oxygen have in the practice of anesthesiology, it is worthwhile to consider how our understanding of respiration came about.

Galen (120-200 AD) and Aristotle (384-322 BC) both thought that the air moving in and out of the lungs served merely to cool the heart, which otherwise became overheated in working to sustain life.[6] In 1678, Robert Hook (1635-1703) attached a bellows to the trachea of a dog with an open chest and demonstrated that the animal could be kept alive by rhythmic and sustained contraction of the bellows. Hook proved that movement of the chest wall was not the essential feature of respiration, but rather it was exposure of fresh air to the blood circulating through the lungs.[7] Richard Lower (1631-1691), who also was the first to transfuse blood from one animal to another, demonstrated in 1669 that the blood absorbed a definite chemical substance necessary for life, that it changed the venous blood from dark blue to red, and that the process was the chief function of the pulmonary circulation.[8]

The nature of the process that takes place in the lungs was misunderstood until the 1780s because of the generally accepted, but erroneous, phlogiston theory promoted by Georg Ernst Stahl (1660-1734).[9] Stahl theorized that combustible substances were composed of *phlogiston* (Greek for "burnt") and *calc* ("ash") and that the phlogiston was released during burning and during respiration. Joseph Priestley (1733-1804) (Fig. 1-1A), a complex individual who was a dissenting minister in Leeds, England and later the "resident intellectual" to the Earl of Shelburne, observed that respiration and combustion had many similarities,[10] because a candle flame would go out and an animal would die if left within a closed space. He thought this was because the air was putrefied with phlogiston. Priestley discovered photosynthesis by showing that placing plants that imbibed the "phlogistic matter" within the contained space could restore this "bad air." By heating mercuric oxide, he generated a gas that would make flames brighter and keep mice alive longer in a closed space. Priestley called it *dephlogisicated air*, and Carl Scheele[11] (1742-1786) in Sweden, who found it earlier but failed to publish, called it *feuer luft* ("fire air"). Priestley thought this process absorbed phlogiston and informed the French chemist Antoine-Laurent Lavoisier (1743-1794) (see Fig. 1-1B) of his discovery.

Lavoisier realized that heating mercuric oxides released a new element and called it oxygen. Lavoisier[12] also showed that sulfur and phosphorus gained weight when burned and thereby produced acid-forming substances— hence the name *oxygen*, which is Greek for "acid producer." When Lavoisier showed that burning some substances caused them to gain weight, the proponents of the phlogiston theory attempted to persist by asserting that phlogiston had a negative weight. Lavoisier was a very wealthy member of the Ferme Generale, the primary tax-collecting agency of the royalist government, but he supported the revolution and was its principal economist. Despite this, he was unceremoniously beheaded at the age of 51 years during the French Revolution. However, his legacy as the father of modern chemistry is without question, and his greatest contribution was to outline the great facts of respiration: absorption of oxygen through the lungs with liberation of carbon dioxide.

Lavoisier thought respiration was accomplished in the lungs, but Humphry Davy (1778-1829) (see Fig. 1-1C), a young English teenager who dropped out of school at the age of 16 years, read the works of Lavoisier and designed his own experiments to study the site of metabolism. Davy heated blood and collected the gases that were produced. By showing these gases were oxygen and carbon dioxide, he surmised that metabolism takes place in the tissues,[13] a conclusion confirmed by Eduard Friedrich Wilhelm Pflüger[14] (1829-1910) 60 years later. Davy also estimated the rates of oxygen consumption and carbon dioxide production, and he measured the total lung and residual volumes.

John S. Haldane (1860-1936) was a pioneer investigator in the study of respiration a century ago. His apparatus for measurement of blood gases was described in 1892.[15] He was the first to promote oxygen therapy for respiratory disease,[15] and in 1905, he discovered that the carbon dioxide tension of the blood was the normal stimulus for respiratory drive.[17] Haldane experimented with self-administration of hypoxic mixtures and coined the ominous phrase that lurks within the inner recesses of the anesthesiologist's mind: "Anoxemia not only stops the machine but wrecks the machinery." He believed until his death, despite experimental evidence, that the lung actively secreted oxygen into the blood from the air. His landmark monograph *Respiration*, published in 1922,[18] summarized his studies on the respiratory system.

At the end of the 19th century, it was known that hemoglobin had a vital role in the transport of oxygen to the tissues. In 1896, Carl Gustav von Hufner (1840-1908) showed that the presence of hemoglobin in the blood greatly enhanced its oxygen carrying capacity, quantifying that 1 g of hemoglobin carried 1.34 mL of oxygen.[19] It was soon observed that delivery of high concentrations of oxygen to patients with advanced pulmonary disease was often inadequate to fully maintain tissue respiration

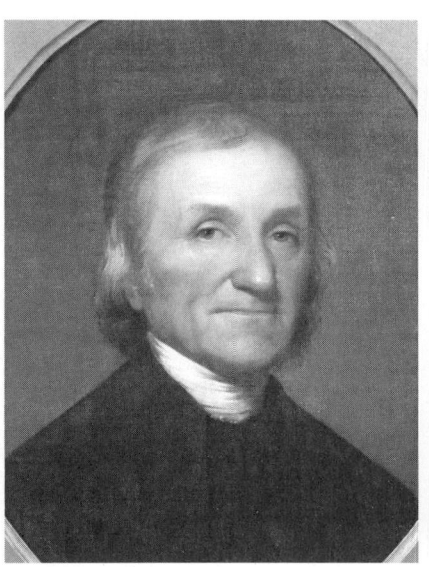 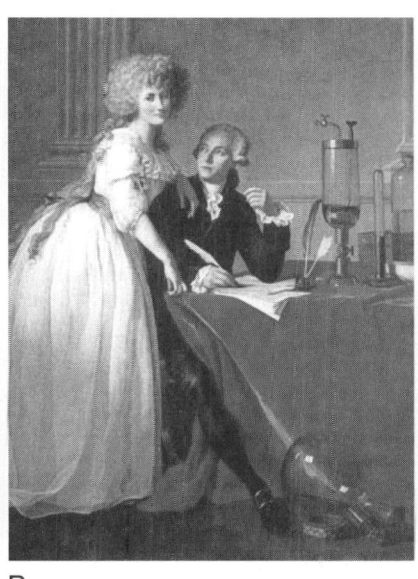 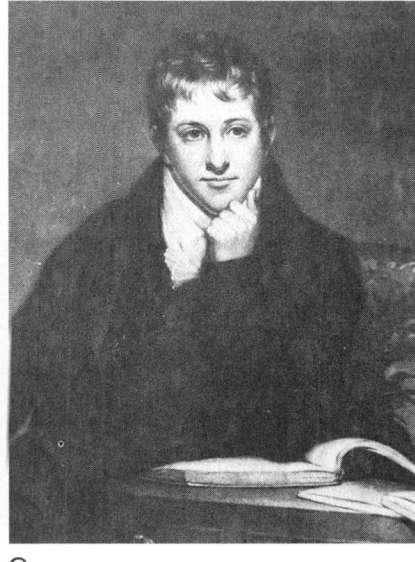

A   B   C

Figure 1–1 A, Joseph Priestley was born in Fieldhead, England, and educated as a minister. His early career was spent as a schoolmaster in Leeds, England. In 1780, he accepted an appointment in Birmingham, as minister, where he joined Erasmus Darwin and James Watt in forming the Lunar Society, which met to discuss the new ideas in chemistry and physics emerging at that time. Because of his political views, his chapel and home were vandalized in 1789. Five years later, he joined his sons in Pennsylvania in the United States, where he died in 1804 at age 70. **B,** The portrait of Lavoisier and his wife, Marie Anne Pierrette Paulz, was painted in 1788 by the famous French artist Jacques Louis David. Marie Paulz, who married Lavoisier when she was only 14 years old, was taught to draw by David, and she drew many of the illustrations in Lavoisier's magnum opus, *Traite Elementaire de Chimie*.[483] Several experimental devices and gasometers are shown on and below the table. **C,** Humphry Davy was born in Cornwall, England, and became apprenticed to a surgeon, J. B. Borlase of Penzance, at age 17. At 20 years of age, he was appointed Superintendent of the Beddoe's Pneumatic Institute, where he studied the effects of nitrous oxide inhalation. His later career in chemistry gained him fame and honors. He directed the Royal Institute and was made a baronet in 1818 at the age of 40. (Courtesy of the Wood Library-Museum of Anesthesiology, Park Ridge, IL.)

and saturate hemoglobin completely. Gradients for inspired, alveolar, and arterial oxygen partial pressures became apparent after the development of the oxygen electrode by Leland C. Clark[20] (1918-) (Fig. 1-2) in 1956. The Clark electrode consisted of a platinum cathode and a silver anode separated from blood by a polyethylene membrane. The platinum was negatively charged to react with any oxygen reaching it through the membrane and was sensitive to the oxygen pressure outside the membrane (i.e., the oxygen tension in the blood).

Further understanding of respiratory physiology arose because of the worldwide polio epidemic that occurred roughly between the years of 1930 and 1960. Thousands of afflicted patients were kept alive with mechanical respirators, but the adequacy of ventilation could not be assessed without some measure of carbon dioxide tension (P_{CO_2}) in the blood. Several methods to measure P_{CO_2} indirectly were made by Donald D. Van Slyke[21] (1883-1971) and Paul B. Astrup (1915-2000), but the modern solution rested on the development of the carbon dioxide electrode. This problem was solved in 1958, when John W. Severinghaus[22] (1922-) (see Fig. 1-2) improved the accuracy of a prototype carbon dioxide electrode produced by Richard Stow (1916-), which measured pH of a thin film of electrolyte separated from the blood by a Teflon membrane through which carbon dioxide could diffuse and equilibrate. Severinghaus and A. F. Bradley (1932-) constructed the first blood gas apparatus by mounting the carbon dioxide electrode and Clark's oxygen electrode in cuvettes in a 37°C bath. To measure blood P_{O_2} accurately, Severinghaus found it necessary to rapidly stir the blood in contact with Clark's electrode because of its high oxygen consumption rate. A pH electrode was added in 1959. Blood gas analysis made possible the rapid assessment of respiratory exchange and acid-base balance. The use of blood gas analysis was rapidly taken up by the anesthesia community and has become one of the most common laboratory tests performed in the modern hospital. The impact of a more in-depth understanding of gas exchange on the practice of anesthesia is summarized by John Nunn in his book *Applied Respiratory Physiology*.[23]

Until the mid-20th century, the saturation of hemoglobin could be determined only by directly measuring a sample of arterial blood, a technique that required an arterial puncture. Oximetry achieves the same measure noninvasively through a finger or ear probe by using optical measures of transmitted light. Glenn Millikan, working in the Johnson Foundation for Medical Physics at the University of Pennsylvania, devised the first ear oximeter in 1942, and it was used to detect hypoxia in pilots, who flew in open cockpits during World War II. Its introduction into anesthesia practice was delayed until the discovery of pulse oximetry by a Japanese engineer, Takuo Aoyagi.[24] Pulse oximetry added the additional measure of heart rate, and it provided assurance that the signal was actually measuring a biologic parameter. A highly successful commercial product, the Nellcor pulse oximeter, was introduced in 1983 and had the unique feature of lowering the pitch of the pulse tone as the saturation dropped.

Intravascular Pressures

The first measurement of the blood pressure was made by Stephen Hales (1677-1761) (Fig. 1-3A), the curate of Middlesex, England, who between sermons occupied himself with experiments on the mechanics of the circulation. He[25] described one of his experiments performed (1733) on an "old mare who was to be killed, as being unfit for service":

> I fixed a brass pipe to the carotid artery of a mare … the blood rose in the tube till it reached to nine feet six inches in height. I then took away the tube from the artery and let out sixty cubic inches of blood, and then replaced the tube to see how high the blood would rise after each evacuation; this was repeated several times until the mare expired. In the three horses, death occurred when the height of the blood in the tube was about two feet.

Hales also discovered that the resistance of a vascular bed could change by mixing alcohol in the blood, which he observed could account for changes in blood pressure brought about by diverse ingested agents. In 1828, Jean L. Poiseuille[26] (1799-1869) repeated these experiments and devised a hemomanometer that used mercury instead of the long blood-filled tubes used by Hales. Poiseuille also showed that the blood pressure varied with respiration.

In 1854, Karl Vierrordt[27] (1818-1884) invented a sphygmograph, acting on the principle that indirect estimation of blood pressure could be accomplished by measuring the counterpressure necessary to obliterate the arterial pulsation. Scipione Riva Rocci's (1863-1937) sphygmomanometer, described in 1896,[28] used the same principle but used a rubber cuff that occluded a major

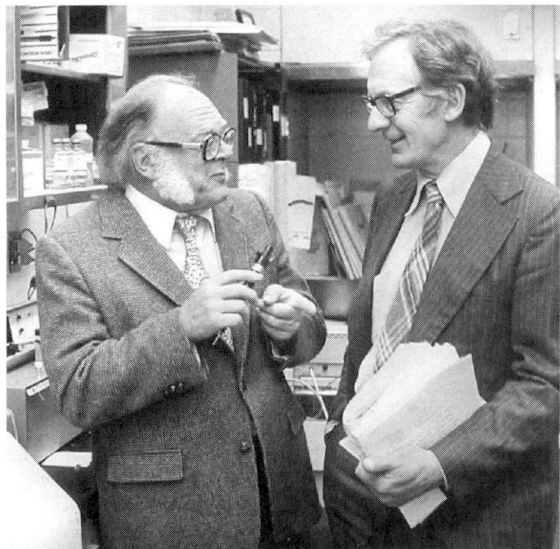

Figure 1–2 This photograph of Leland Clark and John Severinghaus, whose contributions led to modern techniques of blood gas analysis, was taken in Clark's laboratory at the Cincinnati Children's Hospital in 1982. (From Severinghaus JW, Astrup PB: History of Blood Gas Analysis. International Anesthesiology Clinics, Vol. 25, Boston, Little Brown, 1987.)

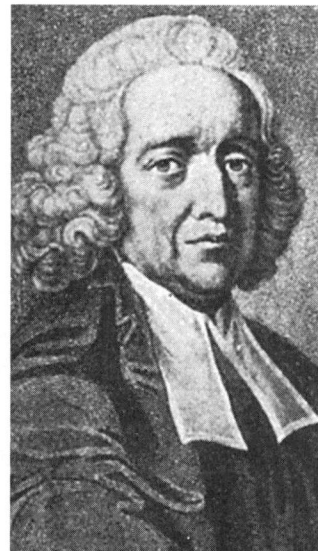

A

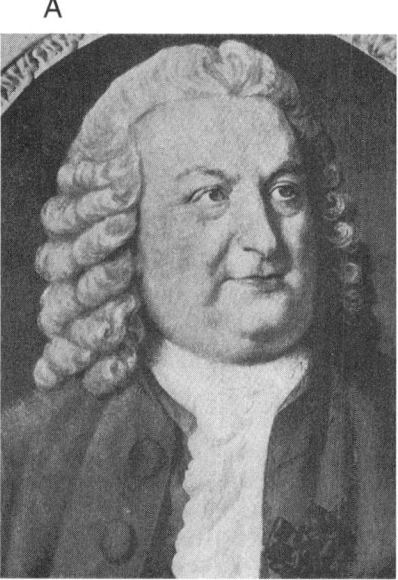

B

Figure 1–3 Two scientists of the Enlightenment era. **A,** Stephen Hales (1677-1761): detail of an oil painting by T. Hudson, 1759, in the National Portrait Gallery, London. Hales was educated at Cambridge University, England and was ordained as a minister in 1703. He spent his career as minister to the parish of Teddington, England. His rudimentary studies on the gas produced by mixing Walton pyrites (i.e., ferric disulfide) and spirit of nitre (i.e., nitric acid) was the spark that prompted Priestley to pursue his studies on nitric oxide, which led to the discovery of nitrous oxide in 1773. Hales was the first to measure blood pressure and cardiac output. He also developed ventilators that brought fresh air into prisons and granaries. **B,** Albrecht von Haller (1708-1777): detail of an engraving by Ambroise Tardieu. Haller was born in Bern, Switzerland. He served as professor of medicine and surgery at the University of Göttingen, Germany, where he began his encyclopedic work, *Physiological Elements of the Human Body,* published in eight volumes between 1757 and 1766. His demonstration that "irritability" was a property of muscle and "sensitivity" was a property of nerves was derived from nearly 600 experiments on live animals. He returned to Bern in 1753, and while there he published a catalog of the scientific literature containing 52,000 references. (Portraits courtesy of the National Library of Medicine, Bethesda, MD.)

arterial vessel and then slowly deflated. In 1905, Nikolai Korotkov[29] (1874-1920) described the sounds produced during auscultation over a distal portion of the artery as the cuff was deflated. The Korotkov sounds resulted in more accurate determinations of systolic and diastolic blood pressures. Oscillometric blood pressure measurements relied on a cuff that sensed the changes in arterial pulsations and was described by H. von Recklinghausen in 1931.[30] Automatic blood pressure devices based on the oscillometric method were developed in the 1970s and have become the standard noninvasive measures of arterial pressure in most hospitals.

The past 50 years have seen a gradual return to direct measurements of arterial blood pressure, which are in principle much the same method used by Stephen Hales nearly 250 years ago. However, the Poiseuille method of using mercury-filled glass tubes was found to be totally inadequate for recording accurate pressures in a dynamic system. In 1876, Herbert Tomlinson[31] introduced the principle of the strain gauge: resistance in a wire increases when it is stretched. It took 70 years after this principle was described before a strain gauge was used to measure blood pressure. In 1947, at the Mayo Clinic in Rochester, Minnesota, E. H. Lambert and E. H. Wood[32] first reported the use of a strain gauge to measure blood pressure continuously in human subjects exposed to acceleration forces. Cannulas placed directly into vessels were first described in 1949,[33] and since then, direct measurements of blood pressure expanded gradually into the operating room and intensive care units.

Venous pressures were of less interest to anesthesiologists until convenient methods for placing cannulas into central vascular structures were described 50 years ago by Sven Seldinger.[34] Werner Forssman (1904-1979), a urologist, described the methods of central venous access and right heart catheterization in humans in 1929,[35] originally experimenting on himself, and was awarded the Nobel Prize in Physiology and Medicine for his work on venous pressures in 1956. The introduction of plastic catheters[36] gradually made it possible to measure central pressures in the clinical setting. Although arm and femoral veins were used initially, subclavian and internal jugular vein cannulation eventually replaced the peripheral sites. Pulmonary artery catheterization with a balloon-tipped, flow-directed catheter was described in 1970[37] and has been used extensively since then by anesthesiologists to measure cardiac outputs using the Fick[38] principle and pulmonary wedge pressures. The pulmonary artery catheter also allowed the clinician to use the well-known pressure-volume relationships of the heart described by Ernest H. Starling (1866-1927) in 1918 to maximize cardiac outputs and oxygen delivery to the tissues.

Transesophageal echocardiography (TEE) was described in 1976[39] and used in anesthesia practice a few years later. One of the original probes used during anesthesia was fashioned from an esophageal stethoscope combined with an M-mode echocardiographic probe and was used to calculate cardiac output and ejection fraction in a 65-year-old woman undergoing mitral valve repair.[40] An improved electronic phased-array transducer was initially applied at the University of California, San Francisco for monitoring regional myocardial function in high-risk surgical patients.[41] Biplane TEE and color flow mapping were introduced in the 1980s and resulted in an explosive growth in TEE applications.[42] With experience and training in TEE, the anesthesiologist can quickly evaluate filling pressures of the heart as well as obtain measures of myocardial contractility and valvular function. TEE has become a routine monitor for certain surgical procedures.

AUTONOMIC NERVOUS SYSTEM AND NEUROHUMORAL TRANSMISSION

Even though the first practitioners of anesthesia had essentially no knowledge of adrenergic or cholinergic transmission, it would be difficult to administer anesthetics today without a thorough understanding of the autonomic nervous system and its neurotransmitters. These concepts are required in part because neuraxial blocks and general anesthetics are known to profoundly alter the ability of the body to respond to fluid losses and stress. Many modern surgical and neurovascular techniques require strict control of arterial and venous pressures, and this control is performed through interventions that alter autonomic tone.

The first hint of involuntary control of glandular and vascular function occurred in the 17th and 18th centuries. Robert Whytt (1714-1766) was the first to describe the reflex nature of many involuntary activities,[43] and Thomas Willis[44] (1621-1675) had described the sympathetic chain as early as 1657. He called it the *intercostal nerve* because it received segmental branches from the spinal cord at each level.

Pourfour du Petit (1664-1741) observed that there was a corresponding miosis and retraction of the nictitating membrane when this nerve was unilaterally cut in the neck of a cat.[45] Winslow gave the intercostal nerve the name of *grand sympathique*, stressing that this nerve brought the various organs of the body into sympathy,[46] a term that was originally coined by the Greek physician Soranus (98-138) in the first century AD (*sym*, "together," and *pathos*, "feeling"). Claude Bernard (1813-1878) observed vasoconstriction and pupillary dilation that followed stimulation of the same intercostal (now called the sympathetic) nerve and then described the vasomotor nerves arising between the cervical and lumbar enlargements of the spinal cord.[47]

In 1889, John N. Langley (1852-1925) began his classic work on sympathetic transmission in autonomic ganglia. He blocked synaptic transmission in the ganglia by painting them with nicotine and then mapped the distribution of the presynaptic and postsynaptic autonomic nerves.[48] He observed the similarity between the effects of injection of adrenal gland extracts and stimulation of the sympathetic nerves.[49] The active principle of adrenal medullary extracts was called *epinephrine* by John J. Abel[50] (1837-1938) in 1897. Abel was one of the first pharmacologists in the United States, and with his discovery of the hormone epinephrine, he uncovered one of the most commonly used lifesaving agents in the anesthesiologist's pharmacopoeia. Although epinephrine is a highly practical agent used by paramedics, emergency room physicians, intensivists, and anesthesiologists, Abel considered himself a "pure scientist." In one of his writings,[51] he made the following comments about the life of an investigator:

> The investigator should freely dare to attack problems not because they give promise of immediate value to the human race, but because they make an irresistible appeal of an inner beauty. ... From this point of view the investigator is a man whose inner life is free in the best sense of the word. In short, there should be in research work a cultural character, an artistic quality, elements that give to painting, music, and poetry their high place in the life of man.

Thomas R. Elliott (1877-1961) postulated that sympathetic nerve impulses release a substance similar to epinephrine and considered this substance to be a chemical step in the process of neurotransmission.[52] George Barger (1878-1939) and Henry H. Dale (1875-1968) then studied the pharmacologic activity of a large series of synthetic amines related to epinephrine and called these drugs *sympathomimetic*.[53] The different effects on end organs produced by adrenal extracts and sympathetic stimulation were analyzed by Walter B. Cannon[54] (1871-1945) and by Ulf Svante von Euler[55] (1905-1983). In a series of papers, these authors demonstrated that the sympathetic nerves released norepinephrine, whereas the adrenal gland released both epinephrine and norepinephrine.

In 1907, Walter E. Dixon[56] (1871-1931) observed that the alkaloid muscarine had the same effect as stimulation of the vagus nerves on various end organs. He proposed that the nerve liberated a muscarine-like chemical that acted as a chemical mediator. In 1914, Henry H. Dale[57] investigated the pharmacologic properties of acetylcholine and was impressed that its effects reproduced the same effects as stimulation of the craniosacral fine myelinated fibers that Walter H. Gaskell[58] (1847-1914) had called the *bulbosacral involuntary nerves* and had by then been called *parasympathetic* by Langley.

The final proof of neurotransmission by acetylcholine through chemical mediation was provided through the elegant experiments of Otto Loewi (1873-1961). He stimulated the neural innervation of the frog heart and then allowed the perfusion fluid to come in contact with a second isolated heart preparation.[59] The resulting bradycardia provided evidence that some substance was released from the donor nerves that slowed the heart rate of the second organ.[59] Loewi and Navrail presented evidence that this substance was acetylcholine, as Dale had suggested. Loewi and Dale were jointly awarded the Nobel Prize in 1936 for their work on chemical neurotransmission.

Theodore Tuffier (1857-1929) first demonstrated the relevance of the sympathetic nervous system to the practice of anesthesia in 1900. In a series of experiments on dogs, he demonstrated the sympatholysis that occurs after spinal anesthesia.[60] Further studies on the sympathectomy resulting from neuraxial block were performed by G. Smith and W. Porter in 1915.[61] Working with cats, they concluded that the fall in blood pressure was secondary to sympathetic paralysis of the vasomotor fibers in the splanchnic vessels. Gaston L. Labat[62] (1877-1934) encouraged the use of sympathetic stimulants such as ephedrine to counter the hypotensive effects of spinal anesthesia.

Reversal of neuromuscular blockade rests on a fundamental understanding of two types of cholinergic receptors, muscarinic and nicotinic, originally described in 1914 by Dale.[57] Physostigmine was isolated from the West African calabar bean by T. R. Fraser (1841-1920) in 1863,[63] and he also demonstrated that atropine blocked its muscarinic side effects. Jacob Pal[64] (1863-1936) discovered the effect of physostigmine to reverse the paralytic effect of curare in 1900. Neostigmine, synthesized in 1931,[65] given alone during reversal of neuromuscular blockade had produced cardiac arrest in several cases before it was learned that a proper dose of antimuscarinic drug should be administered beforehand.[66-68] Atropine was isolated from the plant *Atropa belladonna* by A. Mein[69] in 1831 and blocked peripheral and central nervous system muscarinic receptors. Glycopyrrolate was synthesized in 1960 as an antimuscarinic agent that did not pass the blood-brain barrier.[70] Glycopyrrolate is more titratable, has fewer central nervous system side effects, and has gradually replaced atropine as the preferred anticholinergic during reversal of neuromuscular blockade.

Crucial to the control of arterial blood pressure and heart rate in the perioperative period was the realization that there was more than one type of adrenergic receptor. In 1948, Ahlquist proposed the designations of α- and β-adrenergic receptors,[71] and various subtypes of these two main classes have been characterized since then. Esmolol was introduced in 1985 as a short-acting β-adrenergic antagonist that effectively controls heart rate during anesthesia.[72] Labetalol is a unique agent that was introduced in 1976 and antagonizes α- and β-adrenergic receptors.[73] Agonist activity at the α_2-adrenergic receptor, using agents such as clonidine and dexmedetomidine,[74] may have an expanded role in the practice of anesthesia in the future. The α_2-adrenergic agonist effects produce sedation and analgesia through a central effect and, because they do not induce respiratory depression, may have some advantages over opioids as sedatives in awake subjects.[75]

Manipulation of blood pressure can be achieved by intravenous nitrates, such as nitroglycerin and nitroprusside, which act directly on smooth muscle to allow rapid and more precise control of hemodynamics. Nitroglycerin was synthesized in 1846 by the Italian chemist Ascanio Sobrero (1812-1888) by combining nitric acid and glycerol. The first practical use of the drug was made by Alfred Nobel (1833-1896), who mixed the agent with silica to make dynamite, a highly successful explosive used in building tunnels and canals. A portion of the vast wealth of Nobel was directed by his will to be distributed annually in the form of Nobel Prizes beginning in 1901.[76,77] William Murrell[78] (1853-1912) reported the use of sublingual nitroglycerin in 1879 to treat angina. Intravenous use of the nitrovasodilators during anesthesia was not feasible until the development of continuous arterial monitoring, but for the past 30 years, these agents have been popular for rapid control of hypertensive crisis in the operating room.[79] The mechanism of action of nitrates on smooth muscle, by the release of nitric oxide, was demonstrated by Ferid Murad in 1986.[80] Nitric oxide, considered a toxic gas by Priestley who discovered it and by Humphry Davy who breathed it, has been shown to be a useful inhalation agent when used in a very low dose of 5 to 10 ppm in cases of life-threatening pulmonary hypertension.[81]

HISTORICAL DEVELOPMENT OF THEORIES OF PAIN

An understanding of the mechanism of pain production was not required by the physicians who developed the use of general anesthesia in the second half of the 19th century (see Chapter 73). Although inhalation of vapors produced lack of awareness during surgery, anesthesiologists learned that control of perioperative nociception would require a more thorough understanding of pain. Fortunately, by the beginning of the 20th century, there was already a large body of knowledge on pain mechanisms, dating from the earliest days of medical inquiry.

In antiquity, pain was thought to be an emotion rather than a sensory modality. Pain control was a function of religious authorities and shamans in primitive cultures, and relief of pain was sought through incantations and prayers. Pain was then often considered to be a punishment for committed sins or a form of religious suffering. The word *pain* is derived from the Greek term *poine* ("penalty"). Aristotle thought pain was an emotion emanating from the heart, but Galen correctly observed that the brain was required for pain to be manifested in animals. Galen also proposed that sensation was a property of nervous tissue, but his physiologic system was altogether hampered by his idea that an invisible psychic pneuma traveled within hollow nerves.[6]

The 18th and 19th centuries witnessed considerable progress in understanding the mechanisms of pain. Albrecht von Haller[82] (1708-1777) (see Fig. 1-3B) observed that some tissues in the body have a property that he called *sensibility*: "I call those parts sensible, if the irritation occasions evident signs of pain and disquiet in the animal." Other tissues were insensible, which "if touched occasioned no sign of pain nor convulsion." Some tissues were irritable. "I call that part of the human body irritable, if it becomes shorter upon being touched."

Haller's landmark contribution in 1752[83] concluded that only those parts of the body supplied with nerves possess sensibility, whereas irritability is a property of the muscular fibers. The idea of specific neural pathways for painful sensations began with Charles Bell[84] (1774-1842) and François Magendie[85] (1783-1855), who both demonstrated that the dorsal roots transmitted sensory information and that the ventral roots were for motor transmissions. Johannes Müller (1801-1858), in his 1826 paper entitled "Of the Peculiar Properties on Individual Nerves," proposed that each sense organ gave rise to its own characteristic sensation and to no other; electrical or mechanical stimulation of the optic nerve, for example, gives rise to only to a sensation of light.[86,87] The evidence that pain was a separate and distinct sense with separate end organs was formulated in 1858 by Moritz S. Schiff (1823-1896).[88]

By the end of the 19th century, the idea was firmly established that acute pain was a distinct sensory modality that was susceptible to interruption through conduction block initiated with local anesthetics. Pain as a separate sensation that was transmitted through separate neural fiber tracts was supported by clinical observations after neural blockade. Several investigators found, for example, that acute pain could be abolished with cocaine injections that left some sensory modalities unaffected.[89]

Developments in pain theory led to considerable modifications in the theory that pain was a hard-wired sensory connection between the nociceptor and the brain and that the intensity of the pain was directly proportional the extent of tissue injury. Consider the frightening experience of the missionary, David Livingstone (1813-1873), who spent 16 years in Africa exploring the interior of the continent. He offers this account[90] of his thoughts while being attacked by a lion:

> When in the act of ramming down the bullets I heard a shout, and, looking half round, I saw the lion in the act of springing upon me. He caught me by the shoulder, and we both came to the ground together. Growling horribly, he shook me as a terrier dog does to a rat. The shock produced a stupor similar to that which seems to be felt by a mouse after the first grip of the cat. It caused a sort of dreaminess, in which there was no sense of pain nor feeling of terror, though I was quite conscious of all that was happening.

Livingstone miraculously survived this attack and was left with crushed bones and 11 of the lion's teeth in his arm. It would seem from his account that Livingstone's central nervous system was providing its own powerful analgesic agents, not unlikely in the light of recent evidence that the brain can produce its own opioids that are capable of suppressing nociception. Livingstone compared his experience with what patients describe when partially under the influence of chloroform.

There is evidence that operations undertaken in the battlefield may be associated with less pain compared with similar elective operations performed without anesthesia. The amputation of Lord Horatio Nelson's right arm in the battle at Tenerife, Canary Islands, was performed aboard ship after he sustained a musket shot above the elbow, dividing the artery and shattering the humerus. Nelson complained only that the knife felt cold and thereafter ordered that all knives on board be heated before entering into conflict, because his personal experience had indicated a warm knife would produce almost no discomfort.[91] Henry Beecher[92] (1904-1976) confirmed during World War II that wounded soldiers had surprisingly little pain.

To further explain some of these central influences on nociception, Melzack and Wall proposed the gate control theory of pain in 1965.[93] They proposed that as the nociceptive afferent pain fibers entered the spinal cord, they synapsed in the dorsal horn, where the input was subjected to the modulating influence of a "gate" before it was transmitted rostrally. The theory further suggests that large-fiber inputs tend to close the gate (i.e., inhibit nociceptive transmission), small-fiber inputs open it, and

descending influences from the cortex and midbrain[94] also profoundly influence the gate. Endogenous opioids, first discovered in 1974 by A. Goldstein[95] and later confirmed by J. Hughes[96] in 1975 and S. H. Snyder and coworkers[97] in 1977, are located at diverse sites in the pain pathway, including the dorsal horn, and they can influence the rostral transmission of pain sensations. Several modalities of pain therapy, such as acupuncture and biofeedback, attempt to activate these endogenous systems to suppress chronic pain syndromes.

The gate theory of pain has had considerable influence on the anesthesiologist's management of pain by focusing attention on the unique pharmacology of the dorsal horn of the spinal cord. By using intrathecal and epidural injections,[98] anesthesiologists have learned to suppress nociceptive transmission at the first synaptic relay in the spinal cord. The technique has implications in acute and chronic pain therapy because neuraxially administered drugs can provide analgesia without some of the systemic side effects of intravenously administered drugs. A typically modern view of perioperative pain is to view it as an impediment to recovery. Aggressive methods are often used to minimize pain to facilitate hospital discharge and a rapid return to normal functional activity.[99]

SURGICAL PROCEDURES BEFORE 1846

Greek and Roman surgeons used a variety of surgical instruments that we would recognize today. Drills, saws, syringes, cannulas, probes, and scalpels can all be viewed in the excavations at Herculaneum, Pompeii, and Rheims. Hippocrates (460-377 BC) wrote a treatise on surgery but provided little sympathy for the patient. His advice to the patient was "to accommodate the operator ... and maintain the figure and position of the part operated on ... and avoid sinking down, and shrinking from or turning away."[100] The most famous Roman surgeon was Pedanius Dioscorides (40-90 AD), a Greek physician who served in the armies of Nero. His *Materia Medica,* written in 77 AD, was the authoritative work on pharmacology for more than 15 centuries. In this book, he described the effects of mandragora and wine that produced "anesthesia" in the patient being cut or cauterized. He also described local anesthesia produced by the "stone of Memphis," which "being cut small, and smeared upon the places to be cut or cauterized, it produces anesthesia without danger."[6] Unfortunately, neither Dioscorides nor his students identified this stone so that it could be used by later generations.

During the Middle Ages, attempts were made to use alcohol fumes as an analgesic during surgery (Fig. 1-4B). The *soporific sponge* is mentioned in numerous manuscripts written in the Middle Ages. One example[6] from the 9th century comes from a Benedictine monastery at Monte Cassino, near Salerno, Italy:

> A hypnotic aid, that is a soporific suitable for those who are treated by surgery, so that asleep, they do not feel the pain of cutting. Rx: opium one half ounce, mandragora the juice from the leaves, eight ounces, the juice of fresh hemlock, hyposcyanus

three ounces of the juice together with sufficient water so that it forms a liquor, and then absorb in a fresh dry sponge and dry it carefully. And when thou wouldst employ this sponge, dip it in warm water, place it over the nose and cause the patient to breathe deep until he sleeps. And when thou wouldst wake him up, apply to his nose another sponge well soaked with vinegar and thou willst end the sleep.

The sponge used by Theodoric of Cervia (1205-1296), a member of the Dominican order who practiced in Bologna, contained the same ingredients as the Salernitan sponge. Theodoric was one of the first surgeons to promote methods to ablate pain during surgery (see Fig. 1-4A). A notable German physician of the 15th century, Heinrich von Pfolspeundt, mentioned the same sponge in a book on surgery dating from the year 1460. The effective agents in this sponge were very likely opium and scopolamine.[6]

One of the great physicians of the Renaissance, Theophrastus Bombastus von Hohenheim, otherwise known as Paracelsus (1493-1541), was familiar with the soporific action of sulfuric ether, a compound that had been synthesized from sulfuric acid and alcohol by the chemist Valerius Cordus (1515-1544). Cordus called the flammable, volatile liquid *sweet vitriol*, and in 1740, Frobenius named it *ether* (from the Greek word for "ignite" or "blaze"). Paracelsus described the effect of ether on chickens and stated that it "quiets all suffering without harm, and relieves all pain."[101] Although he was appointed "surgeon to the Danish army" when they besieged Stockholm in 1518, he had little interest in surgery, and these ideas were not expanded into the clinical arena.

Before the mid-19th century, the desire to relieve the pain of surgery was not intense enough for surgeons to develop the idea of general anesthesia. Textbooks on surgery are numerous before 1846, but rarely is there a discussion on the alleviation of pain. One example is Pancoast's *Textbook of Surgery*, which was published in 1844.[102] This text has extensive coverage of surgical procedures that were performed at that time, but no mention is made of methods to provide comfort for the patient. Alcohol, opium, and hypnotism were used, but primarily surgical speed and brute force were required for successful completion of operations. Mesmerism and somnambulism were forms of "animal magnetism" that developed in Europe and were purported to provide relief of pain during surgery. These claims were developed by Franz Anton Mesmer (1734-1815) but were eventually proved fraudulent near the end of the 18th century by a commission set up by the King of France, Louis XVI. This commission was directed by Benjamin Franklin and included Joseph Guillotine, after whom the guillotine was named, and Lavoisier, the discoverer of oxygen. The Mesmerists could, however, be given credit for raising the public's attention to the problem of surgical pain, even though their teachings eventually were proved to be worthless.[103]

Anyone with questions about the dramatic break with the past that occurred in the 1840s has only to examine the accounts written by patients who survived major surgical procedures before that time. One comes from Fanny Burney[104] (1752-1840), a novelist and celebrity of the early part of the 19th century. Here is an abbreviated account of her mastectomy for breast cancer by the surgeon Dominique J. Larrey (1766-1842), the celebrated military surgeon in Napoleon's army, and the date was September 30, 1811:

I mounted the bed and a cambric handkerchief was placed upon my face. The bed was then surrounded by 7 men and my nurse. Through the cambric I saw the glitter of the polished steel knife. A silence ensued. ... Oh what a horrible suspension! ...When the dreadful steel was plunged into the breast,

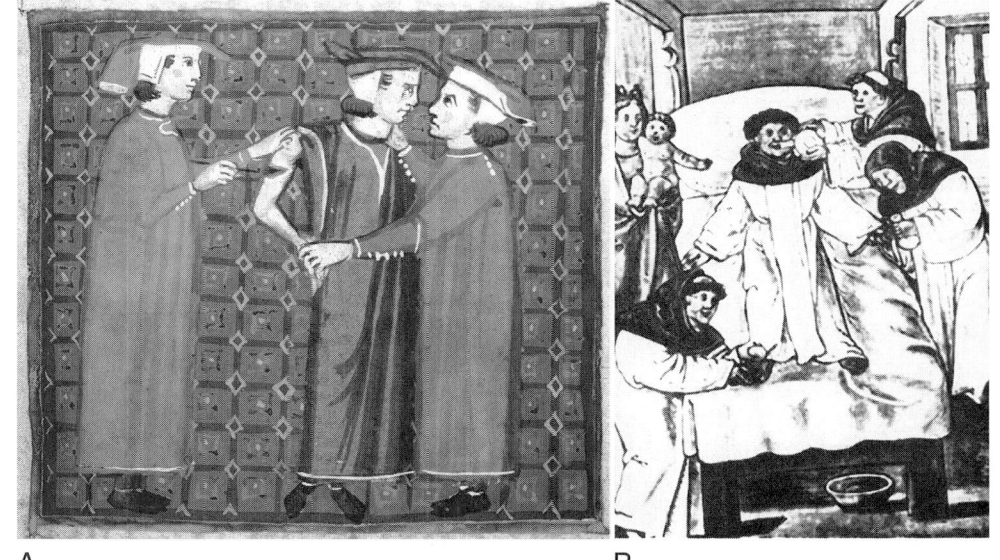

Figure 1–4 A, "Operating on the Upper Arm" is taken from the textbook entitled *Chirurgia* by Theodoric of Cervia. It is noteworthy because it shows an intense focus by the patient directly into the gaze of an assistant. Although hypnosis is a 19th century term and its use for pain relief during surgery was not widely promoted until then, the induction of trances and altered states of being was known to the ancients. Theodoric apparently realized the value of diverting the patient's attention away from pain of surgery. **B,** Inhalation of the vapor of alcohol was tried in the Middle Ages as a method for pain relief during surgery. The inhaler shown here is remarkably similar to that used by William T. G. Morton on October 16, 1846, with ether as the volatile agent (compare with Fig. 1-6).

A   B

I needed no injunctions not to restrain my cries. I began a scream that lasted unintermittently during the whole time of the incision and I almost marvel that it rings not in my ears still, so excruciating was the agony.

Although Fanny Burney lived for another 29 years after this operation, she observed that anything that would recall the surgery to her mind would reactivate the terror of the horrible experience. Apparently, operations performed without anesthesia produced long-lasting emotional and painful side effects. A modern interpretation of this phenomenon could conclude that these patients lacked any form of "preemptive analgesia"[105] and that they therefore experienced lingering side effects after their surgical wounds had healed.

In addition to patients who experienced the terror of an operation, there were countless others who suffered with chronic ailments because the risk of surgery was too high or because they feared death or severe pain during the operation more than they suffered with the chronic condition. For example, even after the introduction of anesthesia in 1846, textbooks on treatment for hernia continued to have extensive descriptions of hernia belts and trusses.[106, 107]

When the old operating room (1830) was recently restored at St. Thomas Hospital in London, the workers found dried poppy seed pods in the rafters. The apparent ineffectiveness of their analgesic methods, which presumably included alcohol and opium, and the clearly religious connotations of pain and suffering can be assumed by a review of the prayer[108] that was read to patients before their departure to the operating theater:

> As sickness is the usual forerunner of death, it should therefore lead you seriously to consider and reflect on your behavior in life. Man's life is but a succession of sorrows and a state of sufferings, that at most it is but of short duration, and at the best, of an uncertain continuance.

INTRODUCTION OF GENERAL ANESTHESIA

Background

In retrospect, a modern person wonders what kind of mental blindness could have prevented physicians from actively pursuing a remedy for the horrors of surgery. Medical historians have stated that the secularization of pain therapy[109] and slowly evolving concepts of disease were the primary influences that determined the introduction of anesthesia in the middle of the 19th century.

Before the Renaissance, disease was considered to result from an imbalance among the four basic fluids within the body: blood, phlegm, yellow bile, and black bile. This theory was slow to dissipate, and remnants of these ideas were still present at the end of the 18th century. However, seminal research studies by Giovanni Battista Morgagni (1682-1771) demonstrated that disease resulted from organ dysfunction and as such was amenable to treatment by various interventions, with

surgical drainage and extirpation among them.[110] Rudolph Virchow (1821-1902), who carried on these concepts of disease in the 19th century,[111] considers that modern medicine began with Morgagni because he pursued the study of disease from a symptom to the organ from which the symptom arose. Occurring at the same time was a trend away from viewing surgical pain as inevitable religious suffering into a more active search for some preventive medical intervention.

Although surgical technique was in development, the patient presented a problem to the surgeon, chiefly because of active physical resistance and because the cries and screams were distracting and often left the patient emotionally and physically exhausted. These factors, combined with the inevitable sepsis, resulted in high mortality rates. No wonder that by the middle of the 19th century there was greater determination by some surgeons to devise ways of improving operating conditions to decrease appalling surgical mortality figures, which in some reports reached nearly 50%. Bold approaches and risks were required, and these factors came together in Boston, Massachusetts, on October 16, 1846, when William T. G. Morton demonstrated the use of ether inhalation for surgical anesthesia.

Gas Inhalation

One perspective on this remarkable discovery is to view it as the culminating event of nearly 75 years of experimentation on the therapeutic use of inhaled gases and vapors. The chemist of the late 16th century was looked on as a blight on society, a person who worked with vile-smelling substances and whose clothes were covered with stains and burns. These attitudes began to change in the 17th and 18th centuries, when the chemists discovered that air was not a simple substance but a combination of different airs, all following certain physical laws. Jean Baptiste van Helmont (1577-1644) invented the word *gas* (from the Greek *chaos*) to describe an uncontrollable substance that was liberated when acid was added to limestone.[112] Robert Boyle[113] (1627-1691), Jacques Charles (1746-1823), and John Dalton (1766-1844) outlined the basic properties of gases, and these laws accelerated the study of combustion, respiration, and the transmission of sound. Of particular importance to our history is the law governing the transfer of gases into liquids, proposed by William Henry[114] (1775-1836) in 1803. Henry's law stated that the amount of gas absorbed by a liquid is proportional to the pressure of the gas above the liquid, provided no chemical reaction occurs.

Joseph Priestley and the Swedish chemist Carl W. Scheele (1742-1786) performed the first investigations on gas inhalation. Scheele, the co-discoverer of oxygen, nearly killed himself by experimenting with inhalation of hydrocyanic acid, one of the several gases he discovered.[11] Priestley played a significant role in the identification of elemental gases and advocated inhalation of "dephlogisicated air" (i.e., oxygen) for various medical conditions. He wrote in 1776 that after inhalation of dephlogisicated air, "I fancied that my breast felt peculiarly light and easy for some time afterwards. Who can tell that in time, this pure air may become a fashionable article in luxury. Hitherto only two mice and myself have had the privilege of breathing it."[10] Unsanitary living conditions in the late 18th century had led to a preoccupation with the evils and disease-producing attributes of putrid air. The corollary was that pure airs, even "fixed air" (i.e., carbon dioxide), the same gas described by van Helmont and rediscovered by Joseph Black[115] (1728-1799), might promote health.

As a result of the growing scientific interest in various types of "airs," popular medical treatments involving gas inhalation evolved. Health resorts were popular attractions and financially successful because of their use by prominent members of society. One important "pneumatic" spa was located at Clifton, near Bristol, England, where Thomas Beddoes[116] (1760-1808) furnished airs for therapeutic use and funded research on the manufacture and use of gases. Nitrous oxide, a gas codiscovered by Priestley and Joseph Black, was by then considered to be a dangerous gas, following the pronouncement by the American chemist Samuel Latham Mitchill that the gas was the "principle of contagion" and if breathed would "spread plague." The young scientist Humphry Davy conducted research on nitrous oxide at the Beddoes institute and, undaunted by these pronouncements, made several important observations. He inhaled nitrous oxide and noticed that it provided relief from the pain caused from an erupting wisdom tooth. In 1800, he wrote: "As nitrous oxide in its extensive operation appears capable of destroying physical pain, it may probably be used with advantage during surgical operations in which no great effusion of blood takes place."[117]

Davy was not a surgeon, and clinicians overlooked his suggestion at the time. He resigned his position at the Beddoes Medical Pneumatic Institute in 1801 and moved to London to lecture at the newly founded Royal Institution of Great Britain. Davy was only 20 years old when he performed the studies on nitrous oxide, and his subsequent, highly successful career took him into other areas of scientific study that led to the discovery of the elements potassium, sodium, calcium, barium, magnesium, strontium, and chlorine. He was knighted in 1812, became President of the Royal Society in 1820, and never returned to develop his promising early thoughts on nitrous oxide analgesia. Regrettably, he left no students to continue these studies, although his successor at the Royal Institute, Michael Faraday (1791-1867), briefly experimented with ether inhalation and observed that its "effects were similar to those occasioned by nitrous oxide."[118]

The first research specifically directed toward an effective method for providing pain-free surgery was made by a physician working in the village of Ludlow, Shropshire in northern England. Henry Hill Hickman (1800-1830) was a practicing surgeon who investigated the use of carbon dioxide to induce insensibility in animals. Because of the widespread interest in inhalation therapy at the beginning of the 19th century, it is not surprising that Hickman used an inhaled gas. Unfortunately for him, he used the wrong gas, because if he had selected nitrous oxide, which was known to produce analgesia, his results might have achieved further attention. Although he published his work in 1824 in a private letter to T. A. Knight,[119]

Hickman failed to find any support from his colleagues in England or France, and he died at an early age without recognition.

Although pneumatic spas such as the Beddoes Institute were short-lived, a lingering interest in gas inhalation persisted in the form of traveling amusement shows that welcomed members of the audience to experience the altered sensations induced by ether or nitrous oxide inhalation. A young ex–merchant marine, Samuel Colt (1814-1862), learned how to produce nitrous oxide from the chief chemist at a textile factory where he had occasional work. Colt needed cash to secure a patent on a new type of handgun that he had invented while at sea. The gun featured a rotating cylinder that advanced up to six new cartridges when the hammer was cocked. In the early 1830s, Colt traveled from village to village along the East Coast of North America selling whiffs of nitrous oxide for 25 cents. The enterprise was highly successful, and he used his accumulated funds to patent his new revolver in 1835. The gun was used by the U.S. military in the U.S.–Mexican War, and during the following decades, the Colt six-shooter became one of the legends of the Wild West of North America and made Samuel Colt one of the wealthiest men of his time.

Beginning of Inhaled Anesthesia

The story of anesthesia continues with another amateur and itinerant chemist, Gardner Quincy Colton (1814-1898) (Fig. 1-5A). Colton had attended 2 years of medical school at the Crosby Street College of Physicians and Surgeons in New York. While in school, he perfected the manufacture of nitrous oxide by heating ammonium nitrate, and after 2 years of study, he proclaimed himself to be a "Professor of Chemistry" and went on the road to lecture on chemistry and present "scientific exhibitions."

On the night of December 10, 1844, Professor Colton presented his exhibit featuring inhalations of nitrous oxide at Union Hall in Hartford, Connecticut. It was at the Colton exhibit that the dentist Horace Wells (1815-1848) originated an idea that culminated in the first successful demonstration of inhalation anesthesia 22 months later. Wells had experimented with mesmerism to relieve the pain of dental extractions and was aware of the work of Humphry Davy. He attended the Colton demonstration and observed a young man, Samuel A. Cooley, sustain a significant leg injury without pain after nitrous oxide inhalation. Here was the answer to the problem of painful tooth extractions that had occupied his mind. He arranged for Colton to administer nitrous oxide to him on the following day for extraction of one of Wells' own teeth by fellow dentist, John M. Riggs. Only a slight tinge of pain was felt, and Wells proceeded to manufacture nitrous oxide according to Colton's instructions and use it for extractions of teeth. He recognized the enormous potential of his discovery and used his connections in Boston to arrange a date at the Harvard Medical School to demonstrate the technique of painless surgery.

Wells' appointment was to administer the gas for a leg amputation. The patient scheduled for this procedure refused to proceed with the anesthetic, and a young male student agreed to breathe nitrous oxide for extraction of a wisdom tooth. During the extraction, the subject moved and groaned, only later to proclaim that little pain was actually felt. Nevertheless, Wells was discredited and became despondent, eventually withdrawing from further public promotions of his methods.

William T. G. Morton (see Fig. 1-5B), a young dentist from Boston, was acquainted with Wells, having been a former student and colleague of his, and had attended the failed demonstration at Harvard. Morton had lingering thoughts about a more suitable agent, in part arising from his interest in promoting his business of selling dentures. He had invented a new method for fitting dentures, but the process was prohibitively painful, and few patients would submit to the procedure. An adequate analgesic could accelerate his business.

Morton was initially trained as a dentist but had enrolled briefly at Harvard Medical School. Because of financial difficulties, he had abandoned these studies and returned to dentistry. In the course of his education, he became acquainted with Charles A. Jackson, a professor of chemistry at Harvard Medical School. On Morton's queries, Jackson advised a trial of sulfuric ether as an alternative to nitrous oxide. Later, Jackson was to claim priority in the discovery of anesthesia based on these consultations, but Morton countered that Jackson's role was negligible. Morton obtained the ether and, after performing experiments on himself and his pet animals, administered the agent successfully on September 30, 1846, to Eben Frost for extraction of an upper bicuspid tooth. Prompted by this success, he promoted use of the agent in his dental practice, thereby gaining the attention of another key figure, Henry J. Bigelow (1818-1890), in the unfolding drama. Bigelow, a prominent young surgeon at the Massachusetts General Hospital, privately witnessed Morton's success with ether and arranged the time and date for its public demonstration.

The events of October 16, 1846, a complete triumph for Morton, have been recounted several times by others, but certain points are of special interest. The patient, George Abbott, whom Morton apparently had never met, was to have a vascular tumor of the neck with large tortuous veins excised in the sitting position by 68-year-old chief surgeon John Collins Warren (1778-1856). Fearing a difficult airway or air embolism, a modern anesthesiologist might seek special equipment for this case, perhaps a special laryngoscope and central venous catheters. Morton, however, had only a poorly designed inhaler and no intravenous access. Close examination of the circumstances surrounding administration of this anesthetic indicates how dangerous this bold endeavor by Morton actually was and how likely it was to fail miserably. With the inhaler that he used, it seems unlikely that the vapor could be administered during the surgical procedure. Fortunately for Morton, the kinetic properties of ether result in a prolonged emergence, and Mr. Abbott responded only briefly at the end of the procedure (Fig. 1-6).

Morton, intending to profit from his discovery, withheld identification of the ether he used and called it *Letheon*. He masked the aroma and appearance of ether by adding a colored dye and additional scents. For a fee,

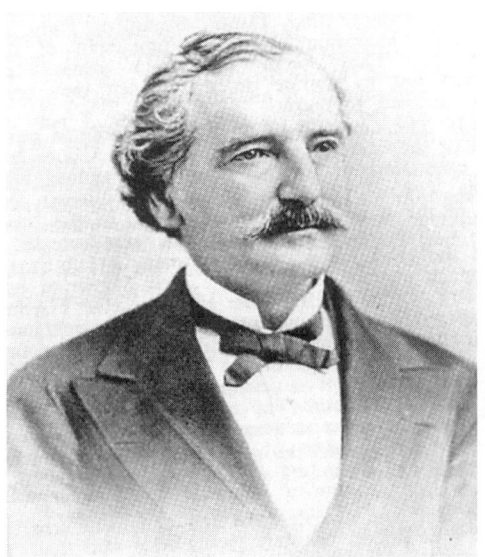

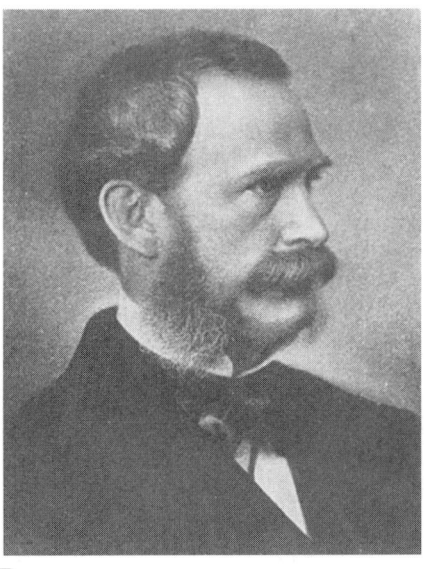

A   B

Figure 1–5 A, Gardner Q. Colton was born in Georgia, Vermont, and studied medicine briefly at the College of Physicians and Surgeons in New York City. His demonstrations of nitrous oxide inhalations were the spark that prompted Horace Wells and William T. G. Morton to use gas inhalation for relief of surgical pain. After a long and adventurous career, he died at age 84 in Rotterdam, Holland. **B,** William T. G. Morton was born in 1819 on a farm near Charlton, Massachusetts. After several business failures, he studied at the Baltimore College of Dental Surgery, and in 1842 entered into a partnership in Boston with another dentist, Horace Wells. This partnership was dissolved within a year on amicable terms. During this association, the two dentists had devised a new method for fitting dentures that required removal of all the diseased teeth, a prohibitively painful procedure for most patients. Morton experimented with laudanum and opium without success, and in proceeding with his investigations, he realized that a greater knowledge of medicine was essential for further success. He briefly entered Harvard Medical School while continuing a part-time dental practice. During the summer of 1844, Morton, on the advice of Charles T. Jackson, used sulfuric ether for painless tooth extractions, and the study of this agent eventually led to his successful demonstration of ether anesthesia at Massachusetts General Hospital on October 16, 1846. The remainder of Morton's life was spent in efforts to patent and receive a monetary recognition for the discovery of ether anesthesia. Broken and despondent, he died of a cerebral hemorrhage in New York City in July 1868. (Images courtesy of the Wood Library-Museum of Anesthesiology, Park Ridge, IL.)

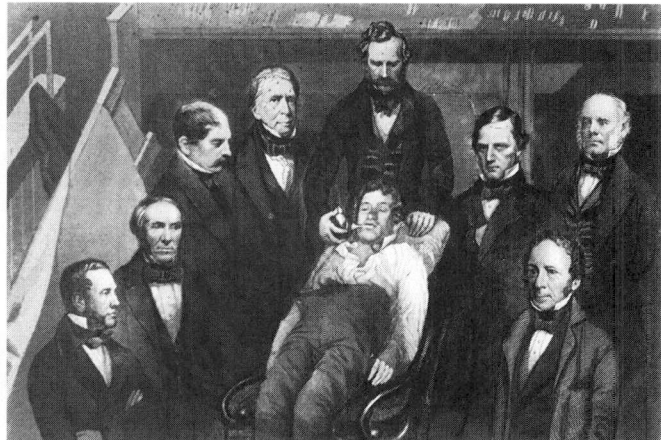

Figure 1–6 Drawing by H. H. Hall in Rice's *Trials of a Public Benefactor* illustrates the first public demonstration of ether anesthesia at Massachusetts General Hospital on October 16, 1846.[482] **From left:** *Henry J. Bigelow* (1818-1890), the earliest advocate and sponsor for William T. G. Morton at the hospital, who also wrote the classic article describing the first experiences with ether anesthesia in the Boston Medical and Surgical Journal. *Augustus A. Gould,* with whom Morton and his wife were boarding and who suggested the design of the first inhaler. Gould also suggested the name Letheon. *Jonathan Mason Warren* (1811-1867), son of John Collins Warren, who later devised new surgical procedures for nasal deformity and cleft lip. Hall erroneously places him at this event. Others (not shown) who were present are George Heywood, house officer, and Eben Frost, who had a tooth pulled by Morton after ether administration on September 30, 1846. *John Collins Warren* (1778-1856), 68-year-old Chief of Surgery at Massachusetts General Hospital who performed the operation that day; *William T. G. Morton,* to whom credit is given for introducing ether anesthesia to the world; *Gilbert Abbott,* 28-year-old house painter and printer with a congenital vascular tumor, visible in the drawing as a tumor below the left mandible; *Samuel Parkman,* Morton's anatomy instructor at Harvard Medical School; and *George Hayward* (1791-1863), 53-year-old senior surgeon at Massachusetts General Hospital, who performed an excision of an arm mass with ether anesthesia the following day, October 17, 1846. His operation for vesicovaginal fistula is considered to be an original procedure. Also present was *Solomon D. Townsend,* one of the prominent surgeons at Harvard Medical School. (Courtesy of the Wood Library-Museum of Anesthesiology, Park Ridge, IL.)

he intended to provide instruction on its safe use. The surgeons at Massachusetts General Hospital then denied continued use of the agent until its true nature was identified. After disclosure of its chemical nature by Morton, further operations were performed with success. Bigelow read his manuscript describing the use of ether for operative surgery on November 3, 1846, before the American Academy of Arts and Sciences and published it (Fig. 1-7) in the November 18, 1846, issue of the *Boston Medical and Surgical Journal.*[120] The name *anesthesia* (Greek for *an,* "without," and *esthesia,* "perception") was suggested by Oliver Wendell Holmes (1809-1894) in a private letter to Morton dated November 21, 1846. Holmes also considered the words *antineurotic, aneuric, neuroleptic, neurolepsia,*

Insensibility During Surgical Operations Produced by Inhalation

Henry Jacob Bigelow, M.D.
Boston Medical and Surgical Journal
1846

It has long been an important problem in medical science to devise some method of mitigating the pain of surgical operations. An efficient agent for this purpose has at length been discovered. A patient has been rendered completely insensible during an amputation of the thigh, regaining consciousness after a short interval. Other severe operations have been performed without the knowledge of the patients. So remarkable an occurrence will, it is believed, render the following details relating to the history and character of the process, not uninteresting.

Figure 1–7 Title and opening paragraph of Henry J. Bigelow's description of the first ether anesthetics.[120]

and *neurostasis,* but he rejected these as being "too anatomical" because the change induced by ether was physiologic.

Aftermath

It is remarkable that without more explicit instructions or an actual demonstration by one of the Boston group, ether anesthesia was adopted so rapidly around the world. Only 63 days after the Morton demonstration, ether was administered in England by James Robinson (1813-1862), a prominent London dentist, for extraction of a deep-seated molar in a 13-year-old girl. Robinson had learned of ether anesthesia through a letter shown to him by a neighboring friend, Francis Boott, who had received the letter from Jacob Bigelow, father of Henry Bigelow, describing the effects of ether inhalation. Robinson devised a new inhaler and wrote the first textbook on anesthesia, which was published in London on March 1, 1847.[121] Two days after Robinson's use of ether, Robert Liston (1794-1847) performed the first operation in England—a leg amputation at University College Hospital, London—with ether as the anesthetic delivered by William Squire. Within a few months, ether anesthesia had spread to the European continent. Nikolai Ivanovitch Pirogoff (1810-1881) used ether in St. Petersburg as early as February 1847, and he wrote a treatise on the subject.[122] Of significant importance for the widespread use of ether was the prestige of the Boston surgeons, who firmly supported its legitimacy.

Many who tried to administer the anesthetic did so without proper preparation, and failures were common. Several questions remained unanswered. Bigelow's article was vague about how it should be administered, simply describing a number of cases with the use of Morton's inhaler. How the ether was supposed to be administered after the loss of consciousness was not addressed.

Nasal breathing or failure to purse the lips around the mouthpiece must have placed a limit on the duration of effective vapor administration. It was another lucky circumstance for Morton that ether was chosen as his agent. Subsequent studies with ether have revealed that it stimulates the sympathetic nervous system at deep levels of anesthesia.[123] This unique property of the drug and its high blood solubility result in a remarkably safe agent, requiring only marginal skills to avoid overdose.

Priority for Discovery

Claims of priority for the discovery of ether anesthesia arose quickly. Wells, Morton, and Jackson all claimed to have discovered anesthesia. The issue of priority was further complicated by a report that a surgeon in Jefferson, Georgia, had used ether anesthesia as early as 1842. Crawford Long (1815-1878) published a manuscript in the *Southern Medical and Surgical Journal* in December 1849, describing his use of ether on March 30, 1842, to excise a tumor from the neck of a young man, James M. Venable.[124]

Numerous monuments have been erected to commemorate the man "who discovered anesthesia." At least 15 have been erected for the group of Morton, Wells, and Long. A chair that Charles Jackson sat in while experimenting with ether inhalation is on display in the Pilgrim Memorial Hall in Plymouth, Massachusetts, with the label "Seated in this chair, Dr. Charles T. Jackson discovered etherization February, 1842." In the Public Gardens of Boston, a monument without a name has been erected to those who discovered anesthesia, suggesting that the introduction of ether anesthesia was the product of several individuals. Howard R. Raper, in his book *Man Against Pain*, analyzed the controversy about "who discovered anesthesia"[2] and suggested that Crawford Long was the discoverer if only the issue of *priority* is considered. However, Long continued to use whiskey and other ineffective means after 1842, indicating his apparent lack of enthusiasm for ether. Wells was the discoverer if the *idea* of inhalation anesthesia is considered, and Morton was the discoverer if the primary consideration is who *introduced* inhalation anesthesia to the world. Historians have generally credited the personality that produces the actual change in medical practice, and that individual was William Thomas Green Morton.

Neither honors nor monetary awards were forthcoming during the remaining lives of Wells or Morton. Wells committed suicide in 1848, unaware that the French Academy of Sciences had just named him as the true discoverer of anesthesia. Morton was unsuccessful in his effort to profit from a patent on his discovery or to secure a financial award from the U.S. government and died, broken and despondent, at age 49. Jackson (1804-1880) was committed to a hospital for the mentally ill at the age of 68 years, where he died 7 years later. Morton was 27 years old when he demonstrated ether anesthesia. The ages of the other participants at the time of their discoveries were as follows: Wells (1815-1848) was 29; Davy (1778-1829) was 22; Hickman (1800-1830) was 24; Jackson (1804-1880) was 41; Long (1815-1878) was 27; and Colton (1814-1898) was 30 years old.

DEVELOPMENT OF INHALATION AGENTS

Chloroform

Within a year after the introduction of ether anesthesia, the search had already begun for other agents that could anesthetize without some of the problems associated with ether. Although ether was a remarkably safe agent, even when administered by untrained hands, there were disadvantages, which included flammability, a prolonged induction, unpleasant odor that was persistent, and a high incidence of nausea and vomiting. James Young Simpson (1811-1870), an obstetrician from Edinburgh, Scotland, used ether in 1846 but was determined to find a better agent. As early as January of 1847, he began experimenting with a variety of different solvents and volatile liquids.[125]

The physician David Waldie, a contemporary of Simpson at Edinburgh Medical School who was practicing in Liverpool, England, suggested chloroform as an alternative agent. Synthesized independently by Samuel Guthrie[126] (1782-1848), Eugene Soubeiran[127] (1787-1858), and Justus von Liebig[128] (1803-1873) in 1831, it had never been tested in humans as an inhaled anesthetic. Marie Jean Flourens[129] (1794-1867) had used chloroform in dogs while studying the stages in the depression of the central nervous system by chloroform and ether. Simpson and a group of friends learned of the surprising potency of chloroform at a dinner party hosted by Simpson on September 4, 1847. Dinner was followed by the experimental inhalation of volatile drugs, and the use of chloroform was followed by stupor and coma by several participants, including Simpson. Simpson promoted chloroform vigorously, and its use was widely accepted in England. As an obstetrician, he advocated its use during labor, promoting, along with others,[130] the employment of analgesics during parturition. Initially, his views conflicted with those of medical authorities who considered it unsafe during labor and with those of religious authorities who opposed it on theologic grounds. Edinburgh had a black history on the issue of pain relief during childbirth. In 1591, a young woman named Euphanie Macalyane was burned alive as punishment for seeking pain relief during labor on direct order from the King of Scotland, James VI.[131] Simpson was not a timid man and met the religious controversy with direct quotations from the Bible that appeared to support his views (Genesis 2, 21: "and the Lord God caused a deep sleep to fall upon Adam, and he slept: and he took one of his ribs, and closed up the flesh instead thereof.").

Chloroform was used widely in England, but controversy developed about its safety, particularly in otherwise healthy subjects, those in whom a physician would not anticipate any difficulties. Various commissions and committees were formed, notably the two Hyderabad commissions (1888 and 1890),[132] to investigate the relative safety of chloroform. In the late 19th century, Hyderabad, a city in the middle of the Indian subcontinent, was the capital of the independent State of Hyderabad, ruled by the Nizam, Mir Mehboob Ali Khan.

The Nizam was persuaded to underwrite an animal investigation into the safety of chloroform anesthesia by Major Edward Lawrie, Principal of the Indian Medical School in Hyderabad. Lawrie had preconceived belief in the safety of chloroform, and the results of his studies understandably concluded that chloroform was entirely safe if given according to his methods. The agent continued in use for several decades, but its slow demise was initiated in 1894, when Leonard G. Guthrie[133] reported on several cases of delayed chloroform hepatotoxicity in children. The future use of chloroform anesthesia was doomed after the studies of A. Goodman Levy[134] (1856-1954), who demonstrated that the combination of light chloroform anesthesia and adrenalin produced fatal ventricular fibrillation in experimental animals, explaining the perplexing sudden demise of several healthy subjects administered chloroform anesthetics.

Nitrous Oxide

Because of the embarrassing public demonstration by Wells in 1863, the revival of nitrous oxide as a surgical anesthetic was delayed until its reintroduction by the same man, Gardner Q. Colton, whose lecture and demonstration Wells had attended in 1844 and from whom he obtained the gas used in his first experiments with inhalation analgesia. Soon after the Wells debacle in 1844, Colton abandoned nitrous oxide demonstrations and joined his brother in California, where he unsuccessfully panned for gold and served briefly as Justice of the Peace for San Francisco. His stay in San Francisco terminated when he was involved in controversial land sales, and he moved to Boston, taking a job as a writer for the *Boston Transcript*.[135] Colton also resumed his "laughing gas" exhibitions, and in 1863, he joined into a partnership with Joseph H. Smith, a dentist in New Haven, Connecticut, for the "painless extraction of teeth." The business thrived, and between 1864 and 1897, the Colton Dental Association had treated nearly 200,000 patients without a fatality. Colton demonstrated nitrous oxide inhalation in Paris at the First International Congress of Medicine in June of 1867, and its wider use in Europe originates from that time. Colton was a unique individual who promoted the continued use of a valuable agent, but he remained ignorant of its true chemical nature. In his writings,[136] he states, for example, the following:

> The gas is composed of half nitrogen and half oxygen and because oxygen is the life giving principle of the air, a person lives a little faster while under its influence. It acts as an exhilarant, as by supplying an extra supply of oxygen to the lungs, the pulse is increased 15 to 20 beats to the minute.

Until 1870, nitrous oxide was administered with air, and the livid appearance of many patients raised the question about whether the analgesic properties of the gas were primarily caused by lack of oxygen. The idea of using nitrous oxide with oxygen is usually credited to Edmund Andrews[137] (1824-1904), a Chicago surgeon, who was able to provide analgesia without cyanosis, therefore confirming the inherent analgesic properties of nitrous oxide. Andrews noticed that the nitrous oxide provided to dentists in gaseous form was often impure and advocated instead the use of liquid nitrous oxide contained in iron flasks. This pure nitrous oxide, when combined with oxygen, provided satisfactory anesthesia without cyanosis for short procedures. Paul Bert[138] (1833-1886), a French physiologist who contributed significantly to an understanding of blood gas tensions at altered barometric pressures, demonstrated that nitrous oxide and oxygen mixtures produced highly satisfactory surgical anesthesia without hypoxia when delivered at pressures greater than 1 atm. Frederick Hewitt[139] (1857-1916) devised the first anesthesia machine to deliver variable portions of nitrous oxide and oxygen. Johnson demonstrated that pupillary dilation, lividity, jactitation, and clonic movements of the extremities after nitrous oxide and air administration were caused by extreme hypoxia, because they could be reproduced exactly by administering nitrogen with only 0.5% oxygen.[140]

These developments led to the reintroduction of nitrous oxide into the operating room, where Horace Wells had predicted it would be used with success. Nitrous oxide and oxygen anesthesia was promoted in the United States by Elmer I. McKesson[141] (1881-1935), Paluel J. Flagg[142] (1886-1970), and F. W. Clement[143] (1892-1970). McKesson's method for induction of anesthesia with 100% nitrous oxide did not survive into the later part of the 20th century. A landmark publication by C. B. Courville described the neuropathologic findings in patients who had sustained hypoxic insults during anesthesia with high concentrations of nitrous oxide.[144] W. D. A. Smith recounts the revival of nitrous oxide after Colton's reintroduction of the agent in an entertaining and informative book on the subject.[145]

Unsatisfactory Inhaled Anesthetics

During the first few decades of the 20th century, practitioners were searching for new and improved anesthetics. An American anesthesia textbook written by James T. Gwathmey (1865-1944) (see Fig. 1-18D) was published in 1914 and briefly discussed more than 600 possible anesthetic agents for the reader to consider.[146] By 1930, all successful anesthetic agents except chloroform and nitrous oxide were explosive. Chloroform by then was thought to be dangerous, and the popularity of nitrous oxide was curtailed by the need for a nearly hypoxic mixture to provide adequate anesthesia. Ethyl chloride was the last agent to be introduced in the 19th century and, like ether, it was flammable. It was a unique agent that was first used as a spray to induce local anesthesia, but if inhaled, it also produced general anesthesia.

In the early 20th century, several unsatisfactory volatile anesthetics were introduced. Ethylene was used clinically in 1923. This agent required high concentrations to achieve anesthesia, had an unpleasant smell, and was explosive.[147] Divinyl ether, developed by Chauncey Leake[148] (1896-1978), had some advantages over ether for induction of anesthesia, but it was also flammable and never widely used. Cyclopropane was introduced in 1934 by Ralph Waters[149] (1884-1979) and was briefly popular, but it was violently explosive. The flammable anesthetics prevented the use of surgical cautery and electronic monitoring. One attempt to produce a nonflammable alternative to ether and cyclopropane was made in 1935, when trichloroethylene was introduced.[150] It was promoted by Christopher L. Hewer[151] (1896-1986) as a nonexplosive agent, but it was eventually withdrawn when it was shown to decompose to the toxic nerve poison dechloroacetylene in the presence of soda lime and to produce phosgene, a severe respiratory irritant, when electrocautery was used. Clearly, new directions were needed.

Fluorinated Anesthetics

In the early 1930s, progress was made in attempts to fluorinate hydrocarbons, and many fluorinated compounds became available commercially, primarily as refrigerants. From a theoretical analysis of hydrocarbon chemistry, it was known that halogenation of the parent hydrocarbon compound would decrease its flammability. One early approach to produce a nonflammable anesthetic was to select a flammable agent and partially fluorinate it. With this in mind, John C. Krantz, Jr., of the University of Maryland took the flammable anesthetic, vinamar, which is ethyl vinyl ether, and produced trifluoroethyl vinyl ether,[152] or fluroxene.

The circumstances surrounding the first anesthetic with fluroxene illustrate the lure of self-experimentation in research related to the advancement of anesthetic practice. Max S. Sadove, an anesthesiologist at the University of Illinois, was a member of the Walter Reed Society, a group of scientists who, following the example of Walter Reed, allowed themselves to be administered the first dose of investigational drugs. Sadove, a close acquaintance of Krantz, insisted that he be given the first fluoride-containing anesthetic, fluroxene, in 1953. Krantz, who had synthesized the drug, was a pharmacologist with no training in anesthesia. Krantz advised Sadove that there was danger that the agent might be administered improperly or might be metabolized to a toxic byproduct. Nevertheless, Sadove was insistent, and on April 10, 1953, Krantz administered open drop fluroxene to Sadove, and recovery was rapid and uneventful.[51]

Fluroxene had marginal success but was eventually withdrawn because of questions about toxicity and the frequent occurrence of postanesthetic nausea and vomiting. Charles Suckling, a chemist at Imperial Chemical Industries, synthesized halothane in 1954 after a theoretical analysis of possible anesthetic halogenated drugs. The pharmacologic properties of halothane were studied by James Raventos[153] (1905-1983), and it was introduced clinically in 1956 by Michael Johnstone.[154] Halothane had definite advantages over ether and cyclopropane because of its more pleasant odor, higher potency, favorable kinetic characteristics, nonflammability, and low toxicity, and it gradually replaced the older agents. Halothane was a highly successful drug and achieved worldwide acceptance, but its unblemished record lasted only a few years before controversy appeared.

In 1958, a case report described a 39-year-old woman who died of fulminant hepatic necrosis 11 days after cholecystectomy with halothane anesthesia.[155] This was followed in 1963 by nine case reports of patients who developed hepatic necrosis after halothane anesthesia.[156] The cases were unique in that hepatic failure often followed minor operations in which other causes of hepatic failure were not apparent. Eventually, the term *halothane hepatitis* became a common clinical diagnosis for patients with postoperative liver failure, even when halothane was not used as the anesthetic agent. A national study, formally entitled The National Halothane Study, was established in 1964 and reported that the incidence of liver failure after halothane anesthesia was no higher than that reported with other agents.[157] Nevertheless, halothane was extensively metabolized in the body, and in some individuals, it seemed that a toxic metabolite might produce liver necrosis. Other halogenated anesthetics were also extensively metabolized, and in the case of methoxyflurane, the metabolism resulted in high levels of fluoride ions. High-output renal failure was an infrequent but potentially morbid side effect of methoxyflurane[158,159] and thought to be related to the rise of the fluoride ion concentration after its use.

Beginning in 1960, the pharmaceutical industry launched new efforts to synthesize the "ideal anesthetic agent." Ross C. Terrell at Ohio Medical Products synthesized more than 700 potential anesthetic compounds between 1960 and 1980. During the same period, Edmund I. Eger II (1930-) began a series of studies that significantly enhanced the rational use of inhalation anesthetics. Eger drew on the work of Seymore S. Kety[160] (1915-2000) and Severinghaus[161] that had previously demonstrated that the end-tidal partial pressure of anesthetic gases at steady state was the same as the brain cerebral partial pressure of those gases. By correlating the end-tidal (alveolar) concentration with the movement response to supramaximal nociceptive stimulation, the concept of minimum alveolar concentration (MAC) was born. By definition, MAC represents the end-tidal concentration for any anesthetic agent at which 50% of patients move in response to a supramaximal stimulus.[162] With this standard measure of potency, new agents could be easily introduced to the anesthesia community. Several further studies by Eger and others on the pharmacokinetics of inhalation anesthetics and the factors that alter MAC[163] accelerated an understanding of volatile anesthetic requirements and significantly enhanced the safe use of these drugs.

Two of the anesthetics developed by Ohio Medical Products, enflurane and isoflurane, were introduced about 30 years ago[164,165] and have been highly successful and used extensively since that time. Desflurane was one of the last volatile anesthetics to be synthesized and required a potentially dangerous explosive method of synthesis. Desflurane had a high vapor pressure and had the added limitation of requiring more than five times the quantity of vapor to produce anesthesia compared with isoflurane. Although desflurane was initially overlooked because of these problems, it was studied thoroughly in animals[166] and first used in humans in 1990.[167] Because of its favorable kinetic properties, it has a more rapid recovery compared with isoflurane and enflurane.

Sevoflurane was synthesized more than 40 years ago at Travenol Laboratories. Recovery is rapid with this agent, but because the compound is unstable in soda lime, it was not introduced until the late 1980s,[168,169] first in Japan and then in the United States. The decision to introduce the product was, as with desflurane, spurred by the emphasis on early discharge after anesthesia. Several million anesthetics have been administered with sevoflurane without apparent complications resulting from the potential by-products arising from contact with carbon dioxide absorbents. Since the introduction of sevoflurane, there have been no additional inhalation anesthetics introduced for clinical use. The inert gas xenon has been under investigation as an anesthetic for several years, but it is expensive and, like nitrous oxide, requires high concentrations to produce anesthesia.

NEEDLES AND SYRINGES

The syringe was known in ancient Greece and appeared sporadically as an aid in various medical treatments before the mid-19th century, when it was popularized by the addition of the fine hollow needle. As one example, a piston syringe used to inject mercurial salts transurethrally for syphilis is on display in the Mary Rose Exhibit in Portsmouth, England. The battleship Mary Rose sank in Portsmouth harbor in 1542, under the shocked gaze of Henry VIII. These early syringes (Fig. 1-8) probably were unreliable and cumbersome to use. Although Christopher Wren experimented with the

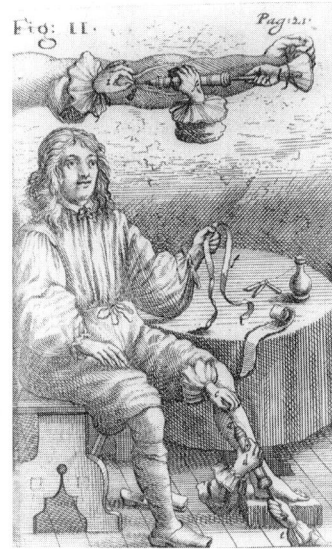

Figure 1–8 Drawing by unknown artist appearing in *Clysmatica Nova*, a book written by Johan S. Elsholtz (1623-1688) and dated 1667. The artist clearly shows that syringes and rudimentary hollow intravenous tubes were used before the 19th century. Although this book was published in Cologne, Germany, most historians credit the first intravenous injections of pharmaceuticals to Christopher Wren and Timothy Clarck in England. (Courtesy of the National Library of Medicine, Bethesda, MD.)

syringe, the device that he used in 1656 to inject opioids intravenously was fashioned from a quill attached to a frog's bladder.

During the first few decades of the 19th century, chemists were active in isolating a number of potent alkaloids from plants. In 1830, Magendie's *Formulary for the Preparation and Employment of Several New Remedies*[170] lists the following newly discovered alkaloids: brucine, morphine, emetine, quinine, piperine, quinine, cinchona, strychnine, and veratrine. The agents were administered to patients for various ailments, often with little or no prior animal experimentation. Strychnine, for example, was used for palsies and paraplegias, often with "temporary relief." Of the alkaloids, morphine (Fig. 1-9A), isolated by the pharmacist Friedrich W. Serturner[171] (1783-1841) in 1817, held the most promise for therapeutic success. Syrups, pills, draughts, and tinctures were used to deliver these drugs because no other effective method of administration was known at the time.

In an attempt to find another route of drug administration, some physicians raised blisters or excoriated the skin and then deposited drugs on the exposed surface of the wound. Francis Rynd[172] (1801-1861) used a lancet to pierce the skin and devised a syringe to insert medication into the wound by gravity. Alexander Wood[173] (1817-1884) invented a hollow needle that would fit on the end of a piston-style syringe made for him by Daniel Ferguson, an instrument maker from London. Wood used the syringe and needle combination to successfully treat painful neuralgias by local morphine injections. The syringe and needle combination became a popular item after these reports, and many practitioners used the device to inject morphine subcutaneously for pain relief. The term *hypodermic injection* was coined by Charles Hunter, who argued with Wood that morphine could be injected any place in the body and achieve the same analgesic effect as that obtained through injection at the site of pain.[174]

The early syringes were inadequate for the work of the developing specialty of regional anesthesia. The rubber or leather plunger cracked or deteriorated after repeated sterilization. During use, the drug contents accumulated proximal to the plunger, or the plunger itself jammed inside the glass barrel. To achieve the fine control required for identification of the epidural space, a more carefully tooled instrument was required. H. Wulfing Luer of Paris introduced the first all-glass syringe in 1896. He sold the patent to Becton, Dickinson and Company in 1898. The Record syringe was made by Dewitt and Herz of Berlin, Germany in 1906,[175] and it consisted of an all-metal plunger with a finely ground glass barrel. The fit between the barrel and plunger was precise and sturdy, and Record syringes nearly 100 years old can still be used for identification of the epidural space.[174]

The first hypodermic needles were made from tempered steel, a metal that rusted easily when in contact with water. A small rusted area might not be observed visually, and defective needles sometimes broke below the skin. Meticulous care was taken to dry each needle after steam sterilization. Specially designed introducers, called rimmers, were used for storage of the needles to prevent rust from developing inside the needle. To avoid

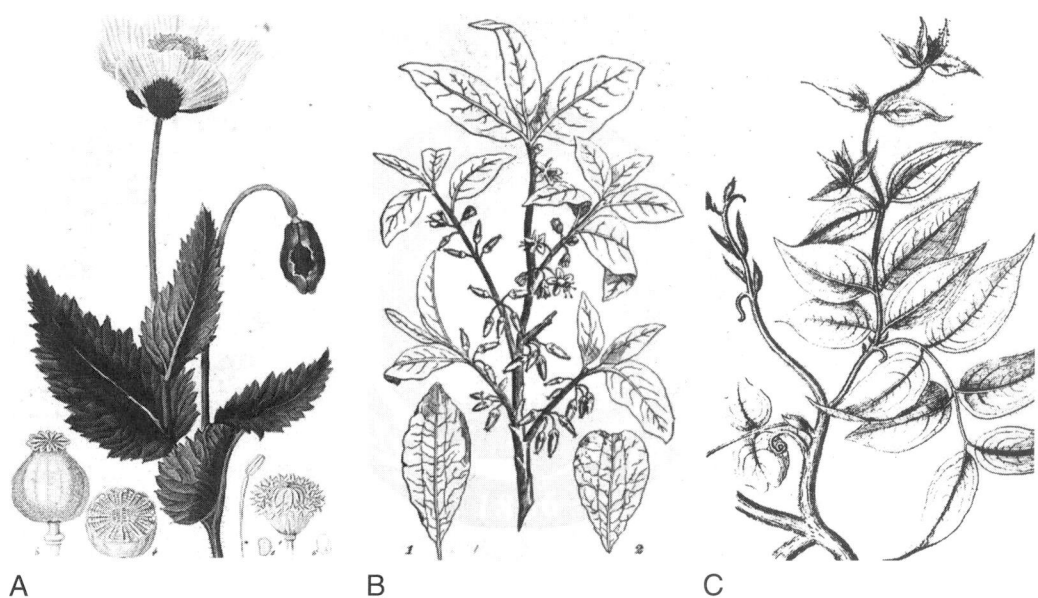

A   B   C

Figure 1–9 Botanical origins of adjuvants used in anesthesiology. **A,** *Papaver somniferum*, from which opium is obtained. *Opium* is the ancient Greek word for juice because the active alkaloids, which include morphine and codeine, are obtained from the juice squeezed from the unripe seed pods. The first undisputed reference to poppy juice is from the writings of Theophrastus (372-287 BC) in the third century BC. **B,** *Erythroxylon coca*, a shrub native to Peru and Bolivia from which cocaine was isolated in 1856. Although the native people of Peru have used the drug for centuries to increase endurance, they may have also used it as a local anesthetic. **C,** *Strychnos toxifera*, a source of curare, as drawn by Robert Schomburgk in 1841.[484] Schomburgk traveled into Guiana following the maps drawn by Waterton and obtained several species containing the active drug. Richard Gill's curare was obtained primarily from Ecuador, and the arrow poisons there were made from *Chondodendron tomentosum*. (Courtesy of the National Library of Medicine, Bethesda, MD.)

the problem with needle breakage, platinum or gold needles were occasionally used. These needles were highly flexible and expensive and never became popular. Stainless steel was produced commercially in 1918, essentially eliminating the problem with rust.[175] Modern needles are usually disposable stainless steel needles, minimizing complications resulting from infection and breakage.

The bevel of the needle was a topic of great discussion in the early 20th century. A long bevel produced less trauma to the tissues, but it allowed a small portion of the needle to lie in the intrathecal space with the proximal portion of the bevel in the epidural space. To increase the success of spinal anesthesia and minimize side effects, short-beveled needles and pencil-point needles were developed by several regional anesthesia specialists, a process that continues to this day. Fine, 25-gauge spinal needles, designed to produce minimal trauma to the dura, reduce the incidence of post-spinal headache.

INTRAVENOUS FLUID THERAPY

An awareness of fluid balance has its beginnings in the writings of Claude Bernard, who in his final published work emphasized the importance of the extracellular fluid in the support of vital functions.[176] In these writings, he stressed that blood and lymph bathe the cells of the body and that these fluids constitute the *milieu interne*, later called the *fluid-matrix* by Walter Cannon.

These researchers pointed out that the organism's freedom from external disturbances such as hunger, thirst, and cold is brought about by mechanisms that maintain uniformity of the bodily fluids. The concept of the steady state maintained in this internal environment became known as *homeostasis* in the Cannon doctrine.[177] During anesthesia, many of the homeostatic mechanisms are abolished or severely blunted, and the anesthesiologist must assume the role of maintaining a favorable milieu interne.

Crystalloids

In the late 19th century, the sodium content of serum was found to be roughly equivalent to an aqueous solution of 0.9% sodium chloride, and this became known as physiologic salt solution. Hartog J. Hamburger (1856-1924) showed a volume change in red blood cells at concentrations above and below 0.9% saline.[178] As a result of these experiments, the value of sodium ions in the maintenance of osmotic pressure in the serum was realized. Ernest H. Starling[179] (1866-1927) extended these observations to explain edema formation on the basis of hydrostatic and colloidal osmotic pressures.

Maintenance of fluid balance was not a priority or even a possibility for those who administered anesthetics during the 19th century. Without intravenous access, there was little the anesthesia provider could do if the surgeon was recklessly losing blood. The importance of intravenously administered salt in patients with dehydration from cholera was observed in 1831 by William B. O'Shaughnessy[180] (1804-1889). Although there were isolated successful attempts to treat the dehydration of cholera with saline infusions, the treatment did not flourish, and the victory over cholera was finally won only through improved sanitary conditions.

The experimental introduction of saline infusions after surgery was based on work performed by Emil Schwarz[181] (1852-1918), who observed that saline infusions could save the lives of bled rabbits. This work was recognized by Johann J. Bischoff[182] (1841-1892), who reported that a salt infusion saved the life of a woman with severe postpartum hemorrhage. Treatment with salt infusions was generally adopted after surgical hemorrhage, but sepsis and failed attempts to revive the bleeding patient soon became apparent.

Alternative solutions to saline originated with Sydney Ringer[183] (1835-1910), Professor of Medicine at University College, London. Ringer observed that saline prepared from distilled water was not as effective as saline made from pipe water in maintaining the contractility of the isolated frog heart. After a careful analysis of the pipe water, he learned that it contained the impurities of calcium and potassium. Adding these cations to the saline made from distilled water proved his hypothesis that these ions played an important role in maintaining normal cardiac function.

In the first decades of the 20th century, there were substantial barriers to the successful use of parenteral electrolyte solutions during surgery. Closed sterile administration sets and intravenous cannulas were slow to develop, and alternative methods therefore were employed. Most patients received several liters of fluid, usually administered rectally; however, salt was administered, if possible, orally or by subcutaneous injection. With these ineffectual methods, the use of saline in the perioperative period fell into decline. In 1944, a syndrome was described as *postoperative salt intolerance*, caused ostensibly by the failure of the kidney to excrete a salt load.[184] These ideas had the support of the influential Francis D. Moore, Chief of Surgery at Peter Bent Brigham Hospital in Boston. When intravenous therapy became more widely available, patients were often administered dextrose and water or dilute sodium-containing solutions. Carl Moyer[185] (1908-1970) presented evidence in 1950 that sodium was avidly retained postoperatively and argued against the use of saline for perioperative fluid maintenance.

The reintroduction of perioperative saline therapy began in 1959, when G. Shires[186,187] and associates reported the redistribution of extracellular fluids into "third space" compartments during extensive surgical procedures. These reports encouraged preoperative fluid administration to compensate for the lack of oral intake and intraoperative sodium-containing fluid administration to replace translocation of extracellular fluid into edematous spaces such as gut and peritoneum. The increased use of saline reduced the incidence of postoperative renal failure and decreased the requirement for blood transfusions. As a result of these studies, fluid replacement today consists of saline-containing fluids, with the addition of colloid and blood when excessive blood loss occurs.[188]

Blood Transfusions

The first blood transfusions were not performed as treatment for blood loss. Jean Baptiste Denis (1625-1704) from Montpellier, France administered lamb's blood[189] to a demented patient with the idea of transferring the attributes of the donating animal to the recipient. Although the first patient survived, a subsequent transfusion resulted in death. Denis was tried for murder, and although he was acquitted, the procedure was condemned and prohibited by the Faculty of Medicine in Paris. Physicians in the 18th and 19th centuries were more prone to remove, rather than administer, blood.

Successful blood transfusions were performed by James Blundell[190] (1790-1877), who experimented with blood transfusions in animals and rejected the idea of animal-to-human transfusions. Blundell recorded 10 human-to-human transfusions between 1818 and 1828 and recognized that acute blood loss was the primary reason for transfusion. Five of those 10 patients died after the transfusion, possibly as a result of incompatible blood.

In 1900, Karl Landsteiner[191] (1868-1943) described three blood groups: A, B, and O; the fourth blood group (AB) was described by A. V. Decastello[192] 2 years later. George W. Crile (1865-1943) performed the first transfusion of human blood after a preceding compatibility test in 1906. Discovery of the Rh antigens was delayed until 1939.

One hundred years ago, the accepted method of transfusing blood was to surgically anastomose the artery of the donor to the vein of the patient. This method required a long and delicate operation, and there was no way to measure the amount of blood transfused. Blood could not be removed from the body without defibrination, a process that often produced serious reactions and air embolization. In 1914, Albert Hustin[193] (1882-1967) noticed that when sodium citrate was added to blood, it prevented coagulation, and with the addition of dextrose by P. Rous and J. R. Turner in 1916,[194] storage of blood products for up to 21 days became a reality.[195] The familiar drip chamber for estimating infusion rates was devised by R. Laurie in 1909.[196] The effect of these advancements in the use of blood products on the practice of anesthesia is apparent by comparing the American textbook by Gwathmey,[146] dated 1914, in which there is no mention of blood administration, with that of John S. Lundy[197] (1894-1972), dated 1945, which contains an extensive chapter on the subject. Lundy was an early proponent of blood transfusions and opened the first blood bank in the United States at the Mayo Clinic in 1935. The effect of two World Wars on the practice of anesthesia in the United States can be appreciated by comparing these two books.

With the rise of hepatitis and human immunodeficiency virus contaminants of homologous blood, a new look at an old technique,[198] autologous transfusion, was begun in 1970. In that year, G. Klebanoff described a disposable autologous transfusion system manufactured by Bentley Laboratories.[199] Klebanoff reported[200] on its use in 53 patients with no deaths if the total volume of blood replaced was less than 3500 mL. Malcolm D. Orr first reported cell-washing techniques in 1975 using the Haemonetics cell-washing system.[201] This system obviated some of the problems when blood was filtered, but not washed, after retrieval from the surgical wound. From these early reports, it became apparent that washed and concentrated red cells obtained from the surgical site could provide safe alternatives to homologous transfusions. The "cell saver" method of autologous blood transfusion has become an integral part of intraoperative fluid management when large volumes of blood loss are anticipated.

Coagulopathies often develop during large-volume blood transfusions, and their diagnosis and prompt treatment significantly contribute to survival during major surgery. Ron Miller and colleagues[202] recognized thrombocytopenia as one of the earliest defects in coagulation after massive blood loss. Advances in specific blood component therapy[203,204] have also contributed to maintenance of normal blood coagulability during large-volume blood loss.

INTRODUCTION OF REGIONAL ANESTHESIA

Early Attempts at Local Anesthesia

The successful development of local anesthesia began in the late 19th century, but the idea of preparing a regional area of reduced sensibility before surgical incision was evident in earlier surgical writings. Ambroise Paré (1510-1590), the noted military surgeon, observed that squeezing a limb before amputation reduced the pain from incision.[131] Benjamin Bell[205] (1749-1806), surgeon to the Royal Infirmary, Edinburgh, described the use of a nerve compressor to reduce pain during amputations in his textbook dated 1796. Napoleon's chief military surgeon Dominique J. Larrey (1766-1842) described performing amputations in cold environments (–19°C) when assistants were nearly unable to hold the instruments. He found it remarkable that under these conditions there was less pain and that the patients recovered rapidly.[131]

In 1876, Benjamin Ward Richardson (1828-1896) observed that rapid evaporation of volatile fluids produced local cooling and insensibility of the underlying skin, and this became the basis for ether (and later ethyl chloride) spray.[206] In his 1864 textbook, Samuel Gross[207] (1805-1884), described local anesthesia produced by the topical application of a mixture of ice and salt, but he found it useless after the first few minutes after incision. The phrase *freeze the skin* is the only contemporary reminder of this early practice.

Cocaine

Although the ineffectual attempts at local anesthesia indicated a growing awareness of local anesthetic methods, the origins of neural blockade as we know it today had already been established in a rudimentary form on the eastern slopes of the Andes in South America for more than 350 years. When the invading Spaniards arrived in Peru in the 16th century (1532-1549), they found an advanced culture, with Cusco as the capital city and people with highly developed engineering and artistic skills. Few historians dispute that the Inca civilization was one of the highest developed cultures in America at the time,

and the Spanish invaders were the means by which the powerful pharmacologic effects of the coca leaf ultimately were revealed to the European community.

Inca priests chewed the dried leaves of a plant, *Erythroxylon coca* (see Fig. 1-9B), as a stimulant and used it as an integral part of religious ceremonies. Cultivation and use of the coca leaves by the Andean Indians date back thousands of years. *Coca* is an indigenous Indian (Aymaran) word meaning "food for the traveler." There is controversy about whether the Incas used the plant as a local anesthetic. Because they had no written language, much of what is known about their civilization is derived from the Spanish chroniclers, whose mention of coca was scanty, perhaps because use of the plant was limited to the priests before the fall of the Incan civilization. There was also no pictorial evidence from Incan pottery or weavings that coca was applied to surgical wounds. The priests did perform painful surgical procedures such as trepanations, and from several sources we learn that the patient chewed coca leaves as well as other native plants, but there is no firm evidence to support the claim that saliva enriched by coca juice was applied to the wound.[131]

The first written account of the coca plant being used as a local anesthetic was by the Spanish Jesuit Bernabe Cobo (1582-1657), who chewed the plant to relieve a toothache and wrote about it in 1544.[208] Albert Niemann (1834-1861) of Göttingen, Germany, who isolated the alkaloid from the dried leaves in 1856, gave the name *cocaine* to the active drug.[209,210] Interest in cocaine in Europe and America was directed initially toward the central effects of the drug when taken systemically. Vasili von Anrep[211] (1852-1918) was the first to remark on its local anesthetic properties, and after animal experiments, he suggested its use as a local anesthetic during surgery. This suggestion went unnoticed, and the drug remained a curiosity. A comprehensive pharmacology textbook from 1883 does not mention cocaine or the plant *E. coca*.[212]

Sigmund Freud (1856-1939), a young house officer at the prestigious Allgemeines Krankenhaus in Vienna, had a unique interest in cocaine and tested the drug as a substitute for opioids on a colleague who was addicted to morphine. Although this research met with little success, he also had noticed its ability to produce numbness of the tongue and provided a small sample to his junior colleague, Carl Koller[213] (1858-1944), an intern who was interested in producing local anesthesia for operations on the eye.

Koller had anticipated a career as a scientist in Vienna. He had taken up this question for his research project because the anesthetic methods of the time were highly unsatisfactory for ophthalmic surgery. General anesthetics presented numerous difficulties for the surgeon, and refrigeration anesthesia, although marginally successful for surgery on the extremities, was clearly inappropriate for the eye. Koller observed that after topical cocaine application, he was able to pinch and prick the cornea of dogs without discomfort to the animals. Self-experimentation confirmed complete analgesia of the corneal surface, and he proceeded to use the agent for superficial surgery on the eye.

Koller arranged to demonstrate the use of topical cocaine analgesia at the Ophthalmologic Congress in Heidelberg, Germany on September 15, 1884. As the time for this presentation approached, he was unable to afford the travel expenses from Vienna, and a colleague from Trieste, Josef Brettauer (1835-1905), presented the three-page manuscript in his absence.[214,215] The presentation and demonstration were followed by an enthusiastically favorable response. Priority for the discovery was briefly confounded by a report on topical cocaine analgesia at an ophthalmologic meeting in October 1884 by Leopold Koenigstein, who did not mention Koller's prior paper, and by other comments that Sigmund Freud had actually originated the idea of cocaine analgesia. Koenigstein later conceded full credit for the discovery to Koller, and Freud eventually rejected all claims to the idea of topical analgesia with cocaine, although many concede that, with his earlier publication on the subject,[216] he was instrumental in reviving interest in a drug that before 1884 was of no interest to pharmacologists.

Koller's career in Vienna seemed secure, but a disagreement arose with another house officer in January 1885. The altercation escalated into a duel with sabers, an activity that was banned in Austria at that time. Koller emerged unscathed from the duel, but the offending party suffered two saber cuts to the face. After this episode, Koller became depressed and ultimately decided to leave Austria. He first immigrated to Holland, and then settled in New York City in 1886. There he built a successful private practice while continuing to contribute occasional clinical articles to the ophthalmologic literature. He died in New York City in 1944, after modestly receiving several awards for his seminal role in the development of local and regional anesthesia.[213]

Regional Blocks

It was not obvious that cocaine would produce blockade of sensation if injected directly into peripheral nerves. In 1880, von Anrep had injected cocaine under the skin of his arm and discovered that it produced insensitivity, but this information did not attract attention. At least one Viennese surgeon, Anton Wölfler, first assistant to Theodore Billroth, had attempted hypodermic cocaine injections without producing analgesia and was convinced that it was effective only on the mucous membranes. The idea of injecting cocaine into nerve trunks is credited to William Halsted (1852-1922) and Alfred Hall, who began their injection experiments as early as 8 weeks after the Heidelberg announcement.

Halsted and Hall had studied in Vienna during 1879 and 1880, but it is unlikely that they met Koller during those years, because Koller did not finish his medical school training until 1882. During those years, Koller was working on a paper about the development of the mesoderm and had not developed his interest in cocaine. In 1884, Halsted was occasionally performing operations in the bedroom of his own house in New York City, and it was there that the two surgeons began their work on regional anesthesia. The first report of their success with injection appeared on December 6, 1884 in the *New York Medical Journal* in a letter written by Hall.[217] In this letter, Hall reports that they first injected 4% cocaine (15 mg) into the forearm and concluded that it blocked transmission in the cutaneous nerves because it provided

analgesia below but not above the point of injection. They then injected 2 mL (80 mg) into the ulnar nerve at the elbow, producing block of the entire ulnar distribution distal to the point of injection. Additional blocks were then performed on the brachial plexus and the infraorbital nerves, inferior dental nerves, and the sciatic nerve, all for operative surgery.[218]

With these large doses, it is not surprising that constitutional symptoms developed. Hall described dizziness and nausea. Both Halsted and Hall became addicted to cocaine; Halsted lived with an occult cocaine or morphine addiction the rest of his life. Hall took a position at Columbia University in New York City, but he later moved to Santa Barbara, California, where he died in 1924.

Carl Schleich[219] (1859-1922) introduced infiltration local anesthesia in 1892 as an alternative to direct injection of nerve trunks. His method was to infiltrate cocaine in dilute concentrations (0.01% to 0.2%) directly into the subcutaneous tissues. James Leonard Corning[220] (1855-1923), a neurologist from New York, observed that placing a tourniquet on the limb could prolong the analgesic effect of infiltration analgesia, and he reasoned that the tourniquet prevented the blood from removing cocaine from its active site. Heinrich F. Braun[221,222] (1862-1934) achieved the same prolonged effect of cocaine by adding epinephrine to the solution, producing a "chemical tourniquet." Braun became the pioneer of the new drug procaine,[223] introduced by Braun in 1905 as a less toxic drug than cocaine. Braun's textbook.[221] first published in 1907, was one of the first devoted to regional anesthesia and went through eight editions, with the last one published in 1933.

Although Halsted was the first to block the brachial plexus, he did not use a percutaneous technique. His method in 1884, and that used by George Crile 13 years later, was to surgically expose the roots and then inject each nerve directly. G. Hirschel[224] produced the first percutaneous brachial plexus block in 1911 through an axillary approach (Fig. 1-10A). The axillary brachial plexus block has been modified by several surgeons, including George Pitkin,[225] and R. H. de Jong,[226] and remains a popular technique today.

D. Kulenkampff introduced the supraclavicular brachial plexus block[227] a few months after Hirschel described the axillary approach (see Fig. 1-10B). Kulenkampff injected his own plexus with 10 mL of procaine at the midclavicular position, lateral to the subclavian artery, obtaining complete anesthesia of the arm. Early reports indicated a high degree of success with this block, but other practitioners soon reported complications such as pneumothorax and mediastinal emphysema. Several modifications of the supraclavicular block have emerged in an effort to avoid pneumothorax. Infraclavicular approaches to the brachial plexus were described by L. Bazy and V. Pauchet[228] in 1917 and later popularized by P. Raj[229] in 1973.

In an attempt to approach the brachial plexus in the neck and thereby avoid pulmonary complications, M. Kappis[230] (1912) attempted to perform the block through a posterior paravertebral approach. Because of a high incidence of failures with the posterior approach, several investigators, including J. Etienne,[231] V. Pauchet, and G. Pitkin, used various anterior approaches to the brachial plexus in the neck. In 1970, Alon P. Winnie[232]

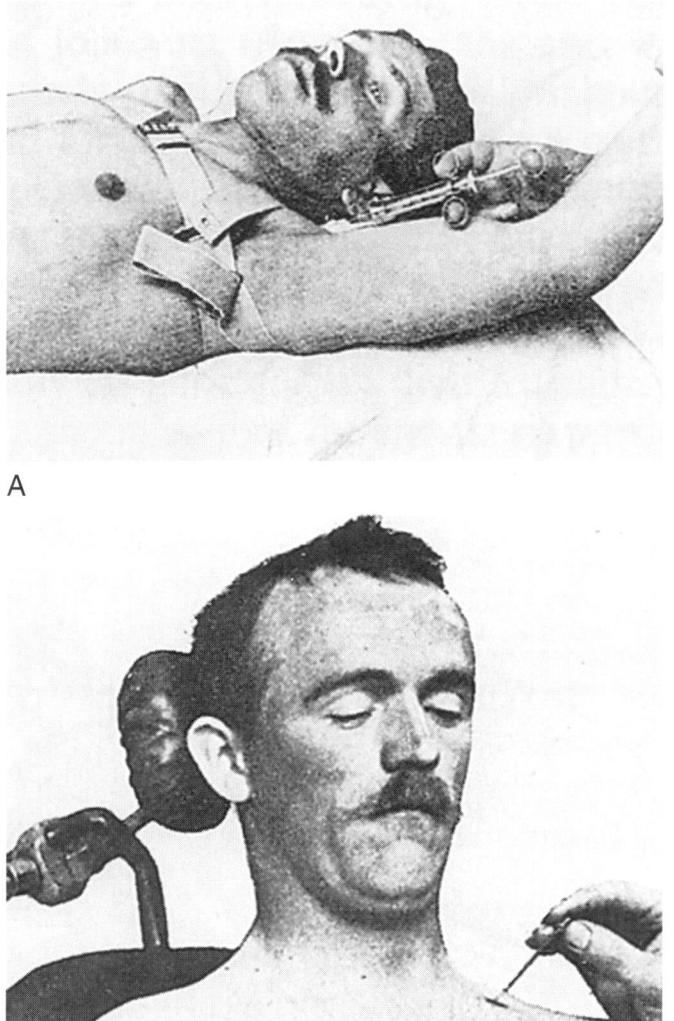

A

B

Figure 1–10 A, Hirschel performed the first percutaneous axillary block with 20 mL of 2% procaine in 1911. He forced a rubber ball under the pectoral muscles and fixed it with elastic bandages to prevent rapid absorption of anesthetic solution, a maneuver that he later abandoned as unnecessary. (From Hirschel G: Die Anasthesierung de Plexus Brachialis fur die Operationen an der oberen Extremitat, Much Med Wochenschr 58:1555-1556, 1911.) **B,** Kulenkampff approached the brachial plexus above the clavicle, just lateral to the subclavian artery. The patients were positioned in the sitting position for the block. An injection of 10 mL of 2% procaine with epinephrine was given only after a paresthesia had been obtained. If the first rib was contacted, the injection was made more medially. (From Kulenkampff D: Anesthesia of the brachial plexus. Zentrabl Chr 38:1337-1340, 1911.)

introduced the interscalene brachial plexus block and emphasized that the scalene muscles are more accurate landmarks to the nerves than the subclavian artery or the midclavicular line. The block has remained popular for operations on the shoulder and upper arm; the nerves are located by paresthesias or direct nerve stimulation. Continuous infusions into the roots of the brachial plexus have been introduced and can provide long-lasting analgesia after operations on the arm and shoulder.

A novel method of producing regional analgesia for operations on the extremities was described by August Bier (1861-1949) (Fig. 1-11A) in 1909.[232,234] Bier first exsanguinated the arm with an Esmarch wrap and, after placement of two tourniquets, injected a dilute solution of procaine intravenously. Analgesia was found to develop within minutes and persist until release of the tourniquet. The technique, known now as intravenous regional anesthesia, has been modified with new agents and remains a useful anesthetic technique for operation on the extremities when a tourniquet is used.

The development of regional anesthesia in the United States was accelerated with the arrival of Gaston Labat at the Mayo Clinic in 1924. Labat had learned regional anesthetic methods from the French authority on injection techniques Victor Pauchet, and expanded on his work while in Rochester, Minnesota. Labat founded the American Society of Regional Anesthesia and was active during its formative years. John Lundy adopted many of the regional techniques introduced by Labat at the Mayo Clinic and continued their use after Labat relocated to the Bellevue Hospital in New York City. Labat's 1922 textbook[62] was one of the first English texts on regional anesthesia and has been followed by several authoritative works on the subject. Labat's influence was also evident in New York City, where his successor, Emery A. Rovenstine, as Chairman of the Department of Anesthesiology at Bellevue Hospital, established the first chronic pain clinic. The commitment of anesthesiologists to chronic pain therapy arose as a natural sequel to their emerging expertise in neuraxial and peripheral nerve blocks. Chronic pain clinics today are often modeled after the multidisciplinary clinic established by John J. Bonica (1917-1994) at the University of Washington in Seattle.[235,236]

The continued success of regional anesthetic techniques can be partially credited to improved local anesthetics with lower toxicities and longer durations of action. Cocaine was highly toxic, addictive, and of short duration. Procaine was synthesized in 1905 by Alfred Einhorn[237] (1856-1917) and was the most commonly used agent until 1932, when tetracaine, a longer-acting agent, became available. Lidocaine, introduced in 1948 by Torsten Gordh[238] (1907-), had several advantages, including lower toxicity and intermediate duration of action, and it is still widely used. Other local anesthetics include chloroprocaine (introduced in 1952), mepivacaine (1957), and bupivacaine (1963). Concerns about therapy-resistant cardiovascular toxicity with bupivacaine[239] led to introduction of the newer agents ropivacaine (1996) and levobupivacaine.[240] Bupivacaine, ropivacaine, and levobupivacaine are popular agents in low concentrations for postoperative pain control and obstetric anesthesia because of their long duration of action.

NEURAXIAL BLOCK AND ACUTE PAIN SERVICE

The first neuraxial block was performed 8 months after the demonstration in Heidelberg of the local anesthetic properties of cocaine (see Chapter 72). James Leonard Corning (1855-1923) was a neurologist who had learned

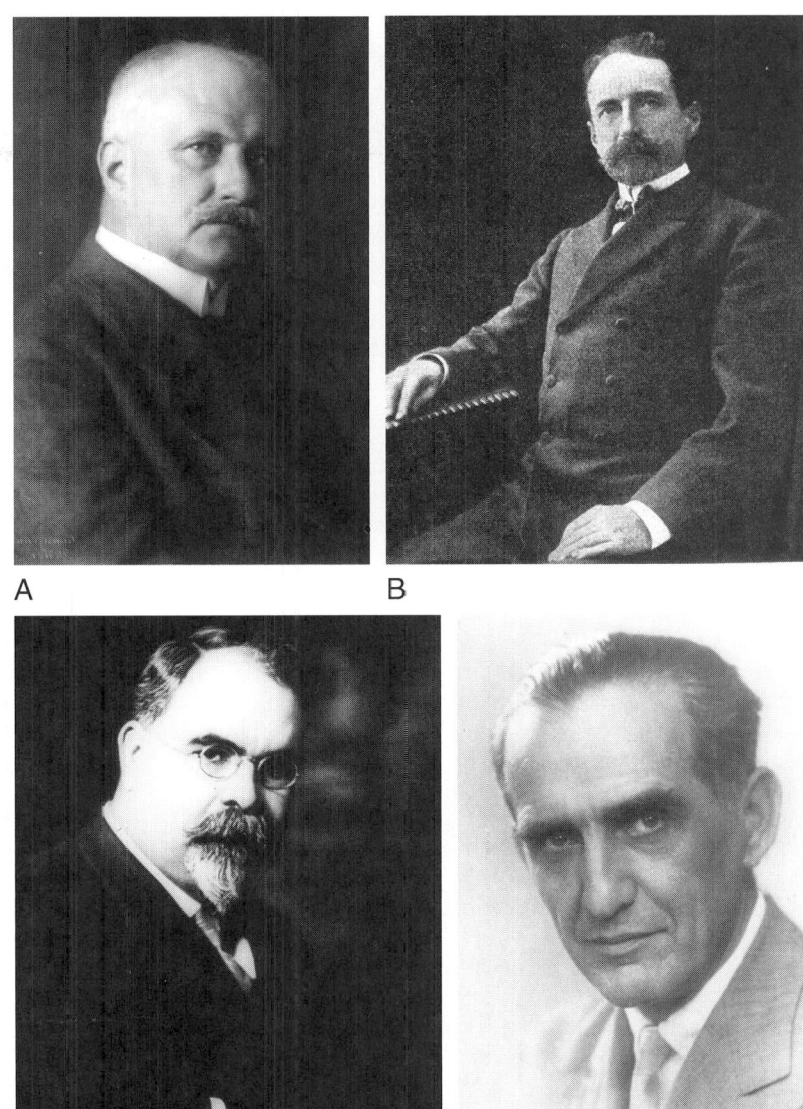

Figure 1–11 Pioneers of neuraxial block: **A,** August K. G. Bier. **B,** Theodore Tuffier. **C,** Rudolph Matas. **D,** Achille M. Dogliotti. (Courtesy of the National Library of Medicine, Bethesda, MD.)

A   B

C   D

of the action of cocaine possibly from observation of Halsted's work in New York City. Corning was interested to know if the blood could carry cocaine to the spinal cord, similar to what had been demonstrated to occur after injection of strychnine between the spinous processes. On October 12, 1885, Corning injected a total of 120 mg of cocaine between the T11 and T12 spinous processes in a 45-year-old man and obtained loss of sensation of the legs and perineum.[241] He concluded that this proved cocaine's action on the spinal cord and suggested its use in certain cases of spinal spasticity and for operations on the genitourinary system.

The consensus is that Corning produced an epidural injection of the drug[242] because 120 mg (60 mg initially and then 60 mg 8 minutes later) of intrathecal cocaine would be expected to produce a total spinal anesthetic or a block extending into the cervical dermatomes. It is not surprising that Corning's method of neuraxial block was not repeated because the technique of consistently injecting into the epidural space had not yet been described. If any investigators had attempted to repeat the Corning experiment with the dose he used, it might have ended in disaster and thereby delayed the development of neuraxial block by several years.

Spinal Analgesia

In Kiel, Germany, during the last decade of the 19th century, preparations were being made for the next major advance in anesthetic practice. At the Kiel University Medical School, Friederich von Esmarch (1823-1908) was the senior surgeon and August Bier one of the junior surgeons. Heinrich I. Quincke (1842-1922) was the leading internist in Kiel and had already contributed several useful clinical observations, among them the Quincke pulse and Quincke's edema, to the medical literature. In 1891, Quincke observed that the dural sac, described by Domenico Cotugno (1736-1822) in 1787, could be punctured by inserting a needle between the lumbar spinous processes.[243] This procedure, independently reported by Walter Wynter[244] (1860-1945) of Leeds, England in the same year, at first was a curiosity without any real purpose. Quincke unsuccessfully attempted to treat hydrocephalus by draining fluid from the dural sac. Microscopic examination of the fluid did have some diagnostic value in cases of inflammation of the central nervous system.

On August 15, 1898, August Bier and his assistant August Hildebrandt (1868-1854) used the Quincke method of entering the intrathecal space and injected between 5 and 15 mg of cocaine to produce spinal anesthesia in six cases for operations on the lower part of the body. They also reported the results of spinal anesthesia given to each other in what has become one of the classic clinical papers in the medical literature.[245] Bier thought it would not replace general anesthesia because of the severity of side effects such as nausea, vomiting, dizziness, and headache. He proposed that these undesirable side effects were caused by escape of cerebrospinal fluid from the dural sac. The method whereby Bier arrived at the correct intrathecal dose of cocaine on the first attempt remains a mystery.

After Bier's report, interest in spinal anesthesia spread rapidly. J. B. Seldowitsch[246] successfully provided spinal anesthesia in St. Petersburg on May 11, 1899; Frederick Dudley Tait (1862-1918) and Guido Caglieri[247] (1871-1951) in San Francisco on October 26, 1899; Theodore Tuffier[248] (see Fig. 1-11B) in Paris on November 9, 1899; and Rudolph Matas[249] (1860-1957) (see Fig. 1-11C) in New Orleans on November 10, 1899. By one report, more than 1000 manuscripts relating to spinal anesthesia had been published within 2 years of the original paper by Bier.[250]

Not all researchers agreed on the technique and indications for spinal anesthesia. Tait and Caglieri suggested the use of cervical intrathecal injections for operating on the upper extremities. A. W. Morton[251] reported success with total spinal anesthesia after lumbar puncture for operations on all parts of the body. Thomas Jonnesco[252] reported no adverse effects from 398 spinal anesthetics administered between the spines of the thoracic and lumbar levels using a novocaine and strychnine mixture. Jonnesco called the method *general spinal anesthesia*. Remarkably, in his series there were 14 operations on the skull, 45 on the face, and 25 on the neck. In 1909, Bier[253] claimed that to be successful with spinal anesthesia, the anesthetist should inject the solution only at body temperature and that tropacocaine was preferable to cocaine.

The early reports of cocaine spinal anesthesia mentioned that after injection, patients often became restless and excitable, often exhibiting a significant rise in body temperature. One of the first physicians to specialize in anesthesia, S. Ormond Goldan, maintained accurate anesthesia records from several cases of spinal anesthesia with cocaine.[254] His records reveal a typical increase in heart rate, pupil size, and body temperature after cocaine spinal anesthesia. Matas reasoned that these effects were secondary to an action of cocaine on the central nervous system. He learned that mixing 1.5 mg of morphine with cocaine was useful in mitigating these symptoms. In his 1900 report on spinal anesthesia, he regarded a mixture of cocaine and morphine as his standard agent. This report by Matas appears to be among the first attempts to use spinal opioids to enhance neuraxial analgesia.[249] The Japanese anesthesiologist Otojiro Kitagawa[255] (1864-1922) used intrathecal morphine (10 mg) in the same year to treat the chronic painful conditions of two patients.

It is not surprising that serious complications from the spinal technique were soon observed. F. Gumprecht[256] reported 15 cases of sudden death from lumbar puncture in 1900. Several investigators observed respiratory arrest after high spinal injections. After the introduction of routine blood pressure measurements by Cushing[257] in 1903, it was observed that severe hypotension could occur after spinal anesthesia.[258]

The scientific study of spinal anesthesia began within a few years after its introduction. Investigations were undertaken by Arthur E. Barker[259] (1850-1916) to determine the factors involved in spread of the local anesthetic within the subarachnoid space. Barker advised meticulous sterile technique and introduced the use of dextrose to produce hyperbaric solutions. His emphasis on gravity as an essential determinant of local anesthetic spread remains an important facet of the spinal technique today.[260] Several researchers reported the dangers of total spinal anesthesia. Gaston Labat[62] and George P. Pitkin[261] contributed clinical observations that improved the safety of spinal anesthesia.

A widely publicized malpractice trial in 1953 had a negative impact on the use of spinal anesthesia.[262] Albert Woolley and Cecil Roe were healthy subjects who received dibucaine spinal anesthetics on the same day at the Chesterfield Royal Hospital in England. Both patients developed permanent painful spastic paraparesis. Although the cause of paresis was inconclusive, it was thought that the injuries were caused by contamination of the spinal solution by phenol, in which the dibucaine ampules had been immersed for sterilization. The Wooley and Roe case was followed by other reports of paralysis after spinal anesthesia.[263] However, in 1954, a reassuring study of 10,098 spinal anesthetics with only 71 minor neuropathies, most unrelated to the block itself, was published in a widely circulated medical journal.[264] Spinal anesthesia then reemerged as a safe anesthetic method provided that attention was directed to meticulous technique.

Consideration has been given to a syndrome characterized by transient paresthesias after lidocaine spinal anesthesia.[265,266] However, with the introduction of disposable spinal kits and improved techniques, the spinal route of drug administration is now firmly established. Research is continuing on new drugs and methods of delivery. Reports of cauda equina syndrome after the introduction of lidocaine through spinal microcatheters[267] emphasize the importance of careful clinical observations when new methods of spinal delivery are introduced.

Post-spinal headache was an annoying problem for the first practitioners and their patients. The exact cause for this reaction was not agreed on for several years.

As late as 1924, Labat had suggested removal of cerebrospinal fluid (CSF) for treatment of spinal headache. However, an extensive study by Leroy Vandam and Robert Dripps (1911-1974) confirmed Bier's original suggestion that leakage of CSF through the dural rent was the causative factor.[268]

The use of small-diameter spinal needles has decreased the incidence of spinal headache after spinal anesthesia. However, inadvertent dural puncture with larger needles can sometimes occur during the placement of epidural catheters. An innovative treatment for headache after dural puncture, the epidural blood patch, was suggested by James B. Gormley[269] in 1960 and further described by Anthony J. DiGiovanni and Burdett S. Dunbar[270] in 1970. The blood patch has been reported to be successful in a high percentage of cases and has withstood the test of time as an effective treatment for this condition.

Epidural Analgesia

Jean Enthuse Sicard[271] (1872-1929) and Fernand Cathelin[272] (1873-1945) independently introduced cocaine through the sacral hiatus in 1901, becoming the first practitioners of caudal (epidural) anesthesia. Sicard was a neurologist and used the technique to treat sciatica and tabes, but Cathelin used the technique for surgical anesthesia. Arthur Läwen[273] (1876-1958), a pupil of Heinrich Braun (1862-1934) and an early proponent of regional anesthesia, successfully used caudal anesthesia with large volumes of procaine for pelvic surgery. It soon became apparent that caudal anesthesia was sufficient for operations on the perineum, but the drug would have to be deposited into the epidural space at higher levels if the surgeon anticipated operating on the abdomen or thorax. Initial attempts to provide epidural anesthesia through needles placed at higher levels were unsuccessful. B. Heile[274] published an extensive study of the epidural space in 1913, but the focus of his final report was on the treatment of neurologic conditions through epidural injections. His unique approach was to enter the epidural space through the intervertebral foramina (a technique that has recently been revived). Tuffier[275] was aware of the need for entry at higher levels but was unable to perfect a reliable technique for lumbar or thoracic epidural injections.

In 1921, Fidel Pagés[276] (1886-1923), a Spanish military surgeon, devised a technique to introduce epidural procaine at all levels of the neuraxis. His method was to use a blunt needle and then feel and hear the entry of the needle through the ligamentum flavum. His report of 43 cases of lumbar and thoracic epidural anesthetics represents a landmark article that went unnoticed because of its publication in an obscure medical journal. Pagés died in an automobile accident soon after his report on epidural analgesia, and no students at the time had learned his technique. Pagés had the idea to produce *segmental anesthesia* through epidural injections, avoiding some of the side effects of complete neuraxial block, which occurred after high subarachnoid administration of local anesthetics. He provided the anesthetics himself and then performed the operations, noting that much time was saved with the epidural technique compared with general anesthesia. Of the 43 cases, it appears that one subject received a total spinal anesthetic but survived after assisted ventilation.

Achille Mario Dogliotti[277] (1897-1966) (see Fig. 1-11D) described epidural injections of local anesthetics in 1931, apparently without prior knowledge of the work of Pagés. Dogliotti performed extensive studies to determine the spread of solutions within the epidural and paravertebral space after injection. His work launched one of the most valuable techniques in the modern practice of anesthesiology. An important innovation was Dogliotti's method of identification of the epidural space. His 1939 textbook illustrates the use of continuous pressure on the plunger of a saline-filled syringe as the needle is advanced through the ligamentous structures. In contrast to the methods of Corning and Pagés, the Dogliotti technique was reproducible and easily learned. Dogliotti also observed the extent and duration of analgesia after injection into various spinal interspaces.

Initial acceptance of epidural analgesia was slow to develop in North America, although it gained early acceptance in Europe and South America. A. Gutierrez of Argentina became an enthusiastic advocate for the epidural method and collected valuable data on a large series of successful epidural anesthetics. He also developed the "hanging drop" sign that is still used by some anesthesiologists to identify the epidural space.[278] Dogliotti's anesthesia textbook[279] was translated into English in 1939 and contained an extensive chapter on epidural analgesia. Textbooks by American authors several years later[197,280] contained only a short description of the technique, treating it as a novelty practiced only by those with special expertise. There were some early practitioners of epidural anesthesia in North America. Charles B. Odom of New Orleans published 285 cases of lumbar epidural anesthesia in 1936 and introduced the concept of a test dose to detect intrathecal injection.[281] In Odom's series, there was one death attributed to the poor condition of the patient. John R. Harger and coworkers[282] of Cook County Hospital in Chicago reported 1000 cases without a fatality using single injections of 45 to 50 mL of 2% procaine. Oral Crawford and colleagues[283] reported more than 600 cases of thoracic epidural analgesia for thoracic surgery in 1951, with two deaths.

One major limitation of the neuraxial techniques was the short duration of procaine. Bier experimented with the addition of rubber and latex to the spinal anesthetic solution in an attempt to prolong the block duration.[253] These ideas were not expanded on because of complications or lack of effect. To deal with the same problem, William Lemmon[284] used a 17-gauge, malleable, silver needle that was connected through a hole in the operating room table to rubber tubing and a syringe. Injections could then be made at intervals to maintain the spinal block for several hours. Edward Tuohy[285] used a ureteral catheter threaded through a large Huber-tipped spinal needle to provide continuous spinal anesthesia. The Tuohy needle was a simple modification of the Huber needle and was used by him to thread the catheter into the subarachnoid space. Beginning in 1947, Manuel Martinez Curbelo[285] of Havana, Cuba used the Tuohy needle and a small ureteral catheter to provide continuous lumbar epidural analgesia. He reported 59 successful cases, and in one case, the catheter remained in place for 4 postoperative days with intermittent injections of local anesthetic.

Caudal anesthesia had a resurgence in popularity after the report by Edwards and Hingson[287] in 1942 that analgesia for labor and delivery could be achieved with caudal injections of tetracaine through a malleable needle left in situ within the sacral canal. Their report was widely publicized, and within months the technique was adopted by several hospitals. Although for many years caudal epidural injections were used for obstetric analgesia, it became apparent that the lumbar approach to the epidural space was more consistent, and it eventually replaced the caudal approach.

Beginning in 1960, coincident with its rising popularity in obstetric anesthesia, the epidural method was taken up by several practitioners in North America. Philip Bromage and John Bonica performed several studies on epidural dose-response relationships and the hemodynamic changes that followed initiation of the block. Textbooks soon followed that introduced epidural analgesia into the operating room.[288-290] Although Dogliotti thought general anesthesia was contraindicated after initiation of epidural block, Bromage, and later Michael Cousins,[291] discussed the advantages of providing general anesthesia during prolonged surgery with epidural analgesia extending throughout the surgical procedure and into the postoperative period. Although lumbar epidurals were widely used for postoperative pain relief, problems with ambulation and inadequate analgesia led to the current practice of placing epidural catheters between the appropriate interspaces to provide selective antinociception along the surgical incision site.

A report in 1979 by J. Wang[292] demonstrated long-lasting analgesia from intrathecal administration of morphine in eight patients with cancer pain. This clinical study had firm groundwork from prior basic studies on the spinal effects of opioids in animals. In 1976, Yaksh[293] had reported that intrathecal morphine produced spinal analgesia in rats. Duggan and associates[294] demonstrated evidence of spinal analgesia after iontophoretic application of morphine into the dorsal horn region of the spinal cords of animals. Autoradiographic studies demonstrated a high density of opioid receptors in the substantia gelatinosa of the spinal cord.[295]

The use of spinal opioids spread rapidly after the initial report by Wang.[292] Samii and colleagues[296] confirmed that selective opioid spinal analgesia occurs in humans. Cousins[297] noticed that 1 to 2 mg of intrathecal morphine injected into the thoracic intrathecal region relieved the pain of breast or lung cancer for more than 24 hours. Behar[298] reported epidural opioid therapy in 1979. The explosive interest in neuraxial opioids that followed these reports was equal to the enthusiasm after the initial report of cocaine spinal anesthesia. The use of epidural catheters to provide long-lasting pain relief after surgery led to the formation of acute pain services.[299] With special attention to drug concentrations and rates of infusion, patients were able to recuperate without pain and ambulate on the first postoperative day, even after extensive thoracic, abdominal, and orthopedic operations. The special advantage of epidural opioids was the synergistic effect they exhibited with local anesthetics, allowing a marked decrease in the dose of both drugs to achieve the same level of analgesia.[300]

INTRAVENOUS ANESTHETICS

The development of intravenous anesthetics has been an important component of anesthetic management for over 70 years (see Chapters 10 and 11). Before the introduction of rapid-acting intravenous agents, induction of general anesthesia necessarily required inhalation of gases or vapors, an unpleasant experience for some patients.

Aristotle thought the arteries contained air, but Galen proved that the arteries and veins contained blood by opening, then ligating, the vessels of live animals. Galen's error was to place the origin of the blood in the liver, from where it flowed outward to the organs. With this arrangement, an intravenous injection would not be expected to produce a systemic effect.

William Harvey (1578-1657) announced his discovery of the circulation of the blood on April 17, 1616, one week before Shakespeare's death, but he did not publish until 1628, when a miserably printed book of 72 pages from Frankfurt, Germany, outlined one of the greatest discoveries in the annals of medicine: Blood flows from the heart to arteries, to veins, and back to the heart.[301] A crucial step in Harvey's analysis of the circulation was that the venous blood flowed to the heart and not to the periphery, opening the possibility of intravenous therapy. Chauncey Leake, a 20th-century pharmacologist who also contributed significantly to the development of anesthetic agents, translated the works of Harvey from Latin to English. The following excerpt from the Leake translation of *De Motu Cordis* concerns the function of the valves in the venous system, previously described by Harvey's teacher, Hieronymus Fabricius Ab Aquapendente (1537-1619) of Padua:

> The discoverer of these valves and his followers did not rightly appreciate their function. It is not to prevent blood from falling by its weight into areas lower down, for there are some in the jugular vein which are directed downwards, and which prevent blood from being carried upwards. They are thus not always looking upwards, but more correctly, always toward the main venous trunks and the heart. ... to this may be added that there are none in the arteries, and that one may note that dogs, oxen, and all such animals have valves at the branches of the crural veins at the top of the sacrum, and in branches from the haunches, in which no such weight effect of an erect stature is to be feared. ... From many experiments it is evident that the function of the valves in the veins is the same as that of the three sigmoid valves placed at the opening of the aorta and pulmonary artery, to prevent, when they are tightly closed, the reflex of blood passing over them.

Between 1656 and 1657, Christopher Wren and Timothy Clarck experimented with the intravenous injection of a variety of substances, including wine, opioids, milk, whey, broths, alcohol, beer, and cathartics, into animals. Christopher Wren was at that time Professor of Astronomy at the University of Oxford, and Timothy Clarck was a physician who attended the King of England, Charles II. Their method was to load the drug into a dissected toad bladder and connect this "syringe" by means of a glass tube or hollow quill into the vein. Summarizing these experiments in 1679, Clarck[302] observed certain occurrences after these injections:

> Various phenomena occurred over and over again which held me in doubt, whether such operations could ever be safely employed ... it would require that previous alteration of the injection should be rendered fit for use.

This final remark might have referred to infectious or other side effects from injecting unsterile or hypertonic solutions.

Pierre-Cyprien Ore[303] (1828-1891) performed the first successful attempt at intravenous anesthesia in 1872 by using chloral hydrate to anesthetize a human subject. Although he believed it superior to chloroform, his contemporaries did not adopt the method. Intravenous paraldehyde was briefly used as an anesthetic during and after World War I. At the same time, the combination of intravenous morphine and scopolamine gained wide popularity, particularly in obstetric anesthesia.[304] The method became known as *twilight sleep*, but this drug combination was slowly abandoned because of unpredictable side effects when given to some patients. Tribromoethanol (Avertin) was originally promoted as a full anesthetic agent to be administered rectally.[305] Although the rectal administration of agents had been promoted by Pirogoff, Gwathmey, and others, the use of rectal tribromoethanol fell into disfavor when rectal ulcerations after use of the agent were reported. Thereafter, tribromoethanol was used briefly an intravenous agent, but because it had a prolonged duration of action and produced profound respiratory depression and probable hepatotoxicity, other suitable intravenous agents were sought.

Adolf von Baeyer discovered the first barbiturate, barbituric acid, in 1864, but the drug had no sedative properties. It is said that Baeyer celebrated the discovery of the compound on Saint Barbara's Day, and he coined the word *barbiturate* as a combination of Barbara with urea, because barbituric acid results from the combination of malonic acid and urea.[306] The first sedative barbiturate was synthesized in 1903 by Emil Fischer[307] (1852-1919) of Berlin, but short-acting intravenous agents such as hexobarbital were not introduced until nearly 30 years later. Helmut Weese[308] (1897-1954), considered by many to be the originator of successful intravenous anesthetic methods, reported several thousand cases of hexobarbital use in 1932. Sodium thiopental followed hexobarbital in 1934, and the first detailed analysis of its use was described by John Lundy of the Mayo Clinic.[309,310] The use of thiopental was a further refinement of his earlier concept of *balanced anesthesia*, whereby anesthesia is administered with the use of multiple agents.[310] According to Lundy, general anesthesia was safer with the use of multiple agents, because the dose of any one particular agent was less and fewer side effects were observed.

It was soon learned that thiopental could be dangerous to administer in certain circumstances. When the drug was used for induction of anesthesia for injured personnel after the bombing of Pearl Harbor in 1941, the frequent occurrence of sudden death emphasized the profound depressant effect this drug has on the cardiovascular system.[311] A later analysis of the use of thiopental at Pearl Harbor, however, did not implicate the drug as the cause of the high mortality rate observed at that time.[312] The only other commonly used short-acting barbiturate is methohexital, an oxybarbiturate that has similar depressant effects on the circulation. Because of its unique proconvulsive effect, methohexital is used as an anesthetic for electroshock therapy.

There have been several attempts to replace the barbiturates with shorter-acting drugs with less cardiovascular depression. Some of these drugs, such as althesin,[313] propanidid, and eltanolone, were withdrawn from clinical use because of unwanted side effects. Etomidate, an intravenous anesthetic used to induce anesthesia that was introduced in 1973, produces only minimal hemodynamic depression and has found use in patients with hypovolemia and in those with significant cardiovascular disease.[314] Etomidate can cause undesirable myoclonic movements during induction in some patients.

The benzodiazepines midazolam, diazepam, and lorazepam are useful intravenous agents that relieve anxiety without the same degree of sedation produced with the barbiturates. Experimental studies on this class of drugs began in 1933 at the University of Kracow in Poland, with the first clinically useful drug, chlordiazepoxide (Librium), introduced in 1960. Diazepam (1963) and midazolam (1978) followed.[315] A specific antagonist can be used to treat overdosage.[316]

Ketamine was introduced as an anesthetic in 1966.[317] It was initially used intravenously or intramuscularly as a complete agent by itself, but reports of postoperative hallucinations led to re-evaluation of its use, and it is now typically used only in combination with other sedative agents. Ketamine is a unique agent in the armamentarium of the anesthesiologist because it does not depress the cardiovascular system, even when used in full anesthetic doses.

Propofol, introduced clinically[313,318] in 1977, is an alkylphenol compound that has some advantages over thiopental. It appears to have antiemetic properties and suppresses laryngeal reflexes to a greater extent than thiopental, allowing easy placement of supraglottic airways. It has achieved widespread use since its introduction, partially because of its rapid recovery profile. Propofol is often administered as a continuous infusion for general anesthesia, with or without the addition of inhalation anesthetics. When combined with analgesic agents such as opioids, propofol can provide all the components of a satisfactory general anesthetic. This method, often called *total intravenous anesthesia* (TIVA), can eliminate the need for any gaseous or volatile agents. Propofol is a profound cardiovascular depressant, and it can produce significant pain on injection.

Although intravenous opioids were once considered unsafe in the private rooms of hospitals, a modality of administration called *patient-controlled analgesia* (PCA) is now routinely used in most hospitals. The rationale is that because pain is a subjective experience, only the patients can assess the need for analgesics and balance that with their experience of side effects. Overdose is obviated by lock-out intervals and by the inability to perform the task of drug administration as somnolence ensues. The methods for intravenous PCA therapy in the postoperative setting were developed by anesthesiologists more than 30 years ago,[319-321] but they are now used by several specialty groups within the hospital.

MUSCLE RELAXANTS

Neuromuscular blocking drugs or muscle relaxants are firmly entrenched as an integral part of everyday anesthetic practice (see Chapter 13). Anesthesia providers practiced for nearly 100 years without these drugs, but it would be difficult to provide the same level of anesthetic service today without their use.

Initial Contact with Arrow Poison

Homer (*Odyssey*, I, 260) and Virgil (*Aeneid*, IX, 772) mention poisoned arrows. The word *toxin* is derived from the Greek root *toxon* ("bow"). Medical fascination with the specific arrow poison now called curare began nearly 500 years ago when the first returning explorers from South America told of a poisoned arrow that was used in warfare and to kill game.[322] In 1505, Pietro Martyr d'Anglera,[323] an Italian monk who visited South America in the early 16th century, wrote the following:

This Indian King layd wait for oure men ... set on them with about seven hundred men armed after theire maner, although they were naked. For only the King and his noblemen were appareled. ... So fiercely assayling oure men with theire venomous arrowes that they slewe of them fortie and seven ... for that poyson is of such force, that albeit the wounds were not great, yet they dyed thereof immediately.

Sir Walter Raleigh[324] (1552-1618) was one of the first to report on the wonders of the drug, which his first lieutenant, Laurence Keymis, called *ourari*, the first English attempt to reproduce the Macusi Indian pronunciation of the poison. Remarkably, the flesh of the poisoned animal was eaten with impunity. The native inhabitants were greatly impressed with gunpowder but noticed that the noise from guns frightened the game, and they preferred the poison-tipped arrow that was sent quietly from a blowgun. Initial reports indicated that the poison was made from a mixture of rat bones and bark.

Charles-Marie de la Condamine[325] (1701-1774) was the first to bring creditable samples back to Europe. His samples were used by Richard Brocklesby (1722-1797) to demonstrate that the heart of a cat continued to beat for 2 hours after it was apparently dead from curare poisoning. The Florentine Abbot, Felix Fontana (1720-1805),

injected the drug directly into the exposed sciatic nerve and observed no effect. He concluded that the curare impaired the irritability of the muscle.[326]

Mechanism of Action

The collaborative project of Benjamin Brodie (1783-1862) (Fig. 1-12A) and Charles Waterton (1783-1865) (see Fig. 1-12B) initiated our modern understanding of muscle relaxants.[327] Benjamin Brodie was the principal figure of English surgery at that time, and Waterton was the eccentric Squire of Walton Hall, near Wakefield, England. Waterton had traveled extensively, including several expeditions into British Guiana, where he owned property and eventually obtained several samples of the arrow poison.

In 1814, Brodie and Waterton[328] demonstrated that an animal could survive a curare injection provided that ventilation was continued after injection. For this famous experiment, it seems that Waterton supplied the curare and the animal—a donkey—and Brodie supplied the experimental idea. They injected the donkey with poison in the shoulder, and it was immobilized within 10 minutes.

An incision was then made in its windpipe, and through it the lungs were inflated for two hours, with a pair of bellows. The ass held up her head, and looked around, but the inflating being discontinued, she sunk once more in apparent death. The artificial respiration was immediately recommenced and continued without intermission for two hours. This saved the ass from final dissolution: she rose up and walked about; she seemed neither in agitation nor pain.

Waterton named the donkey *Wouralia* and nurtured her on his estate, where she died 25 years later. Curiously, in their later correspondence, neither partner mentions the collaboration of the other individual. Waterton's book,[328] entitled *Wanderings in South America* and dated 1879, contains an extensive description of the preparation and use of curare, as well as the manner of use of the blowpipe, which he called the "extraordinary tube of death."

The experiment performed by Claude Bernard[329] (1813-1878) demonstrating the action of curare at the junction between the nerve and muscle was deceptively simple (Fig. 1-13). In his studies with curare, Bernard used the drug to open up a new area of investigation, the physiology and pharmacology of the junction between the nerve and muscle. Experiments on the specialized apparatus where the action of curare is primarily located, the neuromuscular junction, were begun by one of Bernard's students, Willy Kuhne[330] (1837-1900).

Introduction into Clinical Medicine

Waterton suggested the use of his *woraria* for the treatment of tetanus and rabies, and the few successful trials of the small samples of curare that were available then were used to treat these conditions.[331] For the next 175 years in Europe and North America, the drug remained a curiosity with no definite purpose. The medical community

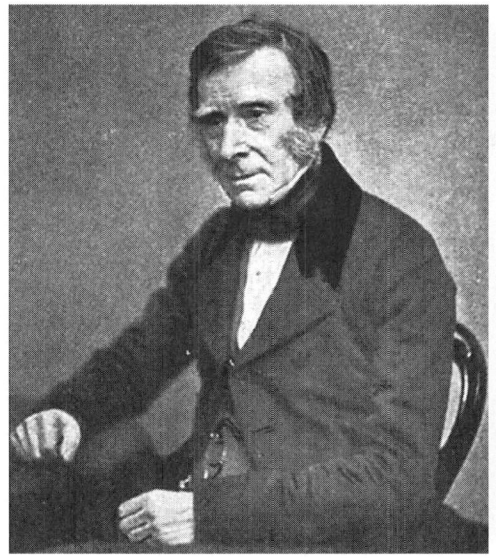
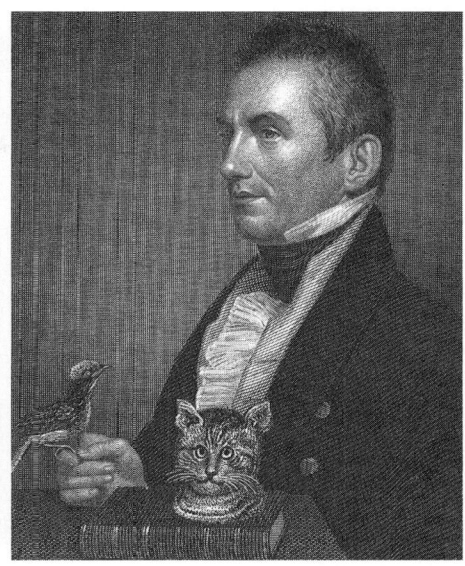

Figure 1–12 Mechanism of curare poisoning. Benjamin Brodie (**A**) and Charles Waterton (**B**) collaborated in demonstrating that animals could survive curare poisoning if artificial ventilation was provided. (Courtesy of the National Library of Medicine, Bethesda, MD.)

A   B

ignored an early report[330] from 1912, suggesting its use to provide muscular relaxation during closure of the abdomen:

> Thus far I have used solution of curarine up to 2% by intramuscular injection. With this dose, closure of the abdominal wall was achieved readily. There is not sufficient curare available, so I have not yet been able to ascertain the correct dose for this purpose.

The active principle was eventually found in several plant species, primarily *Chondodendron tomentosum* and *Strychnos toxifera* (see Fig. 1-9C). King[333] isolated the active compound from the *Chondodendron* species that he called D-tubocurarine in 1935.

The introduction of curare into clinical practice was initiated by several individuals, beginning with Richard C. Gill[334] (1901-1958), whose contributions, like those of Waterton, arose out of a strong sense of wanderlust, combined with an interest in primitive medicine. As a young man growing up in Washington, D. C., Gill was expected to follow his father and older brother into the practice of medicine. Instead, his degree in 1929 from Cornell University was in English, and his career as a teacher was brief. He took a position with a rubber company in Lima, Peru, but with the stock market crash of 1929, he consolidated his savings, and together with his wife Ruth, purchased 750 acres of land in the Ecuadorian jungle. By 1930, Richard and Ruth Gill were the proud owners of a

Figure 1–13 **A,** Claude Bernard (1813-1878) was one of the greatest physiologists of all time and made several contributions to the anesthesia literature. Bernard was born in Saint Julien, France, and was educated in Paris. After his medical training, he became an assistant to François Magendie, the leading physiologist of that era. He never practiced medicine, but his research contributions pervade every field of modern medicine. In 1855, he succeeded Magendie as Professor of Physiology at the College de France. A special Chair of General Physiology was created for him at the Sorbonne. **B,** Experiment by Claude Bernard, illustrating the site of action of curare at the junction of the nerve and muscle. A ligature prevented injected curare (I) from reaching the muscle of the frog's hind limb. After curare injection systemically, Bernard observed that the limb contracted in response to a neural stimulus (N) applied above the ligature. The opposite limb would contract only to direct electric stimulation of the muscle but not to a neural stimulus. He showed that the nerve and muscle were unaffected but that the connection between the nerve and the muscle was blocked.[329] (Courtesy of the National Library of Medicine, Bethesda, MD.)

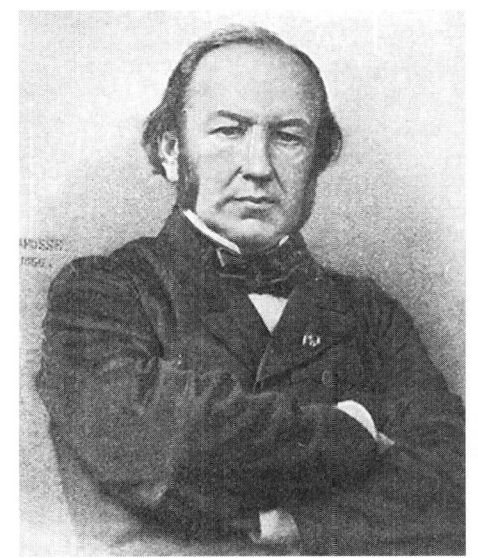
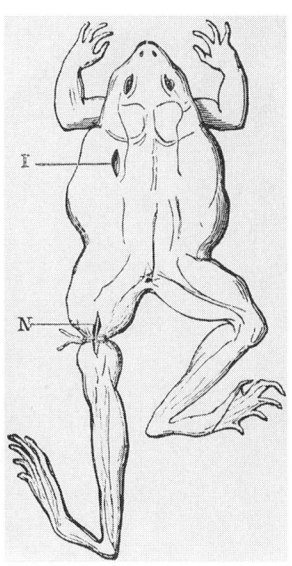

A   B

large hacienda on the Eastern slopes of the Andes,[335] where they raised tropical fruits and vegetables and studied the local Indian customs.

While returning to the United States in 1932 for a brief holiday, Gill fell from his horse and developed a neurologic syndrome, initially thought to be multiple sclerosis, that eventually progressed to a painful spastic disorder. His neurologist Walter Freeman advised him that the arrow poison from South America might help cure his painful spasms, but it was nearly impossible to obtain the drug. Procuring curare and other herbal remedies thereafter became the focus of Gill's life until his death in 1958 at age 57. Gill obtained funding from Sayre Merrill, a wealthy Massachusetts businessman, for an expedition to retrieve indigenous medicinal plants from the Ecuadorian jungle. The primary aim was to retrieve adequate amounts of the crude curare preparation to begin clinical trials with the drug in cases of spasticity. It is noteworthy that Gill was in a unique position to obtain large quantities of curare because the Indian "medicine men," who jealously guarded the secrets of making the poisonous darts, trusted him.

After 4 years of planning, Gill's neurologic condition had improved, and the expedition was launched. In 1938, Richard and Ruth Gill returned with 11 kg of a crude curare mixture and 75 other indigenous medicinal preparations obtained from the Indian shamans. Sadly for the Gills, there was no interest in their jungle remedies. Initially, even the curare failed to generate any interest. Freeman was acquainted with Abram E. Bennett, a psychiatrist at the University of Nebraska who had expressed interest in the drug. Bennett had the crude concoction standardized by the pharmacologist A. R. McIntyre but failed to find any prolonged benefit for it in cases of spasticity (Fig. 1-14A).

Bennett then turned his attention to the use of curare during Metrazol convulsive therapy, which at that time was thought to be therapeutic for depression and mania but was complicated by a high incidence of bone fractures

and joint dislocations. By then, E. R. Squibb and Sons had taken the remainder of Gill's curare and was distributing a small quantity of the drug as Intocostrin, an unpurified form of D-tubocurarine. Bennett[336] reported on the successful use of Intocostrin in cases of Metrazol convulsive therapy in 1940. His method was to administer Intocostrin until a head lift was impossible and then give Metrazol. Surprisingly, he reported no respiratory embarrassment and no complications and thought the patients preferred his new method.

E. R. Squibb and Sons, together with their anesthesiologist consultant, Lewis H. Wright (1894-1974), were convinced that the true home for curare was with the anesthesiologist and in 1940, with some urging, Wright convinced Harold R. Griffith (1894-1985) (see Fig. 1-14B) of Montreal, Canada to use the drug during general anesthesia when muscular relaxation was required by the surgeon. Previous attempts by Wright to generate interest in the drug had failed until Griffith agreed to use Intocostrin during cyclopropane anesthesia. Griffith and his junior colleague Enid Johnson reported the successful use of curare in 43 patients to provide muscular relaxation during surgical anesthesia in 1942.[337] They concluded that the agent provided relaxation without interfering with respiration. This was followed by a study in Iowa by Stuart Cullen[338] (1909-1979), who enthusiastically supported use of the drug to provide muscular relaxation without the need for deep levels of general anesthesia. T. Cecil Gray[339] (1913-) of Liverpool popularized the drug in England and developed an anesthetic technique consisting of profound muscular paralysis and nitrous oxide–oxygen anesthesia. Phyllis Harroun[340,341] used high-dose curare, nitrous oxide, and morphine for thoracic surgery, thereby providing muscular relaxation without the use of flammable agents, a novel technique at the time. In 1947, William Neff[342] used nitrous oxide and oxygen supplemented with meperidine and curare and reported favorable anesthetic conditions. Although Griffith and Cullen had both maintained spontaneous

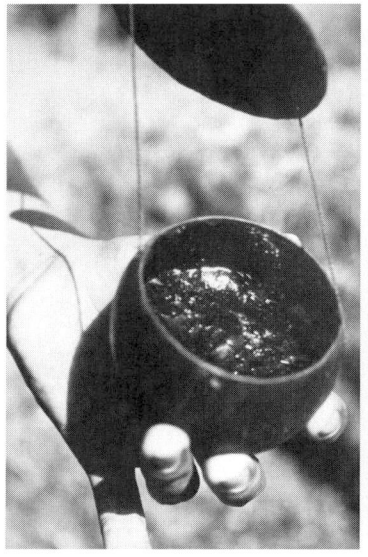
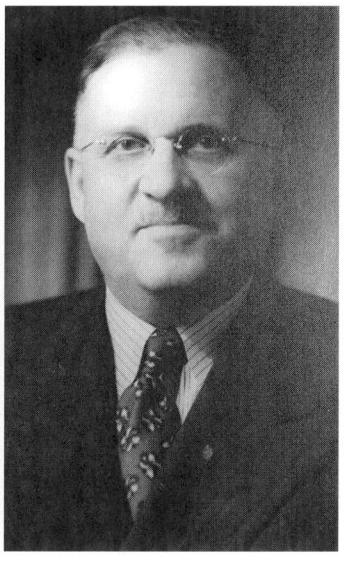

Figure 1–14 A, Richard Gill returned from Ecuador in 1938 with 11 kg of a dark tarlike paste from which Squibb and Sons, Inc., prepared the sterile, injectable solution, Intocostrin. **B,** Harold Griffith and Enid Johnson (not shown) used Intocostrin in 43 cases of abdominal surgery with success in 1942. (Courtesy of the Guedel Memorial Anesthesia Center, San Francisco, CA.)

A   B

respiration, the technique of Harroun, Gray, and Neff provided profound muscular paralysis with controlled respiration.

In a report from 1954, Henry K. Beecher (1907-1976) and D. P. Todd[343] concluded that the use of curare led to a nearly sixfold increase in postoperative complications and deaths. Similar cautionary articles followed their report but were refuted by others. Churchill-Davidson[344] advised in 1952 that a useful technique for monitoring the degree of neuromuscular blockade was to stimulate a peripheral nerve and observe the resulting muscular contraction. Specific devices designed to stimulate the ulnar nerve were promoted in the 1960s.[345,346] Various modifications of the stimulus array have been described since that time to ensure complete return of neuromuscular function before allowing the patient to breathe unassisted.[347]

Since the introduction of curare into anesthesia practice, numerous additional neuromuscular blocking agents have been developed. Gallamine triethiodide was introduced in 1947, but like curare, it had undesirable effects on the autonomic nervous system, which prompted a search for other drugs.[348] Exploration of the structure-activity relationships of the plant alkaloids led to the development of the methonium compounds. In 1949, the neuromuscular blocking activity of one of this class of drugs, succinylcholine, was recognized,[349] and it was introduced clinically soon thereafter.[350] Succinylcholine and other similar agents were shown to depolarize the end plate, preventing additional motor contractions from activity in the motor nerve. Advances in chemistry allowed the synthesis of neuromuscular blocking agents that lacked the autonomic effects of curare. Since the discovery of curare, nearly 50 neuromuscular blocking agents have been introduced, but many of these drugs have been abandoned because of undesirable side effects. Drugs that have maintained favorable safety records are steroid-based synthetic neuromuscular blocking agents such as pancuronium (1966),[351] vecuronium (1980),[352,353] and rocuronium (1991),[354] and they have replaced the older drugs, such as curare and gallamine, in the modern drug armamentarium.

ANESTHESIA APPARATUS

Early Delivery Systems

For the first public demonstration of ether anesthesia, Morton used a specially constructed glass bottle with an attached mouthpiece (see Chapter 9). In England, John Snow developed a new type of ether inhaler and took up the practice of ether anesthesia as a full-time endeavor. His apparatus provided valves to prevent rebreathing, and although he experimented with methods for carbon dioxide absorption, he did not develop it into a clinically useful technique. John Snow was aware of the difficulties associated with the simple mouthpiece that was used with a noseclip by Wells and Morton. In his book on ether published in 1847,[355] he states the following:

> For some of the adult patients, after they lost their consciousness, made such strong instinctive efforts

to breathe by the nostrils, that the air was forced through the lachrymal ducts, and occasionally they held the breath altogether for a short time, and were getting purple in the face, when the nostrils had to be liberated, for a short time, to allow respiration of the external air, and thus a delay was occasioned.

With the introduction of chloroform, several inhalers were developed to administer the agent. Ferdinand Junker[356] (1828-1901) devised a simple inhaler, consisting of a bottle to hold liquid chloroform, an inflow tube into which the anesthetist could squeeze air with a hand pump, and an outflow tube directed into the mask. The Junker inhaler underwent several modifications to improve its safety but was rarely used in the United States. Joseph T. Clover[357,358] (1825-1882), the prominent English anesthetist after John Snow, devised several devices for the administration of nitrous oxide, ether, and chloroform. The Clover bag held more than 16 L of air, with chloroform vapor at approximately 4%. Smaller concentrations could be given by adjusting a valve on the facemask that allowed dilution of the chloroform with air. A clever solution to avoid the problem of high concentrations of chloroform was presented by Augustus Vernon Harcourt (1834-1919) in 1912. This apparatus was one of the several "draw-over" systems that brought the inspired air over a vaporizer heated by a small candle. The chloroform double-necked flask held the liquid chloroform and two beads that rose to the top or sank to the bottom, depending on the temperature of the liquid. Several draw-over chloroform delivery systems are described in Dudley Buxton's 1914 textbook.[359] The problem with these early delivery systems for longer procedures was the potential for hypoxia and partial rebreathing of expired carbon dioxide.

Other types of anesthesia machines were developed to provide anesthesia with the insufflation method, whereby a small catheter was placed with its tip near the carina to deliver air and ether or chloroform. These were continuous-flow machines that did not rely on respiratory movements for oxygenation and were based on the work of Samuel Meltzer (1851-1920) and John Auer (1875-1948) demonstrating its safe use in animals.[360] It was one solution to the problem of pneumothorax and respiratory decompensation during thoracic surgery. C. A. Elsberg's (1871-1948) continuous-flow machine was described in 1911 and went through several modifications.[361] The popular Shipway model was used by Francis E. Shipway (1875-1968) to provide anesthesia to King George V of England for rib resection and drainage of empyema, a feat for which Shipway was knighted. In retrospect, it is clear that these continuous flow machines were not capable of eliminating carbon dioxide in all cases,[362] and anesthesia machines eventually were developed that allowed to-and-fro respiration through one large-bore endotracheal tube.

Compressed Gases and Reducing Valves

Of major importance in the design of the modern anesthesia machine was the compression of gases in metal cylinders. Oxygen and nitrous oxide were available under compression as early as 1885 through the manufacturers S. S. White of Philadelphia and Messrs. Coxeter of London. This allowed the development of compact machines capable of prolonged anesthetic delivery without the cumbersome feature of low-pressure reservoirs. Frederick Hewitt's first anesthetic gas machine designed for giving oxygen and nitrous oxide mixtures had two nitrous oxide cylinders and one oxygen cylinder and were fed into a large breathing bag through a double cylinder yoke.[139] Oxygen concentrations could be adjusted at the stopcock near the mask. His preferred oxygen concentrations were 5% to 8%. With the addition of oxygen, he attempted to "dispense with cyanosis, jerky and irregular breathing, deep stertor and clonic movements of the extremities."

The invention of the reducing valve is accredited to Jay Albion Heidbrink (1857-1957), an anesthesiologist from Minneapolis who observed that the opening from high-pressure cylinders often froze closed as the gases were released. He described a valve that reduced the high tank pressures to working pressures and incorporated this device into his Heidbrink Anesthetizer. In Germany, Heinrich Drager (1847-1917) and his son Bernhard Drager (1870-1928) developed reducing valves to control an even, accurate flow of carbon dioxide gas drawn from beer cylinders, and these valves were later used in the early anesthesia machines. Further refinements to the early machines were added by James T. Gwathmey[363] and H. Edmund G. Boyle[364] (1875-1941) chiefly through the addition of bubble-through heated water baths for estimation of gas flows. The Boyle machine passed various amounts of oxygen through ether with a "water-sight" meter. This flowmeter estimated the flow through the vaporizer from how many of the holes were generating bubbles. Heidbrink further improved the flowmeter by using an inverted float in a tube of varying taper with calibrations marked on the side. Rotating floats, also called rotameters, have slanted grooves cut into the rim, causing them to rotate, and they are more accurate than the ball or nonrotating floats. Rotameters were introduced in 1908 by Karl Kuppers and first used in anesthesia in 1910.[365]

Carbon Dioxide Absorption

Anesthesiologists from the first half of the 20th century were not privileged to visit just one hospital during a day's work. Visits to several institutions might take place in a single day, with the practitioners bringing their own delivery systems and drugs with them as they traveled. Understandably, there was a priority for portability and elimination of waste, because these anesthesiologists paid for the agents themselves. One development that conserved gases and vapors was the use of systems that absorbed expired carbon dioxide and allowed rebreathing of expired gases.

Several ineffectual attempts were made to introduce carbon dioxide absorption methods in the 19th century. John Snow and Alfred Coleman (1828-1902) were motivated to conserve anesthetic gases that escaped into the atmosphere through nonrebreathing valves. Coleman devised a system of absorbing carbon dioxide by passing the expired gases over slaked quick lime.[366,367] The recovered gases were then used for subsequent anesthetics (Fig. 1-15). Franz Kuhn (1866-1929) described soda lime absorption of exhaled carbon dioxide in 1905, but the report did not attract attention.[368]

Dennis Jackson demonstrated the use of soda lime absorption to maintain stable levels of anesthesia for several hours in animals with minimal ether consumption.[369] The animals were given additional oxygen to meet metabolic needs, but the anesthetic gases were rebreathed, resulting in economy and improved maintenance of body temperature and airway humidity. In 1923, Ralph Waters (1884-1979) (see Fig. 1-18B), working then as an anesthesia practitioner in Sioux City, Iowa, contacted Jackson and devised a soda lime canister for clinical use.[370] The canister was attached to a breathing hose close to the face, and although it was cumbersome to use, the device was widely distributed. The in-line soda lime canister launched the academic career of Waters, who later became one of the most prominent figures in anesthesiology during the first half of the 20th century. In 1930, Brian C. Sword[371] altered the Waters canister by attaching it to the chassis of a movable cart with two hoses directed to the airway, one for inspired gases and one for exhaled gases.

Controlled Vaporizers

With the introduction of more potent volatile anesthetics such as halothane it became important to control the concentration of inspired vapor carefully. To solve this problem, Lucien Morris[372] invented the copper kettle to vaporize liquid anesthetics. Its advantage rested on the

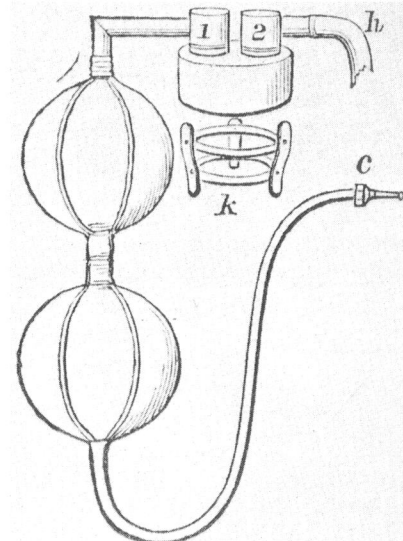

Figure 1–15 Alfred Coleman's economizing device. The anesthetic gases entered the lower bag and passed into the upper bag through a one-way valve. Gases were inhaled and exhaled through the tube (h), passing over a lime container (1, 2) held in frame (k) that eliminated carbon dioxide; (c) is gas inlet. The conserved gas in the upper bag was used during a later anesthetic administration. (From Coleman A: Mr. Coleman's economizing apparatus for re-inhaling the gas. Br J Dent Sci 12:443, 1869.)

fact that as the agent was vaporized, there was little change in the temperature of the anesthetic liquid. The copper kettle could be used with any agent provided that the practitioner was cognizant of the vapor pressure of the agent and the flow rates of the inspired gases. Without the addition of diluent gases such as nitrous oxide or oxygen, the copper kettle could deliver lethal concentrations of vapor. The vaporizers in common use today use bimetallic strips that bend as the temperature drops, permitting more fresh gas to enter the vaporizing chamber. Vaporizers have been designed for all the agents in use today, including halothane, enflurane, isoflurane, desflurane, and sevoflurane. The modern anesthesia machines are also equipped with scavenging systems designed to minimize escape of anesthetic vapors and nitrous oxide into the operating room. Although controversial, some studies have shown that daily exposure to anesthetic vapors in low concentrations can have deleterious side effects.[373]

Ventilators in the Intensive Care Unit

The earliest ventilator, the Fell-O'Dwyer apparatus, was described in 1892.[374] It was used as early as 1896 to provide respiratory support in cases of opium poisoning. Rudolph Matas, a surgeon in New Orleans who contributed significantly to the early development of regional anesthesia in the United States, was one of the first to use the Fell-O'Dwyer ventilator during thoracic surgery.[375] During the polio epidemic, thousands of afflicted patients were kept alive with the Drinker respirator,[376] often referred to as the *iron lung*, a negative-pressure device that surrounded the patient and provided for air movement in and out of the lungs. A Swedish ventilator called the Spiropulsator was introduced in 1934 and modified in 1947 by E. Trier Moerch.[377] This ventilator used a piston pump to deliver a fixed volume of gas. Ventilators today are usually an integral part of the anesthesia machine and direct compressed air into a rigid container containing a bellows that inflates the lungs. Bjørn Ibsen[378] (1915-), a Danish anesthesiologist, initiated the concept of intensive care units in the early 1950s to care for polio patients and guided the transition from iron lungs to modern ventilators. Intensive care units have since become an integral part of the modern hospital, with anesthesiologists actively involved in their daily operation.

STRESS-FREE ANESTHESIA

Procedures before the discovery of anesthesia were necessarily of short duration. Raper relates that surgical cases lasting more than 20 minutes would usually result in the death of the patient, because the stress associated with such intense nociception would exhaust the patient's reserves. Highly stressful procedures such as abdominal surgery were rarely attempted before 1846. Ephraim McDowell[379] (1771-1830), a rural surgeon from Kentucky, performed the first successful intraperitoneal procedure when he excised a 10-kg ovarian cyst from Mrs. Jane Todd Crawford in 1809. McDowell's publication of the case achieved for him a small measure of fame, unusual for a

rural practitioner. However, intraperitoneal procedures are among the most highly stressful operations, and McDowell's accomplishment was rarely repeated. The first successful upper abdominal procedure occurred only after the advent of general anesthesia. Theodor Billroth (1829-1894) performed the first gastrectomy with chloroform anesthesia on January 29, 1881.

The idea that reduction of perioperative stress had a beneficial effect on recovery was championed by George W. Crile (1864-1943), chief surgeon at the Cleveland Clinic at the beginning of the 20th century. Crile's operative technique was to infiltrate all tissues with dilute procaine before incision. Patients were lightly anesthetized with mask inhalation of nitrous oxide and oxygen.[380] He describes these concepts of stress-free anesthesia in his book, *Anoci-Association*, published in 1914.[381]

An early devotee of Crile's ideas was the prominent neurosurgeon Harvey Cushing[382] (1869-1939), who promoted the use of regional blocks before emergence from ether anesthesia to ensue a smooth postoperative course. Cushing was the first surgeon to use blood pressure measurements on his patients after he learned the Rovi-Rocci method in Italy (Fig. 1-16). Accurate anesthetic records were maintained during Cushing's cases[257] and confirmed his opinion that shock could be prevented by careful attention to avoiding the stresses associated with surgery.

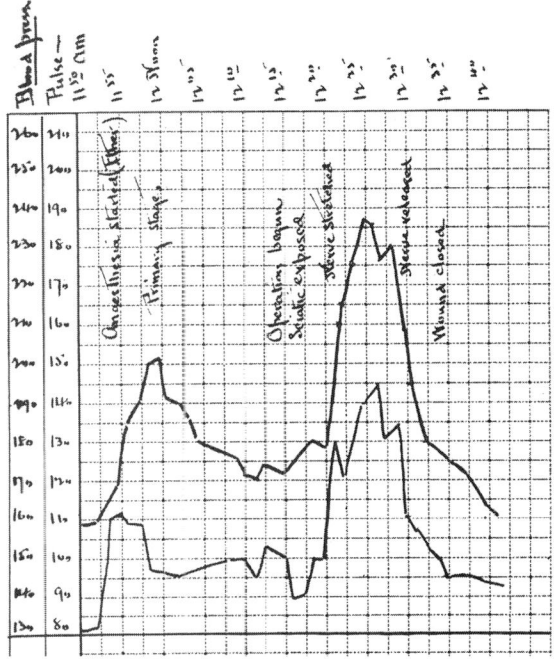

Figure 1–16 One of Harvey Cushing's early anesthesia records shows systolic blood pressure *(top tracing)* and pulse rate *(bottom tracing)*. The first rise in blood pressure occurred during the excitement phase of ether induction, and the second rise occurred during the release of adhesions of the sciatic nerve. Vertical lines take place 2.5 minutes apart. The systolic blood pressure rose to greater than 230 mm Hg during the operation. Cushing was an early proponent of regional anesthesia, possibly stemming from his observations on blood pressure and heart rate.[382] (From Cushing H: On routine determination of arterial tension in operating room and clinic. Boston Med Surg J 148:250-256, 1903.)

Crile's ideas have had significant impact on how the modern anesthesiologist defines *general anesthesia*. In 1957, P. Woodbridge[383] defined general anesthesia as comprising four components: (1) sleep or unconsciousness, (2) blockade of undesirable reflexes, (3) motor blockade, and (4) sensory blockade. These ideas have been discussed and modified by M. Pinsker[384] into three components: (1) paralysis, (2) unconsciousness, and (3) attenuation of the stress response. Lundy's balanced anesthesia[310] is another formulation of the idea that several drugs can be used in combination to produce the state of unconsciousness and analgesia that we define as general anesthesia.

An enduring question during the past century, since Crile's introduction of the concept of stress-free anesthesia, has been how to evaluate the analgesic component of the ideal general anesthetic. Michael Roizen[385] observed in 1981 that general anesthetics did not prevent the increase in sympathetic activity in response to a skin incision, even in concentrations that prevented movement. Surgical stimulation often results in intraoperative hypertension and tachycardia, with the corollary that interventions that prevent these hemodynamic reflexes provide "analgesia." Hemodynamic instability was of marginal significance until surgeons began to operate on patients with significant ischemic heart disease. Studies have demonstrated that perioperative β-adrenergic blockade reduces the risk of perioperative myocardial infarction in patients at risk for this complication.[386]

It became apparent that intravenous opioids were highly successful in ablating the hemodynamic markers of stress. Edward Lowenstein[387] used large doses of morphine to stabilize heart rate and blood pressure during cardiac surgery. In 1967, the short-acting opioid fentanyl was introduced to provide intraoperative hemodynamic stability. Theodore H. Stanley[388] reported its successful use in large doses for cardiac surgery without the side effect of histamine release that sometimes occurs after morphine administration. Other short-acting opioids tailored for the anesthesiologist have been added since that time. Alfentanil, sufentanil, and remifentanil have different pharmacokinetic profiles that make them suitable agents for selected procedures. Naloxone, a specific antagonist for this class of drugs, was first used clinically in 1971.[389] An increased understanding of opioid pharmacology has opened up a new role for anesthesiologists, including acute pain management. Rapid detoxification of opioid addiction by using general anesthesia combined with opioid antagonism is a new technique that, if combined with judicious follow-up, can be a useful treatment for this condition.[390]

The combination of opioids with tranquilizers such as phenothiazines and butyrophenones provides a form of anesthesia called *neuroleptanesthesia*, which was introduced by DeCastro and Mundeleer[391] in 1959. Patients administered this form of anesthesia are immobile and are tranquil and have stable hemodynamics even during major surgical procedures. One goal of this technique is to block the autonomic and endocrine response to stress. This unique method of providing anesthesia is one other method of ablating the stress response, but unless other agents such as nitrous oxide or other intravenous

agents are administered, there can be a high incidence of awareness. Side effects from dopamine antagonism such as dysphoria and uncontrolled extrapyramidal motor movements have limited the widespread use of neuroleptanesthesia.

During the past 30 years, several investigators began a series of studies to measure the markers of the stress response during and after surgery. It was learned that during major surgery, patients anesthetized with traditional vapor anesthetics with or without opioids displayed increased levels of catabolic hormones postoperatively.[99] Significant elevations were observed for the catecholamines and for adrenocorticotropic hormone, cortisol, antidiuretic hormone, and growth hormone. Various methods of preventing postoperative catabolism have been under investigation for several years. The resulting catabolic state is thought by some to delay recovery and, with some operations, can be prevented with the use of neuraxial block.[99,392,393] It is apparent from recent reviews on this subject that the formulations of George Crile are still valid 100 years after he promoted them and likely to be the subject of further studies in the future.

AIRWAY MANAGEMENT AND RESUSCITATION

Masks and Airways

Ventilation during anesthesia was managed without specialized airway devices for more than 50 years after Morton's discovery, and a survey of anesthetic complications during this era attests to the relative safety of inhalation techniques in the spontaneously breathing patient (see Chapters 42 and 78). Deaths occurred during this era, and in some reports the anesthetic death rate was alarmingly high, but an obstructed airway was rarely mentioned as the primary cause of death. Friedrich von Esmarch[394] described the jaw thrust (Fig. 1-17) as a lifesaving maneuver in some cases of airway obstruction that resulted from chloroform or asphyxia:

> Press the lower jaw forwards with both hands by placing the forefingers behind the ascending ramus...by this movement the hyoid bone and root of the tongue, and the epiglottis are drawn forwards, and the entrance to the larynx is thus freed from obstruction.

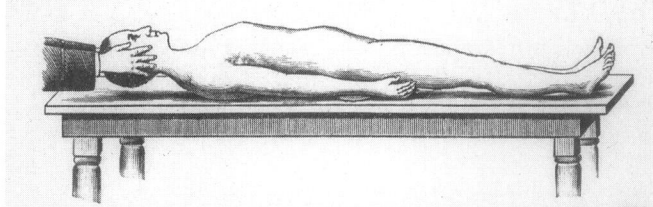

The head should be held as in this cut, extended, and pushed forward in the posture in relation to the trunk of that assumed by a runner.

Figure 1–17 Illustration in a treatise by Von Esmarch[394] shows the technique of maintaining an open airway in an unconscious patient. (From Von Esmarch F: Handbuch der kriegschirurgischen Technik. Hanover, Carl Rumpler, 1877.)

In 1874, the same maneuver had been previously described, but not popularized, by J. Heiberg,[395] a Norwegian surgeon.

Various problems with the Morton inhaler in the United States led to abandonment of inhalers in favor of a simple towel or sponge saturated with ether. In 1850, John Warren,[396] in his address to the American Medical Association, described his preferred technique for ether administration at the Massachusetts General Hospital: (1) no oral intake for at least 3 hours before surgery, (2) a horizontal position for induction, (3) bleeding the patient before surgery for bloodless operations, (4) pulse and respiration watched carefully by an assistant to the anesthetist, (5) ether applied with a large sponge soaked with ether, and (6) avoidance of cautery.

Several wire-frame masks were devised to replace the sponge or folded towel. The popular mask devised by Curl Schimmelbusch (1860-1895) had a trough-shaped rim to prevent liquid chloroform or ether from dropping onto the patient's face. Friederich von Esmarch[394] used a wire mask with a clip that enabled it to be strapped to the patient. The advantages of these masks were low cost, simplicity, and portability. Disadvantages included delivery of vapor throughout the operating room, cooling of the patient, and waste of anesthetic agent.

The development of the modern facemask originated with Francis Sibson[397,398] (1814-1876), who devised a mask made of pliable tinned iron and covered with glove leather. The mask covered the mouth and nose and therefore eliminated the need for noseclips. Snow quickly recognized the superiority of the Sibson mask and incorporated it into his practice.

The first anesthetics were of short duration and rarely required special devices to maintain airway patency. With the increasing complexity and duration of surgical procedures, special devices were fashioned to facilitate an open airway. Frederick Hewitt promoted a simple metal tube that projected through the mouth into the hypopharynx.[399] The commonly used Guedel rubber curved airway was described in 1935.[400] At the same time, cuffs were sometimes used on oral airways,[401] a design that has been resurrected in the form of a modern product, the cuffed oral pharyngeal airway (COPA).

Tracheal Tubes

In the 18th century, tubes were passed into the trachea during resuscitation from drowning, but these tubes were passed without direct visualization and were not for delivery of anesthetic agents. Similarly, the intubations of pediatrician Joseph O'Dwyer (1841-1898) in cases of diphtheria were performed with metal tubes passed blindly.[402] The O'Dwyer metal tube was later attached to a bellows by George Fell (1850-1918) for the treatment of opioid respiratory depression. Placement of tracheal tubes was vigorously opposed by the influential Parisian surgeon Armand Trousseau (1801-1867), who quoted the failures experienced by M. Bouchut in attempting to pass metal tubes for airway obstruction.[403] Bouchut had lost five of seven patients during his procedure, called *le tubage du larynx,* and the other two were rescued only

by tracheotomy.[403] Trousseau was the first to perform a tracheotomy in Paris and wrote a treatise promoting its use during airway compromise in 1851.[403]

John Snow had accomplished administration of chloroform through tracheotomy tubes in animals, and Friedrich Trendelenburg (1844-1924) used the same technique in humans.[406] Sir William Macewen (1848-1924) was the first physician to intubate the trachea orally for the sole purpose of administering anesthesia, and it was done to permit continued administration of chloroform during an operation in the mouth. On July 5, 1878, Macewen[404] performed a blind oral intubation on an awake patient with an ulcerating epithelioma of the tongue. An extensive operation was performed, and the results were excellent. Subsequently, Macewen tracheally intubated three other patients, two for edema of the larynx, and a fourth for another surgical procedure in the mouth. In the fourth case, the pulse was suddenly lost after the chloroform was administered, and the patient died on the table.

The use of tracheal intubation was accelerated to meet the needs of surgeons operating on the face and in the thoracic cavity. To operate within the thoracic cavity, some means was required to avoid respiratory compromise, which followed the inevitable pneumothorax when the chest was opened. Ernst Ferdinand Sauerbruch[407] (1875-1951) studied the problem as a young assistant to Johann von Mickulicz-Radecki (1850-1905) in Breslau, Germany, and his solution, the Sauerbruch Box, elevated him into a position of international prominence at a young age. The Sauerbruch Box was a cumbersome solution to the problem of pneumothorax and entailed placing the surgeon and the patient (below the neck) in a negative-pressure chamber, while the head of the patient and the anesthetist were outside the box at normal atmospheric pressure. The use of such an awkward construction indicates that the surgeons were determined to solve this problem at any cost. The modern solution, endotracheal intubation and controlled ventilation, as it unfolded was relatively simple, but it took several years to become established.

Franz Kuhn[368] (1866-1929) perfected a metal, flexible tube and used blind oral or nasal intubation for anesthetic purposes when the surgeon operated in the mouth. Kuhn's first report was in 1905 and included extensive description of the technique that included carbon dioxide absorption cartridges and 20 illustrations. He proposed but did not use inflatable pharyngeal cuffs to prevent air leaks. Insertion of catheters directly into the trachea to insufflate anesthetic agents was begun in the first decades of the 20th century. With this method, gases were introduced under continuous pressure through catheters that allowed exhalation between the space between the catheter and the tracheal wall.

The use of to-and-fro respiration through one large-bore endotracheal tube is credited to Ivan W. McGill[408] (1888-1986) (Fig. 1-18A) and Edgar S. Rowbotham[409] (1890-1979) to meet the demands of the maxillofacial surgeon. Their technique of blind nasal intubation was to position patients as if they were "sniffing the morning air." Occasional failures of the blind intubation were solved with a special instrument designed by Magill to

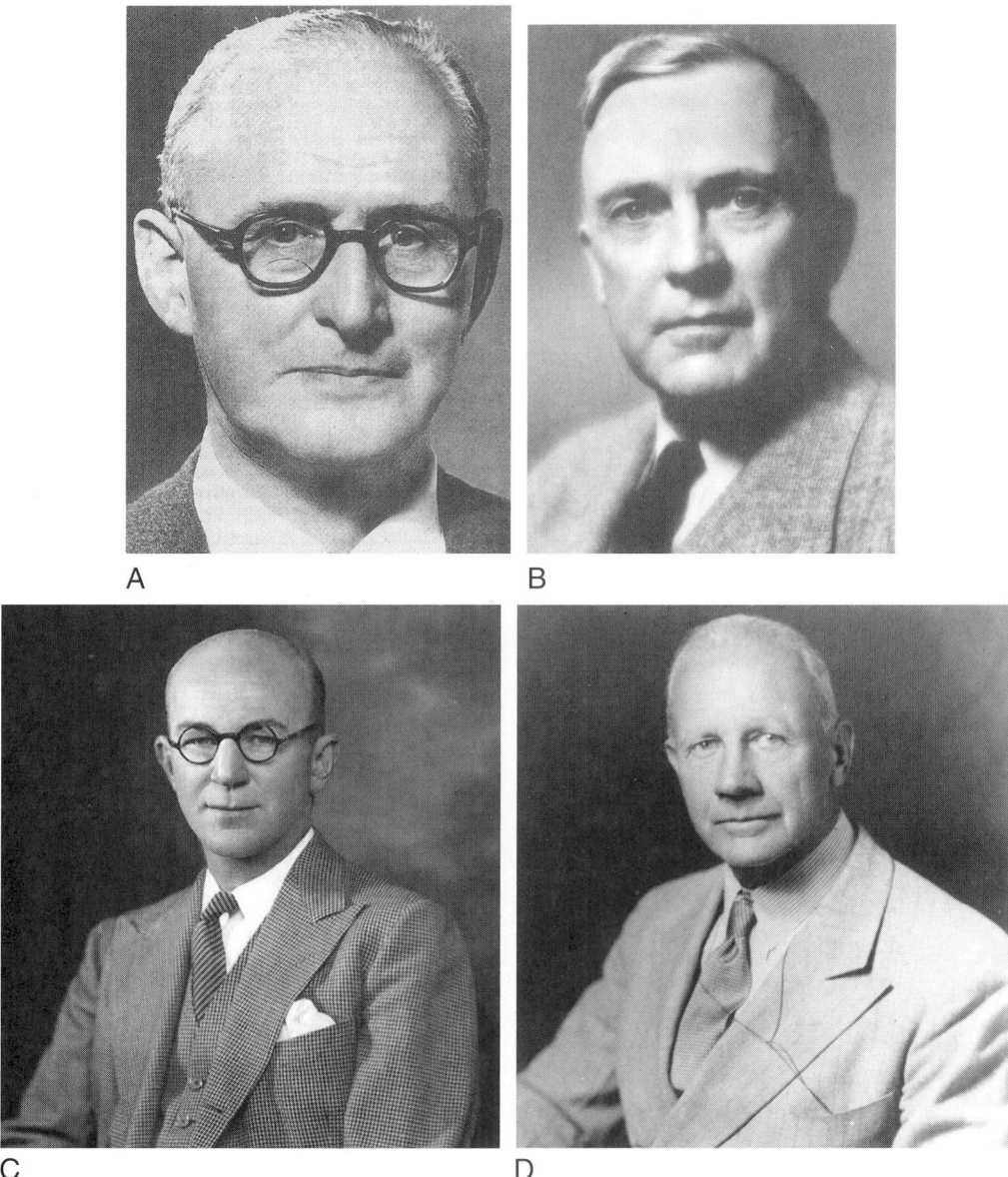

A

B

C

D

Figure 1–18 Prominent anesthesiologists of the 20th century. **A**, Sir Ivan Whiteside Magill (1888-1986) was born in Larne, Northern Ireland. He obtained a medical degree from Queen's University, Belfast, in 1913. During World War I, he served with the Irish Guards in the Medical Corps. After the war, he and Stanley Rowbotham (1890-1979) pioneered the use of large-bore endotracheal tubes to allow plastic surgeons to operate on the facial injuries of wounded soldiers. He designed many pieces of equipment for the anesthesiologist, some of which are still used today. Before his death at the age of 98 years, he received many awards, including a knighthood awarded personally by the Queen of England in 1960 and the Henry Hill Hickman Award. **B**, Ralph M. Waters was born in North Bloomfield, Ohio, and obtained his medical degree from Western Reserve University in Cleveland. He began his career in general practice in Sioux City, Iowa, and specialized in delivering anesthesia in 1916. Waters established the first academic program of anesthesiology in Madison, Wisconsin, in 1927. His contributions were many and included the carbon dioxide absorption method, endobronchial anesthesia for thoracic surgery, and introduction of cyclopropane. His chief legacy is the many residents he trained who then became the leaders within the specialty in the following generation. **C**, Sir Robert R. Macintosh (1897-1989) was born in New Zealand and was a prisoner of war during World War I. He finished medical training after the war in London and began the practice of anesthesia there. In 1937, he was appointed the first Nuffield Professor of Anaesthetics at Oxford University. He was primarily a clinician, and his innovative techniques of airway management were eventually accepted worldwide. He received honorary degrees from universities in several countries and was knighted in 1955. **D**, James T. Gwathmey was born in Roanoke, Virginia, in 1865 and graduated from the Vanderbilt School of Medicine in 1899. In 1903, he limited his practice to the administration of anesthetics, and he is considered one of the first full-time private practice physician anesthesiologists in the United States. He devised several new innovations for the delivery of anesthetic gases and introduced these machines to his European colleagues during World War I. He was an original member of the Long Island Society of Anesthetists, which eventually evolved into the American Society of Anesthesiologists. (Courtesy of the Wood-Library Museum of Anesthesiology, Park Ridge, IL.)

lift the tube off the posterior wall of the pharynx into the glottic opening. The so-called Magill tubes were formed to fit the airway and were made of red mineralized rubber. The cuffed endotracheal tube was promoted by Arthur Guedel (1883-1956) (see Fig. 1-20) and Ralph M. Waters (1883-1979) (see Fig. 1-18B) in 1928,[410] and this refinement allowed the use of intermittent, controlled, positive-pressure ventilation and the potential for one-lung ventilation, introduced by Gale and Waters in 1930.[411] Four years later, McGill introduced the bronchial blocker to confine the secretions of an infected lung to one side. McGill's technique was to pass the blocker before the induction of anesthesia with a specially designed bronchoscope.[412] Double-lumen tubes for bronchospirometry were introduced by Carlens in 1949,[413] but the small lumen size made these tubes inconvenient for anesthetized subjects. The commonly used disposable double-lumen tubes used today are modeled after the Robertshaw tube[414] for the left side and after the Green-Gordon tube[415] for the right side. An opening, called the Murphy eye, on the side of the standard endotracheal tube was suggested in 1941 as an alternative air passage in the event of distal tip occlusion.[416]

Laryngoscopes

Although blind or tactile tracheal intubation of awake patients could be mastered with extensive practice, an improved technique to accomplish tracheal intubation was developed by Alfred Kirstein[417,418] (1863-1922), Chevalier Jackson[419] (1865-1958), and Gustav Killian (1898-1912), all contributors in the introduction of the hand-held laryngoscope. Before the pioneering efforts of these innovators, the only way to visualize the larynx was with indirect laryngoscopy, a technique introduced by the Spanish singing instructor Manuel Garcia (1805-1868). In 1854, Garcia read a paper before the Royal Society entitled "Observations on the Human Voice," wherein he described his use of mirrors to view his student's and his own larynx during vocalization.[420] Alfred Kirstein was charting unknown territory in 1895, when he boldly suggested that the larynx could be directly visualized with instruments similar to the commonly used esophagoscope.[417] Although he abandoned the procedure in 1 year, it was revived 13 years later by Gustav Killian,[421] whose portable laryngoscope was remarkably like the current instrument, but with no light attached.

Direct laryngoscopy did not gain in popularity among anesthesiologists until Chevalier Jackson promoted the use of his hand-held laryngoscope for insertion of tracheal insufflation catheters. Even then, the technique was slow to gain acceptance, but the accelerated use of muscle relaxants eventually required the anesthesiologist to be adept at rapid placement of tubes within the trachea. The first hand-held laryngoscopes, as perfected by Jackson, were U-shaped and had no curve at the tip. A light at the end of the blade was a unique contribution by Jackson that has been retained, with the modification that some instruments today use a fiberoptic bundle in the blade.

Anesthesiologists soon began to design their own laryngoscopes that were more suitable for insertion of endotracheal tubes. Robert A. Miller[422] designed a new blade that

was remarkably similar to Killian's instrument, except for a slight curve at the distal end. Robert R. Macintosh's (1897-1989) (see Fig. 1-18C) improved laryngoscope featured a short, curved blade that elevated, instead of retracted, the epiglottis.[423] This promoted a new concept in laryngoscopy, specifically designed for the anesthesiologist for timely tracheal intubations. Many intubations were then performed without muscle relaxants, and the Macintosh blade was able to expose the glottis without coming into contact with the sensitive posterior surface of the epiglottis. By this time, a detachable joint had been placed between the blade and the handle. The batteries were located in the handle, conveniently avoiding the trailing wires attached to the distal bulb.

Alternatives to the Laryngoscope

Unfortunately, not all patients could be successfully intubated with the hand-held laryngoscope. Several new blades were developed in the 1940s and 1950s to solve the problem of the difficult airway, but none was 100% successful, and it soon became apparent that some airways could not be intubated with any hand-held instrument. In those cases, the few remaining members of the hospital staff who had been trained in blind tactile intubations were called in to secure the airway.

The problem of a difficult or impossible intubation is now solved with a variety of tools, including various modifications of the laryngeal mask airway (LMA) and the flexible laryngoscope, both established tools in the modern anesthesia department. The LMA was developed by A. J. Brain of the Royal Berkshire Hospital, Reading, England, with the commercial product first appearing in 1983.[424] This device is well named, for it is indeed a small mask that covers the glottic opening. The LMA eliminates the need for tracheal intubation in many cases and is useful in managing the difficult airway.

The beginnings of flexible laryngoscopy were rooted in the 19th century. John Tyndall succeeded the more famous Michael Faraday as Superintendent of the Royal Institution in London in 1867 and published his observation in 1854 that light could follow a curved path through a water tube.[425] In 1930, H. Lamm[426] employed this property of light when he introduced the flexible gastroscope, using glass fibers instead of water. S. Ikeda[427] transferred the same technology to a smaller-diameter instrument, introducing flexible bronchofiberoscopy in 1968. The definitive work followed in 1971.[428]

Resuscitation

Resuscitation from drowning was successfully accomplished by a variety of methods as early as 1792, when James Curry[429] used digital intubation of the trachea and forced air into the lungs with a bellows (see Chapter 78). J. Leroy attacked the use of positive pressure with bellows as a dangerous procedure in 1827 by showing it could rupture the alveoli and produce fatal tension pneumothorax.[430] Consequently, several ineffectual techniques developed, such as administration of stimulating vapors, swinging the arms up and down, and pulling the tongue forward in a rhythmic motion,[431] and these futile techniques were slow to dissipate. Largely through the work of O'Dwyer, Tuffier, and Matas, positive-pressure methods were reintroduced in the first few decades of the 20th century. James O. Elam (1918-1995) instinctively demonstrated the efficacy of mouth-to-mouth ventilation in 1946 when ventilators were in short supply during the polio epidemic. Peter Safar (1924-2003) and Elam were influential in converting the teaching of the ineffectual arm-lift method to mouth-to-mouth breathing techniques by demonstrating the proficiency of the later technique on volunteer medical students.[432,433]

Rational methods of resuscitation from full cardiac arrest awaited the development of the electrocardiogram and its interpretation. Augustus Waller[434] (1856-1922) first produced tracings of the electrical activity of the heart in 1887, but Willem Einthoven[435] (1860-1927) is credited with producing the first modern electrocardiogram using a string galvanometer in 1903. Tracings compatible with occlusion of the main coronary vessels were demonstrated first in animals and then confirmed in patients by James B. Herrick[436] (1861-1954) of Chicago. John MacWilliam[437] (1857-1937) described ventricular fibrillation in 1887 and provided a case report showing it to be the cause of death in one subject.[438] In 1899, J. L Prevost and F. Battelli[439] showed that small electrical currents passed across the heart could induce ventricular fibrillation and that larger currents could convert fibrillation to a normal rhythm. Claude Beck[440] performed the first successful use of electric defibrillation in a patient in 1947.

Open cardiac massage was first performed in Norway in 1901[433] and in the following year by Starling,[441] and external massage over the chest was described by W. W. Keen in 1904.[442] Brief anecdotal reports had been presented on closed chest massage as early as 1883 by Franz Koenig of Göttingen, Germany.[443] William B. Kouwenhoven, Dean of the School of Engineering at Johns Hopkins from 1939 to 1953, began his studies on resuscitation from cardiac arrest in 1929 and 31 years later published the full sequence of external cardiac massage, combined with electric countershock, to restore cardiac rhythm.[444] These methods of resuscitation have been promoted by the American Heart Association and, with some modifications, have become the basis for the widely disseminated educational programs of advanced cardiac life support (ACLS).

ANESTHETIC ACCIDENTS AND COMPLICATIONS—PREVENTIVE MEASURES

Anesthetic accidents have occurred since the early days of ether and nitrous oxide administration (see Chapters 23 and 24). Wells and Morton described patients who required resuscitative measures during anesthesia. Several near deaths were reported after the October 1846 demonstration. Bigelow's first description of ether anesthesia provides a case report of a patient who nearly died after ether administration and was resuscitated by cold effusions, ammonia inhalation, and syringing of the ears.[120] Two other cases "failed to be affected by ether." George Hayward[445] (1791-1863) reported a death after ether

inhalation occurring in August 1847. Snow's book[446] on chloroform appeared in 1858 and discusses a number of frightening cases and deaths during administration of anesthesia. The first such tragedy with chloroform struck in 1848, when an anesthetic was given to a 12-year-old girl, Hannah Greener, for a minor surgical procedure. The postmortem examination of this young girl was inconclusive, but the anesthetic was thought to have been administered properly. The controversy surrounding this death has occupied the minds of numerous anesthesiologists for the past 150 years.[447,448]

Most anesthetic deaths were not attributed to the agent or the method of administration but simply resulted from "the patient not taking the anesthetic well." A frequent diagnosis after death during anesthesia was the vague syndrome of "status lymphaticus."[449] Although this was a convenient phrase for the anesthesiologist to use, it thwarted a review of causes that might help to prevent future disasters. A major change occurred in anesthetic practice with the introduction of morbidity and mortality conferences that examined the causes of anesthetic accidents. Originally introduced by Ralph Waters in Madison, Wisconsin, these meetings sought to carefully scrutinize anesthetic complications, thereby shifting the focus of investigation from the patient to the provider and the equipment used to deliver the anesthetic. The postanesthesia care unit, originally designated the recovery room, was promoted for safety reasons by two anesthesiologists from Washington, D. C., in an influential paper in 1951,[450] and these units are now mandated by the accreditation process for all hospitals.

Curtis L. Mendelsohn, an obstetrician from New York City, presented one of the early useful reports of anesthetic complications. In 1945, he reported 66 cases of aspiration of stomach contents during general anesthesia for labor and delivery.[451] He further observed that aspiration of even small volumes of low pH stomach contents in rabbits would result in fatal pulmonary edema. Since his classic descriptions, the syndrome of acid aspiration is often called the Mendelsohn syndrome.

The cuffed endotracheal tube was one solution to the problem of acid aspiration. Authur Guedel and Ralph Waters were motivated to devise a truly closed system of anesthetic administration using carbon dioxide absorption, which would conserve anesthetic gases and body heat. Their 1928 report of the cuffed endotracheal tube[410] achieved these goals with the added benefit of protection of the tracheobronchial tree from aspiration. Others had devised cuffed endotracheal tubes before them,[452] but Guedel and Waters used a novel method to demonstrate and promote the safety features of the cuffed tube. Guedel anesthetized and then intubated his pet dog, appropriately named Airway, with a cuffed endotracheal tube. The dog was submerged in a water tank for several minutes and then removed and awakened unharmed. The demonstration was repeated at several meetings, and this publicity enhanced the rapid acceptance of the new endotracheal tube. The cuffed tube is regarded today as an effective measure for preventing acid aspiration.

In 1961, B. Sellick[453] described the rapid sequence induction for prevention of acid reflux. The method involves the application of firm pressure over the cricoid cartilage, occluding the esophagus during endotracheal intubation. John Hunter[454] had previously described the technique in 1776 for use in resuscitation of individuals "apparently drowned." The rapid sequence induction remains a popular technique for induction of patients at risk for acid aspiration.

Although few defects in apparatus could occur while applying ether onto a folded towel, the increasing complexity of the anesthetic delivery system brought with it the unfortunate side effect of equipment failure. One of the earliest equipment defects occurred with the simple Morton inhaler. George Hayward reported that a defective intake port led to restricted breathing, lividity, and convulsions in an elderly woman having a leg amputated in January 1847.[445] Wrong gas, wrong agent, wrong concentration, sticky or jammed valves, contaminated agents, and hypoxic mixtures—all of these and others were reported as routes to disaster.

Open discussions of these complications led to adjustments in equipment design.[455] Pin indexing of gas cylinders and hoses eliminated the possibility of introducing air or nitrous oxide into the oxygen lines of the gas machine. In-line oxygen analyzers were placed on the inspiratory limb of the breathing circuit. Fail-safe devices prevented the use of any machine that was not supplied with oxygen. Uniform connectors were adopted, thereby providing rapid assembly of breathing circuits. The American Society of Anesthesiologists (ASA) initiated the formation of the Z-79 Committee of the American Standards Institute. This committee recommended safe construction of endotracheal tubes, needles, and connectors. The American Society for Testing and Materials (ASTM), a not-for-profit organization that writes standards for materials and products (through their committee designated F-29), describes the requirements used in the design of safe anesthetic gas machines. The International Standards Organization is also developing global standards for anesthesia equipment.

Further progress in reducing anesthetic related complications resulted from the formation of professional societies, specialty journals, and certification boards. One of the earliest journals limited exclusively to anesthesiology was *Current Research in Anesthesia and Analgesia,* founded in 1922 largely through the efforts of Francis Hoffer McMechan (1879-1939).[456] McMechan was an anesthesiologist who had retired at an early age for health reasons and devoted the remainder of his career to promoting organizational and political causes of anesthesiologists. An independent American Board of Anesthesiology was formed in 1940 and, through its examination process, continues to elevate standards of anesthetic care. Specialty societies of professional anesthesiologists have formed in most countries practicing modern anesthetic techniques. The ASA was founded as the American Society of Anesthetists in 1936 and currently has approximately 38,000 members. *Anesthesiology,* the official journal of the ASA, began publication in 1940. National anesthesia societies promote safe anesthetic practice through annual meetings, refresher courses, and direct communication with members. Practice guidelines for general anesthesia, obstetric anesthesia, and ambulatory surgery are sent annually to each member of the ASA.

Subspecialty societies in cardiac, ambulatory, transplant, pediatric, neurosurgical, and obstetric anesthesia have been formed and strive to improve the anesthetic management of patients within their respective groups.

The Anesthesia Patient Safety Foundation (APSF) was conceived in October 1985, largely through the organizational efforts of Ellison C. Pierce, Jr. This highly successful organization promotes safe anesthesia practice through research grants and periodic mailings to members. As a result of these efforts, anesthesiologists have been recognized as forerunners in promoting agendas that enhance patient safety.[457,458]

Improved monitors have provided the anesthesiologist with methods to fine-tune the anesthetic delivery and detect early signs of danger. Auscultation of the chest, an obligatory skill in the current era, had its beginnings in the early 19th century, when Rene T. Laennec[459] used a cylindrical paper tube to listen to the chest. The term *stethoscope* was a combination of the Greek words *stetho* ("chest") and *scope* ("I see") and was used by anesthesia providers as early as 1896 to monitor cardiac and respiratory sounds. The esophageal stethoscope, introduced in 1954 by C. Smith,[460] has been used extensively to detect breathing circuit disconnects, airway obstruction, and bronchospasm in the anesthetized patient.

A. E. Codman (1869-1940) of Boston introduced the first anesthetic records in 1894, and the practice was encouraged by Harvey W. Cushing (1869-1939), who promoted recordings of blood pressure, pulse, and respiratory rate on all of his cases.[461] Practice guidelines for minimal monitoring standards were first issued[462] at the nine teaching hospitals at Harvard Medical School, and 2 years later, the ASA issued similar standards that included measures of oxygenation, ventilation, circulation, and body temperature. Electronic monitoring has significantly contributed to the safe practice of anesthesiology. Continuous electrocardiography displays, often with ST-segment analysis, are attached to most anesthesia machines. End-tidal gas analysis, using infrared technology developed in the 1940s, is in common use. Thermistors offer a continuous measure of core body temperature, thereby providing an early warning for the rare but potentially lethal syndrome of malignant hyperthermia.[463] An awareness of complications associated with hypothermia in the anesthetized patient and the use of methods to prevent its occurrence have contributed significantly to a safer environment for the surgical patient.[464,465]

Some complications that may seem trivial to the provider can be highly significant for the patient. Surveys have shown, for example, that postoperative nausea and vomiting are feared complications in a large percentage of patients contemplating surgery.[466] Progress has been made in eliminating this complication through the use of agents with less emetogenic potential. An increased understanding of the neurochemical substrates that regulate the vomiting reflex has resulted in specific therapies to prevent or lessen the gastrointestinal side effects of general anesthetics and opioids.[467] Dopamine antagonists and 5-HT$_3$ antagonists have been particularly cost effective.[468]

The increasing use of muscle relaxants by anesthesia providers has led to the terrifying complication of an awake, paralyzed patient who is fully aware of surgical pain. Although early pharmacologic studies of muscle relaxants suggested a central depressant effect of these drugs, this issue was settled when Scott M. Smith[469] allowed himself to receive curare without other agents and reported that no sedation or analgesia was present during complete paralysis. R. S. Blacher[470] noticed that complete paralysis with awareness during surgery could sometimes lead to a postoperative traumatic neurotic syndrome characterized by anxiety, irritability, and repetitive nightmares. Various monitors have been employed to avoid this rare but dreaded complication. Tunstall[471] described the isolated arm technique whereby one arm is excluded from the circulation, allowing the awake, paralyzed patient to follow commands by moving that extremity. The electroencephalogram was described in 1929 by Johannes Hans Berger[472] (1873-1941) and first used during administration of anesthesia by Albert Falconer, Jr.[473] (1911-1985). Within the past 30 years, new technologies have been developed that process the electroencephalographic raw signals and provide a number that is indicative of anesthetic depth. The bispectral index (BIS) monitor is a recent commercial product that analyzes the electroencephalographic pattern and provides some assurance that the paralyzed patient is also asleep.[474] Some exceptions have occurred with this device, with paradoxically low BIS numbers associated with awareness, and solutions to the problem of the awake and paralyzed patient continue to evolve.

Allergic reactions to drugs can be life-threatening. Anaphylaxis (meaning "without protection") is appropriately named, especially for anesthetized patients, because the symptoms of hypotension and bronchospasm can have many causes, and specific treatment can often be delayed. The syndrome was described in 1913 by Charles R. Richet[475] (1850-1935), who was studying the toxicology of various fish poisons and observed the rapid onset of death in dogs that more than 15 days earlier had withstood a much larger dose of the toxin. Richet postulated that an immune response had developed in the interim and produced a fatal reaction to the injection. The role of histamine and vasomotor instability was described in 1932,[476] and this understanding led to the role of vasopressors and antihistamines as treatment.

Even though enormous progress has been achieved toward the goal of zero anesthetic-related morbidity and mortality, no such claim can yet be made at any institution. In part, this is because more extensive procedures are being performed on sicker patients than was the case 100 years ago. In 1914, Gwathmey (see Fig. 1-18D) reported the rate of 0.01% for anesthetic-related mortality with ether anesthesia,[146] a surprisingly low figure considering the anesthetic methods in use at the time. However, in 1914, they did not perform extensive procedures such as liver and heart transplantations on patients with life expectancies (without surgical intervention) of only a few weeks. Anesthesiologists have recently focused on postoperative as well as intraoperative pain, and this extension carries with it additional risks to the anesthesia providers.

The quest for improving the perianesthetic experience is far from over. A physician has only to ask patients about the experience of having a major surgical procedure to conclude that it is far from pleasant, even in the absence of complications. It is futile to attempt to summarize the current hardships a surgical patient must undergo in the modern hospital or even attempt possible solutions. Change will occur—that is certain—and if we can learn anything from the past 150 years, there are possibilities for improvement and modalities of practice that we cannot even imagine today. Some methods in use today will appear nonsensical to future practitioners. As portions of the preceding historical survey demonstrate, one barrier to progress is failure by those entrenched in their routines and biases to recognize a breakthrough when it occurs. Perhaps the smarter we are, the more we fail to see our failures. In 1775, while Joseph Priestley[477] was hopelessly lost in the phlogiston theory of combustion, we find these words written in his classic manuscript, *Experiments and Observations of Different Kinds of Air*: "The more ingenious a man is, the more effectually he is entangled in his errors; his ingenuity only helping him to deceive himself, by evading the force of truth."

Truth in clinical medicine is perhaps even more difficult to recognize than answers to the questions that chemists were contemplating at the end of the 18th century. However, anesthesiology has made remarkable progress in the more than 150 years since the public demonstration of ether anesthesia, and this progress should continue until the safe elimination of all unwanted pain from human experience has been attained.

BIOGRAPHICAL SKETCHES

No history would be complete without brief biographical remarks about a few outstanding figures who spent their lives advancing the art and science of anesthesiology. Although several individuals could be chosen, three are selected, each from a different time period and having different areas of interest.

Virginia Apgar

Virginia Apgar (1909-1974) (Fig. 1-19) was born in Westfield, New Jersey in 1909. She attended Mt. Holyoke College and graduated from Columbia University College of Physicians and Surgeons in 1933. After completion of a surgical internship in 1935, she began training in anesthesiology at Columbia. Further training was obtained in Madison, Wisconsin, with Ralph Waters and at Bellevue Hospital in New York City with Ernest A. Rovenstein (1895-1960). In 1938, she was named director of the Division of Anesthesia at Columbia, one of the first women to hold a prominent leadership position in anesthesiology in the United States. A separate Department of Anesthesiology was created in 1949 with Emanuel M. Papper as Chairman. This allowed her to spend time on her research interests, which were directed toward obstetric anesthesia and perinatal resuscitation.

Her greatest research contribution was the development of a scoring system that evaluated the condition of newborn infants. Presented in 1953 and subsequently

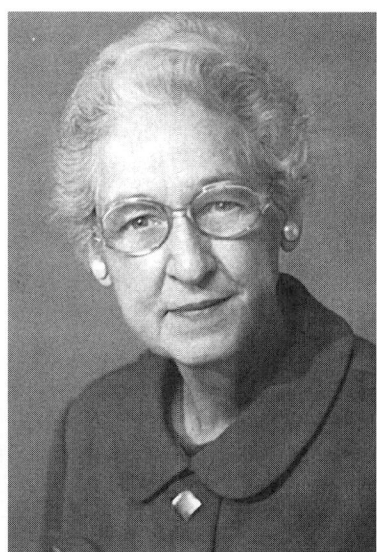

Figure 1–19 Virginia Apgar in a portrait of unknown date but near the end of her career. (Courtesy of Selma H. Calmes, who obtained the photograph from the Apgar family.)

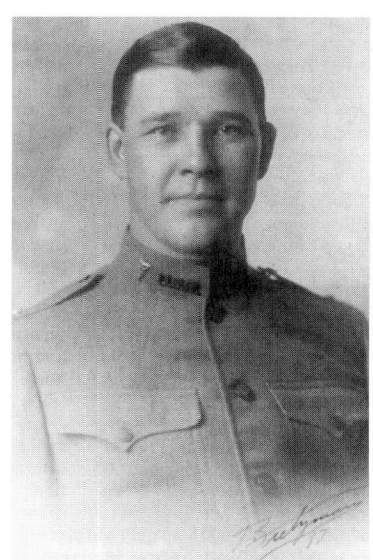

Figure 1–20 Photograph of Arthur Guedel while he was serving in the American Expeditionary Forces in France during World War I. During the war, he was responsible for the safe administration of thousands of anesthetics, often delivered without properly trained personnel. As a guide for teaching nurses and orderlies to administer ether, he devised a wall chart describing the various stages and planes of ether anesthesia that eventually resulted in his classic publication on this topic in 1919. He used a drug sequence of ethyl chloride, chloroform, and ether that prepared the patient for surgery within 2 minutes.[485] (Courtesy of the Guedel Memorial Anesthesia Center, San Francisco, CA.)

named the Apgar score, it is still used worldwide as a routine measure of infant well-being after birth.[483] This scoring system allowed her and others around the world to evaluate the effects of various maternal analgesic methods on the newborn. One of her early observations was that meperidine readily crossed the placenta and was capable of depressing the infant. Volatile anesthetics given to the mother, such as cyclopropane, also depressed the infant, and this work eventually led to the abandonment of general anesthesia for routine vaginal delivery.[479]

She was known as an inspirational teacher, with boundless energy. The research projects that she originated were continued by several of her residents, including Frank Moya and Sol M. Shnider (1929-1994), both leaders in their field. George Gregory (1934-) has continued and greatly expanded her work on neonatal resuscitation.

Although she was an excellent student, early in her training she was discouraged from entering certain specialties because she was a woman. Fortunately, her entry into anesthesia was not barred, but she continued to experience sexual discrimination throughout her life. Partly because of her pioneering efforts and those of people such as Mary Botsford of San Francisco, anesthesiology has become a desirable vocation for women.

Virginia Apgar died in 1974 at the age of 65 years. She received several awards during her life, including being the first woman to be chosen for the Alumni Gold Medal for Distinguished Achievement in Medicine from Columbia University and the Distinguished Service Award from the American Society of Anesthesiologists. In October 1994, a 20-cent stamp was issued in her name in the Great Americans Series from the United States Postal Service.

Arthur E. Guedel

Arthur E. Guedel (1883-1956) (Fig. 1-20) was born in 1883 in Cambridge City, Indiana. Because his family was

poor, he had to work as a young man and was unable to attend high school. His early education was obtained by reading at home, with occasional help from visiting teachers. Through the intervention of the family doctor, he was allowed to take the entrance examination for medical school in his home state. He easily gained admission based on his high scores, and he graduated with honors in 1908.

After a brief trial of general practice, he limited his work solely to anesthesia. His devotion to the specialty was so complete that during his early career he provided anesthetics without pay because "there was nothing else to do." For his first publication, he described the intermittent use of nitrous oxide inhalation to provide analgesia during labor,[480] a method that is still occasionally used.

Guedel served in France during World War I, where he developed an anesthesia training school at Chaumont. During these years, he began a lifelong study of anesthetic depth with ether anesthesia. A profoundly curious individual, he made careful observations on his patients and formulated the various stages and planes of anesthetic depth that have become known as the Guedel signs.[481] These observations were refined throughout his career and published in final form in his book, *Inhalation Anesthesia*, published in 1937.[449]

His era saw the rise of anesthesiology as a profession, a time of remarkable change in how anesthetics are delivered. Guedel's letters are full of ideas, most of which did not work out. His thoughts, revealed in these letters, uncover several bizarre ideas scattered in with ones of true brilliance. He carried on frequent discussions with other members of the Anesthesia Travel Club, which included many of the prominent figures of the specialty during that time. He tried new techniques offered by others and was blunt in his criticisms if they proved useless. His many innovations include the cuffed endotracheal tube, introduction of new anesthetic agents such as divinyl ether and cyclopropane, construction of a new pharyngeal airway,[400] and the introduction of controlled ventilation.

For health reasons, Guedel moved to California in 1928, where he practiced for 12 years before his retirement in 1940. He died of emphysema in 1956 after receiving many awards, including the Henry Hill Hickman Award; he was the first American anesthesiologist to receive this coveted prize. He also received the Distinguished Service Award from the American Society of Anesthesiologists. The Guedel Anesthesia History Center, located in San Francisco, is a repository for his correspondence and other memorabilia relating to the early 20th century developments in anesthesiology.

John Snow

Although William T. G. Morton directed his energy to anesthesia after 1846, he also pursued patent claims and remuneration more often than administration of anesthesia.[482] Most historians therefore suggest that John Snow (Fig. 1-21) was the first full-time anesthesiologist. He promoted anesthesiology as a subject of scientific inquiry and through his own example established it as a worthy profession.

John Snow was born in York, England on June 15, 1813, the oldest child in a farming family. His early years

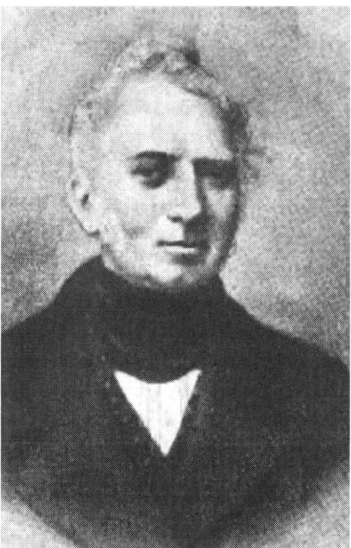

Figure 1–21 John Snow is considered by many to be the first full-time anesthesiologist. His scientific and professional career became a model for future practitioners. (Courtesy of the National Library of Medicine, Bethesda, MD.)

were spent in attendance at a private school in York and working on the family farm. At the age of 14, he became an apprentice to William Hardcastle, a surgeon in Newcastle. Four years later, a cholera epidemic erupted in Newcastle, and while attending those afflicted with this disease, Snow made several observations that proved to be valuable in later years. At 23 years of age, he began the formal study of medicine at the Hunterian School of Medicine in London. This was a short course, and only 1 year later, he passed his examinations and was entered as a member of the Royal College of Surgeons of England.

Benjamin Ward Richardson, who was intimate with Dr. Snow and who wrote a short biography, characterized him as an individual who sought "only the truth, the naked truth for its own sake without consideration of honor or profit." Snow's initial attempts to establish a private general practice were thwarted by his inability to attract paying patients. He would not engage in the common practice of writing prescriptions for neurotic patients. Consequently, his time was spent volunteering at the Charing Cross Hospital and in scientific pursuits and reading. In 1841, at the age of 30, he read his first paper, "Asphyxia and on the Resuscitation of Newborn Children," before the Medical Society of London. This first paper describes positive-pressure ventilation for resuscitation of the depressed newborn and indicates his penchant for matters relating to anesthesia. This interest took firm control of his life after the news from America arrived in London that operations could be performed without pain after the inhalation of sulfuric ether.

Snow took up the exclusive practice of ether administration and within 1 year had written the first of his two landmark books on inhalation anesthesia. When Dr. James Simpson introduced chloroform in October 1847, Snow enthusiastically embraced the new agent. His chloroform inhaler was superior to prior devices in that it used valves to prevent rebreathing. He classified the stages of anesthesia and studied the effect of ether[355] and chloroform on animals and humans to learn the concentrations required for anesthesia at various stages. The precision and detail with which this work was performed was not to be accomplished again for nearly 100 years, when the vapor pressures of inhalation anesthetics necessary for anesthesia were determined. His contemporaries recognized his clinical skills to be of the highest caliber, and he was recommended to provide anesthesia for the delivery of two of Queen Victoria's children. Snow delivered chloroform in 1853 for the birth of Prince Leopold and in 1857 for the birth of Princess Beatrice.

In 1854, a rampant cholera epidemic broke out in the Charing Cross district, and Snow used his prior experience with the disease to analyze the causative factors involved in transmission. His advice to remove the handle of the Broadstreet water pump because of suspected transmission through the water supply was carried out, and the epidemic subsided. His theories on transmission of cholera were published at his own expense in the *London Medical Gazette*. His last treatise, *On Chloroform and Other Anesthetics,*[446] was in its final stages of completion when he died of kidney disease complicated by a stroke on June 14, 1858, at the age of 45.

REFERENCES

1. Fenster J: Ether Day: The Strange Tale of America's Greatest Medical Discovery and the Haunted Men Who Made It. New York, HarperCollins, 2001.
2. Raper H: Man Against Pain: The Epic of Anesthesia. New York, Prentice-Hall, 1945.
3. Robinson V: Victory Over Pain, a History of Anesthesia. New York, Schuman, 1946.
4. Sykes W: Essays on the One Hundred Years of Anesthesia. Edinburgh, Livingstone, 1960.
5. Osler W: Aequanimitas, British Medicine in Greater Britain. Philadelphia, Blakiston's Son, 1904.
6. Major R: A History of Medicine. Springfield, IL, CC Thomas, 1954.
7. Hook R: An account of an experiment made by M Hook of preserving animals alive by blowing through their lungs with bellows. Philos Trans R Soc Lond 2:539-540, 1667.
8. Lower R: Tractatus de Corde. London, Redmayne, 1669.
9. Beck C: Stahl, Georg Ernst. J Chem Educ 37:505-510, 1960.
10. Priestley J: Experiments and Observations on Different Kinds of Air. London, Johnson, 1776.
11. Boklund U: Scheele, CW: His Work and Life. Stockholm, Roos Boktrycherier, 1961.
12. Lavoisier AL: Mémoire sur la nature du principe qui se combine avec les métaux pendant leur calcination, et qui en augmente le poids. Hist Acad R Sci pp 520-526, 1778.
13. Sprigge JS: Sir Humphry Davy: His researches in respiratory physiology and his debt to Antoine Lavoisier. Anaesthesia 57:357-364, 2002.
14. Pflüger E: Zur Gasometrie des Blutes. Zentralbl Med Wiss 4:305-308, 1866.
15. Haldane J: A new form of apparatus for measuring the respiratory exchange of animals. J Physiol 13:419-430, 1892.
16. Haldane J: The therapeutic administration of oxygen. Br Med J 1:181-183, 1917.
17. Haldane J, Priestley J: Lung ventilation. J Physiol 32:225-266, 1905.
18. Haldane J: Respiration. New Haven, Yale University Press, 1922.
19. Hufner C: Über die Quantitat Sauerstoff welche 1 gramm Hamoglobin zu binden vermag. Z Physiol Chem 1:317, 1877.
20. Clark C, Wolf R, Granger D, Taylor Z: Continuous recording of blood oxygen tensions by polarography. J Appl Physiol 6:189-193, 1953.
21. Van Slyke D, Neill J: The determination of gases in blood and other solutions by vacuum extraction and manometric measurement. J Biol Chem 61:523-573, 1924.
22. Severinghaus J, Bradley A: Electrodes for blood P_{O_2} and P_{CO_2} determination. J Appl Physiol 13:515-520, 1958.
23. Nunn J: Nunn's Applied Respiratory Physiology, 4th ed. Oxford, Butterworth-Heinemann, 1993.
24. Severinghaus JW, Honda Y: Pulse oximetry. Int Anesthesiol Clin 25:205-214, 1987.
25. Hales S: Statical Essays, Containing Haemastaticks. London, W Innys & R Manby, 1733.
26. Poiseuille J. Recherches sur la Force du Coeur Aortique. Paris, École Polytechnique, 1828.
27. Vierordt K: Die bildliche Darstellung des menschlichen Arterienpulses. Arch Physiol Heilk 13:284-287, 1854.
28. Riva-Rocci S: Un nuovo sfigmomanometro. Gaz Med Torino 47:981-996, 1896.
29. Korotkov N: On methods of studying blood pressure. Izvest Imp Voyenno Med Akad St Petersburg 11:365, 1905.
30. Von Recklinghausen H: Neue Wege zur Blutdruckmessung. Berlin, Springer-Verlag, 1931.
31. Tomlinson H: On the increase in resistance to the passage of an electric current produced on wires by stretching. Proc R Soc Lond 25:451-453, 1876.
32. Lambert E, Wood E: The use of a resistance wire, strain gauge manometer to measure intraarterial pressure. Proc Soc Exp Biol Med 64:186-190, 1947.
33. Peterson L, Dripps R, Risman G: A method for recording the arterial pressure pulse and blood pressure in man. Am Heart J 37:771-782, 1949.
34. Seldinger S: Catheter replacement of the needle in percutaneous arteriography. Acta Radiol 39:368-376, 1953.
35. Forssmann W: Die Sondierung des rechten Herzens. Klin Wochenschr 8:2085-2087, 1929.
36. Massa D, Lundy JS, Faulconer A Jr: A plastic needle. Mayo Clin Proc 25:413-415, 1950.
37. Swan HJ, Ganz W, Forrester J, et al: Catheterization of the heart in man with use of a flow-directed balloon-tipped catheter. N Engl J Med 283:447-451, 1970.
38. Fick A: Uber die Messung des Blutquantums in den Herzventrikeln. Sitzber Phys Med Ges Wurzburg July 9, 1870. In Fishman AP, Richards DW (eds): Circulation of the Blood: Men and Ideas. New York, Oxford University Press, 1964.
39. Frazin L, Talano JV, Stephandies L: Esophageal echocardiography. Circulation 54:102-108, 1976.
40. Matsumoto M, Oka Y, Lin YT: Transesophageal echocardiography for assessing ventricular performance. N Y State J Med 79:19-21, 1979.
41. Kremer P, Schwartz L, Cahalan M, et al: Intraoperative monitoring of left ventricular performance by transesophageal M-mode and 2D echocardiography. Am J Cardiol 49:956, 1982.
42. Oka Y: The evolution of intraoperative transesophageal echocardiography. Mt Sinai J Med 69:18-20, 2002.
43. Whytt R: An Essay on the Vital and Other Involuntary Motions of Animals. London, Hamilton, Balfour & Neill, 1751.
44. Willis T: Practice of Physik. London, T Dring, C Harper & J Leigh, 1684.
45. Pourfour Du Petit F Mémoire dans lequel il est démontré que les nerfs intercostaux fournissent des rameaux que portent des esprits dans les yeux. Hist Acad R Sci 1727, pp 1-19.
46. Winslow J: Exposition Anatomique de la Structure du Corps Humain. Paris, G Desprez, 1732.
47. Bernard C: Influence du grand sympathique sur la sensibilité et sur la calorification. Comptes rendus Soc Biol 3:163-64, 1852.
48. Langley J, Dickinson W: On the local paralysis of peripheral ganglia, and on the connexion of different classes of nerve fibres with them. Proc R Soc 46:423-431, 1889.
49. Langley J: Observations on the physiological action of extracts of the supra-renal bodies. J Physiol 27:237-256, 1901.
50. Abel J, Crawford A: On the blood-pressure-raising constituent of the suprarenal capsule. Bull Johns Hopkins Hosp 8:151-157, 1897.
51. Krantz J: Historical Medical Classics Involving New Drugs. Baltimore, Williams & Wilkins, 1974.
52. Elliott TR: On the action of adrenalin. J Physiol 31:xx-xxi, 1904.
53. Barger G, Dale H: Chemical structure and sympathomimetic action of amines. J Physiol 41:19-59, 1910.
54. Cannon W, Rosenblueth A: Studies on conditions of activity in endocrine organs. Sympathin e and sympathin i. Am J Physiol 104:557-574, 1933.
55. Euler UV: A specific sympathomimetic ergone in adrenergic nerve fibres (sympathin) and its relations to adrenaline and nor-adrenaline. Acta Physiol Scand 12:73-97, 1946.
56. Dixon W, Hamil P: The mode of action of specific substances with special reference to secretin. J Physiol 38:314-36, 1908-1909.
57. Dale H: The action of certain esters and ethers of choline, and their relation to muscarine. J Pharmacol Exp Ther 6:147-190, 1914.
58. Gaskell W: The involuntary nervous system. Part 1. London, Longmans, Green, 1916.
59. Loewi O: Über humorale Ueebertragbarkeit der Herznervenwirkung. Pflüg Arch Ges Physiol 189:239-242, 1921.
60. Tuffier T: Effets circulatoires des injections sousarachnoidiennes de cocaine dans la region lombaire. Soc Biol 18:897-9, 1900.
61. Smith G, Porter W: Spinal anesthesia in the cat. Am J Physiol 38:107-127, 1915.
62. Labat G: Regional Anesthesia: Its Technic and Clinical Application. Philadelphia, WB Saunders, 1922.
63. Fraser T: On the characters, actions and therapeutical uses of the ordeal bean of Calabar. Edinb Med J 9:36-56, 1863.

64. Pal J: Physostigmin ein Gegengift des Curare. Zentralbl f Physiolog 14:255, 1900.

65. Aeschlimann J, Reinart MJ: The pharmacological action of some analogues of physostigmine. J Pharmacol 43:413, 1931.

66. Clutton Brock J: Death following neostigmine. Br Med J 1:1007, 1949.

67. MacIntosh R: Death following injection of neostigmine. Br Med J 1:852, 1949.

68. Wylie WD, Churchill-Davidson HC: A Practice of Anaesthesia, 2nd ed. Chicago, Year Book Medical Publishers, 1966.

69. Mein A: Ueber die Darstellung des Atropins in weissen Krystallen. Ann Chem Pharm 6:67-72, 1833.

70. Franko B, Lunsford C: Derivatives of 3-pyrrolidinols. III. The chemistry, pharmacology, and toxicology of some N-substituted 3-pyrrolidyl alpha-substituted phenylacetates. J Med Pharm Chem 2:523-540, 1960.

71. Ahlquist R: A study of the adrenotropic receptors. Am J Physiol 153:586-600, 1948.

72. Menkhaus P, Reves JG, Kissin I, et al: Cardiovascular effects of esmolol in anesthetized humans. Anesth Analg 64:327-334, 1985.

73. Scott DB, Buckley FP, Drummond GB, et al: Cardiovascular effects of labetalol during halothane anaesthesia. Br J Clin Pharmacol 3:817-821, 1976.

74. Belleville JP, Ward DS, Bloor BC, Maze M: Effects of intravenous dexmedetomidine in humans. I. Sedation, ventilation, and metabolic rate. Anesthesiology 77:1125-1133, 1992.

75. Kamibayashi T, Maze M: Clinical uses of alpha$_2$-adrenergic agonists. Anesthesiology 93:1345-1349, 2000.

76. Marsh N, Marsh A: A short history of nitroglycerin and nitric oxide in pharmacology and physiology. Clin Exp Pharmacol Physiol 27:313-319, 2000.

77. Ringertz N: Alfred Nobel—his life and work. Nat Rev Mol Cell Biol 2:925-928, 2001.

78. Murrell W: Nitroglycerin in angina pectoris. Lancet 1:80-81, 1879.

79. Siegel P, Moraca PP, Green JR: Sodium nitroprusside in the surgical treatment of cerebral aneurysms and arteriovenous malformations. Br J Anaesth 43:790-795, 1971.

80. Murad F: Cyclic guanosine monophosphate as a mediator of vasodilation. J Clin Invest 78:1-5, 1986.

81. Frostell C, Fratacci MD, Wain JC, et al: Inhaled nitric oxide: A selective pulmonary vasodilator reversing hypoxic pulmonary vasoconstriction. Circulation 83:2038-2047, 1991.

82. Von Haller A: A dissertation on the sensible and irritable parts of animals. London, J Nourse, 1755.

83. Von Haller A: De Partibus Corporis Humani Sensibilibus et Irritabilibus. Comment Soc Reg Sci Gottingen 2:114-158, 1752.

84. Bell SC: Idea of a new anatomy of the brain. London, Strahan & Preston, 1811.

85. Magendie F: Expériences sur les fonctions des racines des nerfs rachidiens. J Physiol Exp Pathol 2:276-279, 366-371, 1822.

86. Müller J: Über die phantastischen Gesichtserscheinungen. Leipzig, J Hölscher, 1826.

87. Müller J: Bestätigung des Bell'schen Lehrsatzes. Notizen aus dem Gebiete der Naturu und Heilkunde 30:113-122, 1831.

88. Dallenbach K: Pain: History and present status. Am J Psychol 52:331, 1939.

89. Gasser H, Erlanger J: The role of fiber size in the establishment of a nerve block by pressure or cocaine. Am J Physiol 88:581-591, 1929.

90. Livingstone D: Missionary Travels and Researches in South Africa. London, John Murray, 1875.

91. Ellis H: Operations That Made History. London, Greenwich Medical Media, 1996.

92. Beecher H: Pain in men wounded in battle. Ann Surg 123:96-105, 1946.

93. Melzack R, Wall P: Pain mechanisms: A new theory. Science 250:971-975, 1965.

94. Reynolds D: Surgery in the rat during electrical analgesia induced by focal brain stimulation. Science 164:444-445, 1969.

95. Goldstein A, Tachibana S, Lowney LI, et al: Dynorphin-(1-13), an extraordinarily potent opioid peptide. Proc Natl Acad Sci U S A 76:6666-6670, 1979.

96. Hughes J: Isolation of an endogenous compound from the brain with pharmacological properties similar to morphine. Brain Res 88:295-308, 1975.

97. Simantov R, Childers SR, Snyder SH: Opioid peptides: Differentiation by radioimmunoassay and radioreceptor assay. Brain Res 135:358-367, 1977.

98. Cousins MJ, Mather LE: Intrathecal and epidural administration of opioids. Anesthesiology 61:276-310, 1984.

99. Kehlet H, Brandt MR, Hansen AP, Alberti KG: Effect of epidural analgesia on metabolic profiles during and after surgery. Br J Surg 66:543-546, 1979.

100. Adams F: The Genuine Works of Hippocrates, On the Surgery. Baltimore, Williams & Wilkins, 1939.

101. Fülöp-Miller R: Triumph Over Pain. Indianapolis, Bobbs-Merrill, 1938.

102. Pancoast J: A Treatise on Operative Surgery. Philadelphia, Carey & Hart, 1844.

103. Dane FJ: Mesmerism. Boston Med Surg J 35:425-428, 1846.

104. Burney F: A Mastectomy, 30 September 1811. In Carey J (ed): Eyewitness to History. Cambridge, Harvard University Press, 1990, pp 272-277.

105. Katz J, Kavanagh BP, Sandler AN, et al: Preemptive analgesia. Clinical evidence of neuroplasticity contributing to postoperative pain. Anesthesiology 77:439-446, 1992.

106. Warren J: A Practical Treatise on Hernia. Boston, Osgood, 1882.

107. Linhart W: Vorlesungen ueber Unterleibs-Hernien. Wurzburg, Stuber's Buchhandlung, 1866.

108. McInnes EM: St Thomas Hospital. London, St Thomas Hospital Press, 1963.

109. Caton D: The secularization of pain. Anesthesiology 62:493-501, 1985.

110. Morgagni G: De Sedibus, et Causis Morborum per Anatomen Indagatis Libri Quinque. Venice, Remondiniani, 1761.

111. Virchow R: Die Cellularpathologie in ihrer Begründung auf physiologische und pathologische Gewebelehre. Berlin, Hirschwald, 1858.

112. Astrup P, Severinghaus JW: The History of Blood Gases: Acids and Bases. Copenhagen, Munksgaard, 1986.

113. Boyle R: New Experiments Physico-mechanicall Touching the Spring of the Air. Oxford, H Hall for T Robinson, 1660.

114. Henry W: Elements of Experimental Chemistry, London, Baldwin, Cradock, and Joy, 1803.

115. Black J: Dissertatio Medica Inauguralis de Humore Acido a Cibis Orto, et Magnesia Alba. Edinburgh, G Hamilton & J Balfour, 1754.

116. Beddoes T, Watts J: Considerations on the Medicinal Use and on the Production of Factitious Airs. Bristol, Bulgin and Rossner, 1795.

117. Davy H: Researches chemical and philosophical chiefly concerning nitrous oxide or dephlogisticated nitrous air, and its respiration. Bristol, Biggs and Cottle, 1800, pp 1-580.

118. Faraday M: Effects of inhaling the vapors of sulphuric ether. Q J Soc Arts Miscellanea 4:158-159, 1818.

119. Hickman H: A letter on suspended animation containing experiments showing that it may be safely employed on animals, with the view of ascertaining its probable utility in surgical operations on the human subject. Ironbridge, W. Smith, 1824.

120. Bigelow HJ: Insensibility during surgical operations produced by inhalation Boston Med Surg J 35:309-317, 379-382, 1846.

121. Robinson J: A treatise on the inhalation of the vapour of ether for the prevention of pain in surgical operations. London, Webster, 1847.

122. Pirogoff N: Researches Practical and Physiological on Etherization. St. Petersburg, Troitzky, 1847.

123. Skovsted P, Price HL: Central sympathetic excitation caused by diethyl ether. Anesthesiology 32:202-209, 1970.

124. Long C: An account of the first use of sulphuric ether by inhalation as an anaesthetic in surgical operations. South Med Surg J 5:705-713, 1849.

125. Simpson SJY: Discovery of a new anaesthetic agent, more efficient than sulphuric ether. Lond Med Gaz 5:934-937, 1847.

126. Guthrie S: New mode of preparing a spirituous solution of chloric ether. Am J Sci Arts 21-22:64-65, 105-160, 1832.

127. Soubeiran E: Recherches sur quelques combinaisons du chlore. Ann Chim 48:113-157, 1831.

128. Liebig JV: Ueber die Verbindungen, welche durch die Einwirkung des Chlors auf Alkohol, Aether, ölbildendes Gas und Essiggeist entstehen. Ann Pharm 1:182-230, 1832.

129. Flourens MJP: Note touchant l'action de l'ether sur les centers nerveux. C R Acad Sci (Paris) 24:340-344, 1847.

130. Channing W: A Treatise on Etherization in Childbirth. Boston, WD Ticknor, 1848.

131. Keys TE: The History of Surgical Anesthesia. New York, Schuman's, 1945.

132. Hyderabad Chloroform Commission: Report of the first Hyderabad Chloroform Commission. Lancet 1:421-429, 1890.

133. Guthrie LG: On some fatal after-effects of chloroform on children. Lancet 1:193-197, 1894.

134. Levy A: Chloroform Anaesthesia. London, John Bales, Sons & Danielsson, 1922.

135. Smith GB, Hirsch NP: Gardner Quincy Colton: Pioneer of nitrous oxide anaesthesia. Anesth Analg 72:382-391, 1991.

136. Colton G: Anaesthesia. Who Made and Developed This Great Discovery? New York, AG Sherwood, 1886.

137. Andrews E: The oxygen mixture, a new anaesthetic combination. Chicago Med Examiner 9:656, 1868.

138. Bert P: Barometric pressure: Researches in experimental physiology. Columbus, College Book Company, 1943.

139. Hewitt FG: Anaesthetics and Their Administration. London, C Griffin, 1893.

140. Johnson G: On the physiology of asphyxia and on the anaesthetic action of pure nitrogen. Lancet 1:814-815, 1891.

141. McKesson EI: Nitrous oxide-oxygen anaesthesia. With a description of a new apparatus. Surg Gynecol Obstet 13:456-462, 1911.

142. Flagg P: The Art of Anesthesia, 6th ed. Philadelphia, JB Lippincott, 1939.

143. Clement F: Nitrous oxide-oxygen anesthesia. Philadelphia, Lea & Febiger, 1939.

144. Courville C: Asphyxia as a consequence of nitrous oxide anesthesia. Medicine (Baltimore) 15:129-245, 1936.

145. Smith WD: Under the Influence: A History of Nitrous Oxide and Oxygen. London, Macmillan, 1982.

146. Gwathmey J: Anesthesia. New York, D Appleton, 1914.

147. Luchhardt A, Carter J: Ethylene as a gas anesthetic; preliminary communication. JAMA 80:1440-1442, 1923.

148. Leake C, Chen M-Y: The anesthetic properties of certain unsaturated ethers. Proc Soc Exp Biol 28:151-154, 1930.

149. Waters R, Schmidt E: Cyclopropane anesthesia. JAMA 103:975-983, 1934.

150. Striker C, Goldblatt S, Warm I, Jackson D: Clinical experiences with the use of trichlorethylene in the production of over 300 analgesias and anesthesias. Curr Res Anal Analg 14:68-71, 1935.

151. Hewer C, Hadfield C: Trichloroethylene as an inhalation anaesthetic. Br Med J 1:924-927, 1941.

152. Krantz JC: Anesthesia. XL. The anesthetic action of trifluoroethyl vinyl ether. J Pharmacol 108:488-495, 1953.

153. Raventós J: The action of Fluothane—A new volatile anaesthetic. Br J Pharmacol 11:394-410, 1956.

154. Johnstone MW: The human cardiovascular response to Fluothane. Br J Anaesth 28:392-410, 1956.

155. Virtue R, Payne KW: Postoperative death after Fluothane. Anesthesiology 19:562-563, 1958.

156. Lindenbaum J, Leifer E: Hepatic necrosis associated with halothane anesthesia. N Engl J Med 268:525-530, 1963.

157. Bunker JP: Final report of the National Halothane Study. Anesthesiology 29:231-232, 1968.

158. Crandell W, Pappas S, Macdonald A: Nephrotoxicity associated with methoxyflurane anesthesia. Anesthesiology 27:591-607, 1966.

159. Mazze RI, Shue GL, Jackson SH: Renal dysfunction associated with methoxyflurane anesthesia: A randomized, prospective clinical evaluation. JAMA 216:278-288, 1971.

160. Kety S, Schmidt C: Nitrous oxide method for quantitative determination of cerebral blood flow in man; theory, procedure and normal values. J Clin Invest 27:476-483, 1948.

161. Severinghaus JW: Methods of measurement of blood and gas carbon dioxide during anesthesia. Anesthesiology 21:717-726, 1960.

162. Eger EI 2nd, Saidman LJ, Brandstater B: Minimum alveolar anesthetic concentration: A standard of anesthetic potency. Anesthesiology 26:756-763, 1965.

163. Quasha A, Eger EI, Tinker J: Determination and applications of MAC. Anesthesiology 53:315-334, 1980.

164. Dobkin AB, Heinrich RG, Israel JS, et al: Clinical and laboratory evaluation of a new inhalation agent: Compound 347 (CHF2-O-CF2-CHF Cl). Anesthesiology 29:275-287, 1968.

165. Stevens WC, Eger EI, Joas TA, et al: Comparative toxicity of isoflurane, halothane, fluroxene and diethyl ether in human volunteers. Can Anaesth Soc J 20:357-368, 1973.

166. Eger EI 2nd, Johnson BH: Rates of awakening from anesthesia with I-653, halothane, isoflurane, and sevoflurane: A test of the effect of anesthetic concentration and duration in rats. Anesth Analg 66:977-982, 1987.

167. Jones RM, Cashman JN, Eger EI 2nd, et al: Kinetics and potency of desflurane (I-653) in volunteers. Anesth Analg 70:3-7, 1990.

168. Katoh T, Ikeda K: The minimum alveolar concentration (MAC) of sevoflurane in humans. Anesthesiology 66:301-303, 1987.

169. Doi M, Ikeda K: Respiratory effects of sevoflurane. Anesth Analg 66:241-244, 1987.

170. Magendie F: Formulary for the Preparation and Employment of Several New Remedies, 6th ed. Joseph Houlton, trans. London, T & G Underwood, 1822.

171. Sertürner F: Ueber das Morphium, eine neue salzfähige Grundlage, und die Mekonsäure als Hauptbestandtheil des Opiums. Gilberts Ann Physik 55:56-89, 1817.

172. Rynd F: Neuralgia—introduction of fluid to the nerve. Dublin Med Press 13:167-168, 1845.

173. Wood A: Treatment of neuralgic pains by narcotic injections. Br Med J 2:721-723, 1858.

174. Howard-Jones N: The origins of hypodermic medication. Sci Am 224:96-102, 1971.

175. Schwidetzky O: History of needles and syringes. Anesth Analg 23:34-38, 1944.

176. Bernard C: Leçons sur les phénoménes de la vie communs aux animaux et aux végétaux. Paris, Baillière, 1879.

177. Cannon W: The Wisdom of the Body. New York, Norton, 1932.

178. Hamburger H: Osmotischer Druck und Ionenlehre in den Medicinischen Wissenschaften. Wiesbaden, JF Bergman, 1902.

179. Starling E: On the absorption of fluids from the connective tissue spaces. J Physiol 19:312-326, 1896.

180. O'Shaughnessy W: Proposal of a new method of treating the blue epidemic cholera by the injection of highly oxygenized salts into the venous system. Lancet 1:366, 1831-1832.

181. Schwarz E: Ueber den Werth der Infusion alcalischer Kochsalzlosung in das Gefasssystem bei acuter Anämie, Dissertation. Halle. Plotzsche Buchsdruckerei, 1888.

182. Astrup P, Bie P, Engell HC: Salt and Water in Culture and Medicine. Copenhagen, Munksgaard, 1993.

183. Ringer S: Regarding the action of hydrate of soda, hydrate of ammonia, and hydrate of potash on the ventricle of the frog's heart. J Physiol 3:195-202, 1880.

184. Coller F, Campbell K, Vaughan H, et al: Postoperative salt intolerance. Ann Surg 119:533-542, 1944.

185. Moyer CA: Acute temporary changes in renal function associated with major surgical procedures. Surgery 27:198-207, 1950.

186. Shires G, Williams J, Brown F: Changing concept of salt water and surgery. Tex State J Med 55:753-756, 1959.

187. Shires G, Brown F, Canizaro P, et al: Distributional changes in extracellular fluid during acute hemorrhagic shock. Surg Forum 11:115-117, 1960.

188. Jenkins M: History of sequestered edema associated with surgical operations and trauma: Fluid and blood therapy in anesthesia. Philadelphia, FA Davis, 1982.

189. Denis JB: A letter concerning a new way of curing sundry diseases by transfusion of blood. Philos Trans R Soc Lond 2:489-504, 1667.

190. Blundell J: Experiments on the transfusion of blood by the syringe. Med Chir Trans 9:56-92, 1818.

191. Landsteiner K: Zur Kenntnis der antifermentativen, lyteschen und agglutinierender Wirkungen des Blutserums und der Lymphek. Centralbl Bakteriol Parasit Infekt 27: 357-362, 1900.

192. Decastello A, Sturli A: Ueber die Isoagglutinine im Serum gesunder und kranker Menschen. Munch Med Wochenschr 49:1090-1095, 1902.

193. Hustin A: Note sur une nouvelle méthode de transfusion. Bull Soc R Sci Med Brux 72:104-111, 1914.

194. Rous P, Turner JR: The preservation of living red blood cells in vitro. J Exp Med 23:219-248, 1916.

195. Loutit J, Mollinson P: Advantages of a disodium-citrate glucose mixture as a blood preservative. Br Med J 2:744-745, 1943.

196. Laurie R: An apparatus for indicating the rate of flow of saline solution in subcutaneous and rectal administration. Lancet 1:248, 1909.

197. Lundy J: Clinical Anesthesia. A Manual of Clinical Anesthesiology. Philadelphia, WB Saunders, 1945.

198. Brown A, Debenham M: Autotransfusion. Use of blood from hemothorax. JAMA 96:1223-1225, 1931.

199. Klebanoff G: Early clinical experience with a disposable unit for the intraoperative salvage of reinfusion of blood loss. Am J Surg 120:718-722, 1970.

200. Klebanoff G, Rogers W: Clinical experience with autotransfusion. Ann Surg 180:269-304, 1974.

201. Orr M: Autotransfusion: The use of washed red cells as an adjunct to component therapy. Surgery 84:728-732, 1978.

202. Miller RD, Robbins TO, Tong MJ, Barton SL: Coagulation defects associated with massive blood transfusions. Ann Surg 174:794-801, 1971.

203. Blajchman MA, Herst R, Perrault RA: Blood component therapy in anaesthetic practice. Can Anaesth Soc J 30: 382-389, 1983.

204. Robblee JA, Crosby E: Transfusion medicine issues in the practice of anesthesiology. Transfus Med Rev 9:60-78, 1995.

205. Bell B: A System of Surgery. Edinburgh, C Elliott, 1796.

206. Richardson B: Reports and lectures on original researches in scientific practical medicine. I. On a new mode of producing local anaesthesia. Med Times Gaz 1:115-117, 1866.

207. Gross SD: A System of Surgery; Pathological, Diagnostic, Therapeutic and Operative, 3rd ed. Philadelphia, Blanchard & Lea, 1864.

208. Cobo B: Historia del Nuevo Mundo. Manuscrito en Lima, Peru, libro 5: capitulo XXIX, 1653.

209. Niemann A: Ueber eine organische Base in der Coca. Ann Chem 124:213, 1860.

210. Niemann A: Sur l'alcaloïde de coca. J Pharm 27:474-475, 1860.

211. Anrep V: Ueber die physiologische Wirkung des cocain. Pflugers Arch Physiol 21:38-77, 1880.

212. Shoemaker J: Materia Medica and Therapeutics, with Reference to the Clinical Application of Drugs. Philadelphia, FA Davis, 1893.

213. Liljestrand G: Carl Koller and the development of local anesthesia. Acta Physiol Scand Suppl 299:3-29, 1967.

214. Koller C: Vorläufige mittheilung über locale anästhesirung am auge. Klin Monatsbl Augenheilk 22:60-63, 1884.

215. Koller C: On the use of cocaine for producing anaesthesia on the eye. Lancet 2:990-994, 1884.

216. Freud S: Ueber Coca. Centralblatt für die gesamte Therapie 2:289-314, 1884.

217. Hall RJ: Hydrochlorate of cocaine, NY Med J 40, 1884.

218. Halsted WS: Practical comments on the use and abuse of cocaine; suggested by its invariably successful employment in more than a thousand minor surgical operations, NY Med J 42:294, 1885.

219. Schleich C: Infiltrationsanästhesie (locale Anästhesie) und ihr Verhältnis zur allgemeinen Narcose (Inhalationsanästhesie), Verhandl D Deutsch Gesellsch F Chir 21:121-127, 1892.

220. Coming JL: On the prolongation of the anaesthetic effect of the hydrochlorate of cocaine, when subcutaneously injected. An experimental study. N Y Med J 42:317-319, 1885.

221. Braun H: Die Lokalanästhesie, ihre wissenschaflichen Grundlagen und praktische Anwendung. Leipzig, Johann Barth, 1907, pp 102-104.

222. Braun H: Ueber den Einfluss der Vitalitat der Gewebe auf die ortlichen und allgemeinen Giftwirkungen localanasthesirender Mittel und ueber die Bedeutung des Adrenalins fur die Localanasthesie. Arch Klin Chir 69:541, 1903.

223. Braun H: Ueber einige neue örtliche Anaesthetica. Deutsche Med 31:1667-1671, 1905.

224. Hirschel G: Anesthesia of the brachial plexus for operations on the upper extremity. Med Med Wochenschr 58:1555-1556, 1911.

225. Pitkin G: Prolonged local or block anesthesia with regulated cell reception. Anesth Analg 21:1-12, 83-95, 1942.

226. de Jong R: Axillary block of the brachial plexus. Anesthesiology 22:215-225, 1961.

227. Kulenkampff D: Anesthesia of the brachial plexus. Zentralbl Chir 38:1337-1340, 1911.

228. Pauchet V, Sourdat P, Tabott G, et al: Regional Anesthesia, 4th ed. Paris, Doin, 1928.

229. Raj P, Montgomery S, Nettles D, Jenkins M: Infraclavicular brachial plexus block—A new approach. Anesth Analg 52:897-904, 1973.

230. Kappis M: Conduction anesthesia of the abdomen, breast, arm and neck with paravertebral injection. Med Wochenschr 59:794-796, 1912.

231. Etienne J. Regional Anesthesia: Its Application in the Surgical Treatment of Cancer of the Breast. Paris, Faculté de Medecine de Paris, 1925.

232. Winnie A: Interscalene brachial plexus block. Anesth Analg 49:455-466, 1970.

233. Bier A: Ueber einen neuen Weg localanasthesie in den gliedmaassen zu erzeugen [On a new technique to induce local anesthesia in extremities]. Langenbecks Archiv Klin Chir 86:1007-1116, 1908.

234. Wulf H: The centennial of spinal anesthesia. Anesthesiology 89:500-506, 1998.

235. Bonica JJ: Basic principles in managing chronic pain. Arch Surg 112:783-788, 1977.

236. Pilowsky I, Chapman CR, Bonica JJ: Pain, depression, and illness behavior in a pain clinic population. Pain 4:183-192, 1977.

237. Einhorn A: Ueber die Chemie der lokalen Anästhetica. Munch. Med Wochenschr 46:1218-1220, 1254-1256, 1899.

238. Holmdahl M: Xylocaine (lidocaine, lignocaine), its discovery and Gordh's contribution to its clinical use. Acta Anaesthesiol Scand Suppl 113:8-12, 1998.

239. Albright GA: Cardiac arrest following regional anesthesia with etidocaine or bupivacaine. Anesthesiology 51:285-287, 1979.

240. Ruetsch YA, Boni T, Borgeat A: From cocaine to ropivacaine: The history of local anesthetic drugs. Curr Top Med Chem 1:175-182, 2001.

241. Coming JL: Spinal anaesthesia and local medication of the cord. N Y Med J 42:483, 1885.

242. Marx GF: The first spinal anesthesia. Who deserves the laurels? Reg Anesth 19:429-430, 1994.

243. Quincke H: Die Lumbalpunktion des Hydrocephalus. Berl Klin Wochenschr 28:929-933, 965-968, 1891.

244. Wynter W: Lumbar puncture. Lancet 1:981-982, 1891.

245. Bier A: Versuche uber Cocainisirung des Ruckenmarkes. Dtsch Z Chir 51:361-369, 1899.

246. Seldowitsch J: Über Kokainisierung des Rückenmarks nach Bier. Centralb Chir 26:1110-1113, 1899.

247. Tait D, Cagliari G: Experimental and clinical notes on the subarachnoid space. Trans Med Soc St Calif:266-271, 1900.

248. Tuffier T: Analgesie Chirurgicale par l'injection sousarachnoidienne lombaire de cocaine. Soc Biol 11:882-884, 1899.

249. Matas R: Local and regional anesthesia with cocaine and other analgesic drugs, including the subarachnoid method,

as applied in general surgical practice. Phila Med J 6:820-843, 1900.

250. Surgical anaesthesia by the injection of cocaine into the lumbar subarachnoid space. Lancet 1:137-138, 1901.

251. Morton A: The subarachnoid injection of cocaine for operations on all parts of the body. Am Med 3:176-179, 1901.

252. Jonnesco T: Remarks on general spinal analgesia. Br Med J 4:1396-1401, 1909.

253. Bier A: Das zurzeit an der Berliner chirurgischen Universitätsklinik übliche Verfahren der Rückenmarksanästhesie. Dtsch Z Chir 95:373-385, 1909.

254. Goldan SO: Intraspinal cocainization for surgical anesthesia. Phil Med J 6:850-857, 1900.

255. Kitagawa O: On spinal anesthesia with cocaine. J Jpn Soc Surg 3:185-191, 1901.

256. Gumprecht F: Gefahren der Lumbalpunktion; plötzliche Todesfalle danach. Dtsch Med Wochenschr 27:386-389, 1900.

257. Cushing H: On routine determinations of arterial tension in operating room and clinic. Boston Med Surg J 148: 250-256, 1903.

258. Gray H, Parsons L: Blood pressure variations associated with lumbar puncture, and the induction of spinal anaesthesia. Q J Med 5:339-367, 1912.

259. Barker A: Clinical experiences with spinal anesthesia in 100 cases. Br Med J 23:665-674, 1907.

260. Lee JA: Arthur Edward James Barker 1850-1916. British pioneer of regional analgesia. Anaesthesia 34:885-891, 1979.

261. Pitkin G: Conduction Anesthesia, 2nd ed. Philadelphia, JB Lippincott, 1953.

262. Cope R: The Wooley and Roe case. Anaesthesia 9:249-270, 1954.

263. Kennedy F, Effron A, Perry G: The grave spinal cord paralysis caused by spinal anesthesia: Surg Gynecol Obstet 91:385-398, 1950.

264. Dripps R, Vandam L: Long term follow-up of patients who received 10,098 spinal anesthetics. Failure to discover major neurological sequelae. JAMA 156:1486-1491, 1954.

265. Schneider M, Ettlin T, Kaufmann M, et al: Transient neurologic toxicity after hyperbaric subarachnoid anesthesia with 5% lidocaine. Anesth Analg 76:1154-1157, 1993.

266. Freedman JM, Li DK, Drasner K, et al: Transient neurologic symptoms after spinal anesthesia: An epidemiologic study of 1,863 patients. Anesthesiology 89:633-641, 1998.

267. Rigler ML, Drasner K, Krejcie TC, et al: Cauda equina syndrome after continuous spinal anesthesia. Anesth Analg 72:275-281, 1991.

268. Vandam L, Dripps R: Long term follow-up of patients who received 10,098 anesthetics. JAMA 161:586-591, 1956.

269. Gormley J: Treatment of post-spinal headache. Anesthesiology 21:565-566, 1960.

270. DiGiovanni AJ, Dunbar BS: Epidural injections of autologous blood for postlumbar-puncture headache. Anesth Analg 49:268-271, 1970.

271. Sicard M: Les injections médicamenteuses extradurales par voie sacro-coccygienne. C R Soc Dev Biol 53:396-398, 1901.

272. Cathelin M: Une nouvelle voie d'injection rachidienne. Methodes des injections epidurales par le precede du canal sacre. Applications a 1'homme. C R Soc Dev Biol 53: 452-453, 1901.

273. Läwen A: Über die Verwertung der Sakralanästhesie fur chirurgische Operationen. Zentralbl Chir 37:708, 1910.

274. Heile B: Der epidurale Raum. Arch Klin Chir 101:845-877, 1913.

275. Tuffier T: Analgesie cocainique par voie extradurale. C R Soc Biol Paris 53:490-492, 1901.

276. Pagés MF: Anestesia metamérica. Rev Sanid Milit 11: 351-365, 389-396, 1921.

277. Dogliotti AM: Eine neue Methode der regionären Anästhesie: Die peridurale segmentäre Anästhesie. Zentralbl Chir 58:3141-3145, 1931.

278. Bromage P: The "hanging drop" sign. Anaesthesia 8:237-241, 1953.

279. Dogliotti AM: Anesthesia. Chicago, SB Debour, 1939.

280. Flagg P: The art of anaesthesia, 7th ed. Philadelphia, JB Lippincott, 1954.

281. Odom C: Epidural anesthesia. Am J Surg 34:547-558, 1936.

282. Harger J, Christofferson EA, Stokes AJ: Peridural anesthesia: A consideration of 1000 cases. Am J Surg 52:24-31, 1941.

283. Crawford O, Buckingham WW, Ottosen P, Brasher CA: Peridural anesthesia in thoracic surgery: A review of 677 cases. Anesthesiology 12:73-84, 1951.

284. Lemmon W: A method for continuous spinal anesthesia: A preliminary report. Ann Surg 111:141-144, 1940.

285. Tuohy E: Continuous spinal anesthesia: Its usefulness and technic involved. Anesthesiology 5:142-148, 1944.

286. Curbelo MM: Continuous peridural segmental anesthesia by means of a ureteral catheter. Anesth Analg 28:13-23, 1949.

287. Edwards WB, Hingson RA: Continuous caudal anesthesia in obstetrics. Am J Surg 57:459-464, 1942.

288. Bromage P: Epidural analgesia. Philadelphia, WB Saunders, 1979.

289. Bonica J: Regional Anesthesia: Recent Advances and Current Status. Philadelphia, Davis, 1969.

290. Moore D: Regional Block. Springfield, IL, CC Thomas, 1953.

291. Cousins M, Bridenbaugh P: Neural Blockade. Philadelphia, JB Lippincott, 1980.

292. Wang JK, Nauss LA, Thomas JE: Pain relief by intrathecally applied morphine in man. Anesthesiology 50:149-151, 1979.

293. Yaksh TL, Rudy TA: Analgesia mediated by a direct spinal action of narcotics. Science 192:1357-1358, 1976.

294. Duggan AW, North RA: Electrophysiology of opioids. Pharmacol Rev 35:219-281, 1983.

295. Atweh S, Kuhar M: Autoradiographic localization of opiate receptors in rat brain. Brain Res 124:53-67, 1977.

296. Samii K, Chauvin M, Viars P: Postoperative spinal analgesia with morphine. Br J Anaesth 53:817-820, 1981.

297. Cousins MJ, Mather LE, Glynn CJ, et al: Selective spinal analgesia. Lancet 1:1141-1142, 1979.

298. Behar M, Magora F, Olshwang D, Davidson JT: Epidural morphine in treatment of pain. Lancet 1:527-529, 1979.

299. Ready LB, Oden R, Chadwick HS, et al: Development of an anesthesiology-based postoperative pain management service. Anesthesiology 68:100-106, 1988.

300. Wang C, Chakrabarti MK, Whitwam JG: Specific enhancement by fentanyl of the effects of intrathecal bupivacaine on nociceptive afferent but not on sympathetic efferent pathways in dogs. Anesthesiology 79:766-773, discussion 25A, 1993.

301. Harvey W: Exercitatio Anatomica de Motu Cordis et Sanguiis in Animalibus. Frankfurt, Fitzeri, 1628.

302. Clarck T: A letter written to the publisher by the learned and experienced Dr. Timothy Clarck, one of his majesties physicians in ordinary, concerning some anatomical inventions and observations, particularly the origin of the injection into veins, the transfusion of blood, and the parts of generation. Philos Trans R Soc 3:672-682, 1668.

303. Oré P: De l'anesthésie produite chez l'homme par les injections de chloral dans les veines. Comptes rendus Acad Sci 78:515-517, 651-654, 1874.

304. Von Steinbüchel G: Die scopolamin-morphium-halbnarkose in der geburtshülfe. Beiträge zur Geburtshilfe und Gynäkologie 1:294-326, 1903.

305. Goerig M: The Avertin story. In Fink B, Morris LE, Stephen CR, et al (eds): The History of Anesthesia. Third International Symposium. Park Ridge, IL, Wood Library-Museum of Anesthesiology, 1992.

306. Harvey S: Hypnotics and Sedatives. In Goodman L, Gilman A, Goodman L, et al (eds): The Pharmacological Basis of Therapeutics, 5th ed. New York, Macmillan, 1975.

307. Fischer E, von Mering J: Ueber eine neue classe von Schlafmitteln. Ther Ggw 44:97-101, 1903.

308. Weese H, Scharpff W: Evipan, ein neuartiges Einschlafmittel. Dtsch Med Wochenschr 58:1205-1207, 1932.

309. Lundy J: Intravenous anesthesia: Preliminary report of the use of two new thiobarbiturates. Proc Mayo Clin 10: 536-543, 1935.

310. Lundy J: Balanced anesthesia. Minn Med 9:399-404, 1926.

311. Halford F: A critique of intravenous anesthesia in war surgery. Anesthesiology 4:67-69, 1943.

312. Bennetts FE: Thiopentone anaesthesia at Pearl Harbor. Br J Anaesth 75:366-368, 1995.

313. Kay B, Stephenson DK: ICI 35868 (Diprivan): A new intravenous anaesthetic. A comparison with Althesin. Anaesthesia 35:1182-1187, 1980.

314. Doenicke A, Kugler J, Penzel G, et al: Cerebral function under etomidate, a new non-barbiturate I.V. hypnotic [author's translation]. Anaesthesist 22:3573-3566, 1973.

315. Sternbach L: Chemistry of 1,4-benzodiazepines and some aspects of the structure-activity relationship. New York, Raven Press, 1973.

316. Hunkeler W, Mohler H, Pieri L, et al: Selective antagonists of benzodiazepines. Nature 290:514-516, 1981.

317. Corssen G, Domino EF: Dissociative anesthesia: Further pharmacologic studies and first clinical experience with the phencyclidine derivative CI-581. Anesth Analg 45:29-40, 1966.

318. Kay B, Rolly G: I.C.I. 35868, a new intravenous induction agent. Acta Anaesthesiol Belg 28:303-316, 1977.

319. Forrest W, Smethurst P, Kienitz M: Self administration of intravenous analgesics. Anesthesiology 33:363-365, 1970.

320. Sechzer PH: Patient-controlled analgesia (PCA): A retrospective. Anesthesiology 72:735-736, 1990.

321. White PF: Use of patient-controlled analgesia for management of acute pain. JAMA 259:243-247, 1988.

322. Thomas K: Curare: Its history and usage. London, Pitman Medicals, 1964.

323. d'Anghera PM: De Orbe Nove. Francis Autustus MacNutt, transl. New York, G P Putnam and Sons, 1912, pp 385-386.

324. Raleigh W: The Discoererie of the Large, Rich and Beautiful Empire of Guina … Performed in the Year 1595 by Walter Raleigh, Captaine of her Maiests's Guard. London, Robert Robinson, 1596.

325. De la Condamine IPJ: Voyagers and Travels. London, Longman, Hurst & Rees, 1813.

326. Betcher A: The civilizing of curare: A history of its development and introduction into anesthesiology. Anesth Analg 56:305-319, 1977.

327. Brodie B: Experiments and observations on the different modes in which death is produced by certain vegetable poisons. Philos Trans R Soc Lond 1:194-195, 1811.

328. Waterton C: Wanderings in South America. London, Macmillan, 1879.

329. Bernard C: Lecons sur les effects des substances toxiques et medicamenteuses. JB Paris, Bailliere, 1857.

330. Kuhne W: Ueber die peripherischen Endorgane der motorischen Nerven. Leipzig, W Engelmann,1862.

331. Wells T: Three cases of tetanus, in which "woorara" was used. Proc R Med Chir Soc Lond 3:142-157, 1859.

332. Läwen A: The combination of local anesthesia with narcosis. Beitr Klin Chir 80:168-189, 1912.

333. King H: Curare. Nature 135:469-470, 1935.

334. Gill R: White water and black magic. New York, Holt, 1940.

335. Gill R: Mrs. Robinson Crusoe in Ecuador. Natl Geog Mag 65:134-150, 1934.

336. Bennett A, McIntyre A, Bennett A: Pharmacologic and clinical investigations with crude curare. JAMA 114:1791, 1940.

337. Griffith H. Johnson G: The use of curare in general anesthesia. Anesthesiology 3:418-420, 1942.

338. Cullen S: The use of curare for improvement of abdominal muscle relaxation during inhalation anesthesia: Report on 131 cases. Surgery 14:261-266, 1943.

339. Gray T, Halton J: A milestone in anaesthesia, d-tubocurarine chloride? Proc R Soc Med 39:400-410, 1946.

340. Harroun P, Beckert F, Hathaway H: Curare and nitrous oxide anesthesia for lengthy operations. Anesthesiology 7:24-28, 1946.

341. Harroun P, Hathaway H: The use of curare in anesthesia for thoracic surgery. Surg Gynecol Obstet 82:229-231, 1946.

342. Neff W, Mayer E, de la Luz Perales M: Nitrous oxide and oxygen anesthesia with curare relaxation. Calif Med 66:67-69, 1947.

343. Beecher HK, Todd DP: A study of the deaths associated with anesthesia and surgery: Based on a study of 599,548 anesthesias in ten institutions 1948-1952. Ann Surg 140:2-34, 1954.

344. Churchill-Davidson H, Richardson AT: Proc R Soc Med 45:179, 1952.

345. Cohen AD: A simple inexpensive nerve stimulator. Anaesthesia 18:534-535, 1963.

346. Katz R: A nerve stimulator for the continuous monitoring of muscle relaxant action. Anesthesiology 26:832-833, 1965.

347. Ali HH, Utting JE, Gray T: Quantitative assessment of residual antidepolarizing block (part II). Br J Anaesth 43:478-485, 1971.

348. Bovet C, Depierre F, Lestrange Y: Propriétés curarisantes des ethers phénoliques à functions ammonium quaternaries. Comptes rendus Acad Sci 225:74-76, 1947.

349. Bovet D: Proprietá farmacodinamiche di alcuni derivati della succinilcolina dotati di azione curarica. Esteri di trialchiletanolammonio di acidi bicarbossilici alifatici. R C Ist Super Sanita 12:106-137, 1949.

350. Thesleff S, von Dardel O, Holmberg F: Succinylcholine iodide. New muscular relaxant. Br J Anaesth 24:238-244, 1952.

351. Baird WL, Reid AM: The neuromuscular blocking properties of a new steroid compound, pancuronium bromide: A pilot study in man. Br J Anaesth 39:775-780, 1967.

352. Durant NN, Marshall IG, Savage DS, et al: The neuromuscular and autonomic blocking activities of pancuronium, Org NC 45, and other pancuronium analogues, in the cat. J Pharm Pharmacol 31:831-836, 1979.

353. Miller RD: Org Nc 45. Br J Anaesth 52(Suppl 1):71S-72S, 1980.

354. Booij LH, Knape HT: The neuromuscular blocking effect of Org 9426. A new intermediately-acting steroidal non-depolarising muscle relaxant in man. Anaesthesia 46:341-343, 1991.

355. Snow J: On the inhalation of the vapour of ether in surgical operations. London, J Churchill, 1847.

356. Junker F: Description of a new apparatus for administering narcotic vapours. Med Times Gaz 2:590, 1867.

357. Clover J: Description of a new double current inhaler for administering ether. Br Med J 1:282-283, 1873.

358. Clover J: On an apparatus for administering nitrous oxide gas and ether, singly or combined. Br Med J 2:74-75, 1876.

359. Buxton D: Anaesthetics, their uses and administration. London, Lewis, 1914.

360. Meltzer S: Continuous respiration without respiratory movements. J Exp Med 11:622-625, 1909.

361. Elsberg C: Anaesthesia by the intratracheal insufflation of air and ether. Ann Surg 53:161-168, 1911.

362. Crafoord C: Pulmonary ventilation and anesthesia in major chest surgery. J Thorac Surg 9:237-253, 1940.

363. Gwathmey J: Anesthesia. New York, Appleton, 1908, p 580.

364. Boyle HEG: Nitrous oxide-oxygen-ether outfit. Proc R Soc Med 11:30, 1917-1918.

365. Neu M: Ein verfahren zur stickoxydulsauerstoffnarkose. Munch Med Wochenschr 57:1873-1875, 1910.

366. Coleman A: Mr. Coleman's economising apparatus for re-inhaling the gas. Br J Den Sci 12:443, 1869.

367. Duncum B: The Development of Inhalation Anesthesia. London, Oxford University Press, 1947.

368. Kuhn F: Perorale Tubagen mit und ohne Druck. Dtsch Chir 76:148-207, 1905.

369. Jackson D: A new method for the production of general analgesia and anaesthesia with a description of the apparatus used. J Lab Clin Med 1:1-12, 1915.

370. Waters R: Clinical scope and utility of carbon dioxide filtration in inhalation anesthesia. Curr Res Anesth Analg 3:20-22, 1924.

371. Sword B: The closed circle method of administration of gas anesthesia. Curr Res Anesth Analg 9:198-202, 1930.

372. Morris L: A new vaporizer for liquid anesthetic agents. Anesthesiology 13:587, 1952.

373. Cohen E: Anesthetic Exposure in the Workplace. New York, MTP Press, 1980.

374. O'Dwyer J: An improved method of performing artificial forcible respiration with exhibition of instruments. Arch Pediatr 9:30-34, 1892.

375. Matas R: Intralaryngeal insufflation for the relief of acute surgical pneumothorax. Its history and methods with

a description of the latest devices for this purpose. JAMA 34:1468-1473, 1900.

376. Drinker P, McKhann C: The use of a new apparatus for the prolonged administration of artificial respiration. I. A fatal case of poliomyelitis. JAMA 92:1658-1660, 1929.

377. Moerch E: Controlled respiration by means of special automatic machines as used in Sweden and Denmark. Proc R Soc Med Lond 40:603-607, 1947.

378. Ibsen B: Anaesthetist's viewpoint on the treatment of respiratory complications in poliomyelitis during the epidemic in Copenhagen, 1952. Proc Roy Soc Med (Lond) 47:72-74, 1954.

379. McDowell E: Three cases of extirpation of diseased ovaria. Med Classics 2:651-653, 1938.

380. Crile G: Nitrous oxide anaesthesia and a note on anoci-association, a new principle in operative surgery. Surg Gynecol Obstet 13:170-173, 1911.

381. Crile G, Lower WE: Anoci-Association. Philadelphia, WB Saunders, 1914.

382. Cushing H: On the avoidance of shock in major amputations by cocainization of large nerve-trunks preliminary to their division. Ann Surg 36:321-345, 1902.

383. Woodbridge P: Changing concepts concerning depth of anesthesia. Anesthesiology 18:536-550, 1957.

384. Pinsker M: Anesthesia: A pragmatic construct. Anesth Analg 65:819-820, 1986.

385. Roizen MF, Horrigan RW, Frazer BM: Anesthetic doses blocking adrenergic (stress) and cardiovascular responses to incision—MAC BAR. Anesthesiology 54:390-398, 1981.

386. Mangano DT, Layug EL, Wallace A, Tateo I: Effect of atenolol on mortality and cardiovascular morbidity after noncardiac surgery. Multicenter Study of Perioperative Ischemia Research Group. N Engl J Med 335:1713-1720, 1996.

387. Lowenstein E, Hallowell P, Levine FH, et al: Cardiovascular response to large doses of intravenous morphine in man. N Engl J Med 281:1389-1393, 1969.

388. Stanley T, Philbin D, Coggins C: Fentanyl oxygen anaesthesia for coronary artery surgery. Cardiovascular and antidiuretic hormone responses. Can Anaesth Soc J 26:168-172, 1979.

389. Clark RB: Transplacental reversal of meperidine depression in the fetus by naloxone. J Ark Med Soc 68:128-130, 1971.

390. Kienbaum P, Thurauf N, Michel MC, et al: Profound increase in epinephrine concentration in plasma and cardiovascular stimulation after mu-opioid receptor blockade in opioid-addicted patients during barbiturate-induced anesthesia for acute detoxification. Anesthesiology 88:1154-1161, 1998.

391. DeCastro J, Mundeleer P: Anesthesie sans sommeil. "La neuroleptanalgesie". Acta Chir Belg 58:689, 1959.

392. Asoh T, Tsuji H, Shirasaka C, Takeuchi Y: Effect of epidural analgesia on metabolic response to major upper abdominal surgery. Acta Anaesthesiol Scand 27:233-237, 1983.

393. Bevan DR: Modification of the metabolic response to trauma under extradural analgesia. Anaesthesia 26:188-191, 1971.

394. Von Esmarch F: Handbuch der Kriegschirurgischen Technik. Hannover, Carl Rumpler, 1877.

395. Heiberg J: A new expedient in administering chloroform. Med Surg Gaz 1:36, 1874.

396. Warren J: Address before the American Medical Association, Boston, John Wilson, 1850, pp 5-65.

397. Sibson F: On the treatment of facial neuralgia by the inhalation of ether. Lond Med Gaz 4:358-364, 1847.

398. Maltby JR: Francis Sibson, 1814-1876. Pioneer and prophet in anaesthesia. Anaesthesia 32:53-62, 1977.

399. Hewitt F: An artificial "airway" for use during anaesthetization. Lancet 1:490-491, 1908.

400. Guedel A: A nontraumatic pharyngeal airway. JAMA 100:1862, 1933.

401. Shipway F: Airway for intranasal operations. Br Med J 2:767, 1935.

402. O'Dwyer J: Fifty cases of croup in private practice treated by intubation of the larynx, with a description of the method and of the dangers incident thereto. Med Rec 32:557-561, 1887.

403. Trousseau A: Du tubage de la glotte et de la tracheotomie, par M Bouchut. Bull Acad Med 24:99, 1858.

404. Macewen W: Clinical observations on the introduction of tracheal tubes by the mouth instead of performing tracheotomy or laryngotomy. Br Med J 2:122-124, 163-165, 1880.

405. Rendell-Baker L: History of thoracic anesthesia. In Mushin WW (ed): Thoracic Anaesthesia. Oxford, Blackwell Scientific, 1963.

406. Trendelenburg F: Beiträge zu den Operationen an den Luftwegen. Arch Klin Chir 12:112-133, 1871.

407. Sauerbruch F: Ueber die physiologischen and physikalischen Grundlagen bei intrathorakalen Eingriffen in meiner pneumatischen Operationskammer. Verh Dtsch Ges Chir 32:105-115, 1904.

408. Magill I: Endotracheal anesthesia. Proc R Soc Med 22:1-6, 1928.

409. Rowbotham E, Magill I: Anaesthetics in the plastic surgery of the face and jaws. Proc R Soc Med 14:17-27, 1921.

410. Guedel A, Waters, RM: A new intratracheal catheter. Anesth & Analg 7:238-239, 1928.

411. Gale J, Waters R: Closed endobronchial anesthesia in thoracic surgery: Preliminary report. Anesth Analg 11:283-287, 1932.

412. MaGill I: Anaesthesia in thoracic surgery, with special reference to lobectomy. Proc R Soc Med 29:649-653, 1936.

413. Carlens E: A new flexible double-lumen catheter for bronchospirometry. J Thorac Surg 18:742-746, 1949.

414. Robertshaw F: Low resistance double-lumen endobronchial tubes. Br J Anaesth 34:576-579, 1962.

415. Green R, Gordon W: Right lung anaesthesia. Anaesthesia 12:86-93, 1957.

416. Murphy F: Two improved intratracheal catheters. Anesth Analg 20:102-105, 1941.

417. Kirstein A: Autoskopie des Larynx und der Trachea. Berl Klin Wochenschr 32:476-478, 1895.

418. Hirsch NP, Smith GB, Hirsch PO: Alfred Kirstein: Pioneer of direct laryngoscopy. Anaesthesia 41:42-45, 1986.

419. Jackson C: Tracheobronchoscopy, Esophagoscopy and Gastroscopy. St Louis, CV Mosby, 1907.

420. Garcia M: Observations on the human voice. Proc R Soc Lond 7:399-410, 1854.

421. Killian G: Ueber directe Brochoskopie. Munch Med Wochenschr 45:844-847, 1898.

422. Miller R: A new laryngoscope. Anesthesiology 2:317-320, 1941.

423. Macintosh R: A new laryngoscope. Lancet 1:205, 1943.

424. Brain A: The laryngeal mask: A new concept in airway management. Br J Anaesth 55:801-805, 1983.

425. Tyndall J: On some phenomena connected with the motion of liquids. Philos Mag 8:74-76, 1854.

426. Lamm H: Biegsame optische Geräte. Z Instrumentenk 50:579-581, 1930.

427. Ikeda S, Yanai N, Ishidawa S: Flexible bronchofiberscope. Keio J Med 17:1-18, 1968.

428. Ikeda S: Atlas of Flexible Bronchofiberoscopy. Baltimore, University Park Press, 1971.

429. Curry J: Popular Observations on Apparent Death from Drowning. Northampton, T Dicey and Co, 1792.

430. Leroy J: Recherches sur l'asphyxie. J Physiol Exp Pathol 7:45-65, 1827.

431. Park R: A Treatise on Surgery, 3rd ed. New York, Lea Brothers, 1901.

432. Elam J, Greene DG, Brown ES, et al: Oxygen and carbon dioxide exchange and energy cost of expired air resuscitation. JAMA 167:328-334, 1958.

433. Lind B: Recent History of Resuscitation in Norway. Anaesthesia—Essays on Its History. Berlin, Springer-Verlag, 1985.

434. Waller A: A demonstration in man of electromotive changes accompanying the heart's beat. J Physiol 8:229-234, 1887.

435. Einthoven W: The string galvanometer and the human electrocardiogram. Proceedings of the Koninklijke Nederlandse Akademie van Wetenschappen, Amsterdam, Section of Sciences. 6:107-115, 1903.

436. Herrick J: Clinical features of sudden obstruction of the coronary arteries. JAMA 59:2015-2020, 1912.

437. MacWilliam J: Fibrillar contraction of the heart. J Physiol 8:296-310, 1887.

438. MacWilliam J: Cardiac failure and sudden death. Br Med J 1:6-8, 1889.

439. Prevost J, Battelli F: La mort par les courants electriques. J Physiol Pathol Gen 1:427, 1899.

440. Beck C, Pritchard W, Feil H: Ventricular fibrillation of long duration abolished by electric shock. JAMA 135:985-986, 1947.

441. Starling E, Lane W: Case report. Lancet 2:1397, 1902.

442. Keen W: A case of total laryngectomy (unsuccessful) and a case of abdominal hysterectomy (successful), in both of which massage of the heart for chloroform collapse was employed, with notes of 25 cases of cardiac massages. Ther Gaz 28:217-230, 1904.

443. Koenig F: Lehrbuch des Allgemeinen. Chirurgie, Göttingen, 1883.

444. Kouwenhoven W, Jude F, Knickerbocker G: Closed chest cardiac massage. JAMA 173:1064-1067, 1960.

445. Hayward G: Surgical Reports and Miscellaneous Papers on Medical Subjects. Boston, Phillips, Sampson, 1855.

446. Snow J: On Chloroform and Other Anaesthetics; Their Action and Administration. London, John Churchill, 1858.

447. Beecher H: The first anesthesia death with some remarks suggested by it on the fields of the laboratory and the clinic in the appraisal of new anesthetic agents. Anesthesiology 2:443-449, 1941.

448. Knight PR 3rd, Bacon DR: An unexplained death: Hannah Greener and chloroform. Anesthesiology 96:1250-1253, 2002.

449. Guedel A: Inhalation anesthesia: A fundamental guide. New York, Macmillan, 1937.

450. Lowenthal PJ, Russell A: Recovery room: Life saving and economical. Anesthesiology 12:470-476, 1951.

451. Mendelson C: The aspiration of stomach contents into the lungs during obstetrical anesthesia. Am J Obstet Gynecol 52:191-205, 1945.

452. Dorrance G: On the treatment of traumatic injuries of the lungs and pleura with the presentation of a new intratracheal tube for use in artificial respiration. Surg Gynecol Obstet 11:160-187, 1910.

453. Sellick B: Cricoid pressure to control regurgitation of stomach contents during induction of anaesthesia. Lancet 2:404-406, 1961.

454. Hunter J: Of persons apparently drowned. Philos Trans R Soc Lond 66:415-425, 1776.

455. Rendell-Baker L: Standards for anesthesia: The issues. Contemp Anesth Pract 8:59-88, 1984.

456. Bacon DR: The promise of one great anesthesia society. Anesthesiology 80:929-935, 1994.

457. Gaba DM, Howard SK: Patient safety: Fatigue among clinicians and the safety of patients. N Engl J Med 347:1249-1255, 2002.

458. Cooper JB, Gaba D: No myth: Anesthesia is a model for addressing patient safety. Anesthesiology 97:1335-1337, 2002.

459. Laennec RT: De l'auscultation mediate. Paris, JA Brosson & JS Chaude, 1819.

460. Smith C: An endo-esophageal stethoscope. Anesthesiology 15:566, 1954.

461. Beecher HK: The first anesthesia records. Surg Gynecol Obstet 71:789, 1940.

462. Eichhorn JH, Cooper JB, Cullen DJ, et al: Standards for patient monitoring during anesthesia at Harvard Medical School. JAMA 256:1017-1020, 1986.

463. Denborough M, Lovell R: Anaesthetic deaths in a family. Lancet 2:45, 1960.

464. Sessler DI: Mild perioperative hypothermia. N Engl J Med 336:1730-1737, 1997.

465. Kurz A, Sessler DI, Lenhardt R: Perioperative normothermia to reduce the incidence of surgical-wound infection and shorten hospitalization. Study of Wound Infection and Temperature Group. N Engl J Med 334:1209-1215, 1996.

466. Orkin F: What do patients want? Preferences for immediate postoperative recovery. Anesth Analg 74:S225, 1992.

467. Watcha M, White P: Postoperative nausea and vomiting—Its etiology, treatment, and prevention. Anesthesiology 77:162-184, 1992.

468. Watcha M, Smith I: Cost-effectiveness analysis of antiemetic therapy for ambulatory surgery. J Clin Anesth 6:370-377, 1994.

469. Smith SM, Brown HO, Toman JEP, et al: The lack of cerebral effects of D-tubocurarine. Anesthesiology 8:1-14, 1947.

470. Blacher R: On awakening paralyzed during surgery. A syndrome of traumatic neurosis. JAMA 234:67-68, 1975.

471. Tunstall ME: Detecting wakefulness during general anaesthesia for caesarean section. Br Med J 1:1321, 1977.

472. Berger J: Über das Elektroenkephalogramm des Menschen. Arch Psychiat Nervenkr 87:527-570, 1929.

473. Falconer AJ, Pender JW, Bickford. RG: The influence of partial pressure of nitrous oxide on the depth of anesthesia and the electro-encephalogram in man. Anesthesiology 10:601-609, 1949.

474. Glass P, Bloom M, Kearse L, et al: Bispectral analysis measures sedation and memory effects of propofol, midazolam, isoflurane, and alfentanil in healthy volunteers. Anesthesiology 86:836-847, 1997.

475. Richet C: De l'anaphysaxie en general et de l'anaphysoxie par la mytilocongestine en particulier. Ann Inst Pasteur 21:497-524, 1907.

476. Dragstedt C, Gebauer-Fuelnegg E: Studies in anaphylaxis. Am J Physiol 102:512-526, 1932.

477. Priestley J: Observations on different kinds of air. Philos Trans R Soc Lond 62:147-264, 1772.

478. Apgar V: A proposal for a new method of evaluation of the newborn infant. Curr Res Anal Analg 32:260-267, 1953.

479. Apgar V, Holaday DA. James LS, et al: Comparison of regional and general anesthesia in obstetrics. JAMA 165:2155-2161, 1957.

480. Guedel A: Nitrous oxide-air anesthesia self administered in obstetrics; a preliminary report. Indianap Med J 14:476-479, 1911.

481. Guedel AE: Third stage of ether anesthesia: A sub-classification regarding the significance of the position and movements of the eyeball. Nat Anesth Res Soc Bull 3:1-4, 1920.

482. Rice N: Trials of a public benefactor, as illustrated in the discovery of etherization. New York, Pudney & Russell, 1858.

483. Lavoisier A: Traite Elementaire de Chimie. Paris, Cuchet, 1789.

484. Schomburgk R: On the Urare, the arrow poison of the Indians of Guiana. Annu Mag Natl Hist 7:407, 1841.

485. Guedel A: Ethyl Chloride-Chloroform-Ether Anesthesia for Rapid Induction and Minor Surgery in War. In McMechan FH (ed): Year Book of Anesthesia and Analgesia 1917-1918. New York, Surgery Publishing Co.

Scientific Principles

CHAPTER
2 Scope of Modern Anesthetic Practice

Fredrick K. Orkin and Stephen J. Thomas

Preoperative Evaluation   56

Operating Room   57

Ambulatory Care   57

Other Sites   58

Postanesthesia Care Unit   58

Critical Care Medicine   59

Pain Management   60

Anesthesia Workforce   60

Value-based Anesthesia
   Care   61

Education   63

Future Directions   64

Since we last opined on the scope of anesthetic practice in the previous edition of this book, published in 1999, the specialty is experiencing a most welcome renewed interest among medical students and a spectacular increase in the demand for services. Nevertheless, many questions about our future, in terms of clinical practices and the best method for the delivery of anesthetic care and the education and research base for that practice have arisen. Politically the world, where now terrorism is feared in every land (see Chapter 64), has changed dramatically. The United States has endured September 11 and its aftermath. We have achieved remarkable military success, invading both Afghanistan and Iraq, toppling and finally capturing Sadaam Hussein. The future plans for these countries remain somewhat vague, manifestly controversial, and incredibly costly. Medically, a crucial issue continues to be medical expenditures. The economy is recovering as the United States has plunged into record-setting deficits from equally impressive surpluses. The impact on federal expenditures to hospitals and clinicians as well as to scientists (the first rumors about the 2005 budget mention reductions in NIH funding) cannot be good. Scientifically, anesthesiology has joined other areas of medicine in the emphasis on outcome studies and on the potential of the new genomic treatment paradigm that promises to treat human disease according to the given patient's genetic individuality.[1]

The organization, financing, and delivery of health care continue to follow the whims of the marketplace. The defeat of the Clinton Health Plan a decade ago ushered in managed care—a cost-containment method of funding and delivering the "commodity" known as health care.[2]

Despite spending almost 15% of the gross domestic product (GDP) on health care, we still managed to leave 15.2% of the population uninsured in 2004. Employer-supplied health care coverage is now undergoing erosion; employee benefits decrease while simultaneously premium contributions increase.[3] Medicare struggles to become more efficient, but efforts to enhance its weak and complicated underlying financing languish.[4] The Medicare bill passed in 2003, supported by most of organized medicine, turns a projected 3.6% decrease in Medicare payment to anesthesiologists into a 1.5% increase for each of the next 2 fiscal years. It also offers a drug benefit, the true effects of which are unclear. What is clear is that the $400 billion price tag when the bill was passed is currently estimated to be $530 billion, a price that would have most likely precluded passage! A mandated push to privatize Medicare (completely unsuccessful to date) and a prohibition on the government from using its incredible purchasing power to negotiate lower drug prices from pharmaceutical companies are further issues. Major legislative, rather than market-based, reform of health care financing in the United States, must await public recognition of an emerging national health care crisis.

The term *scope of practice* has many meanings. Medically, the buzzwords of the day, when referring to anesthesiologists, are "perioperative physician." Anesthesiology seeks to encompass the entire perioperative experience, from preoperative evaluation to intraoperative regional or general anesthesia (given almost anywhere—hospital, ambulatory care center, procedure room, doctor's office) to the post-anesthesia care unit (PACU), intensive care unit (ICU), and, in some pioneering efforts, even the patient's home.[5] The degree to which we will achieve this goal remains problematical, although an anesthesia residency requirement in the United States will increase to 4 years in 2008. As discussed later, preoperative evaluation is largely being done by nurse practitioners, and interest in critical care among anesthesiologists, at least at present, shows no sign of rebound. Our scope of practice also includes many types of management, including clinical-pain, PACU, ICU, and—now administrative—the operating room (OR) (see Chapter 86).

Scientifically, we are still trying to develop new faster-acting drugs of shorter duration, as well as novel approaches to reversing the effects of the drugs that we do have. Other research frontiers include molecular biologic techniques investigating issues ranging from the adrenergic system to mechanisms of anesthesia to outcome studies of the clinical and economic results of our actions. It is significant that the journals *Anesthesia and Analgesia* and *Anesthesiology* both now have separate sections devoted to economics and health services research. This is important not only because of physicians' concerns about their future but also because the economics of our specialty—or at least the perceived economics—resulted in a precipitous decline in interest by American medical students in the latter half of the 1990s, interest which is rebounding as original perceptions and assumptions proved exaggerated (and, perhaps, because the initial zeal for primary care on the part of managed care organizations and deans of medical schools proved misguided). This renewed interest, a boon to all program directors and to practitioners awaiting fresh, well-trained recruits for their expanding practices, appears to be driven by economics (good job, good salary) and by concerns for a "controllable lifestyle."[6]

To better understand the scope of the specialty, it is useful to review how the American Board of Anesthesiology (ABA) defines anesthesiology[7]:

Anesthesiology and perioperative management is defined as a continuity of patient care involving preoperative evaluation, intraoperative and postoperative care and the management of systems and personnel that support these activities.

The ABA exists in order to maintain the highest standards of practice by fostering educational facilities and training in anesthesiology, which the ABA defines as the practice of medicine dealing with but not limited to:

1. Assessment of, consultation for, and preparation of, patients for anesthesia.
2. Relief and prevention of pain during and following surgical, obstetric, therapeutic, and diagnostic procedures.
3. Monitoring and maintenance of normal physiology during the perioperative period.
4. Management of critically ill patients.
5. Diagnosis and treatment of acute, chronic, and cancer-related pain.
6. Clinical management and teaching of cardiac and pulmonary resuscitation.
7. Evaluation of respiratory function and application of respiratory therapy.
8. Conduct of clinical, translational, and basic science research.
9. Supervision, teaching, and evaluation of performance of both medical and paramedical personnel involved in perioperative care.
10. Administrative involvement in health care facilities and organizations and medical schools necessary to implement these responsibilities.

"Scope of practice" also has a distinct political interpretation, encompassing the questions of who can practice anesthesiology and under whose direction. The traditional approaches to delivery of anesthesia care, either by the anesthesiologist alone or as part of an anesthesia care team[8]—including residents and/or Certified Registered Nurse Anesthetists (CRNAs) and/or anesthesia assistants (AAs)—are under increasing political pressure as CRNAs join other advance-practice nurses in seeking independent privileges to practice.[9] The governors of many states have signed "opt-out" requests, under a new rule from the Center for Medicare and Medicaid Services (CMS) that permits CRNAs in those states to administer anesthesia without any physician supervision (and not endanger Medicare reimbursement to their hospitals). This was vigorously opposed by both the American Society of Anesthesiologists (ASA) and individual state societies.

It will not be long before additional data will be available (albeit not prospectively designed and collected) comparing outcomes between physician-directed and CRNA-independent anesthetics to complement recent articles on the subject.[10-12] Many other countries have different types of non-OR specialties, such as emergency medicine in Germany.

PREOPERATIVE EVALUATION

It is ironic that, as our interest, expertise, and knowledge concerning preoperative evaluation (see Chapter 25) is increasing, our ability to meet and talk with patients directly appears to be decreasing. The emphasis on ambulatory surgery (see later; also see Chapter 68) and same-day admissions, regardless of type of surgery, often makes preoperative personal contact with patients, whether in urban or rural settings, difficult. Despite such challenges (as well as those relating to staffing, patient scheduling, and payment), preoperative clinics appear to be increasingly prevalent.[13] They perform the functions of data acquisition, data screening (followed by physician consultation in an unknown percentage of cases), and patient education. Patients are seen, histories and physical examinations are reviewed, appropriate (and only appropriate) laboratory tests are ordered, and additional consultations, if indicated, are requested.[14,15] Explanations of the anesthetic and surgical plans and of the options available for postoperative pain relief decrease patients' anxiety and give them a modicum of control over their own destiny.[15] Evaluation of comorbid conditions is not only directed toward "getting the patient ready for surgery" but also—and more importantly—focuses on the long-term prognosis of specific diseases and may enhance the patient's health status (e.g., initiate β-adrenergic blocker therapy for those at risk for complications of coronary artery disease). Diagnostic, therapeutic, and consultative interventions are then ordered from that perspective. This is especially true in the area of cardiac disease.[17,18]

A primary issue is the staffing of these preoperative clinics. The use of advanced practice nurses appears to be common. A question that arises is whether it is ideal, desirable, and, most importantly, necessary and economically feasible for all patients to talk to an anesthesiologist during the preoperative evaluation. Screening of patient data using various algorithms can determine those whose medical status warrants direct physician consultation. Additionally, even if a patient does talk with an anesthesiologist, it is increasingly likely that it will not be the one who will be directly involved with his or her intraoperative care. This makes review and discussion of the anesthetic plan with the patient on the day of surgery, although occasionally time-consuming and inefficient, mandatory.

Undoubtedly, new options for familiarizing patients about anesthesia and surgery will emerge in the ensuing years. These might, and in some cases already do, include greater family involvement in anesthesia care, especially in the case of pediatric patients, and supplemental videotapes, in-hospital on-demand television, and departmental or hospital-based Web sites accessible from the patient's home.[16] These sites will likely become interactive and a source for data input directly by the patient.

OPERATING ROOM

The OR continues to be the principal focus of the anesthetic practice (see Chapter 86). Whereas the anesthesiologist is comfortable in the OR setting, it can be a hostile environment, both to patients and to other medical personnel. The use of volatile anesthetics and the possible contamination of the environment by those gases are concerns that must be recognized by the anesthesiologist and appropriately monitored. Because anesthesiologists use needles and constantly risk exposing themselves and others to blood and other body fluids, appropriate consideration and thought must be given to how to prevent injury, both to the anesthesia personnel and to others who work in the OR.[19] Unfortunately, not only are physicians and nurses in the OR subject to needlestick injuries, but housekeeping personnel also are at risk because of potential inattention by the medical staff. Certainly, it is in the best interest of the anesthesiologist to exploit creative new ways to administer drugs and monitor patients that will decrease the incidence of contamination of personnel in the OR by body fluids from patients.

It is well recognized that the OR is a major consumer of hospital, physician, and patient resources. It is equally apparent that efficient management of the OR can minimize costs and at the same time maximize patient through-put, contributing to enhanced institutional performance, although not without extraordinary effort and continuing education.[20] Whereas few doubt the wisdom of these observations, fewer still have developed the ideal administrative and operational structure to effect the efficiencies needed in today's cost-constrained environment.[21] Nevertheless, the effort continues, and anesthesiologists, by their temperament, availability, and interest, will be some of the principal players in the game (see Chapter 86). The application of managerial science to the improvement of OR efficiency has already become a scholarly focus in our specialty.[22-24]

Triage is an important aspect of the anesthesiologist's role in the OR. Urgent or emergent cases need to be inserted into operative schedules during normal working hours, and often emergent cases vie for available resources during off-hours. The anesthesiologist must have the broad medical and surgical knowledge to allocate resources and facilitate appropriate treatment of patients in an orderly progression. If this triage responsibility is abdicated, patient care suffers. The anesthesiologist usually has the best overview of the surgical, nursing, and anesthesia personnel necessary to care for the patient.

AMBULATORY CARE

One of the most significant trends affecting health care in the last quarter of the 20th century was the development of ambulatory surgery (see Chapter 68). Indeed, whereas 80% of surgery in the United States was performed on inpatients in 1980, that same percentage of our national surgical workload is now conducted on an ambulatory basis; moreover, the nation's surgery is now estimated to comprise twice as many cases. This trend is expected to continue, albeit at a slower rate (Fig. 2-1).[25] Many factors contribute to this trend, including consumerism, especially because the public is increasingly eager to have an ever-larger decision-making role in medical care; new technologies in anesthesia (fast-acting, short-duration anesthetic drugs and adjuvants) and surgery (tools for minimally invasive surgery such as endoscopic devices and lasers); and changes in health care economics. However, judging from the temporal aspects of the transition depicted in Figure 2-1, economic factors are by far the pivotal factor.

The phase-in of Medicare's prospective payment system, beginning in 1983, limited payments for hospital inpatient care to predetermined resource costs associated with

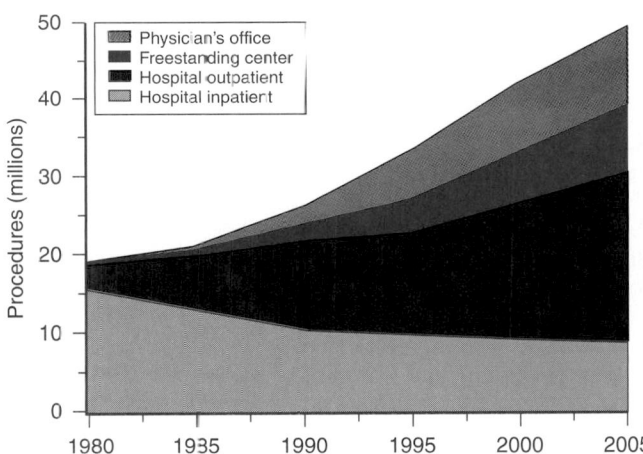

Figure 2–1 The growth of U.S. surgical procedures by site, 1980 to 2005. (Hospital data through 2001 from the American Hospital Association; freestanding surgery center and physician's office data through 1999 and all estimates after 1999 provided by Verispan, LLC, Chicago.)

a surgical procedure's diagnosis-related group. Suddenly, there was a potent financial incentive to perform surgical procedures (and other care) out of the hospital to escape the limitations imposed by these fixed rates. Thus, an increasing amount of surgery was shifted to the hospital's outpatient surgery facilities, where payment was based on the former, uncapped, cost-based system, which allowed the hospital flexibility in setting charges. Once ambulatory care's safety and cost savings became apparent, Medicare and other insurers covered an increasing array of procedures in hospital-independent, freestanding surgery centers, providing a substantial incentive for a further shift of hospital cases into the ambulatory setting.

Increasing cost-consciousness has encouraged the movement of surgery to the setting with the lowest costs: the surgeon's office. What was once only a site for biopsies and dental extractions has matured into freestanding, single-specialty (e.g., hand and cosmetic surgery, cataract extractions, hernia repair) surgery centers. Indeed, the surgeon's office has been the most rapidly growing surgical setting; at present it accounts for about one quarter of the national caseload. Anecdotal data report a similar movement of pain management to freestanding offices.

Although economics, enhanced technology, and a ready and willing public account for the development and flourishing of ambulatory surgical care, the main impetus of this transition in care is its apparent safety. The shift in locus of care could not have occurred unless patient outcomes were at least comparable to those associated with inpatient care, if not better. The corollary is that it behooves anesthesiologists practicing in these various ambulatory sites to maintain the same procedural and institutional safeguards required for high-quality care—including policies and procedures regarding patient and procedure selection as well as practice standards as they pertain to inpatient care. Mishaps occurring to high-profile persons undergoing office-based plastic surgery (usually reported without detail) are evidence of the potential danger of ambulatory procedures.[26] Additionally, catastrophes involving liposuction,[27] sedative drugs, and malignant hyperthermia in ambulatory procedure settings are poignant reminders that high standards must be maintained in all clinical settings. The ASA has prepared an information manual for all anesthesiologists administering anesthesia in an office.[28]

The emphasis on ambulatory procedures has enticed many non-anesthesiologists (emergency medicine and pediatric physicians, specially trained nurses) into the sedation business. Anesthesiologists, however, are responsible for promulgating guidelines for these groups. Burton Epstein, in his 2002 Rovenstein lecture, describes the history and effectiveness of these efforts.[29]

OTHER SITES

The need to provide anesthesia care in myriad non-OR "off-site" locations grows at a furious pace (see Chapter 69). As procedures become "less invasive" and do not need the facilities of an operating room, it is now easier to bring the anesthesia to the patient than the converse. Areas qualifying for the label "off the floor" or "in the outfield" encompass almost every specialty, including in vitro fertilization, lithotripsy, electroshock therapy, cardioversion, and, in the case of children, a variety of procedures for which sedation is often unsatisfactory (e.g., lumbar puncture, bone marrow biopsy, and various radiologic imaging procedures). These environments require special knowledge, equipment, and preparation. Strict adherence to practice standards in these non-surgical settings is critically important, and the ASA has developed a number of relevant standards of care. In this instance, "Guidelines for Nonoperating Room Anesthetizing Locations" (approved in 1994 and amended in 2003) is the appropriate guide.

Interventional neuroradiology, cardiac catheterization, and electrophysiologic laboratories are areas where new procedures seem to appear on a monthly basis. Radiology equipment, the need for shielding, and the fact that many of these laboratories were designed neither for the anesthesiologist nor with the necessary anesthesia equipment often make these procedures a special event. An exception to this is the fact that many of the newly constructed cardiac catheterization laboratories are designed with the ability to be converted to a complete operating room. On the other hand, the magnetic resonance imaging suite continues to be a less-than-hospitable place, whether we are called to care for a child, a trauma victim, or an inconsolable claustrophobic patient.

The cardiac electrophysiologic (EP) laboratory is a continual source of requests for care. Increasing knowledge of conducting systems of the heart permits electrical ablation of specific areas to control arrhythmias. Such procedures are extremely lengthy, and patients often become restless. Providing sedation and/or general anesthesia to these patients may be required. Additionally, the placement of implantable cardioverter-defibrillators, previously performed via a thoracotomy in the OR, is now carried out via the percutaneous route in the EP laboratory. Patients undergoing these procedures often have limited myocardial reserves and are being treated with a variety of antiarrhythmic drugs. Extensive knowledge of drug interactions in such cases is necessary, and the ability to support the circulation may be required.

POSTANESTHESIA CARE UNIT

Requirements for medical direction, nursing education, and the quality of services provided in PACUs are discussed in Chapter 71. With the evolution of new surgical procedures, it is now recognized that the same degree of vigilance that is vital in the OR must continue in the PACU. For example, the widespread use of laparoscopic procedures requires increased vigilance for unrecognized hemorrhage or bowel perforation, as well as early treatment of common emetic responses to the carbon-dioxide insufflating gas used for these procedures (see Chapter 57).

In the past, management of postoperative patients and the resources of the PACU was poorly defined. Now, a medical director must be designated, and it is his or her responsibility to ensure the delivery of appropriate standards of care. This responsibility is gaining importance because of the increasing regulations and severity of illness seen in these settings. The anesthesiologist can effectively manage the PACU to maximize the efficiency of that unit while providing the best possible anesthetic care.

The use of shorter-acting drugs and the prompt institution of effective pain relief, combined with acknowledged standards for PACU admission and discharge, have altered the approach to anesthetic recovery.[30] If a patient meets both anesthetic and surgical PACU criteria for discharge to a second-stage unit, there is no reason not to go directly to the secondary recovery area immediately from the operating room. This type of flexibility, much more than anesthetic drug costs, can influence labor costs crucial to cost containment in the PACU.[31]

It also merits mention that many PACUs serve as mini-ICU's for patients operated upon when the ICU is "full" and the complete panoply of critical care skills is needed to provide postoperative care.

CRITICAL CARE MEDICINE

Bendixen and colleagues, in 1965, reviewed the pathophysiology of respiratory failure and detailed methods of mechanical respiratory support in their seminal book *Respiratory Care*[32] (also see Chapter 75). This documented the beginning of anesthesiology's involvement with care of critically ill patients outside the operating room. Initially, our role was to provide adequate ventilation for a patient and to determine when weaning from mechanical ventilation was feasible. As it became obvious that respiratory function was only one aspect of care of the critically ill, anesthesiologists became knowledgeable in cardiovascular support, nutrition, infection, and various diagnostic procedures needed for these patients (see Chapter 74).

In 1986, the Residency Review Committee for Anesthesiology (RRCA) began to accredit training programs in critical care medicine (CCM) in departments that already had core residency training programs. At the same time, the ABA began examinations in CCM leading to subspecialty certification. This followed fruitless negotiations with the specialties of surgery and pulmonary medicine in attempting to define CCM jointly and to issue only one type of certification. Figure 2-2 demonstrates that there is interest in CCM by anesthesiology residents, although that interest has waned noticeably since publication of the last edition of this book. The number of CCM programs remains stable at around 50, with the number of trainees at a 10-year low of 50. Twenty percent of the programs reported no trainees in 2003, compared to approximately 500 trainees in pulmonary critical care. This is in marked contrast to the positive response following development of programs in pain management. This trend is unfortunate, because hospitals, given the transition to ambulatory care described previously, are devoting more and more of their bed space to intensive care. It also casts doubt on the vision of the anesthesiologist as the perioperative wizard.

One factor that may mitigate this loss of interest in critical care is recent research by Pronovost and colleagues, among others, that demonstrated improved outcomes in patients undergoing abdominal aneurysm resection when a physician specifically trained in critical care made daily rounds and directed postoperative care.[33] This has stimulated the Leapfrog Group, a consortium of corporate purchasers of health care, to specifically request that dedicated intensivists work in the settings with whom they contract. Related cost obstacles are imposing, but the effort continues.

Some hospitals are taking a global approach and forming ICU administration groups that include all relevant physician specialties and jointly decide medical and administrative policies. Critical care, however, is practiced not only in critical care units. With increasing frequency, PACUs are substituting for the inadequate number of critical care beds. Appropriate resources and personnel must therefore be available in the PACU to serve these patients in a manner that is similar to what is available in the ICU.

The ABA, the RRCA, and the Society of Academic Anesthesiology Chairs/ASA Program Directors are discussing a 48-month curriculum for anesthesiology training (to encompass the Clinical Base Year) that emphasizes much more extensive training in critical care.

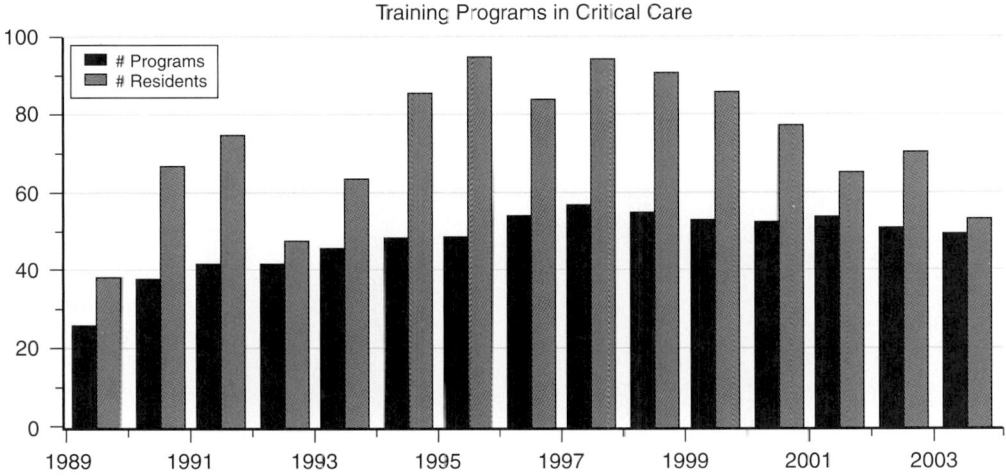

Figure 2–2 The number of critical care medicine programs in departments of anesthesiology and the number of residents in these programs for the years 1989-2003. (Data provided by the American Board of Anesthesiology.)

PAIN MANAGEMENT

John Bonica deserves credit for devoting time, effort, and interest in the understanding, diagnosis, and treatment of pain (see Chapter 73). Despite his entreaties, until recently most anesthesiology departments had devoted few resources—human, financial, or otherwise—to this area. Today, almost every medical facility (community, academic, and governmental) has the capability to treat acute and chronic pain, including cancer pain.

The recent development of acute pain services is yet another example of the expanding role of anesthesiologists in the medical center. We can now offer patients the prospect of a surgical experience that is totally (or almost totally) pain-free. The availability of intravenous patient-controlled analgesia, followed by other modalities such as intrathecal, epidural, and intrapleural infusions and continuous nerve blocks, mandated that acute pain services be developed. The anesthesiologist's role in limiting postoperative pain by the appropriate use of drugs and devices is a very positive aspect of our specialty.

Interest in training in pain management continues to increase (Fig. 2-3) although there was a slight decrease in 2003. About 230 residents are taking an additional year of training in about 100 pain programs. It is notable that 18% of the trainees in the field of pain medicine have their primary certification in Physical Medicine and Rehabilitation.

ANESTHESIA WORKFORCE

The workforce for anesthesia services continues to undergo dramatic change relating to its supply, diversity, and function. Historically an undersupplied specialty, unable to meet clinical demands in even the OR, the specialty of anesthesiology has grown rapidly since 1980.[34] Diverse trends account for this growth, including the increasing sophistication of anesthesia care, itself related to the maturation of subspecialty surgery (e.g., transplantation, cardiothoracic surgery, ambulatory care); increasing

incomes of physician specialists; and a doubling of the number of U.S. medical students graduating each year. Thus, anesthesiologists now work in sites well beyond the OR, including sites outside the hospital, as discussed previously. Indeed, by 1990, anesthesiologists devoted the majority of their professional time to recognized subspecialties (e.g., ambulatory, cardiothoracic, obstetric, and pediatric anesthesia, critical care medicine, and pain management). Clearly, anesthesiology has entered a period of maturation if not sophistication in its professional development.

The growth in the supply of anesthesiologists (208% during the period between 1975 and 2000, compared with 94% for the total physician supply[35]) has markedly altered the mix of anesthesia care providers. In the 1970s there were two nurse anesthetists for every anesthesiologist[36]; by the later 1980s the two provider groups had equal numbers. In 1991, there were about 21,000 nurse anesthetists and 25,000 anesthesiologists[36]; in 2000, there were 24,314 nurse anesthetists[37] and 35,699 anesthesiologists.[35] More than 500 anesthesiologists' assistants have also been trained since two training sites opened in the early 1970s. These personnel are deployed in a highly variable array of configurations, even in the same community, across the United States. Most anesthesia care is delivered by an anesthesia care team composed of an anesthesiologist directing nurse anesthetists and anesthesiology residents, with differing ratios among the provider types reflecting the composition of the care delivered. However, in much of the western part of the United States, anesthesiologists tend to provide direct care, without nurse anesthetists, and in rural areas nurse anesthetists often work in the absence of anesthesiologists.[34,36,38] Overall, there is an almost six-fold variation in the per capita presence of anesthesiologists across the United States (Fig. 2-4), itself suggesting that there is no consensus on the optimal or appropriate mix of anesthesia personnel.

As dramatic as these workforce changes have been, they constitute merely a prelude to future changes. The marked growth in the supply of anesthesiologists peaked by the mid-1990s, when the rate of production of new

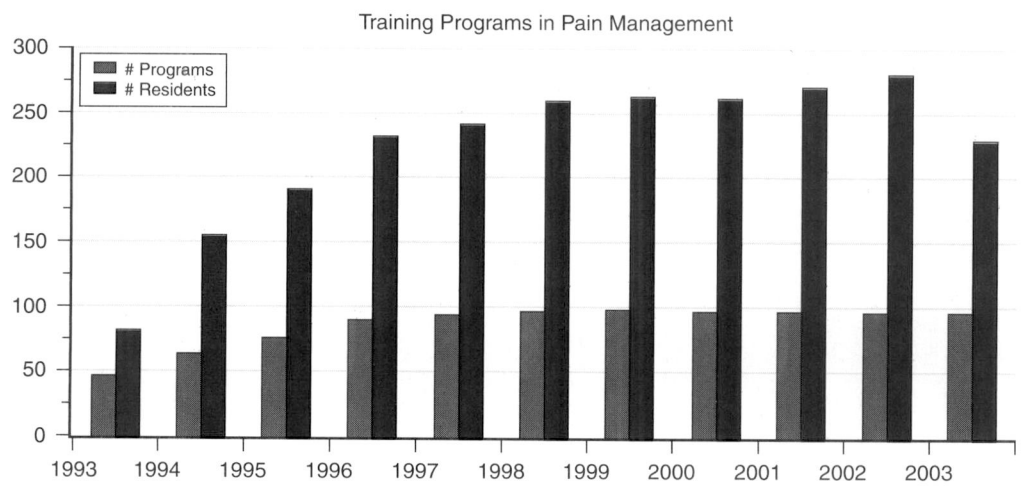

Figure 2–3 The number of pain management programs in departments of anesthesiology and the number of residents in these programs for the years 1993-2003. (Data provided by the American Board of Anesthesiology.)

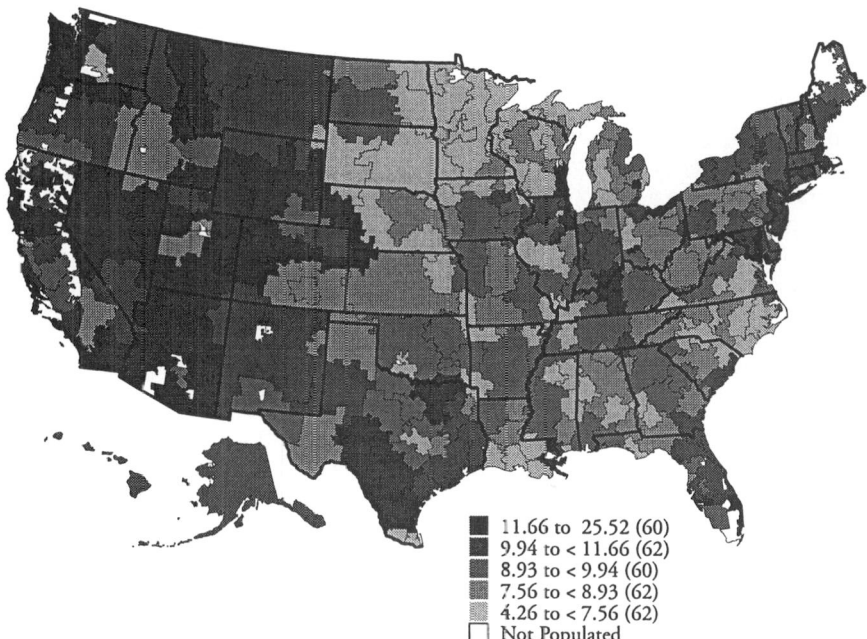

Figure 2–4 The geographic distribution of anesthesiologists per 100,000 population, by hospital referral region in 1996, ranged from 4.3 (Harlingen, Texas) to 25.5 (Hinsdale, Illinois). (From Wennberg and Cooper.[42] Copyright, the Trustees of Dartmouth College, 1997.)

■ 11.66 to 25.52 (60)
■ 9.94 to < 11.66 (62)
■ 8.93 to < 9.94 (60)
■ 7.56 to < 8.93 (62)
□ 4.26 to < 7.56 (62)
□ Not Populated

practitioners was about three times that of attrition.[34] As a result, coupled with marketplace changes related to the accelerating growth of managed care, graduates experienced difficulty finding jobs, medical students shunned the specialty, and new trainee cohorts more closely approximated attrition (perhaps 800 per year). Professional opportunities again seem adequate, but looming on the horizon are diverse factors that are likely to alter the equilibrium if not the practice of anesthesiology.

Among factors that may encourage more students to opt for anesthesiology are the emerging recognition that the shortage of primary care physicians proclaimed early in the decade was either quickly corrected or a forecasting error; further expansion of the anesthesiologist's role and practice sites; and increasing amount and sophistication of surgery for a graying population. As mentioned earlier, the desire of medical students to train in specialties that permit a controllable lifestyle must be appreciated. As an aside, it is interesting that, with the institution of the 80-hour duty limits mandated by the Accreditation Council for Graduate Medical Education (ACGME), general surgery programs have experienced an unprecedented increase in applications. Certain factors may dissuade students from choosing anesthesiology as a specialty. These include the continued political fight to alter Medicare regulations (that are being adopted by private insurers), fostering independent practice by nurse anesthetists; further decreases in federal support of graduate medical education, especially specialist training; continued increases in students' already high loan indebtedness coupled with potential reductions in anesthesiologists' income relative to those of other specialties; new technology that makes some anesthesia services appear so safe that non-anesthesia personnel may provide them (e.g., propofol sedation[39]); and possibly greater instability in professional opportunities in an increasingly competitive health care marketplace. Thus, a grand and most dynamic interplay among diverse factors—far more complex than merely potential numbers of services to be provided and numbers of personnel being trained and lost to attrition—will influence future anesthesia workforce requirements.

VALUE-BASED ANESTHESIA CARE

A feast-and-famine health care marketplace had developed by the early 1990s in the United States. Several decades of runaway escalation of health care costs at two to three times the general economy's inflation rate, coupled with a large uninsured segment of the population and health indices (e.g., life span, infant mortality) below those of countries with lower per capita health care spending, indicated misallocation of resources in the U.S. health care system. When federal reform failed in 1994, the marketplace accelerated the ongoing fundamental restructuring of health care financing and delivery. What has resulted is a payer-dominated, constrained, increasingly competitive health care marketplace that seeks greater value, which may be represented as

$$Value = Quality/Cost$$

Value-based anesthesia care is a neologism advanced to encourage anesthesiologists to look beyond widely misunderstood concepts, such as cost-effectiveness, to focus on enhancing the value of care by providing the best patient outcome achievable at reasonable cost.[40] A large literature documents that perhaps 25% of care is inappropriate,[41] that large variations in resource use for similar care exist across small geographic areas,[42] and that higher utilization of services is not associated with improved health status or quality of care[43,44]; thus it is clear that quality and cost are not tightly linked: Better quality is not necessarily associated with higher cost, nor does spending less (by doing less) necessarily lead to lower quality.

Insights into the relationship between patient outcome (or benefit) and cost may be gleaned by noting the relationship between overall health benefit and incremental inputs to health care (Fig. 2-5A).[45] As in other productive endeavors, the anesthesiologist should continue to add resources (e.g., newer and more costly drugs, special patient monitoring, adjunctive pain management protocols) as long as the result is positive benefits. Beyond "the top of the curve," the point of maximal benefit and thus optimal investment, further investment merely results in negative benefit (e.g., complications,

higher cost without patient benefit). Although it is commonly believed that our health care system has passed the top of the curve, we may "rationalize" our decision-making by reducing investment and moving back to the point of maximal benefit (Fig. 2-5B).[46]

Seemingly arcane, this economic construct applies well to most decisions anesthesiologists face, including drug choice, equipment acquisition, and administrative policies. Common to each decision is choosing the appropriate technology or using technology appropriately. (We must acknowledge that medical technology is not limited to devices such as patient monitors; according to the former congressional Office of Technology Assessment, it also includes drugs, medical and surgical procedures, protocols, support systems, and organizational systems through which health-care professionals deliver care.[47]) The challenge of knowing when we are doing what is "appropriate" (and no more or less) is especially difficult because our knowledge of the effectiveness of our clinical practices, among other complex issues, is incomplete.[41] The quandary is further complicated because of our rudimentary understanding of outcomes and economics, which extend well beyond the purely clinical and financial, to include quality of life, patient preferences, and patient-based assessment of care, among other seemingly subjective topics.[48] Although general[49,50] and anesthesia-specific[48,51,52] guidance is available, few anesthesiologists have sufficient time or expertise to undertake this outcomes-related research. Yet anesthesiologists must develop an appreciation of the considerations when evaluating or planning value-based comparisons of care (Table 2-1).

Once a potential, value-enhancing practice change is identified from the work of others (e.g., an article in a professional journal) or through research in one's own institution, the next challenge is implementation. In truth, there is no shortage of good ideas, but putting

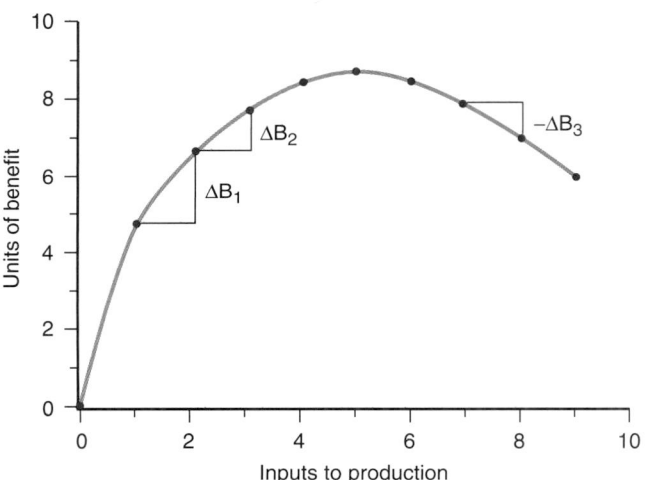

A

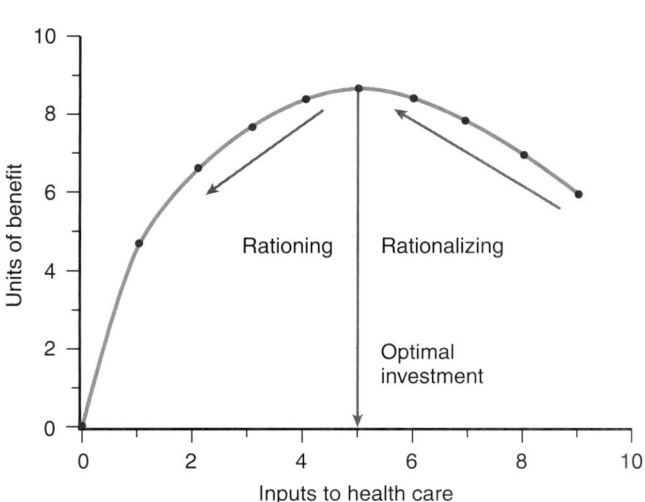

B

Figure 2–5 A, The hypothetical relationship between inputs to a productive process and the benefits derived describes a production function. As investment continues, the net benefit, segment ΔB^n, progressively decreases and then becomes negative, illustrating the law of diminishing returns.
B, Rationalizing rather than rationing health-care technology achieves maximal benefit at "the top of the curve," a level of investment associated with the optimal investment. (**A** is reproduced from Orkin[45]; **B** is modified from Orkin[45] and Reinhardt.[46])

Table 2–1   Considerations in value-based comparisons of care

Include economic considerations in clinical decision-making: it is neither unethical nor immoral.

Be explicit in a comparison; assume nothing, if possible: nothing is "obvious."

Identify all possible benefits and risks associated with alternative clinical approaches.

Focus on costs, not charges (e.g., patient bills).

Capture indirect costs (e.g., patient's out-of-pocket losses) as well as direct costs.

Focus on marginal differences related to alternative approaches rather than on overall cost of care.

Emphasize real outcomes (e.g., myocardial infarction) rather than intermediate or surrogate end points (e.g., myocardial ischemia), unless they are highly associated.

Do not lose sight of implications of early "savings" on events "downstream" in the care process.

Opt for lower-cost approach unless value is demonstrated in higher-cost alternative.

Modified from Orkin.[40]

them into action is often difficult. A major problem is inertia within the institution (e.g., "We always do it this way"). Moreover, even when an improved practice is implemented, the improvement is usually short-lived, due to regression to former practice patterns. (For example, a new departmental policy dictates use of specified lower-cost drugs with similar patient outcomes in each drug class; however, if the full array of drugs remains readily available, backsliding often occurs.) Maintenance of the desired improvement requires fundamental change in practice patterns. As an authority on achieving improvement in institutions notes, "Every system is perfectly designed to get the results it gets."[53] Thus, lasting improvement requires modifying systems and related care processes to sustain desired practice patterns that enhance the value of care.

Substantial cost savings without apparent adverse outcomes are possible through adoption of department-defined pharmaceutical practice guidelines for limiting use of several high-cost drugs.[54] Acceptance ("buy-in") of the guidelines is achieved, in part, through soliciting comments from all anesthesia care providers and including among the guideline committees ardent proponents of particular drugs. Compliance is maintained by several mechanisms, including widely publicizing the department's successes, periodic feedback to each provider on his or her practice patterns, making compliance with the guidelines more convenient than noncompliance, and permitting departures from the guidelines in appropriate circumstances.

Ideally, we want to concentrate our improvement efforts where they will have the greatest effect; however, in many situations we have only vague impressions, in part because the processes of care are themselves so complicated and outcomes are typically not tracked. A variety of sources can guide the focus of improvement efforts: patient complaints, staff suggestions, critical incident reports, accreditation survey results, benchmarking (i.e., comparison with similar institutions), statewide databases, peer review organization results, and articles in professional journals. Figure 2-6 provides a framework for conceptualizing the improvement effort once a focus is chosen. Improving the care requires that we understand the underlying processes, particularly when there may be wasted time and resources.[55] Flowcharting the core processes by a team composed of representatives of the personnel involved intimately in the care helps to identify potential opportunities for improvement. An initiative is adopted and pilot-tested in the care setting, and appropriate outcomes are tracked. Besides the purely clinical, other outcomes include patient satisfaction (e.g., decrease in wait times and delays, adequacy of instructions) and cost (including institutional performance). If improvement is documented, the relevant processes are modified to "hold the gain"; regardless of whether improvement occurs, the team moves on to other improvement opportunities. Although superficially resembling what institutions have been doing to satisfy external requirements (e.g., accreditation) for clinical tracking on a limited number of indicators, this measurement approach is more flexible and serves the need to enhance the value of care.

EDUCATION

The RRCA governs resident training (see also Chapter 85). It is charged by the ACGME with developing standards for residency education, which are reviewed and revised every 5 years, and with inspecting and evaluating all residency programs, both core and subspecialty. The parent organizations for the RRCA are the ABA, the ASA, and the American Medical Association (AMA). In 1998, a resident member was added to the RRCA, bringing the unique and welcome view of a trainee to the discussions.

As mentioned previously and as depicted in Figure 2-7, American medical student interest in the specialty of anesthesiology, which declined dramatically, secondary to the perception that there were few practice opportunities, has rebounded nicely.

Starting on January 1, 2000, the ABA, similar to most other specialty boards, began to issue time-limited certificates (10-year limit). In order to recertify, all diplomates must participate in a developing program called Maintenance of Certification in Anesthesiology (MOCA). Those diplomates whose certificates are not time-limited may participate voluntarily. The MOCA program emphasizes continuous self-improvement—a cornerstone of

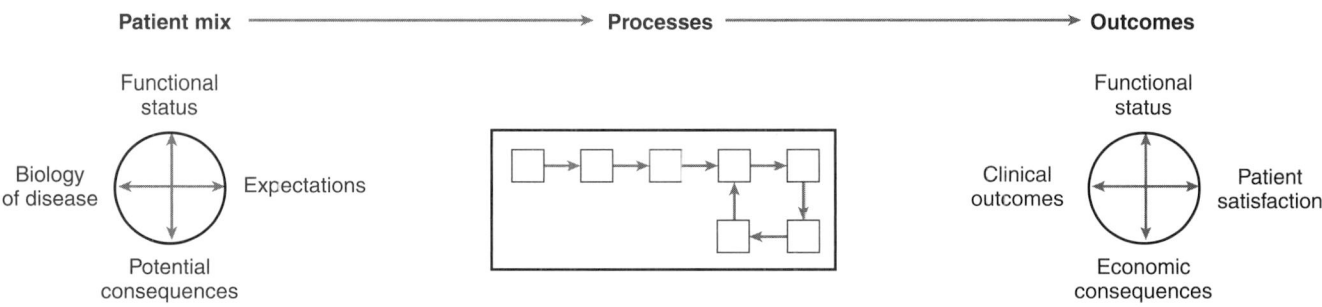

Figure 2–6 General schema for improving the value of health care by applying the clinical value compass model. (Modified from Nelson et al.[55]) Underlying this framework are several assumptions: health is composed of biologic, physical, mental, and social aspects; the aim of health care is to reduce or limit the burden of illness by restoring or improving health functioning; quality health care provides care processes most likely to achieve the health outcomes desired by the patient at a price representing value for that patient; and the value of health care is a function of quality, costs, and volume.

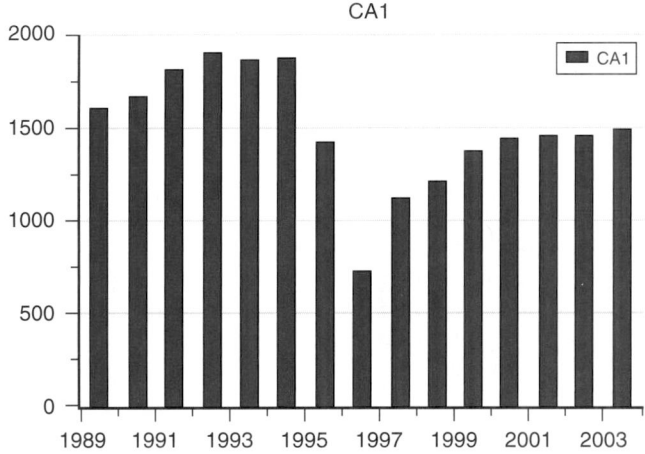

Figure 2–7 Number of first-year residents in anesthesiology registered with the American Board of Anesthesiology over the years 1989-2003. (Data provided by the American Board of Anesthesiology.)

professional excellence—and evaluation of clinical skills and practice performance to assure quality as well as public accountability. The components include a measure of professional standing (unrestricted state licensure), a commitment to lifelong learning (formal and informal continuing medical education), cognitive expertise (taking and passing a secure examination), and evaluation of current practice.

FUTURE DIRECTIONS

Predicting the future is a hazardous business. It is safe to say that the period until the publication of the next edition of this book will be just as tumultuous and challenging for the specialty as the period since the last edition.

The Department of Health and Human Services reported that health care spending for 2002 increased 9.3% to a total of $1.55 trillion, 15% of the GDP. And this is before the baby boomers reach Medicare age![56] Presumably, this will exert further downward influence on patient insurance benefits as well as on physician payment. This—along with continued technological advances, including the development of more rapid-acting, easily controllable, and reversible drugs, more reliable monitoring equipment, and newer less invasive surgical procedures—will mandate review of optimal methods for the delivery of anesthesia care.

In Europe, training schemes for non-physicians vary from as little as one year (for advanced nurses) to supervision ratios as high as 1:6. Are such situations as safe as our current practice? If so, should our role as rescue physicians be expanded? The role of the anesthesiologist in providing moderate sedation will most certainly be reviewed when the issue of "medical necessity" again is posed. Why is an anesthesiologist needed for colonoscopy procedures in New York but not in Iowa City? (Medicare reports a $50 million or 50% increase in this anesthesia code in 2002.) We need to define the best role for ourselves as physicians with unique skill sets.

KEY POINTS

1. Anesthesiology's scope of practice encompasses the entire perioperative experience from preoperative evaluation to intraoperative anesthesia care (in almost any clinical setting, including hospital OR, obstetric suite, ambulatory surgery clinic, procedure room, freestanding ambulatory surgery center, and surgeon's office), to recovery in the postanesthesia care unit or ICU, and even the patient's home. Additional venues for nonsurgical anesthesia care include the obstetrics suite, chronic pain clinic, and intensive care unit. Anesthesiologists also teach resuscitative skills and conduct research to advance future practice.

2. The anesthesiologist's preoperative assessment has multiple objectives, including evaluation of health status, identification of opportunities to enhance health status with the hope of improving patient outcomes, discussion of an anesthetic plan, patient education, and encouragement of greater family involvement in care.

3. Because of their broad medical knowledge and scope of professional activity, anesthesiologists are increasingly involved in management of the OR, to improve efficiency, control costs, enhance institutional performance, and improve quality of care.

4. Anesthesia care is now given throughout the modern hospital in an increasing array of non-OR, alternate site settings: interventional radiology suite, cardiac electrophysiology laboratory, lithotripsy suite, and settings in which cardioversion and electroshock therapy are administered. Patient safety is maintained by adhering to the same clinical practice standards observed in the OR.

5. Among the most significant trends in surgical care since the 1980s is the shift of about 75% of surgery procedures from the inpatient hospital setting to a variety of ambulatory venues, including the hospital outpatient unit, freestanding ambulatory surgery center, and surgeon's office. Maintenance of the specialty's widely recognized success in achieving markedly improved patient safety requires meeting the same high standards of care, regardless of setting.

6. Anesthesiologists were among the pioneers in establishing critical care medicine; the specialty trains substantial numbers of future critical care specialists, and recent research documents that the presence of dedicated critical care specialists is associated with better patient outcomes.

7. Anesthesiologists have been leaders in developing pain management as a subspecialty that improves patient comfort postoperatively and quality of life for those with chronic pain.

8. Anesthesia care is subject to dynamic clinical, social, economic, and political forces that preclude accurate workforce requirement projections beyond a short-term horizon. Workforce needs must be reevaluated periodically as circumstances and assumptions change and evolve.

9. Like other health care practitioners, anesthesiologists face myriad opportunities to improve quality of care and enhance institutional performance through objective evaluation of care practices and patient outcomes and by implementing data-driven quality improvement projects.

REFERENCES

1. Schwinn DA, Booth JV: Genetics infuses new life into human physiology: Implications of the Human Genome Project for anesthesiology and perioperative medicine. Anesthesiology 96:261-263, 2002.
2. Angell M: The American health care system revisited—A new series. N Engl J Med 340:48, 1999.
3. Kutter R: The American health care system: Health insurance coverage. N Engl J Med 340:163-168, 1999.
4. Moon M: Medicare. N Engl J Med 344:928-931, 2001.
5. Klein SM, Greengrass RA, Gleason DH, et al: Major ambulatory surgery with continuous regional anesthesia and a disposable infusion pump. Anesthesiology 19:563-570, 1999.
6. Dorsey ER, Jarjoura D, Rutecki GW: Influence of controllable lifestyle on recent trends in specialty choice by US medical students. JAMA 290:1173-1178, 2003.
7. American Board of Anesthesiology: Booklet of Information. Raleigh, NC: American Board of Anesthesiology, 2004.
8. Abenstein JP, Warner MA: Anesthesia providers, patient outcomes, and costs. Anesth Analg 82:1273-1283, 1996.
9. Zambricki CS: "Anesthesia providers, patient outcomes, and costs": The AANA responds to the Abenstein and Warner article in the June 1996 Anesthesia and Analgesia. AANA J 64:413-463, 1996.
10. Silber JH, Kennedy SK, Even-Shoshan O, et al: Anesthesiologist direction and patient outcomes. Anesthesiology 93:152-153, 2000.
11. Silber JH, Kennedy SK, Even-Shoshan O, et al: Anesthesiologist board certification and patient outcomes. Anesthesiology 96:1044-1052, 2002.
12. Pine M, Holt KD, Lou Y-B: Surgical mortality and type of anesthesia provider. AANA J 71:109-116, 2003.
13. Fischer SP: Development and effectiveness of an anesthesia preoperative evaluation clinic in a teaching hospital. Anesthesiology 85:196-206, 1996.
14. Roizen MF: Cost-effective preoperative laboratory testing. JAMA 271:319-320, 1994.
15. Roizen MF: Preoperative evaluation: A shared vision for change. J Clin Anesth 9:435-463, 1997.
16. Klafta JM, Roizen MF: Current understanding of patients' attitudes toward and preparation for anesthesia: A review. Anesth Analg 83:1314-1321, 1996.
17. Eagle KA, Berger PB, Calkins H, et al: ACC/AHA guideline update for perioperative cardiovascular evaluation for non cardiac surgery—Executive summary. A report of the American College of Cardiology / American Heart Association Task Force on Practice Guidelines (Committee to Update the 1996 Guidelines on Perioperative Cardiovascular Evaluation for Noncardiac Surgery). Anesth Analg 94:1052-1064, 2002.
18. Fleisher LA: Evaluation of the patient with cardiac disease undergoing noncardiac surgery: an update on the original AHA/ACC guidelines. Int Anesthesiol Clin 40:109-120, 2002.
19. Needlestick-prevention devices. Focus on blood collection devices and catheters. Health Devices 27:184-232, 1998.
20. Overdyk FJ, Harvey SC, Fishman RL, Shippey F: Successful strategies for improving operating room efficiency at academic institutions. Anesth Analg 86:896-906, 1998.
21. Truong A, Tessler MJ, Kleiman SJ, Bensimon M: Late operating room starts: Experience with an education trial. Can J Anaesth 43:1233-1236, 1996.
22. Dexter F, Wachtel EE, Yue JCh: Use of discharge abstract databases to differentiate among pediatric hospitals based on operative procedures: Surgery in infants and young children in the state of Iowa. Anesthesiology 99:480-487, 2003.
23. Dexter F, Epstein RH: Scheduling of cases in an ambulatory center. Anesthesiol Clin North Am 21:1387-1402, 2003.
24. Dexter F, Traub RD, Qian F: Comparison of statistical methods to predict the time to complete a series of surgical cases. J Clin Monit Comput 15:45-51, 1999.
25. Surgical Procedures, 1981-2007. Chicago: SMG Marketing Group, Verispan, January 2001.
26. Kaufman L: Olivia Goldsmith Is Dead at 54; Wrote Comic "First Wives Club." New York Times, January 16, 2004.
27. Rao RB, Ely SF, Hoffman RS: Deaths related to liposuction. N Engl J Med 340:1471-1475, 1999.
28. Office-Based Anesthesia—Considerations for Anesthesiologists in Setting Up and Maintaining a Safe Office Anesthesia Environment. The American Society of Anesthesiologists, May 10, 2002.
29. Epstein BS: The American Society of Anesthesiologist's efforts in developing guidelines for sedation and analgesia for nonanesthesiologists. Anesthesiology 98:1261-1269, 2003.
30. Apfelbaum JL, Walawander CA, Grasela TH, et al: Eliminating intensive postoperative care in same-day surgery patients using short-acting anesthetics. Anesthesiology 97:66-74, 2002.
31. Dexter F, Tinker JH: Analysis of strategies to decrease postanesthesia care unit costs. Anesthesiology 82:94-101, 1995.
32. Bendixen HH, Egbert L, Hedley-Whyte J, et al: Respiratory Care. St. Louis: Mosby, 1965.
33. Pronovost PJ, Jenckes MW, Dorman T, et al: Organizational characteristics of intensive care units related to outcomes. JAMA 281:1310, 1999.
34. Orkin FK: Work force planning for anesthesia care. Int Anesthesiol Clin 33:101, 1995.
35. Pasko T, Seidman B: Physician Characteristics and Distribution in the US, 2002-2003. Chicago, American Medical Association, 2002.
36. Rosenbach M, Cromwell J: A profile of anesthesia practice patterns. Health Affairs 7:118-131, 1988.
37. The Registered Nurse Population: Findings from the National Sample Survey of Registered Nurses. Washington: Bureau of Health Professions, Department of Health and Human Services, 2001.
38. Orkin FK: Rural realities. Anesthesiology 88:568-571, 1998.
39. Rex DK, Overly C, Kinser K, et al: Safety of propofol administered by registered nurses with gastroenterologist supervision in 2000 endoscopic cases. Am J Gastroenterology 97:1159-1163, 2002.
40. Orkin FK: Moving toward value-based anesthesia care. J Clin Anesth 5:91-98, 1993.
41. Naylor CD: What is appropriate care? N Engl J Med 338:1918-1920, 1998.
42. Wennberg JE, Cooper MM (eds): The Dartmouth Atlas of Health Care. Chicago, American Hospital Publishing, 1998.
43. Fisher ES, Wennberg DE, Stukel TA, et al: The implications of regional variations in Medicare spending. Part 1: The content, quality, and accessibility of care. Ann Intern Med 138:273-287, 2003.
44. Fisher ES, Wennberg DE, Stukel TA, et al: The implications of regional variations in Medicare spending. Part 2: Health outcomes and satisfaction with care. Ann Intern Med 138:288-298, 2003.
45. Orkin FK: Practice standards: The Midas touch or the emperor's new clothes? [editorial]. Anesthesiology 70:567-571, 1989.
46. Reinhardt U: Health Care Quality Management for the 21st Century. Tampa, FL, American College of Physician Executives, 1991.
47. Office of Technology Assessment, U.S. Congress: Strategies for Medical Technology Assessment, 3rd ed. Washington, DC, U.S. Government Printing Office, 1982.
48. Orkin FK: Outcomes research in anesthesia. Adv Anesthes 16:99-128, 1999.

49. Eisenberg JM: Clinical economics: A guide to the economic analysis of clinical practices. JAMA 262:2879-2886, 1989.

50. Drummond MF, O'Brien B, Stoddart G, et al: Methods for the Economic Evaluation of Health Care Programmes, 2nd ed. New York, Oxford University Press, 1997.

51. Sperry RJ: Principles of economic analysis. Anesthesiology 86:1197-1205, 1997.

52. Watcha MF, White PF: Economics of anesthetic practice. Anesthesiology 86:1170-1196, 1997.

53. Berwick DM: A primer on leading the improvement of systems. Br Med J 312:619-622, 1996.

54. Lubarsky DA, Glass PSA, Ginsburg B, et al: The successful implementation of pharmaceutical practice guidelines: Analysis of associated outcomes and cost savings. Anesthesiology 86:1145-1160, 1997.

55. Nelson EC, Batalden PB, Ryer JC (eds): The Clinical Improvement Action Guide. Oak Brook, IL, Joint Commission on Accreditation of Healthcare Organizations, 1998.

56. Pear R: Health spending rises to 15% of economy, a record level. New York Times, January 9, 2004.

CHAPTER

3 Basic Principles of Pharmacology Related to Anesthesia

Steven L. Shafer and Debra A. Schwinn

Pharmacokinetics 68
Overview 68
Fundamental Pharmacokinetic
Concepts 68
Pharmacokinetic Models 76
Summary of Pharmacokinetics 84

Pharmacodynamics 84
Overview 84
Transduction of Biologic Signals 85

Developments in Molecular Pharmacology 93
Clinical Evaluation of Drug Effects 95

**Variability in Drug
Response 97**
Pharmacogenetics 97
Patient Physiology 100
Drug Interactions 101

Summary 102

Anesthesia involves administration of drugs to produce therapeutic effects while minimizing undesirable side effects or toxicity. Anesthesiologists give drugs to provide analgesia, amnesia, hypnosis, and muscle relaxation; they also administer drugs to manipulate major organ systems pharmacologically to maintain homeostasis and prevent injury. The therapeutic objective is to achieve adequate drug concentrations at specific sites of action to produce the desired effect. The anesthesiologist must select and administer appropriate drugs to provide tissue and receptor concentrations lower than those that produce unacceptable toxicity and higher than those that fail to provide effective therapy (i.e., within the therapeutic window).

The empirical approach to drug administration consists of selecting an initial dose and then titrating subsequent doses based on the clinical responses of the patient. The ability of the anesthesiologist to predict clinical response and to select optimal doses is part of the art of anesthesia. Continued research in the basic and clinical pharmacology of anesthetic drugs has produced guidelines by which the science of anesthesiology can enhance the art.

This chapter is divided into three major sections: pharmacokinetic principles, pharmacodynamic principles, and the principles that underlie variability in drug response. The pharmacokinetics section describes the relationship between drug administration and drug concentration at the site of action. Essential components of pharmacokinetics include volumes of distribution of drug within the tissues, systemic clearance (usually hepatic metabolism for intravenous anesthetics), biologic activity of metabolites, transfer of drugs between plasma and tissues, and binding of drugs to circulating plasma proteins. This section introduces the physiologic processes that determine pharmacokinetics and the mathematical models used to relate dose to concentration.

The pharmacodynamics section explores the relationship between drug concentration and pharmacologic effect. The broad areas of transduction of biologic signals, including fundamental receptor theory and structure, the role of new developments in molecular biology, and clinical evaluation of drug effects are presented.

The third section explores the processes that contribute to variability in drug response. They include pharmacogenetics, influence of the patient's physiology on pharmacokinetics and pharmacodynamics, and drug interactions.

An understanding of fundamental pharmacokinetic and pharmacodynamic principles provides the anesthesiologist with a scientific foundation for using drugs to achieve specific therapeutic objectives. These principles form the basis for the application of pharmacologic science to the practice of anesthesia. Exploring the basics of pharmacogenetics provides state-of-the-art pharmacologic and genetic information to understand important sources of variability in drug response.

PHARMACOKINETICS

Overview

Pharmacokinetics is the relationship between dose and the resulting concentration in plasma or the effect site. The processes of absorption, distribution, and clearance govern this relationship. Absorption is not relevant to intravenously administered drugs, but it is highly relevant to all other routes of drug delivery. The pharmacokinetic profiles of intravenously administered drugs are determined by distribution volumes and the process of clearance. We discuss the physiologic basis of pharmacokinetics and then review basic pharmacokinetic models that relate dose to plasma or tissue concentration.

Fundamental Pharmacokinetic Concepts

Volume of Distribution

The distribution of a drug throughout the plasma and tissues can be viewed as a process of dilution from the highly concentrated solution in the syringe to the dilute concentration in the plasma. This dilution results from mixing of a drug into a larger volume. The pharmacokinetic concept of volume is the apparent size of the tank required to explain the observed drug concentration. Figure 3-1 shows the dilution of administered drug into a tank of fluid. By definition, the concentration in the tank is the amount of drug administered divided by the volume of the tank. If we do not know the volume beforehand but can measure the concentration, we can rearrange the definition of concentration to ascertain the volume of the tank:

$$\text{Volume} = \frac{\text{Amount (or dose)}}{\text{Concentration}} \qquad (1)$$

When the volume of the tank is known, the concentration after any bolus of drug can be calculated as the dose divided by the volume. Just as the tank has a volume with or without drug in it, the volume of distribution of a particular drug is an intrinsic property of the individual with or without drug administration. Unlike the tank in

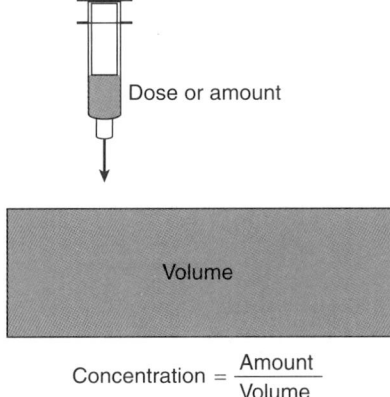

$$\text{Concentration} = \frac{\text{Amount}}{\text{Volume}}$$

Figure 3–1 Volume represents the dilution of drug from the more concentrated form in the syringe to the dilute form in the blood.

Figure 3-1, the volume of distribution also depends on the properties of the drug.

Central Volume of Distribution

If we assume that the drug is injected into an arm vein and that the initial concentration is measured in an artery, the central volume of distribution reflects the volume of the heart and great vessels and the venous volume of the upper arm. It also reflects drug uptake by the lungs. For example, alfentanil is less lipophilic than fentanyl or sufentanil, resulting in less pulmonary uptake of alfentanil than fentanyl or sufentanil. This characteristic results in a smaller central volume for alfentanil than fentanyl or sufentanil. The central volume also reflects any metabolism that occurs between the venous injection site and the arterial sample.

Of the pharmacokinetic concepts introduced in this chapter, the central volume of distribution is the most problematic. The concept is based on an incorrect notion that the plasma concentration after bolus injection instantaneously mixes in this volume, resulting in an instantaneous peak at the moment of injection. However, mixing is not instantaneous, and at the moment of intravenous injection, the arterial drug concentration is 0. The peak concentration is usually seen within 30 to 40 seconds of the injection. This 30- to 40-second delay is of no consequence for most therapeutics outside of anesthesia, but within the field of anesthesia, the pharmacokinetic determinants of anesthetic induction are clinically important. The mathematics of the true time course, including the time delay and recirculatory peaks, have been worked out in detail and are shown in Figure 3-2.[1]

Despite the assumption of instantaneous mixing, the concept of central volume of distribution is useful. The central volume represents the backward (and upward) extrapolation of the concentration versus time curve from its peak at about 30 seconds to the y axis. It can be thought of as the initial concentration if circulation had been infinitely fast. Because of this backward extrapolation, estimates of the central volume are highly influenced by study design. A study with arterial samples has higher initial concentrations and therefore estimates a smaller central volume than a study with venous samples. The timing of blood samples also influences the central volume of distribution. Over the first 2 or 3 minutes after bolus injection, the concentration of anesthetic drugs falls very rapidly. If the first sample is drawn at 30 seconds, the backward extrapolation of the concentration versus time curve to the y axis predicts a high concentration at time 0 and a small central volume. If the first sample is drawn at 5 minutes, the backward extrapolation of the concentration versus time curve to the y axis predicts a much lower concentration and a larger central volume.

Peripheral Volumes of Distribution

Anesthetic drugs distribute extensively into peripheral tissues. This distribution into the periphery is represented pharmacokinetically as additional volumes of distribution that are attached to the central volume. Peripheral volumes are linked to the central compartment (i.e., plasma) by blood flow, a process called *intercompartmental clearance*.

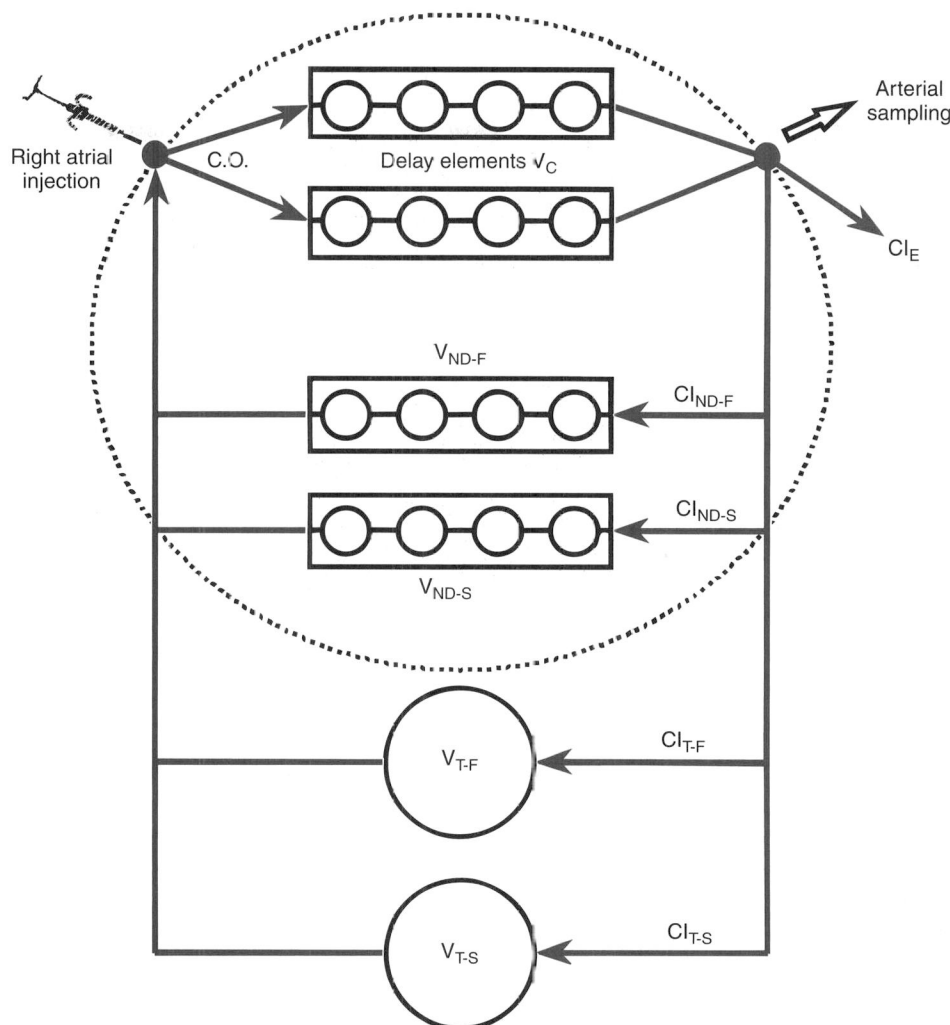

Figure 3–2 A recirculatory model accounting for cardiac output (C.O.), transit delays and pulmonary uptake (Delay elements V_C), and nondistributive mixing pathways (V_{ND} and Cl_{ND}). All components within the *dashed circle* are required to accurately model the central volume of distribution. In most situations, this complexity is not required, and the simpler approach of assuming instantaneous mixing within the central volume is an adequate approximation. Cl_{ND-F} and Cl_{ND-S}, fast and slow nondistributive clearances; Cl_{T-F} and Cl_{T-S}, fast and slow tissue clearances; V_{ND-F} and V_{ND-S}, fast and slow nondistributive volumes; V_{T-F} and V_{T-S}, fast and slow tissue volumes. (From Krejcie TC, Avram MJ, Gentry WB, et al: A recirculatory model of the pulmonary uptake and pharmacokinetics of lidocaine based on analysis of arterial and mixed venous data from dogs. J Pharmacokinet Biopharm 25: 169-190, 1997.)

The linkage of peripheral volumes to a central volume is called a *mammillary model,* a name that refers to the structure of the plumbing: peripheral piglets suckling off a central (mother) pig.

The size of the peripheral volumes of distribution reflects the drug's solubility in tissue relative to blood or plasma. The more soluble a drug is in peripheral tissues relative to blood or plasma, the larger are the peripheral volumes of distribution. Because the tissue solubility of a drug depends on simple physiochemical constants, it would seem likely that peripheral volumes of distribution would be consistent from person to person. However, differences in body habitus and composition influence peripheral volumes of distribution.

Peripheral volumes of distribution explain the apparent dilution of the drug into all body tissues. We usually do not know the actual solubility of drugs in peripheral tissues. For the purpose of calculating drug dosage, a small mass of tissue with high solubility for the drug is indistinguishable from a large mass of tissue with low solubility. The convention in pharmacokinetics is to assume that the solubility of the drug in tissue is the same as the solubility in plasma. This assumption does not compromise the role of peripheral compartments to characterize the dilution of drugs into tissues, but it does lead to very large volumes of distribution for highly soluble drugs (e.g., 5000 L for propofol).

The volume of distribution at steady state is the volume that relates the plasma drug concentration at steady state (i.e., during a very long infusion) to the total amount of drug in the body. By rearranging the definition of concentration, we can calculate the volume of distribution at steady state as the total amount of drug in the body at steady state divided by the plasma drug concentration. The volume of distribution at steady state equals the central volume plus the peripheral volumes.

Clearance

Clearance is the process that removes drug from a volume. Systemic clearance permanently removes drug from the body by elimination or by transforming it into metabolites. Intercompartmental clearance moves drug from the plasma into peripheral tissues. *Clearance* is defined as the volume that is completely cleared of drug per unit of time. The units of clearance are therefore units of flow: volume per unit time (e.g., liters per minute). Clearance is most

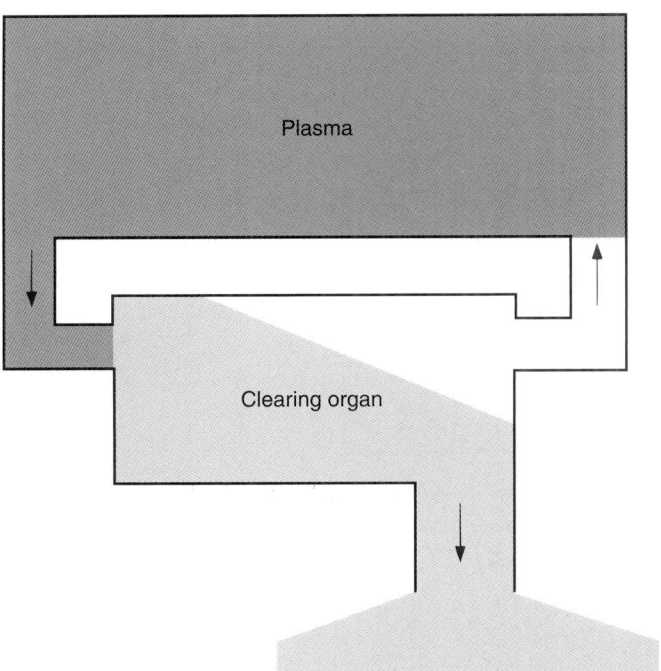

Figure 3–3 Clearance represents the flow of blood or plasma that is completely cleared of drug. If all of the drug is extracted by the clearing organ (i.e., extraction ratio ≈ 1), clearance is the flow to the organ, as illustrated here. (Adapted from Shafer S: Principles of pharmacokinetics and pharmacodynamics. *In* Longnecker DE, Tinker JH, Morgan GE [eds]: Principles and Practice of Anesthesiology, 2nd ed. St. Louis, Mosby–Year Book, 1997.)

easily envisioned as flow to a clearing organ[2] (Fig. 3-3). Clearance describes the body's capacity to remove drug. The actual rate of drug removal is the clearance times the concentration of the drug. If the clearance is 1 L/min, the actual rate of drug elimination is 0 if the concentration is 0, 1 mg/min if the concentration is 1 mg/L, 10 mg/min if the concentration is 10 mg/L, and so on.

Hepatic Clearance

Many drugs are cleared by hepatic biotransformation. The synthetic pathways for biotransformation are covered in detail in many biochemistry texts. Briefly, the liver metabolizes drugs through oxidation, reduction, hydrolysis, or conjugation. Oxidation and reduction occur in the cytochrome P450 system. These enzymes can be induced by exposure to certain drugs, increasing the liver's intrinsic metabolic capacity. Drugs or hepatic disease can also inhibit them. Routes of oxidative metabolism include hydroxylation, dealkylation, deamination, desulfuration, epoxidation, and dehalogenation. Conjugation and hydrolysis often occur outside of the P450 system, although glucuronidation involves the P450 system as well. The effect of conjugation is to transform hydrophobic molecules into water-soluble molecules through addition of polar groups and render the metabolites easier to excrete by the kidneys. The metabolites generated by the liver are generally inactive, although some drugs (e.g., morphine, midazolam) have metabolites that are as potent as the parent drug. Genetic polymorphism can occur in all of these pathways, and this accounts for part of the variability in clearance in the population, as discussed in the last section of this chapter.

Systemic clearance of anesthetic drugs generally occurs by means of hepatic metabolism, although other mechanisms include plasma and tissue ester hydrolysis (e.g., remifentanil, succinylcholine, esmolol), renal elimination (e.g., pancuronium), and nonspecific, "extrahepatic" metabolism for drugs whose clearance exceeds hepatic blood flow (e.g., propofol). The relationship between metabolism and clearance is complex. The following exploration of this relationship assumes hepatic metabolism, although the principles apply to the metabolism of drug in any tissue.

The rate of metabolism for most anesthetic drugs is proportional to the concentration of drug flowing into the liver. This means that metabolic clearance is constant and independent of dose. This is such a common and fundamental assumption for anesthetic pharmacokinetics that we explore the conditions that must be satisfied for it to be valid.

It cannot be true that metabolism is always proportional to concentration because the metabolic capacity of the liver is not infinite. At some rate of drug flow into the liver, the metabolic capacity becomes saturated, and the pharmacokinetic equations cease to behave in a linear manner. To understand the rate of metabolism quantitatively, we start with a simple observation of mass balance: The rate at which drug flows *out* of the liver must be the rate at which drug flows *into* the liver minus the rate of metabolism. The rate at which drug flows into the liver is liver blood flow, $\dot{Q}$, times the concentration of drug flowing in, C_{inflow}. The rate at which drug flows out of the liver is liver blood flow, $\dot{Q}$, times the concentration of drug flowing out, $C_{outflow}$. Putting this together, the rate of hepatic metabolism by the liver, R, is the difference between the drug concentration flowing into the liver and the drug concentration flowing out of the liver times the rate of liver blood flow:

$$\text{Rate of drug metabolism} = R = \dot{Q}(C_{inflow} - C_{outflow}) \quad (2)$$

This relationship is illustrated in Figure 3-4. Because hepatic metabolism does not have infinite capacity, the relationship between the rate of hepatic metabolism, R, and concentration must be saturable. We are carefully inspecting the saturation equation because it shows up repeatedly in pharmacokinetics and pharmacodynamics:

$$\text{Response} = \frac{C}{C_{50} + C} \quad (3)$$

Response in Equation 3 varies from 0 to 1, depending on the value of C. When C is 0, the response is 0. If C is greater than 0 but much less than C_{50}, the response is nearly proportional to C (response $\approx \frac{C}{C_{50}}$). If C equals C_{50}, the response is $\frac{C_{50}}{C_{50} + C_{50}}$, which is 0.5. This is where the term C_{50} comes from; it is the concentration associated with a 50% response. As C becomes much greater

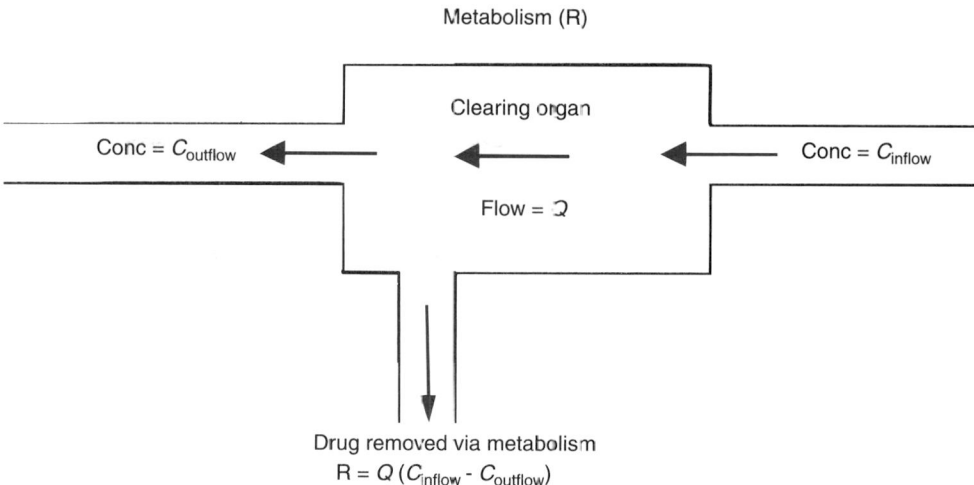

Figure 3–4 The rate of metabolism can be computed as the rate of liver blood flow times the difference between the inflowing and outflowing drug concentrations. This is a common approach to analyzing metabolism or tissue uptake across an organ in mass-balance pharmacokinetic studies.

than C_{50}, the equation approaches $\frac{C}{C}$, which is 1. The shape of this relationship is shown in Figure 3-5. The relationship is linear at low concentrations, but at high concentrations, the response saturates at 1.

We can model the relationship between hepatic metabolism and drug concentration using this equation for saturation. What concentration determines the rate of metabolism: the concentration flowing into the liver, the average concentration within the liver, or the concentration flowing out of the liver? All three have been used, but the most widely used model of metabolism views the rate of metabolism as a function of the concentration flowing out of the liver, $C_{outflow}$. This topic is discussed extensively by Wagner.[3]

We can expand our equation of metabolism to include the observation that the rate of metabolism, R, approaches saturation at the maximum metabolic rate, V_m, as a function of $C_{outflow}$:

$$\text{Rate of drug metabolism} = R$$
$$= \dot{Q}(C_{inflow} - C_{outflow}) \qquad (4)$$
$$= V_m \frac{C_{outflow}}{K_m + C_{outflow}}$$

V_m is the maximum possible metabolic rate. The saturation part of this equation, $\frac{C_{outflow}}{K_m + C_{outflow}}$, determines fraction of the maximum metabolic rate. K_m, also called the *Michaelis constant*, is the outflow concentration at which the metabolic rate is 50% of V_m. This relationship is shown graphically in Figure 3-6. The x axis is $C_{outflow}$ as a fraction K_m, the concentration that yields 50% of the maximum metabolic rate. The y axis is the rate of drug metabolism as a fraction of V_m, the maximum rate of drug metabolism. By normalizing $C_{outflow}$ to K_m and the metabolic rate to V_m, the relationship in Figure 3-6 is true for all values of V_m and K_m. Figure 3-6 shows that as long as the outflow concentration is less than one half of K_m, there is a nearly proportional change in metabolic rate with a proportional change in outflow concentration. For most anesthetic drugs, the clinical concentrations do not exceed one half of K_m, and metabolism of anesthetic drugs is nearly proportional to concentration. We can also interpret Figure 3-6 in terms of the metabolic rate (y axis). As long as the metabolic rate is less than one third of the maximum metabolic capacity, the rate of metabolism increases proportionally with concentration. The clinical message is that the metabolism is proportional to concentration and the pharmacokinetic relationships remain linear, provided the rate of intravenous administration at steady state does not exceed one third of the maximum metabolic capacity.

We have talked about the rate of metabolism but not about hepatic clearance. If the liver could completely extract the drug from the afferent flow, clearance would equal liver blood flow ($\dot{Q}$). However, the liver cannot

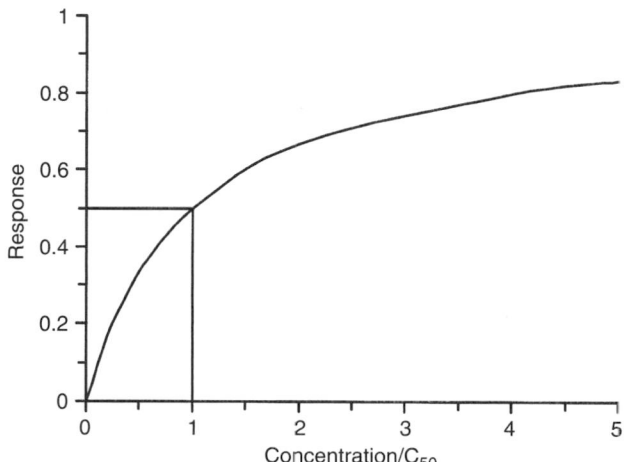

Figure 3–5 The saturation equation, response = $C/(C_{50} + C)$, shows the decreasing incremental response as the system approaches saturation. Variations of this equation show up repeatedly in pharmacokinetics and pharmacodynamics.

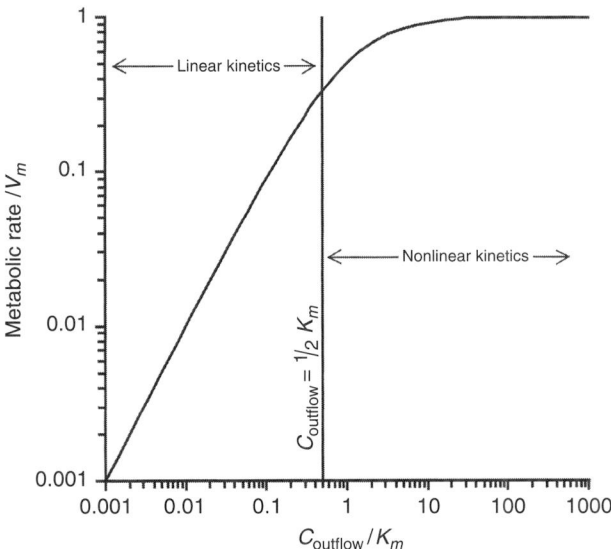

Figure 3–6 The relationship between concentration, expressed as a fraction of K_m (Michaelis constant), and drug metabolism, expressed as a fraction of V_m (maximum rate). As long as the outflow concentration is less than one-half K_m, a change in concentration is matched by a proportional change in metabolic rate. This is true of nearly all anesthetic drugs. (Adapted from Shafer S: Principles of pharmacokinetics and pharmacodynamics. *In* Longnecker DE, Tinker JH, Morgan GE [eds]: Principles and Practice of Anesthesiology, 2nd ed. St. Louis, Mosby–Year Book, 1997.)

remove every drug molecule; there is always some drug in the effluent plasma. The fraction of inflowing drug extracted by the liver is $\dfrac{C_{inflow} - C_{outflow}}{C_{inflow}}$. This is called the *extraction ratio*. Clearance is the volume of blood completely cleared of drug per unit time. We can calculate hepatic clearance as the liver blood flow times the extraction ratio:

$$\text{Clearance} = \dot{Q} \times ER = \dot{Q}\left(\frac{C_{inflow} - C_{outflow}}{C_{inflow}}\right) \quad (5)$$

With this basic understanding of clearance, each part of Equation 4 can be divided by C_{inflow}:

$$\frac{\text{Rate of drug metabolism}}{C_{inflow}} = \frac{R}{C_{inflow}}$$

$$= \dot{Q}\left(\frac{C_{inflow} - C_{outflow}}{C_{inflow}}\right) \quad (6)$$

$$= \frac{C_{outflow}}{C_{inflow}}\left(\frac{V_m}{K_m + C_{outflow}}\right)$$

The third term is clearance: $\dot{Q}$ times the extraction ratio. Because each term must be equivalent to clearance, each brings insight into the process of clearance.

Consider the first term that is equal to clearance: $\dfrac{\text{Rate of drug metabolism}}{C_{inflow}}$. This indicates that clearance is a proportionality constant that relates arterial concentration to the rate of metabolism. If we want to maintain a

given steady-state arterial drug concentration, drug must be infused at the same rate that it is being metabolized. The infusion rate to maintain a given arterial concentration is clearance times the desired arterial concentration.

Consider the third and fourth terms that are equal to clearance: $\dot{Q}\left(\dfrac{C_{inflow} - C_{outflow}}{C_{inflow}}\right)$ and $\dfrac{C_{outflow}}{C_{inflow}}\left(\dfrac{V_m}{K_m + C_{inflow}}\right)$. Taken together, these equations relate clearance to liver blood flow and the extraction ratio[4] (Fig. 3-7). For drugs with an extraction ratio of nearly 1 (e.g., propofol), a change in liver blood flow produces a nearly proportional change in clearance. For drugs with a low extraction ratio (e.g., alfentanil), clearance is nearly independent of the rate of liver blood flow. This makes intuitive sense. If nearly 100% of the drug is extracted by the liver, it implies that the liver has tremendous metabolic capacity for the drug. In this case, the rate-limiting step in metabolism is the flow of drug to the liver, and such drugs are said to be *flow limited*. Any reduction in liver blood flow, such as usually accompanies anesthesia, can be expected to reduce clearance. However, moderate changes in hepatic metabolic function have little impact on clearance because hepatic metabolic capacity is overwhelmingly in excess of demand.

For many drugs (e.g., alfentanil), the extraction ratio is considerably less than 1. For these drugs, clearance is limited by the capacity of the liver to take up and metabolize the drug. These drugs are said to be *capacity limited*. Clearance changes in response to any change in the capacity of the liver to metabolize such drugs, as can be caused by liver disease or enzymatic induction. However, changes in liver blood flow, as can be caused by the anesthetic state itself, usually have little influence on the clearance because the liver handles only a fraction of the drug it makes contact with.

The last two components of equation can also be used to show how the extraction ratio governs the response of clearance to changes in metabolic capacity (V_m). Figure 3-8 shows the clearance for drugs with an extraction ratio ranging from 0.1 to 1, based on a liver blood flow of 1.4 L/min. The extraction ratios were calculated for a $V_m = 1$. Changes in V_m, which can be caused by liver disease (i.e., reduced V_m) or enzymatic induction (i.e., increased V_m), have little effect on drugs with a high extraction ratio. However, drugs with a low extraction ratio have a nearly linear change in clearance with a change in intrinsic metabolic capacity (V_m).

Because V_m and K_m are often unknown, it is occasionally useful to condense them into a single term that summarizes the hepatic metabolic capacity, the *intrinsic clearance*. Returning to the observation that clearance = $\dfrac{C_{outflow}}{C_{inflow}}\left(\dfrac{V_m}{K_m + C_{inflow}}\right)$, consider what happens if hepatic blood flow increases to infinity with no change in hepatic metabolic capacity. $C_{outflow}$ becomes indistinguishable from C_{inflow}, because the finite hepatic capacity metabolizes only an infinitesimal fraction of the drug flowing through the liver. As a result, clearance becomes $\dfrac{V_m}{K_m + C_{inflow}}$. We can solve for this in the *linear range* by finding clearance when

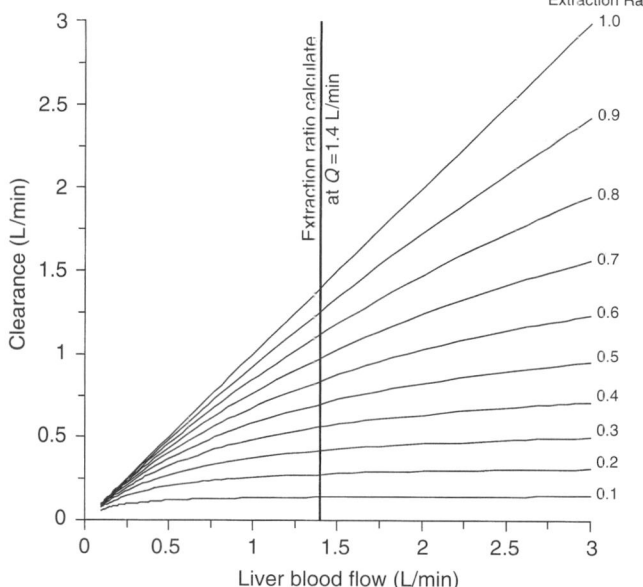

Figure 3–7 Relationships among liver blood flow (Q), clearance, and the extraction ratio. For drugs with a high extraction ratio, clearance is nearly identical to liver blood flow. For drugs with a low extraction ratio, changes in liver blood flow have almost no effect on clearance. (Adapted from Wilkinson GR, Shand DG: Commentary: A physiological approach to hepatic drug clearance. Clin Pharmacol Ther 18:377-390, 1975.)

$C_{inflow} = 0, \dfrac{V_m}{K_m}$. This is the *intrinsic clearance*, Cl_{int}. Without considering the derivation, it can be demonstrated from the definition of Cl_{int} that in the linear range Cl_{int} is directly related to the extraction ratio:

$$\text{Extraction ratio} = \frac{Cl_{int}}{\dot{Q} + Cl_{int}} \tag{7}$$

Combining this with Equation 6 yields the relationship between hepatic clearance and Cl_{int}:

$$\text{Hepatic clearance} = \frac{\dot{Q} \times Cl_{int}}{\dot{Q} + Cl_{int}} \tag{8}$$

The relationship between intrinsic clearance and extraction ratio is shown in Figure 3-9, calculated at a hepatic blood flow of 1400 mL/min. In general, true hepatic clearance and extraction ratio are more useful concepts for anesthetic drugs than the intrinsic clearance. However, intrinsic clearance is introduced here because it is occasionally used in pharmacokinetic analyses of anesthetic drugs.

We have been focusing on linear pharmacokinetics, the pharmacokinetics of drugs whose metabolic rate at clinical doses is less than $V_m/3$. The clearance of such drugs is generally expressed as a constant (e.g., propofol clearance = 1.6 L/min). Some drugs, such as phenytoin, exhibit saturable pharmacokinetics; they have such low V_m values that typical doses exceed the linear portion of Figure 3-6. The clearance of drugs with saturable metabolism is a function of drug concentration, rather than a constant.

Renal Clearance

The kidneys clear drug from plasma by filtration at the glomerulus and direct transport into the tubules. Renal blood flow is inversely correlated with age, as is creatinine clearance, which can be predicted from age and weight according to the equation of Cockroft and Gault[5]:

Men:

$$\text{Creatinine clearance (mL/min)}$$
$$= \frac{(140 - \text{age [yr]}) \times \text{weight (kg)}}{72 \times \text{Serum creatinine (mg/dL)}} \tag{9}$$

Women:
85% of the value for men

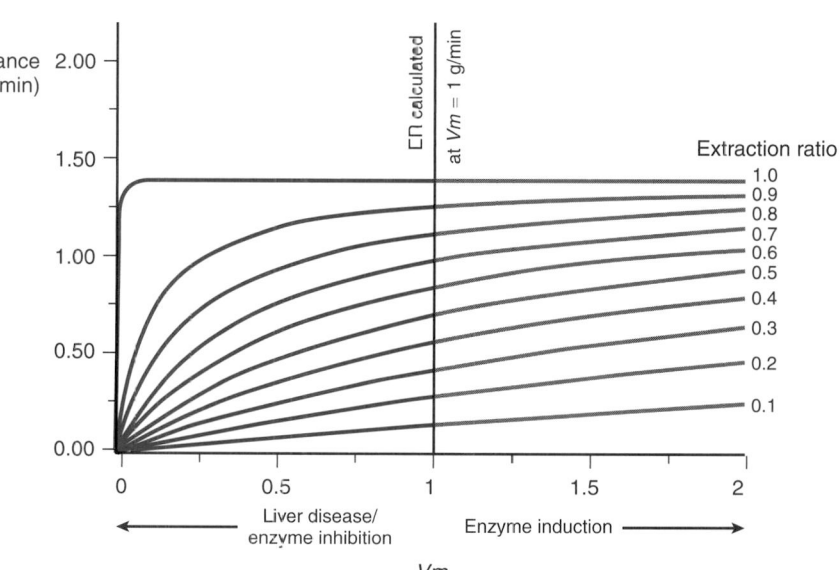

Figure 3–8 Corollary to Figure 3-7, showing the relationships among metabolic capacity, clearance, and the extraction ratio (E.R.). Changes in maximum metabolic velocity (V_m) have little effect on drugs with a high extraction ratio, but they cause a nearly proportional decrease in clearance of drugs with a low extraction ratio.

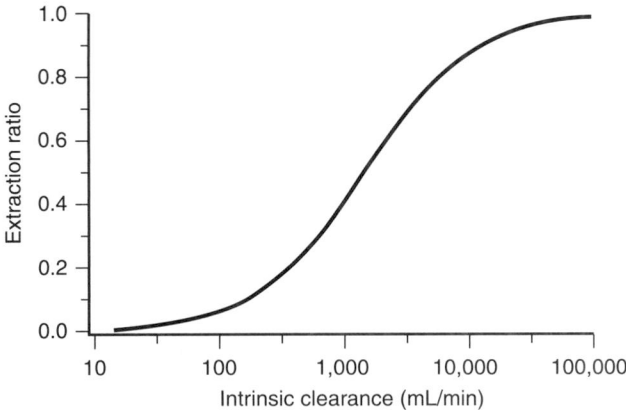

Figure 3–9 The relationship between intrinsic clearance and extraction ratio is calculated for a liver blood flow of 1400 mL/min.

Equation 9 shows that age is an independent factor in predicting creatinine clearance. Elderly people have decreased creatinine clearance, even in the presence of normal serum creatinine levels. Inhaled anesthetics also decrease renal blood flow. Decreased renal clearance delays the offset of effect for renally excreted drugs. For instance, pancuronium is about 85% cleared by the kidneys. The dose of pancuronium should be reduced in elderly patients on the basis of decreased clearance, even though they may have normal serum creatinine levels.

Tissue Clearance

In some cases, anesthetic drugs are cleared in tissues, including blood, muscle, and lungs. For example, remifentanil is cleared by nonspecific esterases located primarily in muscle and intestines, but the lungs, liver, kidneys, and blood contribute minimally to remifentanil clearance. Succinylcholine, mivacurium, and 2-chloroprocaine are metabolized by plasma butyrylcholinesterases (formerly designated pseudocholinesterases). The half-life of succinylcholine, mivacurium, and 2-chloroprocaine in plasma is about 3 minutes, 5 minutes, and 25 seconds, respectively. About one half of atracurium's metabolism is hepatic, and the balance occurs in blood by means of nonspecific cholinesterases (but not by butyrylcholinesterases). Hofmann degradation is a spontaneous process in plasma at normal pH and temperature and does not depend on circulating esterases. Hofmann degradation is a minor route of atracurium metabolism, but it is the major route of metabolism of cisatracurium, an isomer of atracurium. This is an important distinction; unlike atracurium and mivacurium, cisatracurium metabolism is unaffected by disease or genetic variants of cholinesterase metabolism.

Clearance by tissues other than blood can be analyzed using models similar to those for hepatic clearance. Tissue clearance can be flow limited or capacity limited, or both. Clearance within the blood itself cannot be flow limited and therefore depends entirely on the intrinsic metabolic rate and capacity within the blood.

Distribution Clearance

Distribution clearance is the transfer of drug between the blood or plasma and the peripheral tissues. Unlike metabolic clearance, distribution clearance does not permanently remove drug from the body. Distribution clearance is a function of cardiac output, tissue blood flow, and the permeability of the capillary walls to the drug. For a drug that readily crosses into peripheral tissues, such as propofol, the sum of the metabolic clearance and the distribution clearance approaches cardiac output. For drugs such as succinylcholine and remifentanil that are metabolized directly in the plasma or in many peripheral tissues, the sum of metabolic clearance and distribution clearance can exceed cardiac output.

Protein Binding

Many drugs are bound to plasma proteins, particularly to albumin and α_1-acid glycoprotein. The relationship between drugs and their binding proteins can be described as follows:

$$[\text{Free drug}] + [\text{Unbound protein binding sites}]$$
$$\xrightleftharpoons[k_{off}]{k_{on}} [\text{Bound drug}]$$

In this reversible reaction, [Free drug] is the free drug concentration, [Unbound protein binding sites] is the concentration of the available unbound protein binding sites, [Bound drug] is the concentration of drug bound to plasma proteins, k_{on} is the rate constant for binding of drug to plasma protein, and k_{off} is the rate constant for dissociation of bound drug from the plasma proteins. From this relationship, it can be inferred that the rate of formation of bound drug is as follows:

$$\frac{d[\text{Bound drug}]}{dt} = \begin{array}{l} [\text{Free drug}]\,[\text{Unbound protein binding sites}]\,k_{on} \\ -[\text{Bound drug}]\,k_{off} \end{array} \quad (10)$$

At equilibrium (which is nearly instantaneous), d[Bound drug]/dt = 0, permitting us to solve for k, the ratio of k_{on}/k_{off}:

$$k = \frac{k_{on}}{k_{off}} = \frac{[\text{Bound drug}]}{[\text{Free drug}]\,[\text{Unbound protein binding sites}]} \quad (11)$$

Plasma proteins may have more than one binding site. The total number of binding sites is the protein concentration, [Protein], times n, the average number of binding sites per protein molecule. For all of the drugs used in anesthesia, the number of binding sites bound is only a trivial fraction of the total available binding sites, and it is possible to reasonably approximate [Unbound protein binding sites] by n [Protein]. Because the number of binding sites per molecule, n, is constant, we can fold it into the rate constant, k, by defining the association constant, K_a, as follows:

$$K_a = n\frac{k_{on}}{k_{off}} = \frac{[\text{Bound drug}]}{[\text{Free drug}]\,[\text{Protein}]} \quad (12)$$

We can define f_u as the free fraction of drug:

$$f_u = \frac{[\text{Free drug}]}{[\text{Bound drug}] + [\text{Free drug}]} \quad (13)$$

Combining Equations 12 and 13, we can solve for f_u in terms of the unbound drug concentration:

$$f_u = \frac{1}{1 + K_a [\text{Protein}]} \qquad (14)$$

Two observations can be drawn from Equation 14. First, the fraction bound to plasma protein depends only on the protein concentration, not on the drug concentration, within the approximation that [Bound drug] << n[Protein]. This approximation is always true for anesthetic drugs because of their potency. Even for thiopental, possibly the least potent drug used in contemporary anesthesia practice, [Bound drug] << n[Protein], and protein binding is independent of thiopental concentration. Second, if Equation 14 is solved for $f_u = 0.5$, we find the following:

$$K_a = \frac{1}{[\text{Protein}]_{50}} \qquad (15)$$

In Equation 15, $[\text{Protein}]_{50}$ is the concentration of protein at which the drug is one-half bound. Another way of thinking about the association constant is that it is the inverse of the protein concentration associated with 50% binding. If we substitute $\frac{1}{[\text{Protein}]_{50}}$ for K_a in Equation 14, we get the following relationship:

$$f_u = \frac{[\text{Protein}]_{50}}{[\text{Protein}]_{50} + [\text{Protein}]} \qquad (16)$$

This relationship is shown graphically in Figure 3-10. On the left side of Figure 3-10, [Protein] is much smaller than $[\text{Protein}]_{50}$. In this situation, the drug has little affinity for protein binding, and there is far less protein around than required to bind 50% of the drug. The drug is mostly free, and f_u is nearly 1. On the right side of Figure 3-10, [Protein] is much greater than $[\text{Protein}]_{50}$. This means that there is far more protein present than required to

bind 50% of the drug. The result is that drug is mostly bound to plasma proteins, and f_u is nearly 0.

The association constant, K_a, and its inverse, $[\text{Protein}]_{50}$, reflect the affinity of the drug for plasma proteins. They should not change in the presence of disease. However, [Protein] can change with disease, age, or concurrent drugs. Figure 3-11 shows the relationship between changes in protein concentration and changes in the free fraction of drug for drugs with different degrees of protein binding in the normal clinical use. The lines on the graph correspond to different drugs whose free fraction in normal plasma ranges from 1.0 (*horizontal line*) to approximately 0.0 (*straight diagonal line*).

For drugs that are not bound (free fraction = 1.0), there is no relationship between free fraction and protein concentration, as indicated by the horizontal line. For drugs whose free fraction is typically 90%, there is a small change in free drug concentration with changes in protein concentration. For drugs that are highly protein bound, the free drug concentration changes nearly inversely with the change in protein concentration. As the percentage of binding approaches 100% (free drug → 0.0), the relationship between change in protein concentration and change in free fraction becomes inversely proportional. There is never a greater than proportional change in free drug concentration with a change in plasma concentration. For example, the most that a 10% change in protein concentration would produce is a 10% change in free drug concentration, and that would be the case only if the drug were nearly 100% bound to plasma proteins.

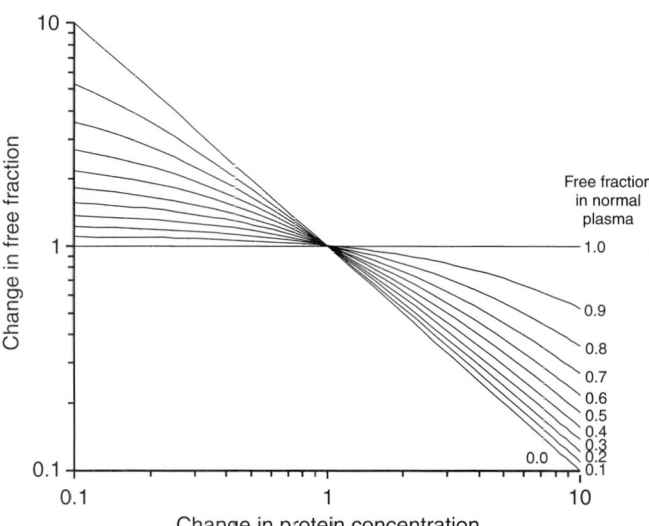

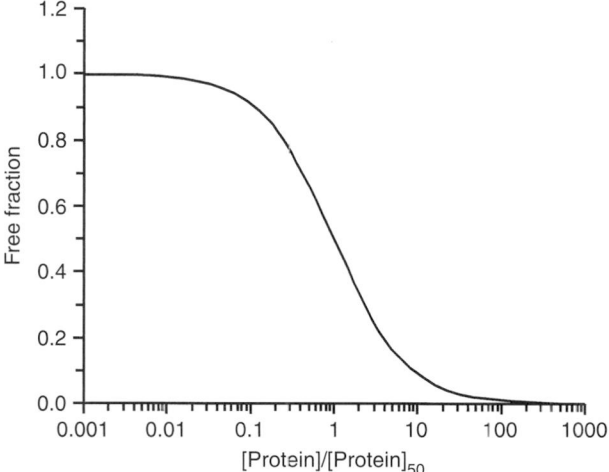

Figure 3–10 Relationship between plasma protein concentration as a fraction of the concentration associated with 50% binding and the fraction of drug that is unbound. This is another example of the saturation equation illustrated in Figure 3-5.

Figure 3–11 The relationship between changes in protein concentration and changes in free fraction depends on the free fraction in normal plasma with typical clinical doses. For a drug that is not bound (free fraction ≈ 1), there is no change in free fraction with a change in protein concentration. For a highly bound drug with a free fraction that is nearly 0, any change in protein causes a nearly inversely proportional change in free fraction. (Adapted from Shafer S: Principles of pharmacokinetics and pharmacodynamics. *In* Longnecker DE, Tinker JH, Morgan GE [eds]: Principles and Practice of Anesthesiology, 2nd ed. St. Louis, Mosby–Year Book, 1997.)

The in vitro observation that changing the protein concentration results in changing the free drug concentration (see Fig. 3-11) does not necessarily apply to the in vivo situation. It is the free (i.e., unbound) drug that equilibrates between the plasma and the tissues. If protein binding decreases, the free drug concentration gradient between the plasma and peripheral tissues increases. As a result, when protein binding decreases, equilibrium is achieved between the plasma and the tissue free drug concentrations at a lower total plasma drug concentration. This lower concentration gives the appearance that the drug has distributed into a larger total space. Decreased protein binding causes an increase in the apparent volume of distribution when referenced to total, rather than free, drug concentration.

This explains why the increased volume of distribution at steady state seen with decreased plasma protein binding is mostly an illusion. If only the unbound drug concentration were measured, there would be almost no change in the apparent volume of distribution of lipophilic drugs (i.e., most of those in anesthesia practice), because it is the partitioning of drug within peripheral tissues that primarily governs the free concentration of lipophilic drugs.

Changes in protein binding may affect the clearance of drugs. If a drug has a high extraction ratio, the liver is going to remove nearly all the drug flowing to it, regardless of the extent of protein binding. However, if the drug has a low hepatic extraction ratio, an increase in the free fraction of drug results in an increase in the driving gradient, with an associated increase in clearance. Protein binding also affects the apparent potency of a drug when referenced to the total plasma drug concentration. An increase in the free fraction increases the driving pressure to the site of drug effect. A change in the free fraction increases the concentration at the effect site. Because of this change in apparent potency, decreased protein binding may decrease the dose required to produce a given drug effect, even in the absence of pharmacokinetic changes.

Stereochemistry

Typical pharmacokinetic analyses describe fictitious drugs. For example, the pharmacokinetics and pharmacodynamics of thiopental, fentanyl, and midazolam describe drugs that do not exist. The reason is that most anesthetic drugs are chiral and are supplied as racemic mixtures. The body is a chiral environment, and drugs interact stereospecifically with enzymes, proteins, and receptors. The pharmacokinetics and pharmacodynamics of the enantiomers may differ. The enantiomers of bupivacaine and ketamine have been particularly well studied, and the levo isomer of bupivacaine, levobupivacaine, is commercially available. Although the importance of studying the pharmacokinetics and pharmacodynamics of individual stereoisomers is widely appreciated, the difficulty of doing such studies has precluded widespread use.

Pharmacokinetic Models

Zero-Order and First-Order Processes

Zero-order processes and first-order processes are the basis of mathematical pharmacokinetic models. Processes such as the flow of a river or a person's consumption of oxygen happen at a constant rate. These are called *zero-order processes*. The rate of change (dx/dt) for a zero-order process is defined by the following equation:

$$\frac{dx}{dt} = k \tag{17}$$

Equation 17 states that the rate of change is constant. If x represents an amount of drug and t represents time, the units of k are amount per time. To find the value of x at time t, x(t), we can compute it as the integral of the equation from time 0 to time t:

$$x(t) = x_0 + k\,t \tag{18}$$

In Equation 18, x_0 is the value of x at time 0. This is the equation of a straight line with a slope of k and an intercept of x_0.

Many processes occur at a rate proportional to the amount. For example, the interest payment on a loan is proportional to the outstanding balance, and the rate at which water drains from a bathtub is proportional to the amount of water in the tub. These are examples of *first-order processes*. The rate of change in a first-order process is only slightly more complex than for a zero-order process:

$$\frac{dx}{dt} = k\,x \tag{19}$$

The units of k are 1/time, because x on the right side already includes the units for the amount. The value of x at time t, x(t) can be computed as the integral from time 0 to time t:

$$x(t) = x_0\,e^{kt} \tag{20}$$

In Equation 20, x_0 is the value of x at time 0. If k is greater than 0, x(t) increases exponentially. If k is less than 0, x(t) decreases exponentially. In pharmacokinetics, k is negative because concentrations decrease over time. For clarity, the minus sign is usually explicit, and k is expressed as a positive number. The identical equation for pharmacokinetics, with the minus sign explicitly written, is:

$$x(t) = x_0\,e^{-kt} \tag{21}$$

Figure 3-12 shows the relationship between x and time as described by Equation 21. In Figure 3-12, x continuously decreases over time, but the slope of the curve continuously increases (i.e., becomes less negative). Taking the natural logarithm of both sides of Equation 21 gives the following:

$$\begin{aligned} \ln\big(x(t)\big) &= \ln\big(x_0\,e^{-kt}\big) \\ &= \ln(x_0) + \ln\big(e^{-kt}\big) \\ &= \ln(x_0) - kt \end{aligned} \tag{22}$$

This is the equation of a straight line, as shown in Figure 3-13, for which the vertical axis is ln(x(t)), the horizontal axis is t, the intercept is ln(x_0), and the slope of the line is −k.

How long does it take for x to go from some value, x_1, to one half of that value, x_1/2. Because k is the slope of a

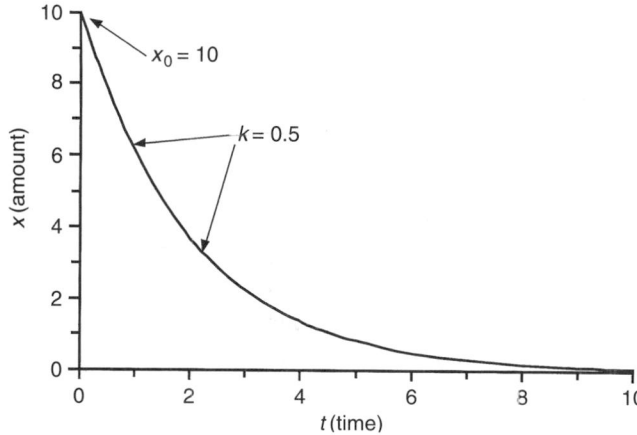

Figure 3–12 Exponential decay curve, as given by $x(t) = x_0 e^{-kt}$, plotted on standard axes, with $x_0 = 10$ and $k = 0.5$.

straight line relating $\ln(x)$ to time, the following is true:

$$k = \frac{\Delta \ln(x)}{\Delta t} = \frac{\ln(x_1) - \ln\left(\dfrac{x_1}{2}\right)}{t_{1/2}} \qquad (23)$$

In Equation 23, $t_{1/2}$ is the half-life, or the time required for a 50% decrease in x. The numerator can be simplified:

$$\ln(x_1) - \ln\left(\frac{x_1}{2}\right) = \ln\left(\frac{x_1}{\left(\dfrac{x_1}{2}\right)}\right) \qquad (24)$$
$$= \ln(2)$$
$$\approx 0.693$$

This succinctly relates slope (or the rate constant, k) to half-life, $t_{1/2}$:

$$k = \frac{0.693}{t_{1/2}} \qquad (25)$$

If we measure the time it takes for x to fall by 50%, $t_{1/2}$, we know the rate constant, k. If the rate constant k is known,

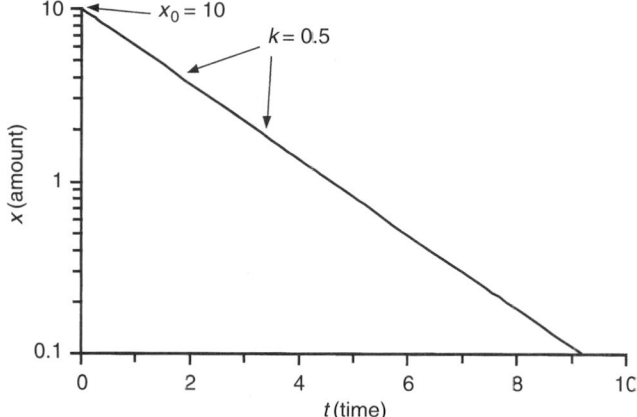

Figure 3–13 The same exponential decay curve, $x(t) = x_0 e^{-kt}$, as in Figure 3-12 is plotted on a log y axis.

we can easily deduce from Equation 25 the time for x to fall by 50%:

$$t_{1/2} = \frac{0.693}{k} \qquad (26)$$

Physiologic Pharmacokinetic Models

It is possible to analyze volumes and clearances for each organ in the body and to construct models of pharmacokinetics by assembling the organ models into physiologically and anatomically accurate models of the entire animal. These models typically assume blood flows throughout the system as zero-order processes and drug transfers between the blood and tissues as first-order processes. Figure 3-14 shows such a model for thiopental in rats.[6] Subsequent studies have shown that individual tissue volumes and blood flows can be scaled up from rats to humans, resulting in accurate models of human pharmacokinetics.[7] This illustrates the potential utility of physiologically based pharmacokinetic models in developing human pharmacokinetic models from animal models.

Models that work with individual tissues are mathematically cumbersome and do not offer a better prediction of plasma drug concentration than models that lump the tissues into a few compartments. If the goal is to determine how to give drugs to obtain therapeutic plasma drug concentrations, all that is needed is to mathematically relate dose to plasma concentration. For this purpose, conventional compartmental models are usually adequate.

Compartmental Pharmacokinetic Models

Compartmental models are built on the same basic concepts as physiologic models, but with gross simplifications. The one-compartment model seen in Figure 3-15 contains a single volume and a single clearance, as though humans were built like buckets. For anesthetic drugs, we resemble several buckets connected by pipes. These situations are usually modeled using two- or three-compartment models (see Fig. 3-15). The volume to the right in the two-compartment model and in the center of the three-compartment model is the central volume. The other volumes are the peripheral volumes, and the sum of all the volumes is the *volume of distribution at steady state*. The clearance leaving the central compartment for the outside is the *central* or *metabolic clearance*. The clearances between the central compartment and the peripheral compartments are the *intercompartmental clearances*.

One-Compartment Model

BOLUS PHARMACOKINETICS. Think of the body as a bucket into which we pour drug. The amount of drug poured into the bucket is x_0 (x at time 0). The initial concentration is x_0/V, and V is the volume of fluid in the bucket. Returning to Equation 1, if we know the concentration we want to achieve, the target concentration, C_T, and the volume in the bucket, V, we can calculate the dose to achieve C_T by rearranging the definition of concentration: Dose $= C_T \times V$. This topic is discussed further in Chapter 12.

We can assume that the fluid is being pumped out of the bucket at a constant rate, which we call *clearance*, Cl. What is the rate, dx/dt, at which drug is flowing out of

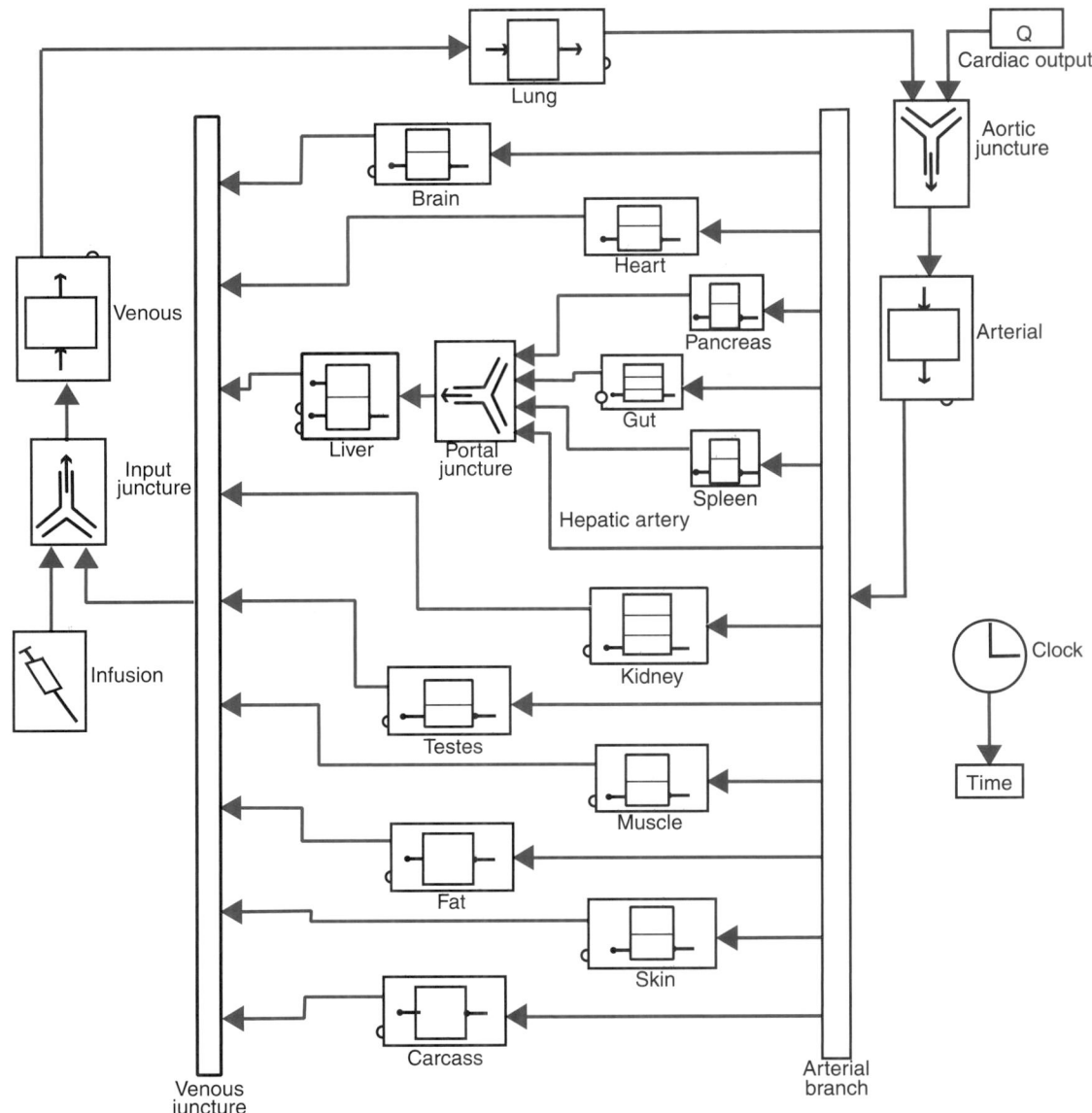

Figure 3–14 Physiologic model for thiopental in rats. The pharmacokinetics of distribution into each organ has been individually determined. The components of the model are linked by zero-order (flow) and first-order (diffusion) processes. (From Ebling WF, Wada DR, Stanski DR: From piecewise to full physiologic pharmacokinetic modeling: Applied to thiopental disposition in the rat. J Pharmacokinet Biopharm 22:259-292, 1994.)

the bucket? Because concentration is x/V and Cl is the rate that the fluid in the bucket is flowing out, the rate at which the drug is flowing out must be x/V × Cl. This rate is a first-order process if and only if it equals a constant, k, times the amount of drug in the bucket. Does it?

$$\frac{dx}{dt} = \frac{x}{V}Cl$$
$$= \frac{Cl}{V}x \qquad (27)$$
$$= kx?$$

The flow out of the bucket, Cl, is constant. The volume, V, is not constant because it is shrinking as fluid flows from the bucket. However, a pipe can be opened to add fluid to the bucket at a rate that matches clearance to keep the volume constant. When V becomes constant, the model looks like physiologic clearance (which does not require exsanguination), as shown in Figure 3-3. Because Cl and V are constants, $\frac{Cl}{V}$ is a constant. Referring to Equation 27, k, a constant by definition of first-order processes, equals $\frac{Cl}{V}$, a constant by the definition of clearance and volume.

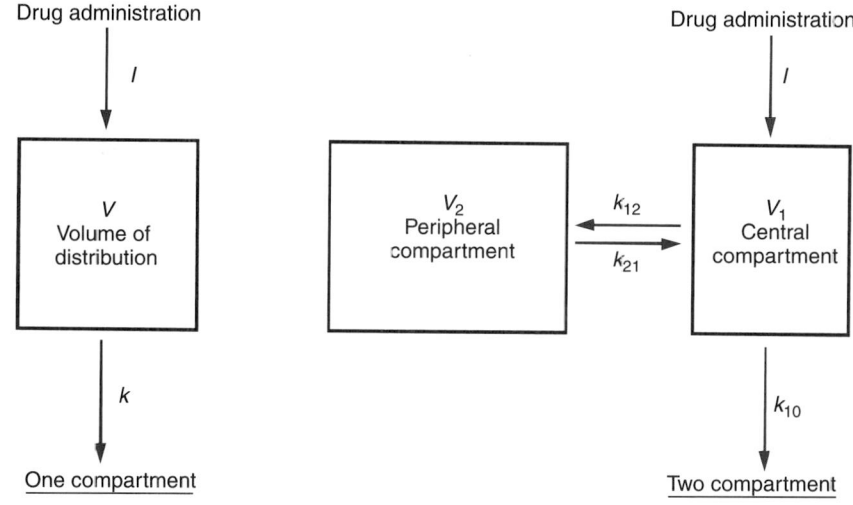

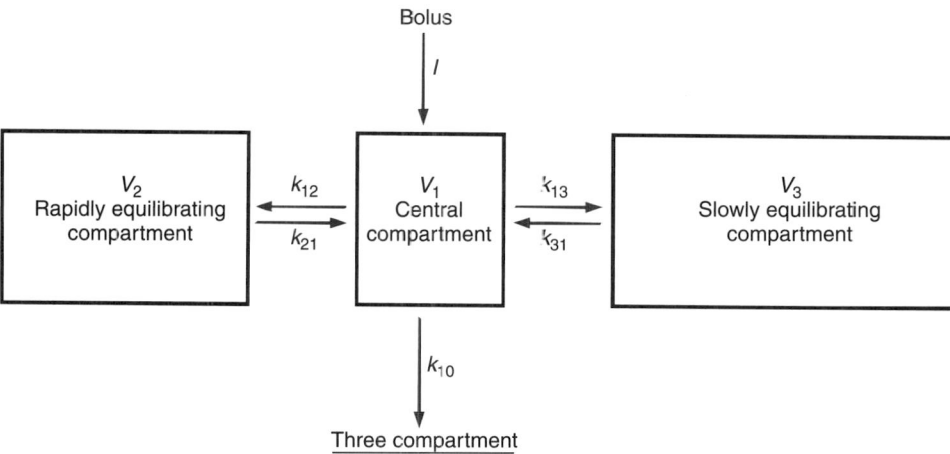

Figure 3–15 One-, two-, and three-compartment mammillary models.

This can be rearranged to yield the fundamental identity of linear pharmacokinetics:

$$Cl \text{ (clearance)} = k \text{ (rate constant)} \\ \times V \text{ (volume of distribution)} \qquad (28)$$

What does this identity reveal about the relationships of half-life, volume, and clearance? Rearranging Equation 28 as $k = \dfrac{Cl}{V}$ and remembering that $t_{1/2} = \dfrac{0.693}{k}$, we can conclude the following:

$$t_{1/2} = 0.693 \frac{V}{Cl} \qquad (29)$$

$$t_{1/2} \propto \frac{V}{Cl}$$

Figure 3-16 shows a one-compartment model with an identical clearance but a bigger volume than that seen in Figure 3-3. Because it takes longer to clear drug from this bigger volume, the half-life increases as predicted by the previous equation. Figure 3-17 shows a one-compartment

model with an identical volume but faster clearance than that seen in Figure 3-3. The concentrations fall more quickly (i.e., shorter half-life) with the larger clearance, as predicted by Equation 29.

Because this is a first-order process, $\dfrac{dx}{dt} = k\,x$, and the integral of this gives the amount of drug at time t in terms of the amount at time 0: $x(t) = x_0\,e^{-kt}$. If we divide both sides by V and remember that x/V is the definition of concentration, we get the equation that relates concentration after an intravenous bolus to time and initial concentration:

$$C(t) = C_0\,e^{-kt} \qquad (30)$$

This equation defines the *concentration over time curve* for a one-compartment model, and it has the log-linear shape seen in Figure 3-13. We can calculate the clearance, Cl, in one of two ways. First, we can calculate V by rearranging the definition of concentration: V = dose/initial concentration = dose/C_0. Referring to Equation 28, if we measure the slope, –k, we can calculate clearance as k × V. A more

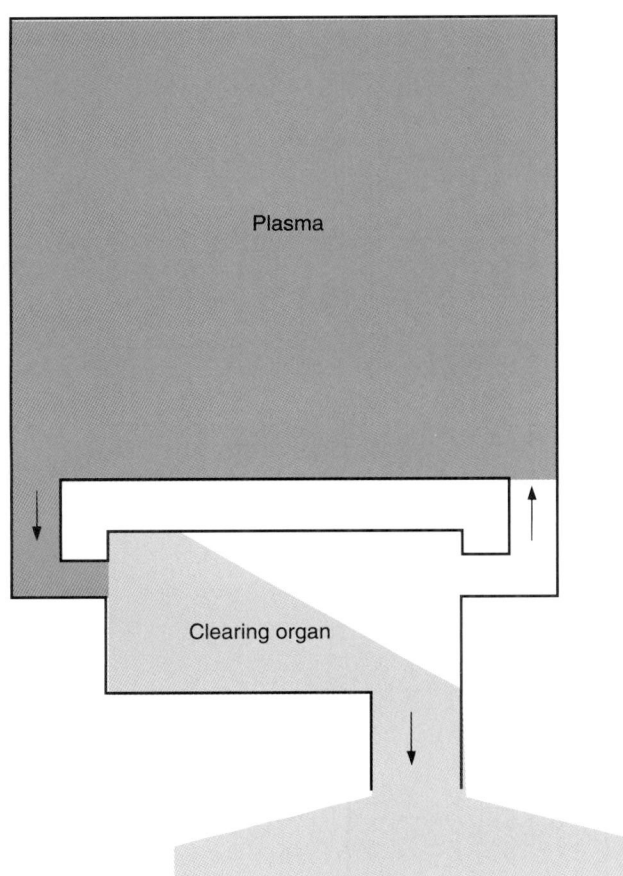

Figure 3–16 A one-compartment model is similar to that in Figure 3-3 but has an increased volume of distribution. After drug administration, concentrations fall more slowly in this model than in the model shown in Figure 3-3.

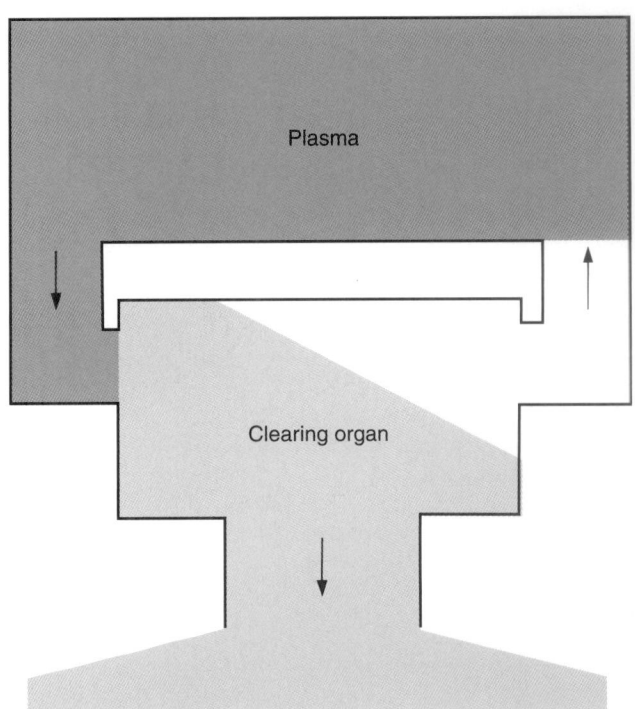

Figure 3–17 A one-compartment model is similar to that in Figure 3-3 but has increased clearance. After drug administration, concentrations fall faster in this model than in the model shown in Figure 3-3.

general solution is to consider the integral of the concentration over time curve (Equation 30), known in pharmacokinetics as the *area under the curve* (AUC):

$$
\begin{aligned}
AUC &= \int_0^\infty C_0\, e^{-kt} dt \\
&= \int_0^\infty \frac{x_0}{V}\left(e^{-\frac{Cl}{V}t}\right) dt \quad \text{(substituting for } C_0 \text{ and k)} \\
&= \frac{x_0}{V} \times \frac{V}{Cl} \quad \text{(evaluating the above integral)} \\
&= \frac{x_0}{Cl}
\end{aligned}
\tag{31}
$$

We can rearrange Equation 31 to solve for clearance, Cl:

$$
Cl = \frac{x_0}{AUC}
\tag{32}
$$

Because x_0 is the dose of drug, clearance equals the dose divided by the AUC. This fundamental property of *linear* pharmacokinetic models applies to one-compartment models, to multicompartment models, and to any type of intravenous drug dosing (provided the *total dose* is used as the numerator). It directly follows that AUC is proportional to dose for linear models (i.e., models in which Cl is constant).

INFUSION PHARMACOKINETICS. When an infusion is given at an input rate of I, the plasma concentration rises as long as the rate of drug going into the body, I, exceeds the rate at which drug leaves the body, $C \times Cl$, in which C is the drug concentration. When $I = C \times Cl$, drug is going in and coming out at the same rate, and drug concentration in the body is at steady state. We can calculate the concentration at steady state by observing that the rate of drug going in must equal the rate of drug coming out. From Equation 6, we know that the rate of drug metabolism at steady state is as follows:

$$
\text{Metabolic rate} = C_\infty\, Cl
\tag{33}
$$

In Equation 33, C_∞ is the arterial concentration at steady state. By definition, the infusion rate at steady state must equal the metabolic rate, and the infusion rate, I, at steady state therefore must be $I = C_\infty\, Cl$. Solving this for the concentration at steady state, C_∞ gives I/Cl. The steady-state concentration during an infusion is the rate of drug input divided by the clearance. It follows that to calculate the infusion rate that can achieve a given target concentration, C_T, at steady state, the infusion rate must be $C_T \times Cl$. This topic is discussed further in Chapter 12.

$C_\infty = \dfrac{I}{Cl}$ is similar in form to the equation describing

the concentration after a bolus injection: $C_0 = \dfrac{x_0}{V}$. Volume is a scalar relating bolus to initial concentration, and clearance is a scalar relating infusion rate to steady-state concentration. It follows that the initial concentration after a bolus is independent of the clearance and that the steady-state concentration during a continuous infusion is independent of the volume.

During an infusion, the rate of change in the amount of drug, x, is the rate of inflow, I, minus the rate of outflow, $k \times x$.

$$\frac{dx}{dt} = I - k\,x \qquad (34)$$

We can calculate x at any time t as the integral from time 0 to time t. Assuming that $x_0 = 0$ (i.e., starting with no drug in the body), the result is this:

$$x(t) = \frac{I}{k}\left(1 - e^{-kt}\right) \qquad (35)$$

As $t \to \infty$, $e^{-kt} \to 0$, and Equation 35 reduces to the following:

$$x_\infty = \frac{I}{k} \qquad (36)$$

How long does it take to reach 50% of the final steady-state concentration (i.e., to reach a concentration of $\frac{x_\infty}{2}$) during an infusion? From Equation 36, we know that $\frac{x_\infty}{2} = \frac{I}{2k}$. Substituting $\frac{I}{2k}$ for x(t) in Equation 35, we obtain the following:

$$\frac{I}{2k} = \frac{I}{k}\left(1 - e^{-kt}\right) \qquad (37)$$

Solving Equation 37 for t, we get $\frac{\ln(2)}{k}$. Equation 26 showed that the half-life, $t_{1/2}$, after a bolus injection was $\frac{\ln(2)}{k}$. Here, we have a parallel between boluses and infusions. During an infusion, it takes one half-life to reach 50% of the steady-state concentration. Similarly, it takes two half-lives to reach 75%, three half-lives to reach 88%, and five half-lives to reach 97% of the steady-state concentration. By four or five half-lives, the patient is typically considered to be at steady state, although the concentrations only asymptotically approach the steady-state value.

ABSORPTION PHARMACOKINETICS. In intravenous drug delivery, all of the drug reaches the systemic circulation. When drugs are given by a different route, such as orally, transdermally, epidurally, or intramuscularly, the drug must first reach the systemic circulation. Oral drugs may be metabolized by first-pass hepatic metabolism before reaching the systemic circulation. Transdermally applied drugs may be sloughed off with the stratum corneum without being absorbed. We cannot assume that the dose given to the patient is the same as the dose that reaches the systemic circulation when working with alternative routes of drug delivery. The dose that reaches the systemic circulation is the administered dose times f, the fraction that is bioavailable.

Alternative routes of drug delivery are often modeled by assuming the drug is absorbed from a reservoir or depot, usually modeled as an additional compartment with a monoexponential rate of transfer to the systemic circulation:

$$A(t) = f\,D_{oral}\,k_a\,e^{-k_a t} \qquad (38)$$

In Equation 38, A(t) is the absorption rate at time t, f is the fraction bioavailable, D_{oral} is the dose taken orally (or intramuscularly or applied to the skin), and k_a is the absorption rate constant. Because the integral of $k_a\,e^{-k_a t}$ is 1, the total amount of drug absorbed is $f \times D_{oral}$. To compute the concentrations over time, we first reduce the problem to differential equations (e.g., Equations 19 and 34) and then integrate. The differential equation for the amount, x, with oral absorption into a one-compartment disposition model follows:

$$\frac{dx}{dt} = \text{inflow} - \text{outflow}$$
$$= A(t) - k\,x = D_{oral}\,f\,k_a\,e^{-k_a t} - k\,x \qquad (39)$$

This is the rate of absorption at time t, A(t), minus the rate of exit, k x. To solve for the amount of drug, x, in the compartment at time t, we integrate this from 0 to time t, knowing that x(0) = 0:

$$x(t) = \frac{D_{oral}\,f\,k_a}{k - k_a}\left(e^{-k_a t} - e^{-kt}\right) \qquad (40)$$

Equation 40 describes the amount of drug in the systemic circulation when absorbed from some depot, such as the stomach, an intramuscular injection, or the skin, or from an epidural dose. To describe the concentrations, rather than amounts of drug, it is necessary to divide both sides of Equation 40 by V, the volume of distribution.

This discussion covers the standard pharmacokinetic equations for one-compartment models. The one-compartment model introduces the concepts of rate constants and half-lives and relates them to the physiologic concepts of volume and clearance. Unfortunately, none of the drugs used in anesthesia can be accurately characterized by one-compartment models. Distribution of anesthetic drugs into and out of peripheral tissues plays a crucial role in the time course of anesthetic drug effect. To describe intravenous anesthetics, we must extend the one-compartment model to account for distribution into tissues.

Multicompartment Models

The plasma concentrations over time after an intravenous bolus resemble the curve in Figure 3-18. In contrast to Figure 3-13, Figure 3-18 is not a straight line even though it is plotted on a log y axis. This curve has the characteristics common to most drugs when given by intravenous bolus. First, the concentrations continuously decrease over time. Second, the rate of decline is initially steep but continuously becomes less steep, until we get to a portion that has a log-linear form.

For many drugs, three distinct phases can be distinguished. There is a *rapid-distribution phase* (see Fig. 3-18, *solid line*) that begins immediately after the bolus injection.

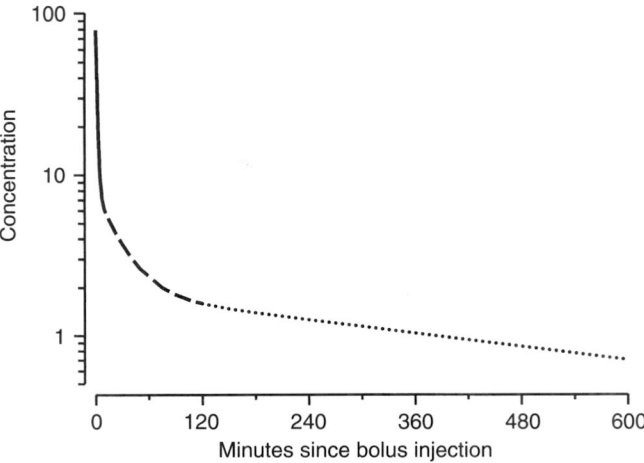

Figure 3–18 Concentration versus time relationship shows a very rapid initial decline after bolus injection. The terminal log-linear portion is seen only after most of the drug has left the plasma. This is characteristic of most anesthetic drugs. Different line types highlight the rapid, intermediate, and slow (log-linear) portions of the curve.

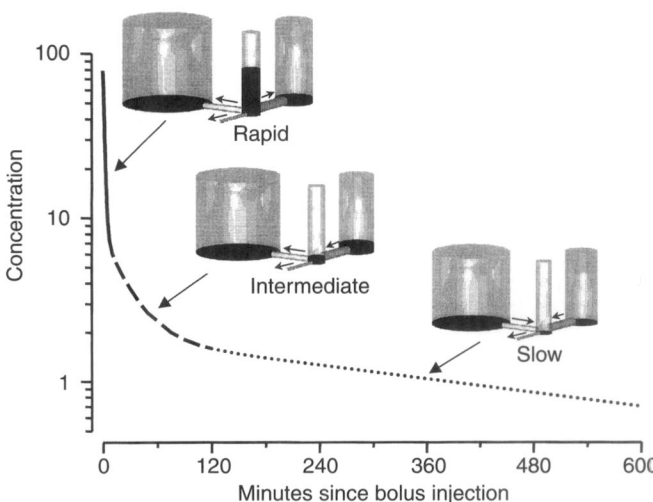

Figure 3–19 Hydraulic model of fentanyl pharmacokinetics. Drug is administered into the central tank, from which it can distribute into two peripheral tanks, or it may be eliminated. The volume of the tanks is proportional to the volumes of distribution. The cross-sectional area of the pipes is proportional to the clearance. (Adapted from Youngs EJ, Shafer SL: Basic pharmacokinetic and pharmacodynamic principles. *In* White PF [ed]: Textbook of Intravenous Anesthesia. Baltimore, Williams & Wilkins, 1997, p 10.)

Very rapid movement of the drug from the plasma to the rapidly equilibrating tissues characterizes this phase. Often, there is a second, *slow-distribution phase* (see Fig. 3-18, *dashed line*) that is characterized by movement of drug into more slowly equilibrating tissues and return of drug to the plasma from the most rapidly equilibrating tissues (i.e., those that reached equilibrium with the plasma during phase 1). The *terminal phase* (see Fig. 3-18, *dotted line*) is a straight line when plotted on a semilogarithmic graph. The terminal phase is often called the *elimination phase* because the primary mechanism for decreasing drug concentration during the terminal phase is drug elimination from the body. The distinguishing characteristic of the terminal elimination phase is that the relative proportion of drug in the plasma and peripheral volumes of distribution remains constant. During this terminal phase, drug returns from the rapid and slow distribution volumes to the plasma and is permanently removed from the plasma by metabolism or excretion.

The presence of three distinct phases after bolus injection is a defining characteristic of a mammillary model with three compartments. It is possible to develop hydraulic models, as shown in Figure 3-19, for intravenous drugs.[8] In this model, there are three tanks, corresponding (see Fig 3-19, *left to right*) with the slowly equilibrating peripheral compartment, the central compartment (i.e., the plasma, into which drug is injected), and the rapidly equilibrating peripheral compartment. The horizontal pipes represent intercompartmental clearance or (for the pipe draining onto the page) metabolic clearance. The volumes of each tank correspond with the volumes of the compartments for fentanyl. The cross-sectional areas of the pipes correlate with fentanyl's systemic and inter-compartmental clearances. The height of water in each tank corresponds to drug concentration.

Using this hydraulic model, we can follow the processes that decrease drug concentration over time after bolus injection. Initially, drug flows from the central compartment to both peripheral compartments through intercompartmental clearance and completely out of the model through metabolic clearance. Because there are three places for drug to go, the central compartment concentration decreases very rapidly. At the transition between the solid line and the dashed line, there is a change in the role of the most rapidly equilibrating compartment. At this transition, the central compartment concentration falls below the concentration in the rapidly equilibrating compartment, and the direction of flow between them is reversed. After this transition (see Fig. 3-19, *dashed line*), drug in the plasma only has two places to go: flow into the slowly equilibrating compartment and be removed by metabolic clearance. These processes are partly offset by the return of drug to the plasma from the rapidly equilibrating compartment. The net effect is that once the rapidly equilibrating compartment has come to equilibration, the central compartment concentration falls far more slowly than before.

After the concentration in the central compartment decreases below those of the rapidly and slowly equilibrating compartments (see Fig. 3-19, *dotted line*), the only method of decreasing the plasma concentration is metabolic clearance. The return of drug from both peripheral compartments to the central compartment greatly slows the rate of decrease in plasma drug concentration.

Curves that continuously decrease over time with a continuously increasing slope (i.e., curves such as those in Figs. 3-18 and 3-19) can be described by a sum of exponentials. In pharmacokinetics, one way of denoting this sum of exponentials is to say that the plasma concentration over time is as follows:

$$C(t) = A e^{-\alpha t} + B e^{-\beta t} + C e^{-\gamma t} \qquad (41)$$

In Equation 41, t is the time since the bolus, C(t) is the drug concentration after a bolus dose, and A, α, B, β, C, and γ are parameters of a pharmacokinetic model. A, B, and C are called *coefficients,* and α, β, and γ are called *exponents.* After a bolus injection, all six of the parameters in Equation 41 are greater than 0.

The main reason that polyexponential equations are used is that they describe the plasma concentrations observed after bolus injection, except for the misspecification in the first minute. Compartmental pharmacokinetics is strictly empirical; the models describe the data, not the processes by which the observations came to be. Fortunately, polyexponential equations permit us to use many of the one-compartment ideas previously developed, with some generalization of the concepts. This involves translating Equation 41 into a model of volumes and clearances that has an appealing, if not necessarily accurate, physiologic flavor.

Equation 41 says that the concentrations over time are the algebraic sum of three separate functions: $Ae^{-\alpha t}$, $Be^{-\beta t}$, and $Ce^{-\gamma t}$. Typically, α > β > γ by about one order of magnitude. We can graph each of these functions separately and their sum, as shown in Figure 3-20. At time 0 (t = 0), Equation 41 reduces to the following:

$$C_0 = A + B + C \qquad (42)$$

The sum of the coefficients A, B, and C equals the concentration immediately after a bolus.

Special significance is often ascribed to the smallest exponent. This exponent determines the slope of the final log-linear portion of the curve. When the medical literature refers to the half-life of a drug, unless otherwise stated, the half-life is the terminal half-life (i.e., 0.693/smallest exponent). However, the terminal half-life for drugs with more than one exponential term is nearly uninterpretable. The terminal half-life is merely the upper limit on the time required for the concentrations to decrease by 50% after drug administration. Usually, the time for a 50% decrease is much faster than that upper limit. This topic is discussed further in Chapter 12.

Constructing pharmacokinetic models represents trade-offs in accurately describing the data, having confidence in the results, and mathematical tractability. Adding exponents to the model usually provides a better description of the observed concentrations. However, adding more exponent terms usually decreases our confidence in how well we know each coefficient and exponential and greatly increases the mathematical burden of the models. This is why most pharmacokinetic models are limited to two or three exponents.

Part of the continuing popularity of polyexponential models of pharmacokinetics is that they can be mathematically transformed from the admittedly unintuitive exponential form in equation to a more easily intuited compartmental form (see Fig. 3-15). Micro rate constants, expressed as k_{ij}, define the rate of drug transfer from compartment i to compartment j. Compartment 0 is a compartment outside the model, and k_{10} is the micro rate constant for processes acting through metabolism or elimination that irreversibly remove drug from the central compartment (i.e., analogous to k for a one-compartment model). The intercompartmental micro rate constants (e.g., k_{12}, k_{21}) describe the movement of drug between the central and peripheral compartments. Each compartment has at least two micro rate constants, one for drug entry and one for drug exit. The micro rate constants for the two- and three-compartment models can be seen in Figure 3-15. The differential equations describing the rate of change for the amount of drugs in compartments 1, 2, and 3 follow directly from the micro rate constants. For the two-compartment model, the differential equations for each compartment are as follows:

$$\frac{dx_1}{dt} = I + x_2\,k_{21} - x_1\,k_{10} - x_1\,k_{12}$$
$$\frac{dx_2}{dt} = x_1\,k_{12} - x_2\,k_{21} \qquad (43)$$

For the three-compartment model, the differential equations for each compartment are as follows:

$$\frac{dx_1}{dt} = I + x_2\,k_{21} + x_3\,k_{31} - x_1\,k_{10} - x_1\,k_{12} - x_1\,k_{13}$$
$$\frac{dx_2}{dt} = x_1\,k_{12} - x_2\,k_{21} \qquad (44)$$
$$\frac{dx_3}{dt} = x_1\,k_{13} - x_3\,k_{31}$$

In Equation 44, I is the rate of drug input. An easy way to model pharmacokinetics is to convert the previous differential equations to difference equations, so that dx becomes Δx and dt becomes Δt. With a Δt of 1 second, the error from linearizing the differential equations is less than 1%. In this way, desktop computers can easily simulate pharmacokinetics using a spreadsheet.

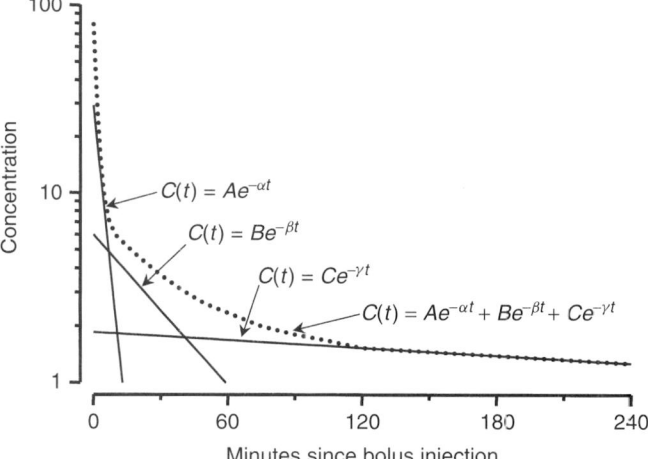

Figure 3–20 The disposition of a three-compartment model (i.e., triexponential model) consists of the sum of three monoexponential functions. The concentrations over time are the algebraic sum of three separate functions, $Ae^{-\alpha t}$, $Be^{-\beta t}$, and $Ce^{-\gamma t}$. Typically, α > β > γ by about one order of magnitude. The functions can be graphed separately *(solid lines)* and as their sum *(dotted line).*

For the one-compartment model, k was both the rate constant and the exponent. For multicompartment models, the relationships are more complex. Interconversion between the micro rate constants and the exponents becomes exceedingly complex as more exponents are added, because every exponent is a function of every micro rate constant and vice versa. These interconversions can be found in the Excel spreadsheet ("convert.xls"), which can be downloaded from http://anesthesia.stanford.edu/pkpd.

The Time Course of Drug Effect

The plasma is not the site of drug effect for anesthetic drugs. There is a time lag between drug concentration in plasma and that in the effect site. For example, one significant difference between fentanyl and alfentanil is the more rapid onset of alfentanil's drug effect. The black bar in the upper graph of Figure 3-21 shows the duration of a fentanyl infusion.[9] Rapid arterial samples document the rise in fentanyl concentration. The time course of electroencephalographic (EEG) effect lags 2 to 3 minutes behind the rapid rise in arterial concentration. This lag is called *hysteresis*. The plasma concentration peaks at the moment the infusion is turned off. After the peak plasma concentration (see Fig. 3-21), the fentanyl concentration rapidly decreases. However, the offset of fentanyl drug effect again lags well behind the decrease in concentration. The lower graph in Figure 3-21 shows the same study design in a patient receiving alfentanil. Because of alfentanil's rapid blood-brain equilibration, there is less hysteresis with alfentanil than with fentanyl.

Typically, the relationship between the plasma and the site of drug effect is modeled with an effect-site model, as shown in Figure 3-22. The site of drug effect is connected to the plasma by a first-order process. The following equation relates effect site concentration to plasma concentration:

$$\frac{dCe}{dt} = k_{e0}\, Cp - k_{e0}\, Ce \qquad (45)$$

In Equation 45, Ce is the effect site concentration, Cp is the plasma drug concentration, and k_{e0} is the rate constant for elimination of drug from the effect site. It is most easily understood in terms of its reciprocal, $0.693/k_{e0}$, the half-time for equilibration between the plasma and the site of drug effect.

The constant k_{e0} has a large influence on the rate of rise of drug effect, the rate of offset of drug effect, and the dose that is required to produce the desired drug effect. The mathematical basis of these relationships is explored in Chapter 12.

Summary of Pharmacokinetics

Pharmacokinetics involves fundamental physiologic processes, including metabolism, protein binding, tissue distribution, and drug transport into the site of drug effect. Pharmacokinetic models are mathematical relationships between dose and concentration in the plasma or at the site of drug effect. Such models can be used to determine how best to give drugs to achieve a therapeutic objective, but only when the relationship between drug concentration and drug effect is understood.

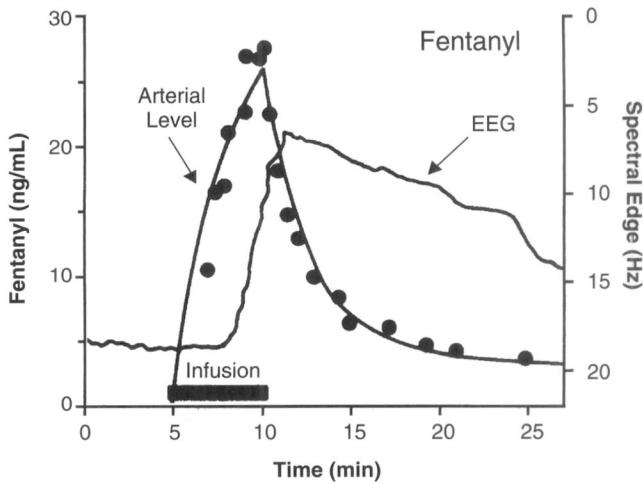

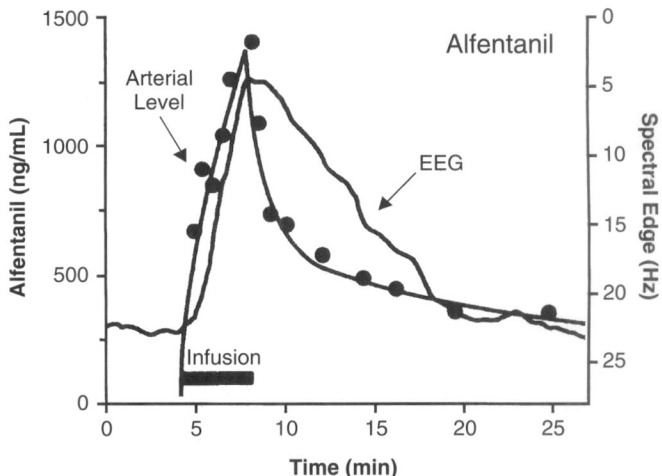

Figure 3–21 Fentanyl and alfentanil arterial concentrations *(circles)* and electroencephalographic (EEG) response *(irregular line)* to an intravenous infusion. With each drug, there is a time lag between the rise and fall in arterial concentration and the EEG response, but the time lag is much greater for fentanyl than for alfentanil. (Adapted from Scott JC, Ponganis KV, Stanski DR: EEG quantitation of narcotic effect: The comparative pharmacodynamics of fentanyl and alfentanil. Anesthesiology 62:234-241, 1985.)

PHARMACODYNAMICS

Overview

Pharmacodynamics describes the relationship between plasma drug concentration and pharmacologic effect. Simply stated, pharmacodynamics attempts to explain what a drug does to the body. Although the study of clinically important drug effects is multifaceted, we divide pharmacodynamics into three general areas: transduction of biologic signals (i.e., receptor theory and structure), developments in molecular pharmacology, and clinical evaluation of drug effects. Each of these aspects of pharmacodynamics is explored in detail in the following sections.

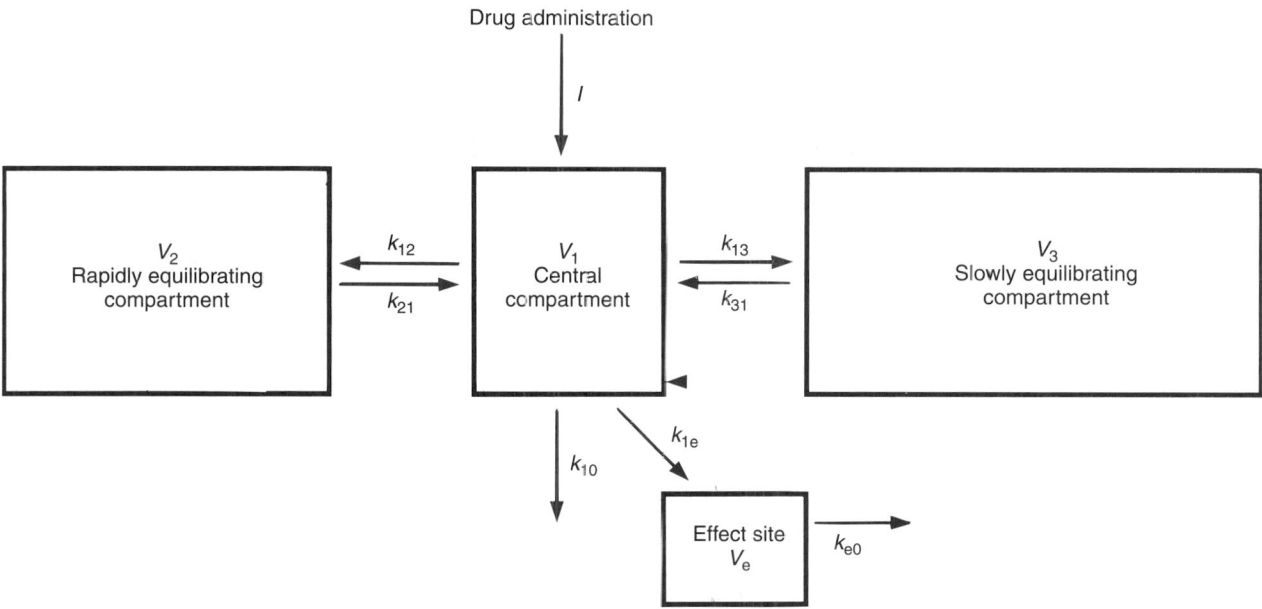

Figure 3–22 A three-compartment model with an added effect site to account for the equilibration delay between the rise and fall of arterial drug concentrations and the onset and offset of drug effect. The effect site is assumed to have a negligible volume.

Transduction of Biologic Signals

Receptor Theory

Definition

In the broadest sense, a receptor is a component of a cell that interacts selectively with an extracellular compound to initiate a cascade of biochemical events that culminate in the observed effects of the compound. Binding of a drug to a receptor determines (1) the quantitative relationship between a given dose of a drug and the resulting effect, (2) the selectivity of a given drug's activity and effect, and (3) an explanation of the pharmacologic activity of receptor agonists, antagonists, and inverse agonists. Receptors therefore mediate or amplify the effect of a drug on the biologic system.

Historical Perspective

Although the overall concept of receptors is generally attributed to Paul Ehrlich (1854-1915), earlier work performed by Claude Bernard (1813-1878) paved the way for receptor theory. This earlier work is of particular interest to anesthesiologists because it elucidated the mechanism of action of curare, an arrow poison. In his experiments, Claude Bernard ligated vessels leading to one hind limb of a frog while leaving nerve input intact; he then administered intravenous curare. Pinching the paralyzed hind limb produced reflex movements in the opposite unparalyzed vessel-ligated hind limb. These experiments and others demonstrated for the first time the separation between sensory and motor nervous systems and revealed that circulating "substances" produced selective effects on organ systems, a concept important in the development of receptor theory.

The concept of selectivity of effect eventually led Paul Ehrlich to his conclusion that "agents cannot act unless they are bound," a cornerstone of receptor theory.

Although Ehrlich is attributed with discovering this concept, his contemporary J. N. Langley (1852-1926) coined the term *receptive substance* (i.e., receptor). Langley extended Claude Bernard's work by showing that nicotine and curare had mutually antagonistic effects on the same receptive substance, which was neither nerve nor muscle. We now recognize this receptive substance as the nicotinic acetylcholine receptor in the neuromuscular junction. Several decades of research have refined the receptor theory, and receptors are now recognized as discrete excitable proteins.

Classic Receptor Theory

The binding of a ligand (i.e., drug molecule) to its receptor follows the laws of chemical reactions (analogous to Michaelis Menten enzyme kinetics) and can be summarized by the following relationship:

$$[L][R] \underset{k_{off}}{\overset{k_{on}}{\rightleftharpoons}} [LR]$$

In this reversible equation, k_{on} is the rate constant for the ligand binding to the receptor, k_{off} is the rate constant for the ligand disassociating from the receptor, [L] is the concentration of the ligand, [R] is the concentration of the unbound receptor, and [LR] is the concentration of the bound receptor. Units for k_{on} are units of [L] multiplied by the units of [R] over time; typically, units of L are nanomoles per liter. The units for k_{off} are the units of [LR] over time. The term K_d, the dissociation constant, mathematically defines characteristics of ligand-receptor interactions at equilibrium:

$$K_d = \frac{[L][R]}{[LR]} = \frac{k_{off}}{k_{on}}$$

The units of K_d are the units of [L], which are units of concentration. When enough drug is administered to occupy exactly 50% of the receptors (i.e., [R] = [LR]), the measured K_d value is equal to the drug concentration. A low K_d value indicates that less drug is required to occupy 50% of the receptors, implying that each molecule of drug is tightly associated with the receptor. A high K_d value indicates that more drug is required to occupy 50% of receptors, implying a weak binding to the receptor. K_d has been determined for many of the drugs administered during anesthesia. The reciprocal of K_d is K_a, the association constant, which is exactly analogous to the K_a defined for protein binding. K_a is a measure of the affinity of the drug for the receptor. A drug with a low K_d value has a high K_a value and therefore high affinity for the receptor.

In practice, it is difficult to measure precise drug-receptor occupancy. It is often assumed that the drug-receptor complex represents an intermediate step in the production of a specific effect. Many investigators apply pharmacodynamic theory to compare a given dose of a drug with a resulting effect. An effect can be any biochemical or physiologic variable that is measurable. A measured effect can be an alteration in a biochemical compound, an enzyme level, a physiologic variable such as heart rate or blood pressure, or a response to any graded input into the biologic system. For example, in evaluating the pharmacodynamics of muscle relaxants, the measured effect is not a direct measurement of drug-receptor complexes, but rather a response to a neuromuscular stimulus as delivered by a nerve stimulator.

From the discussion of pharmacokinetics, the delivery of a drug to a given receptor is clearly time and dose dependent. If the receptor is located within the central compartment, there may be nearly instantaneous equilibration after an intravenous injection, and the peak effect may occur immediately. If drug must cross from the central compartment to the site of drug effect, a delay will occur. The onset of drug effect can also be delayed by the time required for the body to respond to the drug. This delay may occur anywhere on the path between drug-receptor binding and clinical manifestation of drug effect. Examples of post-transduction time delays are drug-receptor complex-induced secondary messenger changes, increased enzyme synthesis, and the time required for physiologic change (e.g., reduced fluid content).

RECEPTOR AGONISTS AND ANTAGONISTS. Drugs that are agonists induce an effect that mimics endogenous hormones or neurotransmitters when bound to a receptor. This effect may be stimulatory or inhibitory. The term *affinity* as related to a given agonist is a measure of the attraction between the given drug and receptor. A drug with low affinity for a given receptor tends not to bind to the receptor and produces little or no effect. An agonist that binds avidly (or with high affinity) to a given receptor produces the receptor-determined effect at a lower given dose.

Full agonists completely activate a receptor, whereas partial agonists only partially activate a receptor, even at very high concentrations (Fig. 3-23). The difference between full and partial agonists results from different intrinsic efficacy for each drug. Efficacy should not be confused with affinity. Two drugs can have identical affinity for a receptor (and therefore bind to the same extent at a given

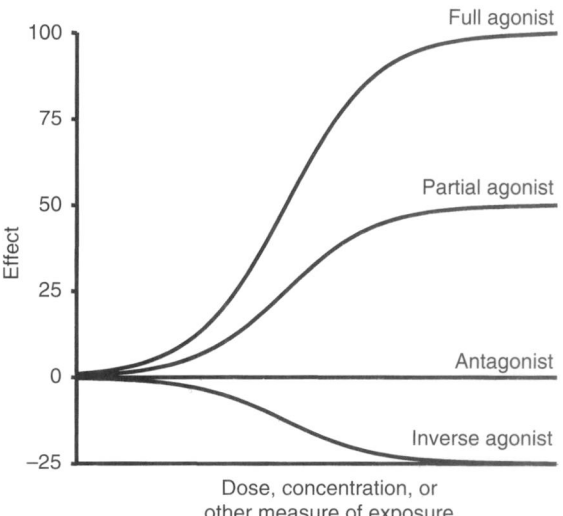

Figure 3–23 Effects of various types of ligands on receptor responses. A full agonist produces complete (100%) activation of a receptor at high concentrations, whereas partial agonist binding results in less than 100% activation, even at very high concentrations. A neutral antagonist has no activity of its own. Inverse agonists can be thought of as "superantagonists" because binding of these ligands produces a response below the baseline response measured in the absence of drug. If the physiologic effect of the baseline levels of activated receptor (R*) is small, antagonists and inverse agonists may not be clinically distinguishable.

drug concentration), but they may produce different levels of activation of the receptor. Both are agonists, but the drug that produces maximal receptor activation is called a *full agonist* and has high efficacy, whereas the drug that produces less than a maximal receptor activation is called a *partial agonist* with less intrinsic efficacy. The mechanisms underlying one drug's producing full versus partial agonist effects remain shrouded in mystery, but they may be related to the ability of the drug to stabilize the high-affinity state of the receptor (see "Receptor States").

Drugs that are antagonists inhibit or prevent receptor-mediated agonist effects by competing for receptor occupancy. A *competitive antagonist* can generally be displaced from the receptor complex by the administration of a large enough concentration of receptor agonist, permitting the agonist to produce the expected effect despite the presence of antagonist. A *noncompetitive antagonist* usually binds irreversibly to the receptor complex, producing loss of the expected effect that cannot be compensated by administration of high concentrations of receptor agonist. For example, vecuronium is a competitive antagonist of acetylcholine (see Chapter 13). Acetylcholine mediates muscle contraction through the postsynaptic nicotinic acetylcholine receptor at the neuromuscular junction. When vecuronium binds to the postsynaptic acetylcholine receptor, acetylcholine agonism is blocked, and neuromuscular transmission is inhibited. The result is flaccid paralysis. Neuromuscular transmission may be reinstated by administering an acetylcholine esterase inhibitor. Acetylcholine esterase inhibitors prevent breakdown of acetylcholine, effectively raising the concentration of the agonist, acetylcholine, at the receptor, which then displaces vecuronium from the receptor complex. When enough vecuronium is displaced, muscle contraction is reinstated. Most antagonist drugs used in clinical medicine are competitive antagonists.

Inverse agonists can be thought of as "superantagonists" because they decrease receptor responses to less than baseline values (see Fig. 3-23). An example of concentration-response relationships for four different benzodiazepines and EEG response[10] is shown in Figure 3-24 (see Chapter 10). In this example, the EEG response represents a surrogate clinical end point for binding of benzodiazepines to the γ-aminobutyric acid (GABA$_A$) ligand-gated ion channel complex with resultant modulations of ion fluxes in the central nervous system (CNS).

RECEPTOR STATES. Classic receptor theory describes interaction between ligand and receptor based on the laws of mass action. At a molecular level, this interaction has been interpreted over the years to suggest that binding of agonist to receptor initiates a change in receptor conformation, changing the receptor from an inactive (R) to an activated (R*) state (Fig. 3-25). In this model, the change in receptor conformation facilitates activated receptor coupling to intermediary proteins (e.g., guanine nucleotide [G] proteins) or second messengers (i.e., effectors [E]), which then initiate a rapid cascade of cellular responses.

Transgenic animal experiments have shed light on ligand and receptor interactions. In an elegant set of experiments in which β$_2$-adrenergic receptors were massively overexpressed in mouse myocardium, second messenger responses were increased in the absence of ligand when compared with normal mouse myocardium. Activity of adenylyl cyclase, the second messenger most commonly studied for β$_2$-adrenergic receptors, is identical at baseline in transgenic animals (in the absence of drug) compared with normal mice stimulated with isoproterenol, a β$_2$-adrenergic-receptor agonist. Isoproterenol stimulation of transgenic animals is unable to increase adenylyl cyclase activity higher than this elevated baseline. This finding suggests that a subpopulation of receptors is already fully activated in these transgenic animals. One way to analyze these findings is to consider that at baseline a small

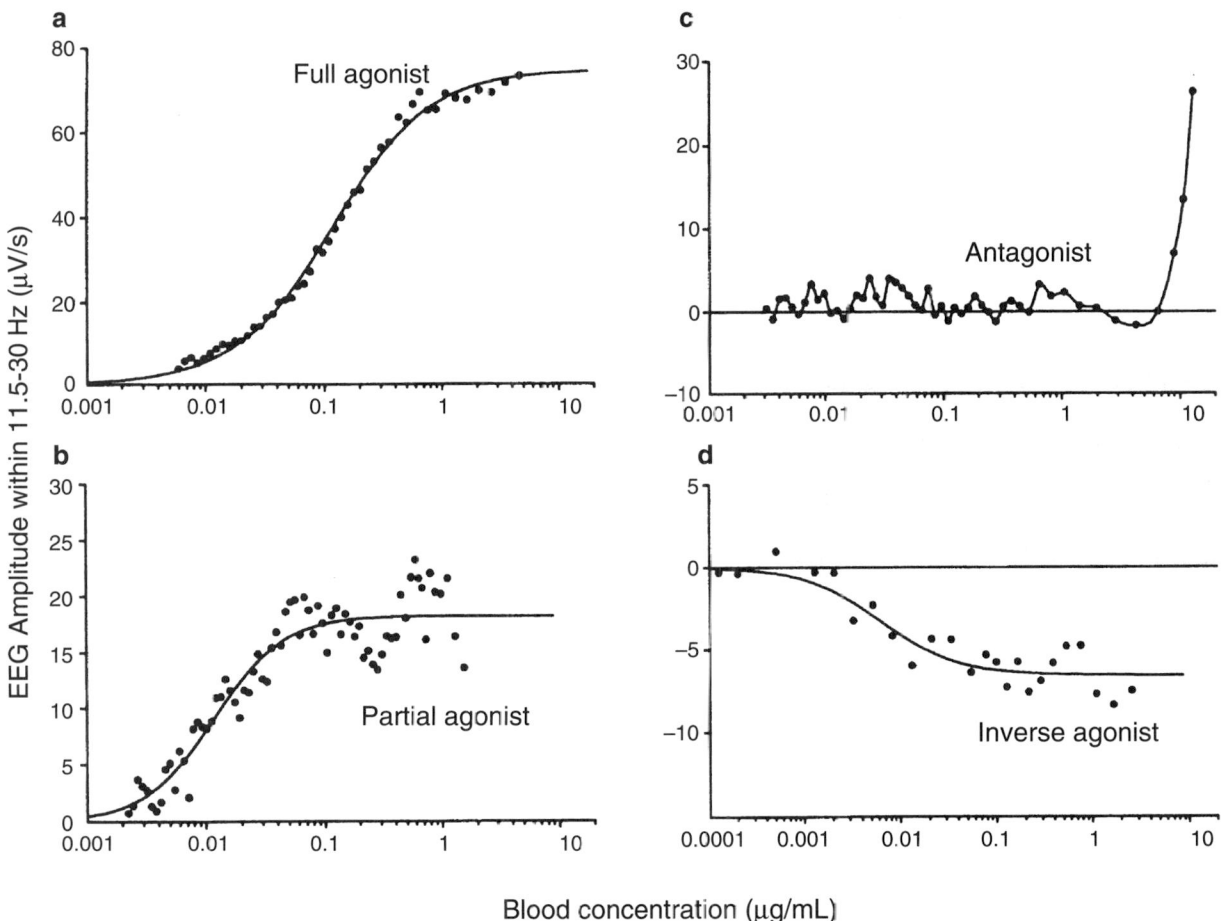

Figure 3–24 The concentration-electroencephalographic (EEG) response relationship for four benzodiazepines: midazolam (full agonist, a), bretazenil (partial agonist, b), flumazenil (antagonist, c), and RO 19-4063 (inverse agonist, d). The maximum effect seen in the EEG response correlates with clinical action (full agonist > partial agonist > antagonist > inverse agonist). (Adapted from Shafer S: Principles of pharmacokinetics and pharmacodynamics. *In* Longnecker DE, Tinker JH, Morgan GE [eds]: Principles and Practice of Anesthesiology, 2nd ed. St. Louis, Mosby–Year Book, 1997, and from Mandema JW, Kuck MT, Danhof M: Differences in intrinsic efficacy of benzodiazepines are reflected in their concentration-EEG effect relationship. Br J Pharmacol 105:164-170, 1992.)

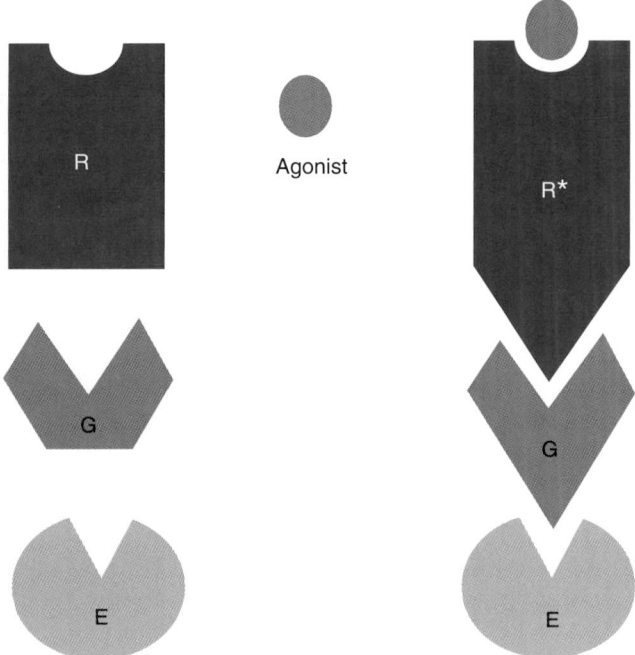

Figure 3–25 Schematic drawing of classic receptor activation. For years, binding of ligand was thought to cause receptors to change from an inactive state (R) to an activated state (R*). The activated receptor interacted with intermediary guanine nucleotide (G) proteins or directly with second messenger cascades (i.e., effectors [E]), or both. Later information suggests a more complicated equilibrium between R and R*, as shown in Figures 2-26 and 2-27.

known to vary among tissues, a finding suggesting that the absolute concentration of R* (and the spontaneous conversion rates between R and R*) may be tissue dependent. This finding is clinically important because inverse agonists, which are known to stabilize R, drive the equation toward the left (i.e., toward R). This decreases responses to less than the clinical baseline value, toward the true baseline in the absence of any receptor activation. The biggest differences between apparent baseline and true baseline are likely to occur in tissues with higher concentrations of spontaneous R*, and inverse agonists are therefore most efficacious in such tissues. Figure 3-24 illustrates a tissue (i.e., CNS) with enough activated GABA$_A$ ligand-gated ion channels (R*) to see EEG changes with an inverse agonist. This finding provides a rationale for the inverse agonist antiepileptic drugs being developed. This discussion assumes only two receptor states, R (completely inactive) and R* (fully activated). Later experimental evidence suggests the existence of intermediate transition states between R and R* (hence the use of curved lines in addition to straight lines in Fig. 3-26). However, in the interest of simplicity, further discussion in this chapter uses only R and R*.

The discovery of spontaneous conversion between R and R* has implications for understanding the action of ligands (i.e., agonists, antagonists, and inverse agonists). Instead of agonists causing conversion from R to R*, it is thought that ligands stabilize a given receptor state. As shown in Figure 3-27, agonists stabilize (or energetically favor) R*, and inverse agonists stabilize R, whereas neutral antagonists bind equally to R and R*. Binding of an agonist to a receptor removes the receptor from the equation because rapid coupling to second messengers occurs, driving (by mass action) the equation toward that specific state (Fig. 3-28). The probability of being in the R* state increases in the presence of an agonist. Conversely, inverse agonists drive the equation to the left, stabilizing the R configuration. Neutral antagonists bind equally to R and R*, preventing agonist binding without altering the equilibrium between R and R*; neutral antagonists do not change the observed baseline response (see Fig. 3-23). Many classic antagonists have been tested and found to be inverse agonists rather than neutral antagonists. For example, among the commonly clinically used β$_2$-adrenergic-receptor (β$_2$AR) antagonists, metoprolol and bisoprolol show significant inverse agonist activity, carvedilol has weaker inverse agonist properties at the β$_2$AR and displays

percentage (e.g., 1%) of receptors spontaneously exists in the activated (R*) state. Because this 1% of activated receptors may be normal in that tissue, the activity of these R* receptors is included as part of the baseline effect measured in the absence of drug. However, after massive overexpression of β$_2$-adrenergic receptors occurs (e.g., in a transgenic animal), 1% of the total receptors becomes a very large number of activated receptors. This mimics the effect of a maximal dose of drug, which would produce similar numbers of receptors in the R* state.

These findings have broad implications for understanding receptor states and drug-receptor interactions. Instead of ligand binding causing a change from R to R* (see Fig. 3-25), these data suggest spontaneous conversion from the R to the R* state (Fig. 3-26). In most tissues, the concentration of R* represents a small fraction of total overall receptor (hence the *large arrow* pointing toward R in Fig. 3-26). However, baseline receptor responses are

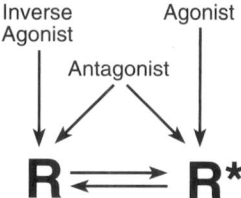

Figure 3–27 Ligand stabilization of receptor states. Agonists stabilize active receptors (R*), inverse agonists stabilize inactive receptors (R), and neutral antagonists bind equally to R and R* without affecting the equilibrium between the two receptor states.

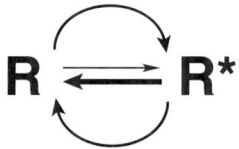

Figure 3–26 Spontaneous conversion of receptors from an inactive (R) to an active (R*) state. In most tissues, R* represents a small fraction of the total receptor population.

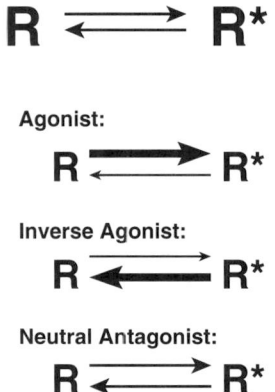

Agonist:

Inverse Agonist:

Neutral Antagonist:

Figure 3–28 Equilibrium between inactive receptors (R) and active receptors (R*) is tissue specific and depends on the type of ligand administered. By stabilizing R*, agonists drive the equilibrium to the right. Inverse agonists stabilize R, driving the equilibrium to the left. Because neutral antagonists bind equally to R and R*, they do not affect tissue-specific equilibrium between R and R*.

neutral antagonist activity at β_1ARs, alprenolol has weaker still (20%) inverse agonist activity at the β_2AR, and xamoterol displays marked partial agonist activity at β_1ARs.[11,12] Because inverse agonists may have theoretical advantages in treating certain diseases (e.g., seizures, congestive heart failure), clinicians should critically evaluate recent pharmacologic data before using an antagonist to distinguish whether the drug is a neutral antagonist or an inverse agonist.

Receptor Structure
General Principles
Receptors are located in many places in the cell—outer cell membrane, cytoplasm, intracellular organelle membranes, and nucleus. The overall physical structure of a receptor depends on the type of receptor considered and its location. For example, membrane receptors have structures different from those of cytoplasmic receptors. In general, cytoplasmic receptors and nuclear receptors bind ligands that readily traverse cell-membrane lipid bilayers to reach the cytoplasm or nucleus. These ligands therefore must contain significant hydrophobic (i.e., lipophilic) components. Examples of cytoplasmic and nuclear receptors include steroid and thyroid hormone receptors. In contrast, most receptors important to the anesthesiologist are excitable cell-membrane proteins, such as membrane receptors, ligand-gated ion channels, and voltage-gated ion channels (Fig. 3-29). Many endogenous hormones and exogenous drugs are water soluble (i.e., hydrophilic and charged) and are unable to cross cell-membrane lipid bilayers. A mechanism is required to transduce drug binding at the extracellular surface into changes in intracellular physiology. Overall, the membrane's receptor structure depends on whether coupling to second messengers through intermediary proteins is required or whether the receptor is part of a larger ion channel complex (e.g., ligand-gated ion channels). Each of these types of membrane receptors has a role in mediating the action of various drugs important in anesthesiology. It is beyond the scope of this chapter to list all identified receptor proteins. However, prototypical examples are used to illustrate important pharmacodynamic principles.

Guanine Nucleotide Protein–Coupled Receptors
One of the most common methods by which membrane receptors translate agonist occupancy into intracellular action is through intermediary G proteins. As a result, G protein–coupled receptors are the most abundant type of receptor known. The overall structure of a G protein–coupled receptor is shown schematically in Figure 3-30. Two-dimensional representation reveals an extracellular amino terminus containing glycosylation sites, an intracellular carboxyl terminus, a fatty acid attachment (usually

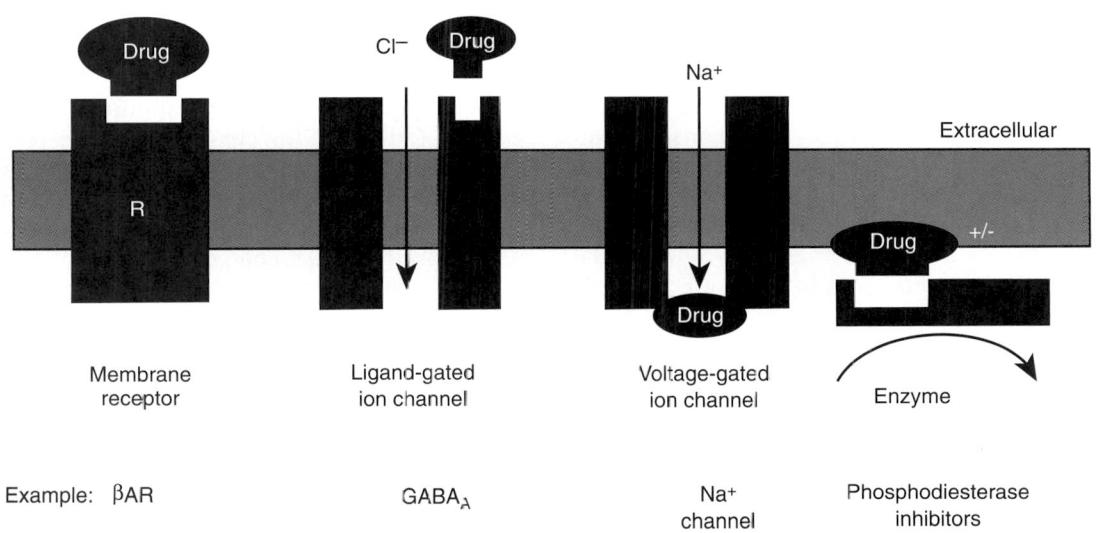

Figure 3–29 Schematic drawing of four types of membrane-associated drug targets: membrane (G protein–coupled) receptor, ligand-gated ion channel, voltage-sensitive ion channel, and an enzyme. Potential sites of drug action are shown. βAR, β-adrenergic receptor; GABA$_A$, γ-aminobutyric acid.

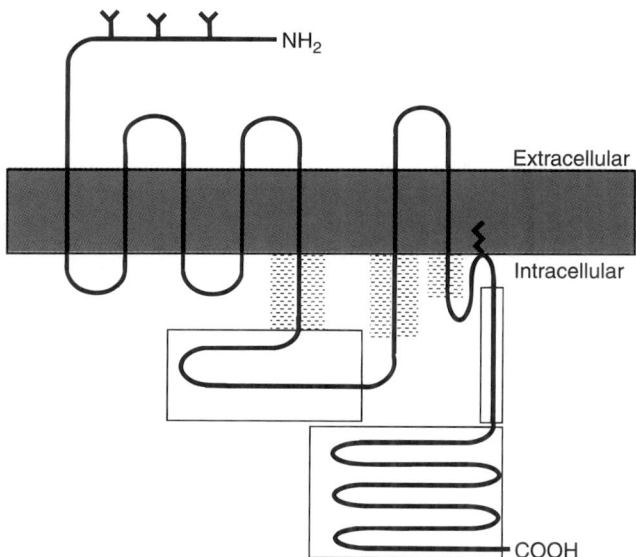

Figure 3–30 Schematic drawing of a G protein–coupled receptor. A two-dimensional version of receptor structure is shown with seven transmembrane domains, an extracellular amino (NH_2) terminus (with associated glycosylation sites [Y]), an intracellular carboxyl (COOH) terminus, palmitoylated cysteine residue (*crooked line* extending into the membrane), three extracellular loops, and four intracellular loops. Major sites of G protein interactions with the receptor are speckled; potential sites of phosphorylation in the third intracellular loop and carboxyl terminus are enclosed in boxes.

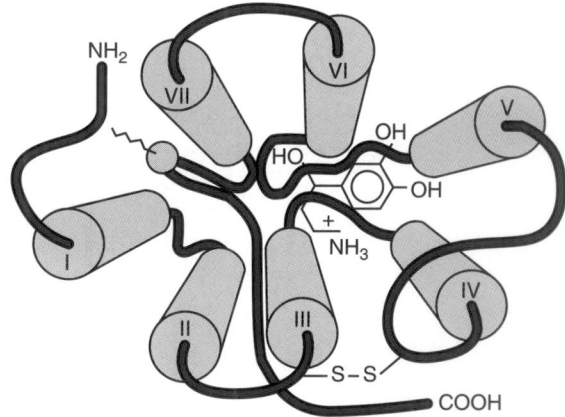

Figure 3–31 Schematic drawing of the three-dimensional structure of the β_2-adrenergic receptor (a prototypical G protein–coupled receptor), looking from the outside of the cell inward. Transmembrane domains (denoted by cylinders and numbered with roman numerals) coalesce to form a binding pocket. The correct orientation of the agonist norepinephrine is shown. Notice that agonist affinity is determined by specific amino acids located in transmembranes III, IV, and VII. These critical sites in transmembrane domains have been determined experimentally using chimeric receptor and mutagenesis approaches combined with sophisticated computer-modeling techniques. Ultimate confirmation of these structures will require crystallographic data, an approach that is being attempted by several laboratories. (Adapted from Stapelfeldt WH: The autonomic nervous system. *In* Schwinn DA [ed]: Scientific Principles of Anesthesia, vol 2. Philadelphia, Current Medicine, 1998.)

through palmitoylation or myristoylation of a carboxyl-terminal cysteine residue), three extracellular loops, and four intracellular loops. Major sites of G protein interactions with the receptor occur in the third and fourth (and to a lesser extent, second) intracellular loops, whereas major sites of phosphorylation, which is often correlated with desensitization (i.e., dampening of receptor responses), generally occur in the third intracellular loop and carboxyl terminus.

Although a two-dimensional schematic is shown in Figure 3-30, it is important to remember that G protein–coupled receptors are three-dimensional structures with transmembrane segments coalescing around a central binding pocket (Fig. 3-31).[13] Although transmembrane amino acids must be hydrophobic overall to be energetically favored in the lipid membrane, side chains on individual amino acids may be charged. Specific amino acids therefore act as counter ions to anchor charged (water-soluble) hormone or drug to the receptor. Structure-activity relationships between drug and the three-dimensional configuration of the receptor's binding site are critically important in determining binding properties. The chemical structure of a drug must match the three-dimensional configuration of the binding area of a receptor. Subtle changes in drug structure may dramatically alter the ability of a drug to bind to a specific receptor population. Two drugs with seemingly unrelated two-dimensional chemical structures may bind to the same receptor if their three-dimensional structures and charged areas are similar. The three-dimensional components of a ligand that interact with ligand-recognition portions of a receptor are referred to as the *pharmacophore.*

Ion Channels

In addition to membrane receptors, pharmacologic agents act on other excitable cell-membrane proteins, such as ion channels. These channels mediate neural signaling by modulating ion permeability in electrically excitable membranes. Because many drugs act directly or indirectly through ion channels, it is important for the anesthesiologist to understand their general function. Classic ion channels such as the sodium channel have charged regions that span the cell membrane. The formation of ion pairs between many positive and negative charges helps to stabilize the channel in the membrane. Voltage-dependent gating of the sodium channel is made possible by the presence of a *voltage sensor*—a collection of charges that moves under the influence of the cell-membrane electrical field (hence the name *voltage-gated ion channels*). During depolarization, these charges presumably move outward, causing conformational changes and rearrangement of ion pairs that result in sodium permeability. Local anesthetics work by blocking voltage-gated sodium channels. This concept is discussed in more detail in Chapter 14.

The combination of a classic receptor protein plus an ion channel results in a ligand-gated ion channel, giving rise to the unique ability of certain drugs to alter membrane permeability to ions directly. Many anesthetic drugs act on ligand-gated ion channels, such as the nicotinic acetylcholine receptor and the GABA$_A$ receptor. The structure of the GABA$_A$ receptor is shown in Figure 3-32.[14,15] Ligand-gated ion channels have hydrophobic and charged

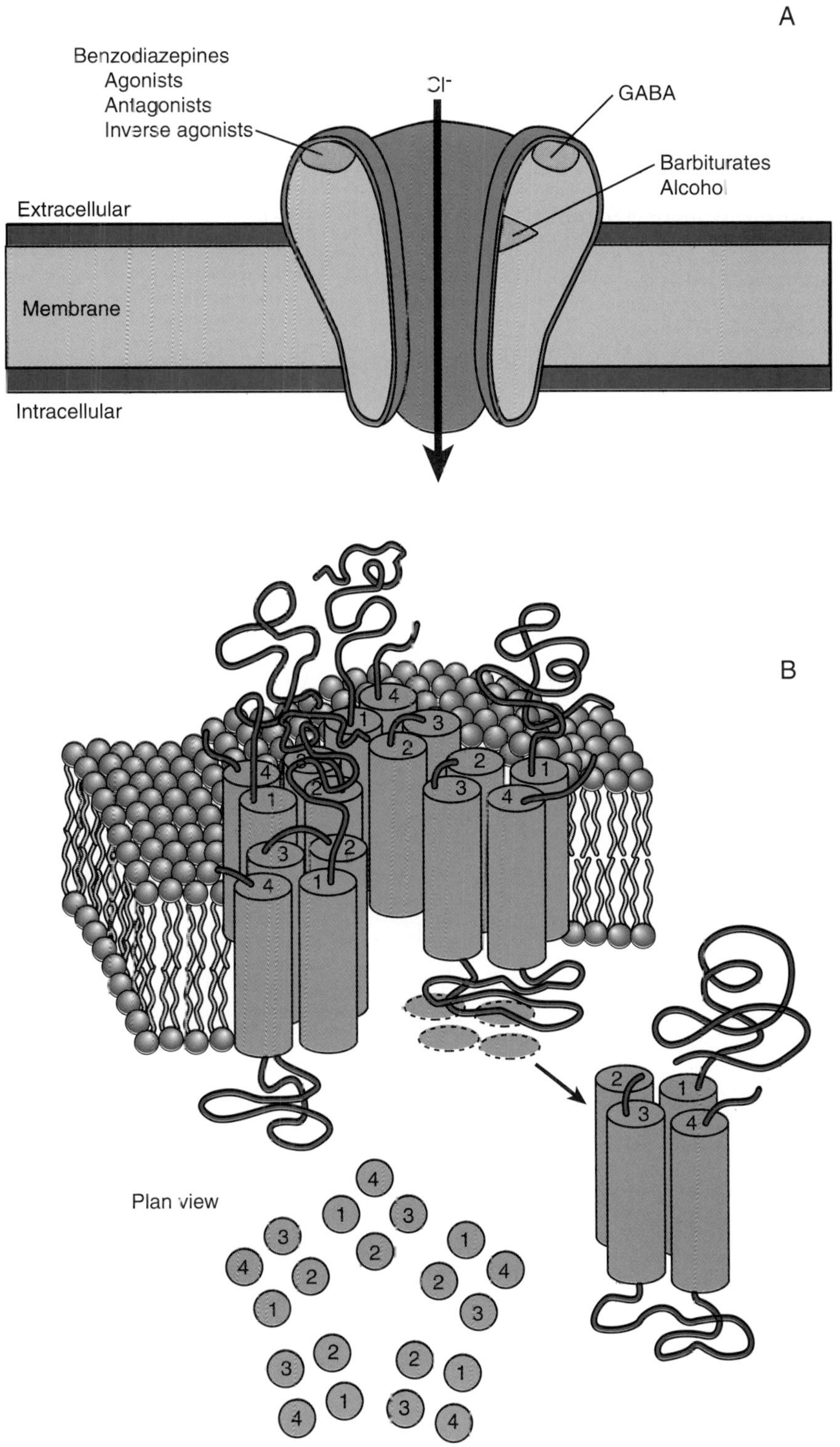

Figure 3–32 Cross-section of a schematized γ-aminobutyric acid (GABA)–benzodiazepine receptor complex, which is a prototypical ligand-gated ion channel complex. Binding of benzodiazepine agonists to the GABA$_A$ ligand–gated ion channel facilitates the action of endogenous GABA. This results in increased inhibitory chloride ion flux in the central nervous system. **A,** Schematic drawing of the GABA$_A$ ligand–gated ion channel complex shows the receptor sites for benzodiazepines and GABA, as well as distinct receptor sites for barbiturates and alcohol. **B,** Model of the GABA$_A$ receptor and chloride ion channel shows that the protein complex is composed of a hetero-oligomer of five subunits, including α, β, γ, and δ or ρ polypeptides. Each subunit has four putative membrane-spanning domains (numbered 1 through 4 and represented by cylinders). (**A,** from Berkowitz DE: Cellular signal transduction. *In* Schwinn DA [ed]: Scientific Principles of Anesthesia, vol 2. Philadelphia, Current Medicine, 1998; **B,** adapted from Firestone L, Quinlan J, Gyulai F: Mechanisms of anesthetic action. *In* Schwinn DA [ed]: Scientific Principles of Anesthesia, vol 2. Philadelphia, Current Medicine, 1998.)

transmembrane regions. The hydrophobic regions stabilize the structure in the membrane, and the centrally charged region serves as the pore for ion flux. The binding of drugs to receptors in ligand-gated ion channel complexes usually enhances or dampens an already existing neurotransmitter-induced ion flux. For example, the neurotransmitter GABA binds to its receptor within the GABA$_A$ ligand-gated ion channel complex and causes the movement of chloride ions intracellularly. This action results in lowered membrane potential, a hallmark of inhibitory neurotransmission. Drugs (e.g. benzodiazepines, barbiturates, alcohols) binding to other receptor sites in the GABA$_A$ ligand-gated ion channel facilitate the action of endogenous GABA. This process results in increased inhibitory chloride ion flux in the CNS (see Fig. 3-32). Most hypnotics (i.e., benzodiazepines, barbiturates, propofol, etomidate, and possibly the hypnotic action of inhaled anesthetics) act through potentiation of endogenous GABA at the $GABA_A$ ligand gated ion channel.

Ion Pumps

Another type of excitable membrane protein is the ion pump. The sodium-potassium–adenosine triphosphatase (ATPase) pump is perhaps the most familiar ion pump to the anesthesiologist because it is inhibited by digitalis. Extracellular fluid has high sodium and low potassium levels, whereas intracellular fluid has high potassium and low sodium concentrations. Because the nerve at rest is selectively permeable to potassium, but not to sodium, potassium moves extracellularly, creating a net positive extracellular charge and a net negative intracellular charge. Action potentials activate sodium channels, allowing sodium to rush intracellularly along chemical and electrical gradients. The sodium-potassium-ATPase pump then rapidly pumps sodium out of the cell in exchange for potassium, returning the cell to its original cation composition and electrical gradient. Drugs that act on ion pumps alter intracellular-extracellular cation ratios, resulting in altered membrane electrical potential.

Digitalis acts by inhibiting the sodium-potassium-ATPase pump. This is of special importance in the myocardial cell, where sodium-potassium-ATPase exchange is replaced by slower sodium-calcium exchange, thereby increasing intracellular calcium concentrations. Because calcium increases myocardial contractility, improved myocardial pump function results. This is the basis of digitalis use in the treatment of congestive heart failure.

Second Messengers

The binding of a hormone or drug to its receptor does not instantly produce clinical effects. Instead, a series of rapid biochemical events couples receptor binding to ultimate clinical effects. These biochemical events are called *second messengers*. Because alterations in second messenger coupling can alter the effectiveness of a drug, it is important that the anesthesiologist understand the general principles of second messenger action.

Many membrane receptors couple to their primary second messenger through G proteins, which are intermediate regulatory molecules. The coupling of G proteins to receptor-hormone complexes requires energy in the form of guanosine triphosphate (GTP). The hydrolysis of G protein–associated GTP to GDP is regulated by another set of proteins, called *RGS proteins*. After the receptor interacts with the G protein, the biochemical reaction in the effector cascade is triggered. There are stimulating (e.g., G_s, G_q) and inhibitory (e.g., G_i, G_o) G proteins, and the physiologic effect is determined by the specific G protein and subsequent cellular response. G proteins are heterotrimeric, composed of three subunits: α, β, and γ. Receptor and G protein interactions result in dissociation of the G protein subunits into α and $\beta\gamma$. The α-subunit of most G proteins confers specificity between receptor and effectors. Although $\beta\gamma$-subunits were originally thought simply to anchor G proteins to the cell membrane, dissociated $\beta\gamma$-subunits are clearly capable of directly

stimulating second messengers. The $\beta\gamma$-subunits play a role in anchoring regulatory kinases to the cell membrane, leading to enhanced phosphorylation of membrane receptors.

One of the best understood second messenger systems is the adenylyl cyclase system. In this system, complexes of stimulatory G protein receptors and hormones increase activity of the enzyme adenylyl cyclase, resulting in increased levels of cyclic adenosine 3′,5′-monophosphate (cAMP) in the cell (Fig. 3-33). Inhibitory G protein–receptor-hormone complexes decrease the activity of adenylyl cyclase, resulting in decreased levels of cellular cAMP. In general, increased levels of intracellular cAMP activate protein kinases that phosphorylate various proteins, ion channels, and second messenger enzymes. For example, β-adrenergic-receptor stimulation results in stimulation of adenylyl cyclase activity, increasing production of intracellular cAMP, which activates protein kinase A, which phosphorylates the L-type calcium channel in myocardium to produce increases in intracellular calcium, ultimately leading to increased inotropy. Examples of drugs or hormones that activate adenylyl cyclase include glucagon and histamine. In contrast, muscarinic (M_2, M_4) agonists, α_2-adrenergic agonists, and adenosine generally inhibit adenylyl cyclase.

Another example of a second messenger system is the phosphatidylinositol system. Hydrolysis of phosphatidyl-inositol-4,5-bisphosphate (PIP_2) in the cell membrane, catalyzed by G_q activation of phospholipase C, generates two main second messenger molecules, inositol-1,4,5-trisphosphate (IP_3) and 1,2-diacylglycerol (DAG). IP_3 then mobilizes intracellular calcium from nonmitochondrial intracellular stores by interacting with distinct IP_3 receptors on the surface of these organelles. The resulting increase in intracellular calcium levels produces biologic effects such as smooth muscle contraction. Examples of drugs that mediate phosphatidylinositol hydrolysis include α_1-adrenergic, endothelin, and muscarinic (M_1, M_3, M_5) agonists.

Stimulation of receptors and second messengers ultimately leads to physiologic effects in a given tissue. The physiologic effects produced depend on the presence of

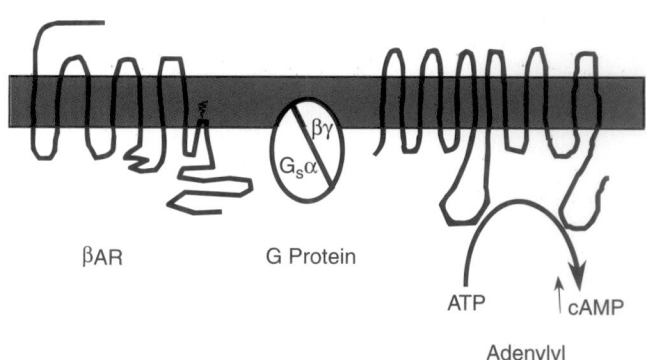

Figure 3–33 Schematic drawing of the signal transduction cascade of the β-adrenergic receptor (βAR). ATP, adenosine triphosphate; $\beta\gamma$, stimulatory G protein $\beta\gamma$ subunit; cAMP, cyclic adenosine monophosphate; $G_s\alpha$, α-subunit of the stimulatory G protein (G_s).

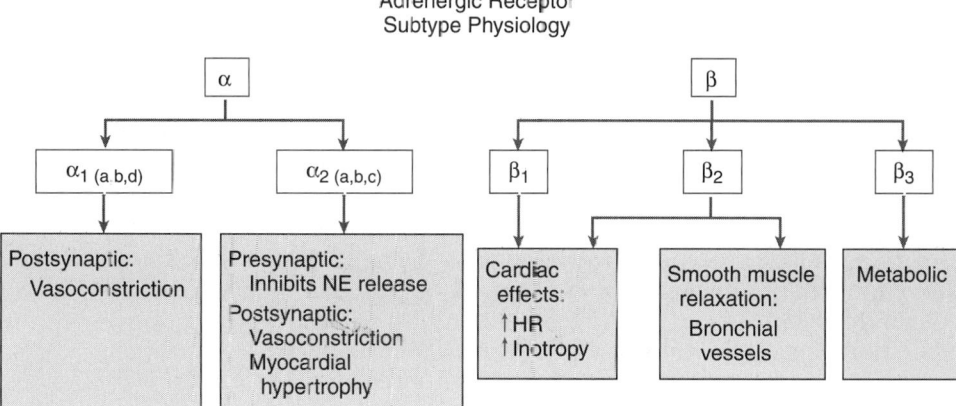

Figure 3–34 Adrenergic receptor subtype physiology. HR, heart rate; NE, norepinephrine.

specific receptor subtypes, G proteins, and second messengers within that tissue. An example of the wide-ranging cardiovascular effects produced by a single hormone—norepinephrine, the predominant sympathetic neurotransmitter—can be seen in Figure 3-34. Effects of sympathetic stimulation vary according to tissue. For example, acute effects of β_2-adrenergic-receptor–mediated vasodilation enhance skeletal muscle blood flow, β-adrenergic-receptor–mediated inotropic effects improve myocardial performance, and adrenergic effects in the CNS result in enhanced alertness; all of these effects enable effective performance during stressful situations. Chronic stimulation of stress responses, however, leads to other adrenergically mediated effects, some maladaptive, such as excessive myocardial hypertrophy, hypertension, and dampening of myocardial function.

Developments in Molecular Pharmacology

The field of molecular pharmacology has advanced our understanding of excitable membrane proteins and their mechanisms of action. Before the advent of molecular biology, most pharmacology research used ligand binding and protein purification techniques to elucidate the structure and mechanism of action of various drugs and receptors. Although important, these studies were tedious because tissues contain more than one receptor subtype, and protein purification of receptors to homogeneity is a lengthy and complicated process. Molecular techniques provide a unique opportunity to study receptors and their structure at the DNA level. Many receptors and receptor subtypes have been discovered, paving the way for more development of receptor-specific pharmacologic agents. We briefly review the general field of molecular pharmacology because future drugs for perioperative use probably will target receptor and receptor subtypes discovered using molecular approaches.

Molecular pharmacology takes advantage of the finding that all proteins, including excitable membrane proteins, are encoded in the human genome as nucleic acids. Every amino acid in a protein is encoded by a specific combination of three nucleotides in DNA. If the DNA sequence that encodes a receptor protein can be determined, the putative primary structure (i.e., amino acid sequence) of the receptor can be deduced. Encoding DNA sequences (i.e., genes) can be inserted into special cells that can express (i.e., manufacture, assemble, and deliver to the appropriate location in the cell) receptor protein in high quantity. This has several advantages.

First, studies on the receptor itself can be performed. By changing (i.e., mutating) nucleotide sequences, an abnormal (i.e., synthetic or "designer") receptor can be created. This abnormal receptor can then be compared with the original receptor to see whether the changes made affect binding of drug to the receptor or its coupling to second messengers. In this manner, the function of each portion of the receptor can be studied. This type of information is often called *structure-activity relationships*. G proteins and second messengers can be investigated in a similar manner. Naturally occurring human receptor variants have been investigated and tested for alterations in pharmacologic properties (see "Pharmacogenetics").

The second advantage of using molecular techniques in pharmacology is that new receptors and receptor subtypes can be discovered by searching the genome for DNA sequences similar to those of known receptors. After these receptors are discovered, they can be easily characterized, because high expression in cells enables them to be screened by various pharmacologic agents. The availability of DNA sequences for the full human genome has accelerated the discovery of receptors through DNA homology searching.

Perhaps the most immediately clinically relevant point is that new investigational drugs can be rapidly screened for effects on various native and variant receptors. In this way, pharmacologic effects of individual receptors can be studied in a controlled manner, isolated from other receptors and receptor subtypes. Such studies have the potential to lead to development of new drugs for use in the perioperative period and for understanding the effects of these drugs in patients with receptor variants.

Although there are many advantages to using molecular approaches to understanding physiologic pathways of individual receptors and in drug discovery, there are also some disadvantages. Cell lines are not integrated organisms, and the function of the receptor protein in a network of physiologic systems cannot be assessed. One approach to understanding the function of a previously identified or new gene product is to develop murine models in which the gene of interest has been eliminated (i.e., knock-out mice) or overexpressed (i.e., transgenic mice). The physiologic consequence of such altered protein expression is then examined. Although details of these technologies are beyond the scope of this chapter, they have become standardized and are widely available at many medical schools, universities, and specialized centers.

The mouse model is robust and useful, but it is important to remember that this scientific model has its own limitations. To interpret data from transgenic and knock-out animals correctly, at least three limitations of this technology should be considered. First, the genetic background of animals created must be carefully examined. If not carefully controlled, altered phenotypes may result from differences in animal strains (or genetic background) rather than from an overexpressed or knocked-out gene product. Second, elimination of specific receptors may be compensated for by alterations of other gene products. In this case, the final phenotype represents the net alteration of several genes; this is of particular concern when elimination of a gene is lethal because surviving progeny by definition have compensated in a way that enhances survival and therefore may not be representative of the results of a single-gene knock-out experiment. Some receptors and proteins have different tissue localizations in humans and other animal species. Results from transgenic and knock-out animal studies should be interpreted cautiously in this circumstance to prevent incorrect conclusions from being drawn regarding the implications for human physiology.

Despite these potential limitations, transgenic and knock-out animal models have proved very important in elucidating novel functions of receptors and proteins. Many unexpected physiologic roles for gene products have been discovered, and important physiologic questions have been answered and confirmed using these approaches. As an example, Table 3-1 lists conclusions drawn from transgenic and knock-out mice based on alterations of adrenergic receptors and their signal transduction cascade. Novel functions for specific adrenergic receptor subtypes (e.g., the role of α_{2a}-adrenergic receptors in sedation and CNS-mediated hypotension, α_{2b}-adrenergic receptors in mediating vasoconstriction, α_{2c}-adrenergic receptors in

Table 3–1 Results of targeting various portions of adrenergic-receptor signaling pathways in knock-out and transgenic mice, with an emphasis on cardiovascular effects

Model	Target	Result
Transgenic	↑β_2AR	↑Basal AC, ↑LV function, ↑atrial contractility, ↑supraventricular premature beats, ↓HR variability
Knock-out	↓β_2AR	No observable effects (except effects of mild exercise)
Transgenic	↑β_1AR	Dilated cardiomyopathy and early death; fibrosis
Knock-out	↓β_1AR	Prenatal death rate of 70%; among survivors: normal AC, ↓ISO-stimulated effects
Transgenic	↑AC-V	↑HR, ↑fractional shortening, no ISO-stimulated effects
Transgenic	↑GRK2	↓AC activity, ↓βARs function, ↓ISO-stimulated effects (rescued with βARK-ct peptide, which inhibits GRK2)
Transgenic	↑GRK5	Enhanced βAR desensitization but not angiotensin II desensitization
Transgenic	↑GRK2 inhibitor (↓GRK2 function)	Enhanced cardiac contractility with ISO
Knock-out	↓GRK2	Lethal phenotype, gestational LV hyperplasia, LVEF <70% in embryos
Transgenic	↑$G_s\alpha$	No change in baseline EF, ↑ISO-stimulated effects, myocardial fibrosis
Knock-out	↓Phospholamban	↓βAR-mediated contractile responses
Transgenic	↑α_{1a}AR	Hypertension, ↑inotropy
Transgenic	↑α_{1b}AR (constitutively active)	Myocardial hypertrophy, hypertension, nociception, memory
Transgenic	↑α_{1b}AR (wild type)	No myocardial hypertrophy or hypertension
Transgenic	↑α_{1d}AR	Nociception, memory
Transgenic	↑G_q	Myocardial hypertrophy (about fourfold overexpression), higher expression produces heart failure
Transgenic	↑G_q inhibitor (↓G_q function)	Prevention of myocardial hypertrophy
Knock-out	↓α_{2a}AR	Presynaptic α_2AR, mediates sedation and hypnosis, ↓BP (central hypotension), analgesia, regulation of DA/5-HT, antiepileptogenic effects of NE
Knock-out	↓α_{2b}AR	Mediates ↑BP (peripheral vasoconstriction)
Knock-out	↓α_{2c}AR	Mediates hypothermia, DA synthesis and metabolism, and presynaptic α_2AR (at low-frequency stimulation)

AC, adenylyl cyclase; AR, adrenergic receptor; βARK, β-adrenergic receptor kinase; BP, blood pressure; DA, dopamine; HR, heart rate; 5-HT, serotonin; ISO, isoproterenol; LV, left ventricle; G, G protein; GRK, G protein–coupled receptor kinase; LVEF, left ventricular ejection fraction; NE, norepinephrine; ↑, increased; ↓, decreased.

temperature control) have been discovered (see Chapter 16). Table 3-1 illustrates that alterations in adrenergic receptor signal transduction pathways and modulating kinases have physiologic consequences in the whole animal.

Clinical Evaluation of Drug Effects

General Principles

After pharmacologic agents have stimulated excitable cell-membrane proteins and have produced a physiologic effect, it is important to evaluate the effect clinically. This section focuses on methods of evaluating drug effects such as dose-response curves, efficacy, potency, the median effective dose (ED$_{50}$), the median lethal dose (LD$_{50}$), and the therapeutic index.

Concentration Versus Response Relationships

The standard comparison of a drug with its clinical effect is the *concentration versus response curve* (Fig. 3-35). The relationship shown is the time-independent relationship between dose, concentration, or some other measure of exposure to the drug (x axis) and the measured effect (y axis). The measured effect can be an absolute response (e.g., twitch height), a normalized response (e.g., percentage of twitch height depression), or a population response (e.g., fraction of subjects moving at incision). The standard equation for this relationship is the *Hill equation*, sometimes called the *sigmoid-E$_{max}$ relationship*:

$$\text{Effect} = E_0 + \left(E_{max} - E_0\right)\frac{C^\gamma}{C_{50}{}^\gamma + C^\gamma} \qquad (46)$$

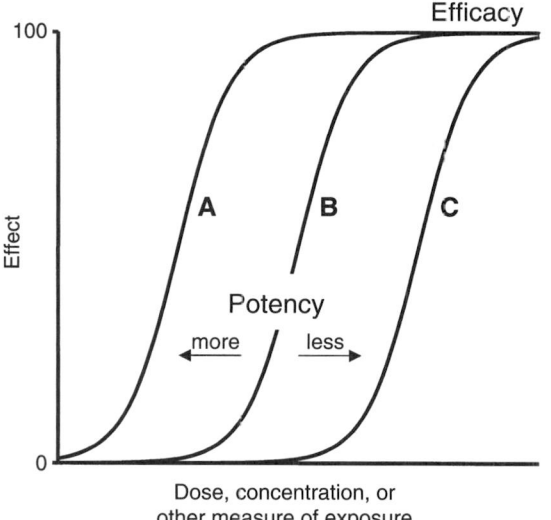

Figure 3–35 Dose or concentration versus response. A sigmoidal concentration-response curve is generated when the log drug concentration is plotted against the clinical response or effect. The concentration-response curve is shifted to the right (B to C) in the presence of a competitive antagonist or desensitization. Curve C may also represent an agonist with a lower receptor affinity (K$_a$) or potency than curve B. Curve A represents an agonist with higher receptor affinity or potency than curve B.

This is another example of the saturation equation shown in Figure 3-5. In Equation 46, E$_0$ is the baseline effect in the absence of drug, and E$_{max}$ is the maximum possible drug effect. C is typically concentration or dose, although other measures of drug exposure (e.g., dose, peak concentration, area under the concentration versus time curve) can be used. C$_{50}$ is the concentration associated with 50% of peak drug effect and is a measure of drug potency. The exponent γ, also called the *Hill coefficient*, is related to the sigmoidicity and steepness of the curve. If γ is less than 1 and the curve is plotted on a standard x axis, the curve appears hyperbolic (see Figure 3-5). If γ is greater than 1, the curve appears sigmoidal, as in Figure 3-35. If the x axis is plotted on a log scale, the curve always appears sigmoidal, regardless of the value of γ.

Potency and Efficacy

Considerable confusion exists about the definition of potency because of competing definitions of the term. One use of potency is to describe the effect of a given dose of the drug. Consider two different oral preparations of an identical drug: one that dissolves quickly in the stomach and is rapidly absorbed, and one that never completely dissolves and is poorly absorbed. A given dose of the rapidly absorbed formulation can produce a more profound drug effect and therefore be considered more potent than an identical dose of the slowly absorbed formulation. From a therapeutic perspective, potency is often defined in terms of the dose versus response relationship.

From a pharmacologic perspective, potency is best described in terms of the concentration versus response relationship. As shown in Figure 3-35, a drug with a left-shifted concentration versus response curve (i.e., lower C$_{50}$) is considered more potent, and a right-shifted dose versus response curve renders it less potent. To be precise, potency should be defined in terms of a specific drug effect (e.g., 50% of maximal effect). This is particularly important if the two drugs have different Hill coefficients or efficacies.

Efficacy is a measure of the intrinsic ability of a drug to produce a given physiologic or clinical effect (Fig. 3-36). For example, in G protein–coupled receptors efficacy is influenced by receptor coupling to G proteins, activation of second messengers, and the ability to generate ultimate physiologic responses. The scale used to describe intrinsic efficacy at a given receptor ranges from 0 to 1. Efficacy for full agonists is 1.0, for neutral antagonists is 0, and for partial agonists ranges between 0 and 1.0. In contrast, the term *potency* refers to the quantity of drug that must be administered to produce a specific effect. Two drugs may have the same efficacy, but if one drug produces the maximum effect at 1 mg and the second drug produces the maximum effect only at 100 mg, the second drug is less potent. The differences between a full agonist and a partial agonist (see Figs. 3-23 and 3-24) represent differences in efficacy.

Effective Dose and Lethal Dose

The ED$_{50}$ is the dose of a drug required to produce a specific effect in 50% of individuals to whom it is administered. The LD$_{50}$ is the dose of a drug required to produce death in 50% of patients (or animals) to whom it is administered. The therapeutic index of a drug is the ratio

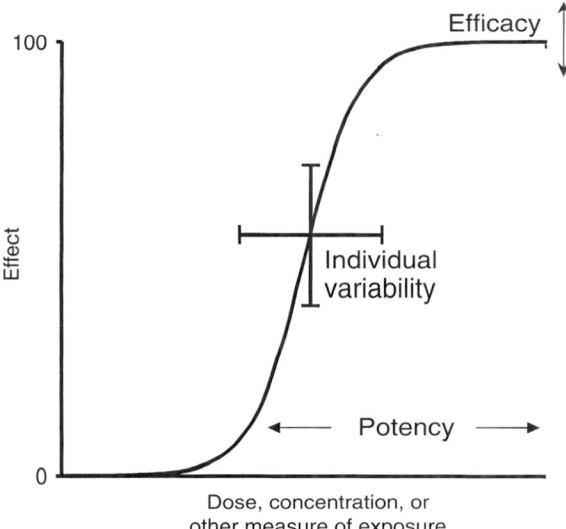

Figure 3–36 Relationships among efficacy, potency, and individual variability as they relate to a typical sigmoidal dose or concentration versus response curve.

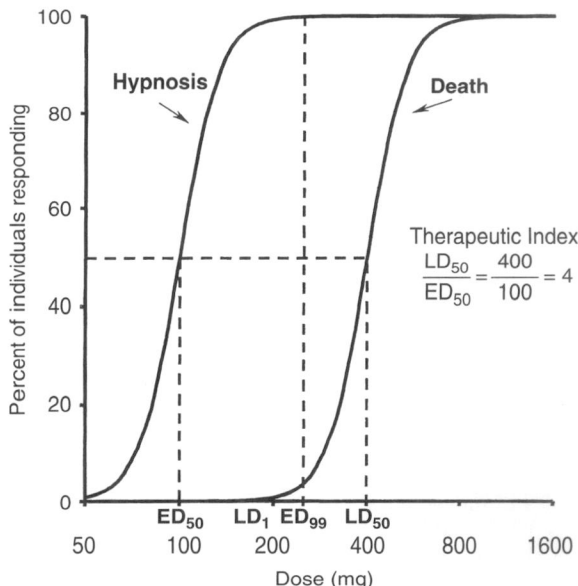

Figure 3–37 Relationships among the median effective dose (ED_{50}), median lethal dose (LD_{50}), and therapeutic index. These curves were generated from data on animals that were injected with various doses of a sedative-hypnotic and the clinical responses determined. ED_{50} is the dose of drug required to produce a specific effect (i.e., hypnosis) in 50% of animals to which it is administered (*left curve*). LD_{50} is the dose of drug required to produce death in 50% of animals to which drug is administered (*right curve*). The therapeutic index of the drug is the ratio between LD_{50} and ED_{50} (LD_{50}/ED_{50}). LD_1 is the lethal dose in 1% of the population, and ED_{99} is the effective dose in 99% of the population. As drawn, $LD_1 < ED_{99}$, which would not be clinically acceptable.

between the LD_{50} and the ED_{50} (LD_{50}/ED_{50}). The larger the therapeutic index of a drug, the safer the drug is for clinical administration because the LD_{50} is far higher than the ED_{50}. The relationships among ED_{50}, LD_{50}, and therapeutic index are shown in Figure 3-37.

Drug Interactions

Actions at the Same Receptor

Agonists and antagonists modify dose-response relationships. If two agonists have an identical affinity (K_a) for a given receptor and identical effectiveness in coupling to second messengers, their resultant dose-response curves should be superimposable. However, if two agonists have different receptor affinities, despite identical effectiveness in coupling to second messengers, their dose-response curves are parallel (with the rightward shifted curve corresponding to the drug with lower receptor affinity) (see Fig. 3-35, curves B and C). When two agonists are administered simultaneously, the clinical effect depends on the total amount of drug-receptor complexes generated.

Full agonists produce maximal responses, whereas partial agonists produce less than maximal response at the same receptor occupancy. The precise molecular mechanism that explains this blunting of the maximal response by partial agonists is unknown, but it may reflect the ability of full agonists to stabilize R* most effectively. Partial agonists shift the dose-response curve of the agonist to the right (see Fig. 3-35, curves B to C).

The addition of a competitive antagonist also shifts the dose-response curve to the right (see Fig. 3-35, B to C). In contrast, the addition of a noncompetitive agonist shifts the dose-response curve to the right and reduces the efficacy of the agonist. This occurs because maximal response cannot be obtained at any agonist dose because blockade of effect (i.e., antagonism) cannot be reversed.

Actions at Different Receptors

Anesthesia is the practice of applied drug interactions. As discussed in Chapter 31, general anesthesia is, at a minimum, a combination of hypnosis and analgesia. There has been extensive work looking at the interaction of hypnotic drugs, which include inhaled anesthetics and GABA agonists (i.e., propofol, barbiturates, etomidate, and benzodiazepines), and analgesic drugs, specifically opioids.

A prototypical study of the relationship between inhaled anesthetics and opioids is the investigation by McEwan and colleagues,[16] who characterized the interaction between isoflurane and fentanyl. The minimum alveolar concentration (MAC) of isoflurane associated with a 50% chance of moving on incision is compared with the plasma fentanyl concentration in Figure 3-38. Initially, the interaction is profound, with a 50% reduction in isoflurane MAC at a plasma fentanyl concentration of 1.7 ng/mL and a 63% reduction in isoflurane MAC associated with a plasma fentanyl concentration of 3 ng/mL. Beyond 3 ng/mL, there is very little benefit from additional fentanyl. The first clinical implication of this interaction is that a modest amount of opioid dramatically reduces the concentrations of inhaled anesthetic required to prevent movement. The second clinical implication is that some hypnotic component must be added to the anesthetic to prevent movement, even with huge doses of opioids.

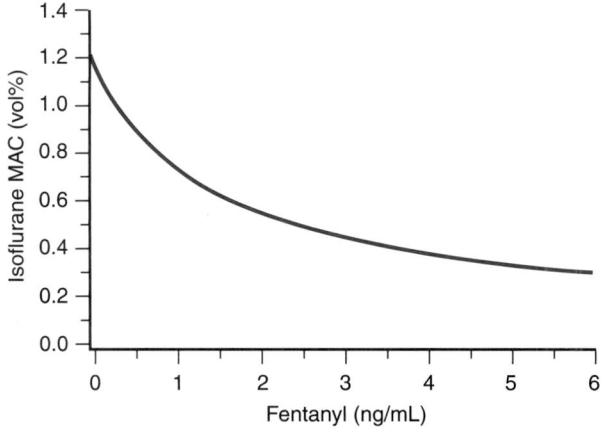

Figure 3–38 Influence of fentanyl on the minimum alveolar concentration (MAC) of isoflurane associated with a 50% probability of movement on incision. Modest amounts of fentanyl greatly reduce the MAC of isoflurane, but a ceiling in MAC reduction is quickly reached. Even with large opioid doses, some isoflurane is required to ablate the movement response. (Adapted from McEwan AI, Smith C, Dyar O, et al: Isoflurane minimum alveolar concentration reduction by fentanyl. Anesthesiology 78:864-869, 1993.)

Similar work has been done for propofol. In a series of elegant studies, Vuyk and colleagues[17] characterized the interaction of propofol with alfentanil. The interaction is markedly synergistic, with modest amounts of alfentanil greatly decreasing the amount of propofol associated with a 50% chance of response to endotracheal intubation or surgical incision (Fig. 3-39). Vuyk and colleagues[17] also documented the interaction of propofol and alfentanil

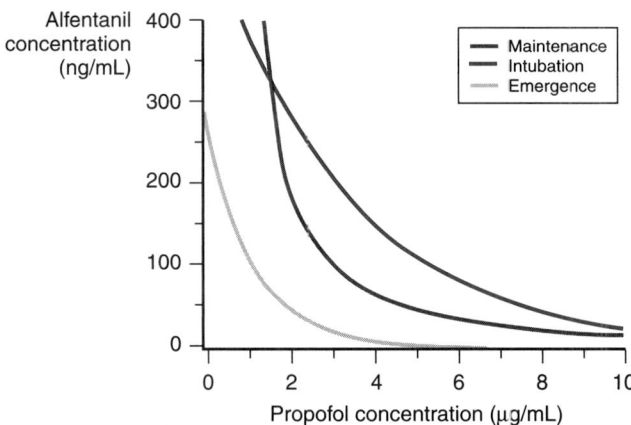

Figure 3–39 Influence of alfentanil on the concentration of propofol associated with a 50% probability of response to intubation and incision, as well as a 50% probability of awakening at the end of surgery. Moderate doses of alfentanil greatly reduce the dose of propofol required to ablate the response to noxious stimulation. However, below propofol concentrations of approximately 2 μg/mL, even large doses of alfentanil cannot reliably ablate the response to noxious stimulation. (Adapted from Vuyk J, Lim T, Engbers FH, et al: The pharmacodynamic interaction of propofol and alfentanil during lower abdominal surgery in women. Anesthesiology 83:8-22, 1995.)

on return of consciousness (see Fig. 3-39). As discussed in Chapters 10 and 11, studies such as these provide the basis for rational selection of opioids and design of optimal opioid infusion regimens.

Classic interaction studies, such as those previously described, examine the concentrations associated with a particular response (e.g., a 50% chance of moving) for two drugs, evaluated separately and in combination. However, a more general view is that any combination of two drugs is associated with a response. This is best viewed as a *response surface* in which the *x* and *y* axes of the surface are concentrations (or doses) of drugs A and B, and the *z* axis is the response to the particular combination. Minto and colleagues[18] proposed a mathematical framework for response surfaces for a variety of interaction surfaces of interest to anesthesiologists. Figure 3-40 shows six examples of response surfaces that apply to a variety of anesthetic drugs.

VARIABILITY IN DRUG RESPONSE

Anesthesiologists observe individual variations in clinical response to administered drugs every day. This variability can result from differences in pharmacokinetic processes such as absorption, distribution, metabolism, and excretion of a drug. Individual variation can also be caused by differences in pharmacodynamics, such as intrinsic differences in end-organ sensitivity, receptor upregulation and down-regulation, and alterations in physiology that affect drug action. The relationship between patient variability and a typical dose-response curve is shown in Figure 3-36. Sources of pharmacokinetic and pharmacodynamic variability include genetics, patient physiology, and drug interactions.

Pharmacogenetics

Overview

The field of pharmacology that describes effects of genetic variation on drug action is called *pharmacogenetics*. Pharmacogenetics refers to the genetic diversity in the body's absorption, metabolism, and distribution of drugs (i.e., inborn pharmacokinetic variability) or in the body's response to the drug, as can be caused by differences in receptor structure or patient physiology (i.e., inborn pharmacodynamic variability). To understand the effect of genetic variation on pharmacokinetics and pharmacodynamics, it is important to first define genetic variants, or polymorphisms.

Genetic polymorphism refers to any type of variation in a gene. More precise language is used to describe each specific type of genetic variant. When one nucleotide is exchanged for another, the resulting variant is called a *single nucleotide polymorphism* (SNP). The rare substituted nucleotide is defined as the minor allele, whereas the more common wild-type nucleotide is defined the major allele. Most SNPs are biallelic, having only two possible nucleotides—the minor or the major allele. In rare cases, SNPs can be triallelic, with two possible minor alleles and three total possible nucleotides. With four total nucleotides

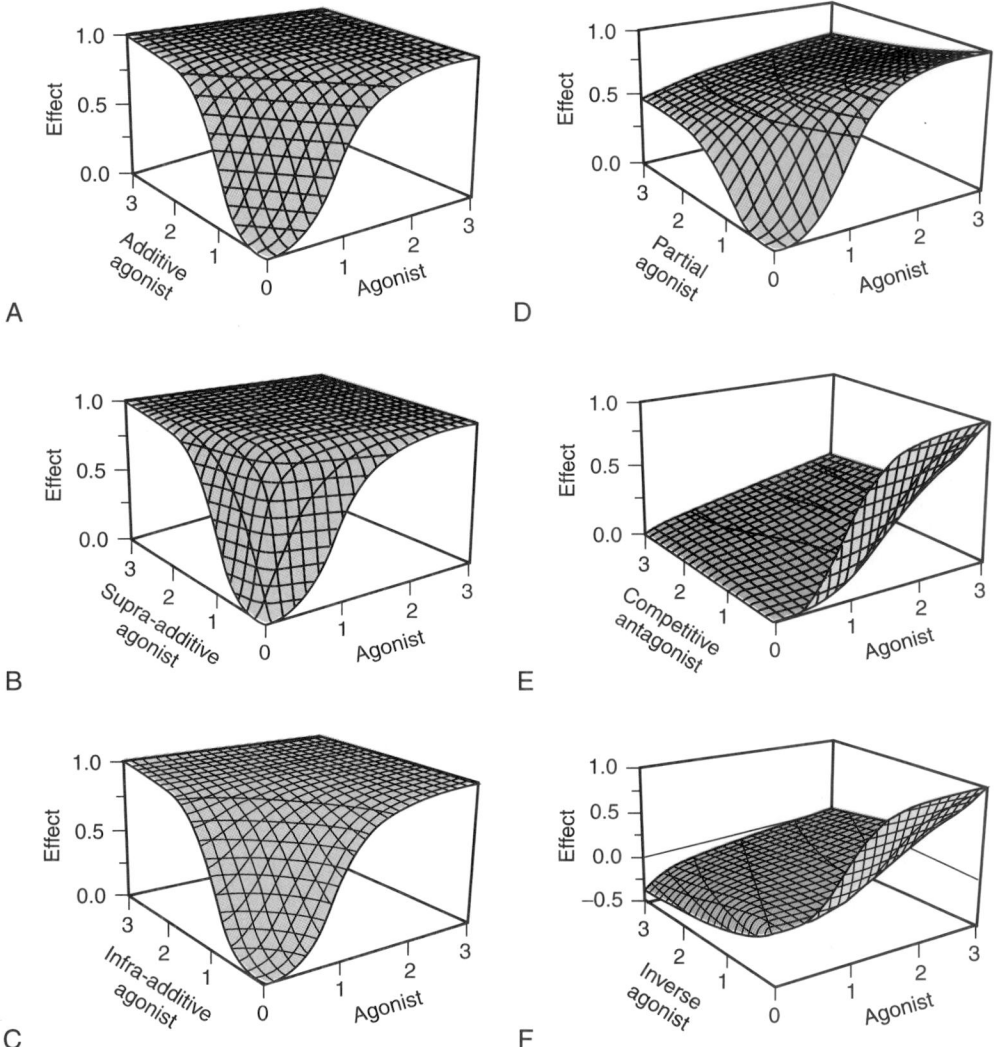

Figure 3–40 Response surfaces for potential pharmacodynamic interactions of anesthetic drugs. **A,** Additive interaction between two agonists that have the same mechanism of action (e.g., fentanyl and alfentanil). **B,** Supra-additive interaction between two agonists (e.g., isoflurane and fentanyl). **C,** Infra-additive interaction between two agonists (i.e., reported for cyclopropane and nitrous oxide). **D,** Partial agonist and full agonist (e.g., hypothetical interaction of nalbuphine and fentanyl). **E,** Competitive antagonist and full agonist (e.g., naloxone and fentanyl). **F,** Inverse agonist and full agonist (e.g., R0 19-4063 and midazolam).

available in DNA, it is possible to have each of the four nucleotides represented, but this almost never happens. We confine our discussion to biallelic SNPs because they are the most common.

Allele frequency refers to the frequency of the minor allele, notated $f(-)$. The frequency of the major allele is therefore $1-f(-)$. Because this is the minor allele, $f(-)$ is by definition less than 0.5. Because individuals have two copies of each allele, there are three possible combinations of biallelic SNPs: AA, Aa, and aa (in which A designates the major allele, and a designates the minor allele). The Hardy-Weinberg equation provides the frequency of each of these combinations based on the generally correct assumption that pairing of alleles is random:

Frequency of aa (homozygous for the minor allele): $f(-)^2$

Frequency of AA (homozygous for the major allele): $[1-f(-)]^2$

Frequency of Aa (heterozygous): $2\,f(-)\,[1-f(-)]$

The sum of these possibilities is 1.

In addition to SNPs, other types of genetic variants include insertions and deletions, in which stretches of genomic DNA are missing or added, and microsatellite repeats, in which several nucleotides repeat (i.e., dinucleotide repeat GCGCGCGC [n = 4 GC repeats] or trinucleotide repeat TACTACTACTACTACTAC [n = 6 TAC repeats]). The number of repeats in a microsatellite correlates with some diseases and can be used in genome-wide scans to identify chromosome regions associated with disease.

Catastrophic DNA changes often include DNA deletions or insertions that are not multiples of three in the coding region. Such changes result in a frameshift in the triplet nucleotide sequence used to encode amino acids in proteins, with the likely result being a nonsense protein. SNPs that change an encoded amino acid to a stop codon may also be catastrophic because they may result in a truncated protein.

Not all genetic variants have biologic consequences. Just as variations in eye color or fingerprint pattern do not have medical consequences, many genetic variants provide "background" variation without overt biologic consequences. Genetic variants with biologic or medical effects represent the minority of all genetic variants known to exist.

The sum total of genetic variation (with and without biologic implications) does provide a unique genetic fingerprint, a fact used in forensic science to identify a specific individual or relatives.

Determining the association between genetic variants and disease, drug therapy, or patient outcome is not straightforward and ideally should involve the help of a statistical geneticist. Clinical covariants and even genetic population structure (loosely defined as genetic variation due to global population movement) must be carefully taken into account in pharmacogenetic studies. Depending on the number of genes to be examined, statistical testing for association ranges from straightforward, simple analyses (e.g., using the chi-square approach to test whether a variant or haplotype [a group of SNPs] is enriched in the target population) to very complicated analyses (e.g., complex modeling, permutation testing, prospective sequential testing). In clinical association studies, it is important to ensure that clinical end-point data are reproducible and ideally include intermediate end points such as protein levels or enzyme activity. As more clinically relevant human genetic variants become known, our knowledge of the role of genetics in drug response and patient outcome should be significantly enhanced. Pharmacogenetics is the wave of the future in clinical studies.

Genetic Variability in Pharmacokinetics

Naturally occurring genetic variants can affect the activity of enzymes responsible for drug metabolism, most often by altering a key amino acid in or near the site of enzymatic action. In practical terms, this enzymatic diversity is rarely evident in the absence of drug therapy. In the presence of drug therapy, pharmacogenetic variation in metabolism is evident as unexpected toxicity, duration of action, or lack of efficacy of administered drugs.

Of particular interest to anesthesiologists is the activity of cytochrome P450 (CYP) 3A4. This is the most abundant cytochrome in the liver and intestines, and it is responsible for the metabolism of almost one half of all drugs, including many important drugs in anesthesia: opioids (e.g., fentanyl, alfentanil, sufentanil, methadone) (see Chapter 11), benzodiazepines (e.g., diazepam, midazolam, alprazolam, triazolam) (see Chapter 10), local anesthetics (e.g., cocaine, lidocaine, ropivacaine) (see Chapter 14), steroids, calcium channel blockers, haloperidol, and halothane. Only two of the many described genetic mutants of the CYP3A4 enzyme alter enzyme activity, with CYP3A4*18 decreasing and CYP3A4*19 increasing drug turnover.[19,20] Most of these CYP3A4 studies have examined only heterozygous (Aa genotype) individuals.

In contrast to the lack of causative CYP3A4 variants, a different story exists for CYP2C19, the enzyme system responsible for metabolizing mephenytoin, omeprazole, diazepam, proguanil, propranolol, and certain antidepressants. Newly described SNPs in this gene, present predominantly in African Americans, appear to decrease metabolism of these drugs in vitro.[21] Effects on drug concentrations in plasma need further testing in prospective human clinical trials.

One of the best-studied pharmacogenetic variants is CYP2D6, also called *debrisoquine hydroxylase* or *sparteine oxygenase*. About 7% to 10% of Caucasians are homozygous for an inactive variant of CYP2D6. This causes altered metabolism of at least 40 drugs. For example, codeine is a prodrug with no intrinsic analgesic efficacy. Codeine, oxycodone, and hydrocodone (Vicodin) all undergo O-demethylation to morphine, oxymorphone, and hydromorphone, their more pharmacologically active metabolites, by means of CYP2D6. Individuals who are homozygous for inactive CYP2D6 have little to no analgesic efficacy from codeine.[22] Such individuals are occasionally accused of malingering after surgery or injury when in fact they have no pain relief and need to be rescued by another analgesic agent. CYP2D6 polymorphisms have also been shown to impair dextromethorphan and metoprolol metabolism. When patients can be assayed for CYP2D6 activity, it will become a useful screen before initiating pain therapy.

Anesthesiologists are familiar with the role of genetics in determining butyrylcholinesterase (pseudocholinesterase) activity. Subjects with abnormal butyrylcholinesterase are at risk for prolonged paralysis from succinylcholine and exaggerated systemic effects from ester-based local anesthetics. Not surprisingly, there are ethnic differences in cholinesterase activity. For example, individuals of Middle Eastern descent are likely to have less butyrylcholinesterase activity than those of European descent. Molecular approaches have permitted extensive characterization of cholinesterase variants in plasma. Most of these variants are not "all or none" types but rather reflect a spectrum of enzymatic activity.

There may be an evolutionary explanation for pharmacogenetic variability in metabolism. It is probable that variability in drug metabolism is a natural adaptive response to an environment that can present a huge variety of toxins. Enzymatic diversity probably is maintained through natural selection to ensure survival when we are confronted with novel environmental toxins.

Genetic Variability in Pharmacodynamics

In addition to variants that affect drug pharmacokinetics, genetic variants can alter drug activity by pharmacodynamic mechanisms. Biologically active genetic polymorphisms have been found in numerous receptors, second messenger systems, and ion channels. One of the most intensively studied receptors in this regard is the β_2-adrenergic receptor (β_2AR) (see Chapter 16). Several β_2AR SNPs have particular relevance to this discussion (Fig. 3-41).[23] One variant, located at −47(T/C) in the 5'-untranslated sequence (referred to as the 5'-leader cistron [5LC]), increases levels of normal (nonvariant) β_2AR mRNA and protein by 72%. This increase in airway wild-type β_2AR expression is protective against methacholine challenge. Another β_2AR SNP present in the amino terminus, Arg16Gly (convention = major allele, amino acid number, minor allele), causes the receptor to have markedly enhanced agonist-promoted downregulation.[24] Because β_2AR stimulation in vessels is important in mediating vasodilation, an SNP such as Arg16 that enhances desensitization (i.e., dampens receptor responsiveness) is not surprisingly associated with a more frequent occurrence of higher arterial blood pressure or hypertension, or both. In contrast, β_2ARs containing Gly16 appear completely resistant to desensitization, and the Glu27 variant has

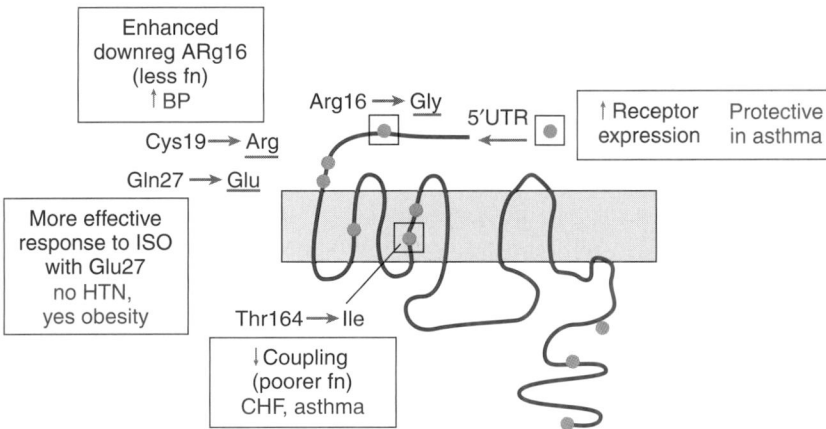

Figure 3–41 Location of some clinically important single nucleotide polymorphisms in the β₂-adrenergic receptor. Amino acid residues identified with a *boxed circle* have the clinical relevance described. BP, blood pressure; CHF, congestive heart failure; HTN, hypertension.

enhanced responsiveness to β₂AR agonists.[24] Cys19Arg and Arg16Gly usually travel together with yet another β₂AR, Gln27Glu, such that Arg19 almost always occurs in the same individual as Glu27, whereas Arg16 rarely occurs with Arg19 or Glu27. This region of the β₂AR is said to be in linkage disequilibrium, with the three SNPs defining a haplotype (i.e., defined regions of DNA that travel together) Gly16, Arg19, Glu27. This has practical implications because only one of the SNPs in the haplotype needs to be genotyped to infer the entire haplotype; this fact greatly enhances power and decreases cost in genetic association studies. Another β₂AR SNP (Thr164Ile), located in the fourth membrane-spanning domain, has altered catecholamine binding (i.e., lower affinity for isoproterenol, epinephrine, and norepinephrine) along with markedly depressed basal and agonist-stimulated adenylyl cyclase activity compared with wild-type Thr164. This poorer coupling appears to result in depressed myocardial function and congestive heart failure, with the variant particularly enriched in heart transplant candidates.

Malignant hyperthermia represents the most striking example of genetic variability in response to commonly used anesthetic drugs (see Chapter 29). Malignant hyperthermia manifests in approximately 1 of 20,000 anesthetic regimens. Various anesthetics, especially halothane, seem to trigger abnormal hypermetabolic responses that result in uncontrolled rise in body temperature, muscle rigidity, metabolic acidosis, hyperkalemia, and hypercapnia. More than 50% of cases of malignant hyperthermia have been positively linked to a series of mutations in the ryanodine receptor protein gene *RYR1*, which leads to altered calcium regulation in the sarcoplasm of muscle tissue. There is evidence of the involvement of the voltage-gated dihydropyridine receptor, which is also involved in sarcoplasmic regulation of calcium, in some cases of malignant hyperthermia not linked to the ryanodine receptor protein.

It is likely that many forms of genetically based variability in response to drugs reflect the interaction of many polymorphisms that subtly affect receptor structure, cellular function, and physiologic response. Understanding the interaction of multiple genes on the variability of drug response presents daunting technical challenges in pharmacogenetic research.

Patient Physiology

Age

Total-body water is decreased in the elderly. One pharmacokinetic result is a reduced initial mixing volume. This smaller central volume of distribution leads to higher peak concentrations after a bolus or during the early part of an infusion. A decreased central volume of distribution partly accounts for the increased sensitivity of elderly patients to many anesthetic drugs (see Chapters 60 and 62).

Aging is also associated with decreased lean body mass and increased body fat. Because the lipid content of elderly patients is higher than that of young patients, elderly patients have more potential for lipophilic drugs to accumulate in peripheral volumes of distribution, leading to increased duration of effect for many anesthetic drugs.

Liver volume, liver blood flow, and hepatic metabolic capacity decrease with advancing age. These changes in hepatic physiology account for the decreased clearance of opioids, hypnotics, benzodiazepines, and muscle relaxants, and they contribute to the increased sensitivity of elderly subjects to anesthetic drugs.

Age only modestly reduces cardiac output in the absence of hypertension, coronary artery disease, valvular heart disease, or other cardiovascular pathology. Advancing age can be expected to modestly reduce intercompartmental clearance for anesthetic drugs. The effect of decreased intercompartmental clearance is to increase initial plasma concentrations during drug administration. After termination of drug administration, the role of decreased intercompartmental clearance is complex. In general, plasma concentrations decrease more rapidly after long infusions when intercompartmental clearance is decreased.

Albumin and α₁-acid glycoprotein are the primary sites of protein binding. Albumin concentration decreases with advancing age, hepatic disease, and malnutrition. In contrast, α₁-acid glycoprotein concentration increases with advancing age and acute disease. The effects of age and disease on protein binding depend on which protein binds the drug. For example, because diazepam primarily binds to albumin, the free fraction of diazepam increases in elderly patients. This may partly explain the increased sensitivity in elderly subjects. In contrast, lidocaine binds primarily to α_1-acid glycoprotein. In elderly patients, an increased level of α_1-acid glycoprotein reduces the free fraction of lidocaine, which may contribute to reduced lidocaine clearance.

Although important age-related pharmacokinetic differences have been investigated in detail, there is a paucity of data addressing pharmacodynamic differences between age groups. Overall, the presence or absence of age-related pharmacodynamic differences appears to depend on the drug. For example, antiepileptic agents and digoxin have been examined in adults and children, and the effective plasma concentration is the same. This finding suggests that no age-related differences in pharmacodynamic responses occur for these two types of drugs. However, many drugs with CNS effects (e.g., thiopental,[25] midazolam,[26] opioids,[27,28] propofol[29]) appear to be intrinsically more potent in the elderly, and this change in potency has been quantitated with pharmacodynamic models. Understanding the biologic basis of increased sensitivity in the elderly to anesthetic and perioperative drugs is an area of active investigation by many researchers.

Disease States

Various diseases contribute to variation in drug response. Although diseases frequently result in pharmacokinetic variations (e.g., decreased liver perfusion in heart failure or decreased elimination in renal failure), pharmacodynamic variation is also observed. Diseases such as diabetes, thyroid disease, adrenal disease, myasthenia gravis, and hypertension alter receptor function and therefore represent pharmacodynamic effects. Some diseases directly affect drug receptors. For example, in patients with myasthenia gravis, antibodies to the postsynaptic nicotinic acetylcholine receptor effectively decrease the number of receptors present. Muscle weakness characterizes the disease. As a result, these patients are exquisitely sensitive to muscle relaxants, which act through the nicotinic acetylcholine receptor. Clinically, the dose of muscle relaxant must be decreased or eliminated in this patient population.

Drug Interactions

Pharmacokinetic Interactions

Historically, certain foods and drugs have been known to inhibit drug metabolism. Among the more dramatic of such interactions is the inhibition of CYP3A4 by grapefruit juice. CYP3A4 is responsible for nearly one half of all drug metabolism. Ingestion of grapefruit juice has been shown to increase the plasma concentration of drugs metabolized by CYP3A4.[30] Many drugs also inhibit CYP3A4, including the antifungal drugs ketoconazole and itraconazole; the protease inhibitors ritonavir, indinavir, and saquinavir; the antibiotics troleandomycin, clarithromycin, and erythromycin; and the selective serotonin reuptake inhibitors (SSRIs) fluoxetine and sertraline. Propofol also inhibits CYP3A4, although it is unclear whether there is any clinical consequence to this. Conversely, several drugs induce CYP3A4, increasing the metabolism of 3A4 substrates. These include rifampin, rifabutin, tamoxifen, glucocorticoids, carbamazepine, barbiturates, and the herb St. Johns Wort.

CYP2D6, responsible for the conversion of codeine to morphine, is also subject to inhibition. Quinidine and the SSRIs fluoxetine and paroxetine produce significant inhibition with standard clinical doses. Codeine, oxycodone, or hydrocodone would be relatively poor analgesic choices for patients on SSRIs.

Anesthetics also interact pharmacokinetically with many drugs by reducing cardiac output and hepatic blood flow. The reduction in cardiac output probably decreases intercompartmental clearance of most drugs, whereas the reduction in hepatic blood flow is expected to decrease metabolic clearance for drugs with high hepatic extraction ratios.

Pharmacodynamic Drug Interactions

Drug-Time Interaction: Desensitization

Desensitization is broadly defined as waning of physiologic responsiveness to a drug over time. For example, acute desensitization (i.e., tachyphylaxis) typically occurs to sodium nitroprusside. It is often necessary to increase the nitroprusside infusion rate over time to maintain the desired amount of vasodilation.

In general, stimulation of receptor pathways results in activation of kinases (e.g., protein kinase A, G protein–coupled receptor kinases, protein kinase C) that phosphorylate specific regions of the receptor, preventing further interaction of the receptor with G proteins or second messengers. Continuous stimulation of a receptor provides a negative-feedback mechanism to receptor stimulation, resulting in desensitization. Although desensitization was initially thought to occur only at the receptor level, it is now recognized that alterations of G proteins and second messengers also occur in response to agonist stimulation. Effectively, desensitization shifts the dose-response curve to the right (see Fig. 3-35, curve B to C) or decreases maximal drug effect, or both. Efficacy and potency can be diminished by desensitization.

Desensitization of receptor responses is a feature of many diseases in the aging population and is therefore relevant to consider during the perioperative period. Common diseases in which desensitization is important include congestive heart failure, hypertension, and diabetes; a hallmark of each of these diseases is elevation of hormone (agonist) concentrations. In the case of congestive heart failure, poor cardiac output induces compensatory sympathetic nervous system stimulation, often resulting in a doubling of circulating catecholamine concentrations (specifically, the sympathetic neurotransmitter norepinephrine). On a long-term basis, this results in desensitization of the myocardial β-adrenergic-receptor signal transduction pathway; specifically, β_1-adrenergic-receptor density and function decrease (75%) with relative sparing of β_2-adrenergic receptors (25%). G_i levels also increase without change in G_s. G protein–coupled receptor kinase concentrations increase, and adenylyl cyclase isoforms are modulated. Physiologic effects of changes important in desensitization of myocardial β-adrenergic receptors have been examined using transgenic and knock-out mice (see Table 3-1 and "Developments in Molecular Pharmacology"). To break the cycle of elevated agonist exposure and resultant desensitization, cardiologists cautiously use long-term, low-dose β-adrenergic-receptor antagonists (approximately one tenth of the usual dose for hypertension or myocardial ischemia) in patients with congestive heart failure. This therapy has been shown to improve functional classification and longevity.

Drug-Time Interaction: Increased Receptor Sensitivity

The opposite of desensitization is increased receptor sensitivity. Long-term exposure to a drug often results in compensatory responses by the receptor system. For example, when a receptor antagonist is administered on a long-term basis, receptor number (density) often increases. If the receptor antagonist is suddenly discontinued, exaggerated responsiveness to agonist may occur. This is the rationale for continuing long-term β-adrenergic-receptor antagonists during the perioperative period. Abrupt discontinuation of these drugs leaves the myocardium vulnerable to exaggerated heart rate and inotropic responses to routine procedures such as tracheal intubation, potentially leading to myocardial ischemia and infarction. Careful consideration should be given before discontinuing a long-term medication before surgery.

A much-feared anesthetic example of increased receptor sensitivity is the upregulation of nictonic receptors at the neuromuscular junction in patients with spinal cord injuries (see Chapter 13). Such patients are hyperreflexic because small releases of acetylcholine generate exaggerated reflex responses. The potential for such patients to have a life-threatening hyperkalemic response to succinylcholine is classically taught to every anesthesia resident.

Drug-Drug Interactions

There is a huge variety of mechanisms by which drugs can interact pharmacodynamically. The nature of pharmacodynamic drug-drug interactions is so diverse that an anesthesiologist can safely assume there is some interaction between anesthetic drugs and virtually all drugs that have action on the CNS or the cardiovascular system.

Some of these drug interactions, such as that between opioids and hypnotics, are fundamental to the practice of anesthesia and were discussed previously. An example of interactions between anesthetics and nonanesthetics is the influence of nonanesthetic drugs on the MAC of inhaled anesthetics (see Chapter 4). Drugs that increase central catecholamines in general increase the MAC. This has been clearly demonstrated for amphetamines (acute exposure), ephedrine, and monoamine oxidase (MAO) inhibitors. Conversely, drugs that decrease central catecholamines decrease the MAC (see Chapter 31). This has been shown for methyldopa, reserpine, and α_2-adrenergic agonists. It has also been demonstrated for chronic amphetamine use.

SUMMARY

This chapter reviewed general pharmacology by examining the basic principles of pharmacokinetics, pharmacodynamics, and sources of pharmacologic variability. Careful consideration of these principles should permit the anesthesiologist to understand drug movement from the site of administration through various body compartments to the site of action and the mechanisms by which drugs act on receptors to bring about the desired clinical effect. Many factors may alter the pharmacokinetic and pharmacodynamic processes by which drugs exert their effects, including genetics, age, disease, and concurrent drug therapy. Understanding basic pharmacologic processes and how they may be altered in individuals should facilitate drug titration for each patient. There is a biologic basis for finding just the right drug, in just the right dose, to provide safe and effective care of the perioperative patient.

KEY POINTS

1. The fundamental pharmacokinetic processes are dilution into volumes of distribution and clearance. These processes are governed by the physical properties of the drug and the metabolic capacity of the patient. Anesthetic drugs tend to be highly bound to protein in plasma and highly bound to lipid in peripheral tissues. Most anesthetic drugs are metabolized in the liver.

2. The pharmacokinetic actions of anesthetic drugs are typically described by mathematical models with a central compartment and one or two peripheral compartments. These compartments do not directly correspond to any anatomic or physiologic structures. Computer simulations can be used to predict the time course of plasma concentration and drug effect.

3. Drugs exert their effects through binding to receptors. The fraction bound is determined by the law of mass action, which yields a sigmoidal relationship between fractional occupancy and drug concentration.

4. Drugs can be agonists, partial agonists, neutral antagonists, or inverse agonists. Receptors exist in activated and inactivated states, and the intrinsic efficacy of a drug is determined by the extent to which it stabilizes the active form of the receptor (i.e., agonists), the inactive form (i.e., inverse agonists), or displaces agonists from the binding site without favoring either form (i.e., neutral antagonists).

5. The four main receptor types are G protein–coupled receptors (e.g., opioids, catecholamines), ligand-gated ion channels (e.g., hypnotics, benzodiazepines, muscle relaxants, ketamine), voltage-gated ion channels (e.g., local anesthetics), and enzymes (e.g., neostigmine, amrinone, caffeine). The first three types are located in cell membranes. Enzymes can be located anywhere.

6. Many drugs act through second messengers, which amplify drug action. Common second messengers are G proteins, which can release stimulating or inhibitory subunits in response to drug binding at the receptor; c-AMP, which is frequently a target of G-protein stimulation or inhibition; IP3 and DAG, also targets of G-protein regulation; and intracellular ions, especially calcium.

7. Advances in molecular pharmacology are helping to identify the specific function of individual receptors and the role of individual amino acids in mediating receptor action. Specific tools include site-directed mutagenesis to create designer receptors and knock-out or knock-down (underexpressed) or transgenic (overexpressed) murine models to understand the physiologic action of individual receptors.

8. The fundamental properties of the concentration versus response relationship are potency and efficacy. Potency is the concentration associated with a 50% drug effect. Efficacy is the maximal possible drug effect.

9. Drugs can interact pharmacokinetically through enzymatic induction or inhibition or pharmacodynamically through synergy or antagonism. Anesthetic techniques typically take advantage of the synergy between hypnotics and opioids to produce the anesthetic state at far lower doses of each drug than would be required if they were used alone.

10. Pharmacogenetics is gradually explaining some of the variability in response to drugs. Genetic variability in pharmacokinetics can be attributed to variability in hepatic cytochromes (e.g., CYP2D6, CYP2C19), circulating enzymes (e.g., pseudocholinesterase), or transporters. Genetic variability in pharmacodynamics can be attributed to alterations in receptors, as has been demonstrated for multiple adrenergic-receptor variants. Malignant hyperthermia has been clearly linked to variability in the ryanodine receptor.

11. Variability in response to drugs can also be attributed to nongenetic causes, such as aging, disease, exposure to environmental toxins, and the pharmacokinetic or pharmacodynamic influence of other drugs. Variability is also introduced through continuous exposure to a single drug, which can trigger desensitization (tolerance) or, if the drug is an antagonist, increased receptor sensitivity to the agonist.

REFERENCES

1. Krejcie TC, Avram MJ, Gentry WB, et al: A recirculatory model of the pulmonary uptake and pharmacokinetics of lidocaine based on analysis of arterial and mixed venous data from dogs. J Pharmacokinet Biopharm 25:169-190, 1997.
2. Shafer S: Principles of pharmacokinetics and pharmacodynamics. In Longnecker DE, Tinker JH, Morgan GE (eds): Principles and Practice of Anesthesiology, 2nd ed. St. Louis, Mosby–Year Book, 1997.
3. Wagner JG: Pharmacokinetics for the Pharmaceutical Scientist. Lancaster, PA, Technomic Publishing, 1993.
4. Wilkinson GR, Shand DG: Commentary: A physiological approach to hepatic drug clearance. Clin Pharmacol Ther 18:377-390, 1975.
5. Cockcroft DW, Gault MH: Prediction of creatinine clearance from serum creatinine. Nephron 16:31-41, 1976.
6. Ebling WF, Wada DR, Stanski DR: From piecewise to full physiologic pharmacokinetic modeling: Applied to thiopental disposition in the rat. J Pharmacokinet Biopharm 22:259-292, 1994.
7. Bjorkman S, Wada DR, Stanski DR: Application of physiologic models to predict the influence of changes in body composition and blood flows on the pharmacokinetics of fentanyl and alfentanil in patients. Anesthesiology 88:657-667, 1998.
8. Youngs EJ, Shafer SL: Basic pharmacokinetic and pharmacodynamic principles. In White PF (ed): Textbook of Intravenous Anesthesia. Baltimore, Williams & Wilkins, 1997, p 10.
9. Scott JC, Ponganis KV, Stanski DR: EEG quantitation of narcotic effect: The comparative pharmacodynamics of fentanyl and alfentanil. Anesthesiology 62:234-241, 1985.
10. Mandema JW, Kuck MT, Danhof M: Differences in intrinsic efficacy of benzodiazepines are reflected in their concentration-EEG effect relationship. Br J Pharmacol 105:164-170, 1992.
11. Engelhardt S, Grimmer Y, Fan G-H, Lohse MJ: Constitutive activity of the human β1-adrenergic receptor in β1-receptor transgenic mice. Mol Pharmacol 60:712-717, 2001.
12. Liu X, Callaerts-Vegh Z, Evans KLJ, Bond RA: Chronic infusion of β-adrenoceptor antagonist and inverse agonists decreases elevated protein kinase A activity in transgenic mice with cardiac-specific overexpression of human β2ARs. J Cardiovasc Pharmacol 40:448-455, 2002.
13. Stapelfeldt WH: The autonomic nervous system. In Schwinn DA (ed): Scientific Principles of Anesthesia, vol 2. Philadelphia, Current Medicine, 1998.
14. Berkowitz DE: Cellular signal transduction. In Schwinn DA (ed): Scientific Principles of Anesthesia, vol 2. Philadelphia, Current Medicine, 1998.
15. Firestone L, Quinlan J, Gyulai F: Mechanisms of anesthetic action. In Schwinn DA (ed): Scientific Principles of Anesthesia, vol 2. Philadelphia, Current Medicine, 1998.
16. McEwan AI, Smith C, Dyar O, et al: Isoflurane minimum alveolar concentration reduction by fentanyl. Anesthesiology 78:864-869, 1993.
17. Vuyk J, Lim T, Engbers FH, et al: The pharmacodynamic interaction of propofol and alfentanil during lower abdominal surgery in women. Anesthesiology 83:8-22, 1995.
18. Minto CF, Schnider TW, Short TG, et al: Response surface model for anesthetic drug interactions. Anesthesiology 92:1603-1616, 2000.
19. Lamba JK, Lin YS, Thummel K, et al: Common allelic variants of cytochrome P4503A4 and their prevalence in different populations. Pharmacogenetics 12:121-132, 2002.
20. Dai D, Tang J, Rose R, et al: Identification of variants of CYP3A4 and characterization of their abilities to metabolize testosterone and chlorpyrifos. J Pharmacol Exp Ther 299:825-831, 2001.
21. Blaisdell J, Mohrenweiser H, Jackson J, et al: Identification and functional characterization of new potentially defective alleles of human CYP2C19. Pharmacogenetics 12:703-711, 2002.
22. Poulsen L, Brosen K, Arendt-Nielsen L, et al: Codeine and morphine in extensive and poor metabolizers of sparteine: Pharmacokinetics, analgesic effect and side effects. Eur J Clin Pharmacol 51:289-295, 1996.
23. Johnson JA, Terra SG: β-Adrenergic receptor polymorphisms: Cardiovascular disease associations and pharmacogenetics. Pharm Res 19:1779-1787, 2002.
24. Dishy V, Sofowora GG, Xie HG, et al: The effect of common polymorphisms of the beta2-adrenergic receptor on agonist-mediated vascular desensitization. N Engl J Med 345:1020-1035, 2002.
25. Homer TD, Stanski DR: The effect of increasing age on thiopental disposition and anesthetic requirement. Anesthesiology 62:714-724, 1985.
26. Bell GD, Spickett GP, Reeve PA, et al: Intravenous midazolam for upper gastrointestinal endoscopy: A study of 800 consecutive cases relating dose to age and sex of patient. Br J Clin Pharmacol 23:241-243, 1987.

27. Scott JC, Stanski DR: Decreased fentanyl and alfentanil dose requirements with age: A simultaneous pharmacokinetic and pharmacodynamic evaluation. J Pharmacol Exp Ther 240:159-166, 1987.

28. Minto CF, Schnider TW, Egan TD, et al: Influence of age and gender on the pharmacokinetics and pharmacodynamics of remifentanil. I. Model development. Anesthesiology 86:10-23, 1997.

29. Schnider TW, Minto CF, Shafer SL, et al: The influence of age on propofol pharmacodynamics. Anesthesiology 90:1502-1516, 1999.

30. Bailey DG, Malcolm J, Arnold O, Spence JD: Grapefruit juice-drug interactions. Br J Clin Pharmacol 46:101-110, 1998.

SUGGESTED READING

Boroujerdi M: Pharmacokinetics. New York, McGraw-Hill, 2002.

Bowdle TA, Horita A, Kharasch ED: The Pharmacologic Basis of Anesthesiology. New York, Churchill Livingstone, 1994.

Chalmers DT, Behan DP: The use of constitutively active GPCRs in drug discovery and functional genomics. Nat Rev Drug Discov 1:599-608, 2002.

Clarke WP, Bond RA: The elusive nature of intrinsic efficacy. Trends Pharmacol Sci 19:270-276, 1998.

Conti-Tronconi BM, McLane KE, Raftery MA, et al: The nicotinic acetylcholine receptor: Structure and autoimmune pathology. Crit Rev Biochem Mol Biol 29:69-123, 1994.

Eckhart AD, Koch WJ: Transgenic studies of cardiac adrenergic receptor regulation. J Pharmacol Exp Ther 299:1-5, 2001.

Eger EI: Anesthetic Uptake and Action. Baltimore, Williams & Wilkins, 1974.

Freedman NJ, Lefkowitz RJ: Desensitization of G protein-coupled receptors. Recent Prog Horm Res 51:319-351, 1996.

Greco WR, Bravo G, Parsons JC: The search for synergy: A critical review from a response surface perspective. Pharmacol Rev 47:331-385, 1995.

Hamm HE: The many faces of G protein signaling. J Biol Chem 273:669-672, 1998.

Jenkinson DH, Barnard EA, Hoyer D, et al: International Union of Pharmacology Committee on Receptor Nomenclature and Drug Classification. IX. Recommendations on terms and symbols in quantitative pharmacology. Pharmacol Rev 47:255-266, 1995.

Kalow W: Pharmacogenetics in biological perspective. Pharmacol Rev 49:369-379, 1997.

Kenakin T: Efficacy at G-protein-coupled receptors. Nat Rev Drug Discov 1:102-110, 2002.

Kenakin T: Inverse, protean, and ligand-selective agonism: Matters of receptor conformation. FASEB J 15:598-611, 2001.

Kenakin T, Onaran O: The ligand paradox between affinity and efficacy: Can you be there and not make a difference? Trends Pharmacol Sci 23:275-280, 2002.

Krumins AM, Barber R: The stability of the agonist beta$_2$-adrenergic receptor–Gs complex: Evidence for agonist-specific states. Mol Pharmacol 52:144-154, 1997.

Lambert JJ, Belelli D, Hill-Venning C, et al: Neurosteroid modulation of native and recombinant GABA$_A$ receptors. Cell Mol Neurobiol 6:155-174, 1996.

Landry Y, Gies JP: Heterotrimeric G proteins control diverse pathways of transmembrane signaling, a base for drug discovery. Mini Rev Med Chem 2:361-372, 2002.

Liu JG, Anand KJ: Protein kinases modulate the cellular adaptations associated with opioid tolerance and dependence. Brain Res Rev 38:1-19, 2001.

Perry SJ, Lefkowitz RJ: Arresting developments in heptahelical receptor signaling and regulation. Trends Cell Biol 12:130-138, 2002.

Pierce KL, Premont RT, Lefkowitz RJ: Seven-transmembrane receptors. Nat Rev Mol Cell Biol 3:639-650, 2002.

Rathz DA, Gregory KN, Fang Y, et al: Hierarchy of polymorphic variation and desensitization permutations relative to beta-1 and beta-2 adrenergic signaling. J Biol Chem 278:10784-10789, 2003.

Rescigno A: Foundations of Pharmacokinetics. New York, Plenum Press, 2003.

Rockman HA, Koch WJ, Lefkowitz RJ: Cardiac function in genetically engineered mice with altered adrenergic receptor signaling. Am J Physiol 272:H1553-H1559, 1997.

Rogers JF, Nafziger AN, Bertino JS Jr: Pharmacogenetics affects dosing, efficacy, and toxicity of cytochrome P450-metabolized drugs. Am J Med 113:746-750, 2002.

Ross EM, Kenakin TP: Pharmacodynamics: Mechanisms of drug action and the relationship between drug concentration and effect. *In* Hardman JG, Limbird LE (eds): The Pharmacological Basis of Therapeutics, 10th ed. New York, McGraw-Hill, 2002, pp 31-43.

Rowland M, Tozer TN: Clinical Pharmacokinetics: Concepts and Applications, 3rd ed. Baltimore, Williams & Wilkins, 1995.

Schwinn DA (ed): Scientific Principles of Anesthesia, vol 2. Philadelphia, Current Medicine, 1997.

Shuldiner AR: Transgenic animals. N Engl J Med 334:653-655, 1996.

Skiba NP, Hamm HE: How Gs$_\alpha$ activates adenylyl cyclase. Nat Struct Biol 5:88-92, 1998.

Svoboda P, Novotny J: Hormone-induced subcellular redistribution of trimeric G proteins. Cell Mol Life Sci 59:501-512, 2002.

Tang WJ, Hurley JH: Catalytic mechanism and regulation of mammalian adenylyl cyclases. Mol Pharmacol 54:231-240, 1998.

Tucek S, Michal P, Vlachova V: Modelling the consequences of receptor–G-protein promiscuity. Trends Pharmacol Sci 23:171-176, 2002.

Vaughan M: Signaling by heterotrimeric G proteins minireview series. J Biol Chem 273:667-668, 1998.

Watson J, Gilman M, Witkowski J, et al: Recombinant DNA, 2nd ed. New York, WH Freeman, 1992.

Weinshilboum R: Inheritance and drug response. N Engl J Med 348:529-537, 2003.

Wilkinson GR: Pharmacokinetics: The dynamics of drug absorption, distribution, and elimination. *In* Hardman JG, Limbird LE (eds): The Pharmacological Basis of Therapeutics, 10th ed. New York, McGraw-Hill, 2002, pp 3-29.

CHAPTER
4 Mechanisms of Action

Donald D. Koblin

Measurement of Anesthetic Potencies—Minimum Alveolar Concentration 107

Alterations in Anesthetic Requirement Pertinent to Theories of Narcosis 108
Effects of Temperature 108
Effects of Pressure 108
Effects of Age 108
Effects of Ion Concentrations 108

Actions of Inhaled Anesthetics in the Central Nervous System 109
Brain 109
Spinal Cord 109
Sites of Central Nervous System Action and Anesthetic End Points 109

Interruption of Neuronal Transmission by Inhaled Anesthetics 109
Peripheral Receptors 109
Highly Sensitive Neurons 110
Axonal Versus Synaptic Transmission 111
Synapses 111

Alterations in Neuroregulators Associated with Anesthesia 112
Acetylcholine 112
Catecholamines 112
Serotonin 113
Adenosine 113
γ-Aminobutyric Acid 113
Glycine 113
Excitatory Amino Acids 113

Cyclic Nucleotides 113
Calcium 114
Endogenous Opiates 114
Nitric Oxide 114

Physicochemical Nature of the Site of Anesthetic Action 114
Hydrophobic Site: The Meyer-Overton Rule 115
Additive Effects of Inhaled Anesthetics 116
Exceptions to the Meyer-Overton Rule 116

The Membrane as the Site of Anesthetic Action 117

Interaction of Inhaled Anesthetics with Membrane Lipids 119
Binding of Anesthetics to Membrane Lipids 119
Effects on Membrane Permeability 119
Alterations in Membrane Dimension 119
Alterations in Membrane Physical State 120

Interaction of Inhaled Agents with Proteins 120
Soluble Proteins 120
Membrane Proteins 120

Animal Models: Attempts to Relate Sustained Alterations in Anesthetic Potency with Neurochemical Composition 123
Dietary Studies 123
Tolerance Studies 123
Genetic Studies 123

Summary 125

Although currently popular inhaled anesthetics include nitrous oxide and the halogenated ethers isoflurane and sevoflurane, a far greater variety of inhaled agents can produce anesthesia (Fig. 4-1). The properties of these anesthetics vary considerably. For example, cyclopropane and diethyl ether are no longer used because of their explosiveness and flammability. Halothane is nonflammable but possesses a permanent dipole moment, can form hydrogen bonds, and is metabolized by the liver. Xenon, an anesthetic more potent than nitrous oxide in humans,[1] is essentially inert and undergoes no known transformation in the body.

The structural diversity of inhaled anesthetics suggests that they all do not interact directly with a single, specific receptor site. However, attempts to find a common (unitary) mechanism of general anesthetic action have

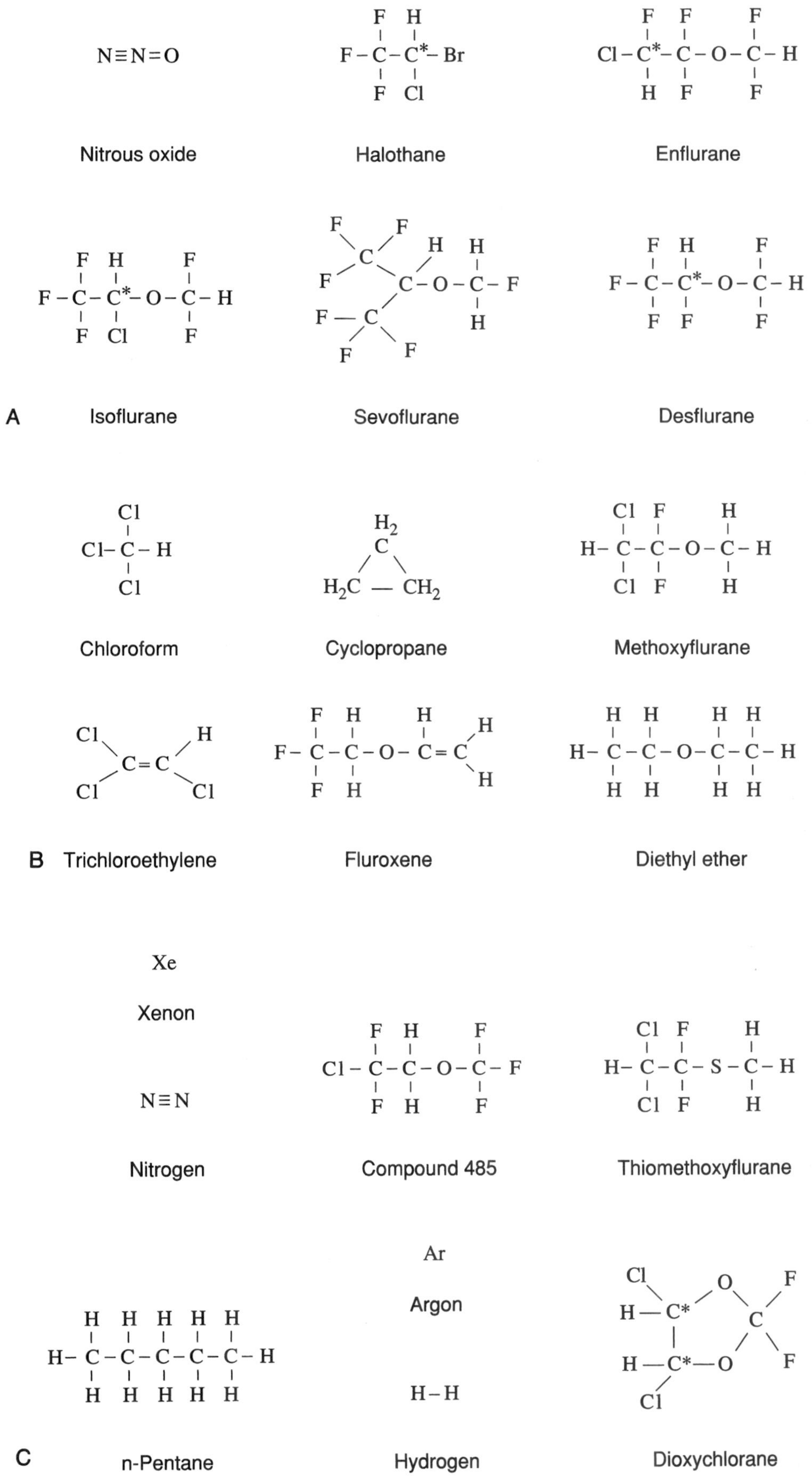

Figure 4–1 Chemical structures of various inhaled anesthetics. **A,** Anesthetics in current clinical use. **B,** Anesthetics in previous clinical use. **C,** Some experimental anesthetics. Anesthetics with asymmetric carbon atoms *(asterisks)* are mixtures of the optical isomers.

sought correlations of the potencies of anesthetics with their physicochemical properties. An example is the striking, albeit imperfect, relationship between anesthetic potency and lipid solubility (see "Physicochemical Nature of the Site of Anesthetic Action"). Although such correlations do not provide a detailed mechanism of anesthesia, they have been helpful in defining the environment in which anesthetics act.

Any molecular hypothesis of anesthesia must explain the effects of anesthetics on the whole organism. For instance, because anesthetic administration can rapidly induce unconsciousness and because awakening can occur quickly after the discontinuation of anesthesia, physical or biochemical changes important to the mechanism of anesthesia must occur within seconds. Similarly, physical or biochemical alterations caused by anesthetics are meaningful only at clinical concentrations and physiologic temperatures and not at high anesthetic levels.[2] High levels may produce toxic effects unrelated to the mechanism by which inhaled anesthetics act. The anesthetic requirement does not change or decreases only slightly with increasing duration of anesthesia.[3] Any physical or biochemical change causally related to the anesthetic state should be stable while an organism is anesthetized and should disappear on emergence from anesthesia.

The mechanisms by which inhaled anesthetics act may overlap the mechanisms of action of intravenous anesthetics (see Chapters 10 and 11), local anesthetics (see Chapter 14), and even of alcohols.[4] This chapter considers only the inhaled agents.

MEASUREMENT OF ANESTHETIC POTENCIES—MINIMUM ALVEOLAR CONCENTRATION

An exploration of the mechanism by which anesthetics act requires knowledge of the relative anesthetic potencies for each of the agents. The best estimate of anesthetic potency is the minimum alveolar concentration (MAC) (at 1 atm) of an agent that produces immobility in 50% of subjects exposed to a noxious stimulus.[5] For determination of the MAC in humans, the stimulus is a surgical skin incision. (Variations on the MAC concept may be used to estimate the potency of other anesthetic end points. For example, lack of response to verbal command [i.e., MAC awake] occurs at lower anesthetic concentrations, and lack of response to endotracheal intubation [i.e., MAC intubation] occurs at higher anesthetic concentrations than those needed to prevent movement to surgical skin incision [see Chapter 31]). In animals, the noxious stimulus is usually produced by clamping the tail or by passing electrical current through subcutaneous electrodes. The advantage of measuring the alveolar concentration is that, after a short period of equilibration, this concentration directly represents the partial pressure of anesthetic in the central nervous system (CNS) and is independent of the uptake and distribution of the agent to other tissues (see Chapters 5 and 31). Another advantage of MAC is its consistency for a given animal or species or between different species or classes

of animals.[5,6] This consistency makes it possible to discern small changes in anesthetic requirement, which may give a clue about how anesthetics act.

The anesthetic concentration that abolishes the righting reflex in 50% of the animals is often used to measure anesthetic potencies in smaller animals; it is an anesthetic with a 50% effective dose (ED_{50}). Because the inspired rather than the alveolar concentrations are measured, the method applies best to rapidly equilibrating (poorly blood-soluble) agents. Only with equilibration can it be assumed that the partial pressure of the inspired gas equals that at the site of action. The use of small animals and inspired concentrations facilitates work with agents at very high pressures (i.e., tens or hundreds of atmospheres). The anesthetic ED_{50} in the mouse, as determined by the rolling response (i.e., the righting reflex), correlates closely with the MAC in humans over a 500-fold change in anesthetic requirements (Fig. 4-2).

The tail-clamp ED_{50} (MAC) and the righting-reflex ED_{50} are not identical. The tail-clamp ED_{50} is higher than the righting-reflex ED_{50}, and the ratio of these measurements averages approximately 2 (Table 4-1). This ratio varies slightly with the anesthetic examined, implying that the righting reflex is depressed, at least in part, by a different mechanism from that which depresses the response to a noxious stimulus.[7-9]

An important action of inhaled anesthetics is the ability to suppress learning and memory. In humans, volatile anesthetic concentrations equivalent to approximately 0.3 MAC are required to suppress learning of auditory or verbal information during nonsurgical conditions. In an animal model, the concentration of volatile anesthetic to suppress learning in rats depends on the conditioned stimulus employed and varies between about 0.2 and 0.6 MAC.[10] The absolute and relative potencies of inhaled anesthetics depend on the end point measured.[11]

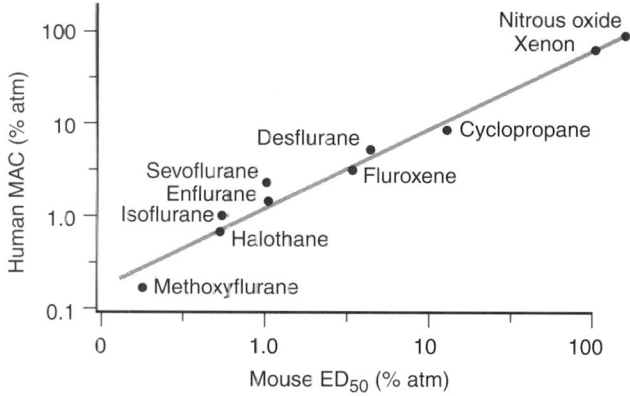

Figure 4-2 A close correlation exists between the minimum alveolar concentration (MAC) of various anesthetics, preventing a response to surgical incision in humans, and the inspired dose of an anesthetic (ED_{50}) required to abolish the righting reflex in the mouse. (Data from references 5, 8, 180, and from Eger EI II, Rutherford, NJ: Desflurane: A Compendium and Reference. Healthpress Publishing Group, 1993, p 13.)

Table 4–1 Ratios of anesthetic potencies: tail-clamp ED_{50}/righting-reflex ED_{50}

Anesthetic	Mouse	Rat
Halothane	1.67	1.74
Sevoflurane	2.71	—
Enflurane	1.91	—
Isoflurane	2.10	2.41
Desflurane	1.78	1.58-2.89
Chloroform	1.61	—
Cyclopropane	1.97	—
Nitrous oxide	1.82	—
Methoxyflurane	1.63-2.08	—
Diethyl ether	—	1.25

Data from references 4, 7, 8, 9, 86, 180 and from Eger EI II, Rutherford, NJ: Desflurane: A Compendium and Reference. Healthpress Publishing Group, 1993, p 13.

ALTERATIONS IN ANESTHETIC REQUIREMENT PERTINENT TO THEORIES OF NARCOSIS

Effects of Temperature

In mammals, the MAC decreases with decreasing body temperatures for all anesthetics, but the reduction (about 2% to 5%) per degree decrease in body temperature varies slightly from agent to agent.[5] Although the gas-phase potencies of inhaled agents increase with decreasing temperature, there is an associated increase in anesthetic solubility with a decrease in temperature so that the aqueous-phase potencies remain relatively constant with changes in temperature (Fig. 4-3).[12] For in vitro experiments involving clinical volatile anesthetics, aqueous concentrations equivalent to 1 MAC range from about 200 to 600 µM.[12]

Effects of Pressure

The exposure of whole organisms to increasing hydrostatic pressures often increases the anesthetic dose required to bring about unresponsiveness, a phenomenon called the *pressure reversal of anesthesia*. In experiments with mammals, pressure is increased by the addition of helium, because helium does not produce anesthesia and possesses little or no inherent anesthetic effect at high pressures.[13] At a total pressure of 100 atm, a 30% to 60% increase in the partial pressure of inhaled anesthetics is required to abolish the righting reflex in the mouse.[14] However, it remains debatable whether pressure reversal represents a specific antagonism at the site of anesthetic action or is simply a generalized phenomenon that counteracts a global depression produced by anesthetics.

Effects of Age

In humans, MACs of volatile agents are maximal in infants at approximately 6 months of age. MAC values gradually decrease with increasing age, and the MAC in the octogenarian is approximately one half that in the infant. The increase in potency (i.e., decrease in MAC) with increasing age is seen for all inhaled anesthetics, and the change averages approximately 6% per decade of age.[15]

Effects of Ion Concentrations

Hypernatremia increases the sodium concentration proportionately in cerebrospinal fluid (CSF) and increases the halothane MAC in dogs by as much as 43%.[5] Conversely, hyponatremia dilutes the CSF sodium level and reduces the halothane MAC.[5] Hyperkalemia in dogs does

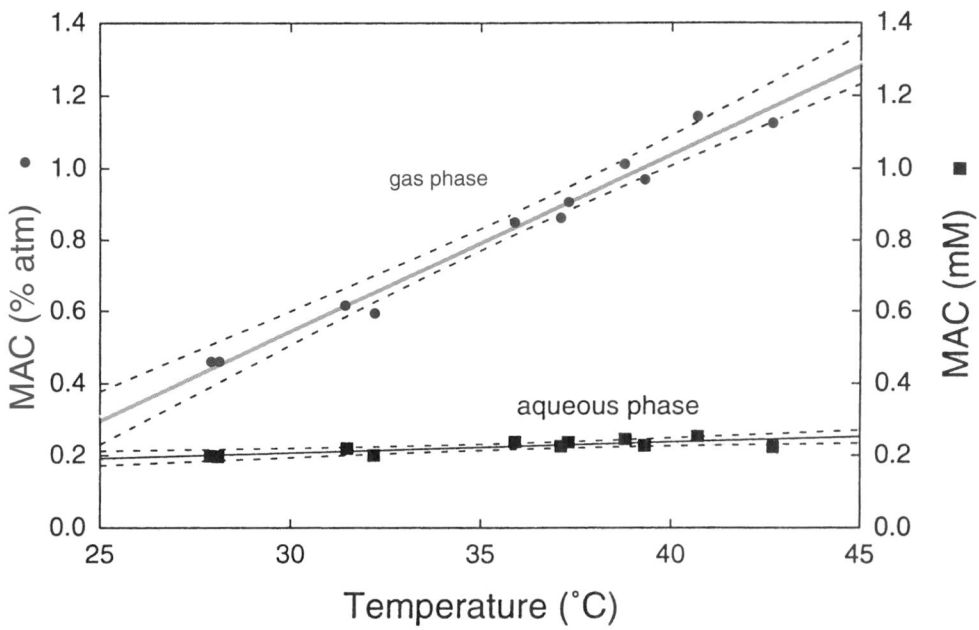

Figure 4–3 Plot of the halothane minimum alveolar concentration (MAC) in dogs versus temperature. When measured as a function of the gas-phase partial pressure, MAC decreases with decreasing temperature. When measured as a function of calculated aqueous concentrations, MAC remains relatively constant with changes in temperature from 28°C to 43°C. (From Franks NP, Lieb WR: Temperature dependence of the potency of volatile general anesthetics. Anesthesiology 84: 716, 1996.)

not alter the CSF potassium level or MAC. Calcium infusions in dogs increase serum and CSF calcium levels by 2.6 and 1.3 times, respectively, without influencing the halothane MAC.[16] A fivefold increase in serum magnesium is associated with a 12% increase in CSF magnesium concentrations in dogs and does not alter the halothane MAC.[16] In rats, a 10-fold increase in plasma magnesium concentration above control levels decreases the halothane MAC by approximately 60%.[17] Alterations in anion concentrations by infusion of hydrochloric acid or sodium bicarbonate have little influence on MAC despite marked changes in arterial pH.[5]

These effects of temperature, pressure, aging, and ion concentrations may be used to test the various models of anesthetic action. Any valid theory of anesthetic action must account for the influence of these physical and physiologic parameters on anesthetic requirement.

ACTIONS OF INHALED ANESTHETICS IN THE CENTRAL NERVOUS SYSTEM

Brain

Inhaled anesthetics may act by altering neuronal activity in selected regions of the CNS. Because the brainstem reticular formation plays a role in altering the state of consciousness and alertness and in regulating motor activity, it is often suggested that this structure is an important site of anesthetic action. Although the idea that anesthesia results from a decrease in "tone" in the ascending reticular system may be correct, it is most likely an oversimplification.[18] The effect of anesthesia on neuronal activity in the reticular formation is variable and can be increased, unchanged, or decreased, depending on the agent and the neuronal unit examined.[19]

General anesthetics interrupt transmission in the CNS at sites other than the reticular formation. Clinical concentrations of inhaled agents may alter spontaneous and evoked activity in the mammalian cerebral cortex and hippocampus. Although inhaled anesthetics usually depress excitability of brain neurons, situations can be found in which anesthetics enhance excitability (Fig. 4-4).[20] Inhibitory transmission may be influenced by volatile agents. For example, halothane, enflurane, isoflurane, and sevoflurane prolong γ-aminobutyric acid (GABA)–induced inhibition in the hippocampus[21,22] in an agent-specific manner. Neuronal pathways between various brain regions and consisting of excitatory and inhibitory components may also be influenced by inhaled agents. The transfer of sensory information from the thalamus to certain cortical regions may be particularly sensitive to anesthetics.[18,23]

Spinal Cord

Excitatory and inhibitory neurotransmissions in mammalian spinal cord may be altered by inhaled anesthetics.[24] Anesthetic effects depend on the concentration of the agent and on the particular spinal cord pathway examined. Inhaled anesthetics alter responses of the spinal dorsal horn (sensory) to noxious and non-noxious stimuli.[24]

Volatile anesthetics also depress spinal motor neurons. Clinical inhaled agents depress the F-wave amplitude, a measure of the excitability of spinal motor neurons, in animals and humans.[25] A reduction in the sensory processing and an inhibition of motor neuron excitation are likely to be involved in the anesthetic-induced lack of movement in response to a noxious stimulus. In addition to a direct action on the spinal cord, inhaled agents may indirectly influence activity of spinal neurons by altering the tonic input received from descending modulatory systems from the brain.[24,26] Conversely, inhaled anesthetics may act in the spinal cord to blunt transmission of noxious inputs to the thalamus and cerebral cortex and thereby indirectly contribute to amnesia and unconsciousness.[27]

Sites of Central Nervous System Action and Anesthetic End Points

Traditionally, most investigators assumed that surgical anesthesia resulted from a supraspinal event. Although it remains probable that an interaction of inhaled anesthetics with various brain structures is required for the production of amnesia, the ability of anesthetics to prevent a motor response to noxious stimulation likely results from a site of action in the spinal cord and not in the brain.

The isoflurane MAC in rats is not altered by bilateral decerebration, including removal of thalamus and hippocampus[28] (Fig. 4-5), nor by high thoracic spinal cord transection and functional separation of the rat brain from the spinal cord.[29] The cerebral blood supply of the goat allows for the preferential anesthetization of its forebrain, which results in an isoflurane MAC that is more than twice the value found when anesthetic is administered through the goat's native circulation.[30] This finding in a second species confirms the importance of extracranial structures in anesthesia as defined by the MAC.

If anesthesia is defined as consisting of at least two components, amnesia and immobility in response to a noxious stimulus, there must be two separate anatomic sites of inhaled anesthetic action: a supraspinal site involved in the production of amnesia and a spinal site involved in the prevention of movement in response to noxious stimuli.[31] Given that the human CNS consists of billions of neurons, each having thousands of synapses, the discovery of the exact nature of these sites of anesthetic action presents a formidable challenge. Attempts to reduce this complexity have led to experiments on isolated neuronal preparations.

INTERRUPTION OF NEURONAL TRANSMISSION BY INHALED ANESTHETICS

Peripheral Receptors

The action of inhaled anesthetics cannot be explained by depression of peripheral receptors. Anesthetizing concentrations of clinical agents do not alter cutaneous receptor responses to touch or movement of hair and can even

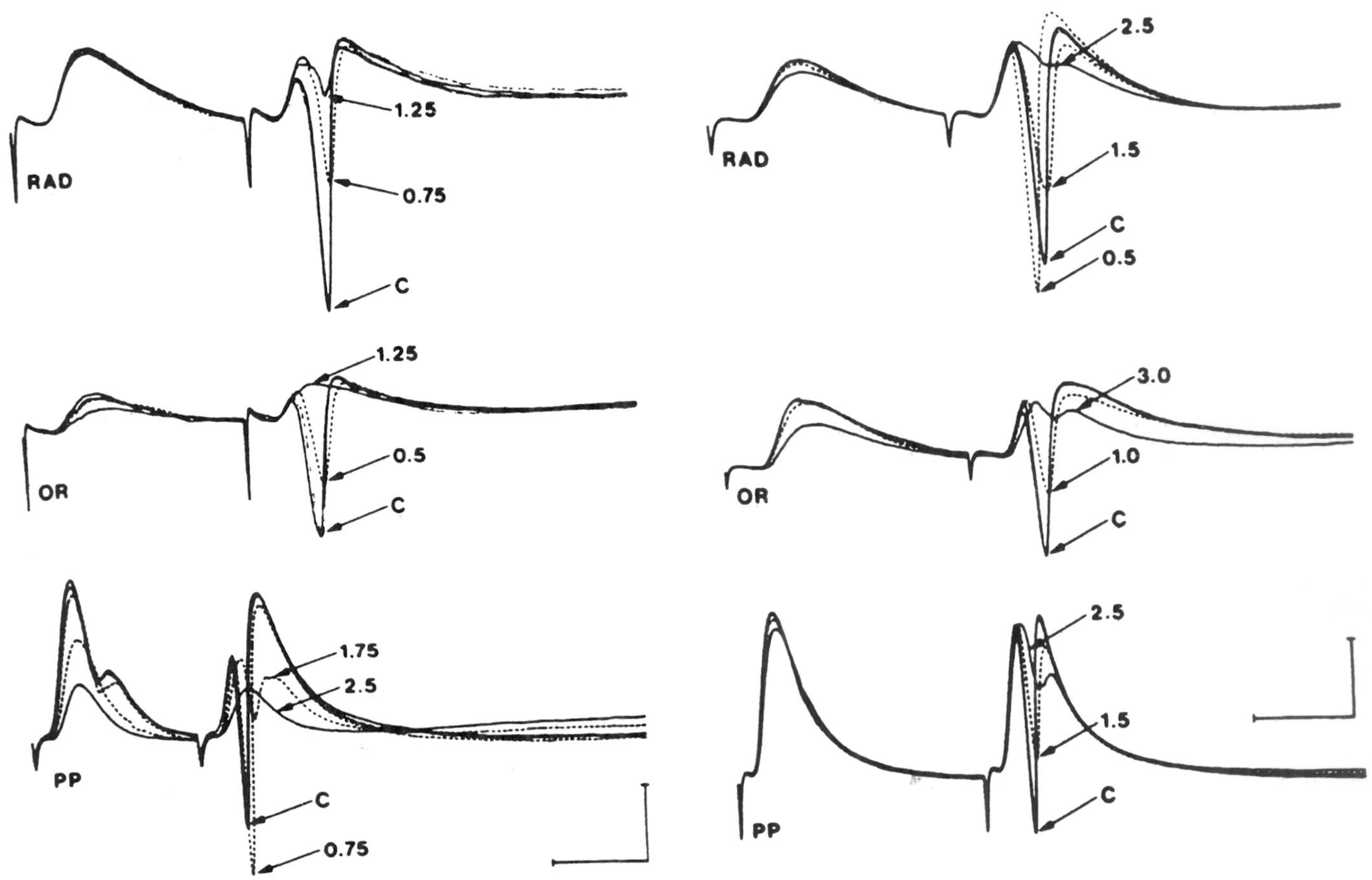

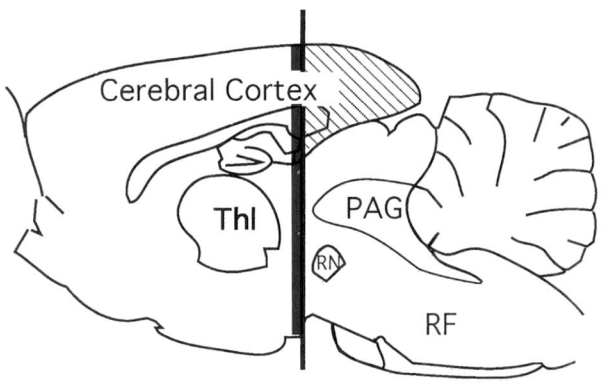

Figure 4–4 The effects of halothane *(left)* and isoflurane *(right)* on three excitatory synaptic pathways in the rat hippocampal slice. The potential recordings were produced from stimulation of three discrete regions of the hippocampal slice: the stratum radiatum (RAD), the stratum oriens (OR), and the perforant path (PP) fibers. Each superimposed series of records shows control (C) responses before *(solid line)* and after washout *(dotted line)* together with two or three concentrations of anesthetic (numbers refer to volume percent). The horizontal calibration bar represents 20 msec, and the vertical calibration bar represents 2.0 mV. These studies demonstrate that the ability of inhaled agents to depress or enhance neuronal excitability depends on the anesthetic, the anesthetic concentration, and the particular brain region examined. (From MacIver MB, Roth SH: Inhalation anaesthetics exhibit pathway-specific and differential actions on hippocampal synaptic responses in vitro. Br J Anaesth 60:680, 1988.)

Figure 4–5 Decerebration does not alter anesthetic requirement, as measured by the minimum alveolar concentration (MAC). Removal of brain tissue rostral to the *heavy black line* does not alter isoflurane MAC in rats. PAG, periaqueductal gray; RF, reticular formation; RN, red nucleus; Thl, thalamus. (Adapted from Rampil IJ, Mason P, Singh H: Anesthetic potency [MAC] is independent of forebrain structures in the rat. Anesthesiology 78:707, 1993.)

sensitize and promote excitation of nociceptors in mammalian A and C fibers.[32] Moreover, a selective perfusion technique allowing for low (about 0.2% atm) isoflurane concentration at the site of peripheral noxious stimulus in dogs while maintaining higher concentrations in the rest of the body results in no change in the isoflurane MAC and demonstrates that the peripheral effects of isoflurane do not influence the response to a noxious stimulus.[33] In humans, peripheral nerve conduction is unaltered by the concentrations of desflurane needed for surgical anesthesia.[25]

Highly Sensitive Neurons

Inhaled agents can alter excitability in many different anatomic regions of the brain or spinal cord. However, within each discrete area of the CNS, there may exist a relatively small number of neurons that are exquisitely sensitive to anesthetics. The existence of such highly sensitive cells is demonstrated in molluscan ganglia having endogenous firing activity.[34,35] The firing activity may be completely inhibited in selected neurons at halothane concentrations of about 1 MAC (Fig. 4-6),[34,35] with other neighboring neurons exhibiting little alteration in neuronal firing activity. There may even exist supersensitive sites in the CNS (i.e., sites that are maximally inhibited at anesthetic concentrations substantially less than MAC) that are related to the anesthetic-induced production of amnesia.[36]

Axonal Versus Synaptic Transmission

Concentrations of inhaled anesthetics that alter synaptic transmission typically have a smaller effect on axonal transmission, with synaptic events being about fivefold more sensitive to inhibition than impulse conduction.[37] Nevertheless, at near-clinical concentrations, inhaled anesthetics may alter transmission through axons, and even a partial decrease in action potential propagation could decrease the amount of neurotransmitter secreted and thereby influence synaptic transmission. An apparent effect at the synapse may simply reflect depression of axonal transmission. Small-diameter axons may exhibit enhanced susceptibility to inhaled anesthetics. In the rat hippocampus, isoflurane (1.4% atm) depresses the activity of thin (0.16-mm) unmyelinated fibers but has little influence on the larger-diameter (1-mm) myelinated fibers.[38]

The frequency at which axons transmit impulses may alter anesthetic potency. At low-impulse frequencies, volatile anesthetics produce a constant level of action potential block, whereas at relatively high frequencies, conduction block by volatile agents increases progressively. The blockade is use dependent.[39] The branch points

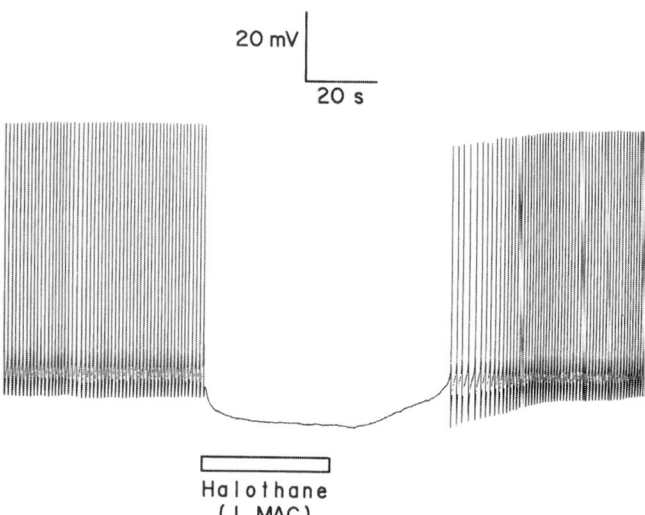

20 mV

20 s

Halothane
(1 MAC)

Figure 4–6 Certain molluscan neurons having endogenous firing activity are extremely sensitive to volatile agents. The figure shows a continuous intracellular recording of membrane potential before, during (*bar*), and after exposure of a sensitive cell to normal saline solution containing halothane at a partial pressure of 0.0080 atm. (From Franks NP, Lieb WR: Volatile general anaesthetics activate a novel neuronal K[+] current. Nature 333:662, 1988.)

of axons may be particularly sensitive to high-frequency conduction block.

Synapses

Anesthetics may disrupt normal synaptic transmission by interfering with the release of neurotransmitter from the presynaptic nerve terminals into the synaptic cleft, by altering the reuptake of neurotransmitter after its release, by changing the binding of neurotransmitter to receptor sites on the postsynaptic membrane, or by influencing the ionic conductance change that follows activation of the postsynaptic receptor by neurotransmitter.[37]

Presynaptic Action

A presynaptic site of inhaled anesthetic action may be inferred from electrophysiologic recordings that compare postsynaptic potentials obtained through presynaptic stimulation compared with those generated by direct application of neurotransmitter. For example, in mouse hippocampal slices, glutamatergic excitatory postsynaptic currents are reduced about 50% by approximately 1 MAC of halothane, whereas halothane (even at concentrations of about 5 MAC) has no effect on the currents induced by bath application of glutamatergic agonists.[40]

A presynaptic site of action is also implied from studies that demonstrate an influence of anesthetics on neurotransmitter release.[37,41] Clinical concentrations of inhaled agents reduce depolarization-evoked release of norepinephrine but not acetylcholine from slices of rat cerebral cortex.[42] In the rat striatum, isoflurane and halothane increase spontaneous dopamine release[43] but decrease nicotine-evoked release of dopamine and have no effect on potassium-induced GABA release.[44] Isoflurane does not alter potassium-evoked glutamate release in cerebral cortex, striatum, or hippocampus, but it inhibits Na[+] channel–mediated glutamate release.[45] The ability of anesthetics to alter neurotransmitter release may depend on the biologic preparation examined, the method employed to evoke neurotransmitter release, the neurotransmitter, and the anesthetic and its concentration.

In addition to an effect on the presynaptic release of neurotransmitters, it is conceivable that inhaled anesthetics may alter the duration of neurotransmitter action by influencing the reuptake of neurotransmitter into the nerve terminal.[41] An anesthetic-induced increase in the uptake of glutamate may decrease excitatory transmission and contribute to the action of some volatile agents.[46]

Postsynaptic Action

Evidence is available for the postsynaptic effects of inhaled anesthetics on excitatory and inhibitory neurons. Postsynaptic sites of anesthetic action may be studied by application of putative neurotransmitters thought to act directly on postsynaptic membrane receptors.[37] Halothane and isoflurane (0.5 to 2.5 MAC) reduce the depolarizing responses to iontophoretic applications of acetylcholine or glutamate to dendrites in guinea pig neocortical slices, with the acetylcholine response being depressed more than the glutamate response.[47] Halothane and isoflurane have little or no effect on the response induced by iontophoretic application of GABA to perikaryons in these neocortical slices,[47] whereas in hippocampal neurons[48] and in neurons dissociated from the nucleus tractus solitarius of the rat,[49] volatile anesthetics enhance the currents produced by application of GABA (Fig. 4-7). In hippocampal neurons, xenon has no measurable effect on GABA-evoked postsynaptic currents but inhibits postsynaptic current at glutamatergic excitatory synapses.[48] Depending on the particular neuronal preparation and neurotransmitter examined, anesthetics may depress, have little influence on, or enhance the postsynaptic response.

A postsynaptic action is also evident from the ability of clinical concentrations of inhaled agents to modulate current flow through a variety of ion channels found on postsynaptic membranes (see "Membrane Proteins").[50]

In summary, inhaled anesthetics act on synaptic regions, including afferent axons at the nerve terminal. Inhaled agents alter axonal and synaptic transmission in isolated monosynaptic and polysynaptic neuronal systems and may have presynaptic and postsynaptic effects. Clinical concentrations of inhaled agents can depress, leave unchanged, or enhance presynaptic neurotransmitter release and the postsynaptic response. The effect depends on the biologic preparation, the frequency of neuronal transmission, the particular neurotransmitter, and the anesthetic examined.

ALTERATIONS IN NEUROREGULATORS ASSOCIATED WITH ANESTHESIA

The list of CNS transmitters is rapidly expanding. In addition to the classic transmitters (e.g., acetylcholine), endogenous amino acids and peptides may act as neurotransmitters or modulate the action of other neurotransmitters. The postsynaptic action of neurotransmitters may result in the formation of second messengers that mediate changes in neuronal transmission. Limited information is available concerning the relationship between the levels of neuroregulators in the CNS and the inhaled anesthetic requirement.

Acetylcholine

Inhaled anesthetics do not alter acetylcholine concentrations in macroscopic structures (e.g., cortex) of rat brain[51] but may increase or decrease[52] acetylcholine content in specific brain nuclei. Inhaled agents decrease acetylcholine turnover rate, and the magnitude of the decrease varies with the brain region examined.[51] Release of acetylcholine into rat cerebral cortex is suppressed by isoflurane and sevoflurane but enhanced by nitrous oxide.[53] Synthesis of acetylcholine in brain is impaired by inhaled agents and is associated with an anesthetic-induced inhibition of choline uptake.[41] Although the direct application of a cholinergic agonist to a discrete nucleus of the rat brainstem reticular formation decreases halothane MAC,[54] intrathecal or intraperitoneal injection of acetylcholine receptor antagonists has little or no influence on isoflurane MAC in rats.[55]

Catecholamines

Rats anesthetized with halothane or cyclopropane have unaltered norepinephrine concentrations in most brain regions but may have an elevated norepinephrine content in the nucleus accumbens, locus ceruleus, and central gray catecholamine areas.[56] Although anesthesia does not deplete brain norepinephrine, a change in norepinephrine availability significantly influences anesthetic requirement. Drugs that decrease central levels of norepinephrine result in a dose-related decrease in the halothane MAC, whereas drugs that elevate central norepinephrine levels increase the anesthetic requirement.[57]

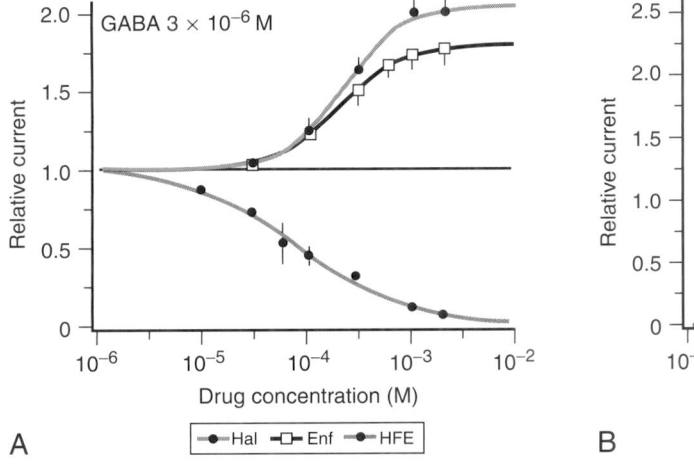
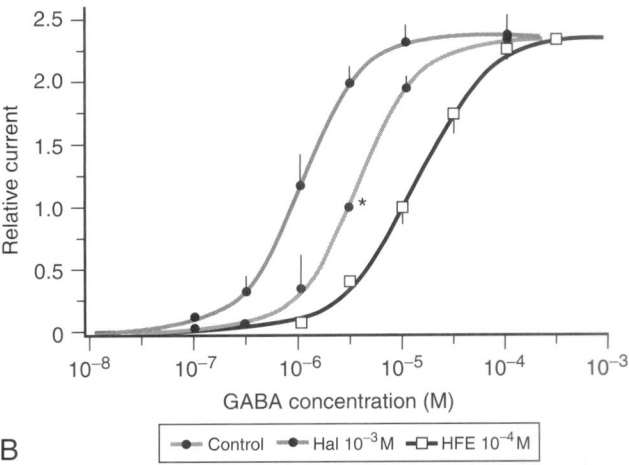

Figure 4–7 A, Effects of halothane (Hal), enflurane (Enf), and the convulsant hexafluorodiethyl ether [flurothyl] (HFE) on current responses evoked by γ-aminobutyric acid (GABA) (3×10^{-6} M) application to dissociated central nervous system neurons of the rat. Responses are normalized to the peak current induced by 3×10^{-6} M GABA alone. **B,** The GABA concentration-response curve is shifted to the left by halothane and to the right by HFE. Peak response was normalized to that evoked by 3×10^{-6} M GABA *(asterisk)*. (Adapted from Wakamori M, Ikemoto Y, Akaike N: Effects of two volatile anesthetics on the excitatory and inhibitory amino acid responses in dissociated CNS neurons of the rat. J Neurophysiol 66:2014, 1991.)

In contrast to those of norepinephrine, central levels of dopamine appear to be inversely related to anesthetic requirement. Administration of levodopa to mice increases striatal dopamine content and decreases the halothane MAC,[58] and an increase in striatal dopamine content is associated with halothane anesthesia.[59] Conversely, chemical destruction of dopaminergic neurons lowers dopamine content and increases the halothane MAC.[58]

The administration of α_2-adrenergic agonists markedly lowers inhaled anesthetic requirement in animals and humans. Dexmedetomidine, an agonist that is more selective than clonidine for the α_2-adrenoreceptor, produces a remarkable decrease in the halothane[60] MAC in dogs to less than 10% of the control value (Fig. 4-8). This effect appears to be highly specific for the α_2-adrenoreceptor, because the optical isomer L-medetomidine does not alter MAC (see Fig. 4-8). The ability of spinally administered α_2-adrenoreceptor antagonists to block the antinociceptive effects of nitrous oxide and isoflurane also suggests an adrenergic mechanism for the analgesic actions of inhaled anesthetics.[61]

Serotonin

Serotonin (5-hydroxytryptamine [5-HT]) levels are unaltered in most brain regions of rats after administration of inhaled agents but may increase in specific brain structures (e.g., substantia nigra, nucleus raphe dorsalis).[62] The inability of ondansetron, a 5-HT_3 receptor antagonist used to treat postoperative nausea, to alter the isoflurane MAC suggests that this particular subtype of serotonergic receptor is not involved in the surgical immobility produced by inhaled anesthetics.[63]

Adenosine

Small alterations of endogenous adenosine concentrations do not substantially alter the anesthetic requirement

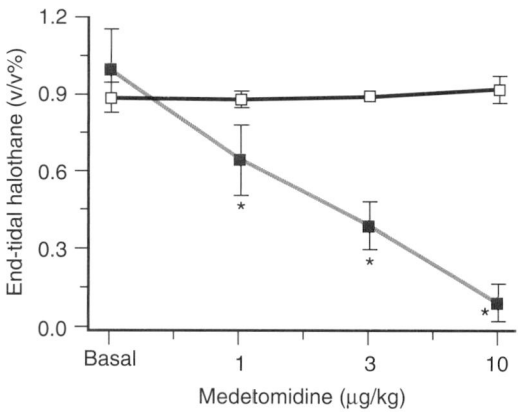

Figure 4–8 The D-stereoisomer (*closed squares*) of the α_2-adrenergic agonist medetomidine causes a dose-dependent decrease in the halothane minimum alveolar concentration (MAC) in dogs, whereas the L-stereoisomer (*open squares*) has little or no influence on halothane MAC. *Asterisks* indicate values that are significantly different from the controls. (Adapted from Vickery RG, Sheridan BC, Segal IS, et al: Anesthetic and hemodynamic effects of the stereoisomers of medetomidine, an α_2-adrenergic agonist, in halothane-anesthetized dogs. Anesth Analg 67:611, 1988.)

in dogs.[64] Exogenous administration of adenosine decreases the halothane MAC in dogs by about 50%,[64] but adenosine (at doses that require vasopressors to maintain blood pressure) does not alter the sevoflurane MAC or sevoflurane MAC-awake in patients.[65] Although adenosine may prove helpful in providing relief from chronic pain, adenosine does not alter response to acute noxious stimulation in humans.[66]

γ-Aminobutyric Acid

Although rats administered 1% to 4% atm halothane for 30 minutes exhibit no change in whole-brain GABA content,[67] anesthesia may alter GABA levels in selected regions of the brain. Treatment of rat cerebral cortex slices with 3% atm halothane inhibits the metabolism and increases the content of the inhibitory transmitter GABA but does not affect the uptake or release of GABA.[68] If the accumulation of GABA in inhibitory neurons is associated with an increase in inhibitory activity, the resulting decrease in synaptic transmission may contribute to the anesthetic state.[68] Consistent with this hypothesis is the reversal of isoflurane-induced suppression of thalamocortical relay neurons by the local iontophoretic application of a GABA_A-receptor antagonist[69] and the ability of GABA_A-receptor antagonists to increase the isoflurane MAC in rats.[70,71]

Glycine

Glycine, a major inhibitory transmitter in the CNS (predominantly in the spinal cord and brainstem), is only slightly increased in whole rat brain at high concentrations of a volatile agent.[67] It seems unlikely that glycine plays a major role in the production of the anesthetic state because massive intravascular infusions of glycine that are occasionally seen as a complication of urologic surgery with the use of a glycine irrigation solution (Chapter 54) do not produce general anesthesia. Nevertheless, the ability of a specific glycine receptor antagonist (e.g., strychnine) to increase the isoflurane MAC implies a partial involvement of glycine receptors in the production of immobility by volatile anesthetics.[71]

Excitatory Amino Acids

A role for excitatory amino acids in anesthesia is indicated by the depression in glutamate-induced neurotransmission by inhaled anesthetics and the decreased requirements for volatile anesthetics after administering inhibitors of excitatory amino acid transmission.[72] Anesthesia does not result from a depletion of excitatory amino acids because rats anesthetized with halothane have an increased whole-brain content of aspartate and glutamate.[67] Volatile anesthetics inhibit postsynaptic excitatory transmission and depress release of excitatory amino acids from nerve terminals.[45,73]

Cyclic Nucleotides

The production of cyclic nucleotides may be influenced by neurotransmitters and anesthetics, and cyclic nucleotides may serve as second messengers in altering neurotransmission. The effect of anesthetics on cyclic adenosine monophosphate (cAMP) content varies with the species and tissues examined.[74] Most studies demonstrate an increase in brain cAMP content of rodents during the administration of volatile anesthetics, with the magnitude of the increase varying among species and among brain regions.[74] In contrast, levels of cyclic guanosine monophosphate (cGMP) in brain are decreased by volatile agents.[75] Nitric oxide activates guanylyl cyclase to form cGMP, and nitric oxide production can be enhanced by excitatory neurotransmitters. It has been suggested that volatile anesthetics decrease brain cGMP by interfering with the neuronal nitric oxide–cGMP pathway.[75] Such alterations in brain cyclic nucleotide content may chemically alter (e.g., through phosphorylation) macromolecules that are important in neurotransmission.

Calcium

Calcium is mentioned as a neuroregulator because there is evidence that inhaled anesthetics alter intracellular concentrations of calcium and because changes in intracellular calcium may influence neuronal excitability (e.g., by a calcium-dependent release of neurotransmitter).[76] Inhaled anesthetics usually increase resting cytoplasmic calcium concentration,[76] and it has been proposed that the depressant action of halothane in rat hippocampal slices involves enhancement of GABA-mediated inhibition through release of intraneuronally stored calcium.[77] In contrast, increases in intraneuronal calcium evoked by various stimuli are often prevented by inhaled agents. The mechanisms for the attenuation of the calcium increase by inhaled anesthetics may depend on the anesthetic and tissue examined and include impairment of calcium influx into cells[76] and modulation of intracellular calcium release through action on inositol triphosphate–dependent pathways.[78]

Endogenous Opiates

In the late 1970s, it was hypothesized that inhaled anesthetics may work through an action on the opiate receptor. Consistent with this hypothesis are the clinical observations and experimental findings that synthetic narcotics partially decrease the requirement for inhaled anesthetics and that the administration of naloxone, a narcotic antagonist, may partially reverse certain actions of inhaled anesthetics. However, high doses of naloxone have little or no influence on anesthetic requirement (e.g., MAC), and any antagonistic effects of naloxone probably result from a general increase in CNS excitation and not by pharmacologic competition for inhaled anesthetics at opiate receptors.[79]

Another prediction of the opiate theory of anesthesia is that inhaled agents may release an endogenous opiate-like substance in the CNS. Data are available both to support and to refute this prediction. Nitrous oxide markedly increases proenkephalin-derived endogenous opioid peptides in canine third ventricle CSF.[80] The lowering of halothane MAC in rats by transcranial electrical stimulation is reversed by naloxone, suggesting that release of endogenous opioids mediated the decrease in halothane requirement.[81] In patients anesthetized with a combination of halothane and nitrous oxide[82] or isoflurane,[83] there is no elevation in the concentration of opioid peptides in CSF. Any contribution of the endogenous opiate system to the production of general anesthesia in humans does not appear to require the release of opioid peptides.

Nitric Oxide

Nitric oxide is recognized as a neuromodulator and has been hypothesized to play a role in mediating consciousness. Although the short half-life (milliseconds to seconds) of nitric oxide makes it a difficult compound to study, administration of nitric oxide synthase inhibitors decreases (by about 30% to 50%) the MAC and righting-reflex ED_{50} of halothane and isoflurane in rodents.[84,85] However, sparing of anesthetic requirement by nitric oxide synthase inhibitors is not found in all experiments.[86] Nitric oxide is involved in cellular communication processes through production of cGMP and various neurotransmitter pathways, processes that may be important to the anesthetic state.[75]

In summary, the predominant effects of inhaled anesthetics are not explained by the depletion, production, or release of a single neuromodulator in the CNS. In all likelihood, the anesthetic state involves a balance between many different neuromodulator systems.

PHYSICOCHEMICAL NATURE OF THE SITE OF ANESTHETIC ACTION

The preceding sections suggest that anesthetics may act at several gross (e.g., spinal cord versus reticular activating system) or microscopic (e.g., presynaptic versus postsynaptic) sites. The varied nature of these sites, however, does not preclude a unique action at a molecular level. For instance, depression of presynaptic neurotransmitter release and blockade of current flow through the postsynaptic membrane may arise from an anesthetic perturbation at an identical molecular site, even though the geographic locations of these sites differ. The concept that all inhaled anesthetics have a common mode of action on a specific molecular structure is called the *unitary theory of narcosis.* The nature of this presumed common site has been explored by correlating the physical properties of anesthetics with their potencies. The rationale behind this approach is that the best correlation between anesthetic potency and a physical property suggests the nature of the anesthetic site of action. For example, the correlation of MAC and lipid solubility implies that the site of action is hydrophobic. The correlations that depend on forces exerted between anesthetic molecules (e.g., the boiling point of an anesthetic) are not important to the study of anesthetic mechanisms; as such, intermolecular forces cannot be representative of a single site of action. These correlations are defined by the interaction of each anesthetic with itself rather than with a common site.

Hydrophobic Site: The Meyer-Overton Rule

The physical property that correlates best with anesthetic potency is lipid solubility (Table 4-2 and Fig. 4-9).[87-89] This correlation is called the *Meyer-Overton rule,* after its two discoverers. For most inhaled agents, the product of the anesthetizing partial pressure and its olive oil–gas partition coefficient varies little over approximately a 100,000-fold range of anesthetizing partial pressures (see Table 4-2 and Fig. 4-9). For the correlation to be perfect, this product would have to be the same for all anesthetics for a given animal. Within a given species, an even better correlation between anesthetic potency and solubility may be obtained with solvents that are better characterized than olive oil, such as lecithin, an amphipathic phospholipid with hydrophobic and polar components.[90] The closeness of this correlation implies a unitary molecular site of action and suggests that anesthesia results when a specific number of anesthetic molecules occupy a crucial hydrophobic region in the CNS. This finding has led many investigators to look for the molecular basis of anesthetic action in cellular hydrophobic regions.

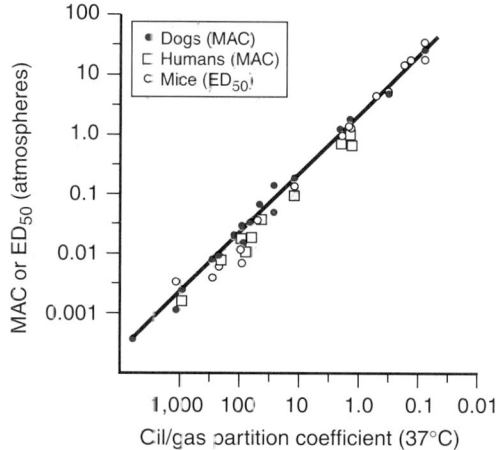

Figure 4–9 Correlation of the minimum alveolar concentration (MAC) in humans and dogs and the righting-reflex 50% effective dose (ED$_{50}$) in mice with lipid solubility (i.e., the olive oil–gas partition coefficient). Values are taken from Table 4-2.

Table 4–2 Oil-gas partition coefficients and potencies of inhaled anesthetics in dogs, humans, and mice

| | | Dogs | | Humans | | Mice | |
| | | MAC (atm) | MAC × Oil-Gas (atm) | MAC (atm) | MAC × Oil-Gas (atm) | Righting Reflex ED$_{50}$ (atm) | Righting Reflex ED$_{50}$ × Oil-Gas (atm) |
Anesthetic	Oil-Gas Partition Coefficient (37°C)						
Thiomethoxyflurane	7230	0.00035	2.53				
Methoxyflurane	970	0.0023	2.23	0.0016	1.55	0.0023	2.23
Dioxychlorane	1286	0.0011	1.41			0.0033	4.24
Chloroform	265	0.0077	2.08			0.00357	0.95
Halothane	224	0.0087	1.95	0.0074	1.66	0.00645	1.45
Enflurane	96.5	0.0267	2.58	0.0168	1.62	0.0123	1.19
Isoflurane	90.8	0.0141	1.28	0.0115	1.04	0.00663	0.60
Compound 485	25.8	0.125	3.23				
Desflurane	18.7	0.072	1.35	0.060	1.12	0.045	0.84
HFClOCHFCF$_3$	96.6	0.0224	2.16				
Iso-Indoklon	27.0	0.460	1.24			0.0265	0.72
Aliflurane	124	0.0184	2.28				
Synthane	95	0.012	1.14				
Diethyl ether	65	0.0304	1.98	0.0192	1.25	0.032	2.08
Fluroxene	47.7	0.0599	2.86	0.034	1.62	0.0345	1.65
Sevoflurane	47.2	0.0236	1.11	0.0205	0.97	0.0116	0.58
Cyclopropane	11.8	0.175	2.06	0.092	1.09	0.142	1.68
Xenon	1.9	1.19	2.26	0.71	1.35	0.95	1.80
Ethylene	1.26			0.67	0.84	1.30	1.64
Nitrous oxide	1.4	1.88	2.63	1.04	1.46	1.54	2.16
Krypton	0.5					4.5	2.25
Sulfur hexafluoride	0.293	4.9	1.44			5.4	1.58
Argon	0.15					15.2	2.28
Carbon tetrafluoride	0.073	26	1.90			18.7	1.36
Nitrogen	0.072	≥43.5	≥3.13			34.3	2.47
Mean ± SE			2.04 ± 0.14		1.30 ± 0.08		1.69 ± 0.19

Additive Effects of Inhaled Anesthetics

The Meyer-Overton rule postulates that it is the number of molecules dissolved at the site of anesthetic action, not the types of molecules present, that causes anesthesia. A 0.5 MAC of one agent and a 0.5 MAC of another agent should have the same effect as a 1.0 MAC of either agent. In general, this prediction has been confirmed for clinically employed agents in animals and humans,[91] although slight antagonistic effects are occasionally observed.

Exceptions to the Meyer-Overton Rule

Isomers

Despite the close correlation between lipid solubility and anesthetic potency, deviations from this correlation do exist. For example, enflurane and isoflurane are structural isomers (see Fig. 4-1) having approximately the same oil-gas partition coefficient, but the anesthetic requirement for enflurane is 45% to 90% greater than that for isoflurane (see Table 4-2). These differences in anesthetic requirements for agents having similar oil-gas partition coefficients suggest that the potency of an agent depends on factors other than lipid solubility.

Several of the commonly used inhaled anesthetics (see Fig. 4-1A) exist as mixtures of two stereoisomers, which are nonsuperimposable compounds that are mirror images of each other, having identical physicochemical properties except for the direction in which they rotate polarized light. For isoflurane stereoisomers in rats, the (+) isomer is 17% to 53% more potent than the (−) isomer.[92] The differential effects of the inhaled anesthetic stereoisomers are relatively modest.

Convulsant Gases

Another apparent exception to the Meyer-Overton rule is the ability of certain lipid-soluble compounds to produce convulsions. Complete halogenation or full halogenation of the end-methyl groups of alkanes and ethers tends to decrease the anesthetic potencies of these agents and to enhance convulsant activity.[93] Flurothyl ($CF_3CH_2OCH_2CF_3$) produces convulsions at concentrations an order of magnitude less than those predicted to be anesthetic by the Meyer-Overton rule.[94] Although loss of the righting reflex in the mouse at very high flurothyl concentrations implies an anesthetic effect, 3% to 4% atm flurothyl only marginally decreases the isoflurane MAC in dogs.[94]

Compound 485 (see Fig. 4-1C) possesses completely halogenated end-methyl groups and is a structural isomer of enflurane and isoflurane. It has occasionally produced convulsions in dogs at concentrations near 6% atm.[95] As an isomer of enflurane and isoflurane, it was predicted to have similar potency and solubility characteristics; however, its MAC was found to be 12.5% atm. This high MAC value was balanced by an approximately fourfold lower oil-gas partition coefficient (see Table 4-2).[95]

Convulsant halogenated ethers have different physical properties from the anesthetic halogenated ethers and have different effects on synaptic transmission. In dissociated rat brain neurons, halothane and enflurane enhance the response to GABA, whereas flurothyl decreases the GABA response (see Fig. 4-7).[49] In contrast to the enhancement of agonist-induced responses at $GABA_A$ receptors by anesthetic ethers, flurothyl acts as a noncompetitive antagonist and decreases current flow through $GABA_A$ receptors.[96]

Cutoff Effect

There has been a long-standing impression that the highly lipid-soluble paraffin hydrocarbon n-decane was nonanesthetic in animals, even though less soluble paraffin homologs such as n-pentane caused anesthesia. This decrease in anesthetic potency in the higher members of a homologous series is known as the *cutoff effect*.[97] However, detailed reexamination of this issue has revealed the cutoff for n-alkanes may be explained by limited delivery of the larger alkanes because of decreasing volatility. Although decane does not anesthetize rats when given alone at its saturated vapor pressure, anesthetic properties are demonstrated by an ability to decrease the requirement for isoflurane.[98] A "true" cutoff exists for the perfluoroalkanes.[99] Perfluoromethane (CF_4) produces anesthesia in rats (MAC ≅ 60 atm), but perfluoroethane (CF_3CF_3) and longer-chain perfluorinated derivatives are nonanesthetic despite being soluble in hydrophobic solvents and in tissues.[99]

Nonanesthetics

In addition to the nonanesthetic perfluoroalkane gases previously discussed, certain volatile polyhalogenated agents that are even more lipid soluble but lack anesthetic properties have also been discovered.[100-102] Examples of such *nonanesthetics* are seen in Figure 4-10. These nonanesthetics do not produce anesthesia when administered alone, even when administered at partial

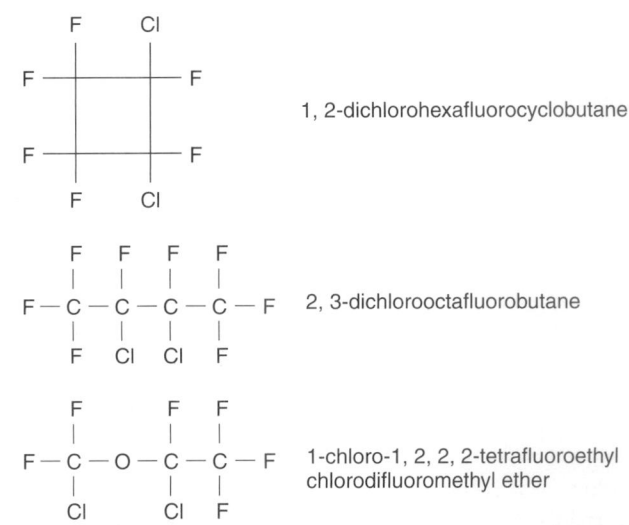

1, 2-dichlorohexafluorocyclobutane

2, 3-dichlorooctafluorobutane

1-chloro-1, 2, 2, 2-tetrafluoroethyl chlorodifluoromethyl ether

Figure 4–10 Examples of nonanesthetics (i.e., nonimmobilizers). Although these compounds have oil-gas partition coefficients (43.5 for 1,2-dichlorohexafluorocyclobutane; 25 for 2,3-dichlorooctafluorobutane; 10.8 for 1-chloro-1,2,2,2-tetrafluoroethyl chlorodifluoromethyl ether) similar to those of conventional anesthetics (see Table 4-2), they completely lack anesthetic properties as determined by minimum alveolar concentration (MAC) measurements.[100,102]

pressures greater than those predicted to have an anesthetic effect by the Meyer-Overton hypothesis, and they do not lower the MAC for conventional anesthetics.[100-102]

These nonanesthetics are not inert. They quickly reach the brain, produce excitable behavior, and typically cause convulsions when administered at high enough partial pressures.[100-103] Because MAC is used as the end point to define a nonanesthetic, it is more appropriate to call these compounds *nonimmobilizers* than nonanesthetics. Although these nonimmobilizers fail to produce immobility in response to a noxious stimulus, they do impair learning and memory and cause amnesia.[31,104]

The nonimmobilizers may be helpful in identifying anesthetic sites and mechanisms of action.[105] Physiologic or biochemical and biophysical changes produced by conventional anesthetics in a model system thought to be important for the anesthetic state (as measured by MAC) should not be produced by the nonimmobilizers.

Hydrophilic Site
The suggestion of a possible nonhydrophobic anesthetic site of action is not new. For example, Pauling[106] suggested that anesthesia might be caused by the ability of anesthetics to precipitate the formation of hydrates. These hydrates are cagelike structures of water molecules surrounding a central anesthetic molecule, and it was speculated that hydrate microcrystals could alter the transmission of electrical charge through a neuron.[106] However, a unitary hydrate theory of anesthesia seems unlikely because there is a poor correlation between the ability of anesthetics to form hydrates and their anesthetic potency.

Another hypothesis is that certain inhaled anesthetics act by disrupting hydrogen bonds.[107] This cannot be a unitary hypothesis because compounds such as xenon and argon are anesthetics but do not form hydrogen bonds. One suggestion is that general anesthetic target sites have, in addition to an overall hydrophobicity, a polar component that is a relatively poor hydrogen bond donor but that accepts a hydrogen bond about as well as water.[107] If hydrogen bonds are important in anesthesia, substitution of hydrogen for deuterium atoms in anesthetic molecules might alter the hydrogen bonding capabilities of a compound and change its anesthetic potency. However, the identical anesthetic potencies of halothane and deuterated halothane[108] do not support this prediction.

Volume Expansion by Inhaled Anesthetics
Although the Meyer-Overton rule postulates that anesthesia occurs when a sufficient number of anesthetic molecules dissolve at a certain site, it does not explain why anesthesia results. One suggestion, called the *critical volume hypothesis*, is that anesthesia occurs when the absorption of anesthetic molecules expands the volume of a hydrophobic region beyond a critical amount. Such an expansion may produce anesthesia by obstructing ion channels or by altering the electrical properties of neurons.

A prediction of the volume expansion hypothesis is that anesthetizing partial pressures of inhaled agents should produce a consistent volume expansion in a model hydrophobic system. Anesthetizing doses of inhaled agents cause hydrophobic solvents to undergo a significant increase in volume.[109] The hypothesis also predicts that anesthesia should be reversed by compressing the volume of the expanded hydrophobic region, and high pressures do reverse many effects of anesthetics in vivo.[14] However, the influence of body temperature on anesthetic requirement (see Fig. 4-3), a nonlinear pressure antagonism for certain anesthetics, and the fact that not all lipid-soluble compounds are anesthetics are findings that are difficult to reconcile with the critical volume hypothesis. Although the critical volume hypothesis is a useful model for estimating the interactions between pressure and inhaled anesthetics, it probably is an oversimplified view of the way in which anesthetics act.

THE MEMBRANE AS THE SITE OF ANESTHETIC ACTION

The electrical activity (i.e., transfer of ions) immediately underlying the transmission of nervous impulses occurs principally at the plasma membranes of nerves. Because inhaled agents disrupt this transmission, synaptic or axonal membranes, or both, are usually assumed to be the primary sites of anesthetic action. A membrane site of action is also consistent with the hydrophobic or amphipathic theories of anesthesia because plasma membranes consist largely of hydrophobic or amphipathic components.

Electrophysiologic studies reveal the effects of anesthetics on the flow of ions through excitable membranes. In isolated axons, the conduction of the nervous impulse requires the sequential flow of sodium and potassium ions through selective transmembrane channels. Excitation produces a rapid increase in sodium conductance to a peak (i.e., activation process) followed by a slower decline in sodium conductance to zero (i.e., inactivation process). Although channels in peripheral neurons tend to be relatively insensitive to anesthetics,[2] clinical concentrations of inhaled anesthetics may decrease the magnitude of sodium[110] and potassium[111] currents in channels isolated from brain.

Electrophysiologic recordings of single membrane channels activated by a neurotransmitter can be obtained by forming a seal between the tip of a glass micropipette and a membrane patch of a few square micrometers. Using this patch-clamp technique, unitary acetylcholine receptor channel currents can be measured in the absence and in the presence of inhaled anesthetics (Fig. 4-11).[112,113] Isoflurane decreases the average open duration of this membrane channel, and such an accelerated decay of the membrane current may decrease the net charge transferred across the membrane and impair transmission (see Fig. 4-11).[112,113]

In contrast to the inhibitory effects of anesthetics on ion flow through membranes described earlier, other experiments suggest that anesthetics may act by enhancing the conductance of certain ions through membranes. Volatile anesthetics enhance the inhibitory current responses produced by GABA (see Fig. 4-7),[49,114] presumably by increasing the flow of chloride ions through GABA receptor–channel complexes in neuronal membranes.[114] Inhaled agents may also enhance potassium conductance, resulting in membrane hyperpolarization

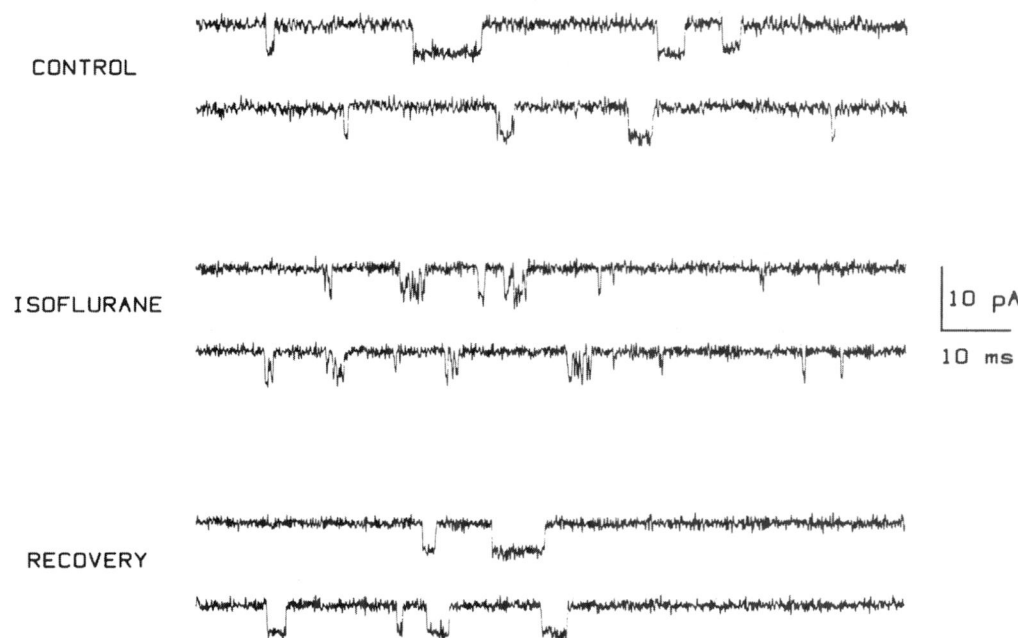

CONTROL

ISOFLURANE

10 pA

10 ms

RECOVERY

Figure 4–11 Examples of unitary acetylcholine receptor channel currents before, during, and after local microperfusion with 5 mM isoflurane. Channel openings are represented by downward directions of the current trace. When isoflurane is removed *(bottom panel)*, the channels are indistinguishable from those observed under control conditions. Notice that pre-equilibrated and 10-fold lower concentrations of isoflurane also decrease the average open duration of acetylcholine receptor channel currents.[113] (From Brett RS, Dilger JP, Yland KF: Isoflurane causes "flickering" of the acetylcholine receptor channel: Observations using the patch clamp. Anesthesiology 69:161, 1988.)

and neuronal inhibition.[115] Molluscan neurons that are highly sensitive to volatile agents (see Fig. 4-6) exhibit a halothane-induced activation of potassium current that is associated with a marked hyperpolarization of the cell membrane and an inability to initiate firing of action potentials.[34,35] However, the finding that anesthetic effects on resting membrane potential are voltage dependent and agent specific[116] indicates that changes in membrane potential are not a universal feature of anesthetic action on CNS neurons.

The requirement of an intact plasma membrane for the transmission of nervous impulses and the abilities of anesthetics to disrupt the flow of ions through plasma membranes point to a membrane site of anesthetic action. Nevertheless, anesthetics could act indirectly at a cytoplasmic site. For example, anesthetics may alter the calcium-accumulating activity of cellular organelles (e.g., mitochondria[76]) and thereby alter the levels of intracellular free calcium. Such alterations in intracellular free calcium could influence the conductance properties of excitable membranes and alter the presynaptic release of neurotransmitters.[76]

This discussion strongly suggests but does not prove that anesthesia results from an association of inhaled agents with the plasma membranes of nerves. If this is so, which components of the plasma membrane are altered by the anesthetics? Biologic membranes consist of a cholesterol-phospholipid bilayer matrix that is approximately 4 nm thick. Peripheral proteins are weakly bound to the exterior hydrophilic membrane, and integral proteins (e.g., ion channels) are deeply embedded in or pass through the lipid bilayer (Fig. 4-12). Synaptic plasma membranes are approximately one-half protein and one-half lipid by weight. If, as implied by the Meyer-Overton rule, inhaled agents bind to hydrophobic sites, anesthetics could act on the nonpolar interior of the lipid bilayer, at hydrophobic pockets in proteins extending outside or embedded into the lipid bilayer, or at the hydrophobic interface between intrinsic membrane proteins and the lipid matrix (see Fig. 4-12).

Attempts to better understand the penetration of inhaled agents into, and their interaction with, membrane sites have led to an examination of isolated membrane components. These experiments were greatly aided by the discovery that phospholipids dispersed in an aqueous medium spontaneously form bilayers comprising the surfaces of spherical structures (i.e., liposomes). These phospholipid bilayers act as a permeability barrier to ions and are similar to those found in biomembranes. In contrast, membrane proteins are often difficult to isolate and purify, and membrane proteins typically exhibit an impaired function unless surrounded by a boundary layer of lipid. Nevertheless, advances have resulted in the biochemical and electrophysiologic characterization of several protein receptor or ionophores thought to permit the passage (i.e., tunneling) of ions through membranes during excitation. However, only limited information is available concerning direct binding of inhaled agents with these membrane protein ionophores, and many experiments that examine anesthetic-protein interactions employ soluble proteins as model systems. Such proteins are easy to prepare in reasonable quantities but may not mimic precisely the natural proteins responsible for ion translocation.

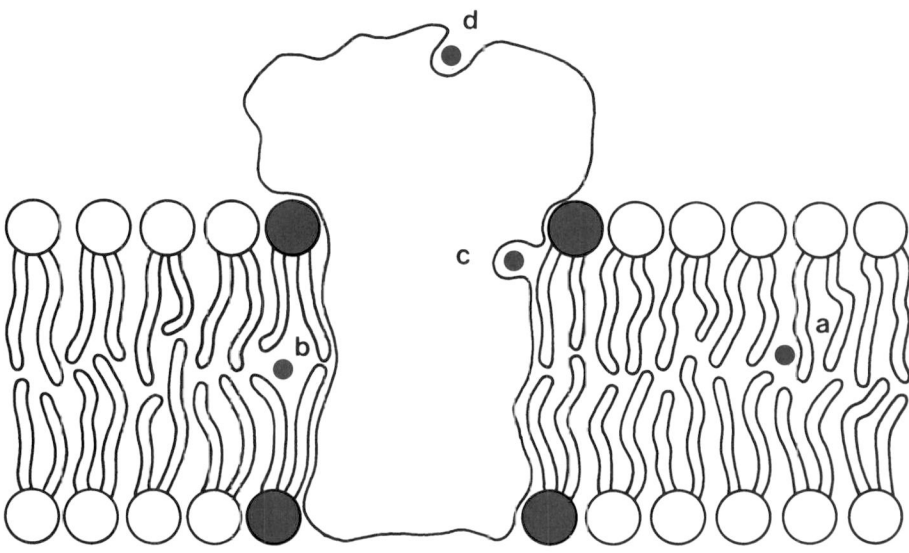

Figure 4–12 Four possible target sites for inhaled anesthetic molecules *(solid circles)* in a neuronal membrane include the lipid bilayer as a whole (a), lipids at a protein-lipid interface (b), a protein site bounded by lipid (c), and a protein site exposed to an aqueous environment (d). (Adapted from Franks NP, Lieb WR: What is the molecular nature of general anesthetic target sites? Trends Pharmacol Sci 8:169, 1987.)

INTERACTION OF INHALED ANESTHETICS WITH MEMBRANE LIPIDS

Binding of Anesthetics to Membrane Lipids

The solubilities of gaseous and volatile agents in membrane lipids tend to correlate with their anesthetic potencies. This correlation is as good[117] as or better[90] than that obtained when olive oil is the model solvent. The incorporation of cholesterol into phospholipid model membranes decreases the partitioning of inhaled agents but does not alter the good correlation between anesthetic potency and lipid membrane solubility.[117] The degree of saturation or length of lipid acyl chains has little effect on the partition coefficient. However, a decrease in temperature increases the partitioning of anesthetics into phospholipid membranes.[117] At anesthetic concentrations close to 1.0 MAC, lipid membranes contain as many as 80 phospholipid molecules for every anesthetic molecule.[89]

The interaction of inhaled agents with membrane lipids is a dynamic process, and anesthetic molecules may rapidly exchange between the membrane and aqueous phases. Although anesthetics may penetrate to all depths of the lipid bilayer, there is a preferential anesthetic distribution at the membrane interface[118,119] where regions of the lipid membrane contact the aqueous environment. In contrast, the nonimmobilizers 1,2-dichlorohexafluorocyclobutane and 2,3-dichlorooctafluorobutane (see Fig. 4-10) exhibit a preferential location in the lipid membrane hydrocarbon core.[118-120] It has been speculated that the interfacial site may be associated with anesthetic-induced immobility in response to noxious stimuli and that the production of amnesia may be associated with anesthetic penetration into the nonpolar interior of a phospholipid bilayer.[31]

Effects on Membrane Permeability

Inhaled anesthetics increase the flow of cations and protons across lipid vesicles.[121] It has been suggested that anesthetics may act by increasing proton permeability across synaptic vesicles, collapsing the pH gradient required for retention of catecholamines in their charged form and thereby depressing neurotransmission by releasing catecholamines from synaptic storage vesicles. However, this hypothesis seems unlikely because marked depletion of brain catecholamines lowers the MAC by a maximum of 40%, clinical concentrations of inhaled agents release only a small fraction of catecholamines trapped in vesicles, and not all anesthetics increase proton conduction across lipid vesicles.[121]

Alterations in Membrane Dimension

Lipid monolayers adsorb inhaled agents, resulting in an increase in the lateral pressure of the monolayer that parallels the potency of the anesthetic. This finding is consistent with the notion that anesthetics may expand membranes and exert pressure on the ionic channels needed for impulse transmission—a variation of the volume expansion theory of anesthesia—and thereby inhibit the opening or accelerate the closure of ionic channels. However, precise volume measurements show only a small (0.1%) expansion when suspensions of membranes in aqueous media are combined with inhaled agents at concentrations near 1.0 MAC.[122] Most studies indicate little or no effect of clinical concentrations of inhaled agents on membrane thickness.[117]

According to the critical volume hypothesis, an increase in pressure or a decrease in temperature should reverse anesthesia because these physical changes should compress membranes. However, a decrease in body temperature consistently decreases MAC (see Fig. 4-3). This apparent contradiction is partly resolved by the increased partitioning of anesthetics into membranes at lower temperatures. Moreover, the expansion of membranes by anesthetics and an increase in temperature may not be equivalent. For example, anesthetics may expand membranes without changing thickness.[117]

Alterations in Membrane Physical State

Further studies of the molecular changes occurring on the insertion of anesthetic molecules into lipid membranes led to the suggestion that anesthetics act by increasing the mobility of membrane components, a proposal called the *fluidization theory of anesthesia*. The ability of an anesthetic to fluidize a lipid bilayer depends on the agent examined, the composition of the lipid bilayer, and the membrane position at which fluidity is measured.[117] The incorporation of cholesterol[117] or gangliosides[123] into neutral phospholipid membranes enhances the membrane-disordering effects by a given partial pressure of inhaled anesthetic. Inhaled anesthetics can produce a small decrease in the fluidity of palmitoyl-oleoylphosphatidylcholine membranes near the head group region and increase fluidity in regions deep in the membrane bilayer.[119] The nonimmobilizers 1,2-dichloro-hexafluorocyclobutane and 2,3-dichlorooctafluorobutane (see Fig. 4-10) do not fluidize membrane lipids.[119,124]

It has been suggested that even small changes in lipid fluidity may profoundly change membrane function. Some investigators have speculated that the increased decay rate of postsynaptic currents and accelerated decay rate of open membrane channels (see Fig. 4-11) caused by inhaled agents may result from an increased fluidity of the postsynaptic membrane, allowing a more rapid relaxation (i.e., return to the closed configuration) of the proteins involved in the conductance change after activation. However, such theories are compromised by the fact that small increases in temperature increase membrane fluidity to approximately the same extent as clinical concentrations of inhaled anesthetics and therefore should, but do not, augment anesthesia.

Other theories of anesthetic action on lipids include anesthetic-induced alterations in membrane electrical properties or membrane pressures. Inhaled agents (at about 1 MAC) can alter dipole potentials at a lipid membrane interface by approximately 10 mV, and it has been suggested that such changes in membrane potential could modulate conformational transitions of membrane channel proteins.[125] Insertion of inhaled anesthetics into a lipid bilayer is predicted to redistribute lateral pressures in the membrane and promote a shift in the conformational equilibrium of ion channels.[126]

INTERACTION OF INHALED AGENTS WITH PROTEINS

Almost all investigators agree that the ultimate action of inhaled anesthetics is on specific neuronal membrane proteins that permit the translocation of ions during membrane excitation. Most believe this occurs by a direct binding of anesthetics to membrane channels, although definitive evidence for direct binding at the atomic level is not yet available. Because of the complexity involved in searching for specific anesthetic binding sites in proteins of whole brain or brain homogenate, attempts have been made to simplify this search by examining the interaction of anesthetics with isolated proteins.

Soluble Proteins

Using x-ray crystallography, distinct anesthetic binding sites have been identified in several soluble proteins, including hemoglobin, myoglobin, and albumin.[88,127,128] Three high-affinity halothane binding sites have been identified on human serum albumin.[129] These discrete binding sites for halothane are preformed amphiphilic pockets on the protein that are capable of binding the natural fatty acid ligands, and the binding of halothane to albumin causes little or no change in structure.[129]

The interaction of inhaled anesthetics with soluble enzymes may be reflected indirectly by changes in enzyme activity. Many enzymes, including several glycolytic enzymes and serum cholinesterase, are resistant to even saturated solutions of volatile agents. However, other soluble enzymes are highly sensitive to clinical anesthetic concentrations. The purified firefly luciferase enzyme combines with its substrate luciferin to produce a photon of light, and a variety of inhaled anesthetics (at about 1.0 MAC) inhibit the activity (i.e., light intensity) of this enzyme by competing with luciferin.[130] However, because luciferin has no anesthetic properties, luciferase is unlikely to represent a good model of the site of anesthetic action.[131]

Membrane Proteins

Two major obstacles are encountered when attempting to study the influence of inhaled anesthetics on the purified protein ionophores involved in the membrane translocation of ions. First, the biochemical purification of such protein ionophores in adequate quantities is a difficult and time-consuming process. Second, even when these membrane proteins can be isolated, they need to be reincorporated into lipids for measurement of their functional ability to translocate ions. This reincorporation of the purified ionophore into a lipid membrane makes it difficult to distinguish whether an anesthetic affects ion flow through a direct action on the membrane protein or through an indirect action on surrounding lipids.

Ligand-Gated Ion Channels

The binding of neurotransmitter alters membrane permeability of ligand-operated channels to specific ions. The muscle-type nicotinic acetylcholine receptor–ionophore complex is the only channel complex that has been isolated in large enough quantities to be studied at the biochemical level with anesthetics.[128] This protein complex is composed of five polypeptide subunits, with each subunit containing four hydrophobic amino acid domains spanning the membrane; the subunits form the wall of the membrane channel. Each subunit of the acetylcholine receptor binds halothane, as measured by a radioligand-binding assay after photoactivation of radioactive halothane.[132] Volatile halogenated anesthetics stabilize the acetylcholine receptor in a conformational form that binds agonists with high affinity and is associated with a desensitized and therefore inactive (closed-channel) state.[133] However, not all anesthetics produce this effect. The nonhalogenated alkane anesthetics cyclopropane and butane do not potentiate agonist actions on the acetylcholine receptor and do not enhance the affinity of agonist to the receptor.[134]

Additional information concerning anesthetic action on the nicotinic acetylcholine receptor ionophore may be made by examining ion flow through channels of defined subunit composition incorporated (through cDNA or mRNA injection) into cellular systems.[50,135] Such studies have revealed a markedly enhanced sensitivity of neuronal (compared with muscular) nicotinic acetylcholine receptors to inhaled anesthetics (Fig. 4-13).[136,137] Because neuronal nicotinic acetylcholine receptors can be inhibited at inhaled anesthetic concentrations as low as 0.1 MAC (see Fig. 4-13), these receptors may play some role in the behavioral and physiologic effects observed at subanesthetic concentrations.[36,136] The ability of specific amino acid mutations between the second and third transmembrane segment of the α-subunit of the neuronal acetylcholine receptor to markedly influence halothane sensitivity suggests that this region of the acetylcholine receptor is important for the transduction of anesthetic binding to channel inhibition.[137]

Other ligand-gated ion channels, including the inhibitory GABA$_A$ and glycine channels (Fig. 4-14A), share a basic structure with the acetylcholine receptor ionophore that consists of five subunits (see Fig. 4-14C), with each subunit containing four transmembrane segments (see Fig. 4-14D).[50,128,135] Interactions of anesthetics with particular subunits of these ligand-gated ion channels can be studied by molecular cloning and expression in cells that do not endogenously contain these receptors.[50,128,135] The dependence of GABA$_A$ receptor subunit composition on the ability of inhaled anesthetics to alter ligand binding[138] or potentiate (see Fig. 4-14B) GABA-activated chloride currents[124,139] implies specific GABA$_A$ subunit binding sites for anesthetics. Selective mutations in the second or third transmembrane domains (see Fig. 4-14D) of GABA$_A$ or glycine subunits removes the ability of anesthetics to potentiate agonist responses at GABA$_A$ and glycine receptors.[140] By using mutagenesis to introduce bulky amino acid substitutions at critical transmembrane sites that control anesthetic sensitivity, it has been estimated that the volume of the anesthetic binding site on the α-subunit of the GABA$_A$ receptor is between 250 and 370 cubic Å.[141]

Inhaled anesthetics have an agent-specific effect on 5-HT$_3$ serotonin receptor function and may potentiate or inhibit 5-HT currents.[142] Inhaled anesthetics produce subunit-selective actions on excitatory glutamate receptors, with GluR3 (AMPA subtype) receptors being inhibited or unaffected by anesthetics, whereas GluR6 (kainate subtype) receptor function is enhanced by volatile agents.[143] Mutations of a specific amino acid located in a transmembrane segment of the GluR6 receptor removes the ability of halothane, isoflurane, and enflurane to enhance GluR6 receptor function.[143]

Gaseous anesthetics may have selective actions on excitatory versus inhibitory receptors compared with volatile anesthetics. Many studies indicate that nitrous oxide and xenon inhibit excitatory N-methyl-D-aspartate (NMDA) glutamate transmission while having little or no effect on GABAergic inhibition,[48,144,145] with volatile anesthetics tending to exert their greatest effects on GABAergic transmission. Moreover, the gaseous anesthetics cyclopropane and butane (at concentrations sufficient to induce anesthesia) fail to potentiate GABAergic transmission.[134] These findings imply different mechanisms of action for gaseous and volatile anesthetics.

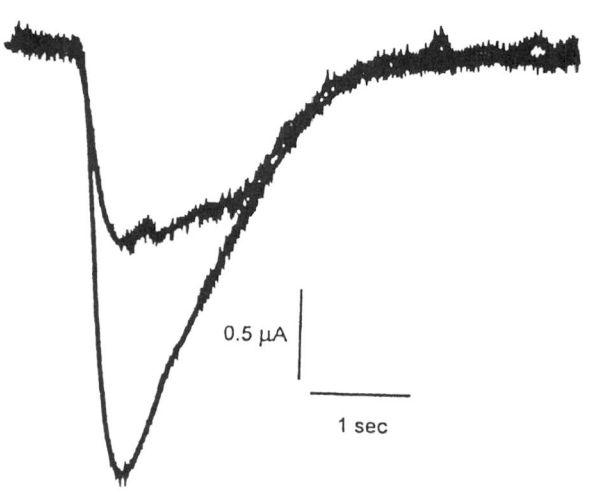
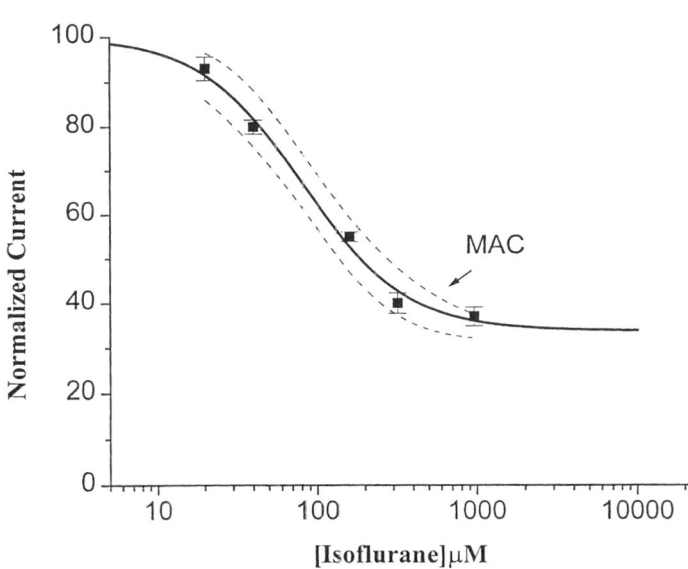

Figure 4–13 The figure on the left shows the current from an oocyte that expresses the predominant nicotinic acetylcholine receptor subtype (α4β2) found in the central nervous system. Isoflurane (320 μM) reduces the peak current obtained in response to 1 μM acetylcholine from 2.4 μA to 1.1 μA (46% of control). The graph on the right shows the dose-response curve of the inhibition of α4β2 receptor subtype current by isoflurane. Notice that some inhibition of receptor function occurs even at an isoflurane concentration of about 0.1 minimum alveolar concentration (MAC). (Adapted from Flood P, Ramirez-Latorre J, Role L: α4β2 Neuronal nicotinic acetylcholine receptors in the central nervous system are inhibited by isoflurane and propofol, but α7-type nicotinic acetylcholine receptors are unaffected. Anesthesiology 86:859, 1997.)

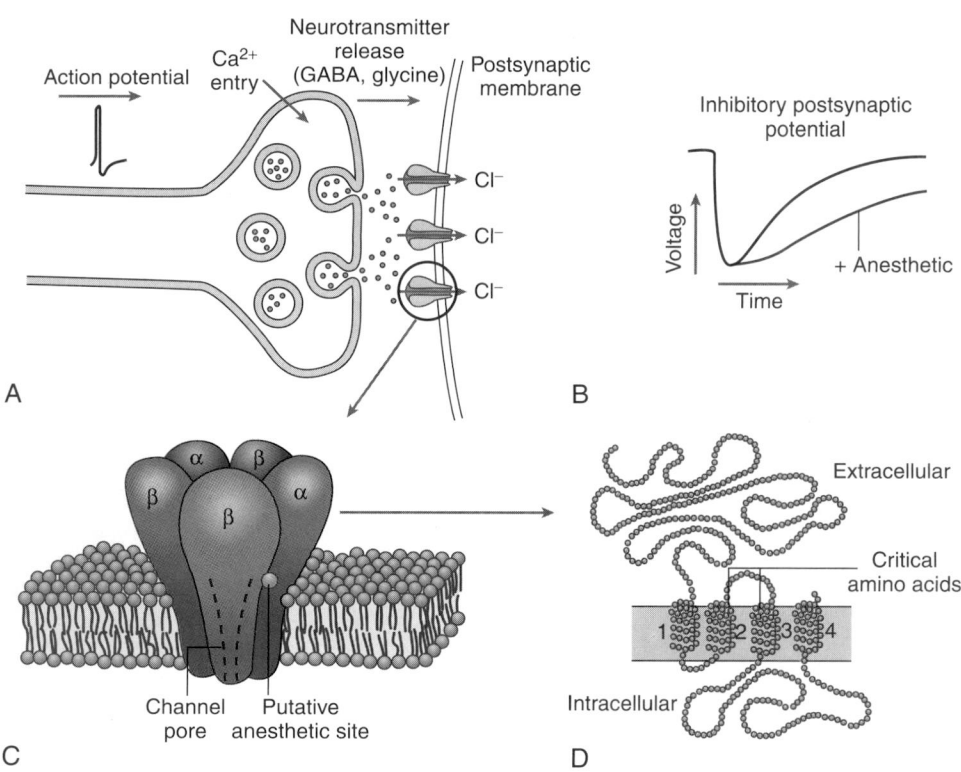

Figure 4–14 A, The neurotransmitters γ-aminobutyric acid (GABA) and glycine are released at inhibitory synapses, bind to their respective receptors, and result in a flow of chloride ions across the postsynaptic membrane. **B,** Inhaled anesthetics potentiate the postsynaptic inhibition produced by GABA or glycine. **C,** Inhibitory receptor-channel complexes, as well as many other ligand-gated channels, typically consist of five subunits embedded in a membrane lipid bilayer. Many subunit combinations may exist for a given receptor-channel complex. **D,** Each of the subunits contains four transmembrane segments, and the second transmembrane segment of each subunit is thought to line a pore (i.e., channel) that extends across the membrane. Anesthetic sensitivity can be altered by mutation of critical amino acids in these transmembrane regions. (Adapted from Franks NP, Lieb WR: Anaesthetics set their sites on ion channels. Nature 389:334, 1997.)

The nonimmobilizers 1,2-dichlorohexafluorocyclobutane and 2,3-dichlorooctafluorobutane (see Fig. 4-10) have little or no effect on GABA, glycine, 5-HT$_3$, and glutamate receptor function.[50,143] However, these nonimmobilizing agents are highly effective in blocking currents through neuronal nicotinic acetylcholine receptors,[146] consistent with the concept that anesthetic action on nicotinic acetylcholine receptors may be important for anesthetic-induced behavioral changes (e.g., amnesia) but not important for preventing response to surgical stimulation.[36,105,136,146]

Voltage-Gated Ion Channels

The flux of ions through voltage-gated ion channels is controlled by the electric field across the membrane. These channels share structural similarities and include sodium and potassium channels involved in the propagation of neuronal action potentials and calcium channels that control neuronal excitability and entry of calcium through presynaptic membranes and eventual neurotransmitter release. Although voltage-gated ion channels are often found to be insensitive to even high anesthetic concentrations,[2,147] it is recognized that pharmacologic effects on a particular channel may vary from tissue to tissue or among channel subtypes. Nitrous oxide inhibits selective (T-type) voltage-gated calcium currents in small sensory neurons at subanesthetic concentrations[148]; volatile anesthetics (but not the nonimmobilizer 1,2-dichlorohexafluorocyclobutane [see Fig. 4-10]) inhibit dorsal root ganglion sodium channels[110]; and clinical concentrations of volatile anesthetics partially inhibit voltage-dependent potassium currents in human potassium channels expressed in a cell line.[111]

Background Potassium Channels

The inhibition of electrical activity by volatile anesthetics in molluscan neurons (see Fig. 4-6) is associated with activation of background (not voltage-gated) potassium channels and membrane hyperpolarization.[34,35] Anesthetic-sensitive background potassium channels are also found in mammals and contain four transmembrane segments with two pore-forming domains.[115] The ability of an inhaled anesthetic to open background potassium channels depends on the subtype of channel examined and is agent specific.[115] Currents through a human potassium channel that is prominent in spinal cord are potentiated by halothane, isoflurane, desflurane, and enflurane, whereas the nonimmobilizer 1,2-dichlorohexafluorocyclobutane (see Fig. 4-10) caused slight inhibition.[149]

Metabotropic Receptors and G Proteins

In contrast to the ionotropic multiple-subunit ligand-gated ion channels where membrane ion permeabilities change within a few milliseconds of agonist binding, metabotropic receptors consist of a single subunit, are coupled to G proteins, and evoke changes in neuronal excitability over hundreds of milliseconds. The ability of halothane but not isoflurane to inhibit muscarinic signaling activated by acetylcholine indicates a variable effect of anesthetics and suggests that muscarinic inhibition may be more relevant to side effects of anesthetics than to anesthetic action per se.[150] The 5-HT type 2A receptor and the metabotropic glutamate receptor mGluR5 are coupled to G proteins and are inhibited by inhaled anesthetics and the nonimmobilizer 1,2-dichlorohexafluorocyclobutane (see Fig. 4-10), implying that these metabotropic receptors are not important for the immobility component of anesthesia but may be associated with anesthetic-induced behavioral changes.[151,152]

G proteins are potential membrane sites where anesthetics exert their functional effects. They are guanine nucleotide–binding neuronal membrane proteins that couple many neurotransmitter receptors to ion channels in the brain. The binding of a neurotransmitter to its receptor can influence the activation state of a G protein, which can control the opening or closing of an ion channel. Although evidence for an anesthetic target site on G proteins is supported by the abilities of volatile anesthetics to reduce the exchange of guanine nucleotides and to promote the interaction of G protein α and $\beta\gamma$ subunits,[153] the use of halothane photoaffinity labeling failed to demonstrate direct anesthetic binding sites on G protein subunits.[154] Alternatively, anesthetic inhibition of metabotropic receptor function may result from a direct action on the coupled ion channel.[147]

Protein Kinase C

Protein kinase C is an enzyme involved in the phosphorylation of proteins and may modulate neurotransmission through effects on transmitter release and conductance of ions through membrane channels.[153] Protein kinase C exists in several isoforms, and anesthetic effects on this enzyme are complicated, with enzyme activity depending on the isoform and tissue examined, the presence of endogenous enzyme activators, and the particular anesthetic and its duration of treatment.[155] The inhibitory actions of inhaled anesthetics on 5-HT type 2A receptors,[151] metabotropic glutamate mGluR5 receptors,[152] substance P receptors,[156] and selected sodium channels[157] are thought to depend on activation of protein kinase C.

ANIMAL MODELS: ATTEMPTS TO RELATE SUSTAINED ALTERATIONS IN ANESTHETIC POTENCY WITH NEUROCHEMICAL COMPOSITION

One approach to the mechanism of anesthetic action is to relate alterations in the anesthetic requirement with biochemical and biophysical changes occurring in the CNS. A correlation between changes in the anesthetic requirement and a structural change in the nervous system may indicate the critical properties of the anesthetic site of action and how anesthetics affect that site.

Dietary Studies

Mice fed diets of different fatty acid composition (saturated versus unsaturated) from birth have large alterations in certain synaptic membrane fatty acid components.[158] The most notable changes occur in the synaptic membrane phosphatidylethanolamine and phosphatidylserine fractions in mice fed the saturated-fat diet; these mice exhibit a relative decrease in docosahexaenoic (22:6ω3) and an increase in eicosatrienoic (20:3ω9) fatty acids. However, these alterations in synaptic membrane fatty acid composition have little or no influence on the righting-reflex ED_{50} for nitrous oxide and isoflurane.[158] In contrast, diet-induced alterations in rat brain fatty acid composition have been correlated with modest alterations in anesthetic potency.[159] Compared with rats on a control diet, rats maintained on a fat-free diet exhibit lower levels of whole-brain arachidonic acid (20:4ω6) and docosahexaenoic acid and an increase in eicosatrienoic acid. The fat-deprived animals exhibited a 10% to 33% decrease in MAC for methoxyflurane, halothane, isoflurane, and cyclopropane compared with control rats.[159]

Tolerance Studies

The inhaled anesthetic requirement can be increased by chronic exposure of mice to subanesthetic levels of nitrous oxide.[160] The maximal increase in the nitrous oxide righting-reflex ED_{50} for mice placed under 40% to 70% nitrous oxide is approximately 0.25 atm and occurs after 2 weeks of continuous exposure.[160,161] No significant differences in membrane order or in the composition of purified synaptic membrane fatty acid, phospholipid, or cholesterol occur in mice tolerant to nitrous oxide.[160,161] Prolonged exposure of rats to nitrous oxide decreases brainstem opiate receptor density by approximately 20% and may in part account for the tolerance to the analgesic action of nitrous oxide.[162]

In humans, an acute tolerance to the analgesic effect of nitrous oxide is seen in some patients within 10 to 60 minutes of administration.[163] A rapidly developing tolerance to gaseous agents is also seen in rodents.[164,165] The mechanistic bases of this acute tolerance remain to be determined.

Genetic Studies

Genetic approaches to anesthetic mechanisms involve the alternatives of forward versus reverse genetics.[166] In forward genetics, untargeted mutations are randomly generated and are chosen for study because they produce lines of animals that are markedly sensitive or resistant to anesthetics. In reverse genetics, the focus is on a particular gene that is thought to be important in the production of anesthesia, with mutations in a cloned copy of the gene resulting in organisms that can be tested for altered anesthetic sensitivities. Most genetic studies have involved three different types of organisms: nematodes (*Caenorhabditis elegans*), fruit flies (*Drosophila*), and rodents. Nematodes and fruit flies are advantageous in genetic studies because of their well-mapped genomes, defined nervous systems, short life cycles, and relatively low cost. However, the behavioral assays used to assess anesthetic potencies in these simpler organisms may be difficult to relate to the anesthetic-induced immobility and amnesia in patients during surgical anesthesia.

Caenorhabditis elegans

The potencies of inhaled anesthetics in wild-type *C. elegans* parallel those found in higher animals.[167] Although certain behavioral end points (e.g., mating, chemotaxis, coordinated movement) are disrupted at clinical anesthetic concentrations, anesthetic-induced immobility of nematodes requires anesthetic concentrations of about 5 to 10 MAC in humans.[167] Mutants of *C. elegans* have been developed that are hypersensitive to clinical anesthetics, with the genes involved encoding a homolog of the human protein stomatin (i.e., controlling sodium and potassium flux across membranes) or encoding a subunit of the electron transport chain.[167] Other mutations in *C. elegans* in genes that encode presynaptic proteins that regulate transmitter release produce resistance to inhaled anesthetics.[168] The similar properties of nonimmobilizing agents (see Fig. 4-10) in *C. elegans* and mammals support the use of *C. elegans* as a model for the study of anesthetic action.[169]

Drosophila

Potencies of inhaled anesthetics in wild-type *Drosophila* (measured by response to mechanical or heat stimuli or disruption of coordinated movement) approximate those required for surgical anesthesia. Mutants have been obtained that are resistant and sensitive to various anesthetics,[170,171] with anesthetic sensitivity depending on the agent examined and the end point measured.[171] Mutations that affect ion channels change the sensitivity of *Drosophila* to volatile anesthetics in a manner suggesting an agent-specific action through different neuronal pathways. For example, genetic inactivation of one class of potassium channel decreases the potency of halothane in a brain circuit of *Drosophila*.[172]

Rodents

A naturally occurring variability in anesthetic potency exists among strains of mice and rats. The antinociceptive effect of nitrous oxide and the development of tolerance vary markedly among different strains of rats.[165] Anesthetic potencies (i.e., MACs) of a given anesthetic (i.e., desflurane, isoflurane, or halothane) measured in 15 mouse strains differed by 39% to 55%.[173] Such findings imply that multiple genes underlie the observed variability in anesthetic potency[173] but do not identify the genetic or biochemical differences between strains that are responsible for the differences in anesthetic requirement.

With selective breeding, use is made of the fact that the anesthetic requirement varies slightly among animals of a given species and that members resistant or vulnerable to anesthesia may be found in a normal population. Mice have been selected from a normal population with consistently high and consistently low nitrous oxide righting-reflex ED_{50}.[174] Repeating the process of selection, breeding, and testing for the nitrous oxide requirement through 15 generations produced two lines of mice with requirements separated by as much as 1 atm (Fig. 4-15).[8,174] Mice resistant to nitrous oxide also have a higher requirement for other inhaled anesthetics, but the separation in righting-reflex ED_{50} values between the two lines is inversely related to the lipid solubility of the anesthetic.[8] The differences in nitrous oxide requirement between these lines of mice could not be explained by an alteration in synaptic membrane fatty acid, phospholipid, or cholesterol composition[174] but is associated with a higher brain norepinephrine content in resistant compared with susceptible mice.[175]

An alternative genetic approach is to knock out a gene in embryonic stem cells thought to be important for the

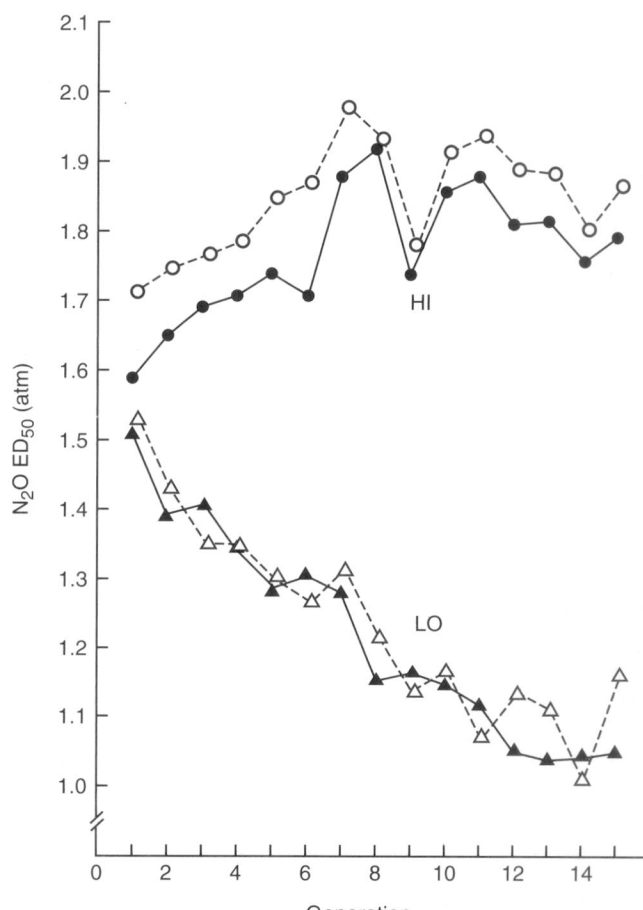

Figure 4–15 The nitrous oxide righting-reflex 50% effective dose (ED_{50}) values for male (*closed symbols*) and female (*open symbols*) offspring of mice selectively bred for resistance (HI group, *circles*) or susceptibility (LO group, *triangles*) to nitrous oxide anesthesia. The nitrous oxide requirements for HI and LO mice became progressively more separated over 15 generations of selective breeding. Standard errors about most points are less than 0.03 atm. Values for generations 1 through 10 are taken from references 8 and 174.

anesthetic state and examine anesthetic sensitivity in mice that lack functional genes. Targeted disruption of the neuronal nitric oxide synthase gene has no influence on isoflurane MAC or isoflurane righting-reflex ED_{50} in knock-out compared with wild-type mice.[84] Unlike wild-type mice, acute administration of nitric oxide synthase inhibitors does not decrease anesthetic requirement in these knock-out mice, suggesting that other non–nitric oxide mechanisms exist in the knock-out mice to compensate for the mutation.[84] Mice lacking the neuronal isoform of the protein kinase C gene demonstrate a small increased resistance to isoflurane but not to halothane or desflurane.[176] The sevoflurane requirement (i.e., MAC) is 20% lower in mice that lack the μ-opioid receptor compared with wild-type control mice.[177] Knock-out mice devoid of functional α_{2A}-adrenoreceptors exhibit reduced isoflurane antinociception, indicating that this receptor subtype at least partially mediates isoflurane antinociception.[61] Mice lacking a particular glutamate receptor subunit (i.e., GluR2) have a decreased requirement for volatile anesthetics to produce loss of the righting reflex, whereas MAC values are unaltered in these animals.[178] Mice with glycine receptor subunit mutations may be more sensitive or resistant to volatile anesthetics, depending on the anesthesia end point and anesthetic examined.[179] Gene knock-out of the α_6-subunit of the GABA receptor does not alter MAC or righting-reflex ED_{50} for enflurane or halothane, implying that this particular subunit of the GABA receptor is not important in the behavioral responses to volatile anesthetics.[180] Mice that lack the β_3-subunit of the $GABA_A$ receptor demonstrate higher MAC values for enflurane and halothane but no change in righting-reflex ED_{50} for these anesthetics.[181] The similar enflurane sensitivity in spinal cords isolated from mice lacking the β_3-subunit of the $GABA_A$ receptor compared with wild-type controls and the decreased role of $GABA_A$ receptors in mediating the actions of enflurane in the mutant mice[182] point out a limitation in the use of knock-out mice. Results from knock-out mice can be difficult to interpret, because mice may adapt to the absence of a gene product by altering the amounts of other receptors or neuroregulators that influence anesthetic requirement. Future genetic approaches to the study of anesthetic mechanisms will involve the use of conditional gene knock-outs selective to specific brain regions or developmental stages and a knock-in technique to introduce a mutation into a specific receptor subunit that alters anesthetic requirement without altering other physiologic functions.

SUMMARY

We remain uncertain about the site of anesthetic action at the macroscopic, microscopic, and molecular levels (Table 4-3). We do know that inhaled anesthetics disrupt neuronal transmission in many areas of the CNS.

They may enhance or depress excitatory or inhibitory transmission through axons or synaptic regions. Presynaptic and postsynaptic effects have been found. Regardless of the macroscopic site of action, the ultimate action of inhaled agents is on neuronal membranes. Although a direct neuronal plasma membrane interaction seems likely, the possibility remains that inhaled anesthetics act indirectly by production of a second messenger. The correlation between lipid solubility and anesthetic potency suggests that anesthetics have a hydrophobic or amphipathic site of action. The discovery of nonimmobilizers, lipid-soluble compounds that do not alter the MAC, implies the site of action is different for different anesthetic end points. Anesthetics bind to and perturb membrane lipids and proteins, but it is uncertain which of these components is most important and how such perturbations may lead to the anesthetic state. Future advances in anesthetic mechanisms will go hand in hand with the development of molecular biology techniques used to clone and characterize excitable membrane channels and biophysical and biochemical advances used to study neuronal interactions. The development of animal models with sustained alterations in anesthetic potency will allow testing of the hypotheses that specific molecular changes in selected regions of the CNS are important in the production of anesthesia.

KEY POINTS

1. The structural diversity of inhaled anesthetics suggests that they all do not interact directly with a single, specific receptor site.
2. Any molecular hypothesis of anesthesia must explain the effects of anesthetics on the whole organism. Physical or biochemical changes important to the

Table 4-3	Possible sites of anesthetic action	
Anatomic Level	**Site of Action**	**Comments**
Macroscopic	Central nervous system (CNS)	
	Brain vs. spinal cord	Anesthetics disrupt transmission throughout the CNS; decerebration does not alter the minimum alveolar concentration (MAC).
Microscopic	Axons vs. synapses	Higher concentrations of inhaled anesthetic are typically required to disrupt axonal than synaptic transmission.
	Excitatory vs. inhibitory synapses	Anesthetics may block excitatory and enhance inhibitory transmission.
Molecular	Presynaptic vs. postsynaptic membrane	Anesthetics may alter release of presynaptic neurotransmitter (perhaps through changes in intracellular Ca^{2+}) and modify flow of ions through postsynaptic channels.
		Meyer-Overton rule implies a hydrophobic site of molecular membrane action. Critical volume hypothesis purports anesthetic action through membrane expansion.
		Possible importance of membrane-aqueous interface.
	Lipid vs. protein	Lipid fluidization theories cannot account for the production of the anesthetic state. Evidence is accumulating for direct binding of anesthetics to excitable membrane proteins.

mechanism of anesthesia must occur within seconds of anesthetic administration and be rapidly reversible on removal of the anesthetic.

3. Potencies of inhaled anesthetics depend on the end point measured. The best-characterized measurement of anesthetic potency is MAC, the minimum alveolar concentration of an agent that produces immobility in 50% of subjects exposed to a noxious stimulus.

4. Inhaled anesthetics have presynaptic and postsynaptic effects in the brain and spinal cord. The ability of anesthetics to prevent a motor response to noxious stimulation results from a site of action in the spinal cord.

5. Many excitatory and inhibitory neurotransmitters and their receptors have an influence on the anesthetic requirement. However, the predominant effects of inhaled anesthetics cannot be explained by the depletion, production, or release of a single neuromodulator in the CNS.

6. The Meyer-Overton rule describes the correlation between lipid solubility and anesthetic potency. Because of this correlation, the search for the molecular bases of anesthetic action has often focused on cellular hydrophobic regions.

7. Clinical concentrations of inhaled anesthetics (i.e., about one anesthetic molecule for every 80 membrane phospholipid molecules) produce only modest changes in membrane lipid structure and function.

8. The Meyer-Overton rule is imperfect, and many exceptions exist. Nonimmobilizers are lipid soluble compounds that fail to produce immobility in response to a noxious stimulus but do impair learning and memory.

9. The ultimate action of inhaled anesthetics is on specific neuronal membrane proteins that permit the translocation of ions during membrane excitation. Although this probably occurs by a direct binding of anesthetics to membrane protein channels or their surrounding lipids, or both, the possibility remains that inhaled anesthetics act indirectly through production of a second messenger.

10. The ability of inhaled anesthetics to modulate ion flow through neurotransmitter receptor-channel complexes can be markedly altered by selective single amino acid mutations in protein channels. These critical amino acids may form the specific binding sites for inhaled anesthetics.

REFERENCES

1. Lynch C, Baum J, Tenbrinck R: Xenon anesthesia. Anesthesiology 92:865, 2000.
2. Franks NP, Lieb WR: Molecular and cellular mechanisms of general anaesthesia. Nature 367:607, 1994.
3. Petersen-Felix S, Zbinden AM, Fischer M, et al: Isoflurane minimum alveolar concentration decreases during anesthesia and surgery. Anesthesiology 79:959, 1993.
4. Firestone LL, Korpi ER, Niemi L, et al: Halothane and desflurane requirements in alcohol-tolerant and -nontolerant rats. Br J Anaesth 85:757, 2000.
5. Quasha AL, Eger EI II, Tinker JH: Determination and applications of MAC. Anesthesiology 53:315, 1980.
6. Travis CC, Bowers JC: Interspecies scaling of anesthetic potency. Toxicol Ind Health 7:249, 1991.
7. Deady JE, Koblin DD, Eger EI II, et al: Anesthetic potencies and the unitary theory of narcosis. Anesth Analg 60:380, 1981.
8. Koblin DD, Deady JE, Eger EI II: Potencies of inhaled anesthetics and alcohol in mice selectively bred for resistance and susceptibility to nitrous oxide anesthesia. Anesthesiology 56:18, 1982.
9. Kissin I, Morgan PL, Smith LR: Anesthetic potencies of isoflurane, halothane, and diethyl ether for various end points of anesthesia. Anesthesiology 58:88, 1983.
10. Dutton RC, Maurer AJ, Sonner JM, et al: The concentration of isoflurane required to suppress learning depends on the type of learning. Anesthesiology 94:514, 2001.
11. Kissin I: A concept for assessing interactions of general anesthetics. Anesth Analg 85:204, 1997.
12. Franks NP, Lieb WR: Temperature dependence of the potency of volatile general anesthetics. Anesthesiology 84:716, 1996.
13. Koblin DD, Fang Z, Eger EI II, et al: Minimum alveolar concentrations of noble gases, nitrogen, and sulfur hexafluoride in rats: Helium and neon as nonimmobilizers (nonanesthetics). Anesth Analg 87:419, 1998.
14. Smith RA, Dodson BA, Miller KW: The interactions between pressure and anaesthetics. Philos Trans R Soc Lond B 304:69, 1984.
15. Eger EI II: Age, minimum alveolar concentration, and minimum alveolar concentration-awake. Anesth Analg 93:947, 2001.
16. Tanifuji Y, Nezu T, Kobayashi K, et al: Effect of brain calcium and magnesium on anesthetic requirement (MAC) in dogs. Jpn J Anesthesiol 29:741, 1980.
17. Thompson SW, Moscicki JC, DiFazio CA: The anesthetic contribution of magnesium sulfate and ritodrine hydrochloride in rats. Anesth Analg 67:31, 1988.
18. Angel A: Central neuronal pathways and the process of anaesthesia. Br J Anaesth 71:148, 1993.
19. Vahle-Hinz C, Detsch O: What can in vivo electrophysiology in animal models tell us about mechanisms of anaesthesia? Br J Anaesth 89:123, 2002.
20. MacIver MB, Roth SH: Inhalation anaesthetics exhibit pathway-specific and differential actions on hippocampal synaptic responses in vitro. Br J Anaesth 60:680, 1988.
21. Banks MI, Pearce RA: Dual actions of volatile anesthetics on GABA_A IPSCs. Dissociation of blocking and prolonging effects. Anesthesiology 90:120, 1999.
22. Nishikawa K, MacIver MB: Agent-selective effects of volatile anesthetics on GABA_A receptor-mediated synaptic inhibition in hippocampal interneurons. Anesthesiology 94:340, 2001.
23. Ries CR, Puil E: Mechanism of anesthesia revealed by shunting actions of isoflurane on thalamocortical neurons. J Neurophysiol 81:1795, 1999.
24. Kendig JJ: In vitro networks: Subcortical mechanisms of anesthetic action. Br J Anaesth 89:91, 2002.
25. Pereon Y, Beernard JC, Tich SNT, et al: The effects of desflurane on the nervous system: From spinal cord to muscles. Anesth Analg 89:490, 1999.
26. Borges M, Antognini JF: Does the brain influence somatic responses to noxious stimuli during isoflurane anesthesia? Anesthesiology 81:1511, 1994.
27. Antognini JF, Carstens E, Sudo M, et al: Isoflurane depresses electroencephalographic and medial thalamic responses to noxious stimulation via an indirect spinal action. Anesth Analg 91:1282, 2000.
28. Rampil IJ, Mason P, Singh H: Anesthetic potency (MAC) is independent of forebrain structures in the rat. Anesthesiology 78:707, 1993.
29. Rampil IJ, Mason P, Singh H: Anesthetic potency is not altered after hypothermic spinal cord transection in rats. Anesthesiology 80:606, 1994.

30. Antognini JF, Schwartz K: Exaggerated anesthetic requirements in the preferentially anesthetized brain. Anesthesiology 79:1244, 1993.
31. Eger EI II, Koblin DD, Harris RA, et al: Hypothesis: Inhaled anesthetics produce immobility and amnesia by different mechanisms at different sites. Anesth Analg 84:915, 1997.
32. MacIver MB, Tanelian DL: Volatile anesthetics excite mammalian nociceptor afferents recorded in vitro. Anesthesiology 72:1022, 1990.
33. Antognini JF, Kien ND: Potency (minimum alveolar anesthetic concentration) of isoflurane is independent of peripheral anesthetic effects. Anesth Analg 81:69, 1995.
34. Franks NP, Lieb WR: Volatile general anaesthetics activate a novel neuronal K+ current. Nature 333:662, 1988.
35. Winegar BD, Owen DF, Yost CS, et al: Volatile general anesthetics produce hyperpolarization of Aplysia neurons by activation of a discrete population of baseline potassium channels. Anesthesiology 85:889, 1996.
36. Evers AS, Steinbach JH: Supersensitive sites in the central nervous system: Anesthetics block brain nicotinic receptors. Anesthesiology 86:760, 1997.
37. Richards CD: Anaesthetic modulation of synaptic transmission in the mammalian CNS. Br J Anaesth 89:79, 2002.
38. Berg-Johnsen J, Langmoen IA: The effect of isoflurane on unmyelinated and myelinated fibers in the rat brain. Acta Physiol Scand 127:87, 1986.
39. Strichartz G: Use-dependent conduction block produced by volatile anesthetic agents. Acta Anaesthesiol Scand 24:402, 1980.
40. Perouansky M, Baranov D, Salman M, et al: Effects of halothane on glutamate receptor-mediated excitatory postsynaptic currents. Anesthesiology 83:109, 1995.
41. Griffiths R, Norman RI: Effects of anaesthetics on uptake, synthesis and release of transmitters. Br J Anaesth 71:96, 1993.
42. Bazil CW, Minneman KP: Clinical concentrations of volatile anesthetics reduce depolarization-evoked release of [3H]norepinephrine, but not [3H]acetylcholine, from rat cerebral cortex. J Neurochem 53:962, 1989.
43. Keita H, Henzel-Rouelle D, Dupont H, et al: Halothane and isoflurane increase spontaneous but reduce the N-methyl-D-aspartate-evoked dopamine release in rat striatal slices: Evidence for direct presynaptic effects. Anesthesiology 91:1788, 1999.
44. Salord F, Keita H, Lecharny JB, et al: Halothane and isoflurane differentially affect the regulation of dopamine and gamma-aminobutyric acid release mediated by presynaptic acetylcholine receptors in the rat striatum. Anesthesiology 86:632, 1997.
45. Lingamaneni R, Birch ML, Hemmings HC: Widespread inhibition of sodium channel-dependent glutamate release from isolated nerve terminals by isoflurane and propofol. Anesthesiology 95:1460, 2001.
46. Vinje ML, Moe MC, Valo ET, et al: The effect of sevoflurane on glutamate release and uptake in rat cerebrocortical presynaptic terminals. Acta Anaesthesiol Scand 46:103, 2002.
47. Puil E, El-Beheiry H: Anaesthetic suppression of transmitter actions in neocortex. Br J Pharmacol 101:61, 1990.
48. de Sousa SLM, Dickinson, Lieb WR, Franks NP: Contrasting synaptic actions of the inhalational general anesthetics isoflurane and xenon. Anesthesiology 92:105, 2000.
49. Wakamori M, Ikemoto Y, Akaike N: Effects of two volatile anesthetics on the excitatory and inhibitory amino acid responses in dissociated CNS neurons of the rat. J Neurophysiol 66:2014, 1991.
50. Yamakura T, Bertaccini E, Trudell JR, Harris RA: Anesthetics and ion channels: Molecular models and sites of action. Annu Rev Pharmacol Toxicol 41:23, 2001.
51. Ngai SH, Cheney DL, Finck AD: Acetylcholine concentrations and turnover in rat brain structures during anesthesia with halothane, enflurane, and ketamine. Anesthesiology 48:4, 1978.
52. Keifer JC, Baghdoyan HA, Lydic R: Pontine cholinergic mechanisms modulate the cortical electroencephalographic spindles of halothane anesthesia. Anesthesiology 84:945, 1996.
53. Shichino T, Murakawa M, Adachi T, et al: Effects of inhalation anaesthetics on the release of acetylcholine in the rat cerebral cortex in vivo. Br J Anaesth 80:365, 1998.
54. Ishizawa Y, Ma HC, Dohi S, et al: Effects of cholinomimetic injection into the brain stem reticular formation on halothane anesthesia and antinociception in rats. J Pharm Exp Ther 293:845, 2000.
55. Eger EI, Zhang Y, Laster M, et al: Acetylcholine receptors do not mediate the immobilization produced by inhaled anesthetics. Anesth Analg 94:1500, 2002.
56. Roizen MF, Kopin KJ, Thoa NB, et al: The effect of two anesthetic agents on norepinephrine and dopamine in discrete brain nuclei, fiber tracts, and terminal regions of the rat. Brain Res 110:515, 1976.
57. Muldoon SM, Cress L, Freas W: Presynaptic adrenergic effects of anesthetics. Int Anesth Clin 27:259, 1989.
58. Segal IS, Walton JK, Irwin I, et al: Modulating role of dopamine on anesthetic requirements. Eur J Pharmacol 186:9, 1990.
59. Miyano K, Tanifuji Y, Eger EI II: The effect of halothane dose on striatal dopamine: An in vivo microdialysis study. Brain Res 605:342, 1993.
60. Vickery RG, Sheridan BC, Segal IS, et al: Anesthetic and hemodynamic effects of the stereoisomers of medetomidine, an α2-adrenergic agonist, in halothane-anesthetized dogs. Anesth Analg 67:611, 1988.
61. Kingery WS, Agashe GS, Guo TZ, et al: Isoflurane and nociception. Spinal α2A adrenoreceptors mediate antinociception while supraspinal α1 adrenoreceptors mediate pronociception. Anesthesiology 96:367, 2002.
62. Roizen MF, Kopin IJ, Palkovits M, et al: The effect of two diverse inhalation anesthetic agents on serotonin in discrete regions of the rat brain. Exp Brain Res 24:203, 1975.
63. Rampil IJ, Laster MJ, Eger EI II: Antagonism of the 5-HT3 receptor does not alter isoflurane MAC in rats. Anesthesiology 95:562, 2001.
64. Seitz PA, Riet MT, Rush W, et al: Adenosine decreases the minimum alveolar concentration of halothane in dogs. Anesthesiology 73:990, 1990.
65. Suzuki A, Katoh T, Ikeda K: The effect of adenosine triphosphate on sevoflurane requirements for minimum alveolar anesthetic concentrations and minimum alveolar anesthetic–awake. Anesth Analg 86:179, 1998.
66. Eisenach JC, Hood DD, Curry R: Preliminary efficacy assessment of intrathecal injection of an American formulation of adenosine in humans. Anesthesiology 96:29, 2002.
67. Arai T, Aoki M, Murakawa M, et al: The effects of halothane on the contents of putative transmitter amino acids in whole rat brain. Neurosci Lett 117:353, 1990.
68. Cheng SC, Brunner EA: Inhibition of GABA metabolism in rat brain slices by halothane. Anesthesiology 55:26, 1981.
69. Vahle-Hinz C, Detsch O, Siemers M, et al: Local GABA_A receptor blockade reverses isoflurane's suppressive effects on thalamic neurons in vivo. Anesth Analg 92:1578, 2001.
70. Zhang Y, Stabernack C, Sonner J, et al: Both cerebral GABA_A receptors and spinal GABA_A receptors modulate the capacity of isoflurane to produce immobility. Anesth Analg 92:1585, 2001.
71. Zhang Y, Wu S, Eger EI II, Sonner J, et al: Neither GABA_A nor strychnine-sensitive glycine receptors are the sole mediators of MAC for isoflurane. Anesth Analg 92:123, 2001.
72. Hudspith MJ: Glutamate: A role in normal brain function, anaesthesia, analgesia and CNS injury. Br J Anaesth 78:731, 1997.
73. Nishikawa K, MacIver BM: Excitatory synaptic transmission mediated by NMDA receptors is more sensitive to isoflurane than are non-NMDA receptor-mediated responses. Anesthesiology 92:228, 2000.
74. Towler SC, Evers AS: Anesthesia and chemical second messenger generation in the adrenergic nervous system. Int Anesth Clin 27:234, 1989.
75. Rengasamy A, Pajewski TN, Johns RA: Inhalational anesthetic effects on rat cerebellar nitric oxide and cyclic guanosine monophosphate production. Anesthesiology 86:689, 1997.

76. Kress HG, Tas WL: Effects of volatile anaesthetics on second messenger Ca^{+2} in neurones and non-muscular cells. Br J Anaesth 71:47, 1993.

77. Mody I, Tanelian DL, MacIver MB: Halothane enhances tonic neuronal inhibition by elevating intracellular calcium. Brain Res 538:319, 1991.

78. Hossain MD, Evers AS: Volatile-anesthetic-induced efflux of calcium from IP_3-gated stores in clonal (GH_3) pituitary cells. Anesthesiology 80:1379, 1994.

79. Kraynack BJ, Gintautas JG: Naloxone: Analeptic action unrelated to opiate receptor antagonism? Anesthesiology 56:251, 1982.

80. Finck AD, Samaniego E, Ngai SH: Nitrous oxide selectively releases Met[5]-enkephalin and Met[5]-enkephalin-Arg[6]-Phe[7] into canine third ventricle cerebral spinal fluid. Anesth Analg 80:664, 1995.

81. Mantz J, Azerad J, Limoge A, et al: Transcranial electrical stimulation with Limoge's currents decreases halothane requirements in rats: Evidence for the involvement of endogenous opioids. Anesthesiology 76:253, 1992.

82. Way WL, Hosobuchi Y, Johnson BH, et al: Anesthesia does not increase opioid peptides in cerebrospinal fluid of humans. Anesthesiology 60:43, 1984.

83. Sjostrom S, Tamsen A, Hartvig P, et al: Cerebrospinal fluid concentrations of substance P and metenkephalin-Arg6-Phe7 during surgery and patient-controlled analgesia. Anesth Analg 67:976, 1988.

84. Ichinose F, Huang PL, Zapol WM: Effects of targeted neuronal nitric oxide synthase gene disruption and nitro[G]-L-arginine methylester on the threshold for isoflurane anesthesia. Anesthesiology 83:101, 1995.

85. Pajewski TN, DiFazio CA, Moscicki JC, et al: Nitric oxide synthase inhibitors, 7-nitro indazole and nitro[G]-L-arginine methyl ester, dose-dependently reduce the threshold for isoflurane anesthesia. Anesthesiology 85:1111, 1996.

86. Ichinose F, Mi W, Miyazaki M, et al: Lack of correlation between the reduction of sevoflurane MAC and the cerebellar cyclic GMP concentrations in mice treated with 7-nitroindazole. Anesthesiology 89:143, 1998.

87. Seeman P: The membrane actions of anesthetics and tranquilizers. Pharmacol Rev 24:583, 1972.

88. Miller KW: The nature of the site of general anaesthesia. Int Rev Neurobiol 27:1, 1985.

89. Franks NP, Lieb WR: What is the molecular nature of general anesthetic target sites? Trends Pharmacol Sci 8:169, 1987.

90. Taheri S, Halsey MJ, Liu J, et al: What solvent best represents the site of action of inhaled anesthetics in humans, rats, and dogs? Anesth Analg 72:627, 1991.

91. Eger EI II: Does 1 + 1 = 2? Anesth Analg 68:551, 1989.

92. Dickinson R, White I, Lieb WR, Franks NP: Stereoselective loss of righting reflex in rats by isoflurane. Anesthesiology 93:837, 2000.

93. Rudo FG, Krantz JC: Anaesthetic molecules. Br J Anaesth 46:181, 1974.

94. Koblin DD, Eger EI II, Johnson BH, et al: Are convulsant gases also anesthetics? Anesth Analg 60:464, 1981.

95. Koblin DD, Eger EI II, Johnson BH, et al: Minimum alveolar concentrations and oil/gas partition coefficients of four anesthetic isomers. Anesthesiology 54:314, 1981.

96. Krasowski MD: Differential modulatory actions of the volatile convulsant flurothyl and its anesthetic isomer at inhibitory ligand-gated ion channels. Neuropharmacology 39:1168, 2000.

97. Raines DE, Miller KW: On the importance of volatile agents devoid of anesthetic action. Anesth Analg 79:1031, 1994.

98. Liu J, Laster MJ, Taheri S, et al: Is there a cutoff in anesthetic potency for the normal alkanes? Anesth Analg 77:12, 1993.

99. Liu J, Laster MJ, Koblin DD, et al: A cutoff in anesthetic potency exists in the perfluoroalkanes. Anesth Analg 79:238, 1994.

100. Koblin DD, Chortkoff BS, Laster MJ, et al: Polyhalogenated and perfluorinated compounds that disobey the Meyer-Overton hypothesis. Anesth Analg 79:1043, 1994.

101. Fang Z, Sonner J, Laster MJ, et al: Anesthetic and convulsant properties of aromatic compounds and cycloalkanes: Implications for mechanisms of narcosis. Anesth Analg 83:1097, 1996.

102. Koblin DD, Laster MJ, Ionescu P, et al: Polyhalogenated methyl ethyl ethers: Solubilities and anesthetic properties. Anesth Analg 88:1161, 1999.

103. Fang Z, Laster MJ, Gong D, et al: Convulsant activity of nonanesthetic gas combinations. Anesth Analg 84:634, 1997.

104. Dutton RC, Maurer AJ, Sonner JM, et al: Short-term memory resists the depressant effect of the nonimmobilizer 1-2-dichlorohexafluorocyclobutane (2N) more than long-term memory. Anesth Analg 94:631, 2002.

105. Borghese CM, Harris RA: Anesthetic-induced immobility: Neuronal nicotinic acetylcholine receptors are no longer in the picture. Anesth Analg 95:509, 2002.

106. Pauling L: A molecular theory of general anesthesia. Science 134:15, 1961.

107. Abraham MH, Lieb WR, Franks NP: Role of hydrogen bonding in general anesthesia. J Pharm Sci 80:719, 1991.

108. Vulliemoz Y, Triner L, Verosky M, et al: Deuterated halothane—Anesthetic potency, anticonvulsant activity, and effect on cerebellar cyclic guanosine 3',5'-monophosphate. Anesth Analg 63:495, 1984.

109. Miller KW: Inert gas narcosis, the high pressure neurological syndrome, and the critical volume hypothesis. Science 185:867, 1974.

110. Ratnakumari L, Vysotskaya TN, Duch DS, et al: Differential effects of anesthetic and nonanesthetic cyclobutanes on neuronal voltage-gated sodium channels. Anesthesiology 92:529, 2000.

111. Friederich P, Benzenberg D, Trellakis, et al: Interaction of volatile anesthetics with human K_v channels in relation to clinical concentrations. Anesthesiology 95:954, 2001.

112. Brett RS, Dilger JP, Yland KF: Isoflurane causes "flickering" of the acetylcholine receptor channel: Observations using the patch clamp. Anesthesiology 69:161, 1988.

113. Dilger JP, Vidal AM, Mody HI: Evidence for direct actions of general anesthetics on an ion channel protein. Anesthesiology 81:431, 1994.

114. Tanelian DL, Kosek P, Mody I, MacIver MB: The role of the $GABA_A$ receptor/chloride channel complex in anesthesia. Anesthesiology 78:757, 1993.

115. Patel AJ, Honore E: Anesthetic-sensitive 2P domain K^+ channels. Anesthesiology 95:1013, 2001.

116. MacIver MB, Kendig JJ: Anesthetic effects on membrane resting potential are voltage-dependent and agent-specific. Anesthesiology 74:83, 1991.

117. Janoff AS, Miller KW: A critical assessment of the lipid theories of general anesthetic action. *In* Chapman D (ed): Biological Membranes. London, Academic Press, 1982, pp 417-476.

118. Tang P, Yan B, Xu Y: Different distribution of fluorinated anesthetics and nonanesthetics in model membrane: A ^{19}F NMR study. Biophys J 72:1676, 1997.

119. North C, Cafiso DS: Contrasting membrane localization and behavior of halogenated cyclobutanes that follow or violate the Meyer-Overton hypothesis of general anesthetic potency. Biophys J 72:1754, 1997.

120. Johansson JS, Zou H: Nonanesthetics (nonimmobilizers) and anesthetics display different microenvironment preferences. Anesthesiology 95:558, 2001.

121. Raines DE, Cafiso DS: The enhancement of proton/hydroxyl flow across lipid vesicles by inhalation anesthetics. Anesthesiology 70:57, 1989.

122. Franks NP, Lieb WR: Is membrane expansion relevant to anaesthesia? Nature 292:248, 1981.

123. Harris RA, Groh GI: Membrane disordering effects of anesthetics are enhanced by gangliosides. Anesthesiology 62:115, 1985.

124. Mihic J, McQuilkin SJ, Eger EI II, et al: Potentiation of γ-aminobutyric acid type A receptor-mediated chloride currents by novel halogenated compounds correlates with their abilities to induce general anesthesia. Mol Pharmacol 46:851, 1994.

125. Qin Z, Szabo G, Cafiso DS: Anesthetics reduce the magnitude of the membrane dipole potential: Measurements in lipid vesicles using voltage-sensitive spin probes. Biochemistry 34:5536, 1995.

126. Cantor RS: Breaking the Meyer-Overton rule: Predicted effects of varying stiffness and interfacial activity on the intrinsic potency of anesthetics. Biophys J 80:2284, 2001.

127. Eckenhoff RG, Johansson JS: Molecular interactions between inhaled anesthetics and proteins. Pharmacol Rev 49:343, 1997.

128. Miller KW: The nature of sites of general anaesthetic action. Br J Anaesth 89:17, 2002.

129. Bhattacharya AA, Curry S, Franks NP: Binding of the general anesthetics propofol and halothane to human serum albumin. J Biol Chem 275:38731, 2000.

130. Dickinson R, Franks NP, Lieb WR: Thermodynamics of anesthetic/protein interactions: Temperature studies on firefly luciferase. Biophys J 64:1264, 1993.

131. Zhang Y, Stabernack CR, Dutton R, et al: Luciferase as a model for the site of inhaled anesthetic action. Anesth Analg 93:1246, 2001.

132. Eckenhoff RG: An inhalational anesthetic binding domain in the nicotinic acetylcholine receptor. Proc Natl Acad Sci U S A 93:2807, 1996.

133. Raines DE, Zachariah VT: Isoflurane increases the apparent agonist affinity of the nicotinic acetylcholine receptor by reducing the microscopic agonist dissociation constant. Anesthesiology 92:775, 2000.

134. Raines DE, Claycomb RJ, Scheller M, Forman SA: Nonhalogenated alkane anesthetics fail to potentiate agonist actions on two ligand-gated ion channels. Anesthesiology 95:470, 2001.

135. Dilger JP: The effects of general anaesthetics on ligand-gated ion channels. Br J Anaesth 89:41, 2002.

136. Flood P, Ramirez-Latorre J, Role L: $\alpha 4\beta 2$ Neuronal nicotinic acetylcholine receptors in the central nervous system are inhibited by isoflurane and propofol, but $\alpha 7$-type nicotinic acetylcholine receptors are unaffected. Anesthesiology 86:859, 1997.

137. Downie DL, Vicente-Agullo F, Campos-Caro A, et al: Determinants of the anesthetic sensitivity of neuronal nicotinic acetylcholine receptors. J Biol Chem 277:10367, 2002.

138. Harris BD, Wong G, Moody EJ, et al: Different subunit requirements for volatile and nonvolatile anesthetics at γ-aminobutyric acid type A receptors. Mol Pharmacol 47:363, 1995.

139. Scheller M, Forman SA: The γ subunit determines whether anesthetic-induced leftward shift is altered by a mutation at $\alpha_1 S270$ in $\alpha_1\beta_2\gamma_{2L}$ GABA$_A$ receptors. Anesthesiology 95:123, 2001.

140. Krasowski MD, Harrison NL: The actions of ether, alcohol and alkane general anaesthetics on GABA$_A$ and glycine receptors and the effects of TM2 and TM3 mutations. Br J Pharmacol 129:731, 2000.

141. Jenkins A, Greenblatt EP, Faulkner HJ, et al: Evidence for a common binding cavity for three general anesthetics within the GABA$_A$ receptor. J Neurosci 21:RC136, 2001.

142. Suzuki T, Koyama H, Sugimoto M, et al: The diverse actions of volatile and gaseous anesthetics on human-cloned 5-hydroxytryptamine3 receptors expressed in *Xenopus* oocytes. Anesthesiology 96:699, 2002.

143. Minami K, Wick MJ, Stern-bach Y, et al: Sites of volatile anesthetic action on kainate (glutamate receptor 6) receptors. J Biol Chem 273:8248, 1998.

144. Jevtovic-Todorovic V, Todorovic SM, Mennerick S, et al: Nitrous oxide (laughing gas) is an NMDA antagonist, neuroprotectant and neurotoxin. Nat Med 4:460, 1998.

145. Yamakura T, Harris RA: Effects of gaseous anesthetics nitrous oxide and xenon on ligand-gated ion channels: Comparison with isoflurane and ethanol. Anesthesiology 93:1095, 2000.

146. Raines DE, Claycomb RJ, Forman SA: Nonhalogenated anesthetic alkanes and perhalogenated nonimmobilizing alkanes inhibit $\alpha 4 2$ neuronal nicotinic acetylcholine receptors Anesth Analg 94:573, 2002.

147. Yamakura T, Lewohl JM, Harris RA: Differential effects of general anesthetics on G protein-coupled inwardly rectifying and other potassium channels. Anesthesiology 95:144, 2001.

148. Todorovic SM, Jevtovic-Todorovic V, Mennerick S, et al: Ca$_v$3,2 channel is a molecular substrate for inhibition of T-type calcium currents in rat sensory neurons by nitrous oxide. Mol Pharmacol 60:603, 2001.

149. Gray AT, Zhao BB, Kindler CH, et al: Volatile anesthetics activate the human tandem pore domain baseline K+ channel KCNK5. Anesthesiology 92:1722, 2000.

150. Durieux ME: Muscarinic signaling in the central nervous system: Recent developments and anesthetic implications. Anesthesiology 84:173, 1996.

151. Minami K, Minami M, Harris RA: Inhibition of 5-hydroxytryptamine type 2A receptor-induced currents by n-alcohols and anesthetics. J Pharm Exp Ther 281:1136, 1997.

152. Minami K, Gereau RW IV, Minami M, et al: Effects of ethanol and anesthetics on type 1 and 5 metabotropic glutamate receptors expressed in *Xenopus laevis* oocytes. Mol Pharmacol 53:148, 1998.

153. Rebecchi MJ, Pentyala SN: Anaesthetic actions on other targets: Protein kinase C and guanine nucleotide-binding proteins. Br J Anaesth 89:62, 2002.

154. Ishizawa Y, Sharp R, Liebman PA, et al: Halothane binding to a G protein coupled receptor in retinal membranes by photoaffinity labeling. Biochemistry 39:8497, 2000.

155. Hemmings HC, Adamo AIB: Effect of halothane on conventional protein kinase C translocation and down-regulation in rat cerebrocortical synaptosomes. Br J Anaesth 78:189, 1997.

156. Minami K, Shiraishi M, Uezono Y, et al: The inhibitory effects of anesthetics and ethanol on substance P receptors expressed in *Xenopus* oocytes. Anesth Analg 94:79, 2002.

157. Patel MK, Mistry D, John JE III, et al: Sodium channel isoform-specific effects of halothane: Protein kinase C co-expression and slow inactivation gating. Br J Pharmacol 130:785, 2000.

158. Koblin DD, Dong DE, Deady JE, et al: Alteration of synaptic membrane fatty acid composition and anesthetic requirement. J Pharmacol Exp Ther 212:546, 1980.

159. Evers AS, Elliott WJ, Lefkowith JB, et al: Manipulation of rat brain fatty acid composition alters volatile anesthetic potency. J Clin Invest 77:1028, 1986.

160. Koblin DD, Dong DE, Eger EI II: Tolerance of mice to nitrous oxide. J Pharmacol Exp Ther 211:317, 1979.

161. Koblin DD, Eger EI II, Smith RA, et al: Chronic exposure of mice to subanesthetic doses of nitrous oxide. *In* Fink BR (ed): Progress in Anesthesiology, vol 2. Molecular Mechanisms of Anesthesia. New York, Raven Press, 1980, pp 157-164.

162. Ngai SH, Finck AD: Prolonged exposure to nitrous oxide decreases opiate receptor density in rat brainstem. Anesthesiology 57:26, 1982.

163. Ramsay DS, Brown AC, Woods SC: Acute tolerance to nitrous oxide in humans. Pain 51:367, 1992.

164. Smith RA, Winter PM, Smith M, et al: Rapidly developing tolerance to acute exposures to anesthetic agents. Anesthesiology 50:496, 1979.

165. Fender C, Fujinaga M, Maze M: Strain differences in the antinociceptive effect of nitrous oxide on the tail flick test in rats. Anesth Analg 90:195, 2000.

166. Nash HA: In vivo genetics of anaesthetic action. Br J Anaesth 89:143, 2002.

167. Humphrey JA, Sedensky MM, Morgan PG: Understanding anesthesia: Making genetic sense of the absence of senses. Hum Mol Genet 11:1241, 2002.

168. van Swinderen B, Metz LB, Shebester LD, et al: Goα regulates volatile anesthetic action in *Caenorhabditis elegans*. Genetics 148:643, 2001.

169. Morgan PG, Radke GW, Sedensky MM: Effects of nonimmobilizers and halothane on *Caenorhabditis elegans*. Anesth Analg 91:1007, 2000.

170. Gamo S, Ogaki M, Nakashima-Tanaka E: Strain differences in minimum anesthetic concentrations in *Drosophila melanogaster*. Anesthesiology 54:289, 1981.

171. Campbell DB, Nash HA: Use of *Drosophila* mutants to distinguish among volatile anesthetics. Proc Natl Acad Sci U S A 91:2135, 1994.

172. Walcourt A, Scott RL, Nash HA: Blockage of one class of potassium channel alters the effectiveness of halothane in a brain circuit of *Drosophila*. Anesth Analg 92:535, 2001.

173. Sonner J, Gong D, Eger EI II: Naturally occurring variability in anesthetic potency among inbred mouse strains. Anesth Analg 91:720, 2000.

174. Koblin DD, Dong DE, Deady JE, et al: Selective breeding alters murine resistance to nitrous oxide without alteration in synaptic membrane lipid composition. Anesthesiology 52:401, 1980.

175. Roizen MF, Koblin DD, Johnson BH, et al: Mechanism of age-related and nitrous oxide-associated anesthetic sensitivity: The role of brain catecholamines. Anesthesiology 69:716, 1988.

176. Sonner J, Gong D, Li J, et al: Mouse strain modestly influences minimum alveolar anesthetic concentration and convulsivity of inhaled compounds. Anesth Analg 89:1030, 1999.

177. Dahan A, Sarton E, Teppema L, et al: Anesthetic potency and influence of morphine and sevoflurane on respiration in μ-opioid receptor knockout mice. Anesthesiology 94:824, 2001.

178. Joo DT, Gong D, Sonner JM, et al: Blockade of AMPA receptors and volatile anesthetics: Reduced anesthetic requirements in GluR2 null mutant mice for loss of the righting reflex and antinociception but not minimum alveolar concentration. Anesthesiology 94:478, 2001.

179. Quinlan JJ, Ferguson C, Jester K, et al: Mice with glycine receptor subunit mutations are both sensitive and resistant to volatile anesthetics. Anesth Analg 95:578, 2002.

180. Homanics GE, Ferguson C, Quinlan JJ, et al: Gene knockout of the α6 subunit of the γ-aminobutyric acid type A receptor: Lack of effect on responses to ethanol, pentobarbital, and general anesthetics. Mol Pharmacol 51:588, 1997.

181. Quinlan JJ, Homanics GE, Firestone LL: Anesthesia sensitivity in mice that lack the β3 subunit of the γ-aminobutyric acid type A receptor. Anesthesiology 88:775, 1998.

182. Wong SME, Cheng G, Homanics GE, et al: Enflurane actions on spinal cords from mice that lack the β3 subunit of the $GABA_A$ receptor. Anesthesiology 95:154, 2001.

5 Uptake and Distribution

Edmond I. Eger II

Inspired-to-Alveolar Anesthetic Relationship 131
Effect of Ventilation 131
Anesthetic Uptake Factors 132
Factors Governing Increases in Alveolar Anesthetic Partial Pressure 134
Concentration Effect 135
Second Gas Effect 135
Percutaneous Anesthetic Loss 135
Metabolism of Anesthetic 136
Intertissue Diffusion 136

Factors Modifying the Ratio of Alveolar Anesthetic Concentration to Inspired Anesthetic Concentration 136
Effect of Ventilatory Changes 136
Effect of Changes in Cardiac Output 138
Effect of Concomitant Changes in Ventilation and Perfusion 139
Ventilation-Perfusion Ratio Abnormalities 139

Effect of Nitrous Oxide on Closed Gas Spaces 140
Volume Changes in Highly Compliant Spaces 140

Pressure Changes in Poorly Compliant Spaces 142

Anesthetic Circuitry 142
Washin of the Circuit 142
Anesthetic Loss to Plastic and Soda Lime 142
Effect of Rebreathing 143

Low-Flow or Closed-Circuit Technique 143
Closed-Circuit Anesthesia 143
Low-Flow Anesthetic Delivery 146

Recovery from Anesthesia 147
General Principles 147
Differences between Induction and Recovery 147
Can I Have My Cake and Eat It Too? 149
Impact of Metabolism 150
Diffusion Hypoxia 150
Impact of the Anesthetic Circuit 151

The modern anesthetist expeditiously develops and then sustains a brain anesthetic concentration sufficient for surgery with agents and techniques that usually permit a rapid recovery from anesthesia. Producing an adequate concentration for surgery requires sufficient but not excessive anesthetic delivery. Knowledge of the factors that govern the relationship between the delivered and brain, heart, or muscle concentrations allows optimal conduct of anesthesia.

INSPIRED-TO-ALVEOLAR ANESTHETIC RELATIONSHIP

Of the steps between delivered and brain anesthetic partial pressures, none is more pivotal than that between the inspired and alveolar gases. The alveolar partial pressure governs the partial pressures of anesthetic in all body tissues; all ultimately approach and equal the alveolar partial pressure. By use of high inflow rates (e.g., a non-rebreathing system), the anesthetist can precisely control the inspired partial pressure of anesthetic.

Effect of Ventilation

Two factors determine the rate at which the alveolar concentration of anesthetic (FA) rises toward the concentration of inspired anesthetic (FI): the inspired concentration (see "Concentration Effect") and alveolar ventilation. The unopposed effect of ventilation on induction rapidly increases the alveolar concentration (i.e., FA/FI ratio quickly approaches 1). This occurs with preoxygenation, which normally produces a 95% or greater washin of oxygen in 2 minutes or less when a non-rebreathing (or high-inflow-rate) system is used (Fig. 5-1).

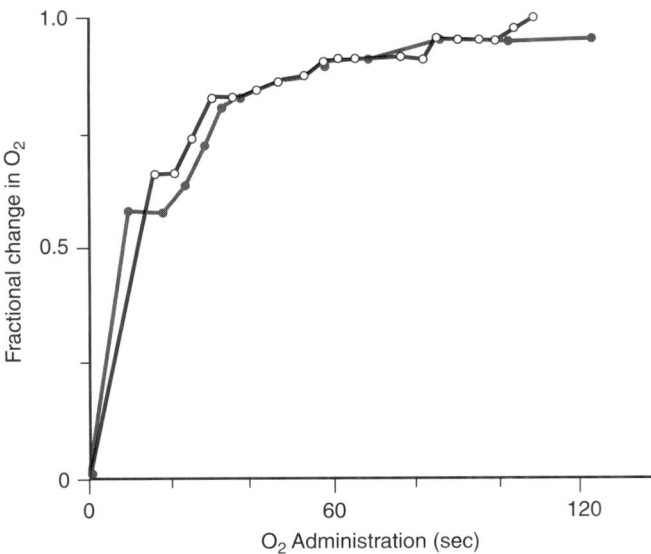

Figure 5–1 The washin of oxygen was determined in two patients breathing from a mask. A 63% change is obtained in about 0.5 minute, an 86% change in about 1 minute, and a 95% to 98% change in 2 minutes. (From Eger EI II, unpublished data, 1992.)

However, the rapid washin of oxygen exceeds that of potent inhaled anesthetics. The solubility of anesthetics far surpasses that of oxygen (or nitrogen), causing uptake of a substantial anesthetic by the pulmonary blood flow. This uptake opposes the effect of ventilation to increase the alveolar anesthetic concentration. A balance between the delivery of anesthetic by ventilation and its removal by uptake determines the FA/FI ratio. The relationship is a simple one. For example, if uptake removes one third of the inspired anesthetic molecules, FA/FI equals 0.67; if uptake removes two thirds of the inspired molecules, FA/FI equals 0.33.

Anesthetic Uptake Factors

The product of three factors determines anesthetic uptake: solubility (λ), cardiac output (Q), and alveolar-to-venous partial pressure difference (PA – Pv).[1]

$$\text{Uptake} = [(\lambda) \times (Q) \times (PA - Pv)]/\text{Barometric pressure}$$

Because uptake is a product of the three factors rather than a sum, if any factor approaches zero, uptake must approach zero, and ventilation rapidly produces an FA/FI of 1.0. If solubility is small (as with oxygen), if cardiac output approaches zero (as in profound myocardial depression or death), or if the alveolar-to-venous difference becomes inconsequential (as can occur after an extraordinarily long anesthetic), uptake would be minimal, and FA/FI would equal 1.0.

Solubility

The blood-gas partition coefficient (i.e., blood solubility [λ]) describes the relative affinity of an anesthetic for two phases and therefore the partitioning of that anesthetic between the two phases at equilibrium. For example, isoflurane has a blood-gas partition coefficient of 1.4, indicating that at equilibrium, isoflurane's concentration in blood is 1.4 times its concentration in the gas (alveolar) phase. *Equilibrium* means that no difference in partial pressure exists (i.e., a blood-gas partition coefficient of 1.4 does not indicate that the partial pressure in blood is 1.4 times that in the gas phase). The partition coefficient indicates the relative capacity of the two phases: a value of 1.4 means that each milliliter of blood holds 1.4 times as much isoflurane as a milliliter of alveolar gas.

A larger blood-gas partition coefficient produces a greater uptake and hence a lower FA/FI ratio. Because the alveolar anesthetic partial pressure is transmitted to the arterial blood and then to all tissues, great blood solubility (as with ether and methoxyflurane [Table 5-1])[1-8] can delay the development of an anesthetizing brain anesthetic partial pressure.[1] Such a delay contributed to the removal of ether and methoxyflurane from anesthetic practice. Even the moderate solubility of enflurane, isoflurane, or halothane would slow induction of anesthesia with these agents if we did not compensate for the uptake of anesthetic by delivering a higher concentration (i.e., overpressure) than we hoped to achieve in the alveoli. For example, anesthesiologists may use 4% to 5% halothane to produce an alveolar concentration of 1%. The use of overpressure can equalize the rate of induction among anesthetics with different solubilities. For example, induction of anesthesia with 5% halothane (6.7 times the minimum alveolar concentration [MAC]) is essentially as rapid as induction with 8% sevoflurane (4.3 MAC), despite a nearly fourfold greater solubility of halothane.[9]

Table 5–1	Partition coefficients at 37°C					
Anesthetic	**Blood-Gas**	**Brain-Blood**	**Liver-Blood**	**Kidney-Blood**	**Muscle-Blood**	**Fat-Blood**
Desflurane	0.45	1.3	1.4	1.0	2.0	27
Nitrous oxide	0.47	1.1	0.8	—	1.2	2.3
Sevoflurane	0.65	1.7	1.8	1.2	3.1	48
Isoflurane	1.4	1.6	1.8	1.2	2.9	45
Enflurane	1.8	1.4	2.1	—	1.7	36
Halothane	2.5	1.9	2.1	1.2	3.4	51
Diethyl ether	12	2.0	1.9	0.9	1.3	5
Methoxyflurane	15	1.4	2.0	0.9	1.6	38

Data from references 1 through 8.

Cardiac Output

Greater pulmonary blood flow removes more anesthetic and thereby lowers the FA/FI ratio. A greater uptake and more rapid delivery to the tissues must accelerate the rise in the tissue anesthetic partial pressure and hasten equilibration of the tissue anesthetic partial pressure with the partial pressure in arterial blood.[10] The more rapid tissue equilibration does not hasten induction of anesthesia because of the lower FA/FI ratio; the accelerated tissue equilibration is to a lower anesthetic partial pressure.

Increased cardiac output has an effect analogous to that of an increased solubility. Doubling solubility doubles the capacity of the same volume of blood to hold anesthetic. Doubling cardiac output also doubles capacity, but in this case by doubling the volume of blood exposed to anesthetic.

Alveolar-to-Venous Anesthetic Gradient

The alveolar-to-venous anesthetic partial pressure difference results from tissue uptake of anesthetic. Were there no tissue uptake, the venous blood returning to the lungs would contain as much anesthetic as the arterial blood that left the lungs. The alveolar (which equals arterial)–to-venous partial pressure difference would be zero.

The factors that determine the fraction of anesthetic removed from blood traversing a given tissue parallel those that govern uptake at the lungs: tissue solubility (i.e., the tissue-blood partition coefficient), tissue blood flow, and arterial-to-tissue anesthetic partial pressure difference. Uptake is the product of these factors. If any factor approaches zero, tissue uptake becomes inconsequential. The capacity of a tissue to hold anesthetic equals the product of the volume of tissue and the solubility of the anesthetic in that tissue.

Blood-gas partition coefficients extend from 0.45 for desflurane to 15 for methoxyflurane (i.e., a 33-fold range) (see Table 5-1). In contrast, tissue-blood partition coefficients for lean tissues range from slightly less than 1 to a maximum of 3.4 (see Table 5-1); different lean tissues have similar capacities per milliliter of tissue relative to blood. Put another way, a given anesthetic has roughly the same affinity for lean tissues and blood. As with blood-gas partition coefficients, tissue-blood partition coefficients define the concentration ratio of anesthetic at equilibrium. For example, a halothane brain-blood partition coefficient of 1.9 means that 1 mL of brain holds 1.9 times more halothane as 1 mL of blood having the same halothane partial pressure.

A larger tissue capacity relative to flow increases the transfer of anesthetic from blood to tissue. However, it takes longer to fill up a tissue with a large capacity relative to blood flow. It takes longer for a tissue such as muscle to equilibrate with the anesthetic partial pressure being delivered in blood, and this sustains the arterial to muscle anesthetic partial pressure difference (and hence uptake) for a longer time. With its high perfusion per gram, brain equilibrates rapidly with the anesthetic partial pressure brought to it in arterial blood. Per milliliter of tissue, muscle has about one-twentieth the perfusion of brain, and muscle takes about 20 times as long as brain to equilibrate. Uptake of anesthetic by muscle continues long after uptake by brain has ceased.

Fat-blood coefficients are significantly greater than 1, particularly those for more potent anesthetics (see Table 5-1) and range from 2.3 (nitrous oxide) to 51 (halothane) to 61 (methoxyflurane). Each milliliter of fat tissue contains 2.3 times more nitrous oxide or 51 times more halothane than a milliliter of blood having the same nitrous oxide or halothane partial pressure. This enormous capacity of fat for anesthetic means that most of the anesthetic contained in the blood perfusing fat is transferred to the fat. Although most of the anesthetic moves from the blood into the fat, the anesthetic partial pressure in fat increases very slowly. The large capacity of fat and its low perfusion per milliliter prolong the time required to narrow the anesthetic partial pressure difference between arterial blood and fat.

Tissue Groups

The algebraic sum of uptake by individual tissues determines the alveolar-to-venous partial pressure difference and therefore uptake at the lungs. However, we do not need to analyze the effect of individual tissues to arrive at the algebraic sum; instead, we can group tissues by their perfusion and solubility characteristics (i.e., features that define the duration of a substantial arterial-to-tissue anesthetic partial pressure difference). Four tissue groups result from such an analysis[1] (Table 5-2).

The brain, heart, splanchnic bed (including liver), kidney, and endocrine glands make up the vessel-rich group (VRG). These organs comprise less than 10% of the body weight but receive 75% of the cardiac output. This great perfusion delivers a relatively large volume of anesthetic and permits an initially large uptake of anesthetic by the VRG. However, the small tissue capacity relative to perfusion produces a rapid equilibration with a time to half-equilibration (i.e., the time at which the VRG anesthetic partial pressure equals one half of that in arterial blood) of 1 minute for nitrous oxide to 2 minutes for halothane (longer for halothane because of its higher tissue-blood partition coefficient and therefore greater capacity) (see Table 5-1).

Characteristic	Tissue Group			
	Vessel-Rich	Muscle	Fat	Vessel-Poor
Percentage of body mass	10	50	20	20
Perfusion as percentage of cardiac output	75	19	6	0

Table 5–2 Tissue group characteristics

Adapted from Eger EI II: Uptake of inhaled anesthetics: The alveolar to inspired anesthetic difference. In Eger EI II: Anesthetic Uptake and Action. Baltimore, Williams & Wilkins, 1974, pp 77-96.

Equilibration of the VRG with the anesthetic in arterial blood is 90% complete in 4 to 8 minutes. After 8 minutes, uptake by the VRG is too small (i.e., the arterial-to-VRG anesthetic partial pressure difference is too small) to significantly influence the alveolar concentration.

For a substantial period after the first 8 minutes, muscle and skin (i.e., the muscle group [MG]) determine uptake. Muscle and skin have similar blood flow and solubility (lean tissue) characteristics. A lower perfusion (about 3 mL of blood per 100 mL of tissue per minute) separates this group from the VRG (70 mL of blood per 100 mL of tissue per minute). Although about one half of the body bulk is muscle and skin, this volume receives only 1 L/min of blood flow at rest; this tissue group receives and initially takes up one fourth of the amount of anesthetic delivered to the VRG. During induction, most of the anesthetic delivered to the MG is removed from its blood flow. Unlike the VRG, the MG continues to remove anesthetic from its blood supply for a long time. The time to half-equilibration ranges from 20 to 25 minutes (nitrous oxide) to 70 to 80 minutes (sevoflurane or halothane). Long after equilibration of the VRG has taken place, muscle continues to take up substantial amounts of anesthetic. MG approaches equilibration in 2 to 4 hours.

After equilibration of the MG, only fat (i.e., the fat group [FG]) serves as an effective depot for uptake. In a normal, lean patient, fat occupies one fifth of the body bulk and receives a blood flow of about 400 mL/min (i.e., perfusion per 100 mL of fat nearly equals the perfusion per 100 mL of resting muscle). During the initial delivery of anesthetic to tissues, the FG has access to only 40% of the anesthetic delivered to the MG (i.e., blood flow to the FG is 40% of that to the MG). Fat also differs from muscle in its higher affinity for anesthetic, and this greatly lengthens the time over which it absorbs anesthetic. The equilibration half-time of the FG ranges from 70 to 80 minutes for nitrous oxide to 30 hours for sevoflurane and halothane.

A fourth tissue group, the vessel-poor group (VPG) consists of ligaments, tendons, bone, and cartilage (i.e., lean tissues that have little or no perfusion). The absence of a significant blood flow means that this group does not participate in the uptake process even though it makes up one fifth of the body mass.

Factors Governing Increases in Alveolar Anesthetic Partial Pressure

Ventilation, solubility, and distribution of blood flow have a combined impact on the increase in the alveolar anesthetic partial pressure (i.e., the rise in the FA/FI ratio). For all agents, FA/FI initially increases rapidly, regardless of agent solubility[11,12] (Fig. 5-2) because of the absence of an alveolar-to-venous anesthetic partial pressure difference (i.e., there is no anesthetic in the lung to create a gradient) and the absence of uptake in the first moment of induction. The capacity of ventilation to increase FA/FI is unopposed. Delivery of anesthetic to the alveoli by ventilation increases the alveolar-to-venous partial pressure difference. The resulting increase in uptake increasingly opposes the effect of ventilation to drive the

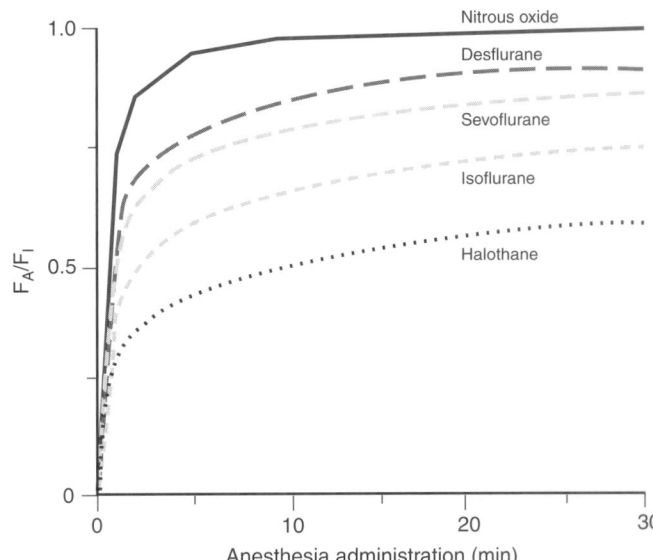

Figure 5–2 The rise in alveolar (FA) anesthetic concentration toward the inspired (FI) concentration is most rapid with the least soluble anesthetics, nitrous oxide and desflurane, and slowest with the most soluble anesthetic, halothane. All data are from human studies. (Data from Yasuda N, Lockhart SH, Eger EI II, et al: Kinetics of desflurane, isoflurane, and halothane in humans. Anesthesiology 74:489-498, 1991, and from Yasuda N, Lockhart SH, Eger EI II, et al: Comparison of kinetics of sevoflurane and isoflurane in humans. Anesth Analg 72:316-324, 1991.)

alveolar concentration upward. Ultimately, removal by uptake balances the input by ventilation. The FA/FI ratio at which the balance is struck depends on the solubility factor in the uptake equation (see earlier equation describing anesthetic uptake). A higher solubility produces more uptake for a given alveolar-to-venous partial pressure difference. Hence, the initially rapid rise in FA/FI halts at a lower level with a more soluble agent. This process results in the first "knee" in the curve, which is higher for desflurane than for sevoflurane, higher for sevoflurane than for isoflurane, and higher for isoflurane than for halothane. The position of nitrous oxide is discussed later (see "Concentration Effect"). The FA/FI ratio indicates the percent of anesthetic removed by uptake. An FA/FI ratio of 0.33 indicates that 67% of the anesthetic is being taken up; an FA/FI ratio of 0.67 indicates that 33% of the anesthetic is being taken up.

The balance struck between ventilation and uptake does not remain constant. FA/FI continues to rise, but at a slower rate than in the first minute. This secondary rise results from the progressive decrease in uptake by the VRG, a decrease to an inconsequential amount after 8 minutes. By about 8 minutes, three fourths of the cardiac output returning to the lungs (i.e., the blood from the VRG) contains nearly as much anesthetic as it had when it left the lungs. The consequent rise in venous anesthetic partial pressure decreases the alveolar-to-venous partial pressure difference and therefore the uptake, allowing ventilation to drive the alveolar concentration upward to a second knee at roughly 8 minutes.

After 8 minutes, the MG and FG become the principal determinants of tissue uptake. The slow decrease in the anesthetic partial pressure difference between arterial blood and MG and FG produces the gradual ascension of the terminal portion of each curve in Figure 5-1, an ascension determined by the progressive equilibration of the MG and, to a lesser extent, the FG with the arterial anesthetic partial pressure. If the graphs were extended for several hours, a third knee would result from equilibration of the MG. Uptake after that time would principally depend on the partial pressure gradient between arterial blood and the FG.

Concentration Effect

The previous analysis ignores the impact of the concentration effect on FA/FI. The inspired anesthetic concentration influences the alveolar concentration that may be attained and the rate at which that concentration may be attained.[13,14] Increasing the inspired concentration accelerates the rise in FA/FI. At an inspired concentration of 100%, the rate of rise is most rapid, dictated solely by the rate at which ventilation washes gas into the lung. At 100% inspired concentration, uptake no longer limits the rise in FA/FI. The cause of this extreme effect is readily perceived. At 100% inspired concentration, the uptake of anesthetic creates a void that draws gas down the trachea. The additional inspiration replaces the gas taken up. Because the concentration of the replacement gas is 100%, uptake cannot modify the alveolar concentration. This explains why FA/FI of nitrous oxide in Figure 5-2 rises more rapidly than that for desflurane despite the identity of their blood-gas partition coefficients.

The concentration effect results from two factors: a concentrating effect and an augmentation of inspired ventilation.[15] Both are illustrated in Figure 5-3. The first rectangle (see Fig. 5-3A) represents a lung containing

80 volumes (80%) nitrous oxide. Uptake of one half of the nitrous oxide yields a residual 40 volumes of nitrous oxide in a total of 60 volumes, a concentration of 67% (see Fig. 5-3B). Uptake of one half of the nitrous oxide does not halve the concentration, because the remaining gases are concentrated in a smaller volume. If the void created by uptake is filled by drawing more gas into the lungs (i.e., augmentation of inspired ventilation), the final concentration equals 72% (see Fig. 5-3C).

This explanation has been criticized as overly simplistic because it ignores the realities of some aspects of ventilation.[16] For example, if ventilation is controlled with a volume-limited respirator, augmentation of inspired ventilation is limited to the period of the expiratory pause. If ventilation is spontaneous, this limitation is minimized. In any event, the anesthesiologist should be aware that although Figure 5-3 describes the basic factors governing the concentration (and second gas effects as discussed later), the actual situation is more complex.

The impact of the concentration effect on FA/FI may be thought of as identical to the impact of a change in solubility[17]; as the inspired concentration increases, the effective solubility decreases. At 50% inspired nitrous oxide, the FA/FI rises as rapidly as the FA/FI of an anesthetic that has one half the solubility of nitrous oxide and is given at 1% inspired concentration, and 75% inspired nitrous oxide acts as does an anesthetic given at 1% that has one fourth the solubility of nitrous oxide.

Second Gas Effect

The factors that govern the concentration effect also influence the concentration of any gas given concomitantly with nitrous oxide (i.e., second gas effect).[15,18] The loss of volume associated with the uptake of nitrous oxide concentrates the second gas (see Fig. 5-3A). Replacement of the gas taken up by an increase in inspired ventilation augments the amount of second gas in the lung (see Fig. 5-3B).

Both the concentration effect and the second gas effect have been demonstrated in dogs[18] and humans.[19] Humans received 4% desflurane in 5% nitrous oxide or 65% nitrous oxide. The FA/FI for nitrous oxide rose more rapidly when 65% nitrous oxide was inspired than when 5% was inspired (i.e., concentration effect) (Fig. 5-4). Similarly, the FA/FI ratio for desflurane rose more rapidly when 65% nitrous oxide was inspired than when 5% was inspired (i.e., second gas effect).

Percutaneous Anesthetic Loss

I have ignored three possible avenues for anesthetic loss: transcutaneous movement, transvisceral movement, and metabolism. Although transcutaneous movement occurs, the movement is small.[20-23] The greatest loss per alveolar anesthetic percent occurs with nitrous oxide. Loss of nitrous oxide may equal 5 to 10 mL/min with an alveolar concentration of 70%. The movement of anesthetic across visceral or pleural surfaces during abdominal or pulmonary surgery is larger than the movement across skin, but such visceral losses are usually small relative to total uptake.[24]

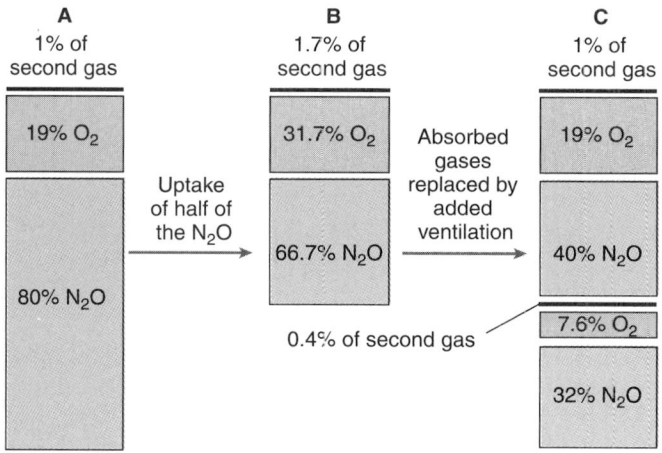

Figure 5–3 A, The rectangle represents a lung filled with 80% nitrous oxide plus 1% of a second gas. B, Uptake of one half of the nitrous oxide does not halve the concentration of nitrous oxide, and the reduction in volume thereby increases the concentration of the second gas. C, Restoration of the lung volume by addition of gas at the same concentration as that contained in A increases the nitrous oxide concentration and adds to the amount of the second gas present in the lung. (Adapted from Stoelting RK, Eger EI II: An additional explanation for the second gas effect: A concentrating effect. Anesthesiology 30:273-277, 1969.)

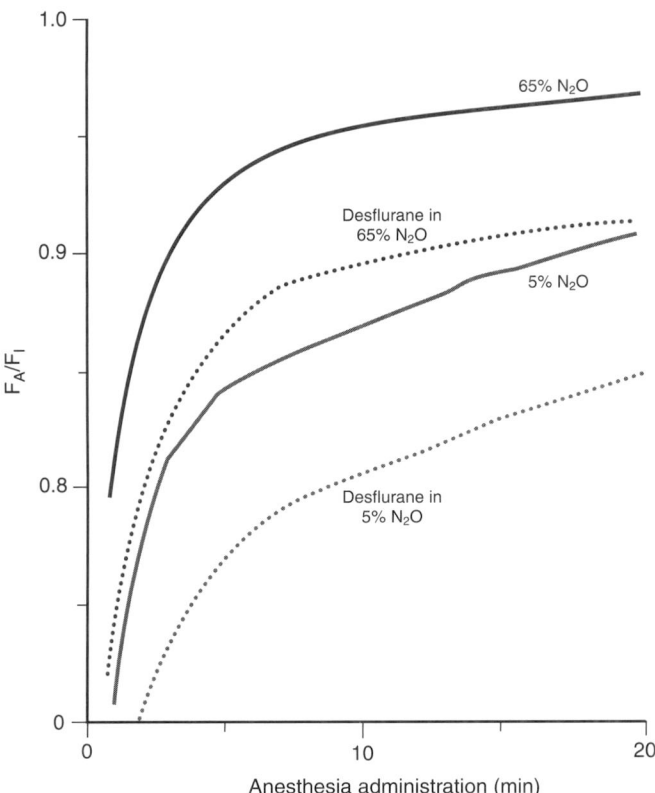

Figure 5–4 In patients, administration of 65% nitrous oxide produces a more rapid rise in the alveolar concentration of anesthetic/concentration of inspired anesthetic (FA/FI ratio) for nitrous oxide than administration of 5% (i.e., concentration effect, *two solid lines*). The FA/FI ratio for 4% desflurane rises more rapidly when given with 65% nitrous oxide than when given with 5% (i.e., second gas effect, *two dotted lines*). (Adapted from Taheri S, Eger EI II: A demonstration of the concentration and second gas effects in humans anesthetized with nitrous oxide and desflurane. Anesth Analg 89:774-780, 1999.)

Metabolism of Anesthetic

Although percutaneous loss of anesthetic may not appreciably affect anesthetic uptake, biodegradation can, particularly with agents that undergo extensive biodegradation. Berman and colleagues[25] found that phenobarbital pretreatment in rats decreased the arterial level of methoxyflurane. In humans, Carpenter and coworkers[26] found that one half of the halothane and three fourths of the methoxyflurane taken up was biodegraded. Such biodegradation explains why the alveolar concentration of halothane decays more rapidly on recovery from anesthesia than the alveolar concentration of isoflurane, an anesthetic significantly less soluble in blood.[27,28] In contrast to halothane or methoxyflurane, isoflurane and desflurane resist biodegradation.[29,30] For all potent inhaled anesthetics, anesthetizing concentrations appear to saturate the enzymes responsible for anesthetic metabolism.[31] Because higher anesthetic partial pressures exist during anesthesia, saturation of enzymes may limit the impact of metabolism more during the washin than the washout of anesthetic. The combined effect of these factors remains to be determined, but it

appears that metabolism is not a significant determinant of FA/FI during anesthesia with isoflurane or desflurane.[11,12] A small influence on the kinetics of sevoflurane may exist, explaining why there is a more substantial difference between the FA/FI for desflurane compared with sevoflurane during induction and maintenance of anesthesia than for the parallel washout curves (FA/FA₀) during recovery.[32]

Intertissue Diffusion

Carpenter and colleagues[27,28] measured the washin and washout of isoflurane, enflurane, halothane, and methoxyflurane given simultaneously for fixed periods to healthy young humans. Washout was examined for several days after discontinuation of anesthetic administration. Analysis suggested that a model with five compartments best explained the resulting data for all the anesthetics (i.e., the model was independent of solubility and anesthetic metabolism). The half-times of four of these compartments were consistent with the model described earlier in this chapter. Four of these compartments could be related to washin and washout of the lungs, the VRG, the MG, and the FG.

An additional important compartment was more difficult to explain. This compartment had a half-time of roughly 300 minutes, which is between those for muscle and for fat. Uptake by highly perfused fat, such as that found in bone marrow, could explain part of this additional compartment, which accounted for almost one third of the anesthetic taken up. However, blood flow to marrow is too small to account for most of the uptake by this compartment. Carpenter and associates[27,28] speculated that this uptake resulted from diffusion of anesthetic from lean tissue to an adjacent thin layer of fat tissue: from the heart to pericardial fat, from the kidney to perirenal fat, from the intestine to mesenteric and omental fat, and from the dermis to subcutaneous fat. Yasuda and associates[11,12] confirmed these findings, extending them to desflurane and sevoflurane.

FACTORS MODIFYING THE RATIO OF ALVEOLAR ANESTHETIC CONCENTRATION TO INSPIRED ANESTHETIC CONCENTRATION

Alteration of factors that govern the rate of delivery of anesthetic to the lungs or its removal from the lungs changes the alveolar concentration of anesthetic. We have seen the importance of differences in solubility (see Fig. 5-2). The following sections examine the impact of differences in ventilation and circulation and the interaction of these differences with factors such as solubility.

Effect of Ventilatory Changes

By augmenting delivery of anesthetic to the lungs, an increased ventilation accelerates the rate of rise of FA/FI (Fig. 5-5).[1,33,34] A change in ventilation produces a greater relative change in FA/FI with a more soluble anesthetic.

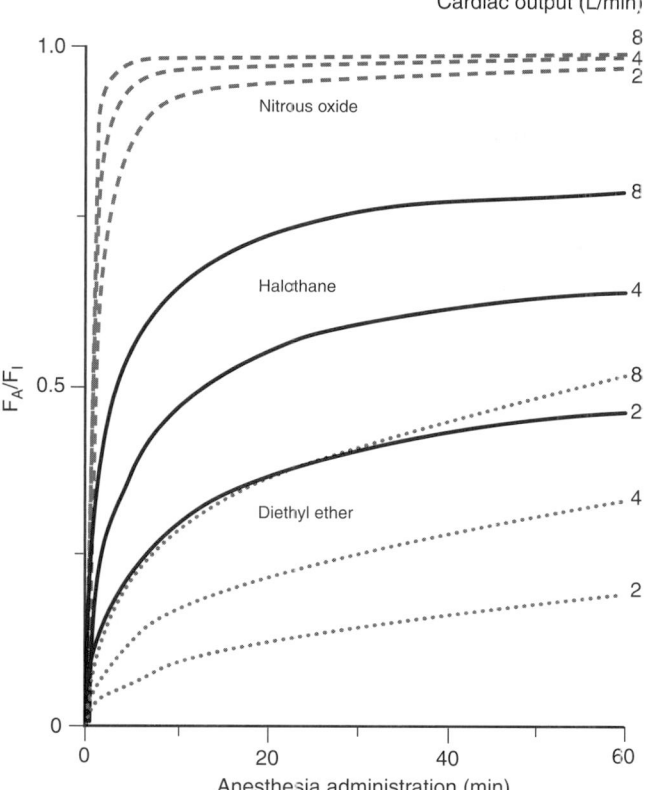

Figure 5–5 The alveolar concentration of anesthetic/concentration of inspired anesthetic (Fᴀ/Fɪ ratio) rises more rapidly if ventilation is increased. Solubility modifies this impact of ventilation; the effect on the anesthetizing partial pressure is greatest with the most soluble anesthetic (ether) and least with the least soluble anesthetic (nitrous oxide). (Adapted from Eger EI II: Ventilation, circulation and uptake. *In* Eger EI II [ed]: Anesthetic Uptake and Action. Baltimore, Williams & Wilkins, 1974, pp 122-145.)

In Figure 5-5, an increase in ventilation from 2 to 8 L/min triples the ether concentration at 10 minutes, only doubles the halothane concentration, and scarcely affects the nitrous oxide concentration.

The impact of solubility may be explained as follows. With a poorly soluble agent, such as nitrous oxide, the rate of rise of Fᴀ/Fɪ is rapid, even with hypoventilation. Because Fᴀ normally cannot exceed Fɪ, augmentation of ventilation can increase Fᴀ/Fɪ but slightly. With a highly soluble agent, such as ether and methoxyflurane, most of the anesthetic delivered to the lungs is taken up, so that if the uptake at 2 L/min ventilation equaled X, the uptake at 4 L/min would approach 2X. If cardiac output is held constant, ventilation of 4 L/min produces an arterial ether concentration that is nearly twice the concentration produced by a ventilation of 2 L/min. Because arterial and alveolar concentrations are in equilibrium, this example suggests that doubling ventilation must nearly double the concentration of a highly soluble anesthetic in lung or blood.

These observations imply that imposed alterations in ventilation (e.g., an increase produced by conversion from spontaneous to controlled ventilation) produce

greater changes in anesthetic effect with more soluble agents. Because such effects include anesthetic depth and depression of circulation, greater caution must be exercised when ventilation is augmented during anesthesia produced with a highly soluble agent.

Anesthetics themselves may alter ventilation and thereby alter their own uptake.[10,35] Modern potent agents (e.g., desflurane, enflurane, halothane, isoflurane, sevoflurane) can profoundly depress respiration, doing so in a dose-related manner.[36-40] At some dose, all inhaled anesthetics produce apnea, a feature that limits the MAC that can be obtained if ventilation is spontaneous.

Anesthetic-induced respiratory depression significantly decreases delivery of anesthetic to the alveoli.[10,41] Doubling the inspired concentration does not double the alveolar concentration attained at a given point in time. At high inspired concentrations, further increases in inspired concentration produce little absolute change in the alveolar concentration (Fig. 5-6). Anesthetics thereby exert a negative feedback effect on their own alveolar concentration, an effect that increases the safety of spontaneous ventilation by limiting the maximum concentration attained in the alveoli.

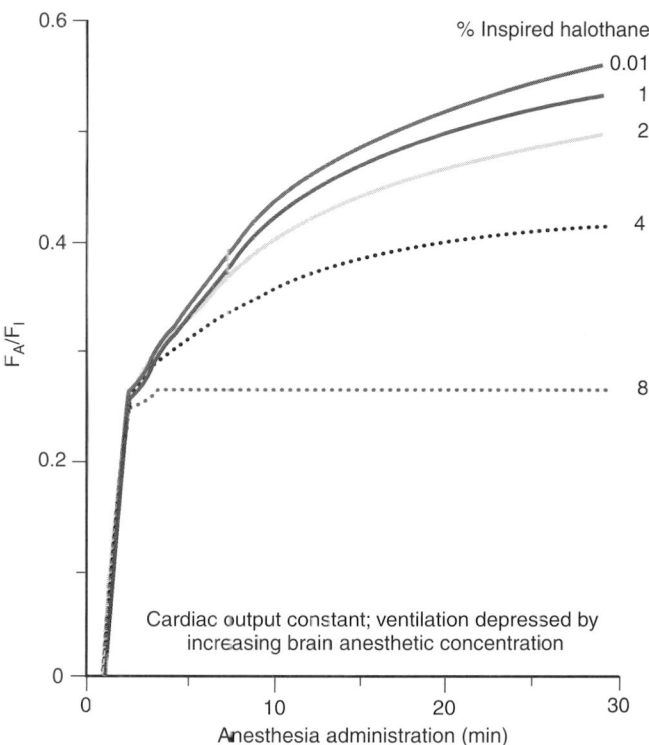

Figure 5–6 An increase in the inspired halothane concentration does not produce a proportional increase in the alveolar concentration because of the progressively greater depression of ventilation that occurs as alveolar halothane is increased. The initial "overshoot" seen with 10% to 20% inspired halothane results from the delay in the transfer of alveolar halothane partial pressure to the brain. Fᴀ/Fɪ is the alveolar concentration of anesthetic/concentration of inspired anesthetic. (Adapted from Munson ES, Eger EI II, Bowers DL: Effects of anesthetic-depressed ventilation and cardiac output on anesthetic uptake. Anesthesiology 38:251-259, 1973.)

Effect of Changes in Cardiac Output

The discussion in the previous section assumed a constant cardiac output and examined the effect of changes in ventilation. This section considers the reverse process. An increased cardiac output augments uptake and thereby hinders the rise in F_A/F_I.[1,42] As with a change in ventilation, a change in cardiac output scarcely affects the alveolar concentration of a poorly soluble agent but considerably influences the alveolar concentration of a highly soluble agent[34] (Fig. 5-7). The reason is similar to the reason explaining the effect of a change in ventilation. A decrease in cardiac output can little increase the F_A/F_I ratio of poorly soluble agents because the rate of rise is rapid at any cardiac output. In contrast, nearly all of a highly soluble agent is taken up, and a halving of blood flow through the lungs must concentrate the arterial (which equals alveolar) anesthetic, nearly doubling its partial pressure in the case of an extremely soluble agent.

This effect of solubility suggests that conditions that lower cardiac output (e.g., shock) can substantially increase the alveolar anesthetic concentrations of highly soluble agents. A higher F_A/F_I ratio should be anticipated and the inspired anesthetic concentration lowered accordingly to avoid further depression of circulation. Shock presents a two-pronged problem: an increase in ventilation usually accompanies a decreased cardiac output, and both of these changes accelerate the rise in F_A/F_I. Perhaps this is why such heavy reliance is placed on the use of nitrous oxide in patients in shock. In contrast to more soluble anesthetics (e.g., halothane), the alveolar concentration of nitrous oxide is influenced little by the associated cardiorespiratory changes.

Anesthetics also affect circulation. Usually, they depress cardiac output,[43,44] although stimulation may occur with some agents (i.e., nitrous oxide and, transiently, desflurane).[45,46] In contrast to the negative feedback that results from respiratory depression, circulatory depression produces a positive feedback; depression decreases uptake, and this increases the alveolar concentration, which further decreases uptake. A potentially lethal acceleration of the rise in F_A/F_I results from the depression of cardiac output[10,35,41] (Fig. 5-8). The impact of this acceleration increases in importance with increasing anesthetic solubility. High inspired concentrations of agents such as enflurane and halothane should be administered with considerable caution, particularly if ventilation is controlled.

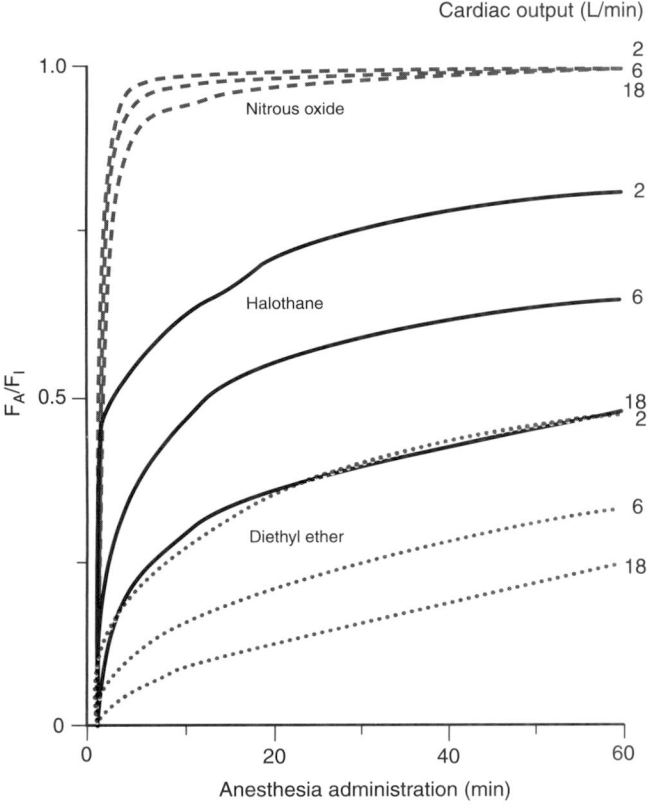

Figure 5–7 If unopposed by a concomitant increase in ventilation, an increase in cardiac output will decrease alveolar anesthetic concentration by augmenting uptake. The resulting alveolar anesthetic change is greatest with the most soluble anesthetic. F_A/F_I is the alveolar concentration of anesthetic/concentration of inspired anesthetic. (Adapted from Eger EI II: Ventilation, circulation and uptake. *In* Eger EI II [ed]: Anesthetic Uptake and Action. Baltimore, Williams & Wilkins, 1974, pp 122-145.)

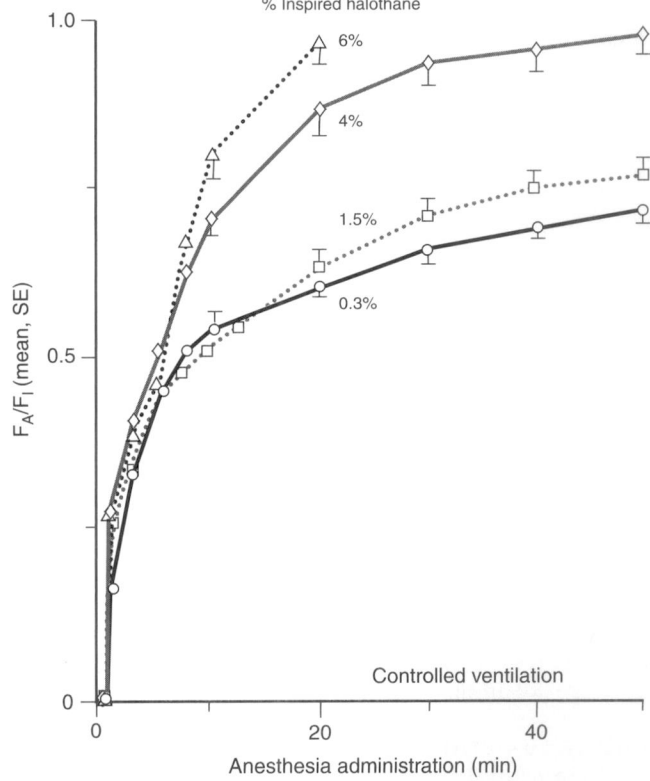

Figure 5–8 Dogs given constant ventilation demonstrate different rates of rise of the alveolar concentration of anesthetic/concentration of inspired anesthetic (F_A/F_I ratio). The rates of rise depend on the inspired halothane concentration. The two higher concentrations accelerated the rate of rise by depressing cardiac output and thereby decreasing uptake. (Adapted from Gibbons RT, Steffey EP, Eger EI II: The effect of spontaneous versus controlled ventilation on the rate of rise of alveolar halothane concentration in dogs. Anesth Analg 56:32-34, 1977.)

Effect of Concomitant Changes in Ventilation and Perfusion

The preceding considerations of the effects of ventilatory and circulatory alterations presume that only one of these variables changed while the other remained constant, but both may change concomitantly. If both ventilation and cardiac output increase proportionately, an intuitive expectation may be that FA/FI would be little altered. After all, uptake equals the product of solubility, the cardiac output, and the alveolar-to-venous anesthetic partial pressure difference (see the earlier anesthetic uptake equation). In the absence of other changes, doubling cardiac output doubles uptake, and this should exactly balance the influence of doubling ventilation on FA/FI. A doubling of both delivery of anesthetic to the lungs and removal of anesthetic from the lungs should produce no net change in the alveolar concentration.

However, this reasoning ignores another factor that defines uptake. By accelerating the rate of tissue equilibration, an increase in cardiac output accelerates the narrowing of the alveolar-to-venous partial pressure difference[47] and thereby reduces the impact of the increase in cardiac output on uptake. A proportional increase in ventilation and cardiac output increases the rate of rise of FA/FI.

The magnitude of the acceleration of rise in FA/FI partly depends on distribution of the increase in cardiac output. If the increase is distributed proportionately to all tissues (e.g., if a doubling of output doubles flow to all tissues), the increase is fairly small[47,48] (Fig. 5-9). Conditions such as hyperthermia and thyrotoxicosis only slightly influence the development of an anesthetizing anesthetic concentration through their influence on FA/FI. However, if the increase in cardiac output primarily flows to the VRG, a greater effect is seen. Perfusion of the VRG is normally high and results in rapid equilibration. Because blood returning from the VRG soon has the same partial pressure as it had when it left the lungs, it cannot remove more anesthetic from the lungs. After a few seconds or minutes, the effect of the increase in cardiac output on uptake cannot match the added delivery of anesthetic by augmented ventilation. The result is a considerable acceleration of the rise in FA/FI. This effect may be seen in a comparison of the FA/FI curves for children and adults (Fig. 5-10). Children (especially infants) have a relatively greater perfusion of the VRG and consequently show a significantly faster rise in FA/FI[6,49-51] (see Chapter 60). A clinical result of this accelerated rise is a more rapid development of anesthesia in young patients. The higher perfusion of the brain further accelerates the development of anesthesia.

Ventilation-Perfusion Ratio Abnormalities

Until this point, I have assumed equality of alveolar and arterial anesthetic partial pressures (i.e., that the alveolar gases completely equilibrate with the blood passing through the lungs). For normal patients, this assumption is approximately correct, but diseases such as emphysema, pneumonia, and atelectasis, as well as congenital cardiac defects, produce substantial deviations from equilibration. The associated ventilation-perfusion ratio abnormality

increases the alveolar (end-tidal) anesthetic partial pressure and decreases the arterial anesthetic partial pressure (i.e., a partial pressure difference appears between alveolar gas and arterial blood). The relative change depends on the solubility of the anesthetic. With a poorly soluble agent, the end-tidal concentration is slightly increased, but the arterial partial pressure is significantly reduced. The opposite occurs with a highly soluble anesthetic.[52]

The considerable decrease in the arterial anesthetic partial pressure that occurs with poorly soluble agents may be explained as follows. Ventilation-perfusion ratio abnormalities increase ventilation relative to perfusion of some alveoli, whereas in other alveoli, the reverse occurs. With a poorly soluble anesthetic, an increase in ventilation relative to perfusion does not appreciably increase the alveolar or arterial anesthetic partial pressure issuing from those alveoli (see Fig. 5-5 for nitrous oxide effect). However, when ventilation decreases relative to perfusion (e.g., with atelectasis), blood emerges from that segment with no additional anesthetic. Such anesthetic-deficient blood then mixes with the blood from the ventilated segments containing a normal complement of anesthetic. The mixture produces an arterial anesthetic partial pressure considerably below normal.

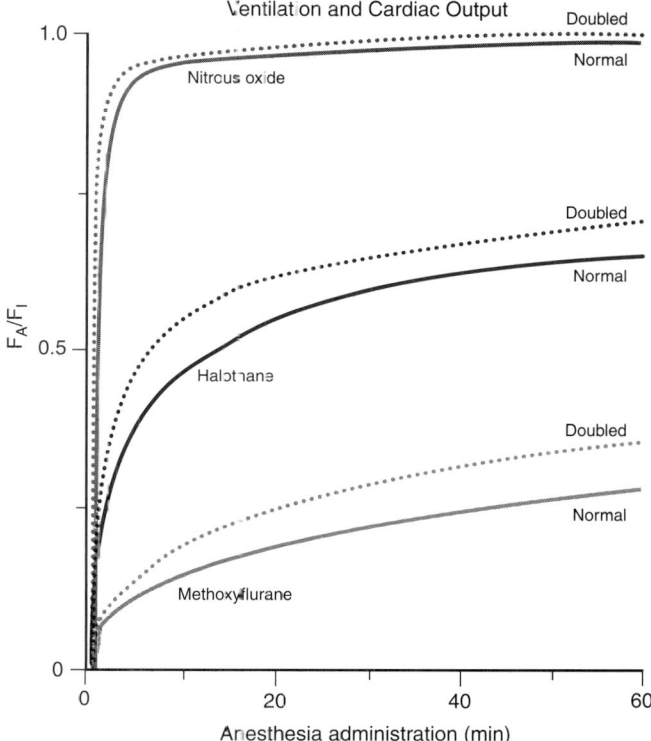

Figure 5–9 Proportional increases in alveolar ventilation (VA) and cardiac output (Q) increase the rate at which the alveolar concentration of anesthetic/concentration of inspired anesthetic (FA/FI ratio) rises. The effect is relatively small if the increase in cardiac output is distributed proportionately to all tissues (i.e., if cardiac output is doubled, all tissue blood flows are doubled). The greatest effect occurs with the most soluble anesthetic. (Adapted from Eger EI II, Bahlman SH, Munson ES: Effect of age on the rate of increase of alveolar anesthetic concentration. Anesthesiology 35:365-372, 1971.)

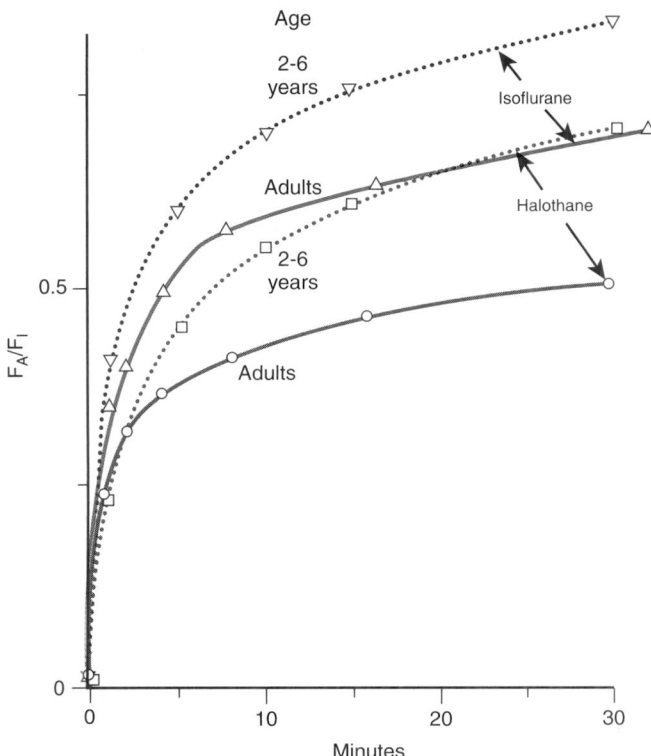

Figure 5–10 The alveolar rate of rise of halothane concentration is more rapid in children *(dashed lines)* than in adults *(solid lines).* The difference probably results from the greater ventilation and perfusion per kilogram of tissue in children and the fact that a disproportionate amount of the increased perfusion is devoted to the vessel-rich tissues. FA/FI is the alveolar concentration of anesthetic/concentration of inspired anesthetic. (Data from references 6, 49, 50, and 51.)

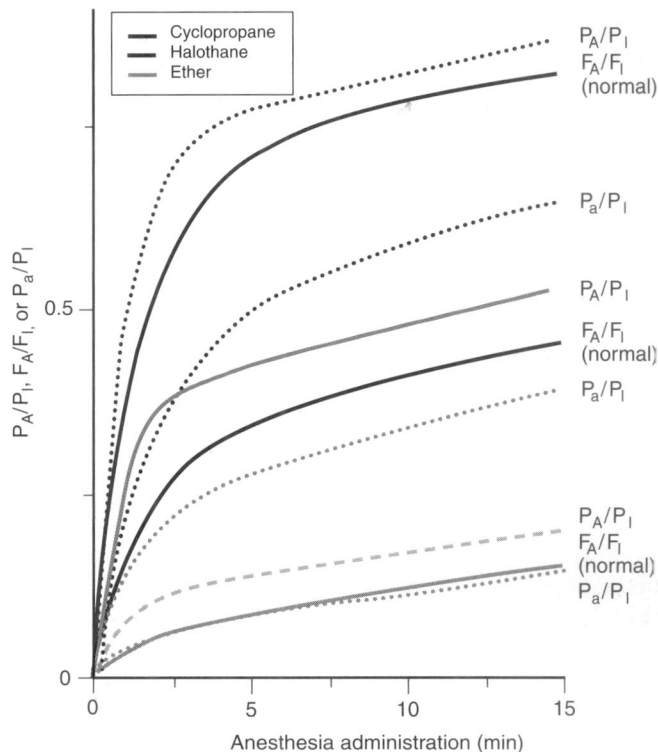

Figure 5–11 When no ventilation-perfusion abnormalities exist, the alveolar (PA) and arterial (Pa) anesthetic partial pressures rise together *(solid lines)* toward the inspired partial pressure (PI). When 50% of the cardiac output is shunted through the lungs, the rate of rise of the end-tidal partial pressure *(dashed lines)* is accelerated, and the rate of rise of the arterial partial pressure *(dotted or dashed lines)* is retarded. The greatest retardation occurs with the least soluble anesthetic, cyclopropane. FA/FI is the alveolar concentration of anesthetic/concentration of inspired anesthetic. (Adapted from Eger EI II, Severinghaus JW: Effect of uneven pulmonary distribution of blood and gas on induction with inhalation anesthetics. Anesthesiology 25:620-626, 1964.)

With highly soluble agents, a different situation results from the same ventilation-perfusion ratio abnormalities. In alveoli receiving more ventilation relative to perfusion, the anesthetic partial pressure increases nearly in proportion to the increase in ventilation (see Fig. 5-5 for effect with diethyl ether). Blood issuing from these alveoli has an increased anesthetic content almost proportional to the increased ventilation. Assuming that overall (total) ventilation remains normal, this increase in the anesthetic contained by blood from the relatively hyperventilated alveoli compensates for the lack of anesthetic uptake in unventilated alveoli.

These effects are illustrated in Figure 5-11 for endobronchial intubation. Direction of all ventilation to one lung produces hyperventilation relative to perfusion. FA/FI for this lung is slightly increased (above that obtained in the absence of endobronchial intubation) with the poorly soluble cyclopropane and greatly increased with the highly soluble ether. The increase with ether compensates for the absence of uptake from the unventilated lung, a compensation that is not available with cyclopropane. The result is that the cyclopropane arterial partial pressure is well below normal, whereas the ether arterial partial pressure is scarcely changed.

These concepts have been confirmed experimentally by comparing the rate of arterial anesthetic rise with

and without endobronchial intubation in dogs.[53] Endobronchial intubation significantly slowed the arterial rate of rise of cyclopropane but did not influence the rise with methoxyflurane. An intermediate result was obtained with halothane (Fig. 5-12). These data suggest that in the presence of ventilation-perfusion ratio abnormalities, the anesthetic effect of agents such as nitrous oxide, desflurane, and sevoflurane may be delayed more than the anesthetic effect of isoflurane or halothane.

EFFECT OF NITROUS OXIDE ON CLOSED GAS SPACES

Volume Changes in Highly Compliant Spaces

During nitrous oxide administration, appreciable volumes of nitrous oxide can move into closed gas spaces within the body. This transfer does not influence FA/FI but may have important functional consequences. There are two types of closed gas spaces in the body: those enclosed by

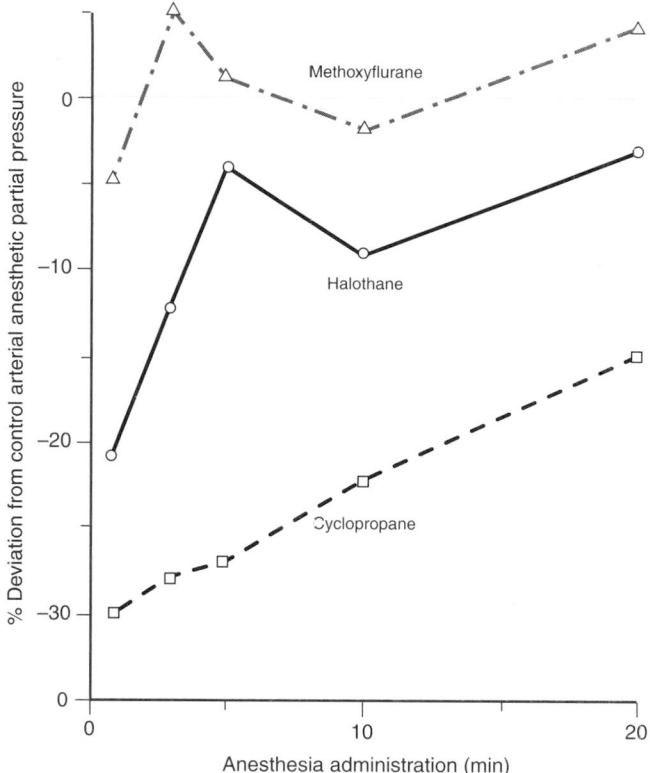

Figure 5–12 In dogs, when only the right lung was ventilated, the rise of the very soluble anesthetic methoxyflurane in arterial blood was normal (i.e., did not deviate from control), but the rise for the poorly soluble anesthetic cyclopropane was significantly slowed. (Adapted from Stoelting RK, Longnecker DE: Effect of right-to-left shunt on rate of increase in arterial anesthetic concentration. Anesthesiology 36:352-356, 1972.)

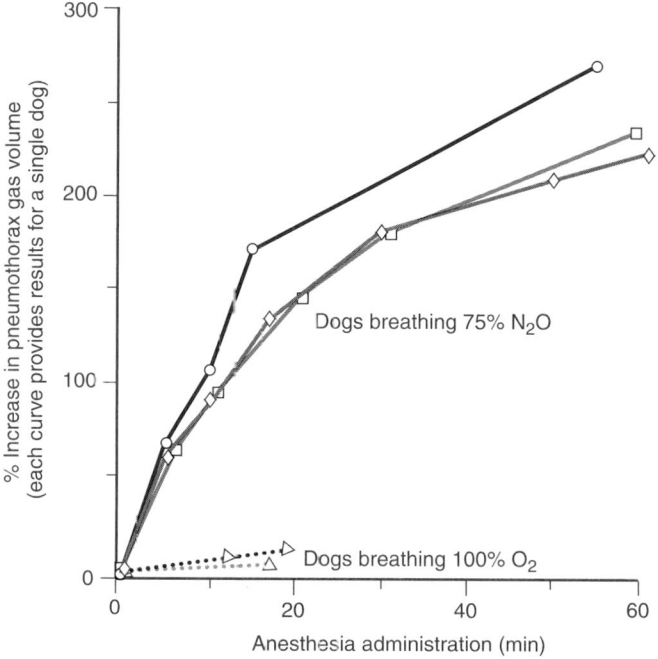

Figure 5–13 The volume of a pneumothorax created by air injection is affected little when oxygen subsequently is breathed (*lower two curves*). However, if 75% nitrous oxide is breathed, the volume doubles in 10 minutes and triples in 0.5 hour (*upper three curves*). (Adapted from Eger EI II, Saidman LJ: Hazards of nitrous oxide anesthesia in bowel obstruction and pneumothorax. Anesthesiology 26:61-66, 1965.)

compliant walls and those enclosed by noncompliant walls. The former (e.g., bowel gas, pneumothorax, or pneumoperitoneum) are subject to changes in volume secondary to the transfer of nitrous oxide into these spaces.[54] These spaces normally contain nitrogen (from air), a gas whose low solubility (blood-gas partition coefficient of 0.015) limits its removal by blood. The entrance of nitrous oxide (whose solubility permits it to be carried to the space in substantial quantities) is not countered by an equal loss, and the result is an increase in volume. The theoretical limit to the increase in volume is a function of the alveolar nitrous oxide concentration, because at equilibrium this concentration must be achieved in the closed gas space. The partial pressure of nitrous oxide in the closed gas space must equal its partial pressure in the alveoli. An alveolar concentration of 50% may double the volume of the gas space, and a 75% concentration may produce a fourfold increase.

These theoretical limits may be approached rapidly in patients with pneumothorax or gas emboli. Administration of 75% nitrous oxide in the presence of a pneumothorax may double the pneumothorax volume by 10 minutes and may triple it by 30 minutes[54] (Fig. 5-13). This increase in volume may seriously impair cardiorespiratory function,[55] and the use of nitrous oxide is contraindicated in the presence of a significant pneumothorax.

A still more rapid expansion of volume occurs if air inadvertently enters the bloodstream in a patient anesthetized with nitrous oxide. Expansion may be complete in seconds rather than minutes. Munson and Merrick[56] demonstrated that breathing nitrous oxide rather than air decreased the lethal volume of an air embolus in animals (Fig. 5-14). The difference could be entirely explained by expansion of the embolus in the animals breathing nitrous oxide (i.e., the predicted total volume of air plus nitrous oxide in the embolus equaled the volume of air needed to produce death in animals breathing only air). These studies suggest caution in the use of nitrous oxide for procedures in which air embolization is a risk (e.g., posterior fossa craniotomies, laparoscopy). They also suggest that nitrous oxide administration should be immediately discontinued if air embolization is suspected. Conversely, a nitrous oxide "challenge" may be used to test whether air embolization has occurred.[57]

The tracheal tube cuff normally is filled with air and is susceptible to expansion by nitrous oxide.[58] The presence of 75% nitrous oxide surrounding such a cuff can double or triple the volume of the cuff. This results from a more rapid diffusion of nitrous oxide than nitrogen across the cuff; the more rapid diffusion occurs because of the greater solubility of nitrous oxide. The result may be an unwanted increase in pressure exerted on the tracheal mucosa. Similarly, nitrous oxide may expand the cuffs of balloon-tipped (e.g., Swan-Ganz) catheters[59,60] when the balloons are inflated with air. The expansion is rapid, and a doubling of volume may occur within 10 minutes.

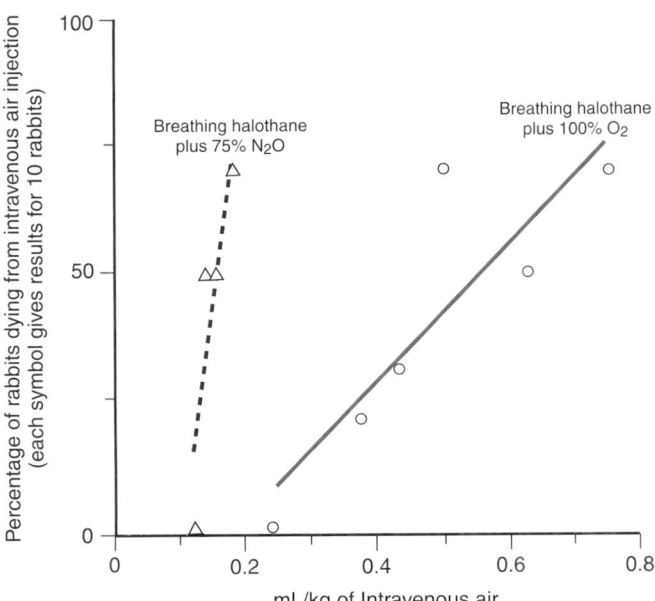

Figure 5–14 An air embolus equaling 0.55 mL/kg killed 50% of rabbits breathing oxygen. If the inspired gas mixture contained 75% nitrous oxide, only 0.16 mL/kg was required to kill one half of the animals. (Adapted from Munson ES, Merrick HC: Effect of nitrous oxide on venous air embolism. Anesthesiology 27:783-787, 1966.)

Pressure Changes in Poorly Compliant Spaces

The entrance of nitrous oxide into gas cavities surrounded by poorly compliant walls can increase the pressure on those walls. Nitrous oxide administration can impose unwanted increases in intraocular pressure after intravitreal sulfur hexafluoride injection.[61] Other examples include the gas space created by pneumoencephalography (now rare as a deliberate procedure) and the natural gas space in the middle ear. Pressures in the head or middle ear may rise by 20 to 50 mm Hg because of the ingress of nitrous oxide at a faster rate than air can be removed.[62,63] Recognition of this problem has decreased the use of nitrous oxide for tympanoplasty because the increased pressure may displace the graft. Increased middle ear pressure may adversely affect postoperative hearing.[64] The capacity of nitrous oxide to expand the gas in the middle ear has also been used to elevate an adherent atelectatic tympanic membrane off the promontory and the ossicles.[65]

ANESTHETIC CIRCUITRY

The previous discussion generally considered that the alveolar anesthetic concentration (F_A) was moving toward a constant inspired anesthetic concentration (F_I). In practice, the inspired concentration is usually not constant because a non-rebreathing system is not used. The rebreathing that results from the use of an anesthetic circuit causes the inspired concentration to be less than that in the gas delivered from the anesthetic machine. The inspired concentration is influenced by the delivered concentration, by the need to "wash in" the circuit, and by the depletion of anesthetic in rebreathed gases produced by uptake of anesthetic.

Washin of the Circuit

To begin anesthesia, the anesthetic must be washed into the volume of the circuit. At inflow rates of 0.5 to 8 L/min and a circuit volume of 7 L (i.e., 3-L bag, 2-L carbon dioxide absorber, and 2 L of corrugated hoses and fittings), the washin of the circuit is 50% to 100% complete in 10 minutes (Fig. 5-15). Higher inflow rates produce a more rapid rise in the inspired concentration, which suggests that induction can be accelerated and made more predictable by use of high inflow rates.

Anesthetic Loss to Plastic and Soda Lime

Uptake of anesthetic by several depots also may hinder the development of an adequate inspired anesthetic concentration. The rubber or plastic components of the circuit may remove agent,[66,67] and this was a significant problem with the obsolete anesthetic methoxyflurane, which has a high solubility in rubber and plastic (Table 5-3). A minor problem exists for halothane and isoflurane, and no problem results from the solution of nitrous oxide, desflurane, or sevoflurane.[68]

Normal (moist) carbon dioxide absorbents containing 13% to 15% water can slightly increase the sevoflurane and, to a lesser extent, halothane requirements by

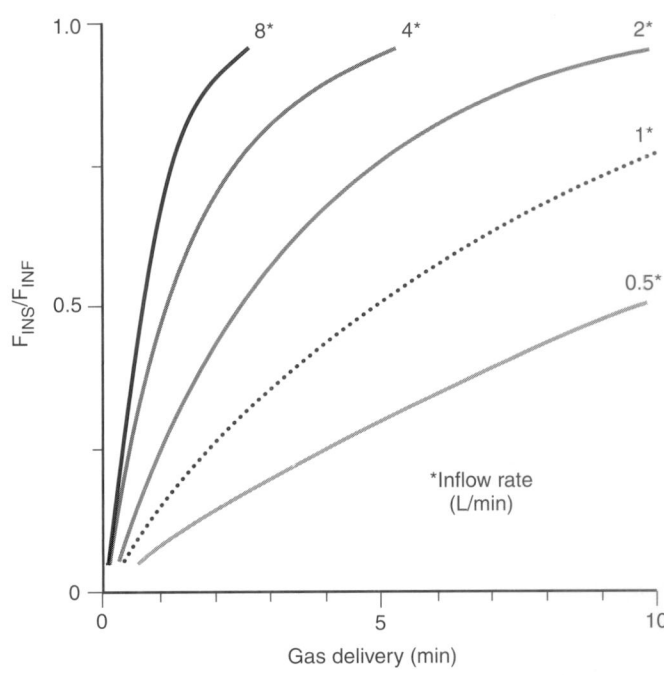

Figure 5–15 The rate at which the inspired anesthetic concentration (F_{INS}) rises toward the inflowing concentration (F_{INF}) is determined by the inflow rate and circuit volume. In the case illustrated, the circuit volume is 7 L. (Adapted from Eger EI II: Effect of anesthetic circuit on alveolar rate of rise. In Eger EI II [ed]: Anesthetic Uptake and Action. Baltimore, Williams & Wilkins, 1974, pp 192-205.)

Table 5–3   Rubber-gas and plastic-gas partition coefficients

Anesthetic	Polyethylene (Circuit Tube)	Rubber (Bag)	Polyvinyl Chloride (Endotracheal Tube)
Nitrous oxide	—	1.2	—
Desflurane	16	19	35
Sevoflurane	31	29	68
Isoflurane	58	49	114
Enflurane	—	74	—
Halothane	128	190	233
Methoxyflurane	118	742	—

Data from references 66, 67, 68, 100, and 101.

degrading each of these anesthetics.[69] Degradation results in the removal of hydrogen fluoride and the production of unsaturated compounds. Nitrous oxide, desflurane, and isoflurane are not materially degraded. For sevoflurane and halothane, degradation is of concern because the unsaturated compounds produced are toxic (e.g., compound A from sevoflurane is nephrotoxic if given for prolonged periods).[70,71]

In contrast to normal (moist) carbon dioxide absorbents, desiccated absorbents materially degrade all potent inhaled anesthetics.[72] Degradation of sevoflurane materially increases anesthetic requirement.[73] Dehydration of Baralyme increases compound A production from sevoflurane, but dehydration of soda lime does the opposite.[73] Desiccated absorbents degrade all anesthetics containing the CHF_2-O- moiety (i.e., desflurane, enflurane, and isoflurane) to carbon monoxide,[72] but degradation by soda lime is minimal at hydrations approximately one tenth of those found in normal soda lime (i.e., it only takes a little water to minimize degradation).

Effect of Rebreathing

Patients breathe two gases from the anesthetic circuit: those delivered from the anesthetic machine and those previously exhaled by the patient and subsequently rebreathed. Because the patient removes (takes up) anesthetic from the rebreathed gas, the amount taken up and the amount rebreathed influence the inspired anesthetic concentration. An increase in uptake or rebreathing lowers the inspired concentration of a highly soluble gas more than the inspired concentration of a poorly soluble gas. Decreasing rebreathing by increasing the inflow rate diminishes this effect of uptake. With a ventilation of 5 L/min, use of a 5-L/min inflow rate essentially abolishes rebreathing.[74]

High inflow rates (≥5 L/min) have the advantage of increasing the predictability of the inspired anesthetic concentration, but they have the disadvantages of being wasteful and of increasing atmospheric pollution. High inflow rates may be unacceptably costly because of the attendant greater consumption of expensive volatile anesthetics. High inflow rates also may result in drier inspired gas and greater difficulty in estimating ventilation from excursions of the rebreathing bag. These several disadvantages promote the use of low-flow techniques.

LOW-FLOW OR CLOSED-CIRCUIT TECHNIQUE

Much of the previous discussion assumed the use of a non-rebreathing system and a fixed inspired concentration of anesthetic. Although this approach does not invalidate the principles described earlier, it also does not reflect the variety of approaches applied in practice. Practice often deviates in two ways. Most anesthetists use lower inflow (fresh gas flow) rates to provide a more economical delivery of anesthesia, and most anesthetists apply a constant alveolar, rather than a constant inspired, concentration because a constant alveolar concentration reflects a constant level of anesthesia.

A low inflow rate results in several advantages and a few disadvantages, with the latter particularly applying to kinetics. The advantages of low inflow administration (i.e., fresh gas flows of less than one half of the minute volume, usually less than 2 L/min) or closed-circuit anesthesia (i.e., delivery of gases in amounts just sufficient to replace the gases—oxygen and anesthetic—removed by the patient) include lower cost, increased humidification, reduced heat loss, decreased release of anesthetic to the environment, and better capacity to assess physiologic variables, such as ventilation. On the debit side, there is more concern about oxygen levels (especially if nitrous oxide is used, but the patient also contributes nitrogen from stores in the body, and such nitrogen can slightly decrease the inspired concentration of oxygen), about increasing concentrations of carbon monoxide, and about rebreathing of toxic products from the breakdown of volatile anesthetics. Regarding this last point, carbon dioxide absorbents can degrade halothane and sevoflurane to toxic unsaturated compounds.[75,76] However, the debit of most immediate concern is the lack of control that low flows and, especially, closed circuits offer.

Closed-Circuit Anesthesia

The use of a closed circuit represents an extreme of anesthetic administration, one infrequently employed because few systems completely eliminate leakage of gas from the circuit. Anesthetists often apply a deliberate leak of approximately 200 mL/min by sampling gases for oxygen, carbon dioxide, and anesthetic analyses.

Usually, closed-circuit anesthesia requires replacement of three gases: oxygen, nitrous oxide, and a potent volatile anesthetic. Each replacement implies somewhat different considerations. Oxygen replacement remains constant unless metabolism changes as a consequence of sympathetic response to stimulation, alteration in body temperature, or shivering. Replacement of nitrous oxide follows a fairly predictable course, in part because the concentration applied does not usually vary. It is also the least soluble of anesthetics, especially in fat, and is the most prone to percutaneous loss (a constant value). Of most interest and potential variability are the uptakes of potent inhaled anesthetics.

Uptake of potent anesthetics may be estimated from the values (constants) obtained by Yasuda and colleagues[11,12] in humans. These values may be applied to obtain uptake at a constant alveolar concentration, such as at an alveolar concentration equal to the MAC. Figure 5-16 reveals parallel shapes for each anesthetic, shapes dictated by the perfusion and solvent characteristics of the three major tissue compartments plus intertissue diffusion. A large initial uptake rapidly decreases to a much lower level in 5 to 10 minutes, reflecting the high initial uptake by the VRG (because of its large perfusion) and the rapid decrease in uptake by the VRG imposed by a low capacity for anesthetics relative to perfusion. The subsequent slower decrease primarily results from the longer time to

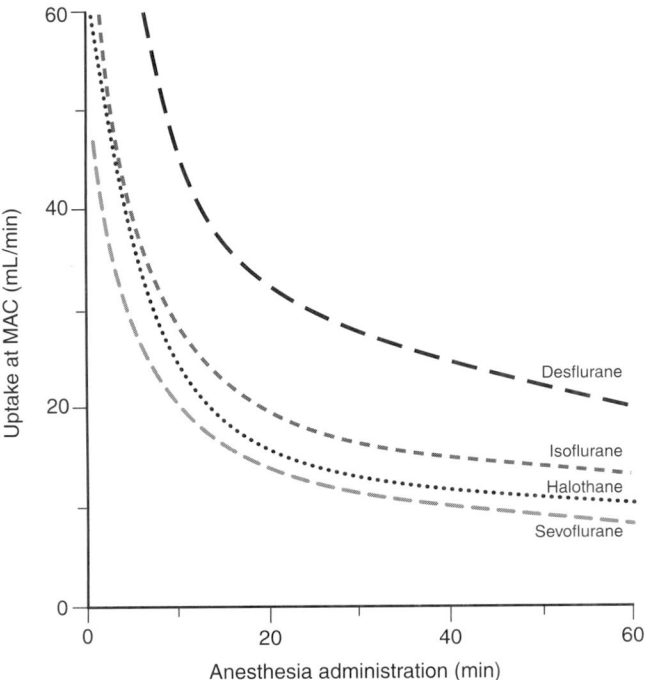

Figure 5–16 The uptake (in milliliters per minute) resulting from the application of the constants calculated by Yasuda and colleagues[11,12] from their measurements in human volunteers. The application assumes that the alveolar concentration equals the minimum alveolar concentration (MAC). Uptake is a function of MAC and solubility of the anesthetic in blood and tissues. The fivefold higher MAC for desflurane compared with isoflurane is offset by a threefold lower solubility, producing less than a twofold difference in uptake at any time. Uptake for all anesthetics initially declines rapidly as a function of the rate at which the vessel-rich tissue group equilibrates. Further decline after 5 to 10 minutes is a function of the approach to equilibration of the muscle group.

fill up the MG, until its uptake declines below that provided by the fourth compartment and FG.

Although the curves for each anesthetic do not differ in shape, they have different positions. The height of each curve (i.e., uptake) is directly proportional to two factors: solubility and MAC. Solubility and MAC tend to move inversely, and this minimizes differences in uptake among anesthetics. For example, although the MAC for desflurane is five times that for isoflurane, desflurane's uptake is less than twice that of isoflurane because of desflurane's lower solubility in both blood and tissues.

Uptake may be estimated from the *square-root-of-time rule*, first proposed by Severinghaus[77] and expanded greatly by Lowe and associates[78,79] in their classic descriptions of closed-circuit anesthesia. This rule states that uptake at any point in time may be estimated as uptake during the first minute of anesthesia divided by the square root of time in minutes. Making certain assumptions permits an estimate of uptake during the first minute. In general, uptake equals the product of blood solubility, cardiac output, and alveolar-to-venous anesthetic partial pressure difference. Several sources supply standard values for solubility and cardiac output, and the alveolar-to-venous anesthetic partial pressure difference may be estimated if we determine what alveolar partial pressure we wish and assume that venous anesthetic partial pressure is inconsequential. An inconsequential venous partial pressure is reasonable because no anesthetic can appear in venous blood before recirculation (about 0.5 minute), and even the anesthetic that appears is small because tissue uptake is maximal during the first minute. Isoflurane uptake in a normal adult can be estimated as $1.4 \times 5400 \times 0.0115$, or 87 mL; 1.4 is the blood-gas partition coefficient, 5400 is a reasonable cardiac output, and 0.0115 is the MAC as a fraction of one atmosphere (1 atm). By 4 minutes, uptake would equal 87 mL/2; by 9 minutes, 87 mL/3; and by 64 minutes, 87 mL/8.

Hendrickx and coworkers[80] questioned the accuracy of the square-root-of-time rule, suggesting that the rule overestimates the decrease in uptake with the passage of time. This matter continues to be debated,[81] but Hendrickx's argument probably is correct: the square-root-of-time rule (an empirical observation) probably provides an imperfect description of uptake.

Replacement of anesthetic taken up may be accomplished by infusion of liquid anesthetic directly into the anesthetic circuit, either continuously or as boluses. A continuous infusion requires a pump of some sort, and an elegant solution uses a computer to direct a progressive decrease in infusion rate as a function of time. Bolus injection from a syringe has a neat simplicity but has two disadvantages. The circuit concentration modestly oscillates, and the anesthetist is required to remember when and how much to inject. A further disadvantage accrues to the injection of desflurane by pump or syringe. The high vapor pressure of desflurane (about 1 atm at room temperature) results in the unpredictable formation of bubbles of desflurane gas and a potential for a marked variability in the rate of infusion or injection, especially when smaller volumes of liquid must be injected.

An alternative solution to injection of liquid applies a conventional vaporizer, one capable of accurate delivery of a range of concentrations at low inflow rates (e.g., 200 mL/min). This solution may not be applicable in the initial delivery of anesthesia, because the demand for vapor may exceed the capability of presently available vaporizers. For example, the maximum output of a conventional isoflurane vaporizer is 5%, and at a 200 mL/min flow of oxygen, only approximately 10 mL of isoflurane vapor can be produced per minute, far less than the 87 mL estimated earlier. Even after 1 hour of anesthesia, an isoflurane vaporizer is barely capable of meeting the demand for anesthetic (Fig. 5-17A). This difficulty may be overcome in several ways. If a concentration less than MAC is acceptable, less delivery of vapor is required. The concurrent use of nitrous oxide or an opioid decreases the demand on the vaporizer. The use of nitrous oxide also requires an increased total fresh gas flow to compensate for the considerable uptake of nitrous oxide. If the fresh gas flow increases to 1500 mL/min, 79 mL of isoflurane vapor can be produced. Another solution is to select an anesthetic having a vaporizer capability closer to demand. Such a solution tends to be available for less soluble anesthetics. For example, we calculate the uptake for desflurane in the first minute of anesthesia to be

$0.45 \times 5400 \times 0.06$, or 146 mL. At a 200-mL/min flow of oxygen, the 18% maximum output of a desflurane vaporizer permits delivery of 44 mL. Although still inadequate to meet demand in the first minute, this figure is 2.6 times closer to meeting that demand than the isoflurane vaporizer, and within 10 minutes, the desflurane vaporizer can supply the required volume (see Fig. 5-17A).

Figure 5-17A suggests one of the major difficulties associated with the closed-circuit approach: control. There is an enormous difference between delivered (i.e., vaporizer dial) and alveolar concentrations. The difference decreases with decreasing anesthetic solubility, but even with an anesthetic such as desflurane and even after the initial high-uptake period is passed, the dialed concentration markedly exceeds the alveolar concentration that it sustains. This means that changes in uptake (e.g., from the increase in cardiac output that may result from surgical stimulation) can cause considerable alterations in alveolar concentration unless the delivered concentration is altered. The alveolar concentration changes for two reasons. First, assuming a constant ventilation, the difference between the alveolar and inspired concentrations varies directly with uptake (e.g., a greater uptake

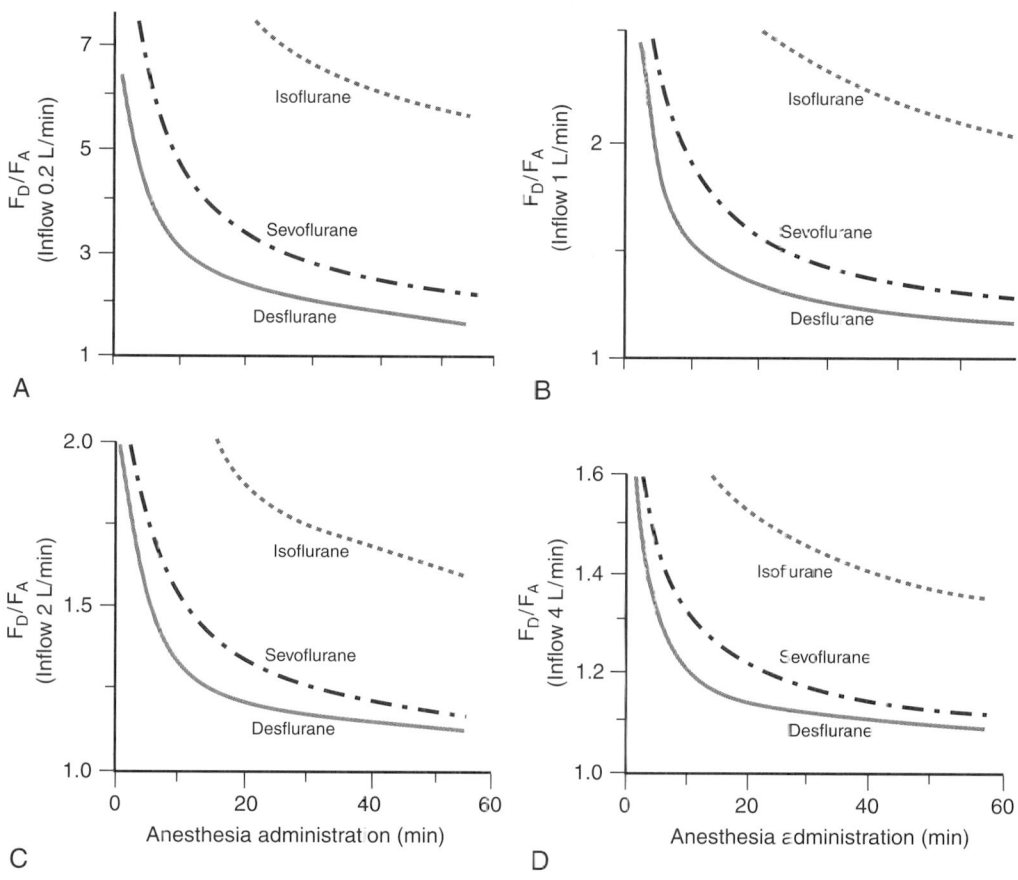

Figure 5–17 The ratio of delivered to alveolar concentrations (F_D/F_A) required to sustain the alveolar concentration constant at, for example, the MAC, is a function of several factors. First, it is determined by uptake (see Fig. 5-16). Second, it is determined by rebreathing. The ratio therefore decreases with increasing inflow rates (**A** to **D**). Although these graphs have the same shape, notice the progressive decrease in the scale on the ordinate as inflow rate increases. The lowest values for any anesthetic result from a non-rebreathing system (i.e., when the inflow rate equals minute ventilation).

increases the difference). Second, because of the rebreathing, the inspired concentration varies inversely with the uptake (e.g., an increased uptake lowers the inspired concentration). The sum of these effects decreases or increases the alveolar concentration. A closed circuit has an inherent element of instability not present in an open circuit.

Low-Flow Anesthetic Delivery

Low-flow anesthetic delivery produces more stability than closed-circuit delivery. Low-flow delivery can provide most of the advantages of closed systems, decreasing instability, while retaining considerable advantages over open systems in economy, maintenance of humidification and temperature, and atmospheric pollution. Relative to closed-circuit delivery, low-flow delivery produces a constancy of oxygen and anesthetic levels and provides greater elimination of carbon monoxide and toxic anesthetic breakdown products.

In a low-flow delivery system, two factors control the relationship between the concentration delivered from a vaporizer (F_D) and that in the alveoli (F_A), a relationship that may best be described by the ratio (F_D/F_A) of the two variables. First, we have already seen that uptake governs this ratio in a closed system (see Fig. 5-17A). F_D/F_A is higher for more soluble anesthetics, and regardless of solubility, the ratio is highest early in anesthetic administration and decreases rapidly in the first 5 to 10 minutes of anesthesia (as uptake by the VRG of tissues decreases to the point of near-equilibration) and more slowly thereafter (as uptake by MG, FG, and the fourth compartment decreases).

Second, inflow rate also governs F_D/F_A. The relationship is inverse: The higher the inflow rate, the lower is the ratio (compare Fig. 5-17B to D with Fig. 5-17A and notice the large scaling differences associated with increasing inflow rate). An increase in inflow rate decreases F_D/F_A by decreasing rebreathing. Rebreathing is important because uptake of anesthetic depletes the anesthetic concentration in rebreathed gases, and the concentration in F_D must be sufficient to compensate for this depletion. The higher the inflow rate, the less compensation is required because rebreathing is reduced.

However, increases in inflow rate do not proportionally decrease F_D/F_A (see Fig. 5-17A to D). The greatest reduction in F_D/F_A comes with only modest increases in inflow rate. A large decrease occurs when the inflow rate is changed from that needed for a closed circuit to an inflow rate of 1 L/min, whereas only a small decrease occurs when the inflow rate is increased from 2 to 4 L/min. After the inflow rate exceeds minute ventilation (i.e., a non-rebreathing system exists), further increases in inflow rate have no effect on F_D/F_A, and F_D/F_A is the same as the ratio of F_I to F_D (i.e., $F_D/F_A = F_I/F_A$).

I use the term *anesthetic tether* as a metaphor for the F_D/F_A ratio.[82] A large ratio equates to a long tether, one permitting considerable freedom or variability in the alveolar concentration. With a long tether, changes in uptake caused by changes in physiologic variables (e.g., an increase in cardiac output consequent to surgical stimulation) can appreciably alter the alveolar concentration

and the level of anesthesia. In the example just cited, there is positive feedback because, by increasing uptake, surgical stimulation decreases the alveolar concentration and thereby increases the perception of that stimulation. Most anesthetists prefer a short anesthetic tether because a short tether provides a tighter control over the level of anesthesia. The use of less soluble anesthetics and higher inflow rates shortens the tether.

Another benefit to a short tether accrues to the anesthetist who does not use an agent-specific analyzer. In the absence of such an analyzer, some anesthetists rely on the dial setting of the vaporizer to indicate the concentration of anesthetic in the patient's lungs (i.e., assume that F_D equals F_A). The vaporizer setting may correlate poorly with the concentration in the lungs under three circumstances: early in anesthesia for all agents, later in anesthesia for closed circuits or very low inflow rates, and later in anesthesia for more soluble agents, such as isoflurane, even at higher inflow rates. The vaporizer setting may correlate well with poorly soluble anesthetics such as sevoflurane and desflurane 30 to 60 minutes after the inception of anesthetic administration. At this time, the delivered concentration from the vaporizer may be less than 20% greater than that in the alveoli (i.e., the F_D/F_A ratio is 1.2), even at inflow rates of 1 to 2 L/min (see Fig. 5-17B and C).

Economic concerns increasingly dictate the practice of anesthesia, and anesthesiologists may wish to appreciate the differences in anesthetic consumption as a function of the choice of inflow rate, the duration of anesthesia, and the choice of anesthetic. The reports by Yasuda and associates[11,12] provide constants that can be used to estimate the uptake of commonly available potent inhaled anesthetics. By using the gas laws and published values for specific gravities, the values for uptake of vapor may be converted to milliliters of liquid taken up. Combining this information with a knowledge of the function of circuit rebreathing systems[74] allows an estimate of the amounts of liquid in milliliters that must be delivered at various inflow rates to provide a constant alveolar concentration equal to the MAC[83] (Table 5-4). The relative costs of anesthesia may be estimated by applying the price of the anesthetic of interest to the number of milliliters needed to sustain anesthesia.

If economy and a low F_D/F_A ratio are desirable, the aforementioned considerations suggest that a good compromise is the use of a low-flow delivery system after an initial period of higher flows. Higher flows (4 to 6 L/min) may be applied early in anesthesia (i.e., at the times of highest uptake) and then decreased progressively as uptake decreases. Flows of 2 to 4 L/min might be given for the period from 5 to 15 minutes after inducing anesthesia, and flows of 1 L/min may be given thereafter. If the average inflow rate were 1 L/min, 1 hour of anesthesia with the four potent anesthetics listed in Table 5-4 would require administration of 6.5 (halothane) to 26.1 (desflurane) mL of liquid. This fourfold range of values is smaller than the eightfold range of potency (MAC) values because the amount of anesthetic delivered must account for more than potency. The amount delivered also must compensate for uptake and losses of anesthetic through the overflow valve. The relatively smaller uptake and

Table 5–4 Milliliters of liquid anesthetic at various inflow rates needed to sustain an alveolar concentration equal to MAC

Anesthetic	Anesthetic Duration (min)	Inflow Rate (Not Including Anesthetic)				
		0.2 L/min	1.0 L/min	2.0 L/min	4.0 L/min	6.0 L/min
Halothane	30	3.0	4.1	5.4	8.0	10.5
	60	4.6	6.5	9.0	13.9	18.8
Isoflurane	30	4.0	5.8	8.0	12.3	16.7
	60	6.3	9.6	13.9	22.3	30.7
Sevoflurane	30	3.3	6.3	10.1	17.6	25.2
	60	4.9	10.9	18.2	33.0	47.8
Desflurane	30	6.7	14.8	25.0	45.2	65.4
	60	10.1	26.1	46.0	85.8	126

Modified from Weiskopf RB, Eger EI II: Comparing the costs of inhaled anesthetics. Anesthesiology 79:1413-1418, 1993.

losses of the less soluble desflurane and sevoflurane are what account for the reduction from eightfold to fourfold. An even smaller range is found at lower inflow rates, decreasing to about twofold for a closed circuit. However, such flows should not be used with sevoflurane because of the greater concentrations of compound A that result.

RECOVERY FROM ANESTHESIA

General Principles

Many factors that govern the rate at which the alveolar anesthetic concentration rises on induction apply to recovery. The immediate decline in the alveolar anesthetic concentration is extremely rapid because the washout of the functional residual capacity by ventilation is as rapid as the washin. Only 2 minutes is required to eliminate 95% to 98% of nitrogen from the lungs when pure oxygen is breathed or to restore the nitrogen concentration when room air is breathed on recovery.

As ventilation sweeps anesthetic from the alveoli during recovery, an anesthetic partial pressure gradient develops between the partial pressure in the returning venous blood and the partial pressure in the alveoli. This gradient drives anesthetic into the alveoli, thereby opposing the tendency of ventilation to lower the alveolar concentration. The solubility of the anesthetic determines part of the capacity of the venous to alveolar gradient to oppose the tendency of ventilation to decrease the alveolar anesthetic partial pressure. A more soluble agent, such as isoflurane (Fig. 5-18C), opposes the elimination produced by ventilation more effectively than does a poorly soluble agent, such as desflurane (see Fig. 5-18A), because a greater reserve exists in blood for the more soluble agent. For a given duration of anesthesia, more isoflurane is available at a given partial pressure for transfer to the alveoli. The fall in the alveolar partial pressure of isoflurane is slower than the fall with sevoflurane, which is less rapid than the fall with desflurane. The rate at which recovery occurs is similarly affected. It is most rapid with desflurane, less rapid with sevoflurane,

and slowest with isoflurane. The rapidity of recovery largely depends on the solubility of the anesthetic.[84]

Differences between Induction and Recovery

Recovery differs from induction in three crucial ways. First, on induction, the effect of solubility to hinder the rise in alveolar anesthetic concentration can be overcome by increasing the inspired anesthetic concentration (i.e., by applying overpressure). No such luxury is available during recovery; the inspired concentration cannot be reduced below zero. Second, on induction, all tissues initially have the same anesthetic partial pressure: zero. On recovery, the tissue partial pressures vary. The VRG has a pressure that usually equals that required for anesthesia; the VRG has come to equilibrium with the alveolar anesthetic partial pressure. The MG may or may not have the same partial pressure as that found in the alveoli. A longer anesthesia duration (2 to 4 hours) may permit equilibrium, but a shorter case would not. The high capacity of fat for all anesthetics except nitrous oxide precludes equilibration of the FG with the alveolar anesthetic partial pressure with hours or even days of anesthesia.

If the muscle and fat have not equilibrated with the alveolar anesthetic partial pressure, these tissues initially cannot contribute to the transfer of anesthetic back to the lungs. As long as an anesthetic partial pressure gradient exists between arterial blood and tissue, the tissue will continue to take up anesthetic. For the first several hours of recovery from halothane anesthesia, fat continues to take up halothane, and by so doing, it accelerates the rate of recovery. Only after the alveolar (which equals arterial) anesthetic partial pressure falls below that in a tissue can the tissue contribute anesthetic to the alveoli.

The failure of several tissues to reach equilibration with the alveolar anesthetic partial pressure means that the rate of decrease of alveolar anesthetic on recovery is more rapid than its rate of increase on induction and that recovery depends in part on the duration of anesthesia[85,86] (see Fig. 5-18). A longer anesthesia duration puts more anesthetic into the slowly filling muscle and fat depots. These reservoirs can supply more anesthetic to the blood returning to the lungs when they are filled

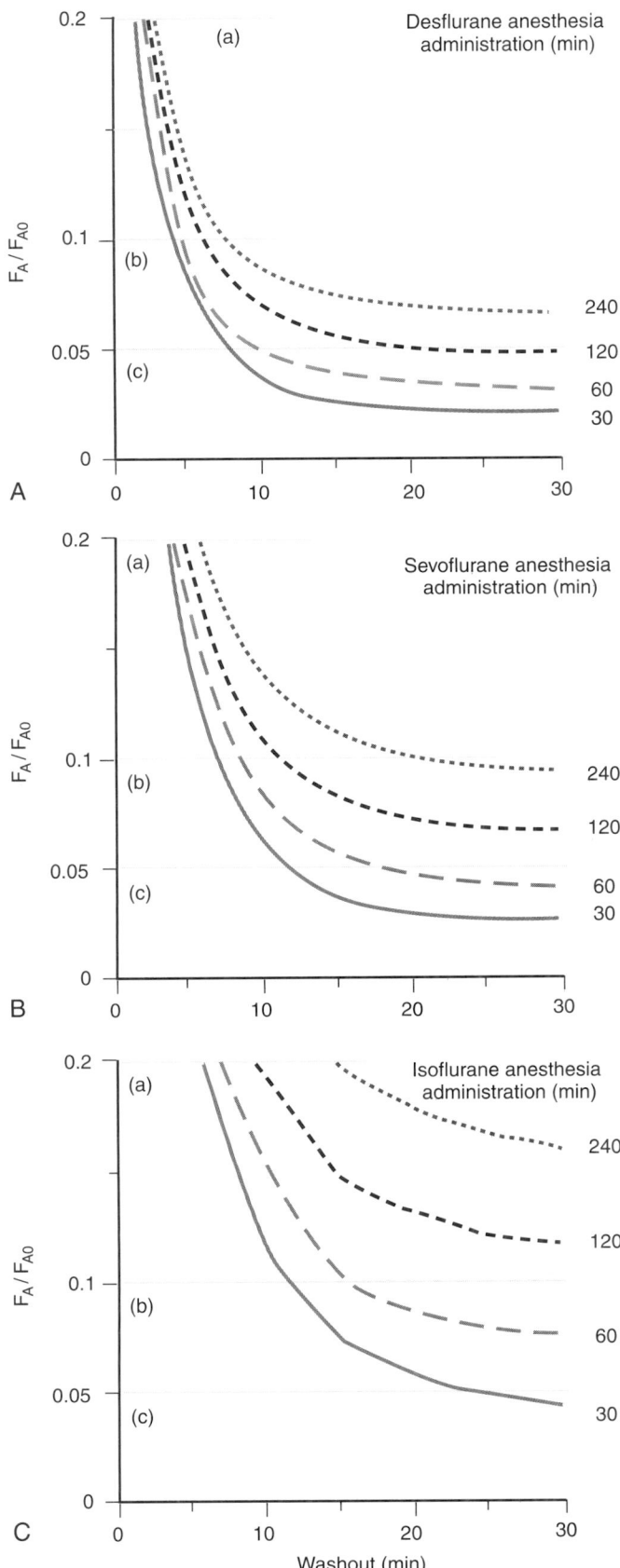

than when they are empty and thereby can prolong the time to recovery.[84]

Solubility influences the effect of duration of anesthesia on the rate at which the alveolar anesthetic partial pressure declines.[86] The decline of the partial pressure of a poorly soluble agent such as desflurane is rapid in any case, and the acceleration imparted by a less than complete tissue equilibration minimally alters the rate of recovery. The approach to equilibration becomes more important with sevoflurane and even more important with isoflurane (see Fig. 5-18). Recovery may be rapid after a short isoflurane anesthetic but may be slow after a prolonged anesthetic. The recovery from anesthesia with desflurane and sevoflurane is quicker than with more soluble agents, such as isoflurane and halothane.[84]

The importance of solubility and of duration of anesthesia to the rate of recovery may be appreciated by the use of context-dependent times to reach particular levels of washout.[87] Regardless of the duration of anesthesia, the alveolar concentrations of poorly soluble anesthetics (e.g., nitrous oxide, desflurane, sevoflurane) and moderately soluble anesthetics (e.g., isoflurane, halothane) decrease by 50% in roughly the same period. If recovery were reached at a 50% decrease, the choice of anesthetic would matter little to the time to recovery from anesthesia. The impact of anesthetic solubility and duration becomes evident if greater levels of washout are required to achieve recovery. If 80% washout is required, increasing duration of anesthesia markedly affects recovery from isoflurane but little affects recovery from desflurane and sevoflurane; notice the differences in concentration intersecting the horizontal line at F_A/F_{A0} of 0.2, as in line (a) in Figure 5-18A, B, and C. If 90% washout is required, as illustrated by F_A/F_{A0} of 0.1 in line (b), or 95% washout is required, as illustrated by F_A/F_{A0} of 0.05 in line (c), increasing duration of anesthesia affects the more soluble anesthetics much more than less soluble anesthetics. After 2, 4, or 8 hours of anesthesia with 1.25 MAC of sevoflurane compared with desflurane, initial (Fig. 5-19) and later (Fig. 5-20) recovery is nearly twice as rapid with desflurane, and the difference between the recovery times appears to increase with increasing duration of anesthesia.[32]

Figure 5–18 Both solubility and duration of anesthesia affect the fall of the alveolar concentration (F$_A$) from its value immediately preceding the cessation of anesthetic administration (F$_{A0}$). A longer anesthetic slows the fall, as does a greater solubility, and the effects are shown for the increasingly soluble desflurane, sevoflurane, and isoflurane (**A** to **C**). The horizontal lines designated (a), (b), and (c) indicate 80%, 90%, and 95% decreases, respectively, in the alveolar concentration from the concentration at the end of anesthesia. (Data from Yasuda N, Lockhart SH, Eger EI II, et al: Kinetics of desflurane, isoflurane, and halothane in humans. Anesthesiology 74:489-498, 1991, and from Yasuda N, Lockhart SH, Eger EI II, et al: Comparison of kinetics of sevoflurane and isoflurane in humans. Anesth Analg 72:316-324, 1991.)

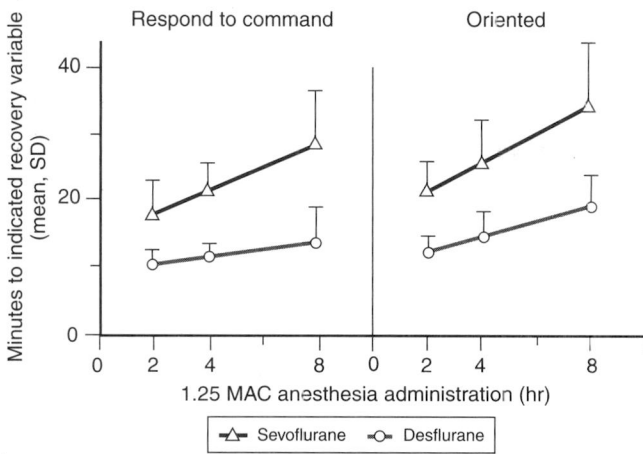

Figure 5–19 Different times to awakening occur after 2, 4, or 8 hours of anesthesia at a 1.25 minimum alveolar concentration (MAC) for desflurane compared with sevoflurane. Awakening to response to command or to orientation is almost twice as rapid after anesthesia with the less soluble desflurane. (Adapted from Eger EI II, Gong D, Koblin DD, et al: Effect of anesthetic duration on kinetic and recovery characteristics of desflurane vs. sevoflurane (plus compound A) in volunteers. Anesth Analg 86:414-421, 1998.)

The third factor affecting recovery is pharmacodynamic rather than kinetic. Anesthesia requires the provision of immobility. If this is accomplished with an inhaled anesthetic, this means that the anesthetist seeks a concentration exceeding MAC. However, recovery sets a different goal: awakening. One measure of this is the return of the capacity to respond to command. *MACawake*, the concentration of anesthetic allowing appropriate

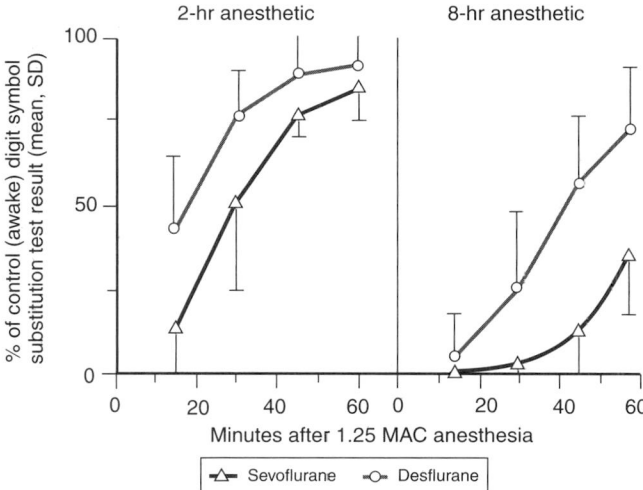

Figure 5–20 The differential suggested by Figure 5-19 extends to measures of more subtle degrees of awakening, such as the digit symbol substitution test (DSST), a measure of judgment and cognition. Notice that there appears to be a greater spread between the results after 2 versus 8 hours of anesthesia. MAC is the minimum alveolar concentration. (Adapted from Eger EI II, Gong D, Koblin DD, et al: Effect of anesthetic duration on kinetic and recovery characteristics of desflurane vs. sevoflurane (plus compound A) in volunteers. Anesth Analg 86:414-421, 1998.)

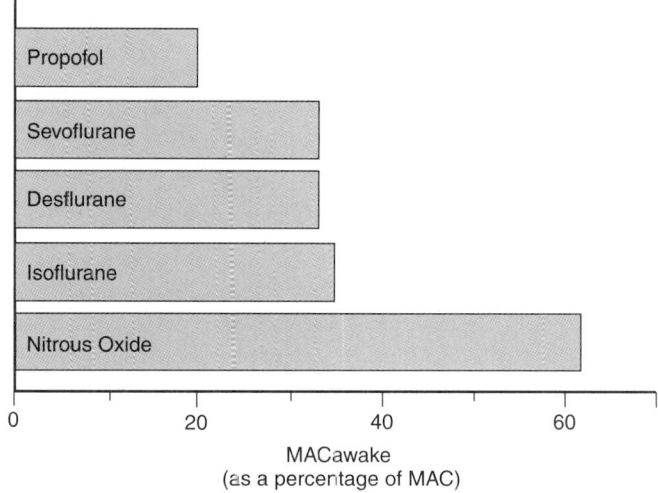

Figure 5–21 As a fraction of the minimum alveolar concentration (MAC), MACawake is greatest for nitrous oxide[89]; less for desflurane,[92] isoflurane,[89] and sevoflurane[90,91]; and least for propofol.[92]

response to command in 50% of subjects,[88] varies among different anesthetics (Fig. 5-21). As a fraction of MAC, the MACawake of nitrous oxide exceeds that for the potent inhaled anesthetics commonly used.[89-91] The MACawake value of propofol is less than that of potent inhaled anesthetics.[92] A lower MACawake value correlates with a greater capacity to provide amnesia; propofol is most potent, and nitrous oxide is least potent. However, a high MACawake means that awakening will be at a higher anesthetic concentration relative to that required for anesthesia. All other factors being equal, awakening from nitrous oxide anesthesia is more rapid than awakening from anesthesia with desflurane or sevoflurane. This argues for the continued use of nitrous oxide.

Can I Have My Cake and Eat It Too?

The less soluble, newer inhaled anesthetics desflurane and sevoflurane offer a more rapid recovery from anesthesia than more soluble older agents, such as isoflurane. However, this rapid recovery comes at a price: The new anesthetics are more expensive. Is it possible to have the best of both worlds by using isoflurane for most of anesthesia, reserving desflurane (or sevoflurane) for the final minutes? Could such an approach provide the economy of isoflurane and the rapid recovery of desflurane? Neumann and colleagues[93] tested this premise. Volunteers were anesthetized for 2 hours on three occasions: once with 1.25 MAC of isoflurane; once with 1.25 MAC of desflurane; and once with 1.5 hours of 1.25 MAC of isoflurane, followed by 0.5 hour of a combination of desflurane and isoflurane (i.e., crossover approach). The combination provided a total of 1.25 MAC (i.e., desflurane was added as the isoflurane was eliminated, with the addition being sufficient to sustain a total of 1.25 MAC). To ensure economy, all anesthetics were delivered at a 2 L/min inflow rate.

Contrary to the premise, recovery after the crossover was no faster than recovery after isoflurane alone (Fig. 5-22).

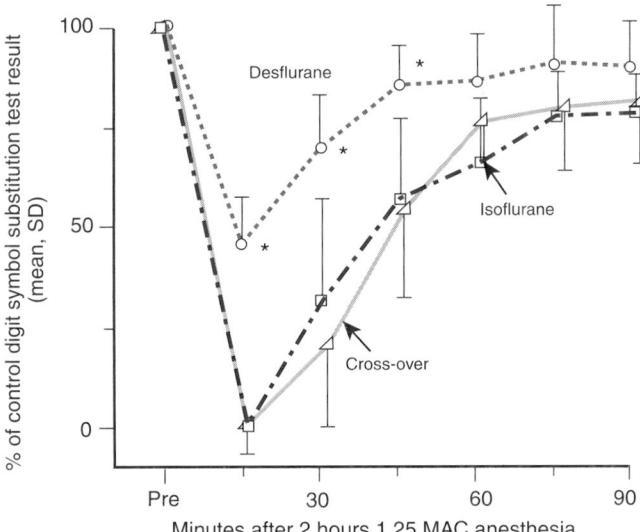

Figure 5–22 Volunteers were anesthetized for 2 hours on three occasions: once with 1.25 minimum alveolar concentration (MAC) of isoflurane; once with 1.25 MAC of desflurane; and once with 1.5 hours of 1.25 MAC isoflurane, followed by 0.5 hour of a combination of desflurane and isoflurane (i.e., crossover administration). The combination provided a total of 1.25 MAC (i.e., desflurane was added as the isoflurane was eliminated, with the addition being sufficient to sustain a total of 1.25 MAC). All anesthetics were delivered at a 2-L/min inflow rate. At the end of 2 hours, anesthetic administration was discontinued and a non-rebreathing system applied. The digit symbol substitution test (DSST) was applied at 15-minute intervals, and the results are displayed as a percentage of the control (preanesthesia) results. Recovery of judgment and cognition as defined by the DSST was more rapid at 15, 30, and 45 minutes with desflurane given alone (*asterisks* indicate significant differences from isoflurane or crossover results). (Data from Neumann MA, Weiskopf RB, Gong DH, et al: Changing from isoflurane to desflurane towards the end of anesthesia does not accelerate recovery in humans. Anesthesiology 88:914-921, 1998.)

Recovery after desflurane alone was considerably faster than recovery after either isoflurane or the crossover from isoflurane to desflurane.

Impact of Metabolism

Saturation of the enzymes responsible for the metabolism of anesthetics may limit the ability of metabolism to significantly alter the rate at which the alveolar anesthetic partial pressure rises. This limitation does not exist on recovery, and metabolism may be an important determinant of the rate at which the alveolar anesthetic partial pressure declines. The importance of metabolism to recovery is implied by results from Munson and coworkers,[51] who showed that the alveolar washout of halothane is more rapid than that of the less soluble enflurane, a result later confirmed by Carpenter and associates.[26,28] This agrees with the relative ease with which these two agents are metabolized: 15% to 20% of the halothane taken up during the course of an ordinary anesthetic can be recovered as urinary metabolites,[94] whereas only 2% to 3% of enflurane can similarly be recovered.[95] Halothane has two

major routes of elimination: ventilation and hepatic metabolism. Enflurane elimination depends primarily on ventilation, which explains why Munson and colleagues[51] found a more rapid fall in alveolar halothane. These results also apply to desflurane, isoflurane, and sevoflurane. Metabolism of desflurane and isoflurane is too small to accelerate their elimination, but metabolism of sevoflurane is sufficient to narrow the difference between its washout and that of desflurane.[32]

Diffusion Hypoxia

The uptake of large volumes of nitrous oxide on induction of anesthesia gives rise to the concentration effect and the second gas effect. On recovery from anesthesia, the outpouring of large volumes of nitrous oxide can produce what Fink[96] called *diffusion anoxia*. These volumes may cause hypoxia (Fig. 5-23) in two ways. First, they may directly affect oxygenation by displacing oxygen.[96-98] Second, by diluting alveolar carbon dioxide, they may decrease respiratory drive and ventilation.[98] Both of these effects require the release of large volumes of nitrous oxide into the alveoli. Because large volumes of nitrous oxide are released only during the first 5 to 10 minutes of recovery, this is the period of greatest concern. The concern is enhanced by the fact that the first 5 to 10 minutes of recovery also may be the time of greatest respiratory depression. For these reasons, many anesthetists administer 100% oxygen for the first 5 to 10 minutes of recovery. This procedure may be particularly indicated in patients with preexisting lung disease or in those in whom postoperative respiratory depression is anticipated (e.g., after a nitrous oxide-narcotic anesthetic).

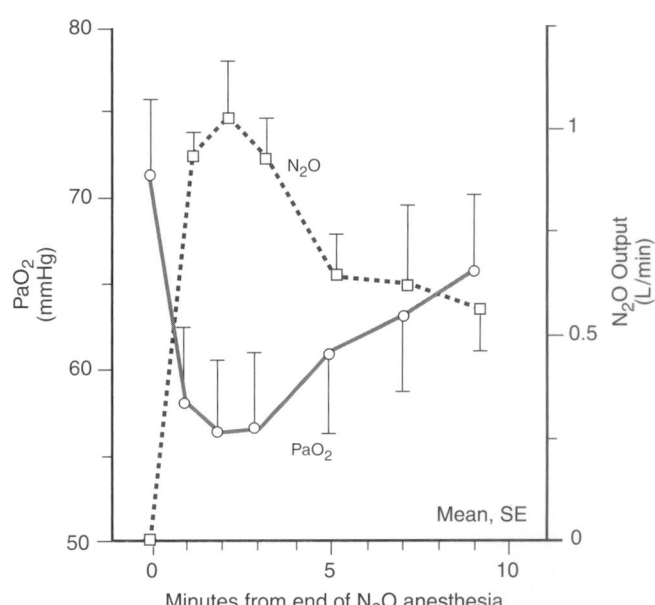

Figure 5–23 At time zero, the inspired gas was changed from 21% oxygen/79% nitrous oxide to 21% oxygen/79% nitrogen. Arterial oxygen subsequently fell in association with the outpouring of nitrous oxide. (Adapted from Sheffer L, Steffenson JL, Birch AA: Nitrous oxide–induced diffusion hypoxia in patients breathing spontaneously. Anesthesiology 37:436-439, 1972.)

Impact of the Anesthetic Circuit

The anesthetic circuit may limit the rate of recovery, just as it limits induction. If the patient is not disconnected from the circuit on cessation of anesthetic delivery, the patient may continue to inspire anesthetic. To reduce the inspired level to zero or almost zero, several factors must be taken into account. The anesthetic within the circuit must be washed out. The rubber or plastic components of the circuit and the soda lime within the circuit have absorbed anesthetic (see Table 5-3) that can be released back into the gas phase,[66] and this anesthetic also must be washed out. The patient's exhaled air contains anesthetic that cannot be rebreathed if the inspired anesthetic concentration is to approach zero. The effect of each of these factors to raise the inspired anesthetic concentration can be overcome by the use of high inflow rates of oxygen (≥ 5 L/min).

KEY POINTS

1. If unopposed, ventilation produces a rapid change (in and out) of gases in the lungs.
2. When the delivered concentration of anesthetic is small (<10%), uptake opposes the effect of ventilation to quickly change the alveolar concentration of anesthetic, and the relationship between the inspired (F_I) and the alveolar (F_A) anesthetic concentrations (i.e., the F_A/F_I ratio) is simple. If uptake removes 80% of the anesthetic delivered by ventilation, the F_A/F_I ratio is 0.2.
3. Uptake from the lungs is the product of three factors: blood solubility, cardiac output, and the partial pressure driving anesthetic from one phase (e.g., lung) into a second phase (e.g., venous blood).
4. Blood solubility (i.e., blood-gas partition coefficient) differs greatly among anesthetics, and solubility is a primary factor that determines the F_A/F_I ratio and clinically relevant issues such as the rates of induction of and recovery from anesthesia: lower solubility, faster recovery.
5. Three tissue groups form depots for anesthetic within the body: the vessel-rich group (VRG), the muscle group (MG), and the fat group (FG). Having the greatest perfusion and limited solubility, the VRG equilibrates rapidly (about 8 minutes). Having a lower perfusion, the MG equilibrates more slowly. Having an enormous capacity (i.e., solubility), the FG equilibrates slowest. The differences in perfusion and equilibration determine the shape of the F_A/F_I ratio.
6. The inspired inhaled anesthetic concentration also determines the rate of rise of the alveolar concentration toward the concentration inspired (i.e., F_A/F_I ratio). The greater the inspired concentration, the more rapid is the rise in the F_A/F_I ratio (i.e., the less the impact of uptake). This is called the *concentration effect*.
7. The concentration effect results from two factors: a concentrating of residual gases and an increase in inspired ventilation. These two factors equally affect other gases given concurrently (i.e., second gas effect).
8. Anesthetic metabolism and intertissue diffusion of anesthetics also influence uptake. Metabolism is minimal for desflurane and isoflurane, modest for sevoflurane, and substantial for halothane.
9. Changes in physiologic variables (e.g., ventilation, circulation, distribution of circulation, ventilation-perfusion abnormalities) influence the F_A/F_I ratio, and the magnitude of this influence is usually governed by solubility.
10. Nitrous oxide presents unique kinetic problems. It increases the volume or pressure within gas-containing spaces in the body.
11. Low fresh gas inflow rates have increasingly become the norm because of the economy associated with their use. They also provide advantages of decreased pollution, heat conservation, and increased humidification. They can, however, increase rebreathing of potentially toxic degradation products.
12. Through rebreathing, anesthetic circuits can exaggerate the impact of differences in solubility on the rate of rise (i.e., F_A/F_I ratio) and required delivered concentration of inhaled anesthetics. Least affected are the least soluble anesthetics.

REFERENCES

1. Eger EI II: Uptake of inhaled anesthetics: The alveolar to inspired anesthetic difference. *In* Eger EI II: Anesthetic Uptake and Action. Baltimore, Williams & Wilkins, 1974, pp 77-96.
2. Eger EI II: Partition coefficients of I-653 in human blood, saline, and olive oil. Anesth Analg 66:971-973, 1987.
3. Eger RR, Eger EI II: Effect of temperature and age on the solubility of enflurane, halothane, isoflurane and methoxyflurane in human blood. Anesth Analg 64:640-642, 1985.
4. Eger EI II, Shargel RO, Merkel G: Solubility of diethyl ether in water, blood and oil. Anesthesiology 24:676-678, 1963.
5. Eger EI II, Shargel R: The solubility of methoxyflurane in human blood and tissue homogenates. Anesthesiology 24:625-627, 1963.
6. Cromwell TH, Eger EI II, Stevens WC, Dolan WM: Forane uptake, excretion and blood solubility in man. Anesthesiology 35:401-408, 1971.
7. Yasuda N, Targ AG, Eger EI II: Solubility of I-653, sevoflurane, isoflurane, and halothane in human tissues. Anesth Analg 69:370-373, 1989.
8. Lerman J, Schmitt-Bantel BI, Gregory GA, et al: Effect of age on the solubility of volatile anesthetics in human tissues. Anesthesiology 65:307-311, 1986.
9. Bacher A, Burton AW, Uchida T, Zornow MH: Sevoflurane or halothane anesthesia: Can we tell the difference? Anesth Analg 85:1203-1206, 1997.
10. Munson ES, Eger EI II, Bowers DL: Effects of anesthetic-depressed ventilation and cardiac output on anesthetic uptake. Anesthesiology 38:251-259, 1973.
11. Yasuda N, Lockhart SH, Eger EI II, et al: Kinetics of desflurane, isoflurane, and halothane in humans. Anesthesiology 74:489-498, 1991.
12. Yasuda N, Lockhart SH, Eger EI II, et al: Comparison of kinetics of sevoflurane and isoflurane in humans. Anesth Analg 72:316-324, 1991.
13. Eger EI II: The effect of inspired concentration on the rate of rise of alveolar concentration. Anesthesiology 24:153-157, 1963.

14. Eger EI II: Application of a mathematical model of gas uptake. *In* Papper EM, Kitz RJ (eds): Uptake and Distribution of Anesthetic Agents. New York, McGraw-Hill, 1963, pp 88-103.

15. Stoelting RK, Eger EI II: An additional explanation for the second gas effect: A concentrating effect. Anesthesiology 30:273-277, 1969.

16. Korman B, Mapleson WW: Concentration and second gas effects: Can the accepted explanation be improved? Br J Anaesth 78:618-625, 1997.

17. Eger EI II, Smith RA, Koblin DD: The concentration effect can be mimicked by a decrease in blood solubility. Anesthesiology 49:282-284, 1978.

18. Epstein RM, Rackow H, Salanitre E, Wolf GL: Influence of the concentration effect on the uptake of anesthetic mixtures: The second gas effect. Anesthesiology 25:364-371, 1964.

19. Taheri S, Eger EI II: A demonstration of the concentration and second gas effects in humans anesthetized with nitrous oxide and desflurane. Anesth Analg 89:774-780, 1999.

20. Stoelting RK, Eger EI II: Percutaneous loss of nitrous oxide, cyclopropane, ether and halothane in man. Anesthesiology 30:278-283, 1969.

21. Cullen BF, Eger EI II: Diffusion of nitrous oxide, cyclopropane, and halothane through human skin and amniotic membrane. Anesthesiology 36:168-173, 1972.

22. Lockhart SH, Yasuda Y, Peterson N, et al: Comparison of percutaneous losses of sevoflurane and isoflurane in humans. Anesth Analg 72:212-215, 1991.

23. Fassoulaki A, Lockhart S, Freire BA, et al: Percutaneous loss of desflurane, isoflurane and halothane in humans. Anesthesiology 74:479-483, 1991.

24. Laster MJ, Tahari S, Eger EI II, et al: Visceral losses of desflurane, isoflurane, and halothane in swine. Anesth Analg 73:209-212, 1991.

25. Berman ML, Lowe HJ, Hagler KT, Bochantin J: Uptake and elimination of methoxyflurane as influenced by enzyme induction in the rat. Anesthesiology 38:352-357, 1973.

26. Carpenter RL, Eger EI II, Johnson BH, et al: The extent of metabolism of inhaled anesthetics in humans. Anesthesiology 65:201-205, 1986.

27. Carpenter RL, Eger EI II, Johnson BH, et al: Pharmacokinetics of inhaled anesthetics in humans: Measurements during and after the simultaneous administration of enflurane, halothane, isoflurane, methoxyflurane, and nitrous oxide. Anesth Analg 65:575-582, 1986.

28. Carpenter RL, Eger EI II, Johnson BH, et al: Does the duration of anesthetic administration affect the pharmacokinetics or metabolism of inhaled anesthetics in humans? Anesth Analg 66:1-8, 1987.

29. Halsey MJ, Sawyer DC, Eger EI II, et al: Hepatic metabolism of halothane, methoxyflurane, cyclopropane, Ethrane and Forane in miniature swine. Anesthesiology 35:43-47, 1971.

30. Sutton TS, Koblin DD, Gruenke LD, et al: Fluoride metabolites following prolonged exposure of volunteers and patients to desflurane. Anesth Analg 73:180-185, 1991.

31. Sawyer DC, Eger EI II, Bahlman SH, et al: Concentration dependence of hepatic halothane metabolism. Anesthesiology 34:230-234, 1971.

32. Eger EI II, Gong D, Koblin DD, et al: Effect of anesthetic duration on kinetic and recovery characteristics of desflurane vs. sevoflurane (plus compound A) in volunteers. Anesth Analg 86:414-421, 1998.

33. Yamamura H, Wakasugi B, Okuma Y, Maki K: The effects of ventilation on the absorption and elimination of inhalation anaesthetics. Anaesthesia 18:427-438, 1963.

34. Eger EI II: Ventilation, circulation and uptake. *In* Eger EI II (ed): Anesthetic Uptake and Action. Baltimore, Williams & Wilkins, 1974, pp 122-145.

35. Fukui Y, Smith NT: Interactions among ventilation, the circulation, and the uptake and distribution of halothane—Use of a hybrid computer multiple model. I. The basic model. Anesthesiology 54:107-118, 1981.

36. Doi M, Ikeda K: Respiratory effects of sevoflurane. Anesth Analg 66:241-244, 1987.

37. Fourcade HE, Stevens WC, Larson CP Jr, et al: The ventilatory effects of Forane, a new inhaled anesthetic. Anesthesiology 35:26-31, 1971.

38. Munson ES, Larson CP Jr, Babad AA, et al: The effects of halothane, fluroxene and cyclopropane on ventilation: A comparative study in man. Anesthesiology 27:716-728, 1966.

39. Calverley RK, Smith NT, Jones CW, et al: Ventilatory and cardiovascular effects of enflurane anesthesia during spontaneous ventilation in man. Anesth Analg 57:610-618, 1978.

40. Lockhart S, Rampil IJ, Yasuda N, et al: Depression of ventilation by desflurane in humans. Anesthesiology 74:484-488, 1991.

41. Gibbons RT, Steffey EP, Eger EI II: The effect of spontaneous versus controlled ventilation on the rate of rise of alveolar halothane concentration in dogs. Anesth Analg 56:32-34, 1977.

42. Yamamura H: The effect of ventilation and blood volume on the uptake and elimination of inhalation anesthetic agents. *In* Progress in Anaesthesiology. Proceedings of the Fourth World Congress of Anesthesiologists. International Congress Series 200. Amsterdam, Excerpta Medica, 1968, pp 394-399.

43. Eger EI II, Smith NT, Stoelting RK, et al: Cardiovascular effects of halothane in man. Anesthesiology 32:396-409, 1970.

44. Calverley RK, Smith NT, Eger EI II: Cardiovascular effects of enflurane anesthesia during controlled ventilation in man. Anesth Analg 57:619-628, 1978.

45. Ebert TJ, Muzi M: Sympathetic hyperactivity during desflurane anesthesia in healthy volunteers. A comparison with isoflurane. Anesthesiology 79:444-453, 1993.

46. Weiskopf RB, Moore M, Eger EI II, et al: Rapid increase in desflurane concentration is associated with greater transient cardiovascular stimulation than with rapid increase in isoflurane concentration in humans. Anesthesiology 80:1035-1045, 1994.

47. Eger EI II, Bahlman SH, Munson ES: Effect of age on the rate of increase of alveolar anesthetic concentration. Anesthesiology 35:365-372, 1971.

48. Wahrenbrock EA, Eger EI II, Laravuso RB, Maruschak G: Anesthetic uptake—Of mice and men (and whales). Anesthesiology 40:19-23, 1974.

49. Salanitre E, Rackow H: The pulmonary exchange of nitrous oxide and halothane in infants and children. Anesthesiology 30:388-394, 1969.

50. Gallagher TM, Black GW: Uptake of volatile anaesthetics in children. Anaesthesia 40:1073-1077, 1985.

51. Munson ES, Eger EI II, Tham MK, Embro WJ: Increase in anesthetic uptake, excretion and blood solubility in man after eating. Anesth Analg 57:224-231, 1978.

52. Eger EI II, Severinghaus JW: Effect of uneven pulmonary distribution of blood and gas on induction with inhalation anesthetics. Anesthesiology 25:620-626, 1964.

53. Stoelting RK, Longnecker DE: Effect of right-to-left shunt on rate of increase in arterial anesthetic concentration. Anesthesiology 36:352-356, 1972.

54. Eger EI II, Saidman LJ: Hazards of nitrous oxide anesthesia in bowel obstruction and pneumothorax. Anesthesiology 26:61-66, 1965.

55. Hunter AR: Problems of anaesthesia in artificial pneumothorax. Proc R Soc Med 48:765-768, 1955.

56. Munson ES, Merrick HC: Effect of nitrous oxide on venous air embolism. Anesthesiology 27:783-787, 1966.

57. Shapiro HM, Yoachim J, Marshall LF: Nitrous oxide challenge for detection of residual intravascular pulmonary gas following venous air embolism. Anesth Analg 61:304-306, 1982.

58. Stanley TH, Kawamura R, Graves C: Effects of nitrous oxide on volume and pressure of endotracheal tube cuffs. Anesthesiology 41:256-262, 1974.

59. Kaplan R, Abramowitz MD, Epstein BS: Nitrous oxide and air-filled balloon-tipped catheters. Anesthesiology 55:71-73, 1981.

60. Eisenkraft JB, Eger EI II: Nitrous oxide anesthesia may double the balloon gas volume of Swan-Ganz catheters. Mt Sinai J Med 49:430-433, 1982.

61. Wolf GL, Capuano C, Hartung J: Nitrous oxide increases intraocular pressure after intravitreal sulfur hexafluoride injection. Anesthesiology 59:547-548, 1983.
62. Thomsen KA, Terkildsen K, Arnfred J: Middle ear pressure variations during anesthesia. Arch Otolaryngol 82:609-611, 1985.
63. Saidman LJ, Eger EI II: Change in cerebrospinal fluid pressure during pneumoencephalography under nitrous oxide anesthesia. Anesthesiology 26:67-72, 1965.
64. Waun JE, Sweitzer RS, Hamilton WK: Effect of nitrous oxide on middle ear mechanics and hearing acuity. Anesthesiology 28:846-850, 1987.
65. Graham MD, Knight PR: Atelectatic tympanic membrane reversal by nitrous oxide supplemented general anesthesia and polyethylene ventilation tube insertion. A preliminary report. Laryngoscope 41:1469-1471, 1981.
66. Eger EI II, Larson CP Jr, Severinghaus JW: The solubility of halothane in rubber, soda lime and various plastics. Anesthesiology 23:356-359, 1962.
67. Titel JH, Lowe HJ: Rubber-gas partition coefficients. Anesthesiology 29:1215-1216, 1968.
68. Targ AG, Yasuda N, Eger EI II: Solubility of I-653, sevoflurane, isoflurane, and halothane in plastics and rubber composing a conventional anesthetic circuit. Anesth Analg 68:218-225, 1989.
69. Eger EI II, Ionescu P, Gong D: Circuit absorption of halothane, isoflurane and sevoflurane. Anesth Analg 86:1070-1074, 1998.
70. Eger EI II, Koblin DD, Bowland T, et al: Nephrotoxicity of sevoflurane vs. desflurane anesthesia in volunteers. Anesth Analg 84:160-168, 1997.
71. Higuchi H, Sumita S, Wada H, et al: Effects of sevoflurane and isoflurane on renal function and on possible markers of nephrotoxicity. Anesthesiology 89:307-322, 1998.
72. Fang ZX, Eger EI II, Laster MJ, et al: Carbon monoxide production from degradation of desflurane, enflurane, isoflurane, halothane, and sevoflurane by soda lime and Baralyme. Anesth Analg 80:1187-1193, 1995.
73. Eger EI II, Ionescu P, Laster MJ, Weiskopf RB: Baralyme dehydration increases and soda lime dehydration decreases the concentration of compound A resulting from sevoflurane degradation in a standard anesthetic circuit. Anesth Analg 85:892-898, 1997.
74. Harper M, Eger EI II: A comparison of the efficiency of three anesthesia circle systems. Anesth Analg 55:724-729, 1976.
75. Sharp JH, Trudell JR, Cohen EN: Volatile metabolites and decomposition products of halothane in man. Anesthesiology 50:2-8, 1979.
76. Morio M, Fujii K, Satoh N, et al: Reaction of sevoflurane and its degradation products with soda lime. Toxicity of the byproducts. Anesthesiology 77:1155-1164, 1992.
77. Severinghaus JW: The rate of uptake of nitrous oxide in man. J Clin Invest 33:1183-1189, 1954.
78. Lowe HJ, Ernst EA: The Quantitative Practice of Anesthesia. Use of Closed Circuit. Baltimore, Williams & Wilkins, 1981, pp 1-234.
79. Titel JH, Lowe HJ, Elam JO, Grosholz JR: Quantitative closed-circuit halothane anesthesia. Anesth Analg 47:560-569, 1968.
80. Hendrickx JFA, Soetens M, VanderDonck A, et al: Uptake of desflurane and isoflurane during closed-circuit anesthesia with spontaneous and controlled mechanical ventilation. Anesth Analg 84:413-418, 1997.
81. Eger EI II: Complexities overlooked: Things may not be what they seem. Anesth Analg 84:239-240, 1997.
82. Eger EI II: Desflurane (Suprane). A Compendium and Reference. Rutherford, NJ, Healthpress Publishing Group, 1993, pp 1-119.
83. Weiskopf RB, Eger EI II: Comparing the costs of inhaled anesthetics. Anesthesiology 79:1413-1418, 1993.
84. Eger EI II, Johnson BH: Rates of awakening from anesthesia with I-653, halothane, isoflurane, and sevoflurane: A test of the effect of anesthetic concentration and duration in rats. Anesth Analg 66:977-982, 1987.
85. Mapleson WW: Quantitative prediction of anesthetic concentrations. In Papper EM, Kitz RJ (eds): Uptake and Distribution of Anesthetic Agents. New York, McGraw-Hill, 1963, pp 104-119.
86. Stoelting RK, Eger EI II: The effects of ventilation and anesthetic solubility on recovery from anesthesia: An in vivo and analog analysis before and after equilibration. Anesthesiology 30:290-296, 1969.
87. Bailey JM: Context-sensitive half-times and other decrement times of inhaled anesthetics. Anesth Analg 85:681-686, 1997.
88. Stoelting RK, Longnecker DE, Eger EI II: Minimal alveolar concentrations on awakening from methoxyflurane, halothane, ether and fluroxene in man: MAC awake. Anesthesiology 33:5-9, 1970.
89. Dwyer R, Bennett HL, Eger EI II, Heilbron D: Effects of isoflurane and nitrous oxide in subanesthetic concentrations on memory and responsiveness in volunteers. Anesthesiology 77:888-898, 1992.
90. Katoh T, Suguro Y, Nakajima R, et al: Blood concentration of sevoflurane and isoflurane on recovery from anaesthesia. Br J Anaesth 69:259-262, 1992.
91. Katoh T, Suguro Y, Ikeda T, et al: Influence of age on awakening concentrations of sevoflurane and isoflurane. Anesth Analg 76:348-352, 1993.
92. Chortkoff BS, Eger EI II, Crankshaw DP, et al: Concentrations of desflurane and propofol that suppress response to command in humans. Anesth Analg 81:737-743, 1995.
93. Neumann MA, Weiskopf RB, Gong DH, et al: Changing from isoflurane to desflurane towards the end of anesthesia does not accelerate recovery in humans. Anesthesiology 88:914-921, 1998.
94. Rehder K, Forbes J, Alter H, et al: Halothane biotransformation in man: A quantitative study. Anesthesiology 28:711-715, 1967.
95. Chase RE, Holaday DA, Fiserova-Bergerova V, et al: The biotransformation of Ethrane in man. Anesthesiology 35:262-267, 1971.
96. Fink BR: Diffusion anoxia. Anesthesiology 16:511-519, 1955.
97. Sheffer L, Steffenson JL, Birch AA: Nitrous oxide–induced diffusion hypoxia in patients breathing spontaneously. Anesthesiology 37:436-439, 1972.
98. Rackow H, Salanitre E, Frumin MJ: Dilution of alveolar gases during nitrous oxide excretion in man. J Appl Physiol 16:723-728, 1961.
99. Eger EI II: Effect of anesthetic circuit on alveolar rate of rise. In Eger EI II (ed): Anesthetic Uptake and Action. Baltimore, Williams & Wilkins, 1974, pp 192-205.
100. Eger EI II, Brandstater B: Solubility of methoxyflurane in rubber. Anesthesiology 24:679-683, 1963.
101. Munson ES, Eger EI II: Methoxyflurane solubility in plastics. Anesthesiology 26:828, 1965.

CHAPTER
6 Pulmonary Pharmacology

Neil E. Farber, Paul S. Pagel, and David C. Warltier

Effects of Inhaled Anesthetics on Bronchomotor Tone   155
Pharmacology of Bronchial Smooth Muscle   155
Inhaled Anesthetics   156
Mechanisms of Action   157
Effects of Inhaled Anesthetics on Bronchomotor Tone   159

Effects of Inhaled Anesthetics on Mucociliary Function   161
Normal Mucociliary Function   161
Specific Effects of Anesthetics   162
Effects of Inhaled Anesthetics on Pulmonary Surfactant   162
Effects of Inhaled Anesthetics on Mucociliary Function   163

Effects of Inhaled Anesthetics on Pulmonary Vascular Resistance   165
Determinants of Pulmonary Vascular Resistance   165
Mechanism of Hypoxic Pulmonary Vasoconstriction   166

Inhaled Anesthetics and Hypoxic Pulmonary Vasoconstriction   166
Effects of Inhaled Anesthetics on Pulmonary Vasculature in Humans   168

Effects of Inhaled Anesthetics on Control of Ventilation   170
Control of Breathing   170
General Ventilatory Effects of Anesthetics   171
Mechanoreceptors and Breathing   171
Lung and Airway Receptors   171
Ventilatory Mechanics and Mechanoreceptors in the Chest Wall   174
Effects of Anesthetics on Ventilatory Response to Chemical Stimuli   177
Responses to Carbon Dioxide   177
Apneic Thresholds   178
Carbon Dioxide Response Curves   178
Ventilatory Responses to Hypoxemia   179
Clinical Implications   180

This chapter describes the physiologic control mechanisms involved in modulating various anatomic components of the lungs and the direct effects of inhaled anesthetics on pulmonary physiology. The lungs are unique in their exposure to a wide variety of physical forces, including ventilation, blood flow, and surface tension. Inhaled anesthetics modulate each of these properties. Specific sections of this chapter focus on airway and PVR, mucociliary function, and ventilatory control.

EFFECTS OF INHALED ANESTHETICS ON BRONCHOMOTOR TONE

Transient increases in airway resistance may be caused, at least in part, by an increase in bronchiolar smooth muscle tone. Retrospective reviews found that patients without recent symptoms of asthma had a very low frequency of perioperative respiratory complications,[1] yet perioperative bronchospasm developed in approximately 6% of patients with asthma.[2,3] Prospective studies have demonstrated that 1.7% of patients with asthma experienced a severe respiratory outcome[4] and that 25% wheezed after the induction of anesthesia.[5] Of the 40 cases of bronchospasm resulting in settled malpractice claims (from the American Society of Anesthesiologists Closed Claims Project),[5a] 88% involved brain damage or death, and only half of these patients had a history of asthma or chronic obstructive pulmonary disease. Significant bronchospasm may occur in normal subjects without underlying lung disease as a result of exposure to a noxious stimulus. Understanding the physiologic effects of inhaled agents on bronchial smooth muscle is clinically important.

Pharmacology of Bronchial Smooth Muscle

Mougdil[6] and Pinto-Pereira and coworkers[7] summarized the mechanisms by which increases in airway resistance might occur. Airway smooth muscle extends as far distally as the terminal bronchioles and is affected by autonomic nervous system activity and nonadrenergic noncholinergic mechanisms. Parasympathetic nerves located in the vagi mediate baseline airway tone and reflex bronchoconstriction. Changes in intracellular calcium (ICa^{2+}) levels and Ca^{2+} influx may be caused by alterations in cyclic nucleotides within bronchial smooth muscle. Agonist-induced contraction is mediated by an increase in myosin light chain kinase activity, phosphorylation of the 20-kd regulatory myosin light chain, and an increase in Ca^{2+} sensitivity.[8] Exogenous administration of acetylcholine or stimulation of the vagus nerve increases the relative amount of cyclic guanosine monophosphate (cGMP) compared with cyclic adenosine monophosphate (cAMP) and results in bronchial smooth muscle contraction. Agonist activation of bronchial smooth muscle cells also involves the second messenger cyclic adenosine diphosphate ribose (cADPR), which indirectly releases Ca^{2+} from the sarcoplasmic reticulum by activating ryanodine channels.[9] Agonist-induced stimulation of particulate guanylyl cyclase relaxes bronchial smooth muscle by decreasing Ca^{2+} current. In contrast, stimulation of soluble guanylyl cyclase by substances such as nitric oxide (NO) reduces intracellular Ca^{2+} concentration and Ca^{2+} sensitivity.[10]

Release of histamine in the airway or various forms of mechanical or chemical stimulation may increase afferent vagal activity to produce reflex bronchoconstriction. This increase in bronchomotor tone is attenuated by the cholinergic antagonist atropine. M_2 and M_3 muscarinic receptors on airway smooth muscle receptors mediate bronchoconstriction by increasing Ca^{2+} sensitivity.[11] Presynaptic M_2 muscarinic receptors have also been identified that inhibit acetylcholine release and cause bronchodilation. Low doses of drugs that preferentially inhibit M_2 receptors (e.g., ipratropium bromide) may paradoxically produce bronchoconstriction.[12]

Adrenergic receptors in bronchial smooth muscle are classified into α and β_2 types. The α–receptors have been characterized in the bronchial tree in humans, but the activity of these receptors appears to be clinically insignificant. In contrast, the β_2-receptor subtypes play an important role in bronchiolar smooth muscle responsiveness. Stimulation of β_2-receptors causes relaxation that is mediated by a relative increase in intracellular cAMP concentration. It appears that asthma, allergic, and methacholine-induced bronchospasm are not genetically linked to a dominant β_2-adrenoceptor gene.[13]

Respiratory epithelium releases substances that modulate bronchial smooth muscle tone. Removal of epithelium enhances contractile responses to acetylcholine, histamine, or serotonin in large airways and decreases relaxation responses to isoproterenol in small airways.[14,15] These actions are analogous to the effect of endothelial damage on vascular smooth muscle tone. However, porcine bronchiolar epithelium-mediated bronchomotor activity is not significantly affected by cardiopulmonary bypass, in contrast to vascular endothelium-mediated smooth muscle dysfunction.[16] Endogenous epithelial factors have been identified, but endothelium-derived relaxing factor (i.e., NO) may play a role in respiratory epithelium similar to that of vascular endothelium. Endothelin-1 is one such potent endogenous bronchoconstrictor that functions by activation of the inositol triphosphate (IP_3) pathway.[17]

Inhaled Anesthetics

Volatile anesthetics are potent bronchodilators. In a retrospective study, Schnider and Papper[2] demonstrated halothane was superior to ether, cyclopropane, and ethylene in decreasing wheezing in 49 patients with symptoms of bronchospasm before anesthesia. Colgan[18] observed an increase in "bronchial distensibility" in dogs anesthetized with halothane, ether, or methoxyflurane. Halothane had the most pronounced effect. Increasing concentrations of halothane also caused a dose-dependent decrease in resting airway resistance in spontaneously breathing dogs.[19] Nevertheless, bronchodilation resulting from hypercarbia associated with deeper planes of anesthesia may have affected the results of these studies. Halothane and diethyl ether caused relaxation of resting tone in isolated guinea pig tracheal strips.[20] These anesthetics also attenuated tracheal muscle constriction produced by acetylcholine, but only halothane accomplished this in clinically relevant doses.

Hickey and colleagues[21] demonstrated the importance of controlled levels of arterial carbon dioxide tension (Pa_{CO_2}) during the evaluation of the effects of drugs on bronchial smooth muscle tone. Halothane and cyclopropane did not alter the resistance of the resting, unstimulated airway in anesthetized, mechanically ventilated, normocapnic dogs. However, 1.5 minimum alveolar concentration (MAC) of halothane produced significant bronchodilation compared with cyclopropane during histamine- or vagal stimulation–induced bronchoconstriction. Halothane and, to a lesser degree, enflurane and methoxyflurane reversed hypocapnia-induced bronchoconstriction in the isolated canine left lower lobe.[22] Halothane also attenuated the bronchoconstricting effects of hypocarbia without affecting the resistive work of breathing (described more fully in "Ventilatory Mechanics") in the unstimulated state in humans undergoing cardiopulmonary bypass.[23] Hypercapnia-induced bronchodilation and hypocapnia-induced bronchoconstriction were shown to be attenuated by isoflurane.[24]

A bronchospasm model developed by Hirshman and Bergman[25] using dogs sensitized to aerosolized *Ascaris* antigen has greatly contributed to our understanding of the effect of anesthetics on airway smooth muscle. Halothane and enflurane (1 MAC) similarly attenuate antigen-induced bronchospasm. Unlike an asthmatic attack during anesthesia, the stimulus to incite bronchospasm in this model is not maintained during experimentation. Isoflurane and halothane (1.5 MAC) produced a similar reduction in airway resistance in this canine model.[26] Similar results were obtained with volatile agents during methacholine-induced airway constriction. Taken together, these data suggest that isoflurane and halothane produce direct bronchodilation and depress airway reflexes. Although isoflurane appears to share significant bronchodilating properties with halothane and enflurane, halothane increased dynamic compliance (a measure of small airway resistance) to a greater extent than did isoflurane. This finding is made more interesting in light of data demonstrating that isoflurane preferentially relaxes the bronchiole rather than the bronchus in vitro.[27] The structure of the respiratory epithelium changes from pseudostratified columnar cells of the large airways to thinner, cuboidal cells of the bronchioles, and it is not surprising that topographic heterogeneity exists between these regions. Park and colleagues[28] demonstrated that isoflurane and halothane dilate fourth-order bronchi at equivalent MAC values. The ability of halothane, isoflurane, sevoflurane, and desflurane to attenuate methacholine-induced bronchoconstriction in open-chest, pentobarbital-anesthetized rats was assessed.[29] These volatile anesthetics produced similar reductions in airway resistance, but they did not cause further effects at concentrations greater than 1 MAC.

Ascaris antigen–induced asthma was associated with increased plasma histamine levels that were not prevented by administration of halothane.[30] Halothane and topical atropine decreased bronchoconstriction during histamine-induced bronchospasm, but these effects were not additive or synergistic.[31]

Using computed tomography (CT), Brown and colleagues[32] showed that halothane causes greater bronchodilation than does isoflurane at low concentrations (Fig. 6-1). Halothane also had a more pronounced relaxing

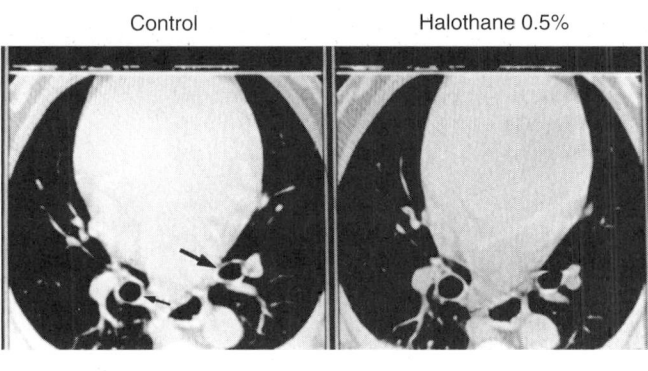

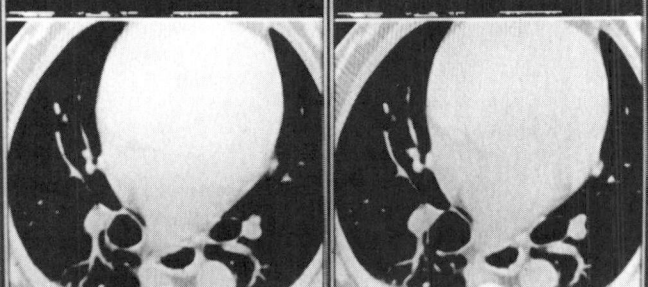

Control   Halothane 0.5%

Halothane 1.0%   Halothane 1.5%

Figure 6–1 High-resolution computed tomography scans from one dog: control *(upper left),* during 0.5% halothane *(upper right),* during 1.0% halothane *(lower left),* and during 1.5% halothane *(lower right).* Notice the progressive dilation of the airways as indicated by the *arrow.* (Adapted from Brown RH, Mitzner W, Zerhouni E, et al: Direct in vivo visualization of bronchodilation induced by inhalational anesthesia using high-resolution computed tomography. Anesthesiology 78:295, 1993.)

effect than did isoflurane at a similar MAC in intact airway smooth muscle as measured by high-resolution CT.[33] All volatile agents, including sevoflurane[34,35] and desflurane,[36] relax airway smooth muscle. Sevoflurane (1 MAC) reduced respiratory system resistance (determined using the isovolume technique) by 15% in patients undergoing elective surgery. In contrast, desflurane did not alter resistance (+5%).[37] Halothane, desflurane, and isoflurane appear to relax distal airways (i.e., bronchioles) to a greater extent than proximal airways (i.e., bronchi).[38] Similarly, isoflurane and sevoflurane had greater inhibitory effects on bronchial than tracheal smooth contraction.[39]

Administration of 1 or 2 MAC of halothane, enflurane, sevoflurane, and isoflurane did not alter baseline pulmonary resistance and dynamic pulmonary compliance. However, these agents significantly attenuated increases in pulmonary resistance and decreases in dynamic pulmonary compliance in response to intravenous histamine. Halothane was most effective in altering indices of bronchodilation, whereas responses to isoflurane, enflurane, and sevoflurane were nearly identical.[35] In contrast, halothane, enflurane, and sevoflurane were found to be equivalent at dilating third- or fourth-generation bronchi as measured directly with a fiberoptic bronchoscope in vivo.[40]

Mechanisms of Action

Volatile anesthetics relax airway smooth muscle by directly depressing smooth muscle contractility. This action appears to result from direct effects on bronchial epithelium and indirect inhibition of reflex neural pathways. The mechanisms responsible for the direct depressant effects of volatile agents are unclear. Halothane was initially believed to exert β–adrenoceptor agonist activity in airway smooth muscle because halothane-induced reduction of airway resistance was blocked by sotalol.[19] However, these effects might have been specific to the drug itself and not attributable to the drug class. Sotalol also might have produced smooth muscle contraction because propranolol did not antagonize the relaxing properties of halothane on acetylcholine-mediated bronchoconstriction.[20] The concentration of ICa^{2+} is an important regulator of smooth muscle reactivity. Several intracellular mediators responsible for Ca^{2+} mobilization are potential sites for the action of volatile anesthetics. Halothane increases cAMP concentrations, which may decrease intracellular free Ca^{2+} in airway smooth muscle.[41] This decrease in Ca^{2+} parallels the inhibitory effects of the volatile anesthetics on airway smooth muscle tension.[39]

Effects of volatile anesthetics on proximal rather than distal airways may be related to differential effects on voltage-dependent calcium channels (VDCs) and the relative distribution of these channels. Long-lasting (L-type) VDCs appear to be the predominant mechanism for Ca^{2+} entry in tracheal smooth muscle, whereas transient (T-type) and L-type VDCs are present in bronchial smooth muscle cells.[39,42] Hypocapnia-induced contraction of tracheal and bronchial smooth muscle appears to be mediated, at least in part, by VDCs.[43] Yamakage and coworkers[39] demonstrated that isoflurane and sevoflurane inhibit both types of VDCs in a dose-dependent fashion, but their effects on T-type VDCs in bronchial smooth muscle were much greater (Fig. 6-2). Early studies proposed that volatile anesthetics relax airway smooth muscles by opening adenosine triphosphate (ATP)–sensitive potassium channels (K_{ATP}). However, halothane had minimal effects on tracheal smooth muscle K_{ATP} channels.[44] Other evidence suggests that the differential effects of volatile anesthetics on tracheal compared with bronchial smooth muscle may be related to various effects on Ca^{2+}-activated chloride channel activity[45] or differential sensitivities of other K^+ channel subtypes.[46]

In addition to effects on VDCs, halothane reduces ICa^{2+} by depleting sarcoplasmic reticulum Ca^{2+}.[47-49] The direct effects of halothane on IP_3 concentrations remain controversial,[47,48] but halothane-induced reductions in sarcoplasmic reticulum Ca^{2+} appear to occur through IP_3 and ryanodine receptor channels.[48] Halothane may reduce free Ca^{2+} in the cytoplasm or limit influx of Ca^{2+} across the cell membrane. Volatile anesthetics also affect the function of G proteins in a variety of tissues. However, halothane-induced depression of airway contractility occurs independent of pertussis toxin–sensitive inhibitory G proteins that attenuate relaxation produced by β-adrenoceptor agonists.[50] Halothane decreased intracellular Ca^{2+} concentration and Ca^{2+} influx during submaximal, but not maximal, muscarinic stimulation.[51] Warner and coworkers[52] suggested that halothane depletes sarcoplasmic reticulum Ca^{2+} stores, but this effect

may not be the primary mechanism by which airway contractility is reduced (Fig. 6-3). Halothane also decreases Ca^{2+} sensitivity of smooth muscle cell myocytes, resulting in a reduced contractile force at a constant Ca^{2+} concentration.[51] Warner's group[53] also demonstrated that halothane attenuates acetylcholine-induced Ca^{2+} sensitization in canine tracheal smooth muscle to a greater extent than does isoflurane or sevoflurane. These findings are analogous to the differential effects of volatile anesthetics on relaxing airway smooth muscle. Alterations in Ca^{2+} sensitivity appear to be mediated by an increase in smooth muscle protein phosphatase[54] and a modulation of G proteins, specifically G_q and G_I, that exert actions on cGMP.[55-58] Halothane suppresses the contraction of dog tracheal smooth muscle initiated by direct and indirect electrical stimulation.[59]

The bronchoconstricting effects of low inhaled concentrations of carbon dioxide were attenuated by inhaled, but not intravenous, halothane.[23] These data suggest that volatile agents produce a direct action on the airway musculature or local neural reflex arcs rather than centrally controlled reflex pathways. Halothane, isoflurane, sevoflurane, and desflurane-induced dilatation of distal bronchial segments partially depends on the presence of bronchial epithelium (Fig. 6-4).[28,60] A prostanoid (e.g., prostaglandin E_2 or I_2) or NO may mediate the bronchodilatory effects of these volatile anesthetics. For example, isoflurane-mediated bronchodilation appears to be more dependent on NO than prostanoids, but the

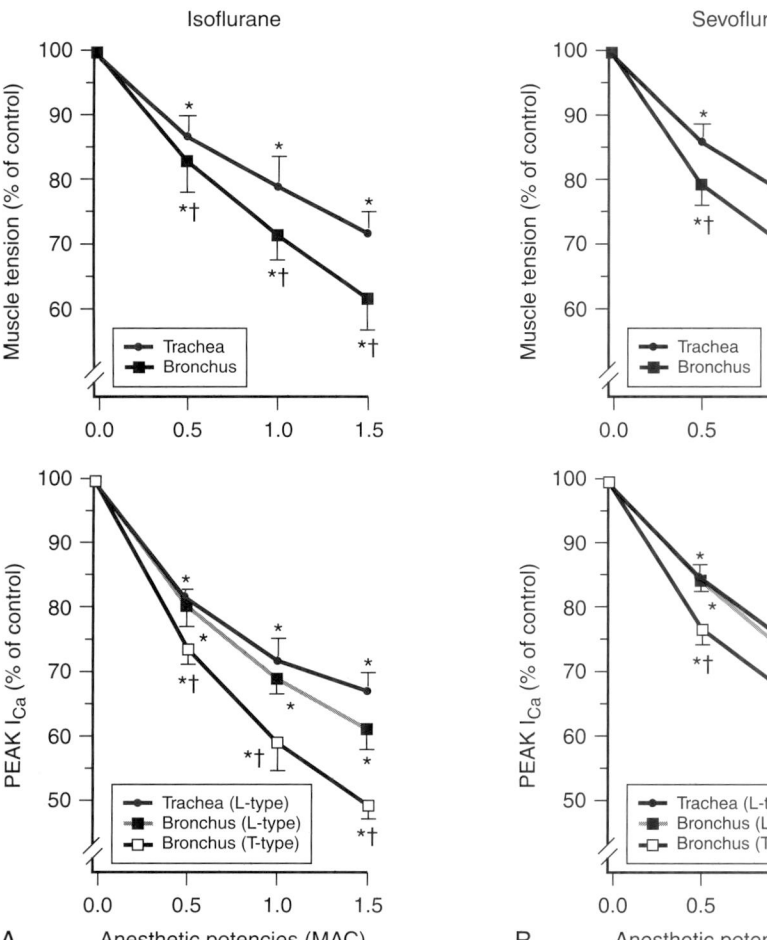

Figure 6–2 Effect of isoflurane (**A**) and sevoflurane (**B**) on porcine tracheal versus bronchial smooth muscle tension or inward Ca^{2+} current (ICa) through T-type and L-type voltage-dependent Ca^{2+} channels (VDCs). There were no differences in the inhibition of L-type VDCs. Both anesthetics had greater inhibitory effects on T-type VDCs in bronchial smooth muscle. Symbols represent the mean ± SD. *$P < .05$ versus 0 MAC. †$P < .05$ versus tracheal smooth muscle in **A** and †$P < .05$ versus L-type VDCs in **B**. (Adapted from Yamakage M, Chen X, Tsuijiguchi N, et al: Different inhibitory effects of volatile anesthetics on T- and L-type voltage-dependent Ca^{2+} channels in porcine tracheal and bronchial smooth muscles. Anesthesiology 94:683, 2001.)

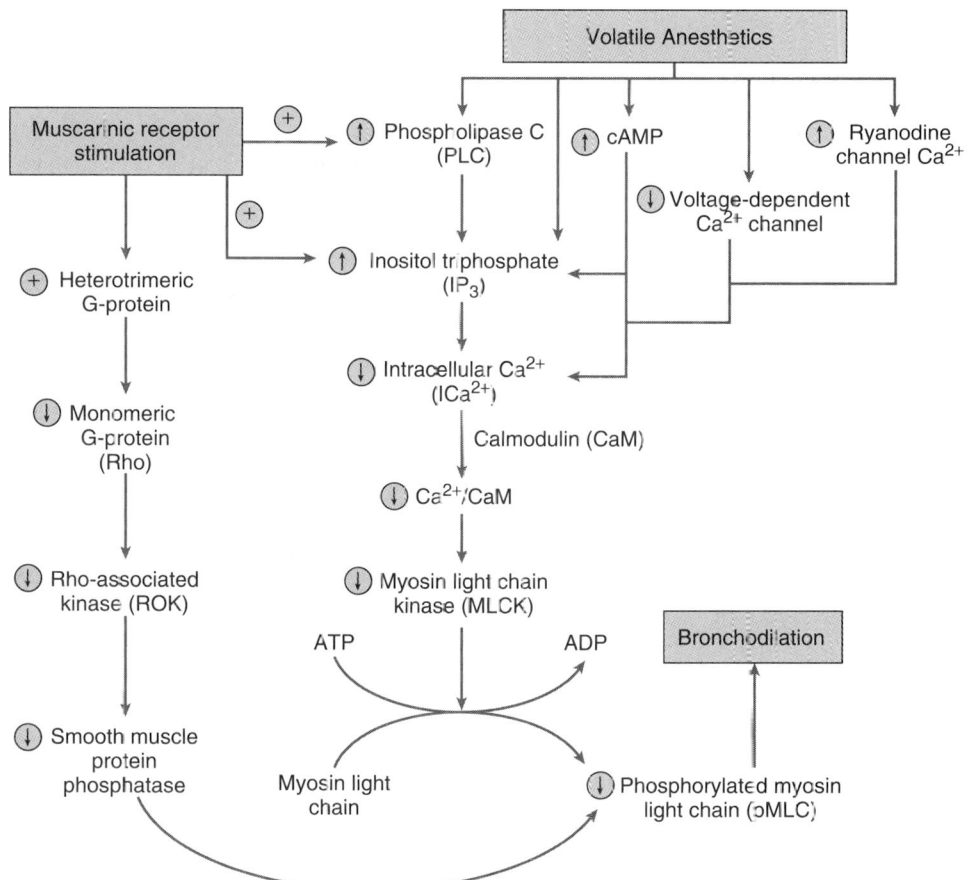

Figure 6–3 Proposed signaling pathways underlying volatile anesthetic (specifically halothane)-induced bronchodilation or inhibition of muscarinic agonist-induced contraction of airway smooth muscle, or both mechanisms. Signal transduction involving Rho protein is supported by work from Warner and coworkers on a role of halothane to decrease Ca^{2+} sensitivity rather than a change in ICa^{2+} content. CaM, calmodulin; ICa^{2+} intracellular Ca^{2+}; IP3, inositol triphosphate; MLC, myosin light chain; MLCK, myosin light chain kinase; pMLC, phosphorylated myosin light chain; Rho, monomeric G protein; ROK, Rho-associated kinase; RyR, ryanodine channels; SMPP, smooth muscle protein phosphatase; SR, sarcoplasmic reticulum; VDC, voltage-dependent Ca^{2+} channels; *encircled plus sign*, excitatory action of muscarinic receptor agonist; *encircled up arrow*, represents activation or increase due to volatile anesthetic; *encircled down arrow*, inhibition or decrease due to volatile anesthetic. (Adapted from Hanazaki M, Jones KA, Perkins WJ, et al: Halothane increases smooth muscle protein phosphatase in airway smooth muscle. Anesthesiology 94:129, 2001 and from Pabelick CM, Prakash YS, Kannan MS, et al: Effects of halothane on sarcoplasmic reticulum calcium release channels in porcine airway smooth muscle cells. Anesthesiology 95:207, 2001.)

converse is true for halothane. Focal epithelial damage or inflammation may occur in distal and small airways in patients with asthma or allergen exposure, and as a consequence, the bronchodilatory response to volatile anesthetics may be reduced.[6] The greatest bronchodilatory action of volatile agents in patients with chronic reactive airway disease occurs primarily in the proximal rather than distal airways.

Stimulation of intrinsic airway nerves in vitro produces a cholinergic contractile response that is inhibited by atropine. In addition to the direct effects previously described, volatile anesthetic-induced bronchodilation occurs by modulation of airway cholinergic neural transmission mediated through prejunctional and postjunctional mechanisms.[59,61,62] The combination of atropine and halothane did not increase airway caliber over that attained with either drug alone. These findings suggest that halothane dilates airways by blocking vagal tone during unstimulated conditions.[63] A nonadrenergic and noncholinergic bronchodilatory neural reflex believed to be mediated by NO[64] was unaffected by halothane at

concentrations of less than 1%.[65] The direct antagonism or release of histamine[30] also does not appear to play a role in volatile anesthetic-induced bronchodilation.

Effects of Inhaled Anesthetics on Bronchomotor Tone

Appropriate anesthetic management of the patient with reactive airway disease has been extensively reviewed.[6,7,66] Volatile anesthetics may be an effective method of treating status asthmaticus when more conventional treatments have failed. Gold and Helrich[67] evaluated the effect of halothane in six intubated patients treated unsuccessfully for status asthmaticus for at least 72 hours with bronchodilators, steroids, and antibiotics. No significant change in airway resistance was recorded during or immediately after halothane exposure, but all patients improved within 3 days of treatment. The lack of a control group in this study confounded the interpretation of the results. Several subsequent studies have demonstrated that the use of inhaled

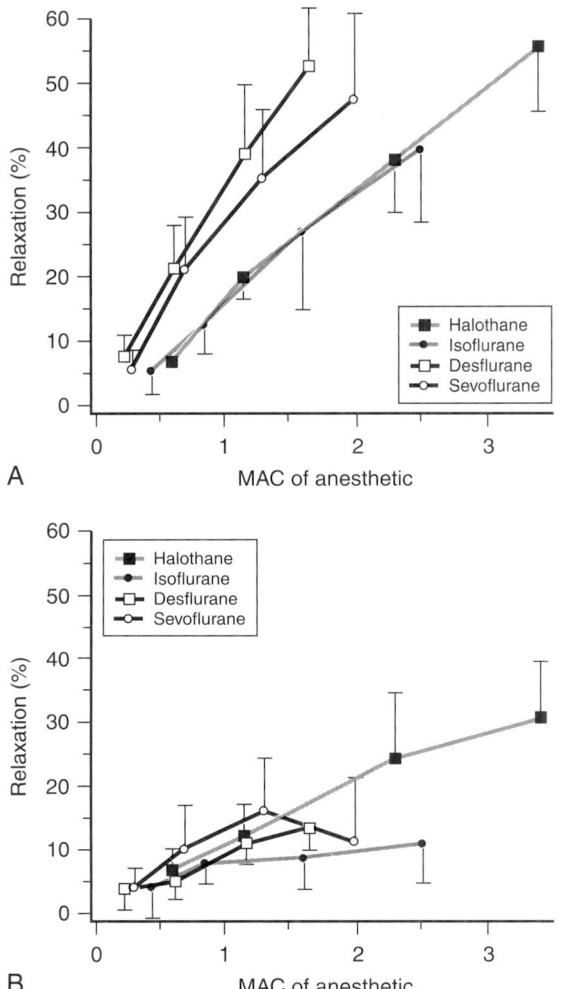

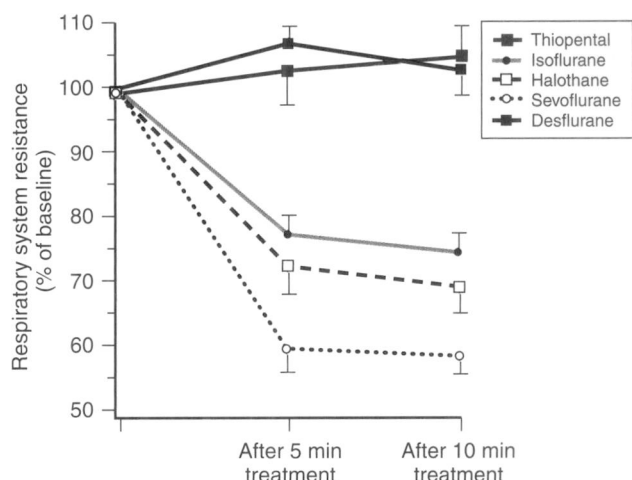

Figure 6–5 The percentage change in respiratory system resistance in patients after 5 and 10 minutes of maintenance anesthesia with 0.25 mg/kg/min thiopental plus 50% nitrous oxide; 1.1 minimum alveolar concentration (MAC) of sevoflurane, halothane, or isoflurane; or approximately 1 MAC of desflurane. All volatile anesthetics except desflurane decreased resistance. Sevoflurane decreased resistance more than isoflurane. (Adapted from Rooke GA, Choi J-H, Bishop MJ: The effect of isoflurane, halothane, sevoflurane, and thiopental/nitrous oxide on respiratory system resistance after tracheal intubation. Anesthesiology 86:1294, 1997 and from Goff MJ, Arain SR, Ficke DJ, et al: Absence of bronchodilation during desflurane anesthesia: A comparison to sevoflurane and thiopental. Anesthesiology 93:404, 2000.)

Figure 6–4 Relaxation of 5-hydroxytryptamine–preconstricted rat bronchial segments with intact (**A**) and disrupted (**B**) epithelium to increasing concentrations of desflurane, sevoflurane, isoflurane, and halothane expressed as minimum alveolar anesthetic concentration (MAC) multiples. Desflurane was a more potent bronchodilator than sevoflurane (**A**), which was more potent than either halothane or isoflurane. Rubbing epithelium significantly blunted the bronchodilatory effects of all anesthetics (**B**). There were no differences between the agents. (Adapted from Park KW, Dai HB, Lowenstein E, et al: Epithelial dependence of the bronchodilatory effect of sevoflurane and desflurane in rat distal bronchi. Anesth Analg 86:646, 1998.)

anesthetics may be beneficial in patients with refractory status asthmaticus.[68-74] Halothane-induced increases in cardiac arrhythmias and depression of myocardial contractility suggest that other agents may be preferred in the treatment of status asthmaticus.[73,75] However, 1% halothane administered to 12 patients in status asthmaticus was associated with a rapid improvement of bronchospasm, a reduced incidence of barotrauma, enhanced arterial blood gas tensions, and the absence of adverse hemodynamic effects including cardiac arrhythmias.[72]

Rooke and associates[76] compared the bronchodilating effects of halothane, isoflurane, sevoflurane, and thiopental or nitrous oxide in 66 healthy patients undergoing induction of anesthesia and tracheal intubation (Fig. 6-5). In contrast to thiopental or nitrous oxide, all volatile anesthetics significantly reduced respiratory system resistance. Equi-MAC sevoflurane and halothane decreased resistance to similar degrees, whereas isoflurane produced substantially less bronchodilation in vivo. Previously described animal studies demonstrating the equal potency of sevoflurane and isoflurane and the relatively greater potency of halothane for bronchodilation must be extrapolated with caution because *Ascaris*- or histamine-mediated experimental bronchospasm may not precisely mimic tracheal intubation-induced bronchospasm in humans. In contrast, Arakawa[75] showed that similar inspired concentrations of halothane, isoflurane, and sevoflurane produced nearly identical reductions in airway resistance in a patient with status asthmaticus.

The noble gas xenon has been used as an inhaled anesthetic for nearly 50 years, and advances in manufacturing technology and scavenging systems are making the use of xenon more economically feasible.[77] The effects of xenon on airway resistance differ markedly from those of volatile anesthetics because this gas has a higher density and viscosity than air.[78-80] In pentobarbital-anesthetized pigs, baseline airway resistance was significantly greater with 70% xenon-oxygen than 70% nitrous oxide–oxygen, although the measured peak and mean airway pressures were unaffected. In contrast, airway pressures and resistance were increased during xenon anesthesia and methacholine-induced bronchoconstriction.[79] The investigators argued that these effects were unlikely to be of significant clinical importance because the changes in airway pressure and resistance were only moderate. Pulmonary resistance during inhalation of 50% xenon was similar to that observed during 50% nitrous oxide or 70% nitrogen in methacholine-treated dogs.[81] A randomized, double-blind comparison of xenon and nitrous oxide showed that although both agents similarly increased expiratory lung resistance, fewer patients receiving xenon experienced decreases in oxygen saturation.[82] In contrast, 33% xenon has been demonstrated to transiently but significantly elevate peak airway pressures in long-term mechanically ventilated patients.[78] This increase in airway pressure was attenuated by a reduction in inspiratory flow rate. The higher density and viscosity of xenon increases the Reynolds number and probably causes the zone of transition from turbulent to laminar gas flow to move distally to smaller airways. However, an increase in flow resistance produced by mechanical loading during anesthesia does not significantly affect pulmonary gas exchange.[83] Other studies have shown that arterial oxygen and arterial carbon dioxide levels are not altered during xenon and nitrous oxide mixtures,[81,84] but some investigators have nonetheless suggested caution when using xenon in patients with bronchospastic or obstructive pulmonary disease.

The effect of albuterol in the presence of halothane on airway reactivity was examined in dogs.[85] Halothane attenuated histamine-induced bronchoconstriction, and albuterol further dilated the airways, indicating an additive or synergistic effect. The dilatory effects of halothane did not adversely affect the ability of isoproterenol to dilate isolated, acetylcholine-preconstricted canine tracheal smooth muscle strips in vitro.[50] These findings support the use of β-adrenoceptor agonists for the treatment of bronchospasm in patients anesthetized with halothane. However, results may differ somewhat with other volatile anesthetics or β-agonists. For example, the β₂-adrenergic agonist fenoterol lowered respiratory system resistance after endotracheal intubation but did not further reduce resistance when administered in the presence of 1.3% isoflurane.[86] However, the technique used to determine respiratory system resistance may be partially responsible for these results, because this index incorporates alterations in lung and chest wall resistance as well as tissue viscosity.

The actions of inhaled anesthetics on bronchomotor tone depend on the agent eliciting contraction in vitro.[33] Relaxation of tracheal smooth muscle by halothane and isoflurane is greatest in the presence of the endogenous mediator serotonin (potentially representing anaphylactoid or immunologic reactions) compared with acetylcholine (representing the neurally derived mediator of reflex bronchospasm). In contrast to the relaxing effects of isoproterenol, the absolute amount of airway smooth muscle relaxation by halothane is independent of the extent of contraction. These findings suggest that inhaled anesthetics remain effective bronchodilators, even in the presence of severe bronchospasm that is refractory to β₂-adrenoceptor therapy.

Volatile anesthetic–induced decreases in bronchomotor tone and neurally mediated airway reflexes may be partially opposed by a simultaneous reduction in functional residual capacity (FRC) in the anesthetized patient. This increase in FRC increases airway resistance.[87] An increased risk for morbidity and mortality has been well established in patients with asthma during the perioperative period that may be partially attributed to these FRC-mediated increases in airway resistance. Exposure of airway smooth muscle to low temperatures may abolish the inhibitory effects of volatile anesthetics on carbachol-induced contraction.[88] These findings suggest that intraoperative hypothermia also may attenuate volatile anesthetic–induced bronchodilation. Future investigations in humans with newer inhaled anesthetics will benefit from advances in knowledge of mechanisms of inhaled anesthetic action on airway smooth muscle under normal and pathophysiologic conditions.

Bronchospasm may occur in respiratory diseases other than asthma. For example, healthy patients undergoing surgical stimulation of pulmonary parenchyma or airways are at risk of developing bronchospasm.[89] Clinically discernible bronchospasm is a common occurrence during stimulation of the trachea by an endotracheal tube in anesthetized patients. The choices of preoperative medication, induction agent, muscle relaxant, and the type of inhaled agent are all important factors in minimizing clinical symptoms in patients with known reactive airway disease.

Halothane may be a more potent bronchodilator than other inhaled anesthetics. The often-profound respiratory irritation produced in the upper airways (i.e., coughing, respiratory secretions, breath-holding, and laryngospasm, especially in the pediatric population) may outweigh the benefit of any direct bronchodilatory action of this agent. Differences in bronchodilating effects between inhaled anesthetics may exist, but of greater clinical importance is avoiding or minimizing airway irritation and maintaining adequate depth of anesthesia with the agent that is chosen.

EFFECTS OF INHALED ANESTHETICS ON MUCOCILIARY FUNCTION

Normal Mucociliary Function

Foreign particulate matter, microorganisms, and dead cells are removed by the upward clearance of mucus from the tracheobronchial tree as a primary pulmonary defense mechanism. Ciliated respiratory epithelium extends throughout the respiratory tract as far as the terminal bronchioles and decreases in density (as do mucus-producing goblet cells and submucous glands) from trachea to alveoli.[90] Ciliary motion consists of a rapid stroke in a cephalad direction, followed by a slower recovery stroke in the opposite direction. Movements of cilia are closely coordinated in a proximal-to-distal direction to move matter toward the trachea efficiently. This resulting wave of motion is known as *metachronism*. The bending of individual cilia results from ATP-dependent sliding of two parallel fibers within the ciliary filament, but it does not appear to involve the autonomic nervous system.

Mucus represents a mixture of water, electrolytes, and macromolecules (e.g., lipids, mucins, enzymes) secreted by goblet cells and mucosal glands. The rheologic properties of mucus influence the rate and efficiency of ciliary function. Thicker layers of mucus slow the removal of surface particles from the airway, whereas low-viscosity mucus promotes the most rapid ciliary transport. The amount and physical properties of the mucous layer may also promote the coordination of ciliary beats.[91] Reid[92] studied the physical and chemical characteristics of mucus in expectorated specimens. However, the volumetric, rheologic, biochemical, and clinical examination of normal respiratory secretions is made somewhat difficult by the contamination by salivary secretions and desiccation of these secretions in sputum.[93] Relatively newer methodologies permit more precise examination of in situ specimens, and some useful information has been garnered from tracheotomized subjects.

Mucociliary function in single cilia or respiratory epithelial tissue cultures may be assessed using high-speed videomicroscopy to examine the ciliary beat frequency. In vivo techniques in experimental animals have employed a tracheal window model. The velocity of mucus movement has been measured with radioactive markers or fiberoptic bronchoscopy in humans. The deposition of inhaled radiopaque or radioactive particles throughout the lung fields, followed by radiographic examinations of clearance of these particles, allows examination of mucociliary function in peripheral and central airways, even in small mammals.[94]

Impaired mucociliary function in the upper airways correlates with low levels of nasal NO, but the clinical significance of this finding remains to be defined.[95] The maintenance of bronchial perfusion is also critically important to the maintenance of normal mucociliary function.[96] Although nervous control of ciliary coordination has not been demonstrated in vertebrates,[93] mucociliary clearance, most likely related to changes in physical characteristics of respiratory secretions, is closely related to autonomic nervous system activity.[91]

Specific Effects of Anesthetics

Postoperative hypoxemia and atelectasis are common causes of perioperative morbidity. Many factors may affect mucociliary function in the mechanically ventilated patient. Poorly humidified inspired gases are known to reduce ciliary movement and desiccate mucus. The flow rates of mucus were maintained in the normal range during a 40-minute exposure to an inspired air temperature greater than 32°C when inspired water vapor content was at least 33 mg/L in dogs.[97] However, 3 hours of inhalation of dry air resulted in a complete cessation of the flow of tracheal mucus, which was restored by subsequent use of inspired gases with 100% relative humidity at 38°C.[98] Other factors that reduce the rate of mucus movement are high inspired oxygen concentration, inflation of an endotracheal tube cuff, and positive-pressure ventilation.[99]

The effects of inhaled anesthetics on mucociliary flow have been determined with scintillation counters measuring radioactive droplet progression in the trachea of dogs (Fig. 6-6).[99-101] Halothane alone, enflurane alone, nitrous oxide with halothane, and nitrous oxide with morphine produced similar dose-dependent decreases in mucociliary movement.[100,101] Clearance of mucus from central and peripheral airways after a 6-hour exposure to

1.2 MAC of halothane was delayed by at least 3 hours.[102] Volatile anesthetics and nitrous oxide may diminish rates of mucus clearance by decreasing ciliary beat frequency, disrupting metachronism, or altering the physical characteristics or quantity of mucus. Exposure to inhaled anesthetic caused dose-related decreases in ciliary activity and cellular mobility of the ciliated protozoan *Tetrahymena pyriformis*.[103] The dose that effectively terminated organism and ciliary movement in 50% of the protozoans closely corresponded to MAC values of the various anesthetics. The mechanism by which cilia were affected was not delineated in this study, but the speed and reversibility of ciliary depression suggested that ATP metabolism was not responsible. Extrapolation from the protozoan to mammalian airway epithelia must be performed with caution. Nevertheless, the results of this interesting study suggest that anesthetics produce a direct inhibitory effect on mucus clearance. High concentrations of halothane (at doses greater than 3%) also depressed ciliary movement in cultures of canine ciliated epithelium.[104] The sensitivity of cilia to halothane appeared to be less pronounced than that observed in *T. pyriformis*.[103] The effects of inhaled anesthetics on ciliary beat frequency in humans have yet to be elucidated.

Effects of Inhaled Anesthetics on Pulmonary Surfactant

Pulmonary surfactant decreases the work of breathing by reducing surface tension at the fluid-gas interface. Similar to mucus, surfactant plays a role in removing foreign particles from airways. Surfactant also enhances the bactericidal actions of alveolar macrophages. The effects of halothane and isoflurane on cultured alveolar type II cells, which secrete surfactant, and the metabolism of phosphatidylcholine, the main lipid component of surfactant, have been investigated.[105,106] Both agents reduced phosphatidylcholine synthesis by alveolar cells in a dose-dependent manner during a 4-hour exposure (Fig. 6-7). This reduction in phosphatidylcholine production was more pronounced with longer durations of exposure to halothane and was reversible within 2 hours after the agent was discontinued. High concentrations of halothane also disrupted the energy metabolism of cultured alveolar cells as indicated by reduced ATP content and enhanced glycolytic metabolism. Halothane and isoflurane potentiated the hydrogen peroxide–mediated reduction of phosphatidylcholine in alveolar type II cells.[105,107] Pretreatment with an inhibitor of H_2O_2-induced oxidation (i.e., nicotinamide) did not attenuate the adverse effects of halothane on alveolar cells. These data suggested a mechanism, possibly related to halothane-specific effects on cell energetics, by which inflammatory lung disease may be worsened during administration of a volatile anesthetic. Clinically relevant concentrations of halothane increase surfactant-associated protein C mRNA in vitro but exert the converse effect in mechanically ventilated rats.[108] Whether effects of halothane on surfactant protein C mRNA are related to similar actions on the actual protein has yet to be established.

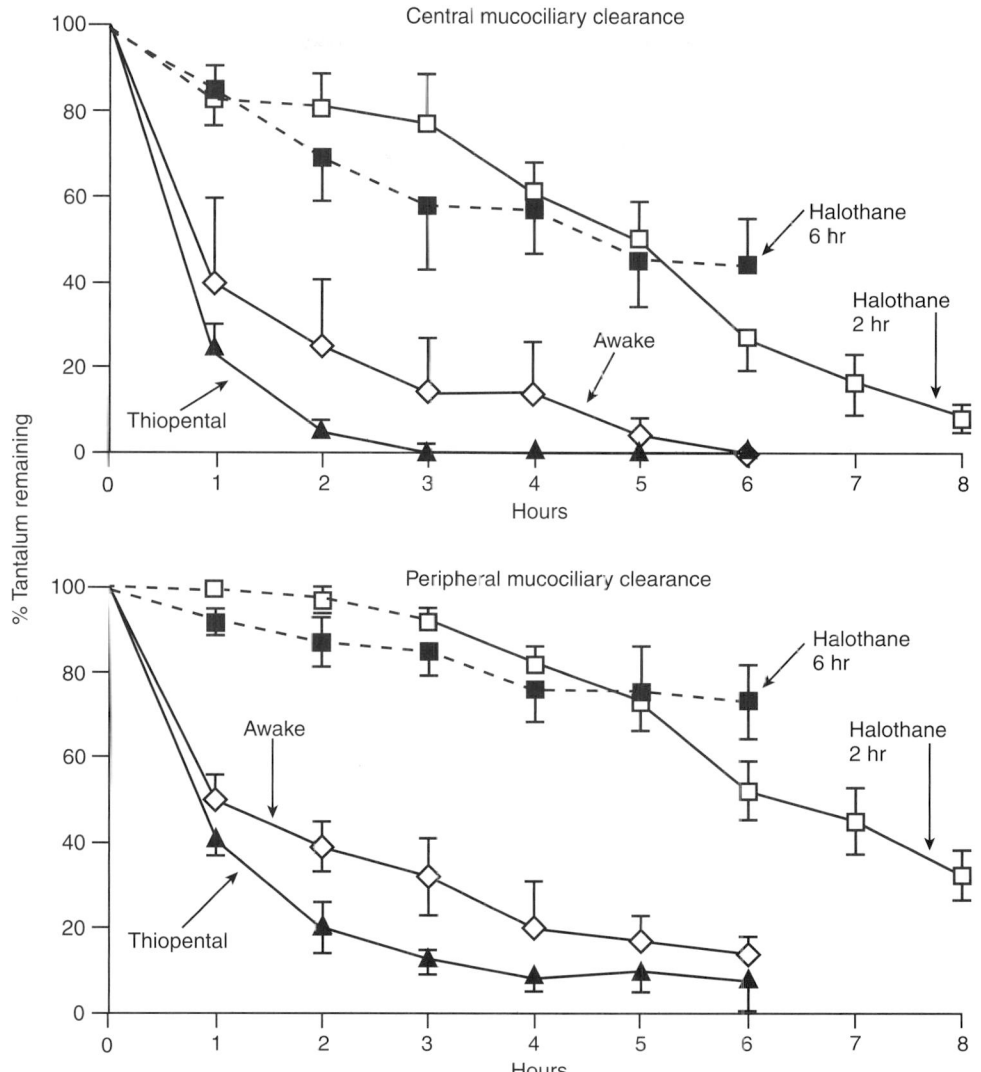

Figure 6–6 Mucociliary clearance measured as tantalum clearance in patients undergoing surgery with general or local anesthesia (i.e., awake). Notice the decrease in mucociliary clearance in the peripheral and central airways during halothane and thiopental anesthesia. (Adapted from Forbes AR, Gamsu G: Mucociliary clearance in the canine lung during and after general anesthesia. Anesthesiology 50:26, 1979.)

Effects of Inhaled Anesthetics on Mucociliary Function

Gamsu and coworkers[109] compared the rate of tantalum clearance from the lungs of postoperative patients who had received general anesthesia for intra-abdominal or lower extremity operations. Patients who underwent lower extremity surgery demonstrated no significant difference in tantalum clearance when compared with a control group measured using tracheography. These patients also did not develop atelectasis. In contrast, retention of tantalum was demonstrated for as long as 6 days after intra-abdominal surgery, with an average retention time three times greater than that observed in the control group. Retention of tantalum was gravity dependent and correlated with the retention of mucus demonstrated in areas of atelectasis. Disappearance of

tantalum from these atelectatic areas occurred only after reexpansion of collapsed lung segments. Teflon disks placed on the tracheal mucosa and observed with fiberoptic bronchoscopy were used to study tracheal mucus velocity in young women undergoing gynecologic surgery.[110] The average velocity of mucus in the awake volunteers was 20 mm/min. Administration of halothane (1% to 2%) and nitrous oxide (60%) rapidly decreased the rate of mucus movement to 7.7 mm/min. Little or no mucus motion was observed after 90 minutes of halothane–nitrous oxide exposure. Inspired gases were humidified, but the use of high inspired concentrations of oxygen, a cuffed endotracheal tube, and positive-pressure ventilation were confounding factors in this study. Bronchial mucosal transport velocity was also determined using radiolabeled albumin microspheres deposited distally in the mainstem bronchi using a

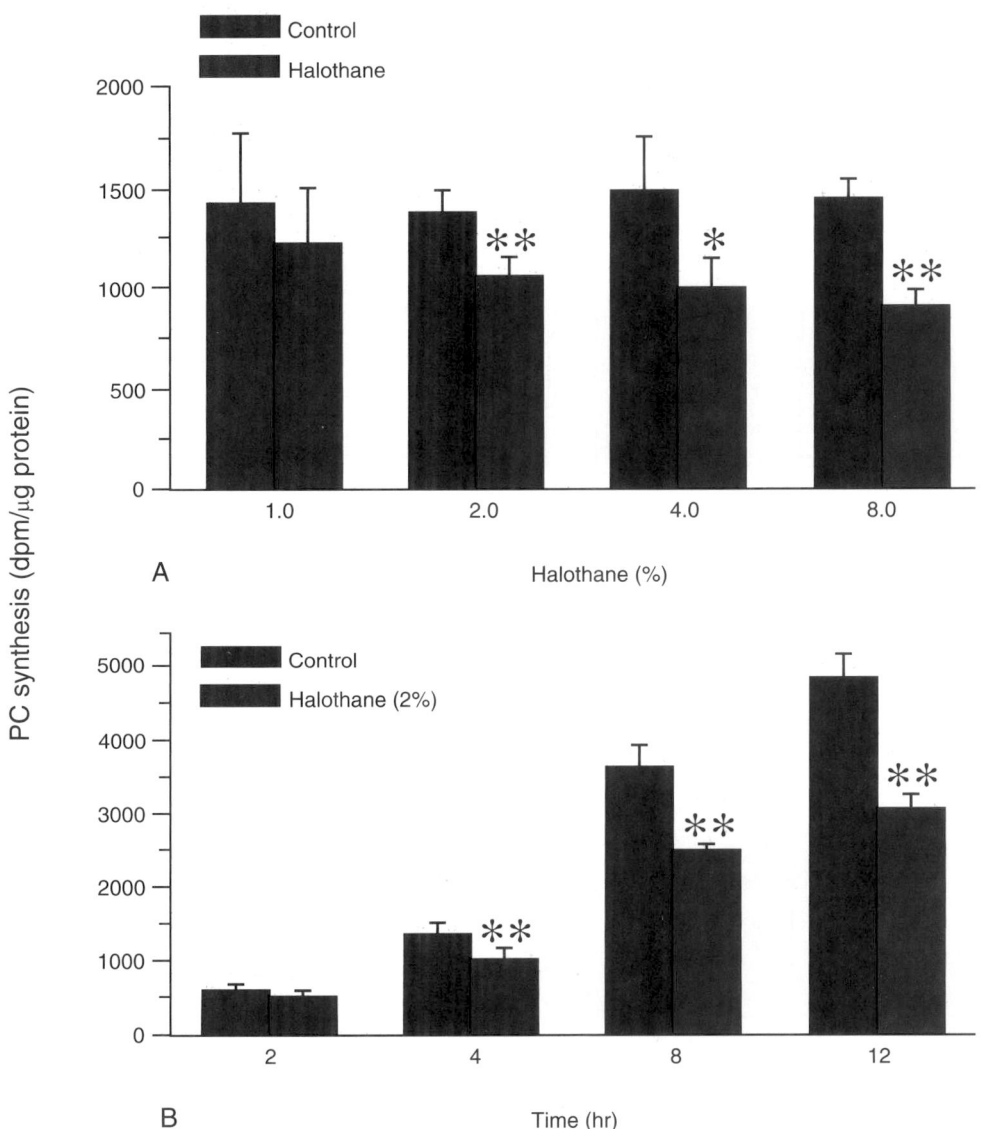

Figure 6–7 Effect of halothane on phosphatidylcholine (PC) synthesis by alveolar type II cells. PC synthesis measured as the incorporation of [^{3}H-methyl]-choline into PC and expressed as disintegrations per minute per microgram of intracellular protein (*$P < .05$, **$P < .01$ versus respective control.) **A**, Effect of increasing halothane concentration with 4-hour exposure. **B**, Effect of increasing exposure time to 2% halothane. (Adapted from Molliex S, Crestani B, Dureuil B, et al: Effects of halothane on surfactant biosynthesis by rat alveolar type II cells in primary culture. Anesthesiology 81:668, 1994.)

fiberoptic bronchoscope in healthy patients.[111] In contrast to the findings of the study with halothane,[110] mucus velocity was unchanged after administration of isoflurane (1.5 MAC). Whether this relative lack of effect of isoflurane on the transport of mucus was specifically related to the type of volatile agent was unclear. However, mucus pooling has been observed during and after anesthesia. The data indicate that vigorous pulmonary therapy directed at enhancing clearance of secretions from the airways should be instituted in the immediate postoperative period, regardless of the type of inhaled anesthetic chosen.

Konrad and coworkers[112] have shown that smokers have significantly slower bronchial mucus transport velocities than nonsmokers in patients undergoing abdominal or thoracic surgery. The investigators postulated that this observation may be related to an increased incidence of postoperative pulmonary complications in smokers.[112] Some evidence exists to support the contention that patients with chronic obstructive pulmonary disease (COPD) receiving regional anesthesia demonstrate a lower incidence of respiratory failure than those having general anesthesia,[113] but other studies have failed to confirm this hypothesis. The consequences of the specific procedure with intrathoracic and intra-abdominal surgery appear to be of greater importance in determining morbidity related to compromised respiratory function compared with peripheral procedures performed under regional anesthesia.

Mucociliary function impairment also occurs after lung transplantation. The mechanism for this dysfunction may be related to alterations in the surface properties of mucus and marked impairment of mucociliary transport distal to bronchial transection and reanastomosis.[114]

Many factors contribute to postoperative pulmonary complications. The specific roles of depressed mucociliary function and alterations in type II alveolar cells in such complications are unclear. Prolonged administration of inhaled anesthetics may produce mucus pooling and adversely alter alveolar cell surfactant metabolism. These actions may result in deleterious effects on pulmonary function including atelectasis and infection. Those at greatest risk appear to include patients with excessive or abnormal mucus or surfactant production (e.g., chronic bronchitis, asthma, cystic fibrosis, chronic mechanical ventilation).

Controlled studies of the effects of inhaled anesthetics on mucociliary function and surfactant metabolism in patients with compromised pulmonary performance have yet to be undertaken, nor has the precise action of inhaled anesthetics on the incidence of pulmonary complications been clearly defined. The specific actions of the newer volatile anesthetics desflurane and sevoflurane on mucociliary function have not been adequately studied, although there are no compelling reasons to suspect a clinically significant difference should exist between these agents and other inhaled anesthetics.

EFFECTS OF INHALED ANESTHETICS ON PULMONARY VASCULAR RESISTANCE

Determinants of Pulmonary Vascular Resistance

Determining the actions of drugs on pulmonary arterial pressures and pulmonary vascular resistance (PVR) is a complicated task because many vasoactive agents have direct effects on the pulmonary circulation and indirect actions mediated by alterations in cardiac output, preload, afterload, and autonomic nervous system activity. Increased vascular-distending pressure may increase the cross-sectional diameter of the pulmonary vascular bed and cause a compensatory reduction in PVR. Similarly, changes in lung volume may alter the dimensions of the pulmonary vasculature and affect resistance. Increases in lung volume above functional residual capacity (FRC) caused by elevated airway pressure and reductions in lung volume below FRC are associated with passive increases in PVR. High lung volumes compress pulmonary vessels, whereas vessels are shorter, narrower, and more tortuous because of loss of supportive tethering of surrounding lung parenchyma at low lung volumes. Resistance of the pulmonary arterial circulation appears to be lowest at a lung volume equivalent to the FRC. Changes in pulmonary arterial pressure and PVR also have significant effects on gas or fluid exchange in the lung. An increase in PVR causes a corresponding increase in pulmonary arterial pressure if cardiac output remains constant. This increase in pulmonary arterial pressure promotes transudation of fluid into the interstitium of the lung. PVR is also increased by positive end-expiratory pressure, alveolar hypoxia and hypercarbia, and critical closing pressure (i.e., a parallel shift in pressure-flow curves).

Inhaled anesthetics tend to reduce lung volume and may therefore have indirect effects on PVR through this mechanism as well.

Direct changes in pulmonary vascular tone alter PVR by altering the slope of pressure-flow relation. Such direct changes may be induced by a rapid rise in ICa^{2+}, alterations in sympathetic nervous system tone, local changes in arterial oxygen and carbon dioxide tension, or alterations in the circulating concentrations of catecholamines. Contractile responses to agonists such as phenylephrine are mediated by Ca^{2+} entry, ICa^{2+} release,[115] and a tyrosine kinase–mediated signal transduction pathway, independent of VDCs.[116] These responses are inhibited by K^+ channel inhibition.[117] Hypercapnia at constant pH (i.e., isohydria) does not alter isolated pulmonary arterial tone, but normocapnic acidosis relaxes isolated pulmonary arteries by an endothelium-independent mechanism.[118] Nevertheless, pulmonary arterial endothelial dysfunction has also been reported to potentiate hypercapnic vasoconstriction.[119]

Vasoactive substances released locally or in blood perfusing the lung also affect vascular tone. NO synthases are widely distributed in the lung and extensively involved in vascular homeostasis.[120] NO synthesis is intimately linked to the pulmonary oxygen environment. For example, a decrease in oxygen tension prolongs the duration of NO action, but conversely provides less substrate for its production.[121-123] NO synthase appears to play little or no role in the regulation of PVR in the healthy, normoxic lung,[120,124] but this substance is a critical mediator of PVR during hypoxia.[125,126] In addition to producing vasodilation in ventilated, normoxic pulmonary regions during one-lung hypoxia, NO may also release an endogenous inhibitor of NO synthase that vasoconstricts nonventilated, hypoxic regions.[127] The action of endogenous NO on PVR and the utility of exogenous NO as a treatment for pulmonary hypertension have been extensively investigated over the past few years.[128] NO may be beneficial in the treatment of high-altitude pulmonary edema[129] and neonatal pulmonary hypertension resulting from a variety of congenital heart diseases, hypoplastic lung, and meconium aspiration.[130] However, NO inhalation during acute bronchospasm may paradoxically worsen hypoxemia.[131] Whether this adverse action is mediated by direct bronchodilatory actions on less-constricted peripheral airways or by worsening intrapulmonary shunt through arterial vasodilation is unclear. Pulmonary endothelial dysfunction after cardiopulmonary bypass impairs endothelium-dependent vasodilation to agents such as acetylcholine and bradykinin.[132] This cardiopulmonary bypass–induced endothelial dysfunction may affect the efficacy of NO administration in this setting to some degree. Nevertheless, use of NO in pediatric and adult cardiac surgical patients has become a common means of reducing PVR in this setting.

Similar to NO, carbon monoxide (CO) is another molecular gas that stimulates guanylyl cyclase and increases cGMP levels in pulmonary arterial vascular smooth muscle cells to regulate vascular tone.[133] Inhaled CO also attenuates hypoxemia-induced increases in PVR through this mechanism.[134]

Regional changes in PVR affect the regional distribution of blood flow within the lung and produce changes in ventilation-perfusion matching and simultaneous alterations in gas exchange. An increase in PVR in an area of atelectasis causes localized tissue hypoxia but optimizes overall gas exchange (e.g., decreases alveolar-arterial oxygen tension gradient [P_{AO_2}–Pa_{O_2}]) by shifting blood flow away from the atelectic segment to a well-ventilated region of the lung. This phenomenon is called *hypoxic pulmonary vasoconstriction* (HPV) and is unique to the pulmonary circulation because other vascular beds (i.e., coronary and cerebral) dilate in response to hypoxia. HPV exerts an important protective effect to maintain oxygenation, and drugs that interfere with HPV may adversely affect gas exchange. For example, administration of a direct pulmonary vasodilator such as sodium nitroprusside attenuates HPV, increases pulmonary shunting, and reduces arterial oxygenation in dogs with oleic acid–induced pulmonary edema.[135] Similarly, isoflurane also increases ventilation-perfusion mismatch and oxygen delivery in mechanically ventilated dogs with experimental lung injury.[136] However, the pulmonary vasodilator effect of inhaled anesthetics is minimal in normal lungs.[137-139] Small decreases in PVR produced by inhaled agents are frequently offset by a concomitant reduction in cardiac output in vivo. The net effect of these actions results in little if any change in pulmonary artery pressure and a small decrease in total pulmonary blood flow. In contrast, nitrous oxide does not substantially affect cardiac output and pulmonary blood flow and causes small increases in PVR.

Mechanism of Hypoxic Pulmonary Vasoconstriction

HPV is a locally mediated phenomenon. HPV may be observed in isolated perfused lungs and experimental animals after autonomic nervous system blockade or catecholamine depletion in vivo. The sympathetic nervous system may play a role in augmenting the HPV response under some conditions, especially during hypoxemia. HPV occurs when alveolar oxygen tension falls to less than 100 mm Hg in the normal lung and is maximal when oxygen tension is approximately 30 mm Hg.[140,141] HPV has been studied in humans with healthy lungs.[142] Unilateral graded or single-step hypoxia ($FI_{O_2} = 0.05$) produced similar reductions in the perfusion of the hypoxic lung to approximately 30% of control. Mixed venous oxygen tension may also influence HPV in the atelectatic lung because alveolar oxygen tension approaches venous oxygen tension in the collapsed lung.[143,144] Hypercapnia-induced acidosis increases PVR in intact animals and isolated, perfused lungs. Acidosis-induced increases in PVR are relatively small at normal alveolar oxygen tensions but are dramatically enhanced during alveolar hypoxia. Local acidosis and increases in alveolar carbon dioxide tension may augment HPV and may further improve arterial oxygenation in healthy lungs. High carbon dioxide concentrations reduce NO levels,[145] but whether this action is responsible for hypercarbia-induced improvements in ventilation and perfusion remains unclear.[146,147]

Inhaled Anesthetics and Hypoxic Pulmonary Vasoconstriction

Several mechanisms contribute to diminished FRC, reduced oxygenation, and increased P_{AO_2}–Pa_{O_2} during anesthesia. Inhaled anesthetics contribute to this process by affecting HPV. The influences of anesthetics on HPV have been examined in a variety of experimental models but have yielded conflicting results.

The effects of inhaled anesthetics on HPV are multifactorial and involve direct actions on the pulmonary vasculature combined with indirect effects mediated by the autonomic nervous system, systemic hemodynamics, and humoral actions. In general, most in vitro studies have demonstrated that inhaled anesthetics attenuate HPV to some degree (Fig. 6-8). Inhibition of HPV has been demonstrated with halothane,[137,148-152] isoflurane[137,138] enflurane,[137,153] sevoflurane,[138] desflurane,[139] and nitrous oxide using isolated perfused lungs or an in situ preparation with constant perfusion.[154-156] Marshall and colleagues[137] examined the effects of halothane, enflurane, and isoflurane on the HPV response to global hypoxia. All three drugs depressed HPV in a dose-dependent fashion. Similar MAC values (approximately 0.6 MAC) of these agents also depressed HPV by 50% in an in vitro preparation using controlled pulmonary perfusion independent of sympathetic nervous system activity. A later study using isolated rat lungs confirmed the depression of HPV by isoflurane and halothane. The addition of verapamil further reduced HPV by an additional 35% to 40%, suggesting that inhaled anesthetics and Ca^{2+} channel antagonists inhibit HPV through different sites of action.[157] Halothane reduced the resistance of the middle vascular segment in an atelectic, hypoxic lung, suggesting a specific, direct action of this agent on small vessels and capillaries.[151,158]

The effect of hypoxia on PVR was assessed by measuring blood flow to an isolated lobe selectively ventilated with a hypoxic gas mixture and comparing it with total pulmonary blood flow with the remainder of the lung ventilated with 100% oxygen.[159,160] A significant decrease in flow to the isolated lobe occurred in the presence of localized alveolar hypoxia during constant pulmonary blood flow (i.e., cardiac output), pulmonary artery pressure, and left atrial pressure. Neither halothane nor nitrous oxide administered to the isolated lobe diminished the magnitude of HPV, but a dose-related inhibition was demonstrated during administration of isoflurane. When these experiments were repeated with the anesthetic administered to the remainder of the lung instead of isolated lobar segment, halothane, isoflurane, and enflurane reduced cardiac output, but the effects on blood flow to the isolated segment were almost identical to those obtained when volatile agents were administered to the isolated lobe alone.

The mechanism of the direct inhibitory action of inhaled anesthetics on HPV is unclear but may be related to enhancement of arachidonic acid metabolism[152,161] or other endothelium-derived vasodilating factors.[162] Conversely, other evidence suggests that inhaled anesthetic-induced inhibition of HPV may occur independent of the presence of pulmonary vascular endothelium, NO, or guanylate cyclase.[163-165]

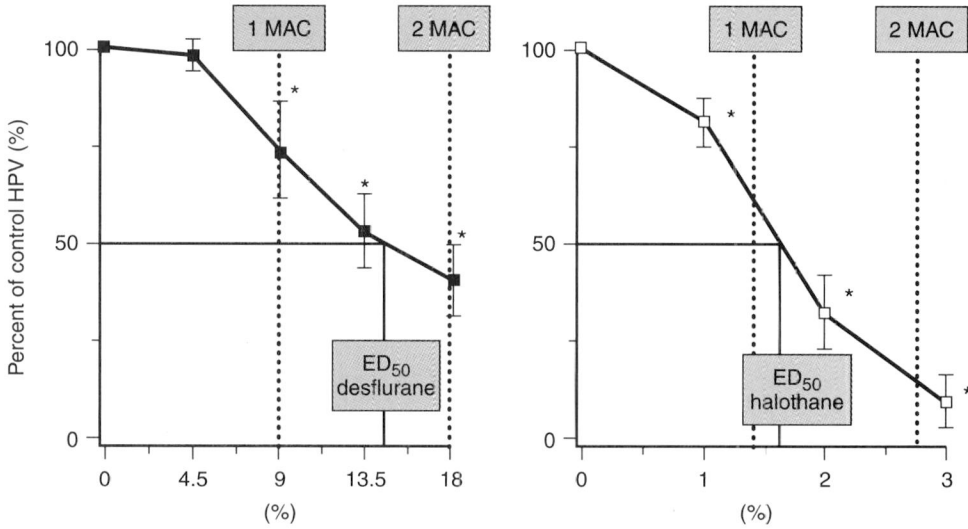

Figure 6–8 Concentration-dependent inhibition of hypoxic pulmonary vasoconstriction (HPV) in isolated rabbit lungs by desflurane *(solid squares)* and halothane *(open squares)*. Values are mean ± SEM and expressed as a percentage of control (*$P < .05$ versus control HPV). The half-maximum inhibiting effect (ED_{50}) values were within the range of 1 to 2 minimum alveolar concentrations (MACs) for rabbits for both agents. (Reproduced from Loer SA, Scheeren TWL, Tarnow J: Desflurane inhibits hypoxic pulmonary vasoconstriction in isolated rabbit lungs. Anesthesiology 83:552, 1995.)

Inhaled anesthetics also disrupt Ca^{2+} homeostasis in vascular smooth muscle and thereby interfere with pulmonary vasoconstriction.[166] Halothane and isoflurane attenuated endothelium-dependent vasodilation by inhibiting accumulation of cGMP[165] and a K_{ATP} channel–mediated interaction between NO and prostacyclin in isolated canine pulmonary artery rings.[167,163] In contrast, isoflurane modulated the HPV response, at least in part through Ca^{2+}-activated and voltage-sensitive K^+ but not K_{ATP} channels in isolated rabbit lungs. Attenuation of HPV by sevoflurane was independent of K^+ channel function.[169] Rats with liver cirrhosis exhibit a blunted HPV response and arterial hypoxemia. These cirrhotic rats demonstrate increased NO and reduced endothelin concentration, but the blunted HPV response observed in these animals does not involve these systems and is mediated instead by activation of Ca^{2+}-activated K^+ channels.[170] Halothane, isoflurane, enflurane, and desflurane also attenuate K_{ATP} channel– and endothelin-mediated pulmonary vasodilation in chronically instrumented dogs,[171-173] in part by inhibiting vasodilatory prostanoids.[167,174] The inhibition of pulmonary vasodilation is not a uniform observation during administration of all volatile agents in all circumstances, because isoflurane and halothane, but not enflurane, enhance isoproterenol-mediated vasodilation.[175,176] Unlike the findings with other volatile agents tested, the sevoflurane-induced pulmonary vasodilation mediated by K_{ATP} channels is also preserved.[173] Isoflurane also attenuates hypotension-induced pulmonary vasoconstriction.[177]

Studies have investigated an apparent biphasic action of volatile anesthetics on isolated pulmonary arterial strips. Dose-dependent increases in force are initially observed with volatile agents after Ca^{2+} release from intracellular stores (associated with protein kinase C activation).

Subsequently, a decrease in force (associated with a Ca^{2+}-calmodulin–dependent protein kinase II activation) occurs (Fig. 6-9).[178-180] Extrapolation of these results in isolated pulmonary artery strips to humans in vivo must be performed cautiously. Nevertheless, the clinical implications of these studies are important and suggest that volatile anesthetics may cause initial pulmonary arterial vasoconstriction before vasodilation. The vasodilatory response may be more profound in patients with low sarcoplasmic reticulum Ca^{2+} stores (i.e., neonates) or those with depressed protein kinase C activity (i.e., primary pulmonary hypertension).

The findings from in vitro studies suggest that volatile anesthetics exert inhibitory actions on HPV, but results from in vivo investigations usually have shown little or no effect. Sykes and associates[181] examined the effects of one-lung hypoxia on relative pulmonary blood flow distribution measured using xenon in dogs. One lung was ventilated with nitrogen, and the other was ventilated with 100% oxygen. A redistribution of flow to the well-oxygenated lung was found consistent with active HPV. This action was preserved during administration of halothane (inspired concentrations = 3%). In contrast, ether and nitrous oxide profoundly affected the redistribution of pulmonary blood flow in response to hypoxia using the same experimental preparation.[182,183] Other in vivo investigations have also verified that nitrous oxide markedly attenuates HPV.[159,160,184] In contrast, clinically relevant concentrations of halothane, isoflurane, enflurane, sevoflurane, and desflurane appear to have minimal effects on HPV in vivo (Fig. 6-10).[159,160,185-191] Lennon and Murray[161] suggested that isoflurane anesthesia may attenuate HPV by inhibiting vasodilatory prostanoids in chronically instrumented dogs. Pulmonary vascular perfusion pressure (determined by the difference between

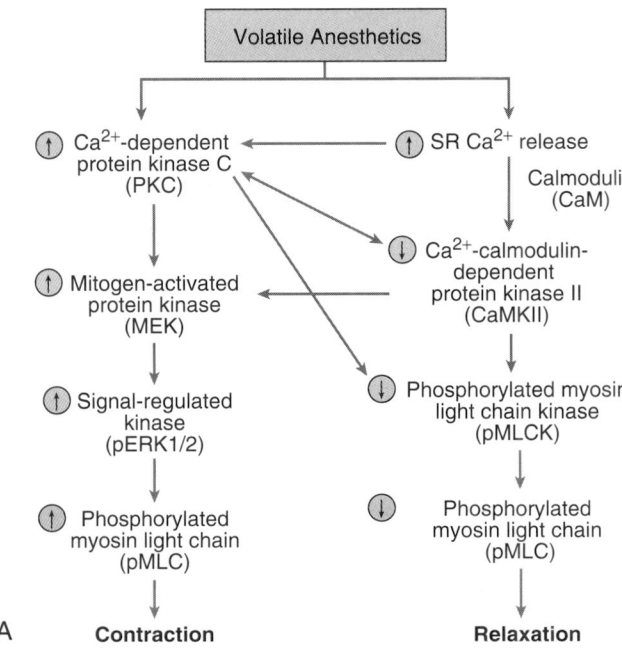

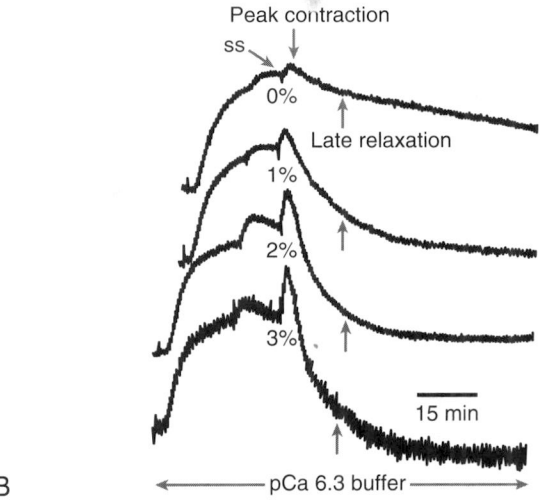

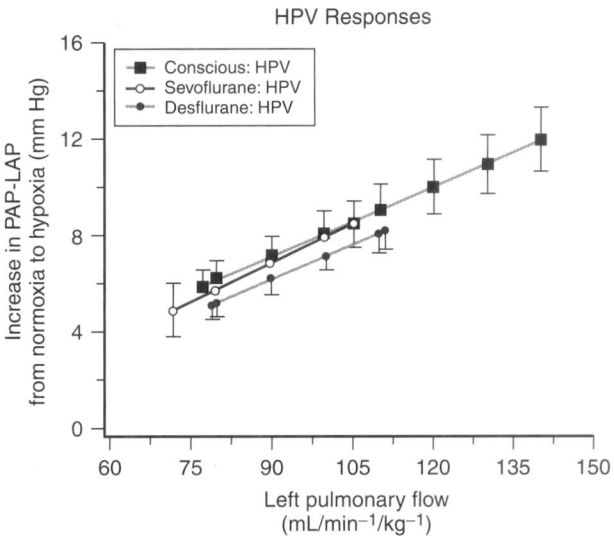

Figure 6–10 Composite hypoxic pulmonary vasoconstriction (HPV) responses as a function of left pulmonary flow in the same seven chronically instrumented dogs in the conscious state and during sevoflurane and desflurane anesthesia. Neither type of anesthesia affected the magnitude of HPV compared with the response in the conscious state. (Adapted from Lesitsky MA, Davis S, Murray PA: Preservation of hypoxic pulmonary vasoconstriction during sevoflurane and desflurane anesthesia compared to the conscious state in chronically instrumented dogs. Anesthesiology 89:1501, 1998.)

Figure 6–9 **A**, Proposed signaling pathways underlying volatile anesthetic (halothane and isoflurane)–induced contraction and relaxation in pulmonary artery smooth muscle. After Ca^{2+} release from intracellular stores, there are dose-dependent increases in force initially (associated with protein kinase C activation), which is followed by a decrease in force (associated with a Ca^{2+}-calmodulin–dependent protein kinase II activation). High concentrations of halothane may activate a protein kinase C–Ca^{2+}-calmodulin–dependent protein kinase II pathway. **B**, Example of biphasic (contraction-relaxation) effect of halothane on pulmonary arterial smooth muscle. Halothane dose-dependently enhanced Ca^{2+}-activated peak force as well as late relaxation. 0%, 1%, 2%, and 3%, halothane concentrations; ss, control force at steady state before halothane. (Adapted from Su JY, Vo AC: Ca^{2+}-calmodulin-dependent protein kinase II plays a major role in halothane-induced dose-dependent relaxation in the skinned pulmonary artery. Anesthesiology 97:207, 2002 and from Zhong L, Su JY: Isoflurane activates PKC and Ca^{2+}-calmodulin-dependent protein kinase II via MAP kinase signaling in cultured vascular smooth muscle cells. Anesthesiology 96:148, 2002.)

pulmonary arterial and left atrial pressures) and blood flow relationships were generated in the absence of baseline anesthesia and acute surgical intervention to demonstrate a flow dependency of the HPV. Inhibition of HPV was not observed using this preparation during sevoflurane or desflurane anesthesia, in contrast to the findings with isoflurane.[190] In animals with a preexisting gas exchange defect due to a pneumoperitoneum, sevoflurane, but not isoflurane, caused more pronounced abnormalities in gas exchange than propofol.[192]

Effects of Inhaled Anesthetics on Pulmonary Vasculature in Humans

One obvious explanation for differences in results between in vitro and in vivo studies is the influence of cardiac output. The direct effects of anesthetics on HPV compared with indirect actions mediated through changes in cardiac output were evaluated using data from several studies.[193] The efficacy of HPV varies inversely with cardiac output (i.e., pulmonary arterial blood flow), and a direct inhibition of HPV by anesthetics may be opposed by a reduction in cardiac output such that HPV may appear to be unaffected. The net HPV response to volatile agents may be unchanged when the cardiac output is reduced, but it may be fully intact or minimally attenuated when cardiac output is maintained (e.g., during administration of nitrous oxide). These data emphasize the flow dependence of HPV in the presence of an inhaled anesthetic.

Isoflurane does not alter pulmonary shunt function in healthy patients even at concentrations that produce systemic hypotension.[194] The effects of diethyl ether and halothane on pulmonary blood flow distribution during nitrogen ventilation of one lung were examined in humans.[185] HPV occurred in the nitrogen-ventilated lung during intravenous anesthesia with barbiturates but disappeared with the inhalation of halothane or diethyl ether in the ventilated lung. Abolition of HPV was accompanied in most patients by a decrease in arterial oxygenation. In contrast to the findings of this study, observations in experimental animals or in patients undergoing single-lung ventilation failed to demonstrate clinically significant attenuation of HPV during administration of halothane or desflurane.[195] Isoflurane, sevoflurane, and desflurane have been shown to impair oxygenation more than intravenous infusions of propofol during single-lung ventilation in pigs and humans.[196,197] However, the differences in oxygenation observed in these studies are small and may be of little clinical relevance. These results differ from other findings demonstrating that shunt fraction is similar in patients receiving propofol or sevoflurane during single-lung ventilation.[198] No significant differences in shunt fraction or arterial oxygen tension were observed when pulmonary gas exchange was compared during intravenous infusions of ketamine (which does not inhibit HPV) and administration of enflurane.[199] Isoflurane and desflurane decreased shunt fraction and did not affect oxygenation during single-lung ventilation.[200] Most clinical thoracic surgery is usually undertaken in the lateral position with an open chest, dramatically altering the relative distribution of ventilation and perfusion. Under these circumstances, a diseased, nondependent lung may substantially affect pulmonary vascular responsiveness to hypoxia, as may surgical manipulation of the lung itself.[201] These well-known observations limit applicability of studies evaluating the effects of inhaled anesthetics on shunt fraction and oxygenation conducted in animals or patients with normal lungs in the absence of surgical intervention.

Benumof and colleagues[202] provided convincing evidence that inhaled anesthetics may be used safely in patients undergoing thoracotomy and single-lung ventilation. Halothane and isoflurane only minimally impair arterial oxygenation under these conditions (Fig. 6-11). The increase in shunt and decrease in oxygenation caused by halothane or isoflurane in this study was consistent with an approximately 20% inhibition of HPV at 1 MAC. Instead of a reduction in pulmonary blood flow of 50% in a hypoxic lung in the absence of a volatile anesthetic, blood flow decreases by 40% during hypoxia in the presence of 1 MAC halothane or isoflurane. This change in flow corresponds to an increase in pulmonary shunt by about 4% of cardiac output.[202] Similar and rather modest changes in shunt fraction and oxygenation were shown to occur with isoflurane, desflurane,[203] and sevoflurane[204] in patients undergoing thoracotomy and single-lung ventilation. The use of total intravenous anesthesia with propofol and alfentanil did not decrease the risk of hypoxemia during single-lung ventilation.[205] Isoflurane appears to be safe to use during single-lung ventilation, and administration of isoflurane before

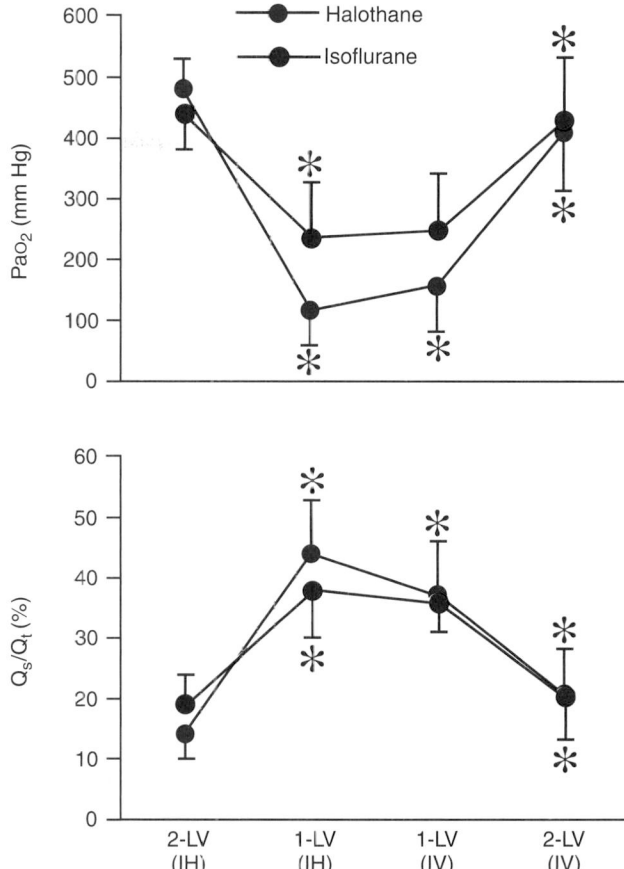

Figure 6–11 Arterial oxygenation (Pao$_2$) and intrapulmonary shunt (Q$_s$/Q$_t$) in patients ventilated with both lungs (2-LV) or with one lung (1-LV). Patients received an inhalational agent (IH) halothane or isoflurane followed by an intravenous (IV) thiopental. Notice the minimal effect on Pao$_2$ and the shunt that occurs in changing from a volatile anesthetic to an IV agent. (Adapted from Benumof JL, Augustine SD, Gibbons JA: Halothane and isoflurane only slightly impair arterial oxygenation during one-lung ventilation in patients undergoing thoracotomy. Anesthesiology 67:910, 1987.)

pulmonary ischemia also protects against ischemia-reperfusion injury as indicated by attenuation of increases in PVR and reductions in the coefficient of filtration and the wet-to-dry ratio.[206]

Important factors that modulate the effects of HPV may also be baseline pulmonary artery blood flow and pressure. High pulmonary artery pressures may tend to cause passive distention of constricted vascular beds and thereby reverse HPV. Alternatively, reflex pulmonary and systemic vasoconstriction in response to hypotension may increase PVR in healthy lung segments, leading to a shift of blood flow to hypoxic areas of lung.

Remarkable increases in pulmonary shunting have been demonstrated by administration of pulmonary vasodilators (e.g., sodium nitroprusside, nitroglycerin) in dogs with oleic acid–induced pulmonary edema.[135] Some volatile anesthetics may produce a similar response in patients with adult respiratory distress syndrome or with other types of pulmonary pathology associated with large right-to-left intrapulmonary shunts, although this hypothesis has yet to be comprehensively examined. Although Lennon and Murray[161] demonstrated an inhibitory effect for isoflurane on HPV in chronically instrumented dogs, these investigators also showed that isoflurane did not attenuate the enhanced pulmonary vasoconstrictor response to sympathetic α-adrenoreceptor activation or influence the pulmonary vascular tone in the presence of increased PVR mediated by increases in plasma endothelin concentrations and endothelin-mediated receptor activation[207] after single-lung transplantation.[208] These results support the hypothesis that the pulmonary circulation after lung transplantation is refractory to conventional pharmacologic therapy. These findings may have significant implications for the intraoperative anesthetic management of patients with similar abnormalities in pulmonary vasoregulation.

The precise effects of inhaled anesthetics on HPV and pulmonary shunts in patients with preexisting pulmonary disease remain to be defined, but the action of these agents on the pulmonary vasculature itself must be considered when evaluating causes of hypoxemia during anesthesia. Additional investigations will be required in humans before the actions of inhaled anesthetics on these determinants of pulmonary function can be precisely predicted.

Clinical observations suggest that inhaled anesthetics exert only modest inhibitory effects on HPV and oxygenation. This relatively minor inhibition of HPV by inhaled anesthetics should not significantly influence clinical decision making, especially given the efficacy of nondependent lung continuous positive pressure in improving oxygenation. The net effect of anesthetics on HPV is multifactorial and depends on a number of other intraoperative factors that commonly occur during anesthesia and surgery.

EFFECTS OF INHALED ANESTHETICS ON CONTROL OF VENTILATION

The most obvious effects of inhaled anesthetics are alterations of minute ventilation. Many different stimuli interact in a complex manner to determine ventilation in humans. The traditional approach to studying effects of drugs on ventilation has been to measure ventilatory responsiveness (e.g., expired minute volume, respiratory frequency, arterial carbon dioxide tension) before and after drug administration. A complete description of ventilatory control is beyond the scope of this chapter, and several excellent reviews of this subject already exist.[209-214] However, an understanding of normal ventilatory responses and control mechanisms is necessary to appreciate the actions of anesthetics and the methods by which these effects are measured.

Control of Breathing

A control system that modulates ventilation is required to maintain stability of arterial blood gas tensions and acid-base status and to integrate respiratory rate and tidal volume to minimize the work of breathing in response to variations in the total ventilatory requirements (Fig. 6-12). The system responsible for receiving and integrating a variety of input signals and ultimately producing movement of air into and out of the lungs is composed of the following elements:

The *sensory system* may be chemical (i.e., peripheral and central chemoreceptors) or mechanical (i.e., distortion receptors located in airways, alveoli, and respiratory muscles).

The *respiratory control system* integrates the signal inputs from the receptor sites, centers of consciousness, and other influences (e.g., pain) and subsequently produces nerve traffic to the muscles of respiration.

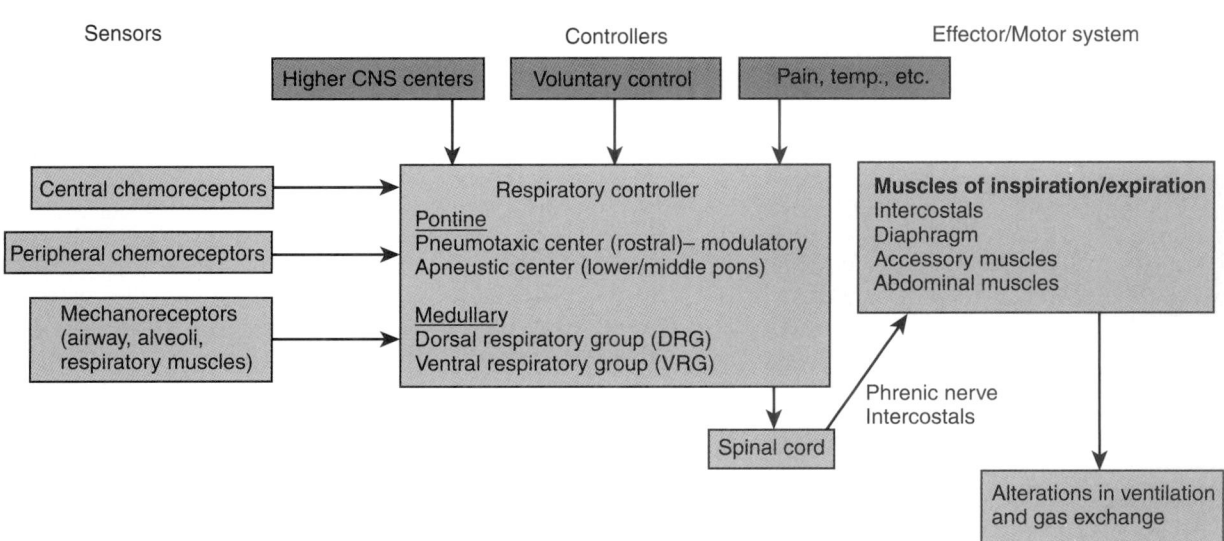

Figure 6–12 Aspects of the reflex control of ventilation. Sensors include central and peripheral chemoreceptors as well as a variety of mechanoreceptors. Inputs from these many sources interact to alter ventilatory controller output from pontomedullary sites to muscles of respiration, altering ventilation and ultimately gas exchange.

The *motor system* is composed of chest wall, intercostal, diaphragmatic, and abdominal muscles, all of which respond to signals from the control center through phrenic and spinal nerves.

The respiratory rhythm generator resides within the brainstem and consists of two primary types of respiratory neurons: the dorsal respiratory group (DRG), composed of cells active during inspiration; and the ventral respiratory group (VRG), containing inspiratory and expiratory neurons. The precise mechanism of rhythm generation remains unknown despite extensive study. Excitatory drive to bulbospinal inspiratory neurons of the caudal ventral respiratory group is mediated by tonic (acting through N-methyl-D-aspartate [NMDA] receptors) and phasic inputs (primarily consisting of non-NMDA glutamate receptors).[215] Neurotransmission in bulbospinal expiratory neurons is mediated through NMDA-type glutamate receptor input and modulated by γ-aminobutyric acid type A (GABA$_A$) receptors.[216,217] The isolated medulla oblongata is capable of generating a rhythmic, albeit abnormal, respiratory pattern.[218] Medullary regions involved in the generation and modulation of respiratory and sympathetic nervous system vasomotor output may also contain neurons functioning as central oxygen detectors.[219] One such central site that may be involved in this process is the retrotrapezoid nucleus of the rostral ventrolateral medulla. However, several other brainstem sites that express FOS during hypercapnia or hypoxia have also been implicated.[220] A particularly useful in vitro neonatal brain slice model was developed by Smith and colleagues.[221] Using this model, a group of pacemaker (self-oscillating) respiratory neurons in the rostral VRG was identified that may represent the elusive rhythm generator at least in the immature animals. The rostral pons contains the pneumotaxic center that involves inspiratory and expiratory neurons and plays a critical modulating role by integrating vagal and chemoreceptive inputs. The inspiratory controller output independent of other mechanical factors may be measured in humans as the pressure developed in the first 0.1 second of inspiration at FRC by acute airway occlusion.[222]

General Ventilatory Effects of Anesthetics

In general, all volatile anesthetics decrease tidal volume. This resultant depression of minute ventilation may be partially offset by a concomitant increase in respiratory rate (Fig. 6-13).[223,224] Early studies demonstrated that isoflurane produced more profound respiratory depression than did halothane, but in contrast to halothane, isoflurane did not progressively increase respiratory rate.[225,226] Like halothane, enflurane reduces tidal volume and minute ventilation concomitant with compensatory tachypnea in a dose-related manner.[227] Prolonged administration (3 to 7 hours) of halothane or enflurane decreased the degree of respiratory depression as indicated by resting arterial carbon dioxide tension.[227,228] Halothane also exerts differential effects on ventilatory timing parameters, including the ratio of occluded-to-unoccluded inspiratory time, in children[229] and infants younger than 2 months of age, depending on postconceptual age.[230]

Desflurane and sevoflurane also exhibit dose-related ventilatory depression, primarily by reducing tidal volume.[231-234] Unlike isoflurane, sevoflurane and desflurane cause dose-related increases in respiratory rate. Desflurane does not significantly reduce minute ventilation at concentrations less than 1.6 MAC. The reduction of respiratory rate produced by desflurane at higher concentrations was less than that caused by halothane. The relative increases in arterial carbon dioxide tension as an index of respiratory depression with volatile anesthetics (<1.24 MAC) are caused by, in order, enflurane, desflurane or isoflurane, and sevoflurane or halothane. Halothane and sevoflurane also cause similar respiratory changes in spontaneously ventilating children.[235,236] Nevertheless, potentially important differences between these two agents have been identified and include reduced minute ventilation and respiratory rate, a delay in the timing of peak inspiratory flow, and an earlier occurrence of peak expiratory flow during sevoflurane compared with halothane anesthesia.[236] The ventilatory depression produced by desflurane and sevoflurane is similar to that produced by enflurane and isoflurane, respectively, at higher concentrations.[224,225,231-234] In spontaneously ventilating dogs, respiratory effects of 1 to 2 MAC sevoflurane are similar to those of isoflurane, greater than those of halothane at 2 MAC, and less than those of enflurane at 1.5 and 2 MAC.[237] Isoflurane-induced respiratory depression is reduced by surgical stimulation (Fig. 6-14).[238] Respiratory depression observed during desflurane or sevoflurane anesthesia is reduced in the presence of nitrous oxide at equi-MAC values.[239] The respiratory depressant effects of xenon were first described in 1955.[240] Unlike other inhaled anesthetics, xenon decreases the respiratory rate and increases tidal volume, resulting in a reduction[241] or an increase in minute ventilation.[242]

Mechanoreceptors and Breathing

Central respiratory control mechanisms regulate tidal volume and inspiratory and expiratory times to achieve adequate ventilation and gas exchange. Input signals emanate from chemoreceptors and from mechanoreceptors in the upper airways, lungs, and chest wall, with signals transmitted by the vagus nerve and spinal nerves. Respiratory muscle function may be assessed by direct measurement of neural activity, electromyography, or mechanical consequences (i.e., tidal volume, minute ventilation, and analysis of motion and pressures generated by specific muscles). Although it was previously believed that inspiratory muscles, including the diaphragm, might fatigue during inspiratory resistance loading, voluntary cessation of loading and carbon dioxide retention occur before muscle fatigue.[210] Upper airway musculature may also be altered by inhaled anesthetics, thereby affecting evaluation of overall respiratory function.

Lung and Airway Receptors

Airway receptors that may be influenced by inhaled anesthetics include laryngeal and pulmonary irritant receptors and pulmonary stretch receptors. It has been suggested

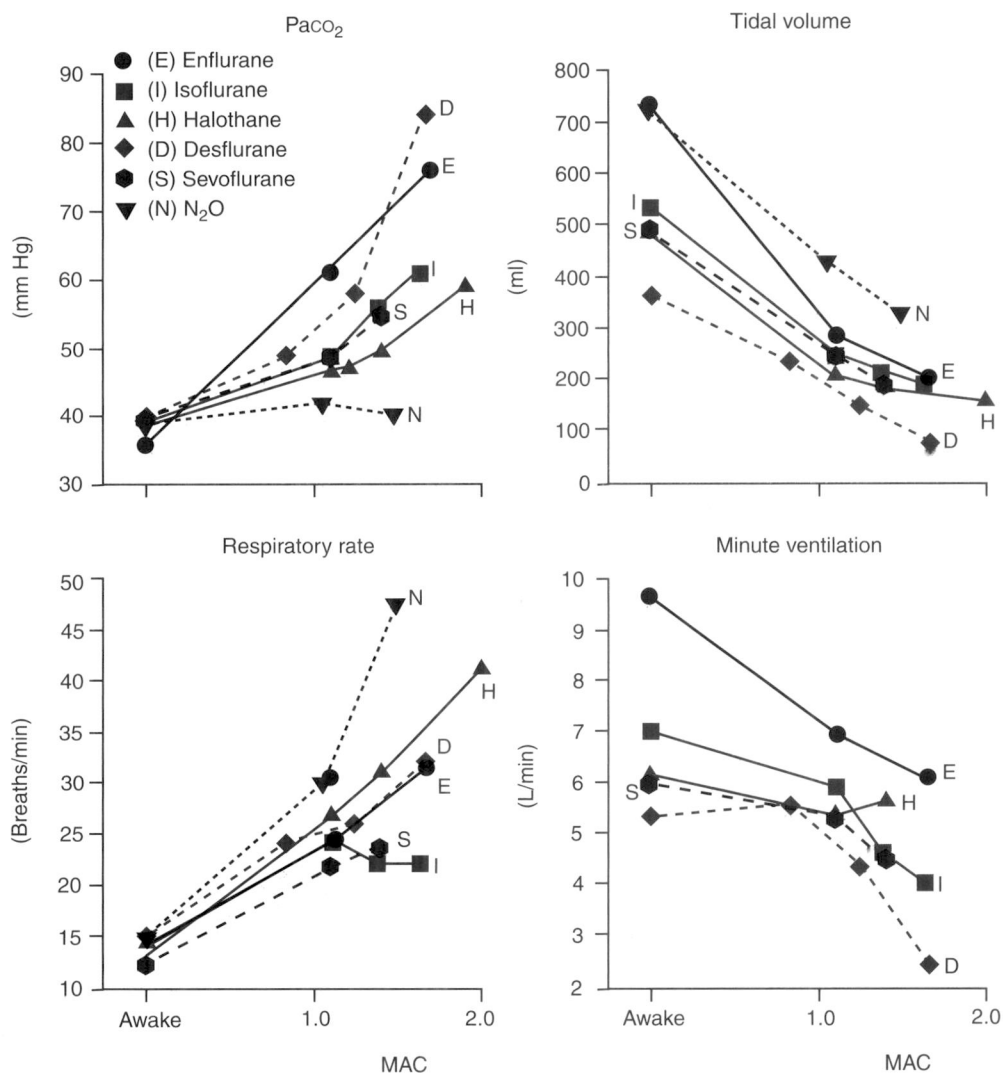

Figure 6–13 Comparison of mean changes in resting $Paco_2$, tidal volume, respiratory rate, and minute ventilation in patients anesthetized with halothane (H), isoflurane (I), enflurane (E), sevoflurane (S), desflurane (D), or nitrous oxide (N). Anesthetic-induced tachypnea compensates in part for the ventilatory depression caused by all volatile anesthetics (i.e., decreased minute ventilation and tidal volume and concomitant increased $Paco_2$). Desflurane results in the greatest increase in $Paco_2$, with corresponding reductions in tidal volume and minute ventilation. Isoflurane, like all other inhaled agents, increases respiratory rate, but isoflurane does not result in dose-dependent tachypnea. (Data from references 224-227, 231, 232.)

that airway receptors do not play a major role in ventilation and breathing control during exercise in normal humans,[243] nor are they involved in the increased respiratory rate that results from an increase in inspiratory flow rate.[244,245] However, these airway receptors are important in the regulation of breathing patterns, laryngeal and pulmonary defense mechanisms, and bronchomotor tone. The sensation of dyspnea is also most likely related to the activation of mechanoreceptors in the respiratory muscles and lungs.[246] Even activation of cold receptors or osmoreceptors located in the nasal mucosa produces protective bronchoconstrictor responses in normal subjects.[247] Chemical and mechanical stimulation of airway receptors causes end-tidal inspiratory activity in diaphragm and parasternal intercostal muscles. These actions contribute to histamine-induced

hyperinflation.[248] Irritant receptors are situated between airway epithelial cells and may mediate rapid reflex responses, including coughing, laryngospasm, bronchoconstriction, and secretion of mucus after the induction of general anesthesia; abrupt increases in the inspired concentration of volatile anesthetics; or sudden mechanical deformation of the laryngotracheobronchial system. The receptors responsible for eliciting protective airway reflexes appear to be non-uniformly distributed. The sensitivity to airway irritation was shown to be greater at the larynx and trachea than at the more peripheral airways in spontaneously breathing anesthetized patients in the presence of a laryngeal mask airway (LMA).[249] Increasing concentrations of sevoflurane had little effect in altering these responses. Similarly, supraglottic airway receptors were shown to be more

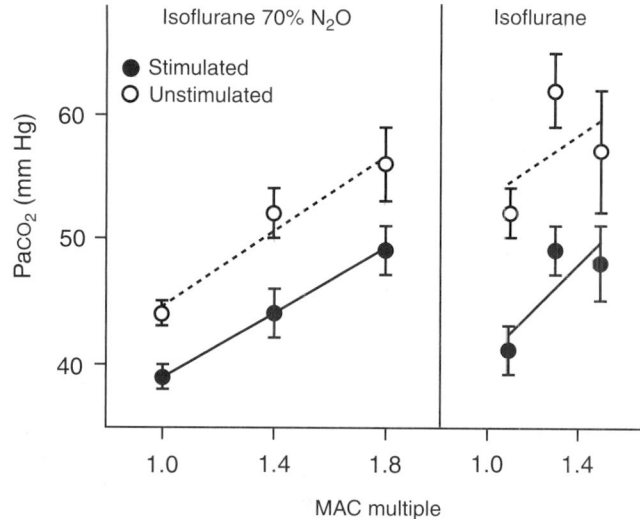

Figure 6–14 The effect of surgical stimulation on the ventilatory depression of inhaled anesthesia with isoflurane in the presence and absence of nitrous oxide. Surgical stimulation increased alveolar ventilation and decreased $PaCO_2$ at all depths of anesthesia examined. (Adapted Eger EI, Dolan WM, Stevens WC, et al: Surgical stimulation antagonizes the respiratory depression produced by Forane. Anesthesiology 36:544, 1972.)

responsible for midlatency afferent information to the somatosensory cortex in response to a brief, negative oral pressure pulse in patients breathing through an LMA.[250] Alterations in airway mechanoreceptor output may also be produced by cooling intrathoracic airways (e.g., filling the pulmonary circulation with cold blood) that subsequently causes tracheal contraction.[251]

Slowly adapting pulmonary stretch receptors are located within small airway smooth muscle and respond to stretching or changes in lung volume. A particularly high concentration of these receptors is located at the carina. Increases in lung volume enhance afferent nerve traffic through the vagus nerve to the respiratory control center and thereby inhibit further inspiration. This phenomenon is known as the Hering-Breuer reflex and appears to be independent of flecainide-sensitive Na^+ channels or 4-aminopyridine–sensitive K^+ channels.[252] The limitation of inspiration elicited by pulmonary stretch receptors may determine the relationship between tidal volume and respiratory frequency in experimental animals, but the Hering-Breuer reflex cannot be demonstrated in the awake, resting human during normal tidal volume breathing. Activation of slow-adapting pulmonary stretch receptors by persistent elevations in end-expiratory lung volumes produced an inhibitory effect on central drive (i.e., an increase in apneic threshold) and an attenuated ventilatory response to progressive hypercapnia.[253] The alteration in ventilatory pattern caused by anesthetics has been attributed to relative sensitization of pulmonary stretch receptors that subsequently produce tachypnea and low tidal volumes. The presence of a volatile anesthetic increased vagal afferent discharge at various lung volumes in decerebrate cats (i.e., sensitization of pulmonary stretch receptors),[254] but

little evidence exists of such a mechanism in humans.[255] There is evidence in the cat that halothane-induced tachypnea is primarily a suprapontine effect, but the mechanism of production of tachypnea with decreased tidal volume in anesthetized humans continues to remain unclear.

The direct effects of halothane, isoflurane, and enflurane on pulmonary and laryngeal irritant receptors and tracheobronchial slow-adapting stretch receptors have been investigated in spontaneously breathing and vagotomized, paralyzed dogs.[256,257] Several types of afferent receptors in the airways have been identified and include pressure, drive, cold, irritant, slowly and rapidly adapting stretch receptors, and C-fibers.[258] Rapidly adapting receptors occur throughout the respiratory tract from the nose to the bronchi. These receptors are characterized by an irregular discharge pattern and rapid adaptation to a stable volume stimulus, but they also display a more gradual adaptation to a chemical stimulus. Rapidly adapting laryngeal (irritant) receptors are most likely responsible for coughing, mucus secretion, and expiratory reflexes including bronchial and laryngeal constriction. Rapidly adapting receptors in the bronchi are more chemosensitive than those located in the more proximal airway but can also cause coughing, mucus secretion, bronchoconstriction, and laryngospasm. Rapidly adapting receptors in the bronchi stimulate hyperventilation.[259]

Volatile anesthetics increase the activity of laryngeal irritant receptors[256] and inhibit pulmonary irritant receptors.[257] Volatile anesthetics also elevate the excitation threshold and increase the sensitivity of low-threshold stretch receptors. Halothane and, to a lesser extent, sevoflurane attenuate end-expiratory discharge frequency of slow-adapting pulmonary receptors.[257,260] These agents may not affect[260] or even augment[257] the inspiratory activity. The clinical implications of these findings have yet to be precisely determined, but these anesthetic-induced changes in slow-adapting receptor function may play a role in the reduction of bronchomotor tone observed with volatile agents.

It has been suggested that volatile anesthesia may result in genioglossus muscle relaxation, causing posterior tongue displacement and consequent upper airway obstruction. However, this hypothesis has not been confirmed.[261-263] Anteroposterior displacement of upper airway structures occurs with changes in head position that occur in the same direction as the mandible. Administration of a volatile anesthetic and a neuromuscular blocker may widen the dimensions of the larynx,[261] but the nasopharyngeal airway decreases in size. During propofol sedation in children, the shape of the upper airway is oblong, and the anterior-posterior diameter is greater than the transverse diameter. This relationship reverses on awakening.[263] Patency of the upper airway during awakening may depend on contraction of pharyngeal dilating muscles that temporally precede diaphragmatic contraction.[264] The increase in thoracic inspiratory activity may also produce caudal traction on the upper airway and assist in expanding the upper airway during inspiration.[265] Central output to the genioglossus muscle and local reflex-mediated activation are important in maintaining upper airway patency, especially during inspiration.[266,267] The major site of airway narrowing is located at the soft palate during conscious sedation.

Volatile anesthetics produce a greater depression of the upper airway electromyogram[268] or nerve activity[269] compared with diaphragmatic activity in anesthetized, spontaneously breathing cats[268] (Fig. 6-15) and paralyzed, ventilated, vagotomized cats.[269] The extent to which this depression of upper airway motor neuron activity occurs as a result of anesthetic-induced inhibition of the reticular activating system is unknown.

The severity of airway hyperreactivity was determined in 123 children breathing through LMAs and receiving isoflurane or sevoflurane anesthesia.[270] Isoflurane was associated with greater airway hyperreactivity than was sevoflurane during LMA removal. The depth of anesthesia during LMA removal did not affect the severity or incidence of airway hyperreactivity during administration of sevoflurane, but LMA removal in the presence of isoflurane was associated with more adverse airway events. Sevoflurane (1 MAC) also provides greater attenuation of moderate to severe responses to tracheal stimulation by inflating the endotracheal tube cuff compared with desflurane.[271] However, higher concentrations (1.8 MAC) of these agents produced similar attenuation of coughing, tachycardia, and hypertension associated with tracheal stimulation.

Ventilatory Mechanics and Mechanoreceptors in the Chest Wall

Induction of general anesthesia reduces FRC. Loss of tonic parasternal intercostal muscle activity,[272-274] development of phasic expiratory activity of respiratory muscles (Fig. 6-16),[274] alteration in diaphragm position,[273] and changes in thoracic blood volume have been proposed as mechanisms responsible for anesthetic-induced decreases in FRC.[274] There is a relative sparing of diaphragmatic activity compared with intercostal muscle function during halothane anesthesia.[272,273] A change in diaphragmatic shape occurs during anesthesia, with dependent regions shifting cephalad and nondependent regions shifting caudad (Fig. 6-17).[275-277] Anesthesia-enhanced expiratory muscle activity results in inward displacement of the rib cage, an action that contributes to the reduction in FRC. In contrast, inspiratory rib cage expansion may remain relatively well preserved because of phasic inspiratory activity of scalene muscles despite the attenuation of parasternal intercostal muscle activity.[273] Areas of atelectasis in dependent lung regions frequently occur in anesthetized, spontaneously ventilating humans, and they may be related to alterations in respiratory muscle tone but not specifically to any single chest wall structure.[275] There is no direct correlation between changes in FRC and anesthesia-induced atelectasis.[277] Atelectasis markedly contributes to gas exchange abnormalities by increasing intrapulmonary shunting and may be reduced by the application of positive end-expiratory pressure or phrenic nerve stimulation of the diaphragm.[278]

The reasons for the differential effects of inhaled anesthetics on inspiratory and expiratory respiratory muscles

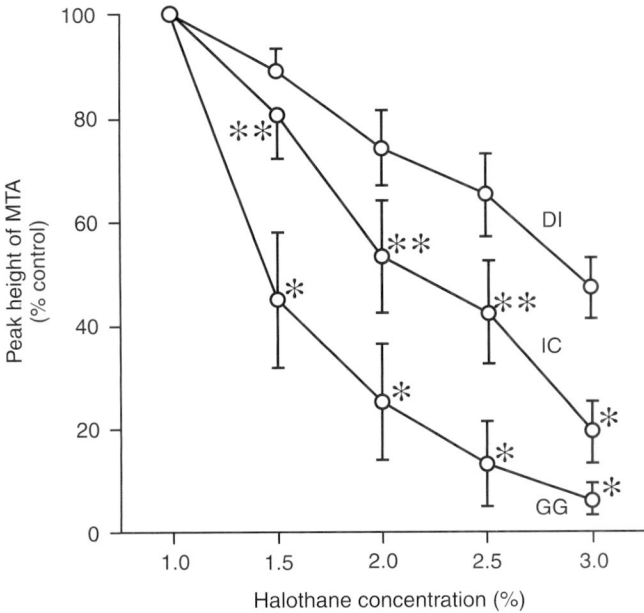

Figure 6–15 Decrease in phasic inspiratory muscle activity, expressed as the peak height of moving time average (MTA), in percent change from control (1% halothane), during halothane anesthesia in adult cats. Values are expressed as the mean ± SEM. The middle curve represents the intercostal muscle (IC) (*$P < .05$ compared with the diaphragm [DI]; **$P < .05$ compared with the genioglossus muscle [GG]). Notice the differential sensitivities of these respiratory muscles. (From Ochiai R, Guthrie RD, Motoyama EK: Effects of varying concentrations of halothane on the activity of the genioglossus, intercostals, and diaphragm in cats: an electromyographic study. Anesthesiology 70:812, 1989.)

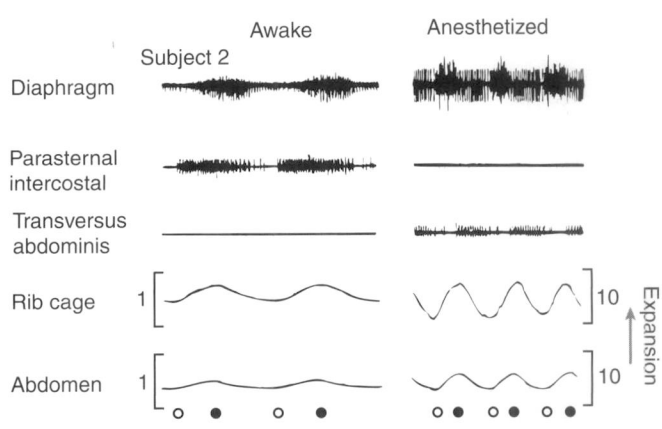

Figure 6–16 Representative record from one subject while awake and during halothane anesthesia. The three *upper tracings* are electromyograms. *Lower tracings* represent ribcage and abdominal dimensions measured by respiratory impedance plethysmography. *Open and solid circles* denote the beginning and end of inspiration, respectively. Notice that the amplitudes of ribcage and abdominal excursions diminish during halothane but that the relationship between their amplitudes is preserved. (From Warner DO, Warner MA, Ritman EL: Human chest wall function while awake and during halothane anesthesia. I. Quiet breathing. Anesthesiology 82:6, 1995.)

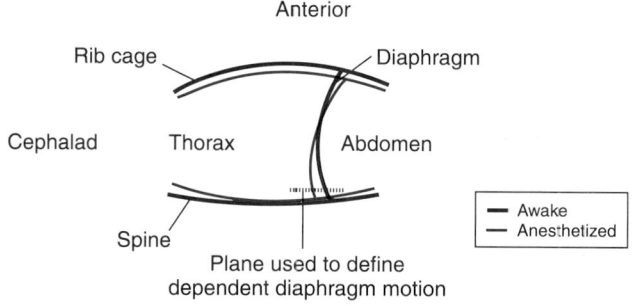

Figure 6–17 Diagram of a midsagittal section of the thorax while awake *(solid lines)* and while anesthetized *(red lines)* with a 1.2 minimum alveolar concentration (MAC) of halothane. Chest wall configuration was determined using images of the thorax obtained by three-dimensional fast computed tomography. (Adapted from Warner DO, Warner MA, Ritman EL: Atelectasis and chest wall shape during halothane anesthesia. Anesthesiology 85:49, 1996.)

are unknown but may be related to direct actions on brainstem control mechanisms or differential sensitivities of premotor neurons and motor neurons. Stuth and coworkers[279-282] showed that bulbospinal respiratory neurons were more resistant to the depressant effects of volatile anesthetics than phrenic nerve activity in vagotomized and decerebrate dogs. The inhibition of expiratory premotor neurons by volatile agents occurs through a presynaptic reduction of glutaminergic excitation and an enhancement of GABA$_A$-ergic inhibitory receptor function (Fig. 6-18).[281,283] Sevoflurane also depressed phrenic nerve activity to a greater extent than did halothane. Increases in carbon dioxide drive only partially compensate for these anesthetic-induced depressant actions. There appears to be less depression of expiratory than inspiratory bulbospinal premotor neurons produced by halothane. These findings suggest that the effects of volatile agents on respiratory muscle function may occur as a result of a relatively greater influence on the motor efferent pathways (including spinal respiratory motor neurons) than brainstem-mediated mechanisms (Fig. 6-19).[280]

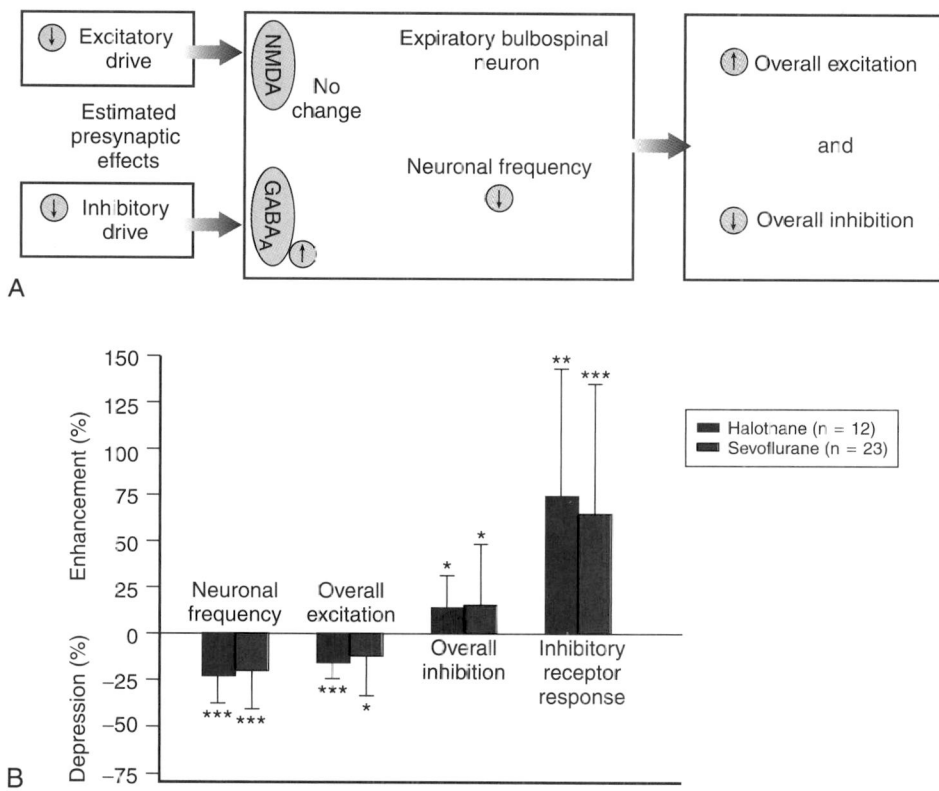

Figure 6–18 A, Schematic diagram of the effects of volatile anesthetics on synaptic transmission to expiratory premotor neurons in the caudal ventral respiratory group. The overall glutaminergic excitatory drive is reduced without effecting NMDA receptor function, and overall inhibition is increased because of an increase in GABA$_A$ receptor function. Presynaptic inhibitory drive is also reduced, leading to a decrease in control discharge frequency of the premotor neuron. *Red arrows* represent anesthetic effects. **B,** Effects of halothane and sevoflurane on excitatory and inhibitory neurotransmission to canine medullary expiratory neurons. Mean changes ± SD are given for neuronal control frequency, overall excitation, overall inhibition and inhibitory receptor response by 1 minimum alveolar concentration (MAC) of halothane and sevoflurane (*$P < .05$, ** $P < .01$, *** $P < .001$ versus no change). (Adapted from Stucke AG, Stuth EAE, Tonkovic-Capin V, et al: Effects of halothane and sevoflurane on inhibitory neurotransmission to medullary expiratory neurons in a decerebrate dog model. Anesthesiology 96:955, 2002.)

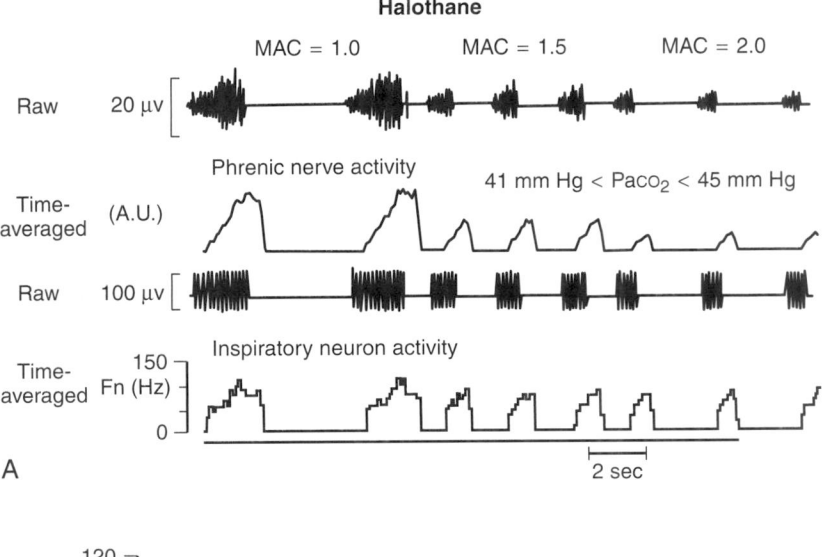

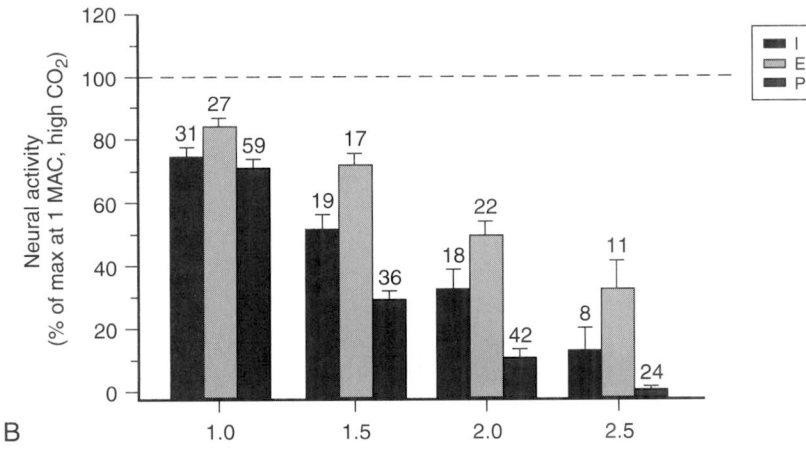

Figure 6–19 Effect of increasing halothane on phrenic nerve and neuron activity. With increasing anesthetic depth, both peak phrenic nerve (PPA) and peak neuron activities are depressed. PPA shows the greatest sensitivity to halothane. **A**, Phrenic nerve activity and the discharge frequency of an inspiratory bulbospinal neuron. Inspiratory (phrenic burst) duration decreases with increasing anesthetic depth. **B**, Peak expiratory neuron (E), peak inspiratory neuron (I) activity, and PPA. Expiratory neuronal activity was most resistant to the effects of halothane. *Bars* show the normalized mean ± SEM, and the numbers above the bars indicate the numbers of neurons studied for each condition. (Adapted from Stuth EAE, Tonkovic-Capin M, Kampine JP, et al: Dose-dependent effects of halothane on expiratory and inspiratory bulbospinal neurons and the phrenic nerve activities in dogs. Anesthesiology 81:1470, 1994.)

Volatile anesthetics also differentially depress neuromuscular transmission and skeletal muscle contractility. Halothane impairs excitation-contraction coupling and neuromuscular transmission to equivalent degrees, whereas isoflurane, sevoflurane, and enflurane depress diaphragmatic contraction primarily through alterations in neuromuscular transmission.[284-286] Isoflurane, enflurane, and sevoflurane depress the tension of the diaphragm in response to phrenic nerve stimulation.[284,287] Although these results may partially explain clinical observations in humans, a wide range of species variations do exist. For example, volatile anesthetics decrease expiratory muscle activity and maintain parasternal intercostal activity in dogs, but converse actions are observed in humans.[273-275] Similar to volatile agents, nitrous oxide affects chest wall function and breathing by changing the distribution and timing of neural drive to the respiratory muscles.[288] Nitrous oxide decreases tidal volume as a result of a reduction in rib cage motion and increased phasic expiratory activity in humans. In contrast, xenon does not affect transdiaphragmatic pressure or diaphragmatic electromyography.[289]

Changes in chest wall positions produce alterations in efferent impulses from stretch receptors in intercostal muscle spindles that act to maintain relatively constant tidal volume during variations in inspiratory resistance. Increases in spindle discharge enhance motor activity to muscle fibers until muscle shortening relieves tension in the spindles. With increased inspiratory resistance, the muscle spindles detect a failure of shortening by the appropriate amount, and afferent signals are subsequently increased to the motor neuron pool. Accessory muscles of inspiration may be recruited as well. This reflex increase in inspiratory effort sustains tidal volume and minute ventilation despite a greater inspiratory resistive load. These and other forces maintain normal ventilation with changes in body position, inspiratory resistance, and compliance. The extrapolation of these data obtained in experimental animals to humans should be approached with caution. For example, tension receptors in the diaphragm, not the muscle spindles, induce reflex inhibition of inspiratory intercostal activity associated with a decrease in inspiratory duration in dogs but not in humans. This effect appears to be mediated at the supraspinal level.[290]

Ventilation is maintained during halothane anesthesia despite increases in resistance produced by partial endotracheal tube occlusion or an acute reduction in lung compliance until a threshold level is reached.[291] Subsequently, minute ventilation falls, and retention of carbon dioxide occurs. Minute ventilation is maintained even during 2 MAC halothane anesthesia by increasing the work of breathing at modest inspiratory resistances as caused by small-diameter endotracheal tubes or humidifiers.[292] The work of breathing is defined as pressure or force multiplied by the tidal volume during inspiration (i.e., expiration in typically passive elastic recoil using stored energy) and is expressed in joules or grams × centimeters. Respiratory work of the lung is further broken down into elastic work (i.e., work required to overcome the elastic recoil of the lung) and resistive work (i.e., overcoming airway flow resistance and viscoelastic resistance of pulmonary tissues, in addition to any imposed work of breathing through an airway apparatus). The work of breathing is usually derived from transpulmonary pressure–tidal volume curves for which the pressure is often measured by esophageal manometry. General anesthetics increase the work of breathing in adults and children.[293-295] Keidan and coworkers[295] have demonstrated that airway devices such as the LMA and mask with an oral airway decrease the work of breathing in spontaneously ventilating, halothane- and nitrous oxide–anesthetized children. Continuous positive airway pressure reduced the work of breathing during use of the LMA or mask (but not with an endotracheal tube). The beneficial effects of continuous positive airway pressure appear to result primarily from the prevention of upper airway collapse and the reduction of upper airway resistance, rather than an increase in FRC.

Expiration is passively affected by the recoil characteristics of the lung during normal breathing. In anesthetized patients, the ventilatory response to expiratory resistance is reduced to a greater extent than is the response to inspiratory resistance. Conscious and anesthetized humans exhibit decreases in respiratory rate during expiratory resistive loads, but only anesthetized subjects develop rib cage–abdominal wall motion asynchrony resulting in less effective ventilation and increases in carbon dioxide.[296] This concept may be particularly important in spontaneously breathing, anesthetized patients who demonstrate expiratory obstruction (e.g., partial breathing circuit occlusion, asthma, emphysema). Patients with COPD who do not retain carbon dioxide in the conscious state display a greater degree of hypoventilation awake than healthy patients during halothane anesthesia, consistent with these observations (Fig. 6-20).[297] Paradoxically, patients with COPD develop less atelectasis and have greater preservation of gas exchange compared with healthy patients, despite similar diaphragmatic displacements during anesthesia.[298] The mechanisms for this observation are unclear, but intrinsic positive end-expiratory pressures, altered patterns of respiratory muscle activation, or altered ventilation-perfusion mismatch may play important roles.[277]

Effects of Anesthetics on Ventilatory Response to Chemical Stimuli

The effects of inhaled anesthetics on respiratory drive are typically characterized by the ventilatory response to alterations in arterial carbon dioxide tension or hypoxia. A complete discussion of chemical control of ventilation may be found in several excellent reviews.[214,299,300] Briefly, central and peripheral chemoreceptors are critical to

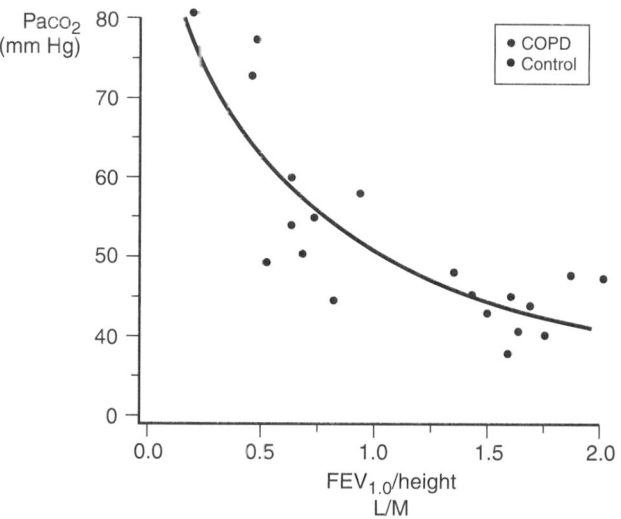

Figure 6–20 Comparison of $Paco_2$ in anesthetized, spontaneously breathing patients relative to preoperative forced expiratory volume in 1 second ($FEV_{1.0}$). Patients with chronic obstructive pulmonary disease (COPD) did not exhibit carbon dioxide retention before anesthesia, but the degree of alveolar hypoventilation is much greater in the more severely obstructed patients. (Adapted from Pietak S, Weenig CS, Hickey RG, et al: Anesthetic effects on ventilation in patients with chronic obstructive pulmonary disease. Anesthesiology 42:160, 1975.)

chemical control of respiration. Central chemoreceptors are located near the ventrolateral medulla and other brainstem locations and respond to changes in hydrogen ion (H^+) concentration in the cerebrospinal fluid but not to arterial carbon dioxide tension or pH. Unlike H^+, carbon dioxide rapidly diffuses through the blood-brain barrier. Central chemoreceptors are more profoundly affected by respiratory alterations than by metabolic alterations in arterial carbon dioxide tensions. In contrast, peripheral chemoreceptors located in the carotid bodies are sensitive to changes in arterial carbon dioxide tension, pH and, most importantly, arterial oxygen tension. The mechanisms by which peripheral chemoreceptive cells respond to hypoxia and hypercapnia appear to be separate and synergistic, because hypoxemia potentiates the chemical drive to a carbon dioxide challenge. Peripheral chemoreceptors appear to contribute about one third to the total resting minute ventilation at normocapnia and normoxia as determined by respiratory functional testing. This contribution falls to 15% during hyperoxic normocapnia, suggesting that central chemoreceptors control 85% of the carbon dioxide drive during hyperoxia. Both stimuli cause membrane depolarization and activation of afferent nerve transmission.[301] Hypercapnia may induce alveolar epithelial cell injury mediated by a NO-dependent pathway.[302] The consequences of these observations on chemoreceptor function are unknown.

Responses to Carbon Dioxide

Changes in ventilation secondary to alterations in arterial carbon dioxide tension are mediated principally at the level of the medulla. Patients whose peripheral chemoreceptors have been denervated by bilateral carotid endarterectomy demonstrate a modestly attenuated increase in ventilation in response to inhaled carbon dioxide.

Apneic Thresholds

The *apneic threshold* is defined as the highest arterial carbon dioxide tension at which a subject remains apneic. The apneic threshold is approximately 4 or 5 mm Hg less than resting arterial carbon dioxide tension achieved during spontaneous ventilation. There are no significant agent-specific or depth-related effects of ether, halothane, or isoflurane on the relationship between apneic thresholds and resting arterial carbon dioxide tension in humans (Fig. 6-21).[303] The difference between resting arterial carbon dioxide tension and apneic threshold is not related to the slope of the carbon dioxide response curves or to the level of resting arterial carbon dioxide tension. This suggests that *assisted* ventilation to a lower arterial carbon dioxide tension less than the apneic threshold during anesthesia ultimately becomes *controlled* ventilation. Another clinically important aspect of this observation is related to the return of spontaneous ventilation in the mechanically hyperventilated patient. Carbon dioxide stores in the body must accumulate to return the arterial carbon dioxide tension toward the apneic threshold after cessation of mechanical ventilation. The duration of apnea required before the patient commences spontaneous ventilation is proportional to anesthetic depth. Continuation of mechanical ventilation

to eliminate inhaled anesthetics and maintenance of higher arterial carbon dioxide tension during ventilation are two commonly employed clinical strategies to reduce the duration of apnea after the anesthetic has been discontinued. These maneuvers decrease the apneic threshold or increase the resting arterial carbon dioxide tension, effectively reducing the time of apnea required to stimulate a return of spontaneous ventilation.

Carbon Dioxide Response Curves

Inspiration of carbon dioxide in normal subjects increases minute ventilation by approximately 3 L/min per 1 mm Hg of arterial carbon dioxide tension. This observation demonstrates a high gain from the central chemoreceptor in response to variations in arterial carbon dioxide tension. The slope of the relationship between minute ventilation and arterial carbon dioxide tension is an index of ventilatory drive provided that hypoxic conditions are avoided to minimize peripheral chemoreceptor stimulation. NO is increased in the carotid bodies during hypoxia,[304] plays an inhibitory role in the peripheral and central chemoreflex pathways during hypoxia,[305] and may act as a respiratory stimulant under normoxic conditions.[306] Experiments determining the relationship between minute ventilation and arterial carbon dioxide tension should be interpreted with these potential confounding variables in mind. All inhaled anesthetics depress the ventilatory response to hypercarbia in a dose-dependent fashion.[224-226,231,232,307] High concentrations of volatile anesthetics may almost

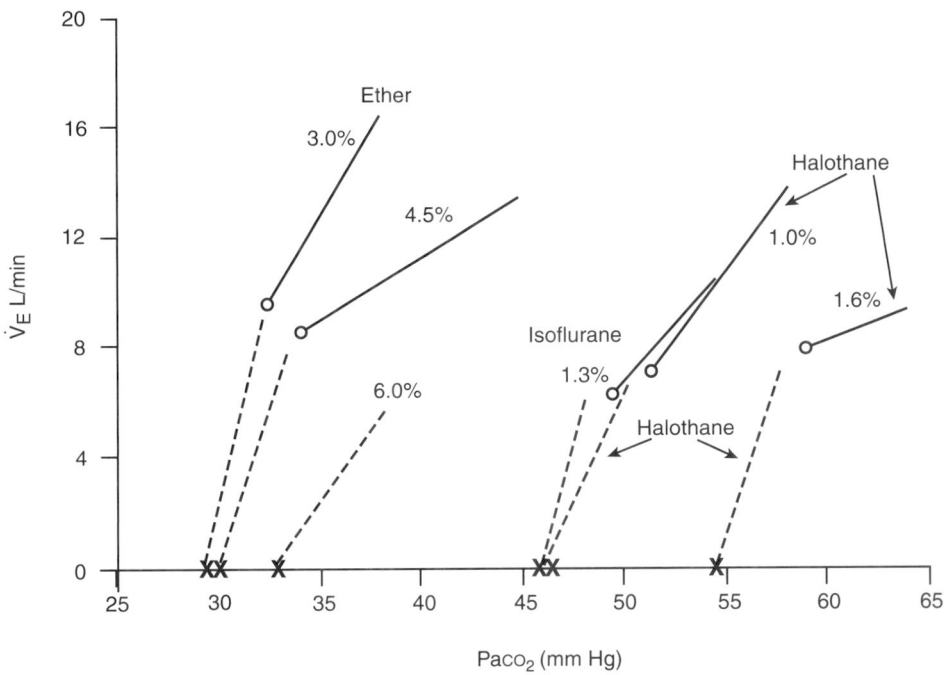

Figure 6–21 Ventilatory responses to increased carbon dioxide and apneic thresholds during ether, isoflurane, and halothane anesthesia in patients. The apneic threshold had a relatively fixed relationship to the resting $Paco_2$. With an increase in ventilatory depression at an increasing depth of anesthesia, resting $Paco_2$ and apneic threshold increased by approximately the same amount. (From Hickey RF, Fourcade HE, Eger EI, et al: The effects of ether, halothane and Forane on apneic threshold in man. Anesthesiology 35:32, 1971.)

entirely eliminate hypercarbia-induced increases in ventilatory drive. Even low concentrations of nitrous oxide may significantly affect responses to hypercapnia.[307] The slope of the minute ventilation–arterial carbon dioxide tension relation returns toward normal after 6 hours of halothane anesthesia, but ventilatory responsiveness to carbon dioxide remains profoundly depressed despite this observation. Studies by Hornbein and coworkers[308] showed that addition of nitrous oxide to halothane depressed ventilation less than an equi-MAC dose of halothane alone. However, such an experimental paradigm does not alter the carbon dioxide ventilatory response slope of desflurane.[231]

The effects of small doses of inhaled anesthetics on ventilatory responses to hypercarbia remain somewhat controversial despite intense investigation. Several studies have demonstrated that subanesthetic concentrations (e.g., 0.1 MAC) of inhaled anesthetics (with the exception of desflurane and nitrous oxide) depress the peripheral chemoreflex loop by approximately 30% to inhibit the ventilatory response to hypercarbia.[309-313] The response was also attenuated during administration of desflurane when a level of sedation comparable with sleep was achieved.[309] At higher concentrations of volatile agents, other sites, including the central chemoreceptors, may also be affected. In marked contrast, results from Pandit and coworkers[314] showed that subanesthetic sevoflurane did not affect the response to acute or sustained hypercapnia.[314] The discrepancies in these results may be related to the sustained nature of the hypercapnic responses or, more likely, to differences in the state of central nervous system arousal under baseline conditions.[312] Unlike the effects of small doses of inhaled anesthetics on peripheral chemoreceptors, the intravenous agent propofol depresses the hypercapnic-induced ventilatory response at the level of the central chemoreceptors.[315]

Depression of ventilatory responsiveness to inhaled carbon dioxide is clinically important. Carbon dioxide accumulation and concomitant acidemia may cause dysfunction in several organs, including the heart, where this condition may produce potentially dangerous arrhythmias. The attenuation of the normal ventilatory responses to elevated arterial carbon dioxide tension makes clinical diagnosis of hypercarbia difficult independent of actual measurement of arterial blood gases or end-tidal carbon dioxide concentration. The respiratory system is less able to compensate for elevations in carbon dioxide tensions that occur in response to rebreathing carbon dioxide from malfunctioning anesthetic circuits or resulting from increased metabolic production of this gas during anesthesia. Reduced ventilatory drive to hypercapnia may also occur in the immediate postoperative period and contribute to significant morbidity. Pietak and associates[297] showed that patients with chronic obstructive pulmonary disease demonstrated a reduced ability to respond to increased arterial carbon dioxide tension during anesthesia.

Experimental studies have shown that carbon dioxide rebreathing recruits expiratory respiratory muscles, including the internal intercostals, but does not reverse the profound depression of parasternal intercostal muscle activity produced by halothane.[316] There is a prolongation of expiration leading to a decrease in respiratory rate during the course of rebreathing. These alterations in individual respiratory muscle control of ventilation during breathing are different in halothane-anesthetized dog than in humans,[317] but these species differences do not necessarily imply that other systems responsible for respiratory control are also dissimilar between species. Halothane depressed the peripheral chemoreceptor transduction (i.e., phrenic nerve response) to an acute, severe carbon dioxide stimulation of the peripheral chemoreceptors in paralyzed, vagotomized dogs in a dose-related manner.[318] Carbon dioxide sensitivity was diminished but not abolished by doses of halothane typically required for surgical anesthesia. It appears that halothane depresses peripheral and central carbon dioxide sensitivities to similar degrees,[319] but the peripheral chemoreceptors contribute only approximately 15% of the total carbon dioxide sensitivity. The response of peripheral chemoreceptors may not initially appear to be of less clinical significance. However, if the peripheral chemoreceptor response to hypoxia is abolished by low concentrations of inhaled anesthetics, this action may contribute to a marked respiratory impairment during the concomitant episodes of hypercarbia and hypoxia that are known to occur in the perioperative period.

Ventilatory Responses to Hypoxemia

Volatile anesthetics and nitrous oxide attenuate the ventilatory response to hypoxia in experimental animals and humans in a dose-dependent manner.[320-324] The peripheral chemoreceptors appear to be the major site of this inhibitory action.[325] Evidence supporting this hypothesis is indicated by the rapid inhibition (30 seconds) of the hypoxic response[326] and the reduction of carotid sinus nerve discharge when the peripheral chemoreceptors are stimulated by a variety of methods during administration of halothane (0.5 to 1.0%) to decerebrate cats.[327] Alternatively, Stuth and colleagues[328] demonstrated that the phrenic nerve response to hypoxia is attenuated but not abolished by halothane in vagotomized dogs. These results also did not indicate a relatively selective depression of peripheral compared with central effects of chemoreflexes in this phenomenon. The cause for these differences may be attributed to the profound degree of hypoxia (arterial oxygen tension <40 mm Hg) conducted in experimental animals, compared with those in human investigations (i.e., $Pa_{O_2} \cong 50$ mm Hg). A significant depression of hypoxia-induced ventilatory responsiveness was observed at 1 MAC of halothane, and the usual synergistic effect of hypoxia and hypercarbia on ventilation was profoundly attenuated. The ventilatory response to hypoxia also depends on the degree to which carbon dioxide exceeds the peripheral chemoreflex threshold rather than its elevation above resting partial pressure[329] and the presence of NO (and presumably, a fully functional pulmonary arterial endothelium).[330] This latter role of NO may be more complicated, because NO is released in the ventrolateral medulla after activation of peripheral chemoreceptors during hypoxia in response to sympathoexcitation.[331]

Humans have a biphasic response to hypoxia. Adults and neonates display a similar initial hypoxia-induced increase in ventilation, but neonates exhibit a more pronounced ventilatory decline in response to prehypoxic oxygen concentration compared with adults. This reaction may represent a balance between active inhibition of brainstem neuronal activities and augmentation of peripheral chemoreceptor function.[332] Halothane also produces a biphasic ventilatory response (similar to that observed in the newborn) in kittens that have previously attained an adult-like hyperventilatory hypoxic response.[325] Whether the cause of this altered response during halothane anesthesia is mediated by peripheral chemoreceptors is unknown, but it is unlikely that activity at the level of the brainstem is solely responsible for this phenomenon.[333] The ventilatory decline occurring during sustained hypoxia is not attenuated by low concentrations of enflurane.[334] Gender-based differences, known to exist within the peripheral but not the central chemoreflex loop in morphine-induced ventilatory depression,[335] do not appear to play a role during sevoflurane-induced reduction in hypoxic drive.[336]

Knill and Gelb[321] demonstrated that peripheral chemoreceptor function was more sensitive to the effects of volatile anesthetics in humans than in dogs. Significant attenuation of the peripheral chemoreceptor response occurred at concentrations of halothane as low as 0.1 MAC. The hypoxic ventilatory response was also proposed to be more sensitive to the effects of inhaled anesthetics than was the response to hypercapnia,[320,321,337] but considerable controversy about the influence of subanesthetic concentrations of volatile agents on hypoxic ventilatory drive has arisen. Several groups have shown that 0.1 MAC of sevoflurane[338] or isoflurane does not affect hypoxic drive in humans[339,340] or animals,[341] but Dahan and coworkers[310,311,342] and others[334,343] confirmed the original findings of Knill and Gelb (Fig. 6-22). As was observed in studies examining the effects of volatile anesthetics on hypercapnia-induced ventilatory responses, the reasons for these disparate findings may be related to differences in techniques and study conditions. Most notably, differences in the state of arousal achieved during each study and the wide variability that may occur by studying subjects on different experimental days might have played important roles.[340] Subanesthetic concentrations of most volatile anesthetics, with the exception of desflurane, depress the ventilatory response to hypoxia in normocapnic resting subjects (Fig. 6-23). However, subanesthetic concentrations of desflurane decrease hypoxic sensitivity during concomitant hypercapnia, suggesting an effect at the peripheral chemoreceptors.[313]

Diffusion hypoxia is a well-known effect and may occur during recovery from nitrous anesthesia. Rapid elimination of nitrous oxide from blood to the alveoli combined with slower nitrogen diffusion reduces alveolar oxygen concentration. However, diffusion hypoxia may not occur during xenon anesthesia, as the blood-gas partition coefficient of xenon (0.12) is similar to that of nitrogen.[84]

Clinical Implications

The profound depression of hypoxic responsiveness produced by inhaled anesthetics suggests that patients may

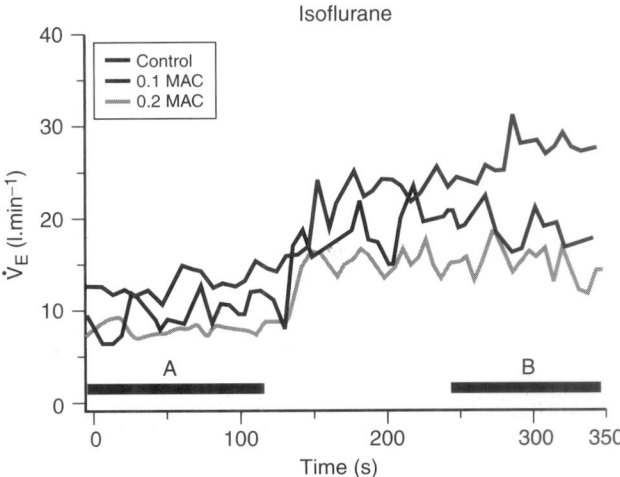

Figure 6–22 The ventilatory responses to acute isocapnic hypoxia (to approximately 44 mm Hg) in one subject during control (i.e., awake) and at 0.1 and 0.2 minimum alveolar concentrations (MACs) of isoflurane. *Solid bars* indicate period A (2-minute period before induction of hypoxia) and period B (minutes 3 and 4 of hypoxia). $\dot{V}_E$, minute ventilation. (Adapted from van den Elsen MJLJ, Dahan A, DeGoede J, et al: Influences of subanesthetic isoflurane on ventilatory control in humans. Anesthesiology 83:478, 1995.)

have a diminished ventilatory response to hypoxemia in the recovery room for some time after the agent has been discontinued. The presence of residual anesthetic (particularly halothane) places the patient at greater risk of hypoventilation in the absence of other stimuli (e.g., pain) or recovery room personnel activity. Stimulation of the postoperative patient may attenuate the effects of low residual concentration of anesthetics

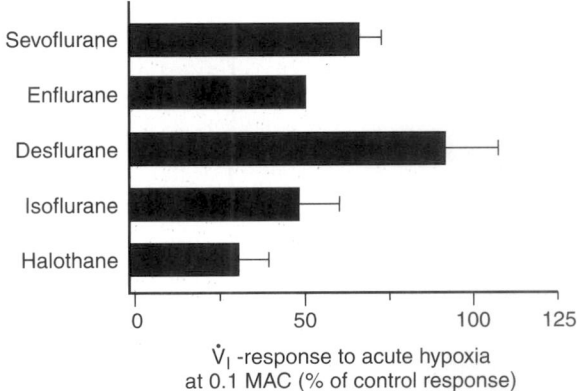

Figure 6–23 Influence of 0.1 minimum alveolar concentration (MAC) of five volatile anesthetic agents on the ventilatory response to a step decrease in end-tidal oxygen concentration. Values are given as the mean ± SD. Subanesthetic concentrations of the volatile anesthetics, except desflurane, profoundly depress the response to hypoxia. (Adapted from Sarton E, Dahan A, Teppema L, et al: Acute pain and central nervous system arousal do not restore impaired hypoxic ventilatory response during sevoflurane sedation. Anesthesiology 85:295, 1996.)

on hypoxic drive. Intraoperative surgical stimulation reduces anesthetic-induced respiratory depression to some degree, but a similar extent of stimulation does not prevent impairment of hypoxia and hypercarbia chemoreflexes during administration of a volatile anesthetic.[344,345] These phenomena may be especially important in patients who depend to some degree on a hypoxic drive to establish their level of ventilation (e.g., those with chronic respiratory failure). Under these circumstances, the ability of patients to maintain adequate spontaneous ventilation during administration of an inhaled anesthetic may be severely impaired. There appear to be few clinically relevant differences between volatile anesthetics in depression hypoxia-induced ventilatory response in these patients.

It has been suggested that volatile anesthetics may augment the inflammatory response during mechanical ventilation.[346,347] However, in normal lungs of isoflurane-anesthetized patients, short-term mechanical ventilation with high tidal volumes caused no clinically relevant increase in systemic proinflammatory or anti-inflammatory cytokines in the lungs of healthy, isoflurane-anesthetized patients.[348] However, whether inhaled agents produce a proinflammatory response in pulmonary parenchyma in the presence of lung disease remains unknown.

SUMMARY

Inhaled anesthetics have potent and clinically significant effects on respiratory function. Volatile anesthetics reduce bronchial smooth muscle tone, adversely affect mucociliary function, and dilate pulmonary vasculature. Volatile anesthetics also alter the activity of respiratory sensors, the central nervous system, and muscles of respiration. These actions are mediated by a variety of mechanisms, including indirect actions on afferent, central, and efferent neural pathways, as well as direct actions on the lungs. The depressant effects of these drugs are further enhanced in patients with pulmonary disorders. An understanding of the multifactorial actions of inhaled anesthetics on the respiratory system is critical to the safe delivery of anesthesia.

KEY POINTS

1. Inhaled anesthetics affect every facet of pulmonary physiology, from the variety of forces controlling ventilation and pulmonary blood flow to surface tension, mucus secretion, and airway smooth muscle tone.
2. Volatile anesthetics are potent bronchodilators in animals and humans. This action occurs through several complex mechanisms that involve a decrease in intracellular calcium concentration and a reduction in calcium sensitivity in the presence of a bronchoconstrictive agent.
3. Volatile anesthetics increase baseline pulmonary dynamic compliance, but these agents are more

effective at attenuating increases in pulmonary airway resistance due to chemical or mechanical stimuli. Inhaled anesthetics also preferentially dilate distal airways rather than proximal airways.

4. Inhaled anesthetics diminish the rate of mucus clearance by decreasing ciliary beat frequency, disrupting metachronism, or altering the characteristics of mucus.
5. Pulmonary surfactant decreases the work of breathing by reducing alveolar surface tension. Volatile anesthetics cause progressive, yet reversible, reductions in phosphatidylcholine, the main lipid component of surfactant. The roles of depressed mucociliary function and alterations in type II alveolar cell function in postoperative pulmonary complications after administration of a volatile agent are unknown.
6. The multiple sites of action of inhaled anesthetics on pulmonary parenchyma and vasculature complicate the direct assessment of anesthetic-induced alterations in PVR. Volatile anesthetics cause a biphasic, contraction-relaxation response in pulmonary vascular smooth muscle that is mediated at multiple sites in a Ca^{2+}-mediated signaling pathway. Overall, the net effect of inhaled anesthetic-induced changes in PVR is relatively small.
7. HPV is an important mechanism by which pulmonary blood is preferentially redistributed away from poorly ventilated lung regions to those with adequate alveolar ventilation. Most inhaled anesthetics attenuate HPV in vitro and exert relatively modest inhibitory effects on HPV, shunting, or oxygenation in vivo.
8. Inhaled anesthetics (with the exception of xenon) reduce tidal volume and minute ventilation and cause tachypnea in a dose-related fashion. The relative increases in arterial carbon dioxide tension (as an index of respiratory depression) occur with these agents in the following order: enflurane, desflurane, isoflurane, sevoflurane, halothane.
9. Inhaled anesthetics affect inspiratory and expiratory respiratory muscles to various degrees, possibly as a result of differential sensitivities of premotor and motor neurons.
10. All inhaled anesthetics depress the ventilatory responses to hypercarbia and hypoxia by altering central and peripheral chemoreceptor function in a dose-dependent fashion. The effects of subanesthetic concentrations of inhaled agents on hypercarbic and hypoxic responses are controversial and seem to depend on the baseline state of central nervous system arousal. Nevertheless, these findings may have important clinical implications during the perioperative period.

REFERENCES

1. Warner DO, Warner MA, Barnes RD, et al: Perioperative respiratory complications in patients with asthma. Anesthesiology 85:460, 1996.

2. Schnider WM, Papper EM: Anesthesia for the asthmatic patient. Anesthesiology 22:886, 1961.

3. Gold MI, Helrich M: A study of the complications related to anesthesia in asthmatic patients. Anesth Analg 42:283, 1963.

4. Forrest JB, Rehder K, Cahalan MK, et al: Multicenter study of general anesthesia. III. Predictors of severe perioperative adverse outcomes. Anesthesiology 76:3, 1992.

5. Pizov R, Brown RH, Weiss YS, et al: Wheezing during induction of general anesthesia in patients with and without asthma. A randomized, blinded trial. Anesthesiology 82:1111, 1995.

5a. Cheney FW, Posner KL, Caplan RA: Adverse respiratory events infrequently leading to malpractice suits. A closed system analysis. Anesthesiology 75:932, 1991.

6. Mougdil GC: The patient with reactive airways disease. Can J Anaesth 44:R77, 1997.

7. Pinto-Pereira LM, Orrett FA, Balbirsingh M: Physiological perspectives of therapy in bronchial hyperreactivity. Can J Anaesth 43:700, 1996.

8. Kai T, Yoshimura H, Jones KA, et al: Relationship between force and regulatory myosin light chain phosphorylation in airway smooth muscle. Am J Physiol Lung Cell Mol Physiol 279:L52, 2000.

9. Prakash YS, Kannan MS, Walseth TF, et al: Role of cyclic ADP ribose in the regulation of $[Ca^{2+}]$ in porcine tracheal smooth muscle. Am J Physiol Cell Physiol 274:C1653, 1998.

10. Rho EH, Perkins WJ, Lorenz RR, et al: Differential effects of soluble and particulate guanylyl cyclase on Ca^{2+} sensitivity in airway smooth muscle. J Appl Physiol 92:257, 2002.

11. Hirshman CA, Lande B, Croxton TL: Role of M2 muscarinic receptors in airway smooth muscle contraction. Life Sci 64:443, 1999.

12. Groeben H, Brown RH: Ipratropium decreases airway size in dogs by preferential M2 muscarinic receptor blockade in vivo. Anesthesiology 85:867, 1996.

13. Emala CW, McQuitty CK, Eleff SM, et al: Asthma, allergy, and airway hyperresponsiveness are not linked to the beta(2)-adrenoceptor gene. Chest 121:722, 2002.

14. Flavahan NA, Aarhus LL, Rimele TJ, et al: Respiratory epithelium inhibits bronchial smooth muscle tone. J Appl Physiol 65:721, 1985.

15. Stuart-Smith K, Vanhoutte PM: Heterogeneity in the effects of epithelium-removal in the canine bronchial tree. J Appl Physiol 63:2510, 1987.

16. Park KW, Sato K, Dai HB, et al: Epithelium-dependent bronchodilatory activity is preserved in pig bronchioles after normothermic cardiopulmonary bypass. Anesth Analg 90:778, 2000.

17. Fehr JJ, Hirshman CA, Emala CW: Cellular signaling by the potent bronchoconstrictor endothelin-1 in airway smooth muscle. Crit Care Med 28:1884, 2000.

18. Colgan FJ: Performance of lungs and bronchi during inhalation anesthesia. Anesthesiology 26:778, 1965.

19. Klide AM, Aviado DM: Mechanism for the reduction in pulmonary resistance induced by halothane. J Pharmacol Exp Ther 158:28, 1967.

20. Fletcher SW, Flacke W, Alper MH: The actions of general anesthetic agents on tracheal smooth muscle. Anesthesiology 29:517, 1969.

21. Hickey RF, Graf PD, Nadel JA, et al: The effects of halothane and cyclopropane on total pulmonary resistance in the dog. Anesthesiology 31:334, 1969.

22. Coon RL, Kampine JP: Hypocapnic bronchoconstriction and inhalation anesthetics. Anesthesiology 43:635, 1975.

23. Patterson RW, Sullivan SF, Malm JR, et al: The effect of halothane on human airway mechanics. Anesthesiology 29:900, 1968.

24. D'Angelo E, Calderini IS, Tavola M: The effects of CO_2 on respiratory mechanics in anesthetized paralyzed humans. Anesthesiology 94:604, 2001.

25. Hirshman CA, Bergman NA: Halothane and enflurane protect against bronchospasm in an asthma dog model. Anesth Analg 57:629, 1978.

26. Hirshman CA, Edelstein G, Pectz S, et al: Mechanism of action of inhalational anesthesia on airways. Anesthesiology 56:107, 1982.

27. Mazzeo AJ, Cheng EY, Stadnicka A, et al: Topographic differences in the direct effects of isoflurane on airway smooth muscle. Anesth Analg 78:948, 1994.

28. Park KW, Dai HB, Lowenstein E, et al: Isoflurane- and halothane-mediated dilation of distal bronchi in the rat depends on the epithelium. Anesthesiology 86:1078, 1997.

29. Habre W, Petak F, Sly PD, et al: Protective effects of volatile agents against methacholine-induced bronchoconstriction in rats. Anesthesiology 94:348, 2001.

30. Hermans JM, Edelstein G, Hanifen JM, et al: Inhalational anesthesia and histamine release during bronchospasm. Anesthesiology 61:69, 1984.

31. Shah MV, Hirshman CA: Mode of action of halothane on histamine-induced airway constriction in dogs with reactive airways. Anesthesiology 65:170, 1986.

32. Brown RH, Zerhouni EA, Hirshman CA: Comparison of low concentrations of halothane and isoflurane as bronchodilators. Anesthesiology 78:1097, 1993.

33. Yamamoto K, Morimoto N, Warner DO, et al: Factors influencing the direct actions of volatile anesthetics on airway smooth muscle. Anesthesiology 78:1102, 1993.

34. Mitsuhata H, Saitoh J, Shimizu R, et al: Sevoflurane and isoflurane protect against bronchospasm in dogs. Anesthesiology 81:1230, 1004.

35. Katoh T, Ikeda K: A comparison of sevoflurane with halothane, enflurane, and isoflurane on bronchoconstriction caused by histamine. Can J Anaesth 41:1214, 1994.

36. Mazzeo AJ, Cheng EY, Bosnjak ZJ, et al: Differential effects of desflurane and halothane on peripheral airway smooth muscle. Br J Anaesth 76:841, 1996.

37. Goff MJ, Arain SR, Ficke DJ, et al: Absence of bronchodilation during desflurane anesthesia: A comparison to sevoflurane and thiopental. Anesthesiology 93:404, 2000.

38. Cheng EY, Mazzeo AJ, Bosnjak ZJ, et al: Direct relaxant effects of intravenous anesthetics on airway smooth muscle. Anesth Analg 83:162, 1996.

39. Yamakage M, Chen X, Tsuijiguchi N, et al: Different inhibitory effects of volatile anesthetics on T- and L-type voltage-dependent Ca^{2+} channels in porcine tracheal and bronchial smooth muscles. Anesthesiology 94:683, 2001.

40. Hashimoto Y, Hirota K, Ohtomo N, et al: In vivo direct measurement of the bronchodilating effect of sevoflurane using a superfine fiberoptic bronchoscope: Comparison with enflurane and halothane. J Cardiothorac Vasc Anesth 10:213, 1996.

41. Yamakage M: Direct inhibitory mechanisms of halothane on canine tracheal smooth muscle contraction. Anesthesiology 77:546, 1992.

42. Janssen LJ: T-type and L-type Ca^{2+} currents in canine bronchial smooth muscle: Characterization and physiological roles. Am J Physiol Cell Physiol 272:C1757, 1997.

43. Lindeman KS, Croxton TL, Lande B, et al: Hypocapnia-induced contraction of porcine airway smooth muscle. Eur Respir J 12:1046, 1998.

44. Fukushima T, Hirasaki A, Jones KA, et al: Halothane and potassium channels in airway smooth muscle. Br J Anaesth 76:847, 1996.

45. Yamakage M, Chen X, Kimura A, et al: The repolarizing effects of volatile anesthetics on porcine tracheal and bronchial smooth muscle cells. Anesth Analg 94:84, 2002.

46. Chen X, Yamakage M, Namiki A: Inhibitory effects of volatile anesthetics on K+ and Cl-channel currents in porcine tracheal and bronchial smooth muscle. Anesthesiology 96:458, 2002.

47. Yamakage M, Kohro S, Matsuzaki T, et al: Role of intracellular Ca^{2+} stores in the inhibitory effect of halothane on airway smooth muscle contraction. Anesthesiology 89:165, 1998.

48. Pabelick CM, Prakash YS, Kannan MS, et al: Effects of halothane on sarcoplasmic reticulum calcium release channels in porcine airway smooth muscle cells. Anesthesiology 95:207, 2001.

49. Pabelick CM, Prakash YS, Kannan MS, et al: Effect of halothane on intracellular calcium oscillations in porcine tracheal smooth muscle cells. Am J Physiol 276:L81, 1999.

50. Morimoto N, Yamamoto K, Jones KA, et al: Halothane and pertussis toxin-sensitive G proteins in airway smooth muscle. Anesth Analg 78:328, 1994.

51. Jones KA, Wong GY, Lorenz RR, et al: Effects of halothane on the relationship between cytosolic calcium and force in airway smooth muscle. Am J Physiol 266:L199, 1994.

52. Warner DO, Jones KA, Lorenz RR: The effects of halothane pretreatment on manganese influx induced by muscarinic stimulation of airway smooth muscle. Anesth Analg 84:1366, 1997.

53. Kai T, Bremerich DH, Jones KA, et al: Drug-specific effects of volatile anesthetics on Ca^{2+} sensitization in airway smooth muscle. Anesth Analg 87:425, 1998.

54. Hanazaki M, Jones KA, Perkins WJ, et al: Halothane increases smooth muscle protein phosphatase in airway smooth muscle. Anesthesiology 94:129, 2001.

55. Kai T, Jones KA, Warner DO: Halothane attenuates calcium sensitization in airway smooth muscle by inhibiting G-proteins. Anesthesiology 89:1543, 1998.

56. Jones KA, Wong GY, Jankowski CJ, et al: cGMP modulation of Ca^{2+} sensitivity in airway smooth muscle. Am J Physiol 276:L35, 1999.

57. Croxton TL, Lande B, Hirshman CA: Role of G proteins in agonist-induced Ca^{2+} sensitization of tracheal smooth muscle. Am J Physiol 275:L748, 1998.

58. Yoshimura H, Jones KA, Perkins WJ, et al: Calcium sensitization produced by G protein activation in airway smooth muscle. Am J Physiol Lung Cell Mol Physiol 281:L631, 2001.

59. Korenaga S, Tekeda K, Ito Y: Differential effects of halothane on airway nerves and muscle. Anesthesiology 60:309, 1984.

60. Park KW, Dai HB, Lowenstein E, et al: Epithelial dependence of the bronchodilatory effect of sevoflurane and desflurane in rat distal bronchi. Anesth Analg 86:646, 1998.

61. Warner DO, Brichant JF, Rehder K: Direct and neurally mediated effects of halothane on pulmonary resistance in vivo. Anesthesiology 72:1057, 1990.

62. Wiklund CU, Lim S, Lindsten U, et al: Relaxation by sevoflurane, desflurane and halothane in the isolated guinea-pig trachea via inhibition of cholinergic neurotransmission. Br J Anaesth 83:422, 1999.

63. Brown RH, Mitzner W, Zerhouni E, et al: Direct in vivo visualization of bronchodilation induced by inhalational anesthesia using high-resolution computed tomography. Anesthesiology 78:295, 1993.

64. Kannan MS, Johnson DE: Nitric oxide mediates the neural nonadrenergic, noncholinergic relaxation in pig tracheal smooth muscle. Am J Physiol 262:L511, 1992.

65. Lindeman KS, Baker SG, Hirshman CA: Interaction between halothane and the nonadrenergic, noncholinergic inhibitory system in porcine trachealis muscle. Anesthesiology 81:641, 1994.

66. Kingstone HGG, Hirshman CA: Perioperative management of the patient with asthma. Anesth Analg 63:844, 1984.

67. Gold MI, Helrich M: Pulmonary mechanics during general anesthesia, status asthmaticus. Anesthesiology 32:422, 1970.

68. Schwartz SH: Treatment of status asthmaticus with halothane. JAMA 251:2688, 1984.

69. Johnston RG, Noseworthy TW, Friesen EG, et al: Isoflurane therapy for status asthmaticus in children and adults. Chest 97:698, 1990.

70. Parnass SM, Feld JM, Chamberlin WH, et al: Status asthmaticus treated with isoflurane and enflurane. Anesth Analg 66:1193, 1987.

71. Echeverria M, Gelb AW, Wexler HR, et al: Enflurane and halothane in status asthmaticus. Chest 89:152, 1986.

72. Saulnier FF, Durocher AV, Deturck RA, et al: Respiratory and hemodynamic effects of halothane in status asthmaticus. Intensive Care Med 16:104, 1990.

73. Maltais F, Sovilj M, Goldberg P, et al: Respiratory mechanics in status asthmaticus. Effects of inhalational anesthesia. Chest 106:1401, 1994.

74. Revich LR, Grinspon SG, Paredes C, et al: Respiratory effects of halothane in a patient with refractory status asthmaticus. Pulm Pharmacol Ther 14:455, 2001.

75. Arakawa H, Takizawa T, Tokuyama K, et al: Efficacy of inhaled anticholinergics and anesthesia in treatment of a patient in status asthmaticus. J Asthma 39:77, 2002.

76. Rooke GA, Choi JH, Bishop MJ: The effect of isoflurane, halothane, sevoflurane, and thiopental/nitrous oxide on respiratory system resistance after tracheal intubation. Anesthesiology 86:1294, 1997.

77. Lynch C III, Baum J, Tenbrinck R: Xenon anesthesia. Anesthesiology 92:865, 2000.

78. Rueckoldt H, Vangerow B, Marx G, et al: Xenon inhalation increases airway pressure in ventilated patients. Acta Anaesthesiol Scand 43:1060, 1999.

79. Calzia E, Stahl W, Handschuh T, et al: Respiratory mechanics during xenon anesthesia in pigs: Comparison with nitrous oxide. Anesthesiology 91:1378, 1999.

80. Fujii Y: Respiratory effects of xenon. Int Anesthesiol Clin 39:95, 2001.

81. Zhang P, Ohara A, Mashimo T, et al: Pulmonary resistance in dogs: A comparison of xenon with nitrous oxide. Can J Anaesth 42, 1995.

82. Lachmann B, Armbruster S, Schairer W, et al: Safety and efficacy of xenon in routine use as an inhalational anaesthetic. Lancet 335:1413, 1995.

83. Moote CA, Knill RL, Clement J: Ventilatory compensation for continuous inspiratory resistive and elastic loads during halothane anesthesia in humans. Anesthesiology 64:582, 1986.

84. Calzia E, Stahl W, Handschuh T, et al: Continuous arterial P(O2) and P(CO2) measurements in swine during nitrous oxide and xenon elimination: Prevention of diffusion. Anesthesiology 90:829, 1999.

85. Tobias JD, Hirshman CA: Attenuation of histamine-induced airway constriction by albuterol during halothane anesthesia. Anesthesiology 72:105, 1990.

86. Wu RSC, Wu KC, Wong TKM, et al: Isoflurane anesthesia does not add to the bronchodilating effect of a beta 2-adrenergic agonist after tracheal intubation. Anesth Analg 83:238, 1996.

87. Lehane JR, Jordan C, Jones JG: Influence of halothane and enflurane on respiratory airflow resistance and specific conductance in anaesthetized man. Br J Anaesth 52:773, 1980.

88. Yamakage M, Tsujiguchi N, Hattori J, et al: Low-temperature modification of the inhibitory effects of volatile anesthetics on airway smooth muscle contraction in dogs. Anesthesiology 93:179, 2000.

89. Bennett DJ, Torda TA, Horton DA, et al: Severe bronchospasm complicating thoracotomy. Arch Surg 101:555, 1970.

90. Leeson TS, Leeson CR: A light and electron microscope study of developing respiratory tissue in the rat. J Anat 98:183, 1964.

91. Lund VJ: Nasal physiology: Neurochemical receptors, nasal cycle, and ciliary action. Allergy Asthma Proc 17:179, 1996.

92. Reid L: Natural history of mucous in the bronchial tree. Arch Environ Health 10:265, 1965.

93. Wanner A: Clinical aspects of mucociliary transport. Am Rev Respir Dis 116:73, 1977.

94. Foster WM, Walters DM, Longphre M, et al: Methodology for the measurement of mucociliary function in the mouse by scintigraphy. J Appl Physiol 90:1111, 2001.

95. Lindberg S, Cervin A, Runer T: Low levels of nasal nitric oxide (NO) correlate to impaired mucociliary function in the upper airways. Acta Otolaryngol 117:728, 1997.

96. Wagner EM, Foster WM: Importance of airway blood flow on particle clearance from the lung. J Appl Physiol 81:1878, 1996.

97. Forbes AR: Temperature, humidity and mucous flow in the intubated trachea. Br J Anaesth 45:874, 1973.

98. Hirsch JA, Tokayer JL, Robinson MJ, et al: Effects of dry air and subsequent humidification on tracheal mucous velocity in dogs. J Appl Physiol 39:242, 1975.

99. Forbes AR, Gamsu G: Lung mucociliary clearance after anesthesia with spontaneous and controlled ventilation. Am Rev Resp Dis 120:857, 1979.

100. Forbes AR: Halothane depresses mucociliary flow in the trachea. Anesthesiology 45:59, 1976.

101. Forbes AR, Horrigan RW: Mucociliary flow in the trachea during anesthesia with enflurane, ether, nitrous oxide, and morphine. Anesthesiology 46:319, 1977.

102. Forbes AR, Gamsu G: Mucociliary clearance in the canine lung during and after general anesthesia. Anesthesiology 50:26, 1979.

103. Nunn JF, Sturrock JE, Wills EJ, et al: The effect of inhalational anaesthetics on the swimming velocity of *Tetrahymena pyriformis*. J Cell Sci 15:537, 1974.

104. Manawadu BR, Mostow SR, LaForce FM: Impairment of tracheal ring ciliary activity by halothane. Anesth Analg 58:500, 1979.

105. Yang T, Li Y, Liu Q, et al: Isoflurane aggravates the decrease of phosphatidylcholine synthesis in alveolar type II cells induced by hydrogen peroxide. Drug Metabol Drug Interact 18:243, 2001.

106. Molliex S, Crestani B, Dureuil B, et al: Effects of halothane on surfactant biosynthesis by rat alveolar type II cells in primary culture. Anesthesiology 81:668, 1994.

107. Patel AB, Sokolowski J, Davidson BA, et al: Halothane potentiation of hydrogen peroxide-induced inhibition of surfactant synthesis: The role of type II cell energy status. Anesth Analg 94:943, 2002.

108. Paugam-Burtz C, Molliex S, Lardeux B, et al: Differential effects of halothane and thiopental on surfactant protein C messenger RNA in vivo and in vitro in rats. Anesthesiology 93:805, 2000.

109. Gamsu G, Singer MM, Vincent HH, et al: Postoperative impairment of mucous transport in the lung. Am Rev Respir Dis 114:673, 1976.

110. Lichtiger M, Landa JF, Hirsch JA: Velocity of tracheal mucus in anesthetized women undergoing gynecologic surgery. Anesthesiology 42:753, 1975.

111. Konrad F, Marx T, Schraag M, et al: Combination anesthesia and bronchial transport velocity. Effects of anesthesia with isoflurane, fentanyl, vecuronium and oxygen-nitrous oxide breathing on bronchial mucus transport. Anaesthesist 46:403, 1997.

112. Konrad FX, Schreiber T, Brecht-Kraus D, et al: Bronchial mucus transport in chronic smokers and nonsmokers during general anesthesia. J Clin Anesth 5:375, 1993.

113. Tarhan S, Moffitt EA, Sessler AD, et al: Risk of anesthesia and surgery in patients with chronic bronchitis and chronic obstructive pulmonary disease. Surgery 74:720, 1973.

114. Rivero DH, Lorenzi-Filho G, Pazetti R, et al: Effects of bronchial transection and reanastomosis on mucociliary system. Chest 119:1510, 2001.

115. Hamada H, Damron DS, Hong SJ, et al: Phenylephrine-induced Ca^{2+} oscillations in canine pulmonary artery smooth muscle cells. Circ Res 81:812, 1997.

116. Doi S, Damron DS, Horibe M, et al: Capacitative Ca^{2+} entry and tyrosine kinase activation in canine pulmonary arterial smooth muscle cells. Am J Physiol Lung Cell Mol Physiol 278:L118, 2000.

117. Doi S, Damron DS, Ogawa K, et al: K+ channel inhibition, calcium signaling, and vasomotor tone in canine pulmonary artery smooth muscle. Am J Physiol Lung Cell Mol Physiol 279:L242, 2000.

118. Sweeney M, Beddy D, Honner V, et al: Effects of changes in pH and CO_2 on pulmonary arterial wall tension are not endothelium dependent. J Appl Physiol 85:2040, 1998.

119. Myers JL, Wizorek JJ, Myers AK, et al: Pulmonary arterial endothelial dysfunction potentiates hypercapnic vasoconstriction and alters the response to inhaled nitric oxide. Ann Thorac Surg 62:1677, 1996.

120. Johns RA: New mechanisms for inhaled NO: Release of an endogenous NO inhibitor? Anesthesiology 95:3, 2001.

121. Rengasamy A, Johns RA: Determination of Km for oxygen of NO synthase isoforms. J Pharmacol Exp Ther 276:30, 1996.

122. Rengasamy A, Johns RA: Characterization of EDRF/NO synthase from bovine cerebellum and mechanism of modulation by high and low oxygen tensions. J Pharmacol Exp Ther 259:310, 1991.

123. Heyman SN, Goldfarb M, Darmon D, et al: Tissue oxygenation modifies nitric oxide bioavailability. Microcirculation 63:199, 1999.

124. Hampl V, Herget J: Role of NO in the pathogenesis of chronic pulmonary hypertension. Physiol Rev 80:1337, 2000.

125. Rocca GD, Passariello M, Coccia C, et al: Inhaled nitric oxide administration during one-lung ventilation in patients undergoing thoracic surgery. J Cardiothorac Vasc Anesth 15:218, 2001.

126. Hermle G, Schutte H, Walmrath D, et al: Ventilation-perfusion mismatch after lung ischemia-reperfusion. Protective effect of nitric oxide. Am J Respir Crit Care Med 160:1179, 1999.

127. Hambraeus-Jonzon K, Chen L, Freden F, et al: Pulmonary vasoconstriction during regional nitric oxide inhalation: Evidence of a blood-borne regulator of nitric oxide synthase activity. Anesthesiology 95:102, 2001.

128. Weinberger B, Heck DE, Laskin DL, et al: Nitric oxide in the lung: Therapeutic and cellular mechanisms of action. Pharmacol Ther 84:401, 1999.

129. Scherrer U, Vollenweider L, Delabays A, et al: Inhaled nitric oxide for high-altitude pulmonary edema. N Engl J Med 334:624, 1996.

130. Roberts JDJ, Fineman JR, Morin FCR, et al: Inhaled nitric oxide and persistent pulmonary hypertension of the newborn. The Inhaled Nitric Oxide Study Group. N Engl J Med 336:605, 1997.

131. Takahashi Y, Kobayashi H, Tanaka N, et al: Worsening of hypoxemia with nitric oxide inhalation during bronchospasm in humans. Respir Physiol 112:113, 1998.

132. Zanaboni P, Murray PA, Simon BA, et al: Selective endothelial dysfunction in conscious dogs after cardiopulmonary bypass. J Appl Physiol 82:1776, 1997.

133. Prabhakar NR: Endogenous carbon monoxide in control of respiration. Respir Physiol 114:57, 1998.

134. Nachar RA, Pastene CM, Herrera EA, et al: Low-dose inhaled carbon monoxide reduces pulmonary vascular resistance during acute hypoxemia in adult sheep. High Alt Med Biol 2:377, 2001.

135. Colley PS, Cheney FWJ, Hlastala MP: Ventilation-perfusion and gas exchange effects of sodium nitroprusside in dogs with normal and edematous lungs. Anesthesiology 50:489, 1979.

136. Putensen C, Rasanen J, Putensen-Himmer G, et al: Effect of low isoflurane concentrations on the ventilation-perfusion distribution in injured canine lungs. Anesthesiology 97:652, 2002.

137. Marshall C, Lindgren L, Marshall BE: Effects of halothane, enflurane, and isoflurane on hypoxic pulmonary vasoconstriction in rat lungs. Anesthesiology 60:304, 1984.

138. Ishibe Y, Gui X, Uno H, et al: Effect of sevoflurane on hypoxic pulmonary vasoconstriction in the perfused rabbit lung. Anesthesiology 79:1348, 1993.

139. Loer SA, Scheeren TWL, Tarnow J: Desflurane inhibits hypoxic pulmonary vasoconstriction in isolated rabbit lungs. Anesthesiology 83:552, 1995.

140. Marshall BE, Clarke WR, Costarino AT, et al: The dose-response relationship for hypoxic pulmonary vasoconstriction. Respir Physiol 96:231, 1994.

141. Marshall BE, Marshall C, Benumof J, et al: Hypoxic pulmonary vasoconstriction in dogs: Effect of lung segment size and oxygen-tension. J Appl Physiol 51:1543, 1981.

142. Hambraeus-Jonzon K, Bindslev L, Mellgard AJ, et al: Hypoxic pulmonary vasoconstriction in human lungs: A stimulus-response study. Anesthesiology 86:308, 1997.

143. Benumof JL, Pirho AF, Johansen I, et al: Interaction of PVO2 with PAO2 on hypoxic pulmonary vasoconstriction. J Appl Physiol 51:871, 1981.

144. Domino KB, Wetstein L, Glasser SA, et al: Influence of mixed venous oxygen tension (PVO2) on blood flow to atelectatic lung. Anesthesiology 59:428, 1983.

145. Adding LC, Agvald P, Persson MG, et al: Regulation of pulmonary nitric oxide by carbon dioxide is intrinsic to the lung. Acta Anaesthesiol Scand 167:167, 1999.

146. Yamamoto Y, Nakano H, Ide H, et al: Role of airway nitric oxide on the regulation of pulmonary circulation by carbon dioxide. J Appl Physiol 91:1121, 2001.
147. Brogan TV, Hedges RG, McKinney S, et al: Pulmonary NO synthase inhibition and inspired CO_2: Effects on V'/Q' and pulmonary blood flow distribution. Eur Respir J 16:288, 2000.
148. Sykes MK, Davies DM, Chakrabarti K, et al: The effects of halothane, trichloroethylene and ether on the hypoxic pressor response and pulmonary vascular resistance in the isolated, perfused cat lung. Br J Anaesth 45:655, 1973.
149. Loh L, Sykes MK, Chakrabarti MK: The effects of halothane and ether on the pulmonary circulation in the innervated perfused cat lung. Br J Anaesth 49:309, 1977.
150. Johnson D, Mayers I, Hurst T: Halothane inhibits hypoxic pulmonary vasoconstriction in the presence of cyclo-oxygenase blockade. Can J Anaesth 37:287, 1990.
151. Johnson D, Mayers I, To T: The effects of halothane in hypoxic pulmonary vasoconstriction. Anesthesiology 72:125, 1990.
152. Marshall C, Kim SD, Marshall BE: The actions of halothane, ibuprofen and BW755C on hypoxic pulmonary vasoconstriction. Anesthesiology 66:537, 1987.
153. Bjertnaes LJ, Mundal R: The pulmonary vasoconstrictor response to hypoxia during enflurane anesthesia. Acta Anaesthesiol Scand 24:252, 1980.
154. Hurtig JB, Tait AR, Loh L, et al: Reduction of hypoxic pulmonary vasoconstriction by nitrous oxide administration in the isolated perfused cat lung. Can Anaesth Soc J 24:540, 1977.
155. Bindlsev L, Cannon D, Sykes MK: Effect of lignocaine and nitrous oxide on hypoxic pulmonary vasoconstriction in the dog constant-flow perfused left lower lobe preparation. Br J Anaesth 58:315, 1986.
156. Bindlsev L, Cannon D, Sykes MK: Reversal of nitrous oxide-induced depression of hypoxic pulmonary vasoconstriction by lignocaine hydrochloride during collapse and ventilation hypoxia of the left lower lobe. Br J Anaesth 58:451, 1986.
157. Kjaeve J, Bjertnaes LJ: Interaction of verapamil and halogenated anesthetics on hypoxic pulmonary vasoconstriction. Acta Anesthesiol Scand 33:193, 1989.
158. Johnson DH, Hurst TS, Mayers I: Effects of halothane on hypoxic pulmonary vasoconstriction in canine atelectasis. Anesth Analg 72:440, 1991.
159. Benumof JL, Wahrenbrock EA: Local effects of anesthetics on regional hypoxic pulmonary vasoconstriction. Anesthesiology 43:525, 1975.
160. Mathers J, Benumof JL, Wahrenbrock EA: General anesthetics and regional hypoxic pulmonary vasoconstriction. Anesthesiology 46:111, 1977.
161. Lennon PF, Murray PA: Attenuated hypoxic pulmonary vasoconstriction during isoflurane anesthesia is abolished by cyclooxygenase inhibition in chronically instrumented dogs. Anesthesiology 84:404, 1996.
162. Johns RA: Endothelium, anesthetics, and vascular control. Anesthesiology 79:1381, 1993.
163. Marshall C, Marshall BE: Endothelium-derived relaxing factor is not responsible for inhibition of hypoxic pulmonary vasoconstriction by inhalational anesthetics. Anesthesiology 73:441, 1990.
164. Marshall C, Marshall BE: Inhalational anesthetics directly inhibit hypoxic pulmonary vasoconstriction. Anesthesiology 79:A1238, 1993.
165. Yoshida K, Tewari S, Kirby T, et al: Halothane attenuates acetylcholine-induced vasorelaxation and cyclic GMP accumulation in human pulmonary artery. Anesthesiology 87:A1104, 1997.
166. Fehr DM, Larach DR, Zangari KA, et al: Halothane constricts bovine pulmonary arteries by release of intracellular calcium. J Pharmacol Exp Ther 277:706, 1996.
167. Gambone LM, Murray PA, Flavahan NA: Isoflurane anesthesia attenuates endothelium-dependent pulmonary vasorelaxation by inhibiting the synergistic interaction between nitric oxide and prostacyclin. Anesthesiology 86:936, 1997.
168. Gambone LM, Murray PA, Flavahan NA: Synergistic interaction between endothelium-derived NO and prostacyclin in pulmonary artery: Potential role for K+ATP channels. Br J Pharmacol 121:271, 1997.
169. Liu R, Ueda M, Okazaki N, et al: Role of potassium channels in isoflurane- and sevoflurane-induced attenuation of hypoxic pulmonary vasoconstriction in isolated perfused rabbit lungs. Anesthesiology 95:939, 2001.
170. Carter EP, Sato K, Morio Y, et al: Inhibition of K(Ca) channels restores blunted hypoxic pulmonary vasoconstriction in rats with cirrhosis. Am J Physiol Lung Cell Mol Physiol 279:L903, 2000.
171. Gambone LM, Fujiwara Y, Murray PA: Endothelium-dependent pulmonary vasodilation is selectively attenuated during isoflurane anesthesia. Am J Physiol Heart Circ Physiol 272:H290, 1997.
172. Seki S, Sato K, Nakayama M, et al: Halothane and enflurane attenuate pulmonary vasodilation mediated by adenosine triphosphate-sensitive potassium channels compared to the conscious state. Anesthesiology 86:923, 1997.
173. Nakayama M, Kondo U, Murray PA: Pulmonary vasodilator response to adenosine triphosphate-sensitive potassium channel activation is attenuated during desflurane but preserved during sevoflurane anesthesia compared with the conscious state. Anesthesiology 88:1023, 1998.
174. Seki S, Horibe M, Murray PA: Halothane attenuates endothelium-dependent pulmonary vasorelaxant response to lemakalim, an adenosine triphosphate (ATP)-sensitive potassium channel agonist. Anesthesiology 87:625, 1997.
175. Lennon PF, Murray PA: Isoflurane and the pulmonary vascular pressure-flow relation at baseline and during sympathetic α- and β-adrenoceptor activation in chronically instrumented dogs. Anesthesiology 82:723, 1995.
176. Sato K, Seki S, Murray PA: Effects of halothane and enflurane anesthesia on sympathetic B-adrenoreceptor-mediated pulmonary vasodilation in chronically instrumented dogs. Anesthesiology 97:478, 2002.
177. Fujiwara Y, Murray PA: Effects of isoflurane anesthesia on pulmonary vascular response to K+ ATP channel activation and circulatory hypotension in chronically instrumented dogs. Anesthesiology 90:799, 1999.
178. Su JY, Vo AC: Role of PKC in isoflurane-induced biphasic contraction in skinned pulmonary arterial strips. Anesthesiology 96:155, 2002.
179. Su JY, Vo AC: Ca^{2+}-calmodulin-dependent protein kinase II plays a major role in halothane-induced dose-dependent relaxation in the skinned pulmonary artery. Anesthesiology 97:207, 2002.
180. Zhong L, Su JY: Isoflurane activates PKC and Ca^{2+}-calmodulin-dependent protein kinase II via MAP kinase signaling in cultured vascular smooth muscle cells. Anesthesiology 96:148, 2002.
181. Sykes MK, Giggs JM, Loh L, et al: Preservation of the pulmonary vasoconstrictor response to alveolar hypoxia during the administration of halothane to dogs. Br J Anaesth 50:1185, 1978.
182. Sykes MK, Hurtig JB, Tait AR, et al: Reduction of hypoxic pulmonary vasoconstriction during diethyl ether anesthesia in the dog. Br J Anaesth 49:293, 1977.
183. Sykes MK, Hurtig JB, Tait AR, et al: Reduction of hypoxic pulmonary vasoconstriction in the dog during administration of nitrous oxide. Br J Anaesth 49:301, 1977.
184. Lejeune P, Brimioulle S, Leeman M, et al: Multipoint pulmonary vascular pressure/flow relationships in hypoxic and in normoxic dogs: Effects of nitrous oxide with and without cyclooxygenase inhibition. Anesthesiology 68:92, 1988.
185. Bjertnaes LJ: Hypoxia-induced pulmonary vasoconstriction in man: Inhibition due to diethyl ether and halothane anesthesia. Acta Anaesthesiol Scand 22:570, 1978.
186. Fargas-Babjak A, Forrest JB: Effect of halothane on the pulmonary vascular response to hypoxia in dogs. Can J Anaesth 26:6, 1979.
187. Naeije RL, Lejeune P, Leeman M, et al: Pulmonary arterial pressure-flow plots in dogs: Effects of isoflurane and nitroprusside. J Appl Physiol 63:969, 1987.

188. Domino KB, Borowec L, Alexander CM, et al: Influence of isoflurane on hypoxic pulmonary vasoconstriction in dogs. Anesthesiology 64:423, 1986.

189. Kerbaul F, Bellezza M, Guidon C, et al: Effects of sevoflurane on hypoxic pulmonary vasoconstriction in anaesthetized piglets. Br J Anaesth 85:440, 1999.

190. Lesitsky MA, Davis S, Murray PA: Preservation of hypoxic pulmonary vasoconstriction during sevoflurane and desflurane anesthesia compared to the conscious state in chronically instrumented dogs. Anesthesiology 89:1501, 1998.

191. Kerbaul F, Guidon C, Stephanazzi J, et al: Sub-MAC concentrations of desflurane do not inhibit hypoxic pulmonary vasoconstriction in anesthetized piglets. Can J Anaesth 48:760, 2001.

192. Kleinsasser A, Lindner KA, Hoermann C, et al: Isoflurane and sevoflurane anesthesia in pigs with a preexistent gas exchange defect. Anesthesiology 95:1422, 2001.

193. Marshall BE, Marshall C: Anesthesia and the pulmonary circulation. *In* Covino BC, Fozzard HA, Rehder K, Strichartz G (eds): Effects of Anesthesia. Clinical Physiology Series. Bethesda, MD, American Physiological Society, 1985, p 121.

194. Nishiwaki K, Nyhan DP, Rock P, et al: *N*-nitro-L-arginine and pulmonary vascular pressure-flow relationship in conscious dogs. Am J Physiol Heart Circ Physiol 262:H1331, 1992.

195. Karzai W, Haberstroh J, Priebe HJ: The effects of increasing concentrations of desflurane on systemic oxygenation during one-lung ventilation in pigs. Anesth Analg 89:215, 1999.

196. Karzai W, Haberstroh J, Priebe HJ: Effects of desflurane and propofol on arterial oxygenation during one-lung ventilation in the pig. Acta Anaesthesiol Scand 42:648, 1998.

197. Abe K, Shimizu T, Takashina M, et al: The effects of propofol, isoflurane and sevoflurane on oxygenation and shunt fraction during one-lung ventilation. Anesth Analg 87:1164, 1998.

198. Beck DH, Doepfmer UR, Sinemus C, et al: Effects of sevoflurane and propofol on pulmonary shunt fraction during one-lung ventilation for thoracic surgery. Br J Anaesth 86:38, 2001.

199. Rees ID, Gaines GY: One lung anesthesia—A comparison of pulmonary gas exchange during anesthesia with ketamine or enflurane. Anesth Analg 63:521, 1984.

200. Schwarzkopf K, Schreiber T, Bauer R, et al: The effects of increasing concentrations of isoflurane and desflurane on pulmonary perfusion and systemic oxygenation during one-lung ventilation in pigs. Anesth Analg 93:1434, 2001.

201. Anderson MW, Benumof JL: Intrapulmonary shunting during one lung ventilation and surgical manipulation. Anesthesiology 45:A377, 1981.

202. Benumof JL, Augustine SD, Gibbons JA: Halothane and isoflurane only slightly impair arterial oxygenation during one-lung ventilation in patients undergoing thoracotomy. Anesthesiology 67:910, 1987.

203. Pagel P, Fu FL, Damask MC, et al: Desflurane and isoflurane produce similar alterations in systemic and pulmonary hemodynamics and arterial oxygenation in patients undergoing one-lung ventilation during thoracotomy. Anesth Analg 87:800, 1998.

204. Abe K, Mashimo T, Yoshiya I: Arterial oxygenation and shunt fraction during one-lung ventilation: A comparison of isoflurane and sevoflurane. Anesth Analg 86:266, 1998.

205. Reid CW, Slinger PD, Lenis S: A comparison of the effects of propofol-alfentanil versus isoflurane anesthesia on arterial oxygenation during one-lung ventilation. J Cardiothorac Vasc Anesth 10:860, 1996.

206. Liu R, Ishibe Y, Ueda M, et al: Isoflurane administration before ischemia and during reperfusion attenuates ischemia/reperfusion-induced injury of isolated rabbit lungs. Anesth Analg 89:561, 1999.

207. Doi S, Smedira N, Murray PA: Pulmonary vasoregulation by endothelin in conscious dogs after left lung transplantation. J Appl Physiol 88:210, 2000.

208. Lennon PF, Murray PA: Pulmonary vascular effects of isoflurane anesthesia after left lung autotransplantation in chronically instrumented dogs. Anesthesiology 85:592, 1996.

209. Forster HV, Pan LG, Lowry TF, et al: Important role of carotid chemoreceptor afferents in control of breathing of adult and neonatal mammals. Respir Physiol 119:199, 2000.

210. Gandevia SC, Allen GM, Butler JE, et al: Human respiratory muscles: Sensations, reflexes and fatigability. Clin Exp Pharmacol Physiol 25:757, 1998.

211. Tobin MJ: Sleep-disordered breathing, control of breathing, respiratory muscles, pulmonary function testing, nitric oxide and bronchoscopy in AJRCCM 2000. Am J Respir Crit Care Med 164:1362, 2001.

212. Georgopoulos D, Roussos C: Control of breathing in mechanically ventilated patients. Eur Respir J 9:2151, 1996.

213. St-John WM: Neurogenesis of patterns of automatic ventilatory activity. Prog Neurobiol 56:97, 1998.

214. Ward DS, Temp JA: Neuropharmacology of the control of ventilation. *In* Yaksh TL, Lynch C III, Zapol WM, et al (eds): Anesthesia: Biologic Foundations. Philadelphia, Lippincott-Raven Publishers, 1997.

215. Krolo M, Stuth EA, Tonkovic-Capin M, et al: Relative magnitude of tonic and phasic synaptic excitation of medullary inspiratory neurons in dogs. Am J Physiol Regul Integr Comp Physiol 279:R639, 2000.

216. Dogas Z, Stuth EAE, Hopp FA, et al: NMDA receptor-mediated transmission of carotid body chemoreceptor input to expiratory bulbospinal neurones in dogs. J Physiol 487:639, 1995.

217. Dogas Z, Krolo M, Stuth EA, et al: Differential effects of $GABA_A$ receptor antagonists in the control of respiratory neuronal discharge patterns. J Neurophysiol 80:2368, 1998.

218. Von Euler C: Neural organization and rhythm generation. *In* Crystal RG, West JB, Barnes PJ, et al (eds): The Lung: Scientific Foundations. New York, Raven Press, 1991, p 1307.

219. Solomon IC: Excitation of phrenic and sympathetic output during acute hypoxia: Contribution of medullary oxygen detectors. Respir Physiol 121:101, 2000.

220. Teppema L, Veening JG, Kranenburg A, et al: Expression of c-fos in the rat brainstem after exposure to hypoxia and to normoxic and hyperoxic hypercapnia. J Comp Neurol 388:169, 1997.

221. Smith JC, Ellenberger HH, Ballanyi K, et al: Pre-Botzinger complex: A brainstem region that may generate respiratory rhythm in mammals. Science 254:726, 1991.

222. Whitelaw WA, Derenne JP, Milic-Emili J: Occlusion pressure as a measure of respiratory center output in conscious man. Respir Physiol 23:181, 1975.

223. Larson CP Jr, Egar EI, Muallem M, et al: The effects of diethyl ether and methoxyflurane on ventilation. Anesthesiology 30:174, 1969.

224. Hickey RF, Severinghaus JW: Regulation of breathing: Drug effects. *In* Hornbein RF (ed): Regulation of Breathing. Lung Biology in Health and Disease, vol 17. New York, Marcel Dekker, 1981.

225. Fourcade HE, Stevens WC, Larson CPJ, et al: The ventilatory effects of Forane, a new inhaled anesthetic. Anesthesiology 35:26, 1971.

226. Eger EI: Isoflurane: A review. Anesthesiology 55:559, 1981.

227. Calverley RK, Smith NT, Jones CW, et al: Ventilatory and cardiovascular effects of enflurane anesthesia during spontaneous ventilation in man. Anesth Analg 57:610, 1978.

228. Fourcade HE, Larson CP, Hickey RF, et al: Effects of time on ventilation during halothane and cyclopropane anesthesia. Anesthesiology 36:83, 1972.

229. Kulkarni P, Brown KA: Ventilatory parameters in children during propofol anaesthesia: A comparison with halothane. Can J Anaesth 43:653, 1996.

230. Brown KA: Pattern of ventilation during halothane anaesthesia in infants less than two months of age. Can J Anaesth 43:121, 1996.

231. Lockhart SH, Rampil IJ, Yasuda N, et al: Depression of ventilation by desflurane in humans. Anesthesiology 74:484, 1991.

232. Doi M, Ikeda K: Respiratory effects of sevoflurane. Anesth Analg 66:241, 1987.

233. Green WB: The ventilatory effects of sevoflurane. Anesth Analg 81(Suppl 6):S23, 1995.

234. Warltier DC, Pagel PS: Cardiovascular and respiratory actions of desflurane: Is desflurane different from isoflurane? Anesth Analg 75:517, 1992.

235. Erb T, Christen P, Kern C, et al: Similar haemodynamic, respiratory and metabolic changes with the use of sevoflurane or halothane in children breathing spontaneously. Acta Anaesthesiol Scand 45:639, 2001.

236. Brown K, Aun C, Stocks J, et al: A comparison of the respiratory effects of sevoflurane and halothane in infants and young children. Anesthesiology 89:86, 1998.

237. Mutoh T, Nishimura R, Kim HY, et al: Cardiopulmonary effects of sevoflurane, compared with halothane, enflurane, and sevoflurane, in dogs. Am J Vet Res 58:885, 1997.

238. Eger EI, Dolan WM, Stevens WC, et al: Surgical stimulation antagonizes the respiratory depression produced by Forane. Anesthesiology 36:544, 1972.

239. Einarsson S, Bengtsson A, Stenqvst O, et al: Decreased respiratory depression during emergence from anesthesia with sevoflurane/N$_2$O than with sevoflurane alone. Can J Anaesth 46:335, 1999.

240. Pittinger CB, Faulconer AJ, Knott JR, et al: Electroencephalographic and other observations in monkeys during xenon anesthesia at elevated pressures. Anesthesiology 16:551, 1955.

241. Winkler SS, Nielsen A, Mesina J: Respiratory depression in goats by stable xenon: Implications for CT studies. J Comput Assist Tomogr 11:496, 1987.

242. Holl K, Nemati N, Kohmura E, et al: Stable-xenon-CT: Effects of xenon inhalation on EEG and cardio-respiratory parameters in the human. Acta Neurochir 87:129, 1987.

243. Krishnan BS, Stockwell MJ, Clemens RE, et al: Airway anesthesia and respiratory adaptations to dead space loading and exercise. Am J Respir Crit Care Med 155:459, 1997.

244. Mitrouska I, Bshouty Z, Younes M, et al: Effects of pulmonary and intercostal denervation on the response of breathing frequency to varying inspiratory flow. Eur Respir J 11:895, 1998.

245. Corne S, Gillespie D, Roberts D, et al: Effect of inspiratory flow rate on respiratory rate in intubated ventilated patients. Am J Respir Crit Care Med 156:304, 1997.

246. Ripamonti C, Bruera E: Dyspnea: Pathophysiology and assessment. J Pain Symptom Manage 13:220, 1997.

247. Fontanari P, Burnet H, Zattara-Hartmann MC, et al: Changes in airway resistance induced by nasal inhalation of cold dry, dry, or moist air in normal individuals. J Appl Physiol 81:1739, 1996.

248. Meessen NE, Van de Grinten CP, Luijendijk SC, et al: Histamine-induced bronchoconstriction and end tidal inspiratory activity in man. Thorax 51:1192, 1996.

249. Nishino T, Kochi T, Ishii M: Differences in respiratory reflex responses from the larynx, trachea, and bronchi in anesthetized female subjects. Anesthesiology 84:70, 1996.

250. Daubenspeck JA, Manning HL, Akay M: Contribution of supraglottal mechanoreceptor afferents to respiratory-related evoked potentials in humans. J Appl Physiol 88:291, 2000.

251. Pisarri TE, Giesbrecht GG: Reflex tracheal smooth muscle contraction and bronchial vasodilation evoked by airway cooling in dogs. J Appl Physiol 82:1566, 1997.

252. Matsumoto S, Ikeda M, Nishikawa T: Effects of sodium and potassium channel blockers on hyperinflation-induced slowly adapting pulmonary stretch receptor stimulation in the rat. Life Sci 67:2167, 2000.

253. Carl ML, Schelegle ES, Hollstein SB, et al: Control of ventilation during lung volume changes and permissive hypercapnia in dogs. Am J Respir Crit Care Med 158:742, 1998.

254. Whittenridge D, Bulbring E: Changes in the activity of pulmonary receptors in anesthesia and their influence on respiratory behavior. J Pharmacol Exp Ther 81:340, 1944.

255. Paskin S, Skovsted P, Smith TC: Failure of the Hering-Breuer reflex to account for tachypnea in anesthetized man: A survey of halothane, fluroxene, methoxyflurane and cyclopropane. Anesthesiology 29:550, 1968.

256. Nishino T, Anderson JW, Sant'Ambrogio G: Effects of halothane, enflurane, and isoflurane on laryngeal receptors in dogs. Respir Physiol 91:247, 1993.

257. Nishino T, Anderson JW, Sant'Ambrogio G: Responses of tracheobronchial receptors to halothane, enflurane, and isoflurane in anesthetized dogs. Respir Physiol 95:281, 1994.

258. Widdicombe J: Airway receptors. Respir Physiol 125:3, 2001.

259. Sant'Ambrogia G, Widdicombe J: Reflexes from airway rapidly adapting receptors. Respir Physiol 125:33, 2001.

260. Moores C, Davies AS, Dallak M: Sevoflurane has less effect than halothane on pulmonary afferent activity in the rabbit. Br J Anaesth 80:257, 1998.

261. Sivarajan M, Joy JV: Effects of general anesthesia and paralysis on upper airway changes due to head position in humans. Anesthesiology 85:787, 1996.

262. Nandi PR, Charlesworth CH, Taylor SJ, et al: Effect of general anesthesia on the pharynx. Br J Anaesth 66:157, 1991.

263. Litman RS, Weissend EE, Shrier DA, et al: Morphologic changes in the upper airway of children during awakening from propofol administration. Anesthesiology 96:607, 2002.

264. Badr MS: Effect of ventilatory drive on upper airway patency in humans during NREM sleep. Respir Physiol 103:1, 1996.

265. van de Graaff WB: Thoracic influence on upper airway patency. J Appl Physiol 65:2124, 1988.

266. Akahoshi T, White DP, Edwards JK, et al: Phasic mechanoreceptor stimuli can induce phasic activation of upper airway muscles in humans. J Physiol 531:677, 2001.

267. Pillar G, Fogel RB, Malhotra A, et al: Genioglossal inspiratory activation: Central respiratory vs mechanoreceptive influences. Respir Physiol 127:23, 2001.

268. Ochiai R, Guthrie RD, Motoyama EK: Effects of varying concentrations of halothane on the activity of the genioglossus, intercostals, and diaphragm in cats: An electromyographic study. Anesthesiology 70:812, 1989.

269. Nishino T, Kohchi T, Yonezawa T, et al: Responses of recurrent laryngeal, hypoglossal, and phrenic nerves to increasing depths of anesthesia with halothane or enflurane in vagotomized cats. Anesthesiology 63:404, 1985.

270. Pappas AL, Sukhani R, Lurie J, et al: Severity of airway hyperreactivity associated with laryngeal mask airway removal: Correlation with volatile anesthetic choice and depth of anesthesia. J Clin Anesth 13:498, 2001.

271. Klock PAJ, Czeslick EG, Klafta JM, et al: The effect of sevoflurane and desflurane on upper airway reactivity. Anesthesiology 94:963, 2001.

272. Tusiewicz K, Bryan AC, Froese AB: Contributions of changing rib cage-diaphragm interactions to the ventilatory depression of halothane anesthesia. Anesthesiology 47:327, 1977.

273. Warner DO, Warner MA, Ritman EL: Mechanical significance of respiratory muscle activity in humans during halothane anesthesia. Anesthesiology 84:309, 1996.

274. Warner DO, Warner MA, Ritman EL: Human chest wall function while awake and during halothane anesthesia. I. Quiet breathing. Anesthesiology 82:6, 1995.

275. Warner DO, Warner MA, Ritman EL: Atelectasis and chest wall shape during halothane anesthesia. Anesthesiology 85:49, 1996.

276. Krayer S, Rehder K, Vettermann J, et al: Position and motion of the human diaphragm during anesthesia-paralysis. Anesthesiology 70:891, 1989.

277. Warner DO: Diaphragm function during anesthesia: Still crazy after all these years. Anesthesiology 97:295, 2002.

278. Hedenstierna G, Tokics L, Lundquist H, et al: Phrenic nerve stimulation during halothane anesthesia: Effects on atelectasis. Anesthesiology 80:751, 1994.

279. Stuth EAE, Tonkovic-Capin M, Kampine JP, et al: Dose-dependent effects of isoflurane on the CO_2 responses of expiratory medullary neurons and the phrenic nerve activities in dogs. Anesthesiology 76:763, 1992.

280. Stuth EAE, Tonkovic-Capin M, Kampine JP, et al: Dose-dependent effects of halothane on expiratory and inspiratory bulbospinal neurons and the phrenic nerve activities in dogs. Anesthesiology 81:1470, 1994.

281. Stucke AG, Stuth EAE, Tonkovic-Capin V, et al: Effects of sevoflurane on excitatory neurotransmission to medullary expiratory neurons and on phrenic nerve activity in a decerebrate dog model. Anesthesiology 95:485, 2001.

282. Stuth EAE, Krolo M, Stucke AG, et al: Effects of halothane on excitatory neurotransmission to medullary expiratory neurons in a decerebrate dog model. Anesthesiology 93:1474, 2000.

283. Stucke AG, Stuth EAE, Tonkovic-Capin V, et al: Effects of halothane and sevoflurane on inhibitory neurotransmission to medullary expiratory neurons in a decerebrate dog model. Anesthesiology 96:955, 2002.

284. Kochi T, Ide T, Isono S, et al: Different effects of halothane and enflurane on diaphragmatic contractility in vivo. Anesth Analg 70:362, 1990.

285. Ide T, Kochi T, Isono S, et al: Diaphragmatic function during sevoflurane anaesthesia in dogs. Can J Anaesth 38:116, 1991.

286. Veber B, Dureuil B, Viires N, et al: Effects of isoflurane on contractile properties of diaphragm. Anesthesiology 70:684, 1989.

287. Ide T, Kochi T, Isono S, et al: Effects of sevoflurane on diaphragmatic contractility in dogs. Anesth Analg 74:739, 1992.

288. Warner DO, Warner MA, Joyner MJ, et al: The effect of nitrous oxide on chest wall function in humans and dogs. Anesth Analg 86:1058, 1998.

289. Hoshi T, Fujii Y, Takahashi S, et al: Effect of xenon on diaphragmatic contractility in dogs. Can J Anaesth 47:819, 2000.

290. De Troyer A, Brunko E, Leduc D, et al: Reflex inhibition of canine inspiratory intercostals by diaphragmatic tension receptors. J Physiol 514:255, 1999.

291. Moote CA, Knill RL, Clement J: Ventilatory compensation for continuous inspiratory resistive and elastic loads during halothane anesthesia in humans. Anesthesiology 64:582, 1986.

292. Slee TA, Sharar SR, Pavlin EG, et al: The effects of airway impedance on work of breathing during halothane anesthesia. Anesth Analg 69:374, 1989.

293. Rheder K, Marsh HM: Respiratory mechanics during anesthesia and mechanical ventilation. *In* Fishman AP, Macklem PT, Mead J, Geiger SR (eds): Handbook of Physiology: The Respiratory System. Mechanics of Breathing, vol 3. Bethesda, MD, American Physiological Society, 1986, p 737.

294. Westbrook PR, Stubbs SE, Sessler AD, et al: Effect of anesthesia and muscle paralysis on respiratory mechanics in normal man. J Appl Physiol 34:81, 1973.

295. Keidan I, Fine GF, Kagawa T, et al: Work of breathing during spontaneous ventilation in anesthetized children: A comparative study among the facemask, laryngeal mask airway and endotracheal tube. Anesth Analg 91:1381, 2000.

296. Isono S, Nishino T, Sugimori K, et al: Respiratory effects of expiratory flow-resistive loading in conscious and anesthetized humans. Anesth Analg 70:594, 1990.

297. Pietak S, Weenig CS, Hickey RG, et al: Anesthetic effects on ventilation in patients with chronic obstructive pulmonary disease. Anesthesiology 42:160, 1975.

298. Kleinman BS, Frey K, VanDrunen M, et al: Motion of the diaphragm in patients with chronic obstructive pulmonary disease while spontaneously breathing versus during positive pressure breathing after anesthesia and neuromuscular blockade. Anesthesiology 97:298, 2002.

299. Berger AJ, Mitchell RA, Severinghaus JW: Regulation of respiration. N Engl J Med 297:92, 1977.

300. Burton MD, Kazemi H: Neurotransmitters in central respiratory control. Respir Physiol 122:111, 2000.

301. Gonzalez C, Almaraz L, Obeso A, et al: Carotid body chemoreceptors from natural stimuli to sensory discharges. Physiol Rev 74:829, 1994.

302. Lang JDJ, Chumley P, Eiserich JP, et al: Hypercapnia induces injury to alveolar epithelial cells via a nitric oxide-dependent pathway. Am J Physiol Lung Cell Mol Physiol 279:L994, 2000.

303. Hickey RF, Fourcade HE, Eger E II, et al: The effects of ether, halothane and Forane on apneic threshold in man. Anesthesiology 35:32, 1971.

304. Fung ML, Ye JS, Fung PC: Acute hypoxia elevates nitric oxide generation in rat carotid body in vitro. Pflugers Archiv 442:903, 2001.

305. Teppema L, Berkenbosch A, Olievier C: Effect of N omega-nitro-L-arginine on ventilatory response to hypercapnia in anesthetized cats. J Appl Physiol 82:292, 1997.

306. Iturriaga R: Nitric oxide and carotid body chemoreception. Biol Res 34:135, 2001.

307. Royston D, Jordan C, Jones JG: Effect of subanesthetic concentrations of nitrous oxide on the regulation of ventilation in man. Br J Anaesth 55:449, 1983.

308. Hornbein TF, Martin WE, Bonica JJ, et al: Nitrous oxide effects on the circulatory and ventilatory responses to halothane. Anesthesiology 31:250, 1969.

309. van den Elsen M, Sarton E, Teppema L, et al: Influence of 0.1 minimum alveolar concentration of sevoflurane, desflurane and isoflurane on dynamic ventilatory response to hypercapnia in humans. Br J Anaesth 80:174, 1998.

310. van den Elsen MJ, Dahan A, DeGoede J, et al: Influences of subanesthetic isoflurane on ventilatory control in humans. Anesthesiology 83:478, 1995.

311. Dahan A, van den Elsen MJ, Berkenbosch A, et al: Effects of subanesthetic halothane on the ventilatory responses to hypercapnia and acute hypoxia in healthy volunteers. Anesthesiology 80:727, 1994.

312. Dahan A, Teppema L: Influence of low-dose anaesthetic agents on ventilatory control: Where do we stand? Br J Anaesth 83:199, 1999.

313. Dahan A, Sarton E, van den Elsen M, et al: Ventilatory response to hypoxia in humans. Influences of subanesthetic desflurane. Anesthesiology 85:60, 1996.

314. Pandit JJ, Manning-Fox J, Dorrington KL, et al: Effects of subanaesthetic sevoflurane on ventilation. 1: Response to acute and sustained hypercapnia in humans. Br J Anaesth 83:204, 1999.

315. Nieuwenhuijs D, Sarton E, Teppema L, et al: Respiratory sites of action of propofol: Absence of depression of peripheral chemoreflex loop by low-dose propofol. Anesthesiology 95:889, 2001.

316. Warner DO, Warner MA: Human chest wall function while awake and during halothane anesthesia. II. Carbon dioxide rebreathing. Anesthesiology 82:20, 1995.

317. Warner DO, Joyner MJ, Ritman EL: Chest wall responses to rebreathing in halothane-anesthetized dogs. Anesthesiology 83:835, 1995.

318. Stuth EAE, Dogas Z, Krolo M, et al: Effects of halothane on the phrenic nerve responses to carbon dioxide mediated by the carotid body chemoreceptors in vagotomized dogs. Anesthesiology 87:1440, 1997.

319. van Dissel JT, Berkenbosch A, Olievier CN, et al: Effects of halothane on the ventilatory response to hypoxia and hypercapnia in cats. Anesthesiology 62:448, 1985.

320. Knill RL, Manninen PH, Clement JL: Ventilation and chemoreflexes during enflurane sedation and anaesthesia in man. Can Anaesth Soc J 26:353, 1979.

321. Knill RL, Gelb AW: Ventilatory responses to hypoxia and hypercapnia during halothane sedation and anesthesia in man. Anesthesiology 49:244, 1978.

322. Weiskopf RB, Raymond LW, Severinghaus JW: Effects of halothane on canine respiratory responses to hypoxia with and without hypercarbia. Anesthesiology 41:350, 1974.

323. Hirshman CA, McCullough RE, Cohen PJ, et al: Depression of hypoxic ventilatory response by halothane, enflurane and isoflurane in dogs. Br J Anaesth 43:957, 1977.

324. Yacoub O, Doell D, Kryger MH, et al: Depression of hypoxic ventilatory response by nitrous oxide. Anesthesiology 45:385, 1976.

325. Morray JP, Nobel R, Bennet L, et al: The effect of halothane on phrenic and chemoreceptor responses to hypoxia in anesthetized kittens. Anesth Analg 83:329, 1996.

326. Knill RL, Clement JL: Site of selective action of halothane on the peripheral chemoreflex pathway in humans. Anesthesiology 61:121, 1984.
327. Davies RO, Edwards MWJ, Lahiri S: Halothane depresses the response to carotid body chemoreceptors to hypoxia and hypercapnia in the cat. Anesthesiology 57:153, 1982.
328. Stuth EAE, Dogas Z, Krolo M, et al: Dose-dependent effects of halothane on the phrenic nerve responses to acute hypoxia in vagotomized dogs. Anesthesiology 87:1428, 1997.
329. Mohan R, Duffin J: The effect of hypoxia on the ventilatory response to carbon dioxide in man. Respir Physiol 108:101, 1997.
330. Kline DD, Yang T, Huang PL, et al: Altered respiratory responses to hypoxia in mutant mice deficient in neuronal nitric oxide synthase. J Physiol 511:273, 1998.
331. Zanzinger J, Czachurski J, Seller H: Nitric oxide in the ventrolateral medulla regulates sympathetic responses to systemic hypoxia in pigs. Am J Physiol Regul Integr Comp Physiol 275:R33, 1998.
332. Fung ML, Wang W, Darnall RA, et al: Characterization of ventilatory responses to hypoxia in neonatal rats. Respir Physiol 103:57, 1996.
333. Maxova H, Vizek M: Ventilatory response to sustained hypoxia in carotid body denervated rats. Physiol Res 50:327, 2001.
334. Nagyova B, Dorrington KL, Poulin MJ, et al: Influence of 0.2 minimum alveolar concentration of enflurane on the ventilatory response to sustained hypoxia in humans. Br J Anaesth 78:707, 1997.
335. Sarton E, Teppema L, Dahan A: Sex differences in morphine-induced ventilatory depression reside within the peripheral chemoreflex loop. Anesthesiology 90:1329, 1999.
336. Sarton E, van de Wal M, Nieuwenhuijs D, et al: Sevoflurane-induced reduction of hypoxic drive is sex-independent. Anesthesiology 90:1288, 1999.
337. Knill RL, Kieraszewicz HT, Dodgson BG: Chemical regulation of ventilation during isoflurane sedation and anaesthesia in humans. Can Anaesth Soc J 30:607, 1983.
338. Pandit JJ, Manning-Fox J, Dorrington KL, et al: Effects of subanaesthetic sevoflurane on ventilation. 2: Response to acute and sustained hypoxia in humans. Br J Anaesth 83:210, 1999.
339. Temp JA, Henson LC, Ward DS: Does a subanesthetic concentration of isoflurane blunt the ventilatory response to hypoxia? Anesthesiology 77:1116, 1992.
340. Temp JA, Henson LC, Ward DS: Effect of a subanesthetic minimum alveolar concentration of isoflurane on two tests of the hypoxic ventilatory response. Anesthesiology 80:739, 1994.
341. Joensen H, Sadler CL, Ponte J, et al: Isoflurane does not depress the hypoxic response of rabbit carotid body chemoreceptors. Anesth Analg 91:480, 2000.
342. van den Elsen MJ, Dahan A, Berkenbosch A, et al: Does subanesthetic isoflurane affect the ventilatory responses to acute isocapnic hypoxia in healthy volunteers? Anesthesiology 81:860, 1994.
343. Nagyova B, Dorrington KL, Robbins PA: Effect of low-dose enflurane on the ventilatory response to hypoxia in humans. Br J Anaesth 72:509, 1994.
344. Sarton E, Dahan A, Teppema L, et al: Acute pain and central nervous system arousal do not restore impaired hypoxic ventilatory response during sevoflurane sedation. Anesthesiology 85:295, 1996.
345. Lam AM, Clement JL, Knill RL: Surgical stimulation does not enhance ventilatory chemoreflexes during enflurane anaesthesia in man. Can Anaesth Soc J 27:22, 1980.
346. Galley HF, DiMatteo MA, Webster NR: Immunomodulation by anaesthetic, sedative and analgesic agents: Does it matter? Intensive Care Med 26:267, 2000.
347. Kotani N, Takahashi S, Sessler DI, et al: Volatile anesthetics augment expression of proinflammatory cytokines in rat alveolar macrophages by mechanical ventilation. Anesthesiology 91:187, 1999.
348. Wrigge H, Zinserling J, Stuber F, et al: Effects of mechanical ventilation on release of cytokines into systemic circulation in patients with normal pulmonary function. Anesthesiology 93:1413, 2000.

CHAPTER
7 Cardiovascular Pharmacology

Paul S. Pagel, Judy R. Kersten, Neil E. Farber, and David C. Warltier

Volatile Anesthetics and Cardiovascular Function 191
Myocardial Contractility 191
Cellular Mechanisms of Myocardial Depression 194
Diastolic Function 195
Left Ventricular–Arterial Coupling and Mechanical Efficiency 196
Left Ventricular Afterload 197
Right Ventricular Function 199
Left Atrial Function 199
Systemic Hemodynamics 201

Volatile Anesthetics and Cardiac Electrophysiology 202
Cardiac Conduction 202
Epinephrine-Induced Arrhythmias 203

Volatile Anesthetics and the Coronary Circulation 203
Coronary Vascular Effects In Vitro 203
Coronary Vascular Effects In Vivo 203
Coronary Vasodilator Reserve and Autoregulation 204
Mechanisms of Volatile Anesthetic–Induced Coronary Vasodilation 205

Volatile Anesthetics and Ischemic Myocardium 205
Volatile Anesthetic–Induced Myocardial Protection 206
Coronary Vascular Effects of Volatile Anesthetics in Humans 210
Myocardial Protection by Volatile Anesthetics in Humans 211

Volatile Anesthetics and Neural Control of the Circulation 211

Nitrous Oxide and Cardiovascular Function 212
Myocardial Contractility and Left Ventricular Diastolic Function 212
Hemodynamics 214

Nitrous Oxide and Cardiac Electrophysiology 214

Nitrous Oxide and the Coronary Circulation 214

Nitrous Oxide and Neural Control of the Circulation 215

Xenon 215

This chapter comprehensively describes the cardiovascular pharmacology of modern volatile anesthetics, nitrous oxide, and xenon. The actions of inhaled anesthetics on cardiovascular function, cardiac electrophysiology, the coronary circulation, and autonomic nervous system control of the circulation are examined in detail.

VOLATILE ANESTHETICS AND CARDIOVASCULAR FUNCTION

Myocardial Contractility

All modern volatile anesthetics, including desflurane and sevoflurane, depress contractile function in normal myocardium in vitro and in vivo.[1] Investigations conducted in the 1960s demonstrated that halothane causes dose-related depression of force-velocity relationships and Frank-Starling curves in isolated cardiac muscle preparations[2,3] and intact, closed-chest dogs,[4] respectively. These findings supported clinical observations of circulatory depression during halothane anesthesia in humans.[5-8] Enflurane[9] and isoflurane[10] produce direct negative inotropic effects, as indicated by decreases in maximal velocity of shortening, peak developed force, and maximal rate of force development during isotonic contraction in isolated feline papillary muscles. These reductions in intrinsic myocardial contractility by enflurane and isoflurane contribute to the cardiovascular depression observed with these agents in humans.[11,12]

The relative degree of myocardial depression produced by different volatile anesthetics in vivo has been more difficult to establish because simultaneous alterations in systemic and pulmonary hemodynamics and autonomic nervous system activity often complicate assessment of left ventricular (LV) systolic function. Early studies using isovolumic and ejection-phase measures of myocardial contractility demonstrated that enflurane and halothane caused similar negative inotropic effects in dogs[13-16] and humans.[11] These findings were subsequently confirmed using the slope (E_{es}) of the LV end-systolic pressure–midaxis diameter relationship as a relatively heart rate– and load-independent index of the inotropic state in chronically instrumented dogs.[17] Equi-anesthetic concentrations of enflurane and halothane depressed myocardial contractility to similar degrees in vivo.[17] In contrast, experimental animal studies have repeatedly demonstrated that isoflurane produces less myocardial depression than does halothane or enflurane. Halothane caused larger reductions in the rate of increase of LV positive pressure (dP/dt) than did isoflurane when equi-anesthetic concentrations were directly compared in the presence and absence of autonomic nervous system function,[16,18,19] suggesting that differences in myocardial depression caused by these anesthetics occurred independent of autonomic nervous system activity.[16] Differences in the negative inotropic effects of halothane and isoflurane have been quantified using the slope (M_w) of the regional preload recruitable stroke work (PRSW) relationship derived from a differentially loaded series of LV pressure–segment length diagrams.[20,21] In these studies conducted in chronically instrumented dogs, isoflurane maintained contractility an average of 20% higher than with equi–minimum alveolar concentrations (MACs) of halothane.[20,21] Differences in the relative degree of myocardial depression produced by halothane and isoflurane in humans have also been inferred using isovolumic and ejection-phase measures of contractile function.[12,22,23] The negative inotropic actions of isoflurane (Fig. 7-1) and halothane are exacerbated by hypocalcemia,[24] calcium ion (Ca^{2+}) channel blockers,[25-27] and β_1-adrenoceptor antagonists[25] and can be reversed by administration of exogenous Ca^{2+},[24,28-30] cardiac phosphodiesterase fraction III inhibitors,[31,32] β_1-adrenoceptor agonists,[1] Ca^{2+} channel agonists,[27] and myofilament Ca^{2+} sensitizers.[33] The differential effects of halothane and isoflurane on myocardial contractility in dogs are maintained during depression or augmentation of an inotropic state produced by these vasoactive drugs.[1]

Desflurane causes systemic and coronary hemodynamic effects that are remarkably similar to those produced by isoflurane.[34] Desflurane and isoflurane have been shown to depress myocardial function to equivalent degrees using isovolumic and ejection-phase measures of contractility in dogs,[16,35] pigs,[36] and humans.[37,38] These observations have been verified using end-systolic pressure-volume relationships and regional and global PRSW (Fig. 7-2) in the presence and absence of autonomic nervous system activity in vivo.[39-41] However, the unique cardiovascular stimulation associated with rapid increases in inspired desflurane concentration in humans[42] may lead to transient increases in myocardial contractility resulting from augmentation of sympathetic nervous system tone.[43-45]

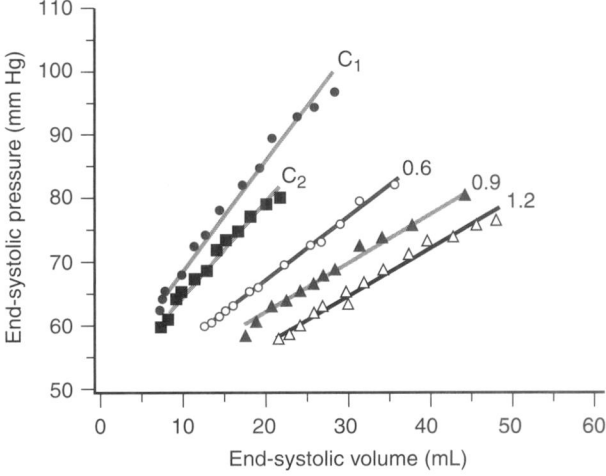

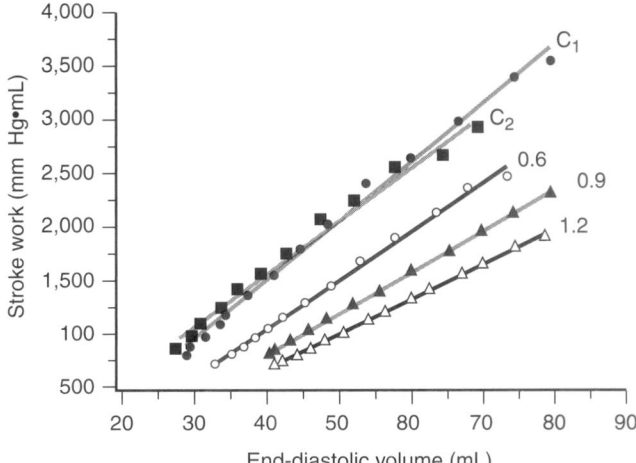

Figure 7–1 End-systolic pressure-volume *(top)* and stroke work versus end-diastolic volume relationships *(bottom)* before (control 1 [C_1]); during 0.6, 0.9, and 1.2 minimum alveolar concentrations (MACs); and after isoflurane (control 2 [C_2]) in an experiment in an open-chest dog. (Adapted from Hettrick DA, Pagel PS, Warltier DC: Desflurane, sevoflurane, and isoflurane impair canine left ventricular-arterial coupling and mechanical efficiency. Anesthesiology 85:403-413, 1996.)

The effects of sevoflurane on myocardial contractility are virtually indistinguishable from those produced by isoflurane in dogs.[46,47] Another study conducted in pigs suggested that sevoflurane may produce less myocardial depression than equi-MACs of halothane.[48] Sevoflurane produces less myocardial depression than does enflurane in volunteers, as assessed by the heart rate–corrected velocity of circumferential fiber shortening versus the LV end-systolic wall stress relationship derived from echocardiography.[49] Sevoflurane decreased contractile function to approximately 40% to 45% of control values at 1.75 MAC in the presence and absence of autonomic nervous system tone using regional PRSW in dogs.[47] This magnitude of myocardial depression agrees with previous data for isoflurane and desflurane using an identical experimental model.[39,40] Volatile anesthetics appear to depress the contractile state in normal ventricular myocardium

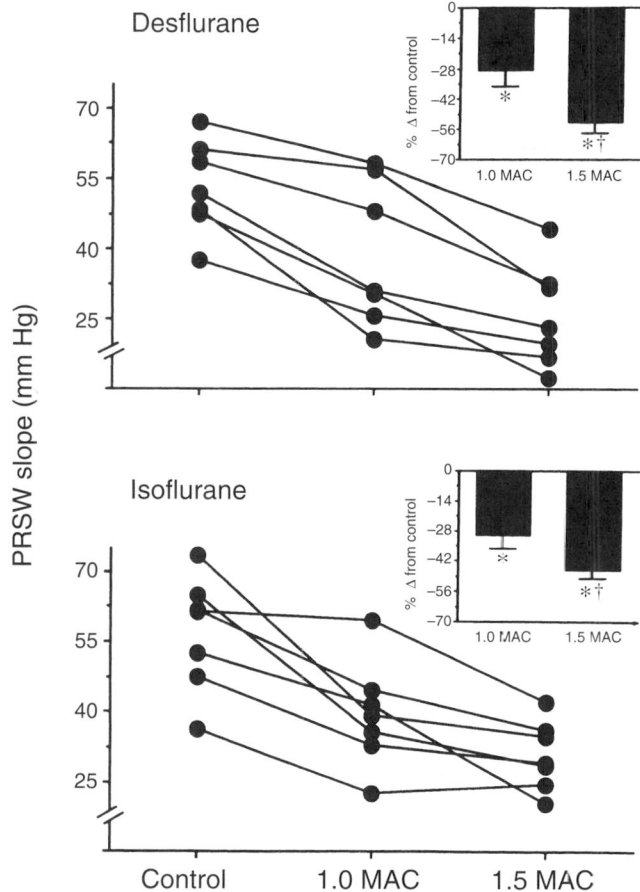

Figure 7–2 Preload recruitable stroke work (PRSW) slope for chronically instrumented dogs during control and at 1.0 and 1.5 end-tidal minimum alveolar concentrations (MAC) of desflurane *(top)* and isoflurane *(bottom)*. *Insets* depict percent changes from control values. *, Significantly (*P* < .05) different from controls; †, significantly (*P* < .05) different from 1.0 MAC. (From Pagel PS, Kampine JP, Schmeling WT, Warltier DC: Influence of volatile anesthetics on myocardial contractility in vivo: Desflurane versus isoflurane. Anesthesiology 74:900-907, 1991.)

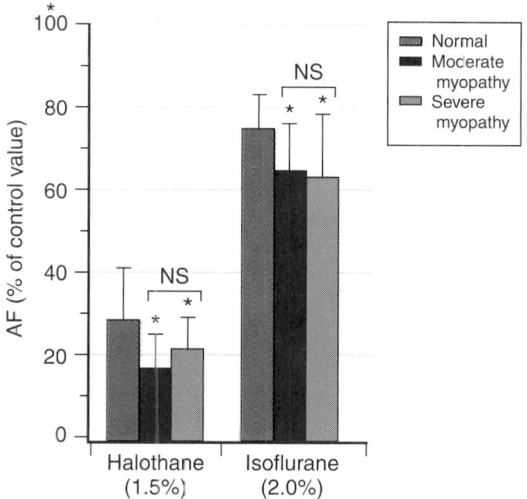

Figure 7–3 Comparison of the effects of halothane *(left)* and isoflurane *(right)* on the isometric active force (AF) of papillary muscles from healthy hamsters *(red bars)* and those with cardiomyopathy *(black and gray bars)*. Probability values refer to between-group differences. *, Significantly (*P* < .05) different from controls. (Adapted from Vivien B, Hanouz J-L, Gueugniaud P-Y, et al: Myocardial effects of halothane and isoflurane in hamsters with hypertrophic cardiomyopathy. Anesthesiology 87:1406-1416, 1997.)

in the following order: halothane = enflurane > isoflurane = desflurane = sevoflurane.

The effects of volatile anesthetics on LV systolic function in animal models or patients with LV dysfunction have not been comprehensively studied. Early in vitro studies demonstrated that isoflurane[10] and enflurane[50] caused larger reductions in maximal shortening velocity and the peak rate of force development in feline papillary muscles from failing hearts subjected to chronic pressure overload than in those from normal hearts. Halothane also produced more pronounced myocardial depression in ischemic than in normal myocardium.[51,52] Isoflurane and halothane caused greater negative inotropic effects in ventricular myocardium obtained from cardiomyopathic hamsters than from normal hamsters (Fig. 7-3).[53] These findings suggested that myocardial depression caused by volatile anesthetics in failing myocardium were accentuated, and they provided indirect evidence that patients with underlying contractile dysfunction might be more sensitive to the negative inotropic effects of

volatile agents. This hypothesis has not been extensively examined in vivo, however.

In experimental models of myocardial ischemia[51] or infarction,[54] volatile anesthetic–induced declines in contractile function were well tolerated and did not precipitate frank systolic dysfunction. Volatile anesthetics can exert important beneficial effects on mechanical function during myocardial ischemia and reperfusion injury. Volatile anesthetics reduce experimental myocardial infarct size,[55,56] preserve metabolic and structural integrity during regional ischemia and reperfusion,[57-59] enhance the functional recovery of stunned myocardium,[60] and improve indices of LV diastolic performance during brief coronary artery occlusion.[61] Halothane and isoflurane also produced beneficial decreases in LV preload and afterload in patients with heart failure and coronary artery disease, respectively.[62-64] These improvements in loading conditions in patients with compromised LV function may serve to partially offset the direct negative inotropic effects of anesthetics[62] and contribute to relative maintenance of cardiac performance by optimizing the operating range of the heart on the Starling curve or by improving LV diastolic function. Isoflurane and halothane can produce dose-related depression of myocardial contractility in a canine model of moderate LV dysfunction induced by chronic, rapid LV pacing (Fig. 7-4).[65] Nevertheless, isoflurane or halothane anesthesia was relatively well tolerated and did not precipitate frank LV failure in dogs with pacing-induced cardiomyopathy. These findings were attributed to simultaneous improvements in LV loading conditions and filling dynamics that contributed to relative maintenance of cardiac output in the setting of moderate LV dysfunction despite concomitant reductions in contractility.[65] The influence of volatile anesthetics on

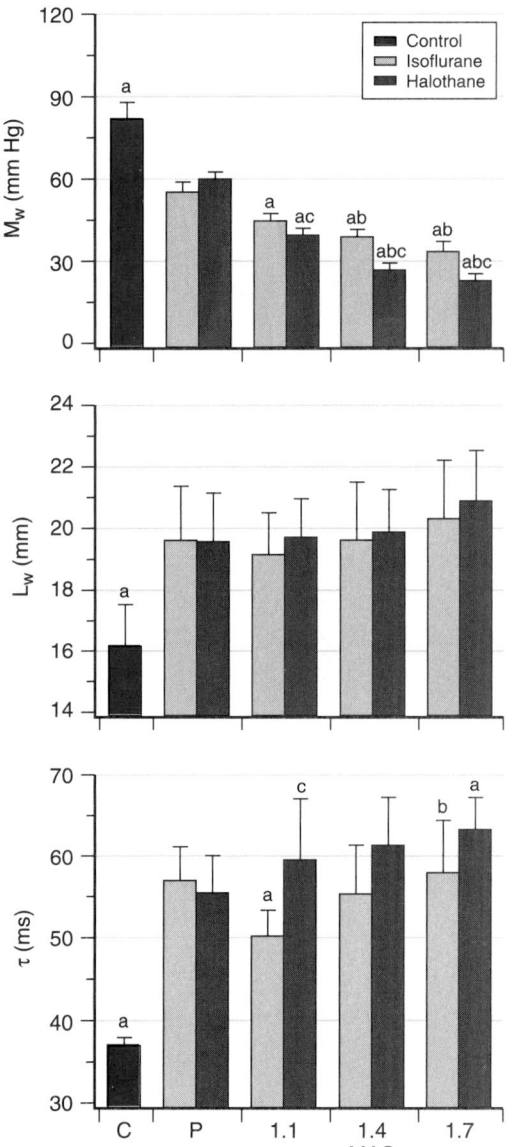

Figure 7–4 Histograms depicting the slope (M_W, *top panel*) and length intercept (L_W, *middle panel*) of the regional preload recruitable stroke work relationship and the time constant for isovolumic relaxation (τ, *bottom panel*) in the conscious state before (C, *red bar*) and after pacing (P) and during 1.1, 1.4, and 1.7 MAC (minimal alveolar concentrations) for isoflurane *(light gray bars)* and halothane *(dark gray bars).* a, Significantly ($P < .05$) different from P; b, significantly ($P < .05$) different from 1.1 MAC; c, significantly ($P < .05$) different from the corresponding isoflurane value. (Adapted from Pagel PS, Lowe D, Hettrick DA, et al: Isoflurane, but not halothane, improves indices of diastolic performance in dogs with rapid ventricular, pacing-induced cardiomyopathy. Anesthesiology 85:644-654, 1996.)

LV systolic function in the presence of overt heart failure remains to be defined. Halothane caused greater depression of contractile function than did isoflurane in cardiomyopathic dogs,[65,66] observations that are similar to those described for normal myocardium in experimental animals and humans. These results contrast with those for isolated ventricular myocardium obtained from cardiomyopathic

hamsters, demonstrating that isoflurane and halothane produce similar negative inotropic effects.[53] Differential actions on autonomic nervous system tone caused by the volatile agents may be responsible for the discrepancy in these findings in vivo and in vitro.

Cellular Mechanisms of Myocardial Depression

Volatile anesthetics depress myocardial contractility through alterations of intracellular Ca^{2+} homeostasis at several subcellular targets in the normal cardiac myocyte.[67,68] Volatile agents cause dose-related inhibition of the transsarcolemmal Ca^{2+} transient[69,70] by affecting L- and T-type Ca^{2+} channels.[69,71-73] Isoflurane causes less pronounced reductions in the intracellular Ca^{2+} transient than does halothane or enflurane,[69] although this contention remains somewhat controversial when equi-anesthetic concentrations of these agents are considered.[74,75] The structural conformation and functional integrity of the voltage-dependent Ca^{2+} channel are directly altered by volatile anesthetics, as indicated by attenuated binding of the dihydropyridine and phenylalkylamine Ca^{2+} channel blockers nitrendipine[76,77] and galopamil,[78] respectively. The partial inhibition of Ca^{2+} influx through sarcolemmal Ca^{2+} channels has several important consequences, including declines in the availability of Ca^{2+} for contractile activation, depression of Ca^{2+}-dependent Ca^{2+} release from the sarcoplasmic reticulum (SR), and reduction of the amount of Ca^{2+} that can be subsequently stored in the SR.[75,79-82] Halothane and enflurane,[80,82] but not isoflurane,[82-84] also stimulate Ca^{2+} release from the SR, a caffeine-like action that may cause transient, modest increases that precede subsequent, more profound reductions in contractility.[80,85,86] Unlike isoflurane, halothane and enflurane directly activate ryanodine-sensitive SR Ca^{2+} release channels,[87,88] thereby reducing SR Ca^{2+} storage. Volatile anesthetics also provoke a nonspecific leak of Ca^{2+} from the SR,[89,90] contributing to further decreases in accumulation of Ca^{2+} available for release during contraction. When combined with decreases in transsarcolemmal Ca^{2+} flux, these alterations in SR function represent important mechanisms by which halothane and enflurane depress the intracellular Ca^{2+} transient and reduce myocardial contractility to a greater extent than equianesthetic concentrations of isoflurane.[69] However, later data suggest that volatile anesthetics inhibit Ca^{2+} transport from the cell through the sarcolemmal Ca^{2+} ATPase.[91] This action may serve to partially offset reductions in SR Ca^{2+} stores. The partial preservation of the myocardial positive frequency staircase effect observed with isoflurane at physiologic excitation rates in vitro[75,92] may also be attributed to the relative maintenance of SR function by this volatile agent, in contrast to halothane and enflurane.

Evidence indicates that volatile anesthetics may also depress contractile function by inhibiting Na^+-Ca^{2+} exchange and reducing intracellular Ca^{2+} concentration independent of the voltage-dependent Ca^{2+} channel in vitro.[93-95] This effect may be particularly important in neonatal myocardium[93] because this tissue has been shown to be more sensitive to the negative inotropic actions of volatile anesthetics than is adult myocardium.[96] However, the relative contribution of Na^+-Ca^{2+} exchanger inhibition to anesthetic-induced depression of myocardial contractility in the intact heart has yet to be defined. Halothane, enflurane, and isoflurane may also exert direct effects on the contractile apparatus and the sensitivity of the myofilaments to activator Ca^{2+}. Volatile anesthetics decrease tension development of skinned cardiac myofibrils[97-99] and directly reduce myofibrillar ATPase activity,[100,101] actions that may contribute to declines in actin-myosin cross-bridge kinetics during contraction.[102,103] Volatile anesthetics do not affect[104] or may decrease[105] the troponin C (TnC) affinity for Ca^{2+}, suggesting that myofilament Ca^{2+} sensitivity is not altered[106,107] or is modestly reduced,[69,107] respectively, by these agents. Nevertheless, although volatile anesthetic–induced reductions in myofilament Ca^{2+} sensitivity have been implicated in some studies,[69,107,108] this mechanism probably plays a relatively minor role in the negative inotropic effects of these agents at clinically relevant concentrations in vivo.[68]

The cellular mechanisms responsible for volatile anesthetic–induced depression of myocardial contractility in failing myocardium have not been extensively studied. It is likely that alterations of intracellular Ca^{2+} regulation produced by volatile anesthetics in normal myocardium also occur at similar subcellular targets in failing myocardium. Profound abnormalities in intracellular Ca^{2+} homeostasis are characteristic features of failing myocardium,[109] and it is likely that volatile anesthetics cause further reductions in contractile function by producing additive or synergistic effects on Ca^{2+} metabolism.

Diastolic Function

Definitions of heart failure based solely on contractile dysfunction have been rendered inadequate by the recognition that LV function during diastole significantly influences overall cardiac performance. The heart serves dual roles, propelling blood into the high-pressure arterial vasculature during systole and collecting blood from the low-pressure venous circulation during diastole. Heart failure may occur from impaired contractility or from altered LV diastolic function. The timing, rate, and extent of LV filling are determined by several major factors, including the rate and degree of myocardial relaxation, the intrinsic mechanical properties of the left ventricle itself and those imposed by external constraints, and the structure and function of the left atrium, the pulmonary venous circulation, and the mitral valve.[110] Although abnormalities in LV diastolic function may be linked to decreases in myocardial contractility, heart failure may result from primary diastolic dysfunction in the absence of or before the appearance of alterations in LV systolic function[111-113] in a variety of pathologic conditions, including ischemic heart disease, pressure- or volume-overload hypertrophy, hypertrophic obstructive cardiomyopathy, and restrictive disease processes.[114,115]

The effects of volatile anesthetics on diastolic function in the normal and diseased heart have been incompletely studied. Volatile agents produce dose-related prolongation of isovolumic relaxation in vivo (Fig. 7-5).[47,116-118] This delay of isovolumic relaxation may be associated with declines in early LV filling[27,30,32,47] but probably is not of sufficient magnitude to affect LV chamber stiffness.

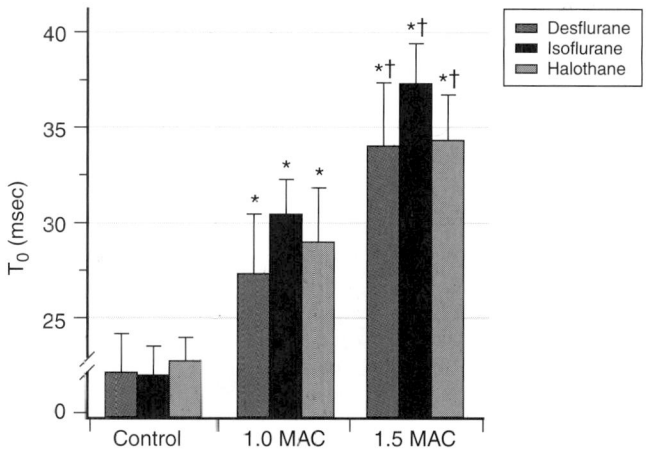

Figure 7–5 Effects of desflurane, isoflurane, and halothane on the time constant of isovolumic relaxation (T_0). *, Significantly ($P < .05$) different from control; †, significantly ($P < .05$) different from 1.0 minimum alveolar concentration (MAC). (Adapted from Pagel PS, Grossman W, Haering JM, Warltier DC: Left ventricular diastolic function in the normal and diseased heart: Perspectives for the anesthesiologist. Anesthesiology 79[Pt 1]:836-854, 1993.)

The significance of anesthetic-induced delays in isovolumic relaxation to early coronary blood flow has not been thoroughly investigated, but coronary blood flow is highest during this phase of diastole, and delays in relaxation lead to impairment of flow during halothane anesthesia.[116] Prolongation of LV relaxation probably occurs as a result of simultaneous depression of myocardial contractility and not because of a direct negative lusitropic effect.[119] Isoflurane, enflurane, and halothane modestly enhance isotonic relaxation of isolated ferret myocardium in vitro.[120]

Volatile anesthetics cause concentration-related decreases in the rate and extent of early LV filling concomitant with negative inotropic effects. Isoflurane and halothane also reduce LV filling associated with atrial systole.[30] Isoflurane, desflurane, and sevoflurane do not alter invasively derived indices of regional myocardial or chamber stiffness, indicating that LV distensibility is unaffected by these volatile agents (Fig. 7-6).[47,118] Although some indirect evidence suggests that halothane affects LV compliance,[121-123] later studies[17,118,124] using invasively derived measures of LV passive elasticity and myocardial stiffness indicate that this is not the case. Halothane increases LV end-diastolic pressure, indicating that the left ventricle operates on a steeper, less compliant region of the LV end-diastolic pressure-volume relationship; however, this volatile agent does not directly alter the intrinsic viscoelastic properties of the myocardium.[1]

The effects of isoflurane and halothane on LV diastolic function in a canine model of dilated cardiomyopathy have been described.[65] In contrast to the findings in dogs with normal LV function, isoflurane improved several indices of LV relaxation and filling in cardiomyopathic dogs despite producing simultaneous negative inotropic effects. Halothane did not exacerbate preexisting diastolic dysfunction inherent to this experimental model.

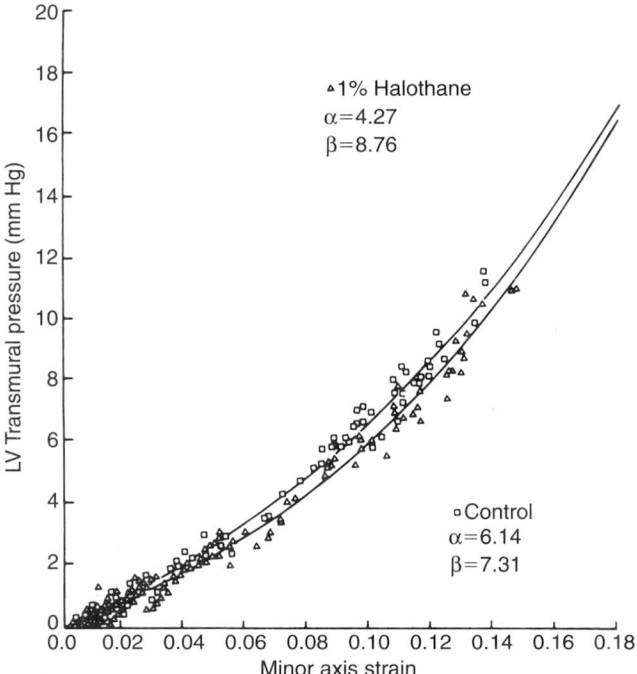

Figure 7–6 Left ventricular (LV) diastolic transmural pressure versus Lagrangian strain relationships in conscious *(squares)* and halothane-anesthetized *(triangles)* dogs. The pressure-strain relationship was not altered by halothane anesthesia, indicating that this volatile anesthetic does not affect intrinsic myocardial stiffness. α, Gain; β, modulus of myocardial stiffness. (Adapted from Van Trigt P, Christian CC, Fagraeus L, et al: The mechanism of halothane-induced myocardial depression: Altered diastolic mechanics versus impaired contractility. J Thorac Cardiovasc Surg 85:832-838, 1983.)

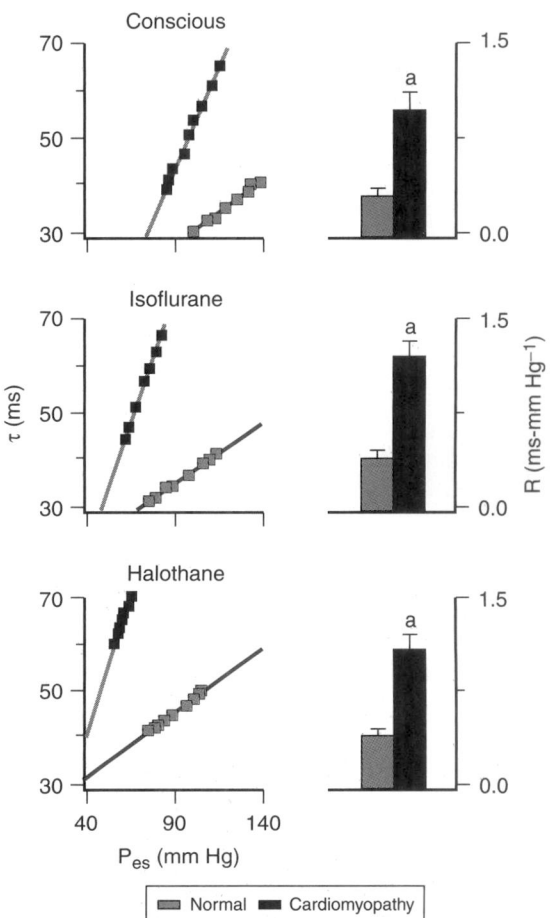

Figure 7–7 Linear relationship between the time constant of isovolumic relaxation (τ) and left ventricular end-systolic pressure (P_{es}) during inferior vena caval occlusion *(left panels)* in a typical dog before *(red squares)* and after *(black squares)* the development of pacing-induced cardiomyopathy in the conscious state and during isoflurane and halothane anesthesia. The histograms illustrate the slope (R) of the τ versus P_{es} relationship in the conscious state *(top right panel)* and during isoflurane *(middle right panel)* and halothane *(bottom right panel)* anesthesia before *(red bars)* and after *(black bars)* pacing. a, Significantly ($P < .05$) different from normal myocardium. (Adapted from Pagel PS, Hettrick DA, Kersten JR, et al: Isoflurane and halothane do not alter the enhanced afterload sensitivity of left ventricular relaxation in dogs with pacing-induced cardiomyopathy. Anesthesiology 87:952-962, 1997.)

The findings with isoflurane and halothane were most likely related to favorable reductions in LV preload produced by these volatile agents and not caused by direct positive lusitropic effects.[65] These data further suggest that isoflurane-induced improvements of LV isovolumic relaxation and filling dynamics may contribute to relative maintenance of cardiac output in the presence of LV dysfunction despite simultaneous reductions in contractility.[65] The findings in cardiomyopathic dogs supported earlier clinical observations[62,64] reporting that patients with severe ischemic heart disease or congestive heart failure tolerated isoflurane or halothane anesthesia without acute hemodynamic decompensation.

Some investigations have demonstrated that the afterload dependence of LV relaxation is markedly enhanced in failing myocardium.[125,126] This observation has important clinical consequences because afterload reduction may increase LV systolic performance by decreasing impedance to LV ejection and may increase the rate of LV relaxation and therefore contribute to improvements in LV diastolic filling and compliance.[127] The effects of isoflurane and halothane on the afterload dependence of LV relaxation have been explored in dogs before and after the development of rapid LV pacing-induced cardiomyopathy.[66] The afterload dependence of LV relaxation was unaffected by isoflurane and halothane anesthesia in dogs with dilated cardiomyopathy (Fig. 7-7), further indicating that these

volatile agents do not exert direct actions on LV isovolumic relaxation in failing myocardium.

Left Ventricular–Arterial Coupling and Mechanical Efficiency

Optimal transfer of stroke volume from the LV to the arterial circulation requires appropriate matching of these mechanical systems. LV-arterial coupling has most often been described using a series elastic chamber model of the cardiovascular system (Fig. 7-8).[128] The elastance of the contracting LV (E_{es}) and the arterial vasculature (E_a) is determined from LV end-systolic pressure-volume and

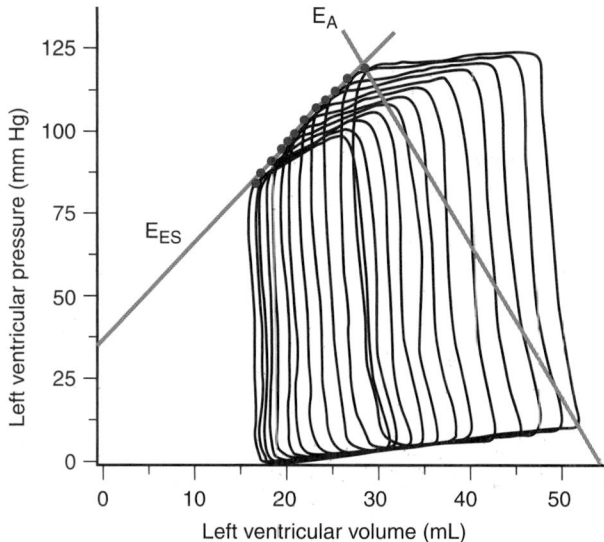

Figure 7–8 Left ventricular (LV) pressure versus LV volume diagrams during inferior vena caval occlusion and the definition of LV-arterial coupling. The LV maximal elastances of each pressure-volume diagram are used to calculate the slope (E_{ES}) of the end-systolic pressure-volume relationship. Effective arterial elastance (E_A) is determined as the ratio of end-systolic arterial pressure and stoke volume during steady-state hemodynamic conditions. In the pressure-volume plane, E_A represents the magnitude of the slope connecting end-systole to end-diastole. (Adapted from Hettrick DA, Pagel PS, Warltier DC: Desflurane, sevoflurane, and isoflurane impair canine left ventricular-arterial coupling and mechanical efficiency. Anesthesiology 85:403-413, 1996.)

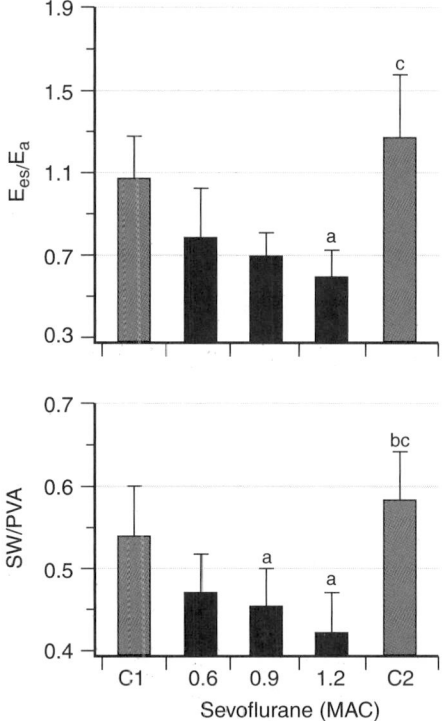

Figure 7–9 Histograms depicting left ventricular–arterial coupling (E_{es}/E_a, *top panel*) and mechanical efficiency (SW/PVA; *bottom panel*) before (control 1 [C1]); during 0.6, 0.9, and 1.2 minimum alveolar concentrations (MAC); and after sevoflurane (control 2 [C2]). a, Significantly ($P < .05$) different from C1; b, significantly ($P < .05$) different from 0.9 MAC of sevoflurane; c, significantly ($P < .05$) different from 1.2 MAC of sevoflurane. (Adapted from Hettrick DA, Pagel PS, Warltier DC: Desflurane, sevoflurane, and isoflurane impair canine left ventricular-arterial coupling and mechanical efficiency. Anesthesiology 85:403-413, 1996.)

end-systolic arterial pressure–stroke volume relationships, respectively.[128-130] The ratio of E_{es} to E_a defines coupling between the LV and the arterial circulation[128,129] and provides a useful technique for assessment of the actions of drug, including volatile anesthetics, on LV-arterial matching in vivo.[131,132] Analysis of the pressure-volume relationship also creates a framework for the study of LV mechanical efficiency defined by the ratio of stroke work (SW) to the pressure-volume area (PVA).[133]

The influence of volatile anesthetics on LV-arterial coupling and mechanical efficiency has been studied in the normal canine cardiovascular system but has not been described in models of heart failure. LV-arterial coupling may theoretically be maintained during anesthesia because declines in LV afterload may balance simultaneous reductions in myocardial contractility. Low concentrations of halothane (1 MAC), but not isoflurane, reduced E_{es}/E_a in barbiturate-anesthetized, acutely instrumented dogs, consistent with depression of mechanical coupling between the LV and arterial circulation.[134] However, isoflurane also decreased E_{es}/E_a at 2 MAC, suggesting that the vasodilating effects of this anesthetic were unable to compensate for the relatively greater declines in contractility. Desflurane, sevoflurane, and isoflurane maintained optimal LV-arterial coupling and mechanical efficiency as evaluated by E_{es}/E_a and SW/PVA at low anesthetic concentrations (0.9 MAC) by producing simultaneous declines in myocardial contractility and LV afterload (Fig. 7-9).[41] However, mechanical matching between the LV and

arterial vasculature and efficiency of total LV energy transfer to external stroke work degenerates at higher anesthetic concentrations, indicating that anesthetic-induced reductions in contractility are not appropriately balanced by declines in afterload. Halothane (<1.0 MAC) has also been shown to reduce the ratio of oscillatory-to-mean hydraulic power in vivo, indicating that this agent decreases LV mechanical efficiency as well.[135] Detrimental alterations in LV-arterial coupling produced by volatile anesthetics contribute to reductions in overall cardiac performance observed with these agents in vivo.

Left Ventricular Afterload

Although a definition of LV afterload that describes the mechanical properties of the arterial vasculature opposing LV ejection is intuitively clear,[136] quantitative evaluation of afterload in vivo remains difficult. Systemic vascular resistance, calculated as the ratio of mean arterial pressure to cardiac output, is the most commonly used estimate of LV afterload. However, systemic vascular resistance inadequately describes LV afterload[137] because this index ignores the mechanical characteristics of the blood and arterial walls, fails to account for the frequency-dependent, phasic nature of arterial blood pressure and blood flow, and does not consider the potential effects of arterial wave reflection. As a result, systemic vascular resistance cannot be used reliably to quantify changes in LV afterload produced by drugs, including volatile anesthetics, or by cardiovascular disease.[138] Aortic input impedance [$Z_{in}(\omega)$] obtained from power spectral or Fourier series analysis of aortic pressure and blood flow waveforms provides a comprehensive description of LV afterload because $Z_{in}(\omega)$ incorporates arterial viscoelasticity, frequency dependence, and wave reflection. However, because analysis of $Z_{in}(\omega)$ is conducted in the frequency domain and not as a function of time, $Z_{in}(\omega)$ is most often interpreted using an electrical three-element Windkessel model of the arterial circulation that describes characteristic aortic impedance (Z_c), total arterial compliance (C), and total arterial resistance (R). Z_c represents aortic resistance to LV ejection, C is determined primarily by the compliance of the aorta and represents the energy storage component of the arterial circulation, and R equals the combined resistances of the remaining arterial vasculature (Fig. 7-10). The three-element Windkessel model has been shown to approximate $Z_{in}(\omega)$ closely under a variety of physiologic conditions.[139,140]

Volatile anesthetics alter $Z_{in}(\omega)$ by affecting the mechanical properties of the arterial vascular tree.[141-144] Isoflurane produced dose-related decreases in R in chronically instrumented dogs consistent with the known effects of this drug on systemic vascular resistance, in contrast to the results obtained with halothane.[143] Isoflurane and halothane also caused similar increases in C and Z_c concomitant with reductions in mean arterial pressure. The major difference between the effects of isoflurane and halothane on LV afterload derived from the Windkessel model of $Z_{in}(\omega)$ was related to R, a property of arteriolar resistance vessels, and not to C or Z_c, the mechanical characteristics of the aorta (Fig. 7-11). A subsequent investigation demonstrated that desflurane, but not sevoflurane, also reduced R in dogs.[144] In contrast to

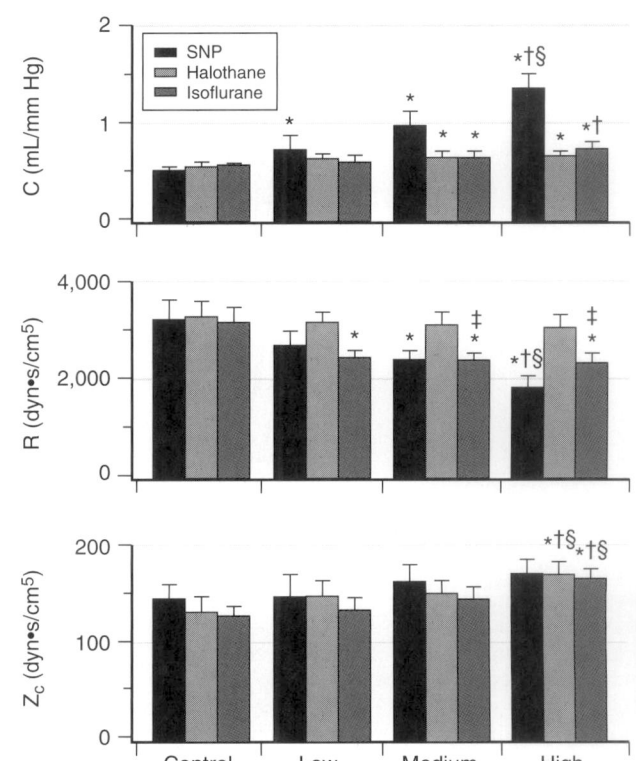

Figure 7–11 Histograms depict the effects of sodium nitroprusside (SNP), halothane, and isoflurane on total arterial compliance (C, *top*), total arterial resistance (R, *middle*), and characteristic aortic impedance (Z_c, *bottom*). The low, medium, and high doses of volatile anesthetics are 1.25, 1.5, and 1.75 minimum alveolar concentrations (MACs), respectively. SNP doses produce comparable changes in mean arterial pressure. *, Significantly (*P* < .05) different from the control; †, significantly (*P* < .05) different from the low dose; §, significantly (*P* < .05) different from the middle dose; ‡, significantly (*P* < .05) different from halothane. (Adapted from Hettrick DA, Pagel PS, Warltier DC: Differential effects of isoflurane and halothane on aortic input impedance quantified using a three-element Windkessel model. Anesthesiology 83:361-373, 1995.)

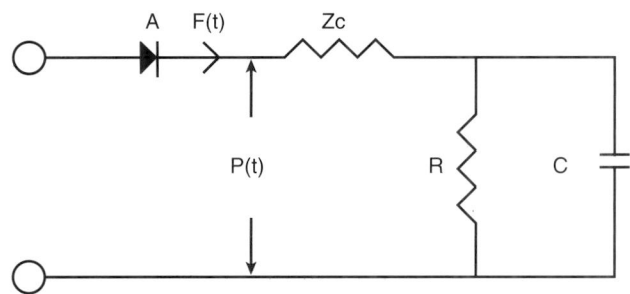

Figure 7–10 Schematic diagram depicting the three-element Windkessel model of the arterial circulation. Diode A represents the aortic valve. Time-dependent blood flow [F(t)] and blood pressure [P(t)] entering the arterial system first encounters the resistance of the ascending aorta (characteristic aortic impedance [Zc]). Further flow is dictated by total arterial resistance (R) and total arterial compliance (C), the energy storage component of the arterial vasculature. (Adapted from Hettrick DA, Pagel PS, Warltier DC: Differential effects of isoflurane and halothane on aortic input impedance quantified using a three-element Windkessel model. Anesthesiology 83:361-373, 1995.)

the findings for isoflurane, desflurane did not affect C and Z_c, suggesting that this agent does not alter the mechanical properties of the aorta. The inverse relationship between C and mean arterial pressure remains unchanged by volatile anesthetics,[143,144] unlike the findings with the arterial vasodilator sodium nitroprusside[143,145] or the intravenous anesthetic propofol.[146]

Isoflurane and halothane produce alterations in $Z_{in}(\omega)$ in cardiomyopathic dogs that are substantially different from those observed in normal dogs.[147] These volatile anesthetics decreased arterial pressure but did not affect C and Z_c in the presence of LV dysfunction. Halothane increased R and isoflurane did not reduce R in dogs with dilated cardiomyopathy. Neither isoflurane nor halothane reduce arterial hydraulic resistance or favorably improve the rectifying properties of the aorta in dogs with pacing-induced cardiomyopathy (Fig. 7-12). The findings suggest that volatile agents do not exert beneficial actions in LV afterload in the presence of failing myocardium.

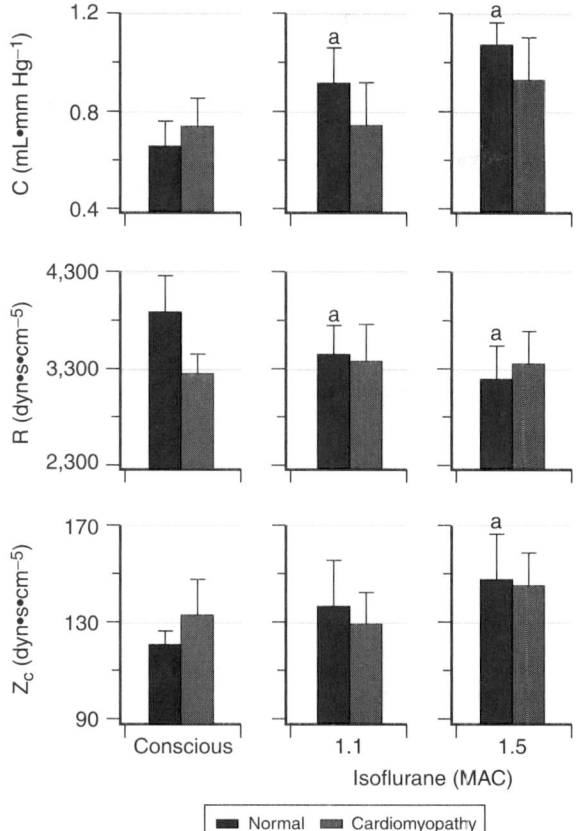

Figure 7–12 Histograms illustrate total arterial compliance (C, *top panel*), total arterial resistance (R, *middle panel*), and characteristic aortic impedance (Z$_C$, *bottom panel*) in the conscious state and during 1.1 and 1.5 minimum alveolar concentrations (MACs) of isoflurane in dogs before *(red bars)* and after *(gray bars)* the development of pacing-induced cardiomyopathy. a, Significantly (*P* < .05) different from normal myocardium. (Adapted from Hettrick DA, Pagel PS, Kersten JR, et al: The effects of isoflurane and halothane on left ventricular afterload in dogs with dilated cardiomyopathy. Anesth Analg 85:979-986, 1997.)

Right Ventricular Function

The crescent-shaped right ventricle is composed of embryologically distinct inflow and outflow tracts[148,149] that differ in their structure and response to autonomic nervous system activity.[150] The sequential contraction of the right ventricular (RV) inflow and outflow tracts establish regional pressure gradients within the right ventricle during systole[151-153] and account for the peristaltic mechanical action of this pump. True isovolumic relaxation does not occur in the right ventricle.[154] Instead, ejection of blood from the outflow tract into the pulmonary artery continues after the inflow tract has begun to relax.[152,154]

The effects of volatile anesthetics on the function and contraction sequence of the RV inflow and outflow tracts have been incompletely studied. Halothane was shown to produce similar depression of contractile function in RV inflow and outflow tracts in dogs using a uniform definition of end systole and end diastole for both regions of the right ventricle.[155] Another investigation conducted in anesthetized pigs[156] demonstrated that halothane caused

dose-related decreases in RV contractility, which was evaluated using regional PRSW derived from RV pressure–segment length diagrams in the RV inflow and outflow tracts in the presence and absence of autonomic nervous system reflexes. Halothane also abolished the normal RV sequential contraction pattern without exerting differential negative inotropic effects in different regions of the right ventricle.[156] These data suggest that volatile anesthetics may alter RV contraction dynamics by adversely affecting cardiac autonomic nervous system activity.

Left Atrial Function

The left atrium serves three major roles that exert a profound effect on LV filling and overall cardiovascular performance. The left atrium is a contractile chamber that actively empties immediately before the onset of LV systole and establishes final LV end-diastolic volume.[157,158] The left atrium is a reservoir that stores pulmonary venous return during LV contraction and isovolumic relaxation after the closure and before the opening of the mitral valve.[159] The left atrium also is a conduit that empties its contents into the left ventricle down a pressure gradient after the mitral valve opens[160] and continues to transfer pulmonary venous blood flow passively during LV diastasis. These contraction, reservoir, and conduit functions of the left atrium mechanically facilitate the transition between the almost continuous flow through the pulmonary venous circulation and the intermittent filling of the left ventricle.[161] Advances in the understanding of left atrial (LA) mechanical function have been reviewed elsewhere.[162]

The negative inotropic effects of halothane and methoxyflurane were initially described by Paradise and colleagues[163-165] in rat atrial myocardium in vitro. Volatile anesthetics also depress the contractile function of atrial myocardium obtained from guinea pigs,[166] rabbits,[81] and humans.[167-169] These actions have been attributed to reductions in transsarcolemmal Ca^{2+} influx through voltage-dependent Ca^{2+} channels and decreases in Ca^{2+} availability from the SR,[81] mechanisms that are similar to those responsible for anesthetic-induced depression of LV myocardium.[170] The negative inotropic effects of volatile agents in the intact left atrium were quantified using pressure-volume analysis (Fig. 7-13).[171] Desflurane, sevoflurane, and isoflurane reduced LA contractility (i.e., E$_{es}$) by approximately 50% at an end-tidal concentration of 1.2 MAC (Fig. 7-14). The magnitude of this effect in LA myocardium was similar to the degree of LV contractile depression produced by these agents as quantified with LV end-systolic pressure-volume relationships.[41] Desflurane, sevoflurane, and isoflurane also impaired LA and LV relaxation to similar degrees. These data indicate that volatile anesthetics produce equivalent alterations in contractility and relaxation in LA myocardium compared with LV myocardium.[171] The magnitude of reductions in LA inotropic and lusitropic states produced by the volatile anesthetics was also similar in the intact left atrium, supporting the results obtained in isolated human atrial myocardium.[169]

Desflurane, sevoflurane, and isoflurane altered LA passive mechanical behavior.[171] LA reservoir function (i.e., V loop area and reservoir volume) was maintained

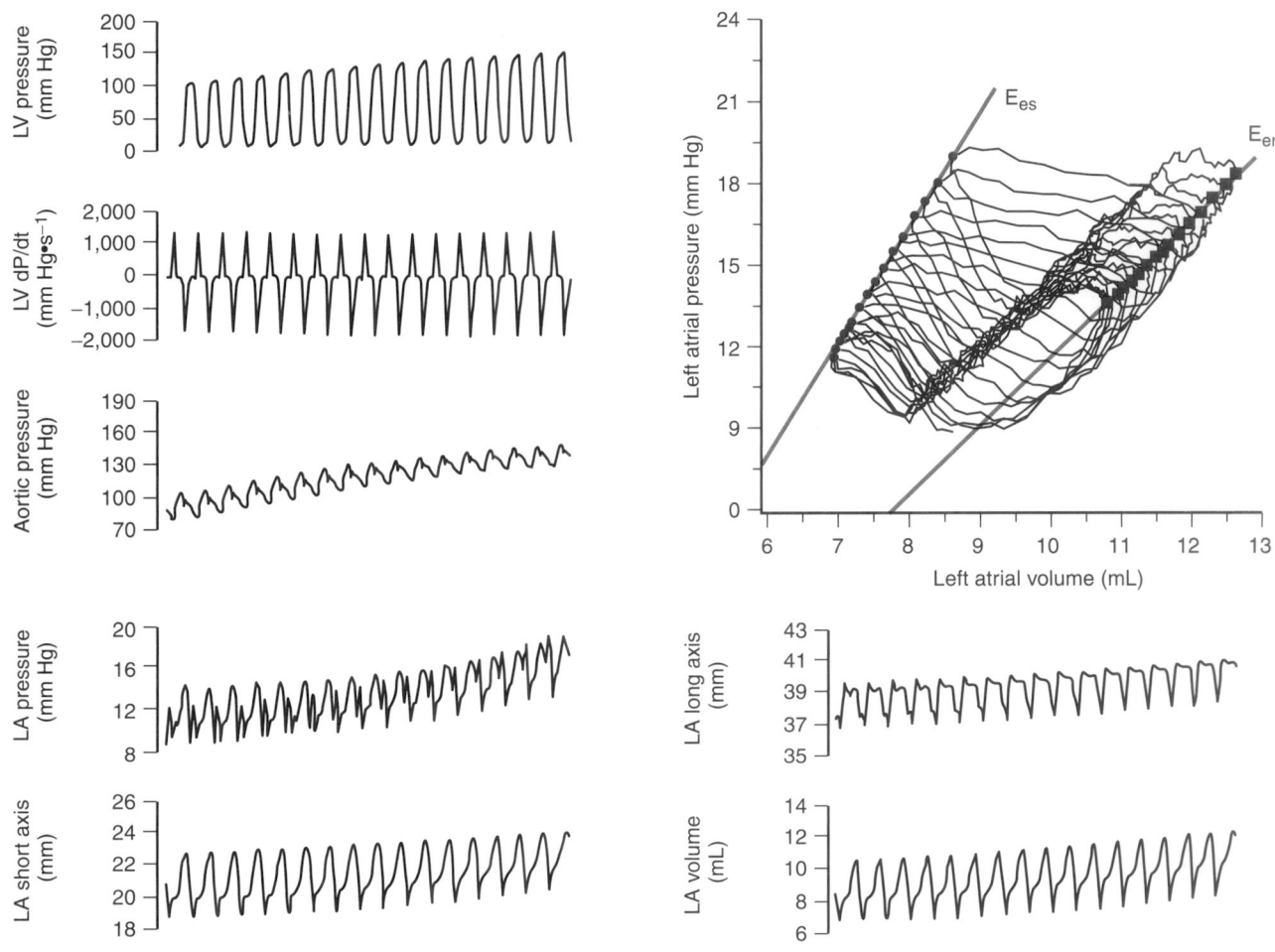

Figure 7–13 Continuous left ventricular (LV) pressure, rate of increase of LV pressure (LV dP/dt), aortic pressure, left atrial (LA) pressure, LA short- and long-axis dimensions, and LA volume wave forms and corresponding LA pressure-volume diagrams resulting from intravenous administration of phenylephrine (200 µg) were observed in a typical experiment. The LA maximum elastance *(solid circles)* and end-reservoir pressure and volume *(solid squares)* for each pressure-volume diagram were used to obtain the slopes (E_{es} and E_{er}) and extrapolated volume intercepts of the LA end-systolic and end-reservoir pressure-volume relationships to quantify myocardial contractility and dynamic chamber stiffness, respectively. (Adapted from Gare M, Schwabe DA, Hettrick DA, et al: Desflurane, sevoflurane, and isoflurane affect left atrial active and passive mechanical properties and impair left atrial–left ventricular coupling in vivo: Analysis using pressure-volume relations. Anesthesiology 95:689-698, 2001.)

during the administration of anesthetic concentrations less than 1.0 MAC (Fig. 7-15). This preservation of reservoir function contributed to the relative maintenance of LV stroke volume[41] by compensating for decreases in LV filling associated with a reduced contribution of LA contraction. The volatile anesthetics also reduced dynamic LA chamber stiffness, an action that most likely contributed to the preservation of reservoir function because the delays in LA relaxation and declines in LV systolic function that also occurred would be expected to decrease reservoir function.[172] However, LA reservoir function was reduced during administration of higher concentrations of the volatile anesthetics because further impairment of LA relaxation and LV contractility occurred. Decreases in the ratio of LA stroke work to total pressure–volume diagram area and the increases in the ratio of LA conduit to total reservoir volume were also produced by desflurane, sevoflurane, and isoflurane. These data indicated that the LA contribution to LV filling becomes less

active and more passive during the administration of the volatile agents.

Desflurane, sevoflurane, and isoflurane decreased the ratio of LA to LV elastance (E_{es}/E_{LV}), consistent with impaired mechanical matching between these chambers (see Fig. 7-14). Volatile anesthetics have been shown to produce LV diastolic dysfunction by delaying LV isovolumic relaxation and impairing early LV filling in association with direct negative inotropic effects.[1] The attenuation of transfer of kinetic energy from the left atrium to the left ventricle probably resulted from the combination of LA contractile depression and LV systolic and diastolic dysfunction. Volatile anesthetic–induced abnormalities in LA-LV matching were greater than analogous impairment of LV-arterial coupling evaluated using a similar series elastic chamber model in a previous investigation[41] because these agents produced beneficial alterations in the determinants of LV afterload[143,144] that partially compensated for simultaneous depression of LV myocardial contractility.

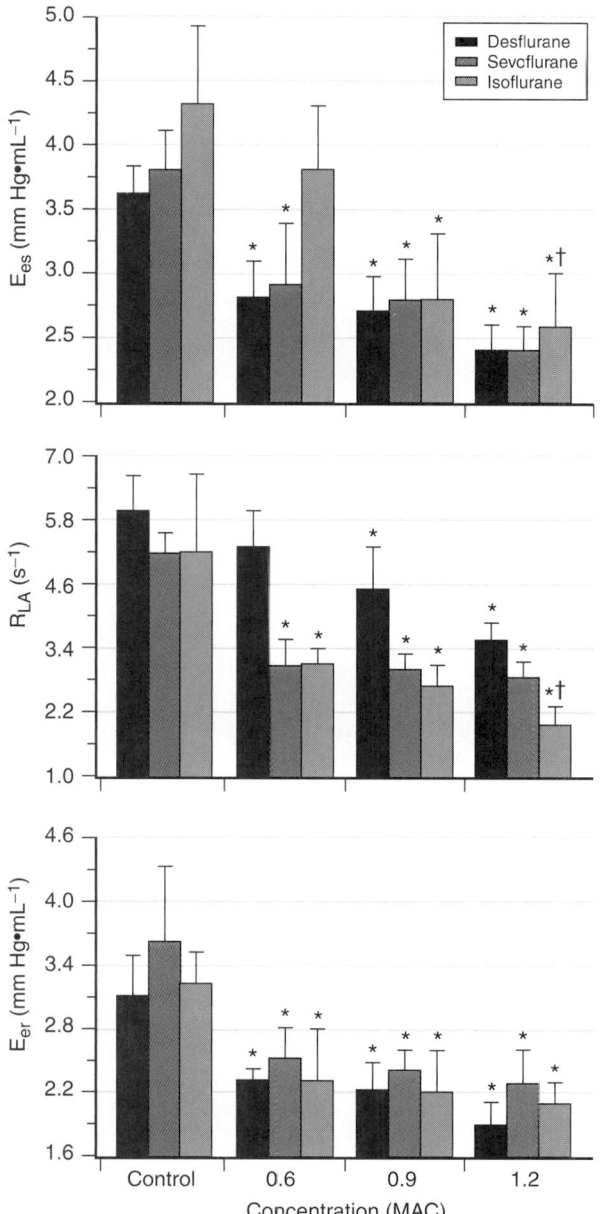

Figure 7–14 Histograms depicting the slope (E_{es}, *top panel*) of the left atrial (LA) end-systolic pressure-volume relationship, LA relaxation (R_{LA}, *middle panel*), and the slope (E_{er}, *bottom panel*) of the LA end-reservoir pressure-volume relationship (i.e., dynamic chamber stiffness) under baseline conditions (Control) and during the administration of 0.6, 0.9, and 1.2 minimum alveolar concentrations (MACs) of desflurane *(black bars)*, sevoflurane *(red bars)*, or isoflurane *(gray bars)*. *, Significantly ($P < .05$) different from the control; †, significantly ($P < .05$) different from 0.6 MAC. (Adapted from Gare M, Schwabe DA, Hettrick DA, et al: Desflurane, sevoflurane, and isoflurane affect left atrial active and passive mechanical properties and impair left atrial-left ventricular coupling in vivo: Analysis using pressure-volume relations. Anesthesiology 95:689-698, 2001.)

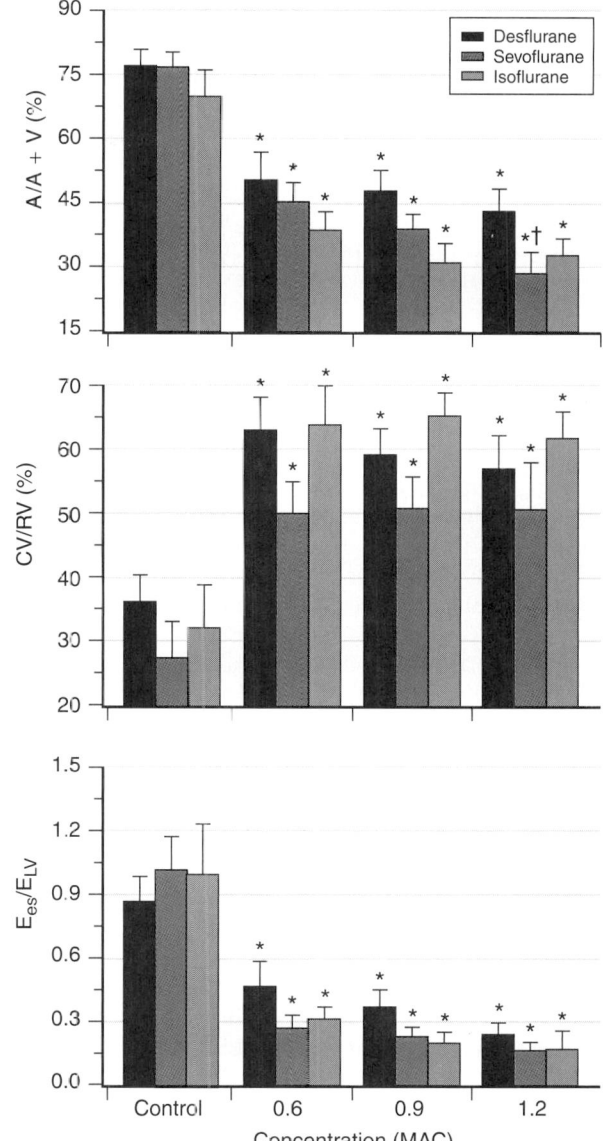

Figure 7–15 Histograms depict the ratio of the left atrial (LA) A loop to the total pressure-volume diagram area (A/A+V, *top panel*), the ratio of LA conduit to total reservoir volume (CV/RV, *middle panel*), and LA–left ventricular coupling (E_{es}/E_{LV}, *bottom panel*) under baseline conditions (Control) and during the administration of 0.6, 0.9, and 1.2 minimum alveolar concentrations (MACs) of desflurane *(black bars)*, sevoflurane *(red bars)*, or isoflurane *(gray bars)*. *, Significantly ($P < .05$) different from the control values; †, significantly ($P < .05$) different from 0.6 MAC. (Adapted from Gare M, Schwabe DA, Hettrick DA, et al: Desflurane, sevoflurane, and isoflurane affect left atrial active and passive mechanical properties and impair left atrial-left ventricular coupling in vivo: Analysis using pressure-volume relations. Anesthesiology 95:689-698, 2001.)

Systemic Hemodynamics

Volatile anesthetics cause direct negative chronotropic actions in vitro by depressing sinoatrial node activity.[173] However, alterations in heart rate in vivo are determined primarily by the interaction of volatile agents and baroreceptor reflex activity.[174,175] Halothane does not appreciably change heart rate in humans[6] because it attenuates baroreceptor reflex responses.[176-178] Heart rate increases to various degrees with enflurane, but these increases may be insufficient to preserve cardiac output.[11,179] Isoflurane increases heart rate in response to simultaneous decreases in arterial pressure.[12] These findings occur with this volatile agent because baroreceptor reflexes are relatively preserved compared with equi-MACs of halothane and enflurane.[175] Desflurane also causes dose-related increases in heart rate in humans.[37,38,180] Desflurane- and isoflurane-induced tachycardia may be more pronounced in pediatric patients or in the presence of vagolytic agents and, conversely, may be attenuated in neonates[181] and geriatric patients or by the concomitant administration of opioids.[182,183] Rapid increases in the inspired desflurane concentration at greater than 1 MAC may be associated with further transient increases in heart rate and arterial pressure resulting from sympathetic nervous system activation.[42,44] Similar increases in heart rate are observed when the inspired isoflurane concentration is rapidly increased.[44] The cardiovascular stimulation induced by rapid increases in desflurane or isoflurane concentration in humans results from activation of tracheopulmonary and systemic receptors[45] and is attenuated by pretreatment with β_1-adrenoceptor antagonists, α_2-adrenoceptor agonists, or opioids.[43] In contrast to the findings with isoflurane and desflurane, sevoflurane neither alters heart rate[184-187] nor causes cardiovascular stimulation during rapid increases in anesthetic concentration in humans.[188]

All modern volatile anesthetics cause concentration-related decreases in arterial pressure.[6,11,12,37,180,184] The mechanism by which these anesthetics reduce arterial pressure differs among anesthetics. Decreases in arterial pressure produced by halothane and enflurane can be primarily attributed to reductions in myocardial contractility and cardiac output.[1] In contrast, decreases in arterial pressure associated with isoflurane, desflurane, and sevoflurane anesthesia occur as a result of reductions in LV afterload,[143,144] whereas myocardial contractility is relatively preserved.[1] Isoflurane, desflurane, and isoflurane maintain cardiac output because these agents produce less pronounced reductions in myocardial contractility and greater decreases in systemic vascular resistance than does halothane or enflurane in humans.[34,186,189] Isoflurane and desflurane may also preserve autonomic nervous system regulation of the circulation to a greater degree than other volatile anesthetics.[42,175,188] The baroreceptor reflex–mediated tachycardia that occurs during isoflurane and desflurane anesthesia maintains cardiac output despite simultaneous declines in myocardial contractility and stroke volume. Declines in arterial pressure produced by volatile anesthetics may be attenuated by surgical stimulation or concomitant administration of nitrous oxide.[38,190] Volatile anesthetics also cause modest, dose-related increases in RA pressure in humans.[34,189] These effects probably occur as a result of direct negative inotropic actions. The vasodilating effects of isoflurane, desflurane, and sevoflurane cause less pronounced increases in right atrial pressure than those observed during halothane or enflurane anesthesia.

The cardiovascular effects of volatile anesthetics are altered by the duration of anesthesia. Increases in myocardial contractility and cardiac output and decreases in LV preload and afterload occur after several hours of constant-MAC anesthesia.[6,12,37,179,191] Heart rate may also increase during prolonged halothane[6,191] or enflurane[179] anesthesia, but arterial pressure remains constant. Recovery from

circulatory depression is greatest during halothane anesthesia[191] and less pronounced during prolonged administration of isoflurane[12] and desflurane.[37] The time-dependent improvements in hemodynamics observed with volatile anesthetics are antagonized by propranolol and may result from enhanced sympathetic nervous system activity.[192]

The systemic hemodynamic effects of volatile agents in the presence of LV dysfunction are similar but not identical to those observed in the normal heart. Volatile anesthetics, including isoflurane, modestly increase or do not affect heart rate in experimental animals with pacing-induced or doxorubicin-induced dilated cardiomyopathy[65,193] and in patients with coronary artery disease and LV dysfunction.[62,64,194,195] These findings may be attributed to altered baroreceptor reflex activity, β_1-adrenoceptor downregulation, and increases in central sympathetic and withdrawal of parasympathetic nervous system tone associated with heart failure.[196] Isoflurane and halothane cause pronounced reductions in LV end-diastolic pressure and chamber dimension in cardiomyopathic dogs concomitant with decreases in mean arterial pressure.[65] These findings support previously observed declines in pulmonary artery pressures during isoflurane, enflurane, and halothane anesthesia in patients with coronary artery disease and heart failure[62,64,194,195] and indicate that venodilation represents a major hemodynamic consequence of these anesthetics in experimental and clinical heart failure. In contrast to the findings in normal dogs, isoflurane did not beneficially influence, and halothane detrimentally affected, the determinants of LV afterload in cardiomyopathic dogs.[147] As a result of these actions and the simultaneous declines in LV preload and myocardial contractility, cardiac output may be more profoundly reduced during isoflurane or halothane anesthesia in the presence of preexisting LV dysfunction.[147]

VOLATILE ANESTHETICS AND CARDIAC ELECTROPHYSIOLOGY

Cardiac Conduction

Volatile anesthetics slow the rate of sinoatrial node discharge by direct and indirect effects on sinoatrial node automaticity.[173,197] These actions may be altered in vivo by vasoactive drugs or autonomic nervous system activity.[198] Halothane, enflurane and, to some extent, isoflurane shorten the cardiac action potential and effective refractory period in normal Purkinje fibers,[197,199,200] but these agents prolong His-Purkinje and ventricular conduction times.[197,200,201] Halothane, enflurane, and isoflurane also prolong atrioventricular conduction time and refractoriness.[200,202,203] When combined with the direct actions of volatile anesthetics on sinoatrial node discharge, the data suggest that volatile anesthetics have the potential to produce bradycardia and atrioventricular conduction abnormalities. However, primary disturbances in atrioventricular conduction leading to second- or third-degree atrioventricular block in humans probably do not occur with volatile anesthetics in the absence of conduction disease or drugs that directly prolong the atrioventricular conduction time.[204,205]

Volatile agents may have proarrhythmogenic or antiarrhythmogenic actions against abnormal cardiac electrophysiologic mechanisms produced by myocardial ischemia or infarction. Halothane, enflurane, and isoflurane have been shown to be cardioprotective against ventricular fibrillation produced by coronary artery occlusion[206,207] and reperfusion.[208] Protective effects against ouabain-induced arrhythmias have also been demonstrated during halothane anesthesia.[209] Volatile anesthetics may also exert antiarrhythmic effects by opposing subsidiary pacemaker activity in infarcted myocardium.[199] Conversely, halothane and, to a lesser extent, isoflurane may be arrhythmogenic in Purkinje fibers in experimental myocardial infarction by facilitating reentrant activity or increasing temporal dispersion of refractory period recovery.[199,210] These actions may be related to inhibition of slow Na^+ current in false tendon fibers and induction of reentry of premature impulses into more refractory Purkinje fibers in the border zone of an ischemic area.[211] Halothane, enflurane, and isoflurane prolong the QT_c interval in humans.[212] These data suggest that patients with idiopathic or acquired long QT syndrome may be at greater risk of developing torsade de pointes tachycardia[213] during anesthesia with these agents.

Epinephrine-Induced Arrhythmias

Halothane and, to a lesser extent, other volatile anesthetics have been shown to sensitize myocardium to the arrhythmogenic effects of epinephrine.[214-216] Sensitization is the interaction between volatile anesthetics and catecholamines that leads to reductions in the threshold for atrial and ventricular arrhythmias. Sequentially escalating doses of epinephrine produce premature ventricular contractions and sustained ventricular tachyarrhythmias during halothane anesthesia.[214] Halothane-epinephrine–induced arrhythmias are attenuated by pretreatment with thiopental,[214] presumably by means of effects on the atrioventricular node or the upper His bundle.[217] A synergistic interaction between α_1- and β-adrenoceptors has been strongly implicated in the pathogenesis of halothane-epinephrine–induced ventricular arrhythmias.[218] Stimulation of the α_{1A}-adrenoceptor in the His-Purkinje system by epinephrine during halothane anesthesia transiently slows Purkinje fiber conduction.[219,220] This proarrhythmogenic effect is mediated by phospholipase C and the intracellular second messenger inositol triphosphate.[220] Evidence indicates that enhanced conduction in the Purkinje-ventricular muscle junction accompanied by simultaneous α_1-adrenoceptor–mediated depression of Purkinje conduction also plays important roles in halothane-epinephrine–induced arrhythmias.[221] The doses of epinephrine required to produce ventricular arrhythmias during desflurane or sevoflurane anesthesia[218,222] are similar to, but significantly less than, those observed during administration of isoflurane and halothane, respectively. Halothane-catecholamine sensitization also promotes abnormal automaticity of dominant and latent atrial pacemakers.[223-226] These effects may produce premature ventricular contractions and arrhythmias originating from the His bundle.[223] Intact sinoatrial node function reduces the incidence of epinephrine-induced ventricular escape during halothane anesthesia and is protective against His bundle arrhythmias.[226]

VOLATILE ANESTHETICS AND THE CORONARY CIRCULATION

Coronary Vascular Effects In Vitro

Volatile anesthetics can produce direct coronary artery vasodilation in vitro, but simultaneous reductions in the determinants of myocardial oxygen consumption (MVO_2), including heart rate, preload, afterload, and an inotropic state, produced by these agents cause coronary vasoconstriction in vivo through metabolic autoregulation. Volatile anesthetic–induced alterations in coronary blood flow also are affected by the reductions in coronary perfusion pressure produced by these agents. The combination of direct and indirect actions ultimately determines the net effect of volatile anesthetics on coronary vascular tone. Halothane, isoflurane, and enflurane cause vasodilation of isolated coronary arteries.[227-234] Halothane produces greater coronary artery dilation than does isoflurane at equivalent MACs[228-230,232,233] in isolated coronary arteries larger than 2000 μm.[228,230-233] In contrast, isoflurane causes vasodilation of predominantly small (<900 μm) canine epicardial coronary arteries.[231] Halothane may produce greater vasodilator effects in large coronary arteries than does isoflurane because halothane causes more pronounced suppression of voltage-dependent Ca^{2+} current.[235]

The direct negative inotropic effects of volatile anesthetics cause a reduction in coronary blood flow in isolated, contracting hearts during precise control of ventricular loading conditions through flow-metabolism coupling.[236] Under these conditions, a decrease in myocardial oxygen demand is accompanied by an increase in coronary vascular resistance, findings that may be incorrectly interpreted as suggesting that volatile agents produce coronary vasoconstriction. However, examination of the actions of volatile anesthetics on myocardial oxygen extraction and the ratio of myocardial oxygen delivery to MVO_2 reveals that inhalational anesthetics are coronary vasodilators. Halothane and isoflurane decrease myocardial oxygen extraction and increase the ratio of oxygen delivery to consumption in isolated, beating hearts.[237-240] These findings indicate that volatile anesthetics produce direct coronary vasodilation in isolated hearts because myocardial oxygen delivery exceeds MVO_2, and coronary sinus oxygen tension increases. Halothane, isoflurane, and sevoflurane cause similar reductions in adenosine-induced coronary flow reserve[241] in tetrodotoxin-arrested, isolated hearts. Because mechanical work is not performed in this preparation, these findings support the hypothesis that volatile agents cause direct coronary vasodilation of similar magnitude.

Coronary Vascular Effects In Vivo

Halothane has variable effects on coronary blood flow and coronary vascular resistance in vivo that occur concomitant with changes in MVO_2.[242-245] Decreases in MVO_2 cause declines in coronary blood flow with relative maintenance or modest increases in coronary vascular resistance during halothane anesthesia.[14,246,247] Despite the decreases in coronary blood flow, halothane increases coronary sinus oxygen tension and decreases oxygen extraction,[243,245] indicating that halothane is a relatively weak coronary vasodilator. Like halothane, isoflurane variably alters coronary blood flow in vivo.[19,248-251] Isoflurane reduces MVO_2 and simultaneously decreases oxygen extraction, indicating direct coronary vasodilation.[249] Isoflurane can also produce mild and transient increases in blood flow independent of changes in MVO_2 and autonomic nervous system activity during inhalational induction of anesthesia.[252] Perfusion of the left anterior descending coronary artery with blood previously equilibrated with isoflurane dramatically increases coronary blood flow,[253] but only mild coronary vasodilation occurs after a period of anesthetic equilibration in a similar experimental model.[250] Isoflurane-induced increases in coronary blood flow are not accompanied by epicardial coronary artery dilation, indicating that isoflurane predominantly dilates small coronary arteries.[254] However, adenosine, a potent coronary vasodilator, causes considerably greater vasodilation in coronary microvessels than does isoflurane.[255] The effects of enflurane on the coronary circulation in vivo are somewhat controversial.[232,238-240] Enflurane produces greater reductions in MVO_2 than does isoflurane concomitant with metabolically determined declines in coronary blood flow.[256,257] However, isoflurane produces more profound decreases in myocardial oxygen extraction than does enflurane, indicating that isoflurane is a more potent coronary vasodilator than its structural isomer.[257]

The influence of the new volatile anesthetics on coronary blood flow in the intact cardiovascular system has been incompletely examined. Desflurane and isoflurane caused similar increases in the ratio of oxygen delivery to consumption and decreases in oxygen extraction, consistent with coronary vasodilation.[258] However, the increases in coronary blood flow produced by desflurane, but not isoflurane, are attenuated by pharmacologic blockade of the autonomic nervous system, suggesting that isoflurane causes greater direct coronary vasodilation in vivo than does desflurane.[16] Sevoflurane does not appear to produce any significant degree of coronary vasodilation,[46,241,259-261] in contrast to the findings with other volatile agents.

Coronary Vasodilator Reserve and Autoregulation

Coronary vasodilator reserve, defined as the ratio of peak coronary blood flow after brief coronary artery occlusion (e.g., reactive hyperemia) and baseline flow, is affected by halothane and isoflurane.[262] Coronary vasodilator reserve is greater during isoflurane than during halothane anesthesia.[262] This observation suggested that halothane may be a more potent coronary vasodilator than isoflurane because greater baseline coronary vasodilation should be accompanied by a reduced ability to increase coronary blood flow further in response to a brief ischemic episode.

However, halothane also reduces the determinants of MVO_2 to a greater degree than does isoflurane in vivo. Peak coronary blood flow during reactive hyperemia and percent flow debt repayment are directly related to the intensity of the ischemic stimulus and the magnitude of oxygen debt accrued during coronary artery occlusion. Differences in coronary vasodilator reserve produced by isoflurane and halothane may reflect differences in the intensity of ischemia during coronary occlusion and not the relative vasodilator efficacy of these volatile anesthetics.[236]

Dilation of coronary arteriolar resistance vessels by volatile anesthetics alters pressure autoregulation in the coronary vasculature.[263] Changes in autoregulation produced by vasoactive drugs, including volatile anesthetics, are typically determined by the slope of the pressure-flow curve generated by progressive constriction of a coronary artery. Changes in these pressure-flow curves demonstrate that autoregulation is disrupted during anesthesia in comparison with the conscious state (Fig. 7-16). Isoflurane produces more profound alterations in autoregulation than does halothane or enflurane, as indicated by greater increases in the slope of the pressure-flow relation. Coronary perfusion pressure also plays a more important role in the determination of coronary blood flow during anesthesia. Although volatile anesthetics impair coronary autoregulation to some degree, these agents do not produce the profound degree of coronary vasodilation and inhibition of autoregulation caused by adenosine or dipyridamole.[250,257,263] In contrast to volatile agents,

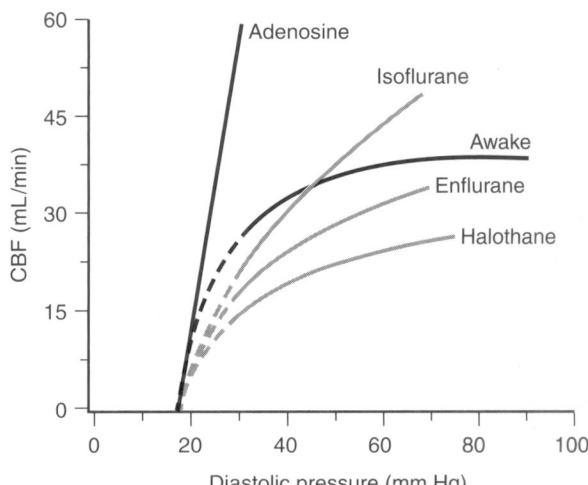

Figure 7–16 A qualitative description of the effects of volatile anesthetics on the coronary blood flow (CBF)–diastolic pressure relationship demonstrates the effect of adenosine-induced maximal coronary vasodilation in awake and anesthetized dogs. *Solid lines* are mean slopes determined by linear regression analysis. *Dashed lines* represent the nonlinear portion of the curve and are estimates. When compared with the findings obtained in awake dogs, the anesthetics affect absolute CBF variably but do not increase the slope of the CBF–diastolic pressure plots. (Adapted from Hickey RF, Sybert PE, Verrier ED, Cason BA: Effects of halothane, enflurane, and isoflurane on coronary blood flow autoregulation and coronary vascular reserve in the canine heart. Anesthesiology 68:21-30, 1988.)

these drugs cause maximal coronary vasodilation and inhibit pressure autoregulation to such a degree that coronary blood flow becomes directly dependent on coronary perfusion pressure. Volatile anesthetics are only weak coronary vasodilators.

Mechanisms of Volatile Anesthetic–Induced Coronary Vasodilation

Volatile anesthetics produce direct coronary artery relaxation by affecting intracellular Ca^{2+} regulation at several locations in the vascular smooth muscle cell.[236] Volatile agents inhibit Ca^{2+} influx through voltage-operated[235] and receptor-operated[227,228,232,233,264] Ca^{2+} channels in coronary vascular smooth muscle. Volatile agents also reduce Ca^{2+} accumulation in, and release by, the coronary vascular smooth muscle SR,[265] inhibit G proteins linked to phospholipase C,[264] and decrease formation of the second messenger inositol triphosphate.[266]

The coronary vasodilating actions of volatile agents probably are not related to the production or release of nitric oxide (i.e., endothelium-dependent relaxing factor). Investigations conducted in isolated coronary[234] and aortic[265,267-269] vascular preparations and in the intact canine coronary circulation[253] demonstrated that volatile anesthetic–induced coronary vasodilation occurs independent of nitric oxide. However, some experimental evidence suggests that the direct coronary vasodilator effects of isoflurane may be mediated by the vascular endothelium.[227,270] Other data indicate that halothane, enflurane, and isoflurane may adversely affect the release or action of nitric oxide.[267-269,271,272] Although nitric oxide–induced formation of cyclic guanylate monophosphate (cGMP) may be attenuated to some degree by halothane,[273] several studies indicate that volatile anesthetics do not affect vasodilation produced by the nitric oxide donors sodium nitroprusside or nitroglycerin.[268,272,274,275] Volatile anesthetics may also reduce the stability of nitric oxide by generating oxygen-derived free radicals[275] while leaving nitric oxide release and its action on vascular smooth muscle unaffected.[271] Whether the results of these later studies conducted in isolated aortic preparations are applicable to the coronary circulation requires further evaluation, but these investigations provide important information about the potential effects of volatile agents on the coronary vasculature.

Halothane and isoflurane cause coronary vasodilation by activation of adenosine triphosphate (ATP)–sensitive potassium (K_{ATP}) channels.[276,277] Increases in coronary blood flow in response to halothane and isoflurane were attenuated by the K_{ATP} channel antagonist glyburide in isolated rat hearts and anesthetized pigs, respectively.[276,277] Glyburide also partially blocked increases in coronary blood flow during intracoronary administration of volatile anesthetic–equilibrated blood in canine hearts in situ.[278] Isoflurane-induced reductions in coronary vascular resistance were attenuated by the selective adenosine$_1$ (A_1)–receptor antagonist 8-cyclopentyl-1,3-dipropylxanthine (DPCPX).[279] These data suggest that coronary vasodilation produced by isoflurane may partially occur as a result of stimulation of A_1 receptors coupled to K_{ATP} channels.[279,280]

Volatile Anesthetics and Ischemic Myocardium

Halothane and isoflurane decrease subendocardial blood flow and myocardial lactate extraction, produce contractile dysfunction, and cause electrocardiographic changes in the presence of a coronary stenosis concomitant with declines in coronary perfusion pressure.[51,281,282] Regional ischemia during isoflurane- or halothane-induced reductions in perfusion pressure is functionally indicated by the appearance of paradoxical systolic lengthening and post-systolic shortening.[51,283] Contractile dysfunction in the region distal to a critical coronary stenosis is more severe during isoflurane anesthesia than during halothane anesthesia, coincident with higher flows in the normal zone and lower flows in the ischemic zone.[282,284] These findings suggest that coronary vasodilation produced by isoflurane may cause a detrimental redistribution of coronary blood flow away from ischemic myocardium if hypotension is allowed to occur.

The adverse effects of volatile anesthetics on ischemic myocardium are avoided if coronary perfusion pressure is restored. Subendocardial blood flow in the perfusion bed distal to a critical coronary stenosis is reduced during isoflurane-induced declines in arterial pressure, but treatment of hypotension with phenylephrine restores subendocardial blood flow to values observed before the administration of isoflurane.[285,286] The transmural distribution of coronary blood flow between the subendocardium and subepicardium (endo/epi ratio) decreases during isoflurane anesthesia despite control of arterial pressure. Administration of phenylephrine to maintain arterial pressure at a constant level increases subepicardial blood flow more than subendocardial flow. This increase in subepicardial perfusion accounts for the decline in the endo/epi ratio in the absence of an absolute reduction in subendocardial flow. Restoration of coronary perfusion pressure to baseline levels during isoflurane anesthesia also increases coronary collateral blood flow and normalizes myocardial oxygen tension in the ischemic zone.[256]

Investigations in dogs with steal-prone anatomy (i.e., complete occlusion of a coronary artery with collateral flow from an adjacent vessel having a critical stenosis) have repeatedly demonstrated that isoflurane and halothane do not alter collateral-dependent or ischemic zone myocardial blood flow,[287-291] endo/epi distribution,[287,288] or the electrocardiogram[287] when diastolic arterial pressure is held constant. Coronary collateral perfusion is unchanged during isoflurane or halothane anesthesia in dogs at a mean arterial pressure of 50 mm Hg.[292] Coronary steal does not occur in a chronically instrumented canine model of coronary artery disease with isoflurane,[289,291] halothane,[290] desflurane,[293] or sevoflurane[294] independent of coronary stenosis severity or coronary collateral development.[288-291] The findings also refute earlier evidence in dogs with amaroid constrictor–induced augmentation of the coronary collateral circulation, suggesting that isoflurane reduces collateral blood flow and causes coronary steal in vivo.[295] These effects of volatile anesthetics are in marked contrast to those obtained with adenosine, a potent coronary vasodilator that produces coronary steal when arterial pressure is maintained at control

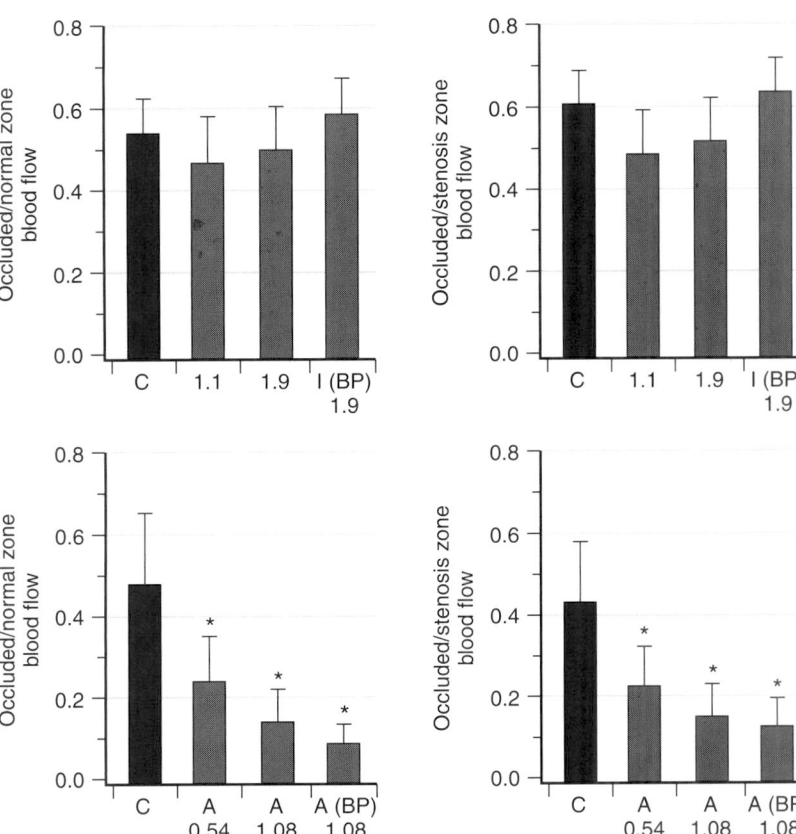

Figure 7–17 Occluded compared with normal and occluded compared with stenotic zone myocardial blood flow in dogs with steal-prone coronary artery anatomy in the conscious state (C), during 1.1 and 1.9 minimum alveolar concentrations (MACs) of isoflurane (I) anesthesia, during adenosine (A) infusions (0.54 and 1.08 mg/min), and during maintenance of heart rate and arterial pressure at conscious values during the highest doses (BP). Isoflurane does not cause coronary steal, in contrast to significant ($P < .05$ [*]) reductions in blood flow to collateral-dependent myocardium produced by adenosine. (Adapted from Hartman JC, Kampine JP, Schmeling WT, Warltier DC: Actions of isoflurane on myocardial perfusion in chronically instrumented dogs with poor, moderate, or well-developed coronary collaterals. J Cardiothorac Anesth 4:715-725, 1990.)

levels in models of multivessel coronary artery disease (Fig. 7-17).[289,291,296]

Volatile Anesthetic–Induced Myocardial Protection

The relatively academic controversy about volatile anesthetic–induced coronary vasodilation and coronary steal has detracted from substantial experimental evidence indicating that volatile agents exert important protective effects during myocardial ischemia and reperfusion injury. Halothane attenuates ST-segment changes caused by brief coronary artery occlusion[297,298] and decreases ST-segment elevation to a greater extent than propranolol and sodium nitroprusside despite producing similar hemodynamic effects.[298] Halothane and isoflurane reduce myocardial infarct size after coronary artery ligation.[55,56,299-301] Enflurane decreases cardiac lactate production in the presence of a critical coronary artery stenosis during artificial control of perfusion pressure.[57] Isoflurane and desflurane produce beneficial actions on LV diastolic mechanics during acute regional myocardial ischemia.[61] Halothane, enflurane, and isoflurane decrease myocardial reperfusion injury and improve functional recovery after global ischemia in isolated hearts.[302-305] Volatile agents also enhance systolic functional recovery of postischemic-reperfused ("stunned") myocardium when these agents are administered before and during,[58,60] but not after,[306,307] brief periods of myocardial ischemia in vivo (Fig. 7-18). These effects are accompanied by

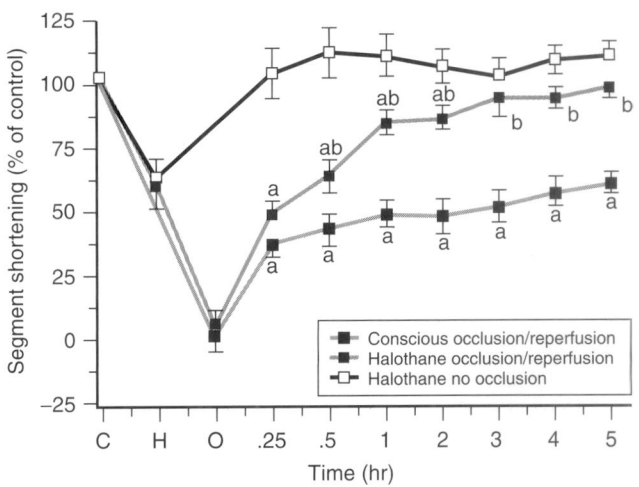

Figure 7–18 Segment shortening data (expressed as a percentage of the control value) during a 15-minute coronary artery occlusion (O) and at various times after reperfusion in the conscious (C) and halothane-anesthetized (H) states. Comparisons are made at various time points with animals anesthetized with halothane for 2.25 hours and allowed to emerge from anesthesia over a 5-hour period but not undergoing coronary artery occlusion and reperfusion. (Adapted from Warltier DC, Al-Wathiqui MH, Kampine JP, Schmeling WT: Recovery of contractile function of stunned myocardium in chronically instrumented dogs is enhanced by halothane or isoflurane. Anesthesiology 69:552-565, 1988.)

preservation of high-energy phosphate levels.[58] Volatile anesthetics attenuate the effect of oxygen-derived free radicals on LV pressure development in isolated hearts.[308] Halothane also preserves contractile function and ultrastructural integrity during reperfusion after normothermic cardioplegic arrest.[59]

Volatile anesthetics may also produce beneficial effects on blood flow to ischemic myocardium. Decreases in collateral blood flow after coronary artery occlusion are less pronounced than declines in flow to normal myocardium in the presence of halothane.[309] The ratio of myocardial oxygen delivery to MVo_2 is also increased in collateral-dependent myocardium during halothane anesthesia.[309] Evidence indicates that sevoflurane actually increases blood flow to collateral-dependent myocardium when arterial pressure is maintained at conscious values.[294] Halothane may inhibit platelet thrombi formation through increases in platelet cAMP concentration and decrease cyclical variations in coronary blood flow associated with a critical coronary artery stenosis.[310] Volatile anesthetics can attenuate the adhesion of neutrophils and platelets in the coronary vasculature after ischemia and reperfusion.[311]

The mechanisms responsible for volatile anesthetic–induced protection during myocardial ischemia and reperfusion are incompletely understood. The beneficial effects of volatile anesthetics may be attributed to a favorable reduction in myocardial oxygen demand required for active contraction with concomitant preservation of energy-dependent vital cellular processes because these anesthetics cause direct negative inotropic, lusitropic, and chronotropic effects and decrease LV afterload. However, halothane also exerts protective effects during complete functional arrest induced by cardioplegia,[59] indicating that preferential alterations in myocardial oxygen supply-demand relationships are not solely responsible for the anti-ischemic actions of this anesthetic. Halothane, enflurane, and isoflurane may significantly lower excessive intracellular Ca^{2+} during reperfusion through a direct decline in the net transsarcolemmal Ca^{2+} transient resulting from partially inhibited Ca^{2+} channel activity[69,71-73] or an indirect reduction of oxygen-derived free radical formation.[308]

Evidence indicates that the protective effects of isoflurane during ischemic injury are mediated by activation of K_{ATP} channels.[280] K_{ATP} channels are heteromultimeric complexes consisting of an inward-rectifying K^+ channel (K_{ir}) and a sulfonylurea receptor (SUR).[312] Pharmacologically distinct K_{ATP} channels have been identified in cardiac sarcolemmal[313] and mitochondrial[314] membranes. It was originally proposed that opening of sarcolemmal K_{ATP} channels protects ischemic myocardium by shortening action potential duration and preventing intracellular Ca^{2+} overload.[313] However, subsequent studies indicated that the beneficial actions of K_{ATP} channel opening occurred independent of the action potential duration.[315,316] Most experimental findings suggest that mitochondrial K_{ATP} channels are the primary mediators of ischemia-induced[317] and anesthetic-induced preconditioning (IPC and APC, respectively). Preservation of mitochondrial bioenergetic function appears to be vital for cellular protection against myocardial ischemia.[318-321]

Mitochondrial K_{ATP} channel openers maintain intracellular Ca^{2+} homeostasis and inhibit mitochondrial Ca^{2+} overload.[320,321] These actions enhance myocyte survival by preventing tissue necrosis or apoptosis.[322] Mitochondrial K_{ATP} channel activation inhibits apoptosis in rat ventricular myocytes[323] by attenuating oxidant stress during reperfusion.[324] Alteration of the mitochondrial oxidation-reduction state by K_{ATP} channel activation may also promote cellular protection.[325] Experiments conducted in isolated cardiac mitochondria[320] indicate that membrane depolarization, matrix swelling, and uncoupling of ATP synthesis occur as a result of increased oxygen consumption, are associated with the opening of mitochondrial K_{ATP} channels, and may mediate cellular viability during IPC.[325] Opening of mitochondrial K_{ATP} channels depolarizes the inner mitochondrial membrane and causes a transient swelling of the mitochondrial matrix,[326] resulting from a shift in the ionic balance.[327] Mitochondrial K_{ATP} channel opening initially reduces ATP production as a result of membrane depolarization[320] but subsequently stimulates a compensatory increase in respiration that optimizes the efficiency of oxidative phosphorylation, in part by regulating energy-dependent matrix volume.[328] A moderate disturbance of mitochondrial homeostasis may promote myocardial tolerance to ischemic stress by altering energetic systems to reduce Ca^{2+} overload, prevent the activation of necrotic or apoptotic pathways, or attenuate oxidant stress.

The endogenous mechanisms involved in APC are strikingly similar to those implicated in IPC. It is hypothesized that a *trigger* (e.g., brief ischemic episode, exposure to a volatile anesthetic) initiates a cascade of signaling events leading to activation of an *end-effector* that is responsible for resistance to injury. K_{ATP} channel activation has been implicated as the end-effector in this protective scheme during APC. Administration of isoflurane and sevoflurane preserved myocyte viability using a cellular model of ischemia compared with cells that were not exposed to a volatile agent.[329] This protective effect was abolished by the selective mitochondrial K_{ATP} channel antagonist 5-hydroxydecanoate (5-HD) but not the selective sarcolemmal K_{ATP} channel antagonist HMR-1098.[329] The nonselective K_{ATP} channel blocker glyburide attenuated the recovery of contractile function produced by isoflurane in stunned myocardium (Fig. 7-19).[279,330] Isoflurane-induced reductions in canine myocardial infarct size[56] (Fig. 7-20) and the ATP-sparing effects of this agent[331] are also abolished by glyburide. 5-HD inhibits preconditioning by isoflurane in rats,[332] rabbits,[333] and isolated human atria.[334,335] HMR-1098 and 5-HD abolished the protective effects of desflurane in dogs,[336] supporting a role for sarcolemmal and mitochondrial K_{ATP} channels in APC. The latter data contrast to some degree with findings that implicate mitochondrial K_{ATP} channels as the predominant mediators of IPC.[317]

Results of in vitro experiments also strongly suggest that volatile anesthetics affect K_{ATP} channel function. Isoflurane stimulated outward K^+ current through sarcolemmal K_{ATP} channels in isolated ventricular myocytes during patch-clamping.[337,338] Volatile anesthetics also reduced sarcolemmal K_{ATP} channel sensitivity to inhibition by ATP, thereby increasing the open-state probability.[339]

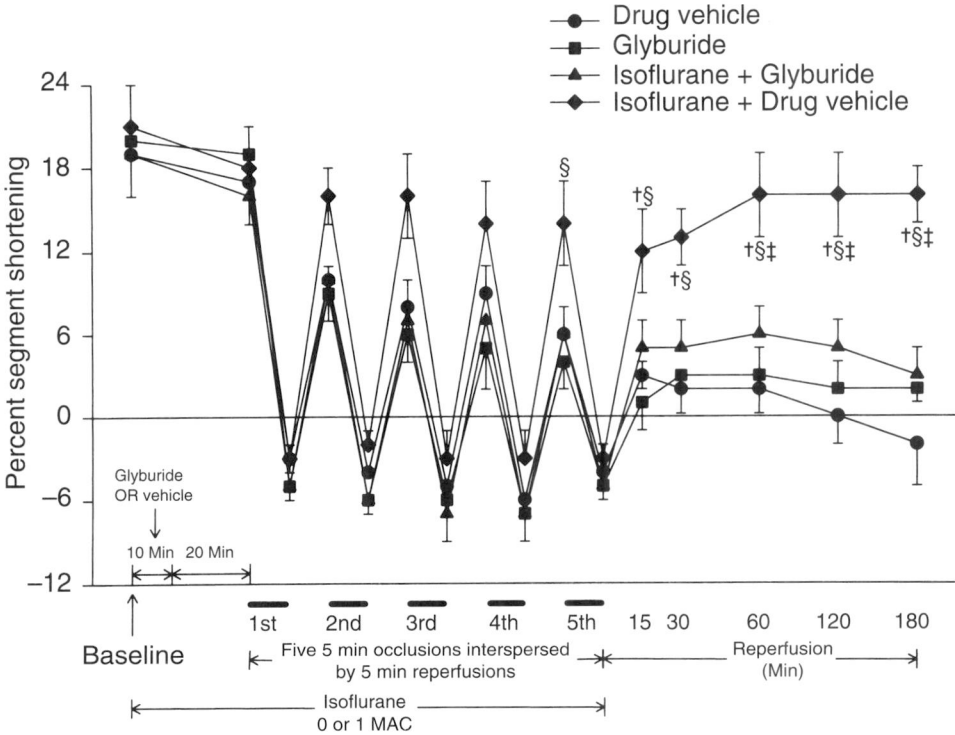

Figure 7–19 Percent segment shortening (%SS) in the intermittently ischemic and reperfused left anterior descending coronary artery (LAD) region. The %SS decreases significantly ($P < .05$) from baseline during each 5-minute LAD occlusion and reperfusion in all groups. Significant decreases in %SS during each 5-minute reperfusion and throughout 180 minutes of final reperfusion are observed in dogs pretreated with glyburide, a K_{ATP} channel antagonist, in the presence or absence of isoflurane. The %SS recovers to baseline values after reperfusion in dogs receiving isoflurane alone. †, Significantly ($P < .05$) different from dogs pretreated with drug vehicle; §, significantly ($P < .05$) different from dogs pretreated with glyburide; ‡, significantly ($P < .05$) different from dogs receiving glyburide and isoflurane. (From Kersten JR, Schmeling TJ, Hettrick DA, et al: Mechanism of cardioprotection by isoflurane: Role of adenosine triphosphate-regulated potassium (KATP) channels. Anesthesiology 85:794-807, 1996.)

Volatile anesthetics enhanced sarcolemmal K_{ATP} channel current by facilitating channel opening after initial activation.[337,338] Isoflurane and sevoflurane increased mitochondrial flavoprotein oxidation, an index of mitochondrial K_{ATP} channel activity, in guinea pig cardiac myocytes, and this increase in fluorescence was inhibited by 5-HD.[340] Isoflurane and sevoflurane also enhanced diazoxide-induced flavoprotein fluorescence in isolated rat ventricular myocytes.[329] Isoflurane failed to augment K_{ATP} channel current in excised membrane patches.[337] These data suggest

that volatile agents may not directly interact with K_{ATP} channels but that they instead act on other intracellular signaling elements that modulate K_{ATP} channel activity. The preponderance of evidence collected suggests that volatile anesthetics may not directly open K_{ATP} channels, but they may instead prime the activation of these channels in sarcolemmal and mitochondrial membranes. This hypothesis is supported by the observation that adenosine facilitates K_{ATP} channel activation through a protein kinase C (PKC)–dependent mechanism during IPC.[341]

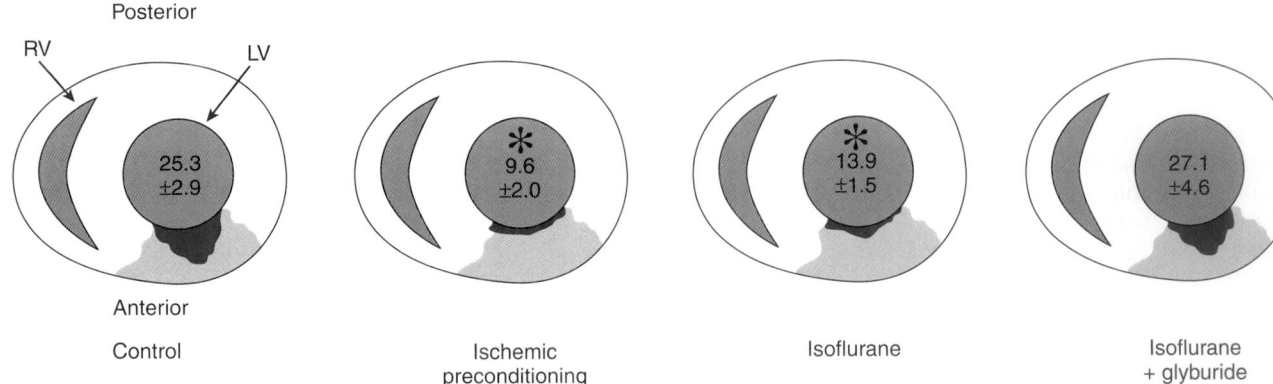

Figure 7–20 Schematic illustration of canine myocardium subjected to a 60-minute coronary artery occlusion and reperfusion and then stained to identify the region of myocardial infarction *(black area)* within the area of myocardium at risk for infarction *(light gray area)*. Isoflurane decreased the extent of myocardial infarction. The protective effect of isoflurane was equivalent to that produced by ischemic preconditioning and was abolished by pretreatment with glyburide. *, Significantly ($P < .05$) different from the control. (Adapted from Kersten JR, Schmeling TJ, Pagel PS, et al: Isoflurane mimics ischemic preconditioning via activation of K_{ATP} channels. Reduction of myocardial infarct size with an acute memory phase. Anesthesiology 87:361-370, 1997.)

Taken as a whole, the experimental results with volatile anesthetics are consistent with previous findings demonstrating that pharmacologic stimulation of K_{ATP} channels with other drugs mimics the conditions present during IPC.[342]

Volatile anesthetics may activate parallel or redundant signal transduction pathways that involve K_{ATP} channel opening to generate a physiologically meaningful cellular response. The sequential activation of several intracellular elements within a given transduction pathway may facilitate signal amplification and interaction between other redundant signaling systems. For example, administration of isoflurane in the presence of the K_{ATP} channel opener nicorandil[333] or diazoxide[343] markedly enhanced protection against ischemic injury beyond that observed with either drug alone. The combination of isoflurane and a selective δ_1-opioid receptor agonist amplified the preconditioning response in the rat.[343] This effect was synergistic and was sensitive to inhibition by glyburide.[343] The combined administration of isoflurane and morphine also markedly reduced infarct size in vivo,[332] and this protective effect was abolished by 5-HD.[332] These data suggest that combined administration of a volatile anesthetic and an opioid capable of agonist action at the δ_1-receptor subtype may stimulate similar or cooperative signaling cascades that amplify K_{ATP} channel activation to profoundly augment myocardial protection beyond that produced by either drug alone.

K_{ATP} channels in vascular smooth muscle cells are essential regulators of coronary vascular tone when ATP production is reduced.[344] Volatile anesthetic–induced coronary vasodilation[278,345-348] is attenuated by glyburide, indicating an important role for K_{ATP} channels in this process. It is possible that the beneficial actions of APC may be partially attributed to increases in myocardial oxygen supply mediated by K_{ATP} channel–dependent coronary vasodilation. However, sevoflurane increases coronary collateral blood flow in the presence of glyburide in vivo, indicating that this volatile anesthetic may enhance coronary collateral blood flow independent of K_{ATP} channel activation.[349] Findings demonstrate that sevoflurane-induced increases in collateral perfusion occur as a result of activation of Ca^{2+}-regulated potassium (BK_{Ca}) and not K_{ATP} channels.[350] Isoflurane and sevoflurane directly activate mitochondrial K_{ATP} channels in isolated cardiac myocytes, and this action is linked to enhanced cell viability.[329] Based on these and other data collected from in vitro studies, it appears highly unlikely that myocardial protection produced by volatile anesthetics is solely related to favorable alterations in coronary vascular tone mediated by K_{ATP} channels.

Several receptor-mediated events and intracellular signaling elements that converge on the K_{ATP} channel have been implicated in APC. Pertussis toxin abolished reductions in infarct size produced by isoflurane (Fig. 7-21), indicating that inhibitory guanine (G_i) nucleotide–binding proteins are linked to the signal transduction pathways that mediate APC.[351] In contrast, pertussis toxin did not prevent the beneficial effects of direct K_{ATP} channel opening produced by nicorandil. These data strongly support the contention that volatile anesthetics modulate K_{ATP} channel activity through a second messenger.

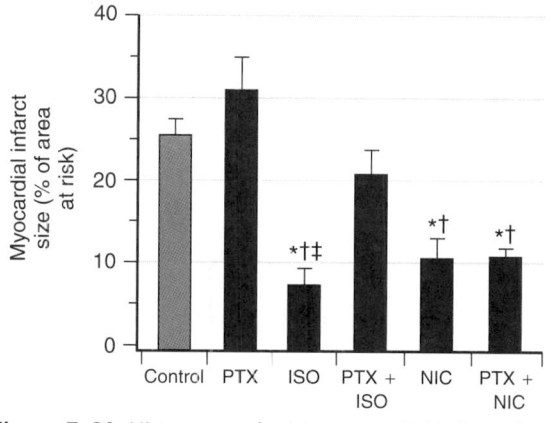

Figure 7–21 Histograms depict myocardial infarct size as a percentage of area at risk in dogs pretreated with vehicle (Control) or pertussis toxin (PTX) in the presence or absence of 1.0 minimum alveolar concentration of isoflurane (ISO) or nicorandil (NIC). *, Significantly ($P < .05$) different from the control; †, significantly ($P < .05$) different from PTX alone; ‡, significantly ($P < .05$) different from PTX plus ISO. (Adapted from Toller WG, Kersten JR, Gross ER, et al: Isoflurane preconditions myocardium against infarction via activation of inhibitory guanine (Gi) nucleotide binding proteins. Anesthesiology 92:1400-1407, 2000.)

Halothane-induced protection against infarction was completely abolished by blockade of the adenosine subtype 1 (A_1) receptor,[300] and a selective A_1-receptor antagonist (i.e., DPCPX) also partially attenuated the beneficial effects of isoflurane in stunned myocardium.[352] Isoflurane eliminated increases in interstitial adenosine during repetitive periods of coronary artery occlusion and reperfusion as demonstrated using a myocardial microdialysis technique.[352] These findings suggest that ATP preservation and a subsequent reduction of adenosine released into the interstitium occur during isoflurane anesthesia. The results are also very similar to findings during IPC[353] and pharmacologic preconditioning produced by bimakalim.[354] The results further indicate that volatile anesthetics may directly activate A_1-receptors or indirectly enhance A_1-receptor sensitivity to diminished endogenous adenosine concentrations.[352] The preservation of cardiac myocyte viability during ischemia produced by volatile anesthetics was also sensitive to adenosine receptor and G_i protein–mediated signaling blockade.[329] Additional findings indicated that the nonselective opioid antagonist naloxone abolishes isoflurane-induced preconditioning in the rat.[332] These intriguing data suggest an important link between volatile anesthetics and another family of G protein–coupled receptors. Evidence reveals that volatile agents competitively inhibited the ligand-binding site of G protein–coupled receptors.[355] APC appears to be associated with the activation of at least two separate receptor-mediated pathways (A_1 and δ_1-opioid) that are linked to G_i proteins.

IPC produces translocation and phosphorylation of several protein kinases, most importantly PKC, involved in signal transduction.[356-358] PKC is an essential component of the signaling pathway involved in protecting myocardium against cell death during ischemia and reperfusion.[359] The diverse PKC isoform family is a large group of serine-threonine protein kinases that are distinguished by variable regulatory domains and cofactors, and they have diverse tissue and species distributions.[360] Volatile anesthetics stimulate PKC translocation and activity,[361] possibly by interacting with the regulatory domain of the enzyme.[362] Inhibition of PKC attenuates isoflurane-induced augmentation of the functional recovery of stunned myocardium in dogs.[363] The beneficial actions of halothane are entirely blocked by selective PKC antagonism in rabbits.[300] Colchicine, a microtubule-depolymerizing drug, prevents isoflurane-induced reductions in myocardial infarct size in rabbits.[364] This interesting result suggests that an intact cytoskeleton may be essential for translocation of these protein kinases to occur. Volatile anesthetic–induced PKC translocation and activation appears to be required to open K_{ATP} channels and produce myocardial protection. For example, the nonselective PKC antagonist chelerythrine abolished sevoflurane-induced increases in mitochondrial K_{ATP} channel activity in rat ventricular myocytes[329] and prevented protection from ischemic damage. Patch-clamp experiments demonstrate that isoflurane enhanced K_{ATP} channel current in a whole-cell configuration concomitant with PKC stimulation.[337] These observations were supported by findings that adenosine and PKC enhance K_{ATP} channel activity during IPC.[343,365-368]

Reperfusion of ischemic myocardium is associated with the release of large quantities of reactive oxygen species (ROS)[369-372] that disrupt intracellular Ca^{2+} homeostasis, cause lipid peroxidation, damage cell membranes, depress contractility, and produce reversible and irreversible tissue injury. Halothane, isoflurane, and enflurane can attenuate the toxic effects of oxygen-derived free radicals on LV pressure development in isolated hearts.[308] Isoflurane decreased hydroxyl radical generation in the ischemic rat heart,[373] and halothane had a similar effect in dogs.[374] The protective effects of sevoflurane were associated with reduced dityrosine formation, an indirect marker of reactive oxygen and nitrogen species.[375] These results support the contention that volatile anesthetics may reduce the release of deleterious quantities of ROS immediately after coronary artery occlusion and reperfusion.

In contrast to the data implicating a pathologic role of large amounts of ROS, newer evidence strongly suggests that a variety of preconditioning stimuli, including brief ischemia, mitochondrial K_{ATP} channel openers, opioids, and volatile anesthetics, stimulate a small burst of ROS that paradoxically appears to initiate downstream signaling events and produce protection from subsequent ischemic injury. The beneficial actions of sevoflurane against ischemic damage were abolished by scavengers of superoxide anion and inhibition of nitric oxide synthase.[375] These results suggest that superoxide anion may act to trigger APC and indicate that nitric oxide may scavenge superoxide anion on reperfusion to reduce injury. ROS scavengers attenuated isoflurane-induced reductions in myocardial infarct size in rabbits.[376,377] Similarly, ROS inhibited the salutary effects of IPC[378,379] or mitochondrial K_{ATP} channel openers.[380] Isoflurane directly increases superoxide formation in vivo independent of ischemia and reperfusion.[377] Volatile anesthetics may be capable of producing small amounts of ROS that exert protective effects during subsequent ischemia. These data provide compelling evidence that small quantities of ROS play a critical role in APC.

Activation of mitochondrial K_{ATP} channels is associated with the ROS generation.[381] Mitochondrial K_{ATP} channel opening produced by selective agonists generated ROS that appeared to be essential for activation of MAP kinase[382] and the subsequent beneficial effects against ischemic injury.[383] Morphine increased the fluorescence intensity of the hydrogen peroxide–sensitive probe 2′,7′-dichlorofluorescin,[384] actions that were blocked by 5-HD. These data also demonstrate a link between activation of mitochondrial K_{ATP} channels by opioids and ROS production. Mitochondria have been hypothesized to be a source of ROS production,[379,385-388] but whether opening of mitochondrial K_{ATP} channels directly contributes to free radical generation remains unclear. Conversely, ROS may also modulate K_{ATP} channel activity.[389] Isoflurane-induced increases in ROS are abolished by the mitochondrial K_{ATP} channel antagonist 5-HD,[390] further suggesting a link between ROS generation and mitochondrial K_{ATP} channel activation during APC.

The identities of the ROS involved in IPC and APC and the signaling pathways that are modulated by these free radicals also remain unclear. ROS have been shown to activate PKC, restore contractility, and limit the extent of myocardial infarction in rabbit hearts.[391] Hydrogen peroxide stimulates tyrosine kinase–dependent activation of phospholipase C in mouse embryonic fibroblasts, rendering these cells resistant to stress.[392] ROS may also directly stimulate PKC activity[393] or indirectly enhance the activity of the enzyme by activation of PLC.[392] Hydrogen peroxide activates G_i and G_o proteins,[394,395] as well as other protein kinases involved in reducing cellular injury.[396,397] Hydrogen peroxide may also be converted to more reactive species that subsequently modify cysteine residues specific to $G_{\alpha i}$ and $G_{\alpha o}$ and selectively activate these proteins.[395] A strong possibility exists that volatile anesthetic–induced production of ROS may directly activate several intracellular mediators of endogenous protection against ischemic injury. However, this tantalizing hypothesis requires further investigation.

Coronary Vascular Effects of Volatile Anesthetics in Humans

Evaluation of the actions of volatile anesthetics on the human coronary circulation is difficult because the methods used to determine coronary blood flow in humans are limited and because the interpretation of clinical findings during anesthesia is complicated by changes in hemodynamics, the impact of surgery, and the use of adjuvant anesthetics or vasoactive drugs. Halothane decreases MVo_2[62,398] and variably alters coronary blood flow in patients with coronary artery disease, but metabolic or electrocardiographic evidence of ischemia has not been observed during halothane anesthesia.[62,398-400] Coronary blood flow may be reduced by halothane or enflurane[401] in some patients concomitant with decreases in MVo_2, but simultaneous declines in oxygen extraction[62,401] reflect relative coronary vasodilation.

In 1983, a report by Reiz and colleagues[63] described the occurrence of myocardial ischemia as indicated by new electrocardiographic changes and abnormal myocardial lactate extraction in 10 of 21 patients anesthetized with isoflurane undergoing major vascular surgery. Five patients were treated with phenylephrine and pacing to return arterial pressure and heart rate to control values, and after these interventions, electrocardiographic and metabolic derangements resolved in two of five patients. Despite the apparent dependence of these new episodes of myocardial ischemia on alterations in systemic hemodynamics, the investigators[63] proposed that isoflurane had caused coronary steal in these patients, even though no specific evidence of blood flow redistribution between normal and collateral-dependent zones was presented. The data of Reiz and colleagues[63] have not been uniformly supported by subsequent studies. Coronary blood flow remains unchanged during isoflurane anesthesia in patients undergoing coronary artery bypass graft (CABG) surgery, but coronary sinus oxygen content increases consistent with modest coronary vasodilation.[402-404] Isoflurane alone does not produce electrocardiographic or metabolic evidence of ischemia.[403] Instead, myocardial ischemia occurring during isoflurane anesthesia is most often associated with tachycardia or hypotension.[64,399,402,404] Isoflurane increases the tolerance to pacing-induced ischemia in patients with coronary artery disease.[405] Comparisons of studies examining the effects of isoflurane on the incidence of intraoperative myocardial ischemia are complicated by differences in patient age, surgical procedure, operative time, and preoperative LV ejection fraction.[406,407] Compelling evidence demonstrating redistribution of coronary blood flow away from ischemic to normal myocardium in humans anesthetized with isoflurane has yet to appear.

The incidence of intraoperative myocardial ischemia in susceptible patients has been difficult to define. Less than 50% of intraoperative ischemic episodes have been linked to alterations in systemic hemodynamics.[408-411] The strongest predictor of intraoperative ischemia remains preexisting ischemia on arrival to the operating room and not anesthetic technique.[408,410] The only hemodynamic event definitively related to intraoperative ischemia in patients undergoing CABG surgery is tachycardia.[410] Evidence[412,413] advocating the perioperative use of β_1-adrenoceptor antagonists to prevent myocardial ischemia strongly supports this contention. Sternotomy causes greater increases in calculated indices of MVO_2,[414] myocardial lactate production,[415] and the incidence of hypertension requiring treatment with vasoactive drugs[415] during morphine compared with halothane anesthesia. In contrast, induction of anesthesia with desflurane in patients undergoing coronary artery bypass surgery may be associated with tachycardia, hypertension, and a greater incidence of ischemia than that occurring during induction with sufentanil.[416] Steal-prone anatomy has been identified in 23% of patients with coronary artery disease enrolled in the Coronary Artery Surgery Study.[417] However, patients with steal-prone coronary anatomy do not have a greater incidence of ischemia during desflurane anesthesia compared with other forms of coronary artery disease.[416] The incidences of myocardial ischemia and adverse cardiac outcomes have been similar for cardiac patients undergoing noncardiac surgery during sevoflurane compared with isoflurane anesthesia.[418] New electrocardiographic changes, incidence of postoperative myocardial infarction, and mortality rates are similar for patients undergoing CABG surgery independent of anesthetic technique[409-411,414-416,419-421] or the presence of steal-prone anatomy.[421] Despite the findings that volatile anesthetics are mild coronary vasodilators, these agents do not cause abnormal redistribution of myocardial perfusion resulting in ischemia when tachycardia and hypotension are avoided.

Myocardial Protection by Volatile Anesthetics in Humans

APC occurs in human myocardium, but evaluation of this process in patients is complicated by simultaneous alterations in systemic and coronary hemodynamics; the use of other anesthetics, analgesics, or vasoactive drugs; preexisting disease states; and the influence of surgery on cardiovascular homeostasis. Isoflurane[335] and desflurane[422] enhanced the recovery of contractile function of human atrial trabeculae by adenosine receptor stimulation and K_{ATP} channel activation. A role for adenosine receptors, MAP kinases,[334] and ROS[423] has been previously demonstrated in other forms of preconditioning in human atrial myocytes concomitant with mitochondrial K_{ATP} channel opening. Isoflurane decreased postoperative release of troponin I and creatine kinase-MB in patients undergoing CABG surgery, suggesting a reduction in the severity of myocardial necrosis.[424] Administration of enflurane before cardioplegic arrest also enhanced postischemic contractile functional recovery in CABG patients.[425] Sevoflurane, but not the intravenous anesthetic propofol, was shown to preserve myocardial function in patients undergoing CABG concomitant with a reduction in troponin I release.[426] These compelling data emphasize that volatile anesthetics may exert beneficial effects against ischemic injury in humans. Volatile anesthetics may represent an important therapeutic modality to reduce the risk of perioperative myocardial ischemia and infarction,[427] although this conclusion has yet to be confirmed in a large-scale, randomized, clinical trial.

VOLATILE ANESTHETICS AND NEURAL CONTROL OF THE CIRCULATION

Volatile anesthetics depress baroreceptor reflex control of arterial pressure in experimental animals to various degrees.[198,428-435] This inhibition of baroreceptor reflex activity occurs as a result of depression of central nervous system integration of afferent baroreceptor input, attenuation of efferent autonomic nervous system activity, and reductions in ganglionic transmission and end-organ response.[198,431,436,437] Volatile anesthetics increase resting afferent nerve traffic and enhance the sensitivity of arterial baroreceptors by a Ca^{2+}-dependent mechanism.[431,436,438]

These anesthetic-induced increases in baroreceptor sensitivity and discharge frequency tonically reduce overall sympathetic nervous system activity and attenuate sympathetic responses to declines in arterial pressure.[439]

Halothane, enflurane, and isoflurane (Fig. 7-22) inhibit preganglionic sympathetic efferent activity at clinically relevant concentrations in vivo.[431,433-436] Volatile agents reduce postganglionic sympathetic nerve activity.[431,436] Postsynaptic nicotinic receptors in the stellate ganglion are also blocked by halothane.[440,441] These findings indicate that attenuation of ganglionic transmission represents a major mechanism by which volatile agents depress sympathetic nerve traffic.[442] Depression of sympathetic outflow caused by volatile anesthetics has also been suggested by examination of endogenous plasma norepinephrine kinetics.[443,444] Halothane, isoflurane, and enflurane decrease plasma concentrations of norepinephrine to various degrees by causing a more pronounced reductions in norepinephrine spillover than clearance.[443,444] Halothane-induced reductions in norepinephrine release from postganglionic sympathetic nerves[445] may also contribute to depression of reflex vasoconstriction in peripheral blood vessels observed with this agent.[446] Volatile anesthetics also attenuate parasympathetic nervous system function. Halothane depresses vagal nerve efferent activity by direct measurement of parasympathetic nerve activity.[435] These findings are supported by the results of several other studies demonstrating that volatile anesthetics inhibit reflex bradycardia in response to increases in arterial pressure.[428,431,436,447] Parasympathetic and sympathetic nervous system outflows appear to be depressed to equivalent degrees during halothane[436,447,448] or isoflurane anesthesia.[431]

The effects of volatile anesthetics on neural control of the cardiovascular system have been incompletely examined in healthy humans and have not been described in patients with autonomic nervous system dysfunction. Halothane[174] and enflurane[449] produce greater attenuation of baroreceptor reflex regulation of heart rate than equi-MACs of isoflurane.[175] Depression of baroreceptor function by these volatile agents may be more profound compared with fentanyl, diazepam, and nitrous oxide anesthesia.[450] Baroreceptor-mediated control of peripheral vascular resistance is also attenuated in young volunteers during halothane anesthesia.[178] Steady-state anesthetic concentrations of sevoflurane have been shown to cause greater depression of sympathetic nerve activity measured directly with microneurography than desflurane at equivalent levels of hypotension.[188] These findings parallel results demonstrating pronounced sympathetic hyperactivity during rapid increases in inspired desflurane concentration in humans (Fig. 7-23).[42,44] The actions of volatile anesthetics on baroreceptor reflex control of the circulation may be profoundly altered during autonomic dysfunction in elderly patients[451] or in those with essential hypertension, diabetes mellitus, or heart failure.[452] Further investigation is required to test these hypotheses.

NITROUS OXIDE AND CARDIOVASCULAR FUNCTION

Myocardial Contractility and Left Ventricular Diastolic Function

Experiments in papillary muscle[453-455] and isolated heart preparations[240] have consistently demonstrated that nitrous oxide produces a direct negative inotropic effect. Conflicting results about the influence of nitrous oxide on contractility have been observed in experimental animals and healthy volunteers. Several problems have contributed to apparently contradictory results in vivo. Observed changes in contractile function may be influenced by the actions of nitrous oxide on the systemic circulation or by autonomic nervous system reflex effects[456,457] because nitrous oxide may increase sympathetic nervous system tone.[458-460] Studies using nitrous oxide alone are difficult to perform and interpret because this gas does not produce total anesthesia at partial pressures less than 1 atmosphere.[461-466] The effects of nitrous oxide on contractile function may be influenced by different baseline anesthetics.[467-473] Lack of use of load-insensitive measures of myocardial contractility has allowed only qualitative assessment of the effects of nitrous oxide on intrinsic inotropic state in the intact heart.

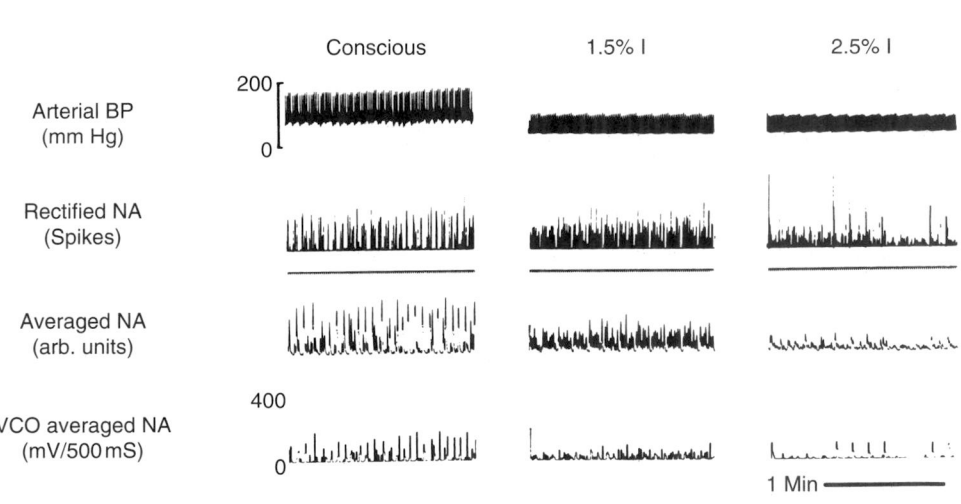

Figure 7–22 Baseline renal sympathetic efferent nerve activity (NA) and arterial blood pressure (BP) recorded in a conscious and isoflurane (I)–anesthetized dog (at 1.5% and 2.5% inspired concentrations). Nerve activity was depressed with the 2.5% inspired isoflurane. (Adapted from Seagard JL, Elegbe EO, Hopp FA, et al: Effects of isoflurane on baroreceptor reflex. Anesthesiology 59:511-520, 1983.)

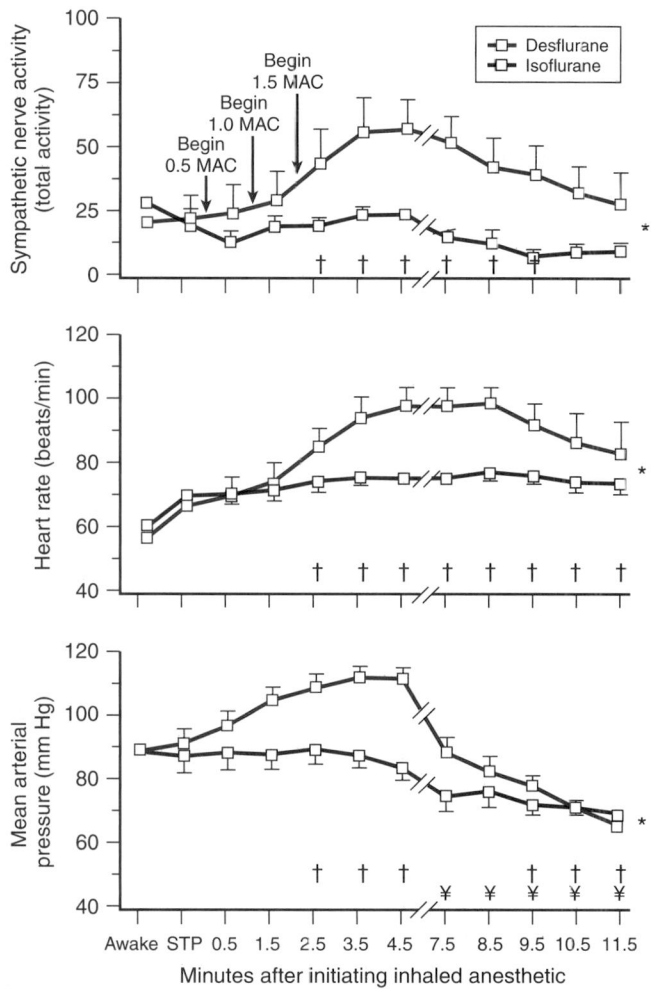

Figure 7–23 Effects of desflurane *(red squares)* and isoflurane *(black squares)* on sympathetic nerve activity *(top)*, heart rate *(middle)*, and mean arterial pressure *(bottom)* in healthy volunteers. Desflurane or isoflurane administration began 2 minutes after anesthetic induction with sodium thiopental (STP). Sympathetic nerve excitation, tachycardia, and hypertension were observed in subjects receiving desflurane. *, Different *(P < .05)* group response; †, desflurane response different *(P < .05)* from STP value; ¥, isoflurane response different *(P < .05)* from STP value. (Adapted from Ebert TJ, Muzi M: Sympathetic hyperactivity during desflurane anesthesia in healthy volunteers: A comparison with isoflurane. Anesthesiology 79:444-453, 1993.)

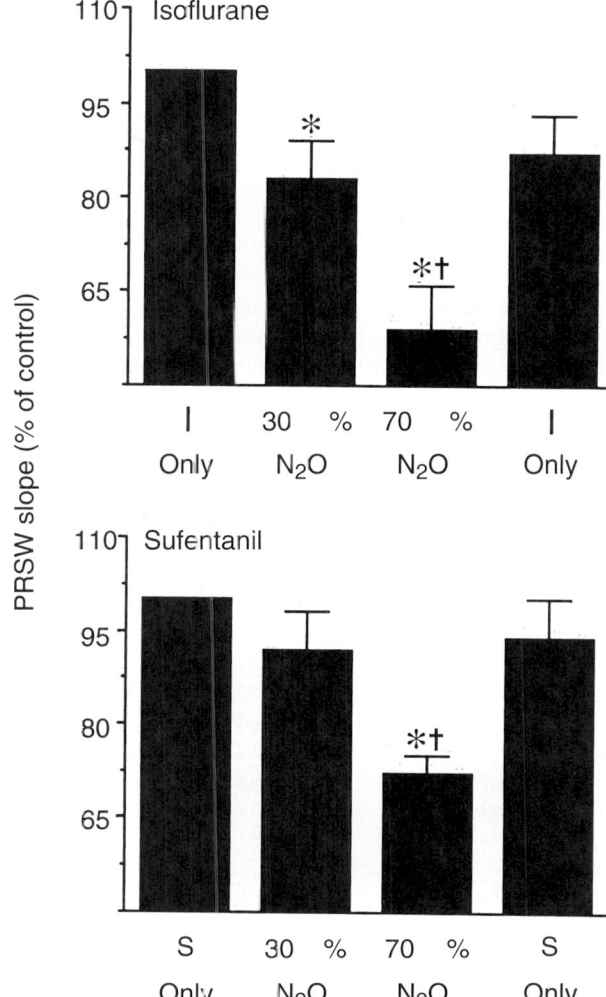

Figure 7–24 Effects of nitrous oxide (N_2O) on the preload recruitable stroke work (PRSW) slope in the presence of isoflurane (I, *top panel*) and sufentanil (S, *bottom panel*) are shown as a percentage of the control (I or S only, respectively). *, Significantly *(P < .05)* different from I or S only; †, significantly *(P < .05)* different from I or S plus 30% nitrous oxide. (Adapted from Pagel PS, Kampine JP, Schmeling WT, Warltier DC: Effects of nitrous oxide on myocardial contractility as evaluated by the preload recruitable stroke work relationship in chronically instrumented dogs. Anesthesiology 73:1148-1157, 1990.)

The regional PRSW relationship demonstrated that nitrous oxide depresses myocardial contractility in dogs anesthetized with isoflurane or sufentanil in the absence of autonomic nervous system activity (Fig. 7-24).[474] Seventy percent nitrous oxide decreased the PRSW slope (M_w) by 28% and 41% during sufentanil and isoflurane anesthesia, respectively. These results indicate that 70% nitrous oxide decreased contractility to approximately the same extent as 1 MAC of isoflurane. Similar findings have been reported using LV end-systolic pressure-dimension relationships in acutely instrumented dogs.[473] These nitrous oxide–induced myocardial depressant effects may be offset by concomitant increases in sympathetic nervous system tone.[459] The negative inotropic actions of

nitrous oxide may be more pronounced in the presence of preexisting LV dysfunction.[475] Nitrous oxide–induced depression of contractile function appears to overcome the mild sympathomimetic effect of this anesthetic gas in patients with coronary artery[465,470,471,476-478] or valvular heart[465,479] disease because increases in baseline sympathetic nervous system activity cannot be further augmented by nitrous oxide in these clinical conditions.

The actions of nitrous oxide on LV diastolic function have been incompletely studied. Modest increases in maximal lengthening velocity and maximal rate of decline of force have been observed in ferret papillary muscle concomitant with decreases in contractile state.[455] No changes in the rate of isometric or isotonic relaxation were observed, indicating that nitrous oxide does not substantially modify myocardial relaxation.[455] Nitrous oxide can modestly increase segmental indices of LV chamber compliance and reduce early LV filling in acutely instrumented dogs.[480] These findings are supported by evidence indicating that nitrous oxide may produce LV diastolic dysfunction after cardiopulmonary bypass in patients undergoing CABG surgery.[478]

Nitrous oxide causes dose-related reductions in the intracellular Ca^{2+} transient in vitro.[455,481] This finding indicates that nitrous oxide–induced depression of myocardial contractility is related to decreases in Ca^{2+} availability for contractile activation. Nitrous oxide does not affect myofibrillar sensitivity to Ca^{2+}[455,482] or Ca^{2+} uptake and release from the SR.[482] The diastolic Ca^{2+} transient is unaffected by nitrous oxide, suggesting that this anesthetic gas does not alter myocardial relaxation kinetics.[481]

Hemodynamics

Assessment of the hemodynamic effects of nitrous oxide in humans is often complicated by concomitant administration of volatile anesthetics, opioids, or other anesthetic adjuvants in the presence or absence of cardiovascular disease. Typical clinical concentrations of nitrous oxide (e.g., 40% to 70%) cause modest increases in heart rate in healthy volunteers.[461,483] Small increases in heart rate also occur when hyperbaric concentrations of nitrous oxide are administered[484] or when this anesthetic gas is added to volatile anesthetics.[485] Declines in heart rate have been observed with nitrous oxide in patients with coronary artery disease anesthetized with isoflurane[194] or halothane.[486] Modest reductions in heart rate have been also reported in patients anesthetized with morphine or fentanyl undergoing cardiac surgery.[465,470,471] Sixty-percent nitrous oxide causes small increases in arterial pressure in humans.[483] Increases in arterial pressure also occur under hyperbaric conditions[484] or during halothane anesthesia in volunteers,[457,467] consistent with a mild sympathomimetic effect. Other studies have also indicated that partial substitution of nitrous oxide for a volatile anesthetic does not affect or modestly increases arterial pressure during enflurane,[472] isoflurane,[469] or desflurane[180] anesthesia in experiments conducted at a constant MAC. In contrast, reductions in arterial pressure have been observed in patients with coronary artery disease receiving nitrous oxide in the presence and absence of opioids.[470,476,487]

Small increases in cardiac output and stroke volume have been observed during administration of 60% nitrous oxide in oxygen in volunteers.[483] However, cardiac output remains unchanged in the presence of hyperbaric nitrous oxide.[484] Cardiac output is greater in volunteers anesthetized with halothane and nitrous oxide than in those receiving halothane alone,[467] concomitant with increases in sympathetic nervous system tone. The addition of nitrous oxide to enflurane, isoflurane, or desflurane anesthesia also modestly increased cardiac output.[37,38,469,472] In contrast, nitrous oxide reduces cardiac output and stroke volume in healthy volunteers[488] and patients with cardiac disease receiving opioids.[465,470,471,486,487] Hyperbaric nitrous oxide (1.5 MAC) caused a modest reduction in systemic vascular resistance.[484] In contrast, systemic vascular resistance is higher during volatile anesthesia in the presence compared with the absence of nitrous oxide.[37,38,467,469,472] Pretreatment with the ganglionic blocker hexamethonium attenuated the relative increase in systemic vascular resistance observed during administration of halothane and nitrous oxide,[457] findings that may be consistent with a reduction in sympathetic nervous system tone. Nitrous oxide–induced increases in systemic vascular resistance have also been reported in volunteers and patients with cardiac disease anesthetized with opioids.[465,488,489]

Nitrous oxide increases venous tone and decreases venous capacitance in conscious volunteers.[461] This anesthetic gas also modestly increases pulmonary artery pressures and pulmonary vascular resistance in patients with coronary artery disease anesthetized with morphine and diazepam[470] or halothane.[490] The combined effects of enhanced venous return, elevated pulmonary vascular resistance, and depressed contractile function probably contribute to the increases in central venous pressure observed with nitrous oxide in humans. Hyperbaric nitrous oxide also enhances central venous pressure in association with increases in pulmonary vascular resistance.[484] Nitrous oxide inhibits norepinephrine uptake by the lung, and subsequent increases in plasma norepinephrine levels detected in the pulmonary vasculature may be partially responsible for the characteristic increases in pulmonary vascular resistance observed during administration of this agent.[491] Nitrous oxide–induced increases in pulmonary vascular resistance may be more pronounced in adults with pulmonary hypertension[490,492] and children with increased pulmonary blood flow.[493] Elevations in pulmonary artery pressures and vascular resistance have also been described during administration of nitrous oxide in neonatal lambs.[494] Such increases in pulmonary vascular resistance may adversely enhance right-to-left atrial or ventricular shunts and compromise arterial oxygenation in patients with congenital heart disease.[495]

NITROUS OXIDE AND CARDIAC ELECTROPHYSIOLOGY

Reversible atrioventricular dissociation has been reported in humans anesthetized with nitrous oxide and volatile or opioid-based anesthetics.[496] Addition of nitrous oxide to halothane anesthesia lowers the threshold at which arrhythmias occur.[497] This observation may result from a combination of sympathetic nervous system stimulation by nitrous oxide and myocardial sensitization by halothane.[498] The incidence of arrhythmias is reduced during combined nitrous oxide–opioid anesthesia compared with halothane anesthesia alone.[499]

NITROUS OXIDE AND THE CORONARY CIRCULATION

Nitrous oxide does not produce direct effects on the coronary vasculature in vitro.[239,500,501] This anesthetic gas alters coronary blood flow concomitant with changes in MVO_2 in dogs.[502,503] Nitrous oxide decreases myocardial segment shortening,[504,505] increases post-systolic shortening,[506] and redistributes transmural coronary blood flow preferentially to the subepicardium (i.e., decreased endo/epi)[505] in experimental models of coronary artery disease. Nitrous oxide also decreases the recovery of contractile function of stunned myocardium.[507] Nitrous oxide–induced sympathetic nervous system activation and imbalances of myocardial oxygen supply and MVO_2 represent potential mechanisms by which this anesthetic gas further delays contractile recovery of stunned myocardium.[508] In the presence of a volatile anesthetic, nitrous oxide decreases MVO_2 and myocardial oxygen extraction[195,486] and may exacerbate myocardial ischemia during concomitant reductions in arterial pressure in patients with coronary artery disease.[194] However, later studies demonstrated that the addition of nitrous oxide to volatile or opioid anesthetics did not increase the incidence of new regional wall motion abnormalities as assessed by transesophageal echocardiography.[195,509]

NITROUS OXIDE AND NEURAL CONTROL OF THE CIRCULATION

Nitrous oxide causes pupillary dilation, diaphoresis, and increases in systemic vascular resistance, central blood volume, and forearm vascular resistance in volunteers during halothane anesthesia,[457] suggesting that nitrous oxide activates the sympathetic nervous system. A subsequent study demonstrated that nitrous oxide does increase sympathetic nerve traffic measured using sympathetic microneurography in human volunteers,[459] especially during the first 15 to 30 minutes of exposure to this anesthetic gas. Although baroreceptor reflex–mediated control of heart rate is impaired during administration of nitrous oxide, regulation of sympathetic outflow to peripheral blood vessels is preserved.[458] This finding suggests nitrous oxide does not alter sympathetic vasoconstrictor-induced maintenance of arterial pressure and may be partially responsible for the relative stability of hemodynamics during nitrous oxide anesthesia.

XENON

The anesthetic properties of the noble gas xenon were first described more than 50 years ago.[510] Xenon has a blood gas partition coefficient less than that of nitrous oxide,[511] does not undergo biotransformation,[512] provides rapid induction and emergence from anesthesia,[513-515] and exerts analgesic effects[516] independent of α_2-adrenergic and opioid receptors.[517] Despite these advantageous properties, xenon has not been routinely used for clinical anesthesia in the United States because it is more expensive than nitrous oxide and volatile anesthetics. More efficient manufacturing techniques and development of low-flow administration and recycling systems have reduced the cost of xenon and rekindled interest in its clinical use.[514,518,519] Many of these issues are succinctly summarized in an excellent review by Lynch and colleagues.[520]

Xenon causes minimal systemic and pulmonary hemodynamic effects in vivo,[513,514,521-523] preserves[513] or very modestly reduces[524] myocardial contractility, and attenuates alterations in hemodynamics and increases in plasma epinephrine and cortisol concentrations associated with surgical stimulation.[521,525,526] Xenon did not alter cardiac function or major ion currents in isolated guinea pig hearts and ventricular myocytes.[527] Similar findings were observed in isolated human atrial myocytes.[528] Xenon exerted modest cardioprotective effects when administered during early reperfusion after regional myocardial ischemia in rabbit hearts.[529] However, the mechanisms responsible for this protective effect are unclear based on data indicating that xenon does not affect the amplitudes of Na^+, L-type Ca^{2+} and inward-rectifier K^- channels in whole-cell patch-clamped myocytes.[527] The effects of xenon on systemic hemodynamics, LV systolic and diastolic function, and the determinants of LV afterload have also been examined in chronically instrumented dogs before and after the development of rapid LV pacing-induced cardiomyopathy.[530] Xenon was remarkably devoid of hemodynamic effects in normal and cardiomyopathic dogs anesthetized with isoflurane. Xenon did not alter isoflurane-induced reductions in the PRSW slope (M_w) in the presence and absence of pacing-induced LV dysfunction (Fig. 7-25). Xenon caused greater increases in the time constant of isovolumic relaxation in isoflurane-anesthetized, cardiomyopathic dogs compared with normal dogs, but indices of early LV filling and chamber compliance remained unchanged, suggesting that xenon does not appreciably influence LV diastolic function during isoflurane anesthesia. Xenon also produced relatively minor alterations in the determinants of LV afterload in dogs before and after pacing. Taken together, these data indicate that xenon produces very subtle cardiovascular effects during isoflurane anesthesia in dogs with and without experimental dilated cardiomyopathy.[530] A level of 56% xenon (end-tidal concentration) depressed sympathetic and parasympathetic nervous system transmission to a greater extent than 0.8 MAC of isoflurane in healthy patients undergoing elective surgery.[531]

SUMMARY

Volatile anesthetics exert profound effects on the cardiovascular system by altering the inotropic, chronotropic, dromotropic, and lusitropic state of the heart. These agents also have significant actions on the preload and afterload systems. The pharmacologic effects cause dramatic changes in hemodynamics that may be accentuated in patients with underlying cardiovascular disease. Less profound but equally important effects are observed with nitrous oxide and xenon. Some of the volatile anesthetics have been shown to be cardioprotective, directly reducing the sequelae of ischemia and reperfusion injury. The use of inhalational anesthetics requires clear understanding of their complex cardiovascular pharmacology.

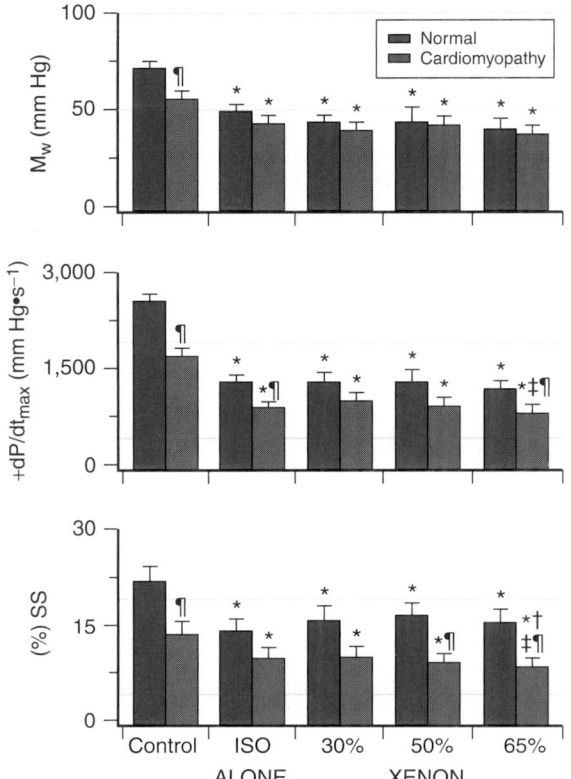

Figure 7–25 Histograms show the effects of isoflurane (ISO) and xenon on the preload recruitable stroke work slope (M_W, *top panel*), the peak rate of increase of left ventricular pressure (+dP/dt$_{max}$, *middle panel*), and percent segment shortening (%SS, *bottom panel*) in normal *(red bars)* and cardiomyopathic *(gray bars)* dogs receiving 1.5 minimum alveolar concentration (MAC) of isoflurane in the presence and absence of 30%, 50%, and 65% xenon. *, Significantly ($P < .05$) different from control; †, significantly ($P < .05$) different from ISO alone; ‡, significantly ($P < .05$) different from ISO and 30% xenon; ¶, significantly ($P < .05$) different from the corresponding value in normal dogs.

KEY POINTS

1. Volatile anesthetics produce dose-related depression of LV, RV, and LA myocardial contractility, LV diastolic function, and LV-arterial coupling in the normal heart.
2. Negative inotropic effects of volatile anesthetics are related to alterations in intracellular Ca^{2+} homeostasis within the cardiac myocyte.
3. Volatile anesthetics affect the determinants of LV afterload to varying degrees in the presence of normal and dysfunctional myocardium.
4. Systemic hemodynamic effects of volatile anesthetics are complex and determined by the interaction of myocardial effects, direct actions on the arterial and venous vasculature, and alterations in autonomic nervous system activity.

5. Volatile anesthetics sensitize myocardium to the arrhythmogenic effects of epinephrine to varying degrees and may prevent or facilitate the development of atrial or ventricular arrhythmias during myocardial ischemia or infarction, depending upon the concentration of the agent, the extent of the injury, and the location affected within the conduction pathway.
6. Volatile anesthetics are relatively weak coronary vasodilators that are not capable of producing coronary steal at typically used clinical concentrations, even in patients with steal-prone coronary anatomy.
7. Volatile anesthetics exert important cardioprotective effects against reversible and irreversible myocardial ischemia in experimental animals and humans by activating intracellular signal transduction pathways involving A_1 receptors, PKC, G_i proteins, mitochondrial or sarcolemmal K_{ATP} channels, and ROS.
8. Volatile agents depress baroreceptor reflex control of arterial pressure to varying degrees.
9. Nitrous oxide causes direct negative inotropic effects, does not substantially affect LV diastolic function, and produces modest increases in pulmonary and systemic arterial pressure via a sympathomimetic effect. These actions are dependent to some degree upon the baseline anesthetic.
10. Xenon is essentially devoid of cardiovascular effects.

REFERENCES

1. Pagel PS, Warltier DC: Anesthetics and left ventricular function. *In* Warltier DC (ed): Ventricular function. Baltimore, Williams & Wilkins, 1995, pp 213-252.
2. Goldberg AH, Ullrick WC: Effects of halothane on isometric contractions of isolated heart muscle. Anesthesiology 28:838-845, 1967.
3. Sugai N, Shimosato S, Etsten BE: Effect of halothane on force-velocity relations and dynamic stiffness of isolated heart muscle. Anesthesiology 29:267-274, 1968.
4. Shimosato S, Li TH, Etsten B: Ventricular function during halothane anesthesia in closed chest dog. Circ Res 12:63-75, 1963.
5. Deutsch S, Linde HW, Dripps RD, Price HL: Circulatory and respiratory actions of halothane in normal man. Anesthesiology 23:631-638, 1962.
6. Eger EI II, Smith NT, Stoelting RK, et al: Cardiovascular effects of halothane in man. Anesthesiology 32:396-409, 1970.
7. Severinghaus JW, Cullen SC: Depression of myocardium and body oxygen consumption with Fluothane. Anesthesiology 19:165-177, 1958.
8. Sonntag H, Donath U, Hillebrand W, et al: Left ventricular function in conscious man and during halothane anesthesia. Anesthesiology 48:320-324, 1978.
9. Shimosato S, Sugai N, Iwatsuki N, Etsten BE: The effect of Ethrane on cardiac muscle mechanics. Anesthesiology 30:513-518, 1969.
10. Kemmotsu O, Hashimoto Y, Shimosato S: Inotropic effects of isoflurane on mechanics of contraction in isolated cat papillary muscles from normal and failing hearts. Anesthesiology 39:470-477, 1973.

11. Calverley RK, Smith NT, Prys-Roberts C, et al: Cardiovascular effects of enflurane anesthesia during controlled ventilation in man. Anesth Analg 57:619-628, 1978.
12. Stevens WC, Cromwell TH, Halsey MJ, et al: The cardiovascular effects of a new inhalation anesthetic, Forane, in human volunteers at constant arterial carbon dioxide tension. Anesthesiology 35:8-16, 1971.
13. Horan BF, Prys-Roberts C, Hamilton WK, Roberts JG: Haemodynamic responses to enflurane anaesthesia and hypovolaemia in the dog, and their modification by propranolol. Br J Anaesth 49:1189-1197, 1977.
14. Merin RG, Kumazawa T, Luka NL: Myocardial function and metabolism in the conscious dog and during halothane anesthesia. Anesthesiology 44:402-415, 1976.
15. Merin RG, Kumazawa T, Luka NL: Enflurane depresses myocardial function, perfusion, and metabolism in the dog. Anesthesiology 45:501-507, 1976.
16. Pagel PS, Kampine JP, Schmeling WT, Warltier DC: Comparison of the systemic and coronary hemodynamic actions of desflurane, isoflurane, halothane, and enflurane in the chronically instrumented dog. Anesthesiology 74:539-551, 1991.
17. Van Trigt P, Christian CC, Fagraeus L, et al: The mechanism of halothane-induced myocardial depression: Altered diastolic mechanics versus impaired contractility. J Thorac Cardiovasc Surg 85:832-838, 1983.
18. Horan BF, Prys-Roberts C, Roberts JG, et al: Haemodynamic responses to isoflurane anaesthesia and hypovolaemia in the dog, and their modification by propranolol. Br J Anaesth 49:1179-1187, 1977.
19. Merin RG: Are the myocardial functional and metabolic effects of isoflurane really different from those of halothane and enflurane? Anesthesiology 55:398-408, 1981.
20. Pagel PS, Kampine JP, Schmeling WT, Warltier DC: Comparison of end-systolic pressure-length relations and preload recruitable stroke work as indices of myocardial contractility in the conscious and anesthetized, chronically instrumented dog. Anesthesiology 73:278-290, 1990.
21. Pagel PS, Nijhawan N, Warltier DC: Quantitation of volatile anesthetic-induced depression of myocardial contractility using a single beat index derived from maximal ventricular power. J Cardiothorac Vasc Anesth 7:688-695, 1993.
22. Graves CL, McDermott RW, Bidwai A: Cardiovascular effects of isoflurane in surgical patients. Anesthesiology 41:486-489, 1974.
23. Tarnow J, Bruckner JB, Eberlein HJ, et al: Haemodynamics and myocardial oxygen consumption during isoflurane (Forane) anaesthesia in geriatric patients. Br J Anaesth 48:669-675, 1976.
24. Hysing ES, Chelly JE, Jacobson L, et al: Cardiovascular effects of acute changes in extracellular ionized calcium concentration induced by citrate and $CaCl_2$ infusions in chronically instrumented dogs, conscious and during enflurane, halothane, and isoflurane anesthesia. Anesthesiology 72:100-104, 1990.
25. Makela VHM, Kapur PA: Amrinone and verapamil-propranolol induced cardiac depression during isoflurane anesthesia in dogs. Anesthesiology 66:792-797, 1987.
26. Merin RG, Chelly JE, Hysing ES, et al: Cardiovascular effects of and interaction between calcium blocking drugs and anesthetics in chronically instrumented dogs. IV. Chronically administered oral verapamil and halothane, enflurane, and isoflurane. Anesthesiology 66:140-146, 1987.
27. Pagel PS, Hettrick DA, Warltier DC: Left ventricular mechanical consequences of dihydropyridine calcium channel modulation in conscious and anesthetized chronically instrumented dogs. Anesthesiology 81:190-208, 1994.
28. Denlinger JK, Kaplan JA, Lecky JH, Wollman H: Cardiovascular responses to calcium administered intravenously to man during halothane anesthesia. Anesthesiology 42:390-397, 1975.
29. Price HL: Calcium reverses myocardial depression caused by halothane: Site of action. Anesthesiology 41:576-579, 1974.
30. Pagel PS, Kampine JP, Schmeling WT, Warltier DC: Reversal of volatile anesthetic-induced depression of myocardial contractility by extracellular calcium also enhances left ventricular diastolic function. Anesthesiology 78:141-154, 1993.
31. Makela VHM, Kapur PA: Amrinone blunts cardiac depression caused by enflurane or isoflurane anesthesia in the dog. Anesth Analg 66:215-221, 1987.
32. Pagel PS, Hettrick DA, Warltier DC: Amrinone enhances myocardial contractility and improves left ventricular diastolic function in conscious and anesthetized chronically instrumented dogs. Anesthesiology 79:753-765, 1993.
33. Pagel PS, Harkin CP, Hettrick DA, Warltier DC: Levosimendan (OR-1259), a myofilament calcium sensitizer, enhances myocardial contractility but does not alter isovolumic relaxation in conscious and anesthetized dogs. Anesthesiology 81:974-987, 1994.
34. Eger EI II: New inhaled anesthetics. Anesthesiology 80:906-922, 1994.
35. Merin RG, Bernard JM, Doursout MF, et al: Comparison of the effects of isoflurane and desflurane on cardiovascular dynamics and regional blood flow in the chronically instrumented dog. Anesthesiology 74:568-574, 1991.
36. Weiskopf RB, Holmes MA, Eger EI II, et al: Cardiovascular effects of I653 in swine. Anesthesiology 69:303-309, 1988.
37. Weiskopf RB, Cahalan MK, Eger EI II, et al: Cardiovascular actions of desflurane in normocarbic volunteers. Anesth Analg 73:143-156, 1991.
38. Cahalan MK, Weiskopf RB, Eger EI II, et al: Hemodynamic effects of desflurane/nitrous oxide anesthesia in volunteers. Anesth Analg 73:157-164, 1991.
39. Pagel PS, Kampine JP, Schmeling WT, Warltier DC: Influence of volatile anesthetics on myocardial contractility in vivo: Desflurane versus isoflurane. Anesthesiology 74:900-907, 1991.
40. Pagel PS, Kampine JP, Schmeling WT, Warltier DC: Evaluation of myocardial contractility in the chronically instrumented dog with intact autonomic nervous system function: Effects of desflurane and isoflurane. Acta Anaesthesiol Scand 37:203-210, 1993.
41. Hettrick DA, Pagel PS, Warltier DC: Desflurane, sevoflurane, and isoflurane impair canine left ventricular-arterial coupling and mechanical efficiency. Anesthesiology 85:403-413, 1996.
42. Ebert TJ, Muzi M: Sympathetic hyperactivity during desflurane anesthesia in healthy volunteers: A comparison with isoflurane. Anesthesiology 79:444-453, 1993.
43. Weiskopf RB, Eger EI II, Noorani M, Daniel M: Fentanyl, esmolol, and clonidine blunt the transient cardiovascular stimulation induced by desflurane in humans. Anesthesiology 81:1350-1355, 1994.
44. Weiskopf RB, Moore MA, Eger EI II, et al: Rapid increase in desflurane concentration is associated with greater transient cardiovascular stimulation than rapid increase in isoflurane concentration in humans. Anesthesiology 80:1035-1045, 1994.
45. Weiskopf RB, Eger EI II, Daniel M, Noorani M: Cardiovascular stimulation induced by rapid increases in desflurane concentration in humans results from activation of tracheopulmonary and systemic receptors. Anesthesiology 83:1173-1178, 1995.
46. Bernard JM, Wouters PF, Doursout M-F, et al: Effects of sevoflurane and isoflurane on cardiac and coronary dynamics in chronically instrumented dogs. Anesthesiology 72:659-662, 1990.
47. Harkin CP, Pagel PS, Kersten JR, et al: Direct negative inotropic and lusitropic effects of sevoflurane. Anesthesiology 81:156-167, 1994.
48. Lerman J, Oyston JP, Gallagher TM, et al: The minumum alveolar concentration (MAC) and hemodynamic effects of halothane, isoflurane, and sevoflurane in newborn swine. Anesthesiology 73:717-721, 1990.
49. Kikura M, Ikeda K: Comparison of effects of sevoflurane-nitrous oxide and enflurane-nitrous oxide on myocardial contractility in humans: Load-independent and noninvasive assessment with transesophageal echocardiography. Anesthesiology 79:235-243, 1993.

50. Kemmotsu O, Hashimoto Y, Shimosato S: The effects of fluroxene and enflurane on contractile performance of isolated papillary muscles from failing hearts. Anesthesiology 40:252-260, 1974.
51. Lowenstein E, Foex P, Francis CM, et al: Regional ischemic ventricular dysfunction in myocardium supplied by a narrowed coronary artery with increasing halothane concentration in the dog. Anesthesiology 55:349-359, 1981.
52. Kissin I, Thomson CT, Smith LR: Effects of halothane on contractile function of ischemic myocardium. J Cardiovasc Pharmacol 5:438-442, 1983.
53. Vivien B, Hanouz J-L, Gueugniaud P-Y, et al: Myocardial effects of halothane and isoflurane in hamsters with hypertrophic cardiomyopathy. Anesthesiology 87:1406-1416, 1997.
54. Prys-Roberts C, Roberts JG, Foex P, et al: Interaction of anesthesia, beta-receptor blockade, and blood loss in dogs with induced myocardial infarction. Anesthesiology 45:326-329, 1976.
55. Davis RF, DeBoer LW, Rude RE, et al: The effect of halothane anesthesia on myocardial necrosis, hemodynamic performance, and regional myocardial blood flow in dogs following coronary artery occlusion. Anesthesiology 59:402-411, 1983.
56. Kersten JR, Schmeling TJ, Pagel PS, et al: Isoflurane mimics ischemic preconditioning via activation of K_{ATP} channels. Reduction of myocardial infarct size with an acute memory phase. Anesthesiology 87:361-370, 1997.
57. Van Ackern K, Vetter HO, Bruckner UB, et al: Effects of enflurane on myocardial ischaemia in the dog. Br J Anaesth 57:497-504, 1985.
58. Kanaya N, Fujita S: The effects of isoflurane on regional myocardial contractility and metabolism in "stunned" myocardium in acutely instrumented dogs. Anesth Analg 79:447-454, 1994.
59. Lochner A, Harper IS, Salie R, et al: Halothane protects the isolated rat myocardium against excessive total intracellular calcium and structural damage during ischemia and reperfusion. Anesth Analg 79:226-233, 1994.
60. Warltier DC, Al-Wathiqui MH, Kampine JP, Schmeling WT: Recovery of contractile function of stunned myocardium in chronically instrumented dogs is enhanced by halothane or isoflurane. Anesthesiology 69:552-565, 1988.
61. Pagel PS, Hettrick DA, Lowe D, et al: Desflurane and isoflurane exert modest beneficial actions on left ventricular diastolic function during myocardial ischemia in dogs. Anesthesiology 83:1021-1035, 1995.
62. Reiz S, Balfors E, Gustavsson B, et al: Effects of halothane on coronary haemodynamics and myocardial metabolism in patients with ischaemic heart disease and heart failure. Acta Anaesthesiol Scand 26:133-138, 1982.
63. Reiz S, Balfors E, Sorensen MB, et al: Isoflurane: A powerful coronary vasodilator in patients with coronary artery disease. Anesthesiology 59:91-97, 1983.
64. Reiz S, Ostman M: Regional coronary hemodynamics during isoflurane-nitrous oxide anesthesia in patients with ischemic heart disease. Anesth Analg 64:570-576, 1985.
65. Pagel PS, Lowe D, Hettrick DA, et al: Isoflurane, but not halothane, improves indices of diastolic performance in dogs with rapid ventricular, pacing-induced cardiomyopathy. Anesthesiology 85:644-654, 1996.
66. Pagel PS, Hettrick DA, Kersten JR, et al: Isoflurane and halothane do not alter the enhanced afterload sensitivity of left ventricular relaxation in dogs with pacing-induced cardiomyopathy. Anesthesiology 87:952-962, 1997.
67. Rusy BF, Komai H: Anesthetic depression of myocardial contractility: A review of possible mechanisms. Anesthesiology 67:745-766, 1987.
68. Lynch C III: Myocardial excitation-contraction coupling. In Yaksh TL, Lynch C III, Zapol WM, et al (eds): Anesthesia: Biologic Foundations. Philadelphia, Lippincott-Raven, 1997, pp 1041-1079.
69. Bosnjak ZJ, Aggarwal A, Turner LA, et al: Differential effects of halothane, enflurane, and isoflurane on Ca^{2+} transients and papillary muscle tension in guinea pigs. Anesthesiology 76:123-131, 1992.
70. Bosnjak ZJ, Kampine JP: Effects of halothane on transmembrane potentials, Ca^{2+} transients, and papillary muscle tension in the cat. Am J Physiol 251:H374-H381, 1986.
71. Eskinder H, Rusch NJ, Supan FD, et al: The effects of volatile anesthetics on L- and T-type calcium channel currents in canine cardiac Purkinje cells. Anesthesiology 74:919-926, 1991.
72. Lynch C III: Effects of halothane and isoflurane on isolated human ventricular myocardium. Anesthesiology 68:429-432, 1988.
73. Hatakeyama N, Momose Y, Ito Y: Effects of sevoflurane on contractile responses and electrophysiologic properties in canine single cardiac myocytes. Anesthesiology 82:559-565, 1995.
74. Bosnjak ZJ, Supan FD, Rusch NJ: The effects of halothane, enflurane, and isoflurane on calcium current in isolated canine ventricular cells. Anesthesiology 74:340-345, 1991.
75. Lynch C III: Differential depression of myocardial contractility by halothane and isoflurane in vitro. Anesthesiology 64:620-631, 1986.
76. Blanck TJJ, Runge S, Stevenson RL: Halothane decreases calcium channel antagonist binding to cardiac membranes. Anesth Analg 67:1032-1035, 1988.
77. Drenger B, Quigg M, Blanck TJJ: Volatile anesthetics depress calcium channel blocker binding to bovine cardiac sarcolemma. Anesthesiology 74:155-165, 1991.
78. Hoehner PJ, Quigg MC, Blanck TJJ: Halothane depresses D600 binding to bovine heart sarcolemma. Anesthesiology 75:1019-1024, 1991.
79. Katsuoka M, Kobayashi K, Ohnishi ST: Volatile anesthetics decrease calcium content of isolated myocytes. Anesthesiology 70:954-960, 1989.
80. Katsuoka M, Ohnishi ST: Inhalation anesthetics decrease calcium content of cardiac sarcoplasmic reticulum. Br J Anaesth 62:669-673, 1989.
81. Komai H, Rusy BF: Direct effect of halothane and isoflurane on the function of the sarcoplasmic reticulum in intact rabbit atria. Anesthesiology 72:694-698, 1990.
82. Wheeler DM, Katz A, Rice RT, Hansford RG: Volatile anesthetic effects on sarcoplasmic reticulum Ca content and sarcolemmal Ca flux in isolated rat cardiac cell suspensions. Anesthesiology 80:372-382, 1994.
83. Wilde DW, Davidson BA, Smith MD, Knight PR: Effects of isoflurane and enflurane on intracellular Ca^{2+} mobilization in isolated cardiac myocytes. Anesthesiology 79:73-82, 1993.
84. Luk HN, Lin CI, Chang CL, Lee AR: Differential inotropic effects of halothane and isoflurane in dog ventricular tissues. Eur J Pharmacol 136:409-413, 1987.
85. Lynch C III, Vogel S, Sperelakis N: Halothane depression of myocardial slow action potentials. Anesthesiology 55:360-368, 1981.
86. Wheeler DM, Rice RT, Lakatta EG: The action of halothane on spontaneous contractile waves and stimulated contractions in isolated rat and dog heart cells. Anesthesiology 72:911-920, 1990.
87. Lynch C III, Frazer MJ: Anesthetic alteration of ryanodine binding by cardiac calcium release channels. Biochim Biophys Acta 1194:109-117, 1994.
88. Connelly TJ, Coronado R: Activation of the Ca^{2+} release channel of cardiac sarcoplasmic reticulum by volatile anesthetics. Anesthesiology 81:459-469, 1994.
89. Casella ES, Suite ND, Fisher YI, Blanck TJ: The effect of volatile anesthetics on the pH dependence of calcium uptake by cardiac sarcoplasmic reticulum. Anesthesiology 67:386-390, 1987.
90. Frazer MJ, Lynch C III: Halothane and isoflurane effects on Ca^{2+} fluxes of isolated myocardial sarcoplasmic reticulum. Anesthesiology 77:316-323, 1992.
91. Hannon JD, Cody MJ: Effects of volatile anesthetics in sarcolemmal calcium transport and sarcoplasmic reticulum calcium content in isolated myocytes. Anesthesiology 96:1457-1464, 2002.
92. Miao N, Lynch C III: Effect of temperature on volatile anesthetic depression of myocardial contractions. Anesth Analg 76:366-731, 1993.
93. Baum VC, Wetzel GT: Sodium-calcium exchange in neonatal myocardium: Reversible inhibition by halothane. Anesth Analg 78:1105-1109, 1994.

94. Haworth RA, Goknur AB, Berkoff HA: Inhibition of Na-Ca exchange by general anesthetics. Circ Res 65:1021-1028, 1989.

95. Haworth RA, Goknur AB: Inhibition of sodium/calcium exchange and calcium channels of heart cells by volatile anesthetics. Anesthesiology 82:1255-1265, 1995.

96. Baum VC, Klitzner TS: Excitation-contraction coupling in neonatal myocardium: Effects of halothane and isoflurane. Dev Pharmacol Ther 16:99-107, 1991.

97. Su JY, Kerrick WG: Effects of halothane on Ca^{2+} activated tension development in mechanically disrupted rabbit myocardial fibers. Pflugers Arch 375:111-117, 1978.

98. Murat I, Ventura-Clapier R, Vassort G: Halothane, enflurane, and isoflurane decrease calcium sensitivity and maximal force in detergent-treated rat cardiac fibers. Anesthesiology 69:892-899, 1988.

99. Tavernier BM, Adnet PJ, Imbenotte M, et al: Halothane and isoflurane decrease calcium sensitivity and maximal force in human skinned cardiac fibers. Anesthesiology 80:625-633, 1994.

100. Merin RG, Kumazawa T, Honig CR: Reversible interaction between halothane and Ca^{2+} on cardiac actomyosin adenosine triphosphatase: Mechanism and significance. J Pharmacol Exp Ther 190:1-14, 1974.

101. Pask HT, England PJ, Prys-Roberts C: Effects of volatile inhalational anesthetic agents on isolated bovine cardiac myofibrillar ATPase. J Mol Cell Cardiol 13:293-301, 1981.

102. Murat I, Lechene P, Ventura-Clapier R: Effects of volatile anesthetics on mechanical properties of rat cardiac skinned fibers. Anesthesiology 73:73-81, 1990.

103. Hannon JD, Cody MJ, Housmans PR: Effects of isoflurane on intracellular calcium and myocardial crossbridge kinetics in tetanized papillary muscles. Anesthesiology 94:856-861, 2001.

104. Blanck TJJ, Chiancone E, Salviati G, et al: Halothane does not alter Ca^{2+} affinity of troponin C. Anesthesiology 76:100-105, 1992.

105. Housmans PR: Negative inotropy of halogenated anesthetics in ferret ventricular myocardium. Am J Physiol 259:H827-H834, 1990.

106. Baele P, Housmans PR: The effects of halothane, enflurane, and isoflurane on the length-tension relation of the isolated papillary muscle of the ferret. Anesthesiology 74:281-291, 1991.

107. Davies LA, Gibson CN, Boyett MR, et al: Effects of isoflurane, sevoflurane, and halothane on myofilament Ca^{2+} sensitivity and sarcoplasmic reticulum Ca^{2+} release in rat ventricular myocytes. Anesthesiology 93:1034-1044, 2000.

108. Jiang Y, Julian FJ: Effects of halothane on $[Ca^{2+}]_i$ transient, SR Ca^{2+} content, and force in intact rat heart trabeculae. Am J Physiol 274:H106-H114, 1998.

109. Morgan JP: Abnormal intracellular modulation of calcium as a major cause of cardiac contractile dysfunction. N Engl J Med 325:625-632, 1991.

110. Pagel PS, Warltier DC: Mechanical function of the left ventricle. In Yaksh TL, Lynch C III, Zapol WM, et al (eds): Anesthesia: Biologic Foundations. Philadelphia, Lippincott-Raven, 1998, pp 1081-1133.

111. Dougherty AH, Naccarelli GV, Gray EL, et al: Congestive heart failure with normal systolic function. Am J Cardiol 54:778-782, 1984.

112. Katz AM, Smith VE: Regulation of myocardial function in the normal and diseased heart. Modification by inotropic drugs. Eur Heart J 3(Suppl D):11-18, 1982.

113. Soufer R, Wohlgelernter D, Vita NA, et al: Intact systolic left ventricular function in clinical congestive heart failure. Am J Cardiol 55:1032-1036, 1985.

114. Pagel PS, Grossman W, Haering JM, Warltier DC: Left ventricular diastolic function in the normal and diseased heart: Perspectives for the anesthesiologist. Anesthesiology 79(Pt 1):836-854, 1993.

115. Pagel PS, Grossman W, Haering JM, Warltier DC: Left ventricular diastolic function in the normal and diseased heart: Perspectives for the anesthesiologist. Anesthesiology 79(Pt 2):1104-1120, 1993.

116. Doyle RL, Foex P, Ryder WA, Jones LA: Effects of halothane on left ventricular relaxation and early diastolic coronary blood flow in the dog. Anesthesiology 70:660-666, 1989.

117. Humphrey LS, Stinson DC, Humphrey MJ, et al: Volatile anesthetic effects on left ventricular relaxation in swine. Anesthesiology 73:731-738, 1990.

118. Pagel PS, Kampine JP, Schmeling WT, Warltier DC: Alteration of left ventricular diastolic function by desflurane, isoflurane, and halothane in the chronically instrumented dog with autonomic nervous system blockade. Anesthesiology 74:1103-1114, 1991.

119. Ihara T, Shannon RP, Komamura K, et al: Effects of anaesthesia and recent surgery on diastolic function. Cardiovasc Res 28:325-336, 1994.

120. Housmans PR, Murat I: Comparative effects of halothane, enflurane, and isoflurane at equipotent anesthetic concentrations on isolated ventricular myocardium of the ferret. II. Relaxation. Anesthesiology 69:464-471, 1988.

121. Goldberg AH, Phear WPC: Halothane and paired stimulation: Effects on myocardial compliance and contractility. J Appl Physiol 28:391-396, 1970.

122. Rusy BF, Moran JE, Vongvises P, et al: The effects of halothane and cyclopropane on left ventricular volume determined by high-speed biplane cineradiography in dogs. Anesthesiology 36:369-373, 1972.

123. Moores WY, Weiskopf RB, Baysinger M, Utley JR: Effects of halothane and morphine sulfate on myocardial compliance following total cardiopulmonary bypass. J Thorac Cardiovasc Surg 81:163-170, 1981.

124. Greene ES, Gerson JI: One versus two MAC halothane anesthesia does not alter the left ventricular diastolic pressure-volume relationship. Anesthesiology 64:230-237, 1986.

125. Ishizaka S, Asanoi H, Wada O, et al: Loading sequence plays an important role in enhanced load sensitivity of left ventricular relaxation in conscious dogs with tachycardia-induced cardiomyopathy. Circulation 92:3560-3567, 1995.

126. Eichhorn EJ, Willard JE, Alvarez L, et al: Are contraction and relaxation coupled in patients with and without congestive heart failure? Circulation 85:2132-2139, 1992.

127. Little WC: Enhanced load dependence of relaxation in heart failure: Clinical implications. Circulation 85:2326-2328, 1992.

128. Sunagawa K, Maughan WL, Burkhoff D, Sagawa K: Left ventricular interaction with arterial load studied in isolated canine ventricle. Am J Physiol 245:H773-H80, 1983.

129. Sunagawa K, Maughan WL, Sagawa K: Optimal arterial resistance for the maximal stroke work studied in isolated canine left ventricle. Circ Res 56:586-595, 1985.

130. Burkhoff D, Sagawa K: Ventricular efficiency predicted by an analytical model. Am J Physiol 250:R1021-R1027, 1986.

131. Little WC, Cheng C-P: Left ventricular-arterial coupling in conscious dogs. Am J Physiol 261:H70-H76, 1991.

132. Starling MR: Left ventricular-arterial coupling relations in the normal human heart. Am Heart J 125:1659-1666, 1993.

133. Suga H: Ventricular energetics. Physiol Rev 70:247-277, 1990.

134. Kawasaki T, Hoka S, Okamoto H, et al: The difference of isoflurane and halothane in ventriculoarterial coupling in dogs. Anesth Analg 79:681-686, 1994.

135. Hettrick DA, Pagel PS, Warltier DC: Isoflurane and halothane produce similar alterations in aortic distensibility and characteristic aortic impedance. Anesth Analg 83:1166-1172, 1996.

136. Milnor WR: Hemodynamics, 2nd ed. Baltimore, Williams & Wilkins, 1989.

137. Lang RM, Borow KM, Neumann A, Janzen D: Systemic vascular resistance: An unreliable index of left ventricular afterload. Circulation 74:1114-1123, 1986.

138. Milnor WR: Arterial impedance as ventricular afterload. Circ Res 36:565-570, 1975.

139. Burkhoff D, Alexander J Jr, Schipke J: Assessment of Windkessel as a model of aortic input impedance. Am J Physiol 255:H742-H53, 1988.

140. Wesseling KH, Jansen JRC, Settels JJ, Schreuder JJ: Computation of aortic flow from pressure in humans using

a nonlinear, three element model. J Appl Physiol 74:2566-2573, 1993.

141. Gersh BJ, Prys-Roberts C, Reuben SR, Schultz DL: The effects of halothane on the interactions between myocardial contractility, aortic input impedance, and left ventricular performance: II. Aortic input impedance, and the distribution of energy during ventricular ejection. Br J Anaesth 44:767-765, 1972.

142. Prys-Roberts C, Gersh BJ, Baker AB, Reuben SR: The effects of halothane on the interactions between myocardial contractility, aortic impedance, and left ventricular performance. 1. Theoretical considerations and results. Br J Anaesth 44:634-649, 1972.

143. Hettrick DA, Pagel PS, Warltier DC: Differential effects of isoflurane and halothane on aortic input impedance quantified using a three element Windkessel model. Anesthesiology 83:361-373, 1995.

144. Lowe D, Hettrick DA, Pagel PS, Warltier DC: Influence of volatile anesthetics on left ventricular afterload in vivo: Differences between desflurane and sevoflurane. Anesthesiology 85:112-120, 1996.

145. Pepine CJ, Nichols WW, Curry RC Jr, Conti CR: Aortic input impedance during nitroprusside infusion: A reconsideration of afterload reduction and beneficial action. J Clin Invest 64:643-654, 1979.

146. Lowe D, Hettrick DA, Pagel PS, Warltier DC: Propofol alters left ventricular afterload as evaluated by aortic input impedance in dogs. Anesthesiology 84:368-376, 1996.

147. Hettrick DA, Pagel PS, Kersten JR, et al: The effects of isoflurane and halothane on left ventricular afterload in dogs with dilated cardiomyopathy. Anesth Analg 85:979-986, 1997.

148. March HW, Ross JK, Lower RR: Observations on the behavior of the right ventricular outflow tract, with reference to its developmental origins. Am J Med 32:835-845, 1962.

149. Armour JA, Pace JB, Randall WC: Interrelationship of architecture and function of the right ventricle. Am J Physiol 218:174-179, 1970.

150. Pace JB, Keefe WF, Armour JA, Randall WC: Influence of sympathetic nerve stimulation on the right ventricular outflow tract pressure in anesthetized dogs. Circ Res 24:397-407, 1969.

151. Meier GD, Bove AA, Santamore WP, Lynch PR: Contractile function in canine right ventricle. Am J Physiol 239:H794-H804, 1980.

152. Pouleur H, Lefevre J, van Mechelen H, Charlier AA: Free wall shortening and relaxation during ejection in the canine right ventricle. Am J Physiol 239:H601-H613, 1980.

153. Tobin JR Jr, Blundell PE, Goodrich RG, Swan HJC: Induced pressure gradients across infundibular zone of right ventricle in normal dogs. Circ Res 16:162-173, 1965.

154. Myhre ESP, Slinker BK, LeWinter MM: Absence of right ventricular isovolumic relaxation in open-chest anesthetized dogs. Am J Physiol 263:H1587-H1590, 1992.

155. Priebe HJ: Effects of halothane on global and regional biventricular performances and on coronary hemodynamics before and during right coronary artery stenosis in the dog. Anesthesiology 78:541-552, 1993.

156. Heerdt PM, Pleimann BE: The dose-dependent effects of halothane on right ventricular contraction pattern and regional inotropy in swine. Anesth Analg 82:1152-1158, 1996.

157. Nolan SP, Dixon SH Jr, Fisher RD, Morrow AG: The influence of atrial contraction and mitral valve mechanics on ventricular filling. A study of instantaneous mitral valve flow in vivo. Am Heart J 77:784-791, 1969.

158. Ruskin J, McHale PA, Harley A, Greenfield JC Jr: Pressure-flow studies in man: Effect of atrial systole on left ventricular function. J Clin Invest 49:472-478, 1970.

159. Grant C, Bunnell IL, Greene DG: The reservoir function of the left atrium during ventricular systole: An angiocardiographic study of atrial stroke volume and work. Am J Med 37:36-43, 1964.

160. Ishida Y, Meisner JS, Tsujioka K, et al: Left ventricular filling dynamics: Influence of left ventricular relaxation and left atrial pressure. Circulation 74:187-196, 1986.

161. Suga H: Importance of atrial compliance in cardiac performance. Circ Res 35:39-43, 1974.

162. Pagel PS, Kehl F, Gare M, et al: Mechanical function of the left atrium: New insights based on analysis of pressure-volume relations and Doppler echocardiography. Anesthesiology 98:975-994, 2003.

163. Paradise RR, Griffith LK: Influence of halothane, chloroform and methoxyflurane on potassium content of rat atria. Anesthesiology 26:195-198, 1965.

164. Ko KC, Paradise RR: The effects of substrates on contractility of rat atria depressed with halothane. Anesthesiology 31:532-539, 1969.

165. Ko KC, Paradise RR: Multiple mechanisms of action of halothane and methoxyflurane on force of contraction of isolated rat atria. Anesthesiology 39:278-284, 1973.

166. Seifen AB, Kennedy RH, Seifen E: Effects of volatile anesthetics on response to norepinephrine and acetylcholine in guinea pig atria. Anesth Analg 73:304-309, 1991.

167. Ko KC, Paradise RR: The effects of substrates on halothane-depressed isolated human atria. Anesthesiology 33:508-514, 1970.

168. Luk HN, Lin CI, Wei J, Chang CL: Depressant effects of isoflurane and halothane on isolated human atrial fibers. Anesthesiology 69:667-676, 1988.

169. Hanouz JL, Massetti M, Guesne G, et al: In vitro effects of desflurane, sevoflurane, isoflurane, and halothane in isolated human right atria. Anesthesiology 92:116-124, 2000.

170. Pagel PS, Farber NE, Warltier DC: Cardiovascular pharmacology. In Miller RD (ed): Anesthesia, 5th ed. Philadelphia, Churchill Livingstone, 2000, pp 96-124.

171. Gare M, Schwabe DA, Hettrick DA, et al: Desflurane, sevoflurane, and isoflurane affect left atrial active and passive mechanical properties and impair left atrial-left ventricular coupling in vivo: Analysis using pressure-volume relations. Anesthesiology 95:689-698, 2001.

172. Barbier P, Solomon SB, Schiller NB, Glantz SA: Left atrial relaxation and left ventricular systolic function determine left atrial reservoir function. Circulation 100:427-436, 1999.

173. Bosnjak ZJ, Kampine JP: Effects of halothane, enflurane, and isoflurane in the SA node. Anesthesiology 58:314-321, 1983.

174. Bristow JD, Prys-Roberts C, Fisher A, et al: Effects of anesthesia on baroreflex control of heart rate in man. Anesthesiology 31:422-428, 1969.

175. Kotrly KJ, Ebert TJ, Vucins E, et al: Baroreceptor reflex control of heart rate during isoflurane anesthesia in humans. Anesthesiology 60:173-179, 1984.

176. Bagshaw RJ, Cox RH: Baroreceptor control of systemic haemodynamics at incremental halothane levels in the dog. Acta Anaesthesiol Scand 25:416-420, 1981.

177. Duke PC, Fownes D, Wade JG: Halothane depresses baroreflex control of heart rate in man. Anesthesiology 46:184-187, 1977.

178. Ebert TJ, Kotrly KJ, Vucins EJ, et al: Halothane attenuates cardiopulmonary baroreflex control of peripheral resistance in humans. Anesthesiology 63:668-674, 1985.

179. Calverley RK, Smith NT, Jones CW, et al: Ventilatory and cardiovascular effects of enflurane anesthesia during spontaneous ventilation in man. Anesth Analg 57:610-618, 1978.

180. Weiskopf RB, Cahalan MK, Ionescu P, et al: Cardiovascular actions of desflurane with and without nitrous oxide during spontaneous ventilation in humans. Anesth Analg 73:165-174, 1991.

181. Murat I, Lapeyre G, Saint-Maurice C: Isoflurane attenuates baroreflex control of heart rate in human neonates. Anesthesiology 70:395-400, 1989.

182. Cahalan MK, Lurz FW, Eger EI II, et al: Narcotics decrease heart rate during inhalational anesthesia. Anesth Analg 66:166-170, 1987.

183. Mallow JE, White RD, Cucchiara RF, Tarhan S: Hemodynamic effects of isoflurane and halothane in patients with coronary artery disease. Anesth Analg 55:135-138, 1976.

184. Holaday DA, Smith FR: Clinical characteristics and biotransformation of sevoflurane in healthy human volunteers. Anesthesiology 54:100-106, 1981.

185. Kasuda H, Akazawa S, Shimizu R: The echocardiographic assessment of left ventricular performance during sevoflurane and halothane anesthesia. J Anesth 4:295-302, 1990.

186. Ebert TJ, Harkin CP, Muzi M: Cardiovascular responses to sevoflurane: A review. Anesth Analg 81:S11-S22, 1995.

187. Frink EJ Jr, Malan TP, Atlas M, et al: Clinical comparison of sevoflurane and isoflurane in healthy patients. Anesth Analg 74:241-245, 1992.

188. Ebert TJ, Muzi M, Lopatka CW: Neurocirculatory responses to sevoflurane in humans: A comparison to desflurane. Anesthesiology 83:88-95, 1995.

189. Eger EI II: The pharmacology of isoflurane. Br J Anaesth 56:71S-99S, 1984.

190. Eger EI II: Nitrous Oxide: N₂O. New York, Elsevier, 1985.

191. Bahlman SH, Eger EI II, Halsey MJ, et al: The cardiovascular effects of halothane in man during spontaneous ventilation. Anesthesiology 36:494-502, 1972.

192. Price HL, Skovsted P, Pauca AL, Cooperman LH: Evidence for β-receptor activation produced by halothane in normal man. Anesthesiology 32:389-395, 1970.

193. Blake DW, Way D, Trigg L, et al: Cardiovascular effects of volatile anesthesia in rabbits: Influence of chronic heart failure and enalaprilat treatment. Anesth Analg 73:441-448, 1991.

194. Reiz S: Nitrous oxide augments the systemic and coronary haemodynamic effects of isoflurane in patients with ischaemic heart disease. Acta Anaesthesiol Scand 27:464-469, 1983.

195. Rydvall A, Haggmark S, Nyhman H, Reiz S: Effects of enflurane on coronary haemodynamics in patients with ischaemic heart disease. Acta Anaesthesiol Scand 28:690-695, 1984.

196. Braunwald E: Pathophysiology of heart failure. In Braunwald E (ed): Heart Disease: A Textbook of Cardiovascular Medicine, 4th ed. Philadelphia, WB Saunders, 1992, pp 393-418.

197. Atlee JL III, Brownlee SW, Burstrom RE: Conscious-state comparisons of the effects of inhalational anesthetics on specialized atrioventricular conduction times in dogs. Anesthesiology 64:703-710, 1986.

198. Seagard JL, Bosnjak ZJ, Hopp FA Jr, et al: Cardiovascular effects of anesthesia. In Covino BG, Fozzard HA, Rehder K, Strichartz G (eds): Effects of Anesthesia. Bethesda, MD, American Physiological Society, 1985, pp 149-177.

199. Turner LA, Bosnjak ZJ, Kampine JP: Actions of halothane on the electrical activity of Purkinje fibers derived from normal and infarcted canine hearts. Anesthesiology 67:619-629, 1987.

200. Atlee JL III, Rusy BF: Atrioventricular conduction times and atrioventricular nodal conductivity during enflurane anesthesia in dogs. Anesthesiology 47:498-503, 1977.

201. Hauswirth O: Effects of halothane on single atrial, ventricular and Purkinje fibers. Circ Res 24:745-750, 1969.

202. Atlee JL III, Rusy BF, Kreul JF, Eby T: Supraventricular excitability in dogs during anesthesia with halothane and enflurane. Anesthesiology 49:407-413, 1978.

203. Atlee JL III, Yeager TS: Electrophysiologic assessment of the effects of enflurane, halothane, and isoflurane on properties affecting supraventricular re-entry in chronically instrumented dogs. Anesthesiology 71:941-952, 1989.

204. Atlee JL III, Bosnjak Z: Mechanisms for cardiac dysrhythmias during anesthesia. Anesthesiology 72:347-374, 1990.

205. Atlee JL III, Bosnjak ZJ, Yeager TS: Effects of diltiazem, verapamil, and inhalation anesthetics on electrophysiologic properties affecting reentrant supraventricular tachycardia in chronically instrumented dogs. Anesthesiology 72:889-901, 1990.

206. MacLeod BA, Augereau P, Walker MJA: Effects of halothane anesthesia compared with fentanyl anesthesia and no anesthesia during coronary ligation in rats. Anesthesiology 58:44-52, 1983.

207. Jang JL, MacLeod BA, Walker MJA: Effects of halogenated hydrocarbon anesthetics on responses to ligation of a coronary artery in chronically prepared rats. Anesthesiology 59:309-315, 1983.

208. Kroll DA, Knight PR: Antifibrillatory effects of volatile anesthetics in acute occlusion/reperfusion arrhythmias. Anesthesiology 61:657-661, 1984.

209. Morrow DH, Townley NT: Anesthesia and digitalis toxicity: An experimental study. Anesth Analg 43:510-519, 1964.

210. Turner LA, Polic S, Hoffmann RG, et al: Actions of halothane and isoflurane on Purkinje fibers in the infarcted canine heart: Conduction, regional refractoriness, and reentry. Anesth Analg 76:718-725, 1993.

211. Turner LA, Polic S, Hoffmann RG, et al: Actions of volatile anesthetics on ischemic and nonischemic Purkinje fibers in the canine heart: Regional action potential characteristics. Anesth Analg 76:726-733, 1993.

212. Schmeling WT, Warltier DC, McDonald DJ, et al: Prolongation of the QT interval by enflurane, isoflurane, and halothane in humans. Anesth Analg 72:137-144, 1991.

213. Hanich RF, Levine JH, Spear JF, Moore EN: Autonomic modulation of ventricular arrhythmia in cesium chloride-induced long QT syndrome. Circulation 77:1149-1161, 1988.

214. Atlee JL III, Malkinson CE: Potentiation by thiopental of halothane-epinephrine-induced arrhythmias in dogs. Anesthesiology 57:285-288, 1982.

215. Joas TA, Stevens WC: Comparison of the arrhythmic doses of epinephrine during Forane, halothane, and fluroxene anesthesia in dogs. Anesthesiology 35:48-53, 1971.

216. Sumikawa K, Ishizaka N, Suzaki M: Arrhythmogenic plasma levels of epinephrine during halothane, enflurane, and pentobarbital anesthesia in the dog. Anesthesiology 58:322-325, 1983.

217. MacCannell KL, Dresel PE: Potentiation by thiopental of cyclopropane-adrenaline cardiac arrhythmias. Can J Physiol Pharmacol 42:627-639, 1964.

218. Hayashi Y, Sumikawa K, Tashiro C, et al: Arrhythmogenic threshold of epinephrine during sevoflurane, enflurane, and isoflurane anesthesia in dogs. Anesthesiology 69:145-147, 1988.

219. Turner LA, Marijic J, Kampine JP, Bosnjak ZJ: A comparison of the effects of halothane and tetrodotoxin on regional repolarization characteristics of canine Purkinje fibers. Anesthesiology 73:1158-1168, 1990.

220. Turner LA, Vodanovic S, Hoffmann RG, et al: A subtype of α₁ adrenoceptor mediates depression of conduction in Purkinje fibers exposed to halothane. Anesthesiology 82:1438-1446, 1995.

221. Vodanovic S, Turner LA, Hoffmann RG, et al: Actions of phenylephrine, isoproterenol, and epinephrine with halothane on endocardial conduction and activation in canine left ventricular papillary muscles. Anesthesiology 87:117-126, 1997.

222. Weiskopf RB, Eger EI II, Holmes MA, et al: Epinephrine-induced premature ventricular contractions and changes in arterial blood pressure and heart rate during I-653, isoflurane, and halothane anesthesia in swine. Anesthesiology 70:293-298, 1989.

223. Woehlck HJ, Vicenzi MN, Bosnjak ZJ, Atlee JL III: Anesthetics and automaticity of dominant and latent pacemakers in chronically instrumented dogs. I. Methodology, conscious state, and halothane anesthesia: Comparison with and without muscarinic blockade during exposure to epinephrine. Anesthesiology 79:1304-1315, 1993.

224. Vicenzi MN, Woehlck HJ, Bosnjak ZJ, Atlee JL III: Anesthetics and automaticity of dominant and latent pacemakers in chronically instrumented dogs. II. Effects of enflurane and isoflurane during epinephrine with and without muscarinic blockade. Anesthesiology 79:1316-1323, 1993.

225. Vicenzi MN, Woehlck HJ, Bajic J, et al: Anesthetics and automaticity of dominant and latent pacemakers in chronically instrumented dogs. III. Automaticity after sinoatrial node excision. Anesthesiology 82:469-478, 1995.

226. Woehlck HJ, Vicenzi MN, Bajic J, et al: Anesthetics and automaticity of dominant and latent pacemakers in chronically instrumented dogs. IV. Dysrhythmias after sinoatrial node excision. Anesthesiology 82:1447-1455, 1995.

227. Blaise G, Sill JC, Nugent M, et al: Isoflurane causes endothelium-dependent inhibition of contractile responses of canine coronary arteries. Anesthesiology 67:513-517, 1987.

228. Bollen BA, Tinker JH, Hermsmeyer K: Halothane relaxes previously constricted isolated porcine coronary artery segments more than isoflurane. Anesthesiology 66:748-752, 1987.

229. Bollen BA, McKlveen RE, Stevenson JA: Halothane relaxes preconstricted small and medium isolated porcine coronary artery segments more than isoflurane. Anesth Analg 75:9-17, 1992.

230. Bollen BA, McKlveen RE, Stevenson JA: Halothane relaxes previously constricted human epicardial coronary artery segments more than isoflurane. Anesth Analg 75:4-8, 1992.

231. Hatano Y, Nakamura K, Yakushiji T, et al: Comparison of the direct effects of halothane and isoflurane on large and small coronary arteries isolated from dogs. Anesthesiology 73:513-517, 1990.

232. Marijic J, Buljubasic N, Coughlan G, et al: Effect of K+ channel blockade with tetraethylammonium on anesthetic-induced relaxation in canine cerebral and coronary arteries. Anesthesiology 77:948-855, 1992.

233. Villeneuve E, Blaise G, Sill JC, et al: Halothane 1.5 MAC, isoflurane 1.5 MAC, and the contractile responses of coronary arteries obtained from human hearts. Anesth Analg 72:454-461, 1991.

234. Witzeling TM, Sill JC, Hughes JM, et al: Isoflurane and halothane attenuate coronary artery constriction evoked by serotonin in isolated porcine vessels and in intact pigs. Anesthesiology 73:100-108, 1990.

235. Buljubasic N, Rusch NJ, Marijic J, et al: Effects of halothane and isoflurane on calcium and potassium channel currents in canine coronary arterial cells. Anesthesiology 76:990-998, 1992.

236. Kersten JR, Warltier DC: The coronary circulation. In Yaksh TL, Lynch C III, Zapol WM, et al (eds): Anesthesia: Biologic Foundations. Philadelphia, Lippincott-Raven, 1997, pp 1169-1192.

237. Larach DR, Schuler HG, Skeehan TM, Peterson CJ: Direct effects of myocardial depressant drugs on coronary vascular tone: Anesthetic vasodilation by halothane and isoflurane. J Pharmacol Exp Ther 254:58-64, 1990.

238. Sahlman L, Henriksson B-A, Martner J, Ricksten SE: Effects of halothane, enflurane, and isoflurane on coronary vascular tone, myocardial performance, and oxygen consumption during controlled changes in aortic and left atrial pressure. Studies on isolated working rat hearts in vitro. Anesthesiology 69:1-10, 1988.

239. Stowe DF, Marijic J, Bosnjak ZJ, Kampine JP: Direct comparative effects of halothane, enflurane, and isoflurane on oxygen supply and demand in isolated hearts. Anesthesiology 74:1087-1095, 1991.

240. Stowe DF, Monroe SM, Marijic J, et al: Comparison of halothane, enflurane, and isoflurane with nitrous oxide on contractility and oxygen supply and demand in isolated hearts. Anesthesiology 75:1062-1074, 1991.

241. Larach DR, Schuler HG: Direct vasodilation by sevoflurane, isoflurane, and halothane alters coronary flow reserve in the isolated rat heart. Anesthesiology 75:268-278, 1991.

242. Smith G, Vance JP, Brown DM, McMillan JC: Changes in myocardial blood flow and oxygen consumption in response to halothane. Br J Anaesth 46:821-826, 1974.

243. Domenech RJ, Macho P, Valdes J, Penna M: Coronary vascular resistance during halothane anesthesia. Anesthesiology 46:236-240, 1977.

244. Weaver PC, Bailey JS, Preston TD: Coronary artery blood flow in the halothane-depressed canine heart. Br J Anaesth 42:678-684, 1970.

245. Wolff G, Claudi B, Rist M, et al: Regulation of coronary blood flow during ether and halothane anaesthesia. Br J Anaesth 44:1139-1149, 1972.

246. Amory DW, Steffenson JL, Forsyth RP: Systemic and regional blood flow changes during halothane anesthesia in the rhesus monkey. Anesthesiology 35:81-90, 1971.

247. Vatner SF, Smith NT: Effects of halothane on left ventricular function and distribution of regional blood flow in dogs and primates. Circ Res 34:155-167, 1974.

248. Brett CM, Teitel DF, Heymann MA, Rudolph AM: The cardiovascular effects of isoflurane in lambs. Anesthesiology 67:60-65, 1987.

249. Crystal GJ, Kim S-J, Czinn EA, et al: Intracoronary isoflurane causes marked vasodilation in canine hearts. Anesthesiology 74:757-765, 1991.

250. Hickey RF, Cason BA, Shubayev I: Regional vasodilating properties of isoflurane in normal swine myocardium. Anesthesiology 80:574-581, 1994.

251. Priebe H-J: Differential effects of isoflurane on regional right and left ventricular performances, and on coronary, systemic, and pulmonary hemodynamics in the dog. Anesthesiology 66:262-272, 1987.

252. Kenny D, Proctor LT, Schmeling WT, et al: Isoflurane causes only minimal increases in coronary blood flow independent of oxygen demand. Anesthesiology 75:640-649, 1991.

253. Crystal GJ, Kim S-J, Salem MR, et al: Nitric oxide does not mediate coronary vasodilation by isoflurane. Anesthesiology 81:209-220, 1994.

254. Sill JC, Bove AA, Nugent M, et al: Effects of isoflurane on coronary arteries and coronary arterioles in the intact dog. Anesthesiology 66:273-279, 1987.

255. Hickey RF, Sybert PE, Verrier ED, Cason BA: Effects of halothane, enflurane, and isoflurane on coronary blood flow autoregulation and coronary vascular reserve in the canine heart. Anesthesiology 68:21-30, 1988.

256. Conzen PF, Hobbhahn J, Goetz AE, et al: Regional blood flow and tissue oxygen pressures of the collateral-dependent myocardium during isoflurane anesthesia in dogs. Anesthesiology 70:442-452, 1989.

257. Habazettl H, Conzen PF, Hobbhahn J, et al: Left ventricular oxygen tensions in dogs during coronary vasodilation by enflurane, isoflurane and dipyridamole. Anesth Analg 68:286-294, 1989.

258. Boban M, Stowe DF, Buljubasic N, et al: Direct comparative effects of isoflurane and desflurane in isolated guinea pig hearts. Anesthesiology 76:775-780, 1992.

259. Conzen PF, Vollmar B, Habazettl H, et al: Systemic and regional hemodynamics of isoflurane and sevoflurane in rats. Anesth Analg 74:79-88, 1992.

260. Crawford MW, Lerman J, Saldivia V, Carmichael FJ: Hemodynamic and organ blood flow responses to halothane and sevoflurane anesthesia during spontaneous ventilation. Anesth Analg 75:1000-1006, 1992.

261. Manohar M, Parks CM: Porcine systemic and regional organ blood flow during 1.0 and 1.5 minimum alveolar concentrations of sevoflurane anesthesia without and with 50% nitrous oxide. J Pharmacol Exp Ther 231:640-648, 1984.

262. Gilbert M, Roberts SL, Mori M, et al: Comparative coronary vascular reactivity and hemodynamics during halothane and isoflurane anesthesia in swine. Anesthesiology 68:243-253, 1988.

263. Conzen PF, Habazettl H, Vollmar B, et al: Coronary microcirculation during halothane, enflurane, isoflurane, and adenosine in dogs. Anesthesiology 76:261-270, 1992.

264. Ozhan M, Sill JC, Atagunduz P, et al: Volatile anesthetics and agonist-induced contractions in porcine coronary artery smooth muscle and Ca2+ mobilization in cultured immortalized vascular smooth muscle cells. Anesthesiology 80:1102-1113, 1994.

265. Su JY, Zhang CC: Intracellular mechanisms of halothane's effect on isolated aortic strips of the rabbit. Anesthesiology 71:409-417, 1989.

266. Sill JC, Eskuri S, Nelson R, et al: The volatile anesthetic isoflurane attenuates Ca2+ mobilization in cultured vascular smooth muscle cells. J Pharmacol Exp Ther 265:74-80, 1993.

267. Brendel JK, Johns RA: Isoflurane does not dilate isolated rat thoracic aortic rings by endothelium-derived relaxing factor or other cyclic GMP-mediated mechanisms. Anesthesiology 77:126-131, 1992.

268. Muldoon SM, Hart JL, Bowen KA, Freas W: Attenuation of endothelium-mediated vasodilation by halothane. Anesthesiology 68:31-37, 1988.

269. Stone DJ, Johns RA: Endothelium-dependent effects of halothane, enflurane, and isoflurane on isolated rat aortic vascular rings. Anesthesiology 71:126-132, 1989.

270. Greenblatt EP, Loeb AL, Longnecker DE: Endothelium-dependent circulatory control—A mechanism for the differing peripheral vascular effects of isoflurane versus halothane. Anesthesiology 77:1178-1185, 1992.

271. Blaise G, To Q, Parent M, et al: Does halothane interfere with the release, action, or stability of endothelium-derived relaxing factor/nitric oxide? Anesthesiology 80:417-426, 1994.

272. Uggeri MJ, Proctor GJ, Johns RA: Halothane, enflurane, and isoflurane attenuate both receptor- and non–receptor-mediated EDRF production in rat thoracic aorta. Anesthesiology 76:1012-1017, 1992.

273. Hart JL, Jing M, Bina S, et al: Effects of halothane on EDRF/cGMP-mediated vascular smooth muscle relaxations. Anesthesiology 79:323-331, 1993.

274. Toda H, Nakamura K, Hatano Y, et al: Halothane and isoflurane inhibit endothelium-dependent relaxation elicited by acetylcholine. Anesth Analg 75:198-203, 1992.

275. Yoshida K-I, Okabe E: Selective impairment of endothelium-dependent relaxation by sevoflurane: Oxygen free radicals participation. Anesthesiology 76:440-447, 1992.

276. Larach DR, Schuler HG: Potassium channel blockade and halothane vasodilation in conducting and resistance coronary arteries. J Pharmacol Exp Ther 267:72-81, 1993.

277. Cason BA, Shubayev I, Hickey RF: Blockade of adenosine triphosphate-sensitive potassium channels eliminates isoflurane-induced coronary artery vasodilation. Anesthesiology 81:1245-1255, 1994.

278. Crystal GJ, Gurevicius J, Salem MR, Zhou X: Role of adenosine triphosphate-sensitive potassium channels in coronary vasodilation by halothane, isoflurane, and enflurane. Anesthesiology 86:448-458, 1997.

279. Kersten JR, Schmeling TJ, Hettrick DA, et al: Mechanism of cardioprotection by isoflurane: Role of adenosine triphosphate-regulated potassium (KATP) channels. Anesthesiology 85:794-807, 1996.

280. Kersten JR, Gross GJ, Pagel PS, Warltier DC: Activation of adenosine triphosphate-regulated potassium channels: Mediation of cellular and organ protection. Anesthesiology 88:495-513, 1998.

281. Hickey RF, Verrier ED, Baer RW, et al: A canine model of acute coronary stenosis: Effects of deliberate hypotension. Anesthesiology 59:226-236, 1983.

282. Priebe H-J, Foex P: Isoflurane causes regional myocardial dysfunction in dogs with critical coronary artery stenoses. Anesthesiology 66:293-300, 1987.

283. Foex P, Francis CM, Cutfield GR, Leone B: The pressure-length loop. Br J Anaesth 60(Suppl 1):65S-71S, 1988.

284. Priebe H-J: Isoflurane causes more severe myocardial dysfunction than halothane in dogs with a critical coronary stenosis. Anesthesiology 69:72-83, 1988.

285. Tatekawa S, Traber KB, Hantler CB, et al: Effects of isoflurane on myocardial blood flow, function, and oxygen consumption in the presence of critical coronary stenosis in dogs. Anesth Analg 66:1073-1082, 1987.

286. Wilton NCT, Knight PR, Ullrich K, et al: Transmural redistribution of myocardial blood flow during isoflurane anesthesia and its effects on regional myocardial function in a canine model of fixed coronary stenosis. Anesthesiology 78:510-523, 1993.

287. Cason BA, Verrier ED, London MJ, et al: Effects of isoflurane and halothane on coronary vascular resistance and collateral myocardial blood flow: Their capacity to induce coronary steal. Anesthesiology 67:665-675, 1987.

288. Hartman JC, Kampine JP, Schmeling WT, Warltier DC: Actions of isoflurane on myocardial perfusion in chronically instrumented dogs with poor, moderate, or well-developed coronary collaterals. J Cardiothorac Anesth 4:715-725, 1990.

289. Hartman JC, Kampine JP, Schmeling WT, Warltier DC: Alterations in collateral blood flow produced by isoflurane in a chronically instrumented canine model of multivessel coronary artery disease. Anesthesiology 74:120-133, 1991.

290. Hartman JC, Kampine JP, Schmeling WT, Warltier DC: Volatile anesthetics and regional myocardial perfusion in chronically instrumented dogs: Halothane versus isoflurane in a single-vessel disease model with enhanced collateral development. J Cardiothorac Anesth 4:588-603, 1990.

291. Hartman JC, Kampine JP, Schmeling WT, Warltier DC: Steal-prone coronary circulation in chronically instrumented dogs: Isoflurane versus adenosine. Anesthesiology 74:744-756, 1991.

292. Moore PG, Kien ND, Reitan JA, et al: No evidence for blood flow redistribution with isoflurane or halothane during acute coronary artery occlusion in fentanyl-anesthetized dogs. Anesthesiology 75:854-865, 1991.

293. Hartman JC, Pagel PS, Kampine JP, et al: Influence of desflurane on the regional distribution of coronary blood flow in a chronically instrumented canine model of multivessel coronary artery obstruction. Anesth Analg 72:289-299, 1991.

294. Kersten JR, Brayer AP, Pagel PS, et al: Perfusion of ischemic myocardium during anesthesia with sevoflurane. Anesthesiology 81:995-1004, 1994.

295. Buffington CW, Romson JL, Levine A, et al: Isoflurane induces coronary steal in a canine model of chronic coronary occlusion. Anesthesiology 66:280-292, 1987.

296. Cheng DCH, Moyers JR, Knutson RM, et al: Dose-response relationship of isoflurane and halothane versus coronary perfusion pressures: Effects on flow redistribution in a collateralized chronic swine model. Anesthesiology 76:113-122, 1992.

297. Bland JHL, Lowenstein E: Halothane-induced decrease in experimental myocardial ischemia in the non-failing canine heart. Anesthesiology 45:287-293, 1976.

298. Gerson JI, Hickey RF, Bainton CR: Treatment of myocardial ischemia with halothane or nitroprusside-propranolol. Anesth Analg 61:10-14, 1982.

299. Davis RF, Sidi A: Effect of isoflurane on the extent of myocardial necrosis and on systemic hemodynamics, regional myocardial blood flow, and regional myocardial metabolism in dogs after coronary artery occlusion. Anesth Analg 69:575-586, 1989.

300. Cope DK, Impastato WK, Cohen MV, Downey JM: Volatile anesthetics protect the ischemic rabbit myocardium from infarction. Anesthesiology 86:699-709, 1997.

301. Cason BA, Gamperl AK, Slocum RE, Hickey RF: Anesthetic-induced preconditioning. Previous administration of isoflurane decreases myocardial infarct size in rabbits. Anesthesiology 87:1182-1190, 1997.

302. Buljubasic N, Stowe DF, Marijic J, et al: Halothane reduces release of adenosine, inosine, and lactate with ischemia and reperfusion in isolated hearts. Anesth Analg 76:54-62, 1993.

303. Coetzee A, Brits W, Genade S, Lochner A: Halothane does have protective properties in the isolated ischemic rat heart. Anesth Analg 73:711-719, 1991.

304. Freedman BM, Hamm DP, Everson CT, et al: Enflurane enhances postischemic functional recovery in the isolated rat heart. Anesthesiology 62:29-33, 1985.

305. Marijic J, Stowe DF, Turner LA, et al: Differential protective effects of halothane and isoflurane against hypoxic and reoxygenation injury in the isolated guinea pig heart. Anesthesiology 73:976-983, 1990.

306. Mattheussen M, Rusy BF, Van Aken H, Flameng W: Recovery of function and adenosine triphosphate metabolism following myocardial ischemia induced in the presence of volatile anesthetics. Anesth Analg 76:69-75, 1993.

307. Belo SE, Mazer CD: Effect of halothane and isoflurane on postischemic "stunned" myocardium in the dog. Anesthesiology 73:1243-1251, 1990.

308. Tanguay M, Blaise G, Dumont L, et al: Beneficial effects of volatile anesthetics on decrease in coronary flow and myocardial contractility induced by oxygen-derived free radicals in isolated rabbit hearts. J Cardiovasc Pharmacol 18:863-870, 1991.

309. Smith G, Rogers K, Thornburn J: Halothane improves the balance of oxygen supply to demand in acute experimental myocardial ischaemia. Br J Anaesth 52:577-583, 1980.

310. Bertha BG, Folts JD, Nugent M, Rusy BF: Halothane, but not isoflurane or enflurane, protects against spontaneous and epinephrine-exacerbated acute thrombus formation in stenosed dog coronary arteries. Anesthesiology 71:96-102, 1989.

311. Kowalski C, Zahler S, Becker BF, et al: Halothane, isoflurane, and sevoflurane redu ce postischemic adhesion of neutrophils in the coronary system. Anesthesiology 86:188-195, 1997.

312. Inagaki N, Gonoi T, Clement JPT, et al: Reconstitution of IKATP: An inward rectifier subunit plus the sulfonylurea receptor. Science 270:1166-1170, 1995.

313. Noma A: ATP-regulated K^+ channels in cardiac muscle. Nature 305:147-148, 1983.

314. Inoue I, Nagase H, Kishi K, Higuti T: ATP-sensitive K^+ channel in the mitochondrial inner membrane. Nature 352:244-247, 1991.

315. Yao Z, Gross GJ: Effects of the K_{ATP} channel opener bimakalim on coronary blood flow, monophasic action potential duration, and infarct size in dogs. Circulation 89:1769-1775, 1994.

316. Hamada K, Yamazaki J, Nagao T: Shortening of action potential duration is not prerequisite for cardiac protection by ischemic preconditioning or a K_{ATP} channel opener. J Mol Cell Cardiol 30:1369-1379, 1998.

317. Sato T, Sasaki N, Seharaseyon J, et al: Selective pharmacological agents implicate mitochondrial but not sarcolemmal K(ATP) channels in ischemic cardioprotection. Circulation 101:2418-2423, 2000.

318. Dos Santos P, Kowaltowski AJ, Laclau MN, et al: Mechanisms by which opening the mitochondrial ATP-sensitive K^+ channel protects the ischemic heart. Am J Physiol Heart Circ Physiol 283:H284-H295, 2002.

319. Dzeja PP, Holmuhamedov EL, Ozcan C, et al: Mitochondria: Gateway for cytoprotection. Circ Res 89:744-746, 2001.

320. Holmuhamedov EL, Jovanovic S, Dzeja PP, et al: Mitochondrial ATP-sensitive K^+ channels modulate cardiac mitochondrial function. Am J Physiol 275:H1567-H1576, 1998.

321. Holmuhamedov EL, Wang L, Terzic A: ATP-sensitive K^+ channel openers prevent Ca^{2+} overload in rat cardiac mitochondria. J Physiol 519(Pt 2):347-360, 1999.

322. Green DR, Reed JC: Mitochondria and apoptosis. Science 281:1309-1312, 1998.

323. Akao M, Ohler A, O'Rourke B, Marban E: Mitochondrial ATP-sensitive potassium channels inhibit apoptosis induced by oxidative stress in cardiac cells. Circ Res 88:1267-1275, 2001.

324. Ozcan C, Bienengraeber M, Dzeja PP, Terzic A: Potassium channel openers protect cardiac mitochondria by attenuating oxidant stress at reoxygenation. Am J Physiol Heart Circ Physiol 282:H531-H539, 2002.

325. Minners J, Lacerda L, McCarthy J, et al: Ischemic and pharmacological preconditioning in Girardi cells and C2C12 myotubes induce mitochondrial uncoupling. Circ Res 89:787-792, 2001.

326. Halestrap AP: The regulation of the matrix volume of mammalian mitochondria in vivo and in vitro and its role in the control of mitochondrial metabolism. Biochim Biophys Acta 973:355-382, 1989.

327. Garlid KD: Cation transport in mitochondria—The potassium cycle. Biochim Biophys Acta 1275:123-126, 1996.

328. Garlid KD: On the mechanism of regulation of the mitochondrial K^+/H^+ exchanger. J Biol Chem 255:11273-11279, 1980.

329. Zaugg M, Lucchinetti E, Spahn DR, et al: Volatile anesthetics mimic cardiac preconditioning by priming the activation of mitochondrial K(ATP) channels via multiple signaling pathways. Anesthesiology 97:4-14, 2002.

330. Kersten JR, Lowe D, Hettrick DA, et al: Glyburide, a K_{ATP} channel antagonist, attenuates the cardioprotective effects of isoflurane in stunned myocardium. Anesth Analg 83:27-33, 1996.

331. Nakayama M, Fujita S, Kanaya N, et al: Blockade of ATP-sensitive K^+ channel abolishes the anti-ischemic effects of isoflurane in dog hearts. Acta Anaesthesiol Scand 41:531-535, 1997.

332. Ludwig LM, Gross GJ, Kersten JR, et al: Morphine enhances pharmacological preconditioning by isoflurane: Role of mitochondrial K_{ATP} channels and opioid receptors. Anesthesiology 98:705-711, 2003.

333. Piriou V, Ross S, Pigott D, et al: Beneficial effect of concomitant administration of isoflurane and nicorandil. Br J Anaesth 79:68-77, 1997.

334. Carroll R, Yellon DM: Delayed cardioprotection in a human cardiomyocyte-derived cell line: The role of adenosine, p38MAP kinase and mitochondrial K_{ATP}. Basic Res Cardiol 95:243-249, 2000.

335. Roscoe AK, Christensen JD, Lynch C 3rd: Isoflurane, but not halothane, induces protection of human myocardium via adenosine A1 receptors and adenosine triphosphate-sensitive potassium channels. Anesthesiology 92:1692-1701, 2000.

336. Toller WG, Gross ER, Kersten JR, et al: Sarcolemmal and mitochondrial adenosine triphosphate-dependent potassium (K_{ATP}) channels. Mechanism of desflurane-induced cardio-protection. Anesthesiology 92:1731-1739, 2000.

337. Fujimoto K, Bosnjak ZJ, Kwok WM: Isoflurane-induced facilitation of the cardiac sarcolemmal K(ATP) channel. Anesthesiology 97:57-65, 2002.

338. Kwok WM, Martinelli AT, Fujimoto K, et al: Differential modulation of the cardiac adenosine triphosphate-sensitive potassium channel by isoflurane and halothane. Anesthesiology 97:50-56, 2002.

339. Han J, Kim E, Ho WK, Earm YE: Effects of volatile anesthetic isoflurane on ATP-sensitive K^+ channels in rabbit ventricular myocytes. Biochem Biophys Res Commun 229:852-856, 1996.

340. Kohro S, Hogan QH, Nakae Y, et al: Anesthetic effects on mitochondrial ATP-sensitive K channel. Anesthesiology 95:1435-1440, 2001.

341. Liu Y, Gao WD, O'Rourke B, Marban E: Priming effect of adenosine on K(ATP) currents in intact ventricular myocytes: Implications for preconditioning. Am J Physiol 273:H1637-H1643, 1997.

342. Yao Z, Mizumura T, Mei DA, Gross GJ: KATP channels and memory of ischemic preconditioning in dogs: Synergism between adenosine and KATP channels. Am J Physiol 272:H334-H342, 1997.

343. Patel HH, Ludwig LM, Fryer RM, et al: Delta opioid agonists and volatile anesthetics facilitate cardioprotection via potentiation of K(ATP) channel opening. FASEB J 16:1468-1470, 2002.

344. Daut J, Maier-Rudolph W, von Beckerath N, et al: Hypoxic dilation of coronary arteries is mediated by ATP-sensitive potassium channels. Science 247:1341-1344, 1990.

345. Cason BA, Shubayev I, Hickey RF: Blockade of adenosine triphosphate–sensitive potassium channels eliminates isoflurane-induced coronary artery vasodilation. Anesthesiology 81:1245-1255, 1994.

346. Novalija E, Fujita S, Kampine JP, Stowe DF: Sevoflurane mimics ischemic preconditioning effects on coronary flow and nitric oxide release in isolated hearts. Anesthesiology 91:701-712, 1999.

347. Crystal GJ, Zhou X, Gurevicius J, et al: Direct coronary vasomotor effects of sevoflurane and desflurane in in situ canine hearts. Anesthesiology 92:1103-1113, 2000.

348. Zhou X, Abboud W, Manabat NC, et al: Isoflurane-induced dilation of porcine coronary arterioles is mediated by ATP-sensitive potassium channels. Anesthesiology 89:182-189, 1998.

349. Kersten JR, Schmeling TJ, Tessmer JP, et al: Sevoflurane selectively dilates coronary collaterals independent of K_{ATP} channels in vivo. Anesthesiology 90:246-256, 1999.

350. Kehl F, Krolikowski JG, Tessmer JP, et al: Increases in coronary collateral blood flow produced by sevoflurane are mediated by calcium-activated potassium (BKCa) channels in vivo. Anesthesiology 97:725-731, 2002.

351. Toller WG, Kersten JR, Gross ER, et al: Isoflurane preconditions myocardium against infarction via activation of inhibitory guanine (Gi) nucleotide binding proteins. Anesthesiology 92:1400-1407, 2000.

352. Kersten JR, Orth KG, Pagel PS, et al: Role of adenosine in isoflurane-induced cardioprotection. Anesthesiology 86:1128-1139, 1997.

353. Van Wylen DGL: Effect of ischemic preconditioning on interstitial purine metabolite and lactate accumulation during myocardial ischemia. Circulation 89:2283-2289, 1994.

354. Mizumura T, Nithipatikom K, Gross GJ: Bimakalim, an ATP-sensitive potassium channel opener, mimics the effects of ischemic preconditioning to reduce infarct size, adenosine release, and neutrophil function in dogs. Circulation 92:1236-1245, 1995.

355. Ishizawa Y, Pidikiti R, Liebman PA, Eckenhoff RG: G protein-coupled receptors as direct targets of inhaled anesthetics. Mol Pharmacol 61:945-952, 2002.

356. Fryer RM, Patel HH, Hsu AK, Gross GJ: Stress-activated protein kinase phosphorylation during cardioprotection in the ischemic myocardium. Am J Physiol Heart Circ Physiol 281:H1184-H1192, 2001.

357. Fryer RM, Pratt PF, Hsu AK, Gross GJ: Differential activation of extracellular signal regulated kinase isoforms in preconditioning and opioid-induced cardioprotection. J Pharmacol Exp Ther 296:642-649, 2001.

358. Fryer RM, Schultz JE, Hsu AK, Gross GJ: Importance of PKC and tyrosine kinase in single or multiple cycles of preconditioning in rat hearts. Am J Physiol 276:H1229-H1235, 1999.

359. Liu H, McPherson BC, Yao Z: Preconditioning attenuates apoptosis and necrosis: Role of protein kinase C epsilon and delta isoforms. Am J Physiol Heart Circ Physiol 281:H404-H410, 2001.

360. Puceat M, Vassort G: Signalling by protein kinase C isoforms in the heart. Mol Cell Biochem 157:65-72, 1996.

361. Hemmings HC Jr, Adamo AI: Activation of endogenous protein kinase C by halothane in synaptosomes. Anesthesiology 84:652-662, 1996.

362. Hemmings HC Jr: General anesthetic effects on protein kinase C. Toxicol Lett 100-101:89-95, 1998.

363. Toller WG, Montgomery MW, Pagel PS, et al: Isoflurane-enhanced recovery of canine stunned myocardium: Role for protein kinase C? Anesthesiology 91:713-722, 1999.

364. Ismaeil MS, Tkachenko I, Hickey RF, Cason BA: Colchicine inhibits isoflurane-induced preconditioning. Anesthesiology 91:1816-1822, 1999.

365. Sato T, O'Rourke B, Marban E: Modulation of mitochondrial ATP-dependent K$^+$ channels by protein kinase C. Circ Res 83:110-114, 1998.

366. Sato T, Sasaki N, O'Rourke B, Marban E: Adenosine primes the opening of mitochondrial ATP-sensitive potassium channels: A key step in ischemic preconditioning? Circulation 102:800-805, 2000.

367. Hu K, Duan D, Li GR, Nattel S: Protein kinase C activates ATP-sensitive K$^+$ current in human and rabbit ventricular myocytes. Circ Res 78:492-498, 1996.

368. Liu Y, Gao WD, O'Rourke B, Marban E: Synergistic modulation of ATP-sensitive K$^+$ currents by protein kinase C and adenosine: Implications for ischemic preconditioning. Circ Res 78:443-454, 1996.

369. Ambrosio G, Zweier JL, Duilio C, et al: Evidence that mitochondrial respiration is a source of potentially toxic oxygen free radicals in intact rabbit hearts subjected to ischemia and reflow. J Biol Chem 268:18532-18541, 1993.

370. Bolli R: Oxygen-derived free radicals and postischemic myocardial dysfunction ("stunned myocardium"). J Am Coll Cardiol 12:239-249, 1988.

371. Bolli R, Patel BS, Jeroudi MO, et al: Demonstration of free radical generation in "stunned" myocardium of intact dogs with the use of the spin trap alpha-phenyl N-tert-butyl nitrone. J Clin Invest 82:476-485, 1988.

372. Zweier JL, Flaherty JT, Weisfeldt ML: Direct measurement of free radical generation following reperfusion of ischemic myocardium. Proc Natl Acad Sci U S A 84:1404-1407, 1987.

373. Nakamura T, Kashimoto S, Oguchi T, Kumazawa T: Hydroxyl radical formation during inhalation anesthesia in the reperfused working rat heart. Can J Anaesth 46:470-475, 1999.

374. Glantz L, Ginosar Y, Chevion M, et al: Halothane prevents postischemic production of hydroxyl radicals in the canine heart. Anesthesiology 86:440-447, 1997.

375. Novalija E, Varadarajan SG, Camara AK, et al: Anesthetic preconditioning: Triggering role of reactive oxygen and nitrogen species in isolated hearts. Am J Physiol Heart Circ Physiol 283:H44-H52, 2002.

376. Mullenheim J, Ebel D, Frassdorf J, et al: Isoflurane preconditions myocardium against infarction via release of free radicals. Anesthesiology 96:934-940, 2002.

377. Tanaka K, Weihrauch D, Kehl F, et al: Mechanism of preconditioning by isoflurane in rabbits: A direct role for reactive oxygen species. Anesthesiology 97:1485-1490, 2002.

378. Tanaka M, Fujiwara H, Yamasaki K, Sasayama S: Superoxide dismutase and N-2-mercaptopropionyl glycine attenuate infarct size limitation effect of ischaemic preconditioning in the rabbit. Cardiovasc Res 28:980-986, 1994.

379. Baines CP, Goto M, Downey JM: Oxygen radicals released during ischemic preconditioning contribute to cardioprotection in the rabbit myocardium. J Mol Cell Cardiol 29:207-216, 1997.

380. Pain T, Yang XM, Critz SD, et al: Opening of mitochondrial K(ATP) channels triggers the preconditioned state by generating free radicals. Circ Res 87:460-466, 2000.

381. Obata T, Yamanaka Y: Block of cardiac ATP-sensitive K$^+$ channels reduces hydroxyl radicals in the rat myocardium. Arch Biochem Biophys 378:195-200, 2000.

382. Samavati L, Monick MM, Sanlioglu S, et al: Mitochondrial K(ATP) channel openers activate the ERK kinase by an oxidant-dependent mechanism. Am J Physiol Cell Physiol 283:C273-C281, 2002.

383. Forbes RA, Steenbergen C, Murphy E: Diazoxide-induced cardioprotection requires signaling through a redox-sensitive mechanism. Circ Res 88:802-809, 2001.

384. McPherson BC, Yao Z: Morphine mimics preconditioning via free radical signals and mitochondrial K(ATP) channels in myocytes. Circulation 103:290-295, 2001.

385. Paraidathathu T, de Groot H, Kehrer JP: Production of reactive oxygen by mitochondria from normoxic and hypoxic rat heart tissue. Free Radic Biol Med 13:289-297, 1992.

386. Vanden Hoek TL, Shao Z, Li C, et al: Mitochondrial electron transport can become a significant source of oxidative injury in cardiomyocytes. J Mol Cell Cardiol 29:2441-2450, 1997.

387. Vanden Hoek TL, Becker LB, Shao Z, et al: Reactive oxygen species released from mitochondria during brief hypoxia induce preconditioning in cardiomyocytes. J Biol Chem 273:18092-18098, 1998.

388. Becker LB, Vanden Hoek TL, Shao ZH, et al: Generation of superoxide in cardiomyocytes during ischemia before reperfusion. Am J Physiol 277:H2240-H2246, 1999.

389. Zhang DX, Chen YF, Campbell WB, et al: Characteristics and superoxide-induced activation of reconstituted myocardial mitochondrial ATP-sensitive potassium channels. Circ Res 89:1177-1183, 2001.

390. Tanaka K, Weihrauch D, Ludwig LM, et al: Mitochondrial adenosine triphosphate-regulated potassium channel opening acts as a trigger for isoflurane-induced preconditioning by generating reactive oxygen species. Anesthesiology 98:935-943, 2003.

391. Tritto I, D'Andrea D, Eramo N, et al: Oxygen radicals can induce preconditioning in rabbit hearts. Circ Res 80:743-748, 1997.

392. Wang XT, McCullough KD, Wang XJ, et al: Oxidative stress-induced phospholipase C-gamma 1 activation enhances cell survival. J Biol Chem 276:28364-28371, 2001.

393. Gopalakrishna R, Jaken S: Protein kinase C signaling and oxidative stress. Free Radic Biol Med 28:1349-1361, 2000.

394. Nishida M, Maruyama Y, Tanaka R, et al: G alpha(i) and G alpha(o) are target proteins of reactive oxygen species. Nature 408:492-495, 2000.

395. Nishida M, Schey KL, Takagahara S, et al: Activation mechanism of Gi and Go by reactive oxygen species. J Biol Chem 277:9036-9042, 2002.

396. Maulik N, Watanabe M, Zu YL, et al: Ischemic preconditioning triggers the activation of MAP kinases and MAPKAP kinase 2 in rat hearts. FEBS Lett 396:233-237, 1996.

397. Dabrowski A, Boguslowicz C, Dabrowska M, et al: Reactive oxygen species activate mitogen-activated protein kinases in pancreatic acinar cells. Pancreas 21:376-384, 2000.

398. Hilfiker O, Larsen R, Sonntag H: Myocardial blood flow and oxygen consumption during halothane-nitrous oxide anaesthesia for coronary revascularization. Br J Anaesth 55:927-932, 1983.

399. Khambatta HJ, Sonntag H, Larsen R, et al: Global and regional myocardial blood flow and metabolism during equipotent halothane and isoflurane anesthesia in patients with coronary artery disease. Anesth Analg 67:936-942, 1988.

400. Sahlman L, Milocco I, Ricksten SE: Myocardial circulatory and metabolic effects of halothane when used to control intraoperative hypertension in patients with coronary artery disease. Acta Anaesthesiol Scand 36:283-288, 1992.

401. Moffitt EA, Imrie DD, Scovil JE, et al: Myocardial metabolism and haemodynamic responses with enflurane anesthesia for coronary artery surgery. Can Anaesth Soc J 31:604-610, 1984.

402. Moffitt EA, Barker RA, Glen JJ, et al: Myocardial metabolism and hemodynamic responses with isoflurane anesthesia for coronary arterial surgery. Anesth Analg 65:53-61, 1986.

403. O'Young J, Mastrocostopoulos G, Hilgenberg A, et al: Myocardial circulatory and metabolic effects of isoflurane and sufentanil during coronary artery surgery. Anesthesiology 66:653-658, 1987.

404. Sahlman L, Milocco I, Appelgren L, et al: Control of intraoperative hypertension with isoflurane in patients with coronary artery disease: Effects on regional myocardial blood flow and metabolism. Anesth Analg 68:105-111, 1989.

405. Tarnow J, Markschies-Hornung A, Schulte-Sasse U: Isoflurane improves the tolerance to pacing-induced myocardial ischemia. Anesthesiology 64:147-156, 1986.

406. Diana P, Tullock WC, Gorcsan J III, et al: Myocardial ischemia: A comparison between isoflurane and enflurane in coronary artery bypass patients. Anesth Analg 77:221-226, 1993.

407. Inoue K, Reichelt W, El-Banayosy A, et al: Does isoflurane lead to a higher incidence of myocardial infarction and perioperative death than enflurane in coronary artery surgery? A clinical study of 1178 patients. Anesth Analg 71:469-474, 1990.

408. Knight AA, Hollenberg M, London MJ, et al: Perioperative myocardial ischemia: Importance of the preoperative ischemia pattern. Anesthesiology 68:681-688, 1988.

409. Pulley DD, Kirvassilis GV, Kelermenos N, et al: Regional and global myocardial circulatory and metabolic effects of isoflurane and halothane in patients with steal-prone coronary anatomy. Anesthesiology 75:756-766, 1991.

410. Slogoff S, Keats AS: Randomized trial of primary anesthetic agents on outcome of coronary artery bypass operations. Anesthesiology 70:179-188, 1989.

411. Tuman KJ, McCarthy RJ, Spiess BD, et al: Does choice of anesthetic agent significantly affect outcome after coronary artery surgery? Anesthesiology 70:189-198, 1989.

412. Wallace A, Layug B, Tateo I, et al: Prophylactic atenolol reduces postoperative myocardial ischemia. Anesthesiology 88:7-17, 1998.

413. Mangano DT, Layug EL, Wallace A, Tateo I: Effect of atenolol on mortality and cardiovascular morbidity after noncardiac surgery. Multicenter Study of Perioperative Ischemia Group. N Engl J Med 335:1713-1720, 1996.

414. Wilkinson PL, Hamilton WK, Moyers JR, et al: Halothane and morphine-nitrous oxide anesthesia in patients undergoing coronary artery bypass operation: Patterns of intraoperative ischemia. J Thorac Cardiovasc Surg 82:372-382, 1981.

415. Moffitt EA, Sethna DH, Bussell JA, et al: Myocardial metabolism and hemodynamic responses to halothane or morphine anesthesia for coronary artery surgery. Anesth Analg 61:979-985, 1982.

416. Helman JD, Leung JM, Bellows WH, et al: The risk of myocardial ischemia in patients receiving desflurane versus sufentanil anesthesia for coronary artery bypass graft surgery. The S.P.I Research Group. Anesthesiology 77:47-62, 1992.

417. Buffington CW, Davis KB, Gillispie S, Pettinger M: The prevelance of steal-prone coronary anatomy in patients with coronary artery disease: An analysis of the Coronary Artery Surgery Study Registry. Anesthesiology 69:721-727, 1988.

418. Ebert TJ, Kharasch ED, Rooke GA, et al: Myocardial ischemia and adverse cardiac outcomes in cardiac patients undergoing noncardiac surgery with sevoflurane and isoflurane. Sevoflurane Ischemia Study Group. Anesth Analg 85:993-999, 1997.

419. Heikkila H, Jalonen J, Arola M, Laaksonen V: Haemodynamics and myocardial oxygenation during anaesthesia for coronary artery surgery: Comparison between enflurane and high-dose fentanyl anaesthesia. Acta Anaesthesiol Scand 29:457-464, 1985.

420. Leung JM, Goehner P, O'Kelly BF, et al: Isoflurane anesthesia and myocardial ischemia: Comparative risk versus sufentanil anesthesia in patients undergoing coronary artery bypass graft surgery. The SPI (Study of Perioperative Ischemia) Research Group. Anesthesiology 74:838-847, 1991.

421. Slogoff S, Keats AS, Dear WE, et al: Steal-prone coronary anatomy and myocardial ischemia associated with four primary anesthetic agents in humans. Anesth Analg 72:22-27, 1991.

422. Hanouz JL, Yvon A, Massetti M, et al: Mechanisms of desflurane-induced preconditioning in isolated human right atria in vitro. Anesthesiology 97:33-41, 2002.

423. Carroll R, Gant VA, Yellon DM: Mitochondrial K(ATP) channel opening protects a human atrial-derived cell line by a mechanism involving free radical generation. Cardiovasc Res 51:691-700, 2001.

424. Belhomme D, Peynet J, Louzy M, et al: Evidence for preconditioning by isoflurane in coronary artery bypass graft surgery. Circulation 100:II340-II344, 1999.

425. Penta de Peppo A, Polisca P, Tomai F, et al: Recovery of LV contractility in man is enhanced by preischemic administration of enflurane. Ann Thorac Surg 68:112-118, 1999.

426. De Hert SG, ten Broecke PW, Mertens E, et al: Sevoflurane but not propofol preserves myocardial function in coronary surgery patients. Anesthesiology 97:42-49, 2002.

427. Warltier DC, Pagel PS, Kersten JR: Approaches to the prevention of perioperative myocardial ischemia. Anesthesiology 92:253-259, 2000.

428. Biscoe TJ, Millar RA: The effects of cyclopropane, halothane and ether on central baroreceptor pathways. J Physiol (Lond) 184:535-559, 1966.

429. Cox RH, Bagshaw RJ: Influence of anesthesia on the response to carotid hypotension in dogs. Am J Physiol 237:H424-H432, 1979.

430. Epstein RA, Wang H-H, Bartelstone HJ: The effects of halothane on circulatory reflexes of the dog. Anesthesiology 29:867-876, 1968.

431. Seagard JL, Elegbe EO, Hopp FA, et al: Effects of isoflurane on baroreceptor reflex. Anesthesiology 59:511-520, 1983.

432. Sellgren J, Biber B, Henriksson BA, et al: The effects of propofol, methohexitone and isoflurane on the baroreceptor reflex in the cat. Acta Anaesthesiol Scand 36:784-790, 1992.

433. Skovsted P, Price HL: The effects of ethrane on arterial pressure, preganglionic sympathetic activity, and barostatic reflexes. Anesthesiology 36:257-262, 1972.

434. Skovsted P, Price ML, Price HL: The effects of halothane on arterial pressure, preganglionic sympathetic activity and barostatic reflexes. Anesthesiology 31:507-514, 1969.

435. Skovsted P, Sapthavichaikul S: The effects of isoflurane on arterial pressure, pulse rate, autonomic nervous activity, and barostatic reflexes. Can Anaesth Soc J 24:304-314, 1977.

436. Seagard JL, Hopp FA, Donegan JH, et al: Halothane and the carotid sinus reflex: Evidence for multiple sites of action. Anesthesiology 57:191-202, 1982.

437. Seagard JL, Hopp FA, Bosnjak ZJ, et al: Sympathetic efferent nerve activity in conscious and isoflurane-anesthetized dogs. Anesthesiology 61:266-270, 1984.

438. Seagard JL, Hopp FA, Bosnjak ZJ, et al: Extent and mechanism of halothane sensitization of the carotid sinus baroreceptors. Anesthesiology 58:432-437, 1983.

439. Ebert TJ, Seagard JL, Hopp FA JR: Autonomic nervous system: Measurement and response under anesthesia. In Yaksh TL, Lynch C III, Zapol WM, et al (eds): Anesthesia: Biologic Foundations. Philadelphia, Lippincott-Raven, 1997, pp 1233-1255.

440. Alper MH, Fleisch JH, Flacke W: The effects of halothane on the responses of cardiac sympathetic ganglia to various stimulants. Anesthesiology 31:429-436, 1969.

441. Christ D: Effects of halothane on ganglionic discharges. J Pharmacol Exp Ther 200:336-342, 1977.

442. Bosnjak ZJ, Seagard JL, Wu A, Kampine JP: The effects of halothane on sympathetic ganglionic transmission. Anesthesiology 57:473-479, 1982.

443. Deegan R, He HB, Wood AJJ, Wood M: Effects of anesthesia on norepinephrine kinetics: Comparison of propofol and halothane anesthesia in dogs. Anesthesiology 75:481-488, 1991.

444. Deegan R, He HB, Wood AJJ, Wood M: Effect of enflurane and isoflurane on norepinephrine kinetics: A new approach to assessment of sympathetic function during anesthesia. Anesth Analg 77:49-54, 1993.

445. Rorie DK, Tyce GM, Mackenzie RA: Evidence that halothane inhibits norepinephrine release from sympathetic nerve endings in dog saphenous vein by stimulation of presynaptic inhibitory muscarinic receptors. Anesth Analg 63:1059-1064, 1984.

446. Cristoforo MF, Brody MJ: The effects of halothane and cyclopropane on skeletal muscle vessels and baroreceptor reflexes. Anesthesiology 29:36-43, 1968.

447. Price HL, Price ML, Morse HT: Effects of cyclopropane, halothane and procaine on the vasomotor "center" of the dog. Anesthesiology 26:55-60, 1965.

448. Price HL, Linde HW, Morse HT: Central nervous actions of halothane affecting the systemic circulation. Anesthesiology 24:770-778, 1963.

449. Morton M, Duke PC, Ong B: Baroreflex control of heart rate in man awake and during enflurane and enflurane–nitrous oxide anesthesia. Anesthesiology 52:221-223, 1980.

450. Kotrly KJ, Ebert TJ, Vucins EJ, et al: Effects of fentanyl-diazepam-nitrous oxide anaesthesia on arterial baroreflex control of heart rate in man. Br J Anaesth 58:406-414, 1986.

451. Gribbin B, Pickering TG, Sleight P, Peto R: Effect of age and high blood pressure on baroreflex sensitivity in man. Circ Res 29:424-431, 1971.

452. Olshan AR, O'Connor DT, Cohen IM, et al: Baroreflex dysfunction in patients with adult-onset diabetes and hypertension. Am J Med 74:233-242, 1983.

453. Goldberg AH, Sohn YZ, Phear WP: Direct myocardial effects of nitrous oxide. Anesthesiology 37:373-380, 1972.

454. Price HL: Myocardial depression by nitrous oxide and its reversal by Ca++. Anesthesiology 44:211-215, 1976.

455. Carton EG, Wanek LA, Housmans PR: Effects of nitrous oxide on contractility, relaxation and the intracellular calcium transient of isolated mammalian ventricular myocardium. J Pharmacol Exp Ther 257:843-849, 1991.

456. Craythorne NW, Darby TD: The cardiovascular effects of nitrous oxide in the dog. Br J Anaesth 37:560-565, 1965.

457. Smith NT, Eger EI II, Stoelting RK, et al: The cardiovascular and sympathomimetic responses to the addition of nitrous oxide to halothane in man. Anesthesiology 32:410-421, 1970.

458. Ebert TJ: Differential effects of nitrous oxide on baroreflex control of heart rate and peripheral sympathetic nerve activity in humans. Anesthesiology 72:16-22, 1990.

459. Ebert TJ, Kampine JP: Nitrous oxide augments sympathetic outflow: Direct evidence from human peroneal nerve recordings. Anesth Analg 69:444-449, 1989.

460. Sellgren J, Ponten J, Wallin BG: Percutaneous recording of muscle nerve sympathetic activity during propofol, nitrous oxide, and isoflurane anesthesia in humans. Anesthesiology 73:20-27, 1990.

461. Eisele JH, Smith NT: Cardiovascular effects of 40 percent nitrous oxide in man. Anesth Analg 51:956-963, 1972.

462. Eriksen S, Johannsen G, Frost N: Effects of nitrous oxide on systolic time intervals. Acta Anaesthesiol Scand 24:74-78, 1980.

463. Falk RB Jr, Denlinger JK, Nahrwold ML, Todd RA: Acute vasodilation following induction of anesthesia with intravenous diazepam and nitrous oxide. Anesthesiology 49:149-150, 1978.

464. Lichtenthal P, Philip J, Sloss LJ, et al: Administration of nitrous oxide in normal subjects. Evaluation of systems of gas delivery for their clinical use and hemodynamic effects. Chest 72:316-322, 1977.

465. Stoelting RK, Gibbs PS: Hemodynamic effects of morphine and morphine-nitrous oxide in valvular heart disease and coronary-artery disease. Anesthesiology 38:45-52, 1973.

466. Thornton JA, Fleming JS, Goldberg AD, Baird D: Cardiovascular effects of 50 percent nitrous oxide and 50 percent oxygen mixture. Anaesthesia 28:484-489, 1973.

467. Bahlman SH, Eger EI II, Smith NT, et al: The cardiovascular effects of nitrous oxide-halothane anesthesia in man. Anesthesiology 35:274-285, 1971.

468. Coetzee A, Fourie P, Bolliger C, et al: Effect of N$_2$O on segmental left ventricular function and effective arterial elastance in pigs when added to a halothane-fentanyl-pancuronium anesthetic technique. Anesth Analg 69:313-322, 1989.

469. Dolan WM, Stevens WC, Eger EI II, et al: The cardiovascular and respiratory effects of isoflurane-nitrous oxide anaesthesia. Can Anaesth Soc J 21:557-568, 1974.

470. Lappas DG, Buckley MJ, Laver MB, et al: Left ventricular performance and pulmonary circulation following addition of nitrous oxide to morphine during coronary-artery surgery. Anesthesiology 43:61-69, 1975.

471. Lunn JK, Stanley TH, Eisele J, et al: High dose fentanyl anesthesia for coronary artery surgery: Plasma fentanyl concentrations and influence of nitrous oxide on cardiovascular responses. Anesth Analg 58:390-395, 1979.

472. Smith NT, Calverley RK, Prys-Roberts C, et al: Impact of nitrous oxide on the circulation during enflurane anesthesia in man. Anesthesiology 48:345-349, 1978.

473. Van Trigt P, Christian CC, Fagraeus L, et al: Myocardial depression by anesthetic agents (halothane, enflurane and nitrous oxide): Quantitation based on end-systolic pressure-dimension relations. Am J Cardiol 53:243-247, 1984.

474. Pagel PS, Kampine JP, Schmeling WT, Warltier DC: Effects of nitrous oxide on myocardial contractility as evaluated by the preload recruitable stroke work relationship in chronically instrumented dogs. Anesthesiology 73:1148-1157, 1990.

475. Messina AG, Yao F-S, Canning H, et al: The effect of nitrous oxide on left ventricular pump performance and contractility in patients with coronary artery disease: Effect of preoperative ejection fraction. Anesth Analg 77:954-962, 1993.

476. Eisele JH, Reitan JA, Massumi RA, et al: Myocardial performance and N$_2$O analgesia in coronary-artery disease. Anesthesiology 44:16-20, 1976.

477. Hohner P, Backman C, Diamond G, et al: Anaesthesia for abdominal aortic surgery in patients with coronary artery disease. Part II. Effects of nitrous oxide on systemic and coronary haemodynamics, regional ventricular function and incidence of myocardial ischaemia. Acta Anaesthesiol Scand 38:793-804, 1994.

478. Houltz E, Caidahl K, Hellstrom A, et al: The effects of nitrous oxide on left ventricular systolic and diastolic performance before and after cardiopulmonary bypass: Evaluation by computer-assisted two-dimensional and Doppler echocardiography in patients undergoing coronary artery surgery. Anesth Analg 81:243-248, 1995.

479. Tempe D, Mohan JC, Cooper A, et al: Myocardial depressant effect of nitrous oxide after valve surgery. Eur J Anaesthesiol 11:353-358, 1994.

480. Marsch SCU, Dalmas S, Philbin DM, et al: Effects and interactions of nitrous oxide, myocardial ischemia, and reperfusion on left ventricular diastolic function. Anesth Analg 84:39-45, 1997.

481. Carton EG, Housmans PR: Role of transsarcolemmal Ca^{2+} entry in the negative inotropic effects of nitrous oxide in isolated ferret myocardium. Anesth Analg 74:575-579, 1992.

482. Su JY, Kerrick WGL, Hill SA: Effects of diethyl ether and nitrous oxide on functionally skinned myocardial cells of rabbits. Anesth Analg 63:451-456, 1984.

483. Kawamura R, Stanley TH, English JB, et al: Cardiovascular responses to nitrous oxide exposure for two hours in man. Anesth Analg 59:93-99, 1980.

484. Winter PM, Hornbein TF, Smith G, et al: Hyperbaric nitrous oxide anesthesia in man: Determination of anesthetic potency (MAC) and cardiorespiratory effects [abstract]. Proceedings of the American Society of Anesthesiologists Annual Meeting, 1972, Boston, pp 103-104.

485. Hornbein TF, Martin WE, Bonica JJ, et al: Nitrous oxide effects on the circulatory and ventilatory responses to halothane. Anesthesiology 31:250-260, 1969.

486. Moffitt EA, Sethna DH, Gary RJ, et al: Nitrous oxide added to halothane reduces coronary flow and myocardial oxygen consumption in patients with coronary disease. Can Anaesth Soc J 30:5-9, 1983.

487. McDermott RW, Stanley TH: The cardiovascular effects of low concentrations of nitrous oxide during morphine anesthesia. Anesthesiology 41:89-91, 1974.

488. Wong KC, Martin WE, Hornbein TF, et al: The cardiovascular effects of morphine sulfate with oxygen and with nitrous oxide in man. Anesthesiology 38:542-549, 1973.

489. Stoelting RK, Reis RR, Longnecker DE: Hemodynamic responses to nitrous oxide-halothane and halothane in patients with valvular heart disease. Anesthesiology 37:430-435, 1972.

490. Schulte-Sasse U, Hess W, Tarnow J: Pulmonary vascular responses to nitrous oxide in patients with normal and high pulmonary vascular resistance. Anesthesiology 57:9-13, 1982.

491. Rorie DK, Tyce GM, Sill JC: Increased norepinephrine release from dog pulmonary artery caused by nitrous oxide. Anesth Analg 65:560-564, 1986.

492. Hilgenberg JC, McCammon RL, Stoelting RK: Pulmonary and systemic vascular responses to nitrous oxide in patients with mitral stenosis and pulmonary hypertension. Anesth Analg 59:323-326, 1980.

493. Landry LD, Emerson CW, Philbin DM, et al: The effect of nitrous oxide on pulmonary vascular resistance in children. Anesth Analg 59:548-549, 1980.

494. Eisele Jr JH, Milstein JM, Goetzman BW: Pulmonary vascular responses to nitrous oxide in newborn lambs. Anesth Analg 65:62-64, 1986.

495. Davidson JR, Chinyanga HM: Cardiovascular collapse associated with nitrous oxide anaesthetic: A case report. Can Anaesth Soc J 29:484-488, 1982.

496. Roizen MF, Plummer GO, Lichtor JL: Nitrous oxide and dysrhythmias. Anesthesiology 66:427-431, 1987.

497. Liu WS, Wong KC, Port JD, Andriano KP: Epinephrine-induced arrhythmias during halothane anesthesia with the addition of nitrous oxide, nitrogen, or helium in dogs. Anesth Analg 61:414-417, 1982.

498. Eisele JH Jr: Cardiovascular effects of nitrous oxide. *In* Eger EI II (ed): Nitrous Oxide: N_2O. New York, Elsevier, 1985, pp 125-156.

499. Puerto BA, Wong KC, Puerto AX, et al: Epinephrine-induced dysrhythmias: Comparison during anaesthesia with narcotics and with halogenated inhalational agents in dogs. Can Anaesth Soc J 26:263-268, 1979.

500. Hughes JM, Sill JC, Pettis M, Rorie DK: Nitrous oxide constricts epicardial coronary arteries in pigs: Evidence suggesting inhibitory effects of endothelium. Anesth Analg 77:232-240, 1993.

501. Stowe DF, Monroe SM, Marijic J, et al: Effects of nitrous oxide on contractile function and metabolism of the isolated heart. Anesthesiology 73:1220-1226, 1990.

502. Dottori O, Haggendal E, Linder E, et al: The haemodynamic effects of nitrous oxide anaesthesia on myocardial blood flow in dogs. Acta Anaesthesiol Scand 20:421-428, 1976.

503. Wilkowski DAW, Sill JC, Bonta W, et al: Nitrous oxide constricts epicardial coronary arteries without effect on coronary arterioles. Anesthesiology 66:659-665, 1987.

504. Cason BA, Demas KA, Mazer CD, et al: Effects of nitrous oxide on coronary pressure and regional contractile function in experimental myocardial ischemia. Anesth Analg 72:604-611, 1991.

505. Nathan HJ: Nitrous oxide worsens myocardial ischemia in isoflurane-anesthetized dogs. Anesthesiology 68:407-415, 1988.

506. Philbin DM, Foex P, Drummond G, et al: Postsystolic shortening of canine left ventricle supplied by a stenotic coronary artery when nitrous oxide is added in the presence of narcotics. Anesthesiology 62:166-174, 1985.

507. Siker D, Pagel PS, Pelc LR, et al: Nitrous oxide impairs functional recovery of stunned myocardium in barbiturate-anesthetized, acutely instrumented dogs. Anesth Analg 75:539-548, 1992.

508. Nathan HJ: Control of hemodynamics prevents worsening of myocardial ischemia when nitrous oxide is administered to isoflurane-anesthetized dogs. Anesthesiology 71:686-694, 1989.

509. Kozmary SV, Lampe GH, Benefiel D, et al: No finding of increased myocardial ischemia during or after carotid endartectomy under anesthesia with nitrous oxide. Anesth Analg 70:591-596, 1990.

510. Lawrence JH, Loomis WF, Tobias CA, Turpin FH: Preliminary observations on the narcotic effect of xenon with a review of values for solubilities of gases in water and oils. J Physiol (Lond) 105:197-204, 1946.

511. Steward A, Allott PR, Cowles AL, Mapleson WW: Solubility coefficients for inhaled anaesthetics in water, oil and biological media. Br J Anaesth 45:282-293, 1973.

512. Kennedy RR, Stokes JW, Downing P: Anaesthesia and the "inert" gases with special reference to xenon. Anaesth Intensive Care 20:66-70, 1992.

513. Luttropp HH, Romner B, Perhag L, Eskilsson J, Fredriksen S, Werner O: Left ventricular performance and cerebral haemodynamics during xenon anaesthesia: A transesophageal echocardiography and transcranial Doppler sonography study. Anaesthesia 48:1045-1049, 1993.

514. Luttropp HH, Thomasson R, Dahm S, et al: Clinical experience with minimal flow xenon anesthesia. Acta Anaesthesiol Scand 38:121-125, 1994.

515. Goto T, Saito H, Shinkai M, et al: Xenon provides faster emergence from anesthesia than does nitrous oxide–sevoflurane or nitrous oxide–isoflurane. Anesthesiology 86:1273-1278, 1997.

516. Yagi M, Mashimo T, Kawaguchi T, Yoshiya I: Analgesic and hypnotic effects of subanaesthetic concentrations of xenon in human volunteers: Comparison with nitrous oxide. Br J Anaesth 74:670-673, 1995.

517. Ohara A, Mashimo M, Zhang P, et al: A comparative study of the antinociceptive action of xenon and nitrous oxide. Anesth Analg 85:931-936, 1997.

518. Saito H, Saito M, Goto T, Morita S: Priming of anesthesia circuit with xenon for closed circuit anesthesia. Artif Organs 21:70-72, 1997.

519. Luttropp HH, Rydgren G, Thomasson R, Werner O: A minimal-flow system for xenon anesthesia. Anesthesiology 75:896-902, 1991.

520. Lynch C III, Baum J, Tenbrinck R: Xenon anesthesia. Anesthesiology 92:865-870, 2000.

521. Boomsma F, Rupreht J, Man in 't Veld AJ, et al: Haemodynamic and neurohumoral effects of xenon anaesthesia: A comparison with nitrous oxide. Anaesthesia 45:273-278, 1990.

522. Marx T, Froeba G, Wagner D, et al: Effects on haemodynamics and catecholamine release of xenon anaesthesia compared to total I.V. anaesthesia in the pig. Br J Anaesth 78:326-327, 1997.

523. Zhang P, Ohara A, Mashimo T, et al: Pulmonary resistance in dogs: A comparison of xenon with nitrous oxide. Can J Anaesth 42:547-553, 1995.
524. Preckel B, Ebel D, Mullenheim J, et al: The direct myocardial effects of xenon in the dog heart in vivo. Anesth Analg 94:545-551, 2002.
525. Nakata Y, Goto M, Saito H, et al: Plasma concentration of fentanyl with xenon to block somatic and hemodynamic responses to surgical incision. Anesthesiology 92:1043-1048, 2000.
526. Nakata Y, Goto T, Morita S: Effects of xenon on hemodynamic responses to skin incision in humans. Anesthesiology 90:406-410, 1999.
527. Stowe DF, Rehmert GC, Kwok WK, et al: Xenon does not alter cardiac function or major cation currents in isolated guinea pig hearts or myocytes. Anesthesiology 92:516-522, 2000.
528. Huneke R, Jugling E, Skasa M, et al: Effects of the anesthetic gases xenon, halothane, and isoflurane on calcium and potassium currents in human atrial cardiomyocytes. Anesthesiology 95:999-1006, 2001.
529. Preckel B, Mullenheim J, Moloschavij A, et al: Xenon administration during early reperfusion reduces infarct size after regional ischemia in the rabbit heart in vivo. Anesth Analg 91:1327-1332, 2000.
530. Hettrick DA, Pagel PS, Kersten JR, et al: Cardiovascular effects of xenon in isoflurane-anesthetized dogs with dilated cardiomyopathy. Anesthesiology 1998; 89:1166-1173, 1998.
531. Ishiguro Y, Goto T, Nakata Y, et al: Effect of xenon on autonomic cardiovascular control—Comparison with isoflurane and nitrous oxide. J Clin Anesth 12:196-201, 2000.

8 Metabolism and Toxicity of Modern Inhaled Anesthetics

Jackie L. Martin, Jr. and Dolores B. Njoku

Drug Metabolism and Biotransformation   231
The Liver and Drug Metabolism   231
Pharmacogenetics of Drug Metabolism   234
Pharmacogenomics of Drug Metabolism   236

Metabolism of Inhaled Anesthetics   236
Nonhalogenated Inhaled Anesthetics   236
Halogenated Inhaled Anesthetics   237

Stereoselective Metabolism of Inhaled Anesthetics   240

Toxicity of Inhaled Anesthetics   240
Hepatitis   240
Fluoride-Associated Nephrotoxicity   248
Toxic Products Formed by Interactions with Carbon Dioxide Absorbents   251
Other Toxicities   256

Summary   262

After a drug is administered, it undergoes the processes of absorption, distribution, target interaction, metabolism, and excretion. Unlike most drugs, inhaled anesthetics are administered in great excess of the amount metabolized. Biotransformation has little effect on the pharmacologic activity of anesthetics but may have a significant effect on anesthetic toxicities. It was once thought that the inhaled anesthetics were chemically inert, but many of these anesthetic agents undergo significant metabolism and, in many cases, biotransformation and chemical breakdown to reactive and potentially toxic intermediates. The metabolic processes are affected by many factors, including age, disease, drug-drug interactions, and perhaps most importantly, genetics. This chapter focuses on the current understanding of mechanisms of anesthetic associated toxicities, particularly liver injury and the role of drug metabolism in many of these processes. The clinical mechanisms, implications, and risks of haloalkene- and carbon monoxide–associated toxicities, as well as other side effects of inhaled anesthetics, are reviewed.

DRUG METABOLISM AND BIOTRANSFORMATION

The Liver and Drug Metabolism

The lipophilic characteristics of drugs that promote their passage through biologic membranes hinder their excretion from the body. Drug metabolism is therefore essential for elimination and termination of biologic activity of lipophilic drugs because it usually results in the formation of more hydrophilic products that are less pharmacologically active and more readily excreted from the body (Fig. 8-1). Drug metabolism sometimes results in the formation of intermediates whose pharmacologic or toxicologic activity are equal to, greater than, or different from the parent drug.[1] Unlike most drugs, the inhaled anesthetics are administered in great excess of the amount metabolized and are excreted mainly by exhalation. Biotransformation has little effect on the pharmacologic activity of anesthetics, but it may have a significant effect

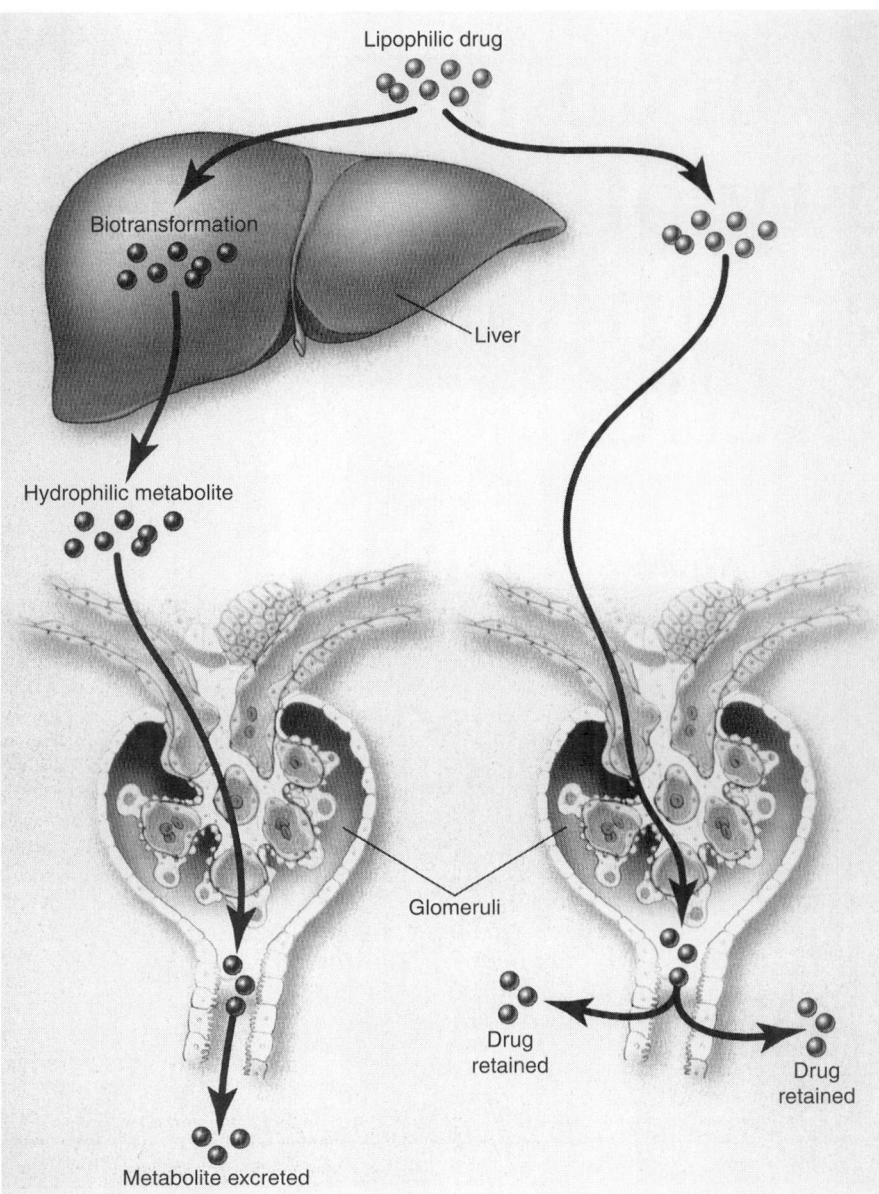

Lipophilic drug

Biotransformation

Liver

Hydrophilic metabolite

Glomeruli

Drug retained

Drug retained

Metabolite excreted

Figure 8–1 Effects of drug metabolism on excretion. Lipophilic (fat-soluble) drugs are metabolized to form relatively more hydrophilic (water-soluble) metabolites than the parent drug, and these metabolites are more easily excreted. (From Weinshilboum R: Inheritance and drug response. N Engl J Med 348:529-537, 2003.)

on the toxicity of these agents.[2] Inhaled anesthetics are absorbed through the respiratory epithelium and mucous membranes of the respiratory tract. Because of the large pulmonary surface area, access to the circulation is rapid, with almost instantaneous absorption of these agents into the blood and avoidance of hepatic first pass metabolism. The pharmacologic effects of inhaled anesthetics are rather rapid and depend less on factors governing the activities of other drugs, such as the amount of drug administered, the extent and rate of absorption, protein binding, excretion, secretion, and metabolism.[3]

The liver is the primary organ of drug metabolism because of its large size, rich concentration of drug-metabolizing enzymes, and unique double blood supply, consisting of 70% of the flow from the portal vein and 30% from the hepatic artery. Blood in the portal vein comes from the alimentary tract, pancreas, and spleen. Toxic materials absorbed from the alimentary tract are

processed by the liver before they enter the systemic circulation. Blood flows through the hepatic sinusoids from the periphery of the hepatic lobule, fed by portal veins and hepatic arteries, to the centrally located hepatic venule or central vein. The hepatocytes, which are bathed by the sinusoidal blood supply, are the major drug-metabolizing cells in the liver and body. Several drug-metabolizing enzyme systems are located within the smooth endoplasmic reticulum of hepatocytes, and others are found in the cytosol of these cells. In addition to the liver, organs with significant drug-metabolizing activity are the gastrointestinal tract, kidneys, and lungs.[4,5]

The major enzymatic reactions biotransforming drugs into metabolites are oxidation, hydrolysis, and conjugation. It is common for a drug to be metabolized into several metabolites. The ratios of various metabolites of a drug depend on enzymatic reaction rates, drug concentration near the enzymes, physicochemical reactions between metabolites and enzymes, competition of multiple drugs or endogenous substrates for the same enzyme, and many other factors.[5] Drug biotransformation reactions are classified broadly as phase 1 functionalization reactions or phase 2 biosynthetic conjugation reactions. The phase 1 reactions are catalyzed by enzymes that introduce or expose a polar functional group such as a hydroxyl or amino moiety in a drug by oxidation or hydrolytic reactions, respectively, whereas phase 2 reactions often lead to the enzymatic conjugation of these polar functional groups to very polar molecules. The net effect of these reactions is the formation of molecules that are more easily excreted into the urine through the kidneys or into the gastrointestinal tract by biliary excretion. *N*-acetylation is the exception, because it leads to the formation of less water-soluble metabolites.

The phase 1 enzymes most relevant to the metabolism of inhaled anesthetics are the cytochromes P450 (CYPs). These enzymes are capable of catalyzing several different types of oxidations reactions, including dehalogenations, *N*- and *O*-dealkylations, *N*- and *S*-oxidations, and deamination reactions. All of these reactions require CYP, oxygen, and NADPH-dependent cytochrome P450 reductase for activity and occur in the endoplasmic reticulum of cells, particularly hepatocytes. Under conditions of low oxygen tension, these enzymes may catalyze reductive reactions. Approximately 50 of the more than 1000 CYPs are functionally active in humans and are categorized into 17 families and subfamilies. Sequences with greater than 40% homology belong to the same family and are identified by an arabic numeral. The sequences of subfamily members are at least 55% identical and are distinguished by a capital letter. An arabic number is used to distinguish individual isoforms within a subfamily. CYP2E1, for example, is a member of the CYP2 family, which is a large family of isozymes that metabolizes many diverse drugs and endogenous compounds.[6] Approximately 10 isoforms in the CYP1, CYP2, and CYP3 families are responsible for most drug metabolism in humans (Fig. 8-2). Most CYP isoforms metabolize multiple drugs, and some overlap in substrate specificity can be seen between the various isoforms. Two or more CYP isoforms may be involved in the overall metabolism of a drug. In human liver, CYP3A4 and CYP3A5 subfamilies account for as much as 60% of the total CYP present. CYP2E1 is particularly important in the oxidative metabolism of halogenated inhaled anesthetics, and like many CYPs, it is concentrated in the perivenular hepatocytes.

In phase 2 reactions, a polar molecule such as glucuronic acid, sulfate, or glycine is conjugated to a drug or its metabolites to produce highly hydrophilic products that are readily excreted into the urine or, in some cases, into the bile and gastrointestinal tract. Glucuronidation is perhaps the most important conjugation reaction, and uridine 5'-diphosphate glucuronosyltransferase (UGT) catalyzes the transfer of glucuronic acid to aromatic and aliphatic alcohols, carboxylic acids, amines, and free sulfhydryl groups to form *O*-, *N*-, and *S*-glucuronides, respectively. UGTs, like CYPs, exist as multiple isoforms with different substrate specificities and are localized in the

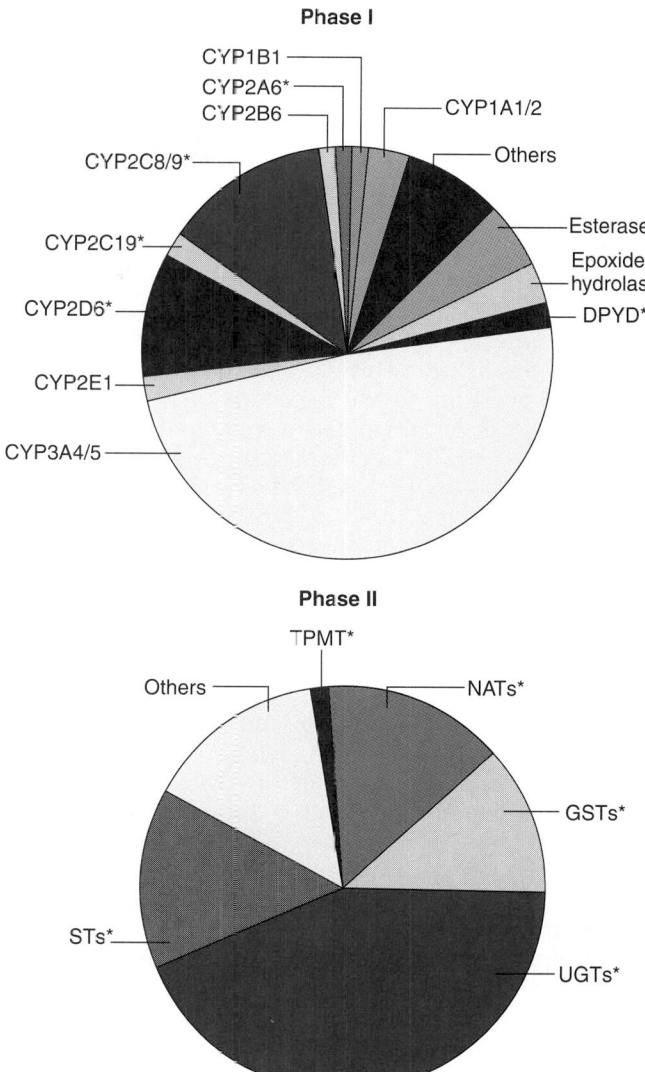

Figure 8–2 Proportion of drugs metabolized by major phase 1 or phase 2 enzymes. The relative size of each pie section indicates the estimated percentage of phase 1 *(left)* or phase 2 *(right)* metabolism that each enzyme contributes to the metabolism of drugs based on literature reports. Enzymes that have functional allelic variants are indicated by an *asterisk*. In many cases, more than one enzyme is involved in a particular drug's metabolism. CYP, cytochrome P450; DPYD, dihydropyridine dehydrogenase; GST, glutathione *S*-transferase; NAT, *N*-acetyltransferase; ST, sulfotransferase; TPMT, thiopurine methyltransferase; UGT, UDP-glucuronosyltransferase. (Adapted from Wilkinson G: Pharmacokinetics: The dynamics of drug absorption, distribution and elimination. *In* Hardman JG, Limbird LE, Goodman GA [eds]: Goodman and Gilman's the Pharmacological Basis of Therapeutics, 10th ed. New York, McGraw-Hill, 2001.)

endoplasmic reticulum, whereas most other phase 2 enzymes are concentrated in the cytosol. Glucuronidation is also important in the elimination of endogenous steroids, bilirubin, bile acids, and fat-soluble vitamins. Cytosolic sulfation is another important conjugation reaction that involves the catalytic transfer by various sulfotransferase members of inorganic sulfate from activated 3'-phosphoadenosine-5'-phosphosulfate to the hydroxyl group of phenols and aliphatic alcohols. Drugs and primary metabolites with a hydroxyl group often form glucuronide and sulfate conjugates. Two *N*-acetyltransferases, NAT1 and NAT2, are involved in the acylation of amines, hydrazines, and sulfonamides (see Fig. 8-2).

Factors Affecting Drug Metabolism

Various factors may affect drug metabolism, including environmental determinants, disease, age, gender, and genetics. The activity of many drug-metabolizing enzymes may be increased (i.e., induced) or decreased (i.e., inhibited) by concomitantly administered drugs. Enzyme induction results from enhanced gene transcription after prolonged exposure to an induction agent or, in some instances, to a decreased rate of enzyme degradation. The induction of CYPs by numerous drugs and environmental agents has been extensively studied by many researchers.[7] Enzyme inducers are often highly lipophilic drugs and environmental chemicals that are metabolized by the CYP isozymes they induce. The inducing properties of a drug are unrelated to the nature of its pharmacologic or toxicologic activity and may vary markedly from those of other drugs in the same class. Induction by drugs such as phenobarbital results in proliferation of the smooth endoplasmic reticulum and an increase in liver weight. With this type of inducer, NADPH–cytochrome P450 reductase and specific CYP isozymes are preferentially increased. Although other inducers increase the synthesis of specific CYP isozymes, they do not affect cytochrome P450 reductase or liver weight. Many classes of drugs and environmental chemicals, including anesthetics, anticonvulsants, insecticides, sedatives, steroids, and tranquilizers, contain one or more compounds considered to be enzyme inducers.[7,8] Even the inhaled anesthetics can induce drug-metabolizing enzymes if exposure is sufficiently prolonged.[9,10] If the parent compound is toxic, enhanced metabolism may decrease toxicity. In contrast, when metabolites are more toxic than the parent compound, metabolism increases toxicity. In many cases involving induction, the dosage of an affected drug must be increased to maintain the therapeutic effect.

Enzyme-inducing agents have the potential to modify acute and chronic toxicities of anesthetics. In view of the current practice of polypharmacy, enzyme induction may be more common in patients undergoing surgery than previously appreciated. Enzyme induction does not necessarily increase the metabolism of all drugs from the same class. For example, unlike methoxyflurane metabolism, enflurane metabolism is not significantly increased in vivo after phenobarbital or phenytoin treatment in humans.[11] Even when anesthetics that are metabolized to toxic metabolites are administered to surgical patients taking enzyme-inducing drugs, significant amounts of toxic metabolites are not necessarily produced.[12,13]

The consequences of enzyme inhibition for therapeutic activity and toxicity can be just as great as those of enzyme induction. This can lead to an increase in the plasma concentration of the parent drug and a reduction in drug metabolites, as well as exaggerated and prolonged pharmacologic effects and an increased chance of toxicity. Many compounds inhibit the activity of the drug-metabolizing enzymes and thereby alter the duration and intensity of pharmacologic action and the severity of toxic effects. There are several mechanisms of inhibition.[14] Protein synthesis inhibitors such as cycloheximide decrease enzyme synthesis and reduce enzyme concentrations. Other agents are reversible inhibitors that compete for the active site of the same enzyme responsible for metabolism of the drug of interest. Still others are irreversible inhibitors that degrade the heme in cytochrome P450. Inhibition of CYP3A is common and important because of the increased expression of CYP3A in the intestinal epithelium and the fact that oral ingestion is the most common route of entry for drugs. There is a potential increase in bioavailability associated with a reduction of first-pass metabolism. Potent CYP3A inhibitors include ritonavir, diltiazem, nicardipine, and verapamil. More general inhibitors of CYPs include amiodarone and cimetidine.

Some sex-related differences in drug-metabolizing activities have been observed, particularly for CYP3A, but such differences are minor relative to previously described factors. An exception is the treatment of seizure patients with phenytoin during pregnancy. Because the liver is the major site of drug metabolism, intrinsic liver disease leading to hepatic dysfunction can impair drug metabolism. Diseases such as hepatitis, primary biliary cirrhosis, alcoholic liver disease, cirrhosis, and hepatocarcinoma can lead to a 50% impairment of enzymatic activity. Severe cardiac failure with decreased hepatic perfusion and impaired metabolism can also occur, as evidenced by the twofold difference in the loading and maintenance doses of lidocaine for dysrhythmia treatment in patients with heart failure. Moreover, viral infections can lead to the inhibition of CYP-mediated reactions.

Developmental Differences in Infants and Children

Phase 1 and phase 2 enzymes begin to mature during the postnatal period, but the levels may be low enough in some case to result in toxicities if drug therapy is not carefully monitored (see Chapter 60). For example, the impairment of bilirubin glucuronidation at birth can lead to hyperbilirubinemia of the newborn and "gray baby" syndrome caused by high levels of the antibiotic chloramphenicol.[15,16] As children age, phase 1 enzymes appear to be affected to a greater degree than phase 2 enzymes. The predominant isoform expressed in fetal liver is CYP3A7, which peaks shortly after birth and then declines rapidly to levels that are undetectable in most adults.[17] Within hours of birth, CYP2E1 activity increases, followed by CYP2D6, CYP3A4, CYP2C9, and CYP2C19. CYP1A2 is the last isoform to appear at about 2 months of age. CYP2C9 and CYP2C19 are responsible for the biotransformation of phenytoin. The apparent half-life of phenytoin is prolonged to about 75 hours in preterm neonates but decreases to about 20 hours in term neonates during the first week of life and 8 hours by the second week of life.[18]

Pharmacogenetics of Drug Metabolism

Although CYPs are most often thought of as being responsible for the deactivation of toxic compounds, they are also responsible for the metabolic activation of drugs and chemicals to toxic forms. Any factor that can influence metabolism has the potential to affect toxicity. Drug biotransformation may be affected by many factors, including route of administration, frequency of administration, exposure to other chemicals, sex, age, diet, and genetics. The concept of *pharmacogenetics* originated from the clinical observation that there were patients with very low or very high plasma or urinary drug levels, followed by the realization that the biochemical traits leading to this variation were inherited. Soon thereafter, drug-metabolizing enzymes were identified, followed by discovery of the genes encoding the proteins and the DNA sequences within the genes. Most of the early pharmacogenetic traits were monogenic, involving a single gene, and most were caused by genetic polymorphism.

The discovery that impairment in the phase 1 hydrolysis of succinylcholine by butyrylcholinesterase was inherited served as an early stimulus for the development of pharmacogenetics. About 1 in 3500 whites are homozygous for a gene encoding an atypical form of butyrylcholinesterase. These individuals have less ability to hydrolyze succinylcholine, prolonging the neuromuscular-blocking effects of this drug.[19,20] Other studies demonstrate that the CYP2D6 enzyme represents one of the best understood examples of pharmacogenetic variation in drug metabolism. Substrates for CYP2D6 include codeine, metoprolol, nortriptyline, dextromethorphan, debrisoquin, and sparteine.[21] Approximately 5% to 10% of white subjects were found to be deficient in their ability to metabolize the antihypertensive drug debrisoquin[21] and the antiarrhythmic drug sparteine,[22] which resulted in low levels of urinary metabolites and high plasma concentrations of the parent compounds. These deficiencies are inherited as an autosomal recessive trait.[22,23] The cDNA for the gene encoding CYP2D6 has been cloned, and a number of genetic variants responsible for the deficient activities of CYP2D6 have been identified. Other subjects have multiple copies of active forms of CYP2D6 that result in rapid elimination of drugs, leading to subtherapeutic levels. Such is the case for the antidepressant nortriptyline (Fig. 8-3). There exist many other examples of poor metabolizers of drugs who have genetic variants of other CYP isoforms. For example, CYP2C9 variants can lead to the poor metabolism of warfarin and phenytoin and subsequent toxic levels of these compounds. Similarly, polymorphisms in the phase 2 metabolizing enzyme N-acetyltransferase (NAT) can lead to bimodal differences in the N-acetylation and inactivation of the antituberculosis drug isoniazid (Fig. 8-4). Molecular cloning studies have shown that there are two NAT genes in humans, *NAT1* and *NAT2*, and the common genotypic polymorphism responsible for the pharmacogenetic variation in isoniazid metabolism involves the *NAT2* gene.[24] The frequency of each acetylation phenotype depends on race but not sex or age. Fast acetylation is found in Inuit and Japanese, and slow acetylation predominates among Scandinavians and North African whites.[25] Another example of the role of genetics in phase 2 metabolism concerns the antineoplastic drug azathioprine, a prodrug that is converted into the active drug, 6-mercaptopurine. Thiopurines such as

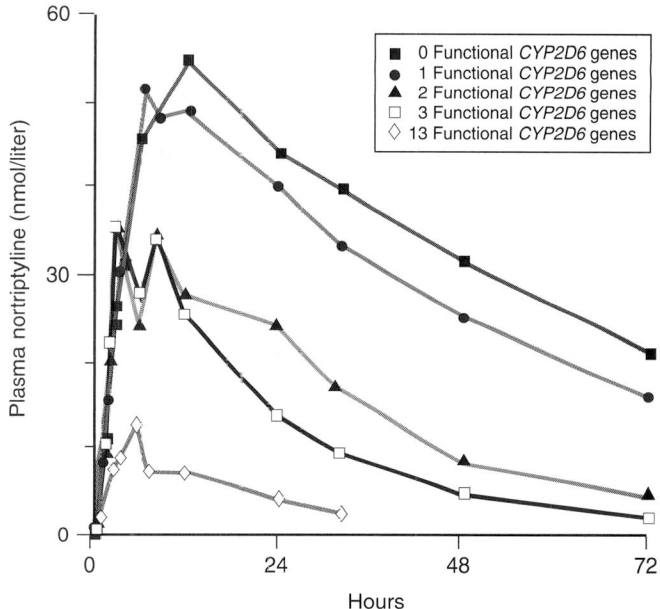

Figure 8–3 Pharmacogenetics of nortriptyline. Mean plasma concentrations of nortriptyline after a single 25-mg oral dose are shown in subjects with 0, 1, 2, 3, or 13 functional *CYP2D6* genes. (Adapted from Weinshilboum R: Inheritance and drug response. N Engl J Med 348:529-537, 2003.)

6-mercaptopurine are metabolized by thiopurine S-methyltransferase (TPMT).[26,27] This enzymatic activity is inherited in an autosomal codominant fashion. Individuals who are homozygous for alleles encoding inactive TPMT and are receiving standard doses of azathioprine are at risk of developing severe pancytopenia.

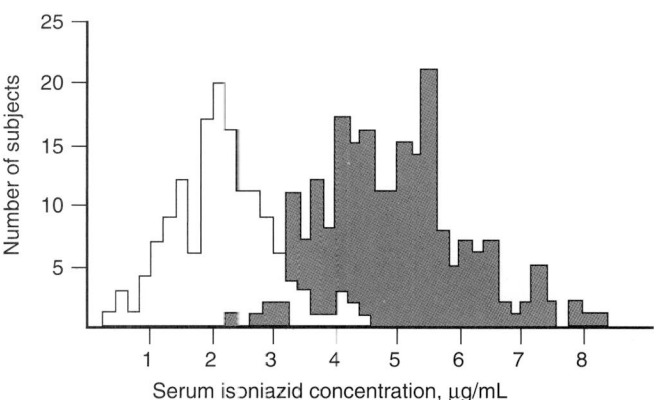

Figure 8–4 Bimodal distribution of serum isoniazid concentrations in a large group of Finnish patients. More than 300 patients were given intravenous injections of 5 mg/kg of isoniazid. Serum drug concentrations were assayed at multiple times after injection. The distribution of serum concentrations of isoniazid is shown for 180 minutes after injection. The red histogram represents rapid inactivators, and the white histogram represents slow inactivators. (From Petri WA Jr: Antimicrobial agents: Drugs used in the chemotherapy of tuberculosis, Mycobacterium complex disease and leprosy. *In* Hardman JG, Limbird LE, Goodman GA [eds]: Goodman and Gillman's the Pharmacological Basis of Therapeutics, 10th ed. New York, McGraw-Hill, 2001.)

Pharmacogenomics of Drug Metabolism

The convergence of pharmacogenetics and human genomics has resulted in the field of *pharmacogenomics*, a term used to describe the influence of DNA-sequence variation on the effect of a drug. The field of pharmacogenomics began with a focus on drug metabolism but has been extended to include the full spectrum of drug disposition, including absorption, transporters, excretion, drug targets, and signal transduction. With the completion of the Human Genome Project, the time is rapidly approaching when the sequences of virtually all genes encoding enzymes that catalyze phase 1 and phase 2 reactions will be known. More than 1.4 million single nucleotide polymorphisms were identified in the initial screening of the human genome, with more than 60,000 in the coding region for genes. Some of these single-nucleotide polymorphisms (SNPs) have already been associated with substantial changes in the metabolism or effects of medications, and some are being used to predict clinical response. The potential exists for pharmacogenomics to yield a powerful set of molecular diagnostic tools with which clinicians can select medications and drug doses for individual patients.

METABOLISM OF INHALED ANESTHETICS

Nonhalogenated Inhaled Anesthetics

Nitrous Oxide

Since the introduction of general anesthesia, a number of nonhalogenated agents have been used as anesthetics (e.g., diethyl ether, ethylene, cyclopropane), but only nitrous oxide (N_2O) remains in clinical use. This drug is not metabolized in human tissue. However, in a physicochemical reaction of N_2O with vitamin B_{12}, N_2O is reductively metabolized by rat and human intestinal bacteria to molecular nitrogen (N_2).[28,29] N_2O reduction in bacteria may occur through a single electron transfer process that results in the formation of nitrogen gas (N_2) and free radicals. The reaction between vitamin B_{12} and N_2O was first reported in 1968, but its clinical relevance was not realized for 10 years.[30] N_2O can oxidize vitamin B_{12} and inhibit its coenzyme function. For example, this reaction could affect the activity of methionine synthase, which catalyses the transmethylation from methyltetrahydrofolate and homocysteine to produce tetrahydrofolate and methionine. The inhibition of methionine synthase can lead to decreased levels of tetrahydrofolate and methionine and subsequent impairment of DNA synthesis and "carbon 1" metabolic reactions, including methylations.

However, such an effect on the activity of vitamin B_{12} probably is inconsequential with the short courses of anesthesia using N_2O.

N_2O can induce hepatic enzyme after prolonged exposure to unspecified concentrations of the drug.[31] Conversely, continuous exposure of rats to 20% N_2O for 14 to 35 days inhibited hepatic drug metabolism and induced pulmonary and testicular metabolism.[32] Exposure of mice to as much as 50% N_2O for 4 hours per day for 14 weeks did not affect hepatic content of cytochrome P450 or the defluorination of enflurane or methoxyflurane.[33] In another study, hexobarbital sleeping time in rats, used as an indicator of drug metabolism, was unchanged after exposure to 50% N_2O for 7 hours per day for 5 days.[34]

Xenon

The noble gases xenon, krypton, and argon are all chemically inert under most circumstances, and all have anesthetic properties. Xenon is of particular interest because it is the only inert gas that is an anesthetic under normobaric conditions. Xenon was first identified as an anesthetic agent in 1951.[35] Although not approved for clinical use, xenon has been submitted for regulatory medical approval in Europe. Xenon is a normal constituent in atmospheric air at a concentration no greater than 0.086 ppm and, unlike all other inhaled anesthetics, is not an environmental pollutant. The gas cannot be manufactured but is recovered in the process of fractional distillation of liquefied air, and after several separation steps, a purity of more than 99.99% can be obtained. The cost of xenon is about $10.00 (U.S.) per liter (i.e., 100 times more expensive than N_2O), and it may be unlikely to enjoy widespread use due to the expense associated with its extraction from air. If this problem could be overcome, xenon would be the most ideal inhaled anesthetic agent, because xenon (minimum alveolar concentration [MAC] = 71%) is more potent than N_2O, can provide surgical anesthesia in 30% oxygen, is very insoluble (blood-gas partition coefficient = 0.14), and has positive medical and environmental effects (Table 8-1). Xenon exhibits minimal cardiovascular and hemodynamic side effects, is not known to be metabolized in the liver or kidney, is not teratogenic, and does not trigger malignant hyperthermia in susceptible swine.[36] Environmental positives are that xenon does not deplete stratospheric ozone nor contribute to global warming and the greenhouse effect. The unique combination of analgesia, hypnosis, and lack of cardiovascular depression in this one agent makes xenon a very attractive choice for patients with limited cardiovascular reserve. Xenon has a density of 5.887 g/L, whereas N_2O and air have densities of 1.53 g/L and 1.00 g/L, respectively. Because of its greater density, xenon does increase

Table 8–1   Anesthetic properties of xenon compared with other anesthetics

	Xenon	Nitrous Oxide	Isoflurane	Desflurane	Sevoflurane
Oil-gas partition coefficient	1.9	1.4	90	18.7	53.4
Blood-gas partition coefficient	0.14	0.47	1.4	0.42	0.6
Minimum alveolar concentration(%)	71	~105	1.15	6.0	1.71

pulmonary resistance,[37] which increases the work of breathing.[38] Xenon should be used with caution in patients with moderate to severe chronic obstructive pulmonary disease, the morbidly obese, premature infants, and any other patient for whom an increase in the work of breathing may have adverse effects.

Xenon was first used successfully for general anesthesia in human volunteers and patients in the 1950s,[35,39] was largely forgotten for 40 years, and rediscovered in 1990.[40] Over the past decade, xenon has been intensely studied in Europe and Japan in a number of clinical trials, with very promising results.[41-43] Lachmann and colleagues[40] showed that patients anesthetized with 70% xenon and 30% oxygen required 80% less supplemental fentanyl than a similar group anesthetized with 70% N_2O and 30% oxygen. In a comparison of 30 American Society of Anesthesiologists (ASA) class I and class II patients undergoing total abdominal hysterectomy and receiving 60% xenon, 60% N_2O with 0.5% isoflurane, or 60% N_2O with 0.7% sevoflurane (all patients had epidurals and received mepivacaine to control heart rate and blood pressure to within 20% of baseline), Goto and coworkers[44] found emergence from xenon anesthesia was two to three times faster than either comparison group. In a randomized, controlled, multicenter trial, a total of 224 patients from six centers received 60% xenon in 40% oxygen or 60% N_2O in 0.5% isoflurane, with 1 µg sufentanil given if indicated by defined criteria.[45] This study demonstrated a significantly faster recovery from xenon anesthesia compared with isoflurane-N_2O anesthesia. It is too early to know whether xenon anesthesia improves clinical outcomes, particularly in high-risk patients, and justifies the additional costs associated with its use in clinical anesthesia.

During xenon anesthesia, nitrogen released from the patient's body accumulates in the anesthesia circuit. Consequently, it is necessary to perform a prolonged denitrogenation before starting xenon to reduce the risk of hypoxia. Another technical challenge lies in the transition from denitrogenation to closed-circuit xenon anesthesia. The anesthesiologist could increase fresh gas flows (too expensive) or add xenon to the circuit as oxygen is consumed by the patient. This second method is too slow because patients typically consume only 200 to 250 mL of oxygen per minute. Several investigators use a second anesthesia machine already primed with 4 L of xenon. Xenon must be given using a rebreathing system, low fresh gas flow, or a closed-circuit system. A closed-circuit system is the most economical technique for the clinical use of xenon. In the study by Goto and coworkers[44] from Japan, the estimated costs of providing anesthesia per patient were $170.00 for xenon ($17.00/L), $57.00 for isoflurane, and $60.00 for sevoflurane. These differences in cost would be different in the United States (xenon = $10.00/L) and would become progressively smaller with longer duration of anesthesia because the rate of xenon consumption declines exponentially as body tissues become saturated in a closed rebreathing system. The total yearly production of xenon is approximately 6 million liters or enough for about 400,000 anesthetic procedures. If delivery systems become available that allow for recycling of anesthetic gases, xenon anesthesia may become more economical and available for selected patients who may benefit from its lack of adverse systemic effects.

Halogenated Inhaled Anesthetics

Halothane

Approximately 25% of administered halothane ($CF_3CHBrCl$) is metabolized to trifluoroacetic acid (CF_3COOH), chloride (Cl^-), and bromide (Br^-) (Fig. 8-5). The major metabolite in humans is trifluoroacetic acid, formed from oxidative metabolism primarily by CYP2E1 and to a lesser extent CYP2A6.[46] The rate-limiting step in oxidative metabolism is breaking of the carbon-hydrogen bond.[47] The first intermediate formed probably is 1,1,1-trifluoro-2-chloro-2-bromoethanol, which would be expected to rapidly decompose to produce hydrogen bromide, and the reactive metabolite, trifluoroacetyl chloride (TFA-Cl). The latter metabolite reacts with water to produce HCl and trifluoroacetic acid, and with phosphatidyl ethanolamine, a membrane phospholipid,[48] to form N-trifluoroacetyl-2-aminoethanol, which has been identified in urine.[49] The TFA-Cl metabolite of halothane also reacts with tissue proteins to form trifluoroacetylated (TFA)–protein adducts (discussed in "Halothane-Associated Immune-Mediated Hepatotoxicity"). Although trifluoroethanol

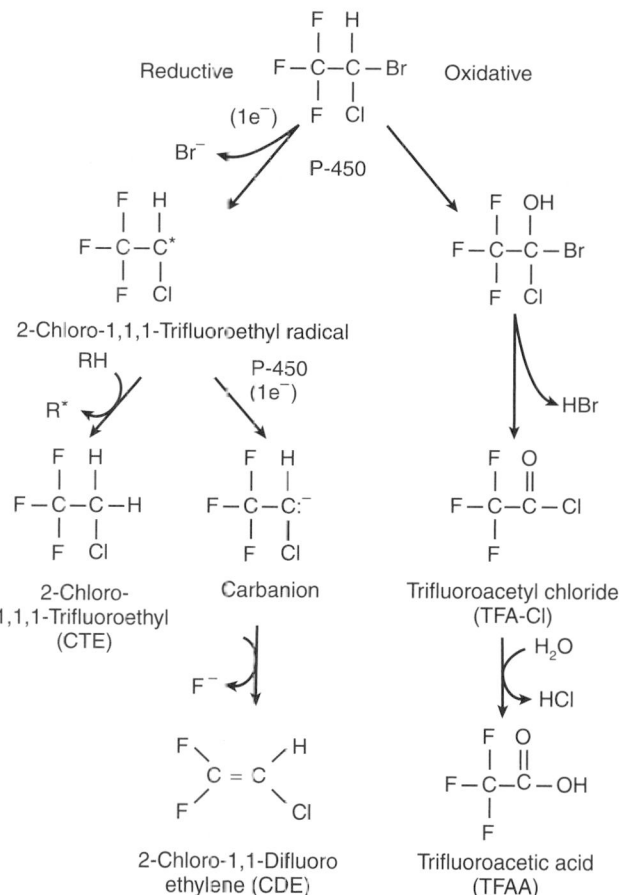

Figure 8-5 Major by-products of oxidative and reductive CYP2E1-catalyzed halothane metabolism.

has been identified in the urine of experimental animals, this metabolite and its glucuronide conjugate have not been found in human urine. Likewise, trifluoroacetalde-hyde, another possible metabolite, has not been isolated from human urine.

An alternative and minor route of halothane metabolism (<1% of absorbed halothane) is by means of a reductive pathway that requires low oxygen tension and can be catalyzed by CYP2A6 and CYP3A4 (see Fig. 8-5).[46] Inorganic Br⁻ and F⁻ are end products of this pathway.[50-52] Two volatile metabolites (2-chloro-1,1-difluoro-ethylene [CDE] and 2-chloro-1,1,1-trifluorethane [CTE]) and a volatile decomposition product of halothane (2-bromo-2-chloro-1,1-difluoroethylene [DBE]) were first identified in the exhaled gases of patients anesthetized with halothane.[53] The formation of CDE and the release of F⁻ probably result from a CYP-mediated, two-electron reduction of halothane, whereas CTE formation and the production of tissue free radicals result from a CYP-mediated, one-electron reduction.[53,54] The suicidal inactivation of CYP observed under hypoxic conditions (<40 torr O_2)[55] is presumably the result of the covalent binding of a reactive intermediate of CTE to CYP formed during the metabolism of CTE by CYP. A major pathway of DBE formation is by the base-catalyzed dehydrofluorination of halothane as a result of its interaction with soda lime.[53,56]

CYP2E1 is inducible by ethanol and by isoniazid and is inhibited by disulfiram.[57] In experimental animals, halothane metabolism is increased after the administration of CYP-inducing agents phenobarbital,[58] Aroclor 1254,[52] and isoniazid.[59] Prolonged exposure to subanesthetic concentrations of halothane results in increased drug metabolism in humans.

Enflurane

Enflurane (CHF_2-O-CF_2-CHClF) is essentially no longer used in the United States, but examination of its metabolism illustrates how relatively minor changes in chemical structure can dramatically affect the extent of metabolism. Approximately 2.5% of absorbed enflurane is metabolized (Fig. 8-6). Initial oxidation and breaking of the carbon-hydrogen bond may occur at the chlorofluoromethyl carbon or at the difluoromethyl carbon. Studies of the metabolism of enflurane with human hepatic microsomes[60] and the isolation of difluoromethoxydifluoroacetic acid from rat liver,[61] human urine,[61,62] human hepatic microsomes, and cDNA-expressed CYP2E1[60] suggest that primary metabolism occurs at the chlorofluoromethyl carbon. Detection of insignificant amounts of chlorofluoroacetic acid further suggests that there is very little metabolism at the difluorormethyl carbon. The reactive intermediate formed from oxidation at the chlorofluoromethyl carbon can hydrolyze to produce difluoromethoxydifluoroacetic acid or acetylate tissue protein to produce an adduct with immunogenic potential.[63] In either case, inorganic F⁻ is a product of these chemical reactions.

Surgical patients treated on a long-term basis with phenobarbital, phenytoin, or diazepam or who consumed ethanol before anesthesia with enflurane did not have elevated serum F⁻ concentrations compared with untreated patients. In contrast, about 50% of surgical patients on chronic isoniazid therapy demonstrated significantly elevated serum F⁻ concentrations.[12] It is unclear why 50% of patients did not significantly defluorinate enflurane. Studies with purified CYP2E1 from rabbits[64] and humans[65] demonstrate that this CYP isoform is predominantly, if not exclusively, responsible for enflurane defluorination in human liver. Isoniazid treatment seems to significantly enhance enflurane metabolism in vitro in rats,[10] rabbits,[64] and humans.[65] In contrast, treatment of rats with phenobarbital[34] phenytoin,[8] or ethanol[64,66] increases enflurane defluorination marginally. As with methoxyflurane, defluorination of enflurane in rats decreases after treatment with the CYP inhibitors SKF-525A or metyrapone.[34] Continuous exposure of rats to subanesthetic concentrations of enflurane significantly decreases hexobarbital sleeping time, indicating that the metabolism of hexobarbital is induced by enflurane.

Isoflurane

Isoflurane (CHF_2-O-CHCl-CF_3), an isomer of enflurane, is metabolized even more slowly (≈0.2%) than halothane or enflurane (see Fig. 8-6). The metabolism of isoflurane results from oxidation of the α-carbon by hepatic CYP2EI.[67,68] The initial hydroxylated intermediate can decompose to produce a reactive TFA-Cl metabolite identical to halothane or a reactive trifluoroacetyl ester intermediate. Both of these products can be expected to react with water to form trifluoroacetic acid or with protein to produce TFA-protein adducts. Very small amounts of inorganic fluoride are expected to be formed during this metabolism. Although phenobarbital[69,70] phenytoin,[71] ethanol,[72] and isoniazid[73,74] pretreatments increase the defluorination of isoflurane, serum F⁻ levels are not clinically significant.[75]

Desflurane

Desflurane (CHF_2-O-CHF-CF_3) is expected to be metabolized in a manner similar to isoflurane, because these two molecules differ by only one atom at the α-carbon position; desflurane has a fluorine atom, and isoflurane has a chlorine atom (see Fig. 8-6). However, the fluorine atom substitution decreases the metabolism at the α-carbon position significantly so that the amount of F⁻ and nonvolatile organic fluorine compounds formed from the metabolism of desflurane is considerably less compared with isoflurane.[76] Peak serum F⁻ concentrations are seen immediately after exposure to desflurane.[77] No increases in serum F⁻ levels above baseline concentrations were measured after volunteers received 7.4 MAC-hours of desflurane. Pretreatment of rats with phenobarbital or ethanol only slightly enhances serum F⁻ concentrations for a brief period.[78]

Sevoflurane

The rate of sevoflurane [CH_2F-O-CH-$(CF_3)_2$] defluorination in vitro is approximately the same as that of methoxyflurane.[79,80] However, serum F⁻ concentrations after sevoflurane administration are significantly less than those after methoxyflurane,[79-81] presumably the result of large differences in blood-gas partition coefficients of the two agents (0.69 for sevoflurane versus 10.2 for methoxyflurane). Approximately 5% of absorbed sevoflurane is biotransformed.[81,82] The fluoromethoxy C-H bond is the site of sevoflurane oxidative metabolism leading to

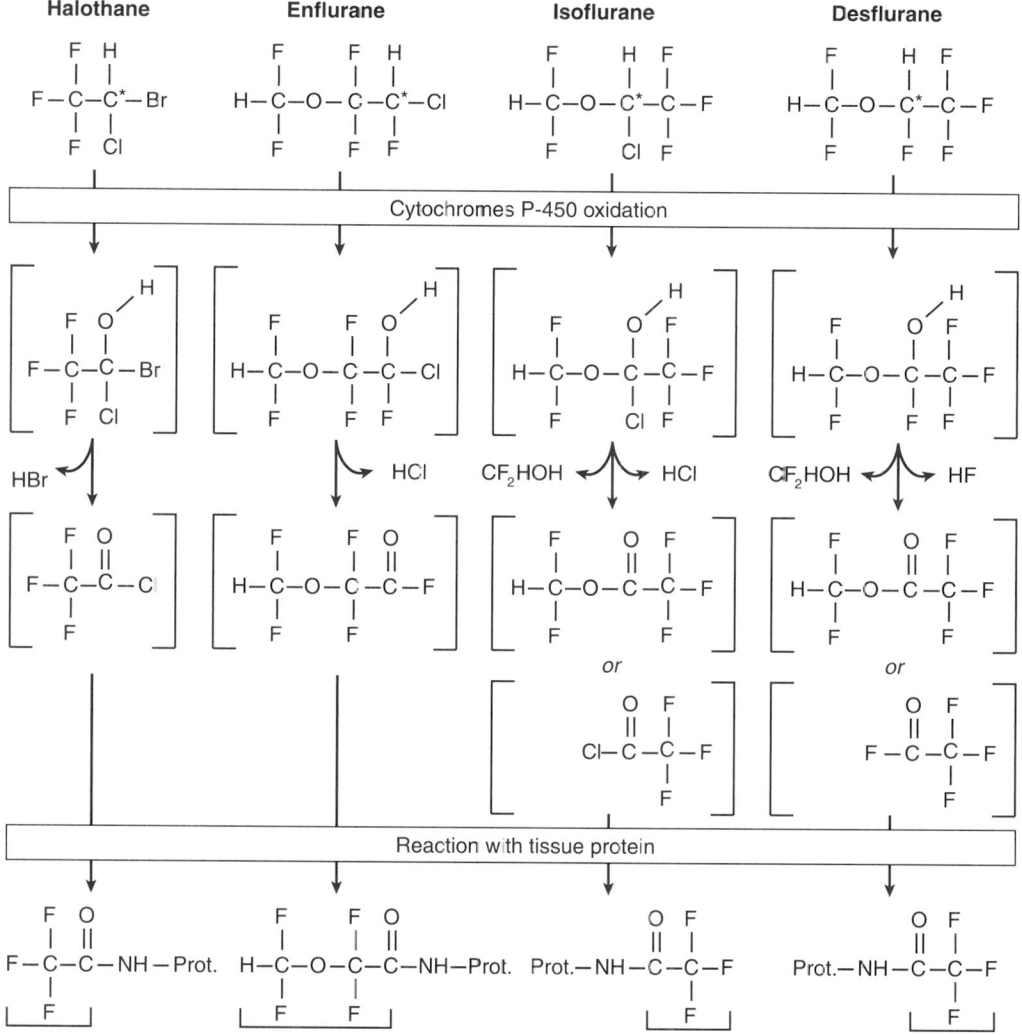

Figure 8–6 Proposed pathways for the CYP2E1-catalyzed metabolism of halothane, enflurane, isoflurane, and desflurane to acylated hepatic proteins. For halothane, isoflurane, and desflurane, the trifluoroacetylated protein adducts are identical in structure, but for enflurane, the adduct is immunologically similar.

the formation of hexafluoroisopropanol and inorganic F^- (Fig. 8-7).[83,84] Experiments using CYP2E1 purified from rabbits[64] and humans confirm the results of in vitro studies with liver microsomes that this isozyme is the predominant, if not the only, CYP participating in sevoflurane oxidation and F^- formation. As with methoxyflurane, the addition of cytochrome b_5 to the reaction mixture significantly enhances metabolism.

In a study of human volunteers, hexafluoroisopropanol accounted for 80% of nonvolatile organic fluorine-containing compounds detected in the blood and urine of volunteers anesthetized with sevoflurane.[81] Hexafluoroisopropanol is not subject to further degradation, but it is conjugated to form a glucuronide conjugate.[64,82] Studies of patients and volunteers have shown that much of the metabolism of sevoflurane to F^- occurs during anesthetic exposure, presumably because of the low tissue solubility of sevoflurane and the stability of its metabolites.[85,86] Peak serum F^- concentrations are reached within a few hours of the end of anesthesia. In rats, phenobarbital pretreatment in vivo increased

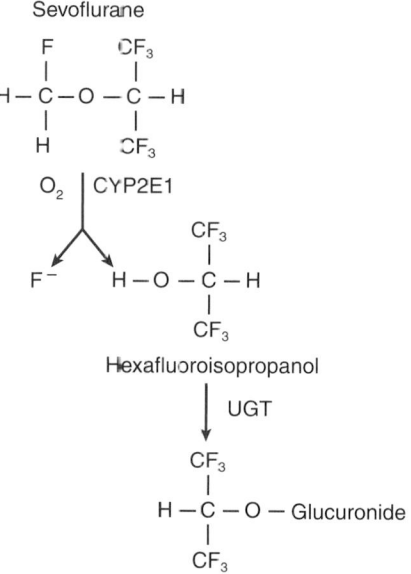

Figure 8–7 In vivo metabolism of sevoflurane to inorganic fluoride (F^-) and hexafluoroisopropanol.

sevoflurane defluorination,[69] as did phenytoin,[71] isoniazid,[73,87] ethanol,[88] and phenobarbital[8,69] pretreatments when sevoflurane defluorination was studied in rat liver microsomes in vitro.

Stereoselective Metabolism of Inhaled Anesthetics

Many drugs, including the fluorinated anesthetics, are prepared and used therapeutically as racemic mixtures. Clinical experience has confirmed that enantiomeric (i.e., non-superimposable mirror image) forms of drugs may differ in their potency, pharmacologic actions, and toxicities.[89-92] Such non-superimposable objects are said to be *chiral*. The most common chiral origin is the presence of an asymmetric center, a carbon atom attached to four different substitute groups. Enantiomers are optically active; a single enantiomeric form rotates the plane of polarized light passing through an aqueous solution of the enantiomer in a clockwise or counterclockwise direction. The International Union of Pure and Applied Chemistry (IUPAC) preferred method for the classification of enantiomers is the Cahn-Perlog-Ingold convention or (R/S) classification. In this system, the four substitutions around the chiral center are assigned priorities depending on atomic number and atomic mass. When looking down the carbon bond to the substituent with the lowest priority, if the other substituents are ordered from higher to lower in a clockwise direction, the assignment is the (R)-configuration; if counterclockwise, the (S)-configuration is designated.

Whether the clinical use of a single stereoisomer provides significant advantages depends on pharmacokinetic and pharmacodynamic properties of the respective enantiomers. For example, (S)-penicillamine is used to treat Wilson's disease, cystinuria, and rheumatoid arthritis because of toxicities associated with the racemic drug.[93] The calcium channel blocker (S)-verapamil is 10 to 20 times more potent than (R)-verapamil and appears to be a better antiarrhythmic, antianginal, and antihypertensive agent.[94] The cardiovascular drug (S)-propranolol is clinically useful as an antihypertensive and antianginal agent, whereas (R)-propranolol, which lacks cardiovascular effects, is useful in the treatment of hypothyroidism.[95,96] Ketamine is provided for clinical use as a racemic mixture, although (S)-ketamine has superior efficacy, faster elimination, and recovery characteristics, with fewer side effects, ranging from restlessness and agitation to emergence reactions, compared with racemic ketamine.[97] (S)-Ketamine is three times more potent than (R)-ketamine as an anesthetic and analgesic agent, and enantiomeric stereoselectivity of hepatic metabolism of ketamine by microsomal enzymes has been demonstrated.[98] Ropivacaine, the (S)-enantiomer of a bupivacaine homolog, and levobupivacaine [i.e., (S)-bupivacaine] were developed as alternatives to racemic bupivacaine because of its known central nervous system and cardiovascular toxicities. Ropivacaine is less potent than (S)-bupivacaine or racemic bupivacaine in blocking sodium channels, although the anesthetic and analgesic effects of the two drugs are similar.[99] Perhaps the most infamous example of enantiomeric differences between optical isomers was observed with the drug thalidomide.

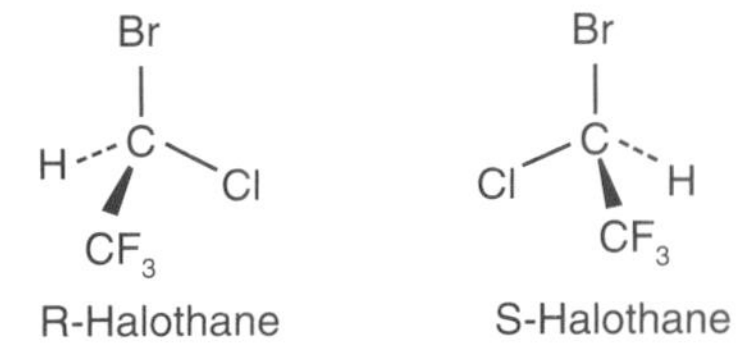

Figure 8–8 (R)- and (S)-enantiomers of halothane.

The (R)- and (S)-isomers of thalidomide and the racemic mixture are equally active hypnotics; however, (S)-thalidomide is transformed into metabolites that proved to be embryogenic and teratogenic.[100]

Commercial halothane is a racemic mixture of the (R)- and (S)-enantiomers (Fig. 8-8). Metabolic studies have shown that racemic halothane undergoes oxidative metabolism catalyzed by CYP2E1 to TFA-Cl, which covalently binds to several hepatic proteins that are believed to be involved in the immune response leading to halothane hepatotoxicity. To investigate whether CYP2E1 catalyzes the metabolism of halothane in a stereoselective fashion, the enantiomers of halothane were prepared and tested in vivo for their ability to form covalently bound TFA-protein adducts in the liver of mice. It was found that halothane underwent stereoselective metabolism, with the (R)-isomer producing significantly greater amounts of TFA-protein adducts in liver than the (S)-isomer[101] (Fig. 8-9). Because the anesthetic potency of the isomers appears to be equal,[102] these findings suggest that the (S)-isomer of halothane may be a safer inhaled anesthetic agent than the (R)-isomer or the racemic mixture. This idea is supported by the observation that the hepatotoxicity caused by halothane, enflurane, isoflurane, and desflurane is related to their relative degree of oxidative metabolism in vivo to reactive acyl halide metabolites (see Fig. 8-6). Because enflurane, isoflurane, and desflurane also contain an asymmetric carbon atom, the potential for stereoselective metabolism exists with these agents. Other researchers have found that the ratio of (R)-enflurane metabolism was 1.9:1 compared with (S)-enflurane metabolism in human liver microsomes.[60] It has also been demonstrated that optical isomers of isoflurane exhibit a significant difference in anesthetic potency,[103] differentially increase sleep time in mice,[104] and exhibit a modest but significant stereoselectivity at the γ-aminobutyric acid A (GABA$_A$) receptor.[105-107] The clinical use of chiral anesthetic drugs as equal mixtures of their enantiomers has been accepted practice in medicine and anesthesia. With increased knowledge and awareness regarding drug toxicities, future anesthetic drugs may be developed and marketed as single, more potent, and potentially less toxic optically active isomers.

TOXICITY OF INHALED ANESTHETICS

Hepatitis

Volatile halogenated anesthetics have been associated with hepatotoxicity since the introduction of chloroform in 1847. Chloroform, carbon tetrachloride, and

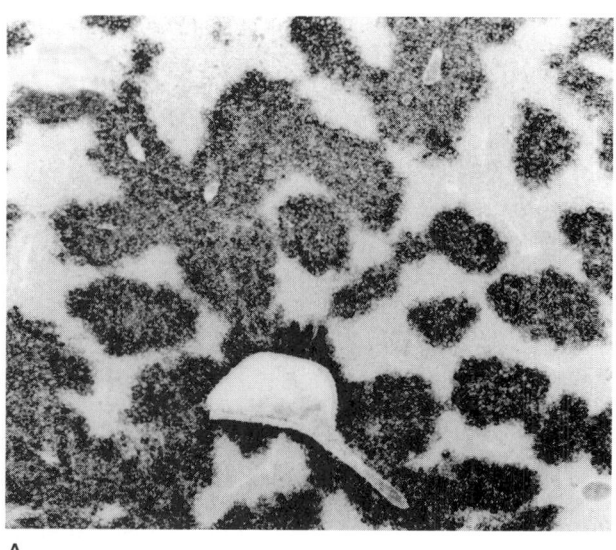 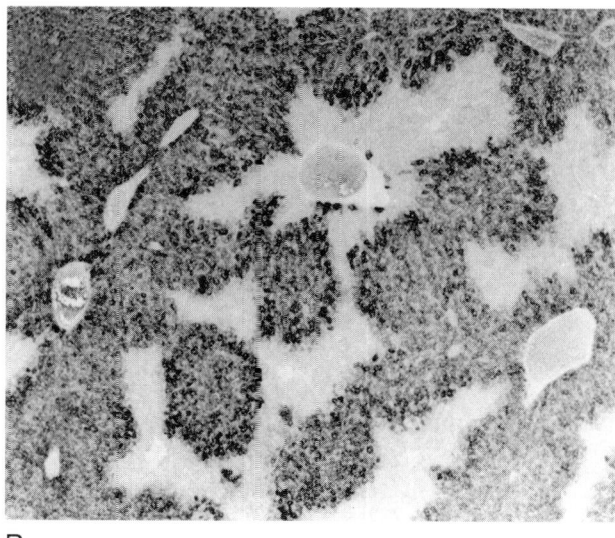

A   B

Figure 8–9 Immunochemical detection of trifluoroacetylated proteins in the livers of mice 24 hours after treatment with (R)- or (S)-halothane. **A,** Mouse treated with (R)-halothane (original magnification ×50). **B,** Mouse treated with (S)-halothane (original magnification ×50). (From Njoku D, Laster MJ, Gong DH, et al: Biotransformation of halothane, enflurane, isoflurane and desflurane to trifluoroacetylated liver proteins: Association between protein acylation and liver injury. Anesth Analg 84:173-178, 1997.)

trichloroethylene were all abandoned as anesthetic agents because of the often observed hepatotoxicity associated with their use. With its introduction into clinical practice in 1956, halothane quickly gained widespread acceptance and use. Halothane was the first of the fluorinated alkane anesthetics and represented a major advance in general anesthetics because it was safe, nonflammable, nonexplosive, and well tolerated by patients. However, within 2 years of its introduction, numerous reports of hepatotoxicity and massive and often fatal hepatic necrosis associated with its use appeared in the medical literature.[108-111] As a result of continuing reports, a large, retrospective analysis, the National Halothane Study, was undertaken under the auspices of the Committee on Anesthesia of the National Academy of Sciences National Research Council.[112] The study compared the mortality and incidence of postoperative hepatic necrosis associated with halothane with that of other general anesthetics, such as ether, cyclopropane, and balanced anesthesia. The study reviewed 865,515 general anesthetics from 1959 to 1962 at 34 medical institutions, identifying 82 cases of fatal hepatic necrosis. Drug-induced hepatic injury was suggested in nine of these cases, and seven of the nine patients had received halothane. Four of the seven patients had received halothane on more than one occasion during the preceding 6 weeks. The study concluded that the mortality rate associated with the use of halothane compared favorably with that of other general anesthetics in use at the time and estimated the incidence of fatal hepatic necrosis associated with halothane at 1 in 10,000 halothane anesthetics. It was further concluded that "unexplained fever and jaundice in a specific patient after the use of halothane should serve as a warning sign to avoid its subsequent use in that patient."[112] These findings provided the impetus for much of the work

done over the past 40 years on the cause of inhaled anesthetic hepatotoxicity, which is now accepted as a distinct clinical entity. Several hundred cases of hepatotoxicity have been attributed to halothane[113-115] and approximately 50 cases to enflurane,[116] whereas hepatotoxicity appears to be rare in cases of isoflurane[117,118] and desflurane.[119]

Drug-induced liver injury may be caused by intrinsic or idiosyncratic mechanisms.[120] Liver injury that is intrinsic to a particular pharmacologic agent is predictable and largely independent of host influences. Acetaminophen and chloroform are examples of pharmacologic agents that cause an intrinsic form of liver injury. The dose threshold for intrinsic toxicities may be achieved because of increased production, altered tissue sequestration, or decreased elimination of toxic metabolites. Moreover, other pharmacologic agents or chemicals, altered physiologic states, or pathologic states may affect the dose threshold for these toxicities. Nonetheless, when the dose threshold is surpassed, tissue injury may result from the direct actions of the metabolite, which may result in inhibition or modification of the enzymatic and structural systems necessary for maintaining cellular integrity.

In contrast to intrinsic mechanisms of toxicity, most pharmacologic agents produce adverse reactions through an idiosyncratic pathway. These reactions are generally host dependent, relatively uncommon, and difficult to produce in animals in which the mechanisms can be systematically studied. Nevertheless, studies done by several laboratories have suggested that many idiosyncratic reactions, including liver injury caused by inhaled anesthetics, may have an allergic or hypersensitivity basis initiated not by the parent drug itself, but instead by drug-protein adducts because small molecules are not immunogenic. These adducts are usually formed from interaction of a reactive metabolite of a drug with tissue

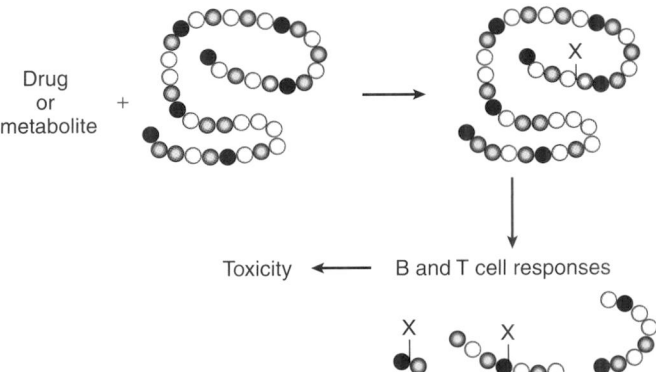

Drug or metabolite +

Toxicity ← B and T cell responses

Figure 8–10 Reactive haptens can covalently bind to a native protein, forming a hapten-protein conjugate. This conjugate can initiate an immune response against the hapten, the native protein, or new antigenic determinants on the carrier molecule induced by the hapten's presence.

proteins because most drugs are not reactive enough to form covalent adducts with tissue macromolecules. After a drug metabolite–protein adduct (i.e., hapten-carrier conjugate) is formed, it may initiate specific antibody or T-cell immune responses against the hapten (i.e., bound drug metabolite), the protein carrier, or an alternate antigenic determinant on the carrier molecule induced by the bound hapten, resulting in immunopathologic injury (Fig. 8-10).

Halothane-Associated, Immune-Mediated Hepatotoxicity

Two distinct types of hepatic injury have been associated with the clinical use of halothane (Table 8-2). A mild injury occurs in 20% of adults who receive halothane, and laboratory tests show mild elevations of alanine aminotransferase (ALT) and aspartate aminotransferase (AST). The second type of injury is the fulminant form, commonly known as *halothane hepatitis*, which is characterized by elevated levels of ALT, AST, bilirubin, and alkaline phosphatase; massive hepatic necrosis; and a fatality rate between 50% and 75%. Because of the potential for halothane-induced hepatitis, halothane is generally not recommended for use in adults. In several medical malpractice cases, the use of halothane resulting in injury or

death of patients has been successfully litigated against anesthesia health care providers. Although there are some indications for the use of halothane in adults, they must be clearly evaluated and written in the medical record before each such use.

Clinical evidence and immunochemical data have suggested that halothane hepatitis may have in some cases an allergic or hypersensitivity basis. Patients often have a history of multiple anesthetic exposures to halothane and one or more symptoms suggestive of on-going immune processes, including fever, rash, arthralgia, and eosinophilia. The first immunochemical evidence suggesting that halothane hepatitis may have an immune-mediated basis was described in 1980, when it was reported that 7 of 11 patients diagnosed with halothane hepatitis had serum antibodies that reacted with the surface of hepatocytes isolated from halothane-exposed rabbits.[121] It was subsequently found that patients with halothane hepatitis often had serum antibodies that recognized native liver microsomal proteins or liver microsomal proteins that were TFA-modified by the TFA-Cl metabolite of halothane[122-130] (see Fig. 8-10). The TFA-protein adducts (Table 8-3), produced by the oxidative metabolism of halothane, are thought to induce humoral or T-cell sensitization, or both, in susceptible individuals that on subsequent exposures to halothane can cause immunopathology[131,132] (Fig. 8-11). Several attempts have been made to develop an animal model of halothane hepatitis that has an immunopathologic basis, but no one has successfully accomplished this task.[133-140] However, studies in guinea pigs have provided important clues regarding the mechanism of halothane hepatitis.

The guinea pig is the only animal studied in which halothane can cause hepatotoxicity without the requirements of extensive pretreatments or other manipulations such as exposing animals to hypoxic conditions.[141] It is thought that the guinea pig is a model of the milder, self-limiting form of liver injury that occurs in approximately 20% of patients administered halothane.[135,136] This form of liver injury, however, may also be a prerequisite for the subsequent development of severe liver damage caused by immunopathologic mechanisms. The reason for this is that injury to hepatocytes would allow adequate levels of the TFA-protein adducts (i.e., neoantigens) to be picked up by professional antigen presenting cells, presumably dendritic cells. These cells may subsequently have a role in activating antigen-specific naive B- and T-cells to produce

Table 8–2   Clinical features of halothane hepatitis

Mild Form	Fulminant Form
Incidence 1:5	Incidence 1:10,000
Repeat exposure not necessary	Multiple exposures
Mild elevation of ALT, AST	Marked elevation of ALT, AST, bilirubin, alkaline phosphatase
Focal necrosis	Massive hepatic necrosis
Self-limited	Mortality rate: 50%
	Antibodies to halothane-altered protein antigens

ALT, alanine aminotransferase; AST, aspartate aminotransferase.

Table 8–3   Halothane antigens

Molecular mass (kd)	Protein
100	Endoplasmin
82	GRP-78
80	ERP-72
63	Calreticulin
59	Carboxylesterase
57	Protein disulfide isomerase
54	Cytochrome P450
58	Protein disulfide isomerase (isoform)

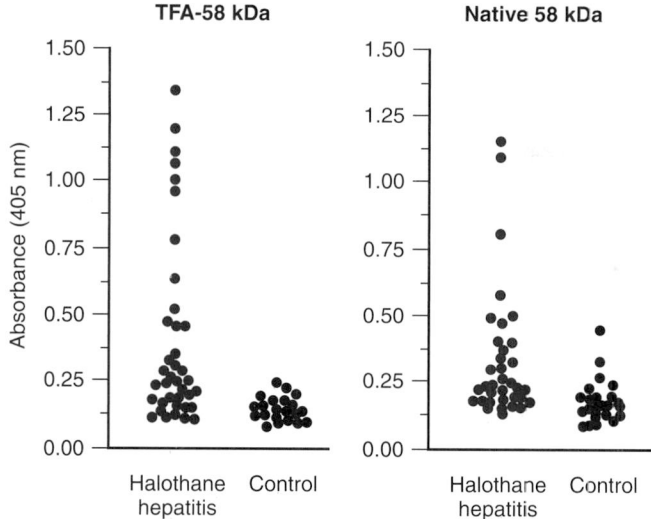

Figure 8–11 ELISA screening of halothane hepatitis patients' sera for antibodies that react with trifluoroacetylated 58-kilodalton and native 58-kilodalton proteins. All sera from 40 halothane hepatitis patients and 32 control patients were assayed at a 1:100 dilution. (Adapted from Martin JL, Reed GF, Pohl LR: Association of anti-58 kDa endoplasmic reticulum antibodies with halothane hepatitis. Biochem Pharmacol 46:1247-1250, 1993.)

pathogenic antibodies or cytotoxic T-cells, in susceptible individuals.[137] Moreover, one study showed that susceptible guinea pigs had higher levels of TFA-protein adducts in their livers than resistant animals and that elevated levels of CYP2A-related protein and not those of CYP2E1 could account for these differences in TFA-protein adduct formation.[140] In susceptible guinea pigs, several intact TFA-protein adducts were released into blood from damaged hepatocytes,[140] where they could be taken in by professional antigen-presenting cells in the liver or at other sites to initiate primary immune reactions against these antigens.

Halothane Hepatitis in the Pediatric Population

The first case of halothane hepatitis in a child was reported in 1959.[142] Since then, there have been numerous reports of hepatotoxicity and massive hepatic necrosis after halothane anesthesia in children.[143-147] Two retrospective studies examined the incidence of halothane-associated hepatotoxicity in children. The first study explored 165,400 halothane anesthetics in a children's hospital in the United Kingdom during the 23-year period from 1957 to 1979 and determined the incidence of halothane hepatitis in children was 1 in 82,000.[148] The second study examined 200,311 cases from 1958 to 1983 in a children's hospital in the United States. Only 1 patient in this study was concluded to have halothane hepatitis.[149] In 1987, data were reported describing halothane hepatitis in seven children between the ages of 11 months and 15 years, all of whom had received multiple halothane anesthetics.[150] The diagnosis in this study was confirmed in all but one child by the presence of serum antibodies that reacted with halothane-altered hepatocyte antigens. There was one fatality in this group, and other causes of liver diseases were excluded by the investigators. These findings indicate that the clinical syndrome of halothane

hepatitis does exist in prepubertal children, although it is much less common than in adults. The reason for the difference in incidence of halothane hepatitis observed between adults and children is not clear because halothane has been found to be metabolized to a similar degree in both groups and because immune competence is known to exist from birth.[151]

Enflurane, Isoflurane, and Desflurane

The incidence of liver injury caused by fluorinated inhaled anesthetics follows the order of halothane > enflurane > isoflurane > desflurane, and it correlates with the extent of their oxidative metabolism (see Fig. 8-6), which is halothane ($\approx$20%), enflurane ($\approx$2.5%), isoflurane ($\approx$0.2%), and desflurane ($\approx$0.01%).[152] Because all of these inhaled anesthetics appear to form protein adducts that are identical or related in structure to those of halothane, it seems possible that they may cause liver injury by a mechanism similar to that of halothane, although at an appreciably lower incidence (Fig. 8-12). The reduced rate results from the lower levels of potentially immunogenic protein adducts formed from these drugs compared with halothane when they are oxidatively metabolized by CYP2E1 (Fig. 8-13).

Enflurane was first used in North America in 1966. Although use of enflurane is much less common today, during the period of its highest use, there were relatively few case reports of liver damage associated with it. In 1986, Eger and associates[153] reviewed 10 published reports and several unpublished reports of liver damage after enflurane administration. Many of the cases were missing critical information on the duration of anesthetic exposure, histologic confirmation of hepatic lesions, and

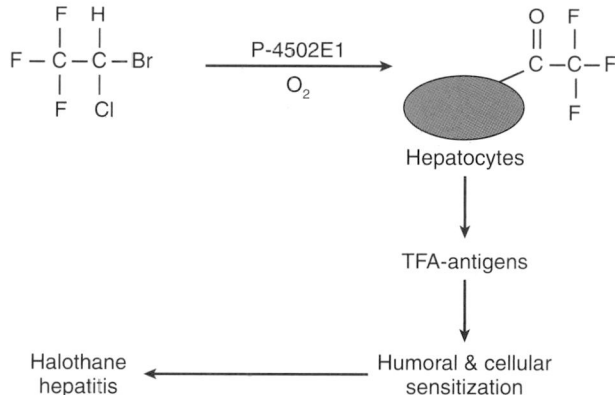

Figure 8–12 Pathway for the generation of the immune response after anesthetic exposure in susceptible patients. Halothane is metabolized to a trifluoroacetylated adduct that binds to liver proteins. The altered protein is seen as nonself, generating an immune response, which on subsequent exposure leads to toxicity and cell death. A similar process may occur after anesthetic exposure to other fluorinated drugs that generate a trifluoroacetylated or similar adduct. TFA, trifluoroacetyl (TFA-Cl). (Adapted from Njoku D, Laster MJ, Gong DH, et al: Biotransformation of halothane, enflurane, isoflurane and desflurane to trifluoroacetylated liver proteins: Association between protein acylation and liver injury. Anesth Analg 84:173-178, 1997.)

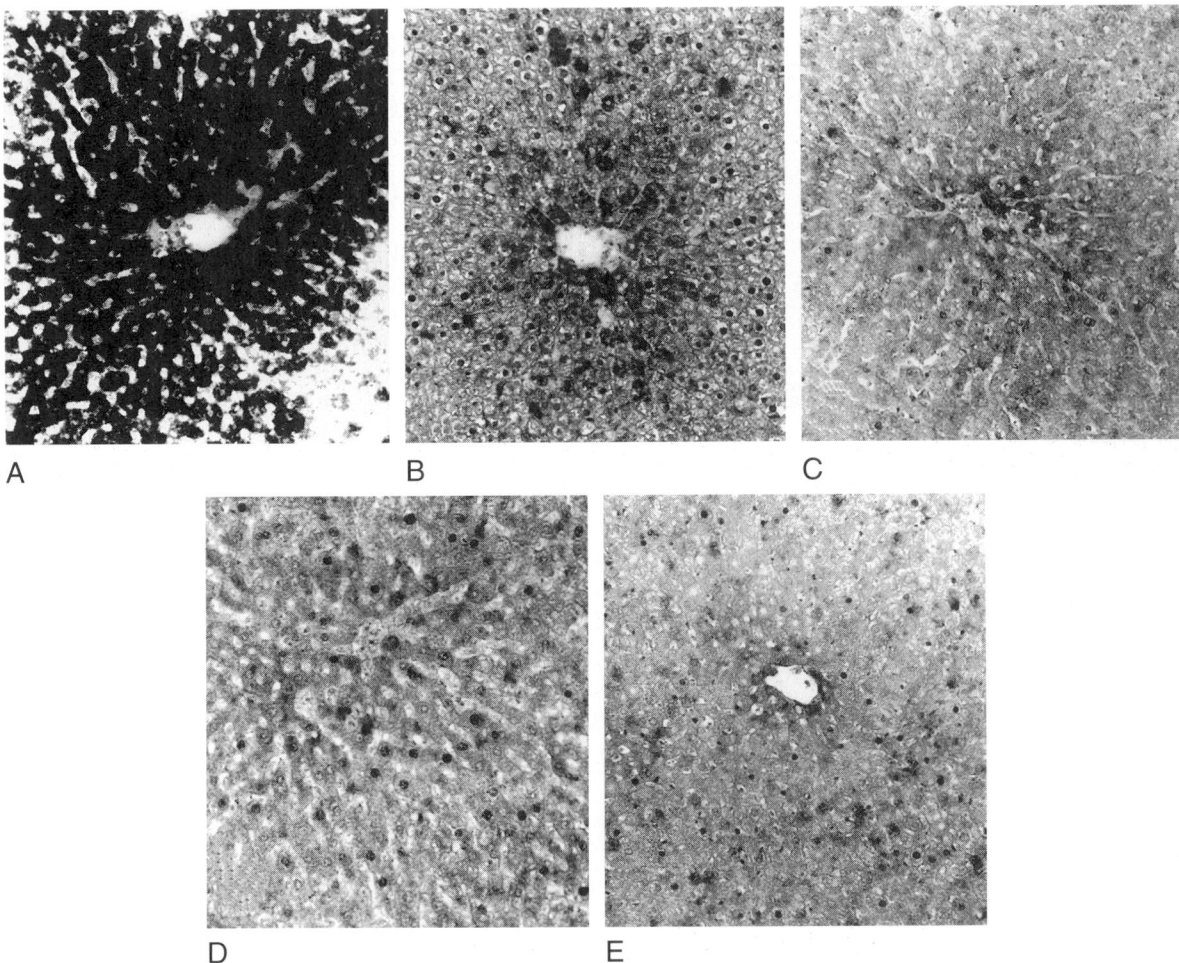

Figure 8–13 Livers from rats exposed to halothane (**A**), enflurane (**B**), isoflurane (**C**), desflurane (**D**), or oxygen (**E**), were incubated with anti-trifluoroacetyl rabbit serum to detect the presence of trifluoroacetylated liver proteins, after anesthetic exposure. Evidence of an immune response to trifluoroacetylated liver proteins can be seen in **A**, **B**, and **C**. No immunoreactivity is evident in **D** or **E**.

previous exposure to hepatic disease and hepatotoxic agents. Several patients had been hypotensive, severely ill, demonstrated signs of shock, and underwent operations with known potential for hepatic dysfunction. The investigators had no choice but to conclude that the evidence did not support the existence of enflurane-associated hepatic dysfunction similar to that seen with halothane. Nevertheless, several case reports suggest that enflurane anesthesia to patients previously anesthetized with or sensitized to halothane can result in hepatotoxicity.[154,155] For example, it was found that protein adducts of halothane and enflurane, which formed in the liver of rats treated separately with these drugs, reacted with serum antibodies from patients diagnosed with halothane hepatitis.[156] This apparent cross-reactivity could be explained by the similarity in structures of the protein adducts of halothane and enflurane (see Fig. 8-6).

Isoflurane, the structural isomer of enflurane, became available clinically in 1981. The combination of its minimal oxidative metabolism and low blood-to-gas solubility contributed to the popularity of this anesthetic agent. For several years after its introduction, there were no published reports of hepatic injury after the administration of this agent. Intrigued by the paucity of cases of hepatic injury after isoflurane, Stoelting and colleagues[157] assessed the contribution of isoflurane to 45 cases of hepatic dysfunction after anesthesia that had been reported to the U.S. Food and Drug Administration. The investigators concluded that the evidence did not support an association between isoflurane and postoperative hepatic dysfunction. However, in 1991, a case report of fulminant hepatic failure after repeated isoflurane exposure was published.[158] In 1993, another case was reported in which a patient with an uneventful initial exposure to isoflurane anesthesia for cecopexy had repeated episodes of hepatitis after subsequent exposures to isoflurane.[158] In the same patient, the second isoflurane anesthetic for pyloroplasty was for a 2-hour period, and the third anesthetic for gastrojejunostomy was 30 minutes of isoflurane, followed by 150 minutes of enflurane. This patient had a far greater serum transaminase and alkaline phosphatase concentration after the second anesthetic than after the third exposure to anesthesia. Unfortunately, as with many other cases, the evidence is suggestive but insufficient to draw firm conclusions. In 2000, a case of fatal hepatotoxicity after isoflurane re-exposure was reported in which histologic evidence of centrilobular injury and microvesicular fatty changes was found.[159]

Similar histopathologic changes were observed in another case of isoflurane liver injury.[160] TFA-protein adducts were detected in the damaged mitochondria by electron microscopy. This finding suggests the TFA-protein adducts may have contributed to the mitochondrial injury by a mechanism that was unrelated to an immunopathologic reaction induced by the TFA-protein adducts.

Although earlier studies of patients and volunteers do not suggest that desflurane is associated with hepatotoxicity in humans,[161,162] there is one report of a patient who developed fulminant hepatitis 12 days after receiving a desflurane anesthetic.[119] Because this patient had been exposed to halothane 10 and 18 years previously, for periods of less than 1 hour, it is possible that the patient may have been sensitized to halothane. After exposure to desflurane, a cross-sensitization reaction may have occurred because both halothane and desflurane can form TFA-protein adducts. A second case report described a weak association between desflurane exposure and hepatotoxicity.[163] Not unexpectedly, because of the limited metabolism of desflurane, animal studies have produced little evidence for hepatotoxicity associated with desflurane.[78]

Several clinical considerations are outlined for the safe and reasonable use of fluorinated anesthetics, which have been associated with the production of acylated liver proteins and liver injury (Table 8-4).

Hydrochlorofluorocarbons

Until the year 2000, the chlorofluorocarbons (CFCs) were widely employed as industrial refrigerants, foam-blowing agents in the manufacture of plastics, aerosol propellants, food preservatives, and cleaning and sterilizing agents. The major source of CFC environmental contamination was the venting of automobile and truck air conditioning units into the atmosphere. CFCs are extremely stable, nontoxic, and nonflammable, and they were first identified as the compounds responsible for stratospheric ozone depletion in 1985.[164] CFC molecules emitted in the lower atmosphere may take up to 7 years to diffuse upward into the stratosphere, where intense ultraviolet radiation liberates chlorine atoms that catalyze reactions that destroy ozone molecules. Once in place, these compounds may persist for 100 years or more. Depletion of stratospheric ozone may have adverse health effects worldwide, such as increases in the incidence of skin

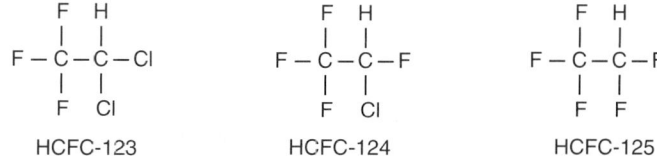

Figure 8–14 Chemical structures of the hydrochlorofluorocarbon (HCFC) analogs of halothane: HCFC-123, HCFC-124, and HCFC-125.

cancer and cataract formation. As a result, recommendations put forth by the Montreal Protocol on Substances That Deplete the Ozone Layer were adopted by the Environmental Protection Agency in the United States and by several other countries.[165] These recommendations called for the total elimination of CFCs by the year 2000.

The addition of hydrogen atoms into CFC molecules to form hydrochlorofluorocarbon (HCFC) molecules (Fig. 8-14) allows degradation of these compounds in the lower atmosphere with little effect on stratospheric ozone. HCFC-123 and -124 are used as CFC replacements. Because of the striking structural similarity between HCFCs and halothane, it seemed possible that the HCFCs would also form TFA-protein adducts similar to that of halothane (Fig. 8-15) and possibly cause liver injury. In studies in rats, the relative concentrations of TFA-protein adducts formed in the liver after administration of these compounds were similar between halothane and HCFC-123, much lower for HCFC-124, and nearly undetectable for HCFC-125.[166] Acute exposure to HCFC-123 has been shown to produce severe hepatotoxicity in guinea pigs, which was enhanced by prior glutathione depletion.[167] In subchronic studies using rats and dogs, increased liver weight, slight focal liver necrosis, induction of peroxisomal activity, and hepatocellular and testicular adenomas have been found.[168,169]

Table 8–4   Clinical considerations
Halothane should not be used in adult patients without a specific, well-documented indication.
In patients experiencing postoperative hepatotoxicity after fluorinated inhaled anesthetics, these anesthetics should be avoided in the future.
Despite reports of halothane hepatitis in children, halothane remains an acceptable anesthetic choice for use in children.
Enflurane, isoflurane, and desflurane remain safer inhaled anesthetics.
Anesthetic-induced hepatitis remains a diagnosis of exclusion.

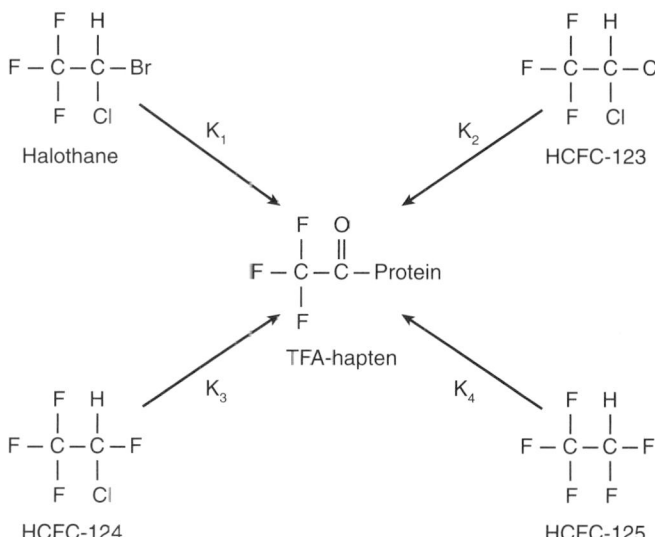

Figure 8–15 Metabolism of halothane and the hydrochlorofluorocarbon (HCFC) replacements, HCFC-123, HCFC-124, and HCFC-125, to an identical trifluoroacetyl (TFA) metabolite.

Human liver microsomes in vitro show a much higher capacity than rat liver microsomes to bioactivate HCFC-123 to reactive metabolites, suggesting that HCFCs may be hepatotoxic to humans. HCFC-123 and HCFC-124 have been implicated in liver injury in humans.[170] In this report, nine workers were accidentally, repeatedly exposed to a mixture of HCFC-123 and HCFC-124. All nine exposed workers were affected to some degree. For one severely affected worker, liver biopsy and immunohisto-chemical staining for the presence of TFA-protein adducts were done. The liver biopsy sample showed hepatocellu-lar necrosis, which was prominent in perivenular zone 3 and focally extended from portal tracts to portal tracts. TFA-adducted proteins were detected in the surviving hepatocytes. Autoantibodies against CYP2E1 or P58 were found in the sera of five of the nine affected workers. This report demonstrates that repeated exposure of human beings to HCFCs-123 and HCFC-124 can result in serious liver injury in a high proportion of the exposed popula-tion. In contrast, halothane hepatitis occurs in only a small fraction of individuals repeatedly anesthetized with this compound. A possible explanation for this difference is that halothane is administered acutely to patients, whereas the injured workers were subchronically exposed to the HCFCs. It is possible that protracted formation of TFA-adducted proteins may result in direct toxicity. Alternatively, on the basis of in vitro metabolic studies with human liver CYP2E1, exposure of human beings to HCFC-123 may result in higher concentrations of TFA-adducted liver proteins than those produced by halothane.[166] The presence of P58 and CYP2E1 autoanti-bodies in the serum of the exposed workers indicates that an immune component may have a role in the patho-genesis of HCFC-induced hepatotoxicity.

Sevoflurane

In several early case reports in the Japanese literature, sevoflurane was associated with postoperative hepatic dysfunction in patients ranging from 11 months to 63 years old.[171,172] However, in all of these reports, the association between sevoflurane exposure and liver injury as manifested by elevations in levels of liver transami-nases is extremely weak. In a single report from the United States,[173] postoperative liver injury was seen after sevoflurane anesthesia for appendectomy. However, this 3-year-old girl was suffering from iatrogenic acetamino-phen intoxication, and her injury might have been the result of acetaminophen rather than sevoflurane.[173] A clinical study of 50 surgical patients showed no signifi-cant changes in serum transaminase levels and hepatic function after 1 to 7 MAC-hours of sevoflurane anesthe-sia.[174] Other studies have shown mild elevations in post-operative levels of liver transaminases after sevoflurane anesthesia.[175-179] Sevoflurane exposure of untreated, phenobarbital-treated, and Aroclor 1254-treated rats also showed no significant changes in the concentrations of serum transaminases, liver triglycerides, or glutathione.[180]

Methoxyflurane

No discussion of immune-mediated hepatotoxicity after inhaled halogenated anesthetics is complete without considering methoxyflurane. Since its introduction into

clinical practice in the United States in 1960, there have been a number of reports of hepatic dysfunction and death from hepatic coma after methoxyflurane exposure. A review of 24 cases of methoxyflurane-associated hepa-titis revealed that a syndrome similar to hepatitis after halothane use may occur.[181] The researchers suggested that a rare and indirect immunologic hepatic injury might have had a direct effect on the liver by interfering with splanchnic circulation. Fortunately, in humans, the minor adverse changes in liver function appear to be reversible and may be related to dose. It is still unclear whether hepatic dysfunction, as measured by bromsul-phalein retention and serum hepatic enzyme elevation, was the result of the depth and duration of the anesthetic exposure, the type of operation, the extent of preexisting hepatic disease, or methoxyflurane itself. Methoxyflurane is rarely used in current anesthesia practice.

Risk Factors

Physiologic effects on the liver caused by the inhaled halogenated anesthetic may affect the susceptibility to hepatic dysfunction after their administration. Inhaled anesthetics can reduce hepatic blood flow to some degree, which may contribute to postoperative hepatic dysfunction. However, studies of healthy volunteers find no evidence of hypoxia or anaerobic metabolism in the liver, but hypoxia or abnormalities in hepatic synthetic function may be manifest in patients with preexisting liver damage or other illnesses. In general, surgical manipula-tion or disturbance of the surgical site appears to be more important in decreasing hepatic blood flow than the anes-thetic agent or technique. Preexisting conditions such as chronic liver disease from alcoholism, viral infection (e.g., viral hepatitis, cytomegalovirus infection), septicemia, severe burns, nutritional deficiency, and previous or con-comitant drug treatment may predispose the patient to postoperative hepatic dysfunction. Unfortunately, the patient demonstrating clinical evidence of hepatic dys-function after exposure to inhaled halogenated anesthet-ics presents a challenge to the anesthesia care provider because clinical tests to assess hepatic function can be nonspecific and reflect only severe hepatic dysfunction. Even so, traditional measures of hepatic function, such as tests for serum enzymes, aminotransferases, proteins, bilirubin, and alkaline phosphatase, are still used to assess liver damage.

The reported mortality rate associated with halothane hepatitis is 40% to 75%. A variety of risk factors are commonly associated with this clinical syndrome[182] (Table 8-5). Numerous studies have demonstrated that the risk of halothane hepatitis is greatly increased with use of an increasing number of anesthetics over a short period.[183,184] Although the basis of this observation is not known, it is possible that increased exposure to TFA-proteins adducts from multiple treatments with halothane promotes the chance of a hypersensitivity reaction. Isoniazid, ethanol, and acetone can stimulate CYP2E1 levels,[185-188] which may result in higher levels of protein adducts of halothane, isoflurane, and desflurane. Some evidence indicates that enzyme induction may play a role in the liver injury observed in patients with halothane hepatitis. A retrospective analysis of 279 patients

Table 8–5   Risk factors for anesthetic-induced hepatitis

Gender
Age
Obesity
Enzyme induction
Prior anesthetic exposure
Genetics

with normal preoperative serum transaminase levels undergoing brain surgery with halothane anesthesia was undertaken.[189] Of the 100 patients taking phenobarbital, 7 suffered postoperative liver injury, and 2 died. Among the 179 patients not taking phenobarbital, there was one case of liver injury and no deaths, suggesting that enzyme induction may play a role in the development of liver injury. Antipyrine clearance is increased in patients after halothane anesthesia; this suggests that halothane can stimulate drug metabolism.[190] Halothane has been demonstrated to induce its own metabolism in mice,[191,192] and it has been suggested that chronic exposure of operating room personnel increases the rate of halothane metabolism in this group.[193] With use of an increasing number of anesthetics, greater amounts of metabolites may be generated, leading to liver toxicity. In a study in which the production of a reductive halothane metabolite was measured (see Fig. 8-5) in children after repeated halothane exposure over short periods, there was no observed trend toward increased reductive metabolism.[194] Phenobarbital can induce the oxidative and reductive metabolism of halothane, whereas phenytoin can induce the generation of reductive halothane metabolites.[195]

Halothane hepatitis may have a hereditary basis in some cases, because this toxic effect has been reported in a mother and daughter, two sisters, and first cousins.[196] Lymphocytes from halothane hepatitis patients and some of their relatives are more susceptible to damage by phenytoin electrophilic intermediates than are lymphocytes from healthy controls.[197] The low incidence of the disease and the decreasing use of halothane make the study of the genetic effects difficult and emphasize the importance of developing an animal model of this disease. Several other associations exist for the development of this disease. There is a clear sex difference observed in halothane hepatitis patients. Approximately twice as many females as males develop the disease.[183,198-200] The reason for this disparity is unclear. Most cases of halothane hepatitis have occurred in middle-aged adults, with relatively few cases reported in prepubertal children,[148,149] and the disease is more common in obese than in nonobese patients.[201] There is no evidence to suggest that the risk of halothane hepatitis is increased in patients with liver disease unrelated to prior halothane exposure. However, because halothane can cause direct hepatotoxicity and other alternatives exist for the provision of general anesthesia, it is prudent to avoid halothane and the other fluorocarbon inhaled anesthetics in patients with preexisting hepatic dysfunction.

Assays to Detect Patients Sensitized to Fluorinated Anesthetics

The diagnosis of halothane hepatitis has always been one of exclusion, in which other potential causes of liver injury such as hepatitis A, hepatitis B, hepatitis C, cytomegalovirus, Epstein-Barr virus, hepatotoxic drugs, hypotension, and hypoxia are systematically excluded as precipitating causes.[124] One of the important goals of halothane hepatitis research is the development of an assay capable of detecting sensitized patients who may be at risk for developing a hypersensitivity response on re-exposure to halothane and detecting patients with the disease (Table 8-6). The assays measure serum antibodies in halothane hepatitis patients, and two general types of immunochemical assays are used. The first method is immunoblotting.[124,202] In this procedure, test antigens are microsomal proteins from halothane-treated rats or rabbits that have been separated into constituent polypeptides by sodium dodecyl sulfate–polyacrylamide gel electrophoresis (SDS-PAGE) and transferred electrophoretically to the surface of nitrocellulose membranes. Using this technique, 42 (62%) of 68 patients with a clinical diagnosis of halothane hepatitis have been found to test positive for the halothane-induced antibodies.[124] Although this approach provides important information about the apparent molecular mass of the neoantigens reacting with the patients' antibodies, it is laborious and time consuming. It also has the potential disadvantage of being inherently less sensitive than other methods because it involves the protein-denaturing conditions of SDS-PAGE. This could lead to a decreased level of response if a patient's antibodies were directed against, at least in part, conformational epitopes of the TFA neoantigens.

The second immunochemical assay that has been employed for the detection of antibodies in the sera of patients with a clinical diagnosis of halothane hepatitis is based on the more rapid, facile, and potentially more sensitive enzyme-linked immunosorbent assay (ELISA) methodology, in which test antigen is applied directly to the wells of a microtiter plate. One reported ELISA procedure uses microsomes from halothane-treated rabbits as test antigen. Employing this approach, investigators have demonstrated the presence of the antibodies in the sera of 16 (67%) of 24 patients[203] and 28 (72%) of 39 patients[203] with a clinical diagnosis of halothane hepatitis. In another ELISA that employs the TFA hapten as test antigen in the form of TFA-rabbit serum, albumin-positive responses from patients with a clinical diagnosis of halothane hepatitis ranged from 2 (33%) of 6 patients[204] to 5 (83%)

Table 8–6   Investigation of postoperative liver dysfunction

History and physical examination
Medications
Prior anesthetic exposure
Intraoperative course
Postoperative course
Clinical tests
Antibody screening

of 6 patients.[205] The purified proteins from rat liver have been used as test antigens in the ELISA. In a study employing three of the purified TFA-protein neoantigens (100 kd, 80 kd, and 57 kd), 79% of a group of 24 patients with halothane hepatitis tested positive by this assay.[206]

Fluoride-Associated Nephrotoxicity

Evidence suggests that inhaled anesthetics may induce differential effects on renal physiology. For example, halothane and enflurane decrease glomerular filtration rate and renal blood flow, whereas isoflurane may also decrease glomerular filtration rate but has minimal effects on renal blood flow. The newest inhaled halogenated anesthetics have minimal effects on renal physiology. Despite these physiologic effects, renal autoregulation protects the kidney from decreases in blood flow that may be caused by the inhaled anesthetic. It has been suggested that decreases in the glomerular filtration rate caused by decreases in arterial pressure return to baseline values when arterial pressure normalizes.[207] These physiologic responses to inhaled halogenated anesthetics should be recognized, but they do not represent true toxic reactions and are not considered further.

The metabolism of certain inhaled halogenated anesthetics can produce inorganic fluoride that may be directly nephrotoxic. We review the potential for fluoride-associated nephrotoxicity after the administration of inhaled halogenated anesthetics.

Methoxyflurane

Methoxyflurane is rarely used in clinical practice today; however, nephrotoxicity from inorganic fluoride released after metabolism of methoxyflurane is discussed as a basis for understanding the nephrotoxic potential of all current and future fluorinated anesthetics. Studies with methoxyflurane demonstrated an association with polyuric renal failure resulting from high levels of inorganic fluoride.[208-210] Patients with levels of inorganic fluoride less than 50 µmol/L had no evidence of renal injury. Levels of 50 to 80 µmol/L (2.5 to 3.0 MAC-hours of methoxyflurane) were associated with moderate injury and levels of 80 to 120 µmol/L (>5 MAC-hours of methoxyflurane) with severe injury. Several patients who had inorganic fluoride levels higher than 120 µmol/L died.

Various mechanisms have been proposed to explain renal injury from inorganic fluoride after methoxyflurane administration. One mechanism involves inorganic fluoride-induced reduction in adenyl cyclase activity and a subsequent effect on antidiuretic hormone.[211] Another mechanism involves effects on the renal countercurrent concentrating system by fluoride-induced increased renal medullary blood flow.[212] Nonetheless, the mechanism involving intrarenal metabolism of methoxyflurane and subsequent intrarenal production of fluoride ion is believed to be a significant cause of methoxyflurane's renal toxicity.[213] The mechanism of methoxyflurane-induced polyuric renal failure has been studied in an animal model. Vasopressin-resistant polyuric renal insufficiency similar to that seen in humans after prolonged methoxyflurane anesthesia can be consistently elicited in male Fischer 344 rats injected with sodium fluoride.[208]

These rats are excellent models for studying inorganic fluoride-induced nephropathy because they demonstrate renal changes after fluoride administration similar to those seen in humans, including polyuria, hypernatremia, and increased serum hyperosmolality. These rats have a serum fluoride threshold for renal dysfunction similar to that of humans.

Despite the overall correlation between nephrotoxicity and peak serum fluoride concentrations, there is individual variability in the level of nephrotoxicity after methoxyflurane administration. Genetic heterogeneity, drug interactions, preexisting renal disease, and a host of other factors may account for the differences observed among patients. For example, enzyme induction is clearly important in Fischer 344 rats[214] with prolonged pretreatment and in human volunteers[215] treated with the enzyme-inducer phenobarbital before methoxyflurane administration, because these subjects show increased defluorination and nephrotoxicity. Other enzyme inducers such as phenytoin,[71] ethanol,[216,217] and diazepam[218] also increase methoxyflurane defluorination in rats. One example of a drug interaction is the additive nephrotoxic effect seen in patients receiving both methoxyflurane and the aminoglycoside antibiotic gentamicin.[219] A similar effect is seen in Fischer 344 rats when concurrent administration of methoxyflurane and gentamicin synergistically promotes greater nephrotoxicity than either drug alone.[220]

Enflurane

In contrast to the renal effects of methoxyflurane, enflurane has been associated with only transient decreases in the renal concentrating ability. These effects are seen after prolonged administration of 9.6 MAC-hours of enflurane.[221,222] Patients rarely show renal dysfunction after the shorter periods of enflurane anesthesia,[221] although postoperative serum F⁻ concentrations are significantly higher than background concentrations. Compared with methoxyflurane, serum fluoride concentrations after enflurane anesthesia peak earlier and fall more rapidly, emphasizing the important role of lipid solubility in determining total fluoride exposure (Fig. 8-16). In one study, peak serum fluoride concentrations from nine surgical patients averaged 22.2 µmol/L after enflurane exposures averaging 2.7 MAC-hours. The only controlled human study to show mild renal dysfunction after enflurane anesthesia involved 11 healthy volunteers.[223] After 9.6 MAC-hours of enflurane, maximum urinary osmolality after antidiuretic hormone administration was reduced from approximately 1050 to 800 mOsm, and the mean serum fluoride concentration was 33.6 µmol/L. The mild impairment of renal-concentrating ability was not associated with hypernatremia, serum hyperosmolality, or increased serum creatinine or urea nitrogen levels and therefore was not regarded as clinically significant.

Some clinicians have speculated that enflurane administered to patients with significant preexisting renal disease could produce additional renal dysfunction. Such fears have not been borne out in clinical or laboratory investigations. Studies of Fischer 344 rats with surgically induced chronic renal insufficiency did not find additional renal dysfunction.[224,225] Results of a study of patients

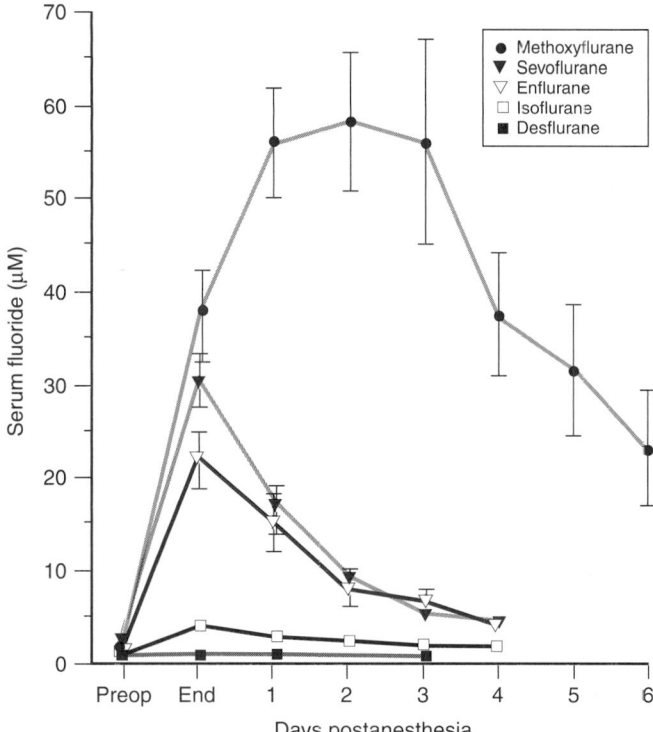

Figure 8–16 Serum inorganic fluoride (F⁻) concentration before and after administration of methoxyflurane, sevoflurane, enflurane, isoflurane, and desflurane anesthesia. After 2 to 3 minimum alveolar concentration (MAC)–hours of methoxyflurane, the mean peak F⁻ concentration was 61 ± 8 mol/L, which slowly declined. Sevoflurane anesthesia of 3.7 MAC-hours resulted in a mean peak F⁻ concentration of 30.6 ± 2 mol/L, which declined more rapidly than methoxyflurane but remained elevated for several days. After 2.7 MAC-hours of enflurane, the mean peak F⁻ concentration was 22.2 ± 2.8 mol/L, which also declined over several days. There was no increase in the F⁻ concentration after desflurane and almost no increase in the F⁻ concentration after isoflurane administration. (Adapted from Baden JM, Rice SA: Metabolism and toxicity of inhaled anesthetics. *In* Miller RD [ed]: Anesthesia, 5th ed. New York, Churchill Livingstone, 2000, p 147.)

with mild to moderate renal insufficiency showed no clinically significant difference between preoperative and postoperative renal function after enflurane or halothane administration.[222] Another concern about enflurane is that fluoride concentrations and the risk of nephrotoxicity may be higher in obese patients. In one study, the peak serum fluoride concentration in an obese patient weighing 130 kg was 52 μmol/L after 5 hours of exposure to enflurane.[221] In another study, peak serum fluoride concentrations averaged 28 μmol/L in morbidly obese patients, compared with 17 μmol/L in nonobese patients.[226] Studies have not been performed in humans to determine whether nephrotoxicity is more common in obese patients receiving enflurane, but this has been the case in obese Fischer 344 rats.[227]

Several investigators have attempted to explain the differences in the nephrotoxic potentials of enflurane and methoxyflurane. One difference may be that enflurane undergoes significantly less oxidative metabolism

than methoxyflurane. Moreover, enzyme induction does not significantly increase enflurane defluorination measured in vitro[69] or in surgical patients[11] receiving common enzyme-inducing drugs such as ethanol, phenobarbital, and phenytoin. In contrast, prior long-term treatment with isoniazid may result in higher than expected serum concentrations of fluoride and a transient urinary-concentrating defect after enflurane anesthesia. Work with Fischer 344 rats has shown that isoniazid significantly increases enflurane defluorination, unlike phenobarbital and phenytoin.[73,228] A study of surgical patients has shown that approximately one half of patients treated with isoniazid on a long-term basis before enflurane anesthesia had significantly higher serum fluoride concentrations than predicted,[229] but these were not sufficiently high or sufficiently sustained to produce clinically significant renal impairment.

Isoflurane

Isoflurane, an isomer of enflurane, is defluorinated much less than enflurane. Peak serum fluoride concentration after 6 hours of isoflurane anesthesia was only 4.4 μmol/L.[230] Isoflurane should not be associated with fluoride-associated nephrotoxicity. However, after prolonged isoflurane anesthesia for about 19 MAC-hours, peak plasma fluoride levels can be much higher after isoflurane administration than after halothane administration.[231] Forty percent of patients administered isoflurane had peak plasma fluoride levels greater than 50 μmol/L. Even so, enzyme induction does not appear to be a problem with isoflurane because phenobarbital pretreatment of rats only slightly enhances isoflurane defluorination and does not produce clinically significant increases in fluoride concentration.[69]

Because of the resistance to defluorination and the decreased likelihood of other toxicities, prolonged isoflurane administration has been investigated for uses outside the operating room. Isoflurane was investigated for its effectiveness in long-term sedation of patients on mechanical ventilation.[232,233] In the first study, the highest serum fluoride concentration was measured for a 2-year-old child who received 73 MAC-hours of isoflurane and had a serum fluoride level of 37.4 μmol/L.[234] In the second study, pediatric patients on mechanical ventilation received isoflurane for 13 to 497 MAC-hours. The highest serum F⁻ concentration was 26.1 μmol/L, with no alterations in serum creatinine or osmolality.[233] From these studies, we can safely conclude that isoflurane can be administered for very long periods without producing clinically significant serum fluoride concentrations; however, influences on metabolism and renal and hepatic functions should be carefully followed.

Sevoflurane

Sevoflurane is defluorinated through oxidative metabolism (see Fig. 8-7) to approximately the same extent as that of enflurane.[235] Clinical studies show that serum fluoride concentrations often peak above 50 μmol/L, even when sevoflurane is administered during surgery of average duration.[235] Because of sevoflurane's low blood-to-gas solubility and its rapid elimination, fluoride concentrations fall very quickly after surgery, and renal toxicities are not expected from sevoflurane administration. Studies in rats have shown that defluorination of sevoflurane is induced with phenobarbital,[80] isoniazid,[73,236] and ethanol. In vivo studies have shown that although peak fluoride levels are comparable to those with enflurane, sevoflurane has less nephrotoxic potential, as measured by maximum urine-concentrating ability and the production of N-acetyl-β-glucosaminidase, an indicator of renal tubular damage.[237-239]

In one study,[239] inorganic fluoride levels were compared after sevoflurane and isoflurane anesthesia. The elimination half-life of fluoride was 8 hours. The mean fluoride levels after sevoflurane were 30 μmol/L, and five of the patients had levels greater than 50 μmol/L. The mean level for isoflurane was significantly lower (3.9 μmol/L). Despite the high levels in five patients, there was no evidence of renal injury detected by blood urea nitrogen (BUN) or creatinine evaluations in this study. A similar study[234] comparing isoflurane with sevoflurane during longer (13.5) MAC-hour exposures resulted in a longer fluoride elimination half-life of about 58 hours in the sevoflurane patients and dramatically higher mean levels of inorganic fluoride (42.5 μmol/L). One half of all sevoflurane-exposed patients had fluoride levels that were higher than 50 μmol/L, but no renal injury was apparent as evidenced by BUN and creatinine measurements. Higuchi and colleagues[240] measured renal concentrating ability after 10.6 MAC-hours of sevoflurane or 8.5 MAC-hours of isoflurane in surgical patients. Mean peak fluoride levels were 41.9 ± 2.5 μM in the sevoflurane group, compared with 5.8 ± 0.4 μM in the isoflurane group.[240] There was no difference in the response to vasopressin between the groups. In a large, multinational, open-label study, patients received low-flow (1 L/min) sevoflurane (n = 98) or isoflurane (n = 90) anesthesia for at least 2 hours. BUN, creatinine, urine glucose, protein, pH, and specific gravity measurements were used to assess renal function up to 3 days after exposure. Peak fluoride levels were higher in the sevoflurane patients (40 ± 16 μM) compared with isoflurane patients (3 ± 2 μM). BUN and creatinine levels decreased in both groups, and no clinically significant differences were found with respect to any measured parameter.[241]

To accurately assess the potential for injury with sevoflurane from inorganic fluoride, more sensitive measures may be needed. These include creatinine clearance, maximal urinary osmolality (Uosmo max), urinary excretion of N-acetyl-β-glucosaminidase (NAG), β₂-microglobulin, and alanine aminopeptidase. One study[242] used several of these parameters and found evidence of transient subclinical nephrotoxicity with sevoflurane. Patients underwent peripheral orthopedic procedures lasting longer than 5 hours and were exposed to isoflurane or sevoflurane. Results were reported for two groups of sevoflurane patients, those with inorganic fluoride levels less than 50 μM/L (sevo_low) and those with levels greater than 50 μM/L (sevo_high). This categorization was based on the levels of inorganic fluoride obtained 1 hour postoperatively: 4.8 μM/L for isoflurane, 36.8 μM/L for the sevo_low group, and 55.8 μM/L for the sevo_high group. BUN, creatinine, and creatinine clearance levels were normal in all groups throughout the study. Maximal urine osmolality

showed a tendency toward injury development in the sevo_high group. NAG levels were twice as high as isoflurane in the sevo_low group and three times higher in the sevo_high group, with the latter group showing evidence of subclinical renal injury. Clinically, a transient loss of renal-concentrating ability occurred among one half of the patients in the sevo_high group. The dysfunction resolved within 6 days. An accompanying editorial suggested that this study raised the possibility of renal injury with sevoflurane in patients with impaired renal function and cautioned against its use in this patient group.[243] A second report of fluoride-induced renal injury in patients after sevoflurane anesthesia has been published.[244] However, a number of clinical reports have demonstrated very high levels of inorganic fluoride in some patients after sevoflurane anesthesia without obvious adverse effects. One report[245] described two such patients with refractory status asthmaticus, both treated with prolonged sevoflurane exposure under non-rebreathing conditions. Despite very high inorganic fluoride levels, no obvious injury followed. It appears that the potential for significant renal impairment or injury after sevoflurane anesthesia in healthy patients due solely to inorganic fluoride is not an important clinical problem.

Whether sevoflurane further affects renal tubular function in patients with impaired renal function is a question investigated by several groups. Cozen and coworkers[246] compared sevoflurane (n = 21) with enflurane (n = 20) at 4 L/min fresh gas flow rates in patients with chronically impaired renal function (creatinine > 1.5 mg/dL). Although peak fluoride levels were significantly higher in the sevoflurane group (25 ± 2.2 μM) than the enflurane group (13.3 ± 1.1 μM), no difference was found in postoperative renal impairment.[246] Tsukamoto and associates[247] compared sevoflurane (n = 7) with isoflurane (n = 7) in patients with moderately impaired renal function (creatinine clearance between 10 and 55 mM/min). Fluoride, urine NAG, γ-GTP, and β₂-microglobulin levels were measured up to 2 weeks after surgery. With the exception of fluoride levels (sevo group >>> iso group), no differences in renal parameters were observed between the groups.[247] In a later study, Morita and colleagues[248] evaluated the effect of sevoflurane (n = 15) and propofol (n = 15) anesthesia on urine concentration and aquaporin-2 (AQP2) levels. AQP2 is an arginine vasopressin–regulated water channel protein localized in the apical region of renal collecting duct cells. In both groups, plasma and urinary concentrations of arginine vasopressin increased, although plasma osmolality remained unchanged. Urinary AQP2 excretion increased in the propofol group along with changes in urinary and plasma arginine vasopressin levels. The urinary AQP2 level was significantly lower at 90 minutes in the sevoflurane group, and urine osmolality showed a transient but significant decrease in parallel with AQP2 suppression, suggesting sevoflurane might have produced transient impairment of the APQ2 response to an increase in intrinsic arginine vasopressin. However, because other inhaled anesthetics were not tested, it is not clear whether this observation applies to sevoflurane alone or is a characteristic effect of other fluorinated inhaled anesthetic agents.

Desflurane

Clinical studies performed with desflurane show no evidence of nephrotoxicity. Desflurane is extremely resistant to defluorination, and serum fluoride concentrations in surgical patients after exposure to desflurane are not increased above background concentrations.[249] From these findings, desflurane does not appear to be nephrotoxic.

Halothane

Halothane is not significantly defluorinated under normal clinical conditions and is not nephrotoxic. In patients who received about 19 MAC-hours of halothane, peak plasma fluoride levels were much higher in the isoflurane group than in the halothane group.[237] Defluorination is enhanced slightly in rats under conditions of hypoxia and enzyme induction, although not to an extent associated with renal damage.

Summary of Fluoride-Induced Nephrotoxicity

Fluoride-induced nephrotoxicity is a well-known entity that is historically associated with methoxyflurane administration and associated with prolonged exposure to enflurane. Surprisingly, during the administration of sevoflurane, serum inorganic fluoride levels can exceed 50 µmol/L, the level known to produce nephrotoxicity, but no correlation with sevoflurane and polyuric renal failure has been documented. Two factors may help to explain the differences seen with methoxyflurane and sevoflurane. First, it is not the peak serum fluoride concentration that determines injury, but rather the duration of the systemic fluoride increase (i.e., the area under the curve for serum fluoride). Sevoflurane is an order of magnitude less soluble than methoxyflurane and is eliminated much more rapidly from the body. Second, the liver is the primary organ of sevoflurane metabolism, whereas both the liver and kidney metabolize methoxyflurane, and it is thought that the high intrarenal fluoride production from methoxyflurane contributes to its nephrotoxicity.

Toxic Products Formed by Interactions with Carbon Dioxide Absorbents

Sevoflurane and Compound A

Several decomposition products are formed during the interaction of sevoflurane with carbon dioxide absorbents, and fluoromethyl-2-2-difluoro-1-(trifluoromethyl) vinyl ether (compound A) is the major degradation product detected[250-252] (Fig. 8-17). The dehydrofluorination of sevoflurane to form compound A is initiated by soda lime abstraction of a proton from the isopropyl group of sevoflurane in a manner that is similar to the base-catalyzed deprotonation of halothane by soda lime to yield difluorobromochloroethylene ($F_2C=CBrCl$, BCDFE). Bito and Ikeda[242] studied patients (n = 16) exposed to sevoflurane at low fresh gas flows (1 L/min) with soda lime or Baralyme as the carbon dioxide absorbent. Soda lime produced individual maximum compound A levels of 23.6 ± 2.9 ppm, and Baralyme produced levels of 32 ± 2.3 ppm.[242] It is now well established that Baralyme is associated with higher compound A production than soda lime.

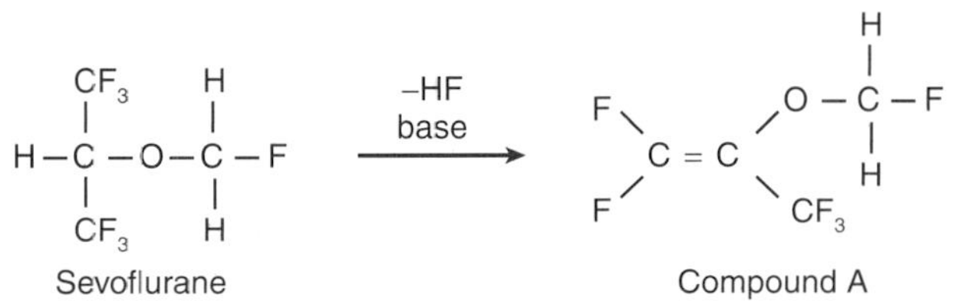

Figure 8–17 Sevoflurane degradation in the presence of a base.

Compound A has been the subject of intense research and debate since the introduction of sevoflurane into clinical practice in the United States in 1995. Morio and colleagues[243] found that high concentrations of compound A could cause renal injury and death in rats. Other investigators confirmed the findings of Morio and coworkers and showed that kidney injury occurred when levels of compound A reached 25 to 50 ppm or greater.[253] Necrosis is found primarily in the proximal tubular cells within the outer strip of the medulla and the percentage of injured cells was lower 4 days after exposure than 1 day after exposure, consistent with repair after renal injury.[254] These and other studies suggest a threshold for renal injury of 150 to 300 ppm-hours of compound A exposure (i.e., 50 ppm of compound A administered for 3 hours).[255,254] Keller and associates[254] reported that compound A inspired concentrations of more than 114 ppm were associated with concentration-dependent increases in BUN and creatinine levels and in the urinary NAG/creatinine ratio. Moderately severe histopathologic changes were seen at 202 ppm, and all chemistry and histopathologic changes reversed within 14 days of exposure. This renal toxicity is dose and time dependent; the higher the exposures over time, the greater is the observed injury. During sevoflurane anesthesia, in a closed or semiclosed system at low fresh gas inflows, patients are routinely exposed to compound A. However, the safe concentration for compound A exposure in humans is unknown.

Several studies enrolling surgical patients and human volunteers have been undertaken to investigate the possible association between sevoflurane anesthesia and renal injury due to compound A exposure during sevoflurane anesthesia. In an early study, Bito and Ikeda[250] exposed 10 patients to sevoflurane for longer than 5 hours under closed-circuit conditions with soda lime as the absorbent. Peak compound A concentrations were 19.5 ± 5.4 ppm, and serum levels of BUN, creatinine, and electrolytes were essentially unchanged. In a follow-up study by the same investigators, 10 patients were exposed to sevoflurane at 1 L/min fresh gas flows for 10 hours. Mean compound A levels were 24.3 ± 2.4 ppm, and routine tests of renal function showed no change from preoperative values.[256] Frink and colleagues[257] measured compound A levels in 16 surgical patients during low-flow sevoflurane anesthesia for 3 hours with soda lime (n = 8) or Baralyme (n = 8) as the absorbent. Maximum compound A concentrations averaged 8.16 ± 2.67 ppm with soda lime and 20.28 ± 8.6 ppm with Baralyme. A compound A concentration of 60.8 ppm was found in the breathing circuit of one of eight subjects to whom sevoflurane was administered using Baralyme. In the same study, no compound A level exceeding 50 ppm was found in the eight volunteers when soda lime was used to scrub carbon dioxide.

In a more comprehensive investigation, Bito and Ikeda[258] studied 100 surgical patients undergoing resection of head and neck tumors for which surgery was expected to last longer than 10 hours. Patients received sevoflurane (n = 50) or isoflurane (n = 50) anesthesia at low fresh gas inflows (1 L/min).[258] The mean peak compound A concentration for the sevoflurane group was 24.6 ± 7.2 ppm. Although bilirubin, AST, and ALT levels increased postoperatively in the sevoflurane and isoflurane groups, there were no significant differences in these parameters between these groups. Preoperative and postoperative BUN and creatinine levels remained unchanged. A number of other reports have evaluated renal function after closed-circuit or low-flow sevoflurane anesthesia using BUN and serum creatinine as markers of renal damage,[259] and none has demonstrated any change in of these markers preoperatively and postoperatively.[258-260]

It has been argued that BUN and creatinine are not sensitive enough tests for detecting renal damage after compound A exposure.[258-261] In an early attempt to address this issue, Kumano and colleagues measured urinary excretion of several renal tubular enzymes as measures of renal injury. Renal excretion of alanine aminopeptidase and NAG (i.e., enzymatic markers of renal integrity) increased 7 days after exposure to 7.6 MAC-hours of enflurane, but no increase was observed in patients receiving 9.6 MAC-hours of sevoflurane. Renal excretion of γ-glutamyl transpeptidase, β_2-microglobulin, BUN, and creatinine were unchanged.[262] Bito and colleagues[263] studied 48 patients undergoing gastrectomy under low-flow (1 L/min) (n = 16) and high-flow (6 to 10 L/min) (n = 16) sevoflurane anesthesia and low-flow isoflurane (1 L/min) (n = 16) anesthesia, looking at BUN, creatinine, creatinine clearance, NAG, and alanine aminopeptidase.[263] The average inspired compound A levels were 20 ppm in the sevo$_{low}$ group, and the average duration of exposure to this concentration was 6.11 hours. The only difference between the sevo$_{low}$ and the sevo$_{high}$ groups was the degree of compound A formation. Postanesthesia laboratory data showed no significant effects of compound A during sevoflurane anesthesia on any markers of renal function. Postanesthesia BUN and creatinine levels decreased, creatinine clearance increased, and urinary excretion of NAG and alanine aminopeptidase increased in all groups compared with preanesthesia values, but there was no significant differences observed between any of the groups. Kharasch and coworkers[264] completed a similar study in which 73 surgical patients received sevoflurane or isoflurane anesthesia at a fresh gas flow of 1 L/min. Anesthetic duration was 3.7 or 3.9 hours, and the maximum inspired compound A concentration was 27 ppm (range, 10 to 67 ppm). Areas under the inspired and expired compound A concentration versus time curves (AUC) were 79 ppm-hours (range, 10 to 223 ppm-hours) and 53 ppm-hours (range, 6 to 159 ppm-hours), respectively. There were no significant differences between anesthetic groups in postoperative BUN, creatinine or urinary excretion of protein, or glucose (i.e., markers of proximal tubular resorptive function) or in NAG, proximal tubular

α-GST, or distal tubular π-GST (i.e., markers of tubular cell necrosis). The investigators concluded that moderate duration of low-flow sevoflurane anesthesia during which compound A formation occurs was as safe as low-flow isoflurane anesthesia.

Nishiyama and associates[265] studied the effect of repeat sevoflurane exposure within 30 to 90 days in neurosurgical patients. Ten patients received sevoflurane at a fresh gas flow rate of 6 L/min on two occasions. Serum inorganic fluoride was measured 1 day after surgery and BUN, creatinine, serum and urine β_2-microglobulin, urine NAG, serum AST, serum ALT, and total bilirubin were measured 7 days postoperatively. Urine β_2-microglobulin, AST, and ALT all increased to abnormal levels after both anesthetics, with no observed differences between the anesthetics. The second sevoflurane exposure did not change the hepatic or renal metabolism of sevoflurane. These changes were indicative of mild hepatic and renal injury. The duration of anesthesia for the first and second anesthetics was 4.3 ± 0.6 hours and 4.0 ± 0.6 hours, respectively.

Cases of humans with renal changes after sevoflurane administration have all occurred under conditions of prolonged sevoflurane exposure. Eger and colleagues[266] and Ebert and associates[267] exposed human volunteers to 8 hours of 1.25 MAC of sevoflurane or desflurane anesthesia at 2 L/min of fresh gas flows and investigated BUN levels, creatinine concentration, and enzymatic markers of urinary function for up to 3 days before or 5 to 7 days after exposure, or both (Table 8-7). Both groups of investigators found no differences in BUN or creatinine levels before and after exposure in either group, but they found significant differences in enzymatic markers of renal integrity (i.e., α-GST and π-GST), albuminuria, and glucosuria in the sevoflurane-exposed group. All renal changes were transient, with normal return of renal function by 4 days after exposure in all but one volunteer, whose renal function was normal 2 weeks after exposure. In Eger's volunteers, rebreathing of sevoflurane produced an average inspired concentration of compound A of 41 ppm, and the total compound A exposure was 328 ppm-hours. In the Ebert study, volunteers were exposed to an average inspired compound A concentration of 27 ppm, and the total exposure was 216 ppm-hours. With the exception or BUN and creatinine, both studies showed significant changes in urinary markers; the Ebert volunteers were lower on the compound A toxicity threshold curve and exhibited less drastic changes in all markers of injury. Goldberg and colleagues[268] replicated Eger's study obtaining lower average compound A levels (253 ppm-hours) and found similar qualitative renal findings. Higuchi and associates[269] found increased excretion of urinary enzymes after average compound A concentrations of 215 ppm-hours. In another study, Higuchi and colleagues[270] found proteinuria in patients (n = 14) given low-flow (1 L/min) sevoflurane anesthesia undergoing orthopedic or dental surgeries but not those (n = 14) given high-flow (6 L/min) sevoflurane or those (n = 14) given low-flow isoflurane. Increased urinary NAG excretion occurred in the low-flow and high-flow sevoflurane groups, whereas levels of BUN, creatinine, and creatinine clearance were unchanged in all groups. In human

Table 8–7   Percent of volunteers with abnormal renal test results after 8 hours of 1.25 minimum alveolar concentration of sevoflurane anesthesia

Determination	Eger Study[266]			Ebert Study[267]		
	Day 1 (%)	Day 2 (%)	Day 3 (%)	Day 1 (%)	Day 2 (%)	Day 3 (%)
Glucose	75	50	80	15		
Albumin	88	60	90	31	31	31
α-GST	43	70	70	54	54	
π-GST	25	38	38	*		
MAC-hr exposure		328 ppm/hr			240 ppm/hr	

*The group mean was significantly increased above baseline. No individual data were reported. BUN and creatinine levels were normal in all patients at all time points.

volunteers exposed to 1.25 MAC of sevoflurane or desflurane for 4 hours (n = 9) or 2 hours (n = 7) at 2 L/min fresh gas flows, Eger and coworkers[271] found average inspired compound A levels of 40 ppm. Relative to desflurane, sevoflurane given for 4 hours resulted in slightly increased levels of urinary albumin and serum creatinine and an increased level of urinary α-GST. In a later study, Ebert and colleagues[272] found that 5 MAC-hours of sevoflurane exposure at 1 L/min fresh gas flows, for which mean peak compound A levels were 39 ppm and total exposure to compound A was 152 ppm-hours, produced no changes in BUN, creatinine, or enzymatic markers of renal or hepatic injury (i.e., AST, ALT, and alkaline phosphatase).

Several studies have examined the use of sevoflurane in the pediatric population. In one report,[273] sevoflurane was compared with halothane anesthesia in children who had a mean age of 6 years. With comparable exposures, the sevoflurane group had significantly higher inorganic fluoride levels. There were no significant differences in BUN and creatinine levels, and there have been no reports of fluoride-associated renal toxicity in pediatric patients after sevoflurane anesthesia. Other tests of renal integrity were not studied. In another study, ASA class I and II children between the ages of 3 months and 7 years received 1 MAC of sevoflurane exposure at a fresh gas flow rate of 2 L/min.[274] The mean anesthetic exposure was 240 minutes, and fresh carbon dioxide absorbent was used for each patient. The soda lime temperature varied from 23°C to almost 41°C, and the inspired and expired compound A concentrations were 5.4 and 3.7 ppm, respectively. There were no differences in clinical chemistry measures, as reflected by AST, ALT, alkaline phosphatase, bilirubin, BUN, and creatinine levels. The maximum soda lime temperature correlated with the maximum compound A concentrations and the body surface area of the child. There have been no reports of markedly abnormal renal chemistry values for pediatric patients after sevoflurane exposure.

There is some concern about pediatric patients related to the major metabolite of sevoflurane, hexafluoroisopropanol (HFIP) because the levels of this metabolite may become relatively high due to a deficiency in UGTs that conjugate glucuronic acid to HFIP (see Fig. 8-7). For example, neonatal rats were found to have high levels of

free HFIP for as long as 21 days after birth after sevoflurane exposure.[275]

It is hypothesized that compound A causes serious injury to kidneys in rats but not humans because of differences in levels of renal cysteine conjugate β-lyase enzymes,[276] which is thought to catalyze the conversion of compound A into a reactive thionoacyl fluoride metabolite that can acylate kidney proteins and cause toxicity (Fig. 8-18). Renal cytosolic and mitochondrial β-lyase enzyme levels in rats are approximately 20 to 30 times higher than those found in humans.[277-279] There is evidence to support the β-lyase theory of compound A–induced nephrotoxicity. Renal β-lyase appears to mediate the renal toxicity produced by several fluorinated alkenes that are structurally similar to compound A,[280-282] and metabolic intermediates of the β-lyase pathway have been identified in the bile and urine of rats and human tissues exposed to compound A.[259,264,278,279,283] Moreover, the glutathione S-conjugate of compound A is nephrotoxic,[284] and the administration of aminooxyacetic acid (AOAA), an inhibitor of the β-lyase (Fig. 8-19), protects against the nephrotoxicity of compound A in rats.[285] However, there is some controversy surrounding the relevance of the β-lyase pathway in compound A–induced renal injury.[283,286,287]

Investigators have reported that pretreatment of rats with AOAA and acivicin (AT-125), inhibitors of the β-lyase pathway (see Fig. 8-19)[286] did not attenuate the nephrotoxicity produced by compound A, but it was instead associated with a nearly threefold increase in renal injury (19% to 53%). These findings suggest that the β-lyase pathway may be a detoxification pathway. In this regard, a report by Kharasch and colleagues[287] showed that pretreatment or rats with AOAA partially protected against compound A–induced diuresis and proteinuria but failed to protect against glucosuria. In another report, AOAA again failed to decrease histologic renal injury, and pretreatment with acivicin significantly increased renal injury.[286] Using an immunochemical approach, other investigators were unable to detect protein adducts of a thionoacyl fluoride metabolite of compound A in kidneys of rats after compound A treatment, suggesting that the β-lyase pathway of compound A metabolism in rats does not occur or is a minor pathway of metabolism. These findings suggest that another pathway of metabolism of

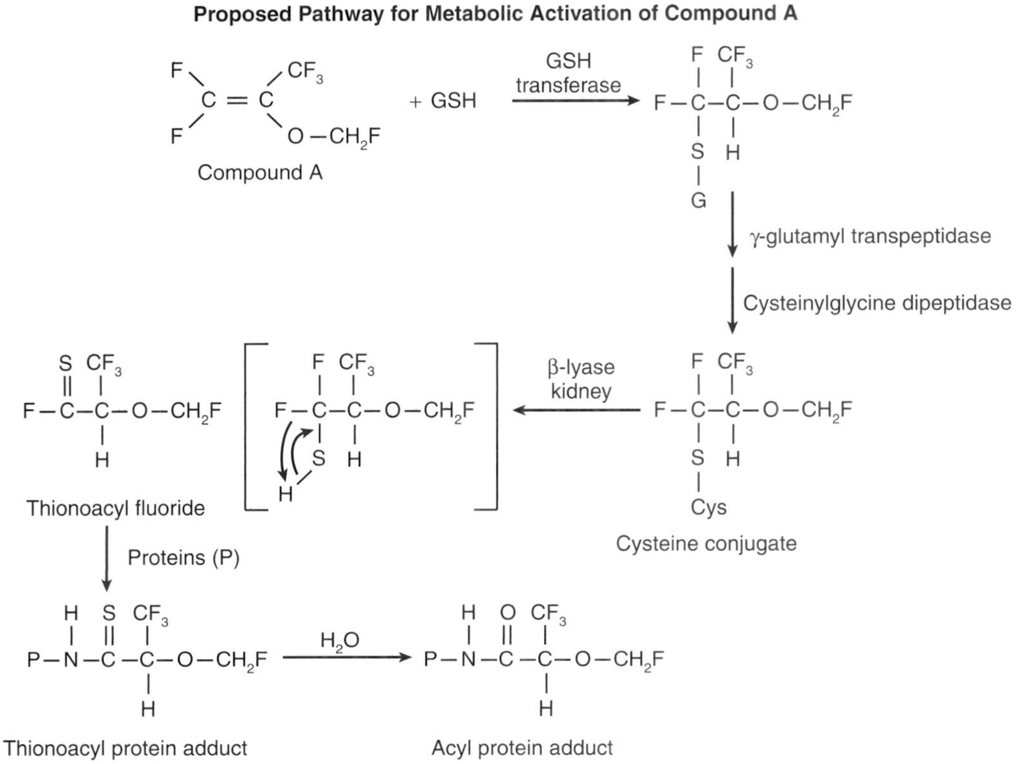

Proposed Pathway for Metabolic Activation of Compound A

Compound A

$+ GSH$ → (GSH transferase) → Cysteine conjugate → (γ-glutamyl transpeptidase) → (Cysteinylglycine dipeptidase) → (β-lyase kidney) → Thionoacyl fluoride → Proteins (P) → Thionoacyl protein adduct → H_2O → Acyl protein adduct

Figure 8–18 Proposed pathway for the metabolic activation of compound A shows formation of an intrahepatic glutathione (GSH) conjugate of compound A that is translocated to the kidney, where γ-glutamyl transpeptidase, cysteinylglycine dipeptidase, and renal cysteine conjugate β-lyase catalyze the formation of a nephrotoxic thiol, which can acylate kidney proteins. (Adapted from Martin JL, Kandel L, Laster MJ, et al: Studies of the mechanism of nephrotoxicity of compound A in rats. J Anesth 11:32-37, 1997.)

compound A may be responsible for the nephrotoxicity of compound A.

Higuchi and associates[288] studied the effect of low-flow sevoflurane or isoflurane anesthesia (1 L/min) on 17 patients with stable moderate renal failure (serum creatinine > 1.5 mg/dL). They found no difference in BUN or creatinine levels up to 14 days after exposure or in creatinine clearance at 7 days after exposure in either group for patient exposures of more than 130 ppm-hours of compound A.[288] In a multicenter, randomized, controlled trial, Conzen and colleagues[289] studied 116 patients with stable renal insufficiency (serum creatinine > 1.5 mg/dL) with low-flow (1 L/min) sevoflurane (n = 59) or isoflurane (n = 57) anesthesia. Total exposure to sevoflurane was 201.3 ± 98 minutes, with an average total compound A exposure of 18.9 ± 7.6 ppm. Isoflurane exposures averaged 213.6 ± 83.4 minutes, and Baralyme was used as the carbon dioxide absorbent. No significant changes above baseline values were found at 24 or 72 hours after exposure for serum creatinine, BUN, creatinine clearance, urine protein, or glucose for either anesthetic.

So what does this all mean, and how does it translate into clinical care of patients? In a rebreathing system with a carbon dioxide absorber in lime (soda lime or Baralyme), patients exposed to sevoflurane will breathe compound A. The typical levels seen under clinical conditions vary and depend upon several factors, the most important being the inspired fresh gas flow. The key factor in determining toxicity from sevoflurane is the total exposure rather than the absolute concentration; exposure is expressed as the product of concentration and time. It appears from the many studies published that the lower threshold for renal changes associated

with sevoflurane exposure and compound A is approximately 150 ppm-hours. At a fresh gas inflow of 2 L/min, these levels would be expected to be seen only under conditions of prolonged sevoflurane exposure and are not of concern for most patients undergoing anesthesia and surgery. Under conditions of prolonged sevoflurane exposure in which renal changes have been observed, these changes have been transient. It appears that compound A is of theoretical concern and academic interest, but no significant clinical renal toxicity has been associated with the use of sevoflurane. It is recommended that patients with preexisting renal disease not be exposed to sevoflurane and that sevoflurane be administered according to approved package labeling guidelines.

Halothane and Bromochlorodifluoroethane

Carbon dioxide absorbents degrade halothane by a dehydrofluorination reaction to form bromochlorotrifluoroethane (BCDFE, $F_2C=CBrCl$). The potential nephrotoxicity of BCDFE was compared with compound A in a study by Eger and colleagues.[290] It was found that BCDFE was 80% less reactive than compound A; halothane degraded to BCDFE 20- to 40-fold less than sevoflurane to compound A in a standard circle system; BCDFE was 75% less nephrotoxic to rats than compound A; and compounds that blocked the renal β-lyase pathway did not change or decreased renal injury from BCDFE, whereas the same blockers did not change or increased renal injury from compound A (see Fig. 8-19), suggesting that BCDFE and compound A may cause kidney injury by different mechanisms. These studies demonstrate that the chance of BCDFE causing nephrotoxicity when halothane is being used as an anesthetic is negligible.

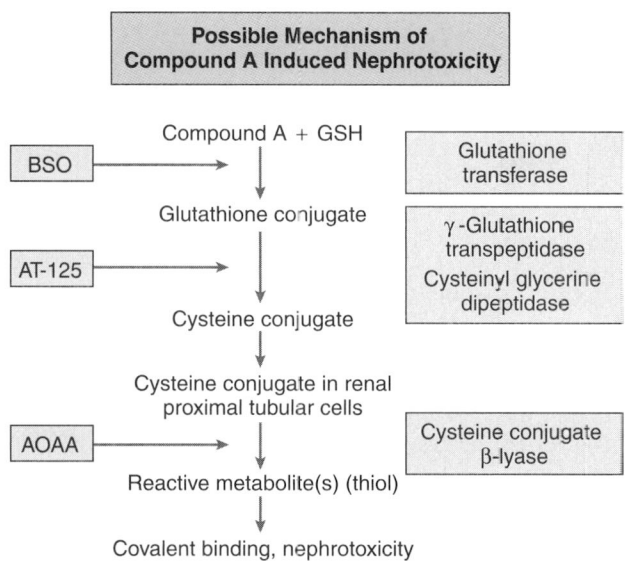

Figure 8–19 Crucial steps in the β-lyase pathway: First, conjugation of compound A with glutathione in the liver is mediated by glutathione S-transferase; this conjugate is then transported to the kidney. Second, the glutathione S-conjugate is converted to a cysteine S-conjugate, a process mediated by γ-glutamyl transpeptidase. Third, the cysteine S-conjugate of compound A is then converted to a reactive thiol, mediated by renal cysteine conjugate β-lyase; DL-buthionine-(S,R)-sulfoximine (BSO) depletes endogenous stores of glutathione in the body, acivicin (AT-125) inhibits the activity of γ-glutamyl transpeptidase, and aminooxyacetic acid (AOAA) inhibits the activity of β-lyase. Compound A, its conjugates, and the reactive thiol have all been postulated to cause the renal necrosis that can occur in rats after the administration of compound A and the glucosuria and enzymuria that can result in rats and humans from compound A administration.

Carbon Monoxide

Carbon monoxide (CO) is an odorless, colorless gas that is poisonous because it displaces oxygen from hemoglobin in the blood, leading to carboxyhemoglobin formation. Its affinity for binding hemoglobin is 250 times greater than that of oxygen. All humans have some CO bound to hemoglobin in their blood; on average, this is 1%, for nonsmokers and as much as 10% for those who smoke. High levels of CO can produce neuropsychiatric problems in patients, and when levels of carboxyhemoglobin reach 50%, death can occur. CO poisonings have been reported during clinical anesthesia.[291-296] The difficulty in monitoring CO levels clinically arises from the fact that pulse oximeters do not distinguish between carboxyhemoglobin and oxyhemoglobin.

All inhaled anesthetics produce some CO as a result of their interaction with strong bases in relatively dry carbon dioxide (CO_2) absorbents.[297] Several factors influence the level of CO production, including the choice of anesthetic agent, the inspired anesthetic concentration, and the type, temperature, and degree of dryness of the CO_2 absorbent.[298] Of the inhaled anesthetics, desflurane produces the most CO, followed in descending order by enflurane and isoflurane, with negligible amounts from sevoflurane and halothane[298,299] (Fig. 8-20). Intraoperative formation of CO has been reported with

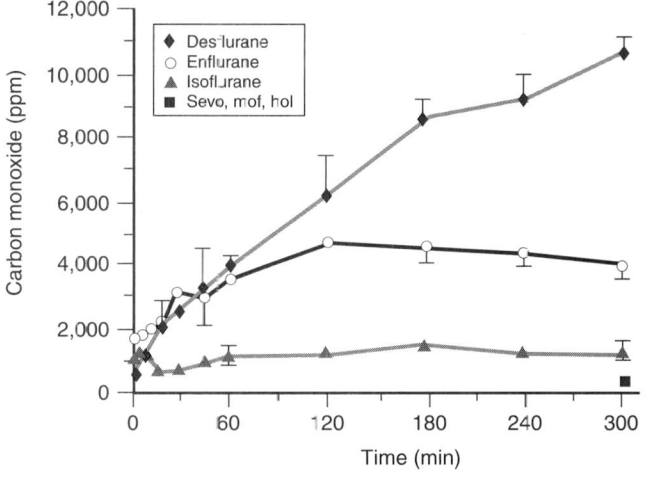

A

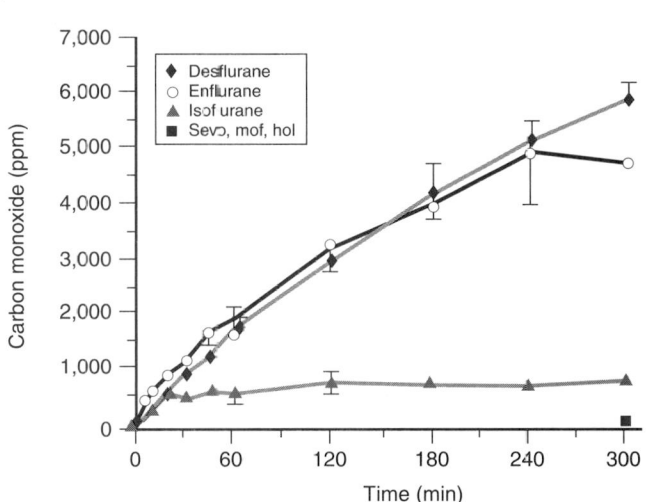

B

Figure 8–20 Anesthetic degradation to carbon monoxide at equi-minimum alveolar concentrations (1.5 MAC) concentrations by (A) barium hydroxide lime and (B) soda lime. Each data point is the mean ± SD (n = 3). The single data point at 300 minutes reflects undetectable carbon monoxide from sevoflurane, methoxyflurane, or halothane. (Adapted from Baxter PJ, Garton K, Kharasch ED: Mechanistic aspects of carbon monoxide formation from volatile anesthetics. Anesthesiology 89:929-941, 1998.)

desflurane, enflurane, and isoflurane, with CO levels exceeding those established as safe by the U.S. Environmental Protection Agency. Desflurane, enflurane, and isoflurane are all difluoromethyl-ethyl ethers; sevoflurane is a monofluoromethyl ether; and halothane is an alkane. The specific mechanism appears to be a base-catalyzed difluoromethoxy proton abstraction from the anesthetic agent[299] (Fig. 8-21). The abstraction of a proton from the difluoromethoxy group is greater with potassium than with sodium hydroxide (NaOH).[299,300] Barium hydroxide [Ba(OH)$_2$] contains 4.6% potassium hydroxide (KOH), whereas soda lime contains only 2.5% KOH and 1.5% NaOH. Unlike KOH and NaOH, Ba(OH)$_2$ does not abstract a proton from the difluoromethoxy moiety and catalyze the formation of

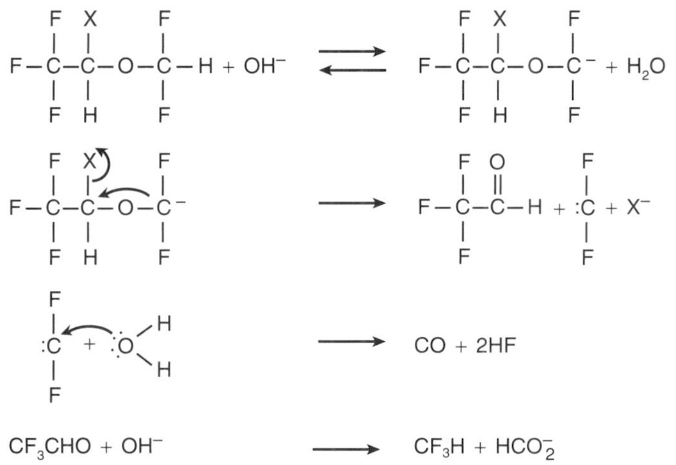

Figure 8–21 Proposed mechanism of carbon monoxide formation from difluoromethyl-ethyl ether anesthetics. The backbone structures for isoflurane (X = Cl) and desflurane (X = F) are shown, along with a putative mechanism for the concomitant formation of trifluoromethane. Water in line 3 may also react as OH⁻. (Adapted from Baxter PJ, Garton K, Kharasch ED: Mechanistic aspects of carbon monoxide formation from volatile anesthetics. Anesthesiology 89:929-941, 1998.)

CO from inhaled anesthetics. Because the divalent $Ca(OH)_2$ and $Ba(OH)_2$ bases are the major active components of the absorbents, the capacity to produce CO is rapidly exhausted while the absorbents retain their capacities to remove CO_2.

Amsorb contains neither NaOH nor KOH and does not degrade inhaled anesthetics to CO or degrade sevoflurane to compound A.[301] Fully hydrated or rehydrated absorbents do not degrade inhaled anesthetics to CO. Soda lime contains 15% water by weight, and only after this level of hydration has been decreased to about 1.4% are appreciable amounts of CO formed. Baralyme contains 13% water by weight, and the threshold of hydration before CO is formed is 4.8%. However, even at these threshold levels, very little CO is produced. Production of large amounts of CO requires complete or nearly complete desiccation of the absorbent, a process that requires high flows of dry gas (10 L) for prolonged periods (1 to 2 days). It has been reported that certain patients had high levels of CO, a situation that was particularly prevalent in the first case on Mondays.[291] This appeared to be related to the practice of flushing the anesthesia machine with high fresh gas flows over the weekend, which dried out the CO_2 absorbent. Higher temperatures are also associated with increased CO production.

In general, CO toxicity has little clinical significance, regardless of the agent used, as long as simple guidelines to minimize or eliminate CO are observed. These include the use of fresh absorbent, the use of soda lime instead of Baralyme, and avoidance of techniques that dehydrate the CO_2 absorbent in the anesthetic circuit. Low fresh gas flows are more economical and limit absorbent desiccation. As a last resort, the absorbent can be rehydrated by adding approximately 1 cup of water (230 mL) per 1.2 kg of absorbent (i.e., standard canister).

Other Toxicities

Hematopoietic and Neurologic Systems

N_2O is the only anesthetic reported to produce hematologic toxicity and neurotoxicity with long-term administration. Both toxicities are the result of the interaction of N_2O with vitamin B_{12} and the disruption of several pathways involved in one-carbon chemistry. The biochemical basis of this effect is the oxidation of the cobalt in vitamin B_{12} by a physicochemical reaction with N_2O, which was previously discussed. The time required to produce megaloblastic hematopoiesis with N_2O exposure varies among patients. In healthy patients undergoing routine surgery, mild megaloblastic bone marrow changes are not seen after 6 hours, but they are seen after about 12 hours of exposure to 50% N_2O; after 24 hours of exposure, the changes are marked.[302] Complete bone marrow failure can be expected after several days of continuous exposure.[303] Limited evidence suggests that N_2O produces bone marrow changes earlier in seriously ill patients.[304] Evidence also suggests that the bone marrow changes are preventable by pretreating patients with large doses of folinic acid.[302] This drug is converted to the 5,10-methylene tetrahydrofolate needed for thymidine synthesis (Fig. 8-22). The neurologic disease, subacute combined degeneration of the spinal cord, develops only after several months of daily exposure to N_2O. The symptoms and signs include numbness and paresthesia in the extremities, loss of balance and unsteady gait, impairment of touch, and muscle weakness. In the late 1970s, the disease was recognized to be similar to vitamin B_{12} deficiency, but treatment with vitamin B_{12} did not alleviate the symptoms or enhance recovery.[305] It occurs in those who abuse N_2O on a long-term basis and rarely in individuals who work for many months in an environment grossly contaminated with the gas. Dental personnel who are occasionally exposed to waste N_2O at levels greater than 1000 ppm in poorly ventilated dental operatories for long periods are particularly at risk. In one study, 3 of 20 dentists exposed to mean concentrations up to 4600 ppm had abnormal bone marrows.[306] Personnel in modem-scavenged operating suites, however, are rarely exposed to such conditions and are not expected to have problems. Epidemiologic surveys confirm that dental, but not operating room, personnel have a higher incidence of neurologic disease, although exposure to waste N_2O has not definitely been shown to be the cause.[307] In humans and animals, there is an irreversible inactivation of the enzyme methionine synthase, which requires vitamin B_{12} in the completely reduced form to act as its coenzyme. Methionine synthase catalyzes the conversion of methyltetrahydrofolate and homocysteine to tetrahydrofolate and methionine. Failure to produce these products has a number of biochemical consequences, including reduced synthesis of thymidine, which is an essential DNA base. The clinical syndrome associated with oxidation of vitamin B_{12} is essentially the same as that seen in pernicious anemia: megaloblastic hematopoiesis and subacute combined degeneration of the spinal cord.

The time required for inactivation of methionine synthase depends on the species. In rats exposed to 50% N_2O, the half-time of inactivation is about 5 minutes.[308]

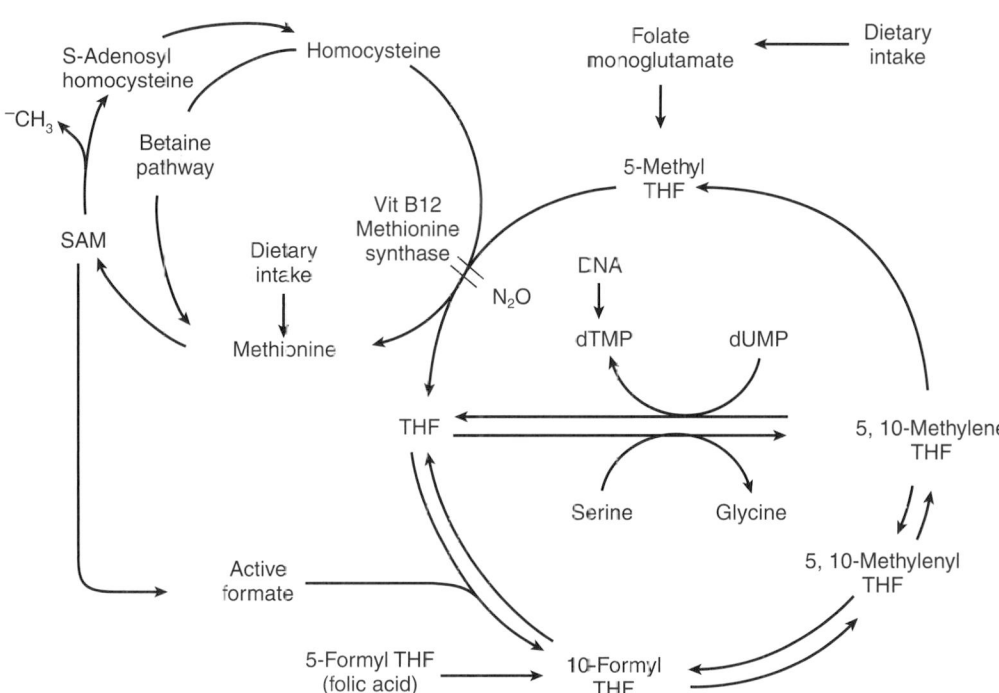

Figure 8–22 Conversion of methyltetrahydrofolate and homocysteine to tetrahydrofolate and methionine. (Adapted from Baden JM, Rice SA: Metabolism and toxicity of inhaled anesthetics. *In* Miller RD [ed]: Anesthesia, 5th ed. New York, Churchill Livingstone, 2000, p 147.)

Recovery of activity takes 3 to 4 days because of oxidation of the vitamin B_{12}, which is irreversible and covalently bound to the enzyme. New enzyme must be synthesized to restore activity. In humans, the half-life of inactivation is much longer than in rats, about 45 minutes.[309] Nevertheless, after several hours of routine anesthesia with N_2O, methionine synthase activity is very low. The decrease of thymidine synthesis takes somewhat longer to develop but also lasts several days. Experimental data suggest that there is a threshold concentration of about 1000 ppm (0.1%), below which N_2O has no biochemical effect.[310]

Reproduction and Development

Inhaled anesthetics present the potential for adverse reproductive and developmental effects for patients administered inhaled anesthetics and health care personnel exposed to waste anesthetic gases. Exposure to waste anesthetic gases occurs because of leaks in the anesthetic system, principally from three sources: masks, high-pressure fittings, and exhalation valves. Good working practices and tracheal intubation results in lower exposure of waste anesthetic gases. Recognition of postoperative exposure to exhaled waste anesthetic gases in the postanesthesia care units (PACUs) and intensive care units (ICUs) represents a new challenge. To control occupational exposure to waste anesthetic gases, it is not sufficient to adopt scavenging systems in operating rooms; working environmental controls and occupational management are required throughout the perioperative process.

In the United States, at least 50,000 pregnant women undergo anesthesia and surgery during gestation for indications unrelated to pregnancy.[310] Operations for ovarian cysts, acute appendicitis, mammary tumors, and repair of incompetent cervix are the most common causes. The risk of unexpected abortion or premature labor is higher

after anesthesia. What is not immediately obvious is whether the patient's disease, surgery, anesthesia, or a combination of these factors is the precipitating cause. Perhaps an even greater concern is that anesthesia during pregnancy may lead to an increased incidence of congenital abnormalities in the offspring of the patient.

To assess the incidence of various anesthesia- and surgery-related hazards occurring during pregnancy, at least five major and several minor studies have been performed.[311-317] The most extensive and thorough study links and analyzes data from three Swedish health care registries—the Medical Birth Registry, the Registry of Congenital Malformations, and the Hospital Discharge Registry—for the years 1973 to 1981.[317] Among the 720,000 pregnant patients whose records were examined, there were 5405 operations performed. The adverse reproductive and developmental outcomes examined were stillbirths, early postnatal deaths, low birth weight, and congenital anomalies. Women who had an operation did not have an increased incidence of stillbirths or of congenital anomalies among offspring. The incidence of postnatal death within 7 days of delivery was increased when an operation occurred during the second or third trimester but not during the first trimester. The incidence of low birth weight and premature delivery was increased regardless of the trimester in which an operation occurred. The cause of these hazards was not determined, although the finding that no particular type of operation or anesthesia was associated with a higher incidence of adverse outcomes suggests that the patient's disease played the major role in determining the outcome.

The increasing popularity of in vitro fertilization has afforded some opportunity to study the effects of anesthetics on ova. Various anesthetic regimens have been examined for their effects on rates of fertilization and cleavage of oocytes, pregnancy, and carriage to term. Results for general anesthesia have been variable, although there is some consensus that regimens that include inhaled anesthetics produce adverse effects.[318,319] In a well-controlled study of in vitro fertilization, no difference in fertilization or pregnancy rates was found between patients having isoflurane anesthesia with or without N_2O, a finding implying that short exposures to N_2O are not harmful.[320] A publication on transvaginal oocyte retrieval and reproductive outcome[321] reported that general anesthesia with N_2O in combination with opiates, barbiturates, and halothane resulted in significantly lower clinical pregnancy rates (14.5%) compared with patients receiving local anesthesia (23.7%) or epidural block (25.8%). There were no adverse effects reported for oocyte collection, embryo yield, or embryo transfer. In vitro test systems of *Drosophila* larvae, sea urchin eggs, and mice embryos have shown significant adverse effects on development.[322] The relevance of these findings to the human situation is unknown, but the amount of anesthetic encountered by these test systems was significantly greater than encountered in scavenged operating rooms.

Several studies have examined the effects of the inhaled anesthetics on sperm. In the only study of human sperm, semen was collected from 46 anesthesiologists who had worked for a minimum of 1 year in a scavenged operating suite.[323] Semen from 26 residents beginning an anesthesia training program was used as controls. The concentration of sperm and the percentage of abnormally shaped sperm were not different between the two groups. Sperm collected from 13 of the 26 residents after they had been working for 1 year was not different from the first sample. Studies of mice and rats under various experimental conditions have provided both positive and negative results, but insufficient information is available to permit extrapolation to humans. Despite some suggestive animal data, inhaled anesthetics have not been shown to have significant effects on sperm in humans. However, the scope of animal and human studies has been limited, and only moderate assurance of no effect has been achieved. Twenty reports have been published of epidemiologic surveys that examined the reproductive performance of operating room and dental personnel exposed to waste gases.[324-343] Table 8-8 lists the overall outcome of these surveys. An evaluation of the merits of each of these studies is beyond the scope of this chapter, which summarizes the outcomes, but a review of the studies is available elsewhere.[344] In a review of many of the studies before 1978, an estimate was made of the relative risks for particular adverse health effects.[345] The magnitude of the relative risk for spontaneous abortion among exposed women was approximately 1.3. The increase was reported to be consistent and statistically significant. For congenital abnormalities among offspring of anesthetic-exposed women, the relative risk was approximately 1.2. The overall data for wives of exposed men and for congenital abnormalities among their offspring were less consistent than the data for spontaneous abortion. For spontaneous abortion and congenital abnormalities, the increases observed were small and could not be attributed to a specific cause. Exposure to waste anesthetic gases, viruses, roentgenograms, a variety of chemicals other than anesthetics, or a combination of these factors might have accounted for the positive results. Most surveys had serious methodologic faults, including failure to verify the medical data supplied by respondents.

To resolve whether there were adverse effects that had not been appropriately acknowledged, in 1985, Buring and colleagues[346] performed a meta-analysis of five studies.[325-327,329,338] The investigators analyzed spontaneous abortion and congenital abnormalities among female physicians and nurses potentially exposed to waste anesthetics. Risk ratios were 1.3 (95% confidence interval [CI]: 1.2-1.4) for spontaneous abortion and 1.2 (95% CI: 1.0-1.4) for congenital abnormalities, both of which were statistically significant. However, response or

Table 8–8 Results of epidemiologic surveys of adverse reproductive effects among personnel exposed to waste anesthetic gases and their spouses

Study (year)	Exposed Women		Wives of Exposed Men	
	Spontaneous Abortion	*Major Anomaly in Offspring*	*Spontaneous Abortion*	*Major Anamoly in Offspring*
Askrog and Harvald (1970)	Negative	—	Positive	—
Cohen et al (1971)	Positive	Negative	—	—
Knill-Jones et al (1972)	Negative	Positive	—	—
Rosenberg and Kirves (1973)	Positive	Negative	—	—
Corbett et al (1974)	—	Positive	—	—
American Society of Anesthesiologists (1974)	Positive	Positive	Negative	Positive
Knill-Jones et al (1975) (1)	Positive	Negative		Negative
(2)	Positive	Positive	Negative	Positive
Cohen et al (1975)	Positive	Positive	Positive	Negative
Pharoah et al (1977)	Positive	Positive	—	—

From Baden JM, Rice SA: Metabolism and toxicity of inhaled anesthetics. In Miller RD (ed): Anesthesia, 5th ed. New York, Churchill Livingstone, 2000, p 147.

recall bias, or both, could explain these significant associations, because most of the studies relied on voluntary responses and self-reported outcomes. One of the acknowledged shortcomings of these studies (i.e., lack of a quantitative measure of exposure) was addressed in two later retrospective studies[343,344] that attempted to quantitate N_2O exposure among female dental assistants. The investigators reported that in unscavenged dental suites, exposure to more than 5 and 3 hours of N_2O per day, respectively, were associated with reduced fertility and increased spontaneous abortion rates.

A retrospective cohort study design, which was subject to selection and recall bias, was used for most of the epidemiologic studies listed in Table 8-8. One of the weakest links in the epidemiologic studies of adverse reproductive and developmental outcomes after occupational anesthetic exposure is the lack of quantification of the extent and duration of anesthetic exposure. Data generally were collected by self-administered questionnaire without verification of exposure or outcome. Because the extent and duration of exposure to waste anesthetics has decreased in recent years, it is difficult to draw conclusions on the likely adverse effects of current anesthetic exposure based on earlier studies at conditions of higher exposure. In the only three studies in which medical records were used to confirm medical data, negative results were obtained for a number of adverse reproductive effects, including spontaneous abortion.[334,339,340]

In addition to problems in quantification of exposure, there is also a problem of identifying the cause of any congenital malformation that is observed. Although human development is remarkably consistent, it is not always perfect, and severe and trivial congenital malformations are found in 2% to 4% of all births in countries in which records are kept.[347] There are many mechanisms involved in abnormal development (Table 8-9). Some, such as mutations that result in specific biochemical abnormalities and chromosomal nondisjunction, are well established. Others, such as interference with abnormal cell membrane states, are less certain mechanisms of teratogenicity. Although the cause of most defects remains unknown, chemical teratogenesis in humans is well established. Because of the difficulty in identifying causes and investigating mechanisms in humans, sophisticated animal studies have been developed over the past 40 years for examining the teratogenicity of chemicals. Complete assessment of a chemical now involves examining its effect on mating behavior, fertility, embryonic and fetal wastage, congenital anomalies, and postnatal survival and behavior. Animal studies provide useful information, but they are limited because of the difficulty of extrapolating animal data to humans and the relatively low statistical power to detect the presence of a weak teratogen.

Developmental effects of the inhaled anesthetics have also been extensively studied in animals in an attempt to control conditions that cannot be controlled in epidemiologic studies. These studies tried to control for the many factors (e.g., genetic variability, environment, diet) that could contribute to the background incidence of congenital malformations in humans. Studies of the inhaled anesthetics on reproductive processes of experimental animals have been conducted at trace and subanesthetic concentrations to simulate occupational exposure and at anesthetic concentrations to simulate surgical exposure. The large number of such studies precludes a complete discussion in this chapter, but several reviews are available.[344,348,349] In general, N_2O is the only inhaled anesthetic that has been convincingly shown to be directly teratogenic to experimental animals, but only under experimental conditions that are considered extreme. High concentrations (50% to 75%) delivered to rats for 24-hour periods during organogenesis and low concentrations (0.1%) delivered to rats continuously throughout pregnancy result in an increased incidence of fetal resorptions and visceral and skeletal abnormalities.[350,351] A particularly interesting abnormality produced by high N_2O exposure is situs inversus, in which there is a disturbance of the left-right body axis, and organs such as the heart are on the wrong side of the body.[352] Although effects in rodents are seen only after extended periods of continuous exposure, it is not known whether humans are more sensitive than rodents and would show effects after shorter periods of exposure.

Table 8–9 Epidemiologic surveys for cancer incidence or deaths among personnel exposed to waste anesthetic gases

Studied Result	Population	Results	Study (year)
Deaths	ASA members	Negative	Bruce et al. (1968)
Incidence	Nurse anesthetists	3.3- fold increase for 1971	Corbett et al. (1973)
Incidence	ASA members	1.3- to 1.9-fold increase for women; negative for men	ASA (1974)
Deaths	ASA members	Negative	Bruce et al. (1974)
Deaths	Anesthetists	Negative	Doll and Peto (1977)
Deaths	Anesthetists and offspring	Negative	Tomlin (1979)
Incidence	Dental personnel	1.5-fold increase for women; negative for men	Cohen et al. (1980)
Deaths	Anesthetists	Negative	Neil et al. (1987)
Incidence	Operating room personnel	Negative	Cuirguis et al. (1990)

ASA, American Society of Anesthesiologists.
From Baden JM, Rice SA: Metabolism and toxicity of inhaled anesthetics. *In* Miller RD (ed): Anesthesia, 5th ed. New York, Churchill Livingstone, 2000, p 147.

The mechanisms that produce teratogenic effects with N_2O are slowly being revealed. The former leading theory was that inhibition of methionine synthase causes critical shortages of intracellular thymidine (and therefore DNA), which is needed by the rapidly growing embryo. Decreased DNA synthesis and decreased total DNA content have been observed in embryos immediately after N_2O exposure.[353,354] It appears that lack of methionine rather than the lack of thymidine plays the critical role in all the adverse reproductive effects other than situs inversus.[355] An entirely different mechanism accounts for the situs inversus: stimulation of α_1-adrenergic receptors by N_2O.[356] The effect is mediated by activation of calmodulin kinase-11 but not phosphokinase C.[357]

N_2O teratogenesis is being actively investigated because of its relevance to patient and occupational safety and because N_2O can be used to determine the importance of vitamin B_{12}, folates, one-carbon chemistry, and the adrenergic system in developmental processes. Halothane, enflurane, isoflurane, desflurane, and sevoflurane are also teratogenic to rodents, but only when they are administered at anesthetizing concentrations for many hours on several days during pregnancy. The consensus is that the teratogenic effects observed in animals exposed to the inhaled anesthetics are caused by physiologic changes associated with anesthesia, rather than by inherent teratologic properties of the anesthetics themselves. Nonetheless, all findings emphasize the potential for anesthetics to interfere with developmental processes, regardless of the mechanism.

Developmental toxicity also encompasses the cognitive and functional deficits that may occur in the absence of observable morphologic changes. Organ systems are most sensitive to chemical teratogens during periods of development (i.e., organogenesis). The central nervous system may be particularly vulnerable during the period of myelination. In humans, this period is from the fourth intrauterine month through the second postnatal year. A chemical or drug may produce behavioral teratogenesis if administered late in gestation or even after birth. Anesthetics have not escaped scrutiny as possible behavioral teratogens. A study of 1-day-old rats exposed to 0.75% or 1.0% halothane with or without 50% or 75% N_2O for 6 hours demonstrated dose-dependent decrements in phosphokinase C activity in growth cone particles isolated from the forebrains.[358] There were no effects at 0.5% halothane or 25% N_2O. Although the anesthetic concentrations causing effects were high, the importance of phosphokinase C in signal transductions in developing brain and the potential disruption by anesthetics cannot be ignored. Although some rodent studies have shown behavioral deficits after exposure to the inhaled anesthetics,[359-361] the mechanism for these changes is unknown, and the applicability to humans is unclear. In general, the anesthetic exposure conditions can be considered extreme relative to any reasonably expected human exposure.

Human studies have generally focused on long-term behavioral effects of maternal obstetric medication, including epidural anesthesia. Claims have been made that the medication given at delivery to the mother produces depressed motor skills and impaired language ability in the infant and child for several years. Such claims, however, are controversial. Behavioral abnormalities of offspring whose mothers received inhaled anesthetics at any time during delivery have not been well studied. Studies have not been done to assess neurobehavioral function of children of operating room personnel who have been exposed to waste anesthetic gases. Firm conclusions about the risk of the occurrence of behavioral teratogenesis among the offspring of exposed personnel or in exposed patients therefore await further investigation.

Long-term occupational exposure to trace concentrations of anesthetic gases is thought to have adverse effects on health of exposed personnel, and there is growing awareness and concern regarding occupational exposure to waste anesthetic gases in the PACUs. Several studies have documented excessive levels of waste anesthetic gases in poorly ventilated PACU areas.[362-365] However, none of these studies has documented any significant, long-term adverse health effects.[362,363] An increased incidence of sister-chromatic exchanges has been found in operating room personnel in three of four studies.[366-369]

DNA, Genetics, and Neoplasia

The potential long-term adverse health effects from occupational exposure to trace concentrations of waste anesthetic gases have been recognized for more than 20 years. Even if inhaled anesthetics have a low potential for causing long-term toxicity, exposure of a large population may represent a considerable public health hazard. In the United States, about 50,000 hospital operating room personnel, including anesthesiologists, nurse anesthetists, and operating room technicians, are exposed daily to waste anesthetic gases.[310] Surgeons, dental personnel, veterinarians, and their technical assistants have a variable but sometimes heavy exposure to waste anesthetics. The total number of exposed or potentially exposed personnel in the United States each year is about 225,000.[310] Of particular concern are reports that inhaled anesthetics possess mutagenic and carcinogenic potentials.

Genotoxicity

Investigators have been interested in the mutagenic potential of inhaled anesthetics for several reasons. First, many chemical carcinogens are also mutagens, although the reverse is not necessarily true. Finding that a particular anesthetic is a mutagen also implies a potential for carcinogenesis that should be evaluated. Second, mutagens may pose a threat to the integrity of the human genome (i.e., the totality of genes and chromosomes). Mutations are heritable changes in genetic information. Unrepaired mutations in germ cells can be passed from generation to generation, and unrepaired mutations in somatic cells can result in diseases, including cancer. The four types of mutations traditionally recognized are base-pair mutations, frameshift mutations, deletions or rearrangements of chromosomal segments, and nondisjunction of chromosomes between daughter cells. A fifth and novel type of mutation has been recognized that involves continuous repeats of three nucleotides at a specific site in a gene.[370]

In vitro assays for mutagenicity require much less time and expense than in vivo tests for carcinogenicity, and these assays have become popular screening methods for detecting carcinogens. A wide variety of test systems has been used to examine the mutagenicity of inhaled anesthetics, including assays with bacteria, yeast, mammalian cells in culture, and intact mammals.

Extensive work has been done with the Ames Salmonella/mammalian hepatic microsome system, which uses several strains of histidine-dependent Salmonella typhimurium as tester organisms. This system is a well-validated assay for mutagenicity and often is regarded as the standard against which other systems are compared. It has been used to test most currently and formerly used anesthetics. Only divinyl ether and fluroxene give unequivocally positive mutagenic responses, whereas trichloroethylene gives a weak mutagenic response. Other anesthetics, including N_2O, halothane, enflurane, isoflurane, sevoflurane, and desflurane are not mutagenic when tested under a wide variety of experimental conditions and anesthetic concentrations. The finding that some mutagenic anesthetic metabolites have a chemical structure reminiscent of vinyl chloride ($CH_2=CHCl$) is consistent with the known high reactivity and mutagenicity of this class of chemicals. Of the many inhaled anesthetic metabolites that have been tested in the Salmonella assay, only 1,1-difluoro-2-bromo-2-chloroethylene ($CF_2=CBrCl$) and 1,1-difluoro-2-chloroethylene ($CF_2=CHCl$) have been found to be even weakly mutagenic. In general, results from numerous studies with other test systems have confirmed those from studies with Salmonella.[33,369] Although there are some anomalous results, the overwhelming evidence from in vitro tests indicates that all currently used and most previously used anesthetics are not mutagens. Compound A has been reported to induce sister chromatic exchanges in Chinese hamster ovary cells.[371] Halothane, enflurane, isoflurane, and desflurane all inhibit the production of nitric oxide, N_2O, nitric oxide synthase (NOS), and messenger RNA for NOS in a dose- and time-dependent manner in a marine macrophage.[372]

Results of genotoxicity studies of humans exposed to inhaled anesthetics have generally been negative. In an early study from 1977,[372] no significant difference in the number of chromosomal aberrations could be detected between the lymphocytes obtained from operating room nurses and those obtained from surgical outpatient nurses. Mutagenic activity was not detected in the Salmonella assay for urine of personnel working in scavenged or unscavenged operating rooms or for urine of anesthesiology residents during the first 15 months of training.[373] Lymphocytes from personnel exposed to waste anesthetic gases for durations up to 312 months had no higher incidence of chromosomal aberrations or sister chromatic exchange compared with lymphocytes from unexposed individuals.[374] The latter study was an extension of previous negative studies by the same investigators of sister chromatic exchanges in lymphocytes of operating room personnel exposed to waste anesthetic gases and of patients anesthetized with halothane, enflurane, or fluroxene. In contrast to these negative results, studies in 1990[375] and 1992[364] showed cytogenic damage

in operating room personnel exposed to waste anesthetic gases. A 1993 study[366] showed DNA single-strand breaks in lymphocytes of patients immediately after anesthesia with isoflurane and N_2O. Why these differences in study results exist is unknown, although positive results could be explained by multiple factors unassociated with the anesthetics. As with the teratogenicity and carcinogenicity studies described elsewhere in this chapter, genotoxicity studies of operating room personnel are more realistically studies of the work environment, which is composed of many chemical and physical agents as well as anesthetic gases.

Inhaled Anesthetics and Carcinogenicity

Chemical carcinogenesis is a multistage, multistep process leading to the formation of malignant tumors. There are two general classes of carcinogens: genotoxic and nongenotoxic. The former type directly interacts with DNA, and the latter type does not. Chemical carcinogenesis consists of three operationally defined stages: initiation, promotion, and progression.

Genotoxic carcinogens are often referred to as initiators because, in interacting with DNA, they initiate the process in normal cells. Initiation is most often accomplished in several steps, the first of which is the metabolic activation of the chemical to a reactive intermediate. The second step consists of the covalent binding of the reactive intermediate to DNA. One or more cell divisions are required to "set" or "fix" the mutation. Before the mutation is fixed, the DNA may still be repaired. Initiation is accomplished only when the mutation is fixed. Once initiation has occurred there is still no guarantee that a cell with defective DNA will survive a sufficiently long period to proceed in the process of carcinogenesis because initiated cells are also subject to apoptosis.

Nongenotoxic carcinogens, unlike genotoxic carcinogens, do not initiate cells. Nongenotoxic agents act through other mechanisms to promote the growth of initiated cells; the term promoter is often applied to these carcinogens. These agents may interact with other cellular components to promote the growth of these cells. A common mechanism is increased rate of cellular proliferation, preventing the normal repair process. One thing in common with these agents is that the promotion of initiated cells into tumors requires the continued presence of the promoter. Without its presence, apoptosis results in the elimination of single initiated cells and natural regression of the preneoplastic tumors.

The terms initiator and promoter are used to indicate the state of carcinogenesis in which a chemical is first active. An initiator may also have activity as a promoter. The phase of progression that results in the appearance of clinically apparent tumors involves additional phenotypic and genotypic changes to cells, resulting in karyotypic instability. These mechanisms are not understood, and many cancers appear to occur over a prolonged period. Covalent binding of reactive intermediates to tissue macromolecules is presumed to be a necessary requirement for initiation of chemical carcinogenesis. Covalent binding, however, is not sufficient for initiation because the binding must be specific to a DNA site that would result in miscoding of a necessary gene product or a regulatory gene. The mutation caused by covalent binding must also be fixed in the DNA by cell division. Current techniques can distinguish specific binding sites, but the older literature did not, giving the impression that any covalent binding was paramount to carcinogenesis.

Structural evaluation of chemicals for similarities to known carcinogens is useful to identify potential mutagens, but minor changes in structure often have profound effects on mutagenic and carcinogenic activity. Methoxyflurane, enflurane, and isoflurane are α-haloethers, as are the nonanesthetic but carcinogenic chemicals bis(chloromethyl)ether, chloromethyl methyl ether, and bis(α-chloroethyl)ether. The anesthetics, however, are not mutagenic. Halothane is a halide, as are the animal carcinogens methyl iodide, butyl bromide, and butyl chloride. Halothane, however, is not mutagenic. Fluroxene and divinyl ether also contain the vinyl moiety similar to vinyl chloride, a human and animal carcinogen. Although the structural similarity between the anesthetics and several chemical carcinogens suggests an association between anesthetics and carcinogenicity, there are no epidemiologic or other data to support that suggestion. Despite the obvious advantage of surveying human populations to determine the carcinogenic risk of exposure to anesthetics, such surveys have provided little information on the carcinogenicity of specific anesthetics. The primary reason is that the doses of anesthetics to which surveyed individuals have been exposed have not been measured and, at best, have been estimated. Nonetheless, the studies performed should indicate whether waste anesthetics are associated with a higher incidence of cancer.

There have been several surveys of cancer incidence among operating room and dental workers[329,335,341,376-380] (see Table 8-9). The largest was an ASA-conducted retrospective survey[48] of 595 operating room personnel working throughout the United States.[333] A 1.3- to 1.9-fold increase in cancer incidence was found for female members of the ASA and the American Association of Nurse Anesthetists compared with unexposed control female groups. No increase in cancer incidence was seen among surveyed mates. In an earlier study, the incidence of cancer among 525 female nurse anesthetists in Michigan was compared with that of women participating in the Connecticut Tumor Registry.[377] The nurse anesthetists had a higher incidence of malignancies diagnosed during 1971 than did all the women of Connecticut during the period of 1966 to 1969.

In another large study, a national survey of health among dental personnel was reported.[336] The study population consisted of 30,650 dentists and 30,547 chairside assistants and was readily divided into those who used or did not use inhaled anesthetics to provide pain relief and sedation of patients. Otherwise, both groups did similar work under similar conditions. An estimate of anesthetic exposure was made by calculating the number of hours per week spent by each respondent in the dental operatory. About 80% of inhaled anesthetics users were exposed to N_2O alone, whereas the remainder was also exposed to potent volatile anesthetics. The cancer incidence among female chairside assistants exposed to waste anesthetics for more than 8 hours per week was 50% greater than among those not exposed, although the increase was not statistically significant ($P = .056$). Analysis of various

types of cancer showed that only cancer of the cervix occurred more frequently ($P = .06$) in exposed women than in unexposed women. However, a 1990 study of health effects associated with waste anesthetic exposure in Ontario hospital personnel did not show an increased cancer incidence for men or women compared with unexposed controls.[341]

Collectively, the foregoing studies of cancer incidence appear to suggest a small risk to women directly exposed to waste anesthetic gases. However, because of problems with study design and the small increase in cancer incidence observed, reviewers have generally been unconvinced of the existence of a hazard to humans.[345,348,349] This lack of conviction is strengthened by the uniformly negative results from surveys of deaths from cancer[335,376,378-380] (see Table 8-9). Problems in interpreting epidemiologic surveys led many investigators to turn to animal studies to provide information on the carcinogenic potential of specific anesthetics. In early studies, chloroform was found to be a rodent carcinogen when the drug was administered in very high doses by oral gavage, but this route of administration is not relevant to inhaled exposure of patients or operating room personnel. It is now recognized that hepatic tumorigenesis in rodents with chloroform is related to high-dose cytotoxicity and the subsequent increased rate of reparative proliferation. At lower doses, at which cytotoxicity is not present, tumors do not form. When halothane, methoxyflurane, enflurane, isoflurane, and N_2O have been administered by inhalation and assessed in adequate studies, results for carcinogenicity have been uniformly negative.[381-386] In none of these studies was there evidence of other types of organ toxicity on histologic examination. The conclusion from animal and human studies is that there is no carcinogenic risk from exposure to the currently used inhaled anesthetics.

Modern fluorinated inhaled anesthetics are not mutagenic, nor are they carcinogenic. N_2O in concentrations greater than 50% is teratogenic in animals, as is exposure to the fluorinated anesthetics for several hours during pregnancy in animals. The analyses of Burning and coworkers,[346] Tannenbaum and Goldberg,[387] and Axelsson and Rylander[338] demonstrate that flawed studies can lead to inaccurate conclusions. In the only long-term, prospective study with or without scavenging of waste anesthetic gases, Spence[388] found no causal relationship between exposure to waste anesthetic gases and adverse health effects. In the dental studies, with no scavenging of waste anesthetic gases and higher levels of N_2O, increased incidences of infertility and spontaneous abortions were observed. Neither animal nor epidemiologic studies have proved that adverse effects are associated with exposure to trace levels of waste fluorinated anesthetic gases such as halothane, enflurane, isoflurane, desflurane, or sevoflurane.

SUMMARY

Volatile anesthetics, like most drugs, undergo metabolism in the body and are sometimes associated with toxic reactions. Scientific investigations and industry research have led to the development of more stable anesthetics with more desirable clinical properties. The inhaled agents that are more heavily metabolized are associated with the greatest numbers of reported toxicities. As with most drugs, these toxicities occur when the anesthetics are given as standard-dose medications (i.e., the appropriate medication and dose are given at the proper time, in the correct manner to the right patient). These associated toxicities under most circumstances meet the definition of adverse drug reactions. For comparison, 51% of approved drugs have serious adverse drug reactions not detected before approval, and adverse drug reactions are responsible for 6% of all hospital admissions, occur in 10% to 20% of hospitalized patients, and are the cause of death of 0.1% of medical and 0.01% of surgical patients. They are the fourth leading cause of death in hospitalized patients (0.32% of hospitalized patients). Compared with most therapeutic agents, the safety of fluorinated inhaled anesthetics is remarkable.

The use of any anesthetic must be based on specific knowledge of its benefits and risks, how it may produce toxicity, and in which patients it may be most safely administered. The perfect anesthetic agent does not exist, and the circumstances of individual patients will continue to dictate the choice and use of inhaled anesthetics in clinical practice. As ongoing research attempts to uncover emerging toxicities, the clinician is challenged to balance new information with current clinical practices and choose the safest, most effective agents for each patient.

KEY POINTS

1. The liver is the major site of endogenous and exogenous drug metabolism. The primary result of drug metabolism is the production of more water-soluble and therefore more easily excreted drug metabolites. Drugs are sometimes biotransformed into more reactive metabolites, which may lead to toxicity.

2. Most drug metabolism is catalyzed by phase 1 or phase 2 enzymes. The predominant phase 1 enzymes are the cytochrome P450 (CYP) monooxygenases. Approximately 50 of the more than 1000 CYPs are functionally active in humans. The predominant isoform catalyzing metabolism of the inhaled anesthetics is CYP2E1. The major phase 2 enzyme is uridine diphosphate glucuronosyltransferase (UGT).

3. Many factors affect drug metabolism. Perhaps the most important are pharmacogenetic factors. Genetic status ultimately determines absorption, distribution, metabolism, and excretion. Other important determinants are environmental factors, age, gender disease states, and other drugs or medications.

4. Pharmacogenomics, or the influence of DNA sequence variation on the effect of a drug, provide a basis for understanding the variations observed in drug responses among patients.

5. N_2O and xenon are nonhalogenated anesthetics. Xenon is not currently approved for clinical use. Other than the expense associated with its use, it may be the most ideal anesthetic agent.

6. Halothane, enflurane, isoflurane, and desflurane are all metabolized to trifluoroacylated hepatic protein adducts, which have been reported to induce liver injury in susceptible patients. The propensity to produce liver injury appears to parallel metabolism of the parent drug: halothane (20%) >>>> enflurane (2.5%) >> isoflurane (0.2%) > desflurane (0.02%). The incidence of halothane hepatitis in the adult population is roughly 1 in 10,000. Sevoflurane does not produce acylated protein adducts.

7. Halothane hepatitis has been reported in the pediatric population. The incidence appears to be approximately 1 in 200,000.

8. Toxicity and liver injury have been reported after repeated exposure on subsequent occasions to different fluorinated anesthetics. This phenomenon of cross-sensitization has also been reported with the chlorofluorocarbon (CFC) replacement agents, the hydrochlorofluorocarbons (HCFCs).

9. Sevoflurane is metabolized to hexafluoroisopropanol, formaldehyde, inorganic fluoride, and carbon dioxide. Although very high fluoride levels have been reported after sevoflurane anesthesia, fluoride-associated renal injury has not been reported.

10. The major base-catalyzed breakdown product of sevoflurane is compound A. Compound A is a nephrotoxic vinyl ether and induces a renal injury that is dose and time dependent. The threshold for renal injury in rats and humans appears to be approximately 150 ppm-hours of compound A exposure (i.e., 50 ppm for 3 hours). The toxic threshold appears to be reached only under clinical conditions of prolonged sevoflurane anesthesia, and observed changes occur in glucosuria and enzymuria. BUN and creatinine levels remain unchanged.

11. Desiccated carbon dioxide absorbents and inhaled anesthetics interactions can lead to the production of CO in the anesthesia circuit (desflurane >>> enflurane > isoflurane). Negligible amounts of CO are formed from halothane and sevoflurane.

12. There appears to be no risk associated with brief periods of low-level occupational exposure to waste anesthetic gases in the operating room, PACU, or ICU. Occupational exposure to high concentrations (10^3 ppm) may be correlated with an increased incidence of abortions and decreased fertility. Individuals with vitamin B_{12} deficiencies may be at risk of neurologic injury from N_2O.

Acknowledgments

The authors wish to acknowledge Jeffrey Baden and Susan Rice, authors of this chapter in the fifth edition of *Anesthesia*, some of whose text has been retained in this edition. We also wish to thank Dr. Lance R. Pohl and Ms. Tami Graf for their critical review and helpful suggestions in the preparation of this chapter.

REFERENCES

1. Wilkinson G: Pharmacokinetics: The dynamics of drug absorption, distribution and elimination. *In* Hardman JG, Limbird LE, Goodman GA (eds): Goodman and Gilman's the Pharmacological Basis of Therapeutics, 10th ed. New York, McGraw-Hill, 2001.
2. Weinshilboum R: Inheritance and drug response. N Engl J Med 348:529-537, 2003.
3. Gibson GG, Skett P: Introduction to drug metabolism. Chelteham, UK, Stanley Thornes Publishers, 1999.
4. Krishna DR, Klotz U: Extra hepatic metabolism of drugs in humans. Clin Pharmacokinet 26:144-160, 1994.
5. Lohr JW, Willsky GR, Acara MA: Renal drug metabolism. Pharmacol Rev 50:107-141, 1998.
6. Koop DR: Oxidative and reductive metabolism by cytochrome P450 2E1. FASEB J 6:724-730, 1992.
7. Guengerich FP: Cytochrome P450 enzymes and drug metabolism. *In* Bridges JAV, Chasseadud LF, Gibson GG (eds): Progress in Drug Metabolism. New York, Taylor & Francis, 1987, p 3.
8. Snyder R, Remmer H: Classes of hepatic microsomal mixed function oxidase inducers. *In* Schenkman JB, Kupfer D (eds): Hepatic Cytochrome P450 Monooxygenase System. New York, Pergamon Press, 1982, p 227.
9. Boobis AR, Davies DS: Human cytochromes P-450. Xenobiotica 14:151-185, 1984.
10. Duvaldestin P, Mazze RI, Nivoche Y, Desmonts JM: Occupational exposure to halothane results in enzyme induction in anesthetists. Anesthesiology 54:57-60, 1981.
11. Dooley JR, Mazze RI, Rice SA, Borel JD: Is enflurane defluorination inducible in man? Anesthesiology 50:213-217, 1979.
12. Mazze RI, Woodruff RE, Heerdt ME: Isoniazid-induced enflurane defluorination in humans. Anesthesiology 57:5-8, 1982.
13. Greene NM: Halothane anesthesia and hepatitis in a high-risk population. N Engl J Med 289:304-307, 1973.
14. Ortiz de Montellano PR, Reich NO: Inhibition of cytochrome P450 enzymes. *In* Ortiz de Montellano PR (ed): Cytochrome P450: Structure, Mechanism, and Biochemistry. New York, Plenum Press, 1986, pp 21-30.
15. Weiss CF, Glazko AJ, Weston JK: Chloramphenicol in the newborn infant. A physiologic explanation of its toxicity when given in excessive doses. N Engl J Med 262:787-794, 1960.
16. Young WS, Lietman PS: Chloramphenicol glucuronyl transferase: Assay, ontogeny and inducibility. J Pharmacol Exp Ther 204:203-211, 1978.
17. Lacroix D, Sonnier M, Moncion A, et al: Expression of CYP3A in the human liver—Evidence that the shift between CYP3A7 and CYP3A4 occurs immediately after birth. Eur J Biochem 247:625-634, 1997.
18. Loughnan PM, Greenwald A, Purton WW, et al: Pharmacokinetic observations of phenytoin disposition in the newborn and young infant. Arch Dis Child 52:302-309, 1977.
19. Kalow W: The Pennsylvania State University College of Medicine 1990 Bernard B. Brodie lecture. Pharmacogenetics: Past and future. Life Sci 47:1385-1397, 1990.
20. Kalow W, Gunn DR: The relation between dose of succinylcholine and duration of apnea in man. J Pharmacol Exp Ther 120:203-214, 1957.
21. Ingelman-Sundberg M, Oscarson M, McLellan RA: Polymorphic human cytochrome P450 enzymes: An opportunity for individualized drug treatment. Trends Pharmacol Sci 20:342-349, 1999.

22. Sata F, Sapone A, Elizondo G, et al: CYP3A4 allelic variants with amino acid substitutions in exons 7 and 12: Evidence for an allelic variant with altered catalytic activity. Clin Pharmacol Ther 67:48-56, 2000.
23. Kuehl P, Zhang J, Lin Y, et al: Sequence diversity in CYP3A promoters and characterization of the genetic basis of polymorphic CYP3A5 expression. Nat Genet 27:383-391, 2001.
24. Blum M, Grant DM, McBride W, et al: Human arylamine *N*-acetyltransferase genes: Isolation, chromosomal localization, and functional expression. DNA Cell Biol 9:193-203, 1990.
25. Lin HJ, Han CY, Lin BK, Hardy S: Slow acetylator mutations in the human polymorphic *N*-acetyltransferase gene in 786 Asians, blacks, Hispanics, and whites: Application to metabolic epidemiology. Am J Hum Genet 52:827-834, 1993.
26. Remy CN: Metabolism of thiopyrimidines and thiopurines: *S*-methylation with *S*-adenosylmethionine transmethylase and catabolism in mammalian tissues. J Biol Chem 238:1078-1084, 1963.
27. Woodson LC, Weinshilboum RM: Human kidney thiopurine methyltransferase, purification and biochemical properties. Biochem Pharmacol 32:819-826, 1983.
28. Banks RGS, Henderson RJ, Pratt JM: Reactions of gases in solution. Some reactions of nitrous oxide with transition metal complexes. J Chem Soc 3(Suppl A):2886, 1968.
29. Hong K, Trudell JR, O'Neil JR, Cohen EN: Metabolism of nitrous oxide by human and rat intestinal contents. Anesthesiology 52:16-19, 1980.
30. Amess JA, Burman JF, Rees GM, et al: Megaloblastic haemopoiesis in patients receiving nitrous oxide. Lancet 2:339-342, 1978.
31. Van Dyke RA: Biotransformation. *In* Chenoweth MB (ed): Handbook of Experimental Pharmacology. New York, Springer-Verlag, 1972, p 354.
32. Rao GS, Meridian DJ, Tong YS, et al: Biochemical toxicology of chronic nitrous oxide exposures. Pharmologist 21:216, 1979.
33. Rice SA, Mazze RI, Baden JM: Effects of subchronic intermittent exposure to nitrous oxide in Swiss Webster mice. J Environ Pathol Toxicol Oncol 6:271-281, 1985.
34. Linde HW, Berman ML: Nonspecific stimulation of drug-metabolizing enzymes by inhalation anesthetic agents. Anesth Analg 50:656-667, 1971.
35. Cullen SC, Gross EG: The anesthetic properties of xenon in animals and human beings, with additional observations on krypton. Science 113:580-582, 1951.
36. Froeba G, Marx T, Pazhur J, et al: Xenon does not trigger malignant hyperthermia in susceptible swine. Anesthesiology 91:1047-1052, 1999.
37. Jaffrin MY, Kesic P: Airway resistance: A fluid mechanical approach. J Appl Physiol 36:354-361, 1974.
38. Zhang P, Ohara A, Mashimo T, et al: Pulmonary resistance in dogs: A comparison of xenon with nitrous oxide. Can J Anaesth 42:547-553, 1995.
39. Morris LE, Knott JR, Pittinger CB: Electro-encephalographic and blood gas observations in human surgical patients during xenon anesthesia. Anesthesiology 16:312-319, 1955.
40. Lachmann B, Armbruster S, Schairer W, et al: Safety and efficacy of xenon in routine use as an inhalational anaesthetic. Lancet 335:1413-1415, 1990.
41. Luttropp HH, Thomasson R, Dahm S, et al: Clinical experience with minimal flow xenon anesthesia. Acta Anaesthesiol Scand 38:121-125, 1994.
42. Hofland J, Gultuna I, Tenbrinck R: Xenon anaesthesia for laparoscopic cholecystectomy in a patient with Eisenmenger's syndrome. Br J Anaesth 86:882-886, 2001.
43. Burov NE, Molchanov IV, Nikolaev LL, Rashchupkin AB: [The method of low-flow xenon anesthesia]. Anesteziol Reanimatol 3:31-34, 2003.
44. Goto T, Saito H, Shinkai M, et al: Xenon provides faster emergence from anesthesia than does nitrous oxide-sevoflurane or nitrous oxide-isoflurane. Anesthesiology 86:1273-1278, 1997.

45. Rossaint R, Reyle-Hahn M, Schulte AM, et al: Multicenter randomized comparison of the efficacy and safety of xenon and isoflurane in patients undergoing elective surgery. Anesthesiology 98:6-13, 2003.

46. Kharasch ED, Hankins DC, Fenstamaker K, Cox K: Human halothane metabolism, lipid peroxidation, and cytochromes P(450)2A6 and P(450)3A4. Eur J Clin Pharmacol 55:853-859, 2000.

47. Lind RC, Gandolfi AJ, Hall PD: The role of oxidative biotransformation of halothane in the guinea pig model of halothane-associated hepatotoxicity. Anesthesiology 70:649-653, 1989.

48. Muller R, Stier A: Modification of liver microsomal lipids by halothane metabolites; a multi nuclear NMR spectroscopic study. Naunyn Schmiedebergs Arch Pharmacol 321:234-237, 1982.

49. Cohen EN, Trudell JR, Edmunds HN, Watson E: Urinary metabolites of halothane in man. Anesthesiology 43:392-401, 1975.

50. Maiorino RM, Sipes IG, Gandolfi AJ, et al: Factors affecting the formation of chlorotrifluoroethane and chlorodifluoroethylene from halothane. Anesthesiology 54:383-389, 1981.

51. Baker MT, Nelson RM, Van Dyke RA: The release of inorganic fluoride from halothane and halothane metabolites by cytochrome P-450, hemin, and hemoglobin. Drug Metab Dispos 11:308-311, 1983.

52. Sipes IG, Brown BR Jr: An animal model of hepatotoxicity associated with halothane anesthesia. Anesthesiology 45:622-628, 1976.

53. Sharp JH, Trudell JR, Cohen EN: Volatile metabolites and decomposition products of halothane in man. Anesthesiology 50:2-8, 1979.

54. Ahr HJ, King LJ, Nastainczyk W, Ullrich V: The mechanism of reductive dehalogenation of halothane by liver cytochrome P450. Biochem Pharmacol 31:383-390, 1982.

55. de Groot H, Harnisch U, Noll T: Suicidal inactivation of microsomal cytochrome P-450 by halothane under hypoxic conditions. Biochem Biophys Res Commun 107:885-891, 1982.

56. Raventos J, Lemon PG: The impurities in Fluothane: Their biological properties. Br J Anaesth 37:716-737, 1965.

57. Kharasch ED, Hankins D, Mautz D, Thummel KE: Identification of the enzyme responsible for oxidative halothane metabolism: Implications for prevention of halothane hepatitis. Lancet 347:1367-1371, 1996.

58. Jee RC, Sipes IG, Gandolfi AJ, Brown BR Jr: Factors influencing halothane hepatotoxicity in the rat hypoxic model. Toxicol Appl Pharmacol 52:267-277, 1980.

59. Rice SA, Maze M, Smith CM, et al: Halothane hepatotoxicity in Fischer 344 rats pretreated with isoniazid. Toxicol Appl Pharmacol 87:411-419, 1987.

60. Garton KJ, Yuen P, Meinwald J, et al: Stereoselective metabolism of enflurane by human liver cytochrome P450 2E1. Drug Metab Dispos 23:1426-1430, 1995.

61. Burke TR Jr, Branchflower RV, Lees DE, Pohl LR: Mechanism of defluorination of enflurane. Identification of an organic metabolite in rat and man. Drug Metab Dispos 9:19-24, 1981.

62. Miller MS, Gandolfi AJ: Enflurane biotransformation in humans. Life Sci 27:1465-1468, 1980.

63. Christ DD, Satoh H, Kenna JG, Pohl LR: Potential metabolic basis for enflurane hepatitis and the apparent cross-sensitization between enflurane and halothane. Drug Metab Dispos 16:135-140, 1988.

64. Hoffman J, Konopka K, Buckhorn C, et al: Ethanol-inducible cytochrome P450 in rabbits metabolizes enflurane. Br J Anaesth 63:103-108, 1989.

65. Thummel KE, Kharasch ED, Podoll T, Kunze K: Human liver microsomal enflurane defluorination catalyzed by cytochrome P-450 2E1. Drug Metab Dispos 21:350-357, 1993.

66. Wrighton SA, Thomas PE, Molowa DT, et al: Characterization of ethanol-inducible human liver N-nitrosodimethylamine demethylase. Biochemistry 25:6731-6735, 1986.

67. Kharasch ED, Thummel KE: Identification of cytochrome P450 2E1 as the predominant enzyme catalyzing human liver microsomal defluorination of sevoflurane, isoflurane, and methoxyflurane. Anesthesiology 79:795-807, 1993.

68. Kharasch ED, Hankins DC, Cox K: Clinical isoflurane metabolism by cytochrome P450 2E1. Anesthesiology 90:766-771, 1999.

69. Hitt BA, Mazze RI: Effect of enzyme induction on nephrotoxicity of halothane-related compounds. Environ Health Perspect 21:179-183, 1977.

70. Mazze RI, Hitt BA, Cousins MJ: Effect of enzyme induction with phenobarbital on the in vivo and in vitro defluorination of isoflurane and methoxyflurane. J Pharmacol Exp Ther 190:523-529, 1974.

71. Caughey GH, Rice SA, Kosek JC, Mazze RI: Effect of phenytoin (DPH) treatment on methoxyflurane metabolism in rats. J Pharmacol Exp Ther 210:180-185, 1979.

72. Van Dyke RA: Enflurane, isoflurane, and methoxyflurane metabolism in rat hepatic microsomes from ethanol-treated animals. Anesthesiology 58:221-224, 1983.

73. Rice SA, Talcott RE: Effects of isoniazid treatment on selected hepatic mixed-function oxidases. Drug Metab Dispos 7:260-262, 1979.

74. Rice SA, Sbordone L, Mazze RI: Metabolism by rat hepatic microsomes of fluorinated ether anesthetics following isoniazid administration. Anesthesiology 53:489-493, 1980.

75. Holaday DA, Fiserova-Bergerova V, Latto IP, Zumbiel MA: Resistance of isoflurane to biotransformation in man. Anesthesiology 43:325-332, 1975.

76. Koblin DD, Eger EI, Johnson BH, et al: I-653 resists degradation in rats. Anesth Analg 67:534-538, 1988.

77. Sutton TS, Koblin DD, Gruenke LD, et al: Fluoride metabolites after prolonged exposure of volunteers and patients to desflurane. Anesth Analg 73:180-185, 1991.

78. Eger EI, Johnson BH, Strum DP, Ferrell LD: Studies of the toxicity of I-653, halothane, and isoflurane in enzyme-induced, hypoxic rats. Anesth Analg 66:1227-1229, 1987.

79. Cook TL, Beppu WJ, Hitt BA, et al: Renal effects and metabolism of sevoflurane in fisher 3444 rats: An in-vivo and in-vitro comparison with methoxyflurane. Anesthesiology 43:70-77, 1975.

80. Cook TL, Beppu WJ, Hitt BA, et al: A comparison of renal effects and metabolism of sevoflurane and methoxyflurane in enzyme-induced rats. Anesth Analg 54:829-835, 1975.

81. Holaday DA, Smith FR: Clinical characteristics and biotransformation of sevoflurane in healthy human volunteers. Anesthesiology 54:100-106, 1981.

82. Kharasch ED, Karol MD, Lanni C, Sawchuk R: Clinical sevoflurane metabolism and disposition. I. Sevoflurane and metabolite pharmacokinetics. Anesthesiology 82:1369-1378, 1995.

83. Kharasch ED, Armstrong AS, Gunn K, et al: Clinical sevoflurane metabolism and disposition. II. The role of cytochrome P450 2E1 in fluoride and hexafluoroisopropanol formation. Anesthesiology 82:1379-1388, 1995.

84. Baker MT, Ronnenberg WC Jr, Ruzicka JA, et al: Inhibitory effects of deuterium substitution on the metabolism of sevoflurane by the rat. Drug Metab Dispos 21:1170-1171, 1993.

85. Kikuchi H, Morio M, Fujii K, et al: Clinical evaluation and metabolism of sevoflurane in patients. Hiroshima J Med Sci 36:93-97, 1987.

86. Frink EJ Jr, Ghantous H, Malan TP, et al: Plasma inorganic fluoride with sevoflurane anesthesia: Correlation with indices of hepatic and renal function. Anesth Analg 74:231-235, 1992.

87. Rice SA, Sbordone L, Mazze RI: Metabolism by rat hepatic microsomes of fluorinated ether anesthetics following isoniazid administration. Anesthesiology 53:489-493, 1980.

88. Van Dyke RA: Enflurane, isoflurane, and methoxyflurane metabolism in rat hepatic microsomes from ethanol-treated animals. Anesthesiology 58:221-224, 1983.

89. Drayer DE: Pharmacodynamic and pharmacokinetic differences between drug enantiomers in humans: An overview. Clin Pharmacol Ther 40:125-133, 1986.

90. Tucker GT, Lennard MS: Enantiomer specific pharmacokinetics. Pharmacol Ther 45:309-329, 1990.

91. Brikett DJ: Racemates or enantiomers: Regulatory approaches. Clin Exp Pharmacol Physiol 16:479, 1989.

92. Ariens EJ, Testa B: Chiral aspects of drug metabolism. Trends Pharmacol 7:60, 1986.

93. Howard-Lock HE, Lock CJ, Mewa A, Kean WF: D-Penicillamine: Chemistry and clinical use in rheumatic disease. Semin Arthritis Rheum 15:261-281, 1986.

94. Satoh K, Yanagisawa T, Taira N: Coronary vasodilator and cardiac effects of optical isomers of verapamil in the dog. J Cardiovasc Pharmacol 2:309-318, 1980.

95. Powell JR, Ambre JJ, Rud TI: Drug stereochemistry. In Wainer IW, Drayer DE (eds): Analytical Methods and Pharmacology. New York, Dekker, 1988, p 245.

96. Buchinger W, Ober O, Uray G, et al: Synthesis and effects on peripheral thyroid hormone conversion of (R)-4-hydroxypropanolol, a main metabolite of (R)-propranolol. Chirality 3:145, 1991.

97. Grisslinger G, Hering W, Thomann P, et al: Pharmacokinetics and pharmacodynamics of ketamine enantiomers in surgical patients using a stereoselective analytical method. Br J Anaesth 70:666-671, 1993.

98. Kharasch ED, Labroo R: Metabolism of ketamine stereoisomers by human liver microsomes. Anesthesiology 77:1201-1207, 1992.

99. Brau ME, Branitzki P, Olschewski A, et al: Block of neuronal tetrodotoxin-resistant Na⁺ currents by stereoisomers of piperidine local anesthetics. Anesth Analg 91:1499-1505, 2000.

100. Blaschke G, Kraft HP, Fickentscher K, Kohler F: Chromatographic separation of racemic thalidomide and teratogenic activity of its enantiomers [author's transl]. Arzneimittelforschung 29:1640-1642, 1979.

101. Martin JL, Meinwald J, Radford P, et al: Stereoselective metabolism of halothane enantiomers to trifluoroacetylated liver proteins. Drug Metab Rev 27:179-189, 1995.

102. Kendig JJ, Trudell JR, Cohen EN: Halothane stereoisomers: Lack of stereospecificity in two model systems. Anesthesiology 39:518-524, 1973.

103. Lysko GS, Robinson JL, Casto R, Ferrone RA: The stereospecific effects of isoflurane isomers in vivo. Eur J Pharmacol 263:25-29, 1994.

104. Harris B, Moody E, Skolnick P: Isoflurane anesthesia is stereoselective. Eur J Pharmacol 217:215-216, 1992.

105. Moody EJ, Harris BD, Skolnick P: Stereospecific actions of the inhalation anesthetic isoflurane at the GABA$_A$ receptor complex. Brain Res 615:101-106, 1993.

106. Jones MV, Harrison NL: Effects of volatile anesthetics on the kinetics of inhibitory postsynaptic currents in cultured rat hippocampal neurons. J Neurophysiol 70:1339-1349, 1993.

107. Harris BD, Moody EJ, Basile AS, Skolnick P: Volatile anesthetics bidirectionally and stereospecifically modulate ligand binding to GABA receptors. Eur J Pharmacol 267:269-274, 1994.

108. Bunker JP, Blumenfeld CM: Liver necrosis after halothane anesthesia: Cause or coincidence? N Engl J Med 268:531-534, 1963.

109. Brody GL, Sweet RB: Halothane anesthesia as a possible cause of massive hepatic necrosis. Anesthesiology 24:29-37, 1963.

110. Gall EA: Report of the Pathology Panel: National Halothane Study. Anesthesiology 29:233-248, 1968.

111. Peters RL, Edmondson HA, Reynolds TB, et al: Hepatic necrosis associated with halothane anesthesia. Am J Med 47:748-764, 1969.

112. Subcommittee on the National Halothane Study of the Committee on Anesthesia, National Academy of Sciences: National Research Council Summary of the National Halothane Study: Possible association between halothane anesthesia and postoperative necrosis. JAMA 197:775, 1966.

113. Davis M, Eddleston AL, Neuberger JM, et al: Halothane hepatitis. N Engl J Med 303:1123-1124, 1980.

114. Van Pelt FN, Straub P, Manns MP: Molecular basis of drug-induced immunological liver injury. Semin Liver Dis 15:283-300, 1995.

115. Baker MT, Van Dyke RA: Hepatotoxicity of halogenated anesthetics. In Rice SA, Fish KJ (eds): Anesthetic Toxicity. New York, Raven Press, 1994, p 73.

116. Lewis JH, Zimmerman HJ, Ishak KG, Mullick FG: Enflurane hepatotoxicity: A clinicopathologic study of 24 cases. Ann Intern Med 98:984-992, 1983.

117. Carrigan TW, Straughen WJ: A report of hepatic necrosis and death following isoflurane anesthesia. Anesthesiology 67:581-583, 1987.

118. Sinha A, Clatch RJ, Stuck G, et al: Isoflurane hepatotoxicity: A case report and review of the literature. Am J Gastroenterol 91:2406-2409, 1996.

119. Martin JL, Plevak DJ, Flannery KD, et al: Hepatotoxicity after desflurane anesthesia. Anesthesiology 83:1125-1129, 1995.

120. Pohl LR, Satoh H, Christ DD, Kenna JG: The immunologic and metabolic basis of drug hypersensitivities. Annu Rev Pharmacol Toxicol 28:367-387, 1988.

121. Vergani D, Mieli-Vergani G, Alberti A, et al: Antibodies to the surface of halothane-altered rabbit hepatocytes in patients with severe halothane-associated hepatitis. N Engl J Med 303:66-71, 1980.

122. Pohl LR, Pumford NR, Martin JL: Mechanisms, chemical structures and drug metabolism. Eur J Haematol Suppl 60:98-104, 1996.

123. Kenna JG: Immunoallergic drug-induced hepatitis: Lessons from halothane. J Hepatol 26(Suppl 1):5-12, 1997.

124. Kenna JG, Satoh H, Christ DD, Pohl LR: Metabolic basis for a drug hypersensitivity: Antibodies in sera from patients with halothane hepatitis recognize liver neoantigens that contain the trifluoroacetyl group derived from halothane. J Pharmacol Exp Ther 245:1103-1109, 1988.

125. Martin JL, Pumford NR, LaRosa AC, et al: A metabolite of halothane covalently binds to an endoplasmic reticulum protein that is highly homologous to phosphatidylinositol-specific phospholipase C-alpha but has no activity. Biochem Biophys Res Commun 178:679-685, 1991.

126. Butler LE, Thomassen D, Martin JL, et al: The calcium-binding protein calreticulin is covalently modified in rat liver by a reactive metabolite of the inhalation anesthetic halothane. Chem Res Toxicol 5:406-410, 1992.

127. Martin JL, Reed GF, Pohl LR: Association of anti-58 kDa endoplasmic reticulum antibodies with halothane hepatitis. Biochem Pharmacol 46:1247-1250, 1993.

128. Martin JL, Kenna JG, Martin BM, et al: Halothane hepatitis patients have serum antibodies that react with protein disulfide isomerase. Hepatology 18:858-863, 1993.

129. Pumford NR, Martin BM, Thomassen D, et al: Serum antibodies from halothane hepatitis patients react with the rat endoplasmic reticulum protein ERp72. Chem Res Toxicol 6:609-615, 1993.

130. Bourdi M, Demady D, Martin JL, et al: CDNA cloning and baculovirus expression of the human liver endoplasmic reticulum P58: Characterization as a protein disulfide isomerase isoform, but not as a protease or a carnitine acyltransferase. Arch Biochem Biophys 323:397-403. 1995.

131. Pohl LR: An immunochemical approach of identifying and characterizing protein targets of toxic reactive metabolites. Chem Res Toxicol 6:786-793, 1993.

132. Gut J, Christen U, Huwyler J: Mechanisms of halothane toxicity: Novel insights. Pharmacol Ther 58:133-155, 1993.

133. Reves JG, McCracken LE Jr: Failure to induce hepatic pathology in animals sensitized to a halothane metabolite and subsequently challenged with halothane. Anesth Analg 55:235-242, 1976.

134. Neuberger JM, Kenna JG, Williams R: Halothane hepatitis: Attempt to develop an animal model. Int J Immunopharmacol 9:123-131, 1987.

135. Chen M, Gandolfi J: Characterization of the humoral immune response and hepatotoxicity after multiple halothane exposures in guinea pigs. Drug Metab Rev 29:103-122, 1997.

136. Lunam CA, Cousins MJ, Hall PD: Guinea-pig model of halothane-associated hepatotoxicity in the absence of enzyme induction and hypoxia. J Pharmacol Exp Ther 232:802-809, 1985.

137. Lind RC, Gandolfi AJ, Hall PD: Covalent binding of oxidative biotransformation intermediates is associated with halothane hepatotoxicity in guinea pigs. Anesthesiology 73:1208-1213, 1990.

138. Furst SM, Luedke D, Gaw HH, et al: Demonstration of a cellular immune response in halothane-exposed guinea pigs. Toxicol Appl Pharmacol 143:245-255, 1997.

139. Palucka K, Banchereau J: Dendritic cells: A link between innate and adaptive immunity. J Clin Immunol 19:12-25, 1999.

140. Bourdi M, Amouzadeh HR, Rushmore TH, et al: Halothane-induced liver injury in outbred guinea pigs: Role of trifluoroacetylated protein adducts in animal susceptibility. Chem Res Toxicol 14:362-370, 2001.

141. Neuberger JM, Kenna JG, Williams R: Halothane hepatitis: Attempt to develop an animal model. Int J Immunopharmacol 9:123-131, 1987.

142. Barton JDM: Jaundice and halothane. Lancet 1:1087, 1959.

143. Crowe GR: Halothane hepatitis in children. Med J Aust 1:794, 1977.

144. Campbell RL, Small EW, Lesesne HR, et al: Fatal hepatic necrosis after halothane anesthesia in a boy with juvenile rheumatoid arthritis: A case report. Anesth Analg 56:589-593, 1977.

145. Psacharopoulos HT, Mowat AP, Davies M, et al: Fulminant hepatic failure in childhood: An analysis of 31 cases. Arch Dis Child 55:252-258, 1980.

146. Smith RM: Anesthesia for Infants and Children, 4th ed. St. Louis, CV Mosby, 1980.

147. Lewis RB, Blair M: Halothane hepatitis in a young child. Br J Anaesth 54:349-354, 1982.

148. Wark HJ: Postoperative jaundice in children: The influence of halothane. Anaesthesia 38:237-242, 1983.

149. Warner LO, Beach TP, Garvin JP, Warner EJ: Halothane and children: The first quarter century. Anesth Analg 63:838-840, 1984.

150. Kenna JG, Neuberger J, Mieli-Vergani G, et al: Halothane hepatitis in children. Br Med J 294:1209-1211, 1987.

151. Barin F, Goudeau A, Denis F, et al: Immune response to hepatitis B vaccine. Lancet 1:251-253, 1982.

152. Njoku D, Laster MJ, Gong DH, et al: Biotransformation of halothane, enflurane, isoflurane, and desflurane to trifluoroacetylated liver proteins: Association between protein acylation and hepatic injury. Anesth Analg 84:173-178, 1997.

153. Eger EI, Smuckler EA, Ferrell LD, et al: Is enflurane hepatotoxic? Anesth Analg 65:21-30, 1986.

154. Sadove MS, Reis L, Askin SH, et al: Hepatitis after use of two different fluorinated anesthetic agents. Anesth Analg 53:336, 1974.

155. Sigurdsson J, Hreidarsson AB, Thjodleifsson B: Enflurane hepatitis: A report of a case with a previous history of halothane hepatitis. Acta Anaesthesiol Scand 29:495-496, 1985.

156. Christ DD, Kenna JG, Kammerer W, et al: Enflurane metabolism produces covalently bound liver adducts recognized by antibodies from patients with halothane hepatitis. Anesthesiology 69:833-838, 1988.

157. Stoelting RK, Blitt CD, Cohen PJ, Merin RG: Hepatic dysfunction after isoflurane anesthesia. Anesth Analg 66:147-153, 1987.

158. Brunt EM, White H, Marsh JW, et al: Fulminant hepatic failure after repeated exposure to isoflurane anesthesia: A case report. Hepatology 13:1017-1021, 1991.

159. Turner GB, O'Rourke D, Scott GO, Beringer TR: Fatal hepatotoxicity after re-exposure to isoflurane: A case report and review of the literature. Eur J Gastroenterol Hepatol 12:955-959, 2000.

160. Njoku DB, Shrestha S, Soloway R, et al: Subcellular localization of trifluoroacetylated liver proteins in association with hepatitis following isoflurane. Anesthesiology 96:757-761, 2002.

161. Jones RM, Koblin DD, Cashman JN, et al: Biotransformation and hepato-renal function in volunteers after exposure to desflurane (I-653). Br J Anaesth 64:482-487, 1990.

162. Wrigley SR, Fairfield JE, Jones RM, Black AE: Induction and recovery characteristics of desflurane in day case patients: A comparison with propofol. Anaesthesia 46:615-622, 1991.

163. Berghaus TM, Baron A, Geier A, et al: Hepatotoxicity following desflurane anesthesia. Hepatology 29:613-614, 1999.

164. Molina DM, Rowland FS: Stratospheric sink for chlorofluoromethanes: Chlorine atom–catalyzed destruction of ozone. Nature 249:810-812, 1974.

165. U.S. Environmental Protection Agency: Report no 53. Federal Register, 1988.

166. Harris JW, Pohl LR, Martin JL, Anders MW: Tissue acylation by the chlorofluorocarbon substitute 2,2-dichloro-1,1,1-trifluoroethane. Proc Natl Acad Sci U S A 88:1407-1410, 1991.

167. Lind RC, Gandolfi AJ, Hall PM: Biotransformation and hepatotoxicity of HCFC-123 in the guinea pig: Potentiation of hepatic injury by prior glutathione depletion. Toxicol Appl Pharmacol 134:175-181, 1995.

168. Rusch GM, Trochimowicz HJ, Malley LJ, et al: Subchronic inhalation toxicity studies with hydrochlorofluorocarbon 123 (HCFC 123). Fundam Appl Toxicol 23:169-178, 1994.

169. Dekant W: Toxicology of chlorofluorocarbon replacements. Environ Health Perspect 104(Suppl 1):75-83, 1996.

170. Hoet P, Graf ML, Bourdi M, et al: Epidemic of liver disease caused by hydrochlorofluorocarbons used as ozone-sparing substitutes of chlorofluorocarbons. Lancet 350:556-559, 1997.

171. Watanabe K, Hatakenaka S, Ikemune K, et al: [A case of suspected liver dysfunction induced by sevoflurane anesthesia.] Masui 42:902-905, 1993.

172. Shichinohe Y, Masuda Y, Takahashi H, et al: [A case of postoperative hepatic injury after sevoflurane anesthesia.] Masui 41:1802-1805, 1992.

173. Bruun LS, Elkjaer S, Bitsch-Larsen D, Andersen O: Hepatic failure in a child after acetaminophen and sevoflurane exposure. Anesth Analg 92:1446-1448, 2001.

174. Frink EJ Jr, Ghantous H, Malan TP, et al: Plasma inorganic fluoride with sevoflurane anesthesia: Correlation with indices of hepatic and renal function. Anesth Analg 74:231-235, 1992.

175. Ray DC, Bomont R, Mizushima A, et al: Effect of sevoflurane anaesthesia on plasma concentrations of glutathione S-transferase. Br J Anaesth 77:404-407, 1996.

176. Taivainen T, Tiainen P, Meretoja OA, et al: Comparison of the effects of sevoflurane and halothane on the quality of anaesthesia and serum glutathione transferase alpha and fluoride in paediatric patients. Br J Anaesth 73:590-595, 1994.

177. Hussey AJ, Aldridge LM, Paul D, et al: Plasma glutathione S-transferase concentration as a measure of hepatocellular integrity following a single general anaesthetic with halothane, enflurane or isoflurane. Br J Anaesth 60:130-135, 1988.

178. Allan LG, Hussey AJ, Howie J, et al: Hepatic glutathione S-transferase release after halothane anaesthesia: Open randomised comparison with isoflurane. Lancet 1:771-774, 1987.

179. Tsujimoto S, Kato H, Minamoto Y, et al: Comparison of postoperative liver dysfunction after halothane and sevoflurane anesthesia in women undergoing mastectomy for cancer. J Anesth 9:129-34, 1995.

180. Lynch S, Martis L, Woods E: Evaluation of hepatoxic potential of sevoflurane in rats. Pharmacologist 21:221, 1979.

181. Joshi PH, Conn HO: The syndrome of methoxyflurane-associated hepatitis. Ann Intern Med 80:395-401, 1974.

182. Martin JL: Halothane hepatitis: A possible immune-mediated hepatitis. In Newcombe DS, Rose NR, Bloom JC (eds): Halothane Hepatitis: A Possible Immune Mediated Hepatitis. New York, Raven Press, 1992, pp 155-175.

183. Bottiger LE, Dalen E, Hallen B: Halothane-induced liver damage: An analysis of the material reported to the Swedish Adverse Drug Reaction Committee, 1966-1973. Acta Anaesthesiol Scand 20:40-46, 1976.
184. Walton B, Simpson BR, Strunin L, et al: Unexplained hepatitis following halothane. Br Med J 1:1171-1176, 1976.
185. Takagi T, Ishii H, Takahashi H, et al: Potentiation of halothane hepatotoxicity by chronic ethanol administration in rat: An animal model of halothane hepatitis. Pharmacol Biochem Behav 18(Suppl 1):461-465, 1983.
186. Ryan DE, Koop DR, Thomas PE, et al: Evidence that isoniazid and ethanol induce the same microsomal cytochrome P-450 in rat liver, an isozyme homologous to rabbit liver cytochrome P-450 isozyme 3a. Arch Biochem Biophys 246:633-644, 1986.
187. Thomas PE, Bandiera S, Maines SL, et al: Regulation of cytochrome P-450j, a high-affinity N-nitrosodimethylamine demethylase, in rat hepatic microsomes. Biochemistry 26:2280-2289, 1997.
188. Gruenke LD, Konopka K, Koop DR, Waskell LA: Characterization of halothane oxidation by hepatic microsomes and purified cytochromes P-450 using a gas chromatographic mass spectrometric assay. J Pharmacol Exp Ther 246:454-459, 1988.
189. Carey RMT, Van Dyke RA: Halothane hepatitis: A critical review. Anesth Analg 51:135-160, 1972.
190. Nimmo WS, Thompson PG, Prescott LF: Microsomal enzyme induction after halothane anaesthesia. Br J Clin Pharmacol 12:433-434, 1981.
191. Cohen EN, Hood N: Application of low-temperature autoradiography to studies of the uptake and metabolism of volatile anesthetics in the mouse. 3. Halothane. Anesthesiology 31:553-559, 1969.
192. Cohen EN: Metabolism of the volatile anesthetics. Anesthesiology 35:193-202, 1971.
193. Cascorbi HF, Vesell ES, Blake DA, Helrich M: Halothane biotransformation in man. Ann N Y Acad Sci 179:244-248, 1971.
194. Plummer JL, Steven IM, Cousins MJ: Metabolism of halothane in children having repeated halothane anaesthetics. Anaesth Intensive Care 15:136-140, 1987.
195. Stenger RJ, Johnson EA: Effects of phenobarbital pretreatment on the response of rat liver to halothane administration. Proc Soc Exp Biol Med 140:1319-1324, 1972.
196. Hoft RH, Bunker JP, Goodman HI, Gregory PB: Halothane hepatitis in three pairs of closely related women. N Engl J Med 304:1023-1024, 1981.
197. Farrell G, Prendergast D, Murray M: Halothane hepatitis. Detection of a constitutional susceptibility factor. N Engl J Med 313:1310-1314, 1985.
198. Carney FM, Van Dyke RA: Halothane hepatitis: A critical review. Anesth Analg 51:135-160, 1972.
199. Inman WH, Mushin WW: Jaundice after repeated exposure to halothane: An analysis of reports to the committee on safety of medicines. Br Med J 1:5-10, 1974.
200. Cousins MJ, Plummer JL, Hall PD: Risk factors for halothane hepatitis. Aust N Z J Surg 59:5-14, 1989.
201. Peters RL, Edmondson HA, Reynolds TB, et al: Hepatic necrosis associated with halothane anesthesia. Am J Med 47:748-764, 1969.
202. Kenna JG, Neuberger J, Williams R: An enzyme-linked immunosorbent assay for detection of antibodies against halothane-altered hepatocyte antigens. J Immunol Methods 75:3-14, 1984.
203. Kenna JG, Neuberger J, Williams R: Specific antibodies to halothane-induced liver antigens in halothane-associated hepatitis. Br J Anaesth 59:1286-1290, 1987.
204. Nomura F, Hatano H, Ohnishi K, et al: Effects of anticonvulsant drugs on halothane-induced liver injury in human subjects and experimental animals. Hepatology 6:952-956, 1986.
205. Hubbard AK, Roth TP, Gandolfi AJ, et al: Halothane hepatitis patients generate an antibody response toward a covalently bound metabolite of halothane. Anesthesiology 68:791-796, 1988.
206. Martin JL, Kenna JG, Pohl LR: Antibody assays for the detection of patients sensitized to halothane. Anesth Analg 70:154-159, 1990.
207. Satoh H, Gillette JR, Takemura T, et al: Investigation of the immunological basis of halothane-induced hepatotoxicity. In Kocsis JI, Jollow DJ, Witmer CM, et al (eds): Biological Reactive Intermediates. New York, Plenum, 1988, pp. 657-673.
208. Crandell WB, Pappas SG, Macdonald A: Nephrotoxicity associated with methoxyflurane anesthesia. Anesthesiology 27:591-607, 1969.
209. Mazze RI, Shue GL, Jackson SH: Renal dysfunction associated with methoxyflurane anesthesia. A randomized, prospective clinical evaluation. JAMA 216:278-288, 1971.
210. Mazze RI, Cousins MJ, Kosek JC: Dose-related methoxyflurane nephrotoxicity in rats: A biochemical and pathologic correlation. Anesthesiology 36:571-587, 1972.
211. Njoku DB: Effects of halogenated inhalation agents on the liver and kidneys. Probl Anesth Curr Issues Pediatr Anesth 10:478-487, 2000.
212. Whitford GM, Taves DR: Fluoride-induced diuresis: Renal-tissue solute concentrations, functional, hemodynamic, and histologic correlates in the rat. Anesthesiology 39:416-427, 1973.
213. Kharasch ED, Hankins DC, Thummel KE: Human kidney methoxyflurane and sevoflurane metabolism. Intrarenal fluoride production as a possible mechanism of methoxyflurane nephrotoxicity. Anesthesiology 82:689-699, 1995.
214. Cousins MJ, Mazze RI, Kosek JC, et al: The etiology of methoxyflurane nephrotoxicity. J Pharmacol Exp Ther 190:530-541, 1974.
215. Smith FA (ed): Handbook of Experimental Pharmacology. Pharmacology of Fluorides. New York, Springer-Verlag, 1970.
216. Van Dyke RA: Enflurane, isoflurane, and methoxyflurane metabolism in rat hepatic microsomes from ethanol-treated animals. Anesthesiology 58:221-224, 1983.
217. Rice SA, Dooley JR, Mazze RI: Metabolism by rat hepatic microsomes of fluorinated ether anesthetics following ethanol consumption. Anesthesiology 58:237-241, 1983.
218. Biermann JS, Rice SA, Gallagher EJ, West JA: Effect of diazepam treatment on hepatic microsomal anesthetic defluorinase activity. Arch Intern Pharmacodyn Ther 283:181-192, 1986.
219. Mazze RI, Cousins MJ: Combined nephrotoxicity of gentamicin and methoxyflurane anaesthesia in man. A case report. Br J Anaesth 45:394-398, 1973.
220. Barr GA, Mazze RI, Cousins MJ, Kosek JC: An animal model for combined methoxyflurane and gentamicin nephrotoxicity. Br J Anaesth 45:306-312, 1973.
221. Cousins MJ, Greenstein LR, Hitt BA, Mazze RI: Metabolism and renal effects of enflurane in man. Anesthesiology 44:44-53, 1976.
222. Mazze RI, Sievenpiper TS, Stevenson J: Renal effects of enflurane and halothane in patients with abnormal renal function. Anesthesiology 60:161-163, 1984.
223. Mazze RI, Calverley RK, Smith NT: Inorganic fluoride nephrotoxicity: Prolonged enflurane and halothane anesthesia in volunteers. Anesthesiology 46:265-271, 1977.
224. Sievenpiper TS, Rice SA, McClendon F, et al: Renal effects of enflurane anesthesia in Fischer 344 rats with pre-existing renal insufficiency. J Pharmacol Exp Ther 211:36-41, 1979.
225. Fish K, Sievenpiper T, Rice SA, et al: Renal function in Fischer 344 rats with chronic renal impairment after administration of enflurane and gentamicin. Anesthesiology 53:481-488, 1980.
226. Bentley JB, Vaughan RW, Miller MS, et al: Serum inorganic fluoride levels in obese patients during and after enflurane anesthesia. Anesth Analg 58:409-412, 1979.
227. Rice SA, Fish KJ: Anesthetic metabolism and renal function in obese and nonobese Fischer 344 rats following enflurane or isoflurane anesthesia. Anesthesiology 65:28-34, 1986.
228. Rice SA, Sbordone L, Mazze RI: Metabolism by rat hepatic microsomes of fluorinated ether anesthetics following isoniazid administration. Anesthesiology 53:489-493, 1980.

229. Mazze RI, Woodruff RE, Heerdt ME: Isoniazid-induced enflurane defluorination in humans. Anesthesiology 57:5-8, 1982.

230. Cousins MJ, Mazze RI: Methoxyflurane nephrotoxicity: A study of dose response in man. JAMA 225:1611, 1973.

231. Murray JM, Trinick TR: Plasma fluoride concentrations during and after prolonged anesthesia: A comparison of halothane and enflurane. Anesth Analg 74:236-240, 1992.

232. Mazze RI, Cousins MJ, Barr GA: Renal effects and metabolism of isoflurane in man. Anesthesiology 40:536, 1974.

233. Arnold JH, Truog RD, Rice SA: Prolonged administration of isoflurane to pediatric patients during mechanical ventilation. Anesth Analg 76:520-526, 1993.

234. Nuscheler M, Conzen P, Peter K: Sevoflurane: Metabolism and toxicity. Anaesthesist 47(Suppl 1):S24-S32, 1998.

235. Kobayashi Y, Ochiai R, Takeda J, et al: Serum and urinary inorganic fluoride concentrations after prolonged inhalation of sevoflurane in humans. Anesth Analg 74:753-757, 1992.

236. Rice SA, Sbordone L, Mazze RI: Metabolism by rat hepatic microsomes of fluorinated ether anesthetics following isoniazid administration. Anesthesiology 53:489-493, 1980.

237. Truog RD, Rice SA: Inorganic fluoride and prolonged isoflurane anesthesia in the intensive care unit. Anesth Analg 69:843, 1989.

238. Hara T, Fukusaki M, Nakamura T, Sumikawa K: Renal function in patients during and after hypotensive anesthesia with sevoflurane. J Clin Anesth 10:539-545, 1998.

239. Frink EJ, Malan TP, Isner J, et al: Renal concentrating function with prolonged sevoflurane or enflurane anesthesia in volunteers. Anesthesiology 80:1019, 1994.

240. Higuchi H, Arimura S, Sumikura H, et al: Urine concentrating ability after prolonged sevoflurane anesthesia. Br J Anaesth 73:239-240, 1994.

241. Groudine SB, Fragen RJ, Kharasch ED, et al: Comparison of renal function following anesthesia with low-flow sevoflurane and isoflurane. J Clin Anesth 11:201-207, 1999.

242. Bito H, Ikeda K: Long-duration, low-flow sevoflurane anesthesia using two carbon dioxide absorbents: Quantification of degradation products in the circuit. Anesthesiology 81:340-345, 1994.

243. Artu AA: Renal effects of sevoflurane during conditions of possible increased risk. J Clin Anesth 10:531-538, 1998.

244. Avery T, Jacobsohn E: A case of nonoliguric renal failure after general anesthesia with sevoflurane and desflurane. Anesth Analg 85:1407-1409, 1997.

245. Mori N, Nagata H, Ohta S, Suzuki M: Prolonged sevoflurane inhalation was not nephrotoxic in two patients with refractory status asthmaticus. Anesth Analg 83:189-191, 1996.

246. Conzen PF, Nuscheler M, Melotte A, et al: Renal function and serum fluoride concentrations in patients with stable renal insufficiency after anesthesia with sevoflurane or enflurane. Anesth Analg 81:569-575, 1995.

247. Tsukamoto N, Hirabayashi Y, Shimizu R, Mitsuhata H: The effects of sevoflurane and isoflurane anesthesia on renal tubular function in patients with moderately impaired renal function. Anesth Analg 82:909-913, 1996.

248. Morita K, Otsuka F, Ogura T, et al: Sevoflurane anaesthesia causes a transient decrease in aquaporin-2 and impairment of urine concentration. Br J Anaesth 83:734-739, 1999.

249. Smiley RM, Ornstein E, Pantuck EJ, et al: Metabolism of desflurane and isoflurane to fluoride ion in surgical patients. Can J Anaesth 38:965-968, 1991.

250. Bito H, Ikeda K: Closed-circuit anesthesia with sevoflurane in humans: Effects on renal and hepatic function and concentrations of breakdown products with soda lime in the circuit. Anesthesiology 80:71-76, 1994.

251. Cunningham DD, Huang S, Webster J, et al: Sevoflurane degradation to compound A in anaesthesia breathing systems. Br J Anaesth 77:537-543, 1996.

252. Bito H, Ikeda K: Degradation products of sevoflurane during low-flow anaesthesia. Br J Anaesth 74:56-59, 1995.

253. Gonoswski BS, Laster MJ, Eger EI, et al: Toxicity of compound A in rats. Anesthesiology 80:550-565, 1994.

254. Keller KA, Callan C, Prokocimer P, et al: Inhalation toxicity study of a haloalkene degradant of sevoflurane, compound A (PIFE), in Sprague-Dawley rats. Anesthesiology 83:1220-1232, 1995.

255. Gonoswski BS, Laster MJ, Eger EI, et al: Toxicity of compound A in rats. Anesthesiology 80:566-573, 1994.

256. Bito H, Ikeda K: Plasma inorganic fluoride and intracircuit degradation product concentrations in long-duration, low-flow sevoflurane anesthesia. Anesth Analg 79:946-951, 1994.

257. Frink EJ Jr, Isner RJ, Malan TP Jr, et al: Sevoflurane degradation product concentrations with soda lime during prolonged anesthesia. J Clin Anesth 6:239-242, 1994.

258. Bito H, Ikeda K: Renal and hepatic function in surgical patients after low-flow sevoflurane or isoflurane anesthesia. Anesth Analg 82:173-176, 1996.

259. Mazze RI, Callan CM, Galvez ST, et al: The effects of sevoflurane on serum creatinine and blood urea nitrogen concentrations: A retrospective, twenty-two-center, comparative evaluation of renal function in adult surgical patients. Anesth Analg 90:683-688, 2000.

260. Kharasch ED, Frink EJ Jr, Artru A, et al: Long-duration low-flow sevoflurane and isoflurane effects on postoperative renal and hepatic function. Anesth Analg 93:1511-1520, 2001.

261. Mazze RI, Jamison RL: Low-flow (1 L/min) sevoflurane: Is it safe? Anesthesiology 86:1225-1227, 1997.

262. Kumano H, Osaka S, Ishimura N, Nishiwada M: [Effects of enflurane, isoflurane, and sevoflurane on renal tubular functions.] Masui 41:1735-1740, 1992.

263. Bito H, Ikeuchi Y, Ikeda K: Effects of low-flow sevoflurane anesthesia on renal function: Comparison with high-flow sevoflurane anesthesia and low-flow isoflurane anesthesia. Anesthesiology 86:1231-1237, 1997.

264. Kharasch ED, Frink EJ Jr, Zager R, et al: Assessment of low-flow sevoflurane and isoflurane effects on renal function using sensitive markers of tubular toxicity. Anesthesiology 86:1238-1253, 1997.

265. Nishiyama T, Hanaoka K: Inorganic fluoride kinetics and renal and hepatic function after repeated sevoflurane anesthesia. Anesth Analg 87:468-473, 1998.

266. Eger EI, Koblin DD, Bowland T, et al: Nephrotoxicity of sevoflurane versus desflurane anesthesia in volunteers. Anesth Analg 84:160-168, 1997.

267. Ebert TJ, Frink EJ Jr, Kharasch ED: Absence of biochemical evidence for renal and hepatic dysfunction after 8 hours of 1.25 minimum alveolar concentration sevoflurane anesthesia in volunteers. Anesthesiology 88:601-610, 1998.

268. Goldberg ME, Cantillo J, Gratz I, et al: Dose of compound A, not sevoflurane, determines changes in the biochemical markers of renal injury in healthy volunteers. Anesth Analg 88:437-445, 1999.

269. Higuchi H, Wada H, Usui Y, et al: Effects of probenecid on renal function in surgical patients anesthetized with low-flow sevoflurane. Anesthesiology 94:21-31, 2001.

270. Higuchi H, Sumita S, Wada H, et al: Effects of sevoflurane and isoflurane on renal function and on possible markers of nephrotoxicity. Anesthesiology 89:307-322, 1998.

271. Eger EI, Gong D, Koblin DD, et al: Dose-related biochemical markers of renal injury after sevoflurane versus desflurane anesthesia in volunteers. Anesth Analg 85:1154-1163, 1997.

272. Ebert TJ, Messana LD, Uhrich TD, Staacke TS: Absence of renal and hepatic toxicity after four hours of 1.25 minimum alveolar anesthetic concentration sevoflurane anesthesia in volunteers. Anesth Analg 86:662-667, 1998.

273. Levine MF, Sarner J, Lerman J, et al: Plasma inorganic fluoride concentrations after sevoflurane anesthesia in children. Anesthesiology 84:348-353, 1996.

274. Frink EJ Jr, Green WB Jr, Brown EA, et al: Compound A concentrations during sevoflurane anesthesia in children. Anesthesiology 84:566-571, 1996.

275. Payne AK, Morgan SE, Gandolfi AJ, Brendel K: Biotransformation of sevoflurane by rat neonate liver slices. Drug Metab Dispos 23:497-500, 1995.

276. Iyer RA, Anders MW: Cysteine conjugate beta-lyase-dependent biotransformation of the cysteine S-conjugates of the sevoflurane degradation product compound A in

human, nonhuman primate, and rat kidney cytosol and mitochondria. Anesthesiology 85:1454-1461, 1996.

277. Spracklin DK, Kharasch ED: Evidence for metabolism of fluoromethyl 2,2-difluoro-1-(trifluoromethyl)vinyl ether (compound A), a sevoflurane degradation product, by cysteine conjugate beta-lyase. Chem Res Toxicol 9:696-702, 1996.

278. Jin L, Baillie TA, Davis MR, Kharasch ED: Nephrotoxicity of sevoflurane compound A [fluoromethyl-2,2-difluoro-1-(trifluoromethyl)vinyl ether] in rats: Evidence for glutathione and cysteine conjugate formation and the role of renal cysteine conjugate beta-lyase. Biochem Biophys Res Commun 210:498-506, 1995.

279. Jin L, Davis MR, Kharasch ED, et al: Identification in rat bile of glutathione conjugates of fluoromethyl-2,2-difluoro-1-(trifluoromethyl)vinyl ether, a nephrotoxic degradate of the anesthetic agent sevoflurane. Chem Res Toxicol 9:555-561, 1996.

280. Commandeur JN, Oostendorp RA, Schoofs PR, et al: Nephrotoxicity and hepatotoxicity of 1,1-dichloro-2,2-difluoroethylene in the rat. Indications for differential mechanisms of bioactivation. Biochem Pharmacol 36:4229-4237, 1987.

281. Vamvakas S, Kremling E, Dekant W: Metabolic activation of the nephrotoxic haloalkene 1,1,2-trichloro-3,3,3-trifluoro-1-propene by glutathione conjugation. Biochem Pharmacol 38:2297-2304, 1989.

282. Green T, Odum J, Nash JA, Foster JR: Perchloroethylene-induced rat kidney tumors: An investigation of the mechanisms involved and their relevance to humans. Toxicol Appl Pharmacol 103:77-89, 1990.

283. Iyer RA, Frink EJ Jr, Ebert TJ, Anders MW: Cysteine conjugate beta-lyase-dependent metabolism of compound A (2-[fluoromethoxy]-1,1,3,3,3-pentafluoro-1-propene) in human subjects anesthetized with sevoflurane and in rats given compound A. Anesthesiology 88:611-618, 1998.

284. Iyer RA, Baggs RB, Anders MW: Nephrotoxicity of the glutathione and cysteine S-conjugates of the sevoflurane degradation product 2-(fluoromethoxy)-1,1,3,3,3-pentafluoro-1-propene (compound A) in male Fischer 344 rats. J Pharmacol Exp Ther 283:1544-1551, 1997.

285. Kharasch ED, Thorning D, Garton K, et al: Role of renal cysteine conjugate beta-lyase in the mechanism of compound A nephrotoxicity in rats. Anesthesiology 86:160-171, 1997.

286. Martin JL, Laster MJ, Kandel L, et al: Metabolism of compound A by renal cysteine-S-conjugate beta-lyase is not the mechanism of compound A-induced renal injury in the rat. Anesth Analg 82:770-774, 1996.

287. Kharasch ED, Hoffman GM, Thorning D, et al: Role of cysteine conjugate β-lyase pathway in inhaled compound A nephrotoxicity in rats. Anesthesiology 88:1624-1633, 1998.

288. Higuchi H, Adachi Y, Wada H, et al: The effects of low-flow sevoflurane and isoflurane anesthesia on renal function in patients with stable moderate renal insufficiency. Anesth Analg 92:650-655, 2001.

289. Conzen PF, Kharasch ED, Czerner SF, et al: Low-flow sevoflurane compared with low-flow isoflurane anesthesia in patients with stable renal insufficiency. Anesthesiology 97:578-584, 2002.

290. Eger EI, Ionescu P, Laster MJ, et al: Quantitative differences in the production and toxicity of $CF_2=BrCl$ versus $CH_2F-O-C(=CF_2)(FC_3)$ (compound A): The safety of halothane does not indicate the safety of sevoflurane. Anesth Analg 85:1164-1170, 1997.

291. Moon RE: Cause of CO poisoning, relation to halogenated agents still not clear. J Clin Monit 11:67-71, 1995.

292. Woehlck HJ, Dunning M III, Connolly LA: Reduction in the incidence of carbon monoxide exposures in humans undergoing general anesthesia. Anesthesiology 87:228-234, 1997.

293. Berry PD, Sessler DI, Larson MD: Severe carbon monoxide poisoning during desflurane anesthesia. Anesthesiology 90:613-616, 1999.

294. Lentz RE: Carbon monoxide poisoning during anesthesia poses puzzles. J Clin Monit 11:66-67, 1995.

295. Baum J, Sachs G, vd Driesch C, Stanke HG: Carbon monoxide generation in carbon dioxide absorbents. Anesth Analg 81:144-146, 1995.

296. Davies MW, Potter FA: Carbon monoxide, soda lime and volatile agents. Anaesthesia 51:90, 1996.

297. Strum DP, Eger EI: The degradation, absorption, and solubility of volatile anesthetics in soda lime depend on water content. Anesth Analg 78:340-348, 1994.

298. Wissing H, Kuhn I, Warnken U, Dudziak R: Carbon monoxide production from desflurane, enflurane, halothane, isoflurane, and sevoflurane with dry soda lime. Anesthesiology 95:1205-1212, 2001.

299. Baxter PJ, Garton K, Kharasch ED: Mechanistic aspects of carbon monoxide formation from volatile anesthetics. Anesthesiology 89:929-941, 1998.

300. Stabernack CR, Brown R, Laster MJ, et al: Absorbents differ enormously in their capacity to produce compound A and carbon monoxide. Anesth Analg 90:1428-1435, 2000.

301. Murray JM, Renfrew CW, Bedi A, et al: Amsorb: A new carbon dioxide absorbent for use in anesthetic breathing systems. Anesthesiology 91:1342-1348, 1999.

302. O'Sullivan H, Jennings F, Ward K, et al: Human bone marrow biochemical function and megaloblastic hematopoiesis after nitrous oxide anesthesia. Anesthesiology 55:645-649, 1981.

303. Lassen HC, Henriksen E, Neukirch F, Kristensen HS: Treatment of tetanus; severe bone-marrow depression after prolonged nitrous-oxide anaesthesia. Lancet 270:527-530, 1956.

304. Amos RJ, Amess JA, Hinds CJ, Mollin DL: Incidence and pathogenesis of acute megaloblastic bone-marrow change in patients receiving intensive care. Lancet 2:835-838, 1982.

305. Layzer RB: Myeloneuropathy after prolonged exposure to nitrous oxide. Lancet 2:1227-1230, 1978.

306. Sweeney B, Bingham RM, Amos RJ, et al: Toxicity of bone marrow in dentists exposed to nitrous oxide. Br Med J 291:567-569, 1985.

307. Brodsky JB, Cohen EN, Brown BW Jr, et al: Exposure to nitrous oxide and neurologic disease among dental professionals. Anesth Analg 60:297-301, 1981.

308. Royston BD, Nunn JF, Weinbren HK, et al: Rate of inactivation of human and rodent hepatic methionine synthase by nitrous oxide. Anesthesiology 68:213, 1988.

309. Sharer NM, Nunn JF, Royston JP, et al: Effects of chronic exposure to nitrous oxide on methionine synthase activity. Br J Anaesth 5:693, 1983.

310. National Institute for Occupational Safety and Health (NOISH). Criteria for a recommended standard for occupation exposure to waste anesthetic gases and vapors. NIOSH publ no 77-140. Washington, DC, NOISH, 1977.

311. Smith BE: Fetal prognosis after anesthesia during gestation. Anesth Analg 42:521-526, 1963.

312. Shnider SM, Webster GM: Maternal and fetal hazards of surgery during pregnancy. Am J Obstet Gynecol 92:891, 1965.

313. Brodsky JB, Cohen EN, Brown BW Jr, et al: Surgery during pregnancy and fetal outcome. Am J Obstet Gynecol 138:1165-1167, 1980.

314. Aldridge LM, Tunstall ME: Nitrous oxide and the fetus: A review and the results of a retrospective study of 175 cases of anaesthesia for insertion of Shirodkar suture. Br J Anaesth 58:1348-1356, 1986.

315. Crawford JS, Lewis M: Nitrous oxide in early human pregnancy. Anaesthesia 41:900-905, 1986.

316. Duncan PG, Pope WDB, Cohen MM, et al: Fetal risk of anesthesia and surgery during pregnancy. Anesthesiology 64:790, 1986.

317. Mazze RI, Kallen B: Reproductive outcome after anesthesia and operation during pregnancy: A registry study of 5405 cases. Am J Obstet Gynecol 161:1178-1185, 1989.

318. Hayes MF, Sacco AG, Savoy-Moore RT, et al: Effect of general anesthesia on fertilization and cleavage of human oocytes in vitro. Fertil Steril 48:975-981, 1987.

319. Critchlow BM, Ibrahim Z, Pollard BJ: General anaesthesia for gamete intra-fallopian transfer. Eur J Anaesthesiol 8:381-384, 1991.
320. Rosen MA, Roizen MF, Eger EI, et al: The effect of nitrous oxide on in vitro fertilization success rate. Anesthesiology 67:42-44, 1987.
321. Gonen O, Shulman A, Ghetler Y, et al: The impact of different types of anesthesia on in vitro fertilization-embryo transfer treatment outcome. J Assist Reprod Genet 12:678-682, 1995.
322. Rice SA: Reproductive and developmental toxicity of anesthetics in animals. *In* Rice SA, Fish KJ (eds): Anesthetic Toxicity. New York, Raven Press, 1994, p 157.
323. Wyrobek AJ, Brodsky J, Gordon L, et al: Sperm studies in anesthesiologists. Anesthesiology 55:527-532, 1981.
324. Askrog V, Harvald B: Teratogenic effects of inhalation anesthetics. Nord Med 83:498, 1970.
325. Cohen EN, Bellville JW, Brown BW Jr: Anesthesia, pregnancy, and miscarriage: A study of operating room nurses and anesthetists. Anesthesiology 35:343-347, 1971.
326. Knill-Jones RP, Rodrigues LV, Moir DD, Spence AA: Anaesthetic practice and pregnancy: Controlled survey of women anaesthetists in the United Kingdom. Lancet 1:1326-1328, 1972.
327. Rosenberg P, Kirves A: Miscarriages among operating theatre staff. Acta Anaesthesiol Scand Suppl 53:37-42, 1973.
328. Corbett TH, Cornell RG, Endres JL, Lieding K: Birth defects among children of nurse-anesthetists. Anesthesiology 41:341-344, 1974.
329. Occupational disease among operating room personnel: A national study. Report of an Ad Hoc Committee on the Effect of Trace Anesthetics on the Health of Operating Room Personnel, American Society of Anesthesiologists. Anesthesiology 41:321-340, 1974.
330. Cohen EN, Brown BW Jr, Bruce DL, et al: A survey of anesthetic health hazards among dentists. J Am Dent Assoc 90:1291-1296, 1975.
331. Knill-Jones RP, Newman BJ, Spence AA: Anesthetic practice and pregnancy. Controlled survey of male anaesthetists in the United Kingdom. Lancet 2:807-809, 1975.
332. Pharoah PO, Alberman E, Doyle P, Chamberlain G: Outcome of pregnancy among women in anaesthetic practice. Lancet 1:34-36, 1977.
333. Rosenberg PH, Vanttinen H: Occupational hazards to reproduction and health in anaesthetists and paediatricians. Acta Anaesthesiol Scand 22:202-207, 1978.
334. Ericson A, Kallen B: Survey of infants born in 1973 or 1975 to Swedish women working in operating rooms during their pregnancies. Anesth Analg 58:302-305, 1979.
335. Tomlin PJ: Health problems of anaesthetists and their families in the West Midlands. Br Med J 1:779-784, 1979.
336. Cohen EN, Gift HC, Brown BW, et al: Occupational disease in dentistry and chronic exposure to trace anesthetic gases. J Am Dent Assoc 101:21-31, 1980.
337. Lauwerys R, Siddons M, Misson CB, et al: Anaesthetic health hazards among Belgian nurses and physicians. Int Arch Occup Environ Health 48:195-203, 1981.
338. Axelsson G, Rylander R: Exposure to anaesthetic gases and spontaneous abortion: Response bias in a postal questionnaire study. Int J Epidemiol 11:250-256, 1982.
339. Hemminki K, Kyyronen P, Lindbohm ML: Spontaneous abortions and malformations in the offspring of nurses exposed to anaesthetic gases, cytostatic drugs, and other potential hazards in hospitals, based on registered information of outcome. J Epidemiol Commun Health 39:141-147, 1985.
340. Johnson JA, Buchan RM, Reif JS: Effect of waste anesthetic gas and vapor exposure on reproductive outcome in veterinary personnel. Am Ind Hyg Assoc J 48:62-66, 1987.
341. Guirguis SS, Pelmear PL, Roy ML, Wong L: Health effects associated with exposure to anaesthetic gases in Ontario hospital personnel. Br J Ind Med 47:490-497, 1990.
342. Rowland AS, Baird DD, Weinberg CR, et al: Reduced fertility among women employed as dental assistants exposed to high levels of nitrous oxide. N Engl J Med 327:993-997, 1992.
343. Rowland AS, Baird DD, Shore DL, et al: Nitrous oxide and spontaneous abortion in female dental assistants. Am J Epidemiol 141:531-538, 1995.
344. Ebi KL, Rice SA: Reproductive and development toxicity of anesthetics in humans. *In* Rice SA, Fish KJ (eds): Anesthetic Toxicity. New York, Raven Press, 1994, p 175.
345. Vessey MP: Epidemiological studies of the occupational hazards of anaesthesia—A review. Anaesthesia 33:430-438, 1978.
346. Buring JE, Hennekens CH, Mayrent SL, et al: Health experiences of operating room personnel. Anesthesiology 62:325-330, 1985.
347. Klingberg MA, Weatherall JA (eds): Epidemiological Methods for Detection of Teratogens. Basel, S Karger, 1979.
348. Ferstandig LL: Trace concentrations of anesthetic gases: A critical review of their disease potential. Anesth Analg 57:328-345, 1978.
349. Baden JM: Chronic toxicity of inhalation anesthetics. *In* Masse RI (ed): Clinics in Anaesthesiology, vol 1. London, WB Saunders, 1983, p 441.
350. Shepard TH, Fink BR: Teratogenic activity of nitrous oxide in rats. *In* Fink BR (ed): Toxicity of Anesthetics. Baltimore, Williams & Wilkins, 1968, p 308.
351. Vieira E, Cleaton-Jones P, Austin JC, et al: Effects of low concentrations of nitrous oxide on rat fetuses. Anesth Analg 59:175-177, 1980.
352. Fujinaga M, Baden JM, Shepard TH, Mazze RI: Nitrous oxide alters body laterality in rats. Teratology 41:131-135, 1990.
353. Mazze RI, Wilson AI, Rice SA, Baden JM: Reproduction and fetal development in rats exposed to nitrous oxide. Teratology 30:259-265, 1984.
354. Fujinaga M, Mazze RI, Baden JM, et al: Rat whole embryo culture: An in vitro model for testing nitrous oxide teratogenicity. Anesthesiology 69:401-404, 1988.
355. Baden JM, Fujinaga M: Effects of nitrous oxide on day 9 rat embryos grown in culture. Br J Anaesth 66:500-503, 1991.
356. Fujinaga M, Maze M, Hoffman BB, Baden JM: Activation of alpha-1 adrenergic receptors modulates the control of left/right sidedness in rat embryos. Dev Biol 150:419-421, 1992.
357. Fujinaga M, Hoffman BB, Baden JM: Receptor subtype and intracellular signal transduction pathway associated with situs inversus induced by alpha 1 adrenergic stimulation in rat embryos. Dev Biol 162:558-567, 1994.
358. Saito S, Fujita T, Igarashi M: Effects of inhalational anesthetics on biochemical events in growing neuronal tips. Anesthesiology 79:1338-1347, 1993.
359. Rice SA: Anaesthesia in pregnancy and the fetus: Toxicological aspects. *In* Reynolds F (ed): Effects on the baby of maternal analgesia and anesthesia. London, WB Saunders, 1993, p 88.
360. Rice SA: Behavioral toxicity of inhalation anesthetic agents. *In* Masse RI (ed): Inhalation Anesthesiology. Oxford, Alden Press, 1983, p 507.
361. Holson RR, Bates HK, LaBorde JB, Hansen DK: Behavioral teratology and dominant lethal evaluation of nitrous oxide exposure in rats. Neurotoxicol Teratol 17:583-592, 1995.
362. Sessler DI, Badgwell JM: Exposure of postoperative nurses to exhaled anesthetic gases. Anesth Analg 87:1083-1088, 1998.
363. McGregor DG, Senjem DH, Mazze RI: Trace nitrous oxide levels in the postanesthesia care unit. Anesth Analg 89:472-475, 1999.
364. Byhahn C, Wilke HJ, Westphal K: Occupational exposure to volatile anaesthetics: Epidemiology and approaches to reducing the problem. CNS Drugs 15:197-215, 2001.
365. Shuhaiber S, Einarson A, Radde IC, et al: A prospective-controlled study of pregnant veterinary staff exposed to inhaled anesthetics and x-rays. Int J Occup Med Environ Health 15:363-373 2002.
366. Sardas S, Cuhruk H, Karakaya AE, Atakurt Y: Sister-chromatid exchanges in operating room personnel. Mutat Res 279:117-120, 1992.

367. Hoerauf K, Lierz M, Wiesner G, et al: Genetic damage in operating room personnel exposed to isoflurane and nitrous oxide. Occup Environ Med 56:433-437, 1999.

368. Hoerauf KH, Wiesner G, Schroegendorfer KF, et al: Waste anaesthetic gases induce sister chromatid exchanges in lymphocytes of operating room personnel. Br J Anaesth 82:764-766, 1999.

369. Bozkurt G, Memis D, Karabogaz G, et al: Genotoxicity of waste anaesthetic gases. Anaesth Intensive Care 30:597-602, 2002.

370. Tschaikowsky K, Ritter J, Schroppel K, Kuhn M: Volatile anesthetics differentially affect immunostimulated expression of inducible nitric oxide synthase: Role of intracellular calcium. Anesthesiology 92:1093-1102, 2000.

371. Frohlich D, Rothe G, Schwall B, et al: Effects of volatile anaesthetics on human neutrophil oxidative response to the bacterial peptide FMLP. Br J Anaesth 78:718-723, 1997.

372. Rosenberg PH, Kallio H: Operating-theatre gas pollution and chromosomes. Lancet 2:452-453, 1977.

373. Baden JM, Kundomal YR, Mazze RI, Kosek JC: Carcinogen bioassay of isoflurane in mice. Anesthesiology 69:750-753, 1988.

374. Husum B, Niebuhr E, Wulf HC, Norgaard I: Sister chromatid exchanges and structural chromosome aberrations in lymphocytes in operating room personnel. Acta Anaesthesiol Scand 27:262-265, 1983.

375. Natarajan D, Santhiya ST: Cytogenetic damage in operation theatre personnel. Anaesthesia 45:574-577, 1990.

376. Bruce DL, Eide KA, Linde HW, Eckenhoff JE: Causes of death among anesthesiologists: A 20-year survey. Anesthesiology 29:565-569, 1968.

377. Corbett TH, Cornefl RG, Lieding K, et al: Incidence of cancer among Michigan nurse anesthetists. Anesthesiology 38:260, 1973.

378. Bruce DL, Eide KA, Smith NJ, et al: A prospective survey of anesthesiologist mortality, 1967-1971. Anesthesiology 41:71-74, 1974.

379. Doll R, Peto R: Mortality among doctors in different occupations. BMJ 1:779, 1977.

380. Neil HA, Fairer JG, Coleman MP, et al: Mortality among male anaesthetists in the United Kingdom, 1957-83. Br Med J 295:360-362, 1987.

381. Eger EI, White AE, Brown CL, et al: A test of the carcinogenicity of enflurane, isoflurane, halothane, methoxyflurane, and nitrous oxide in mice. Anesth Analg 57:678-694, 1978.

382. Baden JM, Kundomal YR, Mazze RI, et al: Carcinogen bioassay of isoflurane in mice. Anesthesiology 69:750, 1988.

383. Baden JM, Mazze RI, Wharton RS, et al: Carcinogenicity of halothane in Swiss/ICR mice. Anesthesiology 51:20, 1979.

384. Baden JM, Egbert B, Mazze RI: Carcinogen bioassay of enflurane in mice. Anesthesiology 56:9, 1982.

385. Baden JM, Kundomal YR, Luttropp ME Jr, et al: Carcinogen bioassay of nitrous oxide in mice. Anesthesiology 64:747, 1986.

386. Coate WB, Ulland BM, Lewis TR: Chronic exposure to low concentrations of halothane-nitrous oxide: Lack of carcinogenic effect in the rat. Anesthesiology 50:306-309, 1979.

387. Tannenbaum TN, Goldberg RJ: Exposure to anesthetic gases and reproductive outcome: A review of the epidemiologic literature. J Occup Med 27:659-668, 1985.

388. Spence AA: Environmental pollution by inhalation anaesthetics. Br J Anaesth 59:96-103, 1987.

CHAPTER
9 Inhaled Anesthetic Delivery Systems*

Russell C. Brockwell and J. Jeff Andrews

Anesthesia Machines and Workstations   273
Standards for Anesthesia Machines and Workstations   274
Generic Anesthesia Machine   274
Pipeline Supply Source   276
Cylinder Supply Source   276
Safety Devices for Oxygen Supply Pressure Failure   276
Flow Meter Assemblies   277
Proportioning Systems   281
Oxygen Flush Valve   283

Vaporizers   284
Physics   284
Variable-Bypass Vaporizers   285
Datex-Ohmeda Tec 6 Vaporizer for Desflurane   289
Datex-Ohmeda Aladin Cassette Vaporizer   292

Anesthetic Circuits   293
Mapleson Systems   293
Traditional Circle Breathing System   295

Carbon Dioxide Absorption   296
Absorber Canister   296
Chemistry of Absorbents   296

Absorptive Capacity   296
Indicators   296
Interactions of Inhaled Anesthetics with Absorbents   297

Anesthesia Ventilators   298
Classification   298
Operating Principles of Ascending Bellows Ventilators   299
Problems and Hazards   300

Newer Anesthesia Workstations   301
Datex-Ohmeda S/5 ADU   301
Dräger Narkomed 6000 and Fabius GS   302

Scavenging Systems   303
Components   304
Hazards   307

Checking Anesthesia Machines   307
Calibration of the Oxygen Analyzer   307
Leak Test for Low-Pressure Circuits   307
Test of the Circle System   310
Machine Self-Tests   310

Summary   310

Appendix 1   315

V10

An anesthesia delivery system consists of various components that communicate with each other during the administration of inhalational anesthetics.[1] System components include the anesthesia machine, the vaporizers, the anesthetic breathing circuit, the ventilator, and the scavenging system. A thorough understanding of these parts is essential to the safe practice of anesthesia. Malpractice claims associated with gas delivery equipment are infrequent but severe and continue to occur, one as recently as 2002.[2,3] This chapter discusses the normal operation, function, and integration of major system components. More importantly, it illustrates some of the problems and hazards associated with each and describes appropriate preoperative checks.

ANESTHESIA MACHINES AND WORKSTATIONS

Anesthesia machines have evolved from simple, pneumatic devices to complex, computer-based, fully integrated

---

*Portions of this chapter have appeared with permission in Andrews JJ, Brockwell RC: Delivery systems for inhaled anesthetics. *In* Barash PG, Cullen BF, Stoelting RK (eds): Clinical Anesthesia, 4th ed. New York, Lippincott-Raven, 2000, pp 567-594.

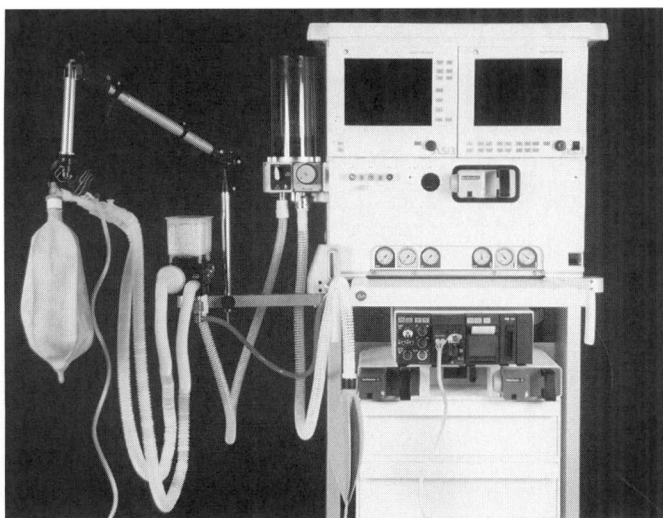

Figure 9–1 Datex-Ohmeda S/5 Anesthesia Delivery Unit (ADU) workstation.

anesthesia workstations (Figs. 9-1 and 9-2). Centralized display integration and functional integration are the hallmarks differentiating simple anesthesia machines from current, sophisticated anesthesia workstations. A few years ago, a rudimentary background in pneumatics sufficed, but today, an understanding of pneumatics, electronics, and even computer science is useful. Even though it is becoming increasingly more difficult for the anesthesiologist to achieve a thorough understanding of a modern anesthesia workstation, understanding the equipment remains essential to the safe practice of anesthesiology. The anesthesiologist must be aware of unique design differences between manufacturers so that appropriate preoperative checks can be performed.

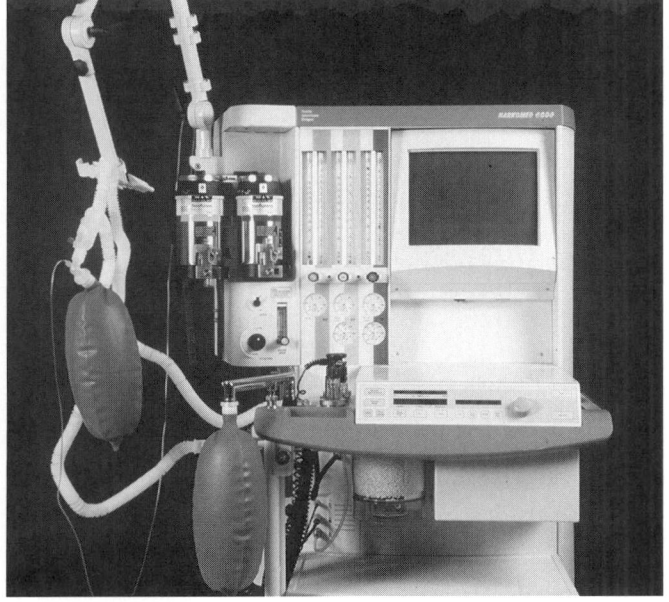

Figure 9–2 Dräger Narkomed 6000 anesthesia workstation.

Standards for Anesthesia Machines and Workstations

Standards for anesthesia machines and workstations provide guidelines to manufacturers regarding their minimum performance, design characteristics, and safety requirements. During the past 2 decades, the progression of anesthesia machine standards has been as follows:

- 1979: American National Standards Institute (ANSI) Z79.8-1979[4]
- 1988: American Society for Testing and Materials (ASTM) F1161-88[5]
- 1994: ASTM F1161-94[6] (reapproved in 1994 and discontinued in 2000)
- 2000: ASTM F1850-00[7]

To comply with the new 2000 ASTM F1850-00 standard, newly manufactured workstations must have monitors that measure the following parameters: continuous breathing system pressure, exhaled tidal volume, ventilatory carbon dioxide concentration, anesthetic vapor concentration, inspired oxygen concentration, oxygen supply pressure, arterial hemoglobin oxygen saturation, arterial blood pressure, and continuous electrocardiogram. The anesthesia workstation must have a prioritized alarm system that groups the alarms into three categories: high, medium, and low priority. These monitors and alarms may be automatically enabled and made to function by turning on the anesthesia workstation, or the monitors and alarms can be manually enabled and made functional by following a checklist before use.[7]

Generic Anesthesia Machine

A diagram of a generic two-gas anesthesia machine is shown in Figure 9-3. The pressures within the anesthesia machine can be divided into three circuits: a high-pressure, an intermediate-pressure, and a low-pressure circuit (see Fig. 9-3). The *high-pressure circuit* is confined to the cylinders and the cylinders' primary pressure regulators. For oxygen, the pressure range of the high-pressure circuit extends from a high of 2200 pounds per square inch gauge (psig) to 45 psig, which is the regulated cylinder pressure. For nitrous oxide in the high-pressure circuit, pressures range from a high of 750 psig in the cylinder to a low of 45 psig. The *intermediate-pressure circuit* begins at the regulated cylinder supply sources at 45 psig, includes the pipeline sources at 50 to 55 psig, and extends to the flow control valves. Depending on the manufacturer and specific machine design, second-stage pressure regulators may be used to decrease the pipeline supply pressures to the flow control valves to even lower pressures, such as 14 or 26 psig within the intermediate-pressure circuit.[8-16] The *low-pressure circuit* extends from the flow control valves to the common gas outlet. The low-pressure circuit includes the flow tubes, the vaporizers, and a one-way check valve on most Datex-Ohmeda machines.[8]

Both oxygen and nitrous oxide have two supply sources: a pipeline supply source and a cylinder supply source. The pipeline supply source is the primary gas source for the anesthesia machine. The hospital piping system provides gases to the machine at approximately 50 psig, which is the normal working pressure of most machines.

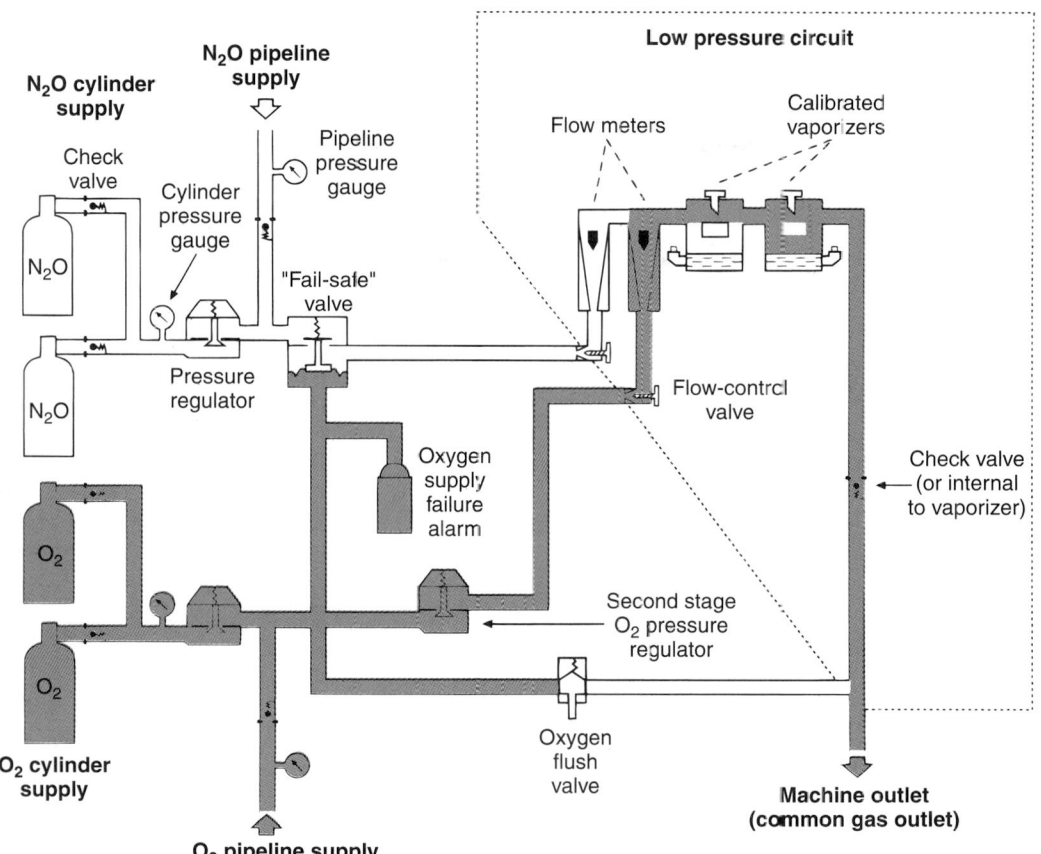

Figure 9–3 Diagram of a generic two-gas anesthesia machine. (Modified from Check-Out, a Guide for Preoperative Inspection of an Anesthesia Machine. Park Ridge, IL, American Society of Anesthesiologists, 1987.)

The cylinder supply source serves as a backup if the pipeline fails. The oxygen cylinder source is regulated from 2200 to approximately 45 psig, and the nitrous oxide cylinder source is regulated from 745 to approximately 45 psig.[8-28]

A safety device traditionally referred to as the *fail-safe valve* is located downstream from the nitrous oxide supply source. It serves as an interface between the oxygen and nitrous oxide supply sources. This valve shuts off or proportionally decreases the supply of nitrous oxide (and other gases) if the oxygen supply pressure decreases. Contemporary machines have an alarm device to monitor the oxygen supply pressure. A high-priority alarm is actuated when the oxygen supply pressure declines to a predetermined threshold, such as 30 psig.[8,9,19,28]

Most Datex-Ohmeda machines have a second-stage oxygen regulator located downstream from the oxygen supply source in the intermediate-pressure circuit. It is adjusted to a precise pressure level, such as 14 psig.[9-16] This regulator supplies a constant pressure to the oxygen flow control valve, regardless of fluctuating oxygen pipeline pressures. For example, the flow from the oxygen flow control valve remains constant if the oxygen supply pressure is greater than 14 psig.

The flow control valves represent an important landmark because they separate the intermediate-pressure circuit from the low-pressure circuit. The low-pressure circuit is the part of the machine that is downstream from the flow control valves. The operator regulates flow entering the low-pressure circuit by adjusting the flow control valves. The oxygen and nitrous oxide flow control valves are linked mechanically or pneumatically by a proportioning system to help prevent delivery of a hypoxic mixture. The flow travels through a common manifold and may be directed to a calibrated vaporizer. Precise amounts of inhaled anesthetic can be added, depending on the setting of the vaporizer control dial. The total fresh gas flow then travels toward the common gas outlet.[8,9]

Many Datex-Ohmeda anesthesia machines have a one-way check valve between the vaporizers and the common gas outlet.[9-14,17,18] Its purpose is to prevent backflow into the vaporizer during positive-pressure ventilation, thereby minimizing the effects of downstream, intermittent pressure fluctuations on inhaled anesthetic concentration (see "Intermittent Backpressure"). The presence or absence of this check valve profoundly influences which preoperative leak test is indicated (see "Checking Anesthesia Machines"). The oxygen flush connection joins the mixed-gas pipeline between the one-way check valve (when present) and the machine outlet. When the oxygen flush valve is activated, the pipeline oxygen pressure has a "straight shot" to the common gas outlet.[8,9]

Pipeline Supply Source

The pipeline supply source is the primary gas source for the anesthesia machine. Most hospitals have a central piping system to deliver medical gases such as oxygen, nitrous oxide, and air to the operating room. The central piping system must supply the anesthesia machine with the correct gases at the appropriate pressure for the anesthesia workstation to function properly. Unfortunately, this does not always occur.

In a survey of approximately 200 hospitals in 1976, 31% reported difficulties with pipeline systems.[29] The most common problem was inadequate oxygen pressure, followed by excessive pipeline pressures. The most devastating reported hazard, however, was accidental crossing of oxygen and nitrous oxide pipelines, which led to several deaths. This problem caused 23 deaths in a newly constructed wing of a general hospital in Sudbury, Ontario, during a 5-month period.[29,30] In 2002, two additional hypoxic deaths were reported in New Haven, Connecticut. These deaths resulted from a medical gas system failure in which a damaged oxygen flow meter was inadvertently connected to a wall supply source for nitrous oxide.[3]

The operator must take two actions if a pipeline crossover is suspected. First, the backup oxygen cylinder should be turned on. Second, the pipeline supply must be disconnected. This step is mandatory because the machine preferentially uses the inappropriate 50 psig pipeline supply source instead of the lower-pressure (45 psig) oxygen cylinder source.

Gas enters the anesthesia machine through the pipeline inlet connections (see Fig. 9-3, *arrows*). The pipeline inlet fittings are gas-specific, Diameter Index Safety System (DISS), threaded-body fittings. The DISS provides threaded, noninterchangeable connections for medical gas lines, which minimize the risk of misconnection. A check valve is located downstream from the inlet. It prevents reverse flow of gases from the machine to the pipeline or the atmosphere.

Cylinder Supply Source

Anesthesia machines have reserve E cylinders if a pipeline supply source is not available or if the pipeline fails. Color-coded cylinders are attached to the anesthesia machine through the hanger yoke assembly. The hanger yoke assembly orients and supports the cylinder, provides a gas-tight seal, and ensures a unidirectional flow of gases into the machine.[8] Each hanger yoke is equipped with the Pin Index Safety System (PISS). The PISS is a safeguard introduced to eliminate cylinder interchanging and the possibility of accidentally placing the incorrect gas on a yoke designed to accommodate another gas. Two pins on the yoke are arranged so that they project into the cylinder valve. Each gas or combination of gases has a specific pin arrangement.[31]

Gas travels from the high-pressure cylinder source to the anesthesia machine when the cylinder is turned on (see Fig. 9-3). A check valve is located downstream from each cylinder if a double-yoke assembly is used. The check valve has several functions. First, it minimizes gas transfer from a cylinder at high pressure to one with lower pressure. Second, it allows an empty cylinder to be exchanged for a full one while gas flow continues from the other cylinder into the machine with minimal loss of gas. Third, it minimizes leakage from an open cylinder to the atmosphere if one cylinder is absent.[8,9] A cylinder gauge indicating supply pressure is located downstream from the check valves. The gauge indicates the pressure in the cylinder having the higher pressure when two reserve cylinders of the same gas are opened at the same time.[25]

Each cylinder supply source has a pressure-reducing valve known as the cylinder's *pressure regulator*. It reduces the high and variable storage pressure in a cylinder to a lower, more constant pressure suitable for use in the anesthesia machine. The oxygen cylinder's pressure regulator reduces the cylinder's oxygen pressure from a high of 2200 psig to approximately 45 psig. The nitrous oxide cylinder's pressure regulator receives pressure of up to 745 psig and reduces it to approximately 45 psig.[8,9]

The cylinders should be turned off except during the preoperative machine checking period or when a pipeline source is unavailable. If left on, the reserve cylinder supply can be silently depleted whenever the pressure inside the machine decreases to a value lower than the regulated cylinder pressure. Oxygen pressure within the machine can decrease below 45 psig with oxygen flushing or with ventilator use, particularly at high peak flow rates. The pipeline supply pressures of all gases can be less than 45 psig if problems exist in the central piping system. If the cylinders are left on, they will eventually become depleted, and no reserve supply will be available if a pipeline failure occurs.[9,32]

Safety Devices for Oxygen Supply Pressure Failure

Oxygen and nitrous oxide supply sources existed as independent entities in older models of anesthesia machines, and they were not pneumatically or mechanically interfaced. Abrupt or insidious oxygen pressure failure could lead to the delivery of a hypoxic mixture. The 2000 ASTM F1850-00 standard states, "The anesthesia gas supply device shall be designed so that whenever oxygen supply pressure is reduced to below the manufacturer specified minimum, the delivered oxygen concentration shall not decrease below 19% at the common gas outlet."[7] Contemporary anesthesia machines have a number of safety devices that act together in a cascade manner to minimize the risk of hypoxia as oxygen pressure decreases. Several of these devices are described in the following sections.

Pneumatic and Electronic Alarm Devices

Many older anesthesia machines have a pneumatic alarm device that sounds a warning when the oxygen supply pressure decreases to a predetermined threshold value such as 30 psig. The 2000 ASTM F1850-00 standard mandates that medium priority alarm shall be activated within 5 seconds when the oxygen pressure decreases below a manufacturer-specified threshold pressure.[7] Electronic alarm devices are used to meet this guideline.

Fail-Safe Valves

A fail-safe valve is present in the gas line supplying each of the flow meters except that for oxygen. Controlled by oxygen supply pressure, the valve shuts off or proportionally decreases the supply pressure of all other gases (e.g., nitrous oxide, air, carbon dioxide, helium, nitrogen) as the oxygen supply pressure decreases. Unfortunately, the misnomer "fail-safe" has led to the misconception that the device prevents administration of a hypoxic mixture. This is not the case. Machines that are not equipped with a flow proportioning system (see "Proportioning Systems") can deliver a hypoxic mixture under normal working conditions. The oxygen flow control valve can be closed intentionally or accidentally. Normal oxygen pressure keeps other gas lines open so that a hypoxic mixture can result.[8,9]

Datex-Ohmeda machines are equipped with a fail-safe valve known as the *pressure sensor's shut-off valve* (Fig. 9-4). The valve operates on a threshold principle, and it is open or closed. Oxygen supply pressure opens the valve, and the valve's return spring closes the valve. Figure 9-4 shows a nitrous oxide pressure sensor's shut-off valve with a threshold pressure of 20 psig.[11,12,14-16] In Figure 9-4A, an oxygen supply pressure greater than 20 psig is exerted on the mobile diaphragm. This pressure moves the piston and pin upward, and the valve opens. Nitrous oxide flows freely to the nitrous oxide flow control valve. In Figure 9-4B, the oxygen supply pressure is less than 20 psig, and the force of the valve's return spring completely closes the valve.[9] Nitrous oxide flow stops at the closed fail-safe valve, and it does not advance to the nitrous oxide flow control valve.

Dräger Medical uses a fail-safe valve known as the *oxygen failure protection device* (OFPD) to interface the oxygen pressure with that of other gases, such as nitrous oxide or other inert gases.[19-21] It differs from Datex-Ohmeda's oxygen pressure sensor's shut-off valve because the OFPD is based on a proportioning principle rather than a threshold principle. The pressure of all gases controlled by the OFPD decreases proportionally with the oxygen pressure. The OFPD consists of a seat-nozzle assembly connected to a spring-loaded piston (Fig. 9-5). The oxygen supply pressure (see Fig. 9-5, left panel) is 50 psig. This pressure pushes the piston upward, forcing the nozzle away from the valve seat. Nitrous oxide and other gases advance toward the flow control valve at 50 psig. The oxygen pressure in the right panel is 0 psig. The spring is expanded and forces the nozzle against the seat, preventing flow through the device. The center panel shows an intermediate oxygen pressure of 25 psig. The force of the spring partially closes the valve. The nitrous oxide pressure delivered to the flow control valve is 25 psig. There is a continuum of intermediate configurations between the extremes (0 to 50 psig) of oxygen supply pressure. These intermediate valve configurations are responsible for the proportional nature of the OFPD.[19] It is important to understand the differences of these fail-safe devices; the Datex-Ohmeda pressure sensor's shut-off valve is an all-or-nothing threshold device, whereas the Dräger OFPD is a variable-flow proportioning system.

Second-Stage Pressure Regulator for Oxygen

Most contemporary Datex-Ohmeda workstations have a second-stage pressure regulator for oxygen that is set at a specific value between 12 and 19 psig.[11-16] The oxygen flow meter's output is constant when the oxygen supply pressure exceeds the threshold value. The Datex-Ohmeda pressure sensor's shut-off valves are set at a higher threshold value (20 to 30 psig). This ensures that oxygen is the last gas flow to decrease if oxygen pressure fails.

Flow Meter Assemblies

The flow meter assembly (Fig. 9-6) precisely controls and measures gas flow to the common gas outlet. With traditional glass flow meter assemblies, the flow control valve regulates the amount of flow that enters a tapered, transparent flow tube known as a *Thorpe tube*. A mobile indicator float inside the flow tube indicates the amount of flow passing through the associated flow control valve. The quantity of flow is indicated on a scale associated with the flow tube.[8,9]

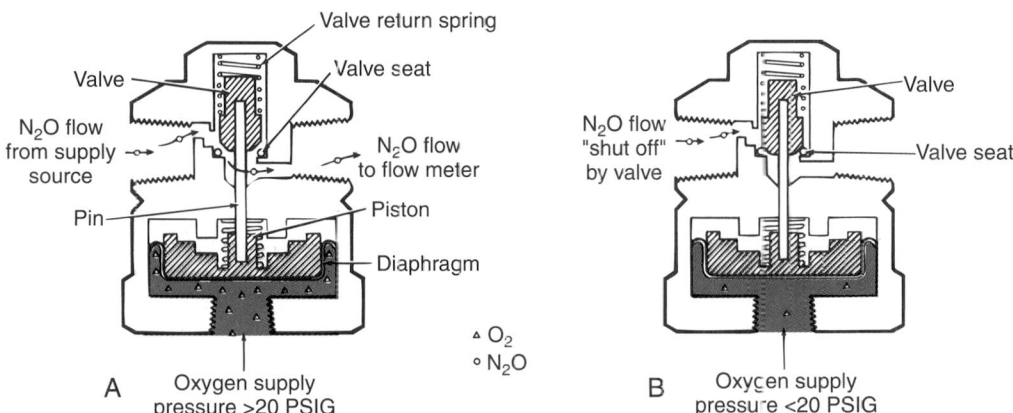

Figure 9–4 Shut-off valve of the pressure sensor. **A,** The valve is open because the oxygen supply pressure is greater than the threshold value of 20 psig. **B,** The valve is closed because of inadequate oxygen pressure. (Adapted from Bowie E, Huffman LM: The Anesthesia Machine: Essentials for Understanding. Madison, WI, Ohmeda, a Division of BOC Health Care, 1985.)

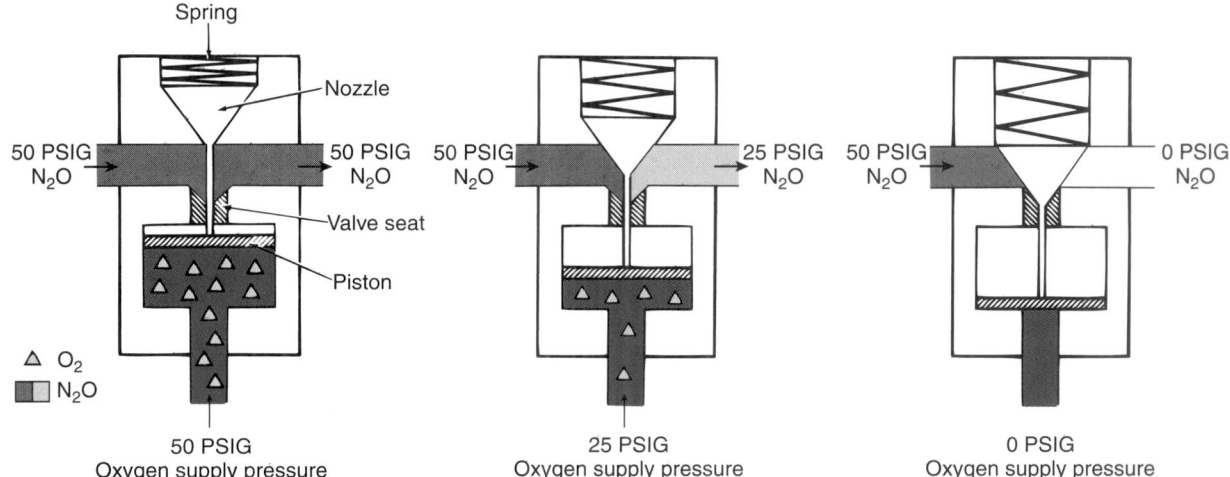

Figure 9–5 The oxygen failure protection device (OFPD) responds proportionally to changes in oxygen supply pressure. The OFPD consists of a seat-nozzle assembly connected to a spring-loaded piston. (Modified with permission from Narkomed 2A Anesthesia System: Technical Service Manual, 6th ed. Telford, PA, North American Dräger, June 1985.)

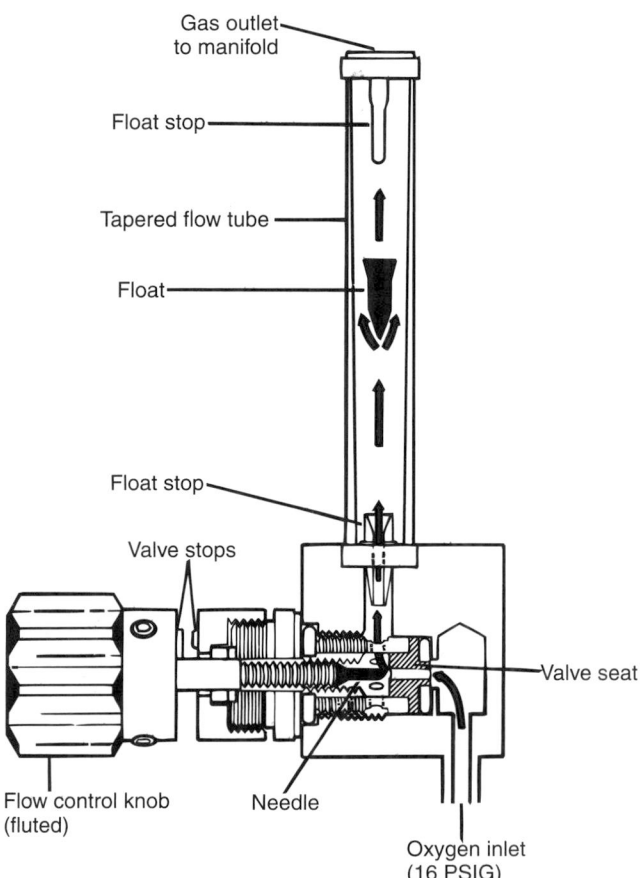

Figure 9–6 Oxygen flow meter assembly. The oxygen flow meter assembly is composed of the flow control valve assembly plus the flow meter subassembly. (Adapted from Bowie E, Huffman LM: The Anesthesia Machine: Essentials for Understanding. Madison, WI, Ohmeda, a Division of BOC Health Care, 1985.)

Physical Principles of Conventional Flow Meters

Opening the flow control valve allows gas to travel through the space between the float and the flow tube. This space is known as the *annular space* (Fig. 9-7). The indicator float hovers freely in an equilibrium position where the upward force resulting from gas flow equals the downward force on the float resulting from gravity at a given flow rate. The float moves to a new equilibrium position in the tube when flow is changed. These flow meters are commonly referred to as *constant-pressure flow meters* because the pressure decrease across the float remains constant for all positions in the tube.[8,32,33]

Flow tubes are tapered, with the smallest diameter at the bottom of the tube and the largest diameter at the top. The term *variable orifice* designates this type of unit because the annular space between the float and the inner wall of the flow tube varies with the position of the float. Flow through the constriction created by the float can be laminar or turbulent, depending on the flow rate (Fig. 9-8). The characteristics of a gas that influence its flow rate through a given constriction are viscosity (i.e., laminar flow) and density (i.e., turbulent flow). Because the annular space is tubular at low flow rates, laminar flow is present, and *viscosity* determines the gas flow rate. The annular space simulates an orifice at high flow rates, and turbulent gas flow then depends predominantly on the *density* of the gas.[8,33]

Components of Flow Meter Assemblies

Flow Control Valve Assembly

The assembly of the flow control valve (see Fig. 9-6) is composed of a flow control knob, a needle valve, a valve seat, and a pair of valve stops.[8] The assembly can receive its pneumatic input directly from the pipeline source (50 psig) or from a second-stage pressure regulator. The location of the needle valve in the valve seat changes to establish different orifices when the flow control valve is adjusted. Gas flow increases when the flow control valve

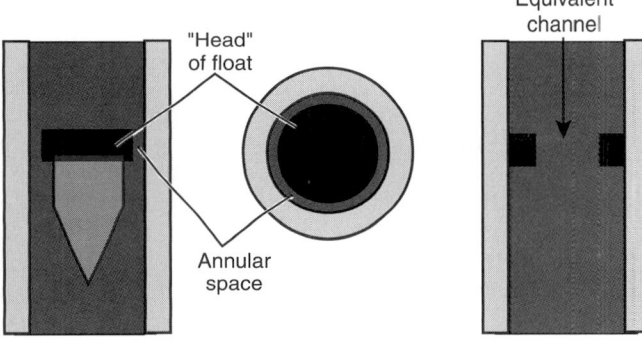

Figure 9–7 The clearance between the head of the float and the flow tube is known as the annular space. It can be considered an equivalent to a circular channel of the same cross-sectional area. (Adapted from Macintosh R, Mushin WW, Epstein HG: Physics for the Anaesthetist, 3rd ed. Oxford, UK, Blackwell Scientific Publications, 1963.)

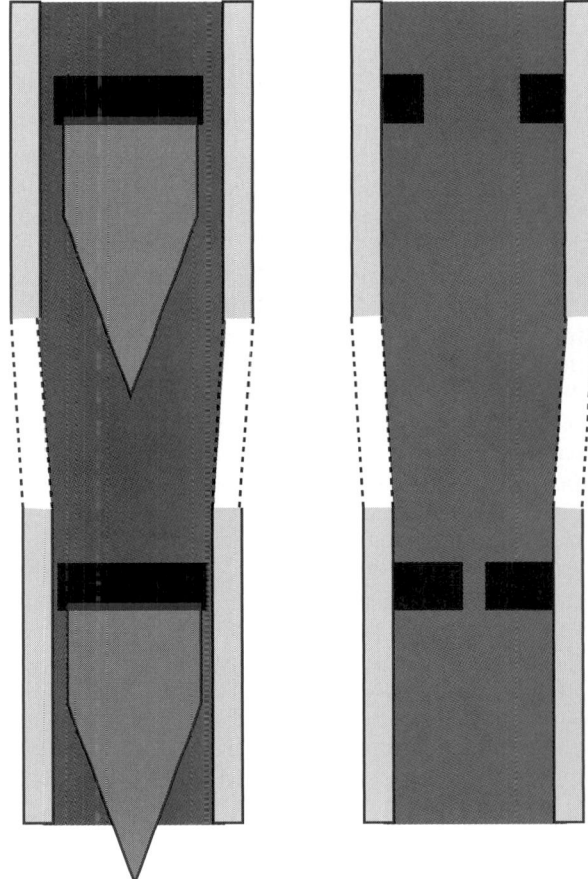

Figure 9–8 Flow tube constriction. The lower portion of the illustration represents the lower portion of two flow tubes. The clearance between the head of the float and the flow tube is narrow. The equivalent channel is tubular because its diameter is less than its length. Viscosity is dominant in determining gas flow rate through this tubular constriction. The upper portion of the illustration represents the upper portion of a flow tube. The equivalent channel is orificial because its length is less than its width. Density is dominant in determining gas flow rate through this orificial constriction. (Adapted from Macintosh R, Mushin WW, Epstein HG: Physics for the Anaesthetist, 3rd ed. Oxford, UK, Blackwell Scientific Publications, 1963.)

is turned counterclockwise, and it decreases when the valve is turned clockwise. Extreme clockwise rotation may result in damage to the needle valve and valve seat. Flow control valves are equipped with valve *stops* to prevent this occurrence.[9]

SAFETY FEATURES. Contemporary assemblies of flow control valves have numerous safety features. The oxygen flow control knob is physically distinguishable from other gas knobs. It is distinctively fluted, projects beyond the control knobs of the other gases, and has a larger diameter than the flow control knobs of other gases. All knobs are color coded for the appropriate gas, and the chemical formula or name of the gas is permanently marked on each. Flow control knobs are recessed or protected with a shield or barrier to minimize inadvertent change from a preset position. If a single gas has two flow tubes, the tubes are arranged in series and are controlled by a single flow control valve.[7]

Flow Meter Subassembly
The flow meter subassembly (see Fig. 9-6) consists of the flow tube, the indicator float with float stops, and the indicator scale.[8]

FLOW TUBES. Contemporary flow tubes are made of glass. Most have a single taper in which the inner diameter of the flow tube increases uniformly from bottom to top. Manufacturers provide double flow tubes for oxygen and nitrous oxide to provide better visual discrimination at low flow rates. A fine flow tube indicates flow from approximately 200 mL/min to 1 L/min, and a coarse flow tube indicates flow from approximately 1 L/min to between 10 and 12 L/min. The two tubes are connected in series and supplied by a single flow control valve. The total gas flow is that shown on the higher flow meter.

INDICATOR FLOATS AND FLOAT STOPS. Contemporary anesthesia machines use several different types of bobbins or floats, including plumb-bob floats[10-12,15,16]; rotating, skirted floats[13,14]; and ball floats.[18-27] Flow is read at the top of plumb-bob and skirted floats and at the center of the ball on the ball-type floats.[8] Flow tubes are equipped with float stops at the top and bottom of the tube. The upper stop prevents the float from ascending to the top of the tube and plugging the outlet. It also ensures that the float is visible at maximum flows instead of being hidden in the manifold. The bottom float stop provides a central foundation for the indicator when the flow control valve is turned off.[8,9]

SCALE. The flow meter scale can be marked directly on the flow tube or located to the right of the tube.[7] Gradations corresponding to equal increments in flow rate are closer together at the top of the scale because the annular space increases more rapidly than does the internal diameter from bottom to top of the tube. Rib guides are used in some flow tubes with ball-type indicators to minimize this compression effect. They are tapered glass ridges that run the length of the tube. There are usually three rib guides that are equally spaced around the inner circumference of the tube. In the presence of rib guides, the annular space from the bottom to the top of the tube increases almost proportionally with the internal diameter. This results in a nearly linear scale.[8] Rib guides are employed on North American Dräger flow tubes.[19,24-25,27]

SAFETY FEATURES. The flow meter subassembly for each gas on the Datex-Ohmeda Modulus I, Modulus II, Modulus II Plus, CD, and Aestiva is housed in an independent, color-coded, pin-specific module. The flow tubes are adjacent to a gas-specific, color-coded backing. The flow scale and the chemical formula or name of the gas are permanently etched on the backing to the right of the flow tube.[10-12,15,16] Flow meter scales are individually hand-calibrated using the specific float to provide a high degree of accuracy. The tube, float, and scale make an inseparable unit. The entire set must be replaced if any component is damaged.[10-12,15,16]

North American Dräger does not use a modular system for the flow meter subassembly. The flow scale, the chemical symbol, and the gas-specific color codes are etched directly onto the flow tube.[19,24-27] The scale in use is obvious when two flow tubes for the same gas are used.

Problems with Flow Meters
Leaks
Flow meter leaks are a substantial hazard because the flow meters are located downstream from all machine safety devices except the oxygen analyzer.[1] Leaks can occur at the O-ring junctions between the glass flow tubes and the metal manifold or in cracked- or broken-glass flow tubes, the most fragile pneumatic component of the anesthesia machine. Even though gross damage to conventional glass flow tubes is usually apparent, subtle cracks and chips may be overlooked, resulting in errors of delivered flows.[34] The elimination of conventional glass flow tubes from some newer anesthesia machines (i.e., Datex-Ohmeda S/5 Anesthesia Delivery Unit [ADU] and the Dräger Fabius) may help to minimize potential sources of leaks[20,21,35,36] (see "Electronic Flow Meters").

In 1963, Eger and colleagues[37] demonstrated that, in the presence of a flow meter leak, a hypoxic mixture is less likely to occur if the oxygen flow meter is located downstream from all other flow meters.[33] Figure 9-9 is

a contemporary version of the figure in Eger's original publication. The air flow tube (not in use) has a large leak. Nitrous oxide and oxygen flow rates are set at a ratio of 3:1. A potentially dangerous arrangement is shown in Figure 9-9A and B because the nitrous oxide flow meter is located in the downstream position. A hypoxic mixture can result because a substantial portion of oxygen flow passes through the leak, and all nitrous oxide is directed to the common gas outlet. A safer configuration is shown in Figure 9-9C and D. The oxygen flow meter is located in the downstream position. A portion of the nitrous oxide flow escapes through the leak, and the remainder goes toward the common gas outlet. A hypoxic mixture is less likely because all the oxygen flow is advanced by the nitrous oxide.[30] North American Dräger flow meters are arranged as in Figure 9-9C, and Datex-Ohmeda flow meters are as in Figure 9-9D.

A leak in the oxygen flow tube can produce a hypoxic mixture even when oxygen is located in the downstream position (Fig. 9-10).[1,34] Oxygen escapes through the leak and nitrous oxide flows toward the common outlet, particularly at high ratios of nitrous oxide to oxygen flow.

Inaccuracy
A flow error can occur even when flow meters are assembled properly with appropriate components. Dirt or static electricity can cause a float to stick, and the actual flow may be higher or lower than that indicated. Sticking is more common with low flow because the annular space is smaller. A damaged float can cause inaccurate readings because the precise relationship between the float and the flow tube is altered. Backpressure from the breathing circuit can cause a float to drop so that it reads less than the actual flow. If flow meters are not aligned properly in the vertical position, readings can be inaccurate because tilting distorts the annular space.[8,36,38]

Ambiguous Scale
Before the standardization of flow meter scales and the widespread use of oxygen analyzers, at least two deaths resulted from confusion created by ambiguous scales.[34,38,39] The operator read the float position beside an adjacent but erroneous scale in both cases. This error

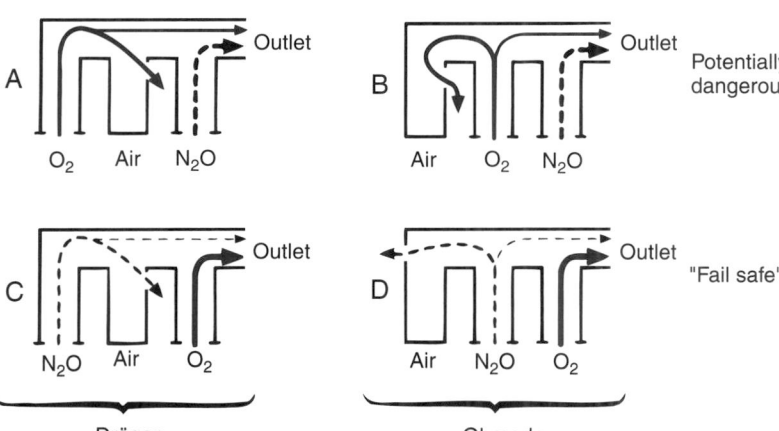

Figure 9-9 The flow meter sequence is a potential cause of hypoxia. **A** and **B,** In the event of a flow meter leak, a potentially dangerous arrangement exists when nitrous oxide is located in the downstream position. **C** and **D,** The safest configuration exists when oxygen is located in the downstream position. (Adapted from Eger EI II, Hylton RR, Irwin RH, et al: Anesthetic flow meter sequence—A cause for hypoxia. Anesthesiology 24:396, 1963.)

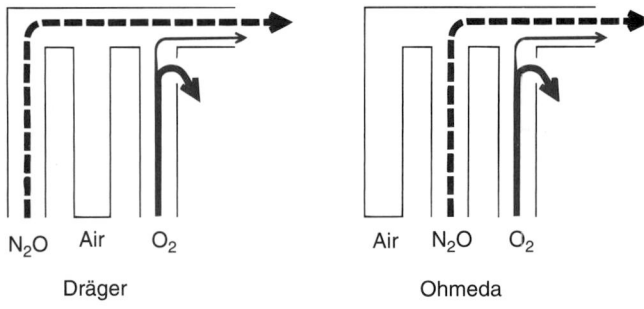

Figure 9–10 An oxygen leak from the flow tube can produce a hypoxic mixture, regardless of the arrangement of the flow tubes.

is less likely to occur now because contemporary flow meter scales are marked directly onto or to the right of the appropriate flow tube.[7] Confusion is minimized when the scale is etched directly onto the tube.

Electronic Flow Meters

Some newer anesthesia machines such as the Datex-Ohmeda S/5 ADU and the North American Dräger Fabius GS have conventional control knobs and flow control valves, but have digital flow meters. The output from the flow control valve is represented graphically or numerically, or both, in liters per minute on the workstation's integrated user interface. These systems depend on electrical power to provide a precise display of gas flow. However, even when electrical power is totally interrupted, because the flow control valves are not electronic, oxygen should continue to flow.[20,35,36] Because these machines do not have individual flow tubes that physically quantitate the flow of each gas, a small, conventional, pneumatic *fresh gas* or *total flow* indicator is provided that indicates the total fresh gas flow from all flow control valves. This miniature flow tube informs the user of the approximate quantity of gas that is leaving the anesthesia workstation's common gas outlet.[20,35-40]

Proportioning Systems

Manufacturers have equipped newer machines with proportioning systems in an attempt to prevent delivery of a hypoxic mixture. Nitrous oxide and oxygen are interfaced mechanically or pneumatically so that the minimum oxygen concentration at the common gas outlet is between 23% and 25%, depending on manufacturer.[12-21,34,35]

Datex-Ohmeda Link-25 Proportion Limiting Control System

Conventional Datex-Ohmeda machines use the Link-25 system. The heart of the system is the mechanical integration of the flow control valves for nitrous oxide and oxygen. It allows independent adjustment of either valve, but automatically intercedes to maintain a minimum 25% oxygen concentration with a maximum nitrous oxide–oxygen flow ratio of 3:1. The Link-25 automatically increases oxygen flow to prevent delivery of a hypoxic mixture.[12-19]

Figure 9-11 shows the Datex-Ohmeda Link-25 system. The nitrous oxide and oxygen flow control valves are identical. A 14-tooth sprocket is attached to the nitrous oxide flow control valve, and a 28-tooth sprocket is attached to the oxygen flow control valve. A chain physically links the sprockets. When the nitrous oxide flow control valve is turned through two revolutions, or 28 teeth, the oxygen flow control valve revolves once because of the 2:1 gear ratio. The final 3:1 flow ratio results because the nitrous oxide flow control valve is supplied by approximately 26 psig, whereas the oxygen flow control valve is supplied by 14 psig. The combination of the mechanical and pneumatic aspects of the system yields the final oxygen concentration.[13,14] The Datex-Ohmeda Link-25 proportioning system can be thought of as a system that *increases oxygen flow* when necessary to prevent delivery of a fresh gas mixture with an oxygen concentration of less than 25%.

A few failures of the Datex-Ohmeda Link-25 system have been described. The authors of these reports describe failures that resulted in an inability to administer oxygen without nitrous oxide or allowed creation of a hypoxic mixture. These reported failures of the Link-25 system on the Datex-Ohmeda Excel series of anesthesia machines should raise the awareness of clinicians to the possibility of a failure of this type of proportioning system.[41-44]

North American Dräger Oxygen Ratio Monitor Controller

North American Dräger's proportioning system, the oxygen ratio monitor controller (ORMC), is used on the North American Dräger Narkomed 2A, 2B, 3, and 4.[19-28]

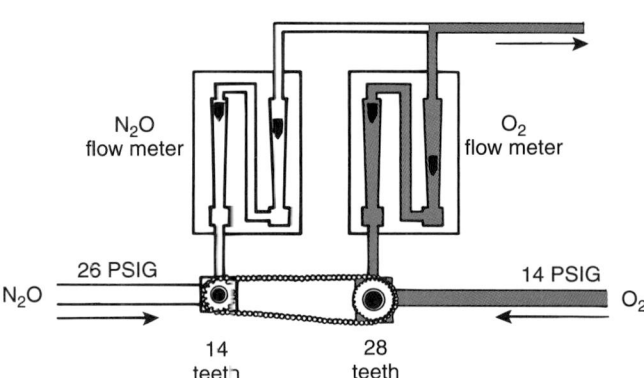

Figure 9–11 In the Ohmeda Link-25 Proportion-Limiting Control System, the nitrous oxide and oxygen flow control valves are identical. A 14-tooth sprocket is attached to the nitrous oxide flow control valve, and a 28-tooth sprocket is attached to the oxygen flow control valve. A chain links the sprockets. The combination of the mechanical and pneumatic aspects of the system yields the final oxygen concentration. The Datex-Ohmeda Link-25 proportioning system can be thought of as a system that increases oxygen flow when necessary to prevent delivery of a fresh gas mixture with an oxygen concentration of less than 25%. (Adapted from Andrews JJ, Brockwell RC: Delivery systems for inhaled anesthetics. *In* Barash PG, Cullen BF, Stoelting RK [eds]: Clinical Anesthesia, 4th ed. New York, Lippincott-Raven, 2000, pp 567-594.)

A virtually identical system known as the sensitive-oxygen ratio controller (S-ORC) is present on some newer Dräger anesthesia workstations such as the Dräger Fabius GS and Narkomed 6000.[20-23] The ORMC and the S-ORC are pneumatic oxygen–nitrous oxide interlock systems designed to maintain a fresh gas oxygen concentration of at least 25% ± 3%. They control the fresh gas oxygen concentration to levels substantially higher than 25% at oxygen flow rates of less than 1 L/min. The ORMC and S-ORC limit nitrous oxide flow to prevent delivery of a hypoxic mixture.[19-27] This approach is unlike that of the Datex-Ohmeda Link-25, which actively increases oxygen flow.

A schematic diagram of the ORMC is shown in Figure 9-12. The system is composed of an oxygen chamber, a nitrous oxide chamber, and a nitrous oxide slave control valve. All are interconnected by a mobile horizontal shaft. The pneumatic input into the device is from the oxygen and the nitrous oxide flow meters. These flow meters are unique because they have specific resistors located downstream from the flow control valves. The resistors create backpressures directed toward the oxygen and nitrous oxide chambers. The value of the oxygen flow tube's resistor is three to four times that of the nitrous oxide flow tube's resistor, and the relative value of these resistors determines the value of the controlled fresh gas concentration of oxygen. The backpressure in the oxygen and nitrous oxide chambers pushes against rubber diaphragms attached to the mobile horizontal shaft. Movement of the shaft regulates the nitrous oxide slave control valve, which feeds the nitrous oxide flow control valve.[1-19,24,28]

If the oxygen pressure is proportionally higher than the nitrous oxide pressure, the nitrous oxide slave control valve opens more widely, allowing more nitrous oxide to flow. As the nitrous oxide flow is increased manually, the nitrous oxide pressure forces the shaft toward the oxygen chamber. The valve opening becomes more restrictive and limits the nitrous oxide flow to the flow meter.

Figure 9-12 illustrates the action of a single ORMC under different sets of circumstances. The backpressure exerted on the oxygen diaphragm (in the upper configuration) is greater than that exerted on the nitrous oxide diaphragm. This causes the horizontal shaft to move to the left, opening the nitrous oxide slave control valve. Nitrous oxide is then able to proceed to its flow control valve and out through the flow meter. In the bottom configuration, the nitrous oxide slave control valve is closed because of inadequate oxygen backpressure.[1-19,24,28] To summarize, in contrast to the Datex-Ohmeda Link-25 system, which actively increases oxygen flow to maintain a fresh gas-oxygen concentration greater than 25%, the Dräger ORMC and S-ORC systems limit nitrous oxide flow to prevent delivery of a fresh gas mixture with an oxygen concentration of less than 25%.

Limitations

Proportioning systems are not foolproof. Machines equipped with proportioning systems still can deliver a hypoxic mixture under certain conditions.

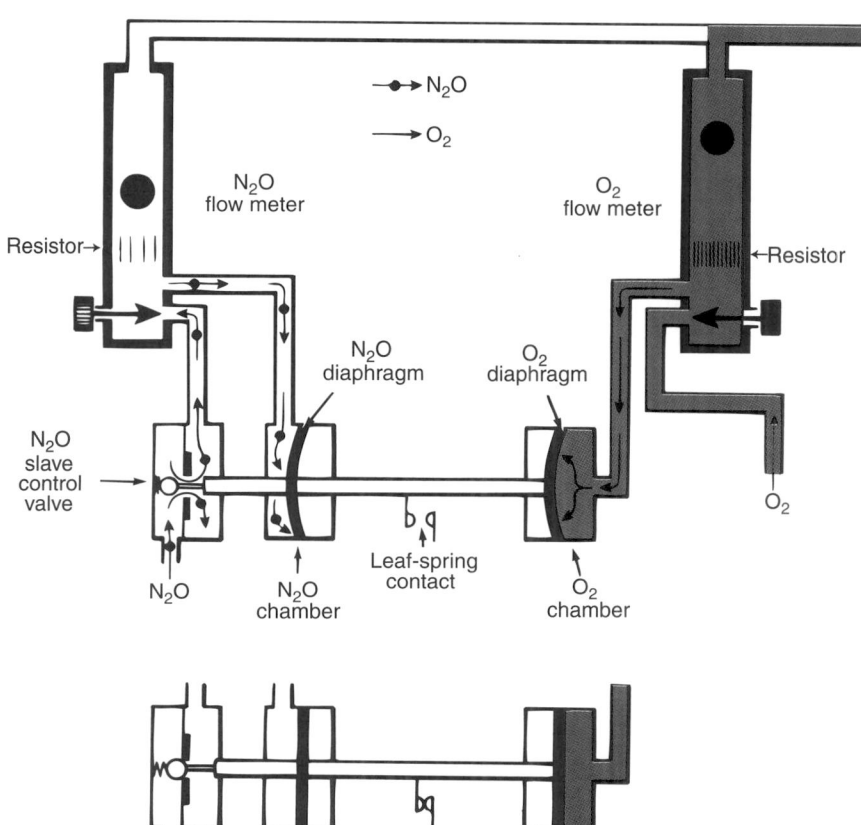

Figure 9–12 A schematic of the North American Dräger Oxygen Ratio Monitor Controller (ORMC) is shown. The ORMC is composed of an oxygen chamber, a nitrous oxide chamber, and a nitrous oxide slave control valve, all of which are interconnected by a mobile horizontal shaft. The pneumatic input into the device is from the oxygen and the nitrous oxide flow meters. These flow meters have resistors located downstream from the flow control valves that create backpressures directed to the oxygen and nitrous oxide chambers. The value of the oxygen flow tube's resistor is three to four times that of the nitrous oxide flow tube's resistor, and the relative value of these resistors determines the value of the controlled fresh gas concentration of oxygen. The backpressure in the oxygen and nitrous oxide chambers pushes against rubber diaphragms attached to the mobile horizontal shaft. Movement of the shaft regulates the nitrous oxide slave control valve, which feeds the nitrous oxide flow control valve. (Adapted from Schreiber P: Safety Guidelines for Anesthesia Systems. Telford, PA, North American Dräger, 1984.)

Wrong Supply Gas

The Datex-Ohmeda Link-25 and the Dräger ORMC/S-ORC can be fooled if a gas other than oxygen is present in the oxygen pipeline. In the Link-25 system, the nitrous oxide and oxygen flow control valves continue to be mechanically linked. Nevertheless, a hypoxic mixture can proceed to the common outlet. The oxygen chamber's rubber diaphragm of the ORMC or S-ORC recognizes adequate supply pressure on the oxygen side, and flow of the wrong gas plus nitrous oxide results. The oxygen analyzer is the only machine monitor besides an integrated multigas analyzer that can detect this condition in either system.

Defective Pneumatics or Mechanics

Normal operation of the Datex-Ohmeda Link-25 and the North American Dräger ORMC/S-ORC is contingent on pneumatic and mechanical integrity.[45] Pneumatic integrity in the Datex-Ohmeda system depends on properly functioning second-stage regulators. A nitrous oxide–oxygen ratio other than 3:1 results if the regulators are not precise. The chain connecting the two sprockets must be intact. A 97% nitrous oxide concentration can occur if the chain is cut or broken.[46] In the North American Dräger system, a functional OFPD is necessary to supply appropriate pressure to the ORMC. The mechanical aspects of the ORMC/S-ORC, such as the rubber diaphragms, the flow tube's resistors, and the nitrous oxide slave control valve, also must be intact.

Leaks Downstream

The ORMC/S-ORC and the Link-25 function at the level of the flow control valves. A leak downstream from these devices, such as a broken oxygen flow tube (see Fig. 9-10), can result in delivery of a hypoxic mixture to the common gas outlet. Oxygen escapes through the leak, and the predominant gas delivered is nitrous oxide. The oxygen monitor and integrated multigas analyzer are the only machine safety devices that can detect the problem.[1] For most of its products, North American Dräger recommends a preoperative positive-pressure leak test to detect such a leak.[19-27] Datex-Ohmeda almost universally recommends a preoperative negative-pressure leak test for its workstations because of the check valve located at the common gas outlet[10-14,16] (see "Checking Anesthesia Machines").

Inert Gas Administration

Administration of a third inert gas, such as helium, nitrogen, or carbon dioxide, can cause a hypoxic mixture because contemporary proportioning systems link only nitrous oxide and oxygen.[12-27,47] Use of an oxygen analyzer is mandatory if the operator uses a third inert gas.

Dilution of Inspired Oxygen Concentration by Volatile Inhaled Anesthetics

Volatile inhaled anesthetics, like inert gases, are added to the mixed gases downstream from the flow meters and the proportioning system. Concentrations of less potent inhaled anesthetics such as desflurane may account for a larger percentage of the total fresh gas than more potent agents. This can be seen when the maximum vaporizer dial settings of the various volatile agents are examined (e.g., desflurane's maximum dial setting of 18% versus isoflurane's maximum dial setting of 5%). Because significant percentages of these inhaled anesthetics may be added downstream of the proportioning system, the resulting gas-vapor mixture may contain an inspired oxygen concentration that is less than 21% despite a functional proportioning system. The anesthesiologist must be aware of this possibility, particularly when high concentrations of lower-potency, inhaled volatile anesthetics are used.

Oxygen Flush Valve

The oxygen flush valve allows direct communication between the oxygen high-pressure circuit and the low-pressure circuit (see Fig. 9-3). Flow from the oxygen flush valve enters the low-pressure circuit downstream from the vaporizers and downstream from the Datex-Ohmeda machine outlet check valve. The spring-loaded oxygen flush valve stays closed until the operator opens it by depressing the oxygen flush button. Actuation of the valve delivers 100% oxygen at a rate of 35 to 75 L/min to the breathing circuit.[9]

The oxygen flush valve can provide a high-pressure oxygen source suitable for jet ventilation when the anesthesia machine is equipped with a one-way check valve positioned between the vaporizers and the oxygen flush valve and when a positive-pressure relief valve exists downstream of the vaporizers; this pressure relief valve must be upstream of the outlet check valve. Because the Ohmeda Modulus II has such a one-way check valve and its positive-pressure relief valve is upstream from the check valve, the entire oxygen flow of 35 to 75 L/min is delivered to the common gas outlet at a high pressure of 50 psig. However, the Ohmeda Modulus II Plus and some Ohmeda Excel machines are not capable of functioning as an appropriate oxygen source for jet ventilation. The Ohmeda Modulus II Plus, which does not have the check valve, provides only 7 psig at the common gas outlet because some oxygen flow travels retrograde through an internal relief valve located upstream from the oxygen flush valve. The Ohmeda Excel 210, which does have a one-way check valve, also has a positive-pressure relief valve downstream from the check valve and is therefore unsuitable for jet ventilation.[16] The older North American Dräger Narkomed 2A, which does not have the check valve, provides an intermediate pressure of 18 psig to the common gas outlet because some oxygen flow travels retrograde through a pop-off valve located in the vaporizers.[48]

The oxygen flush valve is associated with several hazards. A defective or damaged valve can stick in the fully open position, resulting in barotrauma.[49] A valve sticking in a partially open position can result in awareness by the patient because the oxygen flow from the incompetent valve dilutes the inhaled anesthetic.[50] Improper use of normally functioning oxygen flush valves also can result in problems. Overzealous intraoperative oxygen flushing can dilute inhaled anesthetics. Oxygen flushing during the inspiratory phase of positive-pressure ventilation can produce barotrauma in patients if the anesthesia machine does not incorporate fresh gas decoupling or an appropriately adjusted inspiratory pressure limiter. Anesthesia systems (i.e., Dräger Narkomed 6000, Julian, and Fabius GS and Datascope Anestar) with fresh gas decoupling are inherently safer from the standpoint of minimizing the chance of producing barotrauma from inappropriate use of an oxygen flush valve (see "Fresh Gas Decoupling"). With traditional anesthesia breathing circuits, excess volume cannot be vented during the inspiratory phase of mechanical ventilation because the ventilator's relief valve is closed and the adjustable pressure-limiting (APL) valve is "out of circuit" or closed.[51] One caveat is illustrated by the Datex-Ohmeda S/5 ADU and Aestiva. These circle systems use an integrated, adjustable pressure limiter. If this device is properly adjusted, it functions like the APL valve to limit the maximum airway pressure to a safe level, thereby reducing the possibility of barotrauma.[34,35,52] If a machine is equipped with a freestanding vaporizer downstream from the common gas outlet, oxygen flushing can deliver large quantities of inhaled anesthetic to the patient. Inappropriate preoperative use of the oxygen flush to evaluate the low-pressure circuit for leaks can be misleading, particularly on Datex-Ohmeda machines with a one-way check valve at the common outlet.[53] Because backpressure from the breathing circuit closes the one-way check valve air-tight, major leaks in the low-pressure-circuit can go undetected with this leak test (see "Checking Anesthesia Machines").

VAPORIZERS

Through the years, vaporizers have evolved from rudimentary ether inhalers and copper kettles to the present temperature-compensated, variable-bypass vaporizers. In 1993, with the clinical introduction of desflurane, an even more sophisticated vaporizer was introduced to handle the unique physical properties of this agent.

A newer generation of anesthesia vaporizers blending the older, copper kettle–like technology and innovative, computer-controlled technology has emerged in the Datex-Ohmeda Aladin Cassette Vaporizer system. Before the discussion of variable-bypass vaporizers, the Datex-Ohmeda Tec 6 desflurane vaporizer, and the Datex-Ohmeda Aladin cassette vaporizer, certain physical principles are reviewed to facilitate understanding of the operating principles, construction, and design of contemporary vaporizers.

Physics

Vapor Pressure

Contemporary inhaled volatile anesthetics exist in the liquid state below 20°C. When a volatile liquid is in a closed container, molecules escape from the liquid phase to the vapor phase until the number of molecules in the vapor phase is constant. These molecules bombard the wall of the container and create a pressure known as the *saturated vapor pressure*. As the temperature increases, more molecules enter the vapor phase, and the vapor pressure increases (Fig. 9-13). Vapor pressure is independent of atmospheric pressure and is contingent only on the temperature and physical characteristics of the liquid. The boiling point of a liquid is the temperature at which the vapor pressure equals atmospheric pressure.[54-56] At 760 mm Hg, the boiling points for desflurane, isoflurane, halothane, enflurane, and sevoflurane are approximately 22.8°C, 48.5°C, 50.2°C, 56.5°C, and 58.5°C, respectively. Unlike other contemporary inhaled anesthetics, desflurane boils at temperatures that may be encountered in clinical settings such as pediatric and burn operating rooms. This unique physical characteristic alone mandates a special vaporizer design to control the delivery of desflurane. If agent-specific vaporizers are inadvertently misfilled with incorrect liquid anesthetic agents, the resulting mixtures of volatile agents may demonstrate unique properties from those of the individual component agents.

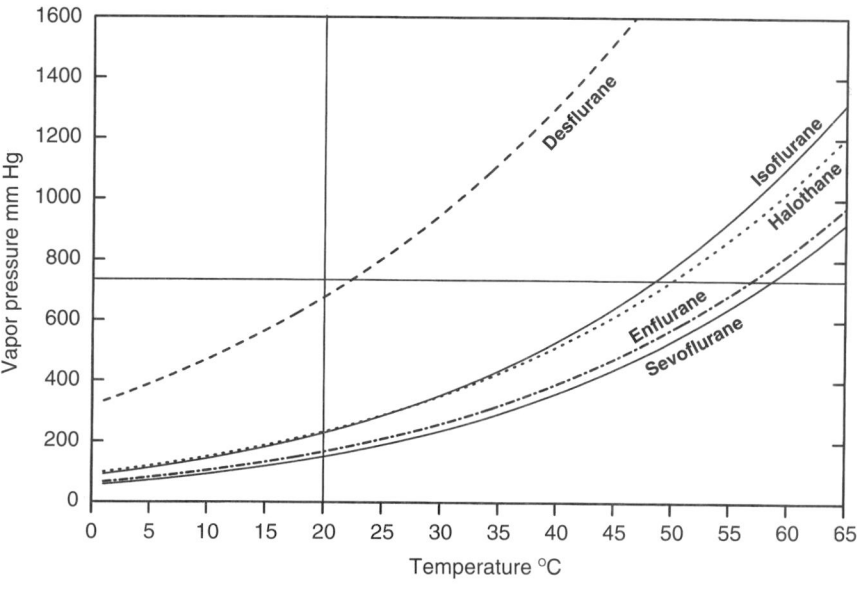

Figure 9–13 Vapor pressure versus temperature curves for desflurane, isoflurane, halothane, enflurane, and sevoflurane. The vapor pressure curve for desflurane is steeper and shifted to higher vapor pressures compared with the curves for other contemporary inhaled anesthetics. (From inhaled anesthetic package insert equations and from Susay SR, Smith MA, Lockwood GG: The saturated vapor pressure of desflurane at various temperatures. Anesth Analg 83:864-866, 1996.)

The altered vapor pressure and other physical properties of the azeotropic mixtures that result from mixing various agents may alter the output of the anesthetic vaporizer[57] (see "Misfilling").

Latent Heat of Vaporization

Energy must be expended to convert a molecule from the liquid to gaseous state because the molecules of a liquid tend to cohere. The *latent heat of vaporization* is defined as the number of calories required to change 1 g of liquid into vapor without a temperature change. The energy for vaporization must come from the liquid itself or from an outside source. The temperature of the liquid decreases during vaporization in the absence of an outside energy source. Energy loss can lead to significant decreases in temperature of the remaining liquid. This temperature drop can greatly decrease vaporization.[54,56,58]

Specific Heat

The *specific heat* of a substance is the number of calories required to increase the temperature of 1 g of a substance by 1°C.[45,49,54] The substance can be solid, liquid, or gas. The concept of specific heat is important to the design, operation, and construction of vaporizers because it is applicable in two ways. First, the specific heat value for an inhaled anesthetic is important because it indicates how much heat must be supplied to the liquid to maintain a constant temperature when heat is lost during vaporization. Second, manufacturers select vaporizer component metals that have a high specific heat to minimize temperature changes associated with vaporization.

Thermal Conductivity

Thermal conductivity is a measure of the speed with which heat flows through a substance. The higher the thermal conductivity, the better the substance conducts heat.[54] Vaporizers are constructed of metals that have relatively high thermal conductivity, which helps maintain a uniform temperature.

Variable-Bypass Vaporizers

The Datex-Ohmeda Tec 4, Tec 5, and Tec 7 and the North American Dräger Vapor 19.n and 20.n vaporizers are classified as variable-bypass, flow-over, temperature-compensated, agent-specific, out-of-breathing-circuit vaporizers.[54] *Variable bypass* refers to the method for regulating output concentration. As gas flow enters the vaporizer's inlet, the setting of the concentration control dial determines the ratio of flow that goes through the bypass chamber and through the vaporizing chamber. The gas channeled to the vaporizing chamber flows over a wick system saturated with the liquid anesthetic and subsequently becomes saturated with vapor. *Flow-over* refers to the method of vaporization and is in contrast to a bubble-through system like that of a copper kettle vaporizer. The Tec 4, the Tec 5, Tec 7 and the Vapor 19.n and 20.n are classified as *temperature-compensated* because they are equipped with an automatic temperature-compensating device that helps maintain a constant vaporizer output over a wide range of temperatures. These vaporizers are *agent specific* and *out of circuit* because they are designed to accommodate a single agent and to be located outside the breathing circuit. Variable-bypass vaporizers are used to deliver halothane, enflurane, isoflurane, and sevoflurane, but not desflurane.

Basic Operating Principles

A diagram of a generic variable-bypass vaporizer is shown in Figure 9-14. Vaporizer components include the concentration control dial, the bypass chamber, the vaporizing chamber, the filler port, and the filler cap. Using the filler port, the operator fills the vaporizing chamber with liquid anesthetic. The maximum safe fill level is predetermined by the position of the filler port, which is positioned to minimize the chance of overfilling. If a vaporizer is overfilled or tilted, liquid anesthetic can spill into the bypass chamber, causing an overdose. The concentration control dial is a variable restrictor, and it

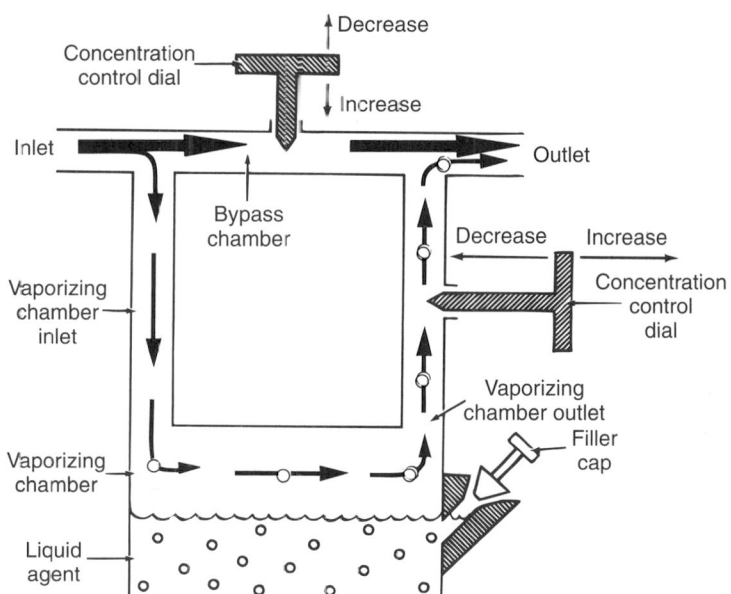

Figure 9–14 Generic variable-bypass vaporizer. Vaporizer components include the concentration control dial, the bypass chamber, the vaporizing chamber, the filler port, and the filler cap. Using the filler port, the operator fills the vaporizing chamber with liquid anesthetic. The maximum safe fill level is predetermined by the position of the filler port, which is positioned to minimize the chance of overfilling. If a vaporizer is overfilled or tilted, liquid anesthetic can spill into the bypass chamber, causing an overdose. The concentration control dial is a variable restrictor, which can be located in the bypass chamber or the outlet of the vaporizing chamber. The function of the concentration control dial is to regulate the relative flow rates through the bypass and vaporizing chambers. (Modified from Andrews JJ, Brockwell RC: Delivery systems for inhaled anesthetics. *In* Barash PG, Cullen BF, Stoelting RK [eds]: Clinical Anesthesia, 4th ed. New York, Lippincott-Raven, 2000, pp 567-594.)

can be located in the bypass chamber or the outlet of the vaporizing chamber. The function of the concentration control dial is to regulate the relative flow rates through the bypass and vaporizing chambers.

Flow from the flow meters enters the inlet of the vaporizer. More than 80% of the flow passes straight through the bypass chamber to the vaporizer outlet, and this accounts for the name *bypass chamber*. Less than 20% of the flow from the flow meters is diverted through the vaporizing chamber. Depending on the temperature and vapor pressure of the particular inhaled anesthetic, the flow through the vaporizing chamber entrains a specific flow of inhaled anesthetic. All three flows—flow through the bypass chamber, flow through the vaporizing chamber, and flow of entrained anesthetic—exit the vaporizer at the outlet. The final concentration of inhaled anesthetic is the ratio of the flow of the inhaled anesthetic to the total gas flow.[54,60]

The vapor pressure of an inhaled anesthetic depends on the ambient temperature (see Fig. 9-13). For example, at 20°C, the vapor pressure of isoflurane is 238 mm Hg, whereas at 35°C, the vapor pressure almost doubles (450 mm Hg). Variable-bypass vaporizers have an internal mechanism to compensate for different ambient temperatures. The temperature-compensating valve of the Datex-Ohmeda Tec–type vaporizer 4 is shown in Figure 9-15.[61] At high temperatures, such as those commonly used in pediatric or burn operating rooms, the vapor pressure inside the vaporizing chamber is high. To compensate for this increased vapor pressure, the bimetallic strip of the temperature-compensating valve leans to the right. This movement allows more flow to pass through the bypass chamber and less flow to pass through the vaporizing chamber. The net effect is a constant vaporizer output. In a cold operating room environment, the vapor pressure inside the vaporizing chamber decreases. To compensate for this decrease in

vapor pressure, the bimetallic strip swings to the left, causing more flow to pass through the vaporizing chamber and less to pass through the bypass chamber. The net effect is a constant vaporizer output.

Factors Influencing Vaporizer Output

The output of an ideal vaporizer with a fixed dial setting would be constant, regardless of varied flow rates, temperatures, backpressures, and carrier gases. Designing such a vaporizer is difficult because, as ambient conditions change, the physical properties of gases and of vaporizers themselves can change.[60] Contemporary vaporizers approach the ideal situation but still have some limitations. Several factors discussed in the following sections can influence vaporizer output.

Flow Rate

With a fixed dial setting, vaporizer output can vary with the rate of gas flowing through the vaporizer. This variation is particularly notable at extremes of flow rates. The output of all variable-bypass vaporizers is less than the dial setting at low flow rates (<250 mL/min). This results from the relatively high density of inhaled volatile anesthetics. Insufficient turbulence is generated at low flow rates in the vaporizing chamber to upwardly advance the vapor molecules. At extremely high flow rates (e.g., 15 L/min), the output of most variable-bypass vaporizers is less than the dial setting. This discrepancy is attributed to incomplete mixing and saturation in the vaporizing chamber. The resistance characteristics of the bypass chamber and the vaporizing chamber can vary as flow increases, and these changes can decrease the output concentration.[60]

Temperature

Because of improvements in design, the output of contemporary temperature-compensated vaporizers is almost

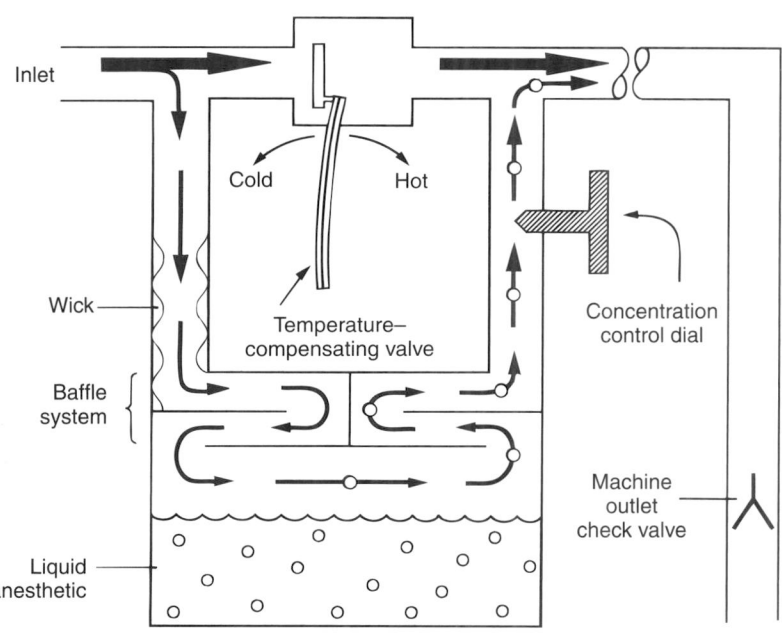

Figure 9–15 Simplified schematic drawing of the Ohmeda Tec–type vaporizer. At high temperatures, the vapor pressure inside the vaporizing chamber is high. To compensate for the increased vapor pressure, the bimetallic strip of the temperature-compensating valve leans to the right, allowing more flow through the bypass chamber and less flow through the vaporizing chamber. The net effect is a constant vaporizer output. In a cold operating room environment, the vapor pressure inside the vaporizing chamber decreases. To compensate for the decreased vapor pressure, the bimetallic strip swings to the left, causing more flow through the vaporizing chamber and less through the bypass chamber. The net effect is a constant vaporizer output. (Modified from Andrews JJ, Brockwell RC: Delivery systems for inhaled anesthetics. *In* Barash PG, Cullen BF, Stoelting RK [eds]: Clinical Anesthesia, 4th ed. New York, Lippincott-Raven, 2000, pp 567-594.)

linear over a wide range of temperatures. Automatic temperature-compensating mechanisms in bypass chambers maintain a constant vaporizer output with varying temperatures.[9,61,62] A bimetallic strip (see Fig. 9-15) or an expansion element (Fig. 9-16) directs a greater proportion of gas flow through the bypass chamber as temperature increases.[60] Wicks are placed in direct contact with the metal wall of the vaporizer to help replace heat used for vaporization. Vaporizers are constructed with metals having relatively high specific heat and high thermal conductivity to minimize heat loss.

Intermittent Backpressure

Intermittent backpressure associated with positive-pressure ventilation or with oxygen flushing can cause higher vaporizer output concentration than the dialed setting. This phenomenon, known as the *pumping effect*,[54,60,63-65] is more pronounced at low flow rates, low dial settings, and low levels of liquid anesthetic in the vaporizing chamber. The pumping effect is increased by rapid respiratory rates, high peak inspired pressures, and rapid drops in pressure during expiration.[61-65] The Datex-Ohmeda Tec 4, Tec 5, and Tec 7 and the North American Dräger Vapor 19.1 and 20.n systems are relatively immune from the pumping effect.[61,62] One proposed mechanism for the pumping effect depends on retrograde pressure transmission from the patient's circuit to the vaporizer during the inspiratory phase of positive-pressure ventilation. Gas molecules are compressed in the bypass and vaporizing chambers. When the backpressure is suddenly released during the expiratory phase of positive-pressure ventilation, vapor exits the vaporizing chamber through the vaporizing chamber outlet and retrograde through the vaporizing chamber inlet. This occurs because the output resistance of the bypass chamber is lower than that of the vaporizing chamber, particularly at low dial settings. The enhanced output concentration results from the increment of vapor that travels in the retrograde direction to the bypass chamber.[60,63-65]

To decrease the pumping effect, the vaporizing chambers of newer systems are smaller than those of older variable-bypass vaporizers such as the Fluotec Mark II (750 mL).[61,62,64] No substantial volumes of vapor can be discharged from the vaporizing chamber into the bypass chamber during the expiratory phase. The North American Dräger Vapor 19.1 and 20.n and the Datex-Ohmeda Tec 5 and Tec 7 (see Fig. 9-16) has a long, spiral tube that serves as the inlet to the vaporizing chamber.[62,64,66] When the pressure in the vaporizing chamber is released, some of the vapor enters this tube but does not enter the bypass chamber because of the tube's length.[64] The Tec 4 (see Fig. 9-15) has an extensive baffle system in the vaporizing chamber, and a one-way check valve has been inserted at the common gas outlet to minimize the pumping effect. This check valve attenuates but does not eliminate the pressure increase because gas still flows from the flow meters to the vaporizer during the inspiratory phase of positive-pressure ventilation.[54,67]

Carrier Gas Composition

Vaporizer output is influenced by the composition of the carrier gas that flows through the vaporizer.[61,62,68-75] When the carrier gas is quickly switched from 100% oxygen to 100% nitrous oxide, there is a rapid transient decrease in vaporizer output followed by a slow increase to a new steady-state value (Fig. 9-17B).[73,74] The transient decrease in vaporizer output is attributed to nitrous oxide's being more soluble than oxygen in halogenated liquid.[73] The quantity of gas leaving the vaporizing chamber is transiently diminished until the anesthetic liquid is totally saturated with nitrous oxide.

The mechanism for the new steady-state output value is less well understood.[75] With contemporary vaporizers such as the North American Dräger Vapor 19.1 and the Ohmeda Tec 4, the steady-state output value is less when nitrous oxide rather than oxygen is the carrier gas (see Fig. 9-17B).[61,62] Conversely, the output of some older vaporizers is enhanced when nitrous oxide is the carrier

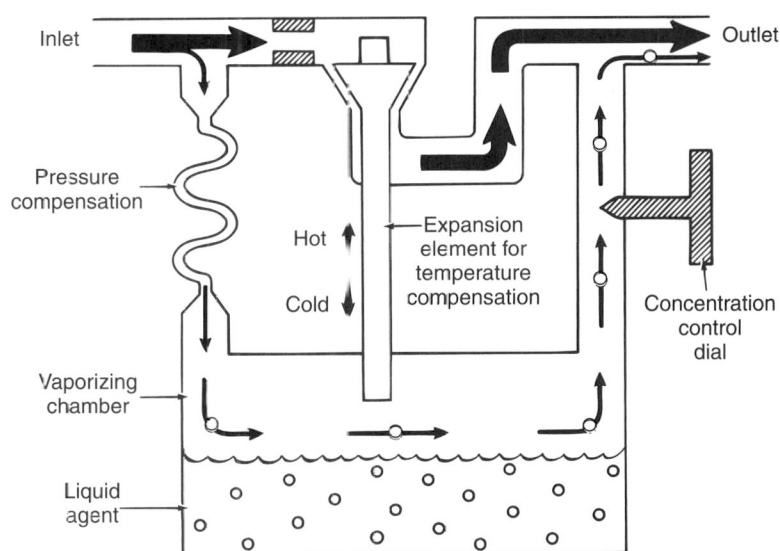

Figure 9–16 Simplified schematic drawing of the North American Dräger Vapor 19.1 vaporizer. Automatic temperature-compensating mechanisms in bypass chambers maintain a constant vaporizer output with varying temperatures. An expansion element directs a greater proportion of gas flow through the bypass chamber as temperature increases. (Modified from Andrews JJ, Brockwell RC: Delivery systems for inhaled anesthetics. *In* Barash PG, Cullen BF, Stoelting RK [eds]: Clinical Anesthesia, 4th ed. New York, Lippincott-Raven, 2000, pp 567-594.)

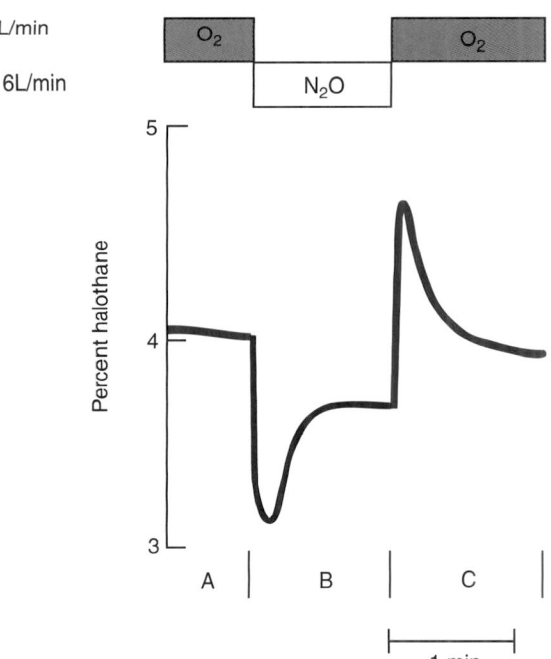

O₂ 6L/min

N₂O 6L/min

Figure 9–17 Halothane output of a North American Dräger Vapor 19.1 vaporizer with different carrier gases. The initial output concentration is approximately 4% halothane when oxygen is the carrier gas at flows of 6 L/min (**A**). When the carrier gas is quickly switched to 100% nitrous oxide (**B**), the halothane concentration decreases to 3% within 8 to 10 seconds. Then, a new steady-state concentration of approximately 3.5% is attained within 1 minute (**C**). (Modified from Gould DB, Lampert BA, MacKrell TN: Effect of nitrous oxide solubility on vaporizer aberrance. Anesth Analg 61:939, 1982.)

gas instead of oxygen.[68,70] The steady-state plateau is achieved more rapidly with increased flow rates, regardless of the ultimate output value.[74] Factors that contribute to the characteristic steady-state response resulting when various carrier gases are used include the viscosity and density of the carrier gas, the relative solubilities of the carrier gas in the liquid anesthetic, the flow-splitting characteristics of the specific vaporizer, and the dial setting.[70,73-75]

Safety Features

The North American Dräger 19.n and 20.n and the Datex-Ohmeda Tec 4, Tec 5, and Tec 7 have safety features that have minimized or eliminated many hazards once associated with variable-bypass vaporizers. Agent-specific, keyed filling devices help prevent filling a vaporizer with the wrong agent. Overfilling of these vaporizers is minimized because the filler port is located at the maximum safe liquid level. Modern vaporizers are firmly secured to the vaporizer manifold, and there is little need to move them. Problems associated with tipping are minimized. Contemporary interlock systems prevent administration of more than one inhaled anesthetic.[61,62,76]

Hazards

Despite many safety features, some hazards are still associated with contemporary variable-bypass vaporizers.

Misfilling

Vaporizers not equipped with keyed fillers occasionally have been misfilled with the wrong anesthetic liquid.[77] A potential for misfilling exists even with contemporary vaporizers equipped with keyed fillers.[78-80]

Contamination

Contamination of anesthetic vaporizer contents has occurred by filling an isoflurane vaporizer with a contaminated bottle of isoflurane. A potentially serious incident was avoided because the operator did not use the contaminated vaporizer after detecting an abnormal acrid odor.[81]

Tipping

Tipping can occur when vaporizers are incorrectly "switched out" or moved. However, tipping is unlikely when a vaporizer is attached to a manifold in the upright position. Excessive tipping can cause the liquid agent to enter the bypass chamber and cause output with extremely high concentration of the agent.[82] The Tec 4 is slightly more immune to tipping than the Vapor 19.1 because of its extensive baffle system. However, if either vaporizer is tipped, it should not be used until it has been flushed for 20 to 30 minutes at high flow rates with the vaporizer set at a low concentration.[54] The Dräger Vapor 2000 series vaporizers have a transport (T) dial setting that helps prevent tipping related problems. When the dial is placed in this position, the vaporizer sump is isolated from the bypass chamber, thereby reducing the likelihood of tipping and a resulting accidental overdose.[83] When one of these vaporizers is moved separate from the anesthesia workstation, the control dial should be placed in the T position. The design of the Aladin cassette system has practically eliminated the possibility of tipping for the Datex-Ohmeda ADU. Because the vaporizer's bypass chamber is physically separated from the cassette and permanently resides in the anesthesia workstation, the possibility of tipping is virtually eliminated barring overturning the entire anesthesia workstation.

Overfilling

Improper filling procedures combined with failure of the vaporizer sight glass can cause overfilling and overdose the patient. Liquid anesthetic enters the bypass chamber, and up to 10 times the intended vapor concentration can be delivered to the common gas outlet.[84]

Underfilling

Just as with overfilling, underfilling of anesthetic vaporizers may be problematic. When a Tec 5 sevoflurane vaporizer is in a low fill state and used under conditions of high fresh gas flow rates (>7.5 L/min) and a high dial setting (e.g., during inhalational inductions), the vaporizer output may abruptly decrease to less than 2%. The causes of this problem are most likely multifactorial, and the exact mechanisms at work are unclear. However, the combination of low vaporizer fill state (<25% full) in combination with the high vaporizing chamber flow can result in a clinically significant and reproducible fall in vaporizer output.[85] Anesthesia care providers must be aware of this phenomenon to avoid problems in their clinical practice.

Simultaneous Administration of Inhaled Anesthetics

Two inhaled anesthetics can be administered simultaneously when the center vaporizer is removed from Datex-Ohmeda machines equipped with the older-style Select-a-Tec vaporizer manifold. The left or right vaporizer should be moved to the central position if the central vaporizer is removed (as indicated by the manifold warning label). The interlock system can then function properly because the two remaining vaporizers are adjacent.[11-13] Later Select-a-Tec vaporizer manifolds have a built-in device that prevents this problem. On these newer systems, a U-shaped plastic device links the vaporizer extension rods even when the vaporizers are not adjacent on the manifold. The manifold plus the vaporizers themselves comprise the *vapor interlock* or *vapor exclusion system*. This system reduces the chances of accidental simultaneous administration of two volatile anesthetic agents.

Leaks

Leaks occur often with vaporizers, and vaporizer leaks can cause awareness by the patient during anesthesia.[54,86-88] A loose filler cap is the most common source of vaporizer leaks. With some key-filled Penlon and Dräger vaporizers, a loose filler screw clamp allows escape of saturated anesthetic vapor.[88] Leaks can occur at the O-ring junction between the vaporizer and its manifold. A vaporizer must be in the on position to detect an internal vaporizer leak. Even though vaporizer leaks in Dräger systems can be detected with a conventional positive-pressure leak test (because of the absence of an outlet check valve), a negative-pressure leak test is more sensitive and allows the user to detect even small leaks. Datex-Ohmeda recommends a negative-pressure leak-testing device (i.e., suction bulb) to detect vaporizer leaks in the Modulus I, Modulus II, Excel, and Aestiva workstations because of the check valve located just upstream of each machine's fresh gas outlet[10-12,14,52] (see "Checking Anesthesia Machines").

Many of the newer anesthesia workstations are capable of performing self-testing procedures, which in some cases may eliminate the need for the conventional negative-pressure leak test. Anesthesia care providers must understand that these machine self-tests cannot detect internal vaporizer leaks on systems with add-on vaporizers. For the self-tests to determine if an internal vaporizer leak is present, the leak test must be repeated with each vaporizer sequentially while its concentration control dial is turned to the on position. When a vaporizer's concentration control dial is set in the off position, it may not be possible to detect even major internal leaks.

Datex-Ohmeda Tec 6 Vaporizer for Desflurane

Controlled vaporization of desflurane requires an electrically heated, pressurized vaporizer because of desflurane's unique physical properties.[89,90] The vapor pressure of desflurane is three to four times that of contemporary inhaled anesthetics, and it boils at 22.8°C,[91] which is near room temperature (see Fig. 9-13). Desflurane has a minimum alveolar anesthetic concentration (MAC) of 6% to 7%.[91] Desflurane is valuable because it has a low

blood gas solubility coefficient of 0.45 at 37°C, and recovery from anesthesia is more rapid than with many other potent inhaled anesthetics.[91]

Unsuitability of Contemporary Variable-Bypass Vaporizers for Controlled Vaporization of Desflurane

Desflurane's high volatility and moderate potency preclude its use with contemporary variable-bypass vaporizers such as Datex-Ohmeda Tec 4, Tec 5, or Tec 7 and the North American Dräger Vapor 19.n or 20.n for two reasons.[89] First, the vapor pressure of desflurane is near 1 atm. The vapor pressures of enflurane, isoflurane, halothane, and desflurane at 20°C are 172, 240, 244, and 669 mm Hg,[91] respectively (see Fig. 9-13). Normal flow through a traditional vaporizer would vaporize many more volumes of desflurane. For example, at 1 atm and 20°C, 100 mL/min passing through the vaporizing chamber entrains 735 mL/min of desflurane versus 29, 46, and 47 mL/min of enflurane, isoflurane, and halothane, respectively.[89] Under these same conditions, the amount of bypass flow necessary to achieve sufficient distribution of anesthetic vapor to produce 1% desflurane output is approximately 73 L/min, compared with 5 L/min or less for the other three anesthetics. Above 22.8°C at 1 atm, desflurane boils. The amount of vapor produced is limited only by the heat energy available from the vaporizer because of its specific heat.[89]

A second reason is that contemporary vaporizers lack an external heat source. Although desflurane has a heat of vaporization approximately equal to that of enflurane, isoflurane, and halothane, its MAC is four to nine times higher than that of the other three inhaled anesthetics. The absolute amount of desflurane vaporized over a given period is considerably higher than with other anesthetics. Supplying desflurane in higher concentrations causes excessive cooling of the vaporizer. In the absence of an external heat source, temperature compensation using traditional mechanical devices would be almost impossible over a broad clinical range of temperatures because of desflurane's steep vapor pressure–versus–temperature curve (see Fig. 9-13).[89]

Operating Principles of the Tec 6

To achieve controlled vaporization of desflurane, Datex-Ohmeda introduced the Tec 6 vaporizer into widespread clinical practice in 1993. This was the first commercially available vaporizer to be electrically heated and pressurized.[92] The physical appearance and operation of the Tec 6 are similar to those of contemporary vaporizers, but some aspects of the internal design and operating principles are radically different. The Tec-6 Plus is a somewhat newer version of the original Tec-6. This device has the same basic Tec-6 design with an enhanced audio alarm system.

A simplified schematic drawing of the Tec 6 vaporizer is shown in Figure 9-18. The vaporizer has two independent gas circuits arranged in parallel. The fresh gas circuit is shown in red, and the vapor circuit is shown in white. The fresh gas from the flow meters enters at the fresh gas inlet, passes through a fixed restrictor (R1), and exits at the vaporizer gas outlet. The vapor circuit originates

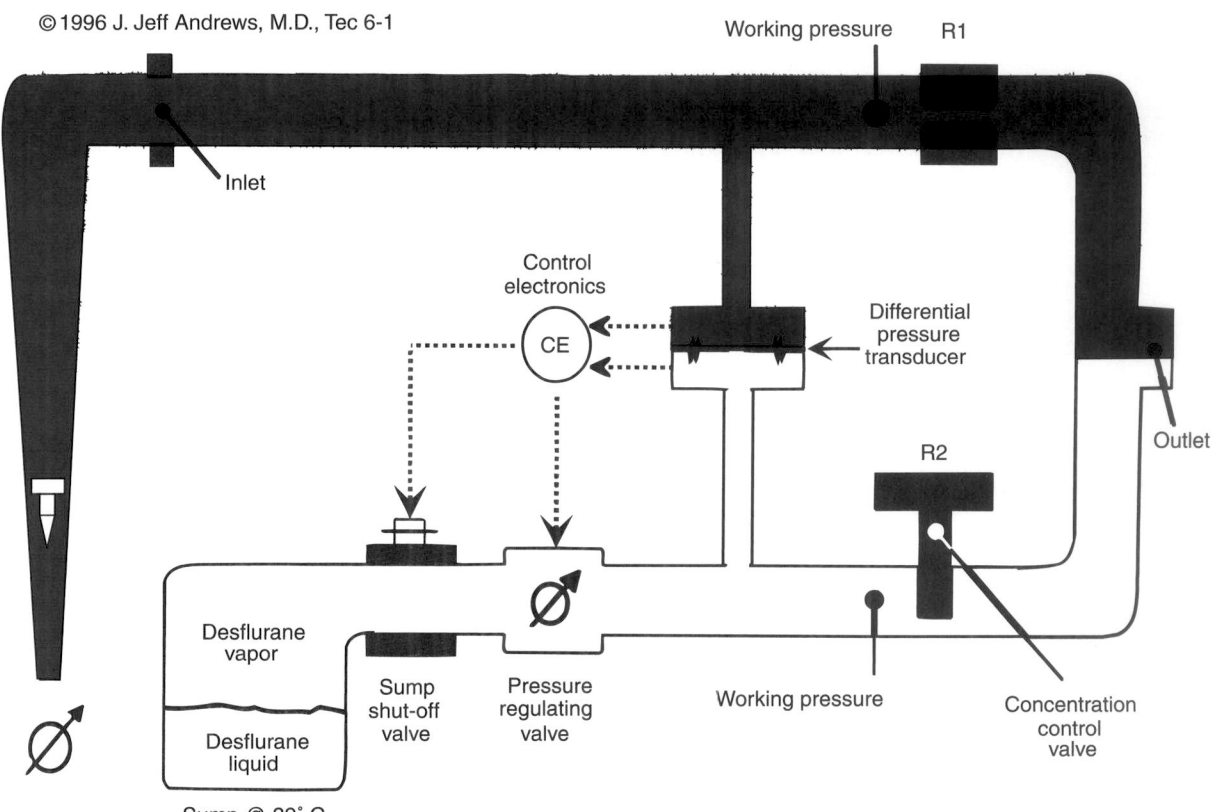

© 1996 J. Jeff Andrews, M.D., Tec 6-1

Figure 9–18 Simplified schematic of the Tec 6 desflurane vaporizer. The vaporizer has two independent gas circuits arranged in parallel. The fresh gas circuit is shown in red, and the vapor circuit is shown in white. The fresh gas from the flow meters enters at the fresh gas inlet, passes through a fixed restrictor (R1), and exits at the vaporizer gas outlet. The vapor circuit originates at the desflurane sump, which is electrically heated and thermostatically controlled to 39°C, a temperature well above desflurane's boiling point. The heated sump assembly serves as a reservoir of desflurane vapor. Downstream from the sump is the shut-off valve. After the vaporizer warms up, the shut-off valve fully opens when the concentration control valve is turned to the on position. A pressure-regulating valve located downstream from the shut-off valve downregulates the pressure. The operator controls desflurane output by adjusting the concentration control valve (R2), which is a variable restrictor. (Adapted from Andrews JJ: Operating Principles of the Ohmeda Tec 6 Desflurane Vaporizer: A Collection of Twelve Color Illustrations. Washington, DC, Library of Congress, 1996.)

at the desflurane sump, which is electrically heated and thermostatically controlled to 39°C, a temperature well above desflurane's boiling point. The heated sump assembly serves as a reservoir of desflurane vapor. At 39°C, the vapor pressure in the sump is approximately 1300 mm Hg absolute,[93] or approximately 2 atm absolute (see Fig. 9-13). Just downstream from the sump is the shut-off valve. After the vaporizer warms up, the shut-off valve fully opens when the concentration control valve is turned to the on position. A pressure-regulating valve located downstream from the shut-off valve downregulates the pressure to approximately 1.1 atm absolute (74 mm Hg gauge) at a fresh gas flow rate of 10 L/min. The operator controls desflurane output by adjusting the concentration control valve (R2), which is a variable restrictor.[89]

The vapor flow through R2 joins the fresh gas flow through R1 at a point downstream from the restrictors. Until this point, the two circuits are physically divorced. They are interfaced pneumatically and electronically, however, through differential pressure transducers, a control electronics system, and a pressure-regulating valve.

When a constant fresh gas flow rate encounters the fixed restrictor, R1, a specific backpressure, proportional to the fresh gas flow rate, pushes against the diaphragm of the control differential pressure transducer. The differential pressure transducer conveys the pressure difference between the fresh gas circuit and the vapor circuit to the control electronics system. The control electronics system regulates the pressure-regulating valve so that the pressure in the vapor circuit equals the pressure in the fresh gas circuit. This equalized pressure supplying R1 and R2 is the *working pressure*, and the working pressure is constant at a fixed fresh gas flow rate. If the operator increases the fresh gas flow rate, more backpressure is exerted on the diaphragm of the control pressure transducer, and the working pressure of the vaporizer increases.[89]

Table 9-1 shows the approximate correlation between fresh gas flow rate and working pressure for a typical vaporizer. At a fresh gas flow rate of 1 L/min, the working pressure is 10 millibars or 7.4 mm Hg gauge. At a fresh gas flow rate of 10 L/min, the working pressure is 100 millibars or 74 mm Hg gauge. There is a linear

Table 9–1   Fresh gas flow rate versus working pressure

Fresh Gas Flow Rate (L/min)	Working Pressure at R1 and R2 by Different Gauges*		
	Millibars	*cm H₂O*	*mm Hg*
1	10	10.2	7.4
5	50	51.0	37.0
10	100	102.0	74.0

*Gas inlet pressure.
R1, fixed restrictor; R2, concentration control valve.
Adapted from Andrews JJ, Johnston RV Jr: The new Tec 6 desflurane vaporizer. Anesth Analg 76:1338, 1993.

relationship between fresh gas flow rate and working pressure. When the fresh gas flow rate is increased 10-fold, the working pressure increases 10-fold.[89]

Two examples are provided to demonstrate the operating principles of the Tec 6.[72] In the first, there is a constant fresh gas flow rate of 1 L/min with an increase in the dial setting. With a fresh gas flow rate of 1 L/min, the working pressure of the vaporizer is 7.4 mm Hg; the pressure supplying R1 and R2 is 7.4 mm Hg. As the operator increases the dial setting, the opening at R2 becomes larger, allowing more vapor to pass through R2. Specific vapor flow values at different dial settings are shown in Table 9-2.

In the second example, there is a constant dial setting with an increase in fresh gas flow from 1 to 10 L/min. At a fresh gas flow rate of 1 L/min, the working pressure is 7.4 mm Hg, and at a dial setting of 6%, the vapor flow rate through R2 is 64 mL/min (see Tables 9-1 and 9-2). With a 10-fold increase in the fresh gas flow rate, there is a concomitant 10-fold increase in the working pressure to 74 mm Hg. The ratio of resistances of R2 to R1 is constant at a fixed dial setting of 6%. Because R2 is supplied by 10 times more pressure, the vapor flow rate through R2 increases 10-fold to 640 mL/min. Vaporizer output is

Table 9–2   Dial setting versus flow through restrictor R2

Dial Setting (Vol %)*	Fresh Gas Flow Rate (L/min)	Approximate Vapor Flow Rate Through R2 (mL/min)
1	1	10
6	1	64
12	1	136
18	1	220

$$\text{*Volume present} = \left(\frac{\text{Vapor flow rate}}{\text{Fresh gas flow rate} + \text{Vapor flow rate}} \right) \times 100\%$$

R2, concentration control valve.
Adapted from Andrews JJ, Johnston RV Jr: The new Tec 6 desflurane vaporizer. Anesth Analg 76:1338, 1993.

constant because both the fresh gas flow and the vapor flow increase proportionally.

Factors that Influence Vaporizer Output
Varied altitude and carrier gas composition influence Tec 6 output.

Varied Altitudes
Unlike contemporary variable-bypass vaporizers, the Tec 6 vaporizer requires manual adjustments of the concentration control dial at altitudes other than sea level to maintain a constant partial pressure of anesthetic. The Tec 6 works at absolute pressures; therefore, altitude makes no difference to the vaporizer's performance. It can accurately deliver the dialed volume percent of desflurane. However, when this gas is brought to ambient atmospheric pressure at high altitudes, the volume percent represents an absolute decrease in the partial pressure of the anesthetic, unlike the contemporary variable-bypass vaporizers, which deliver a constant partial pressure of anesthetic. To compensate for the reduction of partial pressure of vapor at altitude, the Tec 6 rotary valve must be advanced to maintain the required partial pressure of anesthetic. The required dial setting may be calculated using the following formula[92]:

$$\text{Required dial setting} = \text{Normal dial setting (vol \%)} \times 760 \text{ mm Hg/Ambient pressure (mm Hg)}$$

For example, at an altitude of 2000 m or 6564 feet, where the ambient pressure is 608 mm Hg, the operator must advance the concentration control dial from 10% to 12.5% to maintain the required anesthetic partial pressure.[92] In hyperbaric settings, the operator must decrease the dial setting to prevent delivery of an overdose.

Carrier Gas Composition
Vaporizer output approximates the dial setting when oxygen is the carrier gas because the Tec 6 vaporizer is calibrated using 100% oxygen.[92] At low flow rates when a carrier gas other than 100% oxygen is used, a clear trend toward reduction in vaporizer output emerges. This reduction parallels the proportional decrease in viscosity of the carrier gas. Nitrous oxide has a lower viscosity than oxygen, and the backpressure generated by resistor R1 (see Fig. 9-18) is less when nitrous oxide is the carrier gas, and the working pressure is reduced. At low flow rates using nitrous oxide as the carrier gas, vaporizer output is approximately 20% less than the dial setting. This suggests that, at clinically useful fresh gas flow rates, the gas flow across resistor R1 is laminar, and the working pressure is proportional to both the fresh gas flow rate and the viscosity of the carrier gas.[94]

Safety Features
Because desflurane's vapor pressure is near 1 atm, misfilling contemporary vaporizers with desflurane can theoretically cause desflurane overdose and hypoxemia.[95] Datex-Ohmeda has introduced a unique, anesthetic-specific filling system to minimize occurrence of this hazard. The agent-specific filler of the desflurane bottle,

known as the *Saf-T-Fill adapter*, is intended to prevent its use with traditional vaporizers. The filling system also minimizes spillage of liquid or vapor anesthetic by maintaining a "closed system" during the filling process. Each desflurane bottle has a spring-loaded filler cap with an O-ring gasket on the tip. The spring seals the bottle until it is engaged in the filler port of the vaporizer. This anesthetic-specific filling system interlocks the vaporizer and the dispensing bottle, preventing loss of anesthetic to the atmosphere.[92] One case report described misfilling a Tec 6 desflurane vaporizer with sevoflurane, and this error was possible because of similarities between the keyed fillers on the bottles of desflurane and sevoflurane. The desflurane vaporizer detected this error and promptly shut off.[80]

Major vaporizer faults cause the shut-off valve located just downstream from the desflurane sump (see Fig. 9-18) to close, producing a no-output situation. The valve is closed and a no-output alarm is activated immediately if any of the following conditions occur: the anesthetic level decreases to below 20 mL; the vaporizer is tilted; a power failure occurs; or there is a disparity between the pressure in the vapor circuit versus the pressure in the fresh gas circuit exceeding a specified tolerance.[92]

Tec 6 Vaporizer Summary
The Tec 6 vaporizer is an electrically heated, thermostatically controlled, constant-temperature, pressurized, electromechanically coupled, dual-circuit, gas-vapor blender. The pressure in the vapor circuit is electronically regulated to equal the pressure in the fresh gas circuit. At a constant fresh gas flow rate, the operator regulates vapor flow using a conventional concentration control dial. When the fresh gas flow rate increases, the working pressure increases proportionally. At a specific dial setting at different fresh gas flow rates, vaporizer output is constant because the amount of flow through each circuit is proportional.[89]

Datex-Ohmeda Aladin Cassette Vaporizer

The vaporizer system used in the Datex-Ohmeda ADU is unique, and the electronically controlled vaporizer is designed to deliver five different inhaled anesthetics, including halothane, isoflurane, enflurane, sevoflurane, and desflurane. The vaporizer consists of a permanent internal control unit housed within the ADU and an interchangeable Aladin agent cassette that contains anesthetic liquid. The Aladin agent cassettes are color coded for each anesthetic agent, and they are also magnetically coded so that the Datex-Ohmeda ADU can identify which anesthetic cassette has been inserted. The cassettes are filled using agent specific fillers.[54,40]

Although very different in external appearance, the functional anatomy of the Datex-Ohmeda S/5 ADU cassette vaporizer (Fig. 9-19) is very similar to that of the Dräger vapor 19.1 or 20.n and the Datex-Ohmeda Tec 4, Tec 5, or Tec 7 vaporizers, because it is made of a bypass chamber and vaporizing chamber. A fixed restrictor is located in the bypass chamber, and flow-measurement units are located in the bypass chamber and in the outlet of the vaporizing chamber. The heart of the S/5 ADU cassette vaporizer is the electronically controlled flow control valve located in the vaporizing chamber outlet. This valve is controlled by a central processing unit (CPU). The CPU receives input from multiple sources, including the concentration control dial, a pressure sensor located inside the vaporizing chamber, a temperature sensor located inside the vaporizing chamber, a flow-measurement unit located in the bypass chamber, and a flow-measurement unit located in the outlet of the vaporizing chamber. The CPU also receives input from

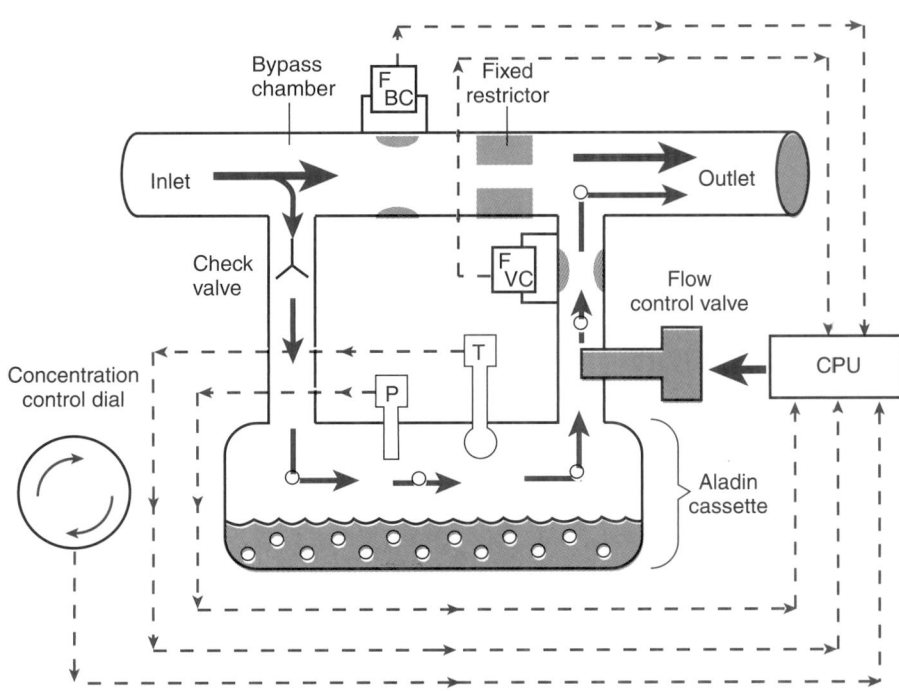

Figure 9–19 Simplified schematic of Datex-Ohmeda Aladin Cassette Vaporizer. The *arrows* represent flow from the flow meters, and the *open circles* represent anesthetic vapor. The heart of the vaporizer is the electronically controlled flow control valve located in the outlet of the vaporizing chamber. CPU, central processing unit, F_{BC}, flow-measurement unit that measures flow through the bypass chamber, F_{VC}, flow-measurement unit that measures flow through the vaporizing chamber, P, pressure sensor, T, temperature sensor. (Modified from Andrews, JJ: Operating Principles of the Datex-Ohmeda Aladin Cassette Vaporizer: A Collection of Color Illustrations. Washington, DC, Library of Congress, 2000.)

the flow meters regarding the composition of the carrier gas. Using data from these multiple sources, the CPU is able to precisely regulate the flow control valve to attain the desired vapor concentration. Appropriate electronic control of the flow control valve is essential to the proper function of this vaporizer.[40,54]

A fixed restrictor is located in the bypass chamber, and it causes the vaporizer inlet flow to split into two portions (see Fig. 9-19). One portion passes through the bypass chamber, and the other portion enters the inlet of the vaporizing chamber and passes through a one-way check valve. The one-way check valve protects against backflow of agent into the bypass chamber, and its presence is crucial when delivering desflurane if the room temperature is greater than the boiling point for desflurane (22.8°C).[54] A precise amount of carrier gas flow and vapor flow passes through the flow control valve, which is regulated by the CPU. This flow then joins the bypass flow to the outlet of the vaporizer.[40,54]

Vaporization of desflurane presents a unique challenge, particularly when the room temperature is greater than the boiling point of desflurane (22.8°C). At higher temperatures, the pressure inside the sump increases, and the sump becomes pressurized. When the sump pressure exceeds the pressure in the bypass chamber, the one-way check valve located in the vaporizing chamber inlet shuts, preventing carrier gas from entering the vaporizing chamber. The carrier gas then passes straight through the bypass chamber. Under these conditions, the electronically controlled flow control valve meters in the appropriate flow of pure desflurane vapor.

When large quantities of anesthetic liquid are vaporized during high fresh gas flow rates and or high dial settings, the vaporizer cools because of the latent heat of vaporization. To offset this cooling effect, the S/5 ADU is equipped with a fan that forces warmed air from an agent-heating resistor across the cassette to raise its temperature when necessary.[35] The fan is activated during two common clinical scenarios: desflurane induction and maintenance and sevoflurane induction.

ANESTHETIC CIRCUITS

Gas exits the anesthesia machine at the common gas outlet and then enters an anesthetic circuit. The function of the anesthesia breathing circuit is to deliver oxygen and anesthetic gases to the patient and to eliminate carbon dioxide. Carbon dioxide can be removed by washout with adequate inflow of fresh gas or by the use of carbon dioxide absorbent media (e.g., soda lime absorption). This discussion is limited to semiclosed rebreathing circuits and the circle system.

Mapleson Systems

In 1954, Mapleson described and analyzed five different semiclosed anesthetic systems, which are classically referred to as the Mapleson systems and designated A to E.[96] Willis and colleagues[97] added the F system to these five original. The Mapleson systems are shown in Figure 9-20. System components can include a facemask, a spring-loaded pop-off valve, reservoir tubing, fresh gas inflow tubing, and a reservoir bag. Three distinct functional groups emerge, and they include the A, the BC, and DEF groups. The Mapleson A, also known as the Magill circuit, has a spring-loaded, pop-off valve located near the facemask, and the fresh gas flow enters the opposite end of the circuit near the reservoir bag. In the B and C systems, the spring-loaded, pop-off valve is located near the facemask, but the fresh gas inlet tubing is located near the patient. The reservoir tubing and breathing bag serve as a blind limb where fresh gas, dead space gas, and alveolar gas can collect. In the Mapleson DEF group, or the T-piece group, the fresh gas enters near the patient, and excess gas is popped off at the opposite end of the circuit.

Even though the component arrangement and components are simple, functional analysis of the Mapleson systems can be complex.[98,99] The amount of carbon dioxide rebreathing associated with each system is multifactorial, and variables that dictate the ultimate carbon dioxide concentration include the following: (1) the fresh gas inflow rate, (2) the minute ventilation, (3) the mode of ventilation (spontaneous or controlled), (4) the tidal volume, (5) the respiratory rate, (6) the inspiratory to expiratory ratio, (7) the duration of the expiratory pause, (8) the peak inspiratory flow rate, (9) the volume of the reservoir tube, (10) the volume of the breathing bag, (11) ventilation by mask, (12) ventilation through an endotracheal tube, and (13) the carbon dioxide sampling site.

Performance of the Mapleson systems is best understood by studying the expiratory phase of the respiratory cycle (see Fig. 9-20).[100] During spontaneous ventilation, the Mapleson A has the best efficiency of the six systems, requiring a fresh gas inflow rate of only one times the minute ventilation to prevent rebreathing of carbon dioxide. However, it has the worst efficiency during controlled ventilation, requiring minute ventilation of as much as 20 L/min to prevent rebreathing. Systems D, E, and F are slightly more efficient than systems B and C. To prevent rebreathing carbon dioxide, systems D to F require a fresh gas inflow rate of approximately 2.5 times the minute ventilation, whereas the fresh gas inflow rates required for systems B and C are somewhat higher.[99]

The following summarizes the relative efficiency of different Mapleson systems with respect to prevention of rebreathing, during spontaneous ventilation: A > DFE > CB. During controlled ventilation, DFE > BC > A.[99,101] The Mapleson A, B, and C systems are rarely used today, but the D, E, and F systems are commonly employed. In the United States, the most popular representative from the DEF group is the Bain circuit.

Bain Circuit

The Bain circuit is a modification of the Mapleson D system. It is a coaxial circuit in which the fresh gas flows through a narrow inner tube within the outer corrugated tubing.[102] The central tube originates near the reservoir bag, but the fresh gas enters the circuit at the patient's end (Fig. 9-21). Exhaled gases enter the corrugated tubing and are vented through the expiratory valve near the reservoir bag. The Bain circuit may be used for spontaneous and controlled ventilation. The fresh gas inflow

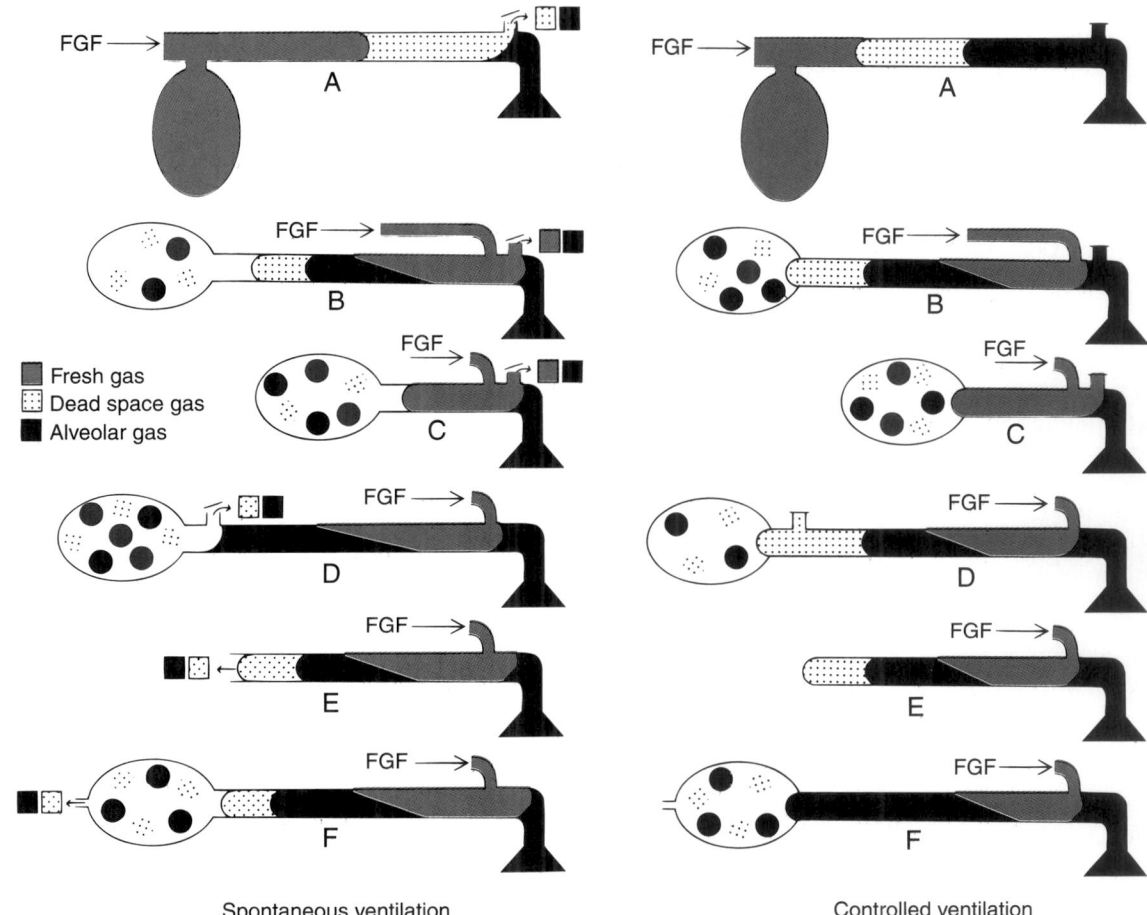

Figure 9–20 Gas disposition at end expiration during spontaneous (*left*) and controlled (*right*) ventilation in circuits A through F. FGF, fresh gas flow. (Adapted from Sykes MK: Rebreathing circuits: A review. Br J Anaesth 40:666, 1968.)

rate necessary to prevent rebreathing is 2.5 times the minute ventilation.

This circuit has many advantages. It is lightweight, convenient, easily sterilized, and reusable. Scavenging of the gases from the expiratory valve is facilitated because the valve is located away from the patient. Exhaled gases in the outer reservoir tubing add warmth to inspired fresh gases. Hazards of the Bain circuit include unrecognized

disconnection or kinking of the inner fresh gas hose. These problems can cause hypercarbia from inadequate gas flow or increased respiratory resistance. An obstructed bacterial filter positioned between the Bain circuit and the endotracheal tube can cause hypoxemia and mimic the signs and symptoms of severe bronchospasm.[103]

The outer tube should be transparent to allow inspection of the inner tube. The integrity of the inner tube can

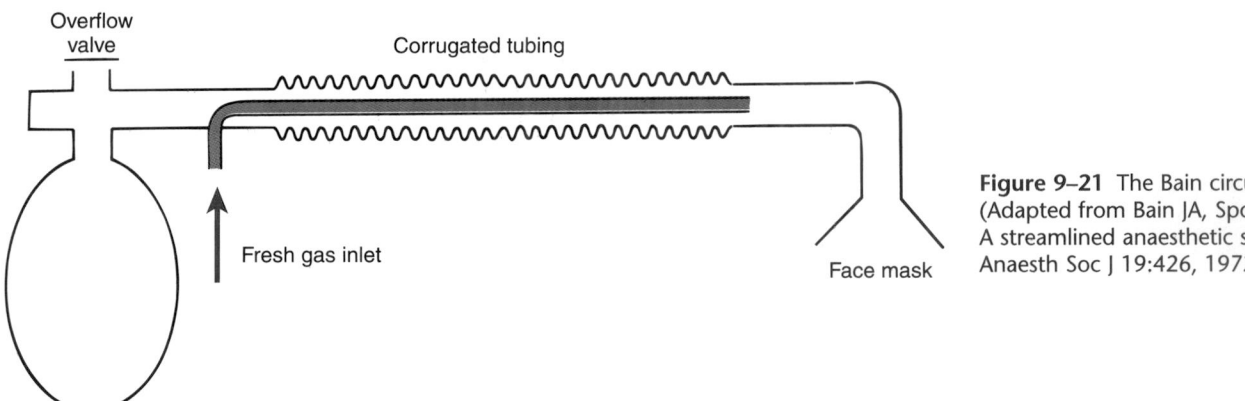

Figure 9–21 The Bain circuit. (Adapted from Bain JA, Spoerel WE: A streamlined anaesthetic system. Can Anaesth Soc J 19:426, 1972.)

be assessed as described by Pethick.[104] High-flow oxygen is fed into the circuit while the patient's end is occluded until the reservoir bag is filled. The patient's end is opened, and oxygen is flushed into the circuit. If the inner tube is intact, the Venturi effect occurs at the patient's end, decreasing pressure within the circuit, and the reservoir bag deflates. Conversely, a leak in the inner tube allows the fresh gas to escape into the expiratory limb, and the reservoir bag remains inflated. This test is recommended as a part of the preanesthesia check if a Bain circuit is used.

Traditional Circle Breathing System

The circle system is the most popular breathing system in the United States. It is so named because its components are arranged in a circular manner. A newer version of the traditional circle system, referred to as a *universal F* or *single-limb circuit*, is growing in popularity. Although these systems appear different externally, they have the same overall functional layout as the traditional circle system and the following discussion is also applicable to them.

The circle system prevents rebreathing of carbon dioxide by use of carbon dioxide absorbents but allows partial rebreathing of other exhaled gases. The extent of rebreathing of the other exhaled gases depends on component arrangement and the fresh gas flow rate. A circle system can be semiopen, semiclosed, or closed, depending on the amount of fresh gas inflow.[105] A semiopen system has no rebreathing and requires a very high flow of fresh gas. A semiclosed system is associated with rebreathing of gases and is the most commonly used system in the United States. A closed system is one in which the inflow gas exactly matches that being consumed by the patient. In a closed system, there is complete rebreathing of exhaled gases after absorption of carbon dioxide, and the overflow (pop-off) valve or relief valve of the ventilator remain closed.

The circle system (Fig. 9-22) consists of seven components: (1) a fresh gas inflow source; (2) inspiratory and expiratory unidirectional valves; (3) inspiratory and expiratory corrugated tubes; (4) a Y-piece connector; (5) an overflow or pop-off valve, referred to as the APL valve; (6) a reservoir bag; and (7) a canister containing a carbon dioxide absorbent. The unidirectional valves are placed in the system to ensure unidirectional flow through the corrugated hoses. The fresh gas inflow enters the circle by a connection from the common gas outlet of the anesthesia machine.

Numerous variations of the circle arrangement are possible, depending on the relative positions of the unidirectional valves, the pop-off valve, the reservoir bag, the carbon dioxide absorber, and the site of fresh gas entry. However, to prevent rebreathing of carbon dioxide in a traditional circle system, three rules must be followed:
1. Unidirectional valves must be located between the patient and the reservoir bag on the inspiratory and expiratory limbs of the circuit.
2. The fresh gas inflow cannot enter the circuit between the expiratory valve and the patient.
3. The overflow (pop-off) valve cannot be located between the patient and the inspiratory valve.

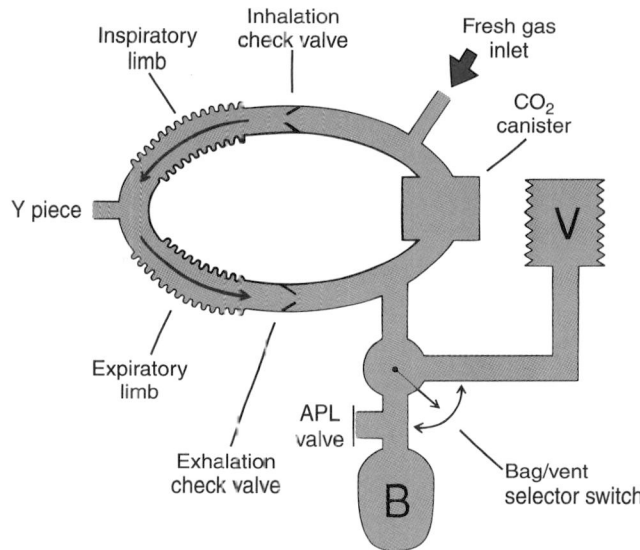

Figure 9–22 Components of the circle system. APL, adjustable pressure limiting; B, reservoir bag; V, ventilator.

If these rules are followed, any arrangement of the other components prevents rebreathing of carbon dioxide.[106] Some newer anesthesia workstations employ less traditional circle breathing systems. Two of these systems are discussed in a later section (see "Newer Anesthesia Workstations").

The most efficient arrangement of the circle system that allows the highest conservation of fresh gases is one with the unidirectional valves near the patient and the pop-off valve just downstream from the expiratory valve. This arrangement conserves dead space gas and preferentially eliminates alveolar gas. A more practical arrangement, the one used on most conventional anesthesia machines (see Fig. 9-22), is somewhat less efficient because it allows alveolar and dead space gas to mix before venting.[106,107]

The advantages of the circle system include a relative stability of inspired gas concentrations, conservation of respiratory moisture and heat, and prevention of operating room pollution. It also can be used for closed system anesthesia or with low oxygen flows. The major disadvantage of the circle system stems from its complex design. The circle system has approximately 10 different connections. Multiple connection sites set the stage for misconnections, disconnections, obstructions, and leaks. In a closed claim analysis of adverse anesthetic outcomes arising from gas delivery equipment, one third (25 of 72) of malpractice claims resulted from misconnections or disconnections of the breathing circuit.[2] Malfunctioning valves can cause serious problems. Rebreathing can occur if the valves stick in the open position, and total occlusion of the circuit can occur if they are stuck closed. If the expiratory valve is stuck shut, breath stacking and tension pneumothorax can occur. Obstructed filters located in the expiratory limb of the circle breathing system have caused increased airway pressures, hemodynamic collapse, and bilateral tension pneumothorax. Obstruction of the expiratory filter may occur because of defective filters, patients' secretions, or albuterol nebulization.[108-110]

The Datex-Ohmeda 7900 SmartVent uses flow transducers on the inspiratory and expiratory limbs of the circle system. Cracked flow-transducer tubing can cause a leak in the circle system that is difficult to detect.[111]

CARBON DIOXIDE ABSORPTION

Different anesthesia systems eliminate carbon dioxide with various degrees of efficiency. The closed and semi-closed circle systems require carbon dioxide absorption. Desirable features of carbon dioxide absorbents include lack of toxicity with common anesthetics, low resistance to airflow, low cost, ease of handling, and efficiency.

Absorber Canister

On modern anesthesia machines, the absorber canister (see Fig. 9-22) is composed of two clear plastic canisters arranged in series. The canisters can be filled with bulk absorbent or with absorbent supplied by the factory in prefilled plastic disposable cartridges called *prepacks*. Free granules from bulk absorbent can create a clinically significant leak if they lodge between the clear plastic canister and the O-ring gasket of the absorber. Leaks have also been caused by defective prepacks that were larger than factory specifications.[112] Prepacks can also cause total obstruction of the circle system if the clear plastic shipping wrapper is not removed before use.[113]

Chemistry of Absorbents

Three formulations of carbon dioxide absorbents are commonly available: soda lime, Baralyme, and calcium hydroxide lime (Amsorb). Of these agents, the most commonly used is soda lime. All serve to eliminate carbon dioxide from the breathing circuit with various degrees of efficiency.

By weight, the approximate composition of "high-moisture" soda lime is 80% calcium hydroxide, 15% water, 4% sodium hydroxide, and 1% potassium hydroxide (an activator). Small amounts of silica are added to produce calcium and sodium silicate. This addition produces a hard compound and reduces dust formation. The efficiency of the soda lime absorption varies inversely with the hardness; therefore, little silicate is used in contemporary soda lime. Sodium hydroxide is the catalyst for the carbon dioxide absorptive properties of soda lime.[114,115] Baralyme is a mixture of approximately 20% barium hydroxide and 80% calcium hydroxide. It may also contain some potassium hydroxide. Calcium hydroxide lime is one of the newest commercially available carbon dioxide absorbents. It consists primarily of calcium hydroxide and calcium chloride and contains two setting agents: calcium sulfate and polyvinylpyrrolidine. The latter two agents enhance the hardness and porosity of the agent.[116] The most significant advantage of calcium hydroxide lime over other agents is its lack of sodium and potassium hydroxides. The absence of these chemicals eliminates the undesirable production of carbon monoxide and the nephrotoxic substance known as compound A.[117]

The size of the absorptive granules has been determined by trial and error, which represents a compromise between resistance to airflow and absorptive efficiency.[118] The smaller the granules, the more surface area is available for absorption. However, air flow resistance increases. The granular size of soda lime and Baralyme in anesthesia practice is between 4 and 8 mesh, a size at which resistance to airflow is negligible. Mesh refers to the number of openings per linear inch in a sieve through which the granular particles can pass. A 4-mesh screen means that there are four 0.25-inch openings per linear inch. An 8-mesh screen has eight 0.125-inch openings per linear inch.[114]

The absorption of carbon dioxide by soda lime is a chemical process, not a physical process. Carbon dioxide combines with water to form carbonic acid. Carbonic acid reacts with the hydroxides to form sodium (or potassium) carbonate and water. Calcium hydroxide accepts the carbonate to form calcium carbonate and sodium (or potassium) hydroxide. The equations for the reaction steps are as follows

1. $CO_2 + H_2O \Leftrightarrow H_2CO_3$
2. $H_2CO_3 + 2NaOH (KOH) \Leftrightarrow Na_2CO_3 (K_2CO_3) + 2H_2O +$ Heat
3. $Na_2CO_3 (K_2CO_3) + Ca(OH)_2 \Leftrightarrow CaCO_3 + 2NaOH (KOH)$

Some carbon dioxide may react directly with $Ca(OH)_2$, but this reaction is much slower.

The reaction with Baralyme differs from that of soda lime because more water is liberated by a direct reaction of barium hydroxide and carbon dioxide.

1. $Ba(OH)_2 + 8H_2O + CO_2 \Leftrightarrow BaCO_3 + 9H_2O +$ Heat
2. $9H_2O + 9CO_2 \Leftrightarrow 9H_2CO_3$

Then by direct reactions and by KOH and NaOH,

3. $9H_2CO_3 + 9Ca(OH)_2 \Leftrightarrow CaCO_3 + 18H_2O +$ Heat

Absorptive Capacity

The maximum amount of carbon dioxide that can be absorbed by soda lime is 26 L of carbon dioxide per 100 g of absorbent. The absorptive capacity of calcium hydroxide lime has been reported at 10.2 L per 100 g of absorbent.[116] However, channeling of gas through granules of soda lime or calcium hydroxide lime may substantially decrease this efficiency and allow only 10 to 20 L or less of carbon dioxide to be absorbed per 100 g of absorbent.[119]

Indicators

Ethyl violet, the pH indicator added to soda lime and Baralyme to help assess the functional integrity of the absorbent, is a substituted triphenylmethane dye with a critical pH of 10.3.[115] Ethyl violet changes in color from colorless to violet when the pH of the absorbent decreases as a result of carbon dioxide absorption. The pH of fresh absorbent exceeds the critical pH, and the dye exists in its colorless form (Fig. 9-23A). As absorbent becomes exhausted, however, the pH decreases below 10.3, and ethyl violet changes to its violet form (see Fig. 9-23B) through alcohol dehydration. Ethyl violet is not always a reliable indicator of the functional status of absorbent. Fluorescent lights can deactivate the dye so

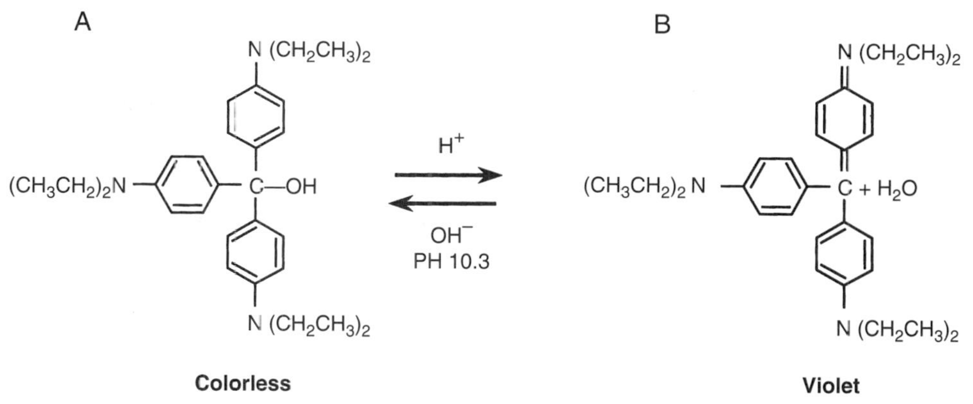

Figure 9–23 Ethyl violet changes from colorless to violet when the pH of the absorbent decreases as a result of carbon dioxide absorption. **A,** The pH of fresh absorbent exceeds the critical level, and the dye exists in its colorless form. **B,** As absorbent becomes exhausted, the pH decreases below 10.3, and ethyl violet changes to its violet form through alcohol dehydration. (Adapted from Andrews JJ, Johnston RV Jr, Bee DE, Arens JF: Photodeactivation of ethyl violet: A potential hazard of Sodasorb. Anesthesiology 72:59, 1990.)

that the absorbent appears white even though it is exhausted.[120]

Interactions of Inhaled Anesthetics with Absorbents

It is important and desirable to have carbon dioxide absorbents that are neither intrinsically toxic nor toxic when exposed to common anesthetics. Soda lime and Baralyme generally fit this description, but inhaled anesthetics do interact with absorbents to some extent. An uncommon anesthetic, trichloroethylene, reacts with soda lime to produce toxic compounds. In the presence of alkali and heat, trichloroethylene degrades into the cerebral neurotoxin dichloroacetylene, which causes cranial nerve lesions and encephalitis. Phosgene, a potent pulmonary irritant, is also produced, and phosgene can cause adult respiratory distress syndrome (ARDS).[121]

Sevoflurane produces degradation products on interaction with carbon dioxide absorbents.[122] The major degradation product produced is an olefin compound known as fluoromethyl-2,2-difluoro-1-(trifluoromethyl) vinyl ether, or compound A. During sevoflurane anesthesia, factors apparently leading to an increase in the concentration of compound A include low-flow or closed-circuit anesthetic techniques, the use of Baralyme rather than soda lime, higher concentrations of sevoflurane in the anesthetic circuit, higher absorbent temperatures, and fresh absorbent.[122-125] Baralyme dehydration increases the concentration of compound A, and soda lime dehydration decreases the concentration of compound A.[126,127] The degradation products apparently do not cause toxic effects in humans, even during low-flow anesthesia,[124] but further studies are needed to verify this.[128-130]

Desiccated soda lime and Baralyme can degrade contemporary inhaled anesthetics to clinically significant concentrations of carbon monoxide, which can produce carboxyhemoglobin concentrations reaching 30% or more.[131] Higher levels of carbon monoxide are more likely after prolonged contact between absorbent and anesthetics and after disuse of an absorber for at least 2 days, especially over a weekend. Case reports describing carbon monoxide poisoning have been most common for patients anesthetized on Monday morning, presumably because continuous flow from the anesthesia machine dehydrated the absorbents over the weekend.[132,133] A fresh gas flow rate of 5 L/min or more through absorbent (without a patient) is sufficient to cause critical drying of the absorbent, particularly if the breathing bag is left off the breathing circuit. Absence of the bag facilitates retrograde flow through the circle system (see Fig. 9-22).[131] Because the inspiratory valve leaflet produces some resistance to flow, the fresh gas flow takes the retrograde path of least resistance through the absorbent and out the 22-mm breathing bag terminal.

Several factors appear to increase the production of carbon monoxide and carboxyhemoglobin:
1. The inhaled anesthetic used (for a given MAC multiple, the magnitude of carbon monoxide production from greatest to least is desflurane ≥ enflurane > isoflurane >> halothane = sevoflurane)
2. The absorbent dryness (completely dry absorbent produces more carbon monoxide than hydrated absorbent)
3. The type of absorbent (at a given water content, Baralyme produces more carbon monoxide than does soda lime)
4. The temperature (a higher temperature increases carbon monoxide production)
5. The anesthetic concentration (more carbon monoxide is produced from higher anesthetic concentrations)[134]
6. Low fresh gas flow rates
7. Reduced animal size[135] per 100 g of absorbent

Interventions have been suggested to reduce the incidence of carbon monoxide exposure in humans undergoing general anesthesia[133]:
1. Educating anesthesia personnel regarding the cause of carbon monoxide production
2. Turning off the anesthesia machine at the conclusion of the last case of the day to eliminate fresh gas flow, which dries the absorbent
3. Changing carbon dioxide absorbent if fresh gas was found flowing during the morning machine check
4. Rehydrating desiccated absorbent by adding water to the absorbent[132]
5. Changing the chemical composition of soda lime (e.g., Dragersorb 800 plus, Sofnolime, Spherasorb) to reduce or eliminate potassium hydroxide
6. Using absorbent materials such as calcium hydroxide lime that are free of sodium and potassium hydroxides

The elimination of sodium and potassium hydroxides from desiccated soda lime diminishes or eliminates degradation of desflurane to carbon monoxide and sevoflurane to compound A but does not compromise carbon dioxide absorption.[117,136]

In late 2003, Abbott Laboratories, North Chicago, IL, makers of sevoflurane, in conjunction with the FDA, published a revised package insert and circulated a letter to anesthesia care providers that explained the potential for fires in the respiratory circuit with the use of sevoflurane. The revised sevoflurane package insert (Abbott Laboratories, reference 58-7208) describes this rare phenomenon occurring when sevoflurane is used in combination with a desiccated carbon dioxide absorbent such as dehydrated Baralyme. A poorly characterized chemical reaction between the sevoflurane and the absorbent reportedly has produced sufficient heat and combustible degradation products to lead to spontaneous generation of fires within the absorber canister subassembly and the breathing circuit. The combination of a rapid color change of the carbon dioxide absorbent (especially Baralyme) and an unusually slow increase in inhaled sevoflurane concentration, compared with the vaporizer concentration control dial setting, may indicate that a decomposition reaction with sevoflurane and the absorbent is occurring. If this happens, the potential for excessive heating or fire may be present within the respiratory circuit. To avoid this, anesthesia care providers should make every effort not to use desiccated carbon dioxide absorbents. Whenever there is a question of whether the absorbent is fresh and adequately hydrated, it should be replaced to avoid the possible occurrence of fire in the respiratory circuit.

ANESTHESIA VENTILATORS

The anesthesia ventilator can substitute for the breathing (reservoir) bag of the circle system, the Bain circuit, and other breathing systems. As recently as the late 1980s, anesthesia ventilators were mere adjuncts to the anesthesia machine, but they have attained a prominent, central role in newer anesthesia workstations. In addition to the nearly ubiquitous role of the anesthesia ventilator in modern anesthesia workstations, many advanced intensive care unit–type ventilation features have been integrated into anesthesia ventilators. This discussion focuses on the classification, operating principles, and hazards of contemporary anesthesia ventilators.

Classification

Ventilators can be classified according to their power source, drive mechanism, cycling mechanism, and bellows type.[137,138] The following section reviews ventilator classification and terminology before the discussion of individual anesthesia machine ventilators.

Power Source
The power source required to operate a mechanical ventilator is provided by compressed gas or electricity, or both. Older pneumatic ventilators required only

a pneumatic power source to function properly. Contemporary electronic ventilators from Dräger, Datex-Ohmeda, and others require an electrical only or electrical and pneumatic power sources.[15,19-27,139,140]

Drive Mechanism and Circuit Designation
Most anesthesia machine ventilators are classified as double-circuit, pneumatically driven ventilators. In a double-circuit system, a driving force (i.e., compressed gas) compresses a bag or bellows, which delivers gas to the patient. The driving gas in the Datex-Ohmeda 7000, 7810, 7100, and 7900 is 100% oxygen.[15,52,139,140] In the North American Dräger AV-E, a Venturi device mixes oxygen and air.[19,21,24-27]

With the introduction of circle breathing systems that integrate fresh gas decoupling, a resurgence has been seen in the use of mechanically driven anesthesia ventilators. These piston-type ventilators use a computer controlled stepper motor instead of compressed drive gas to actuate gas movement in the breathing system. In these systems, rather than having dual circuits with gas for the patient in one and the drive gas in another, there is a single gas circuit for the patient. They are classified as piston-driven, single-circuit ventilators. The piston operates much like the plunger of a syringe to deliver the desired tidal volume or airway pressure to the patient. Sophisticated computerized controls are able to provide advanced types of ventilatory support such as synchronized intermittent mandatory ventilation (SIMV), pressure-controlled ventilation (PCV), and pressure-support ventilation (PSV) in addition to the conventional control-mode ventilation (CMV). Because the patient's mechanical breath is delivered without the use of compressed gas to actuate the bellows, these systems consume less gas during the ventilator's operation than a traditional pneumatic ventilator. This may have clinical significance when the anesthesia workstation is used in a setting where no pipeline gas supply is available (e.g., remote locations, office-based anesthesia practices).

Cycling Mechanism
Most anesthesia machine ventilators are time cycled and provide ventilator support in the control mode. Inspiratory phase is initiated by a timing device. Older pneumatic ventilators use a fluidic timing device. Contemporary electronic ventilators use a solid-state timing device and are classified as time cycled and electronically controlled.

Bellows Classification
The direction of bellows movement during the expiratory phase determines the bellows classification. Ascending (standing) bellows ascend during the expiratory phase (Fig. 9-24B), whereas descending (hanging) bellows descend during the expiratory phase. Older pneumatic ventilators and some new anesthesia workstations use weighted descending bellows, but most contemporary electronic ventilators have an ascending bellows design. Of the two configurations, the ascending bellows design is safer. Ascending bellows do not fill if a total disconnection occurs. The bellows of a descending

Figures 9–24 Inspiratory (**A**) and expiratory (**B**) phases of gas flow in a traditional circle system with an ascending bellows anesthesia ventilator. The bellows physically separates the driving-gas circuit from the patient's gas circuit. The driving-gas circuit is located outside the bellows, and the patient's gas circuit is inside the bellows. During the inspiratory phase (**A**), the driving gas enters the bellows chamber, causing the pressure within it to increase. This causes the ventilator's relief valve to close, preventing anesthetic gas from escaping into the scavenging system, and the bellows to compress, delivering the anesthetic gas within the bellows to the patient's lungs. During the expiratory phase (**B**), the driving gas exits the bellows chamber. The pressure within the bellows chamber and the pilot line declines to zero, causing the mushroom portion of the ventilator's relief valve to open. Gas exhaled by the patient fills the bellows before any scavenging occurs because a weighted ball is incorporated into the base of the ventilator's relief valve. Scavenging happens only during the expiratory phase, because the ventilator's relief valve is open only during expiration. (Adapted from Andrews JJ: The Circle System. A Collection of 30 Color Illustrations. Washington, DC, Library of Congress, 1998.)

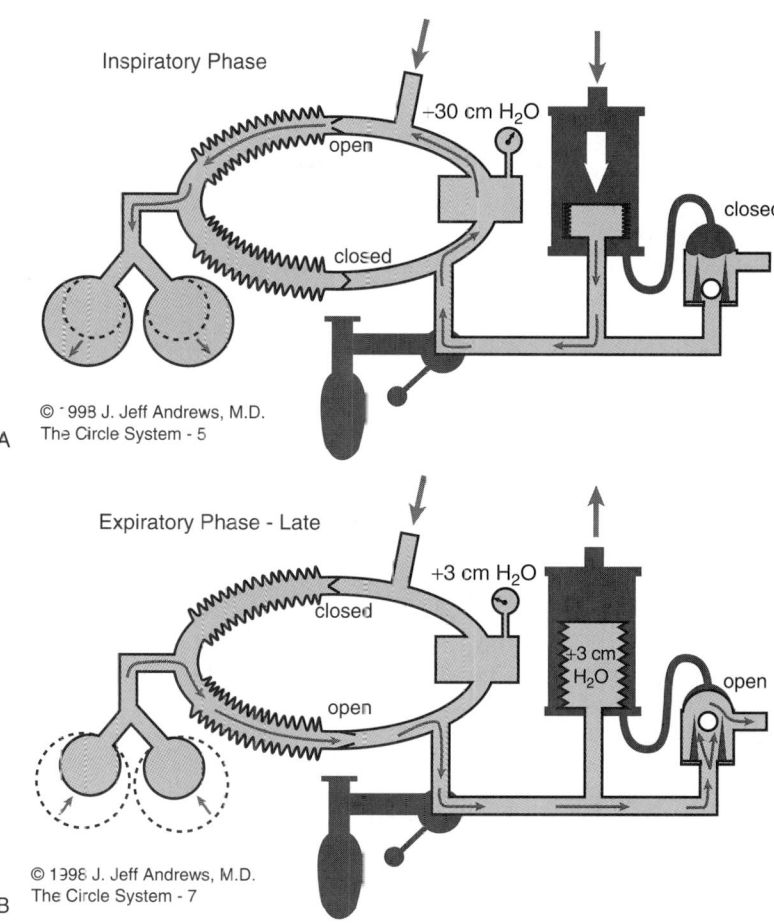

Inspiratory Phase

−30 cm H$_2$O
open
closed
closed

© 1998 J. Jeff Andrews, M.D.
The Circle System - 5

A

Expiratory Phase - Late

+3 cm H$_2$O
closed
+3 cm H$_2$O
open
open

© 1998 J. Jeff Andrews, M.D.
The Circle System - 7

B

bellows ventilator, however, continue upward and downward movement during a disconnection. The driving gas pushes the bellows upward during the inspiratory phase. During the expiratory phase, room air is entrained into the breathing system at the site of the disconnection because gravity acts on the weighted bellows. The disconnection pressure monitor and the volume monitor may be fooled even if a disconnection is complete[1] (see "Breathing Circuit Problems"). Some newer anesthesia systems (i.e., Dräger Julian and Datascope Anestar) have returned to the descending bellows to allow incorporation of fresh gas decoupling. An important safety feature on these descending bellows workstations that should not be considered optional is an integrated carbon dioxide apnea alarm that cannot be disabled while the ventilator is in use.

Operating Principles of Ascending Bellows Ventilators

Contemporary examples of ascending bellows, double-circuit, electronic ventilators include the North American Dräger AV-E and the Datex-Ohmeda 7000, 7800, and 7900 series. A generic ascending bellows ventilator is shown in Figure 9-24. It may be viewed as a breathing bag (i.e., bellows) located within a clear plastic box. The bellows physically separate the driving-gas circuit from the patient's gas circuit. The driving-gas circuit is located outside the bellows, and the patient's gas circuit is inside the bellows. During the inspiratory phase (see Fig. 9-24A),

the driving gas enters the bellows chamber, causing the pressure within it to increase. This increase in pressure is responsible for two events. First, the ventilator's relief valve closes, preventing anesthetic gas from escaping into the scavenging system. Second, the bellows are compressed, and the anesthetic gas within the bellows is delivered to the patient's lungs. This compression action is analogous to the hand of the anesthesiologist squeezing the breathing bag.[51]

During the expiratory phase (see Fig. 9-24B), the driving gas exits the bellows' chamber. The pressure within the bellows' chamber and the pilot line decline to zero, causing the mushroom portion of the ventilator's relief valve to open. Gas exhaled by the patient fills the bellows before any scavenging occurs. This happens because a weighted ball similar to those used in ball-type positive end-expiratory pressure (PEEP) valves is incorporated into the base of the ventilator's relief valve. The ball produces 2 to 3 cm H$_2$O of backpressure; therefore scavenging occurs only after the bellows fill completely and the pressure inside the bellows exceeds this pressure threshold. This design causes all ascending bellows ventilators to produce 2 to 3 cm H$_2$O of PEEP within the breathing circuit. Scavenging occurs only during the expiratory phase because the ventilator relief valve is open only during expiration.[51]

Gas flow from the anesthesia machine into the breathing circuit is continuous and independent of ventilator activity. During the inspiratory phase of mechanical ventilation, the ventilator's relief valve is closed, and the breathing system's APL valve (pop-off valve) is closed or out of circuit. The patient receives a volume from the bellows and flow meters during the inspiratory phase. Factors that influence the correlation between set tidal volume and exhaled tidal volume include the flow meter's settings, the inspiratory time, the compliance of the breathing circuit, external leakage, and the location of the tidal volume sensor.[15,16,139,140] Usually, the volume gained from the flow meters during inspiration is counteracted by the volume lost to the breathing circuit compliance. The set tidal volume generally approximates the exhaled tidal volume. However, oxygen flushing during the inspiratory phase can result in barotrauma because excess volume cannot be vented.[51]

Problems and Hazards

Numerous hazards are associated with anesthesia ventilators, including problems with the breathing circuit, the bellows assembly, and the control assembly.

Traditional Circle System Problems

Disconnection of the breathing circuit is a leading cause of critical incidents in anesthesia practice.[2,141] The most common disconnection site is at the Y-piece. Disconnections can be complete or partial (i.e., leaks). A common source of leaks with older absorbers is failure to close the APL (pop-off) valve on initiation of mechanical ventilation. The bag or ventilator switch on contemporary absorbers helps minimize this problem. Preexisting, undetected leaks can occur in compressed, corrugated, disposable anesthetic circuits. To detect such a leak preoperatively, the circuit must be fully expanded before the circuit is checked for leaks.[142] Disconnections and leaks manifest more readily with the ascending bellows because the bellows will not fill.[1]

Several disconnection monitors exist. The most important monitor is a vigilant anesthesia care provider monitoring breath sounds, chest wall excursion, and mechanical monitors.

Pneumatic and electronic pressure monitors are helpful in diagnosing disconnections. Factors that influence the monitor's effectiveness include the disconnection site, location of the pressure sensor, the threshold-pressure alarm's limit, the inspiratory flow rate, and the resistance of the disconnected breathing circuit.[143,144] Various anesthesia machines and ventilators have different locations for the pressure sensor and different values for the threshold-pressure alarm's limit. The limit for the threshold-pressure alarm may be preset at the factory or adjustable. An audible or visual alarm is actuated if the peak inspiratory pressure of the breathing circuit does not exceed the threshold-pressure alarm's limit. When an adjustable limit for the threshold-pressure alarm is available, such as on the Dräger Narkomed 2A, 2B, 2C, 3, 4, and GS, the operator should set the pressure alarm limit to within 5 cm H_2O of the peak inspiratory pressure.[14-16,19,21,24] Figure 9-25 illustrates how a partial disconnection (i.e., leak) may be unrecognized by the low-pressure monitor if the threshold-pressure alarm's limit is set too low or if the factory preset value is relatively low.

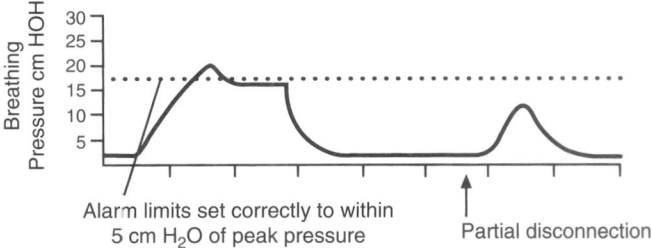

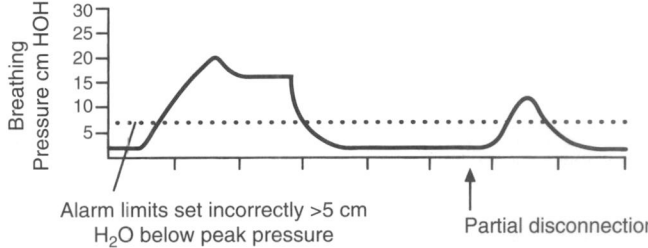

Figure 9–25 The threshold-pressure alarm's limit (*dotted line*) has been set appropriately (*top*). An alarm is actuated when a partial disconnection occurs (*arrow*) because the threshold-pressure alarm's limit is not exceeded by the breathing-circuit pressure. A partial disconnection (*arrow*) is unrecognized by the pressure monitor because the threshold-pressure alarm's limit has been set too low (*bottom*). (Adapted from Baromed Breathing Pressure Monitor. Operator's Instruction Manual. Telford, PA, North American Dräger, August 1986.)

Respiratory volume monitors are useful in detecting disconnections. Volume monitors sense exhaled tidal volume, minute volume, or both. The user should bracket the high and low threshold volumes slightly above and below the exhaled volumes. For example, if the exhaled minute volume of a patient is 10 L/min, reasonable alarm limits are 8 to 12 L/min. Some Datex-Ohmeda ventilators are equipped with sensors to monitor volume that use infrared light and turbine technology. The volume sensor is usually located in the expiratory limb of the breathing circuit, except in the case of the Datex-Ohmeda S/5 ADU (see "Newer Anesthesia Workstations"). Exposure of the infrared-type sensor clip to a direct beam of overhead surgical lighting can cause erroneous volume readings because the surgical beam interferes with the infrared sensor.[145] Other types of expiratory volume sensors can be seen in systems such as the Datex-Ohmeda S/5 ADU, the Aestiva, and other workstations that incorporate the 7100 ventilator or 7900 SmartVent.[35,36,52] These systems generally use differential pressure transduction technology to determine inhaled and exhaled volumes. Still other systems from Dräger measure exhaled volume using ultrasonic or "hot wire" sensor technology.[20]

Carbon dioxide monitors are probably the best devices for revealing disconnections to the patient. Carbon dioxide concentration is measured near the Y-piece directly or by aspiration of a gas sample to the instrument. A drastic change in the difference between the inspiratory and end-tidal carbon dioxide concentration or the absence of carbon dioxide indicates a disconnection, a nonventilated patient, or other problems.[1]

Misconnections of the breathing system are not uncommon, despite efforts by standards committees to eliminate this problem by assigning different diameters to various hoses and terminals. Anesthesia machines, breathing systems, ventilators, and scavenging systems incorporate a multitude of hose terminals. Hoses have been connected to inappropriate terminals and even to various solid, cylindrical protrusions of the anesthesia machine.[1]

Occlusion (i.e., obstruction) of the breathing circuit may occur. Tracheal tubes can become kinked. Hoses throughout the breathing circuit are subject to occlusion by external mechanical forces that can impinge on flow. Blockage of a bacterial filter in the expiratory limb of the circle system has caused a bilateral tension pneumothorax.[109] Incorrect insertion of flow direction-sensitive components can result in a no-flow state.[1] Examples of these components include some PEEP valves and cascade humidifiers. Depending on the location of the occlusion and the pressure sensor, a high-pressure alarm may alert the anesthesiologist to the problem.

Excess inflow to the breathing circuit from the anesthesia machine during the inspiratory phase can cause barotrauma. The best example of this phenomenon is oxygen flushing. Excess volume cannot be vented from the system during inspiration because the ventilator's relief valve is closed and because the APL valve is out of circuit or closed.[51] A high-pressure alarm, if present, may be activated when the pressure becomes excessive. With Dräger systems, audible and visual alarms are actuated when the high-pressure threshold is exceeded.[19-27] In the Modulus II Plus system, the Datex-Ohmeda 7810 ventilator automatically switches from the inspiratory to the expiratory phase when the adjustable peak-pressure threshold is exceeded.[15] This minimizes the possibility of barotrauma if the peak-pressure threshold is set appropriately by the anesthesiologist.

On machines equipped with adjustable inspiratory pressure limiters, such as the Datex-Ohmeda S/5 ADU; Aestiva; Dräger Narkomed 6000, 2C, and GS; and Fabius GS, maximal inspiratory pressure may be set by the user to a desired peak airway pressure. An adjustable pressure relief valve opens when the user-selected pressure is reached to prevent generation of excessive airway pressure. This feature depends on the user setting the appropriate "pop-off" pressure. If it is set too low, insufficient pressure for ventilation may be generated, resulting in inadequate minute ventilation; if set too high, barotrauma may occur. The piston-driven Fabius GS and other systems may also include a factory preset inspiratory pressure safety valve that opens at a preset airway pressure (e.g., 75 cm H_2O) to minimize the risk of barotrauma.[20]

Bellows Assembly Problems

Leaks can occur in the bellows assembly. Improper seating of the plastic bellows housing can result in inadequate ventilation because a portion of the driving gas is vented to the atmosphere. A hole in the bellows can lead to alveolar hyperinflation and possibly barotrauma in some ventilators because high-pressure driving gas can enter the patient's circuit. The value on the oxygen analyzer may increase when the driving gas is 100% oxygen, or it may decrease if the driving gas is composed of an air-oxygen mixture.[146]

The ventilator's relief valve can cause problems. Hypoventilation occurs if the valve is incompetent, because anesthetic gas is delivered to the scavenging system during the inspiratory phase instead of to the patient. Gas molecules preferentially exit into the scavenging system because it represents the path of least resistance, and the pressure within the scavenging system can be subatmospheric. Incompetency of the ventilator's relief valve can result from a disconnected pilot line, a ruptured valve, or a damaged flapper valve.[147,148] A relief valve stuck in the closed position can produce barotrauma. Excessive suction from the scavenging system can draw the ventilator's relief valve to its seat and close the valve during the inspiratory and expiratory phases.[1] Pressure in the breathing circuit escalates because excess anesthetic gas cannot be vented. During the expiratory phase, some newer machines from Datex-Ohmeda (i.e., S/5 ADU, 7100, and 7900 SmartVent) scavenge excess gases from the patient and from the drive gas exhausted from the ventilator. When the ventilator's relief valve opens and waste anesthetic gases are vented from the breathing circuit, the drive gas from the bellows' housing joins with the flow to enter the scavenging system.[35,36,52] Under certain conditions, this could overwhelm the scavenging system, resulting in pollution of the operating room with waste anesthetic gases (see "Scavenging Systems").

Control Assembly Problems

The control assembly can be the source of electrical and mechanical problems. Electrical failure can be total or partial; the former is the more obvious. Some mechanical problems include leaks within the system, faulty regulators, and faulty valves. An occluded muffler on the North American Dräger AV-E can cause barotrauma. Obstructed outflow of the driving gas closes the ventilator's relief valve, and excess gas from the patient cannot be vented.[149]

NEWER ANESTHESIA WORKSTATIONS

With the introduction of new technology often comes the need for adaptation of current technology to successfully allow its incorporation into existing systems. Otherwise, a more comprehensive redesign of an entire anesthesia system may be necessary. One such example of adaptation in the anesthesia workstation can be seen with two new design variations of the circle breathing system. The first of these is found on the Datex-Ohmeda S/5 ADU (see Fig. 9-1), and the second is incorporated into the Dräger Narkomed 6000 and Fabius GS workstations. Because use of the circle system is fundamental to the day-to-day practice for most anesthesiologists, a comprehensive understanding of these new systems is crucial for their safe use.

Datex-Ohmeda S/5 ADU

The Datex-Ohmeda S/5 ADU debuted as the AS/3 ADU in 1998. Along with its more comprehensive safety features and integrated design that eliminated glass flow tubes and conventional anesthesia vaporizers in exchange for a computer screen with digital fresh gas flow scales and the built-in Aladin Cassette Vaporizer system, the machine had a radically different appearance. It is not until closer inspection that the other unique properties of the ADU begin to stand out. The principal difference in the ADU's circle system lies in the incorporation of the specialized "D-lite" flow and pressure transducer fitting into the circle at the level of the Y-connector. On most traditional circle systems, exhaled tidal volume is measured by a spirometry sensor located in proximity to the expiratory valve. The placement of the D-lite fitting at the Y-connector provides a better location to perform exhaled volume measurement, allows airway gas composition and pressure monitoring to be done with a single fitting (instead of multiple fittings) added to the breathing circuit, and allows assessment of inspiratory and expiratory gas flow and therefore generation of complete flow-volume spirometry. The relocation of the spirometer sensor to the Y-connector also makes it possible to move the location of the fresh gas inlet to the "patient's side" of the inspiratory valve without adversely affecting accuracy of exhaled tidal volume measurements.

This atypical arrangement of the circle system, with the fresh gas entering on the patient's side of the inspiratory valve, is advantageous for several reasons. It is likely to be more efficient in delivering fresh gas to the patient while preferentially eliminating exhaled gases. It is less likely to cause desiccation of the carbon dioxide absorbent (see "Interactions of Inhaled Anesthetics with Absorbents"). Other notable changes on the S/5 ADU circle system include a compact proprietary carbon dioxide absorbent canister design that can be changed during ventilation without loss of the circle system's integrity and the relocation of the inspiratory and expiratory unidirectional valves from a horizontal position to a vertical position on the compact block assembly just below the absorbent canister.[35,36,52] Reorientation of the unidirectional valves reduces the breathing circuit's resistance encountered by a spontaneously ventilated patient. The vertically oriented, unidirectional valves only have to be tipped away from the vertical position to be opened, unlike conventional horizontal valve disks, which have to be physically lifted off the valve seat against gravity to be opened.

Drager Narkomed 6000 and Fabius GS

Several important differences exist between the traditional circle breathing systems of the newest Dräger products (see Fig. 9-2). At first glance, the most notable difference lies in the appearance and design of the ventilators used with these systems. From the inconspicuous, horizontally mounted, Divan piston ventilator of the Narkomed 6000 (see Fig. 9-2) to the vertically mounted and visible piston ventilator of the Fabius GS with its absent flow tubes and glowing electronic fresh gas flow indicators, these systems appear drastically different from traditional anesthesia systems. The piston ventilator of the Dräger Narkomed 6000, Dräger Fabius GS, and Dräger Primus anesthesia systems may be classified as electrically powered, piston driven, single circuit, and electronically controlled with fresh gas decoupling.[20,22,23]

The circle breathing systems used by these workstations incorporate a feature known as *fresh gas decoupling* (FGD). Incorporation of this technology to enhance safety for the patient has required a significant redesign of the traditional circle system. A functional schematic of a circle system similar to the one used by the Dräger Narkomed 6000 during the inspiratory and expiratory phases of mechanical ventilation can be seen in Figure 9-26. To understand the operating principles of FGD, it is important to have a good understanding of gas flows in a traditional circle system during the inspiratory and expiratory phases of mechanical ventilation. A complete discussion of this was presented earlier in "Operating Principles of Ascending Bellows Ventilators."

The key concept of the fresh gas–decoupled breathing system can be illustrated during the inspiratory phase of mechanical ventilation. With the traditional circle system, several events are occurring (see Fig. 9-24A): continuous fresh gas flows from the flow meters or the oxygen flush valve, or both, and enters the circle system at the fresh gas inlet; the ventilator is delivering the prescribed tidal volume to the patient's lungs; and the ventilator's relief valve (i.e., ventilator's exhaust valve) is closed, and no gas is escaping the circle system except into the patient's lungs.[150] In a traditional circle system, when these events coincide and fresh gas inflow is coupled directly into the circle system, the total volume delivered to the patient's lungs is the sum of the volume from the ventilator plus the volume of gas that enters the circle through the common gas inlet. In contrast, when FGD is used, during the inspiratory phase (see Fig. 9-26A), the fresh gas coming from the anesthesia machine is diverted into the reservoir bag by a decoupling valve that is between the fresh gas source and the ventilator's circuit. The reservoir (breathing) bag serves as an accumulator for fresh gas until the expiratory phase begins. During the expiratory phase (see Fig. 9-26B), the decoupling valve opens, allowing the accumulated fresh gas in the reservoir bag to be drawn into the circle system to refill the piston ventilator's chamber or descending bellows. Because the ventilator's exhaust valve also opens during the expiratory phase, excess fresh gas and gases exhaled by the patient are allowed to escape to the scavenging system.

Current fresh gas–decoupled systems are designed with piston-type or descending bellows–type ventilators. Because the bellows in either of these systems refill under slight negative pressure, it allows the accumulated fresh gas from the reservoir bag to be drawn into the ventilator for delivery to the patient during the next cycle of the ventilator. Because of this design requirement, it is unlikely that FGD can be used with conventional ascending bellows ventilators, which refill under slight positive pressure.

The most significant advantage of circle systems using FGD is a decreased risk of barotrauma. With a traditional circle system, increases in fresh gas flow from the flow meters or from inappropriate use of the oxygen flush valve may contribute directly to the tidal volume, which if excessive may result in pneumothorax. Because systems with FGD isolate fresh gas from coming into the system from the patient while the ventilator's exhaust valve is closed, the risk of barotrauma is greatly reduced.

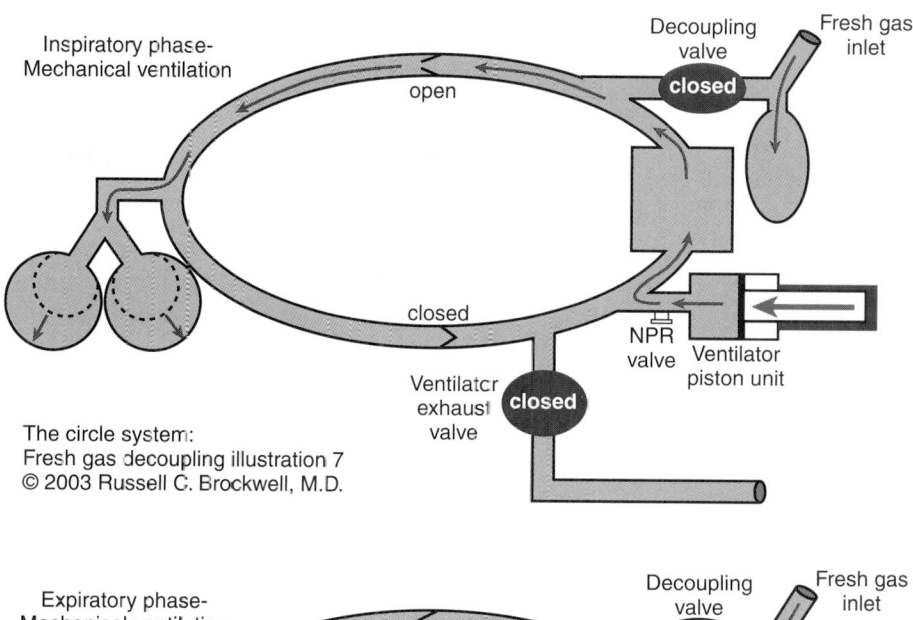

Inspiratory phase-
Mechanical ventilation

The circle system:
Fresh gas decoupling illustration 7
© 2003 Russell C. Brockwell, M.D.

A

Figures 9–26 Inspiratory (**A**) and expiratory (**B**) phases of gas flow in a Dräger-type circle system with a piston ventilator and fresh gas decoupling. NPR valve, negative-pressure relief valve. (Adapted from Brockwell RC: New Circle System Designs: A Collection of 12 Illustrations. Copyright 2003.)

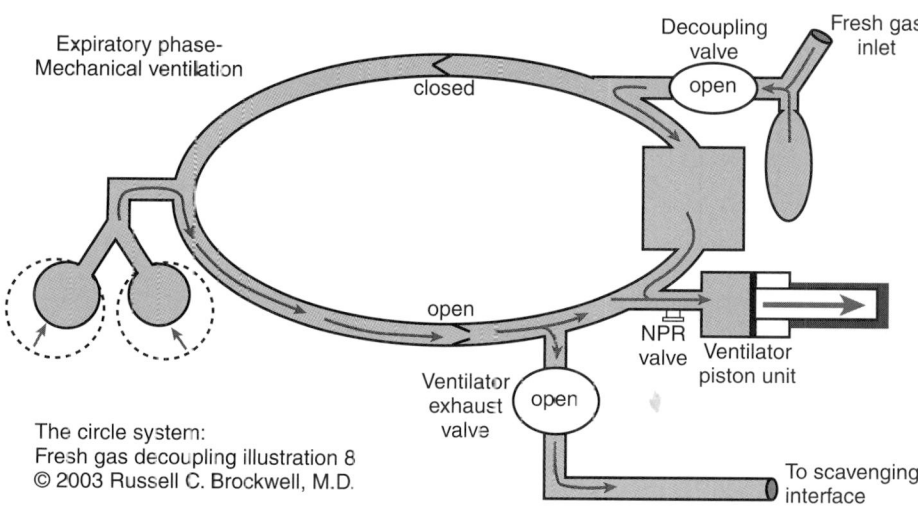

Expiratory phase-
Mechanical ventilation

The circle system:
Fresh gas decoupling illustration 8
© 2003 Russell C. Brockwell, M.D.

B

Possibly the greatest disadvantage to the new anesthesia circle systems that use FGD is the possibility of entraining room air into the patient's gas circuit. The bellows or piston of a circle system with FGD refills under slight negative pressure. If the reservoir bag volume plus the returning volume of gas exhaled from the patient's lungs is inadequate to refill the bellows or piston, negative airway pressures may develop in the patient. To avoid development of negative airway pressure, a negative-pressure relief valve is placed in the breathing system (see Fig. 9-26). If breathing system pressure falls below a preset value, such as −2 cm H_2O, the relief valve opens, and room air is entrained into the patient's gas circuit. If this goes undetected, the entrained atmospheric gases can lead to dilution of both the inhaled anesthetic agents and an enriched oxygen mixture, lowering an enriched oxygen concentration toward 21%.[20] Unchecked, this could lead to intraoperative awareness or hypoxia. High-priority alarms with audio and visual alerts should notify the user that fresh gas flow is inadequate and that room air is being entrained.

Another potential problem with the Dräger-Narkomed 6000–type FGD system lies in its reliance on the reservoir bag to accumulate the incoming fresh gas. If the reservoir bag is removed from the machine during mechanical ventilation or it has a significant leak from poor fit on the bag mount or a perforation, room air may enter the breathing circuit as the ventilator refills during the expiratory phase. This may also result in dilution of both the inhaled anesthetic agents or an enriched oxygen mixture, potentially resulting in awareness of the patient during anesthesia or hypoxia. This type of a disruption can lead to significant pollution of the operating room with nitrous oxide or inhaled anesthetic agents as fresh gases escape into the atmosphere.

SCAVENGING SYSTEMS

Scavenging is the collection and the subsequent removal of vented gases from the operating room.[151] The amount of gas used to anesthetize a patient commonly far exceeds the patient's needs. Scavenging minimizes operating room pollution. In 1977, the National Institute for Occupational Safety and Health (NIOSH) prepared *Criteria for a Recommended Standard: Occupational Exposure to Waste Anesthetic Gases and Vapors*.[152] Although it was maintained that a safe level of exposure could not be defined,

Table 9–3 NIOSH trace gas recommendations, 1977

Anesthetic Gas	Maximum TWA* Concentration (ppm)
Either agent alone	
• Halogenated agent alone	2
• Nitrous oxide	25
Combined halogenated agent and nitrous oxide	
• Halogenated agent	0.5
• Nitrous oxide	25
Dental facilities (nitrous oxide alone)	
• Nitrous oxide	50

*Time-weighted average sampling, also known as time-integrated sampling, is a sampling method that evaluates the average concentration of anesthetic gas over a prolonged period such as 1 to 8 hours.
NIOSH, National Institute for Occupational Safety and Health; ppm, parts per million; TWA, time-weighted average.
Adapted from US Department of Health, Education, and Welfare: Criteria for a Recommended Standard: Occupational Exposure to Waste Anesthetic Gases and Vapors. Washington, DC, US Department of Health, Education, and Welfare, March, 1977.

the NIOSH recommendations are shown in Table 9-3.[152] In 1991, the ASTM released the ASTM F1343-91 standard in a publication called the *Standard Specification for Anesthetic Equipment-Scavenging Systems for Anesthetic Gases.*[153] The document provided guidelines for devices that safely and effectively scavenge excess anesthetic gas to reduce contamination in anesthetizing areas.[153] In 1999, the ASA Task Force on Trace Anesthetic Gases developed a booklet called *Waste Anesthetic Gases: Information for Management in Anesthetizing Areas and the Postanesthesia Care Unit.* This publication addresses analysis of the literature, the role of regulatory agencies, scavenging and monitoring equipment, and recommendations.[154]

The two major causes of waste gas contamination in the operating room are the anesthetic technique employed and equipment issues.[154,155] Several factors related to the anesthetic technique cause operating room contamination: failure to turn off the gas flow control valves at the end of an anesthetic, poorly fitting masks, flushing the circuit, filling anesthetic vaporizers, use of uncuffed endotracheal tubes, and use of breathing circuits such as the Jackson-Rees, which is difficult to scavenge. Equipment failure or lack of understanding the equipment can cause operating room contamination. Leaks can occur in the high-pressure hoses, the mounting for the nitrous oxide tank, the high-pressure circuit and low-pressure circuit of the anesthesia machine, or in the circle system, particularly the carbon dioxide canister. The anesthesia care provider must be certain that the scavenging system is operational and adjusted properly to ensure adequate scavenging. If sidestream carbon dioxide or multigas analyzers are used, the analyzed gas (50 to 250 mL/min) must be directed to the scavenging system or returned to the breathing system.[154,155]

Components

Scavenging systems have five components (Fig. 9-27): (1) the gas-collecting assembly, (2) the transfer means, (3) the scavenging interface, (4) the gas-disposal assembly tubing, and (5) an active or passive gas-disposal assembly.[153] An active system uses a central vacuum to eliminate waste gases. The pressure of the waste gas itself produces flow through a passive system.

Gas-Collecting Assembly

The gas-collecting assembly captures excess anesthetic gas and delivers it to the transfer tubing.[153] Waste anesthetic gases are vented from the anesthesia system through the APL valve or through the ventilator's relief valve. All excess gas from the patient exits the breathing system through these valves, accumulates in the gas-collecting

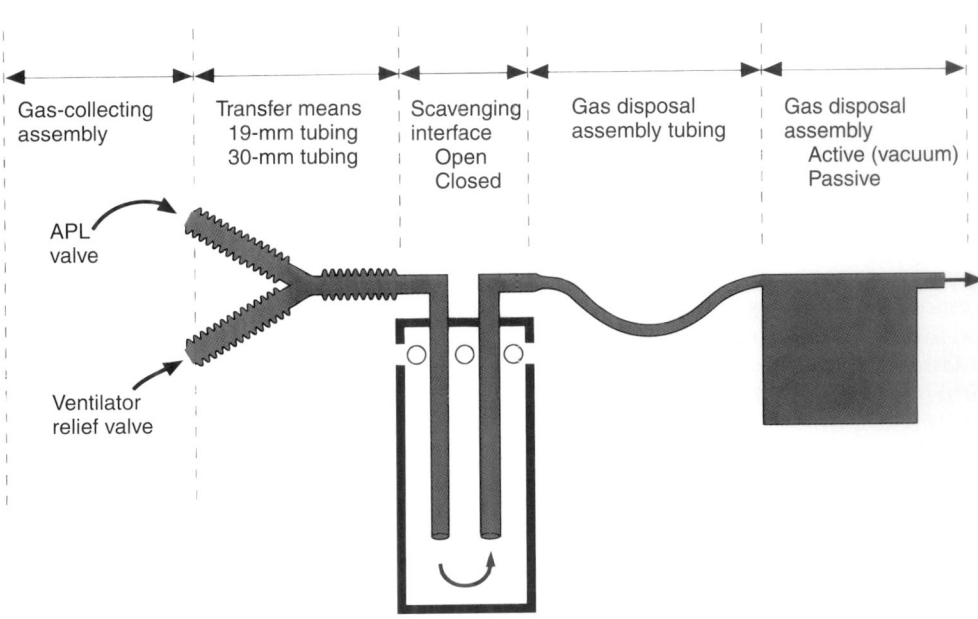

Figure 9–27 Components of a scavenging system. APL valve, adjustable pressure limiting valve. (Modified from Andrews JJ, Brockwell RC: Delivery systems for inhaled anesthetics. *In* Barash PG, Cullen BF, Stoelting RK [eds]: Clinical Anesthesia, 4th ed. New York, Lippincott-Raven, 2000, pp 567-594.)

Gas-collecting assembly

Transfer means
19-mm tubing
30-mm tubing

Scavenging interface
Open
Closed

Gas disposal assembly tubing

Gas disposal assembly
Active (vacuum)
Passive

APL valve

Ventilator relief valve

assembly, and is directed to the transfer means. In some newer Datex-Ohmeda systems that incorporate the 7100 or 7900 ventilators, the ventilator's drive gas is also exhausted into the scavenging system. This is significant, because under conditions of high flows of fresh gas and high minute ventilation, the gases flowing into the scavenging interface may overwhelm the evacuation system. If this occurs, waste anesthetic gases may overflow the system through the positive-pressure relief valve (i.e., closed systems) or through the atmospheric vents (i.e., open systems), polluting the operating room. In contrast, most other pneumatic ventilators from Datex-Ohmeda and Dräger exhaust their drive gas (100% oxygen or oxygen-air mixture) into the atmosphere through a small vent on the back of the ventilator's control housing.

Transfer Means

The transfer means carries excess gas from the gas-collecting assembly to the scavenging interface. The tubing must be 19 or 30 mm, as specified by the ASTM F1343-91 standard.[153] The tubing should be sufficiently rigid to prevent kinking and as short as possible to minimize the chance of occlusion. Some manufacturers color code the transfer tubing with yellow bands to distinguish it from the 22-mm tubing of the breathing system. Many machines have separate transfer tubes for the APL valve and for the ventilator's relief valve. The two tubes frequently merge into a single hose before they enter the scavenging interface. Occlusion of the transfer means can be particularly problematic because it is upstream from the pressure-buffering scavenging interface. If the transfer means is occluded, pressure in the breathing circuit increases, and barotrauma can occur.

Scavenging Interface

The scavenging interface is the most important component of the system because it protects the breathing circuit or ventilator from excessive positive or negative pressure.[151] The interface should limit the pressures immediately downstream from the gas-collecting assembly to between –0.5 and +10 cm H_2O with normal working conditions.[153] Positive-pressure relief is mandatory, irrespective of the type of disposal system used, to vent excess gas in case of occlusion downstream from the interface. If the disposal system is active, negative-pressure relief is necessary to protect the breathing circuit or ventilator from excessive subatmospheric pressure. With active systems, a reservoir is highly desirable because it stores excess waste gas until the evacuation system can eliminate it. Interfaces can be open or closed, depending on the method used to provide positive-pressure and negative-pressure relief.[151]

Open Interfaces

An open interface contains no valves and is open to the atmosphere, allowing positive-pressure and negative-pressure relief. Open interfaces should be used only with active disposal systems that use a central vacuum system. Open interfaces require a reservoir because waste gases are intermittently discharged in surges, whereas flow to the active disposal system is continuous.[151]

Many contemporary anesthesia machines are equipped with open interfaces like those in Figure 9-28.[156] An open canister provides reservoir capacity. The canister volume should be large enough to accommodate a variety of waste gas flow rates. Gas enters the system at the top of the canister and travels through a narrow inner tube to the canister base. Gases are stored in the reservoir

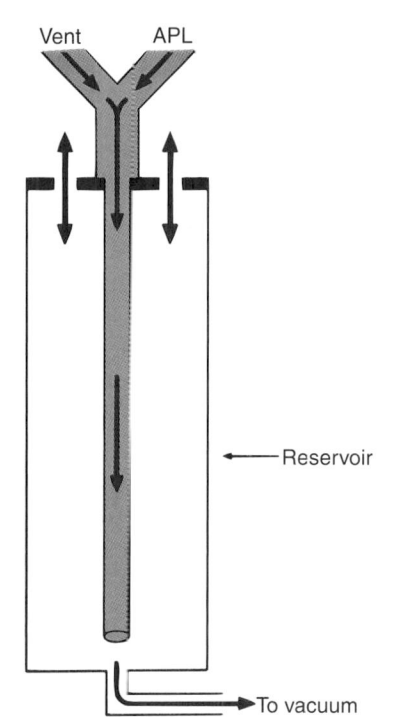
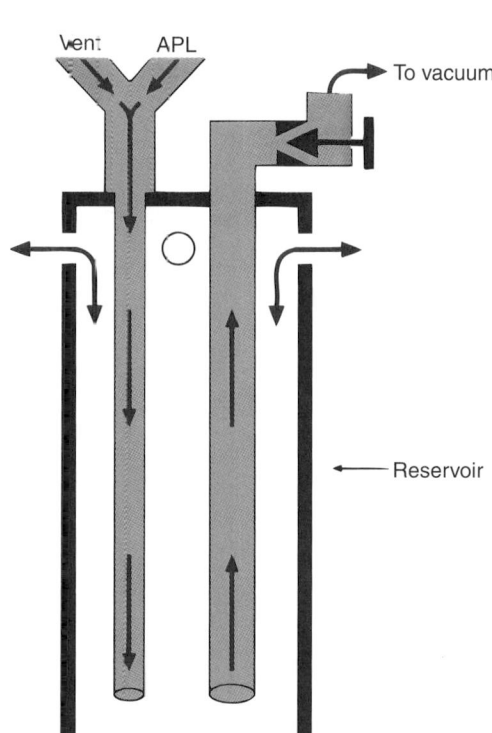

Figure 9–28 Each of the two open scavenging interfaces requires an active disposal system. An open canister provides reservoir capacity. Gas enters the system at the top of the canister and travels through a narrow inner tube to the canister base. Gases are stored in the reservoir between breaths. Relief of positive and negative pressure is provided by holes in the top of the canister. **A** and **B,** The open interface shown in **A** differs somewhat from the one shown in **B.** The operator can regulate the vacuum by adjusting the vacuum control valve shown in **B.** APL, adjustable pressure limiting valve. (Adapted from Dorsch JA, Dorsch SE: Controlling trace gas levels. *In* Dorsch JA, Dorsch SE [eds]: Understanding Anesthesia Equipment, 4th ed. Baltimore, Williams & Wilkins, 1999, p 355.)

between breaths. Positive-pressure and negative-pressure relief is provided by holes in the top of the canister. The open interface shown in Figure 9-28A differs somewhat from the one shown in Figure 9-28B. The operator can regulate the vacuum by adjusting the vacuum control valve shown in Figure 9-28B.[156]

The efficiency of an open interface depends on several factors. The vacuum flow rate per minute must equal or exceed the minute volume of excess gases to prevent spillage. The volume of the reservoir and the flow characteristics within the interface are important. Spillage will occur if the volume of a single exhaled breath exceeds the capacity of the reservoir. Leakage can occur long before the volume of waste gas delivered to the reservoir equals the reservoir volume if large-scale turbulence occurs within the interface.[157]

Closed Interfaces

A closed interface communicates with the atmosphere through valves. All closed interfaces must have a positive-pressure relief valve to vent excess system pressure if obstruction occurs downstream from the interface. A negative-pressure relief valve is mandatory to protect the breathing system from subatmospheric pressure if an active disposal system is used.[151] Two types of closed interfaces are commercially available. One has positive-pressure relief only; the other has positive-pressure and negative-pressure relief. Each type is discussed in the following sections.

POSITIVE-PRESSURE RELIEF ONLY. This interface (Fig. 9-29, left) has a single positive-pressure relief valve that is designed to be used only with passive disposal systems. Waste gas enters the interface at the waste gas inlets. Transfer of the waste gas from the interface to the disposal system relies on the pressure of the waste gas itself because a vacuum is not used. The positive-pressure relief valve opens at a preset value, such as 5 cm H_2O, if an obstruction between the interface and the disposal system occurs.[158] A reservoir bag is unnecessary.

POSITIVE-PRESSURE AND NEGATIVE-PRESSURE RELIEF. This interface has a positive-pressure relief valve, at least one negative-pressure relief valve, and a reservoir bag. It is used with active disposal systems. Figure 9-29 (right) is a schematic drawing of North American Dräger's closed interface for suction systems. A variable volume of waste gas intermittently enters the interface through the waste gas inlets. The reservoir stores transient excess gas until the vacuum system eliminates it. The operator should adjust the vacuum control valve so that the reservoir bag is properly inflated (A) and not over distended (B) or completely deflated (C). Gas is vented to the atmosphere through the positive-pressure relief valve if the system pressure exceeds +5 cm H_2O. Room air is entrained through the negative-pressure relief valve if the system pressure is less than –0.5 cm H_2O. A backup negative-pressure relief valve opens at –1.8 cm H_2O if the primary negative-pressure relief valve becomes occluded.[19]

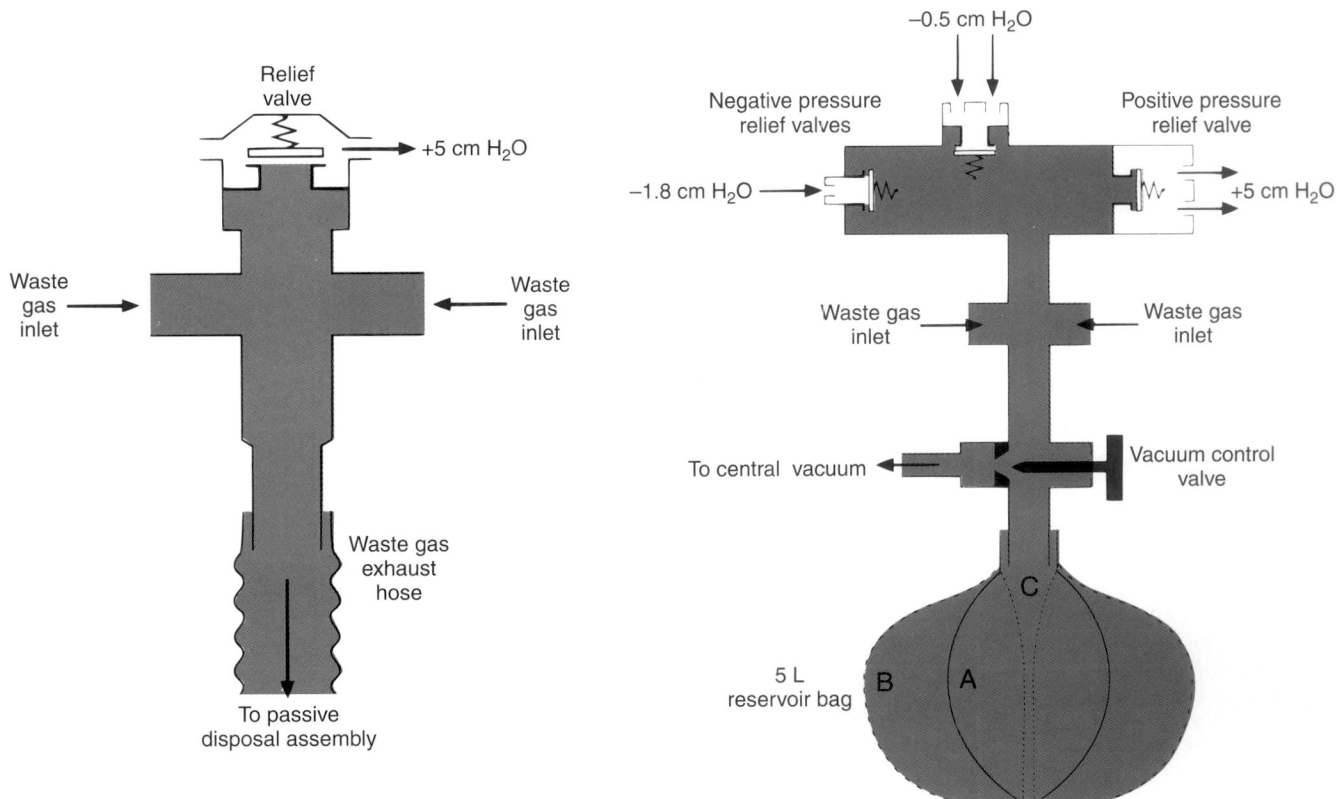

Figure 9–29 Closed scavenging interfaces. Interface used with a passive disposal system (*left*). Interface used with an active system (*right*). (*Left*, Adapted from Scavenger Interface for Air Conditioning: Instruction Manual. Telford, PA, North American Dräger, October 1984; *right*, Adapted from Narkomed 2A Anesthesia System: Technical Service Manual. Telford, PA, North American Dräger, 1985.)

The effectiveness of a closed system in preventing spillage depends on the inflow rate of excess gas, the vacuum flow rate, and the volume of the reservoir. Leakage of waste gases into the atmosphere occurs only when the reservoir bag becomes fully inflated and the pressure increases sufficiently to open the positive-pressure relief valve. The effectiveness of an open system to prevent spillage depends on the volume of the reservoir and on the flow characteristics within the interface.[157]

Tubing for the Gas-Disposal Assembly

The gas-disposal assembly tubing (see Fig. 9-27) conducts waste gas from the scavenging interface to the gas-disposal assembly. It should be collapse-proof and should run overhead, if possible, to minimize the chance of occlusion.[153]

Gas-Disposal Assembly

The gas-disposal assembly ultimately eliminates excess waste gas (see Fig. 9-27). There are two types of disposal systems: active and passive. The most common method of gas disposal is the active assembly, which uses a central vacuum. The vacuum is a mechanical, flow-inducing device that removes the waste gases. An interface with a negative-pressure relief valve is mandatory because the pressure within the system is negative. A reservoir is very desirable, and the larger the reservoir, the lower the suction flow rate needed.[151,157]

A passive disposal system does not use a mechanical, flow-inducing device. Instead, the pressure of the waste gas itself produces flow through the system. Positive-pressure relief is mandatory, but negative-pressure relief and a reservoir are unnecessary. Excess waste gas can be eliminated in several ways, including venting through the wall, ceiling, or floor or venting to the room exhaust grill of a non-recirculating air conditioning system.[151,157]

Hazards

Scavenging systems minimize operating room pollution, but they add complexity to the anesthesia system. A scavenging system extends the anesthesia circuit from the anesthesia machine to the ultimate disposal site. This extension increases the potential for problems. Obstruction of scavenging pathways can cause excessive positive pressure in the breathing circuit, and barotrauma can occur. Excessive vacuum applied to a scavenging system can cause negative pressures in the breathing system.

CHECKING ANESTHESIA MACHINES

A complete anesthesia apparatus checkout procedure should be performed each day before the first case. An abbreviated version should be performed before each subsequent case. Several checkout procedures exist, but the 1993 Food and Drug Administration (FDA) Anesthesia Apparatus Checkout Recommendations reproduced in Appendix 1 is the most popular.[159-163] The FDA checkout procedures serve only as generic guidelines because the designs of different machines vary considerably. Many machines have been modified in the field. Specific

checks must be performed on specific machines. The user must refer to the operator's manual for special procedures and precautions.

The three most important preoperative checks are calibration of the oxygen analyzer, a leak test for the low-pressure circuit, and a test of the circle system. They are discussed in subsequent sections.

Calibration of the Oxygen Analyzer

The oxygen analyzer is the most important machine monitor because it is the only machine safety device that evaluates the integrity of the low-pressure circuit. Other machine safety devices, such as the fail-safe valve, the oxygen supply failure alarm, and the proportioning system, are all upstream from the flow control valves (see Fig. 9-3). The only machine monitor that detects problems downstream from the flow control valves is the oxygen analyzer. Calibration of this monitor is described in step 9 of Appendix 1.

Leak Test for the Low-Pressure Circuit

The low-pressure leak test checks the integrity of the anesthesia machine from the flow control valves to the common outlet. It evaluates the portion of the machine that is downstream from all safety devices except the oxygen analyzer. The components located within this area are precisely the ones most subject to breakage and leaks. Leaks in the low-pressure circuit can cause hypoxia or awareness by the patient.[88,164] Flow tubes, the most delicate pneumatic component of the machine, can crack or break. A typical three-gas anesthesia machine has 16 O-ring gaskets in the low-pressure circuit. Leaks can occur at the interface between the glass flow tube and the manifold, and at the O-ring junction between the vaporizer and its manifold. Loose filler caps on vaporizers are a common source of leaks, and these leaks can cause the patient to become aware while under anesthesia.[88,165]

Several different methods have been used to check the low-pressure circuit for leaks. They include the oxygen flush test, the common gas outlet occlusion test, the traditional positive-pressure leak test, the North American Dräger positive-pressure leak test, the Ohmeda 8000 internal positive-pressure leak test, the Ohmeda negative-pressure leak test, the 1993 FDA universal negative-pressure leak test, and others. One reason for the large number of methods is that the internal design of various machines differs considerably. For example, most Datex-Ohmeda machines have a check valve near the common gas outlet, whereas North American Dräger machines do not. The presence or absence of the check valve profoundly influences which preoperative check is indicated.

Several mishaps have resulted from application of the wrong leak test to a machine.[38,86,166] It is therefore mandatory to perform the appropriate low-pressure leak test before every case. To do this, it is essential to understand the exact location and operating principles of the Datex-Ohmeda check valve. Most Datex-Ohmeda anesthesia machines have a machine outlet check valve located in the low-pressure circuit (Table 9-4). The check

Table 9–4 Check valves and manufacturer-recommended leak test

Anesthesia Machine	Machine Outlet Check Valve	Vaporizer Outlet Check Valve	Low Pressure Leak Test		
			Positive Pressure	Negative Pressure (Suction Bulb)	Self-Test
Dräger Narkomed 2A, 2B, 2C, 3, 4, GS	No	No	Yes		
Dräger Fabius GS	No	No			Yes
Narkomed 6000	No	No			Yes
Ohmeda Unitrol	Yes	Variable		Yes	
Ohmeda 30/70	Yes	Variable		Yes	
Ohmeda Modulus I	Yes	Variable		Yes	
Ohmeda Modulus II	Yes	No		Yes	
Ohmeda Excel series	Yes	No		Yes	
Ohmeda Modulus II Plus	No	No		Yes	
Ohmeda CD	No	No		Yes	
Datex-Ohmeda Aestiva	Yes	No		Yes	
Datex-Ohmeda S5/ADU	No	No			Yes

Data from Ohio Medical Products, Ohmeda, Datex-Ohmeda, North American Dräger, and Dräger Medical.

valve is located downstream from the vaporizers and upstream from the oxygen flush valve (see Fig. 9-3). It is open (Fig. 9-30, left) in the absence of backpressure. Gas flow from the manifold moves the rubber flapper valve off its seat and allows gas to proceed freely to the common outlet. The valve closes (see Fig. 9-30, right) when backpressure is exerted on it.[9] Backpressure sufficient to close the check valve may occur with the following conditions: oxygen flushing, peak pressures in the breathing circuit generated during positive-pressure ventilation, or use of a positive-pressure leak test.

Generally, machines without check valves can be tested using a positive-pressure leak test, and machines with check valves must be tested using a negative-pressure leak test. When performing a positive-pressure leak test, the operator generates positive pressure in the low-pressure circuit using flow from the anesthesia machine or from a positive-pressure bulb to detect a leak. When performing a negative-pressure leak test, the operator creates negative pressure in the low-pressure circuit using a suction bulb to detect leaks. Two leak tests for low-pressure circuits are described in the following sections.

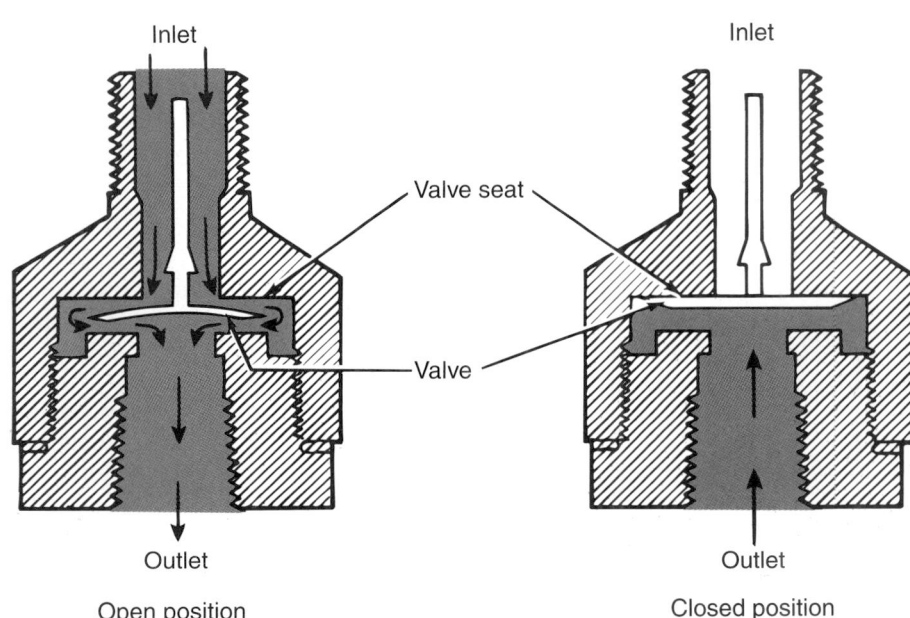

Figure 9–30 Machine outlet check valve. The check valve is located downstream from the vaporizers and upstream from the oxygen flush valve. It is open (*left*) in the absence of backpressure. Gas flow from the manifold moves the rubber flapper valve off its seat and allows gas to proceed freely to the common outlet. The valve closes (*right*) when backpressure is exerted on it. (Adapted from Bowie E, Huffman LM: The Anesthesia Machine: Essentials for Understanding. Madison, WI, Ohmeda, a Division of BOC Health Care, 1985.)

Oxygen Flushing in a Positive-Pressure Leak Test

Historically, older anesthesia machines did not have check valves in the low-pressure circuit. It was common practice to pressurize the breathing circuit and the low-pressure circuit with the oxygen flush valve to test for internal anesthesia machine leaks. Because many modern Datex-Ohmeda machines have check valves in the low-pressure circuit, application of a positive-pressure leak test to these machines can be misleading or even dangerous (Fig. 9-31). Inappropriate use of the oxygen flush valve to evaluate the low-pressure circuit for leaks can lead to a false sense of security despite the presence of huge leaks.[38,53,86,166] Positive pressure from the patient's circuit closes the check valve, and the value on the airway pressure gauge does not decline. The system appears to be tight, but only the circuitry downstream from the check valve is leak free.[32] A vulnerable area exists from the check valve back to the flow control valves because this area is not tested by a positive-pressure leak test.

1993 Food and Drug Administration Universal Negative-Pressure Leak Test

The 1993 FDA universal negative-pressure leak test[163] (see Appendix 1, step 5) was so named because, at that time, it could be used to check all contemporary anesthesia machines, regardless of the presence or absence of check valves in the low-pressure circuit. It remains effective for many anesthesia workstations and can be applied to many Datex-Ohmeda machines, North American Dräger machines, and others. However, some newer machines are not compatible with this test. The American Society of Anesthesiologist's Committee on Equipment and Facilities in conjunction with the FDA is expected to update the 1993 Anesthesia Apparatus Checkout Recommendations soon. Until the new recommendations become available, the 1993 guidelines should continue to be followed as closely as possible, because they remain applicable to most anesthesia workstations in use worldwide.

The 1993 FDA checklist is based on the Datex-Ohmeda negative-pressure leak test (Fig. 9-32). It is performed using a negative-pressure leak-testing device, which is a simple suction bulb. The machine master switch, the flow control valves, and vaporizers are turned off. The suction bulb is attached to the common fresh gas outlet and squeezed repeatedly until it is fully collapsed. This action creates a vacuum in the low-pressure circuitry. The machine is leak-free if the hand bulb remains collapsed for at least 10 seconds. A leak is present if the bulb reinflates during this period. The test is repeated with each vaporizer individually turned to the on position because internal vaporizer leaks can be detected only with the vaporizer turned on.

The FDA universal negative-pressure, low-pressure-circuit leak test has several advantages.[164] It helps eliminate the present confusion regarding exactly which check should be performed on specific machines. The universal test is

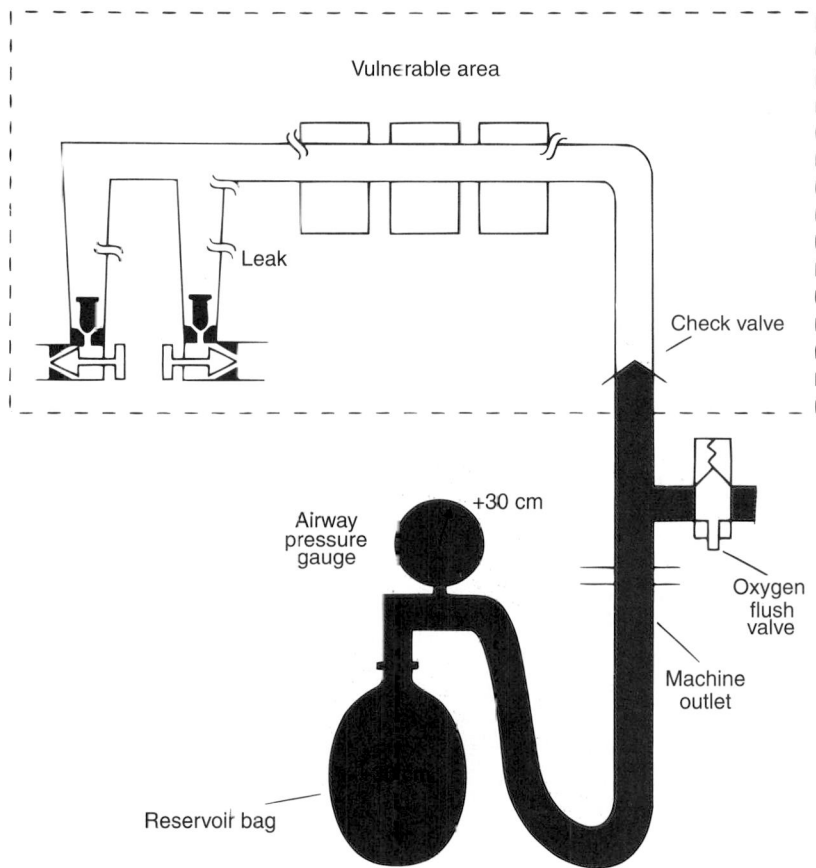

Figure 9–31 Inappropriate use of the oxygen flush valve to check the low-pressure circuit of an Ohmeda machine equipped with a check valve. The area within the rectangle (*dotted line*) is not checked by the inappropriate use of the oxygen flush valve, and the components located within this area are precisely the ones most subject to breakage and leaks. Positive pressure within the patient's circuit closes the check valve, and the value on the airway pressure gauge does not decline despite leaks in the low-pressure circuit. (Adapted from Andrews JJ, Brockwell RC: Delivery systems for inhaled anesthetics. *In* Barash PG, Cullen BF, Stoelting RK [eds]: Clinical Anesthesia, 4th ed. New York, Lippincott-Raven, 2000, pp 567-594.)

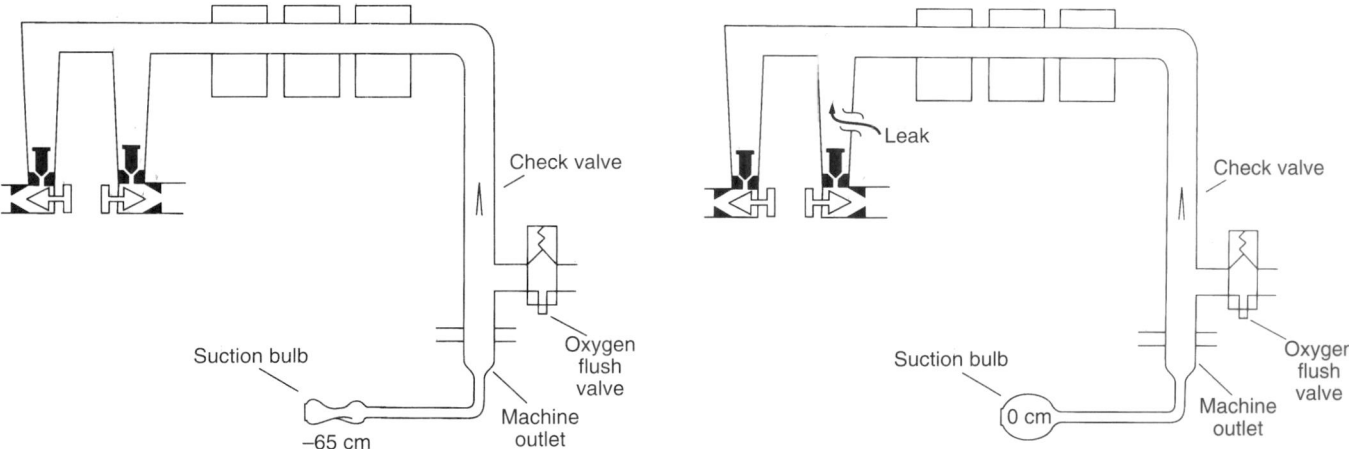

Figure 9–32 The U.S. Food and Drug Administration negative-pressure leak test. A negative-pressure leak-testing device is attached directly to the machine outlet (*left*). Squeezing the bulb creates a vacuum in the low-pressure circuit and opens the check valve. When a leak is present in the low-pressure circuit, room air is entrained through the leak, and the suction bulb inflates (*right*). (Adapted from Andrews JJ: Understanding anesthesia machines. *In* 1988 Review Course Lectures. Cleveland, International Anesthesia Research Society, 1988, p. 78.)

quick and simple to perform. It has an obvious end point, and it isolates the problem. For example, if the bulb reinflates in less than 10 seconds, a leak is present in the low-pressure circuit. It therefore differentiates leaks in the breathing circuit from leaks in the low-pressure circuit. The universal negative-pressure leak test is the most sensitive of all contemporary leak tests because it is not volume dependent; it does not involve a compliant breathing bag or corrugated hoses; and it can detect leaks as small as 30 mL/min. The operator does not need in-depth knowledge about proprietary design differences. If the operator performs the universal test correctly, the leak will be detected.

Test of the Circle System

The circle system test (see Appendix 1, steps 11 and 12) evaluates the integrity of the circle breathing system, which spans from the common gas outlet to the Y-piece (see Fig. 9-22). It has two parts: the leak test and the flow test. To thoroughly check the circle system for leaks, valve integrity, and obstruction, both tests must be performed preoperatively. The *leak test* is performed by closing the pop-off valve, occluding the Y-piece, and pressurizing the circuit to 30 cm H_2O using the oxygen flush valve. The value on the pressure gauge does not decline if the circle system is free of leaks, but this does not ensure valve integrity. The value on the gauge is 30 cm H_2O if the unidirectional valves are stuck shut or if the valves are incompetent.

The *flow test* checks the integrity of the unidirectional valves, and it detects obstruction in the circle system. It can be performed by removing the Y-piece from the circle system and breathing through the two corrugated hoses individually. The valves should be present, and they should move appropriately. The operator should be able to inhale but not exhale through the inspiratory limb. The operator should be able to exhale but not inhale through the expiratory limb. The flow test can also be performed by using the ventilator and a breathing bag

attached to the Y-piece as described in the 1993 FDA Anesthesia Apparatus Checkout Recommendations (see Appendix 1, step 12).[163]

Machine Self-Tests

Many newer anesthesia workstations incorporate technology that allows the machine to automatically or manually go through a series of self-tests to check for functionality of electronic, mechanical, and pneumatic components.[20,22,23,35,36] Tested components commonly include the gas supply system, flow control valves, the circle system, ventilator, and in the case of the Datex-Ohmeda ADU, the Aladin Cassette Vaporizer.[35,36,52] The comprehensiveness of these self-diagnostic tests varies from one model and manufacturer to another. If these tests are to be employed, users must read and strictly follow all of the manufacturer's recommendations. Although a thorough understanding of what the particular workstation's self-tests include is very helpful, this information is often difficult to obtain and may vary greatly between devices.

An important warning is in order for self-tests on systems with add-on vaporizers, such as the Dräger Fabius and Narkomed 6000. An add-on vaporizer does not become a part of an anesthesia workstation's gas flow stream until the concentration control dial is turned to the on position. To detect internal vaporizer leaks on this type of a system, the leak test portion of the self-diagnostic program must be repeated separately with each individual vaporizer turned to the on position. If this precaution is not taken, a large leak, such as that from a loose filler cap or cracked fill indicators, may be undetected.

SUMMARY

Rapid advances in the anesthesia industry make it increasingly difficult for the anesthesia care provider to keep up with anesthesia machine technology. Nevertheless, a thorough understanding of the machine is mandatory for the safe practice of anesthesia. Machines are equipped with dozens of safety features, but none of them is foolproof. The anesthesia care provider still must check the machine preoperatively using appropriate checkout procedures.

KEY POINTS

1. In the event of a pipeline crossover, two actions must be taken. The backup oxygen cylinder must be on, and the wall supply sources must be disconnected.

2. Fail-safe valves and proportioning systems help minimize delivery of a hypoxic mixture, but they are not foolproof. Delivery of a hypoxic mixture can result from the wrong supply gas, a defective or broken safety device, leaks downstream from the safety devices, inert gas administration, and dilution of the inspired oxygen concentration by high concentrations of inhaled anesthetics.

3. Because of desflurane's low boiling point and high vapor pressure, controlled vaporization of desflurane requires special, sophisticated vaporizers such as the Datex-Ohmeda Tec 6 and the Aladin Cassette Vaporizer.

4. Misfilling an empty variable-bypass vaporizer with desflurane could be catastrophic, resulting in delivery of a hypoxic mixture and a massive overdose of inhaled desflurane anesthetic.

5. Inhaled anesthetics can interact with carbon dioxide absorbents and produce toxic compounds. During sevoflurane anesthesia, compound A can be formed, particularly at low rates of fresh gas flow, and during desflurane anesthesia, carbon monoxide can be produced, particularly with desiccated absorbents.

6. Anesthesia ventilators with ascending bellows (i.e., bellows that ascend during the expiratory phase) are safer than those with descending bellows because disconnections readily manifest with ascending bellows.

7. When using anesthesia ventilators with ascending bellows, during the inspiratory phase, fresh gas flow and oxygen flushing contribute to the patient's tidal volume because the ventilator's relief valve is closed. Oxygen flushing during the inspiratory phase can cause barotrauma, particularly in pediatric patients. The anesthesiologist must never activate the oxygen flush during the inspiratory phase of mechanical ventilation.

8. New ventilators that use FGD technology virtually eliminate the possibility of barotrauma by oxygen flushing during the inspiratory phase because fresh gas flow and oxygen flush flow are diverted to the reservoir breathing bag. However, if the breathing bag has a leak or is absent, the patient may become aware while under anesthesia, and a lower than expected oxygen concentration may be delivered because of entrainment of room air.

9. With newer Ohmeda anesthetic ventilators such as the 7100 and 7900 SmartVent, the gas from the patient and the drive gas are scavenged, resulting in substantially increased volumes of scavenged gas. The scavenging systems must be set appropriately to accommodate the increased volume, or pollution of the operating room environment can result.

10. The low-pressure circuit is the vulnerable area of the anesthesia machine because it is most subject to breakage and leaks. The low-pressure circuit is located downstream from all anesthesia machine safety features except the oxygen analyzer, and it is the portion of the machine that is missed if an inappropriate leak test for a low-pressure circuit is performed.

11. It is mandatory to check the low-pressure circuit for leaks before an anesthetic is delivered because leaks in the circuit can cause delivery of a hypoxic mixture or cause the patient to become aware during anesthesia, or both.

12. Because most Ohmeda anesthesia machines have a one-way check valve in the low-pressure circuit, a negative-pressure leak test is required to detect leaks. A positive-pressure leak test cannot detect leaks in the low-pressure circuit of most Datex-Ohmeda products.

13. Internal vaporizer leaks can be detected only with the vaporizer turned on.

14. Before an anesthetic is administered, the circle system must be checked for leaks and for flow. To test for leaks, the circle system is pressurized to 30 cm H_2O, and the circle system's airway pressure gauge is observed (i.e., static test). To check for appropriate flow to rule out obstructions and faulty valves, the ventilator and a test lung (e.g., breathing bag) are used (i.e., dynamic test).

15. Newer anesthesia workstation self-tests do not detect internal vaporizer leaks unless each vaporizer is individually turned on during the self-test.

REFERENCES

1. Schreiber P: Safety Guidelines for Anesthesia Systems. Telford, PA, North American Dräger, 1984.
2. Caplan RA, Vistica MF, Posner KL, Cheney FW: Adverse anesthetic outcomes arising from gas delivery equipment. Anesthesiology 87:741, 1997.
3. Emergency Care Research Institute: Misconnected Flow Meter Leads to Two Deaths. Special Report # SR 0003. Health Devices Alert. 26:A4, January 25, 2002.
4. American National Standards Institute: Minimum Performance and Safety Requirements for Components and Systems of Continuous Flow Anesthesia Machines for Human Use (ANSI Z79.8-1979). New York, American National Standards Institute, 1979.
5. American Society for Testing and Materials: Standard Specification for Minimum Performance and Safety

Requirements for Components and Systems of Anesthesia Gas Machines (ASTM F1161-88). Philadelphia, American Society for Testing and Materials, 1988.

6. American Society for Testing and Materials: Standard Specification for Minimum Performance and Safety Requirements for Components and Systems of Anesthetic Gas Machines (ASTM 1161-94). Philadelphia, American Society for Testing and Materials, 1994.

7. American Society for Testing and Materials: Standard Specification for Particular Requirements for Anesthesia Workstations and Their Components (ASTM F1850-00). West Conshohoken, PA, American Society for Testing and Materials, 2000.

8. Dorsch JA, Dorsch SE: The anesthesia machine. *In* Dorsch JA, Dorsch SE (eds): Understanding Anesthesia Equipment, 4th ed. Baltimore, Williams & Wilkins, 1999, p 75.

9. Bowie E, Huffman LM: The Anesthesia Machine: Essentials for Understanding. Madison, WI, Ohmeda & The BOC Group, 1985.

10. Modulus Anesthesia Gas Machine: Operation Maintenance. Madison, WI, Ohio Medical Products & The BOC Group, 1981.

11. Modulus II Anesthesia System: Operation and Maintenance Manual. Madison, WI, Ohmeda & The BOC Group, 1985.

12. Modulus II Anesthesia System: Service Manual. Madison, WI, Ohmeda, The BOC Group, 1985.

13. Ohmeda 8000 Anesthesia Machine: Operation and Maintenance Manual. Madison, WI, Ohmeda & The BOC Group, 1985.

14. Ohmeda Excel 110 and 210: Operation and Maintenance Manual. Madison, WI, Ohmeda & The BOC Group, 1987.

15. Modulus II Plus Anesthesia System: Operation and Maintenance Manual. Madison, WI, Ohmeda & The BOC Group, 1988.

16. Ohmeda CD Anesthesia System: Operation and Maintenance Manual. Madison, WI, Ohmeda & The BOC Group, 1990.

17. 30/70 Proportionate Anesthesia Machine (Canadian version). Madison, WI, Ohio Medical Products, 1982.

18. Ohmeda Unitrol Anesthesia System: Operation and Maintenance Manual. Madison, WI, Ohmeda & The BOC Group, 1985.

19. Narkomed 2A Anesthesia System: Technical Service Manual, 6th ed. Telford, PA, North American Dräger, 1985.

20. Fabius GS: Anesthesia Workstation: Operator's Instruction Manual. Telford, PA, Dräger Medical, January 15, 2002.

21. Narkomed GS: Anesthesia Workstation: Setup and Installation Manual. Telford, PA, Dräger Medical, January 29, 2002.

22. Narkomed 6000 Anesthesia Workstation: Service Manual, revision H. Telford, PA, Dräger Medical, July 2000.

23. Narkomed 6000 Anesthesia Workstation: Setup and Installation Manual, revision F. Telford, PA, Dräger Medical, July 2000.

24. Narkomed 2A Anesthesia System: Instruction Manual, 7th ed. Telford, PA, North American Dräger, 1985.

25. Narkomed 2B Anesthesia System: Operator's Manual. Telford, PA, North American Dräger, 1988.

26. Narkomed 3 Anesthesia System: Operator's Instruction Manual. Telford, PA, North American Dräger, 1986.

27. Narkomed 4 Anesthesia System: Operator's Instruction Manual. Telford, PA, North American Dräger, 1990.

28. Cicman JH, Jacoby MI, Skibo VF, et al: Anesthesia systems. Part 1. Operating principles of fundamental components. J Clin Monit 8:295, 1992.

29. Feeley TW, Hedley-Whyte J: Bulk oxygen and nitrous oxide delivery systems: Design and dangers. Anesthesiology 44:301, 1976.

30. Pelton DA: Non-flammable medical gas pipeline systems. *In* Wyant GM (ed): Mechanical Misadventures in Anesthesia. Toronto, University of Toronto Press, 1978, p 8.

31. Adriani J: Clinical application of physical principles concerning gases and vapors to anesthesiology. *In* Adriani J (ed): The Chemistry and Physics of Anesthesia, 2nd ed. Springfield, IL, Charles C Thomas, 1962, p 58.

32. Dorsch JA, Dorsch SE: Equipment checking and maintenance. *In* Dorsch JA, Dorsch SE (eds): Understanding

Anesthesia Equipment, 4th ed. Baltimore, Williams & Wilkins, 1999, p 937.

33. Macintosh R, Mushin WW, Epstein HG: Flowmeters. *In* Macintosh R, Mushin WW, Epstein HG (eds): Physics for the Anaesthetist, 3rd ed. Oxford, Blackwell Scientific Publications, 1963, p 196.

34. Eger EI II, Epstein RM: Hazards of anesthetic equipment. Anesthesiology 24:490, 1964.

35. Datex-Ohmeda S5/Anesthesia Delivery Unit: User's Reference Manual. Tewksbury, MA, Datex-Ohmeda, 2000.

36. Datex-Ohmeda S5/Anesthesia Delivery Unit: Technical Reference Manual. Tewksbury, MA, Datex-Ohmeda, 1999.

37. Eger EI II, Hylton RR, Irwin RH, et al: Anesthetic flowmeter sequence—A cause for hypoxia. Anesthesiology 24:396, 1963.

38. Rendell-Baker L: Problems with anesthetic and respiratory therapy equipment. Int Anesthesiol Clin 20:1, 1982.

39. Mazze RI: Therapeutic misadventures with oxygen delivery systems: The need for continuous in-line oxygen monitors. Anesth Analg 51:787, 1972.

40. Datex-Ohmeda AS/3 Anesthesia Delivery Unit: User's Reference Manual. Tewksbury, MA, Datex-Ohmeda, 1998.

41. Cheng CJ, Garewal DS: A Failure of the Chain Link Mechanism of the Ohmeda Excel 210 Anesthetic Machine. Anesth Analg 92:913, 2001.

42. Lohman G: Fault with an Ohmeda Excel 410 Machine [letter and response]. Anaesthesia 46:695, 1991.

43. Kidd AG, Hall I: Fault with an Ohmeda Excel 210 Anesthetic Machine [letter and response]. Anaesthesia 49:83, 1994.

44. Paine GF, Kochan JJ: Failure of the chain link mechanism of the Ohmeda Excel 210 anesthesia machine [letter and response]. Anesth Analg 94:1374, 2002.

45. Richards C: Failure of a nitrous oxide-oxygen proportioning device. Anesthesiology 71:997, 1989.

46. Abraham ZA, Basagoitia B: A potentially lethal anesthesia machine failure. Anesthesiology 66:589, 1987.

47. Neubarth J: Another hazardous gas supply misconnection [letter]. Anesth Analg 80:206, 1995.

48. Gaughan SD, Benumof JL, Ozaki GT: Can an anesthesia machine flush valve provide for effective jet ventilation? Anesth Analg 76:800, 1993.

49. Anderson CE, Rendell-Baker L: Exposed O_2 flush hazard. Anesthesiology 56:328, 1982.

50. Internal leakage from anesthesia unit flush valves. Health Devices 10:172, 1981.

51. Andrews JJ: Understanding your anesthesia machine and ventilator. *In* 1989 Review Course Lectures. Cleveland, OH, International Anesthesia Research Society, 1989, p 59.

52. Datex-Ohmeda Aestiva Operation Manual, Parts 1 & 2. Madison, WI, Datex-Ohmeda, 2000.

53. Dodgson BG: Inappropriate use of the oxygen flush to check an anaesthetic machine. Can J Anaesth 35:336, 1988.

54. Dorsch JA, Dorsch SE: Vaporizers (anesthetic agent delivery devices). *In* Dorsch JA, Dorsch SE (eds): Understanding Anesthesia Machines, 4th ed. Baltimore, Williams & Wilkins, 1999, p 121.

55. Macintosh R, Mushin WW, Epstein HG: Vapor pressure. *In* Macintosh R, Mushin WW, Epstein HG (eds): Physics for the Anaesthetist, 3rd ed. Oxford, Blackwell Scientific Publications, 1963, p 68.

56. Adriani J: Principles of physics and chemistry of solids and fluids applicable to anesthesiology. *In* Adriani J (ed): The Chemistry and Physics of Anesthesia, 2nd ed. Springfield, IL, Charles C. Thomas, 1962, p 7.

57. Korman B, Ritchie IM. Chemistry of halothane-enflurane mixtures applied to anesthesia. Anesthesiology 63:152, 1985.

58. Macintosh R, Mushin WW, Epstein HG: Vaporization. *In* Macintosh R, Mushin WW, Epstein HG (eds): Physics for the Anaesthetist, 3rd ed. Oxford, Blackwell Scientific Publications, 1963, p 26.

59. Macintosh R, Mushin WW, Epstein HG: Specific heat. *In* Macintosh R, Mushin WW, Epstein HG (eds): Physics for the Anaesthetist, 3rd ed. Oxford, Blackwell Scientific Publications, 1963, p 17.

60. Schreiber P: Anaesthetic Equipment: Performance, Classification, and Safety. New York, Springer-Verlag, 1972.

61. Tec 4 Continuous Flow Vaporizer: Operator's Manual. Steeton, UK, Ohmeda & The BOC Group, 1987.
62. Dräger Vapor 19.n Anaesthetic Vaporizer: Instructions for Use, 14th ed. Lubeck, Federal Republic of Germany, Drägerwerk, 1990.
63. Hill DW, Lowe HJ: Comparison of concentration of halothane in closed and semi-closed circuits during controlled ventilation. Anesthesiology 23:291, 1962.
64. Hill DW: The design and calibration of vaporizers for volatile anaesthetic agents. *In* Scurr C, Feldman S (eds): Scientific Foundations of Anaesthesia, 3rd ed. London, William Heineman Medical Books, 1982, p 544.
65. Hill DW: The design and calibration of vaporizers for volatile anaesthetic agents. Br J Anaesth 40:648, 1968.
66. Tec 7 Vaporizer: User's Reference Manual. Madison, WI, Datex-Ohmeda, 2002.
67. Morris LE: Problems in the performance of anesthesia vaporizers. Int Anesthesiol Clin 12:199, 1974.
68. Stoelting RK: The effects of nitrous oxide on halothane output from Fluotec Mark 2 vaporizers. Anesthesiology 35:215, 1971.
69. Diaz PD: The influence of carrier gas on the output of automatic vaporizers. Br J Anaesth 48:387, 1976.
70. Nawaf K, Stoelting RK: Nitrous oxide increases enflurane concentrations delivered by Ethrane vaporizers. Anesth Analg 58:30, 1979.
71. Prins L, Strupat J, Clement J: An evaluation of gas density dependence of anaesthetic vaporizers. Can Anaesth Soc J 27:106, 1980.
72. Lin CY: Assessment of vaporizer performance in low-flow and closed-circuit anesthesia. Anesth Analg 59:359, 1980.
73. Gould DB, Lampert BA, MacKrell TN: Effect of nitrous oxide solubility on vaporizer aberrance. Anesth Analg 61:938, 1982.
74. Palayiwa E, Sanderson MH, Hahn CEW: Effects of carrier gas composition on the output of six anaesthetic vaporizers. Br J Anaesth 55:1025, 1983.
75. Scheller MS, Drummond JC: Solubility of N_2O in volatile anesthetics contributes to vaporizer aberrancy when changing carrier gases. Anesth Analg 65:88, 1986.
76. Tec 5 Continuous Flow Vaporizer: Operation and Maintenance Manual. Steeton, UK, Ohmeda & The BOC Group, 1990.
77. Karis JH, Menzel DB: Inadvertent change of volatile anesthetics in anesthesia machines. Anesth Analg 61:53, 1982.
78. Riegle EV, Desertspring D: Failure of the agent-specific filling device [letter]. Anesthesiology 73:353, 1990.
79. George TM: Failure of keyed agent-specific filling devices. Anesthesiology 61:228, 1984.
80. Broka SM, Gourdange PA, Joucken KL: Sevoflurane and desflurane confusion. Anesth Analg 88:1194, 1999.
81. Lippmann M, Foran W, Ginsburg R et al: Contamination of anesthetic vaporizer contents. Anesthesiology 78:1175, 1993.
82. Munson WM: Cardiac arrest: A hazard of tipping a vaporizer. Anesthesiology 26:235, 1965.
83. DrägerVapor 2000: Operating Instructions. Telford, PA, Drager Medical, 1999.
84. Sinclair A: Vaporizer overfilling. Can J Anaesth 40:77, 1993.
85. Seropian MA, Robins B: Smaller than expected sevoflurane concentrations using the SevoTec 5 vaporizer at low fill states and high fresh gas flows. Anesth Analg 91:834, 2000.
86. Peters KR, Wingard DW: Anesthesia machine leakage due to misaligned vaporizers. Anesth Rev 14:36, 1987.
87. Meister GC, Becker KE Jr: Potential fresh gas flow leak through Dräger vapor 19.1 vaporizer with key-index fill port. Anesthesiology 78:211, 1993.
88. Lewis SE, Andrews JJ, Long GW: An unexpected Penlon sigma elite vaporizer leak. Anesthesiology 90:1221, 1999.
89. Andrews JJ, Johnston RV Jr: The new Tec 6 desflurane vaporizer. Anesth Analg 76:1338, 1993.
90. Weiskopf RB, Sampson D, Moore MA: The desflurane (Tec 6) vaporizer: Design, design considerations and performance evaluation. Br J Anaesth 72:474, 1994.
91. Eger EI: New inhaled anesthetics. Anesthesiology 80:906, 1994.
92. Tec 6 Vaporizer: Operation and Maintenance Manual. Steeton, UK, The BOC Group, 1993.
93. Susay SR, Smith MA, Lockwood GG: The saturated vapor pressure of desflurane at various temperatures. Anesth Analg 83:864, 1996.
94. Johnston RV Jr, Andrews JJ: The effects of carrier gas composition on the performance of the Tec 6 desflurane vaporizer. Anesth Analg 79:548, 1994.
95. Andrews JJ, Johnston RV Jr, Kramer GC: Consequences of misfilling contemporary vaporizers with desflurane. Can J Anaesth 40:71, 1993.
96. Mapleson WW: The elimination of rebreathing in various semiclosed anaesthetic systems. Br J Anaesth 26:323, 1954.
97. Willis BA, Pender JW, Mapleson WW: Rebreathing in a T-piece: Volunteer and theoretical studies of the Jackson-Rees modification of Ayre's T-piece during spontaneous respiration. Br J Anaesth 47:1239, 1975.
98. Rose DK, Froese AB: The regulation of $Paco_2$ during controlled ventilation of children with a T-piece. Canad Anaesth Soc J 26:104, 1979.
99. Froese AB, Rose DK: A detailed analysis of T-piece systems. *In* Steward (ed): Some Aspects of Paediatric Anaesthesia. Amsterdam, Elsevier/North Holland Biomedical Press, 1982, pp 101-136.
100. Sykes MK: Rebreathing circuits: A review. Br J Anaesth 40:666, 1968.
101. Dorsch JA, Dorsch SE: The breathing system II. The Mapleson systems *In* Dorsch JA, Dorsch SE (eds): Understanding Anesthesia Equipment, 2nd ed. Baltimore, Williams & Wilkins, 1984, pp 182-196.
102. Bain JA, Spoerel WE: A streamlined anaesthetic system. Can Anaesth Soc J 19:426, 1972.
103. Aarhus D, Holst-Larsen E, Holst-Larsen H: Mechanical obstruction in the anaesthesia delivery-system mimicking severe bronchospasm. Anaesthesia 52:992, 1997.
104. Pethick SL: Letter to the editor. Can Anaesth Soc J 22:115, 1975.
105. Moyers J: A nomenclature for methods of inhalation anesthesia. Anesthesiology 14:609, 1953.
106. Eger EI II: Anesthetic systems: Construction and function. *In* Eger EI II (ed): Anesthetic Uptake and Action. Baltimore, Williams & Wilkins, 1974, p 206.
107. Eger EI II, Ethans CT: The effects of inflow, overflow and valve placement on economy of the circle system. Anesthesiology 29:93, 1968.
108. Smith CE, Otworth JR, Kaluszyk GSW: Bilateral tension pneumothorax due to a defective anesthesia breathing circuit filter. J Clin Anesth 3:229, 1991.
109. McEwan AI, Dowell L, Karis JH: Bilateral tension pneumothorax caused by a blocked bacterial filter in an anesthesia breathing circuit. Anesth Analg 76:440-442, 1993.
110. Walton JS, Fears R, Burt N, Dorman BH: Intraoperative breathing circuit obstruction caused by albuterol nebulization. Anesth Analg 89:650, 1999.
111. Dhar P, George I, Sloan P: Flow transducer gas leak detected after induction. Anesth Analg 89:1587, 1999.
112. Kshatri AM, Kingsley CP: Defective carbon dioxide absorber as a cause for a leak in a breathing circuit. Anesthesiology 84:475, 1996.
113. Norman PH, Daley MD, Walker JR, Fusetti S: Obstruction due to retained carbon dioxide absorber canister wrapping. Anesth Analg 83:425, 1996.
114. Adriani J: Carbon dioxide absorption. *In* Adriani J (ed): The Chemistry and Physics of Anesthesia, 2nd ed. Springfield, IL, Charles C Thomas, 1962, p 151.
115. Dewey & Almy Chemical Division: The Sodasorb Manual of CO_2 Absorption. New York, WR Grace & Company, 1962.
116. Murray JM, Renfrew CW, Bedi A, et al: A new carbon dioxide absorbent for use in anesthetic breathing systems. Anesthesiology 91:1342, 1999.
117. Versichelen LF, Bouche MP, Rolly G, et al: Only carbon dioxide absorbents free of both NaOH and KOH do not generate compound-A during in vitro closed system sevoflurane: Evaluation of five absorbents. Anesthesiology 95:750, 2001.
118. Hunt HE: Resistance in respiratory valves and canisters. Anesthesiology 16:190, 1955.

119. Brown ES: Performance of absorbents: Continuous flow. Anesthesiology 20:41, 1959.

120. Andrews JJ, Johnston RV Jr, Bee DE, et al: Photodeactivation of ethyl violet: A potential hazard of Sodasorb. Anesthesiology 72:59, 1990.

121. Case History 39: Accidental use of trichloroethylene (Trilene, Trimar) in a closed system. Anesth Analg 43:740, 1964.

122. Morio M, Fujii K, Satoh N, et al: Reaction of sevoflurane and its degradation products with soda lime. Anesthesiology 77:1155, 1992.

123. Kharasch ED, Powers KM, Artru AAl: Comparison of Amsorb, sodalime, Baralyme degradation of volatile anesthetics and formation of carbon monoxide and compound A in swine in vivo. Anesthesiology 96:173, 2002.

124. Frink EJ Jr, Malan TP, Morgan SE, et al: Quantification of the degradation products of sevoflurane in two CO_2 absorbants during low-flow anesthesia in surgical patients. Anesthesiology 77:1064, 1992.

125. Fang ZX, Kandel L, Laster MJ, et al: Factors affecting production of compound A from the interaction of sevoflurane with Baralyme and soda lime. Anesth Analg 82:775, 1996.

126. Eger EI II, Ion P, Laster MJ, Weiskopf RB: Baralyme dehydration increases and soda lime dehydration decreases the concentration of compound A resulting from sevoflurane degradation in a standard anesthetic circuit. Anesth Analg 85:892, 1997.

127. Steffey EP, Laster MJ, Ionescu P, et al: Dehydration of Baralyme increases compound A resulting from sevoflurane degradation in a standard anesthetic circuit used to anesthetize swine. Anesth Analg 85:1382, 1997.

128. Eger EL II, Koblin DD, Bowland T, et al: Nephrotoxicity of sevoflurane versus desflurane anesthesia in volunteers. Anesth Analg 84:160, 1997.

129. Kharasch ED, Frink EJ Jr, Zager R, et al: Assessment of low-flow sevoflurane and isoflurane effects on renal function using sensitive markers of tubular toxicity. Anesthesiology 86:1238, 1997.

130. Bito H, Ikeuchi Y, Ikeda K: Effects of low-flow sevoflurane anesthesia on renal function: Comparison with high-flow sevoflurane anesthesia and low-flow isoflurane anesthesia. Anesthesiology 86:1231, 1997.

131. Berry PD, Sessler DI, Larson MD: Severe carbon monoxide poisoning during desflurane anesthesia. Anesthesiology 90:613, 1999.

132. Baxter PJ, Kharasch ED: Rehydration of desiccated baralyme prevents carbon monoxide formation from desflurane in an anesthesia machine. Anesthesiology 86:1061, 1997.

133. Woehlck HJ, Dunning M, Connolly LA: Reduction in the incidence of carbon monoxide exposures in humans undergoing general anesthesia. Anesthesiology 87:228, 1997.

134. Fang ZX, Eger EI, Laster MJ, et al: Carbon monoxide production from degradation of desflurane, enflurane, isoflurane, halothane, and sevoflurane by soda lime and Baralyme. Anesth Analg 80:1187, 1995.

135. Bonome C, Belda J, Alvarez-Refojo F, et al: Low-flow anesthesia and reduced animal size increase carboxyhemoglobin levels in swine during desflurane and isoflurane breakdown in dried soda lime. Anesth Analg 89:909, 1999.

136. Neumann MA, Laster MJ, Weiskopf RB, et al: The elimination of sodium and potassium hydroxides from desiccated soda lime diminishes degradation of desflurane to carbon monoxide and sevoflurane to compound A but does not compromise carbon dioxide absorption. Anesth Analg 89:768, 1999.

137. Spearman CB, Sanders HG: Physical principles and functional designs of ventilators. *In* Kirby RR, Smith RA, Desautels DA (eds): Mechanical Ventilation. New York, Churchill Livingstone, 1985, p 59.

138. McPherson SP, Spearman CB: Introduction to ventilators. *In* McPherson SP, Spearman CB (eds): Respiratory Therapy Equipment, 3rd ed. St. Louis, CV Mosby, 1985, p 230.

139. 7000 Electronic Anesthesia Ventilator: Operation and Maintenance. Madison, WI, Ohmeda, The BOC Group, 1985.

140. 7000 Electronic Anesthesia Ventilator: Service Manual. Madison, WI, Ohmeda, The BOC Group, 1985.

141. Cooper JB, Newbower RS, Kitz RJ: An analysis of major errors and equipment failures in anesthesia management: Considerations for prevention and detection. Anesthesiology 60:34, 1984.

142. Reinhart DJ, Friz R: Undetected leak in corrugated circuit tubing in compressed configuration. Anesthesiology 78:218, 1993.

143. Raphael DT, Weller RS, Doran DJ: A response algorithm for the low-pressure alarm condition. Anesth Analg 67:876, 1988.

144. Slee TA, Pavlin EG: Failure of low pressure alarm associated with use of a humidifier. Anesthesiology 69:791, 1988.

145. Sattari R, Reichard PS, Riddle RT: Temporary malfunction of the Ohmeda modulus CD series volume monitor caused by the overhead surgical lighting. Anesthesiology 91:894, 1999.

146. Feeley TW, Bancroft ML: Problems with mechanical ventilators. Int Anesthesiol Clin 20:83, 1982.

147. Khalil SN, Gholston TK, Binderman J: Flapper valve malfunction in an Ohio closed scavenging system. Anesth Analg 66:1334, 1987.

148. Sommer RM, Bhalla GS, Jackson JM: Hypoventilation caused by ventilator valve rupture. Anesth Analg 67:999, 1988.

149. Roth S, Tweedie E, Sommer RM: Excessive airway pressure due to a malfunctioning anesthesia ventilator. Anesthesiology 65:532, 1986.

150. Dorsch JA, Dorsch SE: Anesthesia ventilators. *In* Dorsch JA, Dorsch SE (eds): Understanding Anesthesia Equipment, 4th ed. Baltimore, Williams & Wilkins, 1999, p 309-353.

151. Dorsch JA, Dorsch SE: Controlling trace gas levels. *In* Dorsch JA, Dorsch SE (eds): Understanding Anesthesia Equipment, 4th ed. Baltimore, Williams & Wilkins, 1999, p 355.

152. National Institute for Occupational Safety and Health: Criteria for a Recommended Standard: Occupational Exposure to Waste Anesthetic Gases and Vapors. Washington, DC, US Department of Health, Education, and Welfare, March, 1977.

153. American Society for Testing and Materials: Standard Specification for Anesthetic Equipment—Scavenging Systems for Anesthetic Gases (ASTM F1343-91). Philadelphia, American Society for Testing and Materials, 1991.

154. ASA Task Force on Trace Anesthetic Gases, McGregor DG, Chair: Waste Anesthetic Gases: Information for Management in Anesthetizing Areas and the Postanesthesia Care Unit (PACU). Park Ridge, IL, American Society of Anesthesiologists, 1999, pp 3-28.

155. Kanmura Y, Sakai J, Yoshinaka H, Shirao K: Causes of nitrous oxide contamination in operating rooms. Anesthesiology 90:693, 1999.

156. Open Reservoir Scavenger: Operator's Instruction Manual. Telford, PA, North American Dräger, 1986.

157. Gray WM: Scavenging equipment. Br J Anaesth 57:685, 1985.

158. Scavenger Interface for Air Conditioning: Instruction Manual. Telford, PA, North American Dräger, 1984.

159. Cooper JB: Toward prevention of anesthetic mishaps. Int Anesthesiol Clin 22:167, 1984.

160. Spooner RB, Kirby RR: Equipment related anesthetic incidents. Int Anesthesiol Clin 22:133, 1984.

161. Emergency Care Research Institute: Avoiding anesthetic mishaps through pre-use checks. Health Devices 11:201, 1982.

162. US Food and Drug Administration: Anesthesia Apparatus Checkout Recommendations, 8th ed. Rockville, MD, US Food and Drug Administration, 1986.

163. US Food and Drug Administration: Anesthesia Apparatus Checkout Recommendations. Rockville, MD, US Food and Drug Administration, 1993.

164. Myers JA, Good ML, Andrews JJ: Comparison of tests for detecting leaks in the low-pressure system of anesthesia gas machines. Anesth Analg 84:179, 1997.

165. Dorsch JA, Dorsch SE: Hazards of anesthesia machines and breathing systems. *In* Dorsch JA, Dorsch SE (eds): Understanding Anesthesia Equipment, 4th ed. Baltimore, Williams & Wilkins, 1999, p 399.

166. Comm G, Rendell-Baker L: Back pressure check valves: A hazard. Anesthesiology 56:227, 1982.

APPENDIX 1

10 # Anesthesia Apparatus Checkout Recommendations, 1993

This checkout list or a reasonable equivalent should be conducted before administration of anesthesia. These recommendations are valid only for an anesthesia system that conforms to current and relevant standards and that includes an ascending bellows ventilator and at least the following monitors: capnograph, pulse oximeter, oxygen analyzer, respiratory volume monitor (i.e., spirometer), and breathing system pressure monitor with high-pressure and low-pressure alarms. Users are encouraged to modify these guidelines to accommodate differences in equipment design and variations in local clinical practice. Such local modifications should have appropriate peer review. Users should refer to the operator's manual for the manufacturer's specific procedures and precautions, especially the manufacturer's low-pressure leak test (step 5).

EMERGENCY VENTILATION EQUIPMENT

*1. Verify Backup Ventilation Equipment Is Available and Functioning

HIGH-PRESSURE SYSTEM

*2. Check Oxygen Cylinder Supply
    a. Open O_2 cylinder and verify that it is at least half full (about 1000 psi).
    b. Close cylinder.
*3. Check Central Pipeline Supplies
    a. Check that hoses are connected and that pipeline gauges read about 50 psi.

LOW-PRESSURE SYSTEM

*4. Check Initial Status of the Low-Pressure System
    a. Close flow control valves, and turn vaporizers off.
    b. Check the fill level, and tighten the vaporizers' filler caps.
*5. Perform a Leak Check of the Machine's Low-Pressure System
    a. Verify that the machine master switch and flow control valves are OFF.
    b. Attach a suction bulb to the common (fresh) gas outlet.
    c. Squeeze the bulb repeatedly until fully collapsed.
    d. Verify bulb stays *fully* collapsed for at least 10 seconds.
    e. Open one vaporizer at a time, and repeat steps c and d above.
    f. Remove the suction bulb, and reconnect the fresh gas hose.
*6. Turn on the Machine's Master Switch and All Other Necessary Electrical Equipment.
*7. Test Flow Meters
    a. Adjust flow of all gases through their full range, checking for smooth operation of floats and undamaged flow tubes.
    b. Attempt to create a hypoxic O_2/N_2O mixture, and verify correct changes in the flow and/or alarms.

SCAVENGING SYSTEM

*8. Adjust and Check the Scavenging System
    a. Ensure proper connections between the scavenging system and both the adjustable pressure limiting (APL) (pop-off) valve and the ventilator's relief valve.
    b. Adjust the waste gas vacuum (if possible).
    c. Fully open the APL valve and occlude the Y-piece.
    d. With minimum O_2 flow, allow the scavenger reservoir bag to collapse completely, and verify that the absorber pressure gauge reads about zero.
    e. With the O_2 flush activated, allow the scavenger reservoir bag to distend fully, and then verify that absorber pressure gauge reads <10 cm H_2O.

BREATHING SYSTEM

*9. Calibrate the O_2 Monitor
    a. Ensure the monitor reads 21% in room air.
    b. Verify that the low O_2 alarm is enabled and functioning.
    c. Reinstall the sensor in the circuit, and flush the breathing system with O_2.
    d. Verify that monitor now reads greater than 90%.
10. Check Initial Status of Breathing System
    a. Set the selector switch to Bag mode.
    b. Check that the breathing circuit is complete, undamaged, and unobstructed.
    c. Verify that the carbon dioxide absorbent is adequate.
    d. Install the breathing circuit accessory equipment (e.g., humidifier, PEEP valve) to be used during the case.
11. Perform a Leak Check of the Breathing System
    a. Set all gas flows to zero (or minimum).
    b. Close the APL (pop-off) valve, and occlude the Y-piece.
    c. Pressurize the breathing system to about 30 cm H_2O with an O_2 flush.
    d. Ensure that pressure remains fixed for at least 10 seconds.
    e. Open the APL (pop-off) valve, and ensure that the pressure decreases.

MANUAL AND AUTOMATIC VENTILATION SYSTEMS

12. Test the Ventilation Systems and Unidirectional Valves
    a. Place a second breathing bag on the Y-piece.
    b. Set appropriate ventilator parameters for the next patient.
    c. Switch to automatic ventilation mode (i.e., Ventilator).
    d. Turn the ventilator ON, and fill the bellows and breathing bag with an O_2 flush.
    e. Set the O_2 flow to minimum and other gas flows to zero.
    f. Verify that the bellows deliver an appropriate tidal volume during inspiration and that the bellows fill completely during expiration.
    g. Set the fresh gas flow to about 5 L/min.
    h. Verify that the ventilator's bellows and simulated lungs fill *and empty* appropriately without sustained pressure at end expiration.
    i. Check for proper action of unidirectional valves.
    j. Exercise breathing circuit accessories to ensure proper function.
    k. Turn the ventilator off, and switch to manual ventilation mode (i.e., Bag/APL).
    l. Ventilate manually, and ensure inflation and deflation of artificial lungs and appropriate feel of system resistance and compliance.
    m. Remove second breathing bag from the Y-piece.

MONITORS

13. Check, Calibrate, and/or Set Alarm Limits of all Monitors
    a. Capnometer
    b. Oxygen analyzer
    c. Pressure monitor with alarms for high and low airway pressure
    d. Pulse oximeter
    e. Respiratory volume monitor (i.e., spirometer)

FINAL POSITION

14. Check Final Status of the Machine
    a. Vaporizers are off.
    b. APL valve is open.
    c. Selector is switched to Bag mode.
    d. All flow meters are set to zero (or minimum).
    e. Suction level is adequate for the patient.
    f. Breathing system is ready to use.

*If an anesthesia provider uses the same machine in successive cases, these steps need not be repeated or may be abbreviated after the initial checkout.

10 Intravenous Nonopioid Anesthetics

J. G. Reves, Peter S. A. Glass, David A. Lubarsky, and Matthew D. McEvoy

Propofol   318
History   318
Physicochemical Characteristics   318
Metabolism   318
Pharmacokinetics   318
Pharmacology   320
Uses   325
Side Effects and Contraindications   326

Barbiturates   326
History   326
Physicochemical Characteristics   328
Metabolism   329
Pharmacokinetics   329
Pharmacology   330
Uses   332
Side Effects and Contraindications   333

Benzodiazepines   334
History   334
Physicochemical Characteristics   335
Metabolism   335
Pharmacokinetics   336
Pharmacology   337
Uses   340
Side Effects and Contraindications   342
New Benzodiazepines   342

Flumazenil   343
Physicochemical Characteristics   343
Metabolism   343
Pharmacokinetics   344
Pharmacology   344
Uses and Doses   344
Side Effects and Contraindications   345

Phencyclidines (Ketamine)   345
History   345
Physicochemical Characteristics   345
Metabolism   346
Pharmacokinetics   346
Pharmacology   346
Uses   348
Doses and Routes of Administration   350
Side Effects and Contraindications   350

Etomidate   350
History   350
Physicochemical Characteristics   351
Metabolism, Induction, and Maintenance of
   Anesthesia   351
Pharmacokinetics   351
Pharmacology   352
Uses   355

**α_2-Adrenergic Agonists:
   Dexmedetomidine   355**
History   355
Physicochemical Characteristics   356
Metabolism and Pharmacokinetics   356
Pharmacology   356
Uses   358

Droperidol   359
History   359
Metabolism and Pharmacokinetics   360
Pharmacology   360
Uses   360

Summary   361

The introduction of thiopental into clinical practice in 1934 marked the advent of modern intravenous anesthesia. Thiopental and other barbiturates, however, are not ideal intravenous anesthetics, primarily because they provide only hypnosis. The ideal intravenous anesthetic drug would provide hypnosis, amnesia, analgesia, and muscle relaxation without undesirable cardiac and respiratory depression.

Because no single drug is ideal, many other drugs are used, often together, that offer some or all of the desired effects. These drugs were introduced steadily into clinical practice with varying degrees of acceptance. With an increasing number of compounds and superior methods of intravenous anesthetic drug delivery available (see Chapter 9), the use of intravenous anesthetics continues to grow.

The future of anesthetic management involves the simultaneous use of several drugs, including inhaled anesthetics. A 1988 survey of mortality in 100,000 anesthesia cases revealed that the practice of combined anesthetic drug use may be safer than the use of only one or two drugs[1]; the relative odds of dying within 7 days was 2.9 times greater when one or two anesthetic drugs were used than when three or more were used. Although it is exceedingly difficult to interpret these data, the use of several drugs may be beneficial to anesthetic care. Thus, the skillful use of multiple intravenous anesthetics is not only possible but preferable. The purpose of this chapter is to provide information on the major nonopioid intravenous anesthetic drugs available for clinical use today.

PROPOFOL

History

Propofol is the most frequently used intravenous anesthetic today. Work in the early 1970s on substituted derivatives of phenol with hypnotic properties resulted in the development of 2,6-diisopropofol.[2] The first clinical trial, reported by Kay and Rolly[3] in 1977, confirmed the potential of propofol as an anesthetic induction agent. Propofol is insoluble in water and was therefore initially prepared with Cremophor EL (BASF A.G.). Because of anaphylactoid reactions associated with Cremophor EL in this early formulation of propofol,[4] the drug was reformulated as an emulsion. Propofol is used for induction and maintenance of anesthesia, as well as for sedation in and outside the operating room.

Physicochemical Characteristics

Propofol (Fig. 10-1) is one of a group of alkylphenols that have hypnotic properties in animals.[5] The alkylphenols are oils at room temperature and insoluble in aqueous solution, but they are highly lipid soluble. Today, several formulations are presently marketed, and several others are in development. The formulation that followed the removal of Cremophor consists of 1% (weight/volume) propofol, 10% soybean oil, 2.25% glycerol, and 1.2% purified egg phosphatide. Because of concern regarding microbial growth in the emulsion, disodium edetate (0.005%) was added as a retardant of bacterial growth. This formulation has a pH of 7 and appears as a slightly viscous, milky white substance. A second formulation

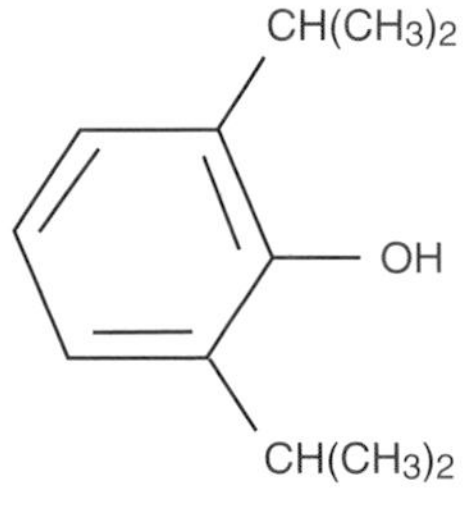

Figure 10–1 Structure of propofol, an alkylphenol derivative.

containing metabisulfite as the antimicrobial has also been introduced for commercial use in the United States. In Europe, a 2% formulation is also available, as well as a formulation in which the emulsion contains a mixture of medium- and long-chain triglycerides. All formulations available commercially are stable at room temperature and are not light sensitive. Changes in the diluent may result in slight changes in pharmacokinetics, cracking of the emulsion, spontaneous degradation of propofol, and possibly changes in pharmacologic effect. If a dilute solution of propofol is required, it is compatible with 5% dextrose in water.

Metabolism

Propofol is rapidly metabolized in the liver by conjugation to glucuronide and sulfate[6] to produce water-soluble compounds, which are excreted by the kidneys.[6] Less than 1% of propofol is excreted unchanged in urine, and only 2% is excreted in feces.[6] The metabolites of propofol are not thought to be active. Because clearance of propofol exceeds hepatic blood flow, extrahepatic metabolism or extrarenal elimination has been suggested. Extrahepatic metabolism has been confirmed during the anhepatic phase of patients receiving a transplanted liver.[7,8] The lungs seem to play an important role in this extrahepatic metabolism. They are responsible for approximately 30% of the uptake and first-pass elimination after a bolus dose.[9] During a continuous infusion of propofol there is a 20% to 30% decrease in propofol concentration measured across the lung in humans and a higher concentration of the metabolite 2,6-diisopropyl-1,4-quinol on the arterial side of the circulation.[10] Other sites of propofol metabolism are also likely. During in vitro studies with human kidney and small intestine, microsomes in these tissues demonstrated an ability to form propofol glucuronide.[11] Propofol itself results in a concentration-dependent inhibition of cytochrome P450 and thus may alter the metabolism of drugs dependent on this enzyme system (e.g., opiates).[12]

Pharmacokinetics

The pharmacokinetics of propofol has been evaluated by numerous investigators after a wide range of doses as well as after continuous infusion,[6,13-18] and it has been described by both two- and three-compartment models (see Table 10-1). After a single bolus injection, whole blood propofol levels decrease rapidly as a result of both redistribution and elimination (Fig. 10-2). The initial distribution half-life of propofol is 2 to 8 minutes.[6,14] In studies using a two-compartment model, the elimination half-life has varied from 1.0 to 3 hours.[6,13,17,18] Studies in which the disposition of propofol was better described by a three-compartment model have yielded initial and slow distribution half-lives of 1 to 8 minutes and 30 to 70 minutes and an elimination half-life of 4 to 23.5 hours.[14-16,18,43] This longer elimination half-life is indicative of a deep compartment with limited perfusion, which results in a slow return of propofol back to the central compartment. Because of rapid clearance of propofol from the central compartment, the slow return of propofol from this deep

Table 10–1 Pharmacokinetic variables of commonly used intravenous anesthetics

Drug	Elimination Half-Life (hr)	Clearance (mL/kg/min)	Vd$_{SS}$ (L/kg)	Reference
Dexmedetomidine	2-3	10-30	2-3	19, 20
Diazepam	20-50	0.2-0.5	0.7-1.7	21
Droperidol	1.7-2.2	14	2.0	22, 23
Etomidate	2.9-5.3	18-25	2.5-4.5	24-28
Flumazenil	0.7-1.3	5-20	0.6-1.6	29, 30
Ketamine	2.5-2.8	12-17	3.1	31
Lorazepam	11-22	0.8-1.8	0.8-1.3	21
Methohexital	2-6	10-15	1.5-3	32, 33
Midazolam	1.7-2.6	6.4-11	1.1-1.7	21
Propofol	4-7	20-30	2-10	34-40
Thiopental	7-17	3-4	1.5-3	33, 41, 42

Vd$_{SS}$, apparent volume of distribution at steady state.

compartment contributes little to the initial rapid decrease in propofol concentration. The context-sensitive half-time of propofol (Fig. 10-3) for infusions lasting up to 8 hours is less than 40 minutes.[44] Because the required decrease in concentration for awakening after anesthesia or sedation with propofol is generally less than 50%, recovery from propofol remains rapid even after prolonged infusions. The volume of distribution of the central compartment has been calculated as 20 to 40 L, and the volume of distribution at steady state has been calculated as 150 to 700 L.[6,13-18] Clearance of propofol is extremely high—1.5 to 2.2 L/min.[6,13-18] As discussed earlier, this clearance exceeds hepatic blood flow, and extrahepatic metabolism has been demonstrated.[7,8] The equilibrium constant (k_{e0}) for propofol based on suppression of the electroencephalogram (EEG) (which is strongly correlated with loss of consciousness) is about 0.3 min^{-1}, and the half-life of equilibrium between the plasma concentration and the EEG effect is 2.5 minutes. The time to

peak effect is 90 to 100 seconds.[45] These values are dependent on the actual pharmacokinetic set from which they are derived. The onset of EEG effect with propofol seems to be independent of age. However, if the measure of effect is systolic blood pressure, its onset is much slower (double the time) and increases with age.[46] For both EEG and hemodynamic end points, the elderly show a concentration-dependent increasing sensitivity.[46,47]

The pharmacokinetics of propofol may be altered by a variety of factors (e.g., gender, weight, preexisting disease, age, concomitant medication).[14,15,18,48,49] Propofol may impair its own clearance by decreasing hepatic blood flow.[50] Of clinical significance is that propofol may alter its own intercompartmental clearance because of its effects on cardiac output. Changes in cardiac output alter

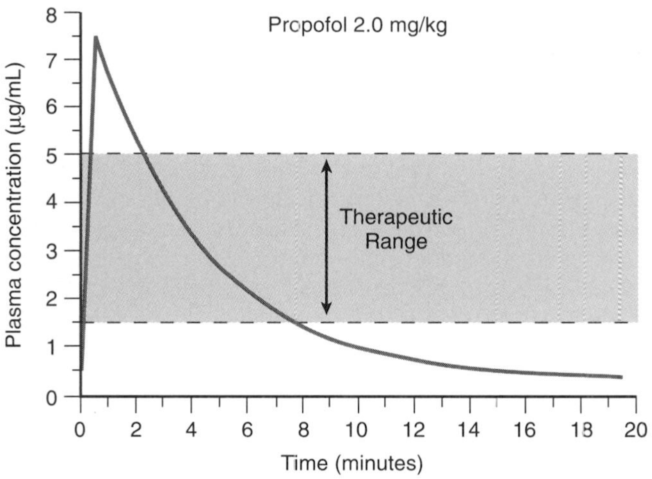

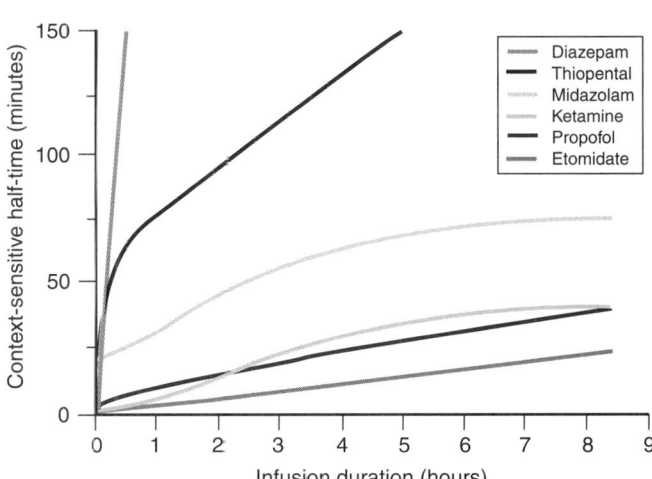

Figure 10–3 The context-sensitive half-times for commonly used intravenous anesthetic drugs are displayed. The context-sensitive half-time is the time for the plasma level of the drug to drop 50% after cessation of infusion. The duration of infusion is plotted on the horizontal axis. Note that the rapidity with which the drug level drops is directly related to the time of infusion (i.e., the longer the drug is infused, the longer the half-time). Also note that etomidate, propofol, and ketamine have significantly shorter half-times than thiopental and diazepam do, which makes them more suitable for prolonged infusion.

Figure 10–2 Simulated time course of whole blood levels of propofol after an induction dose of 2.0 mg/kg. Blood levels required for anesthesia during surgery are 2 to 5 µg/mL, with awakening usually occurring at a blood level lower than 1.5 µg/mL.

propofol concentrations after a bolus dose and during constant infusion. Increasing cardiac output leads to a decrease in propofol plasma concentration and vice versa.[51,52] In a hemorrhagic shock model, propofol concentrations increase up to 20% until uncompensated shock occurs, at which point a rapid and marked increase in propofol concentration occurs.[53] Women have a higher volume of distribution and higher clearance rates, but the elimination half-life is similar for males and females.[14,18] The elderly have decreased clearance rates but a smaller central compartment volume.[15,18] In addition, patients presenting for coronary artery bypass surgery seem to have different pharmacokinetic parameters than other adult populations do. When a patient is placed on a cardiopulmonary bypass machine, the resulting increase in central volume and initial clearance necessitates higher initial infusion rates to maintain the same propofol plasma concentration.[54] Children have a larger central compartment volume (50%) and more rapid clearance (25%).[55] In children older than 3 years, volumes and clearances should be adjusted by weight.[56] Children younger than 3 years also demonstrate weight-proportional pharmacokinetic parameters, but with greater central compartment and systemic clearance values than in adults or older children.[56] This finding explains the higher dosing requirements in this age group.[57] Hepatic disease appears to result in larger steady-state and central compartment volumes; clearance is unchanged, but the elimination half-life is slightly prolonged.[48] The effect of fentanyl administration on the pharmacokinetic parameters of propofol is controversial. Some studies suggest that fentanyl may reduce intercompartmental and total-body clearance rates, as well as volumes of distribution.[58] When propofol was administered with alfentanil at similar infusion rates, the measured propofol concentrations were 22% greater than when propofol was administered alone.[59] A separate study found that fentanyl did not alter propofol pharmacokinetics after a single dose of both drugs.[60] Some of these differences in propofol pharmacokinetics when given with an opioid may be explained by studies in cats in which it was shown that pulmonary uptake of propofol is reduced by 30% when propofol is administered immediately after fentanyl, but not if administered 3 minutes later.[61] In addition, in vitro studies on human hepatocytes have demonstrated that propofol inhibits the enzymatic degradation of both sufentanil and alfentanil in a dose-dependent manner.[62] Propofol kinetics is unaltered by renal disease.[49]

Pharmacology

Effects on the Central Nervous System

Propofol is primarily a hypnotic. The exact mechanism of its action has not yet been fully elucidated; however, evidence suggests that a significant portion of its hypnotic action is mediated by potentiating the γ-aminobutyric acid (GABA)-induced chloride current through binding to the β-subunit of the $GABA_A$ receptor. Sites on the $β_1$ (M 286), $β_2$ (M 286), and $β_3$ (N265) subunits of the transmembrane domains have been shown to be critical for the hypnotic action of propofol.[63,64] The α- and $γ_2$-subtypes also seem to contribute to modulation of the effects of propofol on

the GABA receptor.[65] Through its action on $GABA_A$ receptors in the hippocampus, propofol inhibits acetylcholine release in the hippocampus and prefrontal cortex.[66] This action appears to be important for the sedative effects of propofol.[67] The $α_2$-adrenoreceptor system also seems to play an indirect role in the sedative effects of propofol.[68] Propofol results in widespread inhibition of the N-methyl-D-aspartate (NMDA) subtype of glutamate receptor through modulation of sodium channel gating,[69] an action that may also contribute to the drug's central nervous system (CNS) effects. Studies have demonstrated that propofol has a direct depressant effect on neurons of the spinal cord.[70] In acutely dissociated spinal dorsal horn neurons, propofol acts on both $GABA_A$ and glycine receptors.[71] The hypnotic action of propofol is pressure reversible, and it adheres to the correlation exhibited by other general anesthetics between anesthetic potency and octanol/water distribution coefficient.[72] Unlike barbiturates, propofol is not antianalgesic.[73] At subhypnotic doses, propofol helps in the diagnosis and treatment of central, but not neuropathic pain.[74]

Two interesting side effects of propofol are its antiemetic effect and the sense of well-being noted after administration. Propofol increases dopamine concentrations in the nucleus accumbens (a phenomenon noted with drugs of abuse and pleasure-seeking behavior).[75] Propofol's antiemetic action may be explained by the decrease in serotonin levels that it produces in the area postrema, probably through its action on GABA receptors.[76]

The onset of hypnosis after doses of 2.5 mg/kg is rapid (one arm–brain circulation), with a peak effect seen at 90 to 100 seconds.[77,78] The median effective dose (ED_{50}) of propofol for loss of consciousness is 1 to 1.5 mg/kg after a bolus.[77,79-81] The duration of hypnosis is dose dependent, being 5 to 10 minutes after 2 to 2.5 mg/kg.[77,82] Age markedly affects the induction dose; it is highest at ages younger than 2 years (ED_{95} of 2.88 mg/kg) and decreases with increasing age.[83] The effect of increasing age on decreasing the propofol concentration required for loss of consciousness is shown in Figure 10-4.[84] At subhypnotic doses, propofol provides sedation and amnesia.[85-87] Propofol infusions of at least 2 mg/kg/hr were necessary to provide amnesia in unstimulated volunteers.[88] Awareness during surgery at higher infusion rates has been reported.[89] During surgical procedures, extremely high infusion rates may be necessary to prevent awareness if propofol is used as the sole anesthetic.[90] Propofol alters mood after short surgical procedures to a lesser extent than thiopental does.[91] Propofol also tends to produce a general state of well-being.[91] Hallucinations,[92] sexual fantasies, and opisthotonos[93] have been reported after propofol administration.

The effect of propofol on the EEG as assessed after the administration of 2.5 mg/kg followed by an infusion demonstrates an initial increase in alpha rhythm followed by a shift to gamma and theta frequency. High infusion rates produce burst suppression (see Chapter 31).[94] EEG power analysis indicates that amplitude increases after induction but is thereafter unaltered at propofol blood concentrations of 3 to 8 μg/mL.[95] At propofol concentrations higher than 8 μg/mL, amplitude markedly decreases, with periods of burst suppression.[95] Propofol causes a

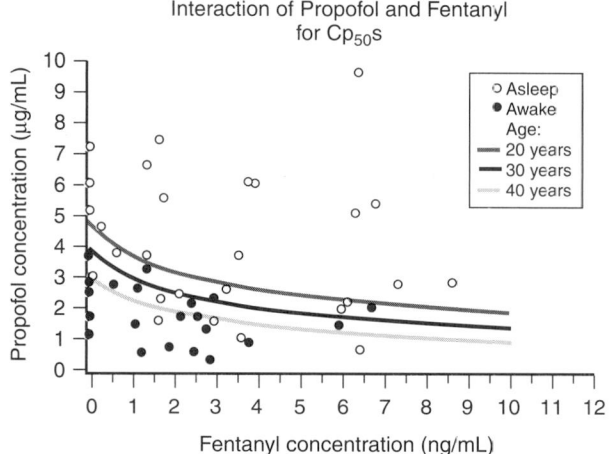

Figure 10–4 Measured arterial propofol and fentanyl concentrations at which patients did and did not respond to a verbal command 10 minutes after the initiation of infusion of these drugs. *Solid lines* denote the modeled concentrations of propofol according to the decade of age when combined with the measured fentanyl concentrations at which 50% of patients did not respond to verbal command ($Cp_{50}s$). (Redrawn from Smith C, McEwan A, Jhaveri R: Reduction of propofol Cp50 by fentanyl. Anesthesiology 81:820-828, 1994.)

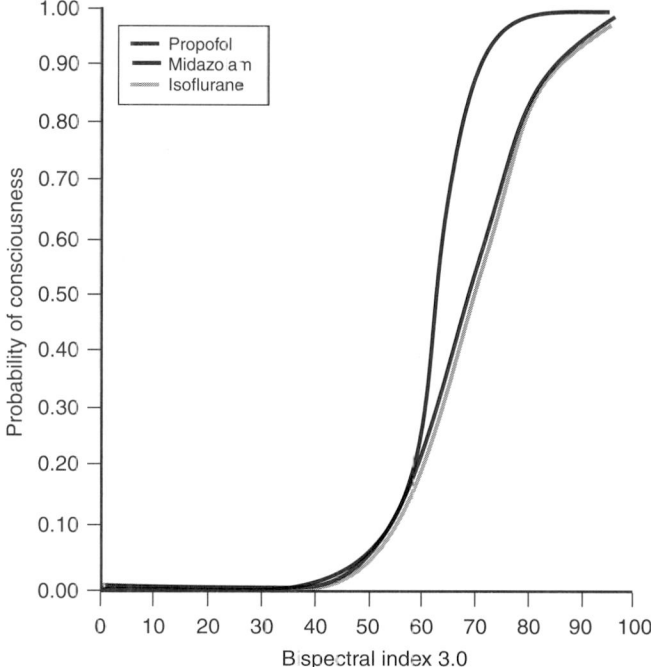

Figure 10–5 Relationship between the bispectral (BIS) index and the probability of consciousness (i.e., response to verbal command) with the use of logistic regression analysis in volunteers receiving propofol, isoflurane, or midazolam. The probability of response was no different for the three anesthetics used. It can also be noted that 95% of the volunteers were unconscious with a BIS index of 50 or less.

concentration-dependent decrease in the bispectral (BIS) index, with 50% and 95% of patients unable to respond to verbal command at BIS values of 63 and 51, respectively (Fig. 10-5). The propofol concentration at which 50% of volunteers failed to respond to verbal command was 2.35 μg/mL. Lack of recall was observed in 95% of patients at a BIS value of 77.[96] Propofol produces a decrease in amplitude of the early components of somatosensory evoked potentials,[97] as well as a small nonsignificant increase in latency of the P_{40} and N_{50} components.[97] Like other intravenous anesthetics, propofol does not alter brainstem auditory evoked potentials.[98] There is, however, a dose-dependent prolongation of latency, as well as a decrease in the amplitude of cortical middle-latency auditory potentials, which are concentration dependent.[98] Auditory evoked potentials show an abrupt change in the auditory evoked potential index between awake and nonresponsive patients. This finding differs from the BIS index, which tends to show a trend toward decreasing BIS values and increasing sedation and loss of consciousness with propofol administration.[99]

The effect of propofol on epileptogenic EEG activity is controversial. Initial studies in mice indicated that propofol neither induces convulsions nor provides anticonvulsant activity.[100] Several more recent reports have shown in a variety of models a direct anticonvulsant effect of propofol that is dose dependent.[101,102] In a few reports, propofol has been used to treat epileptic seizures.[103,104] Propofol also results in a shorter duration of motor and EEG seizure activity after electroconvulsive therapy than methohexital does.[105] Interestingly, propofol has been associated with grand mal seizures and has been used for cortical mapping of epileptogenic foci.[106,107] In 17 patients undergoing cortical resection for intractable epilepsy, 2 mg/kg propofol resulted in markedly reduced or ablated

seizure activity.[108] When propofol was administered at sedative doses to 14 patients with complex seizure disorders, no effect on seizure activity was noted.[109] A few reports have described convulsions after the administration of propofol that occurred several (6) days after anesthesia. Although most of these patients had a history of convulsions, a few did not. The incidence of this adverse effect is very low (≈1 in 50,000 administrations).[110] There have also been reports of tolerance to propofol developing after either repeat anesthesia or prolonged infusion (days),[111,112] but no reports of acute tolerance during a single case of anesthesia. In addition to tolerance, addiction to propofol has been reported.[113] Recently, propofol has been shown to be valuable in the treatment of chronic refractory headache at doses of 20 to 30 mg every 3 to 4 minutes (400 mg maximum).[114]

Propofol decreases intracranial pressure (ICP) in patients with either normal or increased ICP (see Chapter 21).[115-119] In patients with normal ICP, the decrease in ICP (30%) is associated with a small decrease in cerebral perfusion pressure (10%).[118] The administration of small doses of fentanyl and supplemental doses of propofol ablates the rise in ICP secondary to endotracheal intubation.[118] In patients with elevated ICP, the decrease in ICP (30% to 50%) is associated with significant decreases in cerebral perfusion pressure[116,120] and therefore may not be beneficial. Propofol acutely reduces intraocular pressure by 30% to 40%.[121,122] When compared with thiopental, propofol produces a larger decrease in intraocular pressure, and after a small second dose, it is more effective in preventing a rise in intraocular pressure secondary to succinylcholine and endotracheal intubation.[122] Normal cerebral reactivity to carbon dioxide and autoregulation are maintained during propofol infusion.[115,123,124] Propofol reduces the cerebral metabolic oxygen consumption rate ($CMRO_2$) by 36%.[115] With a background of 0.5% enflurane, propofol still reduces $CMRO_2$ by 18%, whereas lactate and glucose metabolism remains unchanged.[119] As determined by measuring the arteriovenous oxygen content difference, cerebral metabolic autoregulation is maintained during burst suppression with propofol.[125]

The neuroprotective effects of propofol remain controversial. Propofol administered to burst suppression results in significantly better neurologic outcomes and less brain tissue injury in an incomplete ischemia model in rats than fentanyl does.[126] Propofol also provides cerebral protective effects after an acute ischemic insult to the same degree that either halothane or thiopental does.[127,128] Propofol administered at sedative concentrations started either immediately or 1 hour after an ischemic insult significantly reduced infarct size when compared with awake controls infused with Intralipid.[129] Pretreatment with propofol fails to protect against focal ischemic insult.[130] In a spinal cord injury model, propofol reduced lipid peroxidation without improving the ultrastructure 1 hour after injury, in contrast to thiopental, which reduced both.[131] The neuronal protective effect of propofol may be due to the attenuation of changes in adenosine triphosphate (ATP), calcium, sodium, and potassium caused by hypoxic injury[132] and its antioxidant action by inhibiting lipid peroxidation.[133] Prolonged propofol sedation in children has been reported to be associated with neurologic sequelae.[134,135] Interestingly, in dissociated cultures of newborn rat cortex, 3-day treatment with propofol caused glial and GABAergic cell death, yet 7-day propofol treatment of intact hippocampal slices produced no lesions.[136]

The steady-state plasma concentration (Cp_{50}) of propofol for loss of response to verbal command in the absence of any other drug is 2.3 to 3.5 µg/mL.[84,137,138] The propofol Cp_{50} (arterial whole blood concentration) to prevent movement on skin incision is 16 µg/mL. This value is markedly reduced by increasing concentrations of fentanyl or alfentanil.[84,137,138] The propofol Cp_{50} for skin incision when combined with benzodiazepine premedication (lorazepam, 1 to 2 mg) and 66% nitrous oxide is 2.5 µg/mL (venous).[139] This concentration is reduced to 1.7 µg/mL when morphine (0.15 mg/kg) rather than lorazepam is used for premedication.[140] The concentration of propofol (when combined with 66% nitrous oxide) required during minor surgery varies from 1.5 to 4.5 µg/mL,[17,18] and that for major surgery varies from 2.5 to 6 µg/mL.[141] Awakening usually occurs at concentrations lower than 1.6 µg/mL,[17,18,82] and orientation is noted at concentrations lower than 1.2 µg/mL,[17,18] when the propofol concentration is falling. However, when equilibration between blood and the effect site is allowed, awakening concentrations (2.2 µg/mL) are much closer to those associated with loss of verbal command.[142] Age also affects (reduces) the propofol concentration required to provide adequate anesthesia.[18]

Effects on the Respiratory System (also see Chapter 17)

Apnea occurs after an induction dose of propofol, the incidence and duration of which appear to be dependent on the dose, speed of injection, and concomitant premedication. An induction dose of propofol results in a 25% to 30% incidence of apnea.[141,143] The duration of apnea occurring with propofol, however, may be prolonged to more than 30 seconds. The incidence of prolonged apnea (>30 seconds) is further increased by the addition of an opiate, either as premedication or just before induction,[141,143,144] and it is more frequent with propofol than with other commonly used intravenous induction agents.[143,145] The onset of apnea is usually preceded by a marked reduction in tidal volume and tachypnea.[144] After a 2.5-mg/kg induction dose of propofol, the respiratory rate is significantly decreased for 2 minutes,[143] and minute volume is significantly reduced for up to 4 minutes, a finding that indicates a more prolonged effect of propofol on tidal volume than on respiratory rate.

A maintenance infusion of propofol (100 µg/kg/min) results in a 40% decrease in tidal volume and a 20% increase in respiratory frequency, with an unpredictable change in minute ventilation.[144] Doubling the infusion rate from 100 to 200 µg/kg/min causes a further moderate decrease in tidal volume (455 to 380 mL) but no change in respiratory frequency.[144] The ventilatory response to carbon dioxide is also decreased during a maintenance infusion of propofol.[144] At 100 µg/kg/min, the slope of the carbon dioxide response curve is reduced by 58%,[144] similar to the 50% depression in carbon dioxide responsiveness measured with 1 minimum alveolar concentration (MAC) of halothane[146] or after a brief infusion of 3 mg/kg/min of thiopental.[147] Doubling the infusion rate (and presumably the blood level) of propofol results in only a minimal further decrease in carbon dioxide responsiveness,[44] in contrast to halothane, for which the use of twice the MAC results in halving the carbon dioxide response.[144] Propofol, 1.5 to 2.5 mg/kg, results in an acute (13% to 22%) rise in $Paco_2$ and a decrease in pH.[148-150] Pao_2 does not change significantly.[148-150] These changes are similar to those seen after an induction dose of thiopental.[149,150] During a maintenance infusion of propofol (54 µg/kg/min), $Paco_2$ is moderately increased from 39 to 52 mm Hg.[151] Doubling this infusion rate does not result in a further increase in $Paco_2$.[151] Propofol (50 to 120 µg/kg/min) also depresses the ventilatory response to hypoxia.[152]

Propofol induces bronchodilation in patients with chronic obstructive pulmonary disease.[153] It does not, however, appear to provide as effective bronchodilating properties as halothane does.[154] Propofol attenuates vagal (at low concentrations) and methacholine (at high concentrations) induced bronchoconstriction[155] and appears to have a direct action on muscarinic receptors. It inhibits the receptor-coupled signal transduction pathway through generation of inositol phosphate and inhibition of Ca^{2+} mobilization.[156] The preservative used with propofol appears to be important in its bronchodilator activity. Propofol with metabisulfite (versus propofol without metabisulfite) does not inhibit vagal- or methacholine-induced bronchoconstriction.[157]

Propofol may also have an impact on the pulmonary pathophysiology of adult respiratory distress syndrome. In an animal model of septic endotoxemia, propofol (10 mg/kg/hr) significantly reduced free radical–mediated and cyclooxygenase-catalyzed lipid peroxidation. In addition, Pao_2 and hemodynamics were maintained closer to baseline.[158] These benefits of propofol have not yet been confirmed in humans. At therapeutic concentrations, propofol also protects mouse macrophages from nitric oxide–induced apoptosis and cell death.[159]

Propofol does not alter basal pulmonary vascular tone or flow in chronically instrumented dogs; however, it does potentiate vasoconstriction when vasomotor tone is increased, but it has no effect when vasomotor tone is pharmacologically decreased. Propofol also attenuates the magnitude of hypoxic pulmonary vasoconstriction.[160] The effect of propofol on pulmonary vasomotor tone appears to result from inhibition of acetylcholine-induced pulmonary vasodilation through nitric oxide and a cytochrome P450 metabolite (probably endothelium-derived hyperpolarizing factor [EDHF]).[161]

Effects on the Cardiovascular System

The cardiovascular effects of propofol have been evaluated after its use for both induction and maintenance of anesthesia[148-151,162-168] (Table 10-2). The most prominent effect of propofol is a decrease in arterial blood pressure during induction of anesthesia. Independent of the presence of cardiovascular disease, an induction dose of 2 to 2.5 mg/kg produces a 25% to 40% reduction in systolic blood pressure.[148-151,162-168] Similar changes are seen in mean and diastolic blood pressure. The decrease in arterial pressure is associated with a decrease in cardiac output/cardiac index ($\approx$15%),[148,151,166-168] stroke volume index ($\approx$20%),[151,167,168] and systemic vascular resistance (15% to 25%).[149,151,167,168] The left ventricular stroke work index is also decreased (by $\approx$30%).[167] When looking specifically at right ventricular function, propofol produces a marked reduction in the slope of the right ventricular end-systolic pressure-volume relationship.[188] In patients with valvular heart disease, pulmonary artery and pulmonary capillary wedge pressure is also reduced, a finding implying that the resultant decrease in pressure is due to a decrease in both preload and afterload.[148] The decrease in systemic pressure after an induction dose of propofol appears to be due to vasodilation and possibly myocardial depression. The direct myocardial depressant effects of propofol are controversial. Most in vitro studies evaluating myocardial function at therapeutic propofol concentrations do not demonstrate a negative inotropic action. This lack of negative inotropic effect is also observed in the hearts of newborn pigs, which may imply some clinical advantage of propofol over volatile anesthetics in this age group.[189] Another mechanism that could account for the decrease in cardiac output after propofol administration may be its action on sympathetic drive to the heart. Propofol at high concentrations (10 μg/mL) abolishes the inotropic effect of α- but not β-adrenoreceptor stimulation and enhances the lusitropic (relaxation) effect of β-stimulation.[190] Clinically, the myocardial depressant effect and the vasodilation appear to be dependent on both the dose and the plasma concentration.[191] The vasodilatory effect of propofol appears to be due to a reduction in sympathetic activity,[192] a direct effect on intracellular smooth muscle calcium mobilization,[193,194] inhibition of prostacyclin synthesis in endothelial cells,[195] reduction of angiotensin II–elicited calcium entry,[196] activation of K^+ ATP channels, and stimulation of nitric oxide. Stimulation of nitric oxide may be modulated by Intralipid rather than propofol.[197]

The heart rate does not change significantly after an induction dose of propofol. It has been suggested that propofol either resets or inhibits the baroreflex, thus reducing the tachycardic response to hypotension.[198,199] Propofol decreases cardiac parasympathetic tone in proportion to the degree of sedation that it produces.[200]

Table 10–2   Hemodynamic changes after induction of anesthesia with nonbarbiturate hypnotics

	Diazepam	Droperidol	Etomidate*	Ketamine	Lorazepam	Midazolam	Propofol
HR	−9%-13%	Unchanged	−5%-10%	0-59%	Unchanged	−14%-12%	−10%-10%
MBP	0%-19%	0%-10%	0-17%	0-40%	−7%-20%	−12%-26%	−10%-40%
SVR	−22%-13%	−5%-15%	−10%-14%	0-33%	−10%-35%	0-20%	−15%-25%
PAP	0%-10%	Unchanged	−9%-8%	44%-47%	—	Unchanged	0-10%
PVR	0-19%	Unchanged	−18%-6%	0-33%	Unchanged	Unchanged	0-10%
PAO	Unchanged	25%-50%	Unchanged	Unchanged	—	0-25%	Unchanged
RAP	Unchanged	Unchanged	Unchanged	15%-33%	Unchanged	Unchanged	0-10%
CI	Unchanged	Unchanged	−20%-14%	0-42%	0-16%	0-25%	−10%-30%
SV	0-8%	0-10%	0-20%	0-21%	Unchanged	0-18%	−10%-25%
LVSWI	0-36%	Unchanged	0-33%	0-27%	—	−28%-42%	−10%-20%
dP/dt	Unchanged	—	0-18%	Unchanged	—	0-12%	Decreased
References	169-174	175, 176	177-180	181-183	184	169, 185-187	148-151, 162

*The larger deviations are in patients with valvular disease.
CI, cardiac index; HR, heart rate; LVSWI, left ventricular stroke work index; MBP, mean blood pressure; PAP, pulmonary artery pressure; PVR, pulmonary vascular resistance; PAO, pulmonary artery occluded pressure; RAP, right atrial pressure; SV, stroke volume; SVR, systemic vascular resistance.

It has minimal direct effect on sinoatrial node function or on normal atrioventricular and accessory pathway conduction.[201] Propofol attenuates the heart rate response to atropine in a dose-dependent manner. During a propofol infusion of 10 mg/kg/hr, a cumulative dose of atropine of 30 µg/kg increased the heart rate above 20 beats per minute in only 20% of subjects versus 100% in the absence of propofol.[202] Interestingly, propofol has been shown to suppress atrial (supraventricular) tachycardias and should probably be avoided during electrophysiologic studies.[203]

During maintenance of anesthesia with a propofol infusion, systolic pressure remains between 20% and 30% below preinduction levels.[151,167] Patients allowed to breathe room air during a maintenance infusion of 100 µg/kg/min of propofol have a significant decrease in systemic vascular resistance (30%), but cardiac index and stroke index are unaltered.[167] In contrast, in patients receiving a narcotic premedication and nitrous oxide with an infusion of propofol (54 and 108 µg/kg/min) for maintenance during surgery, systemic vascular resistance is not significantly decreased from baseline, but cardiac output and stroke volume are decreased.[151] This effect is probably explained by the observation that propofol infusions produce a dose-dependent lowering of sympathetic nerve activity, thereby attenuating the reflex responses to hypotension. In the presence of hypercapnia, the reflex sympathetic responses are better maintained.[204] Increasing the infusion rate of propofol from 54 to 108 µg/kg/min (blood concentration of 2.1 to 4.2 µg/mL) produces only a slightly greater decrease in arterial blood pressure ($\approx$10%).[151] Peak plasma concentrations after a bolus dose are substantially higher than those seen with a continuous infusion. Because the vasodilatory and myocardial depressant effects are concentration dependent, the decrease in blood pressure from propofol during the infusion phase is much less than that seen after an induction bolus. When propofol was compared with midazolam for sedation after coronary revascularization, propofol resulted in a 17% lower incidence of tachycardia, a 28% lower incidence of hypertension, and a 17% greater incidence of hypotension. These differences in hemodynamic parameters resulted in no difference in the number or severity of ischemic events between the two groups.[151]

The heart rate may increase,[150,165] decrease,[148,164] or remain unchanged[163] when anesthesia is maintained with propofol. An infusion of propofol results in a significant reduction in both myocardial blood flow and myocardial oxygen consumption,[162,165] a finding that suggests preservation of the global myocardial oxygen supply-demand ratio. Two recent studies in isolated rat heart preparations demonstrated that propofol provides myocardial protection after ischemia and reperfusion. Propofol attenuated mechanical dysfunction, reduced histologic injury, improved coronary flow, and reduced metabolic derangements.[205,206]

Other Effects

Propofol, like thiopental, does not potentiate the neuromuscular blockade produced by both nondepolarizing and depolarizing neuromuscular blocking drugs.[207,208] Propofol produces no effect on the evoked electromyogram or twitch tension[207]; however, good intubating conditions after propofol alone have been reported.[209] Propofol does not trigger malignant hyperpyrexia and is probably the anesthetic of choice in patients with this condition.[210,211]

After a single dose or a prolonged infusion, propofol does not affect corticosteroid synthesis or alter the normal response to adrenocorticotropic hormone (ACTH) stimulation.[212] In the emulsion formulation propofol does not alter hepatic, hematologic, or fibrinolytic function.[213-215] However, lipid emulsion per se reduces in vitro platelet aggregation.[216] Anaphylactoid reactions to the present formulation of propofol have been reported. In at least some of these patients, the immune response was entirely due to propofol and not to the lipid emulsion. A high percentage of the patients in whom an anaphylactoid response to propofol developed had a previous history of allergic responses. In patients with multiple drug allergies, propofol should be used with caution.[217] Propofol alone in Intralipid does not trigger histamine release.[218]

Propofol also possesses significant antiemetic activity at low (subhypnotic) doses.[219] It has been used successfully to treat postoperative nausea in a bolus dose of 10 mg.[220] It has also been used successfully to treat refractory postoperative nausea and vomiting.[221] The median concentration of propofol that was associated with an antiemetic effect was 343 ng/mL.[222] This concentration can be achieved by a 10- to 20-mg loading dose followed by infusion at 10 µg/kg/min. Propofol used as a maintenance anesthetic during breast surgery was more effective than 4 mg of ondansetron given as prophylaxis in preventing postoperative nausea and vomiting. In the same study, the maintenance propofol infusion was also superior to adding propofol only at the end of the procedure (sandwich technique).[223] The difference in efficacy between the maintenance method and the sandwich technique in preventing postoperative nausea and vomiting is that the propofol concentration drops rapidly below the therapeutic concentration after the sandwich technique whereas with the maintenance technique, although the propofol concentration decreases rapidly to allow awakening, any further decrease is much slower and propofol is maintained above therapeutic concentrations for several hours. Propofol administered as an infusion of 1 mg/kg/hr (17 µg/kg/min) has also provided excellent antiemetic action after anticancer chemotherapy.[224] The antiemetic effect of propofol is not due to action on dopamine DA$_2$ receptors.[225] At subhypnotic doses, propofol has also been reported to relieve cholestatic pruritus and was as effective as naloxone in treating pruritus induced by spinal opiates,[226] although not all studies have confirmed this effect of propofol. Propofol causes a dose-dependent decrease in the thermoregulatory threshold for vasoconstriction, but it has little effect on the sweating threshold.[227]

Propofol decreases polymorphonuclear leukocyte chemotaxis, but not adherence, phagocytosis, and killing. This action contrasts with the effect of thiopental, which inhibits all these chemotactic responses.[228] However, propofol inhibits phagocytosis and killing of

Staphylococcus aureus and *Escherichia coli*.[229] These findings are particularly pertinent in view of the observation of increased life-threatening systemic infections associated with the use of propofol.[225,230] It was also noted that opened vials and syringes of propofol in hospitals where these infections occurred had positive cultures for the offending organisms. The Intralipid that acts as the solvent for propofol is an excellent culture medium. Disodium edetate or metabisulfite has been added to the formulation of propofol in an attempt to retard such bacterial growth. Strict aseptic technique must still be observed.

Propofol also inhibits the ability of cancer cells to invade by modulating Rho A,[231] the clinical implication of which has not yet been ascertained. The administration of propofol has also been associated with the development of pancreatitis, but animal studies have failed to demonstrate this effect.[232]

Uses

Induction and Maintenance of Anesthesia

Propofol is suitable for both induction and maintenance of anesthesia and has also been approved for use in neurologic and cardiac anesthesia (Table 10-3). The induction dose varies from 1.0 to 2.5 mg/kg,[77,233,234] and the ED_{95} in unpremedicated adult patients is 2.25 to 2.5 mg/kg.[233,235] Physiologic characteristics that best determine the induction dose are age, lean body mass, and central blood volume.[236] Premedication with an opiate or a benzodiazepine, or with both, markedly reduces the induction dose.[79,80,237] A dose of 1 mg/kg (with premedication) to 1.75 mg/kg (without premedication) is recommended for inducing anesthesia in patients older than 60 years (also see Chapter 62).[238] To prevent hypotension in sicker patients or those undergoing cardiac surgery, a fluid load should be administered as tolerated, and propofol should be administered in small incremental doses (10 to 30 mg or as an infusion) until the patient loses consciousness. To limit the dose and retain the fastest onset time, an infusion of 80 mg/kg/hr is optimal. Diluting propofol to 0.5 mg/mL further reduces the impact of this induction dose on hemodynamics.[239] The ED_{95} (2.0 to 3.0 mg/kg) for induction is increased in children, primarily because of pharmacokinetic differences (also see Chapter 60).[240,241]

When used for induction of anesthesia in briefer procedures, propofol results in significantly quicker recovery and earlier return of psychomotor function than thiopental or methohexital does, irrespective of the agent used for maintenance of anesthesia.[242-244] The incidence of nausea and vomiting when propofol is used for induction is also markedly lower than after the use of other intravenous induction agents, probably because of the antiemetic properties of propofol.[235,243]

As a result of its pharmacokinetics, propofol provides rapid recovery and is thus superior to barbiturates for maintenance of anesthesia,[244-246] and it appears to be equal to enflurane and isoflurane.[79,242,247] Recovery from desflurane is slightly more rapid than recovery from propofol.[248] Propofol can be given as intermittent boluses or as a continuous infusion for maintenance.[214] After a satisfactory induction dose, a bolus of 10 to 40 mg is needed every few minutes to maintain anesthesia. Because these doses need to be given frequently, it is more suitable to administer propofol as a continuous infusion.

Several infusion schemes have been used to achieve adequate plasma concentrations of propofol (see also Chapter 12).[244,249] After an induction dose, an infusion of 100 to 200 μg/kg/min is usually needed.[79,139,140,188,242,244-246] The infusion rate is then titrated to individual requirements and the surgical stimulus. When combined with propofol, midazolam, clonidine, morphine, fentanyl, sufentanil, alfentanil, or remifentanil reduces its required infusion rate and concentration (see also Chapter 12).[84,137,139,140,250-253] Because opioids alter the concentration of propofol required for adequate anesthesia, the relative dose of either opioid or propofol will markedly affect the time from termination of drug effect to awakening and recovery. The infusion rate required to achieve the combination with the shortest recovery is propofol, 1 to 1.5 mg/kg followed by 140 μg/kg/min for 10 minutes and then 100 μg/kg/min, and alfentanil, 30 μg/kg followed by an infusion of 0.25 μg/kg/min, or fentanyl, 3 μg/kg followed by 0.02 μg/kg/min. Propofol has also been used as a single mixture with alfentanil at 1 mg alfentanil (2 mL) to 400 mg propofol (40 mL). When this mixture was administered at infusion rates commonly used for propofol (i.e., 166 μg/kg/min for 10 minutes, 133 μg/kg/min for 10 minutes, and 100 μg/kg/min thereafter), it provided an outcome equal to that obtained by administering the two drugs as separate infusions.[254]

Increasing age is associated with a decrease in propofol infusion requirements,[255,256] whereas these requirements are higher in children and infants.[55] The blood levels of propofol alone needed to achieve loss of consciousness are 2.5 to 4.5 μg/mL, and the blood levels (when combined with nitrous oxide) required for surgery are 2.5 to 8 μg/mL.[17,18,82,139,140,247] Similar concentrations are necessary when propofol is combined with an opioid for a total intravenous technique. Knowledge of these levels and the pharmacokinetics of propofol has enabled the use of pharmacokinetic model–driven infusion systems to deliver propofol as a continuous infusion for maintenance of anesthesia (see also Chapter 12).[79,139,257,258]

For short (<1 hour) body surface procedures, the advantages of more rapid recovery and decreased nausea and vomiting are still evident.[242] However, if propofol is used only for induction in longer or major procedures, both speed of recovery and the incidence of nausea and vomiting are similar to those after thiopental/isoflurane anesthesia.[79,242]

Table 10–3	Uses and doses of propofol
Induction of general anesthesia	1-2.5 mg/kg IV; dose reduced with increasing age
Maintenance of general anesthesia	50-150 μg/kg/min IV combined with N_2O or an opiate
Sedation	25-75 μg/kg/min IV
Antiemetic	10-20 mg IV; can repeat q5-10min or start infusion of 10 μg/kg/min

Total intravenous anesthesia with propofol plus an opiate results in similar recovery but reduces the incidence of postoperative nausea and vomiting in the first 72 hours by 15% to 20% when compared with an isoflurane-based anesthetic.[259] A meta-analysis of recovery data after either propofol for maintenance or the newer volatile anesthetics indicated only minor differences in times to reach recovery goals; however, the incidence of nausea and vomiting remained significantly lower in patients administered propofol for maintenance.[260]

Several studies have investigated the utility of propofol as a maintenance infusion regimen for cardiac surgery. The use of reduced and titrated doses of propofol for induction and titrated infusion rates of 50 to 200 µg/kg/min combined with an opioid for maintenance provided intraoperative hemodynamic control and ischemic episodes similar to those with either enflurane/opioid or a primary opioid technique.[261-264]

Sedation

Propofol has been evaluated for sedation during surgical procedures[85,86,265,266] and in mechanically ventilated patients in the intensive care unit (ICU).[267-269] Propofol by continuous infusion provides a readily titratable level of sedation and rapid recovery once the infusion is terminated, irrespective of the duration of the infusion.[86,265,268,270] In a study of patients sedated in the ICU for 4 days with propofol, recovery to consciousness was rapid ($\approx$10 minutes). Both the rate of recovery and the decrease in plasma concentration were similar at 24 and 96 hours, when the infusion was discontinued. In addition, the plasma concentrations required for sedation and for awakening were similar at 24 and 96 hours, a finding implying that tolerance to propofol did not occur.[270] As noted earlier, there have been more recent reports of tolerance with propofol. Infusion rates required for sedation to supplement regional anesthesia in healthy patients are half or less than those required for general anesthesia (i.e., 30 to 60 µg/kg/min).[85,265] In elderly patients (older than 65 years) and sicker patients, the infusion rates that are necessary are markedly reduced.[85,267,268] Thus, it is important to titrate the infusion individually to the desired effect. A 1992 report[271] linked propofol with several deaths in children requiring sedation for mechanical ventilation secondary to upper respiratory tract infections. This rare syndrome (see later) may also occur in adults. A potential advantage of propofol for sedation of ICU patients is that it appears to possess antioxidant properties.[272]

Generally, at propofol infusion rates more rapid than 30 µg/kg/min, patients are amnesic.[265,268] When compared with midazolam for maintenance of sedation, propofol provides equal or better control and more rapid recovery.[86,265,268] In mechanically ventilated patients, more rapid recovery translates to more rapid extubation when sedation is terminated.[268] The use of propofol for sedation after cardiac surgery to provide fast tracking has shown that patients can be extubated rapidly with this technique.[273] The incidence of unwanted cardiovascular changes and ischemic events was similar when propofol or midazolam was used for sedation in patients after coronary artery bypass surgery.[188] Propofol has also been used successfully in patient-controlled sedation. It was rated better than midazolam when used by this technique, probably because of its much more rapid onset and offset.[274]

Side Effects and Contraindications

Induction of anesthesia with propofol is associated with several side effects, including pain on injection, myoclonus, apnea, decrease in arterial blood pressure, and rarely, thrombophlebitis of the vein into which propofol is injected. Pain on injection is less than or equal to that with etomidate, equal to that with methohexital, and greater than after thiopental.[213,241,275] Pain on injection is reduced by using a large vein, avoiding veins in the dorsum of the hand, and adding lidocaine to the propofol solution.[213] Myoclonus occurs more frequently after propofol than after thiopental, but less frequently than after etomidate or methohexital.[241] Apnea after induction with propofol is common. The incidence of apnea may be similar to that after thiopental or methohexital; however, propofol produces a greater incidence of apnea lasting longer than 30 seconds.[139,145] The addition of an opiate increases the incidence of apnea, especially prolonged apnea.[139,141]

The most significant side effect on induction is the decrease in systemic blood pressure. Addition of an opiate just before induction of anesthesia appears to augment the decrease in arterial blood pressure.[168] Perhaps slow administration and smaller doses in adequately prehydrated patients may attenuate the decrease in arterial blood pressure. Conversely, the effects of laryngoscopy and endotracheal intubation and the increases in mean arterial pressure, heart rate, and systemic vascular resistance are less significant after propofol than after thiopental.[164,168]

Propofol infusion syndrome is a rare, but lethal syndrome associated with infusion of propofol at 5 mg/kg/hr or greater for 48 hours or longer. It was first described in children but has also subsequently been observed in critically ill adults. Clinical features include cardiomyopathy with acute cardiac failure, metabolic acidosis, skeletal myopathy, hyperkalemia, hepatomegaly, and lipemia.[81,276] Present evidence suggests that this syndrome occurs as a result of failure of free fatty acid metabolism because of inhibition of free fatty acid entry into mitochondria and failure of the mitochondrial respiratory chain.[277]

BARBITURATES

History

Barbituric acid, a combination of urea and malonic acid that is lacking in sedative properties, was first synthesized in 1864 by J.F.W. Adolph von Baeyer, a Nobel Prize–winning organic chemist.[278] Barbital (diethylbarbituric acid), the first barbiturate with sedative properties, was reported by Fischer and von Mering in 1903.[279] This oral hypnotic was very long acting and very popular as a sedative in clinical practice. However, it was not until 1920 with the introduction of Somnifen, a mixture of the barbiturate salts of diethylbarbituratic and diallylbarbituratic acids, that intravenous barbiturates became widely available for clinical use. Somnifen was described by Redonnet in 1920 and was first used in clinical practice by Bardet and Bardet in 1921 on a labor and delivery ward. It was first used in surgical practice in 1924 by Fredet and Perlis, and its use continued for many years in France and Germany.[280,281]

The first ultrashort-acting barbiturate, hexobarbital, was prepared by Kropp and Taub and was introduced into clinical use in July 1932 by H. Weese and W. Scharpff.[282] Although hexobarbital was used widely in Europe, it did not enjoy the same level of success in North America. In 1929, the use of amobarbital (Amytal) was reported by Zerfas and colleagues, and it quickly became the most common intravenous anesthetic in North America.[283]

The thiobarbiturates were first described in 1903. However, because of fatal experiments in dogs, their use was not further explored until the 1930s.[283] In 1935, Tabern and Volwiler synthesized a series of sulfur-containing barbiturates, of which thiopental became the most widely used.[284] Thiopental was introduced clinically by Ralph Waters and John Lundy and became preferred clinically because of its rapid onset of action and short duration, without the excitatory effects of hexobarbital (Fig. 10-6).[283,285]

Though criticized after many casualties during the attack on Pearl Harbor as "the ideal form of euthanasia in war surgery," barbiturates continued to be widely used in clinical practice.[286] Even though many other barbiturate derivatives has been synthesized throughout the past several decades, none has enjoyed the clinical success and popularity of thiopental. Thiopental has survived the test of time as an intravenous anesthetic drug. A more detailed description of the history of the barbiturates in anesthesia is available elsewhere.[278,287,288]

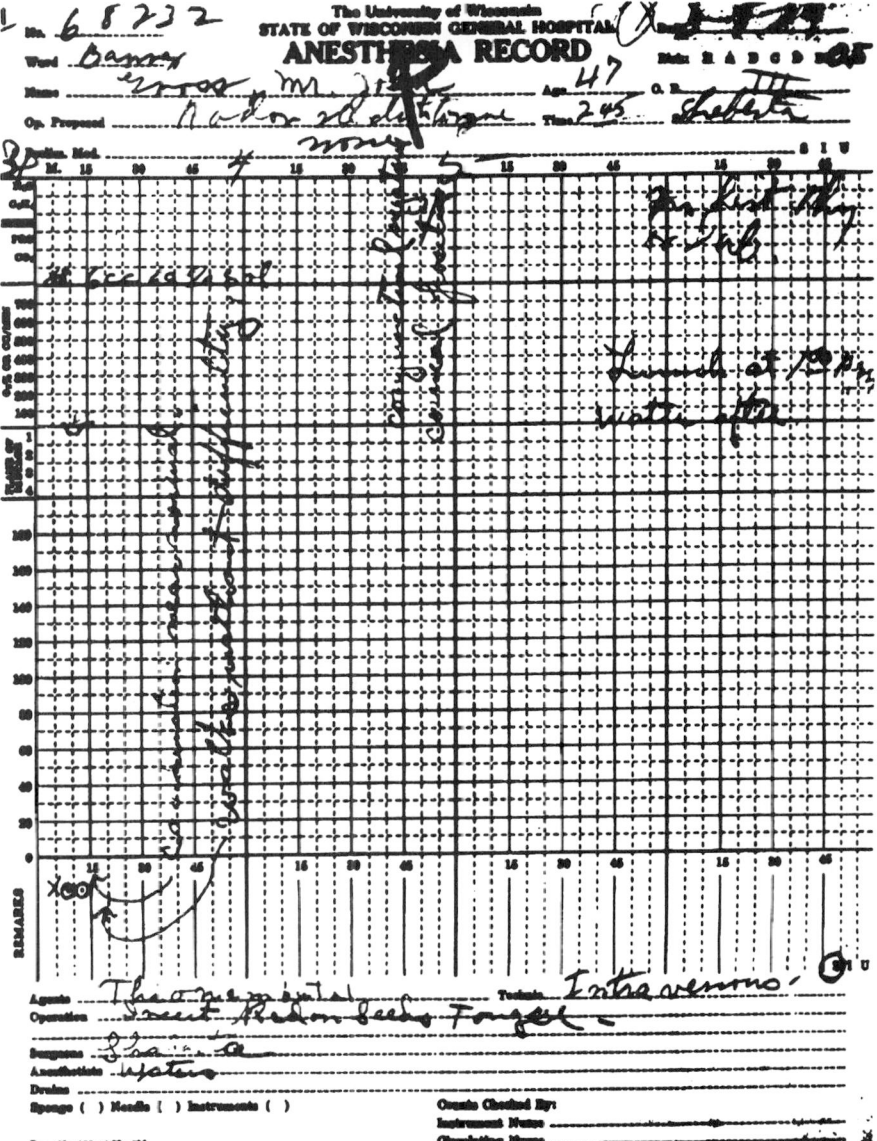

Figure 10–6 Reproduction of the first administration of thiopental by Waters on March 8, 1934. (From Dundee JW, Wyant GM: Intravenous Anaesthesia. Edinburgh, Churchill Livingstone, 1974.)

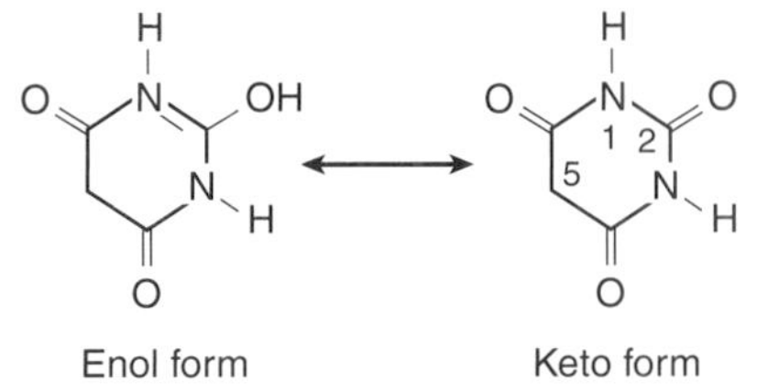

Figure 10–7 The keto and enol tautomeric forms of barbituric acid with the sites of substitution in the hypnotically active barbiturates identified as 1, 2, and 5.

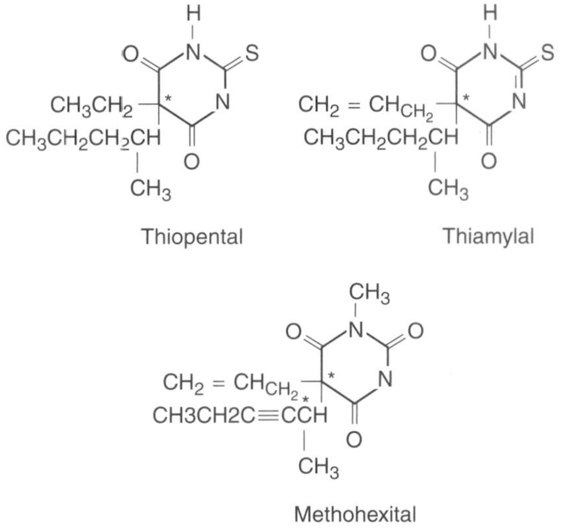

Physicochemical Characteristics

Chemistry and Formulation

Barbiturates are hypnotically active drugs that are derivatives of barbituric acid (2,4,6-trioxohexahydropyrimidine), a hypnotically inactive pyrimidine nucleus formed by the condensation of malonic acid and urea (Fig. 10-7). The two major divisions of barbiturates are those with an oxygen at position 2 (oxybarbiturates) and those with a sulfur at position 2 (thiobarbiturates). Through keto-enol tautomerization, the oxygen or sulfur at position 2 becomes a reactive species in the enol form that allows for the formation of water-soluble barbiturate salts in alkaline solutions. This solubility permits the intravenous use of barbiturates. Although tautomerization to the enol form allows for the creation of salts, it is substitution of the hydrogen attached to the carbon atom in position 5 by aryl or alkyl groups that gives the barbiturates their hypnotic activity. A list of hypnotically active barbiturates can be found in Table 10-4. From this list, only the thiobarbiturates thiopental and thiamylal and the oxybarbiturate methohexital are commonly used for induction of anesthesia (Fig. 10-8).

The formulation of barbiturates involves preparation of them as sodium salts (mixed with 6% anhydrous sodium carbonate by weight) and then reconstitution with either water or normal saline to produce a 2.5% solution of thiopental, a 2.0% solution of thiamylal, or a 1.0% solution of methohexital. Thiobarbiturates are stable for 1 week if refrigerated after reconstitution, and methohexital remains available for use for up to 6 weeks after reconstitution. A decrease in alkalinity of the solution can result in precipitation of barbiturates as free

Figure 10–8 Hypnotically active barbiturates commonly used for induction with their asymmetric centers indicated by an *asterisk*.

acids, which is why they cannot be reconstituted with lactated Ringer's solution or mixed with other acidic solutions. Examples of drugs that are not to be coadministered or mixed in solution with barbiturates are pancuronium, vecuronium, atracurium, alfentanil, sufentanil, and midazolam. Studies have shown that in rapid-sequence induction, mixing of thiopental with vecuronium or pancuronium results in the formation of a precipitate that may occlude the intravenous line.[289]

Structure-Activity Relationships

Substitutions at the 5, 2, and 1 positions confer different pharmacologic activities to the barbiturate nucleus. Substitutions at position 5 with either aryl or alkyl groups produce hypnotic and sedative effects. A phenyl group substitution at C5 produces anticonvulsant activity. An increase in the length of one or both side chains of an alkyl group at C5 increases hypnotic potency. The barbiturates used in clinical practice have either an oxygen or sulfur at C2. Substitution of sulfur at position 2 produces a more rapid onset of action. The addition of a methyl or ethyl group at position 1 may also produce a more rapid onset of action, but excitatory side effects, including tremor, hypertonus, and involuntary movement, may occur with administration. A comparison of the potency, onset of action, length of action, and side effects is presented in Table 10-5.

Stereoisomerism

It has been known since the 1970s that optical isomers of barbiturates can have different anesthetic activities in mammals.[290] Several of the barbiturates, including thiopental, thiamylal, methohexital, secobarbital, and pentobarbital, have asymmetric carbon atoms in at least one of the side chains attached to carbon 5 of the barbiturate ring. The S *(l)* isomers of these barbiturates are roughly twice as potent as the R *(d)* isomers despite their similar access to the CNS.[290-294] The fundamental importance of this fact is that stereoisomers of the same drug

Table 10–4 Hypnotically active barbiturates listed according to duration of action*

Ultrashort Acting	Short Acting	Intermediate Acting	Long Acting
Thiopental	Pentobarbital	Amobarbital	Phenobarbital
Methohexital	Secobarbital	Aprobarbital	Mephobarbital
Thiamylal	Butalbital	Butabarbital	Barbital
	Hexobarbital		Metharbital
			Primidone

*Only the ultrashort-acting drugs are commonly used for induction.

Table 10–5 Relationship of chemical grouping to clinical action and potency of barbiturates

Group	Substituents		Group Characteristics When Given IV
	Position 1	*Position 2*	
Oxybarbiturates	H	O	Delay in onset of action, the degree of which is dependent on the 5 and 5' side chain. Useful as a basal hypnotic. Prolonged action. Excitatory side effects
Methylated thiobarbiturates	CH$_3$	O	Usually rapid acting with fairly rapid recovery. High incidence of excitatory side effects
Thiobarbiturates	H	S	Rapid acting, usually smooth onset of sleep, fairly prompt recovery
Methylated thiobarbiturates	CH$_3$	S	Rapid onset of action and very rapid recovery, but too many excitatory side effects to make clinical use feasible

Modified from Dundee JW, Wyant GM: Intravenous Anaesthesia. Edinburgh, Churchill Livingstone, 1974.

can have different CNS potency and activity, which is suggestive of the existence of chirally active centers on barbiturate receptors rather than nonspecific actions mediated by the drug. For example, the racemic mixture of pentobarbital has isomers that produce different actions in cultured mammalian neurons, with the (+) isomers being primarily excitatory and the (–) isomers being primarily inhibitory. Thus, the overall CNS activity of a particular barbiturate depends on the summation of the effects of the stereoisomers at each point of action and the relative potency of the action at each site. Similarly, the duration of action for any given barbiturate is dependent on the summation of the duration of effects of each isomer at its receptor site.[291]

Metabolism

The barbiturates (with the exception of phenobarbital) are hepatically metabolized. The metabolites that are formed are almost all inactive, water soluble, and excreted in urine. Barbiturates are biotransformed by four processes: (1) oxidation of the aryl, alkyl, or phenyl moiety at C5; (2) N-dealkylation; (3) desulfuration of the thiobarbiturates at C2; and (4) destruction of the barbituric acid ring.[295,296] Oxidation is the most important pathway, and it produces polar (charged) alcohols, ketones, phenols, or carboxylic acids. These metabolites are readily excreted in urine or as glucuronic acid conjugates in bile. The barbituric acid ring is so stable in vivo that hydrolytic cleavage of the ring is a minimal contribution to the total metabolism of barbiturates. Drugs that induce oxidative microsomes enhance the metabolism of barbiturates. Chronic administration of barbiturates will also induce the enzymes.[296] Thus, biotransformation of barbiturates may be enhanced in patients taking drugs that are known to induce hepatic microsomes. The induction of hepatic enzymes by barbiturates is responsible for the recommendation that they not be administered to patients with acute intermittent porphyria. Barbiturates may precipitate an attack by stimulating γ-aminolevulinic acid synthetase, the enzyme responsible for the production of porphyrins.[297]

As mentioned earlier, hepatic metabolism accounts for elimination of all the barbiturates with the exception of phenobarbital. Renal excretion is important in the elimination of phenobarbital and accounts for 60% to 90% of the drug being excreted in unchanged form.[298] Thirty percent of phenobarbital is excreted in urine, but only trivial amounts of other barbiturates are excreted unchanged by the kidney. Alkalinization of urine with bicarbonate enhances the renal excretion of phenobarbital. As the pH of urine increases throughout the tubules, the concentration of the undissociated form of phenobarbital decreases, thereby creating an increased gradient across the lipid tubular epithelium that results in increased flow of the undissociated form of phenobarbital (lipophilic) from the renal parenchyma into the tubular lumen.[298,299]

Methohexital is metabolized in the liver by oxidation to an alcohol; N-dealkylation also occurs. When compared with thiopental, methohexital exhibits similar distribution half-lives, volumes of distribution, and protein binding. A marked difference exists, however, in plasma disappearance and elimination half-lives (4 hours for methohexital and as many as 12 hours for thiopental). This difference is due to the threefold greater rate of hepatic clearance of methohexital, with the mean ranging from 7.8 to 12.5 mL/kg/min.[32] The hepatic extraction ratio of methohexital (clearance/hepatic blood flow) is approximately 0.5, thus indicating that the liver extracts 50% of the drug presented to it. In contrast, the hepatic extraction ratio of thiopental is 0.15.

Pharmacokinetics

The pharmacokinetics of barbiturates has been described in both physiologic and compartmental models, with the latter gaining more support in recent years.[33,41,300,301] Physiologic models of barbiturates describe rapid mixing of the drug with the central blood volume followed by quick distribution of the drug to the highly perfused, low-volume tissues (i.e., brain) and slower redistribution of the drug to lean tissue (muscle), which terminates the effect of the induction dose. In these models, uptake by adipose tissue and metabolic clearance (elimination) play only a minor role in termination of the effects of the induction dose because of the minimal perfusion ratio in comparison to other tissues and the slow rate of removal, respectively. Compartmental model values for thiopental and methohexital, the most commonly used barbiturates for induction, are given in Table 10-1. Both these pharmacokinetic models describe rapid redistribution as the primary mechanism that terminates the action of a single induction dose.[302] The compartmental model explains the delay in recovery when a continuous infusion of a barbiturate is used. This model describes the phenomena whereby the termination of effect becomes increasingly dependent on the slower process of uptake into adipose tissue and elimination or clearance through hepatic metabolism. After prolonged infusions, the pharmacokinetics of barbiturate metabolism is best approximated by nonlinear Michaelis-Menten metabolism.

In usual doses (4 to 5 mg/kg), thiopental exhibits first-order kinetics (i.e., a constant *fraction* of drug is cleared from the body per unit time); however, at very high doses of thiopental (300 to 600 mg/kg) with receptor saturation, zero-order kinetics occurs (i.e., a constant *amount* of drug is cleared per unit time). Because the volume of distribution is slightly larger in female patients, elimination half-lives are longer in this group.[42] Pregnancy also increases the volume of distribution of thiopental, thereby prolonging the elimination half-life.[303] As noted earlier, the clearance rate of thiopental is not altered in patients with cirrhosis because the amount of protein available for the drug to bind to is still adequate even at fairly advanced stages of the disease process.[304]

Because of its affinity for fat, relatively large volume of distribution, and low rate of hepatic clearance, thiopental can accumulate in tissues, especially if given in large doses over a prolonged period. Accumulation of thiopental was shown to occur in studies conducted by Dundee and associates in which the plasma drug level increased when repeat doses of drug were given.[305] Obese patients are likely to have prolonged clearance half-lives of thiopental.[306] Appropriately designed infusion schemes ensure relatively constant blood levels, thus maintaining the hypnotic effect.

Pharmacology

Mechanism of Action

Much research has been conducted to delineate the mechanisms of action of barbiturates on the CNS, but with the exception of their action on the $GABA_A$ receptor, these mechanisms remain largely unknown.[307,308] The selectivity of action of barbiturates on CNS neurophysiologic systems has been grouped into two general categories: (1) enhancement of the synaptic actions of *inhibitory* neurotransmitters and (2) blockade of the synaptic actions of *excitatory* neurotransmitters.[309] GABA is the principal inhibitory neurotransmitter in the mammalian CNS, and the $GABA_A$ receptor is the only site that has been proved to be involved in barbiturate-induced anesthesia.[308] The $GABA_A$ receptor is a chloride ion channel that is composed of at least five subunits with specific sites of action for GABA, barbiturates, benzodiazepines, and other molecules.[285] Binding of barbiturate to the $GABA_A$ receptor both enhances and mimics the action of GABA by increasing chloride conductance through the ion channel, causing hyperpolarization of the cell membrane, and thus increasing the threshold of excitability of the postsynaptic neuron.[310] At low concentrations, barbiturates enhance the effects of GABA by decreasing the rate of dissociation of GABA from its receptor and thus increasing the duration of GABA-activated chloride ion channel opening. This enhancement of the action of GABA is thought to be responsible for the sedative-hypnotic effects of barbiturates. At higher concentrations, barbiturates directly activate chloride channels without binding of GABA, thereby acting as the agonist themselves. The GABA-mimetic effect at slightly higher concentrations may be responsible for what is termed "barbiturate anesthesia."[308,311]

Barbiturates also inhibit the synaptic transmission of excitatory neurotransmitters such as glutamate and acetylcholine.[308] The actions of barbiturates in blocking excitatory CNS transmission are specific for synaptic ion channels. Although these alternate sites have received much attention, their exact role, if any, in the anesthetic effects of barbiturates remains uncertain.[307,312]

Effects on Cerebral Metabolism (also see Chapter 21)

Barbiturates, like other CNS depressants, have potent effects on cerebral metabolism. Several studies in the 1970s demonstrated the effect of barbiturates to be a dose-related depression in $CMRO_2$, which produces progressive slowing of the EEG, a reduction in the rate of ATP consumption, and protection from incomplete cerebral ischemia.[313-315] The relationship of depressed metabolism to drug dosage was shown in dogs in which circulation at high thiopental doses was preserved by an extracorporeal circulation pump.[316] When the results of the EEG became isoelectric, a point at which cerebral metabolic activity is roughly 50% of baseline,[317] no further decrements in $CMRO_2$ occurred. These findings support the hypothesis that metabolism and function are coupled. However, it must be noted that it is the portion of metabolic activity concerned with neuronal signaling and impulse traffic that is reduced by barbiturates, not the portion corresponding to basal metabolic function. The only way to suppress the baseline metabolic activity associated with cellular activity is through hypothermia.[317] Thus, the effect of barbiturates on cerebral metabolism is maximized at a 50% depression of cerebral function in which less oxygen is required as $CMRO_2$ is diminished, with all metabolic energy left for the maintenance of cellular integrity.

With the reduction in $CMRO_2$ comes a parallel reduction in cerebral perfusion, which is seen as decreased cerebral blood flow (CBF) and ICP. With reduced $CMRO_2$, cerebral vascular resistance increases and CBF decreases.[318] The ratio of CBF to $CMRO_2$ is unchanged. Thus, the reduction in CBF after the administration of barbiturates causes a concurrent decrease in ICP. Furthermore, even though mean arterial pressure decreases, barbiturates do not compromise overall cerebral perfusion pressure because cerebral perfusion pressure equals mean blood pressure minus ICP. In this relationship, ICP decreases to a greater extent relative to the decrease in mean arterial pressure after barbiturate use, thus preserving cerebral perfusion pressure.

Pharmacodynamics

Barbiturates produce the clinical effects of sedation and sleep. Sufficient doses produce a CNS depression that is termed *general anesthesia,* which is attended by loss of consciousness, amnesia, and respiratory and cardiovascular depression. The response to pain and other noxious stimulation during general anesthesia appears to be obtunded. However, the results of pain studies reveal that barbiturates may actually decrease the pain threshold.[319] This antalgesic effect occurs only at low blood levels of barbiturates, such as with small induction doses of thiopental or after emergence from thiopental anesthesia when its blood levels are low. The amnesic effect of barbiturates has not been well studied, but it is decidedly less pronounced than that produced by the benzodiazepines.

Onset of Central Nervous System Effects

Barbiturates produce CNS effects when they cross the blood-brain barrier. Several well-known factors help determine the rapidity with which a drug enters the cerebrospinal fluid (CSF) and brain tissue,[299] including the degree of lipid solubility, degree of ionization, level of protein binding, and the plasma drug concentration.

Drugs with high lipid solubility and a low degree of ionization cross the blood-brain barrier rapidly and produce a fast onset of action.[308] Most barbiturates exist in a nonionized form. The degree of lipid solubility of the nonionized form of the drug works in conjunction with the amount of drug that exists in the nonionized form (reflection of pK_a) to determine the rapidity with which a drug crosses the blood-brain barrier. Thiopental and methohexital are more lipid soluble than pentobarbital, which corresponds clinically to the more rapid onset of action of thiopental and methohexital than pentobarbital.[320,321]

Only the nonionized form of a drug can directly traverse the cellular membranes. Thiopental has a pK_a of 7.6. Therefore, approximately 50% of thiopental is nonionized at physiologic pH, which accounts in part for the rapid accumulation of thiopental in the CSF after intravenous administration.[322] Methohexital is 75% nonionized at pH 7.4, a fact that may explain the slightly more rapid effect of this drug than that of thiopental. As pH decreases, for example, with poor perfusion, barbiturates have a larger proportion of nonionized drug available to cross the blood-brain barrier.[321,322] Obvious clinical consequences result: patients with acidosis require the administration of less barbiturate, and patients with alkalosis might require an increased dose to achieve the same level of anesthesia or sedation.

Protein binding also affects the onset of action in the CNS. Barbiturates are highly bound to albumin and other plasma proteins. Because only unbound drug (free drug) can cross the blood-brain barrier, an inverse relationship exists between the degree of plasma protein binding and the rapidity of drug passage across the blood-brain barrier.[302] Drugs have different degrees of protein binding, and in general, the thiobarbiturates are more highly bound than the oxybarbiturates.[323] The degree of protein binding of a drug is influenced by the physiologic pH and disease states that alter the absolute amount of protein. Most barbiturates tend to experience peak protein binding at or around pH 7.5, and slightly fewer drugs have most bound at a more acidic or basic pH. Disease states such as hepatic cirrhosis or chronic renal disease may reduce the total availability of plasma albumin, which could decrease the absolute amount of protein available for binding.[285] However, this situation may be of little clinical significance because most patients have many more protein molecules than drug molecules. Another possible consideration is whether other drugs that are highly protein bound can displace barbiturates from albumin. Again, such displacement is possible in theory, although an important clinical effect is unlikely to occur.

The final factor governing the rapidity of drug penetration of the blood-brain barrier is the plasma drug concentration. Simply because of the concentration gradient, higher drug concentrations in plasma produce greater amounts of drug that diffuses into the CSF and brain. The two primary determinants of the plasma concentration are the *dose* administered and the *rate* (speed) of administration. For example, as the dose of thiopental over the same time is increased, an increased percentage of patients are anesthetized.[324] As regards the absolute dose, 2 mg/kg produced anesthesia in 20% of patients, whereas a dose of 2.4 mg/kg produced anesthesia in 80% of patients. Similarly, the speed of injection influences the effect of thiopental.[325] When a fixed initial dose of thiopental of approximately 2.75 mg/kg was administered, a significantly ($P < .001$) smaller amount of drug was required to produce anesthesia when the dose was delivered over a period of 5 seconds as opposed to 15 seconds. Thus, the dose *and* rate of intravenous administration can profoundly affect the onset of barbiturate CNS effect.

Termination of Effect

Because brain and plasma concentrations are in equilibrium, factors that determine the rate of onset of barbiturate effect also affect their termination. Thus, lipid solubility, the degree of ionization, and the CSF drug concentration affect the movement of drugs from the CSF to plasma. Protein binding is less important because protein is not usually found in CSF, although there is certainly protein in the brain to which barbiturates may be bound. As plasma levels decrease, drug levels in the brain and CSF decrease. The most important factors in the termination of drug effect are those that govern plasma disappearance of the drug. These factors are generally divided into a rapid redistribution phase and a slow metabolic and second redistribution phase. In a classic pharmacologic study, Brodie and coworkers conclusively demonstrated that awakening from thiopental occurred because the plasma level rapidly declined.[326] They further demonstrated that the cause of the rapid plasma decay of thiopental was *not metabolism* of the drug but rather *redistribution* of the drug to other tissues throughout the body (lean tissue). The role of slow-phase distribution to adipose tissue and elimination and clearance from plasma by metabolism was elucidated later.[301,325] The relationship of the plasma drug level to the onset and termination of effect as it relates to drug redistribution is illustrated in Figure 10-9. As time passes, the blood level of barbiturate decreases and the drug is taken up by less well perfused tissues (first muscle and then fat). In addition, the rate of metabolic clearance is constant; the liver biotransforms a constant proportion or fraction (first-order kinetics) of the drug from blood. Clinically, patients awake from a single dose of thiopental 5 to 10 minutes after administration because the drug

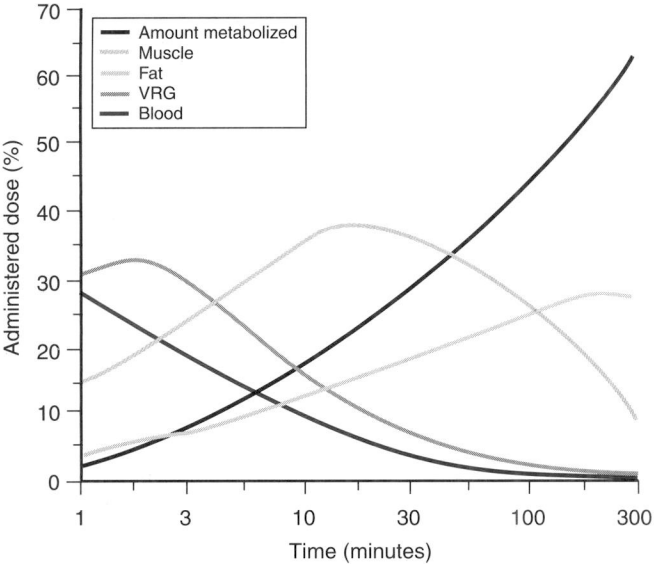

Figure 10–9 After delivery of an intravenous bolus, the percentage of thiopental remaining in blood rapidly decreases as drug moves from blood to body tissues. The time to attainment of peak tissue levels is a direct function of tissue capacity for barbiturate relative to blood flow. Thus, a larger capacity or smaller blood flow is related to a longer time to a peak tissue level. Initially, most thiopental is taken up by the vessel-rich group (VRG) of tissues because of their high blood flow. Subsequently, drug is redistributed to muscle and to a lesser extent to fat. Throughout this period, small but substantial amounts of thiopental are removed and metabolized by the liver. Unlike removal by tissues, this removal is cumulative. Note that the rate of metabolism equals the early rate of removal by fat. The sum of this early removal by fat and metabolism is the same as the removal by muscle. (Redrawn from Saidman LJ: Uptake, distribution and elimination of barbiturates. *In* Eger EI [ed]: Anesthetic Uptake and Action. Baltimore, Williams & Wilkins, 1974.)

level in the brain has decreased (along with the decline in blood level). Drug is redistributed from highly perfused CNS tissues to well-perfused lean tissues. In the case of constant infusion or repeated dosing with saturation of all tissue sites, patients awake at a much delayed rate because first-order hepatic metabolism begins to play a larger role in decreasing plasma levels of barbiturates. In summary, termination of effect after multiple doses or constant infusion is dependent on the drug being eliminated from blood more and more by metabolism than by redistribution and is a function of its context-sensitive decrement time (see Fig. 10-3).

Findings of pharmacokinetic analysis illustrate that awakening from thiopental is related to rapid redistribution.[42] As previously mentioned, awakening is independent of the dose administered, except in the case of continuous infusion, which prolongs recovery. Awakening may be delayed in older patients because of either increased CNS sensitivity, alterations in metabolism, or a decreased central volume of distribution relative to younger adults.[327] The initial volume of distribution is less in elderly patients than young patients, which explains their lower dose requirement for the onset of EEG and hypnotic effects.[327] Pediatric patients (younger than 13 years) seem to have

a greater rate of total clearance and a shorter rate of plasma thiopental clearance than adults do, which theoretically might result in earlier awakening, especially after multiple doses of the drug.[328]

Thiopental and methohexital are not very different with regard to distribution, which may explain the similar wake-up time with these drugs. There is, however, a difference in the rate of total-body clearance, with methohexital being higher. This disparity could explain the difference found in the psychomotor skills of patients and the earlier full recovery after methohexital. Sensitive tests of psychomotor skills tend to show better early performance after methohexital than after thiopental use. A driving test, however, reveals abnormal skills for as long as 8 hours after anesthesia, thus suggesting that despite plasma clearance, residual CNS impairment lasts for about 1 day.[329] Regardless of these residual effects, methohexital is cleared more rapidly than thiopental, which explains why methohexital is preferred for use by some clinicians when rapid awakening is desirable, such as in outpatient anesthesia. This prolongation of both early and late recovery by barbiturates is why they have largely been replaced by propofol.

Uses

Barbiturates are used clinically in the practice of anesthesia for induction and maintenance of anesthesia, as well as for premedication. Less frequently, barbiturates are used to provide cerebral protection to patients at risk for incomplete ischemia. The three barbiturates that are used most commonly in the United States for intravenous anesthesia and maintenance of anesthesia are thiopental, thiamylal, and methohexital.

Thiopental is an excellent hypnotic for use as an intravenous induction agent. The prompt onset (15 to 30 seconds) of action and smooth induction noted with its use make thiopental superior to most other available drugs. The relatively rapid emergence, particularly after single use for induction, was also a reason for the widespread use of thiopental in this setting. Thiopental does not possess analgesic properties and must therefore be supplemented with other analgesic drugs to obtund the reflex responses to noxious stimuli during anesthesia and surgical procedures. Thiopental can be used to maintain general anesthesia because repeated doses reliably sustain unconsciousness and contribute to amnesia. Thiopental is not a perfect choice, however, for use as the hypnotic component during balanced anesthesia.[330] Probably because of thiopental's antanalgesic properties as plasma levels of the drug decrease, analgesic supplementation is required more often with thiopental than with midazolam when used during balanced anesthesia.[331]

Methohexital is the only intravenous barbiturate used for induction that offers a serious challenge to thiopental. At a dose of 1 to 2 mg/kg, induction is swift and so is emergence. Methohexital may also be used as the hypnotic component to maintain anesthesia. Like thiopental, it is not an analgesic. Therefore, additional opioids or volatile anesthetics are required to provide a balanced technique satisfactory for general anesthesia during surgery. Methohexital is cleared more rapidly than thiopental, so it is superior to thiopental for maintenance of anesthesia because accumulation and saturation of peripheral sites take longer. For brief infusion (<60 minutes), recovery from a methohexital infusion titrated to maintain hypnosis (50 to 150 µg/kg/min) is similar to that provided by propofol. The upper limits of safe infusion doses have probably not yet been defined, but seizures have occurred in neurosurgical patients after large doses of methohexital (24 mg/kg).[332] Finally, some clinicians advocate the use of methohexital in pediatric patients as a rectal premedication agent. Methohexital may be given rectally and is absorbed rapidly. Mean peak plasma levels occur within 14 minutes after rectal administration and are associated with a rapid hypnotic effect. The dose recommended for this use is 25 mg/kg by rectal instillation (10% solution through a 14 French catheter, 7 cm into the rectum).[333,334] With this method of administration, onset of sleep is rapid.

Dosing

Doses for the two most commonly used barbiturates are listed in Table 10-6. The usual dose of thiopental (3 to 4 mg/kg) and thiamylal (3 to 4 mg/kg) is about twice that of methohexital (1.0 to 2.0 mg/kg). In dose-response studies, the ED_{50} for thiopental ranged from 2.2 to 2.7 mg/kg, and that for methohexital was 1.1 mg/kg.[324] Because the ED_{50} induces anesthesia in only 50% of a given group of patients, higher doses are needed to reliably induce anesthesia in all patients. Thus, the usual dose of thiopental is 3 to 4 mg/kg given intravenously over a period of 5 to 15 seconds. There is less interpatient variability in the dose response to barbiturates than to benzodiazepines when used for induction of anesthesia, but there is still significant variability in the doses of thiopental required to induce anesthesia.[324] In one large study, the induction dose for healthy patients varied from 2.8 to 9.7 mg/kg.[335] Interpatient dose variability is related to the presence of hemorrhagic shock, the level of cardiac output, lean body mass, obesity, sex, and age. Hemorrhagic shock, lean body mass, age, and obesity contribute to the variability in patient response by decreasing the central volume of distribution. Thus, less blood volume (shock, dehydration) or less lean body mass (obesity, common in the elderly and lower in females than males) decreases the volume in which the drug is diluted or the volume into which it is quickly redistributed, respectively. Finally, patients who have severe anemia or burns, malnutrition, widespread malignant disease, uremia, and ulcerative colitis or intestinal obstruction also require lower induction doses of barbiturate.

Side Effects and Contraindications

The effects of barbiturates on various organ systems have been studied extensively. Some side effects occur in unpredictable, varying proportions of patients, whereas the cardiovascular and pulmonary effects are dose related.[336-338] No important differences have been found between the barbiturates with regard to their effects on the various organ systems (respiratory, cardiovascular, gastrointestinal, hepatic, and renal), but there are differences in other complications with these drugs. Complications of injecting barbiturates include a garlic or onion taste (40% of patients), allergic reactions, local tissue irritation, and rarely, tissue necrosis. An urticarial rash that lasts a few minutes may develop on the head, neck, and trunk. More severe reactions such as facial edema, hives, bronchospasm, and anaphylaxis can also occur. Treatment of anaphylaxis is 1-mL increments of 1:10,000 epinephrine with intravenous fluids. Aminophylline can be given for bronchospasm.

Thiopental and thiamylal produce fewer excitatory symptoms with induction than methohexital does; cough, hiccough, tremors, and twitching are produced approximately five times more often with methohexital. Tissue irritation and local complications may occur more frequently with the use of thiopental and thiamylal than with methohexital. In comparative studies, pain on injection was shown to be greater with methohexital (12%) than with thiopental (9%). Results also show that phlebitis occurs more frequently with methohexital (8%) than with thiopental (1%).[339] Tissue and venous irritation is more common if a 5% solution is used rather than the standard 2% solution.

Rarely, accidental intra-arterial injection can occur, the consequences of which may be severe. The degree of injury is related to the concentration of the drug. Treatment consists of (1) dilution of the drug by the administration of saline into the artery, (2) heparinization to prevent thrombosis, and (3) brachial plexus block.[340] Overall, proper intravenous administration of thiopental is remarkably free of local toxicity.

Cardiovascular System

Cardiovascular depression from barbiturates is a result of both central and peripheral (direct vascular and cardiac) effects.[341] The hemodynamic changes produced by barbiturates have been studied in healthy subjects and patients with heart disease.[342,343] The primary cardiovascular effect of barbiturate induction is peripheral vasodilation resulting in pooling of blood in the venous system.[344] A decrease in contractility is another effect and is related to reduced availability of calcium to myofibrils. In addition, the heart rate is increased.[343] Mechanisms for the decrease in cardiac output include (1) direct negative inotropic action, (2) decreased ventricular filling because

Table 10–6	Recommended doses of barbiturates for induction and maintenance of anesthesia		
Drug	**Induction Dose (mg/kg)*†**	**Onset (sec)**	**IV Maintenance Infusion**
Thiopental	3-4	10-30	50-100 mg q10-12min
Methohexital	1-1.5	10-30	20-40 mg q4-7min

*Adult and pediatric intravenous doses are roughly the same in milligrams per kilogram.

†Methohexital can be given rectally in pediatric patients at 20 to 25 mg/kg per dose.

of increased capacitance, and (3) transiently decreased sympathetic outflow from the CNS.[332,345] The increase in heart rate (10% to 36%) that accompanies thiopental administration probably results from baroreceptor-mediated sympathetic reflex stimulation of the heart in response to the drop in output and pressure. Thiopental produces dose-related negative inotropic effects that appear to result from a decrease in calcium influx into the cells with a resultant diminished amount of calcium at sarcolemma sites. The cardiac index is unchanged or reduced, and mean arterial pressure is maintained or slightly reduced. Thiopental infusions and lower doses tend to be accompanied by smaller hemodynamic changes than those noted with rapid bolus injections. In the dose ranges studied, no relationship between plasma thiopental level and hemodynamic effect has been found. A sympathetic discharge in response to intubation increases the heart rate and blood pressure and can be attenuated by the administration of fentanyl (1 to 3 μg/kg).

Little difference is seen in responses after administration of thiopental and methohexital to heart disease patients. The increase in heart rate (11% to 36%) encountered in patients with coronary artery disease who are anesthetized with thiopental (1 to 4 mg/kg) is potentially deleterious because of the obligatory increase in myocardial oxygen consumption (MV_{O_2}) that accompanies the increased heart rate. Patients who have normal coronary arteries have no difficulty maintaining adequate coronary blood flow to meet the increased MV_{O_2}.[346] When thiopental is given to hypovolemic patients, there is a significant reduction in cardiac output (69%), as well as an important decrease in blood pressure.[347] Patients without adequate compensatory mechanisms may therefore have serious hemodynamic depression with thiopental induction.

Respiratory System

Barbiturates produce dose-related central respiratory depression. In addition, a significant incidence of transient apnea occurs after the administration of barbiturates for induction of anesthesia. The evidence for central depression is a correlation between EEG suppression and minute ventilation. With increased anesthetic effect, minute ventilation is diminished. The time course of respiratory depression has not been fully studied, but it appears that peak respiratory depression (as measured by the slope of CO_2 concentration in blood) and minute ventilation after delivery of thiopental (3.5 mg/kg) occurs 1 to 1.5 minutes after administration. These parameters return to predrug levels rapidly, and within 15 minutes the drug effects are barely detectable.[348] Patients with chronic lung disease are slightly more susceptible to the respiratory depression associated with thiopental. Apnea occurs during induction of anesthesia with thiopental in at least 20% of cases, but the duration of apnea is short, approximately 25 seconds.[349] The usual ventilatory pattern with thiopental induction has been described as "double apnea." The initial apnea that occurs during drug administration lasts a few seconds and is succeeded by a few breaths of reasonably adequate tidal volume, followed by a more lengthy apneic period. During induction of anesthesia with thiopental, ventilation must be assisted or controlled to provide adequate respiratory exchange.

Like other barbiturates, methohexital is a central respiratory system depressant. Induction doses (1.5 mg/kg) significantly decrease the slope of the ventilatory response to carbon dioxide ($VRCO_2$).[350] Maximal reduction in $VRCO_2$ occurred 30 seconds after drug administration and began to approach normal levels within 15 minutes. The peak decrease in tidal volume occurred 60 seconds after methohexital delivery and also returned to baseline within 15 minutes. In contrast to the effects on ventilation, patients were awake within about 5 minutes after the administration of methohexital (1.5 mg/kg). No difference in the duration of ventilatory depression is seen after methohexital or thiopental delivery when the drugs are studied in a similar manner.[348]

Contraindications

Wood has listed the contraindications to intravenous barbiturate use.[351] First, in patients with respiratory obstruction or an inadequate airway, thiopental may worsen respiratory depression. Second, severe cardiovascular instability or shock may preclude its use. Third, status asthmaticus is a condition in which airway control and ventilation may be further worsened by thiopental. Fourth, porphyria may be precipitated or acute attacks may be accentuated by the administration of thiopental. Fifth, without proper equipment for administration (intravenous instrumentation) and airway equipment (means of artificial ventilation), thiopental should not be administered.

BENZODIAZEPINES

History

Benzodiazepines were accidentally discovered to be effective sedative-hypnotic drugs.[352] Sternbach synthesized chlordiazepoxide (Librium) in 1955, but it was discarded without testing because it was considered inert. However, in 1957 the drug was discovered to have entirely unexpected "hypnotic, sedative, and antistrychnine effects in mice."[353] This first benzodiazepine was released for oral use in 1960, and in that year it was clear that in sufficiently large doses, chlordiazepoxide possessed profound hypnotic and amnestic properties, although it was not available in parenteral form for use in anesthesia. However, a patient who was taking chlordiazepoxide was reported to have fallen and fractured her sacrum accidentally[354]; this accident, which was not remembered or painful, suggested the use of benzodiazepines as anesthetics during trauma (surgery). Diazepam (Valium) was synthesized by Sternbach in 1959 while searching for a new and better compound. It was first described for use as an intravenous anesthetic induction agent in 1965.[355] Oxazepam (Serax), a metabolite of diazepam, was synthesized in 1961 by Bell and was marketed by a different pharmaceutical company. Lorazepam (Ativan), a 2'-chloro substitution product of oxazepam, was synthesized in 1971 in an attempt to produce a more potent benzodiazepine. The next major achievement was Walser and colleagues' 1976 synthesis of midazolam (Versed), the first clinically used water-soluble benzodiazepine.[356] It is not

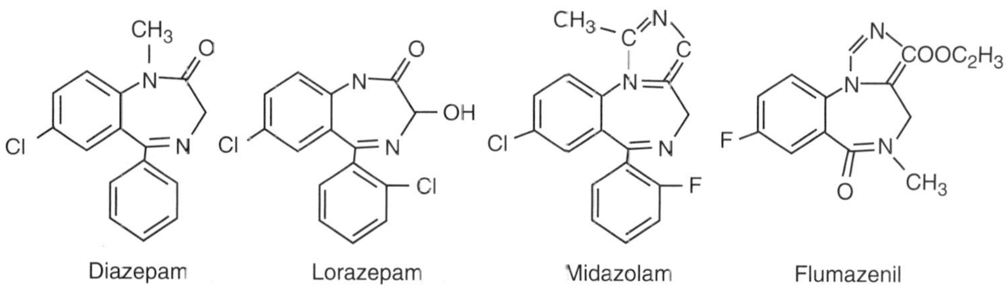

Figure 10–10 The structures of four benzodiazepines used in clinical anesthesia practice.

Diazepam   Lorazepam   Midazolam   Flumazenil

certain when benzodiazepines were initially used to induce anesthesia, but in 1966 several groups reported the use of diazepam for anesthesia.[357,358] Midazolam was the first benzodiazepine that was produced primarily for use in anesthesia.[359]

Benzodiazepines possess many of the characteristics sought by anesthesiologists. They produce their actions by occupying the benzodiazepine receptor, which was first discussed in December 1971 in Milan.[360] Barnett and Fiore[361] postulated a benzodiazepine receptor, and in 1977, specific benzodiazepine receptors were described when ligands were found to interact with a central receptor.[362] Discovery and understanding of the mechanism of the benzodiazepine receptor have enabled chemists to develop many agonist compounds and to even produce a specific antagonist for clinical use.

Physicochemical Characteristics

Three benzodiazepine receptor agonists are commonly used in the practice of anesthesia in the United States: midazolam, diazepam, and lorazepam (Fig. 10-10 and Table 10-7). All these molecules are relatively small and lipid soluble at physiologic pH. Each milliliter of diazepam solution (5 mg) contains 0.4 mL propylene glycol, 0.1 mL alcohol, 0.015 mL benzyl alcohol, and sodium benzoate/benzoic acid in water for injection (pH 6.2 to 6.9). Lorazepam solution (2 or 4 mg/mL) contains 0.18 mL polyethylene glycol with 2% benzyl alcohol as a preservative. Midazolam solution contains 1 or 5 mg/mL midazolam plus 0.8% sodium chloride and 0.01% disodium edetate, with 1% benzyl alcohol used as a preservative. The pH is adjusted to 3 with hydrochloric acid and sodium hydroxide. Midazolam is the most lipid soluble of the three drugs in vivo,[363] but because of its pH-dependent solubility, it is water soluble when formulated in a buffered acidic medium (pH 3.5). The imidazole ring of

midazolam accounts for its stability in solution and rapid metabolism. The high lipophilicity of all three accounts for their rapid CNS effect, as well as their relatively large volumes of distribution.[364]

Metabolism

Biotransformation of the benzodiazepines occurs in the liver. The two principal pathways involve either hepatic microsomal oxidation (N-dealkylation or aliphatic hydroxylation) or glucuronide conjugation.[352,365] The difference in the two pathways is significant because oxidation is susceptible to outside influences and can be impaired by certain population characteristics (e.g., old age), disease states (e.g., hepatic cirrhosis), or the coadministration of other drugs that can impair oxidizing capacity (e.g., cimetidine). Conjugation is less susceptible to these factors.[352] Both midazolam and diazepam undergo oxidation reduction or phase I reactions in the liver.[366] The fused imidazole ring of midazolam is oxidized rapidly by the liver, much more rapidly than the methylene group of the diazepine ring in other benzodiazepines. This rapid oxidation accounts for the greater hepatic clearance of midazolam than diazepam. Lorazepam is less affected by enzyme induction and some of the other factors known to alter the cytochrome P450 and other phase I enzymes. For example, inhibition of oxidative enzyme function by cimetidine impairs the clearance of diazepam,[367] but it has no effect on lorazepam.[366] Age decreases and smoking increases the clearance of diazepam,[34] but neither has a significant effect on midazolam biotransformation.[21] Habitual alcohol consumption increases the clearance of midazolam.[368] Race, because of differences in the isoenzymes responsible for hydroxylation, produces genetic differences in drug metabolism.[369] The high frequency of mutated alleles in Asians in the genes coding for CYP2C19

Table 10–7 Physicochemical characterization of three benzodiazepines

	Diazepam	Lorazepam	Midazolam
Molecular weight (daltons)	284.7*	321.2*	362*
pK_a	3.3 (20°)	11.5 (20°)	6.2 (20°)*
Water soluble	No*	Almost insoluble	Yes†
Lipid soluble	Yes, highly lipophilic*	Yes (relatively less lipophilic, however)	Yes, highly lipophilic†

*Data from Moffet A: Clarke's Isolation and Identification of Drugs, 2nd ed. London, Pharmaceutical Press, 1986.
†pH dependent: pH > 4, lipid soluble; pH < 4, water soluble.

Table 10–8   Pharmacokinetic and pharmacodynamic comparison of midazolam and active metabolites*

	EC$_{50}$ EEG	EC$_{50}$ SVT	Clearance	V$_{SS}$	t$_{1/2}$cl
Midazolam	1.8 ng/mL	0.9 mg/mL	523 mL/min	60 L	98 min
1-Hydroxymidazolam	10.2 ng/mL	5.3 ng/mL	680 mL/min	69 L	69 min

*All values are significantly ($P < .05$) different between midazolam and 1-hydroxymidazolam.
EC$_{50}$, median effective concentration; EEG, peak electroencephalogram change; SVT, saccadic velocity (eye movement);
t$_{1/2}$cl, clearance half-life; V$_{SS}$, volume at steady state.
From Mandema JW, Tuk B, van Steveninck AL, et al: Pharmacokinetic-pharmacodynamic modeling of the central nervous system effects of midazolam and its main metabolite 1-hydroxymidazolam in healthy volunteers. Clin Pharmacol Ther 51:715-728, 1992.

may explain the reduced hepatic biotransformation of diazepam.

The metabolites of benzodiazepines can be important. Diazepam forms two active metabolites, oxazepam and desmethyldiazepam, both of which add to and prolong the drug's effects. Midazolam is biotransformed to hydroxy-midazolams, which have activity and, when given over a longer time, can accumulate.[370] However, these metabolites are rapidly conjugated and excreted in urine. 1-Hydroxymidazolam has an estimated clinical potency that is 20% to 30% that of midazolam.[35] It is excreted largely by the kidneys and can cause profound sedation in patients with renal impairment.[36] The primary hydroxymetabolite is cleared more rapidly[35] than mida-zolam in healthy patients (Table 10-8). Thus, the metabolites are less potent and normally cleared more rapidly than midazolam, so they are of little concern in patients with normal hepatic and renal function. Lorazepam has five metabolites, but the principal one is conjugated to glucuronide. This metabolite is inactive, water soluble, and rapidly excreted by the kidney.

Pharmacokinetics

The three benzodiazepines used in anesthesia are classified as short (midazolam), intermediate (lorazepam), and long lasting (diazepam), according to their metabolism and plasma clearance (see Table 10-1).[21,37] The plasma disappearance curves of all the benzodiazepines can be fitted to a two- or three-compartment model. Protein binding and volumes of distribution are not importantly different among these three benzodiazepines, but their clearance is significantly different. The clearance rate of midazolam ranges from 6 to 11 mL/kg/min, whereas clearance of lorazepam is 0.8 to 1.8 mL/kg/min and that of diazepam is 0.2 to 0.5 mL/kg/min.[21] Because of these differences in clearance, the drugs have predictably different plasma disappearance curves (Figs. 10-11 to 10-13). They also have different context-sensitive half-times (see Fig. 10-3). Although the termination of action of these drugs is primarily a result of redistribution of the drug from the CNS to other tissues after use in anesthesia, after daily (long-term) repeated administration or after prolonged continuous infusion, midazolam blood levels will decrease more rapidly than blood levels of the other drugs because of its greater hepatic clearance. Thus, patients given continuous infusions of midazolam or repeated boluses over days should awaken faster than those given diazepam or lorazepam.

Factors known to influence the pharmacokinetics of benzodiazepines are age, gender, race, enzyme induction, and hepatic and renal disease. Diazepam is sensitive to

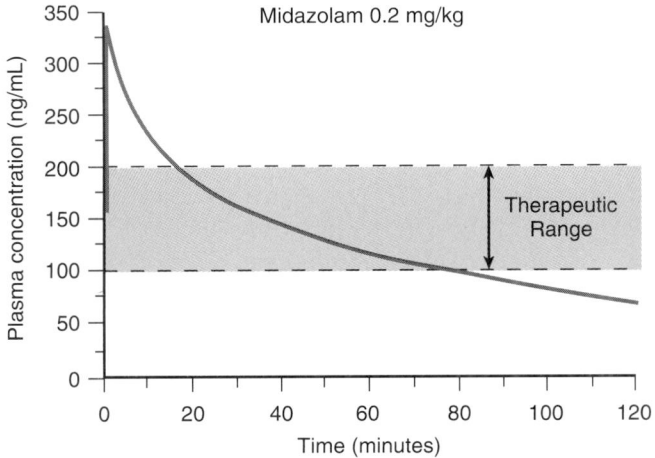

Figure 10–11 Simulated time course of plasma levels of midazolam after an induction dose of 0.2 mg/kg. Plasma levels required for hypnosis and amnesia during surgery are 100 to 200 ng/mL, with awakening usually occurring at levels lower than 50 ng/mL.

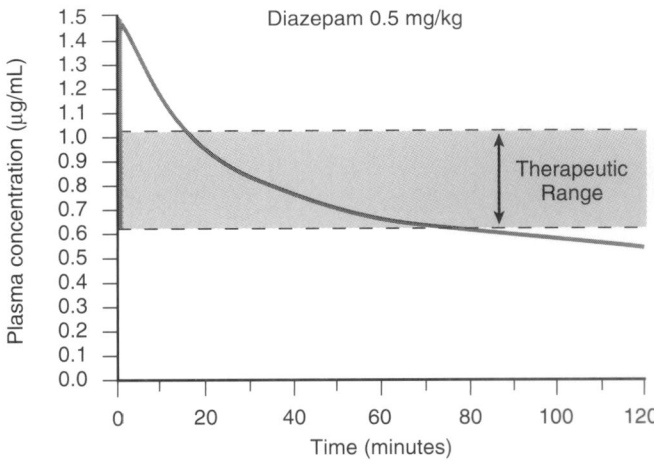

Figure 10–12 Simulated time course of plasma levels of diazepam after an induction dose of 0.5 mg/kg. Plasma levels required for hypnosis and amnesia during surgery are 0.6 to 1.0 µg/mL, with awakening usually occurring at levels lower than 0.5 µg/mL.

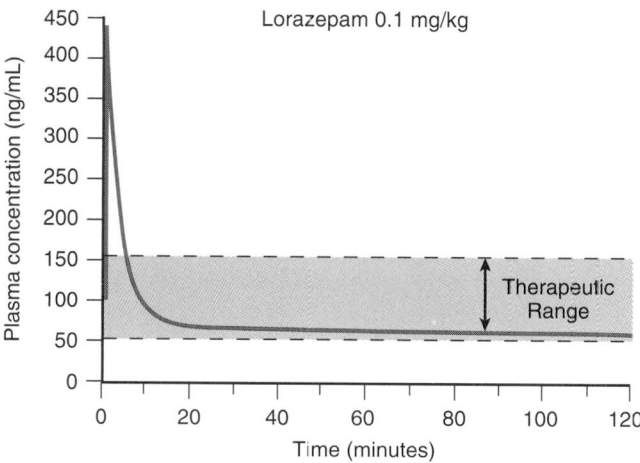

Figure 10–13 Simulated time course of plasma levels of lorazepam after an induction dose of 0.1 mg/kg. Plasma levels required for hypnosis and amnesia during surgery are between 50 and 150 ng/mL, with awakening usually occurring at levels lower than 50 ng/mL.

some of these factors, particularly age. Increasing age tends to reduce the clearance of diazepam[38] significantly and the clearance of midazolam to a lesser degree.[39] Lorazepam is resistant to the effects of age, gender, and renal disease on pharmacokinetics. These drugs are all affected by obesity. The volume of distribution is increased as drug goes from plasma into adipose tissue. Although clearance is not altered, elimination half-lives are prolonged because of delayed return of the drug to plasma in obese persons.[39] In general, sensitivity to benzodiazepines in some groups, such as the elderly, is greater despite relatively modest pharmacokinetic effects; thus, factors other than pharmacokinetics must be considered when these drugs are used.

Pharmacology

All benzodiazepines have hypnotic, sedative, anxiolytic, amnesic, anticonvulsant, and centrally produced muscle relaxant properties. The drugs differ in their potency and efficacy with regard to each of the pharmacodynamic actions. The chemical structure of each drug dictates its particular physicochemical properties and pharmacokinetics, as well as its receptor binding characteristics. Binding of benzodiazepines to their respective receptors is of high affinity and is stereospecific and saturable; the order of receptor affinity (and thus potency) of the three agonists is lorazepam > midazolam > diazepam. Midazolam is approximately 3 to 6 times[40] and lorazepam 5 to 10 times as potent as diazepam.

The mechanism of action of benzodiazepines is reasonably well understood.[371-373] The interaction of ligands with the benzodiazepine receptor represents one of the few examples in which the complex systems of biochemistry, molecular pharmacology, genetic mutations, and clinical behavioral patterns can be explained. More is understood about the mechanism of action of benzodiazepines than about the mechanism of many other general anesthetics. Through recent genetic studies the GABA$_A$ subtypes have

been found to mediate the different effects (amnesic, anticonvulsant, anxiolytic, and sleep).[373] Sedation, anterograde amnesia, and anticonvulsant properties are mediated through α_1-receptors,[373] and anxiolysis and muscle relaxation are mediated by the α_2 GABA$_A$ receptor.[373] Drug effect is a function of the blood level. By using plasma concentration data and pharmacokinetic simulations, it has been estimated that a benzodiazepine receptor occupancy rate of less than 20% may be sufficient to produce the anxiolytic effect. sedation is observed with 30% to 50% receptor occupancy, and unconsciousness requires 60% or higher occupation of benzodiazepine agonist receptors.[374]

It is agreed that benzodiazepines exert their general effects by occupying the benzodiazepine receptor that modulates GABA, the major inhibitory neurotransmitter in the brain. GABA-adrenergic neurotransmission counterbalances the influence of excitatory neurotransmitters. Benzodiazepine receptors are found in highest density in the olfactory bulb, cerebral cortex, cerebellum, hippocampus, substantia nigra, and inferior colliculus, but lower densities are found in the striatum, lower portion of the brainstem, and spinal cord. Although there are two GABA receptors, the benzodiazepine receptor is part of the GABA$_A$ receptor complex on the subsynaptic membrane of the effector neuron. This receptor complex is made up of three protein subunits—α, β, and γ—arranged as a pentameric glycoprotein complex (Fig. 10-14). These proteins contain the various ligand binding sites of the GABA$_A$ receptor, such as the benzodiazepine, GABA, and barbiturate binding sites. The benzodiazepine binding

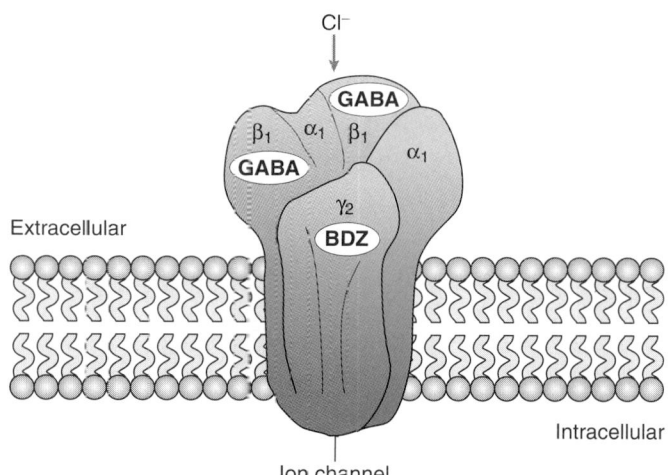

Figure 10–14 Model of the γ-aminobutyric acid (GABA)-benzodiazepine receptor complex. Current data suggest a pentameric protein composed of α-, β-, and γ-subunits; the proposed arrangement of subunits is arbitrary. There are two sites for GABA binding (on the β-subunits) and a single site for benzodiazepine (BDZ) binding (depicted on the γ_2-subunit). Homology between the GABA$_\alpha$ receptor and the nicotinic acetylcholine receptor suggests that the chloride ion channel is formed by contributions from each subunit. (Redrawn with modification from Zorumski CF, Isenberg KE: Insights into the structure and function of GABA-benzodiazepine receptors: Ion channels and psychiatry. Am J Psychiatry 148:162, 1991.)

site is located on the γ_2-subunit,[375,376] and the β-subunit is thought to contain the binding site for GABA. With activation of the GABA$_A$ receptor, gating of the channel for chloride ions is triggered. The cell becomes hyperpolarized and therefore resistant to neuronal excitation. It is now postulated that the hypnotic effects of benzodiazepines are mediated by alterations in the potential-dependent calcium ion flux.[375] The degree of modulation of GABA receptor function has a built-in limitation, which explains the relatively high degree of safety with benzodiazepines.

A fascinating and therapeutically significant discovery regarding the benzodiazepine receptor is that the pharmacologic spectrum of ligands includes three different types or classes[371] that have been termed agonists, antagonists, and inverse agonists (Fig. 10-15), names that connote their actions. Agonists (e.g., midazolam) alter the conformation of the GABA$_A$ receptor complex so that binding affinity for GABA is increased, with resultant opening of the chloride channel. Agonists and antagonists bind to a common (or at least overlapping) area of the receptor by forming differing reversible bonds with the receptor.[377] The well-known effects of an agonist then occur (anxiolysis, hypnosis, and anticonvulsant action). Antagonists (e.g., flumazenil) occupy the benzodiazepine receptor, but they produce no activity and therefore block the actions of both agonists and inverse agonists. Inverse agonists reduce the efficiency of GABA-adrenergic synaptic transmission, and because GABA is inhibitory, the result of decreased GABA is CNS stimulation. The potency of the ligand is dictated by its affinity for the benzodiazepine receptor and the duration of effect by the rate of clearance of the drug from the receptor.

Long-term administration of benzodiazepines produces tolerance, which is defined as a decrease in efficacy of the drug over time.[378] Although the mechanism of chronic tolerance is not fully understood, it appears that long-term exposure to benzodiazepines causes decreased receptor binding and function (i.e., downregulation of the benzodiazepine-GABA$_A$ receptor complex). This decrease would explain the increased dose requirements of benzodiazepines for anesthesia in patients who take them on a long-term basis. Interestingly, it appears that after the cessation of long-term use of benzodiazepines, the receptor complex becomes upregulated,[378] which could mean an increased susceptibility to benzodiazepines during a period after recent use.

The onset and duration of action of a bolus intravenous dose of a benzodiazepine depend on the lipid solubility of the drug, a finding that probably explains the differences in onset and duration of action of the three benzodiazepines used in clinical practice in the United States. Midazolam and diazepam have a more rapid onset of action (usually within 30 to 60 seconds) than lorazepam does (60 to 120 seconds). The half-life of equilibrium between the plasma concentration and the EEG effect of midazolam is approximately 2 to 3 minutes and is not affected by age.[379] This half-life is about two times longer than that of diazepam, but when compared with diazepam, midazolam has sixfold greater intrinsic potency.[40] Similar data

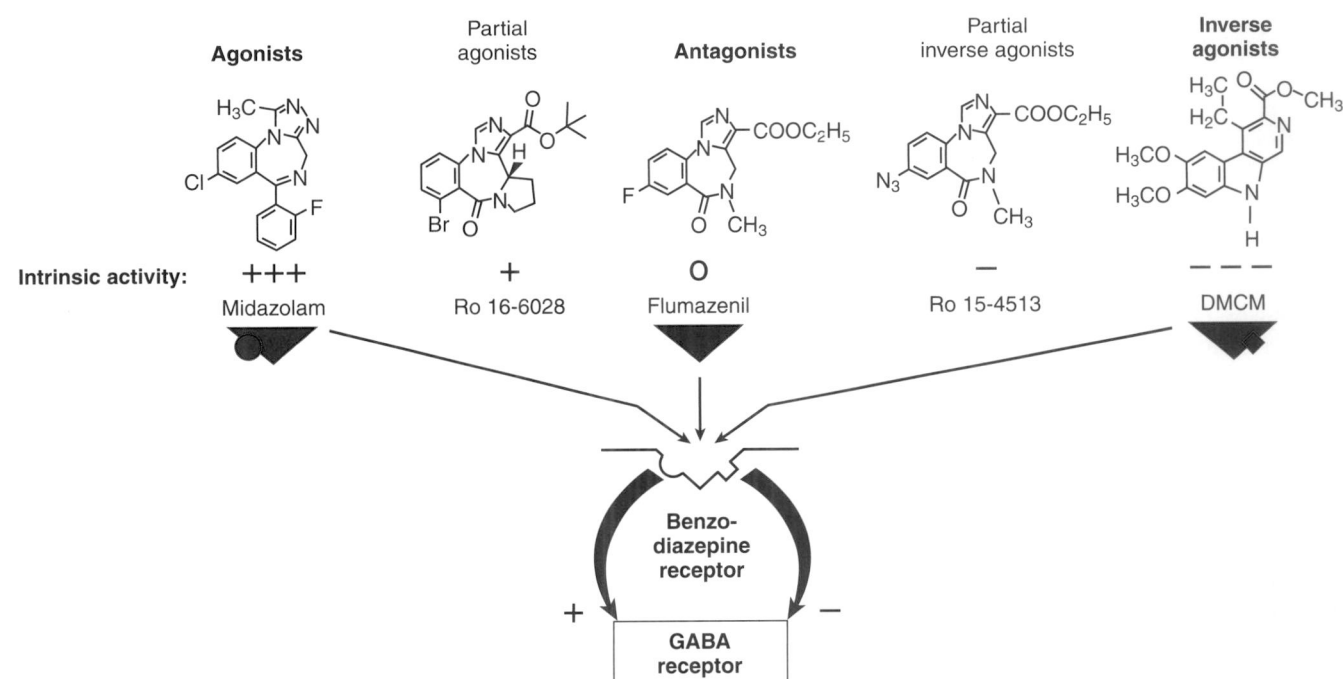

Figure 10–15 Spectrum of the intrinsic activities of benzodiazepine receptor ligands, which range from agonists to inverse agonists. Structures of agonist, partial agonist, antagonist, partial inverse agonist, and inverse agonist compounds are shown. Intrinsic activity is greatest among agonists and is least among inverse agonists. Intrinsic activities are schematically indicated as positive by a *plus sign* and as negative by a *minus sign,* with 0 indicating a lack of intrinsic activity. (Redrawn with modification from Mohler H, Richards JG: The benzodiazepine receptor: A pharmacological control element of brain function. Eur J Anaesthesiol Suppl 2:15-24, 1988.)

for other benzodiazepines are not available. Like onset, the duration of effect is also related to lipid solubility and the blood level.[380] The more rapid redistribution of midazolam and diazepam than that of lorazepam (presumably because of the lower lipid solubility than that of lorazepam)[363] accounts for the shorter duration of their actions.

Effects on the Central Nervous System
(see Chapter 21)

The benzodiazepines reduce $CMRO_2$ and CBF in a dose-related manner. Midazolam and diazepam maintain a relatively normal ratio of CBF to $CMRO_2$. In healthy human volunteers, midazolam, 0.15 mg/kg, induces sleep and reduces CBF by 34% despite a slight increase in $Paco_2$ from 34 to 39 mm Hg.[381] Brown and colleagues[382] studied EEG tracings after 10 mg intravenous midazolam and showed the appearance of rhythmic beta activity at 22 Hz within 15 to 30 seconds of administration in healthy volunteers. Within 60 seconds, a second beta rhythm occurred at 15 Hz. Alpha rhythm started to reappear at 30 minutes; however, after 60 minutes, resistant rhythmic beta activity was noted at 15- to 20-μV amplitude. The EEG changes were similar to the EEG effects with diazepam and were not typical of light sleep, although the patients were clinically asleep. The best method of monitoring depth with midazolam is use of the EEG BIS index.[383]

Midazolam, diazepam, and lorazepam all increase the seizure initiation threshold of local anesthetics and lower the mortality rate in mice exposed to lethal doses of local anesthetics.[384] Midazolam and diazepam induce a dose-related protective effect against cerebral hypoxia, which was demonstrated by extension of mouse survival time when mice were placed in 5% oxygen. The protection afforded by midazolam is superior to that of diazepam but less than that of pentobarbital.[384] Antiemetic effects are not a prominent action of the benzodiazepines.

Effects on the Respiratory System

Benzodiazepines, like most intravenous anesthetics, produce dose-related central respiratory system depression. The respiratory depression may be greater with midazolam than with diazepam and lorazepam, although comparative studies of the three do not exist. Lorazepam (2.5 mg intravenously [IV]) produces a similar, but shorter-lasting decrease in tidal volume and minute ventilation than diazepam (10 mg IV) does in patients with lung disease.[385] The peak decrease in minute ventilation after midazolam (0.15 mg/kg) is almost identical to that produced in healthy patients given diazepam (0.3 mg/kg), as determined by carbon dioxide response data.[386] The slopes of the ventilatory response curves to carbon dioxide are flatter than normal (control) but not shifted to the right, as with opioids. Judging from the plasma level and steepness of the dose-response effect on $Paco_2$ curves (Fig. 10-16),[387] midazolam is about five to nine times as potent as diazepam. The peak onset of ventilatory depression with midazolam (0.13 to 0.2 mg/kg) is rapid (about 3 minutes), and significant depression remains for about 60 to 120 minutes.[348,388] The rate of midazolam administration

affects the time of onset of peak ventilatory depression; the faster the drug is given, the more quickly this peak depression occurs.[388] The respiratory depression associated with midazolam is more pronounced and of longer duration in patients with chronic obstructive pulmonary disease, and the duration of ventilatory depression is longer with midazolam (0.19 mg/kg) than with thiopental (3.3 mg/kg).[348] Lorazepam (0.05 mg/kg) alone does not depress the carbon dioxide response, but when lorazepam is combined with meperidine, predictable respiratory depression occurs.[389] It is probable that benzodiazepines and opioids produce additive or supra-additive (synergistic) respiratory depression, even though they act at different receptors.

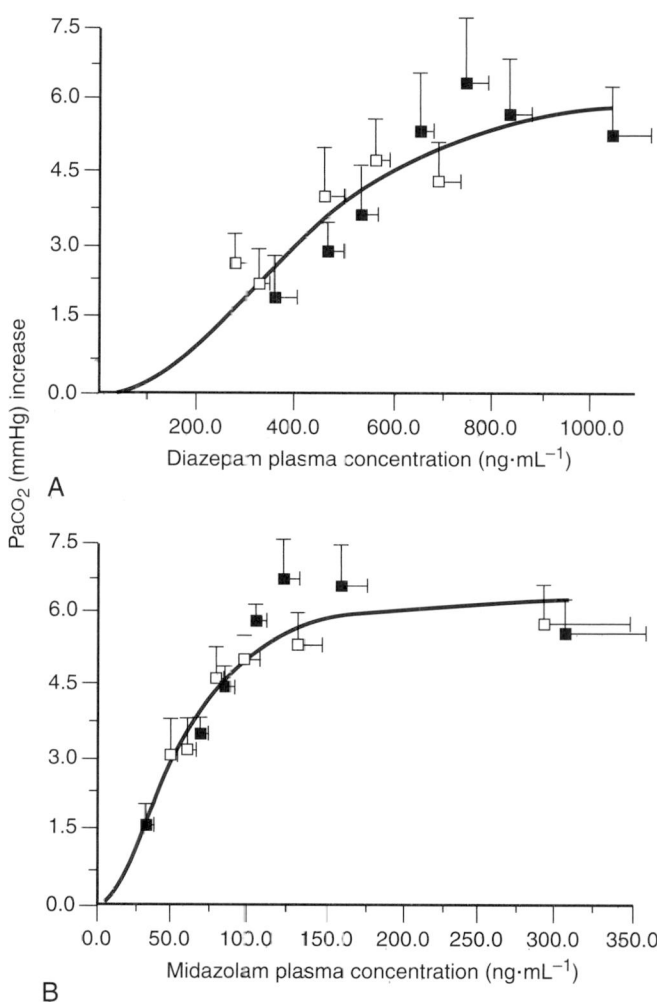

Figure 10–16 A, Increase in $Paco_2$ from baseline versus plasma concentration after three intravenous bolus doses of diazepam (0.15 mg/kg) given at 20-minute intervals. **B,** Increase in $Paco_2$ from baseline versus the midazolam plasma concentration after three intravenous bolus doses of midazolam (0.05 mg/kg) given at 20-minute intervals. The *solid line* represents a best-fit model of the data from the three injections. Mean values are represented as plus or minus standard error of the mean. (Redrawn from Sunzel M, Paalzow L, Berggren L, Eriksson I: Respiratory and cardiovascular effects in relation to plasma levels of midazolam and diazepam. Br J Clin Pharmacol 25:561-569, 1988.)

Apnea occurs with the benzodiazepines. The incidence of apnea after induction of anesthesia with thiopental or midazolam is similar. Apnea occurred in 20% of 1130 patients given midazolam for induction and 27% of 580 patients given thiopental in clinical trials with midazolam.[359] Apnea is related to the dose of the benzodiazepine and is more likely to occur in the presence of opioids. Old age, debilitating disease, and other respiratory depressant drugs probably also increase the incidence and degree of respiratory depression and apnea with benzodiazepines.

Effects on the Cardiovascular System

Used alone, the benzodiazepines have modest hemodynamic effects. The hemodynamic changes reported with anesthetic induction doses of diazepam, midazolam, and lorazepam are shown in Table 10-2. These values represent the peak hemodynamic effect in the first 10 minutes after administration and are derived from studies of both healthy subjects and patients with ischemic and valvular heart disease.[169,170,184,331,390] The predominant hemodynamic change is a slight reduction in arterial blood pressure that results from a decrease in systemic vascular resistance. The mechanism by which benzodiazepines maintain relatively stable hemodynamics involves the preservation of homeostatic reflex mechanisms,[341] but some evidence indicates that the baroreflex is impaired by both midazolam and diazepam.[391] Midazolam causes a slightly greater decrease in arterial blood pressure than the other benzodiazepines do, but the hypotensive effect is minimal and about the same as seen with thiopental.[185] Despite the hypotension, midazolam, even in doses as high as 0.2 mg/kg, is safe and effective for induction of anesthesia even in patients with severe aortic stenosis. The hemodynamic effects of midazolam and diazepam are dose related: the higher the plasma level, the greater the decrease in systemic blood pressure[387]; however, there is a plateau plasma drug effect above which little change in arterial blood pressure occurs. The plateau plasma level for midazolam is 100 ng/mL, and that for diazepam is about 900 ng/mL.[387] Heart rate, ventricular filling pressure, and cardiac output are maintained after induction of anesthesia with the benzodiazepines. In patients with elevated left ventricular filling pressure, diazepam and midazolam produce a "nitroglycerin-like" effect by lowering the filling pressure and increasing cardiac output.

The stresses of endotracheal intubation and surgery are not blocked by midazolam.[169] Thus, adjuvant anesthetics, usually opioids, are often combined with benzodiazepines. The combination of benzodiazepines with opioids and nitrous oxide has been investigated in patients with ischemic and valvular heart disease.[184,392-394] Whereas the addition of nitrous oxide to midazolam (0.2 mg/kg) and diazepam (0.5 mg/kg) has trivial hemodynamic consequences, the combination of benzodiazepines with opioids does have a supra-additive effect.[395] Combinations of diazepam with fentanyl or sufentanil, midazolam with fentanyl[392] or sufentanil,[394] and lorazepam with fentanyl or sufentanil[393] all produce greater decreases in systemic blood pressure than each drug does alone. Presumably, combinations of benzodiazepines with remifentanil will do the same. The mechanism for this synergistic hemodynamic effect is not completely understood, but it is probably related to a reduction in sympathetic tone when the drugs are given together.[396] There is evidence that diazepam and midazolam decrease catecholamines,[391] a finding consistent with this hypothesis.

Uses

Intravenous Sedation

Benzodiazepines are used for sedation as preoperative premedication, intraoperatively during regional or local anesthesia, and postoperatively. The anxiolysis, amnesia, and elevation of the local anesthetic seizure threshold are desirable benzodiazepine actions. The dose of drugs should be titrated for this use; end points of titration are adequate sedation or dysarthria (Table 10-9). The onset of action is more rapid with midazolam, with a peak effect usually reached within 2 to 3 minutes of administration; the time to peak effect is slightly longer with diazepam and is still longer with lorazepam. The duration of action of these drugs depends primarily on the dose used. Although the onset is more rapid with midazolam than with diazepam after bolus administration, recovery is similar,[397] probably because both drugs have similar early plasma decay (redistribution) patterns (see Figs. 10-11 and 10-12). With lorazepam, sedation and particularly amnesia are slower in onset[398] and are longer lasting than with the other two benzodiazepines.[370,399,400] A disparity in the level of sedation versus the presence of amnesia (patients seem conscious and reasonably coherent, yet they are amnesic for events and instructions) is often seen with all three benzodiazepines. Lorazepam is particularly unpredictable with regard to the duration of amnesia, and such unpredictability is undesirable in patients

---

Table 10–9   Uses and doses of intravenous benzodiazepines

	Midazolam	Diazepam	Lorazepam
Induction	0.05-0.15 mg/kg	0.3-0.5 mg/kg	0.1 mg/kg
Maintenance	0.05 mg/kg prn 1.0 µg/kg/min	0.1 mg/kg prn	0.02 mg/kg prn
Sedation*	0.5-1.0 mg repeated 0.07 mg/kg IM	2 mg repeated	0.25 mg repeated

*Incremental doses are given until the desired degree of sedation is obtained.
prn, as required to keep the patient hypnotic and amnestic.

who wish or need to have recall in the immediate post-operative period.[398] The degree of sedation and reliable amnesia, as well as preservation of respiratory and hemodynamic function, are better overall with benzodiazepines than with other sedative-hypnotic drugs used for conscious sedation. When midazolam is compared with propofol for sedation, the two are generally similar except that emergence or wake-up is more rapid with propofol. Propofol requires closer medical supervision because of its respiratory depression.[401,402] Despite the wide safety margin with benzodiazepines, respiratory function must be monitored when these drugs are used for sedation to prevent undesirable degrees of respiratory depression. There may be a slight synergistic action between midazolam and spinal anesthesia with respect to ventilation.[403] Thus, the use of midazolam for sedation during regional and epidural anesthesia requires vigilance with regard to respiratory function, just as when these drugs are given with opioids. Sedation for longer periods, for example, in the ICU, is accomplished with benzodiazepines. Prolonged infusion will result in accumulation of drug and, in the case of midazolam, significant concentration of the active metabolite. Reviews have pointed out concerns as well as advantages of benzodiazepine sedation.[370,404-407] The chief advantages are amnesia and hemodynamic stability, and the disadvantage with respect to propofol is the sometimes longer dissipation of effects when infusions are terminated. Superiority of one drug over the other has not been established; both agents should always be titrated downward to maintain sedation as required. Dosing should not be fixed; instead, it should be reduced over time to avoid the accumulation of parent or metabolites during prolonged infusion.

Oral Sedation

For many years diazepam was given orally for preoperative sedation. It is still used in 5- to 15-mg doses in adults for this purpose. More recently, an oral formulation of midazolam has been used primarily for oral premedication in pediatric patients. The dose is 0.5 mg/kg, and one preparation is from the Roche parenteral formulation of 0.5 mg/mL (Roche Laboratories, Inc., Nutley, NJ) mixed with 10 mg/kg oral acetaminophen (McNeil-PPC, Inc., Fort Washington, PA).[408] Other preparations have been developed, such as strawberry-flavored glucose (pH 4.5) prepared by the pharmacy that is stable for 8 weeks.[409] The 0.5-mg/kg oral dose is rapid acting; it provides reliable amnesia within 10 minutes and effectively sedates children for induction of anesthesia.[408]

Induction and Maintenance of Anesthesia

Midazolam is the benzodiazepine of choice for induction of anesthesia. Although both diazepam and lorazepam have been used for induction of general anesthesia, the faster onset and lack of venous complications make midazolam better suited for this use. With midazolam, induction of anesthesia is defined as unresponsiveness to command and loss of the eyelash reflex. When midazolam is used in appropriate doses (see Table 10-9), induction occurs less rapidly than with thiopental,[359] but the amnesia is more reliable. Numerous factors influence the rapidity

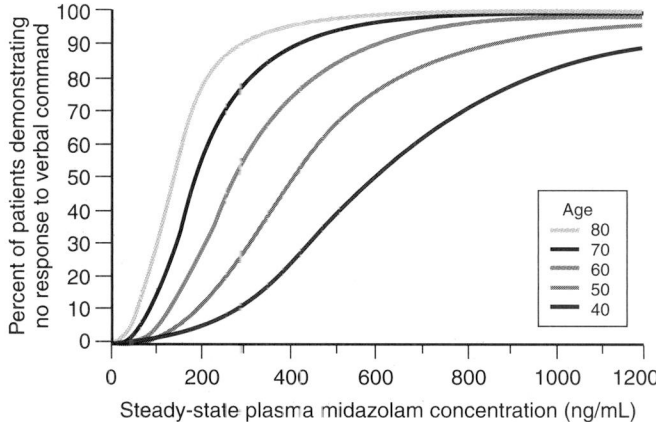

Figure 10–17 Simulated quantal concentration-response curves generated by the parameterized pharmacodynamic model for midazolam. (Redrawn from Jacobs JR, Reves JG, Marty J, et al: Aging increases pharmacodynamic sensitivity to the hypnotic effects of midazolam. Anesth Analg 80:143-148, 1995.)

of action of midazolam and the other benzodiazepines when used for induction of general anesthesia, including the dose, speed of injection, degree of premedication, age, American Society of Anesthesiologists (ASA) physical status, and concurrent anesthetic drugs.[359,410] In a well-premedicated, healthy patient, midazolam (0.2 mg/kg given in 5 to 15 seconds) will induce anesthesia in 28 seconds, whereas with diazepam (0.5 mg/kg given in 5 to 15 seconds), induction occurs in 39 seconds.[169] Elderly patients require lower doses of midazolam than younger patients do (Fig. 10-17).[411,412] Patients older than 55 years and those with ASA physical status higher than class III require a 20% or greater reduction in the induction dose of midazolam.[359] The usual induction dose of midazolam in premedicated patients is between 0.05 and 0.15 mg/kg. When midazolam is used with other anesthetic drugs (coinduction), a synergistic interaction occurs,[382,413,414] and the induction dose is less than 0.1 mg/kg (Fig. 10-18). Synergy is seen when midazolam is used with opioids or other hypnotics such as thiopental and propofol.

Awakening after benzodiazepine anesthesia is a result of redistribution of drug from the brain to other less well perfused tissues. Emergence (defined as orientation to time and place) of young, healthy volunteers who have received 10 mg of intravenous midazolam occurs in about 15 minutes,[382] and after an induction dose of 0.15 mg/kg, it occurs in about 17 minutes.[29] Emergence time is related to the dose of midazolam, as well as the dose of adjuvant anesthetic drugs.[359] Emergence from midazolam (0.32 mg/kg)/fentanyl anesthesia is about 10 minutes longer than that from thiopental (4.75 mg/kg)/fentanyl anesthesia[330] and is more prolonged than with propofol.[30] This difference accounts for some anesthesiologists' preference for propofol induction for short operations.

Benzodiazepines lack analgesic properties and must be used with other anesthetic drugs to provide sufficient analgesia; however, as maintenance anesthetic drugs during general anesthesia, benzodiazepines provide hypnosis and amnesia. Double-blind studies comparing midazolam and thiopental as the hypnotic component of balanced

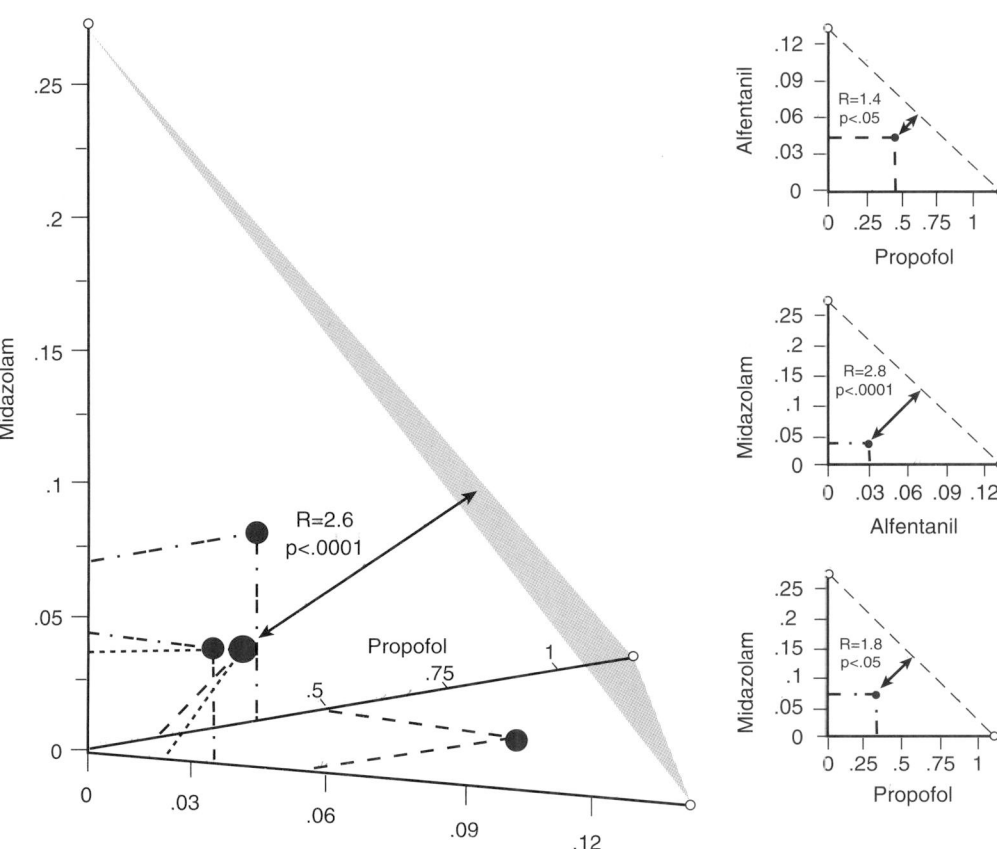

Figure 10–18 Vertical axes all represent drug dose in milligrams per kilogram. On the *right*, median effective dose (ED$_{50}$) isobolograms for the hypnotic interactions among midazolam, alfentanil, and propofol are shown. The *dotted lines* are additive effect lines; note that all combinations fall within the line representing synergism or supra-additive effect. On the *left*, a triple interaction is depicted. The *shaded area* represents an additive plane passing through three single-drug ED$_{50}$ points (*small open circles*). The *largest closed circle* (with *arrows*) is the ED$_{50}$ point for the triple combination. The *smaller closed circles* are ED$_{50}$ points for the binary combinations. R ratios on all graphs represent the interaction (1.0 indicates an additive effect) of the various drug combinations. Note that the combination of midazolam and alfentanil produces the greatest synergism, but the combination of all three is also synergistic. *P* values denote the significance of the additive effects. (Redrawn with modification from Vinik HR, Bradley EL Jr, Kissin I: Triple anesthetic combination: Propofol-midazolam-alfentanil. Anesth Analg 76:S450, 1993.)

anesthesia[330,415] have shown that midazolam is superior for this use because of better amnesia and a smoother hemodynamic course. Opioid requirements are less with midazolam. Midazolam (0.6 mg/kg) lowers the MAC of halothane by 30%[416] and presumably has a similar effect on other inhaled anesthetics. The question of an optimal redosing scheme after induction when midazolam is used as a maintenance hypnotic component of general anesthesia has not been answered. The amnesic period after an anesthetic dose is about 1 to 2 hours. Infusions of midazolam have been used to ensure a constant and appropriate depth of anesthesia.[416] Experience indicates that a plasma level of more than 50 ng/mL when used with adjuvant opioids (e.g., fentanyl) or inhaled anesthetics (e.g., nitrous oxide, volatile anesthetics), or with both, is achieved with a bolus loading dose of 0.05 to 0.15 mg/kg and a continuous infusion of 0.25 to 1 µg/kg/min.[413] This dose is sufficient to keep the patient asleep and amnesic but arousable at the end of surgery. Lower infusion doses may be required in some patients and with certain opioids. Midazolam, as well as diazepam and lorazepam, will accumulate in the blood with repeated bolus administration or with continuous infusion, just as most intravenous anesthetics do on repeated injection. If the benzodiazepines do accumulate with repeated administration, prolonged arousal time can be anticipated. This concern is less of a problem with midazolam than with diazepam and

lorazepam because of the shorter context-sensitive half-time and greater clearance of midazolam.

Side Effects and Contraindications

Benzodiazepines are remarkably safe drugs. They have a relatively high margin of safety, especially when compared with barbiturates. They are also free of allergenic effects and do not suppress the adrenal gland.[414] The most significant problem with midazolam is respiratory depression. The major side effects of lorazepam and diazepam, in addition to respiratory depression, are venous irritation and thrombophlebitis, problems related to aqueous insolubility and the requisite solvents.[359] When used as sedatives or for induction and maintenance of anesthesia, benzodiazepines can produce an undesirable degree or a prolonged interval of postoperative amnesia, sedation, and rarely, respiratory depression. These residual effects can be reversed with flumazenil.

New Benzodiazepines

The primary limitation of midazolam, which is the best suited benzodiazepine for use in anesthesia, is its slightly slower onset and prolonged offset when compared with a hypnotic such as propofol. Other benzodiazepine agonists have been used in clinical trials, but it is unlikely that they will undergo further development. The most welcome new benzodiazepine would be one rapidly metabolized by esterases, as seen with remifentanil, for faster onset and shorter duration. With discovery of the $GABA_A$ subtypes, it is also possible that new specific drugs will be developed to provide certain agonist actions that are devoid of some of the undesirable side effects such as respiratory depression.

FLUMAZENIL

Flumazenil (Anexate, Romazicon) is the first benzodiazepine antagonist approved for clinical use.[338] Preclinical pharmacologic studies with flumazenil revealed it to be a benzodiazepine receptor ligand with high affinity, great specificity, and minimal intrinsic effect by definition.[377] Flumazenil, like the agonists that it replaces at the benzodiazepine receptor, interacts with the receptor in a concentration-dependent manner. Because it is a competitive antagonist at the benzodiazepine receptor, its antagonism is reversible and surmountable. Flumazenil has minimal intrinsic activity,[377,417] which means that its benzodiazepine receptor agonist effects are very weak, significantly less than those of clinical agonists. Flumazenil, like all competitive antagonists at receptors, does not displace the agonist but rather occupies the receptor when an agonist dissociates from the receptor. The half-time (or half-life) of a receptor-ligand bond is a few milliseconds to a few seconds, and new ligand-receptor bonds are then immediately formed. This dynamic situation accounts for the ability of either an agonist or an antagonist to readily occupy the receptor. The proportion of receptors occupied by the agonist in the presence of an antagonist obeys the law of mass action and depends on the affinities and concentrations of the two ligands.[372,377] Equation 1 expresses this relationship[418]:

$$\frac{[R_{Ago}]}{[R_t]} = \frac{1}{1 + \dfrac{K_{Ago}}{[Ago]}\left\{1 + \dfrac{Ant}{K_{Ant}}\right\}} \quad (1)$$

where $[R_{Ago}]$ is the receptor concentration of agonist, $[R_t]$ is the total number of receptors, K_{Ago} is the dissociation constant for agonist, K_{Ant} is the dissociation constant for antagonist, $[Ago]$ is the concentration of agonist at the receptor, and $[Ant]$ is the concentration of antagonist at the receptor.

The ratio of agonist to total receptors produces the effects of the agonist drug, but an antagonist can alter this ratio, depending on its concentration and dissociation constant (see Equation 1). Thus, flumazenil, which is an avid (high-affinity) ligand, will replace a relatively weak agonist such as diazepam as long as it is given in sufficient dose (i.e., high [Ant]). However, flumazenil is cleared relatively rapidly, and the net result is that [Ant] is reduced over time as compared with [Ago]; thus, the proportion of receptors occupied by agonist will increase, and the potential for resedation exists (Fig. 10-19). This situation is less likely to occur when flumazenil is used to reverse midazolam, which has more rapid clearance than other

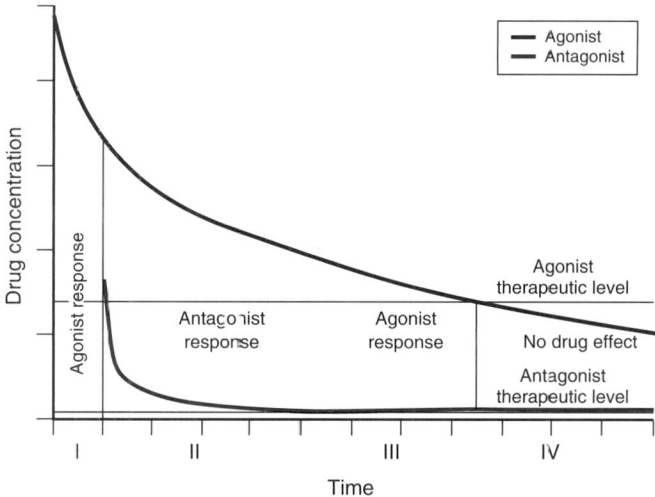

Figure 10-19 Schematic representation of the interaction of a short-acting antagonist with a longer-acting agonist resulting in resedation. The *upper curve* shows disappearance of agonist from blood, and the *lower curve* shows disappearance of antagonist from plasma. Four conditions are represented: I, agonist response; II, antagonist response (the antagonist reverses the agonist effect); III, agonist response (resedation or resumption of agonist response with disappearance of short-lasting antagonist); and IV, no drug effect, with disappearance of both agonist and antagonist (both drugs are below the therapeutic level).

benzodiazepine agonists do.[419] Another important finding is that in the presence of extremely high doses of agonist (e.g., when a mistake in dosing has occurred or suicide is attempted), flumazenil in low dose attenuates the deep CNS depression (loss of consciousness, respiratory depression) by reducing the fractional receptor occupancy by the agonist without decreasing the agonist effects that occur at low fractional receptor occupancy (drowsiness, amnesia). Conversely, high doses of flumazenil in the presence of low doses of agonist completely reverse virtually all the agonist effects. Flumazenil can precipitate withdrawal symptoms in animals or in humans physically dependent on a benzodiazepine receptor agonist.[420] Such symptoms are not a problem when flumazenil is used to reverse benzodiazepine receptor agonists in anesthesia.

Physicochemical Characteristics

Flumazenil, synthesized in 1979, is similar to midazolam and other classic benzodiazepines except for absence of the phenyl group, which is replaced by a carbonyl group (see Fig. 10-10).[421] It forms a colorless, crystalline powder, has a dissociation constant of 1.7, and has weak but sufficient water solubility to permit its preparation in aqueous solution. Its octanol/aqueous buffer partition coefficient is 14, and it demonstrates moderate lipid solubility at pH 7.4.[421]

Metabolism

Flumazenil, like the other benzodiazepines, is metabolized in the liver, is rapidly cleared from plasma, and has three known metabolites, *N*-desmethylflumazenil, *N*-desmethylflumazenil acid, and flumazenil acid.[422] The activities of these metabolites and their corresponding glucuronides are not known at present. The glucuronides are probably excreted in urine.

Pharmacokinetics

Flumazenil is a short-lived compound. Table 10-1 includes a summary of its pharmacokinetics, which has been described in a variety of clinical settings.[422-424] Of particular note is that when compared with benzodiazepine receptor agonists, flumazenil has the highest clearance and shortest elimination half-life. The plasma half-life of flumazenil is about 1 hour—it is the shortest lived of all benzodiazepines used in anesthetic practice. This short half-life means that the potential exists for the antagonist to be cleared, with sufficient concentrations of agonist left at the receptor site to cause resedation.[419] To maintain a constant therapeutic blood level over a prolonged period, either repeated administration or a continuous infusion is required. An infusion rate of 30 to 60 µg/min (0.5 to 1 µg/kg/min) has been used for this purpose.[425] The rapid blood clearance of flumazenil approaches hepatic blood flow, a finding indicating that liver clearance is partially dependent on hepatic blood flow. When compared with other benzodiazepines, flumazenil has a relatively high proportion of unbound drug; its protein binding is low, with the free fraction ranging from 54% to 64%.[423] This property of flumazenil could contribute to its rapid onset and greater clearance, but this hypothesis is unproven.

Pharmacology

When given in the absence of a benzodiazepine receptor agonist, flumazenil has little discernible CNS effect. Although intrinsic (agonist and inverse agonist) effects have been ascribed to flumazenil,[417] they are clinically unimportant. It has been postulated that in low doses a stimulating effect can be seen and in high doses a central depressant effect becomes more likely.[375] When given to volunteers and patients in clinically relevant doses, flumazenil has no effect on the EEG or cerebral metabolism.[424,426,427] In animals, flumazenil has no anticonvulsant properties and in fact reverses the anticonvulsant properties of benzodiazepines in local anesthetic-induced seizures.[428] When administered to patients who have benzodiazepine-induced CNS depression, flumazenil produces rapid and dependable reversal of unconsciousness, respiratory depression, sedation, amnesia, and psychomotor dysfunction.[374,422,429] Flumazenil can be given before, during, or after the agonist to block or reverse the CNS effects of the agonist. The usual clinical need is to reverse the effects of agonists given before flumazenil. Flumazenil has successfully reversed the effects of midazolam, diazepam, lorazepam, and flunitrazepam. Its onset is rapid, with peak effect occurring in 1 to 3 minutes,[374] which coincides with the detection of ^{11}C-flumazenil in human brain.[430] Flumazenil reverses the agonist by replacing it at the benzodiazepine receptor, and its onset and duration are governed by the law of mass action (see Equation 1). A predicted therapeutic plasma level for flumazenil is 20 ng/mL[423]; however, because the relative binding characteristics of agonist and antagonist in part dictate benzodiazepine receptor occupation by the residual agonist, different doses and plasma levels of flumazenil are required to reverse the effects of particular agonists.

The duration of action of flumazenil is determined by its dose, the dose of the agonist, and the specific agonist that is being reversed. The duration is dictated by the factors given in Equation 1. Studies have shown that during a constant infusion of agonist, the duration of flumazenil action is dependent on the dose, but 45 to 90 minutes of antagonism can be expected after an intravenous dose of 3.0 mg or 2 to 3 hours after a dose of 0.8 mg/kg.[34,431] This setting is artificial because in clinical practice, flumazenil is given after the administration of agonist has been discontinued.

Flumazenil is devoid of the respiratory and cardiovascular depressant effects of benzodiazepine receptor agonists. A relatively large dose of flumazenil (0.1 mg/kg) administered to volunteers did not produce significant respiratory depression.[432] However, when flumazenil is given in the presence of agonists, significant respiratory effects occur because it reverses the respiratory depression caused by the agonists (e.g., when given to volunteers made apneic with midazolam).[433] The reversal of midazolam-induced (0.13 mg/kg) respiratory depression with flumazenil (1.0 mg/kg) lasts between 3 and 30 minutes.[388] Other agonists and other doses would have different durations of antagonism of respiratory depression. If the respiratory depression is related to opioid administration, flumazenil will not reverse it.[434] Incremental doses, up to 3 mg intravenously, in patients with ischemic heart disease had no significant effect on cardiovascular variables.[433] Administration of flumazenil to patients given agonists is remarkably free of cardiovascular effects,[374,435] unlike the experience of opioid reversal with naloxone. Of particular interest is the effect of benzodiazepine receptor agonist reversal with flumazenil on plasma catecholamines because this effect on catecholamines is the suspected mechanism of the hyperdynamic response in opioid reversal. Although flumazenil does reverse sedation, it is not associated with significantly higher catecholamine levels than are found in patients receiving saline,[435] but the rise in catecholamines that accompanies arousal is more rapid after flumazenil.[436]

Uses

The relatively few uses for a benzodiazepine antagonist (Table 10-10) include the diagnostic and therapeutic reversal of the effects of benzodiazepine receptor agonists.[437] For diagnostic use in suspected benzodiazepine overdose, flumazenil may be given in incremental intravenous doses of 0.2 to 0.5 mg up to 3 mg. If no change in CNS sedation is noted, it is unlikely that the CNS depression is based solely on benzodiazepine overdose. More commonly in anesthesia, flumazenil is used to reverse the sedation of a patient who remains depressed after the administration of a benzodiazepine for conscious sedation

Table 10–10 Uses and doses of flumazenil

Reversal of benzodiazepines*	0.1-0.2 mg repeated† up to 3.0 mg
Diagnosis in coma	0.5 mg repeated up to 1.0 mg

*The dose required to reverse each benzodiazepine (BZD) depends on the residual amount of BZD and the particular BZD (i.e., higher doses are required for more potent BZDs) (see text).
†The degree of reversal should be titrated by repeating the 0.2-mg increment every 1 to 2 minutes until the desired level of reversal is achieved.

or for general anesthesia. Flumazenil reliably reverses the sedation, respiratory depression, and amnesia induced by benzodiazepines. However, there is now evidence of differential reversal effects on the different agonist actions. Thus, flumazenil tends to reverse the hypnotic and respiratory effects more than the amnesic effects of the agonist benzodiazepines.[434,438,439] Dosage guidelines are presented in Table 10-10, but it must be emphasized that large-scale dosing studies have not yet been completed. The dose varies with the particular benzodiazepine being reversed, and the duration of reversal is dependent on the kinetics of both the agonist and flumazenil. Surveillance is recommended if a long-lasting benzodiazepine is reversed with a single administration of flumazenil because of its relatively short-lived effect. Flumazenil may be administered by continuous infusion to prevent resedation with longer-lasting benzodiazepine receptor agonists. It is postulated that the availability of flumazenil will extend the usefulness of benzodiazepine agonists, although it will not necessarily alter the safety of this class of drugs.

Side Effects and Contraindications

Flumazenil has been given in large oral and intravenous doses with remarkably few toxic reactions.[374] It is free of local or tissue irritant properties, and it has no known organotoxicities. Like all benzodiazepines, it appears to have a high safety margin, probably higher than that of agonists, because it does not produce prominent CNS depression. An important caution is that resedation could occur because of the relatively short half-life of the drug.

PHENCYCLIDINES (KETAMINE)

History

Phencyclidine was the first drug of its class to be used for anesthesia. It was synthesized by Maddox and introduced into clinical use in 1958 by Greifenstein and colleagues[440] and in 1959 by Johnstone and associates.[441] Although phencyclidine proved useful as an anesthetic, it produced unacceptably high adverse psychological effects (hallucinations and delirium) in the postanesthetic recovery period. Cyclohexamine, a congener of phencyclidine, was tried clinically in 1959 by Lear and coworkers,[442] but it was found to be less efficacious than phencyclidine in terms of analgesia and yet had as many adverse psychotomimetic effects. Neither of these drugs is used clinically today, although phencyclidine is available for illicit recreational use. Ketamine (Ketalar) was synthesized in 1962 by Stevens and was first used in humans in 1965 by Corssen and Domino.[443] It was chosen from among 200 phencyclidine derivatives and proved to be the most promising in laboratory animal testing. Ketamine was released for clinical use in 1970 and is still used in a variety of clinical settings. Ketamine is different from most other anesthetic induction agents in that it has significant analgesic effect. It does not usually depress the cardiovascular and respiratory systems,[285,444] but it does possess some of the worrisome adverse psychological effects found with the other phencyclidines. Ketamine consists of two stereoisomers: S-(+) and R-(–). The S-(+)-isomer is more potent and is associated with fewer side effects. Interest in ketamine has recently increased because of its effects on hyperalgesia and opiate tolerance, as well as the availability (in some countries) of S-(+)-ketamine.

Physicochemical Characteristics

Ketamine (Fig. 10-20) has a molecular weight of 238 kd, is partially water soluble, and forms a white crystalline salt with a negative log of the acid ionization constant (pK_a) of 7.5.[285,444] It has a lipid solubility 5 to 10 times that of thiopental.[445] Ketamine is prepared in a slightly acidic (pH 3.5 to 5.5) solution, and the racemic mixture comes in concentrations of 10-, 50-, and 100-mg ketamine base per milliliter of sodium chloride solution containing the preservative benzethonium chloride. The ketamine

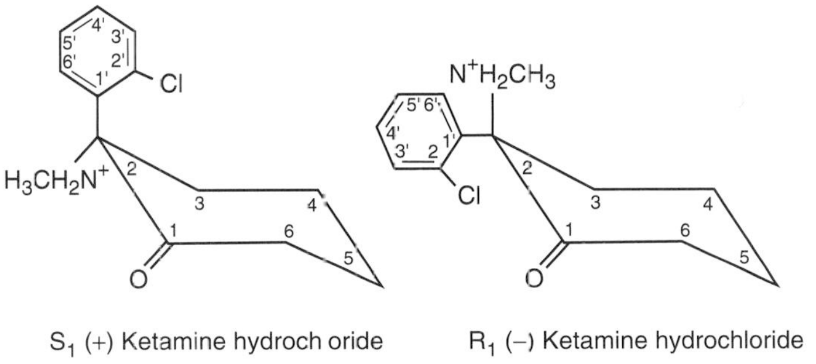

Figure 10–20 Stereoisomers of ketamine as it is formulated.

S_1 (+) Ketamine hydrochloride R_1 (–) Ketamine hydrochloride molecule contains a chiral center and therefore occurs as two resolvable optical isomers or enantiomers. The commercial racemic preparation is a mixture of both enantiomers [S-(+) and R-(–)] in equal amounts.[444] S-(+)-ketamine is available in 5- and 25-mg/mL concentrations.

Metabolism

Ketamine is metabolized by hepatic microsomal enzymes. The major pathway involves N-demethylation to form norketamine (metabolite I), which is then hydroxylated to hydroxynorketamine. These products are conjugated to water-soluble glucuronide derivatives and are excreted in urine.[285,444,446] The activity of the principal metabolites of ketamine has not been well studied, but norketamine has been shown to have significantly less (between 20% and 30%) activity than the parent compound.[447-449] Little is known about the activity of the other metabolites, but it is probable that ketamine is the major active drug.

Pharmacokinetics

The pharmacokinetics of ketamine has not been as well studied as that of many other intravenous anesthetics. Ketamine pharmacokinetics has been examined after bolus administration of anesthetizing doses (2 to 2.5 mg/kg),[31] after a subanesthetic dose (0.25 mg/kg),[31,450] and after continuous infusion (steady-state plasma level of 2000 ng/mL).[451] Regardless of the dose, ketamine plasma disappearance can be described by a two-compartment model. Table 10-1 contains the pharmacokinetic values from bolus administration studies.[31] Of note is the rapid distribution reflected in the relatively brief slow distribution half-life of 11 to 16 minutes (Fig. 10-21). The high lipid solubility of ketamine is reflected in its relatively large volume of distribution, nearly 3 L/kg. Clearance is also relatively high and ranges from 890 to 1227 mL/min, which accounts for the relatively short elimination half-life of 2 to 3 hours. The mean total-body clearance (1.4 L/min)

is approximately equal to liver blood flow, which means that changes in liver blood flow affect clearance. Thus, the administration of a drug such as halothane, which reduces hepatic blood flow, decreases ketamine clearance.[452,453] Low-dose alfentanil increases the volume of distribution and clearance of ketamine, thereby resulting in higher plasma concentrations. In addition, alfentanil increases the distribution of ketamine into the brain.[454]

The pharmacokinetics of the two isomers is different. S-(+)-ketamine has a larger elimination clearance and larger volume of distribution than R-(+)-ketamine does.[455] The S-(+)-enantiomer also appears to be more potent in suppressing the EEG than either S-(–) or the racemic mixture.[456]

Pharmacology

Effects on the Central Nervous System

Ketamine produces dose-related unconsciousness and analgesia. The anesthetized state has been termed *dissociative anesthesia* because patients who receive ketamine alone appear to be in a cataleptic state, unlike other states of anesthesia that resemble normal sleep. Ketamine-anesthetized patients have profound analgesia but keep their eyes open and maintain many reflexes. Corneal, cough, and swallow reflexes may all be present but should not be assumed to be protective.[457] Patients have no recall of surgery or anesthesia, but amnesia is not as prominent with ketamine as with the benzodiazepines. Because ketamine has a low molecular weight, a pK_a near physiologic pH, and relatively high lipid solubility, it crosses the blood-brain barrier rapidly and therefore has an onset of action within 30 seconds of administration. Maximal effect occurs in about 1 minute. After ketamine administration, pupils dilate moderately and nystagmus occurs. Lacrimation and salivation are common, as is increased skeletal muscle tone, often with coordinated but seemingly purposeless movement of the arms, legs, trunk, and head. Despite great interindividual variability, plasma levels of 0.6 to 2.0 µg/mL are considered the minimum concentrations for general anesthesia,[451,452] but children may require slightly higher plasma levels (0.8 to 4.0 µg/mL).[458] The duration of ketamine anesthesia after a single administration of a general anesthetic dose (2 mg/kg IV) is 10 to 15 minutes (see Fig. 10-21),[459] and full orientation to person, place, and time occurs within 15 to 30 minutes.[460]

The S-(+)-enantiomer enables quicker recovery (by a couple of minutes) than the racemic mixture does.[461] This more rapid recovery is thought to be due to the lower dose necessary to produce an equi-anesthetic effect and the 10% faster hepatic biotransformation.[462]

The duration of ketamine anesthesia is determined by the dose; higher doses produce more prolonged anesthesia,[463] and the concurrent use of other anesthetics also prolongs the time of emergence. Because of reasonably good correlation between blood level of ketamine and CNS effect, it appears that ketamine's relatively short duration of action is due to its redistribution from the brain and blood to other tissues in the body. Thus, termination of effect after a single bolus administration of ketamine is a result of drug redistribution from well-perfused to less well perfused tissues. Concomitant administration of a

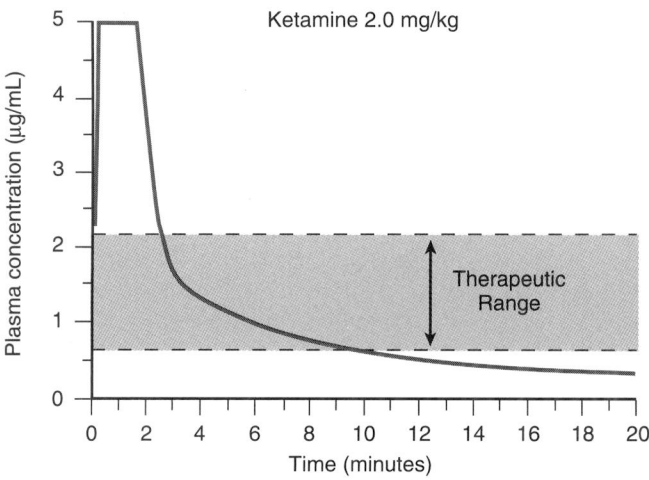

Figure 10–21 Simulated time course of plasma levels of ketamine after an induction dose of 2.0 mg/kg. Plasma levels required for hypnosis and amnesia during surgery are 0.7 to 2.2 µg/mL, with awakening usually occurring at levels lower than 0.5 µg/mL.

benzodiazepine, a common practice, may prolong ketamine's effect.[464] When used in combination with a benzodiazepine, the S-(+)-enantiomer was no different in terms of awareness at 30 minutes, but it was significantly better at 120 minutes than the racemic mixture was.[465] Analgesia occurs at considerably lower blood levels than loss of consciousness does.

Ketamine provides important postoperative analgesia. The plasma level at which pain thresholds are elevated is 0.1 µg/mL or higher,[452] which means that there is a considerable period of postoperative analgesia after ketamine general anesthesia and that subanesthetic doses can be used to produce analgesia. Ketamine has been shown to inhibit nociceptive central hypersensitization.[466] It also attenuates acute tolerance after opiate administration.[467] Ketamine reduces opiate requirements postoperatively when used as a component of a preventive/preemptive analgesia regimen.[468,469]

The primary site of CNS action of ketamine appears to be the thalamoneocortical projection system.[470] The drug selectively depresses neuronal function in parts of the cortex (especially association areas) and thalamus while simultaneously stimulating parts of the limbic system, including the hippocampus. This process creates what is termed functional disorganization[459] of nonspecific pathways in the midbrain and thalamic areas.[471,472] There is also evidence that ketamine depresses the transmission of impulses in the medial medullary reticular formation, which is important for transmission of the affective-emotional components of nociception from the spinal cord to higher brain centers.[473] Blockade of CNS sodium channels has been shown to not be the mechanism of action by which ketamine produces anesthesia.[474] Some evidence indicates that ketamine occupies opiate receptors in the brain and spinal cord, and this property could account for some of the analgesic effects.[285,444,475,476] The S-(+)-enantiomer has been shown to have some opioid µ-receptor activity, which accounts for part of its analgesic effect.[477] NMDA receptor interaction may mediate the general anesthetic effects as well as some analgesic actions of ketamine.[478-480] The spinal cord analgesic effect of ketamine is postulated to be due to inhibition of dorsal horn, wide–dynamic range neuronal activity.[481] Although some drugs have been used to antagonize ketamine, no specific receptor antagonist is yet known that reverses all the CNS effects of ketamine.

Ketamine increases cerebral metabolism, CBF, and ICP. Because of its excitatory CNS effects, which can be detected by generalized EEG development of theta-wave activity,[463] as well as by petit mal seizure–like activity in the hippocampus,[482] ketamine increases $CMRO_2$. Whereas theta-wave activity signals the analgesic activity of ketamine, alpha waves indicate its absence. There is an increase in CBF that appears to be higher than the increase in $CMRO_2$ would mandate. With the increase in CBF as well as the generalized increase in sympathetic nervous system response, there is an increase in ICP after ketamine administration.[483,484] The increase in $CMRO_2$ and CBF can be blocked by the use of thiopental[485] or diazepam.[484,486] Cerebrovascular responsiveness to carbon dioxide appears to be preserved with ketamine; therefore, reducing $Paco_2$ attenuates the rise in ICP after ketamine.[484]

Ketamine has also been shown in animal model of incomplete cerebral ischemia and reperfusion to reduce necrosis and improve neurologic outcome.[487] Decreased sympathetic tone and inhibition of NMDA receptor–mediated ion currents were believed to mediate the reduction in necrotic cell death. Recently, S-(+)-ketamine has been shown to influence the expression of apoptosis-regulating proteins in rat brains 4 hours after cerebral ischemia/reperfusion.[488] Thus, the neuroprotection observed with ketamine may involve antiapoptotic mechanisms in addition to reducing necrotic cell death.

Ketamine, like other phencyclidines, produces undesirable psychological reactions during awakening from anesthesia that are termed *emergence reactions*. Common manifestations of these reactions, which vary in severity and classification, are vivid dreaming, extracorporeal experiences (sense of floating out of one's body), and illusions (misinterpretation of a real, external sensory experience).[489] These incidents of dreaming and illusion are often associated with excitement, confusion, euphoria, and fear.[285] They occur in the first hour of emergence and usually abate within 1 to several hours. It has been postulated that psychic emergence reactions occur secondary to ketamine-induced depression of auditory and visual relay nuclei and thus lead to misperception or misinterpretation (or both) of auditory and visual stimuli.[444] Their incidence ranges from as low as 3% to 5%[285,444] to as high as 100%.[489] A clinically relevant range is probably 10% to 30% of adult patients who receive ketamine as a sole or major part of the anesthetic technique.

Factors that affect the incidence of emergence reactions are age,[490] dose,[285] gender,[491] psychological susceptibility,[492] and concurrent drugs. Playing music during anesthesia does not attenuate the incidence of psychotomimetic reactions.[493] Pediatric patients do not report as high an incidence of unpleasant emergence reactions as adult patients do, nor do men as compared with women. Larger doses and rapid administration of large doses seem to predispose patients to a higher incidence of adverse effects.[494,495] Finally, certain personality types seem to be prone to the development of emergence reactions. Patients who score high in psychoticism on the Eysenck Personality Inventory have a propensity for the development of emergence reactions,[492] and people who commonly dream at home are more likely to have postoperative dreams in the hospital after ketamine.[494] Numerous drugs have been used to reduce the incidence and severity of postoperative reactions to ketamine,[285,444,496] and the benzodiazepines seem to be the most effective group of drugs to attenuate or treat ketamine emergence reactions. Midazolam,[444] lorazepam,[497] and diazepam[498] are useful in reducing reactions to ketamine. The mechanism is not known, but it is probable that both the sedative and amnesic actions of the benzodiazepines make them superior to other sedative-hypnotics. Midazolam has also been shown to reduce the psychotomimetic effect of the S-(+)-enantiomer.[499]

Effects on the Respiratory System

Ketamine has minimal effect on the central respiratory drive as reflected by an unaltered response to carbon dioxide.[500] A transient (1- to 3-minute) decrease in minute ventilation can occur after the bolus administration of an induction dose of ketamine (2 mg/kg IV).[463,501,502] Unusually high doses can produce apnea,[503] but this effect is seldom seen. Arterial blood gas values are generally preserved when ketamine is used alone for anesthesia or analgesia. However, with the use of adjuvant sedatives or anesthetic drugs, respiratory depression can develop. Ketamine has been shown to affect ventilatory control in children and should be considered a possible respiratory depressant when the drug is given to them in bolus doses.[504,505]

Ketamine is a bronchial smooth muscle relaxant. When given to patients with reactive airway disease and bronchospasm, pulmonary compliance is improved.[506,507] Ketamine is as effective as halothane or enflurane in preventing experimentally induced bronchospasm.[508] The mechanism for this effect is probably a result of the sympathomimetic response to ketamine, but isolated bronchial smooth muscle studies have shown that ketamine can directly antagonize the spasmogenic effects of carbachol and histamine.[509] Because of its bronchodilating effect, ketamine has been used to treat status asthmaticus unresponsive to conventional therapy.[510]

A potential respiratory problem, especially in children, is the increased salivation that follows ketamine administration (also see Chapter 60). Such salivation can produce upper airway obstruction, which can be further complicated by laryngospasm. The increased secretions may also contribute to or may further complicate laryngospasm. In addition, although the swallow, cough, sneeze, and gag reflexes are relatively intact after ketamine administration, there is evidence that silent aspiration can occur during ketamine anesthesia.[457]

Effects on the Cardiovascular System

Ketamine also has unique cardiovascular effects; it stimulates the cardiovascular system and is usually associated with increases in blood pressure, heart rate, and cardiac output (see Table 10-2). Other anesthetic induction drugs either cause no change in hemodynamic variables or produce vasodilation with cardiac depression. The S-(+)-enantiomer, despite hope that reducing the dose by half (equi-anesthetic potency) would attenuate its side effects, is equivalent to the racemic mixture regarding hemodynamic response.[499] The increase in hemodynamic variables is associated with increased work and myocardial oxygen consumption. A healthy heart is able to increase oxygen supply by increasing cardiac output and decreasing coronary vascular resistance so that coronary blood flow is appropriate for the increased oxygen consumption.[511] The hemodynamic changes are not related to the dose of ketamine (i.e., there is no hemodynamic difference between the administration of 0.5 and 1.5 mg/kg IV).[512] It is also interesting that a second dose of ketamine produces hemodynamic effects less than or even opposite those of the first dose.[513] The hemodynamic changes after induction of anesthesia with ketamine tend to be the same in healthy patients and those with a variety of acquired or congenital heart diseases.[502,512,514-516] Patients with congenital heart disease do not have any significant changes in shunt direction or fraction[517] or in systemic oxygenation after ketamine induction of anesthesia.[518]

In patients who have elevated pulmonary artery pressure (as with mitral valvular and some congenital lesions), ketamine seems to cause a more pronounced increase in pulmonary than systemic vascular resistance.[516,517,519,520]

The mechanism by which ketamine stimulates the circulatory system remains enigmatic. It does not appear to be a peripheral mechanism such as baroreflex inhibition,[521,522] but rather seems to be central.[523-525] Some evidence indicates that ketamine attenuates baroreceptor function through an effect on NMDA receptors in the nucleus tractus solitarius.[526] Ketamine injected directly into the CNS produces an immediate sympathetic nervous system hemodynamic response.[527] Ketamine also causes the sympathoneuronal release of norepinephrine, which can be detected in venous blood.[528] Blockade of this effect is possible with barbiturates, benzodiazepines, and droperidol.[525,527-529] Ketamine in vitro probably has negative inotropic effects. Myocardial depression has been demonstrated in isolated rabbit hearts,[530] intact dogs,[531] chronically instrumented dogs,[532] and isolated canine heart preparations.[533] However, in isolated guinea pig hearts, ketamine was the least depressant of all the major induction drugs.[534] The finding that ketamine may exert its myocardial effects by acting on myocardial ionic currents (which may exert different effects from species to species or in diverse tissue types) may explain the tissue and animal model variance in direct myocardial action.[535]

The centrally mediated sympathetic responses to ketamine usually override the direct depressant effects of ketamine. Some peripheral nervous system actions of ketamine play an undetermined role in the hemodynamic effects of the drug. Ketamine inhibits intraneuronal uptake of catecholamines in a cocaine-like effect,[536,537] as well as extraneuronal norepinephrine uptake.[538,539]

Stimulation of the cardiovascular system is not always desirable, and certain pharmacologic methods have been used to block ketamine-induced tachycardia and systemic hypertension. Successful methods include the use of adrenergic antagonists (both α and β), as well as a variety of vasodilators[540] and clonidine.[541] However, probably the most fruitful approach has been the administration of benzodiazepines. Modest doses of diazepam, flunitrazepam, and midazolam all attenuate the hemodynamic effects of ketamine. It is also possible to lessen the tachycardia and hypertension caused by ketamine by using a continuous infusion technique with or without a benzodiazepine.[542] Other general anesthetics, particularly the inhaled anesthetics,[543] blunt the hemodynamic effect of ketamine. Ketamine can produce hemodynamic depression in the setting of deep anesthesia when sympathetic responses do not accompany its administration.

Uses

The many unique features of ketamine pharmacology, especially its propensity to produce unwanted emergence reactions, have placed ketamine outside the realm of routine clinical use. Nevertheless, ketamine has an important niche in the practice of anesthesiology when its unique sympathomimetic activity and bronchodilating capability are indicated during induction of anesthesia. It is used for premedication, sedation, induction, and maintenance

Table 10–11 Uses and doses of ketamine

Induction of General Anesthesia*
0.5-2 mg/kg IV
4-6 mg/kg IM
Maintenance of General Anesthesia
0.5-1 mg/kg IV prn with 50% N$_2$O in O$_2$
15-45 µg/kg/min IV with 50%-70% N$_2$O in O$_2$
30-90 µg/kg/min IV without N$_2$O
Sedation and Analgesia
0.2-0.8 mg/kg IV over 2-3 min
2-4 mg/kg IM
Preemptive/Preventive Analgesia
0.15-0.25 mg/kg IV

*Lower doses are used if adjuvant drugs such as midazolam or thiopental are also given.

of general anesthesia (see Table 10-11). There has been increased interest in the routine use of ketamine in small doses (10 to 20 mg) for preventive analgesia and to possibly prevent opiate tolerance and hyperalgesia.

Induction and Maintenance of Anesthesia

Poor-risk patients (ASA class IV) with respiratory and cardiovascular system disorders (excluding ischemic heart disease) represent the majority of candidates for ketamine induction; such induction is particularly appropriate for patients with bronchospastic airway disease or those with hemodynamic compromise based on either hypovolemia or cardiomyopathy (not coronary artery disease). The bronchodilation and profound analgesia that allow the use of high oxygen concentrations make ketamine an excellent choice for induction in patients with reactive airway disease. Otherwise healthy trauma victims whose blood loss is extensive are also candidates for rapid-sequence induction with ketamine.[544] Patients in septic shock may also benefit from ketamine.[545] However, ketamine's intrinsic myocardial depressant effect may become manifested in this situation if trauma or sepsis has caused depletion of catecholamine stores before the patient's arrival in the operating room. The use of ketamine in these patients does not obviate the need for appropriate preoperative preparation, including restoration of blood volume. Other cardiac diseases that can be well managed with ketamine anesthesia are cardiac tamponade and restrictive pericarditis.[546] The finding that ketamine preserves the heart rate and right atrial pressure through its sympathetic stimulating effects makes it an excellent anesthetic induction and maintenance drug in this setting. Ketamine is also often used in patients with congenital heart disease, especially those with a propensity for right-to-left shunting. In addition, the use of ketamine has been reported in a patient susceptible to malignant hyperthermia who had a large anterior mediastinal mass[547] when spontaneous ventilation was required and inhaled anesthetics were contraindicated.[547-549]

Ketamine combined with diazepam or midazolam can be given by continuous infusion to produce satisfactory cardiac anesthesia in patients with valvular and ischemic heart disease. The combination of a benzodiazepine[542] or a benzodiazepine plus sufentanil[550] with ketamine attenuates or eliminates the unwanted tachycardia and hypertension, as well as postoperative psychological derangements. This technique produces minimal hemodynamic perturbations, profound analgesia, dependable amnesia, and an uneventful convalescence. No comparison of this technique with a continuous benzodiazepine-opioid technique has been made.

In patients with known depression, small doses of ketamine administered on induction significantly improved the postoperative depressive state when compared with matched controls.[551]

Low-dose ketamine has been used as an analgesic after thoracic surgery[552]; its lack of respiratory depressant properties and its pain relief equivalent to that of meperidine make it a third choice when one wishes to avoid narcotics because of their respiratory depressant effects and has reason to also avoid nonsteroidal agents such as ketorolac. Additional analgesic use can be considered in asthmatic patients.[553] Ketamine administered in small doses of 10 to 20 mg preoperatively decreases postoperative analgesic consumption. Patients given up to three doses of 0.25 mg/kg ketamine combined with 0.15 mg/kg morphine, or only 0.3 mg/kg morphine, had better visual analog pain scores, were more alert, and experienced less nausea and vomiting.[554] Ketamine administered in a one-to-one combination with morphine and the use of an 8-minute lockout interval provided optimal postoperative analgesia for this combination.[555] Epidural/caudal administration of ketamine (0.5 to 1 mg/kg) is increasingly being reported. Although the efficacy of these doses of ketamine seems to be established, the safety of this technique has not yet received regulatory approval. The preservative in the racemic mixture is potentially neurotoxic, but studies to date indicate that preservative-free S-(+)-ketamine may be safe.[556]

Sedation

Ketamine is particularly suited for the sedation of pediatric patients undergoing procedures away from the operating room. Pediatric patients have fewer adverse emergence reactions[490] than adults do, and this feature makes the use of ketamine in pediatrics more versatile. Ketamine is used for sedation or general anesthesia, or for both, for the following pediatric procedures: cardiac catheterization, radiation therapy, radiologic studies, dressing changes,[557] and dental work.[464] Caution is advised in the use of ketamine for cardiac catheterization in pediatric patients with elevated pulmonary vascular resistance because such resistance can be increased by ketamine.[558]

Ketamine is often used repeatedly in the same patient. Unfortunately, the literature does not provide information on how many times ketamine anesthesia can safely be administered to one individual, whether the frequency of administration is related to tolerance after multiple administrations, and whether frequent/long-term use can produce detrimental effects.

Generally, a subanesthetic dose (≤1.0 mg/kg IV) is used for dressing changes; this dose gives adequate operating conditions but a rapid return to normal function, including the resumption of eating, which is important in maintaining proper nutrition in burn patients.[285,444]

Often, ketamine is combined with premedication consisting of a barbiturate or a benzodiazepine and an antisialagogue (e.g., glycopyrrolate) to facilitate management. Premedication reduces the dose requirement for ketamine, and the antisialagogue reduces the sometimes troublesome salivation.

In adults and children, ketamine can be used as a supplement or an adjunct to regional anesthesia to extend the usefulness of the primary (local anesthetic) form of anesthesia. In this setting, ketamine can be used before the application of painful blocks,[559] but more commonly it is used for sedation or supplemental anesthesia during long or uncomfortable procedures. When used for supplementation of regional anesthesia, ketamine (0.5 mg/kg IV) combined with diazepam (0.15 mg/kg IV) is better accepted by patients and is not associated with more side effects than in unsedated patients.[560] Ketamine in small doses can also be combined with nitrous oxide and propofol for supplementation of conduction or local anesthesia. These techniques of ketamine administration are used in outpatient and inpatient settings, and although patients are comfortable and cooperative, dreams and other unpleasant emergence reactions can occur.[444] In outpatients, premedication with midazolam, concurrent propofol infusion, and intermittent ketamine (for analgesia) in doses less than 3 mg/kg are recommended.[561]

Doses and Routes of Administration

Ketamine has been administered intravenously, intramuscularly, orally, nasally, rectally, and as a preservative-free solution epidurally.[562] Most clinical use involves the intravenous and intramuscular routes, by which the drug rapidly achieves therapeutic levels. The dose depends on the desired therapeutic effect and the route of administration. Table 10-11 contains the general recommended doses for intravenous and intramuscular administration of ketamine for various therapeutic goals.[444] Because of their side effects, most anesthetic drugs require that the dosage be reduced in elderly and seriously ill patients; such a recommendation is probably prudent with ketamine, although data supporting this recommendation are not available. Patients who have been critically ill for a prolonged period may have exhausted their catecholamine stores and may be subject to the circulatory depressant effects of ketamine.[563] Ketamine can be given epidurally and intrathecally for operative and postoperative pain control. An intrathecal dose of 1 mg ketamine combined with 0.15 to 0.2 mg of intrathecal morphine provided effective cancer pain relief compared with 0.4 mg of intrathecal morphine alone. S-(+)-ketamine (0.5 mg/kg) has also been combined with bupivacaine to enhance the duration of analgesia.[565] The peak action after intravenous administration occurs in 30 to 60 seconds. Onset occurs in about 5 minutes, with peak effect occurring approximately 20 minutes after intramuscular administration. An oral dose of 3 to 10 mg/kg generates a sedative effect in 20 to 45 minutes. Continuous infusion of intravenous ketamine with or without concomitant drugs is a satisfactory method to keep blood levels in the therapeutic range (see also Chapter 12). The concomitant use of drugs such as benzodiazepines permits a lower

dose requirement for ketamine while enhancing recovery by reducing emergence reactions. The interaction of ketamine with propofol is strictly additive and not synergistic; thus, the dose of each would be reduced by about half when used together for induction.[566]

For sedation, ketamine may be given intramuscularly if the patient wishes to avoid awareness of intravenous catheter placement. It has also been administered orally in doses of 3 to 10 mg/kg, with 6 mg/kg providing optimal conditions in 20 to 25 minutes in one study and 10 mg/kg providing sedation in 87% of children within 45 minutes in another study.[567,568] In at least one case, deep sleep was produced by a supposedly sedative oral dose.[569]

Side Effects and Contraindications

The common psychological emergence reactions were discussed earlier. Contraindications to ketamine relate to specific pharmacologic actions and patient diseases. Patients with increased ICP and with intracranial mass lesions should not receive ketamine because it can increase ICP and has been reported to cause apnea on this basis.[570] The S-(+)-enantiomer also increases CBF and is probably similarly contraindicated.[571] Additionally, ketamine is contraindicated in patients with an open eye injury or other ophthalmologic disorder, in whom a ketamine-induced increase in intraocular pressure would be detrimental. Because ketamine has a propensity to cause hypertension and tachycardia with a commensurate increase in myocardial oxygen consumption, it is contraindicated as the sole anesthetic in patients with ischemic heart disease.[515] Likewise, it is unwise to give ketamine to patients with vascular aneurysms because of the possible sudden change in arterial pressure. Psychiatric disease such as schizophrenia or a history of adverse reactions to ketamine or one of its congeners also constitutes a contraindication.[285] In addition, one should be cautious in using ketamine when there is a possibility of postoperative delirium from other causes (e.g., delirium tremens, possibility of head trauma) and a ketamine-induced psychomimetic effect would cloud the differential diagnosis.

Other side effects include potentiation of nondepolarizing neuromuscular blockade by an undefined mechanism.[572,573] Finally, because ketamine's preservative, chlorobutanol, has been demonstrated to be neurotoxic, subarachnoid administration is contraindicated.[573] It is probably unwise to administer the drug epidurally for this reason. S-(+)-ketamine is available in a preservative-free solution. The Food and Drug Administration has not approved the use of intrathecal or epidural ketamine.

ETOMIDATE

History

Etomidate (Amidate, Hypnomidate) was synthesized[574] in 1964 and was introduced into clinical practice[575] in 1972. Its properties include hemodynamic stability, minimal respiratory depression, cerebral protection, and pharmacokinetics enabling rapid recovery after either a single dose or a continuous infusion. In animals, etomidate also provides a wider margin of safety (median effective dose/median lethal dose [ED_{50}/LD_{50}]) than thiopental does (26.4 versus 4.6).[576] These beneficial properties led to the widespread use of etomidate for induction, for maintenance of anesthesia, and for prolonged sedation in critically ill patients. Anesthesiologists' enthusiasm for etomidate, however, was tempered by reports that the drug can cause temporary inhibition of steroid synthesis after both single doses and infusions.[338,577,578] This effect, combined with other minor disadvantages (e.g., pain on injection, superficial thrombophlebitis, myoclonus, and a relatively high incidence of nausea and vomiting) led to several editorials[579-581] questioning the role of etomidate in modern anesthetic practice. Use of the drug waned significantly after these editorials, but it has expanded because of rediscovery of etomidate's beneficial physiologic profile combined with a lack of any new reports describing clinically significant adrenocortical suppression after an induction dose or brief infusion.

Physicochemical Characteristics

Etomidate is an imidazole derivative (R-(+)-pentylethyl-1H-imidazole-5 carboxylate sulfate).[576] Its chemical structure is illustrated in Figure 10-22. Etomidate exists as two isomers, but only the (+) isomer is active as a hypnotic.[582] Its molecular weight is 342.36 kd.[582] Etomidate is water insoluble and is unstable in a neutral solution. It therefore has been formulated with several solvents.[583] In the United States it is supplied as a 2-mg/mL propylene glycol (35% by volume) solution with a pH of 6.9 and an osmolality of 4640 mOsm/L. In Europe, a new formulation in a lipid emulsion has been introduced in an attempt to reduce some of the side effects of etomidate.[584] Unlike sodium thiopental, when etomidate is mixed with other commonly used anesthetic agents such as neuromuscular blockers, vasoactive drugs, or lidocaine, it does not cause precipitation.[585]

Metabolism, Induction, and Maintenance of Anesthesia

Etomidate is metabolized in the liver primarily by ester hydrolysis to the corresponding carboxylic acid of etomidate (major metabolite) or by N-dealkylation.[582] The main metabolite is inactive.[585] Only 2% of the drug is excreted unchanged, the rest being excreted as metabolites by the kidney (85%) and in bile (13%).[585]

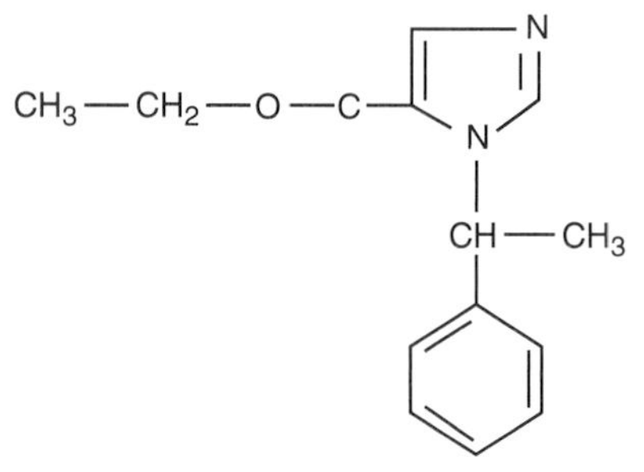

Figure 10–22 Structure of etomidate, an imidazole derivative.

Table 10–12 Uses and doses of etomidate

Induction of general anesthesia	0.2-0.6 mg/kg IV
Maintenance of general anesthesia	10 µg/kg/min IV with N_2O and an opiate
Sedation	5-10 µg/kg/min IV. Prolonged periods of sedation are contraindicated because of inhibition of corticosteroid synthesis

Etomidate has been used for both induction and maintenance of anesthesia (Table 10-12). The induction dose of etomidate varies from 0.2 to 0.6 mg/kg,[575,583,586,587] and it is reduced by premedication with an opiate, a benzodiazepine, or a barbiturate.[575] The onset of anesthesia after a routine induction dose of 0.3 mg/kg etomidate is rapid (one arm–brain circulation) and equivalent to that obtained with an induction dose of thiopental or methohexital.[575,583,588] The duration of anesthesia after a single induction dose is linearly related to the dose—each 0.1 mg/kg administered provides about 100 seconds of loss of consciousness.[589] Repeat doses of etomidate, either by bolus or infusion, prolong the duration of hypnosis. Recovery after multiple doses or an infusion of etomidate is still usually rapid.[575,586,590-594] The addition of small doses of fentanyl with etomidate for short surgical procedures reduces the required dose of etomidate and allows earlier awakening. In children, induction by rectal administration of etomidate has been achieved with 6.5 mg/kg. Hypnosis occurs in 4 minutes. At this dose the drug's hemodynamics is unaltered, and recovery is still rapid.[595]

Various infusion schemes have been devised to use etomidate as a maintenance agent for the hypnotic component of anesthesia (see Chapter 12). Most regimens aim to achieve a plasma level of 300 to 500 ng/mL, which is the concentration necessary for hypnosis.[24,25,596,597] Both two- and three-stage infusions have been used successfully. These regimens consist of an initial rapid infusion of 100 µg/kg/min for 10 minutes followed by 10 µg/kg/min thereafter[597] or 100 µg/kg/min for 3 minutes, 20 µg/kg/min for 27 minutes, and 10 µg/kg/min thereafter.[24] Loss of consciousness with these techniques occurs after 100 to 120 seconds.[24] The infusion is usually terminated 10 minutes before the desired awakening time.[24]

Pharmacokinetics

The pharmacokinetics of etomidate has been calculated after single bolus doses and after continuous infusion (see Table 10-1).[24-27,598] The time course of plasma disappearance after a 0.3-mg/kg bolus is shown in Figure 10-23. The kinetics of etomidate is best described by an open three-compartment model.[26,27,598] The drug has an initial distribution half-life of 2.7 minutes, a redistribution half-life of 29 minutes,[27,598] and an elimination half-life that varies from 2.9 to 5.3 hours.[24-27,598] Clearance of etomidate by the liver is high (18 to 25 mL/kg/min), with a hepatic extraction ratio of 0.5 ± 0.9.[24,26,27,583,598] Thus, drugs affecting hepatic blood flow alter its elimination

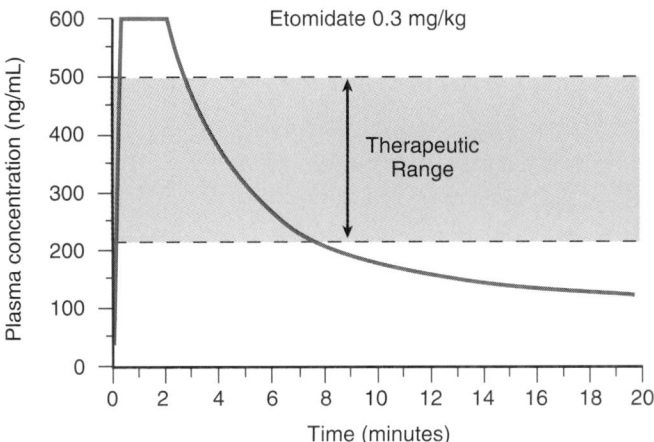

Figure 10–23 Simulated time course of plasma levels of etomidate after an induction dose of 0.3 mg/kg. Plasma levels required for hypnosis during surgery are 300 to 500 ng/mL, with awakening usually occurring at levels lower than 225 ng/mL.

half-life. Because redistribution is the mechanism whereby the effect of a bolus of etomidate is dissipated, hepatic dysfunction should not appreciably alter recovery from its hypnotic effect. The volume of distribution at steady state is 2.5 to 4.5 L/kg.[24-27,598] Etomidate is 75% protein bound.[599] Pathologic conditions that alter serum proteins (e.g., hepatic or renal disease) vary the amount of the free (unbound) fraction and may cause a given dose to have an exaggerated pharmacodynamic effect.[599] A hemorrhagic shock model in pigs bled to a mean pressure of 50 mm Hg did not alter etomidate's pharmacokinetics or pharmacodynamics.[600] This finding contrasts with the marked changes seen in this same model with other intravenous anesthetics.

In patients with cirrhosis, the volume of distribution is doubled, but clearance is normal; the result is an elimination half-life that is twice normal.[601] It is likely that the initial distribution half-life and clinical effect are unchanged. Increasing age is associated with a smaller initial volume of distribution and decreased clearance of etomidate.[602] The relatively short elimination half-life and the rapid clearance of etomidate make it suitable for administration in a single dose, in multiple doses, or in a continuous infusion.

Pharmacology

Effects on the Central Nervous System

The primary action of etomidate on the CNS is hypnosis, which is achieved in one arm–brain circulation after a normal induction dose (0.3 mg/kg).[583,603] Etomidate has no analgesic activity. Plasma levels required during the maintenance of anesthesia are approximately 300 to 500 ng/mL, those required for sedation are 150 to 300 ng/mL, and those for awakening are 150 to 250 ng/mL (see Fig. 10-23).[24,25,597,603] The mechanism by which etomidate produces hypnosis is not fully elucidated; however, it appears to be largely (but not solely) related to the GABA-adrenergic system. Its action may be antagonized by GABA antagonists.[604] In general, the mechanism of action of etomidate appears to be very similar to that established

thus far for propofol (see earlier).[605] For etomidate it appears that the β_2- and β_3-subunits are more important for its hypnotic action than the $GABA_A$ α_1-subunit.[64,606]

At a dose of 0.2 to 0.3 mg/kg, etomidate reduces CBF (by 34%) and $CMRO_2$ (by 45%) without altering mean arterial pressure.[607] Thus, cerebral perfusion pressure is maintained or increased, and there is a beneficial net increase in the cerebral oxygen supply-demand ratio.[607] When given in doses sufficient to produce EEG burst suppression, etomidate acutely lowers ICP by up to 50% in patients with already increased ICP, and ICP returns to almost normal values.[608,609] The decrease in ICP is maintained in the period immediately after intubation (also see Chapter 21).[609] To maintain the effects of etomidate on ICP, high infusion rates (60 µg/kg/min) are necessary.[610] In contrast to the situation with other neuroprotective agents such as thiopental, reduction of ICP and maintenance of burst suppression are not associated with a drop in mean arterial blood pressure.[609] Because cerebral vascular reactivity is still maintained after etomidate administration,[610] hyperventilation may theoretically further reduce ICP when used in conjunction with etomidate. In animals, etomidate has reduced brain disease after an acute cortical ischemic insult.[611] In 1993, Takanobu and coauthors[612] reported the neuroprotective qualities of etomidate to be equal to those of thiopental and superior to those of isoflurane in a rat model. Other investigators disagree on etomidate's neuroprotective qualities.[590] Deeper structures such as the brainstem may not be afforded ischemic protection by etomidate.[613]

A dose of 0.3 mg/kg rapidly reduces intraocular pressure by 30% to 60%.[614] The decrease in intraocular pressure after a single dose lasts 5 minutes, but the reduction may be maintained by an infusion of 20 µg/kg/min (see Chapter 65).[615]

Etomidate produces changes in the EEG similar to those produced by the barbiturates.[616] There is an initial increase in alpha-wave amplitude with sharp beta bursts followed by mixed delta-theta waves, with delta-wave activity predominating before the onset of periodic burst suppression.[616] The absence of beta waves in the initial phase of induction with etomidate is the major difference in the EEG changes induced by thiopental.[616] Etomidate has been associated with grand mal seizures[617,618] and has been shown to produce increased EEG activity in epileptogenic foci. This feature has proved useful for intraoperative mapping of seizure foci before surgical ablation.[618,619] Etomidate is also associated with a high incidence of myoclonic movement.[586,591] Myoclonus is not thought to be associated with seizure-like EEG activity.[616] Giving etomidate to unpremedicated patients caused an increase in EEG activity in 22% of patients versus 17% of those receiving thiopental.[620] The myoclonic movement is believed to result from activity either in the brainstem or in deep cerebral structures.[575]

The effect of etomidate on auditory evoked potentials is similar to that produced by the inhaled anesthetics, with a dose-dependent increase in latency and a decreasing amplitude of the early cortical components (Pa and Nb).[621] The amplitude and latency of upper limb cortical somatosensory evoked potentials are positively affected after 0.4 mg/kg etomidate, which could theoretically obscure neurologic injury during positioning immediately after induction of anesthesia.[622] Brainstem evoked responses are unaltered after etomidate administration.[621] Because the depression in amplitude is less, etomidate may be superior to propofol as an induction agent when monitoring of motor evoked responses to transcranial stimulation is indicated.[623]

Effects on the Respiratory System

Etomidate has minimal effect on ventilation. It does not induce histamine release in either healthy patients or those with reactive airway disease.[624] The ventilatory response to carbon dioxide is depressed by etomidate, but the ventilatory drive at any given carbon dioxide tension is greater than that after an equipotent dose of methohexital.[350] Similarly, the response to occlusion pressure is less depressed after etomidate than after an equivalent dose of methohexital.[625] Induction with etomidate produces a brief period of hyperventilation,[177,626] sometimes followed by a similarly brief period of apnea,[626] which results in a slight ($\approx$15%) increase in $Paco_2$ but no change in Pao_2.[177,178] The incidence of apnea is altered by premedication.[592,627] Hiccups or coughing may accompany etomidate induction, and the incidence is similar to that after methohexital induction.[583]

In laboratory models, etomidate appears to be as effective as propofol in relaxing precontracted tracheal rings, but less effective than propofol in preventing tracheal ring contraction by muscarinic agonists.[628]

Etomidate attenuates the vasorelaxant responses of the pulmonary artery to acetylcholine and bradykinin by inhibiting both nitric oxide– and EDHF-mediated components, probably by inhibiting the endothelial $[Ca^{2+}]_i$ transient in response to receptor activation. These actions on pulmonary vascular tone are similar to those observed with ketamine and propofol.[629]

Effects on the Cardiovascular System

The minimal effect of etomidate on cardiovascular function sets it apart from other rapid-onset induction agents (see Table 10-2).[177-180,627,630] An induction dose of 0.3 mg/kg of etomidate given to cardiac patients for noncardiac surgery results in almost no change in heart rate, mean arterial pressure, mean pulmonary artery pressure, pulmonary capillary wedge pressure, central venous pressure, stroke volume, cardiac index, and pulmonary and systemic vascular resistance.[178] A relatively large dose of etomidate, 0.45 mg/kg (which is 50% larger than a normal induction dose),[627] also produces minimal changes in cardiovascular parameters. In patients with ischemic heart disease or valvular disease,[178,630] etomidate (0.3 mg/kg) produces similar minimal alterations in cardiovascular parameters. In patients with mitral or aortic valve disease, etomidate may produce greater changes in mean arterial pressure (an approximate 20% decrease)[177,631] than in patients without cardiac valvular disease. In isolated strips of myocardial muscle taken from failing and nonfailing hearts, etomidate exerts a dose-dependent negative inotropic effect that is reversible by β-adrenergic stimulation. With clinically therapeutic concentrations of etomidate, the negative inotropic effects noted were minimal and probably of no clinical significance.[632] After induction (18 mg) and

infusion (2.4 mg/min), etomidate produces a 50% decrease in myocardial blood flow and oxygen consumption and a 20% to 30% increase in coronary sinus blood oxygen saturation.[162] The myocardial oxygen supply-demand ratio is thus well maintained.[162,180] It has minimal effect on the QT interval.[633]

The hemodynamic stability seen with etomidate may be due in part to its unique lack of effect on both the sympathetic nervous system and baroreceptor function.[198] However, etomidate, which lacks analgesic efficacy, may not totally ablate the sympathetic response to laryngoscopy and intubation.[588,591] For the least hemodynamic perturbation through the induction/intubation sequence, a low dose (1.5 to 5.0 µg/kg) of fentanyl is often combined with etomidate.[631,634]

In a small study of 30 patients undergoing vascular procedures, etomidate (versus thiopental) resulted in inhibition of platelet function (increased bleeding time and inhibition of adenosine diphosphate and collagen-induced platelet aggregation) with increased blood loss.[635]

Endocrine Effects

The concern surrounding the endocrine effects of etomidate stems from a letter by Ledingham and colleagues[636] in 1983 concerning ICU patients receiving long-term sedative infusions of etomidate while being mechanically ventilated for 5 days or longer. These investigators noted that in this subset of mechanically ventilated, multiple-trauma patients, the mortality rate was higher for 1981 to 1982 than in similar patients treated during 1979 to 1980. The earlier group had received primarily morphine and benzodiazepines for sedation, whereas patients in 1981 to 1982 had received primarily etomidate for sedation. It was postulated that adrenocortical suppression secondary to long-term etomidate infusion was the cause of the increased mortality.[577] Another ICU with similar patients receiving etomidate did not note increased mortality; these patients received high-dose steroids as part of the trauma protocol.[636] This finding helped confirm that hypothesis.

The specific endocrine effects manifested by etomidate are a dose-dependent reversible inhibition of the enzyme 11β-hydroxylase, which converts 11-deoxycortisol to cortisol, and a relatively minor effect on 17α-hydroxylase (Fig. 10-24).[637,638] These effects result in an increase in the cortisol precursors 11-deoxycortisol and 17-hydroxyprogesterone, as well as an increase in ACTH. The blockade of 11β-hydroxylase and, to a lesser extent, 17α-hydroxylase[637] appears to be related to the free imidazole radical of etomidate-binding cytochrome P450.[638-640] Such blockade results in inhibition of ascorbic acid resynthesis, which is required for steroid production in humans.[639,640] Blockade of the cytochrome P450–dependent enzyme 11β-hydroxylase also results in decreased mineralocorticoid production and an increase in intermediaries (11-deoxycorticosterone).[338,578,580] Vitamin C supplementation restores cortisol levels to normal after the use of etomidate.[640] Because minor adrenocortical suppressive effects were shown to follow even single bolus doses,[578,637,641] concern about the use of etomidate for induction of anesthesia arose.[579] No large prospective studies have been conducted, but several smaller studies

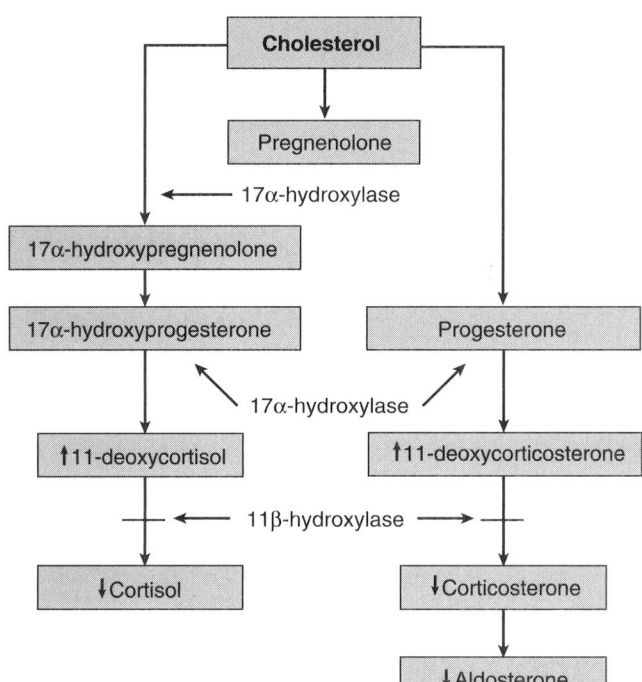

Figure 10–24 Pathway for the biosynthesis of cortisol and aldosterone. The sites at which etomidate affects cortisol-aldosterone synthesis by its action on 11β-hydroxylase (major site) and 17α-hydroxylase (minor site) are illustrated.

have provided some insight into the exact nature of adrenocortical suppression after an induction dose.

Duthie and associates[642] demonstrated that in otherwise healthy patients undergoing minor peripheral surgery, plasma cortisol levels were slightly depressed from preinduction levels for up to 1 hour postoperatively. The nadir of mean cortisol levels did not fall out of the normal range. 11-Deoxycorticosterone, substrate for the etomidate-inhibited 11β-hydroxylase, peaked at very high levels when compared with the thiopental control group.[642] In another study, orthopedic surgical patients underwent etomidate induction followed by an infusion of etomidate (average total dose, 68 mg). Temporary adrenocortical suppression, as measured by a reduced response to ACTH stimulation, was documented for 6 hours postoperatively and returned to normal by 20 hours postoperatively. Postoperative cortisol levels in the etomidate study patients were not significantly different from those in a group that received midazolam induction. As in the study of Duthie and coworkers,[642] mean cortisol levels in the etomidate group remained in the normal range at all times postoperatively.[643] Other studies have shown similar results when evaluating etomidate induction doses; none reported adverse outcomes secondary to short-term adrenocortical suppression.[338,578,637,641-644]

However, in each of the prospective etomidate studies documenting adrenocortical suppression without associated clinical sequelae, a conclusion of safety was not forthcoming. The reason was that these studies did not address high-stress procedures, in which the benefit of a high cortisol level in response to major stress could be desirable and etomidate's blockade of the response to

ACTH could be detrimental. As part of a quality assurance program, we addressed this issue with a small, retrospective analysis of etomidate induction for high-stress procedures (vascular, thoracic, major intra-abdominal, and major retroperitoneal surgery) in 1993. Indices of adrenocortical function and perioperative outcome in patients who received induction doses of etomidate were compared with those in a control group that received thiopental. The incidence of perioperative wound infection, sepsis, miscellaneous infection, myocardial infarction, and hypotension and the need for perioperative vasopressor/inotropic support were evaluated, along with postoperative serum sodium levels. No difference was found between patients receiving etomidate and those receiving other induction agents for these high-stress procedures. In 1994, cortisol levels during and after coronary artery bypass surgery were compared in patients receiving total intravenous anesthesia with etomidate/fentanyl (mean etomidate dose of 87 ± 3 mg) versus midazolam/fentanyl. Except for the first hour after induction, cortisol levels were the same or higher in the etomidate group than in the midazolam group, a finding implying that the body's ability to respond to high surgical stress was still intact despite relatively high doses of etomidate. This study is further proof that etomidate is probably safe for use in major surgery.[645]

In summary, three facts suggest that the issue of temporary adrenocortical suppression after induction doses of etomidate is not clinically significant: (1) there are no known reports of any negative clinical outcome associated with etomidate induction despite millions of uses; (2) after etomidate induction, the nadir of cortisol levels usually remains in the low-normal range, and the adrenocortical suppression is a relatively short-lived phenomenon; and (3) high-stress surgery can overcome the temporary adrenocortical suppression caused by etomidate.

Other Effects

Although etomidate provides stable hemodynamics and minimal respiratory depression, it is associated with several adverse effects when used for induction, including nausea and vomiting, pain on injection, myoclonic movement, and hiccups.[575,583,586,590-593] Etomidate has been associated with a high (30% to 40%) incidence of nausea and vomiting.[586,591-594] In contrast, an incidence of 10% to 20% is reported with methohexital[583,592] and thiopental,[591,646] but some studies have shown no difference.[587,591] More recently, etomidate in a lipid emulsion was associated with an incidence of postoperative nausea equivalent to that of propofol.[647] The addition of fentanyl to etomidate further increases the incidence of nausea and vomiting.[586,591] Nausea and vomiting are the most common reasons for patients to rate anesthesia with etomidate unsatisfactory.[593] It seems prudent to avoid etomidate in patients predisposed to nausea and vomiting.

Superficial thrombophlebitis of the vein used may occur 48 to 72 hours after etomidate injection.[648] The incidence may be as high as 20% when etomidate is given alone through a small (21-gauge) intravenous needle. Intra-arterial injection of etomidate is not associated with local or vascular disease.[575] Pain on injection, similar in incidence to that with propofol,[275] can be essentially eliminated by injecting lidocaine immediately before the injection of etomidate; as little as 20 to 40 mg may be enough.[649] Pain on injection is further reduced by using a large vein.[575,590] Less successful, but somewhat efficacious, is premedication with a benzodiazepine plus a narcotic.[591,594] The incidence of pain on injection varies from 0% to 50%. The lipid formulation of etomidate is also associated with a much lower incidence of pain on injection, thrombophlebitis, and histamine release on injection.[650]

The incidence of muscle movement (myoclonus) and hiccups is also highly variable (0% to 70%), but myoclonus is reduced by premedication with either a narcotic or a benzodiazepine.[594] Both fast and slow injection techniques have also been advocated for reducing myoclonus.[590,594]

Etomidate enhances the neuromuscular blockade of nondepolarizing neuromuscular blockers.[651,652] Hepatic function is unaltered by etomidate.[583,598] In vitro, etomidate inhibits aminolevulinic acid synthetase, but it has been administered to patients with porphyria without inducing an acute attack of porphyria.[646]

The carrier for etomidate, propylene glycol, has also been reported to have some negative effects. Some reports suggest that propylene glycol can be associated with a small degree of hemolysis.[584] Additionally, high-dose prolonged infusion has been reported to result in propylene glycol toxicity (a hyperosmolar state).[653]

Uses

The use of etomidate is most appropriate in patients with cardiovascular disease, reactive airway disease, intracranial hypertension, or any combination of disorders indicating the need for an induction agent with limited or beneficial physiologic side effects. The hemodynamic stability of etomidate is unique among the rapid-onset induction agents.

Etomidate has been primarily used in sick patients. In multiple studies, etomidate has been used for induction in patients with a compromised cardiovascular system who are undergoing coronary artery bypass surgery or valve surgery, in patients requiring induction of general anesthesia for percutaneous transluminal coronary angioplasty, and in other similar situations.[631,634,654] In cardiovascular surgery, particularly surgery for aortic aneurysms, etomidate is an excellent induction anesthetic. When etomidate is used in combination with fentanyl, titrating etomidate up to 0.6 mg/kg maintains blood pressure and heart rate in a narrow range; coronary perfusion pressure is preserved in these patients with probable coronary artery disease while the response to intubation is blunted and unnecessary stress on the aneurysm is avoided. For cardiothoracic procedures, especially cardiac and lung transplantation, the required rapid-sequence induction and hemodynamic stability make etomidate the drug of choice for induction. For patients with concomitant coronary artery disease and reactive airway disease, etomidate induction does not release histamine, and a relatively large dose (0.6 mg/kg) may be titrated to provide a deep level of anesthesia for intubation without compromising hemodynamics and coronary perfusion pressure. For cardioversion, the rapid onset, quick recovery, and maintenance of blood pressure in these sometimes hemodynamically

tenuous patients, combined with continued spontaneous respiration, make etomidate an acceptable choice,[275] although in one report, myoclonus interfered with electrocardiographic evaluation.[655] Even though definitive proof of etomidate's neuroprotective effect in humans is lacking, the combination of animal data and anecdotal reports of successful use of etomidate for neurosurgical procedures such as clipping of giant aneurysms makes etomidate a reasonable choice during neurosurgical induction.[597,609,611,656] In addition, because of its ability to reduce increased ICP, etomidate should be considered when maintenance of cerebral or coronary perfusion pressure is important. Trauma patients with questionable volume status may be well served by induction with etomidate. Although the indirect sympathomimetic effect seen with ketamine induction is absent, there is no direct myocardial depression and no confusion in the differential diagnosis of postoperative delirium. This is especially important in patients whose trauma may be related to drug or alcohol use (or both).

During an infusion, hemodynamic status is well maintained along with adequate spontaneous ventilation.[420,657] The incidence of pain on injection, myoclonus, and thrombophlebitis tends to be less with an infusion technique.[24,596,657] A concentrated form of etomidate used for continuous infusion in Europe is not available in the United States.

Short-term sedation with etomidate is useful in hemodynamically unstable patients, such as those requiring cardioversion,[275] those with acute myocardial infarction or unstable angina who require sedation for a minor operative procedure,[634] or those who require intubation in the emergency room or the ICU. In addition, etomidate has been used to produce short-term sedation for placement of a retrobulbar block and for electroconvulsive therapy, during which maintenance of spontaneous respirations and quick recovery are important features. When used during electroconvulsive therapy, etomidate can produce longer seizures than possible with other hypnotics.[658]

Prolonged sedation for patients in the ICU, though initially popular after the release of etomidate, is now contraindicated because of inhibition of corticosteroid and mineralocorticoid production and a subsequent increase in morbidity.[577,579,636]

α-ADRENERGIC AGONISTS: DEXMEDETOMIDINE

History

Adrenergic receptors were first differentiated into α and β by Ahlquist based on their responses to various amines.[659] α_2-Adrenergic agonists provide sedation, anxiolysis, and hypnosis, as well as analgesia and sympatholysis. The initial impetus for the use of α_2-agonists in anesthesia resulted from observations made in patients during anesthesia who were receiving clonidine therapy.[659-661] This was soon followed by a description of the MAC reduction of halothane by clonidine.[662] Dexmedetomidine is a far more selective α_2-agonist, with 1600-fold greater selectivity

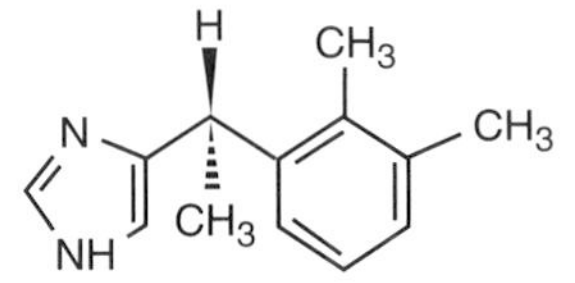

Figure 10–25 Chemical structure of dexmedetomidine.

for the α_2- than the α_1-receptor. It has recently been approved for brief sedation (<24 hours).

Physicochemical Characteristics

Medetomidine is a highly selective α_2-adrenergic agonist. Dexmedetomidine is its specific stereoisomer and is available as a parenteral formulation. Its structure is illustrated in Figure 10-25.

Metabolism and Pharmacokinetics

Dexmedetomidine is rapidly distributed and extensively metabolized in the liver and excreted in both urine and feces. It undergoes conjugation (41%), N-methylation (21%), or hydroxylation followed by conjugation. Dexmedetomidine is 94% protein bound, and its concentration ratio between whole blood and plasma is 0.66. Dexmedetomidine has profound effects on cardiovascular parameters and thus may alter its own pharmacokinetics. At high doses it causes marked vasoconstriction, which probably reduces the drug's volumes of distribution. Thus, in essence, dexmedetomidine displays nonlinear pharmacokinetics.[19] Because it is likely that this drug will be administered only within a narrow therapeutic range of 0.5 to 1.0 ng/mL, it is preferable to describe the pharmacokinetic parameters within this dosage range. Within this range, Dyck and colleagues[19] found that its pharmacokinetics in volunteers is best described by a three-compartment model (see Table 10-1). These pharmacokinetic parameters appear to be unaltered by age, weight, or renal failure, but clearance is a function of height.[19,663] The elimination half-life of dexmedetomidine is 2 to 3 hours, with a context sensitive half-time ranging from 4 minutes after a 10-minute infusion to 250 minutes after an 8-hour infusion. Postoperative patients sedated with dexmedetomidine display pharmacokinetics very similar to that seen in volunteers.[20]

Pharmacology

Effects on the Central Nervous System

α_2-Agonists produce their sedative-hypnotic effect by an action on α_2-receptors in the locus ceruleus and produce their analgesic effect by an action on α_2-receptors within the locus ceruleus and the spinal cord.[664] An interesting observation is that the quality of sedation produced by dexmedetomidine appears to be different from that produced by other sedatives acting through the GABA systems. α_2-Agonists act through the endogenous sleep-promoting pathways to exert their sedative effect. They produce a decrease in activity of the projections of the locus ceruleus to the ventrolateral preoptic nucleus. This action increases GABAergic and galanin release in the tuberomammillary

nucleus and as a result leads to a decrease in histamine release in the cortical and subcortical projections.[665] α_2-Agonists appear to inhibit ion conductance through L- or P-type calcium channels and to facilitate conductance through voltage-gated calcium-activated potassium channels.[666] α_2-Agonists have the advantage that their effects are readily reversible by α_2-adrenergic antagonists (e.g., atipamezole).[667] Like other adrenergic receptors, α_2-agonists also produce tolerance after prolonged administration.[668] However, because dexmedetomidine is approved for only short-term sedation, tolerance, dependence, or addiction does not appear to be a problem. In contrast, dexmedetomidine has been used for rapid opioid detoxification, cocaine withdrawal, and iatrogenic-induced benzodiazepine and opioid tolerance after prolonged sedation.[669] In animals, dexmedetomidine, unlike opioids, does not result in hyperalgesia or allodynia after its withdrawal.[670] Rats rendered tolerant to morphine also show a decrease in efficacy of both the hypnotic and analgesic effects of dexmedetomidine. As tolerance to opioids improves, recovery of the hypnotic effect of dexmedetomidine is more rapid than recovery of its analgesic efficacy.[671] These data would tend to indicate a possible cross-tolerance across receptors.

In animal models of incomplete cerebral ischemia and reperfusion, dexmedetomidine reduces cerebral necrosis and improves neurologic outcome. In a model of focal ischemia in rabbits, dexmedetomidine, administered at doses that reduced the MAC of halothane by 50%, resulted in less cortical neuronal damage than when halothane was administered alone at equi-effective MAC concentrations.[672] Little is known of the effects of dexmedetomidine alone on ICP and CBF. In patients after pituitary surgery, a target concentration of 600 ng/mL dexmedetomidine resulted in no increase in lumbar CSF pressure.[673] In dogs in the presence of volatile anesthetics and dexmedetomidine, CBF was decreased and oxygen consumption was maintained.[674,675] CBF velocity, as measured by transcranial Doppler, decreased with increasing concentrations of dexmedetomidine in parallel with decreasing mean arterial pressure and increasing arterial carbon dioxide.[676] In volunteers, both low (402 to 530 pg/mL) and high concentrations (524 to 732 pg/mL) of dexmedetomidine decreased global CBF by 30%. This decrease persisted for at least 30 minutes after termination of the infusion.[677] In a rat seizure model, dexmedetomidine demonstrated significant proconvulsant action, which is consistent with previous findings that inhibition of central noradrenergic transmission facilitates seizure expression.[678] This finding, however, is in contrast to an anticonvulsant effect shown in rats after kainic acid–induced seizures.[679] As yet, there have been no reports of seizures in humans. Dexmedetomidine is also able to reduce muscle rigidity after high-dose opioid administration.[680] In resting volunteers, dexmedetomidine increased growth hormone secretion in a dose-dependent manner, but it had no effect on other pituitary hormones.[681,682] Dexmedetomidine ablates memory in a dose-dependent manner. In concentrations used for clinical sedation (i.e., 0.7 ng/mL), recall of picture cards is preserved. An increase to concentrations of 2 ng/mL dexmedetomidine largely ablates both recall and recognition of a picture card.[683]

Effects on the Respiratory System

In volunteers, dexmedetomidine at concentrations producing significant sedation reduces minute ventilation but retains the slope of the ventilatory response to increasing CO_2.[684] The changes in ventilation appeared to be very similar to those observed during natural sleep. Ebert and coworkers infused dexmedetomidine up to concentrations of 15 ng/mL in spontaneously breathing volunteers and showed no change in arterial oxygenation or pH. At the very highest concentrations, $Paco_2$ increased by 20%. The respiratory rate increased with increasing concentration from 14 to 25 breaths/min.[683] When dexmedetomidine and propofol were titrated to equal sedative end points (BIS index of 85), both resulted in no change in the respiratory rate.[685] Doses of 1 to 2 μg/kg of dexmedetomidine induce a mild increase in $Paco_2$ (45 mm Hg) and a rightward shift and depression of the carbon dioxide response curves. The changes in respiration are mainly a decrease in tidal volume with little change in respiratory frequency. When combined with alfentanil, dexmedetomidine enhances analgesia without causing further respiratory depression.

Effects on the Cardiovascular System

The basic effects of α_2-agonists on the cardiovascular system are a decreased heart rate, decreased systemic vascular resistance, and indirectly decreased myocardial contractility, cardiac output, and systemic blood pressure.

By developing highly selective α-agonists, it had been hoped that some of these adverse cardiovascular effects would be decreased and the desirable hypnotic-analgesic properties maximized. The hemodynamic effects of a bolus of dexmedetomidine in humans have shown a biphasic response. An acute intravenous injection of 2 μg/kg resulted in an initial increase in blood pressure (22%) and decrease in heart rate (27%) from baseline that occurred 5 minutes after injection. This initial increase in blood pressure is probably due to the effect of dexmedetomidine on peripheral α_2-receptors. The heart rate returned to baseline by 15 minutes, and blood pressure gradually drifted down to approximately 15% below baseline by 1 hour. After an intramuscular injection of the same dose, the initial increase in blood pressure was not seen, and both the heart rate and blood pressure remained within 10% of baseline values.[586] Ebert and colleagues performed a very elegant study in volunteers in which a target-controlled infusion system was used to provide increasing concentrations (0.7 to 15 ng/mL) of dexmedetomidine (Fig. 10-26).[683] The lowest two concentrations produced a decrease in mean arterial pressure (13%) followed by a progressive increase (12%). Increasing concentrations of dexmedetomidine also produce progressive decreases in heart rate (maximum of 29%) and cardiac output (35%).[683] Infusion of dexmedetomidine in volunteers has also been shown to result in a compensated reduction in systemic sympathetic tone without changes in baroreflex sensitivity.

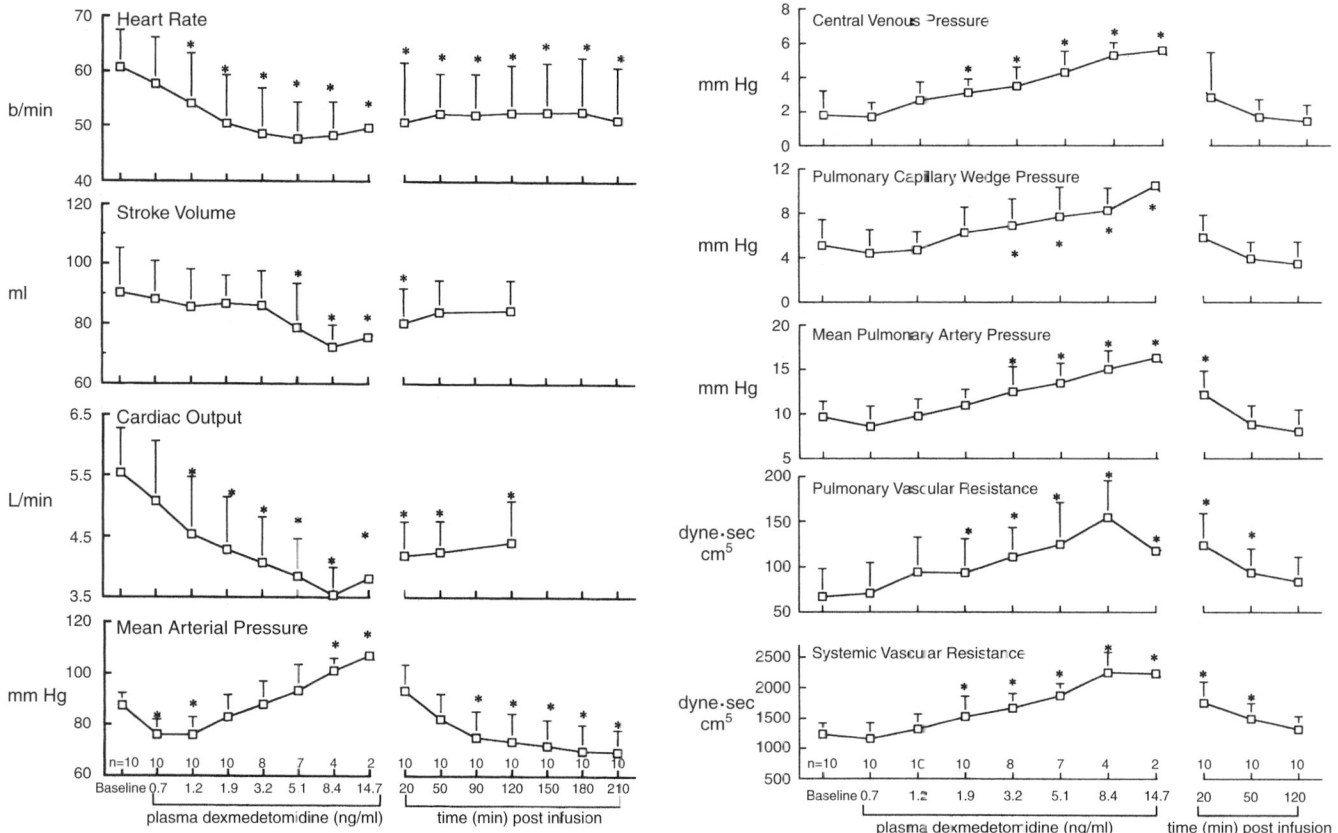

Figure 10–26 Effects of increasing plasma concentrations of dexmedetomidine.

It also blunts the heart rate and the systemic sympathetic response to sweating but is less effective in blunting the cardiac sympathetic response to shivering.[687] In several studies involving both intramuscular and intravenous administration, dexmedetomidine caused profound bradycardia (<40 beats/min) and occasionally sinus arrest/pause in a small percentage of patients. These episodes generally resolved spontaneously or were readily treated by anticholinergics without adverse outcome. It would be expected from its profile that dexmedetomidine would be beneficial to ischemic myocardium. In animal models, dexmedetomidine demonstrated some beneficial effects on the ischemic heart through decreased oxygen consumption and redistribution of coronary flow from nonischemic zones to ischemic zones after acute brief occlusion.[688] Dexmedetomidine also decreased serum lactate levels in a dog model of coronary ischemia with an associated decrease in heart rate and measured catecholamines. In addition, it produced a 35% increase in the endocardial-epicardial blood flow ratio.[689]

Other Effects
A frequently reported side effect of dexmedetomidine has been dry mouth, which is due to a decrease in saliva production.[690]

Uses

Unlike the other drugs described in this chapter, dexmedetomidine is not indicated for induction or maintenance of anesthesia. Its role at present is largely limited to brief (<24 hours) postoperative sedation. It has, however, been described as an adjuvant during anesthesia to reduce the hypnotic and opioid requirements for conscious sedation and may possibly be considered perioperatively in patients at high risk for myocardial ischemia.

Sedation
As a premedicant at intravenous doses of 0.33 to 0.67 µg/kg given 15 minutes before surgery, dexmedetomidine appears to be efficacious while minimizing the cardiovascular side effects of hypotension and bradycardia.[691] Within this dosage range, dexmedetomidine reduces thiopental requirements (by ≈30%) for short procedures,[691,692] reduces the requirements of volatile anesthetics (by ≈25%), and when compared with 2 µg/kg fentanyl, more effectively attenuates the hemodynamic response to endotracheal intubation.[693] Dexmedetomidine has also been evaluated as an intramuscular injection (2.5 µg/kg) with or without fentanyl administered 45 to 90 minutes before surgery. This regimen was compared with intramuscular midazolam plus fentanyl and was found to provide equal anxiolysis, a reduced response to intubation, lower volatile anesthetic requirements, and a lower incidence of postoperative shivering but a higher incidence of bradycardia. Atipamezole, a selective α_2-antagonist, was effective at a dose of 50 µg/kg in reversing the sedation of dexmedetomidine, 2 µg/kg intramuscularly, when used to provide sedation for brief operative procedures.[667] This reversal of effects resulted in a more rapid recovery than occurred after equisedative doses of midazolam.

In several studies dexmedetomidine has demonstrated advantages over propofol for sedation in mechanically ventilated postoperative patients. When both drugs were titrated to equal sedation as assessed by the BIS index (approximately 50) and Ramsay sedation score (5), dexmedetomidine required significantly less alfentanil (2.5 versus 0.8 mg/hr). Heart rates were slower in the dexmedetomidine group, whereas mean arterial pressures were similar. Interestingly, the Pao_2/Fio_2 ratio was significantly higher in the dexmedetomidine group. Time to extubation after discontinuation of the infusion was similar: 28 minutes. Patients receiving dexmedetomidine appeared to have greater recall of their stay in the ICU, but all described it as pleasant overall.[694] Several other studies have confirmed the decreased requirement for opioids (over 50%) when dexmedetomidine is used for sedation versus propofol or benzodiazepines. Most studies also describe more stable hemodynamics during weaning when dexmedetomidine is used for sedation.[695] This finding is of obvious benefit in patients at high risk for myocardial ischemia. For sedation in the ICU, loading doses of 2.5 to 6.0 µg/kg/hr delivered over a 10-minute period have been used. The lower infusion rate has been associated with fewer episodes of severe bradycardia and other hemodynamic perturbations. This dose is followed by infusion rates of 0.1 to 1 µg/kg/hr, which are generally needed to maintain adequate sedation.

When used for intraoperative sedation, dexmedetomidine (1 µg/kg over a 10-minute period) results in a slower onset than propofol (75 µg/kg/min over a 10-minute period) does but similar cardiorespiratory effects when titrated to equal sedation. The average infusion rate of dexmedetomidine intraoperatively to maintain a BIS index value of 70 to 80 was 0.7 µg/kg/hr. Sedation was more prolonged after termination of the infusion, as was recovery of blood pressure. However, lower doses of opioid were needed in the first hour.[685]

Clonidine in doses of 3 to 5 µg/kg orally, usually given 30 to 90 minutes before surgery, similarly reduces the MAC of the potent volatile anesthetics (by 30% to 50%), reduces opioid requirements, attenuates the hemodynamic response to intubation, and generally provides a more stable hemodynamic profile intraoperatively,[659,696,697] although significant bradycardia and hypotension during and immediately after induction have been observed. This reduction in anesthetic requirements also translates into more rapid awakening after surgery.[698] Clonidine also reduces intraocular pressure, perioperative catecholamines, and postoperative analgesic requirements and prevents the usual deterioration in renal function after aortocoronary bypass.[659,698-700] As with clonidine, intraocular pressure is decreased (33%), catecholamine secretion is reduced, perioperative analgesic requirements are less, and recovery is more rapid after dexmedetomidine.[701,702]

Maintenance of Anesthesia
Dexmedetomidine has also been used as a maintenance infusion starting with a loading dose of 170 ng/kg/min for 10 minutes and then followed by an infusion of 10 ng/kg/min. This regimen resulted in a plasma concentration of slightly less than 1 ng/mL. After induction with

thiopental and 70% nitrous oxide, dexmedetomidine reduced isoflurane requirements by 90% when compared with a control group.[703] The interaction of dexmedetomidine, fentanyl, and enflurane on MAC reduction and hemodynamics has been evaluated in dogs. This triple combination is complex, but it appears that dexmedetomidine further enhances the MAC reduction of enflurane by fentanyl. This triple interaction, however, does not seem to reduce the likelihood of hypotension or bradycardia when providing adequate anesthesia.[704] In patients undergoing vascular surgery, three infusion rates of dexmedetomidine were compared with a placebo infusion starting 1 hour before surgery and administered until 48 hours after surgery. In the groups receiving dexmedetomidine, more vasoactive agents were required to maintain hemodynamics intraoperatively, but less tachycardia was noted postoperatively. No other significant differences were noted between the groups.[705]

α_2-Adrenergic agonists possess many important characteristics that are valuable for anesthesia. It would appear, however, that at anesthetic concentrations in humans, the cardiovascular effects (hypotension, bradycardia) of these drugs may be the major drawback that prevents them from being used as the primary anesthetic, and their role is therefore limited to use as an adjuvant for other anesthetic drugs. The exact role of dexmedetomidine either as a premedicant or as an intravenous anesthetic adjuvant is still to be determined. However, dexmedetomidine appears to be a very effective sedative for patients in the ICU, where it may provide advantages over other available sedatives because of its minimal effect on respiration, its analgesic efficacy, and its hemodynamic profile. The use of dexmedetomidine for long-term sedation needs further investigation.

DROPERIDOL

History

General anesthesia with inhaled anesthetics and barbiturates depresses the entire CNS in a nonspecific manner. Laborit and Huguenard[706,707] in the 1950s sought an anesthetic technique that would produce "artificial hibernation" devoid of circulatory and respiratory depression. Their concept was to use drugs that would produce neurovegetative blockade (multifocal inhibition) of the cellular, autonomic, and endocrine mechanisms normally activated in response to stress.[708] The first attempt at developing this concept was the lytic cocktail, which contained an analgesic (meperidine), two tranquilizers (chlorpromazine and promethazine), and atropine. Although this combination of drugs did enjoy widespread use for conscious sedation, it produced respiratory depression and was not used for general anesthesia. Janssen[709] synthesized haloperidol, the first member of the butyrophenones, and it became the primary neuroleptic component in neuroleptanesthesia (NLAN). DeCastro and Mundeleer[710] in 1959 combined haloperidol with phenoperidine (a meperidine derivative also synthesized by Janssen) in a

forerunner to the practice of NLAN. Droperidol, a derivative of haloperidol, and fentanyl, a phenoperidine congener, both synthesized by Janssen, were used by DeCastro and Mundeleer[710] in a combination that they reported to be superior to haloperidol and phenoperidine. This NLAN combination produced more rapid onset of analgesia, less respiratory depression, and fewer extrapyramidal side effects. The fixed combination of droperidol and fentanyl, marketed as Innovar in the United States, was the drug primarily used for NLAN. The use of NLAN has largely disappeared in modern anesthetic practice. The primary use of droperidol in anesthesia has been as an antiemetic and to a lesser extent as a sedative and antipruritic. The present package insert for droperidol in the United States carries a black box warning regarding the potential for fatal arrhythmias and recommendations that it be administered only with continuous electrocardiographic monitoring. However, with the withdrawal of droperidol in certain countries and more stringent labeling regarding potentially lethal dysrhythmias in others, the use of droperidol has decreased tremendously. The validity of the risk of low-dose droperidol causing QT prolongation, dysrhythmias, and death has been challenged by numerous editorials, articles, and letters reviewing the cases that prompted this action.[711-716]

Droperidol is a butyrophenone, a fluorinated derivative of the phenothiazines (Fig. 10-27).[708] Butyrophenones produce CNS depression characterized by marked apparent tranquility and cataleptic immobility. They are potent antiemetics. Droperidol is a potent butyrophenone, and like the others, it produces its action centrally at sites where dopamine, norepinephrine, and serotonin act. It has been postulated that butyrophenones may occupy GABA receptors on the postsynaptic membrane, thereby reducing synaptic transmission and resulting in a build-up of dopamine in the intersynaptic cleft.[708,709] In particular, droperidol results in submaximal inhibition of the α_1-, β_1-, and γ_2-subunits of GABA$_A$ and full inhibition of α_2-acetylcholine receptors. This submaximal inhibition of GABA receptors by droperidol may explain the anxiety, dysphoria, and restlessness that can occur with its administration.[717] An imbalance in dopamine and acetylcholine is thought to occur and result in an alteration in normal transmission of signals in the CNS. The chemoreceptor trigger zone is the emetic center, and "red" astrocytes transport neurolept molecules from the capillary to dopaminergic synapses in the chemoreceptor trigger zone, where they occupy GABA receptors (Fig. 10-28). This is thought to be

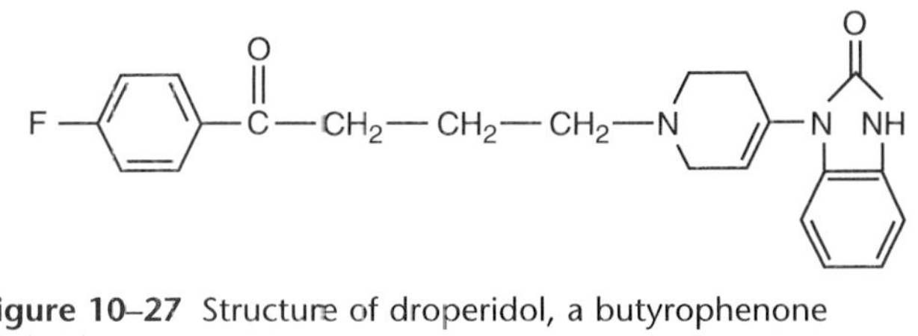

Figure 10–27 Structure of droperidol, a butyrophenone derivative.

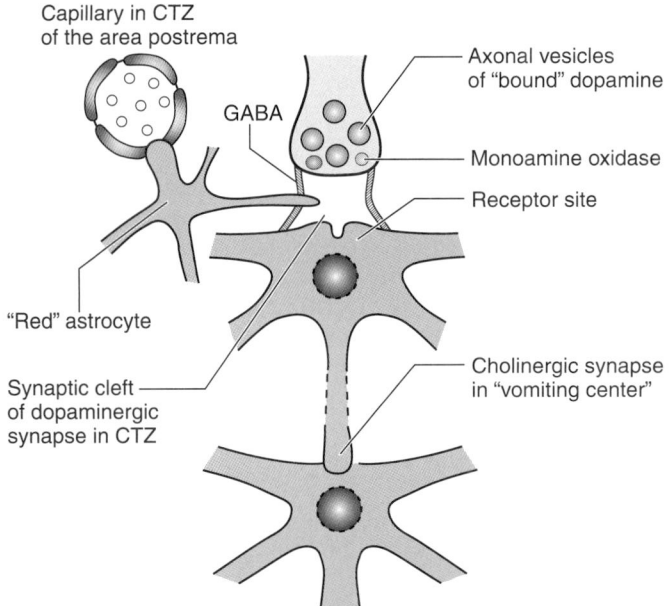

Figure 10–28 Site of action of droperidol. The mode of action of neuroleptanesthetics is at the chemoreceptor trigger zone (CTZ). GABA, γ-aminobutyric acid. (Redrawn with modification from Janssen PAJ: Pharmacological aspects. *In* Bente D, Bradley P [eds]: Neuropsychopharmacology. Amsterdam, Elsevier, 1965, p 151.)

the mechanism by which droperidol exerts its antiemetic effect.[718]

Metabolism and Pharmacokinetics

Droperidol is biotransformed in the liver into two primary metabolites,[719] and its plasma decay can be described by a two-compartment model. Its pharmacokinetics[22] is shown in Table 10-1. Clearance of droperidol is relatively large (14 mL/kg/min), and its elimination half-life is relatively short (103 to 134 minutes).[22,23] Its time course of disappearance from plasma is similar to that of fentanyl, yet the discrepancy in duration of effect of the two has been the subject of criticism because both are formulated together in Innovar. The seemingly longer CNS action of droperidol has prompted some investigators to postulate that droperidol has a propensity to occupy CNS receptors[22] and that it undergoes greater receptor binding than fentanyl does.

Pharmacology

Effects on the Central Nervous System

The effects of neuroleptanesthetics on human CBF and $CMRO_2$ have not been studied. In dogs, droperidol causes potent cerebral vasoconstriction that results in a 40% reduction in CBF. No significant change in $CMRO_2$ occurs during droperidol administration.[720] The EEG in conscious patients shows some reduction in frequency, with occasional slowing.[721] Low-dose droperidol has also been shown to cause balance disturbances at the time of discharge when administered at doses used for antiemetic prophylaxis.[722] Droperidol may produce extrapyramidal

signs and worsens symptoms of Parkinson's disease. It may also rarely precipitate malignant neuroleptic syndrome.

Effects on the Respiratory System

When used alone, droperidol has little effect on the respiratory system.[175] Droperidol (0.044 mg/kg) given to surgical patients produced a slight reduction in respiratory rate,[723] and administration of 3 mg intravenously had no significant effect on tidal volume in volunteers.[176] More detailed respiratory studies are not available.

Effects on the Cardiovascular System

Like most antipsychotics, droperidol may prolong the QT interval by delaying myocardial repolarization and precipitating *torsades de pointes*. This effect appears to be dose dependent and may be of clinical significance when other causes of QT prolongation are also present.[724] Droperidol may also be associated with some antiarrhythmic effects that are much like those of quinidine.[552,725] Droperidol produces vasodilation with a decrease in blood pressure (see Table 10-2). This effect is considered to be a result of moderate α-adrenergic blockade.[719,726,727] Importantly, the dopamine-induced increase in renal blood flow (renal artery flow meter methodology) is not significantly impaired by the administration of droperidol.[728] Droperidol has little effect on myocardial contractility.[725]

Uses

The use of droperidol in the perioperative period is presently largely restricted to its antiemetic and sedative effects. It is an effective antiemetic,[729] the dose for which varies between 10 and 20 μg/kg (0.6 and 1.25 mg for a 70-kg person).[730] These doses of droperidol, given at the start of anesthesia for operations lasting 1 hour, reduce the incidence of nausea and vomiting by about 60%. When given at induction, these doses have little effect on wake-up time, but should they be given at the end of surgery, some residual hypnotic effect could result. Droperidol is also effective in pediatric patients[731] when the drug is given orally (300 μg/kg), and the effect can be enhanced when it is combined with oral metoclopramide (0.15 mg/kg). The overall antiemetic efficacy of droperidol alone is equal to that of ondansetron; it results in an equal number of side effects but is more cost-effective.[732] The efficacy of droperidol as an antiemetic is enhanced when used in combination with serotonin antagonists or dexamethasone, or with both.

A newer use for droperidol is as an antiemetic given as an adjunctive drug intermittently or as a continuous infusion for postoperative pain relief as part of a patient-controlled regimen.[714,733] Droperidol has also been shown to be effective in the treatment and prevention of pruritus secondary to opioid administration. It has been administered both intravenously and into the epidural space for this purpose.[734,735] When used in this fashion, droperidol also effectively reduces nausea, but it does increase sedation. The safety of epidural administration of droperidol, however, has not been fully evaluated, and it is not approved for administration by this route.

SUMMARY

Many different intravenous drugs are available for use in the care of patients requiring general anesthesia. Selection of a particular drug must be based on the individual patient's need for hypnosis, amnesia, and analgesia. Drug selection must match the physiology or the pathophysiology (or both) of the individual patient with the pharmacology of the particular drug. Thus, for example, a patient in shock who requires induction of anesthesia should receive the drug that will produce a rapid onset of effect without causing further hemodynamic compromise. Knowledge of the clinical pharmacology of each of the intravenous anesthetic drugs enables the clinician to induce and maintain sedation or general anesthesia safely and effectively. Because there is no single perfect drug for any particular patient, informed practitioners must wisely use the appropriate drug or drugs in the practice of good anesthesia care.

KEY POINTS

1. The introduction of thiopental into clinical practice in 1934 marked the advent of modern intravenous anesthesia. Today, intravenous anesthetics are used for induction of anesthesia, maintenance of anesthesia, and provision of conscious sedation.

2. The most commonly used intravenous anesthetic is propofol, an alkylphenol presently formulated in a lipid emulsion. Propofol provides rapid onset and offset with context-sensitive decrement times of approximately 10 minutes when infused for less than 3 hours and under 40 minutes when infused for up to 8 hours. Its mechanism of action is thought to be potentiation of GABA-induced chloride currents. At therapeutic doses, propofol produces a moderate depressant effect on ventilation. It causes a dose-dependent decrease in blood pressure primarily through a decrease in cardiac output and systemic vascular resistance. A unique action of propofol is its antiemetic effect, which remains present at concentrations below those producing sedation. The induction dose is 1 to 2 mg/kg for loss of consciousness with a maintenance infusion of 100 to 200 μg/kg/min. For conscious sedation, rates of 25 to 75 μg/kg/min are usually adequate.

3. Until recently, the most commonly used intravenous induction agents were the barbiturates. Thiopental provides rapid onset and offset when used as a single dose, but it accumulates rapidly with prolonged administration and leads to slow recovery. Methohexital has a rapid onset and offset similar to propofol for procedures lasting under 2 hours. The barbiturates are administered as sodium salts diluted in a water base at an alkaline pH. Like propofol, the barbiturates are thought to provide their hypnotic effects largely through action on the GABA$_A$ receptor. Barbiturates provide cerebral protection and are generally used primarily for this purpose. They cause a moderate dose-dependent decrease in blood pressure (primarily as a result of peripheral vasodilation) and respiratory drive. The barbiturates are contraindicated in patients with porphyria. The induction dose of thiopental is 4 mg/kg, and that for methohexital is 2 mg/kg. Methohexital can be used for maintenance of anesthesia at 100 to 200 μg/kg/min or for conscious sedation at 25 to 75 μg/kg/min.

4. The benzodiazepines are used primarily as premedicants for anxiolysis and amnesia or for conscious sedation. The water-soluble benzodiazepine midazolam is the most frequently used intravenously because of its relatively rapid onset and offset and lack of active metabolites when compared with other benzodiazepines (e.g., diazepam). The onset of midazolam is slower than that of both propofol and barbiturates, and its offset, especially when used at higher doses or in a prolonged infusion, is considerably longer than that of propofol or methohexital. The benzodiazepines act through the GABA receptor. Flumazenil is a specific benzodiazepine antagonist. It can be used to reverse the effects of benzodiazepines. In general, the benzodiazepines produce only a mild decrease in blood pressure and mild to moderate respiratory depression. The dose of midazolam for anxiolysis and mild sedation is 0.015 to 0.03 mg/kg intravenously and is generally repeated in 30 to 60 minutes as needed.

5. Ketamine is a phencyclidine derivative that has been used for both induction and maintenance of anesthesia. Ketamine acts primarily, but not entirely, through the NMDA receptor. It provides both a dissociative state of hypnosis and analgesia. Ketamine is associated with significant adverse psychological effects at higher doses, as well as several other side effects. Thus, more recently it is used primarily for its analgesic properties. It has rapid onset and relatively rapid offset, even after an infusion of several hours. It has sympathomimetic action that preserves cardiac function. Ketamine has minimal effect on respiration and tends to preserve autonomic reflexes. The induction dose is 2 to 4 mg intravenously. An infusion of ketamine will provide analgesia and can be given with propofol in a total intravenous anesthesia technique. A dose of 10 to 20 mg preoperatively has been shown to provide preemptive analgesia.

6. Etomidate is an imidazole derivative used primarily for induction of anesthesia, especially in the elderly and patients who are cardiovascularly compromised. It has a rapid onset of effect and a rapid offset even after a continuous infusion. However, prolonged infusion results in inhibition of adrenocortical synthesis and potential mortality in ICU patients. The major advantage of etomidate is its minimal effect on the cardiovascular and respiratory systems. It is associated with a high incidence of burning on injection, thrombophlebitis, and postoperative nausea and vomiting, thus limiting its popularity. The induction dose is 0.2 to 0.3 mg/kg.

7. Dexmedetomidine is the most recently released intravenous anesthetic. It is a highly selective α_2-adrenergic agonist that produces sedation, hypnosis, and analgesia. Dexmedetomidine is presently approved only for brief (<24 hours) postoperative sedation. Its primary action is on α_2-receptors in the locus ceruleus. It has minimal effect on respiration. Dexmedetomidine produces a biphasic effect on blood pressure: at low concentrations mean blood pressure is decreased, and at higher concentrations, blood pressure is increased. Heart rate and cardiac output show a concentration-dependent decrease. Dosing for sedation is a loading dose of 2.5 to 6.0 µg/kg over a 10-minute period, followed by an infusion of 0.1 to 1 µg/kg/hr.

8. Droperidol, a butyrophenone and major tranquilizer, was initially used to produce a state of neuroleptanesthesia. Recent concern regarding its effect on prolonging the QT interval has resulted in its withdrawal in several countries and its limitation to the treatment of postoperative nausea and vomiting with a black box warning in the United States. Prolongation of the QT interval by doses used for postoperative nausea and vomiting (0.625 to 1.25 mg) has been challenged by several editorials, and this effect has not been substantiated by review of the cases reported or any literature. Droperidol at low doses remains one of the most effective antiemetic therapies available.

REFERENCES

1. Cohen MM, Duncan PG, Tate RB: Does anesthesia contribute to operative mortality? JAMA 260:2859-2863, 1988.
2. Fragen R: Diprivan (propofol): A historical perspective. Semin Anesth 7:1, 1988.
3. Kay B, Rolly G: I.C.I. 35868, a new intravenous induction agent. Acta Anaesthesiol Belg 28:303-316, 1977.
4. Briggs LP, Clarke RS, Watkins J: An adverse reaction to the administration of disoprofol (Diprivan). Anaesthesia 37:1099-1101, 1982.
5. James R, Glen JB: Synthesis, biological evaluation, and preliminary structure-activity considerations of a series of alkylphenols as intravenous anesthetic agents. J Med Chem 23:1350-1357, 1980.
6. Simons P, Cockshott I, Douglas E: Blood concentrations, metabolism and elimination after a subanesthetic intravenous dose of (14)C-propofol (Diprivan) to male volunteers [abstract]. Postgrad Med J 61:64, 1985.
7. Veroli P, O'Kelly B, Bertrand F, et al: Extrahepatic metabolism of propofol in man during the anhepatic phase of orthotopic liver transplantation. Br J Anaesth 68:183-186, 1992.
8. Gray PA, Park GR, Cockshott ID, et al: Propofol metabolism in man during the anhepatic and reperfusion phases of liver transplantation. Xenobiotica 22:105-114, 1992.
9. Kuipers JA, Boer F, Olieman W, et al: First-pass lung uptake and pulmonary clearance of propofol: Assessment with a recirculatory indocyanine green pharmacokinetic model. Anesthesiology 91:1780-1787, 1999.
10. Dawidowicz AL, Fornal E, Mardarowicz M, Fijalkowska A: The role of human lungs in the biotransformation of propofol. Anesthesiology 93:992-997, 2000.
11. Raoof AA, van Obbergh LJ, de Ville de Goyet J, Verbeeck RK: Extrahepatic glucuronidation of propofol in man: Possible contribution of gut wall and kidney. Eur J Clin Pharmacol 50:91-96, 1996.
12. Chen TL, Ueng TH, Chen SH, et al: Human cytochrome P450 mono-oxygenase system is suppressed by propofol. Br J Anaesth 74:558-562, 1995.
13. Adam HK, Briggs LP, Bahar M, et al: Pharmacokinetic evaluation of ICI 35 868 in man. Single induction doses with different rates of injection. Br J Anaesth 55:97-103, 1983.
14. Kay NH, Sear JW, Uppington J, et al: Disposition of propofol in patients undergoing surgery. A comparison in men and women. Br J Anaesth 58:1075-1079, 1986.
15. Kirkpatrick T, Cockshott ID, Douglas EJ, Nimmo WS: Pharmacokinetics of propofol (Diprivan) in elderly patients. Br J Anaesth 60:146-150, 1988.
16. Gepts E, Camu F, Cockshott ID, Douglas EJ: Disposition of propofol administered as constant rate intravenous infusions in humans. Anesth Analg 66:1256-1263, 1987.
17. Schuttler J, Stoeckel H, Schwilden H: Pharmacokinetic and pharmacodynamic modeling of propofol ('Diprivan') in volunteers and surgical patients. Postgrad Med J 61(Suppl 3):53-54, 1985.
18. Shafer A, Doze VA, Shafer SL, White PF: Pharmacokinetics and pharmacodynamics of propofol infusions during general anesthesia. Anesthesiology 69:348-356, 1988.
19. Dyck JB, Maze M, Haack C, et al: Computer-controlled infusion of intravenous dexmedetomidine hydrochloride in adult human volunteers. Anesthesiology 78:821-828, 1993.
20. Venn RM, Karol MD, Grounds RM: Pharmacokinetics of dexmedetomidine infusions for sedation of postoperative patients requiring intensive care. Br J Anaesth 88:669-675, 2002.
21. Reves J: Benzodiazepines. In Prys-Roberts CH (ed): Pharmacokinetics of Anesthesia. Boston, Blackwell, 1984, p 157.
22. Fischler M, Bonnet F, Trang H, et al: The pharmacokinetics of droperidol in anesthetized patients. Anesthesiology 64:486-489, 1986.
23. Cressman WA, Plostnieks J, Johnson PC: Absorption, metabolism and excretion of droperidol by human subjects following intramuscular and intravenous administration. Anesthesiology 38:363-369, 1973.
24. Fragen RJ, Avram MJ, Henthorn TK, Caldwell NJ: A pharmacokinetically designed etomidate infusion regimen for hypnosis. Anesth Analg 62:654-660, 1983.
25. Schuttler J, Schwilden H, Stoeckel H: Infusion strategies to investigate the pharmacokinetics and pharmacodynamics of hypnotic drugs: Etomidate as an example. Eur J Anaesthesiol 2:133-142, 1985.
26. Hebron BS, Edbrooke DL, Newby DM, Mather SJ: Pharmacokinetics of etomidate associated with prolonged i.v. infusion. Br J Anaesth 55:281-287, 1983.
27. de Ruiter G, Popescu DT, de Boer AG, et al: Pharmacokinetics of etomidate in surgical patients. Arch Int Pharmacodyn Ther 249:180-188, 1981.
28. Van Hamme MJ, Ghoneim MM, Ambre JJ: Pharmacokinetics of etomidate, a new intravenous anesthetic. Anesthesiology 49:274-277, 1978.
29. Forster A, Gardaz JP, Suter PM, Gemperle M: I.V. midazolam as an induction agent for anaesthesia: A study in volunteers. Br J Anaesth 52:907-911, 1980.
30. Norton AC, Dundas CR: Induction agents for day-case anaesthesia. A double-blind comparison of propofol and midazolam antagonised by flumazenil. Anaesthesia 45:198-203, 1990.
31. Clements JA, Nimmo WS: Pharmacokinetics and analgesic effect of ketamine in man. Br J Anaesth 53:27-30, 1981.
32. Bremier D: Pharmacokinetics of methohexitone following intravenous infusions in humans. Br J Anaesth 48:643, 1976.
33. Hudson RJ, Stanski DR, Burch PG: Pharmacokinetics of methohexital and thiopental in surgical patients. Anesthesiology 59:215-219, 1983.
34. Philip BK, Simpson TH, Hauch MA, Mallampati SR: Flumazenil reverses sedation after midazolam-induced general anesthesia in ambulatory surgery patients. Anesth Analg 71:371-376, 1990.

35. Mandema JW, Tuk B, van Steveninck AL, et al: Pharmacokinetic-pharmacodynamic modeling of the central nervous system effects of midazolam and its main metabolite alpha-hydroxymidazolam in healthy volunteers. Clin Pharmacol Ther 51:715-728, 1992.

36. Bauer TM, Ritz R, Haberthur C, et al: Prolonged sedation due to accumulation of conjugated metabolites of midazolam. Lancet 346:145-147, 1995.

37. Greenblatt DJ, Shader RI, Divoll M, Harmatz JS: Benzodiazepines: A summary of pharmacokinetic properties. Br J Clin Pharmacol 11(Suppl 1):11S-16S, 1981.

38. MacLeod SM, Giles HG, Bengert B, et al: Age- and gender-related differences in diazepam pharmacokinetics. J Clin Pharmacol 19:15-19, 1979.

39. Greenblatt DJ, Abernethy DR, Locniskar A, et al: Effect of age, gender, and obesity on midazolam kinetics. Anesthesiology 61:27-35, 1984.

40. Mould DR, DeFeo TM, Reele S, et al: Simultaneous modeling of the pharmacokinetics and pharmacodynamics of midazolam and diazepam. Clin Pharmacol Ther 58:35-43, 1995.

41. Bischoff KB, Dedrick RL: Thiopental pharmacokinetics. J Pharm Sci 57:1346-1351, 1968.

42. Christensen J, Andreasen F, Jansen J: Pharmacokinetics of thiopentone in a group of young women and a group of young men. Br J Anaesth 52:913-918, 1980.

43. Bailie GR, Cockshott ID, Douglas EJ, Bowles BJ: Pharmacokinetics of propofol during and after long-term continuous infusion for maintenance of sedation in ICU patients. Br J Anaesth 68:486-491, 1992.

44. Hughes MA, Glass PS, Jacobs JR: Context-sensitive half-time in multicompartment pharmacokinetic models for intravenous anesthetic drugs. Anesthesiology 76:334-341, 1992.

45. Dyck J, Varvel J, Hung O: The pharmacokinetics of propofol vs. age. Anesthesiology 75:A315, 1991.

46. Kazama T, Ikeda K, Morita K, et al: Comparison of the effect-site $k(e0)$s of propofol for blood pressure and EEG bispectral index in elderly and younger patients. Anesthesiology 90:1517-1527, 1999.

47. Schnider TW, Minto CF, Shafer SL, et al: The influence of age on propofol pharmacodynamics. Anesthesiology 90:1502-1516, 1999.

48. Servin F, Desmonts JM, Farinotti R, et al: Pharmacokinetics of the continuous infusion of propofol in the cirrhotic patient. Preliminary results [in French]. Ann Fr Anesth Reanim 6:228-289, 1987.

49. Morcos WE, Payne J: The induction of anaesthesia with propofol ('Diprivan') compared in normal and renal failure patients. Postgrad Med J 61(Suppl 3):62-63, 1985.

50. Leslie K, Sessler DI, Bjorksten AR, Moayeri A: Mild hypothermia alters propofol pharmacokinetics and increases the duration of action of atracurium. Anesth Analg 80:1007-1014, 1995.

51. Upton RN, Ludbrook GL, Grant C, Martinez AM: Cardiac output is a determinant of the initial concentrations of propofol after short-infusion administration. Anesth Analg 89:545-552, 1999.

52. Kurita T, Morita K, Kazama T, Sato S: Influence of cardiac output on plasma propofol concentrations during constant infusion in swine. Anesthesiology 96:1498-1503, 2002.

53. Kazama T, Kurita T, Morita K, et al: Influence of hemorrhage on propofol pseudo–steady state concentration. Anesthesiology 97:1156-1161, 2002.

54. Bailey JM, Mora CT, Shafer SL: Pharmacokinetics of propofol in adult patients undergoing coronary revascularization. The Multicenter Study of Perioperative Ischemia Research Group. Anesthesiology 84:1288-1297, 1996.

55. Marsh B, White M, Morton N, Kenny GN: Pharmacokinetic model driven infusion of propofol in children. Br J Anaesth 67:41-48, 1991.

56. Kataria BK, Ved SA, Nicodemus HF, et al: The pharmacokinetics of propofol in children using three different data analysis approaches. Anesthesiology 80:104-122, 1994.

57. Murat I, Billard V, Vernois J, et al: Pharmacokinetics of propofol after a single dose in children aged 1-3 years with minor burns. Comparison of three data analysis approaches. Anesthesiology 84:526-532, 1996.

58. Benoni G, Cuzzolin L, Gilli E: Pharmacokinetics of propofol: Influence of fentanyl administration [abstract]. Eur J Anaesthesiol 183:1457, 1990.

59. Pavlin DJ, Coda B, Shen DD, et al: Effects of combining propofol and alfentanil on ventilation, analgesia, sedation, and emesis in human volunteers. Anesthesiology 84:23-37, 1996.

60. Gill SS, Wright EM, Reilly CS: Pharmacokinetic interaction of propofol and fentanyl: Single bolus injection study. Br J Anaesth 65:760-765, 1990.

61. Matot I, Neely CF, Katz RY, Marshall BE: Fentanyl and propofol uptake by the lung: Effect of time between injections. Acta Anaesthesiol Scand 38:711-715, 1994.

62. Janicki PK, James MF, Erskine WA: Propofol inhibits enzymatic degradation of alfentanil and sufentanil by isolated liver microsomes in vitro. Br J Anaesth 68:311-312, 1992.

63. Krasowski MD, Nishikawa K, Nikolaeva N, et al: Methionine 286 in transmembrane domain 3 of the GABA$_A$ receptor beta subunit controls a binding cavity for propofol and other alkylphenol general anesthetics. Neuropharmacology 41:952-964, 2001.

64. Jurd R, Arras M, Lambert S, Drexler B: General anesthetic actions in vivo strongly attenuated by a point mutation in the GABA$_A$ receptor beta3 subunit. FASEB J 17:250-252, 2003.

65. Lam DW, Reynolds JN: Modulatory and direct effects of propofol on recombinant GABA$_A$ receptors expressed in *Xenopus* oocytes: Influence of alpha- and gamma$_2$-subunits. Brain Res 784:179-137, 1998.

66. Kikuchi T, Wang Y, Sato K, Okumura F: In vivo effects of propofol on acetylcholine release from the frontal cortex, hippocampus and striatum studied by intracerebral microdialysis in freely moving rats. Br J Anaesth 80:644-648, 1998.

67. Pain L, Jeltsch H, Lehmann O, et al: Central cholinergic depletion induced by 192 IgG-saporin alleviates the sedative effects of propofol in rats. Br J Anaesth 85:869-873, 2000.

68. Kushikata T, Hirota K, Yoshida H, et al: Alpha-2 adrenoceptor activity affects propofol-induced sleep time. Anesth Analg 94:1201-1206, 2002.

69. Lingamaneni R, Birch ML, Hemmings HC Jr: Widespread inhibition of sodium channel–dependent glutamate release from isolated nerve terminals by isoflurane and propofol. Anesthesiology 95:1460-1466, 2001.

70. Antognini J, Wang X, Piercy M, Carstens E: Propofol directly depresses lumbar dorsal horn neuronal responses to noxious stimulation in goats. Can J Anaesth 47:273-279, 2000.

71. Dong XP, Xu TL: The actions of propofol on gamma-aminobutyric acid-A and glycine receptors in acutely dissociated spinal dorsal horn neurons of the rat. Anesth Analg 95:907-914, 2002.

72. Tonner PH, Poppers DM, Miller KW: The general anesthetic potency of propofol and its dependence on hydrostatic pressure. Anesthesiology 77:926-931, 1992.

73. Briggs LP, Dundee JW, Bahar M, Clarke RS: Comparison of the effect of diisopropyl phenol (ICI 35,868) and thiopentone on response to somatic pain. Br J Anaesth 54:307-311, 1982.

74. Canavero S, Bonicazzi V, Pagni CA, et al: Propofol analgesia in central pain: Preliminary clinical observations. J Neurol 242:561-567, 1995.

75. Pain L, Gobaille S, Schleef C, et al: In vivo dopamine measurements in the nucleus accumbens after nonanesthetic and anesthetic doses of propofol in rats. Anesth Analg 95:915-919, 2002.

76. Cechetto DF, Diab T, Gibson CJ, Gelb AW: The effects of propofol in the area postrema of rats. Anesth Analg 92:934-942, 2001.

77. Major E, Verniquet AJ, Waddell TK, et al: A study of three doses of ici 35 868 for induction and maintenance of anaesthesia. Br J Anaesth 53:267-272, 1981.

78. Rolly G, Versichelen L, Huyghe L, Mungroop H: Effect of speed of injection on induction of anaesthesia using propofol. Br J Anaesth 57:743-746, 1985.

79. Glass P, Ginsberg B, Hawkins E: Comparison of sodium thiopental/isoflurane to propofol (delivered by means of a pharmacokinetic model–driven device) for the induction, maintenance, and recovery from anesthesia. Anesthesiology 69:A575, 1988.

80. McClune S, McKay AC, Wright PM, et al: Synergistic interaction between midazolam and propofol. Br J Anaesth 68:240-245, 1992.

81. Short TG, Plummer JL, Chui PT: Hypnotic and anaesthetic interactions between midazolam, propofol and alfentanil. Br J Anaesth 69:162-167, 1992.

82. Adam HK, Kay B, Douglas EJ: Blood disoprofol levels in anesthetised patients. Correlation of concentrations after single or repeated doses with hypnotic activity. Anaesthesia 37:536-540, 1982.

83. Aun CS, Short SM, Leung DH, Oh TE: Induction dose-response of propofol in unpremedicated children. Br J Anaesth 68:64-67, 1992.

84. Smith C, McEwan A, Jhaveri R: Reduction of propofol Cp_{50} by fentanyl. Anesthesiology 81:820-828, 1994.

85. Mackenzie N, Grant IS: Propofol for intravenous sedation. Anaesthesia 42:3-6, 1987.

86. Wilson E, Mackenzie N, Grant IS: A comparison of propofol and midazolam by infusion to provide sedation in patients who receive spinal anaesthesia. Anaesthesia 43(Suppl):91-94, 1988.

87. Veselis RA, Reinsel RA, Wronski M, et al: EEG and memory effects of low-dose infusions of propofol. Br J Anaesth 69:246-254, 1992.

88. Zacny JP, Lichtor JL, Coalson DW, et al: Subjective and psychomotor effects of subanesthetic doses of propofol in healthy volunteers. Anesthesiology 76:696-702, 1992.

89. Kelly JS, Roy RC: Intraoperative awareness with propofol-oxygen total intravenous anesthesia for microlaryngeal surgery. Anesthesiology 77:207-209, 1992.

90. Glass PS: Prevention of awareness during total intravenous anesthesia. Anesthesiology 78:399-400, 1993.

91. McDonald NJ, Mannion D, Lee P, et al: Mood evaluation and outpatient anaesthesia. A comparison between propofol and thiopentone. Anaesthesia 43(Suppl):68-69, 1988.

92. Nelson V: Hallucinations after propofol. Anaesthesia 43:170, 1988.

93. Cameron A: Opisthotonos again. Anaesthesia 42:1124, 1987.

94. Hazeaux C, Tisserant D, Vespignani H, et al: Electro-encephalographic changes produced by propofol [in French]. Ann Fr Anesth Reanim 6:261-266, 1987.

95. Yate PM, Maynard DE, Major E, et al: Anaesthesia with ICI 35,868 monitored by the cerebral function analysing monitor (CFAM). Eur J Anaesthesiol 3:159-166, 1986.

96. Glass PS, Bloom M, Kearse L, et al: Bispectral analysis measures sedation and memory effects of propofol, midazolam, isoflurane, and alfentanil in healthy volunteers. Anesthesiology 86:836-847, 1997.

97. Maurette P, Simeon F, Castagnera L, et al: Propofol anaes-thesia alters somatosensory evoked cortical potentials. Anaesthesia 43(Suppl):44-45, 1988.

98. Savoia G, Esposito C, Belfiore F, et al: Propofol infusion and auditory evoked potentials. Anaesthesia 43(Suppl):46-49, 1988.

99. Doi M, Gajraj RJ, Mantzaridis H, Kenny GN: Relationship between calculated blood concentration of propofol and electrophysiological variables during emergence from anaesthesia: Comparison of bispectral index, spectral edge frequency, median frequency and auditory evoked potential index. Br J Anaesth 78:180-184, 1997.

100. Glen JB, Hunter SC, Blackburn TP, Wood P: Interaction studies and other investigations of the pharmacology of propofol ('Diprivan'). Postgrad Med J 61(Suppl 3):7-14, 1985.

101. al-Hader A, Hasan M, Hasan Z: The comparative effects of propofol, thiopental, and diazepam, administered intravenously, on pentylenetetrazol seizure threshold in the rabbit. Life Sci 51:779-786, 1992.

102. Heavner J, Arthur J, Zou J: Propofol vs. thiopental for treating bupivacaine induced seizures in rats. Anesthesiology 77:A802, 1992.

103. Wood P, Browne G, Pugh S: Propofol infusion for the treatment of status epilepticus [letter]. Lancet 1:480, 1988.

104. Chilvers CR, Laurie PS: Successful use of propofol in status epilepticus. Anaesthesia 45:995-996, 1990.

105. Dwyer R, McCaughey W, Lavery J, et al: Comparison of propofol and methohexitone as anaesthetic agents for electroconvulsive therapy. Anaesthesia 43:459-462, 1988.

106. Hodkinson BP, Frith RW, Mee EW: Propofol and the electroencephalogram. Lancet 2:1518, 1987.

107. Committee on Safety of Medicines: Propofol. Curr Probl 20, 1987.

108. Ebrahim ZY, Schubert A, Van Ness P, et al: The effect of propofol on the electroencephalogram of patients with epilepsy. Anesth Analg 78:275-279, 1994.

109. Samra SK, Sneyd JR, Ross DA, Henry TR: Effects of propofol sedation on seizures and intracranially recorded epileptiform activity in patients with partial epilepsy. Anesthesiology 82:843-851, 1995.

110. Anonymous: Convulsions after propofol. Pharm J 249:745, 1992.

111. Deer TR, Rich GF: Propofol tolerance in a pediatric patient. Anesthesiology 77:828-829, 1992.

112. Boyle W, Shear J, White P: Tolerance and hyperlipemia during long term sedation with propofol. Anesthesiology 73:A245, 1990.

113. Follette JW, Farley WJ: Anesthesiologist addicted to propofol. Anesthesiology 77:817-818, 1992.

114. Mendes PM, Silberstein SD, Young WB, et al: Intravenous propofol in the treatment of refractory headache. Headache 42:638-641, 2002.

115. Stephan H, Sonntag H, Schenk HD, Kohlhausen S: Effect of Disoprivan (propofol) on the circulation and oxygen consumption of the brain and CO_2 reactivity of brain vessels in the human [in German]. Anaesthesist 36:60-65, 1987.

116. Hartung HJ: Intracranial pressure in patients with cranio-cerebral trauma after administration of propofol and thiopental [in German]. Anaesthesist 36:285-287, 1987.

117. Hartung HJ: Modification of intracranial pressure by propofol (Disoprivan). Initial results [in German]. Anaesthesist 36:66-68, 1987.

118. Ravussin P, Guinard JP, Ralley F, Thorin D: Effect of propofol on cerebrospinal fluid pressure and cerebral perfusion pressure in patients undergoing craniotomy. Anaesthesia 43(Suppl):37-41, 1988.

119. Vandesteene A, Trempont V, Engelman E, et al: Effect of propofol on cerebral blood flow and metabolism in man. Anaesthesia 43(Suppl):42-43, 1988.

120. Herregods L, Verbeke J, Rolly G, Colardyn F: Effect of propofol on elevated intracranial pressure. Preliminary results. Anaesthesia 43(Suppl):107-109, 1988.

121. Mirakhur R, Shepherd W: Intraocular pressure changes with propofol ('Diprivan'): Comparison with thiopentone. Postgrad Med J 61(Suppl 3):41-44, 1985.

122. Mirakhur RK, Shepherd WF, Darrah WC: Propofol or thiopentone: Effects on intraocular pressure associated with induction of anaesthesia and tracheal intubation (facilitated with suxamethonium). Br J Anaesth 59:431-436, 1987.

123. Enns J, Gelb A, Manninen P: Cerebral autoregulation is maintained during propofol–nitrous oxide anaesthesia in humans. Can J Anaesth 39:A43, 1992.

124. Jansen G, Kagenaar D, Kedaria M: Effects of propofol on the relation between CO_2 and cerebral blood flow velocity. Anesth Analg 76:S163, 1993.

125. Newman MF, Murkin JM, Roach G, et al: Cerebral physio-logic effects of burst suppression doses of propofol during nonpulsatile cardiopulmonary bypass. CNS Subgroup of McSPI. Anesth Analg 81:452-457, 1995.

126. Kochs E, Hoffman WE, Werner C, et al: The effects of propofol on brain electrical activity, neurologic outcome, and neuronal damage following incomplete ischemia in rats. Anesthesiology 76:245-252, 1992.

127. Gelb A, Zhang C, Henderson S: A comparison of the cerebral protective effects of propofol, thiopental, and halothane in temporary feline focal cerebral ischemia. Anesth Analg 76:S115, 1993.

128. Ridenour TR, Warner DS, Todd MM, Gionet TX: Comparative effects of propofol and halothane on outcome from temporary middle cerebral artery occlusion in the rat. Anesthesiology 76:807-812, 1992.

129. Gelb AW, Bayona NA, Wilson JX, Cechetto DF: Propofol anesthesia compared to awake reduces infarct size in rats. Anesthesiology 96:1183-1190, 2002.

130. Bhardwaj A, Castro IA, Alkayed NJ, et al: Anesthetic choice of halothane versus propofol: Impact on experimental perioperative stroke. Stroke 32:1920-1925, 2001.

131. Kaptanoglu E, Sen S, Beskonakli E, et al: Antioxidant actions and early ultrastructural findings of thiopental and propofol in experimental spinal cord injury. J Neurosurg Anesthesiol 14:114-122, 2002.

132. Amorim P, Chambers G, Cottrell J, Kass IS: Propofol reduces neuronal transmission damage and attenuates the changes in calcium, potassium, and sodium during hyperthermic anoxia in the rat hippocampal slice. Anesthesiology 83:1254-1265, 1995.

133. Ergun R, Adkemir G, Sen S, et al: Neuroprotective effects of propofol following global cerebral ischemia in rats. Neurosurg Rev 25:95-98, 2002.

134. Lanigan C, Sury M, Bingham R, et al: Neurological sequelae in children after prolonged propofol infusion. Anaesthesia 47:810-811, 1992.

135. Trotter C, Serpell MG: Neurological sequelae in children after prolonged propofol infusion. Anaesthesia 47:340-342, 1992.

136. Spahr-Schopfer I, Vutskits L, Toni N, et al: Differential neurotoxic effects of propofol on dissociated cortical cells and organotypic hippocampal cultures. Anesthesiology 92:1408-1417, 2000.

137. Vuyk J, Engbers FH, Lemmens HJ, et al: Pharmacodynamics of propofol in female patients. Anesthesiology 77:3-9, 1992.

138. Forrest FC, Tooley MA, Saunders PR, Prys-Roberts C: Propofol infusion and the suppression of consciousness: The EEG and dose requirements. Br J Anaesth 72:35-41, 1994.

139. Turtle MJ, Cullen P, Prys-Roberts C, et al: Dose requirements of propofol by infusion during nitrous oxide anaesthesia in man. II: Patients premedicated with lorazepam. Br J Anaesth 59:283-287, 1987.

140. Spelina KR, Coates DP, Monk CR, et al: Dose requirements of propofol by infusion during nitrous oxide anaesthesia in man. I: Patients premedicated with morphine sulphate. Br J Anaesth 58:1080-1084, 1986.

141. Sanderson JH, Blades JF: Multicentre study of propofol in day case surgery. Anaesthesia 43(Suppl):70-73, 1988.

142. Kazama T, Ikeda K, Morita K, Sanjo Y: Awakening propofol concentration with and without blood–effect site equilibration after short-term and long-term administration of propofol and fentanyl anesthesia. Anesthesiology 88:928-934, 1998.

143. Taylor MB, Grounds RM, Mulrooney PD, Morgan M: Ventilatory effects of propofol during induction of anaesthesia. Comparison with thiopentone. Anaesthesia 41:816-820, 1986.

144. Goodman NW, Black AM, Carter JA: Some ventilatory effects of propofol as sole anaesthetic agent. Br J Anaesth 59:1497-1503, 1987.

145. Gold MI, Abraham EC, Herrington C: A controlled investigation of propofol, thiopentone and methohexitone. Can J Anaesth 34:478-483, 1987.

146. Munson ES, Larson CP Jr, Babad AA, et al: The effects of halothane, fluroxene and cyclopropane on ventilation: A comparative study in man. Anesthesiology 27:716-728, 1966.

147. Knill RL, Clement JL, Gelb AW: Ventilatory responses mediated by peripheral chemoreceptors in anesthetized man. Adv Exp Med Biol 99:67-77, 1978.

148. Aun C, Major E: The cardiorespiratory effects of ICI 35 868 in patients with valvular heart disease. Anaesthesia 39:1096-1100, 1984.

149. Grounds RM, Twigley AJ, Carli F, et al: The haemodynamic effects of intravenous induction. Comparison of the effects of thiopentone and propofol. Anaesthesia 40:735-740, 1985.

150. Al-Khudhairi D, Gordon G, Morgan M, Whitwam JG: Acute cardiovascular changes following disoprofol. Effects in heavily sedated patients with coronary artery disease. Anaesthesia 37:1007-1010, 1982.

151. Coates DP, Monk CR, Prys-Roberts C, Turtle M: Hemodynamic effects of infusions of the emulsion formulation of propofol during nitrous oxide anaesthesia in humans. Anesth Analg 66:64-70, 1987.

152. Blouin R, Seifert H, Conrad P: Propofol significantly depresses hypoxic ventilatory drive during conscious sedation. Anesthesiology 77:A1215, 1992.

153. Conti G, Dell'Utri D, Vilardi V, et al: Propofol induces bronchodilation in mechanically ventilated chronic obstructive pulmonary disease (COPD) patients. Acta Anaesthesiol Scand 37:105-109, 1993.

154. Mehr E, Hirshman C, Lindeman K: The effect of halothane, propofol and thiopental on peripheral airway reactivity. Anesthesiology 77:A1212, 1992.

155. Brown RH, Wagner EM: Mechanisms of bronchoprotection by anesthetic induction agents: Propofol versus ketamine. Anesthesiology 90:822-828, 1999.

156. Lin CC, Shyr MH, Tan PP, et al: Mechanisms underlying the inhibitory effect of propofol on the contraction of canine airway smooth muscle. Anesthesiology 91:750-759, 1999.

157. Brown RH, Greenberg RS, Wagner EM: Efficacy of propofol to prevent bronchoconstriction: Effects of preservative. Anesthesiology 94:851-855, discussion 6A, 2001.

158. Basu S, Mutschler DK, Larsson AO, et al: Propofol (Diprivan-EDTA) counteracts oxidative injury and deterioration of the arterial oxygen tension during experimental septic shock. Resuscitation 50:341-348, 2001.

159. Chang H, Tsai SY, Chang Y, et al: Therapeutic concentrations of propofol protect mouse macrophages from nitric oxide–induced cell death and apoptosis. Can J Anaesth 49:477-480, 2002.

160. Kondo U, Kim SO, Murray PA: Propofol selectively attenuates endothelium-dependent pulmonary vasodilation in chronically instrumented dogs. Anesthesiology 93:437-446, 2000.

161. Horibe M, Ogawa K, Sohn JT, Murray PA: Propofol attenuates acetylcholine-induced pulmonary vasorelaxation: Role of nitric oxide and endothelium-derived hyperpolarizing factors. Anesthesiology 93:447-455, 2000.

162. Larsen R, Rathgeber J, Bagdahn A, et al: Effects of propofol on cardiovascular dynamics and coronary blood flow in geriatric patients. A comparison with etomidate. Anaesthesia 43(Suppl):25-31, 1988.

163. Vermeyen KM, Erpels FA, Janssen LA, et al: Propofol-fentanyl anaesthesia for coronary bypass surgery in patients with good left ventricular function. Br J Anaesth 59:1115-1120, 1987.

164. Patrick MR, Blair I, Feneck RO, Sebel PS: A comparison of the haemodynamic effects of propofol ('Diprivan') and thiopentone in patients with coronary artery disease. Postgrad Med J 61(Suppl 3):23-27, 1985.

165. Stephan H, Sonntag H, Schenk HD, et al: Effects of propofol on cardiovascular dynamics, myocardial blood flow and myocardial metabolism in patients with coronary artery disease. Br J Anaesth 58:969-975, 1986.

166. Coates D, Prys-Roberts C, Spelina K: Propofol ('Diprivan') by intravenous infusion with nitrous oxide: Dose requirements and haemodynamic effects. Postgrad Med J 61(Suppl 3):76-79, 1985.

167. Claeys MA, Gepts E, Camu F: Haemodynamic changes during anaesthesia induced and maintained with propofol. Br J Anaesth 60:3-9, 1983.

168. Van Aken H, Meinshausen E, Prien T, et al: The influence of fentanyl and tracheal intubation on the hemodynamic effects of anesthesia induction with propofol/N_2O in humans. Anesthesiology 68:157-163, 1988.

169. Samuelson PN, Reves JG, Kouchoukos NT, et al: Hemodynamic responses to anesthetic induction with midazolam or diazepam in patients with ischemic heart disease. Anesth Analg 60:802-809, 1981.
170. Rao S, Sherbaniuk RW, Prasad K, et al: Cardiopulmonary effects of diazepam. Clin Pharmacol Ther 14:182-189, 1973.
171. Samuelson PN, Lell WA, Kouchoukos NT, et al: Hemodynamics during diazepam induction of anesthesia for coronary artery bypass grafting. South Med J 73:332-334, 1980.
172. Dhadphale P, Behrendt D, Jackson P: The effect of diazepam on contractility in the intact human heart [abstract]. Paper presented at the annual meeting of the American Society of Anesthesiology, 1977, New Orleans.
173. Prakash R, Thurer R, Vargas A: Cardiovascular effects of diazepam induction in patients for aortocoronary saphenous vein bypass grafts [abstract]. Paper presented at the annual meeting of the American Society of Anesthesiology, 1976.
174. Jackson AP, Dhadphale PR, Callaghan ML, Alseri S: Haemodynamic studies during induction of anaesthesia for open-heart surgery using diazepam and ketamine. Br J Anaesth 50:375-378, 1978.
175. Prys-Roberts C, Kelman GR: The influence of drugs used in neuroleptanalgesia on cardiovascular and ventilatory function. Br J Anaesth 39:134-145, 1967.
176. Israel J, Jansen G, Dobkin A: Circulatory and respiratory response to tilt with pentazocine (Win 20, 228), droperidol (R4749), droperidol-fentanyl (Innovar), and methotrimeprazine in normal healthy male subjects. Anesthesiology 26:253, 1965.
177. Colvin MP, Savege TM, Newland PE, et al: Cardiorespiratory changes following induction of anaesthesia with etomidate in patients with cardiac disease. Br J Anaesth 51:551-556, 1979.
178. Gooding JM, Weng JT, Smith RA, et al: Cardiovascular and pulmonary responses following etomidate induction of anesthesia in patients with demonstrated cardiac disease. Anesth Analg 58:40-41, 1979.
179. Gooding JM, Corssen G: Effect of etomidate on the cardiovascular system. Anesth Analg 56:717-719, 1977.
180. Kettler D, Sonntag H, Donath U, et al: Haemodynamics, myocardial mechanics, oxygen requirement and oxygenation of the human heart during induction of anaesthesia with etomidate [in German]. Anaesthesist 23:116-121, 1974.
181. Tweed WA, Minuck M, Mymin D: Circulatory responses to ketamine anesthesia. Anesthesiology 37:613-619, 1972.
182. Tweed WA, Mymin D: Myocardial force-velocity relations during ketamine anesthesia at constant heart rate. Anesthesiology 41:49-52, 1974.
183. Nishimura K, Kitamura Y, Hamai R, et al: Pharmacological studies of ketamine hydrochloride in the cardiovascular system. Osaka City Med J 19:17-26, 1973.
184. Ruff R, Reves JG: Hemodynamic effects of a lorazepam-fentanyl anesthetic induction for coronary artery bypass surgery. J Cardiothorac Anesth 4:314-317, 1990.
185. Lebowitz PW, Cote ME, Daniels AL, et al: Comparative cardiovascular effects of midazolam and thiopental in healthy patients. Anesth Analg 61:771-775, 1982.
186. Lebowitz P, Cote M, Daniels A: Cardiovascular effects of midazolam and thiopentone for induction of anesthesia in ill surgical patients. Can J Anaesth 30:19-23, 1983.
187. Marty J, Nitenberg A, Blanchet F, et al: Effects of midazolam on the coronary circulation in patients with coronary artery disease. Anesthesiology 64:206-210, 1986.
188. Wahr JA, Plunkett JJ, Ramsay JG, et al: Cardiovascular responses during sedation after coronary revascularization. Incidence of myocardial ischemia and hemodynamic episodes with propofol versus midazolam. Institutions of the McSPI Research Group. Anesthesiology 84:1350-1360, 1996.
189. Graham MR, Thiessen DB, Mutch WA: Left ventricular systolic and diastolic function is unaltered during propofol infusion in newborn swine. Anesth Analg 86:717-723, 1998.
190. Lejay M, Hanouz JL, Lecarpentier Y, et al: Modifications of the inotropic responses to alpha- and beta-adrenoceptor stimulation by propofol in rat myocardium. Anesth Analg 87:277-283, 1998.
191. Pagel PS, Warltier DC: Negative inotropic effects of propofol as evaluated by the regional preload recruitable stroke work relationship in chronically instrumented dogs. Anesthesiology 78:100-108, 1993.
192. Ebert T, Muzi M, Goff D: Does propofol really preserve baroreflex function in humans? Anesthesiology 77:A337, 1992.
193. Xuan YT, Glass PS: Propofol regulation of calcium entry pathways in cultured A10 and rat aortic smooth muscle cells. Br J Pharmacol 117:5-12, 1996.
194. Chang KS, Davis RF: Propofol produces endothelium-independent vasodilation and may act as a Ca^{2+} channel blocker. Anesth Analg 76:24-32, 1993.
195. Yamashita A, Kajikuri J, Ohashi M, et al: Inhibitory effects of propofol on acetylcholine-induced, endothelium-dependent relaxation and prostacyclin synthesis in rabbit mesenteric resistance arteries. Anesthesiology 91:1080-1089, 1999.
196. Samain E, Bouillier H, Marty J, et al: The effect of propofol on angiotensin II–induced Ca(2+) mobilization in aortic smooth muscle cells from normotensive and hypertensive rats. Anesth Analg 90:546-552, 2000.
197. Doursout MF, Joseph PM, Liang YY, et al: Role of propofol and its solvent, Intralipid, in nitric oxide–induced peripheral vasodilatation in dogs. Br J Anaesth 89:492-498, 2002.
198. Ebert TJ, Muzi M, Berens R, et al: Sympathetic responses to induction of anesthesia in humans with propofol or etomidate. Anesthesiology 76:725-733, 1992.
199. Cullen PM, Turtle M, Prys-Roberts C, et al: Effect of propofol anesthesia on baroreflex activity in humans. Anesth Analg 66:1115-1120, 1987.
200. Kanaya N, Hirata N, Kurosawa S, et al: Differential effects of propofol and sevoflurane on heart rate variability. Anesthesiology 98:34-40, 2003.
201. Sharpe MD, Dobkowski WB, Murkin JM, et al: Propofol has no direct effect on sinoatrial node function or on normal atrioventricular and accessory pathway conduction in Wolff-Parkinson-White syndrome during alfentanil/midazolam anesthesia. Anesthesiology 82:888-895, 1995.
202. Horiguchi T, Nishikawa T: Heart rate response to intravenous atropine during propofol anesthesia. Anesth Analg 95:389-392, 2002.
203. Wu M: Propofol and the supraventricular tachydysrhythmias in children. Anesth Analg 86:914, 1998.
204. Ebert TJ, Muzi M: Propofol and autonomic reflex function in humans. Anesth Analg 78:369-375, 1994.
205. Ko SH, Yu CW, Lee SK, et al: Propofol attenuates ischemia-reperfusion injury in the isolated rat heart. Anesth Analg 85:719-724, 1997.
206. Kokita N, Hara A, Abiko Y, et al: Propofol improves functional and metabolic recovery in ischemic reperfused isolated rat hearts. Anesth Analg 86:252-258, 1998.
207. DeGrood P, VanEgmond J, VandeWetering M: Lack of effects of emulsified propofol (Diprivan) on vecuronium pharmacodynamics: Preliminary results in man. Postgrad Med J 61:28, 1985.
208. Nightingale P, Petts NV, Healy TE, et al: Induction of anaesthesia with propofol ('Diprivan') or thiopentone and interactions with suxamethonium, atracurium and vecuronium. Postgrad Med J 61(Suppl 3):31-34, 1985.
209. McKeating K, Bali IM, Dundee JW: The effects of thiopentone and propofol on upper airway integrity. Anaesthesia 43:638-640, 1988.
210. Richardson J: Propofol infusion for coronary artery bypass surgery in a patient with suspected malignant hyperpyrexia. Anaesthesia 42:1125, 1987.
211. Denborough M, Hopkinson KC: Propofol and malignant hyperpyrexia. Lancet 1:191, 1988.
212. Van Hemelrijck J, Weekers F, Van Aken H, et al: Propofol anesthesia does not inhibit stimulation of cortisol synthesis. Anesth Analg 80:573-576, 1995.

213. Stark RD, Binks SM, Dutka VN, et al: A review of the safety and tolerance of propofol (Diprivan). Postgrad Med J 61(Suppl 3):152-156, 1985.

214. Robinson F: Propofol ('Diprivan') by intermittent bolus with nitrous oxide in oxygen for body surface operations. Postgrad Med J 61(Suppl 3):116-119, 1985.

215. Sear JW, Uppington J, Kay NH: Haemotological and biochemical changes during anaesthesia with propofol ('Diprivan'). Postgrad Med J 61(Suppl 3):165-168, 1985.

216. Aviram M, Deckelbaum RJ: Intralipid infusion into humans reduces in vitro platelet aggregation and alters platelet lipid composition. Metabolism 38:343-347, 1989.

217. Laxenaire MC, Mata-Bermejo E, Moneret-Vautrin DA, Gueant JL: Life-threatening anaphylactoid reactions to propofol (Diprivan). Anesthesiology 77:275-280, 1992.

218. Doenicke A, Lorenz W, Stanworth D, et al: Effects of propofol ('Diprivan') on histamine release, immunoglobulin levels and activation of complement in healthy volunteers. Postgrad Med J 61(Suppl 3):15-20, 1985.

219. McCollum JS, Milligan KR, Dundee JW: The antiemetic action of propofol. Anaesthesia 43:239-240, 1988.

220. Borgeat A, Wilder-Smith OH, Saiah M, Rifat K: Subhypnotic doses of propofol relieve pruritus induced by epidural and intrathecal morphine. Anesthesiology 76:510-512, 1992.

221. Schulman SR, Rockett CB, Canada AT, Glass PS: Long-term propofol infusion for refractory postoperative nausea: A case report with quantitative propofol analysis. Anesth Analg 80:636-637, 1995.

222. Gan TJ, Glass PS, Howell ST, et al: Determination of plasma concentrations of propofol associated with 50% reduction in postoperative nausea. Anesthesiology 87:779-784, 1997.

223. Gan TJ, Ginsberg B, Grant AP, Glass PS: Double-blind, randomized comparison of ondansetron and intraoperative propofol to prevent postoperative nausea and vomiting. Anesthesiology 85:1036-1042, 1996.

224. Borgeat A, WilderSmith O, Rifat K: Adjuvant propofol is effective in preventing refractory chemotherapy associated nausea and vomiting. Anesthesiology 77:A344, 1992.

225. Appadu BL, Strange PG, Lambert DG: Does propofol interact with D_2 dopamine receptors? Anesth Analg 79:1191-1192, 1994.

226. Saiah M, Borgeat A, Wilder-Smith OH, et al: Epidural-morphine–induced pruritus: Propofol versus naloxone. Anesth Analg 78:1110-1113, 1994.

227. Leslie K, Sessler DI, Bjorksten AR, et al: Propofol causes a dose-dependent decrease in the thermoregulatory threshold for vasoconstriction but has little effect on sweating. Anesthesiology 81:353-360, 1994.

228. Skoutelis A, Lianou P, Papageorgiou E, et al: Effects of propofol and thiopentone on polymorphonuclear leukocyte functions in vitro. Acta Anaesthesiol Scand 38:858-862, 1994.

229. Krumholz W, Endrass J, Hempelmann G: Propofol inhibits phagocytosis and killing of *Staphylococcus aureus* and *Escherichia coli* by polymorphonuclear leukocytes in vitro. Can J Anaesth 41:446-449, 1994.

230. Bennett SN, McNeil MM, Bland LA, et al: Postoperative infections traced to contamination of an intravenous anesthetic, propofol. N Engl J Med 333:147-154, 1995.

231. Mammoto T, Mukai M, Mammoto A, et al: Intravenous anesthetic, propofol inhibits invasion of cancer cells. Cancer Lett 184:165-170, 2002.

232. Donmez A, Arslan G, Pirat A, Demirhan B: Is pancreatitis a complication of propofol infusion? Eur J Anaesthesiol 16:367-370, 1999.

233. Cummings GC, Dixon J, Kay NH, et al: Dose requirements of ICI 35,868 (propofol, 'Diprivan') in a new formulation for induction of anaesthesia. Anaesthesia 39:1168-1171, 1984.

234. Kay B, Stephenson DK: Dose-response relationship for disoprofol (ICI 35868 Diprivan). Comparison with methohexitone. Anaesthesia 36:863-867, 1981.

235. Rutter DV, Morgan M, Lumley J, Owen R: ICI 35868 (Diprivan): A new intravenous induction agent. A comparison with methohexitone. Anaesthesia 35:1188-1192, 1980.

236. Kazama T, Morita K, Ikeda T, et al: Comparison of predicted induction dose with predetermined physiologic characteristics of patients and with pharmacokinetic models incorporating those characteristics as covariates. Anesthesiology 98:299-305, 2003.

237. Briggs LP, White M: The effects of premedication on anaesthesia with propofol ('Diprivan'). Postgrad Med J 61(Suppl 3):35-37, 1985.

238. Steib A, Freys G, Beller JP, et al: Propofol in elderly high risk patients. A comparison of haemodynamic effects with thiopentone during induction of anaesthesia. Anaesthesia 43(Suppl):111-114, 1988.

239. Kazama T, Ikeda K, Morita K, et al: Investigation of effective anesthesia induction doses using a wide range of infusion rates with undiluted and diluted propofol. Anesthesiology 92:1017-1028, 2000.

240. Purcell-Jones G, Yates A, Baker JR, James IG: Comparison of the induction characteristics of thiopentone and propofol in children. Br J Anaesth 59:1431-1436, 1987.

241. Mirakhur RK: Induction characteristics of propofol in children: Comparison with thiopentone. Anaesthesia 43:593-598, 1988.

242. Doze VA, Shafer A, White PF: Propofol–nitrous oxide versus thiopental-isoflurane–nitrous oxide for general anesthesia. Anesthesiology 69:63-71, 1988.

243. Heath PJ, Kennedy DJ, Ogg TW, et al: Which intravenous induction agent for day surgery? A comparison of propofol, thiopentone, methohexitone and etomidate. Anaesthesia 43:365-368, 1988.

244. Mackenzie N, Grant IS: Propofol ('Diprivan') for continuous intravenous anaesthesia. A comparison with methohexitone. Postgrad Med J 61(Suppl 3):70-75, 1985.

245. Doze VA, Westphal LM, White PF: Comparison of propofol with methohexital for outpatient anesthesia. Anesth Analg 65:1189-1195, 1986.

246. Kay B: Propofol and alfentanil infusion. A comparison with methohexitone and alfentanil for major surgery. Anaesthesia 41:589-595, 1986.

247. Sear JW, Shaw I, Wolf A, Kay NH: Infusions of propofol to supplement nitrous oxide–oxygen for the maintenance of anaesthesia. A comparison with halothane. Anaesthesia 43(Suppl):18-22, 1988.

248. Van Hemelrijck J, Smith I, White PF: Use of desflurane for outpatient anesthesia. A comparison with propofol and nitrous oxide. Anesthesiology 75:197-203, 1991.

249. Roberts FL, Dixon J, Lewis GT, et al: Induction and maintenance of propofol anaesthesia. A manual infusion scheme. Anaesthesia 43(Suppl):14-17, 1988.

250. Thomas VL, Sutton DN, Saunders DA: The effect of fentanyl on propofol requirements for day case anaesthesia. Anaesthesia 43(Suppl):73-75, 1988.

251. Fehr SB, Zalunardo MP, Seifert B, et al: Clonidine decreases propofol requirements during anaesthesia: Effect on bispectral index. Br J Anaesth 86:627-632, 2001.

252. Wilder-Smith OH, Ravussin PA, Decosterd LA, et al: Midazolam premedication reduces propofol dose requirements for multiple anesthetic endpoints. Can J Anaesth 48:439-445, 2001.

253. Hentgen E, Houfani M, Billard V, et al: Propofol-sufentanil anesthesia for thyroid surgery: Optimal concentrations for hemodynamic and electroencephalogram stability, and recovery features. Anesth Analg 95:597-605, 2002.

254. Taylor IN, Kenny GN, Glen JB: Pharmacodynamic stability of a mixture of propofol and alfentanil. Br J Anaesth 69:168-171, 1992.

255. Hilton P, Dev VJ, Major E: Intravenous anaesthesia with propofol and alfentanil. The influence of age and weight. Anaesthesia 41:640-643, 1986.

256. Schuttler J, Kloos S, Roepcke H: Age dependent dose requirements of propofol in total intravenous anesthesia as quantified by closed-loop EEG feedback infusion strategies. Anesthesiology 77:A338, 1992.

257. Schuttler J, Kloos S, Schwilden H, Stoeckel H: Total intravenous anaesthesia with propofol and alfentanil by computer-assisted infusion. Anaesthesia 43(Suppl):2-7, 1988.

258. Tackley R, Lewis G, Prys-Roberts C: Open loop control of propofol infusions [abstract]. Br J Anaesth 59:935, 1987.

259. Visser K, Hassink EA, Bonsel GJ, et al: Randomized controlled trial of total intravenous anesthesia with propofol versus inhalation anesthesia with isoflurane–nitrous oxide: Postoperative nausea with vomiting and economic analysis. Anesthesiology 95:616-626, 2001.

260. Dexter F, Tinker JH: Comparisons between desflurane and isoflurane or propofol on time to following commands and time to discharge. A metaanalysis. Anesthesiology 83:77-82, 1995.

261. Russell GN, Wright EL, Fox MA, et al: Propofol-fentanyl anaesthesia for coronary artery surgery and cardiopulmonary bypass. Anaesthesia 44:205-208, 1989.

262. Mora C, Dudek C, Epstein R: Cardiac anesthesia techniques, fentanyl alone or in combination with enflurane or propofol. Anesth Analg 68:S202, 1989.

263. Underwood SM, Davies SW, Feneck RO, Walesby RK: Anaesthesia for myocardial revascularisation. A comparison of fentanyl/propofol with fentanyl/enflurane. Anaesthesia 47:939-945, 1992.

264. Hall RI, Murphy JT, Moffitt EA, et al: A comparison of the myocardial metabolic and haemodynamic changes produced by propofol-sufentanil and enflurane-sufentanil anaesthesia for patients having coronary artery bypass graft surgery. Can J Anaesth 38:996-1004, 1991.

265. Fanard L, Van Steenberge A, Demeire X, van der Puyl F: Comparison between propofol and midazolam as sedative agents for surgery under regional anaesthesia. Anaesthesia 43(Suppl):87-89, 1988.

266. Gepts E, Claeys MA, Camu F, Smekens L: Infusion of propofol ('Diprivan') as sedative technique for colonoscopies. Postgrad Med J 61(Suppl 3):120-126, 1987.

267. Newman LH, McDonald JC, Wallace PG, Ledingham IM: Propofol infusion for sedation in intensive care. Anaesthesia 42:929-937, 1987.

268. Grounds R, Lalor J, Lumley J: Propofol infusion for sedation in the intensive care unit: Preliminary report. BMJ (Clin Res Ed) 294:397-400, 1987.

269. Beller JP, Pottecher T, Mangin P, et al: Prolonged sedation with propofol in resuscitation. Recovery and pharmacokinetic study. Preliminary results [in French]. Ann Fr Anesth Reanim 6:334-335, 1987.

270. Beller JP, Pottecher T, Lugnier A, et al: Prolonged sedation with propofol in ICU patients: Recovery and blood concentration changes during periodic interruptions in infusion. Br J Anaesth 61:583-588, 1988.

271. Parke TJ, Stevens JE, Rice AS, et al: Metabolic acidosis and fatal myocardial failure after propofol infusion in children: Five case reports. BMJ 305:613-616, 1992.

272. Murphy PG, Myers DS, Davies MJ, et al: The antioxidant potential of propofol (2,6-diisopropylphenol). Br J Anaesth 68:613-618, 1992.

273. Chong JL, Grebenik C, Sinclair M, et al: The effect of a cardiac surgical recovery area on the timing of extubation. J Cardiothorac Vasc Anesth 7:137-141, 1993.

274. Rudkin GE, Osborne GA, Finn BP, et al: Intra-operative patient-controlled sedation. Comparison of patient-controlled propofol with patient-controlled midazolam. Anaesthesia 47:376-381, 1992.

275. Canessa R, Lema G, Urzua J, et al: Anesthesia for elective cardioversion: A comparison of four anesthetic agents. J Cardiothorac Vasc Anesth 5:566-568, 1991.

276. Kang TM: Propofol infusion syndrome in critically ill patients. Ann Pharmacother 36:1453-1456, 2002.

277. Wolf A, Weir P, Segar P, et al: Impaired fatty acid oxidation in propofol infusion syndrome. Lancet 357:606-607, 2001.

278. Dundee JW, McIlroy PD: The history of barbiturates. Anaesthesia 37:726-734, 1982.

279. Ball C, Westhorpe R: The history of intravenous anaesthesia: The barbiturates. Part 1. Anaesth Intensive Care 29:97, 2001.

280. Redonnet T: Recherches comparatives sur l'action pharmacodynamique des derives de l'acide barbiturique. Arch Int Pharmacodyn Ther 25:27, 1920.

281. Bardet G, Bardet D: Contribution a l'etudes des hypnotiques ureiques; action et utilisation du diethyl-diallyl-barbiturate de diethyl-amine. Bull Gen Ther Med Chir Obstet Pharm 172:173, 1921.

282. Weese H, Scharpf W: Evipan; ein neuartiges Einschlafmittel. Dtsch Med Wochenschr 58:1205, 1932.

283. Ball C, Westhorpe R: The history of intravenous anaesthesia: The barbiturates. Part 2. Anaesth Intensive Care 29:219, 2001.

284. Tabern T, Volwiler E: Sulfur-containing barbiturate hypnotics. J Am Chem Soc 57:1961, 1935.

285. Corssen G, Reves J, Stanley T: Dissociative anesthesia. In Corssen G, Reves J, Stanley T (eds): Intravenous Anesthesia and Analgesia. Philadelphia, Lea & Febiger, 1988, p 99.

286. Halford F: A critique of intravenous anaesthesia in war surgery. Anesthesiology 4:67-69, 1943.

287. Adams R: Intravenous Anesthesia. New York, Paul B Hoeber, 1944.

288. Dundee J, Wyant G: Intravenous Anaesthesia. Edinburgh, Churchill Livingstone, 1974.

289. Mahisekar UL, Callan CM, Derasari M, Kirkpatrick AF: Infusion of large particles of thiopental sodium during anesthesia induction. J Clin Anesth 6:55-58, 1994.

290. Wahlstrom G: Differences in anaesthetic properties between optical antipodes of hexobarbital in the rat. Life Sci 5:1781-1790, 1966.

291. Andrews PR, Mark LC: Structural specificity of barbiturates and related drugs. Anesthesiology 57:314-320, 1982.

292. Nguyen KT, Stephens DP, McLeish MJ, et al: Pharmacokinetics of thiopental and pentobarbital enantiomers after intravenous administration of racemic thiopental. Anesth Analg 83:552-558, 1996.

293. Wahlstrom G, Buch H, Buzello W: Unequal anaesthetic potency despite equal brain concentration of hexobarbital antipodes. Acta Pharmacol Toxicol 28:493-498, 1970.

294. Christensen H, Lee I: Anesthetic potency and acute toxicity of optically active disubstituted barbituric acids. Toxicol Appl Pharmacol 26:495-503, 1973.

295. Raventos J: The distribution in the body and metabolic fate of barbiturates. J Pharm Pharmacol 6:217, 1954.

296. Mark L: Metabolism of barbiturates in man. Clin Pharmacol Ther 4:504, 1963.

297. Granik S: Induction of the synthesis of d-amino-levulinic acid synthetase in liver parenchyma cells in culture by chemicals that induce acute porphyria. J Biol Chem 238:PC2247, 1963.

298. Sharpless S: Hypnotics and sedatives. In Goodman LS, Limbird LE, Milinoff PB, et al (eds): The Pharmacological Basis of Therapeutics. New York, MacMillan, 1970.

299. Waddell WJ, Butler TC: The distribution and excretion of phenobarbital. J Clin Invest 36:1217-1226, 1957.

300. Henthorn T, Avram M, Krejcie T: Intravascular mixing and drug distribution: The concurrent disposition of thiopental and indocyanine green. Clin Pharmacol Ther 45:56-65, 1989.

301. Price HL: A dynamic concept of the distribution of thiopental in the human body. Anesthesiology 21:40-45, 1960.

302. Burch P, Stanski D: The role of metabolism and protein binding in thiopental anesthesia. Anesthesiology 58:146-152, 1983.

303. Morgan DJ, Blackman GL, Paull JD, Wolf LJ: Pharmacokinetics and plasma binding of thiopental. II: Studies at cesarean section. Anesthesiology 54:474-480, 1981.

304. Pandele G, Chaux F, Salvadori C, et al: Thiopental pharmacokinetics in patients with cirrhosis. Anesthesiology 59:123-126, 1983.

305. Toner W, Howard PJ, McGowan WA, Dundee JW: Another look at acute tolerance to thiopentone. Br J Anaesth 52:1005-1008, 1980.

306. Jung D, Mayersohn M, Perrier D, et al: Thiopental disposition in lean and obese patients undergoing surgery. Anesthesiology 56:269-274, 1982.

307. Downie DL, Franks NP, Lieb WR: Effects of thiopental and its optical isomers on nicotinic acetylcholine receptors. Anesthesiology 93:774-783, 2000.

308. Tomlin SL, Jenkins A, Lieb WR, Franks NP: Preparation of

barbiturate optical isomers and their effects on GABA(A) receptors. Anesthesiology 90:1714-1722, 1999.

309. Judge S: Effect of general anaesthetics on synaptic ion channels. Br J Anaesth 55:191-200, 1983.

310. Tanelian DL, Kosek P, Mody I, MacIver MB: The role of the GABA$_A$ receptor/chloride channel complex in anesthesia. Anesthesiology 78:757-776, 1993.

311. Snyder SH: Drug and neurotransmitter receptors in the brain. Science 224:22-31, 1984.

312. Sloan T: Anesthesics and the brain. Anesthesiol Clin North Am 20:265-292, 2002.

313. Michenfelder JD, Milde JH, Sundt TM Jr: Cerebral protection by barbiturate anesthesia. Use after middle cerebral artery occlusion in Java monkeys. Arch Neurol 33:345-350, 1976.

314. Michenfelder JD, Theye RA: Cerebral protection by thiopental during hypoxia. Anesthesiology 39:510-517, 1973.

315. Michenfelder JD: The interdependency of cerebral functional and metabolic effects following massive doses of thiopental in the dog. Anesthesiology 41:231-236, 1974.

316. Stullken EH Jr, Milde JH, Michenfelder JD, Tinker JH: The nonlinear responses of cerebral metabolism to low concentrations of halothane, enflurane, isoflurane, and thiopental. Anesthesiology 46:28-34, 1977.

317. Baughman VL: Brain protection during neurosurgery. Anesthesiol Clin North Am 20:315-327, 2002.

318. Albrecht RF, Miletich DJ, Rosenberg R, Zahed B: Cerebral blood flow and metabolic changes from induction to onset of anesthesia with halothane or pentobarbital. Anesthesiology 47:252-256, 1977.

319. Dundee JW: Alterations in response to somatic pain associated with anaesthesia. II: The effect of thiopentone and pentobarbitone. Br J Anaesth 32:407-414, 1960.

320. Pancrazio JJ, Frazer MJ, Lynch C 3rd: Barbiturate anesthetics depress the resting K$^+$ conductance of myocardium. J Pharmacol Exp Ther 265:358-365, 1993.

321. Brodie BB, Kurz H, Schanker LS: The importance of dissociation constant and lipid-solubility in influencing the passage of drugs into the cerebrospinal fluid. J Pharmacol Exp Ther 130:20-25, 1960.

322. Mark LC, Burns JJ, Campomanes CI, et al: The passage of thiopental into brain. J Pharmacol Exp Ther 119:35-38, 1957.

323. Saidman L: Uptake, distribution and elimination of barbiturates. In Eger E (ed): Anesthetic Uptake and Action. Baltimore, Williams & Wilkins, 1974.

324. Stella L, Torri G, Castiglioni CL: The relative potencies of thiopentone, ketamine, propanidid, alphaxalone and diazepam. A statistical study in man. Br J Anaesth 51:119-122, 1979.

325. Way W, Trevor A: Pharmacology of intravenous nonnarcotic anesthetics. In Miller RD (ed): Anesthesia, 2nd ed. New York, Churchill Livingstone, 1986.

326. Brodie B, Mark L, Papper E: The fate of thiopental in man and method for its estimation in biological material. J Pharmacol Exp Ther 98:85, 1950.

327. Homer TD, Stanski DR: The effect of increasing age on thiopental disposition and anesthetic requirement. Anesthesiology 62:714-724, 1985.

328. Sorbo S, Hudson RJ, Loomis JC: The pharmacokinetics of thiopental in pediatric surgical patients. Anesthesiology 61:666-670, 1984.

329. Korttila K, Ghoneim MM, Jacobs L, Lakes RS: Evaluation of instrumented force platform as a test to measure residual effects of anesthetics. Anesthesiology 55:625-630, 1981.

330. Reves JG, Vinik R, Hirschfield AM, et al: Midazolam compared with thiopentone as a hypnotic component in balanced anaesthesia: A randomized, double-blind study. Can Anaesth Soc J 26:42-49, 1979.

331. Reves JG, Samuelson PN, Lewis S: Midazolam maleate induction in patients with ischaemic heart disease: Haemodynamic observations. Can Anaesth Soc J 26:402-409, 1979.

332. Todd MM, Drummond JC, U HS: The hemodynamic consequences of high-dose thiopental anesthesia. Anesth Analg 64:681-687, 1985.

333. Rodriguez E, Jordan R: Contemporary trends in pediatric sedation and analgesia. Emerg Med Clin North Am 20:199-222, 2002.

334. Liu LM, Gaudreault P, Friedman PA, et al: Methohexital plasma concentrations in children following rectal administration. Anesthesiology 62:567-570, 1985.

335. Christensen JH, Andreasen F: Individual variation in response to thiopental. Acta Anaesthesiol Scand 22:303-313, 1978.

336. Dundee J, Wyant G: Intravenous Anaesthesia, 2nd ed. Edinburgh, Churchill Livingstone, 1988.

337. Kaniaris P, Katsilambros N, Castanas E, Theophanidis C: Relation between glucose tolerance and serum insulin levels in man before and after thiopental intravenous administration. Anesth Analg 54:718-721, 1975.

338. Fragen RJ, Shanks CA, Molteni A, Avram MJ: Effects of etomidate on hormonal responses to surgical stress. Anesthesiology 61:652-656, 1984.

339. Kawar P, Dundee JW: Frequency of pain on injection and venous sequelae following the I.V. administration of certain anaesthetics and sedatives. Br J Anaesth 54:935-939, 1982.

340. Bonica J: Intravenous anesthetics. In Bonica JJ, McDonald JS (eds): Principles and Practice of Obstetric Analgesia and Anesthesia. Philadelphia, FA Davis, 1967.

341. Reves J, Gelman S: Cardiovascular effects of intravenous anesthetic drugs. In Covino B, Fozzard H, Rehder K (eds): Effects of Anesthesia. Bethesda, MD, American Physiological Society, 1985, p 179.

342. Tarabadkar S, Kopriva D, Sreenivasan N, et al: Hemodynamic impact of induction in patients with decreased cardiac reserve. Anesthesiology 53:S43, 1980.

343. Seltzer J, Gerson J, Allen F: Comparison of the cardiovascular effects of bolus v. incremental administration of thiopentone. Br J Anaesth 52:527-530, 1980.

344. Eckstein JW, Hamilton WK, McCammond JM: The effect of thiopental on peripheral venous tone. Anesthesiology 22:525-528, 1961.

345. Kissin I, Motomura S, Aultman DF, Reves JG: Inotropic and anesthetic potencies of etomidate and thiopental in dogs. Anesth Analg 62:961-965, 1983.

346. Sonntag H, Hellberg K, Schenk HD, et al: Effects of thiopental (Trapanal) on coronary blood flow and myocardial metabolism in man. Acta Anaesthesiol Scand 19:69-78, 1975.

347. Dundee JW, Moore J: Thiopentone and methohexital: A comparison as main anesthetic agents for a standard operation. Anaesthesia 16:50-61, 1961.

348. Gross JB, Zebrowski ME, Carel WD, et al: Time course of ventilatory depression after thiopental and midazolam in normal subjects and in patients with chronic obstructive pulmonary disease. Anesthesiology 58:540-544, 1983.

349. Wyant GM, Dobkin AD, Aasheim GM: Comparison of seven intravenous anaesthetic agents in man. Br J Anaesth 29:194-209, 1957.

350. Choi SD, Spaulding BC, Gross JB, Apfelbaum JL: Comparison of the ventilatory effects of etomidate and methohexital. Anesthesiology 62:442-447, 1985.

351. Wood M: Intravenous anesthetic agents. In Wood M, Wood AJJ (eds): Drugs and Anesthesia: Pharmacology for Anesthesiologists Baltimore, Williams & Wilkins, 1982.

352. Greenblatt D, Shader R: Benzodiazepines in Clinical Practice. New York, Raven Press, 1974.

353. Randall LO, Schalek W, Heise GA, et al: The psychosedative properties of methaminodiazepoxide. J Pharmacol Exp Ther 129:163-171, 1960.

354. Lemere F: Toxic reactions to chlordiazepoxide. JAMA 174:893, 1960.

355. Stovner J, Endresen R: Diazepam in intravenous anaesthesia. Lancet 2:1298-1299, 1965.

356. Walser A, Benjamin L, Flynn T: Quinazolines and 1,4-benzodiazepines. 84. Synthesis and reactions of imidazo (1,5)(1.4)-benzodiazepines. J Org Chem 43:936, 1978.

357. McClish A: Diazepam as an intravenous induction agent for general anaesthesia. Can Anaesth Soc J 13:562-575, 1966.

358. Stovner J, Endresen R: Intravenous anaesthesia with diazepam. Acta Anaesthesiol Scand Suppl 24:223-227, 1966.

359. Reves JG, Fragen RJ, Vinik HR, Greenblatt DJ: Midazolam: Pharmacology and uses. Anesthesiology 62:310-324, 1985.

360. Haefely W, Hunkeler W: The story of flumazenil. Eur J Anaesthesiol Suppl 2:3-13, 1988.

361. Barnett A, Fiore JW: Acute tolerance to diazepam in cats and its possible relationship to diazepam metabolism. Eur J Pharmacol 13:239-243, 1971.

362. Squires RF, Brastrup C: Benzodiazepine receptors in rat brain. Nature 266:732-734, 1977.

363. Greenblatt DJ, Shader RI, Abernethy DR: Drug therapy. Current status of benzodiazepines. N Engl J Med 309:354-358, 1983.

364. Arendt RM, Greenblatt DJ, deJong RH, et al: In vitro correlates of benzodiazepine cerebrospinal fluid uptake, pharmacodynamic action and peripheral distribution. J Pharmacol Exp Ther 227:98-106, 1983.

365. Elliott HW: Metabolism of lorazepam. Br J Anaesth 48:1017-1023, 1976.

366. Blitt CD: Clinical pharmacology of lorazepam. Contemp Anesth Pract 7:135-145, 1983.

367. Klotz U, Reimann I: Elevation of steady-state diazepam levels by cimetidine. Clin Pharmacol Ther 30:513-517, 1981.

368. Kassai A, Toth G, Eichelbaum M, Klotz U: No evidence of a genetic polymorphism in the oxidative metabolism of midazolam. Clin Pharmacokinet 15:319-325, 1988.

369. Bertilsson L: Geographical/interracial differences in polymorphic drug oxidation. Current state of knowledge of cytochromes P450 (CYP) 2D6 and 2C19. Clin Pharmacokinet 29:192-209, 1995.

370. Barr J, Donner A: Optimal intravenous dosing strategies for sedatives and analgesics in the intensive care unit. Crit Care Clin 11:827-847, 1995.

371. Mohler H, Richards JG: The benzodiazepine receptor: A pharmacological control element of brain function. Eur J Anaesthesiol Suppl 2:15-24, 1988.

372. Amrein R, Hetzel W: Pharmacology of Dormicum (midazolam) and Anexate (flumazenil). Acta Anaesthesiol Scand Suppl 92:6-15, discussion 47, 1990.

373. Mohler H, Fritschy JM, Rudolph U: A new benzodiazepine pharmacology. J Pharmacol Exp Ther 300:2-8, 2002.

374. Amrein R, Hetzel W, Hartmann D, Lorscheid T: Clinical pharmacology of flumazenil. Eur J Anaesthesiol Suppl 2:65-80, 1988.

375. Mendelson WB: Neuropharmacology of sleep induction by benzodiazepines. Crit Rev Neurobiol 6:221-232, 1992.

376. Strange PG: D1/D2 dopamine receptor interaction at the biochemical level. Trends Pharmacol Sci 12:48-49, 1991.

377. Haefely W: The preclinical pharmacology of flumazenil. Eur J Anaesthesiol Suppl 2:25-36, 1988.

378. Miller LG: Chronic benzodiazepine administration: From the patient to the gene. J Clin Pharmacol 31:492-495, 1991.

379. Breimer LT, Burm AG, Danhof M, et al: Pharmacokinetic-pharmacodynamic modelling of the interaction between flumazenil and midazolam in volunteers by aperiodic EEG analysis. Clin Pharmacokinet 20:497-508, 1991.

380. Persson MP, Nilsson A, Hartvig P: Relation of sedation and amnesia to plasma concentrations of midazolam in surgical patients. Clin Pharmacol Ther 43:324-331, 1988.

381. Forster A, Juge O, Morel D: Effects of midazolam on cerebral blood flow in human volunteers. Anesthesiology 56:453-455, 1982.

382. Brown CR, Sarnquist FH, Canup CA, Pedley TA: Clinical, electroencephalographic, and pharmacokinetic studies of a water-soluble benzodiazepine, midazolam maleate. Anesthesiology 50:467-470, 1979.

383. Liu J, Singh H, White PF: Electroencephalogram bispectral analysis predicts the depth of midazolam-induced sedation. Anesthesiology 84:64-69, 1996.

384. de Jong RH, Bonin JD: Benzodiazepines protect mice from local anesthetic convulsions and deaths. Anesth Analg 60:385-389, 1981.

385. Denaut M, Yernault JC, De Coster A: Double-blind comparison of the respiratory effects of parenteral lorazepam and diazepam in patients with chronic obstructive lung disease. Curr Med Res Opin 2:611-615, 1974.

386. Forster A, Gardaz JP, Suter PM, Gemperle M: Respiratory depression by midazolam and diazepam. Anesthesiology 53:494-497, 1980.

387. Sunzel M, Paalzow L, Berggren L, Eriksson I: Respiratory and cardiovascular effects in relation to plasma levels of midazolam and diazepam. Br J Clin Pharmacol 25:561-569, 1988.

388. Brogden RN, Goa KL: Flumazenil. A reappraisal of its pharmacological properties and therapeutic efficacy as a benzodiazepine antagonist. Drugs 42:1061-1089, 1991.

389. Alexander CM, Teller LE, Gross JB: Slow injection does not prevent midazolam-induced ventilatory depression. Anesth Analg 74:260-264, 1992.

390. Elliott HW, Nomof N, Navarro G, et al: Central nervous system and cardiovascular effects of lorazepam in man. Clin Pharmacol Ther 12:468-481, 1971.

391. Marty J, Gauzit R, Lefevre P, et al: Effects of diazepam and midazolam on baroreflex control of heart rate and on sympathetic activity in humans. Anesth Analg 65:113-119, 1986.

392. Heikkila H, Jalonen J, Arola M, et al: Midazolam as adjunct to high-dose fentanyl anaesthesia for coronary artery bypass grafting operation. Acta Anaesthesiol Scand 28:683-689, 1984.

393. Benson KT, Tomlinson DL, Goto H, Arakawa K: Cardiovascular effects of lorazepam during sufentanil anesthesia. Anesth Analg 67:996-998, 1988.

394. Windsor JP, Sherry K, Feneck RO, Sebel PS: Sufentanil and nitrous oxide anaesthesia for cardiac surgery. Br J Anaesth 61:662-668, 1988.

395. Reves J, Croughwell N: Valium-fentanyl interaction. In Reves J, Hall K (eds): Common Problems in Cardiac Anaesthesia. Chicago, Year Book, 1987, p 356.

396. Tomichek R, Rosow C, Schneider R: Cardiovascular effects of diazepam-fentanyl anesthesia in patients with coronary artery disease. Anesth Analg 61:217, 1982.

397. Cole SG, Brozinsky S, Isenberg JI: Midazolam, a new more potent benzodiazepine, compared with diazepam: A randomized, double-blind study of preendoscopic sedatives. Gastrointest Endosc 29:219-222, 1983.

398. George KA, Dundee JW: Relative amnesic actions of diazepam, flunitrazepam and lorazepam in man. Br J Clin Pharmacol 4:45-50, 1977.

399. Fragen RJ, Caldwell N: Lorazepam premedication: Lack of recall and relief of anxiety. Anesth Analg 55:792-796, 1976.

400. McNulty SE, Gratch D, Costello D, et al: The effect of midazolam and lorazepam on postoperative recovery after cardiac surgery. Anesth Analg 81:404-407, 1995.

401. Sanchez-Izquierdo-Riera JA, Caballero-Cubedo RE, Perez-Vela JL, et al: Propofol versus midazolam: Safety and efficacy for sedating the severe trauma patient. Anesth Analg 86:1219-1224, 1998.

402. Vargo JJ, Zuccaro G Jr, Dumot JA, et al: Gastroenterologist-administered propofol versus meperidine and midazolam for advanced upper endoscopy: A prospective, randomized trial. Gastroenterology 123:8-16, 2002.

403. Gauthier RA, Dyck B, Chung F, et al: Respiratory interaction after spinal anesthesia and sedation with midazolam. Anesthesiology 77:909-914, 1992.

404. Shapiro BA, Warren J, Egol AB, et al: Practice parameters for intravenous analgesia and sedation for adult patients in the intensive care unit: An executive summary. Society of Critical Care Medicine. Crit Care Med 23:1596-1600, 1995.

405. Weinbroum AA, Halpern P, Rudick V, et al: Midazolam versus propofol for long-term sedation in the ICU: A randomized prospective comparison. Intensive Care Med 23:1258-1263, 1997.

406. Young C, Knudsen N, Hilton A, Reves JG: Sedation in the intensive care unit. Crit Care Med 28:854-866, 2000.

407. Walder B, Elia N, Henzi I, et al: A lack of evidence of superiority of propofol versus midazolam for sedation in mechanically ventilated critically ill patients: A qualitative and quantitative systematic review. Anesth Analg 92:975-983, 2001.

408. Kain ZN, Hofstadter MB, Mayes LC, et al: Midazolam: Effects on amnesia and anxiety in children. Anesthesiology 93:676-684, 2000.

409. Funk W, Jakob W, Riedl T, Taeger K: Oral preanaesthetic medication for children: Double-blind randomized study of a combination of midazolam and ketamine vs midazolam or ketamine alone. Br J Anaesth 84:335-340, 2000.

410. Kanto J, Sjovall S, Vuori A: Effect of different kinds of premedication on the induction properties of midazolam. Br J Anaesth 54:507-511, 1982.

411. Gamble JA, Kawar P, Dundee JW, et al: Evaluation of midazolam as an intravenous induction agent. Anaesthesia 36:868-873, 1981.

412. Jacobs JR, Reves JG, Marty J, et al: Aging increases pharmacodynamic sensitivity to the hypnotic effects of midazolam. Anesth Analg 80:143-148, 1995.

413. Theil DR, Stanley TE 3rd, White WD, et al: Midazolam and fentanyl continuous infusion anesthesia for cardiac surgery: A comparison of computer-assisted versus manual infusion systems. J Cardiothorac Vasc Anesth 7:300-306, 1993.

414. Nilsson A, Persson MP, Hartvig P, Wide L: Effect of total intravenous anaesthesia with midazolam/alfentanil on the adrenocortical and hyperglycaemic response to abdominal surgery. Acta Anaesthesiol Scand 32:379-382, 1988.

415. Crawford ME, Carl P, Andersen RS, Mikkelsen BO: Comparison between midazolam and thiopentone-based balanced anaesthesia for day-case surgery. Br J Anaesth 56:165-169, 1984.

416. Melvin MA, Johnson BH, Quasha AL, Eger EI 3rd: Induction of anesthesia with midazolam decreases halothane MAC in humans. Anesthesiology 57:238-241, 1982.

417. File SE, Pellow S: Intrinsic actions of the benzodiazepine receptor antagonist Ro 15-1788. Psychopharmacology (Berl) 88:1-11, 1986.

418. Limbird L: Cell Surface Receptors: A Short Course on Theory and Methods. Boston, Kluwer Academic Publishers, 1986, p 42.

419. Lauven PM, Schwilden H, Stoeckel H, Greenblatt DJ: The effects of a benzodiazepine antagonist Ro 15-1788 in the presence of stable concentrations of midazolam. Anesthesiology 63:61-64, 1985.

420. Cumin R, Bonetti EP, Scherschlicht R, Haefely WE: Use of the specific benzodiazepine antagonist, Ro 15-1788, in studies of physiological dependence on benzodiazepines. Experientia 38:833-834, 1982.

421. Hunkeler W: Preclinical research findings with flumazenil (Ro15-1788, Anexate): Chemistry. Eur J Anaesthesiol Suppl 2:37, 1988.

422. Klotz U, Kanto J: Pharmacokinetics and clinical use of flumazenil (Ro 15-1788). Clin Pharmacokinet 14:1-12, 1988.

423. Klotz U: Drug interactions and clinical pharmacokinetics of flumazenil. Eur J Anaesthesiol Suppl 2:103-108, 1988.

424. Breimer LT, Hennis PJ, Burm AG, et al: Pharmacokinetics and EEG effects of flumazenil in volunteers. Clin Pharmacokinet 20:491-496, 1991.

425. Kleinberger G, Grimm G, Laggner A, et al: Weaning patients from mechanical ventilation by benzodiazepine antagonist Ro15-1788. Lancet 2:268-269, 1985.

426. Knudsen L, Cold GE, Holdgard HO, et al: Effects of flumazenil on cerebral blood flow and oxygen consumption after midazolam anaesthesia for craniotomy. Br J Anaesth 67:277-280, 1991.

427. Wolf J, Friberg L, Jensen J, et al: The effect of the benzodiazepine antagonist flumazenil on regional cerebral blood flow in human volunteers. Acta Anaesthesiol Scand 34:628-631, 1990.

428. Yokoyama M, Benson KT, Arakawa K, Goto H: Effects of flumazenil on intravenous lidocaine-induced convulsions and anticonvulsant property of diazepam in rats. Anesth Analg 75:87-90, 1992.

429. Forster A, Juge O, Louis M, Nahory A: Effects of a specific benzodiazepine antagonist (RO 15-1788) on cerebral blood flow. Anesth Analg 66:309-313, 1987.

430. Samson Y, Hantraye P, Baron JC, et al: Kinetics and displacement of [^{11}C]RO 15-1788, a benzodiazepine antagonist, studied in human brain in vivo by positron tomography. Eur J Pharmacol 110:247-251, 1985.

431. Dunton AW, Schwam E, Pitman V, et al: The relationship between dose and duration of action of intravenous flumazenil in reversing sedation induced by a continuous infusion of midazolam. Eur J Anaesthesiol Suppl 2:97-102, 1988.

432. Forster A, Crettenand G, Morel D: Absence of ventilatory agonist or inverse agonist effects of an overdose of Ro15-1788: A specific benzodiazepine antagonist. Anesthesiology 67:A144, 1987.

433. Rouiller M, Forster A, Gemperle M: Assessment of the efficacy and tolerance of a benzodiazepine antagonist (Ro 15-1788) [in French]. Ann Fr Anesth Reanim 6:1-6, 1987.

434. Weinbrum A, Geller E: The respiratory effects of reversing midazolam sedation with flumazenil in the presence or absence of narcotics. Acta Anaesthesiol Scand Suppl 92:65-69, discussion 78, 1990.

435. Duka T, Ackenheil M, Noderer J, et al: Changes in noradrenaline plasma levels and behavioural responses induced by benzodiazepine agonists with the benzodiazepine antagonist Ro 15-1788. Psychopharmacology (Berl) 90:351-357, 1986.

436. Nilsson A: Autonomic and hormonal responses after the use of midazolam and flumazenil. Acta Anaesthesiol Scand Suppl 92:51-54, discussion 78, 1990.

437. White PF, Shafer A, Boyle WA 3rd, et al: Benzodiazepine antagonism does not provoke a stress response. Anesthesiology 70:636-639, 1989.

438. Whitwam JG, Amrein R: Pharmacology of flumazenil. Acta Anaesthesiol Scand Suppl 108:3-14, 1995.

439. Ghoneim MM, Dembo JB, Block RI: Time course of antagonism of sedative and amnesic effects of diazepam by flumazenil. Anesthesiology 70:899-904, 1989.

440. Greifenstein FE, DeVault M, Yoshitake J, Gajewski JE: A study of a 1-aryl cyclo hexyl amine for anesthesia. Anesth Analg 37:283-294, 1958.

441. Johnstone M, Evans V, Baigel S: Sernyl (CI-395) in clinical anaesthesia. Br J Anaesth 31:433-439, 1959.

442. Lear E, Suntay R, Pallin I: Cyclohexamine (CI-400): A new intravenous agent. Anesthesiology 20:330-335, 1959.

443. Corssen G, Domino EF: Dissociative anesthesia: Further pharmacologic studies and first clinical experience with the phencyclidine derivative CI-581. Anesth Analg 45:29-40, 1966.

444. White PF, Way WL, Trevor AJ: Ketamine—its pharmacology and therapeutic uses. Anesthesiology 56:119-136, 1982.

445. Cohen ML, Trevor AJ: On the cerebral accumulation of ketamine and the relationship between metabolism of the drug and its pharmacological effects. J Pharmacol Exp Ther 189:351-358, 1974.

446. Chang T, Glazko AJ: Biotransformation and disposition of ketamine. Int Anesthesiol Clin 12:157-177, 1974.

447. Cheng G: The pharmacology of ketamine. In Ketamine. Berlin, Springer-Verlag, 1969, p 1.

448. White PF, Johnston RR, Pudwill CR: Interaction of ketamine and halothane in rats. Anesthesiology 42:179-186, 1975.

449. Cohen MG, Chan SL, Bhargava HN, Trevor AJ: Inhibition of mammalian brain acetylcholinesterase by ketamine. Biochem Pharmacol 23:1647-1652, 1974.

450. Grant IS, Nimmo WS, Clements JA: Pharmacokinetics and analgesic effects of i.m. and oral ketamine. Br J Anaesth 53:805-810, 1981.

451. Idvall J, Ahlgren I, Aronsen KR, Stenberg P: Ketamine infusions: Pharmacokinetics and clinical effects. Br J Anaesth 51:1167-1173, 1979.

452. Nimmo W, Clements J: Ketamine. In Prys-Robert CH (ed): Pharmacokinetics of Anesthesia. Boston, Blackwell, 1984, p 235.

453. White PF, Marietta MP, Pudwill CR, et al: Effects of halothane anesthesia on the biodisposition of ketamine in rats. J Pharmacol Exp Ther 196:545-555, 1976.

454. Edwards SR, Minto CF, Mather LE: Concurrent ketamine and alfentanil administration: Pharmacokinetic considerations. Br J Anaesth 88:94-100, 2002.

455. Geisslinger G, Hering W, Thomann P, et al: Pharmacokinetics and pharmacodynamics of ketamine enantiomers in surgical patients using a stereoselective analytical method. Br J Anaesth 70:666-671, 1993.

456. Schuttler J, Stanski DR, White PF, et al: Pharmacodynamic modeling of the EEG effects of ketamine and its enantiomers in man. J Pharmacokinet Biopharm 15:241-253, 1987.

457. Taylor PA, Towey RM: Depression of laryngeal reflexes during ketamine anaesthesia. BMJ 2:688-689, 1971.

458. Grant IS, Nimmo WS, McNicol LR, Clements JA: Ketamine disposition in children and adults. Br J Anaesth 55:1107-1111, 1983.

459. Corssen G, Domino EF: Dissociative anesthesia: Further pharmacologic studies and first clinical experience with the phencyclidine derivative CI-581. Anesth Analg 45:29-40, 1966.

460. Corssen G, Miyasaka M, Domino EF: Changing concepts in pain control during surgery: Dissociative anesthesia with CI-581. A progress report. Anesth Analg 47:746-759, 1968.

461. Adams HA, Thiel A, Jung A, et al: Studies using S-(+)-ketamine on probands. Endocrine and circulatory reactions, recovery and dream experiences [in German]. Anaesthesist 41:588-596, 1992.

462. Kharasch ED, Labroo R: Metabolism of ketamine stereoisomers by human liver microsomes. Anesthesiology 77:1201-1217, 1992.

463. Domino E, Chodoff P, Corssen G: Pharmacologic effects of CI-581, a new dissociative anesthetic in man. Clin Pharmacol Ther 6:279-291, 1965.

464. Okamoto GU, Duperon DF, Jedrychowski JR: Clinical evaluation of the effects of ketamine sedation on pediatric dental patients. J Clin Pediatr Dent 16:253-257, 1992.

465. Doenicke A, Kugler J, Mayer M, et al: Ketamine racemate or S-(+)-ketamine and midazolam. The effect on vigilance, efficacy and subjective findings [in German]. Anaesthesist 41:610-618, 1992.

466. Chapman V, Dickenson AH: The combination of NMDA antagonism and morphine produces profound antinociception in the rat dorsal horn. Brain Res 573:321-323, 1992.

467. Kissin I, Bright CA, Bradley EL Jr: The effect of ketamine on opioid-induced acute tolerance: Can it explain reduction of opioid consumption with ketamine-opioid analgesic combinations? Anesth Analg 91:1483-1488, 2000.

468. Menigaux C, Fletcher D, Dupont X, et al: The benefits of intraoperative small-dose ketamine on postoperative pain after anterior cruciate ligament repair. Anesth Analg 90:129-135, 2000.

469. Guignard B, Coste C, Costes H, et al: Supplementing desflurane-remifentanil anesthesia with small-dose ketamine reduces perioperative opioid analgesic requirements. Anesth Analg 95:103-108, 2002.

470. Miyasaka M, Domino E: Neural mechanisms of ketamine-induced anesthesia. Int J Neuropharmacol 7:557-573, 1968.

471. Massopust LC Jr, Wolin LR, Albin MS: Electrophysiologic and behavioral responses to ketamine hydrochloride in the Rhesus monkey. Anesth Analg 51:329-341, 1972.

472. Sparks DL, Corssen G, Aizenman B, Black J: Further studies of the neural mechanisms of ketamine-induced anesthesia in the rhesus monkey. Anesth Analg 54:189-195, 1975.

473. Ohtani M, Kikuchi H, Kitahata LM, et al: Effects of ketamine on nociceptive cells in the medial medullary reticular formation of the cat. Anesthesiology 51:414-417, 1979.

474. Frenkel C, Urban BW: Molecular actions of racemic ketamine on human CNS sodium channels. Br J Anaesth 69:292-297, 1992.

475. Finck A, Ngai S: A possible mechanism of ketamine-induced analgesia. Anesthesiology 51:S34, 1979.

476. Fratta W, Casu M, Balestrieri A, et al: Failure of ketamine to interact with opiate receptors. Eur J Pharmacol 61:389-391, 1980.

477. Freye E, Latasch L, Schmidhammer H: Pharmacodynamic effects of S-(+)-ketamine on EEG, evoked potentials and respiration. A study in the awake dog [in German]. Anaesthesist 41:527-533, 1992.

478. Irifune M, Shimizu T, Nomoto M, Fukuda T: Ketamine-induced anesthesia involves the N-methyl-D-aspartate receptor-channel complex in mice. Brain Res 596:1-9, 1992.

479. Klepstad P, Maurset A, Moberg ER, Oye I: Evidence of a role for NMDA receptors in pain perception. Eur J Pharmacol 187:513-518, 1990.

480. Oye I, Paulsen O, Maurset A: Effects of ketamine on sensory perception: Evidence for a role of N-methyl-D-aspartate receptors. J Pharmacol Exp Ther 260:1209-1213, 1992.

481. Nagasaka H, Nagasaka I, Sato I, et al: The effects of ketamine on the excitation and inhibition of dorsal horn WDR neuronal activity induced by bradykinin injection into the femoral artery in cats after spinal cord transection. Anesthesiology 78:722-732, 1993.

482. Kayama Y, Iwama K: The EEG, evoked potentials, and single-unit activity during ketamine anesthesia in cats. Anesthesiology 36:316-328, 1972.

483. Gardner AE, Dannemiller FJ, Dean D: Intracranial cerebrospinal fluid pressure in man during ketamine anesthesia. Anesth Analg 51:741-745, 1972.

484. Shapiro HM, Wyte SR, Harria AB: Ketamine anaesthesia in patients with intracranial pathology. Br J Anaesth 44:1200-1204, 1972.

485. Dawson B, Michenfelder JD, Theye RA: Effects of ketamine on canine cerebral blood flow and metabolism: Modification by prior administration of thiopental. Anesth Analg 50:443-447, 1971.

486. Thorsen T, Gran L: Ketamine/diazepam infusion anaesthesia with special attention to the effect on cerebrospinal fluid pressure and arterial blood pressure. Acta Anaesthesiol Scand 24:1-4, 1980.

487. Reeker W, Werner C, Mollenberg O, et al: High-dose S(+)-ketamine improves neurological outcome following incomplete cerebral ischemia in rats. Can J Anaesth 47:572-578, 2000.

488. Engelhard K, Werner C, Eberspacher E, et al: The effect of the alpha 2-agonist dexmedetomidine and the N-methyl-D-aspartate antagonist S(+)-ketamine on the expression of apoptosis-regulating proteins after incomplete cerebral ischemia and reperfusion in rats. Anesth Analg 96:524-531, 2003.

489. Garfield JM, Garfield FB, Stone JG, et al: A comparison of psychologic responses to ketamine and thiopental–nitrous oxide–halothane anesthesia. Anesthesiology 36:329-338, 1972.

490. Sussman DR: A comparative evaluation of ketamine anesthesia in children and adults. Anesthesiology 40:459-464, 1974.

491. Dundee JW, Bovill JG, Clarke RS, Pandit SK: Problems with ketamine in adults. Anaesthesia 26:86, 1971.

492. Khorramzadeh E, Lotfy AO: Personality predisposition and emergence phenomena with ketamine. Psychosomatics 17:94-95, 1976.

493. Kumar A, Bajaj A, Sarkar P, Grover VK: The effect of music on ketamine induced emergence phenomena. Anaesthesia 47:438-439, 1992.

494. Hejja P, Galloon S: A consideration of ketamine dreams. Can Anaesth Soc J 22:100-105, 1975.

495. Wulfsohn NL: Ketamine dosage for induction based on lean body mass. Anesth Analg 51:299-305, 1972.

496. Johnstone M: The prevention of ketamine dreams. Anaesth Intensive Care 1:70-74, 1972.

497. Dundee JW, Lilburn JK: Ketamine-lorazepam: Attenuation of the psychic sequelae of ketamine by lorazepam. Anaesthesia 37:312-314, 1977.

498. Kothary S, Zsigmond E: A double-blind study of the effective anti-hallucinatory doses of diazepam prior to ketamine anesthesia. Clin Pharmacol Ther 21:108, 1977.

499. Doenicke A, Angster R, Mayer M, et al: The action of S-(+)-ketamine on serum catecholamine and cortisol. A comparison with ketamine racemate [in German]. Anaesthesist 41:597-603, 1992.

500. Soliman MG, Brinale GF, Kuster G: Response to hypercapnia under ketamine anaesthesia. Can Anaesth Soc J 22:486-494, 1975.

501. Virtue RW, Alanis JM, Mori M, et al: An anesthetic agent: 2-Orthochlorophenyl, 2-methylamino cyclohexanone HCl (CI-581). Anesthesiology 28:823-833, 1967.

502. Stanley V, Hunt J, Willis KW, Stephen CR: Cardiovascular and respiratory function with CI-581. Anesth Analg 47:760-768, 1968.

503. Dillon J: Clinical experience with repeated ketamine administration for procedures requiring anesthesia. In Kreuscher H (ed): Ketamine. Berlin, Springer-Verlag, 1969.

504. Hamza J, Ecoffey C, Gross JB: Ventilatory response to CO_2 following intravenous ketamine in children. Anesthesiology 70:422-425, 1989.

505. Greene CA, Gillette PC, Fyfe DA: Frequency of respiratory compromise after ketamine sedation for cardiac catheterization in patients less than 21 years of age. Am J Cardiol 68:1116-1117, 1991.

506. Huber FC Jr, Gutierrez J, Corssen G: Ketamine: Its effect on airway resistance in man. South Med J 65:1176-1180, 1972.

507. Corssen G, Gutierrez J, Reves JG, Huber FC Jr: Ketamine in the anesthetic management of asthmatic patients. Anesth Analg 51:588-596, 1972.

508. Hirshman CA, Downes H, Farbood A, Bergman NA: Ketamine block of bronchospasm in experimental canine asthma. Br J Anaesth 51:713-718, 1979.

509. Wanna HT, Gergis SD: Procaine, lidocaine, and ketamine inhibit histamine-induced contracture of guinea pig tracheal muscle in vitro. Anesth Analg 57:25-27, 1978.

510. Sarma VJ: Use of ketamine in acute severe asthma. Acta Anaesthesiol Scand 36:106-107, 1992.

511. Sonntag H, Heiss HW, Knoll D, et al: Myocardial perfusion and myocardial oxygen consumption in patients during the induction of anesthesia using dehydrobenzperidol-fentanyl or ketamine [in German]. Z Kreislaufforsch 61:1092-1105, 1972.

512. Zsigmond E, Domino E: Clinical pharmacology and current uses of ketamine. In Aldrete J, Stanley T (eds): Trends in Intravenous Anesthesia. Chicago, Year Book, 1980, p 283.

513. Savege TM, Colvin MP, Weaver EJ, et al: A comparison of some cardiorespiratory effects of althesin and ketamine when used for induction of anaesthesia in patients with cardiac disease. Br J Anaesth 48:1071-1081, 1976.

514. Gooding JM, Dimick AR, Tavakoli M, Corssen G: A physiologic analysis of cardiopulmonary responses to ketamine anesthesia in noncardiac patients. Anesth Analg 56:813-816, 1977.

515. Reves JG, Lell WA, McCracken LE Jr, et al: Comparison of morphine and ketamine anesthetic techniques for coronary surgery: A randomized study. South Med J 71:33-36, 1978.

516. Spotoft H, Korshin JD, Sorensen MB, Skovsted P: The cardiovascular effects of ketamine used for induction of anaesthesia in patients with valvular heart disease. Can Anaesth Soc J 26:463-467, 1979.

517. Morray JP, Lynn AM, Stamm SJ, et al: Hemodynamic effects of ketamine in children with congenital heart disease. Anesth Analg 63:895-899, 1984.

518. Greeley WJ, Bushman GA, Davis DP, Reves JG: Comparative effects of halothane and ketamine on systemic arterial oxygen saturation in children with cyanotic heart disease. Anesthesiology 65:666-668, 1986.

519. Faithfull NS, Haider R: Ketamine for cardiac catheterisation. An evaluation of its use in children. Anaesthesia 26:318-323, 1971.

520. Hickey PR, Hansen DD, Cramolini GM, et al: Pulmonary and systemic hemodynamic responses to ketamine in infants with normal and elevated pulmonary vascular resistance. Anesthesiology 62:287-293, 1985.

521. Slogoff S, Allen GW: The role of baroreceptors in the cardiovascular response to ketamine. Anesth Analg 53:704-707, 1974.

522. Dowdy EG, Kaya K: Studies of the mechanism of cardiovascular responses to CI-581. Anesthesiology 29:931-943, 1968.

523. Chodoff P: Evidence for central adrenergic action of ketamine: Report of a case. Anesth Analg 51:247-250, 1972.

524. Wong DH, Jenkins LC: An experimental study of the mechanism of action of ketamine on the central nervous system. Can Anaesth Soc J 21:57-67, 1974.

525. Iwatsuki K, Aoba Y, Sato K, Iwatsuki N: Clinical study on CI-581, a phencyclidine derivative. Tohoku J Exp Med 93:39-48, 1967.

526. Ogawa A, Uemura M, Kataoka Y, et al: Effects of ketamine on cardiovascular responses mediated by N-methyl-D-aspartate receptor in the rat nucleus tractus solitarius. Anesthesiology 78:163-167, 1993.

527. Ivankovich AD, Miletich DJ, Reimann C, et al: Cardiovascular effects of centrally administered ketamine in goats. Anesth Analg 53:924-933, 1974.

528. Zsigmond E, Kothary S, Matsuki A: Diazepam for prevention of the rise in plasma catecholamines caused by ketamine. Clin Pharmacol Ther 15:223, 1974.

529. Balfors E, Haggmark S, Nyhman H, et al: Droperidol inhibits the effects of intravenous ketamine on central hemodynamics and myocardial oxygen consumption in patients with generalized atherosclerotic disease. Anesth Analg 62:193-197, 1983.

530. Miletich DJ, Ivankovic AD, Albrecht RF, et al: The effect of ketamine on catecholamine metabolism in the isolated perfused rat heart. Anesthesiology 39:271-277, 1973.

531. Valicenti JF Jr, Newman WH, Bagwell EE, et al: Myocardial contractility during induction and steady-state ketamine anesthesia. Anesth Analg 52:190-194, 1973.

532. Pagel PS, Kampine JP, Schmeling WT, Warltier DC: Ketamine depresses myocardial contractility as evaluated by the preload recruitable stroke work relationship in chronically instrumented dogs with autonomic nervous system blockade. Anesthesiology 76:564-572, 1992.

533. Urthaler F, Walker AA, James TN: Comparison of the inotropic action of morphine and ketamine studied in canine cardiac muscle. J Thorac Cardiovasc Surg 72:142-149, 1976.

534. Stowe DF, Bosnjak ZJ, Kampine JP: Comparison of etomidate, ketamine, midazolam, propofol, and thiopental on function and metabolism of isolated hearts. Anesth Analg 74:547-558, 1992.

535. Endou M, Hattori Y, Nakaya H, et al: Electrophysiologic mechanisms responsible for inotropic responses to ketamine in guinea pig and rat myocardium. Anesthesiology 76:409-418, 1992.

536. Hill GE, Wong KC, Shaw CL, et al: Interactions of ketamine with vasoactive amines at normothermia and hypothermia in the isolate rabbit heart. Anesthesiology 48:315-319, 1978.

537. Nedergaard OA: Cocaine-like effect of ketamine on vascular adrenergic neurones. Eur J Pharmacol 23:153-161, 1973.

538. Salt PJ, Barnes PK, Beswick FJ: Inhibition of neuronal and extraneuronal uptake of noradrenaline by ketamine in the isolated perfused rat heart. Br J Anaesth 51:835-838, 1979.

539. Cook DJ, Housmans PR, Rorie DK: Effect of ketamine HCl on norepinephrine disposition in isolated ferret ventricular myocardium. J Pharmacol Exp Ther 261:101-107, 1992.

540. Reves J, Flezzani P, Kissin I: Pharmacology of intravenous anesthetic induction drugs. In Kaplan J (ed): Cardiac Anesthesia. Orlando, FL, Grune & Stratton, 1987, p 125.

541. Munro HM, Sleigh JW, Paxton LD: The cardiovascular response to ketamine: The effects of clonidine and lignocaine. Acta Anaesthesiol Scand 37:75-78, 1993.

542. Hatano S, Keane DM, Boggs RF, et al: Diazepam-ketamine anaesthesia for open heart surgery: A "micro-mini" drip administration technique. Can J Anaesth 23:648-656, 1976.

543. Bidwai AV, Stanley HT, Graves CL, et al: The effects of ketamine on cardiovascular dynamics during halothane and enflurane anesthesia. Anesth Analg 54:588-592, 1975.

544. Corssen G, Reves JG, Carter JR: Neuroleptanesthesia, dissociative anesthesia, and hemorrhage. Int Anesthesiol Clin 12:145-161, 1974.

545. Van der Linden P, Gilbart E, Engelman E, et al: Comparison of halothane, isoflurane, alfentanil, and ketamine in experimental septic shock. Anesth Analg 70:608-617, 1990.

546. Kingston HG, Bretherton KW, Holloway AM, Downing JW: A comparison between ketamine and diazepam as induction agents for pericardiectomy. Anaesth Intensive Care 6:66-70, 1978.

547. Allen GC, Byford LJ, Shamji FM: Anterior mediastinal mass in a patient susceptible to malignant hyperthermia. Can J Anaesth 40:46-49, 1993.
548. Fletcher JE, Rosenberg H, Lizzo FH: Effects of droperidol, haloperidol and ketamine on halothane, succinylcholine and caffeine contractures: Implications for malignant hyperthermia. Acta Anaesthesiol Scand 33:187-192, 1989.
549. Dershwitz M, Sreter FA, Ryan JF: Ketamine does not trigger malignant hyperthermia in susceptible swine. Anesth Analg 69:501-503, 1989.
550. Raza SM, Masters RW, Zsigmond EK: Haemodynamic stability with midazolam-ketamine-sufentanil analgesia in cardiac surgical patients. Can J Anaesth 36:617-623, 1989.
551. Kudoh A, Takahira Y, Katagai H, Takazawa T: Small-dose ketamine improves the postoperative state of depressed patients. Anesth Analg 95:114-118, 2002.
552. Dich-Nielsen JO, Svendsen LB, Berthelsen P: Intramuscular low-dose ketamine versus pethidine for postoperative pain treatment after thoracic surgery. Acta Anaesthesiol Scand 36:583-587, 1992.
553. Jahangir SM, Islam F, Aziz L: Ketamine infusion for postoperative analgesia in asthmatics: A comparison with intermittent meperidine. Anesth Analg 76:45-49, 1993.
554. Weinbroum AA: A single small dose of postoperative ketamine provides rapid and sustained improvement in morphine analgesia in the presence of morphine-resistant pain. Anesth Analg 96:789-795, 2003.
555. Sveticic G, Gentilini A, Eichenberger U, et al: Combinations of morphine with ketamine for patient-controlled analgesia: A new optimization method. Anesthesiology 98:1195-1205, 2003.
556. Eisenach JC, Yaksh TL: Epidural ketamine in healthy children—what's the point? Anesth Analg 96:626, author reply 627, 2003.
557. Groeneveld A, Inkson T: Ketamine. A solution to procedural pain in burned children. Can Nurse 88:28-31, 1992.
558. Wolfe RR, Loehr JP, Schaffer MS, Wiggins JW Jr: Hemodynamic effects of ketamine, hypoxia and hyperoxia in children with surgically treated congenital heart disease residing greater than or equal to 1,200 meters above sea level. Am J Cardiol 67:84-87, 1991.
559. Thompson GE, Moore DC: Ketamine, diazepam, and Innovar: A computerized comparative study. Anesth Analg 50:458-463, 1971.
560. Korttila K, Levanen J: Untoward effects of ketamine combined with diazepam for supplementing conduction anaesthesia in young and middle-aged adults. Acta Anaesthesiol Scand 22:640-648, 1978.
561. Friedberg BL: Propofol-ketamine technique. Aesthetic Plast Surg 17:297-300, 1993.
562. Fuchs C, Schwabe M: Rectal premedication using ketamine-dehydrobenzperidol-atropine in childhood [in French]. Anaesthesiol Reanim 15:322-326, 1990.
563. Waxman K, Shoemaker WC, Lippmann M: Cardiovascular effects of anesthetic induction with ketamine. Anesth Analg 59:355-358, 1980.
564. Yang CY, Wong CS, Chang JY, Ho ST: Intrathecal ketamine reduces morphine requirements in patients with terminal cancer pain. Can J Anaesth 43:379-383, 1996.
565. Weber F, Wulf H: Caudal bupivacaine and s(+)-ketamine for postoperative analgesia in children. Paediatr Anaesth 13:244-248, 2003.
566. Hui TW, Short TG, Hong W, et al: Additive interactions between propofol and ketamine when used for anesthesia induction in female patients. Anesthesiology 82:641-648, 1995.
567. Gutstein HB, Johnson KL, Heard MB, Gregory GA: Oral ketamine preanesthetic medication in children. Anesthesiology 76:28-33, 1992.
568. Tobias JD, Phipps S, Smith B, Mulhern RK: Oral ketamine premedication to alleviate the distress of invasive procedures in pediatric oncology patients. Pediatrics 90:537-541, 1992.
569. Neckel W, Jacobs FE, Tolksdorf W: Oral ketamine as preferred preanesthetic medication of uncooperative patients [in German]. Anasthesiol Intensivmed Notfallmed Schmerzther 27:381-384, 1992.
570. Shapiro HM: Intracranial hypertension: Therapeutic and anesthetic considerations. Anesthesiology 43:445-471, 1971.
571. Thiel A, Adams HA, Fengler G, Hempelmann G: Studies using S-(+)-ketamine on probands. Computerized EEG-analysis and transcranial Doppler ultrasonography [in German]. Anaesthesist 41:604-609, 1992.
572. Tsai SK, Lee C: Ketamine potentiates nondepolarizing neuromuscular relaxants in a primate. Anesth Analg 68:5-8, 1989.
573. Malinovsky JM, Lepage JY, Cozian A, et al: Is ketamine or its preservative responsible for neurotoxicity in the rabbit? Anesthesiology 78:109-115, 1993.
574. Godefroi EF, Janssen PA, Vandereycken CA, et al: DL-1-(1-arylalkyl)imidazole-5-carboxylate esters: A novel type of hypnotic agents. J Med Chem 8:220-223, 1965.
575. Doenicke A: Etomidate, a new intravenous hypnotic. Acta Anaesthesiol Belg 25:307-315, 1974.
576. Janssen P, Niemegeers J, Schellekens K: Etomidate, R-(+)-ethyl-1-(alpha-methyl-benzyl)imidazole-5-carboxylate (R 16659): A potent, short-acting and relatively atoxic intravenous hypnotic agent in rats. Arzneimittelforschung 21:1234-1243, 1971.
577. Ledingham IM, Watt I: Influence of sedation on mortality in critically ill multiple trauma patients. Lancet 1:1270, 1983.
578. Wagner RL, White PF: Etomidate inhibits adrenocortical function in surgical patients. Anesthesiology 61:647-651, 1984.
579. Longnecker DE: Stress free: To be or not to be? Anesthesiology 61:643-644, 1984.
580. Owen H, Spence AA: Etomidate. Br J Anaesth 56:555-557, 1984.
581. Etomidate. Lancet 2:24-25, 1983.
582. Corssen G, Reves J, Stanley T: Etomidate. In Corssen G, Reves J, Stanley T (eds): Intravenous Anesthesia and Analgesia. Philadelphia, Lea & Febiger, 1988, p 285.
583. Nimmo W, Miller M: Pharmacology of etomidate. In Brown B (ed): New Pharmacologic Vistas in Anesthesia. Philadelphia, FA Davis, 1983, p 83.
584. Doenicke A, Roizen MF, Nebauer AE, et al: A comparison of two formulations for etomidate, 2-hydroxypropyl-beta-cyclodextrin (HPCD) and propylene glycol. Anesth Analg 79:933-939, 1994.
585. Hadzija BW, Lubarsky DA: Compatibility of etomidate, thiopental sodium, and propofol injections with drugs commonly administered during induction of anesthesia. Am J Health Syst Pharm 52:997-999, 1995.
586. Fragen RJ, Caldwell N: Comparison of a new formulation of etomidate with thiopental—side effects and awakening times. Anesthesiology 50:242-244, 1979.
587. Carli F, Stribley GC, Clark MM: Etomidate infusion in thoracic anaesthesia. Anaesthesia 38:784-788, 1983.
588. Nauta J, Stanley TH, de Lang S, et al: Anaesthetic induction with alfentanil: Comparison with thiopental, midazolam, and etomidate. Can J Anaesth 30:53-60, 1983.
589. Dundee J, Zacharias M: Etomidate. In Dundee J (ed): Current Topics in Anaesthesia, Series 1. London, Arnold, 1979, p 46.
590. Famewo CE, Odugbesan CO: Further experience with etomidate. Can Anaesth Soc J 25:130-132, 1978.
591. Giese JL, Stockham RJ, Stanley TH, et al: Etomidate versus thiopental for induction of anesthesia. Anesth Analg 64:871-876, 1985.
592. Craig J, Cooper GM, Sear JW: Recovery from day-case anaesthesia. Comparison between methohexitone, Althesin and etomidate. Br J Anaesth 54:447-451, 1982.
593. Wells JK: Comparison of ICI 35868, etomidate and metohexitone for day-case anaesthesia. Br J Anaesth 57:732-735, 1985.
594. Zacharias M, Dundee JW, Clarke RS, Hegarty JE: Effect of preanaesthetic medication on etomidate. Br J Anaesth 51:127-133, 1979.

595. Linton DM, Thornington RE: Etomidate as a rectal induction agent. Part II: A clinical study in children. S Afr Med J 64:309-310, 1983.

596. Schuttler J, Schwilden H, Stoekel H: Pharmacokinetics as applied to total intravenous anaesthesia. Practical implications. Anaesthesia 38(Suppl):53-56, 1983.

597. Sear JW, Walters FJ, Wilkins DG, Willatts SM: Etomidate by infusion for neuroanaesthesia. Kinetic and dynamic interactions with nitrous oxide. Anaesthesia 39:12-18, 1984.

598. Van Hamme MJ, Ghoneim MM, Ambre JJ: Pharmacokinetics of etomidate, a new intravenous anesthetic. Anesthesiology 49:274-277, 1978.

599. Meuldermans WE, Heykants JJ: The plasma protein binding and distribution of etomidate in dog, rat and human blood. Arch Int Pharmacodyn Ther 221:150-162, 1976.

600. Johnson KB, Egan TD, Layman J, et al: The influence of hemorrhagic shock on etomidate: A pharmacokinetic and pharmacodynamic analysis. Anesth Analg 96:1360-1368, 2003.

601. van Beem H, Manger FW, van Boxtel C, van Bentem N: Etomidate anaesthesia in patients with cirrhosis of the liver: Pharmacokinetic data. Anaesthesia 38(Suppl):61-62, 1983.

602. Arden JR, Holley FO, Stanski DR: Increased sensitivity to etomidate in the elderly: Initial distribution versus altered brain response. Anesthesiology 65:19-27, 1986.

603. Doenicke A, Loffler B, Kugler J, et al: Plasma concentration and E.E.G. after various regimens of etomidate. Br J Anaesth 54:393-400, 1982.

604. Evans RH, Hill RG: The GABA-mimetic action of etomidate [proceedings]. Br J Pharmacol 61:484P, 1977.

605. Lingamaneni R, Hemmings HC Jr: Differential interaction of anaesthetics and antiepileptic drugs with neuronal Na$^+$ channels, Ca^{2+} channels, and GABA(A) receptors. Br J Anaesth 90:199-211, 2003.

606. Blednov YA, Jung S, Alva H, et al: Deletion of the alpha1 or beta2 subunit of GABA$_A$ receptors reduces actions of alcohol and other drugs. J Pharmacol Exp Ther 304:30-36, 2003.

607. Cold GE, Eskesen V, Eriksen H, et al: CBF and CMRO$_2$ during continuous etomidate infusion supplemented with N$_2$O and fentanyl in patients with supratentorial cerebral tumour. A dose-response study. Acta Anaesthesiol Scand 29:490-494, 1985.

608. Dearden NM, McDowall DG: Comparison of etomidate and althesin in the reduction of increased intracranial pressure after head injury. Br J Anaesth 57:361-368, 1985.

609. Modica PA, Tempelhoff R: Intracranial pressure during induction of anaesthesia and tracheal intubation with etomidate-induced EEG burst suppression. Can J Anaesth 39:236-241, 1992.

610. Renou AM, Vernhiet J, Macrez P, et al: Cerebral blood flow and metabolism during etomidate anaesthesia in man. Br J Anaesth 50:1047-1051, 1978.

611. Tulleken CA, van Dieren A, Jonkman J, Kalenda Z: Clinical and experimental experience with etomidate as a brain protective agent. J Cereb Blood Flow Metab 2(Suppl 1): S92-S97, 1982.

612. Sano T, Patel PM, Drummond JC, Cole DJ: A comparison of the cerebral protective effects of etomidate, thiopental, and isoflurane in a model of forebrain ischemia in the rat. Anesth Analg 76:990-997, 1993.

613. Drummond JC, Cole DJ, Patel PM, Reynolds LW: Focal cerebral ischemia during anesthesia with etomidate, isoflurane, or thiopental: A comparison of the extent of cerebral injury. Neurosurgery 37:742-748, discussion 748-749, 1995.

614. Guo J, White JA, Batjer HH: Limited protective effects of etomidate during brainstem ischemia in dogs. J Neurosurg 82:278-283, 1995.

615. Thomson MF, Brock-Utne JG, Bean P, et al: Anaesthesia and intra-ocular pressure: A comparative of total intravenous anaesthesia using etomidate with conventional inhalation anaesthesia. Anaesthesia 37:758-761, 1982.

616. Ghoneim MM, Yamada T: Etomidate: A clinical and electroencephalographic comparison with thiopental. Anesth Analg 56:479-485, 1977.

617. Lees NW, Hendry JG: Etomidate in urological outpatient anaesthesia. A clinical evaluation. Anaesthesia 32:592-597, 1977.

618. Ebrahim ZY, DeBoer GE, Luders H, et al: Effect of etomidate on the electroencephalogram of patients with epilepsy. Anesth Analg 65:1004-1006, 1986.

619. Gancher S, Laxer KD, Krieger W: Activation of epileptogenic activity by etomidate. Anesthesiology 61:616-618, 1984.

620. Reddy RV, Moorthy SS, Dierdorf SF, et al: Excitatory effects and electroencephalographic correlation of etomidate, thiopental, methohexital, and propofol. Anesth Analg 77:1008-1011, 1993.

621. Thornton C, Heneghan CP, Navaratnarajah M, et al: Effect of etomidate on the auditory evoked response in man. Br J Anaesth 57:554-561, 1985.

622. McPherson RW, Sell B, Traystman RJ: Effects of thiopental, fentanyl, and etomidate on upper extremity somatosensory evoked potentials in humans. Anesthesiology 65:584-589, 1986.

623. Kalkman CJ, Drummond JC, Ribberink AA, et al: Effects of propofol, etomidate, midazolam, and fentanyl on motor evoked responses to transcranial electrical or magnetic stimulation in humans. Anesthesiology 76:502-509, 1992.

624. Guldager H, Sondergaard I, Jensen FM, Cold G: Basophil histamine release in asthma patients after in vitro provocation with Althesin and etomidate. Acta Anaesthesiol Scand 29:352-353, 1985.

625. Kay B: The measurement of occlusion pressure during anaesthesia. A comparison of the depression of respiratory drive by methohexitone and etomidate. Anaesthesia 34:543-548, 1979.

626. Morgan M, Lumley J, Whitwam JG: Respiratory effects of etomidate. Br J Anaesth 49:233-236, 1977.

627. Criado A, Maseda J, Navarro E, et al: Induction of anaesthesia with etomidate: Haemodynamic study of 36 patients. Br J Anaesth 52:803-806, 1980.

628. Ouedraogo N, Marthan R, Roux E: The effects of propofol and etomidate on airway contractility in chronically hypoxic rats. Anesth Analg 96:1035-1041, 2003.

629. Ogawa K, Tanaka S, Murray PA: Inhibitory effects of etomidate and ketamine on endothelium-dependent relaxation in canine pulmonary artery. Anesthesiology 94:668-677, 2001.

630. Lindeburg T, Spotoft H, Bredgaard Sorensen M, Skovsted P: Cardiovascular effects of etomidate used for induction and in combination with fentanyl-pancuronium for maintenance of anaesthesia in patients with valvular heart disease. Acta Anaesthesiol Scand 26:205-208, 1982.

631. Haessler R, Madler C, Klasing S: Propofol/fentanyl versus etomidate/fentanyl for the induction of anesthesia in patients with aortic insufficiency and coronary artery disease. J Cardiothorac Vasc Anesth 6:173, 1992.

632. Sprung J, Ogletree-Hughes ML, Moravec CS: The effects of etomidate on the contractility of failing and nonfailing human heart muscle. Anesth Analg 91:68-75, 2000.

633. Lischke V, Wilke HJ, Probst S, et al: Prolongation of the QT-interval during induction of anesthesia in patients with coronary artery disease. Acta Anaesthesiol Scand 38:144-148, 1994.

634. de Bruijn NP, Hlatky MA, Jacobs JR, et al: General anesthesia during percutaneous transluminary coronary angioplasty for acute myocardial infarction: Results of a randomized controlled clinical trial. Anesth Analg 68:201-207, 1989.

635. Gries A, Weis S, Herr A, et al: Etomidate and thiopental inhibit platelet function in patients undergoing infrainguinal vascular surgery. Acta Anaesthesiol Scand 45:449-457, 2001.

636. Ledingham I, Finlay W, Watt I: Etomidate and adrenocortical function [letter]. Lancet 2:1434, 1983.

637. Allolio B, Dorr H, Stuttmann R, et al: Effect of a single bolus dose of etomidate upon eight major corticosteroid hormones and plasma ACTH: Clin Endocrinol (Oxf) 22:281-286, 1985.

638. Lamberts SW, Bons EG, Bruining HA, de Jong FH: Differential effects of the imidazole derivatives etomidate, ketoconazole and miconazole and of metyrapone on the secretion of cortisol and its precursors by human adreno-cortical cells. J Pharmacol Exp Ther 240:259-264, 1987.

639. Boidin MP: Steroid response to ACTH and to ascorbinic acid during infusion of etomidate for general surgery. Acta Anaesthesiol Belg 36:15-22, 1985.

640. Boidin MP, Erdmann WE, Faithfull NS: The role of ascorbic acid in etomidate toxicity. Eur J Anaesthesiol 3:417-422, 1986.

641. Wagner RL, White PF, Kan PB, et al: Inhibition of adrenal steroidogenesis by the anesthetic etomidate. N Engl J Med 310:1415-1421, 1984.

642. Duthie DJ, Fraser R, Nimmo WS: Effect of induction of anaesthesia with etomidate on corticosteroid synthesis in man. Br J Anaesth 57:156-159, 1985.

643. Crozier TA, Beck D, Schlaeger M, et al: Endocrinological changes following etomidate, midazolam, or methohexital for minor surgery. Anesthesiology 66:628-635, 1987.

644. Fragen R, Shanks C, Molteni A: Effect on plasma cortisol concentration of a single induction dose of etomidate or thiopentone. Lancet 2:625, 1983.

645. Crozier TA, Schlaeger M, Wuttke W, Kettler D: TIVA with etomidate-fentanyl versus midazolam-fentanyl. The perioperative stress of coronary surgery overcomes the inhibition of cortisol synthesis caused by etomidate-fentanyl anesthesia [in German]. Anaesthesist 43:605-613, 1994.

646. Famewo CE: Induction of anaesthesia with etomidate in a patient with acute intermittent porphyria. Can Anaesth Soc J 32:171-173, 1985.

647. St Pierre M, Dunkel M, Rutherford A, Hering W: Does etomidate increase postoperative nausea? A double-blind controlled comparison of etomidate in lipid emulsion with propofol for balanced anaesthesia. Eur J Anaesthesiol 17:634-641, 2000.

648. Korttila K, Aromaa U: Venous complications after intra-venous injection of diazepam, flunitrazepam, thiopentone and etomidate. Acta Anaesthesiol Scand 24:227-230, 1980.

649. Galloway PA, Nicoll JM, Leiman BC: Pain reduction with etomidate injection. Anaesthesia 37:352-353, 1982.

650. Doenicke AW, Roizen MF, Hoernecke R, et al: Solvent for etomidate may cause pain and adverse effects. Br J Anaesth 83:464-466, 1999.

651. Olkkola KT, Tammisto T: Quantitation of the interaction of rocuronium bromide with etomidate, fentanyl, midazolam, propofol, thiopentone, and isoflurane using closed-loop feedback control of infusion of rocuronium. Eur J Anaesthesiol Suppl 9:99-100, 1994.

652. Olkkola KT, Tammisto T: Quantifying the interaction of rocuronium (Org 9426) with etomidate, fentanyl, midazolam, propofol, thiopental, and isoflurane using closed-loop feedback control of rocuronium infusion. Anesth Analg 78:691-696, 1994.

653. Van de Wiele B, Rubinstein E, Peacock W, Martin N: Propylene glycol toxicity caused by prolonged infusion of etomidate. J Neurosurg Anesthesiol 7:259-262, 1995.

654. Liem TH, Booij LH, Hasenbos MA, Gielen MJ: Coronary artery bypass grafting using two different anesthetic techniques: Part I: Hemodynamic results. J Cardiothorac Vasc Anesth 6:148-155, 1992.

655. Shulman MS, Edelmann R: Use of etomidate for elective cardioversion. Anesthesiology 68:656, 1988.

656. Batjer HH, Frankfurt AI, Purdy PD, et al: Use of etomidate, temporary arterial occlusion, and intraoperative angiography in surgical treatment of large and giant cerebral aneurysms. J Neurosurg 68:234-240, 1988.

657. Lees NW, Glasser J, McGroarty FJ, Miller BM: Etomidate and fentanyl for maintenance of anaesthesia. Br J Anaesth 53:959-961, 1981.

658. Avramov MN, Husain MM, White PF: The comparative effects of methohexital, propofol, and etomidate for electroconvulsive therapy. Anesth Analg 81:596-602, 1995.

659. Maze M, Tranquilli W: Alpha-2 adrenoceptor agonists: Defining the role in clinical anesthesia. Anesthesiology 74:581-605, 1991.

660. Kaukinen S, Kaukinen L, Eerola R: Preoperative and postoperative use of clonidine with neurolept anaesthesia. Acta Anaesthesiol Scand 23:113-120, 1979.

661. Kaukinen S, Pyykko K: The potentiation of halothane anaesthesia by clonidine. Acta Anaesthesiol Scand 23:107-111, 1979.

662. Bloor BC, Flacke WE: Reduction in halothane anesthetic requirement by clonidine, an alpha-adrenergic agonist. Anesth Analg 61:741-745, 1982.

663. De Wolf AM, Fragen RJ, Avram MJ, et al: The pharmacokinetics of dexmedetomidine in volunteers with severe renal impairment. Anesth Analg 93:1205-1209, 2001.

664. Guo TZ, Jiang JY, Buttermann AE, Maze M: Dexmedetomidine injection into the locus ceruleus produces antinociception. Anesthesiology 84:873-881, 1996.

665. Nelson LE, Lu J, Guo T, et al: The alpha2-adrenoceptor agonist dexmedetomidine converges on an endogenous sleep-promoting pathway to exert its sedative effects. Anesthesiology 98:428-436, 2003.

666. Nacif-Coelho C, Correa-Sales C, Chang LL, Maze M: Perturbation of ion channel conductance alters the hypnotic response to the alpha 2-adrenergic agonist dexmedetomidine in the locus coeruleus of the rat. Anesthesiology 81:1527-1534, 1994.

667. Aho M, Erkola O, Kallio A, et al: Comparison of dexmedetomidine and midazolam sedation and antagonism of dexmedetomidine with atipamezole. J Clin Anesth 5:194-203, 1993.

668. Reid K, Hayashi Y, Guo TZ, et al: Chronic administration of an alpha 2 adrenergic agonist desensitizes rats to the anesthetic effects of dexmedetomidine. Pharmacol Biochem Behav 47:171-175, 1994.

669. Maccioli GA: Dexmedetomidine to facilitate drug withdrawal. Anesthesiology 98:575-577, 2003.

670. Davies MF, Haimor F, Lighthall G, Clark JD: Dexmedetomidine fails to cause hyperalgesia after cessation of chronic administration. Anesth Analg 96:195-200, 2003.

671. Hayashi Y, Guo TZ, Maze M: Hypnotic and analgesic effects of the alpha 2-adrenergic agonist dexmedetomidine in morphine-tolerant rats. Anesth Analg 83:606-610, 1996.

672. Maier C, Steinberg GK, Sun GH, et al: Neuroprotection by the alpha 2-adrenoreceptor agonist dexmedetomidine in a focal model of cerebral ischemia. Anesthesiology 79:306-312, 1993.

673. Talke P, Tong C, Lee HW, et al: Effect of dexmedetomidine on lumbar cerebrospinal fluid pressure in humans. Anesth Analg 85:358-364, 1997.

674. Karlsson BR, Forsman M, Roald OK, et al: Effect of dexmedetomidine, a selective and potent alpha 2-agonist, on cerebral blood flow and oxygen consumption during halothane anesthesia in dogs. Anesth Analg 71:125-129, 1990.

675. Zornow MH, Fleischer JE, Scheller MS, et al: Dexmedetomidine, an alpha 2-adrenergic agonist, decreases cerebral blood flow in the isoflurane-anesthetized dog. Anesth Analg 70:624-630, 1990.

676. Zornow MH, Maze M, Dyck JB, Shafer SL: Dexmedetomidine decreases cerebral blood flow velocity in humans. J Cereb Blood Flow Metab 13:350-353, 1993.

677. Prielipp RC, Wall MH, Tobin JR, et al: Dexmedetomidine-induced sedation in volunteers decreases regional and global cerebral blood flow. Anesth Analg 95:1052-1059, 2002.

678. Mirski MA, Rossell LA, McPherson RW, Traystman RJ: Dexmedetomidine decreases seizure threshold in a rat model of experimental generalized epilepsy. Anesthesiology 81:1422-1428, 1994.

679. Halonen P, Kotti T, Tuunanen J, et al: Alpha 2-adrenoceptor agonist, dexmedetomidine, protects against kainic acid–induced convulsions and neuronal damage. Brain Res 693:217-224, 1995.

680. Weinger MB, Segal IS, Maze M: Dexmedetomidine, acting through central alpha-2 adrenoceptors, prevents opiate-induced muscle rigidity in the rat. Anesthesiology 71:242-249, 1989.

681. Scheinin H, Karhuvaara S, Olkkola KT, et al: Pharmacodynamics and pharmacokinetics of intramuscular dexmedetomidine. Clin Pharmacol Ther 52:537-546, 1992.

682. Karhuvaara S, Kallio A, Koulu M, et al: No involvement of alpha 2-adrenoceptors in the regulation of basal prolactin secretion in healthy men. Psychoneuroendocrinology 15:125-129, 1990.

683. Ebert TJ, Hall JE, Barney JA, et al: The effects of increasing plasma concentrations of dexmedetomidine in humans. Anesthesiology 93:382-394, 2000.

684. Yung-Wei H, Robertson K, Young C, et al: Compare the respiratory effects of remifentanil and dexmedetomidine. Anesthesiology 95:A1357, 2001.

685. Arain SR, Ebert TJ: The efficacy, side effects, and recovery characteristics of dexmedetomidine versus propofol when used for intraoperative sedation. Anesth Analg 95:461-466, 2002.

686. Dyck JB, Maze M, Haack C, et al: The pharmacokinetics and hemodynamic effects of intravenous and intramuscular dexmedetomidine hydrochloride in adult human volunteers. Anesthesiology 78:813-820, 1993.

687. Hogue CW Jr, Talke P, Stein PK, et al: Autonomic nervous system responses during sedative infusions of dexmedetomidine. Anesthesiology 97:592-598, 2002.

688. Roekaerts P, Prinzen F, Willingers H: The effect of dexmedetomidine on systemic haemodynamics, regional myocardial function and blood flow during coronary artery stenosis in acute anaesthetized dogs. J Cardiothorac Anesth 8:58, 1994.

689. Willigers HM, Prinzen FW, Roekaerts PM, et al: Dexmedetomidine decreases perioperative myocardial lactate release in dogs. Anesth Analg 96:657-764, 2003.

690. Karhuvaara S, Kallio A, Salonen M, et al: Rapid reversal of alpha 2-adrenoceptor agonist effects by atipamezole in human volunteers. Br J Clin Pharmacol 31:160-165, 1991.

691. Aantaa RE, Kanto JH, Scheinin M, et al: Dexmedetomidine premedication for minor gynecologic surgery. Anesth Analg 70:407-413, 1990.

692. Aantaa R, Kanto J, Scheinin M, et al: Dexmedetomidine, an alpha 2-adrenoceptor agonist, reduces anesthetic requirements for patients undergoing minor gynecologic surgery. Anesthesiology 73:230-235, 1990.

693. Aho M, Lehtinen AM, Erkola O, et al: The effect of intravenously administered dexmedetomidine on perioperative hemodynamics and isoflurane requirements in patients undergoing abdominal hysterectomy. Anesthesiology 74:997-1002, 1991.

694. Venn RM, Grounds RM: Comparison between dexmedetomidine and propofol for sedation in the intensive care unit: Patient and clinician perceptions. Br J Anaesth 87:684-690, 2001.

695. Triltsch AE, Welte M, von Homeyer P, et al: Bispectral index–guided sedation with dexmedetomidine in intensive care: A prospective, randomized, double blind, placebo-controlled phase II study. Crit Care Med 30:1007-1014, 2002.

696. Flacke JW, Bloor BC, Flacke WE, et al: Reduced narcotic requirement by clonidine with improved hemodynamic and adrenergic stability in patients undergoing coronary bypass surgery. Anesthesiology 67:11-19, 1987.

697. Ghignone M, Quintin L, Duke PC, et al: Effects of clonidine on narcotic requirements and hemodynamic response during induction of fentanyl anesthesia and endotracheal intubation. Anesthesiology 64:36-42, 1986.

698. Segal IS, Jarvis DJ, Duncan SR, et al: Clinical efficacy of oral-transdermal clonidine combinations during the perioperative period. Anesthesiology 74:220-225, 1991.

699. Lieper D, Townsend G: Improved hemodynamic and renal function with clonidine in coronary artery bypass grafting. Anesth Analg 70:S240, 1990.

700. Ghignone M, Noe C, Calvillo O, Quintin L: Anesthesia for ophthalmic surgery in the elderly: The effects of clonidine on intraocular pressure, perioperative hemodynamics, and anesthetic requirement. Anesthesiology 68:707-716, 1988.

701. Jaakola ML, Ali-Melkkila T, Kanto J, et al: Dexmedetomidine reduces intraocular pressure, intubation responses and anaesthetic requirements in patients undergoing ophthalmic surgery. Br J Anaesth 68:570-575, 1992.

702. Scheinin B, Lindgren L, Randell T, et al: Dexmedetomidine attenuates sympathoadrenal responses to tracheal intubation and reduces the need for thiopentone and preoperative fentanyl. Br J Anaesth 68:126-131, 1992.

703. Aho M, Erkola O, Kallio A, et al: Dexmedetomidine infusion for maintenance of anesthesia in patients undergoing abdominal hysterectomy. Anesth Analg 75:940-946, 1992.

704. Salmenpera MT, Szlam F, Hug CC Jr: Anesthetic and hemodynamic interactions of dexmedetomidine and fentanyl in dogs. Anesthesiology 80:837-846, 1994.

705. Talke P, Li J, Jain U, et al: Effects of perioperative dexmedetomidine infusion in patients undergoing vascular surgery. The Study of Perioperative Ischemia Research Group. Anesthesiology 82:620-633, 1995.

706. Laborit H, Huguenard P: Practique de l'Hibernotherapie en Chirurgie et en Medicine. Paris, Masson, 1954.

707. Laborit H: Stress and Cellular Function. Philadelphia, JB Lippincott, 1959.

708. Corssen G, Reves J, Stanley T: Neuroleptanalgesia and neurolept-anesthesia. In Corssen G, Reves J, Stanley T (eds): Intravenous Anesthesia and Analgesia. Philadelphia, Lea & Febiger, 1988, p 175.

709. Janssen PA: The pharmacology of haloperidol. Int J Neuropsychiatry 3(Suppl 1):10-18, 1967.

710. De Castro J, Mundeleer P: Anesthesie sans barbituriques: La neuroleptanalgesie (R1407, R1625, hydergine, procain). Anesth Analg 42:1022, 1959.

711. Scuderi PE: Droperidol: Many questions, few answers. Anesthesiology 98:289-290, 2003.

712. Dershwitz M: Droperidol: Should the black box be light gray? J Clin Anesth 14:598-603, 2002.

713. White PF: Droperidol: A cost-effective antiemetic for over thirty years. Anesth Analg 95:789-790, 2002.

714. Gan TJ, Alexander R, Fennelly M, Rubin AP: Comparison of different methods of administering droperidol in patient-controlled analgesia in the prevention of postoperative nausea and vomiting. Anesth Analg 80:81-85, 1995.

715. Gan TJ, White PF, Scuderi PE, et al: FDA "black box" warning regarding use of droperidol for postoperative nausea and vomiting: Is it justified? Anesthesiology 97:287, 2002.

716. Bailey P, Norton R, Karan S: The FDA droperidol warning: Is it justified? Anesthesiology 97:288-289, 2002.

717. Flood P, Coates KM: Droperidol inhibits GABA(A) and neuronal nicotinic receptor activation. Anesthesiology 96:987-993, 2002.

718. Borison HL, Wang SC: Physiology and pharmacology of vomiting. Pharmacol Rev 5:193-230, 1953.

719. Janssen P: Zur Frage des Abbaus und der Ausscheidung der bei Neuroleptanalgesie zur Anwendung kommenden Pharmaka. In Henschel W (ed): Die Neuroleptanalgesie. Berlin, Springer-Verlag, 1966.

720. Michenfelder JD, Theye RA: Effects of fentanyl, droperidol, and Innovar on canine cerebral metabolism and blood flow. Br J Anaesth 43:630-636, 1971.

721. Barker J, Harper A, McDowall D: Cerebral blood flow, cerebrospinal fluid pressure and EEG activity during neuroleptanalgesia induced with dehydrobenzperidol and phenoperidine. Br J Anaesth 40:143, 1968.

722. Song D, Chung F, Yogendran S, Wong J: Evaluation of postural stability after low-dose droperidol in outpatients undergoing gynaecological dilatation and curettage procedure. Br J Anaesth 88:819-823, 2002.

723. Corssen G, Domino EF, Sweet RB: Neuroleptanalgesia and anesthesia. Anesth Analg 43:748-763, 1964.

724. Wooltorton E: Droperidol: Cardiovascular toxicity and deaths. CMAJ 166:932, 2002.

725. Yelnosky J, Katz R, Dietrich EV: A study of some of the pharmacologic actions of droperidol. Toxicol Appl Pharmacol 6:37-47, 1964.

726. Janssen P, Niemegeers C, Schellekens K: The pharmacology of dehydrobenzperidol, a new potent and short acting neuroleptic agent chemically related to haloperidol. Arzneimittelforschung 13:205-211, 1963.

727. Stanley T: Cardiovascular effects of droperidol during enflurane and enflurane–nitrous oxide anaesthesia in man. Can Anaesth Soc J 25:26-29, 1978.

728. Birch AA, Boyce WH: Effects of droperidol-dopamine interaction on renal blood flow in man. Anesthesiology 47:70-71, 1977.

729. Wetchler B, Collins I, Jacob L: Antiemetic effects of droperidol on the ambulatory surgery patient. Anesthesiol Rev 9:23, 1982.

730. Pandit SK, Kothary SP, Pandit UA, et al: Dose-response study of droperidol and metoclopramide as antiemetics for outpatient anesthesia. Anesth Analg 68:798-802, 1989.

731. Kymer PJ, Brown RE Jr, Lawhorn CD, et al: The effects of oral droperidol versus oral metoclopramide versus both oral droperidol and metoclopramide on postoperative vomiting when used as a premedicant for strabismus surgery. J Clin Anesth 7:35-39, 1995.

732. Hill RP, Lubarsky DA, Phillips-Bute B, et al: Cost-effectiveness of prophylactic antiemetic therapy with ondansetron, droperidol, or placebo. Anesthesiology 92:958-967, 2000.

733. McKenzie R, Tantisira B, Jackson D, et al: Antiemetic efficacy of a droperidol-morphine combination in patient-controlled analgesia. J Clin Anesth 7:141-147, 1995.

734. Aldrete JA: Reduction of nausea and vomiting from epidural opioids by adding droperidol to the infusate in home-bound patients. J Pain Symptom Manage 10:544-547, 1995.

735. Kjellberg F, Tramer MR: Pharmacological control of opioid-induced pruritus: A quantitative systematic review of randomized trials. Eur J Anaesthesiol 18:346-357, 2001.

CHAPTER
11 Intravenous Opioid Anesthetics

Kazuhiko Fukuda

Pharmacology of Opioids   380
Classification of Opioid
  Compounds   380
Opioid Receptors   380
Endogenous Opioid Peptides   382
Intracellular Signal Transduction
  Mechanism   383
Mechanism of Analgesia   385
Mood Alterations and Rewarding
  Properties   385
Analysis of Knockout Mice   385
Actions of Opioids on Targets Other Than
  Opioid Receptors   386
The Role of Nociceptin/orphanin FQ in Pain
  Modulation   387

**Neurophysiologic Effects of
  Opioids   387**
Analgesic Action of Opioids   387
Opioids as Anesthetics   387
Electroencephalography   388
Sensory Evoked Potentials   389
Cerebral Blood Flow and Cerebral
  Metabolic Rate   389
Intracranial Pressure   390
Neuroprotection   390
Muscle Rigidity   390
Neuroexcitatory Phenomena   391
Pupil Size   391
Thermoregulation and Shivering   391
Pruritus   392

**Respiratory Effects of
  Opioids   392**
Therapeutic Effects   392
Nontherapeutic Effects   392
Factors Affecting Opioid-induced Respiratory
  Depression   393

**Cardiovascular Effects of
  Opioids   394**
Neurologic Mechanisms   394
Cardiac Mechanisms   394
Hormonal Mechanisms   395
Vascular Mechanisms   396

**Endocrinologic Effects of
  Opioids   396**
Stress Reduction and Outcome   396

Opiate Tolerance and Addiction   397
Management of the Opioid-Dependent
  Patient   397

**Renal and Urodynamic Effects
  of Opioids   397**

**Gastrointestinal Effects of
  Opioids   398**
Biliary and Hepatic Effects   398
Nausea and Vomiting   398

Other Opioid Effects   399
Obstetrics   399
Allergic Reactions   399
Ocular Effects   399
Immune Effects   399

**Pharmacokinetics and
  Pharmacodynamics of Opioids   400**
Physicochemical Properties   400
Common Pharmacokinetic Features
  of Opioids   400
Pharmacokinetic Features of
  Individual Drugs   401
Irrelevance of the Terminal Half-Life   403
Context-Sensitive Half-Time   404
Effect Site and Latency to Peak Effect   404
Slope of the Concentration-Effect
  Relationship   404
Computerized Delivery Methods in
  Clinical Practice   405
Surrogate Measures of Opioid Potency   405
Factors Affecting Pharmacokinetics and
  Pharmacodynamics of Opioids   406

**Anesthetic Techniques Using
  Opioids   410**
Sedation and Analgesia   410
Balanced Anesthesia   410
Neuroleptanalgesia-Anesthesia   412
Total Intravenous Anesthesia   413

Opioid-Based (High-Dose Opioid)
   Anesthesia   414
Other Applications of Opioids   415

Other Opioid Agonists   417

**Agonist-Antagonist Opioid
   Compounds   418**
Pentazocine   419
Butorphanol   419
Buprenorphine   419
Nalbuphine   419
Other Compounds   420

Opioid Antagonists   420
Naloxone   420
Other Opioid Antagonists   421

**Drug Interactions with
   Opioids   421**
General Principles   421
Sedative-Hypnotics   422
Inhaled Anesthetics   423
Muscle Relaxants   423
Miscellaneous   423

The term *opioid* refers broadly to all compounds related to opium. The word "opium" is derived from *opos*, the Greek word for juice, the drug being derived from the juice of the opium poppy, *Papaver somniferum*. Opiates are drugs derived from opium, and include the natural products morphine, codeine, and thebaine and many semisynthetic congeners derived from them.

The first undisputed reference to opium is found in the writings of Theophrastus in third century BC. During the Middle Ages, many of the uses of opium were appreciated. Opium contains more than 20 distinct alkaloids. In 1806, Sertürner reported the isolation of a pure substance in opium that he named morphine, after Morpheus, the Greek god of dreams. By the middle of the nineteenth century, the use of pure alkaloids rather than crude opium preparations began to spread throughout the medical world.

In addition to the remarkable beneficial effects of opioids, the toxic side effects and addictive potential of these drugs also have been known for centuries. Synthetic opioid analgesics without side effects were explored, but many of the synthetic opioids share the side effects of natural opioids. The search for new opioid agonists led to the synthesis of opioid antagonists and compounds with mixed agonist/antagonist properties, which expanded therapeutic options and provided important tools for exploring mechanisms of opioid actions. Furthermore, new methods of opioid administration, including patient-controlled analgesia (PCA) and computer-based infusion techniques, have been developed.

PHARMACOLOGY OF OPIOIDS

Classification of Opioid Compounds

Opioids can be classified as naturally occurring, semisynthetic, and synthetic (Table 11-1). The naturally occurring opioids can be divided into two chemical classes, phenanthrenes (morphine and codeine), and benzylisoquinolines (papaverine). The semisynthetic opioids are morphine derivatives in which one of several changes has been made. Synthetic opioids are classified into four groups, the morphinan derivatives (levorphanol), the diphenyl

or methadone derivatives (methadone, *d*-propoxyphene), the benzomorphans (phenazocine, pentazocine), and the phenylpiperidine derivatives (meperidine, fentanyl, alfentanil, sufentanil, and remifentanil). Structures of opioid compounds are shown in Figure 11-1 and Table 11-2.[1] Opioids can be classified as agonists, partial agonists, mixed agonist-antagonists and antagonists on the basis of their interaction with the opioid receptors.

Opioid Receptors

In 1973, three independent teams of investigators described the presence of opioid binding sites in the nervous system from radioligand binding assays. Based on pharmacological experiments, three types of opioid receptors were postulated. They were named μ for morphine type, κ for the ketocyclazocine type, and σ for the SKF10047 (N-allylnormetazocine) type. In addition, a high-affinity receptor for enkephalins was found in the mouse vas deferens, and named as a δ-receptor. Furthermore, an ε-receptor was proposed as the binding

Table 11–1   Classification of opioid compounds
Naturally occurring
Morphine
Codeine
Papaverine
Thebaine
Semisynthetic
Heroin
Dihydromorphone/morphinone
Thebaine derivatives (e.g., etorphine, buprenorphine)
Synthetic
Morphinan series (e.g., levorphanol, butorphanol)
Diphenylpropylamine series (e.g., methadone)
Benzomorphan series (e.g., pentazocine)
Phenylpiperidine series (e.g., meperidine, fentanyl, sufentanil, alfentanil, remifentanil)

From Bailey PL, Egan TD, Stanley TH: Intravenous opioid anesthetics. *In* Miller RD (ed): Anesthesia, 5th ed. New York, Churchill Livingstone, 2000, p 276.

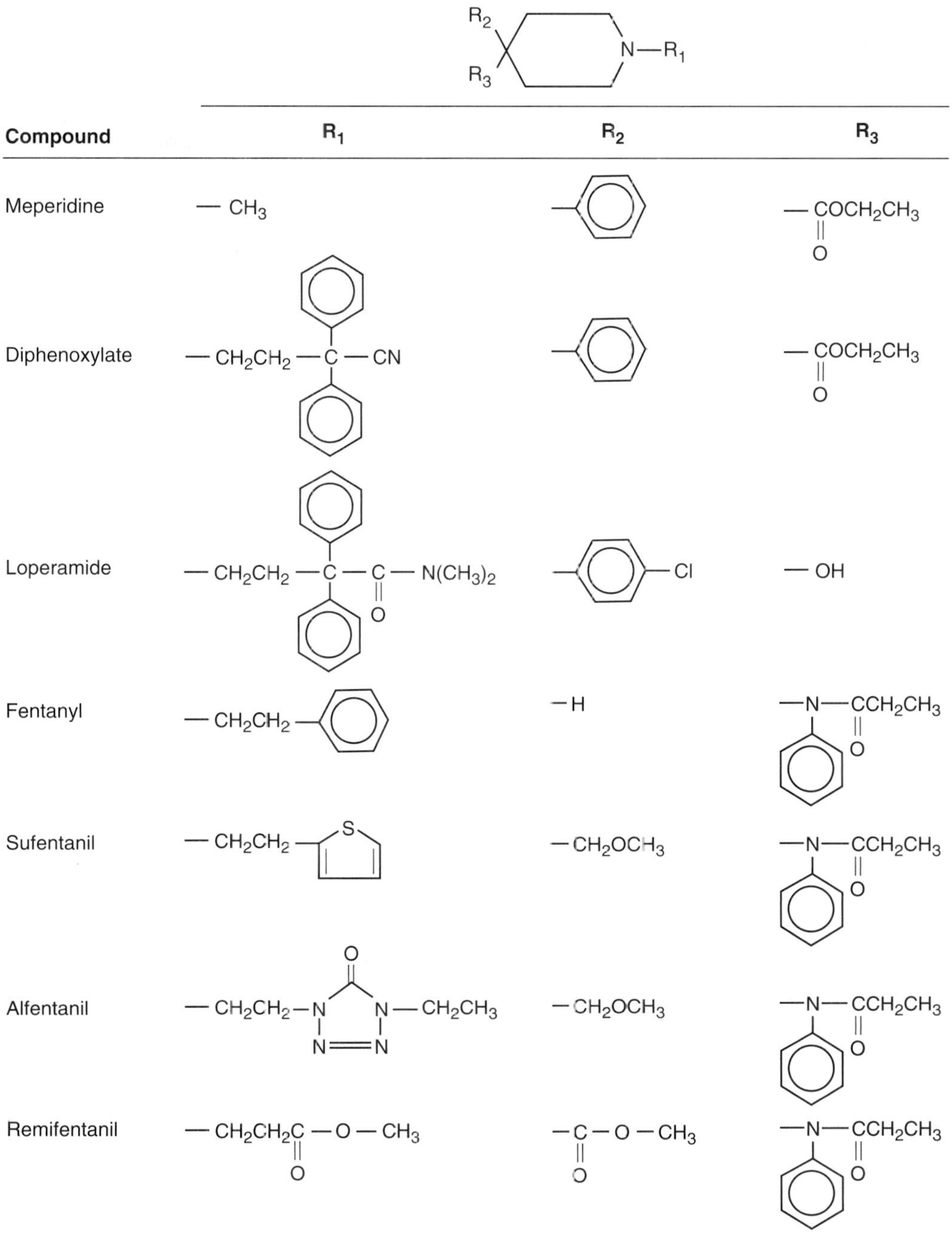

Figure 11–1 Chemical structures of piperidine and phenylpiperidine analgesics. (From Gutstein HB, Akil H: Opioid analgesics. *In* Hardman JG, Limbird LE [eds]: Goodman and Gilman's The Pharmacological Basis of Therapeutics, 10th ed. New York, McGraw-Hill, 2001, pp 569-619.)

site for β-endorphin in the rat vas deferens. Pharmacologic actions of opioids and the involved receptors have been analyzed (Table 11-3).

Biochemical studies attempted to purify the opioid receptor protein but have not been successful. Since the early 1990s, molecular biological studies have elucidated the molecular structures and signal transduction mechanisms of the opioid receptors. Four different types of cDNA have been isolated as the members of the opioid receptor family.[2] It was demonstrated that three of them correspond to the pharmacologically defined μ-, δ-, and κ-opioid receptors. The fourth receptor did not bind with opioid ligands with high affinities. Later, a novel peptide

called nociceptin, or orphanin FQ (see later), was identified as an endogenous agonist of the fourth member of the opioid receptor family.[3,4] The characteristics of three opioid receptors and the nociceptin/orphanin FQ receptor are listed in Table 11-4.

The μ-receptors are located in both the brain and the spinal cord[5] and are thought to mediate a variety of pharmacologic effects of opioids. Further pharmacologic classification of the μ-receptor as μ_1, μ_2, and μ_3 has been proposed. It may be possible that posttranslational modification of the μ-receptor is the molecular basis of μ-receptor subtypes. However, the molecular identity of these receptors remains to be clarified.

Table 11–2 Structures of opioids and opioid antagonists chemically related to morphine

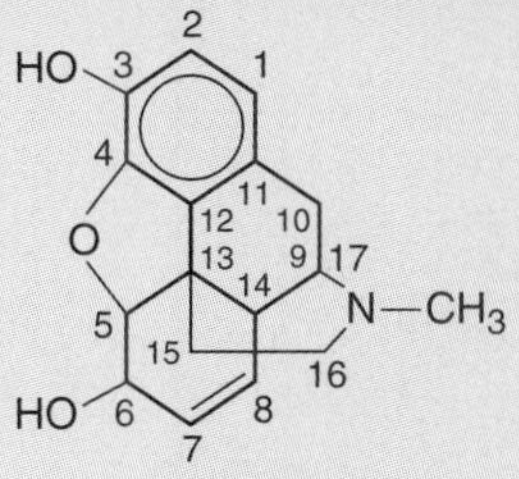

MORPHINE

Nonproprietary Name	Chemical Radicals and Position*			Other Changes†
	3	6	17	
Morphine	—OH	—OH	—CH$_3$	—
Heroin	—OCOCH$_3$	—OCOCH$_3$	—CH$_3$	—
Hydromorphone	—OH	=O	—CH$_3$	(1)
Oxymorphone	—OH	=O	—CH$_3$	(1), (2)
Levorphanol	—OH	—H	—CH$_3$	(1), (3)
Levallorphan	—OH	—H	—CH$_2$CH=CH$_2$	(1), (3)
Codeine	—OCH$_3$	—OH	—CH$_3$	—
Hydrocodone	—OCH$_3$	=O	—CH$_3$	(1)
Oxycodone	—OCH$_3$	=O	—CH$_3$	(1), (2)
Nalmefene	—OH	=CH$_2$	—CH$_2$—▷	(1), (2)
Nalorphine	—OH	—OH	—CH$_2$CH=CH$_2$	—
Naloxone	—OH	=O	—CH$_2$CH=CH$_2$	(1), (2)
Naltrexone	—OH	=O	—CH$_2$—◁	(1), (2)
Buprenorphine	—OH	—OCH$_3$	—CH$_2$—◁	(1), (4)
Butorphanol	—OH	—H	—CH$_2$—◇	(1), (2), (3)
Nalbuphine	—OH	—OH	—CH$_2$—◇	(1), (2)

*The numbers 3, 6, and 17 refer to positions in the morphine molecule, as shown above.
†Other changes in the morphine molecule are as follows:
  (1) Single instead of double bond between C7 and C8.
  (2) OH added to C14.
  (3) No oxygen between C4 and C5.
  (4) Endoetheno bridge between C6 and C14; 1-hydroxy-1,2,2-trimethylpropyl substitution on C7.
From Gutstein HB, Akil H: Opioid analgesics. In Hardman JG, Limbird LE (eds): Goodman and Gilman's The Pharmacological Basis of Therapeutics, 10th ed. New York, McGraw-Hill, 2001, pp 569-619.

Hydropathy analysis of the primary structures of the opioid receptors indicates that opioid receptors possess seven transmembrane domains (Fig. 11-2). This is a characteristic structural feature of the G protein–coupled receptor. The μ-, δ-, and κ-opioid receptors and the nociceptin receptor share ~50% amino acid sequence homology with each other.

Endogenous Opioid Peptides

Enkephalin, β-endorphin, and dynorphin were identified as endogenous agonists for the δ-, μ-, and κ-opioid receptors, respectively. Following purification of these peptides from mammalian tissues, cDNAs for the precursors of these peptides were cloned. cDNA cloning and amino acid determination of preproopiomelanocortin demonstrated that the cleavage of this precursor protein produces not only β-endorphin but also several other neuropeptides, including methionine enkephalin, adrenocorticotropic hormone, and α-melanocyte–stimulating hormone. The amino acid sequencing of preproenkephalin indicates that four methionine enkephalins and one leucine enkephalin are cleaved from this precursor. Furthermore, the primary structure of preprodynorphin, the precursor of dynorphin, was determined by cDNA cloning.

A novel endogenous opioid peptide with a significant sequence homology to dynorphin was isolated in 1995.[3,4] This peptide was called orphanin FQ, or nociceptin, because it lowered the pain threshold under certain conditions, in contrast to the other endogenous opioid peptides. Pharmacologic and physiologic studies have demonstrated that nociceptin/orphanin FQ has behavioral and pain modulatory properties distinct from those of the three classical opioid peptides.[6] Studies of the effects of nociceptin/orphanin FQ on pain sensitivity have produced conflicting results, which may suggest

Table 11–3 Pharmacologic actions of opioids and opioid receptors in animal models

		Actions of	
	Receptor	Agonists	Antagonists
Analgesia			
Supraspinal	μ, δ, κ	Analgesic	No effect
Spinal	μ, δ, κ	Analgesic	No effect
Respiratory function	μ	Decrease	No effect
Gastrointestinal tract	μ, κ	Decrease transit	No effect
Psychotomimesis	κ	Increase	No effect
Feeding	μ, δ, κ	Increase feeding	Decrease feeding
Sedation	μ, κ	Increase	No effect
Diuresis	κ	Increase	
Hormone secretion			
Prolacton	μ	Increase release	Decrease release
Growth hormone	μ and/or δ	Increase release	Decrease release
Neurotransmitter release			
Acetylcholine	μ	Inhibit	
Dopamine	δ	Inhibit	

Intracellular Signal Transduction Mechanism

The opioid receptors belong to the G protein–coupled receptor family. It has been demonstrated that activation of the opioid receptors leads to activation of the pertussis toxin-sensitive G proteins (G_i and/or G_o). Expression of the cloned opioid receptors in cultured cells by transfection of the cloned cDNAs has facilitated the analysis of the intracellular signal transduction mechanisms activated by the opioid receptors (Fig. 11-3).[2] Adenylate cyclase is inhibited by opioid receptor activation, resulting in the reduction of the cellular cyclic adenosine monophosphate (cAMP) content. Electrophysiologically, it was demonstrated that the voltage-gated Ca^{2+} channel is inhibited and that the inwardly rectifying K^+ channels are activated by the opioid receptors. As a result, neuronal excitability is reduced by activation of the opioid receptors. In contrast, it was reported that opioids also stimulate Ca^{2+} influx in neuronal cultured cells.[9] Recently, it was shown that extracellular signal-related kinase, a class of mitogen-activated protein kinases, is activated by opioid receptors.[10] Opioid-induced activation of extracellular signal-related kinase can lead to an increase in arachidonate release[10] and expression of immediate early genes c-fos and jun B.[11]

Chronic exposure of the opioid receptors to agonists induces cellular adaptation mechanisms, which may be involved in opioid tolerance, dependence, and withdrawal symptoms. Several investigators have shown that short-term desensitization probably involves phosphorylation of the opioid receptors via protein kinase C.[12] A number of other kinases also have been implicated, including protein kinase A and β-adrenergic receptor kinase (βARK).[13] βARK selectively phosphorylates agonist-bound receptors, thereby promoting interactions with β-arrestins, which interfere with G protein coupling and promote receptor internalization. Acute morphine-induced analgesia was enhanced in mice lacking β-arrestin 2, suggesting that this protein contributes to regulation of responsivity to opioids in vivo.[14]

Like other G protein–coupled receptors, the opioid receptors can undergo rapid agonist-mediated internalization via a classic endocytic pathway.[15,16] These processes may be induced differentially as a function of the class

that the effects depend on the underlying behavioral state of the animal. Prepronociceptin, the precursor of nociceptin/orphanin FQ, has been cloned, and its amino acid sequence suggested the existence of prepronociceptin-derived neuropeptides other than nociceptin/orphanin FQ.[7]

The search for endogenous ligand binding with the μ receptor with high affinity and high selectivity led to the discovery of a class of novel endogenous opioids termed endomorphin-1 and 2,[8] which are tetrapeptides with the sequence Tyr-Pro-Trp-Phe and Tyr-Pro-Phe-Phe, respectively. An endomorphin gene has yet to be cloned, and much remains to be learned about the anatomic distribution, mode of interaction with the opioid receptors, function in vivo, and potential existence of other related peptides that are highly selective for each of the opioid receptors.

Table 11–4 Characteristics of opioid receptors

	μ	δ	κ	Nociceptin
Tissue bioassay	Guinea pig ileum	Mouse vas deferens	Rabbit vas deferens	
Endogenous ligand	β-Endorphin	Leu-enkephalin	Dynorphin	Nociceptin
	Endomorphin	Met-enkephalin		
Agonist	Morphine	DPDPE	Buprenorphin	
	Fentanyl	Deltorphin	Pentazocine	
	DAMGO		U50 488	
Antagonist	Naloxone	Naloxone	Naloxone	
	Naltrexone	Naltrindole	NorBNI	
Coupled G-protein	$G_{i/o}$	$G_{i/o}$	$G_{i/o}$	$G_{i/o}$
Adenylate cyclase	Inhibition	Inhibition	Inhibition	Inhibition
Voltage-gated Ca^{2+} channels	Inhibition	Inhibition	Inhibition	Inhibition
Inward rectifier K^+ channels	Activation	Activation	Activation	Activation

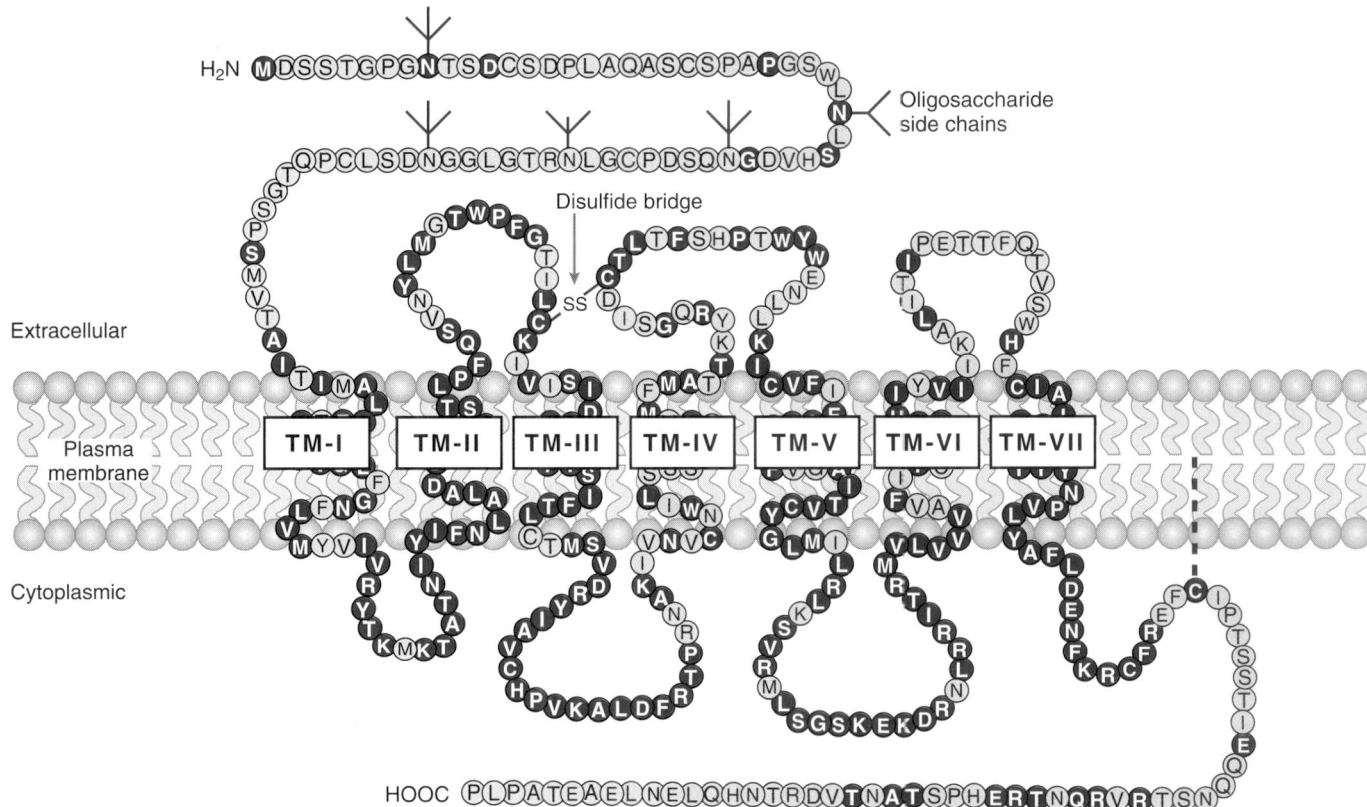

Figure 11–2 Proposed structure of the μ-opioid receptor. *Red circles* indicate amino acid residues identical in the μ- and δ-opioid receptors. TM-I to TM-VII show putative transmembrane segments composed of hydrophobic amino acid residues.

of the ligand. For example, certain agonists, such as etorphine and enkephalins, cause rapid internalization of the μ receptor, whereas morphine, although it decreases adenylyl cyclase activity equally well, does not cause μ receptor internalization.[17] These findings suggest that different ligands may induce different conformational

changes in the receptor, leading to divergent intracellular events. Furthermore, they may provide an explanation for differences in the efficacy and abuse potential of various opioids.

Long-term tolerance to opioids has been thought to be associated with superactivation of adenylyl cyclase

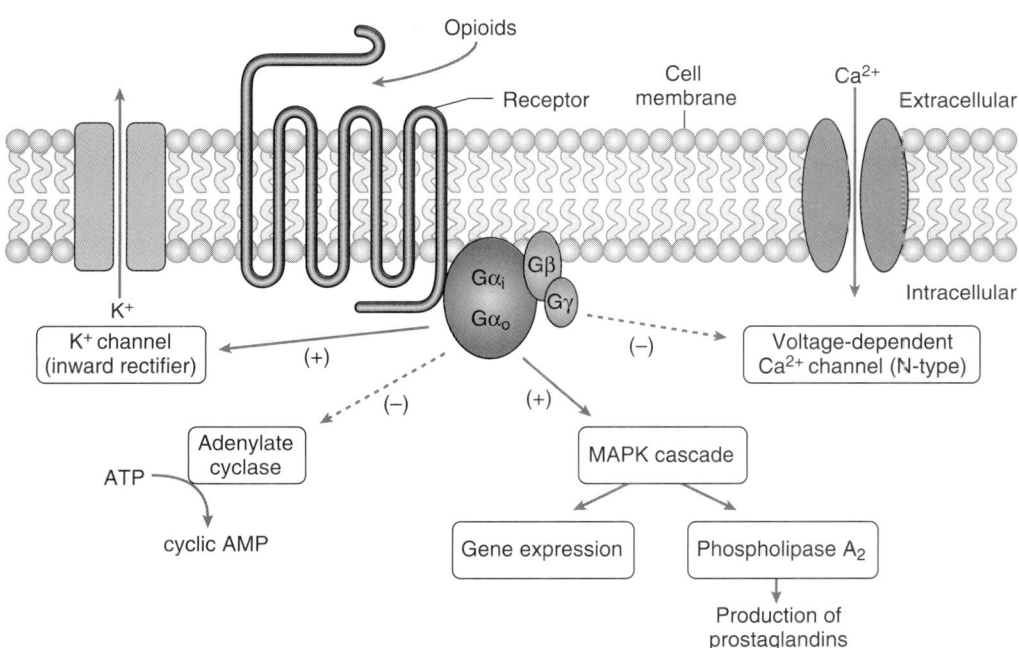

Figure 11–3 Intracellular signal transduction mechanisms linked with the opioid receptors. Opioid agonists bind with the opioid receptors, leading to activation of the G-protein. Activity of adenylate cyclase and the voltage-dependent Ca^{2+} channels is suppressed. On the other hand, inward rectifier K^+ channels and mitogen-activated protein kinase (MAPK) cascade are activated. AMP, adenosine monophosphate; ATP, adenosine triphosphate.

activity—a counter-regulation to the decrease in cAMP levels seen after acute opioid administration.[18] This effect is prevented by pretreatment of cells with pertussis toxin, demonstrating involvement of G proteins (G_i and/or G_o).

Mechanism of Analgesia

Pain control by opioids needs to be considered in the context of brain circuits modulating analgesia and the functions of the various types of receptors in these circuits.[19] It has been well established that the analgesic effects of opioids arise from their ability to inhibit directly the ascending transmission of nociceptive information from the spinal cord dorsal horn[1] and to activate pain control circuits that descend from the midbrain, via the rostral ventromedial medulla (RVM), to the spinal cord dorsal horn.[2]

Immunohistochemical studies and in situ hybridization analysis have demonstrated that opioid receptors are expressed in various areas in the central nervous system (CNS).[5] These include the amygdala, the mesencephalic reticular formation, the periaqueductal gray matter (PAG), and the rostral ventral medulla. However, the role of the opioid receptors in all of these areas has not been completely clarified.

Microinjection of morphine into the PAG or direct electrical stimulation of this area produces analgesia that can be blocked by naloxone. Opioid actions at the PAG influence the RVM, which in turn modulates nociceptive transmission in the dorsal horn of the spinal cord through the action of the descending inhibition pathway. Thus, opioids not only produce analgesia by direct actions on the spinal cord but also produce analgesia by neurally mediated action in the region separated from the site of opioid administration.

The distribution of opioid receptors in descending pain control circuits indicates substantial overlap between μ and κ receptors. Interactions between the κ receptor and the μ receptor may be important for modulating nociceptive transmission from higher nociceptive centers as well as in the spinal cord dorsal horn. The μ receptor produces analgesia within descending pain control circuits, at least in part, by the removal of γ-aminobutyric acid (GABA)ergic inhibition of RVM-projecting neurons in the PAG and spinally projecting neurons in the RVM.[19] The actions of μ-receptor agonists are invariably analgesic, whereas those of κ-receptor agonists can be either analgesic or antianalgesic. The pain-modulating effects of the κ-receptor agonists in the brainstem appear to oppose those of μ-receptor agonists.[20]

Local spinal mechanisms, in addition to descending inhibition, underlie the analgesic action of opioids. In the spinal cord, opioids act at synapses either presynaptically or postsynaptically. Opioid receptors are abundantly expressed in the substantia gelatinosa, where substance P release from the primary sensory neuron is inhibited by opioids.

There is significant opioid-receptor ligand binding, and little detectable receptor mRNA expression in the spinal cord dorsal horn, but high levels of opioid-receptor mRNA in dorsal root ganglia. This distribution suggests that the actions of opioid-receptor agonists relevant to analgesia at the spinal level may be predominantly presynaptic. It is well known that opioids decrease the pain-evoked release of tachykinins from primary afferent nociceptors. However, it was demonstrated that at least 80% of tachykinin signaling in response to noxious stimulation remains intact after the intrathecal administration of large doses of opioids.[21] These results suggest that, while opioid administration may reduce tachykinin release from primary afferent nociceptors, this reduction has little functional impact on the actions of tachykinins on postsynaptic pain-transmitting neurons.

The actions of opioids in bulbospinal pathways are critical to their analgesic efficacy. It is clear that opioid actions in the forebrain contribute to analgesia, because decerebration prevents analgesia when rats are tested for pain sensitivity using the formalin test,[22] and microinjection of opioids into several forebrain regions are analgesic in this test.[23] Analgesia induced by systemic administration of morphine in both the tail flick and formalin tests was disrupted either by lesioning or reversibly inactivating the central nucleus of the amygdala, demonstrating that opioid actions in the forebrain contribute to analgesia in measures of tissue damage as well as acute phasic nociception.[24,25]

Opioids may also produce analgesia through peripheral mechanisms.[26] Immune cells infiltrating the inflammation site may release endogenous opioid-like substances, which act on the opioid receptors located on the primary sensory neuron.[26] However, other studies do not support this conclusion.[27,28]

Mood Alterations and Rewarding Properties

The mechanisms by which opioids produce euphoria, tranquility, and other alterations of mood (including rewarding properties) are not entirely clear. Behavioral and pharmacological evidence points to the role of dopaminergic pathways, particularly involving the nucleus accumbens (NAcc), in drug-induced reward.

The shell of the NAcc is the site that may be involved directly in the emotional and motivational aspects of drug-induced reward. All three opioid receptor types are present on the NAcc and are thought to mediate, at least in part, the motivational effects of opiate drugs.[5] Selective μ- and δ-receptor agonists are rewarding when defined by place preference and intracranial self-administration paradigms. Conversely, selective κ-receptor agonists produce aversive effects. Positive motivational effects of opioids are partially mediated by dopamine release at the level of the NAcc.

The locus caeruleus contains both noradrenergic neurons and high concentrations of opioid receptors and is postulated to play a critical role in feelings of alarm, panic, fear, and anxiety. Neural activity in the locus caeruleus is inhibited by both exogenous opioids and endogenous opioid peptides.

Analysis of Knockout Mice

Physiologic roles of the opioid receptors and endogenous opioid peptides have been investigated mainly by pharmacologic and physiologic methods. However, it has been difficult to analyze functional roles of these proteins. Recently, knockout mice, in which a specific gene is inactivated by molecular biologic methods, have been produced. By analysis of the knockout mice, we can learn the physiological significance of the respective opioid receptors and endogenous opioid peptide precursors.[29]

In the μ-receptor knockout mice, analgesia, reward effect, and withdrawal effect of morphine are lost.[30,31] Morphine-induced respiratory depression was not observed in the μ-receptor knockout mice.[32] Therefore, it was concluded that the μ-receptor is a mandatory component of the opioid system for morphine action. In the μ-receptor knockout mice, ketamine-induced respiratory depression and antinociception are diminished,[33] suggesting that ketamine interacts with the μ-receptor, leading to these phenomena. Furthermore, the minimum alveolar concentration (MAC) of sevoflurane was significantly higher in the μ-receptor knockout mice than in wild-type mice, suggesting involvement of the μ-receptor in anesthetic potency of sevoflurane.[32] The δ-receptor knockout mice display markedly reduced analgesic effect of the opioids selective for the δ-receptors at the spinal cord level.[34] However, at the supraspinal level, analgesia can be induced by δ-receptor agonists in the δ-receptor knockout mice, suggesting the existence of a second δ-like analgesic system. Disruption of the κ-receptor abolishes analgesic, hypolocomotor, and aversive actions of the κ-receptor agonists and induces hyperreactivity in the abdominal constriction test, indicating that the κ-receptor is involved in the perception of visceral chemical pain.[35]

In mice lacking β-endorphin, morphine induces normal analgesia, but naloxone-reversible stress-induced analgesia cannot be observed.[36] The preproenkephalin knockout mice are more anxious than wild-type mice, and males display increased offensive aggressiveness.[37] The mutant mice show marked differences in control in supraspinal, but not in spinal, responses to painful stimuli. Thus, functional roles of individual components of the opioid system have been elucidated by analysis of knockout mice. However, many points remain to be clarified.

Actions of Opioids on Targets Other Than Opioid Receptors

Recent progress in molecular pharmacologic analyses has shown that opioids can interact with molecules other than opioid receptors. In cardiac myocytes, it was shown that morphine can inhibit voltage-dependent Na^+ current in a naloxone-insensitive manner, suggesting the existence of a signal transduction mechanism that is not dependent on the opioid receptors.[38] Meperidine has been classified as an agonist of both μ- and κ-receptors. In addition, it was demonstrated that meperidine can block voltage-dependent Na^+ channels in amphibian peripheral nerves[39] as well as in the *Xenopus* oocyte expression system (Fig. 11-4).[40] Furthermore, meperidine exerts agonist

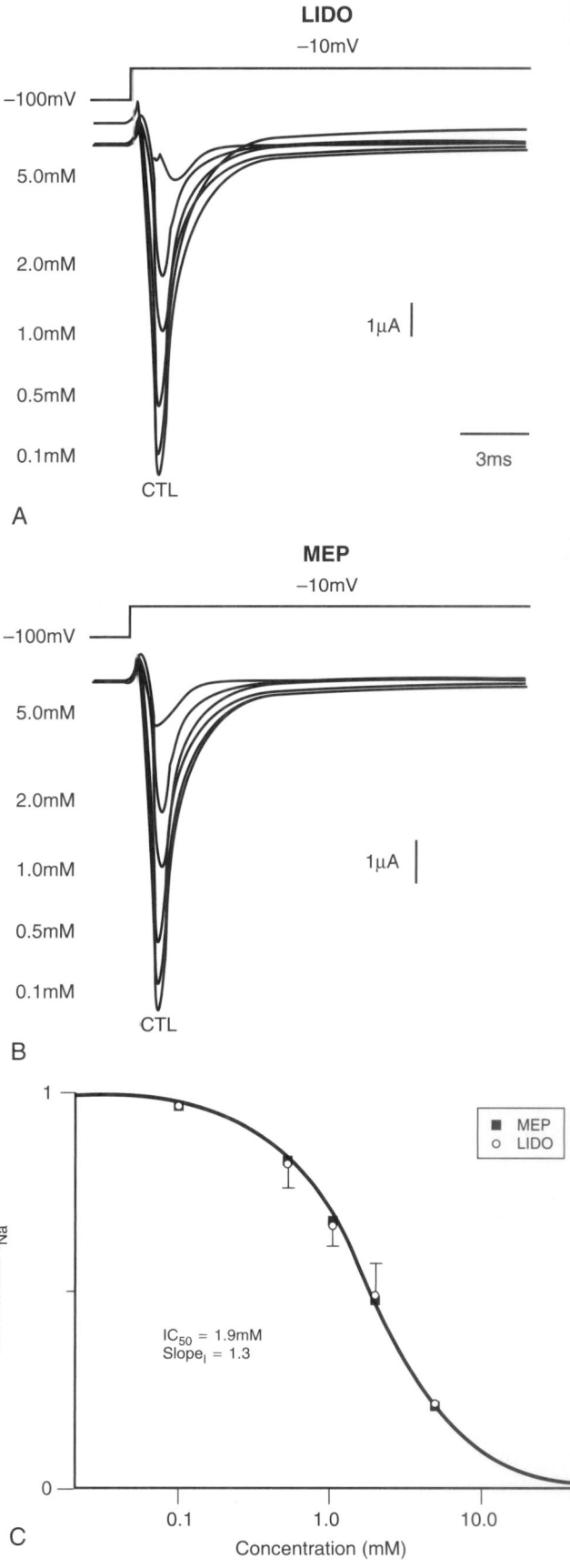

Figure 11–4 Meperidine blocks the Na^+ channels similarly to lidocaine. Na^+ currents induced by voltage jump were recorded from *Xenopus* oocytes expressing the Na^+ channels. Lidocaine (LID; **A**) and meperidine (MEP; **B**) dose-dependently inhibited the current. (From Wagner LE 2nd, Eaton M, Sabnis SS, Gingrich KJ: Meperidine and lidocaine block of recombinant voltage-dependent Na^+ channels: Evidence that meperidine is a local anesthetic. Anesthesiology 91:1481-1490, 1999.)

activity at the α_{2B} adrenoreceptor subtype.[41] Yamakura and colleagues have shown that high concentrations of opioids, including meperidine, morphine, fentanyl, codeine, and naloxone, directly inhibit the N-methyl-D-aspartate (NMDA) receptor expressed in *Xenopus* oocytes.[42]

It remains to be clarified whether these actions of opioids on targets other than the opioid receptor have physiological and/or clinical implications.

The Role of Nociceptin/orphanin FQ in Pain Modulation

Nociceptin/orphanin FQ is a 17-amino-acid peptide, the sequence of which resembles those of opioid peptides (also see Chapters 72 and 73). Nociceptin/orphanin FQ precursor mRNA and peptide are present throughout descending pain control circuits. In the spinal cord, there is stronger nociceptin/orphanin FQ–receptor mRNA expression in the ventral horn than in the dorsal horn, but higher levels of ligand binding in the dorsal horn. Targeted disruption of the nociceptin/orphanin FQ receptor in mice had little effect on basal pain sensitivity in several measures, whereas targeted disruption of the N nociceptin/orphanin FQ precursor consistently elevated basal responses in the tail flick test, suggesting an important role for nociceptin/orphanin FQ in regulating basal pain sensitivity.[43,44] Intrathecal injections of nociceptin/orphanin FQ have been shown to be analgesic[45]; however, supraspinal administration has produced either hyperalgesia, antiopioid effects, or a biphasic hyperalgesic/analgesic response.[46] It was shown that nociceptin/orphanin FQ inhibits both pain-facilitating and analgesia-facilitating neurons in the rostral ventromedial medulla.[47] The effects of nociceptin/orphanin FQ on pain responses appear to depend on the preexisting state of pain in the animal. Yamamoto reported that intrathecal injection of nociceptin/orphanin FQ significantly attenuated the level of mechanical hyperalgesia induced by a skin incision, suggesting the involvement of the nociceptin/orphanin FQ receptor in maintaining postoperative pain.[45] Physiologic implications of nociceptin/orphanin FQ remain to be elucidated.

NEUROPHYSIOLOGIC EFFECTS OF OPIOIDS

Analgesic Action of Opioids

In human beings, morphine-like drugs produce analgesia, drowsiness, changes in mood, and mental clouding. A significant feature of opioid analgesia is that it is not associated with loss of consciousness. When morphine in the same dose is given to a normal, pain-free individual, the experience may be unpleasant. The relief of pain by morphine-like opioids is relatively selective, in that other sensory modalities are not affected. Patients frequently report that the pain is still present, but that they feel more comfortable. It is also important to distinguish between pain caused by stimulation of nociceptive receptors and transmitted over intact neural pathways (nociceptive pain) and pain that is caused by damage to neural

structures, often involving neural supersensitivity (neuropathic pain). Although nociceptive pain usually is responsive to opioid analgesics, neuropathic pain typically responds poorly to opioid analgesics and may require higher doses of drug.[48] Not only is the sensation of pain altered by opioid analgesics, but the affective response is changed as well. It is clear, however, that alteration of the emotional reaction to painful stimuli is not the sole mechanism of analgesia. Intrathecal or epidural administration of opioids can produce profound segmental analgesia without causing significant alteration of motor or sensory function or subjective effects.[49]

The level of antinociception produced by an opioid is determined by the intensity of the nociceptive stimulus and the intrinsic efficacy of the opioid. When opioids are given in combination, the effects can only be predicted on the basis of the nociception when the drugs are administered alone.[50] It has been shown that opioid antinociceptive effects are enhanced in animal models of inflammation. Recently it was shown that the sensitization to opioids is related to a central rather than peripheral site of action.[51]

Animal and human studies indicate the existence of sex-related differences in opioid-mediated behavior.[52] Sarton and associates examined the influence of morphine on experimentally induced pain in healthy volunteers, and demonstrated sex differences in morphine analgesia, with greater morphine potency but slower speed of onset and offset in women.[53] The mechanism of the sex differences remains to be clarified.

Controversies remain about the analgesia produced by peripheral actions of opioids. A recent review concluded from metaanalysis that intraarticularly administered morphine has a definite but mild analgesic effect.[54] It may be dose dependent, and a systemic effect cannot be completely excluded. Addition of opioids in brachial plexus block has been reported to improve success rate and postoperative analgesia.[55,56] In contrast, in another study, addition of sufentanil did not prolong the duration of brachial plexus block.[57] Because of its local anesthetic effect on peripheral nerves, meperidine was tested for intravenous regional anesthesia. However, it was demonstrated that doses of meperidine large enough to produce effective postoperative analgesia caused a significant incidence of side effects.[58]

Opioids as Anesthetics

Whether opioids alone are capable of producing anesthesia was a subject of debate in the past.[59] Reports of patient awareness during high-dose fentanyl anesthesia highlighted the potential for this problem (also see Chapter 31).

The anesthetic potential of opioids was tested by MAC measurement.[60] Studies in rats demonstrate that opioids reduce the MAC of volatile anesthetics to a greater degree than in other animals. Interspecies differences in opioid actions are significant.[61] Fentanyl can reduce the MAC of isoflurane at least 80% at skin incisions in humans (Fig. 11-5).[62] It was shown that the relationship between plasma fentanyl concentration and MAC reduction is not linear, and that a sub-MAC ceiling exists to the effect of fentanyl on isoflurane MAC reduction. The potency ratios for fentanyl, sufentanil, alfentanil, and remifentanil, based

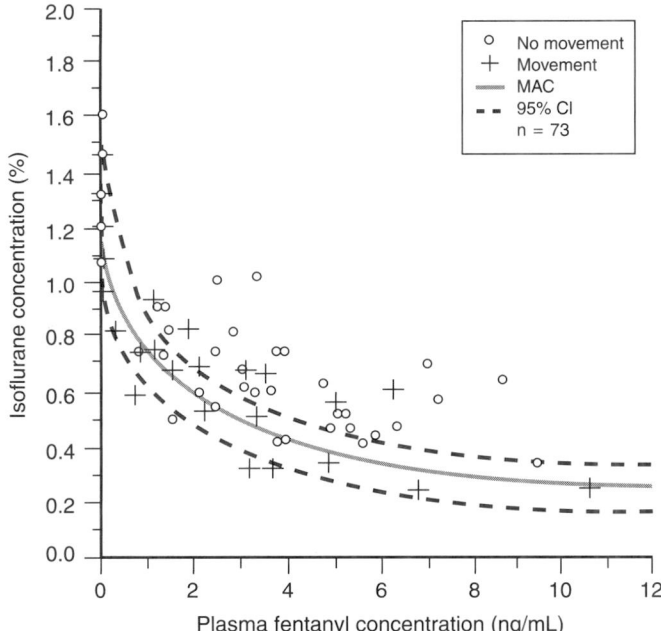

Figure 11–5 Reduction of isoflurane minimum alveolar concentration (MAC) by increasing the concentration of fentanyl. (From McEwan AI, Smith C, Dyar O, et al: Isoflurane minimum alveolar concentration reduction by fentanyl. Anesthesiology 78:864-869, 1993.)

Electroencephalography

Increasing concentrations of inhaled anesthetics produce a continuum of electroencephalography (EEG) changes, eventually resulting in burst suppression and a flat EEG (also see Chapter 31). In contrast, a ceiling effect is reached with opioids. Increasing opioid dosage, once this ceiling has been obtained, does not further affect the EEG.[71] Problems with lead placement and signal processing need to be resolved before EEG analysis can be used as a routine monitor of opioid anesthesia depth. It was reported that emergence from isoflurane but not fentanyl anesthesia is associated with obvious changes in the overall EEG frequency power spectrum.[72]

Although potency and rate of equilibrium between plasma and brain are different among opioids, the effects of fentanyl, alfentanil, sufentanil, and remifentanil are consistent.[73] Small doses of fentanyl (200 µg) produce minimal EEG changes, whereas higher doses (30-70 µg/kg) result in high-voltage slow (delta) waves, suggesting a state consistent with anesthesia. Although transient isolated (usually frontotemporal) sharp wave activity can be observed after large doses of fentanyl and other opioids, it is not generalized. Sufentanil produces EEG changes similar to fentanyl (Fig. 11-6).[74] The effects of alfentanil on the EEG are slightly different from those of fentanyl or sufentanil. Alfentanil (125 µg/kg) produces less synchronization of the EEG and less change in the relative EEG power in the delta band.[75]

As an effect site measure, EEG can be employed to assess onset of drug action and drug potency ratios. It was reported that a lag time between plasma drug concentration and change in the spectral edge is only 1 min for alfentanil and 6 min for fentanyl.[74] The serum concentration ratio that results in a similar EEG pattern is 75:1 for alfentanil and fentanyl,[74] and the lag time is as short for alfentanil as it is for remifentanil (Fig. 11-7).[76] This contrasts with the reported dose ratio in which fentanyl was only three to five times as potent as alfentanil. The serum

on MAC reduction studies in humans, is approximately 1:12:1/16:1.2.[63] Esmolol, a short-acting β₁-receptor antagonist, significantly decreased the MAC of isoflurane in the presence of alfentanil, although it did not significantly affect it in the absence of alfentanil.[64] The mechanism of the interaction is unknown. It was demonstrated that epidural fentanyl infusion reduced the awakening concentration of isoflurane more than intravenous fentanyl infusion, despite the lower plasma concentration, possibly by modulating the afferent nociceptive inputs in the spinal cord.[65] The hypnotic effect of midazolam is also significantly potentiated by alfentanil.[66]

The bispectral index (BIS) has been proposed as a measure of the effects of anesthetics on the brain. In the presence of fentanyl, alfentanil, remifentanil, or sufentanil, loss of consciousness occurred at a lower effect site concentration of propofol and at a higher BIS value compared with propofol alone.[67] This result suggests that the hypnotic effect of propofol is enhanced by analgesic concentrations of opioids without changes in BIS value. On the other hand, it was reported that infusion of remifentanil (effect site target concentration of 0.5, 2.5 and 10 ng/mL), combined with propofol infusion adjusted to BIS ~60, dose-dependently decreased BIS, suggesting a sedative or hypnotic effect of remifentanil.[68]

Although unconsciousness in humans can be produced with high doses of opioids alone, opioid anesthesia can be unpredictable and inconsistent.[69] Whether analgesia and loss of consciousness are produced by opioids through a common mechanism has been questioned. A dual mechanism in the action of opioids has been proposed, and it was demonstrated that the anesthetic action of opioids requires lipid solubility.[70]

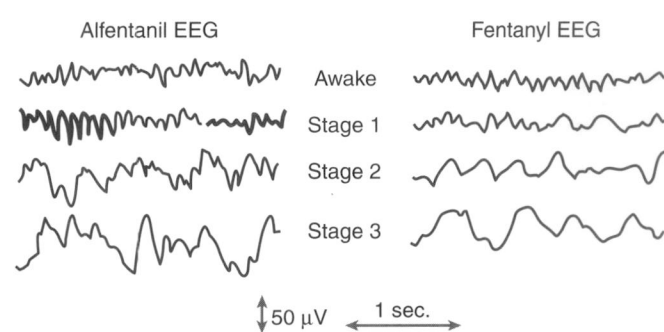

Figure 11–6 Electroencephalography (EEG) stages for fentanyl and alfentanil. Representative 3-second tracings of EEG recordings from fentanyl and alfentanil are shown. Awake = mixed α (8-13 Hz) and β (>13 Hz) activity. Stage 1 = slowing with α spindles. Stage 2 = more slowing, θ activity present (4-7 Hz). Stage 3 = maximal slowing, δ waves present (<4 Hz), with high amplitude. (From Scott JC, Ponganis KV, Stanski DR: EEG quantitation of narcotic effect: The comparative pharmacodynamics of fentanyl and alfentanil. Anesthesiology 62:234-241, 1985.)

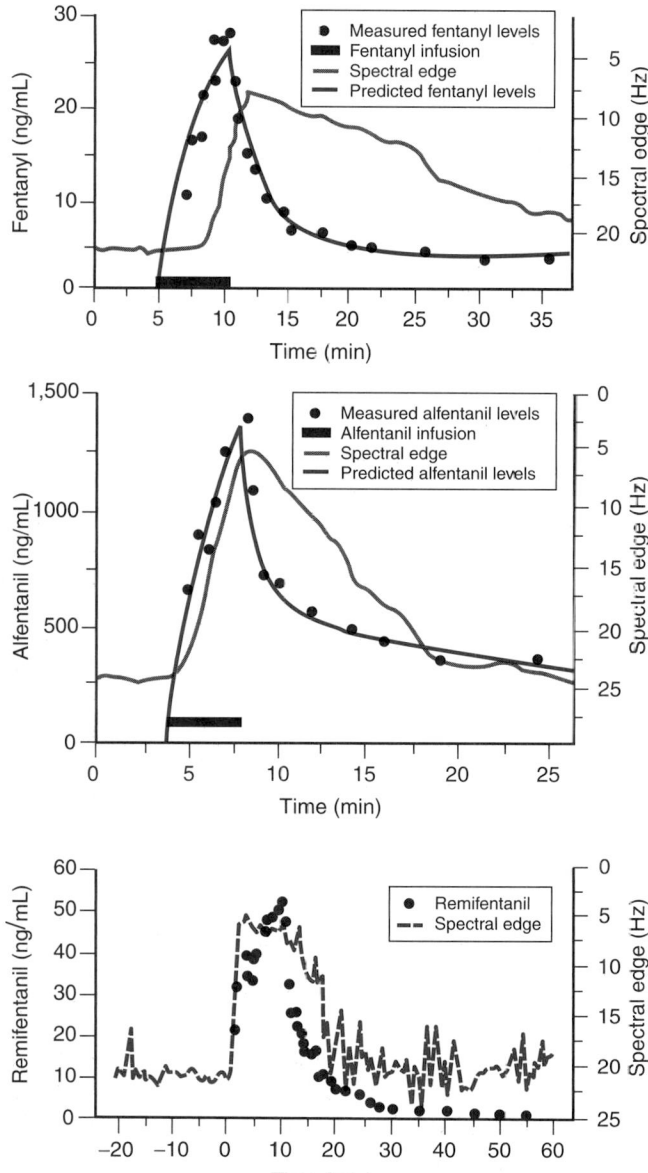

Figure 11-7 Time course of spectral edge and serum opioid concentration. Fentanyl (*top panel*) and alfentanil (*middle panel*) were infused at 150 µg/minute and 1500 µg/minute, respectively. Remifentanil (*bottom panel*) was administered at 3 µg/kg/minute for 10 minutes. The spectral edge changes lag behind the serum concentration changes in the case of fentanyl, whereas the spectral edge and serum concentrations are closely parallel in the cases of alfentanil and remifentanil. (From Scott JC, Ponganis KV, Stanski DR: EEG quantitation of narcotic effect: The comparative pharmacodynamics of fentanyl and alfentanil. Anesthesiology 62:234-241, 1985; and Egan TD, Minto CF, Hermann DJ, Barr J, Muir KT, Shafer SL: Remifentanil versus alfentanil: Comparative pharmacokinetics and pharmacodynamics in healthy adult male volunteers. Anesthesiology 84:821-833, 1996.)

concentration ratio of fentanyl and sufentanil was 12:1 at half-maximal EEG slowing.[77] Similar studies suggest that fentanyl and remifentanil are 75 and 16 times as potent as alfentanil, respectively.[76] Potency ratios based on EEG studies are similar to those obtained from studies determining the plasma drug levels of each opioid necessary to reduce the MAC of isoflurane by 50%. Potency ratios for reduction of the isoflurane MAC for sufentanil:fentanyl: remifentanil:alfentanil are nearly 1:1/10:1/10:1/100.[62,78-80]

Sensory Evoked Potentials

Opioids do not appreciably alter sensory evoked potentials (SEPs) elicited at the posterior tibial or median nerve.[81-84] Therefore, SEP monitoring can be used for spinal cord function monitoring during anesthesia using opioids. Although opioids do not interfere with SEP interpretation, they do inhibit both the velocity and the amplitude of nerve action potential transmission.[85]

Brainstem auditory evoked potentials are also minimally altered by analgesic doses of morphine, fentanyl or sufentanil.[86,87] Remifentanil produced dose-dependent reduction in auditory evoked potentials.[88] Visual evoked potentials during thiopental-fentanyl-N₂O anesthesia show transiently decreased amplitudes and modest but persistent increases in latencies.[89]

Cerebral Blood Flow and Cerebral Metabolic Rate

Opioids generally produce modest decreases in cerebral metabolic rate (CMR) and intracranial pressure (ICP), although the changes are influenced by the concomitant administration of other agents and anesthetics, as well as by patient conditions (also see Chapter 21). When vasodilatation is produced by co-administered anesthetics, opioids are more likely to cause cerebral vasoconstriction. Opioids also decrease cerebral blood flow (CBF) when combined with N_2O. When opioids are administered alone or when the co-administered anesthetics cause cerebral vasoconstriction, opioids usually have no influence or result in a small increase in CBF.

Endogenous opioid activity is present in cerebral arteries, although exogenously administered opioids were found to exert little effect on pial artery diameter in several animal models.[90] Morphine and enkephalins produced dose-dependent pial arterial dilatation.[91] Fentanyl (100 µg/kg) causes dose-related reductions in CBF and $CMRO_2$ in rats receiving N_2O. In the piglet, fentanyl, alfentanil, and sufentanil decrease arteriolar diameter in a dose-dependent naloxone-reversible manner.[92] Fentanyl alone causes little change in CBF in the dog.[93] In human volunteers, positron emission tomography demonstrates that CBF changes induced by fentanyl are regionally heterogeneous.[94]

The effect of sufentanil on CBF in the dog may be dose- and time-dependent. It was reported that sufentanil (20 µg/kg IV) produced 30% to 40% decreases in CBF 5-10 minutes after opioid administration.[95] Another study showed that sufentanil (10-200 µg/kg) produced transient increases in CBF that peaked 2 minutes after drug administration in the dog.[96] In humans, both fentanyl and sufentanil can increase middle cerebral artery blood flow velocity by ~25%.[97] In other reports, it was shown that in healthy volunteers, sufentanil (0.5 µg/kg IV) had no significant effect on CBF.[97] Alfentanil (25 or 50 µg/kg IV), administered to patients receiving isoflurane (0.4%-0.6%)-N_2O anesthesia, produced minimal reductions in middle cerebral artery flow velocity.[98]

In the dog, alfentanil and remifentanil both decreased regional blood flow by 40% to 50% in the cortex, hippocampus, and caudate.[99] A positron emission tomography study in human volunteers showed that remifentanil induced dose-dependent changes in relative regional CBF in areas involved in pain processing, such as lateral prefrontal cortex, inferior parietal cortex, and supplementary motor area.[100] In patients scheduled to undergo supratentorial tumor surgery receiving N_2O, both remifentanil (1 μg/kg/min) and similarly fentanyl (2 μg/kg/min), reduced CBF and did not significantly affect cerebrovascular reactivity to carbon dioxide.[101]

Opioids usually produce mild to moderate decreases in CMR that remain coupled to CBF. However, opioid-induced neuroexcitation and focal seizure activity can cause regional increases in brain metabolism. Regional increases in glucose utilization induced by high doses of alfentanil in the rat were associated not only with epileptiform activity but also with neuropathic lesions.[102] In humans, positron emission tomography evaluation demonstrated that 1-3 μg/kg/min infusions of remifentanil induce significant increases in CMR for glucose.[103]

Intracranial Pressure

Opioids are generally thought to affect ICP minimally. Under background anesthesia (isoflurane-N_2O), opioids do not cause significant increases in ICP during craniotomy for supratentorial space-occupying lesions.[104,105] Under stable anesthesia with isoflurane-N_2O, sufentanil (0.8 μg/kg) or fentanyl (4.5 μg/kg) prior to skull-pin insertion resulted in stable ICP.[106] It was also reported that opioid sedation did not alter ICP in head-injured patients (also see Chapter 53).[107]

However, it has been reported that opioids may produce increases in ICP in patients undergoing craniotomy for excision of supratentorial space-occupying lesions, especially if intracranial compliance is compromised. It was reported that CSF pressure increased by 90% after sufentanil (1 μg/kg) and 20% after alfentanil (50 μg/kg), in contrast to no significant change after fentanyl (5 μg/kg), in patients with brain tumors who were anesthetized with thiopental-N_2O-vecuronium.[108] On the other hand, there was no change in ICP in hydrocephalic children after alfentanil (70 μg/kg).[109] In patients with severe head injury with preserved and impaired autoregulation, morphine (0.2 mg/kg) and fentanyl (2 μg/kg) moderately increased ICP, suggesting that mechanisms other than vasodilatation could be implicated in the opioid-induced ICP elevation.[110]

It is not clear whether these discrepancies in the effects of opioids on ICP are due to different pressure assessment methods or to the effects of other drugs. If opioids do increase ICP, whether cerebrovascular dilatation is directly induced by opioids or results indirectly from opioid-induced decreases in blood pressure is not known. Regional increases in CMR and opioid-induced rigidity may be involved.[111]

Although many studies suggest the possibility of adverse effects of opioids on regional CMR, CBF, and ICP, opioid-based anesthesia in intracranial surgery has an extensive and safe clinical record. The significance of reported opioid-induced changes in CBF and/or ICP and the impact, if any, of such changes on patient outcome is unknown.

Neuroprotection

Although certain early studies suggested potentially adverse effects of μ-opioid agonists on ischemic brain, other studies document that at least certain opioid agents, such as the κ-agonists, can be neuroprotective at least in animal models of focal ischemia.[112,113] Animal studies of neurologic injury suggest that anesthesia with opioids improves neurologic outcome compared with the awake state.[114] It was also shown that activation of δ-opioid receptors increases survival time of mice during lethal hypoxia.[115,116] In addition, spinal cord protection by fentanyl-N_2O anesthesia is equal to that provided by halothane or spinal lidocaine.[114] On the other hand, Charchaflieh et colleagues demonstrated, using the rat hippocampal slice model, that fentanyl is neither neurotoxic nor protective against anoxic injury to neurons when used in concentrations comparable to those produced in clinical practice.[117] In the rat model of focal ischemia, in contrast to isoflurane, fentanyl neither increased nor decreased brain injury compared with awake unanesthetized rats.[118]

Muscle Rigidity

Opioids can increase muscle tone and may cause muscle rigidity. The incidence of rigidity noted with opioid anesthetic techniques varies greatly because of the following: differences in dose and speed of opioid administration, the concomitant use of N_2O, the presence or absence of muscle relaxants, and patient age. Opioid-induced rigidity is characterized by increased muscle tone progressing sometimes to severe stiffness, leading to serious problems (Table 11-5). Clinically significant opioid-induced rigidity usually begins just as, or after, a patient loses consciousness. Mild manifestations of rigidity, such as hoarseness, can occur in conscious patients. Rigidity can decrease pulmonary compliance and functional residual capacity, may diminish or preclude adequate ventilation, and may cause hypercarbia, hypoxia, and an elevated ICP.[119,120] Opioid-induced rigidity also increases pulmonary artery and central venous pressures and pulmonary vascular resistance.[121,122] It has been demonstrated that vocal cord closure is primarily responsible for difficult ventilation with bag and mask that follows opioid administration. Rigidity may rarely occur hours after the last dose of opioid has been administered.[123] Delayed or postoperative rigidity probably is related to second peaks that can occur in plasma opioid concentrations, as may occur in the case of recurrence of respiratory depression. Abnormal muscle movements ranging from extremity flexion to single or multiple extremity tonic-clonic movements or global tonic-clonic motions can also occur after the use of opioids.[124]

The precise mechanism by which opioids may cause muscle rigidity is not clearly understood. Muscle rigidity is not due to a direct action on muscle fibers, because it can be decreased or prevented by pretreatment with muscle relaxants. Mechanisms for opioid-induced muscle rigidity have been sought for in the CNS. The nucleus pontis raphae is reported to be an integral central site concerning

Table 11–5 Potential problems associated with opioid-induced rigidity

System	Problem
Hemodynamic	↑ CVP, ↑ PAP, ↑ PVR
Respiratory	↓ Compliance, ↓ FRC, ↓ ventilation
	Hypercarbia
	Hypoxemia
Miscellaneous	↑ Oxygen consumption
	↑ Intracranial pressure
	↑ Fentanyl plasma levels

CVP, central venous pressure; FRC, functional residual capacity; PAP, pulmonary artery pressure; PVR, pulmonary vascular resistance.
Modified from Bailey PL, Egan TD, Stanley TH: Intravenous opioid anesthetics. *In* Miller RD (ed): Anesthesia, 5th ed. New York, Churchill Livingstone, 2000, p 291.

opioid-induced rigidity.[120] A pharmacologic investigation using selective agonists and antagonists suggested that systemic opioid-induced muscle rigidity is primarily due to the activation of central µ-receptors, whereas supraspinal δ_1 and κ_1 receptors may attenuate this effect.[125] Some aspects of opioid-induced catatonia and rigidity (increased incidence with age, muscle movements resembling extrapyramidal side effects) are similar to Parkinson's disease and suggest similarities in neurochemical mechanisms. Parkinsonian patients, particularly if inadequately treated, may experience reactions like dystonia following opioid administration.[126]

Pretreatment or concomitant use of nondepolarizing muscle relaxants significantly decreases the incidence and severity of rigidity.[124] Induction doses of sodium thiopental and less than anesthetic doses of diazepam and midazolam have also been reported to prevent, attenuate, or successfully treat rigidity. Persisting in an attempt to ventilate a patient with opioid-induced rigidity by mask will likely result in gastric insufflation and inadequate ventilation or oxygenation until a muscle relaxant is administered. Anesthesiologists should anticipate the need for rapid neuromuscular blockade, when doses of opioids are administered that produce rigidity, in order to minimize its occurrence and to allow effective ventilation and airway management.

Neuroexcitatory Phenomena

Fentanyl can cause neuroexcitation ranging from delirium to grand mal seizure-like activity.[127] It was reported that fentanyl causes EEG seizure activity in animals, but EEG evidence of seizure activity after fentanyl, alfentanil, and sufentanil is generally lacking in humans. Remifentanil was reported to induce generalized tonic-clonic seizure-like activity in an otherwise healthy adult.[128]

Animal studies demonstrate that in certain species, opioids cause focal CNS excitation rather than global CNS depression.[129] Focal neuroexcitation (e.g., sharp and spike wave activity) is noted occasionally on EEG in humans after large doses of fentanyl, sufentanil, and alfentanil. Morphine has also been reported to produce tonic-clonic

activity after epidural and intrathecal administration.[130] Meperidine also may cause CNS excitability. The mechanism is related to its N-desmethyl metabolite, normeperidine, which is twice as potent in causing CNS excitation and convulsions as meperidine.[131] Naloxone administration for the CNS adverse effects of meperidine should be avoided, because naloxone can elicit seizures by unmasking the excitatory effects of meperidine when its depressant effects are antagonized.[131]

The mechanisms underlying opioid-induced neuroexcitatory phenomena are not completely clear. More recent work suggests that excitatory opioid actions may be related to their coupling to mitogen-activated protein kinase cascades.[132] Local increases in CBF and metabolism are also of theoretical concern because prolonged seizure activity, even if focal, can lead to neuronal injury and/or cellular death. Fentanyl, alfentanil, and sufentanil in large doses also induce hypermetabolism and histopathologic alterations of the limbic system in rats.[133] In rats, midazolam, naloxone, and phenytoin prevented EEG seizure activity and histologically evident brain damage induced by large-dose fentanyl.[134]

Pupil Size

Morphine and most µ- and κ-receptor agonists cause constriction of the pupil by an excitatory action on the parasympathetic nerve innervating the pupil. Opioids release cortical inhibition of the Edinger-Westphal nucleus, resulting in papillary constriction. It has been demonstrated that alfentanil in a dose-dependent manner attenuates the reflex pupillary dilatation that normally follows noxious stimulation in anesthetized individuals.[135] The time course of the response appears related to plasma opioid levels, even in the presence of potent inhalation agents.[136] The changes in pupil size associated with opioid action may be too small to be of clinical utility in assessing the degree of opioid effect.

Thermoregulation and Shivering

Opioid-based anesthesia probably reduces thermoregulatory thresholds to a degree similar to that of the potent inhaled agents.[137,138] However, meperidine is unique among opioids in its ability to effectively terminate or attenuate shivering in approximately 70% to 80% of patients.[139,140] The antishivering effect of meperidine is primarily related to a reduction in the shivering threshold[141] and seems to be mediated by meperidine's activity on the κ-receptor.[142] However, the relatively specific κ-receptor agonist nalbuphine did not show significant antishivering activity.[143] A recent study has demonstrated that meperidine exerts agonist activity at the α_{2B}-adrenoreceptor subtype, suggesting this as a possible mechanism of this novel action in the antishivering action of meperidine.[41] Alfentanil, morphine, and fentanyl are not as effective as meperidine in the treatment of postoperative shivering, although epidural opioid administration may reduce shivering in obstetric patients receiving regional anesthesia.[144] Tramadol (0.5 mg/kg) suppressed postepidural anesthetic shivering in parturients as effectively as meperidine (0.5 mg/kg).[145] Tramadol had a decreased incidence of somnolence when compared with meperidine.

Pruritus

Histamine release was once thought to underlie this phenomenon; however, non–histamine-releasing opioids also produce pruritus. Intrathecal morphine-induced itching in monkeys was suggested to be mediated by the µ-receptor.[146] Naloxone reverses opioid-induced itching, and this finding supports a receptor-mediated central mechanism for pruritus. However, opioid antagonists are not ideal therapeutic agents against pruritus, because opioid analgesia is also reversed by these agents. Perhaps some mixed opioids, such as nalbuphine and butorphanol, with low to medium efficacy at both µ- and κ-receptors, are useful antipruritics, because they may partially antagonize µ-receptor actions with intact κ-receptor actions and thereby maintain analgesic function.[147,148] Ondansetron has been proposed to treat spinal or epidural morphine-induced pruritus,[149] and tenoxicam, a nonsteroidal anti-inflammatory drug, was reported to be effective for pruritus induced by epidural fentanyl.[150]

Facial itching may not necessarily be a manifestation of direct opioid action at the level of the trigeminal nucleus; rather it may be a reflection of opioid-triggered neural transmission at a distant site. It is not known why the face is prone to pruritus even after spinal opioids. Interestingly, pruritus due to cholestasis is ameliorated by opioid antagonists.[151]

RESPIRATORY EFFECTS OF OPIOIDS

The respiratory-depressant actions of opioids represent their most serious adverse effect. Although significant adverse events related to opioid-induced respiratory depression are presumably preventable, they persist with a perioperative incidence of approximately 0.1% to 1%, no matter what the route of administration.[152]

Morphine has been shown to have a depressant effect on mucociliary flow in the trachea, which is one of the most important defenses against respiratory tract infections.[153] On the other hand, morphine had no effect on nasal cilia beating frequency in vitro.[154] Morphine may have an effect on cilia in vivo because of effects on neural connections that are absent from in vitro preparations.

Therapeutic Effects

Opioids, by decreasing both pain and central ventilatory drive, are effective agents in preventing hyperventilation induced by pain or anxiety.[155,156] The lack of adequate pain relief can also cause postoperative respiratory dysfunction. Opioids can be used as postoperative analgesics to prevent respiratory dysfunction. The antitussive actions of opioids are well known and central in origin. However, fentanyl, sufentanil, and alfentanil curiously elicit a brief cough in up to 50% of patients when injected by intravenous bolus.[157]

Opioids are excellent agents for depressing upper airway, tracheal, and lower respiratory tract reflexes, but the mechanism is not clear. Although opioids can affect the contractile responses of airway smooth muscles, the clinical significance and relevance of opioid-induced effects on airway resistance remains controversial.[158] Opioids blunt or eliminate somatic and autonomic responses to tracheal intubation, allowing patients to tolerate endotracheal tubes without coughing or "bucking." Opioids can also help to avoid increases in bronchomotor tone in asthma. Fentanyl has antimuscarinic, antihistaminergic, and anti-serotoninergic actions and may be more effective than morphine in patients with asthma or other bronchospastic diseases. The relatively slight impact of opioids on hypoxic pulmonary vasoconstriction contributes to their minimal interference with pulmonary gas exchange.

Nontherapeutic Effects

Endogenous opioid peptides are widely distributed in brainstem nuclei regulating respiration. All µ receptor-stimulating opioids cause dose-dependent depression of respiration in humans primarily through a direct action on brainstem respiratory centers.[159] How the various respiratory centers involved with ventilatory drive, respiratory rhythm generation, chemoreception, and neural integration are affected by opioids is unclear.

The stimulatory effect of CO_2 on ventilation is significantly reduced by opioids. The hypercapneic response can be separated into the central component and the peripheral component. Morphine-induced changes in the central component were equal in men and women, whereas changes in the peripheral component were greater in women.[160] In addition, the apneic threshold and resting end-tidal P_{CO_2} are increased by opioids (Fig. 11-8). Opioids also decrease hypoxic ventilatory drive.

The respiratory rate is usually drastically slowed in opioid overdose, although hypoxic CNS insult can counter this effect. The prolonged expiratory time in the respiratory cycle induced by opioids frequently results in greater reductions in respiratory rate than in tidal volume. A recent report demonstrated that monitoring of breath intervals can sensitively detect fentanyl-induced respiratory depression and can be used as a measure of dynamic opioid effect.[161] High doses of opioids usually eliminate spontaneous respirations without necessarily producing unconsciousness. Patients receiving high doses of opioids may still be responsive to verbal commands and often will breathe when directed to do so.

The peak onset of respiratory depression after an analgesic dose of morphine is slower than after comparable doses of fentanyl: 30 ± 15 minutes versus 5 to 10 minutes. Respiratory depression induced by small doses of morphine usually lasts longer than after equipotent doses of fentanyl. Sufentanil (0.1-0.4 µg/kg) produces shorter-lasting respiratory depression and longer-lasting analgesia than fentanyl (1.0-4.0 µg/kg).[162] Plasma fentanyl concentrations of 1.5 to 3.0 ng/mL are usually associated with significant decreases in CO_2 responsiveness. With higher doses of fentanyl (50-100 µg/kg), respiratory depression can persist for many hours. When moderately large (20-50 µg/kg) or greater doses of fentanyl are used, the potential need for postoperative mechanical ventilation should be anticipated. Although adequate spontaneous

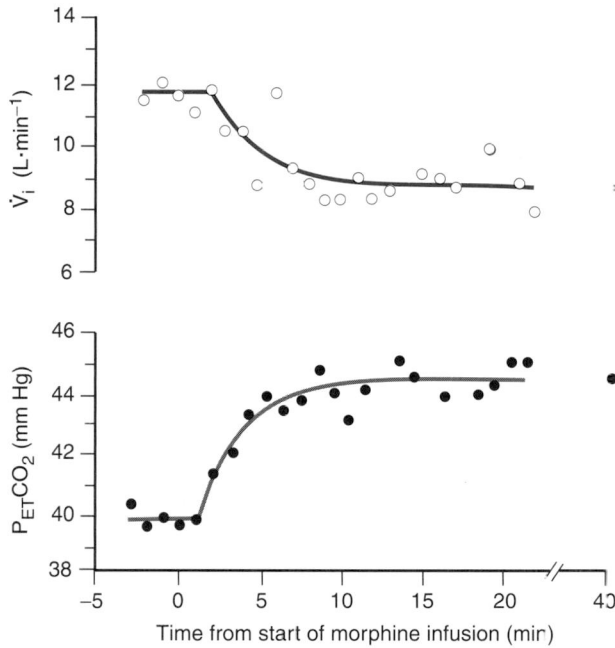

Figure 11–8 Influence of morphine administration (bolus dose of 100 µg/kg given at time 0 minutes, followed by a continuous infusion of 30 µg/kg/hour) on resting inspired minute ventilation and resting pressure of end-tidal CO_2 ($P_{ET}CO_2$) in a single subject. A one-component exponential was fitted to the data. The estimated time constant for the V_i data is 3.0 minutes and for $P_{ET}CO_2$ data is 2.6 minutes. The time delays are between 1 and 2 minutes. (From Sarton E, Teppema L, Dahan A: Sex differences in morphine-induced ventilatory depression reside within the peripheral chemoreflex loop. Anesthesiology 90:1329-1338, 1999.)

Table 11–6 Factors increasing the magnitude and/or duration of opioid-induced respiratory depression

High dose
Sleep
Old age
CNS depressant
    Inhaled anesthetics, alcohol, barbiturates,
      benzodiazepines
Renal insufficiency
Hyperventilation, hypocapnia
Respiratory acidosis
Decreased clearance
    Reduction of hepatic blood flow
Secondary peaks in plasma opioid levels
    Reuptake of opioids from muscle, lung, fat and intestine
Pain

ventilation after alfentanil-N_2O is likely with plasma alfentanil concentrations of less than 200 ng/mL,[163] significant residual respiratory depression can exist at lower levels. The effects of remifentanil, no matter what the dose, are attenuated rapidly and completely within 5 to 15 minutes following termination of its administration. In healthy humans, the EC_{50} for depression of minute ventilation with remifentanil and alfentanil was 1.17 ng/mL and 49.4 ng/mL, respectively[164]

Although the mechanism by which pain modulates ventilatory control is unknown, clinical daily practice provides indirect evidence that pain stimulates ventilation, especially during emergence from anesthesia. Combes and coworkers demonstrated that pain relief with nerve block in patients after knee surgery, who were previously treated with morphine PCA, increases the incidence of abnormal respiratory events associated with oxygen desaturation.[165] Naloxone has been accepted as a standard therapy for opioid-induced respiratory depression. However, there have been reports of naloxone-resistant respiratory depression after intrathecal or epidural opioids.[166,167]

Factors Affecting Opioid-Induced Respiratory Depression

Many factors affect the magnitude and duration of opioid-induced respiratory depression (Table 11-6). Older patients are more sensitive to the anesthetic and respiratory-depressant effects of opioids.[124] Older patients experience higher plasma concentrations of opioids administered on a weight basis. Older patients also have more frequent apnea, periodic breathing, and upper airway obstruction after morphine than young adults.[168] Morphine alone produces greater respiratory depression on a weight basis in neonates than in adults. In neonates and infants with incomplete blood-brain barriers, morphine easily penetrates the brain.

The respiratory-depressant effects of opioids are increased and/or prolonged when administered with other CNS depressants, including the potent inhaled anesthetics, alcohol, barbiturates, benzodiazepines, and most of the intravenous sedatives and hypotics.[162] Exceptions are droperidol, scopolamine, and clonidine, which do not enhance the respiratory-depressant effects of fentanyl or other opioids.[169]

Pain, particularly surgically induced pain, is thought to counteract the respiratory-depressant effects of opioids. However, some investigators have suggested the contrary.[170] Certain postoperative breathing patterns are not predominantly determined by the level or mode of pain relief.[171]

Although opioid action is usually dissipated by redistribution and hepatic metabolism, rather than by urinary excretion, adequacy of renal function may influence the duration of opioid activity. In renal insufficiency, the more potent respiratory-depressant properties of the morphine metabolite morphine-6-glucuronide (M6G) becomes evident as it is accumulated.[172] One study indicates that M6G is a somewhat weaker respiratory depressant than morphine.[173]

Hypocapnic hyperventilation has been shown to enhance and prolong postoperative respiratory depression after fentanyl. Intraoperative hypercarbia produces opposite effects. Possible explanations for these findings include increased brain opioid penetration (increased un-ionized fentanyl with hypocarbia) and removal (decreased CBF with hypocarbia). In patients who hyperventilate because of anxiety and/or pain, even small doses of intravenous opioids can result in transient apnea because of acute shifts in apneic thresholds.

Delayed or recurring respiratory depression has been reported with most opioids. Explanations for this phenomenon are not clear. Numerous investigators have noted the occurrence of significant secondary peaks and fluctuations in plasma opioid levels during the elimination phase.[174] The existence of large peripheral compartments (e.g., skeletal muscle) and the variability in drug uptake from them contributes to and can augment this phenomenon. Mechanisms for renarcotization may include augmented release of fentanyl or other opioids from skeletal muscle into the systemic circulation on rewarming, shivering, motion, or any other condition that enhances muscle perfusion.

CARDIOVASCULAR EFFECTS OF OPIOIDS

Numerous reports have demonstrated that large doses of opioids, administered as the sole or primary anesthetic, result in hemodynamic stability throughout the operative period.

The choice of opioid can affect the perioperative hemodynamic profile. For example, alfentanil is *less* reliable than fentanyl and sufentanil in blocking increases in heart rate and blood pressure during anesthetic induction, sternotomy, sternal spread, and aortotomy in patients with ischemic heart disease who undergo coronary artery surgery.[175,176]

Neurologic Mechanisms

Key areas of the brainstem that integrate cardiovascular responses and maintain cardiovascular homeostasis are the nucleus solitarius, the dorsal vagal nucleus, the nucleus ambiguus, and the parabrachial nucleus. The nucleus solitarius and parabrachial nucleus play an important role in the hemodynamic control of vasopressin secretion. Enkephalin-containing neurons and opioid receptors are distributed in these regions. The direct administration of μ-agonists into the CNS of animals most commonly, but not always, produces hypotension and bradycardia.[177] The ventrolateral periaqueductal gray region, a key central site mediating analgesia, also affects hemodynamic control.[178] Opioids also can modulate the stress response through receptor-mediated actions on the hypothalamic-pituitary-adrenal axis. Most opioids reduce sympathetic and enhance vagal and parasympathetic tone. Patients who are volume-depleted, or individuals depending on high sympathetic tone or exogenous catecholamines to maintain cardiovascular function, are predisposed to hypotension after opioid administration.

Occasionally, opioids produce paradoxic effects. A hyperdynamic cardiovascular response was reported during anesthetic induction with high-dose fentanyl in 10% of one series of patients. It was attributed to central sympathetic activation.[179] Fentanyl increases norepinephrine release from some sympathetic nerve endings, and may also inhibit the neuronal uptake of norepinephrine in dogs.

The predominant and usual effect of opioids on heart rate is to produce bradycardia resulting from stimulation of the central vagal nucleus. Blockade of sympathetic actions may also play a role in opioid-induced bradycardia. Meperidine, in contrast to other opioids, rarely results in bradycardia, but may cause tachycardia. Tachycardia after meperidine may be related to its structural similarity to atropine, to normeperidine (its principal metabolite), or to early manifestations of its toxic CNS effects.

Cardiac Mechanisms

The direct cardiac actions of opioids, and in particular the effects on myocardinal contractile mechanisms, are significantly less than those of many other intravenous and inhalation anesthetics. However, opioid receptors have been demonstrated to exist in cardiac myocytes of several species.

Contractility

Some investigators suggest that opioids produce direct positive inotropic effects on the heart.[180] However, others report negative inotropic actions with some agents (meperidine) and no direct effects with others (morphine).[181] Some investigators suggest that local anesthetic-like effects, and not receptor-related opioid actions, mediate some of the negative inotropic effects of opioids, especially with high drug concentrations.

Morphine decreases Ca^{2+} transients but not cardiac contraction, and enhances myofilament Ca^{2+} sensitivity, through an action on the δ_1 opioid receptor expressed in the heart.[182] On the other hand, it was demonstrated that morphine decreases the isometric force of contraction in atrial muscle samples from non-failing and failing human hearts through a naloxone-insensitive mechanism.[183] Most evidence, however, indicates that fentanyl produces little or no change in myocardial contractility,[184] but it has also been reported that fentanyl has positive inotropic effects. Possible mechanisms of the dose-dependent positive inotropic effects of fentanyl, as well as of sufentanil, include catecholamine release or direct myocardial adrenergic activation. Usually, most hemodynamic variables remain unchanged after large doses of fentanyl. Little or no depression of cardiac index or pump function has been reported after sufentanil in humans.[184] Studies in dogs have demonstrated little change in hemodynamics with moderate doses (160 μg/kg) of alfentanil and transient cardiac stimulation (increases in left ventricular contractility, aortic blood flow velocity, and acceleration) with very large doses (5 mg/kg). In dogs, remifentanil produces hemodynamic effects that include decreases in contractility and cardiac output, as well as decreases in heart rate and blood pressure.[185]

Heart Rate and Rhythm

Opioid-induced bradycardia is primarily mediated by the CNS. However, there have been reports of direct effects of opioids on cardiac pacemaker cells. Asystole may follow opioid-induced bradycardia. Premedication with or concomitant administration of, β-adrenergic or Ca^{2+} entry blockers can exacerbate bradycardias and may result in asystole after opioids. Periods of asystole, 10 to 12 seconds in duration, may resolve on their own, and they usually respond to atropine (0.4-0.8 mg IV).

Cardiac Conduction

Opioids may depress cardiac conduction. Fentanyl slows atrioventricular node conduction, and prolongs the RR interval, the atrioventricular node refractory period and Purkinje fiber action potential duration.[186,187] These effects have been suggested to be mediated by direct membrane actions, as opposed to opioid receptor interactions.[188] Opioids can also prolong the QT interval.[189] However, both sufentanil and alfentanil have been demonstrated to be devoid of electrophysiologic effects on normal or accessory pathways in patients with Wolff-Parkinson-White syndrome.[190,191]

Clinically, cardiac conduction disturbances due to opioids are very rare, but they may be more likely to occur in the presence of Ca^{2+} entry or β-adrenergic blockers.[192] Indeed, the overall effect of opioid anesthesia is anti-arrhythmic.[193] Antifibrillatory effects have been suggested to be produced by fentanyl.[194] Some of the electrophysiologic actions of opioids resemble those of class III anti-arrhythmic drugs. Opioid antagonists appear more antiarrhythmogenic than agonists in rats.[195]

Ischemia

Determining the effects and consequences of opioid action on myocardial ischemia is complex.[196-198] Results can depend on such factors as the species studied and the experimental design. Recently, it has been suggested that opioids can mimic ischemic preconditioning. It was demonstrated that opioid receptor stimulation results in a reduction in infarct size similar to that produced by ischemic preconditioning (Fig. 11-9).[199] It was recently reported that stimulation of the δ_1-opioid receptor generates oxygen radicals via mitochondrial ATP-sensitive K^+ channels, resulting in attenuation of oxidant stress and cell death in cardiomyocytes.[200] Involvement of the adenosine A1 receptor and protein kinase C in the cardioprotective effect of opioids was also suggested.[201,202] Whether the experimental results showing protective effects of opioids against myocardial ischemia will translate into reductions in morbidity and mortality in patients with coronary artery disease has yet to be established by clinical trials.[203]

High doses of opioids can maintain myocardial perfusion and the O_2 supply/demand ratio as well as or better than inhalation-based techniques.[204,205] Among the opioids, alfentanil is associated with more myocardial ischemia (as indicated by reversal of the myocardial lactate extraction to production ratio and the worsening ventricular diastolic compliance) than either fentanyl or sufentanil in patients having coronary artery surgery.[206] Data from a prospective randomized comparison of sufentanil versus enflurane, isoflurane, and halothane for coronary artery surgery revealed no difference in new intraoperative ischemia, the incidence of postoperative myocardial infarction, or death.[207]

Coronary Circulation

Opioids appear to have no significant effect on coronary vasomotion or myocardial metabolism, do not produce steal phenomena, and do not diminish the ability of

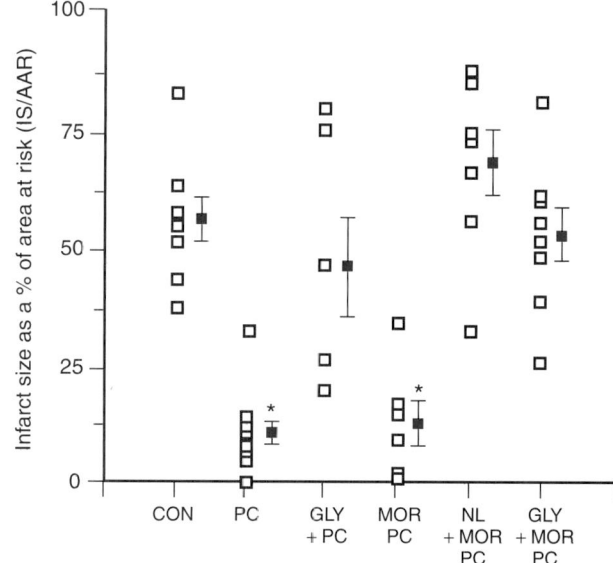

Figure 11–9 Infarct sizes in rat hearts subjected to control conditions (CON), ischemic preconditioning (PC), glibenclamide (0.3 mg/kg IV) given 30 minutes before ischemic PC (GLY + PC), morphine-induced PC (3×100 µg/kg, 5 minutes of IV infusion) (MOR PC), naloxone (3 mg/kg IV) given 10 minutes before morphine-induced PC (NL + MOR PC), and glibenclamide (0.3 mg/kg IV) given 30 minutes before morphine-induced PC (GLY + MOR PC). (From Schultz JE, Hsu AK, Gross GJ: Morphine mimics the cardioprotective effect of ischemic preconditioning via a glibenclamide-sensitive mechanism in the rat heart. Circ Res 78:1100-1104, 1996.)

large coronary arterioles to respond to vasoactive agents.[208] In a study of the effects of opioids and neuroendocrine modulators on porcine coronary arteries, fentanyl (but not sufentanil or morphine) antagonized acetylcholine-induced contractions.[209] The effect of fentanyl was not reversible by naloxone and was thus thought to represent a direct smooth muscle effect.

Baroreception

Potent opioids applied in anesthesia usually produce minimal to no decreases in preload and afterload, and little depression of great vessel and atrial baroreceptors,[210] in contrast to potent inhalation agents such as halothane.[211] Infants, after receiving 10 µg/kg of fentanyl, do demonstrate significant depression of baroreflex responses.[212]

Cardiogenic Reflex

Some authors have suggested that aortic root dissection causes hypertension mediated by serotonin via stimulation of a specific cardiogenic reflex. Although higher doses of fentanyl or sufentanil can decrease the occurrence of intraoperative hypertension, no dose of any opioid has been shown to prevent all hypertensive responses reliably, especially during cardiac surgery in humans.[59]

Hormonal Mechanisms

Morphine (1-3 mg/kg) causes histamine release and sympathoadrenal activation. The release of catecholamines by morphine and meperidine follows and parallels histamine release, which can be marked in some patients.[213]

Increases in plasma histamine after morphine cause dilatation of terminal arterioles and direct positive cardiac chronotropic and inotropic actions. Hormonal alterations contribute to the cardiovascular changes seen after morphine and include an increase in cardiac index and a decrease in arterial blood pressure and systemic vascular resistance.[214] Cardiovascular changes after morphine are similar when patients are pretreated with diphenhydramine (a histamine H_1-antagonist) or cimetidine (a histamine H_2-antagonist). However, in patients pretreated with both H_1- and H_2-antagonists, the cardiovascular responses are significantly attenuated despite comparable increases in plasma histamine concentrations. Meperidine also causes histamine release more frequently than most other opioids. Unlike morphine or meperidine, fentanyl, alfentanil, and remifentanil do not produce increases in plasma histamine, and hypotension is less frequent with these opioids. Although large doses of fentanyl produce significant increases in plasma catecholamines in dogs, large doses of fentanyl (24-75 µg/kg) decrease rather than increase plasma catecholamine and cortisol concentrations in humans.

Opioids also may have direct effects on adrenal secretory mechanisms. Gaumann and coworkers have reported that sufentanil produced 6- to 20-fold increases in adrenal vein concentrations of catecholamines and parallel increases in arterial blood pressures in cats.[215] Although µ-opioid agonists do modulate the adrenal secretory response to pain, the adrenal secretory response to hemorrhage is preserved after sufentanil administration.

Vascular Mechanisms

Morphine selectively impairs certain sympathetic reflexes involving peripheral veins. This response is due to a CNS action of the drug with reduction of sympathetic tone. Vasodilatation after morphine may also result from a direct effect of morphine on vascular smooth muscle. At high doses, morphine inhibits the presynaptic release of norepinephrine in saphenous vein rings and results in a decreased contractile response to electrical stimulation. Pharmacologic studies evaluating alfentanil, fentanyl, and sufentanil in the dog demonstrate direct peripheral vessel smooth muscle relaxation.[216]

ENDOCRINOLOGIC EFFECTS OF OPIOIDS

The main components of the neuroendocrine stress response are the corticotropin-releasing hormone brain centers (e.g., paraventricular hypothalamic nucleus) and the locus caeruleus–norepinephrine secreting areas of the autonomic nervous system.[217] Increased levels of stress hormones are considered undesirable because they promote hemodynamic instability and intraoperative and postoperative metabolic catabolism. In some circumstances, hormonal and metabolic responses to surgery are extreme and are thought to contribute to operative mortality.[218]

Opioids are capable of reducing the stress response by modulating nociception at several different levels of the neuraxis, as well as by influencing centrally mediated neuroendocrine responses. Opioids are potent inhibitors of the pituitary-adrenal axis.[219] Endogenous opioid peptides may serve as stress hormones themselves and not just as modulators of the secretion of other hormones. This activity is suggested by the finding that β-endorphin and adrenocorticotropic hormone (ACTH) are derived from the same precursor preproopiomelanocortin and are cosecreted during stress.

Morphine modifies hormonal responses to surgical trauma in a dose-related fashion. Morphine can prevent ACTH release, suppress surgically induced increases in plasma cortisol, and attenuate the pituitary-adrenal response to surgical stress. Morphine can increase some stress-responding hormones due to increases in plasma histamine release, adrenal medullary release mechanisms, and catecholamine release from sympathetic nerve endings.

Fentanyl and its congeners are more effective than morphine in modifying hormonal responses to surgery. The efficacy of fentanyl in controlling the hormonal manifestations of the stress response can be dose-dependent.[220] Fentanyl, in doses of at least 50 µg/kg, prevents increases in blood glucose, plasma catecholamines, antidiuretic hormone (ADH), renin, aldosterone, cortisol, and growth hormone (GH) concentrations before, but not consistently during or after, cardiopulmonary bypass. Fentanyl doses greater than or equal to 50 µg/kg can help reduce the hyperglycemic response to cardiac surgery in pediatric patients to less than 200 mg/dL throughout operation.[221]

Sufentanil may be superior to fentanyl in modifying the stress response.[222] However, it has been demonstrated that neither fentanyl nor sufentanil alone can completely block sympathetic and hormonal stress responses and that perhaps no dose-response relationship exists for opioid-associated stress response control.[59] The stress response to cardiopulmonary bypass is difficult to suppress with sufentanil, as with fentanyl.

Alfentanil can cause hormone-modifying effects similar to those of sufentanil. Alfentanil can suppress increases in plasma cortisol and catecholamines before but not during cardiopulmonary bypass and may prevent increases in ADH and GH throughout coronary artery bypass surgery. High-dose alfentanil-N_2O anesthesia (150 µg/kg loading dose plus 3 µg/kg/min infusion) better suppresses intraoperative cortisol and glucose elevation than droperidol-fentanyl-N_2O anesthesia in patients undergoing abdominal surgery.[223]

Stress Reduction and Outcome

Some evidence suggests that anesthetic techniques or agents that minimize this stress response may reduce morbidity and mortality in a variety of circumstances.[224] Sufentanil appears to be the most likely opioid to modify stress responses and outcomes successfully.[225,226] Other investigators suggest that neither the opioid administered nor the anesthetic technique has an impact on outcome.[207,227] Anand and colleagues[225] evaluated the impact of sufentanil versus morphine-halothane anesthesia on hormonal and metabolic responses and morbidity and mortality in neonates undergoing cardiac surgery.

Most strikingly, a statistically significant difference in postoperative mortality was observed (0 of 30 given sufentanil versus 4 of 15 given halothane plus morphine). Mangano and associates[226] also reported that, after myocardial revascularization, patients receiving intense postoperative analgesia with sufentanil (1 µg/kg/hour) experience a decrease in the incidence and severity of electrocardiographically documented ischemia compared with patients receiving intermittent intravenous morphine (2.2 ± 2.1 mg/hour) for postoperative analgesia.

Many different hormonal changes induced by surgery have been described. However, the concomitant neural, cellular, immune, and biochemical changes have been less well defined, and little is understood or proven with regard to how modifying hormonal responses alters outcome.[228] Additional studies are necessary for complete elucidation of the relationship between control of surgery-induced hormonal responses and outcome.

OPIATE TOLERANCE AND ADDICTION

The mechanisms of dependence and tolerance involve genetic, molecular, cellular, physiologic, and functional factors. In the locus caeruleus, the major noradrenergic nucleus in the brain, long-term opioid exposure results in inhibition of adenyl cyclase, reduced activity of protein kinase A, and upregulation of the cAMP pathway.[229] Changes in µ-receptor density that occur prior to or during the development of tolerance do not appear to be essential for development of opioid tolerance.[230] Possible mechanisms involve protein kinase signal transduction cascades that link extracellular signals to cellular changes by regulating target gene expression. Much work remains to be done in order to fully elucidate the complex mechanisms of tolerance.[231,232]

Acute administration of opioids results in analgesia and side effects, whereas tolerance and dependence were thought to occur only after chronic administration. However, it has become more recently recognized that tolerance can also develop rapidly after an acute opioid exposure in animals and humans.[233-235] Intraoperative remifentanil infusion (0.3 µg/kg/minute) in patients undergoing major abdominal surgery under desflurane anesthesia increased postoperative pain and morphine requirement compared with low-dose remifentanil (0.1 µg/kg/minute), suggesting the development of acute remifentanil tolerance.[236] In contrast, there is a report that target-controlled infusion of alfentanil and remifentanil for postoperative analgesia does not lead to opioid tolerance.[237] In human volunteers, continuous infusion of remifentanil (0.08 µg/kg/minute) for 3 hours did not decrease the pain threshold.[238] Thus, the development of acute opioid tolerance in humans remains controversial. Opioids can elicit hyperalgesia in experimental models after repeated opioid administration or continuous delivery.[239] This phenomenon seems to be related to opioid tolerance.[240] In rats, thermal hyperalgesia and mechanical allodynia were observed for several days after cessation of morphine administration (40 mg/kg/day for 6 days).[241] The opioid-induced hyperalgesia was shown to be due to spinal sensitization to glutamate and substance P.[242]

Furthermore, cholecystokinin and the NMDA-nitric oxide (NO) system are responsible for the development of acute tolerance to opioids,[243] which is also affected by spinal serotonin activity.[244] There have been reports that opioid-induced hyperalgesia and subsequent acute opioid tolerance can be prevented by ketamine, suggesting the involvement of the NMDA receptor.[245,246]

Peripheral morphine effects have been suggested to be less prone to tolerance.[247] Thus, the method and schedule of drug administration may also affect the development of tolerance.[248] However, modifying an opioid administration schedule to modulate the development of tolerance may not always be useful or effective.[249] Certain patients may appear to be tolerant to opioids, but instead they may suffer from pathophysiologic conditions, such as neuropathies, that are poorly responsive to opioids.[250]

Management of the Opioid-Dependent Patient

Problems in the opioid-addicted patients include cardiopulmonary problems, restrictive lung disease, increased alveolar-arterial O_2 gradients, renal disease and anemia. Long-term morphine administration causes adrenal hypertrophy and impairs corticosteroid secretion. Viral and nonviral hepatitis, acquired immunodeficiency syndrome, osteomyelitis, muscle weakness, and neurologic complications may be found in addicted patients.

Anesthetic management for the opiate-dependent or addicted patient should include adequate premedication with opioids. There is no ideal anesthetic agent or technique to employ in the chronic addict or in the patient with an acute opiate overdose. Cardiovascular and respiratory changes in the patient with acute opioid overdose can be reversed with increments of naloxone (40-80 µg every 1 to 2 minutes IV) until vital signs are adequate. Support of the circulatory system with fluids and monitoring of arterial blood gases and pulmonary function are also important.

Recently, as treatment for opioid addiction, rapid detoxification with high doses of naloxone or naltrexone has been reported. For this treatment, general anesthesia is induced before the start of opioid antagonism and maintained for several hours to prevent the perception of withdrawal symptoms by the patient.[251,252] Blockade of µ-opioid receptors by naloxone (total dose of 12.4 mg) in opioid-addicted patients induces sympathetic neural activation, including increase in plasma catecholamine concentration and cardiovascular stimulation, which is abolished by α_2-agonists.[253]

RENAL AND URODYNAMIC EFFECTS OF OPIOIDS

µ-Receptor activation causes antidiuresis and decreases electrolyte excretion. κ-Receptor stimulation predominantly produces diuresis with little change in electrolyte excretion. The stable dynorphin analogue E-2078 causes κ-receptor mediated diuretic effects in the isolated perfused rat kidney.[254] Indirect actions may involve inhibiting or altering the secretion of ADH and atrial natriuretic peptide.[255]

Kien and associates noted a 25% decrease in renal cortical blood flow that paralleled changes in blood pressure suggesting impairment of autoregulation.[256] However, the absence of increases in plasma ADH, renin, and aldosterone indicates that fentanyl, sufentanil, alfentanil, and probably remifentanil most likely preserve or minimally alter renal function in humans. If renal function does change during opioid anesthesia and surgery, it is probably due to secondary changes in systemic and renal hemodynamics.

Lower urinary tract opioid effects include disturbances of micturition characterized by urinary retention, especially after intrathecal opioid administration. Not all opioid agonists behave similarly, and morphine appears to be particularly potent with regard to producing urodynamic problems.[257] Malinovsky and colleagues. compared the urodynamic effects of intravenously administered morphine (10 mg), buprenorphine (0.3 mg), fentanyl (0.35 mg) and nalbuphine (20 mg).[258] It was shown that all of the opioids altered bladder sensations, but that detrusor contraction decreased only after administration of fentanyl and buprenorphine.

GASTROINTESTINAL EFFECTS OF OPIOIDS

Opioids decrease gastrointestinal motility,[259] and this action underlies their use as antidiarrheal agents. Patients receiving parenteral opioid therapy preoperatively are more likely to have "full stomachs" regardless of their "NPO" status.

Several opioid receptor types can be demonstrated on myenteric neurons, and both κ- and μ-receptor agonists regulate cholinergic transmission in the myenteric plexus. κ-Receptor agonists appear to modulate acetylcholine release more potently than μ-receptor agonists by inhibition of N-type voltage-sensitive Ca^{2+} channels via a pertussis toxin-sensitive G protein in guinea pig ileum.[260]

Opioids alter lower esophageal sphincter activity, resulting in sphincter relaxation.[261] Gastric emptying is delayed by opioids, via supraspinal (vagus nerve–mediated) and spinal, as well as peripheral, mechanisms. Both fentanyl and meperidine reduce antroduodenal motility during balanced anesthesia, but at least partial recovery occurs relatively early (0.5-2.0 hours) postoperatively.[262] Both opioids are also associated with an increase in gastric pH. Tramadol (1.25 mg/kg IV) has a measurable but smaller inhibitory effect on gastric emptying compared with codeine (1 mg/kg IV) or morphine (0.125 mg/kg IV).[263] Opioids administered epidurally as well as intrathecally reduce gastrointestinal motility.[264,265]

Naloxone reverses opioid-induced delays in gastric emptying. Methylnaltrexone, a quaternary naloxone derivative that dose not cross the blood-brain barrier, can attenuate morphine-induced delays in gastric emptying, suggesting that a peripheral mechanism is involved in the opioid effect on the gastrointestinal tract.[259] Intravenous, but not intramuscular, metoclopramide (10 mg) also can reverse morphine-induced delays in gastric emptying.[266]

Opioid effects on the intestine are complex. Transit time from mouth to ileum may not be significantly altered by morphine, because morphine enhances ileal propulsion before decreasing motility. Opioids increase tone and decrease propulsive activity in most of the intestine. Gastrointestinal secretions can be increased by opioids.

The effects of opioids on intestinal circulation are complex and are not completely understood. Fentanyl increases intestinal blood flow in a dose-dependent fashion.

Biliary and Hepatic Effects

All opioid agonists increase biliary duct pressure and sphincter of Oddi (choledochoduodenal sphincter) tone in a dose- and drug-dependent manner through opioid receptor–mediated mechanisms.[267] However, the clinical consequences of opioid-induced biliary tract actions are usually minimal. Increases in biliary pressure caused by opioids are, with the exception of meperidine, reversible with naloxone.

Meperidine has a dual effect on the biliary tract.[268] Low concentrations of meperidine produce an inhibitory effect on the response of the common bile duct to electrical stimulation. Higher concentrations produce an excitatory effect and increase spontaneous contractions. Neither of these responses is affected by naloxone.

Opioids produce mild effects on liver function during anesthesia and surgery. In rats, fentanyl produces a postanesthetic dysfunction of the liver that is independent of the presence of cirrhosis. Alfentanil can reduce hepatic artery blood flow by more than 50% in the dog.[256]

Nausea and Vomiting

Postoperative nausea and vomiting is a serious problem that is a major concern for anesthesiologists.[269,270] The etiology, treatment, and prevention of postoperative nausea and vomiting have been investigated extensively (Fig. 11-10).[271] The intraoperative use of opioids is a well-known risk factor for postoperative nausea and vomiting. Opioids stimulate the chemoreceptor trigger zone in the area postrema of the medulla possibly through δ-receptors, leading to nausea and vomiting. Alfentanil, compared with approximately equipotent doses of fentanyl and sufentanil, is associated with a lower incidence of postoperative nausea and vomiting.[272]

The use of propofol in balanced or total intravenous anesthesia (TIVA) significantly reduces the incidence of opioid-induced nausea and vomiting.[273] The incidence of postoperative nausea and vomiting can be as low as 5% to 20% after propofol-alfentanil anesthesia.

When opioids are employed, antiemetic prophylaxis should be considered, which includes drugs with anticholinergic activity, butyrophenones, dopamine antagonists, serotonin antagonists and acupressure. Ondansetron, a serotonin type 3 receptor antagonist, was proved to be effective for postoperative opioid-induced nausea and vomiting.[274] Cannabinoid receptor agonists have been demonstrated to be effective antiemetics in some clinical settings. Animal experiments have shown that the cannabinoid agonists suppress opioid-induced retching and vomiting by activation of the cannabinoid CB1 receptor.[275]

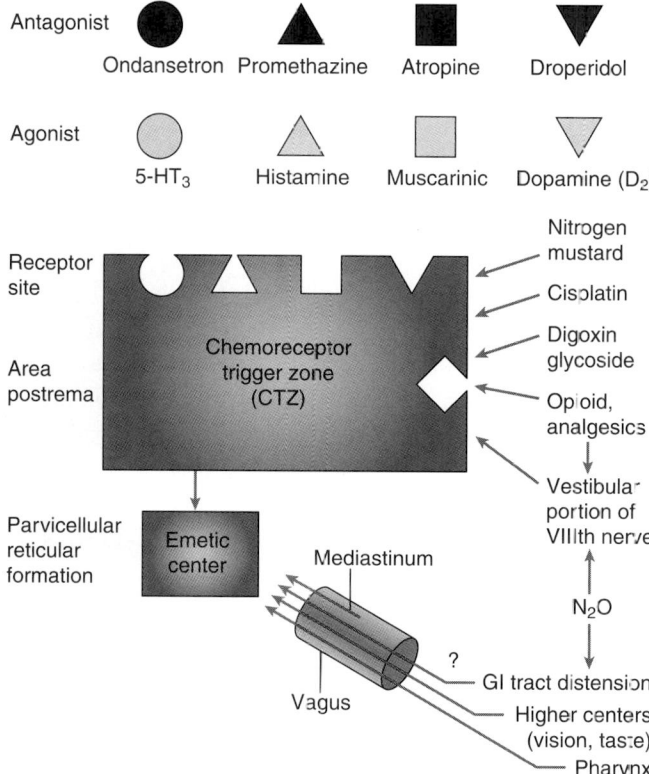

Figure 11–10 The chemoreceptor trigger zone and the emetic center with the agonist and antagonist sites of action of various anesthetic-related agents and stimuli. (From Watcha MF, White PF: Postoperative nausea and vomiting. Its etiology, treatment, and prevention. Anesthesiology 77:162-184, 1992.)

OTHER OPIOID EFFECTS

Obstetrics

Morphine, but not fentanyl, can adversely affect in vitro fertilization of sea urchin eggs. Thus, fentanyl has been recommended as clinically useful during the harvesting of human ova for subsequent in vitro fertilization.[276] Although alfentanil penetrates follicular fluid to a greater extent than fentanyl, it has no effect on cleavage rate and has also been recommended as useful in providing analgesia for oocyte retrieval. The teratogenic actions of opioids, including fentanyl, sufentanil, and alfentanil, at least in animal models, appear to be minimal (also see Chapter 58).[277]

The parenteral administration of opioids prior to vaginal delivery remains a commonly used method of analgesia. Nociception due to uterine cervical distention could be suppressed by μ- and κ-agonists in rats,[278] but the analgesic effect of μ-agonists but not κ-agonists was reduced by estrogen.[279] Aortocaval compression and associated hypotension may be exacerbated by parenteral opioids, especially following morphine or meperidine. Fetal manifestations of maternal opioid administration include decreases in heart rate variability. Adverse neonatal effects can occur after either morphine or meperidine administration to mothers. Fetal acidosis increases opioid transfer from the mother. Attempts to minimize the neonatal

effects of opioids include restricting opioid administration to the first stage of labor. The short-acting opioid alfentanil administered before cesarean delivery attenuated the maternal stress response, but led to slightly reduced Apgar scores.[280]

Morphine has little effect on the pregnant rat uterus, whereas meperidine can increase uterine contractions in a dose-dependent fashion that is not reversible by naloxone.[281] Fentanyl has no effect on uterine blood flow and tone in sheep. Fentanyl (50-100 μg IV every hour), compared with meperidine (25-50 mg IV every 2 to 3 hours), results in less nausea, vomiting, and sedation in the mother and in lower naloxone requirements in newborns.[282]

Morphine and meperidine have been found in the breast milk of mothers receiving intravenous opioid analgesia.[283,284] Although both fentanyl and morphine are concentrated in breast milk in milk-to-plasma ratios of 2 to 3:1, newborn narcosis is reported to be insignificant.

Newborns of addicted mothers can exhibit opioid withdrawal and require observation and appropriate treatment.[285]

Allergic Reactions

True allergic reactions and systemic anaphylactoid reactions to opioids are rare. More commonly, local reactions caused by preservatives or histamine may occur. Wheal and flare responses on intradermal injection of morphine, meperidine, fentanyl, and sufentanil, but not alfentanil, naloxone, and nalbuphine, were greater than those due to saline.[286]

Ocular Effects

The use of fentanyl, sufentanil, and alfentanil during induction of anesthesia can help prevent increases in intraocular pressure. Fentanyl, alfentanil, and sufentanil doses as small as 2.5, 10, and 0.1 μg/kg, respectively, may be sufficient as long as appropriate anesthetic depth is achieved prior to tracheal intubation. Remifentanil (1 μg/kg) combined with propofol (2 mg/kg) or thiopental (5 mg/kg) was reported to be effective for prevention of intraocular pressure changes after succinylcholine and tracheal intubation.[287,288]

Immune Effects

It is now firmly established that opioids influence immune regulation. Direct effects of opioid agonists include modulation of immune cellular activity, as well as that of specific enzymatic degradation and regulation processes.[289] Several immune cell populations, including T cells, macrophages and natural killer (NK) cells, serve as targets for the effects of opioids. It was shown that the maximal effect on NK cell activity, proliferation of splenic T and B cells and interferon-γ production are observed 0.5 to 1 hour after 15 mg/kg morphine injection in rats.[290] The time course was nearly concordant with that of the antinociceptive effect of morphine. Postoperative administration of morphine (10 mg IM) or tramadol (100 mg IM) induced different changes in NK cell activity.[291] More recently, it was reported that intravenously administered fentanyl causes a rapid increase in NK cell cytotoxicity, which was coincident with an increase in the percentage of CD16[+] and CD8[+] cells in peripheral blood.[292] As a potential mechanism for the immunosuppressive effects of opioids, it was demonstrated that NF-κB activation induced by an inflammatory stimulus was inhibited by morphine in a nitric oxide–dependent manner.[293]

PHARMACOKINETICS AND PHARMACODYNAMICS OF OPIOIDS

Humans exhibit substantial intersubject variability in their response to opioids.[294] This variability is at least three- to fivefold and is a function of both pharmacokinetic and pharmacodynamic parameters (Fig. 11-11). Therefore, opioid dosage regimens should be customized for each patient.

With the advent of modern drug assay technology and the widespread availability of computers, it is now possible to analyze pharmacologic data with combined pharmacokinetic-pharmacodynamic models, which separate drug response into pharmacokinetic and pharmacodynamic components. Pharmacokinetic parameters govern the relationship between opioid dose and the opioid concentrations in the blood (or other body fluid). Pharmacodynamic parameters describe the relationship between opioid concentration in blood (or other fluid) and the opioid's pharmacological effect.

Physicochemical Properties

Opioids are weak bases. When dissolved in solution, they are dissociated into protonated and free-base fractions, with the relative proportions depending on the pH and pKa. The free base fraction is more lipid-soluble than the protonated fraction.

High lipid solubility facilitates opioid transport into the biophase or site of action. Therefore, highly lipid-soluble opioids have a more rapid onset of action. However, because the opioid receptor "recognizes" an opioid molecule in the protonated form, the intensity of opioid effects is closely related to the ionized concentration of drug in the biophase (Fig. 11-12).

All opioids are to some extent bound to plasma proteins, including albumin and α_1-acid glycoprotein. It is only the un-ionized, unbound fraction that constitutes the diffusible fraction and provides the concentration gradient that promotes diffusion of opioid from the blood to the tissue of interest. Thus, the speed of onset of opioid effect is influenced by both the lipid solubility and the protein binding.

Common Pharmacokinetic Features of Opioids

Representative pharmacokinetic parameters for the opioids commonly used in anesthesia are displayed in Table 11-7.

After intravenous injection, arterial plasma concentrations of opioids rise to a peak within one circulation time. Thereafter, they exhibit a rapid redistribution phase and a slower elimination phase typical of drugs whose pharmacokinetics are described by compartmental models.[295]

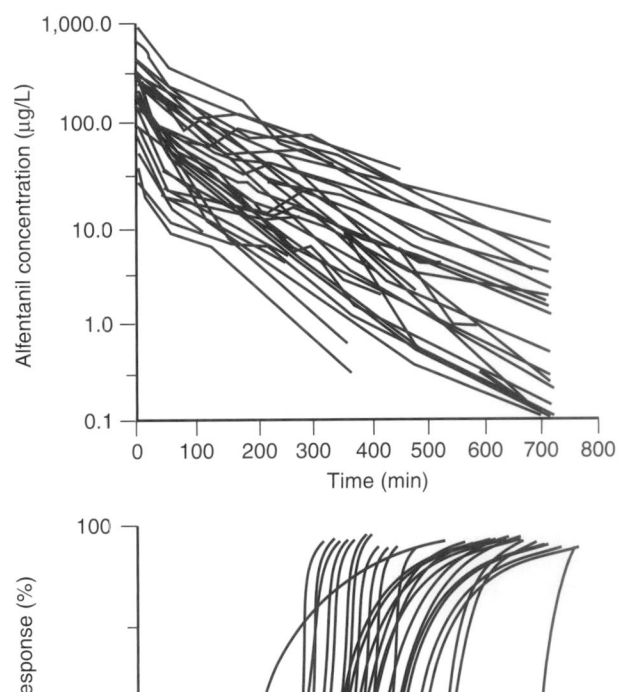

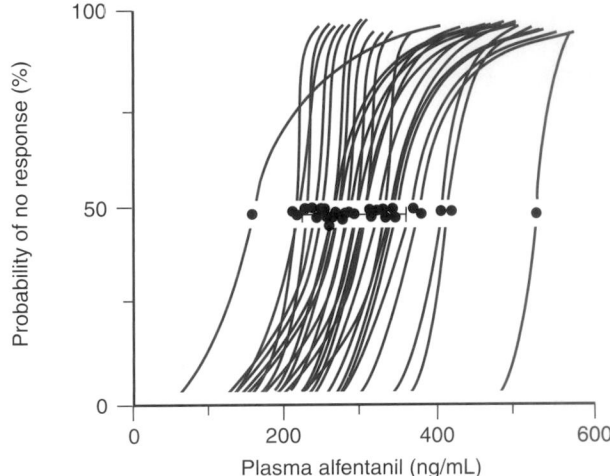

Figure 11–11 Pharmacokinetic and pharmacodynamic variability of the opioid. The *upper panel* demonstrates alfentanil plasma concentration in 45 patients administered with 50 µg/kg alfentanil. The *lower panel* shows dose-response relationships of alfentanil from 34 patients receiving alfentanil and 66% nitrous oxide during intraabdominal surgery. The *black circles* represent the Cp_{50} from each patient. Cp_{50}, the concentration needed to obtund responses to stimuli adequately in 50% of patients. (From Maitre PO, Vozeh S, Heykants J, et al: Population pharmacokinetics of alfentanil: The average dose-plasma concentration relationship and interindividual variability in patients. Anesthesiology 66:3-12, 1987; and Ausems ME, Hug CC Jr, Stanski DR, Burm AG: Plasma concentrations of alfentanil required to supplement nitrous oxide anesthesia for general surgery. Anesthesiology 65:362-367, 1986.)

After administration into a central compartment, opioids are either eliminated from the central compartment (by excretion or biotransformation) or distributed to peripheral compartments. In general, opioids are cleared from the plasma by biotransformation in the liver. However, extrahepatic metabolism is important for some opioids.

As a rule, because of their high lipid solubility, opioids are widely distributed in body tissues. In pharmacokinetic terms, this means that opioids typically have a high apparent volume of distribution at steady state. Because opioids are distributed so widely and so rapidly to various body tissues, redistribution has a prominent impact on

Figure 11–12 Distribution of fentanyl within the body compartments at the extracellular pH of 7.4. The accumulation of fentanyl by the tissue is assumed to be 13-fold. In the extracellular space, an equilibrium exists between the ionized fentanyl (F^+), the free base (F), and the fentanyl molecules bound to macromolecules (F_b). The concentration of ionized fentanyl within the interstitial fluid (encircled F^+) determines the pharmacologic effect, because the opioid receptors are located at the cell surface. Fentanyl as free base readily penetrates into the cells and becomes bound to cytomembranes, lysosomes, and other structures (*thick arrows*) and thus accumulates in the cell. A small decrease of the extracellular pH will shift the equilibrium between F and F^+ toward higher F^+ concentrations and will induce a marked release of fentanyl from the cellular compartment as a result of the decrease of the concentration of F in the interstitium. An increase of the extracellular H^+ concentration by pH 0.2 might roughly double the concentration of ionized fentanyl within the interstitial fluid and accordingly enhance its pharmacologic effect. (From Lullmann H, Martins BS, Peters T: pH-dependent accumulation of fentanyl, lofentanil and alfentanil by beating guinea pig atria. Br J Anaesth 57:1012-1017, 1985.)

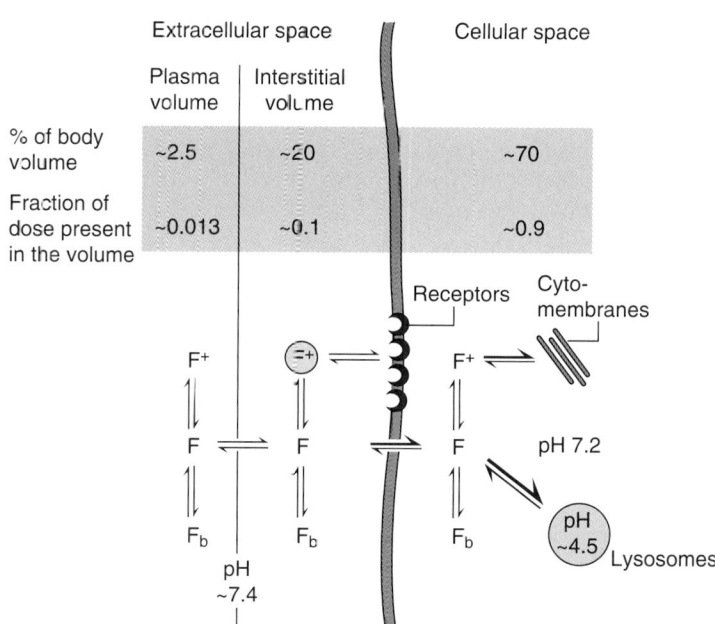

the decline of opioid concentration, particularly in the early period after injection.

Opioid uptake by the lung is a significant implication of opioid pharmacokinetics. The time necessary to reach peak concentration of an opioid is influenced by the percentage of pulmonary uptake. A very substantial proportion of the initial dose of a highly lipophilic opioid such as fentanyl is taken up by the lung (75%) and subsequently is rapidly released.[296]

Pharmacokinetic Features of Individual Drugs

Morphine
Morphine pharmacokinetics are notably different from those of the fentanyl congeners. This difference is in large part due to morphine's comparatively low lipid solubility. There is relatively little transient first-pass uptake of morphine by the lung.[296,297]

The pKa of morphine (8.0) is greater than physiologic pH, and thus, after intravenous injection only a small fraction (10% to 20%) of morphine is un-ionized. Penetration of morphine into and out of the brain is presumably slower compared with that of other opioids. Approximately 20% to 40% of morphine is bound to plasma proteins, mostly albumin.

Morphine is principally metabolized by conjugation in the liver, but the kidney plays a key role in the extrahepatic metabolism of morphine.[298,299] Morphine 3-glucuronide (M3G) is the major metabolite of morphine, but it does not bind to opioid receptors and possesses little or no

Table 11–7 Physicochemical and pharmacokinetic data of commonly used opioid agonists

	Morphine	Meperidine	Fentanyl	Sufentanil	Alfentanil	Remifentanil
pKa	8.0	8.5	8.4	8.0	6.5	7.1
% Un-ionized at pH 7.4	23	<10	<10	20	90	67?
Octanol/H_2O partition coefficient	1.4	39	813	1,778	145	17.9
% Bound to plasma protein	20-40	39	84	93	92	80?
Diffusible fraction (%)	16.8	2.2	1.5	1.6	8.0	13.3?
$t_{1/2\alpha}$ (min)	1-2.5	—	1-2	1-2	1-3	0.5-1.5
$t_{1/2\beta}$ (min)	10-20	5-15	10-30	15-20	4-17	5-8
$t_{1/2\gamma}$ (hr)	2-4	3-5	2-4	2-3	1-2	0.7-1.2
Vd_c (L/kg)	0.1-0.4	1-2	0.4-1.0	0.2	0.1-0.3	0.06-0.08
Vd_{ss} (L/kg)	3-5	3-5	3-5	2.5-3.0	0.4-1.0	0.2-0.3
Clearance (mL/min/kg)	15-30	8.18	10-20	10-15	4-9	30-40
Hepatic extraction ratio	0.6-0.8	0.5-0.7	0.8-1.0	0.7-0.9	0.3-0.5	NA

$t_{1/2}$ α, β, γ are the half-lives of a three-compartment model; Vd_c, volume of distribution of the central compartment; Vd_{ss}, volume of distribution at steady state.
From Bailey PL, Egan TD, Stanley TH: Intravenous opioid anesthetics. *In* Miller RD (ed): Anesthesia, 5th ed. New York, Churchill Livingstone, 2000, p 312.

analgesic activity. M3G may actually antagonize morphine, and this effect may contribute both to variability in response and to resistance to morphine analgesic therapy. Morphine 6-glucuronide (M6G) accounts for nearly 10% of morphine metabolites and is a more potent μ-receptor agonist than morphine, with a similar duration of action. It was reported that M6G contributes substantially to morphine's analgesic effects even in patients with normal renal function.[300] Especially in patients with renal dysfunction, the accumulation of M6G can lead to an increased incidence of adverse effects, including respiratory depression. A recent report suggested that single nucleotide polymorphism at the μ-opioid receptor affects the susceptibility to M6G-related opioid toxicity.[301] Because the hepatic extraction ratio of morphine is high, the bioavailability of orally administered morphine is significantly lower (20% to 30%) than after intramuscular or subcutaneous injection. It appears that M6G is in fact the primary active compound when morphine is administered orally (Fig. 11-13).[302] In contrast to the reports suggesting the high potency of M6G, other studies have shown that short-term intravenous administration of M6G does not provide effective analgesia.[303,304]

Meperidine

Unlike morphine, after intravenous injection first-pass uptake of meperidine by the lungs is approximately 65%.[296] Meperidine is more highly bound to plasma proteins than morphine is, principally (70%) to α_1-acid glycoprotein. As with morphine, a relatively high hepatic extraction ratio results in biotransformation that is dependent on hepatic blood flow. The major metabolite normeperidine has analgesic activity and is roughly twice as potent as meperidine in producing seizures in animals. The elimination half-life of normeperidine is considerably longer than that of meperidine, and thus repeated doses can easily produce accumulation of this toxic metabolite in patients with renal disease, potentially producing seizures.

Fentanyl

A three-compartment model is typically used to describe plasma fentanyl concentration decay. The lungs exert a significant first-pass effect and transiently take up approximately 75% of an injected dose of fentanyl.[296,305] Approximately 80% of fentanyl is bound to plasma proteins, and significant amounts (40%) are taken up by red blood cells.[306] Fentanyl has a relatively long half-life, in large part because of this widespread distribution (i.e., large volume of distribution) in body tissues.

Fentanyl is primarily metabolized in the liver by *N*-dealkylation and hydroxylation. Metabolites begin to appear in the plasma as early as 1.5 minutes after injection. In humans, norfentanyl, the primary metabolite, is detectable in the urine for up to 48 hours after intravenous administration of fentanyl.

Alfentanil

Following intravenous injection, alfentanil plasma concentrations are described by either two-compartment[307] or three-compartment models.[308,309] Alfentanil is bound to plasma proteins (mostly glycoproteins) in higher

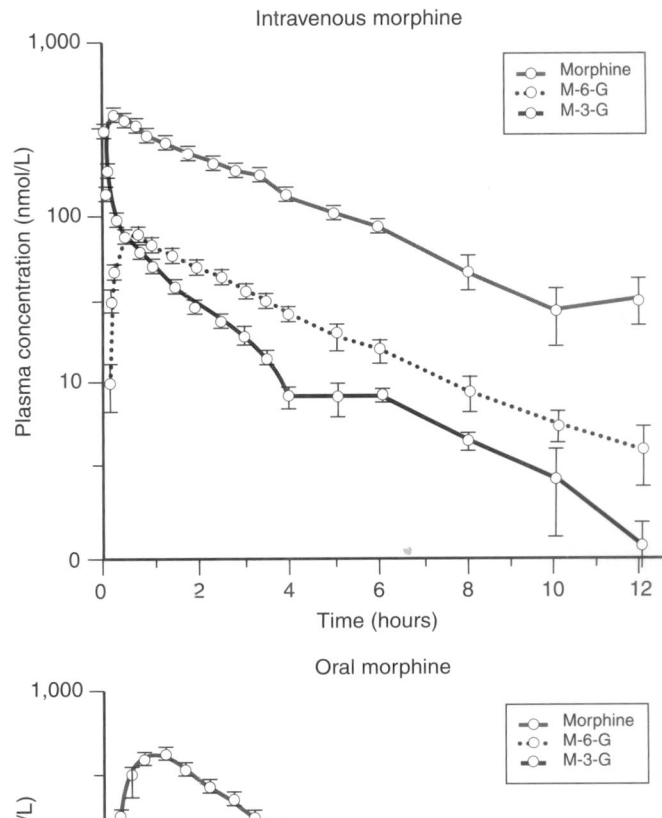

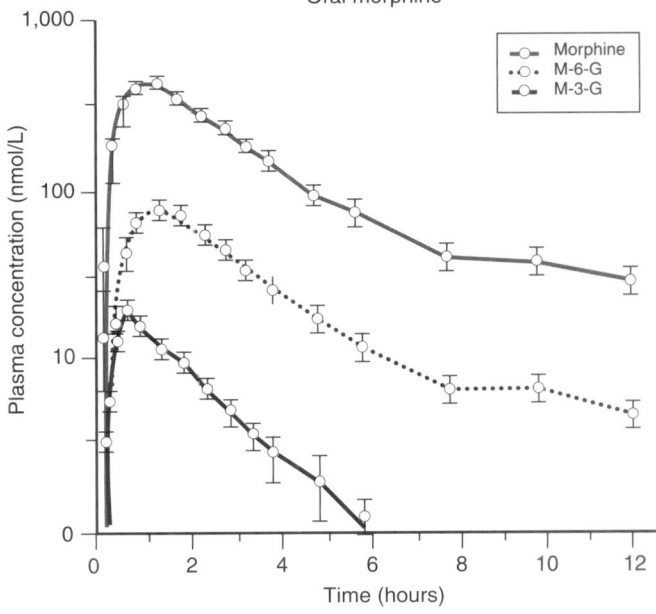

Figure 11–13 Mean plasma concentrations (± SEM) of morphine, morphine-6-glucuronide (M-6-G), and morphine-3-glucuronide (M-3-G) after intravenous and oral administration of morphine. (From Osborne R, Joel S, Trew D, Slevin M: Morphine and metabolite behavior after different routes of morphine administration: demonstration of the importance of the active metabolite morphine-6-glucuronide. Clin Pharmacol Ther 47:12-9, 1990.)

proportions (90%) than fentanyl. At physiologic pH, it is mostly (90%) un-ionized because of its relatively low pKa (6.5). Thus, despite more intense protein binding, the diffusible fraction of alfentanil is higher than that of fentanyl. This explains, in part, its short latency to peak effect after intravenous injection.

The main metabolic pathways of alfentanil are similar to those of sufentanil and include oxidative *N*-dealkylation and *O*-demethylation, aromatic hydroxylation, and ether glucuronide formation.[310] The degradation products of alfentanil have little, if any, opioid activity. Human alfentanil metabolism may be predominantly, if not exclusively, by cytochrome P-450 3A3/4.[311] This enzyme is known to display at least an eightfold range of activity in humans.

Sufentanil

Until recently, the pharmacokinetics of sufentanil had been inadequately characterized because of poor assay sensitivity.[312] Sufentanil's potency is so great that it continues to exert its effects when the concentrations in the plasma are at very low levels. Therefore, it was necessary to develop an assay that could measure sufentanil at low levels in plasma.

The pharmacokinetic properties of sufentanil are adequately described by a three-compartment model.[313] After intravenous injection, first-pass pulmonary extraction, retention, and release are similar to those of fentanyl.[297] The pKa of sufentanil at physiologic pH is the same as that of morphine (8.0) and, therefore, only a small amount (20%) exists in the un-ionized form. Sufentanil is twice as lipid-soluble as fentanyl and is highly bound (93%) to plasma proteins including α_1-acid glycoprotein. The major metabolic pathways of sufentanil include N-dealkylation, oxidative O-demethylation, and aromatic hydroxylation.[314] Major metabolites include N-phenylpropanamide.

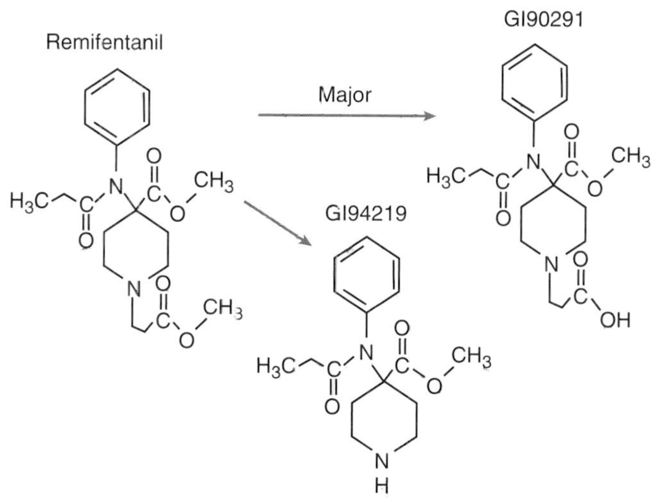

Remifentanil

Although chemically related to the fentanyl congeners, remifentanil is structurally unique because of its ester linkages. Remifentanil's ester structure renders it susceptible to hydrolysis by blood- and tissue-nonspecific esterases, resulting in rapid metabolism. Remifentanil thus constitutes the first "ultrashort"-acting opioid for use as a supplement to general anesthesia.

The pharmacokinetic properties of remifentanil are best described by a three-compartment model.[76,315,316] Its clearance is several times greater than that of normal hepatic blood flow, consistent with widespread extrahepatic metabolism. However, remifentanil is not significantly metabolized or sequestered in the lungs.[317] It is a weak base with a pKa of 7.07. It is highly lipid-soluble with an octanol/water partition coefficient of 19.9 at pH 7.4. Remifentanil is highly bound (70%) to plasma proteins (mostly α_1-acid glycoprotein). The remifentanil free base is formulated as a solution with glycine. Because glycine has been shown to act as an inhibitory neurotransmitter that causes a reversible motor weakness when injected intrathecally in rodents, remifentanil is not approved for spinal or epidural use.[318]

The primary metabolic pathway of remifentanil is de-esterification to form a carboxylic acid metabolite, GI90291 (Fig.11-14),[319] which is 0.001 to 0.003 times as potent as remifentanil. The low in vivo potency of GI90291 can be explained by a low affinity to the μ-receptor in combination with poor brain penetration.[320] Excretion of GI90291 is dependent on renal clearance mechanisms. Evidence from studies in dogs suggests that the remifentanil metabolites are, for practical purposes, completely inactive, even in the face of renal failure. Its pharmacokinetics are not appreciably influenced by renal or hepatic failure.[321,322] In blood, remifentanil is

Figure 11–14 Metabolic pathway of remifentanil. De-esterification by nonspecific plasma and tissue esterases to form a carboxylic acid metabolite (GI90291) that has only 1/300 to 1/1,000 the potency of the parent compound is the primary metabolic pathway. N-dealkylation of remifentanil to GI94219 is a minor metabolic pathway. (From Egan TD, Lemmens HJ, Fiset P, et al: The pharmacokinetics of the new short-acting opioid remifentanil [GI87084B] in healthy adult male volunteers. Anesthesiology 79:881-892, 1993.)

metabolized primarily by enzymes within erythrocytes. Remifentanil is not a substrate for pseudocholinesterase and, therefore, is not influenced by pseudocholinesterase deficiency.[323]

Irrelevance of the Terminal Half-Life

Although the term *half-life* has been popular and often used in pharmacokinetics, it is not a fundamental pharmacokinetic parameter. Because the value of half-life is dependent on the primary pharmacokinetic parameters volume of distribution and clearance, half-life is not independently influenced by changes in patient physiologic states.[295] Although the terminal half-life from multicompartmental models has traditionally been the pharmacokinetic parameter relied on for predictions regarding the duration of opioid effect, it can be grossly misleading. Distribution volumes and clearances can be similarly confusing to apply clinically.

For drugs described by multicompartmental models, numerous half-lives must be considered, along with a host of other parameters. Each half-life contributes variably to the prediction of drug concentration at a given time after drug administration.[324] For most opioids, the terminal elimination half-life has very minimal impact on the overall decline in drug concentration within the range of clinical significance, because most of the concentration decrease is accounted for by other components of the model. The primary shortcoming of half-lives in opioid pharmacology is that they fail to account for the important influence of distribution processes on drug disposition (Fig. 11-15).[325]

For sufentanil, the volume of one of the peripheral compartments is large, and the rate of transfer into it from the central compartment is slow. If the two compartments

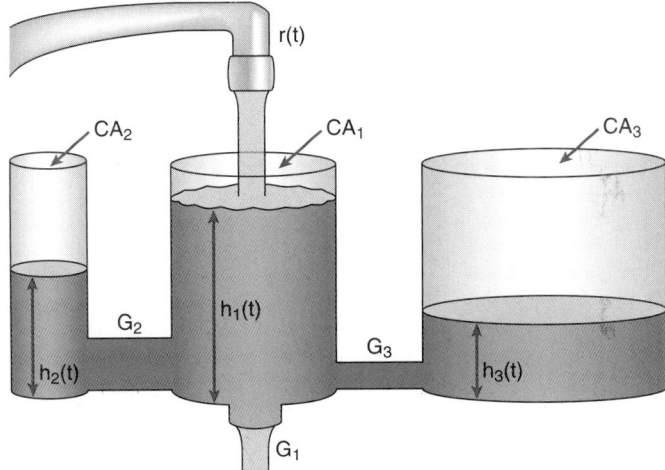

Figure 11–15 Hydraulic model analogy of three-compartment pharmacokinetic model. The height, $h_i(t)$, represents the water level in each compartment. Each bucket is characterized by a cylindrical area, CA_i, and the pipes connecting the buckets to each other or to the outside world are characterized by a conductance, G_i. Water enters bucket 1 at the rate $r(t)$ and leaks irreversibly through G_1. (From Hughes MA, Glass PS, Jacobs JR: Context-sensitive half-time in multicompartment pharmacokinetic models for intravenous anesthetic drugs. Anesthesiology 76:334-341, 1992.)

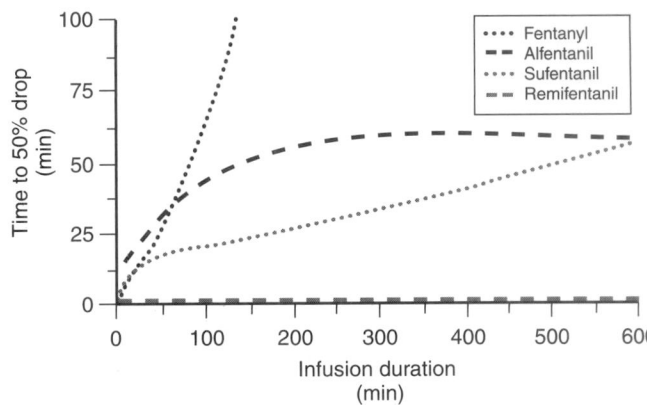

Figure 11–16 A simulation of the time necessary to achieve a 50% decrease in drug concentration in the blood (or plasma) after variable-length intravenous infusions of remifentanil, fentanyl , alfentanil, and sufentanil. (From Egan TD, Lemmens HJ, Fiset P, et al: The pharmacokinetics of the new short-acting opioid remifentanil (GI87084B) in healthy adult male volunteers. Anesthesiology 79:881-892, 1993.)

have reached equilibrium, the peripheral compartment serves as a reservoir of sufentanil that reenters the central compartment after termination of an infusion, thus impeding the decrease in sufentanil concentration produced by elimination from the central compartment.

Context-Sensitive Half-Time

Computer simulation techniques predict "context-sensitive half-time," the time necessary to achieve a 50% decrease in drug concentration after termination of a variable-length continuous infusion at a steady-state drug level (Fig. 11-16).[325,326] Such simulations are intended to provide more clinically relevant meaning to pharmacokinetic parameters. The context-sensitive half-time, more modern pharmacokinetic descriptions, and computer simulations have helped clinicians to select opioids in a more rational fashion.[324,325,327]

Alfentanil does not exhibit a more rapid 50% decrease in plasma concentration compared with sufentanil after termination of a continuous infusion for 8 hours, despite its relatively short terminal elimination half-life. In terms of pharmacokinetic theory, this surprising difference between alfentanil and sufentanil can be explained by the fact that sufentanil's pharmacokinetic model has a large, slowly equilibrating peripheral compartment that continues to fill after termination of an infusion, thus contributing to the faster decrease in sufentanil's central compartment concentration. Remifentanil has a context-sensitive half-time that is markedly shorter than those of the other fentanyl congeners.[315] Remifentanil's context-sensitive half-time is independent of infusion duration.

In cases of very brief duration, the context-sensitive half-times for sufentanil, alfentanil, and fentanyl are

nearly identical. It should be noted that the shapes and relationships of these curves vary depending on the percentage decrease in concentration required.[326]

Effect Site and Latency to Peak Effect

For many opioids, there is a significant time lag between peak concentration in the plasma and peak drug effect. This time lag, or hysteresis, is a function of drug movement into and action within the effect site, or biophase. The time lag is particularly important when giving opioids by bolus administration such as during PCA therapy.

Flow of drug to the effect compartment is a first-order process and can be elucidated by estimating k_{eo}, a first-order rate constant for elimination of drug from the effect compartment. In general, the fentanyl congeners (especially alfentanil and remifentanil) have a short k_{eo} half-life ($t_{1/2}k_{eo}$), whereas morphine's blood-brain equilibration time is much longer. In humans, it was reported that after intravenous administration of sufentanil (10 μg), fentanyl (100 μg) and alfentanil (1 mg) peak brain concentrations were achieved at 45 sec, 5 minutes, and 6 minutes for alfentanil, sufentanil, and fentanyl, respectively (Fig. 11-17).[328] This difference is due to the different times required to reach blood-brain equilibrium. After single bolus administration, alfentanil and remifentanil exhibit rapid speed of offset, because effect-site concentrations begin to fall immediately after achieving a rapid peak.[329]

Slope of the Concentration-Effect Relationship

Although clinicians have traditionally relied on pharmacokinetic parameters in predicting the time course of drug effect, the temporal profile of drug effect is a function of both pharmacokinetic and pharmacodynamic parameters.

For opioids, the concentration-effect relationship is usually described graphically by a sigmoidal maximum-effect curve in which drug concentration in the site of action is plotted against drug effect. This sigmoidal curve is presented mathematically by the following equation.

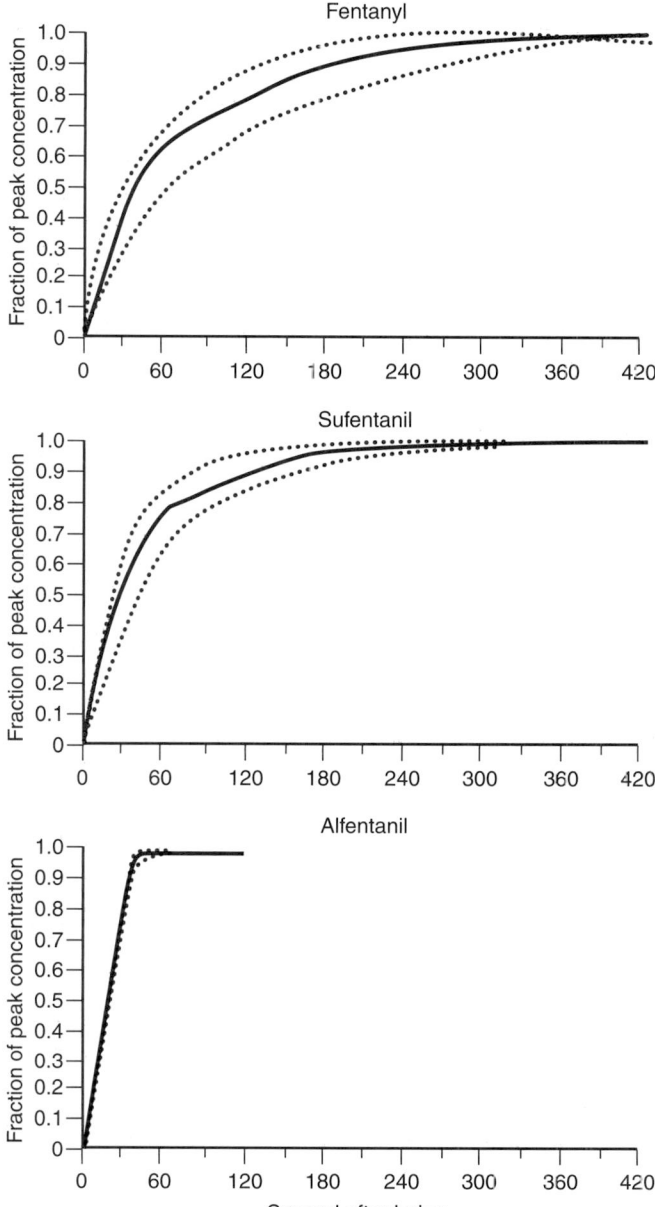

Figure 11–17 Time to reach brain concentration after simultaneous bolus applications of fentanyl, sufentanil, and alfentanil. The fraction of peak brain concentration results from the amount of drug extracted from arterial blood (arterial-jugular bulb concentration difference, integrated over time) plotted as a fraction of the cumulative absorption. Data are presented as the median (*solid lines*) and 50th and 95th percentiles (*dotted lines*) from individual patients. (From Metz C, Gobel L, Gruber M, et al: Pharmacokinetics of human cerebral opioid extraction: A comparative study on sufentanil, fentanyl, and alfentanil in a patient after severe head injury. Anesthesiology 92:1559-1567, 2000.)

$$E = E_0 + \frac{E_{max} / C_e^\gamma}{EC_{50}^\gamma + C_e^\gamma}$$

Where E is the predicted effect, E_0 is the baseline effect, E_{max} is the maximal effect, C_e is the effect site concentration and γ is a measure of curve steepness. EC_{50} is the effect site concentration that produces 50% of maximal effect and can be compared with other drugs as a comparative

measure of drug potency. For drugs such as opioids that have a steep concentration-effect relationship (high γ), the correlation of effect with concentration is often observed to be binary.

Pharmacokinetic parameters cannot be interpreted alone in predicting the duration of drug effect. Although knowledge of the predicted decline in drug concentration based on pharmacokinetic parameters is helpful, it must be interpreted with knowledge about the drug's potency and the steepness of the concentration-effect relationship.[330] The implications of context-sensitive half-time (or 50% decrement time) must thus be interpreted in concert with knowledge of the concentration-effect relationship. The duration of drug effect as predicted by the context-sensitive half-time closely parallels that predicted by the mean effect time when the concentration-effect relationship is shallow. When the concentration-effect relationship is less steep, the context-sensitive half-time may be less useful in predicting the time course of drug effect.

The clinical application of these concepts with regard to opioid pharmacology relates to the steepness of the concentration-effect relationship of opioids. Very small changes in opioid concentration can produce large changes in drug effects. This means that for patients in whom a typical analgesic regimen fails, sometimes very small increases in dosage can result in adequate analgesia.

Computerized Delivery Methods in Clinical Practice

Advances in pharmacokinetic modeling and infusion pump technology have made it possible to administer opioids (and other drugs) via a computer-controlled infusion pump (CCIP).[331] The physician operating a CCIP designates a target concentration to achieve rather than specifying an infusion rate. The CCIP then calculates the necessary infusion rates to achieve the targeted concentration.

Delivery of an opioid via CCIP requires a different approach by clinicians. Rather than setting an infusion rate based on clinical experience and literature recommendations, the anesthesiologist using a CCIP designates a target concentration, and the CCIP calculates the infusion rates necessary to achieve the concentration over time. Successful use of a CCIP thus requires knowledge of the therapeutic concentrations appropriate for the clinical setting.

Surrogate Measures of Opioid Potency

Because a high-resolution measure of analgesia is not available, opioid potencies are usually estimated by some surrogate measures. Reduction of the MAC required to produce lack of movement to skin incision has been a frequently utilized surrogate measure in the estimation of opioid potency (Fig. 11-18).[62,78-80] However MAC is not useful as a surrogate measure of opioid potencies outside the operation room.

The EEG has been another widely utilized surrogate measure in estimating opioid potency.[74,77] The EEG is advantageous, because it is noninvasive and can be used as an effect measure when an experimental subject is unconscious or apneic. When processed by Fourier spectral analysis, the raw EEG changes translate into a significant

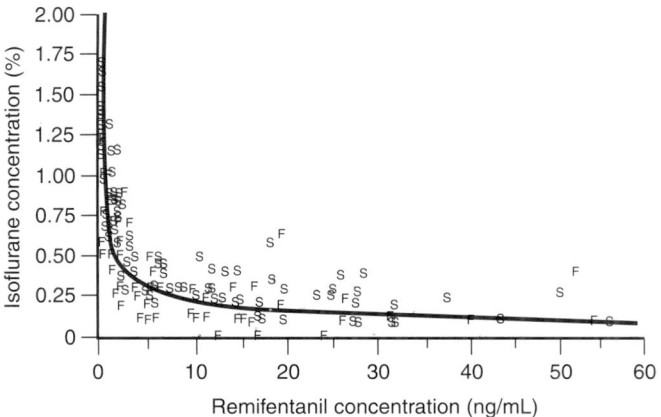

Figure 11–18 The reduction in isoflurane concentration to prevent movement at skin incision in 50% of patients by increasing measured remifentanil whole blood concentrations. F represents a patient who moved and S, a patient who did not move. The solid line is the logistic regression solution for a patient 40 years of age. (From Lang E, Kapila A, Shlugman D, et al: Reduction of isoflurane minimal alveolar concentration by remifentanil. Anesthesiology 85:721-728, 1996.)

decrease in the value of the spectral edge, a parameter that quantitates the frequency below which a given percentage (usually 95%) of the power in the EEG signal is found. Although the clinical meaning of the EEG changes produced by opioids is unclear, the opioid potencies estimated using the EEG as a surrogate measure appear to be clinically reliable because they relate to clinically determined potencies in a proportional, reproducible fashion. For opioids, because the surrogate measures do not always assess the drug effect of clinical interest (analgesia), estimations of potency based on surrogate measures must be interpreted with caution.

Factors Affecting Pharmacokinetics and Pharmacodynamics of Opioids

Age
Pharmacokinetics and pharmacodynamics of opioids can be influenced by age (also see Chapter 62). It is clear that neonates exhibit a reduced rate of elimination of essentially all opioids.[332] This is presumably due to immature metabolic mechanisms, including the cytochrome P-450 system.[333] The prolonged elimination of opioids observed in the neonatal period quickly normalizes toward adult values within the first year of life.[332]

With advanced age, although pharmacokinetic changes may play a minor role, pharmacodynamic differences are primarily responsible for the decreased dose requirement in the elderly. The concentration of fentanyl and alfentanil necessary to produce half to maximal slowing of the EEG (i.e., the EC_{50}) is lower in the elderly compared with younger adults (Fig. 11-19).[334]

Age is inversely correlated with the central volume of distribution, the clearance, and the potency of remifentanil.[335] These combined pharmacokinetic and pharmacodynamic changes mandate a reduction in remifentanil dosage by at least 50% or more in the elderly.

Body Weight
Many opioid pharmacokinetic parameters, especially clearance, appear to be more closely related to lean body mass. This means that opioid dosage regimens may best be based on lean body mass and not total body weight. However, analysis of a large group of patients who received alfentanil suggests that its volume of the central compartment does correlate with total body weight.[336]

Total body weight–based dosing in an obese patient results in much higher remifentanil effect site concentrations than does lean body mass–based dosing.[337] In contrast, for lean patients the concentrations that result from total body weight–based dosing are not much greater than those based on body mass (Fig. 11-20). Clinically, context-sensitive half-times are not significantly different between obese and lean subjects (Fig. 11-21).

There is mounting evidence to suggest that lean body mass is a better predictor of metabolic capacity than total body weight. Ideal body weight, a parameter closely related to lean body mass and one that is perhaps more easily estimated by the clinician, is probably an acceptable alternative.

Renal Failure
Renal failure has implications of major clinical importance with respect to morphine and meperidine (also see

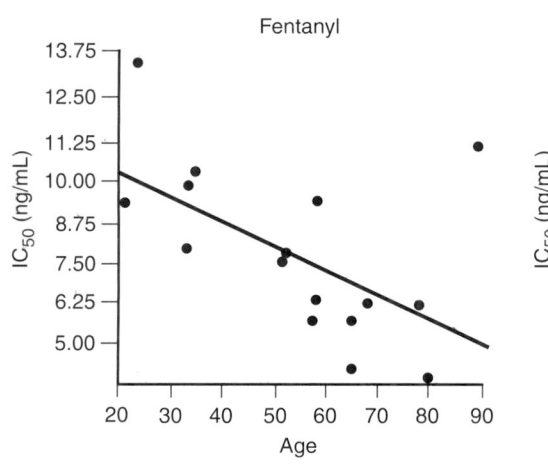

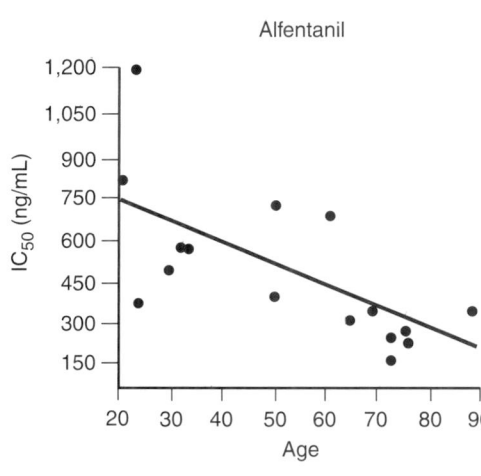

Figure 11–19 Relationship between IC_{50} and age for fentanyl and alfentanil. IC_{50} is the steady-state fentanyl or alfentanil serum concentration that produces half the maximal spectral edge frequency decrease. (From Scott JC, Stanski DR: Decreased fentanyl and alfentanil dose requirements with age. A simultaneous pharmacokinetic and pharmacodynamic evaluation. J Pharmacol Exp Ther 240:159-166, 1987.)

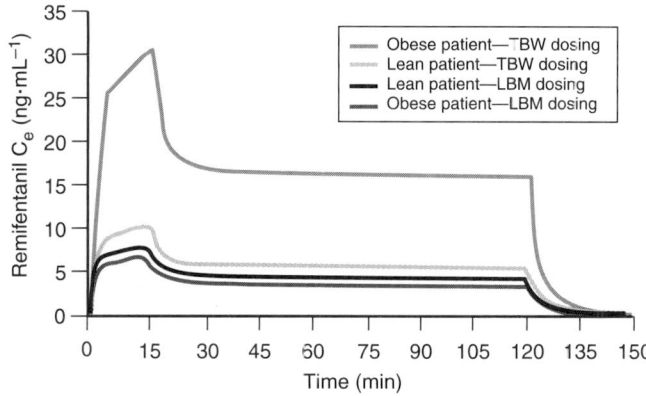

Figure 11–20 A computer simulation of the time course of remifentanil concentration change, when the dosage regimen is calculated based on the lean body mass (LBM) or total body weight (TBW) for both obese and lean patients. Note that TBW-based dosing in an obese patient results in dramatically higher concentrations. (From Egan TD, Huizinga B, Gupta SK, et al: Remifentanil pharmacokinetics in obese versus lean patients. Anesthesiology 89:562-573, 1998.)

Chapter 56). For the fentanyl congeners, the clinical importance of renal failure is less marked.[338]

Morphine is an opioid with active metabolites that are dependent on renal clearance mechanisms for elimination. Morphine is principally metabolized by conjugation in the liver, and the water-soluble glucuronides (M3G and M6G) are excreted via the kidney. The kidney also plays a role in the conjugation of morphine, accounting for nearly 40% of its metabolism.[298] Patients with renal failure can develop very high levels of M6G and life-threatening respiratory depression (Fig. 11-22).[339] In view of these changes induced by renal failure, morphine may not be a good choice in patients with severely altered renal clearance mechanisms.

The clinical pharmacology of meperidine is also significantly altered by renal failure. Normeperidine, the chief metabolite, has analgesic and CNS excitatory effects.[340]

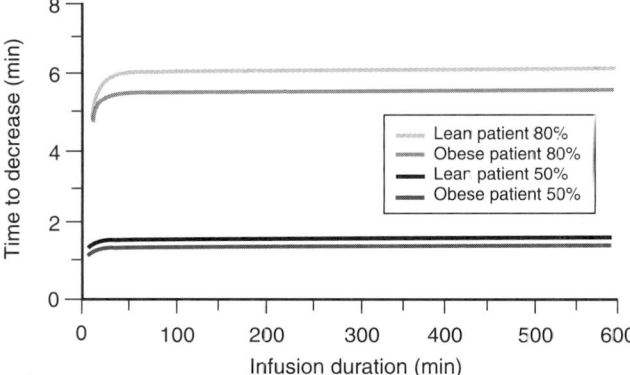

Figure 11–21 A computer simulation of the context-sensitive half-times (50% decrement times) and 80% decrement times of remifentanil in obese versus lean subjects. Note that in clinical terms the curves are not grossly different in obese compared with lean subjects. (From Egan TD, Huizinga B, Gupta SK, et al: Remifentanil pharmacokinetics in obese versus lean patients. Anesthesiology 89:562-573, 1998.)

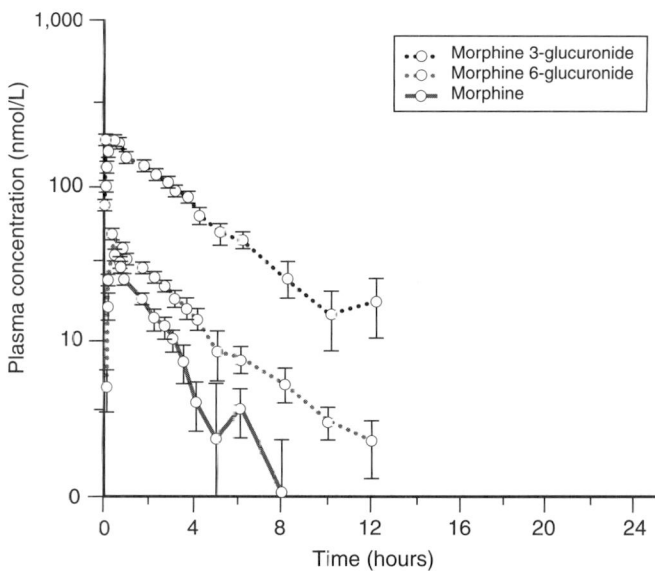

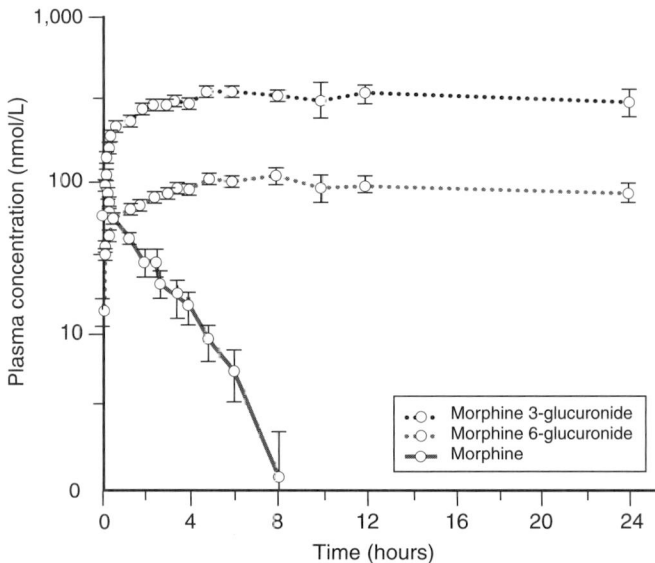

Figure 11–22 Effect of renal failure on pharmacokinetics of morphine. The graphs show the time-dependent change of the serum concentration of morphine and its metabolite in patients with normal renal function *(top graph)* and patients with renal failure *(bottom graph)*, who received 0.1 mg/kg morphine IV. (From Osborne R, Joel S, Grebenik K, et al: The pharmacokinetics of morphine and morphine glucuronides in kidney failure. Clin Pharmacol Ther 54:158-167, 1993.)

Because the active metabolites are subject to renal excretion, this potential CNS toxicity secondary to normeperidine accumulation is especially a concern in patients in renal failure.

The clinical pharmacology of the fentanyl congeners is not grossly altered by renal failure, although a decrease in plasma protein binding may potentially alter the free fraction of the fentanyl class of opioids.[338] Fentanyl clearance is not altered by renal failure. As with fentanyl, sufentanil pharmacokinetics are not altered in any consistent fashion by renal disease, although greater variability exists in its clearance and elimination half-life when patients have impaired renal function.[341] It has been suggested that an increased clinical effect is likely with alfentanil in renal failure because of a decreased initial volume of distribution and an increased free fraction of alfentanil.[342] However, no delay in recovery after alfentanil should be expected. Neither the pharmacokinetics nor the pharmacodynamics of remifentanil are altered by impaired renal function.[322] Levels of GI-90291, the major metabolite, that develop during a remifentanil infusion in patients in renal failure are not likely to produce any clinically significant effects.[322]

Hepatic Failure

Even though the liver is the metabolic organ primarily responsible for opioid biotransformation, the degree of liver failure typically observed in perioperative patients, with the exception of patients undergoing liver transplantation, does not have a major impact on the pharmacokinetics of most opioids (also see Chapter 56) .

In addition to reduced metabolic capacity (i.e., cytochrome P-450 system and conjugation), liver disease may also lead to reductions in hepatic blood flow, hepatocellular mass, and plasma protein binding. The increase in total body water and the edema of advanced liver disease may alter the distribution characteristics of a drug. Finally, enzyme induction such as observed in early alcoholism can actually increase the liver's metabolic capacity.

Morphine pharmacokinetics are relatively unchanged by liver failure because of the substantial extrahepatic metabolism of morphine. A reduction in hepatic blood flow would be expected to slow the decline of morphine plasma concentrations. Meperidine is an opioid whose pharmacokinetics are altered by liver failure. Hepatic cirrhosis is associated with reduced clearance and a longer terminal half-time of meperidine. The disposition of fentanyl is not altered in patients with cirrhosis during general anesthesia.[343] Reductions in liver blood flow that result from either liver disease or some other disorder (e.g., shock) will delay the decline of fentanyl plasma concentrations. As with meperidine, the pharmacokinetics of alfentanil are also altered by hepatic failure. Ferrier and associates reported that patients with alcoholic cirrhosis have reduced alfentanil plasma clearance and prolonged terminal half-times.[344] Children with cholestatic liver disease who were scheduled to undergo orthotopic liver transplantation showed no changes in alfentanil clearance and volume of distribution at steady state. Although liver blood flow does not affect the kinetics of alfentanil as much as those of morphine and fentanyl, decreases in hepatic blood flow can still decrease alfentanil elimination.[345]

Greater elimination half-lives (3.7 ± 2.6 hours) have also been observed for alfentanil in patients undergoing abdominal aortic surgery.[346] The pharmacokinetics of sufentanil appear to be minimally changed in cirrhotic patients. However, major intra-abdominal surgery can increase the volume of distribution at steady state and the elimination half-life of sufentanil.[312] Remifentanil is an opioid whose pharmacokinetics are completely unchanged by liver disease (Fig. 11-23).[321] Its kinetics do not change during the anhepatic phase of orthotopic liver transplantation.[347] It was reported that 0.25-0.5 µg/kg/minute of remifentanil

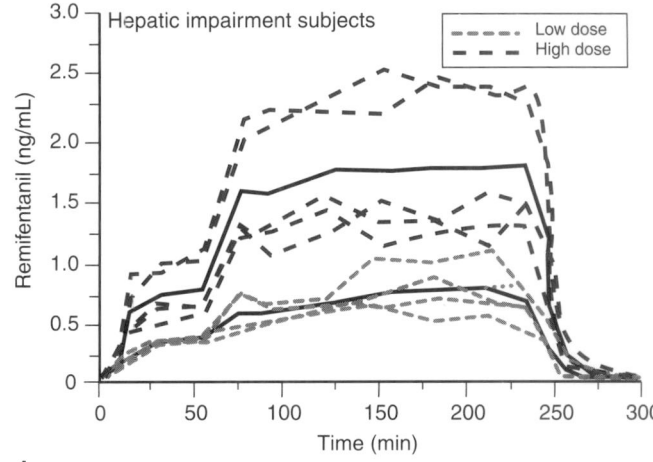

A

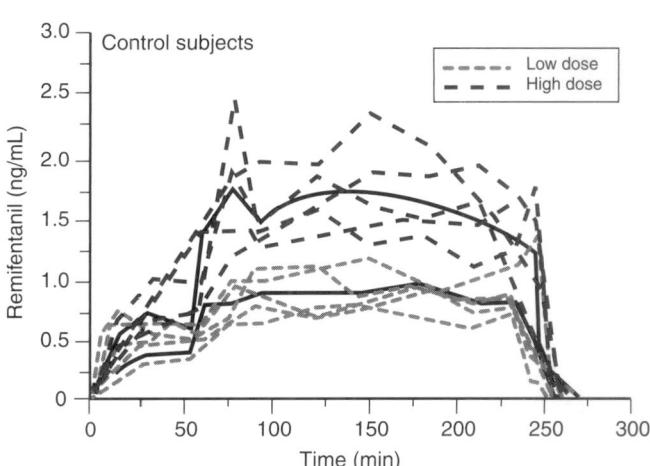

B

Figure 11–23 Time-dependent changes of blood concentration of remifentanil in patients with liver disease *(top graph)* and the control subjects *(bottom graph)*. In the low-dose group, remifentanil was infused at 0.0125 µg/kg/minute for 1 hour followed by 0.025 µg/kg/minute for 3 hours. In the high-dose group, infusion rate of remifentanil was 0.025 µg/kg/minute for 1 hour followed by 0.05 µg/kg/minutes for 3 hours. (From Dershwitz M, Hoke JF, Rosow CE, et al: Pharmacokinetics and pharmacodynamics of remifentanil in volunteer subjects with severe liver disease. Anesthesiology 84:812-820, 1996.)

could provide perioperative analgesia without neurologic deterioration in a patient suffering from chronic hepatic failure with mild encephalopathy.[348]

Cardiopulmonary Bypass

Cardiopulmonary bypass (CPB) produces significant alterations in the pharmacokinetics of most opioids.[349] These alterations are a result of CPB-induced modifications in distribution volumes (secondary to priming), changes in acid-base balance, organ blood flow, plasma protein concentrations and body temperature. The binding of drugs to components of the bypass circuit can also alter opioid pharmacokinetics (also see Chapter 50).

When morphine is given as a premedicant before cardiac anesthesia, its concentrations decline significantly on initiation of CPB.[350] Fentanyl pharmacokinetics are extensively altered by CPB.[351] Some of the initial concentration decline after starting CPB can be attributed to sequestration of fentanyl on components of the bypass circuit, especially the oxygenators.[352] After termination of CPB, there is usually a rise in fentanyl concentration toward pre-bypass levels. Overall, the elimination of fentanyl is prolonged because of increased distribution and decreased clearance. As with fentanyl, elimination of sufentanil is thought to be somewhat prolonged by CPB (Fig. 11-24).[353] Elimination of alfentanil is prolonged by CPB primarily because of increased distribution.[175,354] The free fraction of alfentanil during CPB remains constant despite complex changes in binding protein concentrations.[355] In contrast to fentanyl, alfentanil is not likely to be bound by CPB bypass components.[352] Comparatively little is known about the pharmacokinetics of remifentanil during CPB. However, remifentanil remains a very short-acting drug despite CPB.

Acid-Base Changes

Acid-base changes can affect a variety of aspects of opioid pharmacokinetics.[356] Respiratory acidosis during fentanyl administration has multiple effects including increases in ionization and CBF and decreases in plasma protein binding (also see Chapter 41). More fentanyl in the interstitial compartment will be ionized. More opioid receptors, on cell membranes that interact with ionized fentanyl, are stimulated, producing an enhanced opioid effect. Un-ionized fentanyl is drawn out of the intracellular compartment, further augmenting opioid effects. Increased ionization decreases the amount of fentanyl available for hepatic metabolism or renal excretion.[356] Alfentanil, with a pKa of 6.5, is not as greatly influenced by either pH changes or tissue accumulation as fentanyl.[356]

Brain fentanyl levels are higher with respiratory alkalosis. Alkalosis also increases the lipophilicity of several opioids. Alkalosis favors un-ionized morphine and may enhance brain penetration in spite of decreased CBF and increased plasma protein binding. Thus, both intraoperative respiration alkalosis and respiratory acidosis, especially in the immediate postoperative period, can prolong and exacerbate opioid-induced respiratory depression.

Hemorrhagic Shock

It is a common practice to administer reduced doses of opioids to patients suffering from hemorrhagic shock to minimize adverse hemodynamic consequences and to prevent prolonged opioid effect (also see Chapter 63). This is at least partly attributable to a pharmacokinetic mechanism. Analysis in studies of pigs receiving fentanyl suggested that central clearance and central- and second-compartment distribution volumes were significantly reduced, resulting in higher fentanyl concentrations for any given dosages and a prolonged context-sensitive half-time (Fig. 11-25).[357] Hemorrhagic shock also altered the pharmacokinetics of remifentanil, suggesting that less remifentanil would be required to maintain a target plasma concentration (Fig. 11-26).[358] However, because of its rapid metabolism, changes in context-sensitive half-time are small.

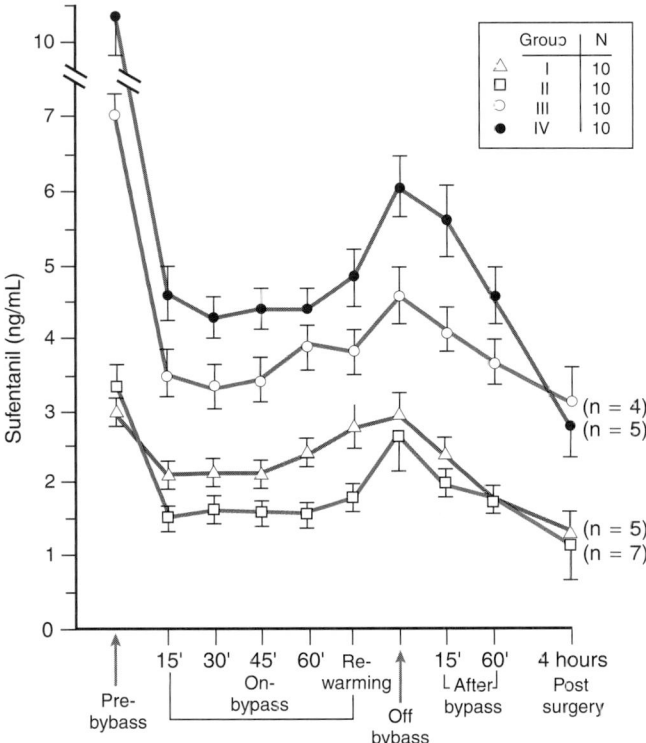

Figure 11-24 Effect of cardiopulmonary bypass on the pharmacokinetics of sufentanil. Sufentanil was administered as a 30 μg/kg bolus (group I), a 10 μg/kg/minute infusion (group II), a 20 μg/kg bolus followed by a 0.1 μg/kg/minute infusion (group III), and a 40 μg/kg bolus followed by a 0.2 μg/kg/minute infusion (group IV). (From Okutani R, Philbin DM, Rosow CE, et al: Effect of hypothermic hemodilutional cardiopulmonary bypass on plasma sufentanil and catecholamine concentrations in humans. Anesth Analg 67:667-670, 1988.)

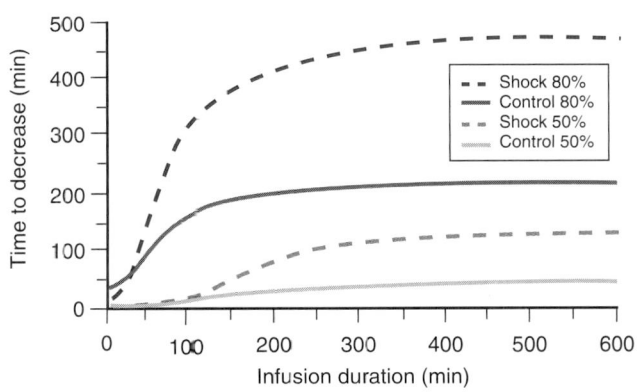

Figure 11-25 A computer simulation of the context-sensitive half-times (50% decrement times) and 80% decrement times of fentanyl in animals with hemorrhagic shock and control animals. (From Egan TD, Kuramkote S, Gong G, et al: Fentanyl pharmacokinetics in hemorrhagic shock: A porcine model. Anesthesiology 91:156-166, 1999.)

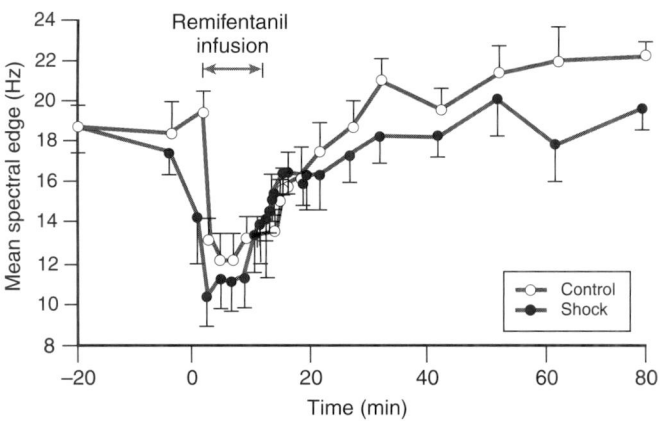

Figure 11–26 Mean spectral edge changes versus time during the remifentanil infusion. The open and closed circles indicate spectral edge measurements for control animals and animals with hemorrhagic shock, respectively. (From Johnson KB, Kern SE, Hamber EA, et al: Influence of hemorrhagic shock on remifentanil: A pharmacokinetic and pharmacodynamic analysis. Anesthesiology 2001; 94:322-332, 2001.)

ANESTHETIC TECHNIQUES USING OPIOIDS

Sedation and Analgesia

Opioids are frequently used to relieve pain during monitored anesthesia care and regional anesthesia. A single bolus administration of opioids can provide significant pain relief. Morphine is slow in onset and does not allow rapid titration to effect. Meperidine (50-100 mg IV) produces variable degrees of pain relief and is not always effective in patients with severe pain. IV boluses of fentanyl (1-3 μg/kg), alfentanil (10-20 μg/kg), or sufentanil (0.1-0.3 μg/kg) can produce potent and short-lasting analgesia. Infusion rates are 0.01 to 0.05 μg/kg/minute for fentanyl, 0.0015 to 0.01 μg/kg/minute for sufentanil, 0.25 to 0.75 μg/kg/minute for alfentanil, and 0.05 to 0.25 μg/kg/minute for remifentanil. Plasma concentrations of opioids necessary for various purposes are listed in Table 11-8.

Changes in the excitability of central neurons play an important role in the establishment of pain. Whether preemptive analgesia can be effectively achieved clinically by the early administration of opioids remains uncertain.[359,360]

However, reductions in postoperative pain and improved recovery have been attributed to preemptive analgesia with either epidural fentanyl or bupivacaine after radical prostatectomy.[361]

PCA with opioids is now a cornerstone of postoperative analgesia. PCA with opioids may improve outcome.[362] Nevertheless, pharmacokinetic optimization of opioid treatment in acute pain is a complex matter.[363] Without considering effect site drug concentrations over time, the choice of opioid and the amount, method, and frequency of administration cannot be optimized.[363] Morphine remains a popular and rational choice for PCA therapy.[364]

Balanced Anesthesia

The term *balanced anesthesia* was introduced by Lundy in 1926. Lundy suggested that a balance of agents and techniques be used to produce the different components of anesthesia (i.e., analgesia, amnesia, muscle relaxation, and abolition of autonomic reflexes with maintenance of homeostasis). Anesthesia with a single agent can require doses that produce excessive hemodynamic depression.[365] The inclusion of an opioid as a component of balanced anesthesia can reduce preoperative pain and anxiety, decrease somatic and autonomic responses to airway manipulations, improve hemodynamic stability, lower requirements for inhaled anesthetics, and provide immediate postoperative analgesia.[366] Although the intent of combining opioids with sedative-hypnotics and/or volatile anesthetics is to produce anesthetic conditions with stable hemodynamics prior to, as well as after, noxious stimulation, this ideal is not always achieved.[367-369]

The administration of an opioid prior to, rather than after, noxious stimulation attenuates physiologic responses. Opioids interact synergistically and markedly reduce the dose of propofol and other sedative-hypnotics required for loss of consciousness and during noxious stimulation such as skin incision.[370] Opioids can ameliorate or eliminate responses to a rapid sequence induction and other noxious stimuli.[371] The heart rate response to laryngoscopy is better controlled with an opioid than with esmolol.[366]

The timing, rate of administration, and dose of supplemental opioid should be tailored to the specific condition of the patient and the expected duration of the operation in order to avoid postoperative pain or respiratory depression. A large dose of any opioid given shortly before the end of surgery is very likely to result in respiratory depression. Analgesic concentrations of opioids,

Table 11–8 Range of approximate plasma (or whole blood for remifentanil) opioid concentration (ng/ml) required for total intravenous anesthesia

	Fentanyl	Sufentanil	Alfentanil	Remifentanil
Predominant agent	15-30	5-10	400-800	—
Major surgery	4-10	1-3	200-400	2-4
Minor surgery	3-6	0.25-1	50-200	1-3
Spontaneous ventilation	1-3	<0.4	<200	0.3-0.6
Analgesia	1-2	0.2-0.4	50-150	0.2-0.4

From Bailey PL, Egan TD, Stanley TH: Intravenous opioid anesthetics. *In* Miller RD (ed): Anesthesia, 5th ed. New York, Churchill Livingstone, 2000, p 330.

however, have little effect on the MAC awake of inhaled anesthetics.[372]

Choice of Opioid

The ideal opioid would permit rapid titration, successfully prevent unwanted responses to noxious stimuli, require little supplementation, not depress cardiovascular function, permit the return of adequate spontaneous ventilation in a timely manner, and produce residual if not complete postoperative analgesia with minimal side effects.

Alfentanil, and remifentanil provide the greatest ability to titrate opioids rapidly because of their extremely rapid time to onset (1 to 2 minutes) of peak effect. Alfentanil, compared with fentanyl, produces greater decreases in heart rate and blood pressure during induction of anesthesia.[373,374] Most studies have found that alfentanil results in a more rapid recovery than fentanyl and a decreased need for naloxone post-anesthetically.[373] Compared with alfentanil, sufentanil provides greater hemodynamic stability and requires less supplementation.[375] Meperidine produced the most side effects, including hypotension, tachycardia, and urticaria, especially during anesthetic induction.

Sufentanil, alfentanil, and remifentanil are arguably superior to fentanyl in many respects. Antagonism of opioid action with naloxone for troublesome respiratory depression is required less frequently after alfentanil and sufentanil compared with fentanyl. Pharmacologic antagonism is rarely required after remifentanil administration.

Fentanyl

Anesthetic induction is usually achieved by combining a loading dose of fentanyl (2-6 µg/kg) with a sedative-hypnotic, most commonly thiopental or propofol, and a muscle relaxant. Maintenance of anesthesia can be achieved with N_2O (60% to 70%) in O_2, low concentrations of potent inhaled anesthetics, and additional fentanyl (intermittent boluses of 25-50 µg every 15 to 30 minutes or a constant infusion of 0.5-5.0 µg/kg/hour), depending on the depth of anesthesia required versus the intensity and duration of surgery.

Fentanyl plasma concentrations of 1.0 to 2.0 ng/mL provide analgesia,[294] but levels of at least 2 to 3 ng/mL are usually required during surgery if the only inhaled agent is N_2O. In unpremedicated patients anesthetized with a fentanyl infusion and N_2O in O_2, the Cp_{50} and the Cp_{50}-BAR (barish autonomic response) for fentanyl at skin incision are 3.26 and 4.17 ng/mL, respectively.[376] The MAC of isoflurane at skin incision can be reduced by 50% and 63% with plasma fentanyl concentrations of 1.67 and 3.0 ng/mL, respectively.[62] Increasing plasma fentanyl concentrations from 3.0 to 10 ng/mL only further reduced the MAC of isoflurane from 63% to 82%. Plasma fentanyl levels associated with adequate analgesia after abdominal surgery have been reported to range fivefold from 0.23 to at least 1.18 ng/mL.[294]

Opioid pharmacokinetics and pharmacodynamics vary considerably among patients. Nevertheless, a balanced technique with fentanyl, titrating the opioid in anticipation of various stimuli and patient responses with pharmacokinetic guidelines in mind, will often result in a stable hemodynamic course and rapid awakening in a relatively pain-free patient. Repeated large doses or continuous infusions of fentanyl at high rates are most likely to result in significant depression of spontaneous ventilation.

Alfentanil

Because alfentanil penetrates the brain so rapidly, equilibration of alfentanil between the plasma and the CNS can be achieved while plasma alfentanil levels are relatively high compared with sufentanil and fentanyl. This property explains how low doses (10-30 µg/kg) of alfentanil, administered just before or simultaneously with a sedative-hypnotic, are effective.

Alfentanil (25-50 µg/kg IV), followed by small titrated sleep doses of any sedative-hypnotic (e.g., 50-100 mg sodium thiopental), is usually successful in preventing significant hemodynamic stimulation from laryngoscopy and intubation. Further opioid supplementation can be achieved with an alfentanil infusion (0.5-2.0 µg/kg/minute) or intermittent boluses of alfentanil (5-10 µg/kg) for shorter procedures. In balanced anesthetic techniques in which potent inhaled anesthetics are also employed, relatively low plasma alfentanil concentrations (e.g., 29 ng/mL) can reduce the MAC of isoflurane by approximately 50%.[78] The Cp_{50}, defined as the concentration needed to obtund responses to stimuli adequately in 50% of patients, is different among various stimuli.[163] It is remarkable that the more intense the stimulus, the greater the variability in the Cp_{50} (Fig. 11-27).

Alfentanil infusions or repeated doses should be reduced 15 to 30 minutes prior to the end of surgery, in order to avoid problematic residual respiratory depression. The alfentanil plasma concentration that permitted the return of spontaneous ventilation was reported to be 223 ± 13 ng/mL.[155] Although alfentanil infusions should be reduced as necessary during balanced anesthesia, they should not be completely terminated until the operation is nearly finished.

Sufentanil

The mean plasma sufentanil concentration reported to be the Cp_{50} for prevention of hemodynamic responses to laryngoscopy and tracheal intubation was 1.08 ng/mL, with a range of 0.73 to 2.55 ng/mL. Maintenance of anesthesia can be achieved with N_2O (60% to 70%) in O_2 and further sufentanil (intermittent boluses, 0.1-0.25 µg/kg, or constant infusion, 0.5-1.5 µg/kg/hour). The Cp_{50} for sufentanil during skin incision is twice as great as that for intubation in unpremedicated patients (2.08 ± 0.62 ng/mL).[377] Cp_{50} value ratios at skin incision for sufentanil, fentanyl, and alfentanil in N_2O-O_2 anesthesia are approximately 1:2:150 and represent different and probably more accurate potency ratios than those traditionally published based on drug dose. In patients undergoing coronary artery bypass grafting, sufentanil >1.25 ± 0.21 ng/mL reduced isoflurane requirements to less than 0.5% through the operation.[378] Sufentanil levels less than 0.25 ng/mL often allow adequate spontaneous ventilation.[379]

Remifentanil

The very short duration of action of remifentanil mandates that an infusion (0.1-1.0 µg/kg/minute) be started prior to or soon after the initial bolus dose to ensure sustained opioid effect. Maintenance infusion rates of

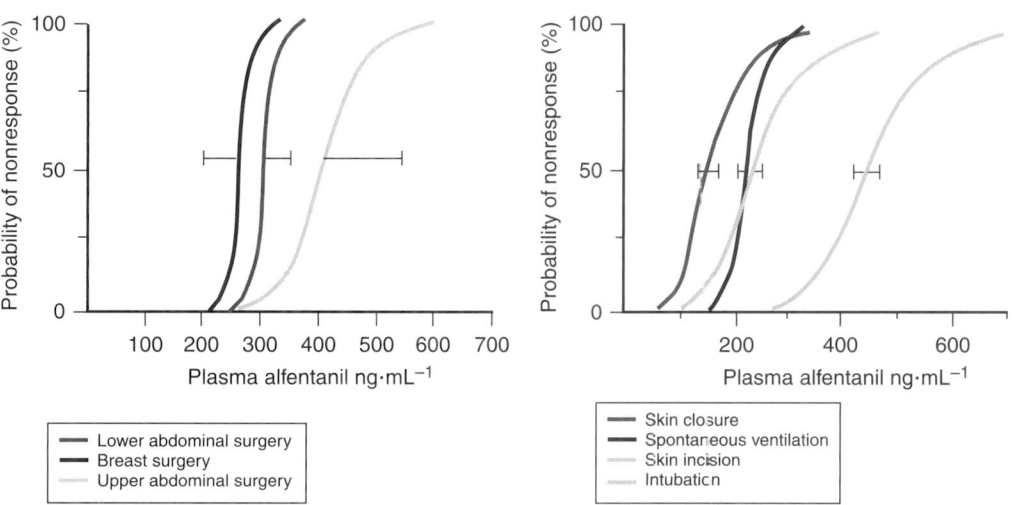

Figure 11–27 Mean alfentanil plasma concentration-effect curves for the intraoperative period in each surgical group of patients, intubation, skin incision, and skin closure (with nitrous oxide), and the relationship between the alfentanil plasma concentration (without nitrous oxide) and the probability of needing naloxone to restore adequate spontaneous ventilation. The Cp_{50} and slope of these curves were determined by averaging the estimates of individual patients. Bars indicate standard deviation of Cp_{50}. Cp_{50}, the concentration needed to obtund responses to stimuli adequately in 50% of patients. (From Ausems ME, Hug CC Jr, Stanski DR, Burm AG: Plasma concentrations of alfentanil required to supplement nitrous oxide anesthesia for general surgery. Anesthesiology 65:362-367, 1986.)

remifentanil range from 0.1 to 1.0 µg/kg/minute for balanced anesthesia. Remifentanil can reliably suppress autonomic, hemodynamic, and somatic responses to noxious stimulation and allows the most predictable and rapid trouble-free emergence from anesthesia.[380]

The use of remifentanil allows a rapid (5 to 15 minutes) emergence without postoperative respiratory depression.[381] Infusion rates of 0.1 ± 0.05 µg/kg/minute should permit the return of spontaneous ventilation and responsiveness with maintenance of analgesia within 10 to 15 minutes. A randomized, double-blind, placebo-controlled study demonstrated that the combination of 0.05-0.1 µg/kg/minute remifentanil infusion and a 2-mg midazolam bolus provided effective sedation and analgesia during outpatient surgical procedures performed under local anesthesia.[382] The administration of remifentanil (1 µg/kg) followed by 0.5 µg/kg/minute with propofol and 66% N_2O provided sufficient anesthesia for craniotomy with stable hemodynamics and rapid tracheal extubation.[383]

Associated with emergence from remifentanil anesthesia, the need for alternative analgesic therapies should be anticipated and administered in a timely fashion prior to or immediately upon emergence from anesthesia. It was reported that perioperative administration of morphine (0.15 or 0.25 mg/kg IV) or fentanyl (0.15 mg) did not provide entirely adequate immediate postoperative pain control after remifentanil-based anesthesia in major abdominal surgery.[384,385] Administration of ketamine (0.15 mg/kg followed by 2 µg/kg/minute) decreased intraoperative remifentanil use during abdominal surgery and postoperative morphine consumption without increasing the incidence of side effects.[386] In children undergoing strabismus surgery, the combination of sevoflurane (2.5%) and remifentanil (1 µg/kg followed by 0.1-0.2 µg/kg/minute) resulted in less frequent postoperative vomiting but higher postoperative pain scores, compared with fentanyl (2 µg/kg followed by 1 µg/kg every 45 minutes).[387]

Postoperative pain relief with low-dose remifentanil infusion has also been achieved successfully. After general anesthesia with propofol (75 µg/kg/minute) and remifentanil (0.5-1.0 µg/kg/minute) for abdominal or thoracic surgery, continuous infusion of remifentanil (0.05 or 0.1 µg/kg/minute) provided adequate analgesia postoperatively.[388]

Neuroleptanalgesia-Anesthesia

In 1949, Laborit and Huygenard introduced the concept of an anesthetic technique that blocked not only cerebrocortical responses but also some cellular, endocrine, and autonomic mechanisms usually activated by surgical stimulation. This state was called "ganglioplegia" or "neuroplegia" (artificial hibernation) and was achieved by the use of a "lytic cocktail" consisting of chlorpromazine, promethazine, and meperidine. From this idea, in 1959, De Castro and Mundeleer derived the concept of neuroleptanalgesia, which involved the combination of a major tranquilizer (usually the butyrophenone droperidol) and a potent opioid analgesic (fentanyl) to produce a detached, pain-free state of immobilization and insensitivity to pain. Neuroleptanalgesia is characterized by analgesia, suppression of motor activity, suppression of autonomic reflexes, maintenance of cardiovascular stability, and amnesia in most patients. The addition of an inhaled agent, usually N_2O, improves amnesia and has been called neuroleptanesthesia.

"Neuroleptic" drugs traditionally include the phenothiazines (e.g., chlorpromazine) and the butyrophenones (e.g., haloperidol and droperidol). Butyrophenones cause sedation, tranquility, immobility, antiemesis, an extrapyramidal syndrome with face and neck dyskinesia, oculogyric crises, torticollis, agitation, and hallucinations. Administering droperidol alone, without analgesics or other sedatives, often produces feelings of discomfort or dysphoria in patients. The cardiovascular effects of droperidol are most often limited to mild hypotension that is thought to be mediated through α-adrenergic blockade. There is little respiratory depression induced by droperidol, although significant variability exists, and occasional respiratory depression may be noted. Droperidol and other butyrophenones may enhance hypoxia-induced increases in ventilation in humans because of their antidopaminergic effects at the carotid body. Droperidol can be used as a premedicant (0.025-0.075 mg/kg IM), an antiemetic (0.01-0.02 mg/kg IV), an adjunct for awake intubations (0.025-0.1 mg/kg IV) and treatment for agitated, belligerent, or psychotic patients (0.05-0.2 mg/kg IV or IM). Neuroleptanalgesia or neuroleptanesthesia is contraindicated in patients receiving monoamine oxidase inhibitors (MAOIs), in those who abuse drugs or alchohol, or those with Parkinson's disease.

Total Intravenous Anesthesia

Although TIVA does not necessarily require an opioid component, especially in minimally stimulating procedures, the fentanyl congeners most often are an important part of TIVA. Numerous advantages exist when drugs are administered by infusion.[389]

Many different intravenous compounds can be employed in a number of combinations to provide TIVA. Most commonly, an opioid is combined with another drug more likely to provide hypnosis and amnesia. For example, the combination of alfentanil and propofol produces excellent TIVA. Alfentanil provides analgesia and hemodynamic stability while blunting responses to noxious stimuli. On the other hand, propofol provides hypnosis and amnesia and is antiemetic. Profound synergism also exists when more than two agents, such as propofol-alfentanil-midazolam, are combined.[390,391] Anesthetic induction with alfentanil (25-50 μg/kg) and propofol (0.5-1.5 mg/kg) followed by infusions of 0.5-1.5 μg/kg/min of alfentanil and 80-120 μg/kg/minute of propofol will produce complete anesthesia in patients ventilated with air and O_2 with or without N_2O for a variety of procedures. It is proposed that alfentanil concentrations as low as 85 ng/mL, when combined with a blood propofol concentration of 3.5 μg/mL, can produce both optimal anesthetic conditions and speed of recovery.[391] Stanski and Shafer suggested that bolus doses and initial infusion rates would be 30 μg/kg and 0.35 μg/kg/minute, respectively, for alfentanil and 0.7 mg/kg and 180 μg/kg/minute, respectively, for propofol.[392] Recognizing that these calculations were

based on EC_{50} data in patients undergoing only moderately painful procedures, anesthesiologists should adjust these doses accordingly. Premedication prior to alfentanil-propofol anesthesia can prolong postoperative recovery and should be avoided if appropriate.[393] In patients undergoing ear-nose-throat surgery, TIVA with remifentanil and propofol provided a more rapid respiratory recovery after brief surgical procedures, compared with TIVA with alfentanil and propofol.[394]

The optimal propofol-opioid concentrations that ensure adequate anesthesia and rapid emergence were determined by computer modeling.[327] The optimal propofol concentration decreases in the order of fentanyl > alfentanil > sufentanil >> remifentanil. A shorter context-sensitive half-time allows the administration of greater amounts of opioid (and less propofol) during anesthesia without creating prolonged opioid effects.

Maintenance infusions vary according to patient condition and surgical stimuli. Propofol (75-125 μg/kg/minute) and alfentanil (1.0-2.0 μg/kg/minute) are initially recommended. Drug infusions should be terminated 10 to 20 minutes prior to end of anesthesia if N_2O is employed. Otherwise, propofol infusions should be terminated 5 to 10 minutes before anticipated patient awakening. Alfentanil infusion rates do not need to be less than 0.25-0.5 μg/kg/minute until surgery is terminated. A multicenter evaluation demonstrated that in patients during elective surgery, remifentanil (1 μg/kg IV followed by 1.0 μg/kg/minute) when combined with propofol (75 μg/kg/minute) effectively controlled responses to tracheal intubation.[381] Remifentanil infusion rate of 0.25 μg/kg/minute after tracheal intubation was also recommended.

Midazolam-opioid combinations can also provide complete anesthesia. However, midazolam-alfentanil TIVA has not been found to compare favorably to propofol-alfentanil TIVA even with flumazenil reversal of benzodiazepine actions.[395] However, TIVA for major (cardiac) and/or long operations may be effectively achieved with the combination of midazolam and sufentanil.[396]

TIVA techniques are especially useful when delivery of inhaled agents is compromised. By keeping the goals of balanced anesthesia in mind, combining modern opioids and other drugs, utilizing infusion pumps, and employing an increased understanding of pharmacokinetics, clinicians can successfully perform a wide variety of TIVA techniques. Approximate opioid doses and infusion rates for TIVA are listed in Table 11-9.

Table 11–9 Approximate opioid loading (bolus) doses, maintenance infusion rates, and additional maintenance doses for total intravenous anesthesia

	Loading Dose (μg/kg)	Maintenance Infusion Rate	Additional Boluses
Alfentanil	25-100	0.5-2 μg/kg/min	5-10 μg/kg
Sufentanil	0.25-2	0.5-1.5 μg/kg/hr	2.5-10 μg
Fentanyl	4-20	2-10 μg/kg/hr	25-100 μg
Remifentanil	1-2	0.1-1.0 μg/kg/min	0.1-1.0 μg/kg

From Bailey PL, Egan TD, Stanley TH: Intravenous opioid anesthetics. *In* Miller RD (ed): Anesthesia, 5th ed. New York, Churchill Livingstone, 2000, p 335.

Opioid-Based (High-Dose Opioid) Anesthesia

Opioids can be administered as the primary or sole anesthetic in opioid-based anesthetic techniques. High-dose opioid anesthesia was introduced as a "stress-free" anesthetic method for cardiac surgery. However, several factors have diminished the popularity of high-dose opioid anesthesia, even in cardiac anesthesia. These include the lack of evidence substantiating any significant outcome benefit associated with the use of large doses of opioids,[207,227] the added drug costs, and the trend toward "fast track" approaches to the cardiac patient that can be impeded by large doses of opioids, especially fentanyl.[226,397] However, opioids, particularly when administered by continuous infusion, are still among the most effective anesthetics for patients undergoing cardiac or other extensive operations.

Fentanyl

High-dose opioid anesthesia was first performed using morphine. However, morphine is no longer recommended, and fentanyl and sufentanil are recommended (Fig.11-28).[398,399] Many different techniques have been used by clinicians and investigators to achieve anesthesia with fentanyl.[397,400,401] Rapid or slow bolus injections of fentanyl range from 5 to 75 µg/kg. These doses will establish sufficient plasma fentanyl concentrations (10-30 ng/mL) that are often sufficient to provide stable hemodynamics throughout the induction/intubation sequence. Continuous infusions of fentanyl for cardiac surgery range from 0.1 to 1.0 µg/kg/minute up to or continuing through CPB. High-dose fentanyl anesthesia has also proved effective and safe in premature infants for repair of patent ductus arteriosus (<50 µg/kg)[402] and for pediatric heart surgery (50-100 µg/kg).[403] A recent report indicated that fentanyl (25-50 µg/kg) combined with isoflurane (0.2%-0.4%) was sufficient to obtund hemodynamic and stress responses in the pre-CPB phase of open heart surgery in infants and young children.[404] On the other hand, high-dose fentanyl 75-100 µg/kg was shown to cause prolonged suppression of NK cell function.[405]

Alfentanil

The induction of anesthesia with large doses of alfentanil has been applied to cardiac surgery.[406] Large doses (150 µg/kg) may be used with or without thiopental to induce anesthesia. Other investigators claim that anesthesia cannot be reliably induced with alfentanil alone, at least in young and healthy adults.[407] Continuous infusions of alfentanil (2-12 µg/kg/minute) have been employed to maintain moderate to very high plasma alfentanil concentrations (<3000 ng/mL) during cardiac surgery. Enthusiasm for high-dose alfentanil anesthesia techniques is limited by the amount (and cost) of drug required and by suggestions that alfentanil anesthesia for cardiac surgery may be inadequate[176] and may be associated with more cardiovascular adverse effects compared with fentanyl and sufentanil.[206] More modest doses of alfentanil have been successfully administered in combination with sedative-hypnotics such as propofol for cardiac anesthesia.[408]

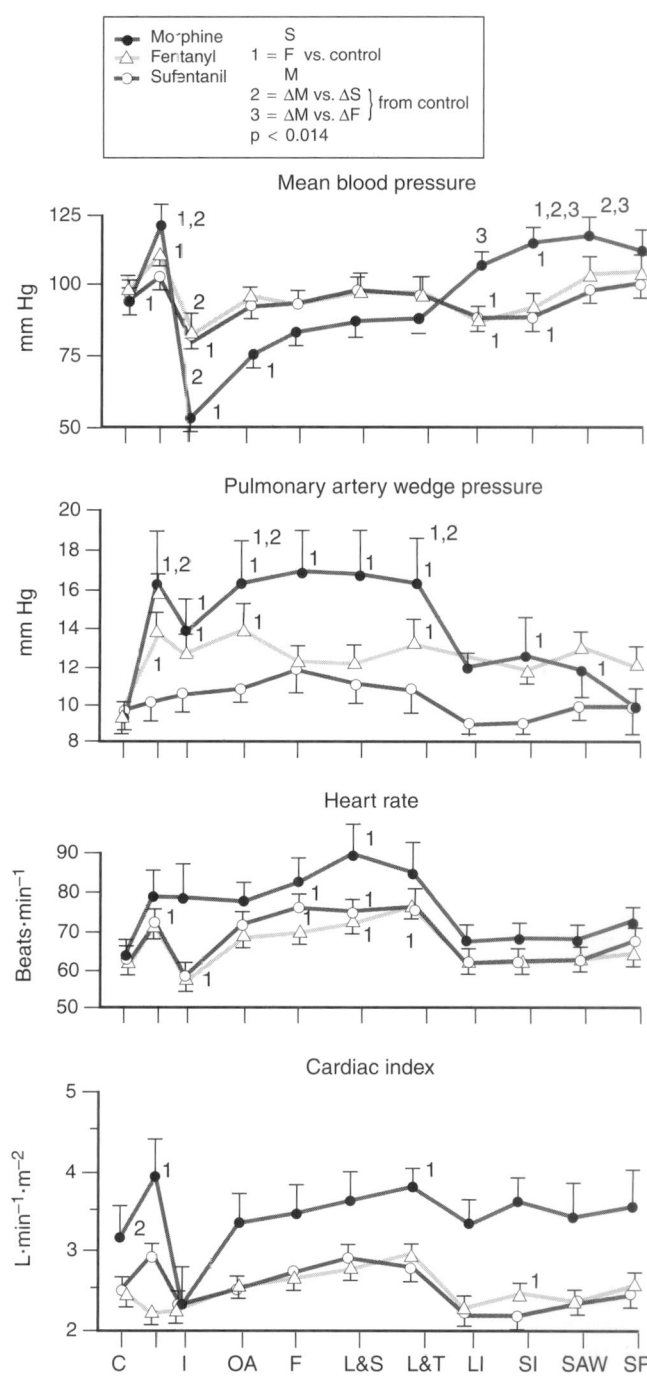

Figure 11–28 Hemodynamic changes during cardiac surgery in patients administered with morphine, fentanyl, or sufentanil. Total doses were 4.4 mg/kg, 95.4 µg/kg and 18.9 µg/kg for morphine, fentanyl and sufentanil, respectively. Cardiovascular variables were analyzed before induction (C), and at the time of maximal (MX) and minimal (MN) systolic arterial pressure change after induction (I), insertion of oral airway (OA), insertion of Foley catheter (F), laryngoscopy + endotracheal lidocaine spray (L&S), laryngoscopy + endotracheal intubation (L&T), leg incision (LI), sternal incision (SI), sternal saw (SAW), and sternal spread (SP). (From Benthuysen JL, Foltz BD, Smith NT, et al: Prebypass hemodynamic stability of sufentanil-O_2, fentanyl-O_2, and morphine-O_2 anesthesia during cardiac surgery: A comparison of cardiovascular profiles. J Cardiothorac Anesth 12:749-757, 1988.)

Sufentanil

Advantages of high-dose sufentanil include more rapid induction of anesthesia, better blunting or elimination of hypertensive episodes, greater reduction in left ventricular stroke work, with higher cardiac outputs, and more stable hemodynamics intraoperatively and/or postoperatively.[184,399,409] Induction doses of sufentanil range from 2 to 20 µg/kg administered as a bolus or infused over 2 to 10 minutes. Total doses of sufentanil employed in high-dose techniques usually range from 15 to 30 µg/kg. However, no additional benefit could be demonstrated in terms of hemodynamic control or EEG signs by increasing the dose of sufentanil from 3 to 15 µg/kg for the induction of anesthesia in patients premedicated with lorazepam.[410] It has been thought that muscle rigidity during induction of anesthesia with high-dose opioid causes difficult ventilation with a mask. It was shown that difficult ventilation during induction of anesthesia with sufentanil 3 µg/kg was due to upper airway closure at the level of the glottis or above.[411]

The amount of sufentanil required can be markedly influenced by the supplements employed concomitantly. For patients undergoing coronary artery surgery, induction (0.4 ± 0.2 µg/kg) and total maintenance (2.4 ± 0.8 µg/kg) doses of sufentanil were used in combination with propofol (1.5 ± 1 mg/kg for induction and 32 ± 12 mg/kg total). Interestingly, sufentanil requirements tripled when midazolam was employed instead of propofol.[412] Etomidate, combined with an opioid, can provide excellent anesthetic conditions with minimal hemodynamic perturbations. Inducing anesthesia with sufentanil (0.5-1.0 µg/kg) and etomidate (0.1-0.2 mg/kg) frequently confers hemodynamic stability. Maintenance of anesthesia, utilizing an infusion of sufentanil (1.0-2.0 µg/kg/hour), in a balanced anesthetic technique, achieves the advantages of an opioid-based anesthetic and avoids prolonged opioid action into the postoperative period.

Remifentanil

Remifentanil has been employed in cardiac anesthesia.[413] The pharmacokinetics of remifentanil were studied in patients undergoing coronary artery bypass grafting with cardiopulmonary bypass.[414] Because the volume of distribution increases by 86% with institution of CPB, and elimination clearance decreases by 6.37% for each degree below 37°C, the infusion rate of remifentanil should be changed to maintain constant plasma remifentanil level. It was shown that induction with remifentanil (2 µg/kg) together with propofol and maintenance with remifentanil at 0.25 or 0.5 µg/kg/min provided appropriate anesthesia for minimally invasive coronary artery bypass surgery with rapid awakening and tracheal extubation (Fig. 11-29).[415]

In an attempt to decrease the costs of cardiac surgery, fast-track programs have been popular. Engoren and coworkers recently reported that the more expensive but shorter-acting opioids sufentanil and remifentanil produced equally rapid extubation, similar stays, and similar costs to fentanyl, indicating that any of these opioids can be recommended for fast-track cardiac surgery.[416]

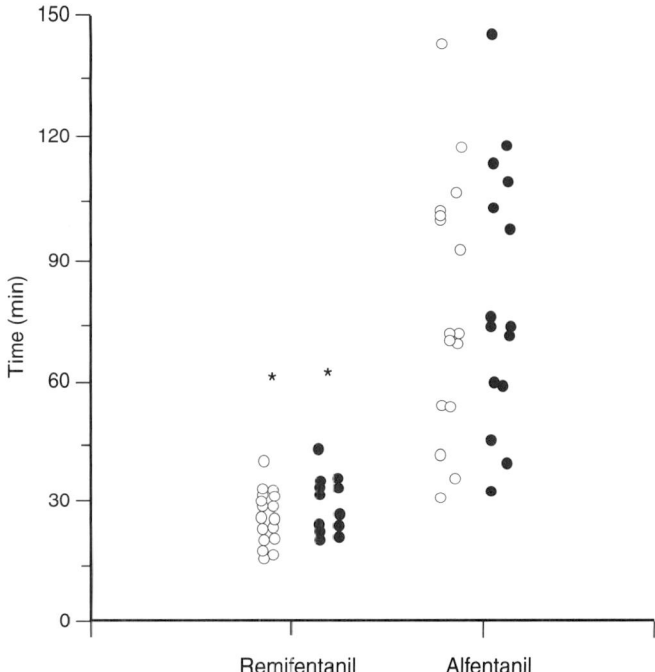

Figure 11–29 Times to awakening *(open circles)* and tracheal extubation *(closed circles)* in patients who underwent minimally invasive direct coronary artery bypass surgery after an intravenous anesthesia with remifentanil-propofol or alfentanil-propofol. (From Ahonen J, Olkkola KT, Verkkala K, et al: A comparison of remifentanil and alfentanil for use with propofol in patients undergoing minimally invasive coronary artery bypass surgery. Anesth Analg 90:1269-1274, 2000.)

Other Applications of Opioids

Transdermal Drug Delivery

Transdermal drug delivery generally requires high solubility in both water and oil, low molecular weight, high potency, and little or no skin irritation. Fentanyl is available in a transdermal delivery system. Potential advantages of delivering fentanyl transdermally include no first-pass drug metabolism by the liver; improved patient compliance, convenience, and comfort; and consistent analgesia. Doses of transdermal fentanyl include 20, 50, 75, and 100 µg/hour and achieve blood levels ranging from less than 1.0 to 2.0 ng/mL, although significant variability exists.[417,418] Plasma fentanyl levels rise and usually reach a plateau within 8 to 16 hours. The half-life for the decline in fentanyl levels after patch removal is high (17 ± 2.3 hour) (Fig. 11-30).[419] Elevated body temperature accelerates either the release of fentanyl from the patch or the distribution from the subcutaneous fat depot.

Results of clinical trials utilizing transdermal fentanyl for postoperative analgesia have demonstrated a high incidence of significant respiratory depression, and this application is not recommended.[417,418,420] Transdermal fentanyl is effective in cancer pain management. Patients should have analgesia provided by faster-acting opioid preparations and then be converted to transdermal fentanyl, with allowances made for drug conversions.

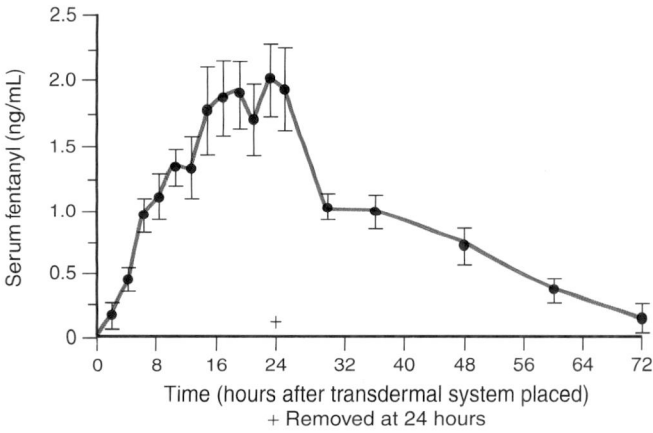

Figure 11–30 Serum fentanyl concentration change after placement of the transdermal fentanyl system. (From Varvel JR, Shafer SL, Hwang SS, et al: Absorption characteristics of transdermally administered fentanyl. Anesthesiology 70:928-934, 1989.)

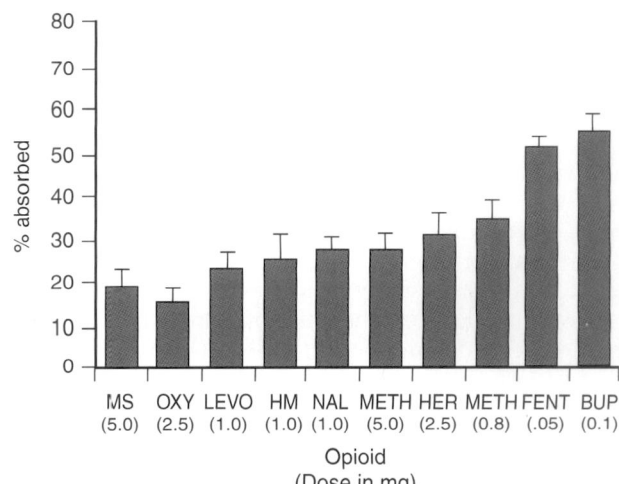

Figure 11–31 The mean absorption of opioids after 10 minutes in the oral cavity of normal subjects. The pH of the dosing solution was 6.5. MS, morphine sulfate; OXY, oxycodone; LEVO, levorphanol; HM, hydromorphone; NAL, naloxone; METH, methadone; HER, heroin; FENT, fentanyl; BUP, buprenorphine. (From Weinberg DS, Inturrisi CE, Reidenberg B, et al: Sublingual absorption of selected opioid analgesics. Clin Pharmacol Ther 44:335-342, 1988.)

Iontophoresis is a technique by which drug passage through the skin is augmented by an external electric current. Clinically significant doses of morphine and fentanyl can be delivered iontophoretically.[421]

Transmucosal Drug Delivery

Similar to transdermal drug delivery, transmucosal delivery through the oropharynx and nasopharynx eliminates hepatic first-pass metabolism (drugs are absorbed directly into the systemic circulation) and improves patient comfort, convenience, and compliance.

Buprenorphine, a potent, synthetic morphine analog with mixed opioid agonist-antagonist properties and a long half-life, is readily absorbed from sublingual mucosal tissues. The portion of the drug that is swallowed is almost completely metabolized by the liver, and only a small fraction can reach the systemic circulation when swallowed. Systemic bioavailability after sublingual buprenorphine is approximately 50% of that following intravenous administration. In several studies, sublingual buprenorphine (0.4 mg) was compared with conventional intramuscular morphine or meperidine and found to provide comparable and satisfactory analgesia.[422]

Initial experience with buccal morphine for postoperative analgesia had been promising. Bell and colleagues demonstrated that buccal morphine has a 50% bioavailability.[423] However, subsequent studies by Fisher and associates questioned the reliability and systemic availability of buccal morphine.[424] The low lipid solubility of morphine makes it an unlikely candidate for effective transmucosal absorption. Opioids with high lipid solubility, such as buprenorphine, fentanyl and methadone are more effectively absorbed sublingually than those with low lipid solubility, such as morphine (Fig. 11-31).[425]

Oral transmucosal fentanyl citrate (OTFC) is a solid dosage form of fentanyl that consists of fentanyl incorporated into a sweetened lozenge on a stick. A portion of fentanyl is absorbed through the oral mucosa, and the rest is swallowed and absorbed through the gastrointestinal tract. Swallowed fentanyl has a low bioavailability because of hepatic first-pass metabolism. The recommended doses range from 5 to 20 µg/kg.[426-430] OTFC should be administered approximately 30 minutes before surgery (or painful procedure) to obtain peak effect. Plasma concentrations after OTFC administration peak at 2.0 ± 0.5 ng/mL, 15 to 30 minutes after OTFC administration, then decline to less than 1 ng/mL an hour later.[431] The elimination half-life of OTFC is 7.7 hours, similar to that for the intravenous route. Unlike transdermal fentanyl, OTFC leaves no significant depot in the mucosal tissues after it is removed. Its systemic bioavailability is 50% and reflects both buccal and gastrointestinal absorption. OTFC bioavailability is similar to that of buprenorphine (55%), but much greater than that of buccal morphine and other opioids with low lipid solubility. Preoperative OTFC was reported to be effective for postoperative analgesia in pediatric tonsillectomy patients.[432] However, it can induce perioperative emesis and respiratory depression. OTFC is also being evaluated for treatment for acute postoperative analgesia and breakthrough cancer pain.[433] It may be ideally suited to treat breakthrough cancer pain, because fentanyl is rapidly absorbed from OTFC and patients can easily self-administer this compound.

Delivery of opioids through the nasal mucosa has also been investigated. Although intranasal sufentanil (1.5, 3.0, 4.5 µg/kg) in children allows easy separation from parents, many of the children cry on drug administration.[434] Side effects of intranasal sufentanil in children include reduced ventilatory compliance (chest wall rigidity), hypoxemia, impaired positive pressure ventilation by mask, and nausea and vomiting.[435,436] In adults, too, 10 to 15 µg of intranasal sufentanil induces moderate sedation with few side effects 20 to 40 minutes after administration.[437] Bioavailability of intranasal sufentanil is 78% of intravenous sufentanil. Butorphanol, a partial µ- and κ-receptor agonist, has also been administered nasally. Transnasal butorphanol provides superior and more prolonged analgesia than similar doses given intravenously for postoperative pain after cesarean section.[438] In human volunteers, transnasal butorphanol (1-2 mg) produced psychomotor, cognitive and subjective effects for 1 to 3 hours.[439] PCA with intranasal fentanyl was demonstrated to be effective for postoperative pain management.[440] It appears that further exploration of the transnasal approach to drug delivery for pain management is merited.

Morphine (10 mg) and fentanyl (300 µg) inhalation produces low plasma drug levels (~10 and 0.2-0.4 ng/mL, respectively) and analgesia that may be disproportionately greater than expected.[441,442] Inhaled liposome-encapsulated fentanyl was also demonstrated to be a noninvasive route of administration with a rapid increase and prolonged maintenance of plasma fentanyl concentration.[443]

The rectal mucosa is another site for transmucosal drug delivery. Morphine is only poorly absorbed from the rectal mucosa of children. However, sustained-release morphine hydrogel suppositories (MHS) may be more promising.[444] Plasma morphine levels after MHS were lower than after intramuscular morphine, but linear analog scales for pain were lower, and the incidence of nausea was reduced after rectal sustained-release therapy.[444] The hydrogel formulation of rectal morphine may be useful for premedication and analgesia in pediatric patients.[445]

Oral Controlled-Release Medications

Despite the high first-pass metabolism of opioid analgesics, morphine has been formulated into an oral, sustained-release tablet (MST) and has been evaluated for premedication,[446] postoperative analgesia,[447,448] and analgesia for chronic cancer pain.[449] MSTs provide unreliable preoperative anxiolysis and postoperative pain relief, possibly because of delayed time to onset of peak effects (3 to 5 hours), which can be increased by impaired gastric emptying and absorption from the small intestine. As an analgesic for chronic cancer pain, MSTs were shown to be an excellent formula.[449] A controlled-release formulation of oxycodone administered every 12 hours was more effective for postoperative analgesia than immediate-release oxycodone in patients undergoing anterior cruciate ligament repair.[450]

OTHER OPIOID AGONISTS

Alphaprodine is a phenylpiperidine derivative that is approximately one fourth as potent as morphine and has a rapid onset and a relatively short duration of action. It has been a popular analgesic for labor pain. It was reported that alphaprodine (39 ± 4 mg IV) produced no effects on neonates when given to parturients 197 ± 96 minutes prior to delivery.[451]

Codeine (methylmorphine) is half as potent as morphine, has a high oral-parenteral potency ratio (2:3) and a plasma half-life of 2 to 3 hours. Codeine has mild to moderate analgesic but strong cough-suppressant properties after oral administration. Cytochrome P-450 2D6 (CYP2D6) is the enzyme responsible for O-demethylation

of codeine to morphine.[452] Intravenous codeine produces profound hypotension and is neither approved nor recommended.[453]

Heroin (diacetylmorphine) is approximately twice as potent as morphine and has a 4- to 5-hour duration of action. Heroin is rapidly hydrolyzed to 6-acetylmorphine and morphine.

Hydromorphone is structurally related to morphine but is approximately five to ten times as potent. Analgesia after hydromorphone lasts 4 to 5 hours.[454] The effects of hydromorphone are essentially indistinguishable from those of heroin.[455] It was recently reported that hydromorphone PCA provided adequate postoperative analgesia with improved mood, and that it can be an alternative to morphine PCA.[456]

Levorphanol is a semisynthetic opioid with a long (12 to 19 hours) half-life. It is five times as potent as morphine with an intramuscular/oral potency ratio of 1:2. Levorphanol may have particular utility in patients with chronic pain and who demonstrate morphine tolerance, perhaps because of differences in opioid receptor activity.

Methadone has an equivalent potency but longer duration of action than morphine.[457] Its major clinical applications are in the prevention of opioid withdrawal symptoms and in the treatment of chronic pain. The plasma half-life of methadone is very long and variable (13 to 100 hours). Despite this property, many patients require dosing every 4 to 8 hours to maintain analgesic effects.

Oxymorphone, also structurally related to morphine, is almost ten times as potent, and has a similar duration of action.

Pentamorphone, a morphinan derivative, is two to eight times as potent as fentanyl and produces analgesia of similar duration without hemodynamic disturbances or increases in plasma histamine.[458] Although respiratory depression may be limited with analgesic doses (0.1 µg/kg), higher doses produce typical opioid-induced respiratory depression.

Phenoperidine is chemically related to meperidine but is 100 times as potent as an analgesic. Onset of its effect is rapid and duration is moderate (2 to 6 hours). Phenoperidine has long been used for sedation in Europe.[459]

Piritramide, a synthetic opioid structurally related to meperidine, is devoid of emetic activity, and is used for postoperative analgesia in several European countries.[460] Pharmacokinetic analysis showed that piritramide is distributed extensively and eliminated slowly, and it is recommended for intermittent bolus administration.[461]

Tramadol is a synthetic 4-phenyl-piperidine analog of codeine with a dual mechanism of action. Tramadol stimulates the µ-receptor, and to a lesser extent the δ- and κ-opioid receptors; like tricyclic antidepressants, it also activates spinal inhibition of pain by decreasing the reuptake of norepinephrine and serotonin.[462] A recent report suggested that tramadol may have a direct serotonin-releasing action.[463] Tramadol is one fifth to one tenth as potent as morphine. In rats, tramadol reduced the MAC of isoflurane in a naloxone-sensitive manner.[464] It was shown that intravenously administered tramadol was effective for post-thoracotomy pain relief.[465] Analgesic doses of tramadol may produce less respiratory depression in part because of its non–opioid receptor–mediated actions.[466] Tramadol has minimal effects on gastrointestinal motor function.[467]

Table 11–10 Dosing data for agonist-antagonist opioids and morphine

	Equianalgesic IM Dose (mg)	Duration of Analgesia (hr)	Oral: IM Efficacy Ratio
Morphine	10	4-5	1:6
Buprenorphine	0.3-0.4	>6	1:2*
Butorphanol	2	3-4	—
Nalbuphine	10	3-6	1:4-5
Pentazocine	40	3	1:3

*Sublingual: IM ratio.

Seizures have been reported in patients taking the drug. Caution should be exercised when combining tramadol with MAOIs, neuroleptic agents, and other drugs that lower the seizure threshold. It was suggested that tramadol may have local anesthetic effects on peripheral nerves when used alone.[468] Tramadol added to lidocaine for intravenous regional anesthesia provided a shorter onset time of sensory block.[469]

Sameridine possesses both local anesthetic and opioid properties. In patients subjected to arthroscopic knee joint surgery, sameridine was administered intrathecally and provided clinically adequate anesthesia.[470] A large intravenous dose of sameridine depressed resting ventilation and the hypercarbic ventilatory response, whereas a smaller clinical dose did not.[471,472]

Morphine-6-glucuronide (M6G) is a potent metabolite of morphine. The molar M6G:morphine potency ratio is approximately 13:1 in rats.[473] In trials using M6G as an analgesic, Osborne and associates. reported that M6G (0.5-4 mg IV) was effective for cancer pain for 2 to 24 hours without nausea and vomiting.[474] M6G (100 µg and 125 µg) given intrathecally provided excellent analgesia after total hip replacement, as did intrathecal morphine sulfate (500 µg).[475]

AGONIST-ANTAGONIST OPIOID COMPOUNDS

Nalorphine, the first agonist-antagonist opioid, was successfully synthesized by Weijland and Erickson in 1942 and was found to be strongly antagonistic to almost all the properties of morphine. Although nalorphine was found to possess strong analgesic actions, it was unsuitable for clinical uses because of its psychotomimetic effects. Nalorphine was used in lower doses as an opioid antagonist.

Agonist-antagonist opioids are usually produced by alkylation of the piperidine nitrogen and addition of a three-carbon side chain such as a propyl, allyl, or methyl allyl to morphine. Buprenorphine is a partial agonist at the µ-receptor. The other compounds are µ-antagonists and full or partial agonists at the κ-receptors. Agonist-antagonist opioids are less prone (but not immune) to abuse because they cause less euphoria and are associated with less drug-seeking behavior and physical dependence.

Dosing data for these compounds are shown in Table 11-10. The agonist-antagonist compounds depress respiration similar to morphine, but ceiling effects exist (Table 11-11). Effects on the cardiovascular system differ among these compounds (Table 11-12).

Table 11–11 Respiratory depressant effects of agonist-antagonists compared with morphine*

Drug	Correlation of Respiratory Depression with Dose
Morphine	Increases proportionally with dose
Buprenorphine	Ceiling effect at 0.15-1.2 mg in adults
Butorphanol	Ceiling effect at 30-60 µg • kg^{-1}
Nalbuphine	Ceiling effect at 30 mg in adults
Pentazocine	Ceiling effect suggested, but difficult to study because of psychotomimetic effects

* Low or moderate naloxone doses readily reverse the respiratory effects produced by therapeutic doses of all drugs listed, except buprenorphine.
From Zola EM, McLeod DC: Comparative effects of analgesic efficacy of the agonist-antagonist opioids. Drug Intell Clin Pharm 17:411, 1983.

Table 11–12 Hemodynamic effects of agonist-antagonist compounds compared with morphine

Drug	Cardiac Workload	Blood Pressure	Heart Rate	Pulmonary Artery Pressure
Morphine	↓	↓	=↓	=↓
Buprenorphine	↓	↓	↓	?
Butorphanol	↑	=↑	=	↑
Nalbuphine	↓	=	=↓	=
Pentazocine	↑	↑	↑	↑

From Zola EM, McLeod DC: Comparative effects of analgesic efficacy of the agonist-antagonist opioids. Drug Intell Clin Pharm 17:411, 1983.

Pentazocine

Analgesia produced by pentazocine is primarily related to κ-receptor stimulation. Pentazocine is one half to one fourth as potent as morphine. Ceilings to both analgesia and respiratory depression occur after 30 to 70 mg of pentazocine. Although the potential for abuse is less than with morphine, prolonged use of pentazocine can lead to physical dependence. Nalorphine-like dysphoric side effects are common, especially after high doses (>60 mg) of pentazocine in the elderly. The dysphoric effects of pentazocine can be reversed with naloxone. Pentazocine depresses myocardial contractility and increases arterial blood pressure, heart rate, systemic vascular resistance, pulmonary artery pressure, and left ventricular work index. Pentazocine also increases blood catecholamine levels.

Pentazocine inhibits gastric emptying and gastrointestinal transit in rats, whereas U50488H, a pure κ-receptor agonist, did not significantly inhibit either.[476] Therefore, it is speculated that pentazocine may affect gastrointestinal function through a mechanism other than the opioid receptors. Because pentazocine is associated with a high incidence of postoperative nausea and vomiting, it provides limited analgesia. It partially antagonizes other opioids, and it can produce undesirable cardiovascular and psychotomimetic effects.

Butorphanol

Butorphanol is an agonist at κ-receptors. Its activity at μ-receptors is either antagonistic or partially agonistic. It is five to eight times as potent as morphine and is only available in parenteral form. After IM injection, onset of effect is rapid, and peak analgesia occurs within 1 hour. Whereas duration of action of butorphanol is similar to that of morphine, its plasma half-life is only 2 to 3 hours. Although butorphanol (10 mg IM) causes as much respiratory depression as the same dose of morphine, higher doses reach a ceiling. Side effects after butorphanol include drowsiness, sweating, nausea and CNS stimulation.

In healthy volunteers, butorphanol (0.03 or 0.06 mg/kg IV) produces minimal cardiovascular changes. However, in patients with cardiac disease, butorphanol causes significant increases in cardiac index, left ventricular end-diastolic pressure and pulmonary artery pressure.

Because butorphanol decreases the MAC for enflurane by only a small fraction, it cannot serve like the fentanyl congeners as an anesthetic agent. Butorphanol does partially antagonize fentanyl-induced respiratory depression.[477] It is subject to less abuse and has less addictive potential than morphine or fentanyl. Acute biliary spasm can occur after butorphanol, but increases in biliary pressure are less than after equipotent doses of fentanyl or morphine.

Buprenorphine

Buprenorphine is a thebaine derivative, μ-receptor partial agonist, and similar in structure to morphine but approximately 33 times more potent. Whereas fentanyl dissociates rapidly from μ-receptors (half-life of 6.8 minutes), buprenorphine has a higher affinity and takes much longer to dissociate (half-life of 166 minutes). Its onset of action is slow, its peak effect may not occur until 3 hours, and its duration of effect is prolonged (>10 hours). The volume of distribution of buprenorphine is 2.8 L/kg and its clearance is 20 mL/kg/min. The metabolites of buprenorphine, buprenorphine-3-glucuronide and norbuprenorphine, are significantly less potent and have lower affinity for the μ-receptor.

The subjective effects (e.g., euphoria) of buprenorphine are similar to those of morphine. Buprenorphine produces respiratory depression with a ceiling after 0.15 to 1.2 mg in adults. Higher doses do not produce further respiratory depression and may actually result in increased ventilation (predominance of antagonistic actions).[478] Reversal with naloxone is limited by high affinity for and slow dissociation from the μ-opioid receptor of buprenorphine.[479] Buprenorphine has been successfully used for premedication (0.3 mg IM), as the analgesic component in balanced anesthesia (4.5 to 12 μg/kg), and for postoperative pain control (0.3 mg IM).[480] Buprenorphine, like the other agonist-antagonist compounds, is not acceptable as a sole anesthetic, and its receptor kinetic profile restricts its usefulness if other μ-agonists are used. Opioid withdrawal symptoms develop slowly (5 to 10 days) after buprenorphine is discontinued following long-term administration.

Nalbuphine

Nalbuphine is an agonist-antagonist opioid that is structurally related to oxymorphone and naloxone. Nalbuphine binds to μ-receptors as well as to κ- and δ-receptors.[481] Nalbuphine acts as an antagonist at the μ-receptor and an agonist at the κ-receptor. Activation of supraspinal and spinal κ-receptors results in limited analgesia, respiratory depression, and sedation.[481] Nalbuphine, like other agonist-antagonist compounds, interferes with the analgesia produced by pure μ-receptor agonists. In rats, coadministration of nalbuphine with morphine dose-dependently blocked the development of morphine tolerance and dependence, without attenuation of the antinociceptive effect of morphine.[482] Nalbuphine is only available for parenteral use. The onset of effect is rapid (5 to 10 minutes), and its duration is long (3 to 6 hours) because of a long plasma elimination half-life (5 hours).

Premedication with nalbuphine (0.1 mg/kg) in patients scheduled for cardiac surgery results in sedation, relief of anxiety, and respiratory depression similar to morphine (0.1 mg/kg), but it causes no significant hemodynamic changes. Nalbuphine (10 mg) caused no significant changes in systemic, pulmonary arterial, and pulmonary capillary wedge pressures in patients experiencing myocardial infarction.

Nalbuphine has been administered as an analgesic supplement for conscious sedation or balanced anesthesia and as an analgesic for postoperative and chronic pain problems. Conscious sedation during monitored anesthesia care has been recommended with a combination of nalbuphine (0.05-0.2 mg/kg) and midazolam (0.05 mg/kg).[483] Balanced anesthesia with nalbuphine as an IV analgesic supplement is effective for surgical procedures not associated with severe pain.[484] Postoperative sedation, dreaming, anxiety, and a longer recovery room stay are more common when nalbuphine (0.3 to 0.5 mg/kg) is used with N_2O for laparoscopy than when fentanyl (1.5 µg/kg) is employed as the opioid.[484] For postoperative patient-controlled epidural analgesia, the combination of hydromorphone (0.075 mg/mL) and nalbuphine (0.04 mg/mL) resulted in lower incidence of nausea and decreased need of bladder catheterization compared with hydromorphone alone.[485] The inability to decrease the MAC of potent inhaled anesthetics by nalbuphine (maximum 10% to 30%) suggests it has little or no role as a sole or primary anesthetic.[486]

Nalbuphine has been extensively evaluated for preservation of analgesia following reversal of opioid-induced respiratory depression. Nalbuphine (0.21 mg/kg) does not reverse and may actually increase respiratory depression after morphine (0.21 mg/kg) (Fig. 11-32).[487] Nalbuphine (20 mg IV) adequately reversed respiratory depression but not analgesia in patients who had received 7 µg/kg of fentanyl and N_2O for general surgery.[488] Unfortunately, other investigators have documented the occurrence of significant pain, hypertension, and tachycardia (often requiring pharmacologic intervention) following opioid reversal with nalbuphine.[489-491] Restoration of spontaneous ventilation using small titrated doses of nalbuphine (2.5 mg IV every 2 to 3 minutes) results in less pain than naloxone (0.08 mg IV every 2 to 3 minutes) after fentanyl (mean dose 25 µg/kg), isoflurane, and N_2O anesthesia.[492]

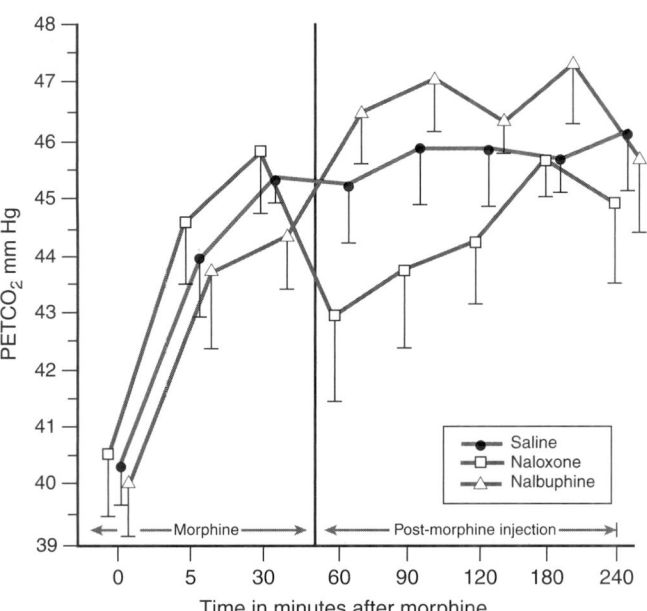

Figure 11–32 Resting end-tidal CO_2 ($PETCO_2$) at baseline; 5 minutes and 30 minutes after morphine (0.21 mg/kg IV); and after nalbuphine (0.21 mg/kg IV), naloxone (0.014 mg/kg IV) and saline given 55 minutes after morphine. (From Bailey PL, Clark NJ, Pace NL, et al: Failure of nalbuphine to antagonize morphine: A double-blind comparison with naloxone. Anesth Analg 65:605-611, 1986.)

Other Compounds

Dezocine

Dezocine is slightly more potent and acts faster than morphine, with a similar duration.[493] Dezocine is a partial agonist at µ- and probably δ-receptors. Side effects are similar to those of morphine. It is more effective in reducing the MAC of potent inhaled anesthetics (<50% with cyclopropane and 58% with enflurane) than other agonist-antagonists.[494] Dezocine can be effective for moderate and severe pain,[495] but it can cause myocardial depression and hypotension.

Meptazinol

Meptazinol has been reported to cause minimal respiratory depression because of its selectivity for μ_1-(high-affinity) receptors.[496] However, meptazinol-induced respiratory depression has been also reported.[497]

There are conflicting reports concerning the efficacy of meptazinol as a postoperative analgesic.[496] Side effects (nausea and vomiting) limit its use to relieve severe pain. Meptazinol, 120 mg, is equianalgesic to 10 mg of morphine.

OPIOID ANTAGONISTS

Naloxone

Clinically, opioid antagonists are used to restore spontaneous ventilation in patients who breathe inadequately after opioid overdoses or opioid anesthesia. In addition, opioid antagonists can reduce or reverse opioid-induced nausea and vomiting, pruritus, urinary retention, rigidity, and biliary spasm associated with numerous therapies employing opioids, such as neuraxial analgesic techniques. It was reported that the potency ratio for naloxone: nalbuphine for antagonism of the pruritic effects of epidural morphine was approximately 40:1.[498]

Morphine requirements were significantly less in patients receiving naloxone, suggesting that naloxone enhanced the analgesic effects of morphine.[499] Proposed possible mechanisms for this apparent paradoxical effect of naloxone include enhanced release of endogenous opioids and opioid receptor upregulation.

Although naloxone is generally considered to be a pure opioid receptor antagonist, it delays gastric emptying of saline or milk, as does morphine in the rat.[500] Furthermore, high doses of naloxone possess partial agonistic activity on the µ- and κ-opioid receptors in cultured cells.[501]

Reversal of Respiratory Depression by Naloxone

In the early 1950s, nalorphine and levallorphan were evaluated as opioid antagonists. They were often found unacceptable because of a high incidence of side effects as well as incomplete reversal. Naloxone was introduced into clinical practice in the late 1960s. There have been reports of side effects (increases in heart rate and blood pressure) and more serious complications (e.g., pulmonary edema).[502,503] Initial naloxone dose recommendations ranged from 0.4 to 0.8 mg. If intravenous access is not available, naloxone, in doses similar to those given intravenously, is effectively absorbed after intratracheal administration.[504]

Several mechanisms produce increases in arterial blood pressure, heart rate, and other significant hemodynamic alterations after naloxone reversal of opioids. These include pain, rapid awakening, and sympathetic activation not necessarily due to pain. When patients receiving naloxone for opioid agonist reversal are hypothermic due to intraoperative heat loss, O_2 consumption and minute ventilation can increase two- to threefold.[505] Such metabolic demands also stress the cardiovascular system, increasing cardiac output. In addition, greater degrees of hypercapnia at the time of opioid antagonism will result in greater degrees of cardiovascular stimulation because of associated sympathetic stimulation. Opioid reversal may be particularly hazardous in patients with pheochromocytoma or chromaffin tissue tumors.[506] Naloxone may also have a nonspecific analeptic effect through activation of a CNS arousal system.[507]

Onset of action of intravenous naloxone is rapid (1 to 2 minutes), and half-life and duration of effect are short, approximately 30 to 60 minutes. Most often, 1.0-2.0 μg/kg titrated in boluses of 0.5-1.0 μg/kg every 2 to 3 minutes will restore adequate spontaneous ventilation.[492] Even smaller doses of naloxone may be adequate after alfentanil.

Recurrence of respiratory depression after naloxone is due to the short half-life of naloxone as well as to the reuptake of opioid from peripheral compartment tissues (e.g., muscle). "Renarcotization" occurs more frequently after the use of naloxone to reverse longer-acting opioids such as morphine. Short-acting opioids such as alfentanil rarely pose a danger of renarcotization, because of a rapid plasma decay curve, less chance of second plasma peaks due to reuptake of drug from peripheral tissues, and weak opioid receptor binding compared with fentanyl and sufentanil.

Naloxone, although active at μ-, δ- and κ-receptors, has the greatest affinity for μ-receptors, which mediate most potent opioid effects, including respiratory depression and analgesia. Careful titration of naloxone often can restore adequate spontaneous ventilation without reversal of adequate analgesia.

Other Applications of Naloxone

Naloxone may be useful in the treatment of postanesthetic apnea in infants, even when exogenous opioids have not been administered.[508]

Although many conflicting reports and opinions exist, high doses of naloxone may reverse the effects of some nonopioid CNS depressants. Reversal of the effects of alcohol, barbiturates, and benzodiazepines by naloxone has been reported. The MAC of potent inhaled anesthetics is unaffected by naloxone. However, pretreatment of rats with naloxone does counteract halothane-induced depression of sympathetic nerve activity, but interestingly, not halothane-induced analgesia.[509] Naloxone may partially antagonize ketamine and N_2O analgesia.

Naloxone increases arterial blood pressure in laboratory animals, primates, and some patients in hypovolemic and septic shock.[510] This effect may be due to centrally mediated increases in sympathetic tone and decreases in

parasympathetic output and/or antagonism of endogenous opioids.

It has been reported that naloxone may ameliorate the neurologic deficit following an ischemic or traumatic neurologic insult in animals. Naloxone may also have a therapeutic role in heat stroke disorders,[511] Alzheimer's disease, schizophrenia, intractable pruritus, and thalamic pain syndrome.

Other Opioid Antagonists

Naltrexone

Naltrexone is a μ-, δ- and κ-opioid receptor antagonist. It is longer acting than naloxone (plasma half-life of 8 to 12 hours versus 0.5 to 1.5 hours), and it is active when taken orally. Oral naltrexone (5-10 mg) reduces the frequency and severity of pruritus, nausea, and vomiting associated with epidural morphine without diminishing analgesia. Naltrexone, like naloxone, can stimulate the cardiovascular system.

Nalmefene

Like naloxone and naltrexone, nalmefene has a greater preference for μ- than for δ- and κ-receptors. Nalmefene is equipotent to naloxone.[512] It is long-acting after oral (0.5-3.0 mg/kg) and parenteral (0.2-2.0 mg/kg) administration. The bioavailability of nalmefene after oral administration is 40% to 50%, and peak plasma concentrations are reached in 1 to 2 hours. The mean terminal elimination half-life of nalmefene is 8.5 hours, compared with 1 hour for naloxone. Prophylactic administration of nalmefene significantly decreased the need for antiemetics and antipruritic medications in patients receiving intravenous patient-controlled analgesia with morphine.[513]

Methylnaltrexone

Methylnaltrexone is the first quaternary ammonium opioid receptor antagonist that does not cross the blood-brain barrier. It can reverse adverse effects of opioid medications mediated by peripheral opioid receptors, whereas the opioid effects mediated by opioid receptors in the CNS, such as analgesia, are not affected. Delayed gastric emptying induced by morphine (0.09 mg/kg) could be attenuated by methylnaltrexone (0.3 mg/kg) in healthy volunteers.[289] It was also reported that methylnaltrexone was effective for reversal of constipation due to chronic methadone use.[514] Because methylnaltrexone does not cross the dura, it might have the potential to reverse the peripherally mediated side effects of epidural opioids.[515]

DRUG INTERACTIONS WITH OPIOIDS

General Principles

Opioids are frequently combined with other anesthetic agents to produce optimal anesthetic conditions. In anesthesia, most concomitantly administered drugs interact. Although some of these interactions are intentionally sought, others are unwanted and adverse. There are three general types of mechanisms of drug interactions: pharmaceutical, pharmacokinetic, and pharmacodynamic.[516]

Pharmaceutical interactions are chemical in nature, as illustrated when an alkaline solution of thiopental and an acidic solution of succinylcholine precipitate when simultaneously administered IV.

Pharmacokinetic interactions occur when the administration of one agent alters the pharmacokinetics or disposition of another. Hemodynamic changes induced by one agent can affect the pharmacokinetic behavior of the other agent. The actions of sufentanil, which has a greater hepatic extraction ratio than alfentanil, are more likely to be affected by decreases in hepatic blood flow. Opioid plasma levels increase in the presence of propofol.[517] Decreased opioid metabolism, by the CYP 3A4 isoform of the cytochrome P-450 enzyme responsible for the oxidative metabolism of more than 50 drugs, may also underlie pharmacokinetic interactions. Liver enzyme induction by alcohol, antiepileptics, and barbiturates can also affect the metabolism of anesthetic drugs.

Pharmacodynamic interactions between opioids and inhaled anesthetics were assessed with classic MAC reduction evaluations in animals and humans. Although marked synergism between opioids and inhaled anesthetics occurs with analgesic doses of opioids, there is a ceiling effect to MAC reduction by opioids. The pharmacodynamic synergism between opioids and sedative-hypnotics such as propofol is profound. Choosing an opioid with a short context-sensitive half-life allows greater doses of that opioid to be administered, along with reduced doses of propofol, without compromising the time for recovery from anesthesia. Thus, the optimal plasma level of propofol is estimated to be approximately 30 percent less when it is combined with remifentanil instead of alfentanil.[517]

The establishment of drug-dosing regimens and plasma concentrations of opioids and sedative-hypnotics needed to provide optimal hemodynamic control during a range of noxious stimuli would be very practical and helpful. However, complicating our understanding of drug interactions is the observation that the same degree of interaction does not apply across different types of stimuli.

Sedative-Hypnotics

Benzodiazepines potentiate the effects of opioids and decrease opioid requirements for loss of consciousness, often in a synergistic fashion.[518,519] On the contrary, concerning the antinociceptive effect, interaction between these two types of drugs may be less than additive.[520,521] Midazolam enhances opioid-induced antinociception at the spinal level but inhibits it at the supraspinal level.[522] Studies have shown that benzodiazepine-opioid interactions for many properties other than analgesia are synergistic (supra-additive).[523] Both the cardiovascular and the respiratory actions of opioids can be significantly altered by the concomitant administration of benzodiazepines.[524] Combinations of benzodiazepines and opioids, although occasionally preserving ventricular function, can cause significant and occasionally profound decreases in blood pressure, cardiac index, heart rate, and systemic vascular resistance.[124,525] Fluid loading may attenuate circulatory depression that occurs when benzodiazepines and opioids are combined.

Either thiopental or propofol can be employed safely in combination with opioids. However, either drug can potentiate or produce hypotension if too large a dose is administered.[526] Hypotension after barbiturate-opioid combinations is due to venodilatation and decreased cardiac filling. Other mechanisms include myocardial depression and decreased sympathetic nervous system activity. Reducing induction doses of barbiturates administered concomitantly with opioids is recommended. The administration of propofol-opioid combinations provides unconsciousness and blocks responses to noxious stimuli, whereas neither drug alone reliably does both. Propofol-fentanyl and propofol-sufentanil anesthesia for coronary artery bypass surgery may provide acceptable conditions, but mean arterial pressure can decrease to levels that may jeopardize coronary perfusion, especially during the induction of anesthesia.[527,528] In healthy volunteers, the addition of alfentanil (effect site concentration of 50 or 100 ng/mL) did not affect the changes in the BIS induced by propofol, but blocked BIS increase induced by painful stimuli.[529] In patients undergoing spine fusion, infusion of fentanyl to blood levels of 1.5 to 4.5 ng/mL reduced the infusion rate of propofol necessary to stabilize mean arterial pressure but delayed spontaneous eye opening and recovery of orientation.[530] In patients undergoing ambulatory gynecologic laparoscopy, the administration of fentanyl (100 µg IV) at the time of anesthetic induction reduced maintenance propofol requirement, but failed to provide effective postoperative analgesia and increased the need for postoperative use of antiemetics.[531]

Other anesthetic induction agents such as etomidate and ketamine can be combined in low doses with opioids with little loss of cardiovascular stability. In patients scheduled for coronary artery bypass grafting, etomidate (0.25 mg/kg) plus fentanyl (6 µg/kg) resulted in less hypotension after induction and intubation than propofol (1 mg/kg) plus fentanyl (6 µg/kg).[532] As described previously, it was reported that opioid-induced hyperalgesia and subsequent acute opioid tolerance can be prevented by ketamine in rats, suggesting the usefulness of a combination of ketamine and opioids for postoperative analgesia. However, it was shown that the combination of ketamine (2.5 or 10 mg IV) and alfentanil (0.25 or 1 mg IV) provided no advantage over a larger dose of either drug alone in relieving pain caused by intradermal capsaicin injection in healthy volunteers.[533] Furthermore, the combination of ketamine (1 mg/mL) and morphine (1 mg/mL) for PCA did not provide benefit to patients undergoing major abdominal surgery.[534] In contrast, Lauretti and associates reported that oral ketamine and transdermal nitroglycerine effectively reduced the daily consumption of oral morphine in patients with cancer pain.[535]

Gabapentin, a structural analog of γ-aminobutyric acid, is a novel anticonvulsant drug, and has analgesic effects on neuropathic pain. One study suggests that both pharmacodynamic and pharmacokinetic interactions between morphine and gabapentin lead to increased analgesic effects.[536] Gamma-aminobutyric acid-A ($GABA_A$) receptors contribute to inhibitory control at the spinal cord level. Intrathecal administration of muscimol or baclofen (the $GABA_A$ and $GABA_B$ receptor agonists, respectively) increased the analgesic action of morphine in intensity and duration.[537]

Inhaled Anesthetics

Cardiovascular function is frequently preserved during N_2O administration. Some reports showed deterioration of cardiac function with N_2O-opioid combinations.[351] Segmental wall motion abnormalities in areas of marginal myocardial perfusion was demonstrated in dogs when N_2O and opioids are combined.[538] However, in clinical studies of patients with ischemic cardiac disease, the addition of N_2O to fentanyl or sufentanil was not to associated with any new ST-segment changes or segmental wall motion abnormalities.[539] It was reported that N_2O produced analgesia that was partially mediated by the release of a proenkephalin-derived family of endogenous opioid peptides.[540] This suggests that interaction between opioids and N_2O is neither synergistic nor additive. Combining N_2O with an opioid in a balanced technique may not best employ drug interaction synergism. Although amnesia and intraoperative conditions may be somewhat improved, N_2O does not produce any effects that are not already produced by either an opioid or a sedative-hypnotic.

Volatile anesthetics are frequently combined in low doses (one third to one half the MAC) with opioids in order to ensure amnesia and to promote immobility and hemodynamic stability.[541] Low concentrations of volatile anesthetics in combination with opioids are usually well tolerated in patients with normal, as well as compromised, ventricular function.[541] Low concentrations of isoflurane have been effectively and safely used to treat intraoperative hypertension during high-dose sufentanil anesthesia for coronary artery surgery.[542,543]

Clinical trials of opioids supplemented with newer volatile anesthetics for cardiac surgery demonstrate well-preserved cardiac output and minimal decreases in mean arterial blood pressure.[544,545] Myocardial ischemia may not, however, always be ameliorated by approaches that combine opioids with potent inhaled agents in spite of apparent "good" hemodynamic control.

Some of the potent inhaled anesthetics can increase sympathetic nervous system activity and may increase the risk of myocardial ischemia in the cardiac patient.[546,547] Prior administration of fentanyl, in doses as low as 1.5 µg/kg, can markedly attenuate such responses.[546] Alfentanil (10 µg/kg) is also effective in attenuating these effects.

Muscle Relaxants

Pancuronium bromide frequently has been used for muscle relaxation during high-dose opioid anesthesia. It was reported that the vagolytic action of pancuronium can attenuate opioid-induced bradycardia and support blood pressure,[548] but other reports cautioned the use of pancuronium with high-dose opioids.[549-551] Many factors may alter the impact of pancuronium and other muscle relaxants on hemodynamics when they are combined with opioids: for example, the dose, timing, and rate of administration of each relaxant, as well as the premedication,

intravascular volume, left ventricular function, and presence of other drugs with autonomic nervous system actions.[548]

Combinations of vecuronium and high doses of opioids produce negative chronotropic and inotropic effects resulting in decreases in heart rate, cardiac output, and blood pressure and increases in the need for vasopressor support.[552,553] Compared with vecuronium (0.15 mg/kg), pancuronium (0.15 mg/kg) produced tachycardia more often (32% versus 7%) in patients undergoing coronary artery surgery.[554] However, pancuronium-induced tachycardia was easily and rapidly treated and caused no differences in ischemia or perioperative myocardial infarction. It was also reported that there is no significant difference in the frequency of intraoperative ischemic events with pancuronium compared with vecuronium.[555]

Metocurine (0.5 mg/kg) alone produces less hemodynamic fluctuation than pancuronium during opioid anesthesia, although high doses (>0.3 mg/kg) may cause hypotension. Doxacurium causes no circulatory changes during sufentanil-midazolam anesthesia.[556] Pipecuronium, in doses as high as three times the ED_{95}, has also been found to be devoid of circulatory actions in patients undergoing coronary artery bypass grafting surgery under midazolam-fentanyl anesthesia.[557] Mivacurium chloride produces modest decreases in blood pressure, probably due to histamine release when larger doses (e.g., twice the ED_{95}) are injected rapidly (<30 seconds).[558,559] Few significant circulatory changes were associated with mivacurium (0.15-0.25 mg/kg over 60 seconds) in patients undergoing coronary artery bypass grafting surgery and receiving sufentanil-midazolam anesthesia.[560]

Miscellaneous

MAOIs can underlie the most serious and potentially fatal interaction of opioids with other drugs. Only meperidine is consistently implicated as capable of this severe interaction.[561,562] Opioid-MAOI interactions are either excitatory or depressive.[562] The excitatory interaction results in agitation, headache, hemodynamic instability, fever, rigidity, convulsions, and coma. This interaction is thought to be due to excessive central serotoninergic activity. Meperidine, but not morphine, blocks neuronal uptake of serotonin. The depressive interaction consists of respiratory depression, hypotension, and coma as a result of MAOI inhibition of hepatic microsomal enzymes and meperidine accumulation.

Because opioids can inhibit voltage-dependent Ca^{2+} channel activity through the activation of G-proteins, it is possible that opioid action is potentiated by Ca^{2+} channel blockers. Numerous animal studies and a few clinical studies have documented that opioid-induced analgesia is potentiated by L-type Ca^{2+} channel blockers. Systemically administered nifedipine was shown to potentiate morphine analgesia in both rats and humans.[563] Furthermore, intrathecal administration of verapamil, diltiazem, and nicardipine enhanced the antinociceptive effect of small doses of morphine in rats.[564] However, there is also a report that L-type Ca^{2+} channel blockers do not potentiate morphine analgesia at clinically relevant doses.[565] N-type Ca^{2+} channels are involved in the release of neurotransmitters from sensory neurons in the spinal cord. It was reported that intrathecal administration of a blocker of this channel, ω-conotoxin GVIA, produced antinociception, and a synergistic interaction with opioids at the spinal cord level.[566]

Erythromycin can inhibit the metabolism of several compounds. It supposedly reduces the oxidizing activity of cytochrome P-450. Alfentanil, but not sufentanil, may have its action prolonged as a result of impaired metabolism in patients receiving erythromycin.[567,568] Cimetidine can prolong opioid effects by decreasing hepatic blood flow and/or diminishing hepatic metabolism. Other drugs that inhibit certain cytochrome systems can decrease endogenous morphine production from codeine.[452]

Magnesium has been shown to have antinociceptive effects probably due to its antagonistic action on the NMDA receptor. Intravenous administration of magnesium sulfate preoperatively (50 mg/kg) and intraoperatively (8 mg/kg/hour) significantly reduced intra- and postoperative fentanyl requirements.[569] However, passage of magnesium across the blood-brain barrier is limited. In patients requesting analgesia for labor, intrathecal administration of fentanyl (25 μg) plus magnesium sulfate (50 mg) provided significantly prolonged analgesia compared with fentanyl alone.[570] It is likely that magnesium can potentiate opioid analgesia by both central and peripheral mechanisms.[571]

Nonsteroidal anti-inflammatory drugs (NSAIDs), such as ibuprofen, diclofenac, and ketorolac, have been perioperatively administered to reduce opioid requirement. The preoperative administration of ibuprofen (2×800 mg) to patients scheduled for lower abdominal gynecologic surgery was shown to reduce postoperative morphine consumption without an increase in side effects.[572] It was also reported that the perioperative administration of diclofenac (75 mg twice daily) reduced morphine consumption and the incidence of adverse side effects such as sedation and nausea after total abdominal hysterectomy.[573] In healthy volunteers, ketoprofen (1.5 mg/kg IV) reduced respiratory depression induced by morphine (0.1 mg/kg).[574]

Diphenhydramine, a histamine H_1 receptor antagonist, is used as a sedative, antipruritic, and antiemetic agent. When administered alone, it modestly stimulates ventilation by augmenting the interaction of hypoxic and hypercarbic ventilatory drives. It was shown that diphenhydramine counteracts the alfentanil-induced decrease in the slope of the ventilatory response to carbon dioxide.[575]

Opioids generally induce nausea and vomiting, the mechanisms of which are clearly identified and now treatable.

3. New pharmacokinetic principles have allowed a more intelligent use of opioids, with more predictable durations of action.

4. Surrogate measures of opioid potency allows more accurate dosing devices for the production of analgesia.

5. During total intravenous anesthesia, the use of opioids is a vital part of providing the analgetic component of anesthesia. Short-acting drugs, such as remifentanil, allow dissipation of total intravenous anesthetic even more rapidly than that from inhaled anesthetics.

6. New opioid delivery systems, such as transdermal fentanyl patches, are continually being developed, which allows more flexibility in providing analgesia, both inside and outside the operating room.

KEY POINTS

1. An increased understanding of the molecular pharmacology of opioid receptors and opioid-induced cellular responses allows utilization of new innovative techniques for analgesia.

2. Regretfully, the opioids have non-opioid effects on many organ systems, such as the cardiovascular system. Proper dosing and monitoring allows these effects to be minimized, when used in humans.

REFERENCES

1. Gutstein HB, Akil H: Opioid analgesics. *In* Hardman JG, Limbird LE (eds): Goodman and Gilman's The Pharmacological Basis of Therapeutics, 10th ed. New York, McGraw-Hill, 2001, pp 569-619.
2. Minami M, Satoh M: Molecular biology of the opioid receptors: structures, functions and distributions. Neurosci Res 23:121-145, 1995.
3. Reinscheid RK, Nothacker HP, Bourson A, et al: Orphanin FQ: A neuropeptide that activates an opioidlike G protein-coupled receptor. Science 270:792-794, 1995.
4. Meunier JC, Mollereau C, Toll L, et al: Isolation and structure of the endogenous agonist of opioid receptor-like ORL1 receptor. Nature 377: 532-535, 1995.
5. Mansour A, Fox CA, Akil H, Watson SJ: Opioid-receptor mRNA expression in the rat CNS: Anatomical and functional implications. Trends Neurosci 18:22-29, 1995.
6. Mogil JS, Pasternak GW: The molecular and behavioral pharmacology of the orphanin FQ/nociceptin peptide and receptor family. Pharmacol Rev 53:381-415, 2001.
7. Nothacker HP, Reinscheid RK, Mansour A, et al: Primary structure and tissue distribution of the orphanin FQ precursor. Proc Natl Acad Sci U S A 93:8677-8682, 1996.
8. Zadina JE, Hackler L, Ge LJ, Kastin AJ: A potent and selective endogenous agonist for the mu-opiate receptor. Nature 386:499-502, 1997.
9. Wandless AL, Smart D, Lambert DG: Fentanyl increases intracellular Ca^{2+} concentrations in SH-SY5Y cells. Br J Anaesth 76:461-463, 1997.
10. Fukuda K, Kato S, Morikawa H, et al: Functional coupling of the delta-, mu-, and kappa-opioid receptors to mitogen-activated protein kinase and arachidonate release in Chinese hamster ovary cells. J Neurochem 67:1309-1316, 1996.
11. Shoda T, Fukuda K, Uga H, et al: Activation of mu-opioid receptor induces expression of c-fos and junB via mitogen-activated protein kinase cascade. Anesthesiology 95:983-989, 2001.
12. Mestek A, Hurley JH, Bye LS, et al: The human mu opioid receptor: Modulation of functional desensitization by calcium/calmodulin-dependent protein kinase and protein kinase C. J Neurosci 15:2396-2406, 1995.
13. Pei G, Kieffer BL, Lefkowitz RJ, Freedman NJ: Agonist-dependent phosphorylation of the mouse delta-opioid receptor: involvement of G protein-coupled receptor kinases but not protein kinase C. Mol Pharmacol 48:73-177, 1995.

14. Bohn LM, Lefkowitz RJ, Gainetdinov RR, et al: Enhanced morphine analgesia in mice lacking beta-arrestin 2. Science 286:2495-2498, 1999.
15. Trapaidze N, Keith DE, Cvejic S, et al: Sequestration of the delta opioid receptor. Role of the C terminus in agonist-mediated internalization. J Biol Chem 271:29279-29285, 1996.
16. Gaudriault G, Nouel D, Dal Farra C, et al: Receptor-induced internalization of selective peptidic mu and delta opioid ligands. J Biol Chem 272:2880-2888, 1997.
17. Keith DE, Murray SR, Zaki PA, et al: Morphine activates opioid receptors without causing their rapid internalization. J Biol Chem 271:19021-19024, 1996.
18. Avidor Reiss T, Nevo I, Levy R, et al: Chronic opioid treatment induces adenylyl cyclase V superactivation. Involvement of G betagamma. J Biol Chem 271:21309-21315, 1996.
19. Fields HL, Heinricher MM, Mason P: Neurotransmitters in nociceptive modulatory circuits. Annu Rev Neurosci 14:219-245, 1991.
20. Pan ZZ, Tershner SA, Fields HL: Cellular mechanism for anti-analgesic action of agonists of the kappa-opioid receptor. Nature 389:382-385, 1997.
21. Trafton JA, Abbadie C, Marchand S, et al: Spinal opioid analgesia: How critical is the regulation of substance P signaling? J Neurosci 19:9642-9653, 1999.
22. Matthies BK, Franklin KB: Formalin pain is expressed in decerebrate rats but not attenuated by morphine. Pain 51:199-206, 1992.
23. Manning BH, Morgan MJ, Franklin KB: Morphine analgesia in the formalin test: Evidence for forebrain and midbrain sites of action. Neuroscience 63:289-294, 1994.
24. Manning BH, Mayer DJ: The central nucleus of the amygdala contributes to the production of morphine antinociception in the rat tail-flick test. J Neurosci 15:8199-8213, 1995.
25. Manning BH, Mayer DJ: The central nucleus of the amygdala contributes to the production of morphine antinociception in the formalin test. Pain 63:141-52, 1995.
26. Stein C: The control of pain in peripheral tissue by opioids. N Engl J Med 332:1685-1690, 1995.
27. Heard SO, Edwards WT, Ferrari D, et al: Analgesic effect of intraarticular bupivacaine or morphine after arthroscopic knee surgery: A randomized, prospective, double-blind study. Anesth Analg 74:822-826, 1992.
28. Picard PR, Tramer MR, McQuay HJ, Moore RA: Analgesic efficacy of peripheral opioids (all except intra-articular): A qualitative systematic review of randomised controlled trials. Pain 72:309-318, 1997.
29. Kieffer BL: Opioids: first lessons from knockout mice. Trends Pharmacol Sci 20:19-26, 1999.
30. Matthes HW, Maldonado R, Simonin F, et al: Loss of morphine-induced analgesia, reward effect and withdrawal symptoms in mice lacking the mu-opioid-receptor gene. Nature 383:819-823, 1996.
31. Sora I, Takahashi N, Funada M, et al: Opiate receptor knockout mice define mu receptor roles in endogenous nociceptive responses and morphine-induced analgesia. Proc Natl Acad Sci U S A 94:1544-1549, 1997.
32. Dahan A, Sarton E, Teppema L, et al: Anesthetic potency and influence of morphine and sevoflurane on respiration in mu-opioid receptor knockout mice. Anesthesiology 94:824-832, 2001.
33. Sarton E, Teppema LJ, Olievier C, et al: The involvement of the mu-opioid receptor in ketamine-induced respiratory depression and antinociception. Anesth Analg 93:1495-1500, 2001.
34. Zhu Y, King MA, Schuller AG, et al: Retention of supraspinal delta-like analgesia and loss of morphine tolerance in delta opioid receptor knockout mice. Neuron 24:243-252, 1999.
35. Simonin F, Valverde O, Smadja C, et al: Disruption of the kappa-opioid receptor gene in mice enhances sensitivity to chemical visceral pain, impairs pharmacological actions of the selective kappa-agonist U-50,488H and attenuates morphine withdrawal. EMBO J 17:886-897, 1998.
36. Rubinstein M, Mogil JS, Japon M, et al: Absence of opioid stress-induced analgesia in mice lacking beta-endorphin by site-directed mutagenesis. Proc Natl Acad Sci U S A 93:3995-4000, 1996.
37. Konig M, Zimmer AM, Steiner H, et al: Pain responses, anxiety and aggression in mice deficient in pre-proenkephalin. Nature 383:535-538, 1996.
38. Hung CF, Tsai CH, Su MJ: Opioid receptor independent effects of morphine on membrane currents in single cardiac myocytes. Br J Anaesth 81:925-931, 1998.
39. Brau ME, Koch ED, Vogel W, Hempelmann G: Tonic blocking action of meperidine on Na$^+$ and K$^+$ channels in amphibian peripheral nerves. Anesthesiology 92:47-55, 2000.
40. Wagner LE 2nd, Eaton M, Sabnis SS, Gingrich KJ: Meperidine and lidocaine block of recombinant voltage-dependent Na$^+$ channels: Evidence that meperidine is a local anesthetic. Anesthesiology 91:1481-1490, 1999.
41. Takada K, Clark DJ, Davies MF, et al: Meperidine exerts agonist activity at the alpha(2B)-adrenoceptor subtype. Anesthesiology 96:1420-1426, 2002.
42. Yamakura T, Sakimura K, Shimoji K: Direct inhibition of the N-methyl-D-aspartate receptor channel by high concentrations of opioids. Anesthesiology 91:1053-1063, 1999.
43. Nishi M, Houtani T, Noda Y, et al: Unrestrained nociceptive response and disregulation of hearing ability in mice lacking the nociceptin/orphanin FQ receptor. EMBO J 16:1858-1864, 1997.
44. Koster A, Montkowski A, Schulz S, et al: Targeted disruption of the orphanin FQ/nociceptin gene increases stress susceptibility and impairs stress adaptation in mice. Proc Natl Acad Sci U S A 96:10444-10449, 1999.
45. Yamamoto T, Nozaki Taguchi N, Kimura S: Analgesic effect of intrathecally administered nociceptin, an opioid receptor-like 1 receptor agonist, in the rat formalin test. Neuroscience 81:249-254, 1997.
46. Grisel JE, Mogil JS, Belknap JK, Grandy DK: Orphanin FQ acts as a supraspinal, but not a spinal, anti-opioid peptide. Neuroreport 7:2125-2129, 1996.
47. Pan Z, Hirakawa N, Fields HL: A cellular mechanism for the bidirectional pain-modulating actions of orphanin FQ/nociceptin. Neuron 26:515-522, 2000.
48. McQuay HJ: Pharmacological treatment of neuralgic and neuropathic pain. Cancer Surv 7:141-159, 1988.
49. Yaksh TL: CNS mechanisms of pain and analgesia. Cancer Surv 7:5-28, 1988.
50. Morgan D, Cook CD, Smith MA, Picker MJ: An examination of the interactions between the antinociceptive effects of morphine and various mu-opioids: the role of intrinsic efficacy and stimulus intensity. Anesth Analg 88:407-413, 1999.
51. Perrot S, Guilbaud G, Kayser V: Differential behavioral effects of peripheral and systemic morphine and naloxone in a rat model of repeated acute inflammation. Anesthesiology 94:870-75, 2001.
52. Kest B, Sarton E, Dahan A: Gender differences in opioid-mediated analgesia Animal and human studies. Anesthesiology 93:539-547, 2000.
53. Sarton E, Olofsen E, Romberg R, et al: Sex differences in morphine analgesia: An experimental study in healthy volunteers [discussion 6A]. Anesthesiology 93:1245-1254, 2000.
54. Gupta A, Bodin L, Holmstrom B, Berggren L: A systematic review of the peripheral analgesic effects of intraarticular morphine. Anesth Analg 93:761-770, 2001.
55. Kapral S, Gollmann G, Waltl B, et al: Tramadol added to mepivacaine prolongs the duration of an axillary brachial plexus blockade. Anesth Analg 88:853-856, 1999.
56. Nishikawa K, Kanaya N, Nakayama M, et al: Fentanyl improves analgesia but prolongs the onset of axillary brachial plexus block by peripheral mechanism. Anesth Analg 91:384-387, 2000.
57. Bouaziz H, Kinirons BP, Macalou D, et al: Sufentanil does not prolong the duration of analgesia in a mepivacaine brachial plexus block: a dose response study. Anesth Analg 90:383-387, 2000.
58. Reuben SS, Steinberg RB, Lurie SD, Gibson CS: A dose-response study of intravenous regional anesthesia with meperidine. Anesth Analg 88:831-835, 1999.
59. Philbin DM, Rosow CE, Schneider RC, et al: Fentanyl and sufentanil anesthesia revisited: how much is enough? Anesthesiology 73:5-11, 1990.

60. Michelsen LG, Salmenpera M, Hug CC Jr, et al: Anesthetic potency of remifentanil in dogs. Anesthesiology 84:865-872, 1996.

61. Steffey EP: Isoflurane-sparing effect of fentanyl in swine. Relevance and importance. Anesthesiology 83:446-448, 1995.

62. McEwan AI, Smith C, Dyar O, et al: Isoflurane minimum alveolar concentration reduction by fentanyl. Anesthesiology 78:864-869, 1993.

63. Glass PS, Gan TJ, Howell S, Ginsberg B: Drug interactions: Volatile anesthetics and opioids. J Clin Anesth 9(Suppl):18-22, 1997.

64. Johansen JW, Schneider G, Windsor AM, Sebel PS: Esmolol potentiates reduction of minimum alveolar isoflurane concentration by alfentanil. Anesth Analg 87:671-676, 1998.

65. Inagaki Y, Tsuda Y: Contribution of the spinal cord to arousal from inhaled anesthesia: Comparison of epidural and intravenous fentanyl on awakening concentration of isoflurane. Anesth Analg 85:1387-1393, 1997.

66. Kissin I, Vinik HR, Castillo R, Bradley EL Jr: Alfentanil potentiates midazolam-induced unconsciousness in subanalgesic doses. Anesth Analg 71:65-69, 1990.

67. Lysakowski C, Dumont L, Pellegrini M, et al: Effects of fentanyl, alfentanil, remifentanil and sufentanil on loss of consciousness and bispectral index during propofol induction of anaesthesia. Br J Anaesth 86:523-527, 2001.

68. Koitabashi T, Johansen JW, Sebel PS: Remifentanil dose/electroencephalogram bispectral response during combined propofol/regional anesthesia. Anesth Analg 94:1530-1533, 2002.

69. Streisand JB, Bailey PL, LeMaire L, Ashburn MA, Tarver SD, Varvel J, Stanley TH: Fentanyl-induced rigidity and unconsciousness in human volunteers. Incidence, duration, and plasma concentrations. Anesthesiology 78:629-634, 1993.

70. Dodson BA, Miller KW: Evidence for a dual mechanism in the anesthetic action of an opioid peptide. Anesthesiology 62:615-620, 1985.

71. Chi OZ, Sommer W, Jasaitis D: Power spectral analysis of EEG during sufentanil infusion in humans. Can J Anaesth 38:275-280, 1991.

72. Long CW, Shah NK, Loughlin C, et al: A comparison of EEG determinants of near-awakening from isoflurane and fentanyl anesthesia. Spectral edge, median power frequency, and delta ratio. Anesth Analg 69:169-173, 1989.

73. Gambus PL, Gregg KM, Shafer SL: Validation of the alfentanil canonical univariate parameter as a measure of opioid effect on the electroencephalogram. Anesthesiology 83:747-756, 1995.

74. Scott JC, Ponganis KV, Stanski DR: EEG quantitation of narcotic effect: The comparative pharmacodynamics of fentanyl and alfentanil. Anesthesiology 62:234-241, 1985.

75. Bovill JG, Sebel PS, Wauquier A, et al: Influence of high-dose alfentanil anaesthesia on the electroencephalogram: Correlation with plasma concentrations. Br J Anaesth 55(Suppl 2):199-209, 1983.

76. Egan TD, Minto CF, Hermann DJ, et al: Remifentanil versus alfentanil: Comparative pharmacokinetics and pharmacodynamics in healthy adult male volunteers. Anesthesiology 84:821-833, 1996.

77. Scott JC, Cooke JE, Stanski DR: Electroencephalographic quantitation of opioid effect: Comparative pharmacodynamics of fentanyl and sufentanil. Anesthesiology 74:34-42, 1991.

78. Westmoreland CL, Sebel PS, Gropper A: Fentanyl or alfentanil decreases the minimum alveolar anesthetic concentration of isoflurane in surgical patients. Anesth Analg 78:23-28, 1994.

79. Brunner MD, Braithwaite P, Jhaveri R, et al: MAC reduction of isoflurane by sufentanil. Br J Anaesth 72:42-46, 1994.

80. Lang E, Kapila A, Shlugman D, et al: Reduction of isoflurane minimal alveolar concentration by remifentanil. Anesthesiology 85:721-728, 1996.

81. McPherson RW, Mahla M, Johnson R, Traystman RJ: Effects of enflurane, isoflurane, and nitrous oxide on somatosensory evoked potentials during fentanyl anesthesia. Anesthesiology 62:626-633, 1985.

82. McPherson RW, Sell B, Traystman RJ: Effects of thiopental, fentanyl, and etomidate on upper extremity somatosensory evoked potentials in humans. Anesthesiology 65:584-589, 1986.

83. Schubert A, Drummond JC, Peterson DO, Saidman LJ: The effect of high-dose fentanyl on human median nerve somatosensory-evoked responses. Can J Anaesth 34:35-40, 1987.

84. Koht A, Schutz W, Schmidt G, et al: Effects of etomidate, midazolam, and thiopental on median nerve somatosensory evoked potentials and the additive effects of fentanyl and nitrous oxide. Anesth Analg 67:435-441, 1988.

85. Pathak KS, Brown RH, Cascorbi HF, Nash CL Jr: Effects of fentanyl and morphine on intraoperative somatosensory cortical-evoked potentials. Anesth Analg 63:833-837, 1985.

86. Samra SK, Krutak Krol H, Pohorecki R, Domino EF: Scopolamine, morphine, and brain-stem auditory evoked potentials in awake monkeys. Anesthesiology 62:437-441, 1985.

87. Samra SK, Lilly DJ, Rush NL, Kirsh MM: Fentanyl anesthesia and human brain-stem auditory evoked potentials. Anesthesiology 61:261-265, 1984.

88. Crabb I, Thornton C, Konieczko KM, et al: Remifentanil reduces auditory and somatosensory evoked responses during isoflurane anaesthesia in a dose-dependent manner. Br J Anaesth 76:795-801, 1996.

89. Chi OZ, Ryterband S, Field C: Visual evoked potentials during thiopentone-fentanyl-nitrous oxide anaesthesia in humans. Can J Anaesth 36:637-640, 1989.

90. Thorogood MC, Armstead WM: Influence of polyethylene glycol superoxide dismutase/catalase on altered opioid-induced pial artery dilation after brain injury. Anesthesiology 84:614-625, 1996.

91. Wahl M: Effects of enkephalins, morphine, and naloxone on pial arteries during perivascular microapplication. J Cereb Blood Flow Metab 5:451-457, 1985.

92. Monitto CL, Kurth CD: The effect of fentanyl, sufentanil, and alfentanil on cerebral arterioles in piglets. Anesth Analg 76:985-989, 1993.

93. Milde LN, Milde JH, Gallagher WJ: Cerebral effects of fentanyl in dogs. Br J Anaesth 63:710-715, 1989.

94. Adler LJ, Gyulai FE, Diehl DJ, et al: Regional brain activity changes associated with fentanyl analgesia elucidated by positron emission tomography. Anesth Analg 84:120-126, 1997.

95. Werner C, Hoffman WE, Baughman VL, et al: Effects of sufentanil on cerebral blood flow, cerebral blood flow velocity, and metabolism in dogs. Anesth Analg 72:177-181, 1991.

96. Milde LN, Milde JH, Gallagher WJ: Effects of sufentanil on cerebral circulation and metabolism in dogs. Anesth Analg 70:138-146, 1990.

97. Mayer N, Weinstabl C, Podreka I, Spiss CK: Sufentanil does not increase cerebral blood flow in healthy human volunteers. Anesthesiology 73:240-243, 1990.

98. Mayberg TS, Lam AM, Eng CC, et al: The effect of alfentanil on cerebral blood flow velocity and intracranial pressure during isoflurane-nitrous oxide anesthesia in humans. Anesthesiology 78:288-294, 1993.

99. Hoffman WE, Cunningham F, James MK, et al: Effects of remifentanil, a new short-acting opioid, on cerebral blood flow, brain electrical activity, and intracranial pressure in dogs anesthetized with isoflurane and nitrous oxide. Anesthesiology 79:107-113, 1993.

100. Wagner KJ, Willoch F, Kochs EF, et al: Dose-dependent regional cerebral blood flow changes during remifentanil infusion in humans: A positron emission tomography study. Anesthesiology 94:732-739, 2001.

101. Ostapkovich ND, Baker KZ, Fogarty-Mack P, et al: Cerebral blood flow and CO_2 reactivity is similar during remifentanil/N_2O and fentanyl/N_2O anesthesia. Anesthesiology 89:358-363, 1998.

102. Kofke WA, Garman RH, Tom WC, et al: Alfentanil-induced hypermetabolism, seizure, and histopathology in rat brain. Anesth Analg 75:953-964, 1992.

103. Kofke WA, Attaallah AF, Kuwabara H, et al: The neuropathologic effects in rats and neurometabolic effects in humans of large-dose remifentanil. Anesth Analg 94:1229-1236, 2002.

104. Warner DS, Hindman BJ, Todd MM, et al: Intracranial pressure and hemodynamic effects of remifentanil versus alfentanil in patients undergoing supratentorial craniotomy. Anesth Analg 83:348-353, 1996.

105. Jamali S, Ravussin P, Archer D, et al: The effects of bolus administration of opioids on cerebrospinal fluid pressure in patients with supratentorial lesions. Anesth Analg 82:600-606, 1996.

106. Jamali S, Archer D, Ravussin P, et al: The effect of skull-pin insertion on cerebrospinal fluid pressure and cerebral perfusion pressure: influence of sufentanil and fentanyl. Anesth Analg 84:1292-1296, 1997.

107. Lauer KK, Connolly LA, Schmeling WT: Opioid sedation does not alter intracranial pressure in head injured patients. Can J Anaesth 44:929-933, 1997.

108. Marx W, Shah N, Long C, et al: Sufentanil, alfentanil, and fentanyl: Impact on cerebrospinal fluid pressure in patients with brain tumors. J Neurosurg Anesth 1:3, 1989.

109. Markovitz BP, Duhaime AC, Sutton L, et al: Effects of alfentanil on intracranial pressure in children undergoing ventriculoperitoneal shunt revision. Anesthesiology 76:71-76, 1992.

110. de Nadal M, Munar F, Poca MA, et al: Cerebral hemodynamic effects of morphine and fentanyl in patients with severe head injury: absence of correlation to cerebral autoregulation. Anesthesiology 92:11-9, 2000.

111. Benthuysen JL, Kien ND, Quam DD: Intracranial pressure increases during alfentanil-induced rigidity. Anesthesiology 68:438-440, 1988.

112. Baskin DS, Widmayer MA, Browning JL, et al: Evaluation of delayed treatment of focal cerebral ischemia with three selective kappa-opioid agonists in cats. Stroke 25:2047-2053, 1994.

113. Takahashi H, Traystman RJ, Hashimoto K, et al: Postischemic brain injury is affected stereospecifically by pentazocine in rats. Anesth Analg 85:353-357, 1997.

114. Cole DJ, Shapiro HM, Drummond JC, Zivin JA: Halothane, fentanyl/nitrous oxide, and spinal lidocaine protect against spinal cord injury in the rat. Anesthesiology 70:967-972, 1989.

115. Mayfield KP, D'Alecy LG: Delta-1 opioid agonist acutely increases hypoxic tolerance. J Pharmacol Exp Ther 268:683-688, 1994.

116. Bofetiado DM, Mayfield KP, D'Alecy LG: Alkaloid delta agonist BW373U86 increases hypoxic tolerance. Anesth Analg 82:1237-1241, 1996.

117. Charchaflieh J, Cottrell JE, Kass IS: The effect of fentanyl on electrophysiologic recovery of CA 1 pyramidal cells from anoxia in the rat hippocampal slice. Anesth Analg 87:68-71, 1998.

118. Soonthon Brant V, Patel PM, Drummond JC, et al: Fentanyl does not increase brain injury after focal cerebral ischemia in rats. Anesth Analg 88:49-55, 1999.

119. Pokela ML, Ryhanen PT, Koivisto ME, et al: Alfentanil-induced rigidity in newborn infants. Anesth Analg 75:252-257, 1992.

120. Blasco TA, Lee D, Amalric M, et al: The role of the nucleus raphe pontis and the caudate nucleus in alfentanil rigidity in the rat. Brain Res 386:280-286, 1986.

121. Comstock MK, Carter JG, Moyers JR, Stevens WC: Rigidity and hypercarbia associated with high dose fentanyl induction of anesthesia. Anesth Analg 60:362-363, 1981.

122. Benthuysen JL, Smith NT, Sanford TJ, et al: Physiology of alfentanil-induced rigidity. Anesthesiology 64:440-446, 1986.

123. Goldberg M, Ishak S, Garcia C, McKenna J: Postoperative rigidity following sufentanil administration. Anesthesiology 63:199-201, 1985.

124. Bailey PL, Wilbrink J, Zwanikken P, et al: Anesthetic induction with fentanyl. Anesth Analg 64:48-53, 1985.

125. Vankova ME, Weinger MB, Chen DY, et al: Role of central mu, delta-1, and kappa-1 opioid receptors in opioid-induced muscle rigidity in the rat. Anesthesiology 85:574-583, 1996.

126. Mets B: Acute dystonia after alfentanil in untreated Parkinson's disease. Anesth Analg 72:557-558, 1991.

127. Crawford RD, Baskoff JD: Fentanyl-associated delirium in man. Anesthesiology 53:168-169, 1980.

128. Haber GW, Litman RS: Generalized tonic-clonic activity after remifentanil administration. Anesth Analg 93:1532-1533, 2001.

129. Tommasino C, Maekawa T, Shapiro HM, et al: Fentanyl-induced seizures activate subcortical brain metabolism. Anesthesiology 60:283-290, 1984.

130. Parkinson SK, Bailey SL, Little WL, Mueller JB: Myoclonic seizure activity with chronic high-dose spinal opioid administration. Anesthesiology 72:743-745, 1990.

131. Armstrong PJ, Bersten A: Normeperidine toxicity. Anesth Analg 65:536-538, 1986.

132. Gutstein HB, Rubie EA, Mansour A, et al: Opioid effects on mitogen-activated protein kinase signaling cascades. Anesthesiology 87:1118-1126, 1997.

133. Kofke WA, Garman RH, Janosky J, Rose ME: Opioid neurotoxicity: Neuropathologic effects in rats of different fentanyl congeners and the effects of hexamethonium-induced normotension. Anesth Analg 83:141-146, 1996.

134. Sinz EH, Kofke WA, Garman RH: Phenytoin, midazolam, and naloxone protect against fentanyl-induced brain damage in rats. Anesth Analg 91:1443-1449, 2000.

135. Larson MD, Kurz A, Sessler DI, et al: Alfentanil blocks reflex pupillary dilation in response to noxious stimulation but does not diminish the light reflex. Anesthesiology 87:849-855, 1997.

136. Woodall NM, Maryniak JK, Gilston A: Pupillary signs during cardiac surgery. Their use in the prediction of major cerebral deficit following cardiopulmonary bypass. Anaesthesia 44:885-888, 1989.

137. Sessler DI, Olofsson CI, Rubinstein EH: The thermoregulatory threshold in humans during nitrous oxide-fentanyl anesthesia. Anesthesiology 69:357-364, 1988.

138. Kurz A, Go JC, Sessler DI, et al: Alfentanil slightly increases the sweating threshold and markedly reduces the vasoconstriction and shivering thresholds. Anesthesiology 83:293-299, 1995.

139. Macintyre PE, Pavlin EG, Dwersteg JF: Effect of meperidine on oxygen consumption, carbon dioxide production, and respiratory gas exchange in postanesthesia shivering. Anesth Analg 66:751-755, 1987.

140. Casey WF, Smith CE, Katz JM, et al: Intravenous meperidine for control of shivering during caesarean section under epidural anaesthesia. Can J Anaesth 35:128-133, 1988.

141. Ikeda T, Sessler DI, Tayefeh F, et al: Meperidine and alfentanil do not reduce the gain or maximum intensity of shivering. Anesthesiology 88:858-865, 1998.

142. Kurz M, Belani KG, Sessler DI, et al: Naloxone, meperidine, and shivering. Anesthesiology 79:1193-1201, 1993.

143. Greif R, Laciny S, Rajek AM, et al: Neither nalbuphine nor atropine possess special antishivering activity. Anesth Analg 93:620-627, 2001.

144. Sevarino FB, Johnson MD, Lema MJ, et al: The effect of epidural sufentanil on shivering and body temperature in the parturient. Anesth Analg 68:530-533, 1989.

145. Tsai YC, Chu KS: A comparison of tramadol, amitriptyline, and meperidine for postepidural anesthetic shivering in parturients. Anesth Analg 93:1288-1292, 2001.

146. Ko MC, Naughton NN: An experimental itch model in monkeys: characterization of intrathecal morphine-induced scratching and antinociception. Anesthesiology 92:795-805, 2000.

147. Cohen SE, Ratner EF, Kreitzman TR, et al: Nalbuphine is better than naloxone for treatment of side effects after epidural morphine. Anesth Analg 75:747-752, 1992.

148. Dunteman E, Karanikolas M, Filos KS: Transnasal butorphanol for the treatment of opioid-induced pruritus unresponsive to antihistamines. J Pain Symptom Manage 12:255-260, 1996.

149. Borgeat A, Stirnemann HR: Ondansetron is effective to treat spinal or epidural morphine-induced pruritus. Anesthesiology 90:432-436,1999.

150. Colbert S, O'Hanlon DM, Chambers F, Moriarty DC: The effect of intravenous tenoxicam on pruritus in patients receiving epidural fentanyl. Anaesthesia 54:76-80, 1999.

151. Jones EA, Bergasa NV: The pruritus of cholestasis and the opioid system. JAMA 268:3359-3362,1992.

152. Etches RC: Respiratory depression associated with patient-controlled analgesia: a review of eight cases. Can J Anaesth 41:125-232, 1994.

153. Forbes AR, Horrigan RW: Mucociliary flow in the trachea during anesthesia with enflurane, ether, nitrous oxide, and morphine. Anesthesiology 46:319-321, 1977.

154. Selwyn DA, Raphael JH, Lambert DG, Langton JA: Effects of morphine on human nasal cilia beat frequency in vitro. Br J Anaesth 76:274-277,1996.

155. Jaeckle KA, Digre KB, Jones CR, et al: Central neurogenic hyperventilation: pharmacologic intervention with morphine sulfate and correlative analysis of respiratory, sleep, and ocular motor dysfunction. Neurology 40:1715-1720,1990.

156. Tobias JD, Heideman RL: Primary central hyperventilation in a child with a brainstem glioma: Management with continuous intravenous fentanyl. Pediatrics 88:818-820, 1991.

157. Bohrer H, Fleischer F, Werning P: Tussive effect of a fentanyl bolus administered through a central venous catheter. Anaesthesia 45:18-21, 1990.

158. Ruiz Neto PP, Auler Junior JO: Respiratory mechanical properties during fentanyl and alfentanil anaesthesia. Can J Anaesth 39:458-465, 1992.

159. Tabatabai M, Kitahata LM, Collins JG: Disruption of the rhythmic activity of the medullary inspiratory neurons and phrenic nerve by fentanyl and reversal with nalbuphine. Anesthesiology 70:489-495, 1989.

160. Sarton E, Teppema L, Dahan A: Sex differences in morphine-induced ventilatory depression reside within the peripheral chemoreflex loop. Anesthesiology 90:1329-1338, 1999.

161. Smart JA, Pallett EJ, Duthie DJ: Breath interval as a measure of dynamic opioid effect. Br J Anaesth 84:735-738, 2000.

162. Bailey PL, Streisand JB, East KA, et al: Differences in magnitude and duration of opioid-induced respiratory depression and analgesia with fentanyl and sufentanil. Anesth Analg 70:8-15, 1990.

163. Ausems ME, Hug CC Jr, Stanski DR, Burm AG: Plasma concentrations of alfentanil required to supplement nitrous oxide anesthesia for general surgery. Anesthesiology 65:362-367, 1986.

164. Glass PS, Iselin-Chaves IA, Goodman D, et al: Determination of the potency of remifentanil compared with alfentanil using ventilatory depression as the measure of opioid effect. Anesthesiology 90:1556-1563, 1999.

165. Combes X, Cerf C, Bouleau D: The effects of residual pain on oxygenation and breathing pattern during morphine analgesia. Anesth Analg 90:156-160, 2000.

166. Knape JT: Early respiratory depression resistant to naloxone following epidural buprenorphine. Anesthesiology 64:382-384, 1986.

167. Krenn H, Jellinek H, Haumer H, et al: Naloxone-resistant respiratory depression and neurological eye symptoms after intrathecal morphine. Anesth Analg 91:432-433, 2000.

168. Arunasalam K, Davenport HT, Painter S, Jones JG: Ventilatory response to morphine in young and old subjects. Anaesthesia 38:529-533, 1983.

169. Furst SR, Weinger MB: Dexmedetomidine, a selective alpha 2-agonist, does not potentiate the cardiorespiratory depression of alfentanil in the rat. Anesthesiology 72:882-888, 1990.

170. Rawal N, Wattwil M: Respiratory depression after epidural morphine—an experimental and clinical study. Anesth Analg 63:8-14, 1984.

171. Nishino T, Hiraga K, Fujisato M, et al: Breathing patterns during postoperative analgesia in patients after lower abdominal operations. Anesthesiology 69:967-972, 1988.

172. Pelligrino DA, Riegler FX, Albrecht RF: Ventilatory effects of fourth cerebroventricular infusions of morphine-6- or morphine-3-glucuronide in the awake dog. Anesthesiology 71:936-940, 1989.

173. Peat SJ, Hanna MH, Woodham M, et al: Morphine-6-glucuronide: effects on ventilation in normal volunteers. Pain 45:101-104, 1991.

174. Koehntop DE, Rodman JH, Brundage DM, et al: Pharmacokinetics of fentanyl in neonates. Anesth Analg 65:227-232, 1986.

175. Robbins GR, Wynands JE, Whalley DG, et al: Pharmacokinetics of alfentanil and clinical responses during cardiac surgery. Can J Anaesth 37:52-57, 1990.

176. Hug CC Jr, Hall RI, Angert KC, et al: Alfentanil plasma concentration vs. effect relationships in cardiac surgical patients. Br J Anaesth 61:435-440, 1988.

177. Feldman PD, Parveen N, Sezen S: Cardiovascular effects of Leu-enkephalin in the nucleus tractus solitarius of the rat. Brain Res 709:331-333, 1996.

178. Keay KA, Crowfoot LJ, Floyd NS, et al: Cardiovascular effects of microinjections of opioid agonists into the 'Depressor Region' of the ventrolateral periaqueductal gray region. Brain Res 762:61-71, 1997.

179. Thomson IR, Putnins CL, Friesen RM: Hyperdynamic cardiovascular responses to anesthetic induction with high-dose fentanyl. Anesth Analg 65:91-95, 1986.

180. Zhang CC, Su JY, Calkins D: Effects of alfentanil on isolated cardiac tissues of the rabbit. Anesth Analg 71:268-274, 1990.

181. Helgesen KG, Ellingsen O, Ilebekk A: Inotropic effect of meperidine: influence of receptor and ion channel blockers in the rat atrium. Anesth Analg 70:499-506, 1990.

182. Nakae Y, Fujita S, Namiki A: Morphine enhances myofilament CA(2+) sensitivity in intact guinea pig beating hearts. Anesth Analg 92:602-608, 2001.

183. Llobel F, Laorden ML: Effects of morphine on atrial preparations obtained from nonfailing and failing human hearts. Br J Anaesth 76:106-110, 1996.

184. Mathews HM, Furness G, Carson IW, et al: Comparison of sufentanil-oxygen and fentanyl-oxygen anaesthesia for coronary artery bypass grafting. Br J Anaesth 60:530-535, 1988.

185. James MK, Vuong A, Grizzle MK, et al: Hemodynamic effects of GI 87084B, an ultra-short acting mu-opioid analgesic, in anesthetized dogs. J Pharmacol Exp Ther 263:84-91, 1992.

186. Royster RL, Keeler DK, Haisty WK, et al: Cardiac electrophysiologic effects of fentanyl and combinations of fentanyl and neuromuscular relaxants in pentobarbital-anesthetized dogs. Anesth Analg 67:15-20, 1988.

187. Blair JR, Pruett JK, Introna RP, et al: Cardiac electrophysiologic effects of fentanyl and sufentanil in canine cardiac Purkinje fibers. Anesthesiology 71:565-570, 1989.

188. Weber G, Stark G, Stark U: Direct cardiac electrophysiologic effects of sufentanil and vecuronium in isolated guinea-pig hearts. Acta Anaesthesiol Scand 39:1071-1074, 1995.

189. Blair JR, Pruett JK, Crumrine RS, Balser JJ: Prolongation of QT interval in association with the administration of large doses of opiates. Anesthesiology 67:442-443, 1997.

190. Sharpe MD, Dobkowski WB, Murkin JM, et al: Alfentanil-midazolam anaesthesia has no electrophysiological effects upon the normal conduction system or accessory pathways in patients with Wolff-Parkinson-White syndrome. Can J Anaesth 39:816-821, 1992.

191. Sharpe MD, Dobkowski WB, Murkin JM, et al: The electrophysiologic effects of volatile anesthetics and sufentanil on the normal atrioventricular conduction system and accessory pathways in Wolff-Parkinson-White syndrome. Anesthesiology 80:63-70, 1994.

192. Schmeling WT, Kampine JP, Warltier DC: Negative chronotropic actions of sufentanil and vecuronium in chronically instrumented dogs pretreated with propranolol and/or diltiazem. Anesth Analg 69:4-14, 1989.

193. Atlee JL, 3rd, Bosnjak ZJ: Mechanisms for cardiac dysrhythmias during anesthesia. Anesthesiology 72:347-374, 1990.
194. Saini V, Carr DB, Hagestad EL, et al: Antifibrillatory action of the narcotic agonist fentanyl. Am Heart J 115:598-605, 1988.
195. McIntosh M, Kane K, Parratt J: Effects of selective opioid receptor agonists and antagonists during myocardial ischaemia. Eur J Pharmacol 210:37-44, 1992.
196. Chinzei M, Morita S, Chinzei T, et al: Effects of isoflurane and fentanyl on ischemic myocardium in dogs: Assessment by end-systolic measurements. J Cardiothorac Vasc Anesth 5:243-249, 1991.
197. Kim YD, Danchek M, Myers AK, et al: Anaesthetic modification of regional myocardial functional adjustments during myocardial ischaemia: Halothane vs fentanyl. Br J Anaesth 68:286-292, 1992.
198. White JL, Myers AK, Analouei A, Kim YD: Functional recovery of stunned myocardium is greater with halothane than fentanyl anaesthesia in dogs. Br J Anaesth 73:214-219, 1994.
199. Schultz JE, Hsu AK, Gross GJ: Morphine mimics the cardioprotective effect of ischemic preconditioning via a glibenclamide-sensitive mechanism in the rat heart. Circ Res 78:1100-1104, 1996.
200. McPherson BC, Yao Z: Signal transduction of opioid-induced cardioprotection in ischemia-reperfusion. Anesthesiology 94:1082-1088, 2001.
201. Kato R, Foex P: Fentanyl reduces infarction but not stunning via delta-opioid receptors and protein kinase C in rats. Br J Anaesth 84:608-614, 2000.
202. Kato R, Ross S, Foex P: Fentanyl protects the heart against ischaemic injury via opioid receptors, adenosine A1 receptors and KATP channel linked mechanisms in rats. Br J Anaesth 84:204-214, 2000.
203. Warltier DC, Pagel PS, Kersten JR: Approaches to the prevention of perioperative myocardial ischemia. Anesthesiology 92:253-259, 2000.
204. Helman JD, Leung JM, Bellows WH, et al: The risk of myocardial ischemia in patients receiving desflurane versus sufentanil anesthesia for coronary artery bypass graft surgery. The S.P.I. Research Group. Anesthesiology 77:47-62, 1992.
205. Leung JM, Goehner P, O'Kelly BF, et al: Isoflurane anesthesia and myocardial ischemia: Comparative risk versus sufentanil anesthesia in patients undergoing coronary artery bypass graft surgery. The SPI (Study of Perioperative Ischemia) Research Group. Anesthesiology 74:838-847, 1991.
206. Miller DR, Wellwood M, Teasdale SJ, et al: Effects of anesthetic induction on myocardial function and metabolism: A comparison of fentanyl, sufentanil and alfentanil. Can J Anaesth 35:219-233, 1988.
207. Slogoff S, Keats AS: Randomized trial of primary anesthetic agents on outcome of coronary artery bypass operations. Anesthesiology 70:179-188, 1989.
208. Blaise GA, Witzeling TM, Sill JC, et al: Fentanyl is devoid of major effects on coronary vasoreactivity and myocardial metabolism in experimental animals. Anesthesiology 72:535-541, 1990.
209. Yamanoue T, Brum JM, Estafanous FG, et al: Effects of opioids on vasoresponsiveness of porcine coronary artery. Anesth Analg 74:889-896, 1992.
210. Nauta J, Stanley TH, de Lange S, et al: Anaesthetic induction with alfentanil: Comparison with thiopental, midazolam, and etomidate. Can Anaesth Soc J 30:53-60, 1983.
211. Ebert TJ, Kotrly KJ, Madsen KE, et al: Fentanyl-diazepam anesthesia with or without N_2O does not attenuate cardiopulmonary baroreflex-mediated vasoconstrictor responses to controlled hypovolemia in humans. Anesth Analg 67:548-554, 1988.
212. Murat I, Levron JC, Berg A, Saint Maurice C: Effects of fentanyl on baroreceptor reflex control of heart rate in newborn infants. Anesthesiology 68:717-722, 1988.
213. Flacke JW, Flacke WE, Bloor BC, et al: Histamine release by four narcotics: A double-blind study in humans. Anesth Analg 66:723-730, 1987.
214. Moss J, Rosow CE: Histamine release by narcotics and muscle relaxants in humans. Anesthesiology 59:330-339, 1983.
215. Gaumann DM, Yaksh TL, Tyce GM, Lucas DL: Opioids preserve the adrenal medullary response evoked by severe hemorrhage: Studies on adrenal catecholamine and met-enkephalin secretion in halothane anesthetized cats. Anesthesiology 68:743-753, 1988.
216. White DA, Reitan JA, Kien ND, Thorup SJ: Decrease in vascular resistance in the isolated canine hind limb after graded doses of alfentanil, fentanyl, and sufentanil. Anesth Analg 71:29-34, 1990.
217. Chrousos GP, Gold PW: The concepts of stress and stress system disorders. Overview of physical and behavioral homeostasis. JAMA 267:1244-1252, 1992.
218. Anand KJ, Hansen DD, Hickey PR: Hormonal-metabolic stress responses in neonates undergoing cardiac surgery. Anesthesiology 73:661-670, 1990.
219. Delitala G, Trainer PJ, Oliva O, et al: Opioid peptide and alpha-adrenoceptor pathways in the regulation of the pituitary-adrenal axis in man. J Endocrinol 141:163-168, 1994.
220. Giesecke K, Hamberger B, Jarnberg PO, et al: High- and low-dose fentanyl anaesthesia: Hormonal and metabolic responses during cholecystectomy. Br J Anaesth 61:575-582, 1988.
221. Ellis DJ, Steward DJ: Fentanyl dosage is associated with reduced blood glucose in pediatric patients after hypothermic cardiopulmonary bypass. Anesthesiology 72:812-815, 1990.
222. Boulton AJ, Wilson N, Turnbull KW, Yip RW: Haemodynamic and plasma vasopressin responses during high-dose fentanyl or sufentanil anaesthesia. Can Anaesth Soc J 33:475-483, 1986.
223. Moller IW, Krantz T, Wandall E, Kehlet H: Effect of alfentanil anaesthesia on the adrenocortical and hyperglycaemic response to abdominal surgery. Br J Anaesth 57:591-594, 1985.
224. Yeager MP, Glass DD, Neff RK, Brinck Johnsen T: Epidural anesthesia and analgesia in high-risk surgical patients. Anesthesiology 66:729-736, 1987.
225. Anand KJ, Hickey PR: Halothane-morphine compared with high-dose sufentanil for anesthesia and postoperative analgesia in neonatal cardiac surgery. N Engl J Med 326:1-9, 1992.
226. Mangano DT, Siliciano D, Hollenberg M, et al: Postoperative myocardial ischemia. Therapeutic trials using intensive analgesia following surgery. The Study of Perioperative Ischemia (SPI) Research Group. Anesthesiology 76:342-353, 1992.
227. Tuman KJ, McCarthy RJ, Spiess BD, et al: Does choice of anesthetic agent significantly affect outcome after coronary artery surgery? Anesthesiology 70:189-198, 1989.
228. Plunkett JJ, Reeves JD, Ngo L, et al: Urine and plasma catecholamine and cortisol concentrations after myocardial revascularization. Modulation by continuous sedation. Multicenter Study of Perioperative Ischemia (McSPI) Research Group, and the Ischemia Research and Education Foundation (IREF). Anesthesiology 86:785-796, 1997.
229. Nestler EJ, Aghajanian GK: Molecular and cellular basis of addiction. Science 278:58-63, 1997.
230. Chan KW, Duttory A, Yoburn BC: Magnitude of tolerance to fentanyl is independent of mu-opioid receptor density. Eur J Pharmacol 319:225-228, 1997.
231. Maze M: Why does insensitivity to opioid narcotics develop? Anesthesiology 87:1033-1034, 1997.
232. Kissin I, Lee SS, Arthur GR, Bradley EL Jr: Time course characteristics of acute tolerance development to continuously infused alfentanil in rats. Anesth Analg 83:600-605, 1996.
233. Kissin I, Brown PT, Robinson CA, Bradley EL Jr: Acute tolerance in morphine analgesia: continuous infusion and single injection in rats. Anesthesiology 74:166-171, 1991.
234. Chia YY, Liu K, Wang JJ, et al: Intraoperative high dose fentanyl induces postoperative fentanyl tolerance. Can J Anaesth 46:872-877, 1999.
235. Vinik HR, Kissin I: Rapid development of tolerance to analgesia during remifentanil infusion in humans. Anesth Analg 86:1307-1311, 1998.

236. Guignard B, Bossard AE, Coste C, et al: Acute opioid tolerance: Intraoperative remifentanil increases postoperative pain and morphine requirement. Anesthesiology 93:409-417, 2000.

237. Schraag S, Checketts MR, Kenny GN: Lack of rapid development of opioid tolerance during alfentanil and remifentanil infusions for postoperative pain. Anesth Analg 89:753-757, 1999.

238. Gustorff B, Nahlik G, Hoerauf KH, Kress HG: The absence of acute tolerance during remifentanil infusion in volunteers. Anesth Analg 94:1223-1228, 2002.

239. Celerier E, Rivat C, Jun Y, et al: Long-lasting hyperalgesia induced by fentanyl in rats: Preventive effect of ketamine. Anesthesiology 92:465-472, 2000.

240. Mao J, Price DD, Mayer DJ: Mechanisms of hyperalgesia and morphine tolerance: A current view of their possible interactions. Pain 62:259-274, 1995.

241. Li X, Angst MS, Clark JD: Opioid-induced hyperalgesia and incisional pain. Anesth Analg 93:204-209, 2001.

242. Li X, Clark JD: Hyperalgesia during opioid abstinence: Mediation by glutamate and substance p. Anesth Analg 95:979-984, 2002.

243. Kissin I, Bright CA, Bradley EL Jr: Acute tolerance to continuously infused alfentanil: The role of cholecystokinin and N-methyl-D-aspartate-nitric oxide systems. Anesth Analg 91:110-116, 2000.

244. Li JY, Wong CH, Huang EY, et al: Modulations of spinal serotonin activity affect the development of morphine tolerance. Anesth Analg 92:1563-1568, 2001.

245. Laulin JP, Maurette P, Corcuff JB, et al: The role of ketamine in preventing fentanyl-induced hyperalgesia and subsequent acute morphine tolerance. Anesth Analg 94: 1263-1269, 2002.

246. Kissin I, Bright CA, Bradley EL Jr: The effect of ketamine on opioid-induced acute tolerance: Can it explain reduction of opioid consumption with ketamine-opioid analgesic combinations? Anesth Analg 91:1483-1488, 2000.

247. Stein C, Pfluger M, Yassouridis A, et al: No tolerance to peripheral morphine analgesia in presence of opioid expression in inflamed synovia. J Clin Invest 98:793-799, 1996.

248. Duttaroy A, Yoburn BC: The effect of intrinsic efficacy on opioid tolerance. Anesthesiology 82:1226-1236, 1995.

249. Ouellet DM, Pollack GM: Pharmacodynamics and tolerance development during multiple intravenous bolus morphine administration in rats. J Pharmacol Exp Ther 281:713-720, 1997.

250. Hanks GW, Forbes K: Opioid responsiveness. Acta Anaesthesiol Scand 41:154-158, 1997.

251. Kienbaum P, Thurauf N, Michel MC, et al: Profound increase in plasma concentration in plasma and cardiovascular stimulation after mu-opioid receptor blockade in opioid-addicted patients during barbiturate-induced anesthesia for acute detoxification. Anesthesiology 88:1154-1161, 1998.

252. Hensel M, Wolter S, Kox WJ: EEG controlled rapid opioid withdrawal under general anaesthesia. Br J Anaesth 84:236-238, 2000.

253. Kienbaum P, Heuter T, Michel MC, et al: Sympathetic neural activation evoked by mu-receptor blockade in patients addicted to opioids is abolished by intravenous clonidine. Anesthesiology 96:346-351, 2002.

254. Salas SP, Roblero JS, Lopez LF, et al: [N-methyl-Tyr1, N-methyl-Arg7-D-Leu8]-dynorphin-A-(1-8)ethylamide, a stable dynorphin analog, produces diuresis by kappa-opiate receptor activation in the rat. J Pharmacol Exp Ther 262:979-986, 1992.

255. Pesonen A, Leppaluoto J, Ruskoaho H: Mechanism of opioid-induced atrial natriuretic peptide release in conscious rats. J Pharmacol Exp Ther 254:690-695, 1990.

256. Kien ND, Reitan JA, White DA, et al: Hemodynamic responses to alfentanil in halothane-anesthetized dogs. Anesth Analg 65:765-770, 1986.

257. Drenger B, Magora F: Urodynamic studies after intrathecal fentanyl and buprenorphine in the dog. Anesth Analg 69:348-353, 1989.

258. Malinovsky JM, Le Normand L, Lepage JY, et al: The urodynamic effects of intravenous opioids and ketoprofen in humans. Anesth Analg 87:456-461, 1998.

259. Murphy DB, Sutton JA, Prescott LF, Murphy MB: Opioid-induced delay in gastric emptying: a peripheral mechanism in humans. Anesthesiology 87:765-770, 1997.

260. Kojima Y, Takahashi T, Fujina M, Owyang C: Inhibition of cholinergic transmission by opiates in ileal myenteric plexus is mediated by kappa receptor. Involvement of regulatory inhibitory G protein and calcium N-channels. J Pharmacol Exp Ther 268:965-970, 1994.

261. Dowlatshahi K, Evander A, Walther B, Skinner DB: Influence of morphine on the distal oesophagus and the lower oesophageal sphincter—a manometric study. Gut 26:802-806, 1985.

262. Schurizek BA, Willacy LH, Kraglund K, et al: Antroduodenal motility, pH and gastric emptying during balanced anaesthesia: Comparison of pethidine and fentanyl. Br J Anaesth 62:674-682, 1989.

263. Crighton IM, Martin PH, Hobbs GJ, et al: A comparison of the effects of intravenous tramadol, codeine, and morphine on gastric emptying in human volunteers. Anesth Analg 87:445-449, 1998.

264. Yukioka H, Tanaka M, Fujimori M: Recovery of bowel motility after high dose fentanyl or morphine anaesthesia for cardiac surgery. Anaesthesia 45:353-356, 1990.

265. Thorn SE, Wickbom G, Philipson L, et al: Myoelectric activity in the stomach and duodenum after epidural administration of morphine or bupivacaine. Acta Anaesthesiol Scand 40:773-778, 1996.

266. McNeill MJ, Ho ET, Kenny GN: Effect of i.v. metoclopramide on gastric emptying after opioid premedication. Br J Anaesth 64:450-452, 1990.

267. Vatashsky E, Haskel Y, Nissan S, Hanani M: Effect of morphine on the mechanical activity of common bile duct isolated from the guinea pig. Anesth Analg 66:245-248, 1987.

268. Goldberg M, Vatashsky E, Haskel Y, et al: The effect of meperidine on the guinea pig extrahepatic biliary tract. Anesth Analg 66:1282-1286, 1987.

269. Fisher DM: The "big little problem" of postoperative nausea and vomiting: Do we know the answer yet? Anesthesiology 87:1271-1273, 1997.

270. Tramer MR, Reynolds DJ, Moore RA, McQuay HJ: Efficacy, dose-response, and safety of ondansetron in prevention of postoperative nausea and vomiting: A quantitative systematic review of randomized placebo-controlled trials. Anesthesiology 87:1277-1289, 1997.

271. Watcha MF, White PF: Postoperative nausea and vomiting. Its etiology, treatment, and prevention. Anesthesiology 77:162-184, 1992.

272. Langevin S, Lessard MR, Trepanier CA, Baribault JP: Alfentanil causes less postoperative nausea and vomiting than equipotent doses of fentanyl or sufentanil in outpatients. Anesthesiology 91:1666-1673, 1999.

273. Raftery S, Sherry E: Total intravenous anaesthesia with propofol and alfentanil protects against postoperative nausea and vomiting. Can J Anaesth 39:37-40, 1992.

274. Rung GW, Claybon L, Hord A, et al: Intravenous ondansetron for postsurgical opioid-induced nausea and vomiting. S3A-255 Study Group. Anesth Analg 84:832-838, 1997.

275. Simoneau, II, Hamza MS, Mata HP, et al: The cannabinoid agonist WIN55,212-2 suppresses opioid-induced emesis in ferrets. Anesthesiology 94:882-887, 2001.

276. Bruce DL, Hinkley R, Norman PF: Fentanyl does not inhibit fertilization or early development of sea urchin eggs. Anesth Analg 64:498-500, 1985.

277. Fujinaga M, Mazze RI, Jackson EC, Baden JM: Reproductive and teratogenic effects of sufentanil and alfentanil in Sprague-Dawley rats. Anesth Analg 67:166-169, 1988.

278. Sandner-Kiesling A, Eisenach JC: Pharmacology of opioid inhibition to noxious uterine cervical distension. Anesthesiology 97:966-971, 2002.

279. Sandner-Kiesling A, Eisenach JC: Estrogen reduces efficacy of mu- but not kappa-opioid agonist inhibition in response

to uterine cervical distension. Anesthesiology 96:375-379, 2002.

280. Gin T, Ngan Kee WD, Siu YK, et al: Alfentanil given immediately before the induction of anesthesia for elective cesarean delivery. Anesth Analg 90:1167-1172, 2000.

281. Sivalingam T, Pleuvry BJ: Actions of morphine, pethidine and pentazocine on the oestrus and pregnant rat uterus in vitro. Br J Anaesth 57:430-433, 1985.

282. Rayburn W, Rathke A, Leuschen MP, et al: Fentanyl citrate analgesia during labor. Am J Obstet Gynecol 161:202-206, 1989.

283. Wittels B, Scott DT, Sinatra RS: Exogenous opioids in human breast milk and acute neonatal neurobehavior: A preliminary study. Anesthesiology 73:864-869, 1990.

284. Spigset O: Anaesthetic agents and excretion in breast milk. Acta Anaesthesiol Scand 38:94-103, 1994.

285. Doberczak TM, Kandall SR, Wilets I: Neonatal opiate abstinence syndrome in term and preterm infants. J Pediatr 118:933-937, 1991.

286. Levy JH, Brister NW, Shearin A, et al: Wheal and flare responses to opioids in humans. Anesthesiology 70:756-760, 1989.

287. Alexander R, Hill R, Lipham WJ, et al: Remifentanil prevents an increase in intraocular pressure after succinylcholine and tracheal intubation. Br J Anaesth 81:606-607, 1998.

288. Ng HP, Chen FG, Yeong SM, et al: Effect of remifentanil compared with fentanyl on intraocular pressure after succinylcholine and tracheal intubation. Br J Anaesth 85:785-787, 2000.

289. Stefano GB, Scharrer B, Smith EM, et al: Opioid and opiate immunoregulatory processes. Crit Rev Immunol 16:109-144, 1996.

290. Nelson CJ, Dykstra LA, Lysle DT: Comparison of the time course of morphine's analgesic and immunologic effects. Anesth Analg 85:620-626, 1997.

291. Sacerdote P, Bianchi M, Gaspani L, et al: The effects of tramadol and morphine on immune responses and pain after surgery in cancer patients. Anesth Analg 90:1411-1414, 2000.

292. Yeager MP, Procopio MA, DeLeo JA, et al: Intravenous fentanyl increases natural killer cell cytotoxicity and circulating CD16+ lymphocytes in humans. Anesth Analg 94:94-99, 2002.

293. Welters ID, Menzebach A, Goumon Y, et al: Morphine inhibits NF-kappa B nuclear binding in human neutrophils and monocytes by a nitric oxide-dependent mechanism. Anesthesiology 92:1677-1684, 2000.

294. Gourlay GK, Kowalski SR, Plummer JL, et al: Fentanyl blood concentration-analgesic response relationship in the treatment of postoperative pain. Anesth Analg 67:329-337, 1988.

295. Egan TD: Pharmacokinetics and rational intravenous drug selection and administration in anesthesia. Adv Anesth 12:363, 1995.

296. Roerig DL, Kotrly KJ, Vucins EJ, et al: First pass uptake of fentanyl, meperidine, and morphine in the human lung. Anesthesiology 67:466-472, 1987.

297. Boer F, Bovill JG, Burm AG, Mooren RA: Uptake of sufentanil, alfentanil and morphine in the lungs of patients about to undergo coronary artery surgery. Br J Anaesth 68:370-375, 1992.

298. Mazoit JX, Sandouk P, Scherrmann JM, Roche A: Extrahepatic metabolism of morphine occurs in humans. Clin Pharmacol Ther 48:613-618, 1990.

299. Merrell WJ, Gordon L, Wood AJ, et al: The effect of halothane on morphine disposition: relative contributions of the liver and kidney to morphine glucuronidation in the dog. Anesthesiology 72:308-314, 1990.

300. Portenoy RK, Thaler HT, Inturrisi CE, et al: The metabolite morphine-6-glucuronide contributes to the analgesia produced by morphine infusion in patients with pain and normal renal function. Clin Pharmacol Ther 51:422-431, 1992.

301. Lotsch J, Zimmermann M, Darimont J, et al: Does the A118G polymorphism at the mu-opioid receptor gene protect against morphine-6-glucuronide toxicity? Anesthesiology 97:814-819, 2002.

302. Osborne R, Joel S, Trew D, Slevin M: Morphine and metabolite behavior after different routes of morphine administration: demonstration of the importance of the active metabolite morphine-6-glucuronide. Clin Pharmacol Ther 47:12-9, 1990.

303. Lotsch J, Kobal G, Stockmann A, et al: Lack of analgesic activity of morphine-6-glucuronide after short-term intravenous administration in healthy volunteers. Anesthesiology 87:1348-1358, 1997.

304. Motamed C, Mazoit X, Ghanouchi K, et al: Preemptive intravenous morphine-6-glucuronide is ineffective for postoperative pain relief. Anesthesiology 92:55-360, 2000.

305. Taeger K, Weninger E, Schmelzer F, et al: Pulmonary kinetics of fentanyl and alfentanil in surgical patients. Br J Anaesth 61:425-434, 1988.

306. Meuldermans WE, Hurkmans RM, Heykants JJ: Plasma protein binding and distribution of fentanyl, sufentanil, alfentanil and lofentanil in blood. Arch Int Pharmacodyn Ther 257:4-19, 1982.

307. Shafer A, Sung ML, White PF: Pharmacokinetics and pharmacodynamics of alfentanil infusions during general anesthesia. Anesth Analg 65:1021-1028, 1986.

308. Bovill JG, Sebel PS, Blackburn CL, Heykants J: The pharmacokinetics of alfentanil (R39209): A new opioid analgesic. Anesthesiology 57:439-443, 1982.

309. Camu F, Gepts E, Rucquoi M, Heykants J: Pharmacokinetics of alfentanil in man. Anesth Analg 61:657-661, 1982.

310. Meuldermans W, Hendrickx J, Lauwers W, et al: Excretion and biotransformation of alfentanil and sufentanil in rats and dogs. Drug Metab Dispos 15:905-913, 1987.

311. Kharasch ED, Thummel KE: Human alfentanil metabolism by cytochrome P450 3A3/4. An explanation for the interindividual variability in alfentanil clearance? Anesth Analg 76:1033-1039, 1993.

312. Hudson RJ, Bergstrom RG, Thomson IR, et al: Pharmacokinetics of sufentanil in patients undergoing abdominal aortic surgery. Anesthesiology 70:426-431, 1989.

313. Gepts E, Shafer SL, Camu F, et al: Linearity of pharmacokinetics and model estimation of sufentanil. Anesthesiology 83:1194-204, 1005.

314. Lavrijsen K, Van Houdt J, Van Dyck D, et al: Biotransformation of sufentanil in liver microsomes of rats, dogs, and humans. Drug Metab Dispos 18:704-710, 1990.

315. Egan TD, Lemmens HJ, Fiset P, et al: The pharmacokinetics of the new short-acting opioid remifentanil (GI87084B) in healthy adult male volunteers. Anesthesiology 79:881-892, 1993.

316. Westmoreland CL, Hoke JF, Sebel PS, et al: Pharmacokinetics of remifentanil (GI87084B) and its major metabolite (GI90291) in patients undergoing elective inpatient surgery. Anesthesiology 79:893-903, 1993.

317. Duthie DJ, Stevens JJ, Doyle AR, et al: Remifentanil and pulmonary extraction during and after cardiac anesthesia. Anesth Analg 84:740-744, 1997.

318. Buerkle H, Yaksh TL: Continuous intrathecal administration of shortlasting mu opioids remifentanil and alfentanil in the rat. Anesthesiology 84:926-935, 1996.

319. Egan TD: Remifentanil pharmacokinetics and pharmacodynamics. A preliminary appraisal. Clin Pharmacokinet 29:80-94, 1995.

320. Cox EH, Langemeijer MW, Gubbens-Stibbe JM, et al: The comparative pharmacodynamics of remifentanil and its metabolite, GR90291, in a rat electroencephalographic model. Anesthesiology 90:535-444, 1999.

321. Dershwitz M, Hoke JF, Rosow CE, et al: Pharmacokinetics and pharmacodynamics of remifentanil in volunteer subjects with severe liver disease. Anesthesiology 84:812-820, 1996.

322. Hoke JF, Shlugman D, Dershwitz M, et al: Pharmacokinetics and pharmacodynamics of remifentanil in persons with renal failure compared with healthy volunteers. Anesthesiology 87:533-541, 1997.

323. Stiller RL, Davis PJ, McGowan FX, et al: In vitro metabolism of remifentanil: The effects of pseudocholinesterase deficiency. Anesthesiology 83:A381, 1995.

324. Shafer SL, Stanski DR: Improving the clinical utility of anesthetic drug pharmacokinetics. Anesthesiology 76:327-330, 1992.

325. Hughes MA, Glass PS, Jacobs JR: Context-sensitive half-time in multicompartment pharmacokinetic models for intravenous anesthetic drugs. Anesthesiology 76:334-341, 1992.

326. Youngs EJ, Shafer SL: Pharmacokinetic parameters relevant to recovery from opioids. Anesthesiology 81:833-842, 1994.

327. Vuyk J, Mertens MJ, Olofsen E, et al: Propofol anesthesia and rational opioid selection: Determination of optimal EC50-EC95 propofol-opioid concentrations that assure adequate anesthesia and a rapid return of consciousness. Anesthesiology 87:1549-1562, 1997.

328. Metz C, Gobel L, Gruber M, et al: Pharmacokinetics of human cerebral opioid extraction: A comparative study on sufentanil, fentanyl, and alfentanil in a patient after severe head injury. Anesthesiology 92:1559-1567, 2000.

329. Shafer SL, Varvel JR: Pharmacokinetics, pharmacodynamics, and rational opioid selection. Anesthesiology 74:53-63, 1991.

330. Bailey JM: Technique for quantifying the duration of intravenous anesthetic effect. Anesthesiology 83:1095-1103, 1995.

331. Egan TD: Intravenous drug delivery systems: toward an intravenous "vaporizer." J Clin Anesth (Suppl 2):8-14, 1996.

332. Olkkola KT, Hamunen K, Maunuksela EL: Clinical pharmacokinetics and pharmacodynamics of opioid analgesics in infants and children. Clin Pharmacokinet 28:385-404, 1995.

333. Mannering GJ: Drug metabolism in the newborn. Fed Proc 44:2302-2308, 1985.

334. Scott JC, Stanski DR: Decreased fentanyl and alfentanil dose requirements with age. A simultaneous pharmacokinetic and pharmacodynamic evaluation. J Pharmacol Exp Ther 240:159-166, 1987.

335. Minto CF, Schnider TW, Egan TD, et al: Influence of age and gender on the pharmacokinetics and pharmacodynamics of remifentanil. I. Model development. Anesthesiology 86:10-23, 1997.

336. Maitre PO, Vozeh S, Heykants J, et al: Population pharmacokinetics of alfentanil: The average dose-plasma concentration relationship and interindividual variability in patients. Anesthesiology 66:3-12, 1987.

337. Egan TD, Huizinga B, Gupta SK, et al: Remifentanil pharmacokinetics in obese versus lean patients. Anesthesiology 89:562-573, 1998.

338. Davies G, Kingswood C, Street M: Pharmacokinetics of opioids in renal dysfunction. Clin Pharmacokinet 31:410-422, 1996.

339. Osborne R, Joel S, Grebenik K, et al: The pharmacokinetics of morphine and morphine glucuronides in kidney failure. Clin Pharmacol Ther 54:158-167, 1993.

340. Schochet RB, Murray GB: Neuropsychiatric toxicity of meperidine. J Intensive Care Med 3:246, 1988.

341. Davis PJ, Stiller RL, Cook DR, et al: Pharmacokinetics of sufentanil in adolescent patients with chronic renal failure. Anesth Analg 67:268-271, 1988.

342. Chauvin M, Lebrault C, Levron JC, Duvaldestin P: Pharmacokinetics of alfentanil in chronic renal failure. Anesth Analg 66:53-56, 1987.

343. Haberer JP, Schoeffler P, Couderc E, Duvaldestin P: Fentanyl pharmacokinetics in anaesthetized patients with cirrhosis. Br J Anaesth 54:1267-1270, 1982.

344. Ferrier C, Marty J, Bouffard Y, Haberer JP, et al: Alfentanil pharmacokinetics in patients with cirrhosis. Anesthesiology 62:480-484, 1985.

345. Chauvin M, Bonnet F, Montembault C, et al: The influence of hepatic plasma flow on alfentanil plasma concentration plateaus achieved with an infusion model in humans: Measurement of alfentanil hepatic extraction coefficient. Anesth Analg 65:999-1003, 1986.

346. Hudson RJ, Thomson IR, Burgess PM, Rosenbloom M: Alfentanil pharmacokinetics in patients undergoing abdominal aortic surgery. Can J Anaesth 38:61-67, 1991.

347. Navapurkar VU, Archer S, Frazer NM, et al: Pharmacokinetics of remifentanil during hepatic transplantation. Anesthesiology 83:A382, 1995.

348. Dumont L, Picard V, Marti RA, Tassonyi E: Use of remifentanil in a patient with chronic hepatic failure. Br J Anaesth 81:265-267, 1998.

349. Gedney JA, Ghosh S: Pharmacokinetics of analgesics, sedatives and anaesthetic agents during cardiopulmonary bypass. Br J Anaesth 75:344-351, 1995.

350. Kentala E, Kaila T, Arola M, et al: Pharmacokinetics and clinical response of hyoscine plus morphine premedication in connection with cardiopulmonary bypass surgery. Eur J Anaesthesiol 8:135-140, 1991.

351. Lunn JK, Stanley TH, Eisele J, et al: High dose fentanyl anesthesia for coronary artery surgery: Plasma fentanyl concentrations and influence of nitrous oxide on cardiovascular responses. Anesth Analg 58:390-395, 1878.

352. Skacel M, Knott C, Reynolds F, Aps C: Extracorporeal circuit sequestration of fentanyl and alfentanil. Br J Anaesth 58:947-949, 1986.

353. Okutani R, Philbin DM, Rosow CE, et al: Effect of hypothermic hemodilutional cardiopulmonary bypass on plasma sufentanil and catecholamine concentrations in humans. Anesth Analg 67:667-670, 1988.

354. Hug CC Jr, Burm AG, de Lange S: Alfentanil pharmacokinetics in cardiac surgical patients. Anesth Analg 78:231-239, 1994.

355. Hynynen M, Hynninen M, Soini H, et al: Plasma concentration and protein binding of alfentanil during high-dose infusion for cardiac surgery. Br J Anaesth 72:571-576, 1994.

356. Lullmann H, Martins BS, Peters T: pH-dependent accumulation of fentanyl, lofentanil and alfentanil by beating guinea pig atria. Br J Anaesth 57:1012-1017, 1985.

357. Egan TD, Kuramkote S, Gong G, et al: Fentanyl pharmacokinetics in hemorrhagic shock: A porcine model. Anesthesiology 91:156-166, 1999.

358. Johnson KB, Kern SE, Hamber EA, et al: Influence of hemorrhagic shock on remifentanil: A pharmacokinetic and pharmacodynamic analysis. Anesthesiology 2001; 94:322-332, 2001.

359. Katz J, Clairoux M, Redahan C, et al: High dose alfentanil pre-empts pain after abdominal hysterectomy. Pain 68:109-118, 1996.

360. Woolf CJ, Chong MS: Preemptive analgesia—treating postoperative pain by preventing the establishment of central sensitization. Anesth Analg 77:362-379, 1993.

361. Gottschalk A, Smith DS, Jobes DR, et al: Preemptive epidural analgesia and recovery from radical prostatectomy: A randomized controlled trial. JAMA 279:1076-1082, 1998.

362. Wasylak TJ, Abbott FV, English MJ, Jeans ME: Reduction of postoperative morbidity following patient-controlled morphine. Can J Anaesth 37:726-731, 1990.

363. Upton RN, Semple TJ, Macintyre PE: Pharmacokinetic optimisation of opioid treatment in acute pain therapy. Clin Pharmacokinet 33:2252-2244, 1997.

364. Plummer JL, Owen H, Ilsley AH, Inglis S: Morphine patient-controlled analgesia is superior to meperidine patient-controlled analgesia for postoperative pain. Anesth Analg 84:794-799, 1997.

365. Andrews DT, Leslie K, Sessler DI, Bjorksten AR: The arterial blood propofol concentration preventing movement in 50% of healthy women after skin incision. Anesth Analg 85:414-419, 1997.

366. Ebert JP, Pearson JD, Gelman S, et al: Circulatory responses to laryngoscopy: The comparative effects of placebo, fentanyl and esmolol. Can J Anaesth 36:301-306, 1989.

367. Vuyk J, Engbers FH, Burm AG, et al: Pharmacodynamic interaction between propofol and alfentanil when given for induction of anesthesia. Anesthesiology 84:288-299, 1996.

368. Billard V, Moulla F, Bourgain JL, et al: Hemodynamic response to induction and intubation. Propofol/fentanyl interaction. Anesthesiology 81:1384-1393, 1994.

369. Kazama T, Ikeda K, Morita K: Reduction by fentanyl of the Cp50 values of propofol and hemodynamic responses to various noxious stimuli. Anesthesiology 87:213-227, 1997.

370. Smith C, McEwan AI, Jhaveri R, et al: The interaction of fentanyl on the Cp50 of propofol for loss of consciousness and skin incision. Anesthesiology 81:820-828, 1994.

371. Van Aken H, Meinshausen E, Prien T, et al: The influence of fentanyl and tracheal intubation on the hemodynamic effects of anesthesia induction with propofol/N₂O in humans. Anesthesiology 68:157-163, 1988.

372. Katoh T, Uchiyama T, Ikeda K: Effect of fentanyl on awakening concentration of sevoflurane. Br J Anaesth 73:322-325, 1994.

373. White PF, Coe V, Shafer A, Sung ML: Comparison of alfentanil with fentanyl for outpatient anesthesia. Anesthesiology 64:99-106, 1986.

374. From RP, Warner DS, Todd MM, Sokoll MD: Anesthesia for craniotomy: a double-blind comparison of alfentanil, fentanyl, and sufentanil. Anesthesiology 73:896-904, 1990.

375. Kuperwasser B, Dahl M, McSweeney TD, Howie MB: Comparison of alfentanil and sufentanil in the ambulatory surgery procedure when used in balanced anesthesia technique. Anesth Analg 67:S122, 1988.

376. Glass PS, Doherty M, Jacobs JR, et al: Plasma concentration of fentanyl, with 70% nitrous oxide, to prevent movement at skin incision. Anesthesiology 78:842-847, 1993.

377. Glass PS, Doherty M, Jacobs JR, et al: Cₚ50 for sufentanil. Anesthesiology 73:A378, 1990.

378. Thomson IR, Henderson BT, Singh K, Hudson RJ: Concentration-response relationships for fentanyl and sufentanil in patients undergoing coronary artery bypass grafting. Anesthesiology 89:852-861, 1998.

379. Marty J, Couderc E, Servin F, et al: Plasma concentration of sufentanil required to suppress hemodynamic responses to noxious stimuli during nitrous oxide anesthesia. Anesthesiology 69:A631, 1988.

380. Patel SS, Spencer CM: Remifentanil. Drugs 52:417-427, 1996.

381. Hogue CW Jr, Bowdle TA, O'Leary C, et al: A multicenter evaluation of total intravenous anesthesia with remifentanil and propofol for elective inpatient surgery. Anesth Analg 83:2792-85, 1996.

382. Avramov MN, Smith I, White PF: Interactions between midazolam and remifentanil during monitored anesthesia care. Anesthesiology 85:1283-1289, 1996.

383. Sneyd JR, Whaley A, Dimpel HL, Andrews CJ: An open, randomized comparison of alfentanil, remifentanil and alfentanil followed by remifentanil in anaesthesia for craniotomy. Br J Anaesth 81:361-364, 1998.

384. Fletcher D, Pinaud M, Scherpereel P, et al: The efficacy of intravenous 0.15 versus 0.25 mg/kg intraoperative morphine for immediate postoperative analgesia after remifentanil-based anesthesia for major surgery. Anesth Analg 90:666-671, 2000.

385. Kochs E, Cote D, Deruyck L, et al: Postoperative pain management and recovery after remifentanil-based anaesthesia with isoflurane or propofol for major abdominal surgery. Remifentanil Study Group. Br J Anaesth 84:169-173, 2000.

386. Guignard B, Coste C, Costes H, et al: Supplementing desflurane-remifentanil anesthesia with small-dose ketamine reduces perioperative opioid analgesic requirements. Anesth Analg 95:103-108, 2002.

387. Eltzschig HK, Schroeder TH, Eissler BJ, et al: The effect of remifentanil or fentanyl on postoperative vomiting and pain in children undergoing strabismus surgery. Anesth Analg 94:1173-1177, 2002.

388. Calderon E, Pernia A, De Antonio P, et al: A comparison of two constant-dose continuous infusions of remifentanil for severe postoperative pain. Anesth Analg 92:715-771, 2001.

389. Ausems ME, Vuyk J, Hug CC Jr, Stanski DR: Comparison of a computer-assisted infusion versus intermittent bolus administration of alfentanil as a supplement to nitrous oxide for lower abdominal surgery. Anesthesiology 68:851-861, 1988.

390. Vinik HR, Bradley EL Jr, Kissin I: Triple anesthetic combination: propofol-midazolam-alfentanil. Anesth Analg 78:354-358, 1994.

391. Vuyk J, Lim T, Engbers FH, Burm AG, et al: The pharmaco-dynamic interaction of propofol and alfentanil during lower abdominal surgery in women. Anesthesiology 83:8-22, 1995.

392. Stanski DR, Shafer SL: Quantifying anesthetic drug interaction. Implications for drug dosing. Anesthesiology 83:1-5, 1995.

393. Richards MJ, Skues MA, Jarvis AP, Prys Roberts C: Total i.v. anaesthesia with propofol and alfentanil: Dose requirements for propofol and the effect of premedication with clonidine. Br J Anaesth 65:157-163, 1990.

394. Wuesten R, Van Aken H, Glass PS, Buerkle H: Assessment of depth of anesthesia and postoperative respiratory recovery after remifentanil- versus alfentanil-based total intravenous anesthesia in patients undergoing ear-nose-throat surgery. Anesthesiology 94:211-217, 2001.

395. Vuyk J, Hennis PJ, Burm AG, et al: Comparison of midazolam and propofol in combination with alfentanil for total intravenous anesthesia. Anesth Analg 71:645-650, 1990.

396. Raza SM, Masters RW, Vasireddy AR, Zsigmond EK: Haemodynamic stability with midazolam-sufentanil analgesia in cardiac surgical patients. Can J Anaesth 35:518-525, 1988.

397. Bell J, Sartain J, Wilkinson GA, Sherry KM: Propofol and fentanyl anaesthesia for patients with low cardiac output state undergoing cardiac surgery: comparison with high-dose fentanyl anaesthesia. Br J Anaesth 73:162-166, 1994.

398. Benthuysen JL, Foltz BD, Smith NT, et al: Prebypass hemodynamic stability of sufentanil-O₂, fentanyl-O₂, and morphine-O₂ anesthesia during cardiac surgery: A comparison of cardiovascular profiles. J Cardiothorac Anesth 12:749-757, 1988.

399. Sanford TJ Jr, Smith NT, Dec Silver H, Harrison WK: A comparison of morphine, fentanyl, and sufentanil anesthesia for cardiac surgery: induction, emergence, and extubation. Anesth Analg 65:259-66, 1986.

400. Weiss Bloom LJ, Reich DL: Haemodynamic responses to tracheal intubation following etomidate and fentanyl for anaesthetic induction. Can J Anaesth 39:780-785, 1992.

401. Howie MB, Black HA, Romanelli VA, et al: A comparison of isoflurane versus fentanyl as primary anesthetics for mitral valve surgery. Anesth Analg 83:941-948, 1996.

402. Walter RR, Kim YD, Macnamara TE, et al: Comparison of isoflurane vs. fentanyl anesthesia in ligation of the patent ductus arteriosus in premature infants. Anesth Analg 65:S165, 1986.

403. Glenski JA, Friesen RH, Berglund NL, Henry DB: Comparison of the cardiovascular effects of sufentanil, fentanyl, isoflurane and halothane during pediatric cardiac surgery. Anesthesiology 65:A438, 1986.

404. Duncan HP, Cloote A, Weir PM, et al: Reducing stress responses in the pre-bypass phase of open heart surgery in infants and young children: a comparison of different fentanyl doses. Br J Anaesth 84:556-564, 2000.

405. Beilin B, Shavit Y, Hart J, et al: Effects of anesthesia based on large versus small doses of fentanyl on natural killer cell cytotoxicity in the perioperative period. Anesth Analg 82:492-497, 1996.

406. Mantz J, Abi Jaoude F, Ceddaha A, et al: High-dose alfentanil for myocardial revascularization: A hemodynamic and pharmacokinetic study. J Cardiothorac Vasc Anesth 5:107-110, 1991.

407. Jhaveri R, Joshi P, Batenhorst R, et al: Dose comparison of remifentanil and alfentanil for loss of consciousness. Anesthesiology 87:253-259, 1997.

408. Roekaerts PM, Gerrits HJ, Timmerman BE, de Lange S: Continuous infusions of alfentanil and propofol for coronary artery surgery. J Cardiothorac Vasc Anesth 9:362-3367, 1995.

409. Howie MB, Smith DF, Reilley TE, et al: Postoperative course after sufentanil or fentanyl anesthesia for coronary artery surgery. J Cardiothorac Vasc Anesth 5:485-489, 1991.

410. Sareen J, Hudson RJ, Rosenbloom M, Thomson IR: Dose-response to anaesthetic induction with sufentanil: Haemodynamic and electroencephalographic effects. Can J Anaesth 44:19-25, 1997.

411. Abrams JT, Horrow JC, Bennett JA, et al: Upper airway closure: A primary source of difficult ventilation with sufentanil induction of anesthesia. Anesth Analg 83:629-632, 1996.

412. Jain U, Body SC, Bellows W, et al: Multicenter study of target-controlled infusion of propofol-sufentanil or sufentanil-midazolam for coronary artery bypass graft surgery. Multicenter Study of Perioperative Ischemia (McSPI) Research Group. Anesthesiology 85:522-535, 1996.

413. Russell D, Royston D, Rees PH, et al: Effect of temperature and cardiopulmonary bypass on the pharmacokinetics of remifentanil. Br J Anaesth 79:456-459, 1997.

414. Michelsen LG, Holford NH, Lu W, et al: The pharmacokinetics of remifentanil in patients undergoing coronary artery bypass grafting with cardiopulmonary bypass. Anesth Analg 93:1100-1105, 2001.

415. Ahonen J, Olkkola KT, Verkkala K, et al: A comparison of remifentanil and alfentanil for use with propofol in patients undergoing minimally invasive coronary artery bypass surgery. Anesth Analg 90:1269-1274, 2000.

416. Engoren M, Luther G, Fenn Buderer N: A comparison of fentanyl, sufentanil, and remifentanil for fast-track cardiac anesthesia. Anesth Analg 93:859-864, 2001.

417. Duthie DJ, Rowbotham DJ, Wyld R, et al: Plasma fentanyl concentrations during transdermal delivery of fentanyl to surgical patients. Br J Anaesth 60:614-618, 1988.

418. Sandler AN, Baxter AD, Katz J, et al: A double-blind, placebo-controlled trial of transdermal fentanyl after abdominal hysterectomy. Analgesic, respiratory, and pharmacokinetic effects. Anesthesiology 81:1169-1180, 1994.

419. Varvel JR, Shafer SL, Hwang SS, et al: Absorption characteristics of transdermally administered fentanyl. Anesthesiology 70:928-934, 1989.

420. Rowbotham DJ, Wyld R, Peacock JE, et al: Transdermal fentanyl for the relief of pain after upper abdominal surgery. Br J Anaesth 63:56-59, 1989.

421. Ashburn MA, Streisand J, Zhang J, et al: The iontophoresis of fentanyl citrate in humans. Anesthesiology 82:1146-1153, 1995.

422. Moa G, Zetterstrom H: Sublingual buprenorphine as postoperative analgesic: A double-blind comparison with pethidine. Acta Anaesthesiol Scand 34:68-71, 1990.

423. Bell MD, Murray GR, Mishra P, et al: Buccal morphine—a new route for analgesia? Lancet 1:71-73, 1985.

424. Fisher AP, Vine P, Whitlock J, Hanna M: Buccal morphine premedication. A double-blind comparison with intramuscular morphine. Anaesthesia 41:1104-1111, 1986.

425. Weinberg DS, Inturrisi CE, Reidenberg B, et al: Sublingual absorption of selected opioid analgesics. Clin Pharmacol Ther 44:335-342, 1988.

426. Stanley TH, Hague B, Mock DL, et al: Oral transmucosal fentanyl citrate (lollipop) premedication in human volunteers. Anesth Analg 69:21-27, 1989.

427. Streisand JB, Stanley TH, Hague B, et al: Oral transmucosal fentanyl citrate premedication in children. Anesth Analg 69:28-34, 1989.

428. Friesen RH, Lockhart CH: Oral transmucosal fentanyl citrate for preanesthetic medication of pediatric day surgery patients with and without droperidol as a prophylactic anti-emetic. Anesthesiology 76:46-51, 1992.

429. Feld LH, Champeau MW, van Steennis CA, Scott JC: Preanesthetic medication in children: A comparison of oral transmucosal fentanyl citrate versus placebo. Anesthesiology 71:374-377, 1989.

430. Goldstein Dresner MC, Davis PJ, Kretchman E, et al: Double-blind comparison of oral transmucosal fentanyl citrate with oral meperidine, diazepam, and atropine as preanesthetic medication in children with congenital heart disease. Anesthesiology 74:28-33, 1991.

431. Streisand JB, Varvel JR, Stanski DR, et al: Absorption and bioavailability of oral transmucosal fentanyl citrate. Anesthesiology 75:223-229, 1991.

432. Dsida RM, Wheeler M, Birmingham PK, et al: Premedication of pediatric tonsillectomy patients with oral transmucosal fentanyl citrate. Anesth Analg 86:66-70, 1998.

433. Ashburn MA, Fine PG, Stanley TH: Oral transmucosal fentanyl citrate for the treatment of breakthrough cancer pain: A case report. Anesthesiology 71:615-617, 1989.

434. Henderson JM, Brodsky DA, Fisher DM, et al: Pre-induction of anesthesia in pediatric patients with nasally administered sufentanil. Anesthesiology 68:671-675, 1988.

435. Karl HW, Keifer AT, Rosenberger JL, et al: Comparison of the safety and efficacy of intranasal midazolam or sufentanil for preinduction of anesthesia in pediatric patients. Anesthesiology 76:209-215, 1992.

436. Zedie N, Amory DW, Wagner BK, O'Hara DA: Comparison of intranasal midazolam and sufentanil premedication in pediatric outpatients. Clin Pharmacol Ther 59:341-348, 1996.

437. Helmers JH, Noorduin H, Van Peer A, et al: Comparison of intravenous and intranasal sufentanil absorption and sedation. Can J Anaesth 36:494-497, 1989.

438. Abboud TK, Zhu J, Gangolly J, et al: Transnasal butorphanol: a new method for pain relief in post-cesarean section pain. Acta Anaesthesiol Scand 35:14-8, 1991.

439. Zacny JP, Lichtor JL, Klafta JM, et al: The effects of transnasal butorphanol on mood and psychomotor functioning in healthy volunteers. Anesth Analg 82:931-935, 1996.

440. Striebel HW, Oelmann T, Spies C, et al: Patient-controlled intranasal analgesia: A method for noninvasive postoperative pain management. Anesth Analg 83:548-551, 1996.

441. Chrubasik J, Wust H, Friedrich G, Geller E: Absorption and bioavailability of nebulized morphine. Br J Anaesth 61:228-230, 1988.

442. Worsley MH, MacLeod AD, Brodie MJ, et al: Inhaled fentanyl as a method of analgesia. Anaesthesia 45:449-451, 1990.

443. Hung OR, Whynot SC, Varvel JR, et al: Pharmacokinetics of inhaled liposome-encapsulated fentanyl. Anesthesiology 83:277-284, 1995.

444. Hanning CD, Vickers AP, Smith G, et al: The morphine hydrogel suppository. A new sustained release rectal preparation. Br J Anaesth 61:221-227, 1988.

445. Lundeberg S, Beck O, Olsson GL, Boreus LO: Rectal administration of morphine in children. Pharmacokinetic evaluation after a single-dose. Acta Anaesthesiol Scand 40:445-451, 1996.

446. Simpson KH, Dearden MJ, Ellis FR, Jack TM: Premedication with slow release morphine (MST) and adjuvants. Br J Anaesth 60:825-830, 1988.

447. Banning AM, Schmidt JF, Chraemmer Jorgensen B, Risbo A: Comparison of oral controlled release morphine and epidural morphine in the management of postoperative pain. Anesth Analg 65:385-388, 1986.

448. Derbyshire DR, Bell A, Parry PA, Smith G: Morphine sulphate slow release. Comparison with i.m. morphine for postoperative analgesia. Br J Anaesth 57:858-865, 1985.

449. Hoskin PJ, Poulain P, Hanks GW: Controlled-release morphine in cancer pain. Is a loading dose required when the formulation is changed? Anaesthesia 44:897-901, 1989.

450. Reuben SS, Connelly NR, Maciolek H: Postoperative analgesia with controlled-release oxycodone for outpatient anterior cruciate ligament surgery. Anesth Analg 88:1286-1291, 1999.

451. Murakawa K, Abboud TK, Yanagi T: Neonatal responses to alphaprodine administered during labor. Anesth Analg 65:392-394, 1986.

452. Caraco Y, Tateishi T, Guengerich FP, Wood AJ: Microsomal codeine N-demethylation: cosegregation with cytochrome P4503A4 activity. Drug Metab Dispos 24:761-764, 1996.

453. Parke TJ, Nandi PR, Bird KJ, Jewkes DA: Profound hypotension following intravenous codeine phosphate. Three case reports and some recommendations. Anaesthesia 47:852-854, 1992.

454. Hill HF, Coda BA, Tanaka A, Schaffer R: Multiple-dose evaluation of intravenous hydromorphone pharmacokinetics in normal human subjects. Anesth Analg 72:330-336, 1991.

455. Wallenstein SL, Houde RW, Portenoy R, et al: Clinical analgesic assay of repeated and single doses of heroin and hydromorphone. Pain 41:5-13, 1990.

456. Rapp SE, Egan KJ, et al: A multidimensional comparison of morphine and hydromorphone patient-controlled analgesia. Anesth Analg 82:1043-1048, 1996.

457. Gourlay GK, Willis RJ, Lamberty J: A double-blind comparison of the efficacy of methadone and morphine in postoperative pain control. Anesthesiology 64:322-327, 1986.

458. Glass PS, Camporesi EM, Shafron D, et al: Evaluation of pentamorphone in humans: A new potent opiate. Anesth Analg 68:302-307, 1989.

459. Papazian L, Albanese J, Thirion X, et al: Effect of bolus doses of midazolam on intracranial pressure and cerebral perfusion pressure in patients with severe head injury. Br J Anaesth 71:267-271, 1993.

460. Morlion B, Ebner E, Weber A, et al: Influence of bolus size on efficacy of postoperative patient-controlled analgesia with piritramide. Br J Anaesth 82:52-55, 1999.

461. Bouillon T, Kietzmann D, Port R, et al: Population pharmacokinetics of piritramide in surgical patients. Anesthesiology 90:7-15, 1999.

462. Halfpenny DM, Callado LF, Hopwood SE, et al: Effects of tramadol stereoisomers on norepinephrine efflux and uptake in the rat locus coeruleus measured by real time voltammetry. Br J Anaesth 83:909-915, 1999.

463. Bamigbade TA, Davidson C, Langford RM, Stamford JA: Actions of tramadol, its enantiomers and principal metabolite, O-desmethyltramadol, on serotonin (5-HT) efflux and uptake in the rat dorsal raphe nucleus. Br J Anaesth 79:352-356, 1997.

464. de Wolff MH, Leather HA, Wouters PF: Effects of tramadol on minimum alveolar concentration (MAC) of isoflurane in rats. Br J Anaesth 83:780-783, 1999.

465. James MF, Heijke SA, Gordon PC: Intravenous tramadol versus epidural morphine for postthoracotomy pain relief: A placebo-controlled double-blind trial. Anesth Analg 83:87-91, 1996.

466. Vickers MD, O'Flaherty D, Szekely SM, et al: Tramadol: Pain relief by an opioid without depression of respiration. Anaesthesia 47:291-296, 1992.

467. Wilder Smith CH, Bettiga A: The analgesic tramadol has minimal effect on gastrointestinal motor function. Br J Clin Pharmacol 43:71-75, 1997.

468. Pang WW, Huang PY, Chang DP, Huang MH: The peripheral analgesic effect of tramadol in reducing propofol injection pain: A comparison with lidocaine. Reg Anesth Pain Med 24:246-249, 1999.

469. Acalovschi I, Cristea T, Margarit S, Gavrus R: Tramadol added to lidocaine for intravenous regional anesthesia. Anesth Analg 92:209-214, 2001.

470. Westman L, Valentin A, Eriksson E, Ekblom A: Intrathecal administration of sameridine to patients subjected to arthroscopic knee joint surgery. Acta Anaesthesiol Scand 42:691-697, 1998.

471. Osterlund Modalen A, Arlander E, Eriksson LI, Lindahl SG: The effects on hypercarbic ventilatory response of sameridine compared to morphine and placebo. Anesth Analg 92:529-534, 2001.

472. Osterlund A, Arlander E, Eriksson LI, Lindahl SG: The effects on resting ventilation of intravenous infusions of morphine or sameridine, a novel molecule with both local anesthetic and opioid properties. Anesth Analg 88:160-165, 1999.

473. Sullivan AF, McQuay HJ, Bailey D, Dickenson AH: The spinal antinociceptive actions of morphine metabolites morphine-6-glucuronide and normorphine in the rat. Brain Res 482:219-224, 1989.

474. Osborne R, Thompson P, Joel S, et al: The analgesic activity of morphine-6-glucuronide. Br J Clin Pharmacol 34:130-138, 1992.

475. Grace D, Fee JP: A comparison of intrathecal morphine-6-glucuronide and intrathecal morphine sulfate as analgesics for total hip replacement. Anesth Analg 83:1055-1059, 1996.

476. Asai T, Mapleson WW, Power I: Effects of nalbuphine, pentazocine and U50488H on gastric emptying and gastrointestinal transit in the rat. Br J Anaesth 80:814-819, 1998.

477. Bowdle TA, Greichen SL, Bjurstrom RL, Schoene RB: Butorphanol improves CO_2 response and ventilation after fentanyl anesthesia. Anesth Analg 66:517-522, 1987.

478. Pedersen JE, Chraemmer Jorgensen B, Schmidt JF, Risbo A: Naloxone—a strong analgesic in combination with high-dose buprenorphine. Br J Anaesth 57:1045-1046, 1985.

479. Gal TJ: Naloxone reversal of buprenorphine-induced respiratory depression. Clin Pharmacol Ther 45:66-71, 1989.

480. Obel D, Hansen LK, Huttel MS, Andersen PK: Buprenorphine-supplemented anaesthesia. Influence of dose on duration of analgesia after cholecystectomy. Br J Anaesth 57:271-274, 1985.

481. De Souza EB, Schmidt WK, Kuhar MJ: Nalbuphine: An autoradiographic opioid receptor binding profile in the central nervous system of an agonist/antagonist analgesic. J Pharmacol Exp Ther 244:391-402, 1988.

482. Lee SC, Wang JJ, Ho ST, Tao PL: Nalbuphine coadministered with morphine prevents tolerance and dependence. Anesth Analg 84:810-815, 1997.

483. Sury MR, Cole PV: Nalbuphine combined with midazolam for outpatient sedation. An assessment of safety in volunteers. Anaesthesia 43:281-284, 1988.

484. Garfield JM, Garfield FB, Philip BK, et al: A comparison of clinical and psychological effects of fentanyl and nalbuphine in ambulatory gynecologic patients. Anesth Analg 66:1303-1307, 1987.

485. Parker RK, Holtmann B, White PF: Patient-controlled epidural analgesia: interactions between nalbuphine and hydromorphone. Anesth Analg 84:757-763, 1997.

486. Murphy MR, Hug CC Jr: The enflurane sparing effect of morphine, butorphanol, and nalbuphine. Anesthesiology 57:489-492, 1982.

487. Bailey PL, Clark NJ, Pace NL, et al: Failure of nalbuphine to antagonize morphine: A double-blind comparison with naloxone. Anesth Analg 65:605-611, 1986.

488. Latasch L, Probst S, Dudziak R: Reversal by nalbuphine of respiratory depression caused by fentanyl. Anesth Analg 63:814-816, 1984.

489. Ramsay JG, Higgs BD, Wynands JE, et al: Early extubation after high-dose fentanyl anaesthesia for aortocoronary bypass surgery: reversal of respiratory depression with low-dose nalbuphine. Can Anaesth Soc J 32:597-606, 1985.

490. Moldenhauer CC, Roach GW, Finlayson DC, et al: Nalbuphine antagonism of ventilatory depression following high-dose fentanyl anesthesia. Anesthesiology 62:647-650, 1985.

491. Jaffe RS, Moldenhauer CC, Hug CC Jr, et al: Nalbuphine antagonism of fentanyl-induced ventilatory depression: A randomized trial. Anesthesiology 68:254-260, 1988.

492. Bailey PL, Clark NJ, Pace NL, et al: Antagonism of postoperative opioid-induced respiratory depression: Nalbuphine versus naloxone. Anesth Analg 66:1109-1114, 1987.

493. Gal TJ, DiFazio CA: Ventilatory and analgesic effects of dezocine in humans. Anesthesiology 61:716-722, 1984.

494. Hall RI, Murphy MR, Szlam F, Hug CC Jr: Dezocine-MAC reduction and evidence for myocardial depression in the presence of enflurane. Anesth Analg 66:1169-2274, 1987.

495. Galloway FM, Varma S: Double-blind comparison of intravenous doses of dezocine, butorphanol, and placebo for relief of postoperative pain. Anesth Analg 65:283-287, 1986.

496. Kaiko RF, Wallenstein SL, Rogers AG, et al: Intramuscular meptazinol and morphine in postoperative pain. Clin Pharmacol Ther 37:589-596, 1985.

497. Wilkinson DJ, O'Connor SA, Dickson GR, Drake HF: Meptazinol—a cause of respiratory depression in general anaesthesia. Br J Anaesth 57:1077-1084, 1985.

498. Kendrick WD, Woods AM, Daly MY, et al: Naloxone versus nalbuphine infusion for prophylaxis of epidural morphine-induced pruritus. Anesth Analg 82:641-647, 1996.

499. Gan TJ, Ginsberg B, Glass PS, et al: Opioid-sparing effects of a low-dose infusion of naloxone in patient-administered morphine sulfate. Anesthesiology 87:1075-1081, 1997.

500. Asai T, Power I: Naloxone inhibits gastric emptying in the rat. Anesth Analg 88:204-208, 1999.

501. Fukuda K, Kato S, Shoda T, et al: Partial agonistic activity of naloxone on the opioid receptors expressed from complementary deoxyribonucleic acids in Chinese hamster ovary cells. Anesth Analg 87:450-455, 1998.

502. Prough DS, Roy R, Bumgarner J, Shannon G: Acute pulmonary edema in healthy teenagers following conservative doses of intravenous naloxone. Anesthesiology 60:485-486, 1984.

503. Partridge BL, Ward CF: Pulmonary edema following low-dose naloxone administration. Anesthesiology 65:709-710, 1986.

504. Kulig K: Initial management of ingestions of toxic substances. N Engl J Med 326:1677-1681, 1992.

505. Just B, Delva E, Camus Y, Lienhart A: Oxygen uptake during recovery following naloxone. Relationship with intraoperative heat loss. Anesthesiology 76:60-4, 1992.

506. Mannelli M, Maggi M, De Feo ML, et al: Naloxone administration releases catecholamines. N Engl J Med 308:654-655, 1983.

507. Kraynack BJ, Gintautas JG: Naloxone: Analeptic action unrelated to opiate receptor antagonism? Anesthesiology 56:251-253, 1982.

508. Beilin B, Vatashsky E, Aronson HB, Weinstock M: Naloxone reversal of postoperative apnea in a premature infant. Anesthesiology 63:317-318, 1985.

509. Delle M, Ricksten SE, Thoren P: The opiate antagonist naloxone counteracts the inhibition of sympathetic nerve activity caused by halothane anesthesia in rats. Anesthesiology 70:309-317, 1989.

510. Skarphedinsson JO, Delle M, Hoffman P, Thoren P: The effects of naloxone on cerebral blood flow and cerebral function during relative cerebral ischemia. J Cereb Blood Flow Metab 9:515-522, 1989.

511. Romanovsky AA, Blatteis CM: Heat stroke: Opioid-mediated mechanisms. J Appl Physiol 81:2565-2570, 1996.

512. Glass PS, Jhaveri RM, Smith LR: Comparison of potency and duration of action of nalmefene and naloxone. Anesth Analg 78:536-541, 1994.

513. Joshi GP, Duffy L, Chehade J, et al: Effects of prophylactic nalmefene on the incidence of morphine-related side effects in patients receiving intravenous patient-controlled analgesia. Anesthesiology 90:1007-1011, 1999.

514. Yuan CS, Foss JF, O'Connor M, et al: Methylnaltrexone for reversal of constipation due to chronic methadone use: A randomized controlled trial. JAMA 283:367-372, 2000.

515. Murphy DB, El Behiery H, Chan VW, Foss JF: Pharmacokinetic profile of epidurally administered methylnaltrexone, a novel peripheral opioid antagonist in a rabbit model. Br J Anaesth 86:120-122, 2001.

516. Bovill JG: Adverse drug interactions in anesthesia. J Clin Anesth 9(Suppl):3S-13S, 1997.

517. Vuyk J: Pharmacokinetic and pharmacodynamic interactions between opioids and propofol. J Clin Anesth 9(Suppl):23-26, 1997.

518. Tverskoy M, Fleyshman G, Ezry J, et al: Midazolam-morphine sedative interaction in patients. Anesth Analg 68:282-285, 1989.

519. Kissin I, Brown PT, Bradley EL Jr, et al: Diazepam–morphine hypnotic synergism in rats. Anesthesiology 70:689-694, 1989.

520. Schwieger IM, Hall RI, Hug CC Jr: Less than additive antinociceptive interaction between midazolam and fentanyl in enflurane-anesthetized dogs. Anesthesiology 74:1060-1066, 1991.

521. Kissin I, Brown PT, Bradley EL Jr: Morphine and fentanyl anesthetic interactions with diazepam: Relative antagonism in rats. Anesth Analg 71:236-241, 1990.

522. Luger TJ, Hayashi T, Weiss CG, Hill HF: The spinal potentiating effect and the supraspinal inhibitory effect of midazolam on opioid-induced analgesia in rats. Eur J Pharmacol 275:153-162, 1995.

523. Vinik HR, Bradley EL Jr, Kissin I: Midazolam-alfentanil synergism for anesthetic induction in patients. Anesth Analg 69:213-217, 1989.

524. Bailey PL, Pace NL, Ashburn MA, et al: Frequent hypoxemia and apnea after sedation with midazolam and fentanyl. Anesthesiology 73:826-830, 1990.

525. Spiess BD, Sathoff RH, el Ganzouri AR, Ivankovich AD: High-dose sufentanil: Four cases of sudden hypotension on induction. Anesth Analg 65:703-705, 1986.

526. Takkunen O, Meretoja OA: Thiopentone reduces the haemodynamic response to induction of high-dose fentanyl-pancuronium anaesthesia in coronary artery surgical patients. Acta Anaesthesiol Scand 32:222-227, 1988.

527. Lepage JY, Pinaud ML, Helias JH, et al: Left ventricular function during propofol and fentanyl anesthesia in patients with coronary artery disease: Assessment with a radionuclide approach. Anesth Analg 67:949-955, 1988.

528. Hall RI, Murphy JT, Moffitt EA, et al: A comparison of the myocardial metabolic and haemodynamic changes produced by propofol-sufentanil and enflurane-sufentanil anaesthesia for patients having coronary artery bypass graft surgery. Can J Anaesth 38:996-1004, 1991.

529. Iselin Chaves IA, Flaishon R, Sebel PS, et al: The effect of the interaction of propofol and alfentanil on recall, loss of consciousness, and the Bispectral Index. Anesth Analg 87:949-955, 1998.

530. Han T, Kim D, Kil H, Inagaki Y: The effects of plasma fentanyl concentrations on propofol requirement, emergence from anesthesia, and postoperative analgesia in propofol-nitrous oxide anesthesia. Anesth Analg 90:1365-1371, 2000.

531. Sukhani R, Vazquez J, Pappas AL, et al: Recovery after propofol with and without intraoperative fentanyl in patients undergoing ambulatory gynecologic laparoscopy. Anesth Analg 83:975-981, 1996.

532. Haessler R, Madler C, Klasing S, et al: Propofol/fentanyl versus etomidate/fentanyl for the induction of anesthesia in patients with aortic insufficiency and coronary artery disease. J Cardiothorac Vasc Anesth 6:173-180, 1992.

533. Sethna NF, Liu M, Gracely R, et al: Analgesic and cognitive effects of intravenous ketamine-alfentanil combinations versus either drug alone after intradermal capsaicin in normal subjects. Anesth Analg 86:1250-1256, 1998.

534. Reeves M, Lindholm DE, Myles PS, et al: Adding ketamine to morphine for patient-controlled analgesia after major abdominal surgery: A double-blinded, randomized controlled trial. Anesth Analg 93:116-120, 2001.

535. Lauretti GR, Lima IC, Reis MP, et al: Oral ketamine and transdermal nitroglycerin as analgesic adjuvants to oral morphine therapy for cancer pain management. Anesthesiology 90:1528-1533, 1999.

536. Eckhardt K, Ammon S, Hofmann U, et al: Gabapentin enhances the analgesic effect of morphine in healthy volunteers. Anesth Analg 91:185-191, 2000.

537. Hara K, Saito Y, Kirihara Y, et al: The interaction of antinociceptive effects of morphine and GABA receptor agonists within the rat spinal cord. Anesth Analg 89:422-427, 1999.

538. Philbin DM, Foex P, Drummond G, et al: Postsystolic shortening of canine left ventricle supplied by a stenotic coronary artery when nitrous oxide is added in the presence of narcotics. Anesthesiology 62:166-174, 1985.

539. Cahalan MK, Prakash O, Rulf EN, et al: Addition of nitrous oxide to fentanyl anesthesia does not induce myocardial ischemia in patients with ischemic heart disease. Anesthesiology 67:925-929, 1986.

540. Finck AD, Samaniego E, Ngai SH: Nitrous oxide selectively releases Met5-enkephalin and Met5-enkephalin-Arg6-Phe7 into canine third ventricular cerebrospinal fluid. Anesth Analg 80:664-670, 1995.

541. Heikkila H, Jalonen J, Arola M, et al: Low-dose enflurane as adjunct to high-dose fentanyl in patients undergoing coronary artery surgery: Stable hemodynamics and maintained myocardial oxygen balance. Anesth Analg 66:111-116, 1987.

542. O'Young J, Mastrocostopoulos G, Hilgenberg A, et al: Myocardial circulatory and metabolic effects of isoflurane and sufentanil during coronary artery surgery. Anesthesiology 66:653-658, 1987.

543. Vermeyen KM, Erpels FA, Beeckman CP, et al: Low-dose sufentanil-isoflurane anaesthesia for coronary artery surgery. Br J Anaesth 63:44-50, 1989.

544. Phillips AS, McMurray TJ, Mirakhur RK, et al: Propofol-fentanyl anesthesia: A comparison with isoflurane-fentanyl anesthesia in coronary artery bypass grafting and valve replacement surgery. J Cardiothorac Vasc Anesth 8:289-296, 1994.

545. Searle NR, Martineau RJ, Conzen P, et al: Comparison of sevoflurane/fentanyl and isoflurane/fentanyl during elective coronary artery bypass surgery. Sevoflurane Venture Group. Can J Anaesth 43:890-899, 1996.

546. Weiskopf RB, Eger EI 2nd, Noorani M, Daniel M: Fentanyl, esmolol, and clonidine blunt the transient cardiovascular stimulation induced by desflurane in humans. Anesthesiology 81:1350-1355, 1994.

547. Ebert TJ, Muzi M: Sympathetic hyperactivity during desflurane anesthesia in healthy volunteers. A comparison with isoflurane. Anesthesiology 79:444-453, 1993.

548. Cote D, Martin R, Tetrault JP: Haemodynamic interactions of muscle relaxants and sufentanil in coronary artery surgery. Can J Anaesth 38:324-329, 1991.

549. Thomson IR, MacAdams CL, Hudson RJ, Rosenbloom M: Drug interactions with sufentanil. Hemodynamic effects of premedication and muscle relaxants. Anesthesiology 76:922-929, 1992.

550. Thomson IR, Putnins CL: Adverse effects of pancuronium during high-dose fentanyl anesthesia for coronary artery bypass grafting. Anesthesiology 62:708-713, 1985.

551. Sethna DH, Starr NJ, Estafanous FG: Cardiovascular effects of non-depolarizing neuromuscular blockers in patients with coronary artery disease. Can Anaesth Soc J 33:280-286, 1986.

552. Paulissian R, Mahdi M, Joseph NJ, et al: Hemodynamic responses to pancuronium and vecuronium during high-dose fentanyl anesthesia for coronary artery bypass grafting. J Cardiothorac Vasc Anesth 5:120-125, 1991.

553. Heinonen J, Salmenpera M, Suomivuori M: Contribution of muscle relaxant to the haemodynamic course of high-dose fentanyl anaesthesia: A comparison of pancuronium, vecuronium and atracurium. Can Anaesth Soc J 33:597-605, 1986.

554. O'Connor JP, Ramsay JG, Wynands JE, et al: The incidence of myocardial ischemia during anesthesia for coronary artery bypass surgery in patients receiving pancuronium or vecuronium. Anesthesiology 70:230-236, 1989.

555. Waldmann CS, Wark KJ, Sebel PS, Feneck RO: Hemodynamic effects of atracurium, vecuronium and pancuronium during sufentanil anesthesia for coronary artery bypass. Acta Anaesthesiol Scand 30:351-356, 1986.

556. Stoops CM, Curtis CA, Kovach DA, et al: Hemodynamic effects of doxacurium chloride in patients receiving oxygen sufentanil anesthesia for coronary artery bypass grafting or valve replacement. Anesthesiology 69:365-370, 1988.

557. Tassonyi E, Neidhart P, Pittet JF, et al: Cardiovascular effects of pipecuronium and pancuronium in patients undergoing coronary artery bypass grafting. Anesthesiology 69:793-795, 1988.

558. Savarese JJ, Ali HH, Basta SJ, et al: The cardiovascular effects of mivacurium chloride (BW B1090U) in patients receiving nitrous oxide-opiate-barbiturate anesthesia. Anesthesiology 70:386-394, 1089.

559. Choi WW, Mehta MP, Murray DJ, et al: Neuromuscular and cardiovascular effects of mivacurium chloride in surgical patients receiving nitrous oxide-narcotic or nitrous oxide-isoflurane anaesthesia. Can J Anaesth 36:641-650, 1989.

560. Stoops CM, Curtis CA, Kovach DA, et al: Hemodynamic effects of mivacurium chloride administered to patients during oxygen-sufentanil anesthesia for coronary artery bypass grafting or valve replacement. Anesth Analg 68:333-339, 1989.

561. Wells DG, Bjorksten AR: Monoamine oxidase inhibitors revisited. Can J Anaesth 36:64-74, 1989.

562. Stack CG, Rogers P, Linter SP: Monoamine oxidase inhibitors and anaesthesia. A review. Br J Anaesth 60:222-227, 1988.

563. Carta F, Bianchi M, Argenton S, et al: Effect of nifedipine on morphine-induced analgesia. Anesth Analg 70:493-498, 1990.

564. Omote K, Sonoda H, Kawamata M, et al: Potentiation of antinociceptive effects of morphine by calcium-channel blockers at the level of the spinal cord. Anesthesiology 79:746-752, 1993.

565. Hasegawa AE, Zacny JP: The influence of three L-type calcium channel blockers on morphine effects in healthy volunteers. Anesth Analg 85:633-638, 1997.

566. Omote K, Kawamata M, Satoh O, et al: Spinal antinociceptive action of an N-type voltage-dependent calcium channel blocker and the synergistic interaction with morphine. Anesthesiology 84:636-643, 1996.

567. Bartkowski RR, Goldberg ME, Huffnagle S, Epstein RH: Sufentanil disposition. Is it affected by erythromycin administration? Anesthesiology 78:260-265, 1993.

568. Bartkowski RR, McDonnell TE: Prolonged alfentanil effect following erythromycin administration. Anesthesiology 73:566-568, 1990.

569. Koinig H, Wallner T, Marhofer P, et al: Magnesium sulfate reduces intra- and postoperative analgesic requirements. Anesth Analg 87:206-210, 1998.

570. Buvanendran A, McCarthy RJ, Kroin JS, et al: Intrathecal magnesium prolongs fentanyl analgesia: A prospective, randomized, controlled trial. Anesth Analg 95:661-666, 2002.

571. Kroin JS, McCarthy RJ, Von Roenn N, et al: Magnesium sulfate potentiates morphine antinociception at the spinal level. Anesth Analg 90:913-917, 2000.

572. Plummer JL, Owen H, Ilsley AH, Tordoff K: Sustained-release ibuprofen as an adjunct to morphine patient-controlled analgesia. Anesth Analg 83:92-96, 1996.

573. Ng A, Parker J, Toogood L, Cotton BR, Smith G: Does the opioid-sparing effect of rectal diclofenac following total abdominal hysterectomy benefit the patient? Br J Anaesth 88:714-716, 2002.

574. Moren J, Francois T, Blanloeil Y, Pinaud M: The effects of a nonsteroidal antiinflammatory drug (ketoprofen) on morphine respiratory depression: A double-blind, randomized study in volunteers. Anesth Analg 85:400-405, 1997.

575. Babenco HD, Blouin RT, Conard PF, Gross JB: Diphenylhydramine increases ventilatory drive during alfentanil infusion. Anesthesiology 89:642-647, 1998.

CHAPTER
12 Intravenous Drug Delivery Systems

Peter S. A. Glass, Steven L. Shafer, and J. G. Reves

Introduction   439

Pharmacokinetic Considerations   440

Pharmacodynamic
   Considerations   444
   The Biophase   444
   Direct Effect Models   445
   Indirect Effect Models   446
   Dose Implications of the Biophase   446
   Drug Potency   446

Designing Dosing Regimens   451
   Bolus Dose Calculations   451
   Maintenance Infusion Rate   452

Recovery from Anesthesia   455

Manual Infusion Schemes for
   Intravenous Anesthetics   458
   Opioids   460
   Hypnotics   461

Infusion Devices   463
   Manual Delivery   463
   Automated Delivery   463

Summary   475

INTRODUCTION

For anesthetic drugs to be effective, they must reach their site of action. In 1628, William Harvey proved in *Exercitatio Anatomica de Motu Cordis et Sanguinis in Animalibus* that venous blood was transported to the arterial circulation and thus to the organs of the body by the heart. It was thus recognized almost immediately that drugs injected into veins could be rapidly carried to the entire body. Indeed, in 1657, Christopher Wren injected opium intravenously by means of a quill and bladder (Fig. 12-1A) in dogs and humans and rendered them unconscious. Eight years later, Sigismund Elsholtz gave an opioid solution for the purpose of rendering subjects insensitive, but it was not until 1874 that Pierre-Cyprien Ore administered chloral hydrate intravenously for a surgical procedure. This landmark occasion followed unsuccessful attempts by the Russian surgeon Pirogoff to administer ether intravenously in 1846, shortly after Crawford Long and William Morton had independently demonstrated the efficacy of ether inhalation for surgery.[1]

Intravenous methods of anesthetic drug delivery have depended on a steady improvement in technology. The quill and bladder used by Wren were not significantly improved on until Alexander Wood used a needle and syringe to administer intravenous medications in 1853. The hollow hypodermic needle was developed by Frances Rynd, and a functional syringe, by Charles Pravaz.[1]

Contemporary needles, catheters, and syringes are descendants of these early devices. The latest technologic development in intravenous anesthesia has been the introduction of computerized pharmacokinetic model–driven continuous-infusion devices (Fig. 12-1B), first published by Helmut Schwilden[2] in 1981. Schwilden demonstrated the ability to attain desired plasma levels of an intravenous anesthetic drug by using a computer-controlled infusion pump driven by the published pharmacokinetics of the drug. These efforts resulted in the release in Europe of the first commercial target-controlled infusion (TCI) device, developed by Zeneca, specifically for the administration of propofol. The March 1998 issue of the journal *Anaesthesia* was devoted entirely to a review of TCI, with a focus on the "Diprifusor" and the role of TCI devices in clinical practice.

The ultimate development in anesthetic delivery systems will be devices for closed-loop administration of intravenous drugs during anesthesia. Systems have been developed for closed-loop administration of sodium nitroprusside[3-7] and muscle relaxants[8-14] (see Chapter 13). The drug effect is easily measured for vasoactive drugs and muscle relaxants, thus facilitating closed-loop control. Until recently, the lack of an unequivocal measure of "anesthetic depth" has hindered the development of closed-loop anesthetic delivery systems. Clinical assessment of anesthetic depth requires integration of the patient's physiology, the drug dosing history, the level of

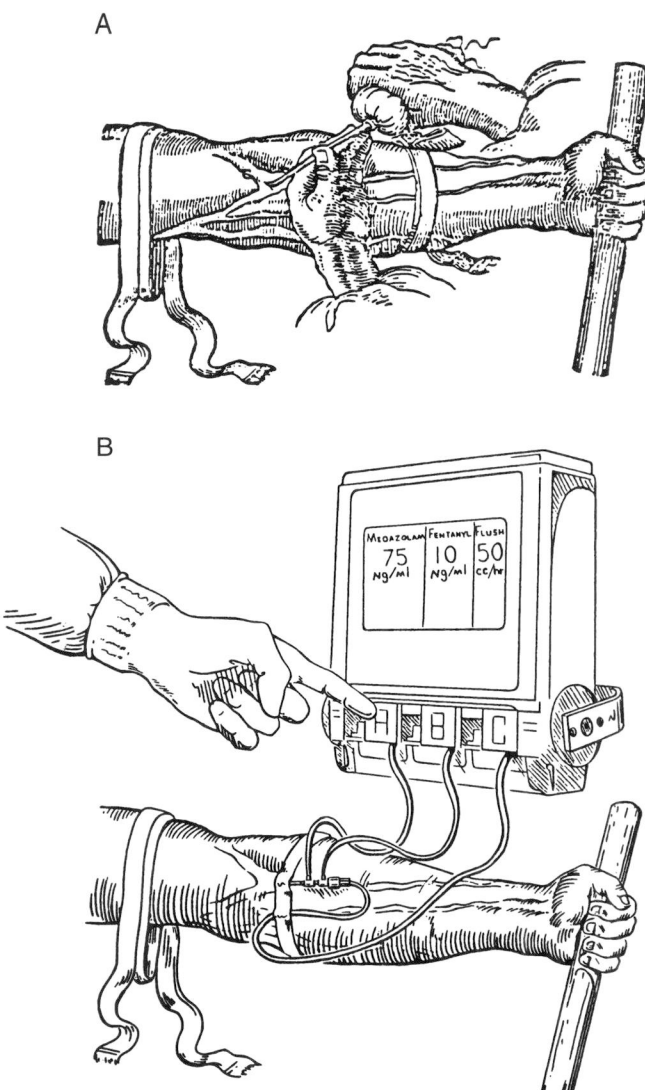

A

B

Figure 12–1 Intravenous drug delivery, past and future. **A,** Depiction of the first intravenous injection of opium with a quill and bladder. **B,** The future of intravenous drug delivery, in which drugs are delivered with the aid of a small, sophisticated infusion pump that permits dosing in terms of plasma drug concentration rather than amount.

noxious stimulation, and measurement of the patient's response to stimulation (hemodynamics, movement, electroencephalogram [EEG], tearing, and so on), as discussed in Chapter 31. Increasing understanding of the physiology involved in providing anesthesia and the development of monitoring devices for specific components of the anesthetic state have resulted in increasing efforts to develop such closed-loop devices. Schwilden and colleagues have developed closed-loop systems for the infusion of methohexital[15,16] and propofol[17] on the basis of the median EEG frequency. Several other investigators have now also developed closed-loop systems based on derivatives of the EEG (e.g., auditory evoked potentials[18] or the bispectral index[19] developed by Aspect Medical Systems[20]).

The development of new techniques has coincided with the development of new drugs. Rapid intravenous induction became popular with the introduction of sodium thiopental in 1934. The pharmacokinetics of thiopental prevented it becoming popular for the maintenance of anesthesia. During the past 50 years, numerous intravenous hypnotics (methohexital, 1957; propanidid, 1957; althesin, 1971; etomidate, 1973; propofol, 1977), anxiolytics (diazepam, 1966; midazolam, 1978), and analgesics (fentanyl, 1959; ketamine, 1966; sufentanil, 1979; alfentanil, 1980; remifentanil, 1996) have been introduced. The general trend in the introduction of these newer drugs has been shorter and shorter times for recovery from drug effect. The newer intravenous anesthetics propofol, etomidate, alfentanil, sufentanil, and remifentanil have all been shown to provide a rapid onset of anesthesia, a stable maintenance phase, and rapid recovery.

Before a review of intravenous anesthesia delivery techniques and devices, we need to review pharmacokinetic and pharmacodynamic principles to understand how to administer intravenous drugs to their best advantage. Therefore, we will develop these concepts and then show how intravenous anesthesia delivery systems can be used to rationally dose the intravenous drugs used in clinical practice. Further discussion of the principles of pharmacokinetics and pharmacodynamics can be found in Chapter 3.

PHARMACOKINETIC CONSIDERATIONS

One objective of anesthetic administration is to produce the clinically desired time course of anesthetic effect, which usually includes rapid onset, smooth maintenance, and rapid recovery after termination of the anesthetic. Conventional pharmacokinetic models assume that a bolus of drug is instantaneously mixed into plasma and produces an immediate peak in the plasma concentration. The concentration then continuously declines until the next bolus. Except for a transient perioperative stimulus (intubation, incision, bowel traction), it is unlikely that the patient's anesthetic requirements follow the saltatory time course of anesthetic effect seen with repeated bolus injections. Thus, the technique of intermittent boluses results in excessive drug effect at the time of the bolus, inadequate drug effect before the next bolus, or both (Fig. 12-2). The technique of giving the entire anesthetic as an initial bolus, as was popular in the early 1980s with massive doses of opioids for cardiac surgery, represents the *reductio ad absurdum* of the intermittent bolus technique. This technique produces a needlessly huge initial peak and, depending on the dose, grossly excessive or possibly subtherapeutic levels later in the procedure. Fortunately, opioids are enormously forgiving drugs in paralyzed patients whose lungs are mechanically ventilated.

The oscillating effect produced by intermittent bolus injection is particularly undesirable for drugs that depress hemodynamics or when prompt emergence is desirable. To produce a time course of drug effect that follows the time course of anesthetic requirement, it is necessary to use a

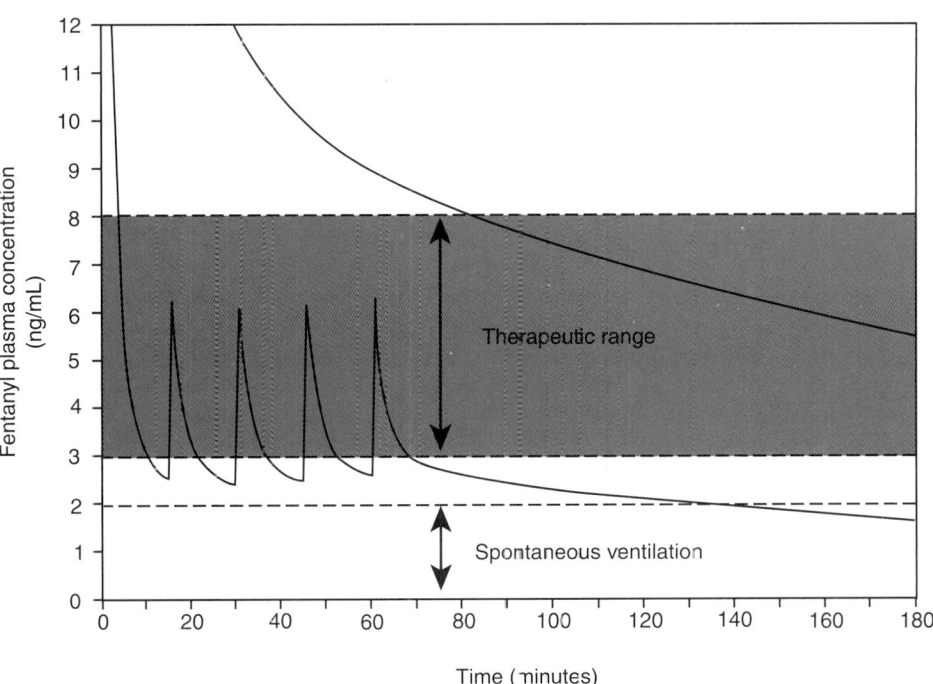

Figure 12–2 Pharmacokinetic simulation of *(upper curve)* a single large bolus of fentanyl (50 μg/kg) and *(lower curve)* a smaller fentanyl bolus (8 μg/kg) followed by intermittent boluses (1.5 μg/kg) every 15 minutes. The single large bolus results in plasma drug concentrations far in excess of those required, whereas the intermittent bolus scheme results in plasma concentrations that periodically fall below the therapeutic range. Ideally, the plasma drug concentration should be continuously within the therapeutic range, which can best be accomplished by a continuous infusion.

continuous infusion titrated to the perceived anesthetic requirement. Ideally, just enough drug is given to achieve the therapeutic blood or plasma drug concentration, which is continuously titrated throughout surgery (Fig. 12-3). This method of drug delivery avoids the peaks and valleys in drug concentration seen with intermittent drug boluses. Theoretical advantages of continuous infusions over intermittent bolus injections include fewer periods of poor anesthetic control, a reduction in the total amount of drug used, and more rapid recovery from anesthesia.[21,22]

The goal of intravenous administration is to produce plasma concentrations yielding the desired time course of drug effect. By the use of pharmacokinetic models, it is possible to calculate the dose of drug needed to produce the desired time course of plasma concentration. The medical literature is replete with articles describing pharmacokinetic models for every intravenous anesthetic drug. These models are of little use without computer simulation. In this chapter we will describe how pharmacokinetic models can be used to develop rational dosing

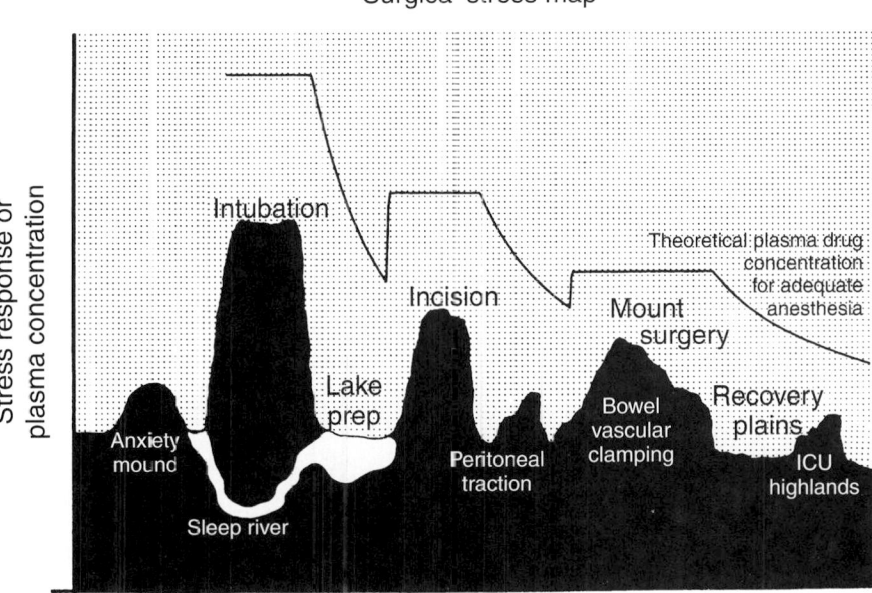

Figure 12–3 Landscape of surgical anesthesia. The stimuli of surgery are not constant; therefore, the plasma concentration of the anesthetic drug should be titrated to match the needs of the patient.

guidelines for use with intravenous infusion systems. We first review some basic pharmacokinetic concepts and define the relevant terminology.

Pharmacokinetic models are mathematical descriptions of how the body "disposes" of drugs. The parameters describing this process are estimated by administering a known dose of the drug and measuring the resulting plasma concentrations. A mathematical model then relates the *input* over time, I(t), with the *concentrations* over time, C(t). These models can take many forms. Figure 12-4 shows the concentrations in plasma over time after a single intravenous bolus of drug at time 0. Drug concentrations continuously decrease after the bolus, and the rate of decrease is approximately proportional to the amount of drug in plasma. Typically, it is convenient to describe this behavior by the use of exponential models. The curve might have a single exponent, in which case the plasma concentration over time might be described by the function C(t) = A e^{-kt}, where

A is the concentration at time 0 and *k* is a constant that describes the rate at which the concentration decreases. The relationship appears to be a straight line when graphed as the log of concentration versus time. The pharmacokinetics of intravenous anesthetic drugs is more complex because after the bolus, one observes a period of rapid decrease before the terminal "log-linear" portion (e.g., the part that is a straight line when graphed as log concentration versus time). We can model this relationship by taking several monoexponential (i.e., one exponent) curves and adding them together. The result is a polyexponential curve. For example, drug concentrations after an intravenous bolus might be described by an equation with two exponents, C(t) = A $e^{-\alpha t}$ + B $e^{-\beta t}$, or an equation with three exponents, C(t) = A $e^{-\alpha t}$ + B $e^{-\beta t}$ + C $e^{-\gamma t}$.

Intravenous anesthetic drugs may be administered by means other than single boluses. A more general way to think of pharmacokinetics is to decompose the input

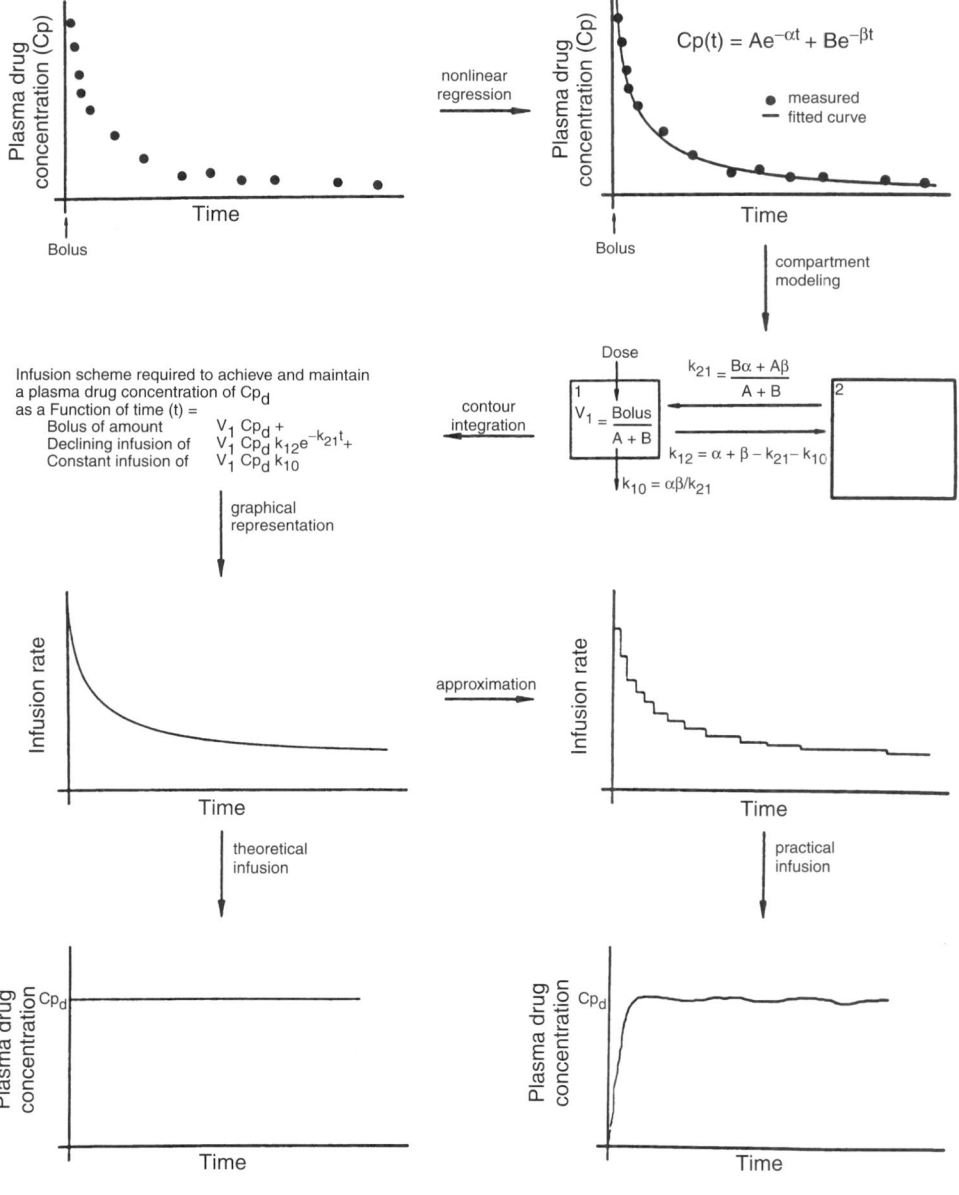

Figure 12–4 Steps involved in a pharmacokinetic model–driven infusion. Typically, pharmacokinetic models are derived from experiments in which plasma drug concentrations are measured at intervals after bolus administration of the drug. Nonlinear regression is used to fit a monoexponential, biexponential, or triexponential curve to the resulting concentration-versus-time data. There is an algebraic relationship between the exponential decay curves and a one-, two-, or three-compartment pharmacokinetic model. The "BET" infusion scheme is developed and consists of a *bolus*, a continuous infusion to replace drug *eliminated* from the body, and an exponentially declining infusion to replace drug *transferred* out of plasma to other body compartments. A BET infusion results in maintenance of a constant specified plasma drug concentration. Practical implementation of the BET scheme with real infusion pumps and infusion rates that change only at discrete intervals results in a plasma drug concentration profile that approximates the profile resulting from a BET infusion.

into a series of bits (boluses) and consider each bit of drug separately. The general pharmacokinetic model of drug disposition commonly used in anesthesia treats each bit of administered drug as though it undergoes polyexponential decay over time. The formal mathematical description of the polyexponential decay of each bit of drug over time is the relationship

$$C(t) = I(t) * \sum_{i=1}^{n} A_i e^{-\lambda_i t} \qquad (1)$$

where $C(t)$ is the plasma concentration at time t and $I(t)$ is the drug input (i.e., a bolus or infusion). The summation after the asterisk (described later) is the function describing how each bit of drug is disposed of (hence its name, the "disposition" function). Note that this function is again a sum of n exponentials, as described in the previous paragraph.

Pharmacokinetic modeling is the process of estimating the parameters within this function. The integer n is the number of exponentials (i.e., compartments) and is usually two or three for the drugs used in anesthesia. Each exponential term is associated with a coefficient A_i and an exponent λ_i. The λ values are inversely proportional to the half-lives (half-life = $0.693/\lambda$), with the smallest λ value representing the longest (terminal) half-life. The A values are the relative contribution of each half-life to overall drug disposition. If a drug has a very long terminal half-life but a coefficient that is much smaller than the other coefficients, the long half-life is likely to be clinically meaningless. The $*$ operator is the mathematical process called convolution, which can be thought of as multiplication, but for functions rather than for simple numbers. For a bolus at time 0, convolution is multiplication. For infusions, the math implied by the $*$ gets more complicated, but the A and λ values estimated are the same.

Constructing pharmacokinetic models represents a trade-off between accurately describing the data, having confidence in the results, and achieving mathematical tractability. It is generally the case that adding exponentials (i.e., increasing n) to the model provides a better description of the data. However, adding exponential terms usually decreases our confidence in how well we know each coefficient and exponential. Additionally, each exponent greatly increases the mathematical burden of pharmacokinetic models, which is why most models of anesthetic drugs are limited to two or three exponents.

The pharmacokinetic model shown has some useful characteristics, thus accounting for its enduring popularity in pharmacokinetic analysis. Most importantly, the model describes observations from studies reasonably well, obviously the *sine qua non* for models. Second, these models have the useful characteristic of linearity. Simply stated, if you double the dose I (e.g., give a bolus twice as large or an infusion twice as fast), you double the concentration.

More generally, linearity implies that the system (i.e., the body acting to produce a plasma drug concentration output from a drug dosage input) behaves in accordance with the principle of superposition. The superposition principle states that the response of a linear system having multiple inputs can be computed by determining the response to each individual input and then summing the individual responses. In other words, when the body treats each bit of drug by polyexponential decay over time, that "disposing" of each bit of drug does not influence the disposing of other bits of drug.

The third reason for the continuing popularity of these models is that they can be mathematically transformed from the admittedly unintuitive exponential form shown earlier to a more easily intuitive compartmental form, as shown in Figure 12-5. The fundamental parameters of the compartment model are the volumes of distribution (central, rapidly equilibrating, and slowly equilibrating peripheral volumes) and clearances (systemic, rapid, and slow intercompartmental). The central compartment (V_1) represents a distribution volume and includes the rapidly

Figure 12–5 Three-compartment model (including the biophase) schematizing the basic pharmacokinetic processes that occur after intravenous drug administration. *I*, dosing scheme as a function of time; k_{10}, rate constant reflecting all processes acting to irreversibly remove drug from the central compartment; k_{ij} intercompartmental rate constants; V_1, central compartment volume, usually expressed in liters or liters per kilogram.

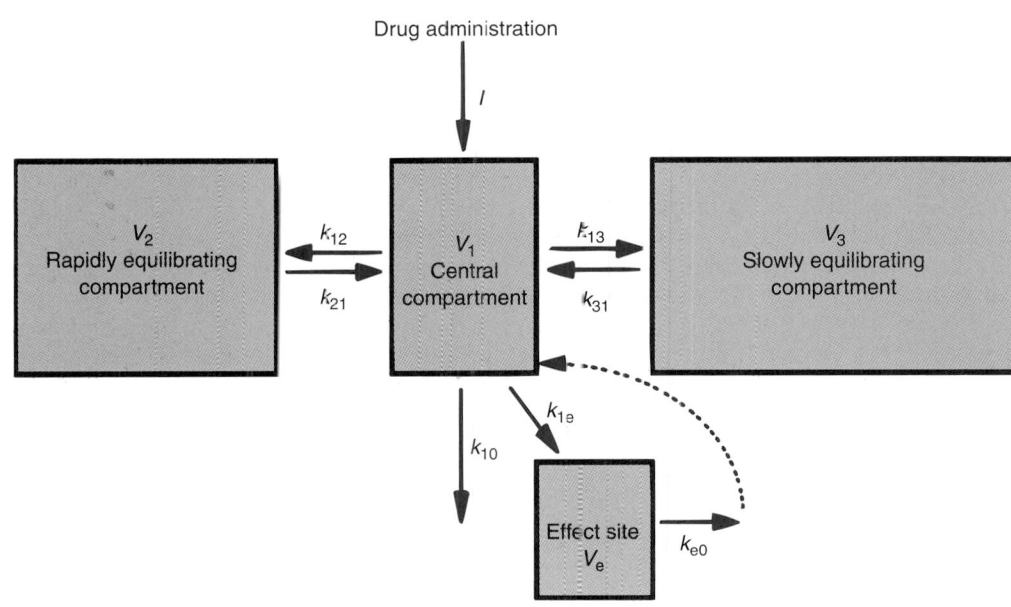

mixing portion of the blood and first-pass pulmonary uptake. The peripheral compartments are composed of tissues and organs that show a time course and extent of drug accumulation (or dissipation) different from that of the central compartment. In the three-compartment model, the two peripheral compartments may correspond roughly to splanchnic and muscle tissue (rapidly equilibrating) and fat stores (slowly equilibrating). The sum of the compartment volumes is the apparent volume of distribution at steady state (Vd_{SS}) and is the proportionality constant relating the plasma drug concentration at steady state to the total amount of drug in the body. The intercompartmental rate constants (k_{12}, k_{21}, and so on) describe the movement of drug between the central and peripheral compartments. The elimination rate constant (k_{10}) encompasses processes acting through biotransformation or elimination that irreversibly remove drug from the central compartment.

Despite their physiologic flavor, compartmental models are simply mathematical transformations of the polyexponential disposition functions computed from observed plasma concentrations. Thus, physiologic interpretation of volumes and clearances, with the possible exception of systemic clearance and Vd_{SS} (the algebraic sum of the volumes), is entirely speculative.

The last reason that these models have been popular is that they can be used to design infusion regimens, which is the point of introducing them in this chapter. If we abbreviate the disposition function

$$\sum_{i=1}^{n} A_i e^{-\lambda_i t} \qquad (2)$$

as simply D(t), we can rewrite the relationship between concentration, dose, and the pharmacokinetic model D(t) as

$$C(t) = I(t) * D(t) \qquad (3)$$

where $*$ is the convolution operator, as noted earlier. In the usual pharmacokinetic study, we know I(t) (the dose we gave the patient), and we measure C(t), the concentrations over time. Our goal is to find D(t), the pharmacokinetic disposition function. Pharmacokinetic analysis can be thought of as a simple rearrangement of Equation 3 to solve for D(t):

$$D(t) = \frac{C(t)}{I(t)} \qquad (4)$$

where the symbol $\divideontimes$ means *deconvolution*, the inverse operation to convolution. Deconvolution is like division, but of functions rather than simple numbers. When we design dosing regimens from known pharmacokinetic models and a desired course for the plasma concentration over time, the known values are D(t) (the pharmacokinetics) and $C_T(t)$ (the desired target concentrations), and the drug dosing scheme is

$$I(t) = \frac{C_T(t)}{D(t)} \qquad (5)$$

Thus, one can calculate the necessary infusion rates, I(t), given the desired target concentrations, $C_T(t)$, and the pharmacokinetics, D(t), by using the same tools used to calculate the original pharmacokinetics. Unfortunately, such a solution might require some negative infusion rates, which are obviously impossible. Because we cannot suck drug out of the body (i.e., give negative infusions), we must restrict ourselves to plasma concentrations over time that can be achieved with non-negative infusion rates.

The standard pharmacokinetic model has one glaring shortcoming. It assumes complete mixing within the central compartment after a bolus injection so that the peak concentration occurs precisely at time 0. It actually takes about 30 to 45 seconds for the drug to make its transit from the venous injection site to the arterial circulation. This model mis-specification of 30 to 45 seconds may not seem significant, but it can cause problems when one is trying to relate the drug effect after a bolus to drug concentrations in the body.[23] Researchers are modifying the standard polyexponential pharmacokinetic models to provide more accurate models of plasma drug concentration in the first minute after a bolus injection.[24]

PHARMACODYNAMIC CONSIDERATIONS

The Biophase

Although the plasma concentration after an intravenous bolus peaks nearly instantaneously, no anesthesiologist would push an intravenous bolus of a hypnotic drug and immediately intubate the patient's trachea. The reason, of course, is that although the plasma concentration peaks almost instantly, additional time is required for the drug concentration in the brain to rise and induce unconsciousness. This delay between peak plasma concentration and peak concentration in the brain is called *hysteresis*. Hysteresis is the clinical manifestation of the fact that the plasma is not the site of anesthetic action, only the mechanism of transport. Drugs exert their pharmacologic effect in the "biophase," which is also called the "effect site." Physically, the biophase is the immediate milieu in which the drug acts on the body, including membranes, receptors, and enzymes.

The concentration of drug in the biophase cannot be measured for two reasons. First, it is usually inaccessible, at least in human subjects. Second, even if we could take tissue samples, the drug concentration in the microscopic environment of the receptive molecules would not be the same as the concentration measured in, for example, homogenated brain. Although it is not possible to actually measure drug concentrations in the biophase, by the use of rapid measures of drug effect we can characterize the time course of drug effect. Knowing the time course of drug effect, we can characterize the rate of drug flow in and out of the biophase (or "effect site") by the use of mathematical models,[25,26] as well as the apparent drug concentration in the biophase, in terms of the steady-state plasma concentration that would produce the same effect.

Measures of effect used to characterize the time course of drug between plasma and the biophase will vary with the drug being evaluated. For neuromuscular blockers, the twitch response is an ideal measure of effect. For opioids and hypnotics, the measure of effect is more challenging. The desired effect for opioids is analgesia, which is a subjective measure that is difficult to monitor and quantify moment by moment. Similarly for hypnotics, until recently there has been no validated monitor of drug effect. For these reasons investigators have turned to the EEG as an objective measure of opioid and hypnotic drug effect. If the EEG did not measure the clinically desired effect of opioids and hypnotics, it was assumed that changes in the EEG would at least reflect the time course of clinical effects. Thus, the time course for equilibration between plasma and the biophase for opioids and hypnotics has largely been defined by using the EEG. The validity of this approach has been confirmed in several studies. Glass and colleagues measured the blood concentration of remifentanil and its analgesic response in volunteers.[27] The time course for equilibration between plasma and the biophase calculated in this study was essentially identical to the time course determined by using the spectral edge of the EEG as the measure of effect.[28] Ludbrook and associates measured propofol concentrations in the carotid artery and jugular bulb to establish propofol movement into and equilibration with the brain.[29] They measured the bispectral index simultaneously and found close correlation between concentrations in the brain (calculated by using mass balance) and changes in the bispectral index.

Direct Effect Models

Just as shown for plasma pharmacokinetics earlier, the biophase concentration is the convolution of an input function (in this case, the plasma drug concentration over time) and the disposition function of the biophase. This relationship can be expressed as

$$C_{biophase}(t) = C_{plasma}(t) * D_{biophase}(t) \qquad (6)$$

The disposition function of the biophase is typically modeled as a single exponential decay:

$$D_{biophase}(t) = k_{e0}e^{-k_{e0}t} \qquad (7)$$

The monoexponential disposition function implies that the effect site is simply an additional compartment in the standard compartmental model that is connected to the plasma compartment (see Fig. 12-5). The effect site is the hypothetical compartment that relates the time course of plasma drug concentration to the time course of drug effect, and k_{e0} is the rate constant of drug elimination from the effect site. By definition, the effect compartment receives such tiny amounts of drug from the central compartment that it has no influence on plasma pharmacokinetics.

We cannot directly measure either $C_{biophase}(t)$ or $D_{biophase}(t)$, but we can measure drug effect. Knowing that the observed drug effect is a function of the drug concentration in the biophase, we can predict the drug effect as

$$\text{Effect} = f_{PD}\left[C_{plasma}(t) * D_{biophase}(t), P_{PD}, k_{e0}\right] \qquad (8)$$

where f_{PD} is a pharmacodynamic model (typically sigmoidal in shape), P_{PD} is the parameters of the pharmacodynamic model, and k_{e0} is the rate constant for

equilibration between plasma and the biophase. Nonlinear regression programs are used to find values of P_{PD} and k_{e0} that best predict the time course of drug effect. Knowledge of these parameters can then be incorporated into dosing regimens that produce the desired time course of drug effect.[30,31]

If a constant plasma concentration is maintained, the time required for the biophase concentration to reach 50% of the plasma concentration ($t^{1}/_{2} k_{e0}$) can be calculated as $0.693/k_{e0}$. After a bolus dose, the time to peak biophase concentration is a function of both plasma pharmacokinetics and k_{e0}. For drugs with a very rapid decline in plasma concentration after a bolus (e.g., adenosine, which has a half-life of several seconds), the effect-site concentration peaks within several seconds of the bolus, regardless of the k_{e0} value. For drugs with a rapid k_{e0} and a slow decrease in concentration after a bolus injection (e.g., pancuronium), the peak effect-site concentration is determined more by k_{e0} than by plasma pharmacokinetics. The time to peak effect and the $t^{1}/_{2} k_{e0}$ for several intravenous anesthetics are listed in Table 12-1.

Indirect Effect Models

Thus far we have been talking about effects that are an instantaneous function of drug concentration at the site of drug effect, as implied by Equation 8. For example, once hypnotics reach the brain or muscle relaxants reach the muscles, the effect is almost instantaneous. Some effects are much more complex. For example, consider the effect of opioids on ventilation. Initially, opioids depress ventilation. As a result of this ventilatory depression, CO_2 accumulates. The accumulation in CO_2 acts to stimulate ventilation, thus partly offsetting the ventilatory depressant effects of opioids. Ventilatory depression is an example in which a direct and an indirect drug effect occurs. The direct effect of the opioid is to depress ventilation, and the indirect effect is to increase CO_2. Modeling the time course of opioid-induced ventilatory depression requires consideration of both components. Bouillon and colleagues developed a model of ventilatory depression that incorporates both direct and indirect effects.[32,33] As is generally the case with indirect effect

Table 12–1 Time to peak effect and $t^{1}/_{2} k_{e0}$ after a bolus dose

Drug	Time to Peak Drug Effect (min)	$t^{1}/_{2} k_{e0}$ (min)
Fentanyl	3.6	4.7
Alfentanil	1.4	0.9
Sufentanil	5.6	3.0
Remifentanil	1.6	1.3
Propofol	2.2	2.4
Thiopental	1.6	1.5
Midazolam	2.8	4.0
Etomidate	2.0	1.5

$t^{1}/_{2} k_{e0}$, rate constant for transfer of drug from the site of drug effect to the environment.

models, characterizing drug-induced ventilatory depression requires considering the entire time course of drug therapy, which is embodied in the following differential equation:

$$\frac{d}{dt} Pa_{CO_2} = k_{e1} \cdot Pa_{CO_2}(0)$$

$$-k_{e1} \cdot \left(1 - \frac{Cp(t)^{\gamma}}{C_{50}{}^{\gamma} + Cp(t)^{\gamma}}\right) \cdot \left(\frac{P_{\text{biophase}}CO_2(t)}{P_{\text{biophase}}CO_2(0)}\right)^{F}$$

$$\cdot Pa_{CO_2}(t) \qquad (9)$$

where Pa_{CO_2} is the arterial CO_2, $P_{\text{biophase}}CO_2$ is the CO_2 in the biophase (i.e., ventilation control centers), k_{el} is the rate constant for CO_2 elimination, C_{50} is the effect-site opioid concentration associated with a 50% reduction in ventilatory drive, and F is the steepness or "gain" of the CO_2 effect on ventilatory drive.

Dose Implications of the Biophase

The delay in onset has important clinical implications. After a bolus, the plasma concentration peaks nearly instantly and then steadily declines. The effect-site concentration starts at zero and increases over time until it equals the descending plasma concentration. The plasma concentration continues to fall, and after that moment of identical concentrations, the gradient between plasma and the effect site favors drug removal from the effect site, and effect-site concentrations decrease. The rate at which the effect-site concentration rises toward the peak after a bolus dictates how much drug must be injected into plasma to produce a given effect. For alfentanil, the rapid plasma effect-site equilibration (large k_{e0}) causes the effect-site concentration to rise rapidly and produce a peak in about 90 seconds. At the time of the peak, about 60% of the alfentanil bolus has been distributed into peripheral tissues or has been eliminated from the body. For fentanyl, the effect-site concentration rises much more slowly and peaks 3 to 4 minutes after the bolus.[34] At the time of the peak, more than 80% of the initial bolus of fentanyl has been distributed into tissues or eliminated. As a result of the slower equilibration with the effect site, relatively more fentanyl than alfentanil must be injected into plasma, which makes the rate of drug offset after a fentanyl bolus slower than after an alfentanil bolus.

This variability in achieving peak effect-site concentration suggests that k_{e0} must be incorporated into dosing strategies. For a rapid onset of effect, a drug with a large k_{e0} (short $t^{1}/_{2}k_{e0}$) should be chosen. For example, for rapid-sequence induction, alfentanil or remifentanil may be the opioid of choice because the peak opioid effect-site concentration coincides with endotracheal intubation. However, for a slower induction in which a nondepolarizing neuromuscular blocking drug is used, it may be appropriate to choose an opioid with a slower onset of drug effect to coincide with the peak effect of the muscle relaxant. In this case, a bolus of fentanyl or sufentanil at the time of induction may be appropriate. The time to peak effect for the commonly used opioids is shown in

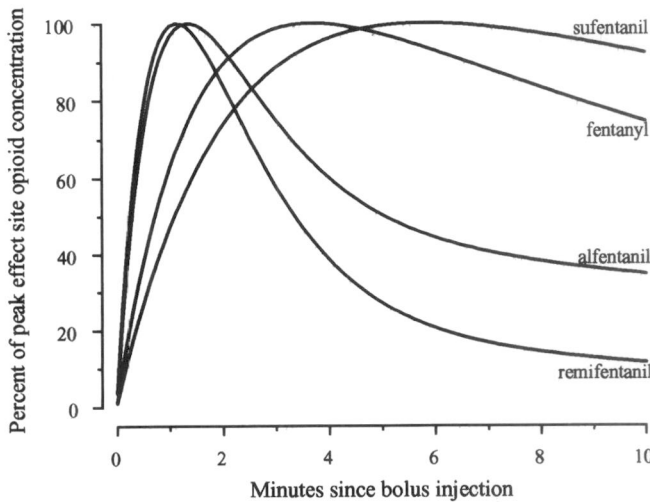

Figure 12–6 Simulated onset and time to peak effect of commonly used opioids based on their k_{e0} and pharmacokinetic parameters. k_{e0}, rate constant for transfer of drug from the site of drug effect to the environment.

Figure 12-6. Knowing the k_{e0} (or time to peak effect) also improves titration of the drug by identifying the time at which the clinician should make an assessment of drug effect. For example, midazolam has a slow time to peak effect, and repeat bolus doses should be spaced at least 3 to 5 minutes apart to avoid inadvertent overdosing.

Drug Potency

Having established that we can produce almost any desired concentration time course at the effect site, what concentration should we choose? The pharmacokinetics and pharmacodynamics of inhaled anesthetics are greatly simplified by the equilibrium established at the alveolar gas/blood interface, which permits measurement of the minimum alveolar concentration (MAC) associated with a 50% likelihood of movement in response to noxious stimulation.[35] Considerable effort has gone into developing a concept equivalent to MAC for intravenous anesthetic drugs.

The pharmacodynamics of intravenous anesthetics are reported in terms of C_{50}, the concentration that produces 50% of the maximum possible drug effect. There are many ways of thinking about C_{50}. It might be the drug concentration that prevents a response (e.g., movement, hypertension, and catecholamine release) to a particular stimulus (e.g., incision, intubation, and sternal spreading) in 50% of patients. In this case, each combination of stimulus and response may have a unique C_{50}. For example, Ausems and colleagues defined the C_{50} of alfentanil in the presence of 66% nitrous oxide for several noxious stimuli.[36] When C_{50} is defined as the drug concentration that produces a given response in 50% of patients, it is also the concentration associated with a 50% probability of response in a given patient. Note that defining C_{50} as the concentration that produces a given effect in 50% of individuals implicitly assumes that the effect can be achieved in all individuals. Some drugs exhibit a ceiling effect.

For example, there appears to be a ceiling on the ability of opioids to suppress the response to noxious stimulation. When a ceiling in drug effect exists, some patients may not exhibit the drug effect even at infinitely high doses. In this case, the C_{50} is not the concentration that causes the drug effect in 50% of patients, but instead the concentration associated with the drug effect in half of whatever fraction of patients are able to respond.

Several studies have been performed to establish appropriate concentrations for intravenous anesthetics. The C_{50} values of alfentanil, fentanyl, and remifentanil in the presence of 70% nitrous oxide have been defined for skin incision (Table 12-2). C_{50} values for loss of consciousness and skin incision have also been defined for the hypnotics thiopental,[37,38] propofol,[39-41] and midazolam (see Table 12-2).[42] Defining the C_{50}, like MAC, provides a measure of relative potency between the intravenous anesthetics.

Another interpretation of C_{50} is the concentration that produces 50% of the maximum possible physiologic response. For example, the C_{50} for an EEG response is the drug concentration that provides 50% of the maximum EEG effect. The C_{50} for EEG response has been measured for the opioids alfentanil,[43] fentanyl,[43] sufentanil.[44] remifentanil,[45-47] and trefentanil.[48] It has also been determined for thiopental,[37,49,50] etomidate,[51] propofol,[52] and benzodiazepines (see Table 12-2).[53]

Although C_{50} values for all combinations of stimuli and measures have not been experimentally determined for each opioid, they can be accurately estimated by scaling the values of C_{50} determined experimentally for other opioids by their relative potency.[54] For example, the C_{50}

of alfentanil for spontaneous ventilation is about 40% of the C_{50} for the EEG response (see Table 12-1). Knowing this, we can estimate the C_{50} of sufentanil for spontaneous ventilation (which has not yet been determined experimentally) as 0.2 to 0.3 ng/mL, that is, 40% of the C_{50} for EEG response (0.7 ng/mL).

To be entirely independent of dosing history, the C_{50} must be determined at steady state, which is rarely possible because most anesthetic drugs do not reach steady state during a continuous infusion until many hours have passed. However, if the drug achieves rapid equilibration between plasma and the effect site and the investigator waits long enough after starting the infusion, this choice can be reasonably satisfactory. For example, Ausems and colleagues[36,55] used a continuous infusion of alfentanil, which equilibrates quickly, in their experiments. They also took their measurements after the effect-site concentration had equilibrated with the plasma concentration.

A second alternative to performing a true steady-state experiment is to use mathematical modeling to calculate the effect-site concentrations of drug at the time of the measurement, as proposed by Hull and colleagues[25] and Sheiner and coworkers.[26] The relationship between effect-site and plasma concentrations is represented graphically in Figure 12-5 and mathematically in Equation 6. Calculating effect-site concentrations is nothing more than attempting to determine the steady-state plasma concentrations that would produce the observed drug effect. Sometimes, when the C_{50} reflects effect-site concentrations, it is represented as Ce_{50} to distinguish it from values of C_{50} that are based on plasma

Table 12-2	**Steady-state concentrations for predefined effects***					
C_{50} Drug	C_{50} for EEG Depression†	C_{50} for Incision or Painful Stimulus‡	C_{50} for Loss of Consciousness§	C_{50} for Spontaneous Ventilation¶	C_{50} for Isoflurane MAC Reduction	MEAC
Alfentanil (ng/mL)	500-600	200-300	—	175-225	50	10-30
Fentanyl (ng/mL)	6-10	4-6	—	2-3	1.67	0.5-1
Sufentanil (ng/mL)	0.5-0.75	(0.3-0.4)	—	(0.15-0.2)	0.145	0.025-0.05
Remifentanil (ng/mL)	10-15	4-6	—	2-3	1.23	0.5-1
Thiopental (µg/mL)	15-20	35-40	8-16	—	—	—
Midazolam (ng/mL)	250-350	—	125-250	—	—	—

*Values in parentheses are estimated by scaling to the alfentanil C_{50} (see text for details).
†The C_{50} for EEG depression is the steady-state serum concentration that causes a 50% slowing of the maximal EEG, except for midazolam, in which the C_{50} is associated with 50% EEG activation.
‡The C_{50} for skin incision is the steady-state plasma concentration that prevents a somatic or autonomic response in 50% of patients.
§The C_{50} for loss of consciousness is the steady-state plasma concentration for absence of a response to a verbal command in 50% of patients.
¶The C_{50} for spontaneous ventilation is the steady-state plasma concentration associated with adequate spontaneous ventilation in 50% of patients.
EEG, electroencephalogram; MAC, minimum alveolar concentration; MEAC, minimum effective plasma concentration providing postoperative analgesia.

concentrations, which are then termed Cp_{50}. However, the distinction is artificial. In both cases, C_{50} is intended to represent the steady-state plasma drug concentration associated with a given drug effect.

A third alternative to performing a steady-state experiment is to establish a pseudo–steady state by the use of computer-controlled drug delivery. This method has become the state-of-the-art means for determining the C_{50} for anesthetic drugs, and many of the C_{50} values referenced earlier were determined at pseudo–steady state by the use of computer-controlled drug delivery. Typically, a constant plasma concentration steady state must be maintained for four to five plasma effect-site equilibration half-lives (e.g., 10 to 15 minutes for fentanyl). Such a long delay is not necessarily required when computer-controlled drug delivery is used. For example, Glass and associates[56] used computer-controlled infusions to achieve initially higher plasma target concentrations to provide more rapid acquisition of the desired effect-site concentration. This process can be automated by having the computer actually target the concentration in the effect site rather than plasma and thereby rapidly establish plasma–effect-site equilibration.[30,31]

Thus, there are several ways to establish C_{50} in terms of steady-state concentrations. C_{50} can be estimated through mathematical effect-site modeling or can be measured experimentally by the use of computer-controlled drug delivery to quickly establish a pseudo–steady state. Either way, when performing studies to define the concentration-effect relationship, equilibrium must exist or be modeled for between the biophase (the site of effect) and plasma or blood (where the concentration is actually measured).

When C_{50} is defined in terms of the concentration associated with a response in half of a population, that same C_{50} is the concentration associated with a 50% probability of response in a typical individual. However, individual patients are not typical individuals but instead will have their own C_{50} values. Expressed in clinical terms, different patients have different anesthetic requirements for the same stimulus. For example, the minimal effective analgesic concentration of fentanyl is 0.6 ng/mL but varies among patients from 0.2 to 2.0 ng/mL.[57] The minimal effective analgesic concentrations of alfentanil[58,59] and sufentanil[60] similarly vary among patients by a factor of 5 to 10. This range encompasses both variability in the intensity of the stimulus and variability in the individual patient. However, this wide range reflects the clinical reality that must be accounted for when dosing regimens are designed. Because of this variability, intravenous anesthetics should be titrated to each patient's unique anesthetic requirement for a given stimulus.

Pharmacodynamic Drug Interactions

A common residency experience for the authors, and perhaps for the reader as well, was an attempt to administer "pure" techniques: pure inhalational anesthesia (e.g., isoflurane/oxygen), pure nitrous/narcotic anesthesia (nitrous oxide/fentanyl/oxygen), pure ketamine anesthesia, and so on. We rapidly discovered that pure hypnotic techniques required huge doses to achieve anything close to a satisfactory anesthetic. The only benefit of struggling with

pure techniques is the appreciation one gets for the essential role of drug interactions in the practice of anesthesia.

Drug interactions cause the C_{50} of one drug to shift in response to administration of a second drug. We have already referred to the ability of opioids to reduce MAC, a clinically useful drug interaction with a long history. In 1901, George Crile suggested that opioids should be administered with supplemental drugs for intravenous anesthesia. In 1959, DeCastro and Mundeleer introduced the term "neurolept anesthesia," which consists of a tranquilizer, opioid, and nitrous oxide. Today, the term coined by John Lundy, "balanced anesthesia," is used to describe the concurrent administration of several anesthetic drugs so that no single drug is given in a dosage sufficient to produce toxicity during or after surgery. Contemporary anesthesia consists of at least two components—analgesia and loss of consciousness. Combining an opioid with a volatile anesthetic or intravenous hypnotic provides both components. The interaction of hypnotics and opioids in producing the anesthetic state is complex but predictable.

Drug interactions are species dependent. Thiopental and opioids show relative antagonism to analgesic end points in rats,[61,62] whereas their effects are synergistic in humans.[63] Just as C_{50} must be defined for very specific end points, drug interactions must also be clearly defined in terms of end points. For example, Kissin and coworkers observed that "the combination of a barbiturate and an opioid gives different outcomes for different endpoints of anesthesia."[62] Often, we differentiate between analgesic end points (i.e., analgesia to noxious stimulation) and hypnotic end points (e.g., sedation and loss of consciousness). In a study of morphine-midazolam interactions on sedation and loss of the righting reflex in rats, Kissin and colleagues[64] observed that "hypnotic" end points differ. Although sedation and loss of the righting reflex appear to be hypnotic end points, these authors found that they were associated with different degrees of synergy between morphine and analgesia, which led to the conclusion that "differences in the outcomes of midazolam-morphine interactions regarding sedation and hypnosis (loss of righting reflex) suggest that underlying mechanisms for these two effects are different. Therefore, they should not be regarded as only increasing depths of the same action."

The MAC of volatile anesthetics appears to be additive when several inhaled anesthetics are administered concurrently.[65,66] The additivity of MAC suggests a uniform mechanism of action for the inhaled anesthetics, although the "unitary theory" of inhalational anesthesia has fallen into disfavor.[67,68] The intravenous anesthetics encompass categories of drugs (hypnotics, opioids, psychotomimetics, anxiolytics, neuroleptics, local anesthetics, and so on) with different receptors and mechanisms of action. In the absence of a uniform mechanism of action, there is no reason to anticipate simple additivity, for example, that maintaining a 30% C_{50} of drug A plus a 40% C_{50} of drug B will produce the same effect as a 70% C_{50} of either drug A or drug B.

The assumption of balanced anesthesia is that drug combinations will be synergistic in anesthetic effect (however defined) but not in toxicity. Such synergism has been demonstrated for a variety of drug combinations but not for others.[69] For example, Smith and colleagues[41] observed minimal synergy between propofol and fentanyl for a hypnotic end point, loss of consciousness, but profound synergy between propofol and fentanyl for an analgesic end point, loss of response to skin incision (Fig. 12-7). More profound synergy for analgesic end points than hypnotic end points has also been demonstrated for the interaction between propofol and alfentanil[40] and sevoflurane and fentanyl.[70] Thus, when anesthetic regimens are designed that rely on synergy to produce the anesthetic state, it is important to distinguish the desired end point—loss of consciousness or ablation of response to noxious stimulation. Different combinations of drugs may be required to achieve each end point.

Vuyk and colleagues characterized the interaction between propofol and alfentanil for several end points: loss of response to intubation, loss of response to intraoperative stimulation, and emergence from anesthesia (Fig. 12-8).[40] The most profound stimulation was tracheal intubation, and abolition of that stimulus required a propofol concentration of at least 2 μg/mL. Vuyk and associates also documented an interaction of propofol and alfentanil on emergence from anesthesia, a sedative end point.

Mean alveolar concentration is defined as the steady-state alveolar concentration of anesthetic gas that inhibits movement during incision in 50% of patients. It is an excellent measure of potency. MAC is also a useful guideline for clinical dosage, provided that the clinician remembers that it is the concentration in 50% of patients that inhibits a movement response and that it is defined in terms of an analgesic end point—loss of movement in

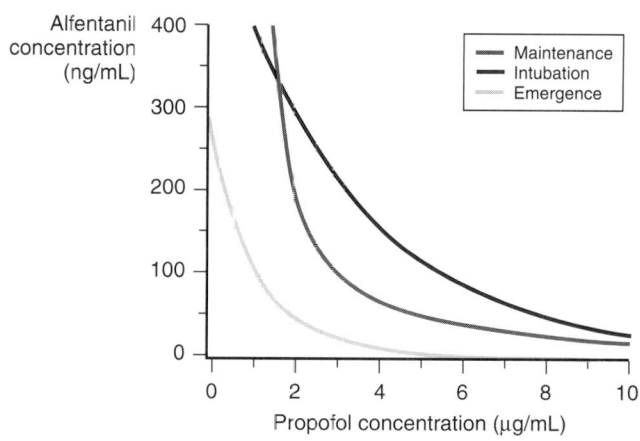

Figure 12–8 Interaction between alfentanil and propofol on three different end points: response to intubation *(red line)*, maintenance of anesthesia *(black line)*, and concentrations associated with emergence from anesthesia *(gray line)*. The *curve* shows the concentrations associated with a 50% probability of the respective end point. (Adapted from Vuyk J, Lim T, Engbers FH, et al: The pharmacodynamic interaction of propofol and alfentanil during lower abdominal surgery in women. Anesthesiology 83:8-22, 1995.)

response to noxious stimulation. To establish the interaction between volatile anesthetics and opioids, the reduction in MAC can be used. When such studies are performed, it is important that both the volatile anesthetic and the opioid be maintained at stable concentrations and have equilibrated with their effect site. For the volatile anesthetic, this objective is readily achieved by the use of a calibrated vaporizer. For the opioid, target-controlled delivery devices described earlier are used to maintain constant opioid concentrations within the effect compartment.

MAC reductions of isoflurane by fentanyl,[71] sufentanil,[72] alfentanil,[73] and remifentanil[74] have all been defined. Concentrations of these opioids that provide a 50% MAC reduction are listed in Table 12-2. Probably the most commonly used combination of anesthetics is isoflurane and fentanyl. McEwan and coworkers[71] demonstrated that the MAC of isoflurane is reduced by 50% at a fentanyl concentration of 1.7 ng/mL (Fig. 12-9), which corresponds to a fentanyl loading dose of 4 μg/kg followed by a 1.75-μg/kg/hr infusion. Because the minimum effective analgesic concentration of fentanyl is 0.6 ng/mL[57] and because clinically significant respiratory depression may occur with plasma fentanyl concentrations above 2 ng/mL,[75] it is fortunate indeed that the steepest reduction in MAC occurred within the useful analgesic range for fentanyl (i.e., 0.6 to 2 ng/mL). In other words, just maintaining fentanyl within an analgesic range reduces MAC by 50%. The study by McEwan and colleagues also demonstrated that beyond a fentanyl plasma concentration of 5 ng/mL, a plateau is seen with a maximal MAC reduction of approximately 80%. The maximal reduction in isoflurane was to a concentration of ±0.3%, that is, a value close to the awake MAC for isoflurane.[76]

Alfentanil,[73] sufentanil,[72] and remifentanil[74] produce similar reductions in isoflurane MAC, with an initial steep

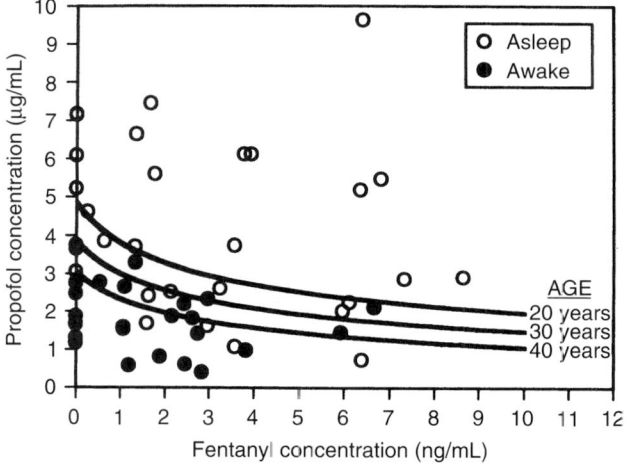

Figure 12–7 The interaction of propofol and fentanyl in providing loss of consciousness. The solid lines represent the concentrations of propofol and fentanyl when administered together that are required to prevent a response to a verbal command in 50% of patients at each decade of age.

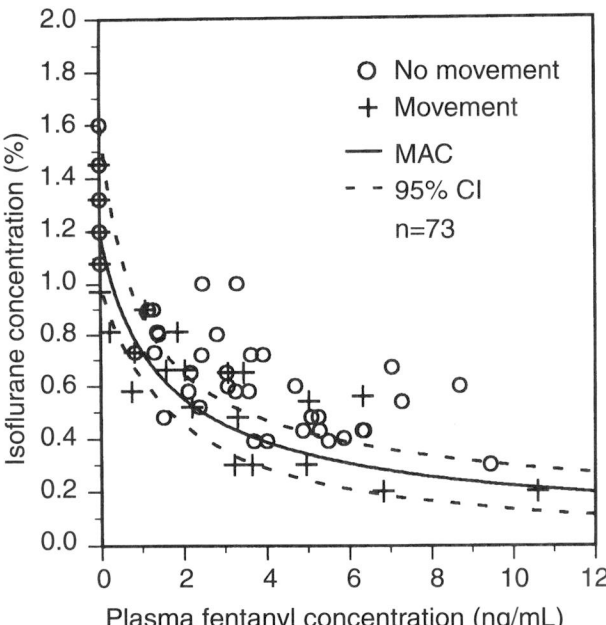

Figure 12–9 Interaction of isoflurane and fentanyl in preventing a somatic response at skin incision (i.e., minimum alveolar concentration [MAC] reduction of isoflurane). The *solid line* represents the concentrations of isoflurane and fentanyl, when administered together, that are required to prevent purposeful movement in 50% of patients at skin incision. The *dashed lines* represent the 95% confidence interval of the MAC at each combination of fentanyl and isoflurane. (From McEwan AI, Smith C, Dyar O, et al: Isoflurane MAC reduction by fentanyl. Anesthesiology 78:864-869, 1993.)

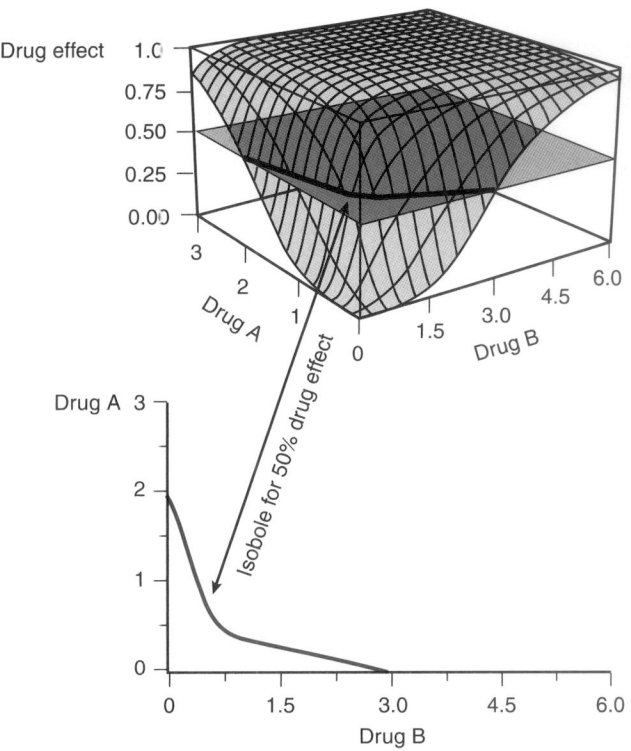

Figure 12–11 Relationship between a response surface and a standard isobologram. Conventional "isobolographic" analysis, whether for doses or concentrations, describes only the concentrations of both drugs that yield a 50% drug effect and thus fails to capture the entire response surface. (From Minto CF, Schnider TW, Short TG, et al: Response surface model for anesthetic drug interactions. Anesthesiology 92:1603-1616, 2000.)

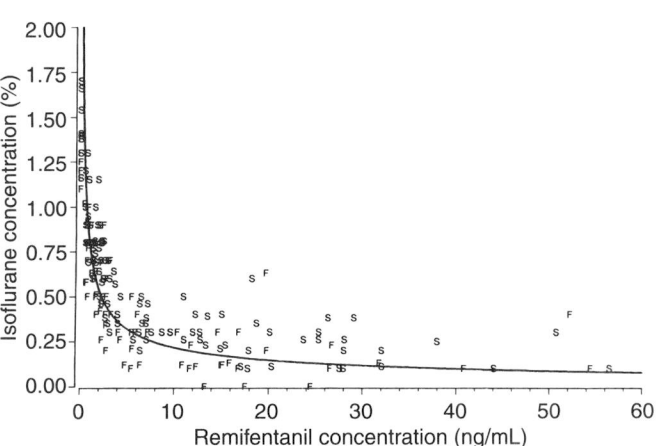

Figure 12–10 Interaction of isoflurane and remifentanil in preventing a somatic response at skin incision (i.e., minimum alveolar concentration reduction of isoflurane). The *solid line* represents the concentrations of isoflurane and remifentanil, when administered together, that are required to prevent purposeful movement in 50% of patients at skin incision. From Lang E, Kapila A, Shlugman D, et al: Reduction of isoflurane minimal alveolar concentration by remifentanil. Anesthesiology 85:721-728, 1996.)

reduction at lower concentrations and a plateau effect at higher concentrations. Because remifentanil is rapidly metabolized,[28] it is possible to give huge doses during MAC studies and still awaken patients after surgery. The MAC reduction of isoflurane by remifentanil is shown in Figure 12-10.[74] Even with enormously high plasma concentrations (>30 ng/mL), a ceiling of opioid effect is observed, and the MAC of isoflurane was not reduced below 0.2% to 0.3%. Little clinical benefit is achieved by administering opioid at concentrations exceeding those that produce a ceiling in MAC reduction, which occurs at a concentration of 3 to 5 ng/mL for fentanyl and remifentanil, 200 to 400 ng/mL for alfentanil, and 0.25 to 0.5 ng/mL for sufentanil. Keeping the opioid dose within an analgesic range prevents the very slow recovery that is associated with high opioid concentrations.

We have examined the relationship between opioids and hypnotics on the C_{50}, the concentration of drug associated with 50% of the maximal effect. It is important to realize that the interaction between two drugs actually describes a surface where each drug has its own axis, and the third axis is the effect from any combination of the two drugs. Figure 12-11 shows the relationship between the three-dimensional response surface and the more commonly shown relationship in two dimensions between the C_{50} of two drugs. Minto and colleagues published "response surfaces" for combinations of midazolam-alfentanil, propofol-alfentanil, and midazolam-propofol

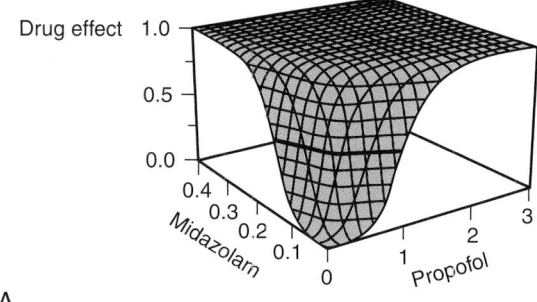

A

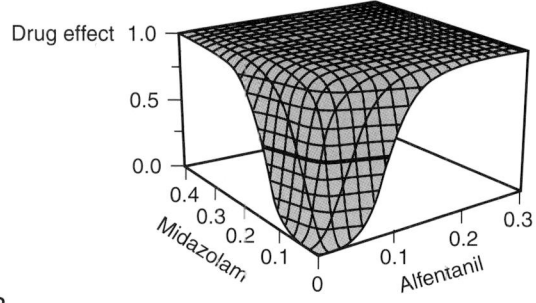

B

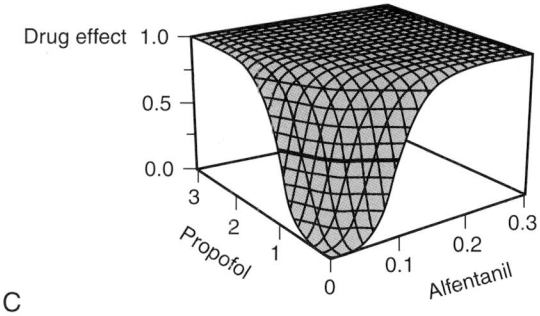

C

Figure 12–12 Response surface for each of the paired interactions between propofol and midazolam (**A**), alfentanil and midazolam (**B**), and alfentanil and propofol (**C**) on the probability of opening eyes to a verbal command. The isoboles for a 10%, 20%, 30%, 40%, 50%, 60%, 70%, 80%, and 90% response are shown. (From Minto CF, Schnider TW, Short TG, et al: Response surface model for anesthetic drug interactions. Anesthesiology 92:1603-1616, 2000.)

Despite this variability, dosing guidelines play an important role in the practice of anesthesia. The concentration ranges of the intravenous anesthetics for anesthesia, sedation, and analgesia are given in Table 12-3. These ranges provide starting estimates on which subsequent titration can be based. They also provide a means of estimating whether the patient is having a typical or an atypical response. If the patient's dosing requirements deviate greatly from established guidelines, it is reasonable to determine whether something else might be going on with either the patient or the drug delivery system.

DESIGNING DOSING REGIMENS

Bolus Dose Calculations

The definition of concentration is amount divided by volume. We can rearrange the definition of concentration to find the amount of drug required to produce any desired concentration for a known volume:

$$\text{Amount} = C_T \times \text{Volume} \qquad (10)$$

where C_T is the desired or "target" concentration. Many introductory pharmacokinetic texts suggest using this formula to calculate the loading bolus required to achieve a given concentration. The problem with applying this concept to anesthetic drugs is that there are several volumes: V_1 (central compartment), V_2 and V_3 (the peripheral compartments), and Vd_{SS}, the sum of the individual volumes. V_1 is usually much smaller than Vd_{SS}, and thus it is tempting to say that the loading dose should be something between $C_T \times V_1$ and $C_T \times Vd_{SS}$.

associated with loss of response to verbal command, as shown in Figure 12-12.[77] They also extended response surface methodology to describe the simultaneous interaction of three drugs. Rendering the full interaction surface for three drugs would require drawing the graph in four dimensions. If the graph is limited to the interaction at a 50% drug effect, it can be rendered in three dimensions, as shown in Figure 12-13.

There is still variability in sensitivity from patient to patient, as well as variability in the level of stimulation associated with different surgical procedures. Thus, each patient is an experiment, with the clinician learning the individual patient's C_{50} for the combination of drugs used during the administration of each anesthetic.

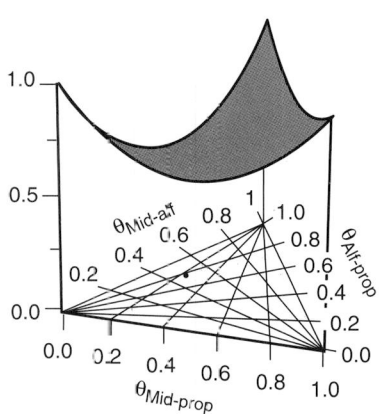

Figure 12–13 Interaction at a 50% drug effect between propofol, midazolam, and alfentanil. Downward deflection of the surface represents synergy, in units of fractional reduction in C_{50}. The three edges represent relative amounts of propofol to midazolam ($\theta_{Mid-Prop}$), alfentanil to midazolam ($\theta_{Mid-Alf}$), and alfentanil to propofol ($\theta_{Alf-Prop}$). The surface between the edges represents the relative synergy of all three drugs taken together. (From Minto CF, Schnider TW, Short TG, et al: Response surface model for anesthetic drug interactions. Anesthesiology 92:1603-1616, 2000.)

Consider the dose of fentanyl required to attenuate the hemodynamic response to intubation when combined with thiopental. The C_{50} for fentanyl, when combined with thiopental for intubation, is approximately 3 ng/mL. The V_1 and Vd_{ss} for fentanyl are 13 and 360 L, respectively. The aforementioned equations can thus be interpreted as suggesting that an appropriate dose of fentanyl to attenuate the hemodynamic response is between 39 µg (3 ng/mL × 13 L) and 1080 µg (3 ng/mL × 360 L). A fentanyl bolus of 39 µg achieves the desired concentration in plasma for an initial instant, but plasma levels almost instantly decrease below the desired target. Levels at the effect site will never be close to the desired target concentration of 3 ng/mL. A fentanyl bolus of 1080 µg, not surprisingly, produces an enormous overshoot in plasma levels that persists for hours (Fig. 12-14). Additionally, it is absurd to use equations to calculate the fentanyl dose if the resulting recommendation is "pick a dose between 39 and 1080 µg."

The usual dosing guidelines for a bolus dose, presented earlier, are designed to produce a specific plasma concentration. Because plasma is not the site of drug effect, it is illogical to base calculation of the initial bolus on a desired plasma concentration. As pointed out previously, by knowing the k_{e0} of an intravenous anesthetic, we can design a dosing regimen that yields the desired concentration at the site of drug effect. If we do not want to overdose the patient, we should select the bolus that produces the desired peak concentration at the effect site.

The decline in plasma concentration between the initial concentration after the bolus (amount/V_1) and the concentration at the time of peak effect can be thought of as a dilution of the bolus into a larger volume than the volume of the central compartment. This approach introduces the concept of Vd_{pe}, the apparent volume of distribution at the time of peak effect,[29,78] or pseudoequilibration between plasma and the site of drug effect.[79] The size of this volume can be readily calculated from the observation that the plasma and effect-site concentrations are the same at the time of peak effect:

$$Vd_{pe} = \frac{\text{Bolus amount}}{C_{pe}} \qquad (11)$$

where C_{pe} is the plasma concentration at the time of peak effect.

Let us assume that our clinical goal is to select the dose required to produce a certain drug effect without producing an overdose. We can rearrange Equation 11 by substituting C_T, the target concentration (which is the same in plasma and the effect site at the moment of peak effect), for C_{pe} to calculate the size of the initial bolus:

$$\text{Loading dose} = C_T \times Vd_{pe} \qquad (12)$$

The Vd_{pe} for fentanyl is 75 L. Producing a peak fentanyl effect-site concentration of 3.0 ng/mL requires 225 µg, which achieves a peak effect in 3.6 minutes. This dosing guideline is much more reasonable than the previous recommendation of picking a dose between 39 and 1080 µg. Table 12-4 lists V_1 and Vd_{pe} for fentanyl, alfentanil, sufentanil, remifentanil, propofol, thiopental, and midazolam. Table 12-1 lists the k_{e0}, $t\frac{1}{2}\ k_{e0}$, and time to peak effect of the commonly used intravenous anesthetics.

Maintenance Infusion Rate

By definition, the rate at which drug exits the body is systemic clearance, Cl_S, times the plasma concentration. To maintain a given target concentration, C_T, drug must be delivered at the same rate that drug is exiting the body. Thus,

$$\text{Maintenance infusion rate} = C_T \times Cl_S \qquad (13)$$

For drugs with multicompartmental pharmacokinetics, which includes all the intravenous drugs used in anesthetic practice, drug is distributed into peripheral tissues as well as cleared from the body. The rate of distribution into tissues changes over time as tissue levels equilibrate with plasma levels. Equation 13 is correct only after the peripheral tissues have fully equilibrated with plasma, which requires many hours. At all other times, this maintenance infusion rate underestimates the infusion rate to maintain a target concentration.

In some situations, this simple maintenance rate calculation may be acceptable. For example, if an infusion at this rate is used along with a bolus dose based on Vd_{pe} and the drug has a long delay between the bolus and peak effect, much of the distribution of drug into tissues may have occurred by the time that the effect-site concentration reaches the target concentration. In this case, the maintenance infusion rate calculated as clearance times target concentration may be fairly accurate because Vd_{pe} is sufficiently higher than V_1 to account for the distribution of drug into peripheral tissues. Unfortunately, most drugs used in anesthesia have sufficiently rapid equilibration between plasma and the effect site that Vd_{pe} does not adequately encompass the distribution process, thus making this approach unsuitable.

Another example of calculating infusion rates for drugs with multicompartmental pharmacokinetics is the two-step approach proposed by Wagner.[80] In this method, two infusions, Q_1 and Q_2, are administered in sequence. The loading infusion, Q_1, is selected on the basis of convenience and the degree of overshoot in plasma concentration that will be clinically acceptable. The second infusion, Q_2, is calculated as $C_T \times Cl_S$, exactly as noted earlier. The Wagner two-step approach does not consider the time course of drug effect and thus is probably not appropriate for most anesthetic drugs.

Having offered to the reader two approaches that do not work very well, we now turn to approaches that are mathematically and clinically sound. Because the net flow of drug into peripheral tissues decreases over time, the infusion rate required to maintain any desired concentration must also decrease over time. If the initial bolus has been based on Vd_{pe}, no infusion need be administered until the effect-site concentrations peak. After the peak in effect-site concentration, the (nearly) correct equation to maintain the desired concentration is

Maintenance infusion rate =

$$C_T \times V_1 \times \left(k_{10} + k_{12}e^{-k_{21}t} + k_{13}e^{-k_{31}t}\right) \quad (14)$$

This equation indicates that a high infusion rate is initially required to maintain C_T. Over time, the infusion rate gradually decreases (see Fig. 12-4). At equilibrium (t = ∞), the infusion rate decreases to $C_TV_1k_{10}$, which is the same as C_TCl_S. Few anesthesiologists would choose to mentally solve such an equation during administration of an anesthetic. Fortunately, some simple techniques can be used in place of solving such a complex expression.

Figure 12-15 is a nomogram in which Equation 14 has been solved, and it shows the infusion rates over time necessary to maintain any desired concentration of fentanyl, alfentanil, sufentanil, and propofol. This nomogram is complex, so we will review it in detail. The y axis represents the target concentration C_T. The x axis is the time since the beginning of the anesthetic (i.e., since the initial bolus). The suggested target initial concentrations (shown in red) are based on the work of Vuyk and colleagues[40] with propofol and alfentanil (see Fig. 12-8) and are scaled to fentanyl and sufentanil based on their relative potencies.[78] The intersections of the target concentration line and the diagonal lines indicate the infusion rate appropriate at each point in time. For example, to maintain a fentanyl concentration of 1.5 ng/mL, the appropriate rates are 4.5 µg/kg/hr at 15 minutes, 3.6 µg/kg/hr at 30 minutes, 2.7 µg/kg/hr at 60 minutes, 2.1 µg/kg/hr at 120 minutes, and 1.5 µg/kg/hr at 180 minutes. Of course, you can select target concentrations and different times of rate adjustment, depending on clinical circumstances

Table 12–3   Plasma drug concentration ranges

Drug*	Skin Incision	Stimulus Minor Surgery	Major Surgery	Spontaneous Ventilation	Awakening	Analgesia or Sedation
Alfentanil (ng/mL)	200-300	250-450	100-300	<200-250	—	50-100
Fentanyl (ng/mL)	3-6	4-8	2-5	<1-2	—	1-2
Sufentanil (ng/mL)	1-3	2-5	1-3	<0.2	—	0.02-0.2
Remifentanil (ng/mL)	4-8	4-8	2-4	<1-3	—	1-2
Propofol (µg/mL)	2-6	2.5-7.5	2-6	—	0.8-1.8	1.0-3.0
Methohexital (µg/mL)	5-10	5-15	5-10	—	1-3	2-5
Thiopental (µg/mL)	7.5-12.5 (with N₂O) 35-45 (without N₂O)	10-20	10-20	—	4-8	7.5-15.0
Etomidate (ng/mL)	400-600	500-1000	300-600	—	200-350	100-300
Midazolam (ng/mL)	—	50-250 (combined with an opioid)	50-250 (combined with an opioid)	—	150-200 (reduced to 20-70 in the presence of an opioid)	40-100
Ketamine (µg/mL)	—	—	1-2	—	—	0.1-1

*Drug levels are when combined with 65% to 70% nitrous oxide (N_2O) unless otherwise stated. Effective plasma concentrations may differ markedly, depending on premedication and intraoperative drug combinations.

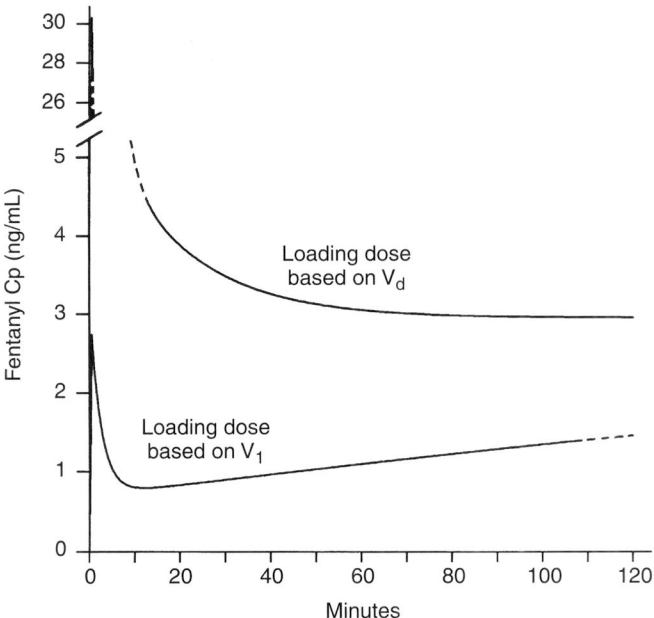

Figure 12–14 Pharmacokinetic simulation demonstrating the limitations of infusion regimens based on simple pharmacokinetic parameters, with fentanyl used as an example. These infusion schemes were designed to achieve a plasma fentanyl concentration of 3 ng/mL. The *upper curve* shows that a regimen using a loading dose based on the volume of distribution followed by a constant infusion based on clearance results in a transient period of extremely high plasma concentrations. If the same maintenance infusion is given but the loading dose is based on the volume of the central compartment, distribution of drug to the peripheral compartments causes the plasma concentration to fall below the desired level until the compartments reach steady-state concentrations, as shown in the *lower curve.* Cp, plasma drug concentration.

and your assessment of how accurately the intravenous drug needs to be titrated.

Another recent approach to manually determining infusion rates for maintenance of anesthesia to a desired target concentration is through the use of concepts used with a slide rule.[81] Figure 12-16 illustrates such a slide rule for propofol. As described by Bruhn and coauthors, "The bolus dose required to reach a given target plasma concentration is the product of the (weight-related) distribution volume

Table 12–4 Volume of distribution at the time of peak effect		
Drug	V_1 **(L)**	Vd_{pe} **(L)**
Fentanyl	12.7	75
Alfentanil	2.19	5.9
Sufentanil	17.8	89
Remifentanil	5.0	17
Propofol	6.7	37
Thiopental	5.6	14.6
Midazolam	3.4	31

V_1, volume of the central compartment; Vd_{pe}, apparent volume of distribution at the time of peak effect.

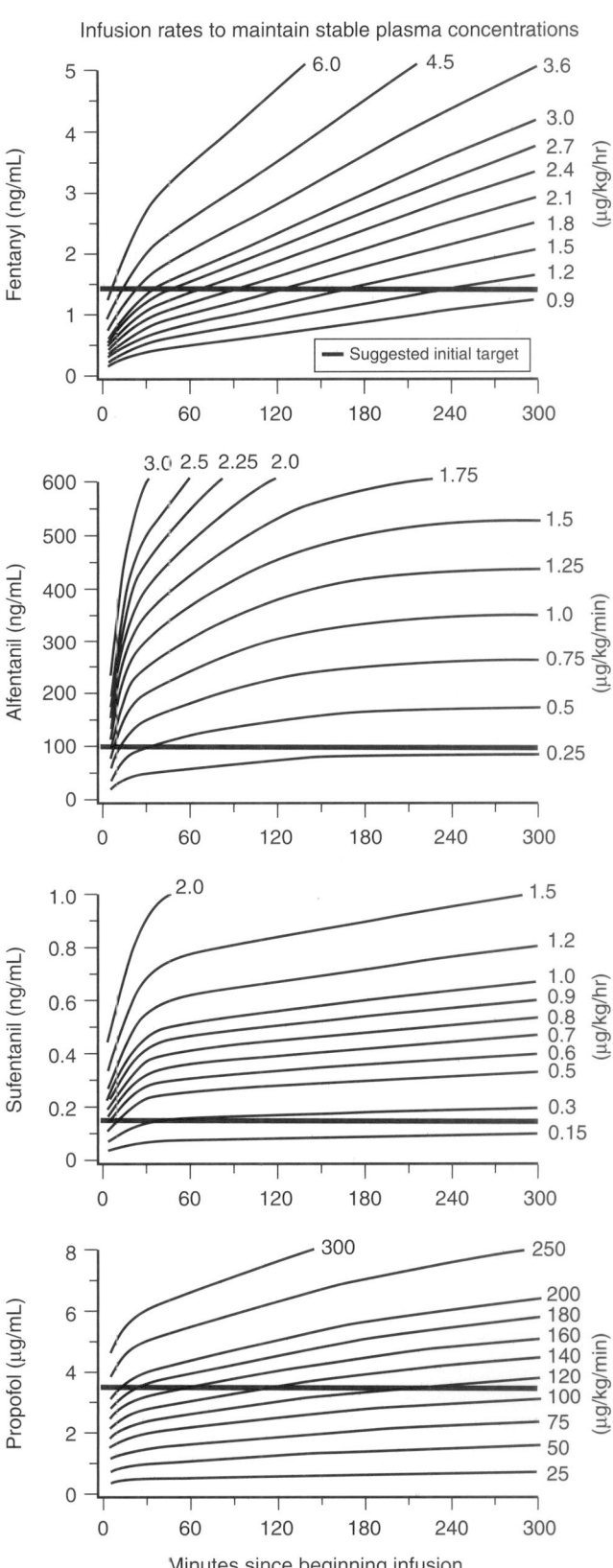

Figure 12–15 Nomogram for calculating maintenance infusion rates to maintain a stable concentration of fentanyl, alfentanil, sufentanil, or propofol. The *y* axis is the desired concentration. The *x* axis is the time relative to the initial bolus. The *diagonal lines* show the infusion rates at different times required to maintain the desired concentration selected on the *y* axis.

Figure 12–16 Slide rule for calculating the maintenance propofol infusion rate from the patient's weight, the desired target concentration, and the elapsed time. (Adapted from Bruhn J, Bouillon TW, Ropcke H, Hoeft A: A manual slide rule for target-controlled infusion of propofol: Development and evaluation. Anesth Analg 96:142-147, 2003.)

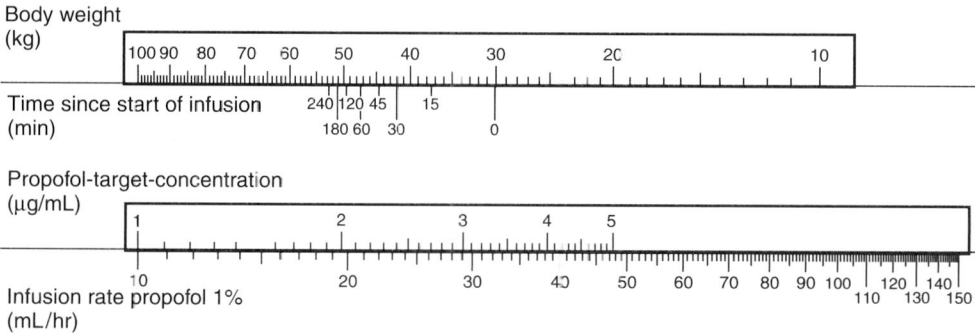

and the required concentration. Similarly, the infusion rate at a particular time point is the product of target concentration, body weight, and a correction factor that depends on the time elapsed from the start of the initial infusion. This factor can be determined for each time point by using a PK simulation program."[81] When compared with computer simulation programs, this manual device performed within an acceptable degree of accuracy (within 7% of the simulated target concentration) for a single target concentration and decreased in accuracy (within 20%) when the device was applied to changing target concentrations.

Recovery from Anesthesia

Recovery from anesthesia is determined by the pharmacokinetic principles that govern the rate of decrease in drug from the effect compartment, once drug administration is terminated, as well as by the pharmacodynamics of the drug. Although the terminal elimination half-life is often interpreted as a measure of how short or long lasting a drug is, the rate at which a drug decreases is dependent on both elimination and redistribution of the drug from the central compartment. The contribution of redistribution and elimination to the rate of decrease in drug concentration varies according to the duration for which the drug has been administered.[78,82]

In 1985, Schwilden[83] developed a mathematical model to relate the time course of offset of the inhaled anesthetics to the duration of anesthetic drug delivery. Similarly, Fisher and Rosen[84] demonstrated how accumulation of muscle relaxants in peripheral volumes of distribution results in slowed recovery with increasing duration of administration. They introduced two measures of the time course of recovery, the time for twitch tension to recover from 5% to 25% and the time for twitch tension to recover from 25% to 75% (also see Chapter 13).

Since then, the time for the plasma concentration to decrease by 50% from an infusion that maintains a constant concentration (e.g., the infusion given by Equation 14) has been termed the "context-sensitive half-time" (Fig. 12-17),[82] with the context being the duration of the infusion. The 50% decrease was chosen both for tradition (e.g., half-lives are the time for a 50% decrease with a one-compartment model) and because, very roughly, a 50% reduction in drug concentration

appears to be necessary for recovery after the administration of most intravenous hypnotics at the termination of surgery. Depending on the circumstances, decreases other than 50% may be clinically relevant. Additionally, sometimes it is the plasma concentration that is of interest, and sometimes it is the effect-site concentration that is of interest. A more general term is the context-sensitive "decrement time,"[85] in which the decrement in concentration is specifically noted, as is the compartment in which the decrease is modeled (plasma or effect site). For example, the relationship between infusion duration and the time required for a 70% decrease in fentanyl effect-site concentration is the "context-sensitive 70% effect-site decrement time."

Context-sensitive effect-site decrement times for varying percent decreases in alfentanil, fentanyl, and remifentanil concentration are illustrated in Figure 12-18. To determine when an infusion should be terminated (to enable awakening of the patient at the end of surgery), the clinician needs to bear in mind the decrease in concentration necessary for recovery, the duration of the infusion (the context), and the context-sensitive effect-site decrement time required for the necessary decrease.

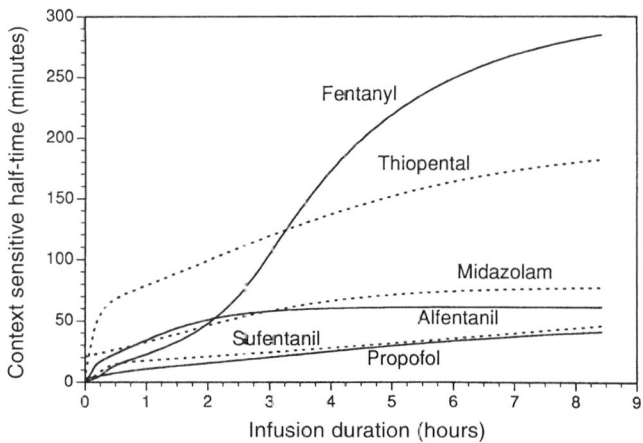

Figure 12–17 Context-sensitive half-times as a function of infusion duration (the "context") derived from pharmacokinetic models of fentanyl, sufentanil, alfentanil, propofol, midazolam, and thiopental. (From Hughes MA, Glass PSA, Jacobs JR: Context-sensitive half-time in multicompartment pharmacokinetic models for intravenous anesthetic drugs. Anesthesiology 76:334-341, 1992.)

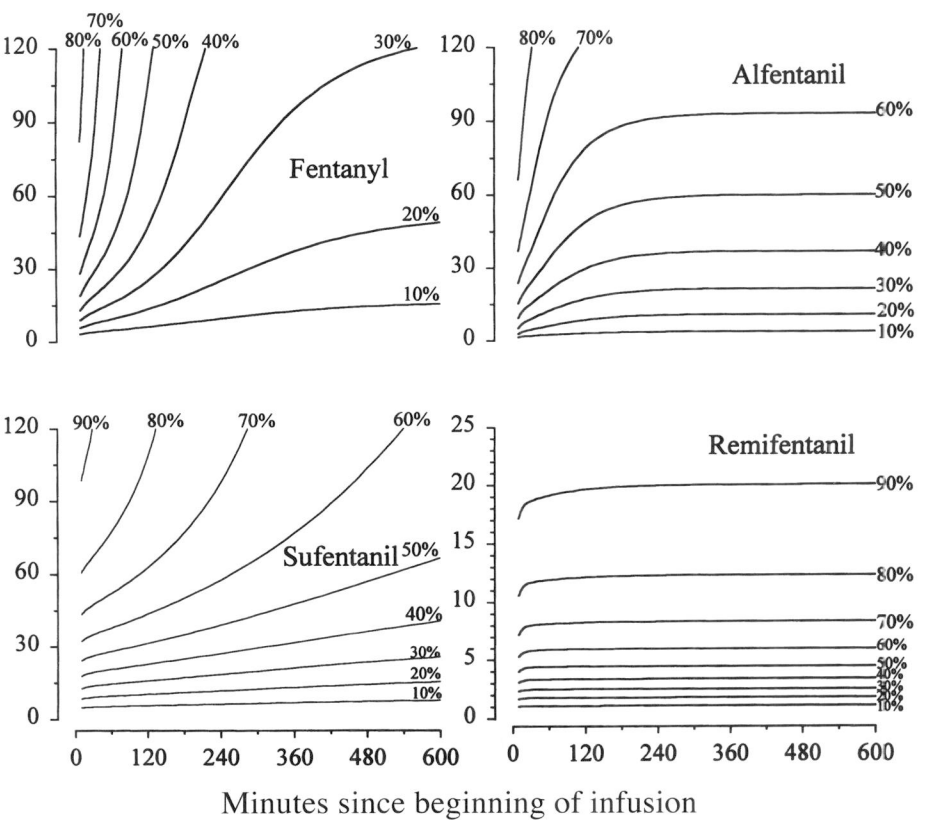

Figure 12–18 Context-sensitive effect-site decrement times for alfentanil, fentanyl, sufentanil, and remifentanil showing the time required for decreases in a given percentage (labeled for each curve) from the maintained effect-site concentration after termination of the infusion.

Context-sensitive decrement times are fundamentally different from the elimination half-life. With monoexponential decay, each 50% decrease in concentration requires the same amount of time, and this time is independent of how the drug was given. Such is not true for the context-sensitive half-time. First, as the name is intended to imply, the time to achieve a 50% decrease is absolutely dependent on how the drug was given, with infusion duration being the context to which the name refers. In addition, small changes in percent decrement can result in surprisingly large increases in the time required. As can be seen from Figure 12-18, in some situations the time required for a 60% decrease in drug concentration can be more than twice the time required for a 50% decrease.

Context-sensitive decrement times are based on the assumption that the plasma or effect-site concentration is maintained at a constant level. This is rarely the case clinically, but maintenance of constant concentrations is a necessary assumption to provide a unique mathematical solution to the time required for a given percent decrement in plasma or effect-site concentration. Because plasma and effect-site concentrations are rarely kept constant, it is important that context-sensitive decrement times be used as general guidelines for interpreting the pharmacokinetics of intravenous drugs and not as absolute predictions for any given case or infusion regimen. Automated drug delivery systems can provide more precise predictions of the time required for the plasma or effect-site concentration to decrease to any desired concentration based on the actual drug dosing in the individual patient. This information provides the clinician with guidance for the most appropriate time to terminate the infusion.

Context-sensitive decrement times focus on the role of pharmacokinetics in recovery from anesthesia. Pharmacodynamics plays an important role in recovery as well. Bailey[86] used integrated pharmacokinetic/pharmacodynamic models to define the "mean effect time" as the average time to responsiveness after maintenance of anesthesia at the 90% probability of unresponsiveness. The mean effect time demonstrates that when drugs have a very shallow concentration-versus-response relationship, concentrations must decrease by a significant fraction to provide adequate emergence, which delays recovery from anesthesia. In contrast, recovery is hastened by a steep concentration-versus-response relationship, in which emergence from anesthesia occurs after a relatively small fractional decrease in concentration. Most intravenous hypnotics have a fairly steep concentration-versus-response relationship.

Pharmacodynamic drug interactions also play a role in recovery from anesthesia. Interaction relationships predict that the same anesthetic state can be achieved by different ratios of two drugs. One way of selecting the best ratio might be the combination that offers the most rapid recovery. For example, when an opioid is combined with a hypnotic, recovery from anesthesia depends on the opioid and hypnotic concentrations, the rate of decrease in both drugs, and the relative synergy between them for loss of response to noxious stimulation (i.e., the state maintained during anesthesia) versus the relative synergy for loss of consciousness. Although the time course of the decrease in opioid and hypnotic concentrations can be approximately described by their respective context-sensitive decrement times for both drugs (Fig. 12-19 and, for propofol/alfentanil, Fig. 12-8), the influence of relative synergy for different end points must be captured by separate models of the interaction of the drugs for adequate anesthesia and emergence from anesthesia.

Vuyk and coworkers[87] modeled the predicted time to awakening when propofol is combined with fentanyl, sufentanil, alfentanil, or remifentanil on the basis of the interaction between propofol and these opioids to provide adequate anesthesia and the interaction between propofol and opioids on emergence from anesthesia, as seen in Figures 12-20 and 12-21. Recovery times vary according to the opioid selected and the relative balance of opioid and propofol during maintenance of anesthesia. For example, in the upper left of Figure 12-20 is a simulation of emergence from a propofol/fentanyl anesthetic of 10 minutes' duration. The simulations assume a steady concentration of fentanyl and propofol throughout the anesthetic, similar to the underlying assumption of context-sensitive decrement times. The red curve in the lower plane is the interaction curve between fentanyl and propofol; it ranges from no fentanyl and 12 µg/mL of propofol on the left to 1.8 µg/mL of propofol and 6 ng/mL of fentanyl on the right. In theory, any point along this curve would provide equivalent maintenance of anesthesia. When the infusion is turned off after 10 minutes of anesthesia, the concentrations of both drugs decrease. The decreasing concentrations of propofol and fentanyl when the infusion is turned off can be found by the upward lines drawn from different points on the interaction curve, with the distance away from the lower plane representing time. Taken together, these upward lines represent a "recovery surface." The red line drawn on the recovery surface shows the points at which the fentanyl-propofol interaction model predicts emergence.

Figure 12-20 shows that after 10 minutes of maintaining 1.8 µg/mL of propofol and 6 ng/mL of fentanyl (right edge of the interaction curve), it takes approximately 12 minutes for the concentrations of both drugs to decrease enough to permit emergence. However, if one maintains concentrations of 3.5 ug/mL of propofol and 1.5 ng/mL of fentanyl (toward the middle of the interaction curve), emergence can be expected just 8 minutes after the infusions are turned off. Examination of the curves for 60, 300, and 600 minutes of fentanyl/propofol anesthesia suggests that the fentanyl target concentration that provides the most rapid emergence is approximately 1.0 to 1.5 ng/mL, which requires a propofol concentration of approximately 3.0 to 3.5 µg/mL to maintain adequate anesthesia. These values are consistent with the earlier observation that most of the MAC reduction benefit of fentanyl occurs within the analgesic range and that exceeding this range is of little benefit during anesthesia. In similar simulations, Vuyk and colleagues demonstrated that maintaining alfentanil and sufentanil concentrations in excess of the analgesic range (i.e., approximately 80 ng/mL for alfentanil and 0.15 ng/mL for sufentanil) is of little clinical benefit but can be expected to delay recovery from anesthesia. A second conclusion from these simulations is that if the patient demonstrates inadequate anesthesia, to prevent prolongation of recovery, it is preferable to increase the hypnotic concentration than to increase the opioid concentration beyond the analgesic range.

The situation is different for remifentanil because of its unusual pharmacokinetic properties (see Fig. 12-21) (also see Chapter 11). The extraordinary clearance of remifentanil results in a very rapid offset of opioid drug effect when a remifentanil infusion is terminated. In Figure 12-21, the lower plane again shows equivalent anesthetic states during maintenance with an opioid, remifentanil, and propofol. High doses of remifentanil permit a modest reduction in the dose of propofol necessary for

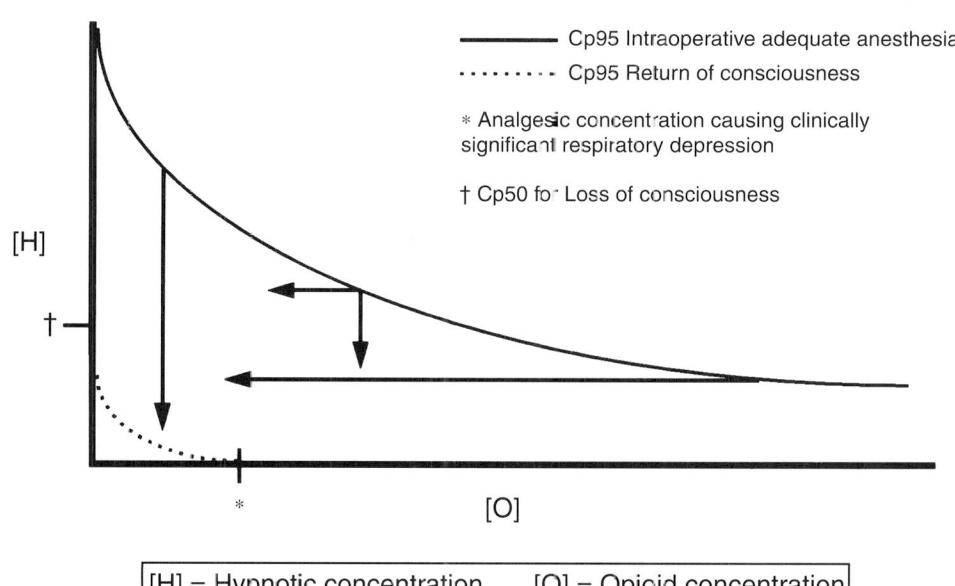

Figure 12–19 Interaction between hypnotics and opioids for prevention of movement after a noxious stimulus and for awakening and adequate spontaneous ventilation at the end of a surgical procedure. From this interaction it can be seen that the time to recover at the end of a procedure is dependent on the concentration of both drugs used during surgery and the time for both to decrease below that required for consciousness and adequate spontaneous ventilation (i.e., their context-sensitive decrement times).

——— Cp95 Intraoperative adequate anesthesia

········· Cp95 Return of consciousness

* Analgesic concentration causing clinically significant respiratory depression

† Cp50 for Loss of consciousness

[H] = Hypnotic concentration   [O] = Opioid concentration

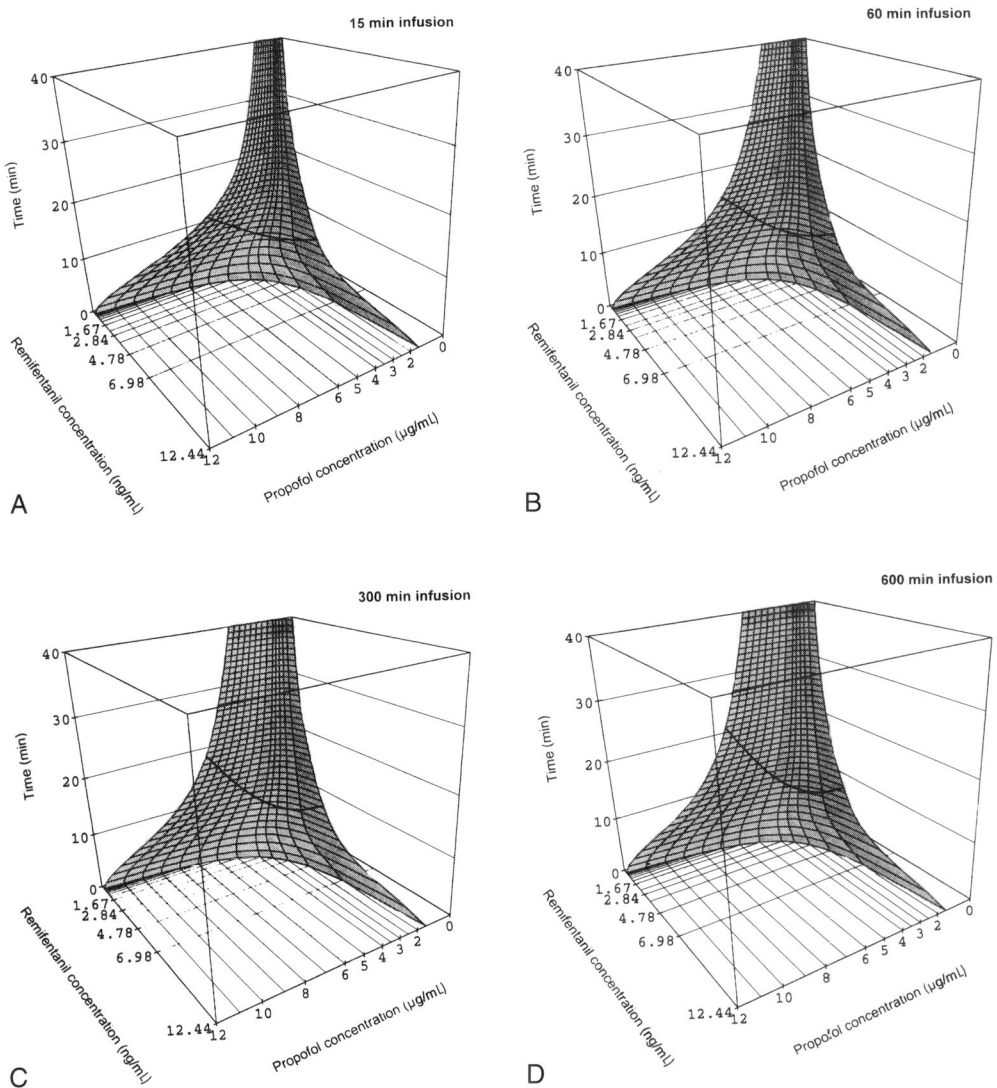

Figure 12–20 Simulation of the interaction of propofol and fentanyl in preventing a somatic response at skin incision and time to recovery. On the *x* axis is the fentanyl concentration, and on the *y* axis, the propofol concentration. The curve in the lower plane shows the propofol-fentanyl interaction required to provide adequate anesthesia. When the infusion is turned off, the concentrations of each drug decrease, as shown on the *z* axis. The curve drawn on the recovery surface shows the time to emergence from anesthesia for combinations of fentanyl and propofol after an anesthetic of 10 minutes' (**A**), 60 minutes' (**B**), 300 minutes' (**C**), or 600 minutes' (**D**) duration. Note that the optimal combination for the most rapid recovery is a propofol concentration of 3.0 to 3.5 μg/mL of propofol combined with 1.5 ng/mL of fentanyl. As the concentration of propofol or fentanyl increases, the time for recovery increases. In addition, the longer the duration of drug infusion, the longer that recovery takes, especially if the optimal combination is not used. Adapted from Vuyk et al.[87]

adequate anesthesia. However, the recovery surfaces show that high doses of remifentanil, with a modest reduction in the propofol dose, permit considerably faster emergence from anesthesia. For example, it takes approximately 12 minutes to awaken from 600 minutes of anesthesia maintained with 3 μg/mL of propofol and 2.5 ng/mL of remifentanil (see Fig. 12-20, lower left graph). If the remifentanil concentration is increased to 5 ng/mL, the propofol concentration can be reduced to 2 to 2.5 μg/mL, and emergence can be anticipated within 6 minutes of discontinuation of the infusions. One might be concerned that such a technique places patients at increased risk for awareness because a propofol concentration of 2 μg/mL is below the C_{50} value for wakefulness.[39,41] Therefore, it is probably reasonable to combine such a technique with intraoperative EEG monitoring to assess anesthetic adequacy.

The offset of effect of isoflurane and sevoflurane is similar to that of propofol. The offset of desflurane effect is slightly quicker than that of propofol. We can draw some logical extrapolations from these propofol/opioid simulations to anesthetics consisting of volatile anesthetics combined with opioids. When fentanyl, alfentanil, or sufentanil is combined with a volatile anesthetic, the most rapid recovery occurs

when the opioid concentration is maintained at an analgesic concentration equivalent to 1 to 1.5 ng/mL of fentanyl (Table 12-5). Concurrently, the volatile anesthetic should be administered at the lowest concentration required to provide adequate anesthesia but no less than an end-tidal concentration of 0.3 MAC, the MAC value for return of consciousness. If the patient demonstrates signs of inadequate anesthesia, it is preferable to increase the volatile anesthetic because this agent has less of an effect on prolonging the wake-up time than does increasing the opioid (with the exception of remifentanil) and is more likely to ensure that awareness does not occur.

MANUAL INFUSION SCHEMES FOR INTRAVENOUS ANESTHETICS

The following infusion schemes are developed from integrated pharmacokinetic-pharmacodynamic models. However, it is the patient's response, demonstrating adequate or inadequate anesthesia, that ultimately determines the rate of drug administration. Individuals vary markedly in their response to a given drug dose or concentration, and it is therefore essential to titrate

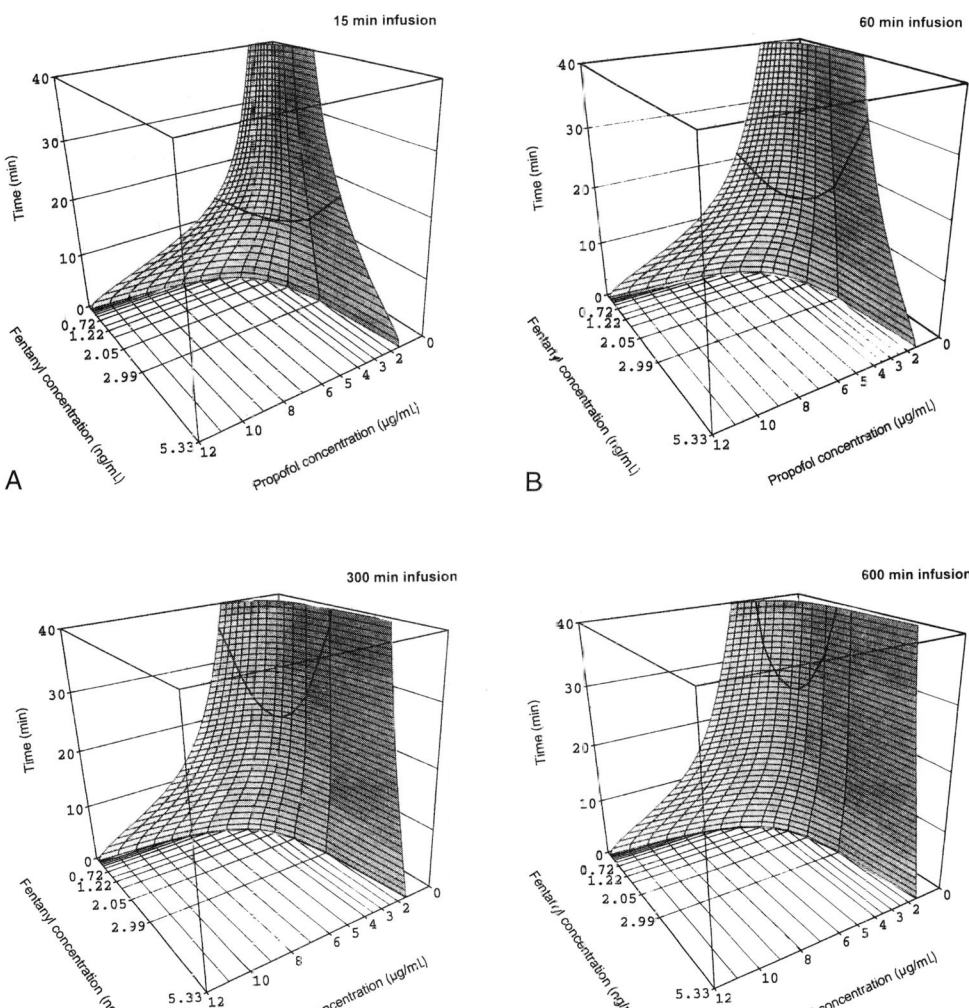

15 min infusion

60 min infusion

300 min infusion

600 min infusion

Figure 12–21 Simulation of the interaction of propofol and remifentanil in preventing a somatic response at skin incision and time to recovery. Note that with remifentanil, the optimal combination is a propofol concentration of 2.5 µg/mL and a remifentanil concentration of 5 to 7 ng/mL and that increasing the duration of the infusion has minimal impact on recovery time if the optimal dose of remifentanil is not used. However, if the propofol dose is increased, recovery is prolonged. (Adapted from Vuyk J, Mertens MJ, Olofsen E, et al: Propofol anesthesia and rational opioid selection: Determination of optimal EC50-EC95 propofol-opioid concentrations that assure adequate anesthesia and a rapid return of consciousness. Anesthesiology 87:1549-1562, 1997.)

to an adequate drug level for each individual patient. Drug concentrations required to provide adequate anesthesia also vary according to the type of surgery (e.g., surface surgery versus upper abdominal surgery). The end of surgery requires lower drug levels, and consequently, titration often involves judicious lowering of the infusion rate toward the end of surgery to facilitate rapid recovery. Common dosing schemes for administering intravenous anesthetics by infusion are given in Table 12-6.

If the infusion rate proves to be insufficient to maintain adequate anesthesia, a further loading (bolus) dose and an increase in infusion are required to rapidly raise the plasma (biophase) drug concentration. Various interventions also require greater drug concentrations, usually for brief periods (e.g., laryngoscopy, endotracheal intubation, skin incision) (see Fig. 12-3). Therefore, the infusion scheme should be tailored to provide peak concentrations during these brief periods of intense stimulation. An adequate drug level for endotracheal intubation is

Table 12–5 Infusion rates for opioids to achieve preset concentrations

Drug	Plasma Target (ng/mL) Concentration	Bolus (µg/kg)	Infusion Rate (µg/kg/min)
Fentanyl	1	3	.020
	4	10	.070
Alfentanil	40	20	0.25
	160	80*	1.00
Sufentanil	0.15	0.15	0.003
	0.50	0.50	0.010
Remifentanil	3	0.5-1*	0.1-0.15
	6	1-2*	0.2-0.3

*Give as a rapid infusion over a period of 1 to 2 minutes.

Table 12–6   Manual infusion schemes*

| Drug | Anesthesia | | Sedation or Analgesia | |
	Loading Dose (μg/kg)	Maintenance Infusion (μg/kg/min)	Loading Dose (μg/kg)	Maintenance Infusion (μg/kg/min)
Alfentanil	50-150	0.5-3	10-25	0.25-1
Fentanyl	5-15	0.03-0.1	1-3	0.01-0.03
Sufentanil	1-5	0.01-0.05	0.1-0.5	0.005-0.01
Remifentanil	0.5-1.0	0.1-0.4	†	0.025-0.1
Ketamine	1500-2500	25-75	500-1000	10-20
Propofol	1000-2000	50-150	250-1000	10-50
Midazolam	50-150	0.25-1.5	25-100	0.25-1
Methohexital	1500-2500	50-150	250-1000	10-50

*After the loading dose, an initially high infusion rate to account for redistribution should be used and then titrated to the lowest infusion rate that will maintain adequate anesthesia or sedation.
†For analgesia or during sedation, an initial loading dose is not required with remifentanil.

often achieved by the initial loading dose, but for procedures such as skin incision, a further bolus dose may be necessary.

Opioids (see Chapter 11)

Alfentanil

As shown by the work of Ausems and associates,[22] the highest alfentanil concentrations (in combination with 70% nitrous oxide) are required for endotracheal intubation. The concentration of alfentanil required for skin closure is less than that required for skin incision or spontaneous ventilation, which allows the opioid to be gradually titrated downward toward the end of the procedure.

Several schemes have been advocated for the infusion of alfentanil when it is used as part of a nitrous-narcotic technique.[88-90] Most schemes vary in the sequence of the initial loading dose, although most provide 100 μg/kg within the first 10 minutes. Thus, the loading dose may be given as an initial rapid infusion of 50 μg/kg/min over a period of 2 minutes or two 50-μg/kg doses given before endotracheal intubation and skin incision or as a slower infusion of 10 μg/kg/min over a 10-minute period. The initial loading dose is followed by an infusion of 0.5 to 2 μg/kg/min. If the plasma concentration needs to be raised, an incremental bolus of 7 to 15 μg/kg with a 0.5- to 1-μg/kg/min increase in the infusion rate is usually successful. For the aforementioned infusion scheme, alfentanil is usually combined with 66% nitrous oxide. If a hypnotic is used with alfentanil to induce anesthesia, the dose of the hypnotic can usually be markedly reduced. Alfentanil can be infused with nitrous oxide or combined with a hypnotic for a total intravenous technique. If combined with midazolam (loading dose, 0.05 to 0.2 mg/kg; maintenance infusion, 0.05 to 0.15 μg/kg/min) or propofol (loading dose, 1 to 2 mg/kg; maintenance infusion, 50 to 150 μg/kg/min), the loading dose and infusion rate of alfentanil can be reduced to 10 to 50 μg/kg followed by 0.5 to 1 μg/kg/min. If given with a potent inhaled anesthetic at 0.3 to 0.5 MAC, both the loading dose and the

infusion rate can be reduced to approximately 30% to 50% of that used with nitrous oxide alone. When alfentanil is combined with a volatile anesthetic or forms part of a total intravenous anesthetic (TIVA) technique, alfentanil is dosed to achieve plasma concentrations of 75 to 150 ng/mL. When these doses are used, the infusion of alfentanil should be discontinued approximately 10 to 20 minutes before the expected end of surgery.

For cardiac anesthesia, in the absence of adjuvant anesthetic drugs, much larger infusion rates are required (also see Chapter 50). An initial infusion of 40 μg/kg/min to loss of consciousness is followed by 10 μg/kg/min until cooling. On patient rewarming, the infusion rate can be restarted at 2.5 μg/kg/min. If inadequate anesthesia occurs, a bolus of 30 μg/kg usually ablates a response. Alfentanil has also been used for sedation in intensive care units. An initial loading dose of 25 μg/kg is followed by 0.25 to 0.5 μg/kg/min for 20 minutes and then titrated according to patient needs (0.1 to 2.0 μg/kg/min). A bolus of 3 μg/kg can be given when further supplementation is needed. In general, doses of alfentanil, as listed earlier, should be reduced in elderly or debilitated patients.

Fentanyl

Infusion of fentanyl has classically been used for cardiac surgery. Again, various schemes have been advocated for the loading dose and vary from a bolus of 50 μg/kg to a rapid infusion of 4 to 5 μg/kg/min for 5 minutes or 2 to 3 μg/kg/min for 10 minutes,[89,90] followed by continuous infusion of 0.1 to 1.0 μg/kg/min. These infusion schemes are designed to obtain a plasma fentanyl concentration of 20 to 40 ng/mL. Such a high dose of fentanyl has not demonstrated any advantage over infusion schemes that provide fentanyl concentrations of 5 to 10 ng/mL and are combined with a low-dose volatile anesthetic or propofol. This approach also facilitates fast tracking of cardiac patients. An initial loading dose of 10 to 20 μg/kg is followed by an infusion of 0.05 to 0.1 μg/kg/min. For noncardiac surgery in which a nitrous-narcotic technique is used, the loading dose can be reduced to 5 to 15 μg/kg, followed by continuous infusion of 0.03 to 0.1 μg/kg/min to provide plasma concentrations of 3 to 10 ng/mL.[56] These concentrations combined with 66% nitrous oxide provide adequate anesthesia for intra-abdominal and body surface surgery but may result in prolonged respiratory depression.

Analgesic concentrations of fentanyl are obtained at a plasma concentration of 1 to 2 ng/mL.[57] This concentration is optimal when combined with an intravenous hypnotic or potent inhaled agent or postoperatively for analgesia and is obtained after a loading dose of 1.5 to 3 µg/kg is administered, followed by continuous infusion of 0.01 to 0.04 µg/kg/min.

Sufentanil

Sufentanil has been successfully administered by infusion during cardiac anesthesia.[89,90] For use in cardiac surgery, an initial loading dose of 15 µg/kg followed by an infusion of 0.75 µg/kg/min is administered. When combined with midazolam (midazolam loading dose, 100 µg/kg; maintenance infusion, 1.0 to 2.5 µg/kg/min), the sufentanil dose is reduced to 2 µg/kg/min for 5 minutes, followed by 0.010 to 0.025 µg/kg/min thereafter. Even smaller doses of midazolam and sufentanil may be adequate for cardiac surgery. Very little has been published on the plasma concentrations or infusion rates of sufentanil required for noncardiac surgery. Several studies have established that in the concentration domain, sufentanil is approximately 10 times more potent than fentanyl. Thus, for noncardiac surgery, infusion rates are based on achieving concentrations approximately one tenth those of fentanyl. When combined with 70% nitrous oxide, a loading dose of 1 to 2 µg/kg of sufentanil followed by an infusion of 0.01 to 0.04 µg/kg/min can be used. As the analgesic component of a total intravenous technique or when combined with a volatile anesthetic, an initial loading dose of 0.2 to 0.5 µg/kg followed by an infusion of 0.005 to 0.01 µg/kg/min of sufentanil is generally appropriate to achieve sufentanil concentrations within the analgesic range of 0.1 to 0.3 ng/mL.

Remifentanil

Remifentanil is the newest µ-agonist available for administration as an analgesic during surgery. Because of its metabolism by general body esterases, the drug is best administered as an infusion. In addition, as a result of this unique metabolism, the decrease in concentration and dissipation of the opioid effect are very rapid after termination of its administration. This property enables the clinician to administer remifentanil at relatively higher analgesic concentrations than is possible with other opioids without the likelihood of prolonged respiratory depression. An initial loading infusion of 0.5 to 1 µg/kg/min is usually administered. This infusion dosage should be reduced by about 50% in the elderly. Moreover, the time to peak effect in the elderly is about 50% longer than in younger patients. Because offset of the drug effect is so rapid, to ablate the response to endotracheal intubation, the infusion should be maintained at 0.1 to 0.3 µg/kg/min until endotracheal intubation has been completed. When it is used in combination with a volatile anesthetic or propofol for noncardiac surgery, the infusion rate can then be reduced to 0.05 to 0.2 µg/kg/min. When it is used as a nitrous-narcotic technique, an infusion rate of 0.1 to 0.5 µg/kg/min is usually necessary. The infusion should be terminated only 5 to 10 minutes before the end of surgery (e.g., at the end of skin closure). If postoperative pain is likely to be present, it is important that the clinician initiate other forms of pain management either before or on termination of the remifentanil infusion. For cardiac surgery, infusion rates of 1 µg/kg/min have been used successfully with marked ablation of the stress response. Infusion rates of 0.5 µg/kg/min combined with low-dose propofol or a volatile anesthetic are also likely to be useful for cardiac surgery. Remifentanil, like all the other opioids, requires lower infusion rates to produce the same effect in elderly subjects.[46,91] In general, by the age of 50 years, the remifentanil infusion rate should be reduced by half of that given to a 21-year-old patient. An 80-year-old patient requires a remifentanil infusion rate that is just one third that required in a 21-year-old patient.

Hypnotics (also see Chapter 10)

Propofol

Propofol is best administered by continuous infusion and is presently the most common intravenous anesthetic used for TIVA and sedation. Plasma concentrations necessary during surgery and for awakening have been established (see Table 12-6).[39-41,92,93] To obtain a plasma level of 3 to 4 µg/mL, a four-stage infusion scheme can be used. This scheme consists of a loading dose of 1 mg/kg over a period of 20 seconds, followed by 170 µg/kg/min (10 mg/kg/hr) for 10 minutes, then 130 µg/kg/min (8 mg/kg/hr) for 10 minutes, and 100 µg/kg/min (6 mg/kg/hr) thereafter. More simply, a loading dose of 1 to 2 mg/kg can be followed by an initial infusion of 150 to 200 µg/kg/min, which is then titrated down to about 100 µg/kg/min. For short surgical procedures, generally higher average infusion rates are required, but for longer procedures, the average infusion rate is 100 to 150 µg/kg/min when combined with nitrous oxide. The reader can also construct propofol infusion regimens for other target concentrations from the nomogram in Figure 12-15.

When propofol is given with an opioid (rather than nitrous oxide) as part of a TIVA technique, the infusion rate of propofol remains similar to that required with nitrous oxide (i.e., an initial induction dose followed by a decreasing infusion rate of 150 to 100 µg/kg/min). Propofol has been combined with alfentanil (loading dose, 10 to 25 µg/kg; maintenance infusion, 0.5 to 1 µg/kg/min), fentanyl (loading dose, 2 to 5 µg/kg; maintenance infusion, 0.02 to 0.06 µg/kg/min), sufentanil (loading dose, 0.2 to 0.5 µg/kg; maintenance infusion, 0.005 to 0.03 µg/kg/min), and remifentanil (loading dose, 1 µg/kg; maintenance infusion, 0.05 to 0.4 µg/kg/min) for total intravenous anesthesia. The required infusion rate of propofol during anesthesia demonstrates a negative correlation with age; that is, elderly patients need lower infusion rates.

For sedation during regional or topical anesthesia, an initial loading infusion of 0.5 mg/kg is given over a 5-minute period, followed by a maintenance infusion of 25 to 75 µg/kg/min. Another technique used by the authors is to give bolus doses of 0.2 mg/kg every 1.5 to 3 minutes until the desired level of sedation is achieved.

Multiply the number of bolus doses by 10 to determine the maintenance infusion rate (in µg/kg/min).

Propofol has been used for up to 2 weeks for continuous sedation of patients in intensive care units.[94] In critically ill patients, a loading dose may not be desirable, and therefore an infusion can be started at 25 to 50 µg/kg/min. This rate is subsequently titrated to the desired level of sedation.

Thiopental

Thiopental is rarely administered by infusion for the maintenance of surgical anesthesia because the context-sensitive half-time is prolonged when an infusion lasting more than just a brief duration is used. Thiopental has been successfully administered by infusion for short body surface procedures in combination with fentanyl.[95] An initial loading dose of 2 to 4 mg/kg is followed by an infusion of 200 to 300 µg/kg/min for the first 20 minutes and 30 to 70 µg/kg/min thereafter. For sedation, an initial loading dose of 2 to 4 mg/kg is followed by an infusion of 30 to 80 µg/kg/min. When thiopental is administered by infusion, its metabolism results in the formation of pentobarbital. It is uncertain, however, whether formation of this barbiturate is of clinical significance.

Methohexital

Methohexital (unlike thiopental) can be used effectively by infusion for the maintenance of anesthesia during surgical procedures lasting up to 2 hours. A loading (induction) dose of 1 to 2 mg/kg is followed by an infusion of 50 to 150 µg/kg/min. Methohexital (at these infusion rates) can be combined with 66% nitrous oxide, an opioid, or both. Methohexital may also be administered by infusion for sedation. A loading dose of 0.5 to 1 mg/kg given over a period of 5 to 10 minutes followed by an infusion of 15 to 25 µg/kg/min usually provides an adequate level of sedation.

Etomidate

The use of etomidate by infusion is controversial (see Chapter 10). Most infusions with etomidate for general anesthesia are designed to provide a plasma etomidate concentration of 500 ng/mL.[96] This concentration may be achieved with either a two- or a three-stage infusion scheme. In the two-stage scheme, etomidate is infused at 100 µg/kg/min for a period of 10 minutes and then at 10 µg/kg/min. In the three-stage regimen, etomidate is infused at 100 µg/kg/min for 3 minutes, 20 µg/kg/min for 27 minutes, and 10 µg/kg/min thereafter. Etomidate is combined with nitrous oxide and usually an opioid given either intermittently or by continuous infusion. Etomidate plus fentanyl (loading dose, 2 to 3 µg/kg; maintenance infusion, 0.02 to 0.06 µg/kg/min) or alfentanil (loading dose, 10 to 20 µg/kg; maintenance infusion, 0.5 to 1 µg/kg/min) can be combined to provide total intravenous anesthesia. The etomidate infusion can usually be terminated 10 to 15 minutes before the anticipated end of the surgical procedure. Etomidate has been administered by infusion for cardiac surgery. An initial loading dose (used for induction) is followed by an infusion of etomidate at 20 µg/kg/min. Such administration

results in a plasma level of 550 to 900 ng/mL. The use of etomidate for prolonged sedation is contraindicated, but it can be administered for brief periods of sedation (i.e., for regional anesthesia). For sedation, a loading dose of 15 to 20 µg/kg/min for 10 minutes is followed by a maintenance infusion of 2.5 to 7.5 µg/kg/min.

Ketamine

Ketamine, although it possesses both hypnotic and analgesic properties, as well as suitable pharmacokinetics, is not a popular agent for maintenance of general anesthesia because of the psychotomimetic action of the currently available racemic mixture. The impact of ketamine on postoperative analgesia may again increase its use, especially at low doses.

When combined with a benzodiazepine, ketamine can provide suitable anesthesia (with or without nitrous oxide). The loading (induction) dose is 1 to 2 mg/kg followed by an infusion of 10 to 50 µg/kg/min.[97] In the absence of nitrous oxide and for more invasive surgery, higher infusion rates of 30 to 100 µg/kg/min may be necessary. Ketamine has also been administered by infusion during cardiac surgery at similar infusion rates. An infusion of ketamine is also useful for analgesia or sedation, or for both. The loading dose can be reduced to 0.2 to 0.75 mg/kg and the infusion to 5 to 20 µg/kg/min. Ketamine has been successfully used with propofol for a TIVA technique. The ketamine infusion consists of a loading dose of 1 to 3 mg/kg followed by an infusion of 5 to 20 µg/kg/min. The propofol infusion is the same regimen used when propofol is combined with nitrous oxide. Like alfentanil, ketamine has been mixed with propofol to provide a single-syringe TIVA technique.

Midazolam

Midazolam can be administered by infusion for sedation or for provision of the hypnotic component of a balanced anesthetic.[98] The effects of an opioid plus a benzodiazepine appear to be synergistic rather than additive for both loss of consciousness and anesthesia.[69,99] The loading (induction) dose of midazolam can therefore be reduced to 0.05 to 0.1 mg/kg when combined with fentanyl (2 to 5 µg/kg) or alfentanil (10 to 25 µg/kg). The midazolam maintenance infusion rate during surgical anesthesia can then be titrated to between 0.25 and 1 µg/kg/min with either fentanyl (maintenance infusion, 0.02 to 0.06 µg/kg/min) or alfentanil (maintenance infusion, 0.5 to 1.5 µg/kg/min). Nitrous oxide, if added to the aforementioned combinations, further decreases the required infusion rates of both midazolam and the opioid. For cardiac surgery, similar doses of midazolam can be combined with slightly larger doses of the chosen opioid.[100] For sedation, a loading dose of 0.02 to 0.1 mg/kg of midazolam is administered. This is best given as 10-µg/kg doses until the desired level of sedation is achieved. The maintenance infusion is then titrated to between 0.25 and 1 µg/kg/min. At the termination of a prolonged (days) infusion, the development of a benzodiazepine withdrawal syndrome is possible. Therefore, the infusion might need to be slowly tapered, or a long-acting benzodiazepine may need to be given.

INFUSION DEVICES

Manual Delivery

When an infusion of an intravenous anesthetic is administered, the infusion regimen can be controlled by a variety of mechanisms. These mechanisms vary from the simple CAIR clamp or Dial-a-Flo (Abbott Laboratories) to complex computer-controlled infusion pumps. Simplicity of mechanical design, however, is not necessarily correlated with ease of use, which has prompted ongoing advances in infusion device technology.

Infusion devices can be classified as either controllers or positive displacement pumps. Explicit in their title, controllers contain mechanisms that control the rate of flow produced by gravity, whereas positive displacement pumps contain active pumping mechanisms.

The most commonly used pumps for the administration of intravenous anesthetics are positive displacement syringe pumps that use a screw mechanism. These pumps are extremely accurate and have the convenience of not requiring specialized tubing. Many of these pumps have features that make them particularly suitable for anesthetic delivery. An important advance has been the introduction of a calculator feature within the pump so that the clinician can set the weight of the patient, the drug concentration, and the infusion rate in dose/unit weight/unit time and the pump then calculates the infusion in volume/unit time. In addition, these pumps allow simple application of a staged infusion scheme (e.g., the two-stage approach of Wagner[80]) by allowing a loading dose and a maintenance infusion rate to be programmed into the pump. Numerous syringe pumps also now include automated recognition of syringe size. These modest advances in pump technology and design enable intravenous anesthetics to be conveniently delivered. However, the only commercially available devices for the delivery of intravenous anesthetics that approach the convenience of the present-day vaporizer are target-controlled infusion devices such as the "Diprifusor," which are available everywhere except North America. These devices go beyond simple calculator pumps to create truly "smart" pumps that use automated drug delivery.

Automated Delivery

Automated drug delivery implies that electronic or mechanical instrumentation performs dose rate adjustments independent of human intervention (in contrast to the manual devices described earlier). The desired target (e.g., drug concentration and clinical response) is still chosen by the clinician. Preprogrammed dosing (either bolus or infusion) is the simplest form of automated drug delivery and consists of a preprogrammed infusion (usually calculated to provide a single target blood or effect concentration) that is automatically implemented by the microprocessor in the pump.[101] Preprogrammed devices are limited in their application for intravenous anesthetic drugs because of their inability to allow the user to vary the target concentration.[102] Generally, two methods may be applied for automated target anesthetic

drug delivery: model-based (a form of open-loop control) and closed-loop systems.

Terms and Definitions

Both model-based and closed-loop systems require a set point (Fig. 12-22).[103] The set point may best be defined as the quantifiable end point (e.g., plasma concentration, percent T1 of the electromyogram, or bispectral index value) related to the clinical objective (e.g., level of anesthesia, neuromuscular blockade). Accordingly, the set point is the value (i.e., target) that the automated system is attempting to maintain. The feedback signal is the measured (e.g., percent T1 of the electromyogram) or predicted (e.g., predicted effect-site concentration from pharmacokinetic simulation) value that has resulted from the automated delivery process.

A closed-loop system is the ideal means of automated drug delivery. Model-based drug delivery, however, provides an important alternative in circumstances in which the feedback signal cannot be measured and an appropriate model is available. A mathematical (e.g., pharmacokinetic) relationship that can simulate the physiology provides the model. Consequently, the accuracy of any model-based control system is dependent on how well the model represents the process under control. The control signal (which for automated drug delivery is the dosing scheme) is the difference between the set point and the model prediction. The control signal directs the actuator (i.e., the infusion pump) to produce the intervention necessary to obtain the set point (i.e., deliver the dosage regimen prescribed by the algorithm to the patient). This intervention results in a new feedback control signal, and the process repeats itself to maintain the patient at the target.

In an adaptive control system, the algorithm is adapted to the individual's unique response to the intervention produced by the actuator. For example, in a closed-loop system to control blood pressure, the algorithm may prescribe a 1-μg/kg/min increase in the infusion of sodium nitroprusside when the blood pressure exceeds 5 mm Hg above the target. Although this prescription may generally be appropriate, a change of this magnitude may cause a much greater drop in blood pressure than desired in a sensitive individual. After experience with the patient, an adaptive controller learns the individual's sensitivity and, by using this sensitivity, changes the

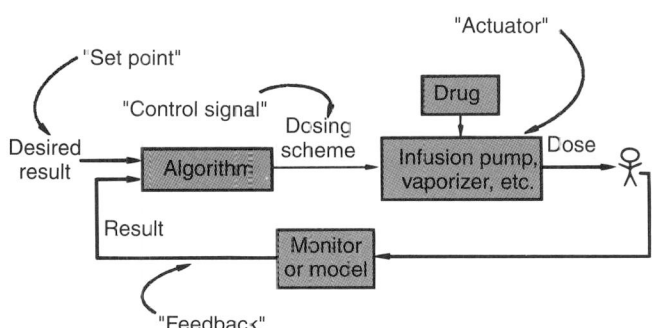

Figure 12–22 Components of a typical automated drug delivery system.

algorithm so that the control signal (dosing scheme) results in an intervention by the actuator that brings the feedback signal more closely to the target.

Target Control Infusion Systems

Devices

In 1968, Kruger-Thiemer[104] described the infusion regimen theoretically required to quickly achieve and maintain a constant plasma concentration of an intravenously administered drug whose kinetics are described by a two-compartment model. This regimen has become known as the "BET scheme" (see Fig. 12-4) and consists of an initial *bolus* of $C_T V_1$, an infusion at a rate of $C_T Cl_S$ to replace drug *eliminated* from the body, and an exponentially decreasing infusion at a rate given by Equation 14 to replace drug *transferred* to the peripheral tissues. The section on designing dosage regimens demonstrates that the bolus portion, calculated as $C_T V_1$, will probably be inadequate for reaching the desired effect-site concentration. Mathematically, the "ET" portion of the BET scheme is identical to the exponentially declining maintenance infusion rate shown in the section on designing dosing regimens. Precise implementation of this complex dosage regimen requires infusion rates that change continuously as a function of time until a steady state is achieved.

More than a decade after publication of Kruger-Thiemer's classic paper, Schwilden and colleagues[2,105,106] interfaced a microcomputer to an infusion pump and demonstrated clinical application of the BET infusion scheme. Many other groups have since implemented either the BET algorithm or modifications of this algorithm on microcomputers connected to infusion pumps. These algorithms are based on the same polyexponential equations or compartment models described previously, and they calculate the infusion rates theoretically required to obtain the desired plasma or effect-site drug concentration. When implementing these algorithms, it is necessary to consider the physical limitations of the system. For example, infusion rates must be positive or zero. Additionally, some pumps have limitations on precision and accuracy that can reduce the accuracy of the infusion.

Despite minor differences in the approaches taken by different investigators using pharmacokinetic model–driven infusion systems, all are conceptually similar. Each consists of a microcomputer interfaced to an infusion pump, as seen in Figure 12-23. The microcomputer executes a program that incorporates the pharmacokinetic model. When using the device, the anesthesiologist enters a target plasma or effect-site drug concentration (Fig. 12-24). This target concentration is based on knowledge of the pharmacokinetic-pharmacodynamic relationship of the drug and the desired effect, as well as on the individual responses of the patient. At frequent intervals (e.g., every 9 to 15 seconds), the program compares the target concentration with the current prediction of the plasma or effect-site drug concentration, which is computed by real-time simulation of a pharmacokinetic model of the drug being infused. The computer calculates the infusion rate required to achieve the desired target concentration and transmits this rate to the pump after adjusting the rate to reflect the physical capabilities of the pump. The pump then delivers drug to the patient at the desired rate.

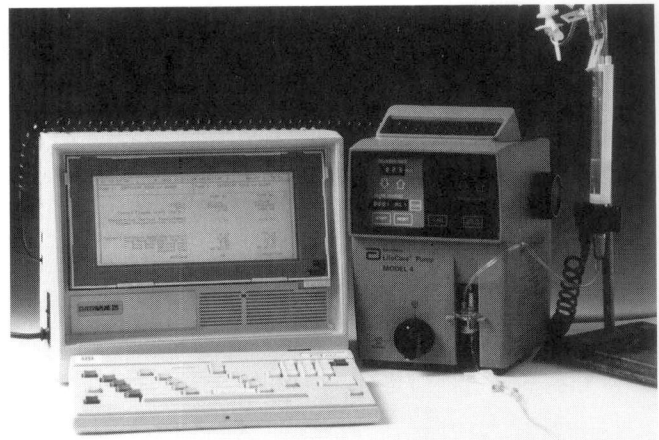

Figure 12–23 The CACI system used at Duke University Medical Center. CACI consists of a laptop computer electronically linked to an infusion pump. The desired drug plasma or effect-site concentration is entered via the keyboard.

At each step, the computer makes sure that the pump has delivered the drug that it was instructed to give and checks for errors reported by the infusion pump (e.g., air in line, out of drug). The computer then calculates what the pump did during the previous interval and updates the internal pharmacokinetic model on the basis of the reported drug delivered. The cycle is completed when the computer calculates the infusion rate required over the next interval to reach the desired target concentration and transmits this rate to the infusion pump. Concurrently, the computer supplies the anesthesiologist with information about the state of the model, the state of the pump, any problems reported by the pump, the anticipated time course for elimination of drug from the patient, the total amount of drug delivered, the current infusion rate, and other information that may be of assistance in providing clinical care.

As a result of the increasing popularity of intravenous anesthesia and continuous-infusion techniques, the inherent reasonableness of pharmacokinetically based drug delivery, and the promising results achieved with automated administration of a variety of drugs by research groups around the world, pharmacokinetic model–driven infusion of propofol has become widely available worldwide, except in North America. This system consists of a commercial pump and the "Diprifusor" software, which provides the control algorithm. Reasons for the lack of availability of these devices in North America are complex but are primarily related to hostility toward computer-controlled drug infusion within the Food and Drug Administration.[107]

Several European device companies are modifying existing infusion pumps, which already contain powerful microprocessors, to provide pharmacokinetic model–driven infusions as a software-selectable option. Pharmacokinetic parameters for various drugs are already programmed into the device, and the devices have the ability to target the concentration at the site of drug effect or in plasma. Such devices are well adapted to the need for rapid titration in anesthesia. The user selects the

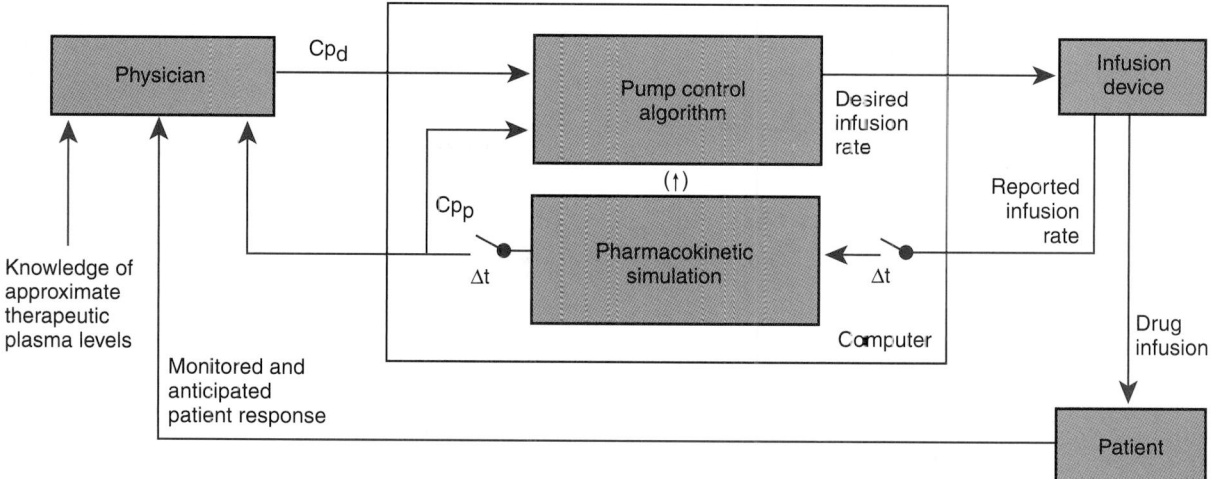

Figure 12–24 Schematic illustration of pharmacokinetic model–driven drug delivery. The physician enters the target plasma or biophase drug concentration (Cp_d). An infusion device control algorithm uses a pharmacokinetic model for the drug being infused to determine what the infusion rate should be for the next infusion interval (e.g., 9 to 15 seconds). The infusion device delivers drug to the patient, and the infusion rate is fed into a simulation of the pharmacokinetic model to compute the current predicted plasma drug concentration (Cp_p). The variables computed in the simulation are available to the infusion algorithm, which then calculates the infusion rate necessary for the next 9 to 15 seconds to achieve the target concentration. On the basis of monitored and anticipated patient response, knowledge of approximate therapeutic plasma drug concentrations (e.g., Cp_{50}), and Cp_p, the physician can titrate Cp_d as necessary.

drug to be infused; enters information about the patient such as weight, age, and gender; and ensures that the infusion setup is primed with drug at a specified concentration. The user then titrates the target concentrations during anesthesia in the same manner that one adjusts the inspired concentration of an inhaled anesthetic.

Pharmacokinetic models may be built into a future generation of anesthesia workstations. These workstations could then control many different brands of infusion pumps and could provide a common platform for implementing precise titration of intravenous anesthetics in the concentration domain.

Evaluation of Target-Controlled Drug Delivery
Acceptance of target-controlled drug delivery of intravenous anesthetics requires evaluation of both accuracy, defined as the difference between the predicted and the measured concentrations, and outcome of patients in whom automated drug delivery has been used. Sources of inaccuracy with pharmacokinetic model–driven devices

include the software, the hardware, and pharmacokinetic variability (Fig. 12-25).

Inaccuracy in the software results from incorrect mathematical implementation of the pharmacokinetic model. Computer simulations can be used to test the infusion rates calculated by a software program, and thus software errors are fairly simple to identify and correct.[108] Drug delivery from the infusion pump is fairly accurate with present syringe-pump technology and thus contributes little to the overall inaccuracy of these devices. The major cause of inaccuracy is biologic variability, which may be due to two sources: (1) the pharmacokinetic model is always wrong, and (2) the patient's pharmacokinetic parameters are never those programmed into the model. The pharmacokinetic model is always wrong because individuals are far more complex than implied by simple compartmental models, and thus no such model can precisely predict the concentrations, even if the pharmacokinetic parameters in the individual were known with absolute precision. However, even if the pharmacokinetic

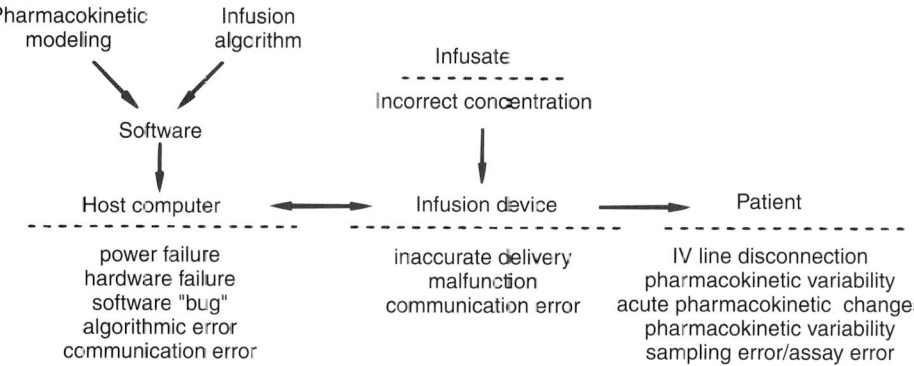

Figure 12–25 Major sources of potential error in pharmacokinetic model–driven drug delivery. In a commercial device, the computer functions would be incorporated into the infusion device itself.

model truly reflected the underlying biology, the parameters of the model would be average parameters for the population and not the parameters in the individual patient. Even if the parameters are modified to reflect the influence of demographic factors such as age, gender, hypovolemia, and coadministration of other drugs, they will still deviate from the true pharmacokinetic parameters in the individual. Thus, biologic variability fundamentally precludes the possibility of precisely achieving the desired target concentration when automated drug delivery devices are used. It is important to realize that biologic variability always exists, no matter how drugs are given, and that this same biologic variability affects all methods of drug delivery.

Optimization of Target-Controlled Drug Delivery

Performance of computer-controlled drug administration must be interpreted in terms of the therapeutic expectations of the clinician. Possible goals include accurately producing a desired concentration in plasma, precisely titrating the plasma drug concentration, producing the desired drug effect, and producing the desired time course of drug effect. Over the past decade, investigators have addressed each of these goals and have refined the performance of automated drug delivery devices in light of these goals.

The ability of an automated drug delivery system to rapidly achieve and then maintain a selected target concentration is a logical measure of the performance of such a device. The difference between the measured and the target concentrations may be expressed in several ways. The simplest means is to either diagram a plot of the target and measured concentration of each sample in each individual patient (Fig. 12-26) or diagram an *xy* plot of the measured to target concentration and observe how much the plots vary from the line of identity (Fig. 12-27).[75] The primary concern is how far the measured concentration is from the predicted one, which is now most frequently described in terms of the performance error, or the difference between the measured and the target concentration as a percentage of the desired target (i.e., [measured − target]/target × 100%).[109] The median value of the performance error for a patient or a population is referred to as the median performance error (MDPE) and represents the average overshoot or undershoot of the system. The median absolute performance error (MDAPE) is the median of the absolute value of all performance errors. The MDAPE is commonly used as a measure of the inaccuracy of an automated drug delivery device. An MDAPE of zero is perfect performance, and an MDAPE of 20% means that half the plasma concentrations will be within 20% of the target and half will be outside that range. A further assessment of accuracy is whether the system maintains a stable target concentration, which is best measured by the wobble of the system. Varvel and coworkers[109] asked a group of clinicians to evaluate the performance of automated drug delivery devices and demonstrated that the MDAPE best predicted the adequacy of performance of the automated delivery device, as judged by experienced clinicians.

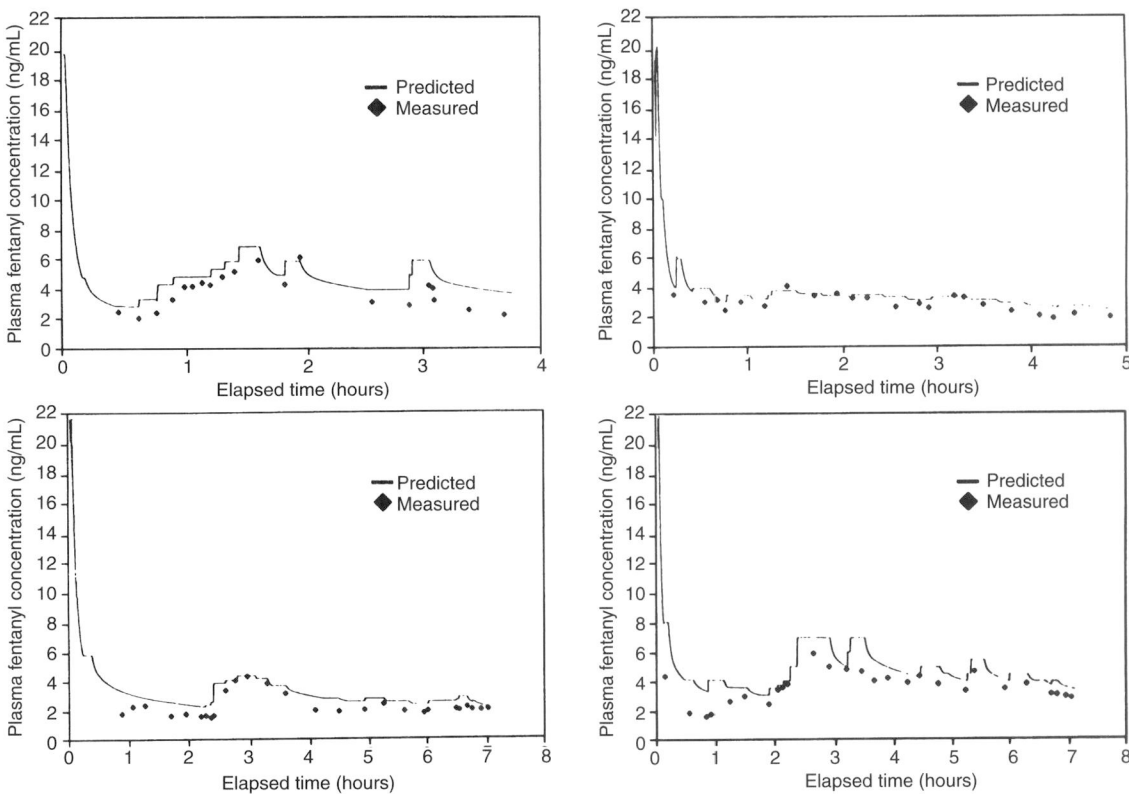

Figure 12–26 Individual plots of the target plasma fentanyl concentration (*solid line*) and measured concentration (*dots*) in four separate patients.

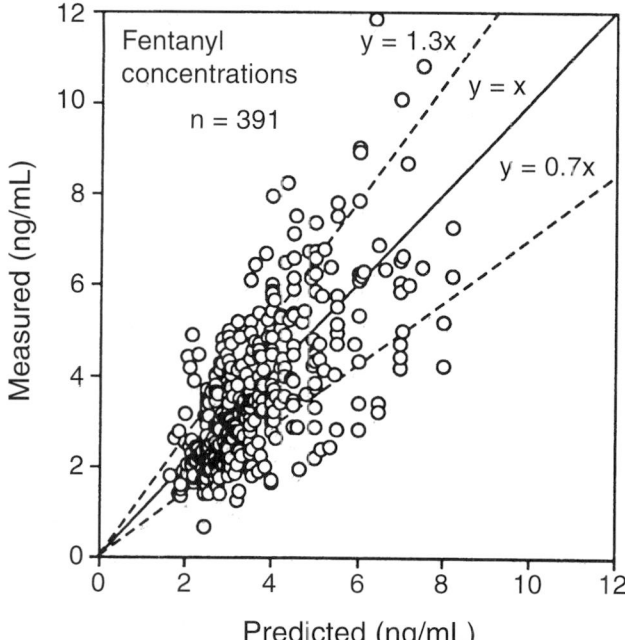

Figure 12–27 Plot of the measured to the predicted concentration of fentanyl administered via CACI in 24 patients. The *solid line* represents the line of identity; that is, the target concentration is equal to the measured concentration. The *dashed lines* represent a bias of ±30%.

As observed earlier, it is not reasonable to expect all performance errors to be zero. However, it would be desirable if positive and negative errors offset each other so that the MDPE of an automated drug delivery device was 0%. The MDPE does not indicate the range of performance errors (because positive and negative performance errors offset each other), but it does indicate whether the plasma concentrations achieved with the device tend to overshoot the desired target (+MDPE) or undershoot the desired target (−MDPE).

Table 12-7 summarizes the accuracy of pharmacokinetic model–driven devices administering several of the intravenous anesthetic drugs.[36,75,101,110-117] It is clear from Table 12-7 that the expected performance of such devices, at best, tends to be around 20% to 30% MDAPE. The pharmacokinetics of propofol has probably been the most frequently tested. Coetzee and colleagues[116] tested the accuracy of three parameter sets and found those of Marsh and associates[117] and Tackley and coworkers[131] to provide the best accuracy in adult patients (Fig. 12-28). To demonstrate the effect of the three different pharmacokinetic parameters on propofol dosing, the infusion rates required to produce a set of target concentrations are plotted in Figure 12-29. The pharmacokinetic parameter set of Marsh is the one included in the Diprifusor software. Better accuracy has been obtained in children[110] because they may have less pharmacokinetic variability as a result of their general lack of chronic disease and more narrow distribution of weight at any given age (than found in adults).

Numerous pharmacokinetic parameter sets have been published for each of the drugs used in anesthesia. The pharmacokinetic parameters within each set may vary considerably, depending on a variety of factors such as the mode of drug administration (e.g., bolus versus infusion), duration of sampling, site of drug sampling (arterial versus venous), sensitivity of the assay, and evaluation of population covariates in determining the model parameters. The implications of such differences are not always obvious, and it is important to test the parameter set to determine whether the parameters provide adequate accuracy for clinical use. If the pharmacokinetic parameters are highly biased, one might expect large errors to occur in performance. Several studies in Table 12-7 show the importance of selecting the proper pharmacokinetic parameters (or at least the cost of selecting the wrong set). Shafer and colleagues[114] examined the performance of a pharmacokinetic model–driven infusion device that used the fentanyl pharmacokinetics described by McClain and Hug[122] and demonstrated an MDAPE of 61% and an MDPE of +61%. The large positive MDPE indicates that nearly all fentanyl concentrations greatly exceeded the target. The performance errors over time with the use of the McClain and Hug pharmacokinetics are shown in Figure 12-30. Shafer and associates also examined the performance of a pharmacokinetic model–driven infusion device by use of the fentanyl pharmacokinetic parameters described by Scott and colleagues.[34] This second parameter set produced an MDAPE of 33% and an MDPE of +19%, as shown in the performance errors over time in Figure 12-30B. Although the measured concentrations tended to be higher than the target concentrations with the Scott and Stanski fentanyl parameter set, the performance was much better than that obtained with the parameter set reported by McClain and Hug. This study demonstrated that selection of the proper parameter set influenced the performance of pharmacokinetic model–driven infusion. Raemer and colleagues[110] demonstrated the same for alfentanil when they compared the performance of the alfentanil pharmacokinetic parameters reported by Maitre and coauthors[119] with the alfentanil pharmacokinetic parameters reported by Scott and coworkers.[34]

Glass and colleagues[75] examined the performance of a pharmacokinetic model–driven infusion device by use of the same fentanyl pharmacokinetics described by McClain and Hug.[122] They demonstrated an MDAPE of 21% and an MDPE of +4% (i.e., an almost completely unbiased performance). It is important to realize that the methodology in the studies by Glass and associates and Shafer and coworkers had major differences, such as arterial versus venous samples, rapid sampling after changes in target concentration versus sampling only when a pseudo–steady state was achieved, and a different set of patients—cardiac versus noncardiac. It is these differences in methodology that result in different investigators reporting differences in the performance of a pharmacokinetic model–driven infusion device using the same pharmacokinetic parameters.

With the goal of improving pharmacokinetic model–driven infusion device performance, Shafer and colleagues recalculated the optimal pharmacokinetic parameters of fentanyl directly from the observed concentrations that were obtained when fentanyl was administered through a pharmacokinetic model–driven infusion device that

Table 12–7   Accuracy of target-controlled infusion devices for intravenous anesthetics using different pharmacokinetic parameter sets

Drug	Author of Pharmacokinetic Parameter Set	Author of Study	Comments	MDAPE* (%)	MDPE* (%)
Alfentanil					
	Schüttler and Stoeckel[118]	Ausems et al[36]			≈22-32
	Schüttler and Stoeckel[118]	Schüttler et al[111]		≈28	≈0
	Maitre et al[119]	Raemer et al[110]		53	+53
	Scott et al[34]	Raemer et al[110]		17	+1
	Estimated	Crankshaw et al[120]		10	+3[†]
	Helmers et al[121]	Lemmens et al[112]		24	+12
Fentanyl					
	McClain and Hug[122]	Alvis et al[115]	Single target	≈20	≈0
	McClain and Hug[122]		Multiple targets	≈26	+11
	McClain and Hug[122]	Glass et al[123]		21	+4
	McClain and Hug[122]	Shafer et al[114]		61	+61
	Scott et al[34]	Shafer et al[114]		33	+19
	Estimated			21[‡]	−13[‡]
	McClain and Hug[122]	Veselis et al[113]		≈40	≈40
Sufentanil					
	Greeley et al[124]	Kern et al[125]	Pre-CPB		49
	Greeley et al[124]	Kern et al[125]	Post-CPB		32
Remifentanil					
	Minto[47]	Mertens et al[126]		20	−15
	Egan[46]	Mertens et al[126]		21	1
Thiopental					
	Ghoneim and Van Hamme[127]	Veselis et al[113]	Volunteers	≈50	≈−50
Midazolam					
	Smith et al[128]	Kern et al[125]	Pre-CPB	44	
	Smith et al[128]	Kern et al[125]	Post-CPB	32	
	Greenblatt et al[129]	Veselis et al[113]	Volunteers	≈100	≈100
Propofol					
	Schüttler et al[111]	Schüttler et al[111]		≈22	≈−12
	Dyck et al[130]	Coetzee et al[116]		20	42
	Tackley et al[131]	Coetzee et al[116]		20	−1
	Marsh et al[117]	Coetzee et al[116]		23	−6
	Marsh et al[117]	Marsh et al[117]	Pediatric patients	25	−18.5
	Estimated	Marsh et al[117]	Pediatric patients	16[§]	+3[§]
	Gepts et al[132]	Veselis et al[113]	Volunteers	≈25	0
	Gepts et al[132]	Glass et al[133]		29	+5

*MDAPE and MDPE were not calculated or only provided as a figure, and thus the reported numbers are approximately inferred from the measure of performance reported by the authors.
†Not model based (see text for details).
‡Retrospectively applied to the same data set.
§Prospectively tested.
CPB, cardiopulmonary bypass; MDAPE, median absolute performance error; MDPE, median performance error.

used the initial pharmacokinetics of McLean and Hug.[122] Figure 12-30C shows the performance errors over time for the optimal fentanyl pharmacokinetics estimated for that population of patients (as compared with those of McLean and Hug[122] and Scott and colleagues[34] in the same group of patients). The optimal pharmacokinetic parameter set still had a median residual error of 21% when retrospectively tested against the same group of patients. This error represents the limit imposed by

pharmacokinetic variability on the possible performance of any fentanyl parameter set for dosing to a similar adult population. In other words, it is unlikely that any fentanyl pharmacokinetic parameter set would produce less than a 21% MDAPE.

Marsh and coworkers[117] took the same approach to optimizing the performance of a pharmacokinetic model–driven infusion device administering propofol to children. They initially used a pharmacokinetic parameter

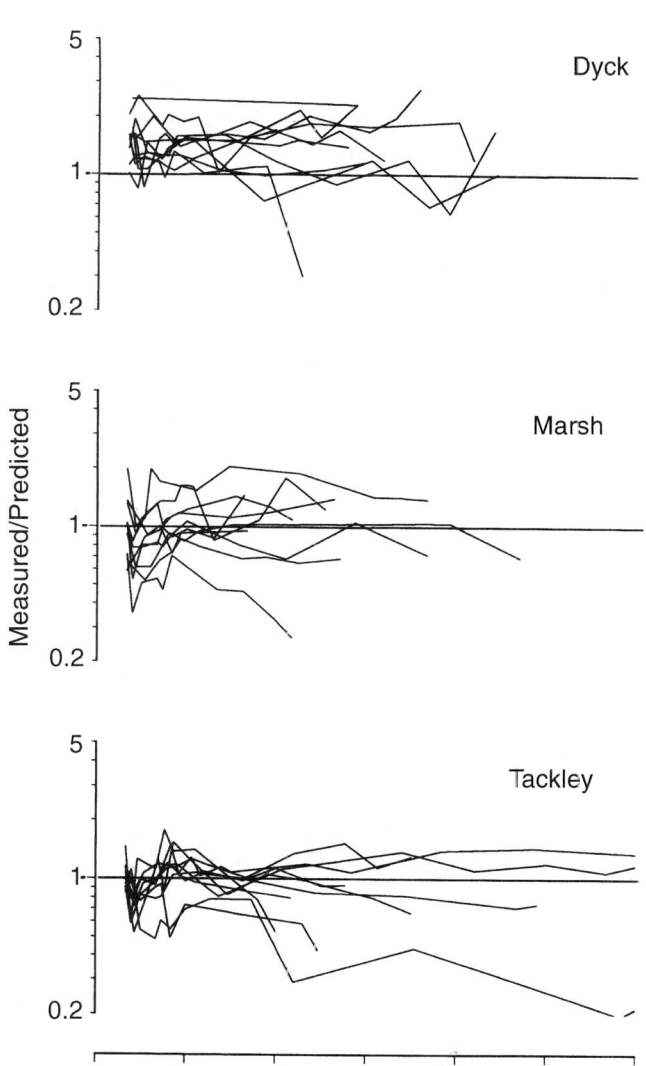

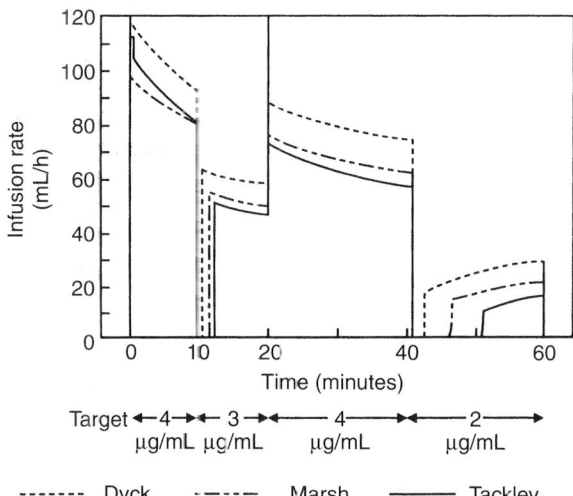

Figure 12–29 Infusion rates (milliliters per hour) calculated to achieve propofol target concentrations of 4 (10 minutes), 3 (10 minutes), 4 (20 minutes), and 2 µg/mL (20 minutes) based on the three pharmacokinetic parameter sets of Dyck, Marsh, and Tackley.

Figure 12–28 Evaluation of three pharmacokinetic parameter sets for propofol. Plotted is the measured-to-predicted concentration ratio for samples obtained during administration of propofol through a target-controlled infusion device programmed with the pharmacokinetics derived by Dyck, Marsh, or Tackley (n = 10 per group). A ratio of 1 means that measured equals predicted. Note that the pharmacokinetic parameters of Dyck provide a consistently positive bias.

set derived from adult subjects in their device and obtained an MDAPE of 25% and an MDPE of –18.5%. They subsequently derived new propofol pharmacokinetics for children and prospectively demonstrated that they had decreased the MDAPE to 16% with a bias of less than 3%. This performance is highly accurate for a model-based device. Ginsberg and colleagues[134] similarly derived a pharmacokinetic set for fentanyl in children, as did Fiset and associates[135] for alfentanil.

Several other studies have also demonstrated that pharmacokinetic parameters vary in certain subsets of patients. For example, the pharmacokinetic parameters of propofol for patients presenting for open heart surgery are different from the previously verified pharmacokinetic parameters of the general population. These new pharmacokinetic parameters for fentanyl also vary both during bypass and after bypass.[136]

Interest has recently focused on what other factors may be responsible for alterations in pharmacokinetic parameters, with the objective of reducing variability and increasing the accuracy of TCI systems. These factors include, among others, the influence of age, gender, hemorrhagic shock, and the administration of a second drug. Numerous studies have investigated the effect of age (both young and old) on pharmacokinetic parameters. For propofol and fentanyl, it has been shown that an adult pharmacokinetic set performs poorly in children and that age-specific parameters improve accuracy.[117,134] Although it is well known that pharmacokinetic parameters are altered in the elderly, it has not been well established whether these changes are sufficiently different to have an impact on the accuracy of the adult parameter sets that are used in a TCI device. The effect of gender on pharmacokinetics has been variable. For propofol, Vuyk and colleagues have recently demonstrated an effect of gender on propofol pharmacokinetic parameters in the elderly.[137] In a pharmacokinetic analysis of several pooled databases of propofol, Schuttler found that gender was not a significant covariate.[138] Similarly, there is no clear indication that gender has a significant effect on opioid pharmacokinetic parameters. Several authors have looked at the effect of hemorrhagic shock on pharmacokinetic parameters. With the use of a pseudo–steady-state model of propofol, compensated hemorrhage increased propofol concentrations by only 20%; however, when uncompensated shock was induced, propofol concentrations increased by 375%.[139]

Using a non–steady-state model, Egan and associates found that hemorrhagic shock reduced central clearance and central volumes of fentanyl[140] and remifentanil[141] and resulted in higher fentanyl concentrations in animals in shock. Investigators have also focused on the impact

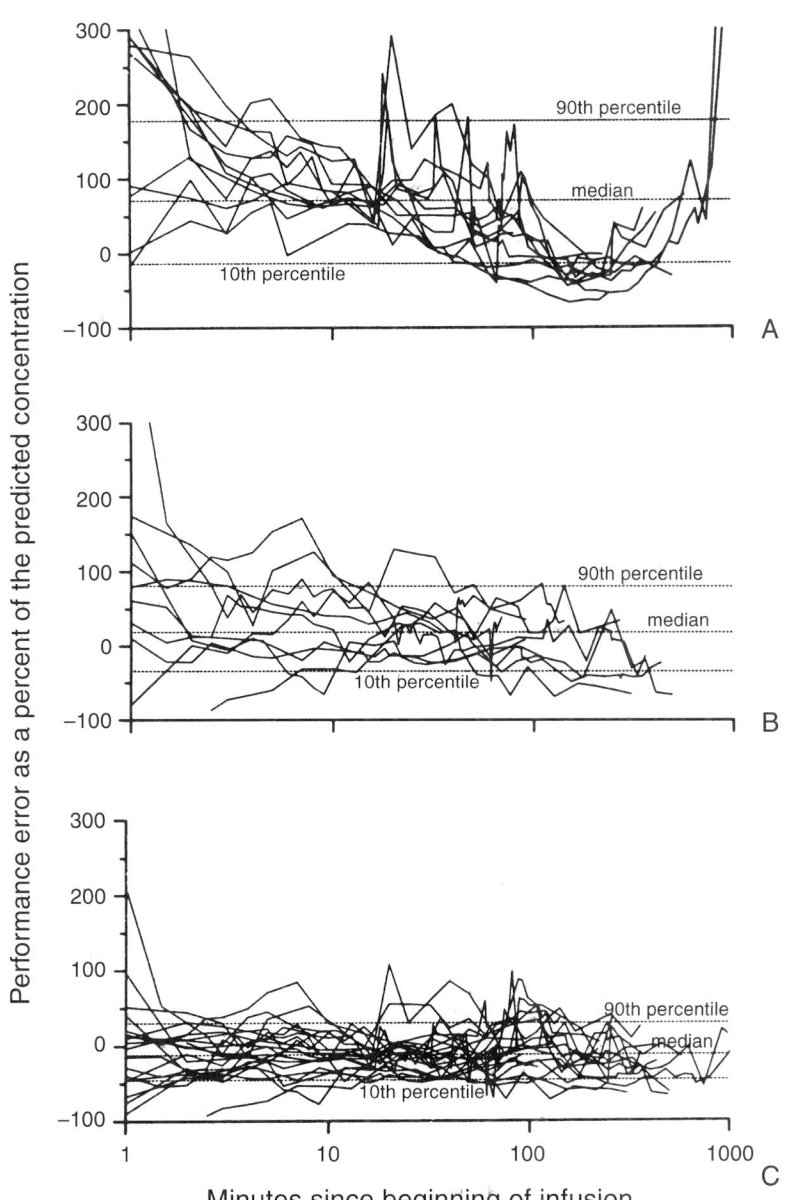

Figure 12–30 Performance errors over time for fentanyl by use of the pharmacokinetics reported by McClain and Hug (**A**) and Scott and Stanski (**B**) and a parameter set derived from these observations (**C**). (From Shafer SL, Varvel SL, Aziz N, et al: The pharmacokinetics of fentanyl administered by computer controlled infusion pump. Anesthesiology 73:1091-1102, 1990.)

of simultaneous administration of a second drug, especially another anesthetic. Propofol, midazolam, and etomidate have been shown in in vitro studies to reduce the clearance of opioids as a result of an interaction on the cytochrome P450 system. In turn, several studies have shown that alfentanil may alter the pharmacokinetic parameters of propofol.[142-144] The exact mechanism of this alteration is unclear. It is unlikely to be related to any interaction with cytochrome P450 systems because the pharmacokinetics of propofol is limited by liver blood flow and thus is not likely to be affected by modest alterations in hepatic metabolic capacity. The differences may result from alterations in cardiac output or reductions in hepatic blood flow. In contrast to alfentanil, remifentanil at concentrations of 0 to 4 ng/mL did not alter the pharmacokinetics of propofol.[145] However, propofol decreased the central volume of distribution and distributional clearance of remifentanil by 41% and the elimination clearance by 15%. Interestingly, in a study of propofol

administration in critically ill patients, two covariates established in the model that best described the pharmacokinetics of these patients were temperature and serum triglyceride concentration for terminal clearance.[146] Not all the factors that have been shown to alter pharmacokinetic parameters have demonstrated a change in outcomes or in the utility of TCI devices. However, some have, and thus in principle, pharmacokinetic sets adapted to the appropriate clinical milieu should be determined for each of the commonly used drugs to enhance the accuracy of TCI drug administration.

Not only is there interindividual variability, but significant intraindividual variability may also occur. Hill and colleagues[147] studied volunteers to learn the individual's own pharmacokinetics for morphine and alfentanil. These investigators then used that volunteer's unique pharmacokinetic values to subsequently control a pharmacokinetic model–driven infusion device. With this technique of personalized pharmacokinetics, they reduced the average error to just less than 20%. It appears that studies that determine the pharmacokinetics of an individual to be used to infuse the same drug to the same individual later result in a bias and MAPE similar to those seen when an optimal pharmacokinetic set derived from the general population is used. The implication of these data is that although highly specific pharmacokinetic sets are desirable, they may not necessarily improve overall accuracy. They also demonstrate that biologic variability precludes obtaining better than approximately 20% error with TCI devices.

It is unlikely that we will have the opportunity to conduct a full pharmacokinetic study on patients *during a single anesthetic procedure*. However, Bayesian forecasting is a statistical technique by which a few measured plasma concentrations from an individual can be incorporated into pharmacokinetic parameters to improve the performance of a pharmacokinetic model–driven infusion device. Maitre and Stanski[148] demonstrated the theoretical improvement in such devices when using Bayesian forecasting for alfentanil. In this study, Maitre and Stanski demonstrated that measurement of a single plasma alfentanil concentration could potentially reduce the inaccuracy by half, to a 14% average performance error. Unfortunately, a rapid assay does not exist for any of the intravenous drugs used in anesthetic practice. However, there are rapid assays for lidocaine, and at least one pharmacokinetic model–driven infusion device (STANPUMP, developed by Shafer and Maitre at Stanford and available at http://anesthesia.stanford.edu/pkpd) performs real-time Bayesian forecasting using measured lidocaine levels for use in coronary care units.

In the absence of rapid assays for anesthetic drugs, the obvious method to decrease variability is to observe the drug effect and adjust the target to the concentration that produces the desired level of drug effect.[30,31] As discussed under "Pharmacodynamic Considerations," by knowing the rate constant k_{e0}, it is possible to model the concentration at the site of drug effect. Figure 12-31 shows the plasma fentanyl concentrations that could theoretically be obtained over the course of a brief operation. Figure 12-31B shows the fentanyl concentrations at the effect site for the same anesthetic shown in Figure 12-31A. Even if the pump produced precisely the concentrations shown in Figure 12-31A (i.e., had perfect performance), the lag between concentrations in plasma and the site of drug effect would, at best, produce a very slurred response because of the equilibration delay between plasma and the effect site. Several pharmacokinetic model–driven infusion devices now simultaneously display both the plasma and the effect-site concentrations. Such devices permit the clinician to target the concentration at the effect site rather than plasma to provide more precise control of drug effect.

By targeting the effect site, an overshoot in the plasma concentration of the drug is produced. The k_{e0} used to model the effect site for intravenous anesthetics has been derived from surrogate measures of effect (i.e., derivatives of the EEG). Thus, it is important to establish for TCI devices targeting the effect site that the k_{e0} value used actually results in the desired effect. Glass and colleagues[149] and Struys and associates[150] conducted similar studies in which they targeted either a plasma or an effect-site concentration of propofol and then observed

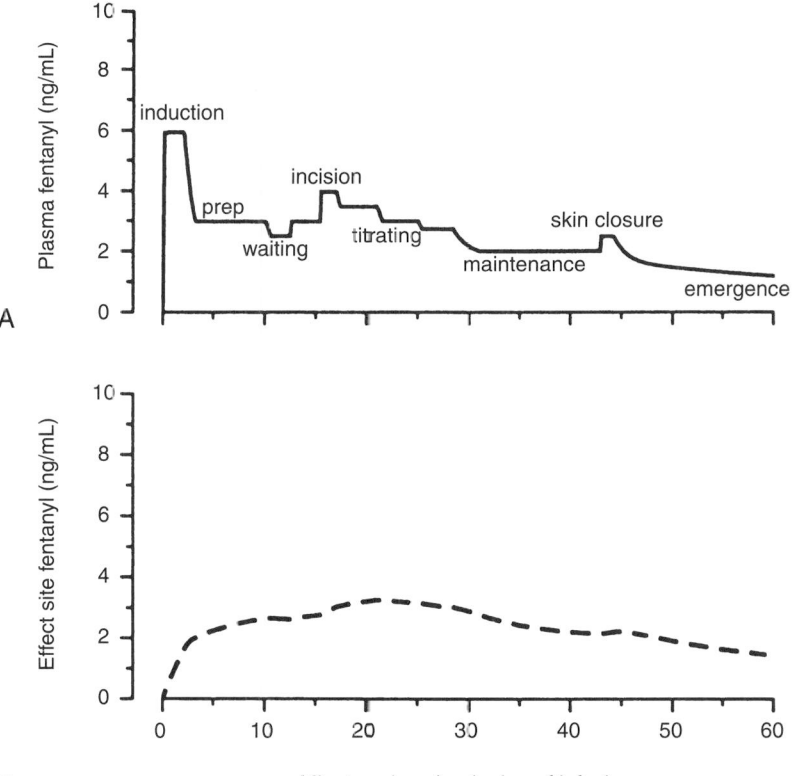

Figure 12–31 Simulated plasma fentanyl concentrations over time for a brief anesthetic showing the rapid rise and fall and impression of precise titration that can be created by a target-controlled drug delivery device (**A**). **B,** Effect-site concentrations for the same anesthetic course demonstrating that precise control of the plasma concentration does not necessarily translate into precise control at the site of drug effect. (Adapted from Shafer SL, Gregg K: Algorithms to rapidly achieve and maintain stable drug concentrations at the site of drug effect with a computer controlled infusion pump. J Pharmacokinet Biopharm 20:147-169, 1992.)

the time and plasma versus effect-site concentration at loss of consciousness. In both studies, regardless of whether the effect-site or plasma concentration was targeted, loss of consciousness occurred when the appropriate *effect-site* concentration for loss of consciousness was achieved, thus validating the concept. Two other important observations were made during these studies. First, the hemodynamics was not different, whether plasma or the effect site was targeted, even though higher plasma concentrations were achieved in the effect-site group. This finding implies, at least for propofol, that the time course for its hemodynamic effects are similar to (or longer than)[151] its anesthetic effects. Second, k_{e0} is very dependent on the pharmacokinetic set from which it is derived.[152] One cannot take a k_{e0} value from one pharmacokinetic set and use it with another pharmacokinetic set. Because various demographics may alter the pharmacokinetics, they may also alter the k_{e0}. Thus, it is desirable to use the k_{e0} best adapted for the clinical milieu.

In summary, automated drug delivery devices appear to be able to achieve and maintain desired plasma concentrations with a median expected error of about 20% to 30% of the target. Although pharmacokinetic analysis after automated drug delivery results in a reduction in the median error to closer to 20% in adults and possibly lower in children, biologic variability sets a limit on the expected accuracy of these devices. More accurate performance could be obtained with Bayesian feedback and the use of rapid intraoperative assays, but this technique is unavailable for the intravenous drugs used in anesthetic practice. However, the equilibration delay between plasma and the effect site is such that an excessive focus on plasma concentrations may be unwarranted. Instead, learning about the pharmacokinetic/pharmacodynamic characteristics of the specific patient by titrating to a readily measured drug effect appears to be the most promising method for optimizing the performance of automated drug delivery devices to the clinical needs of the individual patient.

Outcome

Evaluation of outcome with TCI devices is more difficult than evaluation of accuracy because of the difficulty of precisely measuring patient outcome. Because contemporary anesthetic practice produces very little morbidity, outcome measures are usually based on readily measured variables, such as blood pressure, heart rate, and duration of recovery room stay, rather than on substantive measures of patient morbidity. Evaluation of outcome with automated drug delivery devices requires a comparison of manual methods of administration of the same drug with automated drug delivery of intravenous anesthetics and volatile anesthetics. Numerous studies have now evaluated the administration of intravenous anesthetics by automated drug delivery devices for both brief and complex surgery, in children and adults, for short-term sedation, for prolonged sedation (days), and for chronic pain management. Unfortunately, very few outcome studies comparing automated drug delivery devices and manual delivery systems have thus far been conducted.

Ausems and colleagues[22] compared pharmacokinetic model–driven administration with intermittent bolus administration of alfentanil. Automated drug delivery produced fewer episodes of muscular rigidity, hypotension, and bradycardia on induction. Automated drug delivery during maintenance resulted in significantly fewer hemodynamic response incidents and thus resulted in a greater percentage of anesthesia time within 15% of the desired blood pressure and heart rate. Recovery after TCI was associated with significantly less use of naloxone for adequate ventilation.

Pharmacokinetic model–driven infusion of fentanyl during cardiac surgery resulted in greater hemodynamic control with fewer additional drug interventions and significantly fewer episodes of either hypotension or hypertension than occurred with bolus dose administration.[115] A small study comparing manual alfentanil administration with pharmacokinetic model–driven infusion of alfentanil showed no statistical differences during maintenance or recovery.[123] Theil and coworkers[100] compared double-blind manual administration of fentanyl/midazolam with pharmacokinetic model–driven infusion of these two anesthetics in a small group of patients undergoing cardiac surgery. Both systems were titrated simultaneously (one containing placebo), with the aim of maintaining hemodynamics within 20% of baseline values. Both systems were equally effective in providing hemodynamic control as dictated by the protocol. The most significant difference between the two modes of delivery was the greater variability in drug plasma concentrations in the manual group. This finding suggested that pharmacokinetic model–driven infusion maintained patients within a narrower therapeutic range. The advantages of this mode of infusion would be most important with drugs that have a narrow therapeutic window. This small comparative study, although it did not show many differences in outcome, demonstrated that target-controlled drug delivery was at least equal to manual drug delivery. Many pertinent outcome parameters, such as recovery times, were not measured in this study. Thus, there remains a need to establish which of the theoretical patient benefits will be realized with model-based target-controlled delivery versus manual delivery of intravenous drugs.

Several comparative studies using the commercial TCI device for propofol have been performed. Struys and colleagues[153] ($N = 90$), Russel and associates[154] ($N = 160$), and Servin in a large multicenter study ($N = 562$)[155] found small differences when they compared manual infusion of propofol with TCI administration. Interestingly, in the TCI groups, the maintenance infusion rate tended to be higher but was associated with a lower incidence of movement by patients. Both Servin and Russel and coworkers noted a marked preference of users for the TCI system, even though this was their first use of the device. In contrast, when TCI propofol or manual propofol was titrated to a target bispectral index, no differences were observed between the two groups.[156] Manual versus TCI delivery of remifentanil has also been evaluated in patients undergoing carotid surgery.[157] TCI provided improved hemodynamic control both intraoperatively and postoperatively with less remifentanil and similar propofol infusion rates. As discussed, targeting a plasma concentration does not provide optimal control of effect.

When manual propofol administration has been compared with target effect-site administration, fewer episodes of movement, improved hemodynamic stability, and more rapid recovery occurred.[158]

Pharmacokinetic model–driven infusion of propofol compares favorably with thiopental/isoflurane anesthesia for general surgery lasting several hours.[159] Induction, maintenance, and recovery were similar between the two groups. More recently, Godet and colleagues compared sevoflurane and propofol followed by isoflurane with TCI propofol in patients undergoing carotid surgery. They found minor differences in hemodynamics that tended to favor TCI propofol and no differences in recovery parameters.[160] The results of this study imply that given the appropriate means of administration, intravenous anesthesia can be equal to inhaled anesthetics in providing the objectives of anesthesia, that is, rapid induction and recovery with stable maintenance. Suttner and associates examined cost and the recovery characteristics of target-controlled propofol infusion regimens versus standard methodologies.[161] They found that "target-controlled infusion/total IV anesthesia was associated with the largest intraoperative costs but allowed the most rapid recovery from anesthesia, was associated with fewest postoperative side effects, and permitted earlier discharge from the postanesthesia care unit."

In noncomparative studies, pharmacokinetic model–driven infusion has been used to administer most of the potent opioids, as well as the hypnotics. Different anesthetic techniques have also been tested with pharmacokinetic model–driven infusion devices, including nitrous-narcotic anesthesia, supplementation with volatile anesthetics, total intravenous anesthesia and sedation for monitored anesthesia care, and intensive care unit sedation. In all these studies, outcome, as measured by hemodynamics and recovery, has been within the expectations of normal clinical care. Etomidate, methohexital, midazolam, propofol, thiopental, alfentanil, fentanyl, remifentanil, and sufentanil have all been used with TCI. When these drugs were used with target-controlled drug delivery systems for total intravenous anesthesia or to supplement nitrous oxide or volatile anesthetics, hemodynamics was well maintained during induction and intubation, as well as during maintenance. Recovery milestones were reached at times comparable to those of similar drug combinations used in manual infusion schemes. In none of these numerous studies have authors commented on adverse outcome resulting from target-controlled drug delivery.

The clinical experience with TCI devices is now enormous. A MEDLINE search of "target controlled infusion" generated over 200 articles (May 31, 2003). Clinical experience with TCI devices is now in the millions. It is only in North America that TCI is not a part of routine practice, the unfortunate result of unyielding opposition toward anesthetic drug-device combinations at the U.S. Food and Drug Administration.

Target-controlled infusion devices have also been used to provide patient-controlled analgesia. Hill and colleagues investigated patient-controlled anesthesia devices delivering morphine, fentanyl, or alfentanil[147,162] and the clinical utility of such devices.[163-166] Van den Nieuwenhuyzen and associates[58] demonstrated advantages of such a system with alfentanil over routine morphine patient-controlled anesthesia.

From the body of literature presently available, it appears that automated drug delivery of intravenous anesthetics is at least equal to manual delivery of these drugs. Intravenous drug administration using target-controlled drug delivery is analogous to inhalational vapor delivery using a calibrated vaporizer. Like the vaporizer, pharmacokinetic model–driven infusion facilitates drug delivery based on plasma or biophase concentration rather than drug dosage. Variability occurs with the use of a calibrated vaporizer, including variability in the accuracy of drug delivery with vaporizers, slow equilibration between the fresh gas flow and the circuit at low flow rates, and variable uptake by the patient. This variability does not particularly complicate titration of the inhaled anesthetics. The variability with target-controlled drug delivery is of a similar magnitude, and just as with the vaporizers, the variability associated with target-controlled drug delivery does not particularly complicate titration of intravenous anesthetics. Indeed, the time-varying stresses of surgery and the variability in patient response require that the anesthesiologist titrate the administration of potent inhaled anesthetics by using the calibrated vaporizer as a tool. These same factors require that the anesthesiologist vigilantly titrate the infusion of intravenous anesthetic drugs when using automated drug delivery as a tool.

Target-controlled drug delivery has advantages beyond being a delivery system to simplify the clinical administration of intravenous anesthetics. Probably the most significant contribution of these delivery devices is their use in research. The pseudo–steady state that can be almost instantly achieved with these devices permits the plasma and effect site to rapidly come into equilibrium, which is critically important in studies examining concentration-response relationships (i.e., the C_{50} values) for anesthetic drugs.[22,37,56] In addition, these systems enable interactions involving intravenous drugs to be clearly defined.[71-73] Closed-loop target delivery will eventually enable unbiased and more precise comparisons between drugs. Finally, as noted earlier, target-controlled delivery has provided us with the ability to prospectively test pharmacokinetic parameter sets and modeling approaches and may ultimately provide the most suitable pharmacokinetic parameters for any intravenous drug delivery.[114,117,135,167] Purely as a research tool, automated drug delivery has already had a major impact on anesthetic practice.

Closed-Loop Drug Delivery Systems

The next step in automated drug delivery is to feed the measured drug effect directly back into the automated drug delivery device and permit the model to be updated based on observed measures of drug effect, thus providing a closed-loop system.[4,7,15-19] In this instance, the set point is the measured effect rather than the drug concentration. It has been proposed that closed-loop control of anesthesia may provide several advantages: increased stability of the control variable because of more frequent sampling of the effect and more frequent adjustment of drug delivery, more customized dose delivery that accounts for both interindividual pharmacokinetic and pharmacodynamic differences, and therefore improvement in hemodynamic stability, inadvertent awareness, and recovery.[168]

The simplest form of a closed-loop system is an on-off controller.[169] The infusion pump is programmed to give only one infusion rate. If the effect of the drug reduces the measured effect, the pump will turn on when the measured effect is greater than the set point (positive error) and switch off when the error is negative. Such a system will oscillate around the targeted effect. Several modifications of this simple closed-loop system have been developed that are especially important for their implementation in complex biologic systems. The next engineering modification that has been implemented to improve the performance of closed-loop devices is adjustment of the infusion rate according to the error. A *proportional* controller will adjust the infusion rate in accordance with the size of the error. Depending on the rapidity with which the error changes, this adjustment may also lead to overshooting or undershooting of the target, and thus the *integral* of the error is used to minimize this deviation. This process leads to a reduction in error but may lead to a systemic bias. To prevent such bias, the *derivative* of the error is also used. Most mechanical closed-loop systems are PID controllers. Biologic systems are more complex in that there is a second- or third-order relationship between the infusion dose and the effect and, in addition, sensitivity between individuals may vary by a factor of 10-fold. To deal with these factors, two further modifications in control have been used. The first is that the change in dose, based on the error, is determined by a pharmacokinetic/pharmacodynamic model. Second, as the system learns the sensitivity of the individual, the model "adapts" to that individual. Adaptation may be achieved simply by adjusting the gain, by adjusting the relationship between concentration and effect, or by using fuzzy logic. Several investigators have developed closed-loop target control systems for blood pressure,[4-7,170] neuromuscular blockade,[171] and anesthesia.[15-18,168,172-178] Though not yet commercially available, closed-loop systems for blood pressure and neuromuscular blockade have demonstrated an ability to provide excellent control with zero bias and an MDPE and MDAPE within 10%.

As mentioned earlier, the ability to measure the adequacy of anesthesia is limited. Rather, anesthesia is a composite of several effects: hypnosis or loss of consciousness, amnesia, analgesia, lack of movement, and hemodynamic stability. Several derivatives of the EEG now show a strong correlation with hypnosis/loss of consciousness. Fortunately, amnesia is also reflected by the EEG signal and appears to precede the derived EEG values associated with drug-induced loss of consciousness. The major component of anesthesia for which we do not have a monitor of effect is analgesia. This shortcoming continues to be an impediment to the general application of closed-loop anesthesia. Noxious stimuli during surgery are extremely variable. Intravenous hypnotics (with the exception of ketamine) have limited or no analgesic activity. Thus, a closed-loop system based on a derivative of the EEG may provide perfect hypnosis in the absence of a stimulus, but awakening will occur as soon as a noxious stimulus is administered. To overcome this hurdle, investigators have taken several approaches to test closed-loop systems for anesthesia in patients. They have been used in combination with a regional anesthetic, thereby ablating any painful stimulus reaching the brain. Others have used a low-dose constant opioid concentration for superficial surgery or high-dose opioid for more extensive surgery. Another interesting approach is a combination of an analgesic concentration of opioid and application of a noxious stimulus (e.g., tetany) at regular short intervals, thus minimizing oscillations caused by surgical stimuli.

For maintenance of anesthesia, the question remains whether closed-loop systems actually provide any advantage over either manual or TCI delivery of intravenous anesthetics. Morley and coworkers compared closed-loop administration of isoflurane or a propofol/alfentanil mixture with manual control of these agents to provide a bispectral index of 50.[179] The closed-loop system used a PID control algorithm. The authors were unable to demonstrate any advantage of their closed-loop system over manual control when intraoperative control of the bispectral index, hemodynamic stability, intraoperative drug use, or recovery parameters were used as measures of outcome.

Struys and colleagues also performed a study to determine whether a closed-loop system has any advantages over manual administration of propofol for lower abdominal surgery.[176] Their approach was to have the anesthesiologist performing manual control have clinical criteria of adequate anesthesia as the target of control, whereas for the closed-loop system, the bispectral index was used as the set point. Struys and colleagues also used a model-based adaptive control system. During induction, the system administered staggered increasing propofol concentrations so that it could construct a sigmoid Emax model, thereby "learning" the individuals' concentration-effect relationship. The sigmoid Emax model developed during induction could change based on the degree of noxious stimulation and the opioid concentration. To account for this, the investigators allowed a left or right shift of the Emax curve that corresponded with the new bispectral index value and the predicted concentration. A new target concentration was determined from this new Emax curve, and this concentration was then delivered to return the bispectral index to its target. All patients received 0.5 µg/kg/min of remifentanil. The closed-loop control group achieved statistically significantly better control of both its control variable (bispectral index of 89+, 10%) and systolic pressure (51+, 27%) than did the manual group (bispectral index of 49+, 29%; systolic pressure of 34+, 31%). In addition, recovery was also improved in the closed-loop group (Fig. 12-32). This study does not definitively answer whether closed-loop delivery of anesthesia is better than any manual system, nor does it define what an optimal closed-loop control system is; however, its results are encouraging and should stimulate further work on developing closed-loop anesthetic drug delivery for day-to-day anesthesia.[180]

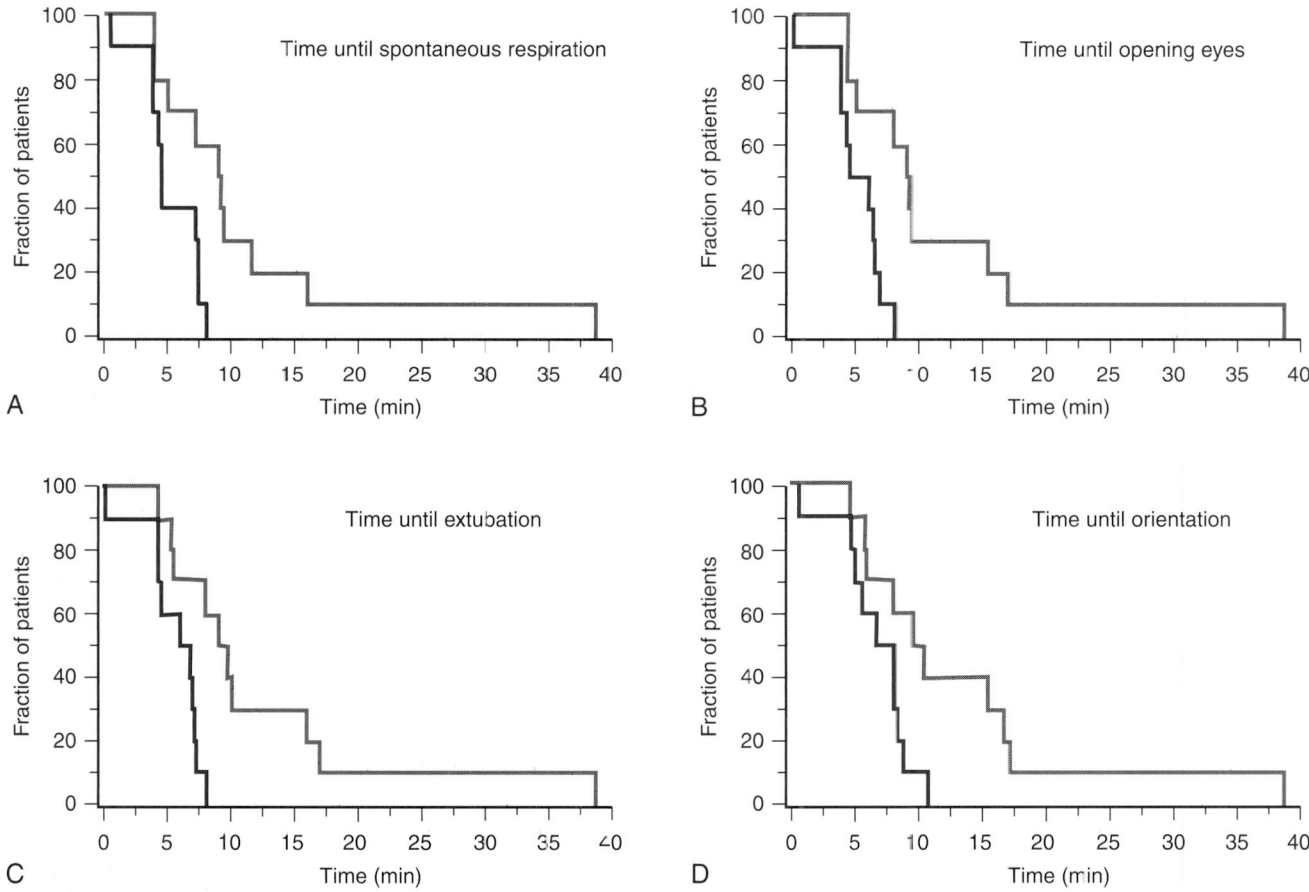

Figure 12–32 Comparison of manual versus closed-loop anesthetic control on the time course of return of spontaneous ventilation (**A**), eye opening (**B**), extubation (**C**), and orientation (**D**). In each case, the more rapid curve is the closed-loop control, and the slower curve is the manual control. (Adapted from Struys MM, De Smet T, Versichelen LF, et al: Comparison of closed-loop controlled administration of propofol using Bispectral Index as the controlled variable versus "standard practice" controlled administration. Anesthesiology 95:6-17, 2001.)

Closed-loop control is also an extremely valuable investigative tool. It can be used to determine the unbiased interaction between two drugs. It has been used extensively with neuromuscular blockers to determine their interaction with various anesthetics.[175,181,182] Similarly, closed-loop control can be used to determine the interaction between opioids and intravenous anesthetics.[183,184] Closed-loop systems may also have the potential to diagnose different pathologic states based on drug dosing. Albrecht and colleagues observed when using closed-loop sedation with propofol that trauma patients required lower EEG set points and needed more propofol to achieve the same level of sedation.[185] As the number of investigators who have access to closed-loop systems for anesthesia increases, the utility of such devices for research is likely to increase substantially.

SUMMARY

When compared with intermittent bolus administration, continuous infusion of intravenous anesthetic drugs provides greater control of anesthetic depth, thus ensuring

(1) better hemodynamic control with fewer episodes of hemodynamic instability, (2) smaller total drug doses, and (3) more rapid return to an awake state. Improved drug administration techniques combined with several new intravenous anesthetic agents have provided greater impetus for the use of intravenous anesthesia in clinical practice. Devices for the administration of intravenous anesthesia are continuing to evolve. The introduction of pumps designed specifically for continuous intravenous anesthetic drug delivery has enhanced intravenous anesthesia. Automated drug delivery is becoming routine in many countries. Pharmacokinetic model–driven infusion has several theoretical advantages over manual infusion systems, such as further improvements in hemodynamic control and a more predictable rapid awakening. Studies comparing outcomes after automated drug delivery of intravenous anesthetics versus manual methods or inhaled anesthesia have either demonstrated improved results or been equivocal. No studies have identified clinical or safety problems with automated anesthetic drug delivery. It thus appears that pharmacokinetic model–driven infusion systems, though limited by the same biologic variability that affects manual drug delivery, are safe and effective in clinical use.

The introduction of commercial TCI systems has grown to an extent that in many institutions, such systems are an everyday part of anesthesia practice. We predict that with the increased emphasis on reducing human error in medicine, especially drug delivery, TCI systems will ultimately replace manual methods. With the advent of monitors of hypnosis and increased understanding of the components of anesthesia, closed-loop drug delivery of anesthesia is showing promise in providing further advantages. Many hurdles still need to be overcome before such devices will come into routine use. However, present knowledge and the results of recent studies are sufficiently encouraging to pursue this goal.

KEY POINTS

1. Anesthetic drugs are described by multicompartmental models. Accurate intravenous drug delivery requires adjusting the dose for drug accumulation in peripheral tissues.

2. The biophase is the site of anesthetic drug action. Initiation, maintenance, and titration of intravenous anesthetics must account for the delay in equilibration between plasma and the site of drug effect.

3. Some drug effects directly reflect the concentration of drug in the biophase (direct effect models). Other drug effects reflect the alteration of feedback systems by anesthetics (indirect effect models). The influence of opioids on ventilation reflects the dynamic influence of opioids on the feedback between ventilation and carbon dioxide and is thus an example of an indirect drug effect.

4. The target concentration in the effect site is the same as the target concentration in plasma at steady state. The target concentration is influenced by patient physiology, surgical stimulation, and concurrent drug administration. Typically, one must set a target concentration for the hypnotic (volatile anesthetic or propofol) and the analgesic (opioid) that properly accounts for the synergy between them.

5. To achieve a target effect concentration, the conventional teaching of administering a loading dose calculated as the target concentration times the volume of distribution, followed by a maintenance rate calculated as the target concentration times clearance, is inaccurate. The initial loading dose may be calculated as the target concentration times the volume of distribution at peak effect. Maintenance rates must initially account for distribution of drug in peripheral tissues and are only turned down to the target concentration times clearance after equilibration with peripheral tissues.

6. The terminal half-life says nothing about the clinical time course of drug concentration. Context-sensitive decrement times are the times for given decrements in drug concentration as a function of the infusion duration for an infusion that maintains a steady plasma concentration. Context-sensitive decrement times properly incorporate the multicompartmental behavior of intravenous anesthetics. The context-sensitive half-time is the time for a 50% decrement in concentration.

7. Alfentanil, fentanyl, sufentanil, remifentanil, propofol, thiopental, methohexital, etomidate, ketamine, and midazolam can all be given by intravenous infusion. Specific caveats, infusion rates, and titration guidelines are given in the text.

8. Target-controlled infusions use pharmacokinetic models to titrate intravenous anesthetics to specified plasma or effect-site drug concentrations. The Diprifusor is a propofol target-controlled infusion system that is available worldwide except in North America.

9. The utility of target-controlled infusions has been demonstrated in 20 years of research experience, well over 100 research publications, and over 8 years of clinical experience with the Diprifusor in millions of patients. Improved patient outcomes have been demonstrated with target-controlled drug delivery.

10. Closed-loop drug delivery systems have used the median EEG frequency, bispectral index, and auditory evoked potentials to control intravenous anesthetic delivery. These systems have generally performed well clinically but remain investigational.

REFERENCES

1. Corssen G, Reves JG, Stanley T: Intravenous Anesthesia and Analgesia. Philadelphia, Lea & Febiger, 1988.
2. Schwilden H: A general method for calculating the dosage scheme in linear pharmacokinetics. Eur J Clin Pharmacol 20:379-386, 1981.
3. Reves JG, Sheppard LC, Wallach R, et al: Therapeutic uses of sodium nitroprusside and an automated method of administration. Int Anesthesiol Clin 16:51-88, 1978.
4. Meline LJ, Westenskow DK, Pace NL, et al: Computer-controlled regulation of sodium nitroprusside infusion. Anesth Analg 64:38, 1985.
5. Reid JA, Kenny GN: Evaluation of closed-loop control of arterial pressure after cardiopulmonary bypass. Br J Anaesth 59:247-255, 1987.
6. Colvin JR, Kenny GN: Development and evaluation of a dual-pump microcomputer-based closed-loop arterial pressure control system. Int J Clin Monit Comput 6:31-35, 1989.
7. Grosmaire EK: Computer-controlled sodium nitroprusside infusions in patients after cardiac surgery. Heart Lung 21:214, 1992.
8. de Vries JW, Ros HH, Booij LH: Infusion of vecuronium controlled by a closed-loop system. Br J Anaesth 58:1100-1103, 1986.
9. Olkkola KT, Schwilden H: Quantitation of the interaction between atracurium and succinylcholine using closed-loop feedback control of infusion of atracurium. Anesthesiology 73:614-618, 1990.
10. O'Hara DA, Derbyshire GJ, Overdyk FJ, et al: Closed-loop infusion of atracurium with four different anesthetic techniques. Anesthesiology 74:258-263, 1991.
11. Schwilden H, Olkkola KT: Use of a pharmacokinetic-dynamic model for the automatic feedback control of atracurium. Eur J Clin Pharmacol 40:293-296, 1991.
12. Uys PC, Morrell DF, Bradlow HS, et al: Self-tuning, microprocessor-based closed-loop control of atracurium-induced neuromuscular blockade. Br J Anaesth 61:685-692, 1988.

13. Wait CM, Goat VA, Blogg CE: Feedback control of neuromuscular blockade: A simple system for infusion of atracurium. Anaesthesia 42:1212-1217, 1987.
14. Webster NR, Cohen AT: Closed-loop administration of atracurium: Steady-state neuromuscular blockade during surgery using a computer controlled closed-loop atracurium infusion. Anaesthesia 42:1085-1091, 1987.
15. Schwilden H, Schüttler J, Stockel H: Closed-loop feedback control of methohexital anaesthesia by quantitative EEG analysis in humans. Anesthesiology 67:341, 1987.
16. Schwilden H, Stoeckel H: Effective therapeutic infusions produced by closed-loop feedback control of methohexital administration during total intravenous anesthesia with fentanyl. Anesthesiology 73:225-229, 1990.
17. Schwilden H, Stoeckel H, Schuttler J: Closed-loop feedback control of propofol anaesthesia by quantitative EEG analysis in humans. Br J Anaesth 62:290-296, 1989.
18. Kenny GNC, Davies FW, Mantzardis H, et al: Closed-loop control of anesthesia. Anesthesiology 77:A328, 1992.
19. Struys M, Desmet T, Audenaert S, et al: Development of a closed loop system for propofol using bispectral analysis and a patient-individual pharmacokinetic-dynamic (PK-PD) model: Preliminary results [abstract]. Br J Anaesth 78(Suppl 1):23, 1997.
20. Sigl JC, Chamoun NG: An introduction to bispectral analysis for the electroencephalogram. J Clin Monit 10:392-404, 1994.
21. White PF: Use of continuous infusion versus intermittent bolus administration of fentanyl or ketamine during outpatient anesthesia. Anesthesiology 59:294, 1983.
22. Ausems ME, Vuyk J, Hug CC, et al: Comparison of a computer-assisted infusion versus intermittent bolus administration of alfentanil as a supplement to nitrous oxide for lower abdominal surgery. Anesthesiology 68:851-861, 1988.
23. Avram MJ, Krejcie TC: Using front-end kinetics to optimize target-controlled drug infusions. Anesthesiology 99:1078-1086, 2003.
24. Krejcie TC, Avram MJ, Gentry WB, et al: A recirculatory model of the pulmonary uptake and pharmacokinetics of lidocaine based on analysis of arterial and mixed venous data from dogs. J Pharmacokinet Biopharm 25:169-190, 1997.
25. Hull CJ, Van Beem HB, McLeod K, et al: A pharmacodynamic model for pancuronium. Br J Anaesth 50:1113-1123, 1978.
26. Sheiner LB, Stanski DR, Vozeh S, et al: Simultaneous modeling of pharmacokinetics and pharmacodynamics: Application to D-tubocurarine. Clin Pharmacol Ther 25:358-371, 1979.
27. Glass PS, Hardman D, Kamiyama Y, et al: Preliminary pharmacokinetics and pharmacodynamics of an ultra-short-acting opioid: Remifentanil (GI87084B). Anesth Analg 77:1031-1040, 1993.
28. Egan TD, Lemmens HJM, Fiset P, et al: The pharmacokinetics of the new short-acting opioid remifentanil (GI87084B) in healthy adult male volunteers. Anesthesiology 79:881-892, 1993.
29. Ludbrook GL, Visco E, Lam AM: Propofol: Relation between brain concentrations, electroencephalogram, middle cerebral artery blood flow velocity, and cerebral oxygen extraction during induction of anesthesia. Anesthesiology 97:1363-1370, 2002.
30. Shafer SL, Gregg K: Algorithms to rapidly achieve and maintain stable drug concentrations at the site of drug effect with a computer controlled infusion pump. J Pharmacokinet Biopharm 20:147-169, 1992.
31. Jacobs JR, Williams EA: Algorithm to control "effect compartment" drug concentrations in pharmacokinetic model–driven drug delivery. IEEE Trans Biomed Eng 40:993-999, 1993.
32. Bouillon T, Schmidt C, Garstka G, et al: Pharmacokinetic-pharmacodynamic modeling of the respiratory depressant effect of alfentanil. Anesthesiology 91:144-155, 1999.
33. Bouillon T, Bruhn J, Radu-Radulescu L, et al: A model of the ventilatory depressant potency of remifentanil in the non–steady state. Anesthesiology 99:779-787, 2003.
34. Scott JC, Ponganis KV, Stanski DR: EEG quantitation of narcotic effect: The comparative pharmacodynamics of fentanyl and alfentanil. Anesthesiology 62:234-241, 1985.
35. Eger EID, Saidman LJ, Brandstater B: Minimum alveolar anesthetic concentration: A standard of anesthetic potency. Anesthesiology 26:756-763, 1965.
36. Ausems ME, Stanski DR, Hug CC: An evaluation of the accuracy of pharmacokinetic data for the computer assisted infusion of alfentanil. Br J Anaesth 57:1217-1225, 1985.
37. Hung OR, Varvel JR, Shafer SL, et al: Thiopental pharmacodynamics II. Quantitation of clinical and electroencephalographic depth of anesthesia. Anesthesiology 77:237-244, 1992.
38. Telford RJ, Glass PSA, Goodman D, et al: Fentanyl does not alter the "sleep" plasma concentration of thiopental. Anesth Analg 75:523-529, 1992.
39. Vuyk J, Engbers FHM, Lemmens HJM, et al: Pharmacodynamics of propofol in female patients. Anesthesiology 77:3-9, 1992.
40. Vuyk J, Lim T, Engbers FH, et al: The pharmacodynamic interaction of propofol and alfentanil during lower abdominal surgery in women. Anesthesiology 83:8-22, 1995.
41. Smith C, McEwan AI, Jhaveri R, et al: Reduction of propofol Cp50 by fentanyl. Anesthesiology 77:A340, 1992.
42. Jacobs JR, Reves JG, Marty J, et al: Aging increases pharmacodynamic sensitivity to the hypnotic effects of midazolam. Anesth Analg 80:143-148, 1995.
43. Scott JC, Stanski DR: Decreased fentanyl and alfentanil dose requirements with age: A simultaneous pharmacokinetic and pharmacodynamic evaluation. J Pharmacol Exp Ther 240:159-166, 1987.
44. Scott JC, Cooke JE, Stanski DR: Electroencephalographic quantitation of opioid effect: Comparative pharmacodynamics of fentanyl and sufentanil. Anesthesiology 74:34, 1991.
45. Egan TD, Lemmens HJ, Fiset P, et al: The pharmacokinetics of the new short-acting opioid remifentanil (GI87084B) in healthy adult male volunteers. Anesthesiology 79:881-892, 1993.
46. Egan TD, Minto CF, Hermann DJ, et al: Remifentanil versus alfentanil: Comparative pharmacokinetics and pharmacodynamics in healthy adult male volunteers. Anesthesiology 84:821-833, 1996.
47. Minto CF, Schnider TW, Egan TD, et al: The influence of age and gender on the pharmacokinetics and pharmacodynamics of remifentanil. I. Model development. Anesthesiology 86:10-23, 1997.
48. Lemmens HJM, Dyck JB, Shafer SL, et al: The application of pharmacokinetics/dynamics and computer simulations to drug development: A3665 versus fentanyl and alfentanil. Anesthesiology 77:A456, 1992.
49. Homer TD, Stanski DR: The effect of increasing age on thiopental disposition and anesthetic requirement. Anesthesiology 62:714-724, 1985.
50. Stanski DR, Maitre PO: Population pharmacokinetics and pharmacodynamics of thiopental: The effect of age revisited. Anesthesiology 72:412-422, 1990.
51. Arden JR, Holley FO, Stanski DR: Increased sensitivity to etomidate in the elderly: Initial distribution versus altered brain response. Anesthesiology 65:19, 1986.
52. Billard V, Gambus PL, Chamoun N, et al: A comparison of spectral edge, delta power, and bispectral index as EEG measures of alfentanil, propofol, and midazolam drug effect. Clin Pharmacol Ther 61:45-58, 1997.
53. Schnider TW, Minto CF, Fiset P, et al: Semilinear canonical correlation applied to the measurement of the electroencephalographic effects of midazolam and flumazenil reversal. Anesthesiology 84:510-519, 1996.
54. Egan TD, Muir KT, Hermann DJ, et al: The electroencephalogram (EEG) and clinical measure of opioid potency: Defining the EEG–clinical potency relationship ("fingerprint") with application to remifentanil. Int J Pharm Med 15:1-9, 2001.
55. Ausems ME, Hug CC Jr, Stanski DR, et al: Plasma concentrations of alfentanil required to supplement nitrous oxide anesthesia for general surgery. Anesthesiology 65:362-373, 1986.

56. Glass PSA, Doherty M, Jacobs JR, et al: Plasma concentration of fentanyl, with 70% nitrous oxide, to prevent movement at skin incision. Anesthesiology 78:842-847, 1993.

57. Gourlay GK, Kowalski SR, Plummer JL, et al: Fentanyl blood concentration–analgesic response relationship in the treatment of postoperative pain. Anesth Analg 67:329-337, 1988.

58. Van den Nieuwenhuyzen MCO, Engbers FHM, Burm AGL, et al: Computer-controlled infusion of alfentanil versus PCA-morphine for postoperative analgesia: A double-blind study. Anesth Analg 40:1112-1118, 1995.

59. Lehmann KA: Patient-controlled analgesia for postoperative pain. Adv Pain Res Ther 14:297, 1990.

60. Lehmann KA, Gerhard A, Horrichs-Haermeyer G, et al: Postoperative patient-controlled analgesia with sufentanil: Analgesic efficacy and minimum effective concentrations. Acta Anaesthesiol Scand 35:221, 1991.

61. Kissin I, Mason JOD, Bradley EL Jr: Morphine and fentanyl interactions with thiopental in relation to movement response to noxious stimulation. Anesth Analg 65:1149-1154, 1986.

62. Kissin I, Mason JO, Bradley EL: Morphine and fentanyl hypnotic interactions with thiopental. Anesthesiology 67:331-335, 1987.

63. Mehta D, Bradley EL Jr, Kissin I: Effect of alfentanil on hypnotic and antinociceptive components of thiopental sodium anesthesia. J Clin Anesth 3:280-284, 1991.

64. Kissin I, Brown PT, Bradley EL Jr: Sedative and hypnotic midazolam-morphine interactions in rats. Anesth Analg 71:137-143, 1990.

65. Ropcke H, Schwilden H: The interaction of nitrous oxide and enflurane on the EEG median of 2-3 Hz is additive, but weaker than at 1.0 MAC [in German]. Anaesthesist 45:819-825, 1996.

66. Gonsowski CT, Eger EI 2nd: Nitrous oxide minimum alveolar anesthetic concentration in rats is greater than previously reported. Anesth Analg 79:710-712, 1994.

67. Deady JE, Koblin DD, Eger EI 2nd, et al: Anesthetic potencies and the unitary theory of narcosis. Anesth Analg 60:380-384, 1981.

68. Targ AG, Yasuda N, Eger EI 2nd, et al: Halogenation and anesthetic potency. Anesth Analg 68:599-602, 1989; see comments.

69. Kissin I: General anesthetic action: An obsolete notion? Anesth Analg 76:215-218, 1993.

70. Katoh T, Ikeda I: The effects of fentanyl on sevoflurane requirements for loss of consciousness and skin incision. Anesthesiology 88:18-24, 1998.

71. McEwan AI, Smith C, Dyar O, et al: Isoflurane MAC reduction by fentanyl. Anesthesiology 78:864-869, 1993.

72. Brunner MD, Braithwaite P, Jhaveri R, et al: The MAC reduction of isoflurane by sufentanil. Br J Anaesth 72:42-46, 1994.

73. Westmoreland C, Sebel PS, Groper A, et al: Reduction of isoflurane MAC by fentanyl or alfentanil. Anesthesiology 77:A394, 1992.

74. Lang E, Kapila A, Shlugman D, et al: Reduction of isoflurane minimal alveolar concentration by remifentanil. Anesthesiology 85:721-728, 1996.

75. Glass PSA, Jacobs JR, Smith RL, et al: Pharmacokinetic model–driven infusion of fentanyl: Assessment of accuracy. Anesthesiology 73:1082-1090, 1990.

76. Dwyer R, Bennett HL, Eger EI 2nd, et al: Isoflurane anesthesia prevents unconscious learning. Anesth Analg 75:107-112, 1992.

77. Minto CF, Schnider TW, Short TG, et al: Response surface model for anesthetic drug interactions. Anesthesiology 92:1603-1616, 2000.

78. Shafer SL, Varvel JR: Pharmacokinetics, pharmacodynamics, and rational opioid selection. Anesthesiology 74:53-63, 1991.

79. Henthorn TK, Krejcie TC, Shanks CA, et al: Time-dependent distribution volume and kinetics of the pharmacodynamic effector site. J Pharm Sci 81:1136, 1992.

80. Wagner JG: A safe method for rapidly achieving plasma concentration plateaus. Clin Pharmacol Ther 16:691-700, 1974.

81. Bruhn J, Bouillon TW, Ropcke H, Hoeft A: A manual slide rule for target-controlled infusion of propofol: Development and evaluation. Anesth Analg 96:142-147, 2003.

82. Hughes MA, Glass PSA, Jacobs JR: Context-sensitive half-time in multicompartment pharmacokinetic models for intravenous anesthetic drugs. Anesthesiology 76:334-341, 1992.

83. Schwilden H: Optimization of the dosage of volatile anesthetics based on pharmacokinetic and dynamic models. Anasthesiol Intensivmed Notfallmed Schmerzther 20:307-315, 1985.

84. Fisher DM, Rosen JI: A pharmacokinetic explanation for increasing recovery time following larger or repeated doses of nondepolarizing muscle relaxants. Anesthesiology 65:286-291, 1986.

85. Youngs EJ, Shafer SL: Pharmacokinetic parameters relevant to recovery from opioids. Anesthesiology 81:833-842, 1994.

86. Bailey JM: Technique for quantifying the duration of intravenous anesthetic effect. Anesthesiology 83:1095-1103, 1995; see comments.

87. Vuyk J, Mertens MJ, Olofsen E, et al: Propofol anesthesia and rational opioid selection: Determination of optimal EC50-EC95 propofol-opioid concentrations that assure adequate anesthesia and a rapid return of consciousness. Anesthesiology 87:1549-1562, 1997.

88. Heykants J, Geerts P, Noorduin H, et al: The pharmacokinetic basis of alfentanil infusion. Eur J Anaesthesiol 1:17, 1987.

89. Moldenhauer CC, Hug CC Jr: Use of narcotic analgesics as anaesthetics. Clin Anaesth 2:107, 1984.

90. Sebel PS, Bovill JG: Opioid analgesics in cardiac anesthesia. In Kaplan JA (ed): Cardiac Anesthesia. Orlando, FL, Grune & Stratton, 1987, p 67.

91. Minto CF, Schnider TW, Shafer SL: Pharmacokinetics and pharmacodynamics of remifentanil. II. Model application. Anesthesiology 86:24-33, 1997.

92. White P: Propofol: Pharmacokinetics and pharmaco-dynamics. Semin Anesth 7:4, 1988.

93. Shafer A, Doze VA, Shafer SL, et al: Pharmacokinetics and pharmacodynamics of propofol infusions during general anesthesia. Anesthesiology 69:348-356, 1988.

94. Barr J, Egan TD, Sandoval NF, et al: Propofol dosing regimens for ICU sedation based upon an integrated pharmacokinetic-pharmacodynamic model. Anesthesiology. 95:324-333, 2001.

95. White PF, Dworsky WA, Horai V, et al: Comparison of continuous infusion fentanyl or ketamine versus thiopental—determining the mean effective serum concentrations for outpatient surgery. Anesthesiology 59:564, 1983.

96. Glass PS, Leiman BC, Reves JG: Etomidate: What is its present role in anesthesia? Semin Anesth 7:143, 1988.

97. White PF, Way WL, Trevor AJ: Ketamine: Its pharmacology and therapeutic uses. Anesthesiology 56:119, 1982.

98. Reves J, Glass PSA, Jacobs J: Midazolam and alfentanil: New anesthetic drugs for continuous infusion and an automated method of administration. Mt Sinai J Med 56:99, 1989.

99. Kissin I, Brown PT, Bradley EL, et al: Diazepam-morphine hypnotic synergism in rats. Anesthesiology 70:689-694, 1989.

100. Theil DR, Stanley TE III, White WD, et al: Midazolam and fentanyl continuous infusion anesthesia for cardiac surgery: A comparison of computer-assisted vs. manual infusion systems. J Cardiothorac Vasc Anesth 7:300-306, 1993.

101. Crankshaw DP, Morgan DJ, Beemer GH, et al: Preprogrammed infusion of alfentanil to constant arterial plasma concentration. Anesth Analg 76:556, 1993.

102. Shafer SL: Constant versus optimal plasma concentrations. Anesth Analg 76:467-469, 1993.

103. Reves JG, Jacobs JR, Glass PSA: Automated drug delivery in anesthesia. ASA Refresher Course in Anesthesiology 19, 1991, p 19.

104. Kruger-Thiemer E: Continuous intravenous infusion and multicompartment accumulation. Eur J Pharmacol 4:317-324, 1968.

105. Schwilden H, Schuttler J, Stoekel H: Pharmacokinetics as applied to total intravenous anaesthesia: Theoretical considerations. Anaesthesia 38(Suppl):51-52, 1983.

106. Schüttler J, Schwilden H, Stoekel H: Pharmacokinetics as applied to total intravenous anaesthesia: Practical implications. Anaesthesia 38(Suppl):53-56, 1983.

107. Bazaral MG, Ciarkowski A: Food and drug administration regulations and computer-controlled infusion pumps. Int Anesthesiol Clin 33:45-63, 1995

108. Shafer SL, Siegel LC, Cooke JE, et al: Testing computer-controlled infusion pumps by simulation. Anesthesiology 68:261-266, 1988.

109. Varvel JR, Donoho DL, Shafer SL: Measuring the predictive performance of computer-controlled infusion pumps. J Pharmacokinet Biopharm 20:63, 1992.

110. Raemer DB, Buschman A, Varvel JR, et al: The prospective use of population pharmacokinetics in a computer-driven infusion system for alfentanil. Anesthesiology 73:66-72, 1990.

111. Schüttler J, Kloos S, Schwilden H, et al: Total intravenous anaesthesia with propofol and alfentanil by computer-assisted infusion. Anaesthesia 43(Suppl):2-7, 1988.

112. Lemmens HJM, Bovill JG, Burm AGL, et al: Alfentanil infusion in the elderly. Anaesthesia 43:850-856, 1988.

113. Veselis RA, Glass P, Dnistrian A, et al: Performance of computer-assisted continuous infusion at low concentrations of intravenous sedatives. Anesth Analg 84:1049-1057, 1997.

114. Shafer SL, Varvel SL, Aziz N, et al: The pharmacokinetics of fentanyl administered by computer controlled infusion pump. Anesthesiology 73:1091-1102, 1990.

115. Alvis JM, Reves JG, Govier AV, et al: Computer assisted continuous infusions of fentanyl during cardiac anesthesia: Comparison with a manual method. Anesthesiology 63:41-49, 1985.

116. Coetzee JF, Glen JB, Wium CA, et al: Pharmacokinetic model selection for target controlled infusions of propofol: Assessment of three parameter sets. Anesthesiology 82:1328-1345, 1995.

117. Marsh B, White M, Morton N, et al: Pharmacokinetic model driven infusion of propofol in children. Br J Anaesth 67:41, 1991.

118. Schüttler J, Stoeckel H: Alfentanil (R39209) ein neues kurzwirkendes opioid. Pharmakokinetik und erste klinische erfahrungen. Anaesthesist 31:10, 1982.

119. Maitre PO, Vozeh S, Heykants J: Population pharmaco-kinetics of alfentanil: The average dose-plasma concentration relationship and interindividual variability in patients. Anesthesiology 66:3-12, 1987.

120. Crankshaw DP, Boyd MD, Bjorksten AR: Plasma drug efflux: A new approach to optimization of drug infusion for constant blood concentration of thiopental and methohexital. Anesthesiology 67:32-41, 1987.

121. Helmers H, Van Peer A, Woestenborghs R, et al: Alfentanil kinetics in the elderly. Clin Pharmacol Ther 36:239-243, 1984.

122. McClain DA, Hug CC Jr: Intravenous fentanyl kinetics. Clin Pharmacol Ther 28:106, 1980.

123. Glass PSA, Jacobs J, Alvis J, et al: Computer assisted continuous infusion of alfentanil during noncardiac anesthesia: A comparison with a manual method. Anesthesiology 65:A546, 1986.

124. Greeley WJ, de Bruijn NP, Davis DP: Sufentanil pharmacokinetics in pediatric cardiovascular patients. Anesth Analg 66:1067-1072, 1987.

125. Kern FH, Ungerleider RM, Jacobs JR, et al: Computerized continuous infusion of intravenous anesthetic drugs during pediatric cardiac surgery. Anesth Analg 72:487-492, 1991.

126. Mertens MJ, Engbers FH, Burm AG, Vuyk J: Predictive performance of computer-controlled infusion of remifentanil during propofol/remifentanil anaesthesia. Br J Anaesth 90:132-141, 2003.

127. Ghoneim MM, Van Hamme MJ: Pharmacokinetics of thiopentone: Effects of enflurane and nitrous oxide anaesthesia and surgery. Br J Anaesth 50:1237-1242, 1978.

128. Smith MT, Eadie MJ, Brophy TO: The pharmacokinetics of midazolam in man. Eur J Clin Pharmacol 19:271-278, 1981.

129. Greenblatt DJ, Abernathy DR, Locniskar A, et al: Effect of age, gender, and obesity on midazolam kinetics. Anesthesiology 61:27-35, 1984.

130. Dyck JB, Varvel J, Hung O, et al: The pharmacokinetics of propofol versus age [abstract]. Can Anaesth J 38(Suppl):A129, 1991.

131. Tackley RM, Lewis GTR, Prys-Roberts C, et al: Computer controlled infusion of propofol. Br J Anaesth 62:46, 1989.

132. Gepts E, Camu F, Cockshott ID, et al: Disposition of propofol administered as constant rate intravenous infusions in humans. Anesth Analg 66:1256-1263, 1987.

133. Glass PSA, Goodman DK, Ginsberg B, et al: Accuracy of pharmacokinetic model–driven infusion of propofol. Anesthesiology 71:A277, 1989.

134. Ginsberg B, Howell S, Glass PSA, et al: Pharmacokinetic model–driven infusion of fentanyl in children. Anesthesiology 85:1268-1275, 1996.

135. Fiset P, Mathers L, Engstrom R, et al: Pharmacokinetics of computer controlled alfentanil administration in children undergoing cardiac surgery. Anesthesiology 83:944-955, 1995.

136. Bailey JM, Mora CT, Shafer SL, et al: Pharmacokinetics of propofol in adult patients undergoing coronary revascularization. Anesthesiology 81:1288-1297, 1996.

137. Vuyk J, Oostwoud CJ, Vletter AA, et al: Gender differences in the pharmacokinetics of propofol in elderly patients during and after continuous infusion. Br J Anaesth 86:183-188, 2001.

138. Schüttler J, Ihmsen H: Population pharmacokinetics of propofol: A multicenter study. Anesthesiology 92:727-738, 2000.

139. Kazama T, Kurita T, Morita K, et al: Influence of hemorrhage on propofol pseudo–steady state concentration. Anesthesiology 97:1156-1161, 2002.

140. Egan TD, Kuramkote S, Gong G, et al: Fentanyl pharmaco-kinetics in hemorrhagic shock: A porcine model. Anesthesiology 91:156-166, 1999.

141. Johnson KB, Kern SE, Hamber EA, et al: Influence of hemorrhagic shock on remifentanil: A pharmacokinetic and pharmacodynamic analysis. Anesthesiology 94:322-332, 2001

142. Pavlin DJ, Coda E, Shen DD, et al: Effects of combining propofol and alfentanil on ventilation, analgesia, sedation, and emesis in human volunteers. Anesthesiology 84:23-37, 1996.

143. Kharasch ED, Russell M, Mautz D, et al: The role of cytochrome P450 3A4 in alfentanil clearance. Anesthesiology 87:36-50, 1997.

144. Vuyk J, Mertens MJ, Vletter AA, et al: Alfentanil modifies the pharmacokinetics of propofol in volunteers. Anesthesiology 87:A300, 1997.

145. Bouillon T, Bruhn J, Radu-Radulescu L, et al: Non–steady state analysis of the pharmacokinetic interaction between propofol and remifentanil. Anesthesiology 97:1350-1362, 2002.

146. Knibbe CA, Zuideveld KP, DeJongh J, et al: Population pharmacokinetic and pharmacodynamic modeling of propofol for long-term sedation in critically ill patients: A comparison between propofol 6% and propofol 1%. Clin Pharmacol Ther 72:670-684, 2002.

147. Hill HF, Saeger L, Bjurstrom R, et al: Steady-state infusions of opioids in human volunteers. I. Pharmacokinetic tailoring. Pain 43:57, 1990.

148. Maitre PE, Stanski DR: Bayesian forecasting improves the prediction of intraoperative plasma concentrations of alfentanil. Anesthesiology 69:652-659, 1988.

149. Wakeling HG, Zimmerman JB, Howell S, Glass PS: Targeting effect compartment or central compartment concentration of propofol: What predicts loss of consciousness? Anesthesiology 90:92-97, 1999.

150. Struys MM, De Smet T, Depoorter B, et al: Comparison of plasma compartment versus two methods for effect compartment–controlled target-controlled infusion for propofol. Anesthesiology 92:399-406, 2000.

151. Kazama T, Ikeda K, Morita K, et al: Comparison of the effect-site k_{e0}s of propofol for blood pressure and EEG bispectral index in elderly and younger patients. Anesthesiology 90:1517-1527, 1999.

152. Minto CF, Schnider TW, Gregg KM, et al: Using the time of maximum effect site concentration to combine pharmacokinetics and pharmacodynamics. Anesthesiology 99:324-333, 2003.

153. Struys M, Versichelen L, Thas O, et al: Comparison of computer-controlled propofol administration with two manual infusion methods [abstract]. Br J Anaesth 76(Suppl 2):87, 1996.

154. Russel D, Wilkes MP, Hunter SC, et al: Manual compared with target-controlled infusion of propofol. Br J Anaesth 75:562-566, 1995.

155. Servin FS: TCI compared with manually controlled infusion of propofol: A multicentre study. Anaesthesia 53(Suppl 1):82-86, 1998.

156. Gale T, Leslie K, Kluger M: Propofol anaesthesia via target controlled infusion or manually controlled infusion: Effects on the bispectral index as a measure of anaesthetic depth. Anaesth Intensive Care 29:579-584, 2001.

157. De Castro V, Godet G, Mencia G, et al: Target-controlled infusion for remifentanil in vascular patients improves hemodynamics and decreases remifentanil requirement. Anesth Analg 96:33-38, 2003.

158. Passot S, Servin F, Allary R, et al: Target-controlled versus manually-controlled infusion of propofol for direct laryngoscopy and bronchoscopy. Anesth Analg 94:1212-1216, 2002.

159. Glass PSA, Ginsberg B, Hawkins ED, et al: Comparison of sodium thiopental/isoflurane to propofol (delivered by means of a pharmacokinetic model–driven device) for the induction, maintenance, and recovery from anesthesia. Anesthesiology 69:A575, 1988.

160. Godet G, Watremez C, El Kettani C, et al: A comparison of sevoflurane, target-controlled infusion propofol, and propofol/isoflurane anesthesia in patients undergoing carotid surgery: A quality of anesthesia and recovery profile. Anesth Analg 93:560-565, 2001.

161. Suttner S, Boldt J, Schmidt C, et al: Cost analysis of target-controlled infusion-based anesthesia compared with standard anesthesia regimens. Anesth Analg 88:77-82, 1999.

162. Hill HF, Chapman CR, Saeger LS, et al: Steady-state infusions of opioids in human. II. Concentration-effect relationships and therapeutic margins. Pain 43:69-79, 1990.

163. Hill HF, Mather LE: Patient-controlled analgesia: Pharmaco-kinetic and therapeutic considerations. Clin Pharmacokinet 24:124-140, 1993.

164. Hill H, Mackie A, Coda B, et al: Evaluation of the accuracy of a pharmacokinetically-based patient-controlled analgesia system. Eur J Clin Pharmacol 43:67-75, 1992.

165. Hill HF, Jacobson RC, Coda BA, et al: A computer-based system for controlling plasma opioid concentration according to patient need for analgesia. Clin Pharmacokinet 20:319-330, 1991.

166. Hill HF, Mackie AM, Coda BA, et al: Patient-controlled analgesic administration: A comparison of steady-state morphine infusions with bolus doses. Cancer 67:873-882, 1991.

167. Schnider TW, Gaeta R, Brose W, et al: Derivation and cross-validation of pharmacokinetic parameters for computer-controlled infusion of lidocaine in pain therapy. Anesthesiology 84:1043-1050, 1996.

168. Absalom AR, Sutcliffe N, Kenny GN: Closed-loop control of anesthesia using Bispectral index: Performance assessment in patients undergoing major orthopedic surgery under combined general and regional anesthesia. Anesthesiology 96:67-73, 2002.

169. O'Hara DA, Bogen DK, Noordergraaf A: The use of computers for controlling the delivery of anesthesia. Anesthesiology 77:563-581, 1992.

170. Westenskow DR, Meline L, Pace NL: Controlled hypotension with sodium nitroprusside: Anesthesiologist versus computer. J Clin Monit 3:80-86, 1987.

171. Olkkola KT, Schwilden H: Quantitation of the interaction between atracurium and succinylcholine using closed-loop feedback control of infusion of atracurium. Anesthesiology 73:614-618, 1990.

172. Struys M, Versichelen L, Byttebier G, et al: Clinical usefulness of the bispectral index for titrating propofol target effect-site concentration. Anaesthesia 53:4-12, 1998.

173. Morley AP, Derrick J, Seed PT, et al: Isoflurane dosage for equivalent intraoperative electroencephalographic suppression in patients with and without epidural blockade. Anesth Analg 95:1412-1418, 2002.

174. Gentilini A, Rossoni-Gerosa M, Frei CW, et al: Modeling and closed-loop control of hypnosis by means of bispectral index (BIS) with isoflurane. IEEE Trans Biomed Eng 48:874-889, 2001.

175. Kansanaho M, Olkkola KT: The effect of halothane on mivacurium infusion requirements in adult surgical patients. Acta Anaesthesiol Scand 41:754-759, 1997.

176. Struys MM, De Smet T, Versichelen LF, et al: Comparison of closed-loop controlled administration of propofol using Bispectral Index as the controlled variable versus "standard practice" controlled administration. Anesthesiology 95:6-17, 2001.

177. Kenny GN, Mantzaridis H: Closed-loop control of propofol anaesthesia. Br J Anaesth 83:223-228, 1999.

178. Sakai T, Matsuki A, White PF, Giesecke AH: Use of an EEG-bispectral closed-loop delivery system for administering propofol. Acta Anaesthesiol Scand 44:1007-1010, 2000.

179. Morley A, Derrick J, Mainland P, et al: Closed loop control of anaesthesia: An assessment of the bispectral index as the target of control. Anaesthesia 55:953-959, 2000.

180. Glass PS, Rampil IJ: Automated anesthesia: Fact or fantasy? Anesthesiology 95:1-2, 2001.

181. Kansanaho M, Olkkola KT, Wierda JM: Dose-response and concentration-response relation of rocuronium infusion during propofol–nitrous oxide and isoflurane–nitrous oxide anaesthesia. Eur J Anaesthesiol 14:488-494, 1997.

182. Meretoja OA, Wirtavuori K, Taivainen T, Olkkola KT: Time course of potentiation of mivacurium by halothane and isoflurane in children. Br J Anaesth 76:235-238, 1996.

183. Milne SE, Kenny GN, Schraag S: Propofol sparing effect of remifentanil using closed-loop anaesthesia. Br J Anaesth 90:623-629, 2003.

184. Schwilden H, Schuttler J: The determination of an effective therapeutic infusion rate for intravenous anesthetics using feedback-controlled dosages [in German]. Anaesthesist 39:603-606, 1990.

185. Albrecht S, Frenkel C, Ihmsen H, Schuttler J: A rational approach to the control of sedation in intensive care unit patients based on closed-loop control. Eur J Anaesthesiol 16:678-687, 1999.

13 Pharmacology of Muscle Relaxants and Their Antagonists

Mohamed Naguib and Cynthia A. Lien

History and Clinical Use   482

Principles of Action of Neuromuscular Blockers at the Neuromuscular Junction   482
Postjunctional Effects   482
Prejunctional Effects   483

Monitoring Neuromuscular Function   484
Peripheral Nerve Stimulation and Clinical Tests   484
Clinical Applications   486

Pharmacology of Succinylcholine   486
Structure-Activity Relationships   486
Pharmacokinetics and Pharmacodynamics   486
Dibucaine Number and Butyrylcholinesterase Activity   487
Dibucaine Number and Atypical Butyrylcholinesterase   488
Side Effects   489
Clinical Uses   491
Interactions with Anticholinesterases   492

Nondepolarizing Neuromuscular Blockers   492
Structure-Activity Relationships   492
Potency of Nondepolarizing Neuromuscular Blockers   497
Pharmacokinetics and Pharmacodynamics   498
Clinical Management   501
Dosage   501
Neuromuscular Blockers and Tracheal Intubation   503
Metabolism and Elimination   505
Adverse Effects of Neuromuscular Blockers   511

Drug Interactions and Other Factors Affecting Response to Neuromuscular Blockers   514
Mechanisms of Drug Interactions   514
Interactions among Nondepolarizing Neuromuscular Blockers   514

Interaction between Succinylcholine and Non-depolarizing Neuromuscular Blockers   515
Inhaled Anesthetics   515
Antibiotics   516
Temperature   516
Magnesium and Calcium   516
Lithium   517
Local Anesthetics and Antidysrhythmics   517
Antiepileptic Drugs   517
Diuretics   517
Other Drugs   518

Recovery from Neuromuscular Blockade   518
Antagonism of Residual Neuromuscular Blockade   519
Major Determinants of Speed and Adequacy of Reversal   519
Clinical Recommendations   522
Other Factors That May Interfere with Antagonism   522
Side Effects of Anticholinesterases   523
Pharmacokinetics of Neostigmine, Pyridostigmine, and Edrophonium   523
Other Antagonists of Nondepolarizing Neuromuscular Blockade   524

Special Populations   525
Pediatric Patients   525
Elderly Patients   526
Obese Patients   527
Severe Renal Disease   527
Hepatobiliary Disease   529
Burns   530
Neuromuscular Blockers and Weakness Syndromes in the Critically Ill   530
Neuromuscular Disorders   533

Economics and Outcome in Practice with Neuromuscular Blocking Drugs   546

HISTORY AND CLINICAL USE

In 1942 Griffith and Johnson[1] suggested that *d*-tubocurarine (dTc) is a safe drug to use during surgery to provide skeletal muscle relaxation. One year later, Cullen[2] described its use in 131 patients who had received general anesthesia for their surgery. In 1954, Beecher and Todd[3] reported a sixfold increase in mortality in patients receiving dTc versus those who had not received a relaxant. The increased mortality was due to a general lack of understanding of the pharmacology of neuromuscular blockers and their antagonism. The impact of residual neuromuscular blockade postoperatively was not appreciated, guidelines for monitoring muscle strength had not been established, and the importance of pharmacologically antagonizing residual blockade was not understood. Since then, the understanding of neuromuscular blocker pharmacology has improved, and relaxants have become an important component of many anesthetics and have facilitated the growth of surgery into new areas with the use of innovative techniques.[4]

Succinylcholine, introduced by Thesleff[5] and by Foldes and colleagues in 1952,[4] changed anesthetic practice drastically. Its rapid onset of effect and ultrashort duration of action allowed for rapid tracheal intubation.

In 1967, Baird and Reid first reported on clinical administration of the synthetic aminosteroid pancuronium.[6] Though similar to dTc, in terms of its duration of action, this compound had an improved cardiovascular side effect profile. It lacked ganglionic-blocking and histamine-releasing properties and was mildly vagolytic. The resulting increases in heart rate and blood pressure were considered significant improvements over its predecessors. Unlike dTc or any of the nondepolarizing neuromuscular blockers previously used, none of which were metabolized, pancuronium underwent some hepatic metabolism through deacetylation of the acetoxy groups.

Development of the intermediate-acting neuromuscular blockers built on compound metabolism and resulted in the introduction of vecuronium,[7] an aminosteroid, and atracurium,[8,9] a benzylisoquinolinium, into practice in the 1980s. These relaxants had little or no dependence on the kidney for elimination. The lack of cardiovascular effects of vecuronium established a benchmark for safety to which newer relaxants are still held.[7] Degradation of atracurium by Hofmann elimination removed any important influence of biologic disorders such as advanced age or organ failure on the pattern of neuromuscular blockade.

Mivacurium, the first short-acting nondepolarizing neuromuscular blocker, was introduced into clinical practice in the 1990s,[10] as was rocuronium,[11] an intermediate-acting nondepolarizing blocker with a rapid onset of effect. Mivacurium, like the intermediate-acting compounds, is extensively metabolized. It is, however, metabolized by butyrylcholinesterase, the same enzyme that is responsible for the metabolism of succinylcholine. In terms of facilitating rapid endotracheal intubation, rocuronium is the first nondepolarizing neuromuscular blocker considered to be a replacement for succinylcholine.

Other neuromuscular blockers have been introduced into clinical practice since the use of dTc was first advocated. These blockers include pipecuronium, doxacurium, cisatracurium, and rapacuronium. Although all do not remain in use, each represented an advance or improvement in at least one aspect over its predecessors. Still other neuromuscular blockers, TAAC3[12] and 430A,[13] are undergoing investigation.

Neuromuscular blockers should be administered only to anesthetized individuals to provide relaxation of skeletal muscles. They should not be administered to stop patient movement because they have no analgesic or amnestic properties. Awareness during surgery[14] and in the intensive care unit (ICU)[15] has been described in multiple publications. Neuromuscular blockers are valuable adjuncts to general anesthetics and should be used as such. As stated by Cullen and Larson, "muscle relaxants given inappropriately may provide the surgeon with optimal [operating] conditions in ... a patient [who] is paralyzed but not anesthetized—a state that [is] wholly unacceptable for the patient."[16] Additionally, "muscle relaxants used to cover up deficiencies in total anesthetic management ... represent an ... inappropriate use of the valuable adjuncts to anesthesia." To administer relaxants for maintenance of neuromuscular blockade intraoperatively, the patient's depth of neuromuscular block must be monitored and the depth of anesthesia continuously assessed.

The use of neuromuscular blockers in the operating room is quite common and has been important in the growth and development of anesthesia and surgery. As stated by Foldes and coauthors,[4] "... [the] first use of ... muscle relaxants ... not only revolutionized the practice of anesthesia but also started the modern era of surgery and made possible the explosive development of cardiothoracic, neurologic and organ transplant surgery." Certainly, neuromuscular blockers are now routinely used to facilitate endotracheal intubation and are commonly used to maintain neuromuscular blockade through any number of different surgical procedures. This chapter will review the pharmacology and clinical use of neuromuscular blockers, as well as anticholinesterases, in the operating room. Diseases of the neuromuscular system are also discussed as regards their influence on the actions of neuromuscular blockers. Finally, the economics of providing neuromuscular blockade is also considered.

PRINCIPLES OF ACTION OF NEUROMUSCULAR BLOCKERS AT THE NEUROMUSCULAR JUNCTION (also see Chapter 22)

Postjunctional Effects

In adult mammalian skeletal muscle, the nicotinic acetylcholine receptor (nAChR) is a pentameric complex of two α-subunits in association with single β-, δ-, and ε-subunits (Fig. 13-1). These subunits are organized to form a transmembrane pore (a channel), as well as the extracellular binding pockets for acetylcholine and other agonists or antagonists.[17] Each of the two α-subunits has an acetylcholine-binding site. These sites are proteins located in pockets approximately 3.0 nm above the surface membrane at the interfaces of the α_H-ε and α_L-δ subunits.[18]

α Subunit

N Terminus   C Terminus

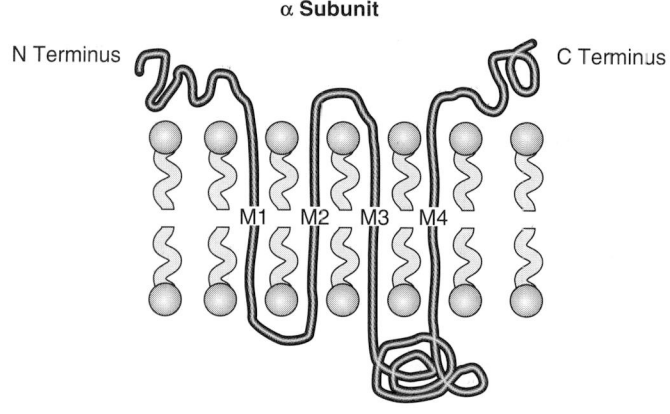

Pentameric complex

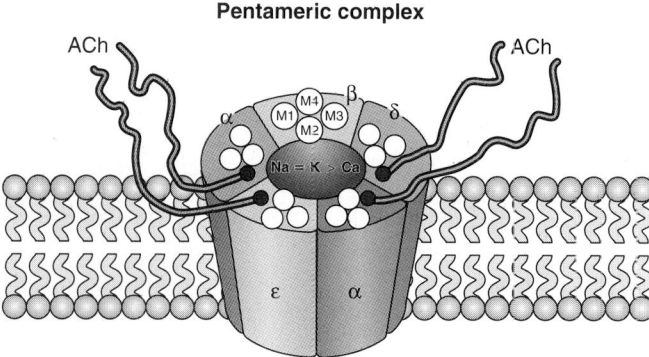

Figure 13–1 Subunit composition of the nicotinic acetylcholine receptor (nAChR) in the end-plate surface of adult mammalian muscle. The adult AChR is an intrinsic membrane protein with five distinct subunits ($\alpha_2\beta\delta\epsilon$). Each subunit contains four helical domains labeled M1 to M4. The M2 domain forms the channel pore. The *upper panel* shows a single α-subunit with its N and C termini on the extracellular surface of the membrane lipid bilayer. Between the N and C termini, the α-subunit forms four helices (M1, M2, M3, and M4) that span the membrane bilayer. The *lower panel* shows the pentameric structure of the nAChR of adult mammalian muscle. The N termini of two subunits cooperate to form two distinct binding pockets for acetylcholine (ACh). These pockets occur at the ε-α and the δ-α subunit interface. The M2 membrane-spanning domain of each subunit lines the ion channel. The doubly liganded ion channel has permeability equal to that of Na^+ and K^+; Ca^{2+} contributes approximately 2.5% to the total permeability. (Redrawn from Naguib M, Flood P, McArdle JJ, et al: Advances in neurobiology of the neuromuscular junction: Implications for the anesthesiologist. Anesthesiology 96:202-231, 2002.)

α_H and α_L indicate the high- and low-affinity binding sites for dTc and probably result from a contribution from the different neighboring subunits.[19,20] For instance, the binding affinity of dTc for the α_H-ε site is approximately 100- to 500-fold higher than that for the α_L-δ site.[18,20,21] Fetal nAChR contains a γ-subunit instead of the adult ε-subunit. Mature nAChR has a shorter burst duration and exhibits higher conductance of Na^+, K^+, and Ca^{2+} than fetal nAChR does.[17,22]

Functionally, the ion channel of the acetylcholine receptor is closed in the resting state. Simultaneous binding of two acetylcholine molecules to the α-subunits[23]

initiates conformational changes that open the channel.[24-26] On the other hand, it is enough for one molecule of a nondepolarizing neuromuscular blocker (a competitive antagonist) to bind to one subunit to produce a block.[27] Paul and coworkers[28] found a correlation between the ED_{50} (the dose that produces 50% depression of twitch tension) and the potency of nondepolarizing blockers at the adult nAChR.

Depolarizing neuromuscular blockers such as succinylcholine produce prolonged depolarization of the end-plate region that results in (1) desensitization of nAChR, (2) inactivation of voltage-gated sodium channels at the neuromuscular junction, and (3) increases in potassium permeability in the surrounding membrane (see Chapter 22 for details).[27] The end result is failure of action potential generation, and block ensues. It should be noted that although acetylcholine produces depolarization, under physiologic conditions it results in muscle contraction because it has a very short (few milliseconds) duration of action.[27] Acetylcholine is rapidly hydrolyzed by acetylcholinesterase[29] to acetic acid and choline. Administration of large doses of acetylcholine in experimental animals, though, produces neuromuscular blockade.[27]

The fetal nAChR is a low-conductance channel, in contrast to the high-conductance channel of adult nAChR. Thus, acetylcholine release causes brief activation and a reduced probability of channel opening.[17] The upregulation of nAChRs that is found in states of functional or surgical denervation is characterized by the spreading of predominantly fetal-type nAChRs. These receptors are resistant to nondepolarizing neuromuscular blockers and more sensitive to succinylcholine.[30] When depolarized, the immature isoform has a prolonged open channel time, which exaggerates K^+ efflux.[31]

Prejunctional Effects

Prejunctional receptors are involved in the modulation of acetylcholine release in the neuromuscular junction. The existence of both nicotinic and muscarinic receptors on motor nerve endings has been described. The prejunctional nicotinic receptor is a pentameric complex composed of $\alpha_3\beta_2$-subunits. Bowman[32] suggested that the prejunctional nicotinic receptors are activated by acetylcholine and function in a positive-feedback control system that serves to maintain the availability of acetylcholine when demand for it is high (e.g., during tetany).[32] Blockage of these receptors by nondepolarizing neuromuscular blockers would explain the fade phenomenon seen with tetanic and train-of-four (TOF) stimulation.[32,33] The G protein–coupled muscarinic receptors are also involved in the feedback modulation of acetylcholine release.[34-36] The prejunctional M_1 and M_2 receptors are involved in facilitation and inhibition of acetylcholine release, respectively, through modulation of Ca^{2+} influx,[37,38] whereas the prejunctional nicotinic receptors are involved in mobilization of acetylcholine, but not in the release process directly.[39] Hence, blockade of prejunctional nicotinic receptors by nondepolarizing neuromuscular blockers prevents acetylcholine from being made available fast enough to support tetanic or TOF stimulation. In contrast, prejunctional muscarinic receptors are involved in upmodulation or downmodulation of the release mechanism. No evidence has indicated that nondepolarizing neuromuscular blockers act on muscarinic receptors.

MONITORING NEUROMUSCULAR FUNCTION

Details of monitoring neuromuscular function are discussed in Chapter 39. In this section, general concepts of monitoring as they relate to the clinical use of neuromuscular blockers are presented.

Peripheral Nerve Stimulation and Clinical Tests

Monitoring of neuromuscular function after the administration of neuromuscular blocking agents is extremely important to appropriately dose these agents and to better guarantee patient safety.[40,41] In the operating room or the ICU, the depth of neuromuscular blockade is typically monitored by observing the response of any superficially located neuromuscular unit to stimulation. Most commonly, contraction of the adductor pollicis associated with stimulation of the ulnar nerve, either at the wrist or at the elbow, is monitored. In certain circumstances, depending on patient positioning where access to the patient's arms may be limited or because of the nature of the injury, the peroneal nerve or the facial nerve may be monitored.

The pattern of response to TOF stimulation (four stimuli delivered over a period of 2 seconds) or a tetanic stimulus varies with the type of neuromuscular blocker administered because the two relaxant types, depolarizing and nondepolarizing, have different mechanisms of action. With a complete block, no response to either mode of stimulation should be seen. However, during partial neuromuscular blockade, different responses are seen to these modes of stimulation, depending on the agent administered. Nondepolarizing neuromuscular blocking agents are competitive inhibitors of the acetylcholine receptor—they compete with acetylcholine for the active, or binding, sites on the α-subunits of the receptor. With repetitive or intense stimulation, the response to stimulation fades over time because of a decrease in the amount of acetylcholine released from the prejunctional nerve terminal with successive stimuli. The fourth response to a TOF stimulus is decreased relative to the first response (Fig. 13-2) because the lesser amount of acetylcholine released into the synaptic cleft with the fourth stimulus cannot overcome the competitive block as readily. Similarly, fade is seen in the response to tetanic stimuli when a partial nondepolarizing neuromuscular block is present. During neuromuscular blockade with nondepolarizing agents, if one administers a TOF stimulus shortly after administering a tetanic stimulus, the response to stimulation is augmented and neuromuscular function appears stronger than it did just a couple of minutes earlier. This presumably occurs because with the tetanic stimuli, acetylcholine is mobilized toward the presynaptic portion of the nerve terminal and then, with subsequent stimulation (TOF), an increased amount of acetylcholine is released into the synaptic cleft and the block imposed by the nondepolarizing agent is

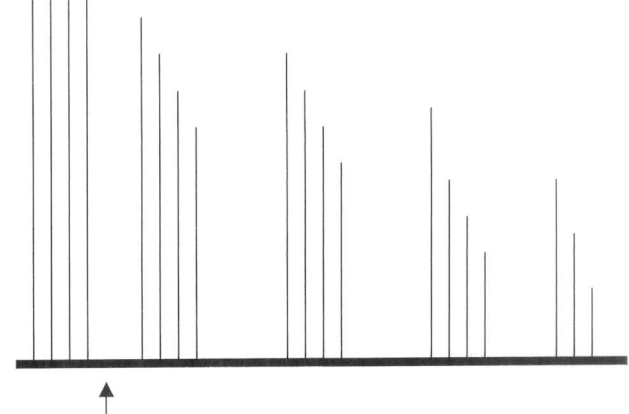

Figure 13–2 Schematic representation of the onset of a neuromuscular block after administration of a nondepolarizing neuromuscular blocking agent at the *arrow*. Neuromuscular function is monitored with repetitive train-of-four (TOF) stimuli (four stimuli of 0.5-msec duration administered over a period of 2 seconds). Note the presence of fade in the response to TOF stimulation.

more readily overcome. It may take from 1 to 10 minutes for recovery to return to pretetanic or baseline values.[42,43] In the case of administration of a depolarizing neuromuscular blocking agent such as succinylcholine, the response that has been classically described is quite different. With repetitive TOF stimuli, after the administration of doses of succinylcholine that cause 100% paralysis, four equal responses are seen with each stimulus, but the response weakens with each successive TOF stimulus (Fig. 13-3). Similarly, no fade or weakening in the response to a tetanic stimulus takes place; however, the entire response will be weaker than it was at baseline. The onset of blockade after the administration of small doses of succinylcholine, 0.05 to 0.3 mg/kg, is accompanied by fade in the TOF response, as has been described for nondepolarizing agents.[44] Interestingly, although one

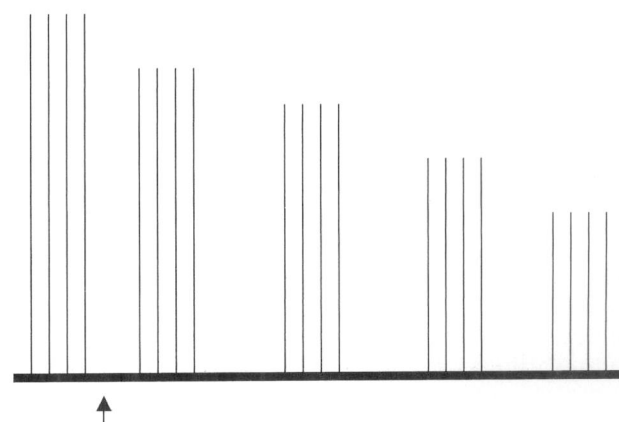

Figure 13–3 Schematic representation of the onset of a neuromuscular block after administration of a depolarizing neuromuscular blocking agent at the *arrow*. Neuromuscular function is monitored with repetitive train-of-four stimuli (four stimuli of 0.5-msec duration administered over a period of 2 seconds).

would not necessarily anticipate that there would be post-tetanic potentiation after the administration of succinylcholine, it has been described.[45] The reason for this observation has yet to be elucidated.

Donati and colleagues[46] and Pansard and associates[47] have demonstrated that neuromuscular blockade develops faster in centrally located muscles, such as the larynx, the jaw, and the diaphragm, than in more peripherally located muscles, such as the adductor pollicis. In addition to developing more quickly, neuromuscular blockade in these regions, at a given dose, is less profound and recovers more quickly (Fig. 13-4) (for details see the section "Neuromuscular Blockers and Tracheal Intubation").[46] Consequently, the choice of monitoring site is important.

To determine the depth of block during maintenance and recovery of neuromuscular function, the response of the adductor pollicis to stimulation of the ulnar nerve should be monitored. If recovery in this neuromuscular unit is complete, recovery in the musculature of the airway should also be complete.[46]

Peripheral nerve stimulation can be used to determine both the magnitude and the depth of neuromuscular blockade. However, the degree of neuromuscular block must be assessed cautiously. Because there is such a wide margin of safety as regards neuromuscular function, with a large number of acetylcholine receptors having to be blocked before weakness becomes detectable, the reduction in contractile response to peripheral nerve stimulation is not proportional to the action of neuromuscular blockers at the receptor. Waud and Waud[48] demonstrated that the twitch response of the tibialis anterior muscle of the cat in response to a single supramaximal stimulus is not reduced unless more than 70% of the receptors are occupied by a nondepolarizing neuromuscular blocker. Twitch is completely eliminated when 90% of the receptors are occupied. Three questions can be answered by observing the response to peripheral nerve stimulation: (1) is the neuromuscular blockade adequate? (2) is the neuromuscular blockade excessive? and (3) can the neuromuscular blockade be antagonized?

Muscle contraction is an all-or-none phenomenon. Each fiber either contracts maximally or does not contract at all.

Therefore, when twitch height, or muscle strength, is reduced, some fibers are contracting normally and others are blocked and remain flaccid. A stronger response indicates that fewer muscle fibers remain flaccid.

Because the interaction of nondepolarizing neuromuscular blockers with acetylcholine receptor binding sites is competitive, neuromuscular blockade can be overcome by increasing—or intensified by reducing—the concentration of acetylcholine. This concept is important in clinical monitoring of neuromuscular blockade. Another important concept is the economy of acetylcholine synthesis, storage, and release. The quantity of acetylcholine released with each nerve action potential is inversely proportional to the number of action potentials reaching the nerve terminal per unit time, or the stimulus frequency. The depth of blockade of evoked neuromuscular responses in the presence of nondepolarizing neuromuscular blockers is directly proportional to the stimulus frequency.

The onset of neuromuscular blockade should be monitored with either single twitch stimuli or TOF stimuli because one is looking for ablation of the twitch response, or its maximal suppression, to determine onset of the block. The depth of block during maintenance of blockade and recovery should be monitored with repeated TOF stimuli, where depending on the surgery and the type of anesthetic administered, the anesthesiologist may want to maintain deeper levels of neuromuscular blockade (one or two twitches in response to TOF stimuli) or lesser degrees of blockade (three to four twitches in response to TOF stimuli). When determining the depth of block to maintain during the course of an anesthetic, it is important to remember that a deep volatile anesthetic will provide some degree of muscle relaxation and patient immobility and that volatile anesthetics potentiate nondepolarizing neuromuscular blockers. Similarly, recovery of neuromuscular function should be monitored with TOF stimuli. Once four responses to stimulation are detectable and fade in the response is no longer detectable, the TOF ratio (the strength of the fourth response in comparison to the strength of the first response to stimulation) may be 40% to 100%. It is difficult to more reliably detect fade in the TOF response[48,49]

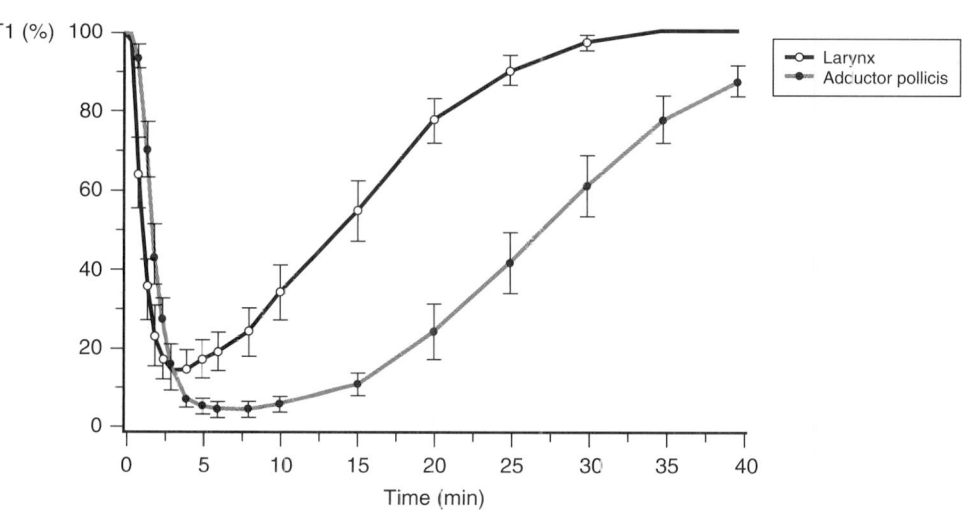

Figure 13–4 Evolution of neuromuscular blockade in the larynx and thumb (adductor pollicis) after 0.07 mg/kg vecuronium. Onset and recovery from the block occur more rapidly in the larynx. (Redrawn from Donati F, Meistelman C, Plaud B: Vecuronium neuromuscular blockade at the adductor muscles of the larynx and adductor pollicis. Anesthesiology 74:833-837, 1991.)

because the middle two responses confuse interpretation of the first and fourth responses. Once fade in response to TOF stimulation is no longer detected, adequacy of recovery should be confirmed with double-burst stimulation. In response to this stimulus, the clinician feels only two responses,[50] thus simplifying interpretation of the relative strength of each response. If no difference in the two responses is apparent, the TOF ratio is at least 0.6.[51,52]

In addition to using monitors of muscle strength, clinical indicators of adequacy of return of neuromuscular function should also be sought. Such clinical tests include a 5-second head lift, handgrip, and in a patient unable to cooperate with simple commands, the ability to bend the legs up off the operating room table. A successful head lift is one done from a flat surface, unaided and maintained for a full 5 seconds. Pavlin and coworkers[53] have shown that if patients can successfully perform a head lift, their maximum inspiratory force is approximately −55 cm H_2O, and if they can lift their legs off a flat surface, their maximum inspiratory force is −50 cm H_2O. With a strong handgrip, clinicians should not be able to pull their fingers from the patient's grip. Even though these tests have long been the mainstay of clinical tests of neuromuscular function, they can be accomplished over a wide range of TOF ratios and must be used with caution. As described by Kopman and coauthors,[54] volunteers with TOF ratios as low as 0.5 are capable of maintaining a 5-second head lift and having a strong handgrip. The ability of patients to oppose their incisors and maintain a tongue blade between them appears to be a more sensitive indicator of the adequacy of muscle strength inasmuch as volunteers were unable to perform this task until their TOF ratios had returned to 0.85. In patients, however, even this ability does not seem to be a sensitive indicator of residual neuromuscular block.[55]

Monitors of respiratory function do not reliably indicate return of muscle strength and function to baseline. Tidal volume is inadequate as a monitor of the adequacy of muscle strength because it is more likely to reflect recovery in the centrally located muscles of respiration and is dependent on diaphragmatic movement only. With a tidal volume of at least 5 mL/kg, 80% of acetylcholine receptors may still be occupied by nondepolarizing neuromuscular blocking drugs. Head lift and handgrip may be 38% and 48% of control, respectively, when both inspiratory and expiratory flow rates are more than 90% of control.[56] Furthermore, inspiratory force may be only 70% of control when vital capacity and the expiratory flow rate are greater than 90% of control values.[57]

Clinical Applications

It is not known what proportion of receptors must be available or how sensitive a test must be to ensure adequate muscle strength to overcome airway obstruction and permit effective coughing and to be free of visual disturbances. The anesthesiologist should not rely on just one test of neuromuscular strength, but should use as many tests as practically possible (Table 13-1). The results of Pavlin and colleagues[53] and the relatively frequent admission of patients to the postanesthesia care unit (PACU) with unacceptable levels of neuromuscular blockade that

was unrecognized by the anesthesiologist[58-60] emphasize the difficulty in ensuring that no residual neuromuscular blockade exists after surgery and anesthesia.

PHARMACOLOGY OF SUCCINYLCHOLINE

Structure-Activity Relationships

All neuromuscular blockers are structurally related to acetylcholine. Neuromuscular blocking agents are quaternary ammonium compounds. Positive charges at these sites in the molecules mimic the quaternary nitrogen atom of the transmitter acetylcholine and are the principal reason for the attraction of these drugs to cholinergic nicotinic receptors at the neuromuscular junction. These receptors are also located at other physiologic sites of acetylcholine in the body, such as the nicotinic receptors in autonomic ganglia and as many as five different muscarinic receptors on both the parasympathetic and sympathetic sides of the autonomic nervous system. In addition, populations of nicotinic and muscarinic receptors are located prejunctionally at the neuromuscular junction.[27]

The depolarizing neuromuscular blocker succinylcholine is composed of two molecules of acetylcholine linked back to back through the acetate methyl groups (Fig. 13-5). As described by Bovet,[61] succinylcholine is a long, thin, flexible molecule. Like acetylcholine, succinylcholine stimulates cholinergic receptors at the neuromuscular junction and at nicotinic (ganglionic) and muscarinic autonomic sites to open the ionic channel in the acetylcholine receptor.

Pharmacokinetics and Pharmacodynamics

Succinylcholine is the only available neuromuscular blocker with a rapid onset of effect and an ultrashort duration of action. The ED_{95} of succinylcholine (the dose causing on average 95% suppression of neuromuscular response) is 0.51 to 0.63 mg/kg.[62,63] Using cumulative dose-response techniques, Smith and coworkers[64] and Kopman and associates[65] have estimated that its potency is far greater with an ED_{95} less than 0.3 mg/kg.

Administration of 1 mg/kg succinylcholine results in complete suppression of response to neuromuscular stimulation in approximately 60 seconds.[66-68] In patients with genotypically normal butyrylcholinesterase (also known as plasma cholinesterase or pseudocholinesterase) activity, recovery to 90% muscle strength after the administration of 1 mg/kg succinylcholine requires from 9 to 13 minutes.[69,70]

The short duration of action of succinylcholine is due to its rapid hydrolysis by butyrylcholinesterase to succinylmonocholine and choline. Butyrylcholinesterase has an enormous capacity to hydrolyze succinylcholine, and only 10% of the administered drug reaches the neuromuscular junction.[71] The initial metabolite (succinylmonocholine) is a much weaker neuromuscular blocking agent than succinylcholine is[72] and is metabolized much more slowly to succinic acid and choline. In dogs,[73] after

Table 13-1 Tests of neuromuscular transmission

	Acceptable Clinical Results to Suggest Normal Function	Approximate Percentage of Receptor Occupied When Response Returns to Normal Value	Comments/Disadvantages/Advantages
Tidal volume	At least 5 mL/kg	80	Insensitive as an indicator of peripheral neuromuscular function
Single twitch	Qualitatively as strong as baseline	75-80	Uncomfortable, need to know twitch strength before relaxant strength as baseline administration. Insensitive as an indicator of recovery, but useful as a gauge of deep neuromuscular blockade
Train-of-four (TOF)	No palpable fade	70-75	Still uncomfortable, but more sensitive as an indicator of recovery than single twitch is. Useful as a gauge of depth of block by counting the number of responses perceptible
Sustained tetanus at 50 Hz for 5 sec	No palpable fade	70	Very uncomfortable, but a reliable indicator of adequate recovery
Vital capacity	At least 20 mL/kg	70	Requires patient cooperation, but is the goal for achievement of full clinical recovery
Double burst	No palpable fade	60-70	Uncomfortable, but more sensitive than TOF as an indicator of stimulation of peripheral function. No perceptible fade indicates TOF recovery of at least 60%
Sustained tetanus at 100 Hz	No palpable fade	50	Very painful, a "stress test" for the neuromuscular junction. It is not always possible to achieve or demonstrate lack of fade at 100 Hz
Inspiratory force	At least −40 cm H_2O	50	Sometimes difficult to perform without endotracheal intubation, but a reliable gauge of normal diaphragmatic function
Head lift	Must be performed unaided with patient supine at 180 degrees and for 5 sec	50	Requires patient cooperation, but remains the standard test of normal clinical function. Must be performed with the patient in a completely supine position
Handgrip	Sustained at a level qualitatively similar to preinduction baseline	50	Sustained strong grip, though also requiring patient cooperation. It is another good gauge of normal function
Sustained bite	Sustained jaw clench on tongue blade	50	Very reliable with patient cooperation. Corresponds to TOF ratio of 0.85

the administration of 0.5 and 1.0 mg/kg, its $t_{1/2}\beta$ is 5 minutes. Its $t_{1/2}\alpha$ is less than 1 minute.[69]

Because little or no butyrylcholinesterase is present at the neuromuscular junction, the neuromuscular block induced by succinylcholine is terminated by its diffusion away from the neuromuscular junction back into the circulation. Butyrylcholinesterase therefore influences the onset and duration of action of succinylcholine by controlling the rate at which the drug is hydrolyzed before it reaches and after it leaves the neuromuscular junction.

Dibucaine Number and Butyrylcholinesterase Activity

Butyrylcholinesterase is synthesized by the liver and is found in plasma. The neuromuscular block induced by succinylcholine is prolonged by a decreased concentration or activity of the enzyme. The activity of the enzyme refers to the number of substrate molecules (µmol) hydrolyzed per unit of time, often expressed in international units (IU). The normal range of butyrylcholinesterase activity is quite large, and as demonstrated by Viby-Mogensen,[69] significant decreases in butyrylcholinesterase activity result in modest increases in the time required to achieve 100% twitch recovery (Fig. 13-6).

Factors that have been found to lower butyrylcholinesterase activity are liver disease,[74] advanced age,[75] malnutrition, pregnancy, burns, oral contraceptives, monoamine oxidase inhibitors, echothiophate, cytotoxic drugs, neoplastic disease, anticholinesterase drugs,[76,77] tetrahydroaminacrine,[78] hexafluorenium,[79,80] and metoclopramide.[81] The histamine type 2 (H_2) receptor antagonists have no effect on butyrylcholinesterase activity or the duration of succinylcholine effect.[82] Bambuterol, a prodrug of terbutaline, produces marked inhibition of butyrylcholinesterase activity and causes prolongation of

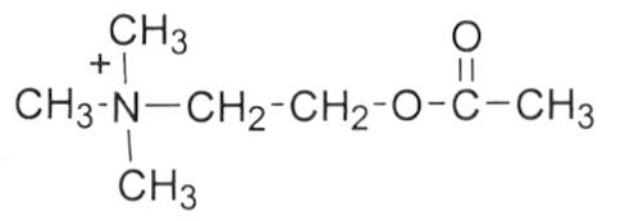

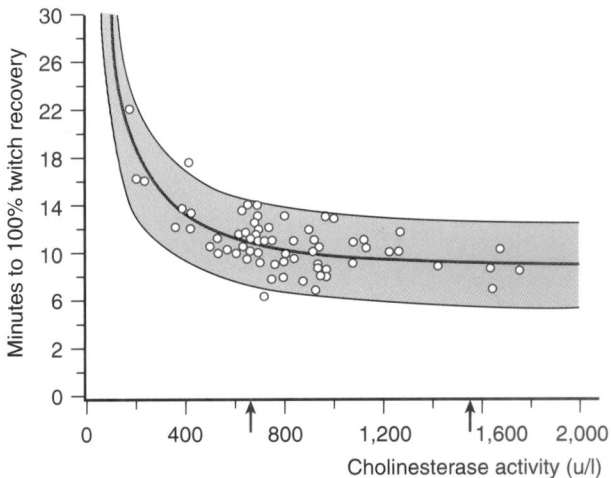

Figure 13–5 Structural relationship of succinylcholine, a depolarizing neuromuscular blocking agent, to acetylcholine. Succinylcholine consists of two acetylcholine molecules linked through the acetate methyl groups. Like acetylcholine, succinylcholine stimulates nicotinic receptors at the neuromuscular junction.

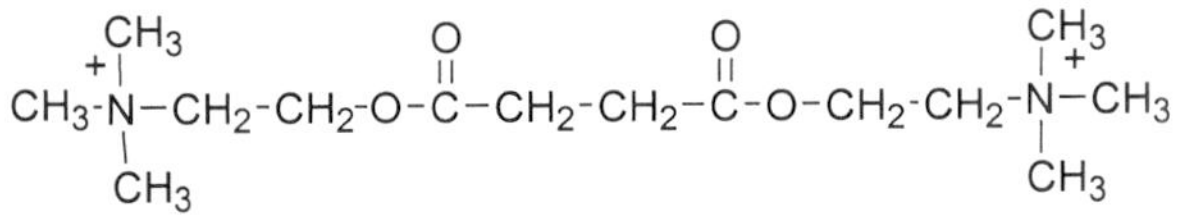

Figure 13–6 Correlation between the duration of succinylcholine neuromuscular blockade and butyrylcholinesterase activity. The normal range of activity lies between the *arrows*. (From Viby-Mogensen J: Correlation of succinylcholine duration of action with plasma cholinesterase activity in subjects with the genotypically normal enzyme. Anesthesiology 53:517-520, 1980.)

succinylcholine-induced blockade.[83,84] The β-blocker esmolol inhibits butyrylcholinesterase but causes only minor prolongation of succinylcholine blockade.[85,86]

Despite all the publications and efforts to identify situations in which normal butyrylcholinesterase enzyme activity may be low, this has not been a major concern in clinical practice because even large decreases in butyrylcholinesterase activity result in only moderate increases in the duration of action of succinylcholine. When butyrylcholinesterase activity is reduced to 20% of normal by severe liver disease, the duration of apnea after the administration of succinylcholine increases from a normal duration of 3 minutes to only 9 minutes. Even when glaucoma treatment with echothiophate decreased butyrylcholinesterase activity from 49% of control to no activity, the increase in duration of neuromuscular blockade varied from 2 to 14 minutes. In no patient did the total duration of neuromuscular blockade exceed 23 minutes.[87]

Dibucaine Number and Atypical Butyrylcholinesterase

Succinylcholine-induced neuromuscular blockade can be significantly prolonged if the patient has an abnormal genetic variant of butyrylcholinesterase. The variant was found by Kalow and Genest[88] to respond to dibucaine differently than normal butyrylcholinesterase does. Dibucaine inhibits normal butyrylcholinesterase to a far greater extent than it does the abnormal enzyme. This observation led

to development of the test for dibucaine number. Under standardized test conditions, dibucaine inhibits the normal enzyme about 80% and the abnormal enzyme about 20% (Table 13-2). Subsequently, many other genetic variants of butyrylcholinesterase have been identified, although dibucaine-resistant variants are the most important. Reviews by Pantuck[89] and by Jensen and Viby-Mogensen[90] can be consulted for more detailed information on this topic.

Although the dibucaine number indicates the genetic makeup of an individual with respect to butyrylcholinesterase, it does not measure the concentration of the enzyme in plasma, nor does it indicate the efficiency of the enzyme in hydrolyzing a substrate such as succinylcholine or mivacurium. Both the latter factors are determined by measuring butyrylcholinesterase activity—which may be influenced by genotype.

The molecular biology of butyrylcholinesterase is well understood. The amino acid sequence of the enzyme is known, and the coding errors responsible for most genetic variations have been identified.[89,90] Most variants are due to a single amino acid substitution error or sequencing error at or near the active site of the enzyme. For example, in the case of the "atypical" dibucaine-resistant (A) gene, a mutation occurs at nucleotide 209, where guanine is substituted for adenine. The resultant change in

Table 13–2 Relationship between dibucaine number and duration of succinylcholine or mivacurium neuromuscular blockade

Type of Butyrylcholinesterase	Genotype	Incidence	Dibucaine Number*	Response to Succinylcholine or Mivacurium
Homozygous typical	UU	Normal	70-80	Normal
Heterozygous atypical	UA	1/480	50-60	Lengthened by about 50%-100%
Homozygous atypical	AA	1/3200	20-30	Prolonged to 4-8 hr

*The dibucaine number indicates the percentage of enzyme inhibited.

this codon causes substitution of glycine for aspartic acid at position 70 in the enzyme. In the case of the fluoride-resistant (F) gene, two amino acid substitutions are possible, namely, methionine for threonine at position 243 and valine for glycine at position 390. Table 13-2 summarizes many of the known genetic variants of butyrylcholinesterase: the amino acid substitution at position 70 is written as Asp ⌀ Gly. New variants of butyrylcholinesterase genotypes continue to be discovered.[91,92]

Side Effects

Cardiovascular Effects

Succinylcholine-induced cardiac dysrhythmias are many and varied. The drug stimulates all cholinergic autonomic receptors: nicotinic receptors on both sympathetic and parasympathetic ganglia[93] and muscarinic receptors in the sinus node of the heart. In low doses, both negative inotropic and chronotropic responses may occur. These responses can be attenuated by previous administration of atropine. With large doses of succinylcholine, these effects may become positive[94] and tachycardia ensues. A prominent clinical manifestation of generalized autonomic stimulation is the development of cardiac dysrhythmias, principally sinus bradycardia, junctional rhythms, and ventricular dysrhythmias. Clinical studies have described these dysrhythmias under various conditions in the presence of the intense autonomic stimulus of tracheal intubation. It is not entirely clear whether the cardiac irregularities are due to the action of succinylcholine alone or due to the added presence of extraneous autonomic stimulation.

Sinus Bradycardia

The autonomic mechanism involved in sinus bradycardia is stimulation of cardiac muscarinic receptors in the sinus node, which is particularly problematic in individuals with predominantly vagal tone, such as children who have not received atropine.[95,96] Sinus bradycardia has also been noted in adults and appears more commonly when a second dose of the drug is given approximately 5 minutes after the first.[97] The bradycardia may be prevented by thiopental,[98,99] atropine,[98] ganglion-blocking drugs, and nondepolarizing neuromuscular blockers.[98,100] The implication from this information is that direct myocardial effects, increased muscarinic stimulation, and ganglionic stimulation may all be involved in the bradycardic response. The higher incidence of bradycardia after a second dose of succinylcholine[100] suggests that the hydrolysis products of succinylcholine (succinylmonocholine and choline) may sensitize the heart to a subsequent dose.

Nodal (Junctional) Rhythms

Nodal rhythms commonly occur after the administration of succinylcholine. The mechanism probably involves relatively greater stimulation of muscarinic receptors in the sinus node and, as a result, suppression of the sinus mechanism and emergence of the atrioventricular node as the pacemaker. The incidence of junctional rhythm is greater after a second dose of succinylcholine but is prevented by previous administration of dTc.[98,100]

Ventricular Dysrhythmias

Under stable anesthetic conditions, succinylcholine lowers the threshold of the ventricle to catecholamine-induced dysrhythmias in the monkey and dog. Circulating catecholamine concentrations increase fourfold and potassium concentrations increase by a third after succinylcholine administration in dogs.[101] Similar increases in catecholamine levels are also observed after the administration of succinylcholine to humans.[102,103] Other autonomic stimuli, such as endotracheal intubation,[104] hypoxia, hypercapnia, and surgery, may be additive to the effect of succinylcholine. The possible influence of drugs such as digitalis, tricyclic antidepressants, monoamine oxidase inhibitors, exogenous catecholamines, and halothane, all of which may lower the ventricular threshold for ectopic activity or increase the arrhythmogenic effect of catecholamines, must be considered as well. Ventricular escape beats may also occur as a result of severe sinus and atrioventricular nodal slowing secondary to succinylcholine administration. The development of ventricular dysrhythmias is further encouraged by the release of potassium from skeletal muscle as a consequence of the depolarizing action of the drug.

Hyperkalemia

The administration of succinylcholine to an otherwise well individual for an elective surgical procedure increases plasma potassium levels by approximately 0.5 mEq/L. This increase in potassium is due to the depolarizing action of the relaxant. With activation of the acetylcholine channels, movement of sodium into the cells is accompanied by movement of potassium out of the cells. This slight increase in plasma potassium levels is well tolerated by individuals and generally does not cause dysrhythmias.

Several early reports suggested that patients in renal failure may be susceptible to a hyperkalemic response to succinylcholine.[105-107] Nevertheless, more controlled studies have shown that renal failure patients are no more susceptible to an exaggerated response to succinylcholine than are those with normal renal function.[108-112] One might postulate that patients who have uremic neuropathy may be susceptible to succinylcholine-induced hyperkalemia, although evidence supporting this view is scarce.[107,112]

Severe hyperkalemia may follow the administration of succinylcholine to patients with severe metabolic acidosis and hypovolemia.[113] In rabbits, the combination of metabolic acidosis and hypovolemia results in a high resting potassium level and an exaggerated hyperkalemic response to succinylcholine.[114] In this situation, the potassium originates from the gastrointestinal tract and not from muscle, as in the classic hyperkalemic response.[115] In patients with metabolic acidosis and hypovolemia, correction of the acidosis by hyperventilation and sodium bicarbonate administration should be attempted before administration of succinylcholine. Should severe hyperkalemia occur, it can be treated with immediate hyperventilation, 1.0 to 2.0 mg calcium chloride intravenously, 1 mEq/kg sodium bicarbonate, and 10 U regular insulin in 50 mL 50% glucose for adults or, for children, 0.15 U/kg regular insulin in 1.0 mL/kg 50% glucose.

Kohlschütter and colleagues[116] found that four of nine patients with severe abdominal infections had an increase in serum potassium concentrations of as much as 3.1 mEq/L above baseline values after succinylcholine administration. These investigators found that in the case of intra-abdominal infections that persist for longer than 1 week, the possibility of a hyperkalemic response to succinylcholine should be considered.

Stevenson and Birch[117] described a single, well-documented case of a marked hyperkalemic response to succinylcholine in a patient with a closed head injury without peripheral paralysis.

In studying soldiers who had undergone trauma during the Vietnam War, Birch and associates[118] found that a significant increase in serum potassium did not occur in 59 patients until about 1 week after the injury, at which time a progressive increase in serum potassium occurred after the infusion of succinylcholine. Three weeks after injury, three of these patients with especially severe injuries showed marked hyperkalemia with an increase in serum potassium of greater than 3.6 mEq/L, sufficient to cause cardiac arrest. Birch and coworkers[118] found that prior administration of 6 mg dTc prevented the hyperkalemic response to succinylcholine. In the absence of infection or persistent degeneration of tissue, a patient is susceptible to the hyperkalemic response probably for at least 60 days after massive trauma or until adequate healing of damaged muscle has occurred.

In addition, patients with any number of conditions that have resulted in the proliferation of extrajunctional acetylcholine receptors, such as those with neuromuscular disease, are likely to have an exaggerated hyperkalemic response after the administration of succinylcholine. The response of these patients to neuromuscular blocking agents is reviewed in detail later in this chapter. Some of these disease states include cerebrovascular accident with resultant hemiplegia or paraplegia, muscular dystrophies, and Guillain-Barré syndrome. The hyperkalemia after administration of succinylcholine may be to such an extent that cardiac arrest ensues. For an in-depth discussion of the clinical and pathophysiologic aspects of succinylcholine-induced hyperkalemia, the reader is referred to a review by Gronert and Theye.[119]

Increased Intraocular Pressure (also see Chapter 65)

Succinylcholine usually causes an increase in intraocular pressure (IOP). The increased IOP is manifested within 1 minute after injection, peaks at 2 to 4 minutes, and subsides by 6 minutes.[120] The mechanism by which succinylcholine increases IOP has not been clearly defined, but it is known to involve contraction of tonic myofibrils or transient dilatation of choroidal blood vessels, or both. Sublingual administration of nifedipine has been reported to attenuate the increase in IOP from succinylcholine, thus suggesting a circulatory mechanism.[121] Despite this increase in IOP, the use of succinylcholine for ophthalmic procedures is not contraindicated unless the anterior chamber is open. Although Meyers and coworkers[122] were unable to confirm the efficacy of precurarization in attenuating increases in IOP after succinylcholine, numerous other investigators have found that previous administration of a small dose of nondepolarizing neuromuscular blocker (such as 3 mg dTc or 1 mg pancuronium) will prevent a succinylcholine-induced increase in IOP.[123] Furthermore, Libonati and coauthors[124] described the anesthetic management of 73 patients with penetrating eye injuries who received succinylcholine with no loss of global contents. Thus, despite the potential concerns of Meyers and coworkers,[122] Libonati and colleagues[124] found that the use of succinylcholine, after pretreatment with a nondepolarizing neuromuscular blocker, in patients with penetrating eye injuries with a carefully controlled rapid-sequence induction of anesthesia is an acceptable technique. Succinylcholine is only one of many factors, such as endotracheal intubation and "bucking" on the endotracheal tube, that may increase IOP.[122] Of prime importance is ensuring that the patient is well anesthetized and is not straining or coughing. Because nondepolarizing neuromuscular blockers with shorter times to onset of effect are now available, providing an anesthetic that allows for the trachea to be intubated rapidly without administering succinylcholine is now an option. Finally, should a patient's anesthesia become too light over the course of intraocular surgery, succinylcholine should not be given to immobilize the patient. Rather, the surgeon should be asked to pause while anesthesia is deepened. If necessary, the depth of neuromuscular blockade can also be increased with nondepolarizing relaxants.[125] In fact, coughing or "bucking" during a vitrectomy may cause serious postoperative eye damage with marked damage to vision.[126] Adequate anesthesia, with or without paralysis, is essential during eye surgery (also see Chapters 65 and 82).

Increased Intragastric Pressure

Unlike the rather consistent increase in IOP, the increase in intragastric pressure (IGP) caused by succinylcholine is quite variable. The increase in IGP from succinylcholine is presumed to be due to fasciculations of abdominal skeletal muscle, which is not surprising because more coordinated abdominal skeletal muscle activity (e.g., straight leg raising) may increase IGP to values as high as 120 cm H_2O. In addition to skeletal muscle fasciculations, the acetylcholine-like effect of succinylcholine may be partly responsible for the observed increases in IGP. Greenan[127] noted consistent increases in IGP of 4 to 7 cm H_2O with direct vagal stimulation.

Miller and Way[128] found that 11 of 30 patients essentially had no increase in IGP after succinylcholine. Nonetheless, 5 of 30 patients had an increase in IGP greater than 30 cm H_2O. The increase in IGP from succinylcholine appeared to be related to the intensity of fasciculations of the abdominal skeletal muscles. Accordingly, when fasciculations were prevented by previous administration of a nondepolarizing neuromuscular blocker, no increase in IGP was observed.

Are the increases in IGP after succinylcholine administration enough to cause incompetence of the gastroesophageal junction? Generally, IGP greater than 28 cm H_2O is required to overcome the competence of the gastroesophageal junction. However, when the normal oblique angle of entry of the esophagus into the stomach is altered, as may occur with pregnancy, an abdomen distended by ascites, bowel obstruction, or a hiatal hernia, the IGP required to cause incompetence of the gastroesophageal junction is frequently less than 15 cm H_2O.[128] In these circumstances, regurgitation of stomach contents after succinylcholine is a distinct possibility, and precautionary measures should be taken to prevent fasciculation. Endotracheal intubation may be facilitated by the administration of a nondepolarizing neuromuscular blocker, or a defasciculating dose of a nondepolarizing relaxant may be administered before succinylcholine.

Apparently, succinylcholine does not increase IGP appreciably in infants and children, possibly because of the minimal or absent fasciculations after administration of succinylcholine in these age groups.[129]

Increased Intracranial Pressure

Succinylcholine has the potential to increase intracranial pressure.[130] The mechanisms and clinical significance of this transient increase are unknown, but the rise in intracranial pressure does not occur after pretreatment with nondepolarizing neuromuscular blockers.[131]

Myalgia

The incidence of muscle pain after administration of succinylcholine varies from 0.2% to 89%.[132] It occurs more frequently after minor surgery, especially in women and ambulatory rather than bedridden patients.[133] Waters and Mapleson[133] postulated that the pain is secondary to damage produced in muscle by the unsynchronized contractions of adjacent muscle fibers just before the onset of paralysis. That damage to muscle may occur has been substantiated by finding myoglobinemia and increases in serum creatine kinase after succinylcholine administration.[134-136] Previous administration of a small dose of a nondepolarizing neuromuscular blocker clearly prevents fasciculations from succinylcholine.[134] However, the efficacy of this approach in preventing muscle pain is questionable. Although some investigators claim that pretreatment with a defasciculating dose of a nondepolarizing neuromuscular blocker has no effect,[132] many believe that the pain from succinylcholine is at least attenuated.[135-137] Pretreatment with a prostaglandin inhibitor (lysine acetylsalicylate) has been shown to be effective in decreasing the incidence of muscle pain after succinylcholine.[138] This finding suggests a possible role for prostaglandins and cyclooxygenases in succinylcholine-induced myalgias. Other investigators have found that myalgias after outpatient surgery occur even in the absence of succinylcholine.[139,140]

Masseter Spasm (also see Chapters 29 and 60)

An increase in tone of the masseter muscle is a frequent response to succinylcholine in adults,[141] as well as children.[142-144] Meakin and associates[142] suggested that the frequent occurrence of spasm in children may be due to an inadequate dose of succinylcholine. In all likelihood, this increase in tone is an exaggerated contractile response at the neuromuscular junction and cannot be used to establish a diagnosis of malignant hyperthermia. Although an increase in tone of the masseter muscle may be an early indicator of malignant hyperthermia,[145] it is not consistently associated with malignant hyperthermia.[145] Currently, there is no indication to change to a "nontriggering" anesthetic in instances of isolated masseter spasm.[143]

Clinical Uses

In spite of its many adverse effects, succinylcholine is still commonly used. Its popularity is probably due to its rapid onset of effect, the profound depth of neuromuscular blockade that it produces, and its short duration of action. Although it may be less commonly used than in the past for routine endotracheal intubation, it is the neuromuscular blocker of choice for rapid-sequence induction of anesthesia. In a study[147] comparing intubating conditions after 1 mg/kg succinylcholine with those after 0.1 mg/kg vecuronium or 0.1 mg/kg pancuronium at 30 seconds after the administration of a relaxant and at 30-second intervals after that for up to 120 seconds, intubation could be accomplished in all patients receiving succinylcholine at 30 seconds, in contrast to the other neuromuscular blockers studied. Furthermore, at all time points studied, up to 90 seconds, intubating conditions were better after the administration of succinylcholine than after either of the other two neuromuscular blockers. Although 1.0 mg/kg succinylcholine has long been recommended to facilitate endotracheal intubation at 60 seconds, recovery of neuromuscular function may not occur quickly enough to prevent hemoglobin desaturation in an apneic patient.[148,149] Recent studies have indicated that 0.5 to 0.6 mg/kg succinylcholine should allow for adequate intubating conditions 60 seconds after administration for nonrapid sequence intubation.[150,151]

A small dose of nondepolarizing neuromuscular blocker is commonly given 2 minutes before administering the intubating dose of succinylcholine. This defasciculating dose of nondepolarizing neuromuscular blocker will attenuate increases in intragastric and intracranial pressure, as well as minimize the incidence of fasciculations in response to succinylcholine. The previous administration of a nondepolarizing agent will render the muscle relatively resistant to succinylcholine, and the succinylcholine dose should therefore be increased by 50%.[152] The use of a defasciculating dose of a nondepolarizing neuromuscular blocker may also slow the onset of succinylcholine and produce less favorable conditions for tracheal intubation.[136,137]

Typically after administering succinylcholine for intubation, a nondepolarizing neuromuscular blocker is given to maintain neuromuscular blockade. Succinylcholine given first may enhance the depth of block induced by a subsequent dose of nondepolarizing neuromuscular blocker.[153-155] However, the effect on duration of action is variable. Succinylcholine has no effect on pancuronium, pipecuronium, or mivacurium,[155,156] but it increases the duration of atracurium and rocuronium.[153,154] The reasons for these differences are not clear.

The changing characteristics of succinylcholine neuromuscular blockade over the course of prolonged administration have been reviewed by Lee and Katz[157] and are summarized in Table 13-3. TOF stimulation is a very safe and useful guide in detecting the transition from a phase 1 to a phase 2 block. A phase 1 block has all the characteristics of a depolarizing block as described previously in the section on monitoring. A phase 2 block has the characteristics of a nondepolarizing block. With the administration of large doses of succinylcholine, the nature of the block, as determined by a neuromuscular blockade

Table 13–3   Clinical characteristics of phase 1 and phase 2 neuromuscular blockade during succinylcholine infusion

Characteristic	Phase 1	Transition	Phase 2
Tetanic stimulation	No fade	Slight fade	Fade
Post-tetanic facilitation	None	Slight	Yes
Train-of-four	No	Moderate fade	Marked fade
Train-of-four ratio	>0.7	0.4-0.7	<0.4
Edrophonium	Augments	Little effect	Antagonizes
Recovery	Rapid	Rapid to slow	Increasingly prolonged
Dose requirements (mg/kg)*	2-3	4-5	>6
Tachyphylaxis	No	Yes	Yes

*Cumulative dosage of succinylcholine by infusion under nitrous oxide anesthesia supplemented with intravenous agents. The dosage requirement to cause a phase 2 block is less in the presence of potent volatile anesthetics (e.g., isoflurane). Adapted from Lee C, Katz RL: Neuromuscular pharmacology. A clinical update and commentary. Br J Anaesth 52:173-188, 1980.

monitor, changes from that of a depolarizing agent to that of a nondepolarizing agent. Clearly, both the dose and the duration of administration of succinylcholine are important variables, although the relative contribution of each has not been established. Practically, if administration of the drug is terminated shortly after TOF fade is clearly evident, rapid return of normal neuromuscular function should ensue. In addition, the decision of whether to attempt antagonism of a phase 2 block has always been controversial. However, if the TOF ratio is less than 0.4, administration of edrophonium or neostigmine should result in prompt antagonism. Ramsey and colleagues[158] recommended that antagonism of a succinylcholine-induced phase 2 block with edrophonium or neostigmine be attempted after spontaneous recovery of the twitch response has been observed for 20 to 30 minutes and has reached a plateau phase with further recovery proceeding slowly. These researchers state that in this situation, edrophonium and neostigmine invariably produce "dramatic" acceleration of the return of the TOF ratio toward normal. Monitoring neuromuscular function with TOF stimuli will help avoid succinylcholine overdose, detect the development of a phase 2 block, observe the rate of recovery of neuromuscular function and assess the effect of edrophonium or neostigmine on recovery.

Interactions with Anticholinesterases

Another interaction with succinylcholine involves neostigmine or pyridostigmine. For example, after dTc has been used for intra-abdominal surgery of long duration and the neuromuscular blockade has been reversed by neostigmine, the surgeon announces that another 15 minutes is needed to retrieve a missing sponge. Succinylcholine should not be administered to reestablish neuromuscular blockade because it produces relaxation that will last up to

60 minutes when given soon after the administration of neostigmine (5 mg). Sunew and Hicks[77] found that the effect of succinylcholine (1 mg/kg) was prolonged from 11 to 35 minutes when it was given 5 minutes after the administration of neostigmine (5 mg). Such prolongation can partly be explained by inhibition of butyrylcholinesterase by neostigmine. Ninety minutes after neostigmine administration, butyrylcholinesterase activity returned to less than 50% of its baseline value.

NONDEPOLARIZING NEUROMUSCULAR BLOCKERS

The use of neuromuscular blocking drugs in anesthesia has its origin in the South American Indians' arrow poisons or curares. Several nondepolarizing neuromuscular blockers are still purified from naturally occurring sources. For example, although dTc can be synthesized, it is still less expensive to isolate it from the Amazonian vine *Chondodendron tomentosum*. Similarly, the intermediates for the production of metocurine and alcuronium, which are semisynthetic, are obtained from *Chondodendron* and *Strychnos toxifera*. Malouetine, the first steroidal neuromuscular blocking drug, was originally isolated from *Malouetia bequaertiana*, which grows in the jungles of Zaire in central Africa. Pancuronium, vecuronium, pipecuronium, rocuronium, rapacuronium, atracurium, doxacurium, mivacurium, cisatracurium, and gallamine are entirely synthetic.

The available nondepolarizing neuromuscular blockers can be classified according to chemical class (steroidal, benzylisoquinolinium, or other compounds) or according to onset or duration of action (long-, intermediate-, and short-acting drugs) of equipotent doses (Table 13-4).

Structure-Activity Relationships

Nondepolarizing neuromuscular blocking drugs were originally classified by Bovet[61] as pachycurares, or bulky molecules having the amine functions incorporated into rigid ring structures. Two extensively studied chemical series of synthetic nondepolarizing neuromuscular blockers are (1) the aminosteroids (steroidal), in which the distance is maintained by an androstane skeleton, and (2) the benzylisoquinolinium series, in which the distance is maintained by linear diester-containing chains or, in the case of curare, by benzyl ethers. For a detailed account of structure-activity relationships, see Lee.[159]

Benzylisoquinolinium Compounds

dTc is a neuromuscular blocker in which the amines are present in the form of two benzyl-substituted tetrahydroisoquinoline structures (Fig. 13-7). The quaternary/tertiary nature of the two amines was initially questioned; however, in nuclear magnetic resonance spectroscopy and methylation/demethylation studies, Everett and colleagues[160] demonstrated that dTc contains only three N-methyl groups. One amine is quaternary (permanently charged with four nitrogen substituents) and the other tertiary (pH-dependent charge with three nitrogen substituents). At physiologic pH, the tertiary

Table 13–4   Classification of nondepolarizing neuromuscular blockers according to duration of action (time to T1 = 25% of control) after 2 × ED$_{95}$ dose

	Clinical Duration			
	Long Acting (>50 min)	Intermediate Acting (20-50 min)	Short Acting (10-20 min)	Ultrashort Acting (<10 min)
Steroidal compounds	Pancuronium Pipecuronium	Vecuronium Rocuronium	Rapacuronium	
Benzylisoquinolinium compounds	d-Tubocurarine Metocurine Doxacurium	Atracurium Cisatracurium	Mivacurium	
Others				
Asymmetric mixed-onium chlorofumarates				430A
Bisquaternary tropinyl diester				TAAC3
Phenolic ether	Gallamine			
Diallyl derivative of toxiferine	Alcuronium			

Most nondepolarizing neuromuscular blockers are bisquaternary ammonium compounds. d-Tubocurarine, vecuronium, rocuronium, and rapacuronium are monoquaternary compounds, and gallamine is a trisquaternary ammonium compound.

nitrogen is protonated to render it positively charged. The structure-activity relationships of bis-benzylisoquinolines (Fig. 13-7) have been described by Waser[161] and by Hill and associates[162] as follows:

1. The nitrogen atoms are incorporated into isoquinoline ring systems. This bulky molecule favors nondepolarizing rather than depolarizing activity.
2. The interonium distance (distance between charged amines) is approximately 1.4 nm.

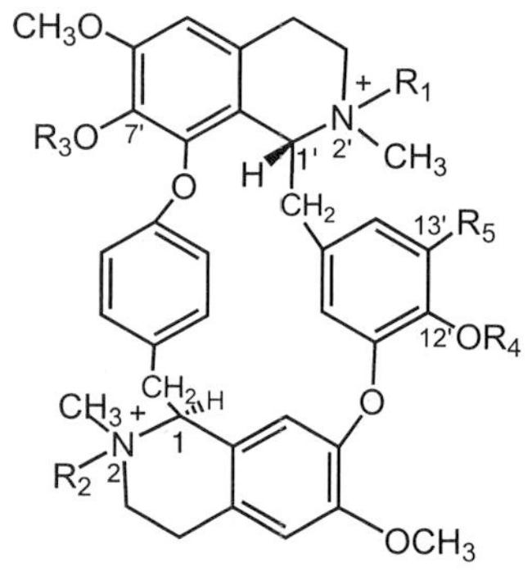

Cyclic benzylisoquinoline

Cyclic benzylisoquinoline derivatives

Name	R$_1$	R$_2$	R$_3$	R$_4$	R$_5$	1	1'
d-Tubocurarine	CH$_3$	H	H	H	H	S	R
Metocurine	CH$_3$	CH$_3$	CH$_3$	CH$_3$	H	S	R
Chondocurine	CH$_3$	CH$_3$	H	H	H	S	R

R and S represent the stereochemical configuration about the designated carbon

Figure 13–7 Chemical structure of d-tubocurarine, metocurine, and chondocurine.

3. Both the ganglion-blocking and the histamine-releasing properties of dTc are probably due to the presence of the tertiary amine function.
4. When dTc is methylated at the tertiary amine and at the hydroxyl groups, the result is metocurine, a compound with greater potency (by a factor of 2 in humans) but much weaker ganglion-blocking and histamine-releasing properties than dTc has (see Fig. 13-7). Metocurine contains three additional methyl groups, one of which quaternizes the tertiary nitrogen of dTc; the other two form methyl ethers at the phenolic hydroxyl groups.
5. Bisquaternary compounds are more potent than their monoquaternary analogs.[163] The bisquaternary derivative of dTc (chondocurine) has more than double the potency of dTc (see Fig. 13-7).
6. Substitution of the methyl groups on the quaternary nitrogen with bulkier groups causes a reduction in both potency and duration of action.

Atracurium is a bis-benzyltetrahydroisoquinolinium with isoquinolinium nitrogens connected by a diester-containing hydrocarbon chain (Fig. 13-8). The presence (in duplicate) of two-carbon separations between quaternary nitrogen and ester carbonyl provides the substrate for a Hofmann degradation reaction.[9,164] In a Hofmann elimination reaction, a quaternary ammonium group is converted into a tertiary amine by cleavage of a carbon-nitrogen bond. This reaction is pH and temperature dependent, with higher pH and temperature favoring elimination. The actual structure of the quaternary centers is the laudanosinium moiety as in metocurine. Atracurium has four chiral centers at each of the adjacent chiral carbons of the two amines. The marketed product has 10 isomers.[164,165] These isomers have been separated into three geometric isomer groups that are designated cis-cis, cis-trans, and trans-trans based on their configuration about the tetrahydroisoquinoline ring system.[164,165] The ratio of the cis-cis, cis-trans, and trans-trans isomers is

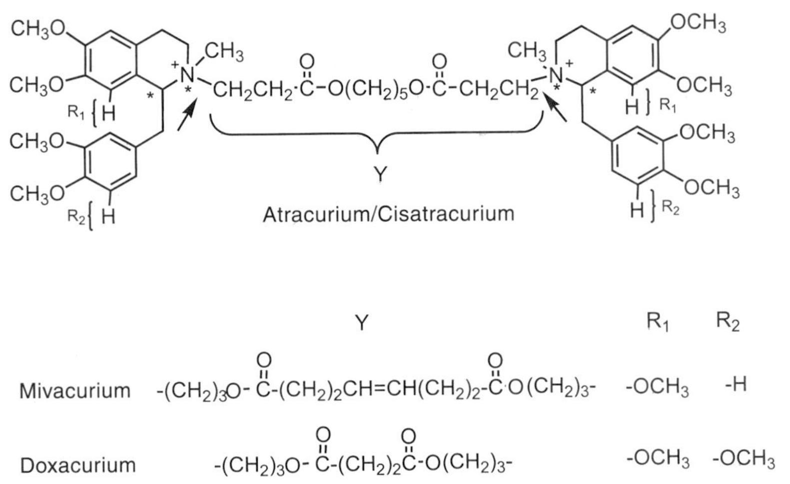

Figure 13–8 Chemical structure of atracurium, cisatracurium, mivacurium, and doxacurium. *Chiral center *arrows* showing the cleavage sites for Hofmann elimination.

approximately 10:6:1, which corresponds to about 50% to 55% *cis-cis*, 35% to 38% *cis-trans*, and 6% to 7% *trans-trans* isomers.[166]

Cisatracurium is the 1R *cis*–1'R *cis* isomer of atracurium and represents about 15% of the marketed atracurium mixture by weight, but more than 50% in terms of potency or neuromuscular blocking activity (see Fig. 13-8). R designates the absolute stereochemistry of benzyltetrahydroisoquinoline rings, and *cis* represents the relative geometry of the bulky dimethoxy and 2-alkyester groups at C(1) and N(1), respectively.[167,168] Cisatracurium is metabolized by Hofmann elimination. It is approximately four times as potent as atracurium, and unlike atracurium, it does not cause histamine release in the clinical dose range.[167,169] This observation indicates that the phenomenon of histamine release may be stereospecific.[167,170] Cisatracurium is the second benzylisoquinolinium (after doxacurium) to be largely free of this side effect.

Mivacurium differs from atracurium by the presence of an additional methylated phenolic group (see Fig. 13-8). When compared with other isoquinolinium neuromuscular blockers, the interonium chain of mivacurium is longer (16 atoms).[162] Mivacurium consists of a mixture of three stereoisomers.[171] The two most active are the *trans-trans* and *cis-trans* isomers (57% and 37% weight per weight [w/w], respectively), which are equipotent; the *cis-cis* isomer (6% w/w) has only a tenth the activity of the others in cats and monkeys.[171] Mivacurium is metabolized by butyrylcholinesterase at about 70% to 88% the rate of succinylcholine to a monoester, a dicarboxylic acid.[10,172]

Doxacurium is a bisquaternary benzylisoquinolinium diester of succinic acid (see Fig. 13-8). The interonium chain is shorter than that in either atracurium or mivacurium. Lee[159] pointed out that the number of methoxy groups on benzylisoquinolinium heads is increased from four (atracurium) and five (mivacurium) to six (doxacurium).[162] This increase was associated with both an increase in potency and a reduction in the propensity to release histamine.[159,162]

Steroidal Neuromuscular Blockers

In the steroidal compounds, it is probably essential that one of two nitrogen atoms in the molecule be quaternized.[173] The presence of acetyl ester (acetylcholine-like moiety) is thought to facilitate its interaction with nAChRs at the postsynaptic muscle membrane.[27,174]

Pancuronium is characterized by the presence of two acetyl ester groups on the A and D rings of the steroidal molecule. Pancuronium is a potent neuromuscular blocking drug with both vagolytic and butyrylcholinesterase-inhibiting properties (Fig. 13-9).[175] Deacetylation of the 3-OH or 17-OH groups decreases its potency.[176]

Vecuronium is an *N*-demethylated derivative of pancuronium in which the 2-piperidine substituent is not methylated (vecuronium lacks the *N*-methyl group at position 2) (see Fig. 13-9).[7,27] At physiologic pH, the tertiary amine is largely protonated similar to dTc. The minor molecular modification in comparison to pancuronium resulted in (1) a slight change in the potency; (2) a marked reduction in vagolytic properties; (3) molecular instability in solution, which explains in part the shorter duration of action of vecuronium than pancuronium; and (4) increased lipid solubility, which results in greater biliary elimination of vecuronium than pancuronium.[27,162]

Pancuronium and vecuronium are very similar in structure, yet vecuronium is prepared as a lyophilized powder. Vecuronium is degraded by the hydrolysis of either (or both) acetyl esters at the C3- and C17-positions. Hydrolysis at the C3-position is the primary degradation product. The acetate at the 3-position is more susceptible to hydrolysis in aqueous solutions. Vecuronium is less stable in solution because the group effect of the adjacent basic piperidine at the 2-position facilitates hydrolysis of the 3-acetate. Therefore, vecuronium cannot be prepared as a ready-to-use solution with a sufficient shelf life, even as a buffered solution.[177] In pancuronium, the 2-piperidine is quaternized and no longer basic. Thus, it does not participate in catalysis of the 3-acetate hydrolysis.[177]

Pipecuronium, like pancuronium, is a bisquaternary compound. Pipecuronium has piperazine rings attached to the A and D rings of the steroid nucleus, whereas pancuronium has piperidine rings (see Fig. 13-9).[162] Pipecuronium is a nonvagolytic substitute for pancuronium. Changes in the quaternary groups, in which the quaternary nitrogen atoms were placed at the distal (4-position) aspect of the 2,16-β substitutions, lessen the vagolytic effects.[162] As a result, pipecuronium is about 10 times less vagolytic than pancuronium.

Rocuronium lacks the acetyl ester that is found in the steroid nucleus of pancuronium and vecuronium in the A ring (see Fig. 13-9). The introduction of cyclic substituents

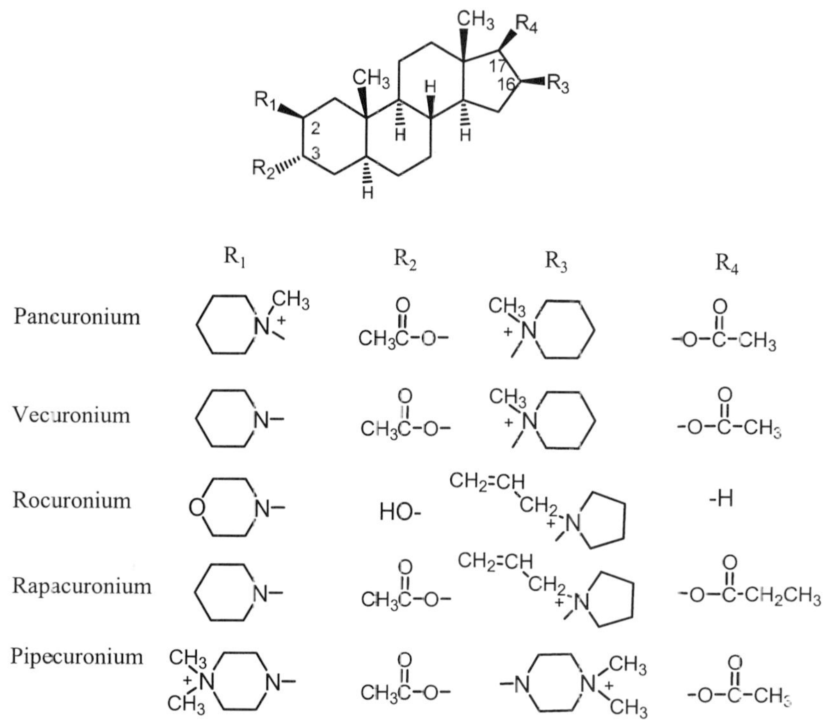

Figure 13–9 Chemical structure of different steroidal neuromuscular blockers.

other than piperidine at the 2- and 16-positions resulted in a fast-onset compound.[178] The methyl group attached to the quaternary nitrogen of vecuronium and pancuronium is replaced by an allyl group in rocuronium and rapacuronium. As a result, rocuronium and rapacuronium are about 6 and 10 times less potent than vecuronium, respectively.[178-180] Replacement of the acetyl ester attached to the A ring by a hydroxy group has made it possible to present rocuronium as a stable solution. At room temperature, rocuronium is stable for 60 days, whereas pancuronium is stable for 6 months. The reason for this difference in shelf life is related to the fact that rocuronium is terminally sterilized in manufacturing and pancuronium is not. Terminal sterilization causes some degree of degradation.[177]

Rapacuronium became available in the United States in 1999 but was withdrawn from the market by the manufacturer in spring 2001 because of a high incidence of respiratory complications.[181-184] Rapacuronium is a monoquaternary compound that has the same basic steroid backbone as the rest of the steroidal neuromuscular blockers (see Fig. 13-9).

Asymmetric Mixed-Onium Chlorofumarates (430A)
The agent 430A (Fig. 13-10) represents a new class of nondepolarizing neuromuscular blockers called asymmetric mixed-onium chlorofumarates. The presence of three methyl groups between the quaternary nitrogen and oxygen atom at each end of the carbon chain suggests that similar to mivacurium, this compound will not undergo Hofmann degradation.[13,185-187] The compound has an ultrashort duration of action in human volunteers and different animal species. A study in anesthetized human volunteers evaluated the onset and recovery profiles of 430A in the thumb and larynx. The pattern of blockade

resembles that of succinylcholine, with fully paralyzing doses (2 to 3 × ED95 or 0.38 to 0.54 mg/kg) producing 100% block of TOF stimulation within 50 to 60 seconds in the larynx. Spontaneous recovery to a TOF of 0.9 develops in the thumb within about 12 to 15 minutes after the administration of doses as large as 0.54 mg/kg (or 3 × ED95). Recovery is accelerated by edrophonium. The cardiovascular changes after rapid (5 second) bolus doses in these volunteers have averaged less than 10% from baseline.[188]

Bisquaternary Tropinyl Diester Derivatives
TAAC3 is a bis[N-(3,4-diacetoxybenzyl)tropanium-3α-yl] glutarate dibromide (Fig. 13-11).[12] No data on this compound in humans have been published. In animals, TAAC3 has a slower onset and shorter duration than succinylcholine has.[189] The short duration of action of TAAC3 is attributed to enzymatic hydrolysis of the acetoxy groups on the quaternary benzyl groups by nonspecific carboxyesterases.[189] At ED90 doses, TAAC3 exhibits a moderate degree of cardiac vagal block, and in large doses of 5 to 10 × ED90, it produces significant hypotension in the dog that is not related to histamine release.[189] The cardiac vagal blocking effect of TAAC3 in equipotent doses is similar to that of rocuronium.[189]

Phenolic Ether Derivative
Gallamine is a trisquaternary substance (Fig. 13-12). Its potent vagolytic activity is due to the presence of three positively charged nitrogen atoms. Gallamine was synthesized originally by Bovet[61] as part of an extensive structure-activity study that helped evolve the concepts of "pachycurares" and "leptocurares." Succinylcholine also evolved from this work, for which Bovet received the Nobel Prize.

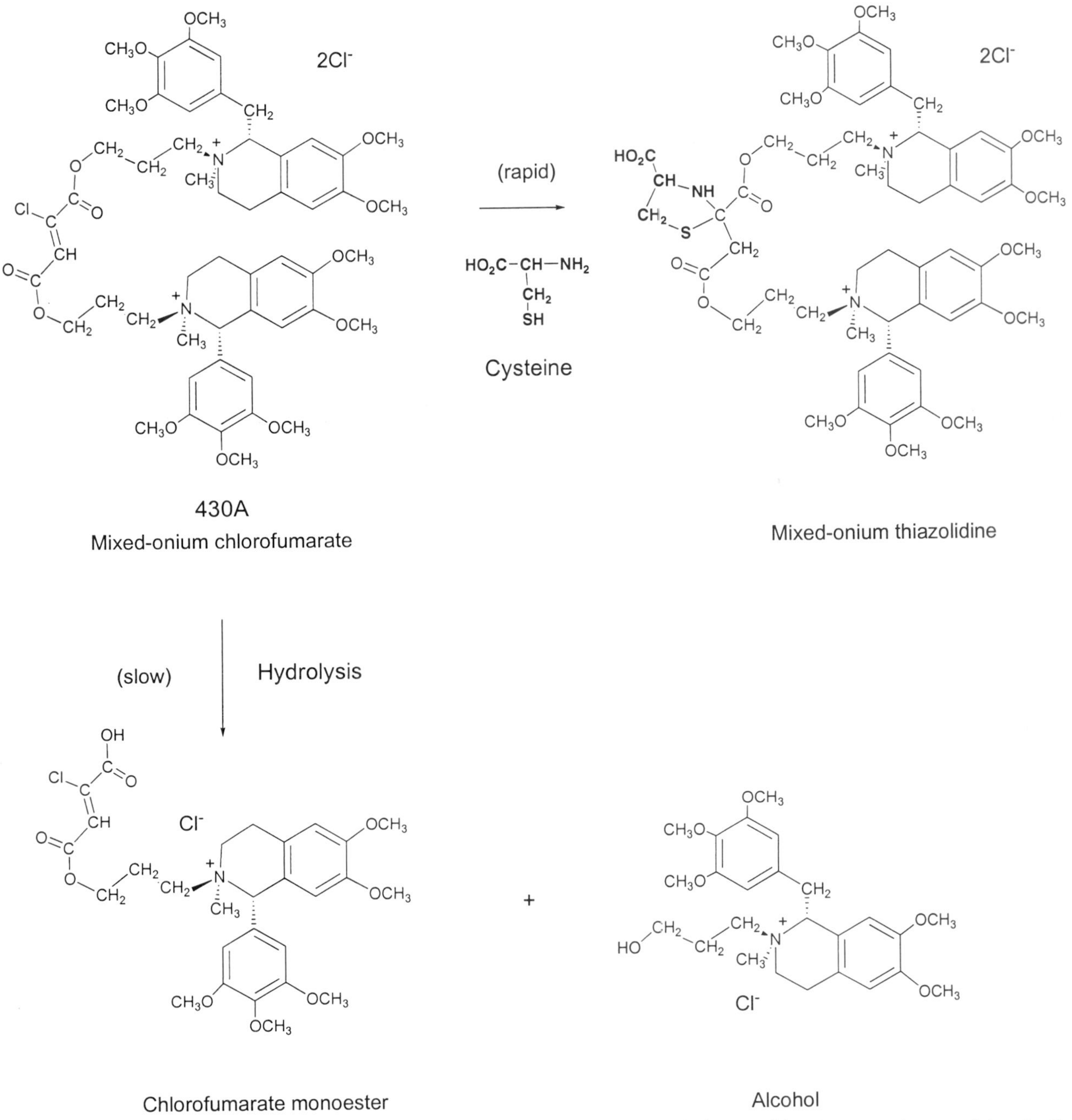

430A

Mixed-onium chlorofumarate

Mixed-onium thiazolidine

Cysteine

(rapid)

(slow) | Hydrolysis

Chlorofumarate monoester

Alcohol

Figure 13–10 Chemical structure of 430A (a mixed-onium chlorofumarate). In whole human blood, two pathways of deactivation occur, neither of which is enzymatic: (1) rapid formation of an apparently inactive cysteine adduction product with cysteine replacing chlorine and (2) slower hydrolysis of the ester bond adjacent to the chlorine substitution to chlorofumarate monoester and alcohol.[187]

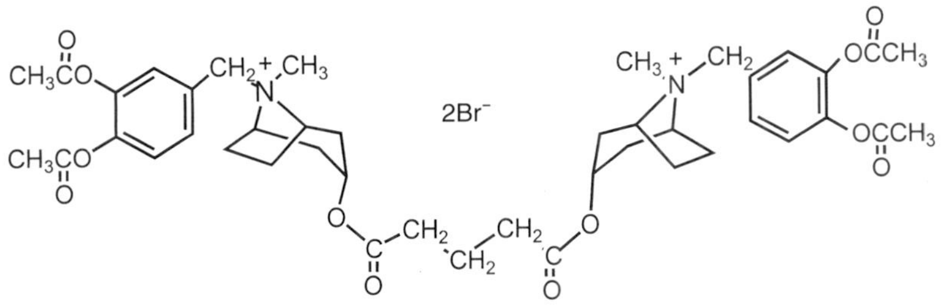

Figure 13–11 Chemical structure of TAAC3.

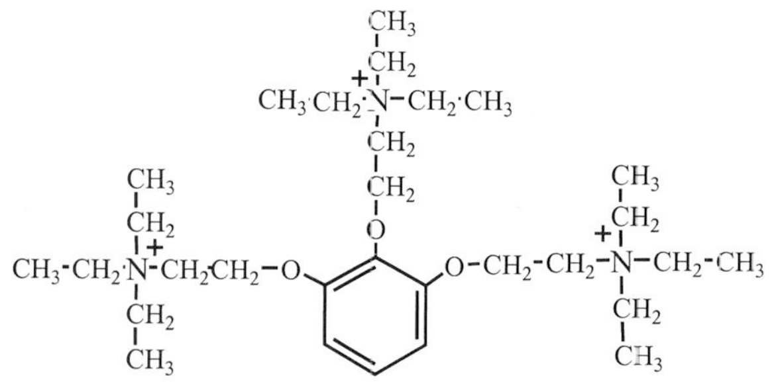

Figure 13–12 Chemical structure of gallamine, a trisquaternary ether of gallic acid. Gallamine is the only trisquaternary compound available. Its strong vagolytic property is probably due to the trisquaternary structure.

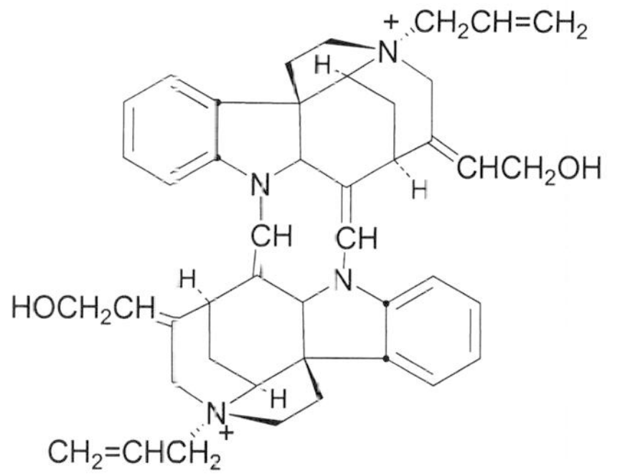

Figure 13–13 Chemica structure of alcuronium, the semisynthetic diallyl derivative of toxiferine. The quaternizing allyl groups actually reduce the potency by a factor of 3 to 5.

Diallyl Derivative of Toxiferine

Introduced in 1964, alcuronium is a long-acting drug that is the semisynthetic diallyl derivative of toxiferine (Fig. 13-13). The latter is purified from *Strychnos toxifera*. Its advantage at the time of its introduction was a relative lack of side effects. It is mildly vagolytic and is excreted unchanged by the kidney with a minor secondary biliary pathway. Alcuronium is moderately popular in Europe, the Far East, and Australia, but it is not available in the United States.

Potency of Nondepolarizing Neuromuscular Blockers

Drug potency is commonly expressed by the dose-response relationship. The dose of a neuromuscular blocking drug required to produce an effect (e.g., 50%, 90%, or 95% depression of twitch height; commonly expressed as ED_{50}, ED_{90}, and ED_{95}, respectively) is taken as a measure of the potency of neuromuscular blockers.[10,179,188,190-220] The drugs have different potencies as illustrated in Table 13-5 and Figure 13-14. For factors affecting the potency of neuromuscular blockers, see the section "Drug Interactions." The dose-response relationship for nondepolarizing neuromuscular blockers is sigmoidal in shape (see Fig. 13-14) and has been derived in a variety of ways. The simplest method is to perform linear regression over the approximately linear portion of a semilogarithmic plot between 25% and 75% neuromuscular block. Alternatively, the curve can be subjected to probit or logit transform to linearize it over its whole length or be subjected to nonlinear regression with the sigmoid Emax model of the form:

$$\text{Effect(e)} = \backslash F(\text{dose}_\epsilon^\gamma, \text{dose}_\epsilon^\gamma + \text{dose}_{e50}^\gamma)$$

Table 13–5   Dose-response relationships of nondepolarizing neuromuscular blocking drugs in human subjects

	ED_{50} (mg/kg)	ED_{90} (mg/kg)	ED_{95} (mg/kg)	References
Long Acting				
Pancuronium	0.036 (0.022-0.042)	0.056 (0.044-0.070)	0.067 (0.059-0.080)	179, 190
Pipecuronium	0.021 (0.013-0.032)	0.032 (0.022-0.033)	0.042 (0.024-0.059)	179, 191-196
d-Tubocurarine	0.23 (0.16-0.26)	0.41 (0.27-0.45)	0.48 (0.34-0.56)	190
Metocurine	0.14 (0.13-0.15)	0.25 (0.24-0.26)	0.30 (0.28-0.32)	190
Doxacurium	0.012 (0.006-0.016)	0.022 (0.021-0.024)	0.024 (0.016-0.033)	197-201
Gallamine	1.30	2.30	2.82	190
Alcuronium	0.11 (0.07-16)	0.18 (0.12-0.25)	0.22 (0.14-0.29)	190
Intermediate Acting				
Rocuronium	0.147 (0.069-0.220)	0.268 (0.200-0.419)	0.305 (0.257-0.521)	179, 202-208
Vecuronium	0.027 (0.015-0.031)	0.042 (0.023-0.055)	0.043 (0.037-0.059)	190
Atracurium	0.12 (0.08-0.15)	0.18 (0.19-0.24)	0.21 (0.13-0.28)	190
Cisatracurium	0.026 (0.015-0.031)	—	0.04 (0.032-0.05)	209-213
Short Acting				
Mivacurium	0.039 (0.027-0.052)	—	0.067 (0.045-0.081)	10, 214-218
Rapacuronium	0.39	—	0.75-1.0	219, 220
Ultrashort Acting				
430A	0.09	—	0.19	188

Data are the median and range of reported values.
ED_{50}, ED_{90}, and ED_{95}, doses of each drug that produce, respectively, a 50%, 90%, and 95% decrease in the force of contraction or amplitude of the electromyogram of the adductor pollicis muscle after ulnar nerve stimulation.

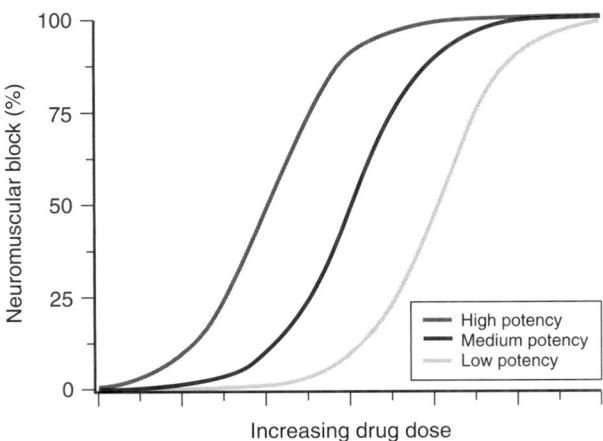

Figure 13–14 Schematic representation of a semilogarithmic plot of muscle relaxant dose versus neuromuscular block. A drug of high potency would be represented by doxacurium, one of medium potency by atracurium, and one of low potency by rocuronium. The graph illustrates that the relative potencies of the muscle relaxants span a range of approximately 2 orders of magnitude.

This equation can be applied to the raw data.[221-223] More complex models that relate the concentration of neuromuscular blockers at the neuromuscular junction to their pharmacologic effect have been developed, and they will be discussed later.[224,225]

Pharmacokinetics and Pharmacodynamics

As defined by Wright,[226] pharmacokinetics and pharmacodynamics are "... empirical mathematical model[s] ... that [describe] drug effect time course after administration." In pharmacokinetic modeling, the concept of "compartments" represents different organs/tissues grouped together on the basis of their blood perfusion (high or low). After injection into the circulation, the concentration of a neuromuscular blocker in plasma decreases rapidly at first, then more slowly (Fig. 13-15). The shape of this curve is determined by the processes of distribution and elimination. Classically, this curve is divided into an initial (distribution) phase and a terminal (elimination) phase. This curve can be represented mathematically by biexponential or triexponential equations[223] in the form

$$\text{Concentration (at time t)} = Ae^{-\alpha t} + Be^{-\beta t} (+ Pe^{-\pi t})$$

These multiexponential equations express the concept of drug being distributed between two or three theoretical compartments.

Figure 13-16 illustrates the classic model whereby drug is administered intravenously into a central compartment with volume V1 and is distributed and eliminated only from this compartment. Drug is distributed very rapidly throughout this central compartment, which includes the plasma volume and the organs of elimination (e.g., in the case of neuromuscular blockers, the kidneys and liver). The "k" terms are the rate constants for drug movement between compartments in the direction of the arrows. The peripheral compartments (usually one or two

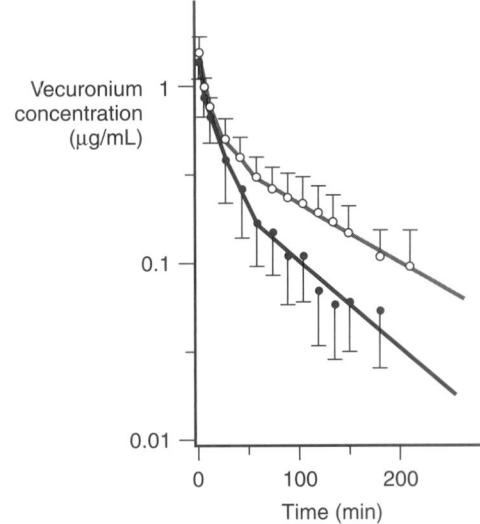

Figure 13–15 Disappearance of vecuronium from plasma after a single bolus dose of 0.2 mg/kg, as illustrated by a semilogarithmic plot of the mean concentration versus time for patients with normal hepatic function *(filled circles)* and cirrhotic patients *(open circles)*. Error bars are the SD for that value. (Redrawn from Lebrault C, Berger JL, D'Hollander AA, et al: Pharmacokinetics and pharmacodynamics of vecuronium [ORG NC 45] in patients with cirrhosis. Anesthesiology 62:601-605, 1985.)

in number, here represented by V2 and V3) can be thought of as the "tissues." The effect compartment, which will be discussed later, is the neuromuscular junction. For computational purposes, it has infinitesimal volume and therefore does not influence overall drug distribution. Drug administration and elimination are unidirectional; distribution is bidirectional.

Initially, the drug concentration in the central compartment (plasma concentration) will exceed that in the peripheral compartment (tissue concentration), and drug

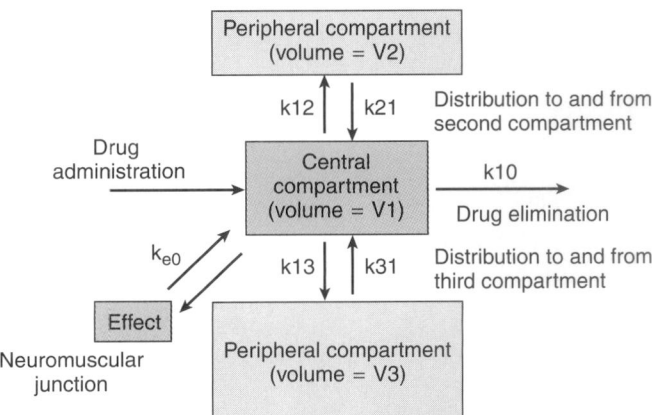

Figure 13–16 Schematic representation of drug disposition into different compartments. These compartments are mathematical concepts only and do not represent real physiologic spaces. The effect compartment in this case would be the neuromuscular junction for computational purposes; it has infinitesimal volume. The terms k_{nm} are the rate constants for drug movement, in the direction of the *arrow*, between these theoretical compartments. See text for further discussion.

will move from plasma to tissues. Later, as the plasma concentration decreases, it becomes less than the tissue concentration, and the net direction of drug movement is now from tissues to plasma. In general, this conceptual model is appropriate for all the neuromuscular blockers, with the exception of atracurium and cisatracurium, which also undergo elimination (by degradation) from tissues.[227] For simplicity, the following discussion will assume only one peripheral compartment.

Volume of distribution is the volume to which the drug has distributed when the processes of distribution and elimination are in equilibrium. Elimination is represented by the variable plasma clearance, that is, the volume of plasma from which drug is irreversibly and completely eliminated per unit time. For most nondepolarizing neuromuscular blockers, the process of distribution is more rapid than that of elimination, and the initial rapid decline in plasma concentration is due primarily to distribution of the drug to tissues. An exception to this rule is mivacurium, which has such rapid clearance, because of metabolism by butyrylcholinesterase, that elimination is the principal determinant of the initial decline in plasma concentration.[228]

After the initial process of drug distribution to tissues, the plasma concentration falls more slowly (terminal phase). The rate of decrease in plasma concentration during this terminal phase is often expressed in terms of elimination half-life, which equals the natural logarithm of 2 divided by the rate constant of decline (i.e., the slope of the terminal phase). During this terminal phase, the tissue drug concentration exceeds that of plasma, and the rate of decrease in plasma concentration is determined by two factors: the rate at which drug can move from tissues back to plasma and clearance of drug from plasma. In classic theory for neuromuscular blockers, drug can move rapidly from tissues to plasma, and elimination from plasma (clearance) is the rate-limiting step. For this reason, the terminal portion of the curve is often termed the elimination phase, even though distribution of drug from tissues to plasma is occurring continually throughout. Volume of distribution can also influence the terminal portion of the curve; the greater the volume of distribution, the slower the decline in plasma concentration.

The neuromuscular blockers are polar drugs, and their volume of distribution is classically thought to be limited to a volume roughly equivalent to a portion of the extracellular fluid space, specifically, 150 to 450 mL/kg (see Tables 13-14 and 13-15).[223] With this model of drug distribution, the potential rate of drug movement from tissues to plasma exceeds the rate of elimination, and plasma clearance is the process that limits the rate of decline in plasma drug concentration. However, some evidence has shown that neuromuscular blockers are distributed more widely, into tissues with low blood flow (e.g., connective tissue),[229] and the true volume of distribution of dTc has been estimated to be as high as 3.4 L/kg and the elimination half-life as long as 40 hours (compare with values in Tables 13-14 and 13-15).[230] Because the rate of drug movement from such tissues is less than that of plasma clearance, this becomes the rate-limiting step in the rate of decline in plasma drug concentration. This phase only becomes obvious when drug is administered

for many days or when sampling is continued for 24 to 96 hours after drug administration. In normal operating room use of neuromuscular blockers, the amount of drug being distributed to this compartment does not affect clinical response to the drug. In conditions in which clearance of the neuromuscular blocker is reduced, such as renal or hepatic disease, it is the terminal portion of the plasma concentration-versus-time curve that is most affected (see Fig. 13-15).[231] The rate of decline in plasma concentration is slowed, and recovery from paralysis is potentially delayed.[231] In conditions associated with an increased distribution volume, such as renal or hepatic disease, early plasma concentrations of drug may be less than those observed when organ function is normal (Fig. 13-17). With a greater volume of distribution, the plasma concentration should be less whereas the total amount of a drug would be greater (see Fig. 13-17). Decreased protein binding of a drug results in a larger distribution volume, but because the degree of protein binding of neuromuscular blockers is low, changes in protein binding will have minimal effect on their distribution.[232]

Recovery of neuromuscular function takes place as plasma concentrations decline. The greater part of this decline occurs primarily because of distribution. Thus, processes that primarily affect elimination of the drug, such as renal failure, may not be associated with a prolonged duration of block.[233,234] However, as recovery comes to rely more on drug elimination than distribution, that is, recovery from 25% to 75% or more or after the administration of larger or repeated doses, the duration of action may be prolonged.[227,235]

After injection of a neuromuscular blocker, the plasma drug concentration immediately starts to decrease. The effect (neuromuscular blockade) takes approximately 1 minute to begin, increases initially, and does not begin to recover for many more minutes despite continually decreasing plasma concentrations of drug. This discrepancy between plasma concentration and drug effect occurs

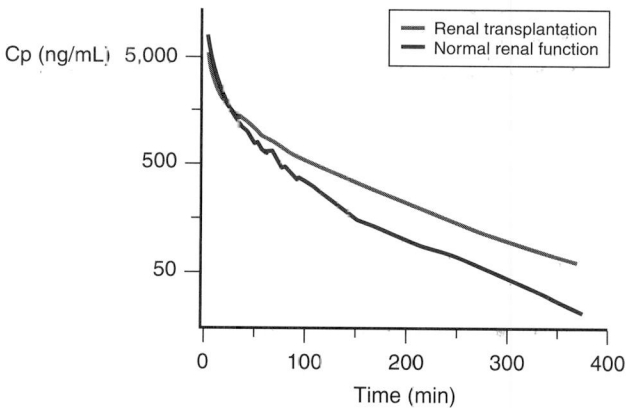

Figure 13–17 "Average" plasma concentration (Cp) versus time after 0.6 mg/kg rocuronium in patients with normal renal function or patients undergoing renal transplantation. (Redrawn from Szenohradszky J, Fisher DM, Segredo V, et al: Pharmacokinetics of rocuronium bromide [ORG 9426] in patients with normal renal function or patients undergoing cadaver renal transplantation. Anesthesiology 77:899-904, 1992.)

because the action of neuromuscular blockers is not in plasma but at the neuromuscular junction. To produce paralysis, the drug must diffuse from plasma to the neuromuscular junction, and the effect is terminated later by drug diffusion back into plasma (see Fig. 13-16). Thus, concentrations at the neuromuscular junction lag behind those in plasma, and they are less during onset of block and greater during recovery. The plasma concentration-effect relationship exhibits hysteresis; that is, for a given level of block, plasma concentrations are greater during onset than during recovery. For this reason, a concentration-effect relationship cannot be obtained simply by directly relating plasma concentration to the level of neuromuscular blockade.

To overcome this problem, pharmacodynamic models have been developed to incorporate a factor for the delay caused by drug diffusion to and from the neuromuscular junction.[153,224,236-247] This factor, k_{e0}, is the rate constant for drug equilibration between plasma and the neuromuscular junction. By measuring plasma drug concentrations and neuromuscular blockade during both the onset and recovery phases and by using the technique of simultaneous pharmacokinetic/pharmacodynamic modeling, it is possible to collapse the hysteresis in the plasma concentration-effect curve, estimate actual neuromuscular junction drug concentrations, and derive true concentration-effect relationships (CE$_{50}$ and k_{e0}) for the neuromuscular blockers (Table 13-6).[224]

Table 13-6 Pharmacodynamic parameters derived from simultaneous pharmacokinetic/pharmacodynamic modeling

	Study Group	Adductor Pollicis		Reference
		CE_{50}* (ng/mL)	k_{e0}† (min⁻¹)	
Mivacurium				
Central link		57	0.169	236
Peripheral link		130	0.101	236
Rocuronium	Adult female	684	0.329	237
	Propofol-remifentanil anesthesia			
	Standard model			
	Recirculatory model	876	0.129	237
	Volunteers	3510	0.405	238
	Propofol-fentanyl anesthesia			
	Infants	1190	0.25	239
	Children	1650	0.32	239
Cisatracurium	Adults	126-158	0.07-0.09	240
0.075-3.0 mg/kg	Propofol-fentanyl anesthesia			
Atracurium	Infants	363	0.19	241
	Children	444	0.16	241
	Young adults	449	0.13	242
	Elderly adults	436	0.12	242
	Standard model	359	0.12	243
	Threshold model	357	0.12	243
	Young adults	669‡	0.07	244
	Burn patients	2270‡	0.10	244
	No succinylcholine	454‡	0.07	153
	After succinylcholine	305‡	0.09	153
Vecuronium	Young adults	94	—	245
	Young adults	92	0.17	246
	Elderly adults	106	0.17	246
d-Tubocurarine	Normal renal function	370	0.13	224
	Renal failure	380	0.16	224
	Halothane 0.5%-0.7%	360‡	0.09‡	247§
	Halothane 1.0%-1.2%	220‡	0.12	247§
	Narcotic anesthesia	600‡	0.15‡	247§
Pancuronium	Young adults	88	—	245

*CE_{50} is the neuromuscular junction concentration (biophase) of each drug that produces a 50% decrease in the force of contraction or amplitude of the electromyogram of the adductor pollicis muscle after ulnar nerve stimulation.
†k_{e0} is the rate constant for equilibration of drug between plasma and the neuromuscular junction.
‡All groups different from each other.
§k_{e0} values calculated as $0.693/t_{1/2}^{ke0}$.

Clinical Management

Neuromuscular blockers are mainly used to facilitate tracheal intubation and provide surgical relaxation. The required intensity of neuromuscular blockade varies with the surgical procedure. In practice, important safety issues with neuromuscular blockers are cardiovascular and respiratory side effects and the adequacy of recovery to normal neuromuscular function.

Several clinical alternatives to neuromuscular blockers are available to provide adequate surgical relaxation. It is important to keep them all in mind to avoid relying only on neuromuscular blockade to achieve a desired degree of relaxation. These options include adjustment of the depth of general anesthesia, regional anesthesia, proper positioning of the patient on the operating table, and proper adjustment of the depth of neuromuscular blockade. The choice of one or several of these options is determined by the estimated remaining duration of surgery, the anesthetic technique, and the surgical maneuver required.

Dosage

General Dosage Guidelines

It is important to select the proper dose of a nondepolarizing neuromuscular blocker to ensure that the desired effect is achieved without excessive overdosage. In addition to a general knowledge of the guidelines, precise practice requires the use of a peripheral nerve stimulator to adjust the relaxant dosage to the individual patient. Overdosage must be avoided for two reasons: (1) to limit the duration of drug effect to match the anticipated length of surgery and (2) to avoid unwanted cardiovascular side effects.

Initial and Maintenance Dosage

The initial dosage is determined by the purpose of administration. Traditionally, doses used to facilitate tracheal intubation are $2 \times ED_{95}$ (this dose also approximates to $4 \times ED_{50}$) (Table 13-7). If the trachea has already been intubated without a nondepolarizing blocker or with succinylcholine and the purpose is simply to produce

Table 13-7 Guide to nondepolarizing relaxant dosage (mg/kg) under different anesthetic techniques*

	ED_{95} under N_2O/O_2	Dose for Intubation	Supplemental Dose after Intubation	Dosage for Relaxation	
				N_2O	Volatile Anesthetic†
Long Acting					
Pancuronium	0.07	0.08-0.12	0.02	0.05	0.03
Metocurine	0.28	0.3-0.4	0.05	0.2	0.1
d-Tubocurarine	0.5	0.5-0.6	0.1	0.3	0.15
Gallamine	3.0	4.0-6.0	0.5	2.0	1.0
Alcuronium	0.25	0.3	0.05	0.2	0.08
Doxacurium	0.025	0.05-0.08	0.005-0.01	0.025	0.02
Pipecuronium	0.05	0.08-0.1	0.01-0.015	0.04	0.03
Intermediate Acting					
Vecuronium	0.05	0.1-0.2	0.02	0.05	0.03
Atracurium	0.23	0.5-0.6	0.1	0.3	0.15
Cisatracurium	0.05	0.15-0.2	0.02	0.05	0.04
Rocuronium	0.3	0.6-1.0	0.1	0.3	0.15
Short Acting					
Mivacurium	0.08	0.2-0.25	0.05	0.1	0.08
Continuous infusions (µg/kg/min) required to maintain 90%-95% twitch inhibition under N_2O/O_2 with intravenous agents					
Mivacurium	3-15				
Atracurium	4-12				
Cisatracurium	1-2				
Vecuronium	0.8-1				
Rocuronium	9-12				

*Suggested dosages provide good intubating conditions under light anesthesia. Satisfactory abdominal relaxation may be achieved at the dosages listed after intubation without a relaxant or with succinylcholine. This table is intended as a general guide to dosage. Individual relaxant requirements should be confirmed with a peripheral nerve stimulator.
†Potentiation of nondepolarizing relaxants by different volatile anesthetics has been reported to vary 20% to 50%. Recent data suggest, however, that this variation may be much less, particularly in the case of intermediate- and short-acting relaxants. Therefore, for the sake of simplicity, this table assumes a potentiation of 40% in the case of all volatile anesthetics.

surgical relaxation, a dose slightly less than the ED_{95} (Table 13-8) should be given, with adjustment upward as indicated by responses evoked by peripheral nerve stimulation. Downward adjustment of the initial dose is necessary in the presence of any of the potent inhaled anesthetics (see the section "Drug Interactions").

To avoid prolonged residual paralysis or inadequate antagonism of residual blockade, or both, the main goal should be to use the lowest possible dose that will provide adequate relaxation for surgery. Management of individual patients should always be guided by monitoring with a peripheral nerve stimulator. In an adequately

Table 13–8 Pharmacodynamic effects of succinylcholine and nondepolarizing neuromuscular blockers

	Anesthesia	Intubating Dose (mg/kg)	Approximate ED_{95} Multiples	Maximum Block (%)	Time to Maximum Block (min)	Clinical Duration* (min)	Reference
Succinylcholine	Narcotic or halothane	0.5	1.7	100	—	6.7	70
Succinylcholine	Desflurane	0.6	2	100	1.4	7.6	151
Succinylcholine	Narcotic or halothane	1.0	3	100	—	11.3	70
Succinylcholine	Desflurane	1.0	3	100	1.2	9.3	151
Succinylcholine	Narcotic	1.0	3	—	1.1	8	248
Succinylcholine	Narcotic	1.0	3	—	1.1	9	249
Succinylcholine	Isoflurane	1.0	3	100	0.8	9	250
Steroidal Compounds							
Rocuronium	Narcotic	0.6	2	100	1.7	36	251
Rocuronium	Isoflurane	0.6	2	100	1.5	37	250
Rocuronium	Isoflurane	0.9	3	100	1.3	53	250
Rocuronium	Isoflurane	1.2	4	100	0.9	73	250
Vecuronium	Isoflurane	0.1	2	100	2.4	41	250
Vecuronium	Narcotic	0.1	2	100	2.4	44	252
Pancuronium	Narcotic	0.08	1.3	100	2.9	86	253, 254
Pancuronium	Narcotic	0.1	1.7	99	4	100	255
Pipecuronium	Narcotic	0.05	1	93	6.3	29	194
Pipecuronium	Narcotic	0.06	1.2	96	5.4	45	256
Pipecuronium	Narcotic	0.08	1.6	99	3.9	74	256
Pipecuronium	Narcotic	0.1	2	100	3.6	94	256
Benzylisoquinolinium Compounds							
Mivacurium	Narcotic	0.15	2	100	3.3	16.8	10
Mivacurium	Narcotic	0.15	2	100	3	14.5	251
Mivacurium	Halothane	0.15	2	100	2.8	18.6	217
Mivacurium	Narcotic	0.2	2.6	100	2.5	19.7	10
Mivacurium	Narcotic	0.25	3.3	100	2.3	20.3	10
Mivacurium	Narcotic	0.25	3.3	—	2.1	21	249
Atracurium	Narcotic	0.5	2	100	3.2	46	209
Cisatracurium	Narcotic	0.1	2	99	7.7	46	257
Cisatracurium	Narcotic	0.1	2	100	5.2	45	209
Cisatracurium	Narcotic	0.2	4	100	2.7	68	209
Cisatracurium	Narcotic	0.4	8	100	1.9	91	209
Doxacurium	Narcotic	0.04	1.6	100	7.6	77.4	198
Doxacurium	Narcotic	0.05	2	100	4.5	125	198
Doxacurium	Narcotic	0.06	2.4	100	4.4	123	198
d-Tubocurarine	Narcotic	0.6	1.2	97	5.7	81	255
Metocurine	Narcotic	0.4	1.3	99	4.1	107	255
Diallyl Derivative of Toxiferine							
Alcuronium	Narcotic	0.25	1.4	100	2.2	54	258

For atracurium and mivacurium, slower injection (30 seconds) is recommended to minimize circulatory effects.
*Time from injection of the intubating dose to recovery of twitch to 25% of control.

anesthetized and monitored patient, there is little reason to completely abolish twitch or TOF responses to peripheral nerve stimulation during maintenance of relaxation. Supplemental (maintenance) doses of neuromuscular blockers should be about a fourth (in the case of intermediate- and short-acting neuromuscular blockers) to a tenth (in case of long-acting neuromuscular blockers) the initial dose and should not be given until clear evidence of initiation of recovery from the previous dose is apparent.

Maintenance of relaxation by continuous infusion of intermediate- and short-acting drugs can be performed and is useful to keep relaxation smooth and to rapidly adjust the depth of relaxation to surgical needs. The depth of block in each patient is kept moderate, if possible, to ensure prompt spontaneous recovery or easy reversal at the end of the procedure. Table 13-7 lists approximate dose ranges that are usually required during infusion to maintain 90% to 95% block of the twitch (one twitch visible on TOF stimulation) under nitrous oxide–oxygen anesthesia supplemented with intravenous anesthetics. The infusion dosage is usually decreased by about 30% to 50% in the presence of potent inhaled anesthetics.

Neuromuscular Blockers and Tracheal Intubation

Speed of onset of a neuromuscular block is one of the requirements to rapidly secure the airway, and it is affected by several factors, including the rate of delivery of the drug to the neuromuscular junction, receptor affinity, plasma clearance, and the mechanism of neuromuscular blockade (depolarizing versus nondepolarizing).[176,259,250] The speed of onset is inversely proportional to the potency of nondepolarizing neuromuscular blockers.[176,259] A high ED_{95} (low potency) is predictive of rapid onset and vice versa (see Table 13-8 and Fig. 13-18). Except for atracurium,[261] molar potency (the ED_{50} or ED_{95} expressed in µM/kg) is highly predictive of a drug's initial rate of onset of effect (at the adductor pollicis).[259] It should be noted that a drug's measured molar potency is the end result of many contributing factors: the drug's intrinsic potency (the CE_{50}, or the biophase concentration resulting in 50% twitch depression), the rate of equilibration between plasma and the biophase (k_{e0}), the initial rate of plasma clearance, and probably other factors as well.[262] Rocuronium has a molar potency ($ED_{95} \approx 0.54$ µM/kg) that is about 13% that of vecuronium and only 9% that of cisatracurium. Thus, rapid onset of rocuronium (at the adductor pollicis) is not unexpected.

Donati and Meistelman[260] proposed a model to explain the inversed potency-onset relationship. Nondepolarizing neuromuscular blockers of low potency (such as rocuronium and rapacuronium) have more molecules to diffuse from the central compartment into the effect compartment. Once in the effect compartment, all molecules act promptly. Weaker binding of low-potency drugs to receptors prevents buffered diffusion,[260] a process that occurs with potent drug. Buffered diffusion causes repetitive binding and unbinding to receptors, thereby keeping potent drugs in the neighborhood of effector sites and potentially lengthening the duration of effect.

The times to 95% block at the adductor pollicis after a $1 \times ED_{95}$ dose of succinylcholine, rocuronium, rapacuronium, vecuronium, atracurium, mivacurium, and cisatracurium are shown in Figure 13-19.[220,259,261] The figure shows that the most potent compound, cisatracurium, has the slowest onset and that the least potent, rocuronium and rapacuronium, are the most rapid (Fig. 13-19).[220,259,261] Bevan[263] also proposed that rapid plasma clearance is associated with a rapid onset of action. The fast onset of succinylcholine is related to its rapid metabolism and plasma clearance.

The onset of neuromuscular blockade is much more rapid in the muscles that are relevant to obtaining optimal intubating conditions (laryngeal adductors, diaphragm, and masseter) than in the muscle typically monitored

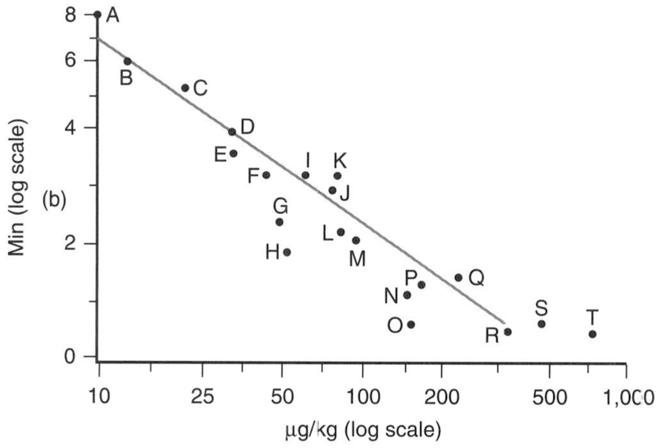

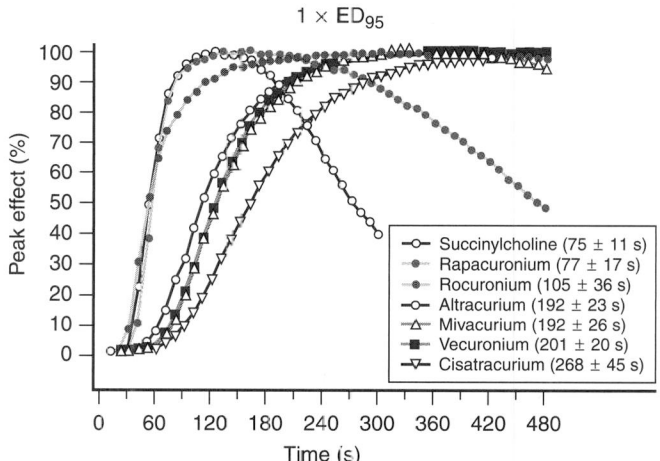

Figure 13–18 Linear regression of the onset of neuromuscular blockade (ordinate) versus potency of a series of steroidal relaxants studied in the cat model by Bowman and colleagues.[176] The data show that onset may be increased in compounds with low potency and encouraged the eventual development of rocuronium and rapacuronium.
A, pipecuronium; C, pancuronium; D, vecuronium.

Figure 13–19 Percentage of peak effect after a $1 \times ED_{95}$ dose of succinylcholine, rapacuronium, rocuronium, atracurium, mivacurium, vecuronium, and cisatracurium at the adductor pollicis muscle. Times (mean ± SD) in seconds to 95% of peak effect are shown in parentheses. (Redrawn from Kopman and associates.[220,259,261])

Table 13–9 Time course of action and peak effect data at the laryngeal adductors and adductor pollicis

Dose (mg/kg)	Anesthesia	Laryngeal Adductors			Adductor Pollicis			Reference
		Onset Time (sec)	Maximum Block (% Depression)	Clinical Duration* (min)	Onset Time (sec)	Maximum Block (% Depression)	Clinical Duration* (min)	
Succinylcholine, 1.0	Propofol-fentanyl	34 ± 12	100 ± 0	4.3 ± 1.6	56 ± 15	100 ± 0	8 ± 2	266
Rocuronium, 0.25	Propofol-fentanyl	96 ± 6	37 ± 8	—	180 ± 18	69 ± 8	—	264
Rocuronium, 0.4	Propofol-fentanyl	92 ± 29	70 ± 15	—	155 ± 40	99 ± 3	24 ± 7	266
Rocuronium, 0.5	Propofol-fentanyl	84 ± 6	77 ± 5	8 ± 3	144 ± 12	98 ± 1	22 ± 3	264
Vecuronium, 0.04	Propofol-fentanyl	198 ± 6	55 ± 8	—	342 ± 12	89 ± 3	11 ± 2	46
Vecuronium, 0.07	Propofol-fentanyl	198 ± 12	88 ± 4	9 ± 2	342 ± 18	98 ± 1	22 ± 2	46
Mivacurium, 0.14	Propofol-alfentanil	137 ± 20	90 ± 7	5.7 ± 2.1	201 ± 59	99 ± 1	16.2 ± 4.6	267
Mivacurium, 0.2	Propofol-alfentanil	89 ± 26	99 ± 4	10.4 ± 1.5	202 ± 45	99 ± 2	20.5 ± 3.9	268

Values are means and SD[266-268] or SEM.[46,264]
*Clinical duration is the time until T1 recovered to 25% of its control value.

(adductor pollicis) (see Fig. 13-4).[264,265] Neuromuscular blockade develops faster, lasts a shorter time, and recovers more quickly in these muscles (Table 13-9).[46,264,266-268] These observations may seem contradictory because there is also convincing evidence that the EC_{50} for almost all drugs studied is between 50% and 100% higher at the diaphragm or larynx than it is at the adductor pollicis. Fisher and coauthors[269] explain this apparent contradiction by postulating more rapid equilibration (shorter $t_{1/2}k_{e0}$) between plasma and the effect compartment at these central muscles. This accelerated rate of equilibrium probably represents little more than differences in regional blood flow. Muscle blood flow rather than intrinsic potency may be more important in determining the onset and offset time of nondepolarizing neuromuscular blockers.[270] More luxuriant blood flow (greater blood flow per gram of muscle) at the diaphragm or larynx would result in the central muscle receiving a higher peak plasma concentration of drug in the brief period before rapid redistribution is well under way.

Onset of block in the larynx occurs 1 to 2 minutes earlier than at the adductor pollicis after the administration of nondepolarizing neuromuscular blocking agents. The pattern of blockade (onset, depth, speed of recovery) in the orbicularis oculi is similar to that in the larynx.[271] By monitoring the onset of neuromuscular blockade at the orbicularis oculi, the quality of intubating conditions can be predicted. The onset of maximal block in the larynx also corresponds to the point at which the adductor pollicis is beginning to show palpable evidence of weakening. Furthermore, return of thumb responses to normal suggests that the efferent muscular arc of protective airway reflexes is intact.

Rapid Tracheal Intubation

Succinylcholine remains the drug of choice when rapid tracheal intubation is needed because it consistently provides muscle relaxation within 60 to 90 seconds. When succinylcholine is considered undesirable or contraindicated, the onset of nondepolarizing neuromuscular blocking drugs can be accelerated by preceding the intubating dose with a priming dose of neuromuscular blocker,[272-275] by the use of high doses of an individual agent,[250,276] or by combinations of neuromuscular blockers.[251,277,278] Although some combinations of mivacurium and rocuronium can achieve rapid onset without undue prolongation of action and without undesirable effects,[251] combination therapy may not consistently result in rapid onset of effect.[277]

The Priming Technique

Since the introduction of rocuronium, the use of priming has significantly decreased. Several groups of investigators have recommended that a small subparalyzing dose of the nondepolarizer (about 20% of the ED_{95} or about 10% of the intubating dose) be given 2 to 4 minutes before administering a second large dose for tracheal intubation.[272-275] This procedure, termed *priming*, has been shown to accelerate the onset of block of most nondepolarizing neuromuscular blockers by about 30 to 60 seconds, with the result that intubation can be performed within approximately 90 seconds after the second dose. However, intubating conditions after priming do not match those after succinylcholine.[279] Moreover, priming carries the risk of aspiration and difficulty swallowing, and the visual disturbances associated with subtle degrees of block are uncomfortable for the patient.[280,281]

High-Dose Regimen for Rapid Tracheal Intubation

Larger doses of neuromuscular blockers are usually recommended when intubation must be accomplished in less than 90 seconds. High-dose regimens, however, are associated with considerable prolongation of the duration of action and potentially increased cardiovascular side effects (see Table 13-8).[250,276,282,283] Increasing the dose of rocuronium from 0.6 ($2 \times ED_{95}$) to 1.2 ($4 \times ED_{95}$) mg/kg shortened the onset time of complete neuromuscular blockade from 89 ± 33 seconds (mean $\pm$ SD) to 55 ± 14 seconds but significantly prolonged the clinical duration (recovery of T1 to 25% of baseline) from 37 ± 15 to 73 ± 32 minutes, respectively.[250]

Whatever technique of rapid-sequence induction of anesthesia and intubation is elected, the following four principles are important: (1) preoxygenation must be performed, (2) an adequate dosage of intravenous drugs must be administered to ensure that the patient is adequately anesthetized, (3) intubation within 60 to 90 seconds must be considered acceptable, and (4) cricoid pressure should be applied subsequent to injection of the induction agent.

Low-Dose Relaxants for Tracheal Intubation

This low-dose technique is not suitable for rapid-sequence induction. Several studies have demonstrated that low doses of neuromuscular blocking drugs can be used for routine tracheal intubation. A low-dose neuromuscular blocker has several advantages: (1) it shortens the time to recovery from neuromuscular blockade, and (2) it reduces the requirement for anticholinesterase drugs. Rocuronium has the shortest onset time of all the nondepolarizing neuromuscular blocking drugs currently available.[264,266] The maximal effect of either 0.25 or 0.5 mg/kg rocuronium at laryngeal muscles was observed after 1.5 minutes.[264] This interval was shorter than the 3.3 minutes reported after the administration of equipotent doses of vecuronium (0.04 or 0.07 mg/kg)[46] and only slightly more than the 0.9 minute reported after 0.25 or 0.5 mg/kg succinylcholine (see Table 13-9).[284]

With a better understanding of the multiple factors that contribute to satisfactory conditions for intubation, it is now possible to take full advantage of the onset profile for rocuronium. Intubating conditions are related more closely to the degree of neuromuscular blockade of the laryngeal adductor muscles than to the degree of blockade typically monitored at the adductor pollicis. Figure 13-20 demonstrates this principle.[262] Complete block at the larynx or diaphragm, or at both, may not be a prerequisite for satisfactory tracheal intubating conditions.

Kopman and colleagues[286] noted that 0.5 mg/kg rocuronium ($1.5 \times ED_{95}$) provided very satisfactory conditions for intubation (25 intubations were rated as excellent and 5 were rated as good) in patients anesthetized with 12.5 µg/kg alfentanil and 2.0 mg/kg propofol if laryngoscopy is delayed for 75 seconds after drug administration. They estimated that a $1.5 \times ED_{95}$ dose (0.5 mg/kg) of rocuronium will produce a 95% block or greater in 98% of the population.[286] Others have reported the same observation.[287] It has also been shown that a similar or lower ED_{95} multiple of rocuronium has a more rapid onset and shorter duration than does either atracurium[288] or

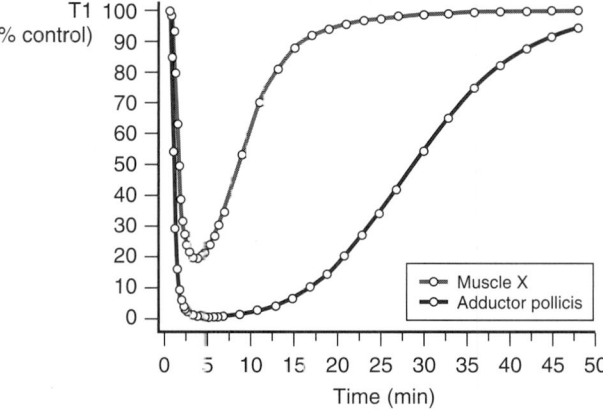

	Muscle X	Adductor pollicis
EC_{50} (µg/mL)	3.00	1.18
$t_{1/2}K_{e0}$ (min)	1.93	3.85
Hill coefficient	4.00	4.50

Figure 13–20 A computer simulation based on Sheiner and colleagues' model[224] and data reported by Wierda et al.[285] The ED_{95} of rocuronium at the adductor pollicis from this model is 0.33 mg/kg. Rocuronium, 0.45 mg/kg, is given as a bolus at time zero. Muscle X represents a muscle (such as the diaphragm or the laryngeal adductors) that is less sensitive to the effects of nondepolarizing relaxants than the adductor pollicis is but has greater blood flow. In this example, the concentration of rocuronium producing a 50% block (EC_{50}) of muscle X is 2.5 times that of the adductor pollicis, but the half-life of transport between plasma and the effect compartment ($t_{1/2}k_{e0}$) of muscle X is only half as long. The rapid equilibration between concentrations of rocuronium in plasma and muscle X results in a more rapid onset of blockade of muscle X than the adductor pollicis. The greater EC_{50} at muscle X explains the faster recovery of this muscle from neuromuscular blockade than the adductor pollicis. Lower blood concentrations of rocuronium must be achieved at the adductor pollicis than at muscle X before recovery begins. (Redrawn from Naguib M, Kopman AF: Low dose rocuronium for tracheal intubation. Middle East J Anesthesiol 17:193-204, 2003.)

cisatracurium.[212,289] The onset of cisatracurium is too slow to provide good conditions for intubation in less than 2 minutes, even after a dose of $2 \times ED_{95}$.[289]

In the vast majority of patients receiving alfentanil, 15 µg/kg, followed by propofol, 2.0 mg/kg, and rocuronium, 0.45 mg/kg, good to excellent conditions for intubation will be present 75 to 90 seconds after the completion of drug administration.[286]

Metabolism and Elimination

The specific pathways of metabolism (biotransformation) and elimination of neuromuscular blocking drugs are summarized in Table 13-10. Of the nondepolarizing neuromuscular blockers listed, pancuronium, pipecuronium, vecuronium, atracurium, cisatracurium, mivacurium, and rapacuronium (ORG 9487) are the only ones that are metabolized or degraded. Nearly all nondepolarizing neuromuscular blocker molecules contain ester linkages, acetyl ester groups, and hydroxyl or methoxy groups. These substitutions, especially the quaternary nitrogen

Table 13–10 Metabolism and elimination of neuromuscular blocking drugs

Drug	Duration	Metabolism (%)	Elimination		Metabolites
			Kidney (%)	Liver (%)	
Succinylcholine	Ultrashort	Butyrylcholinesterase (98%-99%)	<2%	None	Monoester (succinylmonocholine) and choline. The monoester is metabolized much more slowly than succinylcholine is
430A	Ultrashort	Cysteine (fast) and ester hydrolysis (slow)	?	?	Inactive cysteine adduction product, chloroformate monoester and alcohol (see Fig. 13-10)
Mivacurium	Short	Butyrylcholinesterase (95%-99%)	<5%	None	Monoester and quaternary alcohol. The metabolites are inactive. They are most likely not themselves metabolized any further (see Fig. 13-22)
			(Metabolites eliminated in urine and bile)		
Rapacuronium (ORG 9487)	Short	To 3-desacetyl metabolite	20%	Unknown	The 3-OH derivative, ORG 9488, is two to three times more potent than the parent compound and has a longer half-life
Atracurium	Intermediate	Hofmann elimination and nonspecific ester hydrolysis (60%-90%)	10%-40%	None	Laudanosine, acrylates, alcohols, and acids (see Fig. 13-23). Although laudanosine has CNS-stimulating properties, the clinical relevance of this effect is negligible
			(Metabolites eliminated in urine and bile)		
Cisatracurium	Intermediate	Hofmann elimination (77%?)	Renal clearance is 16% of total		Laudanosine and acrylates. Ester hydrolysis of the quaternary monoacrylate occurs secondarily (see Fig. 13-23). Because of the greater potency of cisatracurium, laudanosine quantities produced by Hofmann elimination are 5 to 10 times lower than in the case of atracurium, thus making this a nonissue in practice
Vecuronium	Intermediate	Liver (30%-40%)	40%-50%	50%-60%	The 3-OH metabolite accumulates, particularly in renal failure. It has about 80% the potency of vecuronium and may be responsible for delayed recovery in ICU patients (see Fig. 13-21)
			(Metabolites excreted in urine and bile)		
Rocuronium	Intermediate	None	<10%	>70%	None
Pancuronium	Long	Liver (10%-20%)	85%	15%	The 3-OH metabolite may accumulate, particularly in renal failure. It is about two thirds as potent as the parent compound
d-Tubocurarine	Long	None	80% (?)	20%	None
Pipecuronium	Long	Approximately 10%	>90% (?)	<10%	The 3-OH metabolite is produced in small quantities (≈5%)
Metocurine	Long	None	>98%	<2%	None
Doxacurium	Long	None	>90% (?)	<10%	None
Alcuronium	Long	None	80%-90% (?)	10%-20%	None
Gallamine	Long	None	100%	0%	None

groups, confer a high degree of water solubility with only slight lipid solubility. The hydrophilic nature of relaxant molecules enables easy elimination in urine by glomerular filtration with no tubular resorption or secretion. Therefore, all nondepolarizing neuromuscular blockers show elimination of the parent molecule in urine as a basic route of elimination. Nondepolarizing neuromuscular blockers with a long duration of action are eliminated predominantly in urine and thus have a clearance rate limited by glomerular filtration (1 to 2 mL/kg/min).

Steroidal Compounds

Long-Acting Neuromuscular Blockers

Pancuronium is cleared largely by the kidney.[290] Hepatic uptake of pancuronium is limited.[291] A small amount (15% to 20%) is deacetylated at the 3-position in the liver,[27,292,293] but such deacetylation makes a minimal contribution to its total clearance. Deacetylation also occurs at the 17-position, but to such a small extent that it is clinically irrelevant. The metabolites have been individually studied in anesthetized humans.[253] The 3-OH metabolite is the most potent of the three (approximately half the potency of pancuronium) and the only one present in detectable concentrations in plasma. This metabolite

has pharmacokinetics and duration of action similar to those of pancuronium.[253] The 3-OH metabolite is also most probably excreted largely by the kidney.[253] The parent compound and the 3-OH metabolite are cleared in small amounts through a minor liver pathway.[292] Total clearance is delayed, and the duration of action is significantly lengthened by severe disorders of renal or hepatic function.[233,294-297]

Pipecuronium undergoes very little metabolism. Only a very small amount of the drug (5%) may be deacetylated at the 3-position. The major excretory pathway is the kidney, with the liver possibly being a minor secondary pathway. Excretion is delayed, clearance is decreased, and the elimination half-life is lengthened in the presence of major disorders of renal or hepatic function.[293,298,299]

Intermediate-Acting Neuromuscular Blockers

Vecuronium, the 2-desmethyl derivative of pancuronium, is more lipid soluble than pancuronium because of absence of the quaternizing methyl group at the 2-position. It undergoes two to three times more metabolism than pancuronium does. Vecuronium is taken up into the liver by a carrier-mediated transport system[291,300] and is deacetylated at the 3-position by liver microsomes (Fig. 13-21).[301]

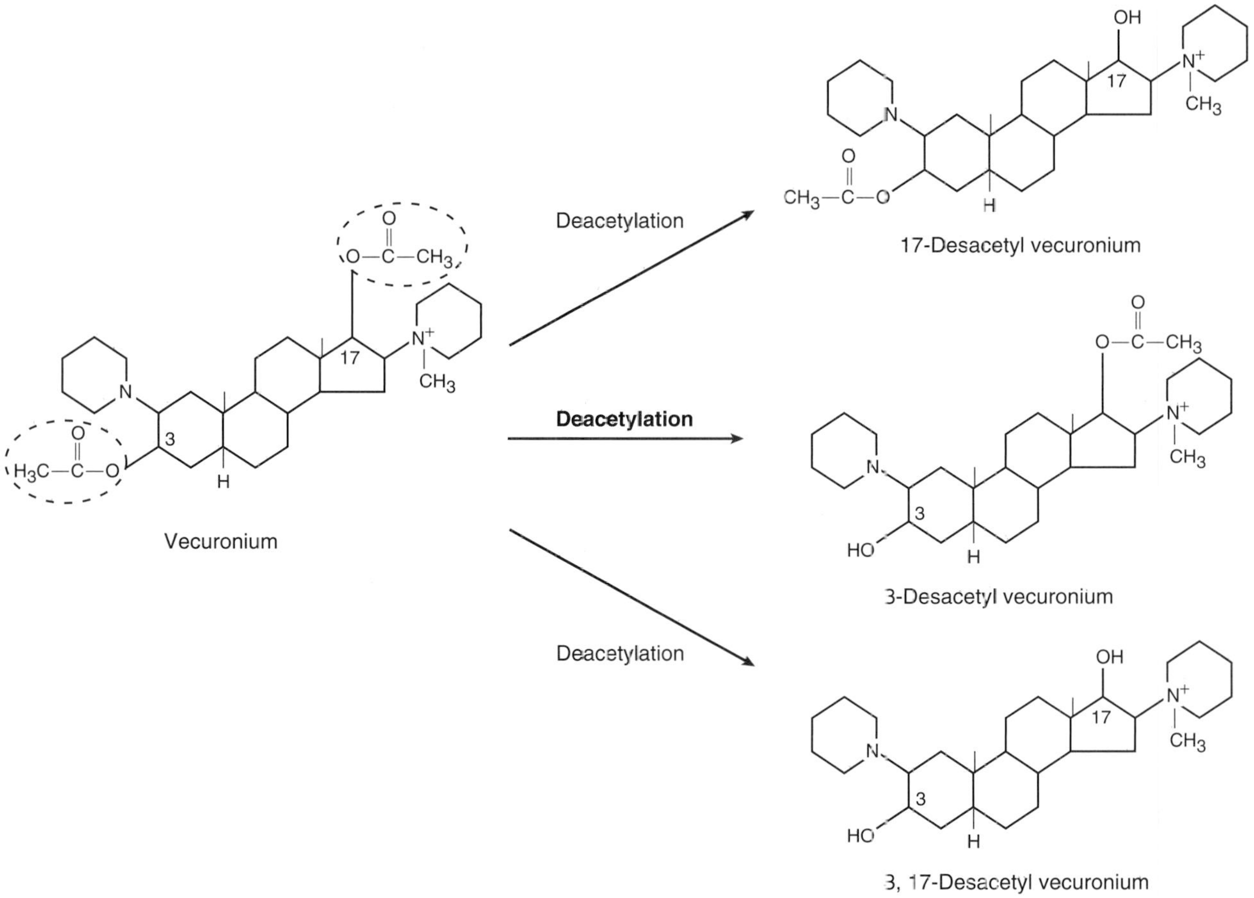

Figure 13–21 Metabolism of vecuronium as it occurs in the liver. About 30% to 40% of an injected dose is deacetylated at the 3- and 17-positions. The major metabolite is 3-OH vecuronium (red arrow). The metabolites are excreted in urine and bile. The 3-OH metabolite is nearly as potent as the parent compound and is probably cleared from blood at a rate slightly slower than that of vecuronium. (Redrawn from Agoston S, Seyr M, Khuenl-Brady KS, et al: Use of neuromuscular blocking agents in the intensive care unit. Anesthesiol Clin North Am 11:345, 1993.)

About 12% of vecuronium clearance is by conversion to 3-desacetylvecuronium,[302] and about 30% to 40% is cleared in bile as the parent compound.[231,303] Although the liver is the principal organ of elimination for vecuronium, the drug also undergoes significant (up to 25%) renal excretion, and this combined elimination gives it a clearance of 3 to 6 mL/kg/min.[302-304]

The principal metabolite of vecuronium, 3-desacetylvecuronium, is a potent (≈80% of vecuronium) neuromuscular blocking drug in its own right. The metabolite, though, has lower plasma clearance and a longer duration of action than vecuronium does.[302] 3-Desacetylvecuronium has a clearance of 3.5 mL/kg/min, and renal clearance accounts for approximately a sixth of its elimination.[302] In patients in the ICU who have renal failure, 3-desacetylvecuronium can accumulate and produce prolonged neuromuscular blockade.[305] Other putative metabolites are 17-desacetylvecuronium and 3,17-bisdesacetylvecuronium, neither of which occurs in clinically significant amounts.[27]

Rocuronium is eliminated primarily by the liver,[306,307] with a small fraction (≈10%) eliminated in urine.[308] It is taken up into the liver by a carrier-mediated active transport system.[309,310] The putative metabolite 17-desacetylrocuronium has not been detected in significant quantities.

Short-Acting Neuromuscular Blockers

Rapacuronium has a clearance of between 8 and 11 mL/kg/min.[219,311] It probably undergoes metabolism to its 3-desacetyl derivative (ORG 9488), which contributes significantly to its neuromuscular blocking effect.[311] The metabolite (ORG 9488) is more potent and shows considerably slower elimination than does the parent compound. Accumulation of the metabolite may be the reason for slower recovery after successive doses of rapacuronium.[311]

Benzylisoquinolinium Compounds

Short-Acting Neuromuscular Blockers

Mivacurium is hydrolyzed in plasma by butyrylcholinesterase to monoester and the amino alcohol (Fig. 13-22).[10,312] These compounds are excreted in urine and bile.[313] The metabolites are positively charged, thus making central nervous system (CNS) entry unlikely. They show less than $1/100$ the neuromuscular blocking activity of the parent compound. They do not affect the autonomic nervous system.[313] Less than 5% is excreted as the parent compound in urine.

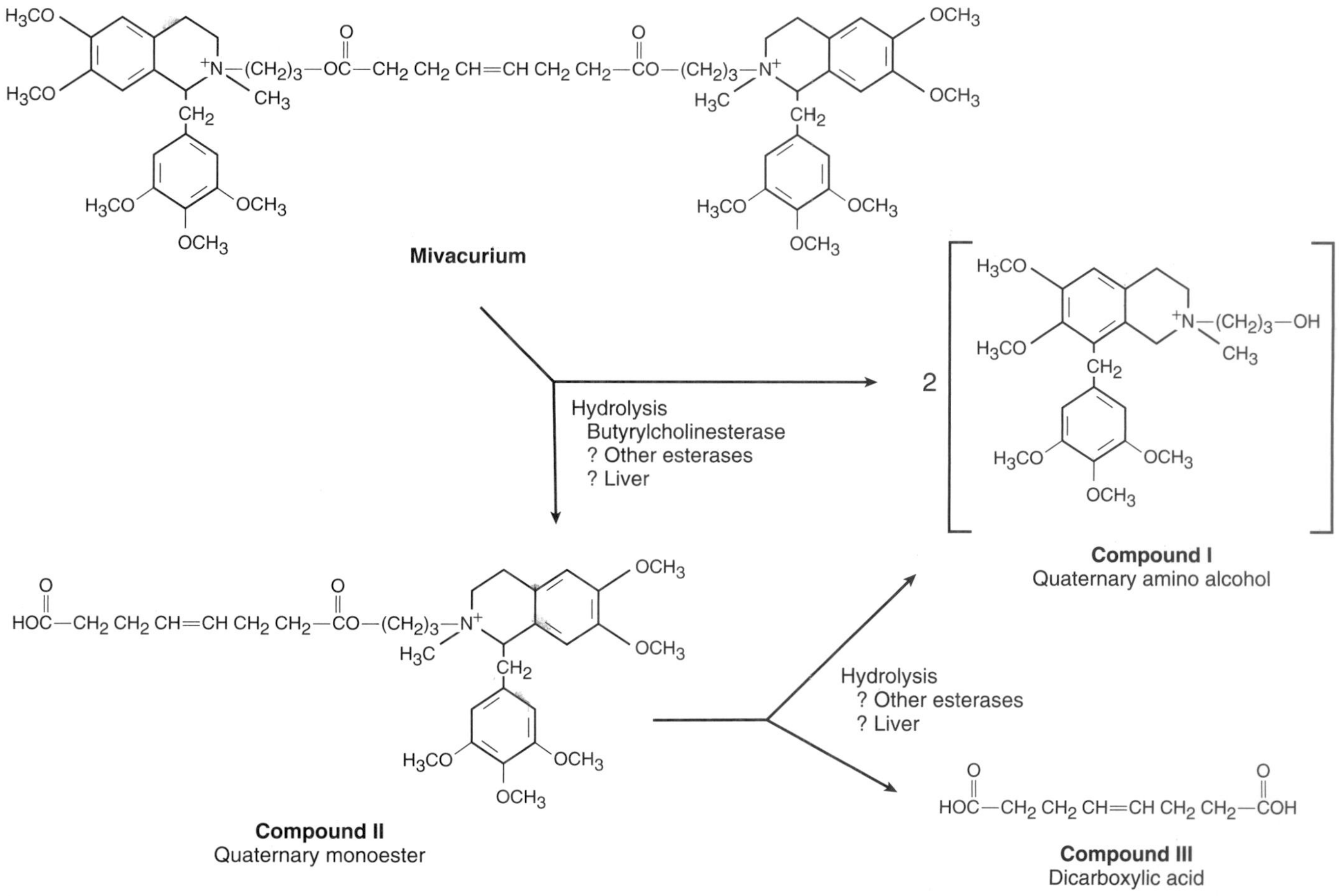

Figure 13–22 Metabolism of mivacurium by butyrylcholinesterase. The reaction occurs at about 70% to 88% of the rate of succinylcholine in vitro. The metabolites are inactive and carry positive charges, thus suggesting minimal central nervous system entry. (Redrawn from Savarese JJ, Ali HH, Basta SJ, et al: The clinical neuromuscular pharmacology of mivacurium chloride [BW B1090U]. A short-acting nondepolarizing ester neuromuscular blocking drug. Anesthesiology 68:723-732, 1988.)

Mivacurium consists of three stereoisomers, and clearance of the two most pharmacologically active isomers, the *cis-trans* and *trans-trans* isomers, is approximately 100 and 50 to 70 mL/kg/min, respectively.[171,172,314] These two isomers have elimination half-lives of 2 to 3 minutes.[171] The third stereoisomer, the *cis-cis* isomer, is present as only 4% to 8% of the mivacurium mixture and has less than 10% of the neuromuscular blocking potency of the other two isomers.[171] Consequently, even though it has a much longer elimination half-life (55 minutes) and lower clearance (≈4 mL/kg/min) than the two other isomers, it does not contribute significantly to the duration of action of mivacurium.[171] This rapid enzymatic clearance of mivacurium accounts for its short duration.[10,171] Mivacurium has a duration of action much shorter than that of vecuronium and atracurium but about twice that of succinylcholine.[315]

When butyrylcholinesterase activity is severely deficient, such as in rare patients (1/3000) who are homozygotes with genetically atypical enzyme, the duration of action of mivacurium is prolonged for up to several hours.[316-320]

Intermediate-Acting Neuromuscular Blockers
Theoretically, atracurium is metabolized through two pathways (see Fig 13-23).[321] The drug undergoes Hofmann elimination and ester hydrolysis by nonspecific esterases. Hofmann elimination is a purely chemical process that results in loss of the positive charges by molecular fragmentation to laudanosine (a tertiary amine) and a monoquaternary acrylate.[322,323] They were thought to have no neuromuscular and little or no cardiovascular activity of clinical relevance.[322,323] Under the proper chemical conditions, these breakdown products may actually be used to synthesize the parent compound.

Because it undergoes Hofmann elimination, atracurium is relatively stable at pH 3.0 and 4°C and becomes unstable when injected into the bloodstream. Early observations of breakdown of the drug in buffer and plasma showed faster degradation in plasma, thus suggesting possible enzymatic hydrolysis of the ester groups.[324] Further evidence suggests that this second pathway, ester hydrolysis, may be of more importance than was originally realized in the breakdown of atracurium.[325] Through the use of pharmacokinetic analysis, Fisher and associates[326] concluded that a significant amount of clearance of atracurium may be accomplished by routes other than ester hydrolysis and Hofmann elimination. Atracurium's metabolism is complicated and may not be completely resolved.[326,327]

Laudanosine, a metabolite of atracurium, has CNS-stimulating properties. Unlike atracurium, laudanosine is dependent on the liver and kidney for elimination and has a long elimination half-life.[328,329] Laudanosine concentrations are elevated in patients with liver disease[330] and those who have received atracurium for many hours in an ICU.[331] Laudanosine freely crosses the blood-brain barrier.[328] Beemer and coworkers[332] found that patients awakened at a 20% higher arterial concentration of thiopental when atracurium had been given; such awakening was attributed to the CNS stimulatory effect of laudanosine. These relatively low concentrations of laudanosine, however, did not influence animal models of epilepsy[333] or lidocaine-induced seizures.[334] In the ICU, blood levels of laudanosine can be as high as 5.0 to

6.0 μg/mL.[331] Though not known in humans, the seizure threshold in animals ranges from 5.0 μg/mL in rabbits[335] to 17 μg/mL in dogs.[336] Thus, adverse effects are unlikely to occur with atracurium use in the operating room or the ICU. Laudanosine also has cardiovascular effects. In dogs, hypotension occurs at a blood concentration of about 6 μg/mL,[328,336] a level higher than usually found in patients in the ICU. However, there is one case report of a patient who had severe hypotension and bradycardia while receiving atracurium, which resolved only when vecuronium was substituted.[337] Laudanosine enhances stimulation-evoked release of norepinephrine,[338,339] a characteristic that may also partly account for its CNS-stimulating effect.

Atracurium is a mixture of 10 optical isomers. Cisatracurium is the 1R *cis*–1'R *cis* isomer of atracurium.[167] Like atracurium, it is metabolized by Hofmann elimination to laudanosine and a monoquaternary alcohol metabolite.[340-342] There is no ester hydrolysis of the parent molecule.[340] Hofmann elimination accounts for 77% of the total clearance of 5 to 6 mL/kg/min.[343] Twenty-three percent of the drug is cleared through organ-dependent means, with renal elimination accounting for 16% of this total.[342] Because cisatracurium is about four to five times as potent as atracurium, about five times less laudanosine is produced, and accumulation of this metabolite is not thought to be of any consequence in clinical practice.

Long-Acting Neuromuscular Blockers
dTc does not undergo active metabolism. The kidney is the major pathway of elimination, with approximately 50% of a dose being eliminated through renal pathways. The liver is probably a secondary route of elimination. The drug is not indicated for use in patients with either renal[234] or hepatic[344] failure because more suitable agents are available.

Metocurine is excreted only by the kidney. It has no alternative biliary pathway, and no metabolism occurs in the liver.[345]

Doxacurium is not metabolized in humans. The drug is excreted in urine and bile as the unchanged parent molecule. Urine is the major route of elimination, with bile being a minor secondary pathway.[346]

Asymmetric Mixed-Onium Chlorofumarates (430A)
430A appears to be degraded by two chemical mechanisms, neither of which is enzymatic: (1) rapid formation of an apparently inactive cysteine adduction product, with cysteine replacing chlorine, and (2) slower hydrolysis of the ester bond adjacent to the chlorine substitution to presumably inactive hydrolysis products (see Fig. 13-10).[187]

Phenolic Ether Derivative
Gallamine is not metabolized and is excreted unchanged in the urine only. It does not have any alternative biliary excretory pathway.[347]

Diallyl Derivative of Toxiferine
Alcuronium undergoes little or no metabolism. Urine is the major excretory pathway, with a small amount of biliary clearance of unchanged drug.[190]

In summary, the long-acting neuromuscular blockers undergo minimal or no metabolism, and they are

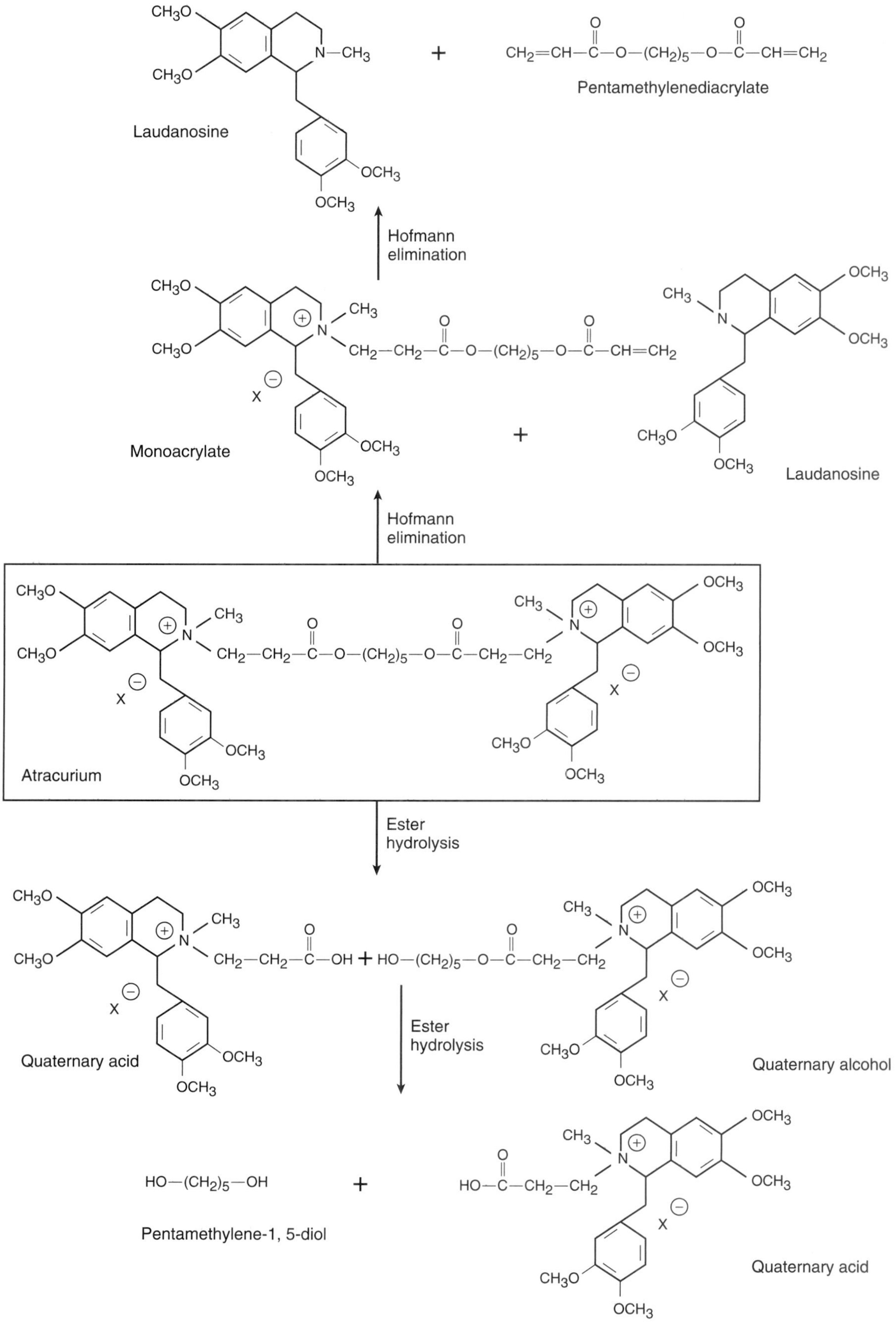

Figure 13–23 Degradation pathways of atracurium. The major metabolite, laudanosine, is excreted in urine and bile. Laudanosine is a tertiary amine that may enter the central nervous system. Less than 10% of atracurium is excreted as the parent compound. (Redrawn from Basta SJ, Ali HH, Savarese JJ, et al: Clinical pharmacology of atracurium besylate [BW 33A]: A new non-depolarizing muscle relaxant. Anesth Analg 61:723-729, 1982.)

eliminated, largely unchanged, mostly by renal excretion. Hepatic pathways are less important.

Neuromuscular blockers of intermediate duration such as vecuronium, rocuronium, atracurium, and cisatracurium have clearances in the range 3 to 6 mL/kg/min because of multiple pathways of degradation, metabolism, and elimination. Atracurium is cleared two to three times more rapidly than the long-acting drugs are.[227,330,348-351] Similar clearance values have been obtained for rocuronium[352-357] and cisatracurium.[341-343,358,359]

The only short-acting neuromuscular blocker currently available for clinical use, mivacurium, is cleared rapidly and almost exclusively through metabolism by butyrylcholinesterase, which results in plasma clearance much greater than that of any other nondepolarizing neuromuscular blocker.[10]

Adverse Effects of Neuromuscular Blockers

Neuromuscular blocking drugs seem to play a predominant role in the occurrence of adverse reactions during anesthesia. The Committee on Safety of Medicines in the United Kingdom reported that 10.8% (218 of 2014) of adverse drug reactions and 7.3% of deaths (21 of 286) were attributable to the neuromuscular blocking drugs.[360]

Autonomic Effects
Neuromuscular blocking drugs interact with nicotinic and muscarinic cholinergic receptors within the sympathetic and parasympathetic nervous systems and at the nicotinic receptors of the neuromuscular junction.

Dose-response ratios comparing the neuromuscular blocking potency of neuromuscular blockers (ED_{95}) with their potencies in blocking vagal (parasympathetic) or sympathetic ganglionic transmission (ED_{50}) can be constructed (Table 13-11). These ratios are termed the autonomic margin of safety of the relaxant in question. The higher the dose ratio, the lower the likelihood or the greater the safety ratio for the occurrence of the particular autonomic effect. The side effect is absent (none) in clinical practice if the safety ratio is greater than 5. The side effect is weak or slight if the safety ratio is 3 or 4, moderate if 2 or 3, and strong or prominent if the ratio is 1 or less.

These autonomic responses are not reduced by slower injection of the relaxant. They are dose related and are additive over time if divided doses are given. If identical to the original dose, subsequent doses will produce a similar response; that is, no tachyphylaxis will occur. Such is not the case when the side effect of histamine release is in question. Cardiovascular responses secondary to histamine release are decreased by slowing the injection rate, and the response undergoes rapid tachyphylaxis. The autonomic effects of neuromuscular blocking drugs are summarized in Table 13-12.

Histamine Release
Quaternary ammonium compounds such as neuromuscular blockers are generally weak histamine-releasing substances relative to tertiary amines such as morphine. Nevertheless, when large doses of certain neuromuscular blockers are administered rapidly, erythema of the face, neck, and upper part of the torso may develop, as well as a brief decrease in arterial pressure and a slight to moderate increase in heart rate. Bronchospasm in this setting is very rare. The clinical effects of histamine are seen when plasma concentrations increase 200% to 300% above baseline values and involve chemical displacement of the contents of mast cell granules containing histamine, prostaglandin, and possibly other vasoactive substances.[361] The serosal mast cell, located in the skin and connective tissue and near blood vessels and nerves, is principally involved in the degranulation process.[361]

Table 13–11	Approximate autonomic margins of safety of nondepolarizing neuromuscular blockers*		
Drugs	**Vagus†**	**Sympathetic Ganglia†**	**Histamine Release‡**
Benzylisoquinolinium Compounds			
Mivacurium	>50	>100	3.0
Atracurium	16	40	2.5
Cisatracurium	>50	>50	None
Doxacurium	>50	>100	>4.0
d-Tubocurarine	0.6	2.0	0.6
Metocurine	3.0	16.0	2.0
Steroidal Compounds			
Rapacuronium	2.0-3.0	? 5-20	? 3.0
Vecuronium	20	>250	None
Rocuronium	3.0-5.0	>10	None
Pancuronium	3.0	>250	None
Pipecuronium	25	>200	None
Others			
Alcuronium	3.0	4.0	None
Gallamine	0.6	>100	None

*Definition: number of multiples of the ED_{95} for neuromuscular blockade required to produce the autonomic side effect (ED_{50}).
†In the cat.
‡In human subjects.

Table 13–12 Clinical autonomic effects of neuromuscular blocking drugs

Drug Type	Autonomic Ganglia	Cardiac Muscarinic Receptors	Histamine Release
Depolarizing Substance			
Succinylcholine	Stimulates	Stimulates	Slight
Benzylisoquinolinium Compounds			
Mivacurium	None	None	Slight
Atracurium	None	None	Slight
Cisatracurium	None	None	None
Doxacurium	None	None	None
d-Tubocurarine	Blocks	None	Moderate
Metocurine	Blocks weakly	None	Slight
Steroidal Compounds			
Rapacuronium*	? None	Blocks moderately	? Slight
Vecuronium	None	None	None
Rocuronium	None	Blocks weakly	None
Pancuronium	None	Blocks moderately	None
Pipecuronium	None	None	None
Others			
Alcuronium	Blocks weakly	Blocks weakly	None
Gallamine	None	Blocks strongly	None

*Has not been extensively studied; may also block calcium channels.

The side effect of histamine release is most often noted after administration of the benzylisoquinolinium class of muscle relaxants, although it has been reported with steroidal relaxants of low potency. The effect is usually of short duration (1 to 5 minutes), is dose related, and is clinically insignificant in healthy patients. Hatano and colleagues[362] showed that the hypotensive cardiovascular response to 0.6 mg/kg dTc in humans is prevented not only by antihistamines but also by nonsteroidal anti-inflammatory drugs (e.g., aspirin). These investigators concluded that the final step in dTc-induced hypotension is modulated by prostaglandins that are vasodilators.[362] The side effect may be reduced considerably by a slower injection rate. It is also attenuated by prophylaxis with combinations of H_1- and H_2-blockers.[363] If a minor degree of histamine release such as just described occurs after an initial dose of neuromuscular blocker, subsequent doses will generally cause no response at all, as long as they are not larger than the original dose. This observation is clinical evidence of tachyphylaxis, an important characteristic of histamine release. A much more significant degree of histamine release occurs during anaphylactic or anaphylactoid reactions, but these reactions are very rare.

Clinical Cardiovascular Manifestations of Autonomic Mechanisms

Hypotension
The hypotension seen with atracurium and mivacurium is due to histamine release. dTc causes hypotension through histamine release and ganglion blockade.[364-367] More than any other neuromuscular blocker, the ganglion-blocking and histamine-releasing effects of dTc occur closer to the dose required to achieve neuromuscular blockade.[219,368] Dowdy and coworkers[369] proposed that

hypotension is not caused by dTc itself but by the preservative in its formulation. However, in anesthetized patients, Stoelting[370,371] disproved this theory. The safety margin for histamine release is about three times greater for atracurium and mivacurium and two times greater for metocurine than for dTc.[215,361,362,367,372] Rapid administration of atracurium in doses greater than 0.4 mg/kg and mivacurium in doses greater than 0.15 mg/kg has been associated with transient hypotension from histamine release (Fig. 13-24).

Tachycardia
Pancuronium causes a moderate increase in heart rate and, to a lesser extent, cardiac output, with little or no change in systemic vascular resistance.[373,374] Pancuronium-induced tachycardia has been attributed to (1) a vagolytic action,[373,375] probably as a result of inhibition of M_2 receptors,[376] and (2) sympathetic stimulation involving both direct (blockade of neuronal uptake of norepinephrine) and indirect (release of norepinephrine from adrenergic nerve endings) mechanisms.[377-380] Vercruysse and associates[381] suggested that both gallamine and pancuronium augment the release of norepinephrine in vascular tissues under vagal control. In studies in humans, Roizen and colleagues[382] surprisingly found a decrease in plasma norepinephrine levels after the administration of either pancuronium or atropine. They postulated that the increase in heart rate or rate-pressure product occurs because pancuronium (or atropine) acts through baroreceptors to reduce sympathetic outflow.[382] More specifically, the vagolytic effect of pancuronium increases the heart rate and, hence, blood pressure and cardiac output, which in turn influence the baroreceptors to decrease sympathetic tone. Support for this concept is provided by

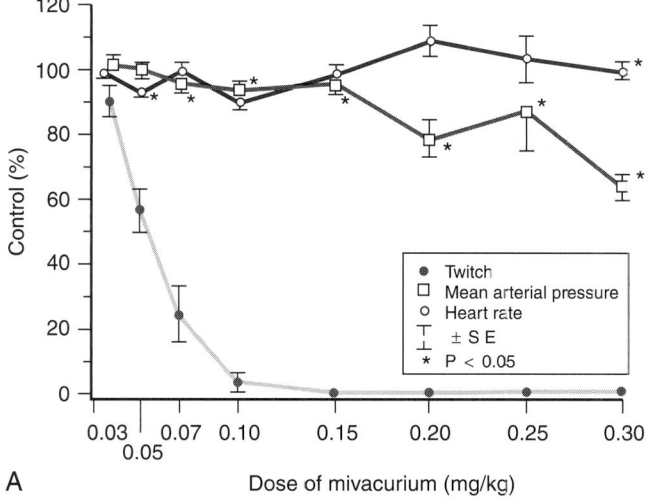

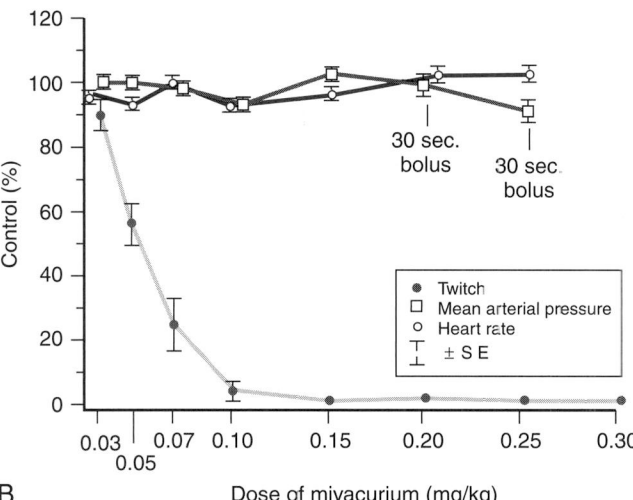

Figure 13–24 Dose response to mivacurium in patients under nitrous oxide–oxygen–opioid anesthesia. Maximum changes at each dose are shown ($n = 9$ subjects per group). **A,** With fast injection, a 15% to 20% decrease in arterial pressure occurred at 2.5 to $3 \times ED_{95}$ (0.20 to 0.25 mg/kg). **B,** The changes were less than 10% when slower injection (30 seconds) was performed. (Redrawn from Savarese JJ, Ali HH, Basta SJ, et al: The cardiovascular effects of mivacurium chloride [BW B1090U] in patients receiving nitrous oxide–opiate–barbiturate anesthesia. Anesthesiology 70:386-394, 1989.)

the fact that previous administration of atropine will attenuate or eliminate the cardiovascular effects of pancuronium.[373] Gallamine increases the heart rate by both a vagolytic effect[375,383] and sympathetic stimulation.[384] Specifically, gallamine releases norepinephrine from adrenergic nerve endings in the heart by an unknown mechanism.[384] However, a positive chronotropic effect that places emphasis on the vagolytic mechanism has not been found in humans.[385] It would not be surprising to ultimately find out that gallamine and pancuronium act by similar mechanisms. The tachycardia seen with benzylisoquinolinium compounds is due to histamine release.

Dysrhythmias

Gallamine, dTc, and succinylcholine actually reduce the incidence of epinephrine-induced dysrhythmias.[386] Possibly because of enhanced atrioventricular conduction,[387] the incidence of dysrhythmias from pancuronium appears to increase during halothane anesthesia.[373] Edwards and collaborators[388] observed a rapid tachycardia (more than 150 beats/min) that progressed to atrioventricular dissociation in two patients anesthetized with halothane who received pancuronium. The only factor common to these two patients was that both were receiving tricyclic antidepressants.

Bradycardia

Several case reports[389,390] have described severe bradycardia and even asystole after vecuronium or atracurium administration. All these cases were associated with opioid administration. Subsequent studies have indicated that vecuronium or atracurium alone does not cause bradycardia.[391] When combined with other drugs that do cause bradycardia (e.g., fentanyl), nonvagolytic relaxants such as vecuronium, cisatracurium, and atracurium allow this mechanism to occur unopposed. The moderate vagolytic effect of pancuronium is often used to counteract opioid-induced bradycardia.

Respiratory Effects

The muscarinic cholinergic system plays an important role in regulating airway function. Five muscarinic receptors have been cloned.[392-394] Cloned m1, m2, m3, and m4 muscarinic receptors correspond to the pharmacologically defined M_1, M_2, M_3, and M_4 receptors, respectively.[392,394,395] Three receptors (M_1 to M_3) exist in the airways.[396,397] M_1 receptors are under sympathetic control and mediate bronchodilation.[398] M_2 receptors are located presynaptically (Fig. 13-25) at the postganglionic parasympathetic nerve endings, and they function in

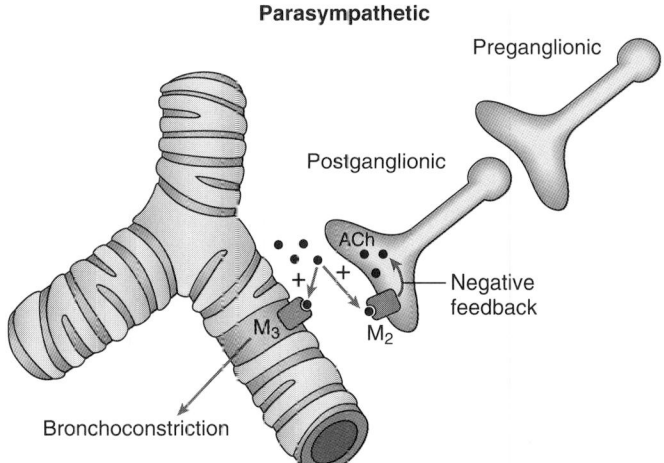

Figure 13–25 Muscarinic (M_3) receptors are located postsynaptically on airway smooth muscle. Acetylcholine (ACh) stimulates M_3 receptors to cause contraction. M_2 muscarinic receptors are located presynaptically at the postganglionic parasympathetic nerve endings, and they function in a negative-feedback mechanism to limit the release of acetylcholine.

a negative-feedback mechanism to limit the release of acetylcholine. M_3 receptors are located postsynaptically (see Fig. 13-25), and they mediate contraction of airway smooth muscles (bronchoconstriction).[398] Nondepolarizing neuromuscular blockers have different antagonistic activities at both the M_2 and M_3 receptors.[376,399,400] Blockage of M_3 muscarinic receptors on airway smooth muscle inhibits vagally induced bronchoconstriction (i.e., causes bronchodilation),[399] whereas blockage of M_2 receptors results in increased release of acetylcholine that will act on M_3 receptors and cause bronchoconstriction. The affinity of rapacuronium to block M_2 receptors is 15 times higher than its affinity to block M_3 receptors,[400] which would explain the high incidence (>9%)[186] of severe bronchospasm[181-184] seen with this drug that resulted in its withdrawal from the market.

Administration of benzylisoquinolinium neuromuscular blocking drugs (with the exception of cisatracurium and doxacurium) is associated with histamine release that may result in an increase in airway resistance and bronchospasm in patients with hyperactive airway disease.[401]

Allergic Reactions

The frequency of life-threatening anaphylactic (immune mediated) or anaphylactoid reactions occurring during anesthesia has been estimated at between 1 in 1000 and 1 in 25,000 anesthetics with an approximately 5% mortality rate.[402-405] Neuromuscular blocking drugs (especially succinylcholine) are the triggering agents in over 50% of these reactions.[360,406] Anaphylactic reactions are mediated through immune responses involving IgE antibodies fixed to mast cells. Anaphylactoid reactions are not immune mediated and represent exaggerated pharmacologic responses in very rare and very sensitive individuals.

Neuromuscular blocking drugs contain two quaternary ammonium ions, which are the epitopes commonly recognized by specific IgE.[407] Cross-reactivity has been reported between neuromuscular blocking drugs and food, cosmetics, disinfectants, and industrial materials.[407] Cross-reactivity is seen in more than 60% of patients with a history of anaphylaxis to a neuromuscular blocking drug.[408]

Steroidal compounds (e.g., rocuronium, vecuronium, pancuronium, or pipecuronium) lack significant histamine release.[367,409] Rocuronium at doses of $4 \times ED_{95}$ (1.2 mg/kg) cause no significant histamine release.[410] Nevertheless, Laxenaire and Mertes[411] have reported a 29.2% (98/336 cases) incidence of anaphylaxis to rocuronium over a 2-year period in France. Rose and Fisher[412] classified rocuronium (and atracurium) as intermediate in risk for causing allergic reactions. They also noted that the increased number of reports of anaphylaxis with rocuronium is in the line with the market share.[412] Watkins[413] stated "The much higher incidence of rocuronium reactions reported in France is currently inexplicable and is likely to remain so if investigators continue to seek a purely antibody-mediated response as an explanation of all anaphylactoid reaction presentations." Currently, there are no standards against which diagnostic tests (skin prick test, intradermal test, or IgE testing) are performed. For instance, Laxenaire and Mertes[411] used a 1:10 dilution of rocuronium for intradermal skin testing, whereas Rose and Fisher[412] used a 1:1000 dilution. Levy and colleagues[414] showed that rocuronium in a 1:10 dilution can produce false-positive results in intradermal testing and suggested that rocuronium be diluted at least 100-fold to prevent false-positive skin tests. Levy and coworkers[414] also found that both rocuronium and cisatracurium at high concentrations ($\geq 10^{-4}$ M) are capable of producing a wheal-and-flare response to intradermal testing associated with mild to moderate mast cell degranulation in the cisatracurium group only.

All neuromuscular blocking drugs can cause noncompetitive inhibition of histamine–N-methyltransferase, but concentrations required for inhibition far exceed those that would be used clinically, except for vecuronium, in which the effect becomes manifested at 0.1 to 0.2 mg/kg.[415,416] This could explain the occurrence of occasional severe bronchospasm in patients after receiving vecuronium.[417-419]

The goals of treatment of anaphylactic reactions are to correct arterial hypoxemia, inhibit further release of chemical mediators, and restore intravascular volume. One hundred percent oxygen and intravenous epinephrine, 10 to 20 µg/kg, should be administered immediately. Early tracheal intubation with a cuffed tracheal tube should be considered in patients with rapidly developing angioedema. Fluids (crystalloid or colloid solutions, or both) must be administered concurrently. Norepinephrine or a sympathomimetic drug (phenylephrine) may also be necessary to maintain perfusion pressure until intravascular fluid volume can be restored. Dysrhythmias should be treated. The use of antihistamines and steroids is controversial.

DRUG INTERACTIONS AND OTHER FACTORS AFFECTING RESPONSE TO NEUROMUSCULAR BLOCKERS

A drug-drug interaction is an in vivo phenomenon that occurs when the administration of one drug alters the effects or kinetics of another drug. In vitro physical or chemical incompatibilities are *not* considered drug interactions.[420]

Mechanisms of Drug Interactions

Pharmacokinetic interactions are interactions in which one drug alters the rate or amount of absorption, distribution, metabolism, or excretion of another drug (or any combination of these processes).

Pharmacodynamic interactions occur when the dose-response relationship of a drug is altered by the coadministration of a second drug. These interactions are generally described as being *synergistic, antagonistic,* or *additive.*

Many drugs have been shown to interact with neuromuscular blockers or their antagonists, or both, and it is beyond the scope of this chapter to review them all. The reader is referred to reviews on drug interactions for more detailed information.[420-423] Some of the more important drug interactions are discussed in the following sections.

Interactions among Nondepolarizing Neuromuscular Blockers

Mixtures of two nondepolarizing neuromuscular blockers are considered to be either (1) additive when the effect is the sum of equipotent doses of either drug given alone or (2) synergistic when the effect of the mixture is greater than the equipotent dose of either drug. Antagonistic interactions have not been reported in this class of drugs.

Additive interactions have been demonstrated after the administration of chemically related agents such as atracurium-mivacurium,[424] atracurium-cisatracurium,[425] or various pairs of steroidal neuromuscular blockers.[179,426-428] On the other hand, combinations of structurally dissimilar (a steroidal with a benzylisoquinolinium) neuromuscular blockers, for example, pancuronium-dTc,[429] pancuronium-metocurine,[429] rocuronium-mivacurium,[251] rocuronium-cisatracurium,[212] and pancuronium-mivacurium,[430] produce a synergistic (potentiating) response.

The administration of two neuromuscular blockers in combination was first introduced by Lebowitz and colleagues[429] in an attempt to reduce the cardiovascular side effects of neuromuscular blockers by giving smaller doses of each drug as a combination.[429] Additional advantage (rapid onset and short duration) is noted for mivacurium-rocuronium combinations.[251] Although the precise mechanisms underlying a synergistic interaction are not known, hypotheses that have been put forward include (1) the existence of multiple binding sites at the neuromuscular junction (presynaptic and postsynaptic receptors)[431] and (2) nonequivalence of binding affinities of the two α-subunits (α_H and α_L) (see the section "Principles of Action of Neuromuscular Blockers at the Neuromuscular Junction"). Furthermore, inhibition of butyrylcholinesterase by pancuronium results in decreased plasma clearance of mivacurium and marked potentiation of neuromuscular blockade.[432]

It should be noted that the pharmacodynamic response after the use of two different nondepolarizing blockers in the course of anesthesia depends not only on the specific drugs used but also on the sequence of their administration. It has been shown that the effect of a maintenance dose of vecuronium given during recovery from an initial dose of either pipecuronium[433] or pancuronium[434,435] is dependent on the neuromuscular blocker that was used initially. Approximately three half-lives will be required for a clinical changeover (so that 95% of the first drug has been cleared) and for the duration of block to begin to take on the characteristics of the second drug. Smith and White[433] noted that the mean duration of a maintenance dose of vecuronium was significantly longer after pipecuronium (40 minutes) than after vecuronium (29 minutes) and was similar to that of pipecuronium after pipecuronium (49 minutes). After pipecuronium, they detected clinically significant prolongation after four maintenance doses of vecuronium.[433] After pancuronium, it has been reported that recovery from the first two maintenance doses of vecuronium is prolonged; however, this effect becomes negligible by the third dose.[434] Similarly, Naguib and coworkers[424] noted that the mean duration of the first maintenance dose of mivacurium to 10% recovery of the first twitch was significantly greater after atracurium (25 minutes) than after mivacurium (14.2 minutes). However, the duration of the second maintenance dose of mivacurium after atracurium (18.3 minutes) was similar to that of mivacurium after mivacurium (14.6 minutes).

The apparent prolongation of action of the first maintenance dose of mivacurium administered after atracurium[424] and those reported with vecuronium after pancuronium[434,435] or pipecuronium[433] is not related to synergism. Combinations of atracurium and mivacurium[424] and combinations of vecuronium and pancuronium or pipecuronium[179,426] are simply additive. However, this prolongation in duration of action could be attributed to the relative concentrations of these drugs at the receptor site. Because most receptors remain occupied by the drug administered initially, the clinical profile depends on the kinetics/dynamics of the drug administered first rather than on that of the second (maintenance) drug. However, with further incremental doses of the second drug, a progressively larger proportion of the receptors are occupied by the second drug, and the clinical profile of that drug becomes evident.

Interaction between Succinylcholine and Nondepolarizing Neuromuscular Blockers

The interaction between succinylcholine and nondepolarizing neuromuscular blockers depends on the order of administration and the doses used.[155,436-438] Administration of small doses of different nondepolarizing neuromuscular blockers before succinylcholine to prevent fasciculations has an antagonistic effect on development of the subsequent depolarizing block produced by succinylcholine.[63,155] Therefore, it is recommended that the dose of succinylcholine be increased after the administration of a defasciculating dose of a nondepolarizing neuromuscular blocker.[63,439]

Studies on the effects of administration of succinylcholine before nondepolarizing neuromuscular blockers have produced conflicting results. Several investigators reported potentiation of the effects of dTc,[440] pancuronium,[437] and vecuronium and atracurium[438,441] by previous administration of succinylcholine. In contrast, others noted the opposite for dTc[436] or found no significant influence of succinylcholine on subsequent administration of pancuronium, doxacurium, pipecuronium, rocuronium, or mivacurium.[155,442-445]

Inhaled Anesthetics

Deep anesthesia with potent volatile anesthetics (in the absence of neuromuscular blockade) may cause a slight reduction in neuromuscular transmission, as measured by depression of sensitive indicators of clinical neuromuscular function such as tetanus and TOF responses.[446] Inhaled anesthetics also potentiate the neuromuscular blocking effect of nondepolarizing neuromuscular blockers. This potentiation results mainly in a decrease in the dosage requirement of the neuromuscular blocker and prolongation of both the duration of action of the relaxant and recovery from neuromuscular blockade.[447,448] The magnitude of potentiation depends on several factors, including the duration of anesthesia,[446,449-452] the specific inhaled anesthetic,[196,453] and the concentration used.[454] The rank of order of potentiation is desflurane > sevoflurane > isoflurane > halothane > nitrous oxide–barbiturate–opioid or propofol anesthesia (Fig. 13-26).[455-458]

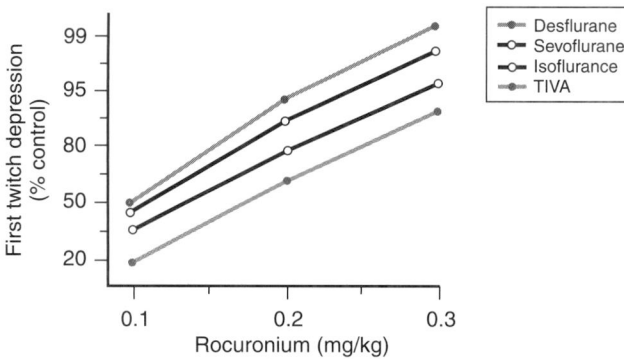

Figure 13–26 Cumulative dose-response curves for rocuronium-induced neuromuscular block during 1.5 MAC anesthesia with desflurane, sevoflurane, isoflurane, and total intravenous anesthesia. (Redrawn from Wulf H, Ledowski T, Linstedt U, et al: Neuromuscular blocking effects of rocuronium during desflurane, isoflurane, and sevoflurane anaesthesia. Can J Anaesth 45:526-532, 1998.)

The more intense clinical muscle-relaxing effect produced by less potent anesthetics is mainly caused by their larger aqueous concentrations.[459] Desflurane and sevoflurane have low blood/gas and tissue/gas solubility, so equilibration between the end-tidal concentration and the neuromuscular junction is reached more rapidly with these agents than with other inhaled anesthetics.[460,461]

The interaction between volatile anesthetics and neuromuscular blockers is a pharmacodynamic (and not a pharmacokinetic) interaction.[247,448] Proposed mechanisms include (1) a central effect on α-motor neurons and interneuron synapses,[462] (2) inhibition of the postsynaptic nAChR,[463-465] and (3) augmentation of the antagonist affinity at the receptor site.[459]

Antibiotics

Most antibiotics can cause neuromuscular blockade in the absence of neuromuscular blocking drugs.[466] The aminoglycoside group of antibiotics, such as polymyxins, lincomycin, and clindamycin, primarily inhibit the prejunctional release of acetylcholine and also depress postjunctional nAChR sensitivity to acetylcholine.[467-469] Tetracyclines, on the other hand, exhibit postjunctional activity only.[468,470-472] When combined with neuromuscular blockers, the aforementioned antibiotics can potentiate neuromuscular blockade.[473,474] Cephalosporins and penicillins have not been reported to potentiate neuromuscular blockade. Antagonism of neuromuscular blockade has been reported to be more difficult after the administration of aminoglycosides.[475,476] Ventilation should be controlled until the neuromuscular blockade terminates spontaneously. Calcium should not be used to hasten recovery of neuromuscular function for two reasons: the antagonism that it produces is not sustained, and it may prevent the antibacterial effect of the antibiotic. Administration of 4-aminopyridine might be of value in these situations.[474]

Temperature

Hypothermia prolongs the duration of action of nondepolarizing neuromuscular blockers.[477-479] The force of contraction of the adductor pollicis decreases by 10% to 16% per degree centigrade decrease in muscle temperature below 35.2°C.[480,481] To maintain muscle temperature above 35.2°C, central temperature must be maintained at 36.0°C.[477] The recovery to 10% twitch height with 0.1 mg/kg vecuronium increases from 28 minutes at a mean central temperature of 36.4°C to 64 minutes at 34.4°C.[477]

The mechanism or mechanisms underlying this prolongation may be pharmacodynamic, pharmacokinetic, or both[479] and include diminished renal and hepatic excretion, changing drug volumes of distribution, altered local diffusion receptor affinity, changes in pH at the neuromuscular junction, and the net effect of cooling on the various components of neuromuscular transmission.[477,482-485] Hypothermia decreases plasma clearance and prolongs the duration of action of rocuronium and vecuronium.[479,486] Temperature-related differences in the pharmacodynamics of vecuronium have been reported. The k_{e0} decreased (0.023/min/°C) with lower temperature, thus suggesting slightly delayed equilibration of drug between the circulation and the neuromuscular junction during hypothermia.[479] The Hofmann elimination process of atracurium is slowed by a decrease in pH and especially by a decrease in temperature.[9,487] In fact, atracurium's duration of action is markedly prolonged by hypothermia.[478] For instance, the duration of action of 0.5 mg/kg atracurium is 44 minutes at 37°C and 68 minutes at 34.0°C.[478] Decreases in temperature also decrease the speed of neural conduction in humans.[488] A decrease in muscle temperature from 35°C to 23.5°C resulted in a 50% reduction in nerve conduction velocity.[488]

Changes in temperature will affect interpretation of the results of monitoring neuromuscular blockade. The duration of action of vecuronium measured in an arm cooled to a skin temperature of 27°C is prolonged, and monitoring by post-tetanic count in that arm is unreliable.[489] In the same patient, TOF responses are different if the arms are at different temperatures, and correlation of responses in the two arms becomes progressively poorer as the temperature difference between the arms increases.[490,491]

The efficacy of neostigmine is not altered by mild hypothermia.[492-494] Hypothermia does not change the clearance, maximum effect, or duration of action of neostigmine in volunteers.[494]

Magnesium and Calcium

Magnesium sulfate, given for the treatment of preeclampsia and eclamptic toxemia, potentiates the neuromuscular block induced by nondepolarizing neuromuscular blockers.[495-500] After a dose of 40 mg/kg magnesium sulfate, the ED_{50} of vecuronium was reduced by 25%, onset time was nearly halved, and recovery time just about doubled.[497] Neostigmine-induced recovery is also attenuated in patients treated with magnesium.[498,501] The mechanisms underlying the enhancement of nondepolarizing blockade by magnesium probably involve both prejunctional and postjunctional effects. High magnesium concentrations inhibit calcium channels at presynaptic nerve terminals that trigger the release of acetylcholine.[17] Furthermore, magnesium ions have an inhibitory effect on postjunctional potentials and cause a decrease in muscle fiber membrane excitability.[502] In patients receiving magnesium, the dose of nondepolarizing neuromuscular blocker must be reduced and carefully titrated by a nerve stimulator to ensure adequate recovery of neuromuscular function at the end of surgery.

The interaction of magnesium with succinylcholine is controversial. Initial studies suggested potentiation of depolarizing blockade[503] or no significant effect.[504] However, one study suggests that magnesium may antagonize the block produced by succinylcholine.[505]

Calcium triggers acetylcholine release from the motor nerve terminal and enhances excitation-contraction coupling in muscle.[17] Increasing calcium concentrations decreased the sensitivity to dTc and pancuronium in a muscle-nerve model.[506] In hyperparathyroidism, hypercalcemia is associated with decreased sensitivity to atracurium and a shortened time course of neuromuscular blockade.[507]

Lithium

Lithium remains the drug of choice for the treatment of bipolar affective disorder (manic-depressive illness). The lithium ion resembles sodium, potassium, magnesium, and calcium ions and may therefore affect the distribution and kinetics of all these electrolytes.[508,509] Lithium enters cells through sodium channels and tends to accumulate within cells.

Lithium, by activation of potassium channels, inhibits neuromuscular transmission presynaptically and muscular contraction postsynaptically.[510] The combination of lithium and pipecuronium resulted in a synergistic inhibition of neuromuscular transmission, whereas the combination of lithium and succinylcholine resulted in an additive inhibition.[510,511] Prolongation of neuromuscular blockade was reported in patients receiving lithium carbonate and both depolarizing[512,513] and nondepolarizing neuromuscular blockers.[513-516] Only one report did not demonstrate prolongation of recovery from succinylcholine in patients receiving lithium.[517] In patients undergoing surgery who are stabilized on lithium therapy, neuromuscular blockers should be administered in incremental and reduced doses and titrated to the degree of block required.

Local Anesthetics and Antidysrhythmics

Local anesthetics have actions on the presynaptic, postsynaptic, and muscle membranes. In large intravenous doses, most local anesthetics block neuromuscular transmission; in smaller doses, they enhance the neuromuscular block from both nondepolarizing and depolarizing neuromuscular blockers.[518,519] The ability of neostigmine to antagonize a combined local anesthetic–neuromuscular blockade has not been studied. Procaine also inhibits butyrylcholinesterase and may augment the effects of succinylcholine and mivacurium by decreasing their hydrolysis by the enzyme.

In small intravenous doses, local anesthetics depress post-tetanic potentiation, and this depression is thought to be a neural, prejunctional effect.[520] At higher doses, local anesthetics block acetylcholine-induced muscular contractions, which suggests that local anesthetics have a stabilizing effect on the postjunctional membrane.[521] Procaine has been shown to displace calcium from the sarcolemma and thus inhibit caffeine-induced contracture of skeletal muscle.[522] Most of these mechanisms of action probably apply to all the local anesthetics.

Several drugs used for the treatment of dysrhythmias augment the block from neuromuscular blockers, particularly that of dTc.[523] Quinidine potentiates the neuromuscular block from both nondepolarizing and depolarizing neuromuscular blockers.[524] Edrophonium is ineffective in antagonizing a nondepolarizing blockade after quinidine. In clinical doses, quinidine appears to act at the prejunctional membrane as judged by its lack of effect on acetylcholine-evoked twitch.

In a rat phrenic-hemidiaphragm preparation, Salvador and coworkers[525] showed substantial potentiation of succinylcholine by diltiazem or verapamil and potentiation of pancuronium by nicardipine. These interactions were not found in humans.[526,527] Clinical reports have suggested potentiation of neuromuscular blockade with verapamil[528] and impaired reversal of vecuronium in a patient receiving disopyramide.[529] The clinical significance of these interactions is probably minor.

Antiepileptic Drugs

Anticonvulsants have a depressant action on acetylcholine release at the neuromuscular junction.[530-533] Patients receiving chronic anticonvulsant therapy demonstrated resistance to nondepolarizing muscle blockers (except mivacurium[534] and probably atracurium as well[533,535]), as evidenced by accelerated recovery from neuromuscular blockade and the need for increased doses to achieve a complete neuromuscular block.[536-538] Vecuronium clearance is increased twofold in patients receiving chronic carbamazepine therapy.[539] Others, however, have attributed this resistance to increased binding (decreased free fraction) of the neuromuscular blockers to α_1-acid glycoproteins or upregulation of neuromuscular acetylcholine receptors, or a combination of both mechanisms.[540] The latter could also explain the hypersensitivity seen with succinylcholine.[541] The slight prolongation of succinylcholine action in patients taking anticonvulsants has few clinical implications. On the other hand, the potential hyperkalemic response to succinylcholine in the presence of receptor upregulation is of concern.

Diuretics

In patients undergoing renal transplantation, the intensity and duration of dTc neuromuscular blockade is increased after a dose of furosemide (1 mg/kg intravenously).[542] Furosemide reduced the concentration of dTc required to achieve 50% depression of twitch tension in the indirectly stimulated rat diaphragm and intensified the neuromuscular blockade produced by dTc and succinylcholine.[543] Furosemide appears to inhibit the production of cyclic adenosine monophosphate. Breakdown of adenosine triphosphate is inhibited and results in reduced output of acetylcholine. Acetazolamide has been found to antagonize the effects of anticholinesterases in the rat phrenic-diaphragm preparation.[544] However, in one report, 1 mg/kg furosemide facilitated recovery of the evoked twitch response after pancuronium.[545] Chronic furosemide treatment had no effect on either dTc- or pancuronium-induced neuromuscular blockade.[546]

By contrast, mannitol appears to have no effect on nondepolarizing neuromuscular blockade. Furthermore, increasing urine output by the administration of mannitol or other osmotic or tubular diuretics has no effect on the rate at which dTc and presumably other neuromuscular blockers are eliminated in urine.[230] However, this lack of effect on excretion of dTc should not be surprising. Urinary excretion of all neuromuscular blockers that are long acting depends primarily on glomerular filtration. Mannitol is an osmotic diuretic that exerts its effects by altering the osmotic gradient within the proximal tubules so that water is retained within the tubules. An increase in urine volume in patients with adequate glomerular filtration therefore would not be expected to increase the excretion of neuromuscular blockers.

Other Drugs

Dantrolene (see Chapter 29), a drug used for the treatment of malignant hyperthermia, prevents Ca^{2+} release from the sarcoplasmic reticulum and blocks excitation-contraction coupling. Although it does not block neuromuscular transmission, the mechanical response to stimulation will be depressed without demonstrating any effect on the electromyogram.[547,548] The effects of nondepolarizing neuromuscular blockers are enhanced by dantrolene.[157]

Azathioprine, an immunodepressant drug used in renal transplantation, has a minor antagonistic action on muscle relaxant–induced neuromuscular blockade.[549,550]

Steroids antagonize the effects of nondepolarizing neuromuscular blockers in humans.[551,552] Animal studies have also demonstrated resistance to the effects of dTc in the presence of prednisolone, dexamethasone, betamethasone, and triamcinolone.[553-555] Possible mechanisms for this interaction include (1) facilitation of acetylcholine release as a result of the effect of steroids on the presynaptic motor nerve terminal[556] or (2) channel blockade of the nAChR.[557] It should be noted that endogenous steroids act noncompetitively on nAChRs.[558] Prolonged treatment—combining corticosteroids with neuromuscular blocking drugs—can result in prolonged weakness (see the section "Neuromuscular Blockers and Weakness Syndromes in the Critically Ill").

Antiestrogenic drugs such as tamoxifen appear to potentiate the effects of nondepolarizing neuromuscular blockers.[559]

RECOVERY FROM NEUROMUSCULAR BLOCKADE

In the 1970s, Ali and coauthors[560,561] described a TOF ratio of 0.60 as being indicative of adequate recovery of neuromuscular strength. As described in the section "Monitoring Neuromuscular Function," with a TOF ratio

of 0.6 to 0.7, patients will have, on average, a vital capacity of 55 mL/kg, a negative inspiratory force of 70 cm H_2O, and a peak expiratory flow of 95% of control values. This degree of recovery should allow for normal respiratory function[57] and maintenance of a patent airway. More recently, though, a TOF ratio of 0.70 in unanesthetized volunteers has been associated with difficulty speaking and swallowing, weakness of the facial musculature, visual disturbances, and an inability to sit up without assistance.[54] Administration of small doses of nondepolarizing neuromuscular blockers (one tenth of an intubating dose) as a defasciculating or precurarizing dose may cause appreciable decreases in the TOF response.[280,562] These small doses of neuromuscular blockers may be associated with general discomfort, malaise, difficulty swallowing, ptosis, and blurred vision. Recent studies in volunteers have shown that TOF ratios of 0.6 to 0.7 are associated with decreased upper esophageal tone and a decrease in coordination of the esophageal musculature during swallowing.[563,564] Fluoroscopic study of these individuals demonstrated significant pharyngeal dysfunction resulting in a fourfold to fivefold increase in the risk of aspiration. With recovery of the TOF ratio to 0.9, esophageal tone and pharyngeal coordination return toward baseline.

Residual paralysis also decreases the hypoxic ventilatory drive (Fig. 13-27).[565,566] This effect appears to be due to inhibition of the carotid body neural response to hypoxia.[567] Vecuronium decreases carotid sinus nerve activity in response to hypoxia in a dose-related fashion, presumably through its interaction with neural nicotinic receptors.

After the administration of nondepolarizing neuromuscular blocking drugs, it is essential to ensure adequate return of normal neuromuscular function. Whether that degree of recovery is a TOF ratio of 0.7, 0.8, or 0.9 is an area of debate.[568] Certainly, the clinician's ability to quantify the degree of residual neuromuscular block is limited (as described in the section "Monitoring Neuromuscular Function"). Kopman and colleagues' work in volunteers demonstrated that when they could oppose their incisors to retain a tongue depressor, their TOF ratio was, on average, 0.8 and at least 0.68.[54] This test of muscle strength, however, would be of limited usefulness in an intubated patient.

Recovery from muscle relaxation caused by nondepolarizing neuromuscular blockers is dependent on several factors. Primarily, it depends on an increase in the acetylcholine concentration relative to that of the relaxant to overcome the competitive neuromuscular block. The relative increase in acetylcholine concentration depends first on the ongoing movement of relaxant from the motor end plate into the central circulation and then on its elimination from the circulating blood volume so that it is not free to move into the synaptic cleft. Ultimately, recovery depends on elimination of the neuromuscular blocker from the body. Neuromuscular blockers may be eliminated from the body through a host of mechanisms, including excretion as unchanged drug in urine, metabolism in the liver, enzymatic hydrolysis, and chemical breakdown. Although it has never been specifically examined, several manuscripts have, through their ranges

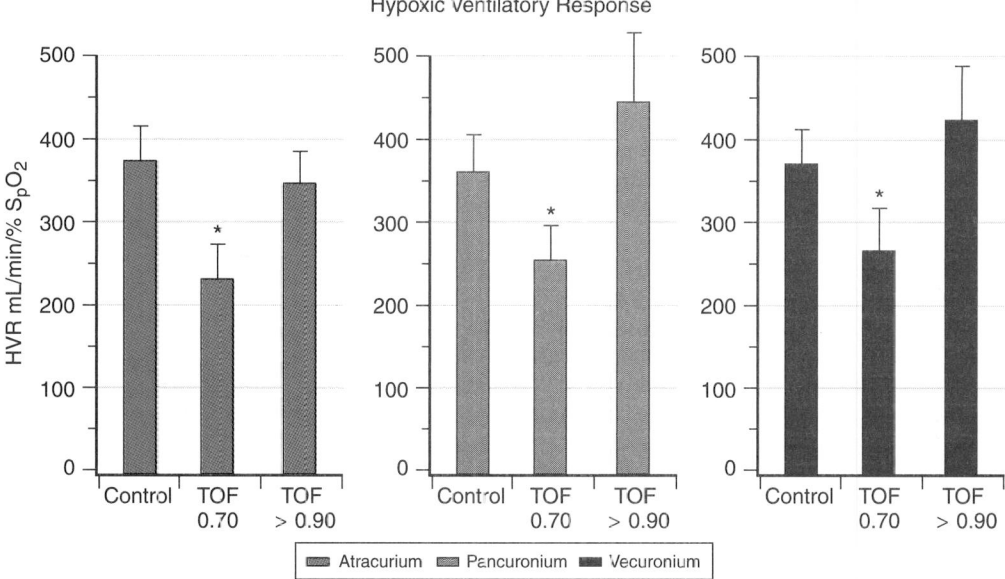

Figure 13–27 Hypoxic ventilatory response (HVR) before (control), during steady-state infusion (train-of-four [TOF] ratio = 0.07) of atracurium, pancuronium and vecuronium, and after recovery (TOF > 0.90). Data are presented as means ± SD. *P < .01. (Redrawn from Eriksson LI: Reduced hypoxic chemosensitivity in partially paralysed man. A new property of muscle relaxants? Acta Anaesthesiol Scand 40:520-523, 1996.)

of recovery parameters, described a wide range of inter-patient variability in spontaneous recovery of neuromuscular function.[569-571] With administration of repeated doses of a drug that relies on the kidney or the liver for its elimination from the body, plasma concentrations of the drug increase during recovery of neuromuscular function.[227,235] This increase is probably due to the fact that recovery of neuromuscular function after administration of these neuromuscular blockers occurs as the relaxant is redistributed to storage sites in the body rather than during elimination of the compound. This mechanism is in contrast to the plasma concentrations of a neuromuscular blocker such as atracurium during recovery of neuromuscular function and subsequent redosing.[227,235] In this case, plasma concentrations of the neuromuscular blocker during recovery consistently return to the same level.

Several factors in addition to coexisting disease will have an impact on the speed of spontaneous recovery of neuromuscular function. The presence of volatile anesthetics will potentiate any existing neuromuscular block and, presumably, render recovery more prolonged.[572] If the anesthesiologist observes no or minimal recovery of neuromuscular function in the presence of a volatile anesthetic, discontinuing or decreasing the concentration of inhaled anesthetic being administered should augment recovery of neuromuscular function.

As will be discussed later, acidosis, hypokalemia, hypothermia, and concomitant medications will all potentiate residual neuromuscular blockade and render pharmacologic antagonism more difficult.

Antagonism of Residual Neuromuscular Blockade

Anticholinesterases act by inhibiting the enzyme acetylcholinesterase. Acetylcholinesterase (enzyme classification 3.1.1.7) is a type B carboxylesterase. At the neuromuscular junction, it occurs in the asymmetric or A12 form, which consists of three tetramers of catalytic subunits covalently linked to a collagen-like tail.[573]

Acetylcholinesterase has a powerful catalytic capacity.[29] It can catalyze 4000 molecules of acetylcholine per active site per second.[29] Nearly half of the released acetylcholine is hydrolyzed across the synaptic cleft before reaching nAChRs. The active site lies deep inside the enzyme protein.[574] For a detailed account of this enzyme, see Soreq and Seidman.[575]

The active surface of acetylcholinesterase is best viewed as having two sites: (1) the anionic site, which is concerned with binding and orienting the substrate molecule, and (2) the esteratic site, which is responsible for the hydrolytic process.[576] A second "anionic" site, known as the "peripheral" anionic site, was also proposed.[577]

Three anticholinesterases, neostigmine, edrophonium, and pyridostigmine, are used to antagonize residual neuromuscular blockade. They exert their effect primarily by increasing the concentration of acetylcholine at the motor end plate by inhibiting acetylcholinesterase. Neostigmine and pyridostigmine are oxydiaphoretic (acid transferring) inhibitors of acetylcholinesterase. Neostigmine and pyridostigmine transfer a carbamate group to the acetylcholinesterase, which forms a covalent bond at the esteratic site. Edrophonium binds to the anionic site on acetylcholinesterase by electrostatic attraction and to the esteratic subsite by hydrogen bonding.[578] In addition, anticholinesterases may also increase the release of acetylcholine from presynaptic nerve terminals, block neural potassium channels, and have a direct agonist effect.[27] Details of the mechanisms of action of these anticholinesterases have been described in review articles.[579,580]

Major Determinants of Speed and Adequacy of Reversal

Antagonism of nondepolarizing blockade is time dependent. Reversal occurs at a rate that depends primarily on five factors: (1) the depth of block at the time of administration of the antagonist, (2) the antagonist administered,

(3) the dose of antagonist, (4) the rate of spontaneous recovery from the neuromuscular blocker, and (5) the concentration of the inhaled anesthetic present during reversal.

Depth of Block

As was shown with the long-acting neuromuscular blocker pancuronium, more time is required to antagonize profound levels of block than lesser levels of block.[254,581,582] Antagonism of pancuronium blockade with 2.5 mg (about 35 μg/kg) of neostigmine shows that the relationship of reversal time to depth of blockade is hyperbolic, with a "knee" in the curve occurring at 80% to 90% twitch inhibition (Fig. 13-28). Lesser degrees of block are associated with more rapid recovery of neuromuscular function. Recovery of single-twitch height from deep levels of neuromuscular blockade requires, as demonstrated in these older studies, 15 to 30 minutes. Recovery of the TOF ratio occurs more slowly than that of a single twitch. Therefore, even more time will be required for recovery to a TOF ratio of more than 0.7 when blockade by long-acting drugs is being antagonized.

Interestingly, a study by Bevan and coworkers[583] demonstrated that antagonism of $1.5 \times ED_{95}$ doses of vecuronium- or rocuronium-induced block occurred at the same rate regardless of the timing of administration of the 70 μg/kg neostigmine. Neostigmine shortened recovery, whether administered at 1%, 10%, or 25% spontaneous recovery, by approximately 40%. As shown in Figure 13-29, the time from administration of the neuromuscular blocker to TOF ratios of 0.7 and 0.9 was not decreased, though, because the extent of spontaneous recovery at the time of neostigmine administration increased. Recovery to TOF ratios of 0.7 and 0.9 required, on average, 25 and 30 minutes, respectively. Recommendations regarding the timing of administration of anticholinesterase remain unclear. However, because the time from administration of the anticholinesterase to full recovery is shortened by waiting for a greater degree of spontaneous recovery before administering the anticholinesterase, it would seem prudent to not administer the anticholinesterase at the earliest

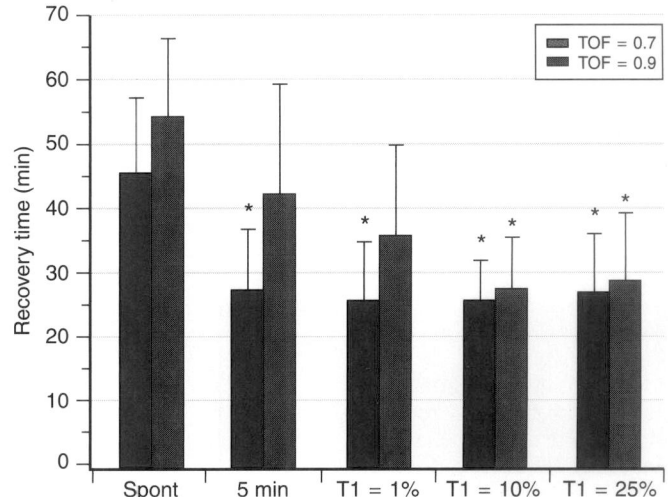

Figure 13–29 Recovery times (mean ± SD) after administration of a single dose of 0.45 mg/kg ($1.5 \times ED_{95}$) rocuronium. In one group (Spont), spontaneous recovery is allowed. In the remaining groups, 70 μg/kg neostigmine is administered 5 minutes after rocuronium or at 1%, 10%, and 25% recovery of the first twitch (T1) from its control value. *$P < 0.01$ versus spontaneous recovery. Note that times to attain a train-of-four ratio of 0.9 are significantly shorter when neostigmine is administered at T1 = 10% or 25% of control tension. (Figure constructed based on data redrawn from Bevan JC, Collins L, Fowler C, et al: Early and late reversal of rocuronium and vecuronium with neostigmine in adults and children. Anesth Analg 89:333-339, 1999.)

degrees of recovery. Kirkegaard and colleagues[584] recently demonstrated that to recover to a TOF ratio of 0.7 within 10 minutes of administering neostigmine, three or four responses to TOF stimulation had to be present at the time of neostigmine administration. If only one response to TOF stimulation were present, recovery to a TOF ratio of 0.7 required up to 23 minutes.

The maximum antagonistic effect of neostigmine occurs in 10 minutes or less.[585,586] If adequate recovery does not occur within this time, subsequent recovery is slow and requires ongoing elimination of the neuromuscular blocker from plasma. For profound vecuronium-induced blockade in which no twitch recovery has occurred, administration of neostigmine, 70 μg/kg, produces an initial reversal that falls far short of adequate recovery.[571] Subsequent recovery is at the same rate as spontaneous recovery and is due to the decrease in plasma concentration of vecuronium as the drug is eliminated.[571,587] Administration of a second dose of neostigmine has no further effect on recovery[571] because acetylcholinesterase is already maximally inhibited.

If the block at the time of neostigmine administration is sufficiently deep that adequate recovery does not occur within 10 minutes, the time at which full recovery of neuromuscular function will occur depends on the inherent duration of action of the neuromuscular blocker.[582] With drugs that have a long duration of action, this period of inadequate neuromuscular function can be 30 to 60 minutes or longer, whereas with drugs that have an intermediate duration of action, it will be much shorter (i.e., 15 to 30 minutes).[60]

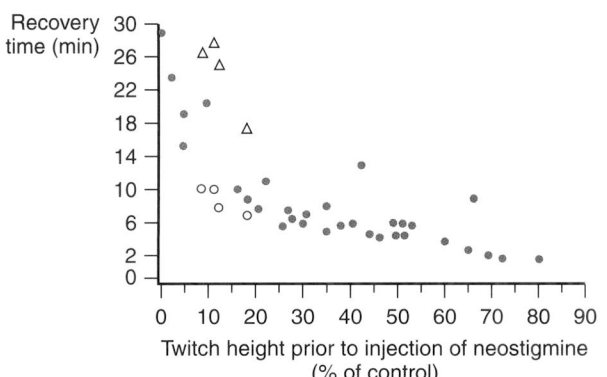

Figure 13–28 Correlation between twitch height when a bolus of neostigmine (2.5 mg) was given intravenously and the time that it took for twitch height to return to its control height. (Redrawn from Katz RL: Clinical neuromuscular pharmacology of pancuronium. Anesthesiology 34:550-556, 1971.)

The Anticholinesterase Administered

Under conditions of moderate depth of blockade (such as two to three twitches palpable by TOF monitoring), the order of rapidity of antagonism of residual blockade by anticholinesterases is edrophonium > neostigmine > pyridostigmine.[585,588] For this reason and because of its lesser atropine requirement, edrophonium regained popularity as an antagonist during the 1980s.[585] However, Rupp and coworkers[589] found that edrophonium is not as effective as neostigmine in antagonizing profound blockade of greater than 90% twitch depression (only one twitch palpable by TOF). Although increasing the edrophonium dose from 0.5 to 1.0 mg/kg increases its efficacy, neostigmine remains capable of more complete antagonism.[589] To be equivalent to 40 µg/kg neostigmine as an antagonist of profound vecuronium blockade, 1.5 mg/kg of edrophonium has to be administered.[590]

The relative potencies of edrophonium and neostigmine differ at various intensities of blockade (Fig. 13-30).[591] Edrophonium becomes less potent with respect to neostigmine as the depth of blockade becomes more intense. In other words, the dose-response curves are not parallel and become increasingly divergent as the depth of blockade intensifies. This difference indicates that edrophonium may be less effective than neostigmine when antagonizing very deep levels of blockade.

The Dose of Anticholinesterase

Larger doses of anticholinesterases should antagonize neuromuscular blockade more rapidly and more completely than smaller doses do. This relationship is true up to the point of the maximum effective dose, beyond which further amounts of anticholinesterase will not produce any further antagonism. For neostigmine, this maximum dosage is in the range 60 to 80 µg/kg[571,592]; for edrophonium, the range is 1.0 to 1.5 mg/kg.[589,590]

Donati and associates[593] studied the reversal of 90% block induced by either dTc or pancuronium to demonstrate the relationship of the dose of neostigmine to the speed of reversal. They showed that increasingly greater amounts of antagonism of neuromuscular block occurred over the course of 10 minutes as the neostigmine dosage was increased from 5 to 50 µg/kg. Even after 50 µg/kg, however, twitch had recovered to only 80% of normal strength 10 minutes after neostigmine administration.

Mixing or combining antagonists is not advisable. Neostigmine and edrophonium do not potentiate each other; in fact, their effects in combination may not even be additive.[594,595] Therefore, when inadequate reversal occurs, one should not be tempted to add a different anticholinesterase but should ensure only that the maximum dose of the original drug has been administered. Ventilation should then be supported until adequate neuromuscular function is achieved.

Rate of Spontaneous Recovery from the Neuromuscular Blocker

After administration of an anticholinesterase, two processes contribute to recovery of neuromuscular function. The first is antagonism induced by the effect of the anticholinesterase at the neuromuscular junction; the second is the natural process of decrease in the plasma concentration of the neuromuscular blocker (and hence the concentration of the neuromuscular blocker at the neuromuscular junction).[582,587] Therefore, the more rapid the elimination of the neuromuscular blocker, the faster the recovery of adequate neuromuscular function after the administration of an antagonist (Fig. 13-31).[596] A clear illustration of this principle is the difference in antagonizing a block induced by neuromuscular blockers with an intermediate versus a long duration of action. Plasma concentrations of drugs with an intermediate duration of action decrease more rapidly than do concentrations of drugs with a long duration of action,[245] and consequently

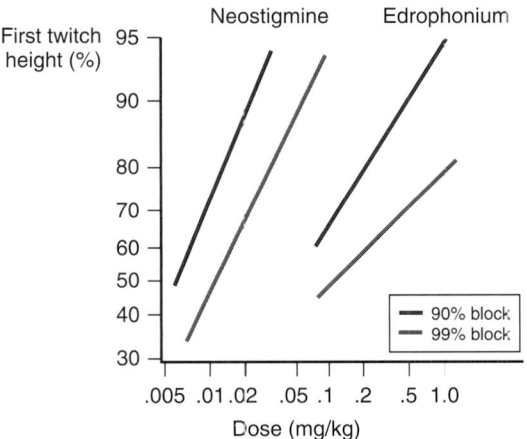

Figure 13–30 First twitch height (logit scale) versus dose (log scale) 10 minutes after administration of neostigmine and edrophonium given at either 1% (99% block) or 10% (90% block) recovery of the first twitch. (Redrawn from Donati F, Smith CE, Bevan DR: Dose-response relationships for edrophonium and neostigmine as antagonists of moderate and profound atracurium blockade. Anesth Analg 68:13-19, 1989.)

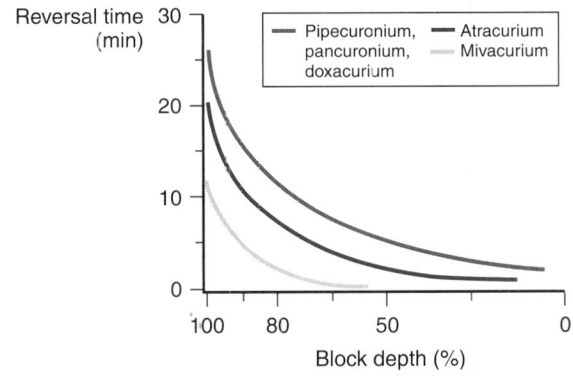

Figure 13–31 Comparative mean speed of antagonism by neostigmine of neuromuscular blockade induced by long-acting drugs (doxacurium, pancuronium, pipecuronium), intermediate-acting drugs (atracurium and others), and the short-acting drug mivacurium. Antagonism is more rapid as processes of clearance increase (see text). (Redrawn from Savarese JJ: Reversal of nondepolarizing blocks: More controversial than ever? Review Course Lectures, 67th Congress, Cleveland, Ohio, International Anesthesia Research Society, 1993.)

recovery of neuromuscular function is more rapid.[586,594,595] The incidence of inadequate neuromuscular function in the postoperative period is less with intermediate-acting than with long-acting neuromuscular blockers.[59,60] Nevertheless, the blocks from *all* intermediate-acting muscle relaxants should be reversed with an anticholinesterase drug.[597] Because of the inability to detect subtle neuromuscular blocks clinically and persistence in the recovery room, pharmacologic reversal should be routine.[598]

The interaction of spontaneous recovery and anticholinesterase-induced reversal of mivacurium is more complex. The rate of spontaneous recovery from mivacurium-induced blockade is more rapid than that from any other nondepolarizing neuromuscular blocker because of its rapid hydrolysis by butyrylcholinesterase. Neostigmine-induced reversal of mivacurium is similar to or faster than that of atracurium.[315,599] During profound (<3% twitch recovery) mivacurium-induced blockade, administration of neostigmine may possibly prolong recovery.[600] Neostigmine has two major effects relevant to mivacurium. First, it inhibits acetylcholinesterase at the neuromuscular junction, thereby effectively increasing the acetylcholine concentration and facilitating recovery. Second, it inhibits butyrylcholinesterase, the enzyme responsible for the metabolism of mivacurium, and slows the normally rapid decrease in plasma concentration of mivacurium.[601,602] In contrast, edrophonium is not as potent an inhibitor of butyrylcholinesterase,[601,603] and it should have little effect on the metabolism of mivacurium. Provided that there is 10% recovery of the twitch response (one twitch in the TOF), either neostigmine, 20 to 40 µg/kg, or edrophonium, 0.3 to 0.5 mg/kg, will accelerate recovery from mivacurium.[579,599,604]

It has been suggested that routine administration of an anticholinesterase may often be omitted because spontaneous recovery from mivacurium is so rapid.[605] However, this strategy may lead to inadequate recovery and postoperative weakness unless at least 20 minutes is allowed for spontaneous recovery.[599,604] As indicated earlier, administration of an anticholinesterase drug should probably be routine.[598]

Because mivacurium is metabolized by butyrylcholinesterase, recovery, in theory, may be made more rapid by the administration of exogenous human butyrylcholinesterase. Administration of purified human cholinesterase does produce some antagonism of mivacurium-induced blockade,[606] but it is ineffective in a profound block[601] and no better than edrophonium alone.[607] It may be justified to administer purified butyrylcholinesterase to patients homozygous for atypical butyrylcholinesterase who have a prolonged block,[320,608] but this therapy has yet to be adequately tested and is expensive.

Concentration of Inhaled Anesthetic

Several studies have documented that antagonism of residual blockade is actually retarded by anesthetizing concentrations of volatile anesthetics.[609-613] For example, Delisle and Bevan[609] showed that pancuronium reversal by neostigmine under enflurane anesthesia occurred more slowly than under nitrous oxide and intravenous anesthetics. It has even been suggested that the effect is different for different anesthetics and that sevoflurane may impede neostigmine-induced antagonism more than isoflurane does.[610] When compared with isoflurane anesthesia, the recovery variables are prolonged during desflurane or sevoflurane anesthesia.[614,615] Withdrawal of the inhaled anesthetic at the end of surgery, with subsequent reduction of its enhancement of neuromuscular blockade, will speed pharmacologic reversal.[572]

Clinical Recommendations

When antagonizing deep levels of neuromuscular blockade (≈10% recovery or one twitch in response to TOF stimulation), larger doses of anticholinesterases should be administered and adequate time allowed for recovery of neuromuscular function. The time required for recovery to a TOF ratio of 0.7 will be approximately 60 minutes for the long-acting neuromuscular blocking drugs and 30 minutes for the intermediate-acting ones. To antagonize lesser degrees of block, smaller doses of anticholinesterases may be administered, with additional anticholinesterase given if adequate recovery has not occurred in 10 minutes.

The maximum dose of neostigmine that should be administered is 70 µg/kg. Giving too much anticholinesterase to antagonize residual neuromuscular blockade may actually render patients weaker,[570,616,617] probably because of the excess of acetylcholine at the neuromuscular junction that remains available to interact with the acetylcholine receptor.

Other Factors That May Interfere with Antagonism

It is not advisable to administer further anticholinesterase if maximal doses of edrophonium (1.5 mg/kg), neostigmine (70 µg/kg), or pyridostigmine (350 µg/kg) fail to antagonize residual blockade.[590,592] These doses inhibit acetylcholinesterase completely, and if they fail to fully antagonize residual blockade, another likely cause of the inadequate antagonism should be sought. Some of these additional potential causes of inadequate antagonism of neuromuscular blockade are described in the following sections.

Acid-Base State

Both metabolic and respiratory acidosis may augment a nondepolarizing neuromuscular blockade, but only respiratory acidosis prevents adequate antagonism.[588,618,619] The probability of achieving adequate antagonism of nondepolarizing neuromuscular blockade in the presence of significant respiratory acidosis ($Paco_2$ greater than 50 mm Hg) is low. Therefore, if a patient hypoventilates, attempts to antagonize a residual block may fail. Administration of narcotics to relieve pain may, by producing hypoventilation, increase the likelihood of this adverse event.

Although metabolic acidosis might also be predicted to prevent antagonism by neostigmine, this theory has not been substantiated.[588,618,619] Metabolic alkalosis, but not metabolic acidosis, prevents neostigmine antagonism of dTc and pancuronium.[588,618,620] These results suggest that the extracellular hydrogen ion concentration (pH) may not be as important as changes in electrolytes and intracellular pH.

Electrolyte Imbalance

Although it has been the subject of review articles,[621] few data are available on the effect of electrolyte imbalance on antagonism of nondepolarizing neuromuscular blockade by neostigmine. Low extracellular concentrations of potassium enhance the blockade from nondepolarizing neuromuscular blockers and diminish the ability of neostigmine to antagonize the blockade. This effect is based on the increase in end-plate transmembrane potential that results from a higher ratio of intracellular to extracellular potassium. Thus, a decrease in extracellular potassium causes hyperpolarization and produces resistance to depolarization. Patients with an imbalance in potassium may have other diseases or injuries that alter their response to neuromuscular blockers (e.g., patients with burns). Cohen[622] and Feldman[621] speculated that in chronic diseases, both intracellular and extracellular potassium is depleted with little net effect on transmembrane potential. Therefore, the response to neuromuscular blockers and their antagonists should be normal. However, muscle transmembrane potentials are changed in patients who are severely ill or bedridden for a few days.[623] In addition, severe dehydration will concentrate the neuromuscular blocker present in plasma, in effect decreasing the volume of distribution and increasing muscle relaxant activity. In an animal model of chronic hypokalemia, cats were given a diuretic without potassium supplementation for 15 days. Less pancuronium was required for neuromuscular blockade and more neostigmine for antagonism.[624] Even though the differences were small, the blockade was always antagonized completely. Assuming that this animal model approximates the clinical situation, changes in potassium appear to be of relatively minor consequence with respect to the clinical question of adequacy of reversal.

Other Factors

The calcium channel blocker verapamil will potentiate nondepolarizing neuromuscular blocking drugs and may make it difficult to achieve adequate reversal of blockade.[625,626] When attempting reversal of neuromuscular blockade in patients receiving verapamil, edrophonium may be more effective than neostigmine.[625,626] Other factors that may interfere with antagonism are hypothermia and the administration of antibiotics, particularly the aminoglycoside or polypeptide classes (see "Drug Interactions").[467-474] In the case of antibiotics, administration of an anticholinesterase may in fact deepen the blockade. Monitoring with a nerve stimulator, if aminoglycosides have been administered,[627] may give misleading results.

Side Effects of Anticholinesterases

Cardiovascular Effects

Because only the nicotinic effects of edrophonium, neostigmine, and pyridostigmine are desired, the muscarinic effects must be blocked by atropine or glycopyrrolate.[27]

Atropine induces its vagolytic effect much more rapidly than glycopyrrolate does. To minimize cardiovascular changes, atropine is better suited for administration with the rapid-acting edrophonium,[27] and glycopyrrolate is better suited for administration with the slower-acting neostigmine and pyridostigmine.[628] In general, 7 to 10 µg/kg of atropine should be given with 0.5 to 1.0 mg/kg of edrophonium.[585] Atropine administration 30 seconds before edrophonium will decrease the ventricular ectopy associated with this anticholinesterase.[629] Glycopyrrolate (7 to 15 µg/kg) should be given with neostigmine (40 to 70 µg/kg). Administration of atropine with pyridostigmine will induce an initial tachycardia,[630] and giving glycopyrrolate with edrophonium may result in an initial bradycardia unless it is administered at least 1 minute earlier.[631] Dysrhythmias can occur,[631-635] and anticholinesterases should be used with caution in patients with autonomic neuropathy.[632] When cardiac dysrhythmias are a concern, glycopyrrolate may be preferable to atropine,[635] and the anticholinesterases and anticholinergics should be administered over a longer period (e.g., 2 to 5 minutes) to reduce the incidence and severity of the disorders of rhythm.

Nausea and Vomiting

Reports on the effect of anticholinesterase administration on postoperative nausea and vomiting are conflicting. Neostigmine administration has been implicated as a cause of postoperative nausea and vomiting.[636,637] It has also been described as having antiemetic properties[638] and as having no impact on postoperative nausea and vomiting.[639] A meta-analysis by Tramer and Fuchs-Bader[640] looked at the results of anticholinesterase administration in over 1100 patients. They found a dose-response relationship for the incidence of nausea and vomiting after the administration of neostigmine. The highest incidence of emesis after the administration of 1.5 mg neostigmine was lower than the lowest incidence of emesis after the administration of 2.5 mg neostigmine. Discrepancies in the other studies may have been at least in part attributable to different dosing regimens. Although emesis will develop in one in three to six patients after the administration of neostigmine, the authors did not recommend letting all patients recover spontaneously because this practice introduced the risk of patients having postoperative residual paralysis. A more recent study demonstrated the hazards of not antagonizing residual neuromuscular blockade at least 2 hours after the administration of two times the ED_{95} of vecuronium, rocuronium, or atracurium.[55] Two hours after administration of these agents, 10% of 526 patients had TOF ratios less than 0.7 and 37% had TOF ratios less than 0.9.

Pharmacokinetics of Neostigmine, Pyridostigmine, and Edrophonium

The pharmacokinetics of edrophonium, neostigmine, and pyridostigmine is summarized in Table 13-13.[641-644] The data indicate several relevant clinical conclusions:
1. Pyridostigmine has a longer elimination half-life than the other anticholinesterases do, which probably accounts for its longer duration of action.[641,642]

Table 13–13 Pharmacokinetics of neostigmine (N), pyridostigmine (P), and edrophonium (E) in patients without and with renal failure

	Without Renal Failure			With Renal Failure		
	N	P	E	N	P	E
Distribution half-life ($t_{1/2}\alpha$, min)	3.4	6.7	7.2	2.5	3.9	7.0
Elimination half-life ($t_{1/2}\beta$, min)	77	113	110	181	379	304
Volume of central compartment (L/kg)	0.2	0.3	0.3	0.3	0.4	0.3
Total plasma clearance (mL/kg/min)	9.1	8.6	9.5	4.8	3.1	3.9

Data from Cronnelly and colleagues[641,642] and Morris and colleagues.[643,644]

2. By comparing elimination half-lives in patients with and without renal failure, renal excretion accounts for about 50% of the excretion of neostigmine and about 75% of that of pyridostigmine and edrophonium. Renal failure decreases the plasma clearance of neostigmine, pyridostigmine, and edrophonium as much as if not more than that of the long-acting neuromuscular blockers. Therefore, if proper doses of anticholinesterase drugs are given and overdoses of neuromuscular blockers are avoided, renal failure should not be associated with "recurarization."[641,642] This remote possibility is further diminished if the clinician restricts relaxant administration to intermediate- or short-acting drugs in patients with renal failure.

3. Edrophonium was once thought to be an unsuitable antagonist in clinical practice because its duration of action was believed to be too short. However, when larger doses (i.e., 0.5 to 1.0 mg/kg) are given, sustained antagonism of a nondepolarizing neuromuscular blockade results.[645,646] In fact, the elimination half-life of edrophonium is similar to that of neostigmine or pyridostigmine (see Table 13-13).[643]

Mild hypothermia (i.e., 34°C to 35°C), as commonly occurs intraoperatively, has an impact on the pharmacokinetics of neostigmine. Its clearance is decreased from 16.2 mL/kg/min at 36.5°C to 13.5 mL/kg/min at 34.5°C.[494] Furthermore, the onset of peak effect of neostigmine is prolonged by mild hypothermia from 4.2 to 5.5 minutes.[494] If hypothermia has any influence on the efficacy of neostigmine-induced reversal, it is more likely to be due to the effect of temperature on the neuromuscular blocker (e.g., prolonged duration of action[477]) than the pharmacology of neostigmine.

The pharmacokinetics of the anticholinesterases depends on several factors, including metabolism as well as distribution and elimination. In the case of neostigmine, a carbamylated complex with acetylcholinesterase is formed,[576,578,647] and it is the rate of dissociation of neostigmine from this complex (i.e., its metabolism) that is probably the major determinant of its duration of action. The decay in its plasma concentration (i.e., its distribution and elimination) may not be as pertinent a determinant of the duration of action of the drug.[648]

Other Antagonists of Nondepolarizing Neuromuscular Blockade

Work is ongoing with a completely novel type of antagonist. This compound, ORG 25969 (Fig. 13-32), is a γ-cyclodextrin.[649-652] It is highly water soluble with a hydrophobic cavity that can encapsulate steroidal neuromuscular blocking drugs.[649-652] ORG 25969 exerts its effect by forming tight complexes with steroidal neuromuscular blocking drugs (rocuronium > vecuronium >> pancuronium),[649-652] and in so doing, the neuromuscular blocker is no longer available to bind with the acetylcholine receptor. ORG 25969 acts as a chelating agent, and it has no effect on acetylcholinesterase. This property eliminates the need for anticholinergic drugs. The compound's efficacy as an antagonist does not appear to rely on renal excretion of the cyclodextrin-relaxant complex.[653] Although a change in acid-base status will affect anticholinesterase activity, it does not appear to influence the efficacy of ORG 25969.[654] In male volunteers, administration of 8 mg/kg ORG 25969 3 minutes after

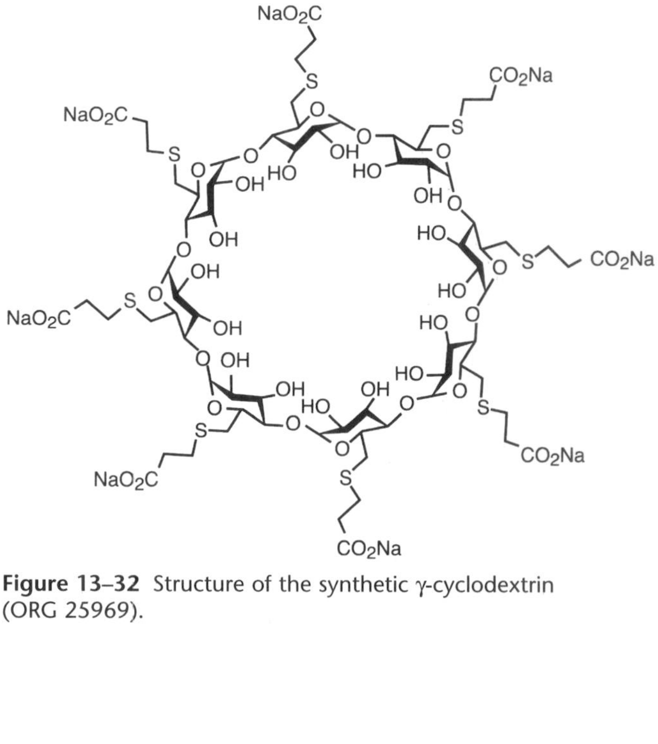

Figure 13–32 Structure of the synthetic γ-cyclodextrin (ORG 25969).

rocuronium (0.6 mg/kg) resulted in recovery of the TOF ratio to 0.9 within 2 minutes.[655]

SPECIAL POPULATIONS

Pediatric Patients

The development of the neuromuscular junction is not complete at birth.[17,656] In humans, maturation of neuromuscular transmission probably occurs after the first 2 months of age.[657] Nonetheless, neuromuscular blockers can be used safely in term and preterm infants.

Routine administration of succinylcholine to healthy children should be discontinued. In apparently healthy children, intractable cardiac arrest with hyperkalemia, rhabdomyolysis, and acidosis may develop after succinylcholine administration, particularly in patients with unsuspected muscular dystrophy of the Duchenne type.[658,659] In response to this potential adverse effect, the U.S. Food and Drug Administration and Glaxo-Wellcome have modified the package insert for succinylcholine by adding a warning against the use of succinylcholine in children except for emergency control of the airway (see the section on complications of succinylcholine; also see Chapter 60).

It is not apparent from older studies whether newborns are more sensitive than adults to nondepolarizing neuromuscular blockers.[660-663] More recent studies by Fisher and colleagues[241,664,665] on the pharmacokinetics and pharmacodynamics of neuromuscular blockers in infants, children, and adults, however, have made it possible to better understand the clinical pharmacology of these drugs in pediatric patients (see Chapter 60). Neonates and infants are more sensitive than adults to the neuromuscular blocking effects of dTc.[664] A lower plasma concentration of this neuromuscular blocker is required to achieve a desired level of neuromuscular blockade in these young patients. However, the dosage should not be decreased because infants have a larger volume of distribution. The increased volume of distribution and slower clearance (Fig. 13-33) contribute to a longer elimination half-life,[664,666] which

means that in infants, dTc may require less frequent dosing (longer dosing intervals) than in older children.

Atracurium, vecuronium, cisatracurium, rocuronium, and mivacurium are commonly administered to children. The popularity of these drugs in children most likely stems from the following points: minimal residual paralysis is seen in the postoperative period,[667,668] and a faster onset of action occurs in children than in adults.

Atracurium and vecuronium, in comparison, show very different kinetic and dynamic patterns in infants. As with the long-acting neuromuscular blockers, the sensitivity of infants to vecuronium is greater than it is in children (ED_{95} of 0.047 versus 0.081 mg/kg, respectively).[669] The increased duration of action in infants is most likely secondary to the increased volume of distribution of vecuronium because its clearance is unchanged.[665,666] Vecuronium therefore acts as a long-acting neuromuscular blocker in neonates.[665,666,670]

In contrast, the duration of action of atracurium is not significantly different in pediatric patients than it is in adults.[671-673] As with vecuronium and dTc, the volume of distribution is increased in infants.[241] However, clearance of atracurium is also more rapid.[241] Therefore, the same dose (0.5 to 0.6 mg/kg) can be used in infants, children, and adults for tracheal intubation without any major difference in its duration of action in the three groups. In children, a dose of 0.1 mg/kg cisatracurium has an onset of just over 2 minutes and a clinical duration of approximately 30 minutes during balanced or halothane anesthesia.[674] The calculated ED_{95} doses of cisatracurium in infants and children are 43 and 47 mg/kg, respectively.[675] The mean infusion rate necessary to maintain 90% to 99% neuromuscular blockade is also similar in infants and children.[676]

Rocuronium in adults is an intermediate-acting neuromuscular blocker with a fast onset of action, and the same is also true in infants and children.[676,677] Its potency is greater in infants than children, but its onset is faster in the latter age group.[677] In children, rocuronium, 0.6 mg/kg, produces better conditions for rapid tracheal intubation than vecuronium, 0.1 mg/kg, or atracurium, 0.5 mg/kg, does.[676] If given by intramuscular

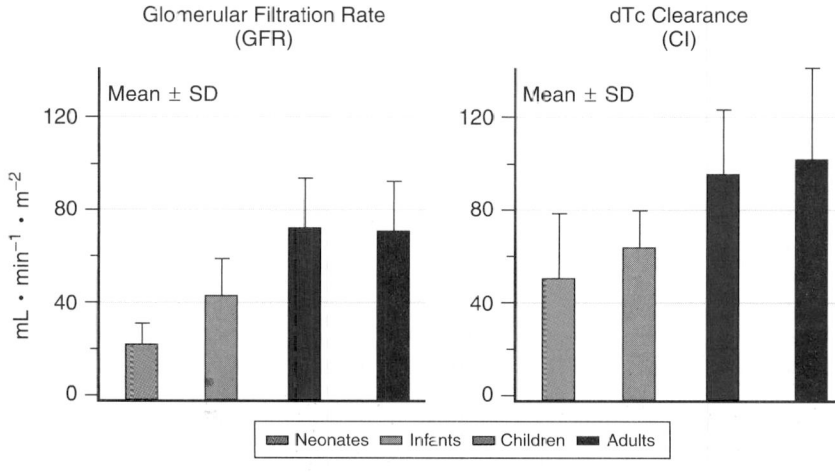

Figure 13–33 Correlation between age, glomerular filtration, and clearance of *d*-tubocurarine (dTc). (Redrawn from Fisher DM, O'Keeffe C, Stanski DR, et al: Pharmacokinetics and pharmacodynamics of *d*-tubocurarine in infants, children, and adults. Anesthesiology 57:203-208, 1982.)

injection into the deltoid (1.0 mg/kg in infants and 1.8 mg/kg in children), rocuronium allows for tracheal intubation in approximately 3 minutes.[678,679] However, intramuscular injection is not recommended as an alternative to rapid-sequence induction.[679] As with adults, for rapid-sequence intubation (60 seconds) in the presence of a full stomach, a 1.2-mg/kg dose of rocuronium is suggested.

The ED_{95} of mivacurium is greater in children than adults (0.10 mg/kg during narcotic anesthesia and 0.09 mg/kg during halothane anesthesia).[680] Children therefore require larger doses of mivacurium than adults do to achieve a given depth of neuromuscular blockade.[680,681] Onset time, as with atracurium[670] and vecuronium,[682] is faster in children than adults, so maximal block is achieved in less than 2 minutes. A dose of 0.25 to 0.30 mg/kg facilitates tracheal intubation in about 90 seconds in children. A dose of twice the ED_{95} (0.2 mg/kg) results in only a 20% increase in the duration of blockade as compared with the ED_{95}.[681] In contrast to adults, large doses have less of a propensity to cause histamine release. Facial flushing and transient hypotension are observed in about 10% to 15% of the pediatric population who receive 0.25 mg/kg mivacurium as a rapid 5- to 10-second injection.[680] Mivacurium's clinical duration of action is shorter in children than adults (12 versus 15 to 20 minutes). Because of its short duration of action, mivacurium is best used as an infusion in children for maintenance of relaxation. Infusion rates required by children (10 to 20 µg/kg/min) are about twice those required by adults, probably because of significantly higher butyrylcholinesterase activity.[683,684]

Antagonism of residual neuromuscular blockade in the case of the various nondepolarizers is similar in children and adults. Fisher and associates[629,685] described some minor variations in the neostigmine and edrophonium dosage for pediatric patients. For example, the ED_{50} of neostigmine for antagonism of a dTc-induced 90% block of the adductor pollicis twitch was 22.9 µg/kg in adults versus 15.5 µg/kg in infants.[629] In the case of edrophonium, the ED_{50} for antagonism of a dTc-induced 90% block was 128 µg/kg in adults. In children, the ED_{50} was 233 µg/kg, and in infants the ED_{50} was 145 µg/kg.[685] The rate of recovery of intermediate- or short-acting neuromuscular blockers is faster than that of long-acting drugs in children.[583,686]

Neostigmine doses of up to 50 to 60 µg/kg or edrophonium doses of 500 to 1000 µg/kg should be used for antagonism of residual neuromuscular blockade in children. In all cases, tests of clinical recovery, such as head lift, leg lift, and cry, should be performed and documented for pediatric patients and adults.

Elderly Patients (also see Chapter 62)

The pharmacodynamics of neuromuscular blockers is altered in elderly patients. A number of physiologic changes accompany the aging process, including decreases in total-body water, increases in total-body fat, decreases in hepatic and renal blood flow, and decreases in cardiac reserve, which account for the altered responses of the elderly to neuromuscular blockers. A number of physiologic

and anatomic changes at the neuromuscular junction also occur with aging. These changes include an increase in the distance between the junctional axon and the motor end plate, flattening of the folds of the motor end plate, a decreased concentration of acetylcholine receptors at the motor end plate, a decrease in the amount of acetylcholine in each vesicle in the prejunctional axon, and decreased release of acetylcholine from the preterminal axon in response to a neural impulse.[687] As shown by Matteo and coworkers,[688] despite these age-related changes, acetylcholine receptor sensitivity to nondepolarizing neuromuscular blockers is not altered by advancing age (Fig. 13-34). That is, the elderly and young adults have similar degrees of neuromuscular blockade at the same plasma concentration of a neuromuscular blocker. Rather, it appears that in the elderly, decreased splanchnic and renal blood flow, decreased glomerular filtration rate, and decreased hepatic function are responsible for the prolonged duration of action of most neuromuscular blockers. The greater depth of blockade with a given dose of relaxant in elderly patients versus young patients may also be due in part to altered volumes of distribution. The impact of aging alone, versus disease states often associated with the aging process, may be difficult to distinguish when identifying mechanisms of altered neuromuscular blocker action in the elderly.

Pancuronium,[688,690] metocurine,[688] dTc,[688] vecuronium,[569,665,691] and rocuronium[354] all show altered pharmacodynamics and pharmacokinetics in the elderly patient population. Decreased clearance of each of these drugs from plasma explains the prolonged duration of action in these patients. These neuromuscular blockers depend on the kidney or the liver (or both) for their metabolism and elimination.

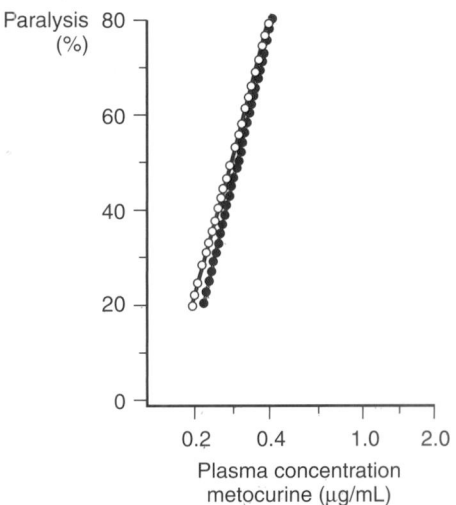

Figure 13–34 Correlation of plasma metocurine concentration versus percent paralysis (twitch depression) in young and elderly patients (*open and closed circles*). Differences are not significant. (Redrawn from Matteo RS, Backus WW, McDaniel DD, et al: Pharmacokinetics and pharmacodynamics of *d*-tubocurarine and metocurine in the elderly. Anesth Analg 64:23-29, 1985.)

Surprisingly, the pharmacokinetics and pharmacodynamics of the long-acting neuromuscular blockers doxacurium[692] and pipecuronium,[693] which rely almost exclusively on the kidney for elimination, do not seem to be significantly different in the elderly. The duration of neuromuscular blockade induced by doxacurium has been found to be more variable in the elderly than in younger patients and tends to be longer. However, clearance and elimination half-lives are the same in the two patient groups. Similarly, recovery from pipecuronium-induced neuromuscular blockade, the volume of distribution, clearance, and the elimination half-life of the drug are the same in young and old patients. Further studies in the elderly with doxacurium and pipecuronium may be needed to better define this issue.

In the case of drugs whose elimination is independent of hepatic or renal blood flow, their pharmacokinetics and pharmacodynamics should be unaffected by age. This is true of atracurium, which depends on Hofmann degradation for its clearance.[242,694] Cisatracurium, which also undergoes Hofmann elimination, has a delayed onset of effect in elderly patients.[343,359] The duration of action of the relaxant, however, appears to not be influenced by advanced age. The prolonged elimination half-life of the drug in the elderly is due to an increased volume of distribution. Clearance is not decreased with advanced age.

Butyrylcholinesterase activity in the elderly, though still in the normal range, is decreased by approximately 26% when compared with that in young adults.[695] Because mivacurium is metabolized by butyrylcholinesterase, its clearance is likely to be slightly reduced in the elderly; as a result, the duration of action is 20% to 25% longer,[696] and the infusion requirement to maintain a stable depth of blockade is decreased.[697]

In general, when maintaining a neuromuscular blockade with nondepolarizing neuromuscular blockers in elderly patients, one can expect that with the exception of atracurium and cisatracurium, the dosing interval will be increased and fewer doses of neuromuscular blocker will be required to maintain the desired depth of neuromuscular blockade. The choice of agent and the use of monitoring of the depth of blockade are exceptionally important in this population because recovery of neuromuscular function is generally delayed in the elderly. Inadequate or incomplete recovery of muscle strength after the use of pancuronium is associated with an increased incidence of perioperative pulmonary complications in this patient population.[60]

Obese Patients

Reports are conflicting concerning the effect of obesity on the pharmacodynamics of nondepolarizing neuromuscular blockade.[698-700] Although the duration of action of pancuronium is unaffected by patient weight,[700] obese patients recover more slowly from doxacurium-,[701] vecuronium-,[702] or rocuronium-induced[703] neuromuscular blockade. These findings imply that elimination of these drugs is decreased. Recovery from atracurium-induced neuromuscular blockade is not affected by obesity,[702] which is most likely secondary to its lack of dependence on end-organ function for elimination.

Neuromuscular blockers should be dosed in obese patients on the basis of about 20% more than lean body mass rather than on actual body weight[704] to ensure that these patients are not receiving relative overdoses.

Severe Renal Disease (also see Chapter 56)

Renal failure influences the pharmacology of nondepolarizing neuromuscular blockers by producing either decreased elimination of the drug or its metabolites via the kidney or decreased activity of butyrylcholinesterase (Table 13-14). Consequently, the duration of action of neuromuscular blockers may be prolonged in patients with renal failure. An early example of prolonged neuromuscular blockade as a result of renal failure was a case of postoperative respiratory failure after gallamine, reported in 1950.[710]

Renal failure does not alter the sensitivity (dose-response relationship) of patients to the neuromuscular blocking action of gallamine,[347] dTc,[711] pancuronium,[234] atracurium,[712] vecuronium,[713] rocuronium,[714] or mivacurium,[715] but it does cause resistance to metocurine.[345]

Gallamine[347] and metocurine,[345] which rely almost exclusively on the kidney for their elimination, have reduced plasma clearance and potentially a very long duration of action in patients with renal failure (see Table 13-14). Pancuronium and dTc are eliminated predominantly by the kidney, and renal failure is associated with reduced plasma clearance and an increased elimination half-life for these drugs as well.[190,716] As a consequence of these pharmacokinetic changes, the duration of neuromuscular blockade produced by these drugs is longer and more variable than in patients with normal renal function.[716] In patients with renal failure, doxacurium has decreased plasma clearance, an increased elimination half-life, and a prolonged duration of action.[346,717] Pipecuronium is eliminated predominantly by the kidney.[293] Its plasma clearance is decreased by one third, and its elimination half-life is increased twofold in patients with renal failure.[298] Because of the potential for prolonged block and the availability of intermediate- and short-acting neuromuscular blockers, there is no longer any reason to recommend the use of long-acting neuromuscular blockers in patients with renal failure.

The pharmacokinetics and duration of action of atracurium are unaffected by renal failure.[705,718,719] This lack of effect is due in part to the fact that Hofmann elimination and ester hydrolysis[340] account for 50% of its total clearance.[326] The elimination half-life of laudanosine, the principal metabolite of atracurium, increases in renal failure.[705,720] Recent evidence suggests, however, that significant concentrations of laudanosine are not achieved during the administration of atracurium in the operating room setting.[705,720]

In patients with chronic renal failure, the duration of action of cisatracurium is not prolonged.[257] Hofmann elimination accounts for 77% of the total clearance of cisatracurium,[342] and renal excretion accounts for 16% of its elimination.[342] Clearance of the drug is slightly decreased by 13% in this patient population.[721]

Vecuronium relies principally on hepatic, not renal mechanisms for its elimination.[303,707] However, its

Table 13–14 Pharmacokinetics of neuromuscular blocking drugs in patients with normal renal function or renal failure

	Plasma Clearance (mL/kg/min)		Volume of Distribution (mL/kg)		Elimination Half-Life (min)		
	Normal Function	Renal Failure	Normal Function	Renal Failure	Normal Function	Renal Failure	Reference
Short-Acting Drugs							
Mivacurium isomers							314
Cis-trans	106	80	278	475	2.0	4.3	
Trans-trans	57	48	211	270	2.3	4.3	
Cis-cis	3.8	2.4*	227	244	68	80	
Intermediate-Acting Drugs							
Atracurium	6.1	6.7	182	224	21	24	348
	5.5	5.8	153	141	19	20	349*†
	10.9	7.8	280	265	17.3	19.7	705
Cisatracurium	5.2	—	31	—	—	—	342
Vecuronium	3.0	2.5	194	239	78	97	706
	3.2	2.6	510	471	117	149	707
	3.6	4.5	242	347	51	68	708
	5.3	3.1*	199	241	53	83*	709
Rocuronium	2.9	2.9	207	264*	71	97*	352
Long-Acting Drugs							
d-Tubocurarine	2.4	1.5	250	250	84	132	224
Metocurine	1.2	0.4*	472	353	300	684*	345
Doxacurium	2.7	1.2*	220	270	99	221*	346
Pancuronium	74	20*	148	236*	97	475*	233†
	1.7	0.9	261	296*	132	257*	295
Pipecuronium	2.4	1.6*	309	442*	137	263*	298
Gallamine	1.20	0.24*	240	280	132	750*	347

*Significant difference between normal renal function and renal failure.
†Values expressed as milliliters per minute, not weight adjusted.

clearance is reduced and its elimination half-life is increased in patients with renal failure.[706,708,709] In one study, the duration of action of vecuronium, 0.1 mg/kg, was both longer and more variable in patients with renal failure than in those with normal renal function.[709] In three other studies, the duration of action of 0.05 to 0.14 mg/kg vecuronium was not prolonged by renal failure, but this result was probably due to the use of relatively small doses or inadequate sample sizes.[303,706,708] The principal metabolite of vecuronium, 3-desacetylvecuronium, has 80% of the neuromuscular blocking activity of vecuronium[302]; it may cause prolonged paralysis in patients with renal failure in the ICU.[305,722] In patients with renal failure, the duration of action and rate of recovery from vecuronium- or atracurium-induced neuromuscular blockade during surgery are similar.[549,723,724]

The plasma clearance of rocuronium may be decreased in patients with renal failure[725] and its distribution volume increased.[352] The duration of action of single and repeated doses, though, is not significantly affected.[714] When rocuronium is administered to patients with renal failure who are undergoing renal transplantation versus patients with normal renal function, plasma clearance is unchanged (2.89 mL/kg/min), the volume of distribution is increased by 28%, and the elimination half-life is lengthened by 37% (see Fig. 13-17).[352,726]

The effect of renal failure on the duration of action and recovery from mivacurium-induced blockade is variable. In some studies, renal failure had no effect,[228] whereas in others, the duration of action and recovery were prolonged and the infusion dose requirements were decreased by renal failure.[727] The effect of renal failure on mivacurium's duration of action is most probably mediated through its effect on butyrylcholinesterase. Renal failure can decrease butyrylcholinesterase activity,[728] and this decrease would be expected to prolong the duration of mivacurium-induced neuromuscular blockade.[320,729] Clearance of the *cis-trans* and *trans-trans* isomers of mivacurium is decreased by approximately 20% in those with renal failure.[314] In the studies in which renal failure had no effect on mivacurium's duration of action, butyrylcholinesterase activity was similar in patients with and without renal failure.[228] In contrast, when patients with renal failure had decreased butyrylcholinesterase activity, the duration of action of mivacurium was longer.[318,727] Because a patient's butyrylcholinesterase activity is not known preoperatively, when mivacurium is used in patients with renal failure, doses should be conservative, and its effect should be carefully monitored.

Hepatobiliary Disease (also see Chapter 56)

Patients with hepatobiliary disease may exhibit prolonged blockade with dTc,[730] pancuronium,[296] doxacurium,[346] vecuronium,[231] rocuronium,[353,357] and mivacurium.[172,228] In the case of pancuronium,[295] vecuronium,[231] and mivacurium,[172,228] this prolonged action is associated with decreased plasma clearance of the drug. However, this relationship is not consistent, and many studies have described a reduction in clearance without a prolonged duration of action. In the case of atracurium, one study even reports increased clearance in patients with cirrhosis, but the duration of action was normal.[330]

The influence of hepatobiliary disease on the pharmacokinetics of neuromuscular blockers is complex (Table 13-15). In most studies, hepatic disease is associated with an increased volume of distribution, and as a result, patients have an apparent resistance to the effect of dTc,[330,735] pancuronium,[297,736] atracurium,[737] and rocuronium.[732] The effect of hepatic disease on the pharmacokinetics of neuromuscular blockers (see Table 13-15) suggests that initial doses may need to be greater than for patients with normal hepatic function but that once the desired level of block has been achieved, subsequent recovery may be slower. This is illustrated in the case of vecuronium, in which doses up to 0.15 mg/kg have a normal duration of action[304,738,739] but a dose of 0.2 mg/kg has prolonged action (see Fig. 13-15).[731,739]

Hepatic disease can alter the elimination of neuromuscular blockers by several mechanisms. The principal route of metabolism of pancuronium and vecuronium is deacetylation at the 3-position.[290,292] This metabolic process is presumed to occur in the liver because 10% to 20% of the total dose of pancuronium and 40% percent of the total dose of vecuronium are found in the liver and bile as both parent drug and metabolite.[290,292,303] In hepatic disease, an increased plasma concentration of bile salts can reduce the hepatic uptake of pancuronium and vecuronium,[290,733] which may be an explanation for the decreased clearance of these drugs observed by some investigators.[294,296,3-6] Excretion of vecuronium is diminished in the presence of decreased hepatic function.[665] The duration of action of vecuronium is longer in these patients, and recovery is slower than in young healthy individuals.

Table 13–15   Pharmacokinetics of neuromuscular blocking drugs in patients with normal liver function or hepatobiliary disease

	Plasma Clearance (mL/kg/min)		Volume of Distribution (mL/kg)		Elimination Half-Life (min)		Hepatic Pathology	Reference
	Normal	Disease	Normal	Disease	Normal	Disease		
Short-Acting Drugs								
Mivacurium isomers							Cirrhosis	172
Cis-trans	95	44*	210	188	1.53	2.48*		
Trans-trans	70	32*	200	199	2.32	11.1*		
Cis-cis	5.2	4.2	266	237	50.3	60.8		
Intermediate-Acting Drugs								
Atracurium	5.3	6.5	159	207*	21	22	Hepatorenal	712
	6.6	8.0*	202	282*	21	25	Cirrhosis	330
Cisatracurium	5.7	6.6*	161	195*	23.5	24.4	Transplantation	
Vecuronium	4.26	2.73*	246	253	58	84*	Cirrhosis	231
	4.30	2.36*	247	206	58	98*	Cholestasis	731
	4.5	4.4	180	220	58	51	Cirrhosis	304
Rocuronium	2.79	2.41	184	234	87.5	96.0	Cirrhosis	353
	217	217	16.4	23.4*	76.4	111.5*	Mixed	356†
	296	189	151	264*	56	98*	Cirrhosis	732†
	3.70	2.66*	211	248	92	143*	Cirrhosis	357
Long-Acting Drugs								
Doxacurium	2.7	2.3	220	290	99	115	Transplantation	346
Pancuronium	123	59*	261	307*	133	267*	Cholestasis	296†
	1.86	1.45*	279	416*	114	208*	Cirrhosis	294
	1.76	1.47	284	425*	141	224*	Cholestasis	732
Pipecuronium	3.0	2.6*	350	452	111	143	Cirrhosis	299
Gallamine	1.22	0.90	237	259	162	220	Cholestasis	733
	1.20	1.21	206	247*	135	160	Cholestasis	734

*Significant difference between normal hepatic function and hepatobiliary disease.
†Values expressed as milliliters per minute, or liters, not weight adjusted.

Atracurium and cisatracurium share organ-independent modes of elimination.[322,323,340-342] As a consequence, their clearance should be little affected by hepatic disease. In fact and in contrast to all other neuromuscular blockers, plasma clearance of atracurium and cisatracurium is slightly increased in patients with liver disease (see Table 13-15).[330,358] Because elimination of atracurium and cisatracurium occurs outside as well as from within the central compartment, it has been suggested that a larger distribution volume should be associated with a larger clearance.[342] In two studies,[330,358] volumes of distribution and clearance of the drugs increased with liver disease, thus lending support to this theory.[342] The increased clearance of the relaxant in patients with liver disease is not reflected in a decrease in the drugs' duration of action.[330,358]

A concern raised about administering atracurium to patients with hepatic disease was the possible accumulation of laudanosine.[339] Although laudanosine relies principally on hepatic mechanisms for elimination, the concentrations encountered during liver transplantation are unlikely to be associated with clinical sequelae.[339,735]

In patients with hepatic disease (most commonly cirrhosis), the distribution volume of rocuronium is increased,[353,356,357,732] and its clearance may be decreased.[357] The duration of action of rocuronium is prolonged in patients with hepatic disease,[353,357,732] and its onset may be prolonged.[353]

In patients with severe liver disease, butyrylcholinesterase activity is decreased because of decreased synthesis of the enzyme in the liver.[228] Consequently, plasma clearance of the isomers of mivacurium is decreased by approximately 50% (see Table 13-15),[172] and its duration of action is prolonged and may be almost tripled.[172,228]

Burns

After a period of immobilization, burn injury causes upregulation of both fetal ($\alpha_2\beta\gamma\delta$) and mature ($\alpha_2\beta\epsilon\delta$) nAChRs.[740-745] Upregulation of nAChRs is usually associated with resistance to nondepolarizing neuromuscular blockers and increased sensitivity to succinylcholine.[746] Causes of upregulation of nAChRs are listed in Table 13-16. A significant increase in the quantal content of evoked acetylcholine release is noted by 72 hours after scald injury in rats.[747] This increased acetylcholine release also contributes to the resistance to nondepolarizing blockers in burn patients. In mice, thermal injury induces changes in diaphragm acetylcholinesterase with respect to total content and specific molecular forms.[748]

Anesthetic Implications

Resistance to the effects of nondepolarizing neuromuscular blocking drugs is usually seen in patients with greater than 25% total–body surface area burns.[244,746] Recovery of neuromuscular function to preburn levels may take several months[749] or even years after the burn injury.[750] The increase in serum potassium that normally follows succinylcholine administration is markedly exaggerated in burned victims.[119,751] Potassium concentrations as high as 13 mEq/L and resulting in ventricular tachycardia,

Table 13–16 Conditions associated with upregulation and downregulation of acetylcholine receptors	
nAChR Upregulation	**nAChR Downregulation**
Spinal cord injury	Myasthenia gravis
Stroke	Anticholinesterase poisoning
Burns	Organophosphate poisoning
Prolonged immobility	
Prolonged exposure to neuromuscular blockers	
Multiple sclerosis	
Guillain-Barré syndrome	

nAChR, nicotinic acetylcholine receptor.
From Naguib M, Flood P, McArdle JJ, et al: Advances in neurobiology of the neuromuscular junction: Implications for the anesthesiologist. Anesthesiology 96:202-231, 2002.

fibrillation, and cardiac arrest have been reported.[751,752] The magnitude of the hyperkalemic response does not appear to closely correlate with the magnitude of the burn injury. Potentially lethal hyperkalemia was seen in a patient with only an 8% total–body surface area burn.[753] Succinylcholine has been safely administered within 24 hours of a burn injury. After this initial 24 hours, however, sufficient alteration in muscle response may have occurred, and the use of succinylcholine is best avoided.

The time course of abnormal muscle membrane function corresponds with that of the healing process. Once normal skin has regrown and any infection has subsided, return of normal acetylcholine receptor populations appears to occur.[754] Normal responses to succinylcholine have been demonstrated in burn patients studied 3 years postinjury.[754] The length of time during which a burn patient may be at risk for a hyperkalemic response is not well defined. A conservative guideline would therefore be to avoid the use of succinylcholine in patients 24 to 48 hours after a thermal injury and for at least 1 to 2 years after the burned skin has healed.

Neuromuscular Blockers and Weakness Syndromes in the Critically Ill (also see Chapters 74 and 75)

Neuromuscular blocking drugs are frequently used in conjunction with sedatives and analgesics in the ICU. Indications for the use of neuromuscular blockers in the ICU are outlined in Table 13-17. Few data support their use, and evidence for a beneficial effect on pulmonary function or patient oxygenation is inconclusive.[755-758] Nonetheless, nondepolarizing neuromuscular blockers are commonly used for weeks in ICU patients, most of the time without monitoring and frequently at doses exceeding those used in the operating room.[759,760] The results of two surveys in the United States, including anesthesiologists and nurses with special certificates of competence in critical care, indicate that 98% of those surveyed use neuromuscular blocking drugs at least occasionally.[759,760]

Table 13–17 Reported indications for use of muscle relaxants in the intensive care unit

Facilitate mechanical ventilation
   Facilitation of endotracheal intubation
   Enable patient to tolerate mechanical ventilation
   High pulmonary inflation pressures, e.g., acute
      respiratory distress syndrome
Hyperventilation for increased intracranial pressure
Facilitate therapeutic or diagnostic procedures
Tetanus
Status epilepticus
Reduce oxygen consumption
   Abolish shivering
   Reduce work of breathing

Table 13–18 Complications of muscle paralysis in the intensive care unit

Short-term use
   Specific, known drug side effects
   Inadequate ventilation in the event of ventilator failure or
      circuit disconnection
   Inadequate analgesia and/or sedation
Long-term use
   Complications of immobility
      Deep venous thrombosis and pulmonary embolism
      Peripheral nerve injuries
      Decubitus ulcers
Inability to cough
   Retention of secretions and atelectasis
   Pulmonary infection
Dysregulation of nicotinic acetylcholine receptors
Prolonged paralysis after stopping relaxant
   Persistent neuromuscular blockade
   Critical illness myopathy
   Critical illness polyneuropathy
   Combination of the above
Unrecognized effects of drug or metabolites
   Succinylcholine and metabolic acidosis/hypovolemia
   3-Desacetylvecuronium and neuromuscular blockade
   Laudanosine and cerebral excitation

Of particular concern in intensive care settings is the risk of paralyzed patients receiving inadequate analgesia and sedation.[761-763] This may be due to the fact that ICU nurses and physicians are unfamiliar with the pharmacology of the neuromuscular blocking drugs.[759,762] For instance, pancuronium was thought to be an anxiolytic by 50% to 70% of ICU nurses and house staff, and 5% to 10% thought that it was an analgesic.[762] In the United Kingdom, the erroneous use of neuromuscular blockers as sedatives in intensive care was not uncommon in the 1980s.[764-766] Approximately 96% of ICU patients received neuromuscular blockers to aid mechanical ventilation in 1980. By 1986, their use had fallen to 16% of ventilated patients.[764-766] This marked reduction followed the publication of patients' ordeals who were paralyzed while conscious in the ICU.[15] In the United States, neuromuscular blockers are used in less than 20% of all patients requiring mechanical ventilation.[759]

Prolonged ICU stay during critical illness is associated with disorders of neuromuscular function that contribute to morbidity, increased length of hospital stay, weaning difficulties, and prolonged rehabilitation.[767,768] Complications of long-term administration of neuromuscular blockers in the ICU are outlined in Table 13-18. In the ICU, the duration of mechanical ventilation, sepsis, dysfunction of two or more organs, female gender, administration of steroids, and hypercapnia are known risk factors for neuromuscular dysfunction.[769-771] Syndromes of weakness in critically ill patients are relatively common and probably polymorphic in origin. In a retrospective study of 92 critically ill patients with clinically diagnosed weakness, electromyographic studies indicated that acute myopathy (critical illness myopathy) is three times as common as acute axonal neuropathy (critical illness neuropathy) (43% versus 13%, respectively).[767] The additional health care cost of one case of persistent weakness was estimated to be approximately $67,000.[772] The differential diagnosis of neuromuscular weakness in the ICU is listed in Table 13-19.

Critical Illness Myopathy

Lacomis and colleagues[773] suggested using the term "critical illness myopathy" (CIM) instead of the current terminology used in the literature such as acute quadriplegic myopathy,[774] acute (necrotizing) myopathy of intensive care,[775] thick filament myopathy, acute corticosteroid myopathy,[776] and critical care myopathy.

Most published reports of CIM in the ICU have focused on patients with status asthmaticus.[777-779] Affected individuals have typically been treated with corticosteroids and nondepolarizing neuromuscular blockers. Nevertheless, myopathy has also been documented in asthmatic patients, in those with chronic lung disease without paralysis who received corticosteroids,[780,781] and in critically ill patients with sepsis who received neither corticosteroids nor nondepolarizing neuromuscular blockers.[782,783] Animal studies found that the number of cytosolic corticosteroid receptors is increased in immobilized muscles relative to contralateral controls.[784] It seems—at least in some patients—that prolonged immobility may be the key risk factor for myopathy in corticosteroid-treated patients[785] and that selective muscle atrophy is a result of changes in glucocorticoid sensitivity.[784]

Sepsis, immobility, and the catabolism associated with negative nitrogen balance may also result in myopathy.[17,768] Skeletal muscle hypoperfusion is noted in patients with severe sepsis despite normal or elevated whole blood oxygen delivery.[786] Antibodies to nAChRs have been demonstrated in a rodent model of sepsis.[787] This myasthenia-like syndrome is also seen in critically ill patients. Evidence of local immune activation by cytokine expression in skeletal muscles was reported in patients with CIM.[788]

The major feature of CIM is flaccid weakness that tends to be diffuse and often includes the facial muscles and the diaphragm.[773] The clinical features of CIM overlap with those of critical illness polyneuropathy (CIP) and prolonged neuromuscular blockade.[773] Electrophysiologic studies and increases in serum creatine kinase concentrations

Table 13–19   Causes of generalized neuromuscular weakness in the intensive care unit

Central nervous system
   Septic or toxic-metabolic encephalopathy
   Brainstem stroke
   Central pontine myelinolysis
   Anterior horn cell disorders (e.g., amyotrophic lateral
      sclerosis)
Peripheral neuropathies
   Critical illness polyneuropathy
   Guillain-Barré syndrome
   Porphyria
   Paraneoplastic
   Vasculitis
   Nutritional and toxic
Neuromuscular junction disorders
   Myasthenia gravis
   Lambert-Eaton myasthenic syndrome
   Botulism
   Prolonged neuromuscular junction blockade
Myopathies
   Critical illness myopathy
   Cachectic myopathy
   Rhabdomyolysis
   Inflammatory and infectious myopathies
   Muscular dystrophies
   Toxic
   Acid maltase deficiency
   Mitochondrial
   Hypokalemia
   Hypermetabolic syndromes with rhabdomyolysis
      (e.g., neuroleptic malignant syndrome)

From Lacomis D: Critical illness myopathy. Curr Rheumatol Rep 4:403-408, 2002.

may differentiate neuropathy from myopathy.[773] Lacomis and coauthors[773] stated that "muscle biopsy should be considered if another myopathic process such as an inflammatory myopathy is suspected or if the histologic findings would affect management."

Critical Illness Polyneuropathy

The polyneuropathy seen in the critically ill has been termed critical illness polyneuropathy. CIP affects both sensory and motor nerves and occurs in 50% to 70% of patients with multisystem organ failure and systemic inflammatory response syndrome (SIRS).[789-792] It has been postulated that SIRS contributes to CIP by releasing cytokines and free radicals that damage the microcirculation of the central and peripheral nervous systems.[788,781] Dysregulation of the microcirculation may render the peripheral nervous system susceptible to injury.[793]

No specific treatment is available for weakness syndromes in critically ill patients other than physical rehabilitation. Intravenous immunoglobulin and nerve growth factors appear to be promising in CIP syndrome.[794,795] Recently, intensive insulin therapy during critical illness has been found to decrease the risk of CIP.[796,797] Maintenance of blood glucose at or below

110 mg/mL in critically ill patients may reduce the risk of CIP.[796,797]

The outcomes from CIM and CIP appear to be similar.[767] The reported mortality rate of patients with CIP syndrome is about 35%.[798] In one study, 100% of the patients (13 of 13) who survived had abnormal clinical or neurophysiologic findings 1 to 2 years after the onset of CIP syndrome.[799] The quality of life was markedly impaired in all patients.[799]

Clinical Implications

Should Succinylcholine Be Used in ICU Patients?
It is likely that upregulation of nAChRs induced by immobilization and by prolonged administration of nondepolarizing neuromuscular blockers[800-802] contributes to (1) the higher incidence of cardiac arrest associated with the use of succinylcholine in ICU patients[803,804] and (2) the increased requirements for nondepolarizing neuromuscular blockers in ICU patients.[802,805-807] Upregulation of nAChRs was noted in the muscles of deceased critically ill adults who had received long-term infusions of vecuronium.[803] Therefore, succinylcholine is best avoided in ICU patients when total-body immobilization exceeds 24 hours.[17] In a recent survey in U.K. ICUs, 68.7% of the respondents indicated that they would use succinylcholine in a clinical scenario suggestive of CIP.[808] This result highlights the lack of awareness of the dangers associated with the use of succinylcholine in these patients.[808]

Should Nondepolarizing Neuromuscular Blockers Be Used in ICU Patients?
Nondepolarizing neuromuscular blocker–associated persistent weakness appears to be a distinct pathologic entity and is not simply a manifestation of weakness syndromes in the critically ill.[789] A prospective study by Kupfer and associates[809] showed a 70% incidence of persistent weakness in ICU patients who received neuromuscular blockers for more than 2 days versus a 0% incidence in similar ICU patients who received no neuromuscular blocker. This study is compelling evidence for the role of nondepolarizing neuromuscular blockers in this complication.

Long-term weakness has been described after all commonly used nondepolarizing neuromuscular blockers.[305,777,779,810,811] The overall incidence of prolonged paralysis after long-term use of neuromuscular blockers is about 5%. Approximately 20% of patients who received neuromuscular blockers for more than 6 days,[810] 15% to 40% of asthmatic patients who also received high-dose steroids,[776,778] and 50% of patients with renal failure who received vecuronium suffered prolonged weakness.[305] Clinically, it appears that prolonged recovery from neuromuscular blockade occurs more frequently when steroidal neuromuscular blockers are used.[305,810]

However, prolonged weakness was also noted after the use of atracurium in ICU patients.[811] Furthermore, the use of atracurium has raised concern regarding its metabolite laudanosine. Laudanosine is also detected in the cerebrospinal fluid (CSF) of ICU patients who receive atracurium.[812] It is an analeptic and can trigger seizures in animals.[813] The toxic dose in humans is not known, but case reports have described patients having seizures while receiving atracurium, and laudanosine has not been ruled out as a cause of these seizures.[814-816] Some evidence has also shown that laudanosine can activate neuronal nicotinic receptors.[817] Cisatracurium is a single isomer of atracurium, and because it is four to five times more potent than atracurium, it is given in smaller doses. Therefore, the risk of laudanosine-related adverse effects should be minimal.[336,818,819]

Nondepolarizing neuromuscular blockers are polar molecules and do not readily cross the blood-brain barrier, but vecuronium and its long-acting active metabolite (3-desacetylvecuronium) have been detected in the CSF of patients in the ICU. The CNS effects of neuromuscular blockers and their metabolites in humans have not been well studied, but in rats, atracurium, pancuronium, and vecuronium injected into the CSF will cause dose-related cerebral excitation culminating in seizures.[813] Cerebral excitation with consequent increased cerebral oxygen demand is undesirable in ICU patients at risk for cerebral ischemia. It has also been suggested that nondepolarizing neuromuscular blockers can gain access to nerves during SIRS and directly result in neurotoxicity.[793,813,820]

Combining corticosteroids and nondepolarizing neuromuscular blockers should be avoided.[821] When nondepolarizing neuromuscular blockers are necessary, the use of a peripheral nerve stimulator is recommended, and periodic return of muscle function should be allowed. However, routine monitoring of neuromuscular function alone is not sufficient to eliminate prolonged recovery and weakness syndromes in ICU patients.[822] Adjusting the dosage of neuromuscular blockers by peripheral nerve stimulation versus standard clinical dosing in critically ill patients reduces drug requirements, produces faster recovery of neuromuscular function, and results in a total cost savings of $738 per patient.[823] A recent study found that daily interruption of sedative drug infusions decreases the duration of mechanical ventilation and length of stay in the ICU.[824] The impact of such an approach on the weakness syndromes in ICU patients is unknown. When nondepolarizing neuromuscular blockers are used, the guidelines in Table 13-20 may help

---

Table 13–20 Recommendations for the use of neuromuscular blockers in the intensive care unit

Avoid the use of neuromuscular blockers by
    Maximal use of analgesics and sedatives
    Manipulation of ventilatory parameters and modes
Minimize the dose of neuromuscular blockers
    Use a peripheral nerve stimulator with train-of-four
      monitoring
    Do not administer for more than 2 days continuously
    Administer by bolus rather than infusion
    Administer only when required and to achieve a
      well-defined goal
    Continually allow recovery from paralysis
Consider alternative therapies
    Avoid vecuronium in female patients with renal failure
    Use isoflurane in place of muscle relaxants in severe
      asthmatics
    Minimize the dose of steroid in asthmatics

---

minimize the incidence of complications. As stated in the clinical practice guidelines for sustained neuromuscular blockade in adult critically ill patients,[758] *"Independent of the reasons for using neuromuscular blockers, we emphasize that all other modalities to improve the clinical situation must be tried, using neuromuscular blockers only as a last resort."*

Neuromuscular Disorders

Demyelinating Diseases
Multiple Sclerosis
Multiple sclerosis (MS), the most common demyelinating disease of the CNS, affects about 1 million people worldwide. The cause of MS is not known. Infectious agents, genetic predisposition, autoimmune reactions to antigens, and channel disease have been implicated in the etiology of MS.[825-830] Recently, it has been hypothesized that MS is a sexually transmitted disease.[828] Paralysis, sensory disturbances, autonomic disturbances, lack of coordination, and visual impairment are common features.[831] Axon loss correlates with permanent functional deficit.[832] It has been demonstrated that the CSF of patients with MS may contain a sodium channel–blocking factor (a local anesthetic–like factor).[833-836] This factor could explain the paresis seen in this disorder.[836] Therefore, it appears that channelopathies play an important role in the pathogenesis of this disorder.[327] In MS, the characteristics of individual skeletal muscles are similar to those observed in disuse myopathy.[837]

ANESTHETIC CONSIDERATIONS. Autonomic dysfunction is seen in a significant number of patients with MS.[838,839] During anesthesia, careful attention should be paid to maintenance of adequate preload, temperature control, postural changes, blood loss, and peak airway pressure during mechanical ventilation. Patients with autonomic dysfunction demonstrate an exaggerated response to α-sympathomimetics.[840]

No conclusive evidence has shown that the stress of surgery and anesthesia may increase the rate of relapse in patients with MS.[841,842] The use of regional anesthesia in MS is more controversial. Both lumbar epidural anesthesia and subarachnoid anesthesia have safely been used in patients with MS.[843] However, some evidence suggests that hyperthermia[842] or higher concentrations of local anesthetic[841] may increase the relapse rate. In one study in which patients received either 0.5% or 0.25% bupivacaine for epidural anesthesia, relapses occurred only in patients receiving the higher dose of local anesthetic.[841]

As with any patient with denervation or disuse, or both, there may be upregulation in nAChR numbers and increased sensitivity to depolarizing neuromuscular blockers.[17] In this case, the patient is at risk for hyperkalemia after the administration of succinylcholine. Paradoxical reports have described increased sensitivity to nondepolarizing neuromuscular blockers in patients with MS, probably because of reduced muscle mass or reduced margin of safety for neuromuscular transmission.[844] Denervation is known to induce a reduction in the resting potential, and this decreased resting potential will significantly contribute to muscle weakness.[17,845,846] In these patients, small doses of short-acting neuromuscular blockers should be used along with adequate monitoring of neuromuscular function.

Motor Neuron Diseases

The motor neuron diseases are a group of diverse disorders characterized by muscle weakness, atrophy, spastic paralysis, or a combination of these findings as a result of involvement of lower or upper motor neurons.[17] Amyotrophic lateral sclerosis (ALS), commonly known as Lou Gehrig's disease, is the most common motor neuron disease and has an incidence of 2 to 4 in 100,000. ALS is a progressive disease characterized by degeneration of cortical, brainstem, and spinal motor neurons.[847] The cognitive and sensory systems are usually spared. Kennedy's disease (spinobulbar muscular atrophy) affects lower motor neurons only. In contrast, hereditary spastic paraplegia involves upper motor neurons.[17]

Several mechanisms have been proposed to account for the progressive motor neuron death evident in ALS, including oxidative stress,[848] neurofilament damage,[849] mitochondrial abnormalities,[850] glutamate-mediated excitotoxicity,[851] and altered responses to hypoxia.[852] A role of oxidative stress has been suggested because mutations in the gene for Cu^{2+}/Zn^{2+} superoxide dismutase (SOD1), which catalyzes conversion of the O_2^- radical to O_2 and H_2O_2, have been identified in some 3% of all ALS cases.[848] In addition, antibodies to voltage-gated Ca^{2+} channels have been identified in ALS patients.[853] Treatment of ALS is aimed at symptomatic support.[847] Stem cell therapy may offer hope in the future.[854]

ANESTHETIC CONSIDERATIONS. Patients with motor neuron disease are at risk for hyperkalemia after the administration of succinylcholine because of upregulation of nAChRs.[855] ALS patients have, in addition, presynaptic impairment of neuromuscular transmission,[856] which explains their hypersensitivity to nondepolarizing neuromuscular blockers.[857]

Respiratory muscle weakness frequently develops in patients with ALS, and most die of pulmonary complications.[858,859] Particularly in late stages of the disease, patients may be cachectic from inadequate nutrition and demonstrate reduced plasma protein binding for many of the anesthetic drugs.[17] These patients have reduced respiratory muscle reserve and abnormal airway protective reflexes and are at increased risk for respiratory depression and aspiration secondary to the use of sedative and anesthetic drugs.[17] Epidural anesthesia has been used in ALS patients without reported untoward effects.[860,861]

ALS is not believed to be associated with significant autonomic dysfunction. There is, however, evidence of sympathetic hyperactivity[862] and autonomic failure[863] accompanied by reduced baroreflex sensitivity.[864]

Guillain-Barré Syndrome

Guillain-Barré syndrome (GBS) is now considered to be a collection of diverse disorders with several clinical manifestations[865,866] and not simply as it was first described—"syndrome of symmetric, rapidly evolving flaccid paralysis and areflexia."[866] In addition to the demyelination seen in GBS, channelopathies have been identified.[827] GBS is not uncommon and has an incidence

of 4 in 10,000.[865] Deaths are usually related to respiratory or autonomic dysfunction.

A sodium channel–blocking factor (a local anesthetic–like factor) has been identified in the CSF of patients with GBS.[833,834,836] This factor could contribute to the paralysis seen in this disorder.[836] There is also strong evidence for an association between certain infections and GBS.[865,867] Bacterial antigens are capable of initiating an immune response that targets similar moieties on nerve fibers[866] or blocks both presynaptic voltage-gated calcium channels[868] and postsynaptic nAChR channels,[869] thereby leading to neuromuscular weakness. GBS patients commonly have symptomatic improvement after plasmapheresis.[870]

ANESTHETIC CONSIDERATIONS. Demyelination or axonal degeneration produces functional denervation of the muscle and upregulation of nAChRs at the postsynaptic membrane. Succinylcholine is contraindicated because of the risk of hyperkalemic cardiac arrest.[871,872] This risk may persist after recovering from the symptomatic neurologic deficit.[873] Increased sensitivity to nondepolarizing neuromuscular blockers is expected in these patients because of the loss of motor units and channels blockade at the neuromuscular junction.[869,872,874]

Autonomic dysfunction is seen in approximately 60% of patients.[875] Asystole was reported after eyeball pressure, carotid sinus massage, and tracheal suction in patients with GBS.[876] During anesthesia, careful attention should be paid to maintenance of adequate preload, temperature control, postural changes, blood loss, and peak airway pressure during mechanical ventilation. Patients with autonomic dysfunction demonstrate an exaggerated response to α-sympathomimetics.[840]

Regional anesthesia is not contraindicated, although patients with GBS are sensitive to local anesthetics,[872,877] probably secondary to the presence of the sodium channel–blocking factor.[833,834,836] Because of the high incidence of autonomic instability, the slower onset of an epidural block may be preferable to the rapid onset of subarachnoid anesthesia.[17] GBS has been reported in four patients 1 to 2 weeks after epidural anesthesia. It was suggested that local trauma to nerve roots may initiate a cascade of immunologic events that result in demyelinating neuropathy in these patients.[878]

Charcot-Marie-Tooth Disease

Charcot-Marie-Tooth disease (CMTD; hereditary motor and sensory demyelinating polyneuropathy) is the most frequently occurring inherited peripheral neuropathy, with an incidence of 1 in 2500.[879] It has diverse genetic (autosomal dominant, X-linked, or autosomal recessive) and clinical manifestations.[880,881] Three genes responsible for CMTD type 1 have been identified: peripheral myelin protein 22 and myelin protein zero for the autosomal dominant form and connexin 32 for the X-linked dominant variant.[882] The latter variant encodes a gap junction protein.[881] Gap junctions are aggregations of channels made of proteins called connexins that are present in the plasma membrane.[883] In the nervous system, gap junctional channels play an essential role in the propagation of action potentials and in allowing rapid exchange of ions and nutrients.[884] Failure of gap junctions leads to impaired Schwann cell function and demyelination.

Peroneal nerve atrophy leading to weakness in the anterior and lateral compartments is the most common clinical manifestation in CMTD, but considerable variability exists in the pattern of atrophy. The sensory disturbance is milder than the motor disturbance.[17] Autonomic disturbances are occasionally reported.[885] Pregnancy may be associated with exacerbations of CMTD, probably because of hormonal changes.[886,887] Respiratory insufficiency has also been described in patients with CMTD.[888]

ANESTHETIC CONSIDERATIONS. CMTD patients have no evidence of a prolonged response to nondepolarizing neuromuscular blockers.[889,890] Although drugs that trigger malignant hyperthermia have been used in CMTD patients without untoward effects,[891,892] episodes of malignant hyperthermia have been reported in these patients.[893,894] Therefore, it is advisable to avoid using drugs known to trigger malignant hyperthermia.[17]

Patients with CMTD have been reported to be sensitive to the effects of thiopental.[885] However, propofol infusion has been safely used in these patients.[889,895] Respiratory insufficiency, vocal cord paresis, and cardiac conduction abnormalities have also been described in patients with CMTD.[888,896-900] Epidural anesthesia has been used successfully for labor and delivery in patients with CMTD.[901,902]

Primary Muscle Diseases

Muscular Dystrophies

Muscular dystrophies are a diverse group of genetically determined disorders of skeletal muscle and in some cases cardiac muscle.[903] They are characterized by muscle fiber necrosis and progressive muscle weakness.[903] The current classification of these disorders relies on molecular, genetic, and protein biochemical characterization (Table 13-21).[903]

In humans, mutations in the gene encoding the dystrophin-glycoprotein complex cause muscular dystrophy.[915] This complex is essential in maintaining the functional integrity of sarcolemma,[915,916] and dystrophic muscles are susceptible to mechanical injury as manifested by repeated necrosis and regeneration of muscle fibers.[917]

Loss of dystrophin and a reduction in neuronal nitric oxide synthase in cardiac muscle have also been implicated in the pathogenesis of cardiomyopathy in these patients.[915,918,919] A reduction in neuronal nitric oxide synthase impairs regulation of the vasoconstrictor response of the affected blood vessels.[920] The distribution of muscle weakness in different types of dystrophy is shown in Figure 13-35.[921] Detailed reviews are available.[903,915,921]

Duchenne's muscular dystrophy is one of the most common genetic diseases in humans, with an incidence of 1 in 3500 male births.[915] It is characterized by progressive proximal weakness beginning in early childhood and progressive cardiomyopathy.[922] Cognitive impairment is also observed and is probably caused by a lack of dystrophin in the neuronal membrane.[923] Death occurs before 30 years of age as result of respiratory or cardiac failure.[922]

Becker's muscular dystrophy is milder and affects 1 in 30,000 male births.[922] Both Duchenne's and Becker's muscular dystrophies are due to an X-linked recessive mutation in the dystrophin gene.[924] In Duchenne's muscular dystrophy, dystrophin is usually absent, whereas in Becker's muscular dystrophy, the protein is present but qualitatively and quantitatively abnormal.[904,925] Onset in childhood may occur as late as 16 years. Cardiomyopathy is present in approximately 15% of patients younger than 16 years and in 75% of those older than 40 years.[922]

Limb-girdle dystrophy is similar to Duchenne's dystrophy and is found most commonly in families in North Africa. Limb-girdle muscular dystrophy may result from autosomal dominant (type 1) or autosomal recessive (type 2) mutations and affects approximately 1 in 20,000 people.[908,915]

Congenital muscular dystrophy has the worst prognosis. Affected infants at birth have hypotonia, weakness, and respiratory and swallowing abnormalities.[909] Fukuyama-type congenital muscular dystrophy, one of the most common (0.7 to 1.2 per 10,000 births) autosomal recessive disorders in Japan, is associated with severe mental retardation and cortical dysgenesis.[926] This syndrome

Table 13–21   Molecular etiology of the muscular dystrophies

Diseases	Mode of Inheritance	Molecular Etiology	Reference
Duchenne	X-linked recessive	Absence of dystrophin	904, 924
Becker	X-linked recessive	Reduced dystrophin	905, 924
Emery-Dreifuss	X-linked recessive	Emerin	906
	Autosomal dominant	Lamin A/C	907
Limb-girdle	Autosomal dominant or recessive	Sarcoglycan deficiency	908
Congenital muscular dystrophy (CMD)	Autosomal recessive		
Classic CMD		Laminin α_2 chain	909
Fukuyama CMD		Fukutin	910
α_7 Integrin congenital myopathy		α_7 Integrin (laminin receptor)	911
Facioscapulohumeral	Autosomal dominant	4q35 rearrangements	912
Myotonic dystrophy (MD)	Autosomal dominant		
MD1		19q13 rearrangements	913
MD2		3q21 rearrangements	914

Modified from Naguib M, Flood P, McArdle JJ, et al: Advances in neurobiology of the neuromuscular junction: Implications for the anesthesiologist. Anesthesiology 96:202-231, 2002.

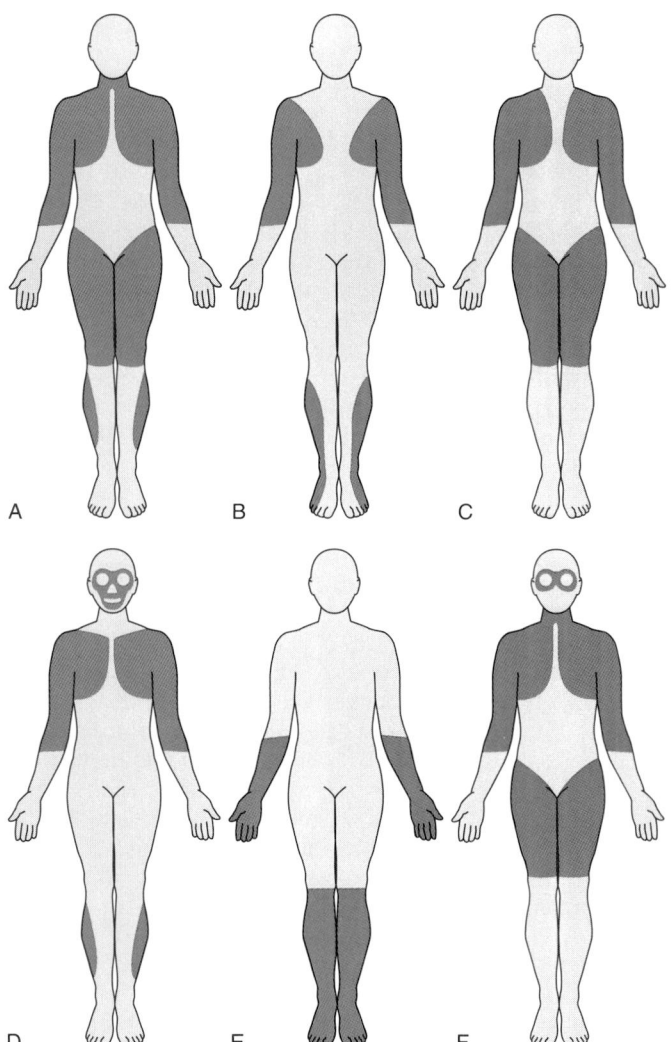

Figure 13–35 Distribution of predominant muscle weakness in different types of dystrophy. **A,** Duchenne type and Becker type; **B,** Emery-Dreifuss; **C,** limb girdle; **D,** facioscapulohumeral; **E,** distal; and **F,** oculopharyngeal. (Redrawn from Emery AE: The muscular dystrophies. BMJ 317:991-995, 1998.)

is caused by lesions in the fukutin gene.[910] Fukutin is a protein involved in formation of the basement membrane.[927]

Recently, it has been possible to rescue dystrophic symptoms in a mouse model of congenital muscular dystrophy by muscle-specific overexpression of an agrin minigene that replaces the missing link between the basement membrane and the muscle fiber.[928] In addition, intravenous injection of stem cells into a mouse model of congenital muscular dystrophy resulted in partial restoration of dystrophin expression in the affected muscle.[929] Therefore, these novel approaches may provide new therapeutic tools to restore muscle function in human muscular dystrophies.

Emery-Dreifuss muscular dystrophy is characterized by early contractures of the elbows and Achilles tendons and wasting in the humeroperoneal muscles; it has an incidence of 1 in 33,000 male births. Cardiomyopathy and conduction blocks are common and can be

life-threatening.[930] Two modes of inheritance exist, X-linked[906] and autosomal dominant.[907] Both forms of the disease are clinically identical.

Facioscapulohumeral muscular dystrophy is a rare variant of muscular dystrophy with an incidence of 10 to 20 cases per million.[931] It is usually manifested in late childhood as facial and scapulohumeral weakness, but cardiac involvement is generally absent. Retinal vasculopathy and sensorineural hearing loss may develop.[912,922] Oculopharyngeal dystrophy is another rare variant of muscular dystrophy that is characterized by progressive dysphagia and ptosis.

Myotonic dystrophy is the most common form of muscular dystrophy in adults, with an incidence of 1 in 8000. It can result from a mutation on either chromosome 19q13 (myotonic dystrophy type 1)[913] or chromosome 3q21 (myotonic dystrophy type 2).[914] Myotonic dystrophy type 1 is caused by a CTG expansion in the 3′ untranslated region of the dystrophia myotonica–protein kinase gene (DMPK).[913,932] DMPK may be involved in cellular Ca^{2+} homeostasis.[933] Abnormalities in sarcoplasmic reticulum Ca^{2+} transport have been noted in muscle fibers with myotonic dystrophy.[934]

Myotonic dystrophy is a dominantly inherited disease characterized by myotonia, progressive myopathy, insulin resistance, defects in cardiac conduction, neuropsychiatric impairment, cataracts, testicular atrophy, and frontal balding in males.[935] Patients with myotonic dystrophy have increased mortality from respiratory complications secondary to aspiration as a result of their muscle weakness, as well as cardiac dysrhythmias. The severity of the symptoms is somewhat related to the number of trinucleotide repeats in DMPK.[936]

ANESTHETIC CONSIDERATIONS. In dystrophic muscle, postsynaptic nAChRs are expressed as a mixture of fetal- and mature-type receptors.[17,937] Expression of fetal nAChR is not a characteristic of dystrophy but a consequence of muscle regeneration.[937] Succinylcholine is contraindicated in these patients because of the risk of hyperkalemic cardiac arrest and rhabdomyolysis.[658,659] This response has led to a Food and Drug Administration–mandated warning against the use of succinylcholine in pediatric patients because of potential mortality in those with clinically inapparent muscular dystrophies. In addition, the incidence of malignant hyperthermia is increased in patients with muscular dystrophies.[938,939]

Resistance to nondepolarizing neuromuscular blockers would be expected on the basis of the reduced sensitivity of fetal nAChRs to competitive antagonists.[17] However, clinically the reverse is seen[940-942] and has been attributed to the underlying muscle wasting and reduced ability to produce contractile force.[943] Other reports, however, indicate a normal response.[944] Buzello and coauthors[945] reported that the response of patients with myotonic dystrophy to neostigmine is unpredictable.[945] Attempts to reverse residual nondepolarizing blockade in one patient with 1.0 mg neostigmine were only partially effective, and the administration of a second dose (0.5 mg) produced long-lasting muscle weakness.[945] A tonic response to neostigmine was noted in another patient with myotonic dystrophy.[945] It is advisable to avoid using anticholinesterases in these patients.

Rhabdomyolysis, with or without cardiac arrest, can occur with inhaled anesthetics, even if succinylcholine is avoided.[946-948] This complication raises major concern regarding the safety of inhaled anesthetics in muscular dystrophy patients.[949,950]

Mathieu and colleagues[951] identified other potential anesthetic problems in patients with myotonic dystrophies, such as glossal hypertrophy, delayed gastric emptying, contractures, spinal deformities, impaired respiratory function, and cardiomyopathy. Therefore, preoperative pulmonary and cardiac status should be evaluated carefully in these patients. The need for a cardiac pacemaker should also be assessed preoperatively in patients with high-degree atrioventricular blocks. Weak ventilatory muscles, velopalatal insufficiency, and delayed gastric emptying are expected to increase the risk of aspiration and pneumonia.[858,952-954] Clinical deterioration may occur in pregnancy, probably because of hormonal changes.[955] Insulin resistance syndrome is also noted in patients with myotonic dystrophy[956] and is probably the result of a lack of insulin receptors in the muscle fiber membrane.[957]

Case reports have described increased sensitivity to thiopental and propofol in myotonic dystrophy patients.[958-960] However, further studies have not confirmed these reports.[950,951,961] In a recent report, neither exaggerated reactions nor hemodynamic instability was observed in 13 patients with myotonic dystrophy anesthetized by continuous propofol infusion, fentanyl, atracurium, and nitrous oxide.[950] The exaggerated physiologic responses to intravenous anesthetics may be related to the severity of the disease.

Regional anesthesia and total intravenous anesthesia with propofol, opioid anesthesia, and a nondepolarizing neuromuscular blocker appear to be safe and effective anesthetic techniques in patients with muscular dystrophy.[942,950,962-964] It is advisable to use short-acting nondepolarizing neuromuscular blockers and monitor neuromuscular function until full recovery to avoid the administration of anticholinesterases in these patients.

Blood loss in patients with Duchenne's muscular dystrophy is significantly greater than in those with spinal muscular atrophy undergoing scoliosis surgery.[965] The difference in blood loss is probably related to an inadequate vasoconstrictive response because of a lack of dystrophin, a reduction in neuronal nitric oxide synthase, and platelet dysfunction.[919,966]

Mitochondrial Myopathies

Mitochondrial myopathies are a clinically and biochemically heterogeneous group of disorders with genetic abnormalities that involve either a mitochondrial or a nuclear gene[967]; the prevalence is 7 per 100,000.[968] This disorder targets metabolically active organs such as the liver, the brain, and skeletal muscles because they contain the largest number of mitochondria.[969,970]

Mitochondrial myopathies are often associated with abnormal proliferation of mitochondria, which accumulate beneath the sarcolemma and between muscle fibers. Histologically, staining affected muscles with Gomori modified trichrome gives the characteristic ragged red fibers. However, ragged red fibers are not pathognomonic of a mitochondrial DNA mutation.[971]

Both isolated myopathies and several multisystem syndromes have been identified. The syndromes, which are defined by characteristic clinical manifestations in addition to mitochondrial myopathy, are chronic progressive external ophthalmoplegia, including Kearns-Sayre syndrome, MELAS syndrome (mitochondrial myopathy, encephalopathy, lactic acidosis, and strokelike episodes), MERRF syndrome (myoclonus epilepsy and ragged red fibers), MNGIE syndrome (myopathy, external ophthalmoplegia, neuropathy, and gastrointestinal encephalopathy), and NARP syndrome (neuropathy, ataxia, and retinitis pigmentosa). Acquired mitochondrial myopathy has been associated with the use of zidovudine, an antiretroviral drug that depletes muscle mitochondrial DNA.[972]

ANESTHETIC CONSIDERATIONS. Patients with mitochondrial disease may have lactic acidosis in the absence of hypoxia or sepsis.[973] Acid-base status should be monitored intraoperatively. Catecholamines, theophylline, nitroprusside, and prolonged infusion of propofol have been reported[974-976] to increase lactate concentrations by inducing transient abnormalities in oxidative phosphorylation.[973] Metabolic acidosis is also noted after exercise, fasting, and short-term use of a new formulation of propofol.[977] The incidence of diabetes mellitus is relatively high in patients with mitochondrial diseases.[978]

Respiratory failure may result from an impaired ventilatory response to hypercapnia and hypoxia,[979] muscle weakness,[980] diaphragmatic paralysis, or any combination of these conditions.[973] Sleep apnea is not uncommon in patients with mitochondrial disease.[981] Hypertrophic cardiomyopathies, cardiac conduction defects, and hypertension are also seen in mitochondrial disorders.[982,983] Bulbar muscle involvement is likely to increase the risk of aspiration in patients with mitochondrial disorders.[984]

Although it has been suggested that mitochondrial myopathy does not involve the neuromuscular junction,[985] increased sensitivity to different nondepolarizing neuromuscular blockers has been demonstrated in patients with mitochondrial myopathies.[986,987] This enhanced sensitivity is of a magnitude similar to that observed in myasthenia gravis.[986] Increased sensitivity to succinylcholine was also noted in these patients.[988] The association between malignant hyperthermia and mitochondrial myopathies is not clear, but published reports indicate a possible association.[989-991] Intrathecal and epidural anesthesia appears to be safe in patients with mitochondrial myopathies.[992,993]

Channelopathies

Cell membranes are composed of two lipid layers, which are not permeable to ions. However, cell membranes have channels that allow ions to diffuse in order to generate an action potential.[994] Siegelbaum and Koester[995] recognized the functions of ion channels as follows: "(1) they conduct ions; (2) they recognize and select among specific ions; and (3) they open and close in response to specific electrical, mechanical or chemical signals." In the neuromuscular junction, different channels are present at the prejunctional and postjunctional sites. These channels play an integral role in maintaining the functional integrity of the neuromuscular junction in health. Disorders of channel function are called channelopathies.[996,997] Most of the channelopathies affecting skeletal muscle will be addressed here, except for malignant hyperthermia (see Chapter 29) and central core disease (for review, see Naguib and coworkers[17]).

Waxman[998] pointed out that there are three main causes of channelopathy and proposed the following classification: (1) acquired (immune mediated and toxic), (2) genetic (caused by mutations in ion channel genes[994]), and (3) transcriptional channelopathies.[998] In immune-mediated and toxic channelopathies, binding of antibodies or toxins to channels alters their function.[866] Examples of acquired (immune mediated) channelopathies affecting the neuromuscular junction are myasthenia gravis (MG), Lambert-Eaton myasthenic syndrome (LEMS), and Isaacs' syndrome or neuromyotonia. A list of hereditary channelopathies that involve the neuromuscular junction is provided in Table 13-22. Waxman[998] pointed out that transcriptional channelopathies are due to "dysregulated expression of non-muted genes." Changes in Na^+ channel transcription have recently been implicated in MS.[999]

The Role of Ion Channels in Neuromuscular Transmission
For a more extensive account of this subject, the reader is referred to reviews by Hoffman,[1010] Cooper and Jan,[1011] Lehmann-Horn and Jurkat-Rott,[1012] and Kleopa and Barchi.[1013] Based on the current evidence,[1010-1012,1014] the role of ion channels in neuromuscular transmission can be summarized as follows:
1. Motor nerve:
   a. Depolarization of the motor nerve will open the voltage-gated Ca^{2+} channels that trigger both mobilization of synaptic vesicles and the fusion machinery in the nerve terminal to release acetylcholine.
   b. Several forms of K^+ channel present in the nerve terminal serve to limit the extent of Ca^{2+} entry and transmitter release (i.e., initiate repolarization of the nerve terminal).[1011]

2. Muscle:
   a. The released acetylcholine binds to α-subunits of the nAChRs. These ligand-gated cation channels allow sodium to enter and depolarize the muscle cell membrane at the neuromuscular junction.[997,1011]
   b. This depolarization activates voltage-gated sodium channels, which mediate the initiation and propagation of action potentials across the surface of the muscle membrane and into the transverse tubules (T-tubules) and thereby result in upstroke of the action potential.[997,1011,1012]
   c. Two types of calcium channels are recognized: the dihydropyridine receptor (DHPR) in the T-tubules and the ryanodine receptor (RyR1) in the sarcoplasmic reticulum (Fig. 13-36). DHPRs act as "voltage sensors,"[1015,1016] are activated by membrane depolarization, and in turn activate RyR1 receptors.
   d. DHPR-RyR1 interaction[1017] releases large amounts of Ca^{2+} from the sarcoplasmic reticulum, which causes muscle contraction. This process is known as excitation-contraction coupling.[1010]
   e. Repolarization of the muscle membrane is initiated by closing of the sodium channels and by opening of the potassium ion channels that conduct an outward K^+ current.[1014]
   f. Return the muscle membrane potential to its resting level (approximately −70 to −90 mV) is achieved by allowing Cl^- to enter the cell through voltage-sensitive chloride channels.[1011]

A list of ion channels mutated in human neuromuscular disease is presented in Table 13-22.

Myasthenic Syndromes
The large number (10,000/μm²) of nAChRs in the postsynaptic muscle membrane is crucial for maintaining normal neuromuscular function and for allowing a margin of safety in neuromuscular transmission.[1018] Although it is now established that MG is due to autoantibodies to

Table 13–22 Channelopathies in neuromuscular diseases

Disease	Ion Channel Subunit	Gene	Reference
Myotonia congenita (dominant and recessive)	Voltage-gated Cl^- channel	CLCN1	1000 1001
Hyperkalemic periodic paralysis	Voltage-gated Na^+ channel	SCN4A	1002
Paramyotonia congenita			1003
Potassium-aggravated myotonia			1004
Hypokalemic periodic paralysis type 1	Voltage-gated Ca^{2+} channel (dihydropyridine receptor)	CACNA1S	1005
Hypokalemic periodic paralysis type 2	Voltage-gated Na^+ channel	SCN4A	1006
Malignant hyperthermia	Ligand-gated Ca^{2+} channel	RYR1	1007
Central core disease			1008
Congenital myasthenic syndromes	nAChR channel	CHRNA1	1009
X-linked Charcot-Marie-Tooth disease	Connexin	GJB1 (Cx32)	882

nAChR, nicotinic acetylcholine receptor.
Modified from Naguib M, Flood P, McArdle JJ, et al: Advances in neurobiology of the neuromuscular junction: Implications for the anesthesiologist. Anesthesiology 96:202-231, 2002.

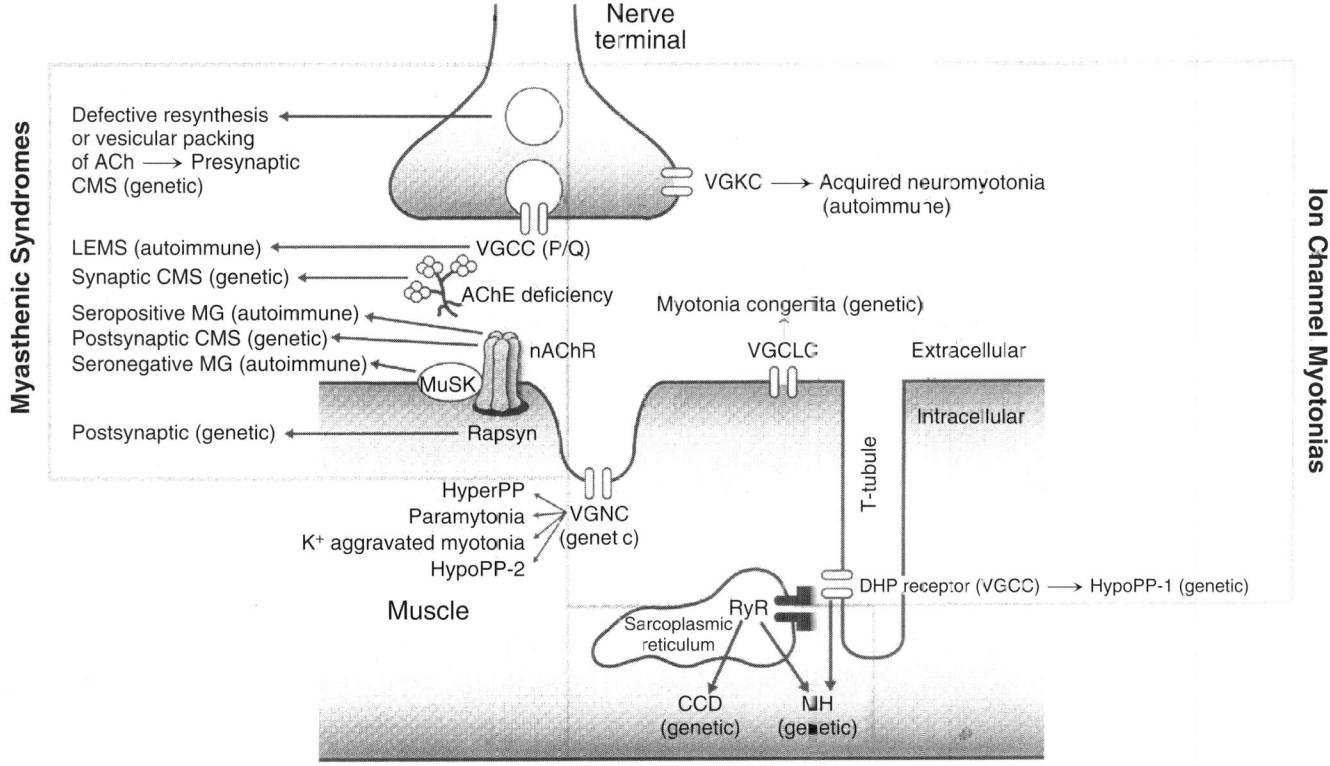

Malignant Hyperthermia

Figure 13–36 Disorders of channel function (channelopathies) that cause myasthenic syndromes, myotonias, malignant hyperthermia (MH), and central core disease (CCD). AChE, acetylcholinesterase; DHP receptor, dihydropyridine receptor; MuSk, muscle-specific kinase; nAChR, nicotinic acetylcholine receptor; RyR, ryanodine receptor; SV, synaptic vesicle; VGCC (P/Q), voltage-gated calcium channel (P/Q type); VGCLC, voltage-gated chloride channel; VGKC, voltage-gated potassium channel; VGNC, voltage-gated sodium channel.

nAChRs, several other autoimmune and genetic myasthenic syndromes have been identified (Fig. 13-36 and Table 13-23).[998] For more extensive accounts, see Vincent and colleagues,[1018,1019] Lindstrom,[1020] and Drachman.[1021]

Myasthenia Gravis

MG is an antibody-mediated autoimmune disease targeted against the α-subunit of nAChRs at the neuromuscular junction; it has a prevalence of 0.25 to 2.00 per 100,000 people.[1018-1021] In MG, the number of functional nAChRs is markedly decreased as a result of (1) cross-linking of antibodies to the receptors[1022] and (2) focal membrane lysis caused by complement fixation.[1021,1023,1024] The condition results in muscular weakness and fatigability.[1021]

Antibodies to the nAChR are present in about 80% of patients with MG.[1025,1026] In the remaining 20% of patients (called seronegative patients), nAChR antibodies are not detectable.[1027] Recently, another form of antibodies has been identified in seronegative MG patients. In about 70% of seronegative (but not seropositive) MG patients, the muscle-specific receptor tyrosine kinase

(MuSK) has been identified as the target for autoantibodies (see Fig. 13-36).[1028] MuSK mediates the agrin-induced clustering of AChRs during synapse formation and is also expressed at the mature neuromuscular junction.[17,1029] Interestingly, antibodies from MG patients do not cross-react with the α_3-subunit of the nAChR that is found principally in the autonomic nervous system or the α_4β_2 nAChRs that occur in the CNS. Perhaps this explains the lack of autonomic and CNS symptoms in typical MG.[1030]

The triggers for the immune response in MG are largely unknown. The thymus has been implicated because approximately 70% of MG patients have thymic lymphoid follicular hyperplasia with germinal centers that produce antibodies to nAChRs.[1020] In a small percentage of MG patients, autoantibodies develop as part of a paraneoplastic syndrome.[1020] About 12% of patients with MG have a thymoma, whereas 30% to 50% of patients with a thymoma suffer from MG.[1020] It is believed that antibodies to nAChRs are produced in other locations because thymectomy does not cure MG and does not protect against the occurrence of MG.[1020,1031] Fetal-type nAChRs,

Table 13–23   Myasthenic syndromes

Syndrome	Location	Mechanism	Etiology
Lambert-Eaton myasthenic syndrome	Presynaptic	Autoimmune	Antibodies to voltage-gated calcium channels at the motor nerve terminal
Congenital myasthenic syndromes		Genetic	
Choline acetyltransferase deficiency	Presynaptic		Mutations in choline acetyltransferase
Acetylcholinesterase deficiency	Synaptic		Mutations in the gene encoding the collagenic tail subunit (ColQ) of the enzyme that anchors acetylcholinesterase in the synaptic cleft
Slow- and fast-channel syndromes	Postsynaptic		Mutations in nAChR genes
nAChR deficiency	Postsynaptic		Mutations in nAChR genes or in rapsyn
Myasthenia gravis	Postsynaptic	Autoimmune	
Seropositive			Antibodies to nAChRs
Seronegative			Antibodies to MuSK

MuSK, muscle-specific kinase; nAChR, nicotinic acetylcholine receptor.

which are normally expressed in extraocular muscles, may be immunogenic as shown by their involvement in MG.[1020] Some evidence also indicates that antibodies generated in response to microbial antigens may be a trigger for MG in certain patients.[1032]

Electron microscopic studies show that the postsynaptic membrane has a simplified appearance with little folds[1033] associated with a marked reduction in the clustering of nAChRs to approximately 30% of those seen in normal neuromuscular junctions.[1040] Although acetylcholine sensitivity is reduced, a compensatory increase in the release of acetylcholine occurs at the neuromuscular junction in both experimental models of MG[1034] and muscle biopsy specimens from patients with MG.[1035]

Improvement in strength after the intravenous injection of edrophonium (Tensilon) helps confirm the diagnosis of MG. After a test dose of 1 to 2 mg, a total dose of 10 mg is administered intravenously. A positive response is expected within 5 minutes. No specific immunotherapy is available for MG. Nonspecific immunosuppression with steroids and other drugs and plasmapheresis are often combined with thymectomy and symptomatic treatment with anticholinesterases.

Lambert-Eaton Myasthenic Syndrome
LEMS is an example of an acquired (immune mediated) channelopathy that results from autoantibodies targeting the presynaptic voltage-gated Ca^{2+} channels and possibly another presynaptic component (such as synaptotagmin), and as a consequence, acetylcholine release is reduced.[1026,1036-1038] Synaptotagmin plays an important role in synaptic vesicle fusion and fast release of acetylcholine.[17,1039] Approximately 60% of LEMS patients show a paraneoplastic response, often in association with small cell carcinoma of the lung.[1026] LEMS is also characterized by weakness and fatigability.

Although both LEMS and MG are autoimmune diseases, they have several differences: (1) in LEMS, the presynaptic site of the neuromuscular junction is the target for autoantibodies, whereas postsynaptic nAChRs are the target in MG; (2) autonomic disturbances are seen in about 30% of patients with LEMS but not in patients with MG; (3) unlike MG, anticholinesterases are of little therapeutic value in LEMS[1036]; (4) improvement in muscle strength is seen after exercise in LEMS as a result of summation of presynaptic Ca^{2+} signals and improved acetylcholine release,[1040] but in MG improvement occurs after rest; (5) LEMS is differentiated from MG by electromyography, in which facilitation of the electromyographic response, rather than fade, occurs during high-frequency (30 to 50 Hz) stimulation; and (6) the two diseases can also be differentiated by antibody titer to specific channels. The acetylcholine contents and the architecture of the neuromuscular junction are normal in diseased nerve endings in LEMS.

Plasmapheresis or intravenous immunoglobulin can often give transient improvement in LEMS.[1041] Treatment with 3,4-diaminopyridine results in significant improvement in symptoms in patients with LEMS.[1042] Pyridostigmine potentiates the response to 3,4-diaminopyridine in many patients.[1042] 3,4-Diaminopyridine blocks potassium channels and thereby prevents potassium efflux. Prevention of potassium efflux increases the action potential duration, which in turn prolongs the activation of voltage-gated Ca^{2+} channels, along with a concomitant increase in intracellular Ca^{2+} concentration and acetylcholine release.

Congenital Myasthenic Syndromes
Congenital myasthenic syndromes (CMSs) are diverse disorders characterized by muscle weaknesses and fatigability (like MG) and caused by congenital defects in different components of the neuromuscular junction (see Fig. 13-36).[994,1043-1045] Inherited mutations are seen in the presynaptic (synaptic vesicles, choline acetyltransferase), synaptic (acetylcholinesterase), or postsynaptic

(nAChRs or rapsyn) component of the neuromuscular junction.[1009,1020,1044-1049] These mutations result in either increasing (gain of function) or decreasing (loss of function) magnitude of response to acetylcholine.[1044] Inheritance of CMSs is either autosomal dominant or autosomal recessive. The most frequent type of postsynaptic CMS is the slow-channel syndrome.[1009,1020,1046-1049] Mutations in the α-, β-, and most frequently the ε-subunit of nAChRs cause slow-channel congenital myasthenic syndromes (SCCMSs).[17] SCCMSs typically show dominant inheritance.

MG and CMSs have several differences: (1) unlike MG, antibodies against the nAChRs are not present and immunosuppressive therapy is not effective in CMSs, and (2) in contrast to neonatal MG, which is caused by passive transfer of anti-nAChR antibodies from a myasthenic mother to the fetus, the mother of a CMS patient does not have myasthenia.

An increase in the affinity of the nAChR for acetylcholine is seen in SCCMSs.[1009] The net effect of such gain-of-function mutations is to prolong the open state of the nAChR.[17] Such prolongation allows what is normally physiologic activation of the neuromuscular junction to overload the postsynaptic region with Ca^{2+} and initiates necrosis.[17] Activation of nitric oxide synthase at the neuromuscular junction can also contribute to free radical damage of the end plate. Nitric oxide synthase inhibitors may be of value in these patients.[1050] Patients with SCCMSs are significantly improved by quinidine sulfate because it normalizes the open duration of slow-channel mutants.[1051]

Loss-of-function mutations, seen in the α- and ε-subunits, decrease the rate of channel opening and increase the closure rate.[1052,1053] This loss of nAChR function reduces the safety factor for synaptic transmission.[17]

ANESTHETIC CONSIDERATIONS. For detailed reviews, see Baraka[1054] and Abel and Eisenkraft.[1055] Preoperative assessment and preparation of an MG patient should include (1) consultation with the patient's neurologist to learn of the recent history and progress of management; (2) preoperative drug therapy (such as pyridostigmine and immunosuppression drugs) and the potential impact of this drug therapy on responses to neuromuscular blockers; (3) counseling and preparation of the patient for possible postoperative endotracheal intubation and mechanical ventilation; and (4) optimization of medical management for myasthenia, which may include preoperative plasmapheresis and continuation of the anticholinesterase therapy. Pyridostigmine therapy should be continued preoperatively.

Patients with bulbar involvement are at increased risk for respiratory depression and aspiration, especially during myasthenic crises.[1056] It has been reported that 25% of myasthenic crisis episodes were associated with radiographic evidence of aspiration pneumonia.[1057] About 33% of the patients in crisis had severe oropharyngeal weakness.[1057] Pulmonary function tests, including flow-volume loops, may be necessary to predict the need for mechanical ventilation postoperatively.[1058]

Because of the decreased number of nAChRs, myasthenic patients are resistant to succinylcholine (Fig. 13-37).[1059] On the other hand, butyrylcholinesterase activity may be

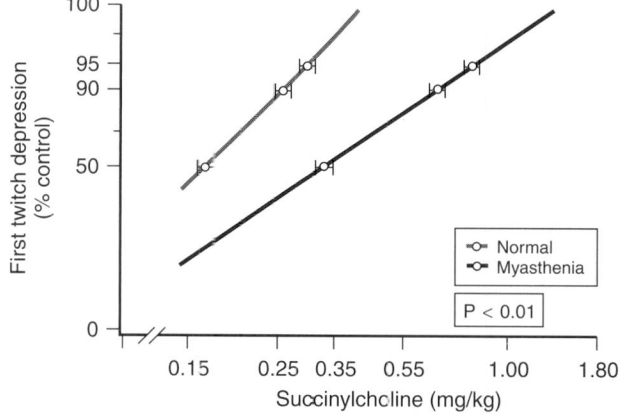

Figure 13–37 Succinylcholine dose-response curves in normal and myasthenic patients. (Redrawn from Eisenkraft JB, Book WJ, Mann SM, et al: Resistance to succinylcholine in myasthenia gravis: A dose-response study. Anesthesiology 69:760-763, 1988.)

decreased in myasthenic patients by preoperative plasmapheresis or by the administration of pyridostigmine (or by both), which would result in potentiation of succinylcholine[1060] or mivacurium-induced blockade.[1061] The interplay between these two factors (resistance to succinylcholine versus reduction in butyrylcholinesterase activity) should be considered when administering succinylcholine to patients with MG (Fig. 13-38). In addition, progression to a phase 2 block is not uncommon in these patients.[1062] Succinylcholine should be avoided in patients with SCCMSs because succinylcholine would be expected to worsen the existent state of excitotoxicity.[17]

The loss of approximately 70% of the postsynaptic nAChRs means that myasthenic patients have a marked reduction or even total loss of the safety margin for neuromuscular transmission. Therefore, it is not unexpected that patients with MG are extremely sensitive to nondepolarizing neuromuscular blockers (Figs. 13-39 and 13-40).[1054,1063-1065] The effective dose of vecuronium is 250% greater in control patients than in MG patients,[1066] but this does not mean that nondepolarizing neuromuscular blockers are contraindicated in these patients. With careful titration and adequate monitoring of neuromuscular function, nondepolarizing agents have been used safely in myasthenic patients undergoing thymectomy.[1054,1058,1063,1064] Long-acting neuromuscular blocking drugs should be avoided in these patients. Intermediate-acting drugs should be used in low dosage as guided by monitoring with a nerve stimulator. About one tenth to one fifth the ED_{95} should be given as a test dose to estimate the patient's requirement. Individual response will vary from extreme sensitivity, such that the test dose is all that is needed, to nearly normal relaxant requirements.

Pyridostigmine will modify the response to relaxants as follows: (1) the sensitivity to nondepolarizers will be diminished, (2) the response to succinylcholine or mivacurium may be prolonged, and (3) reversal of residual block at the end of the procedure may be ineffective because much acetylcholinesterase inhibition already

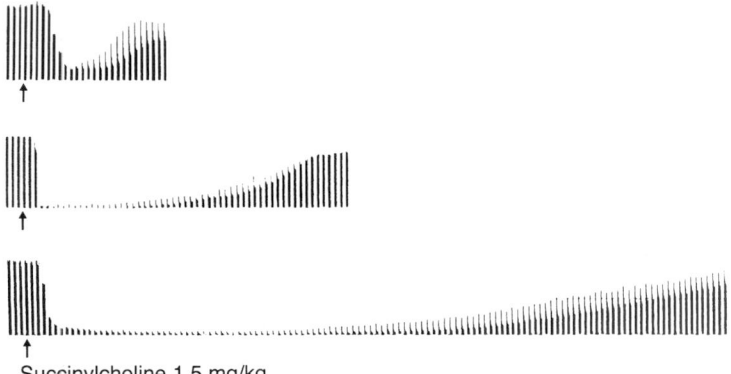

Succinylcholine 1.5 mg/kg

Figure 13–38 Electromyographic response to ulnar nerve stimulation by train-of-four stimulation every 20 seconds. Shown is the effect of 1.5 mg/kg succinylcholine in three myasthenic patients with differing butyrylcholinesterase activity. *Upper tracing,* butyrylcholinesterase = 5.16 U/mL; *middle tracing,* butyrylcholinesterase = 1.45 U/mL; *lower tracing,* butyrylcholinesterase = 0.73 U/mL. (From Baraka A: Suxamethonium block in the myasthenic patient. Correlation with plasma cholinesterase. Anaesthesia 47:217-219, 1992.)

exists as a result of chronic pyridostigmine therapy. Prolonged depolarizing blockade has been documented after reversal of vecuronium with neostigmine (3 mg) was attempted in a myasthenic patient.[1067] Consequently, it may be safer to allow spontaneous recovery from relaxation postoperatively while continuing supportive mechanical ventilation. Atracurium and cisatracurium appear to be the preferred muscle relaxants in myasthenia because their metabolism can obviate the need for reversal.

Different anesthetic techniques have been used in myasthenic patients. Although surgical relaxation can be provided for a myasthenic patient with only a potent inhaled anesthetic without neuromuscular blockers, this technique may be associated with slow recovery from anesthesia. In addition, myasthenic patients are more sensitive than normal to the neuromuscular depressant effects of halothane and isoflurane.[1068-1070] Therefore, it may be safer to intubate the trachea and provide surgical relaxation with the aid of nondepolarizing neuromuscular blockers in these patients than to use deep inhalation anesthesia.

A thoracic epidural anesthetic in combination with balanced general anesthesia provides excellent analgesia both intraoperatively and during the period after transsternal thymectomy.[1071] Regional anesthesia was also used successfully to provide labor analgesia with minimal muscle weakness in a parturient with MG.[1072] However, regional anesthesia is not a risk-free alternative.[1073]

Patients with LEMS are sensitive to both depolarizing and nondepolarizing neuromuscular blockers.[1074] In fact, patients with LEMS have significantly greater sensitivity to nondepolarizing neuromuscular blockers than those with MG do.[1075] In patients with LEMS, neostigmine is ineffective as an antagonist for residual neuromuscular block.[1076] It has been suggested that a combination of an anticholinesterase and 4-aminopyridine might be of value in

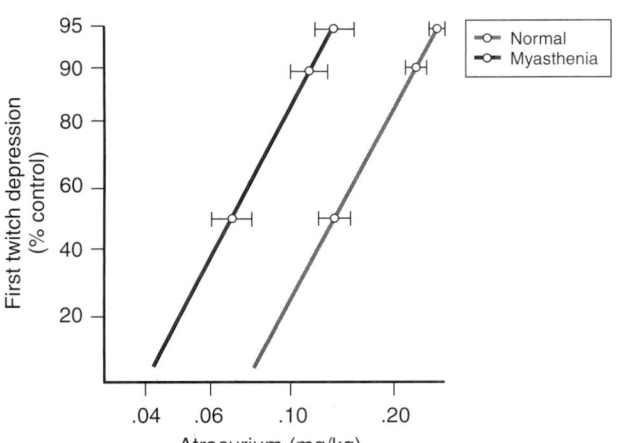

Figure 13–39 Cumulative dose response for atracurium in patients with myasthenia gravis. (Redrawn from Smith CE, Donati F, Bevan DR: Cumulative dose-response curves for atracurium in patients with myasthenia gravis. Can J Anaesth 36:402-406, 1989.)

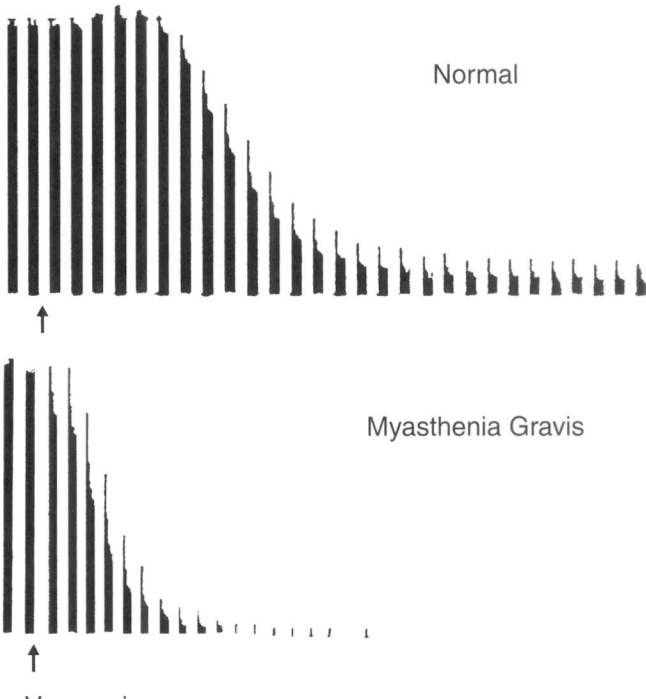

Figure 13–40 Electromyographic response to ulnar nerve stimulation. Injection of 0.1 mg/kg vecuronium in a normal patient resulted in a slow onset of nondepolarizing block *(upper trace),* whereas injecting one tenth the dose (0.01 mg/kg vecuronium) to a myasthenic patient resulted in a rapid onset of block *(lower trace).* (From Baraka A: Onset of neuromuscular block in myasthenic patients. Br J Anaesth 69:227-228, 1992.)

these patients.[1076] Oral 3,4-diaminopyridine should be continued after surgery. The bulbar muscles are usually spared in LEMS patients, but partial weakness and paralysis are not uncommon during recovery from general anesthesia in these patients.[1056]

All myasthenic patients should be closely monitored for neuromuscular weakness postoperatively in the surgical ICU. The differential diagnosis of postoperative weakness in myasthenic patients should include residual effects of neuromuscular blockers or anesthetic drugs, drugs that interfere with neuromuscular transmission (such as aminoglycoside antibiotics, antiarrhythmics, and psychotropics), and myasthenic or cholinergic crisis.

Ion Channel Myotonias

Myotonias are currently differentiated into two different types of disorders. The first type consists of channelopathies (Fig. 13-36 and Table 13-24; also see Table 13-22) and includes acquired neuromyotonia, myotonia congenita, paramyotonia, hyperkalemic periodic paralysis, potassium-aggravated myotonia, and hypokalemic periodic paralysis. The latter is a muscle ion channel disorder without myotonia. The second type includes myotonic dystrophy (see the section "Muscular Dystrophies").

Acquired Neuromyotonia

Neuromyotonia, also known as Isaacs' syndrome or continuous muscle fiber activity syndrome, is a rare peripheral motor neuron disorder. Like MG and LEMS, neuromyotonia is another example of an acquired (immune mediated) channelopathy.[1077-1079] It is believed that autoantibodies target the presynaptic voltage-gated potassium channels (see Fig. 13-36), thereby inhibiting action potential repolarization, enhancing transmitter release, and inducing hyperexcitability.[1026,1077] These antibodies have been detected in neuromyotonia patients.

In contrast to the weaknesses and fatigability seen in MG or LEMS, neuromyotonia is associated with increased activity at the neuromuscular junction that results in severe muscle cramps, stiffness, weakness, and often myokymia (muscular twitching during rest).[1026] Some patients exhibit CNS symptoms such as insomnia, mood changes, and hallucinations.[1077] The association of neuromyotonia with the aforementioned CNS manifestations has been coined "Morvan's syndrome."[1080] A paraneoplastic response often in association with small cell carcinoma or thymoma is seen in about 20% of patients with neuromyotonia.[1081,1082] Neuromyotonia can coexist with MG.[1018]

Drugs that act by increasing the sodium-pumping action of nerve and muscle tissue, such as phenytoin, are effective in treating neuromyotonia.[1083] Plasmapheresis can provide both clinical and electromyographic improvement.[1084] Immunosuppressive therapy with azathioprine may be helpful in severe cases.

ANESTHETIC CONSIDERATIONS. Spinal and epidural anesthesia, as well as succinylcholine and nondepolarizing neuromuscular blockers, are effective in abolishing spontaneous discharge and producing muscle relaxation.[1085,1086] Peripheral nerve blocks are not effective in abolishing myokymia in all patients,[1086] thus suggesting that in some cases the hyperexcitability originates within the distal nerve trunk.[1079] It should be noted that the abnormal muscle fiber activity can persist during sleep and general anesthesia.

Epidural anesthesia was used successfully for labor and delivery in a patient with neuromyotonia.[1087] The clinical effects of general anesthetics and neuromuscular blockers have not yet been reported in these patients. However, resistance to nondepolarizing neuromuscular blockers is expected in neuromyotonia because of (1) the increased acetylcholine release in these patients[1088] and (2) in vitro evidence of resistance to dTc.[1089] Some patients with acquired neuromyotonia may have autonomic and sensory neuropathies.[1077]

Myotonia Congenita

Both dominant (Thomsen) and recessive (Becker) forms of myotonia congenita are caused by mutations in the gene encoding the skeletal muscle voltage-gated chloride channel,[1000,1001,1090] with an estimated prevalence of 1 in 23,000 for recessive myotonia and 1 in 50,000 for dominant myotonia.[1013] As discussed before (see the section "The Role of Ion Channels in Neuromuscular Transmission"), chloride channels are responsible for return of the membrane potential to its resting level.[1011] Mutations in this channel decrease Cl^- conductance into the cell and thereby lead to hyperexcitability of the muscle membrane and muscle stiffness (see Fig. 13-36).[1010,1011,1091] Myotonias are characterized by difficulty initiating muscle movement and delayed muscle relaxation after voluntary contraction. It improves with sustained activity (warm-up phenomenon).

Muscle stiffness responds to Na^+ channels blockers such as local anesthetics and antiarrhythmic drugs.[1091] Although these drugs do not affect the kinetics of Cl^- channels, they decrease cell-membrane excitability.[1092]

ANESTHETIC CONSIDERATIONS. Myotonia may be precipitated by cold, shivering, diathermy, succinylcholine, and anticholinesterases (see Table 13-24).[945,1013,1092] The association between myotonia and malignant hyperthermia is uncertain, probably because of the difficulty in interpretation of the caffeine-halothane contracture test in myotonic patients.[1093,1094] It is prudent, however, to avoid all anesthetic triggering agents in these patients.

Myotonia developing in response to direct surgical activation of muscle is difficult to prevent and treat.[1095] Unlike local anesthetics and antiarrhythmic drugs, nondepolarizing neuromuscular blockers are not effective in alleviating this myotonic response.[1091] Clinical deterioration may occur in pregnancy and is probably due to the associated hormonal changes. Epidural anesthesia is reported to be safe in these patients.[1096]

Hyperkalemic Periodic Paralysis, Paramyotonia Congenita, and Potassium-Aggravated Myotonia

Mutations in the skeletal muscle voltage-gated Na^+ channel gene produce the clinical phenotypes of hyperkalemic periodic paralysis (HyperPP), paramyotonia congenita, and potassium-aggravated myotonia (see Fig. 13-36).[1002,1012] As discussed before (see the section "The Role of Ion Channels in Neuromuscular Transmission"), voltage-gated sodium channels are responsible for amplification and propagation

Table 13–24 Clinical features of ion channel disorders causing myotonia

	Autosomal Dominant Myotonia Congenita (Thomsen)	Autosomal Recessive Myotonia Congenita (Becker)	Potassium-Aggravated Myotonia	Paramyotonia Congenita	Hyperkalemic Periodic Paralysis (HyperPP)	Hypokalemic Periodic Paralysis (HypoPP)
Age at onset	Infancy-early childhood	Late childhood (variable)	First or second decade	First decade	First decade	Second decade (variable)
Initial symptoms	Muscle hypertrophy and generalized myotonia; occasional asymptomatic patients with electrical myotonia	Muscle hypertrophy (legs), generalized myotonia, transient weakness after rest	Myotonia (fluctuans, permanens, painful) affecting facial, eyelid, and paraspinal muscles	Paradoxical eyelid and grip myotonia; focal paralysis common, may overlap with HyperPP	Brief (<1 hr) paralytic attacks; myotonia or paramyotonia (eyelids) between paralytic episodes	Paralytic episodes that last hours-days, tend to remit with age, affect men more than women; no myotonia
Provocative stimuli	Myotonia worsened by rest, improves with exercise ("warm-up" phenomenon)	Myotonia worsened by rest or maintenance of same posture ("warm-up")	Potassium, cold, infection, exercise	Exercise and cold	Rest after exercise; cold and potassium trigger both paralysis and myotonia	Rest after exercise, often when waking up in the morning, after carbohydrate-rich and salty meals
Myopathy	Weakness may develop in older age; biopsy shows mild abnormalities	Possible muscle atrophy and weakness late in life	Rare myopathy, muscle hypertrophy common	Very rare	Infrequent	Possible progressive myopathy (vacuolar in HypoPP-1, tubular aggregates in HypoPP-2)
Therapy	Exercise, antimyotonia therapy (phenytoin, mexiletine)	Exercise, antimyotonia therapy	Acetazolamide, mexiletine, low-potassium diet, flecainide in painful variant	Mild exercise; avoid exposure to cold, mexiletine	Prevention with thiazide diuretics, acetazolamide, sodium restriction, carbohydrate-rich meals; attacks treated with diuretics, calcium gluconate	Prevention with potassium supplements, acetazolamide (worsens HypoPP-2), dichlorphenamide; attacks treated with oral potassium

From Kleopa KA, Barchi RL: Genetic disorders of neuromuscular ion channels. Muscle Nerve 26:299-325, 2002.

of action potentials along the muscle membrane. Mutant channels exhibit sustained Na^+ currents that lead to prolonged membrane depolarization causing myotonia, followed by membrane desensitization (or inactivation) resulting in paralysis.[1010-1013,1097] This is another example of a gain-of-function mutation.

HyperPP is a rare autosomal dominant disorder with a prevalence of 1:100,000.[1012] It is characterized by episodes of muscle weakness associated with hyperkalemia and with signs of myotonia in the interval between attacks.[1010] Respiratory and cardiac muscles are not affected, probably because of the existence of Na^+ channels in these muscles different from those expressed in skeletal muscle.[1013] The attacks of paralysis are frequent, brief, and often precipitated by rest after exertion, stress, ingestion of foods with high potassium content such as bananas, or the administration of potassium. A cold environment, emotional stress, and pregnancy provoke or worsen the attacks.[1014] Increases in serum K^+ up to 5 to 6 mmol/L may be seen during the attack.[1013] Prophylactic treatment with potassium-wasting diuretics can attenuate the frequency and severity of attacks.

The clinical manifestations of HyperPP, paramyotonia congenita, and potassium-aggravated myotonia are similar, which suggest that the three disorders may be allelic (i.e., a single genetic defect is responsible for coinheritance).[1003,1004,1098,1099] Normokalemic periodic paralysis is a variant of HyperPP and has been reported in only a few families.[1100-1102]

ANESTHETIC CONSIDERATIONS. Potassium depletion before surgery, maintenance of carbohydrate stores with dextrose-rich, potassium-free intravenous solutions, maintenance of normothermia, and avoidance of acidosis are essential in the anesthetic management of these patients.[1013,1103] Prewashed packed red blood cells should be used if blood transfusion is required. Careful and frequent monitoring of plasma potassium concentrations and acid-base status is of greatest importance. Succinylcholine should be avoided because it will result in increases in serum potassium concentrations and can cause myotonic symptoms in these patients.[1104] Anticholinesterase drugs should be avoided as well because they may provoke a myotonic reaction.[1105]

An association between malignant hyperthermia and HyperPP in the adult skeletal muscle sodium channel gene has been established.[1106] Patients with HyperPP appear to have a normal response to nondepolarizing neuromuscular blockers.[1103] Hyperkalemia should be considered in the differential diagnosis of postoperative residual weakness. Hyperkalemia should be treated with immediate hyperventilation, calcium chloride, 1.0 to 2.0 mg intravenously, sodium bicarbonate, 1 mEq/kg, and intravenous glucose and insulin (10 U regular insulin in 50 mL 50% glucose or, for children, 0.15 U regular insulin per kilogram in 1.0 mL/kg 50% glucose). Propofol was shown to target and block both normal and mutant voltage-gated sodium channels in a concentration- and voltage-dependent manner.[1107,1108] Therefore, propofol might be beneficial. Spinal anesthesia is reported to be a safe alternative to general anesthesia in these patients.[1109] Cardiac anesthesia poses particular problems. During recovery, special attention should be directed at maintaining normal body temperature and electrolyte and acid-base status.

Hypokalemic Periodic Paralysis

Mutations in the skeletal muscle voltage-gated Ca^{2+} channel gene (DHPR) produce hypokalemic periodic paralysis type 1 (HypoPP-1).[1005] HypoPP-2 is caused by mutations in the gene encoding the voltage-gated Na^+ channel of skeletal muscle (see Fig. 13-36).[1097,1098] Both types have the same clinical features.

HypoPP is a rare autosomal dominant disorder with a prevalence of 1:100,000.[1012] It is characterized by episodic weakness associated with hypokalemia during attacks.[1014] The hypokalemia has been attributed to increased activity of the Na^+-K^+ pump by insulin, which results in shifting of K^+ from the extracellular space into the intracellular compartment.[1111,1112] As discussed before (see the section "The Role of Ion Channels in Neuromuscular Transmission"), repolarization of the membrane in normal muscle is initiated by the outward K^+ current through the potassium ion channel.[1014] The abnormal inward shifting of K^+ (into the cell) in HypoPP causes prolonged depolarization leading to inactivation of both the mutant sodium channels in HypoPP-2 and normal sodium channels and thereby results in muscle weakness and paralysis.[1006,1013,1113,1114] Although this description does not include an explicit role for Ca^{2+} ion channels, the intracellular Ca^{2+} concentration is essential in regulating insulin secretion,[1115,1116] and it appears that mutations of the Ca^{2+} channel in HypoPP-1 may alter this mechanism.[1013,1112] HypoPP is an example of a loss-of-function mutation of Na^+ and Ca^{2+} ion channels.[1014]

In contrast to HyperPP, myotonia is absent in HypoPP, and ventricular dysrhythmias may occur during hypokalemic attacks.[997] HypoPP attacks are triggered by hypothermia, carbohydrate-rich meals, insulin, and vigorous exercise and can be treated by potassium administration (see Table 13-24).[1013] Prophylactic treatment with acetazolamide (a carbonic anhydrase inhibitor) is successful in HypoPP-1 patients, perhaps by producing metabolic acidosis, which decreases the urinary excretion of K^+.[1117] However, acetazolamide should not be used in HypoPP-2 patients because it can induce attacks of weakness and paralysis in this group of patients.[1110]

ANESTHETIC CONSIDERATIONS. Preoperative stress should be adequately alleviated by the administration of anxiolytic drugs such as benzodiazepines. Frequent monitoring of plasma potassium concentrations and acid-base status is required.

A normal response to succinylcholine is noted in these patients,[1118] but an association between HypoPP and malignant hyperthermia has been reported.[1119] There are no reports in the literature on the effects of nondepolarizing neuromuscular blockers in these patients, and their use seem to be safe in HypoPP patients.[1118] In a review of 21 anesthetics administered to members of a family with HypoPP, seven patients suffered from mild or severe postoperative paralysis.[1120] Hypokalemia should be considered in the differential diagnosis of postoperative residual weakness.

Spinal anesthesia and epidural anesthesia are safe alternatives to general anesthesia in these patients.[1121] It should be noted, however, that epidural,[1122] axillary, and intercostal nerve blocks[1123] lower serum potassium 0.3 to

0.7 mmol/L on average. Administration of epinephrine with the local anesthetic accounts for a proportion of this decline.[1122]

ECONOMICS AND OUTCOME IN PRACTICE WITH NEUROMUSCULAR BLOCKING DRUGS

Although the introduction of neuromuscular blocking drugs with intermediate and short durations of action has significantly changed the practice of providing neuromuscular blockade, the acquisition cost of these drugs is considerably greater than that of long-acting drugs such as pancuronium. In recent years, there has been pressure to reduce health care costs by reverting to more widespread use of long-acting neuromuscular blockers.[1124,1125] It is appropriate to remember that the acquisition cost of anesthesia drugs is likely to amount to approximately 0.25% of the total hospital budget and is only a fraction of the cost of running an operating room.[263] Focusing on only drug acquisition costs while trying to reduce health care costs is a simplistic view,[1126] and the impact of the choice of neuromuscular blocker on patient outcome must also be considered. Outcomes that result in increased medical cost must also be included in a patient's total health care costs.[1127]

A prospective trial of anesthesiologists' practices demonstrated that anesthesiologists are not inclined to choose medications based on price alone.[1128] However, price labeling, associated with education regarding the cost of medications in another study, did reduce the cost of acquisition of neuromuscular blockers by 12.5% over a 12-month period. This reduction translated into a savings of just over $47,000.[1129] The decrease in expenses for neuromuscular blockers was accomplished by a 104% increase in the use of pancuronium. However, unless the educational programs are ongoing and the staff remains well motivated, cost savings from this type of practice modification are short lived.[1130]

If a reduction in drug acquisition costs is to be considered an appropriate means of decreasing health care cost, anesthesiologists may look at their own practices. A year-long survey was performed in one hospital for waste of six frequently used or expensive medications. These drugs included thiopental, succinylcholine, rocuronium, atracurium, midazolam, and propofol. The study demonstrated that the total cost of drugs drawn up but not administered amounted to more than $165,000.[1131] Waste of thiopental and propofol accounted for most of this expense. In this practice, rocuronium and atracurium each accounted for 2% of the total expense. Succinylcholine did not significantly contribute to the cost of drug wastage. Although efficiency in the dosing of neuromuscular blockers can be improved, decreasing the amount of neuromuscular blockers drawn up and not administered to patients may not be a truly significant way to decrease health care costs.

The adequacy of recovery of neuromuscular function is crucial because even minor degrees of residual neuromuscular blockade have significant adverse effects.[53,54,563,565]

The muscles of airway protection are very sensitive to residual block,[53] and this predisposes patients to pulmonary aspiration.[563] In addition, residual neuromuscular blockade may compromise a patient's "street readiness" in the postoperative recovery period.[54] Mounting evidence indicates that the standard for acceptable recovery of neuromuscular function is no longer a TOF ratio of 0.7, but in fact greater safety might be achieved at 0.9.[54,563]

The relative incidence of residual neuromuscular blockade in the postoperative period is greater with neuromuscular blockers that have a longer duration of action. In 1979, a study by Viby-Mogensen and colleagues[58] showed that the incidence of residual weakness in the recovery room was higher than 40%. At that time, only long-acting drugs were available. With the introduction of vecuronium and atracurium, the incidence of residual weakness declined significantly to less than 10%.[59] If, however, a TOF ratio of 0.9 is to now be considered adequate, the incidence of unacceptable levels of neuromuscular block on admission to the PACU may be higher.[55]

Residual neuromuscular blockade caused by the administration of long-acting nondepolarizing neuromuscular blockers appears to predispose patients to a greater risk of postoperative pulmonary complications.[60] These complications constitute the greatest potential added expenses, and they accrue as a result of the choice of long-acting neuromuscular blockers over shorter-acting drugs. Delayed discharge from the PACU[1132] also has a significant cost impact. The increased length of stay in the PACU because of long-acting neuromuscular blockers has an estimated cost penalty to the institution of $40 per patient.[1132]

It is argued that the use of long-acting neuromuscular blockers is without adverse effect if strict practice guidelines regarding their use and dosing are implemented and continuously enforced.[1133,1134] However, even with strict regulation, the use of pancuronium rather than an intermediate-acting neuromuscular blocker is associated with a delay (a mean of 3 minutes) in the time from the end of the surgical procedure until the patient reaches the PACU. Much debate has been generated about the importance of this 3-minute delay.

The risks of residual weakness associated with the use of long-acting neuromuscular blockers apply to situations in which the patient's trachea will be extubated at the end of the surgical procedure. After cardiac surgery, for instance, where the tracheal tube will remain in place and the patient's ventilation will be supported postoperatively for hours or days, the use of long-acting neuromuscular blockers does not incur a cost penalty.[1135] In this scenario, the use of intermediate-acting relaxants may decrease the time to extubation of the trachea and the incidence of residual neuromuscular block. They do not, however, shorten the length of ICU stay after bypass surgery.[1136] In the case of relaxant use for shorter surgical procedures, succinylcholine and mivacurium were found to be economically superior to all the other neuromuscular blockers for use during short operations when intense neuromuscular blockade was mandatory.[1137] However, once doses of neuromuscular blockers beyond the initial intubating dose are required, the cost of the use of mivacurium increases, and it becomes more expensive than intermediate-acting neuromuscular blockers.[1138]

The debate regarding cost and neuromuscular blocker use is ongoing. On one side, there is evidence that drug acquisition costs for nondepolarizing neuromuscular blockers can be decreased through physician education. On the other side is evidence suggesting that patients are placed at greater risk for complications associated with residual paralysis when long-acting nondepolarizing neuromuscular blockers are used. As described by Miller,[1139] any savings accrued by using long-acting as opposed to the shorter-acting neuromuscular blockers will be lost with the occurrence of a single adverse event as a result of residual neuromuscular blockade. For example, succinylcholine's side effects render it expensive to use despite its short duration of action. The true cost per dose of succinylcholine from society's perspective is not negligible and is more than 20 times the acquisition cost.[140] Clinicians must constantly assess which neuromuscular blocking drug is best suited for their patients. The decision will be multifaceted and will have to include, in addition to the cost of the neuromuscular blocker, the duration and nature of the surgical procedure, as well as the patient's general health.

KEY POINTS

1. Two different populations of nicotinic acetylcholine receptors are found at the mammalian neuromuscular junction. In the adult, the nicotinic acetylcholine receptor at the postsynaptic (muscular) membrane is composed of $\alpha_2\beta\delta\varepsilon$-subunits. Each of the two α-subunits has an acetylcholine-binding site. The presynaptic (neuronal) nicotinic receptor is also a pentameric complex composed of $\alpha_3\beta_2$-subunits.

2. Nondepolarizing muscle relaxants produce neuromuscular blockade by competing with acetylcholine for the postsynaptic α-subunits. In contrast, succinylcholine produces prolonged depolarization that results in a decrease in sensitivity of the postsynaptic nicotinic acetylcholine receptor and inactivation of sodium channels so that propagation of the action potential across the muscle membrane is inhibited.

3. Different forms of neuromuscular stimulation test for neuromuscular blockade at different areas of the motor end plate. Depression of the response to single-twitch stimulation is probably due to blockade of postsynaptic nicotinic acetylcholine receptors, whereas fade in the response to tetanic and train-of-four stimuli results from blockade of presynaptic nicotinic receptors.

4. Succinylcholine is the only available depolarizing neuromuscular blocker. It has a rapid onset of effect and an ultrashort duration of action because of its rapid hydrolysis by butyrylcholinesterase.

5. The available nondepolarizing neuromuscular blockers can be classified according to chemical class (steroidal, benzylisoquinolinium, or other compounds) or according to onset or duration of action (long-, intermediate-, and short-acting drugs) of equipotent doses.

6. The speed of onset is inversely proportional to the potency of nondepolarizing neuromuscular blocking drugs. With the exception of atracurium, molar potency is highly predictive of a drug's rate of onset of effect. Rocuronium has a molar potency ($ED_{95} \approx 0.54\ \mu M/kg$) that is about 13% that of vecuronium and 9% that of cisatracurium. Its onset of effect is more rapid than that of either of these agents.

7. Neuromuscular blockade develops faster, lasts a shorter time, and recovers more quickly in the more centrally located neuromuscular units (laryngeal adductors, diaphragm, and masseter muscle) than in the more peripherally located adductor pollicis.

8. The long-acting neuromuscular blockers undergo minimal or no metabolism, and they are primarily eliminated, largely unchanged, by renal excretion. Neuromuscular blockers of intermediate duration of action have a more rapid clearance than the long-acting agents do because of multiple pathways of degradation, metabolism, and/or elimination. Mivacurium (a short-acting neuromuscular blocker) is cleared rapidly and almost exclusively by means of metabolism by butyrylcholinesterase.

9. After the administration of nondepolarizing neuromuscular blocking drugs, it is essential to ensure adequate return of normal neuromuscular function. Residual paralysis decreases upper esophageal tone, coordination of the esophageal musculature during swallowing, and the hypoxic ventilatory drive.

10. Defects in ion channels (channelopathies) in the presynaptic (neuronal) or postsynaptic (muscular) membrane of the neuromuscular junction result in a wide spectrum of muscle diseases.

REFERENCES

1. Griffith H, Johnson GE: The use of curare in general anesthesia. Anesthesiology 3:418, 1942.
2. Cullen SC: The use of curare for improvement of abdominal relaxation during cyclopropane anesthesia: Report on 131 cases. Surgery 14:216, 1943.
3. Beecher HK, Todd DP: A study of the deaths associated with anesthesia and surgery: Based on a study of 599,548 anesthesias in ten institutions 1948-1952, inclusive. Ann Surg 140:2-35, 1954.
4. Foldes FF, McNall PG, Borrego-Hinojosa JM: Succinylcholine, a new approach to muscular relaxation in anesthesiology. N Engl J Med 247:596-600, 1952.
5. Thesleff S: Farmakologisks och kliniska forsok med L.T. I. (O,O-succinylcholine jodid). Nord Med 46:1045, 1951.
6. Baird WL, Reid AM: The neuromuscular blocking properties of a new steroid compound, pancuronium bromide. A pilot study in man. Br J Anaesth 39:775-780, 1967.
7. Savage DS, Sleigh T, Carlyle I: The emergence of ORG NC 45,1-[2 beta,3 alpha,5 alpha,16 beta,17 beta-3,17-bis(acetyloxy)-2-(1-piperidinyl)-androstan-16-yl]-1-methylpiperidinium bromide, from the pancuronium series. Br J Anaesth 52(Suppl 1):3S-9S, 1980.
8. Stenlake JB, Waigh RD, Dewar GH, et al: Biodegradable neuromuscular blocking agents. Part 4: Atracurium besylate and related polyalkylylene di-esters. Eur J Med Chem 16:515, 1981.
9. Stenlake JB, Waigh RD, Urwin J, et al: Atracurium: Conception and inception. Br J Anaesth 55(Suppl 1):3S-10S, 1983.

10. Savarese JJ, Ali HH, Basta SJ, et al: The clinical neuromuscular pharmacology of mivacurium chloride (BW B1090U). A short-acting nondepolarizing ester neuromuscular blocking drug. Anesthesiology 68:723-732, 1988.

11. Wierda JM, de Wit AP, Kuizenga K, et al: Clinical observations on the neuromuscular blocking action of Org 9426, a new steroidal non-depolarizing agent. Br J Anaesth 64:521-523, 1990.

12. Gyermek L: Structure-activity relationships among derivatives of dicarboxylic acid esters of tropine. Pharmacol Ther 96:1-21, 2002.

13. Zhu HJ, Sacchetti M: Solid state characterization of a neuromuscular blocking agent—GW280430A. Int J Pharm 234:19-23, 2002.

14. On being aware. Br J Anaesth 51:711-712, 1979.

15. Shovelton DS: Reflections on an intensive therapy unit. BMJ 1:737-728, 1979.

16. Cullen SC, Larson CPJ: Essentials of Anesthetic Practice. Chicago, Year Book, 1974.

17. Naguib M, Flood P, McArdle JJ, et al: Advances in neurobiology of the neuromuscular junction: Implications for the anesthesiologist. Anesthesiology 96:202-231, 2002.

18. Machold J, Weise C, Utkin Y, et al: The handedness of the subunit arrangement of the nicotinic acetylcholine receptor from *Torpedo californica*. Eur J Biochem 234:427-430, 1995.

19. Yu XM, Hall ZW: Extracellular domains mediating epsilon subunit interactions of muscle acetylcholine receptor. Nature 352:64-67, 1991.

20. Willcockson IU, Hong A, Whisenant RP, et al: Orientation of *d*-tubocurarine in the muscle nicotinic acetylcholine receptor–binding site. J Biol Chem 277:42249-42258, 2002.

21. Neubig RR, Cohen JB: Equilibrium binding of [³H]tubocurarine and [³H]acetylcholine by *Torpedo* postsynaptic membranes: Stoichiometry and ligand interactions. Biochemistry 18:5464-5475, 1979.

22. Villarroel A, Sakmann B: Calcium permeability increase of endplate channels in rat muscle during postnatal development. J Physiol (Lond) 496:331-338, 1996.

23. Sine SM, Claudio T, Sigworth FJ: Activation of *Torpedo* acetylcholine receptors expressed in mouse fibroblasts. Single channel current kinetics reveal distinct agonist binding affinities. J Gen Physiol 96:395-437, 1990.

24. Devillers-Thiery A, Galzi JL, Eisele JL, et al: Functional architecture of the nicotinic acetylcholine receptor: A prototype of ligand-gated ion channels. J Membr Biol 136:97-112, 1993.

25. Grosman C, Zhou M, Auerbach A: Mapping the conformational wave of acetylcholine receptor channel gating. Nature 403:773-776, 2000.

26. Grosman C, Salamone FN, Sine SM, et al: The extracellular linker of muscle acetylcholine receptor channels is a gating control element. J Gen Physiol 116:327-340, 2000.

27. Bowman WC: Pharmacology of Neuromuscular Function, 2nd ed. London, Wright, 1990.

28. Paul M, Kindler CH, Fokt RM, et al: The potency of new muscle relaxants on recombinant muscle-type acetylcholine receptors. Anesth Analg 94:597-603, 2002.

29. Rosenberry TL: Acetylcholinesterase. Adv Enzymol Relat Areas Mol Biol 43:103-218, 1975.

30. Martyn JA: Basic and clinical pharmacology of the acetylcholine receptor: Implications for the use of neuromuscular relaxants. Keio J Med 44:1-8, 1995.

31. Kallen RG, Sheng ZH, Yang J, et al: Primary structure and expression of a sodium channel characteristic of denervated and immature rat skeletal muscle. Neuron 4:233-242, 1990.

32. Bowman WC: Prejunctional and postjunctional cholinoceptors at the neuromuscular junction. Anesth Analg 59:935-943, 1980.

33. Prior C, Tian L, Dempster J, et al: Prejunctional actions of muscle relaxants: Synaptic vesicles and transmitter mobilization as sites of action. Gen Pharmacol 26:659-666, 1995.

34. Wessler I, Diener A, Offermann M: Facilitatory and inhibitory muscarine receptors on the rat phrenic nerve: Effects of pirenzepine and dicyclomine. Naunyn Schmiedebergs Arch Pharmacol 338:138-142, 1988.

35. Starke K, Gothert M, Kilbinger H: Modulation of neurotransmitter release by presynaptic autoreceptors. Physiol Rev 69:864-989, 1989.

36. Slutsky I. Silman I, Parnas I, et al: Presynaptic M(2) muscarinic receptors are involved in controlling the kinetics of ACh release at the frog neuromuscular junction. J Physiol 536:717-725, 2001.

37. Slutsky I, Parnas H, Parnas I: Presynaptic effects of muscarine on ACh release at the frog neuromuscular junction. J Physiol 514(Pt 3):769-782, 1999.

38. Slutsky I, Wess J, Gomeza J, et al: Use of knockout mice reveals involvement of M2-muscarinic receptors in control of the kinetics of acetylcholine release. J Neurophysiol 89:1954-1967, 2003.

39. Bowman WC, Prior C, Marshall IG: Presynaptic receptors in the neuromuscular junction. Ann N Y Acad Sci 604:69-81, 1990.

40. Churchill-Davidson HC, Christie TH: Diagnosis of neuromuscular block in man. Br J Anaesth 31:290-295, 1959.

41. Christie TH, Churchill-Davidson HC: St. Thomas' Hospital nerve stimulator in diagnosis of prolonged apnea. Lancet 1:776-778, 1958.

42. Brull SJ, Connelly NR, O'Connor TZ, et al: Effect of tetanus on subsequent neuromuscular monitoring in patients receiving vecuronium. Anesthesiology 74:64-70, 1991.

43. Viby-Mogensen J, Howardy-Hansen P, Chraemmer-Jorgensen B, et al: Posttetanic count (PTC): A new method of evaluating an intense nondepolarizing neuromuscular blockade. Anesthesiology 55:458-461, 1981.

44. Kim SY, Lee JS, Kim SC, et al: Twitch augmentation and train-of-four fade during onset of neuromuscular block after subclinical doses of suxamethonium. Br J Anaesth 79:379-381, 1997.

45. Naguib M: Are fade and sustained post-tetanic facilitation characteristics of typical succinylcholine-induced block? Br J Anaesth 87:522-524, 2001.

46. Donati F, Meistelman C, Plaud B: Vecuronium neuromuscular blockade at the adductor muscles of the larynx and adductor pollicis. Anesthesiology 74:833-837, 1991.

47. Pansard JL, Chauvin M, Lebrault C, et al: Effect of an intubating dose of succinylcholine and atracurium on the diaphragm and the adductor pollicis muscle in humans. Anesthesiology 67:326-330, 1987.

48. Waud BE, Waud DR: The relation between tetanic fade and receptor occlusion in the presence of competitive neuromuscular block. Anesthesiology 35:456-464, 1971.

49. Kopman AF: Tactile evaluation of train-of-four count as an indicator of reliability of antagonism of vecuronium- or atracurium-induced neuromuscular blockade. Anesthesiology 75:588-593, 1991.

50. Engbaek J, Ostergaard D, Viby-Mogensen J: Double burst stimulation (DBS): A new pattern of nerve stimulation to identify residual neuromuscular block. Br J Anaesth 62:274-278, 1989.

51. Connelly NR, Silverman DG, O'Connor TZ, et al: Subjective responses to train-of-four and double burst stimulation in awake patients. Anesth Analg 70:650-653, 1990.

52. Drenck NE, Ueda N, Olsen NV, et al: Manual evaluation of residual curarization using double burst stimulation: A comparison with train-of-four. Anesthesiology 70:578-581, 1989.

53. Pavlin EG, Holle RH, Schoene RB: Recovery of airway protection compared with ventilation in humans after paralysis with curare. Anesthesiology 70:381-385, 1989.

54. Kopman AF, Yee PS, Neuman GG: Relationship of the train-of-four fade ratio to clinical signs and symptoms of residual paralysis in awake volunteers. Anesthesiology 86:765-771, 1997.

55. Debaene B, Plaud B, Dilly MP, et al: Residual paralysis in the PACU after a single intubating dose of nondepolarizing muscle relaxant with an intermediate duration of action. Anesthesiology 98:1042-1048, 2003.

56. Johansen SH, Jorgensen M, Molbeck S: Effect of tubocurarine on respiratory and nonrespiratory muscle power in man. J Appl Physiol 19:990-994, 1964.

57. Ali HH, Wilson RS, Savarese JJ, et al: The effect of tubocurarine on indirectly elicited train-of-four muscle response and respiratory measurements in humans. Br J Anaesth 47:570-574, 1975.
58. Viby-Mogensen J, Jorgensen BC, Ording H: Residual curarization in the recovery room. Anesthesiology 50:539-541, 1979.
59. Bevan DR, Smith CE, Donati F: Postoperative neuromuscular blockade: A comparison between atracurium, vecuronium, and pancuronium. Anesthesiology 69:272-276, 1988.
60. Berg H, Roed J, Viby-Mogensen J, et al: Residual neuromuscular block is a risk factor for postoperative pulmonary complications. A prospective, randomised, and blinded study of postoperative pulmonary complications after atracurium, vecuronium and pancuronium. Acta Anaesthesiol Scand 41:1095-1103, 1997.
61. Bovet D: Some aspects of the relationship between chemical constitution and curare-like activity. Ann N Y Acad Sci 54:407-437, 1951.
62. Chestnut RJ, Healy TE, Harper NJ, et al: Suxamethonium—the relation between dose and response. Anaesthesia 44:14-18, 1989.
63. Szalados JE, Donati F, Bevan DR: Effect of d-tubocurarine pretreatment on succinylcholine twitch augmentation and neuromuscular blockade. Anesth Analg 71:55-59, 1990.
64. Smith CE, Donati F, Bevan DR: Dose-response curves for succinylcholine: Single versus cumulative techniques. Anesthesiology 69:338-342, 1988.
65. Kopman AF, Klewicka MM, Neuman GG: An alternate method for estimating the dose-response relationships of neuromuscular blocking drugs. Anesth Analg 90:1191-1197, 2000.
66. Ferguson A, Bevan DR: Mixed neuromuscular block: The effect of precurarization. Anaesthesia 36:661-666, 1981.
67. Curran MJ, Donati F, Bevan DR: Onset and recovery of atracurium and suxamethonium-induced neuromuscular blockade with simultaneous train-of-four and single twitch stimulation. Br J Anaesth 59:989-994, 1987.
68. Mehta MP, Sokoll MD, Gergis SD: Accelerated onset of non-depolarizing neuromuscular blocking drugs: Pancuronium, atracurium and vecuronium. A comparison with succinylcholine. Eur J Anaesthesiol 5:15-21, 1988.
69. Viby-Mogensen J: Correlation of succinylcholine duration of action with plasma cholinesterase activity in subjects with the genotypically normal enzyme. Anesthesiology 53:517-520, 1980.
70. Katz RL, Ryan JF: The neuromuscular effects of suxamethonium in man. Br J Anaesth 41:381-390, 1969.
71. Gissen AJ, Katz RL, Karis JH, et al: Neuromuscular block in man during prolonged arterial infusion with succinylcholine. Anesthesiology 27:242-249, 1966.
72. Foldes FF, McNall PG, Birch JH: The neuromuscular activity of succinylmonocholine iodide in man. BMJ 1:967-968, 1954.
73. Baldwin KA, Forney R Jr: Correlation of plasma concentration and effects of succinylcholine in dogs. J Forensic Sci 33:470-479, 1988.
74. Foldes FF, Rendell-Baker L, Birch JH: Causes and prevention of prolonged apnea with succinylcholine. Anesth Analg 35:609-633, 1956.
75. Lepage L, Schiele F, Gueguen R, et al: Total cholinesterase in plasma: Biological variations and reference limits. Clin Chem 31:546-550, 1985.
76. Kopman AF, Strachovsky G, Lichtenstein L: Prolonged response to succinylcholine following physostigmine. Anesthesiology 49:142-143, 1978.
77. Sunew KY, Hicks RG: Effects of neostigmine and pyridostigmine on duration of succinylcholine action and pseudocholinesterase activity. Anesthesiology 49:188-191, 1978.
78. Lindsay PA, Lumley J: Suxamethonium apnoea masked by tetrahydroaminacrine. Anaesthesia 33:620-622, 1978.
79. Walts LF, DeAngelis J, Dillon JB: Clinical studies of the interaction of hexafluorenium and succinylcholine in man. Anesthesiology 33:503-507, 1970.
80. Baraka A: Hexafluorenium-suxamethonium interaction in patients with normal versus atypical cholinesterase. Br J Anaesth 47:885-888, 1975.
81. Kao YJ, Tellez J, Turner DR: Dose-dependent effect of metoclopramide on cholinesterases and suxamethonium metabolism. Br J Anaesth 65:220-224, 1990.
82. Woodworth GE, Sears DH, Grove TM, et al: The effect of cimetidine and ranitidine on the duration of action of succinylcholine. Anesth Analg 68:295-297, 1989.
83. Fisher DM, Caldwell JE, Sharma M, et al: The influence of bambuterol (carbamylated terbutaline) on the duration of action of succinylcholine-induced paralysis in humans. Anesthesiology 69:757-759, 1988.
84. Bang U, Viby-Mogensen J, Wiren JE, et al: The effect of bambuterol (carbamylated terbutaline) on plasma cholinesterase activity and suxamethonium-induced neuromuscular blockade in genotypically normal patients. Acta Anaesthesiol Scand 34:596-599, 1990.
85. Barabas E, Zsigmond EK, Kirkpatrick AF: The inhibitory effect of esmolol on human plasmacholinesterase. Can Anaesth Soc J 33:332-335, 1986.
86. Murthy VS, Patel KD, Elangovan RG, et al: Cardiovascular and neuromuscular effects of esmolol during induction of anesthesia. J Clin Pharmacol 26:351-357, 1986.
87. Pantuck EJ: Ecothiopate iodide eye drops and prolonged response to suxamethonium. Br J Anaesth 38:406-407, 1966.
88. Kalow W, Genest K: A method for the detection of atypical forms of human serum cholinesterase: Determination of dibucaine numbers. Can J Med Sci 35:339-346, 1957.
89. Pantuck EJ: Plasma cholinesterase: Gene and variations. Anesth Analg 77:380-386, 1993.
90. Jensen FS, Viby-Mogensen J: Plasma cholinesterase and abnormal reaction to succinylcholine: Twenty years' experience with the Danish Cholinesterase Research Unit. Acta Anaesthesiol Scand 39:150-156, 1995.
91. Primo-Parmo SL, Bartels CF, Wiersema B, et al: Characterization of 12 silent alleles of the human butyrylcholinesterase (BCHE) gene. Am J Hum Genet 58:52-64, 1996.
92. Primo-Parmo SL, Lightstone H, La Du BN: Characterization of an unstable variant (BChE115D) of human butyrylcholinesterase. Pharmacogenetics 7:27-34, 1997.
93. Galindo AHF, Davis TB: Succinylcholine and cardiac excitability. Anesthesiology 23:32-40, 1962.
94. Goat VA, Feldman SA: The dual action of suxamethonium on the isolated rabbit heart. Anaesthesia 27:149-153, 1972.
95. Craythorne NW, Turndorf H, Dripps RD: Changes in pulse rate and rhythm associated with the use of succinylcholine in anesthetized patients. Anesthesiology 21:465, 1960.
96. Leigh MM, McCoy DD: Bradycardia following intravenous administration of succinylcholine chloride to infants and children. Anesthesiology 18:698-702, 1957.
97. Stoelting RK, Peterson C: Heart-rate slowing and junctional rhythm following intravenous succinylcholine with and without intramuscular atropine preanesthetic medication. Anesth Analg 54:705-709, 1975.
98. Schoenstadt DA, Whitcher CE: Observations on the mechanism of succinylcholine-induced cardiac arrhythmias. Anesthesiology 24:358-362, 1963.
99. Badgwell JM, Cunliffe M, Lerman J: Thiopental attenuates dysrhythmias in children: Comparison of induction regimens. Tex Med 86:36-38, 1990.
100. Mathias JA, Evans-Prosser CD, Churchill-Davidson HC: The role of the non-depolarizing drugs in the prevention of suxamethonium bradycardia. Br J Anaesth 42:609-613, 1970.
101. Leiman BC, Katz J, Butler BD: Mechanisms of succinylcholine-induced arrhythmias in hypoxic or hypoxic: hypercarbic dogs. Anesth Analg 66:1292-1297, 1987.
102. Nigrovic V, McCullough LS, Wajskol A, et al: Succinylcholine-induced increases in plasma catecholamine levels in humans. Anesth Analg 62:627-632, 1983.
103. Derbyshire DR: Succinylcholine-induced increases in plasma catecholamine levels in humans. Anesth Analg 63:465-467, 1984.
104. Derbyshire DR, Chmielewski A, Fell D, et al: Plasma catecholamine responses to tracheal intubation. Br J Anaesth 55:855-860, 1983.

105. Roth F, Wuthrich H: The clinical importance of hyper-kalaemia following suxamethonium administration. Br J Anaesth 41:311-316, 1969.

106. Powell JN, Golby MG: Changes in serum potassium following suxamethonium in the uraemic rat. Br J Anaesth 42:804, 1970.

107. Powell JN, Golby M: The pattern of potassium liberation following a single dose of suxamethonium in normal and uraemic rats. Br J Anaesth 43:662-668, 1971.

108. Walton JD, Farman JV: Suxamethonium, potassium and renal failure. Anaesthesia 28:626-630, 1973.

109. Miller RD, Way WL, Hamilton WK, et al: Succinylcholine-induced hyperkalemia in patients with renal failure? Anesthesiology 36:138-141, 1972.

110. Powell DR, Miller R: The effect of repeated doses of succinylcholine on serum potassium in patients with renal failure. Anesth Analg 54:746-748, 1975.

111. Koide M, Waud BE: Serum potassium concentrations after succinylcholine in patients with renal failure. Anesthesiology 36:142-145, 1972.

112. Walton JD, Farman JV: Suxamethonium hyperkalaemia in uraemic neuropathy. Anaesthesia 28:666-668, 1973.

113. Schwartz DE, Kelly B, Caldwell JE, et al: Succinylcholine-induced hyperkalemic arrest in a patient with severe metabolic acidosis and exsanguinating hemorrhage. Anesth Analg 75:291-293, 1992.

114. Antognini JF, Gronert GA: Succinylcholine causes profound hyperkalemia in hemorrhagic, acidotic rabbits. Anesth Analg 77:585-588, 1993.

115. Antognini JF: Splanchnic release of potassium after hemorrhage and succinylcholine in rabbits. Anesth Analg 78:687-690, 1994.

116. Kohlschütter B, Baur H, Roth F: Suxamethonium-induced hyperkalaemia in patients with severe intra-abdominal infections. Br J Anaesth 48:557-562, 1976.

117. Stevenson PH, Birch AA: Succinylcholine-induced hyperkalemia in a patient with a closed head injury. Anesthesiology 51:89-90, 1979.

118. Birch AA Jr, Mitchell GD, Playford GA, et al: Changes in serum potassium response to succinylcholine following trauma. JAMA 210:490-493, 1969.

119. Gronert GA, Theye RA: Pathophysiology of hyperkalemia induced by succinylcholine. Anesthesiology 43:89-99, 1975.

120. Pandey K, Badola RP, Kumar S: Time course of intraocular hypertension produced by suxamethonium. Br J Anaesth 44:191-196, 1972.

121. Indu B, Batra YK, Puri GD, et al: Nifedipine attenuates the intraocular pressure response to intubation following succinylcholine. Can J Anaesth 36:269-272, 1989.

122. Meyers EF, Krupin T, Johnson M, et al: Failure of nondepolarizing neuromuscular blockers to inhibit succinylcholine-induced increased intraocular pressure, a controlled study. Anesthesiology 48:149-151, 1978.

123. Konchigeri HN, Lee YE, Venugopal K: Effect of pancuronium on intraocular pressure changes induced by succinylcholine. Can Anaesth Soc J 26:479-481, 1979.

124. Libonati MM, Leahy JJ, Ellison N: The use of succinylcholine in open eye surgery. Anesthesiology 62:637-640, 1985.

125. Joshi C, Bruce DL: Thiopental and succinylcholine: Action on intraocular pressure. Anesth Analg 54:471-475, 1975.

126. Pollack AL, McDonald RH, Ai E, et al: Massive suprachoroidal hemorrhage during pars plana vitrectomy associated with Valsalva maneuver. Am J Ophthalmol 132:383-387, 2001.

127. Grennan J: The cardio-oesphageal junction. Br J Anaesth 33:432, 1961.

128. Miller RD, Way WL: Inhibition of succinylcholine-induced increased intragastric pressure by nondepolarizing muscle relaxants and lidocaine. Anesthesiology 34:185-188, 1971.

129. Salem MR, Wong AY, Lin YH: The effect of suxamethonium on the intragastric pressure in infants and children. Br J Anaesth 44:166-170, 1972.

130. Minton MD, Grosslight K, Stirt JA, et al: Increases in intracranial pressure from succinylcholine: Prevention by prior nondepolarizing blockade. Anesthesiology 65:165-169, 1986.

131. Stirt JA, Grosslight KR, Bedford RF, et al: "Defasciculation" with metocurine prevents succinylcholine-induced increases in intracranial pressure. Anesthesiology 67:50-53, 1987.

132. Brodsky JB, Brock-Utne JG, Samuels SI: Pancuronium pretreatment and post-succinylcholine myalgias. Anesthesiology 51:259-261, 1979.

133. Waters DJ, Mapleson WW: Suxamethonium pains: Hypothesis and observation. Anaesthesia 26:127-141, 1971.

134. Ryan JF, Kagen LJ, Hyman AI: Myoglobinemia after a single dose of succinylcholine. N Engl J Med 285:824-827, 1971.

135. Maddineni VR, Mirakhur RK, Cooper AR: Myalgia and biochemical changes following suxamethonium after induction of anaesthesia with thiopentone or propofol. Anaesthesia 48:626-628, 1993.

136. McLoughlin C, Elliott P, McCarthy G, et al: Muscle pains and biochemical changes following suxamethonium administration after six pretreatment regimens. Anaesthesia 47:202-206, 1992.

137. Demers-Pelletier J, Drolet P, Girard M, et al: Comparison of rocuronium and d-tubocurarine for prevention of succinylcholine-induced fasciculations and myalgia. Can J Anaesth 44:1144-1147, 1997.

138. Naguib M, Farag H, Magbagbeola JA: Effect of pre-treatment with lysine acetyl salicylate on suxamethonium-induced myalgia. Br J Anaesth 59:606-610, 1987.

139. Zahl K, Apfelbaum JL: Muscle pain occurs after outpatient laparoscopy despite the substitution of vecuronium for succinylcholine. Anesthesiology 70:408-411, 1989.

140. Smith I, Ding Y, White PF: Muscle pain after outpatient laparoscopy—influence of propofol versus thiopental and enflurane. Anesth Analg 76:1181-1184, 1993.

141. Leary NP, Ellis FR: Masseteric muscle spasm as a normal response to suxamethonium. Br J Anaesth 64:488-492, 1990.

142. Meakin G, Walker RW, Dearlove OR: Myotonic and neuromuscular blocking effects of increased doses of suxamethonium in infants and children. Br J Anaesth 65:816-818, 1990.

143. Littleford JA, Patel LR, Bose D, et al: Masseter muscle spasm in children: Implications of continuing the triggering anesthetic. Anesth Analg 72:151-160, 1991.

144. Habre W, Sims C: Masseter spasm and elevated creatine kinase after intravenous induction in a child. Anaesth Intensive Care 24:496-499, 1996.

145. Donlon JV, Newfield P, Sreter F, et al: Implications of masseter spasm after succinylcholine. Anesthesiology 49:298-301, 1978.

146. Van der Spek AF, Fang WB, Ashton-Miller JA, et al: The effects of succinylcholine on mouth opening. Anesthesiology 67:459-465, 1987.

147. Clarke RSJ: Intubating Conditions and Neuromuscular Effects following Vecuronium Bromide. Comparison with Suxamethonium Chloride and Pancuronium Bromide, Clinical Experiences with Norcuron. Amsterdam, Excerpta Medica, 1983.

148. Heier T, Feiner JR, Lin J, et al: Hemoglobin desaturation after succinylcholine-induced apnea: A study of the recovery of spontaneous ventilation in healthy volunteers. Anesthesiology 94:754-759, 2001.

149. Benumof JL, Dagg R, Benumof R: Critical hemoglobin desaturation will occur before return to an unparalyzed state following 1 mg/kg intravenous succinylcholine. Anesthesiology 87:979-982, 1997.

150. Naguib M, Samarkandi A, Riad W, et al: Optimal dose of succinylcholine revisited. Anesthesiology 99:1045-1049, 2003.

151. Kopman AF, Zhaku BA, Lai KS: The "intubating dose" of succinylcholine: The effect of decreasing doses on recovery time. Anesthesiology 99:1050-1054, 2003.

152. Miller RD: The advantages of giving d-tubocurarine before succinylcholine. Anesthesiology 37:568-569, 1972.

153. Donati F, Gill SS, Bevan DR, et al: Pharmacokinetics and pharmacodynamics of atracurium with and without previous suxamethonium administration. Br J Anaesth 66:557-561, 1991.

154. Dubois MY, Lea DE, Kataria B, et al: Pharmacodynamics of rocuronium with and without prior administration of succinylcholine. J Clin Anesth 7:44-48, 1995.

155. Naguib M, Abdulatif M, Selim M, et al: Dose-response studies of the interaction between mivacurium and suxamethonium. Br J Anaesth 74:26-30, 1995.

156. Erkola O, Rautoma P, Meretoja OA: Interaction between mivacurium and succinylcholine. Anesth Analg 80:534-537, 1995.

157. Lee C, Katz RL: Neuromuscular pharmacology. A clinical update and commentary. Br J Anaesth 52:173-188, 1980.

158. Ramsey FM, Lebowitz PW, Savarese JJ, et al: Clinical characteristics of long-term succinylcholine neuromuscular blockade during balanced anesthesia. Anesth Analg 59:110-116, 1980.

159. Lee C: Structure, conformation, and action of neuromuscular blocking drugs. Br J Anaesth 87:755-769, 2001.

160. Everett AJ, Lowe LA, Wilkinson S: Revision of the structures of (+)-tubocurarine chloride and (+)-chondocurine. J Chem Soc D:1020-1021, 1970.

161. Waser PG: Chemistry and pharmacology of natural curare compounds, neuromuscular blocking and stimulating agents. In Cheymol J (ed): International Encyclopedia of Pharmacology and Therapeutics. Oxford, Pergamon, 1972, pp 205-239.

162. Hill SA, Scott RPF, Savarese JJ: Structure-activity relationships: From tubocurarine to the present day. Baillieres Clin Anaesthiol 8:317-348, 1994.

163. Gandiha A, Marshall IG, Paul D, et al: Neuromuscular and other blocking actions of a new series of mono and bisquaternary aza steroids. J Pharm Pharmacol 26:871-877, 1974.

164. Stenlake JB, Waigh RD, Dewar GH, et al: Biodegradable neuromuscular blocking agents. 6. - Stereochemical studies on atracurium and related polyalkylene di-esters. Eur J Med Chem 19:441-450, 1984.

165. Tsui D, Graham GG, Torda TA: The pharmacokinetics of atracurium isomers in vitro and in humans. Anesthesiology 67:722-728, 1987.

166. Nehmer U: Simultaneous determination of atracurium besylate and its major decomposition products and related impurities by reversed-phase high-performance liquid chromatography. J Chromatogr 435:425-433, 1988.

167. Wastila WB, Maehr RB, Turner GL, et al: Comparative pharmacology of cisatracurium (51W89), atracurium, and five isomers in cats. Anesthesiology 85:169-177, 1996.

168. Lien CA: The role of stereoisomerism in neuromuscular blocking drugs. Curr Opin Anesthesiol 9:348-353, 1996.

169. Lien CA, Belmont MR, Abalos A, et al: The cardiovascular effects and histamine-releasing properties of 51W89 in patients receiving nitrous oxide/opioid/barbiturate anesthesia. Anesthesiology 82:1131-1138, 1995.

170. Savarese JJ, Wastila WB: The future of the benzylisoquinolinium relaxants. Acta Anaesthesiol Scand Suppl 106:91-93, 1995.

171. Lien CA, Schmith VD, Embree PB, et al: The pharmacokinetics and pharmacodynamics of the stereoisomers of mivacurium in patients receiving nitrous oxide/opioid/barbiturate anesthesia. Anesthesiology 80:1296-1302, 1994.

172. Head-Rapson AG, Devlin JC, Parker CJ, et al: Pharmacokinetics of the three isomers of mivacurium and pharmacodynamics of the chiral mixture in hepatic cirrhosis. Br J Anaesth 73:613-618, 1994.

173. Buckett WR, Hewett CL, Savage DS: Pancuronium bromide and other steroidal neuromuscular blocking agents containing acetylcholine fragments. J Med Chem 16:1116-1124, 1973.

174. Durant NN, Marshall IG, Savage DS, et al: The neuromuscular and autonomic blocking activities of pancuronium, Org NC 45, and other pancuronium analogues, in the cat. J Pharm Pharmacol 31:831-836, 1979.

175. Stovner J, Oftedal N, Holmboe J: The inhibition of cholinesterases by pancuronium. Br J Anaesth 47:949-954, 1975.

176. Bowman WC, Rodger IW, Houston J, et al: Structure:action relationships among some desacetoxy analogues of pancuronium and vecuronium in the anesthetized cat. Anesthesiology 69:57-62, 1988.

177. Data on file. Organon Inc.

178. Wierda JM, Proost JH: Structure-pharmacodynamic-pharmacokinetic relationships of steroidal neuromuscular blocking agents. Eur J Anaesthesiol Suppl 11:45-54, 1995.

179. Naguib M, Samarkandi AH, Bakhamees HS, et al: Comparative potency of steroidal neuromuscular blocking drugs and isobolographic analysis of the interaction between rocuronium and other aminosteroids. Br J Anaesth 75:37-42, 1995.

180. Goulden MR, Hunter JM: Rapacuronium (Org 9487): Do we have a replacement for succinylcholine? Br J Anaesth 82:489-492, 1999.

181. Naguib M: How serious is the bronchospasm induced by rapacuronium? Anesthesiology 94:924-925, 2001.

182. Kron SS: Severe bronchospasm and desaturation in a child associated with rapacuronium. Anesthesiology 94:923-924, 2001.

183. Meakin GH, Pronske EH, Lerman J, et al: Bronchospasm after rapacuronium in infants and children. Anesthesiology 94:926-927, 2001.

184. Goudsouzian NG: Rapacuronium and bronchospasm. Anesthesiology 94:727-728, 2001.

185. Boros EE, Bigham EC, Boswell GE, et al: Bis- and mixed-tetrahydroisoquinolinium chlorofumarates: New ultra-short-acting nondepolarizing neuromuscular blockers. J Med Chem 42:206-209, 1999.

186. Moore EW, Hunter JM: The new neuromuscular blocking agents: Do they offer any advantages? Br J Anaesth 87:912-925, 2001.

187. Boros EE, Samano V, Ray JA, et al: Neuromuscular blocking activity and therapeutic potential of mixed-tetrahydroisoquinolinium halofumarates and halosuccinates in rhesus monkeys. J Med Chem 46:2502-2515, 2003.

188. Belmont MR, Lien CA, Tjan J, et al: The clinical pharmacology of GW280430A in humans. Anesthesiology (in press).

189. Gyermek L, Lee C, Cho YM, et al: Neuromuscular pharmacology of TAAC3, a new nondepolarizing muscle relaxant with rapid onset and ultrashort duration of action. Anesth Analg 94:879-885, 2002.

190. Shanks CA: Pharmacokinetics of the nondepolarizing neuromuscular relaxants applied to calculation of bolus and infusion dosage regimens. Anesthesiology 64:72-86, 1986.

191. Azad SS, Larijani GE, Goldberg ME, et al: A dose-response evaluation of pipecuronium bromide in elderly patients under balanced anesthesia. J Clin Pharmacol 29:657-659, 1989.

192. Pittet JF, Tassonyi E, Morel DR, et al: Pipecuronium-induced neuromuscular blockade during nitrous oxide–fentanyl, isoflurane, and halothane anesthesia in adults and children. Anesthesiology 71:210-213, 1989.

193. Stanley JC, Mirakhur RK: Comparative potency of pipecuronium bromide and pancuronium bromide. Br J Anaesth 63:754-755, 1989.

194. Wierda JM, Richardson FJ, Agoston S: Dose-response relation and time course of action of pipecuronium bromide in humans anesthetized with nitrous oxide and isoflurane, halothane, or droperidol and fentanyl. Anesth Analg 68:208-213, 1989.

195. Foldes FF, Nagashima H, Nguyen HD, et al: Neuromuscular and cardiovascular effects of pipecuronium. Can J Anaesth 37:549-555, 1990.

196. Naguib M, Seraj M, Abdulrazik E: Pipecuronium-induced neuromuscular blockade during nitrous oxide–fentanyl, enflurane, isoflurane, and halothane anesthesia in surgical patients. Anesth Analg 75:193-197, 1992.

197. Basta SJ, Savarese JJ, Ali HH, et al: Clinical pharmacology of doxacurium chloride. A new long-acting nondepolarizing muscle relaxant. Anesthesiology 69:478-486, 1988.

198. Murray DJ, Mehta MP, Choi WW, et al: The neuromuscular blocking and cardiovascular effects of doxacurium chloride in patients receiving nitrous oxide narcotic anesthesia. Anesthesiology 69 472-477, 1988.

199. Katz JA, Fragen RJ, Shanks CA, et al: Dose-response relationships of doxacurium chloride in humans during anesthesia with nitrous oxide and fentanyl, enflurane, isoflurane, or halothane. Anesthesiology 70:432-436, 1989.

200. Koscielniak-Nielsen ZJ, Law-Min JC, Donati F, et al: Dose-response relations of doxacurium and its reversal with neostigmine in young adults and healthy elderly patients. Anesth Analg 74:845-850, 1992.

201. Maddineni VR, Cooper R, Stanley JC, et al: Clinical evaluation of doxacurium chloride. Anaesthesia 47:554-557, 1992.

202. Booij LH, Knape HT: The neuromuscular blocking effect of Org 9426. A new intermediately-acting steroidal non-depolarising muscle relaxant in man. Anaesthesia 46:341-343, 1991.

203. Foldes FF, Nagashima H, Nguyen HD, et al: The neuromuscular effects of ORG9426 in patients receiving balanced anesthesia. Anesthesiology 75:191-196, 1991.

204. Lambalk LM, De Wit AP, Wierda JM, et al: Dose-response relationship and time course of action of Org 9426. A new muscle relaxant of intermediate duration evaluated under various anaesthetic techniques. Anaesthesia 46:907-911, 1991.

205. Cooper RA, Mirakhur RK, Elliott P, et al: Estimation of the potency of ORG 9426 using two different modes of nerve stimulation. Can J Anaesth 39:139-142, 1992.

206. Bartkowski RR, Witkowski TA, Azad S, et al: Rocuronium onset of action: A comparison with atracurium and vecuronium. Anesth Analg 77:574-578, 1993.

207. Bevan DR, Fiset P, Balendran P, et al: Pharmacodynamic behaviour of rocuronium in the elderly. Can J Anaesth 40:127-132, 1993.

208. Oris B, Crul JF, Vandermeersch E, et al: Muscle paralysis by rocuronium during halothane, enflurane, isoflurane, and total intravenous anesthesia. Anesth Analg 77:570-573, 1993.

209. Belmont MR, Lien CA, Quessy S, et al: The clinical neuromuscular pharmacology of 51W89 in patients receiving nitrous oxide/opioid/barbiturate anesthesia. Anesthesiology 82:1139-1145, 1995.

210. Savarese JJ, Lien CA, Belmont MR, et al: The clinical pharmacology of new benzylisoquinoline-diester compounds, with special consideration of cisatracurium and mivacurium [in German]. Anaesthesist 46:840-849, 1997.

211. Wulf H, Kahl M, Ledowski T: Augmentation of the neuromuscular blocking effects of cisatracurium during desflurane, sevoflurane, isoflurane or total i.v. anaesthesia. Br J Anaesth 80:308-312, 1998.

212. Naguib M, Samarkandi AH, Ammar A, et al: Comparative clinical pharmacology of rocuronium, cisatracurium, and their combination. Anesthesiology 89:1116-1124, 1998.

213. Kim KS, Chung CW, Shin WJ: Cisatracurium neuromuscular block at the adductor pollicis and the laryngeal adductor muscles in humans. Br J Anaesth 83:483-484, 1999.

214. Weber S, Brandom BW, Powers DM, et al: Mivacurium chloride (BW B1090U)-induced neuromuscular blockade during nitrous oxide–isoflurane and nitrous oxide–narcotic anesthesia in adult surgical patients. Anesth Analg 67:495-499, 1988.

215. Choi WW, Mehta MP, Murray DJ, et al: Neuromuscular and cardiovascular effects of mivacurium chloride in surgical patients receiving nitrous oxide–narcotic or nitrous oxide–isoflurane anaesthesia. Can J Anaesth 36:641-650, 1989.

216. Caldwell JE, Kitts JB, Heier T, et al: The dose-response relationship of mivacurium chloride in humans during nitrous oxide–fentanyl or nitrous oxide–enflurane anesthesia. Anesthesiology 70:31-35, 1989.

217. From RP, Pearson KS, Choi WW, et al: Neuromuscular and cardiovascular effects of mivacurium chloride (BW B1090U) during nitrous oxide–fentanyl-thiopentone and nitrous oxide–halothane anaesthesia. Br J Anaesth 64:193-198, 1990.

218. Diefenbach C, Mellinghoff H, Lynch J, et al: Mivacurium: Dose-response relationship and administration by repeated injection or infusion. Anesth Analg 74:420-423, 1992.

219. Wierda JM, Beaufort AM, Kleef UW, et al: Preliminary investigations of the clinical pharmacology of three short-acting non-depolarizing neuromuscular blocking agents, Org 9453, Org 9489 and Org 9487. Can J Anaesth 41:213-220, 1994.

220. Kopman AF, Klewicka MM, Ghori K, et al: Dose-response and onset/offset characteristics of rapacuronium. Anesthesiology 93:1017-1021, 2000.

221. Finney DJ: Probit Analysis, 2nd ed. Cambridge, Cambridge University Press, 1971.

222. Holford NH, Sheiner LB: Understanding the dose-effect relationship: Clinical application of pharmacokinetic-pharmacodynamic models. Clin Pharmacokinet 6:429-453, 1981.

223. Bevan DR, Bevan JC, Donati F: Pharmacokinetic principles. *In* Muscle Relaxants in Clinical Anesthesia. Chicago, Year Book, 1988.

224. Sheiner LB, Stanski DR, Vozeh S, et al: Simultaneous modeling of pharmacokinetics and pharmacodynamics: Application to *d*-tubocurarine. Clin Pharmacol Ther 25:358-371, 1979.

225. Holford NH, Sheiner LB: Kinetics of pharmacologic response. Pharmacol Ther 16:143-166, 1982.

226. Wright PM: Population based pharmacokinetic analysis: Why do we need it; what is it; and what has it told us about anaesthetics? Br J Anaesth 80:488-501, 1998.

227. Fisher DM, Rosen JI: A pharmacokinetic explanation for increasing recovery time following larger or repeated doses of nondepolarizing muscle relaxants. Anesthesiology 65:286-291, 1986.

228. Cook DR, Freeman JA, Lai AA, et al: Pharmacokinetics of mivacurium in normal patients and in those with hepatic or renal failure. Br J Anaesth 69:580-585, 1992.

229. Waser PG, Wiederkehr H, Sin-Ren AC, et al: Distribution and kinetics of ^{14}C-vecuronium in rats and mice. Br J Anaesth 59:1044-1051, 1987.

230. Matteo RS, Nishitateno K, Pua EK, et al: Pharmacokinetics of *d*-tubocurarine in man: Effect of an osmotic diuretic on urinary excretion. Anesthesiology 52:335-338, 1980.

231. Lebrault C, Berger JL, D'Hollander AA, et al: Pharmacokinetics and pharmacodynamics of vecuronium (ORG NC 45) in patients with cirrhosis. Anesthesiology 62:601-605, 1985.

232. Wood M: Plasma drug binding: Implications for anesthesiologists. Anesth Analg 65:786-804, 1986.

233. McLeod K, Watson MJ, Rawlins MD: Pharmacokinetics of pancuronium in patients with normal and impaired renal function. Br J Anaesth 48:341-345, 1976.

234. Miller RD, Matteo RS, Benet LZ, et al: The pharmacokinetics of *d*-tubocurarine in man with and without renal failure. J Pharmacol Exp Ther 202:1-7, 1977.

235. Wright PM, Hart P, Lau M, et al: Cumulative characteristics of atracurium and vecuronium. A simultaneous clinical and pharmacokinetic study. Anesthesiology 81:59-68, 1994.

236. Laurin J, Donati F, Nekka F, et al: Peripheral link model as an alternative for pharmacokinetic-pharmacodynamic modeling of drugs having a very short elimination half-life. J Pharmacokinet Biopharm 28:7-25, 2001.

237. Kuipers JA, Boer F, Olofsen E, et al: Recirculatory pharmacokinetics and pharmacodynamics of rocuronium in patients: The influence of cardiac output. Anesthesiology 94:47-55, 2001.

238. Wright PM, Brown R, Lau M, et al: A pharmacodynamic explanation for the rapid onset/offset of rapacuronium bromide. Anesthesiology 90:16-23, 1999.

239. Wierda JM, Meretoja OA, Taivainen T, et al: Pharmacokinetics and pharmacokinetic-dynamic modelling of rocuronium in infants and children. Br J Anaesth 78:690-695, 1997.

240. Bergeron L, Bevan DR, Berrill A, et al: Concentration-effect relationship of cisatracurium at three different dose levels in the anesthetized patient. Anesthesiology 95:314-323, 2001.

241. Fisher DM, Canfell PC, Spellman MJ, et al: Pharmacokinetics and pharmacodynamics of atracurium in infants and children. Anesthesiology 73:33-37, 1990.

242. Kitts JB, Fisher DM, Canfell PC, et al: Pharmacokinetics and pharmacodynamics of atracurium in the elderly. Anesthesiology 72:272-275, 1990.

243. Parker CJ, Hunter JM: Dependence of the neuromuscular blocking effect of atracurium upon its disposition. Br J Anaesth 68:555-561, 1992.

244. Marathe PH, Dwersteg JF, Pavlin EG, et al: Effect of thermal injury on the pharmacokinetics and pharmacodynamics of atracurium in humans. Anesthesiology 70:752-755, 1989.

245. Cronnelly R, Fisher DM, Miller RD, et al: Pharmacokinetics and pharmacodynamics of vecuronium (ORG NC45) and pancuronium in anesthetized humans. Anesthesiology 58:405-408, 1983.

246. Rupp SM, Castagnoli KP, Fisher DM, et al: Pancuronium and vecuronium pharmacokinetics and pharmacodynamics in younger and elderly adults. Anesthesiology 67:45-49, 1987.

247. Stanski DR, Ham J, Miller RD, et al: Pharmacokinetics and pharmacodynamics of d-tubocurarine during nitrous oxide–narcotic and halothane anesthesia in man. Anesthesiology 51:235-241, 1979.

248. Wierda JM, van den Broek L, Proost JH, et al: Time course of action and endotracheal intubating conditions of Org 9487, a new short-acting steroidal muscle relaxant; a comparison with succinylcholine. Anesth Analg 77:579-584, 1993.

249. Miguel R, Witkowski T, Nagashima H, et al: Evaluation of neuromuscular and cardiovascular effects of two doses of rapacuronium (ORG 9487) versus mivacurium and succinylcholine. Anesthesiology 91:1648-1654, 1999.

250. Magorian T, Flannery KB, Miller RD: Comparison of rocuronium, succinylcholine, and vecuronium for rapid-sequence induction of anesthesia in adult patients. Anesthesiology 79:913-918, 1993.

251. Naguib M: Neuromuscular effects of rocuronium bromide and mivacurium chloride administered alone and in combination. Anesthesiology 81:388-395, 1994.

252. Agoston S, Salt P, Newton D, et al: The neuromuscular blocking action of ORG NC 45, a new pancuronium derivative, in anaesthetized patients. A pilot study. Br J Anaesth 52(Suppl 1):53S-59S, 1980.

253. Miller RD, Agoston S, Booij LH, et al: The comparative potency and pharmacokinetics of pancuronium and its metabolites in anesthetized man. J Pharmacol Exp Ther 207:539-543, 1978.

254. Katz RL: Clinical neuromuscular pharmacology of pancuronium. Anesthesiology 34:550-556, 1971.

255. Savarese JJ, Ali HH, Antonio RP: The clinical pharmacology of metocurine: Dimethyltubocurarine revisited. Anesthesiology 47:277-284, 1977.

256. Sanfilippo M, Fierro G, Vilardi V, et al: Clinical evaluation of different doses of pipecuronium bromide during nitrous-oxide–fentanyl anaesthesia in adult surgical patients. Eur J Anaesthesiol 9:49-53, 1992.

257. Boyd AH, Eastwood NB, Parker CJ, et al: Pharmacodynamics of the 1R cis-1'R cis isomer of atracurium (51W89) in health and chronic renal failure. Br J Anaesth 74:400-404, 1995.

258. Diefenbach C, Kunzer T, Buzello W, et al: Alcuronium: A pharmacodynamic and pharmacokinetic update. Anesth Analg 80:373-377, 1995.

259. Kopman AF, Klewicka MM, Kopman DJ, et al: Molar potency is predictive of the speed of onset of neuromuscular block for agents of intermediate, short, and ultrashort duration. Anesthesiology 90:425-431, 1999.

260. Donati F, Meistelman C: A kinetic-dynamic model to explain the relationship between high potency and slow onset time for neuromuscular blocking drugs. J Pharmacokinet Biopharm 19:537-552, 1991.

261. Kopman AF, Klewicka MM, Neuman GG: Molar potency is not predictive of the speed of onset of atracurium. Anesth Analg 89:1046-1049, 1999.

262. Naguib M, Kopman AF: Low dose rocuronium for tracheal intubation. Middle East J Anesthesiol 17:193-204, 2003.

263. Bevan DR: The new relaxants: Are they worth it? Can J Anaesth 46:R88-R100, 1999.

264. Meistelman C, Plaud B, Donati F: Rocuronium (ORG 9426) neuromuscular blockade at the adductor muscles of the larynx and adductor pollicis in humans. Can J Anaesth 39:665-669, 1992.

265. Cantineau JP, Porte F, d'Honneur G, et al: Neuromuscular effects of rocuronium on the diaphragm and adductor pollicis muscles in anesthetized patients. Anesthesiology 81:585-590, 1994.

266. Wright PM, Caldwell JE, Miller RD: Onset and duration of rocuronium and succinylcholine at the adductor pollicis and laryngeal adductor muscles in anesthetized humans. Anesthesiology 81:1110-1115, 1994.

267. Plaud B, Debaene B, Lequeau F, et al: Mivacurium neuromuscular block at the adductor muscles of the larynx and adductor pollicis in humans. Anesthesiology 85:77-81, 1996.

268. Hemmerling TM, Schmidt J, Hanusa C, et al: Simultaneous determination of neuromuscular block at the larynx, diaphragm, adductor pollicis, orbicularis oculi and corrugator supercilii muscles. Br J Anaesth 85:856-860, 2000.

269. Fisher DM, Szenohradszky J, Wright PM, et al: Pharmacodynamic modeling of vecuronium-induced twitch depression. Rapid plasma-effect site equilibration explains faster onset at resistant laryngeal muscles than at the adductor pollicis. Anesthesiology 86:558-566, 1997.

270. De Haes A, Houwertjes MC, Proost JH, et al: An isolated, antegrade, perfused, peroneal nerve anterior tibialis muscle model in the rat: A novel model developed to study the factors governing the time course of action of neuromuscular blocking agents. Anesthesiology 96:963-970, 2002.

271. Donati F, Meistelman C, Plaud B: Vecuronium neuromuscular blockade at the diaphragm, the orbicularis oculi, and adductor pollicis muscles. Anesthesiology 73:870-875, 1990.

272. Mehta MP, Choi WW, Gergis SD, et al: Facilitation of rapid endotracheal intubations with divided doses of nondepolarizing neuromuscular blocking drugs. Anesthesiology 62:392-395, 1985.

273. Schwarz S, Ilias W, Lackner F, et al: Rapid tracheal intubation with vecuronium: The priming principle. Anesthesiology 62:388-391, 1985.

274. Naguib M, Abdulatif M, Gyasi HK, et al: Priming with atracurium: Improving intubating conditions with additional doses of thiopental. Anesth Analg 65:1295-1299, 1986.

275. Taboada JA, Rupp SM, Miller RD: Refining the priming principle for vecuronium during rapid-sequence induction of anesthesia. Anesthesiology 64:243-247, 1986.

276. Rorvik K, Husby P, Gramstad L, et al: Comparison of large dose of vecuronium with pancuronium for prolonged neuromuscular blockade. Br J Anaesth 61:180-185, 1988.

277. Gibbs NM, Rung GW, Braunegg PW, et al: The onset and duration of neuromuscular blockade using combinations of atracurium and vecuronium. Anaesth Intensive Care 19:96-100, 1991.

278. Motamed C, Donati F: Intubating conditions and blockade after mivacurium, rocuronium and their combination in young and elderly adults. Can J Anaesth 47:225-231, 2000.

279. Baumgarten RK, Carter CE, Reynolds WJ, et al: Priming with nondepolarizing relaxants for rapid tracheal intubation: A double-blind evaluation. Can J Anaesth 35:5-11, 1988.

280. Engbaek J, Howardy-Hansen P, Ording H, et al: Precurarization with vecuronium and pancuronium in awake, healthy volunteers: The influence on neuromuscular transmission and pulmonary function. Acta Anaesthesiol Scand 29:117-120, 1985.

281. Jones RM: The priming principle: How does it work and should we be using it? Br J Anaesth 63:1-3, 1989.

282. Scott RP, Savarese JJ, Basta SJ, et al: Clinical pharmacology of atracurium given in high dose. Br J Anaesth 58:834-838, 1986.

283. Savarese JJ, Ali HH, Basta SJ, et al: The cardiovascular effects of mivacurium chloride (BW B1090U) in patients receiving nitrous oxide–opiate-barbiturate anesthesia. Anesthesiology 70:386-394, 1989.

284. Meistelman C, Plaud B, Donati F: Neuromuscular effects of succinylcholine on the vocal cords and adductor pollicis muscles. Anesth Analg 73:278-282, 1991.

285. Wierda JM, Kleef UW, Lambalk LM, et al: The pharmacodynamics and pharmacokinetics of Org 9426, a new non-depolarizing neuromuscular blocking agent, in patients anaesthetized with nitrous oxide, halothane and fentanyl. Can J Anaesth 38:430-435, 1991.

286. Kopman AF, Klewicka MM, Neuman GG: Reexamined: The recommended endotracheal intubating dose for nondepolarizing neuromuscular blockers of rapid onset. Anesth Analg 93:954-959, 2001.

287. Barclay K, Eggers K, Asai T: Low-dose rocuronium improves conditions for tracheal intubation after induction of anaesthesia with propofol and alfentanil. Br J Anaesth 78:92-94, 1997.

288. Miguel RV, Soto R, Dyches P: A double-blind, randomized comparison of low-dose rocuronium and atracurium in a desflurane anesthetic. J Clin Anesth 13:325-329, 2001.

289. Littlejohn IH, Abhay K, el Sayed A, et al: Intubating conditions following 1R cis, 1′R cis atracurium (51W89). A comparison with atracurium. Anaesthesia 50:499-502, 1995.

290. Agoston S, Vermeer GA, Kertsten UW, et al: The fate of pancuronium bromide in man. Acta Anaesthesiol Scand 17:267-275, 1973.

291. Mol WE, Meijer DK: Hepatic transport mechanisms for bivalent organic cations. Subcellular distribution and hepato-biliary concentration gradients of some steroidal muscle relaxants. Biochem Pharmacol 39:383-390, 1990.

292. Bencini AF, Mol WE, Scaf AH, et al: Uptake and excretion of vecuronium bromide and pancuronium bromide in the isolated perfused rat liver. Anesthesiology 69:487-492, 1988.

293. Wierda JM, Szenohradszky J, De Wit AP, et al: The pharmacokinetics, urinary and biliary excretion of pipecuronium bromide. Eur J Anaesthesiol 8:451-457, 1991.

294. Duvaldestin P, Agoston S, Henzel D, et al: Pancuronium pharmacokinetics in patients with liver cirrhosis. Br J Anaesth 50:1131-1136, 1978.

295. Somogyi AA, Shanks CA, Triggs EJ: The effect of renal failure on the disposition and neuromuscular blocking action of pancuronium bromide. Eur J Clin Pharmacol 12:23-29, 1977.

296. Somogyi AA, Shanks CA, Triggs EJ: Disposition kinetics of pancuronium bromide in patients with total biliary obstruction. Br J Anaesth 49:1103-1108, 1977.

297. Ward ME, Adu-Gyamfi Y, Strunin L: Althesin and pancuronium in chronic liver disease. Br J Anaesth 47:1199-1204, 1975.

298. Caldwell JE, Canfell PC, Castagnoli KP, et al: The influence of renal failure on the pharmacokinetics and duration of action of pipecuronium bromide in patients anesthetized with halothane and nitrous oxide. Anesthesiology 70:7-12, 1989.

299. D'Honneur G, Khalil M, Dominique C, et al: Pharmacokinetics and pharmacodynamics of pipecuronium in patients with cirrhosis. Anesth Analg 77:1203-1206, 1993.

300. Mol WE, Fokkema GN, Weert B, et al: Mechanisms for the hepatic uptake of organic cations. Studies with the muscle relaxant vecuronium in isolated rat hepatocytes. J Pharmacol Exp Ther 244:268-275, 1988.

301. Agoston S, Seyr M, Khuenl-Brady KS, et al: Use of neuromuscular blocking agents in the intensive care unit. Anesthesiol Clin North Am 11:345, 1993.

302. Caldwell JE, Szenohradszky J, Segredo V, et al: The pharmacodynamics and pharmacokinetics of the metabolite 3-desacetylvecuronium (ORG 7268) and its parent compound, vecuronium, in human volunteers. J Pharmacol Exp Ther 270:1216-1222, 1994.

303. Bencini AF, Scaf AH, Sohn YJ, et al: Hepatobiliary disposition of vecuronium bromide in man. Br J Anaesth 58:988-995, 1986.

304. Arden JR, Lynam DP, Castagnoli KP, et al: Vecuronium in alcoholic liver disease: A pharmacokinetic and pharmacodynamic analysis. Anesthesiology 68:771-776, 1988.

305. Segredo V, Caldwell JE, Matthay MA, et al: Persistent paralysis in critically ill patients after long-term administration of vecuronium. N Engl J Med 327:524-528, 1992.

306. Sandker GW, Weert B, Olinga P, et al: Characterization of transport in isolated human hepatocytes. A study with the bile acid taurocholic acid, the uncharged ouabain and the organic cations vecuronium and rocuronium. Biochem Pharmacol 47:2193-2200, 1994.

307. Proost JH, Roggeveld J, Wierda JM, et al: Relationship between chemical structure and physicochemical properties of series of bulky organic cations and their hepatic uptake and biliary excretion rates. J Pharmacol Exp Ther 282:715-726, 1997.

308. Khuenl-Brady K, Castagnoli KP, Canfell PC, et al: The neuromuscular blocking effects and pharmacokinetics of ORG 9426 and ORG 9616 in the cat. Anesthesiology 72:669-674, 1990.

309. Schwarz LR, Watkins JB 3rd: Uptake of taurocholate, a vecuronium-like organic cation, ORG 9426, and ouabain into carcinogen-induced diploid and polyploid hepatocytes obtained by centrifugal elutriation. Biochem Pharmacol 43:1195-1201, 1992.

310. Smit JW, Duin E, Steen H, et al: Interactions between P-glycoprotein substrates and other cationic drugs at the hepatic excretory level. Br J Pharmacol 123:361-370, 1998.

311. van den Broek L, Wierda JM, Smeulers NJ, et al: Pharmacodynamics and pharmacokinetics of an infusion of Org 9487, a new short-acting steroidal neuromuscular blocking agent. Br J Anaesth 73:331-335, 1994.

312. Cook DR, Stiller RL, Weakly JN, et al: In vitro metabolism of mivacurium chloride (BW B1090U) and succinylcholine. Anesth Analg 68:452-456, 1989.

313. Wastila WB: Data on file, Burroughs Wellcome Co., Research Triangle Park, NC.

314. Head-Rapson AG, Devlin JC, Parker CJ, et al: Pharmacokinetics and pharmacodynamics of the three isomers of mivacurium in health, in end-stage renal failure and in patients with impaired renal function. Br J Anaesth 75:31-36, 1995.

315. Caldwell JE, Heier T, Kitts JB, et al: Comparison of the neuromuscular block induced by mivacurium, suxamethonium or atracurium during nitrous oxide–fentanyl anaesthesia. Br J Anaesth 63:393-399, 1989.

316. Goudsouzian NG, d'Hollander AA, Viby-Mogensen J: Prolonged neuromuscular block from mivacurium in two patients with cholinesterase deficiency. Anesth Analg 77:183-185, 1993.

317. Maddineni VR, Mirakhur RK: Prolonged neuromuscular block following mivacurium. Anesthesiology 78:1181-1184, 1993.

318. Mangar D, Kirchhoff GT, Rose PL, et al: Prolonged neuromuscular block after mivacurium in a patient with end-stage renal disease. Anesth Analg 76:866-867, 1993.

319. Ostergaard D, Jensen FS, Jensen E, et al: Mivacurium-induced neuromuscular blockade in patients with atypical plasma cholinesterase. Acta Anaesthesiol Scand 37:314-318, 1993.

320. Naguib M, el-Gammal M, Daoud W, et al: Human plasma cholinesterase for antagonism of prolonged mivacurium-induced neuromuscular blockade. Anesthesiology 82:1288-1292, 1995.

321. Basta SJ, Ali HH, Savarese JJ, et al: Clinical pharmacology of atracurium besylate (BW 33A): A new non-depolarizing muscle relaxant. Anesth Analg 61:723-729, 1982.

322. Neill EA, Chapple DJ, Thompson CW: Metabolism and kinetics of atracurium: An overview. Br J Anaesth 55(Suppl 1):23S-25S, 1983.

323. Chapple DJ, Clark JS: Pharmacological action of breakdown products of atracurium and related substances. Br J Anaesth 55(Suppl 1):11S-15S, 1983.

324. Merrett RA, Thompson CW, Webb FW: In vitro degradation of atracurium in human plasma. Br J Anaesth 55:61-66, 1983.

325. Stiller RL, Cook DR, Chakravorti S: In vitro degradation of atracurium in human plasma. Br J Anaesth 57:1085-1088, 1985.

326. Fisher DM, Canfell PC, Fahey MR, et al: Elimination of atracurium in humans: Contribution of Hofmann elimination and ester hydrolysis versus organ-based elimination. Anesthesiology 65:6-12, 1986.

327. Nigrovic V, Fox JL: Atracurium decay and the formation of laudanosine in humans. Anesthesiology 74:446-454, 1991.

328. Hennis PJ, Fahey MR, Canfell PC, et al: Pharmacology of laudanosine in dogs. Anesthesiology 65:56-60, 1986.

329. Canfell PC, Castagnoli N Jr, Fahey MR, et al: The metabolic disposition of laudanosine in dog, rabbit, and man. Drug Metab Dispos 14:703-708, 1986.

330. Parker CJ, Hunter JM: Pharmacokinetics of atracurium and laudanosine in patients with hepatic cirrhosis. Br J Anaesth 62:177-183, 1989.

331. Yate PM, Flynn PJ, Arnold RW, et al: Clinical experience and plasma laudanosine concentrations during the infusion of atracurium in the intensive therapy unit. Br J Anaesth 59:211-217, 1987.

332. Beemer GH, Bjorksten AR, Dawson PJ, et al: Production of laudanosine following infusion of atracurium in man and its effects on awakening. Br J Anaesth 63:76-80, 1989.

333. Tateishi A, Zornow MH, Scheller MS, et al: Electroencephalographic effects of laudanosine in an animal model of epilepsy. Br J Anaesth 62:548-552, 1989.

334. Lanier WL, Sharbrough FW, Michenfelder JD: Effects of atracurium, vecuronium or pancuronium pretreatment on lignocaine seizure thresholds in cats. Br J Anaesth 60:74-80, 1988.

335. Shi WZ, Fahey MR, Fisher DM, et al: Modification of central nervous system effects of laudanosine by inhalation anaesthetics. Br J Anaesth 63:598-600, 1989.

336. Chapple DJ, Miller AA, Ward JB, et al: Cardiovascular and neurological effects of laudanosine. Studies in mice and rats, and in conscious and anaesthetized dogs. Br J Anaesth 59:218-225, 1987.

337. Powles AB, Ganta R: Use of vecuronium in the management of tetanus. Anaesthesia 40:879-881, 1985.

338. Kinjo M, Nagashima H, Vizi ES: Effect of atracurium and laudanosine on the release of ^{3}H-noradrenaline. Br J Anaesth 62:683-690, 1989.

339. Pittet JF, Tassonyi E, Schopfer C, et al: Plasma concentrations of laudanosine, but not of atracurium, are increased during the anhepatic phase of orthotopic liver transplantation in pigs. Anesthesiology 72:145-152, 1990.

340. Welch RM, Brown A, Ravitch J, et al: The in vitro degradation of cisatracurium, the R, cis-R′-isomer of atracurium, in human and rat plasma. Clin Pharmacol Ther 58:132-142, 1995.

341. Lien CA, Schmith VD, Belmont MR, et al: Pharmacokinetics of cisatracurium in patients receiving nitrous oxide/opioid/barbiturate anesthesia. Anesthesiology 84:300-308, 1996.

342. Kisor DF, Schmith VD, Wargin WA, et al: Importance of the organ-independent elimination of cisatracurium. Anesth Analg 83:1065-1071, 1996.

343. Ornstein E, Lien CA, Matteo RS, et al: Pharmacodynamics and pharmacokinetics of cisatracurium in geriatric surgical patients. Anesthesiology 84:520-525, 1996.

344. Dundee JW, Gray TC: Resistance to d-tubocurarine chloride in the presence of liver damage. Lancet 2:16, 1953.

345. Brotherton WP, Matteo RS: Pharmacokinetics and pharmacodynamics of metocurine in humans with and without renal failure. Anesthesiology 55:273-276, 1981.

346. Cook DR, Freeman JA, Lai AA, et al: Pharmacokinetics and pharmacodynamics of doxacurium in normal patients and in those with hepatic or renal failure. Anesth Analg 72:145-150, 1991.

347. Ramzan MI, Shanks CA, Triggs EJ: Gallamine disposition in surgical patients with chronic renal failure. Br J Clin Pharmacol 12:141-147, 1981.

348. Fahey MR, Rupp SM, Fisher DM, et al: The pharmacokinetics and pharmacodynamics of atracurium in patients with and without renal failure. Anesthesiology 61:699-702, 1984.

349. Ward S, Boheimer N, Weatherley BC, et al: Pharmacokinetics of atracurium and its metabolites in patients with normal renal function, and in patients in renal failure. Br J Anaesth 59:697-706, 1987.

350. Ward S, Wright D: Combined pharmacokinetic and pharmacodynamic study of a single bolus dose of atracurium. Br J Anaesth 55(Suppl 1):35S-38S, 1983.

351. Bion JF, Bowden MI, Chow B, et al: Atracurium infusions in patients with fulminant hepatic failure awaiting liver transplantation. Intensive Care Med 19(Suppl 2):S94-S98, 1993.

352. Szenohradszky J, Fisher DM, Segredo V, et al: Pharmacokinetics of rocuronium bromide (ORG 9426) in patients with normal renal function or patients undergoing cadaver renal transplantation. Anesthesiology 77:899-904, 1992.

353. Khalil M, D'Honneur G, Duvaldestin P, et al: Pharmacokinetics and pharmacodynamics of rocuronium in patients with cirrhosis. Anesthesiology 80:1241-1247, 1994.

354. Matteo RS, Ornstein E, Schwartz AE, et al: Pharmacokinetics and pharmacodynamics of rocuronium (Org 9426) in elderly surgical patients. Anesth Analg 77:1193-1197, 1993.

355. Wierda JM, Proost JH, Schiere S, et al: Pharmacokinetics and pharmacokinetic/dynamic relationship of rocuronium bromide in humans. Eur J Anaesthesiol Suppl 9:66-74, 1994.

356. Magorian T, Wood P, Caldwell J, et al: The pharmacokinetics and neuromuscular effects of rocuronium bromide in patients with liver disease. Anesth Analg 80:754-759, 1995.

357. van Miert MM, Eastwood NB, Boyd AH, et al: The pharmacokinetics and pharmacodynamics of rocuronium in patients with hepatic cirrhosis. Br J Clin Pharmacol 44:139-144, 1997.

358. De Wolf AM, Freeman JA, Scott VL, et al: Pharmacokinetics and pharmacodynamics of cisatracurium in patients with end-stage liver disease undergoing liver transplantation. Br J Anaesth 76:624-628, 1996.

359. Sorooshian SS, Stafford MA, Eastwood NB, et al: Pharmacokinetics and pharmacodynamics of cisatracurium in young and elderly adult patients. Anesthesiology 84:1083-1091, 1996.

360. Anaesthetists and the reporting of adverse drug reactions. BMJ (Clin Res Ed) 292:949, 1986.

361. Basta SJ: Modulation of histamine release by neuromuscular blocking drugs. Curr Opin Anaesth 5:572, 1992.

362. Hatano Y, Arai T, Noda J, et al: Contribution of prostacyclin to D-tubocurarine–induced hypotension in humans. Anesthesiology 72:28-32, 1990.

363. Scott RP, Savarese JJ, Basta SJ, et al: Atracurium: Clinical strategies for preventing histamine release and attenuating the haemodynamic response. Br J Anaesth 57:550-553, 1985.

364. Savarese JJ: The autonomic margins of safety of metocurine and d-tubocurarine in the cat. Anesthesiology 50:40-46, 1979.

365. McCullough LS, Reier CE, Delaunois AL, et al: The effects of d-tubocurarine on spontaneous postganglionic sympathetic activity and histamine release. Anesthesiology 33:328-334, 1970.

366. Munger WL, Miller RD, Stevens WC: The dependence of a d-tubocurarine–induced hypotension on alveolar concentration of halothane, dose of d-tubocurarine, and nitrous oxide. Anesthesiology 40:442-448, 1974.

367. Naguib M, Samarkandi AH, Bakhamees HS, et al: Histamine-release haemodynamic changes produced by rocuronium, vecuronium, mivacurium, atracurium and tubocurarine. Br J Anaesth 75:588-592, 1995.

368. Harrison GA: The cardiovascular effects and some relaxant properties of four relaxants in patients about to undergo cardiac surgery. Br J Anaesth 44:485-494, 1972.

369. Dowdy EG, Holland WC, Yamanaka I, et al: Cardioactive properties of d-tubocurarine with and without preservatives. Anesthesiology 34:256-261, 1971.

370. Stoelting RK: Blood-pressure responses to d-tubocurarine and its preservatives in anesthetized patients. Anesthesiology 35:315-317, 1971.

371. Stoelting RK, Longnecker DE: Effect of promethazine on hypotension following d-tubocurarine use in anesthetized patients. Anesth Analg 51:509-513, 1972.

372. Basta SJ, Savarese JJ, Ali HH, et al: Histamine-releasing potencies of atracurium, dimethyl tubocurarine and tubocurarine. Br J Anaesth 55(Suppl 1):105S-106S, 1983.

373. Miller RD, Eger EI 2nd, Stevens WC, et al: Pancuronium-induced tachycardia in relation to alveolar halothane, dose of pancuronium, and prior atropine. Anesthesiology 42:352-355, 1975.

374. Stoelting RK: The hemodynamic effects of pancuronium and d-tubocurarine in anesthetized patients. Anesthesiology 36:612-615, 1972.

375. Hughes R, Chapple DJ: Effects on non-depolarizing neuromuscular blocking agents on peripheral autonomic mechanisms in cats. Br J Anaesth 48:59-68, 1976.

376. Hou VY, Hirshman CA, Emala CW: Neuromuscular relaxants as antagonists for M2 and M3 muscarinic receptors. Anesthesiology 88:744-750, 1998.

377. Docherty JR, McGrath JC: Sympathomimetic effects of pancuronium bromide on the cardiovascular system of the pithed rat: A comparison with the effects of drugs blocking the neuronal uptake of noradrenaline. Br J Pharmacol 64:589-599, 1978.

378. Domenech JS, Garcia RC, Sastain JM, et al: Pancuronium bromide: An indirect sympathomimetic agent. Br J Anaesth 48:1143-1148, 1976.

379. Quintana A: Effect of pancuronium bromide on the adrenergic reactivity of the isolated rat vas deferens. Eur J Pharmacol 46:275-277, 1977.

380. Ivankovich AD, Miletich DJ, Albrecht RF, et al: The effect of pancuronium on myocardial contraction and cate-cholamine metabolism. J Pharm Pharmacol 27:837-841, 1975.

381. Vercruysse P, Bossuyt P, Hanegreefs G, et al: Gallamine and pancuronium inhibit pre- and postjunctional muscarine receptors in canine saphenous veins. J Pharmacol Exp Ther 209:225-230, 1979.

382. Roizen MF, Forbes AR, Miller RD, et al: Similarity between effects of pancuronium and atropine on plasma norepinephrine levels in man. J Pharmacol Exp Ther 211:419-422, 1979.

383. Eisele JH, Marta JA, Davis HS: Quantitative aspects of the chronotropic and neuromuscular effects of gallamine in anesthetized man. Anesthesiology 35:630-633, 1971.

384. Brown BR Jr, Crout JR: The sympathomimetic effect of gallamine on the heart. J Pharmacol Exp Ther 172:266-273, 1970.

385. Reitan JA, Fraser AI, Eisele JH: Lack of cardiac inotropic effects of gallamine in anesthetized man. Anesth Analg 52:974-979, 1973.

386. Wong KC, Wyte SR, Martin WE, et al: Antiarrhythmic effects of skeletal muscle relaxants. Anesthesiology 34:458-462, 1971.

387. Geha DG, Rozelle BC, Raessler KL, et al: Pancuronium bromide enhances atrioventricular conduction in halothane-anesthetized dogs. Anesthesiology 46:342-345, 1977.

388. Edwards RP, Miller RD, Roizen MF, et al: Cardiac responses to imipramine and pancuronium during anesthesia with halothane or enflurane. Anesthesiology 50:421-425, 1979.

389. Clayton D: Asystole associated with vecuronium. Br J Anaesth 58:937-938, 1986.

390. Starr NJ, Sethna DH, Estafanous FG: Bradycardia and asystole following the rapid administration of sufentanil with vecuronium. Anesthesiology 64:521-523, 1986.

391. Cozanitis DA, Erkola O: A clinical study into the possible intrinsic bradycardic activity of vecuronium. Anaesthesia 44:648-650, 1989.

392. Kubo T, Fukuda K, Mikami A, et al: Cloning, sequencing and expression of complementary DNA encoding the muscarinic acetylcholine receptor. Nature 323:411-416, 1986.

393. Bonner TI, Buckley NJ, Young AC, et al: Identification of a family of muscarinic acetylcholine receptor genes. Science 237:527-532, 1987.

394. Bonner TI, Young AC, Brann MR, et al: Cloning and expression of the human and rat m5 muscarinic acetylcholine receptor genes. Neuron 1:403-410, 1988.

395. Buckley NJ, Bonner TI, Buckley CM, et al: Antagonist binding properties of five cloned muscarinic receptors expressed in CHO-K1 cells. Mol Pharmacol 35:469-476, 1989.

396. Mak JC, Barnes PJ: Autoradiographic visualization of muscarinic receptor subtypes in human and guinea pig lung. Am Rev Respir Dis 141:1559-1568, 1990.

397. Skoogh BE: Parasympathetic ganglia in the airways. Bull Eur Physiopathol Respir 22(Suppl 7):143-147, 1986.

398. Coulson FR, Fryer AD: Muscarinic acetylcholine receptors and airway diseases. Pharmacol Ther 98:59-69, 2003.

399. Okanlami OA, Fryer AD, Hirshman C: Interaction of nonde-polarizing muscle relaxants with M2 and M3 muscarinic receptors in guinea pig lung and heart. Anesthesiology 84:155-161, 1996.

400. Jooste E, Klafter F, Hirshman CA, et al: A mechanism for rapacuronium-induced bronchospasm: M2 muscarinic receptor antagonism. Anesthesiology 98:906-911, 2003.

401. Atracurium. Lancet 1:394-395, 1983.

402. Laxenaire MC, Moneret-Vautrin DA, Watkins J: Diagnosis of the causes of anaphylactoid anaesthetic reactions. A report of the recommendations of the joint Anaesthetic and Immuno-allergological Workshop, Nancy, France: 19 March 1982. Anaesthesia 38:147-148, 1983.

403. Laxenaire MC, Moneret-Vautrin DA, Vervloet D: The French experience of anaphylactoid reactions. Int Anesthesiol Clin 23:145-160, 1985.

404. Laxenaire MC, Moneret-Vautrin DA, Widmer S, et al: Anesthetics responsible for anaphylactic shock. A French multicenter study [in French]. Ann Fr Anesth Reanim 9:501-506, 1990.

405. Fisher MM, More DG: The epidemiology and clinical features of anaphylactic reactions in anaesthesia. Anaesth Intensive Care 9:226-234, 1981.

406. Watkins J: Adverse reaction to neuromuscular blockers: Frequency, investigation, and epidemiology. Acta Anaesthesiol Scand Suppl 102:6-10, 1994.

407. Baldo BA, Fisher MM: Substituted ammonium ions as allergenic determinants in drug allergy. Nature 306:262-264, 1983.

408. Abel M, Book WJ, Eisenkraft JB: Adverse effects of nondepo-larising neuromuscular blocking agents. Incidence, prevention and management. Drug Saf 10:420-438, 1994.

409. Naguib M, Abdulatif M, Absood A: Comparative effects of pipecuronium and tubocurarine on plasma concentrations of histamine in humans. Br J Anaesth 67:320-322, 1991.

410. Levy JH, Davis GK, Duggan J, et al: Determination of the hemodynamics and histamine release of rocuronium (Org 9426) when administered in increased doses under N_2O/O_2-sufentanil anesthesia. Anesth Analg 78:318-321, 1994.

411. Laxenaire MC, Mertes PM: Anaphylaxis during anaesthesia. Results of a two-year survey in France. Br J Anaesth 87:549-558, 2001.

412. Rose M, Fisher M: Rocuronium: High risk for anaphylaxis? Br J Anaesth 86:678-682, 2001.

413. Watkins J: Incidence of UK reactions involving rocuronium may simply reflect market use. Br J Anaesth 87:522, 2001.

414. Levy JH, Gottge M, Szlam F, et al: Weal and flare responses to intradermal rocuronium and cisatracurium in humans. Br J Anaesth 85:844-849, 2000.

415. Futo J, Kupferberg JP, Moss J, et al: Vecuronium inhibits histamine N-methyltransferase. Anesthesiology 69:92-96, 1988.

416. Futo J, Kupferberg JP, Moss J: Inhibition of histamine N-methyltransferase (HNMT) in vitro by neuromuscular relaxants. Biochem Pharmacol 39:415-420, 1990.

417. O'Callaghan AC, Scadding G, Watkins J: Bronchospasm following the use of vecuronium. Anaesthesia 41:940-942, 1986.

418. Durrani Z, O'Hara J: Histaminoid reaction from vecuronium priming: A case report. Anesthesiology 67:130-132, 1987.

419. Holt AW, Vedig AE: Anaphylaxis following vecuronium. Anaesth Intensive Care 16:378-379, 1988.

420. Naguib M, Magboul MM, Jaroudi R: Clinically significant drug interactions with general anesthetics—incidence, mechanism and management. CNS Drugs 8:51-78, 1997.

421. Argov Z, Mastaglia FL: Drug therapy: Disorders of neuromuscular transmission caused by drugs. N Engl J Med 301:409-413, 1979.
422. Miller RD: Factors affecting the action of muscle relaxants. In Katz RL (ed): Muscle Relaxants. Amsterdam, Excerpta Medica, 1975.
423. Feldman S, Karalliedde L: Drug interactions with neuromuscular blockers. Drug Saf 15:261-273, 1996.
424. Naguib M, Abdulatif M, al-Ghamdi A, et al: Interactions between mivacurium and atracurium. Br J Anaesth 73:484-489, 1994.
425. Kim KS, Chun YS, Chon SU, et al: Neuromuscular interaction between cisatracurium and mivacurium, atracurium, vecuronium or rocuronium administered in combination. Anaesthesia 53:872-878, 1998.
426. Ferres CJ, Mirakhur RK, Pandit SK, et al: Dose-response studies with pancuronium, vecuronium and their combination. Br J Clin Pharmacol 18:947-950, 1984.
427. Pandit SK, Ferres CJ, Gibson FM, et al: Time course of action of combinations of vecuronium and pancuronium. Anaesthesia 41:151-154, 1986.
428. Naguib M, Abdulatif M: Isobolographic and dose-response analysis of the interaction between pipecuronium and vecuronium. Br J Anaesth 71:556-560, 1993.
429. Lebowitz PW, Ramsey FM, Savarese JJ, et al: Combination of pancuronium and metocurine: Neuromuscular and hemodynamic advantages over pancuronium alone. Anesth Analg 60:12-17, 1981.
430. Kim S, Shim JC, Kim DW: Interactions between mivacurium and pancuronium. Br J Anaesth 79:19-23, 1997.
431. Paul M, Kindler CH, Fokt RM, et al: Isobolographic analysis of non-depolarising muscle relaxant interactions at their receptor site. Eur J Pharmacol 438:35-43, 2002.
432. Motamed C, Menad R, Farinotti R, et al: Potentiation of mivacurium blockade by low dose of pancuronium: A pharmacokinetic study. Anesthesiology 98:1057-1062, 2003.
433. Smith I, White PF: Pipecuronium-induced prolongation of vecuronium neuromuscular block. Br J Anaesth 70:446-448, 1993.
434. Kay B, Chestnut RJ, Sum Ping JS, et al: Economy in the use of muscle relaxants. Vecuronium after pancuronium. Anaesthesia 42:277-280, 1987.
435. Rashkovsky OM, Agoston S, Ket JM: Interaction between pancuronium bromide and vecuronium bromide. Br J Anaesth 57:1063-1066, 1985.
436. Walts LF, Dillon JB: Clinical studies of the interaction between d-tubocurarine and succinylcholine. Anesthesiology 31:35-38, 1969.
437. Katz RL: Modification of the action of pancuronium by succinylcholine and halothane. Anesthesiology 35:602-606, 1971.
438. Ono K, Manabe N, Ohta Y, et al: Influence of suxamethonium on the action of subsequently administered vecuronium or pancuronium. Br J Anaesth 62:324-326, 1989.
439. Freund FG, Rubin AP: The need for additional succinylcholine after d-tubocurarine. Anesthesiology 36:185-187, 1972.
440. Katz RL, Norman J, Seed RF, et al: A comparison of the effects of suxamethonium and tubocurarine in patients in London and New York. Br J Anaesth 41:1041-1047, 1969.
441. Stirt JA, Katz RL, Murray AL, et al: Modification of atracurium blockade by halothane and by suxamethonium. A review of clinical experience. Br J Anaesth 55(Suppl 1):71S-75S, 1983.
442. Walts LF, Rusin WD: The influence of succinylcholine on the duration of pancuronium neuromuscular blockade. Anesth Analg 56:22-25, 1977.
443. Katz JA, Fragen RJ, Shanks CA, et al: The effects of succinylcholine on doxacurium-induced neuromuscular blockade. Anesthesiology 69:604-607, 1988.
444. Dubois MY, Fleming NW, Lea DE: Effects of succinylcholine on the pharmacodynamics of pipecuronium and pancuronium. Anesth Analg 72:364-368, 1991.
445. Cooper R, Mirakhur RK, Clarke RS, et al: Comparison of intubating conditions after administration of Org 9246 (rocuronium) and suxamethonium. Br J Anaesth 69:269-273, 1992.
446. Kelly RE, Lien CA, Savarese JJ, et al: Depression of neuromuscular function in a patient during desflurane anesthesia. Anesth Analg 76:868-871, 1993.
447. Saitoh Y, Toyooka H, Amaha K: Recoveries of post-tetanic twitch and train-of-four responses after administration of vecuronium with different inhalation anaesthetics and neuroleptanaesthesia. Br J Anaesth 70:402-404, 1993.
448. Cannon JE, Fahey MR, Castagnoli KP, et al: Continuous infusion of vecuronium: The effect of anesthetic agents. Anesthesiology 67:503-506, 1987.
449. Miller RD, Way WL, Dolan WM, et al: The dependence of pancuronium- and d-tubocurarine–induced neuromuscular blockades on alveolar concentrations of halothane and forane. Anesthesiology 37:573-581, 1972.
450. Miller RD, Crique M, Eger EI 2nd: Duration of halothane anesthesia and neuromuscular blockade with d-tubocurarine. Anesthesiology 44:206-210, 1976.
451. Stanski DR, Ham J, Miller RD, et al: Time-dependent increase in sensitivity to d-tubocurarine during enflurane anesthesia in man. Anesthesiology 52:483-487, 1980.
452. Withington DE, Donati F, Bevan DR, et al: Potentiation of atracurium neuromuscular blockade by enflurane: Time-course of effect. Anesth Analg 72:469-473, 1991.
453. Rupp SM, Miller RD, Gencarelli PJ: Vecuronium-induced neuromuscular blockade during enflurane, isoflurane, and halothane anesthesia in humans. Anesthesiology 60:102-105, 1984.
454. Gencarelli PJ, Miller RD, Eger EI 2nd, et al: Decreasing enflurane concentrations and d-tubocurarine neuromuscular blockade. Anesthesiology 56:192-194, 1982.
455. Miller RD, Way WL, Dolan WM, et al: Comparative neuromuscular effects of pancuronium, gallamine, and succinylcholine during forane and halothane anesthesia in man. Anesthesiology 35:509-514, 1971.
456. Wright PM, Hart P, Lau M, et al: The magnitude and time course of vecuronium potentiation by desflurane versus isoflurane. Anesthesiology 82:404-411, 1995.
457. Wulf H, Ledowski T, Linstedt U, et al: Neuromuscular blocking effects of rocuronium during desflurane, isoflurane, and sevoflurane anaesthesia. Can J Anaesth 45:526-532, 1998.
458. Bock M, Klippel K, Nitsche B, et al: Rocuronium potency and recovery characteristics during steady-state desflurane, sevoflurane, isoflurane or propofol anaesthesia. Br J Anaesth 84:43-47, 2000.
459. Paul M, Fokt RM, Kindler CH, et al: Characterization of the interactions between volatile anesthetics and neuromuscular blockers at the muscle nicotinic acetylcholine receptor. Anesth Analg 95:362-367, 2002.
460. Yasuda N, Lockhart SH, Eger EI 2nd, et al: Comparison of kinetics of sevoflurane and isoflurane in humans. Anesth Analg 72:316-324, 1991.
461. Yasuda N, Lockhart SH, Eger EI 2nd, et al: Kinetics of desflurane, isoflurane, and halothane in humans. Anesthesiology 74:489-498, 1991.
462. Pereon Y, Bernard JM, Nguyen The Tich S, et al: The effects of desflurane on the nervous system: From spinal cord to muscles. Anesth Analg 89:490-495, 1999.
463. Brett RS, Dilger JP, Yland KF: Isoflurane causes "flickering" of the acetylcholine receptor channel: Observations using the patch clamp. Anesthesiology 69:161-170, 1988.
464. Franks NP, Lieb WR: Molecular and cellular mechanisms of general anaesthesia. Nature 367:607-614, 1994.
465. Dilger JP, Vidal AV, Mody HI, et al: Evidence for direct actions of general anesthetics on an ion channel protein. A new look at a unified mechanism of action. Anesthesiology 81:431-442, 1994.
466. al Ahdal O, Bevan DR: Clindamycin-induced neuromuscular blockade. Can J Anaesth 42:614-617, 1995.
467. Sanders WE Jr, Sanders CC: Toxicity of antibacterial agents: Mechanism of action on mammalian cells. Annu Rev Pharmacol Toxicol 19:53-83, 1979.
468. Singh YN, Harvey AL, Marshall IG: Antibiotic-induced paralysis of the mouse phrenic nerve–hemidiaphragm preparation, and reversibility by calcium and by neostigmine. Anesthesiology 48:418-424, 1978.

469. Wright JM, Collier B: Characterization of the neuromuscular block produced by clindamycin and lincomycin. Can J Physiol Pharmacol 54:937-944, 1976.

470. Lee C, de Silva AJ: Interaction of neuromuscular blocking effects of neomycin and polymyxin B. Anesthesiology 50:218-220, 1979.

471. Singh YN, Marshall IG, Harvey AL: Depression of transmitter release and postjunctional sensitivity during neuromuscular block produced by antibiotics. Br J Anaesth 51:1027-1033, 1979.

472. Sokoll MD, Gergis SD: Antibiotics and neuromuscular function. Anesthesiology 55:148-159, 1981.

473. Becker LD, Miller RD: Clindamycin enhances a nondepolarizing neuromuscular blockade. Anesthesiology 45:84-87, 1976.

474. Burkett L, Bikhazi GB, Thomas KC Jr, et al: Mutual potentiation of the neuromuscular effects of antibiotics and relaxants. Anesth Analg 58:107-115, 1979.

475. Hasfurther DL, Bailey PL: Failure of neuromuscular blockade reversal after rocuronium in a patient who received oral neomycin. Can J Anaesth 43:617-620, 1996.

476. Martinez EA, Mealey KL, Wooldridge AA, et al: Pharmacokinetics, effects on renal function, and potentiation of atracurium-induced neuromuscular blockade after administration of a high dose of gentamicin in isoflurane-anesthetized dogs. Am J Vet Res 57:1623-1626, 1996.

477. Heier T, Caldwell JE, Sessler DI, et al: Mild intraoperative hypothermia increases duration of action and spontaneous recovery of vecuronium blockade during nitrous oxide–isoflurane anesthesia in humans. Anesthesiology 74:815-819, 1991.

478. Leslie K, Sessler DI, Bjorksten AR, et al: Mild hypothermia alters propofol pharmacokinetics and increases the duration of action of atracurium. Anesth Analg 80:1007-1014, 1995.

479. Caldwell JE, Heier T, Wright PM, et al: Temperature-dependent pharmacokinetics and pharmacodynamics of vecuronium. Anesthesiology 92:84-93, 2000.

480. Heier T, Caldwell JE, Sessler DI, et al: The relationship between adductor pollicis twitch tension and core, skin, and muscle temperature during nitrous oxide–isoflurane anesthesia in humans. Anesthesiology 71:381-384, 1989.

481. Heier T, Caldwell JE, Sessler DI, et al: The effect of local surface and central cooling on adductor pollicis twitch tension during nitrous oxide/isoflurane and nitrous oxide/fentanyl anesthesia in humans. Anesthesiology 72:807-811, 1990.

482. Ham J, Miller RD, Benet LZ, et al: Pharmacokinetics and pharmacodynamics of d-tubocurarine during hypothermia in the cat. Anesthesiology 49:324-329, 1978.

483. Miller RD, Agoston S, van der Pol F, et al: Hypothermia and the pharmacokinetics and pharmacodynamics of pancuronium in the cat. J Pharmacol Exp Ther 207:532-538, 1978.

484. Hubbard JI, Jones SF, Landau EM: The effect of temperature change upon transmitter release, facilitation and post-tetanic potentiation. J Physiol 216:591-609, 1971.

485. Beaufort TM, Proost JH, Maring J, et al: Effect of hypothermia on the hepatic uptake and biliary excretion of vecuronium in the isolated perfused rat liver. Anesthesiology 94:270-279, 2001.

486. Beaufort AM, Wierda JM, Belopavlovic M, et al: The influence of hypothermia (surface cooling) on the time-course of action and on the pharmacokinetics of rocuronium in humans. Eur J Anaesthesiol Suppl 11:95-106, 1995.

487. Stenlake JB, Hughes R: In vitro degradation of atracurium in human plasma. Br J Anaesth 59:806-807, 1987.

488. De Jong RH, Hershey WN, Wagman IH: Nerve conduction velocity during hypothermia in man. Anesthesiology 27:805-810, 1966.

489. Eriksson LI, Viby-Mogensen J, Lennmarken C: The effect of peripheral hypothermia on a vecuronium-induced neuromuscular block. Acta Anaesthesiol Scand 35:387-392, 1991.

490. Thornberry EA, Mazumdar B: The effect of changes in arm temperature on neuromuscular monitoring in the presence of atracurium blockade. Anaesthesia 43:447-449, 1988.

491. Young ML, Hanson CW 3rd, Bloom MJ, et al: Localized hypothermia influences assessment of recovery from vecuronium neuromuscular blockade. Can J Anaesth 41:1172-1177, 1994.

492. Miller RD, Van Nyhis LS, Eger EI: The effect of temperature on a d-tubocurarine neuromuscular blockade and its antagonism by neostigmine. J Pharmacol Exp Ther 195:237-241, 1975.

493. Miller RD, Roderick LL: Pancuronium-induced neuromuscular blockade, and its antagonism by neostigmine, at 29, 37, and 41 c. Anesthesiology 46:333-335, 1977.

494. Heier T, Clough D, Wright PM, et al: The influence of mild hypothermia on the pharmacokinetics and time course of action of neostigmine in anesthetized volunteers. Anesthesiology 97:90-95, 2002.

495. Giesecke AH Jr, Morris RE, Dalton MD, et al: Of magnesium, muscle relaxants, toxemic parturients, and cats. Anesth Analg 47:689-695, 1968.

496. Sinatra RS, Philip BK, Naulty JS, et al: Prolonged neuromuscular blockade with vecuronium in a patient treated with magnesium sulfate. Anesth Analg 64:1220-1222, 1985.

497. Fuchs-Buder T, Wilder-Smith OH, Borgeat A, et al: Interaction of magnesium sulphate with vecuronium-induced neuromuscular block. Br J Anaesth 74:405-409, 1995.

498. Gaiser RR, Seem EH: Use of rocuronium in a pregnant patient with an open eye injury, receiving magnesium medication, for preterm labour. Br J Anaesth 77:669-671, 1996.

499. Ahn EK, Bai SJ, Cho BJ, et al: The infusion rate of mivacurium and its spontaneous neuromuscular recovery in magnesium-treated parturients. Anesth Analg 86:523-526, 1998.

500. Sloan PA, Rasul M: Prolongation of rapacuronium neuromuscular blockade by clindamycin and magnesium. Anesth Analg 94:123-124, 2002.

501. Fuchs-Buder T, Ziegenfuss T, Lysakowski K, et al: Antagonism of vecuronium-induced neuromuscular block in patients pretreated with magnesium sulphate: Dose-effect relationship of neostigmine. Br J Anaesth 82:61-65, 1999.

502. McLarnon JG, Quastel DM: Postsynaptic effects of magnesium and calcium at the mouse neuromuscular junction. J Neurosci 3:1626-1633, 1983.

503. Ghoneim MM, Long JP: The interaction between magnesium and other neuromuscular blocking agents. Anesthesiology 32:23-27, 1970.

504. James MF, Cork RC, Dennett JE: Succinylcholine pretreatment with magnesium sulfate. Anesth Analg 65:373-376, 1986.

505. Tsai SK, Huang SW, Lee TY: Neuromuscular interactions between suxamethonium and magnesium sulphate in the cat. Br J Anaesth 72:674-678, 1994.

506. Waud BE, Waud DR: Interaction of calcium and potassium with neuromuscular blocking agents. Br J Anaesth 52:863-866, 1980.

507. Al-Mohaya S, Naguib M, Abdelatif M, et al: Abnormal responses to muscle relaxants in a patient with primary hyperparathyroidism. Anesthesiology 65:554-556, 1986.

508. Ward ME, Musa MN, Bailey L: Clinical pharmacokinetics of lithium. J Clin Pharmacol 34:280-285, 1994.

509. Price LH, Heninger GR: Lithium in the treatment of mood disorders. N Engl J Med 331:591-598, 1994.

510. Abdel-Zaher AO: The myoneural effects of lithium chloride on the nerve-muscle preparations of rats. Role of adenosine triphosphate–sensitive potassium channels. Pharmacol Res 41:163-178, 2000.

511. Naguib M, Koorn R: Interactions between psychotropics, anaesthetics and electroconvulsive therapy: Implications for drug choice and patient management. CNS Drugs 16:229-247, 2002.

512. Hill GE, Wong KC, Hodges MR: Potentiation of succinylcholine neuromuscular blockade by lithium carbonate. Anesthesiology 44:439-442, 1976.

513. Hill GE, Wong KC, Hodges MR: Lithium carbonate and neuromuscular blocking agents. Anesthesiology 46:122-126, 1977.

514. Reimherr FW, Hodges MR, Hill GE, et al: Prolongation of muscle relaxant effects by lithium carbonate. Am J Psychiatry 134:205-206, 1977.

515. Havdala HS, Borison RL, Diamond BI: Potential hazards and applications of lithium in anesthesiology. Anesthesiology 50:534-537, 1979.

516. Borden H, Clarke MT, Katz H: The use of pancuronium bromide in patients receiving lithium carbonate. Can Anaesth Soc J 21:79-82, 1974.

517. Martin BA, Kramer PM: Clinical significance of the interaction between lithium and a neuromuscular blocker. Am J Psychiatry 139:1326-1328, 1982.

518. Telivuo L, Katz RL: The effects of modern intravenous local analgesics on respiration during partial neuromuscular block in man. Anaesthesia 25:30-35, 1970.

519. Usubiaga JE, Wikinski JA, Morales RL, et al: Interaction of intravenously administered procaine, lidocaine and succinylcholine in anesthetized subjects. Anesth Analg 46:39-45, 1967.

520. Usubiaga JE, Standaert F: The effects of local anesthetics on motor nerve terminals. J Pharmacol Exp Ther 159:353-361, 1968.

521. Kordas M: The effect of procaine on neuromuscular transmission. J Physiol 209:689-699, 1970.

522. Thorpe WR, Seeman P: The site of action of caffeine and procaine in skeletal muscle. J Pharmacol Exp Ther 179:324-330, 1971.

523. Harrah MD, Way WL, Katzung BG: The interaction of d-tubocurarine with antiarrhythmic drugs. Anesthesiology 33:406-410, 1970.

524. Miller RD, Way WL, Katzung BG: The potentiation of neuromuscular blocking agents by quinidine. Anesthesiology 28:1036-1041, 1967.

525. Salvador A, del Pozo E, Carlos R, et al: Differential effects of calcium channel blocking agents on pancuronium- and suxamethonium-induced neuromuscular blockade. Br J Anaesth 60:495-499, 1988.

526. Bell PF, Mirakhur RK, Elliott P: Onset and duration of clinical relaxation of atracurium and vecuronium in patients on chronic nifedipine therapy. Eur J Anaesthesiol 6:343-346, 1989.

527. Kanaya N, Sato Y, Tsuchida H, et al: The effects of nicardipine and verapamil on the recovery time of vecuronium-induced neuromuscular blockade [in Japanese]. Masui 40:246-249, 1991.

528. van Poorten JF, Dhasmana KM, Kuypers RS, et al: Verapamil and reversal of vecuronium neuromuscular blockade. Anesth Analg 63:155-157, 1984.

529. Baurain M, Barvais L, d'Hollander A, et al: Impairment of the antagonism of vecuronium-induced paralysis and intra-operative disopyramide administration. Anaesthesia 44:34-36, 1989.

530. Selzer ME, David G, Yaari Y: Phenytoin reduces frequency potentiation of synaptic potentials at the frog neuromuscular junction. Brain Res 304:149-152, 1984.

531. Selzer ME, David G, Yaari Y: On the mechanism by which phenytoin blocks post-tetanic potentiation at the frog neuromuscular junction. J Neurosci 5:2894-2899, 1985.

532. Jellish WS, Modica PA, Tempelhoff R: Accelerated recovery from pipecuronium in patients treated with chronic anticonvulsant therapy. J Clin Anesth 5:105-108, 1993.

533. Ornstein E, Matteo RS, Schwartz AE, et al: The effect of phenytoin on the magnitude and duration of neuromuscular block following atracurium or vecuronium. Anesthesiology 67:191-196, 1987.

534. Spacek A, Neiger FX, Spiss CK, et al: Chronic carbamazepine therapy does not influence mivacurium-induced neuromuscular block. Br J Anaesth 77:500-502, 1996.

535. Spacek A, Neiger FX, Spiss CK, et al: Atracurium-induced neuromuscular block is not affected by chronic anticonvulsant therapy with carbamazepine. Acta Anaesthesiol Scand 41:1308-1311, 1997.

536. Roth S, Ebrahim ZY: Resistance to pancuronium in patients receiving carbamazepine. Anesthesiology 66:691-693, 1987.

537. Ornstein E, Matteo RS, Weinstein JA, et al: Accelerated recovery from doxacurium-induced neuromuscular blockade in patients receiving chronic anticonvulsant therapy. J Clin Anesth 3:108-111, 1991.

538. Whalley DG, Ebrahim Z: Influence of carbamazepine on the dose-response relationship of vecuronium. Br J Anaesth 72:125-126, 1994.

539. Alloul K, Whalley DG, Shutway F, et al: Pharmacokinetic origin of carbamazepine-induced resistance to vecuronium neuromuscular blockade in anesthetized patients. Anesthesiology 84:330-339, 1996.

540. Kim CS, Arnold FJ, Itani MS, et al: Decreased sensitivity to metocurine during long-term phenytoin therapy may be attributable to protein binding and acetylcholine receptor changes. Anesthesiology 77:500-506, 1992.

541. Melton AT, Antognini JF, Gronert GA: Prolonged duration of succinylcholine in patients receiving anticonvulsants: Evidence for mild up-regulation of acetylcholine receptors? Can J Anaesth 40:939-942, 1993.

542. Miller RD, Sohn YJ, Matteo RS: Enhancement of d-tubocurarine neuromuscular blockade by diuretics in man. Anesthesiology 45:442-445, 1976.

543. Scappaticci KA, Ham JA, Sohn YJ, et al: Effects of furosemide on the neuromuscular junction. Anesthesiology 57:381-388, 1982.

544. Carmignani M, Scoppetta C, Ranelletti FO, et al: Adverse interaction between acetazolamide and anticholinesterase drugs at the normal and myasthenic neuromuscular junction level. Int J Clin Pharmacol Ther Toxicol 22:140-144, 1984.

545. Azar I, Cottrell J, Gupta B, et al: Furosemide facilitates recovery of evoked twitch response after pancuronium. Anesth Analg 59:55-57, 1980.

546. Hill GE, Wong KC, Shaw CL, et al: Acute and chronic changes in intra- and extracellular potassium and responses to neuromuscular blocking agents. Anesth Analg 57:417-421, 1978.

547. Nott MW, Bowman WC: Actions of dantrolene sodium on contractions of the tibialis anterior and soleus muscles of cats under chloralose anaesthesia. Clin Exp Pharmacol Physiol 1:113-122, 1974.

548. Morgan KG, Bryant SH: The mechanism of action of dantrolene sodium. J Pharmacol Exp Ther 201:138-147, 1977.

549. Gramstad L: Atracurium, vecuronium and pancuronium in end-stage renal failure. Dose-response properties and interactions with azathioprine. Br J Anaesth 59:995-1003, 1987.

550. Glidden RS, Martyn JA, Tomera JF: Azathioprine fails to alter the dose-response curve of d-tubocurarine in rats. Anesthesiology 68 595-598, 1988.

551. Meyers EF: Partial recovery from pancuronium neuromuscular blockade following hydrocortisone administration. Anesthesiology 46 148-150, 1977.

552. Reddy P, Guzman A, Robalino J, et al: Resistance to muscle relaxants in a patient receiving prolonged testosterone therapy. Anesthesiology 70:871-873, 1989.

553. Arts WF, Oosterhuis HJ: Effect of prednisolone on neuromuscular blocking in mice in vivo. Neurology 25:1088-1090, 1975.

554. Leeuwin RS, Veldsema-Currie RD, van Wilgenburg H, et al: Effects of corticosteroids on neuromuscular blocking actions of d-tubocurarine. Eur J Pharmacol 69:165-173, 1981.

555. Hall ED: Glucocorticoid modification of the responsiveness of a fast (type 2) neuromuscular system to edrophonium and d-tubocurarine. Exp Neurol 69:349-358, 1980.

556. Parr SM, Robinson BJ, Rees D, et al: Interaction between betamethasone and vecuronium. Br J Anaesth 67:447-451, 1991.

557. Bouzat C, Barrantes FJ: Modulation of muscle nicotinic acetylcholine receptors by the glucocorticoid hydrocortisone. Possible allosteric mechanism of channel blockade. J Biol Chem 271:25835-25841, 1996.

558. Valera S, Ballivet M, Bertrand D: Progesterone modulates a neuronal nicotinic acetylcholine receptor. Proc Natl Acad Sci U S A 89:9949-9953, 1992.

559. Naguib M, Gyasi HK: Antiestrogenic drugs and atracurium—a possible interaction? Can Anaesth Soc J 33:682-683, 1986.

560. Ali HH, Utting JE, Gray TC: Quantitative assessment of residual antidepolarizing block. II. Br J Anaesth 43:478-485, 1971.

561. Ali HH, Kitz RJ: Evaluation of recovery from nondepolarizing neuromuscular block, using a digital neuromuscular transmission analyzer: Preliminary report. Anesth Analg 52:740-745, 1973.

562. Howardy-Hansen P, Moller J, Hansen B: Pretreatment with atracurium: The influence on neuromuscular transmission and pulmonary function. Acta Anaesthesiol Scand 31:642-644, 1987.

563. Eriksson LI, Sundman E, Olsson R, et al: Functional assessment of the pharynx at rest and during swallowing in partially paralyzed humans: Simultaneous videomanometry and mechanomyography of awake human volunteers. Anesthesiology 87:1035-1043, 1997.

564. Sundman E, Witt H, Olsson R, et al: The incidence and mechanisms of pharyngeal and upper esophageal dysfunction in partially paralyzed humans: Pharyngeal videoradiography and simultaneous manometry after atracurium. Anesthesiology 92:977-984, 2000.

565. Eriksson LI: Reduced hypoxic chemosensitivity in partially paralysed man. A new property of muscle relaxants? Acta Anaesthesiol Scand 40:520-523, 1996.

566. Eriksson LI: The effects of residual neuromuscular blockade and volatile anesthetics on the control of ventilation. Anesth Analg 89:243-251, 1999.

567. Igarashi A, Amagasa S, Horikawa H, et al: Vecuronium directly inhibits hypoxic neurotransmission of the rat carotid body. Anesth Analg 94:117-122, 2002.

568. Viby-Mogensen J: Postoperative residual curarization and evidence-based anaesthesia. Br J Anaesth 84:301-303, 2000.

569. Lien CA, Matteo RS, Ornstein E, et al: Distribution, elimination, and action of vecuronium in the elderly. Anesth Analg 73:39-42, 1991.

570. Caldwell JE: Reversal of residual neuromuscular block with neostigmine at one to four hours after a single intubating dose of vecuronium. Anesth Analg 80:1168-1174, 1995.

571. Magorian TT, Lynam DP, Caldwell JE, et al: Can early administration of neostigmine, in single or repeated doses, alter the course of neuromuscular recovery from a vecuronium-induced neuromuscular blockade? Anesthesiology 73:410-414, 1990.

572. Baurain MJ, d'Hollander AA, Melot C, et al: Effects of residual concentrations of isoflurane on the reversal of vecuronium-induced neuromuscular blockade. Anesthesiology 74:474-478, 1991.

573. McMahan UJ, Sanes JR, Marshall LM: Cholinesterase is associated with the basal lamina at the neuromuscular junction. Nature 271:172-174, 1978.

574. Zhou HX, Wlodek ST, McCammon JA: Conformation gating as a mechanism for enzyme specificity. Proc Natl Acad Sci U S A 95:9280-9283, 1998.

575. Soreq H, Seidman S: Acetylcholinesterase—new roles for an old actor. Nat Rev Neurosci 2:294-302, 2001.

576. Wilson IB, Bergmann F: Studies on cholinesterase. VII. The active surface of acetylcholine esterase derived from effects of pH on inhibitors. J Biol Chem 185:479-489, 1950.

577. Bergmann F, Wilson IB, Nachmansohn D: The inhibitory effect of stilbamidine, curare and related compounds and its relationship to the active groups of acetylcholine esterase. Biochim Biophys Acta 6:217-224, 1950.

578. Wilson IB: The interaction of Tensilon and neostigmine with acetylcholinesterase. Arch Int Pharmacodyn 54:204-213, 1955.

579. Bevan DR, Donati F, Kopman AF: Reversal of neuromuscular blockade. Anesthesiology 77:785-805, 1992.

580. Mirakhur RK: Basic pharmacology of reversal agents. Anesthesiol Clin North Am 11:237, 1993.

581. Beattie WS, Buckley DN, Forrest JB: Continuous infusions of atracurium and vecuronium, compared with intermittent boluses of pancuronium: Dose requirements and reversal. Can J Anaesth 39:925-931, 1992.

582. Beemer GH, Goonetilleke PH, Bjorksten AR: The maximum depth of an atracurium neuromuscular block antagonized by edrophonium to effect adequate recovery. Anesthesiology 82:852-858, 1995.

583. Bevan JC, Collins L, Fowler C, et al: Early and late reversal of rocuronium and vecuronium with neostigmine in adults and children. Anesth Analg 89:333-339, 1999.

584. Kirkegaard H, Heier T, Caldwell JE: Efficacy of tactile-guided reversal from cisatracurium-induced neuromuscular block. Anesthesiology 96:45-50, 2002.

585. Cronnelly R, Morris RB, Miller RD: Edrophonium: Duration of action and atropine requirement in humans during halothane anesthesia. Anesthesiology 57:261-266, 1982.

586. Beemer GH, Bjorksten AR, Dawson PJ, et al: Determinants of the reversal of competitive neuromuscular block by anticholinesterases. Br J Anaesth 66:469-475, 1991.

587. Caldwell JE, Robertson EN, Baird WL: Antagonism of vecuronium and atracurium: Comparison of neostigmine and edrophonium administered at 5% twitch height recovery. Br J Anaesth 59:478-481, 1987.

588. Miller RD, Van Nyhuis LS, Eger EI 2nd, et al: Comparative times to peak effect and durations of action of neostigmine and pyridostigmine. Anesthesiology 41:27-33, 1974.

589. Rupp SM, McChristian JW, Miller RD, et al: Neostigmine and edrophonium antagonism of varying intensity neuromuscular blockade induced by atracurium, pancuronium, or vecuronium. Anesthesiology 64:711-717, 1986.

590. Engbaek J, Ording H, Ostergaard D, et al: Edrophonium and neostigmine for reversal of the neuromuscular blocking effect of vecuronium. Acta Anaesthesiol Scand 29:544-546, 1985.

591. Donati F, Smith CE, Bevan DR: Dose-response relationships for edrophonium and neostigmine as antagonists of moderate and profound atracurium blockade. Anesth Analg 68:13-19, 1989.

592. Cronnelly R: Muscle relaxant antagonists. Semin Anesth 4:31, 1985.

593. Donati F, McCarroll SM, Antzaka C, et al: Dose-response curves for edrophonium, neostigmine, and pyridostigmine after pancuronium and d-tubocurarine. Anesthesiology 66:471-476, 1987.

594. Naguib M, Abdulatif M: Priming with anti-cholinesterases—the effect of different priming doses of edrophonium. Can J Anaesth 35:53-57, 1988.

595. Naguib M, Abdulatif M: Priming with anti-cholinesterases—the effect of different combinations of anti-cholinesterases and different priming intervals. Can J Anaesth 35:47-52, 1988.

596. Savarese JJ: Reversal of nondepolarizing blocks: More controversial than ever? Review Course Lectures, 67th Congress, Cleveland, Ohio, International Anesthesia Research Society, 1993.

597. Eriksson LL: Evidence-based practice and neuromuscular monitoring: It's time for routine quantitative assessment. Anesthesiology 98:1037-1039, 2003.

598. Deboene B, Plaud B, Dilly MP, Donati F: Residual paralysis in the PACU after a single intubating dose of nondepolarizing muscle relaxant with an intermediate duration of action. Anesthesiology 98:1042-1048, 2003.

599. Naguib M, Abdulatif M, al-Ghamdi A, et al: Dose-response relationships for edrophonium and neostigmine antagonism of mivacurium-induced neuromuscular block. Br J Anaesth 71:709-714, 1993.

600. Kao YJ, Le ND: The reversal of profound mivacurium-induced neuromuscular blockade. Can J Anaesth 43:1128-1133, 1996.

601. Naguib M, Selim M, Bakhamees HS, et al: Enzymatic versus pharmacologic antagonism of profound mivacurium-induced neuromuscular blockade. Anesthesiology 84:1051-1059, 1996.

602. Szenohradszky J, Lau M, Brown R, et al: The effect of neostigmine on twitch tension and muscle relaxant concentration during infusion of mivacurium or vecuronium. Anesthesiology 83:83-87, 1995.

603. Hart PS, Wright PM, Brown R, et al: Edrophonium increases mivacurium concentrations during constant mivacurium infusion, and large doses minimally antagonize paralysis. Anesthesiology 82:912-918, 1995.

604. Bevan DR, Kahwaji R, Ansermino JM, et al: Residual block after mivacurium with or without edrophonium reversal in adults and children. Anesthesiology 84:362-367, 1996.

605. Mirakhur RK: Spontaneous recovery or evoked reversal of neuromuscular block. Acta Anaesthesiol Scand Suppl 106:62-65, 1995.

606. Naguib M, Daoud W, el-Gammal M, et al: Enzymatic antagonism of mivacurium-induced neuromuscular blockade by human plasma cholinesterase. Anesthesiology 83:694-701, 1995.

607. Naguib M, Samarkandi AH, Bakhamees HS, et al: Edrophonium and human plasma cholinesterase combination for antagonism of mivacurium-induced neuromuscular block. Br J Anaesth 77:424-426, 1996.

608. Ostergaard D, Jensen FS, Viby-Mogensen J: Reversal of intense mivacurium block with human plasma cholinesterase in patients with atypical plasma cholinesterase. Anesthesiology 82:1295-1298, 1995.

609. Delisle S, Bevan DR: Impaired neostigmine antagonism of pancuronium during enflurane anaesthesia in man. Br J Anaesth 54:441-445, 1982.

610. Morita T, Tsukagoshi H, Sugaya T, et al: Inadequate antagonism of vecuronium-induced neuromuscular block by neostigmine during sevoflurane or isoflurane anesthesia. Anesth Analg 80:1175-1180, 1995.

611. Morita T, Kurosaki D, Tsukagoshi H, et al: Sevoflurane and isoflurane impair edrophonium reversal of vecuronium-induced neuromuscular block. Can J Anaesth 43:799-805, 1996.

612. Morita T, Kurosaki D, Tsukagoshi H, et al: Factors affecting neostigmine reversal of vecuronium block during sevoflurane anaesthesia. Anaesthesia 52:538-543, 1997.

613. Reid JE, Breslin DS, Mirakhur RK, et al: Neostigmine antagonism of rocuronium block during anesthesia with sevoflurane, isoflurane or propofol. Can J Anaesth 48:351-355, 2001.

614. Kumar N, Mirakhur RK, Symington MJ, et al: Potency and time course of action of rocuronium during desflurane and isoflurane anaesthesia. Br J Anaesth 77:488-491, 1996.

615. Lowry DW, Mirakhur RK, McCarthy GJ, et al: Neuromuscular effects of rocuronium during sevoflurane, isoflurane, and intravenous anesthesia. Anesth Analg 87:936-940, 1998.

616. Astley BA, Katz RL, Payne JP: Electrical and mechanical responses after neuromuscular blockade with vecuronium, and subsequent antagonism with neostigmine or edrophonium. Br J Anaesth 59:983-988, 1987.

617. Goldhill DR, Wainwright AP, Stuart CS, et al: Neostigmine after spontaneous recovery from neuromuscular blockade. Effect on depth of blockade monitored with train-of-four and tetanic stimuli. Anaesthesia 44:293-299, 1989.

618. Miller RD, Roderick LL: Acid-base balance and neostigmine antagonism of pancuronium neuromuscular blockade. Br J Anaesth 50:317-324, 1978.

619. Biro K: Effects of respiratory and metabolic alkalosis and acidosis on pipecuronium neuromuscular block. Eur J Pharmacol 154:329-333, 1988.

620. Miller RD, Van Nyhuis LS, Eger EI 2nd, et al: The effect of acid-base balance on neostigmine antagonism of d-tubocurarine–induced neuromuscular blockade. Anesthesiology 42:377-383, 1975.

621. Feldman S: Effect of changes in electrolytes, hydration, and pH upon the reactions to muscle relaxants. Br J Anaesth 35:546-551, 1963.

622. Cohen EN: The choice and mode of administration of relaxants. 5. Patients with altered sensitivity. Clin Anesth 2:75-93, 1966.

623. Cunningham JN Jr, Carter NW, Rector FC Jr, et al: Resting transmembrane potential difference of skeletal muscle in normal subjects and severely ill patients. J Clin Invest 50:49-59, 1971.

624. Miller RD, Roderick LL: Diuretic-induced hypokalaemia, pancuronium neuromuscular blockade and its antagonism by neostigmine. Br J Anaesth 50:541-544, 1978.

625. Jones RM, Cashman JN, Casson WR, et al: Verapamil potentiation of neuromuscular blockade: Failure of reversal with neostigmine but prompt reversal with edrophonium. Anesth Analg 64 1021-1025, 1985.

626. Wali FA: Interaction of verapamil with gallamine and pancuronium and reversal of combined neuromuscular blockade with neostigmine and edrophonium. Eur J Anaesthesiol 3:385-393, 1986.

627. Pavlin DJ: T4/T1 does not predict recovery from vecuronium in the presence of gentamicin [abstract]. Anesthesiology 79:A918, 1993.

628. Salem MG, Richardson JC, Meadows GA, et al: Comparison between glycopyrrolate and atropine in a mixture with neostigmine for reversal of neuromuscular blockade. Studies in patients following open heart surgery. Br J Anaesth 57:184-187, 1985.

629. Fisher DM, Cronnelly R, Sharma M, et al: Clinical pharmacology of edrophonium in infants and children. Anesthesiology 61:428-433, 1984.

630. Fogdall RP, Miller RD: Antagonism of d-tubocurarine– and pancuronium-induced neuromuscular blockades by pyridostigmine in man. Anesthesiology 39:504-509, 1973.

631. Dodd P, Day SJ, Goldhill DR, et al: Glycopyrronium requirements for antagonism of the muscarinic side effects of edrophonium. Br J Anaesth 62:77-81, 1989.

632. Triantafillou AN, Tsueda K, Berg J, et al: Refractory bradycardia after reversal of muscle relaxant in a diabetic with vagal neuropathy. Anesth Analg 65:1237-1241, 1986.

633. Naguib M, Gomaa M, Absood GH: Atropine-edrophonium mixture: A dose-response study. Anesth Analg 67:650-655, 1988.

634. Parlow JL, van Vlymen JM, Odell MJ: The duration of impairment of autonomic control after anticholinergic drug administration in humans. Anesth Analg 84:155-159, 1997.

635. van Vlymen JM, Parlow JL: The effects of reversal of neuromuscular blockade on autonomic control in the perioperative period. Anesth Analg 84:148-154, 1997.

636. Rabey PG, Smith G: Anaesthetic factors contributing to postoperative nausea and vomiting. Br J Anaesth 69(7 Suppl 1):40S-45S, 1992.

637. Ding Y, Fredman B, White PF: Use of mivacurium during laparoscopic surgery: Effect of reversal drugs on postoperative recovery. Anesth Analg 78:450-454, 1994.

638. Boeke AJ, de Lange JJ, van Druenen B, et al: Effect of antagonizing residual neuromuscular block by neostigmine and atropine on postoperative vomiting. Br J Anaesth 72:654-656, 1994.

639. Hovorka J, Korttila K, Nelskyla K, et al: Reversal of neuromuscular blockade with neostigmine has no effect on the incidence or severity of postoperative nausea and vomiting. Anesth Analg 85:1359-1361, 1997.

640. Tramer MR, Fuchs-Buder T: Omitting antagonism of neuromuscular block: Effect on postoperative nausea and vomiting and risk of residual paralysis. A systematic review. Br J Anaesth 82:379-386, 1999.

641. Cronnelly R, Stanski DR, Miller RD, et al: Renal function and the pharmacokinetics of neostigmine in anesthetized man. Anesthesiology 51:222-226, 1979.

642. Cronnelly R, Stanski DR, Miller RD, et al: Pyridostigmine kinetics with and without renal function. Clin Pharmacol Ther 28:78-81, 1980.

643. Morris RB, Cronnelly R, Miller RD, et al: Pharmacokinetics of edrophonium in anephric and renal transplant patients. Br J Anaesth 53:1311-1314, 1981.

644. Morris RB, Cronnelly R, Miller RD, et al: Pharmacokinetics of edrophonium and neostigmine when antagonizing d-tubocurarine neuromuscular blockade in man. Anesthesiology 54:399-401, 1981.

645. Kopman AF: Edrophonium antagonism of pancuronium-induced neuromuscular blockade in man: A reappraisal. Anesthesiology 51:139-142, 1979.

646. Bevan DR: Reversal of pancuronium with edrophonium. Anaesthesia 34:614-619, 1979.

647. Barber HE, Calvey TN, Muir KT: The relationship between the pharmacokinetics, cholinesterase inhibition and facilitation of twitch tension of the quaternary ammonium anticholinesterase drugs, neostigmine, pyridostigmine, edrophonium and 3-hydroxyphenyltrimethylammonium. Br J Pharmacol 66:525-530, 1979.

648. Verotta D, Kitts J, Rodriguez R, et al: Reversal of neuromuscular blockade in humans by neostigmine and edrophonium: A mathematical model. J Pharmacokinet Biopharm 19:713-729, 1991.

649. Bom A, Bradley M, Cameron K, et al: A novel concept of reversing neuromuscular block: Chemical encapsulation of rocuronium bromide by a cyclodextrin-based synthetic host. Angew Chem Int Ed Engl 41:266-270, 2002.

650. Adam JM, Bennett DJ, Bom A, et al: Cyclodextrin-derived host molecules as reversal agents for the neuromuscular blocker rocuronium bromide: Synthesis and structure-activity relationships. J Med Chem 45:1806-1816, 2002.

651. Tarver GJ, Grove SJ, Buchanan K, et al: 2-O-substituted cyclodextrins as reversal agents for the neuromuscular blocker rocuronium bromide. Bioorg Med Chem 10:1819-1827, 2002.

652. Cameron KS, Clark JK, Cooper A, et al: Modified gamma-cyclodextrins and their rocuronium complexes. Org Lett 4:3403-3406, 2002.

653. Epemolu O, Bom A, Hope F, Mason R: Reversal of neuromuscular blockade and simultaneous increase in plasma rocuronium concentration after the intravenous infusion of the novel reversal agent Org 25969. Anesthesiology 99:632-637, 2003.

654. Bom A, Mason R, McIndewar I: Org 25060 causes rapid reversal of rocuronium-induced neuromuscular block, independent of acid-base status [abstract]. Anesthesiology 97:A1009, 2002.

655. Gihsenbergh F, Ramael S, De Bruyn S, et al: Preliminary assessment of Org 25969 as a reversal agent for rocuronium in healthy male volunteers [abstract]. Anesthesiology 97:A1008, 2002.

656. Kelly SS: The effect of age on neuromuscular transmission. J Physiol 274:51-62, 1978.

657. Goudsouzian NG: Maturation of neuromuscular transmission in the infant. Br J Anaesth 52:205-214, 1980.

658. Genever EE: Suxamethonium-induced cardiac arrest in unsuspected pseudohypertrophic muscular dystrophy. Case report. Br J Anaesth 43:984-986, 1971.

659. Henderson WA: Succinylcholine-induced cardiac arrest in unsuspected Duchenne muscular dystrophy. Can Anaesth Soc J 31:444-446, 1984.

660. Bennett EJ, Ignacio A, Patel K, et al: Tubocurarine and the neonate. Br J Anaesth 48:687-689, 1976.

661. Goudsouzian NG, Ryan JF, Savarese JJ: The neuromuscular effects of pancuronium in infants and children. Anesthesiology 41:95-98, 1974.

662. Goudsouzian NG, Donlon JV, Savarese JJ, et al: Re-evaluation of dosage and duration of action of d-tubocurarine in the pediatric age group. Anesthesiology 43:416-425, 1975.

663. Bennett EJ, Ramamurthy S, Dalal FY, et al: Pancuronium and the neonate. Br J Anaesth 47:75-78, 1975.

664. Fisher DM, O'Keeffe C, Stanski DR, et al: Pharmacokinetics and pharmacodynamics of d-tubocurarine in infants, children, and adults. Anesthesiology 57:203-208, 1982.

665. Fisher DM, Castagnoli K, Miller RD: Vecuronium kinetics and dynamics in anesthetized infants and children. Clin Pharmacol Ther 37:402-406, 1985.

666. Fisher DM, Miller RD: Neuromuscular effects of vecuronium (ORG NC45) in infants and children during N$_2$O, halothane anesthesia. Anesthesiology 58:519-523, 1983.

667. Meretoja OA, Gebert R: Postoperative neuromuscular block following atracurium or alcuronium in children. Can J Anaesth 37:743-746, 1990.

668. Baxter MR, Bevan JC, Samuel J, et al: Postoperative neuromuscular function in pediatric day-care patients. Anesth Analg 72:504-508, 1991.

669. Meretoja OA, Wirtavuori K, Neuvonen PJ: Age-dependence of the dose-response curve of vecuronium in pediatric patients during balanced anesthesia. Anesth Analg 67:21-26, 1988.

670. Meretoja OA: Is vecuronium a long-acting neuromuscular blocking agent in neonates and infants? Br J Anaesth 62:184-187, 1989.

671. Brandom BW, Woelfel SK, Cook DR, et al: Clinical pharmacology of atracurium in infants. Anesth Analg 63:309-312, 1984.

672. Goudsouzian NG, Liu LM, Cote CJ, et al: Safety and efficacy of atracurium in adolescents and children anesthetized with halothane. Anesthesiology 59:459-462, 1983.

673. Meretoja OA, Kalli I: Spontaneous recovery of neuromuscular function after atracurium in pediatric patients. Anesth Analg 65:1042-1046, 1986.

674. Meretoja OA, Taivainen T, Wirtavuori K: Cisatracurium during halothane and balanced anaesthesia in children. Paediatr Anaesth 6:373-378, 1996.

675. de Ruiter J, Crawford MW: Dose-response relationship and infusion requirement of cisatracurium besylate in infants and children during nitrous oxide–narcotic anesthesia. Anesthesiology 94:790-792, 2001.

676. Scheiber G, Ribeiro FC, Marichal A, et al: Intubating conditions and onset of action after rocuronium, vecuronium, and atracurium in young children. Anesth Analg 83:320-324, 1996.

677. Taivainen T, Meretoja OA, Erkola O, et al: Rocuronium in infants, children and adults during balanced anaesthesia. Paediatr Anaesth 6:271-275, 1996.

678. Reynolds LM, Lau M, Brown R, et al: Intramuscular rocuronium in infants and children. Dose-ranging and tracheal intubating conditions. Anesthesiology 85:231-239, 1996.

679. Kaplan RF, Uejima T, Lobel G, et al: Intramuscular rocuronium in infants and children: A multicenter study to evaluate tracheal intubating conditions, onset, and duration of action. Anesthesiology 91:633-638, 1999.

680. Sarner JB, Brandom BW, Woelfel SK, et al: Clinical pharmacology of mivacurium chloride (BW B1090U) in children during nitrous oxide–halothane and nitrous oxide–narcotic anesthesia. Anesth Analg 68:116-121, 1989.

681. Goudsouzian NG, Alifimoff JK, Eberly C, et al: Neuromuscular and cardiovascular effects of mivacurium in children. Anesthesiology 70:237-242, 1989.

682. Goudsouzian NG, Martyn JJ, Liu LM, et al: Safety and efficacy of vecuronium in adolescents and children. Anesth Analg 62:1083-1088, 1983.

683. Hart PS, McCarthy GJ, Brown R, et al: The effect of plasma cholinesterase activity on mivacurium infusion rates. Anesth Analg 80:760-763, 1995.

684. Markakis DA, Hart PS, Lau M, et al: Does age or pseudocholinesterase activity predict mivacurium infusion rate in children? Anesth Analg 82:39-43, 1996.

685. Fisher DM, Cronnelly R, Miller RD, et al: The neuromuscular pharmacology of neostigmine in infants and children. Anesthesiology 59:220-225, 1983.

686. Bevan JC, Tousignant C, Stephenson C, et al: Dose responses for neostigmine and edrophonium as antagonists of mivacurium in adults and children. Anesthesiology 84:354-361, 1996.

687. Frolkis VV, Martynenko OA, Zamostyan VP: Aging of the neuromuscular apparatus. Gerontology 22:244-279, 1976.

688. Matteo RS, Backus WW, McDaniel DD, et al: Pharmacokinetics and pharmacodynamics of d-tubocurarine and metocurine in the elderly. Anesth Analg 64:23-29, 1985.

689. McLeod K, Hull CJ, Watson MJ: Effects of ageing on the pharmacokinetics of pancuronium. Br J Anaesth 51:435-438, 1979.

690. Duvaldestin P, Saada J, Berger JL, et al: Pharmacokinetics, pharmacodynamics, and dose-response relationships of pancuronium in control and elderly subjects. Anesthesiology 56:36-40, 1982.

691. d'Hollander A, Massaux F, Nevelsteen M, et al: Age-dependent dose-response relationship of ORG NC 45 in anaesthetized patients. Br J Anaesth 54:653-657, 1982.

692. Dresner DL, Basta SJ, Ali HH, et al: Pharmacokinetics and pharmacodynamics of doxacurium in young and elderly patients during isoflurane anesthesia. Anesth Analg 71:498-502, 1990.

693. Ornstein E, Matteo RS, Schwartz AE, et al: Pharmacokinetics and pharmacodynamics of pipecuronium bromide (Arduan) in elderly surgical patients. Anesth Analg 74:841-844, 1992.

694. d'Hollander AA, Luyckx C, Barvais L, et al: Clinical evaluation of atracurium besylate requirement for a stable muscle relaxation during surgery: Lack of age-related effects. Anesthesiology 59:237-240, 1983.

695. Maddineni VR, Mirakhur RK, McCoy EP: Plasma cholinesterase activity in elderly and young adults. Br J Anaesth 72:497, 1994.

696. Maddineni VR, Mirakhur RK, McCoy EP, et al: Neuromuscular and haemodynamic effects of mivacurium in elderly and young adult patients. Br J Anaesth 73:608-612, 1994.

697. Goudsouzian N, Chakravorti S, Denman W, et al: Prolonged mivacurium infusion in young and elderly adults. Can J Anaesth 44:955-962, 1997.

698. Tsueda K, Warren JE, McCafferty LA, et al: Pancuronium bromide requirement during anesthesia for the morbidly obese. Anesthesiology 48:438-439, 1978.

699. Feingold A: Pancuronium requirements of the morbidly obese. Anesthesiology 50:269-270, 1979.

700. Soderberg M, Thomson D, White T: Respiration, circulation and anaesthetic management in obesity. Investigation before and after jejunoileal bypass. Acta Anaesthesiol Scand 21:55-61, 1977.

701. Schmith VD, Fiedler-Kelly J, Abou-Donia M, et al: Population pharmacodynamics of doxacurium. Clin Pharmacol Ther 52:528-536, 1992.

702. Weinstein JA, Matteo RS, Ornstein E, et al: Pharmacodynamics of vecuronium and atracurium in the obese surgical patient. Anesth Analg 67:1149-1153, 1988.

703. Puhringer FK, Khuenl-Brady KS, Mitterschiffthaler G: Rocuronium bromide: Time-course of action in underweight, normal weight, overweight and obese patients. Eur J Anaesthesiol Suppl 11:107-110, 1995.

704. Beemer GH, Bjorksten AR, Crankshaw DP: Effect of body build on the clearance of atracurium: Implication for drug dosing. Anesth Analg 76:1296-1303, 1993.

705. Vandenbrom RH, Wierda JM, Agoston S: Pharmacokinetics and neuromuscular blocking effects of atracurium besylate and two of its metabolites in patients with normal and impaired renal function. Clin Pharmacokinet 19:230-240, 1990.

706. Fahey MR, Morris RB, Miller RD, et al: Pharmacokinetics of Org NC45 (Norcuron) in patients with and without renal failure. Br J Anaesth 53:1049-1053, 1981.

707. Bencini AF, Scaf AH, Sohn YJ, et al: Disposition and urinary excretion of vecuronium bromide in anesthetized patients with normal renal function or renal failure. Anesth Analg 65:245-251, 1986.

708. Meistelman C, Lienhart A, Leveque C, et al: Pharmacology of vecuronium in patients with end-stage renal failure. Eur J Anaesthesiol 3:153-158, 1986.

709. Lynam DP, Cronnelly R, Castagnoli KP, et al: The pharmacodynamics and pharmacokinetics of vecuronium in patients anesthetized with isoflurane with normal renal function or with renal failure. Anesthesiology 69:227-231, 1988.

710. Fairley HB: Prolonged intercostal paralysis due to a relaxant. BMJ 76:1296, 1950.

711. Orko R, Heino A, Rosenberg PH, et al: Dose-response of tubocurarine in patients with and without renal failure. Acta Anaesthesiol Scand 28:452-456, 1984.

712. Ward S, Neill EA: Pharmacokinetics of atracurium in acute hepatic failure (with acute renal failure). Br J Anaesth 55:1169-1172, 1983.

713. Bevan DR, Donati F, Gyasi H, et al: Vecuronium in renal failure. Can Anaesth Soc J 31:491-496, 1984.

714. Khuenl-Brady KS, Pomaroli A, Puhringer F, et al: The use of rocuronium (ORG 9426) in patients with chronic renal failure. Anaesthesia 48:873-875, 1993.

715. Blobner M, Jelen-Esselborn S, Schneider G, et al: Effect of renal function on neuromuscular block induced by continuous infusion of mivacurium. Br J Anaesth 74:452-454, 1995.

716. Ramzan MI, Somogyi AA, Walker JS, et al: Clinical pharmacokinetics of the non-depolarising muscle relaxants. Clin Pharmacokinet 6:25-60, 1981.

717. Cashman JN, Luke JJ, Jones RM: Neuromuscular block with doxacurium (BW A938U) in patients with normal or absent renal function. Br J Anaesth 64:186-192, 1990.

718. Mongin-Long D, Chabrol B, Baude C, et al: Atracurium in patients with renal failure. Clinical trial of a new neuromuscular blocker. Br J Anaesth 58(Suppl 1):44S-48S, 1986.

719. Hunter JM, Jones RS, Utting JE: Use of atracurium in patients with no renal function. Br J Anaesth 54:1251-1258, 1982.

720. Parker CJ, Jones JE, Hunter JM: Disposition of infusions of atracurium and its metabolite, laudanosine, in patients in renal and respiratory failure in an ITU. Br J Anaesth 61:531-540, 1988.

721. Eastwood NB, Boyd AH, Parker CJ, et al: Pharmacokinetics of 1R-*cis* 1'R-*cis* atracurium besylate (51W89) and plasma laudanosine concentrations in health and chronic renal failure. Br J Anaesth 75:431-435, 1995.

722. Segredo V, Matthay MA, Sharma ML, et al: Prolonged neuromuscular blockade after long-term administration of vecuronium in two critically ill patients. Anesthesiology 72:566-570, 1990.

723. Hunter JM, Jones RS, Utting JE: Comparison of vecuronium, atracurium and tubocurarine in normal patients and in patients with no renal function. Br J Anaesth 56:941-951, 1984.

724. Lepage JY, Malinge M, Cozian A, et al: Vecuronium and atracurium in patients with end-stage renal failure. A comparative study. Br J Anaesth 59:1004-1010, 1987.

725. Cooper RA, Mirakhur RK, Wierda JM, et al: Pharmacokinetics of rocuronium bromide in patients with and without renal failure. Eur J Anaesthesiol Suppl 11:43-44, 1995.

726. Szenohradszky J, Caldwell JE, Sharma ML, et al: Interaction of rocuronium (ORG 9426) and phenytoin in a patient undergoing cadaver renal transplantation: A possible pharmacokinetic mechanism? Anesthesiology 80:1167-1170, 1994.

727. Phillips BJ, Hunter JM: Use of mivacurium chloride by constant infusion in the anephric patient. Br J Anaesth 68:492-498, 1992.

728. Ryan DW: Preoperative serum cholinesterase concentration in chronic renal failure. Clinical experience of suxamethonium in 81 patients undergoing renal transplant. Br J Anaesth 49:945-949, 1977.

729. Ostergaard D, Jensen FS, Jensen E, et al: Influence of plasma cholinesterase activity on recovery from mivacurium-induced neuromuscular blockade in phenotypically normal patients. Acta Anaesthesiol Scand 36:702-706, 1992.

730. El-Hakim M, Baraka A: *d*-Tubocurarine in liver disease. Kar-El-Aini 4:99, 1963.

731. Lebrault C, Duvaldestin P, Henzel D, et al: Pharmacokinetics and pharmacodynamics of vecuronium in patients with cholestasis. Br J Anaesth 58:983-987, 1986.

732. Servin FS, Lavaut E, Kleef U, Desmonts JM: Repeated doses of rocuronium bromide administered to cirrhotic and control patients receiving isoflurane. A clinical and pharmacokinetic study. Anesthesiology 84:1092-1100, 1996.

733. Westra P, Vermeer GA, de Lange AR, et al: Hepatic and renal disposition of pancuronium and gallamine in patients with extrahepatic cholestasis. Br J Anaesth 53:331-338, 1981.

734. Ramzan IM, Shanks CA, Triggs EJ: Pharmacokinetics and pharmacodynamics of gallamine triethiodide in patients with total biliary obstruction. Anesth Analg 60:289-296, 1981.

735. Lawhead RG, Matsumi M, Peters KR, et al: Plasma laudanosine levels in patients given atracurium during liver transplantation. Anesth Analg 76:569-573, 1993.

736. Nana A, Cardan E, Leitersdorfer T: Pancuronium bromide. Its use in asthmatics and patients with liver disease. Anaesthesia 27:154-158, 1972.

737. Gyasi HK, Naguib M: Atracurium and severe hepatic disease: A case report. Can Anaesth Soc J 32:161-164, 1985.

738. Bell CF, Hunter JM, Jones RS, Utting JE: Use of atracurium and vecuronium in patients with oesophageal varices. Br J Anaesth 57:160-168, 1985.

739. Hunter JM, Parker CJ, Bell CF, et al: The use of different doses of vecuronium in patients with liver dysfunction. Br J Anaesth 57:758-764, 1985.

740. Kim C, Martyn J, Fuke N: Burn injury to trunk of rat causes denervation-like responses in the gastrocnemius muscle. J Appl Physiol 65:1745-1751, 1988.

741. Kim C, Fuke N, Martyn JA: Burn injury to rat increases nicotinic acetylcholine receptors in the diaphragm. Anesthesiology 68:401-406, 1988.

742. Ward JM, Rosen KM, Martyn JA: Acetylcholine receptor subunit mRNA changes in burns are different from those seen after denervation: The 1993 Lindberg Award. J Burn Care Rehabil 14:595-601, 1993.

743. Nosek MT, Martyn JA: Na+ channel and acetylcholine receptor changes in muscle at sites distant from burns do not simulate denervation. J Appl Physiol 82:1333-1339, 1997.

744. Ibebunjo C, Martyn JA: Thermal injury induces greater resistance to d-tubocurarine in local rather than in distant muscles in the rat. Anesth Analg 91:1243-1249, 2000.

745. Ibebunjo C, Martyn J: Disparate dysfunction of skeletal muscles located near and distant from burn site in the rat. Muscle Nerve 24:1283-1294, 2001.

746. Martyn JA, Szyfelbein SK, Ali HH, et al: Increased d-tubocurarine requirement following major thermal injury. Anesthesiology 52:352-355, 1980.

747. Edwards JP, Hatton PA, Little RA, et al: Increased quantal release of acetylcholine at the neuromuscular junction following scald injury in the rat. Muscle Nerve 22:1660-1666, 1999.

748. Tomera JF, Lilford K, Martyn JA: Diaphragm acetylcholinesterase multimeric forms in mice in response to burn trauma. J Burn Care Rehabil 14:406-419, 1993.

749. Cronan T, Hammond J, Ward CG: The value of isokinetic exercise and testing in burn rehabilitation and determination of back-to-work status. J Burn Care Rehabil 11:224-227, 1990.

750. St-Pierre DM, Choiniere M, Forget R, et al: Muscle strength in individuals with healed burns. Arch Phys Med Rehabil 79:155-161, 1998.

751. Schaner PJ, Brown RL, Kirksey TD, et al: Succinylcholine-induced hyperkalemia in burned patients. 1. Anesth Analg 48:764-770, 1969.

752. Belin RP, Karleen CI: Cardiac arrest in the burned patient following succinyldicholine administration. Anesthesiology 27:516-518, 1966.

753. Viby-Mogensen J, Hanel HK, Hansen E, et al: Serum cholinesterase activity in burned patients. II: Anaesthesia, suxamethonium and hyperkalaemia. Acta Anaesthesiol Scand 19:169-179, 1975.

754. Martyn JA, White DA, Gronert GA, et al: Up-and-down regulation of skeletal muscle acetylcholine receptors. Effects on neuromuscular blockers. Anesthesiology 76:822-843, 1992.

755. Bishop MJ: Hemodynamic and gas exchange effects of pancuronium bromide in sedated patients with respiratory failure. Anesthesiology 60:369-371, 1984.

756. Coggeshall JW, Marini JJ, Newman JH: Improved oxygenation after muscle relaxation in adult respiratory distress syndrome. Arch Intern Med 145:1718-1720, 1985.

757. Conti G, Vilardi V, Rocco M, et al: Paralysis has no effect on chest wall and respiratory system mechanics of mechanically ventilated, sedated patients. Intensive Care Med 21:808-812, 1995.

758. Murray MJ, Cowen J, DeBlock H, et al: Clinical practice guidelines for sustained neuromuscular blockade in the adult critically ill patient. Crit Care Med 30:142-156, 2002.

759. Hansen-Flaschen JH, Brazinsky S, Basile C, Lanken PN: Use of sedating drugs and neuromuscular blocking agents in patients requiring mechanical ventilation for respiratory failure. A national survey. JAMA 266:2870-2875, 1991.

760. Klessig HT, Geiger HJ, Murray MJ, et al: A national survey on the practice patterns of anesthesiologist intensivists in the use of muscle relaxants. Crit Care Med 20:1341-1345, 1992.

761. Parker MM, Schubert W, Shelhamer JH, et al: Perceptions of a critically ill patient experiencing therapeutic paralysis in an ICU. Crit Care Med 12:69-71, 1984.

762. Loper KA, Butler S, Nessly M, et al: Paralyzed with pain: The need for education. Pain 37:315-316, 1989.

763. Hallenberg B, Bergbom-Engberg I, Haljamae H: Patients' experiences of postoperative respirator treatment—influence of anaesthetic and pain treatment regimens. Acta Anaesthesiol Scand 34:557-562, 1990.

764. Merriman HM: The techniques used to sedate ventilated patients. A survey of methods used in 34 ICUs in Great Britain. Intensive Care Med 7:217-224, 1981.

765. Bion JF, Ledingham IM: Sedation in intensive care—a postal survey. Intensive Care Med 13:215-216, 1987.

766. Pollard BJ: Muscle relaxants in critical care. Br J Intensive Care 4:347-353, 1994.

767. Lacomis D, Petrella JT, Giuliani MJ: Causes of neuromuscular weakness in the intensive care unit: A study of ninety-two patients. Muscle Nerve 21:610-617, 1998.

768. Hund EF: Neuromuscular complications in the ICU: The spectrum of critical illness–related conditions causing muscular weakness and weaning failure. J Neurol Sci 136:10-16, 1996.

769. Vianna LG, Koulouris N, Lanigan C, et al: Effect of acute hypercapnia on limb muscle contractility in humans. J Appl Physiol 69:1486-1493, 1990.

770. Coakley JH, Nagendran K, Honavar M, et al: Preliminary observations on the neuromuscular abnormalities in patients with organ failure and sepsis. Intensive Care Med 19:323-328, 1993.

771. De Jonghe B, Sharshar T, Lefaucheur JP, et al: Paresis acquired in the intensive care unit: A prospective multicenter study. JAMA 288:2859-2867, 2002.

772. Rudis MI, Guslits BJ, Peterson EL, et al: Economic impact of prolonged motor weakness complicating neuromuscular blockade in the intensive care unit. Crit Care Med 24:1749-1756, 1996.

773. Lacomis D, Zochodne DW, Bird SJ: Critical illness myopathy. Muscle Nerve 23:1785-1788, 2000.

774. Showalter CJ, Engel AG: Acute quadriplegic myopathy: Analysis of myosin isoforms and evidence for calpain-mediated proteolysis. Muscle Nerve 20:316-322, 1997.

775. Zochodne DW, Ramsay DA, Saly V, et al: Acute necrotizing myopathy of intensive care: Electrophysiological studies. Muscle Nerve 17:285-292, 1994.

776. Douglass JA, Tuxen DV, Horne M, et al: Myopathy in severe asthma. Am Rev Respir Dis 146:517-519, 1992.

777. Kupfer Y, Okrent DG, Twersky RA, et al: Disuse atrophy in a ventilated patient with status asthmaticus receiving neuromuscular blockade. Crit Care Med 15:795-796, 1987.

778. Shee CD: Risk factors for hydrocortisone myopathy in acute severe asthma. Respir Med 84:229-233, 1990.

779. Griffin D, Fairman N, Coursin D, et al: Acute myopathy during treatment of status asthmaticus with corticosteroids and steroidal muscle relaxants. Chest 102:510-514, 1992.

780. Williams TJ, O'Hehir RE, Czarny D, et al: Acute myopathy in severe acute asthma treated with intravenously administered corticosteroids. Am Rev Respir Dis 137:460-463, 1988.

781. Hanson P, Dive A, Brucher JM, et al: Acute corticosteroid myopathy in intensive care patients. Muscle Nerve 20:1371-1380, 1997.

782. Decramer M, de Bock V, Dom R: Functional and histologic picture of steroid-induced myopathy in chronic obstructive pulmonary disease. Am J Respir Crit Care Med 153:1958-1964, 1996.

783. Deconinck N, Van Parijs V, Beckers-Bleukx G, et al: Critical illness myopathy unrelated to corticosteroids or neuromuscular blocking agents. Neuromuscul Disord 8:186-192, 1998.

784. DuBois DC, Almon RR: Disuse atrophy of skeletal muscle is associated with an increase in number of glucocorticoid receptors. Endocrinology 107:1649-1651, 1980.

785. Hund E: Myopathy in critically ill patients. Crit Care Med 27:2544-2547, 1999.
786. Neviere R, Mathieu D, Chagnon JL, et al: Skeletal muscle microvascular blood flow and oxygen transport in patients with severe sepsis. Am J Respir Crit Care Med 153:191-195, 1996.
787. Tsukagoshi H, Morita T, Takahashi K, et al: Cecal ligation and puncture peritonitis model shows decreased nicotinic acetylcholine receptor numbers in rat muscle: Immunopathologic mechanisms? Anesthesiology 91:448-460, 1999.
788. De Letter MA, van Doorn PA, Savelkoul HF, et al: Critical illness polyneuropathy and myopathy (CIPNM): Evidence for local immune activation by cytokine-expression in the muscle tissue. J Neuroimmunol 106:206-213, 2000.
789. Zochodne DW, Bolton CF, Wells GA, et al: Critical illness polyneuropathy. A complication of sepsis and multiple organ failure. Brain 110(Pt 4):819-841, 1987.
790. Berek K, Margreiter J, Willeit J, et al: Polyneuropathies in critically ill patients: A prospective evaluation. Intensive Care Med 22:849-855, 1996.
791. Bolton CF, Breuer AC: Critical illness polyneuropathy. Muscle Nerve 22:419-424, 1999.
792. Tepper M, Rakic S, Haas JA, et al: Incidence and onset of critical illness polyneuropathy in patients with septic shock. Neth J Med 56:211-214, 2000.
793. Bolton CF: Sepsis and the systemic inflammatory response syndrome: Neuromuscular manifestations. Crit Care Med 24:1408-1416, 1996.
794. Mohr M, Englisch L, Roth A, et al: Effects of early treatment with immunoglobulin on critical illness polyneuropathy following multiple organ failure and gram-negative sepsis. Intensive Care Med 23:1144-1149, 1997.
795. Rogers BC: Development of recombinant human nerve growth factor (rhNGF) as a treatment for peripheral neuropathic disease. Neurotoxicology 17:865-870, 1996.
796. van den Berghe G, Wouters P, Weekers F, et al: Intensive insulin therapy in the critically ill patients. N Engl J Med 345:1359-1367, 2001.
797. Lorin S, Nierman DM: Critical illness neuromuscular abnormalities. Crit Care Clin 18:553-568, 2002.
798. Leijten FS, de Weerd AW: Critical illness polyneuropathy. A review of the literature, definition and pathophysiology. Clin Neurol Neurosurg 96:10-19, 1994.
799. Zifko UA: Long-term outcome of critical illness polyneuropathy. Muscle Nerve Suppl 9:S49-S52, 2000.
800. Chang CC, Chuang ST, Huang MC: Effects of chronic treatment with various neuromuscular blocking agents on the number and distribution of acetylcholine receptors in the rat diaphragm. J Physiol 250:161-173, 1975.
801. Berg DK, Hall ZW: Increased extrajunctional acetylcholine sensitivity produced by chronic acetylcholine sensitivity produced by chronic post-synaptic neuromuscular blockade. J Physiol 244:659-676, 1975.
802. Hogue CW Jr, Ward JM, Itani MS, et al: Tolerance and upregulation of acetylcholine receptors follow chronic infusion of d-tubocurarine. J Appl Physiol 72:1326-1331, 1992.
803. Dodson BA, Kelly BJ, Braswell LM, et al: Changes in acetylcholine receptor number in muscle from critically ill patients receiving muscle relaxants: An investigation of the molecular mechanism of prolonged paralysis. Crit Care Med 23:815-821, 1995.
804. Hansen D: Suxamethonium-induced cardiac arrest and death following 5 days of immobilization. Eur J Anaesthesiol 15:240-241, 1998.
805. Callanan DL: Development of resistance to pancuronium in adult respiratory distress syndrome. Anesth Analg 64:1126-1128, 1985.
806. Coursin DB, Klasek G, Goelzer SL: Increased requirements for continuously infused vecuronium in critically ill patients. Anesth Analg 69:518-521, 1989.
807. Kushimo OT, Darowski MJ, Morris P, et al: Dose requirements of atracurium in paediatric intensive care patients. Br J Anaesth 67:781-783, 1991.

808. Hughes M, Grant IS, Biccard B, et al: Suxamethonium and critical illness polyneuropathy. Anaesth Intensive Care 27:636-638, 1999.
809. Kupfer Y, Namba T, Kaldawi E, et al: Prolonged weakness after long-term infusion of vecuronium bromide. Ann Intern Med 117:484-486, 1992.
810. Op de Coul AA, Lambregts PC, Koeman J, et al: Neuromuscular complications in patients given Pavulon (pancuronium bromide) during artificial ventilation. Clin Neurol Neurosurg 87:17-22, 1985.
811. Tousignant CP, Bevan DR, Eisen AA, et al: Acute quadriparesis in an asthmatic treated with atracurium. Can J Anaesth 42:224-227, 1995.
812. Gwinnutt CL, Eddleston JM, Edwards D, et al: Concentrations of atracurium and laudanosine in cerebrospinal fluid and plasma in three intensive care patients. Br J Anaesth 65:829-832, 1990.
813. Szenohradszky J, Trevor AJ, Bickler P, et al: Central nervous system effects of intrathecal muscle relaxants in rats. Anesth Analg 76:1304-1309, 1993.
814. Griffiths RB, Hunter JM, Jones RS: Atracurium infusions in patients with renal failure on an ITU. Anaesthesia 41:375-381, 1986.
815. Beemer GH, Dawson PJ, Bjorksten AR, et al: Early postoperative seizures in neurosurgical patients administered atracurium and isoflurane. Anaesth Intensive Care 17:504-509, 1989.
816. Eddleston JM, Harper NJ, Pollard BJ, et al: Concentrations of atracurium and laudanosine in cerebrospinal fluid and plasma during intracranial surgery. Br J Anaesth 63:525-530, 1989.
817. Chiodini F, Charpantier E, Muller D, et al: Blockade and activation of the human neuronal nicotinic acetylcholine receptors by atracurium and laudanosine. Anesthesiology 94:643-651, 2001.
818. Newman PJ, Quinn AC, Grounds RM, et al: A comparison of cisatracurium (51W89) and atracurium by infusion in critically ill patients. Crit Care Med 25:1139-1142, 1997.
819. Dear GJ, Harrelson JC, Jones AE, et al: Identification of urinary and biliary conjugated metabolites of the neuromuscular blocker 51W89 by liquid chromatography/mass spectrometry. Rapid Commun Mass Spectrom 9:1457-1464, 1995.
820. Kane SL, Dasta JF: Clinical outcomes of critical illness polyneuropathy. Pharmacotherapy 22:373-379, 2002.
821. Kindler CH, Verotta D, Gray AT, et al: Additive inhibition of nicotinic acetylcholine receptors by corticosteroids and the neuromuscular blocking drug vecuronium. Anesthesiology 92:821-832, 2000.
822. Prielipp RC, Coursin DB, Scuderi PE, et al: Comparison of the infusion requirements and recovery profiles of vecuronium and cisatracurium 51W89 in intensive care unit patients. Anesth Analg 81:3-12, 1995.
823. Zarowitz BJ, Rudis MI, Lai K, et al: Retrospective pharmacoeconomic evaluation of dosing vecuronium by peripheral nerve stimulation versus standard clinical assessment in critically ill patients. Pharmacotherapy 17:327-332, 1997.
824. Kress JP, Pohlman AS, O'Connor MF, et al: Daily interruption of sedative infusions in critically ill patients undergoing mechanical ventilation. N Engl J Med 342:1471-1477, 2000.
825. Noseworthy JH: Progress in determining the causes and treatment of multiple sclerosis. Nature 399:A40-A47, 1999.
826. Meinl E: Concepts of viral pathogenesis of multiple sclerosis. Curr Opin Neurol 12:303-307, 1999.
827. Waxman SG: Do 'demyelinating' diseases involve more than myelin? Nat Med 6:738-739, 2000.
828. Hawkes CH: Is multiple sclerosis a sexually transmitted infection? J Neurol Neurosurg Psychiatry 73:439-443, 2002.
829. Oksenberg JR, Barcellos LF: The complex genetic aetiology of multiple sclerosis. J Neurovirol 6(Suppl 2):S10-S14, 2000.
830. Jacobsen M, Schweer D, Ziegler A, et al: A point mutation in PTPRC is associated with the development of multiple sclerosis. Nat Genet 26:495-499, 2000.

831. Steinman L: Multiple sclerosis: A two-stage disease. Nat Immunol 2:762-764, 2001.

832. Lassmann H, Bruck W, Lucchinetti C: Heterogeneity of multiple sclerosis pathogenesis: Implications for diagnosis and therapy. Trends Mol Med 7:115-121, 2001.

833. Aulkemeyer P, Brinkmeier H, Wollinsky KH, et al: The human endogenous local anesthetic–like factor (ELLF) is functionally neutralized by serum albumin. Neurosci Lett 216:37-40, 1996.

834. Brinkmeier H, Seewald MJ, Wollinsky KH, et al: On the nature of endogenous antiexcitatory factors in the cerebrospinal fluid of patients with demyelinating neurological disease. Muscle Nerve 19:54-62, 1996.

835. Brinkmeier H, Wollinsky KH, Seewald MJ, et al: Factors in the cerebrospinal fluid of multiple sclerosis patients interfering with voltage-dependent sodium channels. Neurosci Lett 156:172-175, 1993.

836. Brinkmeier H, Aulkemeyer P, Wollinsky KH, et al: An endogenous pentapeptide acting as a sodium channel blocker in inflammatory autoimmune disorders of the central nervous system. Nat Med 6:808-811, 2000.

837. Kent-Braun JA, Ng AV, Castro M, et al: Strength, skeletal muscle composition, and enzyme activity in multiple sclerosis. J Appl Physiol 83:1998-2004, 1997.

838. Nordenbo AM, Boesen F, Andersen EB: Cardiovascular autonomic function in multiple sclerosis. J Auton Nerv Syst 26:77-84, 1989.

839. Anema JR, Heijenbrok MW, Faes TJ, et al: Cardiovascular autonomic function in multiple sclerosis. J Neurol Sci 104:129-134, 1991.

840. Bannister R, Davies B, Holly E, et al: Defective cardiovascular reflexes and supersensitivity to sympathomimetic drugs in autonomic failure. Brain 102:163-176, 1979.

841. Bader AM, Hunt CO, Datta S, et al: Anesthesia for the obstetric patient with multiple sclerosis. J Clin Anesth 1:21-24, 1988.

842. Siemkowicz E: Multiple sclerosis and surgery. Anaesthesia 31:1211-1216, 1976.

843. Warren TM, Datta S, Ostheimer GW: Lumbar epidural anesthesia in a patient with multiple sclerosis. Anesth Analg 61:1022-1023, 1982.

844. Patten BM, Hart A, Lovelace R: Multiple sclerosis associated with defects in neuromuscular transmission. J Neurol Neurosurg Psychiatry 35:385-394, 1972.

845. Albuquerque EX, McIsaac RJ: Fast and slow mammalian muscles after denervation. Exp Neurol 26:183-202, 1970.

846. McArdle JJ, Michelson L, D'Alonzo AJ: Action potentials in fast- and slow-twitch mammalian muscles during reinnervation and development. J Gen Physiol 75:655-672, 1980.

847. Martin LJ, Price AC, Kaiser A, et al: Mechanisms for neuronal degeneration in amyotrophic lateral sclerosis and in models of motor neuron death (review). Int J Mol Med 5:3-13, 2000.

848. Robberecht W: Oxidative stress in amyotrophic lateral sclerosis. J Neurol 247(Suppl 1):I1-I6, 2000.

849. Rowland LP, Shneider NA: Amyotrophic lateral sclerosis. N Engl J Med 344:1688-1700, 2001.

850. Menzies FM, Ince PG, Shaw PJ: Mitochondrial involvement in amyotrophic lateral sclerosis. Neurochem Int 40:543-551, 2002.

851. Hugon J: ALS therapy: Targets for the future. Neurology 47(6 Suppl 4):S251-S254, 1996.

852. Oosthuyse B, Moons L, Storkebaum E, et al: Deletion of the hypoxia-response element in the vascular endothelial growth factor promoter causes motor neuron degeneration. Nat Genet 28:131-138, 2001.

853. Llinas R, Sugimori M, Cherksey BD, et al: IgG from amyotrophic lateral sclerosis patients increases current through P-type calcium channels in mammalian cerebellar Purkinje cells and in isolated channel protein in lipid bilayer. Proc Natl Acad Sci U S A 90:11743-11747, 1993.

854. Steindler DA, Pincus DW: Stem cells and neuropoiesis in the adult human brain. Lancet 359:1047-1054, 2002.

855. Beach TP, Stone WA, Hamelberg W: Circulatory collapse following succinylcholine: Report of a patient with diffuse lower motor neuron disease. Anesth Analg 50:431-437, 1971.

856. Maselli RA, Wollman RL, Leung C, et al: Neuromuscular transmission in amyotrophic lateral sclerosis. Muscle Nerve 16:1193-1203, 1993.

857. Rosenbaum KJ, Neigh JL, Strobel GE: Sensitivity to nondepolarizing muscle relaxants in amyotrophic lateral sclerosis: Report of two cases. Anesthesiology 35:638-641, 1971.

858. Serisier DE, Mastaglia FL, Gibson GJ: Respiratory muscle function and ventilatory control. I in patients with motor neurone disease. II in patients with myotonic dystrophy. Q J Med 51:205-226, 1982.

859. Arnulf I, Similowski T, Salachas F, et al: Sleep disorders and diaphragmatic function in patients with amyotrophic lateral sclerosis. Am J Respir Crit Care Med 161:849-856, 2000.

860. Kochi T, Oka T, Mizuguchi T: Epidural anesthesia for patients with amyotrophic lateral sclerosis. Anesth Analg 68:410-412, 1989.

861. Hara K, Sakura S, Saito Y, et al: Epidural anesthesia and pulmonary function in a patient with amyotrophic lateral sclerosis. Anesth Analg 83:878-879, 1996.

862. Kawata A, Kato S, Hayashi H, et al: Prominent sensory and autonomic disturbances in familial amyotrophic lateral sclerosis with a Gly93Ser mutation in the SOD1 gene. J Neurol Sci 153:82-85, 1997.

863. Shimizu T, Kawata A, Kato S, et al: Autonomic failure in ALS with a novel SOD1 gene mutation. Neurology 54:1534-1537, 2000.

864. Linden D, Diehl RR, Berlit P: Reduced baroreflex sensitivity and cardiorespiratory transfer in amyotrophic lateral sclerosis. Electroencephalogr Clin Neurophysiol 109: 387-390, 1998.

865. Hughes RA, Hadden RD, Gregson NA, et al: Pathogenesis of Guillain-Barré syndrome. J Neuroimmunol 100:74-97, 1999.

866. Ho TW, McKhann GM, Griffin JW: Human autoimmune neuropathies. Annu Rev Neurosci 21:187-226, 1998.

867. Hahn AF: Guillain-Barré syndrome. Lancet 352:635-641, 1998.

868. Buchwald B, Toyka KV, Zielasek J, et al: Neuromuscular blockade by IgG antibodies from patients with Guillain-Barré syndrome: A macro-patch-clamp study. Ann Neurol 44:913-922, 1998.

869. Buchwald B, Bufler J, Carpo M, et al: Combined pre- and postsynaptic action of IgG antibodies in Miller Fisher syndrome. Neurology 56:67-74, 2001.

870. Rudnicki S, Vriesendorp F, Koski CL, et al: Electrophysiologic studies in the Guillain-Barré syndrome: Effects of plasma exchange and antibody rebound. Muscle Nerve 15:57-62, 1992.

871. Dalman JE, Verhagen WI: Cardiac arrest in Guillain-Barré syndrome and the use of suxamethonium. Acta Neurol Belg 94:259-261, 1994.

872. Brooks H, Christian AS, May AE: Pregnancy, anaesthesia and Guillain Barré syndrome. Ahaesthesia 55:894-898, 2000.

873. Feldman JM: Cardiac arrest after succinylcholine administration in a pregnant patient recovered from Guillain-Barré syndrome. Anesthesiology 72:942-944, 1990.

874. Fiacchino F, Gemma M, Bricchi M, et al: Hypo- and hypersensitivity to vecuronium in a patient with Guillain-Barré syndrome. Anesth Analg 78:187-189, 1994.

875. Zochodne DW: Autonomic involvement in Guillain-Barré syndrome: A review. Muscle Nerve 17:1145-1155, 1994.

876. Minahan RE Jr, Bhardwaj A, Traill TA, et al: Stimulus-evoked sinus arrest in severe Guillain-Barré syndrome: A case report. Neurology 47:1239-1242, 1996.

877. Vassiliev DV, Nystrom EU, Leicht CH: Combined spinal and epidural anesthesia for labor and cesarean delivery in a patient with Guillain-Barré syndrome. Reg Anesth Pain Med 26:174-176, 2001.

878. Steiner I, Argov Z, Cahan C, et al: Guillain-Barré syndrome after epidural anesthesia: Direct nerve root damage may trigger disease. Neurology 35:1473-1475, 1985.

879. Skre H: Genetic and clinical aspects of Charcot-Marie-Tooth's disease. Clin Genet 6:98-118, 1974.

880. Su Y, Brooks DG, Li L, et al: Myelin protein zero gene mutated in Charcot-Marie-Tooth type 1B patients. Proc Natl Acad Sci U S A 90:10856-10860, 1993.
881. Hahn AF, Ainsworth PJ, Naus CC, et al: Clinical and pathological observations in men lacking the gap junction protein connexin 32. Muscle Nerve Suppl 999:S39-S48, 2000.
882. Bergoffen J, Scherer SS, Wang S, et al. Connexin mutations in X-linked Charcot-Marie-Tooth disease. Science 262: 2039-2042, 1993.
883. Evans WH, Martin PE: Gap junctions: Structure and function (review). Mol Membr Biol 19:121-136, 2002.
884. Dermietzel R: Gap junction wiring: A 'new' principle in cell-to-cell communication in the nervous system? Brain Res Brain Res Rev 26:176-183, 1998.
885. Kotani N, Hirota K, Anzawa N, et al: Motor and sensory disability has a strong relationship to induction dose of thiopental in patients with the hypertropic variety of Charcot-Marie-Tooth syndrome. Anesth Analg 82:182-186, 1996.
886. Brian JE Jr, Boyles GD, Quirk JG Jr, et al: Anesthetic management for cesarean section of a patient with Charcot-Marie-Tooth disease. Anesthesiology 66:410-412, 1987.
887. Rudnik-Schoneborn S, Rohrig D, Nicholson G, et al: Pregnancy and delivery in Charcot-Marie-Tooth disease type 1. Neurology 43:2011-2016, 1993.
888. Nathanson BN, Yu DG, Chan CK: Respiratory muscle weakness in Charcot-Marie-Tooth disease. A field study. Arch Intern Med 149:1389-1391, 1989.
889. Naguib M, Samarkandi AH: Response to atracurium and mivacurium in a patient with Charcot-Marie-Tooth disease. Can J Anaesth 45:56-59, 1998.
890. Baraka AS: Vecuronium neuromuscular block in a patient with Charcot-Marie-Tooth syndrome. Anesth Analg 84: 927-928, 1997.
891. Greenberg RS, Parker SD: Anesthetic management for the child with Charcot-Marie-Tooth disease. Anesth Analg 74:305-307, 1992.
892. Antognini JF: Anaesthesia for Charcot-Marie-Tooth disease: A review of 86 cases. Can J Anaesth 39:398-400, 1992.
893. Ducart A, Adnet P, Renaud B, et al: Malignant hyperthermia during sevoflurane administration. Anesth Analg 80:609-611, 1995.
894. Roelofse JA, Shipton EA: Anaesthesia for abdominal hysterectomy in Charcot-Marie-Tooth disease. A case report. S Afr Med J 67:605-606, 1985.
895. Sugino S, Yamazaki Y, Nawa Y, et al: Anesthetic management for a patient with Charcot-Marie-Tooth disease using propofol and nitrous oxide [in Japanese]. Masui 51:1016-1019, 2002.
896. Eichacker PQ, Spiro A, Sherman M, et al: Respiratory muscle dysfunction in hereditary motor sensory neuropathy, type I. Arch Intern Med 148:1739-1740, 1988.
897. Chan CK, Mohsenin V, Loke J, et al: Diaphragmatic dysfunction in siblings with hereditary motor and sensory neuropathy (Charcot-Marie-Tooth disease). Chest 91:567-570, 1987.
898. Tetzlaff JE, Schwendt I: Arrhythmia and Charcot-Marie-Tooth disease during anesthesia. Can J Anaesth 47:829, 2000.
899. Sulica L, Blitzer A, Lovelace RE, et al: Vocal fold paresis of Charcot-Marie-Tooth disease. Ann Otol Rhinol Laryngol 110:1072-1076, 2001.
900. Cuesta A, Pedrola L, Sevilla T, et al: The gene encoding ganglioside-induced differentiation-associated protein 1 is mutated in axonal Charcot-Marie-Tooth type 4A disease. Nat Genet 30:22-25, 2002.
901. Sugai K, Sugai Y: Epidural anesthesia for a patient with Charcot-Marie-Tooth disease, bronchial asthma and hypothyroidism [in Japanese]. Masui 38:688-691, 1989.
902. Scull T, Weeks S: Epidural analgesia for labour in a patient with Charcot-Marie-Tooth disease. Can J Anaesth 43:1150-1152, 1996.
903. Emery AE: The muscular dystrophies. Lancet 359:687-695, 2002.
904. Hoffman EP, Brown RH Jr, Kunkel LM: Dystrophin: The protein product of the Duchenne muscular dystrophy locus. Cell 51:919-928, 1987.
905. Hoffman EP, Fischbeck KH, Brown RH, et al: Characterization of dystrophin in muscle-biopsy specimens from patients with Duchenne's or Becker's muscular dystrophy. N Engl J Med 318:1363-1368, 1988.
906. Bione S, Maestrini E, Rivella S, et al: Identification of a novel X-linked gene responsible for Emery-Dreifuss muscular dystrophy. Nat Genet 8:323-327, 1994.
907. Fenichel GM, Sul YC, Kilroy AW, et al: An autosomal-dominant dystrophy with humeropelvic distribution and cardiomyopathy. Neurology 32:1399-1401, 1982.
908. Moreira ES, Wiltshire TJ, Faulkner G, et al: Limb-girdle muscular dystrophy type 2G is caused by mutations in the gene encoding the sarcomeric protein telethonin. Nat Genet 24:163-165, 2000.
909. Naom I, D'Alessandro M, Sewry CA, et al: Mutations in the laminin alpha2-chain gene in two children with early-onset muscular dystrophy. Brain 123:31-41, 2000.
910. Saito Y, Mizuguchi M, Oka A, et al: Fukutin protein is expressed in neurons of the normal developing human brain but is reduced in Fukuyama-type congenital muscular dystrophy brain. Ann Neurol 47:756-764, 2000.
911. Mayer U, Saher G, Fassler R, et al: Absence of integrin alpha 7 causes a novel form of muscular dystrophy. Nat Genet 17:318-323, 1997.
912. Orrell RW, Tawil R, Forrester J, et al: Definitive molecular diagnosis of facioscapulohumeral dystrophy. Neurology 52:1822-1826, 1999.
913. Brook JD, McCurrach ME, Harley HG, et al: Molecular basis of myotonic dystrophy: Expansion of a trinucleotide (CTG) repeat at the 3' end of a transcript encoding a protein kinase family member. Cell 68:799-808, 1992.
914. Ranum LP, Rasmussen PF, Benzow KA, et al: Genetic mapping of a second myotonic dystrophy locus. Nat Genet 19:196-198, 1998.
915. Durbeej M, Campbell KP: Muscular dystrophies involving the dystrophin-glycoprotein complex: An overview of current mouse models. Curr Opin Genet Dev 12:349-361, 2002.
916. Petrof BJ, Shrager JB, Stedman HH, et al: Dystrophin protects the sarcolemma from stresses developed during muscle contraction. Proc Natl Acad Sci U S A 90:3710-3714, 1993.
917. Pasternak C, Wong S, Elson EL: Mechanical function of dystrophin in muscle cells. J Cell Biol 128:355-361, 1995.
918. Coral-Vazquez R, Cohn RD, Moore SA, et al: Disruption of the sarcoglycan-sarcospan complex in vascular smooth muscle: A novel mechanism for cardiomyopathy and muscular dystrophy. Cell 98:465-474, 1999.
919. Stamler JS, Meissner G: Physiology of nitric oxide in skeletal muscle. Physiol Rev 81:209-237, 2001.
920. Crosbie RH: NO vascular control in Duchenne muscular dystrophy. Nat Med 7:27-29, 2001.
921. Emery AE: The muscular dystrophies. BMJ 317:991-995, 1998.
922. Roland EH: Muscular dystrophy. Pediatr Rev 21:233-237, 2000.
923. Blake DJ, Kroger S: The neurobiology of Duchenne muscular dystrophy: Learning lessons from muscle? Trends Neurosci 23:92-99, 2000.
924. Koenig M, Hoffman EP, Bertelson CJ, et al: Complete cloning of the Duchenne muscular dystrophy (DMD) cDNA and preliminary genomic organization of the DMD gene in normal and affected individuals. Cell 50:509-517, 1987.
925. Brown RH Jr: Dystrophin-associated proteins and the muscular dystrophies. Annu Rev Med 48:457-466, 1997.
926. Fukuyama Y, Osawa M, Suzuki H: Congenital progressive muscular dystrophy of the Fukuyama type—clinical, genetic and pathological considerations. Brain Dev 3:1-29, 1981.
927. Ishii H, Hayashi YK, Nonaka I, et al: Electron microscopic examination of basal lamina in Fukuyama congenital muscular dystrophy. Neuromuscul Disord 7:191-197, 1997.

928. Moll J, Barzaghi P, Lin S, et al: An agrin minigene rescues dystrophic symptoms in a mouse model for congenital muscular dystrophy. Nature 413:302-307, 2001.

929. Gussoni E, Soneoka Y, Strickland CD, et al: Dystrophin expression in the mdx mouse restored by stem cell transplantation. Nature 401:390-394, 1999.

930. Emery AE, Dreifuss FE: Unusual type of benign X-linked muscular dystrophy. J Neurol Neurosurg Psychiatry 29:338-342, 1966.

931. Emery AE: Population frequencies of inherited neuromuscular diseases—a world survey. Neuromuscul Disord 1:19-29, 1991.

932. Aslanidis C, Jansen G, Amemiya C, et al: Cloning of the essential myotonic dystrophy region and mapping of the putative defect. Nature 355:548-551, 1992.

933. Shimokawa M, Ishiura S, Kameda N, et al: Novel isoform of myotonin protein kinase: Gene product of myotonic dystrophy is localized in the sarcoplasmic reticulum of skeletal muscle. Am J Pathol 150:1285-1295, 1997.

934. Damiani E, Angelini C, Pelosi M, et al: Skeletal muscle sarcoplasmic reticulum phenotype in myotonic dystrophy. Neuromuscul Disord 6:33-47, 1996.

935. Harper PS: Myotonic Dystrophy, 3rd ed. London, WB Saunders, 2001.

936. Krivickas LS, Ansved T, Suh D, et al: Contractile properties of single muscle fibers in myotonic dystrophy. Muscle Nerve 23:529-537, 2000.

937. Koltgen D, Franke C: The coexistence of embryonic and adult acetylcholine receptors in sarcolemma of mdx dystrophic mouse muscle: An effect of regeneration or muscular dystrophy? Neurosci Lett 173:79-82, 1994.

938. Brownell AK, Paasuke RT, Elash A, et al: Malignant hyperthermia in Duchenne muscular dystrophy. Anesthesiology 58:180-182, 1983.

939. Ohkoshi N, Yoshizawa T, Mizusawa H, et al: Malignant hyperthermia in a patient with Becker muscular dystrophy: Dystrophin analysis and caffeine contracture study. Neuromuscul Disord 5:53-58, 1995.

940. Buzello W, Huttarsch H: Muscle relaxation in patients with Duchenne's muscular dystrophy. Use of vecuronium in two patients. Br J Anaesth 60:228-231, 1988.

941. Ririe DG, Shapiro F, Sethna NF: The response of patients with Duchenne's muscular dystrophy to neuromuscular blockade with vecuronium. Anesthesiology 88:351-354, 1998.

942. Uslu M, Mellinghoff H, Diefenbach C: Mivacurium for muscle relaxation in a child with Duchenne's muscular dystrophy. Anesth Analg 89:340-341, 1999.

943. Kaufman L: Dystrophia myotonica and succinylcholine [letter]. Anaesthesia 55:929, 2000.

944. Nightingale P, Healy TE, McGuinness K: Dystrophia myotonica and atracurium. A case report. Br J Anaesth 57:1131-1135, 1985.

945. Buzello W, Krieg N, Schlickewei A: Hazards of neostigmine in patients with neuromuscular disorders. Report of two cases. Br J Anaesth 54:529-534, 1982.

946. Sethna NF, Rockoff MA: Cardiac arrest following inhalation induction of anaesthesia in a child with Duchenne's muscular dystrophy. Can Anaesth Soc J 33:799-802, 1986.

947. Sethna NF, Rockoff MA, Worthen HM, et al: Anesthesia-related complications in children with Duchenne muscular dystrophy. Anesthesiology 68:462-465, 1988.

948. Obata R, Yasumi Y, Suzuki A, et al: Rhabdomyolysis in association with Duchenne's muscular dystrophy. Can J Anaesth 46:564-566, 1999.

949. Goresky GV, Cox RG: Inhalation anesthetics and Duchenne's muscular dystrophy. Can J Anaesth 46:525-528, 1999.

950. Bennun M, Goldstein B, Finkelstein Y, et al: Continuous propofol anaesthesia for patients with myotonic dystrophy. Br J Anaesth 85:407-409, 2000.

951. Mathieu J, Allard P, Gobeil G, et al: Anesthetic and surgical complications in 219 cases of myotonic dystrophy. Neurology 49:1646-1650, 1997.

952. Barohn RJ, Levine EJ, Olson JO, et al: Gastric hypomotility in Duchenne's muscular dystrophy. N Engl J Med 319:15-18, 1988.

953. Landrum AL, Eggers GW: Oculopharyngeal dystrophy: An approach to anesthetic management. Anesth Analg 75:1043-1045, 1992.

954. Staiano A, Del Giudice E, Romano A, et al: Upper gastrointestinal tract motility in children with progressive muscular dystrophy. J Pediatr 121:720-724, 1992.

955. Hopkins A, Wray S: The effect of pregnancy on dystrophia myotonica. Neurology 17:166-168, 1967.

956. Moxley RT 3rd, Kingston WJ, Minaker KL, et al: Insulin resistance and regulation of serum amino acid levels in myotonic dystrophy. Clin Sci (Lond) 71:429-436, 1986.

957. Ricker K: Myotonic dystrophy and proximal myotonic myopathy. J Neurol 246:334-338, 1999.

958. Bourke TD, Zuck D: Thiopentone in dystrophy myotonia. Br J Anaesth 29:35, 1957.

959. Speedy H: Exaggerated physiological responses to propofol in myotonic dystrophy. Br J Anaesth 64:110-112, 1990.

960. White DA, Smyth DG: Exaggerated physiological responses to propofol in myotonic dystrophy. Br J Anaesth 64:758-759, 1990.

961. Aldridge LM: Anaesthetic problems in myotonic dystrophy. A case report and review of the Aberdeen experience comprising 48 general anaesthetics in a further 16 patients. Br J Anaesth 57:1119-1130, 1985.

962. Shapiro F, Sethna N, Colan S, et al: Spinal fusion in Duchenne muscular dystrophy: A multidisciplinary approach. Muscle Nerve 15:604-614, 1992.

963. Aldwinckle RJ, Carr AS: The anesthetic management of a patient with Emery-Dreifuss muscular dystrophy for orthopedic surgery. Can J Anaesth 49:467-470, 2002.

964. Shiraishi M, Minami K, Kadaya T: A safe anesthetic method using caudal block and ketamine for the child with congenital myotonic dystrophy. Anesth Analg 94:233, 2002.

965. Noordeen MH, Haddad FS, Muntoni F, et al: Blood loss in Duchenne muscular dystrophy: Vascular smooth muscle dysfunction? J Pediatr Orthop B 8:212-215, 1999.

966. Forst J, Forst R, Leithe H, et al: Platelet function deficiency in Duchenne muscular dystrophy. Neuromuscul Disord 8:46-49, 1998.

967. Schaefer AM, Taylor RW, Turnbull DM: The mitochondrial genome and mitochondrial muscle disorders. Curr Opin Pharmacol 1:288-293, 2001.

968. Chinnery PF, Johnson MA, Wardell TM, et al: The epidemiology of pathogenic mitochondrial DNA mutations. Ann Neurol 48:188-193, 2000.

969. Collombet JM, Coutelle C: Towards gene therapy of mitochondrial disorders. Mol Med Today 4:31-38, 1998.

970. Chinnery PF, Howell N, Andrews RM, et al: Clinical mitochondrial genetics. J Med Genet 36:425-436, 1999.

971. Rifai Z, Welle S, Kamp C, et al: Ragged red fibers in normal aging and inflammatory myopathy. Ann Neurol 37:24-29, 1995.

972. Dalakas MC, Illa I, Pezeshkpour GH, et al: Mitochondrial myopathy caused by long-term zidovudine therapy. N Engl J Med 322:1098-1105, 1990.

973. Clay AS, Behnia M, Brown KK: Mitochondrial disease: A pulmonary and critical-care medicine perspective. Chest 120:634-648, 2001.

974. Parke TJ, Stevens JE, Rice AS, et al: Metabolic acidosis and fatal myocardial failure after propofol infusion in children: Five case reports. BMJ 305:613-616, 1992.

975. Cray SH, Robinson BH, Cox PN: Lactic acidemia and bradyarrhythmia in a child sedated with propofol. Crit Care Med 26:2087-2092, 1998.

976. Stacpoole PW: Lactic acidosis. Endocrinol Metab Clin North Am 22:221-245, 1993.

977. Badr AE, Mychaskiw G 2nd, Eichhorn JH: Metabolic acidosis associated with a new formulation of propofol. Anesthesiology 94:536-538, 2001.

978. van den Ouweland JM, Lemkes HH, Ruitenbeek W, et al: Mutation in mitochondrial tRNA(Leu)(UUR) gene in a large pedigree with maternally transmitted type II diabetes mellitus and deafness. Nat Genet 1:368-371, 1992.

979. Carroll JE, Zwillich C, Weil JV, et al: Depressed ventilatory response in oculocraniosomatic neuromuscular disease. Neurology 26:140-146, 1976.
980. Cros D, Palliyath S, DiMauro S, et al: Respiratory failure revealing mitochondrial myopathy in adults. Chest 101:824-828, 1992.
981. Manni R, Piccolo G, Banfi P, et al: Respiratory patterns during sleep in mitochondrial myopathies with ophthalmoplegia. Eur Neurol 31:12-17, 1991.
982. DiMauro S, Bonilla E, Davidson M, et al: Mitochondria in neuromuscular disorders. Biochim Biophys Acta 1366:199-210, 1998.
983. Wang J, Wilhelmsson H, Graff C, et al: Dilated cardiomyopathy and atrioventricular conduction blocks induced by heart-specific inactivation of mitochondrial DNA gene expression. Nat Genet 21:133-137, 1999.
984. Howell N: Human mitochondrial diseases: Answering questions and questioning answers. Int Rev Cytol 186:49-116, 1999.
985. D'Ambra MN, Dedrick D, Savarese JJ: Kearns-Sayer syndrome and pancuronium-succinylcholine–induced neuromuscular blockade. Anesthesiology 51:343-345, 1979.
986. Naguib M, el Dawlatly AA, Ashour M, et al: Sensitivity to mivacurium in a patient with mitochondrial myopathy. Anesthesiology 84:1506-1509, 1996.
987. Finsterer J, Stratil U, Bittner R, et al: Increased sensitivity to rocuronium and atracurium in mitochondrial myopathy. Can J Anaesth 45:781-784, 1998.
988. Lessell S, Kuwabara T, Feldman RG: Myopathy and succinylcholine sensitivity. Am J Ophthalmol 68:789-796, 1969.
989. Figarella-Branger D, Kozak-Ribbens G, Rodet L, et al: Pathological findings in 165 patients explored for malignant hyperthermia susceptibility. Neuromuscul Disord 3:553-556, 1993.
990. Etcharry-Bouyx F, Sangla I, Serratrice G: Chronic rhabdomyolysis disclosing mitochondriopathy and malignant hyperthermia susceptibility [in French]. Rev Neurol (Paris) 151:589-592, 1995.
991. Fricker RM, Raffelsberger T, Rauch-Shorny S, et al: Positive malignant hyperthermia susceptibility in vitro test in a patient with mitochondrial myopathy and myoadenylate deaminase deficiency. Anesthesiology 97:1635-1637, 2002.
992. Maslow A, Lisbon A: Anesthetic considerations in patients with mitochondrial dysfunction. Anesth Analg 76:884-886, 1993.
993. Rosaeg OP, Morrison S, MacLeod JP: Anaesthetic management of labour and delivery in the parturient with mitochondrial myopathy. Can J Anaesth 43:403-407, 1996.
994. Celesia GG: Disorders of membrane channels or channelopathies. Clin Neurophysiol 112:2-18, 2001.
995. Siegelbaum SA, Koester J: Ion channels. In Kandel ER, Scharrtz JH, Jessel TM (eds): Principles of Neural Science New York, McGraw-Hill, 2000, pp 105-125.
996. Ashcroft FM: Ion Channels and Disease. London, Academic Press, 2000.
997. Jurkat-Rott K, Lerche H, Lehmann-Horn F: Skeletal muscle channelopathies. J Neurol 249:1493-1502, 2002.
998. Waxman SG: Transcriptional channelopathies: An emerging class of disorders. Nat Rev Neurosci 2:652-659, 2001.
999. Black JA, Dib-Hajj S, Baker D, et al: Sensory neuron-specific sodium channel SNS is abnormally expressed in the brains of mice with experimental allergic encephalomyelitis and humans with multiple sclerosis. Proc Natl Acad Sci U S A 97:11598-11602, 2000.
1000. Koch MC, Steinmeyer K, Lorenz C, Ricker K, et al: The skeletal muscle chloride channel in dominant and recessive human myotonia. Science 257:797-800, 1992.
1001. George AL Jr, Crackower MA, Abdalla JA, et al: Molecular basis of Thomsen's disease (autosomal dominant myotonia congenita). Nat Genet 3:305-310, 1993.
1002. Fontaine B, Khurana TS, Hoffman EP, et al: Hyperkalemic periodic paralysis and the adult muscle sodium channel alpha-subunit gene. Science 250:1000-1002, 1990.
1003. Lerche H, Heine R, Pika U, et al: Human sodium channel myotonia: Slowed channel inactivation due to substitutions for a glycine within the III-IV linker. J Physiol (Lond) 470:13-22, 1993
1004. Ricker K, Moxley RT 3rd, Heine R, et al: Myotonia fluctuans. A third type of muscle sodium channel disease. Arch Neurol 51:1095-1102, 1994.
1005. Fontaine B, Vale-Santos J, Jurkat-Rott K, et al: Mapping of the hypokalaemic periodic paralysis (HypoPP) locus to chromosome 1q31-32 in three European families. Nat Genet 6:267-272, 1994.
1006. Jurkat-Rott K, Mitrovic N, Hang C, et al: Voltage-sensor sodium channel mutations cause hypokalemic periodic paralysis type 2 by enhanced inactivation and reduced current. Proc Natl Acad Sci U S A 97:9549-9554, 2000.
1007. Quane KA, Healy JM, Keating KE, et al: Mutations in the ryanodine receptor gene in central core disease and malignant hyperthermia. Nat Genet 5:51-55, 1993.
1008. Zhang Y, Chen HS, Khanna VK, et al: A mutation in the human ryanodine receptor gene associated with central core disease. Nat Genet 5:46-50, 1993.
1009. Sine SM, Ohno K, Bouzat C, et al: Mutation of the acetylcholine receptor alpha subunit causes a slow-channel myasthenic syndrome by enhancing agonist binding affinity. Neuron 15:229-239, 1995.
1010. Hoffman EP: Voltage-gated ion channelopathies: Inherited disorders caused by abnormal sodium, chloride, and calcium regulation in skeletal muscle. Annu Rev Med 46:431-441, 1995.
1011. Cooper EC, Jan LY: Ion channel genes and human neurological disease: Recent progress, prospects, and challenges. Proc Natl Acad Sci U S A 96:4759-4766, 1999.
1012. Lehmann-Horn F, Jurkat-Rott K: Voltage-gated ion channels and hereditary disease. Physiol Rev 79:1317-1372, 1999.
1013. Kleopa KA, Barchi RL: Genetic disorders of neuromuscular ion channels. Muscle Nerve 26:299-325, 2002.
1014. Lehmann-Horn F, Jurkat-Rott K, Rudel R: Periodic paralysis: Understanding channelopathies. Curr Neurol Neurosci Rep 2:61-69, 2002.
1015. Rios E, Pizarro G: Voltage sensor of excitation-contraction coupling in skeletal muscle. Physiol Rev 71:849-908, 1991.
1016. Fill M, Copello JA: Ryanodine receptor calcium release channels. Physiol Rev 82:893-922, 2002.
1017. MacKrill JJ: Protein-protein interactions in intracellular Ca^{2+}-release channel function. Biochem J 337 (Pt 3):345-361, 1999.
1018. Vincent A, Palace J, Hilton-Jones D: Myasthenia gravis. Lancet 357:2122-2128, 2001.
1019. Vincent A: Unravelling the pathogenesis of myasthenia gravis. Nat Rev Immunol 2:797-804, 2002.
1020. Lindstrom JM: Acetylcholine receptors and myasthenia. Muscle Nerve 23:453-477, 2000.
1021. Drachman DB: Myasthenia gravis. N Engl J Med 330:1797-1810, 1994.
1022. Phillips WD, Vladeta D, Han H, et al: Rapsyn and agrin slow the metabolic degradation of the acetylcholine receptor. Mol Cell Neurosci 10:16-26, 1997.
1023. Tzartos SJ, Lindstrom JM: Monoclonal antibodies used to probe acetylcholine receptor structure: Localization of the main immunogenic region and detection of similarities between subunits. Proc Natl Acad Sci U S A 77:755-759, 1980.
1024. Lang TJ, Badea TC, Wade R, et al: Sublytic terminal complement attack on myotubes decreases the expression of mRNAs encoding muscle-specific proteins. J Neurochem 68:1581-1589, 1997.
1025. Lindstrom JM, Seybold ME, Lennon VA, et al: Antibody to acetylcholine receptor in myasthenia gravis. Prevalence, clinical correlates, and diagnostic value. Neurology 26:1054-1059, 1976.
1026. Whitney KD, McNamara JO: Autoimmunity and neurological disease: Antibody modulation of synaptic transmission. Annu Rev Neurosci 22:175-195, 1999.

1027. Vincent A, Newsom-Davis J: Acetylcholine receptor antibody as a diagnostic test for myasthenia gravis: Results in 153 validated cases and 2967 diagnostic assays. J Neurol Neurosurg Psychiatry 48:1246-1252, 1985.

1028. Hoch W, McConville J, Helms S, et al: Auto-antibodies to the receptor tyrosine kinase MuSK in patients with myasthenia gravis without acetylcholine receptor antibodies. Nat Med 7:365-368, 2001.

1029. Valenzuela DM, Stitt TN, DiStefano PS, et al: Receptor tyrosine kinase specific for the skeletal muscle lineage: Expression in embryonic muscle, at the neuromuscular junction, and after injury. Neuron 15:573-584, 1995.

1030. Vernino S, Adamski J, Kryzer TJ, et al: Neuronal nicotinic ACh receptor antibody in subacute autonomic neuropathy and cancer-related syndromes. Neurology 50:1806-1813, 1998.

1031. Hatton PD, Diehl JT, Daly BD, et al: Transsternal radical thymectomy for myasthenia gravis: A 15-year review. Ann Thorac Surg 47:838-840, 1989.

1032. Deitiker P, Ashizawa T, Atassi MZ: Antigen mimicry in autoimmune disease. Can immune responses to microbial antigens that mimic acetylcholine receptor act as initial triggers of myasthenia gravis? Hum Immunol 61:255-265, 2000.

1033. Woolf AL: Morphology of the myasthenic neuromuscular junction. Ann N Y Acad Sci 135:35-59, 1966.

1034. Plomp JJ, van Kempen GT, Molenaar PC: Adaptation of quantal content to decreased postsynaptic sensitivity at single endplates in alpha-bungarotoxin–treated rats. J Physiol 458:487-499, 1992.

1035. Plomp JJ, Van Kempen GT, De Baets MB, et al: Acetylcholine release in myasthenia gravis: Regulation at single end-plate level. Ann Neurol 37:627-636, 1995.

1036. Lambert EH, Eaton LM, Rooke ED: Defect of neuromuscular conduction associated with malignant neoplasm. Am J Physiol 187:612-613, 1956.

1037. Takamori M, Maruta T, Komai K: Lambert-Eaton myasthenic syndrome as an autoimmune calcium-channelopathy. Neurosci Res 36:183-191, 2000.

1038. Leveque C, Hoshino T, David P, et al: The synaptic vesicle protein synaptotagmin associates with calcium channels and is a putative Lambert-Eaton myasthenic syndrome antigen. Proc Natl Acad Sci U S A 89:3625-3629, 1992.

1039. Sudhof TC: The synaptic vesicle cycle: A cascade of protein-protein interactions. Nature 375:645-653, 1995.

1040. Hewett SJ, Atchison WD: Serum and plasma from patients with Lambert-Eaton myasthenic syndrome reduce depolarization-dependent uptake of $^{45}Ca^{2+}$ into rat cortical synaptosomes. Brain Res 566:320-324, 1991.

1041. Sanders DB: Lambert-Eaton myasthenic syndrome: Clinical diagnosis, immune-mediated mechanisms, and update on therapies. Ann Neurol 37(Suppl 1):S63-S73, 1995.

1042. Sanders DB, Massey JM, Sanders LL, et al: A randomized trial of 3,4-diaminopyridine in Lambert-Eaton myasthenic syndrome. Neurology 54:603-607, 2000.

1043. Engel AG, Ohno K, Milone M, et al: Congenital myasthenic syndromes. New insights from molecular genetic and patch-clamp studies. Ann N Y Acad Sci 841:140-156, 1998.

1044. Engel AG, Ohno K, Sine SM: Congenital myasthenic syndromes: Recent advances. Arch Neurol 56:163-167, 1999.

1045. Engel AG, Ohno K, Sine SM: Congenital myasthenic syndromes: Progress over the past decade. Muscle Nerve 27:4-25, 2003.

1046. Engel AG, Walls TJ, Nagel A, et al: Newly recognized congenital myasthenic syndromes: I. Congenital paucity of synaptic vesicles and reduced quantal release. II. High-conductance fast-channel syndrome. III. Abnormal acetylcholine receptor (AChR) interaction with acetylcholine. IV. AChR deficiency and short channel-open time. Prog Brain Res 84:125-137, 1990.

1047. Engel AG, Lambert EH, Gomez MR: A new myasthenic syndrome with end-plate acetylcholinesterase deficiency, small nerve terminals, and reduced acetylcholine release. Ann Neurol 1:315-330, 1977.

1048. Ohno K, Tsujino A, Brengman JM, et al: Choline acetyltransferase mutations cause myasthenic syndrome associated with episodic apnea in humans. Proc Natl Acad Sci U S A 98:2017-2022, 2001.

1049. Ohno K, Engel AG, Shen XM, et al: Rapsyn mutations in humans cause endplate acetylcholine-receptor deficiency and myasthenic syndrome. Am J Hum Genet 70:875-885, 2002.

1050. Jeyarasasingam G, Yeluashvili M, Quik M: Nitric oxide is involved in acetylcholinesterase inhibitor–induced myopathy in rats. J Pharmacol Exp Ther 295:314-320, 2000.

1051. Fukudome T, Ohno K, Brengman JM, et al: Quinidine normalizes the open duration of slow-channel mutants of the acetylcholine receptor. Neuroreport 9:1907-1911, 1998.

1052. Ohno K, Wang HL, Milone M, et al: Congenital myasthenic syndrome caused by decreased agonist binding affinity due to a mutation in the acetylcholine receptor epsilon subunit. Neuron 17:157-170, 1996.

1053. Milone M, Wang HL, Ohno K, et al: Mode switching kinetics produced by a naturally occurring mutation in the cytoplasmic loop of the human acetylcholine receptor epsilon subunit. Neuron 20:575-588, 1998.

1054. Baraka A: Onset of neuromuscular block in myasthenic patients. Br J Anaesth 69:227-228, 1992.

1055. Abel M, Eisenkraft JB: Anesthetic implications of myasthenia gravis. Mt Sinai J Med 69:31-37, 2002.

1056. Nishino T: Swallowing as a protective reflex for the upper respiratory tract. Anesthesiology 79:588-601, 1993.

1057. Cohen MS, Younger D: Aspects of the natural history of myasthenia gravis: Crisis and death. Ann N Y Acad Sci 377:670-677, 1981.

1058. Naguib M, el Dawlatly AA, Ashour M, et al: Multivariate determinants of the need for postoperative ventilation in myasthenia gravis. Can J Anaesth 43:1006-1013, 1996.

1059. Eisenkraft JB, Book WJ, Mann SM, et al: Resistance to succinylcholine in myasthenia gravis: A dose-response study. Anesthesiology 69:760-763, 1988.

1060. Baraka A: Suxamethonium block in the myasthenic patient. Correlation with plasma cholinesterase. Anaesthesia 47:217-219, 1992.

1061. Seigne RD, Scott RP: Mivacurium chloride and myasthenia gravis. Br J Anaesth 72:468-469, 1994.

1062. Baraka A: Anaesthesia and myasthenia gravis. Can J Anaesth 39:476-486, 1992.

1063. Smith CE, Donati F, Bevan DR: Cumulative dose-response curves for atracurium in patients with myasthenia gravis. Can J Anaesth 36:402-406, 1989.

1064. Eisenkraft JB, Book WJ, Papatestas AE: Sensitivity to vecuronium in myasthenia gravis: A dose-response study. Can J Anaesth 37:301-306, 1990.

1065. De Haes A, Proost JH, De Baets MH, et al: Pharmacokinetic-pharmacodynamic modeling of rocuronium in case of a decreased number of acetylcholine receptors: A study in myasthenic pigs. Anesthesiology 98:133-142, 2003.

1066. Nilsson E, Meretoja OA: Vecuronium dose-response and maintenance requirements in patients with myasthenia gravis. Anesthesiology 73:28-32, 1990.

1067. Kim JM, Mangold J: Sensitivity to both vecuronium and neostigmine in a sero-negative myasthenic patient. Br J Anaesth 63:497-500, 1989.

1068. Nilsson E, Paloheimo M, Muller K, et al: Halothane-induced variability in the neuromuscular transmission of patients with myasthenia gravis. Acta Anaesthesiol Scand 33:395-401, 1989.

1069. Nilsson E, Muller K: Neuromuscular effects of isoflurane in patients with myasthenia gravis. Acta Anaesthesiol Scand 34:126-131, 1990.

1070. Rowbottom SJ: Isoflurane for thymectomy in myasthenia gravis. Anaesth Intensive Care 17:444-447, 1989.

1071. Akpolat N, Tilgen H, Gursoy F, et al: Thoracic epidural anaesthesia and analgesia with bupivacaine for transsternal thymectomy for myasthenia gravis. Eur J Anaesthesiol 14:220-223, 1997.

1072. D'Angelo R, Gerancher JC: Combined spinal and epidural analgesia in a parturient with severe myasthenia gravis. Reg Anesth Pain Med 23:201-203, 1998.

1073. de Jose Maria B, Carrero E, Sala X: Myasthenia gravis and regional anaesthesia. Can J Anaesth 42:178-179, 1995.

1074. Small S, Ali HH, Lennon VA, et al: Anesthesia for an unsuspected Lambert-Eaton myasthenic syndrome with autoantibodies and occult small cell lung carcinoma. Anesthesiology 76:142-145, 1992.

1075. Brown JC, Charlton JE: A study of sensitivity to curare in myasthenic disorders using a regional technique. J Neurol Neurosurg Psychiatry 38:27-33, 1975.

1076. Telford RJ, Hollway TE: The myasthenic syndrome: Anaesthesia in a patient treated with 3,4 diaminopyridine. Br J Anaesth 64:363-366, 1990.

1077. Newsom-Davis J, Mills KR: Immunological associations of acquired neuromyotonia (Isaacs' syndrome). Report of five cases and literature review. Brain 116(Pt 2):453-469, 1993.

1078. Vincent A: Understanding neuromyotonia. Muscle Nerve 23:655-657, 2000.

1079. Arimura K, Sonoda Y, Watanabe O, et al: Isaacs' syndrome as a potassium channelopathy of the nerve. Muscle Nerve Suppl 11:S55-S58, 2002.

1080. Lee EK, Maselli RA, Ellis WG, et al: Morvan's fibrillary chorea: A paraneoplastic manifestation of thymoma. J Neurol Neurosurg Psychiatry 65:857-862, 1998.

1081. Hart IK, Waters C, Vincent A, et al: Autoantibodies detected to expressed K$^+$ channels are implicated in neuromyotonia. Ann Neurol 41:238-246, 1997.

1082. Lang B, Vincent A: Autoimmunity to ion-channels and other proteins in paraneoplastic disorders. Curr Opin Immunol 8:865-871, 1996.

1083. Zisfein J, Sivak M, Aron AM, et al: Isaacs' syndrome with muscle hypertrophy reversed by phenytoin therapy. Arch Neurol 40:241-242, 1983.

1084. van den Berg JS, van Engelen BG, Boerman RH, et al: Acquired neuromyotonia: Superiority of plasma exchange over high-dose intravenous human immunoglobulin. J Neurol 246:623-625, 1999.

1085. Ashizawa T, Butler IJ, Harati Y, et al: A dominantly inherited syndrome with continuous motor neuron discharges. Ann Neurol 13:285-290, 1983.

1086. Hosokawa S, Shinoda H, Sakai T, et al: Electrophysiological study on limb myokymia in three women. J Neurol Neurosurg Psychiatry 50:877-881, 1987.

1087. Morgan PJ: Peripartum management of a patient with Isaacs' syndrome. Can J Anaesth 44:1174-1177, 1997.

1088. Shillito P, Molenaar PC, Vincent A, et al: Acquired neuromyotonia: Evidence for autoantibodies directed against K$^+$ channels of peripheral nerves. Ann Neurol 38:714-722, 1995.

1089. Sinha S, Newsom-Davis J, Mills K, et al: Autoimmune aetiology for acquired neuromyotonia (Isaacs' syndrome). Lancet 1991:75-77, 338.

1090. Steinmeyer K, Lorenz C, Pusch M, et al: Multimeric structure of ClC-1 chloride channel revealed by mutations in dominant myotonia congenita (Thomsen). EMBO J 13:737-743, 1994.

1091. Jurkat-Rott K, Lehmann-Horn F: Human muscle voltage-gated ion channels and hereditary disease. Curr Opin Pharmacol 1:280-287, 2001.

1092. Mitchell MM, Ali HH, Savarese JJ: Myotonia and neuromuscular blocking agents. Anesthesiology 49:44-48, 1978.

1093. Heiman-Patterson T, Martino C, Rosenberg H, et al: Malignant hyperthermia in myotonia congenita. Neurology 38:810-812, 1988.

1094. Lehmann-Horn F, Iaizzo PA: Are myotonias and periodic paralyses associated with susceptibility to malignant hyperthermia? Br J Anaesth 65:692-697, 1990.

1095. Ellis FR: Inherited muscle disease. Br J Anaesth 52:153-164, 1980.

1096. Arcas M, Sanchez-Ortega JL, Garcia-Munoz M, et al: Anesthesia for cesarean delivery in a case of myotonia congenita [in Spanish]. Rev Esp Anesthesiol Reanim 43:147-149, 1996.

1097. Cannon SC: Sodium channel defects in myotonia and periodic paralysis. Annu Rev Neurosci 19:141-164, 1996.

1098. Ptacek LJ, George AL Jr, Griggs RC, et al: Identification of a mutation in the gene causing hyperkalemic periodic paralysis. Cell 67:1021-1027, 1991.

1099. McClatchey AI, Van den Bergh P, Pericak-Vance MA, et al: Temperature-sensitive mutations in the III-IV cytoplasmic loop region of the skeletal muscle sodium channel gene in paramyotonia congenita. Cell 68:769-774, 1992.

1100. Poskanzer DC, Kerr DNS: A third type of periodic paralysis, with normokalemia and favourable response to sodium chloride. Am J Med 31:328-342, 1961.

1101. Meyers KR, Gilden DH, Rinaldi CF, et al: Periodic muscle weakness, normokalemia, and tubular aggregates. Neurology 22:269-279, 1972.

1102. Lehmann-Horn F, Rudel R, Ricker K: Non-dystrophic myotonias and periodic paralyses. A European Neuromuscular Center Workshop held 4-6 October 1992, Ulm, Germany. Neuromuscul Disord 3:161-168, 1993.

1103. Ashwood EM, Russell WJ, Burrow DD: Hyperkalaemic periodic paralysis and anaesthesia. Anaesthesia 47:579-584, 1992.

1104. Flewellen EH, Bodensteiner JB: Anesthetic experience in a patient with hyperkalemic periodic paralysis. Anesth Rev 7:44, 1980.

1105. Baur CP, Schara U, Schlecht R, et al: Anesthesia in neuro-muscular disorders. Part 2: Specific disorders [in German]. Anasthesiol Intensivmed Notfallmed Schmerzther 37:125-137, 2002.

1106. Moslehi R, Langlois S, Yam I, et al: Linkage of malignant hyperthermia and hyperkalemic periodic paralysis to the adult skeletal muscle sodium channel (SCN4A) gene in a large pedigree. Am J Med Genet 76:21-27, 1998.

1107. Haeseler G, Stormer M, Mohammadi B, et al: The anesthetic propofol modulates gating in paramyotonia congenita mutant muscle sodium channels. Muscle Nerve 24:736-743, 2001.

1108. Haeseler G, Stormer M, Bufler J, et al: Propofol blocks human skeletal muscle sodium channels in a voltage-dependent manner. Anesth Analg 92:1192-1198, 2001.

1109. Weller JF, Elliott RA, Pronovost PJ: Spinal anesthesia for a patient with familial hyperkalemic periodic paralysis. Anesthesiology 97:259-260, 2002.

1110. Sternberg D, Maisonobe T, Jurkat-Rott K, et al: Hypokalaemic periodic paralysis type 2 caused by mutations at codon 672 in the muscle sodium channel gene SCN4A. Brain 124:1091-1099, 2001.

1111. Minaker KL, Meneilly GS, Flier JS, et al: Insulin-mediated hypokalemia and paralysis in familial hypokalemic periodic paralysis. Am J Med 84:1001-1006, 1988.

1112. Ruff RL: Insulin acts in hypokalemic periodic paralysis by reducing inward rectifier K$^+$ current. Neurology 53:1556-1563, 1999.

1113. Shiang R, Ryan SG, Zhu YZ, et al: Mutations in the alpha 1 subunit of the inhibitory glycine receptor cause the dominant neurologic disorder, hyperexplexia. Nat Genet 5:351-358, 1993.

1114. Quane KA, Healy JM, Keating KE, et al: Mutations in the ryanodine receptor gene in central core disease and malignant hyperthermia. Nat Genet 5:51-55, 1993.

1115. Rasmussen H, Zawalich KC, Ganesan S, et al: Physiology and pathophysiology of insulin secretion. Diabetes Care 13:655-666, 1990.

1116. Osterhoff M, Mohlig M, Schwanstecher M, et al: Ca(2+)/calmodulin-dependent protein kinase II delta(2) regulates gene expression of insulin in INS-1 rat insulinoma cells. Cell Calcium 33:175-184, 2003.

1117. Lehmann-Horn F, Kuther G, Ricker K, et al: Adynamia episodica hereditaria with myotonia: A non-inactivating sodium current and the effect of extracellular pH. Muscle Nerve 10:363-374, 1987.

1118. Siler JN, Discavage WJ: Anesthetic management of hypokalemic periodic paralysis. Anesthesiology 43:489-490, 1975.

1119. Lambert C, Blanloeil Y, Horber RK, et al: Malignant hyperthermia in a patient with hypokalemic periodic paralysis. Anesth Analg 79:1012-1014, 1994.

1120. Horton B: Anesthetic experiences in a family with hypokalemic familial periodic paralysis. Anesthesiology 47:308-310, 1977.

1121. Viscomi CM, Ptacek LJ, Dudley D: Anesthetic management of familial hypokalemic periodic paralysis during parturition. Anesth Analg 88:1081-1082, 1999.

1122. Lofgren A, Hahn RG: Serum potassium levels after induction of epidural anaesthesia using mepivacaine with and without adrenaline. Acta Anaesthesiol Scand 35:170-174, 1991.

1123. Lofgren A, Hahn RG: Hypokalemia from intercostal nerve block. Reg Anesth 19:247-254, 1994.

1124. Durfee DD: A practical approach to achieving a $950,000 cost savings from a joint anesthesia-pharmacy program. Hosp Pharm 30:957-958, 961-963, 1995.

1125. Gora-Harper ML, Hessel E 2nd, Shadick D: Effect of prescribing guidelines on the use of neuromuscular blocking agents. Am J Health Syst Pharm 52:1900-1904, 1995.

1126. Chiu JW, White PF: The pharmacoeconomics of neuromuscular blocking drugs. Anesth Analg 90:S19-S23, 2000.

1127. Souetre EJ, Qing W, Hardens M: Methodological approaches to pharmaco-economics. Fundam Clin Pharmacol 8:101-107, 1994.

1128. Horrow JC, Rosenberg H: Price stickers do not alter drug usage. Can J Anaesth 41:1047-1052, 1994.

1129. Lin YC, Miller SR: The impact of price labeling of muscle relaxants on cost consciousness among anesthesiologists. J Clin Anesth 10:401-403, 1998.

1130. Johnstone RE, Jozefczyk KG: Costs of anesthetic drugs: Experiences with a cost education trial. Anesth Analg 78:766-771, 1994.

1131. Gillerman RG, Browning RA: Drug use inefficiency: A hidden source of wasted health care dollars. Anesth Analg 91:921-924, 2000.

1132. Ballantyne JC, Chang Y: The impact of choice of muscle relaxant on postoperative recovery time: A retrospective study. Anesth Analg 85:476-482, 1997.

1133. Lubarsky DA, Glass PS, Ginsberg B, et al: The successful implementation of pharmaceutical practice guidelines. Analysis of associated outcomes and cost savings. SWiPE Group. Systematic Withdrawal of Perioperative Expenses. Anesthesiology 86:1145-1160, 1997.

1134. Freund PR, Bowdle TA, Posner KL, et al: Cost-effective reduction of neuromuscular-blocking drug expenditures. Anesthesiology 87:1044-1049, 1997.

1135. Butterworth J, James R, Prielipp RC, et al: Do shorter-acting neuromuscular blocking drugs or opioids associate with reduced intensive care unit or hospital lengths of stay after coronary artery bypass grafting? CABG Clinical Benchmarking Data Base Participants. Anesthesiology 88:1437-1446, 1998.

1136. Murphy GS, Szokol JW, Marymont JH, et al: Impact of shorter-acting neuromuscular blocking agents on fast-track recovery of the cardiac surgical patient. Anesthesiology 96:600-606, 2002.

1137. Puura AI, Rorarius MG, Manninen P, et al: The costs of intense neuromuscular block for anesthesia during endolaryngeal procedures due to waiting time. Anesth Analg 88:1335-1339, 1999.

1138. Splinter WM, Isaac LA: The pharmacoeconomics of neuromuscular blocking drugs: A perioperative cost-minimization strategy in children. Anesth Analg 93:339-344, 2001.

1139. Miller RD: How should residual neuromuscular blockade be detected? Anesthesiology 70:379-380, 1989.

1140. Dexter F, Gan TJ, Naguib M, et al: Cost identification analysis for succinylcholine. Anesth Analg 92:693-699, 2001.

CHAPTER
14 Local Anesthetics

Gary R. Strichartz and Charles B. Berde

Basic Pharmacology   573
Chemistry   573
Structure-Activity Relationships and
   Physicochemical Properties   574

Anatomy of the Peripheral Nerve   576
Structure of the Axonal Membrane   576
Physiology of Nerve Conduction   577

**Mechanism of Action of
Local Anesthetics
(Pharmacodynamics)   579**
Active Form   579
The Electrophysiologic Effect of Local
   Anesthetics   580
The Nature of the Local Anesthetic
   Binding Site   581
Neurophysiologic Aspects of Phasic
   Inhibition   581
Summary of Local Anesthetic Mechanisms   582

Clinical Pharmacology   583
General Considerations   583
Factors Influencing Anesthetic
   Activity in Humans   584

**Choice of Local Anesthetic for
Various Regional Anesthetic
Procedures   586**
Infiltration Anesthesia   586
Intravenous Regional Anesthesia   587

Peripheral Nerve Blockade   587
Central Neural Blockade   588
Topical Anesthesia   589
Tumescent Anesthesia   591
Systemic Local Anesthetics for
   Neuropathic Pain   591

Pharmacokinetics   591
Absorption   591
Distribution   592
Biotransformation and Excretion   592
Pharmacokinetic Alterations by
   Patient Status   592

Toxicity   592
Systemic Toxicity   592
Comparative Cardiovascular
   Toxicity   594
Methemoglobinemia   596
Allergies   596
Local Tissue Toxicity   597
Prolonged Infusions of Local
   Anesthetics, Tachyphylaxis, and
   Development of Long-Duration Local
   Anesthetics   598

Local anesthesia, or the blockade of nerve impulses to abolish sensation, may be produced by many tertiary amine bases, certain alcohols, and a variety of other drugs and toxins. However, all currently available clinically useful agents are either aminoesters or aminoamides. These drugs, when applied in sufficient concentration at the site of action, prevent conduction of electrical impulses by the membranes of nerve and muscle. When local anesthetics are given systemically, the functions of cardiac, skeletal, and smooth muscle, as well as the transmission of impulses in the peripheral and central nervous systems and within the specialized conducting system of the heart, may all be altered. Local anesthetics may abolish sensation in various parts of the body by topical application, injection in the vicinity of peripheral nerve endings and major nerve trunks, or instillation within the epidural or subarachnoid space. Toxicity may be local or systemic. The central nervous and cardiovascular systems are most commonly involved in acute clinical toxicity.

BASIC PHARMACOLOGY

Chemistry

The Local Anesthetic Molecule
The typical local anesthetic molecule, exemplified by lidocaine and procaine (Fig. 14-1), contains a tertiary amine attached to a substituted aromatic ring by an intermediate chain. The tertiary amine is a base (proton acceptor). The chain almost always contains either an ester ($-\overset{\overset{\textstyle O}{\|}}{C}-O$)

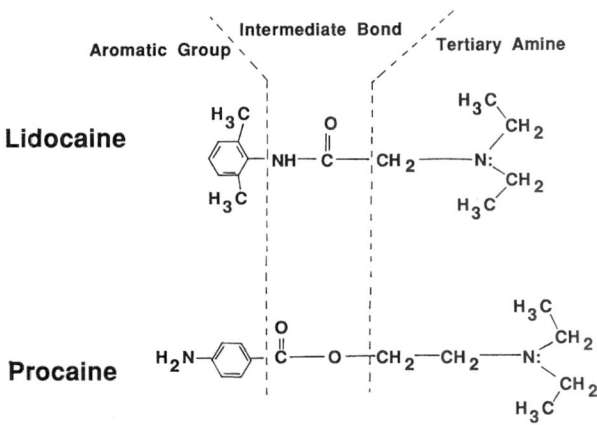

Figure 14–1 Structures of two local anesthetics, the aminoamide lidocaine and the aminoester procaine. In both drugs a hydrophobic aromatic group is joined to a more hydrophilic base, the tertiary amine, by an intermediate amide or ester bond.

or amide ($-NH\overset{\overset{\displaystyle O}{\|}}{C}-$) linkage; local anesthetics may therefore be classified as aminoester or aminoamide compounds. The aromatic ring system gives a lipophilic (membrane-liking) character to its portion of the molecule, whereas the tertiary amine end is relatively hydrophilic, particularly because it is partially protonated and thus bears some positive charge in the physiologic pH range (Fig. 14-2). The structures of commonly administered local anesthetics are given in Table 14-1 and their physicochemical properties in Table 14-2.

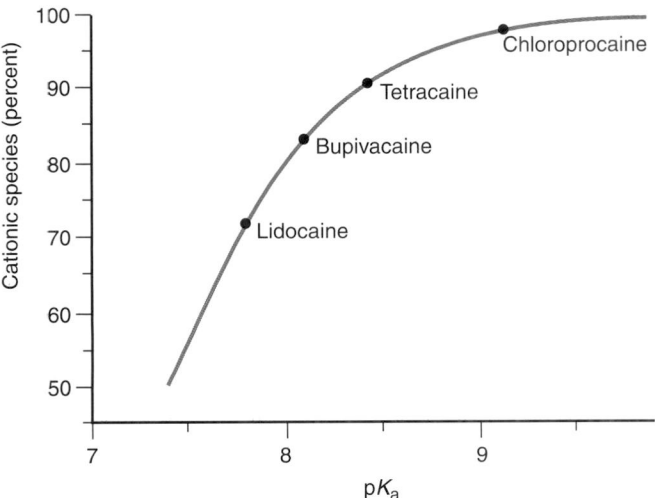

Figure 14–2 The fraction of local anesthetic in the protonated, cationic form in aqueous solution at physiologic pH (7.4) as a function of the pK_a of the drug. The drug with the lowest pK_a, lidocaine, has the smallest fraction of its molecules protonated and the largest in the neutral form, and vice versa for the local anesthetic with the highest pK_a, chloroprocaine. Individual drug molecules become protonated and deprotonated in thousandths of a second in solution.

Structure-Activity Relationships and Physicochemical Properties

The intrinsic potency and duration of action of local anesthetics are clearly dependent on certain features of the molecule.

Lipophilic-Hydrophilic Balance

The lipophilic versus hydrophilic character of local anesthetics depends on the size of the alkyl substituents both on or near the tertiary amine and on the aromatic ring. "Lipophilicity" expresses the tendency of a compound to associate with membrane lipids, which is usually approximated by equilibrium partitioning into a hydrophobic solvent such as octanol.[1] Such octanol/buffer partition coefficients are comparable to membrane/buffer partition coefficients for the uncharged species of local anesthetics but greatly underestimate membrane partitioning for the charged, protonated species, octanol being a poor model for the polar regions near the membrane surface.[2] In this chapter we use the term *hydrophobicity*, expressed by octanol/buffer partitioning, to describe a physicochemical property of local anesthetics.

Compounds with a more hydrophobic nature are obtained by increasing the size of the alkyl substituent or substituents. These agents are more potent and produce longer-lasting blocks than their less hydrophobic congeners do.[3-5] For example, etidocaine, which has three more carbon atoms than lidocaine has in the amine end of the molecule, is four times as potent and five times as long lasting when compared for impulse blockade in the isolated sciatic nerve.

Hydrogen Ion Concentration

Local anesthetics in solution exist in a rapid chemical equilibrium between the basic uncharged form (B) and the charged cationic form (BH⁺). At a certain hydrogen ion concentration ($\log_{10}^{-1}$ [–pH]) specific for each drug, the concentration of local anesthetic base in solution is equal to the concentration of charged cation. This hydrogen ion concentration is called pK_a. The relationship is defined by

$$\frac{[BH^+]}{[B]} = 10^{pK_a - pH} \qquad (1)$$

pK_a values for standard local anesthetics are listed in Table 14-2. The tendency to be protonated also depends on environmental factors, such as temperature and ionic strength, and on the medium surrounding the drug. In the relatively apolar milieu of a membrane, the average pK_a of local anesthetics is lower than in solution.[6] This is chemically equivalent to saying that the membrane concentrates the base form of the local anesthetic more than it concentrates the protonated cation form.

The pH of the medium containing the local anesthetic influences drug activity by altering the relative percentage of the basic or protonated forms. For example, in inflamed tissue, the pH is lower than normal, and local anesthetics are more protonated than in normal tissue and thus penetrate the tissue relatively poorly (see later).

The relationship between pK_a and the percentage of local anesthetic present in the cationic form is shown in

Table 14–1   Representative local anesthetics in common clinical use

Generic* and Common Proprietary Name	Chemical Structure	Approximate Year of Initial Clinical Use	Main Anesthetic Use	Representative Commercial Preparation
Cocaine	$CH_2-CH-CHCOOCH_3$ $NCH_3-CHOOC_6H_5$ $CH_2-CH-CH_2$	1884	Topical	Bulk powder
Benzocaine (Americaine)	H_2N-⬡$-\overset{O}{\underset{}{C}}-OC_2H_5$	1900	Topical Topical	20% ointment 20% aerosol
Procaine (Novocain)	H_2N-⬡$-COOCH_2CH_2N\overset{C_2H_5}{\underset{C_2H_5}{}}$	1905	Infiltration Spinal	10- and 20-mg/mL solutions 100-mg/mL solution
Dibucaine (Nupercaine)	⬡$-N=$, OC_4H_9, $CONHCH_2CH_2N(C_2H_5)_2$	1929	Spinal	0.667-, 2.5-, and 5-mg/mL solutions
Tetracaine (Pontocaine)	$H_9C_4\underset{H}{N}-$⬡$-COOCH_2CH_2N\overset{CH_3}{\underset{CH_3}{}}$	1930	Spinal	Niphanoid crystals—20- and 10-mg/mL solutions
Lidocaine (Xylocaine)	⬡$\overset{CH_3}{\underset{CH_3}{}}-NHCOCH_2N\overset{C_2H_5}{\underset{C_2H_5}{}}$	1944	Infiltration Peripheral nerve blockade Epidural Spinal Topical Topical	5- and 10-mg/mL solutions 10-, 15-, and 20-mg/mL solutions 10-, 15-, and 20-mg/mL solutions 50-mg/mL solution 2.0% jelly, viscous 2.5%, 5.0% ointment
Chloroprocaine (Nesacaine)	H_2N-⬡$\overset{Cl}{}-COOCH_2CH_2N\overset{C_2H_5}{\underset{C_2H_5}{}}$	1955	Infiltration Peripheral nerve blockade Epidural	10-mg/mL solution 10- and 20-mg/mL solutions 20- and 30-mg/mL solutions
Mepivacaine (Carbocaine)	⬡$\overset{CH_3}{\underset{CH_3}{}}-NHCO$⬡$N-CH_3$	1957	Infiltration Peripheral nerve blockade Epidural	10-mg/mL solution 10- and 20-mg/mL solutions 10-, 15-, and 20-mg/mL solutions
Prilocaine (Citanest)	⬡$\overset{CH_3}{}-NHCOCH-NH-C_3H_7$ CH_3	1960	Infiltration Peripheral nerve blockade Epidural	10- and 20-mg/mL solutions 10-, 20-, and 30-mg/mL solutions 10-, 20-, and 30-mg/mL solutions
Bupivacaine (Marcaine)	⬡$\overset{CH_3}{\underset{CH_3}{}}-NHCO$⬡$N-C_4H_9$	1963	Infiltration Peripheral nerve blockade Epidural Spinal	2.5-mg/mL solution 2.5- and 5-mg/mL solutions 2.5-, 5-, and 7.5-mg/mL solutions 5- and 7.5-mg/mL solutions
Ropivacaine (Naropin)	⬡$\overset{CH_3}{\underset{CH_3}{}}-NHCO$⬡$N-C_3H_7$	1992	Infiltration Peripheral nerve blockade Epidural	2.5- and 5-mg/mL solutions 5- and 10-mg/mL solutions 5- and 7.5-mg/mL solutions

*USP nomenclature
Modified from Covino B, Vassallo H: Local Anesthetics: Mechanisms of Action and Clinical Use. Orlando, FL, Grune & Stratton, 1976.

Table 14-2   Relative in vitro conduction-blocking potency and physicochemical properties of local anesthetics

		Physicochemical Properties	
Drug	Relative Conduction-Blocking Potency*	pK_a†	Hydrophobicity†
Low-potency procaine	1	8.9	100
Intermediate potency			
Mepivacaine	1.5	7.7	130
Prilocaine	1.8	8.0‡	129
Chloroprocaine	3	9.1	810
Lidocaine	2	7.8	366
High potency			
Tetracaine	8	8.4	5822
Bupivacaine	8	8.1	3420
Etidocaine	8	7.9	7320

*Data derived from C fibers of isolated rabbit vagus and sciatic nerve.
†pK_a and hydrophobicity at 36°C; hydrophobicity equals the octanol buffer partition coefficient of the base. Values are ratios of concentrations.
‡Values at 25°C.
From Strichartz GR, Sanchez V, Arthur GR, et al: Fundamental properties of local anesthetics. II. Measured octanol:buffer partition coefficients and pKa values of clinically used drugs. Anesth Analg 71:158–170, 1990.

Figure 14-2. As described later, pH has dual effects on clinical effectiveness, depending on the location at which the local anesthetic is injected and the importance of the base form for tissue penetration.

ANATOMY OF THE PERIPHERAL NERVE

Each peripheral nerve axon possesses its own cell membrane, the axolemma. Nonmyelinated nerves, such as autonomic postganglionic efferent and nociceptive afferent C fibers, contain many axons encased in a single Schwann cell sheath. Most large motor and sensory fibers are enclosed in many layers of myelin, which consists of plasma membranes of specialized Schwann cells that wrap themselves around the axon during axonal outgrowth. Myelin greatly increases the speed of nerve conduction by insulating the axolemma from the surrounding conducting salt medium and forcing the action current to flow through the axoplasm to the nodes of Ranvier, which are periodic interruptions in the myelin sheath where action currents are regenerated (Fig. 14-3). The Na^+ channels that serve impulse generation and propagation are highly concentrated at the nodes of Ranvier of myelinated fibers,[7] but they are distributed all along the axon of nonmyelinated fibers (Fig. 14-3). A classification of peripheral nerves according to fiber size and physiologic properties is presented in Table 14-3.

A typical peripheral nerve consists of several axon bundles, or fascicles. Each fiber has its own connective tissue covering, the endoneurium. Each fascicle of axons is encased by a second connective tissue layer, the epithelial-like perineurium, and the entire nerve is wrapped in a loose outer sheath called the epineurium (Fig. 14-4). To reach its site of action (the nerve axon), a local anesthetic molecule must traverse four or five layers of connective tissue or lipid membranous barriers, or both.

Structure of the Axonal Membrane

Biologic membranes consist of a molecular lipid bilayer containing proteins adsorbed on the surface, as well as embedded in or spanning the hydrocarbon core (Fig. 14-5). The bilayer character is imposed by the amphiphilic phospholipids, which have long hydrophobic fatty acyl tails that lie in the center of the membrane, and polar hydrophilic head groups composed of zwitterionic

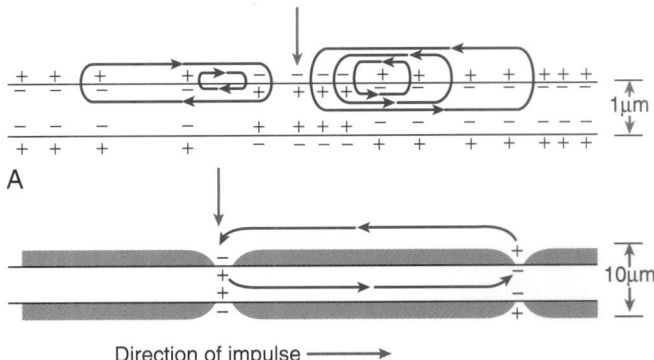

Figure 14-3 Pattern of "local circuit currents" flowing during impulse propagation in a nonmyelinated C fiber's axon (**A**) and a myelinated axon (**B**). During propagation of impulses, from left to right, current entering the axon at the initial rising phase of the impulse (gray downpointing arrows) passes through the axoplasm (local circuit current, red loops) and depolarizes the adjacent membrane. Plus and minus signs adjacent to the axon membrane indicate the polarization state of the axon membrane: negative inside at rest, positive inside during active depolarization under the action potential, and less negative in the regions where local circuit currents flow. This ionic current passes relatively uniformly across a nonmyelinated axon, but in a myelinated axon it is restricted to entry at the nodes of Ranvier, several of which are simultaneously depolarized during a single action potential.

Table 14–3   Classification of peripheral nerves according to anatomy, physiology, and function

Fiber Class	Subclass	Myelin	Diameter (μm)	Conduction Velocity (m/sec)	Location	Function	Susceptibility to Local Anesthetic Block
A	α	+	6-22	30-120	Efferent to muscles	Motor	++
	β	+	6-22	30-120	Afferent from skin and joints	Tactile, proprioception	++
	γ	+	3-6	15-35	Efferent to muscle spindles	Muscle tone	++++
	δ	+	1-4	5-25	Afferent sensory nerves	Pain, cold temperature, touch	+++
B		+	<3	3-15	Preganglionic sympathetic	Various autonomic functions	++
C	sC	−	0.3-1.3	0.7-1.3	Postganglionic sympathetic	Various autonomic functions	++
	dγC	−	0.4-1.2	0.1-2.0	Afferent sensory nerves	Various autonomic functions; pain, warm temperature, touch	+

Modified from Bonica JJ: Principles and Practice of Obstetric Anesthesia and Analgesia. Philadelphia, FA Davis, 1967.

(containing positive and negative charges) components that project into the cytoplasm or extracellular fluid. Within the membrane, both lateral and rotational diffusion occurs, which allows lipids and certain proteins to migrate in a fluid mosaic, but most membrane proteins are fixed within specific regions of a membrane, anchored by connections to specific proteins of the cell's cytoskeleton.[7]

A dynamic interaction exists between the cell's membrane and cytoplasm. Although we focus here on the channel-blocking actions of local anesthetics, it is noteworthy that many other cellular activities, including both metabolic and signal transduction pathways, are inhibited by these drugs.

Physiology of Nerve Conduction

The neural membrane is able to maintain a voltage difference of 60 to 90 mV between its inner and outer aspects because at rest it is relatively impermeable to sodium ions but selectively permeable to potassium ions. An active, energy-dependent mechanism, the Na⁺/K⁺ pump, sustains the ion gradients that drive this potential difference by constant extrusion of sodium from within the cell in exchange for a net uptake of potassium by using adenosine triphosphate as an energy source. Although the membrane is relatively permeable to potassium ions, an intracellular-to-extracellular potassium ratio of 150 to 5 mM, or 30:1, is maintained because of both the membranes'

Figure 14–4 Transverse sections of a peripheral nerve (**A**) showing the outermost epineurium; the inner perineurium, which collects nerve axons in fascicles; and the endoneurium, which surrounds each myelinated fiber. Each myelinated axon (**B**) is encased in the multiple membranous wrappings of myelin formed by one Schwann cell, each of which stretches longitudinally over approximately 100 times the diameter of the axon. The narrow span of axon between these myelinated segments, the node of Ranvier, contains the ion channels that support action potentials. Nonmyelinated fibers (**C**) are enclosed in bundles of 5 to 10 axons by a chain of Schwann cells that tightly embrace each axon with but one layer of membrane.

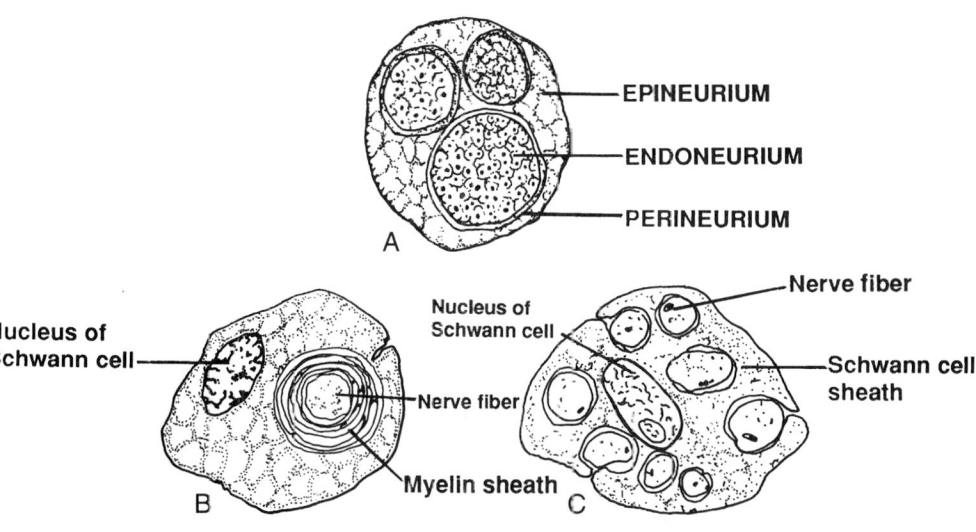

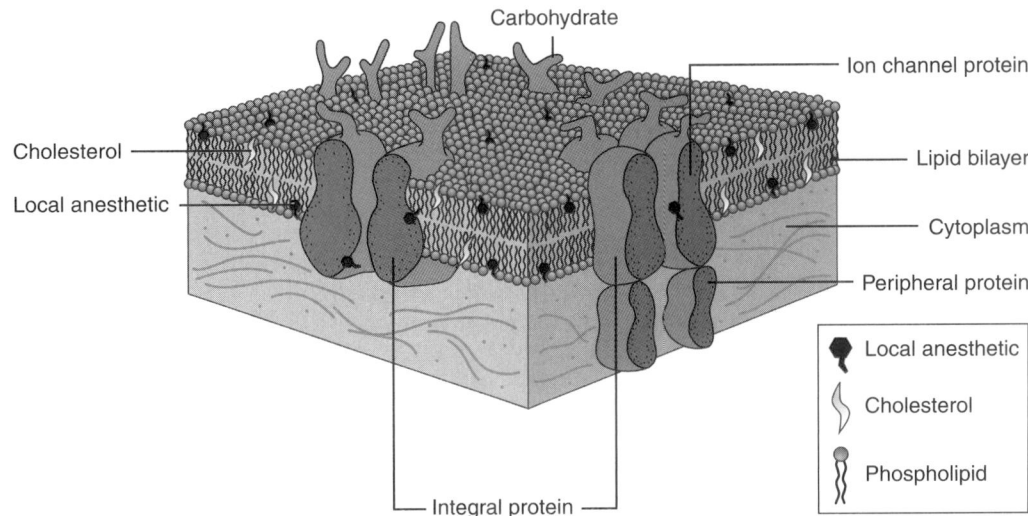

Figure 14–5 A typical plasma membrane has at its core the lipid bilayer, which is composed of phospholipids and cholesterol molecules (in about a 5:1 ratio) embedding the membrane integral proteins. These proteins are most often glycosylated by extracellular carbohydrates and include receptors and ion channels essential for intercellular communication. "Peripheral proteins" regulate the functions of membrane proteins, chaperone them to the plasma membrane, and stabilize them in the cell through interactions with both the cytoskeleton and the extracellular matrix. Probable membrane locations and protein sites for local anesthetics are also shown.

impermeability to other, potentially cotransported ions and the active removal of extracellular potassium.

The nerve at rest behaves largely as a "potassium electrode," according to the Nernst equation:

$$E_m \approx E_K = \left(\frac{-RT}{F} \right) \ln \left(\frac{[K^+]_i}{[K^+]_o} \right) \qquad (2)$$

where E_m is the membrane potential, E_K is the potassium equilibrium potential, R is the gas constant, T is temperature (Kelvin), F is Faraday's constant, and $[K^+]$ is the potassium ion concentration inside (i) and outside (o) the cell. For potassium, therefore,

$$E_K = -58 \log 30, \text{ or } -85.7 \text{ mV}$$

An opposite situation exists for Na^+, which is at higher concentration outside the cell and has a Nernst potential, E_{Na}, of about +60 mV. During an action potential the nerve membrane transiently switches its permeability from K^+ selective to Na^+ selective, thus changing the membrane potential from negative to positive, and back again.[8] The progress of this potential change and the underlying events are graphed in Figure 14-6. They provide a basis for understanding local anesthetic conduction block.

Ion permeation through membranes occurs by means of special proteins called ion channels.[9] The conformation of these channels is often sensitive to the membrane potential; both Na^+ and K^+ channels in nerve membranes are activated to an open conformation by membrane depolarization. Sodium channels, in addition, close to an inactivated conformation after their initial activation. A small membrane depolarization, one that extends along an axon from a region of excited membrane, for example, will begin to open both Na^+ and K^+ channels. The Na^+ channels open faster, however, and because the membrane potential is initially much further

from the Nernst potential for Na^+ than for K^+, the inwardly directed Na^+ current is larger (Fig. 14-6). Sodium ions thus entering the nerve depolarize it further, which leads to the opening of more Na^+ channels and thereby increases the current even further (Fig. 14-7). This sequence of events continues in the positive feedback of the depolarizing phase until some of the Na^+ channels have become inactivated and enough of the potassium channels have opened to change the balance of current and result in a net outward current that produces membrane repolarization (Fig. 14-7). After one action potential, the concentrations of Na^+ and K^+ have changed very little. The very small amount of Na^+ entering and K^+ leaving the cell as a result of this process is restored by the Na^+/K^+ pump.[10]

Depolarizations too weak to activate enough Na^+ channels to produce a net inward current are below the membrane's excitability threshold. The precise value of the threshold varies among different regions of the cell and also changes with activity. Directly after an impulse, when some Na^+ channels are still inactivated and some K^+ channels are still activated, the threshold is above its resting value and the membrane is "refractory" to stimulation. In the immediately repolarized membrane, as Na^+ inactivation decays and K^+ channels return to their closed conformation, the original threshold value is progressively restored.

The impulse is a wave of depolarization that is propagated along the axon by continuous coupling between excited and nonexcited regions of the membrane. Ionic current (the action current) entering the axon in the excited, depolarized region flows down the axoplasm and exits through the surrounding membrane, thus passively depolarizing the adjacent region (see Fig. 14-3). Although this local circuit current spreads away from the excited zone in both directions, the region behind the impulse, having just been depolarized, is absolutely refractory, and impulse propagation is thus unidirectional.

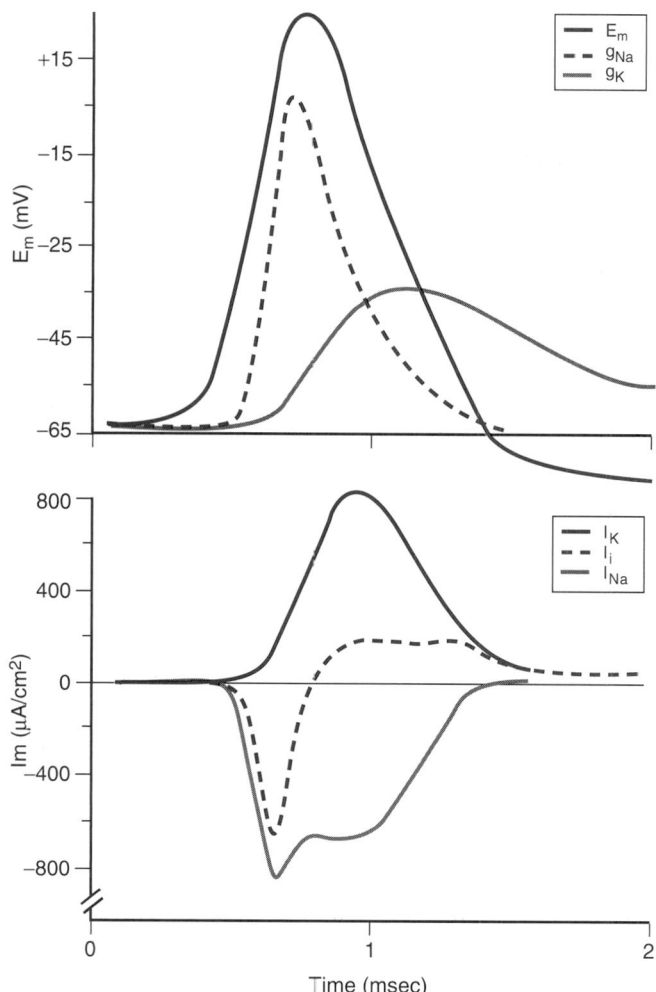

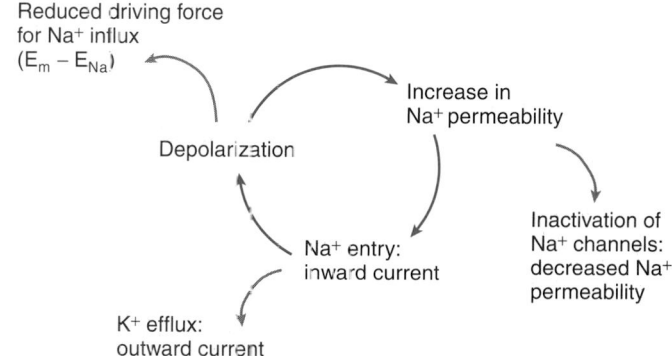

Figure 14–7 The action potential can be understood in terms of the cyclic relationships between factors contributing to the regenerative, depolarizing phase and the passive repolarizing phase. Positive factors *(red arrows)* increase the rate of depolarization in a "positive-feedback loop," with each element in the cycle favoring the subsequent one. Negative factors *(gray arrows)* decrease the depolarization rate by reducing or opposing the related positive factor, with K^+ efflux eventually dominating the ionic flow and repolarizing the membrane.

Figure 14–6 The membrane potential (E_m) and the voltage-gated ionic conductance of sodium (g_{Na}) and potassium (g_K) that determine the corresponding membrane currents (I_{Na} and I_K) during a propagated action potential. Modeled from the original studies of Hodgkin and Huxley on the squid giant axon (see Hodgkin[8]), these relationships hold for almost all invertebrate and vertebrate nerve fibers. The direction of the total ionic current (I_i), which is the sum of I_{Na} and I_K, is inward (negative values) for the depolarizing phase of the action potential and outward (positive values) for the repolarizing phase.

The local circuit current spreads rapidly along a length of insulated internode in a myelinated axon (Fig. 14-3), and many nodes of Ranvier in sequence are depolarized to threshold with little intervening delay. Single impulses do not jump from node to node as separate, discrete events, but instead, active depolarization occurs simultaneously along several centimeters of the largest axons[11] (see Fig. 14-10). Indeed, the local circuit current is so robust that it can skip past two completely nonexcitable nodes and successfully stimulate a third.[12] If nodal excitability is partially reduced, for example, by inhibition of some of the Na^+ channels, the amplitude of impulses in successive nodes falls decrementally, a process that can continue for many centimeters.[13] This situation probably occurs during certain phases of local anesthesia, as discussed later. However, when enough of the Na^+ channels are blocked, the

local circuit current fails to bring the adjacent resting region to threshold, and the impulse is extinguished.

MECHANISM OF ACTION OF LOCAL ANESTHETICS (PHARMACODYNAMICS)

Active Form

Local anesthetic bases are poorly to sparingly soluble in water but are soluble in relatively hydrophobic organic solvents. Therefore, as a matter of convenience, most of these drugs are marketed as the hydrochloride salts. The pK_a of the drug and tissue pH determine the amount of drug that exists in solution as free base or as positively charged cation when injected into living tissue (see earlier). Furthermore, uptake of the drug by the tissue, largely as a result of lipophilic adsorption, will also alter its activity, both by shifting the effective pK_a downward and thereby favoring the neutral base form and by limiting diffusion of the anesthetic away from the site of injection. Moderately hydrophobic local anesthetics will act more rapidly than either hydrophilic or highly hydrophobic ones when delivered at the same concentration for the following reasons. Moderately hydrophilic local anesthetics, such as lidocaine, are less bound to tissues than very hydrophobic drugs (e.g., tetracaine), but are still more membrane permeant than very hydrophilic ones (e.g., chloroprocaine). Highly hydrophobic local anesthetics also have higher intrinsic potencies (see Table 14-2); therefore, they are used in lower concentrations, and their rate of onset is correspondingly reduced.

Which form of the local anesthetic, charged cation or neutral base, is actually responsible for impulse blockade? More alkaline solutions of local anesthetics more effectively block nerve conduction.[14] In a desheathed nerve and in an isolated single axon, the rate of inhibition by tertiary amine anesthetics is greater at alkaline than at neutral external pH[15,16] because membrane penetration and transport, highly favored by base over cation species, are essential for controlling the rate of access to the binding site. Direct control of axoplasmic pH[17] (or internal perfusion with permanently charged quaternary amine homologs) shows that the dominant potency is derived from the cationic species acting from the cytoplasmic surface.[18,19] The uncharged base also has intrinsic pharmacologic activity, however, and in addition to molecules with tertiary amine moieties, those having hydroxyl (alcohols) or alkyl groups (e.g., benzocaine) can also inhibit Na^+ channels and block impulses.[16,20-22]

To obtain a clear picture of the fundamental blocking mechanism, knowledge of the channel-binding kinetics of the drug is necessary, but it is almost impossible to measure the rate of binding of local anesthetics to the receptor after their addition to a bathing solution. Drug diffusion through the unstirred layer of solution next to the membrane and through the membrane itself present steps that limit the rate of access to the receptor site.[16,23] However, once the drug has equilibrated with membranes and solutions, it is possible to perturb the channels by depolarizing the membrane and follow the "phasic" inhibition by local anesthetics to clarify the details of the binding reaction, as described later.

The Electrophysiologic Effect of Local Anesthetics

The resting membrane potential of a nerve is little affected by local anesthetics.[24] As the concentration of local anesthetic applied to a nerve is raised, a decrease in the rate and degree of impulse-associated depolarization is produced until the impulse is abolished. It is not possible, however, to derive direct data on the binding of local anesthetics to Na^+ channels from measurement of the changes in nerve impulses.

By using a "voltage-clamp" procedure, Na^+ currents and their inhibition by local anesthetics can be directly assayed (Fig. 14-8A). When the membrane of isolated neurons is rapidly depolarized to a constant value, the time course of ionic currents is observed. Sodium currents during one initial depolarization are reduced by subclinical doses of local anesthetic (e.g., 0.2 mM lidocaine) and totally abolished by clinical doses (e.g., 1% lidocaine, which equals about 40 mM). If the test depolarization is repeatedly applied, for example, at frequencies above 5 Hz (5 pulses per second), the partially depressed (tonically inhibited) Na^+ current is further reduced, incrementally for each pulse, until a new steady-state level of inhibition is reached.[19,24] This frequency-dependent inhibition, also called phasic inhibition, is reversed when stimulation is slowed or stopped and currents return to the level of tonic inhibition observed in the resting nerve. Paralleling the phasic inhibition of Na^+ currents in voltage-clamped membranes is a "use-dependent" blockade of action potentials during normal physiologic function (Fig. 14-8B). The ability of local anesthetics to produce both tonic and phasic inhibition is similarly dependent on their structure, hydrophobicity, and pK_a.[24,25] At its simplest, there appears to be a single binding site for local anesthetics on the Na^+ channel, with

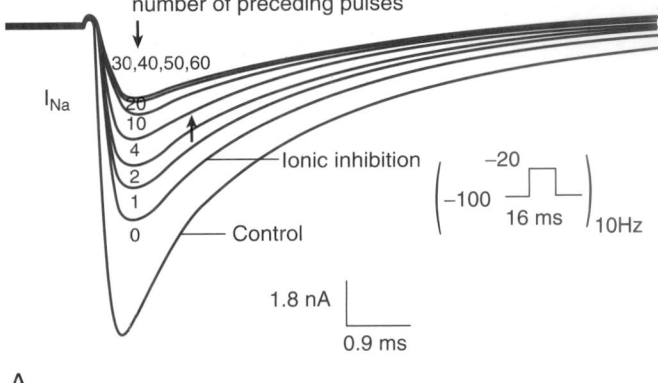

0.2mM Lidocaine

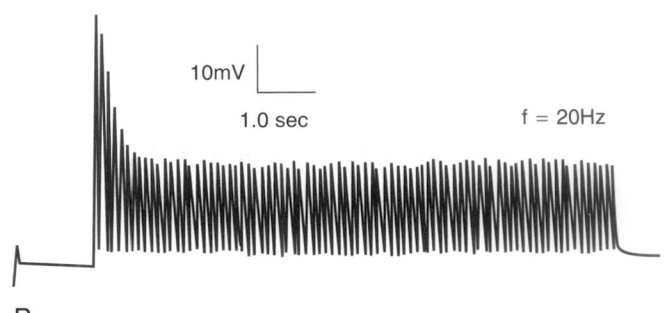

0.8mM Lidocaine

Figure 14–8 "Use-dependent" actions of local anesthetics on excitable membrane properties. **A,** Ionic Na^+ currents measured by voltage clamp are transiently activated by brief steps of depolarization applied infrequently ("tonic" test) or in a train at 10 times per second ("phasic" test, see E_m pattern in parentheses). After equilibration with 0.2 mM (0.005%) lidocaine, the currents measured tonically are reduced by about 30% from control currents. Application of the "phasic" train of depolarizations results in a dynamic reduction in currents after each depolarization, with a steady-state value of phasic inhibition reached during the train in 75% of control currents. Recovery of currents to the tonic value occurs within a few seconds when phasic testing stops (not shown). **B,** Action potentials are also inhibited in a phasic manner by local anesthetics. After equilibration with 0.8 mM lidocaine (0.02%), the action potential is tonically reduced by about 20% from its amplitude in drug-free solution (not shown). Stimulation by a train at 20 stimuli per second induces phasic inhibition, which further reduces the amplitude to about 30% of the control value. As with ionic currents (**A**), phasic inhibition of the action potential recovers rapidly when high-frequency stimulation stops.

a "tonic" affinity at rest and increased "phasic" affinity occurring as a result of depolarization. The phasic blocking mode can thus be used to reveal the true kinetics of local anesthetic binding to the functional receptor, the Na^+ channel itself.

Phasic actions are a manifestation of the selective affinity of local anesthetics for conformations of the Na^+ channel that occur during depolarization. Both "open" and "inactivated" states of the channel bind local anesthetics more avidly than the resting state does. Repeated depolarizations thus increase the fraction of drug-bound channels; dissociation of these bound drug molecules is usually a slower process than the normal recovery from inactivation (see earlier), which results in the use-dependent accumulation of channels in the blocked condition and the phenomenon of phasic block.

By its selective binding to a channel state, the local anesthetic stabilizes that state. During phasic block, therefore, more inactivated channels become drug bound, and reciprocally, less activation can occur. This relationship between state-dependent affinities and modification of transitions among states through drug binding is known as the "modulated receptor" model. Thus, overall binding of anesthetic is increased by membrane depolarization for two reasons: more binding sites become accessible during activation (the "guarded receptor" model), and drug dissociation from inactivated channels is slower than from resting channels (the modulated receptor model).

The specific binding rates and affinities for the different conformations of the sodium channel depend on the particular local anesthetic drug. When the details of this dependence are correlated with the physicochemical properties of the drug and with the experimental conditions, they provide insight into the molecular features of the local anesthetic binding site.

The Nature of the Local Anesthetic Binding Site

Mutation of specific amino acids of the Na^+ channel has allowed definition of the regions that interact with local anesthetics. The major functional protein of the Na^+ channel (the α-subunit) is composed of four homologous "domains" (DI to DIV), each of which contains six helical regions (S1 to S6) that span the core of the membrane (Fig. 14-9A). Each domain also has a loop, termed the "P region," that links the extracellular ends of its S5 and S6 segments; P regions extend inward between the transmembrane regions such that when the α-subunit folds together, each P loop contributes a quarter of the cylindrical, ion "selectivity pore," the narrowest passage of an open channel (Fig. 14-9B). Voltage sensitivity is derived from the positively charged S4 segments, which slide or swing "outward" in response to membrane depolarization. By linkages still unknown, this movement of S4 results in a rearrangement of the S6 segments to form the inner, cytoplasmic entry to the channel. Closed to open channel gating results from S6's movements, whereas inactivation gating appears to result from binding of the cytoplasmic loop between D-3 and D-4 to the cytoplasmic opening.

Local anesthetics bind in the "inner vestibule" of the Na^+ channel (Fig. 14-9C). Mutations of amino acids in the S6 segments of D-1, D-3, and D-4 all modify local anesthetic action, thus suggesting that these regions can form a pharmacophere small enough to simultaneously contact the drug or that the local anesthetic molecule rapidly moves among these three segments. Mutation of loci on the Na^+ channel closer to the external opening also modify local anesthetic blockade, consistent with the ability of extracellular Na^+ ions to antagonize blockade by these drugs and the ability of extracellular H^+ to protonate them and thus prolong and potentiate the drug-bound states.

The blocking rate constant for local anesthetics is higher for the more hydrophobic molecules, which suggests that drug molecules can reach the binding site (and depart from it) through a "hydrophobic" pathway. This pathway could be from the membrane phase laterally, into the channel, or through hydrophobic amino acid residues that limit access through the closed pore pathway. The slow blockade of closed and inactivated channels appears to use such a hydrophobic access, thus accounting for tonic inhibition.

In brief, hydrophobicity delivers the drug to the receptor, and charge keeps it there.

Neurophysiologic Aspects of Phasic Inhibition

Different fiber types in the nerve are affected differently during local anesthesia. At least part of this difference arises from pharmacokinetic factors. At the onset and during recovery from clinical block, in particular, longitudinal and radial diffusion of drug will produce concentration variations within and along the nerve. This variation is superimposed on the dynamic use-dependent inhibition to provide variable propagation that depends on a fiber's geometry, position within the nerve, and functional as well as electrophysiologic properties.

Different fiber types are also differentially sensitive to local anesthetic blockade. In vivo experiments involving equilibration of local anesthetics by continuous superfusion of peripheral nerves, as well as experiments using percutaneous bolus injection analogous to clinical peripheral nerve block, show unequivocally that small myelinated axons (Aγ motor and Aδ sensory fibers) are the most susceptible to impulse annihilation. Next in order of block are the large myelinated (Aα and Aβ) fibers, and the least susceptible are the small, nonmyelinated C fibers. In fact, among this last group, impulses in the slowest conducting population (conduction velocity = 0.5 to 0.8 $msec^{-1}$) are the most resistant to local anesthetic.[26] The generalized notion "that local anesthetics block the smallest fibers first or most" is clearly wrong.

Selective Susceptibility of Na^+ Channel Isoforms

Ten different Na^+ channels have been physiologically identified and biochemically sequenced. At least four of them are found in peripheral neurons, some exclusively associated with nociceptive afferents. Obviously, it would be clinically advantageous to selectively inhibit these channels and thus prevent or reduce pain while sparing other functions. Unfortunately, as of this writing (2003), no such selective compounds have been reported, either because the local anesthetic pharmacophore is too similar among the different channel isoforms or because the same drug features that favor inhibition of "therapeutic" target channels also result in blockade of "toxic" target channels (e.g. cardiac Na^+ channels).

On the other hand, the aberrant impulses that are often considered the hallmark of various diseases of excitable membranes, such as abnormal repetitive firing in neuropathic pain from sites of peripheral nerve injury, are unusually susceptible and are abolished by systemic lidocaine doses that do not block normal propagating impulses. The conditions for such sensitivity to these local anesthetics (i.e., lidocaine) appear to result from the

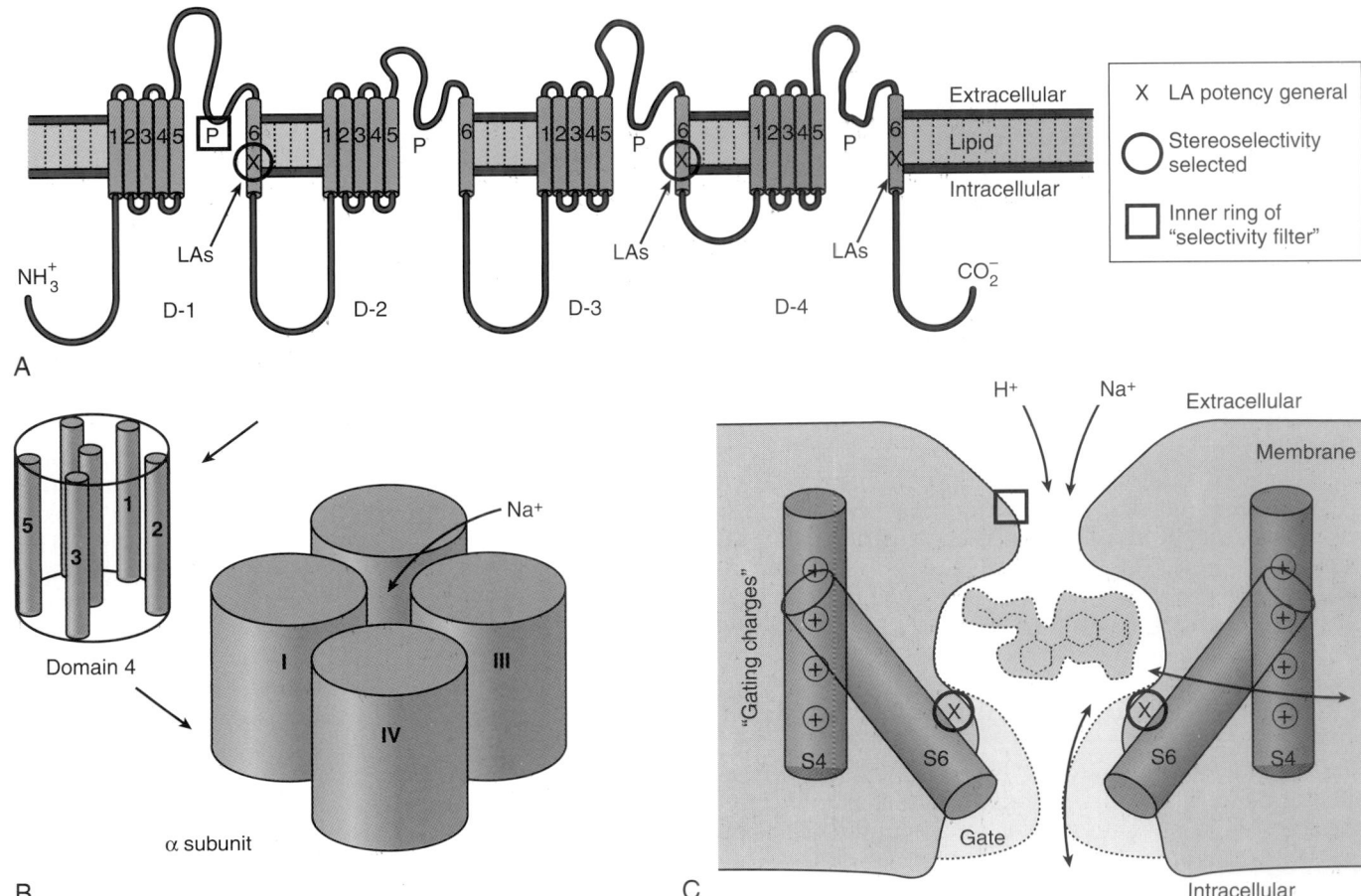

A

B

C

Figure 14–9 Structural features of the Na+ channel that determine local anesthetic (LA) interactions. **A,** Consensus arrangement of the single peptide of the Na+ channel α-subunit in a plasma membrane. Four domains with homologous sequences (D-1 through D-4) each contain six α-helical segments that span the membrane (S1 to S6). Each domain folds within itself to form one cylindrical bundle of segments, and these bundles converge to form the functional channel's quaternary structure (**B**). Activation gating that leads to channel opening results from primary movement of the positively charged S4 segments in response to membrane depolarization (see panel **C**). Fast inactivation of the channel follows binding to the cytoplasmic end of the channel of part of the small loop that connects D-3 to D-4. Ions travel through an open channel along a pore defined at its narrowest dimension by the P region formed by partial membrane penetration of the four extracellular loops of protein connecting S5 and S6 in each domain. Intentional, directed mutations of different amino acids on the channel indicate residues that are involved in LA binding in the inner vestibule of the channel (X, on S6 segments) and at the interior regions of the ion-discriminating "selectivity filter (⊏, square, on the P region), and they are also known to influence stereoselectivity for phasic inhibition (O, also on S6 segments). **C,** Schematic cross section of the channel speculating on the manner in which S6 segments, which form a "gate," may realign during activation to open the channel and allow entry and departure of a bupivacaine molecule by the "hydrophilic" pathway. The closed (inactivated) channel has a more intimate association with the LA molecule, whose favored pathway for dissociation is no longer between S6 segments (the former pore), but now, much more slowly, laterally between segments and then through the membrane, the "hydrophobic" pathway. Na+ ions entering the pore will compete with the LA for a site in the channel, and H+ ions, which pass very slowly through the pore, can enter and leave from the extracellular opening, thereby protonating and deprotonating a bound LA molecule and thus regulating its rate of dissociation from the channel.

patterns of impulses and membrane depolarizations caused by abnormal expression of Na+ channels rather than from selective sensitivity of certain subtypes of channels (Fig. 14-10).

Summary of Local Anesthetic Mechanisms

Impulse blockade by local anesthetics may be summarized by the following chronology[4]:

1. Solutions of local anesthetic are deposited near the nerve. Diffusion of drug molecules away from this locus is a function of tissue binding, removal by the circulation, and local hydrolysis of aminoester anesthetics.

The net result is penetration of the nerve sheath by the remaining drug molecules.

2. Local anesthetic molecules then permeate the nerve's axon membranes and reside there and in the axoplasm. The speed and extent of these processes depend on a particular drug's pK_a and the lipophilicity of its base and cation species.

3. Binding of local anesthetic to sites on voltage-gated Na+ channels prevents opening of the channels by inhibiting the conformational changes that underlie channel activation. Local anesthetics bind in the channel's pore and also occlude the path of Na+ ions.

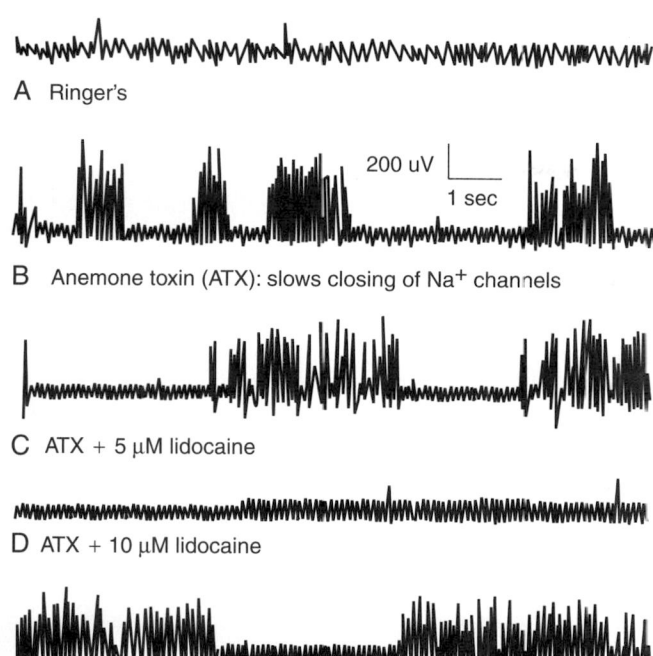

A Ringer's

200 uV

1 sec

B Anemone toxin (ATX): slows closing of Na$^+$ channels

C ATX + 5 μM lidocaine

D ATX + 10 μM lidocaine

↑

E ATX + Ringer's after lidocaine washout

Figure 14–10 Spontaneous ectopic impulses in "abnormal" nerves are blocked by very low concentrations of local anesthetics. When 10% to 20% of the Na$^+$ channels close very slowly, as caused here by the addition of a peptide neurotoxin (ATX), but otherwise an intrinsic property of channels that are upregulated after nerve injury, spontaneous impulses appear (trace B). Occurring as bursts of action potentials separated by quiet periods, these impulses appear similar to the ectopic discharges in a peripheral nerve after injury. Very low concentrations of lidocaine, equal to plasma levels during intravenous infusions that can reverse neuropathic pain, strongly suppress (C) and eventually abolish (D) these spontaneous discharges, an effect that is reversed when lidocaine is removed from the nerve (E). In contrast, electrically stimulated action potentials are unaffected by such low lidocaine concentrations (e.g., see Fig 14-8B). (From Persaud N, Strichartz G: Micromolar lidocaine selectively blocks propagating ectopic impulses at a distance from their site of origin. Pain 99:333-340, 2002.)

4. During onset and recovery from local anesthesia, impulse blockade is incomplete, and partially blocked fibers are further inhibited by repetitive stimulation, which produces an additional, use-dependent binding to Na$^+$ channels.

5. One local anesthetic binding site on the Na$^+$ channel may be sufficient to account for the drug's resting (tonic) and use-dependent (phasic) actions. Access to this site may potentially involve multiple pathways, but for clinical local anesthetics, the primary route is the hydrophobic approach from within the axon membrane.

6. The clinically observed rates of onset and recovery from blockade are governed by the relatively slow diffusion of local anesthetic molecules into and out of the whole nerve, not by their much faster binding and dissociation to ion channels.

A clinically effective block that may last for hours can be achieved with local anesthetic drugs that dissociate from Na$^+$ channels in a few seconds.

CLINICAL PHARMACOLOGY

The successful use of regional anesthesia requires knowledge of the pharmacologic properties of the various local anesthetics, as well as technical skill in performance of the nerve block. Local anesthetic requirements vary considerably and depend on factors such as the type of block, the surgical procedure, and the physiologic status of the patient.

Commonly used aminoester local anesthetics include procaine, chloroprocaine, tetracaine, and cocaine. Commonly used aminoamides include lidocaine, mepivacaine, prilocaine, bupivacaine (racemic and its levo enantiomer), ropivacaine, and etidocaine. The ester and amide local anesthetics differ in their chemical stability, locus of biotransformation, and allergic potential. Amides are extremely stable, whereas esters are relatively unstable in solution. The aminoesters are hydrolyzed in plasma by cholinesterase enzymes, whereas the amide compounds undergo enzymatic degradation in the liver. Two exceptions to this trend include cocaine, an ester that is metabolized predominantly by hepatic carboxylesterase, and articaine, an amide local anesthetic widely used in dentistry that is inactivated by plasma carboxyesterase-induced cleavage of a methyl ester on the aromatic ring.

p-Aminobenzoic acid is one of the metabolites of ester-type compounds that can induce allergic-type reactions in a small percentage of patients. The aminoamides are not metabolized to *p*-aminobenzoic acid, and reports of allergic reactions to these agents are extremely rare.

General Considerations

The clinically important properties of the various local anesthetics include potency, speed of onset, duration of anesthetic action, and differential sensory/motor blockade. As previously indicated, the profile of the individual drugs is determined by their physicochemical characteristics (Table 14-2).

Anesthetic Potency

Hydrophobicity appears to be a primary determinant of intrinsic anesthetic potency[5,28-30] because the anesthetic molecule must penetrate the nerve membrane and bind at a partially hydrophobic site on the Na$^+$ channel. Clinically, however, the correlation between hydrophobicity and anesthetic potency is not as precise as in an isolated nerve. For example, etidocaine is more potent than bupivacaine in an isolated nerve, but it is actually less potent than bupivacaine in vivo.[31-33] Differences between in vitro and in vivo potency may be related to a number of factors, including local anesthetic charge and hydrophobicity (which influence partitioning into and transverse diffusion across biologic membranes) and vasodilator or vasoconstrictor properties (which influence the initial rate of vascular uptake from injection sites into the central circulation).

Onset of Action

The onset of conduction block in isolated nerves is related to the physicochemical properties of the individual drugs. In vivo latency is also dependent on the dose or concentration of local anesthetic used. For example, 0.25% bupivacaine possesses a rather slow onset of action, but increasing the concentration to 0.75% results in a significant acceleration of anesthetic effect.[33] Chloroprocaine demonstrates a rapid onset of action in humans despite the fact that its pK_a is approximately 9; its proportion of charged molecules is high (97%), and thus its onset of action in isolated nerves is relatively slow.[34] However, the low systemic toxicity of this drug allows its use in high concentrations (e.g., 3%). Therefore, the rapid onset of chloroprocaine in vivo may be related simply to mass diffusion as a result of the large number of molecules placed in the vicinity of peripheral nerves. In humans, 1.5% lidocaine produces a more rapid onset of epidural anesthesia than 1.5% chloroprocaine does[35]; however, 3% chloroprocaine results in more rapid onset than 2% lidocaine does.

Duration of Action

The duration of action of the various local anesthetics differs markedly. Procaine and chloroprocaine have a short duration of action. Lidocaine, mepivacaine, and prilocaine produce a moderate duration of anesthesia, whereas tetracaine, bupivacaine, and etidocaine have the longest durations. For example, with procaine the duration of brachial plexus blockade is 30 to 60 minutes, whereas up to approximately 10 hours of anesthesia has been reported for brachial plexus blockade induced by bupivacaine or etidocaine.[36]

In humans, the duration of anesthesia is markedly influenced by the peripheral vascular effects of the local anesthetic. Many local anesthetics have a biphasic effect on vascular smooth muscle: at low concentrations they tend to cause vasoconstriction, whereas at larger, clinically administered concentrations, they cause vasodilation.[37,38] However, differences exist in the degree of vasodilator activity of the various drugs. For example, lidocaine is a more potent vasodilator than mepivacaine or prilocaine. Although little difference in the rate of recovery from conduction block is apparent between these agents in an isolated nerve, in vivo, the anesthesia produced by lidocaine is of shorter duration than that produced by mepivacaine or prilocaine. In the spinal cord, the pial vessels are dilated by bupivacaine but constricted by ropivacaine, thus suggesting a stereoselective effect on vascular tone independent of nerve block per se.[39]

Effects of local anesthetics on vascular tone and regional blood flow are complex and vary according to concentration, time, and the particular vascular bed near the site of application, among other factors. As a practical example, the topical local anesthetic formulation EMLA (eutectic mixture of the local anesthetics lidocaine and prilocaine) vasoconstricts cutaneous vessels initially and throughout most of the first hour of application, but vasodilation is observed after 2 or more hours of application.

Differential Sensory/Motor Blockade

Another important clinical consideration is the ability of local anesthetics to cause differential inhibition of sensory and motor activity. Bupivacaine became popular in the 1980s for epidural blockade because it was better than previously available drugs in producing adequate antinociception without profound inhibition of motor activity, particularly when dilute solutions are used. Bupivacaine and etidocaine provide an interesting contrast in their differential sensory- and motor-blocking activity, although they are both potent, long-acting anesthetics.[40] Bupivacaine is widely used epidurally for obstetric analgesia and postoperative pain management because it can provide acceptable analgesia with only mild muscle weakness, particularly when used for infusions in concentrations of 0.125% or less (also see Chapters 43-45 and 58). When given by epidural bolus dosing, bupivacaine produces more effective sensory than motor blockade over a concentration range from 0.25% to 0.75%, whereas etidocaine produces almost equal effective sensory and motor blockade over this concentration range.

Traditional texts often state that small-diameter axons, such as C fibers, are more susceptible to local anesthetic blockade than larger-diameter fibers are. However, when careful measurements are made of single-impulse annihilation in individual nerve fibers, exactly the opposite differential susceptibility is seen (see earlier).[41,42] Repetitive stimulation, such as occurs during propagation of trains of impulses, produces a further, phasic inhibition of excitability, but it is unclear how this inhibition will effect a functionally selective failure of impulses. The length of drug-exposed nerve in the intrathecal space, imposed by anatomic restrictions, can perhaps explain clinically documented differential spinal or epidural blockade[43] because longer drug-exposed regions yield block by lower concentrations of local anesthetic.[44] However, this reasoning does not explain the functionally differential loss from peripheral nerve block. Other factors may include actual spread of the drug along the nerve[45] or its selective ability to inhibit Na^+ channels over K^+ channels,[46] which in itself can produce a differential block because these channels are present in very different proportions in different types of nerves.[47] Because of these confounding factors, clinicians should be discouraged from making conclusions about fiber-type involvement in chronic pain syndromes based on the dose or concentration needed for pain relief in diagnostic nerve blockade.[48]

Factors Influencing Anesthetic Activity in Humans

Dosage of Local Anesthetic

As the dosage of local anesthetic is increased, the probability and duration of satisfactory anesthesia increase and the time to onset of blockade is shortened. The dosage of local anesthetic can be increased by administering either a larger volume or a more concentrated solution. For example, increasing the concentration of epidurally administered bupivacaine from 0.125% to 0.5% while maintaining the same volume of injectate (10 mL) results in shorter latency, an improved incidence of satisfactory analgesia, and a longer duration of sensory analgesia.[49] The volume of anesthetic solution per se probably influences the spread of anesthesia. For example, 30 mL of 1% lidocaine administered into the epidural space produces a level of anesthesia that is 4.3 dermatomes higher than that achieved when 10 mL of 3% lidocaine is given.[50]

Addition of Vasoconstrictors

Vasoconstrictors, usually epinephrine (5 µg/mL or 1:200,000), are frequently included in local anesthetic solutions to decrease the rate of vascular absorption, thereby allowing more anesthetic molecules to reach the nerve membrane and thus improving the depth and duration of anesthesia, as well as providing a marker for inadvertent intravascular injection.[51] Epinephrine in a concentration of 1:200,000 has been reported to provide the optimal degree of vasoconstriction when used with lidocaine for epidural or intercostal application.[45] Other vasoconstrictors such as norepinephrine and phenylephrine have been used but do not appear to be superior to epinephrine. For example, equipotent concentrations, for vasoconstriction, of epinephrine and phenylephrine prolong the duration of spinal anesthesia produced by tetracaine to a similar extent.[52]

The extent to which epinephrine prolongs the duration of anesthesia depends on the specific local anesthetic used and the site of injection. Epinephrine will significantly extend the duration of both infiltration anesthesia and peripheral nerve blocks with shorter-duration drugs (e.g., lidocaine).[53,54] Epinephrine does not markedly prolong the duration of motor blockade by epidural bupivacaine or etidocaine; however, it does modestly extend sensory blockade by these epidural drugs.[40] The depth and duration of epidural analgesia in obstetric patients were improved slightly when epinephrine 1:300,000 was added to 0.25% bupivacaine.[55] α-Adrenergic receptors in the spinal cord are known to activate endogenous analgesic mechanisms,[56] and the increased depth of analgesic action produced by epinephrine and the α_2-agonist clonidine with both epidural and intrathecal local anesthetics may arise both from this pharmacodynamic mechanism and from the pharmacokinetic (vasoconstrictive) action.

Site of Injection

The most rapid onset but the shortest duration of action occurs after intrathecal or subcutaneous administration of local anesthetics. The longest latencies and durations are observed after brachial plexus blocks. For example, intrathecal bupivacaine will usually produce anesthesia within 5 minutes that will persist for 3 to 4 hours. However, when bupivacaine is administered for brachial plexus blockade, the time of onset is approximately 20 to 30 minutes, and the duration of anesthesia (or at least analgesia) averages 10 hours. These differences in the onset and duration of anesthesia and analgesia are due in part to the particular anatomy of the area of injection, which will influence the rates of diffusion and vascular absorption and, in turn, affect the amount of drug used for various types of regional anesthesia. In the subarachnoid space, for example, the lack of a nerve sheath around the spinal cord and deposition of the local anesthetic solution in the immediate vicinity of the spinal cord are responsible for the rapid onset of action, whereas the relatively small amount of drug used for spinal anesthesia probably accounts for the short duration of conduction block.

On the other hand, the onset of brachial plexus blockade is slow because the anesthetic is usually deposited at some distance from the nerve and must diffuse through various tissue barriers before reaching the nerve membrane. The prolonged block with brachial plexus blockade may be related to several factors, including comparatively slow rates of vascular absorption from the brachial plexus sheath, larger doses of drug required for this regional anesthetic technique, and comparatively long segments of nerves exposed to local anesthetic.

Carbonation and pH Adjustment of Local Anesthetics

The addition of bicarbonate:carbon dioxide to a solution of local anesthetic applied to an isolated nerve accelerates the onset and decreases the minimum concentration (C_m) required for conduction blockade.[57-59] Although the effect of carbon dioxide on local anesthetic activity is easily demonstrable in isolated nerve,[57,58] controversy exists concerning the clinical utility of carbonated local anesthetic solutions. For example, some studies have failed to demonstrate a significantly more rapid onset of action for lidocaine carbonate than for lidocaine hydrochloride when used for epidural blockade,[60] whereas others have reported a significant reduction in the time of onset of epidural blockade with lidocaine carbonate.[61] Although the effect of carbon dioxide on accelerating the onset of epidural sensory and motor blockade has been equivocal, carbonated solutions appear to improve the depth of sensory and motor blockade.[60,61] In addition, these solutions may produce a more complete blockade of the radial, median, and ulnar nerves when used for brachial plexus blockade.[62]

The addition of sodium bicarbonate to local anesthetic solutions has also been reported to decrease the time of onset of conduction blockade.[62,63] An increase in the pH of the local anesthetic solution increases the amount of drug in the uncharged base form, which should enhance the rate of diffusion across the nerve sheath and nerve membrane and result in a more rapid onset of anesthesia. Alkalinization of solutions of bupivacaine or lidocaine accelerated the onset of brachial plexus and epidural blockade in some studies,[62,63] but not others.[64] Comparison among studies is difficult because of lack of uniform reporting on the pH or buffering capacity of the injected solutions and because inclusion of vasoconstrictors may strongly modify the actions of added bicarbonate.

Mixtures of Local Anesthetics

Mixtures of local anesthetics for regional anesthesia are sometimes used in an effort to compensate for the short duration of action of certain rapidly acting agents such as chloroprocaine and lidocaine and the long latency of longer-acting agents such as tetracaine and bupivacaine. Mixtures of chloroprocaine and bupivacaine theoretically offer significant clinical advantages because of the rapid onset and low systemic toxicity of chloroprocaine and the long duration of action of bupivacaine. A mixture of 3% chloroprocaine and 0.5% bupivacaine was reported to produce a short latency and prolonged duration of brachial plexus blockade.[65] However, subsequent studies indicated that the duration of epidural anesthesia produced by a mixture of chloroprocaine and bupivacaine was significantly shorter than that obtained with bupivacaine alone, whereas the time to onset was longer than that of chloroprocaine alone.[66] At present, there appear to be few, if any, clinically significant advantages to the use of mixtures of local anesthetics. Etidocaine and bupivacaine provide clinically acceptable onsets of action and prolonged durations of anesthesia. In addition, the use of catheter techniques for many forms of regional anesthesia makes it possible to indefinitely extend the duration of action of rapidly acting agents such as chloroprocaine or lidocaine. Conversely, clinicians should be cautioned to not use maximum doses of two local anesthetics in combination in the mistaken belief that their toxicities are independent.[67] In the absence of additional data, the toxicities should be presumed to be additive.

Pregnancy (also see Chapter 58)

The spread and depth of epidural and spinal anesthesia are reported to be greater in pregnant than nonpregnant women.[68] This difference was originally attributed to mechanical factors associated with pregnancy (that is, dilated epidural veins decrease the volume of the epidural and subarachnoid spaces). Hormonal alterations probably play a more important role in the apparent increase in local anesthetic sensitivity during pregnancy because a greater spread of epidural anesthesia occurs during the first trimester of pregnancy, before any gross change in vascular dimensions within the epidural or subarachnoid space.[69] A correlation appears to exist between progesterone concentrations in cerebrospinal fluid and the milligrams-per-segment requirement of lidocaine for spinal anesthesia in pregnant and nonpregnant patients. Lidocaine's block of sciatic nerve functions in pregnant rats significantly outlasts that in age-matched nonpregnant female or male rats,[70] although pregnancy does not influence lidocaine uptake kinetics into nerves.[70] These results suggest that the hormonal changes associated with pregnancy enhance the apparent potency of local anesthetics; thus, the dosage should probably be reduced in patients in all stages of pregnancy.

CHOICE OF LOCAL ANESTHETIC FOR VARIOUS REGIONAL ANESTHETIC PROCEDURES (also see Chapters 43-45, 58, 72, and 73)

On the basis of anatomic considerations, regional anesthesia may be divided into infiltration anesthesia, intravenous regional anesthesia, peripheral nerve blockade (including plexus blockade), central neural blockade, and topical anesthesia. An additional method of local anesthetic injection, tumescent anesthesia, is included because it is widely used in office plastic surgery practice.

Infiltration Anesthesia

Any local anesthetic may be used for infiltration anesthesia. The onset of action is almost immediate for all agents after intradermal or subcutaneous administration; however, the duration of anesthesia varies (Table 14-4). Epinephrine will prolong the duration of infiltration anesthesia by all local anesthetics, although this effect is most pronounced when epinephrine is added to lidocaine. The choice of a specific drug for infiltration anesthesia largely depends on the desired duration of action.

The dosage of local anesthetic required for adequate infiltration anesthesia depends on the extent of the area to be anesthetized and the expected duration of the surgical procedure. When large surface areas have to be anesthetized, large volumes of dilute anesthetic solutions should be used. These considerations are particularly important when performing infiltration anesthesia in infants and smaller children. As an example, consider a 4-kg infant receiving infiltration anesthesia with the maximum safe dose of lidocaine, 5 mg/kg. Dosing to 5 mg/kg × 4 kg permits the administration of 20 mg, which is 1 mL of a 2% solution or 4 mL of a 0.5% solution. Lidocaine is effective for infiltration anesthesia in concentrations as dilute as 0.3% to 0.5%, so the more dilute solution can be used to more safely anesthetize a larger area.

Patients frequently experience pain immediately after the subcutaneous injection of local anesthetic solutions,[71] in part because of the acidic nature of these solutions.[72,73]

Table 14-4 Infiltration anesthesia

Drug	Plain Solution			Epinephrine-Containing Solution	
	Concentration (%)	Maximum Dose (mg)	Duration (min)	Maximum Dose (mg)	Duration (min)
Short Duration					
Procaine	1.0-2.0	400	20-30	600	30
Chloroprocaine	1.0-2.0	800	15-30	1000	30
Moderate Duration					
Lidocaine	0.5-1.0	300	30-60	500	120
Mepivacaine	0.5-1.0	300	45-90	500	120
Prilocaine	0.5-1.0	500	30-90	600	120
Long Duration					
Bupivacaine	0.25-0.5	175	120-240	225	180
Etidocaine	0.5-1.0	300	120-180	400	180

Doses listed refer to 70-kg adults. Doses should be reduced, as detailed in Chapter 45, for children and for patients with specific risk factors.

For example, neutralization of lidocaine solutions by the addition of sodium bicarbonate reduces pain on skin infiltration and may improve the onset of action (see earlier).

Intravenous Regional Anesthesia

Intravenous regional anesthesia involves the intravenous administration of a local anesthetic into a tourniquet-occluded limb (i.e., Bier block). The local anesthetic diffuses from the peripheral vascular bed to nonvascular tissue such as axons and nerve endings. Both the safety and efficacy of this regional anesthetic procedure depend on the interruption of blood flow to the involved limb and gradual release of the occluding tourniquet. Intravenous regional anesthesia has been used primarily for surgical procedures on the upper limbs. Shorter procedures on the foot can also be successfully performed under intravenous regional anesthesia. If a lower leg tourniquet is used, it should be applied well below the fibular neck to avoid pressure over the superficial peroneal nerve; in general, use of an upper leg tourniquet is preferred over lower leg tourniquets.

Lidocaine has been the drug used most frequently for intravenous regional anesthesia, but prilocaine, mepivacaine, chloroprocaine, procaine, bupivacaine, and etidocaine have also been used successfully. One might suppose a safety advantage with the aminoester-linked compounds because of their hydrolysis in blood; however, thrombophlebitis has been reported in several patients in whom chloroprocaine was used.[74] Cardiovascular collapse has been reported after the use of bupivacaine for intravenous regional anesthesia, and this use of bupivacaine is therefore discouraged.[75]

In general, approximately 3 mg/kg (40 mL of a 0.5% solution) of preservative-free lidocaine without epinephrine is used for upper extremity procedures. For surgical procedures on the lower limbs, 50 to 100 mL of 0.25% lidocaine has been used.

Peripheral Nerve Blockade
(also see Chapters 44 and 45)

Regional anesthetic procedures that inhibit conduction in fibers of the peripheral nervous system can be classified together under the general category of peripheral nerve blockade. This form of regional anesthesia has been arbitrarily subdivided into minor and major nerve blocks. Minor nerve blocks are defined as procedures involving single nerve entities such as the ulnar or radial nerve, whereas major nerve blocks involve the blockade of two or more distinct nerves or a nerve plexus.

Most local anesthetics can be used for minor nerve blocks. The onset of blockade is rapid with most drugs, and the choice of drug is determined primarily by the required duration of anesthesia. A classification of the various drugs according to their duration of action is shown in Table 14-5. The duration of both sensory analgesia and motor blockade is prolonged significantly when epinephrine is added to the various local anesthetic solutions.

In 1986 a technique of intrapleural regional analgesia was described as an alternative to multiple intercostal nerve blocks.[76] This procedure involves the administration of local anesthetic solution into the pleural space, either by percutaneous administration or by placement through the open chest by the surgeon. With percutaneous administration, an epidural needle is inserted into the pleural space, usually by way of the fourth to the ninth intercostal space. An epidural catheter is then passed into the pleural space approximately 5 to 10 cm beyond the tip of the needle and directed posteriorly, superiorly, and medially. The needle is removed, and the local anesthetic is administered through the catheter. The risk of pneumothorax has varied in published case series. Intrapleural analgesia can also be administered by the surgeon through the open chest during thoracotomy. Although interpleural analgesia appeared useful for unilateral postoperative analgesia after cholecystectomy, mastectomy, and nephrectomy,[77,78] its efficacy for post-thoracotomy pain is doubtful.[79] In the original case series, 22 to 30 mL of 0.5% bupivacaine with epinephrine was used in this technique; the duration of analgesia was reported to average approximately 8 hours with a range of 4 to 24 hours. The advantage of the technique is the ability to administer subsequent injections of local anesthetics by catheter to provide long-lasting analgesia without subjecting patients to repeated multiple intercostal nerve blocks. Caution is advised, however, because this technique has been associated with extremely high

		Plain Solution		Epinephrine-Containing Solution	
Drug	Usual Concentration (%)	Usual Volume (mL)	Dosage (mg)	Average Duration (min)	Average Duration (min)
Procaine	2	5-20	100-400	15-30	30-60
Chloroprocaine	2	5-20	100-400	15-30	30-60
Lidocaine	1	5-20	50-200	60-120	120-180
Mepivacaine	1	5-20	50-200	60-120	120-180
Prilocaine	1	5-20	50-200	60-120	120-180
Bupivacaine	0.25	5-20	12.5-50	180-360	240-480
Etidocaine	0.5	5-20	25-100	120-240	180-420

Table 14-5   Minor nerve blocks*

*Also see Chapter 45.
Doses listed refer to 70-kg adults. Doses should be reduced for children (see Chapter 45) and for patients with specific risk factors.

Table 14–6 Major nerve blocks

Drug with Epinephrine 1:200,000	Usual Concentration (%)	Usual Volume (mL)	Maximum Dose (mg)	Usual Onset (min)	Usual Duration (min)
Lidocaine	1-2	30-50	500	10-20	120-240
Mepivacaine	1-1.5	30-50	500	10-20	180-300
Prilocaine	1-2	30-50	600	10-20	180-300
Bupivacaine	0.25-0.5	30-50	225	15-30	360-720
Etidocaine	0.5-1.0	30-50	400	10-20	360-720
Tetracaine	0.25-0.5	30-50	200	20-30	300-600

Doses listed refer to 70-kg adults receiving epinephrine-containing solutions. Doses should be reduced, as detailed in Chapter 45, for children, for patients with specific risk factors, and when non–epinephrine-containing solutions are used.

plasma concentrations of anesthetic and an associated risk of convulsions.[76] Interpleural analgesia has also been used to provide analgesia for chronic pain conditions as diverse as upper extremity complex regional pain syndromes, pancreatitis, and cancer of the thorax and abdomen. In many centers, interpleural analgesia has largely been supplanted by thoracic epidural analgesia for most thoracic and abdominal procedures.

Two related approaches for unilateral somatic blockade in the thorax are continuous extrapleural catheters (placed through the chest by the surgeon dorsal to the parietal pleura) and continuous thoracic paravertebral somatic blockade. One advantage of these two latter approaches over interpleural analgesia is that very little of the administered solution leaks out of the chest into the chest tubes.

Brachial plexus blockade for upper limb surgery is the most common major peripheral nerve block technique. A significant difference exists between the time of onset of various drugs when these blocks are used (Table 14-6). In general, drugs with intermediate potency exhibit more rapid onset than the more potent compounds do. Onset times of approximately 14 minutes for lidocaine and mepivacaine have been reported, as opposed to approximately 23 minutes for bupivacaine.[80] Etidocaine may be an exception in that it produces a relatively rapid onset and a long duration of blockade. A variety of approaches to the brachial plexus are available; the choice of approach is dictated by several factors, including the site of surgery and the ability of the patient to tolerate spillover to other nerves, such as the phrenic nerve. Similarly, the lumbar plexus can be approached by several routes, including a posterior approach, an anterior perivascular "3 in 1" approach, and an anterior fascia iliaca compartment approach.[81]

Epinephrine will prolong the duration of most local anesthetics used for brachial plexus blockade, but it is less effective with drugs that have intrinsically longer durations of action. The variation in duration of anesthesia after brachial plexus blockade is also considerably greater than that observed with other types of conduction block. For example, durations of anesthesia varying from 4 to 30 hours have been reported for bupivacaine. It would be prudent to forewarn patients who are to be given a major nerve block about the possibility of prolonged sensory and motor block in the involved region, particularly when drugs such as bupivacaine and etidocaine are used. Knowledge shapes expectation and can often relieve anxiety over unusual sensations and thus increase comfort and reduce distress.

Central Neural Blockade (also see Chapter 43)

Any of the local anesthetics may be used for epidural anesthesia (Table 14-7), although procaine and tetracaine are rarely used because of their long onset times. Drugs with intermediate potency produce surgical anesthesia of 1 to 2 hours' duration, whereas the long-acting drugs usually produce 3 to 4 hours of anesthesia. The duration of short- and intermediate-acting drugs is significantly

Table 14–7 Epidural anesthesia*

Drug with Epinephrine 1:200,000	Usual Concentration (%)	Usual Volume (mL)	Total Dose (mg)	Usual Onset (min)	Usual Duration (min)
Chloroprocaine	2-3	15-30	300-900	5-15	30-90
Lidocaine	1-2	15-30	150-500	5-15	
Mepivacaine	1-2	15-30	150-500	5-15	60-180
Prilocaine	1-3	15-30	150-600	5-15	
Bupivacaine	0.25-0.75	15-30	37.5-225	10-20	180-300
Etidocaine	1.0-1.5	15-30	150-300	5-15	

Doses listed refer to 70-kg adults receiving epinephrine-containing solutions. Doses should be reduced, as detailed in Chapter 45, for children, for patients with specific risk factors, and when non–epinephrine-containing solutions are used.
*Also see Chapter 43.

Table 14–8   Spinal anesthesia*

Drug	Usual Concentration (%)	Usual Volume (mL)	Total Dose (mg)	Baricity	Glucose Concentration (%)	Usual Duration (min)
Procaine	10.0	1-2	100-200	Hyperbaric	5.0	30-60
Lidocaine	1.5, 5.0	1-2	30-100	Hyperbaric	7.5	30-90
Mepivacaine	4	1-2	40-80	Hyperbaric	9.0	30-90
Tetracaine	0.25-1.0	1-4	5-20	Hyperbaric	5.0	75-150
	0.25	2-6	5-20	Hypobaric	0	75-150
	1.0	1-2	5-20	Isobaric	0	75-150
Dibucaine	0.25	1-2	2.5-5.0	Hyperbaric	5.0	75-180
	0.5	1-2	5-10	Hypobaric	0	75-180
	0.06	5-20	3-12	Isobaric	0	75-180
Bupivacaine	0.5	3-4	15-20	Isobaric	0	75-150
	0.75	2-3	15-22.5	Hyperbaric	8.25	75-150

*Also see Chapter 43.

Doses listed refer to 70-kg adults. Doses should be modified as detailed in Chapters 44 and 45 for children, during pregnancy, and for elderly subjects.

prolonged by the addition of epinephrine (1:200,000), but the long-acting drugs benefit little from its addition. The onset of lumbar epidural anesthesia occurs within 5 to 15 minutes after the administration of chloroprocaine, lidocaine, mepivacaine, and prilocaine. Bupivacaine has a slower onset of action.

Bupivacaine at 0.125% produces adequate analgesia with only mild motor deficits. Such solutions of bupivacaine are useful for labor epidural analgesia and postoperative analgesia. Bupivacaine at 0.25% may be used for more intense analgesia (particularly during combined epidural–light general anesthesia) with moderate degrees of motor blockade. At concentrations of 0.5% to 0.75%, bupivacaine is associated with a more profound degree of motor block, which makes these solutions most suitable for major surgical procedures, particularly when epidural anesthesia is not combined with general anesthesia. Etidocaine produces adequate sensory analgesia and profound, long-lasting motor block and is primarily useful for surgical procedures in which muscle relaxation is required.

Drugs that can be used for subarachnoid administration are shown in Table 14-8. Tetracaine is available both as crystals and as a 1% solution, which may be diluted with 10% glucose to obtain a 0.5% hyperbaric solution.

Hypobaric solutions of tetracaine (tetracaine in sterile water) may be used for specific operative situations, such as anorectal or hip surgery. Isobaric tetracaine, obtained by mixing 1% tetracaine with cerebrospinal fluid or normal saline, is useful for lower limb surgical procedures. Bupivacaine is widely used as a spinal anesthetic, either as a hyperbaric solution at a concentration of 0.75% with 8.25% dextrose or by using the nearly isobaric 0.5% solution.

Intrathecal bupivacaine has an anesthetic profile similar to that of tetracaine.[82,83] However, differences do exist between the two drugs. Although two-segment regression of anesthesia is similar for bupivacaine and tetracaine, the total duration of sensory anesthesia is significantly longer after the subarachnoid administration of tetracaine. The depth and duration of motor blockade are also greater with tetracaine than with bupivacaine. On the other hand, bupivacaine has been reported in some studies to

be associated with less hypotension. In addition, the frequency of tourniquet pain in the lower limbs during certain orthopedic surgical procedures has been reported to be significantly reduced when bupivacaine instead of tetracaine is used for spinal anesthesia.[84,85]

Whereas tetracaine and bupivacaine are considered to be drugs of long duration, lidocaine provides a short duration of spinal anesthesia. The onset of spinal anesthesia is extremely rapid with a drug such as lidocaine. The addition of vasoconstrictors may prolong the duration of spinal anesthesia; for example, the addition of 0.2 to 0.3 mg of epinephrine to tetracaine solutions will produce a 50% or greater increase in duration. The duration of spinal anesthesia produced by tetracaine can also be increased to a similar extent by adding 1 to 5 mg of phenylephrine. The addition of epinephrine to bupivacaine or lidocaine may not significantly prolong the duration of spinal anesthesia in thoracic segments,[86,87] although the total duration of anesthesia (e.g., in the lumbosacral roots) will be significantly increased. Even though lidocaine has long been used for spinal anesthesia as a 5% solution, recent studies of local anesthetic neurotoxicity have led some to question this practice; this issue is discussed later in the chapter in the section on neurotoxicity of local anesthetics.

Topical Anesthesia

A number of local anesthetic formulations are available for topical anesthesia (Table 14-9), with lidocaine, dibucaine, tetracaine, and benzocaine being the drugs most commonly used. In general, these preparations provide effective, but relatively short durations of analgesia when applied to mucous membranes or abraded skin. In addition, lidocaine and tetracaine sprays have been used for endotracheal anesthesia before intubation. The topical anesthetic formulation EMLA, which is a eutectic mixture of 2.5% lidocaine base and 2.5% prilocaine base, is widely used for cutaneous analgesia through intact skin.[88] Clinical studies have demonstrated that this preparation can decrease the pain associated with the percutaneous insertion of intravenous needles and cannulas.[89]

Table 14–9 Various preparations for topical anesthesia

Anesthetic Ingredient	Concentration (%)	Pharmaceutical Application Form	Intended Area of Use
Benzocaine	1-5	Cream	Skin and mucous membrane
	20	Ointment	Skin and mucous membrane
	20	Aerosol	Skin and mucous membrane
Cocaine	4	Solution	Ear, nose, throat
Dibucaine	0.25-1	Cream	Skin
	0.25-1	Ointment	Skin
	0.25-1	Aerosol	Skin
	0.25	Solution	Ear
	2.5	Suppositories	Rectum
Lidocaine	2-4	Solution	Oropharynx, tracheobronchial tree, nose
	2	Jelly	Urethra
	2.5-5	Ointment	Skin, mucous membrane, rectum
	2	Viscous	Oropharynx
	10	Suppositories	Rectum
	10	Aerosol	Gingival mucosa
Tetracaine	0.5-1	Ointment	Skin, rectum, mucous membrane
	0.5-1	Cream	Skin, rectum, mucous membrane
	0.25-1	Solution	Nose, tracheobronchial tree
EMLA	Lidocaine 2.5 Prilocaine 2.5	Cream	Intact skin
TAC	Tetracaine 0.5 Epinephrine 1:200,000 Cocaine 11.8	Solution	Cut skin
LET	Lidocaine 4 Epinephrine 1:200,000 Tetracaine 0.5	Solution	Cut skin

EMLA, eutectic mixture of lidocaine and prilocaine; LET, lidocaine-epinephrine-tetracaine; TAC, tetracaine-epinephrine-cocaine.
Modified from Covino B, Vassallo H: Local Anesthetics: Mechanisms of Action and Clinical Use. Orlando, FL, Grune & Stratton, 1976.

In addition, EMLA has been successfully used for cutaneous anesthesia in skin-grafting procedures.[90] This preparation must be applied under an occlusive bandage for 45 to 60 minutes to obtain effective cutaneous anesthesia; longer application times increase the depth and reliability of skin analgesia. EMLA appears to be quite safe in neonates, and methemoglobinemia is exceedingly uncommon after the application of prilocaine. EMLA is more effective for newborn circumcision than placebo is, but less effective than dorsal penile nerve block.[91] Several alternative topical local anesthetic formulations are also in use, including tetracaine gel[92] and liposomal lidocaine. Physical methods to accelerate local anesthetic transit across skin are also under study, including iontophoresis, local heating, and electroporation.

Topical anesthesia through cut skin is commonly used in pediatric emergency departments for liquid application into lacerations that require suturing. Historically, such anesthesia has been provided by a mixture of tetracaine, epinephrine (adrenaline), and cocaine, known as TAC. TAC is usually supplied as 0.5% tetracaine, 1:2,000 epinephrine, and 10% to 11.8% cocaine, although studies suggest that more dilute concentrations may be almost equally effective and less likely to cause toxicity. The generally recommended safe maximum dose is 3 to 4 mL for adults and 0.05 mL/kg for children. TAC is ineffective through intact skin; in contrast, it can be absorbed rapidly from mucosal surfaces and lead to toxic reactions. There is a report of a fatal reaction after application to a nasal laceration, with presumed dripping into the mouth and rapid mucosal absorption.[93,94]

Because of concern regarding cocaine toxicity and the potential for diversion and abuse, several groups have investigated alternative cocaine-free topical preparations. Tetracaine-phenylephrine and lidocaine-epinephrine-tetracaine (LET) preparations are as effective as TAC.[95] Over the past 5 years, non–cocaine-containing formulations, especially LET, have largely supplanted TAC. Similarly, cocaine has in the past been widely administered by otolaryngologists as a solution or aerosol into the nasal passages because it provides both mucosal analgesia and vasoconstriction. In recent years, cocaine has been increasingly replaced for nasal application by combined use of an adrenergic agonist (oxymetazoline or phenylephrine) and a local anesthetic such as 2% to 4% lidocaine; more dilute solutions are recommended for infants and children. Systemic absorption of phenylephrine can cause severe hypertension and reflex bradycardia; oxymetazoline is associated with much less systemic effect and has a considerably wider margin of safety.

Tumescent Anesthesia

A technique of local anesthesia most commonly used by plastic surgeons during liposuction procedures involves the subcutaneous injection of large volumes of dilute local anesthetic in combination with epinephrine and other agents. Total doses of lidocaine ranging from 35 to 55 mg/kg have been reported to produce safe plasma concentrations, which may peak more than 8 to 12 hours after infusion. Despite these seemingly huge doses, very good outcomes have been reported in several case series.[96] Conversely, there have been several recent case series of cardiac arrest and death during plastic surgical procedures in which multiple risk factors, including high local anesthetic concentrations, may have contributed to the patients' instability and deterioration. The factors governing uptake and clearance from this method of local anesthetic delivery deserve further study. Clinicians should use great caution when administering additional local anesthetics by infiltration or other routes for at least 12 to 18 hours after the use of this technique.

Systemic Local Anesthetics for Neuropathic Pain
(also see Chapter 72)

A broad variety of local anesthetics, antiarrhythmics, anticonvulsants, and other Na$^+$ channel blockers are administered intravenously and orally to relieve neuropathic pain. Allodynia, causalgia, and other sensory disturbances from nerve injury, diabetes, and herpes infection have all been treated by such drugs, but with variable success. Clinical results are unpredictable. Although successful responses to intravenous lidocaine are often taken as a positive indication for oral mexiletine, many patients find mexiletine difficult to tolerate. When the signs of neuropathic pain are reversed by lidocaine infusion, normal nociception and other sensory modalities are unaffected, thus suggesting that the neurophysiologic correlate of the disease or diseases has an unusually high susceptibility to these drugs, which are present in plasma at concentrations 50 to 100 times lower than those required to block normal impulses in peripheral fibers. Laboratory studies suggest that the ectopic impulse activity that arises at an injury site or elsewhere (e.g., the dorsal root ganglion) contributes to neuropathic pain and that such impulses are particularly sensitive to use-dependent Na$^+$ channel blockers. It is noteworthy that relief of preexisting neuropathic pain, both clinically and in animal models,[97] can in some cases persist for days, weeks, or months after a single intravenous infusion of drug (e.g., lidocaine), far beyond the lifetime of the drug in vivo or of any nerve block that it might effect. The mechanism of this remarkable action remains a mystery.

PHARMACOKINETICS

The concentration of local anesthetics in blood is determined by the amount injected, the rate of absorption from the site of injection, the rate of tissue distribution, and the rate of biotransformation and excretion of the specific drug. Patient-related factors such as age, cardiovascular status, and hepatic function influence the physiologic disposition and the resultant blood concentration of local anesthetics.

Absorption

The systemic absorption of local anesthetics is determined by the site of injection, the dosage and volume, the addition of a vasoconstrictor agent, and the pharmacologic profile of the agent itself. A comparison of the blood concentration of local anesthetics after various routes of administration reveals that the anesthetic drug level is highest after intercostal nerve blockade, followed in order of decreasing concentration by injection into the caudal epidural space, lumbar epidural space, brachial plexus, and subcutaneous tissue.[98] When a local anesthetic solution is distributed to an area of greater vascularity, a greater rate and degree of absorption occur. This relationship is of clinical significance because the use of a fixed dose of a local anesthetic may be potentially toxic in one area of administration but not in others. For example, the use of 400 mg of lidocaine without epinephrine for an intercostal nerve block results in an average peak venous plasma level of approximately 7 µg/mL, which is sufficiently high to cause symptoms of central nervous system (CNS) toxicity in some patients.[98] By comparison, this same dose of lidocaine used for brachial plexus block yields a mean maximum blood level of approximately 3 µg/mL, which is rarely associated with signs of toxicity.

The maximum blood level of local anesthetics is related to the total dose of drug administered for any particular site of administration. For most drugs, a proportionality exists between the amount of drug administered and the resultant peak anesthetic blood levels.[99] Higher blood levels also follow from the administration of larger volumes of a correspondingly dilute solution than from the same dose in a smaller volume.

Local anesthetic solutions frequently contain a vasoconstrictor, usually epinephrine, in concentrations varying from 5 to 20 µg/mL. Epinephrine decreases the rate of vascular absorption of certain drugs from various sites of administration and thus lowers their potential systemic toxicity. A 5-µg/mL dose of epinephrine (1:200,000) significantly reduces the peak blood levels of lidocaine and mepivacaine, irrespective of the site of administration. Peak blood levels of bupivacaine and etidocaine are minimally influenced by the addition of a vasoconstrictor after injection into the lumbar epidural space.[100] However, epinephrine will significantly reduce the rate of vascular absorption of these drugs when used for peripheral nerve blocks such as brachial plexus blockade.[101]

Differences also exist in the rate of absorption of various local anesthetics. For example, a comparison of drugs of similar anesthetic profile reveals that lidocaine is absorbed more rapidly after brachial plexus blockade than prilocaine is, whereas bupivacaine is absorbed more rapidly than etidocaine is.

Distribution

The systemic distribution of local anesthetics can be described sufficiently by a two-compartment model.[102] The rapid disappearance phase is believed to be related to uptake by rapidly equilibrating tissues (i.e., tissues that have high vascular perfusion). The slower phase of disappearance from blood is mainly a function of the particular compound (Table 14-10).[103] The half-lives of lidocaine and mepivacaine are similar, but a comparison of bupivacaine and etidocaine reveals that etidocaine has a more rapid rate of tissue redistribution and biotransformation than bupivacaine does.[104]

Local anesthetics are distributed throughout all body tissues, but the relative concentration in different tissues varies. In general, more highly perfused organs show higher concentrations of local anesthetic than less well perfused organs do. Local anesthetics are rapidly extracted by lung tissue, so the whole-blood concentration of local anesthetics decreases markedly as they pass through the pulmonary vasculature.[105,106] The highest percentage of an injected dose of a local anesthetic is found in skeletal muscle. Although this tissue does not have any particular affinity for this class of drugs, the mass of skeletal muscle makes it the largest reservoir for local anesthetics.

Biotransformation and Excretion

The pattern of metabolism of local anesthetics varies according to their chemical classification. Ester, or procaine-like, drugs undergo hydrolysis in plasma by pseudocholinesterase enzymes. Chloroprocaine has the fastest rate, 4.7 mol/mL/hr, versus rates of 1.1 mol/mL/hr for procaine and 0.3 mol/mL/hr for tetracaine.[107,108]

The aminoamide drugs undergo enzymatic degradation primarily in the liver. Lidocaine is metabolized somewhat more rapidly than mepivacaine,[108] and bupivacaine is metabolized more slowly than either lidocaine or mepivacaine.[109] Some degradation of the amide-type compounds may take place in tissues other than liver; in particular, the metabolism of lidocaine is discussed in detail elsewhere.[108]

Excretion of the metabolites of amide-type anesthetics occurs through the kidney. Less than 5% of the unchanged drug is excreted by the kidney into urine.

Pharmacokinetic Alterations by Patient Status

Patient age may influence the physiologic disposition of local anesthetics. The half-life of lidocaine after intravenous administration averaged 80 minutes in human volunteers ranging in age from 22 to 26 years, whereas volunteers aged 61 to 71 years demonstrated a significantly prolonged lidocaine half-life that averaged 138 minutes.[110]

Newborn infants have immature hepatic enzyme systems and prolonged elimination of lidocaine and bupivacaine.[111,112] Prolonged elimination is particularly an issue for continuous infusions of local anesthetics in infants, and seizures have been associated with rapid bupivacaine infusion rates.[113,114] Based on analysis of these cases, a maximum infusion rate of 0.4 mg/kg/hr for prolonged bupivacaine infusions has been proposed for children and adults, whereas prolonged infusion rates for neonates and young infants should not exceed 0.2 mg/kg/hr.[115] Even at 0.2 mg/kg/hr, plasma bupivacaine concentrations were found to be rising toward a toxic range in some younger infants after 48 hours.[116] Similarly, prolonged lidocaine infusions in neonates should not exceed 0.8 mg/kg/hr. Chloroprocaine may offer unique advantages for epidural infusion in neonates because it is cleared rapidly from plasma, even in preterm neonates.[117]

Decreased hepatic blood flow or impaired hepatic enzyme function can produce substantially elevated blood levels of the aminoamide local anesthetics. An average lidocaine half-life of 1.5 hours was reported in volunteers with normal hepatic function, whereas patients with liver disease had an average half-life of 5.0 hours.[118] The rate of lidocaine disappearance from blood has also been shown to be markedly prolonged in patients with congestive heart failure.[119]

TOXICITY

Local anesthetics are relatively safe if administered in an appropriate dosage and in the correct anatomic location. However, systemic and localized toxic reactions can occur, usually as a result of accidental intravascular or intrathecal injection or administration of an excessive dose. In addition, specific adverse effects are associated with the use of certain drugs, such as allergic reactions to the aminoester drugs and methemoglobinemia after the use of prilocaine.

Systemic Toxicity (also see Chapters 43-45 and 58)

Systemic reactions to local anesthetics primarily involve the CNS and the cardiovascular system. In general, the CNS is more susceptible to the actions of systemic local anesthetics than the cardiovascular system is, and thus the dose and blood level of local anesthetic required to produce CNS toxicity are usually lower than that resulting in circulatory collapse.

Table 14-10 Pharmacokinetic properties of various amide local anesthetics

Agent	$t_{1/2\alpha}$ (min)	$t_{1/2\beta}$ (min)	V_{dss} (L)	$t_{1/2\gamma}$ (hr)	Cl (L/min)
Prilocaine	0.5	5.0	261	1.5	2.84
Lidocaine	1.0	9.6	91	1.6	0.95
Mepivacaine	0.7	7.2	84	1.9	0.78
Bupivacaine	2.7	28.0	72	3.5	0.47
Etidocaine	2.2	19.0	133	2.6	1.22

Cl, clearance; V_{dss}, volume of distribution at steady state.

Central Nervous System Toxicity

The initial symptoms of local anesthetic–induced CNS toxicity are feelings of lightheadedness and dizziness, followed frequently by visual and auditory disturbances such as difficulty focusing and tinnitus. Other subjective CNS symptoms include disorientation and occasional feelings of drowsiness. Objective signs of CNS toxicity are usually excitatory in nature and include shivering, muscular twitching, and tremors initially involving muscles of the face and distal parts of the extremities. Ultimately, generalized convulsions of a tonic-clonic nature occur. If a sufficiently large dose or a rapid intravenous injection of a local anesthetic is administered, the initial signs of CNS excitation are rapidly followed by a state of generalized CNS depression. Seizure activity ceases, and respiratory depression and ultimately respiratory arrest may occur. In some patients, CNS depression without a preceding excitatory phase is seen, particularly if other CNS depressant drugs have been administered.

CNS excitation may be the result of an initial blockade of inhibitory pathways in the cerebral cortex by local anesthetics,[120] but it can also result from the net stimulation of glutamate release, an excitatory amino acid neurotransmitter. Blockade of the inhibitory pathways allows facilitatory neurons to function in an unopposed fashion, which results in an increase in excitatory activity leading to convulsions. An increase in the dose of local anesthetic leads to inhibition of the activity of both inhibitory and facilitatory circuits and thereby results in a generalized state of CNS depression. Persistent glutamate release can result in receptor desensitization or transmitter depletion, both of which will depress the CNS.

In general, a correlation exists between the anesthetic potency and intravenous CNS toxicity of various drugs. For example, in cats the dose of intravenous procaine required to cause convulsions is approximately seven times greater than the convulsive dose of bupivacaine.[121] However, bupivacaine is also approximately eight times more potent than procaine as a local anesthetic.[122] Intravenous infusion studies in human volunteers have also demonstrated an inverse relationship between the intrinsic anesthetic potency of various drugs and the dosage required to induce premonitory signs of CNS toxicity.[122,123] Convulsions from an inadvertent intravenous bolus of local anesthetic can generally be terminated by small intravenous doses of benzodiazepines, such as midazolam, or by small intravenous doses of thiopental.

Respiratory or metabolic acidosis increases the risk of CNS toxicity from local anesthetics in animals and patients. In cats, the convulsive threshold of various local anesthetics was inversely related to the arterial Pco_2 level.[121] An increase in $Paco_2$ from 25 to 40 mm Hg to 65 to 81 mm Hg decreases the convulsive threshold of procaine, mepivacaine, prilocaine, lidocaine, and bupivacaine by approximately 50%.

An elevation in $Paco_2$ enhances cerebral blood flow, and as a result, anesthetic is delivered more rapidly to the brain. In addition, diffusion of carbon dioxide into neuronal cells decreases intracellular pH, which facilitates conversion of the base form of the drugs to the cationic form. The cationic form does not diffuse well across the nerve membrane, so ion trapping will occur, which will increase the apparent CNS toxicity of local anesthetics.

Hypercapnia or acidosis (or both) also decreases the plasma protein binding of local anesthetics.[124,125] Accordingly, an elevation in $Paco_2$ or a decrease in pH will increase the proportion of free drug available for diffusion into the brain. On the other hand, acidosis increases the cationic form of the local anesthetic, which should decrease the rate of diffusion through lipoid barriers.

The clinical implication of this effect of hypercapnia and acidosis on toxicity deserves emphasis. Seizures produce hypoventilation and a combined respiratory and metabolic acidosis, which further exacerbates the CNS toxicity. In the setting of local anesthetic toxic reactions, it is essential to provide prompt assisted ventilation and circulatory support as needed to prevent or correct hypercapnia and acidosis, as well as prevent or correct hypoxemia, which also exacerbates CNS toxicity. Based on the discussion just presented, it should be apparent that clinicians performing major conduction blockade should make a routine practice of having the following ready at hand: monitoring equipment; an oxygen tank or wall oxygen outlet; airway equipment, including at minimum a bag-mask circuit for delivery of positive-pressure ventilation; and drugs to terminate convulsions, such as midazolam, lorazepam, diazepam, or thiopental.

Cardiovascular System Toxicity

Local anesthetics can exert direct actions on both the heart and peripheral blood vessels, as well as indirect actions on the circulation by blockade of sympathetic or parasympathetic efferent activity.

Direct Cardiac Effects

The primary cardiac electrophysiologic effect of local anesthetics is a decrease in the rate of depolarization in the fast-conducting tissues of Purkinje fibers and ventricular muscle.[120,121] This reduction in rate is believed to be due to a decrease in the availability of fast sodium channels in cardiac membranes. Action potential duration and the effective refractory period are also decreased by local anesthetics.[126] However, the ratio of the effective refractory period to the duration of the action potential is increased in both Purkinje fibers and ventricular muscle.

The electrophysiologic effects of various agents differ qualitatively. Bupivacaine depresses the rapid phase of depolarization ($\dot{V}max$) in Purkinje fibers and ventricular muscle to a greater extent than lidocaine does.[126] In addition, the rate of recovery from a use-dependent block is slower in bupivacaine-treated papillary muscles than in lidocaine-treated muscles.[127] This slow rate of recovery results in incomplete restoration of Na^+ channel availability between action potentials, particularly at high heart rates. In contrast, recovery from lidocaine is complete, even at rapid heart rates. These differential effects of lidocaine and bupivacaine have been advanced as explanations of the antiarrhythmic properties of lidocaine and the arrhythmogenic potential of bupivacaine.

Electrophysiologic studies in intact dogs and in humans have shown that high blood levels of local anesthetics will prolong the conduction time through various

Table 14–11 Comparative effect of various local anesthetics on cardiac contractility and cardiac output

Drug	Relative Anesthetic Potency	Isolated Guinea Pig Atria (50% ↓) (μg/mL)	Cardiac Output in Dogs (50% ↓) (mg/kg)
Procaine	1	277	100
Chloroprocaine	1	102	30
Cocaine	2	56	—
Lidocaine	2	67	30
Prilocaine	2	42	40
Mepivacaine	2	55	40
Etidocaine	6	—	20
Bupivacaine	8	6	10
Tetracaine	8	6	20

parts of the heart, as indicated on the electrocardiogram (ECG) by an increase in the PR interval and duration of the QRS complex. Extremely high concentrations of local anesthetics depress spontaneous pacemaker activity in the sinus node, thereby resulting in sinus bradycardia and sinus arrest.

All local anesthetics exert a dose-dependent negative inotropic action on cardiac muscle.[128,129] This depression of cardiac contractility is proportional to the conduction-blocking potency of the various drugs in isolated nerves[129] and in dogs[130-132] (Table 14-11). Thus, bupivacaine and tetracaine are more potent cardiodepressants than lidocaine, which in turn is a more potent cardiodepressant than chloroprocaine.

Local anesthetics may depress myocardial contractility by affecting calcium influx and triggered release. For example, procaine blocks the intracellular release of calcium in isolated sarcoplasmic reticulum preparations.[133] However, in the isolated guinea pig heart, an increase in the extracellular concentration of calcium failed to reverse the negative inotropic action of bupivacaine or lidocaine.[134]

Voltage-clamp studies show that lidocaine inhibits cardiac sarcolemmal Ca^{2+} currents as well as Na^+ currents.[135] This action alone should be antagonized by an increase in extracellular Ca^{2+}, so it is likely that the negative inotropy of local anesthetics involves several mechanisms, not just the blockade of inward currents.

Direct Peripheral Vascular Effects
Local anesthetics exert a biphasic effect on peripheral vascular smooth muscle. Low concentrations of lidocaine and bupivacaine produce vasoconstriction in the cremaster muscle of rats, whereas high concentrations increase arteriolar diameter, indicative of vasodilation.

In vivo studies have also demonstrated that small doses of local anesthetics decrease peripheral arterial flow without any change in arterial blood pressure whereas larger doses increase blood flow.[136] Cocaine is the only local anesthetic that consistently causes vasoconstriction at all concentrations because of its ability to inhibit the uptake of norepinephrine by premotor neurons and thus potentiate neurogenic vasoconstriction.[137,138]

Some studies in anesthetized animals and in isolated heart-lung preparations have found increases in pulmonary vascular resistance after infusion of local anesthetic.[131,132] The addition of lidocaine to cultured smooth muscle cells acutely elevates intracellular Ca^{2+} and could be a mechanism for local vasoconstriction. It has not been determined to what degree these pulmonary vascular effects in vivo are direct actions on pulmonary vascular smooth muscle or to what degree they reflect responses to circulatory or respiratory depression from drug acting on the CNS.

Comparative Cardiovascular Toxicity
(also see Chapters 43-45 and 58)

In recent years, the more potent drugs (i.e., bupivacaine and etidocaine) have been reported to cause rapid and profound cardiovascular depression.

The cardiotoxicity of the more potent drugs such as bupivacaine appears to differ from that of lidocaine in the following manner[139]:
1. The ratio of the dosage required for irreversible cardiovascular collapse (CC) and the dosage that will produce CNS toxicity (convulsions) (i.e., the CC/CNS ratio) is lower for bupivacaine and etidocaine than for lidocaine.
2. Ventricular arrhythmias and fatal ventricular fibrillation may occur more often after rapid intravenous administration of a large dose of bupivacaine but far less frequently with lidocaine.
3. A pregnant animal or patient may be more sensitive than a nonpregnant animal or patient to the cardiotoxic effects of bupivacaine.
4. Cardiac resuscitation is more difficult after bupivacaine-induced cardiovascular collapse.
5. Acidosis and hypoxia markedly potentiate the cardiotoxicity of bupivacaine.

CC/CNS Ratio
In sheep, the CC/CNS dose and blood level ratios for bupivacaine and etidocaine were found to be lower than those for lidocaine.[140] A CC/CNS dose ratio of 7.1 ± 1.1 was found for lidocaine, which indicates that seven times as much drug was required to induce irreversible cardiovascular collapse as was needed to produce convulsions. The CC/CNS dose ratio for bupivacaine was 3.7 ± 0.5 whereas that for etidocaine was 4.4 ± 0.9, and the CC/CNS blood level ratio for lidocaine was 3.6 ± 0.3 versus 1.6 to 1.7 for bupivacaine and etidocaine. At the time of cardiovascular collapse, higher concentrations of bupivacaine and etidocaine than lidocaine were present in the myocardium, which suggests that some of the enhanced cardiac toxicity of these more potent drugs is due to greater myocardial uptake.

Ventricular Arrhythmias
Bupivacaine and to a lesser degree etidocaine may induce severe cardiac arrhythmias, including ventricular fibrillation, in various animal species.[134,141-145] Ventricular arrhythmias were rarely seen with lidocaine, mepivacaine, or tetracaine.[146] These electrophysiologic effects of bupivacaine may result in conduction abnormalities leading

to a reentrant type of arrhythmia similar to torsades de pointes arrhythmias.[142] Although the cardiac arrhythmias observed in bupivacaine-treated animals are due in part to a direct cardiac effect, injection of bupivacaine directly into certain regions of the brain resulted in the development of cardiac arrhythmias, which may indicate a relationship between the CNS and cardiotoxic effects of bupivacaine.[147,148]

Enhanced Cardiotoxicity in Pregnancy
(also see Chapter 58)
A number of the cardiotoxic reactions that have been reported after the use of bupivacaine occurred in pregnant patients. As a result, the 0.75% solution is no longer recommended for use in obstetric anesthesia in the United States. In studies of pregnant and nonpregnant sheep, the CC/CNS dose ratio of bupivacaine decreased from 3.7 ± 0.5 in nonpregnant to 2.7 ± 0.4 in pregnant animals.[140] However, little difference was observed in the CC/CNS blood level ratio, which varied from 1.6 ± 1.0 in nonpregnant animals to 1.4 ± 0.1 in pregnant ewes. The blood level of bupivacaine at which circulatory collapse occurred was lower in pregnant animals, but no difference in the myocardial uptake of bupivacaine in pregnant and nonpregnant sheep was observed at the time of cardiovascular collapse.

Cardiac Resuscitation (also see Chapter 78)
Studies in acidotic and hypoxic sheep have demonstrated that cardiac resuscitation after bupivacaine-induced toxicity is difficult.[149] Studies in cats and hypoxic dogs rendered toxic with bupivacaine indicate that resuscitation is possible if massive doses of epinephrine and atropine are administered.[150,151] In addition, bretylium but not lidocaine could raise the ventricular tachycardia threshold that was lowered by bupivacaine.[152] Other drugs have also been tested for their effects on resuscitation from bupivacaine cardiotoxicity. Amrinone was found to be effective in two studies in dogs but ineffective in a study in rats. Case reports have suggested that either bretylium or phenytoin[153] may be effective.

The clinical implications for cardiac resuscitation after an intravascular injection or overdose of local anesthetic are the following:

1. No medications are uniformly effective in facilitating resuscitation from bupivacaine-induced cardiac arrest or severe ventricular tachycardia. The basic principles of cardiopulmonary resuscitation should be emphasized first, including attention to securing the airway, providing oxygenation and ventilation, and instituting chest compressions if needed. Epinephrine remains a first-line choice of medication in the event of circulatory collapse.

2. Because resuscitation after local anesthetic–induced circulatory collapse is so difficult, prevention of massive intravascular injection or excessive dosing is crucial.

3. Negative aspiration of the syringe does not always exclude intravascular placement. Incremental, fractionated dosing should be the rule for all patients undergoing major conduction blockade. Although changes in the ECG are not always present before circulatory collapse, they often are, and continuous

attention to the ECG (including changes in QRS morphology, rate, rhythm, or ectopy) may be life-saving by terminating injection before a lethal dose is administered.

Ropivacaine
In response to reports of cardiovascular toxicity from accidental intravenous injection of bupivacaine,[75] a new long-lasting amide local anesthetic was developed. Ropivacaine (Naropin) differs from bupivacaine both in the substitution of a propyl for the butyl group on the piperidine ring's tertiary nitrogen atom and the fact that it consists of a single enantiomer, the (S)-stereoisomer (see Fig. 14-2). Commercial bupivacaine is a racemic mixture of both isomers, whereas lidocaine, which lacks a chiral center, has no stereosymmetry. With these designed changes in molecular structure, it was hoped that ropivacaine would be less intrinsically cardiotoxic. The hope that it would be cleared more rapidly from the circulation if injected intravenously has, however, been confounded by evidence that the (S)-enantiomers of mepivacaine and bupivacaine are metabolized by the liver more slowly than the corresponding (R)-enantiomers, as well as having a slower rate of total-body clearance.[154,155]

The cardiovascular toxicity of local anesthetics is complex and involves direct effects on the myocardium,[129] on vascular tissue[138] (both smooth muscle and its neuronal supply), and on the central innervation of the heart.[147,156] In both neuronal and cardiac Na^+ channels, the (S)-isomers of these piperidine-containing local anesthetics are less potent than the (R)-isomers,[157,158] but the stereopotency of the cardiovascular effects mediated through vascular tissue and the CNS is not known. Because of the smaller propyl substituent, (S)-ropivacaine is slightly less potent than (S)-bupivacaine in its effect on single sodium channels[159] and isolated nerve action potentials. More germane to the direct cardiotoxic actions is that the very slow reversal of Na^+ channel blockade after a cardiac action potential, which is a hallmark of bupivacaine, is considerably faster with ropivacaine.[160] Such slow drug reversal has been related to persistent conduction slowing, reentry circuits, and the development of ventricular tachycardias leading to fibrillation.[127] In addition to these electrical differences, the negative inotropic potency of ropivacaine on isolated cardiac tissue appears to be considerably less than that of bupivacaine.[160,161] Both electrical and mechanical differences in the toxic profiles may arise from the selective inhibition of Ca^{2+} currents by bupivacaine.[128,146,162]

Do the data thus far support the claim of a greater therapeutic index for ropivacaine than bupivacaine, particularly with regard to cardiotoxicity? In clinical studies comparing potencies of ropivacaine and bupivacaine administered for brachial plexus[163] or lumbar epidural block,[164,165] the anesthetic profiles of the drugs were almost identical. A third study comparing lumbar epidural 0.5% bupivacaine with 0.75% ropivacaine also found no significant differences in motor or sensory effects between the drugs at these different concentrations.[166] Overall, it appears that ropivacaine is slightly less potent than (1:1.3 to 1:1.5) or equally as potent as bupivacaine for regional anesthesia. In some laboratory animal studies and in some human studies, ropivacaine also produced blocks of shorter duration than bupivacaine did.[165,167,168] Other studies in animals[169] and humans have found equal durations of sensory and motor blockade for the two drugs.

At the projected equipotent doses for nerve block, are the drugs equally toxic? The overall impression is that ropivacaine is less cardiotoxic than bupivacaine. Studies in animals have generally found that bupivacaine more readily produces conduction disturbances, cardiac collapse, or ventricular fibrillation than ropivacaine does.

Chirality rather than the difference between the propyl- and butyl-N-piperidine substituent may account for the greater safety of ropivacaine, for many fewer cardiotoxic events also occur when (S)-bupivacaine (levobupivacaine) rather than racemic bupivacaine is administered to sheep. In contrast, death from ventricular arrhythmias is comparable between ropivacaine and bupivacaine at equipotent doses in sheep. Convulsant doses of ropivacaine are larger than those of bupivacaine but less than those of lidocaine.[170,171] Levobupivacaine has been developed for clinical use,[172] and studies are in progress to determine whether it will have unique clinical benefits.

Perhaps the most notable difference between ropivacaine and bupivacaine is that aggressive cardiac resuscitation after an intentional intravenous bolus in dogs led to effective reversal of the toxic effects far more frequently with ropivacaine than with bupivacaine.[173] Furthermore, intravenous ropivacaine is cleared from the circulation more rapidly than intravenous bupivacaine.[174] This feature will enhance the safety of ropivacaine relative to bupivacaine when the drugs are used for repeated dosing or by infusion. In contrast to bupivacaine, the cardiotoxic profile of ropivacaine in pregnant ewes is the same as the corresponding profile in nonpregnant ewes.[175] These studies would suggest that ropivacaine may have slightly greater safety than bupivacaine for local and regional anesthesia.

Acidosis and Hypoxia

Hypercapnia, acidosis, and hypoxia potentiate the negative chronotropic and inotropic action of lidocaine and bupivacaine in isolated cardiac tissue, and the combination of hypoxia and acidosis markedly potentiates the cardiodepressant effects of bupivacaine. Hypoxia and acidosis also increased the frequency of cardiac arrhythmias and the mortality rate in sheep after the intravenous administration of bupivacaine.[149,176] Hypercapnia, acidosis, and hypoxia occur very rapidly in some patients after seizure activity induced by the rapid accidental intravascular injection of local anesthetics.[177] Thus, the cardiovascular depression observed in some patients after the accidental intravenous injection of bupivacaine may be related in part to the severe acid-base changes that occur during toxic reactions to this drug.

Indirect Cardiovascular Effects

High levels of spinal or epidural blockade can produce severe hypotension. In a review of closed claims of patients who suffered perioperative cardiac arrest, a series of cases were identified that involved generally healthy patients undergoing spinal anesthesia.[178] Common features of these cases and subsequent case series[179] included high dermatomal levels of spinal anesthesia, liberal use of sedatives, and hypotension accompanied by bradycardia. The authors noted that adverse outcomes seemed to be associated with delays in recognition of the problem, delays in instituting airway support (particularly in sedated patients), and delays in administration of direct-acting combined α- and β-adrenergic agonists such as epinephrine. Although mild degrees of hypotension generally respond well to indirect-acting sympathomimetics such as ephedrine or incremental dosing of phenylephrine, the combination of severe hypotension and significant bradycardia under spinal anesthesia should in most clinical settings be treated promptly with incremental dosing of epinephrine.

Methemoglobinemia

A unique systemic side effect associated with a specific local anesthetic is the development of methemoglobinemia after the administration of large doses of prilocaine.[180] A dose-response relationship exists between the amount of prilocaine administered epidurally and the degree of methemoglobinemia; in general, 600-mg doses are required for the development of clinically significant levels of methemoglobin in adults. The metabolism of prilocaine in the liver results in the formation of O-toluidine, which is responsible for the oxidation of hemoglobin to methemoglobin.[181] The methemoglobinemia associated with the use of prilocaine is spontaneously reversible or may be treated by the intravenous administration of methylene blue. With increased use of EMLA (which contains prilocaine) in neonates and young infants, there has been concern regarding the risk of methemoglobinemia.[182] Standard dosing of EMLA in term newborns produced minimal amounts of methemoglobin, and EMLA should be regarded as very safe in the great majority of newborns. Risk may be increased in rare newborns made more susceptible by metabolic disorders and concomitant administration of other drugs that impair the reduction of methemoglobin.[182]

Allergies

Although patients receiving local anesthetics may experience a range of local and systemic symptoms, prospective studies indicate that very few of these reactions are confirmed as allergic reactions.[183] Aminoester drugs such as procaine may produce allergic-type reactions.[184] These drugs are derivatives of p-aminobenzoic acid, which is known to be allergenic. Aminoamide local anesthetics are not derivatives of p-aminobenzoic acid, and allergic reactions to these drugs are extremely rare. Although the aminoamide anesthetics appear to be relatively free of allergic-type reactions, solutions of these drugs may contain a preservative, methylparaben, whose chemical structure is similar to that of p-aminobenzoic acid. Contamination of vials with latex antigen has been suspected in some allergic reactions, although such contamination has been difficult to confirm.[185] In the very rare patient for whom confirmed allergy to both aminoamides and aminoesters precludes their use for spinal anesthesia, meperidine can be considered as an alternative.[186]

Local Tissue Toxicity

All the clinically used aminoamide and aminoester local anesthetics can produce direct toxicity to nerves if they achieve sufficiently high intraneural concentrations. Conversely, in the great majority of clinical applications, no damage to nerves occurs. Although local anesthetics are usually packaged and injected at concentrations well above their physiologically effective range, in the process of delivery they are usually diluted sufficiently that no harm is done. If such dilution does not occur, however, long-term or permanent neural deficits do result. Thus, the application of 5% (200 mM) lidocaine in viscous, dense solutions through narrow intrathecal catheters has been associated with a high frequency of cases of cauda equina syndrome.[187] Laboratory investigations have shown that such high concentrations of local anesthetics alone applied directly to bare nerve fibers produce irreversible conduction block in less than 5 minutes.[188] Indeed, previous studies on ensheathed peripheral nerves in vivo had shown neurologic and histologic changes after infiltration of the space surrounding the nerve with local anesthetics at concentrations as low as 1% to 2%. Clinicians should be aware that the concentrations of formulated local anesthetic solutions are neurotoxic per se and that dilution of them, in situ or in tissue, is essential for safe use.

Concentrations of lidocaine required to produce irreversible conduction blockade in isolated desheathed peripheral nerves slightly overlap the concentrations used clinically (e.g., 2%), but these concentrations are applied clinically to ensheathed nerve in situ embedded in drug-absorbing tissue. Irreversible block in desheathed nerve by lidocaine has a threshold of 20 mM (0.5%) and a 50% effective concentration (EC_{50}) of 45 mM (1.1%) versus an EC_{50} of 1 mM for reversible impulse blockade in vivo.[189] The intrathecal administration of tetracaine or etidocaine in rabbits resulted in histopathologic spinal cord changes after the use of 2% tetracaine, which exceeds the maximum concentration of 1% used for spinal anesthesia in humans.[190]

In the late 1970s and early 1980s, prolonged sensory and motor deficits were reported in some patients after the epidural or subarachnoid injection of large doses of chloroprocaine.[191,192] Studies in animals have proved somewhat contradictory regarding the potential neurotoxicity of chloroprocaine.[193-198] The results of these studies suggest that the combination of low pH, sodium bisulfite, and inadvertent intrathecal dosing is responsible in part for the neurotoxic reactions observed after the use of large amounts of chloroprocaine solution. Chloroprocaine itself at high concentrations may also be neurotoxic,[198] but these concentrations are not achieved during properly positioned epidural anesthesia. The currently available commercial solutions of chloroprocaine do not contain sodium bisulfite. Sodium bisulfite was initially replaced by ethyleneglycoltetraacetic acid (EGTA), a preservative and high-affinity calcium chelator that was occasionally reported to cause local muscle spasm after

epidural administration. More recently, chloroprocaine has become available in an entirely preservative-free preparation. Chloroprocaine has unique utility in situations in which rapid plasma clearance is required to prevent excessive systemic accumulation of local anesthetic. Chloroprocaine has been administered by epidural infusion in young infants in settings in which lidocaine and bupivacaine could not provide an effective therapeutic index.[117]

Concern regarding local anesthetic–associated neurotoxicity was increased after studies of continuous spinal anesthesia administered by microcatheter.[187] In a number of patients in these initial studies, transient or longer-term radicular irritation or, in some cases, cauda equina syndrome developed. Investigations suggested that microcatheters may facilitate localized injection of high concentrations of drug that are inadequately dispersed and diluted in cerebrospinal fluid, thereby leading to high intraneural drug concentrations around the sacral roots and subsequent toxicity.

Related investigations showed that single-shot spinal anesthesia with commonly recommended doses and concentrations of local anesthetics can produce more limited and transient neurologic symptoms (back pain, paresthesias, radicular pain, or hypoesthesia).[199-202] Transient neurologic symptoms have since been observed with many different local anesthetics. Some studies have found that mepivacaine and lidocaine at a range of dilutions cause more frequent symptoms than bupivacaine does. The risk of transient neurologic symptoms after spinal anesthesia was not diminished by dilution of lidocaine from 5% to 1-2%. Differences in study design, method of questioning, and criteria for inclusion may be partially responsible for differences in the prevalence of radicular sequelae in different studies. Despite these differences in study design, a recent meta-analysis concluded that the pooled relative risk for transient neurologic symptoms after spinal anesthesia with lidocaine was 6.7-fold higher than with bupivacaine and 5.5-fold higher than with prilocaine.[203] The addition of vasoconstrictors to local anesthetic solutions may also increase the risk.[204] Neurotoxicity appears to be unrelated to conduction block per se because tetrodotoxin, a highly potent blocker of sodium channels, can produce intense conduction blockade without histologic or behavioral signs of nerve injury.[205]

Intraoperative positioning also appears to be a risk factor. Patients undergoing surgery in the lithotomy position seem to have an increased risk for neurologic symptoms after either spinal or epidural anesthesia. It is unknown at present why this association produces increased risk; nerve compression or stretch or reduced perfusion pressure in the vasa nervorum may possibly exacerbate toxicity from local anesthetics. The lithotomy position per se can produce neurologic sequelae and lower extremity compartment syndromes, particularly with prolonged surgery and use of the Trendelenburg position.[206-208]

Skeletal muscle changes have been observed after the intramuscular injection of local anesthetics such as lidocaine, mepivacaine, prilocaine, bupivacaine, and etidocaine.[209-211] In general, the more potent, longer-acting agents bupivacaine and etidocaine appear to cause more localized skeletal muscle damage than do the less potent, shorter-acting drugs lidocaine and prilocaine. This effect on skeletal muscle is reversible, and muscle regeneration occurs rapidly and is complete within 2 weeks after the injection of local anesthetics. Furthermore, such skeletal muscle processes have not been associated with overt signs of local irritation and probably cannot account for the transient neurologic syndromes.

Prolonged Infusions of Local Anesthetics, Tachyphylaxis, and Development of Long-Duration Local Anesthetics
(see also Chapters 72 and 73)

Local anesthetics are increasingly being administered by continuous infusion for several days after surgery or for periods of weeks to months for the treatment of chronic malignant and nonmalignant pain. With prolonged infusions, there is potential for delayed systemic accumulation and toxicity. Continuous infusions of bupivacaine of up to 30 mg/hr in adults for up to 2 weeks produced no overt CNS or cardiac toxicity despite total plasma bupivacaine concentrations in the range of 2 to 5 µg/mL in several patients.[212]

Apparent reductions in the effectiveness of local anesthetic infusions may be due to a number of causes unrelated to tolerance per se, including dislodgement of epidural catheters and changes in the dermatomal origin or intensity of nociceptive input. In obstetric patients receiving epidural bolus injections, recurrence of pain before the next injection resulted in a reduction in the intensity and duration of blockade, whereas repeat injection before the return of pain prevented this rapidly occurring form of tolerance, or tachyphylaxis.[73] In postoperative patients, the coadministration of systemic opioids prevented regression of segmental blockade in patients receiving thoracic epidural bupivacaine infusions.[213] Studies in rats suggest that both pharmacokinetic and pharmacodynamic mechanisms are involved. In a rat model, tachyphylaxis was linked to the development of hyperalgesia,[214] and drugs that inhibited hyperalgesia, including N-methyl-D-aspartate receptor antagonists[215] and nitric oxide synthase inhibitors,[216] also prevented tachyphylaxis. Conversely, repeated sciatic injections of lidocaine produced reduced intraneural lidocaine content along with a reduced duration of block.[99]

Several methods are under investigation to produce long-duration nerve blockade. Liposomal encapsulation can prolong blockade, depending on the dose and the physical properties of the liposome (surface charge, size, lamellar structure).[217,218] Local anesthetics can be incorporated into biodegradable polymer microspheres for sustained release. These preparations produce peripheral nerve block in animal models[219] ranging from 2 to 8 days, depending on the dose, site, and species.[220] Prolonged-duration local anesthesia also appears to be feasible with the use of site 1 sodium channel toxins in combination with either local anesthetics or adrenergics.[221] Other drugs have been examined for use as local anesthetics, including tricyclic antidepressants.[222]

It remains to be determined whether local anesthetics with prolonged duration will receive widespread use in clinical practice. If they prove safe and effective, they may have potential use in intercostal blockade and wound infiltration, particularly for surgery on the thorax and abdomen, where protective sensation is comparatively less important than for limb surgery. If drugs can be developed that last for weeks or longer, they may have additional applications in the management of chronic pain and cancer pain.

KEY POINTS

1. Local anesthetics block voltage-gated sodium channels by interrupting the initiation and propagation of impulses in axons, but they have a wide variety of other biologic actions, both desirable and undesirable.

2. The currently available local anesthetics are of two chemical classes: aminoesters and aminoamides.

3. The low potency and lack of specificity of the available local anesthetics are due in part to the structural constraint that they must have high solubility and diffuse rapidly in both aqueous environments and the lipid phases of biologic membranes.

4. Reversible protonation of the tertiary amine group makes local anesthetics uncharged at basic pH and charged at acid pH; the base forms are more soluble in lipid environments, whereas the acid forms are more soluble in aqueous environments.

5. Aminoesters are primarily metabolized by plasma esterases; aminoamides are metabolized primarily by hepatic cytochrome P450–linked enzymes.

6. The principal systemic toxicities of local anesthetics involve the heart (including atrioventricular conduction block, arrhythmias, myocardial depression, and cardiac arrest) and the brain (including irritability, lethargy, seizures, and generalized CNS depression). Hypoxemia and acidosis exacerbate these toxicities. Resuscitation after bupivacaine overdose is particularly difficult. Therefore, prevention of intravascular injection or overdose is crucial, and major nerve blockade should involve incremental, fractionated dosing.

7. Local anesthetics are directly toxic to nerve at the concentrations supplied in commercial solutions. Intraneural concentrations during regional anesthesia are generally (but not always) below the threshold for toxicity because of spread of solutions through tissues and diffusion gradients from injection sites into nerve. Injection into a constrained tissue space increases the risk of local toxicity.

8. Optimal use of local anesthetics in regional anesthesia requires an understanding of the individual patient's clinical situation; the location, intensity, and duration of regional anesthesia and analgesia required; anatomic factors affecting the deposition of drug near nerves; proper drug selection and dosing; and ongoing assessment of clinical effects after administration of local anesthetics.

9. Recent efforts have led to the development of several new formulations for topical anesthesia. Single-stereoisomer (as opposed to a racemic mixture) formulations have been developed in an effort to reduce systemic toxicity and improve sensory selectivity.

10. Local anesthetics are increasingly being used for postoperative infusion and local and systemic administration in the management of chronic pain. Further research and development may lead to safe, more selective agents that can facilitate more prolonged administration in the setting of acute or chronic pain.

REFERENCES

1. Sanchez V, Arthur GR, Strichartz GR: Fundamental properties of local anesthetics. I. The dependence of lidocaine's ionization and octanol:buffer partitioning on solvent and temperature. Anesth Analg 66:159-165, 1987.
2. Sanchez V, Ferrante F, Cibotti N, et al: Partitioning of tetracaine base and cation into phospholipid membranes: Relevance to anesthetic potency. Reg Anesth 13(Suppl):81, 1988.
3. Gissen AJ, Covino BG, Gregus J: Differential sensitivities of mammalian nerve fibers to local anesthetic agents. Anesthesiology 53:467-474, 1980.
4. Courtney KR: Structure-activity relations for frequency-dependent sodium channel block in nerve by local anesthetics. J Pharmacol Exp Ther 213:114-119, 1980.
5. Courtney K, Strichartz G: Structural elements which determine local anesthetic activity. In Strichartz G (ed): Handbook of Experimental Pharmacology: Local Anesthetics. Heidelberg, Springer-Verlag, 1987, p 53.
6. Schreier S, Frezzatti WA Jr, Araujo PS, et al: Effect of lipid membranes on the apparent pK of the local anesthetic tetracaine. Spin label and titration studies. Biochim Biophys Acta 769:231-237, 1984.
7. Ritchie JM, Rogart RB: Density of sodium channels in mammalian myelinated nerve fibers and nature of the axonal membrane under the myelin sheath. Proc Natl Acad Sci U S A 74:211-215, 1977.
8. Hodgkin A: The Conduction of the Nervous Impulse. Springfield, IL, Charles C Thomas, 1964.
9. Hille B: Ionic Channels of Excitable Membranes. Sunderland, MA, Sinauer Associates, 1991.
10. Skou J: Enzymatic basis for active transport of Na$^+$ and K$^+$ across cell membrane. Physiol Rev 45:596-617, 1965.
11. Rushton W: A theory of the effects of fibre size in medullated nerve. J Physiol (Lond) 115:101, 1951.
12. Tasaki I: Nervous Transmission. Springfield, IL, Charles C Thomas, 1953.
13. Condouris GA, Goebel RH, Brady T: Computer simulation of local anesthetic effects using a mathematical model of myelinated nerve. J Pharmacol Exp Ther 196:737-745, 1976.
14. Trevan J, Boock E: The relation of hydrogen ion concentration to the action of local anesthetics. Br J Exp Pathol 8:307, 1927.
15. Ritchie JM, Ritchie B, Greengard P: The effect of the nerve sheath on the action of local anesthetics. J Pharmacol Exp Ther 150:160-164, 1965.
16. Hille B: The pH-dependent rate of action of local anesthetics on the node of Ranvier. J Gen Physiol 69:475-496, 1977.
17. Narahashi T, Frazier T, Yamada M: The site of action and active form of local anesthetics. I. Theory and pH experiments with tertiary compounds. J Pharmacol Exp Ther 171:32-44, 1970.
18. Frazier DT, Narahashi T, Yamada M: The site of action and active form of local anesthetics. II. Experiments with quaternary compounds. J Pharmacol Exp Ther 171:45-51, 1970.
19. Strichartz GR: The inhibition of sodium currents in myelinated nerve by quaternary derivatives of lidocaine. J Gen Physiol 62:37-57, 1973.
20. Hille B: Local anesthetics: Hydrophilic and hydrophobic pathways for the drug-receptor reaction. J Gen Physiol 69:497-515, 1977.
21. Ritchie JM, Ritchie BR: Local anesthetics: Effect of pH on activity. Science 162:1394-1395, 1968.
22. Chernoff DM, Strichartz GR: Tonic and phasic block of neuronal sodium currents by 5-hydroxyhexano-2',6'-xylide, a neutral lidocaine homologue. J Gen Physiol 93:1075-1090, 1989.
23. Ulbricht W: Kinetics of drug action and equilibrium results at the node of Ranvier. Physiol Rev 61:785-828, 1981.
24. Courtney KR, Kendig JJ, Cohen EN: The rates of interaction of local anesthetics with sodium channels in nerve. J Pharmacol Exp Ther 207:594-604, 1978.
25. Chernoff D: Kinetics of Anesthetic Binding to Sodium Channels: Role of pKa. Boston, Massachusetts Institute of Technology, 1988.
26. Gokin AP, Philip B, Strichartz GR: Preferential block of small myelinated sensory and motor fibers by lidocaine: In vivo electrophysiology in the rat sciatic nerve. Anesthesiology 95:1441-1454, 2001.
27. Brzezinski MR, Spink BJ, Dean RA, et al: Human liver carboxylesterase hCE-1: Binding specificity for cocaine, heroin, and their metabolites and analogs. Drug Metab Dispos 25:1089-1096, 1997.
28. Pindel EV, Kedishvili NY, Abraham TL, et al: Purification and cloning of a broad substrate specificity human liver carboxylesterase that catalyzes the hydrolysis of cocaine and heroin. J Biol Chem 272:14769-14775, 1997.
29. Bokesch PM, Post C, Strichartz G: Structure-activity relationship of lidocaine homologs producing tonic and frequency-dependent impulse blockade in nerve. J Pharmacol Exp Ther 237:773-781, 1986.
30. Wildsmith JA, Gissen AJ, Gregus J, et al: Differential nerve blocking activity of amino-ester local anaesthetics. Br J Anaesth 57:612-620, 1985.
31. Wildsmith JA, Gissen AJ, Takman B, et al: Differential nerve blockade: Esters v. amides and the influence of pKa. Br J Anaesth 59:379-384, 1987.
32. Gissen AJ, Covino BG, Gregus J: Differential sensitivity of fast and slow fibers in mammalian nerve. III. Effect of etidocaine and bupivacaine on fast/slow fibers. Anesth Analg 61:570-575, 1982.
33. Scott DB, McClure JH, Giasi RM, et al: Effects of concentration of local anaesthetic drugs in extradural block. Br J Anaesth 52:1033-1037, 1980.
34. Rosenberg PH, Heinonen E, Jansson SE, et al: Differential nerve block by bupivacaine and 2-chloroprocaine. An experimental study. Br J Anaesth 52:1183-1189, 1980.
35. Galindo A, Benavides O, De Munos SO, et al: Comparison of anesthetic solutions used in lumbar and caudal peridural anesthesia. Anesth Analg 57:175-179, 1978.
36. Covino BG: Pharmacology of local anaesthetic agents. Br J Anaesth 58:701-716, 1986.
37. Johns RA, DiFazio CA, Longnecker DE: Lidocaine constricts or dilates rat arterioles in a dose-dependent manner. Anesthesiology 62:141-144, 1985.
38. Johns RA, Seyde WC, DiFazio CA, et al: Dose-dependent effects of bupivacaine on rat muscle arterioles. Anesthesiology 65:186-191, 1986.
39. Iida H, Watanabe Y, Dohi S, et al: Direct effects of ropivacaine and bupivacaine on spinal pial vessels in canine. Assessment with closed spinal window technique. Anesthesiology 87:75-81, 1997.
40. Sinclair CJ, Scott DB: Comparison of bupivacaine and etidocaine in extradural blockade. Br J Anaesth 56:147-153, 1984.
41. Fink BR, Cairns AM: Differential slowing and block of conduction by lidocaine in individual afferent myelinated and unmyelinated axons. Anesthesiology 60:111-120, 1984.
42. Fink BR, Cairns AM: Lack of size-related differential sensitivity to equilibrium conduction block among mammalian

myelinated axons exposed to lidocaine. Anesth Analg 66:948-953, 1987.

43. Fink BR: 1992 Labat Lecture. Toward the mathematization of spinal anesthesia. Reg Anesth 17:263-273, 1992.

44. Raymond SA, Steffensen SC, Gugino LD, et al: The role of length of nerve exposed to local anesthetics in impulse blocking action. Anesth Analg 68:563-570, 1989.

45. Braid DP, Scott DB: The systemic absorption of local analgesic drugs. Br J Exp Anaesth 37:394-404, 1965.

46. Drachman D, Strichartz G: Potassium channel blockers potentiate impulse inhibition by local anesthetics. Anesthesiology 75:1051-1061, 1991.

47. Kocsis J: Functional characteristics of potassium channels of normal and pathological mammalian axons. *In* Ritchie J, Keynes R, Bolis L (eds): Ion Channels in Neural Membranes. New York, Alan R Liss, 1986, p 123.

48. Hogan QH, Abram SE: Neural blockade for diagnosis and prognosis. A review. Anesthesiology 86:216-241, 1997.

49. Littlewood D, Buckley P, Covino B, et al: Comparative study of various local anaesthetic solutions in extradural block in labour. Br J Anaesth 51:475, 1979.

50. Erdemir H, Soper L, Sweet R: Studies of factors affecting peridural anesthesia. Anesth Analg 44:400, 1965.

51. Moore DC, Batra MS: The components of an effective test dose prior to epidural block. Anesthesiology 55:693-696, 1981.

52. Concepcion M, Maddi R, Francis D, et al: Vasoconstrictors in spinal anesthesia with tetracaine—a comparison of epinephrine and phenylephrine. Anesth Analg 63:134-138, 1984.

53. Swerdlow M, Jones R: The duration of action of bupivacaine, prilocaine and lignocaine. Br J Anaesth 42:335-339, 1970.

54. Albert J, Lofstrom B: Bilateral ulnar nerve blocks for the evaluation of local anesthetic agents. 3. Tests with a new agent, prilocaine, and with lidocaine in solutions with and without epinephrine. Acta Anaesthesiol Scand 9:203-211, 1965.

55. Eisenach JC, Grice SC, Dewan DM: Epinephrine enhances analgesia produced by epidural bupivacaine during labor. Anesth Analg 66:447-451, 1987.

56. Eisenach JC, Lysak SZ, Viscomi CM: Epidural clonidine analgesia following surgery: Phase I. Anesthesiology 71:640-646, 1989.

57. Gissen A, Covino B: Differential sensitivity of fast and slow fibres in mammalian nerve. IV. Effect of carbonation of local anesthetics. Reg Anesth 10:68, 1985.

58. Bokesch PM, Raymond SA, Strichartz GR: Dependence of lidocaine potency on pH and PCO_2. Anesth Analg 66:9-17, 1987.

59. Wong K, Strichartz GR, Raymond SA: On the mechanisms of potentiation of local anesthetics by bicarbonate buffer: Drug structure-activity studies on isolated peripheral nerve. Anesth Analg 76:131-143, 1993.

60. Morison DH: A double-blind comparison of carbonated lidocaine and lidocaine hydrochloride in epidural anaesthesia. Can Anaesth Soc J 28:387-389, 1981.

61. Nickel P, Bromage PR, Sherrill D: Comparison of hydrochloride and carbonated salts of lidocaine for epidural analgesia. Reg Anesth 11:62, 1986.

62. Hilgier M: Alkalinization of bupivacaine for brachial plexus block. Reg Anesth 10:59, 1985.

63. DiFazio CA, Carron H, Grosslight KR, et al: Comparison of pH-adjusted lidocaine solutions for epidural anesthesia. Anesth Analg 65:760-764, 1986.

64. Bedder MD, Kozody R, Craig DB: Comparison of bupivacaine and alkalinized bupivacaine in brachial plexus anesthesia. Anesth Analg 67:48-52, 1988.

65. Cunningham NL, Kaplan JA: A rapid-onset, long-acting regional anesthetic technique. Anesthesiology 41:509-511, 1974.

66. Cohen SE, Thurlow A: Comparison of a chloroprocaine-bupivacaine mixture with chloroprocaine and bupivacaine used individually for obstetric epidural analgesia. Anesthesiology 51:288-292, 1979.

67. Badgwell JM, Heavner JE, Kytta J: Cardiovascular and central nervous system effects of co-administered lidocaine and bupivacaine in piglets. Reg Anesth 16:89-94, 1991.

68. Bromage PR: Spread of analgesic solutions in the epidural space and their site of action. Br J Anaesth 34:161-178, 1962.

69. Fagraeus L, Urban BJ, Bromage PR: Spread of epidural analgesia in early pregnancy. Anesthesiology 58:184-187, 1983.

70. Popitz-Bergez FA, Leeson S, Thalhammer JG, et al: Intraneural lidocaine uptake compared with analgesic differences between pregnant and nonpregnant rats. Reg Anesth 22:363-371, 1997.

71. Morris R, McKay W, Mushlin P: Comparison of pain associated with intradermal and subcutaneous infiltration with various local anesthetic solutions. Anesth Analg 66:1180-1182, 1987.

72. McKay W, Morris R, Mushlin P: Sodium bicarbonate attenuates pain on skin infiltration with lidocaine, with or without epinephrine. Anesth Analg 66:572-574, 1987.

73. Bromage PR, Pettigrew RT, Crowell DE: Tachyphylaxis in epidural analgesia: I. Augmentation and decay of local anesthesia. J Clin Pharmacol 9:30-38, 1969.

74. Harris WH, Slater EM, Bell HM: Regional anesthesia by the intravenous route. JAMA 194:1273-1276, 1965.

75. Albright GA: Cardiac arrest following regional anesthesia with etidocaine or bupivacaine. Anesthesiology 51:285-287, 1979.

76. Reiestad F, Stromskag KE: Interpleural catheter in management of post-operative pain: A preliminary report. Reg Anesth 11:89, 1986.

77. Brismar B, Pettersson N, Tokics L, et al: Postoperative analgesia with intrapleural administration of bupivacaine-adrenaline. Acta Anaesthesiol Scand 31:515-520, 1987.

78. Stromskag KE, Reiestad F, Holmqvist EL, et al: Intrapleural administration of 0.25%, 0.375%, and 0.5% bupivacaine with epinephrine after cholecystectomy. Anesth Analg 67:430-434, 1988.

79. Rosenberg PH, Scheinin BM, Lepantalo MJ, et al: Continuous intrapleural infusion of bupivacaine for analgesia after thoracotomy. Anesthesiology 67:811-813, 1987.

80. Bromage PR, Gertel M: An evaluation of two new local anaesthetics for major conduction blockade. Can Anaesth Soc J 17:557-564, 1970.

81. Dalens B, Vanneuville G, Tanguy A: Comparison of the fascia iliaca compartment block with the 3-in-1 block in children. Anesth Analg 69:705-713, 1989.

82. Rocco A, Mallampati S, Boon J, et al: Double blind evaluation of intrathecal bupivacaine and tetracaine. Reg Anesth 9:183, 1984.

83. Bigler D, Hjortso NC, Edstrom H, et al: Comparative effects of intrathecal bupivacaine and tetracaine on analgesia, cardiovascular function and plasma catecholamines. Act Anaesthesiol Scand 30:199-203, 1986.

84. Concepcion MA, Lambert DH, Welch KA, et al: Tourniquet pain during spinal anesthesia: A comparison of plain solutions of tetracaine and bupivacaine. Anesth Analg 67:828-832, 1988.

85. Stewart A, Lambert DH, Concepcion MA, et al: Decreased incidence of tourniquet pain during spinal anesthesia with bupivacaine. A possible explanation. Anesth Analg 67:833-837, 1988.

86. Chambers WA, Littlewood DG, Logan MR, et al: Effect of added epinephrine on spinal anesthesia with lidocaine. Anesth Analg 60:417-420, 1981.

87. Chambers WA, Littlewood DG, Scott DB: Spinal anesthesia with hyperbaric bupivacaine: Effect of added vasoconstrictors. Anesth Analg 61:49-52, 1982.

88. Evers H, von Dardel O, Juhlin L, et al: Dermal effects of compositions based on the eutectic mixture of lignocaine and prilocaine (EMLA). Studies in volunteers. Br J Anaesth 57:997-1005, 1985.

89. Hallen B, Uppfeldt A: Does lidocaine-prilocaine cream permit pain free insertion of IV catheters in children? Anesthesiology 57:340-342, 1982.

90. Ohlsen L, Englesson S, Evers H: An anaesthetic lidocaine/prilocaine cream (EMLA) for epicutaneous application tested for cutting split skin grafts. Scand J Plast Reconstr Surg 19:201-209, 1985.

91. Butler-O'Hara M, LeMoine C, Guillet R: Analgesia for neonatal circumcision: A randomized controlled trial of EMLA cream versus dorsal penile nerve block. Pediatrics 101:E5, 1998.

92. Browne J, Awad I, Plant R, et al: Topical amethocaine (Ametop) is superior to EMLA for intravenous cannulation. Eutectic mixture of local anesthetics. Can J Anaesth 46:1014-1018, 1999.

93. Bonadio WA, Wagner V: TAC (tetracaine, adrenaline, cocaine) for the repair of minor dermal lacerations. Pediatr Emerg Care 4:82, 1988.

94. Bonadio WA: TAC: A review. Pediatr Emerg Care 5:128-130, 1989.

95. Smith GA, Strausbaugh SD, Harbeck-Weber C, et al: New non–cocaine-containing topical anesthetics compared with tetracaine-adrenaline-cocaine during repair of lacerations. Pediatrics 100:825-830, 1997.

96. Choi RH, Birknes JK, Popitz-Bergez FA, et al: Pharmacokinetic nature of tachyphylaxis to lidocaine: Peripheral nerve blocks and infiltration anesthesia in rats. Life Sci 61:PL177-PL84, 1997.

97. Araujo MC, Sinnott CJ, Strichartz GR: Multiple phases of relief from experimental mechanical allodynia by systemic lidocaine: Responses to early and late infusions. Pain 103:21-29, 2003.

98. Covino B: Pharmacokinetics of local anesthetic drugs. In Prys-Roberts C, Hug CJ (eds): Pharmacokinetics of Anesthesia. Oxford, Blackwell Scientific, 1984, p 202.

99. Covino B, Vassallo H: Local Anesthetics: Mechanisms of Action and Clinical Use. Orlando, FL, Grune & Stratton, 1976.

100. Abdel-Salam AR, Vonwiller JB, Scott DB: Evaluation of etidocaine in extradural block. Br J Anaesth 47:1081-1086, 1975.

101. Wildsmith JA, Tucker GT, Cooper S, et al: Plasma concentrations of local anaesthetics after interscalene brachial plexus block. Br J Anaesth 49:461-466, 1977.

102. Tucker GT, Mather LE: Pharmacology of local anaesthetic agents. Pharmacokinetics of local anaesthetic agents. Br J Anaesth 47:213-224, 1975.

103. Tucker GT, Mather LE: Clinical pharmacokinetics of local anesthetics. Clin Pharmacokinet 4:241-278, 1979.

104. Tucker GT: Pharmacokinetics of local anesthetics. Br J Anaesth 58:717-731, 1986.

105. Lofstrom JB, Alm BE, Bertler A, et al: Lung uptake of lidocaine [proceedings]. Acta Anaesthesiol Scand Suppl 70:80-82, 1978.

106. Lofstrom JB: Tissue distribution of local anesthetics with special reference to the lung. Int Anesthesiol Clin 16:53-71, 1978.

107. Strichartz GR, Sanchez V, Arthur GR, et al: Fundamental properties of local anesthetics. II. Measured octanol:buffer partition coefficients and pKa values of clinically used drugs. Anesth Analg 71:158-170, 1990.

108. Boyes RN: A review of the metabolism of amide local anaesthetic agents. Br J Anaesth 47:225-230, 1975.

109. Tucker GT, Wiklund L, Berlin-Wahlen A, et al: Hepatic clearance of local anesthetics in man. J Pharmacokinet Biopharm 5:111-122, 1977.

110. Nation RL, Triggs EJ, Selig M: Lignocaine kinetics in cardiac patients and aged subjects. Br J Clin Pharmacol 4:439-448, 1977.

111. Mazoit J, Denson D, Samii K: Pharmacokinetics of bupivacaine following caudal anesthesia in infants [abstract]. Anesthesiology 63:A465, 1992.

112. Yaster M, Aronoff D, Kornhauser D, et al: The pharmacokinetics of lidocaine during caudal anesthesia in children [abstract]. Anesthesiology 63:A465, 1985.

113. Agarwal R, Gutlove DP, Lockhart CH: Seizures occurring in pediatric patients receiving continuous infusion of bupivacaine. Anesth Analg 75:284-286, 1992.

114. McCloskey JJ, Haun SE, Deshpande JK: Bupivacaine toxicity secondary to continuous caudal epidural infusion in children. Anesth Analg 75:287-290, 1992.

115. Berde CB: Convulsions associated with pediatric regional anesthesia. Anesth Analg 75:164-166, 1992.

116. Larsson BA, Lonnqvist PA, Olsson GL: Plasma concentrations of bupivacaine in neonates after continuous epidural infusion. Anesth Analg 84:501-505, 1997.

117. Henderson K, Sethna NF, Berde CB: Continuous caudal anesthesia for inguinal hernia repair in former preterm infants. J Clin Anesth 5:129-133, 1993.

118. Stenson RE, Constantino RT, Harrison DC: Interrelationships of hepatic blood flow, cardiac output, and blood levels of lidocaine in man. Circulation 43:205-211, 1971.

119. Thomson PD, Melmon KL, Richardson JA, et al: Lidocaine pharmacokinetics in advanced heart failure, liver disease, and renal failure in humans. Ann Intern Med 78:499-508, 1973.

120. Wagman IH, De Jong RH, Prince DA: Effects of lidocaine on the central nervous system. Anesthesiology 28:155-172, 1967.

121. Englesson S: The influence of acid-base changes on central nervous system toxicity of local anaesthetic agents. I. An experimental study in cats. Acta Anaesthesiol Scand 18:79-87, 1974.

122. Scott DB: Evaluation of clinical tolerance of local anaesthetic agents. Br J Anaesth 47:328-331, 1975.

123. Arthur GR, Scott DH, Boyes RN, et al: Pharmacokinetic and clinical pharmacological studies with mepivacaine and prilocaine. Br J Anaesth 51:481-485, 1979.

124. Burney RG, DiFazio CA, Foster JA: Effects of pH on protein binding of lidocaine. Anesth Analg 57:478-480, 1978.

125. Apfelbaum JL, Shaw LM, Gross JB, et al: Modification of lidocaine protein binding with CO_2. Can Anaesth Soc J 32:468-471, 1985.

126. Moller RA, Covino BG: Cardiac electrophysiologic effects of lidocaine and bupivacaine. Anesth Analg 67:107-114, 1988.

127. Clarkson CW, Hondeghem LM: Mechanism for bupivacaine depression of cardiac conduction: Fast block of sodium channels during the action potential with slow recovery from block during diastole. Anesthesiology 62:396-405, 1985.

128. Lynch C 3rd: Depression of myocardial contractility in vitro by bupivacaine, etidocaine, and lidocaine. Anesth Analg 65:551-559, 1986.

129. Block A, Covino B: Effect of local anesthetic agents on cardiac conduction and contractility. Reg Anesth 6:55, 1982.

130. Stewart DD, Rogers WP, Mahaffey JE, et al: Effect of local anesthetics on the cardiovascular system in the dog. Anesthesiology 24:620-624, 1963.

131. Liu P, Feldman H, Covino B, et al: Acute cardiovascular toxicity of procaine, chloroprocaine and tetracaine in anesthetized ventilated dogs. Reg Anesth 7:14, 1982.

132. Liu P, Feldman HS, Covino BM, et al: Acute cardiovascular toxicity of intravenous amide local anesthetics in anesthetized ventilated dogs. Anesth Analg 61:317-322, 1982.

133. Chamberlain BK, Volpe P, Fleischer S: Inhibition of calcium-induced calcium release from purified cardiac sarcoplasmic reticulum vesicles. J Biol Chem 259:7547-7553, 1984.

134. Tanz RD, Heskett T, Loehning RW, et al: Comparative cardiotoxicity of bupivacaine and lidocaine in the isolated perfused mammalian heart. Anesth Analg 63:549-556, 1984.

135. Josephson IR: Lidocaine blocks Na, Ca and K currents of chick ventricular myocytes. J Mol Cell Cardiol 20:593-604, 1988.

136. Blair MR: Cardiovascular pharmacology of local anaesthetics. Br J Anaesth 47:247-252, 1975.

137. MacMillan W: A hypothesis concerning the effect of cocaine on the action of sympathomimetic amines. Br J Pharmacol 14:385, 1959.

138. Lofstrom JB: 1991 Labat Lecture. The effect of local anesthetics on the peripheral vasculature. Reg Anesth 17:1-11, 1992.

139. Rocco AG, Raymond SA, Murray E, et al: Differential spread of blockade of touch, cold, and pinprick during spinal anesthesia. Anesth Analg 64:917-923, 1985.

140. Morishima HO, Pedersen H, Finster M, et al: Bupivacaine toxicity in pregnant and nonpregnant ewes. Anesthesiology 63:134-139, 1985.

141. de Jong RH, Ronfeld RA, DeRosa RA: Cardiovascular effects of convulsant and supraconvulsant doses of amide local anesthetics. Anesth Analg 61:3-9, 1982.

142. Kotelko DM, Shnider SM, Dailey PA, et al: Bupivacaine-induced cardiac arrhythmias in sheep. Anesthesiology 60:10-18, 1984.

143. Kasten G: High serum bupivacaine concentrations produce rhythm disturbances similar to torsades de pointes in anesthetized dogs. Reg Anesth 11:20, 1986.

144. Sage D, Feldman H, Arthur G, et al: The cardiovascular effects of convulsant doses of lidocaine and bupivacaine in the conscious dog. Reg Anesth 10:175, 1985.

145. Reiz S, Nath S: Cardiotoxicity of local anaesthetic agents. Br J Anaesth 58:736-746, 1986.

146. Coyle DE, Sperelakis N: Bupivacaine and lidocaine blockade of calcium-mediated slow action potentials in guinea pig ventricular muscle. J Pharmacol Exp Ther 242:1001-1005, 1987.

147. Heavner JE: Cardiac dysrhythmias induced by infusion of local anesthetics into the lateral cerebral ventricle of cats. Anesth Analg 65:133-138, 1986.

148. Thomas RD, Behbehani MM, Coyle DE, et al: Cardiovascular toxicity of local anesthetics: An alternative hypothesis. Anesth Analg 65:444-450, 1986.

149. Rosen MA, Thigpen JW, Shnider SM, et al: Bupivacaine-induced cardiotoxicity in hypoxic and acidotic sheep. Anesth Analg 64:1089-1096, 1985.

150. Chadwick HS: Toxicity and resuscitation in lidocaine- or bupivacaine-infused cats. Anesthesiology 63:385-390, 1985.

151. Kasten GW, Martin ST: Successful cardiovascular resuscitation after massive intravenous bupivacaine overdosage in anesthetized dogs. Anesth Analg 64:491-497, 1985.

152. Kasten GW, Martin ST: Bupivacaine cardiovascular toxicity: Comparison of treatment with bretylium and lidocaine. Anesth Analg 64:911-916, 1985.

153. Maxwell LG, Martin LD, Yaster M: Bupivacaine-induced cardiac toxicity in neonates: Successful treatment with intravenous phenytoin. Anesthesiology 80:682-686, 1994.

154. Mather LE: Disposition of mepivacaine and bupivacaine enantiomers in sheep. Br J Anaesth 67:239-246, 1991.

155. Rutten AJ, Mather LE, McLean CF: Cardiovascular effects and regional clearances of i.v. bupivacaine in sheep: Enantiomeric analysis. Br J Anaesth 67:247-256, 1991.

156. Bernards CM, Artu AA: Hexamethonium and midazolam terminate dysrhythmias and hypertension caused by intra-cerebroventricular bupivacaine in rabbits. Anesthesiology 74:89-96, 1991.

157. Vanhoutte F, Vereecke J, Verbeke N, et al: Stereoselective effects of the enantiomers of bupivacaine on the electro-physiological properties of the guinea-pig papillary muscle. Br J Pharmacol 103:1275-1281, 1991.

158. Lee-Son S, Wang GK, Concus A, et al: Stereoselective inhibition of neuronal sodium channels by local anesthetics. Evidence for two sites of action? Anesthesiology 77:324-335, 1992.

159. Wang GK: Binding affinity and stereoselectivity of local anesthetics in single batrachotoxin-activated Na+ channels. J Gen Physiol 96:1105-1127, 1990.

160. Arlock P: Actions of three local anaesthetics: Lidocaine, bupivacaine and ropivacaine on guinea pig papillary muscle sodium channels (Vmax). Pharmacol Toxicol 63:96-104, 1988.

161. Pitkanen M, Feldman HS, Arthur GR, et al: Chronotropic and inotropic effects of ropivacaine, bupivacaine, and lidocaine in the spontaneously beating and electrically paced isolated, perfused rabbit heart. Reg Anesth 17:183-192, 1992.

162. Moller R, Covino BG: Cardiac electrophysiologic properties of bupivacaine and lidocaine compared with those of ropivacaine, a new amide local anesthetic. Anesthesiology 72:322-329, 1990.

163. Hickey R, Hoffman J, Ramamurthy S: A comparison of ropivacaine 0.5% and bupivacaine 0.5% for brachial plexus block. Anesthesiology 74:639-642, 1991.

164. Brown DL, Carpenter RL, Thompson GE: Comparison of 0.5% ropivacaine and 0.5% bupivacaine for epidural anesthesia in patients undergoing lower-extremity surgery. Anesthesiology 72:633-636, 1990.

165. Kerkkamp HE, Gielen MJ, Edstrom HH: Comparison of 0.75% ropivacaine with epinephrine and 0.75% bupivacaine with epinephrine in lumbar epidural anesthesia. Reg Anesth 15:204-207, 1990.

166. Katz JA, Knarr D, Bridenbaugh PO: A double-blind comparison of 0.5% bupivacaine and 0.75% ropivacaine administered epidurally in humans. Reg Anesth 15:250-252, 1990.

167. Feldman HS, Covino BG: Comparative motor-blocking effects of bupivacaine and ropivacaine, a new amino amide local anesthetic, in the rat and dog. Anesth Analg 67:1047-1052, 1988.

168. Nolte H, Fruhstorfer H, Edstrom HH: Local anesthetic efficacy of ropivacaine (LEA 103) in ulnar nerve block. Reg Anesth 15:118-124, 1990.

169. Kohane DS, Sankar WN, Shubina M, et al: Sciatic nerve blockade in infant, adolescent, and adult rats: A comparison of ropivacaine with bupivacaine. Anesthesiology 89:1199-1208, discussion 10A, 1998.

170. Feldman HS, Arthur GR, Covino BG: Comparative systemic toxicity of convulsant and supraconvulsant doses of intravenous ropivacaine, bupivacaine, and lidocaine in the conscious dog. Anesth Analg 69:794-801, 1989.

171. Rutten AJ, Nancarrow C, Mather LE, et al: Hemodynamic and central nervous system effects of intravenous bolus doses of lidocaine, bupivacaine, and ropivacaine in sheep. Anesth Analg 69:291-299, 1989.

172. Lerman J, Nolan J, Eyres R, et al: Efficacy, safety, and pharmacokinetics of levobupivacaine with and without fentanyl after continuous epidural infusion in children: A multicenter trial. Anesthesiology 99:1166-1174, 2003.

173. Feldman HS, Arthur GR, Pitkanen M, et al: Treatment of acute systemic toxicity after the rapid intravenous injection of ropivacaine and bupivacaine in the conscious dog. Anesth Analg 73:373-384, 1991.

174. Arthur GR, Feldman HS, Covino BG: Comparative pharmacokinetics of bupivacaine and ropivacaine, a new amide local anesthetic. Anesth Analg 67:1053-1058, 1988.

175. Santos AC, Pedersen H, Harmon TW, et al: Does pregnancy alter the systemic toxicity of local anesthetics? Anesthesiology 70:991-995, 1989.

176. Sage DJ, Feldman HS, Arthur GR, et al: Influence of lidocaine and bupivacaine on isolated guinea pig atria in the presence of acidosis and hypoxia. Anesth Analg 63:1-7, 1984.

177. Moore DC, Crawford RD, Scurlock JE: Severe hypoxia and acidosis following local anesthetic–induced convulsions. Anesthesiology 53:259-260, 1980.

178. Caplan RA, Ward RJ, Posner K, et al: Unexpected cardiac arrest during spinal anesthesia: A closed claims analysis of predisposing factors. Anesthesiology 68:5-11, 1988.

179. Gelfin B, Shapiro L: Sinus bradycardia and asystole during spinal and epidural anesthesia: A report of 13 cases. J Clin Anesth 10:278-285, 1998.

180. Lund PC, Cwik JC: Propitocaine (Citanest) and methemoglobinemia. Anesthesiology 26:569-571, 1965.

181. Hjelm M, Holmdahl M: Biochemical effects of aromatic amines. II. Cyanosis, methaemoglobinaemia and Heinz-body formation induced by a local anaesthetic agent (prilocaine). Acta Anaesthesiol Scand 2:99-120, 1965.

182. Taddio A, Stevens B, Craig K, et al: Efficacy and safety of lidocaine-prilocaine cream for pain during circumcision. N Engl J Med 336:1197-1201, 1997.

183. Baluga JC, Casamayou R, Carozzi E, et al: Allergy to local anaesthetics in dentistry. Myth or reality? Allergol Immunopathol 30:14-19, 2002.

184. Sidhu SK, Shaw S, Wilkinson JD: A 19-year retrospective study on benzocaine allergy in the United Kingdom. Am J Contact Dermat 10:57-61, 1999.

185. Shojaei AR, Haas DA: Local anesthetic cartridges and latex allergy: A literature review. J Can Dent Assoc 68:622-626, 2002.

186. Norris MC, Honet JE, Leighton BL, et al: A comparison of meperidine and lidocaine for spinal anesthesia for postpartum tubal ligation. Reg Anesth 21:84-88, 1996.

187. Rigler ML, Drasner K, Krejcie TC, et al: Cauda equina syndrome after continuous spinal anesthesia. Anesth Analg 72:275-281, 1991.

188. Lambert LA, Lambert DH, Strichartz GR: Irreversible conduction block in isolated nerve by high concentrations of local anesthetics. Anesthesiology 80:1082-1093, 1994.

189. Bainton CR, Strichartz GR: Concentration dependence of lidocaine-induced irreversible conduction loss in frog nerve. Anesthesiology 81:657-667, 1994.

190. Adams HJ, Mastri AR, Eicholzer AW, et al: Morphologic effects of intrathecal etidocaine and tetracaine on the rabbit spinal cord. Anesth Analg 53:904-908, 1974.

191. Ravindran RS, Bond VK, Tasch MD, et al: Prolonged neural blockade following regional analgesia with 2-chloroprocaine. Anesth Analg 59:447-451, 1980.

192. Reisner LS, Hochman BN, Plumer MH: Persistent neurologic deficit and adhesive arachnoiditis following intrathecal 2-chloroprocaine injection. Anesth Analg 59:452-454, 1980.

193. Barsa J, Batra M, Fink BR, Sumi SM: A comparative in vivo study of local neurotoxicity of lidocaine, bupivacaine, 2-chloroprocaine, and a mixture of 2-chloroprocaine and bupivacaine. Anesth Analg 61:961-967, 1982.

194. Rosen MA, Baysinger CL, Shnider SM, et al: Evaluation of neurotoxicity after subarachnoid injection of large volumes of local anesthetic solutions. Anesth Analg 62:802-808, 1983.

195. Ravindran RS, Turner MS, Muller J: Neurologic effects of subarachnoid administration of 2-chloroprocaine-CE, bupivacaine, and low pH normal saline in dogs. Anesth Analg 61:279-283, 1982.

196. Wang BC, Hillman DE, Spielholz NI, et al: Chronic neurological deficits and Nesacaine-CE—an effect of the anesthetic, 2-chloroprocaine, or the antioxidant, sodium bisulfite? Anesth Analg 63:445-447, 1984.

197. Gissen A, Datta S, Lambert D: The chloroprocaine controversy II. Is chloroprocaine neurotoxic? Reg Anesth 9:135, 1984.

198. Taniguchi M, Bollen AW, Drasner K: Sodium bisulfite: Scapegoat for chloroprocaine neurotoxicity? Anesthesiology 100:85-91, 2004.

199. Freedman JM, Li DK, Drasner K, et al: Transient neurologic symptoms after spinal anesthesia: An epidemiologic study of 1,863 patients [erratum appears in Anesthesiology 1998 Dec;89(6):1614]. Anesthesiology 89:633-641, 1998.

200. Hampl KF, Heinzmann-Wiedmer S, Luginbuehl I, et al: Transient neurologic symptoms after spinal anesthesia: A lower incidence with prilocaine and bupivacaine than with lidocaine. Anesthesiology 88:629-633, 1998.

201. Pollock JE: Transient neurologic symptoms: Etiology, risk factors, and management. Reg Anesth Pain Med 27:581-586, 2002.

202. Zaric D, Christiansen C, Pace NL, Punjasawadwong Y: Transient neurologic symptoms (TNS) following spinal anaesthesia with lidocaine versus other local anaesthetics Cochrane Database Syst Rev CD003006, 2003.

203. Eberhart LH, Morin AM, Kranke P, et al: Transient neurologic symptoms after spinal anesthesia. A quantitative systematic overview (meta-analysis) of randomized controlled studies [in German]. Anaesthesist 51:539-546, 2002.

204. Sakura S, Sumi M, Sakaguchi Y, et al: The addition of phenylephrine contributes to the development of transient neurologic symptoms after spinal anesthesia with 0.5% tetracaine. Anesthesiology 87:771-778, 1997.

205. Sakura S, Bollen AW, Ciriales R, et al: Local anesthetic neurotoxicity does not result from blockade of voltage-gated sodium channels. Anesth Analg 81:338-346, 1995.

206. Keld DB, Hein L, Dalgaard M, et al: The incidence of transient neurologic symptoms (TNS) after spinal anaesthesia in patients undergoing surgery in the supine position. Hyperbaric lidocaine 5% versus hyperbaric bupivacaine 0.5%. Acta Anaesthesiol Scand 44:285-290, 2000.

207. Warner MA, Warner DO, Harper CM, et al: Lower extremity neuropathies associated with lithotomy positions. Anesthesiology 93:938-942, 2000.

208. Anema JG, Morey AF, McAninch JW, et al: Complications related to the high lithotomy position during urethral reconstruction. J Urol 164:360-363, 2000.

209. Libelius R, Sonesson B, Stamenovic BA, et al: Denervation-like changes in skeletal muscle after treatment with a local anaesthetic (Marchaine). J Anat 106:297-309, 1970.

210. Benoit PW, Belt WD: Destruction and regeneration of skeletal muscle after treatment with a local anaesthetic, bupivacaine (Marcaine). J Anat 107:547-656, 1970.

211. Benoit PW, Belt WD: Some effects of local anesthetic agents on skeletal muscle. Exp Neurol 34:264-278, 1972.

212. Denson DD, Raj PP, Saldahna F, et al: Continuous perineural infusion of bupivacaine for prolonged analgesia: Pharmacokinetic considerations. Int J Clin Pharmacol Ther Toxicol 21:591-597, 1983.

213. Lund C, Mogensen T, Hjortso NC, et al: Systemic morphine enhances spread of sensory analgesia during postoperative epidural bupivacaine infusion. Lancet 2:1156-1157, 1985.

214. Lee KC, Wilder RT, Smith RL, et al: Thermal hyperalgesia accelerates and MK-801 prevents the development of tachyphylaxis to rat sciatic nerve blockade. Anesthesiology 81:1284-1293, 1994.

215. Sholas M, Wilder RT, Berde CB: Tachyphylaxis to sciatic nerve blockade persists in spinalized rats [abstract]. Anesthesiology 81:A964, 1994.

216. Wilder RT, Sholas MG, Berde CB: NG-nitro-L-arginine methyl ester (L-NAME) prevents tachyphylaxis to local anesthetics in a dose-dependent manner. Anesth Analg 83:1251-1255, 1996.

217. Boogaerts JG, Lafont ND, Carlino S, et al: Biodistribution of liposome-associated bupivacaine after extradural administration to rabbits. Br J Anaesth 75:319-325, 1995.

218. Mowat JJ, Mok MJ, MacLeod BA, et al: Liposomal bupivacaine. Extended duration nerve blockade using large unilamellar vesicles that exhibit a proton gradient. Anesthesiology 85:635-643, 1996.

219. Kopacz DJ, Lacouture PG, Wu D, et al: The dose response and effects of dexamethasone on bupivacaine microcapsules for intercostal blockade (T9 to T11) in healthy volunteers. Anesth Analg 96:576-582, 2003.

220. Curley J, Castillo J, Hotz J, et al: Prolonged regional nerve blockade. Injectable biodegradable bupivacaine/polyester microspheres. Anesthesiology 84:1401-1410, 1996.

221. Kohane DS, Yieh J, Lu NT, et al: A re-examination of tetrodotoxin for prolonged duration local anesthesia. Anesthesiology 89:119-131, 1998.

222. Sudoh Y, Cahoon EE, Gerner P, et al: Tricyclic antidepressants as long-acting local anesthetics. Pain 103:49-55, 2003.

15 Complementary and Alternative Therapies

Michael Ang-Lee, Chun-Su Yuan, and Jonathan Moss

Herbal Medicines   605
Preoperative Assessment and
   Management   606
Echinacea *(Echinacea purpurea)*   606
Ephedra *(Ephedra sinica)*   608
Garlic *(Allium sativum)*   609
Ginkgo *(Ginkgo biloba)*   610
Ginseng *(Panax ginseng* and *Panax*
   quinquefolius)   610
Kava *(Piper methysticum)*   610
Saw Palmetto *(Serenoa repens)*   611

St. John's Wort *(Hypericum perforatum)*   611
Valerian *(Valerian officinalis)*   611
Nonherbal Dietary Supplements   612

Acupuncture   612
Mechanism and General Practice   612
Acupuncture for Postoperative Nausea and
   Vomiting   612

Music   613

Summary   613

Complementary and alternative medicine (CAM) has implications for physicians in general but has particular importance for perioperative physicians because of complications associated with the use of certain therapies and their roles as anesthesia adjuvants. The rapidly rising number of patients using CAM therapies mandates knowledge of them by anesthesiologists. In 1997, 42.1% of Americans used CAM therapies, a significant increase from 33.8% in 1990.[1] Visits to CAM practitioners now exceed those to American primary care physicians,[1] and CAM is even more widely used in Europe, where herbal medicines are more frequently prescribed than conventional drugs in many situations. Of particular relevance for anesthesiologists is that patients undergoing surgery appear to use CAM more than the general population.[2]

Despite the public enthusiasm for CAM, scientific knowledge in this area is still incomplete and often confusing for practitioners and patients. Recommendations for clinicians are often based on small clinical trials, case reports, animal studies, predictions derived from known pharmacology, and expert opinion. Research is essential because CAM therapies are often widely adopted by the public before there are adequate data to support their safety and efficacy. In 1991, Congress established the Office of Alternative Medicine, which became the National Center for Complementary and Alternative Medicine within the National Institutes of Health in 1998. In 2001, nearly three times as many CAM-related English-language research articles were published as in 1991.

The practices encompassed by CAM are heterogeneous and are evolving as CAM therapies are integrated into conventional medicine (e.g., diet, exercise, behavioral medicine). CAM practices can be classified into five general categories[3] (Table 15-1). This chapter is not intended as a comprehensive review of CAM. Specific therapies relevant to anesthesia are discussed, and we focus primarily on herbal medicines. Nonherbal dietary supplements, acupuncture, and music are also examined.

HERBAL MEDICINES

Preoperative use of herbal medicines has been associated with adverse perioperative events.[2] Surveys estimate that 22% to 32% of patients having surgery use herbal medicines.[4-6] As pharmacologically active agents, herbal medicines may affect the perioperative period through several mechanisms: direct effects (i.e., intrinsic pharmacologic effects), pharmacodynamic interactions (i.e., alteration of the action of conventional drugs at effector sites), and pharmacokinetic interactions (i.e., alteration of the absorption, distribution, metabolism, and elimination of conventional drugs). Because approximately one half of herbal medicine users take multiple herbs concomitantly,[5] adverse effects are difficult to predict and attribute. For example, PC-SPES, a commercially available combination of eight herbs used by patients with prostate cancer, has been associated with thrombotic (i.e., deep venous thrombosis and pulmonary embolism) and hemorrhagic (i.e., anticoagulation from phytocoumarins) complications.[7]

Table 15–1 Five major categories of complementary and alternative medicine

1. Alternative medical systems (e.g., homeopathic medicine, naturopathic medicine, traditional Chinese medicine, Ayurveda)
2. Mind-body interventions (e.g., meditation; prayer; art, music, or dance therapy)
3. Biologically based treatments (e.g., herbal medicines, dietary supplements)
4. Manipulative and body-based methods (e.g., chiropractic manipulation, osteopathic manipulation, massage)
5. Energy therapies (e.g., acupuncture, electromagnetic fields, Reiki, qi gong)

Adapted from the National Center for Complementary and Alternative Medicine.
http://nccam.nih.gov/health/whatiscam/ Accessed August 15, 2003.

Herbal medicines are associated with problems not usually found with conventional drugs.[8] Because herbal medicines are classified as dietary supplements, they are not subject to preclinical animal studies, premarketing controlled clinical trials, or postmarketing surveillance. Under current law, the burden is shifted to the U.S. Food and Drug Administration (FDA) to prove products unsafe before they can be withdrawn from the market. Commercial herbal medicine preparations may have unpredictable pharmacologic effects resulting from inaccurate labeling, misidentified plants, adulterants, natural potency variations, and unstandardized processing methods.

In this chapter, we discuss the preoperative assessment and management of patients who use herbal medicines and examine nine herbal medicines that have the greatest impact on perioperative patient care: echinacea, ephedra, garlic, ginkgo biloba, ginseng, kava, saw palmetto, St. John's wort, and valerian (Table 15-2). These nine account for 50% of the herbal medicines sold in the United States[9] (Table 15-3). Print and Internet resources for additional information on herbal medicines are provided in Table 15-4.

Preoperative Assessment and Management

The preoperative assessment should address the use of herbal medicines (see Chapter 25). More than 70% of patients are not forthcoming about their herbal medicine use during routine preoperative assessment.[5] When a positive history of herbal medicine use is obtained, one of five patients is unable to properly identify the preparation being taken.[13] Patients should be asked to bring their herbal medicines and other dietary supplements with them at the time of the preoperative evaluation. A positive history of herbal medicine use should also prompt anesthesiologists to suspect the presence of undiagnosed disorders causing symptoms leading to self-medication. Patients who use herbal medicines may be more likely than those who do not to avoid conventional diagnosis and therapy.[14]

Herbal medicines should be discontinued preoperatively. When pharmacokinetic data for the active constituents in an herbal medication are available, the timeframe for preoperative discontinuation can be tailored. For other herbal medicines, 2 weeks is recommended.[15] However, because many patients require nonelective surgery, are not evaluated until the day of surgery, or are noncompliant with instructions to discontinue herbal medications preoperatively in clinical practice, they may take herbal medicines until the day of surgery. In this common situation, anesthesia can usually proceed safely at the discretion of the anesthesiologist, who should be familiar with commonly used herbal medicines to avoid or recognize and treat complications that may arise. For instance, recent use of herbal medicines that inhibit platelet function (e.g., garlic, ginseng, ginkgo biloba) may warrant specific strategies in the face of procedures with substantial intraoperative blood loss (e.g., platelet transfusion) and those that alter the risk-benefit ratio of using certain anesthetic techniques (e.g., neuraxial blockade).

Preoperative discontinuation of all herbal medicines may not eliminate complications related to their use. Withdrawal of regular medications is associated with increased morbidity and mortality after surgery.[16] In alcoholics, preoperative abstinence may result in poorer postoperative outcome than continued preoperative drinking.[17] The danger of abstinence after long-term use may be similar with herbal medicines such as valerian, which has the potential to produce acute withdrawal after long-term use.

Echinacea (Echinacea purpurea)

Echinacea is used in the prophylaxis and treatment of viral, bacterial, and fungal infections, particularly those of upper respiratory origin. However, compelling evidence supporting its use in upper respiratory infections is lacking.[18] Patients may also use echinacea as an immunostimulant after chemotherapy and radiation therapy, an adjunct in cancer treatment, and a topical promoter of wound healing.

Echinacea contains alkylamides, alkaloids, caffeic acid esters, polysaccharides, flavonoids, polyacetylenes, and essential oils. Pharmacologic activity cannot be attributed to a single compound, although the lipophilic fraction, which contains the alkylamides (primarily the dodeca-2,4,8,10-tetraenoic acid isobutylamides), polyacetylenes, and essential oil appears to be more active than the hydrophilic fraction.

Echinacea has a number of immunomodulatory effects. In vitro, it activated immune cells, increased cytokine production, and inhibited hyaluronidase.[19] In vivo, it activated natural killer cells in humans[20] and increased production of immunoglobulins G and M in rats.[21]

Echinacea's immunostimulatory effects may diminish the effectiveness of immunosuppressive medications. Patients awaiting or post–organ transplantation should avoid echinacea. Patients with asthma, atopy, or allergic rhinitis should also avoid this herbal medicine because it is associated with allergic reactions, including one reported case of anaphylaxis.[22] If taken for more than 8 weeks, echinacea may cause immunosuppression, which may

Table 15–2 Clinically important effects, perioperative concerns, and recommendations for perioperative discontinuation of nine commonly used herbal medicines

Herbs (Common Names)	Important Pharmacologic Effects	Perioperative Concerns	Preoperative Discontinuation
Echinacea Purple coneflower root	Activation of cell-mediated immunity	Allergic reactions Decreased effectiveness of immunosuppressants Potential for immunosuppression with long-term use	No data
Ephedra (ma huang)	Increased heart rate and blood pressure through direct and indirect sympathomimetic effects	Risk of myocardial ischemia and stroke from tachycardia and hypertension Ventricular arrhythmias with halothane Long-term use depletes endogenous catecholamines and may cause intraoperative hemodynamic instability Life-threatening interaction with MAO inhibitors	At least 24 hours before surgery
Garlic (ajo)	Inhibition of platelet aggregation (may be irreversible) Increased fibrinolysis Equivocal antihypertensive activity	May increase risk of bleeding, especially when combined with other medications that inhibit platelet aggregation	At least 7 days before surgery
Ginkgo (duck-foot tree, maidenhair tree, silver apricot)	Inhibition of platelet-activating factor	May increase risk of bleeding, especially when combined with other medications that inhibit platelet aggregation	At least 36 hours before surgery
Ginseng (American ginseng, Asian ginseng, Chinese ginseng, Korean ginseng)	Lowers blood glucose Inhibition of platelet aggregation (may be irreversible) Increased PT/PTT in animals Many other diverse effects	Hypoglycemia May increase risk of bleeding May decrease anticoagulant effect of warfarin	At least 7 days before surgery
Kava (awa, intoxicating pepper, kawa)	Sedation Anxiolysis	May increase sedative effect of anesthetics Ability to increase anesthetic requirements with long-term use unstudied	At least 24 hours before surgery
Saw palmetto (dwarf palm, sabal)	Inhibition of 5-α reductase Inhibition of cyclooxygenase	May increase risk of bleeding	No data
St. John's wort (amber, goat weed, hardhay, hypericum, Klamath weed)	Inhibition of neurotransmitter reuptake MAO inhibition is unlikely	Induction of cytochrome P450 enzymes, affecting cyclosporin, warfarin, steroids, and protease inhibitors and possibly affecting benzodiazepines, calcium channel blockers, and many other drugs Decreased serum digoxin levels Delayed emergence	At least 5 days before surgery
Valerian (all heal, garden heliotrope, vandal root)	Sedation	May increase sedative effect of anesthetics Benzodiazepine-like acute withdrawal May increase anesthetic requirements with long-term use	No data

MAO, monoamine oxidase; PT, prothrombin time; PTT, partial thromboplastin time.

Table 15–3 Most commonly used herbal medicines in 2001

1. Echinacea*
2. Ginkgo biloba*
3. Garlic*
4. Ginseng*
5. Saw palmetto*
6. Noni *(Morinda)*
7. St. John's wort*
8. Soy
9. Ephedra (ma huang)*
10. Milk thistle
11. Valerian*
12. Kava*
13. Grape seed extract
14. Green tea
15. Goldenseal
16. Primrose
17. Black cohosh root
18. Aloe
19. Bilberry
20. Cranberry

*Reviewed in this chapter.
Adapted from the Nutritional Business Journal's herbal and botanical U.S. consumer sales.[9]

increase the risk of certain postsurgical complications such as poor wound healing and opportunistic infections.[23] The pharmacokinetics of echinacea have not been studied.

Ephedra *(Ephedra sinica)*

The predominant active constituent in ephedra, also known as ma huang in Chinese medicine, is ephedrine. Its sympathomimetic effects are used, often in combination with caffeine, to promote weight loss, increase energy, and treat respiratory conditions such as asthma and bronchitis. In 1998, 2% of obese Americans and 1% of the general population took over-the-counter weight loss products containing ephedra.[24] Current usage rates of ephedra are probably higher in light of an FDA proposal in 2001 to withdraw approval of phenylpropanolamine, another popular over-the-counter weight loss agent.

Ephedra is far less safe than other commonly used herbal medications. It has been associated with numerous adverse events, including fatal cardiac and central nervous system complications.[25] Hypertension, tachycardia, vasoconstriction, and vasospasm are the putative causes of myocardial infarction and stroke in these patients.[26] Ephedra may also affect cardiovascular function by causing myocarditis.[27] Many of these adverse events are reported in healthy patients taking typical doses of ephedra (Table 15-5). Long-term use results in

Table 15–4 Printed and world wide web sources of herbal medicine information

Source	Comments
Physicians' Desk Reference for Herbal Medicines[10]	
Commission E Monographs[11]	
Textbook of Complementary and Alternative Medicine[12]	
Center for Food Safety and Applied Nutrition, Food and Drug Administration: http://vm.cfsan.fda.gov/~dms/supplmnt.html	Clinicians should use this site to report adverse events associated with herbal medicines and other dietary supplements. Sections also contain safety, industry, and regulatory information.
National Center for Complementary and Alternative Medicine, National Institutes of Health: http://nccam.nih.gov/	This site contains fact sheets about alternative therapies, consensus reports, and databases.
Agricultural Research Service, United States Department of Agriculture: www.ars-grin.gov/duke	The site contains an extensive phytochemical database with search capabilities.
Quackwatch: www.quackwatch.com	Although this site addresses all aspects of health care, there is a considerable amount of information covering complementary and herbal therapies.
National Council Against Health Fraud: www.ncahf.org	This site focuses on health fraud with a position paper on over-the-counter herbal remedies.
HerbMed: www.herbmed.org	This site contains information on numerous herbal medications, with evidence for activity, warnings, preparations, mixtures and mechanisms of action. There are short summaries of important research publications with Medline links.
ConsumerLab: www.consumerlab.com	This site is maintained by a corporation that conducts independent laboratory investigations of dietary supplements and other health products.

Table 15–5   Adverse events associated with ephedra in 11 patients

Patient No.	Age/ Sex	Estimated Dose of Ephedra Alkaloids (mg/day)	Duration of Use	Adverse Event	Outcome	Preexisting Conditions or Concurrent Risks
1	35/F	45	1 wk	Subarachnoid hemorrhage	Permanent disability	None
2	22/M	20-60	Unknown	Arrhythmia Cardiac arrest	Permanent disability	Asthma
3	28/F	21	1 day	Cardiac arrest	Permanent disability	None
4	43/M	60	7 mo	Cardiac arrest	Death	Family history of coronary artery disease
5	37/F	36	1 wk	Severe hypertension Cardiac arrest Hypokalemia	Death	None
6	59/F	36	3 wk	Acute myocardial infarction	Coronary artery bypass surgery	Hypertension
7	38/M	20	1 yr	Arrhythmia Cardiac arrest	Death	None
8	47/F	44-65	9 mo	Hypertension Bilateral lacunar infarctions	Permanent disability	Concomitant ingestion of caffeine and ethanol
9	29/M	30	2 wk	Stroke	Permanent disability	Concomitant use of dehydroepiandrosterone and androstenedione
10	39/M	Unknown	Unknown	Hemorrhagic stroke	Permanent disability	None
11	47/M	Unknown	3 wk	Hemorrhagic stroke	Permanent disability	Possible hypertension

From Haller CA, Benowitz NL: Adverse cardiovascular and central nervous system events associated with dietary supplements containing ephedra alkaloids. N Engl J Med 343:1833, 2000.

tachyphylaxis from depletion of endogenous catecholamine stores and may contribute to intraoperative hemodynamic instability. In these situations, direct-acting sympathomimetics are the first-line therapy for hypotension and bradycardia. Halothane should be avoided in patients who have recently taken ephedra because of the increased risk of ventricular arrhythmias. Concomitant use of ephedra and monoamine oxidase inhibitors can result in life-threatening hyperpyrexia, hypertension, and coma. Heavy ephedra use can result in nephrolithiasis, which by some estimates accounts for 0.06% of all kidney stones.[28,29]

The pharmacokinetics of ephedrine have been studied in humans.[30,31] The elimination half-life of ephedrine (5.2 hours) is approximately the same whether given as an alkaloid in ephedra or as purified ephedrine hydrochloride. However, absorption may be slower (absorption rate constant of 0.49/hour versus 1.73/hour) when ephedrine is consumed as part of an herbal medication. Given this information, ephedra should be discontinued at least 24 hours before surgery.

Garlic (Allium sativum)

Garlic is used for its potential to prevent atherosclerosis by reducing blood pressure, thrombus formation, and serum lipid and cholesterol levels. It is also used in the treatment and prevention of cancer and infectious diseases. The most compelling evidence of its therapeutic efficacy is in lowering serum cholesterol, but this effect appears to be modest.[32] The development of concentrated garlic preparations has made it possible for patients to take otherwise unachievable high doses, which may increase the risk of adverse effects.[33]

The pharmacologic effects of garlic are primarily attributed to organosulfur compounds, particularly allicin and its transformation products. Several of these compounds inhibit platelet aggregation in a dose-dependent manner.[34-37] The inhibition of platelet aggregation by one of these compounds, ajoene, appears to be irreversible and may potentiate the effect of other compounds such as prostacyclin, forskolin, indomethacin, and dipyridamole.[38] The mechanism by which these effects occur is unknown, although some investigators have implicated the cyclooxygenase pathway.[39] Others have found a direct interaction with the platelet fibrinogen receptor.[40] The exogenous adenosine in garlic[41] and inhibition of endogenous adenosine deamination and cyclic AMP phosphodiesterase may also play a role.[39]

The clinical significance of garlic's antiplatelet activity is uncertain. In volunteers, inhibition of platelet aggregation to 5-hydroxytryptamine was transient but potent[42]; another study showed no such activity.[43] Inconsistent experimental findings may be explained by differences in garlic preparations. Garlic may also increase the risk of bleeding by promoting fibrinolysis, a finding that has been demonstrated in volunteers.[44] There is one case in the literature of an octogenarian who developed a spontaneous epidural hematoma that was attributed to heavy use of garlic.[45] Although data are unreliable, bleeding times were significantly elevated when the patient was hospitalized and returned to normal 3 days after the discontinuation of garlic.

Although there are insufficient pharmacokinetic data for the constituents of garlic, the potential for irreversible inhibition of platelet function warrants the discontinuation of garlic at least 7 days before surgery, especially if intraoperative or postoperative bleeding is a special concern or other platelet inhibitors are used.

Ginkgo *(Ginkgo biloba)*

Ginkgo is used by patients with cognitive disorders, peripheral vascular disease, age-related macular degeneration, vertigo, tinnitus, erectile dysfunction, and altitude sickness. Ginkgo may stabilize or improve cognitive performance in patients with Alzheimer's disease and multi-infarct dementia[46,47] but not in healthy patients.[48]

The compounds believed to be responsible for ginkgo's pharmacologic effects are the terpenoids (i.e., bilobalide and ginkgolides A, B, C and J) and flavonoids (i.e., kaempferol, quercetin, and isorhamnetin derivatives). These compounds alter vasoregulation,[49] act as antioxidants,[50] modulate neurotransmitter and receptor activity,[51,52] and inhibit platelet-activating factor (PAF).[53] Of these effects, the inhibition of PAF is the most worrisome given the potential for inhibition of platelet function. Clinical trials enrolling a small number of patients have not demonstrated bleeding complications, but one case of postoperative bleeding after laparoscopic cholecystectomy,[54] four reported cases of spontaneous intracranial bleeding,[55-58] and one case of spontaneous hyphema[59] have been attributed to ginkgo use. Ginkgo also has been associated with seizures.[60]

Elimination half-lives of bilobalide and ginkgolides A and B after oral administration are 4.5, 10.6, and 3.2 hours, respectively.[61] Based on the pharmacokinetic data and the risk of bleeding, ginkgo should be discontinued at least 36 hours before surgery.

Ginseng *(Panax ginseng* and *Panax quinquefolius)*

Ginseng has been labeled an *adaptogen* because it reputedly protects the body against stress and restores homeostasis.[62]

It has been used for virtually every purpose, including to promote health, immune function, endocrine function, athletic performance, and cognitive function and to treat cardiovascular disease, diabetes mellitus, cancer, impotence, and viral infections.[63] Although ginseng has measurable pharmacologic activity, compelling evidence to support its use for any specific indication is lacking.[64] Other "varieties" of ginseng, such as Siberian ginseng (*Eleutherococcus senticosus*) and Brazilian ginseng (*Pfaffia paniculata*) are unique plants with different pharmacologic effects that may nevertheless be included in commercially available ginseng preparations.

Most pharmacologic effects of ginseng are attributed to the ginsenosides, a group of compounds known as steroidal saponins that act as steroid hormones. It is not known, however, whether long-term use of ginseng can cause the well-described complications of long-term steroid use. The broad but incompletely understood pharmacologic profile of ginseng can be attributed to the many heterogeneous and sometimes opposing effects of different ginsenosides.[63] Actions on virtually every organ system have been described, but the neuroendocrine and hematologic effects have the greatest implications for anesthesiologists. *Panax quinquefolius* lowers postprandial blood glucose in healthy subjects and in patients with type 2 diabetes mellitus.[65,66] Although this effect may have therapeutic potential, it may also create unintended hypoglycemia, particularly in patients fasting preoperatively. Another potential clinical issue surrounding the use of this herb is its effects on coagulation pathways. Ginsenosides inhibit platelet aggregation in vitro[67,68] and prolong the thrombin time and activated partial thromboplastin time in rats.[69] Results from one preliminary study suggest that the antiplatelet activity of panaxynol, a constituent of ginseng, may be irreversible in humans.[70] Although ginseng may inhibit the coagulation cascade, ginseng use was associated with a significant decrease in warfarin anticoagulation in one reported case.[71]

The pharmacokinetics of ginsenosides Rg1, Re, and Rb2 have been investigated in rabbits.[72] The elimination half-lives of these three ginsenosides ranged from 0.8 hour for ginsenoside Re to 7.4 hours for ginsenoside Rb2. These data suggest that patients should discontinue ginseng use at least 24 hours before surgery, but discontinuation at least 7 days before surgery is preferred because of the potential for irreversible platelet inhibition.

Kava *(Piper methysticum)*

Kava is a popular herbal anxiolytic and sedative.[73] Because of its psychomotor effects, it was one of the first herbal medications expected to interact with anesthetics. The kavalactones (i.e., kawain, dihydrokawain, methysticin, dihydromethysticin, yangonin, and desmethoxyyangonin) appear to be the source of kava's pharmacologic activity.[74]

Kava acts by potentiating γ-aminobutyric acid (GABA) inhibitory neurotransmission.[75] Kavalactones and pentobarbital produce a synergistic effect on [³H]muscimol binding to GABA. This effect probably explains why kava increased barbiturate sleep time in laboratory animals.[76,77] Prolonged sedation with alprazolam and kava was reported in one patient.[78] Although kava may have abuse potential, whether long-term use can result in addiction, tolerance, and acute withdrawal after abstinence has not been satisfactorily investigated. With heavy use, kava produces *kava dermopathy*, characterized by reversible scaly cutaneous eruptions. Increasing evidence of kava hepatotoxicity has caused its withdrawal in some countries.[79] This may have important implications in patients with hepatic dysfunction.

Plasma levels peak 1.8 hours after an oral dose, and the elimination half-life of kavalactones is 9 hours.[74] These pharmacokinetic data and the possibility of potentiation of the sedative effects of anesthetics suggest that kava should be discontinued at least 24 hours preoperatively.

Saw Palmetto (Serenoa repens)

Saw palmetto is used to treat symptoms associated with benign prostatic hypertrophy (BPH), a condition found in approximately 40% of men in their 50s and 90% of men in their 80s.[80] In Europe, it is often used as first-line treatment for BPH.[81] The major constituents of saw palmetto are fatty acids and their glycerides (i.e., triacylglycerides and monoacylglycerides), carbohydrates, steroids, flavonoids, resin, pigment, tannin, and volatile oil. The pharmacologic activity of saw palmetto has not been attributed to a single compound.

The mechanism of action of saw palmetto is not known, but multiple mechanisms based on available research have been proposed.[82] In vitro data support the widely held belief that saw palmetto extract, like finasteride, inhibits 5α-reductase.[83] However, in vivo studies have been inconsistent.[82] Another hypothesis is that saw palmetto exerts its effects by inhibiting dihydrotestosterone binding to the androgen receptors in the prostate.[84] Other proposed mechanisms are inhibition of estrogen receptors,[85] blocking prolactin receptor signal transduction,[86] interference with fibroblast proliferation,[87] induction of apoptosis,[88] inhibition of α_1-adrenergic receptors,[89] and anti-inflammatory effects.[90,91]

In a patient undergoing a craniotomy, saw palmetto was associated with excessive intraoperative bleeding that required termination of the procedure.[92] This complication was attributed to saw palmetto's anti-inflammatory effects, specifically the inhibition of cyclooxygenase and subsequent platelet dysfunction. Because there are no pharmacokinetic data for saw palmetto, specific recommendations for preoperative discontinuation cannot be made.

St. John's Wort (Hypericum perforatum)

St. John's wort is used for the short-term treatment of mild to moderate depression.[93,94] It is not effective in the treatment of major depression.[95,96] It is used for other psychiatric complaints such as anxiety, but little evidence supports its use for conditions other than depression. The six classes of key compounds in St. John's wort are the naphthodianthrones (i.e., hypericin and pseudohypericin), acylphloroglucinols (i.e., hyperforin and adhyperforin), flavonol glycosides, biflavones, proanthocyanidins, and phenylpropanes. Although hypericin was long thought to be the primary active compound,

evidence suggests that hyperforin may be more important in the antidepressant effects.[97]

St. John's wort inhibits serotonin, norepinephrine, and dopamine reuptake.[98,99] Early in vitro data implicated monoamine oxidase inhibition as a possible mechanism of action,[100] but subsequent data showed this was not the mechanism.[97,101,102] The use of St. John's wort with or without serotonin-reuptake inhibitors may create a syndrome of central serotonin excess.[103] More importantly, St. John's wort can significantly increase the metabolism of many concomitantly administered drugs through the induction of cytochrome P450 microsomal enzymes, roughly doubling their metabolic activity.[104] The most affected enzyme appears to be CYP3A4, which is responsible for the metabolism of more than 50% of conventional medications subject to oxidative metabolism by cytochrome P450. Interactions with the CYP3A4 substrates indinavir,[105] ethinyl estradiol,[106] and cyclosporin have been reported. In a series of 45 organ transplant recipients, cyclosporin levels decreased an average of 49% after St. John's wort was taken.[107] Two cases of acute heart transplant rejection have also been associated with this particular pharmacokinetic interaction.[108] Other CYP3A4 substrates used in the perioperative period include alfentanil, midazolam hydrochloride, lidocaine, calcium channel blockers, and serotonin receptor antagonists, and it is reasonable to assume that metabolism of these drugs would also be increased. St. John's wort induces CYP2C9, substrates of which include nonsteroidal anti-inflammatory drugs, phenytoin, and warfarin. The anticoagulant effect of warfarin was reduced in seven reported cases.[106] St. John's wort also lowers digoxin levels by induction of the P-glycoprotein transporter.[109]

The effect of St. John's wort on drug pharmacokinetics makes its preoperative discontinuation important in many patients. Discontinuation is crucial in certain patients awaiting or after organ transplantation because of the risk of rejection. Also included are patients receiving warfarin during the perioperative period for prophylaxis against thrombotic complications because typical warfarin doses may not provide adequate anticoagulation for patients who take St. John's wort preoperatively. Management of drug dosing in the immediate postoperative period may be difficult as the metabolic function of cytochrome P450 enzymes normalize after discontinuation. A case of delayed emergence has been attributed to St. John's wort.[110]

The single-dose and steady-state pharmacokinetics of hypericin, pseudohypericin, and hyperforin have been determined in humans.[111,112] After oral administration, peak plasma levels of hypericin, pseudohypericin, and hyperforin are obtained in 6.0, 3.0, and 3.5 hours, respectively. The median elimination half-lives of hypericin, pseudohypericin, and hyperforin are 43.1, 24.8, and 9.0 hours, respectively. These pharmacokinetic data suggest that St. John's wort should be discontinued at least 5 days preoperatively.

Valerian (Valerian officinalis)

Valerian is used as a sedative, particularly in the treatment of insomnia. Virtually all commercial herbal sleep aids contain valerian.[113] Valerian contains many compounds acting synergistically, but sesquiterpenes are the primary source of the pharmacologic effects.

Valerian produces dose-dependent sedation and hypnosis.[114] These effects appear to be mediated through modulation of GABA neurotransmission and receptor function.[115] Valerian increased barbiturate sleep time in experimental animals.[116] Valerian also mediated benzodiazepine withdrawal in rats.[117] In one patient, valerian withdrawal appeared to mimic an acute benzodiazepine withdrawal syndrome characterized by delirium and cardiac complications after surgery with symptoms attenuated by benzodiazepine administration.[118] Based on these findings, valerian should be expected to potentiate the sedative effects of anesthetics that act at the GABA receptor.

The pharmacokinetics of valerian's constituents have not been studied, although their effects are thought to be short lived. Abrupt discontinuation in patients who may be physically dependent on valerian risks benzodiazepine-like withdrawal. In these individuals, it may be prudent to taper this herbal medication with close medical supervision over the course of several weeks before surgery. If this is not feasible, physicians can advise patients to continue taking valerian up until the day of surgery. Benzodiazepines should be used to treat withdrawal symptoms if they develop in the postoperative period.

NONHERBAL DIETARY SUPPLEMENTS

Herbal medicines fall into the broader category of dietary supplements that also includes vitamins, minerals, amino acids, enzymes, and animal extracts. Data on the safety of these agents in the perioperative period are scant. High-dose vitamin use, particularly of the fat-soluble vitamins (i.e., A, D, E, and K) can be associated with acute and chronic toxicity. Glucosamine and chondroitin sulfate, which are used for joint disorders by many patients having orthopedic procedures, have not been associated with perioperative complications, although chondroitin sulfate belongs to the same group of glycosaminoglycan molecules as heparin and may have minor anticoagulant effects.[119] Whether long-term chondroitin sulfate use can cause thrombocytopenia is unknown. Creatine, a dietary supplement used by athletes to enhance performance, has been associated with renal dysfunction in at least one case.[120] There are preliminary data that exogenous melatonin, a hormone produced by the pineal gland, may be useful in preventing and treating postoperative delirium.[121]

ACUPUNCTURE

Mechanism and General Practice

Increasing evidence supports the use of acupuncture, particularly in areas of relevance to anesthesia. In 1998, a National Institutes of Health (NIH) Consensus Panel reported that acupuncture showed promise in reducing postoperative and chemotherapy-related nausea and postoperative dental pain.[122]

Acupuncture is the stimulation of anatomic locations on the skin by a variety of techniques that can be classified as invasive (e.g., needles, injections) or noninvasive (e.g., transcutaneous electrical stimulation, pressure, laser). Needles inserted into the skin can be stimulated by manual manipulation, moxibustion (i.e., burning a substance to produce heat), pressure, laser, and electricity. There are Chinese, Japanese, Korean, French, and other acupuncture systems for identifying acupuncture points, but there is little research comparing these different systems. As a result, there are no standard or optimal acupuncture points. Practitioners consider acupuncture an art as much as a science.

The traditional theory of acupuncture is that it corrects disruptions in the flow of energy (i.e., qi) and restores the balance of dual forces (i.e., ying-yang) in the body. Data suggest that there is a scientific basis for acupuncture. Acupuncture stimulates high-threshold, small-diameter nerves leading to activation of spinal cord, brainstem (i.e., periaqueductal gray area), and hypothalamic (i.e., arcuate) neurons, which trigger endogenous opioid mechanisms.[123] The effect of acupuncture analgesia can be reversed by naloxone.[124] Functional magnetic resonance imaging[125,126] and positron emission tomography[127,128] have demonstrated that acupuncture stimulation produces identifiable effects in the human brain. Other mechanisms such as modulation of immune function,[129] inhibition of the inflammatory response,[130] regulation of neuropeptide gene expression,[131] and alterations in hormonal levels[132] have been proposed.

Although many clinical acupuncture studies have been published, many are of poor quality, suffering from insufficient sample sizes, high dropout rates, inadequate follow-up, and poorly defined illnesses, enrollment criteria, and outcome measures.[123] Acupuncture studies suffer from inherent methodologic difficulties that include difficulties blinding patients and acupuncturists, using placebo or sham acupuncture, and choosing between different acupuncture techniques. One of the most promising indications for acupuncture is to prevent postoperative nausea and vomiting (PONV).

Acupuncture for Postoperative Nausea and Vomiting

PONV remains a significant problem that results in patient dissatisfaction, delayed discharge, unanticipated hospital admission, and the use of resources (see Chapter 68). Pharmacologic agents are the mainstay of management. However, they have limited effectiveness, are associated with side effects, and can be costly. There is considerable interest in acupuncture for its potential to prevent PONV with minimal side effects and expense.

Available evidence suggests that acupuncture prevents PONV compared with placebo (e.g., sham acupuncture, no treatment).[133-143] Acupuncture appears to prevent PONV to approximately the same extent as pharmacologic agents, including metoclopramide, droperidol, prochlorperazine, and ondansetron. A meta-analysis of studies published before 1998 reached the conclusion that acupuncture and related techniques prevent PONV in adults with a calculated absolute risk reduction of 20% to 25% (i.e., for every four or five patients treated, one case of PONV is avoided).[144] This meta-analysis also concluded that acupuncture was not effective in children. Since the meta-analysis was published, however, several randomized, controlled trials suggest that acupuncture also may prevent PONV in the pediatric population.[139-142]

Most PONV acupuncture studies use the P6 (i.e., Nei-guan or pericardium) acupuncture point, which is located between the palmaris longus and flexor carpi radialis muscle tendons, 4 cm proximal to the distal wrist crease and 1 cm below the skin (Fig. 15-1). Korean hand acupuncture may be equally effective.[136] Studies often differ on the acupuncture method: duration and timing of stimulation, unilateral versus bilateral stimulation, and type of stimulation (i.e., needles with or without additional stimulation, acupressure, transcutaneous electrical stimulation, cutaneous laser stimulation, or injection of 50% dextrose solution). Data to compare the effectiveness, safety, and costs of different methods of stimulation are inadequate. It is recommended that stimulation of the acupuncture point be initiated before induction of anesthesia,[145] although in children, stimulation immediately before emergence and in the recovery room has been effective. Some anesthesiologists anecdotally report taping a small needle cap or other piece of smooth plastic over the P6 point as an effective means of acupressure stimulation.

MUSIC

Music may decrease preoperative anxiety, reduce intraoperative sedative and analgesic requirements, and increase patient satisfaction. Patient-selected music reduced patient-controlled sedative requirements during spinal anesthesia and analgesic requirements during lithotripsy.[146] Preoperative music reduces anxiety without

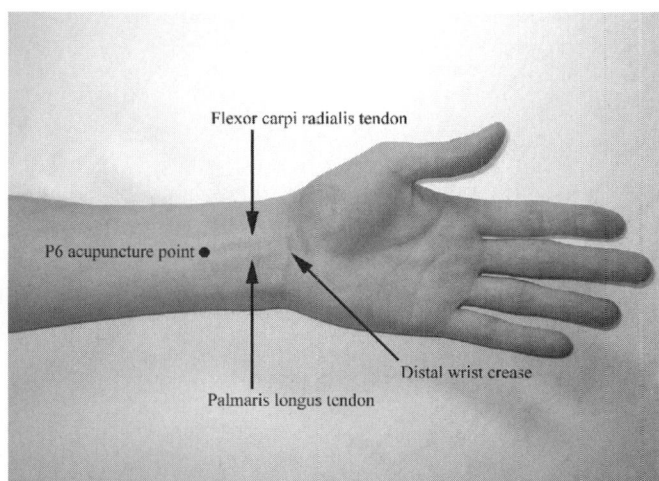

Figure 15-1 The P6 acupuncture point is located between the palmaris longus and flexor carpi radialis muscle tendons, 4 cm proximal to the distal wrist crease and 1 cm below the skin.

affecting physiologic measures of stress.[147] Music may be part of a low sensory stimulation strategy to reduce anxiety and increase cooperation in children undergoing induction of anesthesia.[148] Music increased patient satisfaction and reduced systolic blood pressure during cataract surgery using retrobulbar block.[149]

SUMMARY

One of the fastest changing aspects of health care is the growing public and scientific interest in CAM. When taken preoperatively, some herbal medicines may adversely affect patient care. Surgery and anesthesia can usually proceed safely if potential complications are predicted and can be avoided. Preliminary data suggest that acupuncture and music may be useful adjuncts in the perioperative period. Although medical schools are beginning to incorporate CAM into their curriculums, it is difficult but important for anesthesiologists in practice to stay informed about these practices.

KEY POINTS

1. Despite lack of federal oversight, herbal medication use has increased dramatically in the overall population and particularly in preoperative patients.
2. Patients may not volunteer information unless they are specifically queried about herbal medication use.
3. Many commonly used herbs have side effects that affect drug metabolism, bleeding, and neuronal function.
4. Although stopping herbs up to 2 weeks preoperatively can eliminate many of these problems, patients often present for surgery without a visit 2 weeks before surgery. Knowledge of specific interactions and metabolism of these herbs can provide practical guidelines to facilitate care.
5. Other complementary therapies, including acupuncture and music therapy, have become increasingly popular, although less is known about their effectiveness.

REFERENCES

1. Eisenberg DM, Davis RB, Ettner SL, et al: Trends in alternative medicine use in the United States, 1990-1997. JAMA 280:1569, 1998.
2. Ang-Lee MK, Moss J, Yuan CS: Herbal medicines and perioperative care. JAMA 286:208, 2001.
3. National Center for Complementary and Alternative Medicine. http://nccam.nih.gov/health/whatiscam/ Accessed August 15, 2003.
4. Tsen LC, Segal S, Pothier M, et al: Alternative medicine use in presurgical patients. Anesthesiology 93:148, 2000.
5. Kaye AD, Clarke RC, Sabar R, et al: Herbal medications: Current trends in anesthesiology practice—A hospital survey. J Clin Anesth 12:468, 2000.
6. Leung JM, Dzankic S, Manku K, et al: The prevalence and predictors of the use of alternative medicine in presurgical

patients in five California hospitals. Anesth Analg 93:1062, 2001.

7. Weinrobe MC, Montgomery B: Acquired bleeding diathesis in a patient taking PC-SPES. N Engl J Med 347:1213, 2001.

8. De Smet P: Herbal remedies. N Engl J Med 347:2046, 2002.

9. NBJ's herbal and botanical U.S. consumer sales. http://store.yahoo.com/nbj/new2019top75.html/Accessed November 24, 2003.

10. Gruenwald J (ed): Physicians' Desk Reference for Herbal Medicines, 2nd ed. Montvale, NJ, Medical Economics, 2000.

11. Blumenthal M, Busse WR, Goldberg A for the German Federal Institute for Drugs and Medical Devices Commission E, American Botanical Council, and Integrative Medical Communications (eds): The Complete German Commission E Monographs: Therapeutic Guide to Herbal Medicines. Boston, Integrative Medicine Communications, 1998.

12. Yuan CS, Bieber EJ (eds): Textbook of Complementary and Alternative Medicine. New York, Parthenon, 2003.

13. Kassler WJ, Blanc P, Greenblatt R: The use of medicinal herbs by human immunodeficiency virus-infected patients. Arch Intern Med 151:2281, 1991.

14. Cirigliano M, Sun A: Advising patients about herbal therapies. JAMA 280:1565, 1998.

15. Leak JA: Herbal medicines: What do we need to know? ASA Newsletter 64:6-7, 2000.

16. Kennedy JM, van Rij AM, Spears GF, et al: Polypharmacy in a general surgical unit and consequences of drug withdrawal. Br J Clin Pharmacol 49:353, 2000.

17. Tonnesen H, Rosenberg J, Nielsen HJ, et al: Effect of preoperative abstinence on poor postoperative outcome in alcohol misusers: Randomized controlled trial. BMJ 318:1311, 1999.

18. Melchart D, Linde K, Fischer P, Kaesmayr J: Echinacea for preventing and treating the common cold [review]. Cochrane Database Syst Rev 2:CD000530, 2000.

19. Pepping J: Echinacea. Am J Health Syst Pharm 56:121, 1999.

20. See DM, Broumand N, Sahl L, et al: In vitro effects of echinacea and ginseng on natural killer and antibody-dependent cell cytotoxicity in healthy subjects and chronic fatigue syndrome or acquired immunodeficiency syndrome patients. Immunopharmacology 35:229, 1997.

21. Rehman J, Dillow JM, Carter SM, et al: Increased production of antigen-specific immunoglobulins G and M following in vivo treatment with the medicinal plants Echinacea angustifolia and Hydrastis canadensis. Immunol Lett 68:391, 1999.

22. Mullins RJ: Echinacea-associated anaphylaxis. Med J Aust 168:170, 1998.

23. Boullata JI, Nace AM: Safety issues with herbal medicine. Pharmacotherapy 20:257, 2000.

24. Blanck HM, Khan LK, Serdula MK: Use of nonprescription weight loss products. JAMA 286:930, 2001.

25. Bent S, Tiedt TN, Odden MC, et al: The relative safety of ephedra compared with other herbal products. Ann Intern Med 138:468, 2003.

26. Haller CA, Benowitz NL: Adverse cardiovascular and central nervous system events associated with dietary supplements containing ephedra alkaloids. N Engl J Med 343:1833, 2000.

27. Zaacks SM, Klein L, Tan CD, et al: Hypersensitivity myocarditis associated with ephedra use. J Toxicol Clin Toxicol 37:485,1999.

28. Blau JJ: Ephedrine nephrolithiasis associated with chronic ephedrine abuse. J Urol 160:825, 1998.

29. Powell T, Hsu FF, Turk J, et al: Ma-huang strikes again: Ephedrine nephrolithiasis. Am J Kidney Dis 32:153, 1998.

30. White LM, Gardner SF, Gurley BJ, et al: Pharmacokinetics and cardiovascular effects of ma-huang (Ephedra sinica) in normotensive adults. J Clin Pharmacol 37:116, 1997.

31. Gurley BJ. Gardner SF, White LM, et al: Ephedrine pharmacokinetics after the ingestion of nutritional supplements containing Ephedra sinica (ma huang). Ther Drug Monit 20:439, 1998.

32. Stevinson C, Pittler MH, Ernst E: Garlic for treating hypercholesteremia: A meta-analysis of randomized clinical trials. Ann Intern Med 133:420, 2000.

33. Agarwal KC: Therapeutic actions of garlic constituents. Med Res Rev 16:111, 1996.

34. Mohammad SF, Woodward SC: Characterization of a potent inhibitor of platelet aggregation and release reaction isolated from Allium sativum (garlic). Thromb Res 44:793, 1986.

35. Srivastava KC: Evidence for the mechanism by which garlic inhibits platelet aggregation. Prostaglandins Leukot Med 22:313, 1986.

36. Ariga T, Oshiba S, Tamada T: Platelet aggregation inhibitor in garlic. Lancet 1:150, 1981.

37. Boullin DJ: Garlic as a platelet inhibitor. Lancet 1:776, 1981.

38. Apitz-Castro R, Escalante J, Vargas R, et al: Ajoene, the antiplatelet principle of garlic, synergistically potentiates the antiaggregatory action of prostacyclin, forskolin, indomethacin and dipyridamole on human platelets. Thromb Res 42:303, 1986.

39. Ali M, Al-Qattan KK, Al-Enezi F, et al: Effect of allicin from garlic powder on serum lipids and blood pressure in rats fed with a high cholesterol diet. Prostaglandins Leukot Essent Fatty Acids 62:253, 2000.

40. Apitz-Castro R, Ledezma E, Escalante J, et al: The molecular basis of the antiplatelet action of ajoene: Direct interaction with the fibrinogen receptor. Biochem Biophys Res Commun 141:145, 1986.

41. Makheja AN, Bailey JM: Antiplatelet constituents of garlic and onion. Agents Actions 29:360, 1990.

42. Gebhardt R: Multiple inhibitory effects of garlic extracts on cholesterol biosynthesis in hepatocytes. Lipids 28:613, 1993.

43. Harenberg J, Giese C, Zimmermann R: Effect of dried garlic on blood coagulation, fibrinolysis, platelet aggregation and serum cholesterol level in patients with hyperlipoproteinemia. Atherosclerosis 74:247, 1988.

44. Chutani SK, Bordia A: The effect of fried versus raw garlic on fibrinolytic activity in man. Atherosclerosis 38:417, 1981.

45. Rose KD, Croissant PD, Parliamet CF, et al: Spontaneous spinal epidural hematoma with associated platelet dysfunction from excessive garlic ingestion: A case report. Neurosurgery 26:880, 1990.

46. Le Bars PL, Katz MM, Berman N, et al: A placebo-controlled, double-blind, randomized trial of an extract of Ginkgo biloba for dementia. JAMA 278:1327, 1997.

47. Oken BS, Storzbach DM, Kaye JA: The efficacy of Ginkgo biloba on cognitive function in Alzheimer disease. Arch Neurol 55:1409, 1998.

48. Solomon PR, Adams F, Silver A, et al: Ginkgo for memory enhancement: A randomized controlled trial. JAMA 288:835, 2002.

49. Jung F, Mrowietz C, Kiesewetter H, et al: Effect of Ginkgo biloba on fluidity of blood and peripheral microcirculation in volunteers. Arzneimittelforschung 40:589, 1990.

50. Maitra I, Marcocci L, Droy-Lefaix MT, et al: Peroxyl radical scavenging activity of Ginkgo biloba extract EGb 761. Biochem Pharmacol 49:1649, 1995.

51. Hoyer S, Lannert H, Noldner M, et al: Damaged neuronal energy metabolism and behavior are improved by Ginkgo biloba extract (EGb 761). J Neural Transm 106:1171, 1999.

52. Huguet F, Tarrade T: Alpha 2-adrenoceptor changes during cerebral aging. The effect of Ginkgo biloba extract. J Pharm Pharmacol 44:24,1992.

53. Chung KF, Mccusker M, Page CP, et al: Effect of a ginkgolide mixture (BN 52063) in antagonizing skin and platelet responses to platelet activating factor in man. Lancet 1:248, 1987.

54. Fessenden JM, Wittenborn W, Clarke L: Ginkgo biloba: A case report of herbal medicine and bleeding postoperatively from a laparoscopic cholecystectomy. Am Surg 67:33, 2001.

55. Rowin J, Lewis SL: Spontaneous bilateral subdural hematomas associated with chronic Ginkgo biloba ingestion. Neurology 46:1775, 1996.

56. Vale S: Subarachnoid haemorrhage associated with Ginkgo biloba. Lancet 352:36, 1998.

57. Gilbert GJ: Ginkgo biloba. Neurology 48:1137, 1997.

58. Matthews MK: Association of Ginkgo biloba with intracerebral hemorrhage. Neurology 50:1933, 1998.

59. Rosenblatt M, Mindel J: Spontaneous hyphema associated with ingestion of Ginkgo biloba extract. N Engl J Med 336:1108, 1997.

60. Gregory PJ: Seizure associated with *Ginkgo biloba*. Ann Intern Med 134:344, 2001.
61. Mills S, Bone K (eds): Ginkgo. *In* Principles and Practice of Phytotherapy. New York, Churchill Livingstone, 2000.
62. Brekham II, Dardymov IV: New substances of plant origin which increase nonspecific resistance. Annu Rev Pharmacol 9:419, 1969.
63. Attele AS, Wu JA, Yuan CS: Ginseng pharmacology: Multiple constituents and multiple actions. Biochem Pharmacol 58:1685, 1999.
64. Vogler BK, Pittler MH, Ernst E: The efficacy of ginseng. A systematic review of randomized clinical trials. Eur J Clin Pharmacol 55:567, 1999.
65. Attele AS, Zhou YP, Xie JT, et al: Antidiabetic effects of *Panax ginseng* berry extract and the identification of an effective component. Diabetes 51:1851, 2002.
66. Vuksan V, Sievenpiper JL, Koo V, et al: American ginseng (*Panax quinquefolius L*) reduces postprandial glycemia in nondiabetic subjects and subjects with type 2 diabetes mellitus. Arch Intern Med 160:1009, 2000.
67. Kimura Y, Okuda H, Arichi S: Effects of various ginseng saponins on 5-hydroxytryptamine release and aggregation in human platelets. J Pharm Pharmacol 40:838, 1988.
68. Kuo SC, Teng CM, Lee JC, et al: Antiplatelet components in *Panax ginseng*. Planta Med 56:164, 1990.
69. Park HJ, Lee JH, Song YB, et al: Effects of dietary supplementation of lipophilic fraction from *Panax ginseng* on cGMP and cAMP in rat platelets and on blood coagulation. Bio Pharm Bull 19:1434, 1996.
70. Teng CM, Kuo SC, Ko FN, et al: Antiplatelet actions of panaxynol and ginsenosides isolated from ginseng. Biochim Biophys Acta 990:315, 1989.
71. Janetzky K, Morreale AP: Probable interaction between warfarin and ginseng. Am J Health Syst Pharm 54:692, 1997.
72. Chen SE, Sawchuk RJ, Staba EJ: American ginseng. III. Pharmacokinetics of ginsenosides in the rabbit. Eur J Drug Metab Pharmacokinet 5:161, 1980.
73. Pittler MH, Ernst E: Efficacy of kava extract for treating anxiety: Systematic review and meta-analysis. J Clin Psychopharmacol 20:84, 2000.
74. Pepping J: Kava: *Piper methysticum*. Am J Health Syst Pharm 56:957, 1999.
75. Yuan CS, Dey L, Wang A, et al: Kavalactones and dihydrokavain modulate GABAergic activity in a rat gastric-brainstem preparation. Planta Med 68:1092, 2002.
76. Jamieson DD, Duffield PH, Cheng D, et al: Comparison of the central nervous system activity of the aqueous and lipid extract of kava *(Piper methysticum)*. Arch Int Pharmacodyn 301:66, 1989.
77. Keledjian J, Duffield PH, Jamieson DD, et al: Uptake into mouse brain of four compounds present in the psychoactive beverage kava. J Pharm Sci 77:1003, 1988.
78. Almeida JC, Grimsley EW: Coma from the health food store: Interaction between kava and alprazolam. Ann Intern Med 125:940, 1996.
79. Ernst E: Second thoughts about kava. Am J Med 113:347, 2002.
80. Berry SL, Coffey DS, Walsh PC, et al: The development of human benign prostatic hyperplasia with age. J Urol 132:474, 1984.
81. Buck A: Phytotherapy for the prostate. Br J Urol 78:325, 1996.
82. Gerber GS: Saw palmetto for the treatment of men with lower urinary tract symptoms. J Urol 163:1408, 2000.
83. Iehle C, Delos S, Guirou O, et al: Human prostatic steroid 5 alpha-reductase isoforms: A comparative study of selective inhibitors. J Steroid Biochem Mol Biol 54:273, 1995.
84. Plosker GL, Brogden RN: *Serenoa repens* (Permixon). A review of its pharmacology and therapeutic efficacy in benign prostatic hyperplasia. Drugs Aging 9:379, 1996.
85. Di Silverio F, D'Eramo G, Lubrano C, et al: Evidence that *Serenoa repens* extract displays an antiestrogenic activity in prostatic tissue of benign prostatic hypertrophy patients. Eur Urol 21:309, 1992.
86. Vacher P, Prevarskaya N, Skyrma R, et al: The lipidosterolic extract from *Serenoa repens* interferes with prolactin receptor signal transduction. J Biomed Sci 2:357, 1995.
87. Paubert-Braquet M, Cousse H, Raynaud JP, et al: Effect of the lipidosterolic extract of *Serenoa repens* (Permixon) and its major components on basic fibroblast growth factor-induced proliferation of cultures of human prostate biopsies. Eur Urol 33:340, 1998.
88. Vacherot F, Azzouz M, Gil-Diez-de-Medina S, et al: Induction of apoptosis and inhibition of cell proliferation by the lipidosterolic extract of *Serenoa repens* (LSESr, Permixon) in benign prostatic hyperplasia. Prostate 45:259, 2000.
89. Goepel M, Hecker U, Krege S, et al: Saw palmetto extracts potently and noncompetitively inhibit human alpha-1-adrenoceptors in vitro. Prostate 38:208, 1999.
90. Brue W, Hagenlocer M, Redl K, et al: Anti-inflammatory activity of sabal fruit extracts prepared with supercritical carbon dioxide. In vitro antagonists of cyclooxygenase and 5-lipooxygenase metabolism. Arzneimittelforschung 42:547, 1992.
91. Paubert-Braquet M, Mencia Huerta JM, Cousse H, et al: Effect of the lipidic lipidosterolic extract of *Serenoa repens* (Permixon) on the ionophore A23187-stimulated production of leukotriene B4 (LTB4) from human polymorphonuclear neutrophils. Prostaglandins Leukot Essent Fatty Acids 57:299, 1997.
92. Cheema P, El-Mefty O, Jazieh AR: Intraoperative haemorrhage associated with the use of extract of saw palmetto herb: A case report and review of literature. J Intern Med 250:167, 2001.
93. Gaster B, Holroyd J: St. John's wort for depression: A systematic review. Arch Intern Med 160:152, 2000.
94. Lecrubier Y, Clerc G, Didi R, et al: Efficacy of St. John's wort extract WS 5570 in major depression: A double-blind, placebo-controlled trial. Am J Psychiatry 159:1361, 2002.
95. Shelton RC, Keller MB, Gelenberg A, et al: Effectiveness of St. John's wort in major depression. JAMA 285:1978, 2001.
96. Hypericum Depression Trial Study Group: Effect of *Hypericum perforatum* (St. John's wort) in major depressive disorder: A randomized controlled trial. JAMA 287:1807, 2002.
97. Muller WE, Singer A, Wonnemann M, et al: Hyperforin represents the neurotransmitter reuptake-inhibiting constituent of *Hypericum* extract. Pharmacopsychiatry 31(Suppl 1):16, 1998.
98. Neary JT, Bu Y: Hypericum LI 160 inhibits uptake of serotonin and norepinephrine in astrocytes. Brain Res 816:358, 1999.
99. Franklin M, Chi J, McGavin C, et al: Neuroendocrine evidence for dopaminergic actions of *Hypericum* extract (PI 160) in healthy volunteers. Biol Psychiatry 46:581, 1999.
100. Suzuki O, Katsumata Y, Oya M, et al: Inhibition of monoamine oxidase by hypericin. Planta Med 50:272, 1984.
101. Yu PH: Effect of the *Hypericum perforatum* extract on serotonin turnover in the mouse brain. Pharmacopsychiatry 33:60, 2000.
102. Muller WE, Rolli M, Schafer C, et al: Effects of *Hypericum* extract (LI 160) in biochemical models of antidepressant activity. Pharmacopsychiatry 30(Suppl 2):102, 1997.
103. Lantz MS, Buchalter E, Giambanco V: St. John's wort and antidepressant drug interactions in the elderly. J Geriatr Psychiatry Neurol 12:7, 1999.
104. Ernst E: Second thoughts about safety of St. John's wort. Lancet 354:2014, 1999.
105. Piscitelli SC, Burstein AH, Chaitt D, et al: Indinavir concentrations and St. John's wort. Lancet 355:547, 2000.
106. Yue QY, Bergquist C, Gerden B: Safety of St. John's wort. Lancet 355:576, 2000.
107. Breidenbach T, Hoffmann MW, Becker T, et al: Drug interaction of St. John's wort with cyclosporine. Lancet 355:1912, 2000.
108. Ruschitzka F, Meier PJ, Turina M, et al: Acute heart transplant rejection due to Saint John's wort. Lancet 355:548, 2000.
109. Johne A, Brockmoler J, Bauer S, et al: Pharmacokinetic interaction of digoxin with an herbal extract from St. John's wort *(Hypericum perforatum)*. Clin Pharmacol Ther 66:338, 1999.

110. Crowe S, McKeating K: Delayed emergence and St. John's wort. Anesthesiology 96:1025, 2002.
111. Kerb R, Brockmoller J, Staffeldt B, et al: Single-dose and steady-state pharmacokinetics of hypericin and pseudo hypericin. Antimicrob Agents Chemother 40:2087, 1996.
112. Biber A, Fischer H, Romer A, et al: Oral bioavailability of hyperforin from *Hypericum* extracts in rats and human volunteers. Pharmacopsychiatry 31(Suppl 1):36, 1998.
113. Houghton PJ: The scientific basis for the reputed activity of valerian. J Pharm Pharmacol 51:505, 1999.
114. Hendriks H, Bos R, Allersma DP, et al: Pharmacological screening of valerenal and some other components of essential oil of *Valeriana officinalis*. Planta Med 42:62, 1981.
115. Ortiz JG, Nieves-Natal J, Chavez P: Effects of *Valeriana officinalis* extracts on [3H] flunitrazepam binding, synaptosomal [3H]GABA uptake, and hippocampal [3H]GABA release. Neurochem Res 24:1373, 1999.
116. Leuschner J, Muller J, Rudmann M: Characterization of the central nervous depressant activity of a commercially available valerian root extract. Arzneimittelforschung 43:638, 1993.
117. Andreatini R, Leite JR: Effect of valepotriates on the behavior of rats in the elevated plus-maze during diazepam withdrawal. Eur J Pharmacol 260:233, 1994.
118. Garges HP, Varia I, Doraiswamy PM: Cardiac complications and delirium associated with valerian root withdrawal. JAMA 280:1566, 1998.
119. Bjornsson TD, Nash PV, Schaten R: The anticoagulant effect of chondroitin-4-sulfate. Thromb Res 27:15, 1982.
120. Pritchard NR, Kalra PA: Renal dysfunction accompanying oral creatine supplements. Lancet 351:1252, 1998.
121. Hanania M, Kitain E: Melatonin for treatment and prevention of postoperative delirium. Anesth Analg 94:338, 2002.
122. NIH Consensus Conference. Acupuncture [review]. JAMA 280:1518, 1998.
123. Kaptchuk TJ: Acupuncture: Theory, efficacy, and practice. Ann Intern Med 136:374, 2002.
124. Tsunoda Y, Sakahira K, Nakano S, et al: Antagonism of acupuncture analgesia by naloxone in unconscious man. Bull Tokyo Med Dent Univ 27:89, 1980.
125. Wu MT, Hsieh JC, Xiong J, et al: Central nervous pathway for acupuncture stimulation: Localization of processing with functional MR imaging of the brain—Preliminary experience. Radiology 212:133, 1999.
126. Hui KK, Liu J, Makris N, et al: Acupuncture modulates the limbic system and subcortical gray structures of the human brain: Evidence from fMRI studies in normal subjects. Hum Brain Mapp 9:13, 2000.
127. Hsieh JC, Tu CH, Chen FP, et al: Activation of the hypothalamus characterizes the acupuncture stimulation at the analgesic point in human: A positron emission tomography study. Neurosci Lett 307:105, 2001.
128. Biella G, Sotgiu ML, Pellegata G, et al: Acupuncture produces central activations in pain regions. Neuroimage 14:60, 2001.
129. Mori H, Nishijo K, Kawamura H, et al: Unique immunomodulation by electro-acupuncture in humans possibly via stimulation of the autonomic nervous system. Neurosci Lett 320:21, 2002.
130. Son YS, Park HJ, Kwon OB, et al: Antipyretic effects of acupuncture on the lipopolysaccharide-induced fever and expression of interleukin-6 and interleukin-1 beta mRNAs in the hypothalamus of rats. Neurosci Lett 319:45, 2002.
131. Guo HF, Tian J, Wang X, et al: Brain substrates activated by electroacupuncture (EA) of different frequencies (II): Role of Fos/Jun proteins in EA-induced transcription of pre-proenkephalin and preprodynorphin genes. Brain Res Mol Brain Res 43:167, 1996.
132. Gerhard I, Postneek F: Auricular acupuncture in the treatment of female infertility. Gynecol Endocrinol 6:171, 1992.
133. Agarwal A, Bose N, Gaur A, et al: Acupressure and ondansetron for PONV after laparoscopic cholecystectomy. Can J Anaesth 49:554, 2002.
134. Alkaissi A, Evertsson K, Johnsson VA, et al: P6 acupressure may relieve nausea and vomiting after gynecological surgery: An effectiveness study in 410 women. Can J Anaesth 49:1034, 2002.
135. Alkaissi A, Stalnert M, Kalman S: Effect and placebo effect of acupressure P6 on nausea and vomiting after outpatient gynaecological surgery. Acta Anaesthesiol Scand 43:270, 1999.
136. Boehler M, Mitterschiffthaler G, Schlager A: Korean hand acupressure reduces postoperative nausea and vomiting after gynecological laparoscopic surgery. Anesth Analg 94:872, 2002.
137. Harmon D, Gardiner J, Harrison R, et al: Acupressure and the prevention of nausea and vomiting after laparoscopy. Br J Anaesth 82:387, 1999.
138. Harmon D, Ryan M, Kelly A, et al: Acupressure and prevention of nausea and vomiting during and after spinal anesthesia for caesarean section. Br J Anaesth 84:463, 2000.
139. Rusy LM, Hoffman GM, Weisman SJ: Electroacupuncture prophylaxis of postoperative nausea and vomiting following pediatric tonsillectomy with or without adenoidectomy. Anesthesiology 96:300, 2002.
140. Schlager A, Boehler M, Puhringer F: Korean hand acupressure reduces postoperative nausea and vomiting in children after strabismus surgery. Br J Anaesth 85:267, 2000.
141. Schlager A, Offer T, Baldissera I: Laser stimulation of acupuncture point P6 reduces postoperative vomiting in children undergoing strabismus surgery. Br J Anaesth 81:529, 1998.
142. Wang SM, Kain ZN: P6 acupoint injections are as effective as droperidol in controlling early postoperative nausea and vomiting in children. Anesthesiology 97:359, 2002.
143. Zarate E, Mingus M, White PF, et al: Use of transcutaneous acupoint electrical stimulation for preventing nausea and vomiting after laparoscopic surgery. Anesth Analg 92:629, 2001.
144. Lee A, Done ML: The use of nonpharmacologic techniques to prevent postoperative nausea and vomiting: A meta-analysis. Anesth Analg 88:1362, 1999.
145. Dundee JW, Ghaly RG: Does the timing of P6 acupuncture influence its efficacy as a postoperative antiemetic? Br J Anaesth 63:630, 1989.
146. Koch ME, Kain ZN, Ayoub C, et al: The sedative and analgesic sparing effect of music. Anesthesiology 89:300, 1998.
147. Wang SM, Kulkarni L, Dolev J, et al: Music and preoperative anxiety: A randomized, controlled study. Anesth Analg 94:1489, 2002.
148. Kain ZN, Wang SM, Mayes LC, et al: Sensory stimuli and anxiety in children undergoing surgery: A randomized, controlled trial. Anesth Analg 92:897, 2001.
149. Cruise CJ, Chung F, Yogendran S, et al: Music increases satisfaction in elderly outpatients undergoing cataract surgery. Can J Anaesth 44:43, 1997.

CHAPTER
16 The Autonomic Nervous System

Jonathan Moss and David Glick

Background 617
History and Definitions 617
New Concepts of Transmitter Action 618

Functional Anatomy 621
Sympathetic Nervous System 621
Parasympathetic Nervous System 622
Enteric Nervous System 624

Function 625
Organization and Integration 625
Adrenergic Function 625
Cholinergic Function 627

Pharmacology 630
Adrenergic Pharmacology 630
Cholinergic Pharmacology 640
Ganglionic Pharmacology 644

**Drugs and the Autonomic Nervous
System 645**
Drugs Affecting Adrenergic
Transmission 646
Drugs Affecting the Renin-Angiotensin
System 659
Cholinergic Drugs 659
Ganglionic Drugs 662

Autonomic Dysfunction 663
Assessment of Autonomic
Function 663
Plasma Catecholamines 663
Clinical Syndromes 664
Autonomic Changes with Aging 664
Autonomic Changes in Spinal Cord
Transection 664

BACKGROUND

Much of the action of the body in maintaining cardio-vascular, gastrointestinal, and thermal homeostasis occurs through the autonomic nervous system (ANS). The ANS is also our primary defense against challenges to that homeostasis. It provides involuntary (i.e., outside of consciousness) control and organization of maintenance and stress responses. In the words of Claude Bernard, "... nature thought it provident to remove these important phenomena from the capriciousness of an ignorant will." Activation of the sympathetic nervous system elicits what is traditionally called the *fight or flight response*, including redistribution of blood flow from the viscera to skeletal muscle, increased cardiac function, sweating, salivation, and pupillary dilation. The parasympathetic system governs activities of the body more closely associated with maintenance of function, such as digestive and genitourinary functions. A major goal of anesthetic administration is maintaining optimum homeostasis in the patient despite powerful challenges to a sometimes tenuous physiologic balance. The intelligent administration of anesthetic care to patients requires knowledge of ANS pharmacology to achieve desirable interactions of anesthetics with the involuntary control system and to avoid responses or interactions with deleterious effects. Disease states may impair ANS function to a significant extent and may thereby alter the expected responses to surgery and anesthesia. Possible negative effects of the human stress response have long been appreciated, and considerable effort has been expended in examining the possibility that modification or ablation of the stress response may improve perioperative outcome.

History and Definitions

Initially, nerves were thought to be connected in a giant syncytium. Claude Bernard, a student of Magendie, postulated the theory of chemical synapse transmission. Later, Sherrington initiated a systemic study of reflexes and described some characteristics of reflex function. A chemist, J.J. Abel, first synthesized epinephrine in 1899, and his student Langley demonstrated that it caused the same effect as stimulating postganglionic sympathetic neurons. When the nerve was cut and epinephrine was injected, Langley found that there was a more profound effect, demonstrating denervation supersensitivity. From these observations, the concept of chemical transmission in the ANS developed. Sir Henry Dale isolated choline and studied an ester, acetylcholine, in animals. He demonstrated that it caused a marked decrease in blood pressure and vasodilation, mimicking parasympathetic activity.

Nerves are traditionally classified by the chemical transmitters they contain. Nerves containing acetylcholine are called *cholinergic*, whereas those containing norepinephrine or epinephrine are called *adrenergic*. In addition to classifying nerves, the term *cholinergic* refers to other structures or functions that relate in some way to acetylcholine. For instance, cholinergic receptors (i.e., cholinoceptors) are proteins in cell membranes that react with acetylcholine and cause the cell to respond in a characteristic way (e.g., muscles contract, glands secrete). *Cholinergic agonists* are drugs that act like acetylcholine on cholinoceptors to cause the cell to react in its characteristic way. They are sometimes referred to as *cholinomimetic drugs*. *Cholinergic antagonists* are drugs that react with cholinoceptors to block the access by acetylcholine and thereby prevent its action. These drugs may also be referred to as *cholinolytic*, *cholinergic-blocking*, or *anticholinergic drugs*.

Because muscarine, a chemical isolated from a mushroom, causes effects similar to those produced by activation of the parasympathetic nervous system, it was thought to be the endogenous parasympathetic transmitter. Since then, drugs that mimic the effects of muscarine on the parasympathetically innervated structures, including the heart, smooth muscles, and glands, have been called *muscarinic drugs*.

In the early 1900s, nicotine was found to act on ganglionic and skeletal muscle synapses and on nerve membranes and sensory endings. Accordingly, drugs that act on these parts of the cholinergic system are called *nicotinic drugs*. Nicotinic drugs that are more specific in their action have been discovered and are referred to by the name of the system they affect, such as *ganglionic drugs* or *neuromuscular drugs*. Agonists and antagonists exist in each category, with little crossover of effect between drugs acting at the ganglia and those acting at the neuromuscular junction.

For purposes of this chapter, cholinergic nerves include the following (Fig. 16-1):
1. All the motor nerves that innervate skeletal muscle
2. All postganglionic parasympathetic neurons
3. All preganglionic parasympathetic and sympathetic neurons
4. Some postganglionic sympathetic neurons, such as those that innervate sweat glands and certain blood vessels
5. Preganglionic sympathetic neurons that arise from the greater splanchnic nerve and innervate the adrenal medulla
6. Central cholinergic neurons

Drugs mimicking the action of norepinephrine are referred to as *sympathomimetic*, whereas drugs inhibiting these effects of norepinephrine are called *sympatholytic*. Norepinephrine is the transmitter acting at adrenergic nerves, whereas epinephrine and norepinephrine are released by the adrenal medulla.

Adrenergic receptors have been identified and subdivided into α- and β-receptors and further subdivided into α_1, α_2, β_1, β_2, and other types. α_2-Adrenergic receptors are primarily located on the presynaptic membrane, whereas α_1-adrenergic receptors mediate smooth muscle vasoconstriction. The β_1-adrenergic receptors are found primarily on cardiac tissue, and β_2-adrenergic receptors mediate smooth muscle relaxation in some organs. We define adrenergic neurons as follows:
1. Postganglionic sympathetic neurons
2. Some interneurons
3. Certain central neurons

New Concepts of Transmitter Action

Until recently, nervous control of the vasculature was considered predominantly in terms of classic transmitters: norepinephrine and acetylcholine. For many years, they were the only transmitters recognized in perivascular nerves.

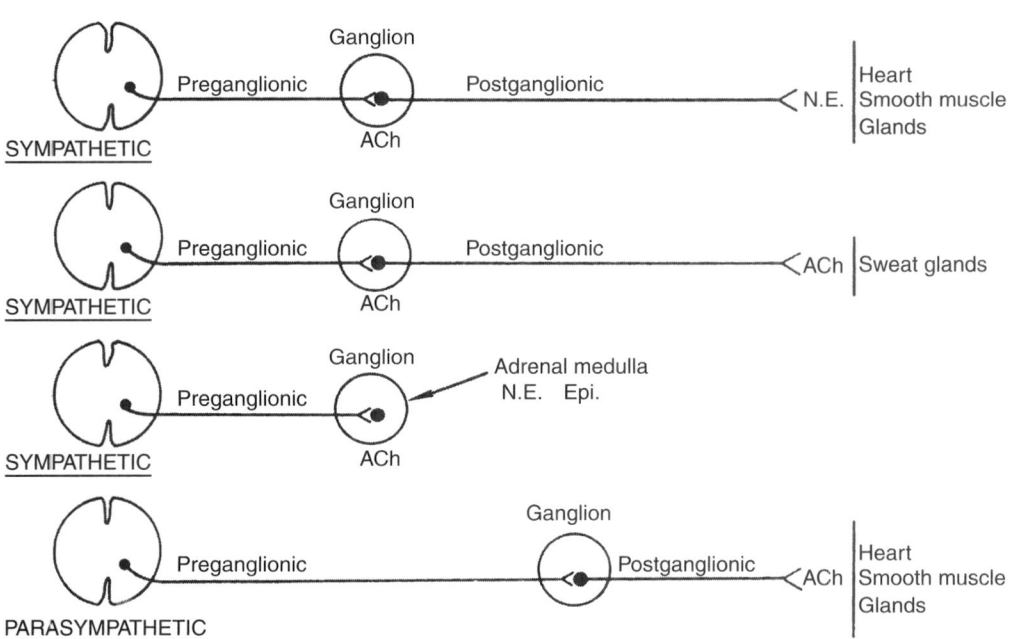

Figure 16–1 Autonomic nervous system neurotransmission. ACh, acetylcholine; Epi, epinephrine; NE, norepinephrine.

Beginning in the early 1960s, various other compounds, including monoamines, purines, amino acids, and polypeptides, were identified that fulfilled the criteria of functional neurotransmitters.[1,2] As reviewed by Burnstock,[3] nonadrenergic, noncholinergic components are part of the ANS. Other transmitter candidates demonstrated in perivascular nerves using histochemical and immunohistochemical techniques include adenosine 5'-triphosphate (ATP), vasoactive intestinal polypeptide (VIP), substance P, 5-hydroxytryptamine (5-HT), neuropeptide Y (NPY), and calcitonin gene–related peptide (CGRP). Immunocytochemical studies show that more than one transmitter or putative transmitter may be colocalized in the same nerve. The most common combinations of transmitters in perivascular nerves are norepinephrine, ATP, and NPY in sympathetic nerves; acetylcholine and VIP in parasympathetic nerves; and substance P, CGRP, and ATP in sensory-motor nerves. Many of these putative transmitters act through *cotransmission,* which is the synthesis, storage, and release of more than one transmitter by a nerve.[4] Initially, the multiplicity of transmitters released in various combinations appeared random and bewildering, but a pattern is emerging that clarifies the situation. Autonomic nerves exhibit *chemical coding*—individual neurons serving a specific physiologic function contain distinct combinations of transmitter substances.[5]

The concepts of cotransmission and neuromodulation have become accepted mechanisms in autonomic nervous control. To establish that transmitters coexisting in the same nerves act as cotransmitters, it is necessary to demonstrate that, on release, each substance acts postjunctionally on its own specific receptor to produce a response.

For many perivascular sympathetic nerves, there is evidence that norepinephrine and ATP act as cotransmitters and are released from the same nerves but act on α_1-adrenoceptors and P_2-purinoceptors, respectively, to produce vasoconstriction[6,7] (Fig. 16-2). ATP, once thought to act only as an electrical buffer for the charged norepinephrine, is believed to mediate contraction through P_{2x}-receptors by voltage-dependent calcium channels.[8] The fast component of contraction appears to be mediated by these purinoceptors, whereas norepinephrine sustains contraction of muscle by acting on the α_1-adrenoreceptor through receptor-operated calcium channels. Specific drugs have been designed to interact with this purinergic component.[9]

Neuromodulators modify the process of neurotransmission. They may be circulating neurohormones, local agents, or neurotransmitter substances released from the same nerves or from others nearby. Neuromodulation can occur prejunctionally by decreasing or increasing the amount of transmitter released during transmission or

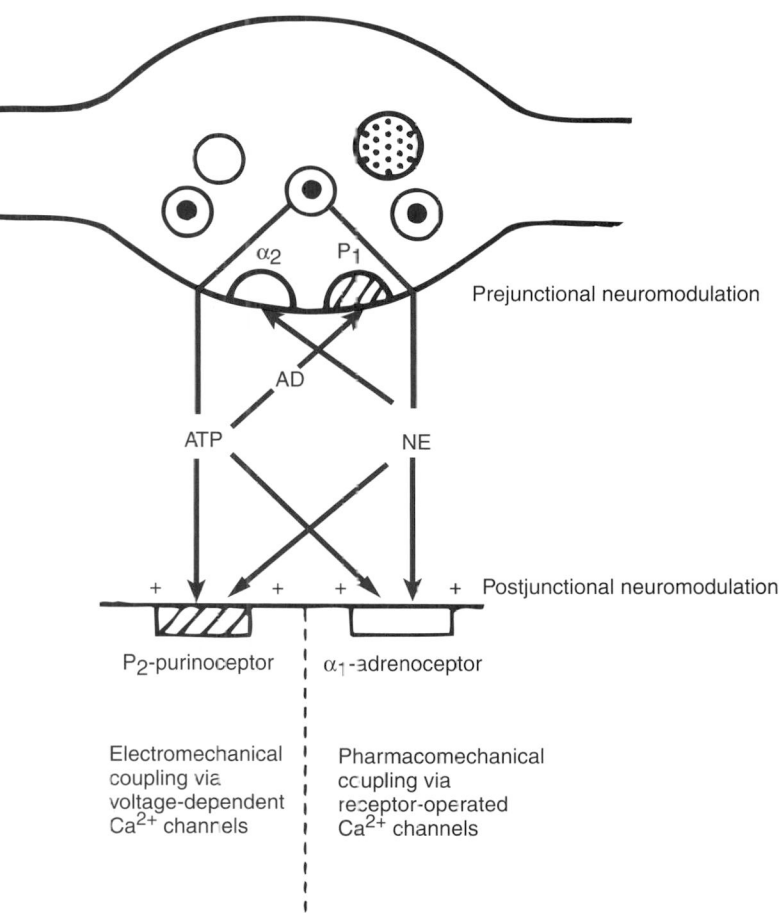

Figure 16–2 The diagram shows that adenosine triphosphate (ATP) and norepinephrine (NE) are released as cotransmitters from the sympathetic nerves supplying the vas deferens and some blood vessels. ATP acts on P_2-purinoceptors on the smooth muscles to initiate excitatory junction potentials, action potentials, and a fast initial contraction involving electromechanical coupling through voltage-dependent calcium (Ca^{2+}) channels. NE acts on α_1-adrenoceptors to produce the second, slower phase of the contraction by pharmacomechanical (or at least spike-independent) coupling through receptor-operated Ca^{2+} channels. Prejunctional α_2-adrenoceptors and P_1-purinoceptors can reduce transmitter release when activated by NE and adenosine (AD), respectively (i.e., prejunctional neuromodulation), whereas NE and ATP enhance each other's actions (i.e., postjunctional neuromodulation). (Adapted from Burnstock G: Local mechanisms of blood flow control by perivascular nerves and endothelium. J Hypertens Suppl 8:S95, 1990.)

postjunctionally by altering the extent or time course of neurotransmitter effect. In all known examples in which prejunctional and postjunctional neuromodulation occurs, these substances act in concert to attenuate or to augment effective transmission. The rationale for such effects may reflect the variable geometry of the autonomic neuroeffector junction.[10,11] Unlike the neuromuscular junction, the autonomic neuroeffector junction exists in a dynamic state and manifests only modest postjunctional specialization. Biogenic amines often must traverse wide distances. Given the short half-lives of these chemicals, neuromodulation provides a biologic mechanism for augmentation and prolongation of their action.[12]

NPY is also colocalized with norepinephrine and ATP. However, in some vessels, NPY has little or no direct action; instead, NPY acts as a neuromodulator prejunctionally to inhibit the release of norepinephrine from the nerve or postjunctionally to enhance the action of norepinephrine (Fig. 16-3A).[13,14] In other vessels, notably those of the spleen, skeletal muscle, and cerebral and coronary vasculature, NPY has direct vasoconstrictor actions. In the heart and brain, local intrinsic (nonsympathetic) neurons use NPY as the principal transmitter (see Fig. 16-3B). In the spleen, NPY appears to act as a genuine cotransmitter with norepinephrine in perivascular sympathetic nerves (see Fig. 16-3C).[15] The frequency of stimulation determines which vesicles are mobilized to release their transmitters.

A classic transmitter such as acetylcholine coexists with VIP in the parasympathetic nerves of many organs, but in this instance, the two transmitters are stored in separate vesicles. They can be released differentially at different stimulation frequencies, depending on where they are located.[16,17] For example, in the salivary gland, they can act independently on acinar cells and glandular blood vessels (Fig. 16-4).[7] Cooperation is achieved by the selective release of acetylcholine at low frequencies and of VIP at high frequencies of stimulation. Elements of prejunctional and postjunctional modulation have also been described. It is becoming increasingly apparent that in many biologic states, including pregnancy,[18]

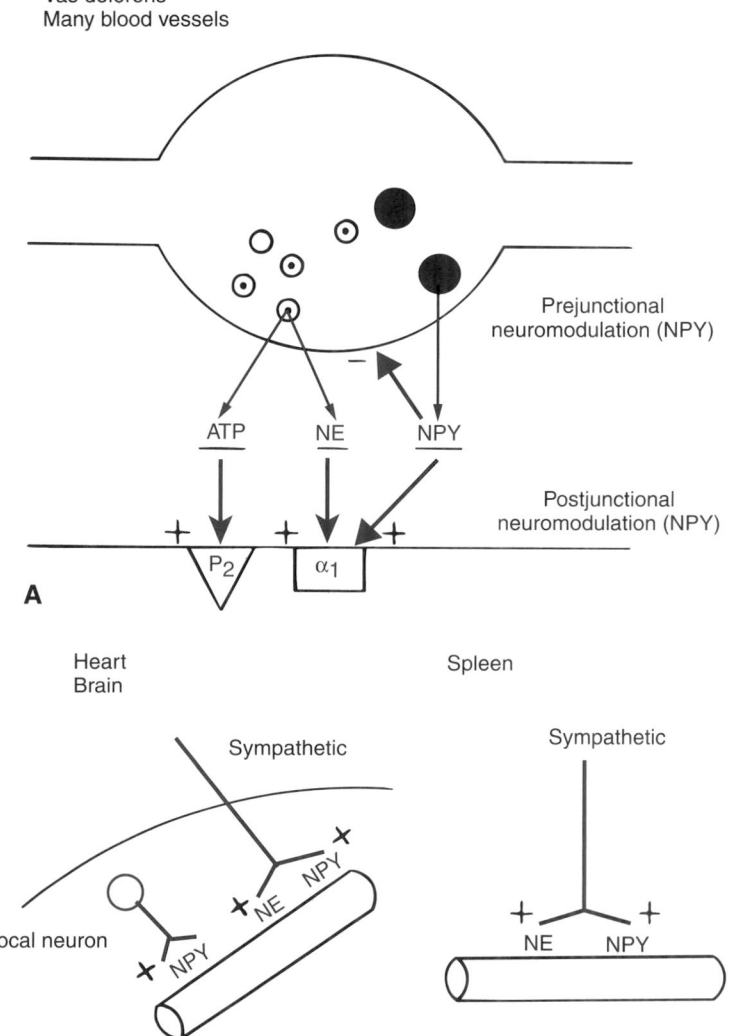

A

B

C

Figure 16–3 Schematic representation of different interactions that occur between neuropeptide Y (NPY) and adenosine triphosphate (ATP), and norepinephrine (NE) released from single sympathetic nerve varicosities. **A,** Diagram shows what occurs in the vas deferens and many blood vessels, where NE and ATP, probably released from small granular vesicles, act synergistically to contract (+) the smooth muscle through α_1-adrenoceptors and P_2-purinoceptors, respectively. **B** and **C,** Sympathetic neurotransmission in the heart and brain (**B**) and spleen (**C**). (From Lincoln J, Burnstock G: Neural-endothelial interactions in control of local blood flow. *In* Warren J [ed]: The Endothelium: An Introduction to Current Research. New York, Wiley-Liss, 1990, p 21.)

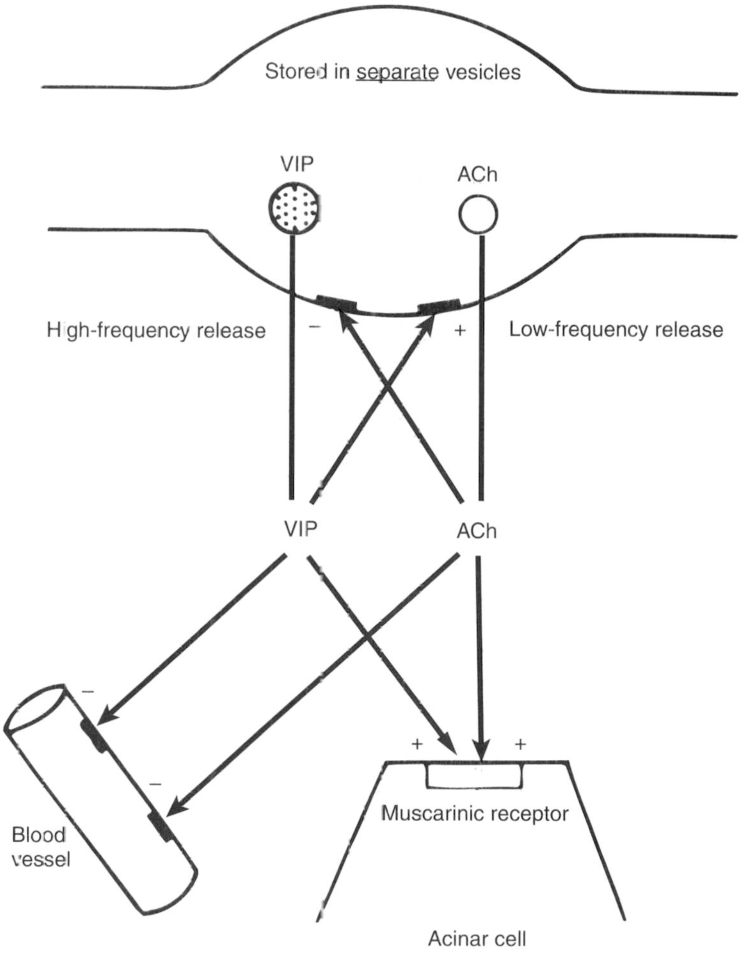

Figure 16–4 A classic transmitter, acetylcholine (ACh), coexists with vasoactive intestinal polypeptide (VIP) in parasympathetic nerves supplying the cat salivary gland. ACh and VIP are stored in separate vesicles; they can be released differentially at different stimulation frequencies to act on acinar cells and glandular blood vessels. Cooperation is achieved by the selected release of ACh at low impulse frequencies and of VIP at high frequencies. Prejunctional and postjunctional modulation is indicated. (From Burnstock G: Local mechanisms of blood flow control by perivascular nerves and endothelium. J Hypertens Suppl 8:S95, 1990.)

hypertension, and aging, the relationships among cotransmitters may be an important determinant of a compensatory response, allowing finer control of important physiologic function.

FUNCTIONAL ANATOMY

Each branch of the ANS exhibits a different anatomic motif, which is recapitulated on a cellular and molecular level. The underlying theme of the sympathetic nervous system is an *amplification response*, whereas that of the parasympathetic nervous system is a *discrete and narrowly targeted response*. The enteric nervous system is arranged nontopographically, as would be appropriate for the viscera, and relies on the mechanism of chemical coding to differentiate between nerves serving different functions.

Sympathetic Nervous System

The sympathetic nervous system originates from the spinal cord in the thoracolumbar region, from the first thoracic through the second or third lumbar segment. The preganglionic sympathetic neurons have cell bodies within the horns of the spinal gray matter (i.e., the intermediolateral columns). Nerve fibers from these cell bodies extend to three types of ganglia, grouped as paired sympathetic chains, various unpaired distal plexuses, or terminal or collateral ganglia near the target organ.

The 22 paired ganglia lie along either side of the vertebral column. Nerve trunks connect these ganglia to each other, and gray rami communicantes connect the ganglia to the spinal nerves. The preganglionic fibers leave the cord in the anterior nerve roots, join the spinal nerve trunks, and enter the ganglion at that level through the white (myelinated) ramus. Leaving the ganglion, postsynaptic fibers reenter the spinal nerve through the gray (unmyelinated) ramus and then go on to innervate pilomotor and sudomotor (sweat gland) effectors and blood vessels of the skeletal muscle and skin (Fig. 16-5). Sympathetic innervation of the trunk and limbs is carried by the spinal nerves.

The sympathetic distribution to the head and neck, enabling and mediating vasomotor, pupillodilator, secretory, and pilomotor functions, comes from the three ganglia of the cervical sympathetic chain. Preganglionic fibers of these cervical structures originate in the upper thoracic segments. In 80% of people, the stellate ganglion is formed by the fusion of the inferior cervical ganglion with the first thoracic ganglion on each side.

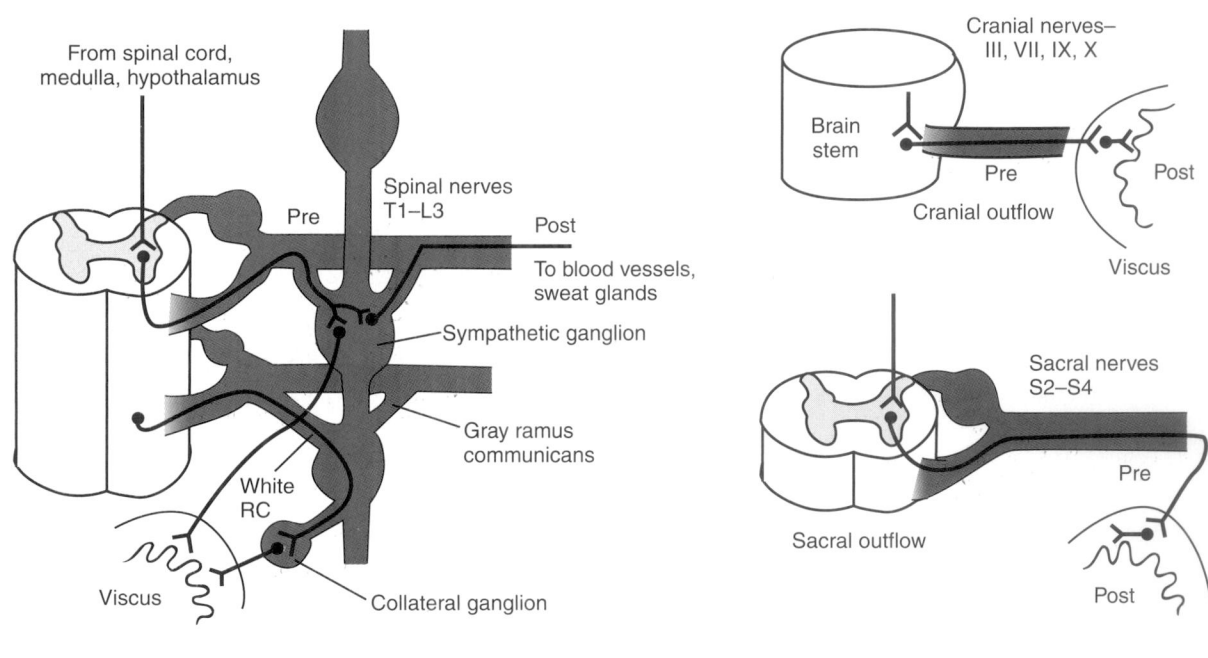

Figure 16–5 Autonomic nervous system. Post, postganglionic neuron; pre, preganglionic neuron; RC, ramus communicans. (From Ganong W: The autonomic nervous system. *In* Ganong W [ed]: Review of Medical Physiology, 15th ed. Norwalk, CT, Appleton & Lange, 1991, p 210.)

The unpaired prevertebral ganglia reside in the abdomen and pelvis anterior to the vertebral column and are primarily the celiac, superior mesenteric, aorticorenal, and inferior mesenteric ganglia. The celiac ganglion is innervated by T5 through T12 and innervates the liver, spleen, kidney, pancreas, small bowel, and proximal colon. Many preganglionic fibers from T5 to T12 may pass through the paired paravertebral ganglia to form the splanchnic nerves; most do not synapse until in the celiac ganglion, whereas others innervate the adrenal medulla. The superior mesenteric ganglion innervates the distal colon, and the inferior mesenteric ganglion serves the rectum, bladder, and genitals (Fig. 16-6). Postganglionic fibers arising from the synaptic links of upper thoracic sympathetic fibers in vertebral ganglia form terminal cardiac, esophageal, and pulmonary plexuses. These fibers also innervate the viscera of the abdomen and pelvis. Ganglia of the third type, the terminal or collateral ganglia, are small, few in number, and near their target organs. The adrenal medulla and other chromaffin tissue are homologous to sympathetic ganglia, and all are derived embryonically from neural crest cells; unlike sympathetic ganglia, the adrenal medulla releases epinephrine and norepinephrine.

Sympathetic preganglionic fibers are relatively short because sympathetic ganglia are generally close to the central nervous system (CNS), but they are distant from the effector organs; therefore, postganglionic fibers run a long course before innervating effector organs (see Fig. 16-1). The distribution is also diffuse and is capable of amplification. Preganglionic sympathetic fibers may pass through multiple ganglia before synapsing, and terminal fibers may contact large numbers of postganglionic neurons. Terminal fibers of preganglionic axons may synapse with more than 20 ganglia, and one cell may be supplied by several preganglionic fibers. Sympathetic nerves need not synapse solely in the ganglion of their origin, but they can course up and down the paired ganglia of the spinal cord. Sympathetic response is not confined to segments from which the stimulus originates. This allows for a more dramatic response, with diffuse discharge of the sympathetic system.

Autonomic reflexes remain after transection of the spinal cord. The autonomic reflexes are normally inhibited by supraspinal feedback, but this supraspinal inhibition is lost with the division of the spinal tracts. After transection, trivial stimuli may elicit an exaggerated sympathetic discharge (see "Autonomic Dysfunction").

Parasympathetic Nervous System

The parasympathetic nervous system arises from cranial nerves III, VII, IX, and X, as well as from sacral segments. Unlike in the sympathetic nervous system, the ganglia of the parasympathetic nervous system are proximal to or within the innervated organ. This location of ganglia makes the parasympathetic nervous system more targeted and less robust than the sympathetic nervous system.

Preganglionic fibers of the parasympathetic nervous system originate in three areas of the CNS: the midbrain, the medulla oblongata, and the sacral part of the spinal cord. Fibers arising in the Edinger-Westphal nucleus of the oculomotor nerve course in the midbrain to synapse in the ciliary ganglion. This pathway innervates the

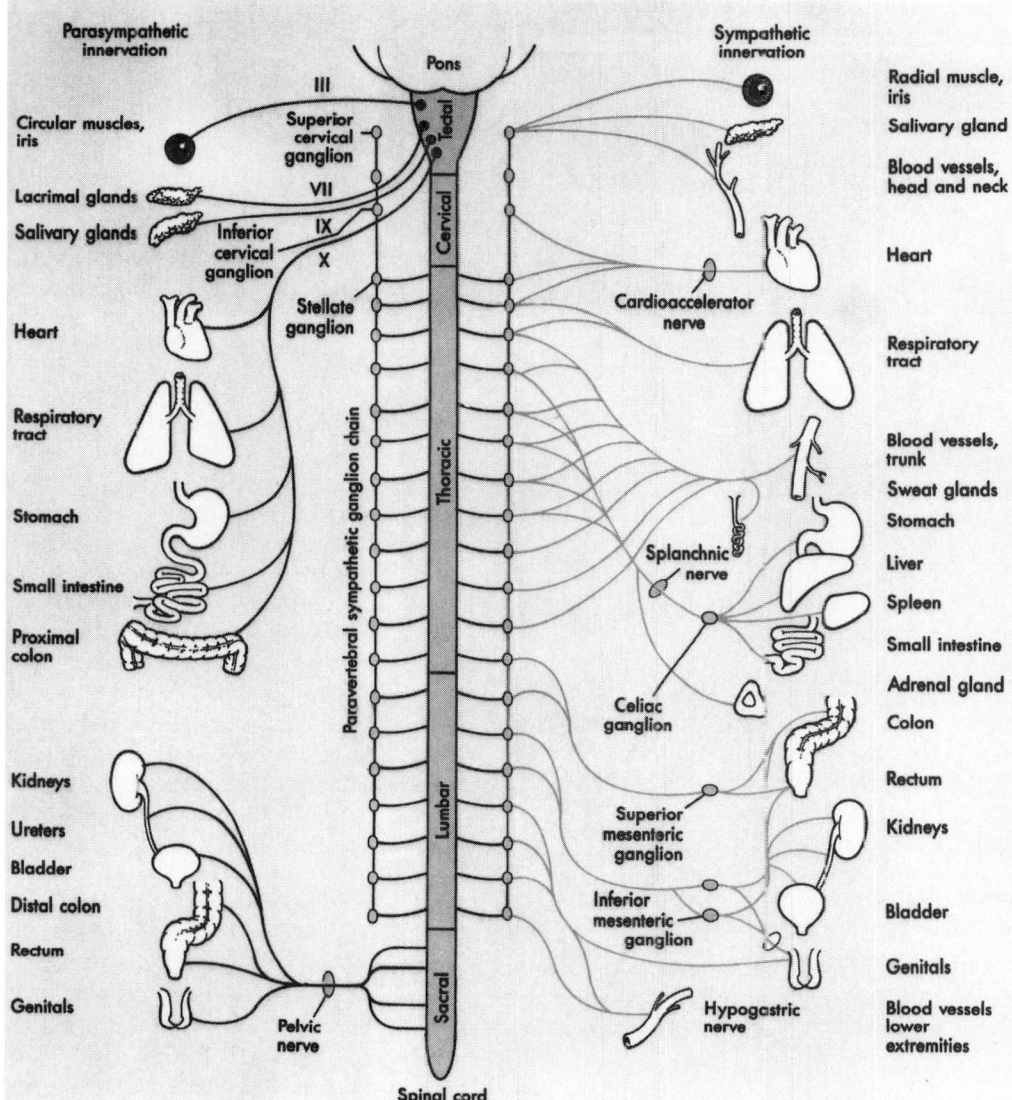

Figure 16–6 Schematic representation of the autonomic nervous system depicting the functional innervation of peripheral effector organs and the anatomic origin of peripheral autonomic nerves from the spinal cord. Although both paravertebral sympathetic ganglia chains are presented, the sympathetic innervation to the peripheral effector organs is shown only on the right part of the figure, whereas the parasympathetic innervation of peripheral effector organs is depicted on the left. The roman numerals on nerves originating in the tectal region of the brainstem refer to the cranial nerves that provide parasympathetic outflow to the effector organs of the head, neck, and trunk. (From Ruffolo R: Physiology and biochemistry of the peripheral autonomic nervous system. In Wingard L, Brody T, Larner J, et al [eds]: Human Pharmacology: Molecular to Clinical. St. Louis, Mosby–Year Book, 1991, p 77.)

smooth muscle of the iris and the ciliary muscle. In the medulla oblongata lie parasympathetic components of the facial (lacrimatory nucleus), glossopharyngeal, and vagus (dorsal nucleus) nerves. The facial nerve gives off parasympathetic fibers to the chorda tympani and greater superficial petrosal nerve, which subsequently synapse in the ganglia of the submaxillary or sublingual glands and the sphenopalatine ganglion, respectively. The glossopharyngeal nerve synapses in the otic ganglion. These postganglionic fibers innervate the mucous, salivary, and lacrimal glands; they also carry vasodilator fibers.

The vagus is unquestionably the most important of the parasympathetic nerves. The vagus transmits fully three fourths of the traffic of the parasympathetic nervous system. It supplies the heart, tracheobronchial tree, liver, spleen, kidney, and the entire gastrointestinal tract except the distal colon. The preganglionic fibers of the vagus are long, whereas the postganglionic fibers are short. Most vagal fibers do not synapse until they arrive at small ganglia on and about the thoracic and abdominal viscera. Although the parasympathetic nerves may synapse with a 1:1 ratio of nerve to effector cells, the vagal innervation of the Auerbach plexus may connect one nerve fiber to 8000 cells.

The second through fourth sacral segments contribute the nervi erigentes, or pelvic splanchnic nerves. They synapse in terminal ganglia associated with the rectum and genitourinary organs.

Enteric Nervous System

Given the importance of clinical phenomena such as nausea, vomiting, and alterations in bowel and bladder function associated with anesthesia, it is surprising how little is understood about the third branch of the ANS. The enteric nervous system is the system of neurons and their supporting cells found within the walls of the gastrointestinal tract, including the neurons within the pancreas and gallbladder.[19] The history of this system is as rich as its innervation: Meissner (1829-1903) and Auerbach (1828-1897) first described the ganglionated plexus of the system; Dogiel (1852-1922) recognized and classified the unique morphologies of enteric neurons and correctly predicted that differences in shape would indicate differences in function; Bayliss (1860-1924) and Starling (1866-1927) showed the existence of polarized reflexes operating in the intestine independent of extrinsic influences; and John Langley defined the unusual features of the enteric nervous system and classified it as the "third division of the autonomic nervous system." The enteric nervous system contains as many nerve cells as the spinal cord. It is derived from neuroblasts of the neural crest that migrate to the gastrointestinal tract along the vagus nerve.

One major difference between the enteric nervous system and the sympathetic and parasympathetic branches of the ANS is its extraordinary degree of local autonomy. Digestion and peristalsis occur after spinal cord transection or during spinal anesthesia, although sphincter function may be impaired.

Although functionally discrete, the gut is influenced by sympathetic and parasympathetic activity. The sympathetic preganglionic fibers from T5 through L1 inhibit gut action; a spinal or epidural anesthetic to the midthoracic levels removes this inhibition, yielding a contracted small intestine that may afford superior surgical conditions in combination with the profound muscle relaxation of a spinal anesthetic.[20] The sphincters are relaxed, and peristalsis is normally active.

Norepinephrine within the gut is the transmitter of postganglionic sympathetic neurons to the gut. For example, if the contents of the upper intestine become overly acidic or hypertonic, an adrenergically mediated enterogastric reflex reduces the rate of gastric emptying. The adrenergic neurons, which run to the myenteric ganglia of the gastrointestinal tract from the thoracic and lumbar spinal segments, are usually inactive in the resting individual. Reflex pathways within and external to the alimentary tract cause discharge of these neurons. During abdominal surgery, when the viscera are handled, a reflex firing of the adrenergic inhibitory nerves inhibits the motor activity of the intestine for an extended period. This adrenergic inhibition is thought to be the basis of the common condition known as *postoperative ileus*. Loss of parasympathetic nervous control usually decreases bowel tone and peristalsis, but over time, the increased activity of the enteric plexus compensates for the loss. Spinal cord lesions may remove sacral parasympathetic input, but cranial parasympathetics may still be carried by the branches of the vagus nerve down to the end-organ ganglia; colonic dilation and fecal impaction (which may precipitate hypertension in autonomic dysreflexia) occur more often than small intestinal dysfunction.

Enteric neurons can be sensory, monitoring tension in the wall of the intestine or its chemical contents; associative, acting like interneurons; or motor, contracting intestinal muscles, dilating vessels, or transporting water and electrolytes. The motor neurons in the enteric nervous system may be excitatory or inhibitory.

Certain plexuses play important roles in the enteric nervous system. The myenteric plexus, also called the Auerbach plexus, is a network of nerve strands and small ganglia lying in the plane between the external longitudinal and circular muscle coats of the intestine. The submucous plexus (Meissner plexus) consists of nerve cell bodies, glial cells, and glial and neuronal processes, but it does not contain connective tissue or blood vessels. Within the ganglia, many neuronal processes contain vesicles that store neurotransmitters.

What is the organizational pattern of these neurons, which can contain up to a dozen neurotransmitters? Unlike the sympathetic and parasympathetic nervous systems, in which geographic location can confer selective action, this is anatomically impossible in the gut, and an alternative pattern of chemical coding for function assumes an important organizational role. The combination of amines and peptides within the enteric neuron is thought to code for its function.

Acetylcholine is the principal excitatory trigger of the nonsphincteric portion of the enteric nervous system, causing muscle contraction. Cholinergic neurons have several roles in the enteric nervous system, including excitation of external muscle, activation of motor neurons augmenting water and electrolyte secretion, and stimulation of gastric cells. Neural control of gastrointestinal motility is mediated through two types of motor neurons: excitatory and inhibitory. These neurons act in concert on the circular smooth muscle layer on sphincteric and nonsphincteric regions throughout the digestive tract, and they supply the muscle of the biliary tree and the muscularis mucosae. Although excitatory motor neurons supply the external longitudinal muscle, it is not well established that all regions of the longitudinal muscle are supplied by inhibitory motor neurons. Enteric motor neurons to the circular muscle of the small and large intestine are activated by local reflex pathways contained within the wall of the intestine. Distention evokes polarized reflexes, including contraction orally and relaxation anally, which in synchrony constitute peristalsis. Nicotinic antagonists abolish enteric reflexes, suggesting that the sensory neurons or interneurons in the pathway are cholinergic. In cases of cholinergic overload, such as insecticide poisoning or "overreversal" of muscle relaxants, there is a tendency for the gut (in which cholinesterase is inhibited) to become hyperreactive.

There are, however, many other compounds that participate in intestinal function, including substance P, a variety of opiate peptides, VIP, and a growing population of peptide hormones. There is evidence for nonadrenergic, noncholinergic (NANC) neurons in the small intestine and for similar cells that mediate gastrin release. Evidence also indicates that nitric oxide (NO), the same compound that dilates the vasculature and is secreted by the endothelial cells, may be an important component of interneurons and may be cosecreted with VIP. (NO-containing NANC neurons also mediate penile erection.[21]) In the sphincters, substance P, opioid peptides, and acetylcholine may be involved in excitatory transmission, although their relative roles may vary from sphincter to sphincter.

FUNCTION

Organization and Integration

The sympathetic system, in response to internal or external challenges, acts to increase heart rate, blood pressure, and cardiac output; to dilate the bronchial tree; and to shunt blood away from the intestines and other viscera to voluntary muscles. Teleologically, the body is then better prepared to deal with the challenge. Parasympathetic nervous input acts primarily to conserve energy and maintain organ function and to support the vegetative processes.

Most organs of the body exhibit dual innervation, with input from the sympathetic and parasympathetic systems frequently mediating opposing effects[22] (Table 16-1). Stimulation of one system may have an excitatory effect on the end organ, whereas stimulation of the other system may have an inhibitory effect. The eye, heart, bronchial tree, and gastrointestinal and genitourinary systems are innervated. For example, sympathetic stimulation acts on the heart to increase rate and vigor of contraction and to enhance conduction through the atrioventricular node, whereas parasympathetic stimulation acts to decrease rate and contractility and to slow conduction through the atrioventricular node. One of the two systems normally dominates the organ's function, providing its "resting tone" (Table 16-2). In a few organs, the sympathetic system alone provides innervation; certain blood vessels, the spleen, and piloerector muscles are examples.

Table 16–1   Responses elicited in effector organs by stimulation of sympathetic and parasympathetic nerves

Effector Organ	Adrenergic Response	Receptor Involved	Cholinergic Response	Dominant Response (A or C)
Heart				
Rate of contraction	Increase	β_1	Decrease	C
Force of contraction	Increase	β_1	Decrease	C
Blood vessels				
Arteries (most)	Vasoconstriction	α_1		A
Skeletal muscle	Vasodilation	β_2		A
Veins	Vasoconstriction	α_2		A
Bronchial tree	Bronchodilation	β_2	Bronchoconstriction	C
Splenic capsule	Contraction	α_1		A
Uterus	Contraction	α_1	Variable	A
Vas deferens	Contraction	α_1		A
Prostatic capsule	Contraction	α_1		A
Gastrointestinal tract	Relaxation	α_2	Contraction	C
Eye				
Radial muscle, iris	Contraction (mydriasis)	α_1		A
Circular muscle, iris			Contraction (miosis)	C
Ciliary muscle	Relaxation	β	Contraction (accommodation)	C
Kidney	Renin secretion	β_1		A
Urinary bladder				
Detrusor	Relaxation	β	Contraction	C
Trigone and sphincter	Contraction	α_1	Relaxation	A, C
Ureter	Contraction	α_1	Relaxation	A
Insulin release from pancreas	Decrease	α_2		A
Fat cells	Lipolysis	β_1		A
Liver glycogenolysis	Increase	α_1		A
Hair follicles, smooth muscle	Contraction (piloerection)	α_1		A
Nasal secretion			Increase	C
Salivary glands	Increase secretion	α_1	Increase secretion	C
Sweat glands	Increase secretion	α_1	Increase secretion	C

A, adrenergic; C, cholinergic.
From Ruffolo R: Physiology and biochemistry of the peripheral autonomic nervous system. In Wingard L, Brody T, Larner J, et al (eds): Human Pharmacology: Molecular to Clinical. St. Louis, Mosby–Year Book, 1991, p 77.

Table 16–2   Usual sympathetic or parasympathetic dominance at specific effector sites

Site	Predominant Tone
Ciliary muscle	Parasympathetic
Iris	Parasympathetic
Sinoatrial node	Parasympathetic
Arterioles	Sympathetic
Veins	Sympathetic
Gastrointestinal tract	Parasympathetic
Uterus	Parasympathetic
Urinary bladder	Parasympathetic
Salivary glands	Parasympathetic
Sweat glands	Sympathetic (cholinergic)

To predict the effects of drugs, the interaction of the sympathetic and parasympathetic system in different organs must be understood. Blockade of sympathetic function unmasks preexisting parasympathetic activity, and the converse relation also is true. For example, administration of atropine blocks the resting muscarinic tone of the parasympathetically dominated heart, and unopposed sympathetic tone then causes tachycardia. Autonomic denervation, which may occur with neuraxial anesthesia, diabetes, and myocardial infarction (MI), can be assessed by traditional methods, such as orthostatic hypotension, or by changes in the time interval between successive heart beats (i.e., beat-to-beat or heart rate variability) as a measure of sympathovagal balance.[23]

Adrenergic Function

Overview of the Effects of Epinephrine
The adrenergic neurons influence many bodily functions, but the effects on circulation and respiration are among the most important. The effects of sympathetic nervous stimulation on the body's physiology are designed to facilitate fight or flight (Table 16-3). Ventilation is increased by a central effect on the ventilatory centers and by bronchodilation. Cardiac output is increased through an increase in the contractile force of the heart and the rate of contraction, and perfusion pressure for vital organs is increased by constriction of vessels to nonvital organs. Function of the gastrointestinal and genitourinary systems is decreased as a result of a relaxation of the smooth muscle in these organs and contraction of their sphincters. Gastrointestinal secretory activity is inhibited, and adrenal medullary output is increased. Metabolism is generally stimulated to provide more fuel for bodily function in the form of glucose and fatty acids.

The endogenous catecholamines, norepinephrine and epinephrine, possess α- and β-receptor agonistic activity. Norepinephrine has minimal β_2-receptor activity, whereas epinephrine stimulates the β_1- and β_2-receptors (Table 16-4). Fundamental differences exist between the infusion of exogenous catecholamines and release of endogenous catecholamines. For example, infused norepinephrine can elicit bradycardia, but when released in response to stress, it evokes tachycardia.

The physiologic responses mediated by α-adrenoceptors are wide ranging and important. α-Receptor-mediated activity is responsible for most of the sympathetically induced smooth muscle contraction throughout the body, including the ciliary muscle of the eye and vascular, bronchial, and ureteral smooth muscle.[24] The gastrointestinal and genitourinary sphincter mechanisms are stimulated by α-adrenergic receptors. α-Receptor agonism also mediates sympathetic nervous system control of pancreatic insulin secretion. In the peripheral vasculature, postjunctional α_1- and α_2-receptors are found on arteries and veins and act to mediate vasoconstriction independent of nerve supply.

β-Receptor agonism appears to be primarily responsible for sympathetic stimulation of the heart, relaxation of vascular and bronchial smooth muscle, stimulation of renin secretion by the kidney, and several metabolic

Table 16–3   Effects of sympathetic nervous system activation

Site of Action	Stimulation	Inhibition
Heart	Rate, conduction, contractility	
Blood vessels	Vasoconstriction (skin, gut, liver, heart, kidney)	Vasodilation (skeletal muscle, heart, brain)
Respiration	Respiratory center Bronchodilation	
Gastrointestinal tract	Sphincters	Smooth muscle
Genitourinary tract	Sphincters	Ureteral and uterine muscle
Metabolic and endocrine effects	Glycogenolysis (muscle, liver) Lipolysis Gluconeogenesis Insulin release (β_1) Renin release ADH release	Insulin release (α stimulation or β_1 antagonism)

ADH, antidiuretic hormones or arginine vasopressin.

Table 16–4   Adrenergic-receptor differentiation

Receptor	Stimulation	Inhibition
Alpha		
Heart		
Blood vessels	Vasoconstriction (skin, gut, kidney, liver, heart)	
Gastrointestinal tract	Sphincters	
Genitourinary tract	Sphincters	
Metabolic and endocrine effects		Insulin release
Beta		
Heart	(1) Rate, conduction contractility	
Blood vessels		(2) Vasodilation (skeletal muscle, heart, brain)
Respiration	(?) Respiratory center	
	(2) Bronchodilation	
Gastrointestinal tract		(2) Smooth muscle
Genitourinary tract		(2) Ureteral and uterine muscle
Metabolic and endocrine effects	(2) Glycogenolysis (muscle, liver)	
	(1) Lipolysis	
	(2) Gluconeogenesis	
	(1) Insulin release	
	(?) Renin release	
	(?) Antidiuretic hormone release	

1, mediated by β_1-receptors: 2, mediated by β_2-receptors: ?, controversial.

consequences, including lipolysis and glycogenolysis. The β_1-receptor mechanism is thought to be primarily involved in the cardiac effects[25] and release of fatty acids and renin, whereas the β_2-receptors are primarily responsible for smooth muscle relaxation and hyperglycemia. In specialized circumstances, however, β_2-receptors may also mediate cardiac activity. Although acute changes in blood pressure or heart rate can be caused by norepinephrine or epinephrine, chronic hypertension does not appear to be related to levels of these hormones.[26] It is estimated that 85% of resting blood pressure is controlled by renin (Fig. 16-7). An additional important effect of epinephrine includes increasing gap junctions in bone, causing an increase in circulating blood elements.[27,28]

Psychological and physical stimuli may evoke different compensatory responses. Whereas public speaking activates the adrenal gland and the sympathetic nervous system, physical exercise elicits primarily a sympathetic response.[29] The stress response should not be conceived of as a uniform response; it can vary in intensity and manifestations.

Blood Glucose

Catecholamines are released to mobilize glucose in the face of systemic hypoglycemia and to normalize glucose values, providing cells with energy. Overall, sympathetic nervous stimulation through β-receptor stimulation increases glycogenolysis in liver and muscle and liberates free fatty acids from adipose tissue, ultimately increasing blood glucose levels. In neonates, epinephrine plays an additional role in the exothermic breakdown of brown fat to maintain body temperature (i.e., nonshivering thermogenesis).

The α_2- and β_2-receptors also are present in the pancreas. α_2-Receptor activation suppresses insulin secretion by pancreatic islets and inhibits lipolysis; blockade of these receptors may increase insulin release and may be associated with significant lowering of blood glucose levels. β-Receptor stimulation increases glucagon and insulin secretion.[30]

Potassium Shift

Plasma epinephrine also regulates serum potassium concentration. β-Adrenergic stimulation can initiate transient hyperkalemia as potassium shifts out of hepatic cells with the glucose efflux produced by β_2-adrenergic stimulation. This effect is followed by a more prolonged hypokalemia as β_2-adrenergic stimulation drives potassium into red blood cells and muscle cells. Exogenously administered or endogenously released epinephrine stimulates the β_2-receptors of red blood cells, activating adenylate cyclase and the sodium-potassium ATPase, driving potassium into cells. This leads to a reduction in serum potassium concentration and may contribute to the cardiac dysrhythmias accompanying MI and other stresses. β_2-Adrenergic blockade has the theoretical advantage of inhibiting this potassium shift. However, the selective and nonselective β-blockers have been shown to be equivalent in protecting the postinfarction heart against arrhythmias.[31-35]

Cholinergic Function

Overview of the Effects of Acetylcholine

In contrast to the diffuse discharge of the sympathetic nervous system that constitutes the fight or flight

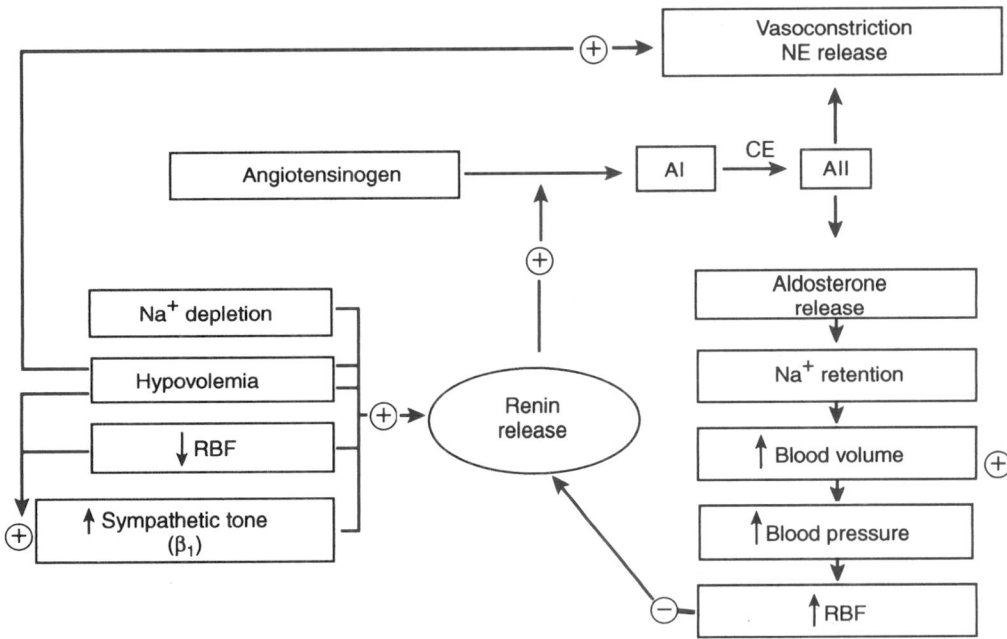

Figure 16–7 The interactions of the renin-angiotensin-aldosterone and sympathetic nervous systems in maintaining blood pressure and volume. AI, angiotensin I; AII, angiotensin II; CE, converting enzyme; NE, norepinephrine; RBF, renal blood flow; +, stimulating effects; –, inhibiting effects.

response, the parasympathetic system is anatomically and functionally more localized in its effects. Parasympathetic activation conserves energy and maintains organ function. A massive parasympathetic response would only prostrate the organism, leaving it helplessly salivating, weeping, wheezing, vomiting, urinating, defecating, and seizing. Although the sympathetic system is needed for the emergency response to stressful situations, it is not necessary for survival; the parasympathetic system is, however, essential for the maintenance of life.

Acetylcholine release is the hallmark of parasympathetic activation. The actions of acetylcholine are almost diametrically opposed to those of norepinephrine and epinephrine. In general, the muscarinic effects of acetylcholine are qualitatively the same as the effects of vagal stimulation. Acetylcholine is the only endogenous compound that causes simultaneous bradycardia and hypotension.

The dose of acetylcholine determines the effect or effects. A small intravenous dose causes generalized vasodilation (including the coronary and pulmonary circulation), whereas a larger dose is required to demonstrate negative chronotropic and dromotropic effects. Significant numbers of muscarinic receptors exist in these vascular beds despite the apparent absence of cholinergic nerve supply to most vessels. A second mechanism of vessel relaxation by acetylcholine is inhibition of norepinephrine release from adrenergic nerve terminals.

Acetylcholine decreases the rate of cardiac contraction, the velocity of conduction in the sinoatrial and atrioventricular nodes, and contractility (although not as marked as the increase produced by sympathetic stimulation) of the atria. In the sinoatrial node, acetylcholine causes

membrane hyperpolarization, delaying resumption of the threshold potential and the ability to generate another action potential. This action slows the heart rate. Although the duration of the action potential and the effective refractory period are increased, the rate of conduction through atrial myocardium is unchanged. In the atrioventricular node, acetylcholine decreases conduction velocity and increases the effective refractory period. This decrease in nodal conduction usually accounts for the complete heart block seen when large amounts of cholinergic agonists are given. In the ventricle, acetylcholine decreases the Purkinje system automaticity, thereby increasing the fibrillation threshold. In the heart, presynaptic and postsynaptic muscarinic receptors are involved in these effects. Acetylcholine inhibits adrenergic stimulation of the heart presynaptically by inhibiting the release of norepinephrine from sympathetic nerve endings and postsynaptically by opposing the effects of catecholamines on the myocardium.

Parasympathetic activation has many effects outside the cardiovascular system. Acetylcholine stimulates the chemoreceptors of the carotid and aortic bodies. Cholinergic stimulation causes smooth muscle constriction, including that of bronchial walls. In the gastrointestinal and genitourinary tracts, smooth muscle in the walls constricts, but sphincter muscles relax. Topically administered acetylcholine constricts the smooth muscle of the iris, causing miosis.

Signs and symptoms of cholinergic overload reflect all these effects, with nausea and vomiting, intestinal cramps, belching, urination, and urgent defecation. All parasympathetic glands are stimulated to produce secretions, including the lacrimal, tracheobronchial, salivary, digestive, and exocrine glands.

Local Control of Vascular Tone

In addition to the pharmacologic effects of acetylcholine that are mediated by the parasympathetic nervous system, acetylcholine has a significant effect on blood vessels, dilating virtually all vessels in vivo. In 1980, Furchgott and Zawadzki[36] observed that blood vessels with intact endothelium dilated when acetylcholine was applied. If the endothelial cells were damaged, the vessels constricted. Endothelial cells respond to acetylcholine stimulation by producing one or more endothelium-derived relaxing factors (EDRFs).[37] It now appears that the endothelial cells have receptors to numerous agonists, including serotonin, adenosine, histamine, and catecholamines (Fig. 16-8). The radical NO is the first identified EDRF. It is produced by the endothelial cells in minute quantities, but it acts to relax vascular smooth muscle cells and to limit or modify the actions of many vasoconstrictors. Nitroglycerin is degraded to NO in the vascular myocyte. The mechanism of this vasodilator action is mediated through activation of guanylate cyclase by means of a protein phosphorylation cascade to phosphorylate actinomyosin directly. When the endothelium is damaged, as in atherosclerosis, production of EDRF diminishes and constriction increases. This change explains why patients with damaged or diseased vessels react differently.

The biology of NO appears to be important.[38] This simple compound, the mechanism of whose storage and release is still poorly understood, plays a prominent role in signal transduction and is a neurotransmitter in the gut and cerebellum (N-methyl-D-aspartate [NMDA] induces release of NO in the cerebellum).[39,40] NO is produced during the conversion of arginine to citrulline by a class of enzymes known as NO synthases (NOS). Five isoforms of this family of enzymes have been identified, and the most common form, found in the cerebellum, has been cloned.[41] There is a requirement for flavins, reduced nicotinamide adenine dinucleotide phosphate (NADPH), and calmodulin. Some isoforms are inducible, and in septic (but not traumatic) shock or during chemotherapy, there is evidence that NO causes hypotension.[42] Other isoforms of the enzyme, such as those in the brain, are constitutive and appear to reside in a population of cells that are tonically active. Curiously, the structure of NOS closely resembles that of cytochrome P450.[43] The head of the enzyme contains the NOS function, and the tail contains an NADPH diaphorase function. Preclinical studies with NOS inhibitors suggest that the systemic vasculature is in a state of constant active vasodilation.[44]

Endothelial cells control the circulation in addition to producing NO. Endothelial cells metabolize many vasoactive amines, convert angiotensin I to angiotensin II, and secrete NO, prostacyclin, and the vasoconstrictive peptide endothelin-1 (ET-1). NO, ET-1, and prostacyclin are local hormones released by endothelial cells to influence their immediate microenvironment. Prostacyclin and NO relax underlying smooth muscle on the abluminal side, whereas in the lumen, they act separately or in concert to prevent platelets from clumping onto the endothelium. There is clear synergism between the anti-aggregating effect of prostacyclin and subthreshold concentrations of NO. Substances that activate prostacyclin generally stimulate NO release. Shear stress increases NO as an adaptive mechanism to dilate the circulation actively. NO works by the guanylate cyclase mechanism; prostacyclin works by activation of adenylate cyclase. Although they work in concert, they activate different second messengers.[45]

Although prostacyclin and NO are short-lived vasodilators, injection of the vasoconstrictor ET-1 causes a powerful and long-lasting pressor effect. ET-1, which consists of 21 amino acids bound by two disulfide bonds,

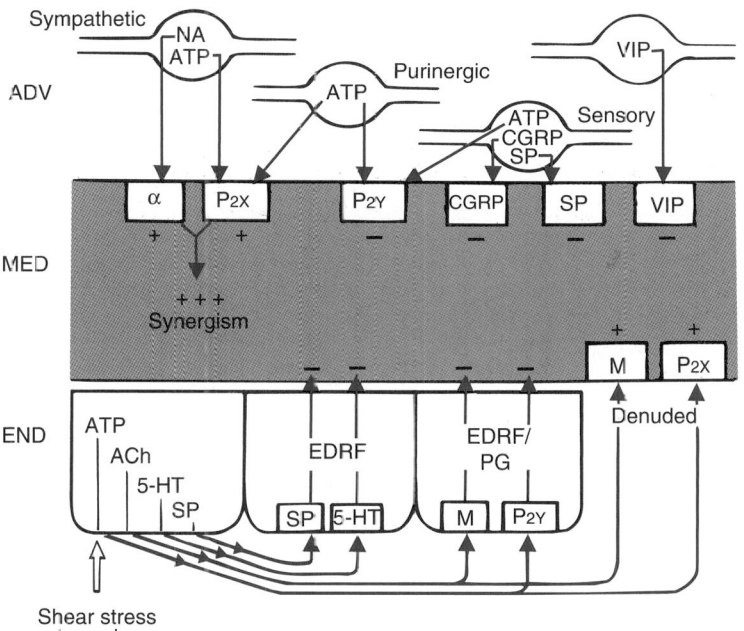

Figure 16–8 Schematic representation of potential modes of regulation of vascular tone by endothelial cell–related mechanisms. Norepinephrine (NA), adenosine triphosphate (ATP), calcitonin gene–related peptide (CGRP), substance P (SP), and vasoactive intestinal polypeptide (VIP) can be released from nerves in the adventitia (ADV) to act on their respective receptors in the media (MED) to cause vasoconstriction or vasodilation. ATP, acetylcholine (ACh), 5-hydroxytryptamine (5-HT), and SP released from endothelial cells (END) by shear stress or hypoxia act on their receptors on endothelial cells to cause release of endothelium-derived relaxing factors (EDRF) or prostaglandins (PG), which act on smooth muscle to cause relaxation. In areas denuded of endothelial cells, opposite effects may be produced by receptors on the smooth muscle. α, noradrenaline receptor; M, muscarinic receptor; P_{2x}, P_{2x}-purinoceptor; P_{2y}, P_{2y}-purinoceptor. (From Lincoln J, Burnstock G: Neural-endothelial interactions in control of local blood flow. In Warren J [ed]: The Endothelium: An Introduction to Current Research. New York, Wiley-Liss, 1990, p 21.)

is enzymatically generated from the 39–amino acid ET-1 precursor, known as *big ET-1*. The vasoconstrictor action of ET-1 results from activation of endothelium receptors on smooth muscle.[46]

NO, prostacyclin, and ET-1 appear to be operative in local control of the circulation. The prostacyclin system may be a mechanism reserved to reinforce the NO system in the presence of endothelial damage. Acting together, these two dilators are a strong defense mechanism against intravascular thrombosis. ET-1 can be produced locally in response to trauma such as wounds to the vessel wall. Long-term functions of these local hormones are of considerable interest in the pathophysiology of many disease states, including septic shock, pulmonary hypertension, and renal failure.[47-49]

PHARMACOLOGY

Adrenergic Pharmacology

Synthesis of Norepinephrine

Norepinephrine is synthesized from tyrosine, which is actively transported into the varicosity of the postganglionic

sympathetic nerve ending (Fig. 16-9). Tyrosine is synthesized from phenylalanine. It is therefore expected that in phenylketonuric patients, who lack phenylalanine hydroxylase, there would be a significant defect in the ANS. However, tyrosine is available from the diet as well as from phenylalanine, and no autonomic defect exists in phenylketonuric patients. In hypertensive rats, tyrosine may increase central adrenergic transmission, decreasing peripheral sympathetic outflow.[50] In hypotensive (hemorrhaged) rats, tyrosine may increase peripheral synthesis and release of catecholamines. Precursors are taken up in greater amounts in shock and may have beneficial effects on the efforts of the sympathetic nervous system to maintain perfusion pressure.

A series of steps results in the conversion of tyrosine to norepinephrine and epinephrine (in the adrenal medulla). The first of these steps involves tyrosine hydroxylase (TH). This cytoplasmic enzyme is the rate-controlling step for norepinephrine biosynthesis. High levels of norepinephrine inhibit TH, and low levels stimulate the enzyme. During sympathetic nervous system stimulation, an increased supply of tyrosine also increases synthesis of norepinephrine. TH activity is modified by phosphorylation. TH depends on a pteridine

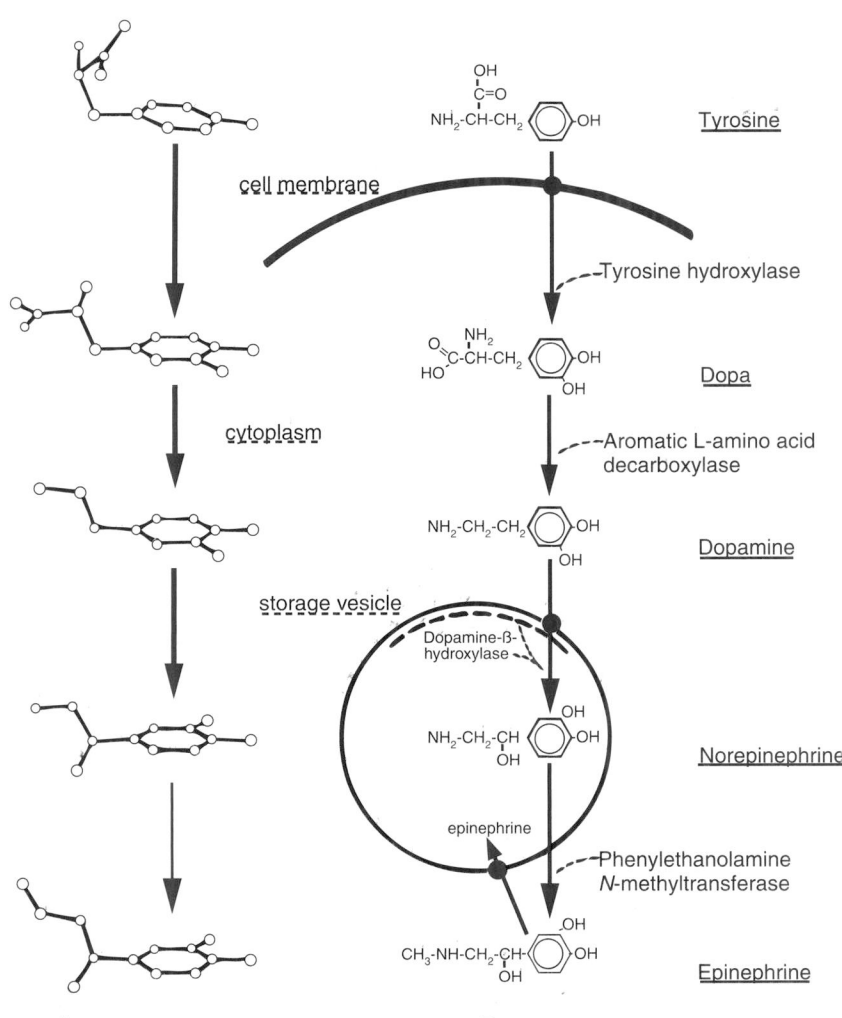

Figure 16–9 Biosynthesis of norepinephrine and epinephrine in sympathetic nerve terminal (and adrenal medulla). **A,** Perspective view of molecules. **B,** Enzymatic processes. (From Tollenaeré JP: Atlas of the Three-Dimensional Structure of Drugs. Amsterdam, Elsevier North-Holland, 1979 as modified by Vanhoutte PM: Adrenergic neuroeffector interaction in the blood vessel wall. Fed Proc 37:181, 1978.)

A

B

cofactor and the presence of molecular oxygen. Molecular oxygen, when in reduced quantity, may significantly reduce norepinephrine synthesis and may account for changes in wakefulness. Whereas acute control of TH occurs by altering enzyme activity, chronic stress can elevate TH levels by stimulating synthesis of new enzyme. Tyrosine is converted by the enzyme TH to dihydroxyphenylalanine (DOPA), which is decarboxylated to dopamine by aromatic amino acid decarboxylase (DOPA decarboxylase), a relatively promiscuous enzyme in its substrate specificity. In Parkinson's disease, dopaminergic function is impaired. Although some of the most troubling chronic problems of Parkinson's disease are attributable to central dopamine depletion, peripheral sympathetic defects also have been recognized. Imaging procedures have demonstrated decreased neuronal uptake, release, turnover, and synthesis of norepinephrine in the myocardium, with a nearly complete loss of sympathetic terminal innervation in the hearts of patients with Parkinson's disease–associated autonomic dysfunction. Sympathetic denervation of the heart was present in 50% of the Parkinson's patients who had no clinical signs of autonomic failure on provocative testing. Administration of DOPA attempts to improve dopaminergic function in the brain, because DOPA, but not dopamine, crosses the blood-brain barrier.

Dopamine can and does act as a neurotransmitter in some cells, but in most adrenergic neurons, dopamine is catabolized quickly by the enzyme monoamine oxidase (MAO), found particularly in mitochondria. Subsequently, dopamine is β-hydroxylated within the vesicles to norepinephrine by the enzyme dopamine β-hydroxylase (DBH). In the adrenal medulla and to a limited extent in discrete regions of the brain, another enzyme, phenylethanolamine N-methyl transferase (PNMT), methylates about 85% of the norepinephrine to epinephrine. Glucocorticoids from the adrenal cortex pass through the adrenal medulla and can activate the system, and stress-induced steroid release can increase epinephrine production. This local circulation amplifies the effects of glucocorticoid release.[51]

Storage of Norepinephrine

Norepinephrine is stored within large, dense-core vesicles. Electron microscopy demonstrates that the dense cores in these vesicles are not filled with norepinephrine but perhaps with other binding proteins. The vesicles also contain calcium and a variety of peptides and ATP. Depending on the nature and frequency of physiologic stimuli, the ATP can be selectively released for an immediate postsynaptic effect through purinoreceptors.

Synaptic vesicles are heterogeneous and exist within functionally defined compartments. There appears to be an actively recycling population of synaptic vesicles and a reserve population of vesicles that is mobilized only on extensive stimulation. Newly synthesized or taken up transmitters are preferentially incorporated into the actively recycling vesicles and are preferentially released on stimulation. Drugs that mimic the neurotransmitter and are taken up presynaptically may be disproportionately represented in release. Functionally, norepinephrine is stored in compartments, of which 10% is readily releasable. In general, 1% of stored norepinephrine is released with each depolarization, implying a significant functional reserve. On stimulation, the contents of the vesicle are released into the synaptic cleft. Approximately 10% of stored norepinephrine is resistant to depletion, such as occurs with reserpine.

Synaptic vesicles have two fundamentally different functions: They take up and store neurotransmitters, and they fuse with and bud from the presynaptic plasma terminal membrane. The proteins of synaptic vesicles can be divided into two functionally discrete classes. The first class, transport proteins, provides the channels and pumps for the uptake and storage of neurotransmitters. The second class of proteins directs movement and docking reactions of the synaptic vesicle membrane.

Release of Norepinephrine

There are several different processes by which the contents of the vesicle enter the synaptic cleft. In exocytosis, the dominant physiologic mechanism of release, the vesicle responds to the entry of calcium by initiating vesicle docking, fusion, and endocytosis (the process by which vesicular membrane and proteins are recaptured) (Fig. 16-10).[49] The entire contents of the vesicle are liberated on nerve stimulation. The biology of vesicular release is not a random event, but a highly differentiated process. The fact that exocytosis is so highly conserved from species to species indicates its biologic importance. Angiotensin II, prostacyclin, and histamine may potentiate release, whereas acetylcholine and prostaglandin E inhibit release. Because of its generalized importance in neurotransmitter release, the process of exocytosis has been extensively investigated.

In this model, the vesicle merges with the cell membrane, a process that depends on microfilaments and influenced by calcium. A widely accepted view of the role of synaptic vesicles in transmitter release is as follows. When an action potential reaches a nerve terminal, the presynaptic plasma membrane depolarizes, and the voltage-gated calcium channels open at the active zone. Although only small amounts of calcium are required to initiate the process, the concentration of calcium in the specialized zones of active release, nanodomains, is very high. This concept of calcium nanodomains is postulated to represent the biologic explanation underlying augmentation and post-tetanic potentiation[52] in that the gradual diffusion of these high calcium levels from the nanodomains recruits new vesicles for release on subsequent stimulations (see Chapter 22). That calcium levels cause this phenomenon appears to be well accepted.[53] The ensuing rise in intracellular calcium triggers exocytosis of synaptic vesicles, resulting in the release of neurotransmitters.[54] The synaptic vesicle membranes are reclaimed from the plasma membrane by endocytosis, and the vesicles eventually refill with neurotransmitters. A diagram of this process can be seen in Figure 16-11.[55]

Various specific soluble and membrane-bound proteins have been identified that participate in docking, fusion, and endocytosis. Synaptotagmin serves as the intermediary between calcium entry and docking, because it binds calcium.[56] Microinjection of this protein participates in

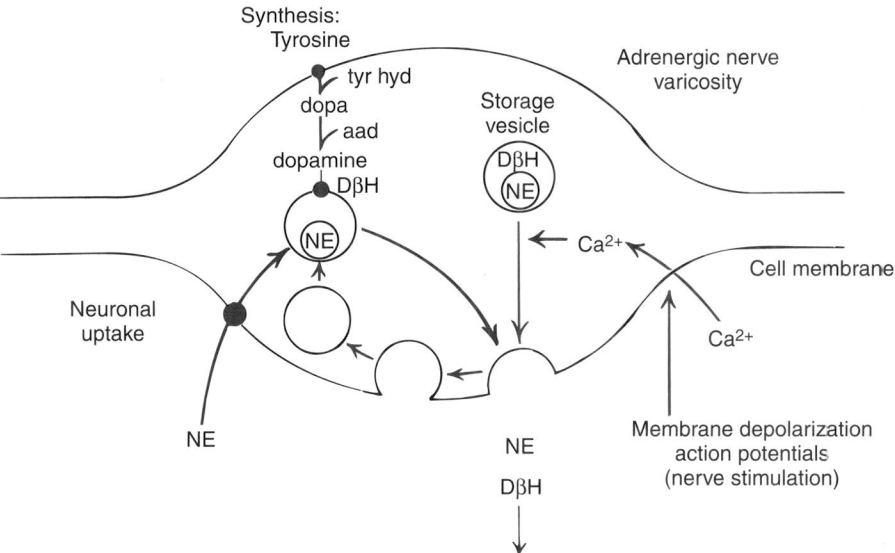

Figure 16–10 Release and reuptake of norepinephrine at sympathetic nerve terminals. aad, aromatic L-amino decarboxylase: DβH, dopamine β-hydroxylase; dopa, L-dihydroxyphenylalanine; NE, norepinephrine; tyr hyd, tyrosine hydroxylase; *solid circle, active carrier.* (From Vanhoutte PM: Adrenergic neuroeffector interaction in the blood vessel wall. Fed Proc 37:181, 1978 as modified by Shepherd J, Vanhoutte P: Neurohumoral regulation. In Shepherd S, Vanhoutte P [eds]: The Human Cardiovascular System: Facts and Concepts. New York, Raven Press, 1979, p 107.)

the step between docking and fusion,[57] and in transgenic mice deficient in this protein, neurotransmitter release was attenuated.[58] Although the mechanism of docking and fusion is still incompletely understood, it appears to be a highly differentiated process in which a pair of soluble binding proteins—soluble N-ethyl maleimide sensitive factor (NSF) attachment proteins (SNAPs) and soluble NSF receptors (SNAREs)—interact.[59,60] Evidence for the biologic relevance of these proteins is derived from observations that tetanus toxin and botulinus toxin block

vesicular release by binding to the docking and fusion proteins,[61] whereas microinjection of SNAP into neurons enhances exocytosis.[56,62] In vesicular docking and release, a subpopulation of vesicles is tethered to the active zone of the prejunctional neuron. Some of these vesicles, called *readily releasable vesicles,* are primed for fusion in response to Ca^{2+} influx.[55,63,64] The short latency between presynaptic excitation and vesicle release[65] has functional implications, particularly in facilitating rapid transmission in the sympathetic nervous system.

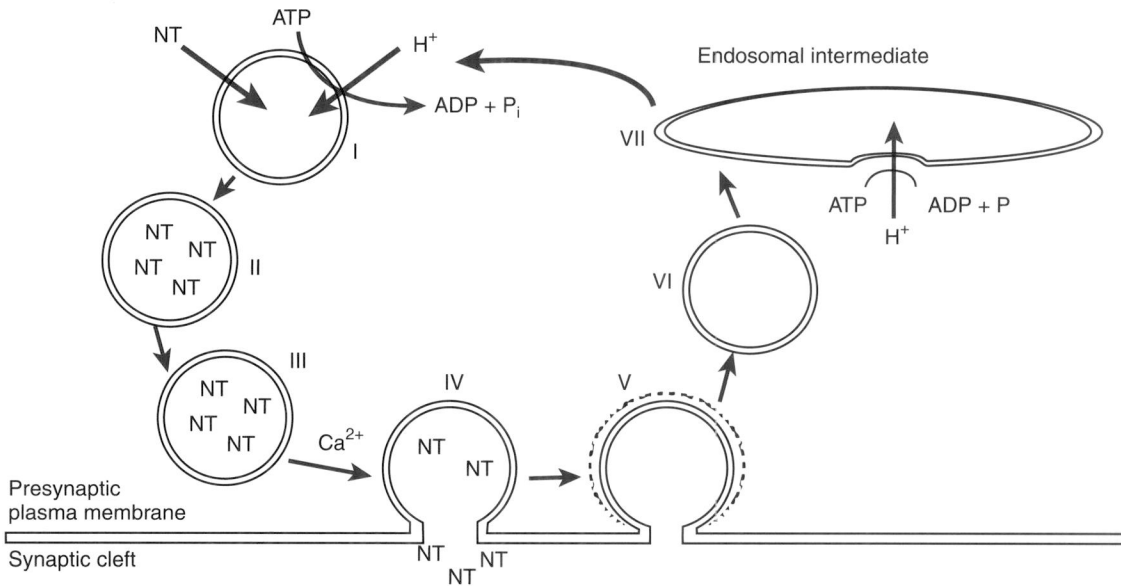

Figure 16–11 Pathway of synaptic vesicle movement in the nerve terminal. Synaptic vesicles accumulate neurotransmitters (NT) by active transport (stage I) and then move to the plasma membrane (stage II), where they become docked at the active zone (stage III). Calcium (Ca^{2+}) influx after membrane depolarization triggers synaptic vesicle exocytosis and release of neurotransmitters (stage IV), after which the empty synaptic vesicles are endocytosed by clathrin-coated pits (stage V) and recycled (stage VI) by means of an endosomal intermediate (stage VII). Stages V and VII have not been definitely proved but are probable on the basis of morphologic observations. (From Südhof TC, Jahn R: Proteins of synaptic vesicles involved in exocytosis and membrane recycling. Neuron 6:665, 1991.)

Exocytosis is distinct from the generalized secretory process in that it is far faster and independent of organelles such as the Golgi apparatus. The entire process of exocytosis, endocytosis, and vesicular reconstitution occurs in seconds.[66-69] Neurotransmitters from a single nerve terminal can be released 50 times per second, requiring a coordinated and tightly linked regulation of underlying biochemical processes. Proof for exocytosis as the dominant mechanism of release is derived from elegant experiments in which nerve stimulation caused release of the biosynthetic enzyme dopamine β-hydroxylase and norepinephrine in the same proportions that are contained within the vesicles.

Exocytosis accounts for most norepinephrine release, although leakage is continuous from the cytoplasm into the neuroeffector junction. Release is indirect with drugs such as ephedrine or bretylium, which displace norepinephrine from the vesicles. Drugs that inhibit vesicular uptake, such as reserpine, also facilitate indirect release. Norepinephrine leakage from storage vesicles into the axoplasm exceeds leakage into the presynaptic cleft by 100-fold and presynaptic reuptake by 10-fold, which explains the initial hypertensive effect of drugs such as reserpine that cause release of neurotransmitter from this compartment.[70] Another hypothesis of vesicular release called *kiss and run* was proposed by Stevens and Williams.[71] Although this mechanism is thought to account for less than 15% of the total release of norepinephrine, it may be functionally important in facilitating immediacy of transmission. Studies of cultured hippocampal cells found a resting pool of 180 vesicles and a recycling pool of approximately 25 vesicles, of which only 5 to 8 were in the readily releasable subset.[72] This results in a very small active pool and a large inactive reserve pool.[60,71] After release, the fusion pores seal rapidly, and the vesicles immediately refill with transmitters, the so-called kiss and run subset.[73]

Although chromaffin cells in the adrenal medulla synthesize epinephrine and norepinephrine, the two compounds are stored in and secreted from distinct chromaffin cell subtypes. Pharmacologic differences between cells containing norepinephrine and epinephrine have been described, and data suggest that there may be a preferential release from one or another form of chromaffin cell contingent on the nature of the stimulus.[74] Nicotinic agonists or depolarizing agents may cause the preferential release of norepinephrine, whereas histamine elicits predominantly epinephrine release.[75-77] Protein kinase C plays an important role in regulating catecholamine secretion from norepinephrine-containing chromaffin cells.[78]

Inactivation

Most of the norepinephrine released is rapidly removed from the synaptic cleft by an amine mechanism (i.e., uptake-1 mechanism) or by nonneuronal tissue (i.e., uptake-2 mechanism). If a transmitter is to exert fine control over an effector system, as when norepinephrine controls blood pressure through the baroreceptor reflex, its half-life in the biophase (i.e., the extracellular space close to the receptor) must be very short. The uptake-1 mechanism represents the first and most important step in the inactivation of released norepinephrine. Most released norepinephrine is transported into the storage vesicle for reuse. This neurotransmitter uptake into synaptic vesicles is driven by an electrochemical proton gradient across the synaptic vesicle membrane. The vacuolar proton pump is a large, hetero-oligomeric complex, containing eight to nine different subunits. After reuptake, the small amounts of norepinephrine not taken up into the vesicle are deaminated by MAO. There are several organ-specific forms of this enzyme.

Since its isolation and cloning in 1991, considerable information on the human norepinephrine transporter has been developed.[79,80] The pharmacologic characteristics of this binding protein identify it as the cocaine binding site, although tricyclic antidepressants (i.e., desipramine and nortriptyline) were also potent antagonists.

Uptake of norepinephrine into the nerve varicosity and its return to the storage vesicle, albeit efficient, is not specific for the neurotransmitter. Some compounds structurally similar to norepinephrine may enter the nerve by the same mechanism and may result in depletion of the neurotransmitter. These false transmitters can be of great clinical importance. Moreover, some drugs that block reuptake into the vesicle or into the synaptic ending itself may enhance response to catecholamines; that is, more norepinephrine is available to receptors. These drugs include cocaine and tricyclic antidepressants (Table 16-5).

Activity of the uptake-1 system varies greatly among different tissues. Because of anatomic barriers, peripheral blood vessels have almost no reuptake of norepinephrine, but they have the highest rate of synthesis in the body. The highest rate of reuptake is found in the heart. Drugs or disease states that alter biosynthesis or storage (e.g., methyldopa decreases storage) would be expected to have a more profound effect on blood pressure; those that affect reuptake (e.g., cocaine) would be expected to affect cardiac rate and rhythm.

Typically, the lungs remove 25% of the norepinephrine that passes through their circulation, whereas epinephrine and dopamine pass through unchanged. Pulmonary uptake of norepinephrine appears to be a sodium-dependent, facilitated-transport process in the endothelial cells of precapillary and postcapillary vessels and pulmonary veins. There is no significant uptake by nerve endings. Pulmonary hypertension diminishes norepinephrine uptake, presumably because of concomitant thickening of the pulmonary vasculature.[81] Uptake is diminished in patients with primary or secondary pulmonary hypertension and elevated pulmonary vascular resistance. Although the functional significance of the endothelial uptake mechanism of the pulmonary vasculature is unknown, uptake of other powerful vasoactive compounds suggests that the pulmonary endothelium functions to protect the left heart.

Defects in the ANS are common in patients with congestive heart failure (CHF). The heart is depleted of catecholamines, and the reuptake of norepinephrine is decreased.[82] Sustained sympathoexcitation results in increased neuronal release of norepinephrine.[83] Cardiac norepinephrine spillover rates differ widely, even among patients with end-stage heart failure awaiting cardiac transplantation, but some studies suggest that plasma

Table 16–5 Comparison of direct- and indirect-acting sympathomimetics

	Response of Effector Organ To	
Pretreatment	Direct Sympathomimetic (e.g., epinephrine): Acts at Receptor	Indirect Sympathomimetics (e.g., tyramine): Causes NE Release after Its Uptake by Uptake 1

Denervation
    Loss of uptake-1 sites
    Receptor upregulation
	Increased	Reduced

Reserpine
    Blocks vesicular uptake
    Depletes NE
    May cause upregulation
	Slightly increased	Reduced

Cocaine
    Blocks uptake 1
    Depletes NE
	Increased	Reduced

NE, norepinephrine.
Adapted from Moore K: Drugs affecting the sympathetic nervous system. *In* Wingard L, Brody T, Larner J, et al (eds): Human Pharmacology: Molecular to Clinical. St. Louis, Mosby–Year Book, 1991, p 114.

catecholamine levels may provide a better guide to prognosis than traditional cardiovascular indices.[84,85] Because augmentation of catecholamine release is markedly impaired in patients with CHF, compensation for further decreases in systemic vascular resistance requires activation of the renin-angiotensin system. Together, these events result in increased adrenergic drive, desensitization of β-receptors, and depletion of norepinephrine stores, which contribute to insufficient inotropic function.[86,87]

Metabolism

During storage and reuptake, a small amount of norepinephrine escapes uptake into the nerve ending and enters the circulation, where it is metabolized by MAO or catechol-O-methyl transferase (COMT), or both, in the blood, liver, and kidney (Fig. 16-12).[88]

Epinephrine, which is released by the adrenal medulla, is inactivated by the same enzymes. The final metabolic product of inactivation is vanillylmandelic acid (VMA). The two catabolic enzymes and the vigorous uptake system account for an efficient clearance of catecholamines. Because of this rapid clearance, the half-life of norepinephrine (and most biogenic amines) in plasma is very short, less than 1 minute. This short half-life necessitates administration of these agents by infusion. Another consequence of their short half-life is that a more ideal measure of catecholamine production may be metabolic products, rather than catecholamines themselves. For example, screening for a norepinephrine-producing pheochromocytoma is frequently done by measuring urine metanephrine and VMA. Only a small percentage of norepinephrine appears in the urine for assay.

Inhibition of MAO would be expected to have a great impact on the sympathetic function of a patient. MAO inhibitors (MAOIs) are generally well tolerated, but the stability of the patient belies the fact that amine handling is fundamentally changed. Clinically important, life-threatening drug interactions are discussed in "Drugs and the Autonomic Nervous System."

Other compounds can be metabolized by catabolic enzymes to produce *false transmitters*. Although it is not used therapeutically, tyramine is the prototypic drug studied. Tyramine is present in many foods, particularly aged cheese and wines, and it can be synthesized from tyrosine. Tyrosine is decarboxylated in the liver and gut. Tyramine enters the sympathetic nerve terminal through the uptake-1 mechanism, displacing norepinephrine from the vesicles into the cytoplasm. Released norepinephrine leaks out from the cytoplasm and is responsible for the sympathomimetic effect of tyramine. However, a secondary effect can occur. In the vesicle, tyramine is converted by DBH into octopamine, which is eventually released as a false transmitter in place of norepinephrine, but without the expected effects, because it has only 10% of the potency of norepinephrine.[89] Sodium plays a key role in the transport of norepinephrine into the cell.[90]

Adrenergic Receptors

Ahlquist originally identified α- and β-adrenergic receptors by their different responses to pharmacologic agents. Initially, α-adrenergic receptors were distinguished from β-adrenergic receptors by their greater response to epinephrine and norepinephrine than to isoproterenol.[24] The development of α- and β-antagonists further supported the existence of separate α-receptors. The advent of radioligand binding techniques signaled an era of pharmacology in which subtypes of receptors could be more readily assessed.

Traditionally, adrenergic receptors have been classified as α or β and more recently as α_1, α_2, β_1, or β_2 based on available drugs. With the advent of molecular biology, classification evolved to three major subtypes and nine sub-subtypes[91] (Fig. 16-13). Justification for such a scheme is derived from pharmacologic analyses of drug-affinity patterns, functional differences in signal transduction

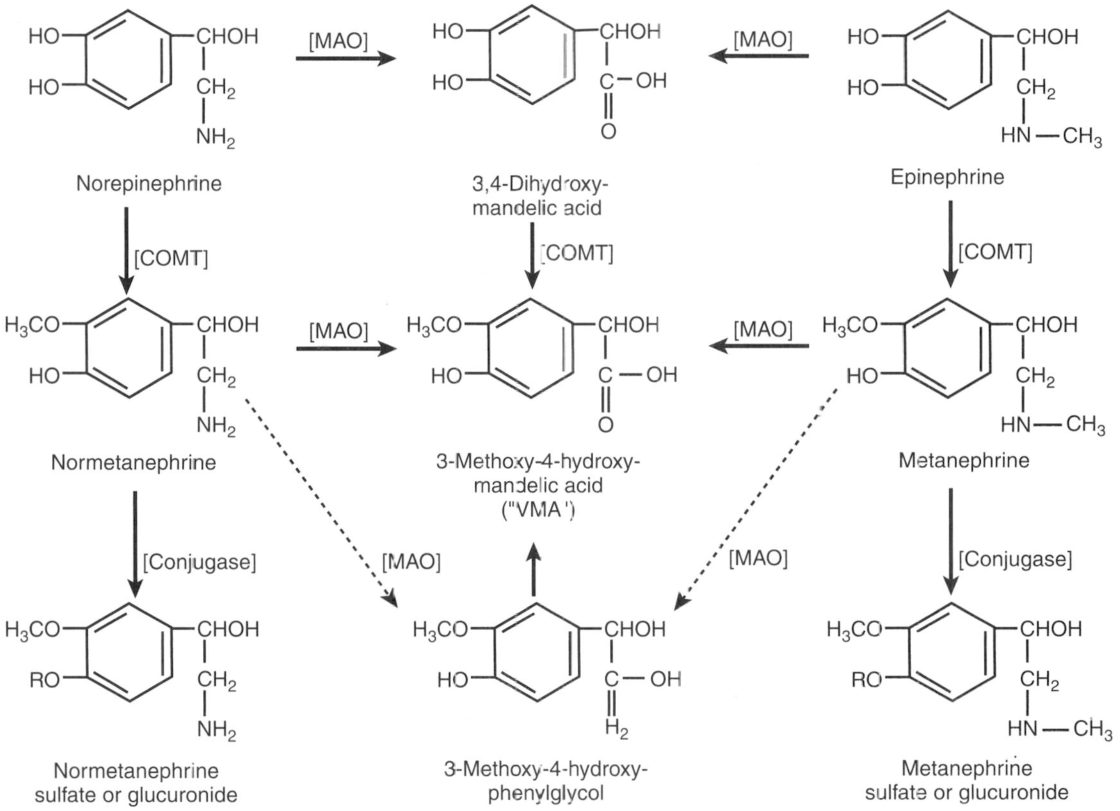

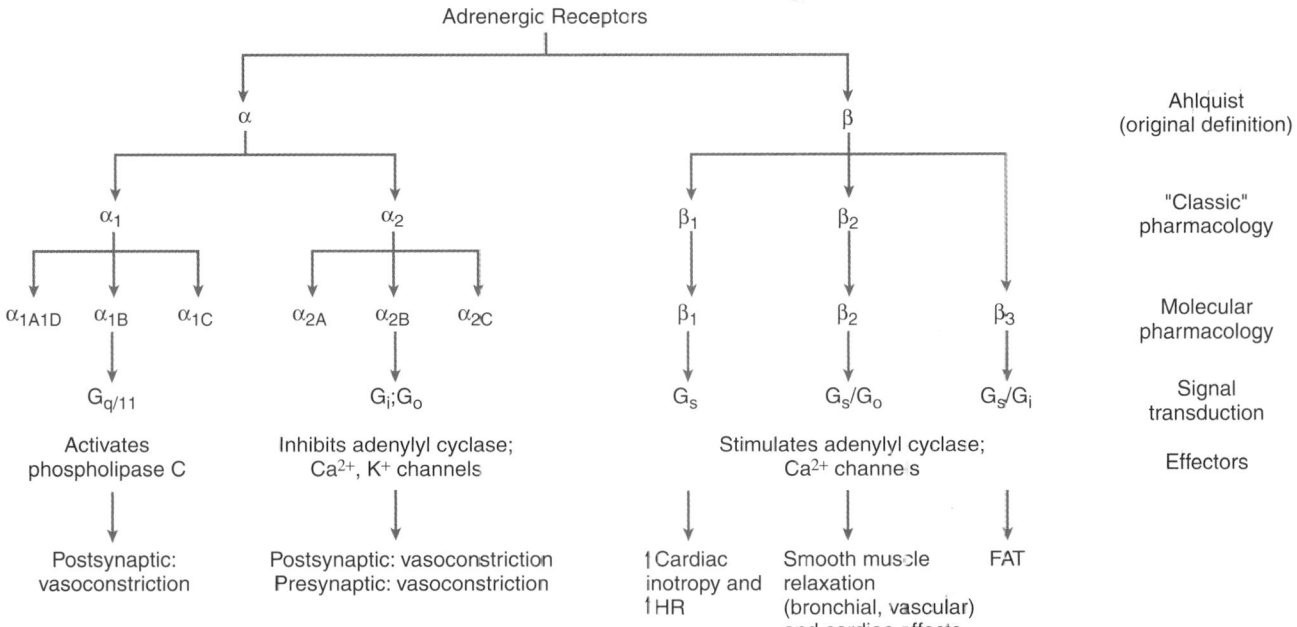

Figure 16–12 Metabolism of catecholamines. (From Lake CR, Chernow B, Feuerstein G, et al: The sympathetic nervous system in man, its evaluation and the measurement of plasma norepinephrine. *In* Ziegler M, Lake C [eds]: Frontiers of Clinical Neuroscience, vol 2. Baltimore, Williams & Wilkins, 1984, p 1.)

Figure 16–13 Classification of adrenergic receptors. HR, heart rate.

mechanisms, and primary structural differences in the receptors. Although such a classification is consistent with the available scientific evidence, the drugs available for clinical use may still be classified in the more traditional pattern. Table 16-6 describes the distribution, response, typical agonists, and antagonists of the α_1-, α_2-, β_1-, and β_2-receptors.

α-Adrenergic Receptors

Radioligand binding affinities have shown that at the α_1-receptor prazosin is more potent than yohimbine; the reverse is true at α_2-receptors. Functional and binding assays and molecular biologic methods have unequivocally confirmed the classification of α-adrenoceptors into subtypes.[92] Within α_1-adrenergic receptors, $\alpha_{1A/D}$-, α_{1B}-, and α_{1C}-receptors have been characterized. Several α_2-isoreceptors (α_{2A}, α_{2B}, and α_{2C}) have been described. The α_2-receptors can be expressed presynaptically or even in non-neuronal tissue. The α_2-receptors are found in the peripheral nervous system, in the CNS, and in a variety of organs, including platelets, liver, pancreas, kidney, and eyes, where specific physiologic functions have been identified.[93] Later, the predominant α_2-receptor of the human spinal cord was identified as the α_{2A}-subtype.[91,94] It appears that mammalian genomes contain two sets of at least three unique genes encoding the α-adrenoceptors. The genes encoding α_2-receptors have been localized in chromosomes 2, 4, and 10.

There is more than theoretical relevance in subclassification of receptors.[95] For example, the α-adrenergic receptors in the prostate gland are predominantly α_{1A}. Therapy with selective α_{1A}-antagonists for benign prostatic hypertrophy may avoid some of the postural hypotension and other deleterious effects that occur with less specific α-antagonists. Localization of β_3-receptors to fat cells suggests a new therapy for obesity. Polymorphism of this β-receptor subtype is associated with obesity and the potential for the development of diabetes.[96-98] Point mutations in genes encoding β_2-receptors are correlated with decreased downregulation of β-receptors and nocturnal asthma.[99,100] Of particular clinical interest to anesthesiologists is the demonstration that mutations that decrease α_{2C} presynaptic function and enhance β_1 receptor linkage cause adrenergic hyperactivity and predispose to CHF.[101,102]

Amino acid sequence comparisons indicate that α-receptors are members of the seven transmembrane segment gene superfamily using G protein for signal transduction. A core of 175 amino acids constitutes the seven transmembrane regions that are highly conserved among different family members.[103] The plethora of receptor subtypes remains incompletely explained, although the observation that different signal transduction mechanisms are used suggests finer control and physiologic significance. It may be important that there is considerable variability in α-adrenergic receptor subtypes among species.[104]

Receptors can be presynaptic as well as postsynaptic. Presynaptic receptors may act as heteroreceptors or autoreceptors. An *autoreceptor* is a presynaptic receptor that reacts with the neurotransmitter released from its own nerve terminal, providing feedback regulation. A *heteroreceptor* is a presynaptic receptor that responds to substances other than the neurotransmitter released from that specific nerve terminal. This regulatory scheme is present throughout the nervous system but is particularly important in the sympathetic nervous system.[105]

Although several presynaptic receptors have been identified, the α_2-receptor may be of the greatest clinical import. Presynaptic α_2-receptors regulate the release of norepinephrine and ATP through a negative-feedback mechanism.[106] Activation of presynaptic α_2-receptors by norepinephrine inhibits subsequent norepinephrine release in response to nerve stimulation. Clonidine is a prototype α_2-agonist. In the human brain, ligand studies reveal a high density of α_2-receptors, particularly in cerebral cortex and medulla.[107] This latter distribution may account for the bradycardiac and hypotensive responses to α_2-agonist drugs. In summary, presynaptic α_2-receptors and cholinergic receptors inhibit release, and presynaptic β-receptors stimulate release of norepinephrine.

β-Adrenergic Receptors

The structure of the β-adrenergic receptor was among the first to be ascertained and is well characterized. Like the α-receptor, the β-receptor is one of the superfamily of proteins that have seven helices woven through the cellular membrane. These *transmembrane domains* are labeled M_1 through M_7; antagonists have specific binding sites, whereas agonists are more diffusely attached to hydrophobic membrane-spanning domains (Fig. 16-14). The extracellular portion of the receptor ends in an amino group. A carboxyl group occupies the intracellular terminus, where phosphorylation occurs. At these cytoplasmic domains, there is interaction with G proteins and kinases, including β-adrenergic receptor kinase. The β-receptor has

Table 16–6	Distribution of α- and β-receptors			
Receptor	**Distribution**	**Response**	**Agonist**	**Antagonist**
α_1	Smooth muscle	Constriction	Methoxamine Phenylephrine	Prazosin
α_2	Presynaptic	Inhibit norepinephrine release	Clonidine Dexmedetomidine	Yohimbine
β_1	Heart	Inotropy Chronotropy	Dobutamine	Metoprolol
β_2	Smooth muscle	Dilation Relaxation	Terbutaline	

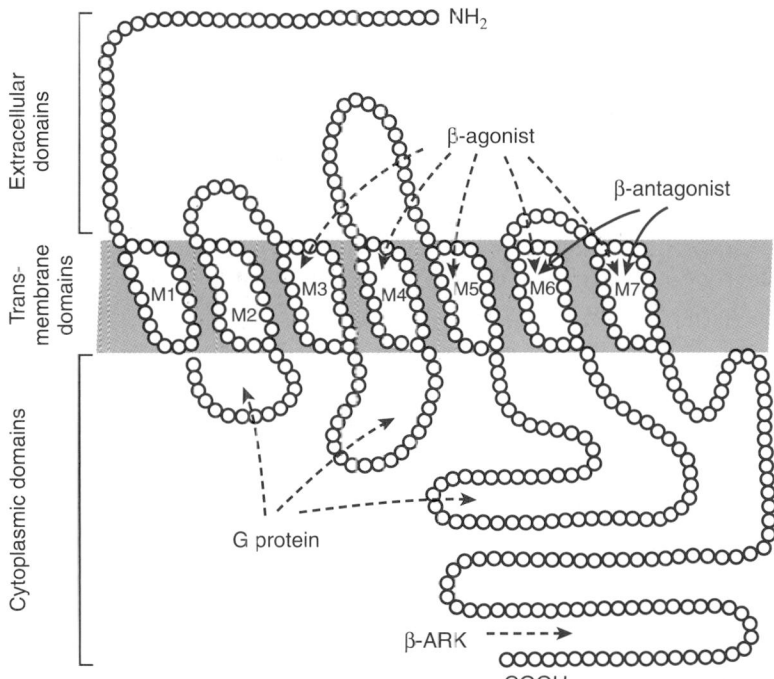

Figure 16–14 Molecular structure of the β-adrenergic receptor. Notice the three domains. The transmembrane domains act as a ligand-binding pocket. Cytoplasmic domains can interact with G proteins and kinases, such as β-adrenergic receptor kinase (β-ARK). The latter can phosphorylate and desensitize the receptor. (From Opie L: Receptors and signal transduction. *In* Opie LH [ed]: The Heart: Physiology and Metabolism. New York, Raven Press, 1991.)

mechanistic and structural similarities with muscarinic, but not nicotinic, receptors, primarily in the transmembrane sections. Muscarinic receptors and β-receptors are coupled to adenylate cyclase through G proteins, and both can initiate the opening of ion channels.

β-receptors have been further divided into β_1-, β_2-, and β_3-subtypes, all of which increase cyclic adenosine monophosphate (cAMP) through adenylate cyclase and the mediation of G proteins.[108,109] Traditionally, the β_1-receptors were thought to be isolated to cardiac tissue, and β_2-receptors were believed to be restricted to vascular and bronchial smooth muscle. Although this model of distribution is still useful because it reflects the primary clinical effects of pharmacologic manipulation of the β_1- and β_2-receptor subtypes, β_2-receptors are more important in cardiac function than indicated by this model. The β_2-receptor population in human cardiac tissue is substantial, accounting for 15% of the β-receptors in the ventricles and 30% to 40% in the atria.[110] β_2-receptors may help to compensate for disease by maintaining response to catecholamine stimulation when β_1-receptors are downregulated during chronic catecholamine stimulation and in CHF.[111] The β_2-population is almost unaffected in end-stage congestive cardiomyopathy.[112] In addition to positive inotropic effects, β_2-receptors in the human atria participate in the regulation of heart rate. The generation of cAMP in the human heart appears to be mediated primarily by β_2-receptors, although this may be an artifact related to lability of β_1-receptors.[112] The β_2-agonism may have significant effects on cardiac contractility and rate.[111]

Dopamine Receptors

Dopamine exists as an intermediate in norepinephrine biosynthesis, and it exerts α- or β-adrenergic effects (depending on the dose administered). Goldberg and Rajfer[113] demonstrated physiologically distinct dopamine type 1 (DA_1) and dopamine type 2 (DA_2) receptors, the most important of the five dopamine receptors cloned (Fig. 16-15). DA_1 receptors are postsynaptic and act on renal, mesenteric, splenic, and coronary vascular smooth muscle to mediate vasodilation through stimulated adenylate cyclase and increased cAMP production. The vasodilatory effect tends to be strongest in the renal arteries. It is for this action, particularly the redistribution of renal blood flow, that dopamine is most frequently used. Additional renal DA_1 receptors located in the tubules modulate natriuresis through the sodium-potassium ATPase pump and the sodium-hydrogen exchanger.[113-116] The DA_2 receptors are presynaptic; they may inhibit norepinephrine and perhaps acetylcholine release. There are also central DA_2 receptors that may mediate nausea and vomiting. The antiemetic activity of droperidol is thought to be related to its DA_2 activity.

G Proteins

After adrenergic receptor stimulation, the extracellular signal is transformed into an intracellular signal by a process known as *signal transduction* in which α_1- and β-receptors are coupled to G proteins. When activated, the G proteins can modulate the synthesis or the availability of intracellular second messengers (Fig. 16-16). The activated second messenger diffuses through the cytoplasm and stimulates an enzymatic cascade. The sequence of first messenger → receptor → G protein → effector → second messenger → enzymatic cascade is found in a wide variety of cells; the specific entities that fulfill the separate roles vary from cell to cell.[117] G proteins located on the inner surface of the cell membrane can also directly modify the activity of transmembrane ion channels.

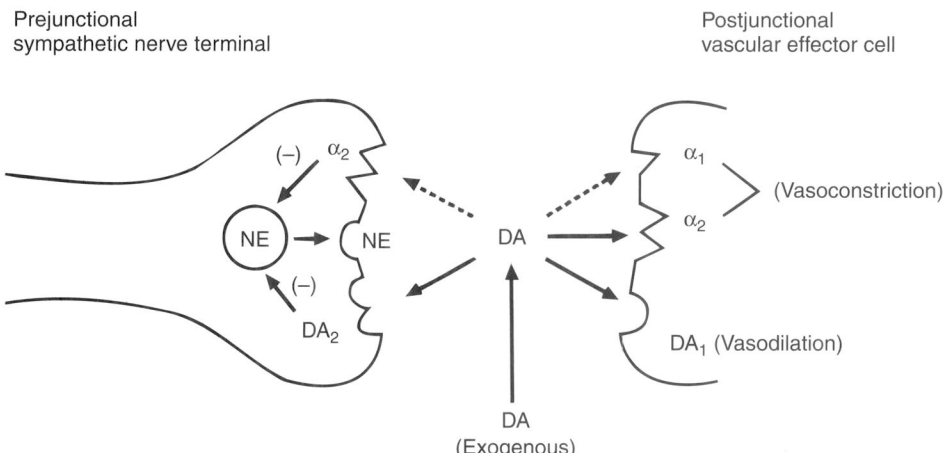

Figure 16–15 Location of dopamine-1 (DA_1) receptors, α_1- and α_2-adrenoceptors on postganglionic vascular effector cells, and DA_2 receptors and α_2-adrenoceptors on the prejunctional sympathetic nerve terminal. When dopamine is administered, activation of DA_1 receptors causes vasodilation, whereas activation of DA_2 receptors causes inhibition (−) of norepinephrine (NE) release from storage granules. A larger dose of dopamine activates α_1- and α_2-adrenoceptors on the postjunctional effector cells to cause vasoconstriction and on α_2-adrenoceptors on the prejunctional sympathetic terminal to inhibit release of NE. NE released from the prejunctional sympathetic terminal also acts on α_1- and α_2-adrenoceptors. (From Goldberg LI, Rajfer SI: Dopamine receptors: Applications in clinical cardiology. Circulation 72:245, 1985.)

The structure of G proteins has been the subject of intense scrutiny. Three types of subunits (α, β, and γ) have been described. The α-subunit is most variable and determines the activity of the protein, whether it is stimulatory (G_s), inhibitory (G_i), G_o, or $G_{q/11}$.[118,119] The α-subunit may split off and behave independently, whereas the β- and γ-subunits remain together. Although 20 α-subunits, 5 β-subunits, and 6 γ-subunits have been cloned, the constellation of G proteins used by any individual receptor is more limited. Each class of adrenergic receptor couples to a different major subfamily of G proteins, which are linked to different effectors. The major subtypes of α_1-, α_2-, and β-receptors are linked to G_q, G_i, and G_s, respectively, which are linked to phospholipase C activation (α_1), adenylyl cyclase inhibition (α_2), or adenylyl cyclase stimulation (β) (see Fig. 16-13). The pertussis-resistant G_q protein was identified in 1991[119] and subsequently was observed to mediate α_1-adrenergic receptor signal transduction by activation of phospholipase C and generation of inositol triphosphate and diacylglycerol.[120] The physiologic relevance of the subunits is all the more important because the pharmacologic tools for dissecting signal transduction are associated with diseases that have been scourges of humankind (e.g., *Bordetella pertussis*, *Vibrio cholerae*, *Clostridium botulinum*).

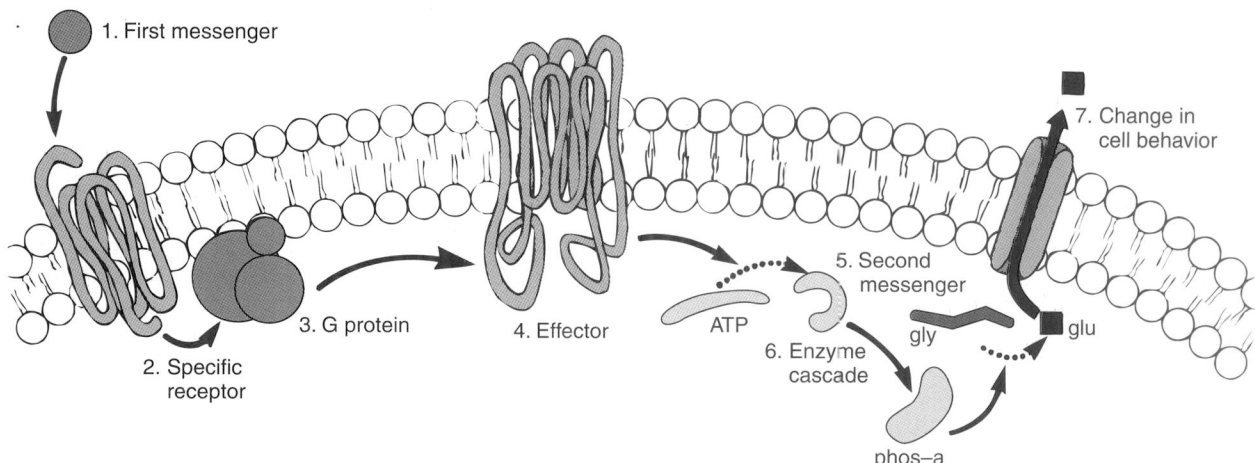

Figure 16–16 Epinephrine-stimulated glycogenolysis in a liver cell demonstrates the role of G proteins in cellular function. The first messenger (epinephrine) binds to its specific receptor, stimulating the G protein (in this case, Gs) to activate the effector, adenylyl cyclase. This enzyme converts adenosine triphosphate (ATP) to cyclic adenosine monophosphate (cAMP), the second messenger, which then triggers a cascade of enzymatic reactions that stimulates the enzyme phosphorylase (phos-a) to convert glycogen into glucose, which the cell extrudes. (From Linder ME, Gilman AG: G Proteins. Sci Am 267:56, 1992.)

In its resting state, the G protein is bound to guanosine diphosphate (GDP) and is not in contact with the receptor. When the receptor is activated by the first messenger, it stimulates the G protein to release GDP and bind GTP to its α-subunit, activating itself. The bound GTP signals the G protein to split into two parts consisting of the α-GTP structure and the βγ-subunit. The released α-subunit binds to the effector and activates it, and then converts its attached GTP to GDP, returning itself to the resting state. The α-subunit joins with the βγ-unit, and the reconstructed G protein again waits at the inner membrane.

β-Receptor stimulation activates G proteins, enhancing adenylate cyclase activity and cAMP formation. The briefest encounter of plasma membrane β-adrenergic receptors with epinephrine or norepinephrine results in profound increases (up to 400-fold higher than the basal level within minutes) in the intracellular levels of cAMP. Increased cAMP synthesis activates protein kinases, which phosphorylate target proteins. Phosphorylation elicits various cellular responses that complete the path between receptor and effect. Stimulation of α_2-receptors results in G_i inhibition of the adenylate cyclase. There is a relative abundance of G proteins, resulting in amplification of receptor agonism at the signal transduction step. The number of G protein molecules greatly exceeds the number of β-adrenergic receptors and adenylate cyclase molecules. It is the receptor concentration and ultimately adenylate cyclase activity that limit the response to catecholamines, perhaps explaining the efficacy of phosphodiesterase inhibitors.[121,122]

Other transduction pathways are known. The α_{13}-receptor acts through G proteins, but it activates phospholipase C in the inner cell membrane, which then increases hydrolysis of the diphosphate form of phosphoinositol to the triphosphate and diacylglycerol. These two compounds then mobilize intracellular calcium stores from the sarcoplasmic reticulum and probably the subsarcolemma, which markedly increases intracellular calcium ion concentration. Ultimately, the calcium ions bind to calmodulin. This calcium-sensitive intracellular protein then activates a myosin light chain kinase that phosphorylates the myosin light chain and facilitates the interaction between actin and myosin, resulting in the contraction of the smooth muscle. In other cells, calmodulin stimulates different kinases, eliciting different effector activity.

Myocardial cells respond to receptor stimulation differently depending on the identity of the first messenger. Two opposing effects, inhibition or stimulation of contractility, are produced by the sequence of receptor → G protein → effector → enzymatic cascade, but the identity of the chemicals in the sequence differs.[123] Norepinephrine causes myocardial cells to contract with more vigor when the α-subunit of the stimulatory protein (G_s) activates adenylate cyclase. The α-subunits of this protein cause potassium channels to open and permit efflux of potassium ion. The force of contraction is diminished when acetylcholine acts as a first messenger, stimulating its receptor to activate the inhibitory protein G_i or G_o. Clinically important, second-to-second changes in heart rate can be explained by the simultaneous activation of G_s and G_o. The current caused by G_o is larger

than that of G_s, which explains the clinical impression that vagal inhibition of heart rate is augmented in the presence of sympathetic stimulation, such as may occur in unpremedicated patients.[123]

Interaction of anesthetics with G proteins has been suggested as a mechanism for the negative inotropic effects of halothane and other volatile anesthetics. Halothane attenuates neurotransmitter release from peripheral sympathetic neurons,[124-127] but other important postsynaptic effects may be involved in its negative inotropic action.[128-132]

Although the changes in cAMP formation caused by halothane would be a plausible explanation for halothane's negative inotropic effects, studies suggest that this alteration is unrelated to adenylate cyclase.[133] Halothane blocks slow calcium channels in the heart,[134,135] alters calcium fluxes in sarcoplasmic reticulum,[136,137] and inhibits cAMP-dependent protein kinase.[129] It appears that the negative inotropic effect of inhaled anesthetics occurs at several sites.

Upregulation and Downregulation

The β-adrenergic receptors are not fixed; they change significantly in dynamic response to the amount of norepinephrine present in the synaptic cleft or in plasma. For β-adrenergic receptors, this response is fast; within 30 minutes of denervation or adrenergic blockade, the number of receptors increases. This upregulation may explain why sudden discontinuation of β-adrenergic receptor blocking drugs causes rebound tachycardia and increases the incidence of MI and ischemia. Many chronic phenomena, such as varicose veins[138] or aging, can decrease adrenergic receptor number or responsiveness systemically.

Clinically and at the cellular level, responses to many hormones and neurotransmitters wane rapidly despite continuous exposure to adrenergic agonists.[139] This phenomenon, called *desensitization*, has been particularly well studied for the stimulation of cAMP levels by plasma membrane β-adrenergic receptors.[103] Mechanisms postulated for desensitization include uncoupling (e.g., phosphorylation), sequestration, and downregulation. The molecular mechanisms underlying rapid β-adrenergic receptor desensitization do not appear to require internalization of the receptors, but rather an alteration in the functioning of β-receptors themselves that uncouples the receptors from the stimulatory G_s protein. Agonist-induced desensitization involves phosphorylation of G protein–coupled receptors by two classes of serine-threonine kinases. One of these initiates receptor-specific or homologous desensitization. The other works through second messenger–dependent kinases, mediating a general cellular hyporesponsiveness, called *heterologous desensitization*. Ultimately, an inhibitory arrestin protein binds to the phosphorylated receptor, causing desensitization by blocking signal transduction. Because enzymatic phosphorylation occurs only in the activated state, transient β-blockade has been used in states of receptor desensitization such as CHF or cardiopulmonary bypass to achieve a "a receptor holiday."[12,104,140] Regeneration of a functional β-adrenergic receptor is contingent on sequestration of the receptor, with dephosphorylation and presumed recycling. There has been some evidence that the arrestins contribute to desensitization by uncoupling signal transduction and by contributing to the process of receptor internalization.[141,142] Receptor populations can change rapidly with such sequestration, which does not require protein synthesis. Downregulation may be distinguished from these rapid mechanisms because it occurs after hours of exposure to an agonist (as in chronic stress or CHF), and receptors are destroyed. New receptors must be synthesized before a return to a baseline state is possible.

Chronic CHF is one of the most important and best-studied pathophysiologic situations in which tolerance or downregulation occurs. It was initially observed that the density of cardiac β-receptors decreased markedly in patients with terminal heart failure in response to the elevated plasma catecholamine levels. This finding explained why administration of exogenous β-agonists was relatively ineffectual in this syndrome. With the demonstration that β_1- and β_2-receptors coexisted in human ventricles, Bristow and coworkers,[143] using radioligand techniques, documented that β_1-receptor density decreased without change in the density of β_2-receptors in human ventricles affected by CHF. Consequently, β_2-agonism accounted for 60% of the total inotropic response stimulated by isoproterenol in the failing heart, compared with 40% in the nonfailing heart.[144] Receptor polymorphisms associated with decreased α_{2C} presynaptic function and enhanced β_1–G protein linkage lead to adrenergic hyperactivity and predispose to the development of CHF.[102]

Another disease in which adrenergic receptor function is altered is hyperthyroidism. The activity of the thyroid gland influences the receptor density, with hyperthyroidism increasing density and hypothyroidism decreasing density. There is some evidence that corticosteroids decrease receptor density.[25] Consequently, the reaction of the body to well-characterized sympathetic agonists may be considerably different, depending on the pathologic and environmental circumstances.[145] However, the structural similarity of thyroid hormone and tyrosine suggests that false transmitters may play a role.[146]

Cholinergic Pharmacology

Acetylcholine Synthesis

Many of our presumptions about cholinergic pharmacology are drawn from what is known about the neuromuscular junction, for which detailed electrophysiologic information on cholinergic transmission is readily available. Acetylcholine is synthesized intraneurally from acetyl coenzyme A and choline through the enzyme choline acetyl transferase in the synaptosomal mitochondria (Fig. 16-17).[147] Despite the presence of this enzyme, choline is not made in the brain, but it appears to be transported. Sources of choline include dietary phospholipids, hepatic synthesis of phosphatidylcholine from dietary precursors such as ethanolamines, and choline released by hydrolysis of acetylcholine. Most choline originates in the liver. Choline is transported as

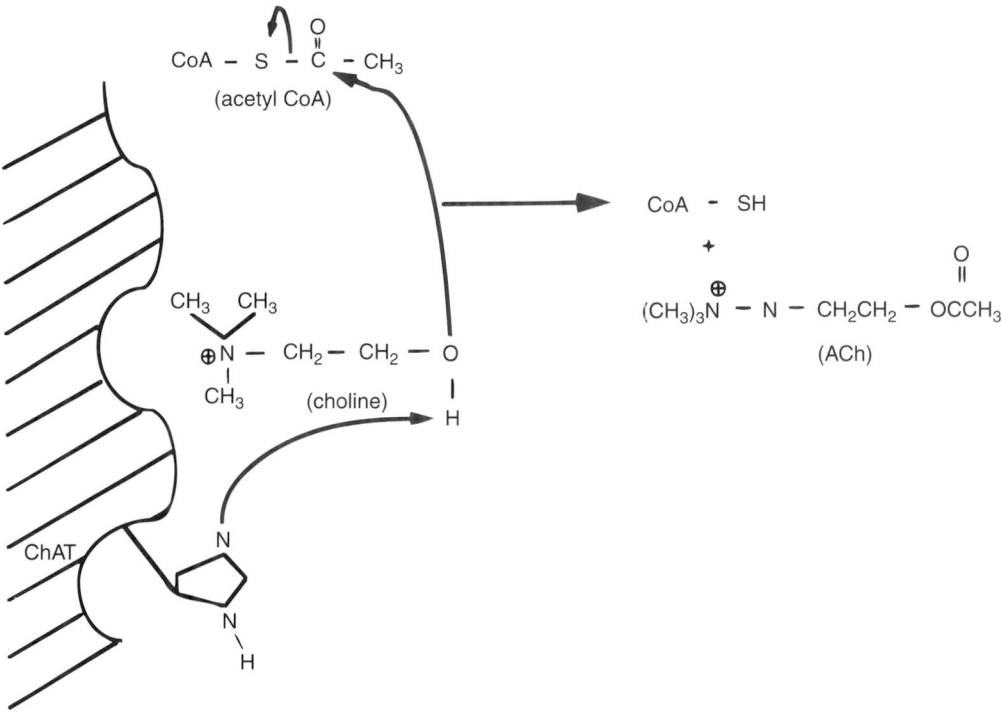

Figure 16–17 Synthesis of acetylcholine (ACh). Choline and acetyl coenzyme A (CoA) bind to the surface of choline acetyltransferase (ChAT). An imidazole on ChAT promotes proton removal and generates a more nucleophilic choline, facilitating condensation with the acetyl group of acetyl-CoA. The products of the reaction are coenzyme A and ACh, which are rapidly packaged in vesicles for immediate release on proper stimulation. ChAT also catalyzes the reverse reaction between ACh and CoASH, although at a much slower rate than the forward reaction. (From Doukas PH: Drugs affecting the parasympathetic nervous system. *In* Wingard L, Brody T, Larner J, et al [eds]: Human Pharmacology: Molecular to Clinical. St. Louis, Mosby–Year Book, 1991.)

the phospholipid and is taken up by a high-affinity transport system. This system appears to be largely responsible for determining acetylcholine levels, although there is some evidence that precursor availability may limit cholinergic activity. The level of circulating choline can affect the release of acetylcholine when rapid firing is taking place at cholinergic motor neurons. In one interesting experiment, plasma choline levels were measured in marathon runners before and immediately after a race; running a marathon decreased choline levels to well below those usually seen in fasting individuals, potentially lowering performance ability by possibly decreasing acetylcholine release at the neuromuscular junction or cholinergic sites.[148] Choline analogs are being developed to enhance neuromuscular performance and to treat Alzheimer's disease.

Storage and Release

The neuromuscular junction includes the nerve ending, the muscle, and the synaptic cleft, which is a space between the nerve and the muscle. On the nerve or presynaptic side, the nerve ending contains many synaptic vesicles (i.e., quanta) that contain acetylcholine. On the muscle membrane, there are many infoldings of the postjunctional membrane. There are presynaptic release sites located opposite the junctional folds at the shoulders

of the junctional folds. Vesicles containing acetylcholine move toward these specific release sites and then fuse with the presynaptic membrane and open, spilling their contents across the synaptic cleft onto the receptors on the postsynaptic membrane (Fig. 16-18).[149]

Acetylcholine is stored in vesicles approximately 300 μm in diameter, with each containing 10,000 molecules of the chemical. Central cholinergic transmission is different from the neuromuscular model in that few vesicles are present in the presynaptic terminal. These vesicles appear clear on electron microscopy.

The spontaneous release of the acetylcholine in one vesicle causes a miniature end-plate potential of 0.5 millivolts (mV), and 2000 channels open in the membrane of a muscle cell, permitting sodium influx and potassium efflux. Twelve thousand ions enter the postsynaptic cell each millisecond that each channel is open.

When a nerve impulse arrives at the presynaptic nerve terminal, it causes an influx of calcium ions across the membrane. This induces 100 to 300 synaptic vesicles to fuse with the presynaptic membrane at specific release sites at the active zone, resulting in the liberation of acetylcholine from vesicles into the synaptic cleft.

Although the original hypothesis proposed by Katz, of calcium as the exocytotic trigger, has stood the test of time, calcium entrance is necessary but not sufficient; the

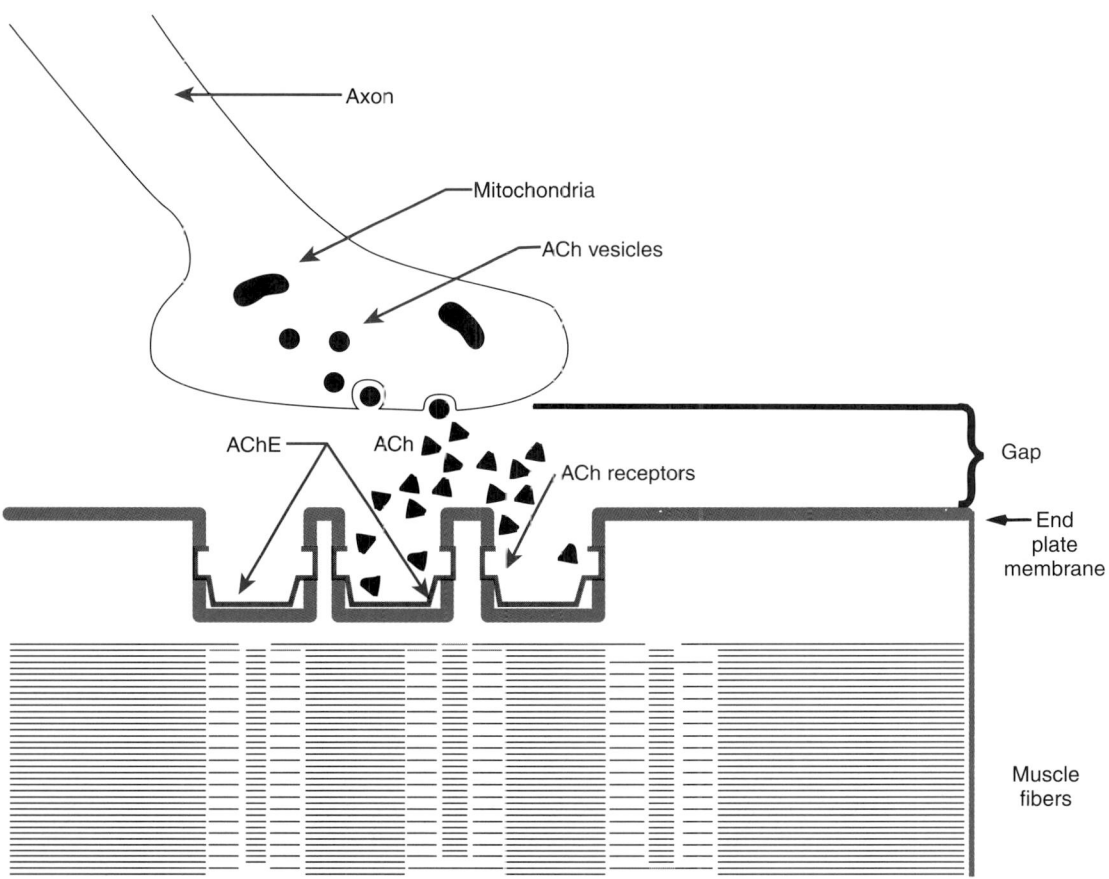

Figure 16–18 Acetylcholine (ACh) release, diffusion across the synaptic cleft, binding to receptors on the end-plate membrane, and hydrolysis by acetylcholine esterase (AChE) in the absence of blocking drugs. (From Stiller R: Neuromuscular blocking agents. *In* Wingard L, Brody T, Larner J, et al [eds]: Human Pharmacology: Molecular to Clinical. St. Louis, Mosby–Year Book, 1991.)

presynaptic terminal must also be depolarized. With sodium entering the cell and potassium leaving, ion flow gives rise to an electrical current and changes the normal resting potential of –90 mV. This nerve impulse–induced brief depolarization of 100 to 300 vesicles is known as an *end-plate potential* (EPP), but it is also a synaptic potential or an *excitatory postsynaptic potential* (EPSP), terms used to describe synaptic transmission in general. The EPP (50 to 100 mV) triggers a muscle action potential.

Normally, in the absence of a nerve impulse, a series of miniature end-plate potentials (MEPPs) results from the spontaneous release of one quantum of acetylcholine (10,000 molecules, or the contents of one vesicle). Each opened channel produces a depolarization of 0.00022 mV. The MEPP involves 1500 ion channels being opened and causes a deflection of 0.5 mV. The EPP, which is summated, involves 500,000 ion channels opening and represents a depolarization of 50 to 100 mV.

Inactivation

Acetylcholine is an ester that hydrolyzes spontaneously in alkaline solutions into acetate and choline, neither of which has significant pharmacologic action. In vivo, the rate of hydrolysis is increased enormously by enzymatic catalysis. The two most important enzymes are acetylcholinesterase and butyrylcholinesterase.

Sometimes called *tissue esterase* or *true esterase*, acetylcholinesterase is a membrane-bound enzyme that is present in all cholinergic synapses, where it functions to destroy the neurotransmitter released from the nerve endings. Acetylcholinesterase is one of the most efficient of enzymes and destroys acetylcholine, terminating transmission within milliseconds after its release. The enzyme also is present in tissues that are not innervated, such as erythrocytes. Its function in these tissues is not known.

Butyrylcholinesterase, sometimes called *plasma esterase* or *pseudocholinesterase,* is a soluble enzyme that is made primarily in the liver and circulates in the blood. Its function in normal situations is not known; individuals who are genetically incapable of making the enzyme are normal in all other regards.

Of these two enzymes, acetylcholinesterase is the more important in terms of the function of acetylcholine. It is present in all cholinergic synapses, where it destroys neurally released acetylcholine, and it is the more efficient of the two enzymes. The substrate turnover is 2500 molecules per second, and one catalytic event lasts 40 μsec. Butyrylcholinesterase is important for the destruction of some cholinergic drugs, many of which are not destroyed by acetylcholinesterase.

Both forms of cholinesterase have been cloned. It is of more than passing interest that the first example of gene amplification in humans occurred in this enzyme system. The offspring of Israeli farmers exposed to insecticide expressed abnormal cholinesterase.[150,151]

Traditionally, the catalytic part of the enzyme has been thought to contain two areas: an anionic site, which carries a strong negative charge, and an esteratic site, which contains electrophilic amino acids. It has been believed that acetylcholine during its hydrolysis is attracted to the enzyme because the negative charge of the anionic site attracts the positive charge in the quaternary nitrogen of acetylcholine. The ester group of acetylcholine aligns with the esteratic site of the enzyme. After an electrophilic attack on the molecule, the acetate link is transferred from the choline to an amino acid in the enzyme. The choline drifts away, leaving a covalently bound, acetylated enzyme. The acetate link is subsequently attacked and broken by a hydroxyl group from water. The acetate drifts away, and the regenerated enzyme is ready to interact with another molecule of acetylcholine.

However, the atomic structure of acetylcholinesterase is different from what had been previously thought, and our understanding of the binding of acetylcholine to its hydrolytic enzyme has altered.[152] The new model predicts that the quaternary ammonium binds to some of the 14 aromatic amino acids lining a deep gorge in the enzyme.

Inhibition of acetylcholinesterase prevents the destruction of acetylcholine in cholinergic synapses and can activate all cholinergic systems simultaneously. In addition to their therapeutic use, cholinesterase inhibitors are the active ingredients in insecticides and many nerve gases.

Cholinergic Receptors

Traditionally, cholinergic receptors have been organized into two major subdivisions, nicotinic and muscarinic, that predict most clinical effects. Muscarinic receptors are present mostly in peripheral visceral organs; nicotinic receptors are found on parasympathetic and sympathetic ganglia and on the neuromuscular junctions of skeletal muscle.

Although these two structurally and functionally distinct classes of receptors have significantly different responses to acetylcholine, the chemical itself exhibits no specificity. However, specific antagonists can exploit the difference between the muscarinic and nicotinic receptors. As a result, structure-activity relationships have emerged. All cholinergic agonists appear to need a quaternary ammonium group as well as an atom capable of forming a hydrogen bond through an unshared pair of electrons. The distance between the two may determine whether the agonism is nicotinic or muscarinic. With muscarinic agonists, the distance appears to be about 4.4 Å, whereas for nicotinic agonists, the distance is 5.9 Å.

The nicotinic receptors on ganglia and motor end plates differ, and they are blocked by different drugs. D-Tubocurarine predominantly blocks the neuromuscular junction, whereas hexamethonium acts to block the ganglionic receptors. Methonium compounds were developed to explore the structure-activity relationships of the curare alkaloids. The most potent depolarizing neuromuscular blocking structure contains 10 carbon atoms (i.e., decamethonium); in contrast, the structure containing six carbon atoms (i.e., hexamethonium) is an active ganglionic blocking agent but has little effect at the neuromuscular junction. There is some evidence that ganglionic nicotinic acetylcholine receptors are far more sensitive to anesthetics than receptors in the neuromuscular junction but the clinical significance is unclear.[153] The identification of a new class of acetylcholine-binding proteins released from glial cells suggests another functional difference between central and peripheral cholinergic transmission.[154]

Acetylcholine receptors on the neuromuscular junctions of mature mammals belong to the superfamily of receptor-gated ion channels, which includes glutamate and glycine. The nicotinic receptors are pentameric membrane proteins, which form nonselective cation channels. There are two α-units (each 40 kd) and one each of the β-, ε-, and δ-units (Fig. 16-19). Although different subunits may be expressed developmentally, the α-subunits represent the binding sites for acetylcholine or nicotinic antagonists. At birth, a γ-subunit occupies the position that will be taken by the ε-subunit within the first 2 weeks of life. This change in subunits converts the receptor from one with a low conductance and a relatively long duration of opening to a receptor with a high conductance but a brief duration of opening.[155] There are functional differences in acetylcholine receptors during development, but the important drug-binding subunits remain constant.

These five subunits surround each ion channel through which sodium or calcium may enter the cell or potassium may exit. Each ion has its own separate channel, a unique characteristic of the neuromuscular junction. For the channel to open, acetylcholine must occupy a receptor site on each of the two α-subunits. If only one site is occupied and the other is empty, the channel remains closed, and there is no flow of ions and no change in electrical potential. If one site is occupied by acetylcholine and the other site is occupied by an antagonist such as D-tubocurarine, or if both sites are occupied by D-tubocurarine, the channel also remains closed. The ion channel response to acetylcholine is instantaneous and usually lasts only a few milliseconds because acetylcholine is rapidly destroyed by acetylcholinesterase in the synapse. This time course lends a rapidity and flexibility of response of motor end plates to neural stimulation that contributes profoundly to the viability of an organism and to its ability to control its own movements precisely.

In addition to binding of the α-subunit binding site by competing, nonacetylcholine structures, there are two types of channel block: open and closed. With open-channel block, a drug enters a channel opened by acetylcholine but cannot travel all the way through the channel. It impedes ionic flow and prevents depolarization. Because only an open channel may be entered, the intensity of this block depends on how often the channels are open and how active the system is; it is therefore use dependent. Open-channel blockade is driven by the electrical potential difference across the membrane and the charge inherent in the molecular structure. Drugs penetrating an open channel may temporarily bind at some point on the wall of the channel, and the duration of effect therefore partially depends on the identity of the molecule. Closed-channel blockade is harder to study and is less well understood. In this case, a drug may react with the mouth of a closed channel and prevent ion flow. Channel opening is not required, and blockade is therefore not use dependent. Because block does not occur at the acetylcholine receptor site, closed-channel block is not caused by a competitive antagonism of acetylcholine. The classic agents that inhibit cholinesterase may not be completely effective.

In adult skeletal muscle and postganglionic cells, cholinoceptors and their associated ion channels are present only in the immediate synaptic area and are absent from the rest of the cell membrane. The high density (10,000 molecules/μm^2) of nicotinic acetylcholine receptors at the motor end plate is central to accomplishing successful neuromuscular transmission. Studies have demonstrated that agrin, a nerve-derived extracellular protein in the basal lamina, provides the signal that directs formation of presynaptic terminals[156,157] and results in a 1000-fold increase in nicotinic receptors in the motor end plate within hours of the arrival of the

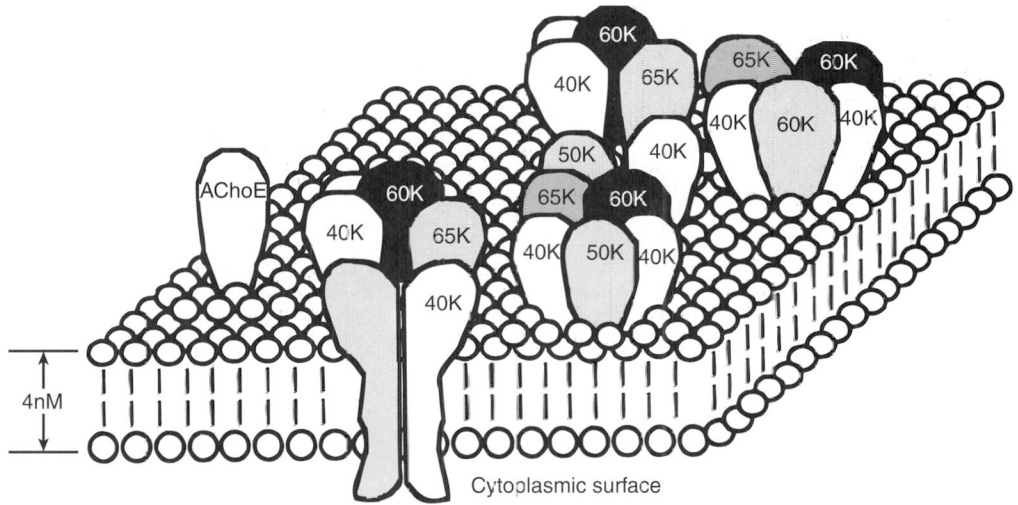

Figure 16–19 Sketch of postjunctional nicotinic acetylcholine receptors with an acetylcholinesterase (AChoE) molecule nearby. (From Standaert F: Donuts and holes: Molecules and muscle relaxants. *In* Katz R [ed]: Muscle Relaxants: Basic and Clinical Aspects. Orlando, FL, Grune & Stratton, 1984.)

presynaptic terminals at the myocyte. A series of acetylcholine receptor–associated proteins has been identified, but the precise way in which these extracellular[158] (i.e., agrin, laminin, and dystroglycan) and intracellular (i.e., utrophin and syntrophin) membrane-associated proteins maintain the necessary acetylcholine receptor clustering and integrity of motor end plate and bind to the cytoskeleton is unclear. Only the synaptic area is depolarized by acetylcholine. Depolarization usually leads to the generation of action potentials that spread along the whole membrane of the cell and cause muscles to contract or neurons to transmit. However, if acetylcholine action is prolonged, such as by inhibition of acetylcholinesterase or if a long-acting cholinomimetic drug is administered, the initial activation is quickly followed by blockade of transmission. This biphasic effect occurs because sodium channels in the membrane around the synapse, which are unaffected by acetylcholine, accommodate to the continued depolarization of the synaptic membrane. They become inactivated and will not open again until the synaptic potential disappears. Propagated action potentials cannot be generated without sodium flow across the membrane, and the message sent across the synapse is blocked from propagating through the postsynaptic cell.

Compared with adrenergic receptors, the cholinergic receptors turn over slowly. When a nerve to a muscle is transected, it takes 1 to 3 days to increase the number of cholinergic receptors. In the diaphragm, the number may increase eightfold. These new receptors are no longer confined to the motor end plate, and that change has important clinical ramifications, especially in burn-induced denervation.

In contrast to the ion-gated nicotinic receptors, muscarinic receptors belong to the superfamily of G protein–coupled receptors. Muscarinic receptors have a greater homology to α- and β-adrenergic receptors than to nicotinic receptors. Like the other members of the family of receptors with seven helices (i.e., α_2, β_1, β_2, serotonin, rhodopsin, and opsin), muscarinic receptors use G proteins for signal transduction. Five muscarinic receptors (i.e., M_1 through M_5) exist with the primary structural variability residing in a huge cytoplasmic loop between the fifth and sixth membrane-spanning domains. Although molecular studies have described five forms, of which four are defined pharmacologically (i.e., M_1, M_2, M_3, and M_4), selective muscarinic drugs are not available. The M_2-cholinergic postjunctional receptor predominates in visceral organs. M_2 and M_3 receptors have been identified in the airway smooth muscle of many species. In vitro studies reveal that the M_3 receptor mediates the contractile and secretory response. However, the excess of M_2 receptors could explain the relative ineffectiveness of β-adrenergic agonists in reversing cholinergic bronchoconstriction.[159]

The muscarinic receptors have diverse signal transduction mechanisms. The odd-numbered receptors (i.e., M_1, M_3, and M_5) work predominantly through the hydrolysis of polyphosphoinositide, whereas the even-numbered receptors work primarily through G_i proteins to regulate adenylate cyclase.[160]

When the M_3 muscarinic receptor is activated, G_q activates phospholipase C, which catalyzes the hydrolysis of phosphatidylinositol biphosphate into diacylglycerol and inositol triphosphate. Receptors in the muscarinic series are coupled to second messenger systems, such as cyclic nucleotides or phosphoinositides. These are coupled to ion channels. In other cases, the influx of a cation is the trigger for cellular response. In some cases, however, an influx of calcium ions acts as messengers that react with and open other ion channels. The nature of the response is determined by the specific cation. If calcium or sodium is permitted to flow, the membrane depolarizes; if only potassium is permitted to flow, the membrane hyperpolarizes. In addition to affecting ion channels, the messenger calcium can stimulate various intracellular proteins to alter cell activity. In cardiac atria, activation of muscarinic receptors leads to the efflux of potassium and hyperpolarization of the cell membrane. This efflux slows conduction and slows or stops pacemakers. In glands, an influx of calcium or sodium, or both, activates intracellular events and causes the cells to secrete. Similarly, the influx of these ions into smooth muscle cells causes them to contract.

Muscarinic receptors are found on central and peripheral neurons; a single neuron may have muscarinic receptors with excitatory as well as inhibitory effects. Prejunctional autoreceptors are perhaps not as well studied in the parasympathetic nervous system as in the sympathetic nervous system. Exogenous α_2-agonists may act on prejunctional cholinergic receptors to decrease acetylcholine release. As in the sympathetic system, presynaptic inhibition is of clinical relevance. Presynaptic muscarinic receptors may inhibit the release of acetylcholine from postganglionic parasympathetic neurons; prejunctional nicotinic receptors may increase its release.

Because of the complex coupling, the response of the muscarinic system is sluggish; no response is seen for seconds to minutes after the application of acetylcholine. Similarly, the effect long outlives the presence of the agonist. Even though the transmitter is destroyed rapidly, the train of events it initiates causes the cellular response to continue for many minutes. Muscarinic receptors are desensitized through agonist-dependent phosphorylation in a mechanism similar to that described earlier for β-adrenergic receptors.

Ganglionic Pharmacology

Ganglia serve far more complex functions than that of a simple connection between the nerve process of one cell and the cell body of its next connection. Integrative and processing functions may contribute to the subtlety of response and organization of the ANS. The electrophysiology of ganglionic stimulation is complex, with at least four different types of responses to electrical stimulation[161,162] (Table 16-7).

The central event at the ganglion is the excitatory postsynaptic potential (EPSP) when acetylcholine interacts with a nicotinic receptor to rapidly depolarize the postsynaptic membrane. Depolarization results primarily from the influx of sodium ions through the nicotinic receptor channel, and it is sensitive to nondepolarizing nicotinic blocking drugs such as hexamethonium. The other changes in electrical potential are related to secondary

Table 16–7   Fast and slow responses of postganglionic neurons in sympathetic ganglia

Potential	Duration	Mediator	Receptor
Fast EPSP	30 msec	Acetylcholine	Nicotinic cholinergic
Slow IPSP	2 sec	Dopamine	D_2
Slow EPSP	30 sec	Acetylcholine	M_1-cholinergic
Late slow EPSP	4 min	GnRH	GnRH

D_2, dopamine receptor inhibiting adenylate cyclase through inhibitory G protein; EPSP, excitatory postsynaptic potential; GnRH, gonadotropin-releasing hormone; IPSP, inhibitory postsynaptic potential. Adapted from Ganong W: The autonomic nervous system. *In* Ganong W (ed): Review of Medical Physiology, 15th ed. Norwalk, CT, Appleton & Lange, 1991, p 210.

or subsidiary pathways that augment or suppress; these pathways are insensitive to classic nicotinic antagonists.

Secondary pathways are indicated by the following changes in potential elicited by electrical stimulation of the ganglia: (1) slow EPSP, (2) late slow EPSP, and (3) inhibitory postsynaptic potential (IPSP).

The slow EPSP is slower in onset than the EPSP and lasts 30 to 60 seconds because of a decrease in potassium ion conductance. The interaction of acetylcholine with nicotinic receptors leads to closing of a potassium channel (i.e., M channel). The slow EPSP is associated with the reduction or suppression of a potassium current through this channel. This wave is initiated by muscarinic receptor agonists and can be blocked by atropine and the selective M_1-muscarinic antagonists.

Like the slow EPSP, the late slow EPSP is caused by a decrease in potassium ion conductance. It lasts for several minutes after being initiated by peptides in specialized ganglia. Peptides have special properties as neurotransmitters, showing prolonged stability and extending their influence to other postsynaptic sites, not just those in the immediate vicinity of the nerve ending. Depolarization of the membrane activates the potassium channel; the conductance of potassium ion has been labeled the *M current* and appears to act to regulate the cell's response to repetitive fast depolarizations.

The IPSP is inhibitory because the membrane is hyperpolarized and therefore resistant to depolarization. The slow IPSP seems to be mediated by the activation of an interneuron interposed between the preganglionic fiber and the ganglionic cell. The preganglionic nerve ending releases acetylcholine, which stimulates the catecholamine-containing interneurons to release dopamine and norepinephrine. Catecholamine released by the interneuron then hyperpolarizes the ganglion cell membrane, causing an IPSP. M_2 receptors appear to be involved, as are small, intensely fluorescent (SIF) cells. IPSP and catecholamine-induced hyperpolarization are blocked by adrenergic blocking drugs. IPSP is not affected by classic nicotinic blocking agents but is frequently sensitive to block by atropine.

The impact of the secondary pathways on the initial EPSP and the identity of the involved neurotransmitter vary among ganglia and differ between the parasympathetic and sympathetic ganglia. Many peptides identified in the ganglia are released on stimulation of preganglionic

nerves, including gonadotropin-releasing hormone, substance P, angiotensin, VIP, NPY, and the enkephalins. The peptides are associated primarily with the late slow EPSP and inhibition of the M current; 5-HT and γ-aminobutyric acid (GABA) modify ganglionic transmission.

Autonomic ganglia may be stimulated by two groups of drugs, the nicotinic and muscarinic agonists. Nicotinic agonists cause the rapid onset of excitatory effects, mimic the initial EPSP, and are blocked by classic nondepolarizing ganglionic blocking drugs. Muscarinic agonists delay onset of excitatory effects, are blocked by atropine, and mimic the slow EPSP.

Blockade of ganglionic transmission results primarily from action at the nicotinic receptor to stop or inhibit transmission. Two groups of drugs block ganglionic transmission. The first group is classically represented by nicotine and initially stimulates the receptor but then blocks it. This action is similar to the action of persistent depolarization. The second group causes no prior stimulation of the ganglia or change in ganglionic potentials and includes the drugs hexamethonium, trimethaphan, and mecamylamine. Trimethaphan acts by competing with acetylcholine at the cholinergic receptor sites on the ganglia; hexamethonium blocks the channel when it is open. Either mechanism blocks the initial EPSP and ganglionic transmission.

Muscarinic antagonists or α-agonists are incapable of completely blocking transmission, but they may inhibit normal modulation of the nerve impulse. β-Adrenergic stimulation facilitates nicotinic and muscarinic transmission, whereas α-adrenergic stimulation inhibits it. 5-HT is mostly facilitative, but it can be inhibitory in certain areas. Dopamine may also be inhibitory through stimulation of the IPSP. The adrenal medulla is a specialized ganglionic synapse and is therefore under influences similar to those arising on the autonomic ganglia.

DRUGS AND THE AUTONOMIC NERVOUS SYSTEM

The structure and function of the sympathetic and parasympathetic systems are discussed in the preceding sections. Pharmacologic manipulation of autonomic function is the basis of therapy in many acute and chronic illnesses. The complex pharmacology allows many points for intervention, including enhancement or inhibition of synthesis, storage, or receptor-mediated activity[161] (Table 16-8). In the following sections, specific autonomic drugs of interest to anesthesiologists and the mechanisms by which they work are discussed.

Drugs Affecting Adrenergic Transmission

Endogenous Catecholamines

The endogenous sympathetic transmitters norepinephrine, epinephrine, and dopamine are catecholamines, an important subclass of the sympathomimetic drugs (Fig. 16-20). The parent compound of this sympathomimetic group is β-phenylethylamine, the structure of which includes a benzene ring and ethylamine side chain. Substitution of hydroxyl groups at the 3 and 4 positions of the benzene ring converts benzene to catechol, and these compounds are known as *catecholamines*. Although synthetic, isoproterenol and dobutamine are also catecholamines. Noncatecholamine drugs may also act as sympathomimetics and have a similar structure.

The catecholamines are primarily metabolized by COMT. The loss of either hydroxyl group enhances oral effectiveness and duration of action because the drug is no longer metabolized by COMT. Noncatecholamines are primarily metabolized by MAO. The noncatecholamines that have a substituted α-carbon have a longer duration of action because they are not metabolized by COMT or MAO.[163]

Epinephrine

Epinephrine is used intravenously in life-threatening circumstances, including the treatment of cardiac arrest, circulatory collapse, and anaphylaxis, but it is also commonly used locally to limit the spread of local anesthetics or to reduce blood loss. The systemic effects of epinephrine are variable and are related to blood levels. The choice of dosing and the route of administration are determined by the indication for use and its urgency.

Table 16–8 Some drugs and toxins that affect autonomic activity

Site of Action	Compounds that Augment Autonomic Activity	Compounds that Depress Autonomic Activity*

Sympathetic and parasympathetic ganglia	Stimulate postganglionic neurons
	  Nicotine
	Inhibit AChE
	  Physostigmine (Eserine)
	  Neostigmine (Prostigmin)
	  Parathion
		Block conduction
		  Hexamethonium (C-6)
		  Mecamylamine (Inversine)
		  Trimethaphan (Arfonad)
		  High concentrations of ACh
		  Anticholinesterase drugs

Endings of postganglionic noradrenergic neurons	Release NE
	  Tyramine
	  Ephedrine
	  Amphetamine
		Block NE synthesis
		  Metyrosine (Demser)
		Interfere with NE storage
		  Reserpine
		  Guanethidine (Ismelin)
		Prevent NE release
		  Bretylium (Bretylol)
		  Guanethidine (Ismelin)
		Form false transmitters
		  Methyldopa (Aldomet)

α-Receptors	Stimulate α_1-receptors
	  Methoxamine (Vasoxyl)
	  Phenylephrine (Neo-Synephrine)
	Stimulate α_2-receptors
	  Clonidine† (Catapres)
		Block α-receptors
		  Phenoxybenzamine
		    (Dibenzyline)
		  Phentolamine (Regitine)
		  Prazosin (Minipres) (blocks α_1)
		  Yohimbine (blocks α_2)

β-Receptors	Stimulate β-receptors
	  Isoproterenol (Isuprel)
	  Dobutamine (Dobutrex)
		Block β-receptors
		  Propranolol (Inderal) and
		    others (block β_1 and β_2)
		  Atenolol (Tenormin) and
		    others (block β_1)

ACh, acetylcholine; NE, norepinephrine; AChE, acetylcholinesterase.

*Only the principal actions are listed. Guanethidine is believed to have two principal actions.

†Clonidine stimulates α_2-receptors in the periphery, but along with other α_2-agonists that cross the blood-brain barrier, it also stimulates α_2-receptors in the brain that decrease sympathetic output. Therefore, the overall effect is decreased sympathetic discharge.

Adapted from Ganong W: The autonomic nervous system. *In* Ganong W (ed): Review of Medical Physiology, 15th ed. Norwalk, CT, Appleton & Lange, 1991, p 210.

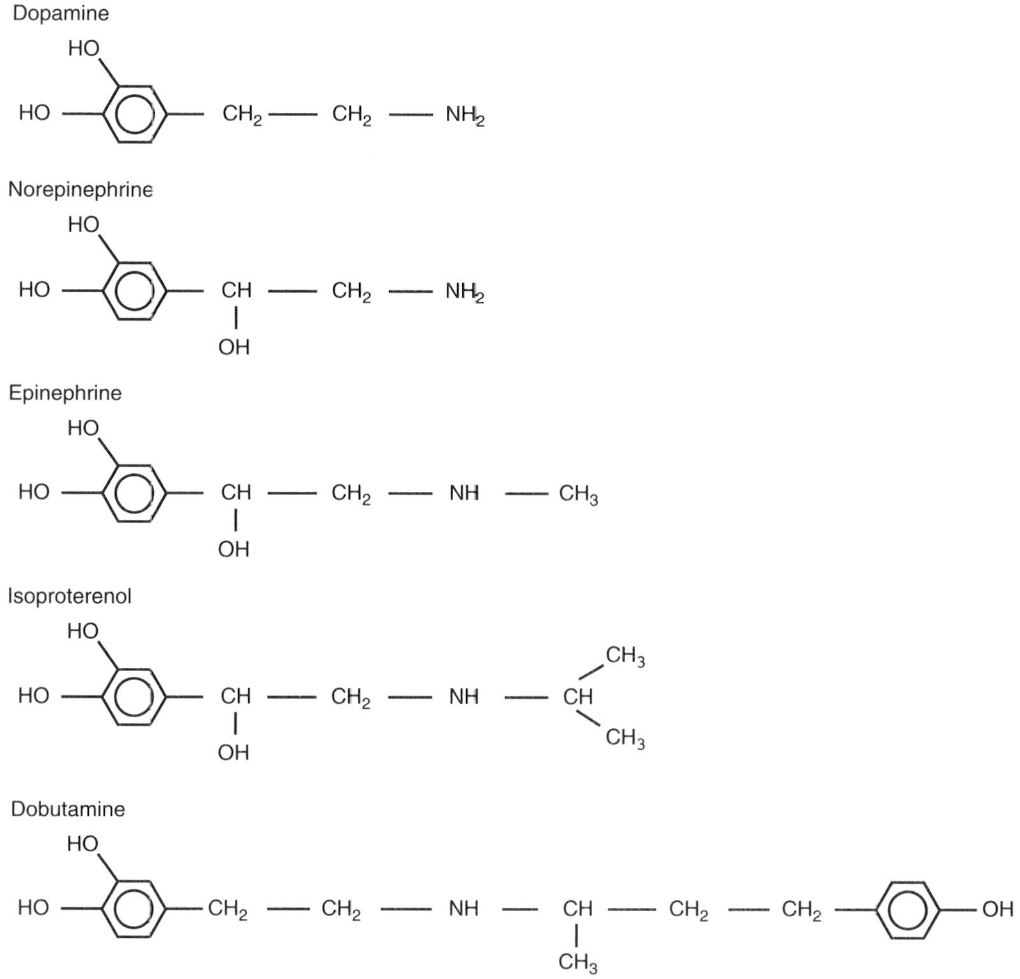

Dopamine

Norepinephrine

Epinephrine

Isoproterenol

Dobutamine

Figure 16–20 Catecholamine structures. A benzene ring with two adjacent hydroxyl groups forms the catechol nucleus.

Epinephrine activates all adrenergic receptors: α_1, α_2, β_1, β_2, and β_3. Potential therapeutic effects of epinephrine include positive inotropy, chronotropy, and enhanced conduction in the heart (β_1); smooth muscle relaxation in the vasculature and bronchial tree (β_2); and vasoconstriction (α_1). With vasoconstriction, aortic diastolic pressure is increased, promoting coronary flow during cardiac arrest, which may be the single most important determinant of survival.[164] Endocrine and metabolic effects of epinephrine include increased levels of glucose, lactate, and free fatty acids (see Table 16-1).

Epinephrine may be given intravenously as a bolus or by infusion. Usual bolus doses for pressure support begin at 2 to 8 μg given intravenously; 0.02 mg/kg or approximately 1.0 mg is given for cardiovascular collapse, asystole, ventricular fibrillation, electromechanical dissociation, or anaphylactic shock. The higher dose range is recommended in these critical situations to maintain myocardial and cerebral perfusion through peripheral vasoconstriction. High-dose epinephrine (0.1 to 0.2 mg/kg) has been studied in resuscitation from cardiac arrest, but it does not appear to improve rates of survival in adults. High-dose epinephrine may be given in adults if usual doses fail to generate a response.[155]

In pediatric patients, outcome after asystole and pulseless cardiac arrest is abysmal, and the current recommendation is that high-dose epinephrine (0.1 mg/kg) be administered within 3 to 5 minutes after the initial dose (0.01 mg/kg) and repeated every 3 to 5 minutes throughout resuscitative attempts.[166] Doses as large as 0.2 mg/kg may be effective.[167] Endotracheal or intraosseous administration is an option in urgent situations such as cardiac arrest while intravenous access is obtained. Endotracheal doses should be at least tripled and diluted in 10 mL of normal saline in adult patients.[168] In pediatric patients, 10 times the intravenous dose may be needed.[166] When continued cardiovascular support is required, infusion rates can be adjusted to elicit specific receptor stimulation. Epinephrine should not be administered in alkaline solutions, because it is rapidly degraded to its biologically inactive metabolite, adrenochrome. If adrenochrome is present, the vial will have a pink hue and should be discarded.[163]

Patients vary tremendously in their response to these agents, and given rates of infusion cannot guarantee the expected serum levels in all patients; the "pressors" therefore should be carefully titrated, and measures to monitor renal, cerebral, and myocardial perfusion are more critical than adherence to a rigid dosing scheme (Table 16-9). A rate of 1 to 2 µg/min, although rarely used, should predominantly activate β$_2$-receptors, with resulting vascular and bronchial smooth muscle relaxation. A rate of 2 to 10 µg/min (25 to 120 ng/kg/min) increases heart rate, contractility, and conduction through the atrioventricular node and decreases the refractory period. Doses in excess of 10 µg/min (100 ng/kg/min) cause marked α-adrenergic stimulation with resultant generalized vasoconstriction. Epinephrine is a potent renal vasoconstrictor acting directly by α-receptor stimulation and indirectly by stimulation of renin release. It is frequently used in combination with "renal-dose" dopamine in an attempt to avoid renal ischemia. Although low-dose epinephrine increases heart rate by direct β$_1$-adrenergic stimulation, reflex bradycardia is seen with higher doses, because of marked elevation of blood pressure through peripheral vasoconstriction.

In the past, inhaled epinephrine was used in a 1% (1 g/100 mL) solution to treat bronchospasm, but it has been largely supplanted by β$_2$-specific agonists. Racemic epinephrine (i.e., mixture of the levorotary and dextrorotary isomers) constricts edematous mucosa and is used in the treatment of severe croup[169] and of postextubation and traumatic airway edema. A 2.25% solution (MicroNefrin or Vaponefrin) is diluted with water or saline in a 1:8 ratio and is nebulized. Treatments may be given as frequently as every 2 hours, with effects lasting 30 to 60 minutes; the patient should remain under observation for at least 2 hours, because initial improvement may be followed by rebound swelling up to 2 hours after administration.[163] Although it is common clinical practice to use the racemic form of epinephrine for these clinical applications, data show that L-epinephrine is 15 to 30 times more potent than the mixture[170,171] and is equally effective and less expensive in treating these clinical complications.[172]

Bronchospasm may also be treated by subcutaneous administration of epinephrine in doses of 300 µg every 20 minutes up to three doses. In addition to its direct bronchodilatory effects, epinephrine may decrease antigen-induced release of endogenous bronchospastic substances from mast cells and is particularly useful in anaphylactic reactions.[173] Relative contraindications include advanced age, significant tachycardia, hypertension, and coronary occlusive disease. Absorption of subcutaneous epinephrine is extremely slow because of intense local vasoconstriction, and the effect of a very large subcutaneous dose of 0.5 to 1.5 mg is roughly equivalent to an intravenous infusion of 10 to 30 µg/min.[163] Intravenous injection of epinephrine in a dose appropriate for subcutaneous administration can result in life-threatening ventricular arrhythmias, hypertension, and cerebral hemorrhage. Sus-Phrine, a sustained-release form of epinephrine, may be used in children by subcutaneous injection but should never be given intravenously.

Epinephrine is often applied locally to mucosal surfaces to decrease bleeding in the operative site. It is mixed with local anesthetics for infiltration into tissues or intrathecal injection. The α-mediated vasoconstriction decreases bleeding in the area and slows vascular uptake of local anesthetic, prolonging the duration of effect and decreasing the peak serum level of the local anesthetic. Although clinicians express concern about the systemic effects of such injections, several studies have shown that, barring intravascular injection, the elevations in plasma levels from vascular uptake are relatively modest and are substantially less than levels seen during psychological stress.[29,174]

Drug interactions with epinephrine are often predictable. Cocaine and other uptake inhibitors enhance the effect and duration of exogenous epinephrine. Preexisting α$_1$-blockade can cause the paradoxic phenomenon of *epinephrine reversal* as the β$_2$-vasodilating effects are unmasked. Patients receiving nonselective β-blockers may demonstrate unopposed α-responses. Cardioselective (β$_1$) blockade does not have this effect.[175]

Table 16–9 Dose-dependent actions of inotropes and chronotropes

Drug* (Proprietary Name)	Receptors	Usual Infusion Rate
Epinephrine (Adrenalin)	β$_2$	1–2 µg/min
	β$_1$ + β$_2$	2–10 µg/min
	α$_1$	≥10 µg/min[†] (bolus: 2–10 µg; 0.5–1.0 mg[‡])
Norepinephrine (Levophed)	α$_1$, β$_1$, ≫ β$_2$	4–12 µg/min[†]
Dopamine (Intropin)	Dopaminergic	0–3 µg/kg/min
	β	3–10 µg/kg/min
	α	>10 µg/kg/min[†]
Dobutamine (Dobutrex)	β$_1$ ≫ β$_2$, α	2.5–10 µg/kg/min[†]
Isoproterenol (Isuprel)	β$_1$ > β$_2$	0.5–10 µg/min
Amrinone (Inocor)	Increase cyclic adenosine monophosphate through phosphodiesterase inhibition	0.75 mg/kg/load over 2–3 min; 5–10 µg/kg/min infusion

*All agents have elimination half-lives of a few minutes, except amrinone (t$_{1/2}$, 3.6 hours; 5.8 hours in congestive heart failure).
[†]Much higher doses have been used in clinical practice.
[‡]With anaphylaxis or cardiac arrest.
Data from Hoffman BB, Lefkowitz RJ: Catecholamines and sympathetic drugs. *In* Goodman A, Rall T, Nies A, et al (eds): Goodman and Gilman's the Pharmacological Basis of Therapeutics, 8th ed. New York, Pergamon Press, 1990, p 187.

Halothane sensitizes the heart to catecholamines, and the potential for troublesome arrhythmias under light inhalational anesthesia has long been appreciated by clinicians. Epinephrine decreases the refractory period, rendering the heart more susceptible to arrhythmias. In adults, the epinephrine dose required to produce three premature ventricular contractions in 50% of patients (ED_{50}) at 1.25 minimum alveolar concentration (MAC) was 2.1 µg/kg for halothane, 6.7 µg/kg for isoflurane, and 10.9 µg/kg for enflurane.[176] Children appear to tolerate higher doses than do adults. It has been suggested that children receiving a halothane anesthetic can receive a maximum of 10 to 15 µg/kg of epinephrine subcutaneously every 10 minutes.[169] Hypocapnia potentiates this drug interaction.

Norepinephrine

Norepinephrine differs structurally from epinephrine only in its lack of a methyl group. Like epinephrine, norepinephrine acts at α- and β-receptors, but it is typically used for its potent α-agonism. It is frequently the pressor of last resort in supporting the systemic vascular resistance. Because of its short half-life of 2.5 minutes, a continuous infusion is preferred. Whereas less than 2 µg/min (30 ng/kg/min) may uncover the effects of β_1-adrenergic stimulation, the usual infusion rates of greater than 3 µg/min (50 ng/kg/min) elicit peripheral vasoconstriction from α-adrenergic stimulation.[177]

Peripheral vasoconstriction increases blood pressure and may cause reflex bradycardia. Venous return is increased by the powerful venoconstriction. Cardiac output is frequently unchanged or decreased; oxygen consumption is markedly increased. Pulmonary vascular resistance may be increased, and norepinephrine should be used with caution in patients with pulmonary hypertension.[178]

Like epinephrine, norepinephrine is a potent constrictor of the renal and mesenteric vascular beds and can cause renal failure, mesenteric infarction, and peripheral hypoperfusion. The decrease in hepatic flow is of clinical relevance because plasma levels of hepatically metabolized drugs (e.g., lidocaine) are markedly increased.[179] To ameliorate the renal effects, a low-dose dopamine infusion may be added to norepinephrine.[180] Extravasation of norepinephrine can cause tissue necrosis and may be treated with local infiltration of phentolamine. Prolonged infusion has caused gangrene of the digits. The potential for profound vasoconstriction makes careful patient selection and close monitoring mandatory.

Dopamine

Dopamine acts at α-adrenergic, β-adrenergic, and dopaminergic receptors; it also acts to release norepinephrine and therefore has mixed direct and indirect effects. Although dopamine is a precursor of norepinephrine, its most important effect may be to cause peripheral vasodilation. Improvement of blood flow through the renal and mesenteric beds in shocklike states is expected through its action at dopamine receptors on the postjunctional membrane. It is rapidly metabolized by MAO and COMT and has a half-life of about 1 minute. Like other endogenous catecholamines, it is given as a continuous intravenous infusion and without a loading dose. At low doses (0.5 to 2.0 µg/kg/min), DA_1 receptors are stimulated, and renal and mesenteric vascular beds dilate.[181] In addition to an improvement in renal blood flow, glomerular filtration rate and sodium excretion increase. With an infusion rate of 2 to 10 µg/kg/min, β_1-receptors are stimulated, which increases cardiac contractility and output. Rates higher than 5 µg/kg/min stimulate release of endogenous norepinephrine, which contributes to cardiac stimulation. In larger doses (10 to 20 µg/kg/min), α- and β_1-receptors are stimulated, the α-adrenergic vasoconstrictive effect predominates, and the benefit to renal perfusion may be lost.[182] Patients' responses to dopamine are extremely variable, and dosages must be individualized. Monitoring to ensure organ and peripheral perfusion is critical. The dose should be significantly decreased in patients treated previously with an MAOI or tricyclic antidepressant.

Dopamine is frequently the initial agent used in the treatment of shock, particularly in vasodilated states such as sepsis; it is often used to protect the kidney and to aid in diuresis, especially in patients with severe CHF.[183] Infusion in combination with dobutamine for the therapy of cardiogenic shock may be more effective than either agent given alone.[184]

Dopexamine hydrochloride (Dopacard), an inotropic vasodilator, is a synthetic parenteral dopamine analog that may be of use in CHF. Dopexamine is approximately 60 times more potent at β_2-adrenergic receptors than dopamine, one third as potent at DA_1 receptors, and one seventh as potent at DA_2 receptors.[185,186] Unlike dopamine, it shows no α-adrenergic effects and negligible β_1-adrenergic effects and is therefore devoid of vasoconstrictive activity.[185,187] Dopexamine has a reported half-life of 3 to 7 minutes in healthy patients and approximately 11 minutes in patients with low cardiac output.[188] β_2-Agonism produces systemic vasodilation and indirect inotropic activity (through inhibition of neuronal uptake of norepinephrine).[185-187,189,190] The stimulation of dopaminergic receptors produces selective vasodilation of renal and splanchnic vessels and increases glomerular filtration rate, diuresis, and natriuresis.[186,191-194]

The use of dopexamine is preferable when vascular resistance is high. Within the dose range of 1 to 6 µg/kg/min, the combined inotropic, vasodilative, diuretic, and natriuretic effects have shown benefit in the management of CHF[195-198] but an indeterminate outcome in the treatment of septic shock.[197,199-203] Use of this agent has been limited by dose-dependent tachycardia, mainly at doses higher than 4 µg/kg/min.[204,205] The effects of dopexamine on intestinal mucosal and hepatic perfusion remain controversial.[206-211] In general, systemic vasodilation appears more pronounced with dopexamine, and positive inotropic effects appear more marked with dopamine[212] and dobutamine.[213]

Fenoldopam is a selective DA_1 agonist and potent vasodilator (i.e., six to nine times as potent as dopamine) that enhances natriuresis, diuresis, and renal blood flow.[214-218] Because of its poor bioavailability and varied results in clinical trials, fenoldopam is no longer being investigated as a candidate for therapy of chronic hypertension or CHF. Instead, intravenous fenoldopam, given by infusion at rates of 0.1 to 0.8 µg/kg/min with incremental titration at 0.1 µg/kg/min, has been approved to treat severe hypertension. It is an alternative to sodium nitroprusside, with potentially fewer side effects (i.e., no thiocyanate toxicity, rebound effect, or coronary steal) and improved renal function. Its peak effects occur within 15 minutes.[219,220]

Noncatecholamine Sympathomimetic Amines

Whereas the β-agonist isoproterenol and the α-agonists phenylephrine and methoxamine act predominantly at only one type of receptor, most of the sympathomimetic drugs act at α- and β-receptors. Most noncatecholamine sympathomimetic amines act at α- and β-receptors because they have two mechanisms of action: directly at a receptor and indirectly by releasing endogenous norepinephrine.

Mephentermine (Wyamine), ephedrine, and metaraminol (Aramine) are mixed-acting drugs. Ephedrine increases blood pressure and has a positive inotropic effect. Because it does not have detrimental effects on uterine blood flow, ephedrine is widely used as a pressor in the hypotensive parturient patient.[221] Because of its β_1-adrenergic stimulating effects, ephedrine is helpful in treating moderate hypotension, particularly if accompanied by bradycardia. It also has some direct β_2-adrenergic stimulating effects and has been used orally as a bronchodilator. The usual dose is 2.5 to 25 mg given intravenously or 25 to 50 mg administered intramuscularly. Mephentermine is similar to ephedrine in its effects, whereas metaraminol has relatively stronger direct α_1-adrenergic stimulating effects and may be associated with reflex bradycardia.

Tachyphylaxis to the indirect effect may develop through depletion of norepinephrine stores. Although all sympathomimetic amines are capable of producing tolerance or tachyphylaxis, the mechanism has been best studied with metaraminol. Metaraminol is taken up into the sympathetic nerve ending, displacing norepinephrine and producing the sympathomimetic effect. However, after some time, the drug acts as a false transmitter, and subsequent sympathetic nerve stimulation results in much less effect. Consequently, the drug probably should not be used widely when other, more effective drugs are available. Indirect action is attenuated in the presence of long-term reserpine or cocaine use, but these drugs may still be efficacious at higher doses. Although indirect-acting agents are widely used as a first-line therapy for intraoperative hypotension, epidemiologic studies of adverse reactions under anesthesia suggest that dependence on these agents in life-threatening events may contribute to morbidity.[222]

α-Receptor Agonists

Phenylephrine and methoxamine are selective α_1-agonists. These drugs are commonly used when peripheral vasoconstriction is needed and cardiac output is adequate, as in the hypotension that may accompany spinal anesthesia, and in patients with coronary artery disease or aortic stenosis to increase coronary perfusion pressure without chronotropic side effects. Phenylephrine (Neo-Synephrine) has a rapid onset and a relatively short duration of action (5 to 10 minutes) when given intravenously. It may be given by bolus doses of 40 to 100 µg or by infusion at a starting rate of 10 to 20 µg/min. Higher doses of up to 1 mg are used to slow supraventricular tachycardia through reflex action. Phenylephrine is also used as a mydriatic and nasal decongestant. In anesthetic practice, it is applied topically, alone or mixed with local anesthetic gel, to prepare the nose for intubation. It is also added to local anesthetic to prolong subarachnoid block. In contrast, methoxamine (Vasoxyl) is a much longer-acting drug (30 to 60 minutes).[223] In larger doses, methoxamine possesses some membrane-stabilizing and β-blocking properties.

The α_2-agonists are assuming greater importance as anesthetic adjuvants and analgesics. Their primary effect is sympatholytic. They reduce peripheral norepinephrine release by stimulation of prejunctional inhibitory α_2-adrenoreceptors. They inhibit central neural transmission in the dorsal horn by presynaptic and postsynaptic mechanisms and directly in spinal preganglionic sympathetic neurons. Traditionally, they have been used as antihypertensive drugs, but uses based on sedative, anxiolytic, and analgesic properties are being developed.

Clonidine, the prototypic drug of this class (Table 16-10), is a selective partial agonist for α_2-adrenoreceptors, with a ratio of approximately 200:1 (α_2 to α_1). Its antihypertensive effects are caused by central and peripheral attenuation of sympathetic outflow and central activation of nonadrenergic imidazoline-preferring receptors.[176,224-226] The decrease in central sympathetic outflow reduces activity in peripheral sympathetic neurons without

Table 16–10 α_2-Agonists dosing

Drug	Route	Bolus	Continuous Infusion	References
Clonidine	Oral	150 µg, 4–5 µg/kg		230, 231, 234, 291, 304
	Intramuscular	2 µg/kg		272
	Intravenous	150 µg, 4–8 µg/kg	2 µg/kg/hr	266, 273, 305
	Epidural	150–450 µg, 6–8 µg/kg	12.5–70 µg/hr, 1–2 µg/kg/hr	240-243, 270, 272, 282-286, 306-309
	Intrathecal	30–225 µg	8–400 µg/day	244-249, 301-303, 310-317
Dexmedetomidine	Intravenous	1 µg/kg over 10 min	0.4–0.7 µg/kg/hr	261

affecting baroreceptor reflexes.[227] Arterial blood pressure is thereby decreased without the accompanying orthostatic hypotension produced by many antihypertensive drugs.[228] Because clonidine is lipid soluble, it penetrates the blood-brain barrier to reach the hypothalamus and medulla and, unlike methyldopa, it does not require transformation into another substance.[229] Clonidine withdrawal may precipitate hypertensive crises, and clonidine should be continued throughout the perioperative period (perhaps by patch) or at the least replaced by close monitoring of blood pressure and ready ability to treat hypertension. The administration of nonselective β-blockers during clonidine withdrawal can worsen hypertension by leaving α_1-receptor–mediated vasoconstriction unopposed. Labetalol has been used to treat this withdrawal syndrome.

Although α_2-agonists have not been used as sole anesthetic agents in humans, these drugs reduce the anesthetic requirement and provide a more stable cardiovascular course, presumably because of their sympatholytic effect and the need for lower doses of cardioactive anesthetic.[230-232] Clonidine reduced the halothane MAC by up to 50% in a dose-dependent fashion,[233] limited by α_1-adrenoreceptor activation at higher concentrations. Data suggest that oral, intravenous, epidural, and intrathecal administration of clonidine potentiates the anesthetic action of other agents, volatile or injectable, and reduces general and regional anesthetic requirements with correspondingly fewer side effects,[230,231,233-254] although perioperative ischemia was not reduced.[255] Clonidine also attenuates the rise in intraocular pressure associated with laryngoscopy and endotracheal intubation.[256-258]

Another α_2-agonist, dexmedetomidine, which has a half-life of 2.3 hours and has a 1600:1 preference for α_2-receptors relative to α_1-receptors,[259] was introduced into clinical practice as an adjunct to regional, local, and general anesthetics.[260] Dexmedetomidine decreases the halothane MAC by more than 95% in animals.[233,261,262] In healthy volunteers, dexmedetomidine increases sedation, analgesia, and memory loss and decreases heart rate, cardiac output, and circulating catecholamines in a dose-dependent fashion.[259] The purported MAC-reducing sedative and analgesic effects in preclinical and volunteer studies have been largely borne out in clinical practice. Dexmedetomidine infusions attenuate the hemodynamic lability of induction, maintenance, and emergence, but they require careful down titration of other agents to prevent overdosing[263,264] because requirements for other anesthetics may decrease.[256] Another use for this drug is to provide sedation for mechanically ventilated patients during weaning from the ventilator.[265] Dexmedetomidine is administered as a loading dose of 1 µg/kg over 10 to 20 minutes followed by an infusion at 0.4 to 0.7 µg/kg/hour.

In addition to their use in the operative setting, α_2-agonists provide effective analgesia for acute and chronic pain, particularly as adjuncts to local anesthetics and opioids. The addition of clonidine increased duration of analgesia and reduced doses of each component.[240,242,243,266-280] Epidural clonidine is indicated for the treatment of intractable pain, which is the basis for approval of parenteral clonidine in the United States as an orphan drug.[281] Patients with intractable pain that is unresponsive to maximum doses of oral or epidural opioids benefit from oral, patch, intramuscular, and neuraxial administration of clonidine,[282-286] as do patients with reflex sympathetic dystrophy[287] and neuropathic pain.[283,288] The intrinsic analgesic effects of α_2-agonists have been demonstrated with large doses of clonidine alone, administered intrathecally (as much as 450 µg) or epidurally (1 to 2 µg/kg/hour) to control intraoperative and postoperative pain. Clonidine decreases postoperative oxygen consumption and adrenergic stress response.[289,290] Despite dose-dependent adverse effects such as hypotension and sedation and idiosyncratic adverse effects such as bradycardia, clonidine does not induce profound respiratory depression and only mildly potentiates opiate-induced respiratory depression.[291-293]

Aside from its role as an anesthetic adjuvant and antihypertensive agent, clonidine has been used to treat panic disorder[294]; symptoms of opiate, benzodiazepine, and ethanol withdrawal[295,296]; cigarette craving after smoking cessation[297-299]; and emesis in cancer chemotherapeutic regimens. Its use in diabetic diarrheas is based on the presence of α_2-receptors on gut epithelial cells. Normally, stimulation of ileal mucosal α_2-receptors by epinephrine promotes sodium chloride absorption and inhibits bicarbonate secretion. Intractable diarrhea can be a major problem in diabetes because mucosal norepinephrine stores are depleted, and denervation hypersensitivity increases the numbers of postsynaptic α_2-receptors. Clonidine may increase blood glucose concentrations by inhibiting insulin release.[300] Unlike spinal opioids, clonidine does not cause urinary retention and may hasten the time to first micturition after spinal anesthesia.[300-303]

β-Receptor Agonists

Nonselective β-Receptor Agonists

DOBUTAMINE. Although at clinical doses it can act at β_2- and α_1-receptors, dobutamine, a synthetic analog of dopamine, has predominantly β_1-adrenergic effects. Compared with isoproterenol, it is reported to affect inotropy more than chronotropy, but it increases conduction velocity through nodal tissue to the same extent.[318] It exerts less β_2-type effect than isoproterenol and less α_1-type effect than norepinephrine. Unlike dopamine, it does not directly release endogenous norepinephrine, nor does it act at dopaminergic receptors.

Dobutamine is particularly useful in CHF and MI complicated by a low-output state, although in cases of severe hypotension, it may not be effective because it lacks significant α_1-pressor effect. Although dobutamine increases cardiac contractility in the failing heart, its ability to lower filling pressures contrasts with the effects of dopamine and norepinephrine. It is relatively safe to use in myocardial ischemia without increasing the size of the infarct or causing arrhythmias.[319] Doses less than 20 µg/kg/min do not produce tachycardia, but in especially severe CHF, significant tachycardia is the primary adverse effect. Because dobutamine directly stimulates β_1-receptors, it does not rely on norepinephrine stores and may still be effective in catecholamine-depleted states such as chronic CHF. However, in severe chronic CHF, the downregulation of β-adrenergic receptors may hamper its effectiveness.

The $β_2$-vasodilating effects of dobutamine are almost exactly offset by its $α_1$-constricting effects, which experimentally can be revealed by administering a nonselective β-blocking drug.[320] Its modest ability to dilate the peripheral vasculature is probably more closely connected with its ability to relieve the high-adrenergic state of decompensated CHF than to specific $β_2$-mediated vasodilation.[321] Clinical situations that call for distinct afterload reduction may be better served by an agent such as nitroprusside.

Prolonged treatment with dobutamine causes downregulation of β-receptors; tolerance to its hemodynamic effects is significant after 3 days and may be temporarily offset by increasing the rate of infusion.[322] Intermittent infusions of dobutamine have been used in the long-term treatment of heart failure and have improved exercise tolerance[323] but not survival.[324]

ISOPROTERENOL. Isoproterenol (Isuprel) provides relatively pure nonselective β-adrenergic stimulation with no significant effect at α-receptors. Its $β_1$-adrenergic stimulation is significantly stronger than $β_2$, but it still causes more $β_2$-adrenergic activity than dobutamine. Since the development of other inotropes, its popularity has declined because of its adverse effects of tachycardia and arrhythmias. Isoproterenol historically was used in bradycardia or heart block resistant to atropine, but it is not included in the most recent American Heart Association Advanced Cardiac Life Support protocol. Its primary use at this time is as a chronotropic agent in patients after heart transplantation. These patients are unable to generate an endogenous sympathetic response to challenges because the sympathetic fibers are divided when the native heart is removed. The availability of superior pharmacologic options for most clinical indications has led to Isuprel's removal from many hospital formularies. Infusion rates start at 0.5 to 5 μg/min for adults. Because it is not taken up into adrenergic nerve endings, its duration of action is slightly longer than that of the natural catecholamines.

Selective $β_2$-Receptor Agonists

In the past, isoproterenol was used in the treatment of bronchospasm for its $β_2$-adrenergic stimulating properties, but unpleasant and dangerous $β_1$-mediated adverse effects limited its use. The development of $β_2$-selective agents has made β-stimulants a cornerstone of the treatment of bronchospasm. However, this $β_2$-selectivity is only relative, and it may be lost at higher doses; in addition, $β_2$-receptors in the sinoatrial node may cause tachycardia when stimulated. The structures of these drugs have also been modified to slow their metabolism, prolonging therapeutic benefit and enabling oral administration. In particular, the addition of bulky structures on the catecholamine amino group increases $β_2$-selectivity, decreases affinity for α-receptors, and protects against metabolism by COMT. These agents are aerosolized and given by inhaler for rapid onset and to minimize systemic drug levels and adverse effects.

An increase in the annual number of deaths from asthma has been well documented, and it has been suggested that this increase may be related to $β_2$-agonist use.[325-327] A susceptibility to arrhythmia caused by these agents by direct cardiac stimulation or by $β_2$-induced hypokalemia is one suggested mechanism. It has also been hypothesized that the long-term use of these drugs may increase airway hyperreactivity. Nonetheless, their safe use in many thousands of patients is well documented.

Commonly used drugs include metaproterenol (Alupent, Metaprel), terbutaline (Brethine, Bricanyl), and albuterol (Proventil, Ventolin). Metaproterenol is probably less $β_2$-selective than albuterol or terbutaline. Terbutaline is the only $β_2$-selective agent that can be given subcutaneously and therefore may have particular use in status asthmaticus. The normal subcutaneous dose is 0.25 mg, which may be repeated after 15 to 30 minutes.

The $β_2$-agonists are also used to treat premature labor.[328] Ritodrine (Yutopar) has been marketed for this purpose. $β_1$-Adrenergic adverse effects are common, particularly when the drugs are used intravenously. The other $β_2$-selective drugs have also been used as tocolytics, and all have been associated with significant $β_1$-adrenergic adverse effects and the occasional incidence of pulmonary edema.[329] Their use for this purpose has recently been questioned.[330]

α-Receptor Antagonists

$α_1$-Antagonists have long been used clinically as antihypertensives, but they have become less popular over the years. An $α_1$-blockade vasodilates by blocking the effect of endogenous catecholamines on arterial and venous constriction. The effects are potentiated when standing or in the presence of hypovolemia. Reflex tachycardia and fluid retention can ensue. The $α_2$-antagonists may act presynaptically to release norepinephrine.

Phenoxybenzamine (Dibenzyline) is the prototypical $α_1$-antagonist, although it irreversibly binds to $α_1$- and $α_2$-receptors. New receptors must be synthesized before complete offset of its effects occurs. Its half-life after oral administration is unknown, but that after an intravenous dose is about 24 hours. Phenoxybenzamine decreases peripheral resistance and increases cardiac output; blood flow to skin and viscera is increased. As expected, its primary adverse effect is orthostatic hypotension; nasal stuffiness may occur. In addition to receptor blockade, phenoxybenzamine inhibits neuronal and extraneuronal uptake of the catecholamines. Phenoxybenzamine is used in the treatment of pheochromocytoma; with extended use, it establishes a "chemical sympathectomy" preoperatively that aids in blood pressure control, permits correction of the contracted plasma volume, and protects against catecholamine-induced cardiac damage. Phenoxybenzamine treatment allows for a smoother perioperative course. The total daily dose is 40 to 120 mg in two or three divided doses. When exogenous sympathomimetics are administered after $α_1$-receptor blockade, their vasoconstrictive effects are inhibited. The effect of phenylephrine is completely blocked, whereas that of norepinephrine is limited to its $β_1$-adrenergic effect of cardiac stimulation. Potential epinephrine reversal caused by unopposed $β_2$-agonism manifests as severe hypotension and tachycardia. Despite its irreversible binding to the receptor, the recommended treatment for overdosage of phenoxybenzamine is norepinephrine infusion, because some receptors remain free of the drug.[331]

Phentolamine (Regitine) is a shorter-acting drug that blocks α_1- and α_2-receptors. Historically used to treat pulmonary hypertension, it has been largely supplanted by nitroglycerin and nitroprusside. It is also used to treat hypertension associated with clonidine withdrawal or with tyramine ingestion during MAOI therapy, but few data have been collected on its efficacy and safety for these indications. The dose is 1 to 5 mg of phentolamine given intramuscularly or slowly intravenously. Its plasma half-life is 19 minutes after intravenous administration. Phentolamine has also been infiltrated into affected tissues after extravasation of agents such as norepinephrine in an attempt to relax vasoconstriction; for this purpose, 5 to 10 mg is diluted in 10 mL of saline. Adverse effects of phentolamine include hypotension and gastrointestinal distress; reflex tachycardia and arrhythmias may result from action at α_2-receptors. Coronary artery disease and peptic ulcer disease are relative contraindications. As in phenoxybenzamine overdosage, severe hypotension may require treatment with norepinephrine rather than epinephrine. Tolazoline (Priscoline) is a related drug used in persistent pulmonary hypertension of the newborn.[331]

Prazosin (Minipress) is a potent selective α_1-adrenergic blocker often used as a prototypic antagonist in pharmacologic experiments. It antagonizes the vasoconstrictor effects of norepinephrine and epinephrine, causing a decline in peripheral vascular resistance and venous return to the heart. Although heart rate does not normally increase, orthostatic hypotension is a major problem. Unlike other antihypertensive drugs, prazosin improves lipid profiles, lowering low-density lipid levels while raising the level of high-density lipids. It is primarily used to treat hypertension. It has also been used in CHF, but unlike the angiotensin-converting enzyme inhibitors (ACEIs), prazosin does not prolong life. It is metabolized by the liver. Supplied as 1-, 2-, and 5-mg tablets, its starting dose is usually 0.5 to 1 mg, given at bedtime because of the orthostatic hypotension. Eventually, it can be given twice daily.[331]

α_2-Antagonists, such as yohimbine, increase sympathetic outflow by enhancing release of norepinephrine. These drugs have proved to be of little clinical utility in anesthesia, although they are used in urology.

β-Receptor Antagonists
Pharmacology
The β-adrenergic receptor antagonists (i.e., β-blockers) are among the most commonly prescribed drugs and are frequently taken by patients presenting for surgery. Current indications for the use of β-blockade include ischemic heart disease, postinfarction management, arrhythmias, hypertrophic cardiomyopathy, hypertension, heart failure, and prophylaxis for migraine headache. Concern that patients treated with β-blockers would be hemodynamically unstable under anesthesia has proved to be largely unjustified. These drugs are an important part of the armamentarium of the anesthesiologist in the ongoing attempt to limit stress responses perioperatively and

to protect the cardiovascular system. A comprehensive analysis by the Agency for Healthcare Research and Quality found that use of β-blockers perioperatively reduced the morbidity and mortality in noncardiac surgery for patients at risk.[332] Several well-known clinical trials[333-337] and the widespread use and safety of these drugs in heart failure[338] have made β-blockade an evolving standard.

A wide spectrum of β-adrenergic blockers is available to the clinician. The most important properties to consider when choosing a β-blocker for long-term use are cardioselectivity, intrinsic sympathomimetic activity, and lipid solubility.[339,340] In anesthetic practice, cardioselectivity, duration of action, and a formulation suitable for intravenous use are crucial factors (Table 16-11). The β-antagonists resemble isoproterenol in structure and bind competitively to the β-receptor, blocking access by more potent β-agonists (Fig. 16-21).[331] Competitive inhibition at the β-receptor can be overcome by increasing the available concentration of β-agonist. The potency of a β-blocker is often determined by its ability to inhibit induction of tachycardia by isoproterenol. Propranolol is assigned a potency of 1, and the other drugs are evaluated in relation to it.

Nonselective β-adrenergic blockers act at the β_1- and β_2-receptors. The nonselective β-blockers include propranolol, nadolol, pindolol, sotalol, oxprenolol, penbutolol, and timolol.[321, 340] Cardioselective β-blockers have a stronger affinity for β_1-adrenergic receptors than for β_2-adrenergic receptors, and the predominant effects therefore are cardiac. Velocity of atrioventricular conduction, heart rate, and cardiac contractility are decreased, as is the release of renin by the juxtaglomerular apparatus and lipolysis at the adipocytes. With larger doses, the relative selectivity for β_1-adrenergic receptors is lost, and β_2-receptors are also blocked,[341] with potential bronchoconstriction, peripheral vasoconstriction, and decreased glycogenolysis. Cardioselective drugs include atenolol, betaxolol, bevantolol, esmolol, and metoprolol.[321,340] These drugs may be preferable for patients with obstructive pulmonary disease, peripheral vascular disease, Raynaud's phenomenon, and diabetes mellitus. Although previously a matter of controversy, a meta-analysis concluded that cardioselective β-blockers can be given safely to patients with chronic obstructive pulmonary disease.[342] Nevertheless, because the selectivity is only relative and may be lost at conventional clinical doses, extreme care should be used in administering a β-blocker in the presence of pulmonary disease. Some β-antagonists also have vasodilatory effects, making them particularly useful in the treatment of hypertension[321] and CHF.[343,344] Labetalol vasodilates by blocking α_1-receptors and by direct β_2-receptor agonism.

β-Blockers exerting a partial agonist effect at the receptor while blocking access by more potent agonists possess intrinsic sympathomimetic activity (ISA). Agents with ISA include acebutolol, carteolol, celiprolol, dilevalol, oxprenolol, penbutolol, and pindolol.[340] Of these, acebutolol and pindolol are most often used in the United States, but neither is commonly used in anesthetic practice. These agents lower blood pressure with less decrease in resting heart rate and left ventricular function.

Table 16–11 Pharmacokinetics and pharmacology of selected β-adrenoceptor blockers

Characteristic	Atenolol	Metoprolol	Propranolol HCl	Labetalol	Esmolol	Carvedilol
Proprietary name	Tenormin	Lopressor	Inderal Ipran	Trandate Normodye	Brevibloc	Coreg
Relative β sensitivity	+	+	0	0	+	0
Intrinsic sympathetic activity	0	0	0	+	0	0
Membrane-stabilizing activity	0	0	++	0	0	—*
Lipophilicity[†]	Low	Moderate	High	Low	Low	High
Predominant route of elimination	RE (mostly unchanged)	HM	HM	HM	Hydrolysis by RBC esterase	HM
Drug accumulation in renal disease	Yes	No	No	No	No	No
Elimination half-life (hr)	6 to 9	3 to 4	3 to 4	≈6	9 min	2 to 8
Usual maintenance dose PO	50–100 mg qd	50–100 mg qid	60 mg qid	100–600 mg bid	N/A	25–50 mg bid
Usual IV dose (caution)		5 mg q 5 min × 3	0.1 mg/kg (maximum)	1–2 mg/kg	50–300 µg/kg/min infusion	15 mg

*Data not available.
[†]Determined by the distribution ratio between octanol and water.
HM, hepatic metabolism; N/A, not applicable; RE, renal excretion; 0, no effect; +, mild effect; ++, moderate effect.

When sympathetic activity is high, such as during exercise, these drugs behave more like conventional β-blockers. The partial β$_2$-agonism of pindolol induces bronchodilation.[345] ISA may therefore be useful if β-blockade is required in a patient with bradycardia, peripheral vascular disease, or very mild hyperreactive airway disease. The β-blockers with ISA appear not to have the adverse effects on triglyceride and high-density lipoprotein levels of the other agents, although the clinical significance of this finding is unclear.[346] Agents with ISA may not be as effective in controlling symptoms in severe angina or in reducing mortality after MI.[347] ISA may protect against β-blocker withdrawal syndrome.[348]

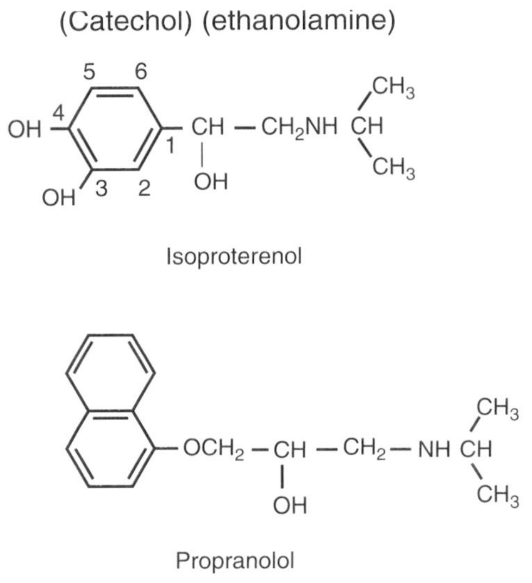

The degree of lipid solubility greatly affects absorption and metabolism. Propranolol, metoprolol, and pindolol, the most lipid-soluble agents, are readily absorbed from the gastrointestinal tract and metabolized in the liver, undergoing extensive first-pass metabolism. Propranolol and metoprolol are given in a much lower dose intravenously than orally because up to 70% of the orally administered drug is removed on the first pass of portal blood through the liver.[339] Altered hepatic function may have a profound effect on plasma levels. The oral or intravenous dose of these agents required to reach a clinical end point varies greatly between patients. Because of a relatively short half-life, lipid-soluble agents are usually given at least twice each day.[340] The extremely short half-life of esmolol, however, results from its metabolism by esterases.

The non–lipid-soluble, or hydrophilic, drugs are atenolol, sotalol, and nadolol. They are not as readily absorbed from the gastrointestinal tract or as extensively metabolized, and they are excreted unchanged by the kidneys. Because of a relatively long half-life, daily dosing may be adequate. There is less interpatient variability in plasma drug levels and clinical effects because of the lack of hepatic metabolism and first-pass effect.[340] Because the lipid-insoluble drugs are slower to cross the blood-brain barrier, they may avoid the CNS adverse effects associated

Figure 16–21 Structures of isoproterenol and propranolol. (From Tollenaeré JP: Atlas of the Three-Dimensional Structure of Drugs. Amsterdam, Elsevier North-Holland, 1979.)

with β-blocker therapy (i.e., depression, sleep disturbances, nightmares, and fatigue). However, the relationship between lipid solubility and the occurrence of these symptoms is not consistent.[349,350]

Propranolol and acebutolol possess membrane-stabilizing activity (MSA), also referred to as the quinidine-like or local anesthetic effect. This effect reduces the rate of rise of the cardiac action potential. The MSA of propranolol may explain the decrease in the oxygen affinity of hemoglobin[351] when it is administered.[352] However, MSA is seen only at concentrations 10 times that required for blockade of β-receptors[353] and is probably of little clinical consequence. Overdose with agents with MSA is associated with a higher incidence of fatality.[354]

Indications for Use

PERIOPERATIVE β-BLOCKADE. β-Adrenergic antagonists have been used to establish perioperative β-blockade (see Chapter 25). Compelling results from the multicenter study of a perioperative ischemia research group[330] have shown that β-blockade improves outcomes. Atenolol was given before and after surgery and continued for the duration of the hospitalization. In this study, patients were randomly allocated to receive atenolol or placebo preoperatively, intraoperatively, and until discharge; follow-up lasted more than 2 years. The overall mortality rate after discharge from the hospital was significantly less for the treated group. Surprisingly, this difference in survival persisted at the 2-year point (68% survival in the placebo group and 83% in the atenolol group). A meta-analysis of this and subsequent studies has confirmed that β-antagonists have a significant role in preventing perioperative cardiac morbidity, particularly in patients at risk for cardiac events.[355]

The safety of continuing β-blockade perioperatively is well established, and initial concerns regarding interaction with general anesthesia have not been confirmed.[356] Attempts to discontinue β-blockers increase the risk of rebound tachycardia (with or without atrial fibrillation) and myocardial ischemia in patients with coronary disease. These drugs should be given up to the time of surgery, and intravenous forms in appropriate dosages should be used whenever gastrointestinal absorption may be in question. Doses for intravenous administration vary less among patients because of the absence of first-pass hepatic effects. If β-blockers have been omitted from the preoperative regimen, esmolol or labetalol may be used acutely to blunt tachycardia and hypertension. Cardioselective and nonselective β-blockers appear effective in blocking chronotropic effects of endotracheal intubation and surgical stress.[357]

MYOCARDIAL ISCHEMIA. Propranolol was initially introduced for treatment of myocardial ischemia 3 decades ago, and β-blocking drugs remain an important part of drug therapy for myocardial ischemia (see Chapter 50). This class of drugs reduces oxygen demand by decreasing heart rate and cardiac contractility. Cardioselective and nonselective β-blockers are effective. Atenolol, metoprolol, nadolol, and propranolol have been approved in the United States for the treatment of angina; metoprolol and atenolol are the only β-blockers approved for intravenous use in acute MI.[340] Although initially there was

concern that β₂-receptor blockade could worsen ischemia through unopposed α-mediated vasoconstriction, this phenomenon is rarely seen, even in patients with variant angina. In usual clinical practice, the dose is increased until the heart rate is 60 to 80 beats/min at rest and until there is no tachycardia with exercise. In theory, a nonselective antagonist may seem a better choice in acute MI because the blockade of β₂-receptors may protect against stress-induced potassium shifts and hypokalemia-associated arrhythmias, but cardioselective and nonselective drugs appear equally useful.[321] Agents with ISA are not as beneficial in this situation.[321] The β-antagonists are used in treating acute MI and on a long-term basis in patients after infarction to reduce reinfarction and mortality.[358-361] Early administration of intravenous β-blocking agents to patients receiving thrombolytic therapy appears to lower the incidence of ischemia and reinfarction[362] and may reduce the incidence of serious ventricular arrhythmias.[363] The long-term use of β-blockers (i.e., timolol, propranolol, metoprolol, and atenolol) has been shown unequivocally to decrease mortality after MI.

CONGESTIVE HEART FAILURE. Over the past 5 years, β-blockers have become first-line agents for the treatment of CHF of ischemic and nonischemic origin. Clinicians had been disinclined to use β-blockers for heart failure patients because of the drugs' negative chronotropic and inotropic effects. These effects have not turned out to be significant concerns in clinical practice. Early studies demonstrated a significant decrease in all-cause mortality for heart failure patients treated with metoprolol[343] or bisoprolol.[344] Several large studies[364,365] were stopped because the decrease in mortality in treated patients with moderate to severe heart failure was so pronounced. The benefits of β-blockers in patients with heart failure have been attributed to normalization and remodeling of the ventricle that begins after 1 month of β-blockade,[366] to decreased norepinephrine-related cardiomyocyte apoptosis in the presence of β₁-blockade,[367] and to decreased sudden cardiac death because of the β-blockers' antiarrhythmic activity. To avoid worsening a patient's heart failure symptoms and to minimize negative inotropic effects, β-blockers are started at very low doses and titrated to the target dose.[368] The only β-blocker approved for treatment of CHF by the U.S. Food and Drug Administration is carvedilol, and its efficacy in patients with severe (i.e., New York Heart Association class IV) heart failure is still being studied. If decompensation occurs with the β-blocker, the phosphodiesterase inhibitors are the inotropes of choice because their effects are not antagonized by β-blockade.[369]

HYPERTENSION. Although β-blockers are recognized by the Joint National Council of the USA Guidelines as one of the first-line therapies for hypertension,[370] the mechanisms by which β-antagonists treat hypertension are incompletely understood. Blood pressure reduction is specific to hypertensive patients because long-term treatment of normotensive individuals does not lower blood pressure. Reduced cardiac output and renin release have been suggested as mechanisms. In hypertensive patients, β-antagonists without ISA may cause a 15% to 20% reduction in cardiac output and a 60% reduction in renin release. However, pindolol, which has ISA and minimal effect on renin, is also successful in treating hypertension.[371] Maximum renin suppression precedes significant changes in arterial blood pressure.[372] Initially, β-blockade increases peripheral vascular resistance and then over time lowers it.[373] The decrease in cardiac output and eventual lowering of peripheral resistance may account for much of the antihypertensive efficacy of these drugs. However, this too is an incomplete explanation because labetalol is an effective antihypertensive despite its lack of effect on cardiac output. A primary CNS effect is not likely to be a major mechanism because antihypertensive efficacy of lipophilic and hydrophilic compounds is similar. Generally, β-blockade is ineffective as monotherapy in hypertensive African American patients older than 60 years.

CARDIAC ARRHYTHMIAS. The β-blockers are widely used in the therapy of tachyarrhythmias as class II agents (see Chapter 32). Two possible mechanisms of action are blockade of catecholamine effects and MSA, although the latter is most likely not clinically significant because antiarrhythmic effects are present in agents without MSA.[374] β-Antagonists slow the rate of depolarization of the sinus node and any ectopic pacemakers, slow conduction through atrial tissue and the atrioventricular node, and increase the refractory period of the atrioventricular node. These drugs can convert atrial arrhythmias to sinus rhythm,[375] but β-blockade is primarily used to slow the ventricular response. Reentrant tachyarrhythmias and those associated with Wolff-Parkinson-White syndrome, mitral valve prolapse, and prolonged QT interval may also respond to these drugs.[353] Care should be exercised if an atrioventricular block is present, as in digitalis toxicity, although these drugs are useful in the treatment of digitalis-associated tachyarrhythmias.[353] Sotalol, a β-blocker with added class III activity, is effective against ventricular tachyarrhythmias; however, in a trial comparing racemic sotalol with D-sotalol in post-MI patients to protect against ventricular fibrillation, mortality increased with D-sotalol.[376] The trial was terminated when patients at lowest risk for arrhythmic events after MI had an increased mortality rate with this drug.[377]

TACHYCARDIA. β-Antagonists are frequently used as adjuvants to moderate the reflex tachycardia associated with vasodilators. This tachycardia can limit the effectiveness of blood pressure control or may cause myocardial ischemia. It is crucial that appropriate β-blockade be administered during vasodilator therapy of aortic dissection. In addition to potentiating blood pressure reduction, β-blockade also reduces the velocity of left ventricular ejection (dp/dt) to attenuate the shearing force associated with the increased velocity of ventricular contraction when nitroprusside is used without concomitant β-blockade.[378] Labetalol has been particularly useful in this situation.[379]

THYROTOXICOSIS. Cardiac complications are a primary cause of morbidity in thyrotoxicosis (see Chapter 27). β-Blockade can suppress the tachycardia and rhythm disturbances, although very large doses may be required. β-Antagonists also may be combined with digitalis for their synergistic effect on atrioventricular node conduction. Propranolol inhibits conversion of thyroxine to the active form, triiodothyronine, in the periphery.[380]

MISCELLANEOUS CONDITIONS. Timolol (Timoptic) and betaxolol (Betoptic) are β-blocking drugs used topically in the eye to treat glaucoma. They reduce the production of aqueous humor. Even topical use of these agents has been associated with significant systemic effects of β-blockade. The β-blockers are used in idiopathic hypertrophic subaortic stenosis to reduce the dynamic obstruction to left ventricular outflow. The drugs are also effective in prophylaxis, but not therapy, of migraine headaches and in controlling acute panic symptoms and essential tremor.

Adverse Effects

The adverse effects of most concern are those involving cardiopulmonary function. Severe noncardiopulmonary reactions such as cutaneous reactions or anaphylaxis are rare. Life-threatening bradycardia, even asystole, may occur, and decreased contractility may precipitate CHF in vulnerable individuals. In patients with bronchospastic lung disease, β_2-blockade may be fatal. CNS effects, although an appropriate consideration in long-term therapy, are not a concern in the usual anesthetic use of these agents. Diabetes mellitus is a relative contraindication to the long-term use of β-antagonists, because hypoglycemia in the face of sympathetic blockade is not accompanied by warning signs such as tachycardia and tremor, and compensatory glycogenolysis is blunted. However, most non–insulin-dependent diabetic patients can tolerate these drugs, although β-blockade may cause insulin resistance in rare cases. In addition to the potential worsening of peripheral perfusion by β_2-blockade in patients with peripheral vascular disease, the Raynaud phenomenon may be triggered in susceptible patients. Sudden withdrawal of β-blockers may cause myocardial ischemia and possibly infarction, although this is less of a problem with β-blockers with ISA such as pindolol.[368,381,382] Although β-antagonists may reduce renal blood flow and glomerular filtration rate, these agents can be used in renal failure. For these patients, the doses of lipid-insoluble drugs should be reduced. To avoid worsening of hypertension, use in pheochromocytoma should be avoided unless α-receptors have previously been blocked. Nonselective agents may elicit hypertensive responses in cases of high sympathetic stimulation.[383]

Undesirable drug interactions are possible with β-blockers.[331,340] The rate and contractility effects of verapamil are additive to those of the β-blockers,[384,385] and care should be taken in combining these agents, especially the intravenous forms in acute situations such as supraventricular tachycardia. The combination of digoxin and β-blockers can have powerful effects on heart rate and conduction and should be used with special care. Pharmacokinetic interactions are predictable from the degree of lipid solubility of the drug. Cimetidine and hydralazine may reduce hepatic perfusion, thereby increasing plasma levels and half-lives of the lipid-soluble β-antagonists. Barbiturates, phenytoin, rifampin, and smoking may induce hepatic enzymes, enhancing metabolism. Propranolol may reduce hepatic clearance of lidocaine, increasing the risk of toxicity.

Overdose of β-blocking drugs may be treated with atropine, but isoproterenol, dobutamine, or glucagon infusions (or some combination) may be required along with cardiac pacing to ensure an adequate rate of contraction.

Specific Drugs

The drugs propranolol, metoprolol, labetalol, and esmolol are particularly useful in anesthetic practice because they are widely available in intravenous formulation and have well-characterized effects. If the drug the patient has taken on a long-term basis is propranolol, metoprolol, or labetalol, it may be continued in intravenous form if the clinical situation is relatively stable. In deciding which intravenous β-blocker to substitute in a patient taking a β-blocker on a long-term basis, the need for cardioselectivity is a primary consideration. Cardioselectivity is provided by metoprolol or esmolol. If the long-term agent has ISA, oxprenolol and acebutolol have intravenous forms, but they are not readily available. In many situations, esmolol may be substituted and titrated to effect, with the expectation that its effects will fade relatively rapidly in case it is not well tolerated.

PROPRANOLOL. Propranolol (Inderal, Ipran) is the prototypic β-blocker, and its actions and its use are well characterized.[374] It is a nonselective β-blocking drug with MSA but no ISA.[340] It readily penetrates the CNS. Because of its high lipid solubility, it is extensively metabolized in the liver, but metabolism varies greatly from patient to patient. Its effective dose is extremely variable: 10 mg to as much as 320 mg may be given orally each day. Clearance of the drug can be affected by liver disease or altered hepatic blood flow. Renal impairment does not require adjustment of dosing. Despite its half-life of 4 hours, its antihypertensive effect persists long enough to permit dosing once or twice daily.[374,386] Inderal LA is a sustained-release formulation given once daily.[331]

Propranolol is available in an intravenous form; although initially used as bolus or infusion, the infusion has been largely supplanted by esmolol. For bolus administration, doses of 0.1 mg/kg may be given, although most practitioners initiate therapy with much smaller doses, typically 0.25 to 0.5 mg, and titrate to effect. Propranolol shifts the oxyhemoglobin dissociation curve to the right, perhaps accounting for its efficacy in vasospastic disorders.[387-389]

METOPROLOL. Metoprolol (Lopressor) is approved for the treatment of angina pectoris and is the only intravenous β-blocker formally approved by the U.S. Food and Drug Administration for treatment of acute MI. Lacking ISA and MSA, it is cardioselective. Because it is metabolized in the liver by the monooxygenase system, doses need not be adjusted in the presence of renal failure.[340] The usual oral dose is 100 to 200 mg/day, once or twice daily for hypertension and twice daily for angina pectoris. It may be administered intravenously in doses of 2.5 to 5 mg every 2 to 5 minutes up to about 15 mg, titrating to heart rate and blood pressure.

LABETALOL. Labetalol (Trandate, Normodyne) is representative of a class of drugs that act as competitive antagonists at the α_1- and β-adrenergic receptors. Labetalol consists of four isomers that block the α_1-, β_1-, and β_2-receptors; inhibit neuronal uptake of norepinephrine (uptake-1); act as a partial agonist at β_2-receptors; and possibly have some direct dilating abilities.[331]

The potency of the mixture for β-blockade is 5- to 10-fold that for α-blockade.[390] The usual oral dose of labetalol is 200 to 400 mg twice daily, although much larger doses have been used. It is metabolized by the liver, and clearance is affected by hepatic perfusion. The dose need not be adjusted for renal dysfunction.[340] Labetalol may be given intravenously every 5 minutes in 5- to 10-mg doses or up to a 2-mg/min infusion. It significantly blunts cardiovascular responses to tracheal intubation.[391] It can be effective in treatment of aortic dissection,[379] hypertensive emergencies,[392,393] and postoperative cardiac surgical patients,[394] particularly because vasodilation is not accompanied by tachycardia. It may be used in pregnancy to treat hypertension on a long-term basis and in more urgent situations.[395] Uterine blood flow is not affected even with a significant reduction of blood pressure.[396]

CARVEDILOL. Carvedilol, a mixed α- and β-antagonist, has been introduced as therapy for mild or moderate hypertension,[397-405] for management of stable or unstable angina, and after acute MI.[406-410] Clinical trials of carvedilol use in the treatment of controlled CHF (New York Heart Association class II-IV) suggest a significant reduction in mortality,[364,365,411,412] especially for patients with diabetes.[413]

ESMOLOL. Because of its hydrolysis by esterases, esmolol (Brevibloc) has a uniquely short half-life of 9 to 10 minutes, which makes it particularly useful in anesthetic practice. It is administered when β-blockade of short duration is desired or in critically ill patients for whom adverse effects of bradycardia, heart failure, or hypotension may necessitate rapid withdrawal of the drug. Peak effects of a loading dose are seen within 5 to 10 minutes and diminish rapidly (within 20 to 30 minutes). It is cardioselective. It may be given as a bolus of 0.5 mg/kg to blunt cardiovascular responses to tracheal intubation. If used as an infusion for the treatment of supraventricular tachycardia, 500 µg/kg is given over 1 minute, followed by an infusion of 50 µg/kg/min for 4 minutes. If the rate is not controlled, a repeat loading dose followed by a 4-minute infusion of 100 µg/kg/min is given, and this sequence is repeated, increasing the infusion in 50-µg/kg/min increments, up to 200 or 300 µg/kg/min if needed. The effect may persist for 20 to 30 minutes after discontinuation of the infusion. Compared with verapamil, esmolol is more likely to convert atrial fibrillation to sinus rhythm.[375] Esmolol is safe and effective in treatment of intraoperative and postoperative hypertension and tachycardia.[414-416] If continuous use is required, it may be reasonably replaced by a longer-lasting cardioselective drug such as intravenous metoprolol. It has been used safely even in patients with compromised left ventricular function.[417,418]

Drugs that Inhibit Synthesis, Storage, or Release of Norepinephrine

Some early antihypertensive drugs acted by replacing norepinephrine in the nerve ending with a much less potent false transmitter. Methyldopa (Aldomet) is such a drug and was the most popular nondiuretic antihypertensive used before the development of β-blockers.[339] Like DOPA, methyldopa enters the biosynthetic pathway for norepinephrine (see Fig. 16-9). It is then decarboxylated to α-methylnorepinephrine. Initially, this chemical was thought to act as a false transmitter, but it was found to be almost as potent as norepinephrine. In the CNS, methyldopa may be further metabolized to α-methylepinephrine,[419] and it acts at α2-receptors to decrease sympathetic outflow,[420] reducing blood pressure. Because of its sedating qualities, fluid retention, postural hypotension, and occasional reports of hepatic necrosis, methyldopa is now used much less often.[339]

Methylparatyrosine (metyrosine, Demser) is a potent inhibitor of tyrosine hydroxylase, which catalyzes the formation of DOPA from tyrosine (see Fig. 16-9). Because this is the rate-limiting step in the biosynthesis of norepinephrine, the drug significantly decreases levels of endogenous catecholamines and is useful in treating inoperable or malignant pheochromocytomas.[421]

Reserpine affects the uptake of norepinephrine not at the neuronal membrane but at the vesicular membrane, thereby inhibiting transport and storage of norepinephrine and dopamine. Eventually, norepinephrine stores are depleted, and postsynaptic receptors increase in number, which may increase the effects of epinephrine in patients who have been given reserpine (see Table 16-5). When patients who take reserpine require a sympathomimetic drug, direct-acting agents are more useful than mixed-acting drugs, which are efficacious only at higher doses, if at all. Reserpine has central effects that lead to sedation and depression; peripheral effects are responsible for its utility as an antihypertensive drug.

Guanethidine (Ismelin) acts initially by blocking the release of norepinephrine, and then it is taken up into adrenergic nerve endings by the uptake-1 mechanism and depletes norepinephrine stores. It is used to treat hypertension, usually after many other drugs have been tried. Its inability to cross the blood-brain barrier accounts for its lack of sedative effects. Guanadrel (Hylorel) is similar to guanethidine, but it has a faster onset and shorter duration of action.

Bretylium, a class III antiarrhythmic used parenterally to treat life-threatening ventricular tachyarrhythmias, is now largely of historical interest. Like guanethidine, it is taken up into adrenergic nerve terminals, but its mechanism of action is otherwise quite different. Bretylium initially causes norepinephrine release and subsequently blocks that release by decreasing sympathetic nerve excitability. Unlike guanethidine, bretylium does not deplete norepinephrine stores.[422] The initial catecholamine release may worsen some arrhythmias, such as those associated with digitalis toxicity and myocardial ischemia.[353] As a consequence, bretylium, which had been part of the advanced cardiac life support protocols for treating ventricular arrhythmias, has been dropped from the algorithms.

MAO and COMT are enzymes important in degradation of the catecholamines. MAOIs bind irreversibly to the enzyme and increase amine concentration within the presynaptic terminal. This increase is associated with antihypertensive, antidepressant, and antinarcoleptic effects.[423] MAOIs are thought to exert their antihypertensive effect through a false transmitter mechanism. Tyramine is usually oxidatively deaminated in the gut by MAO. With administration of an MAOI, tyramine levels rise. When tyramine is taken up into the sympathetic nerve terminal by the uptake-1 mechanism, it enters the varicosities and is transformed by DBH into octopamine. On its subsequent release in place of norepinephrine, octopamine is only weakly reactive at sympathetic receptors, resulting in a lowering of blood pressure. The MAOIs are no longer used as antihypertensives because many other drugs with better risk-benefit profiles have been developed.

MAOIs are primarily used in psychiatric practice. The use of MAOIs as antidepressants is based on the theory that depression is caused by decreased amine in the synapses of the CNS. Inhibition of MAO makes more amine available for release. MAOIs available for treatment of depression include isocarboxazid (Marplan), phenelzine sulfate (Nardil), and tranylcypromine sulfate (Parnate).

Based on substrate specificity, there are at least two forms of MAO. MAO-A acts on 5-HT, norepinephrine, and dopamine, whereas MAO-B is specific for tyramine. A specific MAO-B inhibitor, selegiline hydrochloride (deprenyl), has been developed for the treatment of Parkinson's disease, in hope that by blocking central dopamine breakdown, more dopamine will be preserved in the affected areas.[424]

Drug and food reactions have been of great concern in patients taking MAOIs. Tyramine-containing foods such as red wine and aged cheese must be avoided by patients taking these drugs. Consumption delivers a huge amount of tyramine to the adrenergic nerve terminal, with a subsequent massive release of norepinephrine. This release is manifest clinically as a hypertensive crisis with the potential for MI, cerebral hemorrhage, and death. Any intake of biogenic amine precursors can be expected to increase catecholamine levels greatly, as seen with the concurrent administration of levodopa with MAOIs. The effects of sympathomimetic amines, particularly the indirectly acting drugs, are enhanced.[423] Narcotics, particularly meperidine, have been associated with hyperpyrexic coma and death in patients treated with MAOIs. The depressant effects of agents such as sedatives, alcohol, and general anesthetics are enhanced in these patients. Interactions between MAOI and tricyclic antidepressants can be disastrous.[423] Anesthetic interactions with deprenyl have not been reported, but experience with this drug is limited.[424] Great concern has been expressed that patients receiving long-term therapy with an MAOI risk life-threatening drug interactions during anesthesia. Emergency surgery in patients given an MAOI can be punctuated by marked hemodynamic instability. Severe reactions to narcotics and indirect-acting sympathomimetics, as well as altered metabolism of endogenous and exogenous catecholamines, make these patients potentially difficult to manage. Because of the possibly dangerous interactions of many drugs with MAOIs, controversy exists about the best way to anesthetize these patients.[425,426] It has been suggested that the level of concern expressed over the years may be excessive. Although prudence and custom dictate discontinuation of an MAOI at least 2 weeks in advance of elective procedures, there appear to be rational anesthetic choices based on pharmacology and risk-benefit considerations for patients when surgery cannot be delayed.

Drugs Affecting the Renin-Angiotensin System

The renin-angiotensin system maintains blood pressure and fluid balance (see Fig. 16-7). The major end product of the system, angiotensin II, is a potent vasoconstrictor that also stimulates the release of aldosterone from the adrenal cortex. Aldosterone causes salt and water retention by the kidney. The mechanism by which angiotensin II is produced is as follows. The juxtaglomerular cells of the renal cortex secrete the proteolytic enzyme renin, which cleaves angiotensinogen, a protein produced in the liver, producing the decapeptide angiotensin I. Angiotensin I is converted almost immediately to angiotensin II by ACE. This converting enzyme is located predominantly in the endothelial tissue of the lung. In addition to its direct vasoconstrictive activity, angiotensin II enhances the prejunctional release of norepinephrine from the adrenergic nerve ending and increases efferent sympathetic nerve activity. Angiotensin II also affects sodium and water homeostasis by directly decreasing tubular reabsorption of sodium, increasing antidiuretic and adrenocorticotropic hormone secretion, and stimulating the secretion of aldosterone. ACE is also a kinase that degrades the vasodilator bradykinin. ACE inhibition blocks angiotensin II formation and delays bradykinin breakdown along with effects on associated prostaglandins.[427]

A few patients with hypertensive vascular disease have high circulating plasma renin levels, but many more, 70% of patients, respond to the antihypertensive effects of ACEIs, and there is no dramatic difference in hypertensive response among patients with low or high renin levels.[339] The ACEIs have proved to be useful in the treatment of hypertension and CHF and have decreased mortality after MI.[428] Captopril (Capoten), was the first active oral agent available, followed by enalapril (Vasotec) and lisinopril (Prinivil, Zestril). Four new ACEIs have been marketed: benazepril (Lotensin), fosinopril (Monopril), quinapril (Accupril), and ramipril (Altace). The ACEIs affect the renin-angiotensin-aldosterone system by inhibiting ACE activity.[427,429,430] Enalapril is the only ACEI available in a parenteral dosage at this time. Lisinopril offers once-daily dosing.

Although all the ACEIs are approved for the treatment of hypertension, only captopril and enalapril are approved for the treatment of CHF. Both agents can decrease morbidity and mortality in patients with CHF. Captopril is associated with more frequent adverse effects than enalapril, may have a few more drug interactions, and has a dosing regimen of two or three times daily, compared with enalapril, which has a dosing regimen of once or twice daily.

Some adverse effects observed with ACEIs are common to the entire class, such as cough, angioedema, acute renal failure, and hyperkalemia. Angioedema, especially after the first dose, affects the face, extremities, lips, mucous membranes, tongue, glottis, or larynx.[427,431,432] Some occurrences may be fatal.[427,431-433] Rash and taste disturbance are more frequent with captopril than with the other ACEIs. Because impairment of renal function with an ACEI is usually reversible after withdrawal of the drug, renal function must be monitored,[431,432] and because hyperkalemia may result from inhibition of aldosterone secretion, serum potassium levels should be monitored.[427,430-432] ACEIs can cause fetal morbidity and mortality in humans. These agents should not be used at all during the second or third trimester of pregnancy.[433] The adverse effect profile of the ACEIs has led to the development of angiotensin II receptor antagonists. Losartan was the first of this new class of antihypertensive agents that now includes candesartan, irbesartan, olmesartan, and valsartan. Initial trials have not demonstrated angiotensin II receptor antagonists to be superior to ACEIs; however, the addition of these agents during chronic ACEI therapy reduced all-cause mortality and hospitalization in patients with heart failure.[434]

Cholinergic Drugs

Overview of Mechanisms of Action

The cholinergic drugs act by mimicking, amplifying, or inhibiting the effects of acetylcholine. Cholinergic drugs do not behave exactly as does acetylcholine; their drug action is more specific, affecting fewer sites than acetylcholine, and their duration of action is generally longer than that of acetylcholine.

Unlike adrenergic pharmacology, in which the clinician can select from a wide choice of drugs, there is a relative paucity of drugs that influence parasympathetic function. In general, drugs that affect the parasympathetic system act in one of four ways:

1. As an agonist, stimulating cholinergic receptors
2. As an antagonist, blocking or inhibiting the actions mediated by the cholinergic receptor
3. Blocking or stimulating receptors on autonomic ganglia
4. Inhibiting the metabolism of acetylcholine, thereby increasing and prolonging its effect

There are no effective clinically used drugs that act through mechanisms affecting synthesis of acetylcholine (by inhibiting choline acetyltransferase) or by causing indirect release of acetylcholine (because tyramine, ephedrine, and amphetamine may release norepinephrine). Hemicholinium, which interferes with choline uptake and could deplete acetylcholine stores, is not used clinically. Adenosine may inhibit the release of acetylcholine by decreasing the affinity of binding sites for calcium ions; aminoglycoside antibiotics may compete with calcium for membrane calcium channels, as does magnesium ion. Exocytotic release of acetylcholine is inhibited by botulinum toxin; this toxin is sometimes given by local injection to treat strabismus and blepharospasm. Botulinum toxin has also been used for trigger point injections in pain clinics and to treat age lines. The popularity of off-label uses of this toxin increases the chances of botulism poisoning. In a full-blown botulism-poisoning syndrome, fatalities may result from muscle weakness and respiratory failure.

Cholinergic Agonists

Cholinergic agonists have limited therapeutic use because of their detrimental effects. As a result of its diffuse, nonselective actions and rapid hydrolysis by acetylcholinesterase and butyrylcholinesterase, acetylcholine has had almost no therapeutic use other than as an intraocular medication for transient constriction of the pupil during ophthalmic surgery.

Cholinergic agonists in clinical use have been derived from acetylcholine, but they resist hydrolysis by cholinesterase, permitting a useful duration of action. The different systemic effects of the cholinergic agonists are more quantitative than qualitative, but some limited organ selectivity is useful therapeutically, as is seen with the synthetic choline esters bethanechol and carbachol. Methacholine and bethanechol are primarily muscarinic agonists; carbachol has significant nicotinic and muscarinic effects. The simple maneuver of adding a methyl group to the β-position of the choline in acetylcholine produces methacholine, which is almost purely muscarinic and is almost totally resistant to hydrolysis by either of the cholinesterases. An intravenous infusion of methacholine causes hypotension and bradycardia; a small subcutaneous dose causes transient hypotension with a reflex increase in heart rate. The sole current use of methacholine (Provocholine) is as a provocative agent in diagnosing hyperreactive airways, making positive use of the deleterious bronchoconstrictive effect of muscarinic agonists. It is administered only by inhalation; serious adverse effects include gastrointestinal symptoms, chest pain, hypotension, loss of consciousness, and complete heart block when the drug is given orally or parenterally. Excessive bronchoconstrictive response should be treated by an inhaled β-agonist; coexisting β-blockade is considered a contraindication to the use of methacholine.

The carbamate derivative of methacholine, bethanecol (Urecholine), is occasionally used postoperatively to reinstitute peristaltic activity in the gut or to force the extrusion of urine from an atonic bladder. It is administered subcutaneously or orally to avoid effects in other organ systems.

Carbachol is used topically or intraocularly to constrict the pupil for long-term treatment of wide-angle glaucoma. When used topically, it is often better tolerated than the ophthalmic anticholinesterase agents, and it may be effective in patients resistant to pilocarpine and physostigmine. The rapid pupillary constriction is caused by the combination of ganglionic block and muscarinic effects. Another natural alkaloid, pilocarpine, was used to treat glaucoma until the advent of more modern drugs.

Muscarinic Antagonists

Muscarinic antagonists are the active ingredients in some common plants used since antiquity for medicinal and poisonous effects. It has been suggested that atropine poisoning figures in the American classic, *The Scarlet Letter*.[435] Despite their age, muscarinic antagonists still represent important drugs in anesthesia and critical care.

Muscarinic antagonists compete with neurally released acetylcholine for access to muscarinic cholinoceptors and block its effects. They also antagonize the actions of muscarinic agonists at noninnervated, muscarinic cholinoceptors. Presynaptic muscarinic receptors on the adrenergic nerve terminal may inhibit norepinephrine release, and muscarinic antagonists may enhance sympathetic activity. With the exception of quaternary ammonium compounds that do not readily cross the blood-brain barrier and have few CNS actions, there is no significant specificity of action among these drugs; they block all muscarinic effects with equal efficacy, although some quantitative differences in effect may be seen (Table 16-12). Research has revealed several subtypes of muscarinic receptors, and agonists and antagonists have been synthesized that bind preferentially to one or another. None of these selective agents is yet available commercially, but with this rapidly developing area of research, there will soon be drugs that selectively act on one site or another, such as the heart, bronchial system, smooth muscle, gastric mucosa, or specific areas of the CNS.

Historically, these drugs were used in peptic ulcer disease, various forms of spastic bowel syndrome, upper respiratory illness, and asthma. However, with the availability of the specific histamine (H₂)–blocking drugs such as cimetidine for peptic ulcer disease, these uses have markedly decreased. Atropine, once used to treat bronchospasm, was displaced with the introduction of β₂-agonist drugs that did not dry secretions or diminish ciliary motility. Topical use of atropine analogs in ophthalmologic practice to dilate the pupil is still common.

The addition of a muscarinic anticholinergic drug to anesthetic premedication to decrease secretions and to prevent harmful vagal reflexes was mandatory in the era of ether anesthesia, but it is no longer necessary with modern inhaled agents. Scopolamine combined with an opiate, usually morphine, is still used by cardiac anesthesiologists to sedate a patient while minimizing cardiorespiratory effects. Routine preoperative use of these drugs as antisialagogues continues in some pediatric and otorhinolaryngologic cases or when fiberoptic intubation is planned.

Atropine has a tertiary structure that easily crosses the blood-brain barrier (Fig. 16-22). CNS effects have been seen with the relatively large doses (1 to 2 mg) given to block the muscarinic adverse effects of the anticholinesterase drugs

Table 16–12	Muscarinic anticholinergic drugs			
Drug	**Duration**	**Central Nervous System***	**Antisialagogue**	**Heart Rate**
Atropine	Short	Stimulation	+	++
Glycopyrrolate	Long	0	++	+
Scopolamine	Short	Sedation	++	0/+

*Effects of atropine are limited with usual clinical doses, but they can be significant in the elderly.
0, no effect; +, mild effect, ++, moderate effect.

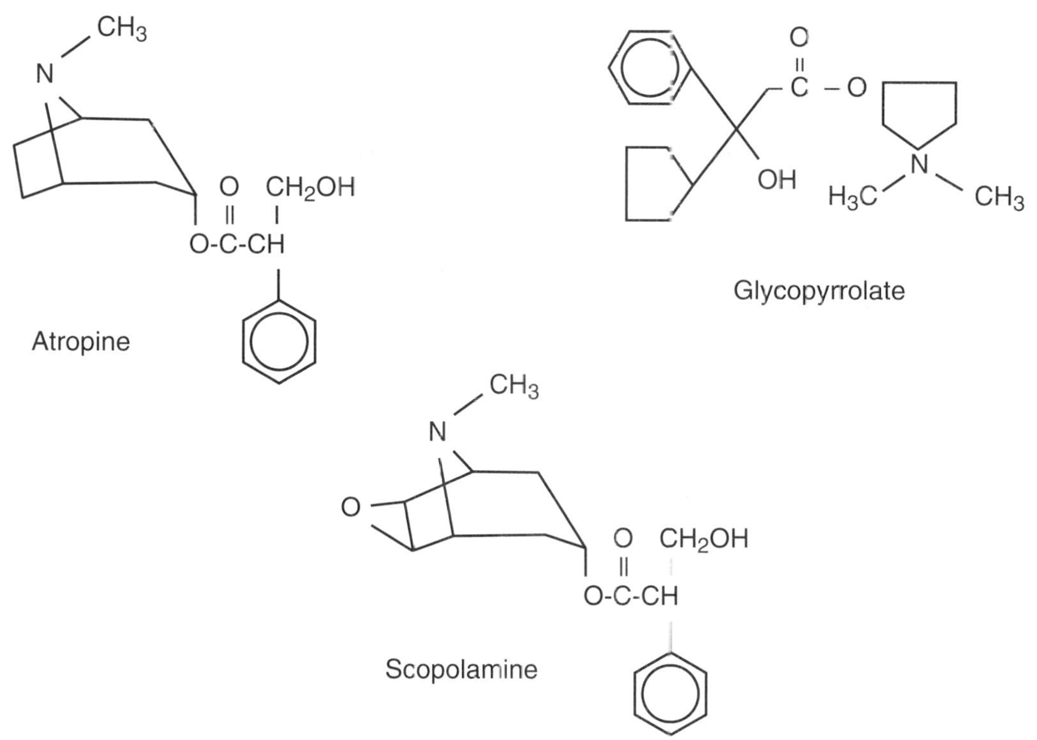

Figure 16–22 Structural formulas of the clinically useful antimuscarinic drugs.

that reverse neuromuscular blockade (see Chapter 13). In contrast, one of the synthetic antimuscarinic drugs, glycopyrrolate (Robinul), does not cross the blood-brain barrier and has gained popularity for this use. Glycopyrrolate has a longer duration of action than atropine.

Scopolamine, which resembles the others of this class in peripheral actions, has pronounced CNS effects. It is the active ingredient in most over-the-counter preparations sold as soporifics, and it is effective in preventing motion sickness. The patch preparation of scopolamine can be used prophylactically for motion sickness and for postoperative nausea and vomiting, but like oral and parenteral forms, it may be associated with eye, bladder, skin, and psychological adverse effects.[436,437]

The development of ipratropium (Atrovent) reestablished antimuscarinic drugs for the treatment of asthma and bronchospastic disorders.[438] Although ipratropium is structurally similar to atropine and has essentially the same effects when administered parenterally, an important difference is that ipratropium is a quaternary ammonium compound. It is very poorly absorbed when inhaled and has few extrapulmonary effects, even in extremely large doses by this route. Ninety percent of inhaled drug is swallowed, but only 1% of the total dose is absorbed systemically.

When administered to normal volunteers, ipratropium provides almost complete protection against bronchospasm induced by a variety of provocative agents. However, in asthmatic patients, results vary. The bronchospastic effects of some agents, such as methacholine or sulfur dioxide, are completely blocked, whereas there is little effect on leukotriene-induced bronchoconstriction.

The onset of bronchodilation is slow, and the maximum effect is less than that seen with β-agonists. Unlike atropine, ipratropium has no negative effect on ciliary clearance. In general, therapeutic effect from antimuscarinics, including ipratropium, is greater in patients with chronic obstructive pulmonary disease than in asthmatic patients.[438,439] Ipratropium is supplied as a metered-dose inhaler dispensing 18 μg per puff. Dosage is two puffs orally four times each day. Maximum bronchodilation occurs in 30 to 90 minutes and may last 4 hours.[439]

The toxic effects of the muscarinic antagonists come from the blockade of muscarinic cholinoceptors in the periphery and the CNS. The peripheral effects (e.g., dry mouth) may be irritating but are not life threatening in healthy adults. However, children depend more than adults on sweating for thermoregulation and easily become dangerously hyperthermic. Moreover, older individuals may not be able to tolerate the cardiac, ocular, or urinary effects of muscarinic blockade.

The CNS effects are the usual cause of death or injury. Increasing doses of atropine or scopolamine cause greater distortions of mentation, progressing from thought disorders to hallucinations, delusions, delirium, and severe psychoses. These effects are reversible, but the mental dysfunction can persist for weeks. Left alone, the intoxicated individual will die of starvation, dehydration, or trauma. Those who have received more than 500 mg of atropine, which is more than 1000 times the usual dose, and have been disabled for weeks have recovered fully.

Small doses of atropine (0.05 mg) can evoke bradycardia, a finding that has led some clinicians to increase the dose in children. It was thought that a CNS effect of atropine could be responsible, but the time course and the fact that bradycardia occurred in vagotomized animals cast doubt on this explanation. Whether this paradoxic bradycardia is a central or peripheral effect, or both, and the role of muscarinic subtypes are still subjects of debate.[440]

Atropine and scopolamine toxicity have been treated for decades by the use of the naturally occurring alkaloid physostigmine (Antilirium), which is an anticholinesterase that penetrates the blood-brain barrier.[441] The use of this drug in doses of 1 to 2 mg given intravenously to treat the postoperative CNS effects of intravenous atropine or scopolamine has been successful. Physostigmine may also reverse the CNS effects of other compounds with anticholinergic activity, including the tricyclic antidepressants, several major tranquilizers, and antihistamine drugs.[442] Physostigmine also may antagonize the sedative effects of the benzodiazepines, but a specific benzodiazepine antagonist, flumazenil (Romazicon), has supplanted physostigmine for this use.[443,444] Physostigmine must be administered with care because of its potentially lethal nicotinic effects, which are not prevented by the muscarinic antagonists, and because its half-life rarely matches that of the intoxicant.

Cholinesterase Inhibitors

Anticholinesterase drugs are a common means of producing sustained, systemic cholinergic agonism. These drugs are used to reverse neuromuscular blockade, to treat myasthenia gravis, and to treat certain tachyarrhythmias.

The first anticholinesterase agent available was physostigmine. There are three chemical classes of compounds used as cholinesterase inhibitors: carbamates, organophosphates, and quaternary ammonium alcohols. Neostigmine was first used as a gastrointestinal tract stimulant and later as a treatment for myasthenia gravis.

Physostigmine, neostigmine, and pyridostigmine are carbamates, whereas edrophonium is a quaternary ammonium alcohol. The cholinesterase enzyme is inhibited so long as the esteratic site is bound to an acetate, carbamate, or phosphate. Carbamate and phosphate bonds are much more resistant to attack by hydroxyl groups than are acetate bonds. The acetylated form lasts for only microseconds, whereas the carbamylated form lasts for 15 to 20 minutes. Organophosphates include diisopropyl fluorophosphate, parathion, Malathion, soman, sarin, VX, and a variety of other compounds used as insecticides. Although the toxicity of the organophosphate insecticides is primarily related to their anticholinesterase activity, the mechanism of this effect is different from the clinically used anticholinesterase drugs. The organophosphates produce an irreversible enzyme inhibition and have CNS effects.[445] Consequently, treatment of organophosphate insecticide poisoning relies on chemical compounds capable of displacing the insecticides from the enzyme to reactivate the cholinesterase activity. The best documented of these chemicals is pralidoxime (2-PAM). Physostigmine and most of the organophosphates are not quaternary ammonium compounds and have major effects on cholinergic functions in the CNS.

Edrophonium is unique in that it lacks an acetate, carbamate, or phosphate group. It acts because the positive charge of the nitrogen is attracted strongly by the anionic site and physically blocks the esteratic site. The edrophonium molecule is postulated to be held in place only by an ionic bond. The duration of inhibition provided by each molecule is short (milliseconds), but because they are not changed in the reaction, the molecules can hop onto and off the enzyme repeatedly to render the enzyme unavailable to acetylcholine.

Aside from reversal of neuromuscular blockade, there are few other therapeutic uses of these compounds. Because these compounds can increase the effect and duration of neurally released acetylcholine, they are useful in situations in which such release is deficient, such as myasthenia gravis. Anticholinesterase drugs are occasionally used to stimulate intestinal function and used topically in the eye as a miotic. An irreversible organophosphate anticholinesterase that is used clinically is echothiophate iodide (Phospholine), which is available as topical drops for the treatment of glaucoma. Its major advantage over other topical agents is its prolonged duration of action. Because this chemical also inactivates plasma cholinesterase, it may prolong the action of succinylcholine. Although prudence dictates discontinuation of echothiophate for 1 week before surgery, there are numerous case reports of successful anesthesia performed without discontinuation of echothiophate under emergency conditions.

Ganglionic Drugs

Ganglionic Agonists

The ganglionic agonists are essential for analyzing the mechanism of ganglionic function, but they have no therapeutic use. Nicotine is the classic ganglionic agonist, and its effects have been well described.[446]

Parasympathetic drugs stimulate ganglia, but this action is usually masked by the other parasympathomimetic effects. Experimentally, relatively large doses of acetylcholine administered intravenously after blockade of muscarinic receptors by atropine causes ganglionic stimulation and release of epinephrine by the adrenal medulla.[446]

Ganglionic Antagonists

The ganglionic antagonists were the first effective therapy for the management of hypertension and were used extensively during the 1950s and 1960s. However, because of interference with transmission through sympathetic and parasympathetic ganglia, antihypertensive action was accompanied by numerous undesirable effects. Hexamethonium, the prototypic drug of this class, has minimal neuromuscular and muscarinic activity. Paton[447] provided a vivid description of the clinical effects of chronic ganglionic blockade with his "hexamethonium man." The systemic effects of ganglionic blockade are determined by the resting tone of a specific body system before the application of ganglionic blockade (see Table 16-2). With the disappearance of trimethaphan from clinical use, these drugs are largely of historic value.

AUTONOMIC DYSFUNCTION

Assessment of Autonomic Function

The increased operative risk of patients with autonomic dysfunction that may occur with aging and diabetes[448] makes the diagnosis of autonomic neuropathy extremely important. A panel of five tests of cardiovascular function has been developed to evaluate autonomic function in diabetic patients.[449] The tests include heart rate responses to the Valsalva maneuver, standing up, and deep breathing and blood pressure responses to standing up and sustained handgrip. The tests involving changes in heart rate measure injury to the parasympathetic system and precede changes in the measures of blood pressure that reflect sympathetic injury. *Early autonomic dysfunction* is defined as a single abnormal or two borderline-abnormal results on the tests involving changes in heart rate. Definite involvement comes when two of the tests of changes in heart rate are abnormal. *Severe dysfunction* is defined as abnormalities in the blood pressure assessments. The application of these standards requires that the investigator understand the proper techniques for performing the five tests and the expected results in patients without autonomic neuropathy (Table 16-13). If patients demonstrate an increase in heart rate of more than 20 beats/min with a vigorous handgrip, it can be assumed they are incompletely β-blocked. The simplicity and effectiveness of this clinical assessment has led to its use in the evaluation of patients with nondiabetic causes of autonomic dysfunction.

Plasma Catecholamines

Accurate and sensitive techniques for measuring plasma catecholamines have existed for 3 decades, but interpretation of the data they yield has been controversial. Normal plasma epinephrine and norepinephrine levels are typically in the range of 100 to 400 pg/mL, and they can increase sixfold or more with stress.

Plasma concentrations of epinephrine, which reflect adrenal medullary activity[450] if not overall sympathetic activity, are labile. The uncontrolled stress experienced by experimental subjects has clouded the meaning of measured levels. Significant isolated adrenal medullary secretion results from certain stressful situations, such as public speaking.[29] Moreover, venous samples may reflect the epinephrine kinetics in the organ being sampled rather than in the whole body, and arterial samples may be more reliable.[451]

The significance of norepinephrine concentration in plasma is even more controversial. Although the adrenal

Table 16–13 Noninvasive tests for assessing the autonomic nervous system

Clinical Examination	Technique	Normal Value
Parasympathetic		
HR response to Valsalva	The seated subject blows into a mouthpiece (maintaining a pressure of 40 mm Hg) for 15 seconds. The Valsalva ratio is the ratio of the longest R-R interval (which comes shortly after the release) to the shortest R-R interval (which occurs during the maneuver).	Ratio of >1.21
HR response to standing	HR is measured as the subject moves from a resting supine position to standing. Normal tachycardic response is maximal around the 15th beat after rising. A relative bradycardia follows that is most marked around the 30th beat after standing. The response to standing is expressed as the 30:15 ratio and is the ratio of the longest R-R interval around the 30th beat to the shortest R-R interval around the 15th beat.	Ratio of >1.04
HR response to deep breathing	The subject takes six deep breaths in 1 minute. The maximum and minimum heart rates during each cycle are measured, and the mean of the differences (maximum HR-minimum HR) during three successive breathing cycles is taken as the maximum-minimum HR.	Mean difference >15 BPM
Sympathetic		
BP response to standing	The subject moves from resting supine to standing, and the standing SBP is subtracted from the supine SBP.	Difference <10 mm Hg
BP response to sustained handgrip	The subject maintains a handgrip of 30% of the maximum squeeze for up to 5 minutes. The blood pressure is measured every minute, and the initial DBP is subtracted from the DBP just before release.	Difference >16 mm Hg

BP, blood pressure; BPM, beats per minute; DBP, diastolic blood pressure; HR, heart rate; SBP, systolic blood pressure.

medulla secretes some norepinephrine, levels in plasma generally reflect spillover from sympathetic stimulation because most of the norepinephrine released at the nerve ending is taken up again by the nerve terminal. Although reuptake may be tissue specific and markedly influenced by alterations in physiology or diseases, this spillover in humans is 10% to 20% of the norepinephrine synthesis rate at baseline and may be greatly enhanced in periods of sympathetic activation.[452] The most compelling argument for use of plasma norepinephrine as a marker for sympathetic activity comes from animal studies in which plasma norepinephrine levels directly mirrored nerve stimulation.[453] Many important studies have correlated elevations in plasma catecholamines with acute and chronic stress and have led to the concept of stress-free anesthesia. A striking relationship between mortality rates for patients with CHF and elevated plasma norepinephrine levels resulted in the use of β-adrenergic antagonists to treat ventricular dysfunction.[454,455]

The development of experimental radiotracer techniques to assess the in vivo kinetics of catecholamines has provided additional information that is of clinical importance, particularly in relation to regional kinetics. For example, studies relying only on arterial and venous catecholamines suggested that the hepatomesenteric bed contributed significantly to the total body clearance of catecholamines but only minimally (<8%) to the spillover. However, later studies of regional norepinephrine kinetics demonstrated that the gut release of norepinephrine (≤25% of the total body) was largely obscured by efficient extraction (>80%) in the liver. Similarly, selective elevations in norepinephrine release from the heart, which may be associated with ischemia, the early onset of CHF, and tachyarrhythmias, may not be apparent in measured arterial or venous levels.[456] Observations involving regional spillover led to the realization that although stress may activate a generalized sympathetic response, there may be different patterns contingent on the stimulus. It is possible that the lack of association of plasma norepinephrine levels in the presence of clinically significant sympathetic activation may be a function of the measurement technique or the particular stressor. Although many anesthetic techniques, including inhaled, opiate, and regional anesthetics, can attenuate the stress response, whether attenuation represents a benefit or liability in patient care remains a matter of controversy.[457,458] Until recently, there were few data to suggest that the attenuation of the stress response altered outcome, with the exception of prolonged postoperative epidural anesthesia or special surgical situations. However, results of several studies in infants and adults undergoing heart surgery suggest that the use of high-dose opiates or other strategies to diminish perioperative stress may improve outcome.[459-462] In the past 5 to 10 years, studies have reported that neuraxial analgesia can decrease ischemic and thrombotic complications by attenuating the sustained increase in perioperative catecholamines associated with surgery and general anesthesia.[463-465]

It is our belief that, given the effects of age, posture, and hydration, small changes in plasma catecholamine levels correlate poorly with hemodynamic changes and merit cautious interpretation, whereas significant increases (>1000 pg/mL) in levels are good markers of sympathetic nervous system activation.

Clinical Syndromes

Surgical Stress Response

Surgical stress, particularly associated with major operations, results in profound metabolic and endocrine responses. The combination of autonomic, hormonal, and catabolic changes that accompany surgery has been called the *surgical stress response*.[466] Despite the widespread clinical intuition that attenuation of the stress response is beneficial, there has been a long-standing debate about whether such a strategy does affect outcome. Three separate lines of evidence suggest that attenuation of the surgical stress response can lead to improved outcomes. In a series of studies, interruption of the sympathetic response to surgery markedly reduced surgical stress intraoperatively and postoperatively.[467] The use of continuous thoracic epidural infusions of local anesthetics minimized the rise in plasma catecholamines, cortisol, and glucagon and improved outcome. Improved outcome was independent of the patient's level of pain because metabolic and endocrine responses to surgery were not similarly reduced in patients receiving other methods of pain relief, including nonsteroidal anti-inflammatory drugs and opioids.[467] Continuation of epidural infusions well into the postoperative period was regarded as essential to improving outcome. Inflammatory and immunologic responses, which are necessary for infection control and wound healing, appear to be unaffected. Using similar techniques and other stress-reducing maneuvers, faster and more complete recoveries were achieved in elderly patients undergoing colon resections.[468]

A separate line of evidence supporting the hypothesis that long-term attenuation of the stress response alters outcome comes from the pediatric literature. When neonates with complex congenital heart disease underwent cardiac surgery, those who received high-dose sufentanil infusions intraoperatively and for the first 24 hours postoperatively to reduce the stress response had lower β-endorphin, norepinephrine, epinephrine, glucagon, aldosterone, and cortisol levels compared with controls.[459] The mortality rate in the opiate group was significantly lower than in the study or historical controls. Anesthetic techniques can have profound effects on the metabolic and endocrine responses to surgery, and effective management of these reflexes can alter outcomes.

A third line of evidence involves the results from the multicenter study of the perioperative ischemia research group (see "Perioperative β-Blockade").[334] The ability to alter overall survival at 2 years by a perioperative regimen of β-blockade has been validated by several other studies,[335,336,338] has provided compelling evidence of the benefit of attenuating the stress response, and has altered clinical practice for patients at risk for cardiac morbidities.

Diabetes Mellitus

Diabetic autonomic neuropathy is the most common form of autonomic neuropathy and the most extensively investigated (see Chapter 27). It occurs in 20% to 40% of all insulin-dependent diabetic patients. The symptoms associated with diabetic autonomic neuropathy confer an increased risk during anesthesia and surgery by direct and secondary mechanisms. Common manifestations of diabetic autonomic neuropathy include impotence, postural hypotension, gastroparesis, diarrhea, and sweating abnormalities.[469] Early small-fiber damage is revealed by loss or impairment of vagally controlled normal heart rate variability, decreased peripheral sympathetic tone with subsequent increase in blood flow, and diminished sweating. In the diabetic neuropathic foot, the senses of pain and temperature are lost before loss of touch or vibration. With sympathetic denervation, sympathetic nerves normally found supplying small arterioles are entirely absent or are abnormally distant from their effector sites. When impotence or diarrhea is the sole manifestation, there is little effect on survival; however, with postural hypotension or gastroparesis, 5-year mortality rates are greater than 50%.

Most clinicians recognize that diabetic patients with autonomic neuropathy may be at additional risk in general anesthesia.[470] Gastroparesis is probably caused by vagal degeneration and is of clinical relevance because awake or rapid-sequence intubation may be required. Systemic injury to the vasa vasorum in patients with postural hypotension increases the risk of hemodynamic instability and cardiovascular collapse in the perioperative period. Mechanisms that maintain normal standing blood pressure are altered, and normal precapillary vasoconstriction in the foot on standing may be diminished. When healthy people stand, roughly 700 mL of the blood volume may pool in the legs and splanchnic circulation, with an associated 20% decrease in cardiac output. Baroreceptors in the carotid sinus and aortic arch, which normally detect the decrease and mediate sympathetic impulses to the heart and blood vessels, are compromised by diabetic neuropathy. Diabetic patients with orthostatic hypotension usually have lower norepinephrine levels.

Even in seemingly minor surgery, diabetic autonomic neuropathy can lead to significant complications. In a series of ophthalmologic procedures requiring general anesthesia, diabetics with autonomic neuropathy had a significantly greater decline in blood pressure with induction and a greater need for vasopressors than did diabetic patients without autonomic dysfunction.[470] Page and Watkins[471] reported five cases of unexpected cardiorespiratory arrest in young diabetic patients, all of whom had symptoms of autonomic neuropathy. In a large, prospective study of diabetic autonomic neuropathy using the five evocative clinical tests discussed earlier, parasympathetic dysfunction preceded sympathetic failure in 96% of the patients.[472] This battery of autonomic tests identifies patients with autonomic neuropathy and is highly predictive of mortality[469] and perioperative risk.[448]

Autonomic Changes with Aging

Aging is associated with alterations in vascular reactivity manifesting clinically as exaggerated changes in blood pressure—hypertension and orthostatic hypotension (see Chapter 62). Orthostatic hypotension is quite common (about 20%) in the elderly and may result largely from diminished baroreceptor responsiveness. Heart rate response to changes in blood pressure, Valsalva maneuver, and the respiratory cycle are blunted with aging.[473-477]

Resting and exercise-induced norepinephrine levels increase with age in healthy subjects (by about 13% per decade),[478] in part because of decreased clearance.[478,479] Previously a matter of controversy, it now appears that besides the well-documented reduction in vagal function associated with aging,[480,481] the primary autonomic defect in aging is an impairment in norepinephrine reuptake, perhaps as a function of decreased nerve density. Although there is no apparent age-dependent decrement in nerve firing rates from sympathetic efferents in skeletal muscle,[482] kinetic studies reveal selective and dramatic increases in cardiac norepinephrine spillover attributable to decreased reuptake in elderly patients subjected to mental stress or exercise.[452] The augmented synaptic concentration of norepinephrine in the setting of age-related reduction in vagal function can precipitate clinical complications (i.e., arrhythmogenesis and sudden cardiac death) in patients with cardiac disease. However, end-organ responsiveness is blunted by compensatory downregulation of the β_1-adrenoreceptors (i.e., decreased receptor density and affinity) and uncoupling of β_2-adrenoreceptors through decreased G_s activity.[483-485] Despite increased cardiac spillover, cardiac oxygen consumption was not altered.[486]

Attenuation of presynaptic α_2-adrenoreceptor–mediated inhibition of neuronal norepinephrine release[487-489] also accounts for increased norepinephrine levels observed with age. Reduced postsynaptic α-adrenoreceptor activity decreases contractile responses and further attenuates vasoconstrictor tone. In a seemingly vicious cycle, the increase in circulating norepinephrine levels is associated with downregulation of platelet α_2-adrenoreceptor density and responsiveness.[490] The loss of adrenergic control through the reduction of α_2- and β-receptor–mediated responses with age causes a loss in the efficacy of the sympathetic system to control cardiovascular responsiveness, implying a relationship with or an explanation of the increased incidence of cardiovascular disorders such as CHF in the elderly.

Autonomic Changes in Spinal Cord Transection

The most drastic of all alterations in the ANS that an anesthesiologist may encounter is complete spinal cord transection (see Chapter 53). Spinal cord transection affects motor and sensory function, and it also may result in profound changes in autonomic activity that can alter anesthetic care. As is obvious from the anatomy of the sympathetic and parasympathetic outflow, spinal cord injuries or transection can cause various degrees of autonomic dysfunction, depending on the site, extent, and timing of the lesion. Many autonomic reflexes are inhibited by supraspinal feedback that is lost after spinal cord transection. In paraplegic patients, small stimuli can evoke exaggerated sympathetic discharges.

In patients with cervical spinal cord transection, sympathetic and parasympathetic outflows are detached from central control mechanisms. In addition to expected motor and sensory changes, there are profound abnormalities altering the cardiovascular, thermoregulatory, gastrointestinal, and urinary systems. The autonomic consequences of transection are not always apparent because the distal portion of the spinal cord may retain some function, resulting in unanticipated autonomic abnormalities.

There are fundamental differences between the acute and chronic effects of spinal cord transection. Initially, a transient state of decreased excitability occurs. This phenomenon, known as *spinal shock,* usually occurs immediately after the lesion and may last days to weeks. In these patients, the periphery is generally atonic, and the peripheral blood vessels are dilated. Investigators have suggested that methylprednisolone may be of some use in treating this phase of spinal shock.[491] In patients with high thoracic lesions who have sustained recent injury, the basal supine blood pressure is usually low and accompanied by plasma catecholamine levels that are approximately 35% of normal.[492] Patients with recent low spinal injuries may exhibit compensatory tachycardia from intact parts of the ANS.

Patients with high spinal lesions may fail to respond to hypovolemia with an increased heart rate and may exhibit bradycardia. The only intact efferent component of baroreflex pathways in quadriplegic patients is the vagus. Bradycardia occurs with changes in position and with Valsalva maneuvers or increased intrathoracic pressure.[493]

One aspect of care that is frequently overlooked is the effect of tracheal suctioning on patients with high spinal transection. Given that many of these patients depend on artificial respiration because of their respiratory muscle paralysis, unopposed vagal stimuli may contribute to profound bradycardia. This vagal response is particularly accentuated during hypoxemia.

Because the sympathetic nervous system may be dysfunctional in these patients, the renin-angiotensin-aldosterone system compensates for the maintenance of blood pressure. Patients who have spinal cord transection may be exquisitely sensitive to ACEIs, even with modest changes in intravascular volume or posture. The release of renin may be independent of sympathetic stimulation and may be caused by renal baroreceptor stimulation that accompanies the decline in renal perfusion pressure.

Although pressure stimuli above the lesion do not usually change blood pressure, the phenomenon of autonomic dysreflexia can occur with stimulation below the lesion. Bladder or bowel distention can elicit the so-called mass reflex. This autonomic reflex includes a dramatic rise in blood pressure, a marked reduction in flow to the periphery, and flushing and sweating in areas above the lesion. The patient's heart rate may decline as a reflex. Surprisingly, evidence from microneurography studies indicates that there is only a modest rise in sympathetic nerve activity during activation of the mass reflex,[494] and plasma levels increase only modestly. Speculation has arisen that the exaggerated blood pressure response may be caused by supersensitivity of adrenoreceptors.

As anticipated, there is an increase in sensitivity to exogenously administered pressors in quadriplegic patients.[492] Blood pressure in quadriplegic patients may increase 5- to 10-fold in response to the exogenous administration of angiotensin and to catecholamines. Impairment of descending inhibitory reflex pathways that are activated during hypertension may contribute to the supersensitivity. This hypothesis is supported by the finding that sensitivity is rarely increased when the lesion is below T5. There is apparently a normal level of adrenoreceptors in these patients, even those with long-standing quadriplegia.

The management of autonomic dysreflexia is of clinical importance. Although the anesthesiologist may be tempted to opt for minimal anesthesia in a patient without sensory or motor function, significant visceral reflexes can be evoked. The anesthesiologist may use spinal anesthesia, general anesthesia, or a vasodilator such as nitroprusside or nitroglycerin to attenuate this reflex even if pain is not appreciated. There has been some enthusiasm for using clonidine prophylactically to diminish this response.

An additional problem arising from the autonomic denervation of spinal cord transection is thermogenesis. In these patients, hypothermia may result from cutaneous vasodilation and the inability to shiver. Similarly, hyperthermia can occur because the normal sweating mechanism is impaired. It is therefore important to monitor temperature assiduously in these patients during the course of anesthesia.

KEY POINTS

1. The ANS works in concert with renin, cortisone, and other hormones to respond to internal and external stresses.
2. The hallmark of the sympathetic nervous system is amplification; the hallmark of the parasympathetic nervous system is targeted response.
3. Inhaled and intravenous anesthetics can alter hemodynamics by influencing autonomic function.
4. β-Adrenergic blockade has emerged as an important prophylaxis for ischemia and as therapy for hypertension, MI, and CHF.
5. The sympathetic nervous system demonstrates acute and chronic adaptation to stress presynaptically and postsynaptically (e.g., biosynthesis, receptor regulation).
6. Presynaptic α-receptors play an important role in regulating sympathetic release.
7. Many therapies for the treatment of hypertension are based on direct or indirect effects of sympathetic function.
8. The vagus nerve is the superhighway of parasympathetic function, accommodating 75% of parasympathetic traffic.
9. Aging and many disease states (e.g., diabetes, spinal cord injury) are accompanied by important changes in autonomic function.

REFERENCES

1. Burnstock G: The first von Euler lecture in physiology: The changing face of autonomic neurotransmission. Acta Physiol Scand 126:67, 1986.
2. Burnstock G: Autonomic neuromuscular junctions: Current developments and future directions. J Anat 146:1, 1986.
3. Burnstock G: Sympathetic purinergic transmission in small blood vessels. Trends Pharmacol Sci 9:116, 1988.
4. Burnstock G: Do some nerve cells release more than one transmitter? Neuroscience 1:239, 1976.
5. Bartfai T, Iverfeldt K, Fisone G, et al: Regulation of the release of coexisting neurotransmitters. Annu Rev Pharmacol Toxicol 28:285, 1988.
6. Von Kügelgen I, Starke K: Noradrenaline-ATP co-transmission in the sympathetic nervous system. Trends Pharmacol Sci 12:319, 1991.
7. Burnstock G: Local mechanisms of blood flow control by perivascular nerves and endothelium. J Hypertens Suppl 8:S95, 1990.
8. Ralevic V, Burnstock G: Receptors for purines and pyrimidines. Pharmacol Rev 50:413, 1998.
9. Jacobson KA, Trivedi BK, Churchill PC, et al: Novel therapeutics acting via purine receptors. Biochem Pharmacol 41:1399, 1991.
10. Burnstock G: Overview: Purinergic mechanisms. Ann N Y Acad Sci 603:1, 1990.
11. Goncalves J, Guimaraes S: Influence of neuronal uptake on pre- and postjunctional effects of α-adrenoceptor agonists in tissues with noradrenaline: ATP cotransmission. Naunyn Schmiedebergs Arch Pharmacol 344:532, 1991.
12. Hirst G, Bramich N, Edwards F, et al: Transmission at autonomic neuroeffector junctions. Trends Neurosci 15:40, 1992.
13. Walker P, Grouzmann E, Burnie M, et al: The role of neuropeptide Y in cardiovascular regulation. Trends Pharmacol Sci 12:111, 1991.
14. Lincoln J, Burnstock G: Neural-endothelial interactions in control of local blood flow. In Warren J (ed): The Endothelium: An Introduction to Current Research. New York, Wiley-Liss, 1990, p 21.
15. Lundberg JM, Rudehill A, Sollevi A, et al: Frequency- and reserpine-dependent chemical coding of sympathetic transmission: Differential release of noradrenaline and neuropeptide Y from pig spleen. Neurosci Lett 63:96, 1986.
16. Bloom S, Edwards A: Vasoactive intestinal polypeptide in relation to atropine resistant vasodilatation in the submaxillary gland of the cat. J Physiol 300:41, 1980.
17. Lundberg JM: Evidence for coexistence of vasoactive intestinal polypeptide (VIP) and acetylcholine in neurons of cat exocrine glands: Morphological, biochemical and functional studies. Acta Physiol Scand Suppl 496:1, 1981.
18. Mione M, Cavanagh J, Lincoln J, et al: Pregnancy reduces noradrenaline but not neuropeptide levels in the uterine artery of the guinea pig. Cell Tissue Res 259:503, 1990.
19. Furness JB, Costa M: The Enteric Nervous System. New York, Churchill Livingstone, 1987.
20. Bridenbaugh PO, Greene NM: Spinal (subarachnoid) neural blockade. In Cousins M, Bridenbaugh P (eds): Neural Blockade in Clinical Anesthesia and Pain Management, 2nd ed. Philadelphia, JB Lippincott, 1988, p 213.
21. Rajfer J, Aronson WJ, Bush PA, et al: Nitric oxide as a mediator of relaxation of the corpus cavernosum in response to nonadrenergic, noncholinergic neurotransmission. N Engl J Med 326:90, 1992.
22. Ruffolo R: Physiology and biochemistry of the peripheral autonomic nervous system. In Wingard L, Brody T, Larner J, et al (eds): Human Pharmacology: Molecular to Clinical. St. Louis, Mosby–Year Book, 1991, p 77.
23. Fleisher LA, Frank SM, Shir Y, et al: Cardiac sympathovagal balance and peripheral sympathetic vasoconstriction: Epidural versus general anesthesia. Anesth Analg 79:165, 1994.
24. Lefkowitz R, Hoffman B, Taylor P: Drugs acting at synaptic and neuroeffector junctional sites. In Gilman A, Rall T, Nies A, et al (eds): Goodman and Gilman's the Pharmacological Basis of Therapeutics, 8th ed. New York, Pergamon Press, 1990, p 84.
25. Hoffman B, Lefkowitz R: Adrenergic receptors in the heart. Annu Rev Physiol 44:475, 1982.
26. Goldstein DS, Ziegler MG, Lake CR: Plasma norepinephrine in essential hypertension. In Ziegler M, Lake C (eds): Frontiers of Clinical Neuroscience, vol 2. Baltimore, Williams & Wilkins, 1984, p 389.
27. Ottolenghi D: Su i nervi del midollo delle ossa. Atti R Accad Sci Torino 36:939, 1903.
28. Radu A, Dahl G, Loewenstein WR: Hormonal regulation of cell junction permeability: Upregulation by catecholamine and prostaglandin E_1. J Membr Biol 70:239, 1982.
29. Dimsdale J, Moss J: Plasma catecholamines in stress and exercise. JAMA 243:340, 1980.
30. Philipson LH: β-Agonists and metabolism. J Allergy Clin Immunol 110(Suppl 6):S313, 2001.
31. Kharasch ED, Bowdle T: Hypokalemia before induction of anesthesia and prevention by beta 2 adrenoceptor antagonism. Anesth Analg 72:216, 1991.
32. Williams ME, Gervino EV, Rosa RM, et al: Catecholamine modulation of rapid potassium shifts during exercise. N Engl J Med 312:823, 1985.
33. Struthers AD, Reid JL: The role of adrenal medullary catecholamines in potassium homoeostasis. Clin Sci 66:377, 1984.
34. Brown M: Hypokalemia from β2-receptor stimulation by circulating epinephrine. Am J Cardiol 56:3D, 1985.
35. Vincent HH, Man in't Veld AJ, Boomsma F, Schalekamp MA: Prevention of epinephrine-induced hypokalemia by nonselective beta blockers. Am J Cardiol 56:10D, 1985.
36. Furchgott RF, Zawadzki JV: The obligatory role of endothelial cells in the relaxation of arterial smooth muscle by acetylcholine. Nature 288:373, 1980.
37. Johns RA: EDRF/nitric oxide: The endogenous nitrovasodilator and a new cellular messenger. Anesthesiology 75:927, 1991.
38. Snyder SH, Bredt DS: Biological roles of nitric oxide. Sci Am 266:68, 1992.
39. Bredt DS, Hwang PM, Snyder SH: Localization of nitric oxide synthase indicating a neural role for nitric oxide. Nature 347:768, 1990.
40. Bredt DS, Snyder S: Nitric oxide, a novel neuronal messenger. Neuron 8:3, 1992.
41. Forstermann U, Schmidt H, Pollock J, et al: Isoforms of nitric oxide synthase: Characterization and purification from different cell types. Biochem Pharmacol 42:1849, 1991.
42. Petros A, Bennett D, Vallance P: Effect of nitric oxide synthase inhibitors on hypotension in patients with septic shock. Lancet 338:1557, 1991.
43. Bredt DS, Hwang PM, Glatt CE, et al: Cloned and expressed nitric oxide synthase structurally resembles cytochrome P-450 reductase. Nature 351:714, 1991.
44. Rees DD, Palmer R, Moncada S: Role of endothelium-derived nitric oxide in the regulation of blood pressure. Proc Natl Acad Sci U S A 86:3375, 1989.
45. Koesling D, Böhme D, Schultz G: Guanylyl cyclases, a growing family of signal-transducing enzymes. FASEB J 5:2785, 1991.
46. Sakurai T, Yanagisawa M, Masaki T: Molecular characterization of endothelin receptors. Trends Pharmacol Sci 13:103, 1992.
47. Nava E, Palmer R, Moncada S: Inhibition of nitric oxide synthesis in septic shock: How much is beneficial? Lancet 338:1555, 1991.
48. Moore K, Wendon J, Frazer M, et al: Plasma endothelin immunoreactivity in liver disease and the hepatorenal syndrome. N Engl J Med 327:1774, 1992.
49. Shepherd J, Vanhoutte P: Neurohumoral regulation. In Shepherd S, Vanhoutte P (eds): The Human Cardiovascular System: Facts and Concepts. New York, Raven Press, 1979, p 107.
50. Conlay L, Maher TJ, Wurtman RJ: Tyrosine increases blood pressure in hypotensive rats. Science 212:559, 1981.
51. Nussdorfer GG: Paracrine control of adrenal cortical function by medullary chromaffin cells. Pharmacol Rev 48:495, 1996.

52. Kamiya H, Zucker RS: Residual Ca^{2+} and short-term synaptic plasticity. Nature 371:603, 1994.
53. Zucker RS: Exocytosis: A molecular and physiological perspective. Neuron 17:1049, 1996.
54. Katz B: Nerve, Muscle, and Synapse. New York, McGraw-Hill, 1966.
55. Südhof TC, Jahn R: Proteins of synaptic vesicles involved in exocytosis and membrane recycling. Neuron 6:665, 1991.
56. DeBello WM, O'Connor V, Dresbach T, et al: SNAP-mediated protein-protein interactions essential for neurotransmitter release. Nature 373:626, 1995.
57. Bommert K, Charlton MP, DeBello WM, et al: Inhibition of neurotransmitter release by C2-domain peptides implicates synaptotagmin in exocytosis. Nature 363:163, 1993.
58. Geppert M, Goda Y, Hammer RE, et al: Synaptotagmin I: A major Ca^{2+} sensor for transmitter release at a central synapse. Cell 79:717, 1994.
59. Jahn R, Sudhof TC: Membrane fusion and exocytosis. Annu Rev Biochem 68:863, 1999.
60. Sudhof TC: The synaptic vesicle cycle revisited. Neuron 28:317, 2000.
61. Schiavo G, Rossetto O, Montecucco C: Clostridial neurotoxins as tools to investigate the molecular events of neurotransmitter release. Semin Cell Biol 5:221, 1994.
62. Morgan A, Burgoyne RD: A role for soluble NSF attachment proteins (SNAPs) in regulated exocytosis in adrenal chromaffin cells. EMBO J 14:232, 1995.
63. Bennett MK, Scheller RH: A molecular description of synaptic vesicle membrane trafficking. Annu Rev Biochem 63:63, 1994.
64. Rothman JE: Mechanisms of intracellular protein transport. Nature 372:55, 1994.
65. Katz B, Miledi R: The effect of temperature on the synaptic delay at the neuromuscular junction. J Physiol 181:656, 1965.
66. Betz WJ, Bewick GS: Optical monitoring of transmitter release and synaptic vesicle recycling at the frog neuromuscular junction. J Physiol 460:287, 1993.
67. Ryan TA, Smith SJ: Vesicle pool mobilization during action potential firing at hippocampal synapses. Neuron 14:983, 1995.
68. Ryan TA, Reuter H, Wendland B, et al: The kinetics of synaptic vesicle recycling measured at single presynaptic boutons. Neuron 11:713, 1993.
69. Von Gersdorff H, Matthews G: Dynamics of synaptic vesicle fusion and membrane retrieval in synaptic terminals. Nature 367:735, 1994.
70. Eisenhofer G: In vivo kinetics of catecholamines. J Auton Pharmacol 14:7, 1994.
71. Stevens CF, Williams JH: "Kiss and run" exocytosis at hippocampal synapses. Proc Natl Acad Sci U S A 97:12828, 2000.
72. Murthy VN, Stevens CF: Reversal of synaptic vesicle docking at central synapses. Nat Neurosci 2:503, 1999.
73. Pyle JL, Kavalali ET, Piedras-Renteria ES, Tsien RW: Rapid reuse of readily releasable pool vesicles at hippocampal synapses. Neuron 28:221, 2000.
74. Moro MA, Lopez MG, Gandia L, et al: Separation and culture of living adrenaline and noradrenaline-containing cells from bovine adrenal medulla. Anal Biochem 185:243, 1990.
75. Livett BG, Marley PD: Effects of opioid peptides and morphine on histamine-induced catecholamine secretion from cultured, bovine adrenal chromaffin cells. Br J Pharmacol 89:327, 1986.
76. Marley PD, Livett BG: Differences between the mechanism of adrenaline and noradrenaline secretion from isolated, bovine, adrenal chromaffin cells. Neurosci Lett 77:81, 1987.
77. Owen PJ, Plevin R, Boarder MR: Characterization of bradykinin-stimulated release of noradrenaline from cultured bovine adrenal chromaffin cells. J Pharmacol Exp Ther 248:1231, 1989.
78. Cahill A, Perlman RL: Phorbol esters cause preferential secretion of norepinephrine from bovine chromaffin cells. J Neurochem 58:768, 1992.
79. Pacholczyk T, Blakely RD, Amara SG: Expression cloning of a cocaine- and antidepressant-sensitive human noradrenaline transporter. Nature 350:350, 1991.
80. Eisenhofer G: The role of neuronal and extraneuronal plasma membrane transporters in the inactivation of peripheral catecholamines. Pharmacol Ther 91:35, 2001.
81. Sole MJ, Drobac M, Schwartz L, et al: The extraction of circulating catecholamines by the lungs in normal man and in patients with pulmonary hypertension. Circulation 60:160, 1979.
82. Moss J, Lappas D, Slater E: Role of the renin catecholamine system in hemodynamic performance in man. In Usdin E, Kvetnansky R, Kopin IJ (eds): Catecholamines and Stress: Recent Advances in Neurosciences. New York, Elsevier, 1980, p 513.
83. Kaye DM, Lambert GW, Lefkovits J, et al: Neurochemical evidence of cardiac sympathetic activation and increased central nervous system norepinephrine turnover in severe congestive heart failure. J Am Coll Cardiol 23:570, 1994.
84. Cohn J, Levine T, Olivari M, et al: Plasma norepinephrine as a guide to prognosis in patients with chronic congestive heart failure. N Engl J Med 311:819, 1984.
85. Bristow M: The adrenergic nervous system in heart failure [editorial]. N Engl J Med 311:850, 1984.
86. Eisenhofer G, Friberg P, Rundqvist B, et al: Cardiac sympathetic nerve function in congestive heart failure. Circulation 93:1667, 1996.
87. Port JD, Gilbert EM, Larrabee P, et al: Neurotransmitter depletion compromises the ability of indirect-acting amines to provide inotropic support in the failing human heart. Circulation 81:929, 1990.
88. Lake CR, Chernow B, Feuerstein G, et al: The sympathetic nervous system in man, its evaluation and the measurement of plasma norepinephrine. In Ziegler M, Lake C (eds): Frontiers of Clinical Neuroscience, vol 2. Baltimore, Williams & Wilkins, 1984, p 1.
89. Kopin IJ: False neurochemical transmitters and the mechanism of sympathetic blockade by monoamine oxidase inhibitors. J Pharmacol Exp Ther 147:186, 1965.
90. Trendelenburg U: Functional aspects of the neuronal uptake of noradrenaline. Trends Pharmacol Sci 12:334, 1991.
91. Lawhead R, Blaxall H, Bylund D: $\alpha 2A$ is the predominant $\alpha 2$-adrenergic receptor subtype in human spinal cord. Anesthesiology 77:983, 1992.
92. Bylund DB: Subtypes of $\alpha 1$- and $\alpha 2$-adrenergic receptors. FASEB J 6:832, 1992.
93. Szabo B, Hedler L, Starke K: Peripheral presynaptic and central effects of clonidine, yohimbine and rauwolscine on the sympathetic nervous system in rabbits. Naunyn Schmiedebergs Arch Pharmacol 340:648, 1989.
94. Ongioco RR, Richardson CD, Rudner XL, et al: Alpha2-adrenergic receptors in human dorsal root ganglia: Predominance of alpha2b and alpha2c subtype mRNAs. Anesthesiology 92:968, 2000.
95. Michelotti GA, Price DT, Schwinn DA: Alpha 1-Adrenergic receptor regulation: Basic science and clinical implications. Pharmacol Ther 88:281, 2000.
96. Walston J, Silver K, Bogardus C, et al: Time of onset of non-insulin-dependent diabetes mellitus and genetic variation in the $\beta 3$-adrenergic-receptor gene. N Engl J Med 333:343, 1995.
97. Widen E, Lehto M, Kanninen T, et al: Association of a polymorphism in the $\beta 3$-adrenergic receptor gene with features of the insulin resistance syndrome in Finns. N Engl J Med 333:348, 1995.
98. Clement K, Vaisse C, Manning BSF, et al: Genetic variation in the $\beta 3$-adrenergic receptor and an increased capacity to gain weight in patients with morbid obesity. N Engl J Med 333:352, 1995.
99. Hall IP, Wheatley A, Wilding P, et al: Association of Glu27 $\beta 2$-adrenoceptor polymorphism with lower airway reactivity in asthmatic subjects. Lancet 345:1213, 1995.
100. Turki J, Pak J, Green SA, et al: Genetic polymorphisms of the $\beta 2$-adrenergic receptor in nocturnal and non-nocturnal asthma: Evidence that Gly 16 correlates with the nocturnal phenotype. J Clin Invest 95:1635, 1995.

101. Mason DA, Moore JD, Green SA, et al: A gain-of-function polymorphism in a G-protein coupling domain of the human beta 1-adrenergic receptor. J Biol Chem 274:12670, 1999.

102. Small KM, Wagoner LE, Levin AM, et al: Synergistic polymorphisms of β1- and α2c-adrenergic receptors and the risk of congestive heart failure. N Engl J Med 347:1135, 2002.

103. Hausdorff WP, Caron MG, Lefkowitz RJ: Turning off the signal: Desensitization of β-adrenergic receptor function. FASEB J 4:2881, 1990.

104. Michel MC, Kenny B, Schwinn DA: Classification of α1-adrenoceptor subtypes. Naunyn Schmiedebergs Arch Pharmacol 352:1, 1995.

105. Boehm S, Kubista H: Fine tuning of sympathetic transmitter release via ionotropic and metabotropic presynaptic receptors. Pharmacol Rev 54:43, 2002.

106. Szabo B, Schramm A, Starke K: Effect of yohimbine on renal sympathetic nerve activity and renal norepinephrine spillover in anesthetized rabbits. J Pharmacol Exp Ther 260:780, 1992.

107. Limberger N, Singer EA, Starke K: Only activated but not non-activated presynaptic α2-autoreceptors interfere with neighboring presynaptic receptor mechanisms. Naunyn Schmiedebergs Arch Pharmacol 338:62, 1988.

108. Opie L: Receptors and signal transduction. In Opie LH (ed): The Heart: Physiology and Metabolism. New York, Raven Press, 1991.

109. Raymond J, Hnatowich M, Lefkowitz R, et al: Adrenergic receptors: Models for regulation of signal transduction processes. Hypertension 15:119, 1990.

110. Vanhees L, Aubert A, Fagard R, et al: Influence of β1- versus β2-adrenoceptor blockade on left ventricular function in humans. J Cardiovasc Pharmacol 8:1086, 1986.

111. Opie L: Ventricular overload and heart failure. In Opie LH (ed): The Heart: Physiology and Metabolism, 2nd ed. New York, Raven Press, 1991, p 386.

112. Brodde O: The functional importance of β1- and β2-adrenoceptors in the human heart. Am J Cardiol 62:24C, 1988.

113. Goldberg LI, Rajfer SI: Dopamine receptors: Applications in clinical cardiology. Circulation 72:245, 1985.

114. Bertorello A, Aperia A: Both DA1 and DA2 receptor agonists are necessary to inhibit Na+/K+ ATPase activity in proximal tubules from the rat kidney. Acta Physiol Scand 132:441, 1988.

115. Bertorello A, Aperia A: Regulation of Na+/K+ ATPase activity in kidney proximal tubules: Involvement of GTP binding proteins. Am J Physiol 256:F57, 1989.

116. Gesek FA, Schoolwerth AC: Hormonal interactions with the proximal Na+/H+ exchanger. Am J Physiol 258:F514, 1990.

117. Linder ME, Gilman AG: G Proteins. Sci Am 267:56, 1992.

118. Pang IH, Sternweis PC: Purification of unique α subunits of GTP-binding regulatory proteins (G proteins) by affinity chromatography with immobilized βγ subunits. J Biol Chem 265:18707, 1990.

119. Blank JL, Ross AH, Exton JH: Purification and characterization of two G-proteins that activate the β1 isozyme of phosphoinositide-specific phospholipase C. J Biol Chem 266:18206, 1991.

120. Gutowski S, Smrcka A, Nowak L, et al: Antibodies to the αq subfamily of guanine nucleotide-binding regulatory protein α subunits attenuate activation of phosphatidylinositol 4,5-bisphosphate hydrolysis by hormones. J Biol Chem 266:20519, 1991.

121. Alousi AA, Jasper JR, Insel PA, et al: Stoichiometry of receptor Gs-adenylate cyclase interactions. FASEB J 5:2300, 1991.

122. Post SR, Hilal-Dandan R, Urasawa K, et al: Quantification of signaling components and amplification in the β-adrenergic receptor-adenylate cyclase pathway in isolated adult rat ventricular myocytes. Biochem J 311:75, 1995.

123. Yatani A, Okabe K, Codina J, et al: Heart rate regulation by G proteins acting on the cardiac pacemaker channel. Science 249:1163, 1990.

124. Roizen M, Horrigan R, Frazier B: Anesthetic doses blocking adrenergic stress and cardiovascular responses to incision: MAC BAR. Anesthesiology 54:390, 1981.

125. Roizen MF, Thoa NB, Moss J, et al: Inhibition by halothane of release of norepinephrine, but not of dopamine-β-hydroxylase, from guinea pig vas deferens. Eur J Pharmacol 31:313, 1975.

126. Rorie DK, Tyce GM, Mackenzie RA: Evidence that halothane inhibits norepinephrine release from sympathetic nerve endings in dog saphenous vein by stimulation of presynaptic inhibitory muscarinic receptors. Anesth Analg 63:1059, 1984.

127. Lunn JJ, Rorie DK: Halothane-induced changes in the release and disposition of norepinephrine at adrenergic nerve endings in dog saphenous vein. Anesthesiology 61:377, 1984.

128. Bernstein KJ, Gangat Y, Verosky M, et al: Halothane effect on β-adrenergic receptors in canine myocardium. Anesth Analg 60:401, 1981.

129. Bernstein K, Verosky M, Triner L: Halothane inhibition of canine myocardial adenylate cyclase: Modulation by endogenous factors. Anesth Analg 63:285, 1984.

130. Gangat Y, Vulliemoz Y, Verosky M, et al: Action of halothane on myocardial adenylate cyclase of rat and cat. Proc Soc Exp Biol Med 160:154, 1979.

131. Narayanan TK, Confer RA, Dennison RL, et al: Halothane attenuation of muscarinic inhibition of adenylate cyclase in rat heart. Biochem Pharmacol 37:1219, 1988.

132. Vulliemoz V, Verosky M, Triner L: Effect of halothane on myocardial cyclic AMP and cyclic GMP content of mice. J Pharmacol Exp Ther 236:181, 1986.

133. Thurston T, Glusman S: Halothane myocardial depression: Interactions with the adenylate cyclase system. Anesth Analg 75:63, 1993.

134. Terrar DA, Victory JG: Effects of halothane on membrane currents associated with contraction in single myocytes from guinea pig ventricle. Br J Pharmacol 94:500, 1988.

135. Lynch C, Vogel S, Sperelakis N: Halothane depression of myocardial slow action potentials. Anesthesiology 55:360, 1988.

136. Komai H, Rusy BF: Direct effect of halothane and isoflurane on the function of the sarcoplasmic reticulum in intact rabbit atria. Anesthesiology 72:694, 1990.

137. Su JY, Kerrick WG: Effects of halothane on caffeine-induced tension transients in functionally skinned myocardial fibers. Pflugers Arch 380:29, 1979.

138. Blochl-Daum B, Schuller-Petrovic S, Wolzt M, et al: Primary defect in α-adrenergic responsiveness in patients with varicose veins. Clin Pharmacol Ther 49:49, 1991.

139. Insel PA: Adrenergic receptors: Evolving concepts and clinical implications. N Engl J Med 334:580, 1996.

140. Bristow MR, Ginsburg R, Minobe W, et al: Decreased catecholamine sensitivity and β-adrenergic receptor density in failing human hearts. N Engl J Med 307:205, 1982.

141. Menard L, Ferguson SS, Zhang J, et al: Synergistic regulation of β2-adrenergic receptor sequestration: Intracellular complement of β-adrenergic receptor kinase and β-arrestin determine kinetics of internalization. Mol Pharmacol 51:800, 1997.

142. Ferguson SS, Barak LS, Zhang J, et al: G-protein-coupled receptor regulation: Role of G-protein-coupled receptor kinases and arrestins. Can J Physiol Pharmacol 74:1095, 1996.

143. Hedberg A, Kemp F Jr, Josephson ME, et al: Co-existence of β1- and β2-adrenergic receptors in the human heart: Effects of treatment with receptor antagonists or calcium entry blockers. J Pharmacol Exp Ther 234:561, 1985.

144. Bristow M, Ginsburg R, Umans V, et al: β1- and β2-adrenergic receptor subpopulations in non-failing and failing human ventricular myocardium: Coupling of both receptor subtypes to muscle contraction and selective β1 receptor downregulation in heart failure. Circ Res 59:297, 1986.

145. Hedberg A: Adrenergic receptors: Methods of determination and mechanisms of regulation. Acta Med Scand Suppl 672:7, 1983.

146. Dratman M, Crutchfield F, Axelrod J, et al: Localization of triiodothyronine in nerve ending fractions of rat brain. Proc Natl Acad Sci U S A 73:941, 1976.

147. Doukas PH: Drugs affecting the parasympathetic nervous system. *In* Wingard L, Brody T, Larner J, et al (eds): Human Pharmacology: Molecular to Clinical. St. Louis, Mosby–Year Book, 1991.

148. Conlay L, Wurtman RJ, Blusztaj K, et al: Decreased plasma choline concentrations in marathon runners. N Engl J Med 86:892, 1986.

149. Stiller R: Neuromuscular blocking agents. *In* Wingard L, Brody T, Larner J, et al (eds): Human Pharmacology: Molecular to Clinical. St. Louis, Mosby–Year Book, 1991.

150. Soreq H, Zakut H: Amplification of butyrylcholinesterase and acetylcholinesterase genes in normal and tumor tissues: Putative relationship to organophosphorus poisoning. Pharm Res 7:1, 1990.

151. Prody CA, Dreyfus P, Zamir R, et al: De novo amplification within a "silent" human cholinesterase gene in a family subjected to prolonged exposure to organophosphorus insecticides. Proc Natl Acad Sci U S A 86:690, 1989.

152. Sussman JL, Harel M, Frolow F, et al: Atomic structure of acetylcholinesterase from Torpedo californica: A prototypic acetylcholine-binding protein. Science 253:872, 1991.

153. Tassonyi E, Charpantier E, Muller D, et al: The role of nicotinic acetylcholine receptors in the mechanisms of anesthesia. Brain Res Bull 57:133, 2002.

154. Smit AB, Syed NI, Schaap D, et al: A glia-derived acetylcholine-binding protein that modulates synaptic transmission. Nature 411:261, 2001.

155. Martinou J-C, Falls DL, Fischbach GD, et al: Acetylcholine receptor-inducing activity stimulates expression of the ε-subunit gene of the muscle acetylcholine receptor. Proc Natl Acad Sci U S A 87:7669, 1991.

156. McMahan UJ, Horton SE, Werle MJ, et al: Agrin isoforms and their role in synaptogenesis. Curr Opin Cell Biol 4:869, 1992.

157. Nastuk MA, Fallon JR: Agrin and the molecular choreography of synapse formation. Trends Neurosci 16:72, 1993.

158. Apel ED, Merlie JP: Assembly of the postsynaptic apparatus. Curr Opin Neurobiol 5:62, 1995.

159. Eglen RM, Hedge SS, Watson N: Muscarinic receptor subtypes and smooth muscle function. Pharmacol Rev 48:531, 1996.

160. Hosey MM: Diversity of structure, signaling and regulation within the family of muscarinic cholinergic receptors. FASEB J 12:845, 1992.

161. Ganong W: The autonomic nervous system. *In* Ganong W (ed): Review of Medical Physiology, 15th ed. Norwalk, CT, Appleton & Lange, 1991, p 210.

162. Glusman S: Electrophysiology of ganglionic transmission in the sympathetic nervous system. Int Anesthesiol Clin 27:273, 1989.

163. Hoffman BB, Lefkowitz RJ: Catecholamines and sympathetic drugs. *In* Goodman A, Rall T, Nies A, et al (eds): Goodman and Gilman's the Pharmacological Basis of Therapeutics, 8th ed. New York, Pergamon Press, 1990, p 187.

164. Paradis NA, Martin GB, Rivers EP, et al: Coronary perfusion pressure and the return of spontaneous circulation in human cardiopulmonary resuscitation. JAMA 263:1106, 1990.

165. Emergency Cardiac Care Committee: Guidelines for cardiopulmonary resuscitation and emergency cardiac care. III. Adult advanced cardiac life support. JAMA 268:2199, 1992.

166. Emergency Cardiac Care Committee: Guidelines for cardiopulmonary resuscitation and emergency cardiac care. VI. Pediatric advanced life support. JAMA 268:2262, 1992.

167. Goetting M, Paradis N: High-dose epinephrine improves outcome from pediatric cardiac arrest. Ann Emerg Med 20:22, 1991.

168. Aitkenhead A: Drug administration during CPR: What route? Resuscitation 22:191, 1991.

169. Berry F: Clinical pharmacology of inhalational anesthetic, muscle relaxants, vasoactive agents, and narcotics, and techniques of general anesthesia. *In* Berry F (ed): Anesthetic Management of Difficult and Routine Pediatric Patients, 2nd ed. New York, Churchill Livingstone, 1990, p 64.

170. Ziment I: Pharmacology of sympathomimetic agents. *In* Ziment I (ed): Respiratory Pharmacology and Therapeutics. Philadelphia, WB Saunders, 1978.

171. Waisman Y, Klein BL, Boenning DA, et al: Prospective randomized double blind study comparing L-epinephrine and racemic epinephrine aerosols in the treatment of laryngotracheitis (croup). Pediatrics 89:302, 1992.

172. Nutman J, Brooks LJ, Deakins KM, et al: Racemic versus L-epinephrine aerosol in the treatment of postextubation laryngeal edema: Results from a prospective, randomized double-blind study. Crit Care Med 22:1591, 1994.

173. Bochner BS, Lichtenstein L: Anaphylaxis. N Engl J Med 324:1785, 1991.

174. Donlon J, Moss J: Plasma catecholamine levels during local anesthesia for cataract operations. Anesthesiology 51:471, 1979.

175. Houben H, Thien T, van't Laar A: Effect of low-dose epinephrine on hemodynamics after selective and nonselective beta-blockade in hypertension. Clin Pharmacol Ther 31:685, 1982.

176. Johnston R, Eger E, Wilson C: A comparative interaction of epinephrine with enflurane, isoflurane, and halothane in man. Anesth Analg 55:709, 1976.

177. Zaritsky A, Chernow B: Catecholamines, sympathomimetics. *In* Chernow B, Lake C (eds): The Pharmacologic Approach to the Critically Ill Patient. Baltimore, Williams & Wilkins, 1983, p 481.

178. O'Neill MJ Jr, Pennock JL, Seaton JF, et al: Regional endogenous plasma catecholamine concentrations in pulmonary hypertension. Surgery 84:140, 1978.

179. Benowitz N, Forsyth RP, Melman KL, et al: Lidocaine disposition kinetics in monkey and man: Effects of hemorrhage and sympathomimetic drug administration. Clin Pharmacol Ther 16:19, 1974.

180. Schafer G, Fink M, Parillo J: Norepinephrine alone versus norepinephrine plus low dose dopamine: Enhanced renal blood flow with combination pressor therapy. Crit Care Med 13:492, 1985.

181. Goldberg L: Dopamine: Clinical uses of an endogenous catecholamine. N Engl J Med 291:707, 1974.

182. Goldberg LI, Hsieh Y-Y, Resnekov L: Newer catecholamines for treatment of heart failure and shock: An update on dopamine and a first look at dobutamine. Prog Cardiovasc Dis 19:327, 1977.

183. Maskin C, Ocken S, Chadwick B, et al: Comparative systemic and renal effects of dopamine and angiotensin-converting enzyme inhibitor with enalapril in patients with heart failure. Circulation 72:846, 1985.

184. Richard C, Ricome J, Rimailho A, et al: Combined hemodynamic effects of dopamine and dobutamine in cardiogenic shock. Circulation 67:620, 1983.

185. Brown RA, Dixon J, Farmer JB, et al: Dopexamine: A novel agonist at peripheral dopamine receptors and β2-adrenoceptors. Br J Pharmacol 85:599, 1985.

186. Foulds RA: Clinical development of dopexamine hydrochloride (Dopacard) and an overview of its hemodynamic effects. Am J Cardiol 62:41C, 1988.

187. Smith GW, O'Connor SE: An introduction to the pharmacologic properties of Dopacard (dopexamine hydrochloride). Am J Cardiol 62:9C, 1988.

188. Fitton A, Benfield P: Dopexamine hydrochloride: A review of its pharmacodynamic and pharmacokinetic properties and therapeutic potential in acute cardiac insufficiency. Drugs 39:308, 1990.

189. Smith GW, Hall JC, Farmer JB, et al: The cardiovascular actions of dopexamine hydrochloride, an agonist at dopamine receptors and β2-adrenoceptors in the dog. J Pharm Pharmacol 39:636, 1987.

190. Mitchell PD, Smith GW, Wells E, et al: Inhibition of uptake 1 by dopexamine hydrochloride in vitro. Br J Pharmacol 92:265, 1987.

191. Lokhandwala MF: Renal actions of dopexamine hydrochloride. Clin Intensive Care 1:163, 1990.

192. Vyas SJ, Lokhandwala MF: Role of tubular dopamine-1 receptors in the natriuretic and diuretic response to dopexamine. Pharmacologist 31:378, 1989.
193. Bass AS: Contrasting effects of dopexamine hydrochloride on electrolyte excretion in canine kidneys. J Pharmacol Exp Ther 253:798, 1990.
194. Chintala MS, Lokhandwala MF, Jandhyala BS: Protective effects of dopexamine hydrochloride in renal failure after acute hemorrhage in anesthetized dogs. J Auton Pharmacol 10(Suppl):S95, 1990.
195. Leier CV, Binkley PF, Carpenter J, et al: Cardiovascular pharmacology of dopexamine in low output congestive heart failure. Am J Cardiol 62:94, 1988.
196. Baumann G, Felix SB, Filcek SAL: Usefulness of dopexamine hydrochloride versus dobutamine in chronic congestive heart failure and the effects on hemodynamics and urine output. Am J Cardiol 65:748, 1990.
197. Colardyn FC, Vandenbogaerde FE: Use of dopexamine hydrochloride in intensive care patients with low-output left ventricular heart failure. Am J Cardiol 62:68C, 1988.
198. Friedel N, Wenzel R, Matheis G, et al: Haemodynamic effects of different doses of dopexamine hydrochloride in low cardiac output states following cardiac surgery. Eur Heart J 13:1271, 1992.
199. Bredle DL, Cain SM: Systemic and muscle oxygen uptake delivery after dopexamine infusion in endotoxic dogs. Crit Care Med 19:198, 1991.
200. Cain SM, Curtis SE: Systemic and regional oxygen uptake and delivery and lactate flux in endotoxic dogs infused with dopexamine. Crit Care Med 19:1552, 1991.
201. Colardyn FC, Vandenbogaerde JF, Vogelaers DP, et al: Use of dopexamine hydrochloride in patients with septic shock. Crit Care Med 17:999, 1989.
202. Preiser JC, Arminstead C, Le Minh T, et al: Increase in oxygen supply during experimental septic shock: The effects of dobutamine versus dopexamine. J Crit Care 4:40, 1989.
203. Webb AR, Moss RF, Tighe D, et al: The effects of dobutamine, dopexamine and fluid on hepatic histological response to porcine faecal peritonitis. Intensive Care Med 17:487, 1991.
204. Hakim M, Foulds R, Latimer RD, et al: Dopexamine hydrochloride, a β2-adrenergic and dopaminergic agonist Haemodynamic effects following cardiac surgery. Eur Heart J 9:853, 1988.
205. Macgregor DA, Butterworth JF IV, Zaloga GP, et al: Hemodynamic and renal effects of dopexamine and dobutamine in patients with reduced cardiac output following coronary artery bypass grafting. Chest 106:835, 1994.
206. Smithies M, Yee TH, Jackson L, et al: Protecting the gut and the liver in the critically ill: Effects of dopexamine. Crit Care Med 22:789, 1994.
207. Lund N, de Asla RJ, Papadakos PJ, et al: Dopexamine hydrochloride in septicemia: Effects on gut, liver and muscle oxygenation [abstract]. Crit Care Med 20(Suppl 4):46, 1992.
208. Trinder TJ, Lavery GG, Fee JPH, et al: Correction of splanchnic oxygen deficit in the intensive care unit: Dopexamine and colloid versus placebo. Anaesth Intensive Care 23:178, 1995.
209. Kuhly P, Oschmann G, Specht M, et al: Dopexamine hydrochloride does not improve gastric and sigmoid mucosal acidosis in patients with sepsis [abstract]. Br J Anesth 74(Suppl 1):121, 1995.
210. Schmidt H, Secchi A, Wellmann R, et al: Dopexamine maintains intestinal villus blood flow during endotoxemia in rats. Crit Care Med 24:1233, 1996.
211. Maynard N, Bihari D, Dalton RN, et al: Increasing splanchnic blood flow in the critically ill. Chest 108:1648, 1995.
212. Jackson NC, Taylor SH, Frais MA: Hemodynamic comparison of dopexamine hydrochloride and dopamine in ischemic left ventricular dysfunction. Am J Cardiol 62:73, 1988.
213. Tan LB, Littler WA, Murray RG: Comparison of the haemodynamic effects of dopexamine and dobutamine in patients with severe congestive heart failure. Int J Cardiol 30:203, 1991.
214. Young JB, Leon CA: Fenoldopam. In Messerli FH (ed): Cardiovascular Drug Therapy. Philadelphia, WB Saunders, 1990.
215. Lokhandwala MF: Pre-clinical and clinical studies on the cardiovascular and renal effects of fenoldopam: A DA-1 receptor agonist. Drug Dev Res 10:123, 1987.
216. Goldberg LI: Dopamine and new dopamine analogs: Receptors and clinical applications. J Clin Anesth 1:66, 1988.
217. Aronson S, Goldberg L, Roth S, et al: Preservation of renal blood flow during hypotension induced with fenoldopam in dogs. Can J Anaesth 37:380, 1990.
218. Aronson S, Goldberg LI, Roth S, et al: Effects of fenoldopam on renal blood flow and systemic hemodynamics during isoflurane anesthesia in dogs. J Cardiothorac Vasc Anesth 5:29, 1991.
219. Shusterman NH, Elliott WJ, White WB: Fenoldopam, but not nitroprusside, improves renal function in severely hypertensive patients with impaired renal function. Am J Med 95:161, 1993.
220. Pilmer BL, Green JA, Panacek EA, et al: Fenoldopam mesylate versus sodium nitroprusside in the acute management of severe system hypertension. J Clin Pharmacol 33:549, 1993.
221. Shnider S, Levinson G, Cosmi E: Obstetric anesthesia and uterine blood flow. In Schnider S, Levinson G (eds): Anesthesia for Obstetrics, 3rd ed. Baltimore, Williams & Wilkins, 1993, p 29.
222. Caplan R, Ward R, Posner K, Cheney F: Unexpected cardiac arrest during spinal anesthesia: A closed claims analysis of predisposing factors. Anesthesiology 68:5, 1988.
223. Shibata S, Seriguchi DG, Iwadare S, et al: The regional and species differences on the activation of myocardial α-adrenoreceptors by phenylephrine and methoxamine. Gen Pharmacol 11:173, 1980.
224. DeVos H, Bricca G, DeKeyser J, et al: Imidazoline receptors, non-adrenergic idazoxan binding sites and α2-adrenoceptors in the human central nervous system. Neuroscience 59:589, 1994.
225. Hamilton CA: The role of imidazoline receptors in blood pressure regulation. Pharmacol Ther 54:231, 1992.
226. Guyenet PG, Cabot JB: Inhibition of sympathetic preganglionic neurons by catecholamines and clonidine: Mediation by an α-adrenergic receptor. J Neurosci 1:908, 1981.
227. Ruffolo RR Jr: Distribution and function of peripheral α-adrenoceptors on the cardiovascular system. Pharmacol Biochem Behav 22:827, 1985.
228. Muzi M, Goff D, Kampine J, et al: Clonidine reduces sympathetic activity but maintains baroreflex responses in normotensive humans. Anesthesiology 77:864, 1992.
229. Aho M, Erkola O, Korttila K: α2-Adrenergic agonists in anaesthesia. Curr Opin Anaesthesiol 5:481, 1992.
230. Flacke J, Bloor BC, Flacke WE, et al: Reduced narcotic requirement by clonidine with improved hemodynamic and adrenergic stability in patients undergoing coronary bypass surgery. Anesthesiology 67:11, 1987.
231. Ghignone M, Quintin L, Duke P, et al: Effects of clonidine on narcotic requirements and hemodynamic response during induction of fentanyl anesthesia and endotracheal intubation. Anesthesiology 64:36, 1986.
232. Maze M, Tranguilli W: α2-Adrenoreceptor agonists: Defining the role in clinical anesthesia. Anesthesiology 74:581, 1991.
233. Bloor BC, Flacke WE: Reduction in halothane anesthetic requirement by clonidine, an α2 adrenergic agonist. Anesth Analg 61:741, 1982.
234. Ghignone M, Calvillo O, Quintin L: Anesthesia and hypertension: The effect of clonidine on perioperative hemodynamics and isoflurane requirements. Anesthesiology 67:3, 1987.
235. Orko R, Pouttu J, Ghignone M: Effect of clonidine on hemodynamic responses to endotracheal intubation and gastric acidity. Acta Anaesthesiol Scand 31:325, 1987.
236. Aantaa R, Jaakola ML, Kallio A, et al: A comparison of dexmedetomidine, an α2-adrenoceptor agonist, and midazolam as i.m. premedication for minor gynaecological surgery. Br J Anaesth 67:402, 1991.

237. Aantaa RE, Kanto JH, Scheinin M: Dexmedetomidine premedication for minor gynecologic surgery. Anesth Analg 70:407, 1990.

238. Aantaa RE, Kanto JH, Scheinin M: Dexmedetomidine, an alpha 2-adrenoceptor agonist, reduces anesthetic requirements for patients undergoing minor gynecologic surgery. Anesthesiology 73:230, 1990.

239. Richards MJ, Skues MA, Jarvis AP, Prys-Roberts C: Total i.v. anaesthesia with propofol and alfentanil: Dose requirements for propranolol and the effect of premedication with clonidine. Br J Anaesth 65:157, 1990.

240. Bonnet F, Brun-Buisson V, Saada M: Dose-related prolongation of hyperbaric tetracaine spinal anesthesia by clonidine in humans. Anesth Analg 68:619, 1989.

241. Murga G, Samso E, Valles J, et al: The effect of clonidine on intra-operative requirements of fentanyl during combined epidural/general anesthesia. Anaesthesia 49:999, 1994.

242. Klimscha W, Chiari A, Drafft P, et al: Hemodynamic and analgesic effects of clonidine added repetitively to continuous epidural and spinal blocks. Anesth Analg 80:322, 1995.

243. Delaunay L, Leppert C, Dechaubry V, et al: Epidural clonidine decreases postoperative requirements for epidural fentanyl. Reg Anesth 18:176, 1993.

244. Bonnet F, Diallo A, Saada M, et al: Prevention of tourniquet pain by spinal isobaric bupivacaine with clonidine. Br J Anaesth 63:93, 1989.

245. Racle JP, Benkhadra A, Poy JY, Bleizal B: Prolongation of isobaric bupivacaine spinal anesthesia with epinephrine and clonidine for hip surgery in the elderly. Anesth Analg 66:442, 1987.

246. Bonnet F, Catoire P, Brun-Buison V, et al: Effects of oral and subarachnoid clonidine on spinal anesthesia with bupivacaine. Reg Anesth 15:211, 1990.

247. Fogarty DJ, Carabine UA, Milligan KR: Comparison of the analgesic effects of intrathecal clonidine and intrathecal morphine after spinal anesthesia in patients undergoing total hip replacement. Br J Anaesth 71:661, 1993.

248. Niemi L: Effects of intrathecal clonidine on duration of bupivacaine spinal anaesthesia, haemodynamics, and postoperative analgesia in patients undergoing knee arthroscopy. Acta Anaesthesiol Scand 38:724, 1994.

249. Fukuda T, Dohi S, Naito H: Comparisons of tetracaine spinal anesthesia with clonidine or phenylephrine in normotensive and hypertensive humans. Anesth Analg 78:106, 1994.

250. Singelyn FJ, Dangoisse M, Bartholomee S, Gouverneur JM: Adding clonidine to mepivacaine prolongs the duration of anesthesia and analgesia after axillary brachial plexus block. Reg Anesth 17:148, 1992.

251. Macaire P, Bernard JM, LeRoux D, et al: Dose-ranging study of clonidine added to lidocaine for axillary plexus block in outpatients [abstract]. Anesthesiology 83:A774, 1995.

252. Singelyn FJ, Muller G, Gouverneur JM: Adding fentanyl and clonidine to mepivacaine results in a rapid onset and prolonged anesthesia and analgesia after brachial plexus blockade [abstract]. Anesthesiology 75:A653, 1991.

253. Bartholomee S, Singelyn FJ, Broka S, Gouverneur JM: Clonidine added to mepivacaine for brachial plexus blockade: Its minimal effective dose prolonging the duration of both anesthesia and analgesia [abstract]. Anesthesiology 75:A1084, 1991.

254. Tschernko E, Benditte H, Kritzinger M, et al: Clonidine added to the anesthetic solution prolongs analgesia and improves arterial oxygen tension after intercostal nerve blockade [abstract]. Anesthesiology 83:A846, 1995.

255. Breslow MJ: The role of stress hormones in perioperative myocardial ischemia. Int Anesthesiol Clin 30:81, 1992.

256. Ghignone MC, Cavillo O, Quintin L: Anesthesia for ophthalmic surgery in the elderly: The effects of clonidine on intraocular pressure, perioperative hemodynamics, and anesthesia requirement. Anesthesiology 68:707, 1988.

257. Jaakola ML, Ali-Melkkila T, Kanto J: Dexmedetomidine reduces intraocular pressure, intubation responses and anaesthetic requirements in patients undergoing ophthalmic surgery. Br J Anaesth 68:570, 1992.

258. Kumar A, Bose S, Phattacharya A: Oral clonidine premedication for elderly patients undergoing intraocular surgery. Acta Anaesthesiol Scand 36:159, 1992.

259. Ebert TJ, Hall JE, Barney JA, et al: The effects of increasing plasma concentrations of dexmedetomidine in humans. Anesthesiology 93:382, 2000.

260. Arain SR, Ebert TJ: The efficacy, side effects, and recovery characteristics of dexmedetomidine versus propofol when used for intraoperative sedation. Anesth Analg 95:461, 2002.

261. Segal IS, Vickery RG, Walton JK: Dexmedetomidine diminishes halothane anesthetic requirements in rats through a postsynaptic α2-adrenergic receptor. Anesthesiology 69:818, 1988.

262. Vickery RG, Sheridan BS, Segal IS, Maze M: Anesthetic and hemodynamic effects of the stereoisomers of medetomidine, an α2-adrenergic agonist, in halothane-anesthetized dogs. Anesth Analg 67:611, 1988.

263. Talke P, Chen R, Thomas B, et al: The hemodynamic and adrenergic effects of perioperative dexmedetomidine infusion after vascular surgery. Anesth Analg 90:834, 2000.

264. Peden CJ, Cloote AH, Stratford N, et al: The effect of intravenous dexmedetomidine premedication on the dose requirement of propofol to induce loss of consciousness in patients receiving alfentanil. Anaesthesia 56:408, 2001.

265. Triltsch AE, Welte M, von Homeyer P, et al: Bispectral index-guided sedation with dexmedetomidine in intensive care: A prospective, randomized, double blind, placebo-controlled phase II study. Crit Care Med 30:1007, 2002.

266. DeKock M, Pichon G, Scholtes JL: Intraoperative clonidine enhances postoperative morphine patient-controlled analgesia. Can J Anaesth 39:537, 1992.

267. Motsh J, Graber E, Ludwig K: Addition of clonidine enhances postoperative analgesia from epidural morphine: A double blind study. Anesthesiology 73:1066, 1990.

268. Bernard JM, Hommeril JL, Passuti N, Pinaud M: Postoperative analgesia by intravenous clonidine. Anesthesiology 75:577, 1991.

269. Carabine UA, Milligan KR, Moore J: Extradural clonidine and bupivacaine for postoperative analgesia. Br J Anaesth 68:132, 1992.

270. Carabine UA, Milligan KR, Mulholland D, Moore J: Extradural clonidine infusions for analgesia after total hip replacement. Br J Anaesth 68:338, 1992.

271. Rostaing S, Bonnet F, Levron JC: Effect of epidural clonidine on analgesia and pharmacokinetics of epidural fentanyl in postoperative patients. Anesthesiology 75:420, 1991.

272. Bonnet F, Boico O, Rostaining S: Clonidine-induced analgesia in postoperative patients: Epidural versus intramuscular administration. Anesthesiology 72:423, 1990.

273. Tryba M, Zenz M, Strumpf M: Clonidine i.v. is equally effective as morphine i.v. for postoperative analgesia–A double blind study [abstract]. Anesthesiology 75:A1085, 1991.

274. DeKock M, Crochet B, Morimont C, Scholtes JL: Intravenous or epidural clonidine for intra- and postoperative analgesia. Anesthesiology 79:525, 1993.

275. Mogensen T, Eliasen K, Ejlersen E, et al: Epidural clonidine enhances postoperative analgesia from a combined low-dose epidural bupivacaine and morphine regimen. Anesth Analg 75:607, 1992.

276. Vercauteren M, Lauwers E, Meert T, et al: Comparison of epidural sufentanil plus clonidine with sufentanil alone for postoperative pain relief. Anaesthesia 45:531, 1990.

277. Rockemann MG, Seeling W, Brinkmann A, et al: Analgesic and hemodynamic effects of epidural clonidine, clonidine/morphine and morphine after pancreatic surgery: A double-blind study. Anesth Analg 80:869, 1995.

278. O'Meara ME, Gin T: Comparison of 0.125% bupivacaine with 0.125% bupivacaine and clonidine as extradural analgesia in the first stage of labour. Br J Anaesth 71:651, 1993.

279. Brichant JF, Bonhomme V, Mikulski M, et al: Admixture of clonidine to epidural bupivacaine for analgesia during labor: Effect of varying clonidine doses [abstract]. Anesthesiology 81:A1136, 1994.

280. Cigarini I, Kaba A, Bonnet F, et al: Epidural clonidine combined with bupivacaine for analgesia in labor: Effects on mother and neonate. Reg Anesth 20:113, 1995.

281. Eisenach JC, DePen S, Dubois M, et al: Epidural clonidine study group: Epidural clonidine anesthesia for intractable cancer pain. Pain 61:391, 1995.

282. Petros AJ, Wright RMB: Epidural and oral clonidine in domiciliary control of deafferentation pain. Lancet 1:1034, 1987.

283. Eisenach JC, Rauck RL, Buzzanell C, Lysak S: Epidural clonidine analgesia for intractable cancer pain: Phase I. Anesthesiology 71:647, 1989.

284. Ferit PA, Aydinli I, Akra S: Management of cancer pain with epidural clonidine [abstract]. Reg Anesth 17(Suppl 3S):173, 1992.

285. Lund C, Hansen O, Kehlet H: Effect of epidural clonidine on somatosensory evoked potentials to dermatomal stimulation. Eur J Anaesth 6:207, 1989.

286. Strube PJ, Lavies NG, Rubin J: Epidural clonidine [letter]. Anaesthesia 39:834, 1984.

287. Marruecos I, Roglan A, Frati ME, Artigas A: Clonidine overdose. Crit Care Med 11:959, 1988.

288. Zeigler D, Lynch SA, Muir J: Transdermal clonidine versus placebo in painful diabetic neuropathy. Pain 48:403, 1992.

289. Slogoff S: Perioperative ischemia. Semin Anesth 9:107, 1990.

290. Quintin L, Viale JP, Annat G: Oxygen uptake after major abdominal surgery: Effect of clonidine. Anesthesiology 74:236, 1991.

291. Bailey PL, Sperry RJ, Johnson GK, et al: Respiratory effects of clonidine alone and combined with morphine in humans. Anesthesiology 74:43, 1991.

292. Ooi R, Pattison J, Feldman SA: The effects of intravenous clonidine on ventilation. Anaesthesia 46:632, 1991.

293. Rauck RL, Eisenach JC, Jackson K, et al: Epidural clonidine treatment for refractory reflex sympathetic dystrophy. Anesthesiology 79:1163, 1993.

294. Uhde TW, Stein MB, Vittone BJ, et al: Behavioral and physiologic effects of short-term and long-term administration of clonidine in panic disorder. Arch Gen Psychiatry 46:170, 1989.

295. Gold MS, Pottash AC, Sweeney DR, Klever HD: Opiate withdrawal using clonidine. A safe, effective, and rapid nonopiate treatment. JAMA 243:343, 1980.

296. Franz DN, Hare BD, McCloskey KL: Spinal sympathetic neurons: Possible sites of opiate-withdrawal suppression by clonidine. Science 215:1643, 1982.

297. Davison R, Kaplan K, Fintel D, et al: The effect of clonidine on the cessation of cigarette smoking. Clin Pharmacol Ther 44:265, 1988.

298. Glassman AH, Stetner F, Walsh BT: Heavy smokers, smoking cessation, and clonidine. Results of a double-blind, randomized trial. JAMA 259:2863, 1988.

299. Hughes JR: Clonidine, depression, and smoking cessation. JAMA 259:2901, 1988.

300. Metz SA, Halter JB, Robertson RP: Induction of defective insulin secretion and impaired glucose tolerance by clonidine. Selective stimulation of metabolic α-adrenergic pathways. Diabetes 27:554, 1978.

301. Gentili M, Bonnet F: Incidence of urinary retention after spinal anesthesia: Comparison of morphine and clonidine [abstract]. Anesthesiology 81:A945, 1994.

302. Gentili M, Mamelle JC, Le Foll G: Combination of low-dose bupivacaine and clonidine for unilateral spinal anesthesia in arthroscopic knee surgery. Reg Anesth 20:169, 1995.

303. Kapral S, Kocek S, Krafft P, et al: Intrathecal clonidine delays motor onset of bupivacaine [abstract]. Anesthesiology 81:A935, 1994.

304. Ota K, Namiki A, Ujike Y, Takahashi I: Prolongation of tetracaine spinal anesthesia by oral clonidine. Anesth Analg 75:262, 1992.

305. DeKock M, Lavandhomme P, Scholtes JL: Intraoperative and postoperative analgesia using intravenous opioid, clonidine and lignocaine. Anaesth Intensive Care 22:15, 1994.

306. Mendez R, Eisenach JC, Kashtan K: Epidural clonidine analgesia after cesarean section. Anesthesiology 73:848, 1990.

307. Filos KS, Goudas LC, Patroni O, Polyzou V: Intrathecal clonidine as a sole analgesic for pain relief after cesarean section. Anesthesiology 77:267, 1990.

308. Bernard JM, Kick O, Bonnet F: Comparison of intravenous and epidural clonidine for postoperative patient-controlled analgesia. Anesth Analg 81:706, 1995.

309. Huntoon M, Eisenach JC, Boese P: Epidural clonidine after cesarean section: Appropriate dose and effect of prior local anesthetic. Anesthesiology 76:187, 1992.

310. Bouguet D: Caudal clonidine added to local anesthetics enhances post-operative analgesia after anal surgery in adults [abstract]. Anesthesiology 81:A942, 1994.

311. Coombs DW, Saunders RL, Fratkin JD, et al: Continuous intrathecal hydromorphone and clonidine for intractable cancer pain. J Neurosurg 64:890, 1986.

312. van Essen EJ, Bovill JG, Ploeger EJ, Beerman H: Intrathecal morphine and clonidine for control of intractable cancer pain. A case report. Acta Anaesthiol Belg 39:109, 1988.

313. Hardy PAJ, Wells JCD: Pain after spinal intrathecal clonidine. An adverse interaction with tricyclic antidepressants? Anaesthesia 43:1026, 1988.

314. Grace D, Milligan KR, Morrow BJ, Fee JPH: Co-administration of pethidine and clonidine: A spinal anaesthetic technique for total hip replacement. Br J Anaesth 73:628, 1994.

315. Boico O, Bonnet F, Bazoit JX: Effects of epinephrine and clonidine on plasma concentrations of spinal bupivacaine. Acta Anaesthesiol Scand 36:684, 1992.

316. Grace D, Bunting H, Milligan KR, Fee JPH: Postoperative analgesia after co-administration of clonidine and morphine by the intrathecal route in patients undergoing hip replacement. Anesth Analg 80:86, 1995.

317. Sucu Y, Kanbak O, Gogus N, Aksu C: Comparison of intrathecal clonidine and alfentanil [abstract]. Br J Anaesth 74(Suppl 1):131, 1995.

318. Sonnenblick EH, Frishman WH, LeJemtel TH: Dobutamine: A new synthetic cardioactive sympathetic amine. N Engl J Med 300:17, 1979.

319. Gillespie T, Ambos H, Sobel B, Roberts R: Effects of dobutamine in patients with acute myocardial infarction. Am J Cardiol 39:588, 1977.

320. Ruffolo RR Jr, Yaden E: Vascular effects of the stereoisomers of dobutamine. J Pharmacol Exp Ther 224:46, 1983.

321. Opie L, Sonnenblick E, Kaplan N, Thadani V: Beta-blocking agents. In Opie LH: Drugs for the Heart, 3rd ed. Philadelphia, WB Saunders, 1991.

322. Unverferth DV, Blanford M, Kates RE, et al: Tolerance to dobutamine after a 72-hour continuous infusion. Am J Med 69:262, 1980.

323. Leier CV, Huss P, Lewis RP, Unverferth DV: Drug-induced conditioning in congestive heart failure. Circulation 65:1382, 1982.

324. Krell MJ, Kline EM, Bates ER, et al: Intermittent, ambulatory dobutamine infusions in patients with severe congestive heart failure. Am Heart J 112:787, 1986.

325. Spitzer W, Suissa S, Ernst P, et al: The use of β-agonists and the risk of death and near death from asthma. N Engl J Med 326:501, 1992.

326. Robin E, McCauley R: Sudden cardiac death in bronchial asthma, and inhaled β-adrenergic agonists. Chest 101:1699, 1992.

327. Ziment I: Infrequent cardiac deaths occur in bronchial asthma. Chest 101:1703, 1992.

328. Caritis SN, Edelstone DI, Mueller-Heubach E: Pharmacologic inhibition of preterm labor. Am J Obstet Gynecol 133:557, 1979.

329. Wagner JM, Morton MJ, Johnson KA, et al: Terbutaline and maternal cardiac function. JAMA 246:2697, 1981.

330. The Canadian Preterm Labor Investigators Group: Treatment of preterm labor with the β-adrenergic agonist ritodrine. N Engl J Med 327:308, 1992.

331. Hoffman B, Lefkowitz R: Adrenergic receptor antagonists. In Gilman A, Rall T, Nies A, Taylor P (eds): Goodman and Gilman's the Pharmacological Basis of Therapeutics, 8th ed. New York, Pergamon Press, 1990, p 221.

332. Shojania KG, Duncan BW, McDonald KM, et al: Making health care safer: A critical analysis of patient safety practices. Evidence report/technology assessment no. 43. Prepared by the University of California at San Francisco-Stanford University Evidence-based Practice Center under Contract No. 290-97-0013, AHRQ publication no. 01-E058. Rockville, MD, Agency for Healthcare Research and Quality, July 2001.

333. Stone JG, Foex P, Sear JW, et al: Myocardial ischemia in untreated hypertensive patients: Effect of a single small oral dose of a beta-adrenergic blocking agent. Anesthesiology 68:495, 1988.

334. Mangano DT, Layug EL, Wallace A, et al: Effect of atenolol on mortality and cardiovascular morbidity after noncardiac surgery. Multicenter Study of Perioperative Ischemia Research Group. N Engl J Med 335:1713, 1996.

335. Poldermans D, Boersma E, Bax JJ, et al: The effect of biso-prolol on perioperative mortality and myocardial infarction in high-risk patients undergoing vascular surgery. Dutch Echocardiographic Cardiac Risk Evaluation Applying Stress Echocardiography Study Group. N Engl J Med 341:1789, 1999.

336. Raby KE, Brull SJ, Timimi F, et al: The effect of heart rate control on myocardial ischemia among high-risk patients after vascular surgery. Anesth Analg 88:477, 1999.

337. Urban MK, Markowitz SM, Gordon MA, et al: Postoperative prophylactic administration of beta-adrenergic blockers in patients at risk for myocardial ischemia. Anesth Analg 90:1257, 2000.

338. Stevenson LW: Beta-blockers for stable heart failure. N Engl J Med 346:1346, 2002.

339. Kaplan N: Treatment of hypertension: Drug therapy. *In* Kaplan N (ed): Clinical Hypertension, 5th ed. Baltimore, Williams & Wilkins, 1990, p 182.

340. Rutherford J, Braunwald E: Chronic ischemic heart disease. *In* Braunwald E (ed): Heart Disease, A Textbook of Cardiovascular Medicine. Philadelphia, WB Saunders, 1992, p 1292.

341. Conolly ME, Kersting F, Dollery CT: The clinical pharmacology of β-adrenoreceptor blocking drugs. Prog Cardiovasc Dis 19:203, 1976.

342. Salpeter SS, Ormiston T, Salpeter E, et al: Cardioselective beta-blockers for chronic obstructive pulmonary disease. Cochrane Database Syst Rev 2:CD003566, 2002.

343. MERIT-HF Study Group: Effect of metoprolol CR/XL in chronic heart failure: Metoprolol CR/XL Randomized Intervention Trial in Congestive Heart Failure (MERIT-HF). Lancet 353:2001, 1999.

344. CIBIS-II Investigators and Committees: The Cardiac Insufficiency Bisoprolol Study II (CIBIS-II): A randomized trial. Lancet 353:9, 1999.

345. Kostis JB, Frishman W, Hosler MH, et al: Treatment of angina pectoris with pindolol: The significance of intrinsic sympathomimetic activity of beta-blockers. Am Heart J 104:496, 1982.

346. Miller N: Effects of adrenoceptor-blocking drugs on plasma lipoprotein concentrations. Am J Cardiol 60:17E, 1987.

347. Furberg C: Secondary prevention trials after acute myocardial infarction. Am J Cardiol 60:28A, 1987.

348. Rango R, Langlois S: Comparison of withdrawal phenomena after propranolol, metoprolol, and pindolol. Am Heart J 104:437, 1982.

349. Streufert S, DePadova A, McGlynn T, et al: Impact of β-blockade on complex cognitive functioning. Am Heart J 116:311, 1988.

350. Gengo FM, Huntoor L, McHugh WB: Lipid-soluble and water-soluble beta-blockers. Comparison of the central nervous system depressant effect. Arch Intern Med 147:39, 1987.

351. Fortier NL, Snyder LM, Palek J, et al: Effect of propranolol on normal human erythrocytes. J Lab Clin Med 89:41, 1977.

352. Oski FA, Miller LD, Delivoria-Papadopoulos M, et al: Oxygen affinity in red cells: Changes induced in vivo by propranolol. Science 175:1372, 1972.

353. Zipes DG: Management of cardiac arrhythmias: Pharmacological, electrical and surgical techniques. *In* Braunwald E (ed): Heart Disease: A Textbook of Cardiovascular Medicine, 4th ed. Philadelphia, WB Saunders, 1992, p 628.

354. Henry J, Cassidy S: Membrane stabilizing activity: A major cause of fatal poisoning. Lancet 1:1414, 1986.

355. Auerbach AD, Goldman L: ß-Blockers and reduction of cardiac events in noncardiac surgery: Scientific review. JAMA 287:1435, 2002.

356. Viljoen JF, Estafanous G, Kellner GA: Propanolol and cardiac surgery. J Thorac Cardiovasc Surg 64:826, 1972.

357. DeBruijn N, Reves JG, Croughnell N, Knopes K: Comparison of hemodynamic responses to isoproterenol infusion and surgical stress in patients given cardioselective and non-cardioselective β-adrenergic antagonists. Anesth Analg 66:637, 1987.

358. Olsson G, Rehnqvist N, Sjogren A, et al: Long-term treatment with metoprolol after myocardial infarction: Effect on 3-year mortality and morbidity. J Am Coll Cardiol 5:1428, 1985.

359. Yusuf S: Interventions that potentially limit myocardial infarct size: Overview of clinical trials. Am J Cardiol 60:11A, 1987.

360. ISIS-1 (First International Study of Infarct Survival) Collaborative Group: Randomized trial of intravenous atenolol among 16,027 cases of suspected acute myocardial infarction: ISIS-1. Lancet 1:57, 1986.

361. Yusuf S, Peto R, Lewis J, et al: Beta blockade during and after myocardial infarction: An overview of the randomized trials. Prog Cardiovasc Dis 27:335, 1985.

362. The TIMI Study Group: Comparison of invasive and conservative strategies after treatment with intravenous tissue plasminogen activator in acute myocardial infarction. N Engl J Med 320:618, 1989.

363. Ryden L, Ariniego R, Arnman K, et al: A double-blind trial of metoprolol in acute myocardial infarction. Effects on ventricular tachyarrhythmias. N Engl J Med 308:614, 1983.

364. Bristow MR, Gilbert EM, Abraham WT, et al: Carvedilol produces dose-related improvements in left ventricular function and survival in subjects with chronic heart failure. MOCHA Investigators. Circulation 94:2807, 1996.

365. Packer M, Colucci WS, Sackner-Bernstein JD, et al: Double blind, placebo-controlled study of the effects of carvedilol in patients with moderate to severe heart failure. The PRECISE Trial: Prospective Randomized Evaluation of Carvedilol on Symptoms and Exercise. Circulation 94:2793, 1996.

366. Eichhorn EJ, Bristow MR: Medical therapy can improve the biological properties of the chronically failing heart. A new era in the treatment of heart failure. Circulation 94:2285, 1996.

367. Communal C, Singh K, Sawyer D, et al: Opposing effects of β1- and β2-adrenergic receptors on cardiac myocyte apopto-sis: Role of a pertussis toxin-sensitive G protein. Circulation 100:2210, 1999.

368. Eichhorn EJ, Bristow MR: Practical guidelines for initiation of beta-adrenergic blockade in patients with chronic heart failure. Am J Cardiol 79:794, 1997.

369. Bristow MR: β-Adrenergic receptor blockade in chronic heart failure. Circulation 101:558, 2000.

370. Joint National Committee on Detection, Evaluation and Treatment of High Blood Pressure: The fifth report of the Joint National Committee on Detection, Evaluation and Treatment of High Blood Pressure (JNC-V). Arch Intern Med 153:154, 1993.

371. Frishman W: Pindolol: A new β-adrenoceptor antagonist with partial agonist activity. N Engl J Med 308:940, 1983.

372. Van den Meiracker AH, Man in't Veld AJ, Ritsema van Eck HJ, et al: Hemodynamic and hormonal adaptations to β-adrenoceptor blockade: A 24-hour study of acebutolol, atenolol, pindolol, and propranolol in hypertensive patients. Circulation 78:957, 1988.

373. Man in't Veld AJ, Van den Meiracker AH, Schalekamp MA: Do beta-blockers really increase peripheral vascular resistance? Review of the literature and new observations under basal conditions. Am J Hypertens 1:91, 1988.

374. Shand D: Propanolol. N Engl J Med 293:280, 1975.

375. Platia E, Fitzpatrick P, Wallis D, et al: Esmolol vs verapamil for the treatment of recent-onset atrial fibrillation/flutter. J Am Coll Cardiol 11:170A, 1988.

376. Waldo AL, Camm AJ, deRuyter H, et al: Effect of D-sotalol on mortality in patients with left ventricular dysfunction after recent and remote myocardial infarction. Lancet 348:7, 1996.

377. Doggrell SA, Brown L: D-Sotalol: Death by the SWORD or deserving of further consideration for clinical use? Expert Opin Invest Drugs 9:1625, 2000.

378. DeSanctis RW, Doroghazi RM, Austen WG, Buckley MJ: Aortic dissection. N Engl J Med 317:1060, 1987.

379. Grubb BP, Sirio C, Zelis R: Intravenous labetalol in acute aortic dissection. JAMA 258:78, 1987.

380. Wiersinga WM, Touber JL: The influence of β-adrenergic blocking agents on plasma thyroxine and triiodothyronine. J Clin Endocrinol Metab 45:293, 1977.

381. Miller RR, Olson HG, Amsterdam EA, Mason OT: Propanolol-withdrawal rebound phenomenon: Exacerbation of coronary events after abrupt cessation of antianginal therapy. N Engl J Med 292:416, 1975.

382. Psaty B, Koepsell T, Wagner E, et al: The relative risk of incident coronary heart disease associated with recently stopping the use of β-blockers. JAMA 263:1653, 1990.

383. Cleophas T, Kauw F: Pressor responses from non-cardioselective beta-blockers. Angiology 39:587, 1988.

384. Strauss W, Parisi A: Combined use of calcium-channel and β-adrenergic blockers for the treatment of chronic stable angina. Ann Intern Med 109:570, 1988.

385. Wayne VS, Harper RW, Laufer E, et al: Adverse interaction between β-adrenergic blocking drugs and verapamil: Report of three cases. Aust N Z J Med 12:285, 1982.

386. Douglas-Jones A, Baber N, Lee A: Once daily propranolol in the treatment of mild to moderate hypertension: A dose range finding study. Eur J Clin Pharmacol 14:163, 1978.

387. Lichtman M, Cohen J, Murphy M, et al: Effect of propranolol on oxygen binding to hemoglobin in vitro and in vivo. Circulation 49:881, 1974.

388. Schrumpf JD, Sheps DS, Wolfson S, et al: Altered hemoglobin-oxygen affinity with long-term propranolol therapy in patients with coronary artery disease. Am J Cardiol 40:76, 1977.

389. Pendleton RG, Newman DJ, Sherman SS, et al: Effect of propranolol upon the hemoglobin-oxygen dissociation curve. J Pharmacol Exp Ther 180:647, 1972.

390. Hoffman BB, Lefkowitz RJ: Catecholamines, sympathomimetic drugs, and adrenergic receptor antagonists. In Hardman JG, Limbird LE, Molinoff PB, et al (eds): Goodman and Gilman's The Pharmacological Basis of Therapeutics. New York, McGraw-Hill, 1996.

391. Bernstein JS, Ebert TJ, Stowe DF, et al: Partial attenuation of hemodynamic responses to rapid sequence induction and intubation with labetalol. J Clin Anesth 1:444, 1989.

392. Huey J, Thomas JP, Hendricks DR, et al: Clinical evaluation of labetalol for the treatment of hypertensive urgency. Am J Hypertens 1:284S, 1988.

393. Gabrielson G, Lingham R. Dimich I, et al: Comparative study of labetalol and hydralazine in the treatment of postoperative hypertension [abstract]. Anesth Analg 66:S63, 1987.

394. Skrobic J, Cruise C, Webster R, et al: Labetalol vs nitroprusside in hypertension post coronary-bypass surgery. Am J Hypertens 2:1295, 1989.

395. Lavies NG, Meiklejohn BH, May AE, et al: Hypertensive and catecholamine response to tracheal intubation in patients with pregnancy-induced hypertension. Br J Anaesth 63:429, 1989.

396. Jouppilla P, Kirkinen P, Koivula A: Labetalol does not alter the placental and fetal blood flow or maternal prostanoids in pre-eclampsia. Br J Obstet Gynaecol 93:543, 1986.

397. Dupont AG, Van der Niepen P, Taeymans Y, et al: Effect of carvedilol on ambulatory blood pressure, renal hemodynamics, and cardiac function in essential hypertension. J Cardiovasc Pharmacol 10(Suppl 1):S130, 1987.

398. Eggertsen R, Sivertsson R, Adren L, et al: Haemodynamic effects of carvedilol, a new β-adrenoceptor blocker and precapillary vasodilator in essential hypertension. J Hypertens 2:529, 1984.

399. Leonetti G, Sempieri L, Cuspidi C, et al: Resting and postexercise hemodynamic effects of carvedilol, a β-adrenergic blocker and precapillary vasodilator in hypertensive patients. J Cardiovasc Pharmacol 10(Suppl 1):S94, 1987.

400. Omvik P, Lund-Johansen P: Acute haemodynamic effects of carvedilol in essential hypertension at rest and during exercise. Eur Heart J 12:736, 1991.

401. Cervantes Escarcega JL, Ruiz de Chavez A, Guadalajara Boo J: Double blind study of the efficacy and tolerability of carvedilol vs nifedipine S.R. in uncomplicated essential hypertension [in Spanish]. Invest Med Int 19:142, 1992.

402. Ostergren J, Storstein L, Karlberg BE, et al: Quality of life in hypertensive patients treated with either carvedilol or enalapril. Blood Press 5:41, 1996.

403. Ruilope LM, Group CS: Comparison of a new vasodilating beta blocker, carvedilol, with atenolol in the treatment of mild to moderate essential hypertension. Am J Hypertens 7:129, 1994.

404. Weber K, Bohmeke T, van der Does R, et al: Comparison of the hemodynamic effects of metoprolol and carvedilol in hypertensive patients. Cardiovasc Drug Ther 10:113, 1996.

405. Albergati F, Paterno E, Venuti RP, et al: Comparison of the effects of carvedilol and nifedipine in patients with essential hypertension and non-insulin-dependent mellitus. J Cardiovasc Pharmacol 19(Suppl 1):S86, 1992.

406. Louis WJ, Krum H, Conway EL: A risk-benefit assessment of carvedilol in the treatment of cardiovascular disorders. Drug Saf 11:86, 1994.

407. van der Does R, Eberhardt R, Derr I, et al: Efficacy and safety of carvedilol in comparison with nifedipine sustained-release in chronic stable angina. J Cardiovasc Pharmacol 19(Suppl 1):S122, 1992.

408. Basu S, Senior R, van der Does R, et al: Carvedilol reduces adverse cardiac events following acute myocardial infarction [abstract]. Circulation 92(Suppl 1):1, 1995.

409. Senior R, Basu S, Lahiri A: Carvedilol prevents remodeling and improves prognosis in patients with left ventricular dysfunction following acute myocardial infarction [abstract]. J Am Coll Cardiol 27(Suppl A):319A, 1996.

410. Zehender M, Faber T, Schnabel P, et al: Benefits and hazards of carvedilol in unstable angina: A double-blind placebo controlled, randomized study [abstract]. Circulation 92(Suppl 1):I, 1995.

411. Cohn JN, Fowler MB, Bristow MA, et al: Effect of carvedilol in severe chronic heart failure [abstract]. J Am Coll Cardiol 27(Suppl A):169A, 1996.

412. Colucci WS, Packer M, Bristow MR, et al: Carvedilol inhibits clinical progression in patients with mild symptoms of heart failure. Circulation 94:2800, 1996.

413. Bristow MR, Gilbert EM, Abraham WT, et al: Effects of carvedilol on LV function and mortality in diabetic versus nondiabetic patients with ischemic or nonischemic dilated cardiomyopathy [abstract]. Circulation 94(Suppl 1):I, 3879, 1996.

414. Gray R, Bateman T, Czer L, et al: Comparison of esmolol and nitroprusside for acute post-cardiac surgical hypertension. Am J Cardiol 59:887, 1987.

415. Reves JG, Croughwell ND, Hawkins E, et al: Esmolol for treatment of intraoperative tachycardia and/or hypertension in patients having cardiac operations, bolus loading technique. J Thorac Cardiovasc Surg 100:221, 1990.

416. Oxorn D, Knox JW, Hill J: Bolus doses of esmolol for the prevention of perioperative hypertension and tachycardia. Can J Anaesth 37:206, 1990.

417. Wallis DE, Littman WJ, Scanlon PJ: Safety and efficacy of esmolol for unstable angina pectoris. Am J Cardiol 62:1033, 1988.

418. Kirshenbaum JM, Kloner RJ, McGowan N, Antman EM: Use of an ultrashort-acting β-receptor blocker (esmolol) in patients with acute myocardial ischemia and relative contraindications to beta-blockade therapy. J Am Coll Cardiol 12:773, 1988.

419. Beart PM, Rowe PR, Louis WJ: Alpha methyl adrenaline is a central metabolite of α-methyldopa. J Pharm Pharmacol 35:519, 1980.

420. Tung C-S, Goldberg MR, Hollister AS, et al: Central and peripheral cardiovascular effects of α-methylepinephrine. J Pharmacol Exp Ther 227:484, 1983.

421. Triner L, Baer L, Gallagher R, et al: Use of metyrosine in the anesthetic management of patients with catecholamine-secreting tumors. Br J Anaesth 54:1333, 1982.

422. Bigger J, Hoffman B: Antiarrhythmic drugs. In Gilman A, Rall T, Nies A, Taylor P (eds): Goodman and Gilman's the Pharmacological Basis of Therapeutics, 8th ed. New York, Pergamon Press, 1990, p 840.

423. Baldessarini R: Drugs and the treatment of psychiatric disorders. In Gilman A, Rall T, Nies A, Taylor P (eds): Goodman and Gilman's the Pharmacological Basis of Therapeutics. New York, Pergamon Press, 1990.

424. The Parkinson Study Group: Effect of deprenyl on the progression of disability in early Parkinson's disease. N Engl J Med 321:1364, 1989.

425. Roizen MF: Monoamine oxidase inhibitors: Are we condemned to relive history, or is history no longer relevant [letter]? J Clin Anesth 2:293, 1990.

426. Doyle DJ: Ketamine induction and monoamine oxidase inhibitors. J Clin Anesth 2:324, 1990.

427. Materson BJ: Adverse effects of angiotensin-converting enzyme inhibitors in antihypertensive therapy with focus on quinapril. Am J Cardiol 69:46C, 1992.

428. ISIS-4 (Fourth International Study of Infarct Survival) Collaborative Group: A randomized factorial trial assessing early oral captopril, oral mononitrate, and intravenous magnesium sulphate in 58,050 patients with suspected acute myocardial infarction. Lancet 345:669, 1995.

429. Nash DT: Comparative properties of angiotensin-converting enzyme inhibitors: Relations with inhibition of tissue angiotensin-converting enzyme and potential clinical implications. Am J Cardiol 69:26C, 1992.

430. Raia JJ Jr, Barone JA, Byerly WG, Lacy CR: Angiotensin-converting enzyme inhibitors: A comparative review. DICP 24:506, 1990.

431. Weber MA: Safety issues during antihypertensive treatment with angiotensin converting enzyme inhibitors. Am J Med 84(Suppl 4A):16, 1988.

432. Warner JN, Rush JE: Safety profiles of the angiotensin-converting enzyme inhibitors. Drugs 35(Suppl 5):89, 1988.

433. Ferner RE: Adverse effects of angiotensin-converting-enzyme inhibitors. Adverse Drug React Acute Poisoning Rev 141:528, 1990.

434. Jong P, Demers C, McKelvie RS, et al: Angiotensin receptor blockers in heart failure: Meta-analysis of randomized controlled trials. J Am Coll Cardiol 39:463, 2002.

435. Khan JA: Atropine poisoning in Hawthorne's The Scarlet Letter. N Engl J Med 311:414, 1984.

436. Ziskind A: Transdermal scopolamine-induced psychosis. Postgrad Med 84:73, 1988.

437. Wilkinson JA: Side-effects of transdermal scopolamine. J Emerg Med 5:389, 1987.

438. Gross NJ: Ipratropium bromide. N Engl J Med 319:486, 1988.

439. Brown JH: Atropine, scopolamine and related antimuscarinic drugs. In Gilman A, Rall T, Nies A, Taylor P (eds): Goodman and Gilman's the Pharmacological Basis of Therapeutics, 8th ed. New York, Pergamon Press, 1990, p 150.

440. Alcalay M, Izraeli S, Wallach-Kapon R, et al: Paradoxical pharmacodynamic effect of atropine on parasympathetic control: A study by spectral analysis of heart rate fluctuations. Clin Pharmacol Ther 52:518, 1992.

441. Cromwell EB, Ketchum JS: The treatment of scopolamine-induced delirium with physostigmine. Clin Pharmacol Ther 8:409, 1967.

442. Heiser JF, Wilbert D: Reversal of delirium induced by tricyclic antidepressant drugs with physostigmine. Am J Psychiatry 131:1275, 1974.

443. Bidwai AV, Stanley TH, Rogers C, et al: Reversal of diazepam-induced post-anesthetic somnolence with physostigmine. Anesthesiology 51:256, 1979.

444. Ghoneim MM, Dembo JB, Block RI: Time course of antagonism of sedative and amnesic effects of diazepam by flumazenil. Anesthesiology 70:899, 1989.

445. Flacke WE, Flacke JE: Cholinergic and anticholinergic agents. In Smith NT, Corbasci A (eds): Drug Interactions in Anesthesia, 2nd ed. Philadelphia, Lea & Febiger, 1986, p 160.

446. Taylor P: Agents acting at the neuromuscular junction and autonomic ganglia. In Gilman A, Rall T, Nies A, Taylor P (eds): Goodman and Gilman's the Pharmacological Basis of Therapeutics, 8th ed. New York, Pergamon Press, 1990.

447. Paton W: The principles of ganglionic block. In Scientific Basis of Medicine. London, Athlone Press, London, 1954.

448. Charlson ME, MacKenzie CR, Gold JP: Preoperative autonomic function abnormalities in patients with diabetes mellitus and patients with hypertension. J Am Coll Surg 179:1, 1994.

449. Ewing DJ, Martyn CN, Young RJ: The value of cardiovascular autonomic function tests: 10 years' experience in diabetes. Diabetes Care 8:491, 1985.

450. Thomas J, Fouad FM, Tarazi RC, et al: Evaluation of plasma catecholamines in humans. Correlation of resting levels with cardiac responses to beta-blocking and sympatholytic drugs. Hypertension 5:858, 1983.

451. Best JD, Halter JB: Release and clearance rates of epinephrine in man: Importance of arterial measurements. J Clin Endocrinol Metab 55:263, 1982.

452. Esler M, Thompson J, Kaye D, et al: Effects of aging on the responsiveness of the human cardiac sympathetic nerves to stressors. Circulation 91:351, 1995.

453. Yamaguchi I, Kopin IJ: Plasma catecholamine and blood pressure responses to sympathetic stimulation in pithed rats. Am J Physiol 237:H305, 1979.

454. Adams K: Current perspectives on β-receptor antagonists in the treatment of symptomatic ventricular dysfunction. Pharmacotherapy 16(Pt 2):69S, 1996.

455. Eichhorn EJ: Do β-blockers have a role in patients with congestive heart failure? Cardiol Clin 12:133, 1994.

456. Rundqvist B, Eisenhofer G, Elam M, Friberg P: Attenuated cardiac sympathetic responsiveness during dynamic exercise in patients with heart failure. Circulation 95:940, 1997.

457. Klassen G, Bramwell R, Bromage P, Zborowska-Sluis D: Effect of acute sympathectomy by epidural anesthesia on the canine coronary circulation. Anesthesiology 52:8, 1980.

458. Bland J, Lowenstein E: Halothane-induced decrease in experimental myocardial ischemia in the non-failing canine heart. Anesthesiology 45:287, 1976.

459. Anand K, Hickey P: Halothane-morphine compared with high dose sufentanil for anesthesia and postoperative analgesia in neonatal cardiac surgery. N Engl J Med 326:1, 1992.

460. Roizen MF, Lampe GH, Benefiel DJ, et al: Is increased operative stress associated with worse outcome [abstract]? Anesthesiology 67:A1, 1987.

461. Scott NB, Kehlet H: Regional anaesthesia and surgical morbidity. Br J Surg 75:299, 1988.

462. Yeager M, Glass D, Neff R, Brinck-Johnsen T: Epidural anesthesia and analgesia in high-risk surgical patients. Anesthesiology 66:729, 1987.

463. Breslow MJ, Jordan DA, Christopherson R, et al: Epidural morphine decreases postoperative hypertension by attenuating hypertension by attenuating sympathetic nervous system hyperactivity. JAMA 261:3577, 1989.

464. Christopherson R, Beattie C, Frank SM, et al: Perioperative morbidity in patients randomized to epidural or general anesthesia for lower extremity vascular surgery. Anesthesiology 79:422, 1993.

465. Parker SD, Breslow MJ, Frank SM, et al: Catecholamine and cortisol responses to lower extremity revascularization: Correlation with outcome variables. Crit Care Med 23:1954, 1995.

466. Selye H: Forty years of stress research: Principal remaining problems and misconceptions. Can Med Assoc J 115:53, 1976.
467. Kehlet H: Manipulation of the metabolic response in clinical practice. World J Surg 24:690, 2000.
468. Bardram L, Funch-Jensen P, Jensen P, et al: Recovery after laparoscopic colonic surgery with epidural analgesia, and early oral nutrition and mobilization. Lancet 345:763, 1995.
469. Ewing DJ, Campbell IW, Clarke BF: The natural history of diabetic autonomic neuropathy. Q J Med 49:95, 1980.
470. Burgos LG, Ebert TJ, Asiddao C, et al: Increased intraoperative cardiovascular morbidity in diabetics with autonomic neuropathy. Anesthesiology 70:591, 1989.
471. Page MM, Watkins PJ: Cardiorespiratory arrest and diabetic autonomic neuropathy. Lancet 1:14, 1978.
472. Ewing DJ, Clarke BF: Diagnosis and management of diabetic autonomic neuropathy. BMJ 285:916, 1982.
473. Davies HEF: Respiratory change in heart rate, sinus arrhythmia in the elderly. Gerontol Clin 17:96, 1975.
474. Gribbin B, Pickering TG, Sleight P, et al: Effect of age and high blood pressure on baroreflex sensitivity in man. Circ Res 29:424, 1971.
475. Kalbfleish JH, Stowe DF, Smith JJ: Evaluation of the heart rate response to the Valsalva maneuver. Am Heart J 95:707, 1978.
476. Rothbaum DA, Shaw DJ, Angell CS, et al: Cardiac performance in the unanesthetized senescent male rat. J Gerontol 28:287, 1974.
477. Sato I, Hasegawa Y, Takahashi N, et al: Age-related changes of cardiac control function in man. With special reference to heart rate control at rest and during exercise. J Gerontol 36:564, 1981.
478. Esler M, Skews H, Leonard P, et al: Age-dependence of noradrenaline kinetics in normal subjects. Clin Sci Lond 60:217, 1981.
479. Esler MD, Turner AG, Kaye DM, et al: Aging effects on human sympathetic neuronal function. Am J Physiol 268:R278, 1995.
480. Nafelski LA, Brown CFG: Action of atropine on the cardiovascular system in normal persons. Arch Intern Med 86:898, 1950.
481. Mancia G, Ferrari A, Gregorini L, et al: Blood pressure and heart rate variabilities in normotensive and hypertensive human beings. Circ Res 53:96, 1983.
482. Ng AV, Callister R, Johnson DG, et al: Sympathetic neural reactivity to stress does not increase with age in healthy humans. Am J Physiol 267:H344, 1994.
483. White M, Roden R, Minobe W, et al: Age-related changes in β-adrenergic neuroeffector systems in the human heart. Circulation 90:1225, 1994.
484. Guaneri T, Filburn CR, Zitnik G, et al: Contractile and biochemical correlates of β-adrenergic stimulation of the aged heart. Am J Physiol 239:H501, 1980.
485. Krall JF, Connelly M, Weisbart R, Tuck ML: Age-related elevation of plasma catecholamine concentration and reduced responsiveness of lymphocyte adenylate cyclase. J Clin Endocrinol Metab 52:863, 1981.
486. Vaz M, Rajkumar C, Wong J, et al: Oxygen consumption in the heart, hepatomesenteric bed, and brain in young and elderly human subjects, and accompanying sympathetic nervous activity. Metabolism 45:1487, 1996.
487. Buchholz J, Duckles SP: Effect of age on prejunctional modulation of norepinephrine release. J Pharmacol Exp Ther 252:159, 1990.
488. Hyland L, Docherty JR: Further examination of the effects of aging on the adrenoceptor responsiveness of the rat vas deferens. Eur J Pharmacol 110:241, 1985.
489. Fernandes F, Salaices CF, Sanchez-Ferrer JL, et al: Effect of aging and hypertension on [3H]noradrenaline release in rat mesenteric artery. J Hypertens 10(Suppl 4):S65, 1992.
490. Supiano MA, Neubig RR, Linares OA, et al: Effects of low-sodium diet on regulation of platelet α2-adrenergic receptors in young and elderly humans. Am J Physiol 256:E339, 1989.
491. Bracken MB, Shepard MJ, Collins WF, et al: A randomized, controlled trial of methylprednisolone or naloxone in the treatment of acute spinal-cord injury. N Engl J Med 322:1405, 1990.
492. Mathias CJ, Christensen NJ, Frankel HL, et al: Cardiovascular control in recently injured tetraplegics in spinal shock. Q J Med 48:273, 1979.
493. Van Lieshout JJ, Imholz BPM, Wesseling KH, et al: Singing-induced hypotension: A complication of high spinal cord lesion. Neth J Med 38:75, 1991.
494. Stjernberg L, Blumberg H, Wallin B: Sympathetic activity in man after spinal cord injury: Outflow to muscle below the lesion. Brain 109:695, 1986.
495. Tollenaeré JP: Atlas of the Three-Dimensional Structure of Drugs. Amsterdam, Elsevier North-Holland, 1979.
496. Vanhoutte PM: Adrenergic neuroeffector interaction in the blood vessel wall. Fed Proc 37:181, 1978.
497. Standaert F: Donuts and holes: Molecules and muscle relaxants. In Katz R (ed): Muscle Relaxants: Basic and Clinical Aspects. Orlando, FL, Grune & Stratton, 1984.

17 Respiratory Physiology and Respiratory Function during Anesthesia

William C. Wilson and Jonathan L. Benumof

Respiratory Physiology   679
   Normal (Gravity-Determined) Distribution of
      Perfusion, Ventilation, and the Ventilation-
      Perfusion Ratio   679
   Nongravitational Determinants of Pulmonary
      Vascular Resistance and Blood Flow
      Distribution   683
   Other (Nongravitational) Important
      Determinants of Pulmonary Compliance,
      Resistance, Lung Volume, and
      Ventilation   689
   Oxygen and Carbon Dioxide Transport   697
   Pulmonary Microcirculation, Pulmonary
      Interstitial Space, and Pulmonary
      Interstitial Fluid Kinetics (Pulmonary
      Edema)   703

**Respiratory Function during
Anesthesia   705**
   Effect of Anesthetic Depth on Respiratory
      Pattern   705
   Effect of Anesthetic Depth on Spontaneous
      Minute Ventilation   706
   Effect of Preexisting Respiratory Dysfunction on
      the Respiratory Effects of Anesthesia   707
   Effect of Special Intraoperative Conditions on
      the Respiratory Effects of Anesthesia   707
   Mechanisms of Hypoxemia during
      Anesthesia   707
   Mechanisms of Hypercapnia and Hypocapnia
      during Anesthesia   714
   Physiologic Effects of Abnormalities in
      Respiratory Gases   715

RESPIRATORY PHYSIOLOGY

Anesthesiologists require an extensive knowledge of respiratory physiology to care for patients in the operating room and the intensive care unit. Mastery of the normal respiratory physiologic processes is a prerequisite to understanding the mechanisms of impaired gas exchange that occur during anesthesia and surgery and with disease. This chapter is divided into two sections. The first section reviews the normal (gravity-determined) distribution of perfusion and ventilation, the major nongravitational determinants of resistance to perfusion and ventilation, transport of respiratory gases, and the pulmonary reflexes and special functions of the lung. In the second section of this chapter, these processes and concepts are discussed in relation to the general mechanisms of impaired gas exchange during anesthesia and surgery. The text has been updated to reflect recent developments in cellular physiology and molecular biology (e.g., the mechanisms

of hypoxic pulmonary vasoconstriction). The interested reader is referred to other chapters in this book to review the topics of pulmonary function testing (Chapter 26) and pulmonary pharmacology (including control of breathing and effects of anesthetic gases—Chapter 6).

Normal (Gravity-Determined) Distribution of Perfusion, Ventilation, and the Ventilation-Perfusion Ratio

Distribution of Pulmonary Perfusion

Contraction of the right ventricle imparts kinetic energy to the blood in the main pulmonary artery. As the kinetic energy in the main pulmonary artery is dissipated in climbing a vertical hydrostatic gradient, the absolute pressure in the pulmonary artery (Ppa) decreases by 1 cm H_2O per centimeter of vertical distance up the lung (Fig. 17-1). At some height above the heart, Ppa becomes zero (atmospheric), and still higher in the lung, Ppa becomes negative.[1]

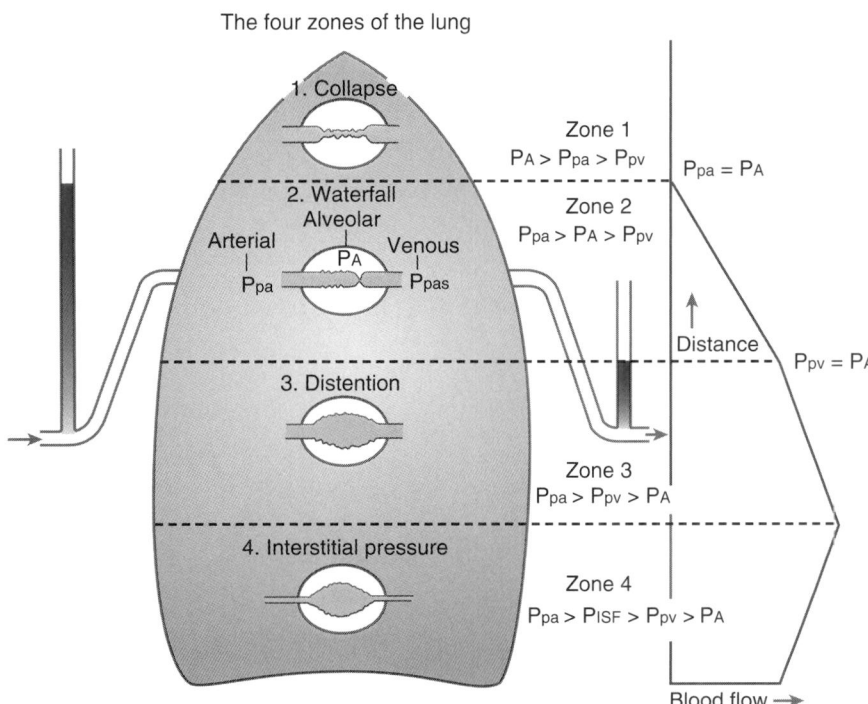

The four zones of the lung

1. Collapse

Zone 1
$P_A > P_{pa} > P_{pv}$

$P_{pa} = P_A$

2. Waterfall

Alveolar

Zone 2
$P_{pa} > P_A > P_{pv}$

Arterial   Venous

P_A

P_{pa} P_{pas}

Distance

$P_{pv} = P_A$

3. Distention

Zone 3
$P_{pa} > P_{pv} > P_A$

4. Interstitial pressure

Zone 4
$P_{pa} > P_{ISF} > P_{pv} > P_A$

Blood flow →

Figure 17–1 Schematic diagram showing the distribution of blood flow in the upright lung. In zone 1, alveolar pressure (P_A) exceeds pulmonary artery pressure (P_{pa}), and no flow occurs because the intra-alveolar vessels are collapsed by the compressing alveolar pressure. In zone 2, P_{pa} exceeds P_A, but P_A exceeds pulmonary venous pressure (P_{pv}). Flow in zone 2 is determined by the P_{pa}-P_A difference ($P_{pa} - P_A$) and has been likened to an upstream river waterfall over a dam. Because P_{pa} increases down zone 2 whereas P_A remains constant, perfusion pressure increases, and flow steadily increases down the zone. In zone 3, P_{pv} exceeds P_A, and flow is determined by the P_{pa}-P_{pv} difference ($P_{pa} - P_{pv}$), which is constant down this portion of the lung. However, transmural pressure across the wall of the vessel increases down this zone, so the caliber of the vessels increases (resistance decreases), and therefore flow increases. Finally, in zone 4, pulmonary interstitial pressure becomes positive and exceeds both P_{pv} and P_A. Consequently, flow in zone 4 is determined by the Ppa–interstitial pressure difference ($P_{pa} - P_{ISF}$). (Redrawn with modification from West JB: Ventilation/Blood Flow and Gas Exchange, 4th ed. Oxford, Blackwell Scientific, 1970.)

In this region, alveolar pressure (P_A) then exceeds P_{pa} and pulmonary venous pressure (P_{pv}), which is very negative at this vertical height. Because the pressure outside the vessels is greater than the pressure inside the vessels, the vessels in this region of the lung are collapsed, and no blood flow occurs (zone 1, $P_A > P_{pa} > P_{pv}$). Because there is no blood flow, no gas exchange is possible, and the region functions as alveolar dead space, or "wasted" ventilation. Little or no zone 1 exists in the lung under normal conditions,[2] but the amount of zone 1 lung may be greatly increased if P_{pa} is reduced, as in oligemic shock, or if P_A is increased, as in the application of excessively large tidal volumes or levels of positive end-expiratory pressure (PEEP) during positive-pressure ventilation.

Further down the lung, absolute P_{pa} becomes positive, and blood flow begins when P_{pa} exceeds P_A (zone 2, $P_{pa} > P_A > P_{pv}$). At this vertical level in the lung, P_A exceeds P_{pv}, and blood flow is determined by the mean $P_{pa} - P_A$ difference rather than by the more conventional $P_{pa} - P_{pv}$ difference (see later).[3] The zone 2 blood flow–alveolar pressure relationship has the same physical characteristics as a waterfall flowing over a dam. The height of the upstream river (before reaching the dam) is equivalent to P_{pa}, and the height of the dam is equivalent to P_A. The rate of water flow over the dam is proportional to only the difference between the height of the upstream river and the dam ($P_{pa} - P_A$), and it does not matter how far below the dam the downstream riverbed (P_{pv}) is. This phenomenon has various names, including the waterfall, Starling resistor, weir (dam made by beavers), and "sluice" effect. Because mean P_{pa} increases down this region of the lung but mean P_A is relatively constant, the mean driving pressure ($P_{pa} - P_A$) increases linearly, and therefore mean blood flow increases linearly. However, respiration and pulmonary blood flow are cyclic phenomena. Therefore, absolute instantaneous P_{pa}, P_{pv}, and P_A are changing continuously, and the relationships among P_{pa}, P_{pv}, and P_A are dynamically determined by the phase lags between the cardiac and respiratory cycles. Consequently, a given point in zone 2 may actually be in either a zone 1 or a zone 3 condition at a given moment, depending on whether the patient is in respiratory systole or diastole or in cardiac systole or diastole.

Still lower in the lung, there is a vertical level at which P_{pv} becomes positive and also exceeds P_A. In this region, blood flow is governed by the pulmonary arteriovenous pressure difference ($P_{pa} - P_{pv}$) (zone 3, $P_{pa} > P_{pv} > P_A$), for here both these vascular pressures exceed P_A, and the capillary systems are thus permanently open and blood flow is continuous. In descending zone 3, gravity causes both absolute P_{pa} and P_{pv} to increase at the same rate, so perfusion pressure ($P_{pa} - P_{pv}$) is unchanged. However, the pressure outside the vessels, namely, pleural pressure (P_{pl}), increases less than P_{pa} and P_{pv}, so the transmural distending pressures ($P_{pa} - P_{pl}$ and $P_{pv} - P_{pl}$) increase down zone 3, the vessel radii increase, vascular resistance decreases, and blood flow therefore increases further.

Finally, whenever pulmonary vascular pressure (PVR) is extremely high, as it is in a severely volume-overloaded patient, in a severely restricted and constricted pulmonary vascular bed, in an extremely dependent lung (far below the vertical level of the left atrium), and in patients with pulmonary embolism or mitral stenosis, fluid may transude out of the pulmonary vessels into the pulmonary interstitial compartment. In addition, pulmonary interstitial edema can be caused by extremely negative Ppl and perivascular hydrostatic pressure, such as may occur in a vigorously spontaneously breathing patient with an obstructed airway (upper airway masses [tumors, hematoma, abscess, edema], laryngospasm [most common], strangulation, infectious processes [epiglottitis, pharyngitis, croup], and vocal cord paralysis), by rapid re-expansion of lung and by the application of very negative Ppl during thoracentesis.[4,5] Transuded pulmonary interstitial fluid may significantly alter the distribution of pulmonary blood flow.

When the flow of fluid into the interstitial space is excessive and cannot be cleared adequately by the lymphatics, it accumulates in the interstitial connective tissue compartment around the large vessels and airways and forms peribronchial and periarteriolar edema fluid cuffs. The transuded pulmonary interstitial fluid fills the pulmonary interstitial space and may eliminate the normally present negative and radially expanding interstitial tension on the extra-alveolar pulmonary vessels. Expansion of the pulmonary interstitial space by fluid causes pulmonary interstitial pressure (PISF) to become positive and exceed Ppv (zone 4, Ppa > PISF > Ppv > PA).[6,7] In addition, the vascular resistance of extra-alveolar vessels may be increased at a very low lung volume (i.e., residual volume); at such volumes the tethering action of the pulmonary tissue on the vessels is also lost, and as a result, PISF increases positively (see the lung volume discussion later).[8,9] Consequently, zone 4 blood flow is governed by the arteriointerstitial pressure difference (Ppa – PISF), which is less than the Ppa – Ppv difference, and therefore zone 4 blood flow is less than zone 3 blood flow. In summary, zone 4 is a region of the lung from which a large amount of fluid has transuded into the pulmonary interstitial compartment or is possibly at a very low lung volume. Both these circumstances produce positive interstitial pressure, which causes compression of extra-alveolar vessels, increased extra-alveolar vascular resistance, and decreased regional blood flow.

It should be evident that as Ppa and Ppv increase, three important changes take place in the pulmonary circulation, namely, recruitment or opening of previously unperfused vessels, distention or widening of previously perfused vessels, and transudation of fluid from very distended vessels.[10,11] Thus, as mean Ppa increases, zone 1 arteries may become zone 2 arteries, and as mean Ppv increases, zone 2 veins may become zone 3 veins. The increase in both mean Ppa and Ppv distends zone 3 vessels according to their compliance and decreases the resistance to flow through them. Zone 3 vessels may become so distended that they leak fluid and become converted to zone 4 vessels. In general, recruitment is the principal change as Ppa and Ppv increase from low to moderate levels, distention is the principal change as Ppa and Ppv increase from moderate to high levels, and finally, transudation is the principal change when Ppa and Ppv increase from high to very high levels.

Distribution of Ventilation

Gravity also causes differences in vertical Ppl, which in turn causes differences in regional alveolar volume, compliance, and ventilation. The vertical gradient of Ppl can best be understood by imagining the lung as a plastic bag

filled with semifluid contents; in other words, it is a viscoelastic structure. Without the presence of a supporting chest wall, the effect of gravity on the contents of the bag would cause the bag to bulge outward at the bottom and inward at the top (it would assume a globular shape). With the lung inside the supporting chest wall, the lung cannot assume a globular shape. However, gravity still exerts a force on the lung to assume a globular shape; this force creates relatively more negative pressure at the top of the pleural space (where the lung pulls away from the chest wall) and relatively more positive pressure at the bottom of the lung (where the lung is compressed against the chest wall) (Fig. 17-2). The density of the lung determines the magnitude of this pressure gradient. Because the lung has about one fourth the density of water, the gradient of Ppl (in cm H_2O) is about one fourth the height of the upright lung (30 cm). Thus, Ppl increases positively by 30/4 = 7.5 cm H_2O from the top to the bottom of the lung.[12]

Because PA is the same throughout the lung, the Ppl gradient causes regional differences in transpulmonary distending pressure (PA – Ppl). Ppl is most positive (least negative) in the dependent basilar lung regions, so alveoli in these regions are more compressed and are therefore considerably smaller than the superior, relatively noncompressed apical alveoli (there is an approximately fourfold volume difference).[13] If regional differences in alveolar volume are translated to a pressure-volume curve for normal lung (Fig. 17-3), the dependent small alveoli are on the midportion and the nondependent large alveoli are on the upper portion of the S-shaped pressure-volume curve.

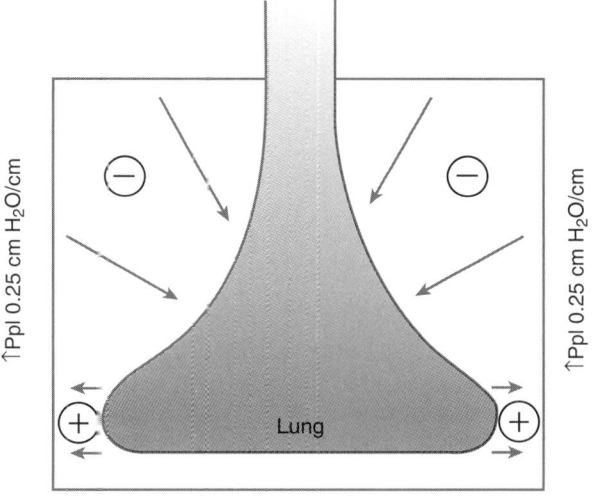

Chest wall

Figure 17–2 Schematic diagram of the lung within the chest wall showing the tendency of the lung to assume a globular shape because of gravity and the lung's viscoelastic nature. The tendency of the top of the lung to collapse inward creates a relatively negative pressure at the apex of the lung, and the tendency of the bottom of the lung to spread outward creates a relatively positive pressure at the base of the lung. Thus, alveoli at the top of the lung tend to be held open and are larger at end-exhalation, whereas those at the bottom tend to be smaller and compressed at end-exhalation. Pleural pressure increases by 0.25 cm H_2O per centimeter of lung dependency.

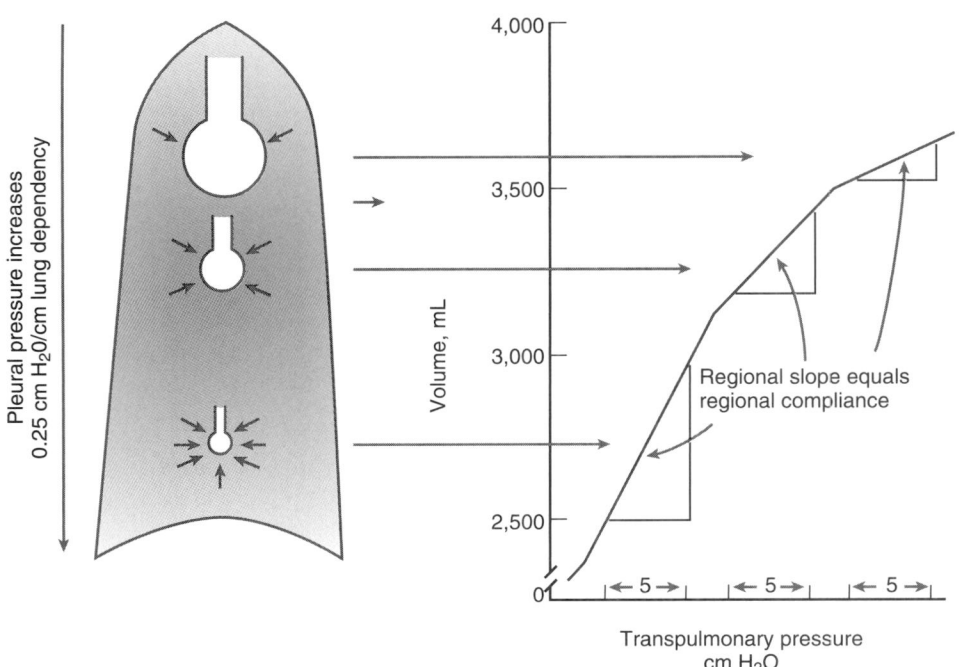

Figure 17–3 Pleural pressure increases by 0.25 cm H_2O every centimeter down the lung. The increase in pleural pressure causes a fourfold decrease in alveolar volume from the top of the lung to the bottom. The caliber of the air passages also decreases as lung volume decreases. When regional alveolar volume is translated over to a regional transpulmonary pressure–alveolar volume curve, small alveoli are on a steep (large slope) portion of the curve, and large alveoli are on a flat (small slope) portion of the curve. Because the regional slope equals regional compliance, the dependent small alveoli normally receive the largest share of the tidal volume. Over the normal tidal volume range (lung volume increases by 500 mL from 2500 mL [normal functional residual capacity] to 3000 mL), the pressure-volume relationship is linear. The lung volume values in this diagram are derived from the upright position.

Because the different regional slopes of the composite curve are equal to the different regional lung compliance values, dependent alveoli are relatively compliant (steep slope), and nondependent alveoli are relatively noncompliant (flat slope). Thus, most of the tidal volume (V_T) is preferentially distributed to dependent alveoli because they expand more per unit pressure change than nondependent alveoli do.

Distribution of the Ventilation-Perfusion Ratio

Both blood flow and ventilation (both on the left-hand vertical axis of Fig. 17-4) increase linearly with distance down the normal upright lung (horizontal axis, reverse polarity).[14] Because blood flow increases from a very low value and more rapidly than ventilation does with distance down the lung, the ventilation-perfusion ($\dot{V}_A/\dot{Q}$) ratio (right-hand vertical axis) decreases rapidly at first and then more slowly.

The $\dot{V}_A/\dot{Q}$ ratio best expresses the amount of ventilation relative to perfusion in any given lung region. Thus, alveoli at the base of the lung are overperfused in relation to their ventilation ($\dot{V}_A/\dot{Q} < 1$). Figure 17-5 shows the calculated ventilation ($\dot{V}_A$) and blood flow ($\dot{Q}$) in liters per minute, the $\dot{V}_A/\dot{Q}$ ratio, and the alveolar partial pressure of oxygen (P_{AO_2}) and partial pressure of carbon dioxide (P_{ACO_2}) in mm Hg for horizontal slices from the top (7% of lung volume), middle (11% of lung volume), and bottom (13% of lung volume) of the lung.[15] P_{AO_2} increases by more than 40 mm Hg from 89 mm Hg at the base to 132 mm Hg at the apex, whereas P_{CO_2} decreases by 14 mm Hg from 42 mm Hg at the bottom to 28 mm Hg at the top. Thus, in keeping with the regional $\dot{V}_A/\dot{Q}$ ratio, the bottom of the lung is relatively hypoxic and hypercapnic as compared with the top of the lung.

$\dot{V}_A/\dot{Q}$ inequalities have different effects on arterial P_{CO_2} (Pa_{CO_2}) than on arterial P_{O_2} (Pa_{O_2}). Blood passing through

underventilated alveoli tends to retain its CO_2 and does not take up enough O_2; blood traversing overventilated alveoli gives off an excessive amount of CO_2 but cannot take up a proportionately increased amount of O_2 because of the flatness of the oxygen-hemoglobin (oxy-Hb) dissociation

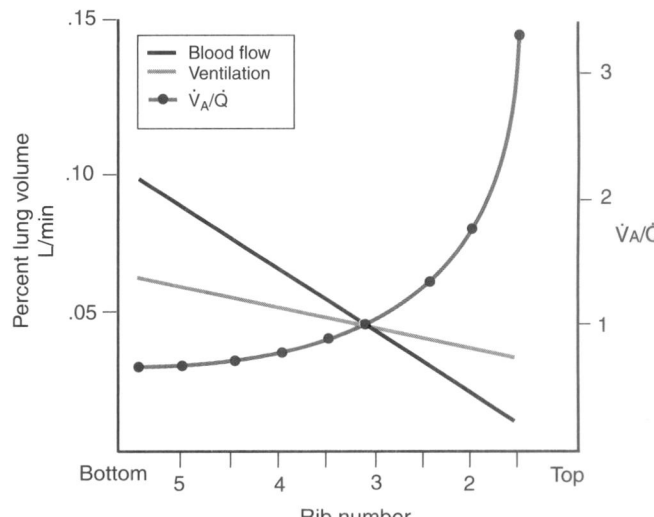

Figure 17–4 Distribution of ventilation and blood flow (left-hand vertical axis) and the ventilation-perfusion ratio ($\dot{V}_A/\dot{Q}$, right-hand vertical axis) in normal upright lung. Both blood flow and ventilation are expressed in liters per minute per percentage of alveolar volume and have been drawn as smoothed-out linear functions of vertical height. The *closed circles* mark the $\dot{V}_A/\dot{Q}$ ratios of horizontal lung slices (three of which are shown in Fig. 17-5). A cardiac output of 6 L/min and a total minute ventilation of 5.1 L/min were assumed. (Redrawn with modification from West JB: Ventilation/Blood Flow and Gas Exchange, 4th ed. Oxford, Blackwell Scientific, 1970.)

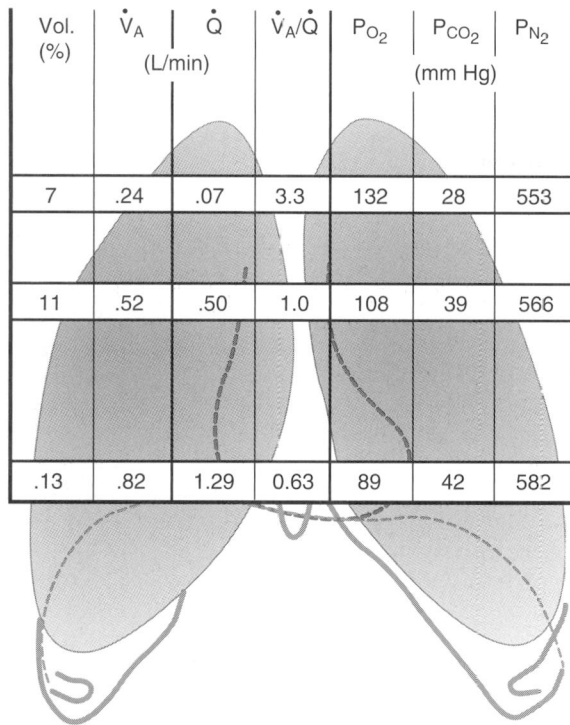

Vol. (%)	$\dot{V}_A$ (L/min)	$\dot{Q}$	$\dot{V}_A/\dot{Q}$	P_{O_2}	P_{CO_2}	P_{N_2}
					(mm Hg)	
7	.24	.07	3.3	132	28	553
11	.52	.50	1.0	108	39	566
	.13	.82	1.29	0.63	89	42	582

Figure 17–5 Ventilation-perfusion ratio ($\dot{V}_A/\dot{Q}$) and the regional composition of alveolar gas. Values for regional flow ($\dot{Q}$), ventilation ($\dot{V}_A$), P_{O_2}, and P_{CO_2} were derived from Figure 17-4. P_{N_2} was obtained by what remains from total gas pressure (which, including water vapor, equals 760 mm Hg). The volumes [Vol. (%)] of the three lung slices are also shown. When compared with the top of the lung, the bottom of the lung has a low $\dot{V}_A/\dot{Q}$ ratio and is relatively hypoxic and hypercapnic. (Redrawn from West JB: Regional differences in gas exchange in the lung of erect man. J Appl Physiol 17:893, 1962.)

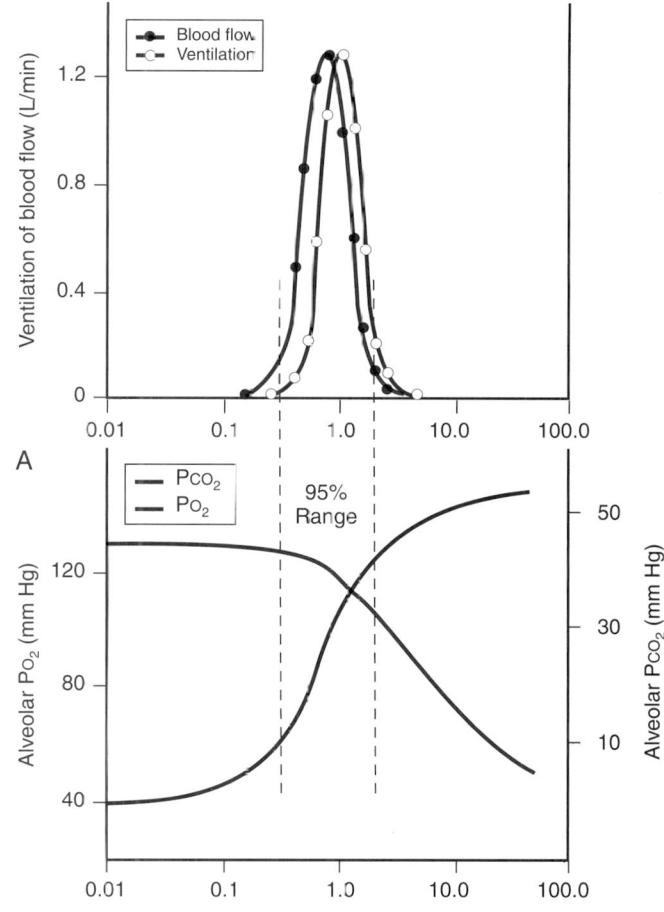

Figure 17–6 A, Average distribution of ventilation-perfusion ratios ($\dot{V}_A/\dot{Q}$) in normal young semirecumbent subjects. The 95% range covers from 0.3 to 2.1 (between *dashed lines*). **B,** Corresponding variations in P_{O_2} and P_{CO_2} in alveolar gas. (Redrawn from West JB: Blood flow to the lung and gas exchange. Anesthesiology 41:124, 1974.)

curve in this region (see Fig. 17-25). Hence, a lung with uneven $\dot{V}_A/\dot{Q}$ relationships can eliminate CO_2 from the overventilated alveoli to compensate for the underventilated alveoli. Thus, with uneven $\dot{V}_A/\dot{Q}$ relationships, Pa_{CO_2}-to-Pa_{CO_2} gradients are small, and Pa_{O_2}-to-Pa_{O_2} gradients are usually large.

In 1974, Wagner and colleagues[16] described a method of determining the continuous distribution of $\dot{V}_A/\dot{Q}$ ratios within the lung based on the pattern of elimination of a series of intravenously infused inert gases. Gases of differing solubility are dissolved in physiologic saline solution and infused into a peripheral vein until a steady state is achieved (20 minutes). Toward the end of the infusion period, samples of arterial and mixed expired gas are collected, and total ventilation and cardiac output ($\dot{Q}_T$) are measured. For each gas, the ratio of arterial to mixed venous concentration (retention) and the ratio of expired to mixed venous concentration (excretion) are calculated, and retention-solubility and excretion-solubility curves are drawn. The retention- and excretion-solubility curves can be regarded as fingerprints of the particular distribution of $\dot{V}_A/\dot{Q}$ ratios that give rise to them.

Figure 17-6 shows the type of distributions found in young, healthy subjects breathing air in the semirecumbent position.[17] The distributions of both ventilation and blood flow are relatively narrow. The upper and lower 9% limits shown (vertical interrupted lines) correspond to $\dot{V}_A/\dot{Q}$ ratios of 0.3 and 2.1, respectively. Note that these young, healthy subjects had no blood flow perfusing areas with very low $\dot{V}_A/\dot{Q}$ ratios, nor did they have any blood flow to unventilated or shunted areas ($\dot{V}_A/\dot{Q} = 0$) or unperfused areas ($\dot{V}_A/\dot{Q} = 8$). Figure 17-6 also shows Pa_{O_2} and Pa_{CO_2} in respiratory units with different $\dot{V}_A/\dot{Q}$ ratios. Within the 95% range of $\dot{V}_A/\dot{Q}$ ratios (0.3 to 2.1), P_{O_2} ranges from 60 to 123 mm Hg, whereas the corresponding P_{CO_2} range is 44 to 33 mm Hg.

Nongravitational Determinants of Pulmonary Vascular Resistance and Blood Flow Distribution

Passive Processes (Cardiac Output and Lung Volume)

Cardiac Output

The pulmonary vascular bed is a high-flow, low-pressure system in health. As $\dot{Q}_T$ increases, pulmonary vascular pressures increase minimally.[18] However, increases in $\dot{Q}_T$ distend open vessels and recruit previously closed vessels.

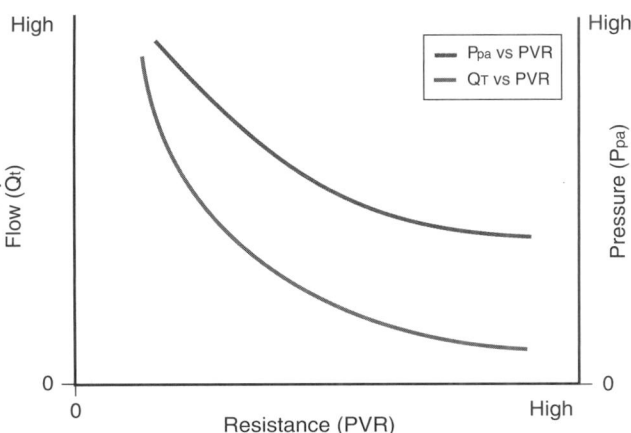

Figure 17–7 Passive changes in pulmonary vascular resistance (PVR) as a function of pulmonary artery pressure (Ppa) and pulmonary blood flow ($\dot{Q}T$) (PVR = Ppa/$\dot{Q}T$). As $\dot{Q}T$ increases, Ppa also increases, but to a lesser extent, and PVR decreases. As $\dot{Q}T$ decreases, Ppa also decreases, but to a lesser extent, and PVR increases. (Redrawn with modification from Fishman AP: Dynamics of the pulmonary circulation. *In* Hamilton WF [ed]: Handbook of Physiology, section 2. Circulation, vol 2. Baltimore, Williams & Wilkins, 1963, p 1667.)

Accordingly, PVR drops because the normal pulmonary vasculature is quite distensible (and partly because of the addition of previously unused vessels to the pulmonary circulation). As a result of the distensibility of the normal pulmonary circulation, an increase in Ppa increases the radius of the pulmonary vessels, which causes PVR to decrease (Fig. 17-7). Conversely, the opposite effect occurs within the pulmonary vessels during a decrease in $\dot{Q}T$. As $\dot{Q}T$ decreases, pulmonary vascular pressures decrease, the radii of the pulmonary vessels are reduced, and PVR consequently increases. The pulmonary vessels of patients with significant pulmonary hypertension are less distensible and act more like rigid pipes. In this setting, Ppa increases much more sharply with any increase in $\dot{Q}T$ because PVR in these stiff vessels does not decrease significantly due to minimal expansion of their radii.

Understanding the relationship among Ppa, PVR, and $\dot{Q}T$ during passive events is a prerequisite to recognition of active vasomotion in the pulmonary circulation (see the next section). Active vasoconstriction occurs whenever $\dot{Q}T$ decreases and Ppa remains either constant or increases. Increased Ppa and PVR have been found to be "a universal feature of acute respiratory failure."[19] Active pulmonary vasoconstriction can increase Ppa and Ppv, thereby contributing to the formation of pulmonary edema, and in that way has a role in the genesis of adult respiratory distress syndrome (ARDS). Active vasodilation occurs whenever $\dot{Q}T$ increases and Ppa either remains constant or decreases. When deliberate hypotension is achieved with sodium nitroprusside, $\dot{Q}T$ often remains constant or increases, but Ppa decreases, and therefore so does PVR.

Lung Volume
Lung volume and PVR have an asymmetric U-shaped relationship because of the varying effect of lung volume on intra- and extra-alveolar vessels, which in both cases

is minimal at functional residual capacity (FRC). FRC is defined as the amount of volume (gas) in the lungs at end-exhalation during normal tidal breathing. Ideally, this means that the patient is inspiring a normal VT, with minimal or no muscle activity or pressure difference between the alveoli and atmosphere at end-exhalation. Total PVR is increased when lung volume is either increased or decreased from FRC[20-22] (Fig. 17-8). The increase in total PVR above FRC is due to alveolar compression of small intra-alveolar vessels, which results in an increase in small-vessel PVR (i.e., creation of zone 1 or zone 2).[24] As a relatively small mitigating or counterbalancing effect to the compression of small vessels, the large extra-alveolar vessels may be expanded by the increased tethering of interstitial connective tissue at high lung volumes (and with spontaneous ventilation only—the negativity of perivascular pressure at high lung volumes). The increase in total PVR below FRC is due to an increase in the PVR of large extra-alveolar vessels (passive effect). The increase in large-vessel PVR is partly due to mechanical tortuosity or kinking of these vessels (passive effect). However, small or grossly atelectatic lungs become hypoxic, and it

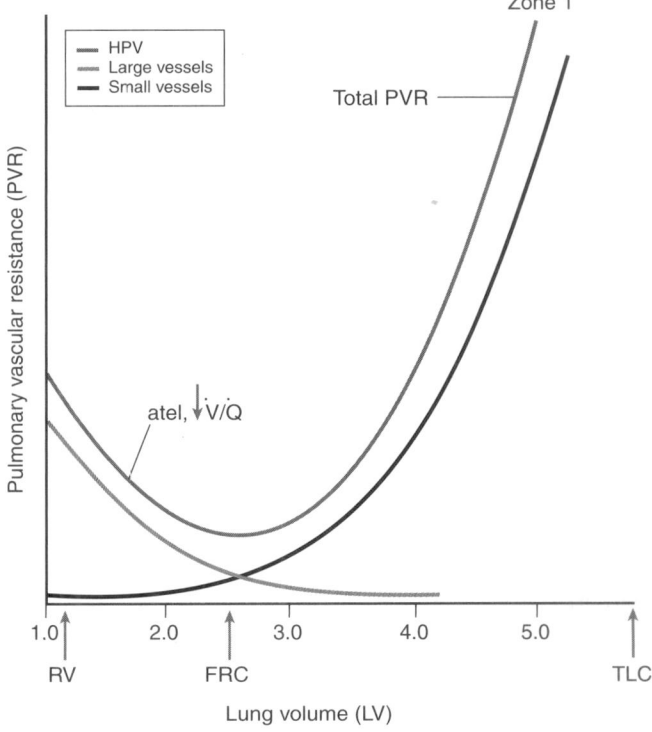

Figure 17–8 Total pulmonary vascular resistance relates to lung volume as an asymmetric U-shaped curve. The trough of the curve occurs when lung volume equals functional residual capacity (FRC). Total pulmonary resistance is the sum of the resistance in small vessels (increased by increasing lung volume) and the resistance in large vessels (increased by decreasing lung volume). The end point for increasing lung volume (toward total lung capacity [TLC]) is the creation of zone 1 conditions, and the end point for decreasing lung volume (toward residual volume [RV]) is the creation of low ventilation-perfusion ($\dot{V}A/\dot{Q}$) and atelectatic (atel) areas that demonstrate hypoxic pulmonary vasoconstriction (HPV). The curve represents a composite of data from references 20, 21, and 23.

has been shown that the mechanism of increased large-vessel PVR in these lungs is due mainly to an active vasoconstrictive mechanism known as hypoxic pulmonary vasoconstriction (HPV).[23] The effect of HPV (discussed in greater detail in the next section) is significant whether the chest is open or closed and whether ventilation is by positive pressure or spontaneous.[25]

Active Processes

Four major categories of active processes affect the pulmonary vascular tone of normal patients: (1) local tissue (endothelial and smooth muscle)-derived autocrine/paracrine products, which act on smooth muscle (Table 17-1); (2) alveolar gas concentrations (chiefly hypoxia), which also act on smooth muscle; (3) neural influences; and (4) humoral (or hormonal) effects of circulating products within the pulmonary capillary bed. The neural and humoral effects work by means of either receptor-mediated mechanisms involving the autocrine/paracrine molecules listed in Table 17-1 or related mechanisms ultimately affecting the smooth muscle cell.[26] These four interrelated systems, each affecting pulmonary vascular tone, will be briefly reviewed in sequence.

Tissue (Endothelial and Smooth Muscle Derived) Products
The pulmonary vascular endothelium synthesizes, metabolizes, and converts a multitude of vasoactive mediators and plays a central role in the regulation of PVR. However, the main effecter site of pulmonary vascular tone is the pulmonary vascular smooth muscle cell (which both senses and produces multiple pulmonary vasoactive compounds).[27] The autocrine/paracrine molecules listed in Table 17-1 are all actively involved in the regulation of pulmonary vascular tone during various conditions. Numerous additional compounds bind to receptors on the endothelial or smooth muscle cell membranes and modulate the levels (and effects) of these vasoactive molecules.

Nitric oxide (NO) is the predominant (but not the only) endogenous vasodilatory compound. It was discovered to be the long-sought-after endothelial-derived relaxant factor (EDRF) over a decade ago by Moncada and Palmer.[28] Since then, a massive amount of laboratory and clinical research has demonstrated the ubiquitous nature of NO and its predominant role in vasodilation of both pulmonary and systemic blood vessels.[29] In the pulmonary endothelial cell, L-arginine is converted to L-citrulline

(by means of NO synthase [NOS]) to produce the small, yet highly reactive NO molecule.[30] Because of its small size, NO can freely diffuse across membranes into the smooth muscle cell, where it binds to the heme moiety of guanylate cyclase (which converts guanosine triphosphate to cyclic guanosine monophosphate [cGMP]).[30] cGMP activates protein kinase G, which dephosphorylates the myosin light chains of pulmonary vascular smooth muscle cells and thereby causes vasodilatation.[30] NOS exists in two forms: constitutive (cNOS) and inducible (iNOS). cNOS is permanently expressed in some cells, including pulmonary vascular endothelial cells, and produces short bursts of NO in response to changing levels of calcium and calmodulin and sheer stress. The cNOS enzyme is also stimulated by linked membrane-based receptors that bind numerous molecules in the blood (e.g., acetylcholine, bradykinin).[30] In contrast, iNOS is usually only produced as a result of inflammatory mediators and cytokines and, when stimulated, will produce large quantities of NO for an extended duration.[30] There is now ample and long-standing evidence that NO is produced in normal lungs and contributes to the maintenance of low PVR.[31,32]

Endothelin-1 (ET-1) is a recently discovered pulmonary vasoconstrictor.[33] The endothelins are 21–amino acid peptides produced by a variety of cells. ET-1 is the only family member produced in pulmonary endothelial cells, and it is also produced in vascular smooth muscle cells.[33] ET-1 exerts its major vascular effects through activation of two distinct G protein–coupled receptors (ETA and ETB). ETA receptors are found in the medial smooth muscle layers of the pulmonary (and systemic) blood vessels and in atrial and ventricular myocardium.[33] When stimulated, ETA receptors induce vasoconstriction and cellular proliferation by increasing intracellular calcium.[34] ETB receptors are localized on endothelial cells and some smooth muscle cells.[35] Activation of ETB receptors stimulates the release of NO and prostacyclin, thereby promoting pulmonary vasodilation and inhibiting apoptosis.[36] Additionally, the ET-1 receptor antagonist bosentan showed modest improvement in the treatment of pulmonary hypertension.[37] Recently, the more selective ETA receptor antagonist sitaxsentan showed additional benefit in improving pulmonary hypertension.[38] However, both ET-1 receptor antagonists (bosentan and sitaxsentan) are associated with an increased risk of liver toxicity.[39] In summary, it appears that there is a normal

Table 17–1   Local tissue (autocrine/paracrine) molecules involved in active control of pulmonary vascular tone

Molecule	Subtype (Abbreviation)	Site of Origin	Site of Action	Response
Nitric oxide	NO	Endothelium	Sm. muscle	Vasodilation
Endothelin	ET-1	Endothelium	Sm. muscle (ETA receptor)	Vasoconstriction
	ET-1	Endothelium	Endothelium (ETB receptor)	Vasodilation
Prostaglandin	PGI$_2$	Endothelium	Endothelium	Vasodilation
Prostaglandin	PGF$_2\alpha$	Endothelium	Sm. muscle	Vasoconstriction
Thromboxane	TXA$_2$	Endothelium	Sm. muscle	Vasoconstriction
Leukotriene	LTB$_4$-LTE$_4$	Endothelium	Sm. muscle	Vasoconstriction

ETA receptor, endothelin-1 receptor located on the smooth muscle cell membrane; ETB receptor, endothelin-1 receptor located on the endothelial cell membrane; Sm. muscle, pulmonary arteriole smooth muscle cell.

balance between NO and ET-1, with a slight predominance toward NO production and vasodilation in health.

Similarly, various eicosanoids are elaborated by the pulmonary vascular endothelium, with a balance toward the vasodilatory compounds in health. Prostaglandin I_2 (PGI_2), now known as epoprostenol (previously known as prostacyclin), causes vasodilation and is continuously elaborated in small amounts in healthy endothelium. In contrast, thromboxane A_2 and leukotriene B_4 are elaborated under pathologic conditions and are thought to be involved in the pathophysiology of pulmonary artery hypertension (PAH) associated with sepsis and reperfusion injury.[40]

Therapeutically, epoprostenol has been successfully used to decrease PVR in patients with chronic PAH when infused[41] or inhaled.[42] Currently, the synthetic PGI_2 iloprost is now the most commonly used inhaled eicosanoid for reduction of PVR in patients with PAH.[43] Interestingly, most patients with chronic PAH are unresponsive to an acute vasodilator challenge with short-acting agents such as epoprostenol, adenosine, or NO.[44] However, long-term administration of epoprostenol has been shown to decrease PVR in these patients despite their initial non-responsiveness.[45] Furthermore, some patients with previously severe PAH have been weaned off epoprostenol after long-term administration, with dramatically decreased PVR and improved exercise tolerance.[44] The vascular remodeling required to provide such a dramatic reduction in PVR is probably due to mechanisms besides simple local vasodilation, as predicted by Fishman in an editorial in 1998.[46] One such mechanism that appears important is the fact that long-term epoprostenol administration increases the clearance of ET-1 (a potent vasoconstrictor and mitogen).[47]

Alveolar Gases (Chiefly Hypoxia)

Hypoxia-induced vasoconstriction in pulmonary vessels constitutes a fundamental difference from all other systemic blood vessels (which vasodilate in the presence of hypoxia). Alveolar hypoxia of in vivo and in vitro whole lung, unilateral lung, lobe, or lobule of lung all result in localized pulmonary vasoconstriction. This phenomenon is widely referred to as "hypoxic pulmonary vasoconstriction" and was first described nearly 60 years ago by Von Euler and Liljestrand.[48] The HPV response is present in all mammalian species and serves as an adaptive mechanism for diverting blood flow away from poorly ventilated to better ventilated regions of the lung and thereby improving $\dot{V}A/\dot{Q}$ ratios.[49] The HPV response is also critical for fetal development by minimizing perfusion of the unventilated lung.

The HPV response occurs primarily in pulmonary arterioles of about 200-μm internal diameter in humans (60- to 700-μm internal diameter, depending on the species).[50] These vessels are advantageously situated anatomically in close relation to small bronchioles and alveoli, which permits rapid and direct detection of alveolar hypoxia. Indeed, blood may actually become oxygenated in small pulmonary arteries because of the ability of oxygen to directly diffuse across the small distance between the contiguous air spaces and vessels.[51] This direct access that gas in the airways has to small arteries makes possible a rapid and localized vascular response to changes in gas composition.

The oxygen tension at the HPV stimulus site (PsO_2) is a function of both PAO_2 and mixed venous O_2 pressure ($P\bar{v}O_2$).[52] The PsO_2-HPV response is sigmoid, with a 50% response when PAO_2, $P\bar{v}O_2$, and PsO_2 are approximately 30 mm Hg. Usually, PAO_2 has a much greater effect than $P\bar{v}O_2$ does because O_2 uptake is from the alveolar space to the blood in the small pulmonary arteries.[52]

Over the last 50 years, numerous theories were developed to explain the mechanism of HPV.[48,53-55] Many vasoactive substances have been proposed as mediators of HPV (e.g., leukotrienes, prostaglandins, catecholamines, serotonin, histamine, angiotensin, bradykinin, and ET-1), but none has been identified as the primary mediator. In 1992, Xuan proposed that NO has a pivotal role in modulating PVR.[56] NO has involvement, but not precisely the way that Xuan first proposed. There are multiple sites of oxygen sensing with variable contributions from the NO, ET-1, and eicosanoid systems (described earlier). In vivo, HPV is currently thought to result from the synergistic action of molecules produced in both endothelial cells and smooth muscle cells.[57] However, HPV can proceed in the absence of intact endothelium, thus suggesting that the primary oxygen sensor is in the smooth muscle cell and that endothelial-derived molecules modulate only the primary HPV response.

The precise mechanism of HPV is still under investigation. However, current data support a mechanism involving the smooth muscle mitochondrial electron transport chain as the HPV sensor (Fig. 17-9).[58] Additionally, reactive oxygen species (possibly H_2O_2 or superoxide) are released from complex III of the electron transport chain and probably serve as second messengers to increase calcium in pulmonary artery smooth muscle cells during acute hypoxia.[59] However, alternative (less likely) mechanisms are still being investigated.[60] One alternative hypothesis suggests that smooth muscle microsomal reduced nicotinamide adenine dinucleotide phosphate (NADPH) oxido-reductase or sarcolemmal NADPH oxidase is the sensing mechanism.[60] Another, previously popular theory posited that voltage-sensitive potassium (K_V) channels were required for the HPV response. However, K_V channels are no longer believed to be "obligate" but instead are thought to be attenuators because a recent study demonstrated that inhibition of K_V channels failed to inhibit the HPV response.[60]

In summary, HPV is probably due to a direct action of alveolar hypoxia on pulmonary smooth muscle cells, sensed by mitochondrial ETC, with reactive oxygen species (probably H_2O_2 or superoxide) serving as second messengers to increase calcium and smooth muscle vasoconstriction. The endothelial-derived products serve to both potentiate (ET-1) and attenuate (NO, PGI_2) the HPV response. Additional mechanisms (humoral, neurogenic influences) may also modulate the baseline pulmonary vascular tone and affect the magnitude of the HPV response.

Elevated $PaCO_2$ has a pulmonary vasoconstrictor effect. Both respiratory and metabolic acidosis will augment HPV, whereas alkalosis (both respiratory and metabolic) causes pulmonary vasodilation and serves to reduce HPV.

The clinical effects of HPV can be classified under three basic mechanisms in humans. First, life at high altitude

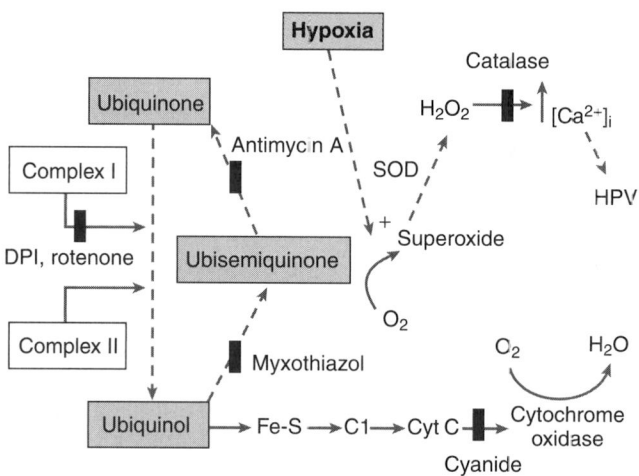

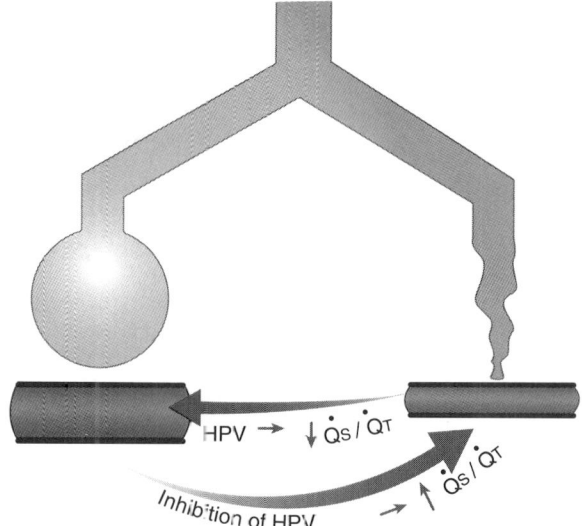

Figure 17–9 Schematic model of the mitochondrial O_2-sensing and effector mechanism probably responsible for hypoxic pulmonary vasoconstriction (HPV). In this model, reactive O_2 species (ROS) are released from electron transport chain complex III and act as second messengers in the hypoxia-induced calcium (Ca^{2+}) increase and resultant HPV. The *solid arrows* represent electron transfer steps; *solid bars* show sites of electron chain inhibition. Normal mitochondrial electron transport involves the movement of reducing equivalents generated in the Krebs cycle through complex I or II and then through complex III (ubiquinone) and IV (cytochrome oxidase). The Q cycle converts the dual electron transfer in complex I and II into a single electron transfer step used in complex IV. The ubisemiquinone (a free radical) created in this process can generate superoxide, which in the presence of superoxide dismutase (SOD) produces H_2O_2, the probable mediator of the hypoxia-induced increased Ca^{2+} and HPV. This process is amplified during hypoxia. (DPI, diphenyleneiodonium. DPI, rotenone, and myxothiazol [not shown in figure] are inhibitors of the proximal portion of the electron transport chain.) (From Waypa GB, Marks JD, Mack MM, et al: Mitochondrial reactive oxygen species trigger calcium increases during hypoxia in pulmonary artery myocytes. Circ Res 91:719-726, 2002.)

Figure 17–10 Schematic drawing of regional hypoxic pulmonary vasoconstriction (HPV); one-lung ventilation is a common clinical example of regional HPV. HPV in the hypoxic atelectatic lung causes redistribution of blood flow away from the hypoxic lung to the normoxic lung, thereby diminishing the amount of shunt flow ($\dot{Q}s/\dot{Q}T$) that can occur through the hypoxic lung. Inhibition of hypoxic lung HPV causes an increase in the amount of shunt flow through the hypoxic lung, thereby decreasing Pao_2.

or whole-lung respiration of a low inspired concentration of O_2 (Fio_2) increases Ppa. This is true for newcomers to high altitude, for the acclimatized, and for natives.[55] The vasoconstriction is considerable, and in healthy people breathing 10% O_2, Ppa doubles whereas pulmonary wedge pressure remains constant.[61] The increased Ppa increases perfusion of the apices of the lung (recruitment of previously unused vessels), which results in gas exchange in a region of lung not normally used (i.e., zone 1). Thus, with a low Fio_2, Pao_2 is greater and the alveolar-arterial O_2 tension difference and the Vd/Vt ratio are less than would be expected or predicted on the basis of a normal (sea level) distribution of ventilation and blood flow. High-altitude pulmonary hypertension is an important component in the development of mountain sickness subacutely (hours to days) and cor pulmonale chronically (weeks to years).[62] In fact, there is now good evidence that in patients with chronic obstructive pulmonary disease, even nocturnal episodes of arterial O_2 desaturation (caused by episodic hypoventilation) are accompanied by elevations in Ppa and may account for or lead to sustained pulmonary hypertension and cor pulmonale.[53]

Second, hypoventilation (low $\dot{V}a/\dot{Q}$ ratio), atelectasis, or nitrogen ventilation of any region of the lung (one lung, lobe, lobule) generally causes a diversion of blood flow away from the hypoxic to the nonhypoxic lung (40% to 50%, 50% to 60%, 60% to 70%, respectively) (Fig. 17-10).[64] The regional vasoconstriction and blood flow diversion are of great importance in minimizing transpulmonary shunting and normalizing regional $\dot{V}a/\dot{Q}$ ratios during disease of one lung, one-lung anesthesia (see Chapter 49), inadvertent intubation of a main stem bronchus, and lobar collapse. Third, in patients who have chronic obstructive pulmonary disease, asthma, pneumonia, or mitral stenosis but not bronchospasm, administration of pulmonary vasodilator drugs such as isoproterenol, sodium nitroprusside, and nitroglycerin causes a decrease in Pao_2 and PVR and an increase in right-to-left transpulmonary shunting.[65] The mechanism for these changes is thought to be deleterious inhibition of preexisting and, in some lesions, geographically widespread HPV without concomitant and beneficial bronchodilation.[65] In accordance with the latter two lines of evidence (one-lung or regional hypoxia and vasodilator drug effects on whole-lung or generalized disease), HPV is thought to divert blood flow away from hypoxic regions of the lung, thereby serving as an autoregulatory mechanism that protects Pao_2 by favorably adjusting regional $\dot{V}a/\dot{Q}$ ratios. Factors that inhibit regional HPV are extensively discussed elsewhere.[66]

Neural Influences on Pulmonary Vascular Tone
The three systems used to innervate the pulmonary circulation are the same ones that innervate the airways: the sympathetic, parasympathetic, and nonadrenergic noncholinergic (NANC) systems.[40]

Sympathetic (adrenergic) fibers originate from the first five thoracic nerves and enter the pulmonary vessels as branches from the cervical ganglia, as well as from a plexus of nerves arising from the trachea and main stem bronchi. These nerves act mainly on pulmonary arteries down to a diameter of 60 μm.[40] Sympathetic fibers cause pulmonary vasoconstriction through α_1-receptors. However, the pulmonary arteries also contain vasodilatory α_2-receptors and β_2-receptors. The α_1-adrenergic response predominates during sympathetic stimulation, as occurs during pain, fear, and anxiety.[40]

The parasympathetic (cholinergic) nerve fibers originate from the vagus nerve and cause pulmonary vasodilation through an NO-dependent process.[40] Binding of acetylcholine to a muscarinic (M_3) receptor on the endothelial cell increases intracellular calcium and stimulates cNOS.[40]

NANC nerves cause pulmonary vasodilation through NO-mediated systems by using vasoactive intestinal peptide as the neurotransmitter. The functional significance of this system is still under investigation.[40]

Humoral Influences on Pulmonary Vascular Tone

Numerous molecules are released into the circulation that either affect pulmonary vascular tone (by binding to pulmonary endothelial receptors) or are acted on by the pulmonary endothelium and subsequently become activated or inactivated (Table 17-2). The entire topic of nonrespiratory function of the lung is fascinating, but beyond the scope of this chapter. Here, we will highlight the effects that circulating molecules have on pulmonary vascular tone.

Although we understand the basic effect that various circulating factors have on pulmonary vascular tone, it is unlikely that these compounds are modulators of normal pulmonary vascular tone. However, they have marked effects on pulmonary vascular tone during disease (e.g., ARDS, sepsis).

Endogenous catecholamines (epinephrine and norepinephrine) bind to both α_1 (vasoconstrictor) and β_2 (vasodilator) receptors on the pulmonary endothelium but, when elaborated in high concentration, have a predominant α_1 (vasoconstrictor) effect. The same is true for exogenously administered catecholamines.

Other amines (e.g., histamine, serotonin) are elaborated systemically or locally after various challenges and have variable effects on PVR. Histamine can be released from mast cells, basophils, and elsewhere. When histamine binds directly to H_1 receptors on endothelium, NO-mediated vasodilation occurs (as seen after epinephrine-induced pulmonary vasoconstriction). Direct stimulation of H_2 receptors on smooth muscle cell membranes also causes vasodilation. In contrast, stimulation of H_1 receptors on the smooth muscle membrane results in vasoconstriction. Serotonin (5-hydroxytryptamine [5-HT]) is a potent vasoconstrictor that can be elaborated from activated platelets (e.g., after pulmonary embolism) and lead to acute severe pulmonary hypertension.[67]

Numerous peptides circulate and cause either pulmonary vasodilation (e.g., substance P, bradykinin, and vasopressin [a systemic vasoconstrictor]) or vasoconstriction (e.g., neurokinin A and angiotensin). These peptides produce clinically detectable effects on PVR only when administered in high concentration (e.g., exogenous administration or in disease).

Two other classes of molecules must be mentioned for completeness, eicosanoids (vasoactive effects discussed earlier) and purine nucleosides (which are similarly highly vasoactive).[40] Adenosine is a pulmonary vasodilator in normal subjects, whereas adenosine triphosphate (ATP) has a variable "normalizing effect," depending on baseline pulmonary vascular tone.[68]

Alternative (Nonalveolar) Pathways of Blood Flow through the Lung

Blood can use several possible pathways to travel from the right side of the heart to the left without being fully

---

Table 17–2 Effect on hormones by passage through the pulmonary circulation

Molecule	Effect of Compounds Passing through Pulmonary Circulation		
	Activated	*Unchanged*	*Inactivated*
Amines		Dopamine	5-Hydroxytryptamine
		Epinephrine	Norepinephrine
		Histamine	
Peptides	Angiotensin I	Angiotensin II	Bradykinin
		Oxytocin	Atrial natriuretic peptide
		Vasopressin	Endothelins
Eicosanoids	Arachidonic acid	PGI_2	PGD_2
		PGA_2	PGE_1, PGE_2
			$PGF_{2\alpha}$
			Leukotrienes
Purine derivatives			Adenosine
			ATP, ADP, AMP

ADP, adenosine diphosphate; AMP, adenosine monophosphate; ATP, adenosine triphosphate; PG, prostaglandin.
Modified from Lumb AB: Non-respiratory functions of the lung. *In* Lumb AB (ed): Nunn's Applied Respiratory Physiology, 5th ed. London, Butterworths, 2000, p 309.

oxygenated or oxygenated at all. Blood flow through poorly ventilated alveoli (low-$\dot{V}_A/\dot{Q}$ regions at an $F_{IO_2} < 0.3$ have a right-to-left shunt effect on oxygenation) and blood flow through nonventilated alveoli (atelectatic or consolidated regions; $\dot{V}_A/\dot{Q} = 0$ at all F_{IO_2} values) are sources of right-to-left shunting. Low-$\dot{V}_A/\dot{Q}$ and atelectatic lung units occur in conditions in which FRC is less than the closing capacity (CC) of the lung (see the section "Lung Volumes, Functional Residual Capacity, and Closing Capacity").

Several right-to-left blood flow pathways through the lungs and heart do not pass by or involve the alveoli at all. The bronchial and pleural circulations originate from systemic arteries and empty into the left side of the heart without being oxygenated; these circulations constitute the 1% to 3% true right-to-left shunt normally present. With chronic bronchitis, the bronchial circulation may carry 10% of the cardiac output, and with pleuritis, the pleural circulation may carry 5% of the cardiac output. Consequently, as much as a 10% and a 5% obligatory right-to-left shunt may be present, respectively, under these conditions. Intrapulmonary arteriovenous anastomoses are normally closed, but in the face of acute pulmonary hypertension, such as may be caused by a pulmonary embolus, they may open and result in a direct increase in right-to-left shunting. The foramen ovale is patent in 20% to 30% of individuals, but it normally remains functionally closed because left atrial pressure exceeds right atrial pressure. However, any condition that causes right atrial pressure to be greater than left atrial pressure may produce a right-to-left shunt, with resultant hypoxemia and possible paradoxical embolization. Such conditions include the use of high levels of PEEP, pulmonary embolization, pulmonary hypertension, chronic obstructive pulmonary disease, pulmonary valvular stenosis, congestive heart failure, and postpneumonectomy states.[69] Indeed, even such common events as mechanical ventilation[70] and reaction to the presence of an endotracheal tube during the excitement phase of emergence from anesthesia[71] have caused right-to-left shunting across a patent foramen ovale and severe arterial desaturation (with the potential for paradoxical embolization).[71]

Transesophageal echocardiography (TEE) has been demonstrated to be the most sensitive modality for diagnosing a patent foramen ovale in anesthetized patients with elevated right atrial pressure.[72] Esophageal to mediastinal to bronchial to pulmonary vein pathways have been described and may explain in part the hypoxemia associated with portal hypertension and cirrhosis. There are no known conditions that selectively increase thebesian channel blood flow (thebesian vessels nourish the left ventricular myocardium and originate and empty into the left side of the heart).

Other (Nongravitational) Important Determinants of Pulmonary Compliance, Resistance, Lung Volume, and Ventilation

Pulmonary Compliance

For air to flow into the lungs, a pressure gradient (ΔP) must be developed to overcome the elastic resistance of the lungs and chest wall to expansion. These structures are arranged concentrically, and their elastic resistance is therefore additive. The relationship between ΔP and the resultant volume increase (ΔV) of the lungs and thorax is independent of time and is known as total compliance (C_T), as expressed in the following equation:

$$C_T \text{ (L/cm } H_2O) = \Delta V \text{ (L)}/\Delta P \text{ (cm } H_2O) \qquad (1)$$

The C_T of lung plus chest wall is related to the individual compliance of the lungs (C_L) and chest wall (C_{CW}) according to the following expression:

$$1/C_T = 1/C_L + 1/C_{CW} \qquad (2)$$
$$[\text{or } C_T = (C_L)(C_{CW})/C_L + C_{CW}]$$

Normally, C_L and C_{CW} each equal 0.2 L/cm H_2O; thus, $C_T = 0.1$ L/cm H_2O. To determine C_L, ΔV and the transpulmonary pressure gradient ($P_A - P_{pl}$, the ΔP for the lung) must be known; to determine C_{CW}, ΔV and the transmural pressure gradient ($P_{pl} - P_{ambient}$, the ΔP for the chest wall) must be known; and to determine C_T, ΔV and the transthoracic pressure gradient ($P_A - P_{ambient}$, the ΔP for the lung and chest wall together) must be known. In clinical practice, only C_T is measured, which can be done dynamically or statically, depending on whether a peak or plateau inspiratory ΔP (respectively) is used for the C_T calculation.

During a positive- or negative-pressure inspiration of sufficient duration, transthoracic ΔP first increases to a peak value and then decreases to a lower plateau value. The peak transthoracic pressure value is due to the pressure required to overcome both elastic and airway resistance (see the section "Airway Resistance"). Transthoracic pressure decreases to a plateau value after the peak value because with time, gas is redistributed from stiff alveoli (which expand only slightly and therefore have only a short inspiratory period) into more compliant alveoli (which expand a great deal and therefore have a long inspiratory period). Because the gas is redistributed into more compliant alveoli, less pressure is required to contain the same amount of gas, which explains why the pressure decreases. In practical terms, dynamic compliance is the volume change divided by the peak inspiratory transthoracic pressure, and static compliance is the volume change divided by the plateau inspiratory transthoracic pressure. Therefore, static C_T is usually greater than dynamic C_T because the former calculation uses a smaller denominator (lower pressure) than the latter. However, if the patient is receiving PEEP, this pressure must first be subtracted from the peak or plateau pressure before calculating thoracic compliance (i.e., compliance = volume delivered/peak or plateau pressure – PEEP).

P_A deserves special comment. The alveoli are lined with a layer of liquid. The lining of a curved surface (sphere or cylinder, such as the alveoli, bronchioles, and bronchi) with liquid creates a surface tension that tends to make the surface area that is exposed to the atmosphere as small as possible. Simply stated, water molecules crowd much closer together on the surface of a curved layer of water than elsewhere in the fluid. As lung or alveolar size decreases, the degree of curvature and the retractive surface tension increase.

According to the Laplace expression (Equation 3), the pressure in an alveolus (P, in dynes per square centimeter) is higher than ambient pressure by an amount that depends on the surface tension of the lining liquid (T, in dynes per centimeter) and the radius of curvature of the alveolus (R, in centimeters). This relationship is expressed in the following equation:

$$P = 2T/R \qquad (3)$$

Although surface tension contributes to the elastic resistance and retractive forces of the lung, two difficulties must be resolved. First, the pressure inside small alveoli should be higher than that inside large alveoli, a conclusion that stems directly from the Laplace equation (R in the denominator). From this reasoning, one would expect a progressive discharge of each small alveolus into a larger one until eventually only one gigantic alveolus would be left (Fig. 17-11A). The second problem concerns the relationship between lung volume and transpulmonary ΔP (PA – Ppl). Theoretically, the retractive forces of the lung should increase as lung volume decreases. If this were true, lung volume should decrease in a vicious circle, with an increasingly progressive tendency to collapse as lung volume diminishes.

These two problems are resolved by the fact that the surface tension of the fluid lining the alveoli is variable and decreases as its surface area is reduced. The surface tension of alveolar fluid can reach levels that are well below the normal range for body fluids such as water and plasma. When an alveolus decreases in size, the surface tension of the lining fluid falls to an extent greater than the corresponding reduction in radius, and as a result, the transmural pressure gradient (equal to 2T/R) diminishes. This explains why small alveoli do not discharge their contents into large alveoli (Fig. 17-11B) and why the elastic recoil of small alveoli is less than that of large alveoli.

The substance responsible for the reduction (and variability) in alveolar surface tension is secreted by the intra-alveolar type II pneumocyte and is a lipoprotein called surfactant, which floats as a 50-Å-thick film on the surface of the fluid lining the alveoli. When the surface film is reduced in area and the concentration of surfactant at the surface is increased, the surface-reducing pressure is increased and counteracts the surface tension of the fluid lining the alveoli.

Airway Resistance

For air to flow into the lungs, ΔP (pressure gradient) must also be developed to overcome the nonelastic airway resistance of the lungs to airflow. The relationship between ΔP and the rate of airflow ($\dot{V}$) is known as airway resistance (R):

$$R \,(cm\,H_2O\,/\,L\,/\,sec) = \frac{\Delta P \,(cm\,H_2O)}{\Delta \dot{V} \,(L\,/\,sec)} \qquad (4)$$

The ΔP along the airway depends on the caliber of the airway and the rate and pattern of airflow. There are three main patterns of airflow. Laminar flow occurs when the gas passes down parallel-sided tubes at less than a certain critical velocity. With laminar flow, the pressure drop down the tube is proportional to the flow rate

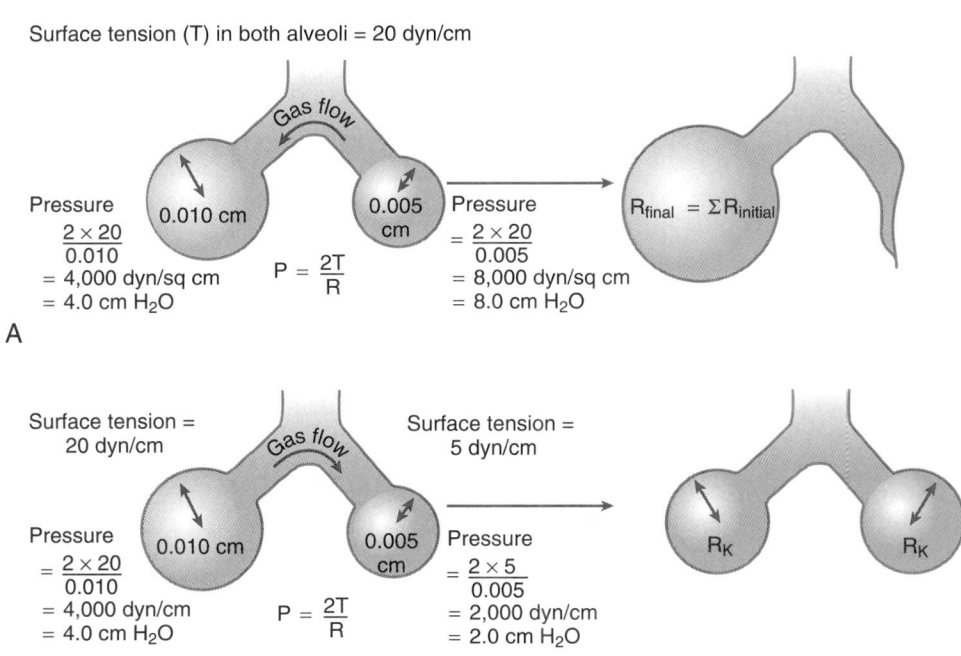

A

B

Figure 17–11 Relationship between surface tension (T), alveolar radius (R), and alveolar transmural pressure (P). The *left* side of the diagrams shows the starting condition. The *right* side of the diagrams shows the expected result in alveolar size (using the Laplace equation to calculate the starting pressure). In the upper example (**A**), the surface tension in the fluid lining both the large and the small alveolus is the same (no surfactant). Accordingly, the direction of gas flow is from the higher-pressure small alveolus to the lower-pressure large alveolus, which results in one large alveolus ($R_{final} = \Sigma R_{initial}$). In the bottom example (**B**), the expected changes in surface tension when surfactant lines the alveoli are shown (less tension in the smaller alveolus). The direction of gas flow is from the larger alveolus to the smaller alveolus until the two alveoli are of equal size and are volume stable (R_K). K, constant; ΣR, sum of all individual radii.

and may be calculated from the equation derived by Poiseuille:

$$\Delta P = \dot{V} \times 8L \times \mu / \pi r^4 \qquad (5)$$

In Equation 5, ΔP is the pressure drop (in cm H_2O), $\dot{V}$ is the volume flow rate (in mL/sec), μ is viscosity (in poises), L is the length of the tube (in cm), and r is the radius of the tube (in cm).

When flow exceeds the critical velocity, it becomes turbulent. The significant feature of turbulent flow is that the pressure drop along the airway is no longer directly proportional to the flow rate but is proportional to the square of the flow rate according to Equation 6 for turbulent flow:

$$\Delta P = \dot{V}^2 pfL / 4\pi^2 r^5 \qquad (6)$$

In Equation 6, p is the density of the gas (or liquid), and f is a friction factor that depends on the roughness of the tube wall.[73] Thus, with increases in turbulent flow (and/or orifice flow; see the next paragraph), ΔP increases much more than $\dot{V}$, and therefore airway resistance (R) increases more also, as predicted by Equation 4.

Orifice flow occurs at severe constrictions such as a nearly closed larynx or a kinked endotracheal tube. In these situations, the pressure drop is also proportional to the square of the flow rate, but density replaces viscosity as the important factor in the numerator. This explains why a low-density gas such as helium diminishes the resistance to flow (by threefold in comparison to air) in severe obstruction of the upper airway.

Because the total cross-sectional area of the airways increases as branching occurs, the velocity of airflow decreases distal in the airways; laminar flow is therefore chiefly confined to the airways below the main bronchi. Orifice flow occurs at the larynx, and flow in the trachea is turbulent during most of the respiratory cycle. By viewing the components that constitute each of the preceding airway pressure equations one can see that many factors may obviously affect the pressure drop down the airways during respiration. However, variations in diameter of the smaller bronchi and bronchioles are particularly critical (bronchoconstriction may convert laminar flow to turbulent flow), and the pressure drop along the airways may become much more closely related to the flow rate.

Different Regional Lung Time Constants

Thus far, the compliance and airway resistance properties of the chest have been discussed separately. In the following analysis, pressure at the mouth is assumed to increase suddenly to a fixed positive value[74] (Fig. 17-12) that overcomes both elastic and airway resistance and to be maintained at this value during inflation of the lungs. The ΔP required to overcome nonelastic airway resistance is the difference between the fixed mouth pressure and the instantaneous height of the dashed line in Figure 17-12 and is proportional to the flow rate during most of the respiratory cycle. Thus, the ΔP required to overcome nonelastic airway resistance is maximal initially but then decreases exponentially (Fig. 17-12A, hatched lines).

The rate of filling therefore also declines in an approximately exponential manner. The remainder of the pressure gradient overcomes the elastic resistance (the instantaneous height of the dashed line in Fig. 17-12A) and is proportional to the change in lung volume. Thus, the ΔP required to overcome elastic resistance is minimal initially but then increases exponentially, as does lung volume. Alveolar filling ceases (lung volume remains constant) when the pressure resulting from the retractive

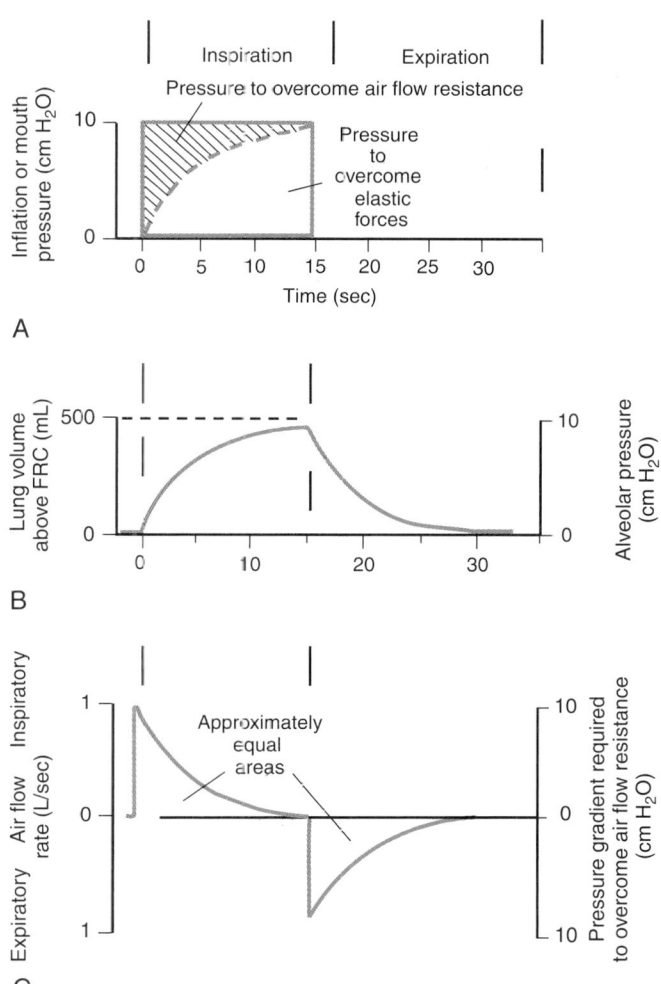

Figure 17–12 Artificial ventilation by intermittent application of constant pressure (square wave) followed by passive expiration. The pressure required to overcome airway resistance (*hatched lines,* **A**) and the airflow rate (of Equation 4, **C**) are proportional to one another and decrease exponentially (assuming that resistance to airflow is constant). The pressure required to overcome the elastic forces (height of the *dashed line,* **A**) and lung volume (**B**) are proportional to one another and increase exponentially. Values shown are typical for an anesthetized supine paralyzed patient: total dynamic compliance, 50 mL/cm H_2O; pulmonary resistance, 3 cm H_2O/L/sec; apparatus resistance, 7 cm H_2O/L/sec; total resistance, 10 cm H_2O/L/sec; time constant, 0.5 second. (Redrawn from Lumb AB: Artificial ventilation. *In* Lumb AB [ed]: Nunn's Applied Respiratory Physiology, 5th ed. London, Butterworths, 2000, p 590.)

elastic forces balances the applied (mouth) pressure (see Fig. 17-12A, dashed line).

Because only a finite time is available for alveolar filling and because alveolar filling occurs in an exponential manner, the degree of filling obviously depends on the duration of the inspiration. The rapidity of change in an exponential curve can be described by its time constant τ, which is the time required to complete 63% of an exponentially changing function if the total time allowed for the function change is unlimited ($2\tau = 87\%$, $3\tau = 95\%$, and $4\tau = 98\%$). For lung inflation, $\tau = C_T \times R$; normally, $C_T = 0.1$ L/cm H_2O, R = 2.0 cm H_2O/L/sec, $\tau = 0.2$ second, and $3\tau = 0.6$ second.

When this equation is applied to individual alveolar units, the time taken to fill such a unit clearly increases as airway resistance increases. The time to fill an alveolar unit also increases as compliance increases because a greater volume of air will be transferred into a more compliant alveolus before the retractive force equals the applied pressure. The compliance of individual alveoli differs from top to bottom of the lung, and the resistance of individual airways varies widely depending on their length and caliber. Therefore, various time constants for inflation exist throughout the lung.

Pathways of Collateral Ventilation

Collateral ventilation is another nongravitational determinant of the distribution of ventilation. Four pathways of collateral ventilation are known. First, interalveolar communications (pores of Kohn) exist in most species; they may range from 8 to 50 per alveolus and may increase with age and with the development of obstructive lung disease. Their precise role has not been defined, but they probably function to prevent hypoxia in neighboring, but obstructed lung units. Second, distal bronchiolar to-alveolar communications are known to exist (channels of Lambert), but their function in vivo is speculative (may be similar to the pores of Kohn). Third, respiratory bronchiole–to–terminal bronchiole connections have been found in adjacent lung segments (channels of Martin) in healthy dogs and in humans with lung disease. Fourth, interlobar connections exist; the functional characteristics of interlobar collateral ventilation through these connections have been described in dogs,[75] and they have been observed in humans as well.[76]

Work of Breathing

The pressure-volume characteristics of the lung also determine the work of breathing. Because

$$\text{Work} = \text{Force} \times \text{Distance} \qquad (7)$$
$$\text{Force} = \text{Pressure} \times \text{Area}$$
$$\text{Distance} = \text{Volume/Area}$$

work is defined by the equation

$$\text{Work} = (\text{Pressure} \times \text{Area})(\text{Volume/Area})$$
$$\text{Work} = \text{Pressure} \times \text{Volume} \qquad (8)$$

and ventilatory work may be analyzed by plotting pressure against volume.[77] In the presence of increased airway resistance or decreased C_L, increased transpulmonary pressure is required to achieve a given V_T with a consequent increase in the work of breathing. The metabolic cost of the work of breathing at rest constitutes only 1% to 3% of the total O_2 consumption in healthy subjects, but it is increased considerably (up to 50%) in patients with pulmonary disease.

Two different pressure-volume diagrams are shown in Figure 17-13. During normal inspiration (left graph), transpulmonary pressure increases from 0 to 5 cm H_2O while 500 mL of air is drawn into the lung. Potential energy is stored by the lung during inspiration and is expended during expiration; as a consequence, the entire expiratory cycle is passive. The hatched area plus the triangular area ABC represents pressure multiplied by volume and is the work of breathing. Line AB is the lower section of the pressure-volume curve of Figure 17-13. The triangular area ABC is the work required to overcome elastic forces (C_T), whereas the hatched area is the work required to overcome airflow or frictional resistance (R). The graph on the right applies to an anesthetized patient with diffuse obstructive airway disease resulting from the accumulation of mucous secretions. There is a marked

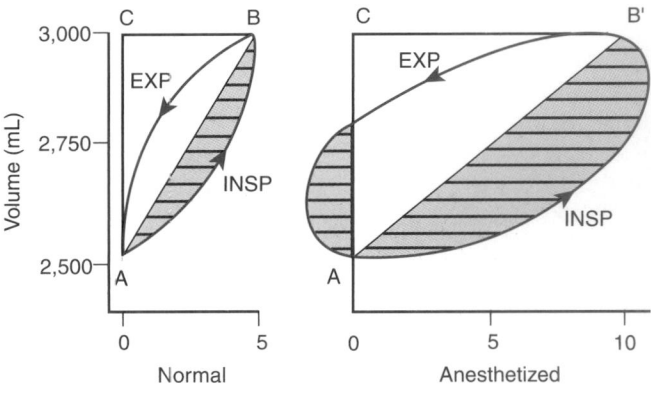

Figure 17-13 Lung volume plotted against transpulmonary pressure in a pressure-volume diagram for an healthy awake (normal) and an anesthetized patient. The lung compliance of the awake patient (slope of line AB = 100 mL/cm H_2O) equals that shown for the small dependent alveoli in Figure 17-3. The lung compliance of the anesthetized patient (slope of line AB′ = 50 mL/cm H_2O) equals that shown for the medium midlung alveoli in Figure 17-3 and for the anesthetized patient in Figure 17-12. The total area within the *oval* and *triangles* has the dimensions of pressure multiplied by volume and represents the total work of breathing. The *hatched area* to the right of lines AB and AB′ represents the active inspiratory work necessary to overcome resistance to airflow during inspiration (INSP). The *hatched area* to the left of the triangle AB′C represents the active expiratory work necessary to overcome resistance to airflow during expiration (EXP). Expiration is passive in the healthy subject because sufficient potential energy is stored during inspiration to produce expiratory airflow. The fraction of total inspiratory work necessary to overcome elastic resistance is shown by the triangles ABC and AB′C. The anesthetized patient has decreased compliance and increased elastic resistance work (triangle AB′C) when compared with the healthy patient's compliance and elastic resistance work (triangle ABC). The anesthetized patient shown in this figure has increased airway resistance to both inspiratory and expiratory work.

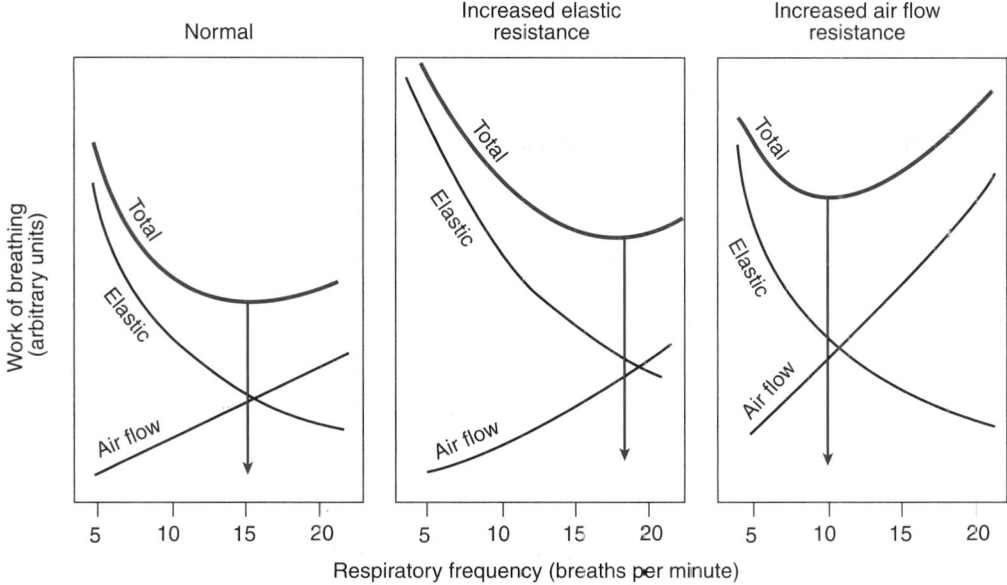

Normal

Increased elastic resistance

Increased air flow resistance

Respiratory frequency (breaths per minute)

Work of breathing (arbitrary units)

Figure 17–14 The diagrams show the work done against elastic and airflow resistance separately and summated to indicate the total work of breathing at different respiratory frequencies. The total work of breathing has a minimum value at about 15 breaths/min under normal circumstances. For the same minute volume, minimum work is performed at higher frequencies with stiff (less compliant) lungs and at lower frequencies when airflow resistance is increased. (Redrawn with modification from Lumb AB: Pulmonary ventilation: Mechanisms and the work of breathing. *In* Lumb AB [ed]: Nunn's Applied Respiratory Physiology, 5th ed. London, Butterworths, 2000, p 128.)

increase in both the elastic (triangle AB′C) and airway (hatched area) resistive components of respiratory work. During expiration, only 250 mL of air leaves the lungs during the passive phase when intrathoracic pressure reaches the equilibrium value of 0 cm H_2O. Active effort-producing work is required to force out the remaining 250 mL of air, and intrathoracic pressure actually becomes positive.

For a constant minute volume, the work done against elastic resistance is increased when breathing is deep and slow. On the other hand, the work done against airflow resistance is increased when breathing is rapid and shallow. If the two components are summated and the total work is plotted against respiratory frequency, there is an optimal respiratory frequency at which the total work of breathing is minimal (Fig. 17-14).[78] In patients with diseased lungs in which elastic resistance is high (pulmonary fibrosis, pulmonary edema, infants), the optimum frequency is increased, and rapid, shallow

breaths are favored. As with other muscles, respiratory muscles can become fatigued, especially with rapid shallow breathing.[79] When airway resistance is high (asthma, obstructive lung disease), the optimum frequency is decreased, and slow, deep breaths are favored. Although the optimum frequency is slow (allowing for a prolonged expiratory phase), a rapid shallow breathing pattern also develops in these patients when fatigued and further exacerbates their primary (airway resistance) problem.[79]

Lung Volumes, Functional Residual Capacity, and Closing Capacity

Lung Volumes and Functional Residual Capacity
FRC is defined as the volume of gas in the lung at the end of a normal expiration when there is no airflow and PA equals ambient pressure. Under these conditions, expansive chest wall elastic forces are exactly balanced by retractive lung tissue elastic forces (Fig. 17-15).[80]

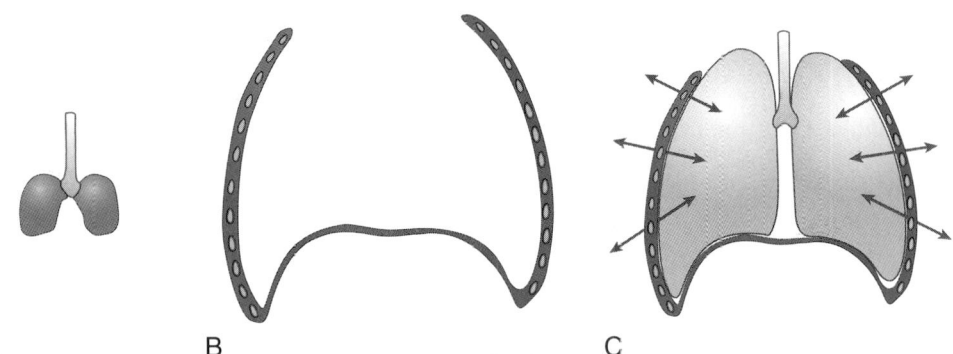

A   B   C

Figure 17–15 A, The resting state of normal lungs when they are removed from the chest cavity; that is, elastic recoil causes total collapse. **B,** The resting state of a normal chest wall and diaphragm when the thoracic apex is open to the atmosphere and the thoracic contents are removed. **C,** The lung volume that exists at the end of expiration is the functional residual capacity (FRC). At FRC, the elastic forces of the lung and chest walls are equal and in opposite directions. The pleural surfaces link these two opposing forces. (Redrawn with modification from Shapiro BA, Harrison RA, Trout CA: The mechanics of ventilation. *In* Clinical Application of Respiratory Care, 3rd ed. Chicago, Year Book, 1985, p 57.)

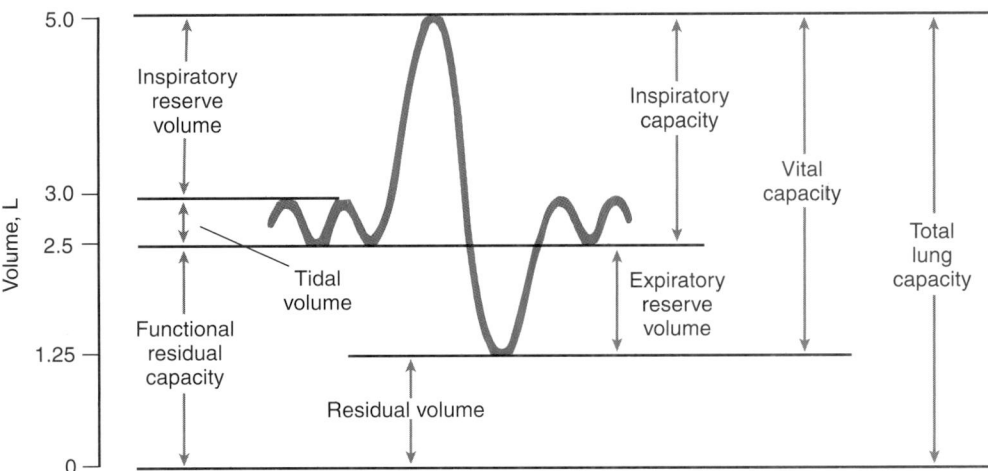

Figure 17–16 The dynamic lung volumes that can be measured by simple spirometry are tidal volume, inspiratory reserve volume, expiratory reserve volume, inspiratory capacity, and vital capacity. The static lung volumes are residual volume, functional residual capacity, and total lung capacity. Static lung volumes cannot be measured by simple spirometry and require separate methods of measurement (e.g., inert gas dilution, nitrogen washout, or whole-body plethysmography).

The expiratory reserve volume is part of FRC; it is that additional gas beyond the end-tidal volume that can be consciously exhaled and result in the minimum volume of lung possible, known as residual volume. Thus, FRC equals residual volume plus the expiratory reserve volume (Fig. 17-16). With regard to the other lung volumes shown in Figure 17-16, V_T, vital capacity, inspiratory capacity, inspiratory reserve volume, and expiratory reserve volume can all be measured by simple spirometry. Total lung capacity (TLC), FRC, and residual volume all contain a fraction (residual volume) that cannot be measured by simple spirometry. However, if one of these three volumes is measured, the others can easily be derived because the other lung volumes, which relate these three volumes to one another, can be measured by simple spirometry.

Residual volume, FRC, and TLC can be measured by any of three techniques: (1) nitrogen washout, (2) inert gas dilution, and (3) total-body plethysmography. The first method, the nitrogen washout technique, is based on measuring expired nitrogen concentrations before and after breathing pure O_2 for several minutes and thus calculating the total quantity of nitrogen eliminated. Thus, if 2 L of nitrogen is eliminated and the initial alveolar nitrogen concentration was 80%, the initial volume of the lung was 2.5 L. The second method, the inert gas dilution technique, uses the wash-in of an inert tracer gas such as helium. If 50 mL of helium is introduced into the lungs and, after equilibration, the helium concentration is found to be 1%, the volume of the lung is 5 L. The third method, the total-body plethysmography technique, uses Boyle's law (i.e., $P_1V_1 = P_2V_2$), where P_1 = initial pressure, V_1 = initial volume). The subject is confined within a gas-tight box (plethysmograph) so that changes in the volume of the body during respiration may be readily determined as a change in pressure within the sealed box. Although each technique has technical limitations, all are based on sound physical and physiologic principles and provide accurate results in normal patients. Disparity between FRC as measured in the body plethysmograph and by the helium dilution method is often used as a way of detecting large, nonventilating air-trapped blebs.[81] Obviously, there are difficulties in applying the body plethysmograph to anesthetized patients.

Airway Closure and Closing Capacity

As discussed earlier in the section on the distribution of ventilation, Ppl increases from the top to the bottom of the lung and determines regional alveolar size, compliance, and ventilation. Of even greater importance to the anesthesiologist is the recognition that these gradients in Ppl may lead to airway closure and collapse of alveoli.

AIRWAY CLOSURE IN PATIENTS WITH NORMAL LUNGS. Figure 17-17A illustrates the normal resting end-expiratory (FRC) position of the lung–chest wall combination. The distending transpulmonary and the intrathoracic air passage transmural ΔP is 5 cm H_2O, and the airways remain patent. During the middle of a normal inspiration (Fig. 17-17B), there is an increase in transmural ΔP (to 6.8 cm H_2O) that encourages distention of the intrathoracic air passages. During the middle of a normal expiration (Fig. 17-17C), expiration is passive; PA is attributable only to the elastic recoil of the lung (2 cm H_2O), and there is a decrease (to 5.2 cm H_2O), but still a favorable (distending) intraluminal transmural ΔP. During the middle of a severe forced expiration (Fig. 17-17D), Ppl increases far higher than atmospheric pressure and is communicated to the alveoli, which have a pressure that is still higher because of the elastic recoil of the alveolar septa (an additional 2 cm H_2O). At high gas flow rates, the pressure drop down the air passage is increased, and there will be a point at which intraluminal pressure equals either the surrounding parenchymal pressure or Ppl; that point is termed the equal pressure point (EPP). If the EPP occurs in small intrathoracic air passages (distal to the 11th generation, the airways have no cartilage and are called bronchioles), they may be held open at that particular point by the tethering effect of the elastic recoil of the immediately adjacent or surrounding lung parenchyma. If the EPP occurs in large extrathoracic air passages (proximal to the

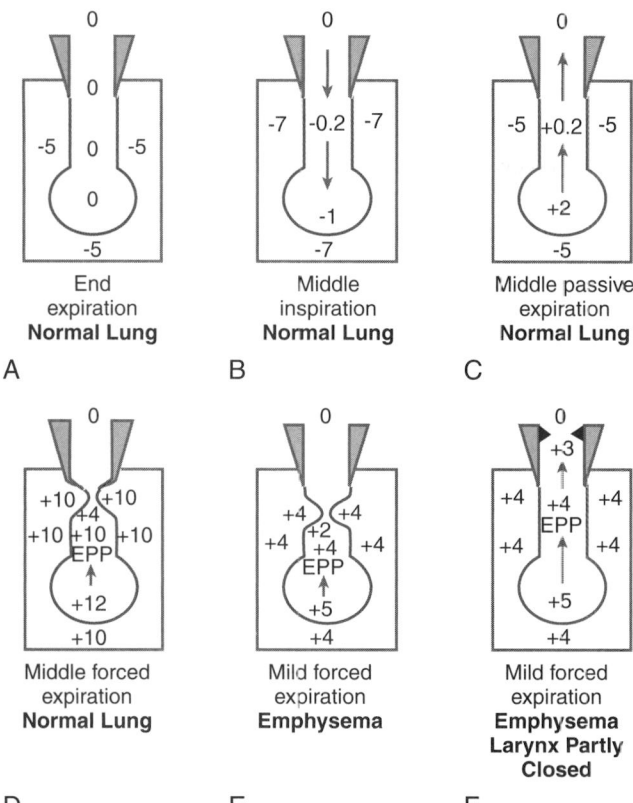

Figure 17–17 Pressure gradients across the airways. The airways consist of a thin-walled intrathoracic portion (near the alveoli) and a more rigid (cartilaginous) intrathoracic and extrathoracic portion. During expiration, the pressure from elastic recoil is assumed to be +2 cm H_2O in normal lungs (**A-D**) and +1 cm H_2O in abnormal lungs (**E** and **F**). The total pressure inside the alveolus is pleural pressure plus elastic recoil. The *arrows* indicate the direction of airflow. EPP, equal pressure point. See the text for an explanation. (Redrawn with modification from Benumof JL: Anesthesia for Thoracic Surgery, 2nd ed. Philadelphia, WB Saunders, 1995, Chapter 8.)

11th generation, the airways have cartilage and are called bronchi), they may be held open at that particular point by their cartilage. Downstream of the EPP (in either small or large airways), transmural ΔP is reversed (−6 cm H_2O), and airway closure occurs. Thus, the patency of airways distal to the 11th generation is a function of lung volume, and the patency of airways proximal to the 11th generation is a function of intrathoracic (pleural) pressure. In extrathoracic bronchi with cartilage, the posterior membranous sheath appears to give first by invaginating into the lumen.[82] If lung volume were abnormally decreased (for example, because of splinting) and expiration were still forced, the caliber of the airways would be relatively reduced at all times, which would cause the EPP and point of collapse to move progressively from larger to smaller air passages (closer to the alveolus).

In adults with normal lungs, airway closure may still occur even if exhalation is not forced, provided that residual volume is approached closely enough. Even in patients with normal lungs, as lung volume decreases toward residual volume during expiration, small airways

(0.5 to 0.9 mm in diameter) show a progressive tendency to close, whereas larger airways remain patent.[83,84] Airway closure occurs first in the dependent lung regions (as directly observed by computed tomography)[85] because the distending transpulmonary pressure is less and the volume change during expiration is greater. Airway closure is most likely to occur in the dependent regions of the lung whether the patient is in the supine or the lateral decubitus position[85] and whether ventilation is spontaneous or positive-pressure ventilation.[86,87]

AIRWAY CLOSURE IN PATIENTS WITH ABNORMAL LUNGS. Airway closure occurs with milder active expiration, lower gas flow rates, and higher lung volumes and occurs closer to the alveolus in patients with emphysema, bronchitis, asthma, and pulmonary interstitial edema. In all four conditions, the increased airway resistance causes a larger decrease in pressure from the alveoli to the larger bronchi, thereby creating the potential for negative intrathoracic transmural ΔP and narrowed and collapsed airways. In addition, the structural integrity of the conducting airways may be diminished because of inflammation and scarring, and therefore these airways may close more readily for any given lung volume or transluminal ΔP.

In emphysema, the elastic recoil of the lung is reduced (to 1 cm H_2O in Fig. 17-17E), the air passages are poorly supported by the lung parenchyma, the point of airway resistance is close to the alveolus, and transmural ΔP can become negative quickly. Therefore, during only a mild forced expiration in an emphysematous patient, the EPP and the point of collapse are near the alveolus (see Fig. 17-17E). The use of pursed-lip or grunting expiration (the equivalents of partly closing the larynx during expiration), PEEP, and continuous positive airway pressure in an emphysematous patient restores a favorable (distending) intrathoracic transmural air ΔP (Fig. 17-17F). In bronchitis, the airways are structurally weakened and may close when only a small negative transmural ΔP is present (as with mild forced expiration). In asthma, the middle-sized airways are narrowed by bronchospasm, and if expiration is forced, they are further narrowed by a negative transmural ΔP. Finally, with pulmonary interstitial edema, perialveolar interstitial edema compresses the alveoli and acutely decreases FRC; the peribronchial edema fluid cuffs (within the connective tissue sheaths around the larger arteries and bronchi) compress the bronchi and acutely increase closing volume.[88-90]

MEASUREMENT OF CLOSING CAPACITY. CC is a sensitive test of early small-airway disease and is performed by having the patient exhale to residual volume (Fig. 17-18).[91] As inhalation from residual volume toward TLC is begun, a bolus of tracer gas (xenon 133, helium) is injected into the inspired gas. During the initial part of this inhalation from residual volume, the first gas to enter the alveolus is the VD gas and the tracer bolus. The tracer gas will enter only alveoli that are already open (presumably the apices of the lung) and does not enter alveoli that are already closed (presumably the bases of the lung). As the inhalation continues, the apical alveoli complete filling and the basilar alveoli begin to open and fill, but with gas that does not contain any tracer gas.

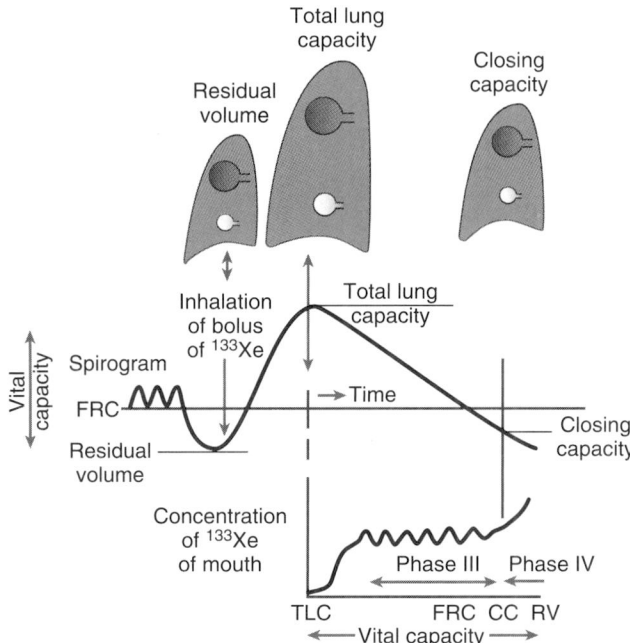

Figure 17–18 Measurement of closing capacity with the use of a tracer gas such as xenon 133 (^{133}Xe). The bolus of tracer gas is inhaled near residual volume and, because of airway closure in the dependent lung, is distributed only to nondependent alveoli whose air passages are still open (shown as *crosshatched* in diagram). During expiration, the concentration of tracer gas becomes constant after the dead space is washed out. This plateau (phase 3) gives way to a rising concentration of tracer gas (phase 4) when there is once again closure of the dependent airways because the only contribution made to expired gas is by the nondependent alveoli with a high ^{133}Xe concentration. CC, closing capacity; FRC, functional residual volume; RV, residual volume; TLC, total lung capacity. (Redrawn with modification from Lumb AB: Respiratory system resistance: Measurement of closing capacity. *In* Lumb AB [ed]: Nunn's Applied Respiratory Physiology, 5th ed. London, Butterworths, 2000, p 79.)

A differential tracer gas concentration is thus established, with the gas in the apices having a higher tracer concentration (see Fig. 17-18) than that in the bases (see Fig. 17-18). As the subject exhales and the diaphragm ascends, a point is reached at which the small airways just above the diaphragm start to close and thereby limit airflow from these areas. The airflow now comes more from the upper lung fields, where the alveolar gas has a much higher tracer concentration, which results in a sudden increase in the tracer gas concentration toward the end of exhalation (phase IV of Fig. 17-18).

Closing volume (CV) is the difference between the onset of phase IV and residual volume; because it represents part of a vital capacity maneuver, it is expressed as a percentage of vital lung capacity. CV plus residual volume is known as CC and is expressed as a percentage of TLC. Smoking, obesity, aging, and the supine position increase CC.[92] In healthy individuals at a mean age of 44 years, CC = FRC in the supine position, and at a mean age of 66 years, CC = FRC in the upright position.[93]

RELATIONSHIP BETWEEN FUNCTIONAL RESIDUAL CAPACITY AND CLOSING CAPACITY. The relationship between FRC and CC is far more important than consideration of FRC or CC alone because it is this relationship that determines whether a given respiratory unit is normal or atelectatic or has a low $\dot{V}_A/\dot{Q}$ ratio. The relationship between FRC and CC is as follows. When the volume of the lung at which some airways close is greater than the whole of V_T, lung volume never increases enough during tidal inspiration to open any of these airways. Thus, these airways stay closed during the entire tidal respiration. Airways that are closed all the time are equivalent to atelectasis (Fig. 17-19). If the CV of some airways lies within V_T, then as lung volume increases during inspiration, some previously closed airways will open for a short time until lung volume recedes once again below the CV of these airways. Because these opening and closing airways are open for a shorter time than normal airways are, they have less chance or time to participate in fresh gas exchange, a circumstance equivalent to a low-$\dot{V}_A/\dot{Q}$ region. If the CC of the lung is below the whole of tidal respiration, no airways are closed at any time during tidal respiration; this is a normal circumstance. Anything that decreases FRC relative to CC or increases CC relative to FRC will convert normal areas to low-$\dot{V}_A/\dot{Q}$ and atelectatic areas,[94] which causes hypoxemia.

Mechanical intermittent positive-pressure breathing (IPPB) may be efficacious because it can take a previously spontaneously breathing patient with a low-$\dot{V}_A/\dot{Q}$ relationship (in which CC is greater than FRC but still within V_T, as depicted in Fig. 17-20, right panel) and increase the amount of inspiratory time that some previously closed (at end-exhalation) airways spend in fresh gas exchange and thereby increase the $\dot{V}_A/\dot{Q}$ relationship (Fig. 17-20, middle panel). However, if PEEP is added to IPPB, PEEP increases FRC to or above a lung volume greater than CC,

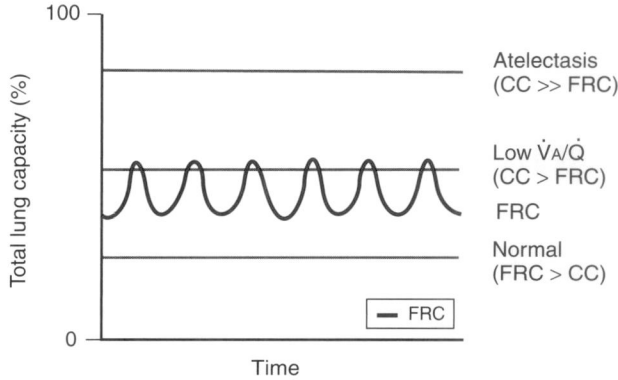

Figure 17–19 Relationship between functional residual capacity (FRC) and closing capacity (CC). FRC is the amount of gas in the lungs at end-exhalation during normal tidal breathing, shown by the level of each trough of the sine wave tidal volume. CC is the amount of gas that must be in the lungs to keep the small conducting airways open. This figure shows three different CCs, as indicated by the three different *straight lines*. See the text for an explanation of why the three different FRC-CC relationships depicted result in normal or low ventilation-perfusion ($\dot{V}_A/\dot{Q}$) relationships or atelectasis. The abscissa is time. (Redrawn from Benumof JL: Anesthesia for Thoracic Surgery, 2nd ed. Philadelphia, WB Saunders, 1995, Chapter 8.)

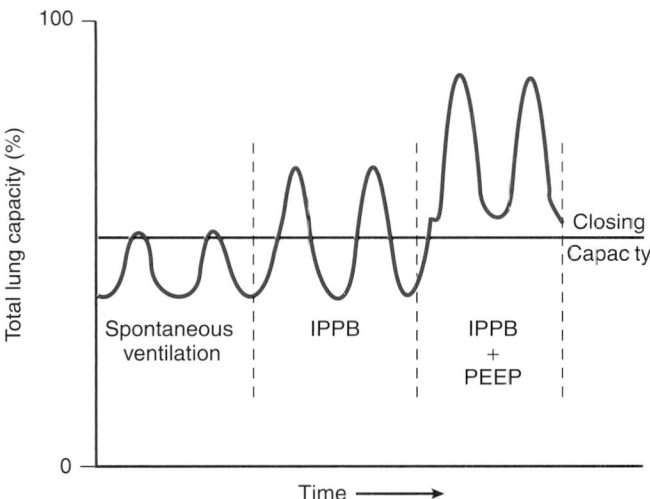

Figure 17–20 Relationship of functional residual capacity (FRC) to closing capacity (CC) during spontaneous ventilation, intermittent positive-pressure breathing (IPPB), and IPPB and positive end-expiratory pressure (IPPB + PEEP). See the text for an explanation of the effect of the two ventilatory maneuvers (IPPB and PEEP) on the relationship of FRC to CC. TLC, total lung capacity. The abscissa is time.

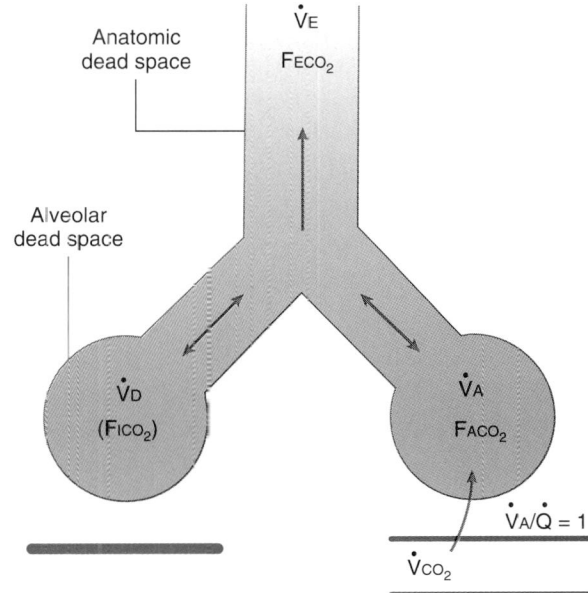

V_D = Total dead space
    = Anatomic + alveolar dead space

Figure 17–21 Two-compartment model of the lung in which the anatomic and alveolar dead space compartments have been combined into the total (physiologic) dead space (V_D). F_{ACO_2} = alveolar CO_2 fraction; F_{ECO_2} = mixed expired CO_2 fraction; F_{ICO_2} = inspired CO_2 fraction; $\dot{V}_A$ = alveolar ventilation; $\dot{V}_A/\dot{Q}$ = 1 means ventilation and perfusion are equal in liters per minute; $\dot{V}_{CO_2}$ = carbon dioxide production; $\dot{V}_E$ = expired minute ventilation. Normally, the amount of CO_2 eliminated at the airway ($\dot{V}_E \times F_{ECO_2}$) equals the amount of CO_2 removed by alveolar ventilation ($\dot{V}_A \times F_{ACO_2}$) because there is no CO_2 elimination from alveolar dead space (F_{ICO_2} = 0).

thereby restoring a normal FRC-to-CC relationship so that no airways are closed at any time during the tidal respiration depicted in Figure 17-20 (left panel) (IPPB + PEEP). Thus, anesthesia-induced atelectasis (computed tomography shows crescent-shaped densities) in the dependent regions of patients' lungs has not been reversed with IPPB alone but has been reversed with IPPB plus PEEP (5 to 10 cm H_2O).[85]

Oxygen and Carbon Dioxide Transport

Alveolar and Dead Space Ventilation and Alveolar Gas Tensions

In normal lungs, approximately two thirds of each breath reaches perfused alveoli to take part in gas exchange. This constitutes the effective or alveolar ventilation ($\dot{V}_A$). The remaining third of each breath takes no part in gas exchange and is therefore termed the total (or physiologic) dead space ventilation (V_D). The relationship is as follows: alveolar ventilation ($\dot{V}_A$) = frequency (f) ($V_T - V_D$). The physiologic (or total) dead space ventilation ($V_{D_{physiologic}}$) may be further divided into two components: a volume of gas that ventilates the conducting airways, the anatomic dead space ($V_{D_{anatomic}}$), and a volume of gas that ventilates unperfused alveoli, the alveolar dead space ($V_{D_{alveolar}}$). Clinical examples of $V_{D_{alveolar}}$ ventilation include zone 1, pulmonary embolus, and destroyed alveolar septa, and such ventilation therefore does not participate in gas exchange. Figure 17-21 shows a two-compartment model of the lung in which the anatomic and alveolar dead space compartments have been combined into the total (physiologic) dead space compartment; the other compartment is the alveolar ventilation compartment, whose idealized $\dot{V}_A/\dot{Q}$ ratio is 1.0.

The anatomic dead space varies with lung size and is approximately 2 mL/kg of body weight (150 mL in a 70-kg adult). In a normal healthy adult lying supine, anatomic dead space and total (physiologic) dead space are approximately equal to each other because alveolar dead space is normally minimal. In the erect posture, the uppermost alveoli may not be perfused (zone 1), and alveolar dead space may increase from a negligible amount to 60 to 80 mL.

Figure 17-21 illustrates that in a steady state, the volume of CO_2 entering the alveoli ($\dot{V}_{CO_2}$) is equal to the volume of CO_2 eliminated in the expired gas ($\dot{V}_E$)(F_{ECO_2}). Thus $\dot{V}_{CO_2}$ = ($\dot{V}_E$)(F_{ECO_2}). However, the expired gas volume consists of alveolar gas ($\dot{V}_A$)(F_{ACO_2}) and $\dot{V}_D$ gas ($\dot{V}_D$)(F_{ICO_2}). Thus, $\dot{V}_{CO_2}$ = ($\dot{V}_A$)(F_{ACO_2}) + ($\dot{V}_D$)(F_{ICO_2}). Setting the first equation equal to the second equation and using the relationship $\dot{V}_L = \dot{V}_A + \dot{V}_D$, subsequent algebraic manipulation, including setting P_{ACO_2} equal to P_{aCO_2}, results in the modified Bohr equation:

$$V_D/V_T = (P_{aCO_2} - P_{ECO_2})/P_{aCO_2} \qquad (9)$$

The P_{ECO_2} value may be obtained by measuring exhaled CO_2 in a large (Douglas) bag, or more commonly, end-tidal P_{CO_2} (P_{ETCO_2}) can be used as a surrogate. In severe lung disease, physiologic V_D/V_T provides a useful expression of the inefficiency of ventilation. In a healthy adult, this ratio is usually less than 30%; that is, ventilation is more than 70% efficient. In a patient with obstructive airway disease, V_D/V_T may increase to 60% to 70%. Under these conditions, ventilation is obviously grossly inefficient. Figure 17-22 shows the relationship between minute ventilation ($\dot{V}_E$) and Pa_{CO_2} for several V_D/V_T values. As $\dot{V}_E$ decreases, Pa_{CO_2} increases for all V_D/V_T values. As V_D/V_T increases, a given decrease in $\dot{V}_E$ causes a much greater increase in Pa_{CO_2}. If Pa_{CO_2} is to remain constant while V_D/V_T increases, $\dot{V}_E$ must increase.

The alveolar concentration of a gas is equal to the difference between the inspired concentration of a gas and the ratio of the output (or uptake) of the gas to $\dot{V}_A$. Thus, for gas X during dry conditions, $P_{AX} = (P_{dry\ atm})(F_{IX}) \pm \dot{V}_X$ (output or uptake)$/\dot{V}_A$, where P_{AX} = alveolar partial pressure of gas X, F_{IX} = inspired concentration of gas X, $P_{dry\ atm}$ = dry atmospheric pressure = $P_{wet\ atm} - P_{H_2O} = 760 - 47 = 713$ mm Hg, $\dot{V}_X$ = output or uptake of gas X, and $\dot{V}_A$ = alveolar ventilation.

For CO_2, $Pa_{CO_2} = 713(F_{ICO_2} + \dot{V}_{CO_2}/\dot{V}_A)$. Because $F_{ICO_2} = 0$ and using standard conversion factors:

$$Pa_{CO_2} = 713[\dot{V}_{CO_2}\ (mL/min\ STPD)/\dot{V}_A \\ (L/min/BTPS)(0.863)] \qquad (10)$$

For example, 36 mm Hg = (713)(200/4000).
For O_2,

$$P_{AO_2} = 713[F_{IO_2} - \dot{V}_{O_2}\ (mL/min)/\dot{V}_A\ (mL/min)] \qquad (11)$$

For example, 100 mm Hg = 713(0.21 − 225/3200).

Figure 17-23 shows the hyperbolic relationships expressed in Equations 10 and 11 between Pa_{CO_2} and $\dot{V}_A$ (see Fig. 17-22) and between P_{AO_2} and $\dot{V}_A$ for different levels of $\dot{V}_{CO_2}$ and $\dot{V}_{O_2}$, respectively. Pa_{CO_2} is substituted for P_{ACO_2} because P_{ACO_2}-to-Pa_{CO_2} gradients are small (as opposed to P_{AO_2}-to-Pa_{O_2} gradients, which can be large). Note that as $\dot{V}_A$ increases, the second term of the right side of Equations 10 and 11 approaches zero and the composition of the alveolar gas approaches that of the inspired gas. In addition, it should be noted from Figures 17-22 through 17-24 that because anesthesia is usually administered with an oxygen-enriched gas mixture, hypercapnia is a more common result of hypoventilation than hypoxemia is.

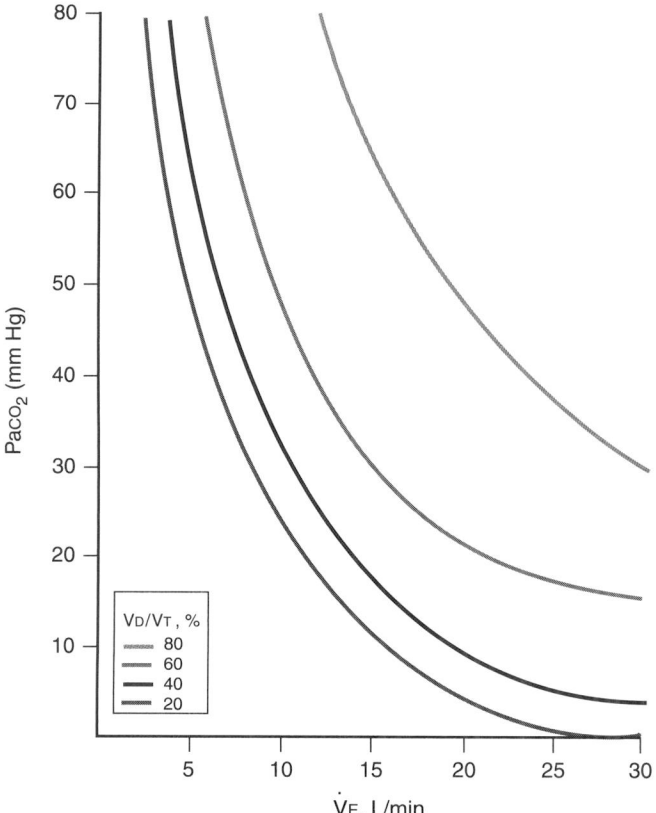

Figure 17–22 Relationship between minute ventilation ($\dot{V}_E$, L/min) and Pa_{CO_2} for a family of ratios of total dead space to tidal volume (V_D/V_T). These *curves* are hyperbolic (see Equation 10) and rise steeply at low $\dot{V}_E$ values.

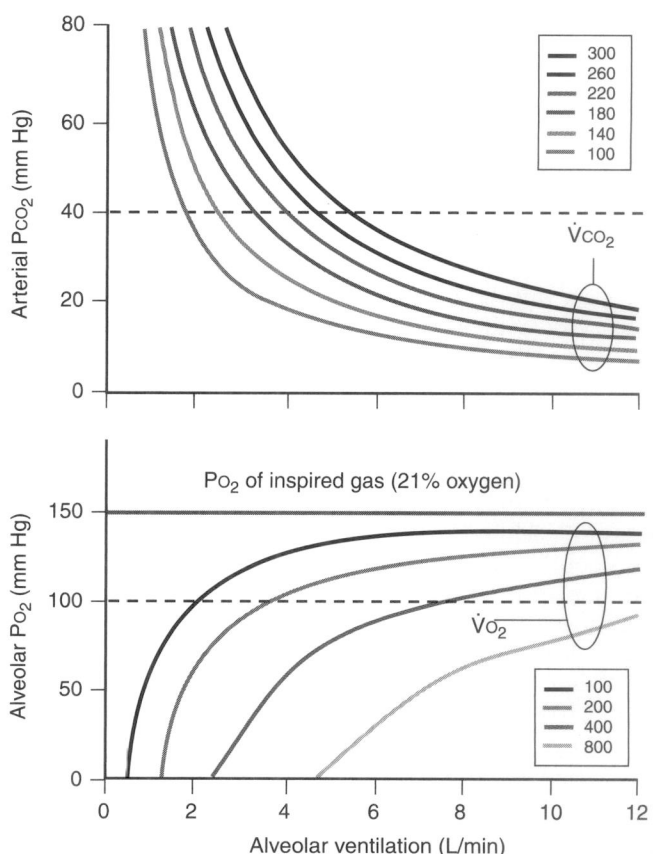

Figure 17–23 The relationship between alveolar ventilation and P_{AO_2} and Pa_{O_2} for a group of different O_2 consumption ($\dot{V}_{O_2}$) and CO_2 production ($\dot{V}_{CO_2}$) values is derived from Equations 10 and 11 in the text and is hyperbolic. As alveolar ventilation increases, P_{AO_2} and Pa_{CO_2} approach inspired concentrations. Decreases in alveolar ventilation to less than 4 L/min are accompanied by precipitous decreases in P_{AO_2} and increases in Pa_{CO_2}.

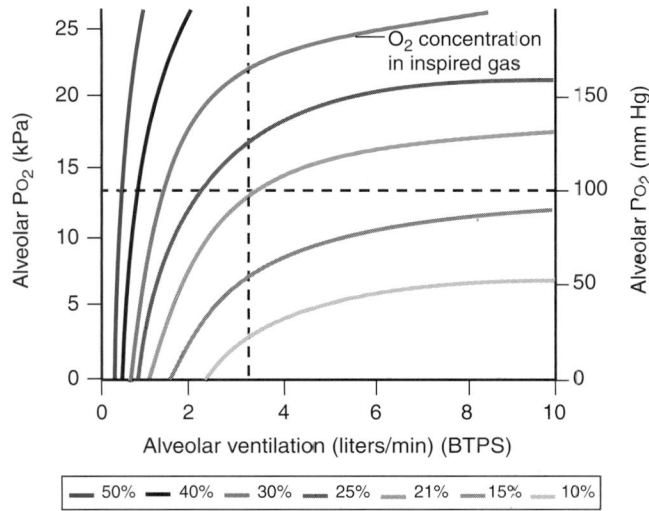

50%	40%	30%	25%	21%	15%	10%

Figure 17–24 For any given O_2 concentration in inspired gas, the relationship between alveolar ventilation and Pao_2 is hyperbolic. As the inspired O_2 concentration is increased, the amount that alveolar ventilation must decrease to produce hypoxemia is greatly increased. BTPS, body temperature, ambient pressure, saturated. (Redrawn from Lumb AB: Respiratory system resistance: Measurement of closing capacity. In Lumb AB [ed]: Nunn's Applied Respiratory Physiology, 5th ed. London, Butterworths, 2000, p 79.)

Oxygen Transport

Overview of Oxygen Transport

The principal function of the heart and lungs is supporting O_2 delivery to and CO_2 removal from the tissues in accordance with metabolic requirements while maintaining arterial blood O_2 and CO_2 partial pressures within a narrow range. The respiratory and cardiovascular systems are series-linked to accomplish this function over a wide range of metabolic requirements, which may increase 30-fold from rest to heavy exercise. The functional links in the oxygen transport chain are as follows: (1) ventilation and distribution of ventilation with respect to perfusion, (2) diffusion of O_2 into blood,

(3) chemical reaction of O_2 with Hb, (4) $\dot{Q}_T$ of arterial blood, and (5) distribution of blood to tissues and release of O_2 (Table 17-3). The system is seldom stressed except at exercise, and the earliest symptoms of cardiac or respiratory diseases are often seen only during exercise.

The maximum functional capacity of each link can be determined independently. Table 17-3 lists these measured functional capacities for healthy, young men. Because theoretical maximal O_2 transport at the ventilatory step or the diffusion and chemical reaction steps (about 6 L/min in healthy humans at sea level) exceeds the O_2 transportable by the maximum cardiac output and distribution steps, the limit to O_2 transport is the cardiovascular system. Respiratory diseases would not be expected to limit maximum O_2 transport until functional capacities are reduced nearly 40% to 50%.

Oxygen-Hemoglobin Dissociation Curve

As a red blood cell (RBC) passes by the alveolus, O_2 diffuses into plasma and increases Pao_2. As Pao_2 increases, O_2 diffuses into the RBC and combines with Hb. Each Hb molecule consists of four heme molecules attached to a globin molecule. Each heme molecule consists of glycine, α-ketoglutaric acid, and iron in the ferrous (Fe^{2+}) form. Each ferrous ion has the capacity to bind with one O_2 molecule in a loose, reversible combination. As the ferrous ions bind to O_2, the Hb molecule begins to become saturated.

The oxy-Hb dissociation curve relates the saturation of Hb (rightmost y axis in Fig. 17-25) to Pao_2. Hb is fully saturated (100%) by a Po_2 of about 700 mm Hg. The normal arterial point on the right side and flat part of the oxy-Hb curve in Figure 17-25 is 95% to 98% saturated by a Pao_2 of about 90 to 100 mm Hg. When Po_2 is less than 60 mm Hg (90% saturation), saturation falls steeply, and the amount of Hb uncombined with O_2 increases greatly for a given decrease in Po_2. Mixed venous blood has a Po_2 ($P\bar{v}o_2$) of about 40 mm Hg and is approximately 75% saturated, as indicated by the middle of the three points on the oxy-Hb curve in Figure 17-25.

Table 17–3 Functional capacities and potential maximum O_2 transport of each link in the O_2 transport chain in normal humans* at sea level

Link in Chain	Functional Capacity in Normal Humans	Theoretical Maximum O_2 Transport Capacity
Ventilation	200 L/min (MVV)	$0.030 \times MVV = 6.0$ L O_2/min
Diffusion and chemical reaction	$87 \dfrac{\text{mL } O_2/\text{min}}{\text{mm Hg } O_2 \text{ gradient}}$	$D_{LO_2} = 6.1$ L O_2/min
CO	20 L/min	
O_2 extraction	75%	$0.16 \times CO = 3.2$ L O_2/min
(a-v O_2 difference)	(16 mL O_2/100 mL or 0.16)	

*Hemoglobin = 15 g/dL; physiologic dead space in percentage of tidal volume = 0.25; partial alveolar pressure of oxygen > 110 mm Hg.
CO = cardiac output; MVV = maximum voluntary ventilation.
From Cassidy SS: Heart-lung interactions in health and disease. Am J Med Sci 30:451-461, 1987.

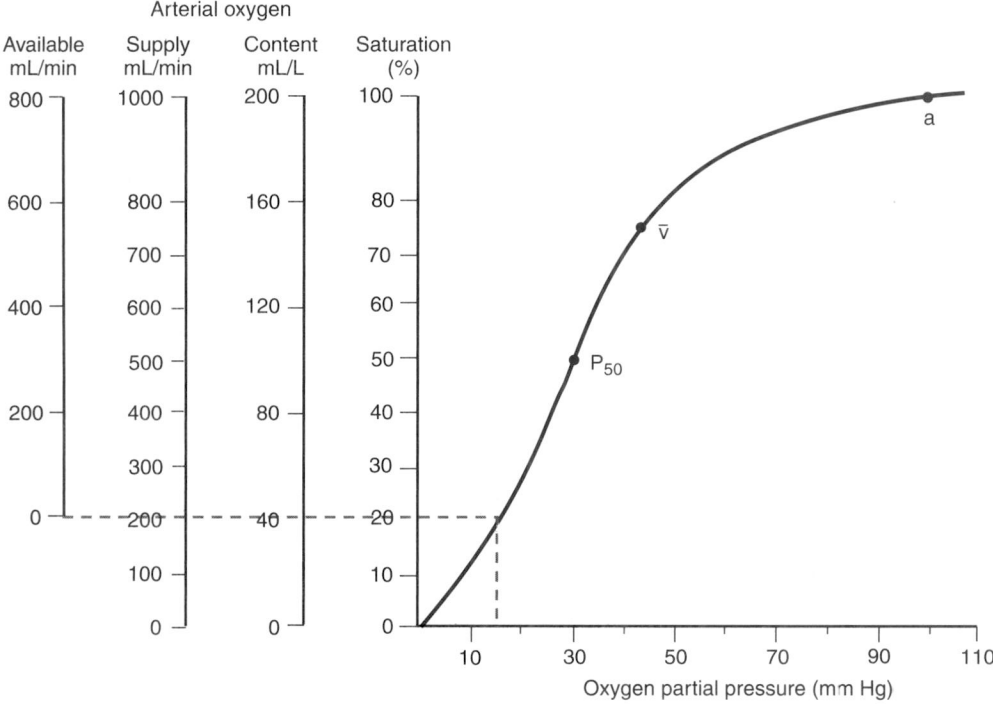

Figure 17–25 Oxygen-hemoglobin dissociation curve. Four different ordinates are shown as a function of oxygen partial pressure (the abscissa). In order from right to left, they are saturation (%); O_2 content (mL of O_2/0.1 L of blood); O_2 supply to peripheral tissues (mL/min); and O_2 available to peripheral tissues (mL/min), which is O_2 supply minus the approximately 200 mL/min that cannot be extracted below a partial pressure of 20 mm Hg. Three points are shown on the curve: a, normal arterial pressure; $\bar{v}$, normal mixed venous pressure; and P_{50}, the partial pressure (27 mm Hg) at which hemoglobin is 50% saturated.

The oxy-Hb curve can also relate the O_2 content (Co_2) (vol%, mL of O_2/0.1 L of blood; second most right y axis in Fig. 17-25) to Po_2. Oxygen is carried in solution in plasma, 0.003 mL of O_2/mm Hg Po_2/0.1 L, and is combined with Hb, 1.39 mL of O_2/g of Hb, to the extent (percentage) that Hb is saturated. Thus,

$$Co_2 = (1.39)(Hb)(\text{percent saturation}) + 0.003(Po_2) \quad (12)$$

For a patient with an Hb content of 15 g/0.1 L, Pao_2 of 100 mm Hg, and $P\bar{v}o_2$ of 40 mm Hg, the arterial O_2 content (Cao_2) = (1.39)(15)(1) + (0.003)(100) = 20.9 + 0.3 = 21.2 mL of O_2/0.1 L; the mixed venous O_2 content ($C\bar{v}o_2$) = (1.39)(15)(0.75) + (0.003)(40) = 15.6 + 0.1 = 15.7 mL of O_2/0.1 L. Thus, the normal arteriovenous O_2 content difference is approximately 5.5 mL/0.1 L.

Note that Equation 12 uses the constant 1.39, which means that 1 g of Hb can carry 1.39 mL of oxygen. Controversy exists over the magnitude of this number. Originally, 1.34 had been used,[95] but with determination of the molecular weight of Hb (64,458), the theoretical value of 1.39 became popular.[96] After extensive human studies, Gregory[97] observed in 1974 that the applicable value was 1.31 mL O_2/g of Hb in human adults. The reason that the clinically measured Co_2 is lower than the theoretical 1.39 is probably due to the small amount of methemoglobin (Met-Hb) and carboxyhemoglobin (CO-Hb) normally present in blood.

The oxy-Hb curve can also relate O_2 transport (L/min) to the peripheral tissues (see the third most right y axis in Fig. 17-25) to Po_2. This value is obtained by multiplying the O_2 content by $\dot{Q}T$ (O_2 transport = $\dot{Q}T \times Cao_2$). To do this multiplication, one must convert the content unit of mL/0.1 L to mL/L by multiplying the usual O_2 content by 10 (results in mL of O_2/L of blood); subsequent multiplication of mL/L against $\dot{Q}T$ in L/min yields mL/min. Thus, if $\dot{Q}T$ = 5 L/min and Cao_2 = 20 mL of O_2/0.1 L, the arterial point corresponds to 1000 mL O_2/min going to the periphery, and the venous point corresponds to 750 mL O_2/min returning to the lungs, with $\dot{V}o_2$ = 250 mL/min.

The oxy-Hb curve can also relate the O_2 actually available to the tissues (see leftmost y axis in Fig. 17-25) as a function of Po_2. Of the 1000 mL/min of O_2 normally going to the periphery, 200 mL/min of O_2 cannot be extracted because it would lower Po_2 below the level (see the rectangular dashed line in Fig. 17-25) at which organs such as the brain can survive; the O_2 available to tissues is therefore 800 mL/min. This amount is approximately three to four times the normal resting $\dot{V}o_2$. When $\dot{Q}T$ = 5 L/min and arterial saturation is less than 40%, the total flow of O_2 to the periphery is reduced to 400 mL/min; the available O_2 is now 200 mL/min and O_2 supply just equals O_2 demand. Consequently, with low arterial saturation, tissue demand can be met only by an increase in $\dot{Q}T$ or, in the longer term, by an increase in Hb concentration.

The affinity of Hb for O_2 is best described by the Po_2 level at which Hb is 50% saturated (P_{50}) on the oxy-Hb curve. The normal adult P_{50} is 26.7 mm Hg (see the point on the left side and steep portion of the oxy-Hb curve in Fig. 17-24).

The effect of a change in Po_2 on Hb saturation is related to both P_{50} and the portion of the oxy-Hb curve at which the change occurs.[98] In the region of normal Pao_2 (75 to 100 mm Hg), the curve is relatively horizontal, so shifts of the curve have little effect on saturation. In the region of mixed venous Po_2, where the curve is relatively steep, a shift of the curve leads to a much greater difference in saturation. A P_{50} lower than 27 mm Hg describes a left-shifted oxy-Hb curve, which means that at any given Po_2, Hb has a higher affinity for O_2 and is therefore more saturated than normal. This lower P_{50} may require higher than normal tissue perfusion to produce the normal amount of O_2 unloading. Causes of a left-shifted oxy-Hb curve are alkalosis (metabolic and respiratory—the Bohr effect), hypothermia, abnormal and fetal Hb, carboxyhemoglobin, methemoglobin, and decreased RBC 2,3-diphosphoglycerate (2,3-DPG) content (which may occur with the transfusion of old acid-citrate-dextrose–stored blood; storage of blood in citrate-phosphate-dextrose minimizes changes in 2,3-DPG with time).[98]

A P_{50} higher than 27 mm Hg describes a right-shifted oxy-Hb curve, which means that at any given PO_2, Hb has a low affinity for O_2 and is less saturated than normal. This higher P_{50} may allow a lower tissue perfusion than normal to produce the normal amount of O_2 unloading. Causes of a right-shifted oxy-Hb curve are acidosis (metabolic and respiratory—the Bohr effect), hyperthermia, abnormal Hb, increased RBC 2,3-DPG content, and inhaled anesthetics (see later).[98]

Abnormalities in acid-base balance result in alteration of 2,3-DPG metabolism to shift the oxy-Hb curve to its normal position. This compensatory change in 2,3-DPG requires between 24 and 48 hours. Thus, with acute acid-base abnormalities, O_2 affinity and the position of the oxy-Hb curve change. However, with more prolonged acid-base changes, the reciprocal changes in 2,3-DPG levels shift the oxy-Hb curve and therefore O_2 affinity back toward normal.[98]

Many inhaled anesthetics have been shown to shift the oxy-Hb dissociation curve to the right.[99] Isoflurane shifts P_{50} to the right by 2.6 ± 0.07 mm Hg at a vapor pressure of approximately 1 minimum alveolar concentration (MAC) (1.25%).[100] On the other hand, high-dose fentanyl, morphine, and meperidine do not alter the position of the curve.

Effect of $\dot{Q}s/\dot{Q}T$ on Pao_2

PAO_2 is directly related to Fio_2 in normal patients. PAO_2 and Fio_2 also correspond to Pao_2 when there is little to no right-to-left transpulmonary shunt ($\dot{Q}s/\dot{Q}T$). Figure 17-26 shows the relationship between Fio_2 and Pao_2 for a family of right-to-left transpulmonary shunts ($\dot{Q}s/\dot{Q}T$); the calculations assume a constant and normal $\dot{Q}T$ and $Paco_2$. With no $\dot{Q}s/\dot{Q}T$, a linear increase in Fio_2 results in a linear increase in Pao_2 (solid straight line). As the shunt is increased, the $\dot{Q}s/\dot{Q}T$ lines relating Fio_2 to Pao_2 become progressively flatter.[101] With a shunt of 50% of $\dot{Q}T$, an increase in Fio_2 results in almost no increase in Pao_2. The solution to the problem of hypoxemia secondary to a large shunt is not increasing the Fio_2, but rather causing a reduction in the shunt (fiberoptic bronchoscopy, PEEP, patient positioning, antibiotics, suctioning, diuretics).

Effect of $\dot{Q}T$ and $\dot{V}o_2$ on Cao_2

In addition to an increased $\dot{Q}s/\dot{Q}T$, Cao_2 is decreased by decreased $\dot{Q}T$ (for a constant $\dot{V}o_2$) and by increased $\dot{V}o_2$ (for a constant $\dot{Q}T$). In either case (decreased $\dot{Q}T$ or

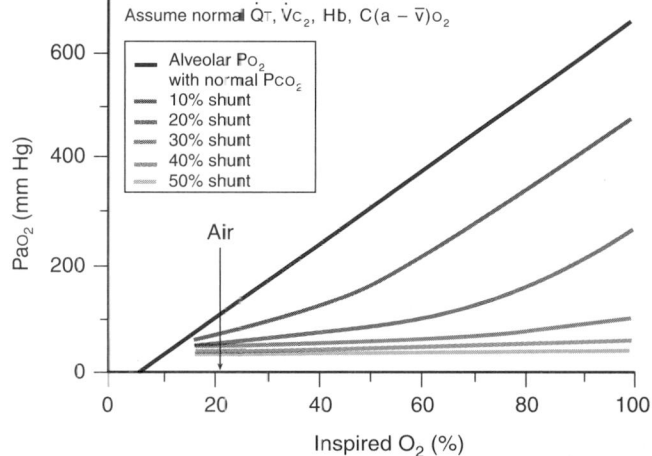

Figure 17–26 Effect of changes in inspired oxygen concentration on Pao_2 for various right-to-left transpulmonary shunts. Cardiac output ($\dot{Q}T$), hemoglobin (Hb), oxygen consumption ($\dot{V}o_2$), and arteriovenous oxygen content differences [$C(a - v)o_2$] are assumed to be normal.

increased $\dot{V}o_2$), along with a constant right-to-left shunt, the tissues must extract more O_2 from blood per unit blood volume, and therefore, $C\bar{v}o_2$ must primarily decrease (Fig. 17-27). When blood with lower $C\bar{v}o_2$ passes through whatever shunt exists in the lung and remains unchanged

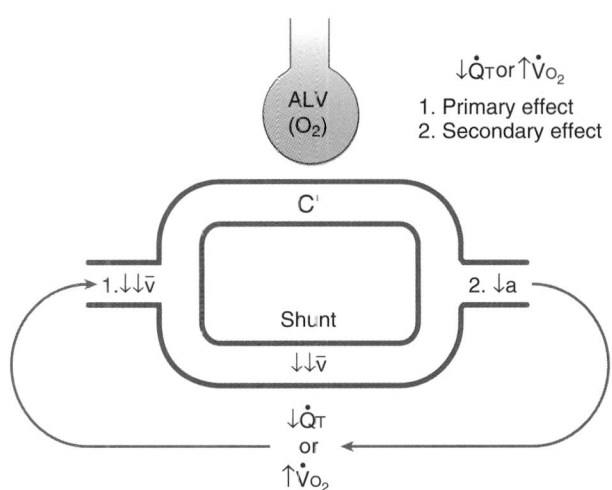

Figure 17–27 Effect of a decrease in cardiac output or an increase in oxygen consumption on mixed venous and arterial oxygen content. Mixed venous blood ($\bar{v}$) either perfuses ventilated alveolar (ALV O_2) capillaries and becomes oxygenated end-pulmonary capillary blood (c') or perfuses whatever true shunt pathways exist and remains the same in composition (desaturated). These two pathways must ultimately join together to form mixed arterial (a) blood. If cardiac output ($\dot{Q}T$) decreases or oxygen consumption ($\dot{V}o_2$) increases, or both, the tissues must extract more oxygen per unit volume of blood than under normal conditions. Thus, the primary effect of a decrease in $\dot{Q}T$ or an increase in $\dot{V}o_2$ is a decrease in mixed venous oxygen content. The mixed venous blood with a decreased oxygen content must flow through the shunt pathway as before (which may remain constant in size) and lower the arterial content of oxygen. Thus, the secondary effect of a decrease in $\dot{Q}T$ or an increase in $\dot{V}o_2$ is a decrease in arterial oxygen content.

in its $\dot{V}O_2$, it must inevitably mix with oxygenated end-pulmonary capillary blood (c' flow) and secondarily decrease CaO_2 (see Fig. 17-27).

The amount of O_2 flowing through any given particular lung channel per minute, as depicted in Figure 17-27, is a product of blood flow times the O_2 content of that blood. Thus, from Figure 17-27, $\dot{Q}T \times CaO_2 = \dot{Q}c' \times Cc'O_2 + \dot{Q}s \times C\bar{v}O_2$. With $\dot{Q}c' = \dot{Q}T - \dot{Q}s$ and further algebraic manipulation,[102]

$$\dot{Q}s/\dot{Q}T = Cc'O_2 - CaO_2/Cc'O_2 - C\bar{v}O_2 \qquad (13)$$

The larger the intrapulmonary shunt, the greater is the decrease in CaO_2 because more venous blood with lower $C\bar{v}O_2$ can admix with end-pulmonary capillary blood (see Fig. 17-37).[103,104] Thus, $P(A - a)O_2$ is a function both of the size of the $\dot{Q}s/\dot{Q}T$ and of what is flowing through the $\dot{Q}s/\dot{Q}T$, namely, $C\bar{v}O_2$, and $C\bar{v}O_2$ is a primary function of $\dot{Q}T$ and $\dot{V}O_2$.

Figure 17-28 shows the equivalent circuit of the pulmonary circulation in a patient with a 50% shunt, a normal $C\bar{v}O_2$ of 15 vol%, and a moderately low CaO_2 of 17.5 vol%. Decreasing $\dot{Q}T$ or increasing $\dot{V}O_2$, or both, causes a larger primary decrease in $C\bar{v}O_2$ to 10 vol% and a smaller, but still significant secondary decrease in CaO_2 to 15 vol%; the ratio of change in $C\bar{v}O_2$ to CaO_2 in this example of 50% $\dot{Q}s/\dot{Q}T$ is 2:1.

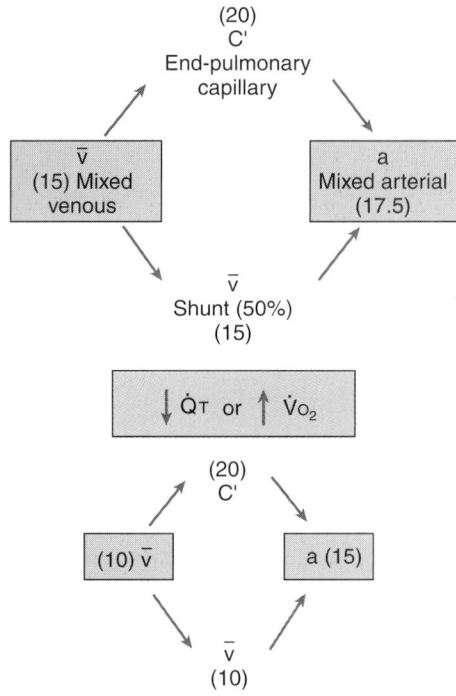

Figure 17–28 The equivalent circuit of the pulmonary circulation in a patient with a 50% right-to-left shunt. Oxygen content is in mL/100 mL of blood (vol%). A decrease in cardiac output ($\dot{Q}T$) or an increase in O_2 consumption ($\dot{V}O_2$) can cause a decrease in mixed venous oxygen content (from 15 to 10 vol% in this example), which in turn will cause a decrease in the arterial content of oxygen (from 17.5 to 15.0 vol%). In this 50% shunt example, the decrease in mixed venous oxygen content was twice the decrease in arterial oxygen content.

If a decrease in $\dot{Q}T$ or an increase in $\dot{V}O_2$ is accompanied by a decrease in $\dot{Q}s/\dot{Q}T$, there may be no change in PaO_2 (a decreasing effect on PaO_2 is offset by an increasing effect on PaO_2) (Table 17-4). These changes sometimes occur in diffuse lung disease. If a decrease in $\dot{Q}T$ or an increase in $\dot{V}O_2$ is accompanied by an increase in $\dot{Q}s/\dot{Q}T$, PaO_2 may be greatly decreased (a decreasing effect on PaO_2 is compounded by another decreasing effect on PaO_2) (see Table 17-4). These changes sometimes occur in regional ARDS and atelectasis.[105]

Fick Principle
The Fick principle allows calculation of $\dot{V}O_2$ and states that the amount of O_2 consumed by the body ($\dot{V}O_2$) is equal to the amount of O_2 leaving the lungs ($\dot{Q}T$)(CaO_2) minus the amount of O_2 returning to the lungs ($\dot{Q}T$)($C\bar{e}O_2$). Thus

$$\dot{V}O_2 = (\dot{Q}T)(CaO_2) - (\dot{Q}T)(C\bar{v}O_2) = \dot{Q}T(CaO_2 - C\bar{v}O_2)$$

Condensing the content symbols yields the usual expression of the Fick equation:

$$\dot{V}O_2 = (\dot{Q}T)[C(a - v)O_2] \qquad (14)$$

This equation states that O_2 consumption is equal to $\dot{Q}T$ times the arteriovenous O_2 content difference. Normally, (5 L/min)(5.5 mL)/0.1 L = 0.27 L/min (see the section "Oxygen-Hemoglobin Dissociation Curve").

$$\dot{V}O_2 = \dot{V}E(FIO_2) - \dot{V}E(FEO_2) = \dot{V}E(FIO_2 - FEO_2) \qquad (15)$$

Similarly, the amount of O_2 consumed by the body ($\dot{V}O_2$) is equal to the amount of O_2 brought into the lungs by ventilation ($\dot{V}I$)(FIO_2) minus the amount of O_2 leaving the lungs by ventilation ($\dot{V}E$)(FEO_2), where $\dot{V}E$ is expired minute ventilation and FEO_2 is the mixed expired O_2 fraction.

Thus, $\dot{V}O_2 = (\dot{V}I)(FIO_2) - (\dot{V}E)(FEO_2)$. Because the difference between $\dot{V}I$ and $\dot{V}E$ is due to the difference between $\dot{V}O_2$ (normally 250 mL/min) and $\dot{V}CO_2$ (normally 200 mL/min) and is only 50 mL/min (see later), $\dot{V}I$ essentially equals $\dot{V}E$.

Normally, $\dot{V}O_2 = 5.0$ L/min (0.21 − 0.16) = 0.25 L/min. In determining $\dot{V}O_2$ in this way, $\dot{V}E$ can be measured with a spirometer, FIO_2 can be measured with an O_2 analyzer or from known fresh gas flows, and FEO_2 can be measured by collecting expired gas in a bag for a few minutes.

Table 17–4 Cardiac output ($\dot{Q}T$), shunt ($\dot{Q}s/\dot{Q}T$), and venous ($P\bar{v}O_2$) and arterial (PaO_2) oxygenation

Changes	Clinical Situation
If $\dot{Q}T \downarrow \rightarrow \downarrow P\bar{v}O_2$ and $\dot{Q}s/\dot{Q}T =$ K $\rightarrow PaO_2 \downarrow$	Decreased cardiac output, stable shunt
If $\dot{Q}T \downarrow \rightarrow \downarrow P\bar{v}O_2$ and $\dot{Q}s/\dot{Q}T \downarrow \rightarrow PaO_2 =$ K	Application of PEEP in ARDS
If $\dot{Q}T \downarrow \rightarrow \downarrow P\bar{v}O_2$ and $\dot{Q}s/\dot{Q}T \uparrow \rightarrow PaO_2 \downarrow\downarrow$	Shock combined with ARDS or atelectasis

ARDS, adult respiratory distress syndrome; K, constant; PEEP, positive end expiratory pressure; ↓, decrease; ↑, increase.

A sample of the mixed expired gas is used to measure P_{EC_2}. To convert P_{EO_2} to F_{EO_2}, simply divide P_{EO_2} by dry atmospheric pressure: $P_{EO_2}/713 = F_{EO_2}$.

Additionally, the Fick equation is useful in understanding the impact of changes in $\dot{Q}_T$ on Pa_{O_2} and $P\bar{v}_{CO_2}$. If $\dot{V}_{O_2}$ remains constant (K) and $\dot{Q}_T$ decreases ($\downarrow$), the arteriovenous O_2 content difference has to increase ($\uparrow$):

$$\dot{V}_{O_2} = K = (\downarrow)\dot{Q}_T \times (\uparrow)C(a - \bar{v})O_2.$$

The $C(a - \bar{v})O_2$ difference increases because a decrease in $\dot{Q}_T$ causes a much larger and primary decrease in $C\bar{v}_{O_2}$ versus a smaller and secondary decrease in Ca_{O_2}:

$$(\uparrow)C(a - \bar{v})O_2 = C(\downarrow a - \downarrow\downarrow\bar{v})O_2{}^{103}$$

Thus, $C\bar{v}_{O_2}$ (and $P\bar{v}_{O_2}$) are much more sensitive indicators of $\dot{Q}_T$ because they change more with changes in $\dot{Q}_T$ than Ca_{O_2} (or Pa_{O_2}) does (see Figs. 17-27 and 17-37).

Carbon Dioxide Transport

The amount of CO_2 circulating in the body is a function of both CO_2 elimination and production. Elimination of CO_2 depends on pulmonary blood flow and alveolar ventilation. Production of CO_2 ($\dot{V}_{CO_2}$) parallels O_2 consumption ($\dot{V}_{O_2}$) according to the respiratory quotient (R):

$$R = \frac{\dot{V}_{CO_2}}{\dot{V}_{O_2}} \qquad (16)$$

Under normal resting conditions, R is 0.8; that is, only 80% as much CO_2 is produced as O_2 is consumed. However, this value changes as the nature of the metabolic substrate changes. If only carbohydrate is used, the respiratory quotient is 1.0. Conversely, with the sole use of fat, more O_2 combines with hydrogen to produce water, and the R value drops to 0.7.

CO_2 is transported from mitochondria to the alveoli in a number of forms. In plasma, CO_2 exists in physical solution, hydrated to carbonic acid (H_2CO_3), and as bicarbonate (HCO_3^-). In the RBC, CO_2 combines with Hb as carbaminohemoglobin (Hb-CO_2). The approximate relative values of H_2CO_3 ($H_2O + CO_2$), HCO_3^-, and Hb-CO_2 to the total CO_2 transported are 7%, 80%, and 13%, respectively.

In plasma, CO_2 exists both in physical solution and as H_2CO_3:

$$H_2O + CO_2 \Leftrightarrow H_2CO_3 \qquad (17)$$

The CO_2 in solution can be related to Pco_2 by the use of Henry's law[106]:

$$Pco_2 \times \alpha = [CO_2] \text{ in solution} \qquad (18)$$

where α is the solubility coefficient of CO_2 in plasma (0.03 mmol/L/mm Hg at 37°C). However, the major fraction of CO_2 produced passes into the RBC. As in plasma, CO_2 combines with water to produce H_2CO_3. However, unlike the slow reaction in plasma, in which the equilibrium point lies toward the left, the reaction in an RBC is catalyzed by the enzyme carbonic anhydrase. This zinc-containing

enzyme moves the reaction to the right at a rate 1000 times faster than in plasma. Furthermore, nearly 99.9% of the H_2CO_3 dissociates to HCO_3^- and hydrogen ions (H^+):

$$H_2O + CO_2 \xrightarrow{\text{carbonic anhydrase}} H_2CO_3$$
$$H_2CO_3 \rightarrow H^+ + HCO_3^- \qquad (19)$$

The H^- produced from H_2CO_3 in the production of HCO_3^- is buffered by Hb ($H^- + Hb \Leftrightarrow HHb$). The HCO_3^- produced passes out of the RBC into plasma to perform its function as a buffer. To maintain electrical neutrality within the RBC, chloride ion (Cl^-) moves in as HCO_3^- moves out (Cl^- shift). Finally, CO_2 can combine with Hb in the erythrocyte (to produce Hb-CO_2). Again, as in HCO_3^- release, an H^+ ion is formed in the reaction of CO_2 and Hb. This H^+ ion is also buffered by Hb.

Bohr and Haldane Effects

Just as the percent saturation of Hb with O_2 is related to Po_2 (described by the oxy-Hb curve), so is the total CO_2 in blood related to Pco_2. Additionally, Hb has variable affinity for CO_2; it binds more avidly in the reduced state than as oxy-Hb.[98] The Bohr effect describes the effect of Pco_2 and [H^+] ions on the oxy-Hb curve. Hypercapnia and acidosis both shift the curve to the right (reducing the oxygen-binding affinity of hemoglobin), and hypocapnia and alkalosis both shift the curve to the left. Conversely, the Haldane effect describes the shift in the CO_2 dissociation curve caused by oxygenation of Hb. Low Po_2 shifts the CO_2 dissociation curve to the left so that the blood is able to pick up more CO_2, as occurs in capillaries of rapidly metabolizing tissues). Conversely, oxygenation of Hb (as occurs in the lungs) reduces the affinity of Hb for CO_2, and the CO_2 dissociation curve is shifted to the right, thereby increasing CO_2 removal.

Pulmonary Microcirculation, Pulmonary Interstitial Space, and Pulmonary Interstitial Fluid Kinetics (Pulmonary Edema)

The ultrastructural appearance of an alveolar septum[107] is schematically depicted in Figure 17-29. Capillary blood is separated from alveolar gas by a series of anatomic layers: capillary endothelium, endothelial basement membrane, interstitial space, epithelial basement membrane, and alveolar epithelium (of the type I pneumocyte).

On one side of the alveolar septum (the thick, upper [see Fig. 17-29], fluid- and gas-exchanging side), the epithelial and endothelial basement membranes are separated by a space of variable thickness containing connective tissue fibrils, elastic fibers, fibroblasts, and macrophages. This connective tissue is the backbone of the lung parenchyma; it forms a continuum with the connective tissue sheaths around the conducting airways and blood vessels. Thus, the pericapillary perialveolar interstitial space is continuous with the interstitial tissue space that surrounds terminal bronchioles and vessels, and both spaces constitute the connective tissue space of the lung. There are no lymphatics in the interstitial space of the alveolar septum. Instead, lymphatic capillaries first appear in the interstitial space surrounding terminal bronchioles, small arteries, and veins.[108]

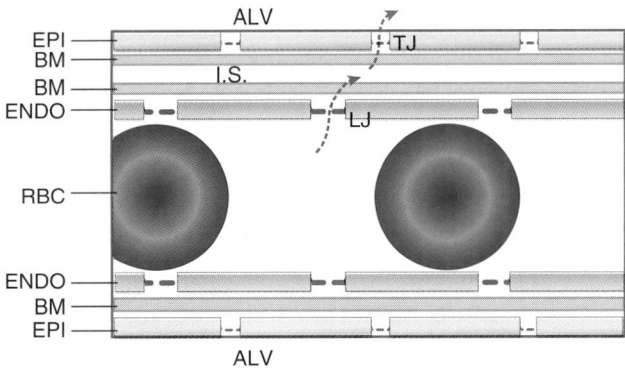

Figure 17–29 Schematic summary of the ultrastructure of a pulmonary capillary. The upper side of the capillary has the endothelial and epithelial basement membranes separated by an interstitial space, whereas the lower side contains only fused endothelial and epithelial basement membranes. The *dashed arrows* indicate a potential pathway for fluid to move from the intravascular space to the interstitial space (through loose junctions in the endothelium) and from the interstitial space to the alveolar space (through tight junctions in the epithelium). ALV, alveolus; BM, basement membrane; ENDO, endothelium; EPI, epithelium; IS, interstitial space; LJ, loose junction; RBC, red blood cell; TJ, tight junction. (Redrawn from Fishman AP: Pulmonary edema: The water-exchanging function of the lung. Circulation 46:390, 1972.)

The opposite side of the alveolar septum (the thin, down [see Fig. 17-29], gas-exchanging-only side) contains only fused epithelial and endothelial basement membranes. The interstitial space is thus greatly restricted on this side because of fusion of the basement membranes. Interstitial fluid cannot separate the endothelial and epithelial cells from one another, and as a result, the space and distance barrier to fluid movement from the capillary to the alveolar compartment is reduced and composed of only the two cell linings with their associated basement membranes.[109]

Between the individual endothelial and epithelial cells are holes or junctions that provide a potential pathway for fluid to move from the intravascular space to the interstitial space and finally from the interstitial space to the alveolar space. The junctions between endothelial cells are relatively large and are therefore termed loose; the junctions between epithelial cells are relatively small and are therefore termed tight. Pulmonary capillary permeability (K) is a direct function of and essentially equivalent to the size of the holes in the endothelial and epithelial linings.

To understand how pulmonary interstitial fluid is formed, stored, and cleared, it is necessary to first develop the concepts that (1) the pulmonary interstitial space is a continuous space between the periarteriolar and peribronchial connective tissue sheath and the space between the endothelial and epithelial basement membranes in the alveolar septum and (2) the space has a progressively negative distal-to-proximal ΔP.

The concepts of a continuous connective tissue sheath–alveolar septum interstitial space and a negative interstitial space ΔP are prerequisite to understanding interstitial fluid kinetics (Fig. 17-30). After entering the

lung parenchyma, both the bronchi and arteries run within a connective tissue sheath that is formed by an invagination of the pleura at the hilum and ends at the level of the bronchioles (Fig. 17-30A). Thus, there is a potential perivascular and peribronchial space, respectively, between the arteries and the bronchi and the connective tissue sheath. The negative pressure in the pulmonary tissues surrounding the perivascular connective tissue sheath exerts a radial outward traction force on the sheath. This radial traction creates negative pressure within the sheath that is transmitted to the bronchi and arteries and tends to hold them open and increase their diameters (see Fig. 17-30).[109] The alveolar septum

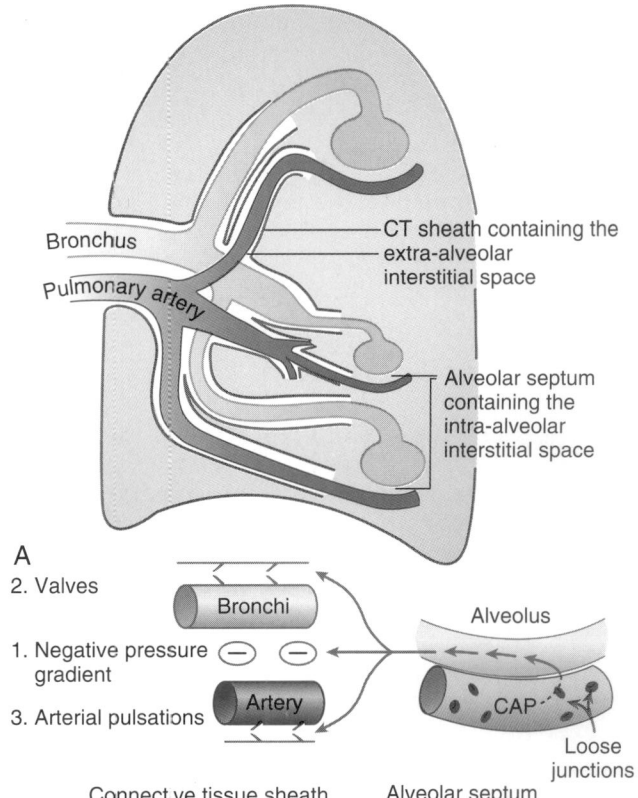

Figure 17–30 A, Schematic diagram of the concept of a continuous connective tissue (CT) sheath–alveolar septum interstitial space. The entry of the main stem bronchi and pulmonary artery into the lung parenchyma invaginates the pleura at the hilum and forms a surrounding connective tissue sheath. The connective tissue sheath ends at the level of the bronchioles. The space between the pulmonary arteries and bronchi and the interstitial space is continuous with the alveolar septum interstitial space. The alveolar septum interstitial space is contained within the endothelial and epithelial basement membranes of the capillaries and alveoli, respectively. **B,** Schematic diagram showing how interstitial fluid moves from the alveolar septum interstitial space (no lymphatics) to the connective tissue interstitial space (lymphatic capillaries first appear). The mechanisms are a negative-pressure gradient (sump), the presence of one-way valves in the lymphatics, and the massaging action of arterial pulsations. (Redrawn with modification from Benumof JL: Anesthesia for Thoracic Surgery, 2nd ed. Philadelphia, WB Saunders, 1995, Chapter 8.)

interstitial space is the space between the capillaries and alveoli (or more precisely, the space between the endothelial and epithelial basement membranes) and is continuous with the interstitial tissue space that surrounds the larger arteries and bronchi (see Fig. 17-30A). Studies indicate that the alveolar interstitial pressure is also uniquely negative, but not as much as the negative interstitial space pressure around the larger arteries and bronchi.[110]

The forces governing net transcapillary–interstitial space fluid movement are as follows. The net transcapillary flow of fluid (F) out of pulmonary capillaries (across the endothelium and into the interstitial space) is equal to the difference between pulmonary capillary hydrostatic pressure (P_{inside}) and interstitial fluid hydrostatic pressure ($P_{outside}$) and the difference between capillary colloid oncotic pressure (π_{inside}) and interstitial colloid oncotic pressure ($\pi_{outside}$). These four forces produce a steady-state fluid flow (F) during a constant capillary permeability (K) as predicted by the Starling equation:

$$F = K[(P_{inside} - P_{outside}) - (\pi_{inside} - \pi_{outside})] \qquad (20)$$

K is a capillary filtration coefficient expressed in mL/min/mm Hg/100 g. The filtration coefficient is the product of the effective capillary surface area in a given mass of tissue and the permeability per unit surface area of the capillary wall to filter the fluid. Under normal circumstances and at a vertical height in the lung that is at the junction of zones 2 and 3, intravascular colloid oncotic pressure ($\approx$26 mm Hg) acts to keep water in the capillary lumen, and working against this force, pulmonary capillary hydrostatic pressure ($\approx$10 mm Hg) acts to force water across the loose endothelial junctions into the interstitial space. If these were the only operative forces, the interstitial space and, consequently, the alveolar surfaces would be constantly dry, and there would be no lymph flow. In fact, alveolar surfaces are moist, and lymphatic flow from the interstitial compartment is constant ($\approx$500 mL/day). This can be explained in part by $\pi_{outside}$ ($\approx$8 mm Hg) and in part by the negative $P_{outside}$ (−8 mm Hg). Negative (subatmospheric) interstitial space pressure would promote, by suction, a slow loss of fluid across the endothelial holes.[111] Indeed, extremely negative pleural (and perivascular hydrostatic) pressure, such as may occur in a vigorously, spontaneously breathing patient with an obstructed airway, can cause pulmonary interstitial edema (Table 17-5).[112] Relative to the vertical level of the junction of zones 2 and 3, as lung height decreases (lung dependency), absolute P_{inside} increases, and fluid has a propensity to transudate; as lung height increases (lung nondependency), absolute P_{inside} decreases, and fluid has a propensity to be reabsorbed. However, fluid transudation induced by an increase in P_{inside} is limited by a concomitant dilution of proteins in the interstitial space and therefore a decrease in $\pi_{outside}$.[113] Any change in the size of the endothelial junctions, even if the foregoing four forces remain constant, changes the magnitude and perhaps even the direction of fluid movement; increased size of endothelial junctions (increased permeability) promotes transudation, whereas decreased size of

Table 17–5 Causes of extremely negative pulmonary interstitial fluid pressure ($P_{outside}$) in pulmonary edema

Vigorous spontaneous ventilation against an obstructed airway
    Laryngospasm
    Infection, inflammation, edema
    Upper airway mass (tumor, hematoma, abscess, foreign body, etc.)
    Vocal cord paralysis
    Strangulation
Rapid re-expansion of lung
Vigorous pleural suctioning (thoracentesis, chest tube)

endothelial junctions (decreased permeability) promotes reabsorption.

No lymphatics are present in the interstitial space of the alveolar septum. The lymphatic circulation starts as blind-ended lymphatic capillaries, first appearing in the interstitial space sheath surrounding terminal bronchioles and small arteries, and ends at the subclavian veins. Interstitial fluid is normally removed from the alveolar interstitial space into the lymphatics by a sump (pressure gradient) mechanism, which is caused by the presence of more negative pressure surrounding the larger arteries and bronchi.[114,115] The sump mechanism is aided by the presence of valves in the lymph vessels. In addition, because the lymphatics run in the same sheath as the pulmonary arteries, they are exposed to the massaging action of arterial pulsations. The differential negative pressure, the lymphatic valves, and the arterial pulsations all help propel the lymph proximally toward the hilum through the lymph nodes (pulmonary to bronchopulmonary to tracheobronchial to paratracheal to scalene and cervical nodes) to the central venous circulation depot (Fig. 17-30B). An increase in central venous pressure, which is the backpressure for lymph to flow out of the lung, would decrease lung lymph flow and perhaps promote pulmonary interstitial edema.

If the rate of entry of fluid into the pulmonary interstitial space exceeds the capability of the pulmonary interstitial space to clear the fluid, the pulmonary interstitial space will fill with fluid; the fluid, now under an increased and positive driving force (P_{ISF}), will cross the relatively impermeable epithelial wall holes and the alveolar space will fill. Intra-alveolar edema fluid will additionally cause alveolar collapse and atelectasis, thereby promoting further accumulation of fluid.

RESPIRATORY FUNCTION DURING ANESTHESIA

Arterial oxygenation is impaired in most patients during anesthesia with either spontaneous or controlled ventilation.[116-121] In otherwise normal patients, it is generally accepted that the impairment in arterial oxygenation during anesthesia is more severe in the elderly,[122,123] the obese,[124] and smokers.[125] In various studies of healthy young to middle-aged patients under general anesthesia, venous admixture (shunt) has been found to average 10%, and the scatter in $\dot{V}_A/\dot{Q}$ ratios is small to moderate,[123,126] whereas in patients with a more marked deterioration in preoperative pulmonary function, general anesthesia causes considerable widening of the $\dot{V}_A/\dot{Q}$ distribution and large increases in both low-$\dot{V}_A/\dot{Q}$ ($0.005 < \dot{V}_A/\dot{Q} < 0.1$) (underventilated) regions and shunting.[122,125,127] The magnitude of shunting correlates closely with the degree of atelectasis.[122,127]

In addition to the foregoing generalizations concerning respiratory function during anesthesia, the effect of a given anesthetic on respiratory function depends on the depth of general anesthesia, the patient's preoperative respiratory condition, and the presence of special intraoperative anesthetic and surgical conditions.

Effect of Anesthetic Depth on Respiratory Pattern

The respiratory pattern is altered by the induction and deepening of anesthesia. When the depth of anesthesia is inadequate (less than MAC), the respiratory pattern may vary from excessive hyperventilation and vocalization to breath-holding. As anesthetic depth approaches or equals MAC (light anesthesia), irregular respiration progresses to a more regular pattern that is associated with a larger than normal V_T. However, during light but deepening anesthesia, the approach to a more regular respiratory pattern may be interrupted by a pause at the end of inspiration (a "hitch" in inspiration), followed by a relatively prolonged and active expiration in which the patient seems to exhale forcefully rather than passively. As anesthesia deepens to moderate levels, respiration becomes faster and more regular, but shallower. The respiratory pattern is a sine wave losing the inspiratory hitch and lengthened expiratory pause. There is little or no inspiratory or expiratory pause, and the inspiratory and expiratory periods are equivalent. Intercostal muscle activity is still present, and there is normal movement of the thoracic cage with lifting of the chest during inspiration. The respiratory rate is generally slower and the V_T larger with nitrous oxide–narcotic anesthesia than with anesthesia involving halogenated drugs. During deep anesthesia with halogenated drugs, increasing respiratory depression is manifested by increasingly rapid and shallow breathing (panting). On the other hand, with deep nitrous oxide–narcotic anesthesia, respirations become slower but may remain deep. In the case of very deep anesthesia with all inhaled drugs, respirations often become jerky or gasping in character and irregular in pattern. This situation results from loss of the active intercostal muscle contribution to inspiration. As a result, a rocking boat movement occurs in which there is out-of-phase depression of the chest wall during inspiration, flaring of the lower chest margins, and billowing of the abdomen. The reason for this type of movement is that inspiration is dependent solely on diaphragmatic effort. Independent of anesthetic depth, similar chest movements may be simulated by upper and lower airway obstruction and by partial paralysis.

Effect of Anesthetic Depth on Spontaneous Minute Ventilation

Despite the variable changes in respiratory pattern and rate as anesthesia deepens, overall spontaneous $\dot{V}_E$ progressively decreases. The normal awake response to breathing CO_2 (the x axis in Fig. 17-31 shows an increasing end-tidal concentration of CO_2) causes a linear increase in $\dot{V}_E$ (see the y axis in Fig. 17-31). In Figure 17-31 the slope of the line relating $\dot{V}_E$ to the end-tidal CO_2 concentration in awake individuals is 2 L/min/mm Hg. (In healthy individuals, the variation in the slope of this response is large.) Figure 17-31 also shows that increasing halothane concentration displaces the end-tidal CO_2 ventilation-response curve progressively to the right (meaning that at any CO_2 concentration, ventilation is less than before), decreases the slope of the curve, and shifts the apneic threshold to a higher end-tidal CO_2 concentration level.[128] Similar alterations are observed with narcotics and other halogenated anesthetics.[129] Figures 17-22 to 17-24 show that decreases in $\dot{V}_E$ cause increases in Pa_{CO_2} and decreases in Pa_{O_2}. The relative increase in Pa_{CO_2} caused by depression of $\dot{V}_E$ (<1.24 MAC) by halogenated anesthetics is enflurane > desflurane = isoflurane > sevoflurane > halothane. At higher concentrations, desflurane causes increasing ventilatory depression and becomes similar to enflurane, and sevoflurane becomes similar to isoflurane (see Chapter 6 for additional further study).

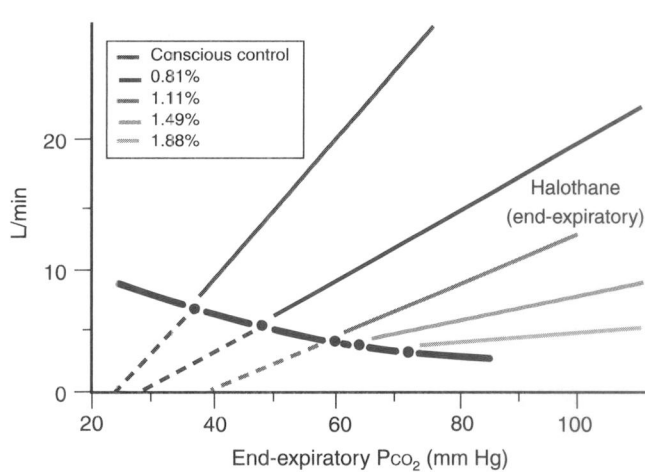

Figure 17–31 In conscious controls *(heavy solid line)*, increasing end-expiratory P_{CO_2} increases pulmonary minute volume. The *dashed line* is an extrapolation of the CO_2 response curve to zero ventilation and represents the apneic threshold. An increase in anesthetic (halothane) concentration (end-expiratory concentration) progressively diminishes the slope of the CO_2 response curve and shifts the apneic threshold to a higher P_{CO_2}. The *heavy line interrupted by dots* shows the decrease in minute ventilation and the increase in P_{CO_2} that occur with increasing depth of anesthesia. (Redrawn with modification from Munson ES, Larson CP Jr, Babad AA, et al: The effects of halothane, fluroxene and cyclopropane on ventilation: A comparative study in man. Anesthesiology 27:716, 1966.)

Effect of Preexisting Respiratory Dysfunction on the Respiratory Effects of Anesthesia

Anesthesiologists are frequently required to care for (1) patients with acute chest disease (pulmonary infection, atelectasis) or systemic diseases (sepsis, cardiac and renal failure, multiple trauma) who require emergency operations, (2) heavy smokers with subtle pathologic airway and parenchymal conditions and hyperreactive airways, (3) patients with classic emphysematous and bronchitic problems, (4) obese people prone to decreases in FRC during anesthesia,[130] (5) patients with chest deformities, and (6) extremely old patients.

The nature and magnitude of these preexisting respiratory conditions determine, in part, the effect of a given standard anesthetic on respiratory function. For example, in Figure 17-32, the FRC-CC relationship is depicted for normal, obese, bronchitic, and emphysematous patients.

In a healthy patient, FRC exceeds CC by approximately 1 L. In the latter three respiratory conditions, CC is 0.5 to 0.75 L less than FRC. If anesthesia causes a 1-L decrease in FRC, a healthy patient will have no change in the qualitative relationship between FRC and CC. In patients with special respiratory conditions, a 1-L decrease in FRC will cause CC to exceed FRC and will change the previous marginally normal FRC-CC relationship to either a grossly low $\dot{V}A/\dot{Q}$ or an atelectatic FRC-CC relationship. Similarly, patients with chronic bronchitis, who have copious airway secretions, may suffer more from an anesthetic-induced decrease in mucus velocity flow than other patients. Finally, if an anesthetic inhibits HPV, the drug may increase shunting more in patients with preexisting HPV than in those without preexisting HPV. Thus, the effect of a standard anesthetic can be expected to produce varying degrees of respiratory change in patients who have different degrees of preexisting respiratory dysfunction.

Effect of Special Intraoperative Conditions on the Respiratory Effects of Anesthesia

Some special intraoperative conditions (such as surgical position, massive blood loss, and surgical retraction on the lung), may cause impaired gas exchange. For example, some of the surgical positions (i.e., the lithotomy, jackknife, and kidney rest positions) and surgical exposure requirements may decrease QT, may cause hypoventilation in a spontaneously breathing patient, and may reduce FRC. The type and severity of preexisting respiratory dysfunction, as well as the number and severity of special intraoperative conditions that can embarrass respiratory function, will magnify the respiratory depressant effects of any anesthetic.

Mechanisms of Hypoxemia during Anesthesia

Malfunction of Equipment
Mechanical Failure of Anesthesia Apparatus to Deliver Oxygen to the Patient
Hypoxemia resulting from mechanical failure of the O_2 supply system (also see Chapter 9) or the anesthesia machine is a recognized hazard of anesthesia. Disconnection of the patient from the O_2 supply system (usually at the juncture of the endotracheal tube and the elbow connector) is by far the most common cause of mechanical failure to deliver O_2 to the patient. Other reported causes of failure of the O_2 supply during anesthesia include the following: an empty or depleted O_2 cylinder, substitution of a nonoxygen cylinder at the O_2 yoke because of absence or failure of the pin index, an erroneously filled O_2 cylinder, insufficient opening of the O_2 cylinder (which hinders free flow of gas as pressure decreases), failure of gas pressure in a piped O_2 system, faulty locking of the piped O_2 system to the anesthesia machine, inadvertent switching of the Schrader adapters on piped lines, crossing of piped lines during construction, failure of a reducing valve or gas manifold, inadvertent disturbance of the setting of the O_2 flow meter, use of the fine O_2 flow meter instead of the coarse flow meter, fractured or sticking

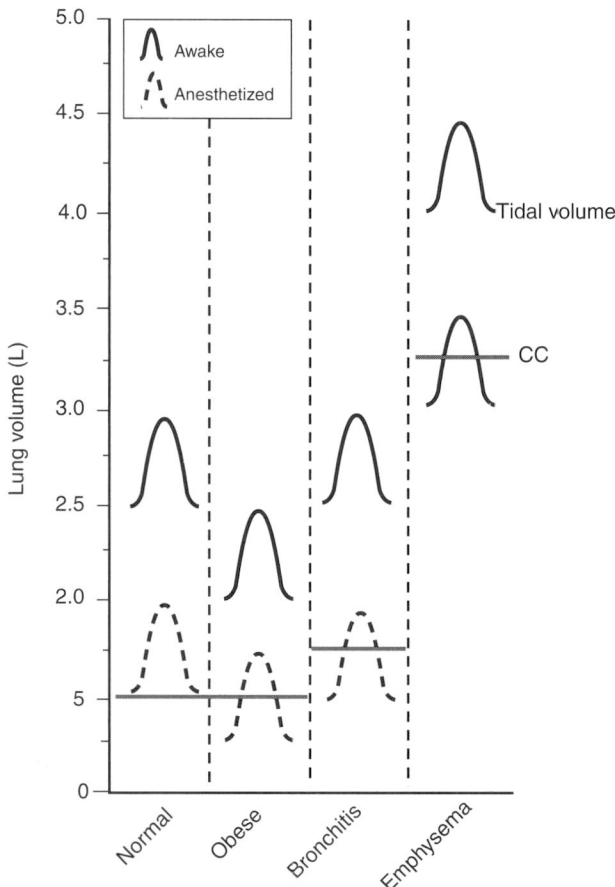

Figure 17–32 The lung volume (ordinate) at which tidal volume is breathed decreases (by 1 L) from the awake state to the anesthetized state. Functional residual capacity (FRC), which is the volume of lung existing at the end of tidal volume, therefore also decreases (by 1 L) from the awake to the anesthetized state. In healthy, obese, bronchitic, and emphysematous patients, the awake FRC considerably exceeds the closing capacity (CC). In obese, bronchitic, and emphysematous patients, the anesthetized state causes FRC to be less than CC. In healthy patients, anesthesia causes FRC to equal CC.

flow meters, transposition of rotameter tubes, erroneous filling of a liquid O_2 reservoir with nitrogen, and disconnection of the fresh gas line from machine to in-line hosing.[131-135] Monitoring of the inspired O_2 concentration with an in-line FiO_2 analyzer and monitoring of airway pressure should detect most of these causes of failure to deliver O_2 to the patient.[131-135]

Mechanical Failure of the Endotracheal Tube: Intubation of the Main Stem Bronchus

Esophageal intubation results in almost no ventilation. Virtually all other mechanical problems (except disconnection) with endotracheal tubes (such as kinking, blockage of secretions, and herniated or ruptured cuffs) cause an increase in airway resistance that may result in hypoventilation. Intubation of a main stem bronchus (also see Chapter 42) results in the absence of ventilation of the contralateral lung. Though potentially minimized by HPV, some perfusion to the contralateral lung always remains, and shunting increases and PaO_2 decreases. A tube previously well positioned in the trachea may enter a bronchus after the patient or the patient's head is turned or moved into a new position.[136] Flexion of the head causes the tube to migrate deeper (caudad) into the trachea, whereas extension of the head causes cephalad (outward) migration of the endotracheal tube.[136] A high incidence of main stem bronchial intubation after the institution of a 30-degree Trendelenburg position has been reported.[137] Cephalad shift of the carina and mediastinum during the Trendelenburg position caused the previously "fixed" endotracheal tube to migrate into a main stem bronchus. Main stem bronchial intubation may obstruct the ipsilateral upper lobe in addition to the contralateral lung.[138,139] Infrequently, the right upper bronchus or one of its segmental bronchi branches from the lateral wall of the trachea and may be occluded by a properly positioned endotracheal tube.

Hypoventilation (Decreased Tidal Volume)

Patients under general anesthesia may have a reduced spontaneous V_T for two reasons. First, increased work of breathing can occur during general anesthesia as a result of increased airway resistance and decreased C_L. Airway resistance may be increased because of reduced FRC, endotracheal intubation, the presence of external breathing apparatus and circuitry, and possible airway obstruction in patients whose tracheas are not intubated.[140-142] C_L is reduced as a result of some (or all) of the factors that can decrease FRC.[143] Second, patients may have a decreased drive to breathe spontaneously during general anesthesia (decreased chemical control of breathing) (see Fig. 17-31).

Decreased V_T may cause hypoxemia in two ways.[116] First, shallow breathing may promote atelectasis and cause a decrease in FRC (see the section "Ventilation Pattern").[144,145] Second, decreased $\dot{V}_E$ decreases the overall $\dot{V}_A/\dot{Q}$ ratio of the lung, which decreases PaO_2 (see Figs. 17-23 and 17-24).[116] This is likely to occur with spontaneous ventilation during moderate to deep levels of anesthesia, in which the chemical control of breathing is significantly altered.

Hyperventilation

Hypocapnic alkalosis (hyperventilation) may result in decreased PaO_2 by several mechanisms: decreased $\dot{Q}_T$[102,103] and increased $\dot{V}O_2$[146,147] (see the section "Decreased Cardiac Output and Increased Oxygen Consumption"), a left-shifted oxy-Hb curve (see the section "Oxygen-Hemoglobin Dissociation Curve"), decreased HPV[148] (see the section "Inhibition of Hypoxic Pulmonary Vasoconstriction"), and increased airway resistance and decreased compliance[149] (see the section "Increased Airway Resistance").

Decrease in Functional Residual Capacity

Induction of general anesthesia is consistently accompanied by a significant (15% to 20%) decrease in FRC,[85,94,150] which usually causes a decrease in compliance.[143] The maximum decrease in FRC appears to occur within the first few minutes of anesthesia[85,151,152] and, in the absence of any other complicating factor, does not seem to decrease progressively during anesthesia. During anesthesia, the reduction in FRC is of the same order of magnitude whether ventilation is spontaneous or controlled. Conversely, in awake patients, FRC is only slightly reduced during controlled ventilation.[152] In obese patients, the reduction in FRC is far more pronounced than in normal patients, and the decrease is inversely related to the body mass index (BMI).[153] The reduction in FRC continues into the postoperative period.[154] For individual patients, the reduction in FRC correlates well with the increase in the alveolar-arterial PO_2 gradient during anesthesia with spontaneous breathing,[155] during anesthesia with artificial ventilation,[152] and in the postoperative period.[154] The reduced FRC may be restored to normal or above normal by the application of PEEP.[84,156] The following discussion considers all possible causes of reduced FRC.

Supine Position

Anesthesia and surgery are usually performed with the patient in the supine position (see Chapter 28). In changing from the upright to the supine position, FRC decreases by 0.5 to 1.0 L[85,94,150] because of a 4-cm cephalad displacement of the diaphragm by the abdominal viscera (Fig. 17-33). Pulmonary vascular congestion may also contribute to the decrease in FRC in the supine position, particularly in patients who experienced orthopnea preoperatively. These FRC changes are magnified in obese patients, with the decrement directly related to BMI.[153]

Induction of General Anesthesia: Change in Thoracic Cage Muscle Tone

At the end of a normal (awake) exhalation, there is slight tension in the inspiratory muscles and no tension in the expiratory muscles. Thus, at the end of a normal exhalation, there is a force tending to maintain lung volume and no force decreasing lung volume. After induction of general anesthesia, there is a loss of inspiratory tone and an appearance of end-expiratory tone in the abdominal expiratory muscles at the end of exhalation. The end-expiratory tone in the abdominal expiratory muscles increases intra-abdominal pressure, forces the diaphragm cephalad, and decreases FRC[151,157] (see Fig. 17-33).

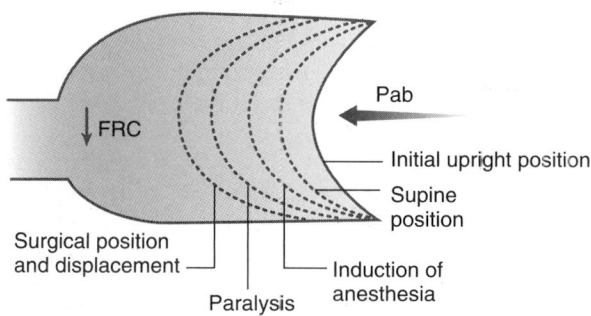

Progressive Cephalad Displacement of the Diaphragm

Figure 17–33 Anesthesia and surgery may cause a progressive cephalad displacement of the diaphragm. The sequence of events involves assumption of the supine position, induction of anesthesia, establishment of paralysis, assumption of several surgical positions, and displacement by retractors and packs. Cephalad displacement of the diaphragm results in decreased functional residual capacity ($\downarrow$ FRC). P$_{ab}$, pressure of abdominal contents. (Redrawn with modification from Benumof JL: Anesthesia for Thoracic Surgery, 2nd ed. Philadelphia, WB Saunders, 1995, Chapter 8.)

Thus, after the induction of general anesthesia, there is loss of the force tending to maintain lung volume and gain of the force tending to decrease lung volume. Indeed, Innovar (droperidol and fentanyl citrate) may increase tone in expiratory muscles to such an extent that the reduction in FRC with Innovar anesthesia alone is greater than that with Innovar plus paralysis induced by succinylcholine.[157,158]

With emphysema, exhalation may be accompanied by pursing the lips or grunting (partially closed larynx). An emphysematous patient exhales in either of these ways because both these maneuvers cause an expiratory retardation that produces PEEP in the intrathoracic air passage and decreases the possibility of airway closure and a decrease in FRC (see Fig. 17-17F). Endotracheal intubation bypasses the lips and glottis and may abolish the normally present pursed-lip or grunting exhalation and in that way contributes to airway closure and loss of FRC in some spontaneously breathing patients.

Paralysis

In an upright subject, FRC and the position of the diaphragm are determined by the balance between lung elastic recoil pulling the diaphragm cephalad and the weight of the abdominal contents pulling it caudad.[159] There is no transdiaphragmatic pressure gradient.

The situation is more complex in the supine position. The diaphragm separates two compartments of markedly different hydrostatic gradients. On the thoracic side, pressure increases by approximately 0.25 cm H_2O/cm of lung height,[6,7] and on the abdominal side, it increases by 1.0 cm H_2O/cm of abdominal height,[159] which means that in horizontal postures, progressively higher transdiaphragmatic pressure must be generated toward dependent parts of the diaphragm to keep the abdominal contents out of the thorax. In an unparalyzed patient, this tension is developed either by passive stretch and changes in

shape of the diaphragm (causing an increased contractile force) or by neurally mediated active tension. With acute muscle paralysis, neither of these two mechanisms can operate, and a shift of the diaphragm to a more cephalad position occurs (see Fig. 17-33).[160] The latter position must express the true balance of forces on the diaphragm, unmodified by any passive or active muscle activity.

The cephalad shift in the FRC position of the diaphragm as a result of expiratory muscle tone during general anesthesia is equal to the shift observed during paralysis (awake or anesthetized patients).[151,161] The equal shift suggests that the pressure on the diaphragm caused by an increase in expiratory muscle tone during general anesthesia is equal to the pressure on the diaphragm caused by the weight of the abdominal contents during paralysis. It is quite probable that the magnitude of these changes in FRC due to paralysis also depends on body habitus.

Light or Inadequate Anesthesia and Active Expiration

Induction of general anesthesia can result in increased expiratory muscle tone,[157] but the increased expiratory muscle tone is not coordinated and does not contribute to the exhaled volume of gas. In contrast, spontaneous ventilation during light general anesthesia usually results in a coordinated and moderately forceful active exhalation and larger exhaled volumes. Excessively inadequate anesthesia (relative to a given stimulus) results in very forceful active exhalation, which may produce exhaled volumes of gas equal to an awake expiratory vital capacity.

As during an awake expiratory vital capacity maneuver, forced expiration during anesthesia raises intrathoracic and alveolar pressure considerably above atmospheric pressure (see Fig. 17-17). This increase in pressure results in rapid outflow of gas, and because part of the expiratory resistance lies in the smaller air passages, a drop in pressure occurs between the alveoli and the main bronchi. Under these circumstances, intrathoracic pressure rises considerably above the pressure within the main bronchi. Collapse will occur if this reversed pressure gradient is sufficiently high to overcome the tethering effect of the surrounding parenchyma on the small intrathoracic bronchioles or the structural rigidity of cartilage in the large extrathoracic bronchi. Such collapse occurs in a normal subject during a maximal forced expiration and is responsible for the associated wheeze in both awake and anesthetized patients.[162]

In a paralyzed, anesthetized patient, the use of a subatmospheric expiratory pressure phase is analogous to a forced expiration in a conscious subject; the negative phase may set up the same adverse ΔP, which can cause airway closure, gas trapping, and a decrease in FRC. An excessively rapidly descending bellows of a ventilator during expiration has caused subatmospheric expiratory pressure and resulted in wheezing.[163]

Increased Airway Resistance

The overall reduction in all components of lung volume during anesthesia results in reduced airway caliber, which increases airway resistance and any tendency toward airway collapse (Fig. 17-34). The relationship between airway resistance and lung volume is well established (Fig. 17-35).

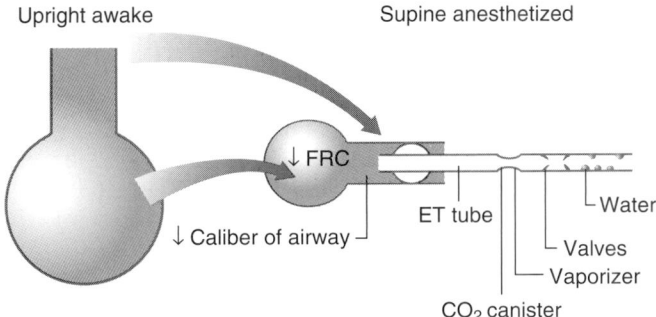

Figure 17–34 An anesthetized patient in the supine position has increased airway resistance as a result of decreased functional residual capacity (FRC), decreased caliber of the airways, endotracheal intubation, and connection of the endotracheal tube (ET) to the external breathing apparatus and circuitry. (Redrawn with modification from Benumof JL: Anesthesia for Thoracic Surgery, 2nd ed. Philadelphia, WB Saunders, 1995, Chapter 8.)

The decreases in FRC caused by the supine position (≈0.8 L) and induction of anesthesia (≈0.4 L) are often sufficient to explain the increased resistance seen in a healthy anesthetized patient.[140]

In addition to this expected increase in airway resistance in anesthetized patients, there are a number of additional special potential sites of increased airway resistance, including the endotracheal tube (if present), the upper and lower airway passages, and the external anesthesia apparatus. Endotracheal intubation reduces the

size of the trachea, usually by 30% to 50% (see Fig. 17-34). Pharyngeal obstruction, which can be considered to be a normal feature of unconsciousness, is most common. A minor degree of this type of obstruction occurs in snoring. Laryngospasm and obstructed endotracheal tubes (secretions, kinking, herniated cuffs) are not uncommon and may be life threatening.

The respiratory apparatus often causes resistance that is considerably higher than the resistance in the normal human respiratory tract (see Fig. 17-34).[91] When certain resistors such as those shown in Figure 17-34 are joined in a series to form an anesthetic gas circuit, they generally add to produce larger resistance (as with resistance in series in an electrical circuit). The increase in resistance associated with commonly used breathing circuits and endotracheal tubes may impose an additional work of breathing that is two to three times normal.[142]

Supine Position, Immobility, and Excessive Intravenous Fluid Administration

Patients undergoing anesthesia and surgery are often kept supine and immobile for long periods. Thus, some of the lung may be continually dependent and below the left atrium and therefore in zone 3 or 4 condition. Being in a dependent position, the lung is predisposed to accumulation of fluid. Coupled with excessive fluid administration, conditions sufficient to promote transudation of fluid into the lung are present and will result in pulmonary edema and decreased FRC. When mongrel dogs were placed in a lateral decubitus position and anesthetized for several hours (Fig. 17-36, bottom horizontal axis), expansion of the extracellular space with fluid (top horizontal axis) caused the P_{O_2} (left-hand axis) of blood draining the dependent lung (closed circles) to

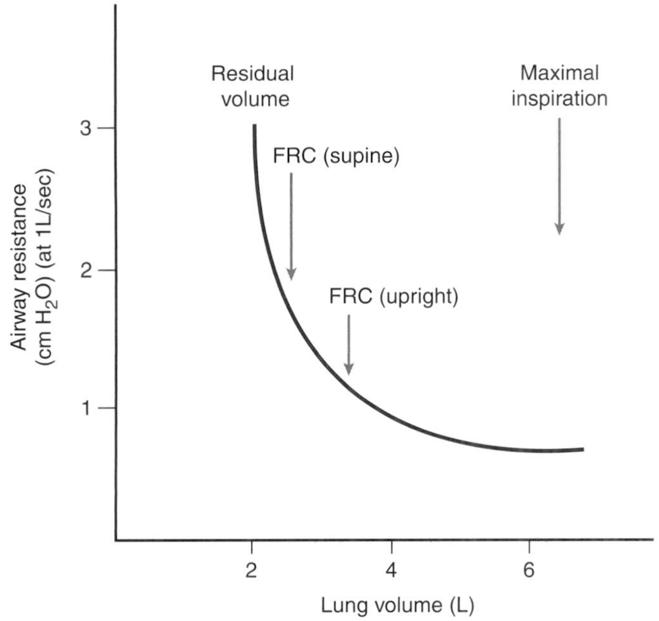

Figure 17–35 Airway resistance is an increasing hyperbolic function of decreasing lung volume. Functional residual capacity (FRC) decreases when changing from the upright to the supine position. (Redrawn with modification from Lumb AB: Respiratory system resistance. In Lumb AB [ed]: Nunn's Applied Respiratory Physiology, 5th ed. London, Butterworths, 2000, p 67.)

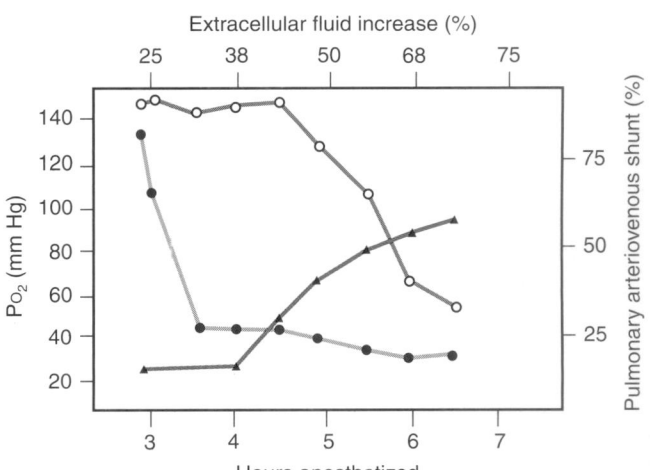

Figure 17–36 Mongrel dogs anesthetized with pentobarbital (bottom axis), placed in a lateral decubitus position, and subjected to progressive extracellular fluid expansion (top axis) have a marked decrease in the P_{O_2} (left vertical axis) of blood draining the dependent lung (solid circles) and a smaller, much slower decrease in the P_{O_2} of blood draining the nondependent lung (open circles). The pulmonary arteriovenous shunt (right vertical axis) rises progressively (triangles). (Redrawn from Ray JF, Yost L, Moallem S, et al: Immobility, hypoxemia, and pulmonary arteriovenous shunting. Arch Surg 109:537, 1974.)

decrease precipitously to mixed venous levels (no O_2 uptake).[164] Blood draining the nondependent lung maintained its P_{O_2} for a period, but in the face of the extracellular fluid expansion, it also suffered a decline in P_{O_2} after 5 hours. Transpulmonary shunting (right-hand axis) progressively increased. If the animals were turned every hour (and received the same fluid challenge), only the dependent lung, at the end of each hour period, suffered a decrease in oxygenation. If the animals were turned every half-hour and received the same fluid challenge, neither lung suffered a decrease in oxygenation. In patients who undergo surgery in the lateral decubitus position (e.g., pulmonary resection, in which they have or will have a restricted pulmonary vascular bed) and receive excessive intravenous fluids, the risk of the dependent lung becoming edematous is certainly increased. These considerations also explain, in part, the beneficial effect of a continuously rotating (side-to-side) bed on the incidence of pulmonary complications in critically ill patients.[165]

High Inspired Oxygen Concentration and Absorption Atelectasis

General anesthesia is usually administered with an increased F_{IO_2}. In patients who have areas of moderately low $\dot{V}_A/\dot{Q}$ ratios (0.1 to 0.01), administration of F_{IO_2} greater than 0.3 adds enough O_2 into the alveolar space in these areas to eliminate the shuntlike effect that they have, and total measured right-to-left shunting decreases. However, when patients with a significant amount of blood flow perfusing lung units with very low $\dot{V}_A/\dot{Q}$ ratios (0.01 to 0.0001) have a change in F_{IO_2} from room air to 1.0, the very low $\dot{V}_A/\dot{Q}$ units virtually disappear, and a moderately large right-to-left shunt appears.[16,17,166] In these studies, the increase in shunting was equal to the amount of blood flow previously perfusing the areas with low $\dot{V}_A/\dot{Q}$ ratios during the breathing of air. Thus, in these studies the effect of breathing O_2 was to convert units that had low $\dot{V}_A/\dot{Q}$ ratios into shunt units. The pathologic basis for this data is the conversion of low-$\dot{V}_A/\dot{Q}$ units into atelectatic units.

The cause of the atelectatic shunting during O_2 breathing is presumably a large increase in O_2 uptake by lung units with low $\dot{V}_A/\dot{Q}$ ratios.[166,167] A unit that has a low $\dot{V}_A/\dot{Q}$ ratio during breathing of air will have a low P_{AO_2}. When an enriched O_2 mixture is inspired, P_{AO_2} rises, and the rate at which O_2 moves from alveolar gas to capillary blood increases greatly. The O_2 flux may increase so much that the net flow of gas into blood exceeds the inspired flow of gas, and the lung unit will become progressively smaller. Collapse is most likely to occur if F_{IO_2} is high, the $\dot{V}_A/\dot{Q}$ ratio is low, the time of exposure of the unit with low $\dot{V}_A/\dot{Q}$ to high F_{IO_2} is long, and $C_{\bar{v}O_2}$ is low. Thus, given the right $\dot{V}_A/\dot{Q}$ ratio and time of administration, an F_{IO_2} as low as 50% can produce absorption atelectasis.[166,167] This phenomenon is of considerable significance in the clinical situation for two reasons. First, enriched O_2 mixtures are often used therapeutically, and it is important to know whether this therapy is causing atelectasis. Second, the amount of shunt is often estimated during breathing of 100% O_2, and if this maneuver results in additional shunt, the measurement will be hard to interpret.

Surgical Position

In the supine position, the abdominal contents force the diaphragm cephalad and reduce FRC (see Chapter 28).[94,151,157,161] The Trendelenburg position allows the abdominal contents to push the diaphragm further cephalad so that the diaphragm must not only ventilate the lungs but also lift the abdominal contents out of the thorax. The result is a predisposition to decreased FRC and atelectasis.[168] The Trendelenburg position–related decrease in FRC is exacerbated in obese patients.[153] Increased pulmonary blood volume and gravitational force on the mediastinal structures are additional factors that may decrease pulmonary compliance and FRC. In the steep Trendelenburg position, most of the lung may be below the left atrium and therefore in a zone 3 or 4 condition. As such, the lung may be susceptible to the development of pulmonary interstitial edema. Thus, patients with elevated Ppa, such as those with mitral stenosis, do not tolerate the Trendelenburg position well.[169]

In the lateral decubitus position, the dependent lung experiences a moderate decrease in FRC and is predisposed to atelectasis, whereas the nondependent lung may have increased FRC. The overall result is usually a slight to moderate increase in total-lung FRC.[170] The kidney and lithotomy positions also cause small decreases in FRC above that caused by the supine position. The prone position may increase FRC moderately.[170]

Ventilation Pattern (Rapid Shallow Breathing)

Rapid shallow breathing is often a regular feature of anesthesia. Monotonous shallow breathing may cause a decrease in FRC, promote atelectasis, and decrease compliance.[144,145,171] These changes with rapid shallow breathing are probably due to progressive increases in surface tension.[171] Initially, these changes may cause hypoxemia with normocapnia and may be prevented or reversed (or both) by periodic large mechanical inspirations, spontaneous sighs, PEEP, or a combination of these techniques.[171-173]

Decreased Removal of Secretions (Decreased Mucociliary Flow)

Tracheobronchial mucous glands and goblet cells produce mucus, which is swept by cilia up to the larynx, where it is swallowed or expectorated. This process clears inhaled organisms and particles from the lungs. The secreted mucus consists of a surface gel layer lying on top of a more liquid sol layer in which the cilia beat. The tips of the cilia propel the gel layer toward the larynx (upward) during the forward stroke. As the mucus streams upward and the total cross-sectional area of the airways diminishes, absorption takes place from the sol layer to maintain a constant depth of 5 mm.[174]

Poor systemic hydration and low inspired humidity reduce mucociliary flow by increasing the viscosity of secretions and slowing the ciliary beat.[175-177] Mucociliary flow varies directly with body or mucosal temperature (low inspired temperature) over a range of 32°C to 42°C.[178,179] High F_{IO_2} decreases mucociliary flow.[180] Inflation of an endotracheal tube cuff suppresses tracheal mucus velocity,[181] an effect that occurs within 1 hour, and apparently it does not matter whether a low- or high-compliance cuff is used. Passage of an uncuffed tube through the vocal cords and keeping it in situ for several hours does not affect tracheal mucus velocity.[181]

The mechanism for suppression of mucociliary clearance by the endotracheal tube cuff is speculative. In the report of Sackner and colleagues,[181] mucus velocity was decreased in the distal portion of the trachea, but the cuff was inflated in the proximal portion. Thus, the phenomenon cannot be attributed solely to damming of mucus at the cuff site. One possibility is that the endotracheal tube cuff caused a critical increase in the thickness of the layer of mucus proceeding distally from the cuff. Another possibility is that mechanical distention of the trachea by the endotracheal tube cuff initiated a neurogenic reflex arc that altered mucous secretions or the frequency of ciliary beating.

Other investigators have shown that when all the foregoing factors are controlled, halothane reversibly and progressively decreases, but does not stop mucus flow over an inspired concentration of 1 to 3 MAC.[182] The halothane-induced depression of mucociliary clearance was probably due to depression of the ciliary beat, an effect that caused slow clearance of mucus from the distal and peripheral airways. In support of this hypothesis is the finding that cilia are morphologically similar throughout the animal kingdom, and in clinical dosages, inhaled anesthetics, including halothane, have been found to cause reversible depression of the ciliary beat of protozoa.[183]

Decreased Cardiac Output and Increased Oxygen Consumption

Decreased $\dot{Q}_T$ in the presence of constant O_2 consumption ($\dot{V}_{O_2}$), increased $\dot{V}_{O_2}$ in the presence of a constant $\dot{Q}_T$, or decreased $\dot{Q}_T$ and increased $\dot{V}_{O_2}$ must all result in lower $C\bar{v}_{O_2}$. Venous blood with lowered $C\bar{v}_{O_2}$ then flows through whichever shunt pathways exist, mixes with the oxygenated end-pulmonary capillary blood, and lowers Ca_{O_2} (see Figs. 17-27 and 17-28). Figure 17-37 shows these relationships quantitatively for several different intrapulmonary shunts.[103,104] The larger the intrapulmonary shunt, the greater the decrease in Ca_{O_2} because more venous blood with lower $C\bar{v}_{O_2}$ can admix with end-pulmonary capillary blood. Decreased $\dot{Q}_T$ may occur with myocardial failure and hypovolemia; the specific causes of these two conditions are beyond the scope of this chapter. Increased $\dot{V}_{O_2}$ may occur with excessive stimulation of the sympathetic nervous system, hyperthermia, or shivering and can further contribute to impaired oxygenation of arterial blood.[184]

Inhibition of Hypoxic Pulmonary Vasoconstriction

Decreased regional Pa_{O_2} causes regional pulmonary vasoconstriction, which diverts blood flow away from hypoxic regions of the lung to better ventilated normoxic regions. The diversion of blood flow minimizes venous admixture from the underventilated or nonventilated lung regions. Inhibition of regional HPV could impair arterial oxygenation by permitting increased venous admixture from hypoxic or atelectatic areas of the lung (see Fig. 17-9).

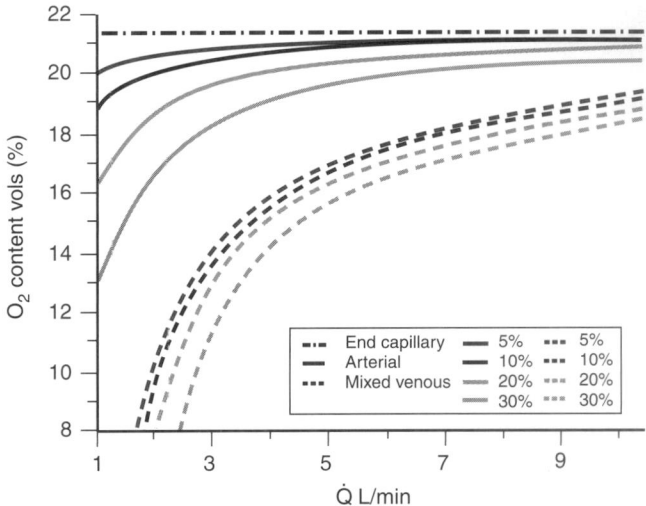

Figure 17–37 Effects of changes in cardiac output ($\dot{Q}$) on the O_2 content of end-pulmonary capillary, arterial, and mixed venous blood for a group of different transpulmonary right-to-left shunts. The magnitude of the right-to-left shunt is indicated by the various numbered percent symbols for arterial *(solid line)* and mixed venous *(dashed line)* blood; the oxygen content of end-capillary blood is unaffected by the degree of shunting. Note that a decrease in $\dot{Q}$ results in a greater decrease in the arterial content of O_2 the larger the shunt. (Redrawn from Kelman GF, Nunn JF, Prys-Roberts C, et al: The influence of the cardiac output on arterial oxygenation: A theoretical study. Br J Anaesth 39:450, 1967.)

Because the pulmonary circulation is poorly endowed with smooth muscle, any condition that increases the pressure against which the vessels must constrict (i.e., Ppa) will decrease HPV. Numerous clinical conditions can increase Ppa and therefore decrease HPV. Mitral stenosis,[185] volume overload,[185] low (but greater than room air) Fi_{O_2} in nondiseased lung,[186] a progressive increase in the amount of diseased lung,[186] thromboembolism,[186] hypothermia,[187] and vasoactive drugs[188] can all increase Ppa. Direct vasodilating drugs (such as isoproterenol, nitroglycerin, and sodium nitroprusside),[61,188] inhaled anesthetics,[189] and hypocapnia[148,188] can directly decrease HPV. The selective application of PEEP to only the nondiseased lung can selectively increase PVR in the nondiseased lung and may divert blood flow back into the diseased lung.[190]

Paralysis

In the supine position, the weight of the abdominal contents pressing against the diaphragm is greatest in the dependent or posterior part of the diaphragm and least in the nondependent or anterior part of the diaphragm. In an awake patient breathing spontaneously, active tension in the diaphragm is capable of overcoming the weight of the abdominal contents, and the diaphragm moves the most in the posterior portion (because the posterior of the diaphragm is stretched higher into the chest, it has the smallest radius of curvature, and therefore it contracts most effectively) and least in the anterior portion. This circumstance is healthy because the greatest amount of ventilation occurs in areas with the most perfusion (posteriorly or dependently), and the least amount occurs in areas with the least perfusion (anteriorly or nondependently). During paralysis and positive-pressure breathing, the passive diaphragm is displaced by the positive pressure preferentially in the anterior nondependent portion (where there is the least resistance to diaphragmatic movement) and is displaced minimally in the posterior dependent portion (where there is the most resistance to diaphragmatic movement). This circumstance is unhealthy because the greatest amount of ventilation now occurs in areas with the least perfusion, and the least amount occurs in areas with the most perfusion.[161] However, the magnitude of the change in the diaphragmatic motion pattern with paralysis varies with body position.[191,192]

Right-to-Left Interatrial Shunting

Acute arterial hypoxemia from a transient right-to-left shunt through a patent foramen ovale (PFO) has been described, particularly during emergence from anesthesia.[193] However, unless a real-time technique of imaging the cardiac chambers is used (e.g., TEE with color flow Doppler imaging),[72] it is difficult to document an acute and transient right-to-left intracardiac shunt as a cause of arterial hypoxemia. Nonetheless, right-to-left shunting through a PFO has been described in virtually every conceivable clinical situation that afterloads the right side of the heart and increases right atrial pressure. When right-to-left shunting through a PFO is identified, administration of inhaled NO can decrease PVR and functionally close the PFO.[194]

Involvement of Mechanisms of Hypoxemia in Specific Diseases

In any given pulmonary disease, many of the mechanisms of hypoxemia listed earlier may be involved.[116] Pulmonary embolism (air, fat, thrombi) (Fig. 17-38) (see Chapter 53) and the evolution of ARDS (see Chapter 75) (Fig. 17-39) will be used to illustrate this point. A significant pulmonary embolus can cause severe increases in pulmonary artery pressure, and these increases can result in right-to-left transpulmonary shunting through opened arteriovenous anastomoses and the foramen ovale (possible in 20% of patients), pulmonary edema in nonembolized regions of the lung, and inhibition of HPV. The embolus may cause hypoventilation via increased dead space ventilation. If the embolus contains platelets, serotonin may be released, and such release can cause hypoventilation as a result of bronchoconstriction and pulmonary edema as a result of increased pulmonary capillary permeability. Finally, the pulmonary embolus can increase PVR (by platelet-induced serotonin release,[26] among other etiologies) and decrease cardiac output.

After major hypotension, shock, blood loss, sepsis, and other conditions, noncardiogenic pulmonary edema may occur and lead to acute respiratory failure or ARDS[195] (described more fully in Chapters 74 and 75). The syndrome can evolve during and after anesthesia and has the hallmark characteristics of decreased FRC and compliance and hypoxemia. After shock and trauma, plasma levels of serotonin, histamine, kinins, lysozymes, reactive oxygen species, fibrin degradation products, products of complement metabolism, and fatty acids increase.

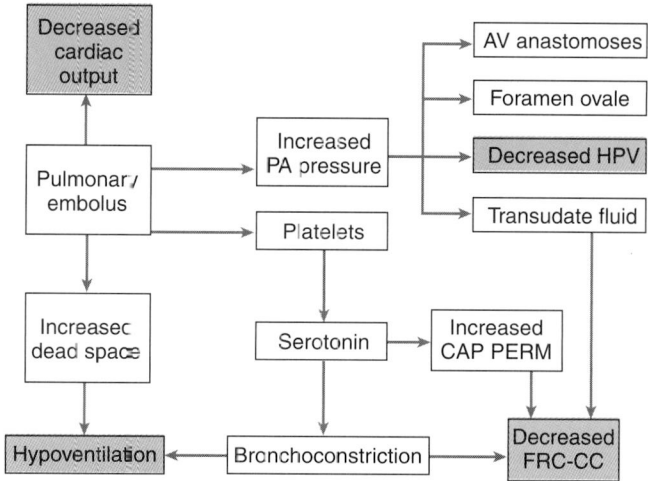

Figure 17–38 Mechanisms of hypoxemia during pulmonary embolism. See the text for an explanation of the pathophysiologic flow diagram. AV, arteriovenous; CAP PERM, capillary permeability; CC, closing capacity; FRC, functional residual capacity; HPV, hypoxic pulmonary vasoconstriction; PA, pulmonary artery. (Redrawn with modification from Benumof JL: Anesthesia for Thoracic Surgery, 2nd ed. Philadelphia, WB Saunders, 1995, Chapter 8.)

Sepsis and endotoxemia may be present. Increased levels of activated complement activate neutrophils into chemotaxis in patients with trauma and pancreatitis; activated neutrophils can damage endothelial cells. These factors, along with pulmonary contusion (if it occurs), may individually or collectively increase pulmonary capillary permeability. After shock, acidosis, increased circulating catecholamines and sympathetic nervous system activity, leukotriene and prostaglandin release, histamine release, microembolism (with serotonin release), increased intracranial pressure (with head injury), and alveolar

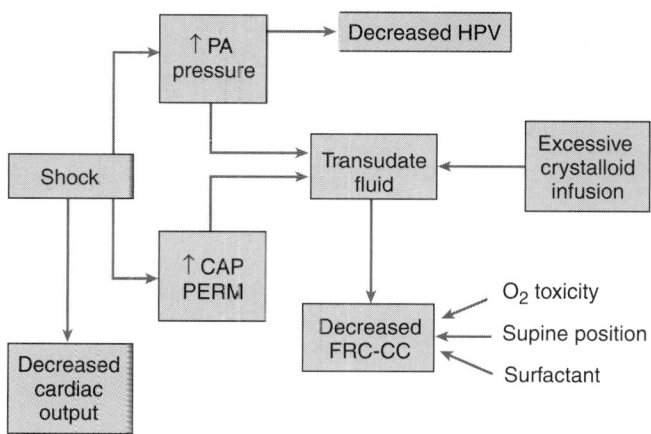

Figure 17–39 Mechanisms of hypoxemia during adult respiratory distress syndrome. See the text for an explanation of the pathophysiologic flow diagram. CAP PERM, capillary permeability; CC, closing capacity; FRC, functional residual capacity; HPV, hypoxic pulmonary vasoconstriction; PA, pulmonary artery. (Redrawn with modification from Benumof JL: Anesthesia for Thoracic Surgery, 2nd ed. Philadelphia, WB Saunders, 1995, Chapter 8.)

hypoxia may occur and may individually or collectively, particularly after resuscitation, cause a moderate increase in Ppa. After shock, the normal compensatory response to hypovolemia is movement of a protein-free fluid from the interstitial space into the vascular space to restore vascular volume. Dilution of vascular proteins by protein-free interstitial fluid can cause decreased capillary colloid oncotic pressure. Increased pulmonary capillary permeability and Ppa along with decreased capillary colloid oncotic pressure will result in fluid transudation and pulmonary edema. Additionally, decreased $\dot{Q}_T$, inhibition of HPV, immobility, the supine position, excessive fluid administration, and an excessively high F_{IO_2} can contribute to the development of ARDS.

Mechanisms of Hypercapnia and Hypocapnia during Anesthesia

Hypercapnia

Hypoventilation, increased dead space ventilation, increased CO_2 production, and inadvertent switching off of a CO_2 absorber can all cause hypercapnia (Fig. 17-40).

Hypoventilation

Patients spontaneously hypoventilate during anesthesia because it is more difficult to breathe (abnormal surgical position, increased airway resistance, decreased compliance) and they are less willing to breathe (decreased respiratory drive because of anesthetics). Hypoventilation results in hypercapnia (see Figs. 17-22 and 17-23).

Increased Dead Space Ventilation

A decrease in Ppa, as during deliberate hypotension,[196] may cause an increase in zone 1 and alveolar dead space ventilation. An increase in airway pressure (as with PEEP) may also cause an increase in zone 1 and alveolar dead space ventilation. Pulmonary embolism, thrombosis, and

vascular obliteration (kinking, clamping, blocking of the pulmonary artery during surgery) may increase the amount of lung that is ventilated but unperfused. Vascular obliteration may be responsible for the increase in dead space ventilation with age ($V_D/V_T\% = 33 + age/3$). Rapid short inspirations may be distributed preferentially to non-compliant (short time constant for inflation) and badly perfused alveoli, whereas slow inspiration allows time for distribution to more compliant (long time constant for inflation) and better perfused alveoli. Thus, rapid, short inspirations may have a dead space ventilation effect.

The anesthesia apparatus increases total dead space (V_D/V_T) for two reasons. First, the apparatus simply increases the anatomic dead space. Inclusion of normal apparatus dead space increases the total V_D/V_T ratio from 33% to about 46% in intubated patients and to about 64% in patients breathing through a mask.[197] Second, anesthesia circuits cause rebreathing of expired gases, which is equivalent to dead space ventilation. The rebreathing classification by Mapleson is widely accepted. The order of increasing rebreathing (decreasing clinical merit) during spontaneous ventilation with Mapleson circuits is A (Magill), D, C, and B. The order of increasing rebreathing (decreasing clinical merit) during controlled ventilation is D, B, C, and A. There will be no rebreathing in system E (Ayre's T-piece) if the patient's respiratory diastole is long enough to permit washout with a given fresh gas flow (common event) or if the fresh gas flow is greater than the peak inspiratory flow rate (uncommon event).

The effects of an increase in dead space can usually be counteracted by a corresponding increase in the respiratory $\dot{V}_E$. If, for example, the $\dot{V}_E$ is 10 L/min and the V_D/V_T ratio is 30%, alveolar ventilation will be 7 L/min. If a pulmonary embolism occurred and resulted in an increase in the V_D/V_T ratio to 50%, $\dot{V}_E$ would need to be increased to 14 L/min to maintain an alveolar ventilation of 7 L/min (14 L/min × 0.5).

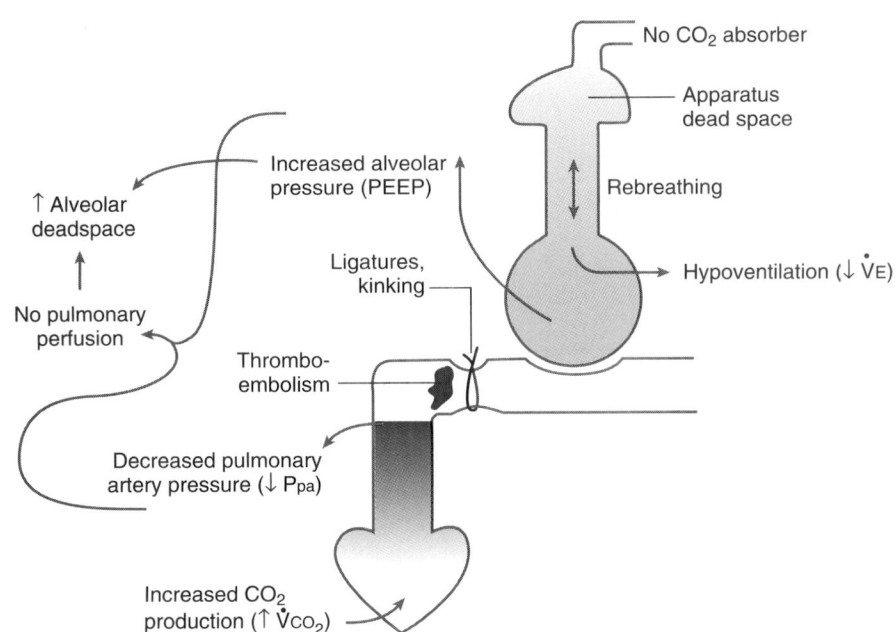

Figure 17–40 Schematic diagram of the causes of hypercapnia during anesthesia. An increase in carbon dioxide (CO_2) production ($\dot{V}_{CO_2}$) will increase Pa_{CO_2} with a constant minute ventilation ($\dot{V}_E$). Several events can increase alveolar dead space: a decrease in pulmonary artery pressure (Ppa), the application of positive end-expiratory pressure (PEEP), thromboembolism, and mechanical interference with pulmonary arterial flow (ligatures and kinking of vessels). A decrease in $\dot{V}_E$ causes an increase in Pa_{CO_2} with a constant $\dot{V}_{CO_2}$. It is possible for some anesthesia systems to cause rebreathing of CO_2. Finally, the anesthesia apparatus may increase the anatomic dead space, and inadvertent switching off of a CO_2 absorber in the presence of low fresh gas flow can increase Pa_{CO_2}. (Redrawn with modification from Benumof JL: Anesthesia for Thoracic Surgery, 2nd ed. Philadelphia, WB Saunders, 1995, Chapter 8.)

Increased Carbon Dioxide Production

All the causes of increased O_2 consumption also increase CO_2 production: hyperthermia, shivering, catecholamine release (light anesthesia), hypertension, and thyroid storm. If $\dot{V}E$, total dead space, and $\dot{V}A/\dot{Q}$ relationships are constant, an increase in CO_2 production will result in hypercapnia.

Inadvertent Switching Off of a Carbon Dioxide Absorber

Many factors, such as patient ventilatory responsiveness to CO_2 accumulation, fresh gas flow, circle system design, and CO_2 production, determine whether hypercapnia will result from accidental switching off or depletion of a circle CO_2 absorber (see Chapter 9). However, high fresh gas flows (>–5 L/min) minimize the problem with almost all systems for almost all patients.

Hypocapnia

The mechanisms of hypocapnia are the reverse of those that produce hypercapnia. Thus, all other factors being equal, hyperventilation (spontaneous or controlled ventilation), decreased VD ventilation (change from a mask airway to an endotracheal tube airway, decreased PEEP, increased Ppa, or decreased rebreathing), and decreased CO_2 production (hypothermia, deep anesthesia, hypotension) will lead to hypocapnia. By far the most common mechanism of hypocapnia is passive hyperventilation by mechanical means.

Physiologic Effects of Abnormalities in Respiratory Gases

Hypoxia

The end products of aerobic metabolism (oxidative phosphorylation) are CO_2 and water, both of which are easily diffusible and lost from the body. The essential feature of hypoxia is the cessation of oxidative phosphorylation when mitochondrial PO_2 falls below a critical level. Anaerobic pathways, which produce energy (ATP) inefficiently, are then used. The main anaerobic metabolites are hydrogen and lactate ions, which are not easily excreted. They accumulate in the circulation, where they may be quantified in terms of the base deficit and the lactate-pyruvate ratio.

Because the various organs have different blood flow and O_2 consumption rates, the manifestations and clinical diagnosis of hypoxia are usually related to symptoms arising from the most vulnerable organ. This organ is

generally the brain in an awake patient and the heart in an anesthetized patient (see later), but in special circumstances it may be the spinal cord (aortic surgery), kidney (acute tubular necrosis), liver (hepatitis), or limb (claudication, gangrene).

The cardiovascular response to hypoxemia[198-200] is a product of both reflex (neural and humoral) and direct effects (Table 17-6). The reflex effects occur first and are excitatory and vasoconstrictive. The neuroreflex effects result from aortic and carotid chemoreceptor, baroreceptor, and central cerebral stimulation, and the humoral reflex effects result from catecholamine and renin-angiotensin release. The direct local vascular effects of hypoxia are inhibitory and vasodilatory and occur late. The net response to hypoxia in a subject depends on the severity of the hypoxia, which determines the magnitude and balance between the inhibitory and excitatory components; the balance may vary according to the type and depth of anesthesia and the degree of preexisting cardiovascular disease.

Mild arterial hypoxemia (arterial saturation less than normal but still 80% or higher) causes general activation of the sympathetic nervous system and release of catecholamines. Consequently, the heart rate, stroke volume, $\dot{Q}T$, and myocardial contractility (as measured by a shortened pre-ejection period [PEP], left ventricular ejection time [LVET], and a decreased PEP/LVET ratio) are increased (Fig. 17-41).[201] Changes in systemic vascular resistance are usually slight. However, in patients under anesthesia with β-blockers, hypoxia (and hypercapnia when present) may cause circulating catecholamines to have only an α-receptor effect, the heart may be unstimulated (even depressed by a local hypoxia effect), and systemic vascular resistance may be increased. Consequently, $\dot{Q}T$ may be decreased in these patients. With moderate hypoxemia (arterial O_2 saturation of 60% to 80%), local vasodilation begins to predominate and systemic vascular resistance and blood pressure decrease, but the heart rate may continue to be increased because of a systemic hypotension-induced stimulation of baroreceptors. Finally, with severe hypoxemia (arterial saturation less than 60%), local depressant effects dominate and blood pressure falls rapidly, the pulse slows, shock develops, and the heart either fibrillates or becomes asystolic. Significant preexisting hypotension will convert a mild hypoxemic hemodynamic profile into a moderate hypoxemic hemodynamic profile and convert a moderate hypoxemic hemodynamic profile into a severe hypoxemic

Table 17–6	Cardiovascular response to hypoxemia					
	Hemodynamic Variable					
O_2 Saturation (%)	*HR*	*BP*	*SV*	*CO*	*SVR*	**Predominant Response**
>80	↑	↑	^	↑	No change	Reflex, excitatory
60-80	↑Baroreceptor	↓	No change	No change	↓	Local, depressant > reflex, excitatory
<60	↓	↓	↓	↓	↓	Local, depressant

BP, systemic blood pressure; CO, cardiac output; HR, heart rate; SV, stroke volume; SVR, systemic vascular resistance; ↑, increase; ↓ = decrease.

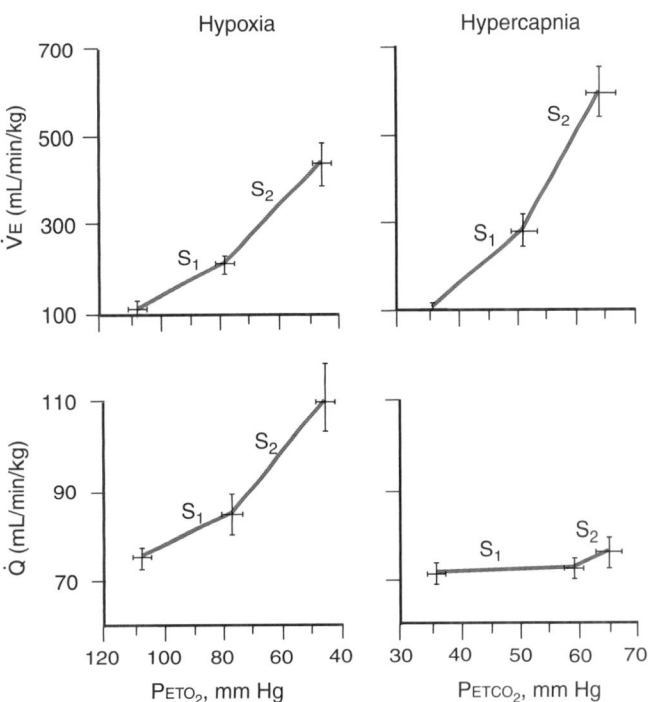

Figure 17–41 Changes in the minute ventilation and the circulation of healthy awake humans during progressive isocapnic hypoxia and hyperoxic hypercapnia. P_{ETCO_2}, end-tidal P_{CO_2}; P_{ETO_2}, end-tidal P_{O_2}; $\dot{Q}$, cardiac output; S_1, slope during the first phase of slowly increasing ventilation and/or circulation; S_2, slope during the second phase of sharply increasing ventilation and/or circulation. $\dot{V}_E$, expired minute ventilation. (Redrawn from Serebrovskaya TV: Comparison of respiratory and circulatory human responses to progressive hypoxia and hypercapnia. Respiration 59:35, 1992.)

hemodynamic profile. Similarly, in well-anesthetized or sedated patients (or both), early sympathetic nervous system reactivity to hypoxemia may be reduced and the effects of hypoxemia may be expressed only as bradycardia with severe hypotension and, ultimately, circulatory collapse.[202]

Hypoxemia may also promote cardiac arrhythmias, which may in turn potentiate the already mentioned deleterious cardiovascular effects. Hypoxemia-induced arrhythmias may be caused by multiple mechanisms; the mechanisms are interrelated because they all cause a decrease in the myocardial O_2 supply-demand ratio, which in turn increases myocardial irritability. First, arterial hypoxemia may directly decrease the myocardial O_2 supply. Second, early tachycardia may result in increased myocardial O_2 consumption, and decreased diastolic filling time may lead to decreased myocardial O_2 supply. Third, early increased systemic blood pressure may cause an increased afterload on the left ventricle, which increases left ventricular O_2 demand. Fourth, late systemic hypotension may decrease myocardial O_2 supply because of decreased diastolic perfusion pressure. Fifth, coronary blood flow reserve may be exhausted by a late, maximally increased coronary blood flow as a result of maximal coronary vasodilation.[203] The level of hypoxemia that will cause cardiac arrhythmias cannot be predicted with certainty

because the myocardial O_2 supply-demand relationship in a given patient is not known (i.e., the degree of coronary artery atherosclerosis may not be known). However, if a myocardial area (or areas) become hypoxic or ischemic, or both, unifocal or multifocal premature ventricular contractions, ventricular tachycardia, and ventricular fibrillation may occur.

The cardiovascular response to hypoxia includes a number of other important effects. Cerebral blood flow increases (even if hypocapnic hyperventilation is present). Ventilation will be stimulated no matter why hypoxia exists (see Fig. 17-41). The pulmonary distribution of blood flow is more homogeneous because of increased pulmonary artery pressure. Chronic hypoxia causes an increased Hb concentration and a right-shifted oxy-Hb curve (as a result of either an increase in 2,3-DPG or acidosis), which tends to raise tissue P_{O_2}.

Hyperoxia (Oxygen Toxicity)

The dangers associated with the inhalation of excessive O_2 are multiple (see Chapter 70). Exposure to high O_2 tension clearly causes pulmonary damage in healthy individuals.[204,205] A dose-time toxicity curve for humans is available from a number of studies.[204-206] Because the lungs of normal human volunteers cannot be directly examined to determine the rate of onset and the course of toxicity, indirect measures such as the onset of symptoms have been used to construct dose-time toxicity curves. Examination of the curve indicates that 100% O_2 should not be administered for more than 12 hours, 80% O_2 should not be administered for more than 24 hours, and 60% O_2 should not be administered for more than 36 hours.[204-206] No measurable changes in pulmonary function or blood-gas exchange occur in humans during exposure to less than 50% O_2, even for long periods.[206] Nevertheless, it is important to note that in the clinical setting, these dose-time toxicity relationships are often generally obscured[207] because of the complex multivariable nature of the clinical setting.

The dominant symptom of O_2 toxicity in human volunteers is substernal distress, which begins as mild irritation in the area of the carina and may be accompanied by occasional coughing.[208] As exposure continues, the pain becomes more intense, and the urge to cough and to deep-breathe also becomes more intense. These symptoms will progress to severe dyspnea, paroxysmal coughing, and decreased vital capacity when the FiO_2 has been 1.0 for longer than 12 hours. At this point, recovery of mechanical lung function usually occurs within 12 to 24 hours, but more than 24 hours may be required in some individuals.[206] As toxicity progresses, other pulmonary function studies such as compliance and blood gases deteriorate. Pathologically, in animals, the lesion progresses from tracheobronchitis (exposure for 12 hours to a few days), to involvement of the alveolar septa with pulmonary interstitial edema (exposure for a few days to 1 week), to pulmonary fibrosis of the edema (exposure for more than 1 week).[209]

Ventilatory depression may occur in patients who, by reason of drugs or disease, have been ventilating in response to a hypoxic drive. By definition, ventilatory depression resulting from removal of a hypoxic drive by increasing the inspired O_2 concentration will cause hypercapnia but does not necessarily produce hypoxia (because of the increased FIO_2).

Absorption atelectasis was presented earlier (see the section "High Inspired Oxygen Concentration and Absorption Atelectasis"). Retrolental fibroplasia, an abnormal proliferation of the immature retinal vasculature of a prematurely born infant, can occur after exposure to hyperoxia. Extremely premature infants are most susceptible to retrolental fibroplasia (i.e., those less than 1.0 kg in birth weight and 28 weeks' gestation). The risk of retrolental fibroplasia exists whenever FIO_2 causes PaO_2 to be more than 80 mm Hg for more than 3 hours in an infant whose gestational age plus life age combined is less than 44 weeks. If the ductus arteriosus is patent, arterial blood samples should be drawn from the right radial artery (umbilical or lower extremity PaO_2 is lower than the PaO_2 to which the eyes are exposed because of ductal shunting of unoxygenated blood).

The mode of action of O_2 toxicity in tissues is complex, but interference with metabolism seems to be widespread. Most importantly, many enzymes, particularly those with sulfhydryl groups, are inactivated by O_2-derived free radicals.[207] Neutrophil recruitment and release of mediators of inflammation occur next and greatly accelerate the extent of endothelial and epithelial damage and impairment of the surfactant systems.[207] The most acute toxic effect of O_2 in humans is a convulsive effect, which occurs during exposure to pressures in excess of 2 atm absolute.

High inspired O_2 concentrations can be of use therapeutically. Clearance of gas loculi in the body may be greatly accelerated by the inhalation of 100% O_2. Inhalation of 100% O_2 creates a large nitrogen gradient from the gas space to the perfusing blood. As a result, nitrogen leaves the gas space and the space diminishes in size. Administration of O_2 to remove gas may be used to ease intestinal gas pressure in patients with intestinal obstruction, decrease the size of an air embolus, and aid in the absorption of pneumoperitoneum, pneumocephalus, and pneumothorax.

Hypercapnia

The effects of CO_2 on the cardiovascular system are as complex as those of hypoxia. Like hypoxemia, hypercapnia appears to cause direct depression of both cardiac muscle and vascular smooth muscle, but at the same time it causes reflex stimulation of the sympathoadrenal system, which compensates to a greater or lesser extent for the primary cardiovascular depression (see Fig. 17-41).[200,203] With moderate to severe hypercapnia, a hyperkinetic circulation results with increased $\dot{Q}T$ and systemic blood pressure (see Fig. 17-41).[201] Even in patients under halothane anesthesia, plasma catecholamine levels increase in response to increased CO_2 levels in much the same way as in conscious subjects. Thus, hypercapnia, like hypoxemia, may cause increased myocardial O_2 demand (tachycardia, early hypertension) and decreased myocardial O_2 supply (tachycardia, late hypotension).

Table 17-7 summarizes the interaction of anesthesia with hypercapnia in humans; increased $\dot{Q}T$ and decreased systemic vascular resistance should be emphasized.[210,211] The increase in $\dot{Q}T$ is most marked during anesthesia with drugs that enhance sympathetic activity and least marked with halothane and nitrous oxide. The decrease in systemic vascular resistance is most marked during enflurane anesthesia and hypercapnia. Hypercapnia is a potent pulmonary vasoconstrictor even after the inhalation of 3% isoflurane for 5 minutes.[210]

Arrhythmias have been reported in unanesthetized humans during acute hypercapnia, but they have seldom been of serious import. A high $PaCO_2$ level is, however, more dangerous during general anesthesia. With halothane anesthesia, arrhythmias frequently occur above a $PaCO_2$ arrhythmic threshold that is often constant for a particular patient. Furthermore, halothane, enflurane, and isoflurane have been shown to prolong the QT_C interval in humans, thereby increasing the risk for *torsades de pointes* ventricular tachycardia, which in turn is notorious for decompensating into ventricular fibrillation.[212]

The maximum stimulatory respiratory effect is attained by a $PaCO_2$ of about 100 mm Hg. With a higher $PaCO_2$, stimulation is reduced, and at extremely high levels, respiration is depressed and later ceases altogether. The PCO_2 ventilation-response curve is generally displaced to the right, and its slope is reduced by anesthetics and other depressant drugs.[213] With profound anesthesia, the response curve may be flat or even sloping downward, and CO_2 then acts as a respiratory depressant. In patients with ventilatory failure, CO_2 narcosis occurs when $PaCO_2$ rises to more than 90 to 120 mm Hg. A 30% CO_2

Table 17–7   Cardiovascular responses to hypercapnia ($PaCO_2$ = 60 to 83 mm Hg) during various types of anesthesia (1 MAC equivalent except for nitrous oxide)*

Anesthesia	Heart Rate	Contractility	Cardiac Output	Systemic Vascular Resistance
Conscious	++	++	+++	−
Nitrous oxide	0	+	++	−−
Halothane	0	+	+	−
Enflurane	+	+	++	−−−
Isoflurane	++	++	+++	−

*The increase in the partial arterial pressure of carbon dioxide ($PaCO_2$) in conscious subjects was 11.5 mm Hg from a normal level of 38 mm Hg.
+, <10% increase; ++, 10% to 25% increase; +++, >25% increase; 0, no change; − <10% decrease; −− 10% to 25% decrease; −−−, >25% decrease; MAC, minimum alveolar concentration for adequate anesthesia in 50% of subjects.

concentration is sufficient for the production of anesthesia, and this concentration causes total, but reversible flattening of the electroencephalogram.[214] As expected, hypercapnia causes bronchodilation in both healthy persons and patients with lung disease.[215]

Quite apart from the effect of CO_2 on ventilation, it exerts two other important effects that influence the oxygenation of the blood.[116] First, if the concentration of nitrogen (or other inert gas) remains constant, the concentration of CO_2 in alveolar gas can increase only at the expense of O_2, which must be displaced. Thus, PAO_2 and PaO_2 may decrease. Second, hypercapnia shifts the oxy-Hb curve to the right, thereby facilitating tissue oxygenation.[98]

Chronic hypercapnia results in increased resorption of bicarbonate by the kidneys, which further raises the plasma bicarbonate level and constitutes a secondary or compensatory metabolic alkalosis. The decrease in renal resorption of bicarbonate in patients with chronic hypocapnia results in a further fall in plasma bicarbonate and produces a secondary or compensatory metabolic acidosis. In each case, arterial pH returns toward the normal value, but the bicarbonate ion concentration departs even further from normal.

Hypercapnia is accompanied by leakage of potassium from cells into plasma. Much of the potassium comes from the liver, probably from glucose release and mobilization, which occur in response to the rise in plasma catecholamine levels.[216] Because the plasma potassium level takes an appreciable time to return to normal, repeated bouts of hypercapnia at short intervals result in a stepwise rise in plasma potassium. Finally, hypercapnia can predispose the patient to other complications in the operating room (e.g., the oculocephalic response is far more common during hypercapnia than during eucapnia).[217]

Hypocapnia

In this section, hypocapnia is considered to be produced by passive hyperventilation (by the anesthesiologist or ventilator). Hypocapnia may cause a decrease in $\dot{Q}T$ by three separate mechanisms. First, if it is present, an increase in intrathoracic pressure will decrease cardiac output. Second, hypocapnia is associated with withdrawal of sympathetic nervous system activity, and such withdrawal can decrease the inotropic state of the heart. Third, hypocapnia can increase pH, and the increased pH can decrease ionized calcium, which may in turn decrease the inotropic state of the heart. Hypocapnia with alkalosis also shifts the oxy-Hb curve to the left, which increases Hb affinity for O_2 and thus impairs O_2 unloading at the tissue level. The decrease in peripheral flow and the impaired ability to unload O_2 to the tissues are compounded by an increase in whole-body O_2 consumption as a result of increased pH-mediated uncoupling of oxidation from phosphorylation.[218] A $PaCO_2$ of 20 mm Hg will increase tissue O_2 consumption by 30%. Consequently, hypocapnia may simultaneously increase tissue O_2 demand and decrease tissue O_2 supply. Thus, to have the same amount of O_2 delivery to the tissues, $\dot{Q}T$ or tissue perfusion has to increase at a time when it may not be possible to do so. The cerebral effects of hypocapnia may be related to a state of cerebral acidosis and hypoxia because hypocapnia may cause a selective reduction in cerebral blood flow and also shifts the oxy-Hb curve to the left.[219]

Hypocapnia may cause $\dot{V}A/\dot{Q}$ abnormalities by inhibiting HPV or by causing bronchoconstriction and decreased CL. Finally, passive hypocapnia promotes apnea.

REFERENCES

1. West JB, Dollery CT, Naimark A: Distribution of blood flow in isolated lung: Relation to vascular and alveolar pressures. J Appl Physiol 19:713, 1964.
2. Puri GD, Venkataranan RK, Singh H, et al: Physiological dead space and arterial to end-tidal CO_2 difference under controlled normocapnic ventilation in young anaesthetized subjects. Indian J Med Res 94:41, 1991.
3. Permutt S, Bromberger-Barnea B, Bane HN: Alveolar pressure, pulmonary venous pressure and the vascular waterfall. Med Thorac 19:239, 1962.
4. McConkey PP: Postobstructive pulmonary oedema: A case series and review. Anaesth Intensive Care 28:72-76, 2000.
5. Bhavani-Shankar K, Hart NS, Mushlin PS: Negative pressure induced airway and pulmonary injury. Can J Anaesth 44:78-81, 1997.
6. West JB, Dollery CT, Heard BE: Increased pulmonary vascular resistance in the dependent zone of the isolated dog lung caused by perivascular edema. Circ Res 17:191, 1965.
7. West JB (ed): Regional Differences in the Lung. Orlando, FL, Academic Press, 1977.
8. Hughes JMB, Glazier JB, Maloney JE, et al: Effect of lung volume on the distribution of pulmonary blood flow in man. Respir Physiol 4:58, 1968.
9. Hughes JM, Glazier JB, Maloney JE, et al: Effect of extra-alveolar vessels on the distribution of pulmonary blood flow in the dog. J Appl Physiol 25:701, 1968.
10. Permutt S, Caldini P, Maseri A, et al: Recruitment versus distensibility in the pulmonary vascular bed. In Fishman AP, Hecht H (eds): The Pulmonary Circulation and Interstitial Space. Chicago, University of Chicago Press, 1969, p 375.
11. Maseri A, Caldini P, Harward P, et al: Determinants of pulmonary vascular volume: Recruitment versus distensibility. Circ Res 31:218, 1972.
12. Hoppin FG Jr, Green ID, Mead J: Distribution of pleural surface pressure. J Appl Physiol 27:863, 1969.
13. Milic-Emili J, Henderson JAM, Dolovich MB, et al: Regional distribution of inspired gas in the lung. J Appl Physiol 21:749, 1966.
14. West JB: Ventilation/Blood Flow and Gas Exchange, 4th ed. Oxford, Blackwell Scientific, 1970.
15. West JB: Regional differences in gas exchange in the lung of erect man. J Appl Physiol 17:893, 1962.
16. Wagner PD, Saltzman HA, West JB: Measurement of continuous distributions of ventilation-perfusion ratios: Theory. J Appl Physiol 36:588, 1974.
17. West JB: Blood flow to the lung and gas exchange. Anesthesiology 41:124, 1974.
18. Fishman AP: Dynamics of the pulmonary circulation. In Hamilton WF (ed): Handbook of Physiology, section 2. Circulation, vol 2. Baltimore, Williams & Wilkins, 1963, p 1667.
19. Zapol WM, Snider MT: Pulmonary hypertension in severe acute respiratory failure. N Engl J Med 296:476, 1977.
20. Simmons DH, Linde CM, Miller JH, et al: Relation of lung volume and pulmonary vascular resistance. Circ Res 9:465, 1961.
21. Burton AC, Patel DJ: Effect on pulmonary vascular resistance of inflation of the rabbit lungs. J Appl Physiol 12:239, 1958.

22. Wittenberger JL, McGregor M, Berglund E, et al: Influence of state of inflation of the lung on pulmonary vascular resistance. J Appl Physiol 15:878, 1960.
23. Benumof JL: Mechanism of decreased blood flow to the atelectatic lung. J Appl Physiol 46:1047, 1978.
24. Benumof JL, Rogers SN, Moyce PR, et al: Hypoxic pulmonary vasoconstriction and regional and whole lung PEEP in the dog. Anesthesiology 52:503, 1979.
25. Pirlo AF, Benumof JL, Trousdale FR: Atelectatic lobe blood flow: Open vs. closed chest, positive pressure vs. spontaneous ventilation. J Appl Physiol 50:1022, 1981.
26. Barnes PJ, Liu SF: Regulation of pulmonary vascular tone. Pharmacol Rev 47:87-131, 1995.
27. Aaronson PI, Robertson TP, Ward JP: Endothelium-derived mediators and hypoxic pulmonary vasoconstriction. Respir Physiol Neurobiol 132:107-120, 2002.
28. Palmer RM, Ferrige AG, Moncada A: Nitric oxide release accounts for the biological activity of endothelium-derived relaxing factor. Nature 327:524-526, 1987.
29. Wang T, El Kebir D, Blaise G: Inhaled nitric oxide in 2003: A review of its mechanisms of action: Can J Anaesth 50:839-846, 2003.
30. Moncada S, Higgs A: The L-arginine–nitric oxide pathway. N Engl J Med 329:2002-2012, 1993.
31. Cooper CJ, Landzberg MJ, Anderson TJ, et al: Role of nitric oxide in the regulation of pulmonary vascular resistance in humans. Circulation 93:266-271, 1996.
32. Stamler JS, Loh E, Roddy M-A, et al: Nitric oxide regulated basal systemic and pulmonary vascular resistance in healthy humans. Circulation 89:2035-2040, 1994.
33. Hosada K, Nakao K, Arai H, et al: Cloning and expression of human endothelin-1 receptor cDNA. FEBS Lett 287:23-26, 1991.
34. Yang Z, Krasniei N, Lüscher TF: Endothelin-1 potentiates human smooth muscle cell growth to PDGF: Effects of ETA and ETB receptor blockade. Circulation 100:5-8, 1999.
35. Ogawa Y, Nakao K, Arai H, et al: Molecular cloning of a non–isopeptide-selective human endothelin receptor. Biochem Biophys Res Commun 178:248-255, 1991.
36. Niwa Y, Nagata N, Oka M, et al: Production of nitric oxide from endothelial cells by 31-amino-acid length endothelin-1, a novel vasoconstrictive product by human chymase. Life Sci 67:1103-1109, 2000.
37. Channick RN, Simonneau G, Sitbon O, et al: Effects of the dual endothelin-receptor antagonist bosentan in patients with pulmonary hypertension: A randomized placebo-controlled study. Lancet 358:1119-1123, 2001.
38. Barst RJ, Rich S, Widlitz A, et al: Clinical efficacy of sitaxsentan, an oral endothelin-A receptor antagonist, in patients with pulmonary arterial hypertension. Chest 121:1860-1868, 2002.
39. Rich S, McLaughlin VV: Endothelin receptor blockers in cardiovascular disease. Circulation 108:2184, 2003.
40. Barnes PJ, Liu SF: Regulation of pulmonary vascular tone. Pharmacol Rev 47:87-131, 1995.
41. Barst RJ, Rubin LJ, Long WA, et al: A comparison of continuous intravenous epoprostenol (prostacyclin) with conventional therapy for primary pulmonary hypertension. The Primary Pulmonary Hypertension Study Group. N Engl J Med 334:296-302, 1996.
42. Olschewski H, Ghofrani HA, Walmrath D, et al: Inhaled prostacyclin and iloprost in severe pulmonary hypertension secondary to lung fibrosis. Am J Respir Crit Care Med 160:600-607, 1999.
43. Olschewski H, Rohde B, Behr J, et al: Pharmacodynamics and pharmacokinetics of inhaled iloprost, aerosolized by three different devices, in severe pulmonary hypertension. Chest 124:1294-1304, 2003.
44. Kim NH, Channick RN, Rubin LJ: Successful withdrawal of long-term epoprostenol therapy for pulmonary arterial hypertension. Chest 124:1612-1615, 2003.
45. McLaughlin VV, Genthner DE, Panella MM, et al: Reduction in pulmonary vascular resistance with long-term epoprostenol (prostacyclin) therapy in primary pulmonary hypertension. N Engl J Med 338:273-277, 1998.
46. Fishman AP: Pulmonary hypertension—beyond vasodilator therapy. N Engl J Med 338:321-322, 1998.
47. Langleben D, Barst RJ, Badesch D, et al: Continuous infusion of epoprostenol improves the net balance between pulmonary endothelin-1 clearance and release in primary pulmonary hypertension. Circulation 99:3266-3271, 1999.
48. Von Euler US, Liljestrand G: Observations on the pulmonary arterial blood pressure in the cat. Acta Physiol Scand 12:301-320, 1946.
49. Dawson CA: The role of pulmonary vasomotion in physiology of the lung. Physiol Rev 64:544-616, 1984.
50. Weir EK, Archer SL: The mechanism of acute hypoxic pulmonary vasoconstriction: The tail of two channels. FASEB J 9:183-189, 1995.
51. Reid L: Structural and functional reappraisal of the pulmonary arterial system. In The Scientific Basis of Medicine Annual Reviews. London, Athlone Press, 1968.
52. Marshall C, Marshall BE: Site and sensitivity for stimulation of hypoxic pulmonary vasoconstriction. J Appl Physiol 55:711, 1983.
53. Benumof JL, Mathers JM, Wahrenbrock EA: The pulmonary interstitial compartment and the mediator of hypoxic pulmonary vasoconstriction. Microvasc Res 15:69, 1978.
54. Bohr D: The pulmonary hypoxic response. Chest 71(Suppl):244, 1977.
55. Fishman AP: Hypoxia on the pulmonary circulation: How and where it works. Circ Res 38:221, 1976.
56. Xuan DAT: Endothelial modulation of pulmonary vascular tone. Eur Respir J 5:757, 1992.
57. Gurney AM: Multiple sites of oxygen sensing and their contributions to hypoxic pulmonary vasoconstriction. Respir Physiol Neurobiol 132:43-53, 2002.
58. Waypa GB, Schumacker PT: O2 sensing in hypoxic pulmonary vasoconstriction: The mitochondrial door re-opens. Respir Physiol Neurobiol 132:81-91, 2002.
59. Waypa GB, Marks JD, Mack MM, et al: Mitochondrial reactive oxygen species trigger calcium increases during hypoxia in pulmonary artery myocytes. Circ Res 91:719-726, 2002.
60. Sham JSK: Hypoxic pulmonary vasoconstriction: Ups and downs of reactive oxygen species. Circ Res 91:649-651, 2002.
61. Doyle JT, Wilson JS, Warren JV: The pulmonary vascular responses to short-term hypoxia in human subjects. Circulation 5:263, 1952.
62. Fishman AP: State of the art: Chronic cor pulmonale. Am Rev Respir Dis 114:775, 1976.
63. Boysen PG, Block AJ, Wynne JW, et al: Nocturnal pulmonary hypertension in patients with chronic obstructive pulmonary disease. Chest 76:536, 1979.
64. Zasslow MA, Benumof JL, Trousdale FR: Hypoxic pulmonary vasoconstriction and the size of the hypoxic compartment. J Appl Physiol 53:626, 1982.
65. Benumof JL: Hypoxic pulmonary vasoconstriction and sodium nitroprusside perfusion. Anesthesiology 50:481, 1979.
66. Benumof JL: Anesthesia for Thoracic Surgery, 2nd ed. Philadelphia, WB Saunders, 1995, Chapters 4 and 8.
67. Elliott CG: Pulmonary physiology during pulmonary embolism. Chest 101:163S-171S, 1992.
68. Reid PG, Fraser A, Watt A, et al: Acute haemodynamic effects of adenosine in conscious man. Eur Heart J 11:1018-1028, 1990.
69. Hagen PT, Scholz DG, Edwards WD: Incidence and size of patent foramen ovale during the first ten decades of life: An autopsy study of 965 normal hearts. Mayo Clin Proc 59:17, 1984.
70. Jaffe RA, Pinto FJ, Schnittger I, et al: Intraoperative ventilator-induced right-to-left intracardiac shunt. Anesthesiology 75:153, 1991.
71. Moorthy SS, Haselby KA, Caldwell RL, et al: Transient right-left interatrial shunt during emergence from anesthesia: Demonstration by color flow Doppler mapping. Anesth Analg 68:820, 1989.
72. Dittrich HC, McCann HA, Wilson WC, et al: Identification of interatrial communication in patients with elevated right atrial pressure using surface and transesophageal contrast echocardiography. J Am Coll Cardiol 21(Supp):135A, 1993.

73. Sykes MK: The mechanics of ventilation. *In* Scurr C, Feldman S (eds): Scientific Foundations of Anesthesia. Philadelphia, FA Davis, 1970, p 174.

74. Lumb AB: Artificial ventilation. *In* Lumb AB (ed): Nunn's Applied Respiratory Physiology, 5th ed. London, Butterworths, 2000, p 590.

75. Scanlon TS, Benumof JL: Demonstration of interlobar collateral ventilation. J Appl Physiol 46:658, 1979.

76. Kent EM, Blades B: The surgical anatomy of the pulmonary lobes. J Thorac Surg 12:18, 1941.

77. Peters RM: Work of breathing following trauma. J Trauma 8:915, 1968.

78. Lumb AB: Pulmonary ventilation: Mechanisms and the work of breathing. *In* Lumb AB (ed): Nunn's Applied Respiratory Physiology, 5th ed. London, Butterworths, 2000, p 128.

79. Moxham J: Respiratory muscle fatigue: Mechanisms, evaluation and therapy. Br J Anaesth 65:43-53, 1990.

80. Shapiro BA, Harrison RA, Trout CA: The mechanics of ventilation. *In* Clinical Application of Respiratory Care, 3rd ed. Chicago, Year Book, 1985, p 57.

81. Comroe JH, Forster RE, Dubois AB, et al: The Lung, 2nd ed. Chicago, Year Book, 1962.

82. Macklem PT, Fraser RG, Bates DV: Bronchial pressures and dimensions in health and obstructive airway disease. J Appl Physiol 18:699, 1983.

83. Craig DB, Wahba WM, Don HF, et al: "Closing volume" and its relationship to gas exchange in seated and supine positions. J Appl Physiol 31:717, 1971.

84. Burger EJ Jr, Macklem P: Airway closure: Demonstration by breathing 100% O_2 at low lung volumes and by N_2 washout. J Appl Physiol 25:139, 1968.

85. Brismer B, Hedenstierna G, Lundquist H, et al: Pulmonary densities during anesthesia with muscular relaxation: A proposal of atelectasis. Anesthesiology 62:422, 1985.

86. Strandberg A, Hedenstierna G, Tokics L, et al: Densities in dependent lung regions during anaesthesia: Atelectasis or fluid accumulation? Acta Anaesthesiol Scand 30:256, 1986.

87. Strandberg A, Tokics L, Brismar B, et al: Atelectasis during anaesthesia and in the postoperative period. Acta Anaesthesiol Scand 30:154, 1986.

88. Hales CA, Kazemi H: Small airways function in myocardial infarction. N Engl J Med 290:761, 1974.

89. Harken AH, O'Connor NE: The influence of clinically undetectable edema on small airway closure in the dog. Ann Surg 184:183, 1976.

90. Biddle TL, Yu PN, Hodges M, et al: Hypoxemia and lung water in acute myocardial infarction. Am Heart J 92:692, 1976.

91. Lumb AB: Respiratory system resistance: Measurement of closing capacity. *In* Lumb AB (ed): Nunn's Applied Respiratory Physiology, 5th ed. London, Butterworths, 2000, p 79.

92. Rehder K, Marsh HM, Rodarte JR, et al: Airway closure. Anesthesiology 47:40, 1977.

93. Leblanc P, Ruff F, Milic-Emili J: Effects of age and body position on "airway closure" in man. J Appl Physiol 28:448, 1970.

94. Craig DB, Wahba WM, Don HF, et al: "Closing volume" and its relationship to gas exchange in seated and supine positions. J Appl Physiol 31:717, 1971.

95. Föex P, Prys-Roberts C, Hahn CEW, et al: Comparison of oxygen content of blood measured directly with values derived from measurement of oxygen tension. Br J Anaesth 42:803, 1970.

96. Sykes MK, Adams AP, Finley WEI, et al: The cardiorespiratory effects of hemorrhage and overtransfusion in dogs. Br J Anaesth 42:573, 1970.

97. Gregory IC: The oxygen and carbon monoxide capacities of foetal and adult blood. J Physiol 236:625, 1974.

98. Hsia CCW: Respiratory function of hemoglobin. N Engl J Med 338:239-247, 2003.

99. Gilles IDS, Bard BD, Norman J: The effect of anesthesia on the oxyhemoglobin dissociation curve. Br J Anaesth 42:561, 1970.

100. Kambam JR: Effect of isoflurane on P_{50} and on Po_2 measurement. Anesthesiol Rev 14:40, 1987.

101. Lawler PGP, Nunn JF: A re-assessment of the validity of the iso-shunt graph. Br J Anaesth 56:1325, 1984.

102. Kelman GF, Nunn JF, Prys-Roberts C, et al: The influence of the cardiac output on arterial oxygenation: A theoretical study. Br J Anaesth 39:450, 1967.

103. Philbin DM, Sullivan SF, Bowman FO, et al: Post-operative hypoxemia: Contribution of the cardiac output. Anesthesiology 32:136, 1970.

104. Berggren SM: The oxygen deficit of arterial blood caused by non-ventilating parts of the lung. Acta Physiol Scand Suppl 4:11, 1942.

105. Cheney FW, Colley PS: The effect of cardiac output on arterial blood oxygenation. Anesthesiology 52:496, 1980.

106. Henry W: Experiments on the quantity of gases absorbed by water at different temperatures and under different pressures. Philos Trans R Soc 93:29, 1803.

107. Fishman AP: Pulmonary edema: The water-exchanging function of the lung. Circulation 46:390, 1972.

108. Mallick A, Bodenham AR: Disorders of the lymph circulation: Their relevance to anesthesia and intensive care. Br J Anaesth 91:265-272, 2003.

109. Weibel ER: Morphological basis of alveolar-capillary gas exchange. Physiol Rev 53:419, 1973.

110. Guyton AC: A concept of negative interstitial pressure based on pressures in implanted perforated capsules. Circ Res 12:399, 1963.

111. Smith-Erichsen N, Bo G: Airway closure and fluid filtration in the lung. Br J Anaesth 51:475, 1979.

112. Oswalt CE, Gates GA, Holmstrom EMG: Pulmonary edema as a complication of acute airway obstruction. Rev Surg 34:364, 1977.

113. Staub NC: Pulmonary edema: Physiologic approaches to management. Chest 74:559, 1978.

114. Permutt S: Effect of interstitial pressure of the lung on pulmonary circulation. Med Thorac 22:118, 1965.

115. Staub NC: "State of the art" review: Pathogenesis of pulmonary edema. Am Rev Respir Dis 109:358, 1974.

116. Wilson WC, Shapiro B: Perioperative hypoxia: The clinical spectrum and current oxygen monitoring methodology. Anesthesiol Clin North Am 19:769-812, 2001.

117. Marshall BE, Wyche MO: Hypoxemia during and after anesthesia. Anesthesiology 37:178, 1972.

118. Nunn JF, Bergman NA, Coleman AJ: Factors influencing the arterial oxygen tension during anaesthesia with artificial ventilation. Br J Anaesth 37:898, 1965.

119. Sykes MK, Young WE, Robinson BE: Oxygenation during anaesthesia with controlled ventilation. Br J Anaesth 37:314, 1965.

120. Lumb AB: Anaesthesia. *In* Lumb AB (ed): Nunn's Applied Respiratory Physiology, 5th ed. London, Butterworths, 2000, p 420.

121. Hedenstierna G: Gas exchange during anaesthesia. Br J Anaesth 64:507, 1990.

122. Gunnarsson L, Tokics L, Gustavsson H, et al: Influence of age on atelectasis formation and gas exchange impairment during general anesthesia. Br J Anaesth 66:423, 1991.

123. Lumb AB: Anaesthesia: Ventilation/perfusion relationships: Effect of age. *In* Lumb AB (ed): Nunn's Applied Respiratory Physiology, 5th ed. London, Butterworths, 2000, p 445.

124. Vaughan RW, Wise L: Intraoperative arterial oxygenation in obese patients. Ann Surg 184:35, 1976.

125. Dueck R, Young I, Clausen J, et al: Altered distribution of pulmonary ventilation and blood flow following induction of inhalational anesthesia. Anesthesiology 52:113, 1980.

126. Rehder K, Knopp TH, Sessler AD, et al: Ventilation-perfusion relationships in young healthy awake and anesthetized-paralyzed man. J Appl Physiol 47:745, 1979.

127. Tokics L, Hedenstierna G, Strandberg A, et al: Lung collapse and gas exchange during general anesthesia: Effects of spontaneous breathing, muscle paralysis and positive end-expiratory pressure. Anesthesiology 66:157, 1987.

128. Munson ES, Larson CP Jr, Babad AA, et al: The effects of halothane, fluroxene and cyclopropane on ventilation: A comparative study in man. Anesthesiology 27:716, 1966.

129. Green Jr WB: The ventilatory effects of sevoflurane. Anesth Analg 81:S23, 1995.

130. Couture J, Picken J, Trop D, et al: Airway closure in normal, obese, and anesthetized supine subjects. FASEB J 29:269, 1970.

131. Ward CS: The prevention of accidents associated with anesthetic apparatus. Br J Anaesth 40:692, 1968.

132. Mazze RI: Therapeutic misadventures with oxygen delivery systems: The need for continuous in-line oxygen monitors. Anesth Analg 51:787, 1972.

133. Epstein RM, Rackow H, Lee ASJ, et al: Prevention of accidental breathing of anoxic gas mixture during anesthesia. Anesthesiology 23:1, 1962.

134. Sprague DH, Archer GW: Intraoperative hypoxia from an erroneously filled liquid oxygen reservoir. Anesthesiology 42:360, 1975.

135. Eger EI II, Epstein RM: Hazards of anesthetic equipment. Anesthesiology 25:490, 1964.

136. Martin JT: Positioning in Anesthesia and Surgery. Philadelphia, WB Saunders, 1978.

137. Heinonen J, Takki S, Tammisto T: Effect of the Trendelenburg tilt and other procedures on the position of endotracheal tubes. Lancet 1:850, 1969.

138. Seto K, Goto H, Hacker D, et al: Right upper lobe atelectasis after inadvertent right main bronchial intubation. Anesth Analg 62:851, 1983.

139. Halpern NA, Siegal RE, Papadakos PJ, et al: Right upper lobe collapse following uneventful endotracheal intubation. J Cardiothorac Vasc Anesth 3:620, 1989.

140. Mead J, Agostoni E: Dynamics of breathing. In Fenn WO, Rahn H (eds): Handbook of Physiology, section 3. Respiration, vol 1. Baltimore, Williams & Wilkins, 1964, p 411.

141. Wright PE, Marini JJ, Bernard GR: In vitro versus in vivo comparison of endotracheal tube airflow resistance. Am Rev Respir Dis 140:10, 1989.

142. Bersten AD, Rutten AJ, Vedig AE, et al: Additional work of breathing imposed by endotracheal tube, breathing circuits and intensive care ventilators. Crit Care Med 17:671, 1989.

143. Lumb AB: Respiratory system resistance. In Lumb AB (ed): Nunn's Applied Respiratory Physiology, 5th ed. London, Butterworths, 2000, p 67.

144. Bendixen HH, Hedley-Whyte J, Chir B, et al: Impaired oxygenation in surgical patients during general anesthesia with controlled ventilation. N Engl J Med 269:991, 1963.

145. Bendixen HH, Bullwinkel B, Hedley-Whyte J, et al: Atelectasis and shunting during spontaneous ventilation in anesthetized patients. Anesthesiology 25:297, 1964.

146. Cain SM: Increased oxygen uptake with passive hyperventilation of dogs. J Appl Physiol 28:4, 1970.

147. Karetzky MS, Cain SM: Effect of carbon dioxide on oxygen uptake during hyperventilation in normal man. J Appl Physiol 28:8, 1970.

148. Benumof JL, Mathers JM, Wahrenbrock EA: Cyclic hypoxic pulmonary vasoconstriction induced by concomitant carbon dioxide changes. J Appl Physiol 41:466, 1976.

149. Cutillo A, Omboni E, Perondi R, et al: Effect of hypocapnia on pulmonary mechanics in normal subjects and in patients with chronic obstructive lung disease. Am Rev Respir Dis 110:25, 1974.

150. Don H: The mechanical properties of the respiratory system during anesthesia. Int Anesthesiol Clin 15:113, 1977.

151. Don HF, Wahba M, Cuadrado L, et al: The effects of anesthesia and 100 percent oxygen on the functional residual capacity of the lungs. Anesthesiology 32:521, 1970.

152. Westbrook PR, Stubbs SE, Sessler AD, et al: Effects of anesthesia and muscle paralysis on respiratory mechanics in normal man. J Appl Physiol 34:81, 1973.

153. Pelosi P, Croci M, Ravagnan I, et al: The effects of body mass on lung volumes, respiratory mechanics, and gas exchange during general anesthesia. Anesth Analg 87:654-660, 1998.

154. Alexander JI, Spence AA, Parikh RK, et al: The role of airway closure in postoperative hypoxemia. Br J Anaesth 45:34, 1973.

155. Hickey RF, Visick W, Fairley HB, et al: Effects of halothane anesthesia on functional residual capacity and alveolar-arterial oxygen tension difference. Anesthesiology 38:20, 1973.

156. Wyche MQ, Teichner RL, Kallos T, et al: Effects of continuous positive-pressure breathing on functional residual capacity and arterial oxygenation during intra-abdominal operation. Anesthesiology 38:68, 1973.

157. Freund F, Roos A, Dodd RB: Expiratory activity of the abdominal muscles in man during general anesthesia. J Appl Physiol 19:693, 1964.

158. Kallos T, Wyche MQ, Garman JK: The effect of Innovar on functional residual capacity and total chest compliance. Anesthesiology 39 558, 1973.

159. Campbell EJM, Agostini E, David JN: The Respiratory Muscles: Mechanics and Neural Control, 2nd ed. Philadelphia, WB Saunders, 1970.

160. Milic-Emili J, Mead J, Tanner JM: Topography of esophageal pressure as a function of posture in man. J Appl Physiol 19:212, 1964.

161. Froese AB, Bryan CA: Effects of anesthesia and paralysis on diaphragmatic mechanics in man. Anesthesiology 41:242, 1974.

162. Dekker E, Defares JG, Heemstra H: Direct measurement of intrabronchial pressure: Its application to the location of the check-valve mechanism. J Appl Physiol 13:35, 1958.

163. Ward CF, Gagnon RL, Benumof JL: Wheezing after induction of general anesthesia: Negative expiratory pressure revisited. Anesth Analg 58:49, 1979.

164. Ray JF, Yost L, Moallem S, et al: Immobility, hypoxemia, and pulmonary arteriovenous shunting. Arch Surg 109:537, 1974.

165. Gentilello L, Thompson DA, Tonnesen AS, et al: Effect of a rotating bed on the incidence of pulmonary complications in critically ill patients. Crit Care Med 16:783-786, 1988.

166. Wagner PD, Laravuso RB, Uhl RR, et al: Continuous distributions of ventilation-perfusion ratios in normal subjects breathing air and 100% O_2. J Clin Invest 54:54, 1974.

167. Briscoe WA, Cree EM, Filler J, et al: Lung volume, alveolar ventilation and perfusion interrelationships in chronic pulmonary emphysema. J Appl Physiol 15:785, 1960.

168. Slocum HC, Hoeflich EA, Allen CR: Circulatory and respiratory distress from extreme positions on the operating table. Surg Gynecol Obstet 84:1065, 1947.

169. Laver MB, Hallowell P, Goldblatt A: Pulmonary dysfunction secondary to heart disease: Aspects relevant to anesthesia and surgery. Anesthesiology 33:161, 1970.

170. Lumb AB, Nunn JF: Respiratory function and ribcage contribution to ventilation in body positions commonly used during anesthesia. Anesth Analg 73:422, 1991.

171. Huang YC, Weinmann GG, Mitzner W: Effect of tidal volume and frequency on the temporal fall in lung compliance. J Appl Physiol 65:2040, 1988.

172. Tweed WA, Phua WT, Chong KY, et al: Large tidal volume ventilation improves pulmonary gas exchange during lower abdominal surgery in Trendelenburg's position. Can J Anaesth 38:989, 1991.

173. Grim PS, Freund FR, Cheney FW: Effect of spontaneous sighs on arterial oxygenation during isoflurane anesthesia in humans. Anesth Analg 66:839, 1987.

174. Yeaker H: Tracheobronchial secretions. Am J Med 50:493, 1971.

175. Forbes AR: Humidification and mucous flow in the intubated trachea. Br J Anaesth 45:874, 1973.

176. Bang BG, Bang FB: Effect of water deprivation on nasal mucous flow. Proc Soc Exp Biol Med 106:516, 1961.

177. Hirsch JA, Tokayer JL, Robinson MJ, et al: Effects of dry air and subsequent humidification on tracheal mucous velocity in dogs. J Appl Physiol 39:242, 1975.

178. Dalhamn T: Mucous flow and ciliary activity in the tracheas of rats exposed to respiratory irritant gases. Acta Physiol Scand Suppl 36:123, 1956.

179. Hill L: The ciliary movement of the trachea studies in vitro. Lancet 2:802, 1928.

180. Sackner MA, Landa J, Hirsch J, et al: Pulmonary effects of oxygen breathing. Ann Intern Med 82:40, 1975.

181. Sackner MA, Hirsch J, Epstein S: Effect of cuffed endotracheal tubes on tracheal mucous velocity. Chest 68:774, 1975.

182. Forbes AR: Halothane depresses mucociliary flow in the trachea. Anesthesiology 45:59, 1976.

183. Nunn JF, Sturrock JE, Wills EJ, et al: The effect of inhalation anaesthetics on the swimming velocity of *Tetrahymena pyriformis*. J Cell Sci 15:537, 1974.

184. Prys-Roberts C: The metabolic regulation of circulatory transport. *In* Scurr C, Feldman S (eds): Scientific Foundation of Anesthesia. Philadelphia, FA Davis, 1970, p 87.

185. Benumof JL, Wahrenbrock EA: Blunted hypoxic pulmonary vasoconstriction by increased lung vascular pressures. J Appl Physiol 38:846, 1975.

186. Scanlon TS, Benumof JL, Wahrenbrock EA, et al: Hypoxic pulmonary vasoconstriction and the ratio of hypoxic lung to perfused normoxic lung. Anesthesiology 49:177, 1978.

187. Benumof JL, Wahrenbrock EA: Dependency of hypoxic pulmonary vasoconstriction on temperature. J Appl Physiol 42:56, 1977.

188. Benumof JL: Anesthesia for Thoracic Surgery, 2nd ed. Philadelphia, WB Saunders, 1995, Chapter 4.

189. Benumof JL: Anesthesia for Thoracic Surgery, 2nd ed. Philadelphia, WB Saunders, 1995, Chapter 8.

190. Benumof JL: One lung ventilation: Which lung should be PEEPed? Anesthesiology 56:161, 1982.

191. Krayer S, Rehder K, Vettermann J, et al: Position and motion of the human diaphragm during anesthesia-paralysis. Anesthesiology 70:891, 1989.

192. Froese AB: Anesthesia-paralysis and the diaphragm: In pursuit of an elusive muscle. Anesthesiology 70:887, 1989.

193. Moorthy SS, Haselby KA, Caldwell RL, et al: Transient right-left interatrial shunting during emergence from anesthesia: Demonstration by color flow Doppler mapping. Anesth Analg 68:820, 1989.

194. Fellahi JL, Mourgeon E, Goarin JP, et al: Inhaled nitric oxide–induced closure of a patent foramen ovale in an adult patient with acute respiratory distress syndrome and life-threatening hypoxemia. Anesthesiology 83:635-638, 1995.

195. Ware LB, Matthay MA: Acute respiratory distress syndrome. N Engl J Med 342:1334-1349, 2000.

196. Eckenhoff JE, Enderby GEH, Larson A, et al: Pulmonary gas exchange during deliberate hypotension. Br J Anaesth 35:750, 1963.

197. Kain ML, Panday J, Nunn JF: The effect of intubation on the dead space during halothane anaesthesia. Br J Anaesth 41:94, 1969.

198. Heistad DD, Abboud FM: Circulatory adjustments to hypoxia: Dickinson W. Richards Lecture. Circulation 61:463, 1980.

199. Roberts JG: The effect of hypoxia on the systemic circulation during anaesthesia. *In* Prys-Roberts E (ed): The Circulation in Anaesthesia: Applied Physiology and Pharmacology. Oxford, Blackwell Scientific, 1980, p 311.

200. Rothe CF, Flanagan AD, Maass-Moreno R: Reflex control of vascular capacitance during hypoxia, hypercapnia, or hypoxic hypercapnia. Can J Physiol Pharmacol 68:384, 1990.

201. Serebrovskaya TV: Comparison of respiratory and circulatory human responses to progressive hypoxia and hypercapnia. Respiration 59:35, 1992.

202. Dohzaki S, Ohtsuka H, Yamamura T, et al: Comparative effects of volatile anesthetics on the sympathetic activity to acute hypoxemia or hypercarbia in dogs. Anesth Analg 70:S87, 1990.

203. Lehot JJ, Leone BJ, Föex P: Effects of altered Pao_2 and $Paco_2$ on left ventricular function and coronary hemodynamics of sheep. Anesth Analg 72:737, 1991.

204. Winter PM, Smith G: The toxicity of oxygen. Anesthesiology 37:210, 1972.

205. Lambertsen CJ: Effects of oxygen at high partial pressure. *In* Fenn WO, Rahn H (eds): Handbook of Physiology, section 3. Respiration, vol 2. Baltimore, Williams & Wilkins, 1965, p 1027.

206. Clark JM: Pulmonary limits of oxygen tolerance in man. Exp Lung Res 14:897, 1988.

207. Klein J: Normobaric pulmonary oxygen toxicity. Anesth Analg 70:195, 1990.

208. Montgomery AB, Luce JM, Murray JF: Retrosternal pain is an early indicator of oxygen toxicity. Am Rev Respir Dis 139:1548, 1989.

209. Nash G, Blennerhasset JB, Pontoppidan H: Pulmonary lesions associated with oxygen therapy and artificial ventilation. N Engl J Med 276:368, 1967.

210. Magnus L, Wattwil T, Olsson JG: Circulatory effects of isoflurane during acute hypercapnia. Anesth Analg 66:1234, 1987.

211. Prys-Roberts C: Hypercapnia. *In* Gray TC, Nunn JF, Utting JE (eds): General Anaesthesia, 4th ed. London, Butterworths, 1980, p 435.

212. Schmeling WT, Warltier DC, McDonald DJ, et al: Prolongation of the QT interval by enflurane, isoflurane, and halothane in humans. Anesth Analg 72:137, 1991.

213. Severinghaus JW, Larson CP: Respiration in anesthesia. In Fenn WO, Rahn H (eds): Handbook of Physiology, section 3. Respiration, vol 2. Baltimore, Williams & Wilkins, 1965, p 1219.

214. Clowes GHA, Hopkins AL, Simeone FA: A comparison of the physiological effects of hypercapnia and hypoxia in the production of cardiac arrest. Ann Surg 142:446, 1955.

215. Parson PE, Grunstein MM, Fernandez E: The effects of acute hypoxia and hypercapnia on pulmonary mechanics in normal subjects and patients with chronic pulmonary disease. Chest 96:96, 1989.

216. Fenn WO, Asano T: Effects of carbon dioxide inhalation on potassium liberation from the liver. Am J Physiol 185:567, 1956.

217. Kil HK: Hypercapnia is an important adjuvant factor of oculocardiac reflex during strabismus surgery. Anesth Analg 91:1044, 2000.

218. Patterson RW: Effect of $Paco_2$ on O_2 consumption during cardiopulmonary bypass in man. Anesth Analg 55:269, 1976.

219. Brian JE Jr: Carbon dioxide and the cerebral circulation. Anesthesiology 88:1365-1386, 1998.

CHAPTER
18 Cardiac Physiology

Lena S. Sun and Johanna Schwarzenberger

Introduction   723

Physiology of the Intact Heart   723
Cardiac Cycle   723
Ventricular Structure and Function   724
Cardiac Output   728

Cellular Cardiac Physiology   729
Cellular Anatomy   729

Cardiomyocyte Structure and Function   729

Control of Cardiac Function   735
Neural Regulation of Cardiac
Function   735
Hormones Affecting Cardiac
Function   737
Cardiac Reflexes   738

INTRODUCTION

The modern concept of circulation and that the heart is the generator for the circulation was initially advanced by Harvey in 1628. Since that time, the field of cardiac physiology has developed to now include the physiology of the heart as a pump, cellular and molecular biology of the cardiomyocyte, and regulation of cardiac function by neural and humoral factors. Moreover, we now appreciate that physiology of the heart is only a component of the interrelated and integrated cardiovascular and circulatory physiology. This chapter will discuss only the physiology of the heart. It begins with the physiology of the intact heart. The second part of the chapter focuses on cellular cardiac physiology. Finally, we will briefly discuss the various factors that regulate cardiac function.

The basic anatomy of the heart consists of two atria and two ventricles providing two separate circulations in series. The pulmonary circulation, a low-resistance and high-capacitance vascular bed, receives output from the right side of the heart, and its chief function is bidirectional gas exchange. The left side of the heart provides the output for the systemic circulation. It functions to deliver oxygen and nutrients and remove CO_2 and metabolites from various tissue beds.

PHYSIOLOGY OF THE INTACT HEART

To understand the mechanical performance of the intact heart, it is important to have knowledge of the phases of the cardiac cycle and determinants of ventricular function.

Cardiac Cycle

The cardiac cycle is the sequence of electrical and mechanical events during the course of a single heartbeat.

Figure 18-1 illustrates (1) the electrical events of a single cardiac cycle represented by the electrocardiogram (ECG) and (2) the mechanical events of a single cardiac cycle represented by left atrial and left ventricular pressure pulses correlated in time with aortic flow and ventricular volume.[1]

The cardiac cycle begins with initiation of the heartbeat. Intrinsic to the specialized cardiac pacemaker tissues is automaticity and rhythmicity. The sinoatrial (SA) node is usually the pacemaker; it can generate impulses at the greatest frequency and is the natural pacemaker.

Electrical Events and the Electrocardiogram
Electrical events of the pacemaker and the specialized conduction system are represented by the ECG at the body surface (also see Chapter 34). It is the result of electrical potential differences generated by the heart at sites of the surface recording. The action potential initiated at the SA node is propagated to both atria by specialized conduction tissue, and it leads to atrial systole (contraction) and the P wave of the ECG. At the junction of the interatrial and interventricular septa, specialized atrial conduction tissue converges at the atrioventricular (AV) node, which is connected distally to the His bundle. The AV node is an area of relatively slow conduction, and a delay between atrial and ventricular contraction normally occurs at this locus. The PR interval can be used to measure the delay between atrial and ventricular contraction at the level of the AV node. From the distal His bundle, an electrical impulse is propagated through large left and right bundle branches and finally to the Purkinje system fibers, which are the smallest branches of the specialized conduction system. Finally, electrical signals are transmitted from the Purkinje system to the individual ventricular cardiomyocytes. The spread of depolarization to the ventricular myocardium is manifested as the QRS complex on the ECG. Depolarization is followed by ventricular repolarization and appearance of the T wave on the ECG.[2]

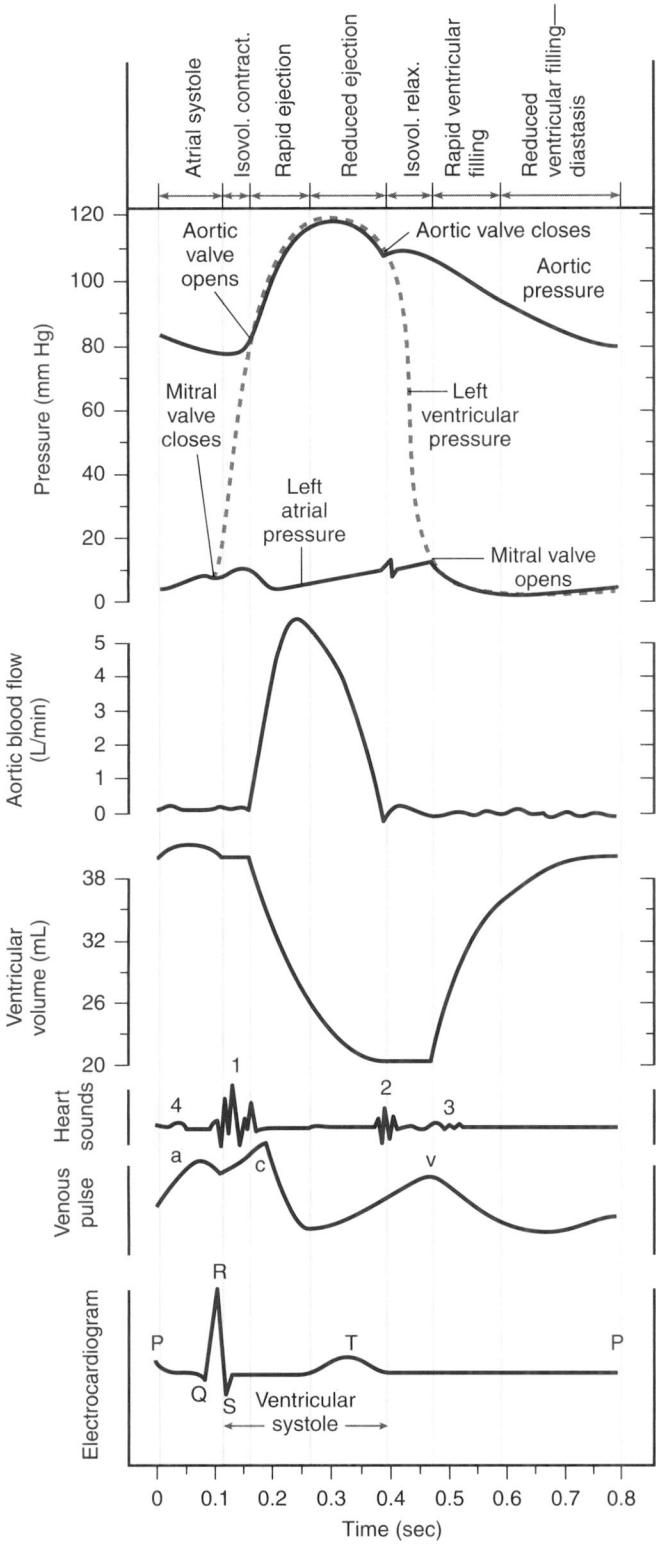

Figure 18–1 The electrical and mechanical events during a single cardiac cycle are depicted. Shown are pressure curves of aortic blood flow, ventricular volume, venous pulse, and the electrocardiogram. (From Berne RM, Levy MN: The cardiac pump. *In* Cardiovascular Physiology, 8th ed. St Louis, Mosby, 2001, pp 55-82.)

Mechanical Events

The mechanical events of a cardiac cycle begin with return of the blood to the right and left atria from the systemic and pulmonary circulation, respectively. As blood accumulates in the atria, atrial pressure increases until it exceeds the pressure within the ventricle, and the AV valve opens. Blood first flows passively into the ventricular chambers, and such flow accounts for approximately 75% of total ventricular filling.[3] The remainder of the blood flow is by active atrial contraction or systole, known as the atrial "kick." The onset of atrial systole is coincident with depolarization of the sinus node and the P wave. While the ventricles fill, the AV valves are displaced upward and ventricular contraction (systole) begins with closure of the tricuspid and mitral valves, which corresponds to the end of the R wave on the ECG. The first part of ventricular systole is known as isovolumic or isometric contraction. The electrical impulse traverses the AV region and passes through the right and left bundle branches into the Purkinje fibers. This leads to contraction of ventricular myocardium and a progressive increase in intraventricular pressure. When intraventricular pressure exceeds pulmonary artery and aortic pressure, the pulmonic and aortic valves open and ventricular ejection occurs, which is the second part of ventricular systole.

Ventricular ejection can be further separated into the rapid ejection phase and the reduced ejection phase. During the rapid ejection phase, forward flow is maximal, and pulmonary artery and aortic pressure is maximally developed. In the reduced ejection phase, flow and great artery pressure taper with progression of systole. Pressure in both ventricular chambers falls as blood is ejected from the heart, and ventricular diastole begins with closure of the pulmonic and aortic valves. The initial period of ventricular diastole consists of the isovolumic/ isometric relaxation phase. This phase is concomitant with repolarization of the ventricular myocardium and corresponds to the end of the T wave on the ECG. The final portion of ventricular diastole involves a rapid decrease in intraventricular pressure until it falls below that of the right and left atria, at which point the AV valve reopens, ventricular filling occurs, and the cycle repeats itself.

Ventricular Structure and Function

Ventricular Structure

The specific architectural order of the cardiac muscles provides the basis for the heart to function as a pump. The ellipsoid shape of the left ventricle (LV) is a result of the laminar layering of spiraling bundles of cardiac muscles (Fig. 18-2). The orientation of the muscle bundle is longitudinal in the subepicardial myocardium and circumferential in the middle segment and again becomes longitudinal in the subendocardial myocardium. Because of the ellipsoid shape of the LV, there are regional differences in wall thickness that result in corresponding variations in the cross-sectional radius of the LV chamber. These regional differences may serve to accommodate the variable loading conditions of the LV.[4] In addition, such anatomy allows the LV to eject blood in a corkscrew-type

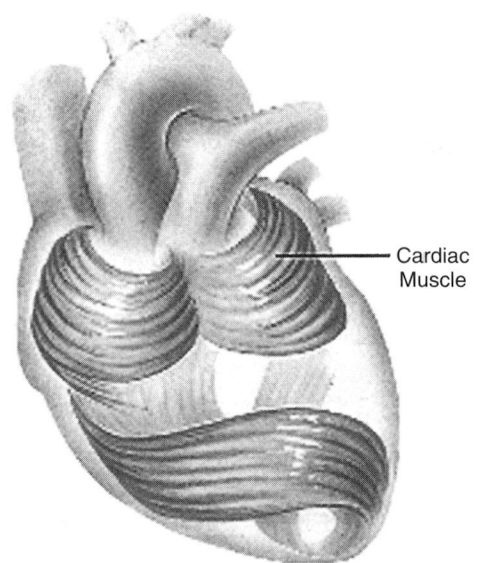

Figure 18–2 Muscle bundles. (From Marieb EN: Human Anatomy & Physiology, 5th ed. San Francisco, Peason Benjamin Cummings, 2001, p 684.)

motion beginning from the base and ending at the apex. The architecturally complex structure of the LV thus allows for maximal shortening of myocytes, which results in increased wall thickness and generation of force during systole. Moreover, release of the twisted LV may provide a suction mechanism for LV filling during diastole. The LV free wall and the septum have similar muscle bundle architecture. As a result, the septum moves inward during systole in a normal heart. Regional wall thickness is a commonly used index of myocardial performance that can be assessed clinically, for example, by perioperative echocardiography or magnetic resonance imaging.

Unlike the LV, which needs to pump against the higher-pressure systemic circulation, the right ventricle (RV)

pumps against a much lower pressure circuit in the pulmonary circulation. Consequently, wall thickness is considerably less in the RV. In contrast to the ellipsoidal form of the LV, the RV is crescent shaped, as a result of which the mechanics of RV contraction are more complex. Inflow and outflow contraction is not simultaneous, and much of the contractile force seems to be recruited from interventricular forces of the LV-based septum.

An intricate matrix of collagen fibers form a scaffold of support for the heart and adjacent vessels. This matrix provides enough strength to resist tensile stretch. The collagen fibers are made up of mostly the thick collagen type I fiber, which cross-links with the thin collagen type III fiber, the other major type of collagen.[5] In close proximity to the collagen fibers are elastic fibers that contain elastin. They account for the elasticity of the myocardium.[6]

Systolic Function

The heart provides the driving force to deliver blood throughout the cardiovascular system to supply nutrients and remove metabolic waste. Because of the complexity of RV anatomy, the traditional description of systolic function is usually limited to the left ventricle. Systolic performance of the heart is dependent on loading conditions and contractility. Preload and afterload are two interdependent factors extrinsic to the heart that govern cardiac performance.

Preload and Afterload

Preload is defined as the ventricular load at the end of diastole, before contraction has started. First described by Starling, a linear relationship exists between sarcomere length and myocardial force (Fig. 18-3). In clinical practice, surrogate representatives of left ventricular volume such as pulmonary wedge pressure or central venous pressure are used to estimate preload.[3]

Afterload is defined as systolic load on the LV after contraction has begun. Aortic compliance is an additional

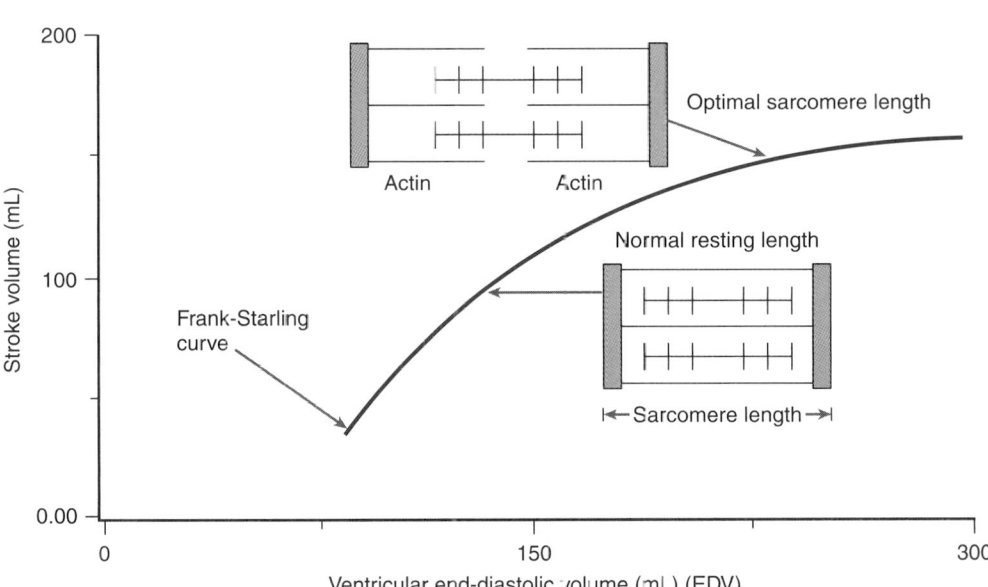

Figure 18–3 Frank-Starling relationship. The relationship between sarcomere length and tension developed in cardiac muscles is shown. In the heart, an increase in end-diastolic volume is the equivalent of an increase in myocardial stretch; therefore, according to Starling's law, increased stroke volume is generated.

determinant of afterload.[1] Aortic compliance is the ability of the aorta to give way to systolic forces from the ventricle. Changes in the aortic wall (dilatation or stiffness) can alter aortic compliance and thus afterload. Examples of pathologic conditions that alter afterload are aortic stenosis and chronic hypertension. Both impede ventricular ejection, thus increasing afterload. Aortic impedance, or aortic pressure divided by aortic flow at that instant, is an accurate means to gauge afterload. However, clinical measurement of aortic impedance is invasive. Echocardiography can estimate aortic impedance noninvasively by determining aortic blood flow at the time of its maximal increase. In more general clinical practice, measurement of systolic blood pressure is adequate to approximate afterload, provided that aortic stenosis is not present.

Preload and afterload can be considered as the wall stress that is present at the end of diastole and during LV ejection, respectively. Wall stress is a useful concept because it includes preload, afterload, and the energy required to generate contraction. Wall stress and heart rate are probably the two most relevant indices that account for changes in myocardial oxygen demand. The law of Laplace states that wall stress (σ) is the product of pressure (P) and radius (R) divided by wall thickness (h)[3]:

$$\sigma = P \times R/2h$$

The ellipsoid shape of the LV allows for the least amount of wall stress such that as the ventricle changes its shape from ellipsoid to spherical, wall stress is increased. By using the ratio of the long axis to the short axis as a measure of the ellipsoid shape, a decrease in this ratio would signify a transition from ellipsoid to spherical.

Thickness of the LV muscle is an important modifier of wall stress. For example, in aortic stenosis, afterload is increased. The ventricle has to generate far higher pressure to overcome the increased load opposing systolic ejection of blood. To generate such high performance, the ventricle increases its wall thickness (LV hypertrophy). By applying Laplace's law, increased LV wall thickness will decrease wall stress despite the necessary increase in LV pressure to overcome the aortic stenosis (Fig. 18-4).[7] In a failing heart, the radius of the LV increases, thus increasing wall stress.

Frank-Starling Relationship

The Frank-Starling relationship is an intrinsic property of myocardium by which stretching of the myocardial sarcomere results in enhanced myocardial performance for subsequent contractions (see Fig. 18-3). Otto Frank first noted in 1895 that in skeletal muscle, the change in tension was directly related to its length and that in the heart, as pressure changed, a corresponding change in volume occurred.[8] E. H. Starling, using an isolated heart-lung preparation as a model, observed in 1914 that "the mechanical energy set free on passage from the resting to the contracted state is a function of the length of the muscle fiber."[9] If a strip of cardiac muscle is mounted in a muscle chamber under isometric conditions and stimulated at a fixed frequency, an increase in sarcomere length results in an increase in twitch force. Starling

concluded that the increased twitch force was the result of a greater interaction of muscle bundles.

Electron microscopy has demonstrated that sarcomere length (2.0 to 2.2 μm) is positively related to the amount of actin and myosin cross-bridging and that there is an optimal sarcomere length at which the interaction is maximal. This concept is based on the assumption that the increase in cross-bridging is equivalent to an increase in muscle performance. Although this theory continues to hold true for skeletal muscle, the force-length relationship in cardiac muscle is more complex. When comparing force-strength relationships between skeletal and cardiac muscle, it is noteworthy that the reduction in force is only 10% even if cardiac muscle is at 80% sarcomere length.[8] The cellular basis of the Frank-Starling mechanism is still being investigated and will be briefly discussed later. A common clinical application of Starling's law is the relationship of left ventricular end-diastolic volume (LVEDV) and stroke volume. The Frank-Starling mechanism may remain intact even in a failing heart.[10] However, ventricular remodeling after injury or in heart failure may modify the Frank-Starling relationship.

Contractility

Each Frank-Starling curve specifies a level of contractility or the inotropic state of the heart, which is defined as the work performed by cardiac muscle at any given end-diastolic fiber. Factors that modify contractility will create a family of Frank-Starling curves with different contractility (Fig. 18-5).[7] Among the factors that are

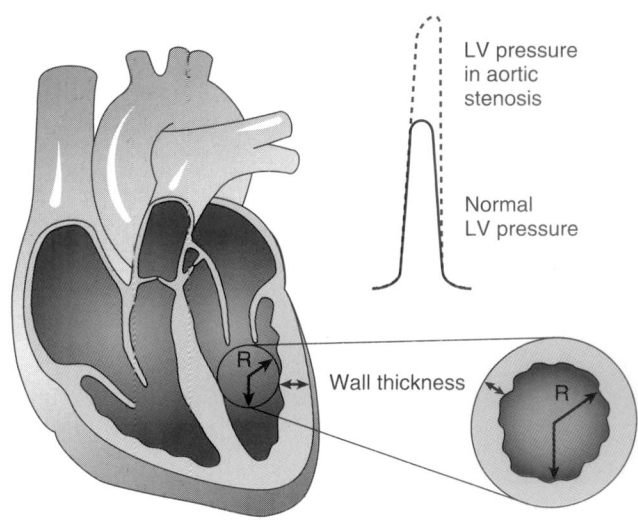

Laplace Law

$$\text{Wall stress} = \frac{\text{pressure} \times \text{radius}}{2(\text{wall thickness})}$$

Figure 18–4 In response to aortic stenosis, left ventricular pressure increases. To maintain wall stress at control levels, compensatory left ventricular hypertrophy develops. According to Laplace's law, wall stress = pressure × radius ÷ (2 × wall thickness). Therefore, the increase in wall thickness offsets the increased pressure and wall stress is maintained at control levels. (From Opie LH: Ventricular function. *In* The Heart. Physiology from Cell to Circulation, 3rd ed. Philadelphia, Lippincott-Raven, 1998, pp 343-389.)

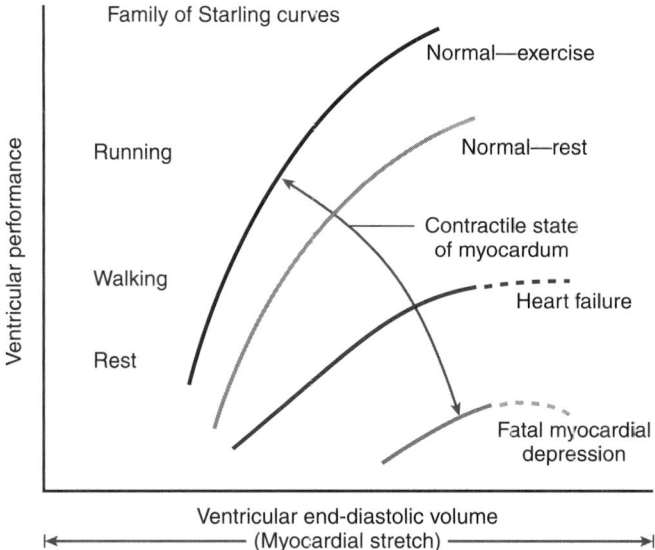

Figure 18–5 A family of Starling curves is shown. A leftward shift of the curve denotes enhancement of the inotropic state, whereas a rightward shift denotes decreased inotropy. (From Opie LH: Ventricular function. *In* The Heart. Physiology from Cell to Circulation, 3rd ed. Philadelphia, Lippincott-Raven, 1998, pp 343-389.)

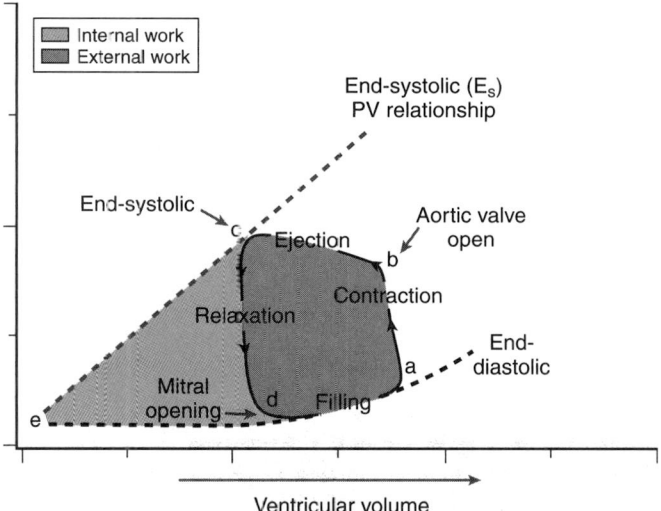

Figure 18–6 Pressure-volume loop. Point *a* depicts the start of isovolumic contraction. The aortic valve opens at point *b*, and ejection of blood follows (*b*→*c*). The mitral valve opens at *d*, and ventricular filling ensues. External work is defined by *a, b, c,* and *d* and internal work by *e, d,* and *c*. The pressure-volume area is the sum of external and internal work. (From Opie LH: Ventricular function. *In* The Heart. Physiology from Cell to Circulation, 3rd ed. Philadelphia, Lippincott-Raven, 1998, pp 343-389.)

known to modify contractility are exercise, adrenergic stimulation, changes in pH, temperature, and drugs such as digitalis. The ability of the LV to develop and generate pressure and sustain the pressure for the ejection of blood is the intrinsic inotropic state of the heart.

In isolated muscle, the maximal velocity of contraction, or Vmax, is defined as the maximal velocity of ejection at zero load. Vmax is obtained by plotting the velocity of muscle shortening in isolated papillary muscle at varying degrees of force. Although this relationship can be replicated in isolated myocytes, Vmax cannot be measured in an intact heart because complete unloading is impossible. To measure the intrinsic contractile activity of an intact heart, several strategies have been attempted with varying success. Pressure-volume loops, albeit requiring catheterization of the left side of the heart, are currently the best way to determine contractility in an intact heart (Fig. 18-6).[7] The pressure-volume loop represents an indirect measure of the Starling relationship between force (pressure) and muscle length (volume). Clinically, the most commonly used noninvasive index of ventricular contractile function is the ejection fraction, which is assessed by echocardiography, angiography or radionucleotide ventriculography.

Ejection fraction = (LVEDV − LVESV)/LVEDV,

where LVESV is left ventricular end-systolic volume.

Cardiac Work
The work of the heart can be divided into external and internal work. External work is expended to eject blood under pressure, whereas internal work is expended within the ventricle to change the shape of the heart and prepare the heart for ejection. Internal work contributes

to inefficiency in performance of the heart. Wall stress is directly proportional to the internal work of the heart.[11]

External work or stroke work is a product of the stroke volume (SV) and pressure (P) developed during ejection of the stroke volume.

Stroke work = SV × P or (LVEDV − LVESV) × P

The external work and internal work of the ventricle both consume O_2. The clinical significance of internal work is illustrated in the case of a poorly drained LV during cardiopulmonary bypass. Although external work is provided by the roller pump during bypass, myocardial ischemia can still occur because poor drainage of the LV creates tension on the LV wall and increases internal work.

The efficiency of cardiac contraction is estimated by the following formula[12]:

Cardiac efficiency = External work/Energy equivalent of oxygen consumption

The corkscrew motion of the heart for the ejection of blood is the most favorable in terms of work efficiency based on the architecture in a normal LV (with the cardiac muscle bundles arranged so that a circumferentially oriented middle layer is sandwiched by longitudinally oriented outer layers). In heart failure, ventricular dilation reduces cardiac efficiency because it increases wall stress, which in term increases oxygen consumption.[11]

Heart Rate and Force-Frequency Relationship
In isolated cardiac muscle, an increase in the frequency of stimulation induces an increase in the force of contraction. This relationship is termed the "treppe"

(Treppe in German means staircase) phenomenon or the force-frequency relationship.[12,13] Between 150 and 180 stimuli per minute, maximal contractile force is reached in an isolated heart muscle at a fixed muscle length. Thus, an increased frequency incrementally increases inotropy, whereas stimulation at lower frequency decreases contractile force. However, when the stimulation becomes extremely rapid, the force of contraction decreases. In the clinical context, pacing-induced positive inotropic effects may be effective only up to a certain heart rate based on the force-frequency relationship. In a failing heart, the force-frequency relationship may be much less effective in producing a positive inotropic effect.[12]

Diastolic Function

Diastole is ventricular relaxation, and it occurs in four distinct phases: (1) isovolumic relaxation; (2) the rapid filling phase, that is, the LV chamber filling at variable LV pressure; (3) slow filling, or diastasis; and (4) final filling during atrial systole. The isovolumic relaxation phase is energy dependent. During the auxotonic relaxation phases (phases 2 through 4), ventricular filling occurs against pressure. It encompasses a period during which the myocardium is unable to generate force and filling of the ventricular chambers takes place. The isovolumic relaxation phase does not contribute to ventricular filling. The vast amount of ventricular filling occurs in the second phase, whereas the third phase adds only about 5% of the total diastolic volume and the final phase provides 15% of ventricular volume from atrial systole.

To assess diastolic function, several indices have been developed. The most widely used index for examining the isovolumic relaxation phase of diastole is to calculate the peak instantaneous rate of LV pressure decline ($-dP/dt$) or the time constant of isovolumic LV pressure decline (τ). The aortic closing–mitral opening interval or the isovolumic relaxation time and the peak rate of LV wall thinning as determined by echocardiography have both been used to estimate diastolic function during auxotonic relaxation. Ventricular compliance can be evaluated by pressure-volume relationships to determine function during the auxotonic phases of diastole.[12,14]

Many different factors influence diastolic function: systolic volume load, passive chamber stiffness, elastic recoil of the ventricle, the diastolic interaction between the two ventricular chambers, atrial properties, and catecholamines. Whereas systolic dysfunction is a reduced ability of the heart to eject, diastolic dysfunction is a decreased ability of the heart to fill. Abnormal diastolic function is now being recognized as the predominant cause of the pathophysiology of congestive heart failure.[15]

Ventricular interactions during systole and diastole are internal mechanisms that function as internal feedback to modulate stroke volume. Systolic ventricular interaction involves the effect of the interventricular septum on the function of both ventricles. Because the interventricular septum is anatomically linked to both ventricles, it will be part of the load against which each ventricle has to work. Therefore, any changes in one ventricle will also be present in the other. In diastolic ventricular interaction, dilatation of either the LV or RV will have an impact on effective filling of the contralateral ventricle and thereby modify function.

Cardiac Output

Cardiac output is the amount of blood pumped by the heart per unit time ($\dot{Q}$) and is determined by four factors: two factors that are intrinsic to the heart—*heart rate* and *myocardial contractility*—and two factors that are extrinsic to the heart but functionally couple the heart and the vasculature—*preload* and *afterload*.

Heart rate is defined as the number of beats per minute and is influenced mainly by the autonomic nervous system. Increases in heart rate increase cardiac output as long as ventricular filling is adequate during diastole. Contractility can be defined as the intrinsic level of contractile performance that is independent of loading conditions. Contractility is difficult to define in an intact heart because it cannot be separated from loading conditions.[12,13] For example, the Frank-Starling relationship is defined as the change in intrinsic contractile performance based on changes in preload. Measurement of cardiac output in a living organism can be determined by using the Fick principle, a schematic depiction of which is illustrated in Figure 18-7.[1]

The Fick principle is based on the concept of conservation of mass such that the O_2 delivered from pulmonary

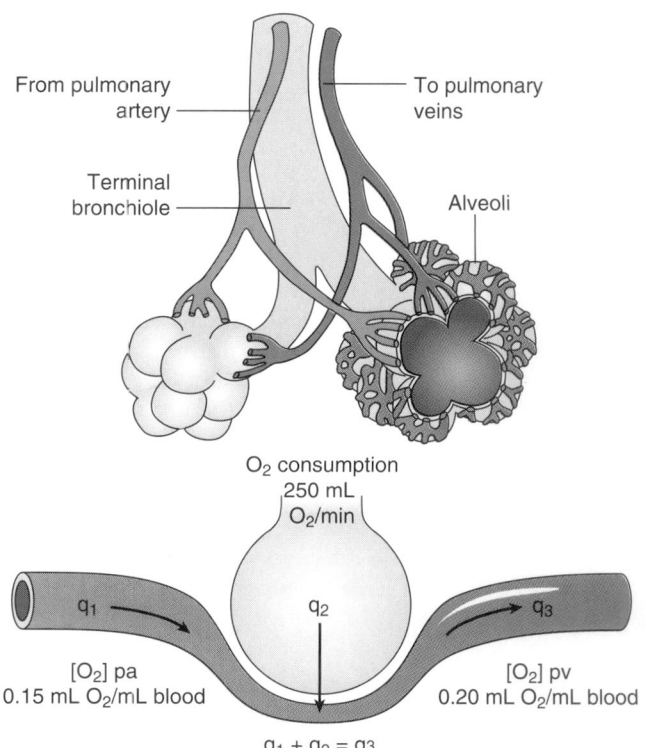

Figure 18–7 Illustration demonstrating the principle of determination of cardiac output according to Fick's equation. If the O_2 concentration of the pulmonary artery ($Cpao_2$), the O_2 concentration of the pulmonary vein ($Cpvo_2$), and O_2 consumption are known, cardiac output can be calculated. (From Berne RM, Levy MN: The cardiac pump. *In* Cardiovascular Physiology, 8th ed. St Louis, CV Mosby, 2001, pp 55-82.)

venous blood (q_3) is equal to the total O_2 delivered to pulmonary capillaries through the pulmonary artery (q_1) and the alveoli (q_2).

The amount of O_2 delivered to the pulmonary capillaries by way of the pulmonary arteries (q_1) equals the total pulmonary arterial blood flow ($\dot{Q}$) times the O_2 concentration in pulmonary arterial blood ($Cpao_2$):

$$q_1 = \dot{Q} \times Cpao_2$$

The amount of O_2 carried away from the pulmonary venous blood (q_3) is equal to the total pulmonary venous blood flow ($\dot{Q}$) times the O_2 concentration in pulmonary venous blood ($Cpvo_2$):

$$q_3 = \dot{Q} \times Cpvo_2$$

The pulmonary arterial O_2 concentration is the mixed systemic venous O_2, and the pulmonary venous O_2 concentration is the peripheral arterial O_2. O_2 consumption is the amount of O_2 delivered to the pulmonary capillaries from the alveoli (q_2). Because $q_1 - q_2 = q_3$,

$$\dot{Q}(Cpao_2) + q_2 = \dot{Q}(Cpvo_2)$$
$$q_2 = \dot{Q}(Cpvo_2) - \dot{Q}(Cpao_2)$$
$$q_2 = \dot{Q}(Cpvo_2) - Cpao_2$$
$$\dot{Q} = q_2/(Cpvo_2 - Cpao_2)$$

Thus, if the O_2 concentration in the pulmonary artery ($Cpao_2$), the O_2 concentration in the pulmonary vein ($Cpvo_2$), and O_2 consumption (q_2) are known, cardiac output can be determined.

The indicator dilution technique is another method of determining cardiac output, and it is also based on the law of conservation of mass. The two most commonly used indicator dilution techniques are the dye dilution and the thermodilution methods. Figure 18-8 illustrates the principles of the dye dilution method.[1]

CELLULAR CARDIAC PHYSIOLOGY

Cellular Anatomy

At the cellular level, the heart consists of three major components: cardiac muscle tissue (contracting cardiomyocytes), conduction tissue (conducting cells), and extracellular connective tissue. A group of cardiomyocytes with its connective tissue support network or extracellular matrix make up a myofiber (Fig. 18-9). Adjacent myofibers are connected by strands of collagen. The extracellular matrix is the synthetic product of fibroblasts and is made up of collagen, which is the main determinant of myocardial stiffness, and other major matrix proteins. One of the matrix proteins, elastin, is the chief constituent of elastic fibers. The elastic fibers account for, in part, the elastic properties of the myocardium.[6] Other matrix proteins include the glycoproteins or proteoglycans and matrix metalloproteins. Proteoglycans are proteins with short sugar chains, and

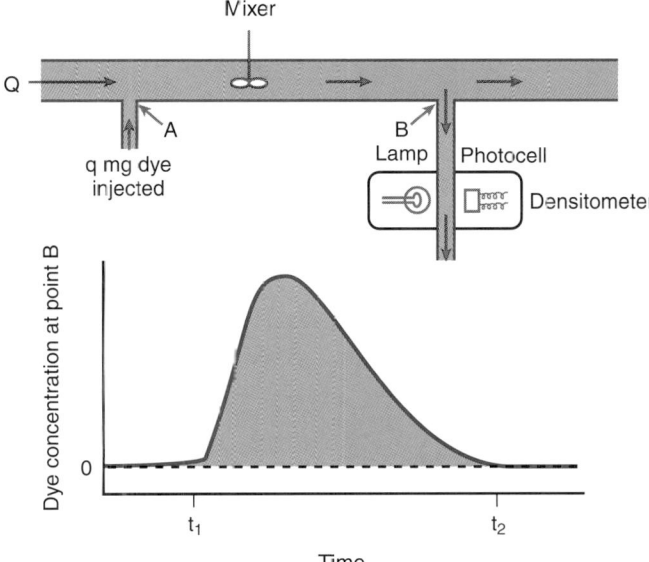

Figure 18–8 Illustration demonstrating the principle of determination of cardiac output by using the indicator dilution technique. This model assumes that there is no recirculation. A known amount of dye (q) is injected at point A into a stream flowing at $\dot{Q}$ (mL/min). A mixed sample of the fluid flowing past point B is withdrawn at a constant rate through a densitometer. The change in dye concentration over time is depicted in a *curve.* Flow may be measured by dividing the amount of indicator injected upstream by the area under the downstream concentration curve. (From Berne RM, Levy MN: The cardiac pump. *In Cardiovascular Physiology,* 8th ed. St Louis, CV Mosby, 2001, pp 55-82.)

they include heparan sulfate, chondroitin, fibronectin, and laminin. Matrix metalloproteins are enzymes that degrade collagen and other extracellular proteins. The balance between accumulation of extracellular matrix proteins by synthesis and their breakdown by matrix metalloproteins contributes to the mechanical properties and function of the heart.[6]

Cardiomyocyte Structure and Function

Individual contracting cardiomyocytes are large cells between 20 μm (atrial cardiomyocytes) and 140 μm

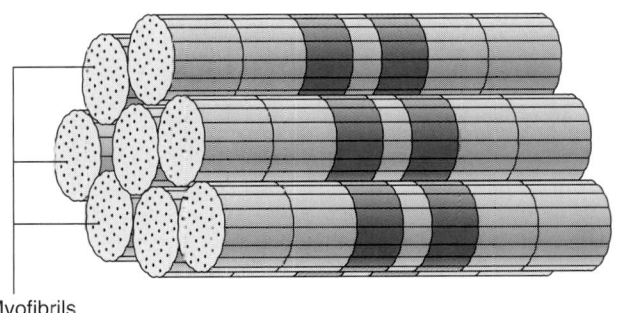

Myofibrils

Figure 18–9 Organization of cardiomyocytes. Fifty percent of cardiomyocyte volume is made up of myofibrils; the remainder consists of mitochondria, nucleus, sarcoplasmic reticulum, and cytosol.

(ventricular cardiomyocytes) in length. Approximately 50% of the cell volume in a contracting cardiomyocyte is made up of myofibrils, and the remainder consists of mitochondria, nucleus, sarcoplasmic reticulum (SR), and the cytosol. The myofibril is the rodlike bundle that forms the contractile elements within cardiomyocytes. Within each contractile element are contractile proteins, regulatory proteins, and structural proteins. Contractile proteins make up about 80% of the myofibrillar protein, with the remainder being regulatory and structural proteins.[16,17] The basic unit of contraction is the sarcomere, which will be described later.

The sarcolemma, or the outer plasma membrane, separates the intracellular and extracellular space. It surrounds the cardiomyocyte and invaginates into the myofibrils through an extensive tubular network known as transverse or T tubules, and it also forms specialized intercellular junctions between cells.[18,19]

Transverse or T tubules are in close proximity to an intramembrane system and the SR, which plays an important role in calcium metabolism that is critical in excitation-contraction coupling of the cardiomyocyte. The SR can be further divided into the longitudinal (or network) and the junctional SR. The longitudinal SR is involved in the uptake of calcium for initiation of relaxation. The junctional SR contains the large calcium release channels (ryanodine receptors) that release SR calcium stores in response to depolarization-stimulated calcium influx through the sarcolemmal calcium channels. The ryanodine receptors not only are calcium release channels but also form the scaffolding proteins that anchor many of the key regulatory proteins.[20]

Mitochondria are found immediately beneath the sarcolemma, wedged between myofibrils within the cell. They contain enzymes that promote the generation of adenosine triphosphate (ATP), and they are the energy powerhouse for the cardiomyocyte. In addition, mitochondria can also function to accumulate calcium and thereby contribute to regulation of the cytosolic calcium concentration. Nearly all of the genetic information is found within the centrally located nucleus. The cytosol is the fluid-filled microenvironment within the sarcolemma, exclusive of the organelles and the contractile apparatus and proteins.

Cardiac muscle cells contain three different types of intercellular junctions: gap junctions, "spot" desmosomes, and "sheet" desmosomes (or fasciae adherens) (Fig. 18-10).[19,21] Gap junctions are responsible for electrical coupling and transfer of small molecules between cells, whereas desmosome-like junctions provide mechanical linkage. The adhesion sites formed by "spot" desmosomes anchor the intermediate filament cytoskeleton of the cell; those formed by the fasciae adherens anchor the contractile apparatus. Gap junctions consist of clusters of plasma membrane channels directly linking the cytoplasmic compartments of neighboring cells. Gap junction channels are constructed from connexins, a multigene family of conserved proteins. The principal connexin isoform of the mammalian heart is connexin 43; other connexins, notably connexin 40, 45, and 37, are also expressed, but in smaller quantities.[20,21]

The conducting cardiomyocytes, or Purkinje cells, are specialized cells for conducting propagated action potentials. These cells have a low content of myofibrils and a prominent nucleus and contain an abundance of gap junctions. Cardiomyocytes can be functionally separated into (1) the excitation system, (2) excitation-contraction-coupling, and (3) the contractile system.

Excitation System

The cellular action potential originating in the specialized conduction tissue is propagated to individual cells where it initiates the intracellular event that leads to contraction of the cell through the sarcolemmal excitation system.

Action Potential

Ion fluxes across plasma membranes result in depolarization (attaining a less negative membrane potential) and repolarization (attaining a more negative membrane potential). They are mediated by membrane proteins with ion-selective pores. Because these ion channel proteins open and close the pores in response to changes in membrane potential, the channels are voltage gated. In the heart, sodium, potassium, calcium, and chloride channels have been found to contribute to the action potential.

The types of action potential in the heart can be separated into two categories: fast-response action potentials, which are found in the His-Purkinje system and atrial or ventricular cardiomyocytes, and slow-response action potentials, which are found in the pacemaker cells in the SA and AV nodes. A typical tracing for an action potential

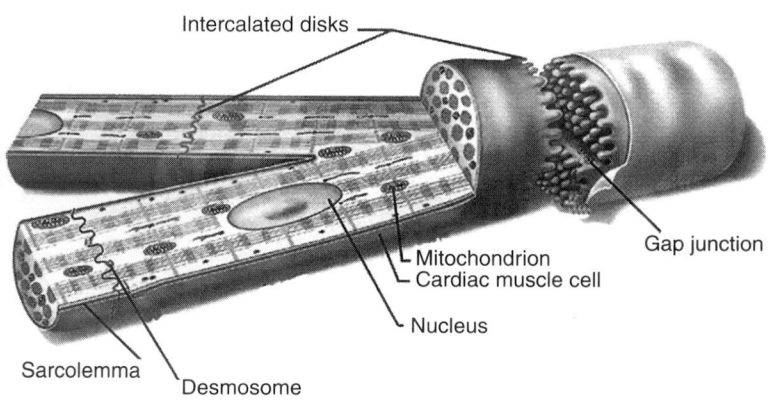

Figure 18–10 Sarcolemma that envelops cardiomyocytes becomes highly specialized to form the intercalated disks where ends of neighboring cells are in contact. The intercalated disks consist of gap junctions and "spot" and "sheet" desmosomes.

in the His-Purkinje system is depicted in Figure 18-11.[12] The electrochemical gradient for potassium across the plasma membrane is the determinant for the resting membrane potential. Mostly as a result of the influx of Na^+, the membrane potential becomes depolarized, which leads to an extremely rapid upstroke (phase 0). As the membrane potential reaches a critical level, or threshold, during depolarization, the action potential is propagated. The rapid upstroke is followed by a transient repolarization (phase 1). Phase 1 is a period of brief and limited repolarization that is largely due to the activation of a transient outward potassium current, i_{to}. The plateau phase (phase 2) occurs with a net influx of Ca^{2+} through L-type calcium channels and efflux of K^+ through several potassium channels: the inwardly rectifying I_k, the delayed rectifier i_{K1}, and i_{to}. Repolarization (phase 3) is brought about when the efflux of K^+ from the three outward potassium currents exceeds the influx of Ca^{2+}, thus returning the membrane to the resting potential. Very little ionic flux occurs during diastole (phase 4) in a fast-response action potential.

In contrast, during diastole (phase 4), pacemaker cells that show slow-response action potentials have the capability of spontaneous diastolic depolarization and generate the automatic cardiac rhythm. Pacemaker currents during phase 4 are the result of an increase in the three inward currents and a decrease in the two outward currents. The three inward currents that contribute to spontaneous pacemaker activity include two carried by calcium, i_{CaL} and i_{CaT}, and one that is a mixed cation current, I_f. The two outward currents are the delayed rectifier potassium current i_k and the inward rectifying potassium current i_{k1}. When compared with the fast-response action potential, phase 0 is much less steep, phase 1 is absent, and phase 2 is indistinct from phase 3 in the slow-response action potential.[22]

During the cardiac action potential, movement of Ca^{2+} into the cell and Na^+ out of the cell creates an ionic imbalance. The Na^+-Ca^{2+} exchanger restores cellular ionic balance by actively transporting Ca^{2+} out of the cell against a concentration gradient while moving Na^+ into the cell in an energy-dependent manner.

Excitation-Contraction Coupling

The structures that participate in cardiac excitation-contraction coupling (ECC) include the sarcolemma, transverse tubules, SR, and the myofilaments (Fig. 18-12A).[23] The process of ECC begins with depolarization of the plasma membrane and the spread of electrical excitation along the sarcolemma of cardiomyocytes. Calcium enters through plasma membrane channels concentrated at the T tubules, and such entry triggers the release of calcium from the SR, which in turn stimulates myofibrillar contraction.[24]

The ubiquitous second messenger calcium is the key player in cardiac ECC (Fig. 18-12B).[23] The cycling of calcium within the structures that participate in ECC initiates and terminates contraction. Activation of the contractile system depends on the increase in free cytosolic calcium and its subsequent binding to contractile proteins. The influx of calcium through the voltage-gated L-type calcium channels (dihydropyridine receptors) causes an initial small increase in intracellular calcium. The local increase in Ca^{2+} concentration as a result of the entry of Ca^{2+} through the voltage-gated L-type calcium channels activates the calcium release channels (ryanodine receptors), induces further release of calcium from the subsarcolemmal cisternae in the SR, and thus leads to a large increase in intracellular calcium. The increase in intracellular calcium, however, is transient inasmuch as calcium is removed by (1) active uptake by the SR calcium pump adenosine triphosphatase (ATPase), (2) extrusion of calcium from the cytosol by the Na^+-Ca^{2+} exchanger, and (3) binding of calcium to proteins.[25]

The SR provides the anatomic framework and is the major organelle for the cycling of calcium. It is the depot for intracellular calcium stores. The cyclic release plus reuptake of calcium by the SR regulates the cytosolic calcium concentration and couples excitation to contraction. The physical proximity between the L-type calcium channels and the ryanodine receptors at the SR membrane makes calcium-induced calcium release occur easily. The "foot" region of the ryanodine receptor is the part that extends from the SR membrane to the T tubules, where the L-type calcium channels are located.[16,25,26]

The SR is also concerned with the reuptake of calcium that initiates relaxation or terminates contraction. Sarcoplasmic reticulum ATPase (SERCA) is the ATP-dependent pump that actively pumps the majority of the calcium back into the SR after its release. SERCA makes up

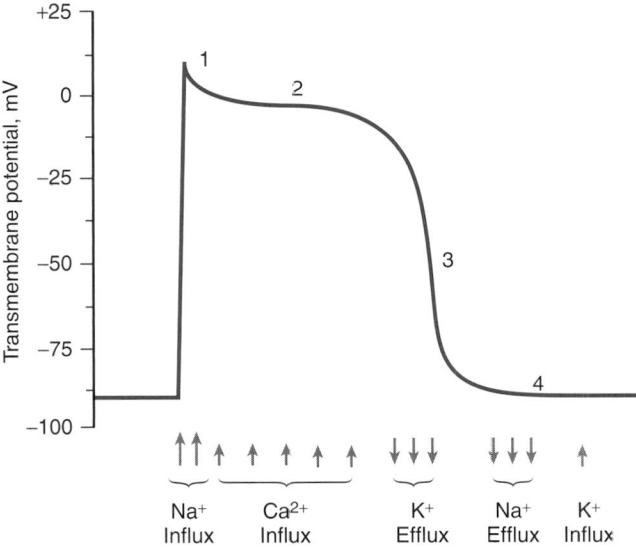

Figure 18–11 Phases of cellular action potentials and major associated currents in ventricular myocytes. The initial phase zero spike and overshoot (1) are caused by a rapid inward Na current, the plateau phase (2) by a slow Ca current through L-type Ca channels, and repolarization (phase 3) by outward K currents. Phase 4, the resting potential (Na efflux, K influx), is maintained by Na-K-ATPase. The Na-Ca exchanger is mainly responsible for Ca extrusion. In specialized conduction system tissue, spontaneous depolarization takes place during phase 4 until the voltage resulting in opening of the Na channel is reached. (From LeWinter MM, Osol G: Normal physiology of the cardiovascular system. *In* Fuster V [ed]: Hurst's The Heart, 10th ed. New York, McGraw-Hill, 2001, pp 63-94.)

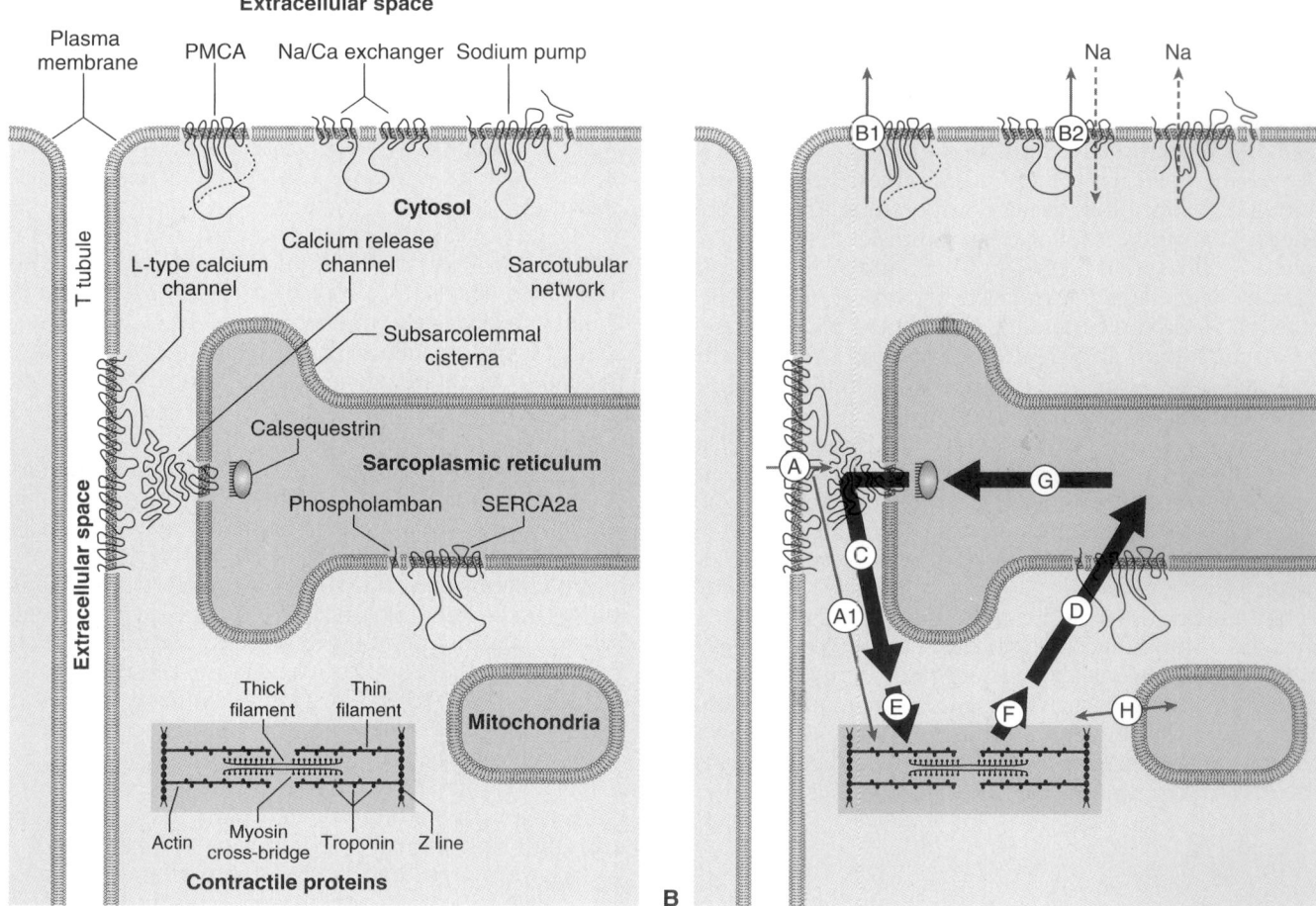

Figure 18–12 A, Diagram depicting the components of cardiac excitation-contraction coupling. Calcium pools are noted in bold letters. **B,** Extracellular (*arrows A, B1, B2*) and intracellular calcium flux (*arrows C, D, E, F, G*) is shown. The thickness of the *arrows* indicates the magnitude of the calcium flux, the vertical orientations describe their energetics: *downward-pointing arrows* represent passive calcium flux, and *upward pointing arrows* represent energy-dependent calcium transport. Calcium entering the cell from extracellular fluid through L-type calcium channels triggers calcium release from the sarcoplasmic reticulum (SR). Only a small portion directly activates the contractile proteins (A1). *Arrow B1* depicts active transport of calcium into the extracellular fluid by means of the plasma membrane pump ATPase and the Na^+-Ca^{2+} exchanger. Sodium that enters the cell in exchange for calcium (*dashed line*) is pumped out of the cytosol by the sodium pump. SR regulates calcium efflux from the subsarcolemmal cisternae (*arrow C*) and calcium uptake into the sarcotubular network (*arrow D*). *Arrow G* represents calcium that diffuses within the SR. Calcium binding to (*arrow E*) and dissociation from (*arrow F*) high-affinity calcium binding sites of troponin C activate and inhibit interactions of the contractile proteins. *Arrow H* depicts calcium movement into and out of mitochondria to buffer the cytosolic calcium concentration. (From Katz AM: Calcium fluxes. *In* Physiology of the Heart, 3rd ed. Philadelphia, Lippincott-Raven, 2001, pp 232-233.)

close to 90% of all of the SR proteins, and it is inhibited by the phosphoprotein phospholamban at rest. Phospholamban is an SR membrane protein that is active in the dephosphorylated form. Phosphorylation by a variety of kinases as a result of β-adrenergic stimulation or other stimuli inactivates phospholamban and releases its inhibitory action on SERCA. Positive feedback ensues and leads to further phospholamban phosphorylation and greater SERCA activity. The active reuptake of calcium by SERCA then promotes relaxation.[16,25,26]

Once taken up into the SR, calcium is stored until it is released during the next cycle. Calsequestrin and calreticulin are two storage proteins in the SR. Calsequestrin is a highly charged protein located in the cisternal component of the SR near the T tubules. Because it lies close to the calcium release channels, the stored calcium can be quickly discharged for release once the calcium release channels are stimulated.

Cytosolic calcium can also be removed by extrusion through the sarcolemmal calcium pump and the activity of the sodium-calcium exchanger. An important "sensor" and regulator of intracellular calcium is the protein calmodulin.[18]

Contractile System
Contractile Elements
The basic working unit of contraction is the sarcomere. A sarcomere is defined as the distance between Z lines (Z is an abbreviation for the German *Zuckung*, or "contraction"), which join the sarcomeres in series. Each sarcomere consists of a central A band that is separated by half of an I band from the Z lines on each side because the

Z line bisects the I band. A schematic representation is depicted in Figure 18-13.[12] Within each sarcomere are two principal contractile proteins (see the next section) and one noncontractile protein, titin.[25] The two contractile proteins are actin, the thin filament, and myosin, the thick filament. Actin filaments and titin are both tethered to the Z line, but myosin filaments do not actually reach the Z lines. The third filament protein titin tethers the myosin thick filament to the Z line. The Z lines at the two ends of the sarcomere are brought closer together during contraction as the thick myosin filament heads interact with the thin actin filaments and slide over each other.[27,28]

Familial hypertrophic cardiomyopathy is an inherited autosomal dominant sarcomeric disease[29] that is the most common cause of sudden death in otherwise healthy individuals. Its clinical features are left ventricular hypertrophy and myocyte/myofibrillar disarray. Mutations in at least eight different genes encoding sarcomere proteins have been identified to be the molecular basis for the disorder. These genes are β-cardiac myosin heavy chain, cardiac troponin T, α-tropomyosin, cardiac myosin binding protein C, essential or regulatory myosin light chain, cardiac troponin I, α-cardiac actin, and titin.[29]

Contractile Proteins

The contractile apparatus within the cardiomyocyte consists of contractile and regulatory proteins.[18,30,31] The thin filament actin and the thick filament myosin are the two principal contractile proteins. Actin contains two helical chains. Tropomyosin, a double-stranded α-helical regulatory protein, winds around the actin array and forms the backbone for the actin thin filament. The myosin thick filament is made up of 300 myosin molecules. Each myosin molecule has two functional domains: the body or filament and the bilobar myosin head. The myosin head is composed of one heavy chain and two light chains. The heavy head chain has two domains: the larger one interacts with actin at the actin cleft and has an ATP-binding pocket where myosin

ATPase is located, and the other smaller one is flexible and attached to the two light chains. The regulatory troponin heterotrimer complex is found at regular intervals along tropomyosin. The heterotrimer troponins are made up of troponin C (TnC), the Ca^{2+} receptor; troponin I (TnI), an inhibitor of actin-myosin interaction; and troponin T, which links the troponin complex to tropomyosin. Tropomodulin is another regulatory protein. It is located at the end of the actin thin filament and caps the end to prevent any excessive elongation of the thin filament.[27,28]

Myocyte Contraction and Relaxation

At rest, cross-bridge cycling and generation of force do not occur because either the myosin heads are blocked from physically reacting with the thin filament or they are only weakly bound to actin (Fig. 18-14).[16] Cross-bridge cycling is initiated on binding of calcium to TnC, which increases the TnC-TnI interaction and decreases the inhibitory TnI-actin interaction. These events that ensue from the binding of Ca^{2+} to TnC lead to conformational changes in tropomyosin and permit attachment of the myosin head to actin. Cross-bridging involves detachment of the myosin head from actin and reattachment of myosin to another actin on hydrolysis of ATP by myosin ATPase. ATP binding to the nucleotide pocket of the myosin head leads to the activation of myosin ATPase,[26-28] ATP hydrolysis, and changes in the configuration of the myosin head, thus facilitating the binding of myosin head to actin and generation of the power stroke of the myosin head. Based on this model, it is apparent that the rate of cross-bridge cycling is dependent on the activity of myosin ATPase.[31] The turnoff of cross-bridge cycling is largely initiated by the fall in cytosolic calcium.

Myocyte relaxation is an energy-dependent process because the restoration of cytosolic calcium to resting levels requires the expenditure of ATP. The fall in cytosolic calcium occurs through the active reuptake of calcium into the SR by SERCA and extrusion of calcium by the Na^+-Ca^{2+} exchanger. This activity results in the release of Ca^{2+} binding from TnC and separation of the myosin-actin cross-bridge. Myocyte relaxation is dependent on the kinetics of cross-bridge cycling, the affinity of Ca^{2+} for TnC, and the activity of the calcium reuptake mechanisms. Relaxation is enhanced by increased kinetics of cross-bridge cycling, decreased Ca^{2+} affinity for TnC, and increased activity of calcium reuptake mechanisms.[25]

Titin is a giant stringlike protein that acts as the third filament within the sarcomere. A single titin molecule spans half the sarcomere. Structurally, titin consists of an inextensible anchoring segment and an extensible elastic segment. Its two main functions involve muscle assembly and elasticity. Titin is the principal determinant of the passive properties of the myocardium at low ventricular volume.[32]

The Frank-Starling relationship states that an increase in end-diastolic volume results in enhanced systolic function.[33,34] At the cellular level, the key component for the Frank-Starling relationship is a length-dependent shift in Ca^{2+} sensitivity.[35-37] Several possible mechanisms for this change in Ca^{2+} sensitivity have been implicated,

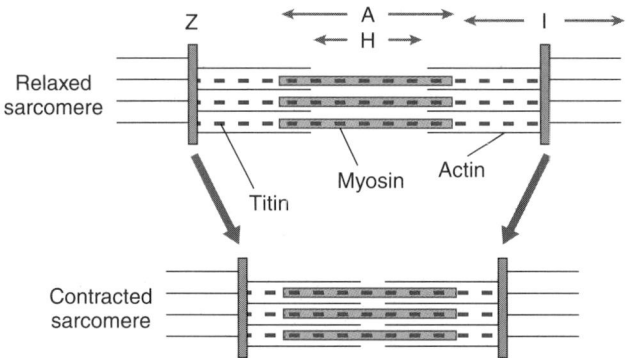

Figure 18–13 The basic unit for contraction is the sarcomere. A contracted and a relaxed sarcomere is depicted. Z lines are located at the ends of the sarcomere. The A band is the site of overlap between myosin and actin filaments. The I band is located on either side of the A band and contains only actin filament. The H zone is located in the center of the A band, and only myosin is present.

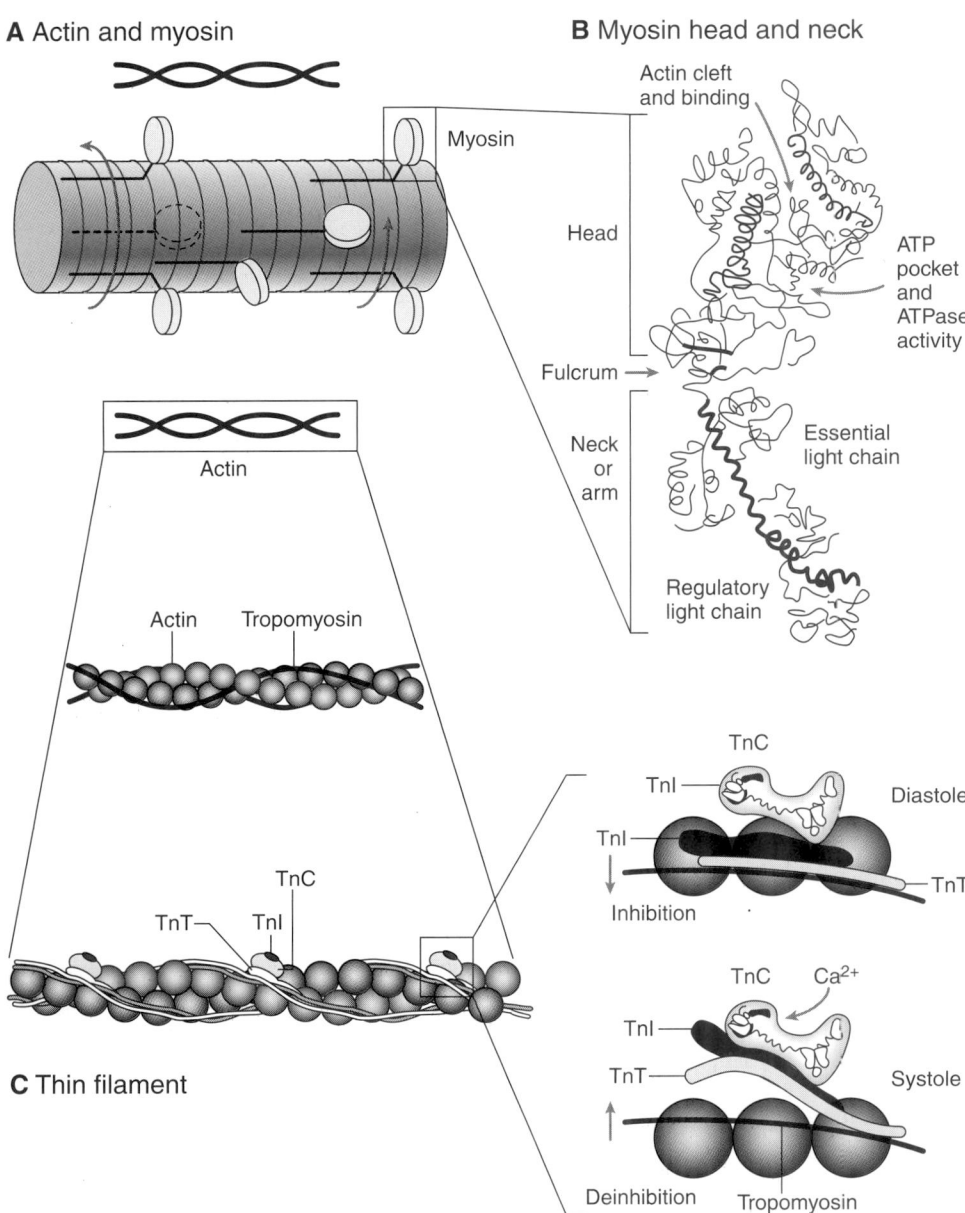

A Actin and myosin

Myosin

B Myosin head and neck

Actin cleft and binding

Head

ATP pocket and ATPase activity

Fulcrum →

Neck or arm

Essential light chain

Regulatory light chain

Actin

Actin   Tropomyosin

TnC

TnT— TnI

C Thin filament

TnC

TnI

TnI

Diastole

TnT

Inhibition

TnC   Ca²⁺

TnI

TnT

Systole

Deinhibition   Tropomyosin

D Troponin I and T

Figure 18–14 Molecules of the contractile system. (From Opie LH: Myocardial contraction and relaxation. *In* The Heart. Physiology from Cell to Circulation, 3rd ed. Philadelphia, Lippincott-Raven, 1998, pp 209-231.)

including (1) Ca^{2+} sensitivity as a function of myofilament lattice spacing, (2) Ca^{2+} sensitivity involving positive cooperativity in cross-bridge binding to actin, and (3) dependence of Ca^{2+} sensitivity on strain of the elastic protein titin.[31,36]

Cytoskeleton Proteins

The cytoskeleton is the protein framework within the cytoplasm that links, anchors, or tethers structural components inside the cell.[17,18] Microfilament (actin filament), microtubules, and intermediate filaments are three classes of cytoskeleton proteins found in the cytoplasm. Microfilament proteins are actin filaments, either sarcomeric or cortical, depending on their location. Sarcomeric actin filaments are the thin filaments in the contractile machinery that have already been described. Cortical actin filaments are found below the plasma membranes at the cell surface and are linked to several other microfilament

proteins, including dystrophin, vinculin, and ankyrin. Microtubules assemble by polymerization of the α- and β-dimers of tubulin. They play a major role in intracellular transport and cell division.[38] Attachment of the ends of microtubules to cellular structures causes the microtubules to expand and contract, thereby pulling and pushing these structures around the cell. The intermediate filaments are relatively insoluble. They have been demonstrated to be important in normal mitochondrial function and behavior. The desmin intermediate filament in cardiomyocytes connects the nucleus to the plasma membrane and is important in transmission of the stress and strain of contractile force between cells.[39] The cytoskeleton provides the organization of microenvironments within the cell for enzyme/protein activity and interaction.

Whereas familial hypertrophic cardiomyopathy is a genetic sarcomeric disease, familial dilated cardiomyopathy

(FDCM) is a disease of cytoskeleton proteins. The genetic basis for FDCM includes two genes for X-linked FDCM (dystrophin, G4.5) and four genes for the autosomal dominant form (actin, desmin, lamin A/C, δ-sarcoglycan).[17]

CONTROL OF CARDIAC FUNCTION

Neural Regulation of Cardiac Function

The two limbs of the autonomic nervous system provide opposing input to regulate cardiac function.[40] The neurotransmitter of the sympathetic nervous system is norepinephrine, which provides positive chronotropic (heart rate), inotropic (contractility), and lusitropic (relaxation) effects. The parasympathetic nervous system has a more direct inhibitory effect in the atria and has a negative modulatory effect in the ventricles. The neurotransmitter of the parasympathetic nervous system is acetylcholine. Norepinephrine and acetylcholine both bind to seven-transmembrane-spanning G protein–coupled receptors to transduce their intracellular signals and effect their functional responses (Fig. 18-15).[41] At rest, the heart has a tonic level of parasympathetic cardiac nerve firing and little, if any sympathetic activity. Therefore, the major influence on the heart is parasympathetic at rest. During exercise or stress, however, the sympathetic neural influence becomes more prominent.

Parasympathetic innervation of the heart is through the vagal nerve. Supraventricular tissue receives much greater vagal innervation than the ventricles do. The principal parasympathetic target neuroeffectors are the muscarinic receptors in the heart.[42,43] Activation of muscarinic receptors reduces pacemaker activity, slows AV conduction, decreases the atrial contractile force directly, and exerts inhibitory modulation of ventricular contractile force. A total of five muscarinic receptors have been cloned.[44] The M_2 receptors are the predominant subtype found in the mammalian heart. In the coronary circulation, M_3 receptors have been identified. Moreover, non-M_2 receptors have also been reported to exist in the heart. In general, for intracellular signaling, M_1, M_3, and M_5 receptors couple to $G_{q/11}$ protein and activate the phospholipase C–diacylglycerol–inositol phosphate system. On the other hand, the M_2 and M_4 receptors couple to the pertussis toxin–sensitive G protein $G_{i/o}$ to inhibit adenylyl cyclase. M_2 receptors can couple to certain K^+ channels and can influence the activity of calcium channels, I_f current, phospholipase A_2, phospholipase D, and tyrosine kinases.

In contrast to vagal innervation, sympathetic innervation of the heart is more predominant in the ventricle than the atrium. Norepinephrine released from sympathetic nerve terminals stimulates adrenergic receptors (adrenoreceptors [ARs]) located in the heart. The two major classes of adrenoceptors are α and β, both of which are G protein–coupled receptors that transduce their intracellular signals by means of specific signaling cascades (Fig. 18-16).

β-ARs can be further divided into subpopulations of $β_1$, $β_2$, and $β_3$.[43,45] Although most mammalian hearts contain $β_1$- and $β_2$-ARs, $β_3$-ARs have also been demonstrated in many mammalian ventricular tissues. The relative contribution of each β-AR subtype to the modulation of cardiac function varies among species. In humans, $β_1$-ARs are the predominant subtype in both the atria and ventricle, but a substantial proportion of $β_2$-ARs are located in the atria and approximately 20% $β_2$-ARs are found in the LV. Much less is known about $β_3$-ARs, but their existence has been documented in the human ventricle. Despite the fact that the $β_1$-AR population is greater than the $β_2$-AR population, the cardiostimulant effect is not proportional to the relative densities of these two subpopulations, which is largely attributable to the tighter coupling of $β_2$-AR to the cyclic adenosine monophosphate (cAMP) signaling pathway in comparison to $β_1$-ARs. Both $β_1$- and $β_2$-ARs activate a pathway that involves the stimulatory G protein (G_s), activation of adenylyl cyclase, accumulation of cAMP, stimulation of cAMP-dependent protein kinase A, and phosphorylation of key target proteins, including L-type calcium channels, phospholamban, and TnI.

Although traditional teaching is that both $β_1$- and $β_2$-ARs are coupled to the G_s-cAMP pathway, more recent experimental evidence has indicated that $β_2$-ARs also couple to the inhibitory G protein G_i to activate non–cAMP-dependent signaling pathways. Additionally, $β_2$-ARs can also couple to G protein–independent pathways to modulate cardiac function. β-AR stimulation increases both contraction and relaxation, as summarized in Figure 18-17.

The two major subpopulations of α-ARs are $α_1$ and $α_2$. The $α_1$- and $α_2$-ARs can be further subdivided into different subtypes. $α_1$-ARs are G protein–coupled receptors and include the $α_1$A, $α_1$B, and $α_1$D subtypes. The $α_1$-AR subtypes are products of separate genes and differ in structure, G protein coupling, tissue distribution, signaling, regulation, and function. Both $α_1$A and $α_1$B ARs mediate positive inotropic responses. However, the positive inotropic effect mediated by $α_1$-ARs is believed to be of minor importance in the heart. $α_1$-ARs are coupled to phospholipase C, phospholipase D, and phospholipase A_2; they increase intracellular Ca^{2+} and myofibrillar sensitivity to Ca^{2+}.

Cardiac hypertrophy is primarily mediated by $α_1$A ARs.[46,47] Cardiac hypertrophic responses to $α_1$-AR agonists involve activation of protein kinase C and mitogen-activated protein kinase through G_q signaling mechanisms. Three subtypes of $α_2$-ARs are recognized: $α_2$A, $α_2$B, and $α_2$C ARs. In the mammalian heart, $α_2$-ARs in the atrium play a role in the presynaptic inhibition of norepinephrine release. These prejunctional $α_2$-ARs are believed to belong to the $α_2$C subtype.

Neural regulation of cardiac function involves a complex interaction between the different classes and

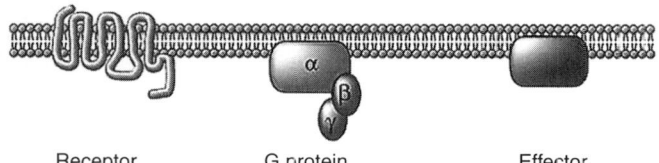

Figure 18–15 A general scheme for a G protein–coupled receptor consisting of receptor, the heterotrimeric G protein, and the effector unit is shown. (Reprinted by permission from Bers DM: Cardiac excitation-contraction coupling. Nature 415:198-205, 2002. Copyright © MacMillan Magazines Ltd.)

Receptor   G protein   Effector

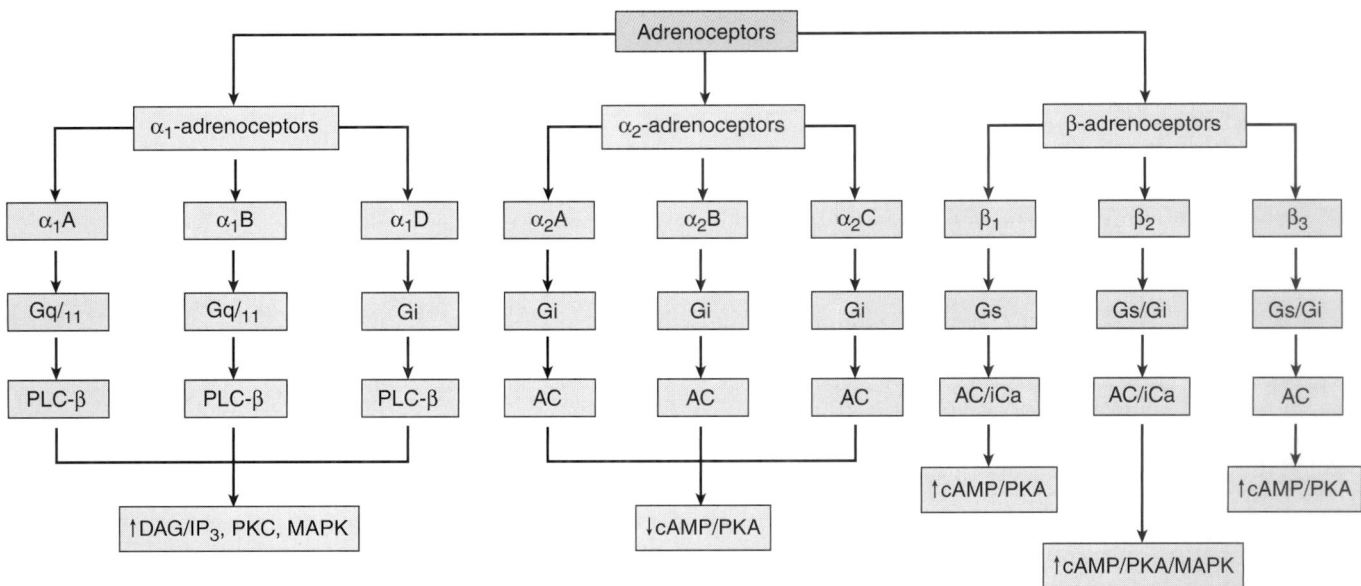

Figure 18–16 Adrenoceptor signaling cascades. G proteins and effectors (AC, adenylyl cyclase; iCA$_L$, L-type calcium current; PLC-β, phospholipase β) are the primary G protein and effectors in the heart. The intracellular signals are DAG (diacylglycerol), IP$_3$ (inositol triphosphate), PKC (protein kinase C), cAMP (cyclic adenosine monophosphate), PKA (protein kinase A), and MAPK (mitogen-activated protein kinase).

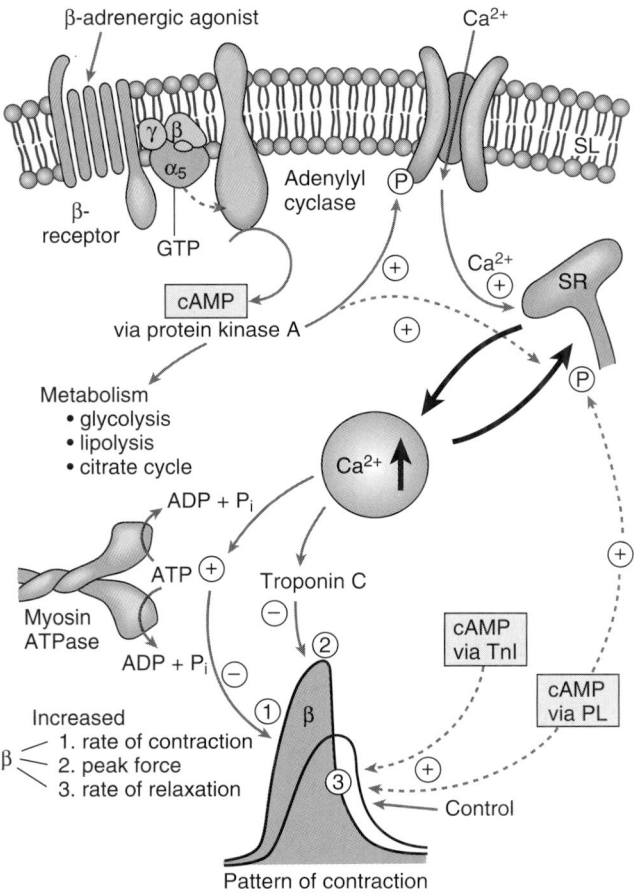

Figure 18–17 The β-adrenoceptor signaling system leads to an increased rate and force of contraction and increased relaxation. SL, sarcolemma; SR, sarcoplasmic reticulum. (From Opie LH: Receptors and signal transduction. *In* The Heart. Physiology from Cell to Circulation, 3rd ed. Philadelphia, Lippincott-Raven, 1998, p 195.)

subpopulations of adrenoceptors and their signaling pathways. Targeted therapeutics in cardiovascular medicine will involve the clinical application and manipulation of our basic understanding of adrenoceptor pharmacology.

Hormones Affecting Cardiac Function

Many hormones have direct and indirect actions on the heart (Table 18-1). Hormones with cardiac actions can be synthesized and secreted by cardiomyocytes or produced by other tissues and delivered to the heart. They act on specific receptors expressed in cardiomyocytes. The great majority of these hormone receptors are plasma membrane G protein-coupled receptors (GPCRs). Non-GPCRs include the natriuretic peptide receptors, which are guanylyl cyclase–coupled receptors, and glucocorticoid/ mineralocorticoid receptors, which bind androgens and aldosterone and are nuclear zinc finger transcription factors. Hormones can have activity in normal cardiac physiology or are active only in pathophysiologic conditions, or both situations can apply. Much of the understanding that has been gained over the past decade on the action of hormones in the heart has been derived from the endocrine changes associated with chronic heart failure.

Cardiac hormones are polypeptides secreted by cardiac tissues into the circulation in the normal heart. Natriuretic peptides,[51,52] aldosterone,[53] and adrenomedullin[54] are hormones that are secreted by cardiomyocytes. Angiotensin II, the effector hormone in the renin-angiotensin system, is also produced by cardiomyocytes.[55,56] The renin-angiotensin system is one of the most important regulators of cardiovascular physiology. It is a key modulator of cardiac growth and function. Angiotensin II stimulates two separate receptor subtypes, AT_1 and AT_2, both of which are present in the heart. AT_1 receptors are the predominant subtype expressed in the normal adult human heart. Stimulation of AT_1 receptors induces a positive chronotropic and inotropic effect. Angiotensin II also mediates cell growth and proliferation in cardiomyocytes and fibroblasts and induces release of the growth factors aldosterone and catecholamines through stimulation of AT_1 receptors. Activation of AT_1 receptors is directly involved in the development of cardiac hypertrophy

and heart failure, as well as adverse remodeling of the myocardium. In contrast, AT_2 receptor activation is counter-regulatory and is generally antiproliferative. Expression of AT_2 receptors, however, is relatively scant in the adult heart because it is most abundant in the fetal heart and declines with development. In response to injury and ischemia, AT_2 receptors become upregulated. The precise role of AT_2 receptors in the heart remains to be defined.

The beneficial effects of blockade of the renin-angiotensin system by using angiotensin-converting enzyme inhibitors in the treatment of heart failure have been attributed to inhibition of AT_1 receptor activity. In addition to the renin-angiotensin system, other cardiac hormones that have been shown to play pathogenic roles in the promotion of cardiomyocyte growth and cardiac fibrosis, the development of cardiac hypertrophy, and the progression of congestive heart failure include aldosterone,[53] adrenomedullin,[57-59] natriuretic peptides,[51,52] angiotensin,[60,61] endothelin,[52] and vasopressin.[63,64]

Increased stretch of the myocardium stimulates the release of atrial natriuretic protein (ANP) and B-type natriuretic protein (BNP) from the atria and ventricles, respectively. Both ANP and BNP bind to natriuretic peptide receptors to generate the second messenger cyclic guanosine monophosphate and represent part of the cardiac endocrine response to hemodynamic changes caused by pressure or volume overload. They also participate in cardiac organogenesis of the embryo heart and cardiovascular system.[51,52] In patients with chronic heart failure, elevation of serum ANP and BNP levels has been documented to be a predictor of mortality.

Adrenomedullin is a recently discovered cardiac hormone that was originally isolated from pheochromocytoma tissues. Adrenomedullin increases accumulation of cAMP and has direct positive chronotropic and inotropic effects.[54,57,58] Adrenomedullin, with interspecies and regional variations, has also been shown to increase nitric oxide production and functions as a potent vasodilator.

Aldosterone is one of the cardiac-generated steroids, although its physiologic significance remains to be defined. It binds to mineralocorticoid receptors and can increase the expression or activity (or both) of cardiac

Table 18-1	Actions of hormones on cardiac function		
Hormone	**Receptor**	**Cardiac Action**	**Increase with CHF**
Adrenomedullin	GPCR	+Inotropy/+chronotropy	+
Aldostereone	MR	?	+
Angiotensin	GPCR	+Inotropy/+chronotropy	+
Endothelin	GPCR	?	+
Natriuretic peptides	GCCR		
ANP (ANF)			+
BNP			+
Neuropeptide Y[48,49]	GPCR	−Inotropy	+
Vasopressin	GPCR	+Inotropy/+chronotropy	+
Vasoactive intestinal peptide[50]	GPCR	+Inotropy	No

ANF, atrial natriuretic factor; ANP, atrial natriuretic peptide; BNP, B-type natriuretic peptide; CHF, congestive heart failure; GCCR, guanylyl cyclase–coupled receptor; GPCR, G protein–coupled receptor; MR, cytosolic or nuclear mineralocorticoid receptor.

proteins, such as cardiac Na^+-K^+-ATPase, Na^+-K^+ cotransporter, Cl^--HCO_3^{2-}, and the Na-H antiporter, involved in ionic homeostasis or regulation of pH.[53] Aldosterone modifies cardiac structure by inducing cardiac fibrosis in both ventricular chambers and thereby leads to impairment of cardiac contractile function.

Cardiac Reflexes

Cardiac reflexes are fast-acting reflex loops between the heart and the central nervous system (CNS) that contribute to the regulation of cardiac function and maintenance of physiologic homeostasis. Specific cardiac receptors elicit their physiologic responses by various pathways. Cardiac receptors are linked to the CNS by myelinated or unmyelinated afferent fibers that travel along the vagus nerve. Cardiac receptors can be found in the atria, ventricles, pericardium, and coronary arteries. Extracardiac receptors are located in the great vessels and the carotid artery. Sympathetic and parasympathetic nerve inputs are processed in the CNS. After central processing, efferent fibers to the heart or the systemic circulation will provoke a particular reaction. The response of the cardiovascular system to efferent stimulation varies with age and duration of the underlying condition that elicited the reflex in the first instance.

Baroreceptor Reflex (Carotid Sinus Reflex)
The baroreceptor reflex is responsible for the maintenance of blood pressure. This reflex is capable of regulating arterial pressure around a preset value through a negative feedback loop (Fig. 18-18).[65,66] In addition, the baroreceptor reflex is capable of establishing a prevailing set point for blood pressure when the preset value has been reset because of chronic hypertension. Changes in blood pressure are monitored by circumferential and longitudinal stretch receptors located in the carotid sinus and aortic arch. The nucleus solitarius located in the cardiovascular center of the medulla receives impulses from these stretch receptors through afferents of the glossopharyngeal and the vagus nerves. The cardiovascular center in the medulla consist of two functionally different areas: the area responsible for increasing blood pressure is located laterally and rostrally, whereas the area responsible for lowering blood pressure is located centrally and caudally. The latter area also integrates impulses from the hypothalamus and the limbic system. Typically, stretch receptors are activated if systemic blood pressure is greater than 170 mm Hg. The response of the depressor system includes decreased sympathetic activity leading to a decrease in cardiac contractility, heart rate, and vascular tone. In addition, activation of the parasympathetic system further decreases the heart rate and myocardial contractility. Reverse effects are elicited with the onset of hypotension.

The baroreceptor reflex plays an important role during acute blood loss and shock. However, the reflex arch loses its functional capacity at a blood pressure less than 50 mm Hg. Hormonal status and therefore sex differences have been implicated in altered baroreceptor responses.[67] Furthermore, volatile anesthetics (in particular, halothane) inhibit the heart rate component of this reflex.[68]

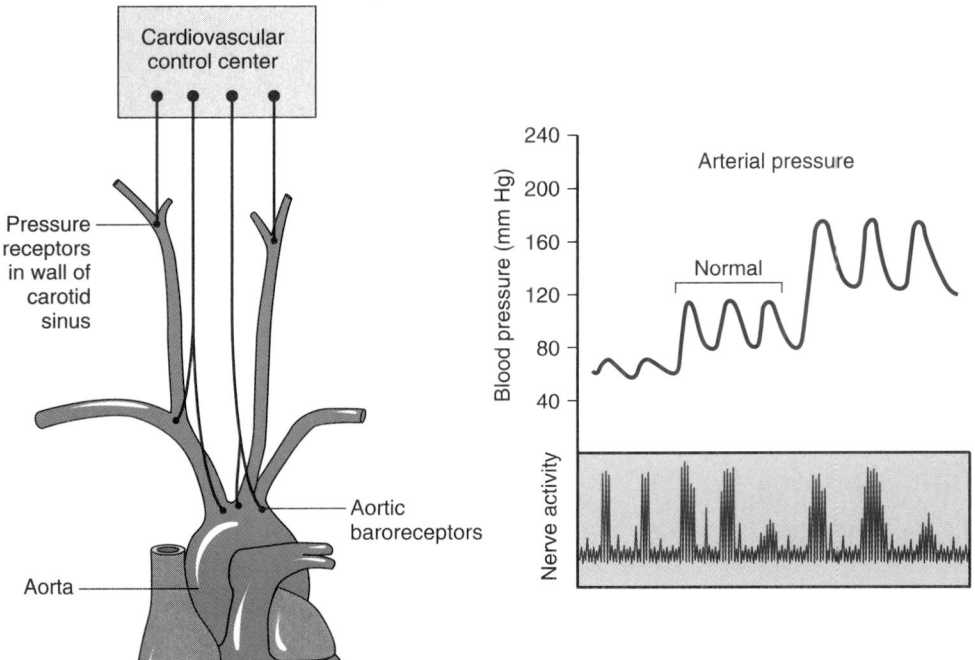

Figure 18–18 Anatomic configuration of the baroreceptor reflex. Pressure receptors in the wall of the carotid sinuses and aorta detect arterial pressure changes in the circulation. These signals are conveyed to afferent receptive regions of the medulla through the Hering and vagus nerves. Output from effector portions of the medulla modulates peripheral tone and heart rate. The increase in blood pressure results in increased activation of the reflex (*right*), which effects a decrease in blood pressure. (From Campagna JA, Carter C: Clinical relevance of the Bezold-Jarisch reflex. Anesthesiology 98:1250-1260, 2003.)

Concomitant use of calcium channel blockers, angiotensin-converting enzyme inhibitors, or phosphodiesterase inhibitors will lessen the cardiovascular response of raising blood pressure through the baroreceptor reflex. This lessened response is achieved by either their direct effects on the peripheral vasculature or, more importantly, their interference with CNS signaling pathways (calcium, angiotensin).[69] Patients with chronic hypertension often exhibit perioperative circulatory instability as a result of a decrease in their baroreceptor reflex response.

Chemoreceptor Reflex

Chemosensitive cells are located in the carotid bodies and the aortic body. These cells respond to changes in pH status and blood oxygen tension. At an arterial partial oxygen pressure (Pao_2) of less than 50 mm Hg or in conditions of acidosis, the chemoreceptors send their impulses along the sinus nerve of Hering (a branch of the glossopharyngeal nerve) and the 10th cranial nerve to the chemosensitive area of the medulla. This area responds by stimulating the respiratory centers and thus increasing the ventilatory drive. In addition, activation of the parasympathetic system ensues and leads to a reduction in heart rate and myocardial contractility. In the case of persistent hypoxia, the CNS will be directly stimulated, with a resultant increase in sympathetic activity.

Bainbridge Reflex

The Bainbridge reflex is elicited by stretch receptors located in the right atrial wall and the cavoatrial junction. An increase in right-sided filling pressure sends vagal afferent signals to the cardiovascular center in the medulla. These afferent signals inhibit parasympathetic activity, thus increasing the heart rate. Acceleration of the heart rate also results from a direct effect on the SA node by stretching the atrium. The changes in heart rate are dependent on the underlying heart rate before stimulation.

Bezold-Jarisch Reflex

The Bezold-Jarisch reflex responds in the triad of hypotension, bradycardia, and coronary artery dilatation to noxious ventricular stimuli sensed by chemoreceptors and mechanoreceptors within the LV wall.[66] The activated receptors communicate along unmyelinated vagal afferent type C fibers. These fibers reflexively increase parasympathetic tone. Because it invokes bradycardia, the Bezold-Jarisch reflex is thought of as a cardioprotective reflex. This reflex has been implicated in the physiologic response to a range of cardiovascular conditions such as myocardial ischemia or infarction, thrombolysis, or revascularization and syncope. Natriuretic peptide receptors stimulated by endogenous ANP or BNP may modulate the Bezold-Jarisch reflex. Thus, the Bezold-Jarisch reflex may be less pronounced in patients with cardiac hypertrophy or atrial fibrillation.[70]

Valsalva Maneuver

Forced expiration against a closed glottis produces increased intrathoracic pressure, increased central venous pressure, and decreased venous return. Cardiac output and blood pressure will be decreased after this (Valsalva) maneuver. This decrease will be sensed by baroreceptors and reflexively result in an increase in heart rate and myocardial contractility through sympathetic stimulation. When the glottis opens, venous return increases and causes the heart to respond by vigorous contraction and an increase in blood pressure. This increase in blood pressure will in turn be sensed by baroreceptors, thus stimulating the parasympathetic efferent pathways to the heart.

Cushing's Reflex

The Cushing reflex is a result of cerebral ischemia caused by increased intracranial pressure. Cerebral ischemia at the medullary vasomotor center induces an initial activation of the sympathetic nervous system. Such activation will lead to an increase in heart rate, blood pressure, and myocardial contractility in an effort to improve cerebral perfusion. As a result of the high vascular tone, reflex bradycardia mediated by baroreceptors will ensue.

Oculocardiac Reflex

The oculocardiac reflex is provoked by pressure applied to the globe of the eye or traction on the surrounding structures. Stretch receptors are located in the extraocular muscles. Once activated, stretch receptors will send afferent signals through the short and long ciliary nerves. The ciliary nerves will merge with the ophthalmic division of the trigeminal nerve at the ciliary ganglion. The trigeminal nerve will carry these impulses to the gasserian ganglion, thereby resulting in increased parasympathetic tone and subsequent bradycardia. The incidence of this reflex during ophthalmic surgery ranges from 30% to 90%. Administration of an antimuscarinic drug such as glycopyrrolate or atropine reduces the incidence of bradycardia during eye surgery (also see Chapter 65).

KEY POINTS

1. The cardiac cycle is the sequence of electrical and mechanical events during the course of a single heartbeat.
2. Cardiac output is determined by the heart rate, myocardial contractility, and preload and afterload.
3. The majority of cardiomyocytes consist of myofibrils, which are rodlike bundles that form the contractile elements within the cardiomyocyte.
4. The basic working unit of contraction is the sarcomere.
5. Gap junctions are responsible for electrical coupling of small molecules between cells.
6. Action potentials have four phases in the heart.
7. The key player in cardiac excitation-contraction coupling is the ubiquitous second messenger calcium.
8. β-Adrenoreceptors stimulate chronotropy, inotropy, lusitropy, and dromotropy.
9. Hormones with cardiac action can be synthesized and secreted by cardiomyocytes or produced by other tissues and delivered to the heart.
10. Cardiac reflexes are fast-acting reflex loops between the heart and the CNS that contribute to regulation of cardiac function and maintenance of physiologic homeostasis.

REFERENCES

1. Berne RM, Levy MN: The cardiac pump. *In* Cardiovascular Physiology, 8th ed. St Louis, CV Mosby, 2001, pp 55-82.
2. Berne RM, Levy MN: Electrical activity of the heart. *In* Cardiovascular Physiology, 8th ed. St Louis, CV Mosby, 2001, pp 7-32.
3. Katz AM: The heart as a muscular pump. *In* Physiology of the Heart, 3rd ed. Philadelphia, Lippincott-Raven, 2001, pp 408-417.
4. Takayama Y, Costa KD, Covell JW: Contribution of laminar myofiber architecture to load-dependent changes in mechanics of LV myocardium. Am J Physiol Heart Circ Physiol 282:H1510-1520, 2002.
5. Katz AM: Structure of the heart. *In* Physiology of the Heart, 3rd ed. Philadelphia, Lippincott-Raven, 2001, pp 1-38.
6. Opie LH: Heart cells and organelles. *In* The Heart. Physiology from Cell to Circulation, 3rd ed. Philadelphia, Lippincott-Raven, 1998, pp 43-68.
7. Opie LH: Ventricular function. *In* The Heart. Physiology from Cell to Circulation, 3rd ed. Philadelphia, Lippincott-Raven, 1998, pp 343-389.
8. Frank O: Zur Dynamik des Herzmuskels. Z Biol 32:370, 1895.
9. Starling EH: Linacre Lecture on the Law of the Heart. London, Longmans Green, 1918.
10. Holubarsch C, Ruf T, Goldstein D, et al: Existence of the Frank-Starling mechanism in the failing human heart. Circulation 94:683-689, 1996.
11. Katz AM: The working heart. *In* Physiology of the Heart, 3rd ed. Philadelphia, Lippincott-Raven, 2001, pp 418-443.
12. LeWinter MM, Osol G: Normal physiology of the cardiovascular system. *In* Fuster V (ed): Hurst's The Heart, 10th ed. New York, McGraw-Hill, 2001, pp 63-94.
13. Opie LH: Mechanisms of cardiac contraction and relaxation. *In* Braunwald E (ed): Heart Disease, 6th ed. Philadelphia, WB Saunders, 2001, pp 443-478.
14. Little WC: Assessment of normal and abnormal cardiac function. *In* Braunwald E (ed): Heart Disease, 6th ed. Philadelphia, WB Saunders, 2001, pp 479-502.
15. Zile MR, Brutsaert DL: New concepts in diastolic dysfunction and diastolic heart failure. Circulation 105:1387-1393, 2002.
16. Opie LH: Myocardial contraction and relaxation. *In* The Heart. Physiology from Cell to Circulation, 3rd ed. Philadelphia, Lippincott-Raven, 1998, pp 209-231.
17. Roberts R: Principles of molecular cardiology. *In* Fuster V (ed): Hurst's The Heart, 10th ed. New York, McGraw-Hill, 2001, pp 95-112.
18. Katz AM: Contractile proteins and cytoskeleton. *In* Physiology of the Heart, 3rd ed. Philadelphia, Lippincott-Raven, 2001, pp 123-150.
19. Severs NJ: The cardiac muscle cell. Bioessays 22:188-199, 2000.
20. Yeager M: Structure of cardiac gap junction intercellular channels. J Struct Biol 121:231-245, 1998.
21. Severs NJ: Intercellular junctions and the cardiac intercalated disk. Adv Myocardiol 5:223-242, 1985.
22. Fill M, Copello JA: Ryanodine receptor calcium release channels. Physiol Rev 82:893-922, 2002.
23. Kumar NM, Gilula NB: The gap junction communication channel. Cell 84:381-388, 1996.
24. Katz AM: The cardiac action potential. *In* Physiology of the Heart, 3rd ed. Philadelphia, Lippincott-Raven, 2001, pp 478-516.
25. Katz AM: Calcium fluxes. *In* Physiology of the Heart, 3rd ed. Philadelphia, Lippincott-Raven, 2001, pp 232-233.
26. Bers DM: Cardiac excitation-contraction coupling. Nature 415:198-205, 2002.
27. de Tombe PP: Cardiac myofilaments: Mechanics and regulation. J Biomech 36:721-730, 2003.
28. Opie LH: Excitation-contraction coupling. *In* The Heart. Physiology from Cell to Circulation, 3rd ed. Philadelphia, Lippincott-Raven, 1998, pp 149-171.
29. Bonne G, Carrier L, Richard P, et al: Familial hypertrophic cardiomyopathy, from mutations to functional defect. Circ Res 83:580-593, 1998.
30. Solaro RJ, Rarick HM: Troponin and tropomyosin. Circ Res 83:417-480, 1998.
31. Fuchs F, Smith SH: Calcium, cross-bridges, and the Frank-Starling relationship. News Physiol Sci 16:5-10, 2001.
32. Trinick J, Tskhovrebova L: Titin: A molecular control freak. Trends Cell Biol 9:377-380, 1999.
33. Moss RL, Fitzsimons DP: Frank-Starling relationship. Circ Res 90:11-13, 2002.
34. Alvarez BV, Perez NG, Ennis IL, et al: Mechanisms underlying the increase in force and Ca^{2+} transient that follow stretch of cardiac muscle. Circ Res 85:716-722, 1999.
35. Fukuda N, Sasaki D, Ishiwata S, Kurihara S: Length dependence of tension generation in rat skinned cardiac muscle. Circulation 104:1639-1645, 2001.
36. Konhilas JP, Irving TC, de Tombe PP: Myofilament calcium sensitivity in skinned rat cardiac trabeculae. Circ Res 90:59-65, 2002.
37. Konhilas JP, Irving TC, de Tombe PP: Length-dependent activation in three striated muscle types of the rat. J Physiol 544:225-236, 2002.
38. Capetanaki Y: Desmin cytoskeleton: A potential regulator of muscle mitochondrial behavior and function. Trends Cardiovasc Med 12:339-348, 2002.
39. Howard J, Hyman AA: Dynamics and mechanics of the microtubule plus end. Nature 422:753-758, 2003.
40. Opie LH: Receptors and signal transduction. *In* The Heart. Physiology from Cell to Circulation, 3rd ed. Philadelphia, Lippincott-Raven, 1998, p 195.
41. Rockman HA, Koch WJ, Lefkowitz RJ: Seven-transmembrane-spanning receptors and heart function. Nature 415:206-212, 2002.
42. Mendelowitz D: Advances in parasympathetic control of heart rate and cardiac function. News Physiol Sci 14:155-161, 1999.
43. Brodde OE, Michel MC: Adrenergic and muscarinic receptors in the human heart. Pharm Rev 51:651-689, 1999.
44. Dhein S, Van Koppen CJ, Brodde OE: Muscarinic receptors in the mammalian heart. Pharm Res 44:161-182, 2001.
45. Kaumann AJ, Molenaar P: Modulation of human cardiac function through 4 β-adrenoceptor populations. Naunyn Schmiedebergs Arch Pharmacol 355:667-681, 1997.
46. Endoh M: Cardiac α_1-adrenoceptors that regulate contractile function: Subtypes and subcellular signal transduction mechanisms. Neurochem Res 21:217-229, 1996.
47. Artega GM, Kobayashi T, Solaro RJ: Molecular actions of drugs that sensitize cardiac myofilaments to Ca^{2+}. Ann Med 34:248-258, 2002.
48. Maisel AS, Scott NA, Motulsky HJ, et al: Elevation of plasma neuropeptide Y levels in congestive heart failure. Am J Med 86:43-48, 1989.
49. Grundemar L, Hakanson R: Multiple neuropeptide Y receptors are involved in cardiovascular regulation. Peripheral and central mechanisms. Gen Pharmacol 24:785-796, 1993.
50. Henning RJ, Sawmiller DR: Vasoactive intestinal peptide: Cardiovascular effects. Cardiovasc Res 49:27-37, 2001.
51. de Bold AJ, Bruneau BG, Kuroski de Bold M: Mechanical and neuroendocrine regulation of the endocrine heart. Cardiovasc Res 31:7-18, 1996.
52. Cameron VA, Ellmers LJ: Minireview: Natriuretic peptides during development of the fetal heart and circulation. Endocrinology 144:2191-2194, 2003.
53. Delcayre C, Silvestre JS: Aldosterone and the heart: Towards a physiological function? Cardiovasc Res 42:7-12, 1999.
54. Martinez A: Biology of adrenomedullin. Microsc Res Tech 57:1-2, 2002.
55. Schuijt MP, Jan Danser AH: Cardiac angiotensin II: An intracrine hormone? Am J Hypertens 15:1109-1116, 2002.
56. Dinh DT, Frauman AG, Johnston CI, Fabiani ME: Angiotensin receptors: Distribution, signalling and function. Clin Sci 100:481-492, 2001.

57. Kitamura K, Kangawa K, Eto T: Adrenomedullin and PAMP: Discovery, structures, and cardiovascular functions. Microsc Res Tech 57:3-13, 2002.

58. Minamino N, Kikumoto K, Isumi Y: Regulation of adrenomedullin expression and release. Microsc Res Tech 57:28-39, 2002.

59. Smith DM, Coppock HA, Withers DJ, et al: Adrenomedullin: Receptor and signal transduction. Biochem Soc Trans 30:432-437, 2002.

60. Opie LH, Sack MN: Enhanced angiotensin II activity in heart failure. Circ Res 88:654-658, 2001.

61. De Mello WC: Cardiac arrhythmias: The possible role of the renin-angiotensin system. J Mol Med 79:103-108, 2001.

62. Kramer BK, Ittner KP, Beyer ME, et al: Circulatory and myocardial effects of endothelin. J Mol Med 75:886-890, 1997.

63. Walker BR, Childs ME, Adamas EM: Direct cardiac effects of vasopressin: Role of V_1 and V_2 vasopressinergic receptors. Am J Physiol 255:H261-H265, 1988.

64. Chandrashekhar Y, Prahash AJ, Sen A, et al: The role of arginine vasopressin and its receptors in the normal and failing rat heart. J Mol Cell Cardiol 35:495-504, 2003.

65. Parlow JL, Bégou G, Sagnard P, et al: Cardiac baroreflex during the postoperative period in patients with hypertension. Anesthesiology 90:681-692, 1999.

66. Campagna JA, Carter C: Clinical relevance of the Bezold-Jarisch reflex. Anesthesiology 98:1250-1260, 2003.

67. Huikuri HV, Pikkujamsa SM, Airaksinen KE, et al: Sex-related differences in autonomic modulation of heart rate in middle-aged subjects. Circulation 94:122-125, 1996.

68. Keyl C, Schneider A, Hobbhan, et al: Sinusoidal neck suction for evaluation of baroreflex sensitivity during desflurane and sevoflurane anesthesia. Anesth Analg 95:1629-1636, 2002.

69. Devlin MG, Angus JA, Wilson KM, et al: Acute effects of L- and T-type calcium channel antagonists on cardiovascular reflexes in conscious rabbits. Clin Exp Pharmacol Physiol 29:372-380, 2002.

70. Thomas CJ, Woods RL: Guanylyl cyclase receptors mediate cardiopulmonary vagal reflex actions of ANP. Hypertension 41:279-285, 2003.

19 Hepatic Physiology and Pathophysiology

Phillip S. Mushlin and Simon Gelman

Hepatic Anatomy and Circulation   743
Hepatic Blood Flow   743
Microcirculation: The Liver Acinus   744
Intrinsic Regulation of Hepatic Blood Flow   745
Extrinsic Regulation of Hepatic Blood Flow   746

Functions of the Liver   747
Protein Metabolism   747
Carbohydrate Metabolism   747
Lipid Metabolism   748
Bile Metabolism   748
Coagulation   749
Erythropoiesis: Heme and Bilirubin Metabolism   749
Endocrine Function   750
Immune Function and Inflammation   750
Metabolism of Drugs (Xenobiotics)   750

Evaluation of the Liver   752
Clinical Assessment   752
Biochemical Tests   753
Quantitative Tests   756
Measurement of Liver Blood Flow   756
Radiologic and Endoscopic Techniques   756

Hepatic Pathophysiology   757
Mechanisms of Cell Death   757
Oxidative Stress and the Glutathione System   757
Ischemia/Reperfusion Injury   758
Bacterial, Viral, and Immune Injury   758
Drug- and Toxin-Induced Damage   758
Ethanol-Induced Liver Disease   759
Cirrhosis and Portal Hypertension   760
Cholestatic Disease   763

HEPATIC ANATOMY AND CIRCULATION

Surface anatomy shows the liver to have four distinct topographical lobes: left, right, caudate, quadrate (Fig. 19-1).[1] The physiologic anatomy, however, reveals eight functionally independent segments, collectively referred to as the French (Couinaud) system (Fig. 19-2). Each segment has its own vascular flow and biliary drainage. Couinaud anatomy simplifies efforts to preserve healthy tissue and extirpate diseased regions, and has resulted in improved clinical outcomes for patients undergoing hepatic surgery for neoplasms or trauma-induced injuries.[2-4]

The liver accounts for about 2% of body weight in adults (1.5 kg per 70 kg) and 5% in neonates.[5] The liver holds around 10% to 15% of the total blood volume and serves as an important blood reservoir for the body.[6] About 20% of blood is in arteries, 10% is in capillaries, and 70% is in veins.[7] The hepatic venous circulation directly affects intravascular fluid homeostasis.[8,9] Even small increases in hepatic venous pressure can shift large volumes of plasma into the lymphatics or peritoneal cavity (through Glisson's capsule). The transudated fluid has a protein concentration similar to that of plasma.

Hepatic Blood Flow

Roughly 25% of the cardiac output passes through the liver (1 mL blood per 1 g liver). The blood supply to the liver is from the hepatic artery and portal vein (Fig. 19-3; also see Fig. 19-1).[1,10] After branching from the celiac axis, the common hepatic artery divides into the gastroduodenal and proper hepatic arteries. The latter artery provides 25% to 30% of the total hepatic blood flow and 45% to 50% percent of the oxygen consumed by the liver. The portal vein—a valveless nutrient vessel that transports the pooled effluent of pre-portal splanchnic beds—delivers 70% to 75% of the total blood flow to the liver and 50% to 55% of the hepatic oxygen consumption.[7]

The hepatic artery and portal vein enter the liver at its hilum (porta hepatis) and course through the liver in parallel, ramifying into consecutively smaller branches, which end as terminal portal venules and hepatic arterioles. These terminal branches drain into the hepatic sinusoids

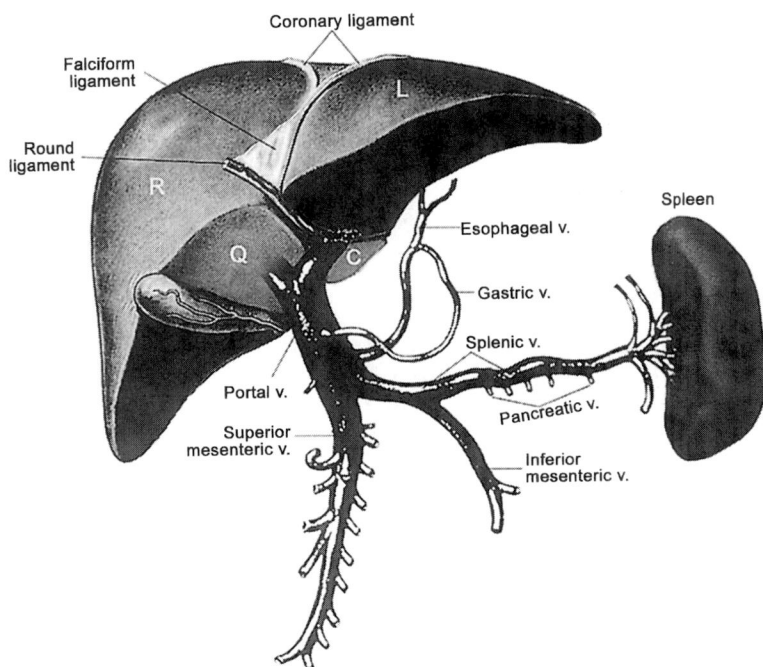

Figure 19–1 Lobar anatomy of the liver. R, right lobe; L, left lobe; Q, quadrate lobe; C, caudate lobe; v, vein. (From Mushlin PS, Gelman S: Anesthesia and the liver. *In* Barash PG, Cullen BF, Stoelting RK [eds]: Clinical Anesthesia, 4th ed. Philadelphia, Lippincott Williams & Wilkins, 2001, pp 1067-1101.)

(i.e., capillaries of the liver), which are the main conduits for perfusing hepatocytes (Fig. 19-4).[11] Lining the sinusoids are Kupffer cells, hepatic stellate cells (formerly called lipid-storing or Ito cells), and fenestrated endothelial cells. Constituents of blood pass through these fenestrations into the space of Disse, gaining direct access to hepatic parenchymal cells. Blood leaves the sinusoids through the central veins (i.e., terminal hepatic venules) and flows into sublobular, lobular, and major hepatic veins (right, middle, and left, respectively). These veins, and many smaller vessels, drain into the inferior vena cava (Fig. 19-5).[5]

Microcirculation: The Liver Acinus

The acinus is the functional microvascular unit of the liver. It forms around a vertical axis (the portal canal) which consists of a hepatic arteriole, a portal venule, a bile ductule, as well as lymph vessels and nerves. Blood flow is vertical to the portal triads and directed radially toward the central veins.

The acinus has three circulatory zones (Fig. 19-6),[5] which reflect the closeness of hepatocytes to the portal axis or central vein. Zone 1 (periportal zone) cells are closest to the portal axis (i.e., origin of the sinusoid) and receive blood that is rich in oxygen and nutrients. Zone 2 (midzonal region) is the arbitrary intermediary transition zone. Zone 3 (pericentral zone) cells occupy the margin of the acinus, and receive blood that has exchanged gases and metabolites with cells in zones 1 and 2.

This microvascular architecture creates metabolic diversity among the three zones. Compartmentalization of metabolic pathways in acinar zones can promote the efficient use and clearance of metabolic by-products.[12,13] Nitrogen metabolism provides an example. Zone 1 and zone 2 hepatocytes are the chief producers of ammonia,

which is formed when amino acids are converted to ketoacids. These hepatocytes contain the enzymes of the urea cycle—a high-capacity, low-affinity cyclical pathway that eliminates ammonia by incorporating it into urea. If ammonia molecules get through zone 2, they encounter glutamine synthetase in zone 3. This enzyme is expressed only in zone 3 and acts to recapture ammonia in the form of glutamine substrate. If the enzyme were present in zones 1 or 2, ammonia excretion via the urea cycle would be compromised. However, its presence in zone 3 empowers pericentral hepatocytes to be important scavengers of ammonia and prevents this toxic substance from reaching the central circulation.[12]

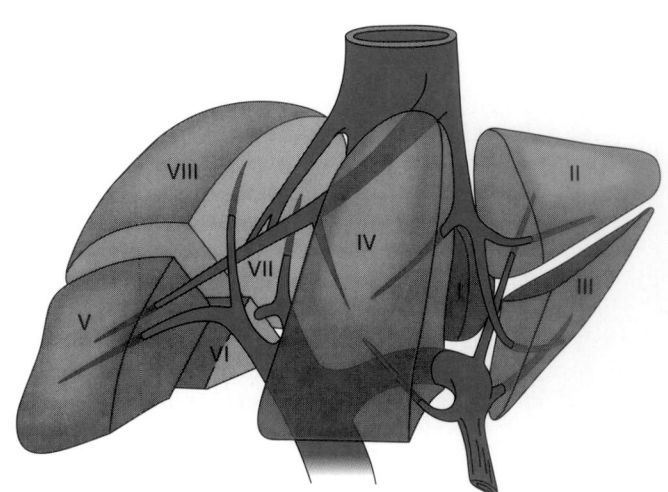

Figure 19–2 Segmental divisions of the liver, with Couinaud's nomenclature. (Reprinted with permission from Parks RW, Chrysos E, Diamond T: Br J Surg 86:1121, 1999.)

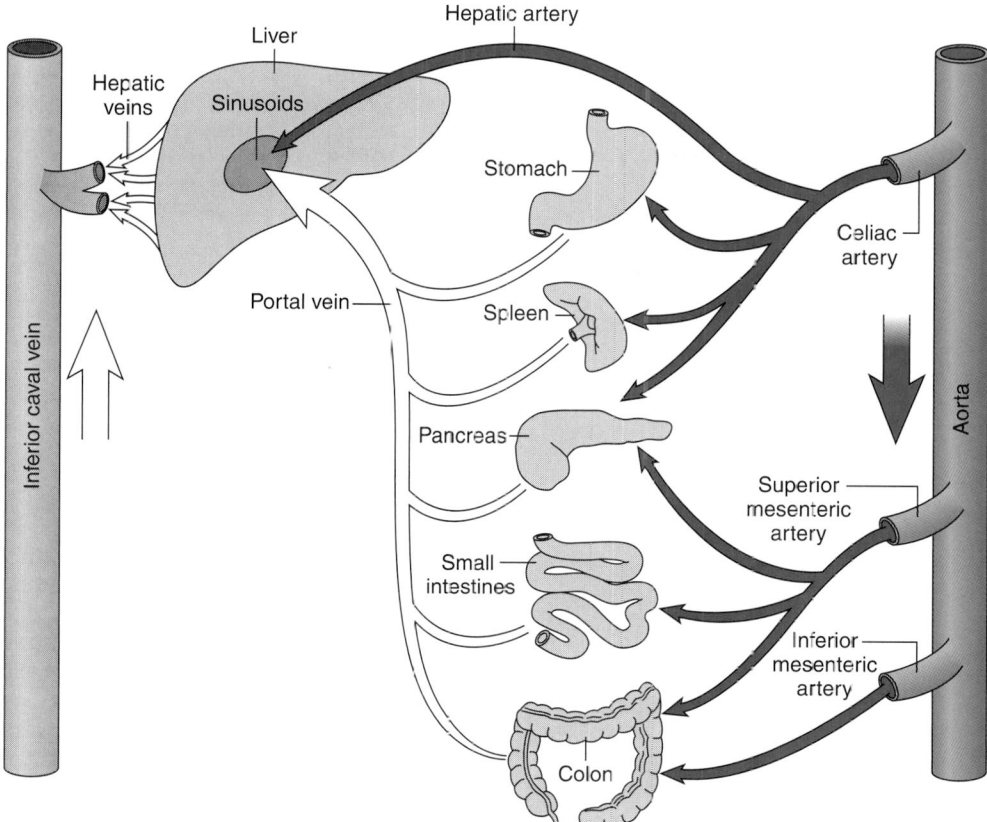

Figure 19–3 The splanchnic circulation. (Redrawn with permission from Gelman S, Mushlin PS: Catecholamine induced changes in the splanchnic circulation affecting systemic hemodynamics. Anesthesiology 100:434-439, 2004.)

Zone 1 hepatocytes have a high proportion of mitochondria and are the major contributors to oxidative metabolism and glycogen synthesis. In contrast, zone 3 hepatocytes have large amounts of smooth endoplasmic reticulum, reduced nicotinamide adenine dinucleotide phosphate (NADPH), and cytochrome P-450 proteins, and are specialized for anaerobic metabolism and biotransforming xenobiotics. Centrilobular hepatocytes are therefore the most likely to be injured by toxic intermediates of xenobiotic metabolism or circulatory disturbances (i.e., ischemia, hypoxia, passive congestion). Thus, ischemic events often induce decreases of drug metabolism.

Intrinsic Regulation of Hepatic Blood Flow

The control of hepatic blood flow involves both intrinsic and extrinsic mechanisms. Intrinsic regulation, which works independently of neurohumoral influences, includes pressure-flow autoregulation, metabolic control, and the hepatic arterial buffer response.

Pressure-Flow Autoregulation
Pressure-flow autoregulation involves myogenic responses of vascular smooth muscle to stretching and acts to keep local blood flow constant, despite changes in systemic arterial pressure. Within limits, an increase in transmural pressure raises myogenic tone, causes vasoconstriction, and prevents hypertension-induced elevations of local blood flow. Conversely, a decrease in transmural pressure lowers myogenic tone, causing vasodilation, which helps preserve organ perfusion during systemic hypotension.

Pressure-flow autoregulation of the hepatic artery is present to a certain extent in metabolically active liver (postprandial) but is usually absent in the fasted state.[14] Because pressure-flow autoregulation does not exist in the portal circulation, decreases in systemic blood pressure beget proportional decreases in portal venous blood flow.[15,16] Thus, pressure-flow autoregulation is unlikely to have an important influence on hepatic blood flow intraoperatively, with the possible exception of emergency procedures performed on patients in the fed state.

Metabolic Control
Constituents of blood can influence hepatic arterial and portal venous blood flow.[17] Decreases in the pH or oxygen tension of the portal blood are often associated with increases in hepatic arterial flow. Postprandial hyperosmolarity increases both the hepatic arterial and the portal venous flow.[17] Changes in metabolic or respiratory status, such as hypercarbia, alkalosis, or arterial hypoxemia, can also influence liver blood flow.

Hepatic Arterial Buffer Response
The hepatic arterial buffer response acts to ensure that changes in portal venous flow induce reciprocal changes in hepatic arterial flow.[18] This reciprocal relation helps

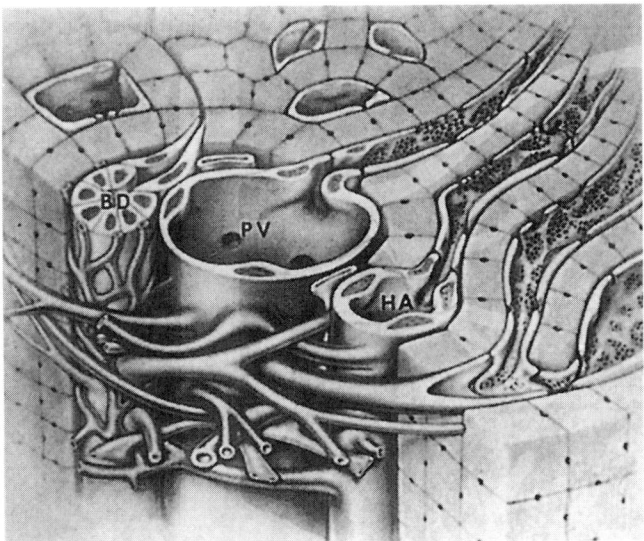

Figure 19–4 Relationship of branches of the portal vein (PV), hepatic artery (HA), and bile duct (BD). Notice the peribiliary capillary plexus that envelops the bile ducts. These three structures constitute a portal triad, which is a transverse section of a portal canal. (Reprinted with permission from Jones AL: Anatomy of the normal liver. *In* Zakim D, Boyer T [eds]: Hepatology: A Textbook of Liver Disease, 3rd ed. Philadelphia, WB Saunders, 1996, p 3.)

balance hepatic needs for oxygen and blood flow. The buffer response works through the synthesis and washout of adenosine (i.e., a vasodilator) from the periportal region.[19] As portal venous flow decreases, adenosine builds up in the periportal region; increases in periportal adenosine cause arteriolar resistance to fall and hepatic

arterial flow to rise. Conversely, an increase in portal venous flow washes out adenosine from the periportal region, which raises arteriolar resistance and lowers hepatic arterial flow. Neural, myogenic, or metabolic influences (e.g., portal venous oxygen content or pH) may alter the buffer response.[20] Although the buffer response can substantially increase hepatic arterial flow, it cannot preserve total hepatic blood flow when portal venous flow falls precipitously. Furthermore, pathophysiologic states, such as endotoxemia and splanchnic hypoperfusion, may decrease or even abolish the buffer response.[21,22]

Extrinsic Regulation of Hepatic Blood Flow

Neural Control

Branches of the splanchnic nerves (postganglionic sympathetic fibers from T6-11), vagus nerve, and phrenic nerve enter the liver with the major blood vessels and bile ducts. These nerve fibers form an intercommunicating plexus, with synapses on the terminal arterioles and venules. Sympathetic innervation of the hepatic and splanchnic vasculature plays a major role in regulating the volume of whole blood stored in, and expelled from, the hepatic reservoir. Studies in a canine model have shown that sympathoadrenal stimulation (e.g., hypercarbia, pain, hypoxia) can abruptly decrease hepatic blood flow and splanchnic vascular capacitance. Within seconds, splanchnic nerve stimulation can autotransfuse up to 80% of the hepatic blood (400-500 mL) into the central circulation.[7,23] Other studies have shown that vagal stimulation alters the tone of presinusoidal sphincters[24] and influences blood flow distribution within the liver rather than total hepatic blood flow.

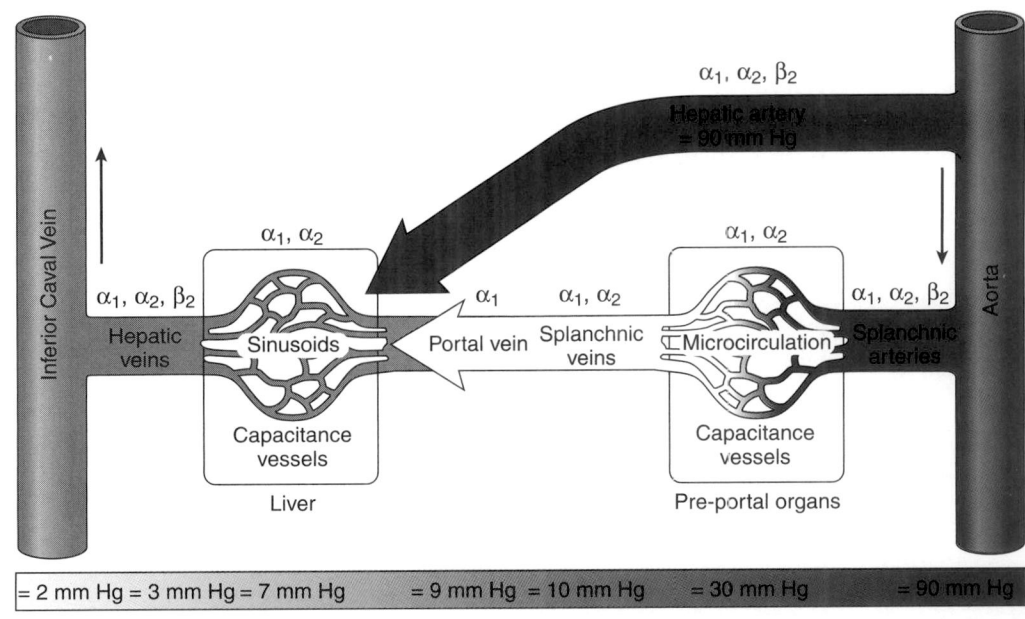

Figure 19–5 Adrenoceptor subtypes (α_1, α_2, β_2) and intravascular pressures throughout the splanchnic circulation. *Splanchnic arteries* represent all arterial vessels of the pre-portal organs; *splanchnic veins* represent the pooled venous blood from all these organs. (Redrawn with permission from Gelman S, Mushlin PS: Catecholamine induced changes in the splanchnic circulation affecting systemic hemodynamics. Anesthesiology 100:434-439, 2004.)

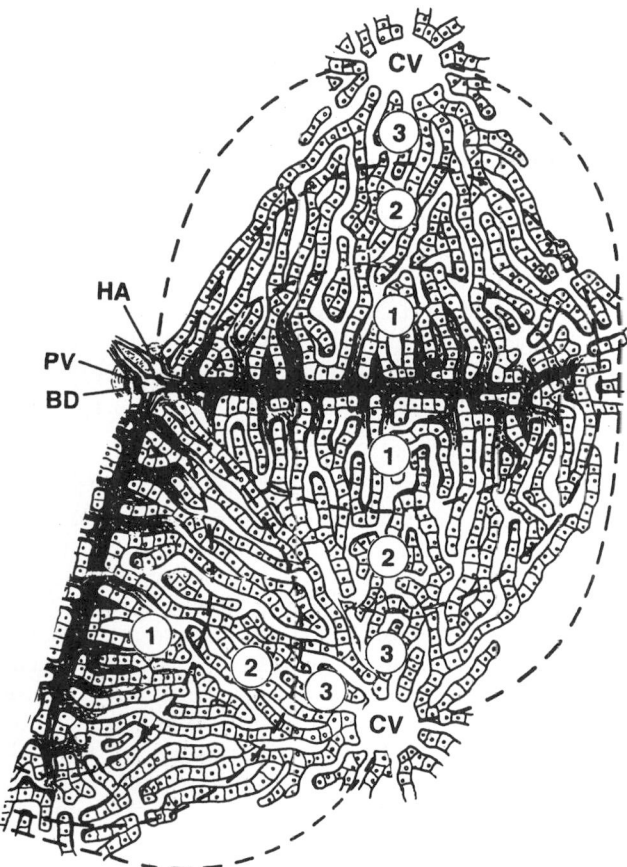

Figure 19–6 Blood supply of the simple liver acinus. The oxygen tension and the nutrient level of the blood in sinusoids decrease from Zone 1 through Zone 3. Note that the lower left side of the figure also depicts Zones 1, 2, and 3 in a portion of an adjacent acinar unit. BD, bile duct; HA, hepatic artery; PV, portal vein; CV, central vein. (Reprinted with permission from Jones AL: Anatomy of the normal liver. *In* Zakim D, Boyer T [eds]: Hepatology: A Textbook of Liver Disease, 3rd ed. Philadelphia, WB Saunders, 1996, p 3.)

Humoral Control

The hepatic arterial bed has α_1-, α_2-, and β_2-adrenergic receptors, whereas the portal vein has only α-receptors (see Fig. 19-5).[25] Of the adrenergic mediators, epinephrine induces the most consequential changes in the hepatic circulation. When injected directly into the hepatic artery, epinephrine initially causes vasoconstriction (α-receptor stimulation), followed by vasodilation (β-receptor stimulation). When injected into the portal vein, however, epinephrine causes only vasoconstriction (α-receptor stimulation). Dopamine is unlikely to influence the hepatic circulation during sympathoadrenal activation; its vasoactive effects are weak and dwarfed by those of epinephrine and norepinephrine.[17,25]

Glucagon induces dose-dependent relaxation of hepatic arterial smooth muscle and antagonizes vasoconstrictor responses of the hepatic artery to various physiologic stimuli-including increases in sympathoadrenal tone.[26] Angiotensin II severely constricts hepatic arterial and portal venous beds, and markedly decreases both mesenteric blood flow and portal venous flow; blood flow to the liver may plummet.[27] In comparison, vasopressin

intensely constricts the splanchnic arterial bed, but it also lowers portal venous resistance. Therefore, vasopressin can be an effective treatment for portal hypertension.[28]

FUNCTIONS OF THE LIVER

Protein Metabolism

The liver is the hub for protein metabolism. It synthesizes and degrades an enormous variety of proteins and peptides and has an essential role in the production and breakdown of amino acids. Hepatocytes convert amino acids to keto acids, glutamine, and ammonia via transamination and oxidative deamination reactions. Removal of ammonia and other nitrogen-containing molecules from the body usually involves the Krebs-Henseleit cycle, which captures nitrogen in the form of urea. Thus, with a failing liver (and normal renal function), the blood urea nitrogen (BUN) concentration typically remains low, whereas nitrogenous wastes (e.g., ammonia) collect in blood and other tissues and may contribute to hepatic encephalopathy.[29]

Hepatically synthesized proteins affect every organ in the body. Included among these proteins are coagulant factors, acute phase reactants, precursors of hormones, and transport proteins. Albumin accounts for about 15% of the protein made by the liver. Healthy adults make between 12 to 15 g of albumin each day, and have an albumin pool containing about 0.50 kg.[30] The daily production ranges from 120 to 300 mg per kg of body weight, and is highest in the neonate.[30-33] The rate of albumin production is influenced by dietary amino acids,[34,35] hormonal balance,[36] and plasma oncotic pressure.[37] Plasma oncotic pressure regulates the intravascular albumin concentration. Albumin also has importance as a plasma transport protein: it binds to many different substances (e.g., drugs, hormones, metals, metabolites, unconjugated bilirubin, free fatty acids), influencing their biologic actions and kinetics of elimination.

Alpha-fetoprotein (AFP) is genetically similar to albumin. In early life, AFP synthesis occurs in the yolk sac, fetal hepatocyte, and cells of the fetal gastrointestinal tract.[38] Important roles of AFP include preserving oncotic pressure and binding free fatty acids. By the time an infant is 1 year of age, serum albumin has replaced most of the AFP. After that, increases of plasma AFP usually signal hepatocellular proliferation. With acute hepatitis, plasma AFP levels rise in nearly all patients (97%).[39] The largest increases occur in patients with hepatic neoplasms. AFP levels that exceed 400 ng/mL and progressively increase suggest hepatocellular carcinoma.[38,39]

Carbohydrate Metabolism

The liver plays an important role in the homeostasis of blood glucose, especially after a carbohydrate meal, diurnal fast, or prolonged exercise.[40-90] Whether the liver consumes or produces glucose depends on (1) the glucose concentration in the sinusoidal blood and (2) hormonal influences—primarily insulin, catecholamines, and glucagon.[13] The rate at which the liver takes up or releases glucose relates directly to the degree of hyperglycemia or hypoglycemia. A reciprocal relation exists between the hepatic synthesis of glucose and glycogen. In the fed state, the liver converts glucose to glycogen. Conversely, carbohydrate deprivation prompts the liver to increase glucose production. This initially involves breaking hepatic glycogen down to glucose and releasing it into the blood. Two rate-limiting enzymes control hepatic glycogen metabolism: (1) glycogen synthase promotes polymer formation from uridine diphosphate (UDP) glucose, and (2) glycogen phosphorylase helps cleave glycogen to glucose-1-phosphate, one residue at a time.

When hepatic glycogen stores have been drained (e.g., as a result of starvation for 24 to 48 hours or prolonged exercise), gluconeogenesis is the sole pathway for producing glucose. Substrates for this pathway include lactate, glycerol (from hydrolysis of triglycerides), and glucogenic amino acids (alanine, glutamine) supplied by muscle.[13,91] Glucagon stimulates gluconeogenesis by activating cyclic adenosine monophosphate (cAMP)–dependent protein kinase; catecholamines stimulate this pathway by cAMP-dependent and -independent mechanisms.[92,93] In contrast, insulin inhibits hepatic gluconeogenesis and antagonizes the effects of both catecholamines and glucagon on this pathway.

Lipid Metabolism

The major sources of fatty acids in the liver include (1) de novo lipogenesis, (2) lipoproteins taken up by the liver, (3) exogenous (plasma) free fatty acids, and (4) the hydrolysis of cytoplasmic triglycerides.[94-105] With its glycogen stores full, the liver will efficiently convert glucose to fatty acids and triglycerides. Dietary fatty acids absorbed from the intestines reach the liver by the lymph and blood, mostly in the form of chylomicrons. The nutritional and hormonal status determines whether the liver oxidizes, stores, or releases free fatty acids.[94,106,107]

The liver uses two major pathways for dispensation of fatty acids: esterification and beta-oxidation. Esterification of fatty acids and glycerol produces triglycerides (fat). The liver either stores this fat or incorporates it into lipoproteins—principally very-low-density lipoproteins (VLDLs) for transport to other tissues. Free fatty acids regulate VLDL production, whereas nutritional and hormonal signals regulate VLDL secretion. Insulin and estrogens, for example, stimulate the hepatic secretion of VLDLs.[94,108] The beta-oxidation pathway in mitochondria sequentially degrades fatty acids to acetyl coenzyme A (CoA). Glucagon markedly stimulates beta-oxidation, whereas insulin inhibits it.

Acetyl-CoA is central to lipid metabolism; it plays key roles in both synthetic (triglycerides, phospholipids, cholesterol, lipoproteins) and catabolic (e.g., tricarboxylic acid cycle) pathways. Mitochondria oxidize acetyl groups to adenosine triphosphate (ATP), carbon dioxide, and water. High rates of fatty acid oxidation produce more acetyl-CoA than the tricarboxylic acid cycle can efficiently metabolize.[13] One result of this is ketogenesis—the formation of ketone bodies; namely acetoacetate, beta-hydroxybutyrate, and acetone. However, the catabolism of ketones requires ketoacyl-CoA transferase (also called acetoacetate:succinyl-CoA transferase), an enzyme present in all tissues except liver.[12] Being unable to extract energy from ketones, the liver releases the ketones into the bloodstream, providing an important energy source for extrahepatic tissues during prolonged starvation. Starvation-induced ketosis is self-limited because ketones promote the release of insulin from the pancreas. Insulin inhibits lipolysis in adipose tissue[109] and cuts off the hepatic supply of fatty acids for ketone synthesis.[91] Without insulin, this feedback loop cannot work, and diabetic ketoacidosis occurs.[13]

Bile Metabolism

The liver synthesizes bile acids and is chiefly responsible for excreting sterols from the body. Roughly 600 to 800 mL of bile is produced each day. Bile contains lipids, electrolytes, organic anions, and most importantly the bile acids (also called bile salts), which account for 85% of biliary solids.[110] The body works to conserve bile acids; the enterohepatic circulation recycles them 20 to 30 times a day, relying on specific transmembrane transporters (on apical and basolateral hepatocellular surfaces) and binding proteins in hepatocytes and enterocytes. Also, a unique sodium-dependent bile acid transporter prevents loss of bile acids in the stool.

Bile acids are natural ionic detergents and play key roles in absorbing, transporting, solubilizing, and secreting lipids.[111,112] They activate lipases (bile acid–dependent) and enable fat micelles to form in the gut; these micelles are needed for the intestinal absorption of cholesterol, fat-soluble vitamins, and other lipids. The liver relies on bile acids for excreting most endogenous (e.g., bilirubin, cholesterol, amphipathic steroid hormonal derivatives) and exogenous (e.g., drugs, xenobiotics) substances. Bile acids regulate the expression of specific genes by binding to, or activating, members of the sterol nuclear receptor family, such as the farnesoid X receptor (FXR). They are the chief regulators of pathways for metabolizing and excreting sterols, including cholesterol. Bile acids also regulate lipoprotein receptors, which control the uptake of lipoprotein cholesterol by hepatocytes[110,113] and directly influence 3-hydroxyl-3-methylglutaryl coenzyme A (HMG-CoA) reductase, the rate-limiting step in cholesterol biosynthesis.

Unlike the kidney, which secretes small, hydrophilic molecules, the liver secretes a wide range of organic anions with higher molecular weights. Because the hydrostatic pressure within bile ducts exceeds that within the sinusoidal space, hydrostatic pressure cannot drive bile formation. Instead, the energy is from an osmotic pressure gradient, caused by the active secretion of solutes across apical hepatocellular membranes and bile duct epithelium. Primary active transporters, powered by the hydrolysis of ATP, create bile by pumping solutes against their concentration gradients into the canalicular space. This canalicular bile is alkalinized and diluted as it courses through the ductular collecting system.[110] Opioids (μ-agonists) may interfere with biliary flow by increasing the pressure in the common bile duct or inducing spasm in the sphincter of Oddi.[114] Many different agents antagonize these effects, including volatile anesthetics, μ-antagonists (e.g., naloxone), smooth muscle relaxants (e.g., nitroglycerin), antimuscarinic agents (e.g., atropine), and glucagon.

Coagulation

Coagulant Factors and Procoagulants

The liver synthesizes all coagulant factors, except for factors III (tissue thromboplastin), IV (Ca), and VIII (von Willebrand factor). It also makes proteins that modulate fibrinolysis and clotting, such as plasminogen activator inhibitor, antithrombin III, protein C, and protein S. Protein C and protein S, for example, work together to inactivate VIIIa and Va complexes. Thus, severe liver disease not only decreases the synthesis of clotting factors but also increases their consumption.[115]

Vitamin K as a Cofactor

Vitamin K–dependent proteins include coagulant factors II, VII, IX, and X, protein C, and protein S. Each of these proteins undergoes γ-carboxylation, which is a unique, post-translational modification involving vitamin K–dependent insertion of carboxyl groups into the γ-position of specific glutamic acid residues at the amino terminus.[91,116] This modification enables the proteins to bind to divalent cations (calcium), which is required for their activation by phospholipids or plasma membranes.[117] In other words, the liver normally releases γ-carboxylated pro-coagulants (vitamin K–dependent zymogens), whose activation in plasma (to serine proteases) enables their involvement in the clotting cascade.[91,118]

The γ-carboxylation pathway is complex, involving a series of reactions that use O_2, CO_2, NADPH, and vitamin K cofactor.[118] There are two major steps. First, γ-carboxylation occurs, a process that uses vitamin K–dependent carboxylase and oxidizes (via microsomal enzymes) vitamin K cofactor (naptho-hydroquinone) to 2,3-epoxide vitamin K. Second, microsomal or cytoplasmic reductases regenerate vitamin K cofactor from the epoxide.[119-122] Warfarin works by blocking the second step; through inhibition of hepatic vitamin K epoxidase, warfarin exhausts the supply of vitamin K cofactor. Although this inhibitory action is rapid, the clinical effect of warfarin takes much longer to develop because it requires a decline in the serum prothrombin complex (of clotting factors), which has a half-life of about 14 hours.

The responses of patients to vitamin K administration can help uncover the cause of a prolonged prothrombin time (PT). When PT is prolonged solely because of warfarin or malnutrition, it should be readily corrected by oral or parenteral vitamin K. When the cause is intestinal malabsorption (e.g., cholestasis), the efficacy of vitamin K therapy is dependent on the route of administration, parenteral being superior to enteral. With severe hepatocellular dysfunction (acute hepatitis, cirrhosis), vitamin K therapy is ineffective because the problem is insufficient synthesis of vitamin K–dependent factors, not a shortage of vitamin K.

Erythropoiesis: Heme and Bilirubin Metabolism

The liver is the primary erythropoietic organ of the fetus between the 9th and 24th week of gestation. It continues to be a major site of hematopoiesis until an infant is about 2 months of age. Recognizable hematopoietic cells normally disappear from the liver as the bone marrow develops. With certain diseases, however, they may persist (e.g., congenital hemolytic anemias) or reappear (e.g., bone marrow failure or myeloproliferative disorders).

In healthy adults, the liver is responsible for about 20% of heme production; bone marrow makes the rest. The two organs use nearly identical pathways to synthesize heme, although the regulatory mechanisms differ slightly.[112,123-126] The focus here is on the hepatocellular pathway. Heme synthesis begins in mitochondria. In the first step, which is rate-limiting in the synthesis of heme, 5-aminolevulinic acid (ALA) synthase condenses glycine and succinyl-CoA, to produce ALA. Heme is the main (feedback) inhibitor of ALA synthase. ALA diffuses from mitochondria into the cytoplasm, where ALA dehydratase links two ALA molecules together to produce porphobilinogen (PBG). The linear arrangement of PBG molecules by PBG deaminase yields hydroxymethylbilane (HMB). HMB is transformed to uroporphyrinogen III, which is converted to coproporphyrinogen III. Mitochondria take up coproporphyrinogen III and convert it to protoporphyrin IX through the actions of coproporphyrinogen oxidase and protoporphyrin oxidase. In the final step of the pathway, ferrochelatase adds ferrous iron to protoporphyrin IX, creating heme. In other words, heme is a complex of ferrous iron and protoporphyrin IX. Subjecting porphyrinogens to oxygen rapidly oxidizes them to matching porphyrins.

Porphyrias

Porphyrias are uncommon disorders of heme synthesis (porphyrin metabolism). Usually, the disorder remains subclinical until an endogenous or exogenous stress triggers a porphyric crisis.[127] Clinical features of acute porphyrias include recurrent, dramatic, and potentially fatal neurologic reactions. Most patients develop abdominal pain (90%) and dark urine (80%). Neurotoxicity may result from increased plasma and tissue levels of porphyrin precursors (particularly ALA and PBG), which have chemical structures resembling the inhibitory neurotransmitter γ-aminobutyric acid (GABA). The most common of the acute porphyrias is acute intermittent porphyria (AIP). Its prevalence is about 1 in 10,000 in the general population and may be as high as 1 in 500 among patients with psychiatric disorders. Women are five times more likely than men to have AIP. Among the triggers of porphyric crises are sex hormones, glucocorticoids, cigarette smoking, and medications,[112,128,129] including certain anesthetic agents (e.g., barbiturates, etomidate, enflurane, pentazocine).[129] Barbiturates and other inducers of cytochrome P-450 (CYP) stimulate the synthesis of cytochrome protein; incorporating heme into newly forming hemoproteins causes the intracellular heme concentration to decline.[129-132] The decrease in heme reduces the inhibitory influence on ALA synthetase, which is rate-limiting, and thus porphyrin (heme) synthesis speeds up.[133,134]

Hemoglobin Metabolism and Bilirubin

The metabolism of hemoglobin produces bilirubin.[112] About 300 mg of bilirubin is formed daily, mostly from the destruction of senescent erythrocytes by macrophages of the reticuloendothelial system. These macrophages (mainly in the spleen, liver, and bone marrow) extract the protein portion of hemoglobin and then catabolize heme in a two-step process. First, heme oxygenase cleaves the porphyrin macrocycle of heme, in a reaction that consumes molecular oxygen and produces carbon monoxide, ferrous iron, and a linear tetrapyrrole (biliverdin). Second, cytoplasmic reductases rapidly convert biliverdin to bilirubin.[135]

The bilirubin is released into the bloodstream and binds tightly to albumin. Hepatic parenchymal cells avidly extract protein-bound bilirubin and conjugate it, using glucuronic acid and bilirubin UDP-glucuronosyltransferase. Hepatocytes secrete bilirubin conjugates into the canalicular bile, which flows into the alimentary tract. Most conjugated bilirubin undergoes intestinal excretion, with little returning to the liver in the enterohepatic circulation. In healthy individuals, only a small fraction of conjugated bilirubin enters the plasma by direct (from hepatic sinusoids) or indirect (absorption from bile ducts or lymphatics) routes.[136]

Endocrine Function

The liver plays a central role in the metabolism of hormones and hormone-binding proteins.[115] It synthesizes (angiotensinogen, thrombopoietin, insulin-like growth factor 1[137]) and inactivates (aldosterone, estrogens, androgens, antidiuretic hormone) a wide variety of hormones. Nearly half the insulin produced by the pancreas never reaches the systemic circulation because it is degraded during a single passage through the liver.[138,139] Thyroxine (T_4), the major secretory product of the thyroid gland, is actively taken up by the liver and converted to triiodothyronine (T_3) or inactivated.

Immune Function and Inflammation

The liver is the largest of the reticuloendothelial organs and has a prominent role in host defense. Kupffer cells account for nearly 10% of the hepatic mass. These cells filter splanchnic venous blood before it reaches the central circulation, phagocytizing and processing antigens and other substances absorbed from the gastrointestinal tract.[140] In sepsis, Kupffer cells are responsible for scavenging bacteria, inactivating bacterial products, and clearing inflammatory mediators.[141] Kupffer cell activation (e.g., by inflammatory stimuli) produces or triggers the release of proinflammatory substances (reduced oxygen species, nitro-radicals, leukotrienes, proteases), including cytokines and chemokines, which recruit neutrophils to the liver and heighten the inflammatory response.[141] Although Kupffer cells are essential for defending the body against foreign intrusions, their activation can also harm the liver when they induce, or exacerbate, hepatocellular injury in diseases involving the liver.[141-145] During oxidative stress, endothelial cells of the hepatic sinusoids or terminal hepatic veins are vulnerable to toxic injury because of their low glutathione content.[146] These cells may be a pathogenic focus of drug-induced vascular injury. Hepatic stellate cells are the principal liver cell type involved in matrix deposition and hepatic fibrosis. Activated stellate cells (as occurs in methotrexate-induced hepatic fibrosis) may be transformable by certain drugs into collagen-synthesizing myofibroblasts.

Metabolism of Drugs (Xenobiotics)

OVERVIEW. Drugs and other xenobiotics typically contain lipophilic moieties, which promote gastrointestinal absorption, penetration of membranes, and retention by the body. The kidney does not readily excrete lipophilic substances for two reasons: (1) lipophilic molecules bind to plasma proteins, and therefore escape glomerular filtration, and (2) if filtered, their lipophilicity increases their reabsorption through the renal tubules. Biotransforming such molecules to hydrophilic metabolites hastens their elimination from the body. The lung, kidney, intestines, skin, and other tissues can all metabolize xenobiotics, but the liver is clearly the chief drug-metabolizing organ. Although biotransformation generally causes pharmacologic deactivation, metabolites are occasionally more active than parent compounds. The metabolism of xenobiotics occasionally produces reactive intermediates that cause liver damage directly or indirectly (by inducing immunopathologic events, as occurs with halothane hepatitis).[147,148]

PATHWAYS OF DRUG METABOLISM. The enzymatic pathways that contribute to the hepatic clearance of drugs can be partitioned into three broad categories or phases. Phase 1 reactions typically work through cytochrome P450 (CYP) and increase the polarity of drugs. Phase 2 reactions are conjugations between the drug or a metabolite and an endogenous hydrophilic substance. Phase 3 reactions involve drug elimination via energy-dependent transporter systems. The hepatic clearance of a drug may occur in one or more of these phases.[147,149-151]

Phase 1 Reactions (Metabolism)

Phase 1 reactions alter the parent drug by inserting or unmasking a polar group (e.g., OH, NH_2, SH). The major classes of reactions are oxidations, reductions, and hydrolysis. Compared with parent drugs, metabolites of phase 1 reactions are more hydrophilic and more readily excreted in the bile or urine. These metabolites may also be substrates for phase 2 conjugations.

Microsomal Oxidases and Cytochrome P-450

Microsomal drug oxidases catalyze more than 90% of drug biotransformation reactions. Most of these reactions involve hemoproteins of the cytochrome P-450 (CYP) gene superfamily. The human liver has more than 20 different CYP enzymes[147,149-152]; many of these isozymes contribute to the oxidation of drugs, environmental toxins, steroid hormones, lipids, and bile acids. Hepatocytes of zone 3 have the highest content of CYP proteins. The locations of specific CYP proteins are often responsible for the patterns of liver damage that are characteristic of certain drugs and toxins.

Acetaminophen (at toxic doses), for example, causes centrilobular necrosis because of its metabolism by CYP2E—an isozyme of CYP localized in pericentral hepatocytes.[147]

In the CYP reaction cycle, oxygen binds to heme iron. Oxygen becomes activated after receiving an electron from a flavoprotein reductase—specifically, NADPH:hemoprotein oxidoreductase (CYP).[149-152] The incorporation of activated oxygen into lipophilic molecules produces substrates for mixed function oxidases. These oxidases take an oxygen atom from O_2 and transfer it to a substrate (e.g., parent drug), and get a second substrate (e.g., NADPH) to supply electrons to reduce the remaining oxygen atom (from O_2) to water. Intermediates of mixed function oxidase reactions include free radicals and various reduced oxygen species (ROS); these are highly reactive molecules that induce oxidative stress and can cause hepatocellular injury.[153]

A multitude of chemicals—including drugs, insecticides, organic solvents, carcinogens, and environmental contaminants—stimulate microsomal drug metabolism.[154] Some compounds, such as phenobarbital and phenytoin, increase the expression of several different CYP proteins,[149-152] whereas others selectively induce a specific CYP. Examples of the latter include smoke from cigarettes or cannabis, which induces CYP1A2,[155] and isoniazid, which is a powerful inducer of CYP2E1. Hypericum, the active ingredient of St. John's wort, and rifampicin are potent inducers of CYP3A4.[156] Alcohol induces both CYP2E1 and CYP3A4.[147,157] Inducers of CYP not only affect their own metabolism, but also influence the metabolism and biologic actions of many other substances. Furthermore, CYP inducers, by activating nuclear orphan receptor transcriptional regulators, can increase the expressions of alkaline phosphatase and γ-glutamyl transpeptidase (GGTP), which are part of the "hepatic adaptation" to chronic drug administration.[147]

Molecular Genetic Basis of CYP Induction

Studies on CYP3A4—the predominant CYP isoform in human liver—provide insight into the molecular genetics of CYP induction.[158] Inducers of CYP3A4 (rifampin, hypericum) interact with and activate the pregnane x-receptor (PXR). PXR is a transcriptional regulator in the orphan nuclear receptor family.[159] When activated, PXR and the analogous constitutive androstane receptor (CAR) bind to cognate nucleotide sequences located upstream to the CYP3A4 structural gene, within a "xenobiotic responsive enhancer module" (XREM).[158,160] The binding of PXR and CAR activates the CYP3A4 promoter (downstream) and induces the synthesis of the mRNA for CYP3A4 protein. Other CYP pathways are similarly regulated, including those involved in bile acid synthesis, where the nuclear receptors include the FXR.[158,160]

Phase 2 Reactions (Metabolism)

Phase 2 reactions create conjugates of parent compounds (or their metabolites) and endogenous, hydrophilic substrates, such as glucuronic acid, acetate, sulfates, amino acids, and glutathione.[147,161] These conjugations often involve glucuronic acid and UDP-glucuronosyltransferase in the endoplasmic reticulum. Other enzymes that catalyze phase 2 reactions include sulfatases, glutathione S-transferases, acetyl N-transferases, and amino acid N-transferases. In comparison with their precursors, conjugated metabolites are typically less efficacious, less toxic, more hydrophilic, and more readily excreted in bile or urine.

Phase 3 Reactions (Elimination)

Phase 3 elimination reactions involve ATP-binding cassette (ABC) transport proteins. These proteins use the energy of ATP hydrolysis to drive molecular transport, and are essential for excreting many endogenous and exogenous substances. Included among the ABC proteins are the cystic fibrosis transmembrane conductance regulator (CFTR), canalicular and intestinal copper transporters, multidrug resistance protein (MDR), and multidrug resistance related protein (MRP). MDRs (or MDR-1, formerly termed p-glycoprotein), which are on apical (canalicular) hepatocellular surfaces, play an important role in the transport of cationic compounds (e.g., many anticancer drugs) into the bile.[162,163]

Another family of ABC proteins (MRP) excretes conjugated molecules. MRP-1, which is on the lateral hepatocellular surfaces, transports drug conjugates into the sinusoids. MRP-2 (formerly termed canalicular multispecific organic anion transporter [cMOAT]), on canalicular membranes, pumps drug conjugates and endogenous substances (bilirubin diglucuronide, leukotriene-glutathionyl conjugates) into bile. Dysfunction of ABC transport proteins hinders the flow of bile, predisposing to drug accumulation in the body, and cholestatic liver injury.[164,165]

Determinants of Drug Metabolism

Genetic and environmental influences (including drugs) are the most important of the variables affecting drug metabolism. The genetic makeup controls the expression of CYP enzymes and is chiefly responsible for the more than fourfold differences in rates of drug metabolism among healthy subjects. Many different drugs and chemicals can either stimulate or inhibit drug biotransformation.[147,149-151] Nutritional status and disease states influence CYP proteins.[166] Both obesity and fasting increase CYP2E1,[147,149-151] whereas CYP may be inhibited by infusions of nitrogen-free[167] or nitrogen-rich solutions,[168] systemic inflammatory disorders,[169] or fever.[170] Diseases that affect specific CYP isozymes include diabetes mellitus (increases CYP2E1), hypothyroidism (decreases CYP1A), and hypopituitarism (decreases CYP3A4).[149-151] Advanced cirrhosis lowers both total CYP and hepatic perfusion and results in significantly reduced clearances of many substances.[149-151]

In hepatic drug metabolism, sex and age are relatively unimportant variables. Women express CYP3A4 and CYP2E1 to a greater extent than men, but drug metabolism by these CYP proteins (erythromycin, chlordiazepoxide, midazolam) is just slightly greater in women than men.[147] It is only at the extremes of the life cycle that age has an impact on biotransformation reactions. In newborns, the hepatic content of certain CYP proteins is only 25% of the adult level; therefore clearances of drugs with a low extraction ratio may be much lower than in adults.

Phase 2 reactions proceed slowly; the delayed development of bilirubin-UDP-glucuronosyltransferase predisposes to neonatal hyperbilirubinemia, which occurs often. In the geriatric population, CYP protein contents may decrease by up to 10%,[171] which causes only minor decreases in intrinsic hepatic clearance. When the elimination half-life of a drug increases because of aging, it is more often a result of an increased volume of distribution than a decreased intrinsic hepatic clearance. Pharmacodynamic changes with advancing age can also be important clinically (e.g., with benzodiazepines). However, the age-related physiologic change with the greatest impact pharmacologically is the progressive decline in the excretory capacity of the kidney.[172-174] In geriatric medicine, it is important to downwardly adjust dosages of drugs whose clearance depends mainly on renal elimination.

Anesthetic agents and techniques that decrease hepatic blood flow should be expected to reduce clearances of substances with a high extraction ratio (perfusion-dependent clearance). During halothane anesthesia, decreases in liver blood flow account for the reduced clearances of agents such as fentanyl, verapamil, and propranolol.[175] However, some anesthetics may also affect hepatic clearance by altering CYP and glucuronosyltransferase activity.[176] Ketamine induces its own metabolism, which may contribute to the tolerance that develops to this agent.[177] Diazepam can increase or decrease its own metabolism.[178] Halothane-induced decreases of metabolism may be responsible for reduced clearances of certain drugs, such as phenytoin,[179] warfarin,[180] and ketamine.[181] Both halothane and enflurane cause concentration-dependent decreases in the metabolism of acetaminophen, antipyrine, and sulfanilamide in isolated rat hepatocytes. Halothane inhibits enflurane metabolism, possibly by competing for drug-metabolizing sites on CYP.[182] In contrast to effects of brief treatments, persistent exposure to halothane can induce CYP (e.g., cytochrome c reductase) and stimulate drug metabolism[183]; this may explain the 29% increase in antipyrine metabolism in people exposed to trace amounts of halothane for prolonged periods.[184]

Pharmacokinetics

Perfusion models of drug elimination incorporate the major determinants of hepatic drug disposition, namely hepatic blood flow, intrinsic hepatic clearance, and protein binding. The extraction ratio (ER) is a measure of the relative efficiency with which the liver extracts or eliminates a given drug (ER = intrinsic hepatic clearance of the drug / hepatic blood flow).[185-189] Table 19-1 presents a compilation of drugs with high and low extraction ratios. Generally speaking, the liver efficiently extracts calcium channel blockers, β-adrenoceptor antagonists (except atenolol), opioid analgesics, tricyclic antidepressants, and organic nitrates. Poorly extracted compounds include warfarin, aspirin, alcohol, and many anticonvulsants. Changes in intrinsic hepatic clearance or protein binding affect the elimination of drugs with a low ER (i.e., capacity-limited elimination), whereas changes in hepatic blood flow are inconsequential. Conversely, only changes in hepatic blood flow affect the elimination of drugs with

a high intrinsic hepatic clearance (i.e., flow-dependent elimination); changes in protein binding or drug metabolizing enzymes do not (Table 19-2).

Using pharmacokinetic data as the primary basis for clinical decision-making has important limits. For example, laboratory data show that changes in protein binding do not affect the hepatic elimination of highly extracted drugs. Such changes, however, can alter pharmacologic activity by changing the free fraction (active form), volume of distribution, and elimination of drugs. Furthermore, various diseases alter the pharmacokinetics and pharmacodynamics of many drugs. The pathophysiologic changes of advanced liver disease (e.g., hepatic encephalopathy) or renal failure (e.g., uremic encephalopathy) markedly alter the relation between plasma concentrations and pharmacologic responses to certain drugs. In such settings, ensuring efficacy and minimizing toxicity involves adjusting standard drug dosages, based on an analysis of all relevant pharmacologic information.

Table 19–1   Drugs that are efficiently and poorly extracted from blood flowing through the liver

Efficiently Extracted Drugs	Poorly Extracted Drugs
Amitriptyline	Acetaminophen
Desipramine	Amobarbital
Imipramine	Antipyrine
Labetalol	Aspirin
Lidocaine	Clindamycin
Meperidine	Diazepam
Metoprolol	Digitoxin
Morphine	Ethanol
Nortriptyline	Hexobarbital
Pentazocine	Phenobarbital
Propoxyphene	Phenytoin
Propranolol	Tolbutamide
Ranitidine	Valproic acid
Verapamil	Warfarin
Zidovudine	

EVALUATION OF THE LIVER

Clinical Assessment

Detecting liver disease often requires special attention to detail. The only manifestations may be mild, nonspecific symptoms, such as loss of appetite, easy fatigability, malaise, altered sleep patterns, or subtle changes in personality. Even long-standing, severe hepatic disorders may elude detection until peripheral edema, overt ascites, or encephalopathy develops. The history should probe for causes of liver disease, including alcoholism, illicit drug use, sexual promiscuity, exposure to harmful chemicals or toxins, and blood transfusions. It should also seek to identify clinical features of hepatobiliary disease, including pruritus, abdominal pain, indigestion, changes in color of the stool or urine, and prior bouts of jaundice (particularly after anesthesia). Occasionally, it is

Table 19–2 Flow-dependent versus capacity-limited elimination of drugs by the liver

Type of Hepatic Elimination	Extraction Ratio (ER)	Rate of Hepatic Drug Metabolism
Flow-dependent elimination	*High ER*: At clinically relevant concentrations, most of the drug in the afferent hepatic blood is eliminated on first pass through the liver.	*Rapid*: Because drugs with a high ER are metabolized so rapidly, their hepatic clearances roughly equal their rates of transport to the liver (i.e., hepatic blood flow).
Capacity-limited elimination (also referred to as dose-dependent, nonlinear, saturable, or zero-order elimination)	*Low ER*: The hepatic elimination of these drugs is determined by their plasma concentration.	*Slow*: When the capacity of the liver to eliminate a drug is less than the dosing rate, a steady state is unachievable; plasma levels of drug will continue to rise unless the dosing rate is decreased. Drug clearance has no real meaning in such settings.

useful to inquire about heritable diseases such as hemochromatosis, α_1-antitrypsin deficiency, and Wilson's disease. The physical examination should focus on stigmata of advanced liver disease, including icterus, jaundice, ascites, collateral portal circulation, spider angiomata, palmar erythema, xanthelasma, encephalopathy, and fetor hepaticus.

Biochemical Tests

A wide variety of biochemical tests are available for the detection and differential diagnosis of hepatobiliary disorders (Table 19-3).[30,190] Most of these tests lack utility for diagnosing a specific liver disease. Instead, they help identify and classify pathologic changes that involve the liver and biliary tree, particularly hepatocellular injury, hepatocellular synthetic dysfunction, and cholestasis.

Hepatocellular Injury
Aminotransferases
Hepatocellular injury leads to increased serum levels of aspartate aminotransferase (AST; formerly serum glutamic oxaloacetic transaminase [SGOT]) and alanine aminotransferase (ALT; formerly serum glutamic pyruvic transaminase [SGPT]). These enzymes take part in gluconeogenesis, in which an amine group is transferred to α-ketoglutarate via AST or ALT, yielding glutamate plus either oxaloacetate or pyruvate. AST isozymes are present in both cytoplasm and mitochondria, but ALT is only a cytoplasmic enzyme. ALT is relatively specific to the liver, whereas considerable amounts of AST are present in extrahepatic tissues, including the heart, skeletal muscle, brain, kidney, pancreas, adipose, and blood. Rarely, muscle diseases may be the source of elevated levels of both AST and ALT.[190]

Table 19–3 Liver blood tests and the differential diagnosis of hepatobiliary disorders

	Predominant Abnormality		
Blood Test	*Bilirubin Overload (Hemolysis)*	*Hepatocellular Injury*	*Cholestasis*
Aminotransferases	Normal	Increased—may be normal or decreased in advanced stages	Normal—may be increased in advanced stages
Serum albumin	Normal	Decreased—may be normal with acute fulminant hepatic failure	Normal—may be decreased in advanced stages
Prothrombin time (PT)*	Normal	Prolonged	Normal—may be prolonged in advanced stages
Bilirubin (main form present)	Unconjugated (also mild increase of conjugates)	Conjugated	Conjugated
Alkaline phosphatase	Normal	Normal—may be increased by hepatic infiltrative disease	Increased
γ-Glutamyl transpeptidase 5'-nucleotidase	Normal	Normal	Increased
Blood urea nitrogen	Normal—may be increased by renal dysfunction	Normal—may be decreased by severe liver disease and normal kidney	Normal
BSP/ICG (dye)	Normal	Retention of dye	Normal—or retention of dye

*Used interchangeably with INR (International Normalized Ratio).
BSP/ICG, bromsulphalein/indocyanine green.

Mild increases in aminotransferases (<250 IU/L) can result from almost any pathologic process that causes hepatocellular injury. Examples include hepatic steatosis, alcohol- or drug-induced liver disease, chronic viral hepatitis, cirrhosis, hemochromatosis, previous jejunoileal bypass, cholestasis, and neoplasms. Moderately raised levels of aminotransferases (250-1000 IU/L) result from disorders that produce hepatocellular necrosis. Common causes include acute viral hepatitis, drug-induced hepatitis, and exacerbations of chronic hepatitis (e.g., alcoholic hepatitis). Large elevations of AST and ALT (above 1000 IU/L) often reflect viral or drug-induced liver damage superimposed on alcoholic liver disease, or autoimmune hepatitis. Extreme elevations (over 2000 IU/L) suggest massive hepatic necrosis, usually from drugs (acetaminophen, halothane hepatitis), toxins, ischemic hepatitis ("shock liver"), or acute viral hepatitis and rarely from acute biliary obstruction or autoimmune hepatitis.[190]

The AST/ALT ratio may be of value in the differential diagnosis of hepatic disorders. When the ratio is increased and ALT is normal, the increase in AST is likely to be from an extrahepatic source. When AST and ALT both increase, a ratio above 4 suggests Wilsonian hepatitis; a ratio between 2 and 4 suggests alcoholic liver disease; and a ratio below 1 suggests nonalcoholic steatosis or hepatitis (without cirrhosis). When AST and ALT are below 300 IU/L and the ratio exceeds 2, the likely diagnosis is alcoholic liver disease or cirrhosis of any etiology.[190]

Although ALT and AST are helpful for identifying hepatocellular injury, these tests provide no information about hepatic dysfunction or the extent of liver damage. For example, a severely jaundiced patient with a markedly prolonged PT can have normal aminotransferase levels, reflecting liver damage so massive that few hepatocytes remain to release enzymes into the blood. Furthermore, chronic, indolent diseases such as hepatitis C can destroy much of the liver without significantly increasing ALT or AST. Thus, interpretations of aminotransferase levels should incorporate clinical findings and results of other tests, such as blood urea nitrogen, creatinine, ammonia, and bilirubin. Liver-specific enzymes, including ornithine carbamoyl transferase and alcohol dehydrogenase, have been used experimentally but are not widely available for clinical application.[30,190]

Lactate Dehydrogenase
Increased serum levels of lactate dehydrogenase (LDH) may reflect acute or chronic liver injury. A massive but transient elevation of LDH suggests ischemic hepatitis (shock liver) or severe hemolysis associated with acute liver damage. A sustained increase in LDH and alkaline phosphatase is consistent with malignant infiltration of the liver. However, large increases in LDH can also occur in various disorders in the absence of liver disease. Included among these disorders are hemolysis, renal infarction, acute stroke, myocardial damage, and skeletal muscle injury. Thus, LDH rarely yields information beyond that provided by aminotransferases and is not a useful diagnostic test for liver disease.[30,190]

Glutathione S-Transferase
Glutathione S-transferase (GST) is a relatively sensitive and specific test for detecting drug-induced hepatocellular damage.[191] This enzyme has a brief plasma half-life (90 minutes) and is rapidly released into the circulation following hepatocellular injury. Measurements of plasma GST may therefore reveal the time course of hepatocellular injury, from onset to resolution. Unlike AST and ALT, which reside in the periportal region (zone 1), GST is localized in the centrilobular region (zone 3),[192] where the hepatocytes are most susceptible to injuries from hypoxia and reactive drug metabolites. For detecting such injuries (e.g., centrilobular necrosis), GST may be a more sensitive test than either AST or ALT.

Hepatic Synthetic Capacity
Serum Albumin
Serum albumin can provide useful information about hepatocellular function in certain clinical settings. Because plasma albumin has a half-life of nearly 3 weeks, the hepatic synthesis of albumin can have ceased for days before hypoalbuminemia results. Thus, serum albumin is an insensitive test for rapidly developing liver dysfunction. On the other hand, it can be helpful for gauging the severity and course of chronic liver diseases in which changes in serum albumin mainly reflect decreases in albumin synthesis. Patients with cirrhosis and ascites characteristically have a low plasma albumin concentration, although the total mass of albumin in the exchangeable pool is often normal. It is important to be aware that hypoalbuminemia has many causes, including expansion of the plasma volume, maldistribution of albumin, increased degradation of albumin, and loss of this protein from the kidney (e.g., nephrotic syndrome).[193]

Prothrombin Time
In contrast to serum albumin, liver-derived coagulation factors have short half-lives (ranging from 4 hours for factor VII to 4 days for fibrinogen), so their concentrations begin to decline shortly after the liver begins to fail. Thus, the PT, or international normalized ratio (INR), can be useful for detecting rapidly declining liver function. Although a prolonged INR may result from decreases of many of the hepatic coagulants, it usually reflects a lack of factor VIIa, which is the most rapidly cleared coagulation factor.[190] The INR provides useful prognostic information for hepatotoxin-induced liver failure[194] and for surgical interventions in the presence of severe liver disease.[195]

Cholestatic Disorders
Alkaline Phosphatase
Serum alkaline phosphatase (AP) is a useful screening test for diseases of the liver or biliary tree, including acute hepatitis, malignancies, and cholestatic disorders. AP makes up a group of at least 11 isoenzymes that occur in plasma membranes throughout the body.[190] Sources of serum AP include liver, bone, placenta, intestine, kidney, leukocytes, and various neoplasms. Increases of metabolism in these tissues may cause elevations in serum AP. Fatty meals can also raise the serum AP level by releasing

isozymes of AP from the small bowel. On routine laboratory testing, up to one third of individuals will have mild, transient increases of AP. Thus, serum AP lacks specificity as a test for liver or biliary disease.

Increases in serum AP usually reflect increases in AP production (and release), rather than decreased AP clearance. In cholestatic disorders, bile acids may act to solubilize membranes and promote the release of AP. On the other hand, AP may be normal for a day or two after biliary obstruction develops, until more AP synthesis (and release) occurs. Because of its half-life of nearly a week, serum AP may remain elevated for days after bile flow is restored.[190] Extreme increases in AP suggest a major block in biliary flow (primary biliary cirrhosis, choledocholithiasis) or a hepatic malignancy (primary or metastatic tumors) that is compressing small intrahepatic bile ducts. Occasionally, multifocal obstructions of intrahepatic ducts increase serum AP without increasing serum bilirubin. Conversely, AP may remain normal despite extensive hepatic metastasis or large duct obstruction. Thus, serum AP does not reliably distinguish between intrahepatic and extrahepatic duct obstruction or hepatic infiltration.[190]

5'-Nucleotidase and Gamma-Glutamyl-Transpeptidase

An increased AP level should prompt consideration of AP sources besides the hepatobiliary tree. These sources include (1) placenta, usually during the third trimester of pregnancy; (2) normal bone, when growing rapidly around puberty; (3) diseased bone in Paget's disease, rickets, or osteomalacia; and (4) intestines (see Table 19-3). Specific biochemical tests such as 5'-nucleotidase (5'-NT) or leucine aminopeptidase (LAP) and gamma-glutamyl-transpeptidase (GGTP) are helpful for discovering whether increases in AP are the result of a hepatobiliary disorder.

For several reasons, 5'-NT can be a useful test for distinguishing between hepatic and extrahepatic sources of AP. First, the test is sensitive (similar to AP) and specific for detecting hepatobiliary disorders. Although 5'-NT is present in many extrahepatic tissues (placenta, bone, brain, intestine, heart, blood vessels, endocrine pancreas), most of the 5'-NT in plasma is from the biliary system. Releasing 5'-NT from hepatocellular plasma membranes may require the detergent action of bile acids. Second, normal pregnancy, bone growth, and bone diseases do not affect 5'-NT. Third, in patients with hepatobiliary disease, changes in AP are usually followed by similar changes in 5'-NT.[190]

During the onset and resolution of biliary disease, the time courses of AP and 5'-NT often differ. For example, with acute interruption of biliary flow, 5'-NT may remain unaltered for days, whereas AP and GGTP progressively increase.[190] Nonetheless, using GGTP to evaluate an increased AP has certain limits. Because GGTP is an inducible microsomal enzyme (e.g., by alcohol, anticonvulsants, warfarin), plasma GGTP levels may vary unpredictably. GGTP is also less specific than 5'-NT as a marker for hepatobiliary disease. Unlike 5'-NT, GGTP may be released from many sites (kidney, spleen, pancreas, heart, lung, brain) besides the hepatobiliary tree. However, bone, which is an important source of AP, has little GGTP.

Thus, GGTP is useful for distinguishing between hepatic and osseous sources of AP.[190]

Serum Bilirubin

Serum bilirubin is the most useful test for assessing the excretory function of the liver. In the absence of hepatobiliary disease, total bilirubin is usually below 1 mg/dL. Benign, unconjugated hyperbilirubinemia is present in up to 10% of healthy adults. Most of these individuals have Gilbert's syndrome, which probably represents activities of bilirubin UDP-glucuronosyltransferase within the lowermost tail of the normal distribution curve. A serum bilirubin level above 4 mg/dL produces jaundice (yellowish discoloration of body tissues). When natural light is used, scleral icterus is detectable at bilirubin levels below 3 mg/dL.[190,196]

Conjugated hyperbilirubinemia mainly results from obstructed biliary flow or inadequate transport of bilirubin conjugates into the bile. The bilirubin load from massive hemolysis typically causes unconjugated hyperbilirubinemia. However, plasma levels of conjugated bilirubin rise when hepatocytes produce more bilirubin conjugates than the hepatocellular transporters can excrete into the bile. The presence of bilirubin in the urine usually reflects conjugated hyperbilirubinemia. The kidneys can readily excrete bilirubin conjugates, whereas the unconjugated form, which binds tightly to plasma albumin, is neither filtered nor excreted by normal kidneys.[190,196]

Markers of Specific Diseases: Special Tests

Specific tests are essential for diagnosing and managing certain hepatic or biliary diseases. Examples include (1) serologic profiles that detect viral, microbial, and autoimmune diseases; (2) chemistry panels and genetic tests that identify metabolic disorders; and (3) tumor markers that detect hepatocellular carcinoma. The characteristic time-related changes in viral antigens and antibodies in serum usually provide the key to the diagnosis of hepatotropic viral infections (HAV, HBV, and HCV).[38] Serologic tests can also help identify other pathogenic agents (cytomegalovirus, Epstein-Barr virus, spirochetes, parasites) and various inflammatory diseases affecting the liver and biliary tree.[197-199]

An increased serum γ-globulin level is a marker for chronic severe hepatic disease. HBV and HCV infections are often associated with immunologic abnormalities—particularly increases in anti-smooth muscle antibodies, antinuclear antibodies, and mixed cryoglobulins.[38,200] Anti-asialoglycoprotein receptor antibodies occur with HAV infections and autoimmune hepatitis. Distinct serological features also help to characterize autoimmune cholangitides.[201] For example, nearly all patients with primary biliary cirrhosis have antimitochondrial antibodies.[199,202-208] These antibodies are typically absent in patients with primary sclerosing cholangitis, but other autoantibodies often appear, including anti-smooth muscle and antinuclear antibodies.[199,209-211]

Special tests are needed for diagnosing inborn errors of metabolism. With α_1-antitrypsin (α_1-AT) deficiency, which is the most common metabolic disease affecting the liver, important diagnostic tests include phenotype analysis and measurements of the serum α_1-AT level. Typical findings in Wilson's disease (an autosomal recessive disorder of copper overload) include a low serum ceruloplasmin and a high urinary copper level, especially after penicillamine administration.

Serum tumor markers are useful for detecting hepatic malignancies. As a test for hepatocellular carcinoma, alpha-fetoprotein (AFP) is 90% specific and between 50% and 90% sensitive, depending on population subgroups.[115] Hepatocellular carcinoma produces coagulant factors without adequately γ-carboxylating them.[212,213] Up to 91% of patients with hepatocellular carcinoma have increased levels of non–γ-carboxylated, vitamin K–dependent factors. More than two thirds of these patients have levels above 300 ng/mL, far exceeding values found in cirrhosis or acute hepatitis. After resection of hepatocellular tumors, serum levels of des-γ-carboxylated factors decrease, and the levels increase with tumor recurrence.[214] Thus, des-γ-carboxylated prothrombin and AFP are useful serum markers for hepatocellular carcinoma.[115,212,215,216]

Quantitative Tests

Many complex techniques are available for quantitatively assessing specific hepatocellular functions. For example, measuring the clearance of substances that the liver avidly extracts—such as bromsulphalein, indocyanine green (ICG), and rose bengal—may provide information about the mass of working hepatocytes.[217] However, the body may retain such substances without losing any hepatocytes. Retention may reflect decreases in hepatic blood flow or abnormalities in hepatocellular uptake, intracellular binding, metabolic transformation, or hepatobiliary excretion of these substances. Various tests provide a measure of hepatic drug metabolizing capacity. Included among these tests are galactose elimination capacity, aminopyrine breath test (ABT), antipyrine clearance, monoethylglycinexylidide (MEGX), and caffeine clearance.[190,218-223] MEGX, a lidocaine metabolite, is measured in a blood sample taken 15 minutes after an intravenous injection of lidocaine (1 mg/kg).

Noninvasive methods can be used to determine caffeine clearance. This involves sequential measurements of caffeine metabolites in saliva for up to 24 hours after an oral dose of caffeine (150-300 mg). Such quantitative tests have been mainly limited to research centers. Generally, they are more expensive, invasive, or time-consuming than conventional biochemical tests, without compelling evidence of being superior, either diagnostically or prognostically. Thus, the role of quantitative tests in managing patients with liver disease remains to be determined.

Measurement of Liver Blood Flow

Methods for measuring hepatic blood flow fit into three broad categories: clearance techniques, indicator dilution techniques, and direct measurements.

Clearance Techniques
Hepatic clearance depends on both hepatic blood flow and the liver's intrinsic ability to eliminate the molecule.

Certain substances are selectively and extensively extracted from the circulation by the liver; their total clearances are nearly equal to the hepatic blood flow. When using such molecules, the indirect Fick principle can be used to compute hepatic blood flow. Substances with a very high intrinsic clearance include propranolol, lidocaine, ICG, and colloidal particles. ICG, for example, is taken up almost exclusively by hepatocytes and excreted unchanged in the bile. Despite the limited stability of this dye, a constant infusion of ICG may be the most reliable extraction method for determining liver blood flow. Kupffer cells avidly phagocytose radiolabeled colloidal particles such as gold-198. The area under the initial curve of radioactivity versus time provides a useful measure of hepatic blood flow when the reticuloendothelial system is functioning normally.[224]

Clearance techniques, however, do not reliably reflect hepatic blood flow in the presence of liver disease. With severe liver diseases, decreased clearances may reflect a combination of factors, including the loss of hepatocyte mass, a reduction in the capacity of hepatocytes to eliminate substances, and a decrease in hepatic blood flow.[225]

Indicator Dilution Techniques
Unlike with clearance techniques, liver blood flow measurements by indicator dilution methods are unaffected by hepatic function. A radiolabeled marker (e.g., iodinated albumin) is injected into the spleen, and hepatic flow is determined from indicator dilution curves; these curves are obtained by sampling continuously from one of the hepatic veins or by external γ-scintillation counting. For this technique to be valid, the indicator must be resistant to clearance by the liver and uniformly mixed upon injection.[226]

Direct Measurements
Electromagnetic flow probes provide direct measurements of blood flow through the hepatic artery or portal vein.[227] Procedures for implanting the probes can themselves alter hepatic blood flow. If the probes are left in place after the implantation procedure, flow can be measured telemetrically, either in the absence or presence of anesthesia.

Radiologic and Endoscopic Techniques

Interventional techniques for evaluating the hepatobiliary system include percutaneous transhepatic cholangiography and endoscopic retrograde cholangiopancreatography. The former is useful when bile ducts are dilated, whereas the latter can help with preoperative localization of biliary tract disease. Improved imaging techniques such as nuclear magnetic resonance may obviate endoscopic examination of biliary ducts. Nevertheless, endoscopy remains a useful mode for delivering therapy. For example, papillotomy via endoscopy can eliminate the need for operative removal of common bile duct stones.[228] Esophagogastroscopy is a reliable and simple method for detecting and treating submucosal varices in the upper digestive tract. If portal hypertension is present, measurement of hepatic venous pressure may localize anatomic sites of increased resistance to blood flow.

Splenoportography may be useful for delineating abnormalities in the splenic and portal veins. Using three-dimensional computed tomography (with multi-detector row) helps create vascular maps whose quality equals or exceeds those from classic angiography.[229] This technique is useful for performing portal venography in patients with cirrhosis. The images can show the extent and location of portosystemic collateral communications (left gastric, short gastric, paraumbilical, and abdominal wall veins; esophageal varices; splenorenal and gastrorenal shunts). Radionuclide and ultrasonic scanning are useful for detecting space-occupying lesions of the hepatobiliary tree.[228,230]

HEPATIC PATHOPHYSIOLOGY

Mechanisms of Cell Death

Death of hepatic parenchymal cells occurs in almost all forms of liver disease, but the mechanisms are often poorly understood. Hepatocellular degeneration and mechanisms of cell death are discussed in detail in the literature.[143,211,231,232]

Necrosis

Hypoxia or anoxia is the most common cause of cellular death in humans. This is usually the result of a circulatory derangement that critically compromises oxygen delivery to tissues. The immediate effect is a decrease in intracellular ATP, which stimulates glycogenolysis and glycolysis, causes lactate to accumulate, and reduces intracellular pH. Precipitous decreases of high-energy phosphates induce subcellular events that lead inexorably to hepatocellular necrosis. The energy-dependent ion pumps that preserve intracellular fluid and electrolyte balance fail abruptly. The plasma membrane loses integrity; hepatocytes swell rapidly and rupture. Necrosis releases various substances into the surrounding tissues, including hepatocellular enzymes and macromolecular breakdown products such as lipid peroxides, aldehydes, and eicosanoids. Some of these molecules are chemoattractants for circulating neutrophils, recruiting them to engage in the hepatic inflammatory response.

Apoptosis

Unlike necrosis, apoptosis requires energy. This is a genetically programmed form of cell death that advances in an orderly sequence. Hepatic injuries from various causes (toxic, viral, immune) can trigger apoptosis by activating pro-apoptotic intracellular signaling pathways or pro-apoptotic cell surface receptors. These receptors include Fas, tumor necrosis factor receptor (TNFR), and other members of the TNFR superfamily.[233-237]

Apoptosis produces the following characteristic ultrastructural features: (1) a shrunken cell and nucleus; (2) condensed, marginated nuclear chromatin; (3) blebs on plasma membrane; and (4) cellular fragmentation into membrane-bound bodies that contain intact organelles. Epithelial and mesenchymal cells engulf these apoptotic bodies, and lysosomes help to digest and recycle them. Thus, apoptosis conserves cellular fragments (intact mitochondria, nucleic acids) and minimizes the release of bioactive substances. In its purest form, apoptosis does not incite an inflammatory tissue reaction. The seeming dichotomy between apoptosis and necrosis probably represents the ends of a spectrum of overlapping morphologic and mechanistic cell death processes.[143,233]

Oxidative Stress and the Glutathione System

Mitochondrial respiration and microsomal redox reactions continuously produce reactive oxygen species within hepatocytes. Molecular oxygen[02] usually undergoes tetravalent reduction to water (during aerobic metabolism). Small quantities of oxygen, however, undergo univalent and divalent reactions, to yield superoxide and hydrogen peroxide.[238] Besides hepatic parenchyma, other types of cells within the liver produce reactive radicals. For example, Kupffer cells, endothelial cells, polymorphonuclear leukocytes, and macrophages, when activated, produce significant quantities of reduced oxygen species and nitro-radicals.[144,239-241]

The liver has various defense mechanisms for preserving intracellular oxidants within a safe range, below the micromolar level.[147,242] These defenses involve (1) thiol-rich peptides, such as glutathione (γ-glutamyl-cysteine-glycine); (2) micronutrients, such as vitamin E and vitamin C; (3) metal-sequestering proteins, such as ferritin; (4) enzymes for detoxifying reactive oxygen species, such as catalase and superoxide dismutase; and (5) enzymes that detoxify lipid peroxides, such as glutathione peroxidase. Of the antioxidant defenses, the single most important one is glutathione.[233,243-247]

Glutathione is an essential cofactor for many antioxidant pathways, including glutathione peroxidase and thiol/disulfide exchange reactions. Glutathione peroxidase detoxifies organic peroxides and free radicals and has a higher affinity for hydrogen peroxide than does catalase. Glutathione S-transferase forms conjugates between electrophilic substances and the free thiol of reduced glutathione (GSH). GSH also takes part in nonenzymatic reactions, yielding products such as oxidized glutathione (GSSG) and mixed disulfides of glutathione and protein. Hepatocytes, which are the main site of glutathione synthesis, contain high cytoplasmic concentrations of glutathione, ranging from 5 to 10 mmol/L.[147] Mitochondria actively take up glutathione; disruption of this transport (e.g., secondary to chronic ethanol exposure) leads to mitochondrial damage.[233]

Under normal conditions, most glutathione exists as GSH. GSH plays a critical role in preserving the redox capacity of the cell. Oxidative stresses deplete GSH, converting it to GSSG. Glutathione reductase reverses this reaction, regenerating GSH and restoring the redox state. Synthesis of NADPH, the cofactor for glutathione reductase, requires ATP. Therefore, the capacity of hepatocytes to withstand oxidative stress is dependent on hepatocellular energy production.[243]

Adverse conditions (malnutrition, ischemia and reperfusion, toxic radical production) can rapidly exhaust glutathione substrate, making hepatocytes highly susceptible to oxidative injury. In this setting, it may be important to treat patients with thiol-rich agents, such as cysteamine (mercaptoethylamine) or *N*-acetylcysteine (glutathione precursor), to increase glutathione synthesis and refill the pool of reduced glutathione. This therapy restores the capacity of hepatocytes to detoxify intracellular electrophiles.[243]

Ischemia/Reperfusion Injury

Injury induced by ischemia and reperfusion results from (1) oxygen deprivation during the ischemic period and (2) cytotoxic events during reperfusion.[240,248-250] Following brief periods of ischemia, reperfusion is the main cause of cellular injury. Reperfusion stimulates the production of highly reactive molecules (superoxide, hydrogen peroxide, hydroxyl radicals), which can induce apoptosis or necrosis. As the ischemic period lengthens, oxygen deprivation causes an increasing proportion of the ischemia/reperfusion injury.

Role of Xanthine Dehydrogenase/Xanthine Oxidase

The highest specific activities of xanthine dehydrogenase/xanthine oxidase (XDH/XO) in humans occur in the liver and intestines.[251] In healthy tissue, XDH catalyzes the rate-limiting step in nucleic acid degradation. XDH uses nicotinamide adenine dinucleotide (rather than O_2) as the electron acceptor and therefore does not produce oxygen radicals. Ischemic conditions, however, transform XDH to XO, which is a significant generator of reactive radicals. During reperfusion, XO-derived oxidants stimulate the production and release of leukotriene B_4 and platelet-activating factor, which promote neutrophil adherence and migration. These neutrophils can damage the microvascular circulation by releasing proteases and physically disrupting the endothelial barrier. Pretreatment with allopurinol, an inhibitor of xanthine oxidase, markedly decreases reperfusion-induced increases in microvascular permeability and epithelial cell necrosis.[252,253]

A pathologically important result of hepatocellular damage—from ischemia, orthotopic transplantation, acute hepatitis, cholestasis—is the release of XO and other hepatocellular substances into the central circulation.[238,242,254-259] Circulating XO binds to vascular endothelial cells in various organs.[251,260-262] The endothelial cells produce superoxide, which reacts with nitric oxide (NO·) to form peroxynitrite (OONO⁻).[239,263] Peroxynitrite is a reactive molecule that can further damage hepatic and extrahepatic tissues. Experimental data suggest that various interventions may confer protection against reperfusion injury, including (1) antioxidants; (2) oxygen radical scavengers, such as superoxide dismutase and dimethyl sulfoxide; (3) inhibitors of XO; and (4) inhibitors of leukocyte adherence and migration.[253,264-266]

Hepatic Injury During Transplantation

PRESERVATION INJURY. Paradoxically, solutions used to preserve the liver can eventually make the transplanted liver susceptible to injury. For example, storing livers in the University of Wisconsin solution for more than 24 hours increases the likelihood of microcirculatory disturbances, leukocyte and platelet adhesion, and a systemic inflammatory response after graft implantation. Over time this "preservation" method exhausts the hepatic supply of antioxidants, contributing to the excessive production of reactive molecules on reperfusion of the transplanted liver.[252]

The pathogenesis of ischemia and reperfusion injury is complex.[267-270] It involves (1) activated Kupffer cells[271,272]; (2) formation of xanthine oxidase[259,273]; (3) production of reactive oxygen and nitrogen species, including superoxide, nitric oxide, peroxynitrite, and hydroxyl radicals; (4) release of proinflammatory cytokines[274]; and (5) endothelial cell destruction.[275-278] Hypothermic preservation solutions can induce apoptotic changes in endothelial cells, which may later cause their destruction. Improvements in graft survival may be achieved by downregulating Kupffer cells with calcium channel blockers, pentoxifylline, or gadolinium. Similarly, flushing grafts after storage with Carolina rinse solution (antioxidants, adenosine, calcium channel blocker, energy substrates, glycine, and pH 6.5) reduces Kupffer cell activation and endothelial cell killing and improves graft survival.[279]

Bacterial, Viral, and Immune Injury

Bacterial products such as endotoxins injure and kill hepatocytes. Endotoxins refer to lipopolysaccharide complexes that are integral to the outer membrane of Gram-negative bacteria. Bacterial lysis releases these endotoxins, which consist of two polysaccharide regions (a bacterial strain-specific O-antigen and more constant core R-antigen) and a common lipid part (lipid A). Lipid A binds to high-density lipoproteins in blood and to other tissues, and mediates the biologic reactions common to endotoxins. Endotoxins bind more extensively to Kupffer cells than to hepatocytes. Thus, endotoxins can damage hepatocytes both directly and indirectly. Indirect hepatocellular or cholestatic damage involves Kupffer cell stimulation. Activated Kupffer cells produce and release proinflammatory mediators, including cytokines and ecosanoids.[280] Viruses may similarly cause hepatocellular injury through direct and indirect mechanisms. Viral infections can stimulate the production of cytokines that induce lymphocyte- or macrophage-dependent cytotoxicity, which is typical of hepatotropic viruses and certain herpesviruses. Antigens on hepatocellular membranes may be primary targets of cell-mediated injury. Antibodies to such antigens selectively increase in patients with autoimmune hepatitis and primary biliary cirrhosis. Other potential antigenic focuses for cell-mediated cytotoxicity include liver-specific lipoproteins and hepatic lectins, which may be important targets in hepatitis B and other liver diseases.

Drug- and Toxin-Induced Damage

Xenobiotics can cause hepatocellular injuries by several different mechanisms, including (1) covalently binding to and inactivating key enzymes, (2) peroxidation of membrane lipids, (3) depletion of intracellular antioxidants, and (4) induction of immunopathologic responses. Certain substances are toxic enough to damage organelles (e.g., plasma membrane, mitochondria), interrupt energy production, disrupt ion gradients, and destroy the physical integrity of the cell. However, the hepatotoxic effects of most clinically or environmentally relevant compounds occur because of CYP, and involve reactive metabolites such as carbon-based radicals, nitro-radicals, and reduced oxygen species. For example, CYP oxidizes carbon tetrachloride to a toxic intermediate, trichloromethyl radical, which causes centrilobular necrosis. Similarly, hepatic damage from nitrofurantoin and other aromatic molecules involves free radical intermediates formed during their metabolism.

Similar to CYP of the smooth endoplasmic reticulum, enzymes of the mitochondrial electron transport pathway involved in xenobiotic metabolism may produce reactive intermediates. For example, cocaine or nitrofurantoin metabolism yields nitro-radicals,[147,233] which can transfer an electron to molecular oxygen via flavoprotein reductases, forming superoxide and other reactive oxygen species. Reactive intermediates can arise by many other mechanisms, including redox cycling reactions, as occurs with anthracycline chemotherapeutics or imidazole antimicrobial agents.

Various drugs can damage the liver by weakening antioxidant defense mechanisms. Examples include acetaminophen and bromobenzene, which cause extensive liver necrosis by draining hepatocellular stores of reduced glutathione.[281,282] Further oxidative stresses can damage important proteins and enzymes, phospholipids in membranes, and nucleotides by activating proteases, phospholipases, and endonucleases. Oxidative stress causes pathologic increases in cytosolic Ca^{2+} by allowing excessive uptake of Ca^{2+} into cells and stimulating Ca^{2+} release from intracellular storage pools (from the endoplasmic reticulum or mitochondria). These events can induce apoptosis, necrosis, or both.

Occasionally, conjugation pathways produce reactive intermediates, such as acyl glucuronides (metabolites of carboxylate drugs), which can damage the liver.[153,283-285] Injury typically occurs when intermediates covalently bind to and inactivate essential molecules—particularly nucleophiles, thiol-rich proteins, and nucleic acids. Intermediates can also damage the liver through depletion of antioxidant stores (oxidative stress) or by inducing neoantigens and autoantigen formation, which subsequently trigger immunopathologic responses.

Drug-Induced Apoptosis

Drugs that induce oxidative stress and mitochondrial injury can trigger intracellular apoptotic pathways.[233,236,243] The following events may be involved: (1) CYP produces reactive drug metabolites; (2) these metabolites deplete glutathione; (3) mitochondria are injured, with cytochrome c release and operation of the mitochondrial membrane permeability transition; (4) capsaicin is activated; and (5) apoptosis occurs.[236,286-288] Enzymes in mitochondria are likely to be a pathogenically important target of the acetaminophen metabolite N-acetyl-p-benzoquinone imine (NAPQI). The characteristic hepatic pathology of Reye's syndrome may reflect mitochondrial injury induced by drugs such as tetracycline, aspirin, valproic acid, and certain nucleoside analogs (e.g., zidovudine).[288]

Whether mitochondrial injury causes apoptosis or necrosis depends on the energy state of the cell as well as on the acuteness and severity of the injury.[233] When ATP levels decline slowly, apoptosis may occur, whereas rapid energy depletion causes necrosis.

Immunopathology

Immunopathology often underlies idiosyncratic adverse drug reactions that affect the liver. Halothane hepatitis provides a prototypic example. The clinical features of such reactions characteristically include (1) a delayed onset after the first drug exposure and a hastened onset following later challenges; (2) fever, rash, or lymphadenopathy; and (3) eosinophilia and inflammatory infiltrates in the liver. Immunopathologic events may involve (1) production of antibodies that lyse hepatocytes via molecular mimicry with host enzymes[289]; (2) antibody-dependent cell-mediated immunity, such as occurs with diclofenac[290]; and (3) dysregulation of the immune system or drug-induced autoimmunity.[291,292]

According to the altered antigen concept, drug metabolites alter cellular proteins, causing drug-protein adducts or neoantigens to form. For example, trifluoroacylated (TFA) adducts form after exposure to halothane or other halogenated anesthetics.[293] Antibodies directed against TFA protein adducts are often present in patients recovering from halothane-induced liver injury. However, the specificity and pathogenicity of these antibodies remain unclear,[293] because only a tiny fraction of the patients that make these antibodies suffer hepatic injury. Tissue-damaging immune responses seem to require a chain of events. For example, Kupffer cells, in association with mixed histocompatibility complex (MHC), process the adduct molecules. Responsive CD4+ T cells induce the immune response, and the target cells express drug-derived antigen and a class II MHC molecule, which attracts CD8+ (cytotoxic) T cells. The development of autoimmune disease may involve genetic predisposition through anomalies of immune tolerance. Dysregulation of the immune system induces autoantibodies to form. Some autoantibodies are organ-specific, like the liver-kidney microsomal (LKM) antibodies that target microsomal enzymes (after halothane hepatitis, LKM antibodies are directed at CYP2El), whereas others lack tissue specificity, such as antinuclear and smooth muscle antibodies.

Ethanol-Induced Liver Disease

Alcoholism (>5 g of alcohol or about five drinks per day) causes several types of liver injury, including steatosis (fatty liver), alcoholic hepatitis, and cirrhosis. Although almost all people who chronically abuse alcohol develop steatosis, only 10% to 20% develop cirrhosis.[294] Chronic liver disease is notoriously difficult to detect by a brief history and physical examination. The clinical presentation correlates poorly with hepatic pathology, because physiologic compensatory mechanisms can mask extensive liver disease. Identifying patients with severe alcoholic liver disease is important, as their risk for perioperative morbidity may be increased two- to threefold.[295] The most frequent perioperative complications are bleeding, infections, and cardiopulmonary disorders.

Contributing factors to such complications include malnutrition, immune incompetence, fluid and electrolyte imbalances, alcohol abstinence, and cardiac failure (alcoholic or cirrhotic cardiomyopathy).

Clinical studies and laboratory experiments have shown that alcoholism produces a multitude of subcellular disturbances, including: (1) acetaldehyde-induced lesions, (2) metabolic perturbations, (3) microvascular hypoxia, (4) increased production of oxygen and nitrogen radicals, and (5) depletion of antioxidant defenses. The metabolism of ethanol plays an integral role in the pathogenesis of alcoholic liver disease.[296-302] Alcohol dehydrogenase (ADH), a zinc metalloenzyme, catalyzes the rate-limiting step in the ethanol metabolism. Although this enzyme is present in many tissues,[300,303] more than 95% of ethanol metabolism occurs in the liver. Cytoplasmic ADH is chiefly responsible for oxidizing ethanol to acetaldehyde. However, when ADH activity decreases, as occurs in alcoholic liver disease, microsomal ethanol-oxidizing enzymes (e.g., ethanol-induced CYP2E1) and catalase in peroxisomes become important contributors to ethanol metabolism.[304,305]

ADH is polymorphic; there are more than 20 different isozymes, with widely varying kinetic properties.[294,306] It seems likely that genetic polymorphisms of ethanol-metabolizing enzymes affect susceptibility to alcoholic liver disease.[306-308] Polymorphisms at the ADH2 gene locus (increased frequency of B allele), for example, have been linked to the development of cirrhosis.[309] Sustained liver injury can diminish the mitochondrial capacity to metabolize acetaldehyde to acetate via aldehyde dehydrogenase (ALDH).[305,307,310] When this occurs, acetaldehyde increases in plasma and tissues and probably contributes to the intra- and extra-hepatic toxicities of ethanol.[311] Acetaldehyde may induce injury in several ways. It forms adducts with intracellular proteins,[312] binds to glutathione, and depletes the antioxidant pool.[313] It also triggers the release of chemotactic substances (e.g., leukotriene B_4) that attract neutrophils to the liver,[314] induces changes in plasma membranes to augment superoxide production,[315,316] and stimulates collagen production and fibroplasia.[317]

Similarities in Hepatic Injuries from Hypoxia and Ethanol

There is notable similitude in liver injuries caused by hypoxia and ethanol. Laboratory studies have shown that ethanol markedly increases hepatic oxygen consumption, which is associated with liver injury.[294,318] The injury is mainly in the centrilobular region (zone 3), where ADH activity is localized, and the oxygen supply is already tenuous.[147,304,305,319,320] Further, prolonged administration of ethanol increases NO· synthase expression and NO· production. This effect on the NO· pathway, and the resultant vasodilation, may represent a compensatory response to chronic ethanol-induced vasoconstriction in the hepatic microcirculation.[321,322] Hypoxic liver injury promotes the release of proinflammatory cytokines, tumor necrosis factor-α (TNF-α), and interleukins 1 and 6. These substances increase the expression of adhesion molecules, decrease leukocyte velocity, increase margination and platelet adherence, and reduce hepatic blood flow.[323]

Complement, cytokines, and xanthine oxidase intensify inflammation, and may contribute to pulmonary and cardiac injuries from hepatoenteric ischemia and reperfusion.[238,242,324,325] Similar increases in proinflammatory mediators occur in alcoholic liver disease.[326]

There is much evidence, both indirect (lipid peroxidation)[327] and direct (electron spin resonance data),[328] that alcoholism causes a significant oxidant stress. Prolonged ethanol intake can simultaneously weaken antioxidant defenses and increase oxidant production; thus the liver damage is progressive.[302,327] Antioxidants decrease because their consumption increases and/or their synthesis decreases, owing to malnutrition or reduced expression of genes for antioxidant-producing enzymes.[329] The oxidant stress may involve cytosolic oxidases (aldehyde oxidase, xanthine oxidase) and microsomal ethanol oxidation, which produce superoxide and other reactive species. The activation of inflammatory cells, including Kupffer cells,[330] can increase nitric oxide synthetase (iNOS) expression in hepatocytes, macrophages, endothelial cells, and vascular myocytes,[331] and stimulate peroxynitrite formation.[263] This unstable anion (formed when NO· reacts with $O_2\cdot^-$) oxidizes sulfhydryl groups as well as nitrating and oxidizing lipids, proteins, and other substances.[332-337] The depletion of glutathione and α-tocopherol aggravates oxygen radical–mediated ethanol toxicity.[327,338,339]

Cirrhosis and Portal Hypertension

Persistent or repeated intermittent hepatic injuries can lead to hepatic cirrhosis. Alcoholism and chronic viral hepatitis (B and C) are the most common causes of cirrhosis in the United States.[340] Because of the large physiologic reserves of the liver, low-grade hepatic inflammation diseases (like hepatitis C) may remain subclinical while they are destroying much of the liver. Pathologic changes in the liver may include cellular hypertrophy, fatty metamorphosis, mitochondrial and lysosomal dysfunction, and disruption of transport and storage processes. Eventually, significant fibroplasia occurs, and, as hepatocytes become encircled by fibrous tissue, the liver becomes cirrhotic.[341] The progression of cirrhosis induces portal hypertension. Patients typically have a hyperdynamic circulation with extensive arteriovenous communications, and a decreased effective plasma volume. The characteristic clinical features of cirrhosis and portal hypertension include weakness, anorexia, nausea, vomiting, abdominal discomfort, jaundice, spider nevi, ascites, splenomegaly, a firm liver, esophageal varices, hepatorenal syndrome, and portosystemic encephalopathy. Advanced liver disease affects nearly every organ in the body and poses complex challenges to the health care team.[342] The multiple severe pathophysiologic derangements set the stage for devastating complications, including life-threatening hemorrhage, infection, renal failure, coma, and death.

Pulmonary Dysfunction

Advanced liver disease often causes pulmonary dysfunction and hypoxemia.[343-345] Various pathologic changes, such as increased intrapulmonary arteriovenous communications, may induce hypoxemia. Other influences include (1) disruption of hypoxic pulmonary vasoconstriction due to endogenous vasodilators such as NO·, glucagon, adenosine, and prostacyclin; and (2) a rightward shift of the oxyhemoglobin dissociation curve owing to increased erythrocyte 2,3-diphosphoglycerate levels. Also, restrictive lung pathology or atelectasis, secondary to ascites and pleural effusions, causes ventilation/perfusion mismatching. Hepatic hydrothorax (pleural effusions without cardiopulmonary disease) occurs in up to 10% of patients with cirrhosis.[346]

Renal Dysfunction

Portal hypertension combined with cirrhosis causes two major changes in renal function: avid sodium retention and decreased glomerular filtration rate (GFR). Renal function decreases progressively despite the absence of overt renal injury (e.g., no histopathology) or tubular dysfunction. The urinalysis typically is normal, and the urine sodium concentration is low. Prerenal disorders are chiefly responsible for the most severe renal complications of advanced liver disease—acute renal failure (ARF) and the hepatorenal syndrome.[29,347-349]

In patients with advanced liver disease, poor renal perfusion is the major cause of both prerenal ARF and acute tubular necrosis (ATN). Renal hypoperfusion is usually the result of intravascular volume depletion, hypotension, or type 1 hepatorenal syndrome (HRS). Common causes of intravascular volume depletion include hemorrhage (e.g., variceal bleeding), ascites formation, sequestration of blood volume in the splanchnic vasculature, and increased loss of fluid from the kidneys (e.g., vigorous diuretic therapy) and gastrointestinal tract. Restoring renal blood flow—which involves identifying and treating the specific cause of the hypoperfusion—is the key to correcting prerenal ARF.

Proper fluid replacement is effective in most cases of "non-HRS" prerenal failure. ATN is usually a sequela of prolonged renal hypoperfusion (prerenal ARF), which eventually causes renal tubular ischemia. Other potential causes of ATN are nonsteroidal anti-inflammatory drugs and intravascular radiocontrast agents. There is no specific treatment for ATN; care is mainly supportive.[350] For type 1 HRS, when the expected short-term survival rate is low, liver transplantation is the preferred treatment. Type 2 HRS (the more stable form of HRS) usually occurs in patients with preserved hepatic function. Treatments that may transiently improve renal performance include (1) intravenous vasoconstrictors such as terlipressin, noradrenaline, and midodrine, in combination with octreotide; (2) molecular adsorbent recirculating system (MARS); and (3) transjugular intrahepatic portosystemic shunt (TIPS).[350]

Hematologic Dysfunction

Hematologic and hemostatic abnormalities are common in severe liver disease.[115] Anemia may occur because of plasma volume expansion, gastrointestinal bleeding, malnutrition, vitamin deficiencies, hemolysis, hypersplenism, or bone marrow depression. As the synthesis of vitamin K–dependent factors decreases, coagulopathies develop. The factor VII level must decrease by roughly 60% to 70% before the prothrombin time becomes prolonged. Thrombocytopenia and thrombopathy usually coexist with overt portal hypertension (ascites, splenomegaly). Causes of these abnormalities include splenic sequestration syndrome, bone marrow suppression (from alcohol or interferon or other medications), and immune-mediated platelet destruction (platelet-associated IgG). Dysfibrinogenemia (activation of fibrinolysis) is not uncommon. In this disorder, increases in fibrin degradation products and D-dimer occur but fibrinogen levels may be normal. The presence of overt disseminated intravascular coagulation, however, should prompt a rigorous pursuit of various reversible causes, such as endotoxemia.

Gastrointestinal Complications

Patients with cirrhosis and portal hypertension are at high risk for developing esophagogastric varices and portal hypertensive gastropathy. The prevalence of this latter condition parallels the severity of portal hypertension and liver dysfunction. Severe bleeding as a result of this gastropathy seldom occurs.[351] In contrast, hemorrhage from ruptured esophagogastric varices accounts for about one third of the deaths in this patient population. Generally, gastric varices bleed less often but more severely than esophageal varices. Variceal size is the most important predictor of variceal bleeding. The rates of variceal formation and enlargement parallel the degree of liver dysfunction. In patients with cirrhosis and portal hypertension, the incidence of variceal bleeding at 2 years ranges from 20% to 30%.[351] The first episode of variceal hemorrhage is acutely lethal in about 7% of cases; the 6-week mortality rate approaches 30%. Rebleeding is a major concern. Survivors of a variceal hemorrhage, if untreated, have a 60% risk of rebleeding within 2 years; the associated death rate is around 40% to 50%. Because of this poor prognosis, it is important to begin therapy promptly to prevent rebleeding.

Endocrinopathies

Advanced liver disease produces several endocrine abnormalities. For example, increased plasma concentrations of growth hormone and glucagon contribute to insulin resistance. Decreased plasma concentrations of insulin-like growth factor 1 (IGF-1) adversely affect normal growth and development.[137] Gonadal dysfunction occurs in both men and women secondary to abnormal metabolism of sex hormones. Men undergo feminization, developing gynecomastia, testicular atrophy, infertility, and impotence. In women, oligomenorrhea, amenorrhea and infertility are common.

Central Nervous System Dysfunction

Hepatic encephalopathy is a complex neuropsychiatric syndrome, occurring in 50% to 70% of patients with cirrhosis.[29] The pathogenesis is complex and involves decreased hepatocellular function, reduced hepatic blood flow, and diversion of portal flow through extrahepatic collateral vessels (i.e., portacaval blood flow). Various chemical substances may contribute to the encephalopathy, including ammonia and various gut-derived molecules—short-chain fatty acids, mercaptans, phenols, and manganese. False neurotransmitters, such as octopamine, may be produced, which decrease central excitability; also, endogenous ligands (activators of γ-aminobutyric acid benzodiazepine receptors) may be formed, which increases central inhibitory outflow. Other influences that may contribute to encephalopathy include abnormalities of cerebral energy metabolism and disruptions of the blood-brain barrier. The pathogenesis and management of hepatic encephalopathy are described in detail elsewhere.[29,115,352]

Cardiovascular Dysfunction

Advanced liver disease induces a hyperdynamic cardiovascular system characterized by increased cardiac output and low systemic vascular resistance.[353] Heart rate is often mildly increased, systemic arterial pressure is slightly decreased, and central filling pressures are normal. The increase in cardiac output leads to an increase in mixed venous O_2 saturation and a decrease in the arteriovenous O_2 content gap. Overall, the clinical and pathophysiologic changes resemble those of a peripheral arteriovenous fistula. These changes are mainly a result of widespread arteriovenous communications within the splanchnic organs, lungs, muscle, and skin. Vasodilatory substances, including glucagon, NO·, ferritin, and vasoactive intestinal polypeptide (VIP), may contribute to the high blood flow through these collateral vessels.[354-360]

Increases in endogenous vasodilators may also explain the decreases in cardiovascular responsiveness to physiologic (e.g., epinephrine) and pharmacologic vasoconstrictors in patients with advanced liver disease.[361] Laboratory investigations suggest that NO· could mediate the quintessential cardiovascular and renal changes of cirrhosis and portal hypertension.[362,363] In animal models of chronic portal hypertension (partial portal vein ligation, CCl_4-induced cirrhosis), NO· induces cyclic guanosine monophosphate (cGMP) elevations that correlate directly with peripheral arterial dilation.[363,364] Also, inhibition of NO· synthase (1) prevents the increase in cardiac output and the decrease in total peripheral resistance; (2) restores plasma aldosterone and arginine vasopressin levels; and (3) corrects the derangements of sodium and water excretion. Clinical investigations of healthy subjects and patients with cirrhosis have shown a positive correlation between the partial pressure of exhaled NO· and the cardiac index.[365]

Pathogenesis of Portal Hypertension

The pathogenesis of portal hypertension includes one or more of the following influences: (1) increased pre-portal blood flow, (2) increased resistance to intrahepatic flow, and (3) increased flow through the portacaval collaterals. The classic "backward theory" proposes that proliferating fibrotic tissue induces cirrhosis and increases portal venous resistance, which causes portal pressure to rise. However, many observations are inconsistent with this theory. For example, experimental narrowing of the portal vein induces portal hypertension and the following effects: (1) increased mesenteric vascular resistance, (2) decreased mesenteric flow, (3) decreased splanchnic venous oxygen saturation, and (4) increased mesenteric arteriovenous oxygen content gap. This is the exact opposite of what happens in patients with cirrhosis and portal hypertension.

The "forward theory" addresses clinical and pathophysiologic features not well explained by the "backward theory."[366] According to the forward theory, endogenous vasodilators (e.g., NO·, glucagon, prostacyclin, adenosine) stimulate arteriovenous fistulae to form in the intestine and spleen. Splanchnic blood flow and cardiac output both increase, whereas portal venous flow decreases substantially. Hepatic arterial flow remains unchanged or may increase. The hepatic oxygen supply is preserved despite a decrease in total hepatic blood flow.

Control of Circulatory Volume

When volume receptors detect decreases in effective plasma volume, they activate the sympathetic nervous system.[367] This stimulates the kidney to release renin, which increases angiotensin II and aldosterone production. Increases in aldosterone and sympathoadrenal tone cause the renal tubules to avidly resorb sodium. There is an inverse relation between plasma norepinephrine level and blood flow to the kidney—suggesting a key role for sympathoadrenal activation in the renal retention of sodium. Vasoconstrictive effects of norepinephrine and angiotensin II redistribute intrarenal blood flow, which increases sodium uptake by the kidney. The kallikrein-kinin system also modulates sodium retention. Patients with cirrhosis and ascites have increased levels of endothelin, a potent vasoconstrictor and a likely contributor to the renal dysfunction. When cirrhosis and ascites coexist, vasodilatory prostaglandins are important for preserving renal blood flow. Inhibitors of prostaglandin synthesis decrease renal plasma flow and GFR and may therefore cause acute renal injury.

Pathogenesis of Ascites

Patients with cirrhosis and portal hypertension develop edema, ascites, and increases in total body water because the kidneys avidly retain sodium (Fig. 19-7).[1,368,369] The pathogenesis of the sodium retention remains unclear. For instance, it is unknown whether severe liver disease mainly produces abnormal mediators that promote excessive sodium retention, or whether it decreases effective blood volume and therefore causes normal kidneys to avidly retain sodium.[367]

The first idea—the "overflow theory"—presumes that the kidney will hold on to sodium and water despite an overfilled intravascular compartment, whereas the second hypothesis—the "underfill theory"—simply reflects the normal homeostatic response to intravascular volume depletion (sodium and water retention). According to the overflow theory, sodium and water retention expands the intravascular volume and lowers plasma oncotic pressure. Expansion of the plasma volume increases portal hydrostatic pressure, which eventually causes portal hypertension. Portal hypertension and low oncotic pressure together cause edema and ascites. Proof for this theory will require identifying a primary pathogenic agent or process that causes the kidney to retain sodium when the plasma volume is increased.

According to the underfill theory, cirrhosis causes a decrease in the effective plasma volume, which stimulates

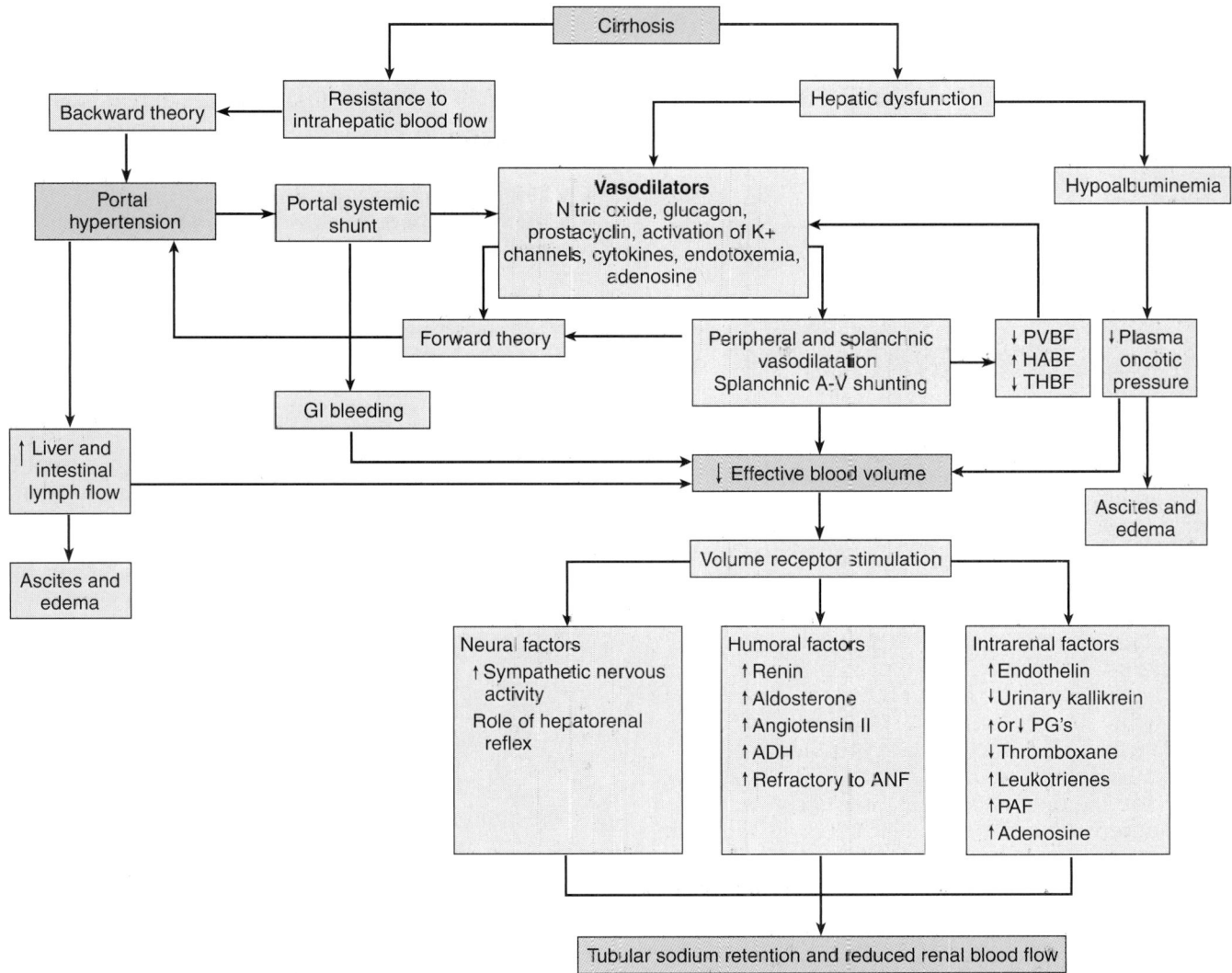

Figure 19–7 Schematic of pathways for cirrhosis-induced portal hypertension: the forward and backward theories. Cirrhosis and portal hypertension induce circulatory changes that decrease the effective blood volume. This activates volume receptors and stimulates neurohumoral and intrarenal reflexes to decrease renal blood flow and to increase renal retention of sodium. PVBF, portal venous blood flow; HABF, hepatic arterial blood flow; THBF, total hepatic blood flow; A-V, arteriovenous; PG's, prostaglandins; ADH, antidiuretic hormone; ANF, atrial natriuretic factor; PAF, platelet activating factor. (Reprinted with permission from Mushlin PS, Gelman S: Anesthesia and the liver. *In* Barash PG, Cullen BF, Stoelting RK [eds]: Clinical Anesthesia, 4th ed. Philadelphia, Lippincott Williams & Wilkins, 2001, p. 1088.)

homeostatic reflex responses to retain sodium. Physiologically, negative feedback loops, involving neuroendocrine reflexes and the kidney, tightly regulate intravascular volume. Schrier and Abraham[367] state that the "integrity of the arterial circulation, as determined by cardiac output and peripheral arterial resistance, is the primary determinant of renal sodium and water excretion." Thus, the normal response to a decrease in arterial volume—whether from arterial dilation or decreased cardiac output—is activation of homeostatic reflexes that stimulate renal retention of sodium and water. This response can correct the "underfilling" problem as well as increasing total plasma volume and total body water. In cirrhosis, decreases in effective plasma (or arterial) volume result from arterial dilation and losses of intravascular fluid. Massive fluid transudation (through the hepatic

sinusoids and splanchnic capillaries) occurs in response to unbalanced Starling forces.

The mechanisms underlying the overflow and underfill theories are not mutually exclusive. Each could play a role in various stages of cirrhosis. For example, in the early stages, a primary defect in sodium excretion could play the more critical role, whereas with more advanced disease, a decrease in circulating plasma volume could be the more important cause.[368]

Cholestatic Disease

Cholestasis is defined as impaired biliary flow. Dysfunction of the bile transporter is the main cause of intrahepatic cholestasis (inherited or acquired), whereas mechanical obstructions to bile flow is the chief cause of extrahepatic cholestasis. Pruritus is an early symptom of cholestasis, which results from retained bile salts.[370-373] As cholestasis progresses, jaundice develops and increases in severity.[370,374] The stool becomes lighter in color and the urine darkens, because bile pigments are diverted from the gastrointestinal tract to the kidney for excretion. Laboratory tests show increased blood levels of the major constituents of bile: namely, bile acids, cholesterol, bilirubin, hepatic enzymes in bile (AP, GGTP, 5′-NT, leucine aminopeptidase) and immunoglobulin A. Unconjugated bilirubin is the most toxic of the biliary substances. It disrupts essential metabolic pathways (e.g., oxidative phosphorylation, tricarboxylic acid cycle, glycogenesis) and, at high concentrations, causes membrane dysfunction.

The pathogenesis of cholestatic disorders is complex,[371,375-377] and the etiology is vast (Table 19-4).[165,373,378-405] Cholestatic disorders can induce pathologic changes throughout the body, variably affecting elimination and pharmacokinetics.[406-410] For many drugs, their alpha-phase of disposition increases and their initial elimination decreases.[411,412] Treatments for the symptoms of cholestasis have been reviewed elsewhere.[379,383,384,413,414]

Coagulation Disorders

Coagulopathy may develop after brief periods of disrupted biliary flow. Enteric absorption of fat-soluble vitamins, such as vitamin K, depends on the presence of bile in the gut and an intact enterohepatic circulation. Patients with obstructive jaundice or receiving warfarin therapy usually produce vitamin K–dependent factors at the normal rate, but the factors lack the γ-carboxyl glutamic acid residues needed for coagulant activity. If a coagulopathy is purely cholestatic, it should be correctable by parenteral vitamin K. Failure of vitamin K therapy implies severe liver disease, which can be caused by prolonged biliary obstruction. In such settings, particularly when surgery is urgently needed, the hemostatic abnormality can usually be corrected by giving fresh frozen plasma (and platelets, if needed).[115]

Renal Dysfunction

Hepatocellular disease and obstructive jaundice impede the transfer of blood from the splanchnic to the central circulation. Changes in the splanchnic vasculature and decreases in effective plasma volume predispose to renal hypoperfusion. Mild-to-moderate hemorrhage is likely to cause severe hypotension (see following discussion of cardiovascular dysfunction). The risk of prerenal ARF therefore increases. Prolonged tubular ischemia can cause ATN. Bilirubin, which is toxic to renal tubules, may play a role in the pathogenesis of ATN in jaundiced patients.

Cardiovascular Dysfunction

The hemodynamic changes associated with cholestasis are qualitatively similar to those induced by cirrhosis, but usually not as severe. These changes often include (1) increased cardiac output, owing to decreased total peripheral vascular resistance; (2) decreased portal venous flow, secondary to increased portal venous resistance; and (3) decreased vascular responsiveness to endogenous vasoconstrictors (e.g., catecholamines) and vasopressor therapy.[415]

The mechanisms by which cholestasis induces cardiovascular changes remain unclear, and clarifying them is not trivial. Bile is a complex mixture of chemicals, with various types, amounts, and proportions of bilirubins and bile salts. Biliary constituents may affect cardiovascular performance directly or indirectly by modulating reflexes that preserve circulatory homeostasis. Furthermore, disease-specific pathophysiologic changes (e.g., primary biliary cirrhosis vs. choledocholithiasis) may influence cardiovascular responses to the constituents of bile. Thus, it is not surprising that laboratory studies have yet to provide a coherent view of the cardiovascular effects of cholestasis.

The cardiac effects of bile salts (primary, conjugated, and secondary) have been studied in isolated rat ventricular muscle preparations, using bile salt concentrations similar to those in patients with cholestatic jaundice. Bile salts were noted to decrease peak tension, rate of rise of tension, contractile duration, and action potential duration. In voltage clamp experiments in rat ventricular myocytes, sodium taurocholate decreases the slow inward current and slightly increases the outward potassium current. Thus, negative inotropic effects of bile salts may result from altered membrane currents.[416]

Laboratory studies have also shown that increased concentrations of bile salts in blood (cholemia) can depress cardiovascular function and blunt cardiovascular responses to norepinephrine, angiotensin II, and isoproterenol.[415-418] However, other experiments have demonstrated that acute cholestasis can rapidly depress the heart without altering the responsiveness of cardiac β-adrenoceptors.[417] For example, rats subjected to bile duct ligation displayed cardiomyopathic changes 3 days later.[417] After a 3-day period of extrahepatic cholestasis, the rats were pithed; subsequent experiments revealed intact β–adrenoceptors despite global decreases of myocardial contractility.

Subsequent studies in animals show that cholestasis markedly decreases homeostatic reflex responses to losses of intravascular blood volume.[418] In normal rats, a 10% loss of blood volume does not decrease arterial pressure, whereas the same blood loss in the presence of cholestasis causes a 50% decline in blood pressure. Normal animals compensate for the blood loss by mobilizing 15% of the blood volume from their pulmonary and splanchnic vascular beds. However, animals with cholestasis mobilize

---

Table 19–4 Etiology of intrinsic cholestatic disorders

Drugs[165,382-386]
Alcoholism[387]
Pregnancy[378-381]
Inflammation[373,390]
Sepsis[391-393]
Parenteral nutrition[388,389]
Primary biliary cirrhosis[394]
Primary sclerosing cholangitis[395-398]
Genetic cholestatic liver diseases[399-405]

only 7% of the pulmonary blood volume and none of the splanchnic blood volume.[418] Thus, cholestasis can decrease the ability of the major physiologic blood reservoirs (splanchnic and pulmonary vasculatures) to transfer blood to the central circulation. Mild-to-moderate hypovolemia may therefore cause marked arterial hypotension. If these experimental findings are clinically relevant, patients with obstructed biliary flow would need rapid replacement of perioperative fluid losses to avert severe hypotension. The anesthesiologist should also be aware that biliary decompression can cause severe cardiovascular collapse.[419]

KEY POINTS

1. The liver receives roughly one fourth of the cardiac output in healthy adults at rest. The portal vein delivers nearly 75% of the hepatic blood flow, and the hepatic artery provides the rest. Each of these vessels supplies about half of the O_2 consumed by the liver. Blood enters the hepatic sinusoids (capillaries of the liver) by terminal portal venules and hepatic arterioles and exits through hepatic venules (often called "central veins"). Hepatic veins (downstream to the sinusoids) are the major source of intravascular resistance within the liver.

2. The acinus (the functional microvascular unit of the liver) has three circulatory zones, defined by relative distances of hepatocytes from the portal axis. Hepatocytes in zone 1 (periportal region) receive oxygen- and nutrient-rich blood, whereas the blood that perfuses zone 3 (centrilobular region) delivers less oxygen and contains metabolites from zone 1 and zone 2 (midzonal region). Centrilobular hepatocytes have the greatest density of cytochrome P450 proteins and are the most vulnerable to ischemia, hypoxia, venous congestion, and reactive drug metabolites.

3. The hepatic arterial buffer response is the main intrinsic regulator of hepatic blood flow. Arterial hypotension causes portal venous flow to decrease since pressure-flow autoregulation is absent in the liver (i.e., in the fasted state). When this occurs, the buffer response increases hepatic arterial flow, which helps preserve the hepatic oxygen supply. Advanced liver disease disrupts the buffer response, increasing the risk that protracted hypotension (e.g., from controlled hypotensive anesthetic techniques) will cause hypoxic liver damage.

4. The liver is an essential part of the splanchnic circulation. In normovolemic adults, sympathoadrenal stimulation rapidly transfers roughly a liter of splanchnic blood to the systemic circulation. Splanchnic reservoir dysfunction, such as occurs in patients with advanced liver disease, will worsen hypotensive responses to sudden losses of intravascular volume.

5. A 12- to 24-hour fast exhausts liver glycogen stores, making the production of blood glucose dependent on hepatic gluconeogenesis. Starvation stimulates lipolysis, beta-oxidation of fatty acids, and ketone synthesis by the liver. Ketones promote the pancreatic release of insulin, which decreases lipolysis and fatty acid oxidation. Starvation- or stress-induced ketosis is therefore self-limited—except in insulin-deficient states, when diabetic ketoacidosis ensues.

6. Albumin accounts for 15% of the protein made by the liver and plays key roles in maintaining plasma oncotic pressure and transporting endogenous (e.g., bilirubin, free fatty acids) and exogenous substances to the liver. Hepatocytes convert amino acids to ammonia and intermediary metabolites and transform ammonia and other nitrogenous compounds to urea. Thus, in patients with severe liver disease (and normal renal function), the blood urea nitrogen (BUN) level typically remains low, whereas nitrogenous wastes increase in blood and other tissues.

7. The liver makes most coagulant factors (except III, IV, and VIII) and inserts γ-carboxylate groups into many of them (II, VII, IX, X, protein C, protein S) in vitamin K–dependent, post-translational reactions. γ-Carboxylation enables activation of these zymogens in plasma.

8. Bile acids are produced by hepatocytes and facilitate the gastrointestinal absorption of many lipophilic molecules, including vitamin K. In cholestatic disorders, the liver synthesizes, but does not γ-carboxylate, clotting factors. Parenteral vitamin K therapy will rapidly correct the resultant coagulopathy, unless liver failure supervenes. In such cases, patients need frozen plasma because the γ-carboxylation pathway is dysfunctional.

9. The liver is the major organ for metabolizing and removing a wide variety of substances through phase 1 (mostly oxidations with cytochrome P450), phase 2 (conjugations), and phase 3 (ATP transport proteins) reactions. The major pharmacokinetic parameters of hepatic drug clearance are liver blood flow, protein binding, intrinsic clearance, and extraction ratio (ER). Generally, decreases in liver blood flow only lower the hepatic clearances of drugs that have a high ER, whereas decreases in drug metabolizing capacity or increases in protein binding only lower hepatic clearances of drugs that have a low ER.

10. The liver filters venous blood from the gastrointestinal tract. Porto-systemic shunting—whether caused by intrinsic liver disease or a procedure to decompress portal hypertension—circumvents the hepatic filter. Shunting decreases the hepatic clearance of drugs, nitrogenous wastes, and toxins and therefore increases the concentrations of such substances in arterial blood (greater bioavailability) and their effects on the body (e.g., hepatic encephalopathy).

11. The panel of biochemical tests typically used to evaluate the liver (liver function tests) will not reveal specific hepatic diseases. Rather, these tests identify broad categories of pathology: namely hepatocellular injury, hepatobiliary dysfunction, and hepatic synthetic dysfunction. A sudden decrease in the ability of the liver to synthesize proteins is detectable within days as a prolongation of the PT owing to the short half-life of factor VII. Serum albumin concentration is useful for evaluating the status of chronic, but not acute, liver dysfunction because plasma albumin has a half-life of 3 weeks.

12. Kupffer cells, which account for nearly 10% of the hepatic mass, phagocytose and process antigens absorbed from the gastrointestinal tract. In sepsis, these cells scavenge bacteria, inactivate toxins, and remove inflammatory mediators. When activated, Kupffer cells produce reactive oxygen species, nitro-radicals, leukotrienes, proteases, and cytokines and recruit neutrophils to the liver to augment the inflammatory response. Activated Kupffer cells also play a role in the pathogenesis of hepatocellular disease.

13. Portal hypertension is responsible for severe complications of advanced liver disease, such as variceal bleeding, hepatic encephalopathy, and renal failure. Cirrhosis and portal hypertension cause a hyperdynamic circulatory state characterized by high cardiac output, low total peripheral resistance, and low-normal arterial blood pressure. Pathophysiologic hallmarks include extensive arteriovenous communications, hypervolemia within the splanchnic vasculature, and hypovolemia of the extrasplanchnic circulation (decreased effective plasma volume). The cardiovascular responsiveness to vasopressors decreases, which usually reflects increased concentrations of endogenous vasodilators and occasionally myocardial dysfunction (e.g., cirrhotic cardiomyopathy).

REFERENCES

1. Mushlin PS, Gelman S: Anesthesia and the liver. *In* Barash PG, Cullen BF, Stoelting RK (eds): Clinical Anesthesia, 4th ed. Philadelphia, Lippincott Williams & Wilkins, 2001, pp 1067-1101.
2. Gazelle GS, Lee MJ, Muelle PR: Cholangiographic segmental anatomy of the liver. Radiographics 14(5):1005-1013, 1994.
3. Heriot AG, Karanjia ND: A review of techniques for liver resection. Ann R Coll Surg Engl 84(6):371-380, 2002.
4. Parks RW, Chrysos E, Diamond T: Management of liver trauma [comment]. Br J Surg 86(9):1121-1135, 1999.
5. Jones AL: Anatomy of the normal liver. In Zakim D, Boyer T (eds): Hepatology: a Textbook of Liver Disease, 3rd ed. Philadelphia, WB Saunders, 1996, pp 3-32.
6. Campra JL, Reynolds TB: The hepatic circulation. *In* Arias IM, Jakoby WB, Popper H, et al (eds): The Liver: Biology and Pathobiology, 2nd ed. New York, Raven Press, 1988, pp 911.
7. Greenway C, Lautt W: Hepatic Circulation: Handbook of Physiology—The Gastrointestinal System, Motility and Circulation. Bethesda, American Physiology Society, 1989, pp 1519-1564.
8. Gelman S, Mushlin PS: Catecholamine induced changes in the splanchnic circulation affecting systemic hemodynamics. Anesthesiology 100(2):434-439, 2004.
9. Greenway CV, Innes IR, Scott GD: Pre- and post-sinusoidal origin of hepatic exudate in anesthetized cats. Can J Physiol Pharmacol 69(12):1914-1916, 1991.
10. Gelman S: Effects of anesthetics on splanchnic circulation. *In* Altura BM, Halvey S (eds): Cardiovascular Action of Anesthetics and Drugs Used in Anesthesia, 1st ed. Basel, Karger, 1986, pp 127.
11. Rappaport AM: Hepatic blood flow: Morphologic aspects and physiologic regulation. Int Rev Physiol 21:1-63, 1980.
12. Cooper AJL: Role of the liver in amino acid metabolism. *In* Zakim D, Boyer T (eds): Hepatology: A Textbook of Liver Disease, 3rd ed. Philadelphia, WB Saunders, 1996, pp 563-604.
13. Zakim D: Metabolism of glucose and fatty acids by the liver. *In* Zakim D, Boyer TD (eds): Hepatology: A Textbook of Liver Disease, 3rd ed. Philadelphia, WB Saunders, 1996, pp 58-92.
14. Norris CP, Barnes GE, Smith EE, et al: Autoregulation of superior mesenteric flow in fasted and fed dogs. Am J Physiol 237(2):H174-177, 1979.
15. Richardson PD, Withrington PG: Liver blood flow. II. Effects of drugs and hormones on liver blood flow. Gastroenterology 81(2):356-375, 1981.
16. Richardson PD, Withrington PG: Liver blood flow. I. Intrinsic and nervous control of liver blood flow. Gastroenterology 81(1):159-173, 1981.
17. Richardson PD: Physiological regulation of the hepatic circulation. Fed Proc 41(6):2111-2116, 1982.
18. Lautt WW: Mechanism and role of intrinsic regulation of hepatic arterial blood flow: Hepatic arterial buffer response. Am J Physiol 249(5 Pt 1):G549-556, 1985.
19. Lautt WW: The 1995 Ciba-Geigy Award Lecture. Intrinsic regulation of hepatic blood flow. Can J Physiol Pharmacol 74(3):223-233, 1996.
20. Gelman S, Ernst EA: Role of pH, PCO_2, and O_2 content of portal blood in hepatic circulatory autoregulation. Am J Physiol 233(4):E255-262, 1977.
21. Jakob SM: Splanchnic blood flow in low-flow states. Anesth Analg 96(4):1129-1138, 2003.
22. Jakob SM: Clinical review: Splanchnic ischaemia [comment]. Crit Care 6(4):306-312, 2002.
23. Carneiro JJ, Donald DE: Change in liver blood flow and blood content in dogs during direct and reflex alteration of hepatic sympathetic nerve activity. Circ Res 40(2):150-158, 1977.
24. Rappaport AM, Schneiderman JH: The function of the hepatic artery. Rev Physiol Biochem Pharmacol 76:129-175, 1976.
25. Richardson PD, Withrington PG: The role of beta-adrenoceptors in the responses of the hepatic arterial vascular bed of the dog to phenylephrine, isoprenaline, noradrenaline and adrenaline. Br J Pharmacol 60(2):239-249, 1977.
26. Richardson PD, Withrington PG: Glucagon inhibition of hepatic arterial responses to hepatic nerve stimulation. Am J Physiol 233(6):H647-654, 1977.
27. Cohen MM, Sitar DS, McNeill JR, et al: Vasopressin and angiotensin on resistance vessels of spleen, intestine, and liver. Am J Physiol 218(6):1704-1706, 1970.
28. Richardson PD, Withrington PG: The effects of intra-arterial and intraportal injections of vasopressin on the simultaneously perfused hepatic arterial and portal venous vascular beds of the dog. Circ Res 43(4):496-503, 1978.
29. Jalan R, Hayes PC: Hepatic encephalopathy and ascites. Lancet 350(9087):1309-1315, 1997; see comments.
30. Friedman LS, Martin P, Munoz SJ: Liver function tests and the objective evaluation of the patient with liver disease. *In* Zakim D, Boyer TD (eds): Hepatology: A Textbook of Liver Disease, 3rd ed. Philadelphia, WB Saunders, 1996, pp 791-832.
31. Rothschild MA, Oratz M, Schreiber SS: Albumin synthesis. Int Rev Physiol 21:249-274, 1980.
32. Rothschild MA, Oratz M, Schreiber SS: Albumin synthesis. 1. N Engl J Med 286(14):748-757, 1972.

33. Rothschild MA, Oratz M, Schreiber SS: Albumin synthesis (second of two parts). N Engl J Med 286(15):816-821, 1972.

34. Kirsch RE, Saunders SJ, Frith L, et al: Plasma amino acid concentration and the regulation of albumin synthesis. Am J Clin Nutr 22(12):1559-1562, 1969.

35. Kirsch R, Frith L, Black E, et al: Regulation of albumin synthesis and catabolism by alteration of dietary protein. Nature 217(128):578-579, 1968.

36. Kelman L, Saunders SJ, Frith L, et al: Effects of amino acids and hormones on the fractional catabolic rate of albumin by the isolated perfused rat liver. J Nutr 102(8):1045-1048, 1972.

37. Schreiber G, Urban J: The synthesis and secretion of albumin. Rev Physiol Biochem Pharmacol 82:27-95, 1978.

38. Seeff LB: Diagnosis, therapy, and prognosis of viral hepatitis. *In* Zakim D, Boyer TD (eds): Hepatology: A Textbook of Liver Disease, 3rd ed. Philadelphia, WB Saunders, 1996, pp 1067-1145.

39. Kew MC: Hepatic tumors and cysts. *In* Feldman M, Friedman LS, Sleisenger MH (eds): Sleisenger & Fordtran's Gastrointestinal and Liver Disease: Pathophysiology/ Diagnosis/Management, 7th ed. Philadelphia, WB Saunders, 2002, pp 1577-1602.

40. Moore MC, Burish MJ, Farmer B, et al: Chronic hepatic artery ligation does not prevent liver from differentiating portal vs. peripheral glucose delivery. Am J Physiol Endocrinol Metab 285(4):E845-853, 2003.

41. Gustavson SM, Chu CA, Nishizawa M, et al: Glucagon's actions are modified by the combination of epinephrine and gluconeogenic precursor infusion. Am J Physiol Endocrinol Metab 285(3):E534-544, 2003.

42. Nishizawa M, Moore MC, Shiota M, et al: Effect of intraportal glucagon-like peptide-1 on glucose metabolism in conscious dogs. Am J Physiol Endocrinol Metab 284(5):E1027-1036, 2003.

43. Gustavson SM, Chu CA, Nishizawa M, et al: Interaction of glucagon and epinephrine in the control of hepatic glucose production in the conscious dog. Am J Physiol Endocrinol Metab 284(4):E695-707, 2003.

44. Chu CA, Galassetti P, Igawa K, et al: Interaction of free fatty acids and epinephrine in regulating hepatic glucose production in conscious dogs. Am J Physiol Endocrinol Metab 284(2):E291-301, 2003.

45. Cherrington AD, Sindelar D, Edgerton D, et al: Physiological consequences of phasic insulin release in the normal animal. Diabetes 51(Suppl 1):S103-108, 2002.

46. Edgerton DS, Cardin S, Pan C, et al: Effects of insulin deficiency or excess on hepatic gluconeogenic flux during glycogenolytic inhibition in the conscious dog. Diabetes 51(11):3151-3162, 2002.

47. Igawa K, Mugavero M, Shiota M, et al: Insulin sensitively controls the glucagon response to mild hypoglycemia in the dog. Diabetes 51(10):3033-3042, 2002.

48. Cardin S, Walmsley K, Neal DW, et al: Involvement of the vagus nerves in the regulation of basal hepatic glucose production in conscious dogs. Am J Physiol Endocrinol Metab 283(5):E958-964, 2002.

49. Goldstein RE, Rossetti L, Palmer BA, et al: Effects of fasting and glucocorticoids on hepatic gluconeogenesis assessed using two independent methods in vivo. Am J Physiol Endocrinol Metab 283(5):E946-957, 2002.

50. Dunning BE, Moore MC, Ikeda T, et al: Portal glucose infusion exerts an incretin effect associated with changes in pancreatic neural activity in conscious dogs. Metabolism 51(10):1324-1330, 2002.

51. Jetton TL, Shiota M, Knobel SM, et al: Substrate-induced nuclear export and peripheral compartmentalization of hepatic glucokinase correlates with glycogen deposition [comment]. Int J Exp Diabetes Res 2(3):173-186, 2001.

52. Satake S, Moore MC, Igawa K, et al: Direct and indirect effects of insulin on glucose uptake and storage by the liver. Diabetes 51(6):1663-1671, 2002.

53. Shiota M, Moore MC, Galassetti P, et al: Inclusion of low amounts of fructose with an intraduodenal glucose load markedly reduces postprandial hyperglycemia and hyperinsulinemia in the conscious dog. Diabetes 51(2):469-478, 2002.

54. Chu CA, Sherck SM, Igawa K, et al: Effects of free fatty acids on hepatic glycogenolysis and gluconeogenesis in conscious dogs.[erratum appears in Am J Physiol Endocrinol Metab 2002 Oct;283(4):section E following table of contents]. Am J Physiol Endocrinol Metab 282(2):E402-411, 2002.

55. Moore MC, Satake S, Baranowski B, et al: Effect of hepatic denervation on peripheral insulin sensitivity in conscious dogs. Am J Physiol Endocrinol Metab 282(2):E286-296, 2002.

56. Moore MC, Davis SN, Mann SL, et al: Acute fructose administration improves oral glucose tolerance in adults with type 2 diabetes. Diabetes Care 24(11):1882-1887, 2001.

57. Edgerton DS, Cardin S, Emshwiller M, et al: Small increases in insulin inhibit hepatic glucose production solely caused by an effect on glycogen metabolism. Diabetes 50(8):1872-1882, 2001.

58. Shiota M, Postic C, Fujimoto Y, et al: Glucokinase gene locus transgenic mice are resistant to the development of obesity-induced type 2 diabetes. Diabetes 50(3):622-629, 2001.

59. Cardin S, Jackson PA, Edgerton DS, et al: Effect of vagal cooling on the counterregulatory response to hypoglycemia induced by a low dose of insulin in the conscious dog. Diabetes 50(3):558-564, 2001.

60. Flattem N, Igawa K, Shiota M, et al: Alpha- and beta-cell responses to small changes in plasma glucose in the conscious dog. Diabetes 50(2):367-375, 2001.

61. Jackson PA, Cardin S, Coffey CS, et al: Effect of hepatic denervation on the counterregulatory response to insulin-induced hypoglycemia in the dog. Am J Physiol Endocrinol Metab 279(6):E1249-1257, 2000.

62. Moore MC, Hsieh PS, Neal DW, et al: Nonhepatic response to portal glucose delivery in conscious dogs. Am J Physiol Endocrinol Metab 279(6):E1271-1277, 2000.

63. Chu CA, Wiernsperger N, Muscato N, et al: The acute effect of metformin on glucose production in the conscious dog is primarily attributable to inhibition of glycogenolysis. Metabolism 49(12):1619-1626, 2000.

64. Moore MC, Cherrington AD, Mann SL, et al: Acute fructose administration decreases the glycemic response to an oral glucose tolerance test in normal adults. J Clin Endocrinol Metab 85(12):4515-4519, 2000.

65. Connolly CC, Holste LC, Aglione LN, et al: Alterations in basal glucose metabolism during late pregnancy in the conscious dog. Am J Physiol Endocrinol Metab 279(5): E1166-1177, 2000.

66. Chu CA, Sindelar DK, Igawa K, et al: The direct effects of catecholamines on hepatic glucose production occur via alpha(1)- and beta(2)-receptors in the dog. Am J Physiol Endocrinol Metab 279(2):E463-473, 2000.

67. Hsieh PS, Moore MC, Neal DW, et al: Importance of the hepatic arterial glucose level in generation of the portal signal in conscious dogs. Am J Physiol Endocrinol Metab 279(2):E284-292, 2000.

68. Shiota M, Jackson P, Galassetti P, et al: Combined intraportal infusion of acetylcholine and adrenergic blockers augments net hepatic glucose uptake. Am J Physiol Endocrinol Metab 278(3):E544-552, 2000.

69. Cardin S, Emshwiller M, Jackson PA, et al: Portal glucose infusion increases hepatic glycogen deposition in conscious unrestrained rats. J Appl Physiol 87(4):1470-1475, 1999.

70. Hsieh PS, Moore MC, Marshall B, et al: The head arterial glucose level is not the reference site for generation of the portal signal in conscious dogs. Am J Physiol 277(4 Pt 1):E678-684, 1999.

71. McGuinness OP, Snowden RT, Moran C, et al: Impact of acute epinephrine removal on hepatic glucose metabolism during stress hormone infusion. Metabolism 48(7):910-914, 1999.

72. Galassetti P, Chu CA, Neal DW, et al: A negative arterial-portal venous glucose gradient increases net hepatic glucose uptake in euglycemic dogs. Am J Physiol 277(1 Pt 1):E126-134, 1999.

73. Galassetti P, Coker RH, Lacy DB, et al: Prior exercise increases net hepatic glucose uptake during a glucose load. Am J Physiol 276(6 Pt 1):E1022-1029, 1999.

74. Hsieh PS, Moore MC, Neal DW, et al: Rapid reversal of the effects of the portal signal under hyperinsulinemic

conditions in the conscious dog. Am J Physiol 276(5 Pt 1):E930-937, 1999.

75. Cherrington AD: Banting Lecture 1997. Control of glucose uptake and release by the liver in vivo. Diabetes 48(5): 1198-1214, 1999.

76. Nordlie RC, Foster JD, Lange AJ: Regulation of glucose production by the liver. Annu Rev Nutr 19:379-406, 1999.

77. Fanelli CG, Pampanelli S, Porcellati F, et al: Rate of fall of blood glucose and physiological responses of counterregulatory hormones, clinical symptoms and cognitive function to hypoglycaemia in Type I diabetes mellitus in the postprandial state. Diabetologia 46(1):53-64, 2003.

78. Hallsten K, Yki-Jarvinen H, Peltoniemi P, et al: Insulin- and exercise-stimulated skeletal muscle blood flow and glucose uptake in obese men. Obes Res 11(2):257-265, 2003.

79. De Feo P, Pampanelli S, Porcellati F, et al: Adrenaline vs glucagon in the primacy of glucose counterregulation. Diabetes Nutr Metab 15(5):323-327; discussion 328, 2002.

80. Bolli GB: Clinical strategies for controlling peaks and valleys: Type 1 diabetes. Int J Clin Pract Suppl (129):65-74, 2002.

81. Owens DR, Zinman B, Bolli GB: Insulins today and beyond. [erratum appears in Lancet 2001 Oct 20;358(9290):1374]. Lancet 358(9283):739-746, 2001.

82. Bolli GB, Fanelli CG: Physiology of glucose counterregulation to hypoglycemia. Endocrinol Metab Clin North Am 28(3): 467-493, v, 1999.

83. Seywert AJ, Tappy L, Gremion G, et al: Effect of a program of moderate physical activity on mental stress-induced increase in energy expenditure in obese women. Diabetes Metab 28(3):178-183, 2002.

84. Tappy L, Cayeux MC, Gillet M, et al: Measurement of the whole body clearance of infused glycerol as a test of liver function after major hepatectomy. Clin Physiol Funct Imaging 22(4):266-270, 2002.

85. Minehira K, Tappy L, Chiolero R, et al: Fractional hepatic de novo lipogenesis in healthy subjects during near-continuous oral nutrition and bed rest: A comparison with published data in artificially fed, critically ill patients. Clin Nutr 21(4):345-350, 2002.

86. Dirlewanger M, Schneiter P, Jequier E, et al: Effects of fructose on hepatic glucose metabolism in humans. Am J Physiol Endocrinol Metab 279(4):E907-911, 2000.

87. Seematter G, Battilana P, Tappy L: Effects of dexamethasone on the metabolic responses to mental stress in humans. Clin Physiol Funct Imaging 22(2):139-144, 2002.

88. Seematter G, Dirlewanger M, Rey V, et al: Metabolic effects of mental stress during over- and underfeeding in healthy women. Obes Res 10(1):49-55, 2002.

89. Tappy L, Minehira K: New data and new concepts on the role of the liver in glucose homeostasis. Curr Opin Clin Nutr Metab Care 4(4):273-277, 2001.

90. Tirone TA, Brunicardi FC: Overview of glucose regulation. World J Surg 25(4):461-467, 2001.

91. Stolz A: Liver physiology and metabolic function. In Feldman M, Friedman LS, Sleisenger MH (eds): Sleisenger & Fordtran's Gastrointestinal and Liver Disease: Pathophysiology/Diagnosis/Management, 7th ed. Philadelphia, WB Saunders, 2002, pp 1202-1226.

92. Riou JP, Claus TH, Pilkis SJ: Stimulation of glucagon of in vivo phosphorylation of rat hepatic pyruvate kinase. J Biol Chem 253(3):656-659, 1978.

93. Sharma RJ, Rodrigues LM, Whitton PD, et al: Control mechanisms in the acceleration of hepatic glycogen degradation during hypoxia. Biochim Biophys Acta 630(3):414-424, 1980.

94. Lewis GF: Fatty acid regulation of very low density lipoprotein production. Curr Opin Lipidol 8(3):146-153, 1997.

95. Lewis GF, Vranic M, Harley P, et al: Fatty acids mediate the acute extrahepatic effects of insulin on hepatic glucose production in humans. Diabetes 46(7):1111-1119, 1997.

96. Lamarche B, Lewis GF: Atherosclerosis prevention for the next decade: Risk assessment beyond low density lipoprotein cholesterol. Can J Cardiol 14(6):841-851, 1998.

97. Lewis GF, Vranic M, Giacca, A: Role of free fatty acids and glucagon in the peripheral effect of insulin on glucose production in humans. Am J Physiol 275(1 Pt 1): E177-186, 1998.

98. Adeli K, Taghibiglou C, Van Iderstine SC, et al: Mechanisms of hepatic very low-density lipoprotein overproduction in insulin resistance. Trends Cardiovasc Med 11(5):170-176, 2001.

99. Rashid S, Shi ZQ, Niwa M, et al: Beta-blockade, but not normoglycemia or hyperinsulinemia, markedly diminishes stress-induced hyperglycemia in diabetic dogs. Diabetes 49(2):253-262, 2000.

100. Lewis GF: Lipid metabolism. Curr Opin Lipidol 13(1):97-99, 2002.

101. Lewis GF, Carpentier A, Adeli K, et al: Disordered fat storage and mobilization in the pathogenesis of insulin resistance and type 2 diabetes. Endocr Rev 23(2):201-229, 2002.

102. Carpentier A, Taghibiglou C, Leung N, et al: Ameliorated hepatic insulin resistance is associated with normalization of microsomal triglyceride transfer protein expression and reduction in very low density lipoprotein assembly and secretion in the fructose-fed hamster. J Biol Chem 277(32):28795-28802, 2002.

103. Taghibiglou C, Rashid-Kolvear F, Van Iderstine SC, et al: Hepatic very low density lipoprotein-ApoB overproduction is associated with attenuated hepatic insulin signaling and overexpression of protein-tyrosine phosphatase 1B in a fructose-fed hamster model of insulin resistance. J Biol Chem 277(1):793-803, 2002.

104. Lam TK, Carpentier A, Lewis GF, et al: Mechanisms of the free fatty acid-induced increase in hepatic glucose production. Am J Physiol Endocrinol Metab 284(5): E863-873, 2003.

105. Carpentier A, Zinman B, Leung N, et al: Free fatty acid-mediated impairment of glucose-stimulated insulin secretion in nondiabetic Oji-Cree individuals from the Sandy Lake community of Ontario, Canada: A population at very high risk for developing type 2 diabetes. Diabetes 52(6):1485-1495, 2003.

106. Lutz TA, Tschudy S, Mollet A, et al: Dopamine D(2) receptors mediate amylin's acute satiety effect. Am J Physiol Regul Integr Comp Physiol 280(6):R1697-1703, 2001.

107. Scharrer E: Control of food intake by fatty acid oxidation and ketogenesis. Nutrition 15(9):704-714, 1999.

108. Chan L, Jackson RL, O'Malley BW, et al: Synthesis of very low density lipoproteins in the cockerel. Effects of estrogen. J Clin Invest 58(2):368-379, 1976.

109. Miles JM, Haymond MW, Gerich JE: Suppression of glucose production and stimulation of insulin secretion by physiological concentrations of ketone bodies in man. J Clin Endocrinol Metab 52(1):34-37, 1981.

110. Fitz JG: Cellular mechanisms of bile secretion. In Zakim D, Boyer TD (eds): Hepatology: A Textbook of Liver Disease, 3rd ed. Philadelphia, WB Saunders, 1996, pp 362-376.

111. Dawson PA: Bile secretion and the enterohepatic circulation of bile acids. In Feldman M, Friedman LS, Sleisenger MH (eds): Sleisenger & Fordtran's Gastrointestinal and Liver Disease: Pathophysiology/Diagnosis/Management, 7th ed. St. Louis, WB Saunders, 2002, pp 1051-1064.

112. Leonis MA, Balistreri WF: Inherited metabolic disorders of the liver. In Feldman M, Friedman LS, Sleisenger MH (eds): Sleisenger & Fordtran's Gastrointestinal and Liver Disease: Pathophysiology/Diagnosis/Management, 7th ed. Philadelphia, WB Saunders, 2002, pp 1240-1260.

113. Vlahcevic ZR, Heuman DM, Hylemon PB: Physiology and pathophysiology of enterohepatic circulation of bile acids. In Zakim D, Boyer TD (eds): Hepatology: A Textbook of Liver Disease, 3rd ed. Philadelphia, WB Saunders, 1996, pp 376-417.

114. Radnay PA, Duncalf D, Novakovic M, et al: Common bile duct pressure changes after fentanyl, morphine, meperidine, butorphanol, and naloxone. Anesth Analg 63(4):441-444, 1984.

115. Fitz JG: Hepatic encephalopathy, hepatopulmonary syndromes, hepatorenal syndrome, coagulopathy, and

endocrine complications of liver disease. *In* Feldman M, Friedman LS, Sleisenger MH (eds): Sleisenger & Fordtran's Gastrointestinal and Liver Disease: Pathophysiology/ Diagnosis/Management, 7th ed. St. Louis, WB Saunders, 2002, pp 1543-1567.

116. Nelsestuen GL, Shah AM, Harvey SB: Vitamin K–dependent proteins. Vitam Horm 58:355-389, 2000.

117. Sunnerhagen M, Drakenberg T, Forsen S, et al: Effect of Ca^{2+} on the structure of vitamin K–dependent coagulation factors. Haemostasis 26(Suppl 1):45-53, 1996.

118. Berkner KL: The vitamin K–dependent carboxylase. J Nutr 130(8):1877-1880, 2000.

119. Dowd P, Ham SW, Naganathan S, et al: The mechanism of action of vitamin K. Annu Rev Nutr 15:419-440, 1995.

120. Furie BC, Furie, B: Structure and mechanism of action of the vitamin K–dependent gamma-glutamyl carboxylase: recent advances from mutagenesis studies. Thromb Haemost 78(1):595-598, 1997.

121. Suttie JW: Synthesis of vitamin K–dependent proteins. FASEB J 7(5):445-452, 1993.

122. Sugiura I, Furie B, Walsh CT, et al: Propeptide and glutamate-containing substrates bound to the vitamin K–dependent carboxylase convert its vitamin K epoxidase function from an inactive to an active state. Proc Natl Acad Sci U S A 94(17):9069-9074, 1997.

123. Fujita H: Molecular mechanism of heme biosynthesis. Tohoku J Exp Med 183(2):83-99, 1997.

124. Ponka P: Cell biology of heme. Am J Med Sci 318(4):241-256, 1999.

125. Ferreira GC, Gong J: 5-Aminolevulinate synthase and the first step of heme biosynthesis. J Bioenerg Biomembr 27(2):151-159, 1995.

126. Sassa S: Regulation of the genes for heme pathway enzymes in erythroid and in non-erythroid cells. Int J Cell Cloning 8(1):10-26, 1990.

127. Daniell WE, Stockbridge HL, Labbe RF, et al: Environmental chemical exposures and disturbances of heme synthesis. Environ Health Perspect 105(Suppl 1):37-53, 1997.

128. Anderson KE: The porphyrias. *In* Zakim D, Boyer TD (eds): Hepatology: A Textbook of Liver Disease, 3rd ed. Philadelphia, WB Saunders, 1996, pp 417-465.

129. Jensen NF, Fiddler DS, Striepe V: Anesthetic considerations in porphyrias[comment]. Anesth Analg 80(3):591-599, 1995.

130. Ashley EM: Anaesthesia for porphyria. Br J Hosp Med 56(1):37-42, 1996.

131. James MF, Hift RJ: Porphyrias. Br J Anaesth 85(1):143-153, 2000.

132. Baker SD, Taylor B: Anaesthesia is also risky in patients with porphyria [comment]. BMJ 321(7267):1023, 2000.

133. Marks GS, McCluskey SA, Mackie JE, et al: Disruption of hepatic heme biosynthesis after interaction of xenobiotics with cytochrome P-450. FASEB J 2(12):2774-2783, 1988.

134. Marks GS: Exposure to toxic agents: The heme biosynthetic pathway and hemoproteins as indicator. Crit Rev Toxicol 15(2):151-179, 1985.

135. Shibahara S, Kitamuro T, Takahashi K: Heme degradation and human disease: Diversity is the soul of life. Antioxid Redox Signal 4(4):593-602, 2002.

136. Schmid R: Bilirubin metabolism: State of the art. Gastroenterology 74(6):1307-1312, 1978.

137. Moller S, Becker U: Insulin-like growth factor 1 and growth hormone in chronic liver disease. Dig Dis 10(4):239-248, 1992.

138. Rojdmark S, Bloom G, Chou MC, et al: Hepatic extraction of exogenous insulin and glucagon in the dog. Endocrinology 102(3):806-813, 1978.

139. Rojdmark S, Bloom G, Chou MC, et al: Hepatic insulin and glucagon extraction after their augmented secretion in dogs. Am J Physiol 235(1):E88-96, 1978.

140. Laskin DL: Nonparenchymal cells and hepatotoxicity. Semin Liver Dis 10(4):293-304, 1990.

141. Dhainaut JF, Marin N, Mignon A, et al: Hepatic response to sepsis: Interaction between coagulation and inflammatory processes. Crit Care Med 29(7 Suppl):S42-47, 2001.

142. Bosch-Morell F, Flohe L, Marin N, et al: 4-Hydroxynonenal inhibits glutathione peroxidase: Protection by glutathione. Free Radic Biol Med 26(11-12):1383-1387, 1999.

143. Lemasters JJ: V. Necrapoptosis and the mitochondrial permeability transition: Shared pathways to necrosis and apoptosis. Am J Physiol 276(1 Pt 1):G1-6, 1999.

144. Bautista AP, Spitzer JJ: Role of Kupffer cells in the ethanol-induced oxidative stress in the liver. Front Biosci 4:D589-595, 1999.

145. Bailey SM, Reinke LA: Antioxidants and gadolinium chloride attenuate hepatic parenchymal and endothelial cell injury induced by low flow ischemia and reperfusion in perfused rat livers. Free Radic Res 32(6):497-506, 2000.

146. DeLeve LD, McCuskey RS, Wang X, et al: Characterization of a reproducible rat model of hepatic veno-occlusive disease. Hepatology 29(6):1779-1791, 1999.

147. Farrell GC: Liver disease caused by drugs, anesthetics, and toxins. *In* Feldman M, Friedman LS, Sleisenger MH (eds): Sleisenger & Fordtran's Gastrointestinal and Liver Disease: Pathophysiology/Diagnosis/Management, 7th ed. St. Louis, WB Saunders, 2002, pp 1403-1447.

148. Vessey DA: Metabolism of xenobiotics by the human liver. *In* Zakim D, Boyer TD (eds): Hepatology: A Textbook of Liver Disease, 3rd ed. Philadelphia, WB Saunders, 1996, pp 257-306.

149. Estabrook R: An introduction to the cytochrome P450s. Mol Aspects Med 20(1-2):5-12, 13-137, 1999.

150. Murray M: Mechanisms and significance of inhibitory drug interactions involving cytochrome P450 enzymes [review]. Int J Mol Med 3(3):227-238, 1999.

151. Murray M: Induction and inhibition of CYPs and implications for medicine. Mol Aspects Med 20(1-2):24-33, 34-137, 1999.

152. Hasle JA: Pharmacogenetics of cytochromes P450. Mol Aspects Med 20(1-2):12-24, 25-137, 1999.

153. Sies H: Oxidative stress: from basic research to clinical application. Am J Med 91(3C):31S-38S, 1991.

154. Conney AH: Pharmacological implications of microsomal enzyme induction. Pharmacol Rev 19(3):317-366, 1967.

155. Sesardic D, Boobis AR, Edwards RJ, et al: A form of cytochrome P450 in man, orthologous to formed in the rat, catalyses the O-deethylation of phenacetin and is inducible by cigarette smoking. Br J Clin Pharmacol 26(4):363-372, 1988.

156. Moore LB, Goodwin B, Jones SA, et al: St. John's wort induces hepatic drug metabolism through activation of the pregnane X receptor. Proc Natl Acad Sci U S A 97(13):7500-7502, 2000.

157. Sinclair JF, Szakacs JG, Wood SG, et al: Acetaminophen hepatotoxicity precipitated by short-term treatment of rats with ethanol and isopentanol: Protection by triacetyloleandomycin. Biochem Pharmacol 59(4):445-454, 2000.

158. Goodwin B, Hodgson E, Liddle C: The orphan human pregnane X receptor mediates the transcriptional activation of CYP3A4 by rifampicin through a distal enhancer module. Mol Pharmacol 56(6):1329-1339, 1999.

159. Moore LB, Parks DJ, Jones SA, et al: Orphan nuclear receptors constitutive androstane receptor and pregnane X receptor share xenobiotic and steroid ligands. J Biol Chem 275(20):15122-15127, 2000.

160. del Castillo-Olivares A, Gil G: Role of FXR and FTF in bile acid-mediated suppression of cholesterol 7 alpha-hydroxylase transcription. Nucleic Acids Res 28(18):3587-3593, 2000.

161. Meech R, Mackenzie PI: Structure and function of uridine diphosphate glucuronosyltransferases. Clin Exp Pharmacol Physiol 24(12):907-915, 1997.

162. Lee J, Boyer JL: Molecular alterations in hepatocyte transport mechanisms in acquired cholestatic liver disorders. Semin Liver Dis 20(3):373-384, 2000.

163. Trauner M, Meier PJ, Boyer JL: Molecular pathogenesis of cholestasis. N Engl J Med 339(17):1217-1227, 1998.

164. Huang L, Smit JW, Meijer DK, et al: Mrp2 is essential for estradiol-17beta(beta-D-glucuronide)-induced cholestasis in rats. Hepatology 32(1):66-72, 2000.

165. Stieger B, Fattinger K, Madon J, et al: Drug- and estrogen-induced cholestasis through inhibition of the hepatocellular bile salt export pump (Bsep) of rat liver. Gastroenterology 118(2):422-430, 2000.

166. George J, Byth K, Farrell GC: Influence of clinicopathological variables on CYP protein expression in human liver. J Gastroenterol Hepatol 11(1):33-39, 1996.

167. Alvares AP, Anderson KE, Conney AH, et al: Interactions between nutritional factors and drug biotransformations in man. Proc Natl Acad Sci U S A 73(7):2501-2504, 1976.

168. Pantuck EJ, Pantuck CB, Weissman C, et al: Effects of parenteral nutritional regimens on oxidative drug metabolism. Anesthesiology 60(6):534-536, 1984.

169. Whitehouse MW, Beck FJ: Impaired drug metabolism in rats with adjuvant-induced arthritis: A brief review. Drug Metab Dispos 1(1):251-255, 1973.

170. Elin RJ, Vesell ES, Wolff SM: Effects of etiocholanolone-induced fever on plasma antipyrine half-lives and metabolic clearance. Clin Pharmacol Ther 17(4):447-457, 1975.

171. George J, Byth K, Farrell GC: Age but not gender selectively affects expression of individual cytochrome P450 proteins in human liver. Biochem Pharmacol 50(5):727-730, 1995.

172. Turnheim K: Drug dosage in the elderly. Is it rational? Drugs Aging 13(5):357-379, 1998.

173. Hammerlein A, Derendorf H, Lowenthal DT: Pharmacokinetic and pharmacodynamic changes in the elderly. Clinical implications. Clin Pharmacokinet 35(1):49-64, 1998.

174. Dodds C: Anaesthetic drugs in the elderly. Pharmacol Ther 66(2):369-386, 1995.

175. Reilly CS, Wood AJ, Koshakji RP, et al: The effect of halothane on drug disposition: contribution of changes in intrinsic drug metabolizing capacity and hepatic blood flow. Anesthesiology 63(1):70-76, 1985.

176. Aune H, Bessesen A, Olsen H, et al: Acute effects of halothane and enflurane on drug metabolism and protein synthesis in isolated rat hepatocytes. Acta Pharmacol Toxicol (Copenh) 53(5):363-368, 1983.

177. Livingston A, Waterman AE: The development of tolerance to ketamine in rats and the significance of hepatic metabolism. Br J Pharmacol 64(1):63-69, 1978.

178. Kanto J, Iisalo E, Lehtinen V, et al: The concentrations of diazepam and its metabolites in the plasma after an acute and chronic administration. Psychopharmacologia 36(2):123-131, 1974.

179. Karlin JM, Kutt H: Acute diphenylhydantoin intoxication following halothane anesthesia. J Pediatr 76(6):941-944, 1970.

180. Ghoneim MM, Delle M, Wilson WR, et al: Alteration of warfarin kinetics in man associated with exposure to an operating-room environment. Anesthesiology 43(3):333-336, 1975.

181. White PF, Johnston RR, Pudwill CR: Interaction of ketamine and halothane in rats. Anesthesiology 42(2):179-186, 1975.

182. Fish KJ, Rice SA: Halothane inhibits metabolism of enflurane in Fischer 344 rats. Anesthesiology 59(5):417-420, 1983.

183. Dale O, Nielsen K, Westgaard G, et al: Drug metabolizing enzymes in the rat after inhalation of halothane and enflurane. Different pattern of response in liver, kidney and lung and possible implications for toxicity. Br J Anaesth 55(12):1217-1224, 1983.

184. Duvaldestin P, Mazze RI, Nivoche Y, et al: Occupational exposure to halothane results in enzyme induction in anesthetists. Anesthesiology 54(1):57-60, 1981.

185. Wilkinson GR, Schenker S: Drug disposition and liver disease. Drug Metab Rev 4(2):139-175, 1975.

186. Wilkinson GR, Shand DG: Commentary: A physiological approach to hepatic drug clearance. Clin Pharmacol Ther 18(4):377-390, 1975.

187. Williams RL, Mamelok RD: Hepatic disease and drug pharmacokinetics. Clin Pharmacokinet 5(6):528-547, 1980.

188. Williams RL: Drug administration in hepatic disease. N Engl J Med 309(26):1616-1622, 1983.

189. Adedoyin A, Branch RA: Pharmacokinetics. *In* Zakim D, Boyer TD (eds): Hepatology: A Textbook of Liver Disease, 3rd ed. Philadelphia, WB Saunders, 1996, pp 307-322.

190. Davern TJ, Scharschmidt BF: Biochemical liver tests. *In* Feldman M, Friedman LS, Sleisenger, MH (eds): Sleisenger & Fordtran's Gastrointestinal and Liver Disease: Pathophysiology/Diagnosis/Management, 7th ed. St. Louis, WB Saunders, 2002, pp 1227-1239.

191. Hussey AJ, Aldridge LM, Paul D, et al: Plasma glutathione S-transferase concentration as a measure of hepatocellular integrity following a single general anaesthetic with halothane, enflurane or isoflurane. Br J Anaesth 60(2):130-135, 1988.

192. Redick JA, Jakoby WB, Baron J: Immunohistochemical localization of glutathione S-transferases in livers of untreated rats. J Biol Chem 257(24):15200-15203, 1982.

193. Rothschild MA, Oratz M, Zimmon D, et al: Albumin synthesis in cirrhotic subjects with ascites studied with carbonate-14C. J Clin Invest 48(2):344-350, 1969.

194. Sussman NL: Fulminant hepatic failure. *In* Zakim D, Boyer TD (eds): Hepatology: A Textbook of Liver Disease, 3rd ed. Philadelphia, WB. Saunders, 1996, pp 618-650.

195. Aranha GV, Greenlee HB: Intra-abdominal surgery in patients with advanced cirrhosis. Arch Surg 121(3):275-277, 1986.

196. Roy-Chowdhury J, Jansen PLM: Bilirubin metabolism and its disorders. *In* Zakim D, Boyer TD (eds): Hepatology: A Textbook of Liver Disease, 3rd ed. Philadelphia, WB Saunders, 1996, pp 323-362.

197. Drygiannakis D, Lionis C, Drygiannakis I, et al: Low prevalence of liver-kidney microsomal autoantibodies of type 1 (LKM1) in hepatitis C seropositive subjects on Crete, Greece. BMC Gastroenterol 1(1):4, 2001.

198. Zamanou A, Tsirogianni A, Terzoglou C, et al: Anti-smooth muscle antibodies (ASMAs) and anti-cytoskeleton antibodies (ACTAs) in liver diseases: A comparison of classical indirect immunofluorescence with ELISA. J Clin Lab Anal 16(4):194-201, 2002.

199. Strassburg CP, Manns MP: Autoimmune tests in primary biliary cirrhosis. Baillieres Best Pract Res Clin Gastroenterol 14(4):585-599, 2000.

200. Nocente R, Ceccanti M, Bertazzoni G, et al: HCV infection and extrahepatic manifestations. Hepatogastroenterology 50(52):1149-1154, 2003.

201. Invernizzi P, Crosignani A, Battezzati PM, et al: Comparison of the clinical features and clinical course of antimitochondrial antibody-positive and -negative primary biliary cirrhosis. Hepatology 25(5):1090-1095, 1997.

202. Long SA, Van de Water J, Gershwin ME: Antimitochondrial antibodies in primary biliary cirrhosis: The role of xenobiotics. Autoimmun Rev 1(1-2):37-42, 2002.

203. Jones DE: Autoantigens in primary biliary cirrhosis. J Clin Pathol 53(11):813-821, 2000.

204. Mondelli MU, Manns M Ferrari, C: Does the immune response play a role in the pathogenesis of chronic liver disease? Arch Pathol Lab Med 112(5):489-497, 1988.

205. Nishio A, Bass NM, Luketic VA, et al: Primary biliary cirrhosis: from induction to destruction. Semin Gastrointest Dis 12(2):89-102, 2001.

206. Sasaki M, Ansari AA, Nakanuma Y, et al: The immunopathology of primary biliary cirrhosis: thoughts for the millennium. Arch Immunol Ther Exp (Warsz) 48(1):1-10, 2000.

207. Okolicsanyi L, Fabris L: Diagnostic approach to primary sclerosing cholangitis: open questions. Ital J Gastroenterol 23(7):436-441, 1991.

208. Tanaka A, Miyakawa H, Luketic, VA et al: The diagnostic value of anti-mitochondrial antibodies, especially in primary biliary cirrhosis. Cell Mol Biol (Noisy-le-grand) 48(3):295-299, 2002.

209. Lacerda MA, Ludwig J, Dickson ER, et al: Antimitochondrial antibody-negative primary biliary cirrhosis. Am J Gastroenterol 90(2):247-249, 1995.

210. Czaja A: Autoimmune liver disease. *In* Zakim D, Boyer T (eds): Hepatology: A Textbook of Liver Disease, 3rd ed. Philadelphia, WB Saunders, 1996, pp 1259-1292.

211. Czaja AJ: Autoimmune hepatitis. In Feldman M, Friedman LS, Sleisenger MH (eds): Sleisenger & Fordtran's Gastrointestinal and Liver Disease: Pathophysiology/ Diagnosis/Management, 7th ed. St. Louis, WB Saunders, 2002, pp 1462-1474.

212. Ajisaka H, Shimizu K, Miwa K: Immunohistochemical study of protein induced by vitamin K absence or antagonist II in hepatocellular carcinoma. J Surg Oncol 84(2):89-93, 2003.

213. Sugimoto H, Takeda S, Inoue S, et al: Des-gamma-carboxy prothrombin (DCP) ratio, a novel parameter measured by monoclonal antibodies MU-3 and 19B7, as a new prognostic indicator for hepatocellular carcinoma. Liver Int 23(1): 38-44, 2003.

214. Yamanaka J, Yamanaka N, Nakasho K, et al: Clinicopathologic analysis of stage II-III hepatocellular carcinoma showing early massive recurrence after liver resection. J Gastroenterol Hepatol 15(10):1192-1198, 2000.

215. Fujioka M, Nakashima Y, Nakashima O, et al: Immunohistologic study on the expressions of alpha-fetoprotein and protein induced by vitamin K absence or antagonist II in surgically resected small hepatocellular carcinoma. Hepatology 34(6):1128-1134, 2001.

216. Cui R, He J, Zhang F, et al: Diagnostic value of protein induced by vitamin K absence (PIVKAII) and hepatoma-specific band of serum gamma-glutamyl transferase (GGTII) as hepatocellular carcinoma markers complementary to alpha-fetoprotein. Br J Cancer 88(12):1878-1882, 2003.

217. Barnes P, Lunzer M, O'Halloran M: Comparative sensitivity of serum cholylglycine concentration and bromsulphalein retention in patients with early and late alcoholic liver disease. Aust N Z J Med 16(6):785-787, 1986.

218. Denaro CP, Jacob P 3rd, Benowitz NL: Evaluation of pharmacokinetic methods used to estimate caffeine clearance and comparison with a Bayesian forecasting method. Ther Drug Monit 20(1):78-87, 1998.

219. Jover R, Carnicer F, Sanchez-Paya J, et al: Salivary caffeine clearance predicts survival in patients with liver cirrhosis. Am J Gastroenterol 92(10):1905-1908, 1997.

220. Lewis FW, Rector WG JR: Caffeine clearance in cirrhosis. The value of simplified determinations of liver metabolic capacity [comment]. J Hepatol 14(2-3):157-162, 1992.

221. McDonagh JE, Nathan VV, Bonavia IC, et al: Caffeine clearance by enzyme multiplied immunoassay technique: A simple, inexpensive, and useful indicator of liver function. Gut 32(6):681-684, 1991.

222. Wahllander A, Mohr S, Paumgartner, G: Assessment of hepatic function. Comparison of caffeine clearance in serum and saliva during the day and at night. J Hepatol 10(2):129-137, 1990.

223. Schnegg M, Lauterburg BH: Quantitative liver function in the elderly assessed by galactose elimination capacity, aminopyrine demethylation and caffeine clearance. J Hepatol 3(2):164-171, 1986.

224. Szabo G, Benyo I, Sandor J, et al: Estimation of the hepatic blood flow in the dog with the Xe133 and hydrogen wash-out Au190-colloid uptake techniques and with the electromagnetic flowmeter. Res Exp Med (Berl) 169(1):69-76, 1976.

225. Kraul H, Truckenbrodt J, Sigusch H, et al: [Comparison of ICG elimination with biotransformation of model substances and histological features of liver biopsy in liver diseases]. Gastroenterol J 51(3-4):123-128, 1991.

226. Huet PM, Lavoie P, Viallet A: Simultaneous estimation of hepatic and portal blood flows by an indicator dilution technique. J Lab Clin Med 82(5):836-846, 1973.

227. Hopkinson BR, Schenk WG JR: The electromagnetic measurement of liver blood flow and cardiac output in conscious dogs during feeding and exercise. Surgery 63(6):970-975, 1968.

228. Whitcomb DC: Hereditary and childhood disorders of the pancreas, including cystic fibrosis. In Feldman M, Friedman LS, Sleisenger MH (eds): Sleisenger & Fordtran's Gastrointestinal and Liver Disease: Pathophysiology/ Diagnosis/Management,7th ed. St. Louis, WB Saunders, 2002, pp 881-912.

229. Kang HK, Jeong YY, Choi JH, et al: Three-dimensional multi-detector row CT portal venography in the evaluation of portosystemic collateral vessels in liver cirrhosis. Radiographics 22(5):1053-1061, 2002.

230. Ostroff JW, LaBerge JM: Endoscopic and radiologic treatment of biliary disease. In Feldman M, Friedman LS, Sleisenger MH (eds): Sleisenger & Fordtran's Gastrointestinal and Liver Disease: Pathophysiology/ Diagnosis/Management, 7th ed. St. Louis, WB Saunders, 2002, pp 1167-1192.

231. Toledo-Pereyra LE, Suzuki S: Cellular and biomolecular mechanisms of liver ischemia and reperfusion injury. Transplant Proc 26(1):325-327, 1994.

232. Kurokawa T, Nonami T, Harada A, et al: Mechanism and prevention of ischemia-reperfusion injury of the liver. Semin Surg Oncol 12(3):179-182, 1996.

233. Kaplowitz N: Mechanisms of liver cell injury. J Hepatol 32(1 Suppl):39-47, 2000.

234. Galle PR: Apoptosis in liver disease. J Hepatol 27(2):405-412, 1997.

235. Patel T, Steer CJ, Gores GJ: Apoptosis and the liver: A mechanism of disease, growth regulation, and carcinogenesis. Hepatology 30(3):811-815, 1999.

236. Patel T: Apoptosis in hepatic pathophysiology. Clin Liver Dis 4(2):295-317, 2000.

237. Kaplowitz N: Cell death at the millennium. Implications for liver diseases. Clin Liver Dis 4(1):1-23, v, 2000.

238. Nielsen VG, McCammon AT, Tan S, et al: Xanthine oxidase inactivation attenuates postocclusion shock after descending thoracic aorta occlusion and reperfusion in rabbit. J Thorac Cardiovasc Surg 110(3):715-722, 1995.

239. Jaeschke H, Gores GJ, Cederbaum AI, et al: Mechanisms of hepatotoxicity. Toxicol Sci 65(2):166-176, 2002.

240. Carden DL, Granger DN: Pathophysiology of ischaemia-reperfusion injury. J Pathol 190(3):255-266, 2000.

241. Arai M, Thurman RG, Lemasters JJ: Ischemic preconditioning of rat livers against cold storage-reperfusion injury: Role of nonparenchymal cells and the phenomenon of heterologous preconditioning [comment]. Liver Transpl 7(4):292-299, 2001.

242. Weinbroum A, Nielsen VG, Tan S, et al: Liver ischemia-reperfusion increases pulmonary permeability in rat: Role of circulating xanthine oxidase. Am J Physiol 268(6 Pt 1):G988-996, 1995.

243. Kaplowitz N, Tsukamoto H: Oxidative stress and liver disease. Prog Liver Dis 14:131-159, 1996.

244. Ursini F, Maiorino M, Roveri A: Phospholipid hydroperoxide glutathione peroxidase (PHGPx): More than an antioxidant enzyme? Biomed Environ Sci 10(2-3):327-332, 1997.

245. Doroshow JH, Akman S, Chu FF, et al: Role of the glutathione-glutathione peroxidase cycle in the cytotoxicity of the anticancer quinones. Pharmacol Ther 47(3):359-370, 1990.

246. Michiels C, Raes M, Toussaint O, et al: Importance of Se-glutathione peroxidase, catalase, and Cu/Zn-SOD for cell survival against oxidative stress. Free Radic Biol Med 17(3):235-248, 1994.

247. Luo GM, Ren XJ, Liu JQ, et al: Towards more efficient glutathione peroxidase mimics: substrate recognition and catalytic group assembly. Curr Med Chem 10(13):1151-1183, 2003.

248. Kim JS, Qian T, Lemasters JJ: Mitochondrial permeability transition in the switch from necrotic to apoptotic cell death in ischemic rat hepatocytes. Gastroenterology 124(2):494-503, 2003.

249. Sawaya DE Jr, Brown M, Minardi A, et al: The role of ischemic preconditioning in the recruitment of rolling and adherent leukocytes in hepatic venules after ischemia/reperfusion. J Surg Res 85(1):163-170, 1999.

250. Kurose I, Argenbright LW, Wolf R, et al: Ischemia/ reperfusion-induced microvascular dysfunction: role of oxidants and lipid mediators. Am J Physiol 272(6 Pt 2): H2976-2982, 1997.

251. Yokoyama Y, Beckman JS, Beckman TK, et al: Circulating xanthine oxidase: potential mediator of ischemic injury. Am J Physiol 258(4 Pt 1):G564-570, 1990.

252. Adkison D, Hollwarth ME, Benoit JN, et al: Role of free radicals in ischemia-reperfusion injury to the liver, Acta Physiol Scand Suppl 548:101-107, 1986.

253. Toledo-Pereyra LH: Liver preservation: experimental and clinical observations. Transplant Proc 20(5):965-968, 1988.

254. Nielsen VG, Tan S, Weinbroum A, et al: Lung injury after hepatoenteric ischemia-reperfusion: Role of xanthine oxidase. Am J Respir Crit Care Med 154(5):1364-1369, 1996.

255. Nielsen VG, Tan S, Baird MS, et al: Gastric intramucosal pH and multiple organ injury: impact of ischemia-reperfusion and xanthine oxidase. Crit Care Med 24(8):1339-1344, 1996.

256. Nielsen VG, Tan S, Baird MS, et al: Xanthine oxidase mediates myocardial injury after hepatoenteric ischemia-reperfusion. Crit Care Med 25(6):1044-1050, 1997.

257. Nielsen VG, Tan S, Kirk KA, et al: Halothane and xanthine oxidase increase hepatocellular enzyme release and circulating lactate after ischemia-reperfusion in rabbits. Anesthesiology 87(4):908-917, 1997.

258. Nielsen VG, Tan S, Brix AE, et al: Hextend (hetastarch solution) decreases multiple organ injury and xanthine oxidase release after hepatoenteric ischemia-reperfusion in rabbits. Crit Care Med 25(9):1565-1574, 1997.

259. Pesonen EJ, Linder N, Raivio KO, et al: Circulating xanthine oxidase and neutrophil activation during human liver transplantation. Gastroenterology 114(5):1009-1015, 1998.

260. Tan S, Yokoyama Y, Dickens E, et al: Xanthine oxidase activity in the circulation of rats following hemorrhagic shock. Free Radic Biol Med 15(4):407-414, 1993.

261. Radi R, Rubbo H, Bush K, et al: Xanthine oxidase binding to glycosaminoglycans: Kinetics and superoxide dismutase interactions of immobilized xanthine oxidase-heparin complexes. Arch Biochem Biophys 339(1):125-135, 1997.

262. Adachi T, Fukushima T, Usami Y, et al: Binding of human xanthine oxidase to sulphated glycosaminoglycans on the endothelial-cell surface. Biochem J 289(Pt 2):523-527, 1993.

263. Beckman JS, Koppenol WH: Nitric oxide, superoxide, and peroxynitrite: The good, the bad, and ugly. Am J Physiol 271(5 Pt 1):C1424-1437, 1996.

264. Jamieson NV, Sundberg R, Lindell S, et al: The 24- to 48-hour preservation of canine liver by simple cold storage using UW lactobionate solution. Transplant Proc 21(1 Pt 2):1292-1293, 1989.

265. Marsh DC, Vreugdenhil PK, Mack VE, et al: Glycine protects hepatocytes from injury caused by anoxia, cold ischemia and mitochondrial inhibitors, but not injury caused by calcium ionophores or oxidative stress. Hepatology 17(1):91-98, 1993.

266. den Butter G, Marsh DC, Lindell SL, et al: Amino acids to suppress reperfusion injury after liver preservation. Transplant Proc 23(5):2378-2379, 1991.

267. Jaeschke H, Lemasters JJ: Apoptosis versus oncotic necrosis in hepatic ischemia/reperfusion injury. Gastroenterology 125(4):1246-1257, 2003.

268. Sindram D, Rudiger, HA, Upadhya AG, et al: Ischemic preconditioning protects against cold ischemic injury through an oxidative stress dependent mechanism. J Hepatol 36(1):78-84, 2002.

269. Lehnert M, Artee GE, Smutney OM, et al: Dependence of liver injury after hemorrhage/resuscitation in mice on NADPH oxidase-derived superoxide. Shock 19(4): 345-351, 2003.

270. Schemmer P, Connor HD, Arteel GE, et al: Reperfusion injury in livers due to gentle in situ organ manipulation during harvest involves hypoxia and free radicals. J Pharmacol Exp Ther 290(1):235-240, 1999.

271. Lee YG, Lee SH, Lee SM: Role of Kupffer cells in cold/warm ischemia-reperfusion injury of rat liver. Arch Pharm Res 23(6):620-625, 2000.

272. Schauer RJ, Bilzer M, Kalmuk S, et al: Microcirculatory failure after rat liver transplantation is related to Kupffer cell-derived oxidant stress but not involved in early graft dysfunction. Transplantation 72(10):1692-1699, 2001.

273. Radi R, Cassina A, Hodara R: Nitric oxide and peroxynitrite interactions with mitochondria. Biol Chem 383(3-4):401-409, 2002.

274. Warle MC, Farhan A, Metselaar HJ, et al: In vitro cytokine production of TNFalpha and IL-13 correlates with acute liver transplant rejection. Hum Immunol 62(11):1258-1265, 2001.

275. Imamura H, Sutto F, Brault A, et al: Role of Kupffer cells in cold ischemia/reperfusion injury of rat liver [comment]. Gastroenterology 109(1):189-197, 1995.

276. Kerkweg U, Jacob M, De Groot H, et al: Cold-induced apoptosis of rat liver endothelial cells: contribution of mitochondrial alterations. Transplantation 76(3):501-508, 2003.

277. Doeppner TR, Grune T, de Groot H, et al: Cold-induced apoptosis of rat liver endothelial cells: involvement of the proteasome. Transplantation 75(12):1946-1953, 2003.

278. Sindram D, Porte RJ, Hoffman MR, et al: Platelets induce sinusoidal endothelial cell apoptosis upon reperfusion of the cold ischemic rat liver. Gastroenterology 118(1):183-191, 2000.

279. Lemasters JJ, Thurman RG: Reperfusion injury after liver preservation for transplantation. Annu Rev Pharmacol Toxicol 37:327-338, 1997.

280. Shedlofsky SI, Israel BC, McClain CJ, et al: Endotoxin administration to humans inhibits hepatic cytochrome P450-mediated drug metabolism. J Clin Invest 94(6):2209-2214, 1994.

281. Gerson RJ, Casini A, Gilfor D, et al: Oxygen-mediated cell injury in the killing of cultured hepatocytes by acetaminophen. Biochem Biophys Res Commun 126(3):1129-1137, 1985.

282. Casini A, Giorli M, Hyland RJ, et al: Mechanisms of cell injury in the killing of cultured hepatocytes by bromobenzene. J Biol Chem 257(12):6721-6728, 1982.

283. Tang W, Stearns RA, Bandiera SM, et al: Studies on cytochrome P-450-mediated bioactivation of diclofenac in rats and in human hepatocytes: Identification of glutathione conjugated metabolites. Drug Metab Dispos 27(3):365-372, 1999.

284. Wang M, Dickinson RG: Disposition and covalent binding of diflunisal and diflunisal acyl glucuronide in the isolated perfused rat liver. Drug Metab Dispos 26(2):98-104, 1998.

285. Tang W, Borel AG, Abbott FS: Conjugation of glutathione with a toxic metabolite of valproic acid, (E)-2-propyl-2,4-pentadienoic acid, catalyzed by rat hepatic glutathione-S-transferases. Drug Metab Dispos 24(4):436-446, 1996.

286. Fau D, Lekehal M, Farrell G, et al: Diterpenoids from germander, an herbal medicine, induce apoptosis in isolated rat hepatocytes [comment]. Gastroenterology 113(4):1334-1346, 1997.

287. Haouzi D, Lekehal M, Moreau A, et al: Cytochrome P450-generated reactive metabolites cause mitochondrial permeability transition, caspase activation, and apoptosis in rat hepatocytes. Hepatology 32(2):303-311, 2000.

288. Lewis W, Dalakas MC: Mitochondrial toxicity of antiviral drugs. Nat Med 1(5):417-422, 1995.

289. Gut J, Christen U, Huwyler J, et al: Molecular mimicry of trifluoroacetylated human liver protein adducts by constitutive proteins and immunochemical evidence for its impairment in halothane hepatitis. European Journal of Biochemistry 210(2):569-576, 1992.

290. Kretz-Rommel A, Boelsterli UA: Cytotoxic activity of T cells and non-T cells from diclofenac-immunized mice against cultured syngeneic hepatocytes exposed to diclofenac. Hepatology 22(1):213-222, 1995.

291. Bourdi M, Larrey D, Nataf J, et al: Anti-liver endoplasmic reticulum autoantibodies are directed against human cytochrome P-450IA2. A specific marker of dihydralazine-induced hepatitis. J Clin Invest 85(6):1967-1973, 1990.

292. Lecoeur S, Bonierbale E, Challine D, et al: Specificity of in vitro covalent binding of tienilic acid metabolites to human liver microsomes in relationship to the type of hepatotoxicity: comparison with two directly hepatotoxic drugs. Chem Res Toxicol 7(3):434-442, 1994.

293. Mushlin PS, Gelman S: Liver dysfunction after anesthesia. *In* Benumof JL, Saidman LJ (eds): Anesthesia and Perioperative Complications, 2nd ed. St. Louis, Mosby, 1999, pp 441-470.

294. Bardag-Gorce F, French BA, Li J, et al: The importance of cycling of blood alcohol levels in the pathogenesis of experimental alcoholic liver disease in rats. Gastroenterology 123(1):325-335, 2002.

295. Tonnesen H, Kehlet H: Preoperative alcoholism and postoperative morbidity. Br J Surg 86(7):869-874, 1999.

296. Nanji AA, Su GL, Laposata M, et al: Pathogenesis of alcoholic liver disease—recent advances. Alcohol Clin Exp Res 26(5):731-736, 2002.

297. Lieber CS: S-adenosyl-L-methionine: Its role in the treatment of liver disorders. Am J Clin Nutr 76(5):1183S-1187S, 2002.

298. Lieber CS: Alcoholic liver injury: Pathogenesis and therapy in 2001. Pathol Biol 49(9):738-752, 2001.

299. Lieber CS: Alcoholic liver disease: New insights in pathogenesis lead to new treatments. J Hepatol 32(1 Suppl):113-128, 2000.

300. Lieber CS: Microsomal ethanol-oxidizing system (MEOS): The first 30 years (1968-1998)—a review. Alcohol Clin Exp Res 23(6):991-1007, 1999.

301. Lieber CS: Cytochrome P-4502E1: Its physiological and pathological role. Physiol Rev 77(2):517-544, 1997.

302. Zima T, Fialova L, Mestek O, et al: Oxidative stress, metabolism of ethanol and alcohol-related diseases. Biomed Sci 8(1):59-70, 2001.

303. Saleem MM, Al-Tamer YY, Skursky L, et al: Alcohol dehydrogenase activity in the human tissues. Biochem Med 31(1):1-9, 1984.

304. Dow J, Krasner N, Goldberg A: Ethanol oxidizing enzyme activities in liver disease. Br J Clin Pharmacol 3(3):461-467, 1976.

305. Panes J, Soler X, Pares A, et al: Influence of liver disease on hepatic alcohol and aldehyde dehydrogenases. Gastroenterology 97(3):708-714, 1989.

306. Bosron WF, Li TK: Genetic polymorphism of human liver alcohol and aldehyde dehydrogenases, and their relationship to alcohol metabolism and alcoholism. Hepatology 6(3):502-510, 1986.

307. Ehrig T, Bosron WF, Li TK: Alcohol and aldehyde dehydrogenase. Alcohol Alcohol 25(2-3):105-116, 1990.

308. Ramchandani VA, Bosron WF, Li TK: Research advances in ethanol metabolism. Pathol Biol 49(9):676-682, 2001.

309. Sherman DI, Ward RJ, Warren-Perry M, et al: Association of restriction fragment length polymorphism in alcohol dehydrogenase 2 gene with alcohol induced liver damage [comment]. BMJ 307(6916):1388-1390, 1993.

310. Poupon RE, Nalpas B, Coutelle C, et al: Polymorphism of alcohol dehydrogenase, alcohol and aldehyde dehydrogenase activities: Implication in alcoholic cirrhosis in white patients. The French Group for Research on Alcohol and Liver [comment]. Hepatology 15(6):1017-1022, 1992.

311. Crabb DW, Edenberg HJ, Bosron WF, et al: Genotypes for aldehyde dehydrogenase deficiency and alcohol sensitivity. The inactive ALDH2(2) allele is dominant. J Clin Invest 83(1):314-316, 1989.

312. Thiele GM, Miller JA, Klassen LW, et al: Long-term ethanol administration alters the degradation of acetaldehyde adducts by liver endothelial cells. Hepatology 24(3):643-648, 1996.

313. Shaw S, Rubin KP, Lieber CS: Depressed hepatic glutathione and increased diene conjugates in alcoholic liver disease. Evidence of lipid peroxidation. Dig Dis Sci 28(7):585-589, 1983.

314. Roll FJ, Bissell DM, Perez HD: Human hepatocytes metabolizing ethanol generate a non-polar chemotactic factor for human neutrophils. Biochem Biophys Res Commun 137(2):688-694, 1986.

315. Williams AJ, Barry RE: Superoxide anion production and degranulation of rat neutrophils in response to acetaldehyde-altered liver cell membranes. Clin Sci (Lond) 71(3):313-318, 1986.

316. Lewis KO, Paton A: Could superoxide cause cirrhosis? Lancet 2(8291):188-189, 1982.

317. Holt K, Bennett M, Chojkie, M: Acetaldehyde stimulates collagen and noncollagen protein production by human fibroblasts. Hepatology 4(5):843-848, 1984.

318. Mezey E: Commentary on the hypermetabolic state and the role of oxygen in alcohol-induced liver injury. Recent Dev Alcohol 2:135-141, 1984.

319. Ito D, Ishii H, Kato S, et al: Significance of alcohol dehydrogenase (ADH) as a marker of hepatic centrilobular injury: A biochemical and immunohistochemical study. Alcohol Alcohol Suppl(1):523-527, 1987.

320. Nanji AA, Zakim D: Alcoholic liver disease. *In* Zakim D, Boyer TD (eds): Hepatology: A Textbook of Liver Disease, 3rd ed. Philadelphia, WB Saunders, 1996, pp 891-961.

321. Oshita M, Takei Y, Kawano S, et al: Endogenous nitric oxide attenuates ethanol-induced perturbation of hepatic circulation in the isolated perfused rat liver. Hepatology 20(4 Pt 1):961-965, 1994.

322. Nanji AA, Greenberg SS, Tahan SR, et al: Nitric oxide production in experimental alcoholic liver disease in the rat: Role in protection from injury. Gastroenterology 109(3):899-907, 1995.

323. Granger DN, Korthuis RJ: Physiologic mechanisms of postischemic tissue injury. Annu Rev Physiol 57:311-332, 1995.

324. Carden DL, Young JA, Granger DN: Pulmonary microvascular injury after intestinal ischemia-reperfusion: Role of P-selectin. J Appl Physiol 75(6):2529-2534, 1993.

325. Mulligan MS, Smith CW, Anderson DC, et al: Role of leukocyte adhesion molecules in complement-induced lung injury. J Immunol 150(6):2401-2406, 1993.

326. McClain C, Hill D, Schmidt J, et al: Cytokines and alcoholic liver disease. Semin Liver Dis 13(2):170-182, 1993.

327. Nordmann R: Alcohol and antioxidant systems. Alcohol Alcohol 29(5):513-522, 1994.

328. Reinke LA, Kotake Y, McCay PB, et al: Spin-trapping studies of hepatic free radicals formed following the acute administration of ethanol to rats: In vivo detection of 1-hydroxyethyl radicals with PBN. Free Radic Biol Med 11(1):31-39, 1991.

329. Nanji AA, Griniuviene B, Sadrzadeh SM, et al: Effect of type of dietary fat and ethanol on antioxidant enzyme mRNA induction in rat liver. J Lipid Res 36(4):736-744, 1995.

330. Rosser BG, Gores GJ: Liver cell necrosis: Cellular mechanisms and clinical implications. Gastroenterology 108(1):252-275, 1995.

331. Wang JF, Greenberg SS, Spitzer JJ: Chronic alcohol administration stimulates nitric oxide formation in the rat liver with or without pretreatment by lipopolysaccharide. Alcohol Clin Exp Res 19(2):387-393, 1995.

332. Skinner KA, White CR, Patel R, et al: Nitrosation of uric acid by peroxynitrite. Formation of a vasoactive nitric oxide donor. J Biol Chem 273(38):24491-24497, 1998.

333. Beckman JS: Protein tyrosine nitration and peroxynitrite [comment]. FASEB J 16(9):1144, 2002.

334. Beckman JS: -OONO: Rebounding from nitric oxide [comment]. Circ Res 89(4):295-297, 2001.

335. Reiter CD, Teng RJ, Beckman JS: Superoxide reacts with nitric oxide to nitrate tyrosine at physiological pH via peroxynitrite. J Biol Chem 275(42):32460-32466, 2000.

336. Beckmann JS, Ye YZ, Anderson PG, et al: Extensive nitration of protein tyrosines in human atherosclerosis detected by immunohistochemistry. Biol Chem Hoppe Seyler 375(2):81-88, 1994.

337. Beckman JS, Beckman TW, Chen J, et al: Apparent hydroxyl radical production by peroxynitrite: Implications for endothelial injury from nitric oxide and superoxide. Proc Natl Acad Sci U S A 87(4):1620-1624, 1990.

338. Lieber CS, Leo MA, Mak KM, et al: Choline fails to prevent liver fibrosis in ethanol-fed baboons but causes toxicity. Hepatology 5(4):561-572, 1985.

339. Lauterburg BH, Davies S, Mitchell JR: Ethanol suppresses hepatic glutathione synthesis in rats in vivo. J Pharmacol Exp Ther 230(1):7-11, 1984.

340. Quinn PG, Johnston DE: Detection of chronic liver disease: Costs and benefits. Gastroenterologist 5(1):58-77, 1997.

341. McCaughan GW, Gorrell MD, Bishop GA, et al: Molecular pathogenesis of liver disease: An approach to hepatic inflammation, cirrhosis and liver transplant tolerance. Immunol Rev 174:172-191, 2000.

342. Chung RT, Jaffe DL, Friedman LS: Complications of chronic liver disease. Crit Care Clin 11(2):431-463, 1995.

343. Rakela J, Krowka MJ: Cardiovascular and pulmonary complications of liver disease. In Zakim D, Boyer, TD (eds): Hepatology: A Textbook of Liver Disease, 3rd ed. Philadelphia, WB Saunders, 1996, pp 675-685.

344. Castro M, Krowka MJ, Schroeder DR, et al: Frequency and clinical implications of increased pulmonary artery pressures in liver transplant patients. Mayo Clin Proc 71(6):543-551, 1996.

345. Daoud FS, Reeves JT, Schaefer JW: Failure of hypoxic pulmonary vasoconstriction in patients with liver cirrhosis. J Clin Invest 51(5):1076-1080, 1972.

346. Lazaridis KN, Frank JW, Krowka MJ, et al: Hepatic hydrothorax: Pathogenesis, diagnosis, and management. Am J Med 107(3):262-267, 1999.

347. Arroyo V, Gines P: Mechanism of sodium retention and ascites formation in cirrhosis. J Hepatol 17(Suppl 2):S24-28, 1993.

348. Moreau R: Hepatorenal syndrome in patients with cirrhosis. Gastroenterol Hepatol 17(7):739-747, 2002.

349. Moore KP, Wong F, Gines P, et al: The management of ascites in cirrhosis: Report on the consensus conference of the International Ascites Club. Hepatology 38(1):258-266, 2003.

350. Moreau R, Lebrec D: Acute renal failure in patients with cirrhosis: Perspectives in the age of MELD. Hepatology 37(2):233-243, 2003.

351. de Franchis R, Primignani M: Natural history of portal hypertension in patients with cirrhosis. Clin Liver Dis 5(3):645-663, 2001.

352. Gitlin N: Hepatic encephalopathy. In Zakim D, Boyer T (eds): Hepatology: A Textbook of Liver Disease, 3rd ed. Philadelphia, WB Saunders, 1996, pp 605-618.

353. Vaughan RB, Chin-Dusting JP: Current pharmacotherapy in the management of cirrhosis: Focus on the hyperdynamic circulation. Expert Opin Pharmacother 4(5):625-637, 2003.

354. Geraghty JG, Angerson WJ, Carter DC: Splanchnic haemodynamics and vasoactive agents in experimental cirrhosis. HPB Surg 8(2):83-87; discussion 87-88, 1994.

355. Iwao T, Toyonaga A, Sato M, et al: Effect of posture-induced blood volume expansion on systemic and regional hemodynamics in patients with cirrhosis. J Hepatol 27(3):484-491, 1997; see comments.

356. Silva G, Navasa M, Bosch J, et al: Hemodynamic effects of glucagon in portal hypertension. Hepatology 11(4):668-673, 1990.

357. Cerini R, Koshy A, Hadengue A, et al: Effects of glucagon on systemic and splanchnic circulation in conscious rats with biliary cirrhosis. J Hepatol 9(1):69-74, 1989.

358. Moller S, Bendtsen F, Henriksen JH: Vasoactive substances in the circulatory dysfunction of cirrhosis. Scand J Clin Lab Invest 61(6):421-429, 2001.

359. Moller S, Bendtsen F, Henriksen JH: Splanchnic and systemic hemodynamic derangement in decompensated cirrhosis. Can J Gastroenterol 15(2):94-106, 2001.

360. Cahill PA, Redmond EM, Sitzmann JV: Endothelial dysfunction in cirrhosis and portal hypertension. Pharmacol Ther 89(3):273-293, 2001.

361. Bomzon A, Blendis LM: Vascular reactivity in experimental portal hypertension. Am J Physiol 252(2 Pt 1):G158-162, 1987.

362. Martin PY, Gines P, Schrier RW: Nitric oxide as a mediator of hemodynamic abnormalities and sodium and water retention in cirrhosis. N Engl J Med 339(8):533-541, 1998.

363. Martin PY, Ohara M, Gines P, et al: Nitric oxide synthase (NOS) inhibition for one week improves renal sodium and water excretion in cirrhotic rats with ascites [published erratum appears in J Clin Invest 1998 Aug 1;102(3) inside back cover]. J Clin Invest 101(1):235-242, 1998.

364. Niederberger M, Martin PY, Gines P, et al: Normalization of nitric oxide production corrects arterial vasodilation and hyperdynamic circulation in cirrhotic rats. Gastroenterology 109(5):1624-1630, 1995.

365. Matsumoto A, Ogura K, Hirata Y, et al: Increased nitric oxide in the exhaled air of patients with decompensated liver cirrhosis. Ann Intern Med 123(2):110-113, 1995.

366. Witte CL, Witte MH: Splanchnic circulatory and tissue fluid dynamics in portal hypertension. Fed Proc 42(6):1685-1689, 1983.

367. Schrier RW, Abraham WT: Hormones and hemodynamics in heart failure. N Engl J Med 341(8):577-585, 1999.

368. Heneghan MA, Harrison PM: Pathogenesis of ascites in cirrhosis and portal hypertension. Med Sci Monit 6(4):807-816, 2000.

369. Levy M, Wexler MJ: Renal sodium retention and ascites formation in dogs with experimental cirrhosis but without portal hypertension or increased splanchnic vascular capacity. J Lab Clin Med 91(3):520-536, 1978.

370. Basso D, Fabris C, Plebani M, et al: Alterations in bilirubin metabolism during extra- and intrahepatic cholestasis. Clinical Investigator 70(1):49-54, 1992.

371. Kullak-Ublick GA, Meier PJ: Mechanisms of cholestasis. Clin Liver Dis 4(2):357-385, 2000.

372. Glasova H, Beuers U: Extrahepatic manifestations of cholestasis. J Gastroenterol Hepatol 17(9):938-948, 2002.

373. Trauner M, Fickert P, Stauber RE: Inflammation-induced cholestasis. J Gastroenterol Hepatol 14(10):946-959, 1999.

374. Berk PD, Javitt NB: Hyperbilirubinemia and cholestasis, Am J Med 64(2):311-326, 1978.

375. Strazzabosco M: Transport systems in cholangiocytes: Their role in bile formation and cholestasis. Yale J Biol Med 70(4):427-434, 1997.

376. Shaffer EA: Cholestasis: The ABCs of cellular mechanisms for impaired bile secretion—transporters and genes. Can J Gastroenterol 16(6):380-389, 2002.

377. Elferink RO: Cholestasis. Gut 52(Suppl 2):ii42-48, 2003.

378. Tan LK: Obstetric cholestasis: current opinions and management. Ann Acad Med Singapore 32(3):294-298, 2003.

379. Mullally BA, Hansen WF: Intrahepatic cholestasis of pregnancy: Review of the literature. Obstet Gynecol Surv 57(1):47-52, 2002.

380. Germain AM, Carvajal JA, Glasinovic JC, et al: Intrahepatic cholestasis of pregnancy: An intriguing pregnancy-specific disorder. J Soc Gynecol Investig 9(1):10-14, 2002.

381. Reyes H, Sjovall J: Bile acids and progesterone metabolites in intrahepatic cholestasis of pregnancy. Ann Med 32(2):94-106, 2000.

382. Erlinger S: Drug-induced cholestasis. J Hepatol 26(Suppl 1):1-4, 1997.

383. Velayudham LS, Farrell GC: Drug-induced cholestasis. Expert Opin Drug Saf 2(3):287-304, 2003.

384. Levy C, Lindor KD: Drug-induced cholestasis. Clin Liver Dis 7(2):311-330, 2003.

385. Chitturi S, Farrell GC: Drug-induced cholestasis. Semin Gastrointest Dis 12(2):113-124, 2001.

386. Malaguarnera M, Santangelo N, Motta M, et al: Danazol induced cholestasis: Pathogenetic hypothesis. Panminerva Med 39(3):244-247, 1997.

387. Tung BY, Carithers RL Jr: Cholestasis and alcoholic liver disease. Clin Liver Dis 3(3):585-601, 1999.

388. Sandhu IS, Jarvis C, Everson GT: Total parenteral nutrition and cholestasis. Clin Liver Dis 3(3):489-508, viii, 1999.

389. Teitelbaum DH, Tracy T: Parenteral nutrition-associated cholestasis. Semin Pediatr Surg 10(2):72-80, 2001.

390. Hilzenrat N, Lamoureux E, Sherker A, et al: Cholestasis in Crohn's disease: A diagnostic challenge. Can J Gastroenterol 11(1):35-37, 1997.

391. Gilroy RK, Mailliard ME, Gollan JL: Gastrointestinal disorders of the critically ill. Cholestasis of sepsis. Baillieres Best Pract Res Clin Gastroenterol 17(3):357-367, 2003.

392. Hirata K, Ikeda S, Honma T, et al: Sepsis and cholestasis: Basic findings in the sinusoid and bile canaliculus. J Hepatobiliary Pancreat Surg 8(1):20-26, 2001.

393. Moseley RH: Sepsis and cholestasis. Clin Liver Dis 3(3): 465-475, 1999.
394. Jansen PL: The pathophysiology of cholestasis with special reference to primary biliary cirrhosis. Baillieres Best Pract Res Clin Gastroenterol 14(4):571-583, 2000.
395. Bayraktar Y, Arslan S, Saglam F, et al: What is the association of primary sclerosing cholangitis with sex and inflammatory bowel disease in Turkish patients? Hepatogastroenterology 45(24):2064-2072, 1998.
396. Harrison PM: Prevention of bile duct cancer in primary sclerosing cholangitis. Ann of Oncol 10(Suppl 4):208-211, 1999.
397. Casali AM, Carbone G, Cavalli G: Intrahepatic bile duct loss in primary sclerosing cholangitis: A quantitative study. Histopathology 32(5):449-453, 1998.
398. van Milligen de Wit AW, van Deventer SJ, Tytgat GN: Immunogenetic aspects of primary sclerosing cholangitis: Implications for therapeutic strategies. Am J Gastroenterol 90(6):893-900, 1995.
399. Luketic VA, Shiffman ML: Benign recurrent intrahepatic cholestasis. Clin Liver Dis 3(3):509-528, viii, 1999.
400. Trauner M, Fickert P, Stauber RE: Hepatocellular bile salt transport: Lessons from cholestasis. Can J Gastroenterol 14(Suppl D):99D-104D, 2000.
401. Jansen PL, Muller M: Genetic cholestasis: Lessons from the molecular physiology of bile formation. Can J Gastroenterol 14(3):233-238, 2000.
402. Knisely AS: Progressive familial intrahepatic cholestasis: A personal perspective. Pediatr Dev Pathol 3(2):113-125, 2000.
403. Karpen SJ: Update on the etiologies and management of neonatal cholestasis. Clin Perinatol 29(1):159-180, 2002.
404. Emerick KM, Whitington PF: Molecular basis of neonatal cholestasis. Pediatr Clin North Am 49(1):221-235, 2002.
405. Thompson R, Strautnieks S: BSEP: Function and role in progressive familial intrahepatic cholestasis. Semin Liver Dis 21(4):545-550, 2001.
406. Carulli N, Manenti F, Ponz de Leon M, et al: Alteration of drug metabolism during cholestasis in man. Eur J Clin Invest 5(6):455-462, 1975.
407. Richter E, Breimer DD, Zilly W: Disposition of hexobarbital in intra- and extrahepatic cholestasis in man and the influence of drug metabolism-inducing agents. Eur J Clin Pharmacol 17(3):197-202, 1980.
408. Miguet JP, Vuitton D, Deschamps JP, et al: Cholestasis and hepatic drug metabolism. Comparison of metabolic clearance rate of antipyrine in patients with intrahepatic or extrahepatic cholestasis. Dig Dis Sci 26(8):718-722, 1981.
409. Kawata S, Imai Y, Inada M, et al: Selective reduction of hepatic cytochrome P450 content in patients with intrahepatic cholestasis. A mechanism for impairment of microsomal drug oxidation. Gastroenterology 92(2):299-303, 1987.
410. Chen J, Farrell GC: Bile acids produce a generalized reduction of the catalytic activity of cytochromes P450 and other hepatic microsomal enzymes in vitro: Relevance to drug metabolism in experimental cholestasis. J Gastroenterol Hepatol 11(9):870-877, 1996.
411. Harrison LI, Gibaldi M: Influence of cholestasis on drug elimination: Pharmacokinetics. J Pharm Sci 65(9): 1346-1348, 1976.
412. Lebrault C, Duvaldestin P, Henzel D, et al: Pharmacokinetics and pharmacodynamics of vecuronium in patients with cholestasis. Br J Anaesth 58(9):983-987, 1986.
413. Jenkins JK, Boothby LA: Treatment of itching associated with intrahepatic cholestasis of pregnancy. Ann Pharmacother 36(9):1462-1465, 2002.
414. Palma J, Reyes H, Ribalta J, et al: Ursodeoxycholic acid in the treatment of cholestasis of pregnancy: A randomized, double-blind study controlled with placebo. J Hepatol 27(6):1022-1028, 1997.
415. Better OS: Renal and cardiovascular dysfunction in liver disease [clinical conference]. Kidney Int 29(2):598-607, 1986.
416. Binah O, Rubinstein I, Bomzon A, et al: Effects of bile acids on ventricular muscle contraction and electrophysiological properties: Studies in rat papillary muscle and isolated ventricular myocytes. Naunyn Schmiedebergs Arch Pharmacol 335(2):160-165, 1987.
417. Jacob G, Nassar N, Hayam G, et al: Cardiac function and responsiveness to beta-adrenoceptor agonists in rats with obstructive jaundice. Am J Physiol 265(2 Pt 1):G314-320, 1993.
418. Bomzon A, Monies-Chass I, Kamenetz L, et al: Anesthesia and pressor responsiveness in chronic bile-duct-ligated dogs. Hepatology 11(4):551-556, 1990.
419. Tamakuma S, Wada N, Ishiyama M, et al: Relationship between hepatic hemodynamics and biliary pressure in dogs: Its significance in clinical shock following biliary decompression. Jpn J Surg 5(4):255-268, 1975.

20 Renal Physiology

Robert N. Sladen

Introduction 777
Glomerulus (Renal Corpuscle) 777
Tubule 781
Regulatory Mechanisms in Salt
and Water Reabsorption 784

Renal Function Tests 784
Renal Clearance Techniques 784
Tubular Function Tests 789
Investigational Tests of Renal Function 789

**Neurohormonal Regulation of
Renal Function 791**
Systems Promoting Vasoconstriction
and Salt Retention 791
Systems Promoting Vasodilation
and Salt Excretion 794

**Pharmacologic Renal
Protection 798**
Dopaminergic Agonists 798
Prostaglandins 799
Calcium Channel Blockers 799
Natriuretic Peptides 800

**Perioperative Ischemic and
Nephrotoxic Injury 800**
Anesthetic Drugs 800
Positive-Pressure Ventilation 801
Induced Hypotension 802
Aortic Cross-Clamping 802
Cardiopulmonary Bypass 802
Nephrotoxic Insults 803
Sepsis 805

INTRODUCTION

The kidneys contain approximately 2×10^6 nephrons, each of which consists of a glomerulus and a tubule, which empties into a collecting duct. These functional units collectively enable the kidneys to maintain a remarkably stable interior milieu despite large fluctuations in fluid and solute intake. Together, they regulate intravascular volume, osmolality, and acid-base and electrolyte balance and excrete the end products of metabolism and drugs. Urine is formed by the combination of glomerular ultrafiltration and tubular reabsorption and secretion. The nephron also elaborates hormones that contribute to fluid homeostasis (renin, prostaglandins, kinins), bone metabolism (1,25-dihydroxycholecalciferol), and hematopoiesis (erythropoietin). The function of the nephron is closely integrated with the vascular supply of the kidney (Fig. 20-1).

Glomerulus (Renal Corpuscle)

The glomerulus consists of five distinct components: capillary endothelium, glomerular basement membrane, visceral epithelium (which together make up the filtration barrier), parietal epithelium (Bowman's capsule), and mesangium (interstitial cells).[1,2] The glomerular tuft, a highly convoluted series of capillary loops, is fed by the afferent arteriole and drains into the efferent arteriole (Fig. 20-2).

The capillary endothelium has fenestrations about 70 to 100 nm in diameter and lies atop the glomerular basement membrane, which has a total cross section of about 350 nm. The visceral epithelium, which is applied to the underside of the basement membrane, consists of podocytes with filamentous, interdigitating foot processes that contain contractile actin filaments. Filtration slits form 25- to 60-nm gaps between the foot processes and are bridged by a membranous slit diaphragm, whose size and permeability are altered by contraction of the foot processes.

The blind parietal epithelial sac of the renal tubule is invaginated around the capillary tuft as Bowman's capsule and meets the visceral epithelium at the vascular pole of the glomerulus. Bowman's space, between the visceral and parietal layers of the capsule, becomes the lumen of the proximal tubule at the urinary pole of the glomerulus, and the parietal endothelium merges with the cuboidal cells of the proximal tubule.

The central or interstitial mesangial cells are specialized pericytes with numerous functions, including structural support, matrix elaboration, and phagocytosis. They contain myofilament-like threads of actin and myosin. Mesangial contraction in response to vasoactive substances such as angiotensin II restricts blood flow to fewer capillary loops. The mesangial cells thereby regulate the

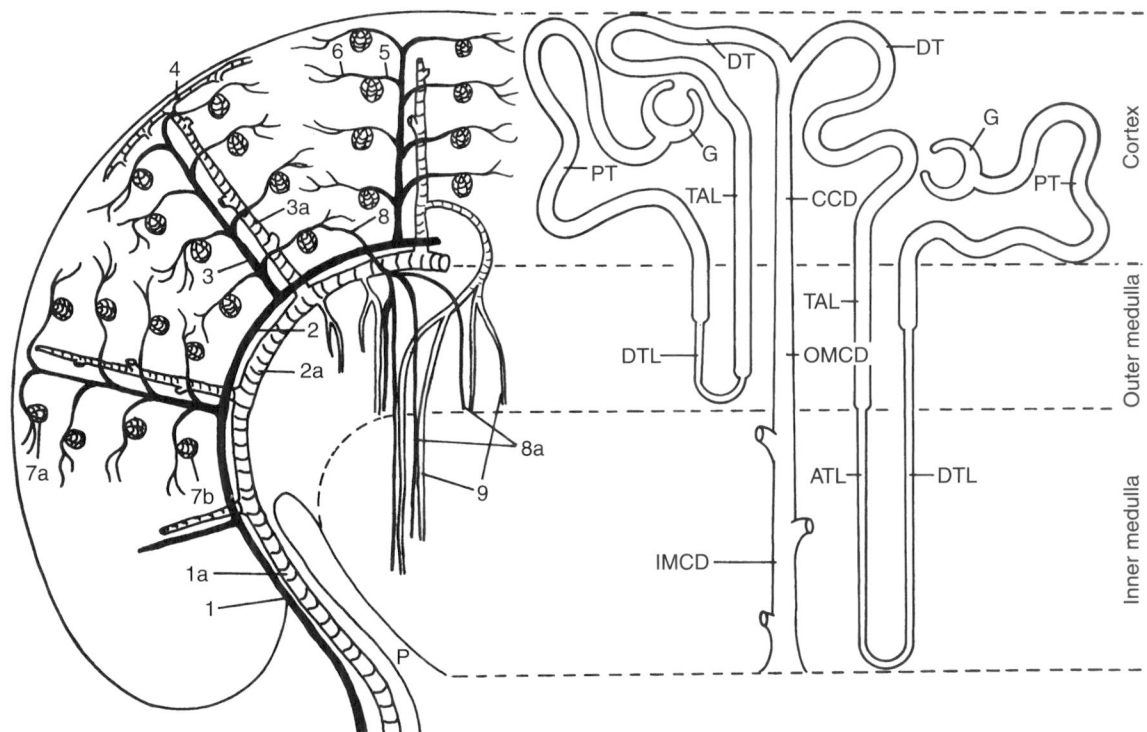

Figure 20–1 Anatomic relationships of the nephron and the renal vasculature. The *left* side of the diagram represents the renal vasculature as distributed through the inner medulla, outer medulla, and cortex. Arteries are drawn as *solid lines,* veins as *hollow tubes.* The renal artery divides serially into interlobar arteries (1), arcuate arteries (2), and interlobular arteries (3). The afferent arterioles (5) branch off laterally and provide the capillary tufts of the renal glomeruli in the outer cortex (7a), whose efferent arterioles (6) supply the cortical capillary network (not shown). In the juxtamedullary zone (7b), the efferent arterioles become the vasa recta, which are closely applied to the long loops of Henle (8, 8a, 9). The venous drainage consists of stellate veins (4), interlobular veins (3a), arcuate veins (2a), and interlobar veins (1a). The *right* side of the diagram represents two nephrons. On the *left* is the more numerous superficial cortical nephron with a short loop of Henle. On the *right* is the juxtamedullary nephron with a long loop of Henle, which dives deep into the inner medulla to generate the hyperosmotic interstitium required for tubular urine concentration. ATL, ascending thin loop of Henle; CCD, cortical collecting duct; DT, distal tubule; DTL, descending thin loop of Henle; G, glomerulus; IMCD, inner medullary collecting duct; OMCD, outer medullary collecting duct; PT, proximal tubule; TAL, thick ascending loop. (Used with permission from Kriz W: A standard nomenclature for structures of the kidney. Kidney Int 33:1-7, 1988.)

effective glomerular surface area for filtration and, as a consequence, glomerular permeability.[3]

Formation of the Glomerular Ultrafiltrate

To cross the filtration barrier between plasma and tubular fluid, a molecule must pass in succession through the endothelial fenestrations, the glomerular basement membrane, and the epithelial slit diaphragm. The capillary endothelium restricts the passage of cells, but the basement membrane filters plasma proteins. All three layers contain negatively charged glycoproteins that retard the passage of other negatively charged proteins. Thus, the filtration barrier is both size and charge selective.[2] Molecules with an effective radius of less than 1.8 nm (e.g., water, sodium, urea, glucose, inulin) are freely filtered. Molecules larger than 3.6 nm (e.g., hemoglobin, albumin) are not filtered. Filtration of molecules between 1.8 and 3.6 nm depends on their electrical charge. Cations are filtered, whereas anions are not. In glomerulonephritis, the negatively charged glycoproteins are destroyed, polyanionic proteins are filtered, and proteinuria ensues.

Glomerular ultrafiltration is governed by the balance of Starling's forces regulating fluid flux across the filtration barrier.[2] The glomerular filtration rate (GFR) depends on the permeability of the filtration barrier and the net difference between hydrostatic forces pushing fluid into Bowman's space and osmotic forces keeping fluid in plasma:

$$GFR = K_{uf} \left[(P_{gc} - P_{bs}) - (\pi_{gc} - \pi_{bs}) \right] \qquad (1)$$

where uf = ultrafiltration, gc = glomerular capillary, and bs = Bowman's space.

The ultrafiltration coefficient K_{uf} reflects capillary permeability and the glomerular surface area. Renal arterial pressure determines the hydrostatic pressure in the glomerular capillary (P_{gc}). Afferent arteriolar plasma flow determines plasma oncotic pressure (π_{gc}): rapid blood flow washes out osmotically effective molecules and lowers π_{gc}, and vice versa.

The Juxtaglomerular Apparatus

The juxtaglomerular apparatus provides a remarkable integration of tubular and glomerular structure and function (Fig. 20-3). A modified portion of the thick ascending limb, the macula densa, is applied to the glomerulus

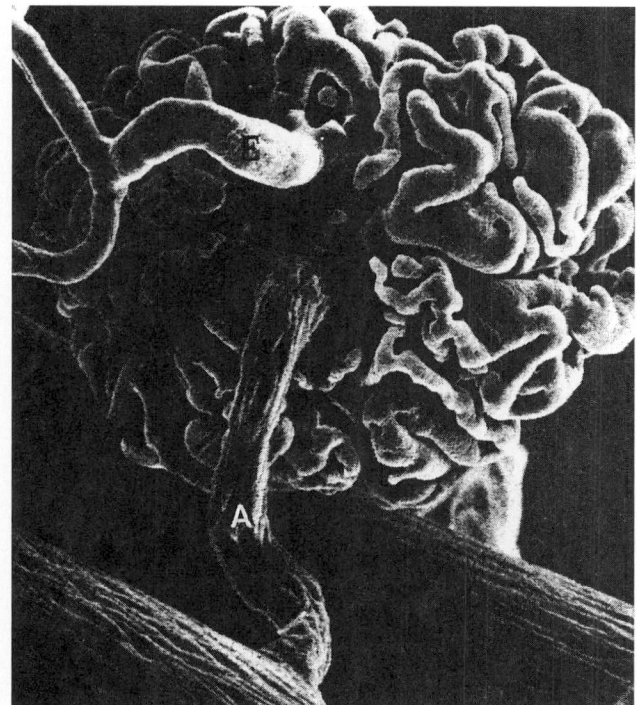

Figure 20–2 Photomicrograph of a cast of a glomerulus without Bowman's capsule. At the *lower left,* the afferent arteriole (A) originates from an interlobular artery and enters the glomerulus with its many capillary loops. At the *upper left,* the efferent arteriole (E) leaves the glomerulus and branches to form the peritubular capillary plexus (magnification ×300). (From Tisher CC, Madsen KM: Anatomy of the kidney. *In* Brenner BM [ed]: Brenner & Rector's The Kidney, 6th ed. Philadelphia, WB Saunders, 2000, pp 3-67.)

at the vascular pole between the afferent and efferent arterioles.[2] The cells of the macula densa are chemoreceptors that sense the tubular concentration of sodium chloride (NaCl). The juxtaposed segments of the afferent and efferent arterioles contain modified smooth muscle cells (granular cells) that produce renin. The arterioles are innervated by sympathetic nerve fibers and contain baroreceptors that respond to changes in intraluminal blood pressure. Renin catalyzes the formation of angiotensin, which modulates efferent and afferent arteriolar tone and the GFR (see later). The relationship of the juxtaglomerular apparatus to the sympathoadrenal system is discussed later in the section "Neurohormonal Regulation of Renal Function."

Afferent and Efferent Arteriolar Control Mechanisms

A primary determinant of the GFR is glomerular filtration pressure, which depends not only on renal artery perfusion pressure but also on the balance between afferent and efferent arteriolar tone. In the face of decreased afferent arteriolar pressure or blood flow, low levels of catecholamines, angiotensin, and arginine vasopressin (AVP) induce preferential efferent arteriolar constriction, which maintains glomerular filtration pressure. This adaptive response is reflected by an increase in the calculated filtration fraction (FF), which is the GFR expressed as

a fraction of renal plasma flow (RPF): FF = GFR/RPF. High levels of catecholamines and angiotensin (but not AVP) increase afferent arteriolar tone and decrease glomerular filtration pressure (and GFR) out of proportion to RPF, and FF decreases (Fig. 20-4). These mechanisms are described in more detail later.

Tubuloglomerular Feedback

Tubuloglomerular feedback may be a primary mechanism in renal autoregulation.[2] When the GFR is increased, distal tubular NaCl delivery is enhanced. The increase in chloride is sensed by the macula densa, which triggers the release of renin from the adjacent afferent arteriole. Angiotensin is elaborated and arteriolar constriction ensues, which decreases the GFR.

It may also be a compensatory mechanism to prevent polyuria in acute renal failure ("acute renal success"). When the thick ascending loop becomes ischemic, reabsorption of NaCl ceases, the ability of the tubule to concentrate urine is lost, and theoretically, intractable polyuria should result. Thurau and Boylan[4] suggested that the increased delivery of NaCl to the macula densa triggers angiotensin-mediated arteriolar constriction, which decreases the GFR, induces oliguria, conserves intravascular volume, and protects the organism from dehydration—so-called acute renal success.

Renal Autoregulation

Autoregulation enables the kidney to maintain solute and water regulation independently of wide fluctuations in arterial blood pressure. In 1951, the classic dog studies of Shipley and Study[5] demonstrated that the kidney maintains a constant renal blood flow (RBF) and GFR through an arterial pressure range of 80 to 180 mm Hg (Fig. 20-5). It is noteworthy that the urinary flow rate is not subject to autoregulation. Tubular water reabsorption determines the urinary flow rate and is closely related to hydrostatic pressure in the peritubular capillaries. Hypotension, whether induced or inadvertent, results in a decreased urinary flow rate that may be correctable only when arterial blood pressure is restored toward normal.

The precise mechanism of renal autoregulation is not yet defined. Renal vascular resistance appears to be mediated by variable resistance of the preglomerular afferent arteriole. As mean arterial pressure decreases, renal vascular resistance decreases and RBF is maintained. The most plausible explanation is a myogenic response in which the arterioles constrict in response to increased arterial pressure and vice versa. Tubuloglomerular feedback by way of the juxtaglomerular apparatus may also play a role.[6] When arterial pressure increases through the autoregulatory range, it enhances delivery of sodium chloride to the cells of the macula densa, which induces afferent arteriolar constriction and decreased RBF and GFR.[2] The opposite effect occurs when arterial pressure declines.

Though not abolished by most anesthetic agents, autoregulation appears to be impaired in severe sepsis,[7] in acute renal failure,[8] and possibly during cardiopulmonary bypass (CPB).[9] In these situations, RBF declines strikingly during hypotension. It is restored by normalization of renal perfusion pressure, even if such normalization is achieved by vasoconstrictor therapy.

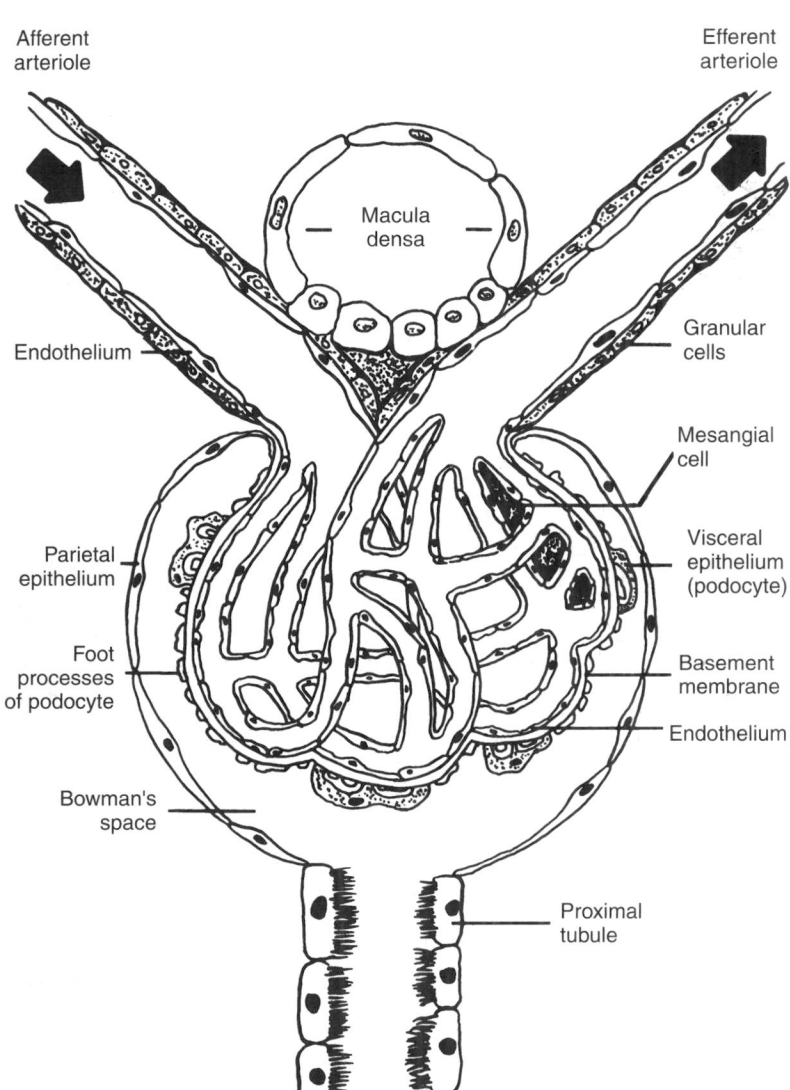

Afferent
arteriole

Efferent
arteriole

Macula
densa

Endothelium

Granular
cells

Mesangial
cell

Parietal
epithelium

Visceral
epithelium
(podocyte)

Foot
processes
of podocyte

Basement
membrane

Endothelium

Bowman's
space

Proximal
tubule

Figure 20–3 The juxtaglomerular apparatus. (From Stanton BA, Koeppen BM: Elements of renal function. *In* Berne RM, Levy MN [eds]: Physiology, 4th ed. St Louis, CV Mosby, 1998, pp 677-698.)

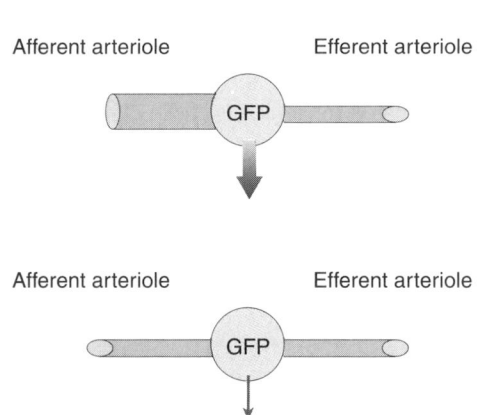

Afferent arteriole

Efferent arteriole

GFP

Afferent arteriole

Efferent arteriole

GFP

Figure 20–4 Afferent and efferent arteriolar control mechanisms. GFP, glomerular filtration pressure. (Redrawn from Sladen RN, Landry D: Renal blood flow regulation, autoregulation, and vasomotor nephropathy. Anesthesiol Clin North Am 18:791-807, 2000.)

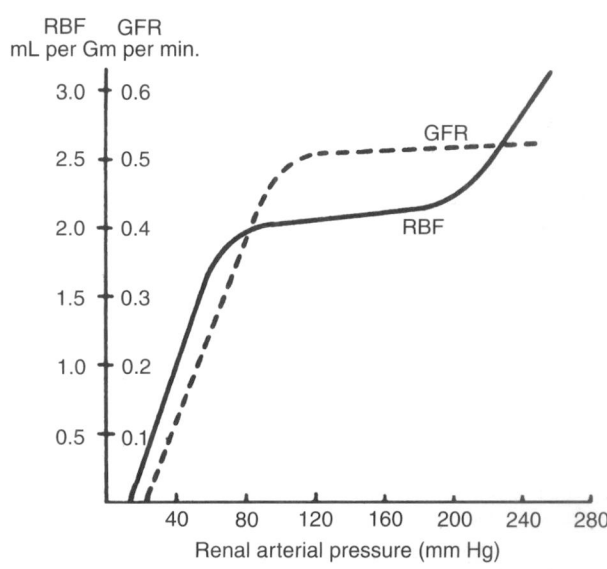

RBF   GFR
mL per Gm per min.

GFR

RBF

Renal arterial pressure (mm Hg)

Figure 20–5 Autoregulation of the glomerular filtration rate (GFR) and renal blood flow (RBF), based on the original work of Shipley and Study.[5] GFR and RBF remain constant between a renal arterial pressure of 80 and 180 mm Hg. (From Pitts RF: Physiology of the Kidney and Body Fluids. Chicago, Year Book, 1974.)

Tubule

The tubule has four distinct segments: the proximal tubule, the loop of Henle, the distal tubule, and the connecting segment. The loop of Henle itself is divided into the pars recta (the straight portion of the proximal tubule), the descending and ascending thin limb segments, and the thick ascending limb. Each distal tubule drains into a collecting duct, which courses through the cortex, outer medulla, and inner medulla before entering the renal pelvis at the papilla (see Fig. 20-1).

Nephrons may be classified as cortical or juxtamedullary nephrons. Cortical nephrons populate the outer and middle renal cortex, are far more numerous, receive about 85% of RBF, and have short loops of Henle. Their efferent arterioles drain into a peritubular capillary plexus. The juxtamedullary nephrons populate the inner renal cortex, receive about 10% of RBF, and have larger glomeruli and long loops of Henle that dive deeply into the inner medulla.[1] Their efferent arterioles drain into elongated vascular conduits, the vasa recta, which are closely applied to the loops of Henle. Although the vasa recta receive less than 1% of RBF, they play an important role in generating the countercurrent mechanism for medullary hypertonicity and renal concentrating ability (see later).

Tubular Reabsorption and Secretion

The tubule has an enormous capacity for reabsorption of water and NaCl. Each day, 180 L of protein-free glomerular ultrafiltrate is formed, of which almost 99% of the water and 99% of the sodium is reabsorbed.

Many other filtered substances are completely reabsorbed, but some, such as glucose, have a maximal rate of tubular reabsorption (tubular maximum). Tubular reabsorption of glucose increases at a rate equal to that of the filtered load. If the GFR is constant, the rate is directly proportional to the plasma glucose concentration. Once plasma glucose exceeds the tubular maximum (375 mg/dL), no further glucose is reabsorbed, and glycosuria results. Thereafter, the amount of glucose excreted in urine increases in direct proportion to the filtered load.

Many important endogenous and exogenous solutes are secreted into the tubular lumen from capillary blood. Some also have a tubular maximum for secretion, such as para-aminohippurate (PAH), which is used to calculate RPF. This topic is discussed further in the section "Renal Function Tests."

A striking relationship exists between the structure and function of the different segments of the tubule (Fig. 20-6). The most metabolically active components of the tubule are the proximal tubule, the thick ascending loop of Henle, and the first part of the distal tubule.

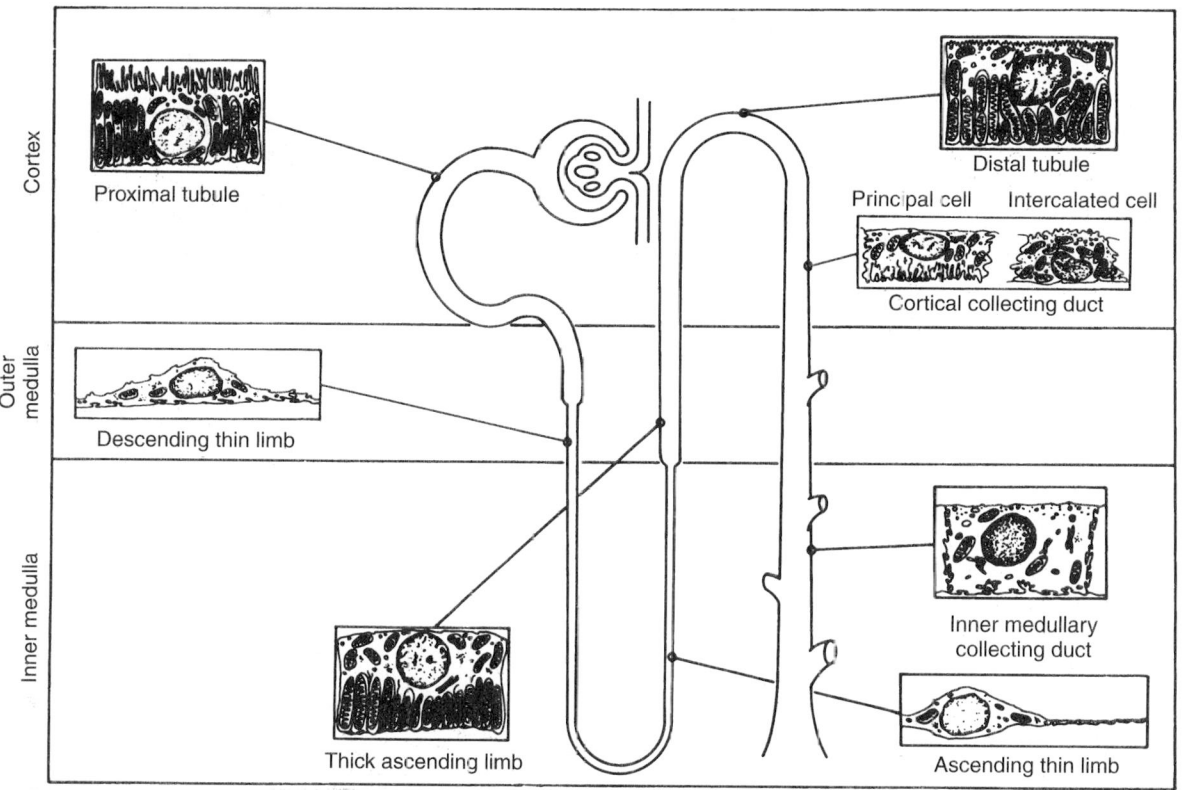

Figure 20–6 Structure-function relationships in the renal tubule. The most metabolically active components of the tubule are the proximal tubule, the thick ascending loop of Henle, and the first part of the distal tubule. Their cells are large, and the capillary surface (basolateral membrane) has many invaginations rich in mitochondria. The cells of the proximal tubule have a brush border on the luminal surface (apical cell membrane), whereas the cells of the descending and thin ascending loops of Henle are flattened with few mitochondria. The second part of the distal tubule and collecting duct are intermediate in nature. The intercalated cells of the distal tubule have many mitochondria, whereas the principal cells have few. (From Stanton BA, Koeppen BM: Elements of renal function. *In* Berne RM, Levy MN [eds]: Physiology, 4th ed. St Louis, CV Mosby, 1998, pp 677-698.)

Figure 20-7 illustrates a tubular cell in the thick ascending loop of Henle that encompasses all the major mechanisms of reabsorption and secretion. The tubular lumen abuts the apical cell membrane, which joins adjacent cells at the tight junctions. The remainder of the cell is lined by the basolateral cell membrane, which interfaces with the lateral interstitial spaces on either side and with the peritubular capillary at its base. A number of protein-based active transport systems exist, the most important of which is the sodium-potassium–adenosine triphosphatase (Na-K–ATPase) system, situated in the basolateral membrane. It pumps sodium out of the tubular cell into the interstitial fluid (and capillary blood) against a concentration and an electrical gradient in exchange for potassium from inside the tubular cell. The consequent decrease in intracellular sodium concentration facilitates passive reabsorption of sodium from the tubular lumen into the cell. The transport of virtually all solutes is coupled to that of sodium.

Active transport systems that move solutes in the same direction into or out of the cell are called *symporter* systems, whereas those that move solutes in opposite directions are called *antiporter* systems. Solutes are transported by active and passive mechanisms, but water always diffuses passively along an osmotic gradient.

Proximal Tubule

The first part of the proximal tubule reabsorbs about 100% of the filtered glucose, lactate, and amino acids, as well as some phosphate, by coupling with sodium symporter systems.[2] Hydrogen ions are extruded into the tubule by a sodium-H+ antiporter system in exchange for bicarbonate. The absorption of organic anions and bicarbonate in the first part of the proximal tubule results in a relatively high chloride concentration downstream that promotes the passive ingress of chloride. As a consequence, the tubular fluid is positively charged relative to

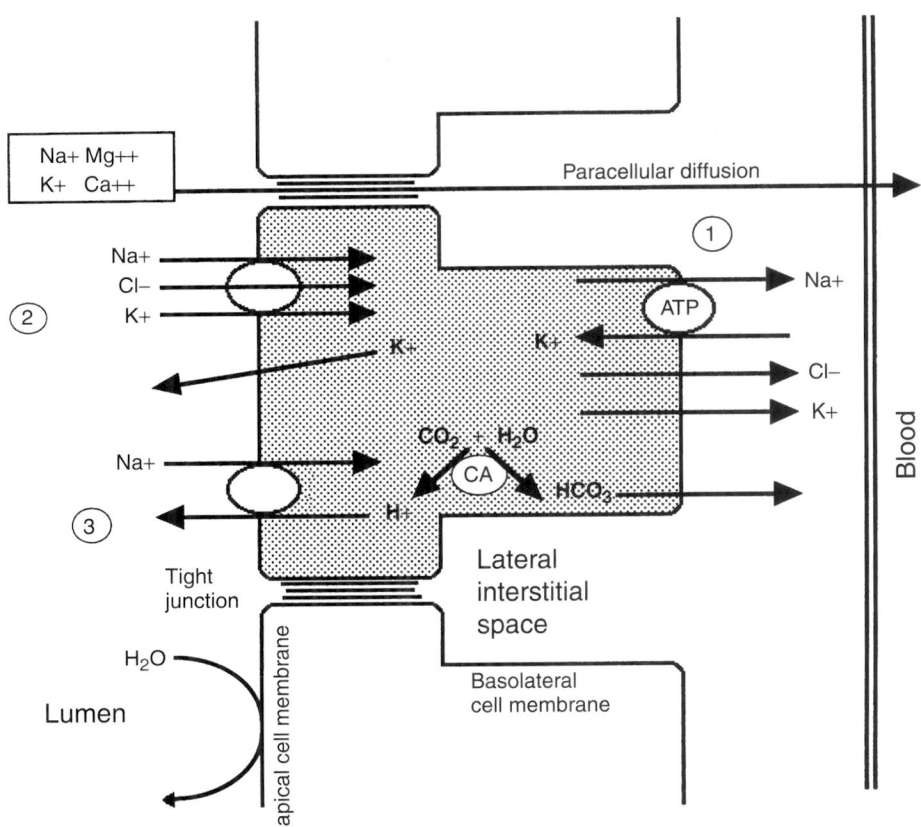

Figure 20–7 Mechanisms of tubular secretion and reabsorption. This tubular cell in the thick ascending loop of Henle encompasses the major mechanisms of secretion and reabsorption, one or more of which is used by various segments of the tubule. The most ubiquitous and important transport mechanism is the energy-requiring Na-K–ATPase pump in the basolateral cell membrane (1), which pumps sodium out into the interstitium against its concentration gradient and maintains a low intracellular concentration. This mechanism favors inward movement of sodium from the tubular lumen, facilitated by a sodium chloride symporter system on the apical cell membrane (2), which creates enough potential energy to draw in potassium against its concentration gradient and is the primary inhibitory site of action of loop diuretics. A sodium-H+ antiporter system on the apical cell membrane (3) aids sodium reabsorption and extrudes H+, thereby promoting the reaction of water with carbon dioxide to form H+ and bicarbonate ion under the influence of carbonic anhydrase (CA). Bicarbonate diffuses out into the capillary. Sodium reabsorption is thereby coupled to H+ loss and bicarbonate reabsorption. The transport proteins create a positive charge in the lumen, which drives ions such as sodium, calcium, potassium, and magnesium passively through the tight junctions by paracellular diffusion. The thick ascending loop of Henle is uniquely highly water impermeable, so luminal osmolality progressively falls to less than 150 mOsm/kg (the "diluting segment"). (Modified from Stanton BA, Koeppen BM: Elements of renal function. *In* Berne RM, Levy MN [eds]: Physiology, 4th ed. St Louis, CV Mosby, 1998, pp 677-698.)

blood, which further promotes the movement of sodium from the tubular fluid into the cell.

Most NaCl is absorbed transcellularly by a sodium-H^+ and chloride-based antiporter system in the apical cell membrane. The Na-K–ATPase system pumps sodium into the interstitial space, and a potassium-chloride symporter system pumps chloride. The resulting increase in osmolality draws water across as well. In all, about two thirds of the filtered water, chloride, and potassium are reabsorbed by the proximal tubule, coupled with and strongly influenced by sodium absorption.[2]

The proximal tubule is also an important site of secretion of many endogenous anions (bile salts, urate), cations (creatinine, dopamine), and drugs (diuretics, penicillin, probenecid, cimetidine). Organic ions compete with each other for protein transport systems. Thus, administration of probenecid impairs the tubular secretion of penicillin and prolongs its action. In chronic renal insufficiency, organic acids accumulate and compete with drugs such as furosemide for secretor proteins, thereby conferring an apparent "resistance" to loop diuretics.

Thick Ascending Loop of Henle

The metabolically active component of the loop of Henle is the thick ascending loop, which reabsorbs about 20% of the filtered sodium, chloride, potassium, and bicarbonate. Only the descending loop is permeable to water. In the water-impermeable thick ascending loop, sodium is actively reabsorbed, but water remains. In this so-called diluting segment of the kidney, tubular fluid osmolality decreases to less than 150 mOsm/kg H_2O.

As in the proximal tubule, the Na-K–ATPase pump in the basolateral membrane is the engine that drives the resorptive capacity of the thick ascending loop.[2] Sodium moves from the tubular lumen by passive diffusion along its concentration gradient. A sodium-H^+ antiporter system in the apical cell membrane mediates the net secretion of H^+ and reabsorption of bicarbonate.

An important symporter protein system couples the reabsorption of sodium, chloride, and potassium (the latter against its concentration gradient) across the apical membrane. Blockade of this system is the major mechanism of action of loop diuretics in inhibiting NaCl reabsorption in the thick ascending loop of Henle.

Oxygen Balance in the Medullary Thick Ascending Loop

The kidneys receive 20% of the total cardiac output but extract relatively little oxygen. The renal arteriovenous oxygen difference ($\Delta a - \Delta vO_2$) is only 1.5 mL/dL. However, there is a marked discrepancy between the renal cortex and medulla with regard to blood flow, oxygen delivery, and oxygen consumption (Table 20-1). The medulla receives only 6% of RBF and has an average oxygen tension (Po_2) of 8 mm Hg. Thus, it is possible that severe hypoxia could develop in the medulla despite a relatively adequate total RBF, and the metabolically active medullary thick ascending loop of Henle is particularly vulnerable.[10]

The medullary thick ascending loop is also a potential site for nephrotoxic injury. Intrarenal blood flow is regulated by endogenous vasoactive compounds. In the

Table 20–1 Distribution of renal blood flow between the cortex and medulla

	Cortex	Medulla
Percent renal blood flow	94	6
Blood flow (mL/min/g)	5.0	0.03
Po_2 (mm Hg)	50	8
O_2 extraction ratio (Vo_2/Do_2)	0.18	0.79

The renal medulla receives only a small fraction of the total renal blood flow, and flow rates are extremely slow. As a result, tissue oxygen tension is extremely low, and the medulla extracts almost 80% of the oxygen delivered to it. A very mild reduction in total and cortical renal blood flow may therefore induce ischemia and hypoxia in the renal medulla.
Do_2, oxygen delivery; Po_2, oxygen tension; Vo_2, oxygen consumption.
Data from Brezis M, Rosen S: Hypoxia of the renal medulla—its implications for disease. N Engl J Med 332:647-655, 1995.

outer cortex, adenosine induces vasoconstriction (at variance with its vasodilator actions elsewhere). In the deep juxtamedullary zone, endogenous prostaglandins and nitric oxide promote vasodilation. The net effect is to direct as much available blood flow to the medulla as possible. Drugs that inhibit prostaglandin synthesis, such as nonsteroidal anti-inflammatory drugs (NSAIDs), can upset this compensatory mechanism and result in medullary ischemia.

Stress (pain, trauma, hemorrhage, hypoperfusion, sepsis, congestive heart failure) activates the sympathoadrenal system and results in renal cortical constriction and potential tubular ischemia. The kidney is relatively devoid of β_2 receptors, so epinephrine release induces predominantly vasoconstriction through α receptor or angiotensin activation.

In hemodynamically mediated renal injury, the initial response to renal hypoperfusion is increased active NaCl absorption in the thick ascending limb. Such absorption increases oxygen consumption in the face of decreased oxygen delivery. Subsequent sympathoadrenal responses and renal cortical vasoconstriction may be a compensatory attempt to redistribute blood flow to the medulla. Ultimately, adenosine triphosphate (ATP) stores become depleted and active NaCl reabsorption winds down. This increases the NaCl concentration in tubular fluid reaching the macula densa in the distal tubule and thereby results in angiotensin release and afferent arteriolar constriction (i.e., tubuloglomerular feedback). Teleologically, the resultant decrease in GFR benefits renal oxygen balance by decreasing solute reabsorption and oxygen consumption in the medullary thick ascending loop of Henle.[10]

This hypothesis implies that ischemic or nephrotoxic insults to the renal tubules could be alleviated by the administration of loop diuretics or dopaminergic agents. These drugs inhibit active sodium reabsorption in the thick ascending limb, thereby decreasing oxygen consumption and enhancing tubular oxygen balance.

Distal Tubule and Collecting Duct

The proximal segment of the distal tubule is structurally and functionally similar to the thick ascending loop. Sodium reabsorption is mediated by an apical cell membrane NaCl symporter system, which is the site of action of thiazide diuretics.[2]

The last part of the distal tubule is composed of two types of cells. Principal cells reabsorb sodium and water and secrete potassium via the Na-K–ATPase pump, and intercalated cells secrete H^+ and reabsorb bicarbonate by means of an H^+-ATPase pump in the apical cell membrane.

Regulatory Mechanisms in Salt and Water Reabsorption

Osmotic Equilibrium

The ability of the kidney to concentrate urine is dependent on the interaction of at least three processes: (1) the generation of a hypertonic medullary interstitium by the countercurrent mechanism and urea recycling, (2) concentration and then dilution of tubular fluid in the loop of Henle, and (3) the action of antidiuretic hormone (now known as AVP) in increasing water permeability in the last part of the distal tubule and collecting ducts.

The medullary interstitium is rendered hypertonic by the countercurrent multiplier effect of the loop of Henle. The primary mechanism is separation of solute from water (the single effect) by the combination of NaCl reabsorption and water impermeability in the ascending limb. This results in an increased NaCl concentration and osmolality in the medullary interstitium. The descending limb is freely permeable to water, which diffuses into the interstitium along the osmotic gradient, and the tubular fluid becomes progressively hyperosmotic at the bend of the loop.

The vasa recta, which are closely applied to the long loops of Henle of juxtamedullary nephrons, maintain this condition by removing water and adding solute as they pass through the medullary interstitium. A standing osmotic gradient is thereby set up between the cortex (300 mOsm/kg), juxtamedullary zone (600 mOsm/kg), and deep medulla (1200 mOsm/kg). This process is enhanced by the passive recycling of urea, which diffuses out of the inner medullary collecting duct into the interstitium and thence into the distal loop of Henle. These processes are summarized in Figure 20-8.

Tubular Concentration and Dilution

Hypovolemia

Contraction of the extracellular volume (hypovolemia) activates a series of vasoconstrictor, salt-retaining neurohormonal systems: the sympathoadrenal system, the renin-angiotensin-aldosterone axis, and AVP. Initially, the GFR and the filtered load of sodium decrease. Sodium reabsorption in the proximal tubule is increased from about 66% to 80% by sympathetic activity and angiotensin II, as well as by the decline in peritubular capillary pressure induced by renal vasoconstriction. Sodium delivery to the thick ascending loop of Henle, distal tubule, and collecting duct is decreased, but aldosterone promotes reabsorption of sodium at these sites. Under the influence of AVP, water is also avidly reabsorbed in the collecting duct so that the urine becomes highly concentrated (osmolality, 600 mOsm/kg), but with virtually no sodium (10 mEq/L).

Diuretic agents abolish the kidney's ability to concentrate urine by washing out the hypertonic medulla. They do this either by an osmotic effect that prevents water reabsorption (e.g., mannitol) or by inhibition of active NaCl transport in the thick ascending loop (e.g., furosemide) or the first part of the distal tubule (e.g., hydrochlorothiazide). An early and important manifestation of acute tubular necrosis is the loss of urinary concentrating ability caused by breakdown of the energy-requiring Na-K-ATPase pump in the thick ascending loop of Henle.

Hypervolemia

Expansion of the extracellular volume, or hypervolemia, is controlled by a series of vasodilator, salt-excreting neuropeptides, of which atrial natriuretic peptide (ANP) is predominant. The GFR and filtered sodium load increase because of a combination of reflex decreases in sympathetic and angiotensin II activity and the release of ANP. Together with the increase in peritubular capillary hydrostatic pressure, these responses cause sodium reabsorption in the proximal tubule to decrease from 67% to 50%. The decline in plasma aldosterone decreases sodium absorption from the thick ascending loop of Henle to the collecting duct. The presence of ANP and absence of AVP impairs water absorption at the collecting duct so that dilute urine (osmolality, 300 mOsm/kg) with abundant sodium (80 mEq/L) is produced.

It is noteworthy that loop diuretics, which depress tubular resorptive capacity, and acute tubular necrosis, which abolishes it completely, may generate an identical urinary profile (low osmolality, high urinary sodium), even in the presence of hypovolemia.

RENAL FUNCTION TESTS

Renal hemodynamic function is defined by RBF, RPF, intrarenal distribution of flow, FF, and renal vascular resistance. Glomerular function is defined by the GFR. Tubular functions include concentrating ability, water conservation, and sodium conservation. For practical purposes, however, clinical tests of renal function can be described as those based on clearance techniques (the most commonly used) and those that test tubular function. A number of tests are also primarily used for clinical and laboratory investigation.

Renal Clearance Techniques

Renal function is indirectly assessed by clearance techniques,[11] which are based on the Fick principle. The amount of substance x excreted by the kidney equals the amount delivered in the arterial supply minus the amount in venous return:

$$Excretion_x = Delivery_x - Return_x \qquad (2)$$

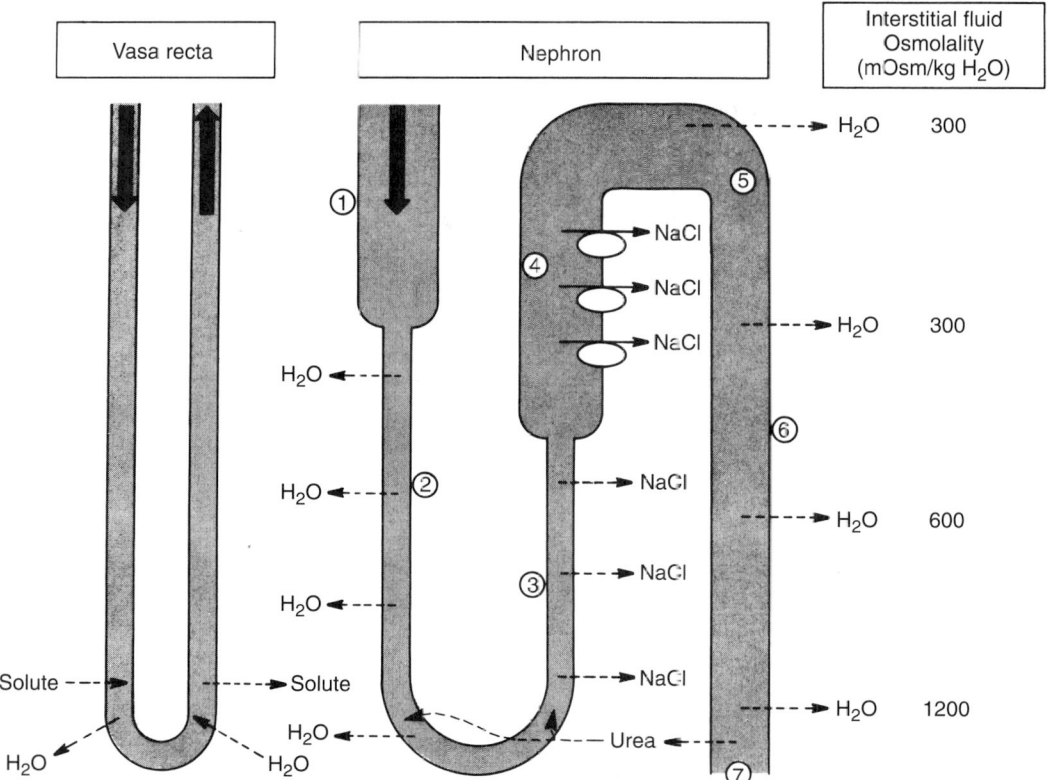

Figure 20–8 Tubular concentration of urine. The juxtamedullary nephrons have long loops of Henle associated with the vasa recta. *Dashed arrows* represent passive movement of fluid or solutes along concentration or osmolar gradients; *solid arrows* represent active transport. Tubular fluid enters the distal proximal tubule iso-osmotic with plasma (300 mOsm/kg) (1). In the descending limb of Henle (2), water rapidly diffuses out into the increasingly hypertonic medulla and is removed by the vasa recta, and as a consequence, the tubular fluid becomes hypertonic, largely because of concentration of sodium chloride (NaCl). Urea diffuses in from the hypertonic interstitium, further increasing tubular fluid osmolality (1200 mOsm/kg). In the thin ascending loop of Henle (3), NaCl passively diffuses into the interstitium along its concentration gradient, but water s trapped in the water-impermeable tubule, which progressively decreases tubular fluid osmolality. Urea passively diffuses into the tubular fluid (urea recycling). Tubular dilution is accelerated by active reabsorption of NaCl in the thick ascending loop (the diluting segment) and proximal distal tubule (4). The fluid entering the distal tubule is quite hypo-osmotic (100 mOsm/kg). In the collecting segment (5), the osmolality of the tubular fluid returns to that of plasma (300 mOsm/kg), but unlike the contents of the proximal tubule, the solute component consists largely of urea, creatinine, and other excreted compounds. Increased plasma antidiuretic hormone (ADH) renders the cortical and medullary collecting ducts (6) permeable to water, which passively diffuses into the hypertonic medullary interstitium. Even though some urea diffuses out into the medulla, the maximal osmolality of concentrated urine (7) approaches that of the hypertonic medullary interstitium, about 1200 mOsm/kg. In the absence of ADH, the collecting ducts remain impermeable to water, and the urine is diluted. (From Stanton BA, Koeppen BM: Control of body fluid osmolality and volume. *In* Berne RM, Levy MN [eds]: Physiology, 4th ed. St Louis, CV Mosby, 1998, pp 715-743.)

Therefore

$$\text{Delivery}_x = \text{Return}_x + \text{Excretion}_x \qquad (3)$$

The amount of substance x delivered to the kidney is the product of the arterial plasma concentration (Pa_x) and RBF. The amount returning from the kidney is the product of the venous plasma concentration (Pv_x) and RBF. The urinary excretion rate of substance x is the product of its urinary concentration (U_x) and the urine flow rate in milliliters per minute (V).

Therefore,

$$(Pa_x \times RBF) = (Pv_x \times RBF) + (U_x \times V) \qquad (4)$$

However, in practice, RBF and venous return are not measured. Instead, the removal of substance x from plasma by the kidney is expressed in the concept of clearance.

Clearance (C) is defined as the virtual volume of plasma cleared of substance x per unit time, in milliliters per minute. This term allows the urinary excretion rate of x to be equated to its renal arterial plasma concentration:

$$Pa_x \times C = U_x \times V \qquad (5)$$

If the assumption is made that the concentration of x in renal arterial and venous plasma is identical, clearance of substance x may be calculated by using a urine sample, arm venous sample, and measured urinary flow rate:

$$C_x = (U_x \times V)Pa_x \qquad (6)$$

Para-Aminohippurate Clearance

PAH is an organic anion that is almost completely cleared from plasma in a single pass through the kidney by a combination of glomerular filtration and proximal tubular secretion. Calculated clearance of PAH (C_{PAH}) therefore represents RPF. To obtain maximal PAH extraction, a steady state with a low plasma PAH level must be achieved by giving an intravenous loading dose followed by an infusion to maintain a plasma PAH concentration of about 2 mg/dL.[11] A carefully timed catheter urine collection is required. Because only 90% of RPF enters the peritubular capillaries surrounding the proximal tubule, PAH clearance underestimates true renal plasma flow, and it is known as the effective renal plasma flow (eRPF).

$$eRPF = C_{PAH} = (U_{PAH} \times V)/P_{PAH} \qquad (7)$$

The normal eRPF is 660 mL/min/1.73 m^2.

Effective renal blood flow (eRBF) may be derived if the hematocrit level (Hct) is known and expressed as a decimal (i.e., 35% = 0.35):

$$eRBF = eRPF/(1 - Hct) \qquad (8)$$

In a number of circumstances C_{PAH} provides misleading information about RPF. If the plasma PAH concentration exceeds the tubular maximum for reabsorption of 12 mg/dL, the excess PAH is returned to the renal vein, the secreted fraction declines, and RPF is underestimated.[2] About 80% of PAH is cleared by tubular secretion, so if proximal tubule function deteriorates, PAH clearance declines and again underestimates RPF.

These errors can be overcome if arterial (Pa) and renal vein (Pv) PAH levels are accessible. The renal extraction of PAH (E_{PAH}) can be calculated and provides an assessment of proximal tubule function:

$$E_{PAH} = (Pa_{PAH} - Pv_{PAH})/Pa_{PAH} \qquad (9)$$

When renal function is normal, renal vein PAH is close to zero and PAH extraction approaches 1.0. As proximal tubule function declines, the concentration of PAH in the renal vein increases, and PAH extraction progressively decreases below 1.0. True RPF is calculated by dividing PAH clearance by PAH extraction:

$$RPF = C_{PAH}/E_{PAH} \qquad (10)$$

In the presence of hypovolemia and oliguria, PAH is sequestered in the kidney. Even with the use of extraction techniques, PAH clearance may misrepresent RPF under these conditions. Despite its relative convenience as an experimental tool, PAH clearance may be an unreliable indicator of RBF during the perturbations induced by anesthesia and surgical stress.

Inulin Clearance
Inulin is an inert polyfructose sugar that is completely filtered by the glomerulus and is neither secreted nor reabsorbed by the renal tubules. The volume in milliliters of plasma cleared of inulin per minute represents the GFR (mL/min). Inulin clearance is measured identically to PAH clearance. After an intravenous loading dose of 30 to 50 mg/kg, a continuous infusion of inulin is given to establish a steady-state plasma concentration of

15 to 20 mg/dL. The bladder is usually flushed with air to eliminate any pooled urine. A very carefully timed urine collection is then made, which can be as short as 30 minutes. It is generally accepted that inulin clearance (C_{In}) provides the most accurate available determination of GFR:

$$GFR = C_{In} = (U_{In} \times V)/P_{In} \qquad (11)$$

Although inulin clearance is the "gold standard" for measurement of GFR, it is seldom used clinically because its accurate measurement is laborious and requires meticulous attention to detail. The inulin assay is time consuming, and inulin itself is in short supply because of lack of demand. Inulin meets all the criteria of an ideal filtration marker, but large changes in blood glucose during the test may interfere with its measurement, and its accuracy in reflecting the GFR cannot be directly assessed, only inferred. The predicted variability of inulin clearance is 20% when measurements are compared at two different times in the same individual and 40% when measurements are compared between two individuals.[11] Normal values for inulin clearance are 110 to 140 mL/min/1.73 m^2 (males) and 95 to 125 mL/min/1.37 m^2 (females).

Filtration Fraction
FF is the fraction of RPF that is filtered by the glomerulus:

$$FF = GFR/RPF = C_{In}/C_{PAH} \qquad (12)$$

Normally, the GFR is about 125 mL/min and RPF is about 660 mL/min, so FF approximates 125/660, or about 0.2. Changes in FF are thought to represent changes in periglomerular arteriolar tone (see the earlier section "Afferent and Efferent Arteriolar Control Mechanisms"). An increase in FF indicates that the GFR is increased relative to RPF. This increase could be achieved by efferent arteriolar constriction or afferent arteriolar dilation and maintains glomerular filtration pressure in the face of decreased RPF. Conversely, a decrease in FF implies that the GFR is decreased relative to RPF by afferent arteriolar constriction or efferent arteriolar dilation.

Creatinine Clearance
Creatinine, the endogenous end product of creatine phosphate metabolism, is normally generated from muscle at a very uniform rate and is handled by the kidney in a manner similar to that of inulin. Thus, creatinine clearance (C_{Cr}) provides a simple, inexpensive bedside estimate of GFR. A single blood sample is drawn at the midpoint of a carefully timed urine collection:

$$GFR = C_{Cr} = (U_{Cr} \times V)/P_{Cr} \qquad (13)$$

Bedside use of creatinine clearance has been restricted by the belief that a prolonged (12- to 24-hour) urine collection is necessary to eliminate error induced by residual urine in the bladder neck after spontaneous voiding, a practice both tedious and cumbersome. The estimated creatinine clearance depends on when the blood sample is drawn, so if serum creatinine changes rapidly during the time of urine collection, a misleading result may be obtained.

The precise timing, not the duration, of the urine collection is the critical issue.[12] If a brisk urine flow is induced by diuresis and care is taken to empty the bladder, the variability in creatinine clearance is no greater with a 1-hour urine collection than with a 24-hour collection. In catheterized patients with urine flow rates greater than 15 mL/hr, creatinine clearance obtained with a 2-hour urine collection gives values equivalent to those obtained with a 12- to 24-hour collection.[13] Moreover, a short urine collection enables rapid, repeated estimates of GFR to be obtained. This not only makes 2-hour creatinine clearance a viable bedside test in critically ill patients but also implies that a changing GFR can be closely tracked by serial estimations of creatinine clearance (Figs. 20-9 to 20-11). For example, in trauma patients, a 1-hour creatinine clearance of less than 25 mL/min determined within 6 hours of surgery reliably predicted postoperative acute renal failure despite the absence of oliguria.[14]

Considerable variation in the normal range of creatinine clearance has been noted. Tobias and coauthors[12] reported a variation in creatinine clearance between 88 and 148 mL/min and in serum creatinine between 0.9 and 1.5 mg/dL in a single healthy individual over a period of 5 years. There is also a diurnal variation, with higher values in the afternoon and a variance of up to 25% around mean values.[15] It is prudent to obtain short-collection creatinine clearance estimates at the same time each day to minimize diurnal variability. "Normal" creatinine clearance is related to body surface area and weight, so values may fluctuate widely in patients with cachexia or edema.

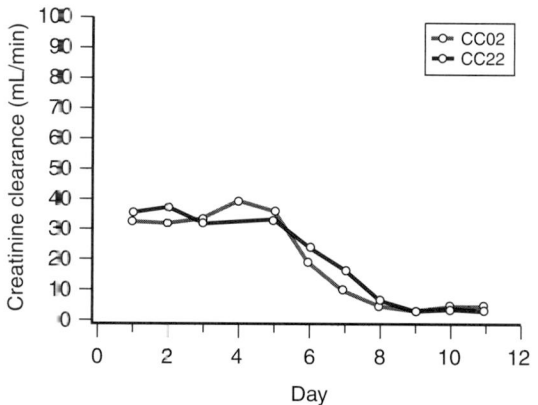

Figure 20–10 New-onset acute renal failure. In a patient in whom acute renal failure is developing in the intensive care unit, the exponential decline in creatinine clearance is tracked equally well whether a 2-hour (CC02) or a 22-hour (CC22) urine collection is used. However, data from the 2-hour collection are available well before those from the 22-hour collection.

Creatinine clearance has a number of inherent limitations even if collection error is carefully avoided. The creatinine generation rate varies with muscle mass, physical activity, protein intake, and catabolism. The most commonly used serum creatinine assay is the Jaffé reaction, which is based on the red color of the creatinine complex with alkaline picrate. It also measures other normally occurring chromogens, such as glucose, protein, ketones, and ascorbic acid, which represent about 14% of total creatinine when renal function is normal, though substantially less when serum creatinine is elevated. Ketoacidosis, barbiturates, and cephalosporin antibiotics may artifactually increase serum creatinine by as much as 100% and falsely decrease measured creatinine clearance.

Unlike inulin, about 20% of creatinine is secreted by the proximal tubule, so creatinine clearance overestimates

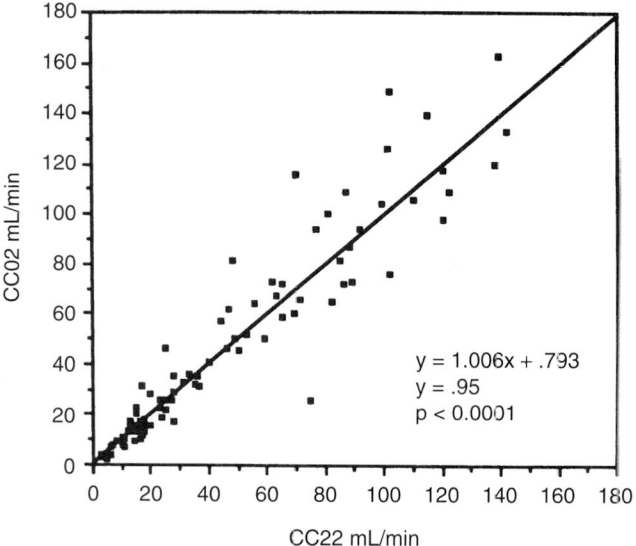

Figure 20–9 Creatinine clearance: 2- versus 22-hour values. There is a close and significant correlation in creatinine clearance estimates from a 2-hour and 22-hour urine collection. CC02, 2-hour urine collection; CC22, 22-hour urine collection. (From Sladen RN, Endo E, Harrison T: Two-hour versus 22-hour creatinine clearance in critically ill patients. Anesthesiology 67:1013-1016, 1987.)

$$y = 1.006x + .793$$
$$y = .95$$
$$p < 0.0001$$

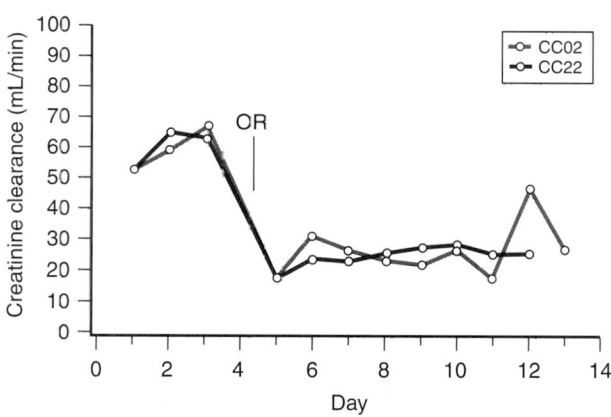

Figure 20–11 Renal revascularization in a patient with renovascular hypertension and renal insufficiency admitted to the intensive care unit for preoperative monitoring and stabilization. Bilateral renal revascularization was performed, and after return from the operating room, a substantial decline in renal function was noted. These changes were tracked equally well by creatinine clearance derived from a 2-hour (CC02) and a 22-hour (CC22) collection.

the GFR, and the ratio between the clearance of creatinine and inulin is 1.2:1. As the GFR declines, tubular secretion of creatinine increases. When the GFR is less than 40 mL/min/1.73 m², a creatinine-inulin clearance ratio as high as 1.8:1 to 2.5:1 may be achieved.[16] In patients with normal renal function, the underestimation of GFR induced by the Jaffé reaction is balanced by the overestimation of GFR induced by tubular creatinine secretion, and creatinine clearance provides a reasonable representation of the GFR. However, widely used drugs such as trimethoprim, H_2 receptor antagonists, and salicylates block the tubular secretion of creatinine and may elevate serum creatinine and decrease creatinine clearance. When serum levels of creatinine are very high, it is excreted into the gut and undergoes extrarenal metabolism by intestinal organisms.

For all these reasons, an isolated creatinine clearance estimate may not be diagnostic of lesser degrees of renal dysfunction. Nonetheless, serial estimates of creatinine clearance provide a useful clinical guide to alterations in renal function and prognosis. The variability of creatinine clearance diminishes as the GFR declines; in fact, loss of variability is a clue to deteriorating renal function. If the GFR is rapidly declining, creatinine clearance alerts the physician earlier and more compellingly than serum creatinine does because it reflects the creatinine excretion rate (i.e., urine creatinine content times urine flow rate [$U_{Cr} \times V$]). Directional changes between creatinine clearance and inulin clearance show good agreement.[16] At low GFR levels, a creatinine-inulin clearance ratio as high as 2:1 (e.g., 12 versus 6 mL/min) would induce little actual difference in clinical management.

Serum Creatinine

Serum creatinine is a useful marker of stable renal function, but it is unreliable when the GFR is rapidly changing.[17] The serum creatinine concentration depends on its volume of distribution (total-body water), creatinine generation rate (muscle mass and rate of catabolism), and creatinine excretion rate (GFR). Perioperative fluid administration increases total body water and dilutes serum creatinine, which underestimates renal dysfunction. In a cachectic patient with very low muscle mass, creatinine generation may be so feeble that the serum creatinine level remains subnormal even in the face of a markedly decreased GFR. In some patients with a serum creatinine concentration of less than 0.9 mg/dL, creatinine clearance may be less than 25 mL/min.[18]

The relationship between serum creatinine and GFR is inverse and exponential. A doubling of serum creatinine implies a halving of the GFR. An increase in serum creatinine from 0.8 to 1.6 mg/dL may not generate much attention, but it indicates a 50% decrease in the GFR. A much larger increase from 4 to 8 mg/dL also represents a 50% decrease in GFR, but by this time renal insufficiency is well established (Fig. 20-12). After a transient renal insult (e.g., suprarenal aortic cross-clamping), serum creatinine may increase for a few days while the GFR is actually recovering.[19] In oliguric acute renal failure, serum creatinine is directly proportional to the creatinine generation rate. Creatinine clearance is reliably low but is associated with wide variability in serum creatinine.

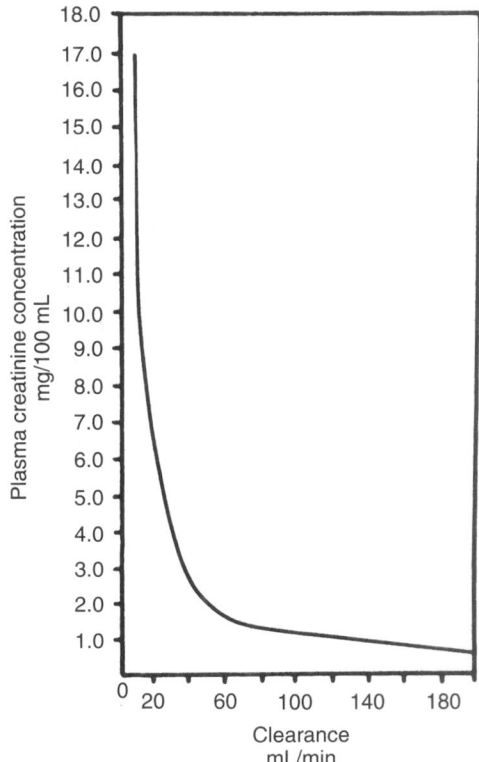

Figure 20–12 Relationship between serum creatinine and glomerular filtration rate (GFR). The relationship between serum creatinine and GFR as measured by creatinine clearance is reciprocal and exponential. Doubling of serum creatinine corresponds to halving of the GFR. Relatively large declines in GFR from normal are associated with small increases in serum creatinine until the GFR decreases below 60 mL/min; further decrements are associated with large increases in serum creatinine. (From Alfrey AC, Chan L: Chronic renal failure: Manifestations and pathogenesis. *In* Schrier RW [ed]: Renal and Electrolyte Disorders, 4th ed. Boston, Little, Brown, 1992, p 541.)

Serum Creatinine–Based Nomograms

Cockroft and Gault[20] formulated a nomogram for rapid estimation of creatinine clearance without urine collection. The nomogram was based on population studies incorporating serum creatinine, age, weight, and gender.

For males,

$$C_{Cr} = (140 - Age) \times \text{Weight in kg} / (\text{Serum creatinine} \times 72) \quad (14)$$

For females, the derived creatinine clearance is multiplied by 0.85.

In these formulas, the body weight that is used may substantially alter the derived creatinine clearance. In obese or edematous patients, total body weight is much greater than the lean body mass from which creatinine is derived, and creatinine clearance is overestimated. In cachectic patients with depleted lean body mass, creatinine production is so low that serum creatinine is frequently less than 1.0 mg/dL and overestimates the true GFR. Robert and associates[21] adjusted the Cockroft-Gault equation to incorporate ideal body weight from a nomogram and serum creatinine corrected to 1.0 mg/dL (if less than

1.0 mg/dL). With this modification they found that single measurements in hemodynamically stable patients correlate more closely with inulin clearance than either a 30-minute or a 24-hour creatinine clearance.

When renal function is rapidly changing, serum creatinine–based nomograms are subject to the same limitations as serum creatinine itself. Rapid alterations in GFR are reflected by rapid changes in the creatinine excretion rate, which is incorporated into measured creatinine clearance as $U_{CR} \times V$. Serum creatinine itself changes much more slowly and depends on the equilibrium point between creatinine production and excretion. In fact, serum creatinine does not begin to increase above normal levels until the GFR declines below 50 mL/min/1.73 m^2, and occasionally it will remain normal even when the GFR dips as low as 20 to 40 mL/min/1.73 m^2.

Tubular Function Tests

Tests of renal tubular function essentially measure urinary concentrating ability and sodium handling. As such, they can distinguish oliguria caused by dehydration (prerenal syndrome) from that attributable to tubular injury (acute tubular necrosis). In prerenal oliguria, tubular function is preserved, in fact "switched on" to concentrate urine and conserve sodium. It is reset by restoration of hemodynamic status to normal. In established acute tubular necrosis, concentrating ability and sodium conservation are lost and are not reestablished by restoration of normal RBF. However, in nonoliguric renal failure, which accounts for as much as 75% of cases of acute tubular necrosis encountered clinically, the changes in tubular function are less distinct from those of prerenal syndrome. In addition, any potent diuretic may override the tubular conserving function and generate a diuresis and natriuresis despite intravascular hypovolemia. These agents include loop diuretics, osmotic diuretics, and natriuretic vasodilators such as low-dose dopamine, fenoldopam, prostaglandin E_1 (PGE$_1$), and ANP.

Urinary Concentrating Ability
Concentrating ability is a very sensitive index of tubular function. In prerenal states, the urinary osmolar concentration is markedly increased. In acute tubular necrosis, the ability to concentrate urine may be lost 24 to 48 hours before serum creatinine or blood urea nitrogen (BUN) starts to increase.

Urine-to-Plasma Osmolar Ratio
The normal tubular response to dehydration or hypovolemia is to generate a urine-to-plasma osmolar ratio (U:P$_{Osm}$) of 1.5 or greater. Isosthenuria (U:P$_{Osm}$ = 1.0) in the presence of oliguria implies loss of tubular function and established acute renal failure. However, isosthenuria can occur in a prerenal state when it is induced by diuretic administration (see earlier).

Free Water Clearance
Free water clearance (CH$_2$O) attempts to represent the degree of urinary concentration or dilution in the tubules by distinguishing the renal clearance of solute from that of free water. Solute or osmolar clearance (C$_{Osm}$) is calculated by standard methods that entail the use of urine osmolality in mOsm/kg (U$_{Osm}$), plasma osmolality in mOsm/kg (P$_{Osm}$), and urine flow in mL/min (V):

$$C_{Osm} = (U_{Osm} \times V)/P_{Osm} \text{ (mL/min)} \qquad (15)$$

Then, osmolar clearance is subtracted from the urine flow rate to give free water clearance:

$$C_{H_2O} = V - C_{Osm} \text{ (mL/min)} \qquad (16)$$

When the urine is isosmotic with plasma (i.e., U$_{Osm}$ = P$_{Osm}$), osmolar clearance equals the urine flow rate (i.e., C$_{Osm}$ = V) and CH$_2$O is zero. Dilute urine reflects a hypo-osmotic state in which the urine flow rate exceeds osmolar clearance, and free water clearance has a positive value. Concentrated urine reflects a hyperosmotic state in which the urine flow rate is less than osmolar clearance. This situation results in negative free water clearance (i.e., free water retention), also known as tubular conservation of water (TCH$_2$O). Conceptually, TCH$_2$O represents the volume of fluid that would have to be added to urine to make its osmolality equivalent to that of plasma.[22]

With the onset of acute tubular necrosis and loss of concentrating ability, the urine becomes isosmotic, and CH$_2$O approaches zero ($\pm$0.25 mL/min). However, in distinguishing between prerenal and intrarenal oliguria, CH$_2$O does not really provide any more information about concentrating ability than U:P$_{Osm}$ does, and in addition, it requires a timed urine collection.

The concept of free water excretion emphasizes that renal regulation of solute and water balance occur independently of each other. The kidney has an enormous range in its ability to handle water. The maximal excretion of water, or positive free water clearance, is 18 L/day, about 10% of the GFR. The maximal conservation of water, or negative free water clearance, is 8 L/day.[22]

Water Conservation
Urine-to-Plasma Creatinine Ratio
The urine-to-plasma creatinine ratio (U:P$_{Cr}$) represents the proportion of water filtered by the glomerulus that is abstracted by the distal tubule. Normally, about 98% of water is abstracted, and urine creatinine is much greater than plasma creatinine. The ratio can increase a hundredfold in severe prerenal states. When tubular function is lost, the ratio declines to less than 20:1. For example, two patients have a serum creatinine of 2.0 mg/dL. In one, urine creatinine is 100 mg/dL, which implies a prerenal state (U:P$_{Cr}$, 50:1). In the other, urine creatinine is 20 mg/dL, which suggests acute tubular necrosis (U:P$_{Cr}$, only 10:1). Similar information may be obtained during the performance of an inulin clearance test by calculating the urine-to-plasma inulin ratio.

Sodium Conservation
Urine Sodium
During dehydration or hypovolemia, the tubules intensely reabsorb sodium so that the urinary sodium

concentration (U_{Na}) declines to less than 20 mEq/L. In established acute renal failure, the ability to conserve sodium and protect the intravascular volume is lost, and U_{Na} exceeds 60 to 80 mEq/L. Diuretic therapy overcomes tubular sodium conservation, so a high U_{Na} value does not necessarily imply loss of tubular function. However, a low U_{Na} value in the face of diuretic therapy implies the existence of an intense prerenal state.[23]

Fractional Excretion of Sodium

Fractional excretion of sodium (FE_{Na}) expresses sodium clearance as a percentage of creatinine clearance:

$$FE_{Na} = (Sodium\ clearance/Creatinine\ clearance) \times 100\%$$

Based on the relationship expressed in Equation 5,

$$FE_{Na} = [(U_{Na} \times V)/P_{Na}]/[(U_{Cr} \times V)/P_{Cr}] \times 100\%$$

The urine flow rate (V) is identical in the numerator and denominator and thus cancels out:

$$FE_{Na} = (U_{Na}/P_{Na})/(U_{Cr}/P_{Cr}) \times 100\% \qquad (17)$$

Thus, FE_{Na} may be calculated from a spot sample of blood and urine without requiring a timed urine collection.

During dehydration or hypovolemia, sodium clearance and FE_{Na} are decreased to less than 1% of creatinine clearance. When tubular ability to conserve sodium is lost in acute renal failure, FE_{Na} increases to more than 3%. However, FE_{Na} increases with normal tubular function after diuretic therapy and during postoperative sodium mobilization. Sequential increases in FE_{Na} associated with a declining creatinine clearance provide a more reliable indicator of deteriorating renal function than an isolated high FE_{Na} value does.

Investigational Tests of Renal Function

Glomerular Filtration Rate
Radioisotopic Filtration Markers

The use of intravascularly injected radiolabeled compounds to define the GFR is potentially simpler and more precise than the methods discussed earlier because it involves detection of decay in radiation and avoids the necessity for a timed urine collection. These compounds include sodium iothalamate (^{125}I), diethylenetriamine penta-acetic acid (DTPA) (^{99m}Tc), and ethylenediamine tetra-acetic acid (EDTA) (^{51}Cr). However, none of these compounds is inherently superior to inulin in its renal handling, the tests require great attention to detail and quality control, and there is the constant risk, albeit low, of radiation exposure.[11]

Total Renal Blood Flow
Flow Probes

Flow measurement by electromagnetic flow probes is based on the creation of a magnetic field around the circumference of the vessel. The field is disrupted by blood flow, and a voltage output proportional to blood velocity is generated. Ultrasonic flow probes use the Doppler technique in which high-frequency sound is transmitted across the lumen of the vessel. A shift in sound frequency is created by the movement of blood and is proportional to blood velocity.

$$Flow\ (mL/min) = Blood\ velocity\ (cm/min) \\ \times Area\ of\ vessel\ (cm^2)$$

Flow probe placement is invasive and requires direct surgical exposure of the renal arteries. Probes must be calibrated in vitro before and after measurements. However, they are generally very accurate.

Thermodilution Estimation of Renal Vein Effluent

Schaer and colleagues[24] used a double-lumen pigtail catheter with a thermistor placed in the renal vein of dogs under direct vision or fluoroscopy. RBF was calculated by thermodilution with cold saline, which allowed repeated measurements in conscious animals. The effect of the presence of the probe itself on RBF is unknown. A similar technique was used by Haywood and coworkers[25] to measure RBF for the assessment of renal oxygen delivery and consumption during septic shock in pigs.

Contrast Ultrasonography

Aronson and associates[26] attempted to measure RBF in vivo by contrast ultrasound. They injected sonicated albumin microspheres into the aorta of anesthetized dogs and then recorded simultaneous ultrasonographic images of the kidney and aorta and calculated RBF with a mathematical model. RBF was altered by means of a renal artery occluder or vasoactive drugs (dopamine or fenoldopam), and the results were compared with direct measurements by electromagnetic flow probe. Although the correlation between ultrasonography and flow probe measurements of RBF was reasonable (0.84), there was a large bias (in many cases greater than 200 mL/min) and variance. Ultrasonography tended to overestimate RBF, especially when cardiac output was changing. The authors concluded that this method allows estimation of trends in RBF and may be helpful in the qualitative assessment of regional distribution of blood flow between the renal cortex and medulla.

Intrarenal Blood Flow Distribution
Diffusible Gas Tracers

Considerable supposition about the intrarenal distribution of RBF within and between the renal cortex and medulla was based on studies using the radioactive gases ^{133}Xe and [85]Kr. The gases are injected into the renal artery, and radioactivity is counted externally. Renal radioactivity disappears faster the higher the blood flow, and flow is calculated mathematically from washout curves. In 1963, Thorburn and colleagues[27] extrapolated four monoexponential components from these curves, said to represent the outer renal cortex (zone I), juxtamedullary cortex (zone II), medulla (zone III), and perihilar fat (zone IV). Blood flow was greatest in zone I and progressively diminished through zones II to IV.

During the next decade, gas tracer studies such as those by Hollenberg and associates[28] suggested that ischemia and stress cause intrarenal redistribution of blood flow from zones I to II. Juxtamedullary nephrons are relatively salt retaining and have loops of Henle that penetrate the hypertonic medulla. Thus, this finding explained the retention of NaCl and edema observed during states of relative renal cortical hypoperfusion. However, the shortcomings of gas tracer techniques have generated skepticism about the validity of these studies.[29] The washout curves have not been matched to any specific anatomic area; ^{133}Xe itself decreases RBF, and the inert gases may diffuse out into the interstitium, especially in pathologic states.

Radioactive Microspheres

This terminal experimental procedure consists of the injection of radioactive microspheres—radiolabeled polystyrene beads 9 to 50 μm in diameter—into the central circulation. It is presumed that the microspheres are distributed to and within organs proportional to blood flow. The animal is then sacrificed, the organs are removed and dissected, and radioactivity is counted.

$$RBF = [Renal\ radioactivity\ (counts/min) \times Cardiac\ output]/$$
$$Total\ radioactivity\ of\ injected\ microspheres$$

Intrarenal localization of the microspheres truly represents regional blood flow. However, certain assumptions are made—that the injection itself does not interfere with renal hemodynamics and that all microspheres come to rest in the glomeruli without passing through the kidney or plugging arteries. It is also possible for this method to overestimate outer cortical blood flow because inner cortical afferent arterioles run at right angles to the interlobular arteries and microspheres may bypass through axial streaming.

NEUROHORMONAL REGULATION OF RENAL FUNCTION

The role of the kidney in controlling the interior milieu is modulated by a complex set of interactions. Two mutually dependent, but opposing neurohormonal systems maintain blood pressure, intravascular volume, and salt and water homeostasis (Fig. 20-13). The sympathoadrenal axis, the renin-angiotensin-aldosterone system, and AVP defend against hypotension and hypovolemia by promoting vasoconstriction and salt and water retention. The prostaglandins, bradykinins, and ANPs defend against hypertension and hypervolemia by promoting vasodilation and salt and water excretion (Fig. 20-14).

Anesthesia does not perturb these systems to any substantial degree. A considerable body of work suggests that in an intact organism, anesthetics affect renal function through extrarenal circulatory changes rather than by direct actions on the kidney.[30] Surgical or traumatic injury, on the other hand, induces profound vasoconstriction and salt and water retention, which may persist for several days. The clinical sequela is postoperative oliguria and edema. Renal vasoconstriction also predisposes the kidney to further perioperative ischemic and nephrotoxic insults. Elucidation of the role of ANP enhances the concept that these changes can be prevented or modified by maintenance of normal or increased intravascular (and thereby atrial) volume.

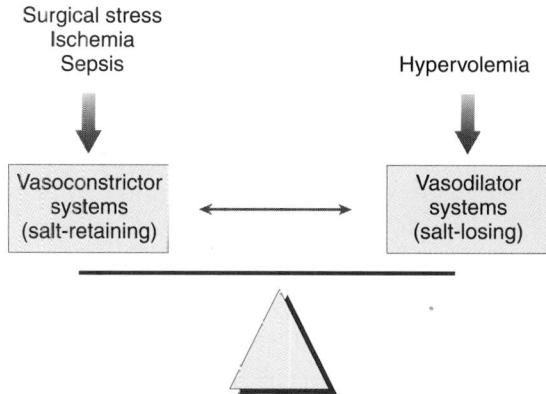

Figure 20-13 Neurohormonal regulation of renal function. Normally, a balance is present between systems promoting renal vasoconstriction and sodium retention versus systems promoting renal vasodilation and sodium excretion. Surgical stress, ischemia, and sepsis tip the balance in favor of vasoconstriction and sodium retention. On the other hand, hypervolemia (or induction of atrial stretch) tips the balance in favor of vasodilation and sodium excretion.

Systems Promoting Vasoconstriction and Salt Retention

Sympathoadrenal Axis

Sympathetic effects on the kidney are mediated by circulating epinephrine and neuronal release of norepinephrine. The renal cortex has a dense plexus of autonomic nerve fibers derived from the T12 to L4 spinal segments by way of the celiac plexus. The primary stimulus to the sympathetic response is a decrease in arterial blood pressure sensed by baroreceptors in the aortic arch, carotid sinus, and afferent arteriole. Afferent fibers travel by means of the vagus nerve and decrease the impulse transmission rate to the mediating centers in the hypothalamus, which results in increased adrenergic nerve activity. The kidney does not have any parasympathetic innervation.

A G protein–coupled phospholipase C receptor populates vascular smooth muscle and the mesangium and responds to α-adrenergic stimulation by epinephrine

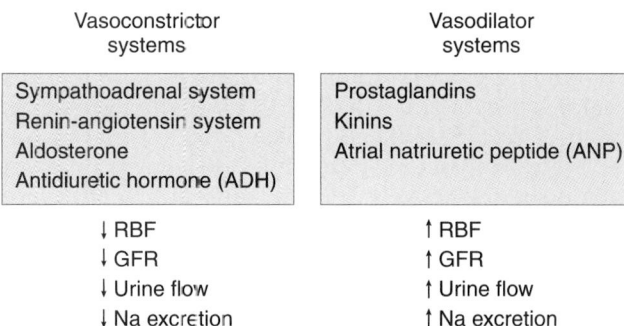

Figure 20-14 Neurohormonal renal regulatory systems. GFR, glomerular filtration rate; RBF, renal blood flow. (Modified from Sladen RN: Effect of anesthesia and surgery on renal function. Crit Care Clin 3:380, 1987. © 1987, The Williams and Wilkins Company, Baltimore.)

and norepinephrine. It also mediates vasoconstriction induced by a variety of other hormones and peptides, including angiotensin II, vasopressin, endothelin, platelet-activating factor, and leukotrienes.[3] The receptor subunit in the cell membrane is coupled through G_q protein to phospholipase C, which hydrolyzes phosphatidylinositol biphosphate (PIP_2) to inositol triphosphate (IP_3) and diacylglycerol (DAG). In turn, DAG activates protein kinase, which opens up a calcium channel in the membrane, and IP_3 triggers the release of calcium from the sarcoplasmic or endoplasmic reticulum. Both mechanisms bring about a rapid increase in intracellular calcium, and this increased intracellular calcium binds with calmodulin and thereby activates myosin light chain kinase, which results in smooth muscle contraction. The calcium-calmodulin complex simultaneously activates phospholipase A_2, and such activation results in the production of vasodilator prostaglandins (see later).

Mild α-adrenergic stimulation appears to cause preferential efferent arteriolar constriction, which preserves the FF. Severe α-adrenergic stimulation causes predominant afferent arteriolar constriction and decreases the FF.[31] Thus, the adrenergic response to a moderate decrease in renal perfusion (e.g., general anesthesia) favors preservation of the GFR. In contrast, the adrenergic response to shock exacerbates the decrease in GFR already induced by renal hypoperfusion (see Fig. 20-4).

Adrenergic nerves also supply the proximal tubule, thick ascending limb of Henle, and collecting duct, and their stimulation enhances NaCl reabsorption at these sites. Gas tracer studies suggested that sympathetic activation causes sodium retention by intrarenal redistribution of RBF from the outer cortex to salt-retaining juxtamedullary nephrons, but this effect was not confirmed by microsphere studies.[28,29]

A close relationship has been found between sympathetic stimulation and activation of the renin-angiotensin system. Adrenergic stimulation releases renin from the juxtaglomerular apparatus, and adrenergically induced vasoconstriction can be blocked by angiotensin-converting enzyme (ACE) inhibitor drugs such as captopril.

The effects of the administration of exogenous adrenergic agonists depend on their agonist activity. Drugs with predominantly α-adrenergic effects, such as norepinephrine, epinephrine, phenylephrine, and high-dose dopamine (>10 μg/kg/min), exacerbate the endogenous sympathetic responses to hypotension (see also Chapter 16). Drugs with predominantly $β_1$- and $β_2$-adrenergic activity, such as dobutamine or isoproterenol, cause marked increases in cardiac output and thus RBF, but it is difficult to ascertain their intrarenal effects. Dopaminergic agonists, such as low-dose dopamine (<3 μg/kg/min), dopexamine, and fenoldopam, selectively increase RBF and may oppose α-adrenergic renal vasoconstriction.[24] They induce a quite different response in the kidney and will be discussed separately.

Renin-Angiotensin-Aldosterone System

Renin and Angiotensin

The juxtaglomerular apparatus consists of three groups of specialized tissue. In the afferent arteriole, modified fenestrated endothelial cells produce renin; in the juxtaposed distal tubule, cells of the macula densa act as chemoreceptors; and in the glomerulus, mesangial cells have contractile properties (see Fig. 20-3). Together, these cells provide an important regulating system for blood pressure, salt, and water homeostasis.[32]

Renin secretion is stimulated by actual hypovolemia (hemorrhage, diuresis, sodium loss or restriction) or effective hypovolemia (positive-pressure ventilation, congestive heart failure, sepsis, or cirrhosis with ascites). Its release is controlled by several mechanisms. A decrease in renal artery perfusion pressure triggers baroreceptors in the afferent arterioles. Sympathetic nerve stimulation and circulating catecholamines act on β-adrenergic receptors in the afferent arterioles. An increase in chloride concentration in the distal tubular fluid activates cells of the macula densa, which trigger renin release from the afferent arteriole. This tubuloglomerular feedback appears to play a role in modulating GFR during normal and abnormal renal function through a continuous feedback loop.[4,22]

Renin acts on angiotensinogen, a large circulating glycoprotein released from the liver, and cleaves off a decapeptide, angiotensin I. In the kidney and the lung, angiotensin I is further cleaved by endothelial-based ACE to form an octapeptide, angiotensin II, a potent vasoconstrictor (Fig. 20-15). Renin is the rate-limiting enzyme in the production of angiotensin II.[33]

Activation of modest amounts of angiotensin II causes renal cortical vasoconstriction predominantly at the level of the efferent arterioles (see Fig 20-4). This vasoconstriction acts to maintain the glomerular FF in the face of mild to moderate decreases in RBF or perfusion pressure. The importance of this protective mechanism is emphasized by the deterioration in GFR that occurs when ACE inhibitors are administered to patients with hypotension, renal insufficiency, or unilateral renal artery stenosis.[34,35] Severe stress induces the release of high levels of angiotensin II, which constricts the glomerular mesangial cells and decreases the glomerular FF. Angiotensin II promotes systemic vasoconstriction at about one tenth of its renal effect, yet systemic arterial pressure and vascular resistance can be markedly decreased by ACE inhibitors such as captopril and enalapril or angiotensin receptor antagonists.

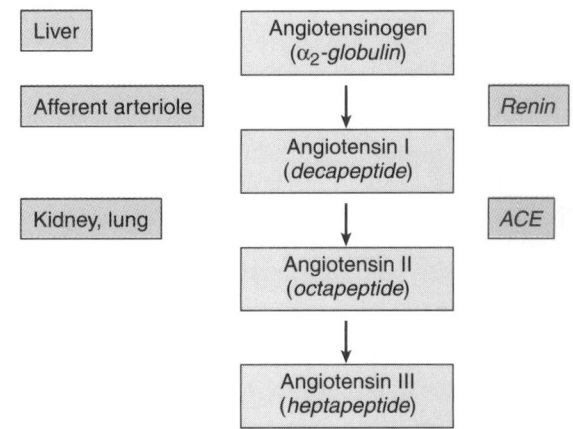

Figure 20–15 Renin-angiotensin system. For an explanation, see the text. ACE, angiotensin-converting enzyme.

The effect of angiotensin II in causing salt and water retention is enhanced by its actions in stimulating aldosterone secretion by the adrenal cortex, AVP secretion by the posterior pituitary, and NaCl reabsorption by the proximal tubule.[32]

Angiotensin II triggers a number of responses that modulate or oppose its own actions. It inhibits renin secretion by a negative feedback mechanism. Blockade of angiotensin formation by ACE inhibitors causes vasodilation but increases plasma renin levels. Angiotensin II activates phospholipase A_2, which triggers the synthesis of intrarenal prostaglandins. Vasodilator prostaglandins modulate the action of angiotensin II and may be responsible for its preferential activity on the efferent arteriole at low plasma levels.[33] Angiotensin-induced vasoconstriction increases atrial pressure and releases ANP, which opposes the renin-angiotensin-aldosterone system.

The consequences of ACE inhibition on renal function depend on the patient's volume status, systemic hemodynamics, and baseline renal perfusion. In the long-term treatment of hypertension and congestive heart failure, especially in diabetics, the administration of ACE inhibitors such as captopril, enalapril, or lisinopril decreases renal vascular resistance and appears to benefit renal function. Short-term pretreatment with captopril may prevent a decrease in RBF and GFR and preserve sodium excretion during CPB.[36] However, deterioration in renal function and hyperkalemia have been reported with the use of ACE inhibitors in patients with hypotension, renal insufficiency, or unilateral renal artery stenosis, probably related to the blockade of compensatory angiotensin-mediated efferent arteriolar constriction.[35] It may be prudent to avoid their use in patients with unstable hemodynamics in the immediate perioperative period.

Aldosterone

Aldosterone is a steroid hormone secreted by the zona glomerulosa of the adrenal cortex in response to hyperkalemia or hyponatremia. Angiotensin II and adrenocorticotropic hormone also trigger its release. It acts at the thick ascending limb of the loop of Henle, the principal cells of the distal tubule, and the collecting duct to increase active absorption of sodium and passive absorption of water, thus culminating in an expanded blood volume. Sodium retention in vessel walls appears to enhance their response to vasoconstrictor agents.

In contrast to the immediate sympathetic angiotensin II response to hypovolemia, there is a delay of about 1 to 2 hours from the secretion of aldosterone to its action on sodium reabsorption. As illustrated in Figure 20-16, aldosterone forms a complex with a receptor at the cell membrane in the principal cells of the distal tubule. The aldosterone-receptor complex travels to the cell nucleus, where it induces cytoplasmic transcription of mRNA. Such transcription fosters the synthesis of proteins that form sodium channels in the apical cell membrane and thus enhances the Na-K–ATPase pump in the basolateral cell membrane.[37] Sodium is transported from the tubular fluid into the peritubular capillary in exchange for potassium. Long-standing stimulation of aldosterone secretion, characteristically induced by the intravascular

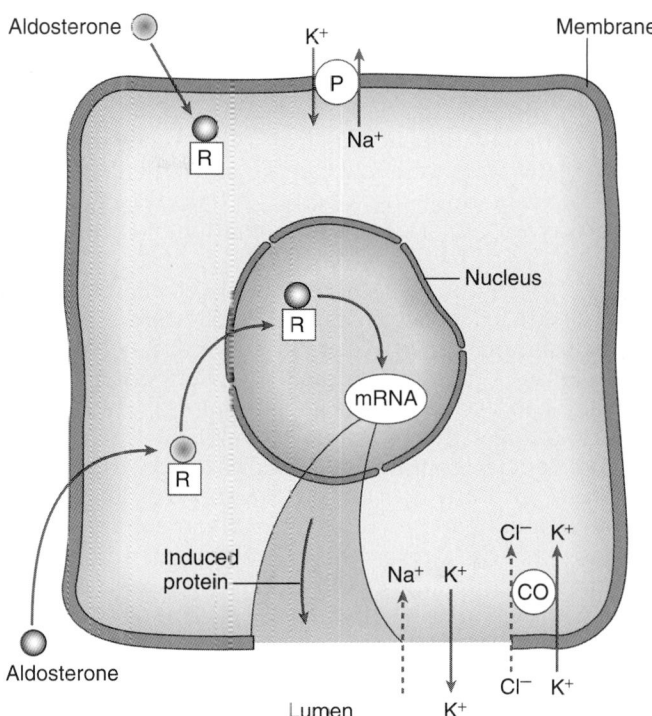

Figure 20–16 Action of aldosterone. Aldosterone enters the distal tubular cytoplasm, attaches to a receptor, and then migrates to the nucleus, where it induces the formation of messenger RNA (mRNA). The mRNA in turn induces the synthesis of a protein that enhances the permeability of the apical (luminal) membrane to sodium and potassium. Reabsorption of sodium stimulates the basolateral membrane Na-K-ATPase pump, the intracellular concentration of potassium rises, and it follows its concentration gradient out into the lumen. The net effect of aldosterone's action is sodium reabsorption and potassium loss. CO, cotransporter (= symporter); P, sodium-potassium-ATPase pump; R, receptor. (Redrawn from Wingard LB, Brody TM, Larner J, Schwartz A: Diuretics: Drugs that increase excretion of water and electrolytes. In Wingard LB, Brody TM, Larner J, Schwartz A [eds]: Human Pharmacology: Molecular-to-Clinical. London, Wolfe, 1991, p 249.)

volume depletion of chronic ascites, culminates in potassium depletion and hypokalemic alkalosis.

Arginine Vasopressin

AVP, previously known as antidiuretic hormone, regulates urinary volume and osmolality and controls diuresis and antidiuresis. It is a nine–amino acid peptide, 8-arginine-vasopressin, that is synthesized in the supraoptic and paraventricular nuclei of the anterior hypothalamus.[37] These nuclei are essentially the cell bodies of neurons whose axons extend down into nerve terminals in the posterior pituitary, together constituting the neurohypophysis. When AVP is synthesized, it undergoes neuroaxonal transport to the posterior pituitary gland, where it is stored in granules. Neural stimulation of the cell bodies triggers exocytosis of AVP from the terminal vesicles into the circulation.

AVP acts on specific V_2 receptors in the collecting ducts to induce water reabsorption and a decreased flow of concentrated urine. It also increases NaCl reabsorption from the thick ascending loop of Henle into the medullary interstitium, which maintains its hypertonicity and facilitates movement of water out of the collecting duct along the osmotic gradient. Such reabsorption results in tubular conservation of water and free water retention (i.e., negative free water clearance). The net effect is that AVP increases urine osmolality and decreases plasma osmolality without a significant alteration in excretion of solute.

The V_2 receptor on the basolateral cell membrane of the collecting duct responds to AVP through a receptor mechanism analogous to the β-adrenergic receptor.[37] By activation of G protein–coupled adenylyl cyclase, ATP is converted to cyclic adenosine monophosphate (cAMP). In turn, cAMP activates a protein kinase that causes pre-formed vesicles containing water channels to migrate and fuse with the apical cell membrane. This action results in a dramatic increase in membrane permeability to water, which is reabsorbed into the cell and thence into the peritubular capillary. This process is rapidly reversed when plasma AVP levels decline (the plasma half-life of AVP is between 5 and 15 minutes).

Regulation of AVP Secretion

Hypothalamic osmoreceptors are sensitive to increases in serum osmolality of as little as 1% above normal. As illustrated in Figure 20-17A, the threshold for AVP secretion (and the sensation of thirst) is between 280 and 290 mOsm/kg. Once this threshold is exceeded, the secretion rate has a very steep gain.[38] Even mild dehydration results in rapid antidiuresis, and urine osmolality can increase from 300 to 1200 mOsm/kg as plasma AVP levels rise from 0 to 5 pg/mL (see Fig. 20-17B).

Decreases in intravascular volume also stimulate AVP secretion mediated by stretch receptors with vagal afferents in the left atrium and pulmonary veins. Hypovolemia-induced secretion of AVP overrides the osmolar responses and contributes to the perioperative syndrome of inappropriate antidiuretic hormone secretion (SIADH): fluid retention, hypo-osmolality, and hyponatremia.[39] The situation is exacerbated by the administration of large volumes of hypotonic solutions that decrease serum osmolality. Psychic stress, through cortical input, also induces AVP release and can override osmotic and volume sensors.

By far the most potent trigger for AVP release is systemic arterial hypotension mediated by aortic and carotid baroreceptors. It overrides all other triggers, and plasma AVP may reach levels 10- to a 1000-fold greater than normal (see Fig. 20-17C). At these concentrations AVP acts as a vasoconstrictor, especially in the outer renal cortex. It does so by stimulating the V_1 receptor, which is found on vascular smooth muscle cells, glomerular mesangial cells, and cells of the vasa recta and promotes vasoconstriction through the phosphatidylinositol pathway.[38] AVP maintains effective glomerular filtration pressure because it is an extremely potent constrictor of the efferent arteriole, and unlike catecholamines and angiotensin, it has little effect on the afferent arteriole, even at high plasma levels.[40]

Anesthetic agents have little direct effect on AVP secretion, except through the changes that they induce in

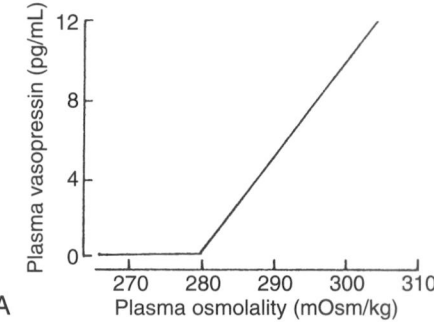

A

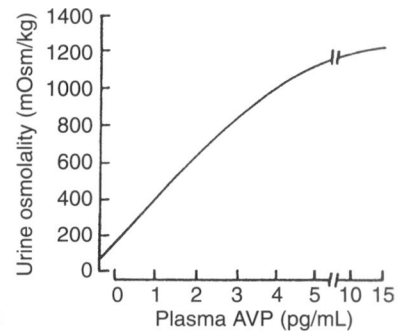

B

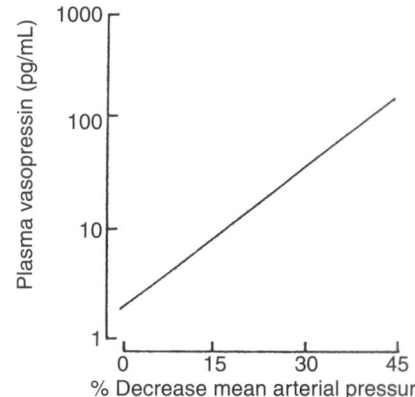

C

Figure 20–17 Physiologic regulation of arginine vasopressin (AVP). For an explanation, see the text. (From Landry DW: Vasopressin deficiency and hypersensitivity in vasodilatory shock: Discovery of a new clinical syndrome. P & S Med Rev 3:3-7, 1996.)

arterial blood pressure, venous volume, and serum osmolality. Surgical trauma is a major stimulus to AVP secretion. This stress response, whether mediated by pain or by intravascular volume changes, is profound and lasts at least 2 to 3 days after the surgical procedure.

Systems Promoting Vasodilation and Salt Excretion

Prostaglandins and Kinins

Prostaglandins

Intrarenal prostaglandins play an important role in endogenous renal protection, largely by vasodilating juxtamedullary blood vessels and maintaining inner cortical blood flow.[41] Prostaglandins are called autocoids because unlike true hormones, they are produced in minute amounts and have a local, evanescent action. They are also referred to as eicosanoids because their structure is based on a 20-carbon fatty acid (*eicosa* is 20 in Greek). The synthesis of intrarenal prostaglandins is summarized in Figure 20-18.

Phospholipase A_2, which resides in the inner lipid layer of the cell membrane, controls prostaglandin production through its formation of the prime precursor arachidonic acid. It is stimulated by ischemia and hypotension and also by norepinephrine, angiotensin II, and AVP. Thus, the factors that induce and mediate the stress response simultaneously activate prostaglandins, which defend the kidney against their actions. Cyclooxygenase-1 (COX-1) acts on arachidonic acid to form PGG_2, the precursor of the family of vasodilator prostaglandins that includes PGD_2, PGE_2, and PGI_2 (prostacyclin). They induce vasodilation through activation of cAMP, which blocks distal tubule sodium reabsorption, and they oppose the actions of norepinephrine, angiotensin II, and AVP. Prostaglandins may be particularly important in decreasing the vasoconstrictor activity of angiotensin II on the afferent arteriole and glomerular mesangial cells.[33] Production of prostaglandins promotes renal vasodilation, maintains intrarenal hemodynamics, and enhances sodium and water excretion. The renal vasodilator response to mannitol during hypoperfusion appears to be mediated through prostaglandin activation.[42] At the same time, prostaglandins also stimulate renin secretion, so a constant "yin and yang" occurs between the two systems.[43]

COX-2 forms derivatives of arachidonic acid that induce inflammation and renal vasoconstriction, and these derivatives are thus important in pathologic states. Thromboxane A_2 is derived from cyclic endoperoxides by the action of thromboxane synthetase. It induces vasoconstriction and platelet aggregation, and in the kidney it causes mesangial cell contraction, which decreases the GFR by diminishing the effective glomerular surface area and filtration constant (K_f). Renal levels of thromboxane are increased in experimental acute renal failure and sepsis. In animal experiments, the administration of a specific thromboxane synthetase inhibitor prevents the deterioration in renal function induced by the injection of endotoxin.[44] Another vasoconstrictor prostaglandin, PGF_2, which acts on the thromboxane receptor, is formed when arachidonic acid is oxidized by free radicals liberated by leukostasis during acute inflammation. The leukotrienes, arachidonic acid derivatives formed by lipoxygenase, are also released from endotoxin-activated leukocytes. Like thromboxane, leukotrienes C_4 and D_4 induce mesangial cell contraction and decrease the GFR.

Kinins
Kinins act as vasodilators that interact with and enhance the action of prostaglandins while modulating the renin-angiotensin system.[45] For example, kinins stimulate phospholipase A_2, and kininase (which controls the intrarenal kinin concentration) is blocked by ACE inhibitors. Two important intrarenal kinins, bradykinin and kallidin, appear to decrease the renal vasoconstriction induced by adrenergic hormones and angiotensin II.

Atrial Natriuretic Peptide
The potential role of an endogenous natriuretic hormone was postulated for many years before ANP was identified. In 1972, Gorfinkel and coworkers[46] demonstrated a profound difference in the canine renal response to shock in that it depended on concomitant atrial pressure. Hypovolemic shock resulted in a rapid diminution in RBF

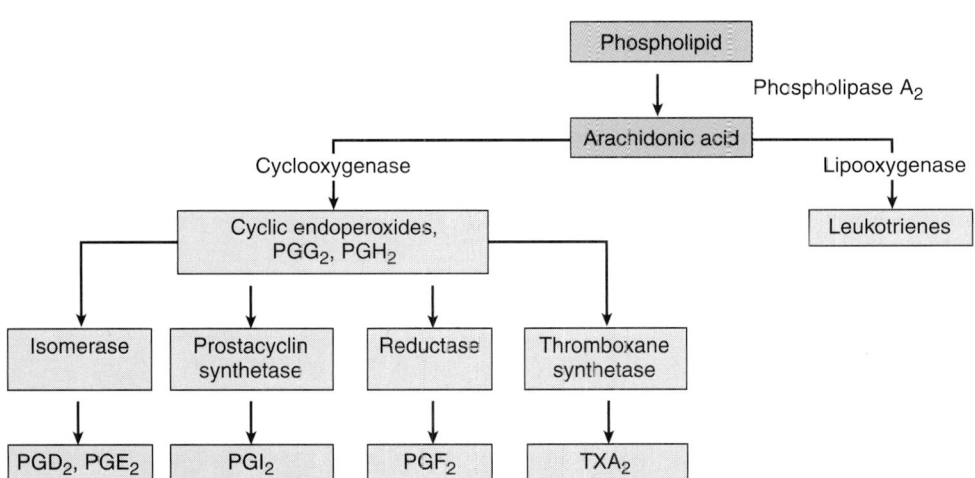

Figure 20–18 Synthesis of renal prostaglandins. Phospholipase A_2 is stimulated by ischemia, norepinephrine, and angiotensin II and cleaves arachidonic acid from its bond with membrane phospholipid. Cyclooxygenase acts on arachidonic acid to form evanescent cyclic endoperoxides (PGG_2 and PGH_2). The action of isomerase and prostacyclin synthetase culminates in formation of the vasodilator prostaglandins PGD_2, PGE_2, and PGI_2 (prostacyclin), which oppose the action of the renin-angiotensin system on the kidney and protect against ischemic stress. Inhibition of cyclooxygenase by nonsteroidal anti-inflammatory drugs predisposes the kidney to damage. Under hypoxic or ischemic conditions, cyclic endoperoxides undergo reduction to the vasoconstrictor PGF_2, which acts on thromboxane receptors. Endotoxin increases the activity of leukocyte lipoxygenase and thromboxane synthetase. Leukotrienes (especially C_4 and D_4) and thromboxane (TXA_2) induce renal vasoconstriction and contribute to the vasomotor nephropathy of sepsis.

to 10% of control, whereas in cardiogenic shock, RBF was preserved at 75% of control. The primary difference was that in cardiogenic shock, atrial pressure was elevated, thus suggesting that atrial distention caused the release of a renal protective hormone. In 1981, de Bold and colleagues[47] confirmed the existence of ANP by demonstrating that an extract of atrial tissue caused natriuresis in rats. In the subsequent decades the important actions of ANP on renal hemodynamics and sodium excretion have been well characterized.[48]

Indeed, an entire series of peptides with a similar precursor have been identified, with a core of 25 to 32 amino acids required for ANP-like activity. ANP is now referred to as human A-type natriuretic peptide in recognition of the existence of B-type natriuretic peptide (BNP) released from brain and cardiac ventricles and C-type natriuretic peptide released from the endothelium of major vessels.[49] Urodilatin is a natriuretic peptide produced in the lower urinary tract. Analogs have been developed and produced in recombinant form for exogenous administration, such as anaritide (derived from ANP) and nesiritide (derived from BNP). All these compounds induce arterial and venous dilation, increase RBF and GFR, and suppress the action of norepinephrine, angiotensin, and endothelin.

ANP is released from electron-dense granules in atrial myocytes in response to local wall stretch and increased atrial volume.[33] It dilates vascular smooth muscle through activation of guanylate cyclase and the formation of cyclic guanosine monophosphate (cGMP). At the phospholipase C–linked receptor, ANP competitively blocks norepinephrine and noncompetitively blocks angiotensin II, thus reversing vascular smooth muscle constriction. ANP causes a prompt, sustained increase in GFR and the glomerular filtration fraction, even when RBF is not increased or when arterial pressure is decreased. This effect suggests that it causes afferent arteriolar dilation with or without efferent arteriolar constriction. The increased GFR increases the filtered load of sodium, but natriuresis may be due to increased medullary blood flow, which washes out the concentration gradient.[50]

ANP appears to have a mutually antagonistic interaction with endothelin, the endogenous vasoconstrictor peptide produced by vascular endothelium.[33] It opposes the renin-angiotensin-aldosterone system on several fronts (Fig. 20-19). ANP inhibits renin secretion and decreases angiotensin-stimulated aldosterone release. It also inhibits aldosterone release directly at the zona glomerulosa of the adrenal cortex and blocks the salt-retaining action of aldosterone at the distal tubule and collecting duct. Through cGMP activation, it inhibits NaCl reabsorption at the medullary portion of the collecting duct.[22] ANP also promotes diuresis by inhibiting AVP secretion from the posterior pituitary and antagonizing its effect on the antidiuretic V_2 receptor in the collecting duct.

The renal protective role of endogenous ANP was further elucidated by Shannon and associates,[51] who noticed that patients undergoing mitral valve replacement had lower urine output after cardiac surgery than did those undergoing aortic valve replacement or coronary revascularization. They discovered that patients whose postoperative mean left atrial pressure declined by more than 7 mm Hg from

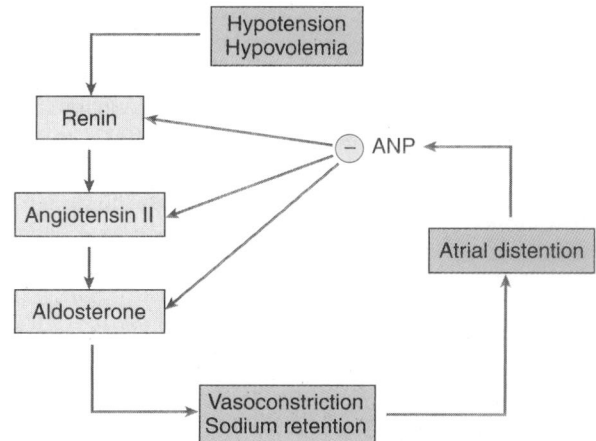

Figure 20–19 Interactions between atrial natriuretic peptide (ANP) and the renin-angiotensin-aldosterone system. Hypotension or hypovolemia triggers the release of renin from the afferent arteriole, thereby causing the formation of angiotensin II, which stimulates the release of aldosterone from the adrenal cortex. Angiotensin II and aldosterone cause vasoconstriction and sodium retention, ultimately resulting in re-expansion of intravascular volume; this volume re-expansion causes atrial distention, which triggers the release of ANP. ANP inhibits the release of renin, renin's action on angiotensinogen to form angiotensin II, angiotensin-induced vasoconstriction, stimulation of aldosterone secretion by angiotensin II, and the action of aldosterone on the collecting duct. Thus, the actions of ANP promote vasodilation and sodium excretion. Therapeutic administration of fluids to distend the atrium and release ANP is an important intervention to curtail renal vasoconstriction and sodium retention.

preoperative values (which commonly occurs with correction of mitral valve disease) had a significantly decreased postoperative urine sodium excretion and flow rate. Furthermore, a direct correlation was found between the quantitative decrease in left atrial pressure and the postoperative decline in circulating ANP levels (Fig. 20-20). In other words, patients with mitral valve disease and high left atrial pressure have a constant stimulus to ANP release. Valve replacement or repair results in decreased left atrial pressure, decreased ANP, and therefore decreased sodium excretion and urinary flow rate.

Dopaminergic System

The dopaminergic (DA) receptor has two subtypes (Table 20-2).[52] At the end organ, DA_1 receptors occur not only on the renal and splanchnic vasculature but also on the proximal tubule itself.[53] Stimulation of the DA_1

Table 20–2   Dopamine and its analogs

Receptor	DA_1	DA_2	β_1	β_2	α_1
Dopamine	+++	++	++	±	+++
Dobutamine	0	0	+++	++	±
Dopexamine	++	+	±	+++	0
Fenoldopam	++++	0	0	0	0

DA, dopamine; 0, no activity; ±, minimal activity; ++-++++, increasing potency of adrenergic action.

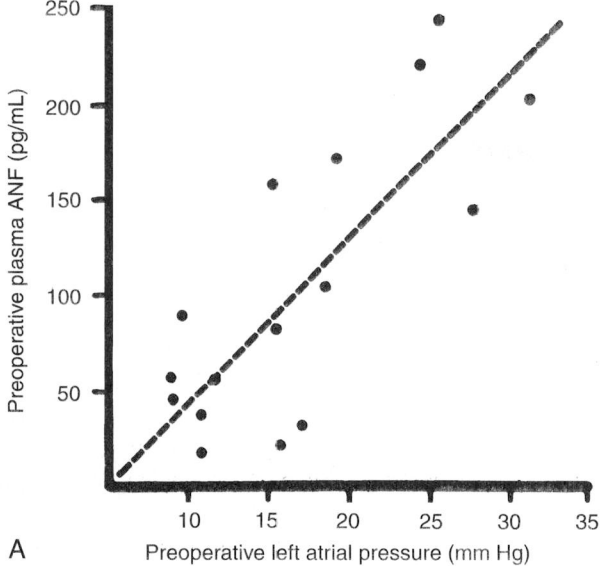

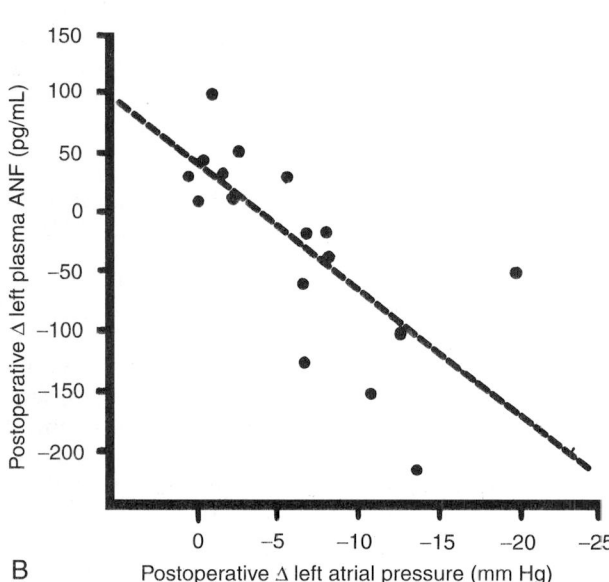

Figure 20–20 Correlation between left atrial pressure and plasma atrial natriuretic peptide (ANP) in a group of patients undergoing cardiac surgery. **A**, Significant correlation ($r = 0.8$, $P < .001$) between absolute preoperative left atrial pressure and plasma ANP. **B**, Significant correlation ($r = 0.72$, $P < .002$) between the postoperative decrease in left atrial pressure and the postoperative decrease in plasma ANP. ANF, atrial natriuretic factor (synonymous with ANP); Δ, change. (From Shannon RP, Libby E, Elahi D, et al: Impact of acute reduction in chronically elevated left atrial pressure on sodium and water excretion. Ann Thorac Surg 46:430-437, 1988.)

receptor activates cAMP and induces renal vasodilation, increased RBF and GFR, natriuresis, and diuresis. However, natriuresis can occur independently of increases in RBF and GFR and is abolished by specific D_1 receptor antagonists.[54] In the proximal tubule, dopamine inhibits the sodium-hydrogen antiporter system at the brush border membrane. In the medullary thick ascending limb, it also inhibits the Na-K–ATPase pump at the basolateral membrane.[54]

Neuronal DA_2 receptors are found on the presynaptic terminal of postganglionic sympathetic nerves. Stimulation inhibits the release of norepinephrine from presynaptic vesicles, a mechanism analogous to stimulation of the presynaptic α_2-adrenergic receptor. Through inhibition of norepinephrine, DA_2 receptor activation facilitates vasodilation.

Dopaminergic receptors form an integral component of the endogenous vasodilator-natriuresis system and are involved in maintenance of normal blood pressure. Endogenous dopamine appears to constitutively activate the DA_2 receptor, which synergistically enhances activation of the DA_1 receptor.[55] It acts as an autocrine and paracrine natriuretic factor by inhibiting tubular Na$^+$-K$^+$–ATPase activity, especially when sodium intake is increased.[56] It also opposes the antinatriuretic effects of norepinephrine and angiotensin II. Some evidence indicates that endogenous ANP also acts through the renal dopamine system by recruiting "silent" DA_1 receptors from the interior of the cell toward the plasma membrane.[56] It has been suggested that decreased dopaminergic activity contributes to the pathogenesis of idiopathic edema, which is manifested as retention of salt and water in the upright position.[57]

Nitric Oxide

Endogenous formation of nitric oxide is controlled by the enzyme nitric oxide synthase (NOS). NOS catalyzes hydroxylation of the nonessential amino acid L-arginine to L-citrulline.[58] Most actions of nitric oxide are mediated through its activation of soluble guanylate cyclase, which catalyzes the conversion of guanidine triphosphate to cGMP. cGMP has two major actions: relaxation of vascular smooth muscle and suppression of the inflammatory response. It inhibits leukocyte adhesion, platelet activation and aggregation, and cellular proliferation. cGMP is converted to GMP by phosphodiesterase I and V. Thus, the local action of nitric oxide can be enhanced by the administration of a selective phosphodiesterase V inhibitor such as sildenafil. Nitric oxide itself is rapidly inactivated by binding to intracellular heme and heme proteins (oxyhemoglobin, oxymyoglobin, guanylate cyclase, COX, cytochrome P450).

Nitric Oxide Synthase

NOS has several distinct subtypes that determine the site and function of nitric oxide synthesis. Constitutive NOS is calcium and calmodulin dependent and releases small amounts of nitric oxide for short periods ("tonic" release). Constitutive NOS has two subtypes: neuronal NOS, which acts as a peripheral neurotransmitter and induces cerebral vasodilation, and endothelial NOS, which is found in the vascular endothelium and mediates the activity previously ascribed to endothelium-derived relaxing factor. The latter is an important modulator of systemic and pulmonary vascular resistance. In the kidney, endogenous nitric oxide preserves blood flow to the oligemic juxtamedullary cortex[59] and may also provide endogenous protection against ischemic and nephrotoxic renal insults.[60]

Inducible NOS is calcium and calmodulin independent and is induced by cytokines predominantly in inflammatory cells (macrophages, granulocytes) but also in vascular smooth muscle cells. At low levels of activation, inducible NOS enhances the response to infection and promotes inflammation and wound healing. In severe sepsis, inducible NOS produces huge amounts of nitric oxide for protracted periods ("phasic" release) and is largely responsible for the characteristically profound systemic vasodilation that is refractory to norepinephrine.[61] High levels of nitric oxide and its reactive products nitrogen dioxide and peroxynitrite induce lipid peroxidation and denaturation of proteins, which drives the systemic inflammatory response syndrome and its attendant acute renal injury.

Duality of Nitric Oxide in Renal Function and Injury

Goligorsky and Noiri[62] have framed the hypothesis that an imbalance between the expression and activity of constitutive and inducible NOS plays an important role in the pathophysiology of acute renal failure. In experimental models of sepsis, nonselective inhibitors of both constitutive and inducible NOS improve blood pressure but worsen overall perfusion, including renal perfusion. Selective inhibitors of inducible NOS show promise in suppressing severe inflammation and vasodilation while maintaining tonic perfusion to vital organs, including the kidneys.[63]

Renal Adenosine System

Adenosine Receptors

Adenosine, the endogenous degradation product of ATP, is produced by every mammalian cell type and is normally thought of as a potent vasodilator. However, in the kidney, it plays an essential role in regulating intrarenal blood flow by inducing outer cortical vasoconstriction and preserving juxtamedullary perfusion. This variance in function is explained by the identification of at least four subtypes of adenosine receptor: A_1, A_{2a}, A_{2b}, and A_3 (Table 20-3).[64] Activation of the A_1 adenosine receptor induces outer cortical vasoconstriction; it also decreases renin release and inhibits diuresis and natriuresis. In contrast, A_{2a} adenosine receptors increase medullary RBF and enhance renin release, diuresis, and natriuresis.

Table 20-3 Adenosine receptor subtypes and functions

Receptor	Agonist Function	Ischemic Injury
A_1	Outer cortical vasoconstriction Decreased renin release Inhibition of diuresis and natriuresis	Highly protective
A_{2a}	Juxtamedullary vasodilation Increased renin release Promotion of diuresis and natriuresis	Highly protective
A_{2b}	Unknown	
A_3	Unknown	Potentiates injury

Ischemic Preconditioning and Adenosine

In a series of studies in an in vivo rat model of ischemic acute renal failure, Lee and Emala[65] characterized the role of adenosine and its receptor subtypes in ischemic preconditioning. Pre-ischemic administration of adenosine as well as a selective A_1 adenosine receptor agonist protected the kidney against global renal ischemic reperfusion injury. In contrast, pretreatment with selective A_3 receptor activation potentiated ischemic injury. A selective A_{2a} adenosine receptor agonist had the greatest renal protective effects, even if its administration was delayed until the early reperfusion period after termination of renal ischemia.[66]

It is conceivable that A_1 adenosine receptor stimulation decreases renal oxygen consumption through a decrease in cortical blood flow, GFR, and sympathetic tone and that A_2 adenosine receptor stimulation increases renal oxygen delivery through increased medullary blood flow. In addition, adenosine has cytoprotective properties, is the key mediator of ischemic preconditioning in the heart and brain, and is known to increase cellular resistance to ischemia in these organ systems. Pharmacologic development of a safe, specific A_{2a} adenosine receptor agonist might provide specific protection against renal ischemic injury.

PHARMACOLOGIC RENAL PROTECTION

Based on the physiology described in the preceding sections, an increasing number of pharmacologic agents have been used or promoted as protective agents. Although short-term benefits (increased urine flow, improved GFR) are commonly encountered, few definitive data have demonstrated differences in outcome measures such as acute renal failure, dialysis requirement, or mortality. Some of these agents will be discussed here, whereas others will be related to specific high-risk situations in the next section.

Dopaminergic Agonists

Dopamine

Dopaminergic agonists and antagonists may be classified on the basis of their selective or nonselective action on DA_1 and DA_2 receptors (see Table 20-2). Haloperidol,[67] a nonselective dopaminergic antagonist, and metoclopramide, a selective DA_1 antagonist,[68] inhibit the effects of dopamine in vitro and are used to categorize receptor activity. Their clinical impact on dopaminergic stimulation is not well studied.

The "triphasic" effects of dopamine have been well characterized by Olsen and colleagues, who performed a dose-response (1 to 12 µg/kg/min) study with dopamine in hydrated, salt-loaded normal subjects.[69] Mean arterial pressure decreased at 1 to 2 µg/kg/min, thus suggesting predominantly vasodilator dopaminergic effects. eRPF peaked at 3 µg/kg/min at 50% above baseline, but the GFR did not increase at any dose. An increase in cardiac output occurred at a dose of 5 µg/kg/min, consistent with a predominantly β-adrenergic inotropic effect. Mean arterial pressure increased progressively above 7.5 µg/kg/min, presumably reflecting increasing α-adrenergic-induced vasoconstriction.

Dopamine-induced natriuresis appears to be caused by increased proximal tubular outflow and diminished distal reabsorption.[69] At higher doses, saluresis actually increases, which suggests a pressure-dependent natriuretic effect. In a study comparing equi-inotropic doses of dopamine and dobutamine after cardiac surgery, the two agents had similar effects on GFR, RBF, renal vascular resistance, and FF. However, dopamine results in a greater urine flow rate, natriuresis, FE_{Na}, and potassium excretion, thus indicating a diuretic effect independent of changes in RBF and GFR.[70]

Dopamine may theoretically benefit renal function by selectively increasing RBF and inducing saluresis (DA_1 effects) or by increasing cardiac output and renal perfusion (β-adrenergic effects). It has been demonstrated to increase RBF in the face of norepinephrine-induced vasoconstriction.[24] However, dopamine's effectiveness is limited by its mixed adrenergic activity, with overlapping dose-response curves. Moreover, in a pharmacokinetic study on normal volunteers, MacGregor and associates found a 30-fold intersubject variability in plasma dopamine levels.[71] Some subjects given an infusion of "low-dose" dopamine had plasma levels consistent with those associated with doses in the high α-adrenergic range. The wide range in dopamine disposition may account for the variable and unpredictable responses observed when dopamine is administered in clinical practice. Even at low doses it can cause unwanted tachycardia. At doses above 10 μg/kg/min, dopamine has increasing activity on the $α_1$-adrenergic receptor, in part because of its biotransformation to norepinephrine. The net effect is progressive renal vasoconstriction and a diminished urine flow rate.

Perhaps because of the constraints just enumerated, few data are available to support the prophylactic administration of low-dose dopamine for renal protection in surgery, trauma, or sepsis. Low-dose dopamine did not improve RBF, GFR, or urine flow during canine thoracic aortic cross-clamping.[72] It does not significantly increase GFR or RBF in chronic renal insufficiency when the baseline GFR is less than 50 mL/min/1.73 m^2.[73] In a controlled prospective study on patients undergoing orthotopic liver transplantation, prophylactic low-dose dopamine had no significant benefit on intraoperative urine flow, postoperative creatinine clearance, acute renal failure, or mortality.[74] In a randomized, prospective study on cadaveric kidney graft recipients, dopamine at 2 μg/kg/min increased urine flow but did not alter postoperative creatinine clearance or the requirement for dialysis.[75] It was noted to frequently cause tachycardia.

Given this evidence, one concludes that dopamine should be restricted to therapeutic use as an inotropic agent with diuretic activity. If oliguria persists despite intravascular volume repletion, especially when associated with hypotension, dopamine can enhance blood pressure, cardiac output, and RBF and is useful in promoting urine flow.

Dopexamine

Dopexamine is a synthetic analog of dopamine. It is a potent $β_2$ receptor agonist and nonselective dopaminergic agonist, with about a third of dopamine's effect on the renal vasculature.[76] Its effects are predominantly chronotropic, with a moderate inotropic effect coupled with intense arterial vasodilation (inodilation). Potential advantages include improved myocardial efficiency through its lusitropic actions (enhanced diastolic relaxation and decreased wall stress) and promotion of renal perfusion. Used in the dose range of 1 to 5 μg/kg/min, it provides left and right ventricular afterload reduction in acute and chronic heart failure while augmenting RBF.[77] Tachycardia is common, but tachyarrhythmias are not. In a sense, dopexamine provides the pharmacologic profile of a phosphodiesterase inhibitor such as milrinone, but with the rapid onset and offset of action of a catecholamine.

Fenoldopam

Fenoldopam, a benzodiazepine dopamine analog, is a selective DA_1 receptor agonist and is devoid of DA_2, β-adrenergic, or α-adrenergic activity. When administered between 0.03 and 0.3 μg/kg/min, it causes a dose-related increase in RBF and natriuresis. In vitro, it antagonizes norepinephrine-induced vasoconstriction. It is rapidly metabolized with a half-life of 10 minutes, and when administered by intravenous infusion, it has a rapid onset and offset of effect.

In 1998 fenoldopam was approved for the short-term parenteral treatment of severe hypertension. Fenoldopam is as effective as sodium nitroprusside in controlling severe renovascular hypertension, but unlike nitroprusside, it induces significant increases in GFR, urine flow, and saluresis without rebound hypertension.[78] The selective DA_1 receptor agonist activity of fenoldopam suggests that it may confer protection against nephrotoxic or ischemic renal insults without the β-adrenergic side effects of dopamine.[79] At present, it appears that fenoldopam may have a role only in the realm of attenuation of contrast-induced nephropathy (see later).

Prostaglandins

The ability of vasodilator prostaglandins to counteract the vasoconstrictor effects of norepinephrine and angiotensin and to maintain inner cortical perfusion has led to considerable research on their renal protective effects. Exogenous infusion of synthetic prostaglandins such as PGE_1 prevents ischemia-induced acute renal failure in animals and may have a role in preservation of the donor kidney in renal transplantation.[80]

Calcium Channel Blockers

Calcium channel blockers prevent ischemic renal injury by a number of mechanisms, including prevention of reflow-induced vasoconstriction after ischemia, inhibition of angiotensin action in the glomerulus, and reduction of circulating interleukin-2 receptors.[81] They may reduce the accumulation of oxygen free radicals and reperfusion injury through prevention of intracellular calcium influx and the calcium/calmodulin-dependent conversion of xanthine dehydrogenase to xanthine oxidase.

However, calcium blockers may overcome renal autoregulation and worsen renal function when they induce hypotension. Administration of nifedipine to patients with renal insufficiency has been reported to cause nonoliguric renal failure that improved when use of the drug was discontinued.[82] In contrast, in hypertensive patients, diltiazem and nifedipine promote natriuresis and increase RBF and GFR.[83]

Calcium channel blockers confer important protection against nephrotoxins such as cyclosporine, cisplatin, and radiocontrast dyes (see later).

Natriuretic Peptides

Exogenous administration of ANP or its analog anaritide decreases systemic blood pressure through arterial and venous dilation. Nesiritide (human recombinant BNP), the only natriuretic peptide thus far approved by the Food and Drug Administration (FDA) for exogenous administration, is effective in the parenteral treatment of end-stage congestive heart failure. Its use promotes diuresis and relieves symptoms related to pulmonary congestion and edema. Urodilatin, an ANP congener produced by the kidney and excreted in urine, lacks the systemic vasodilator effects of the parent compound but has similar action on renal function.

Considerable interest has arisen regarding the ability of infused ANP to reverse established acute renal failure ("renal rescue"). Animal studies of both ischemic[84] and nephrotoxic[85] acute tubular necrosis have demonstrated that ANP infusion improves RBF and GFR, induces natriuresis, and decreases azotemia and renal histologic damage. In a controlled pilot study[86] involving 53 patients with established intrinsic acute renal failure, ANP infusion doubled creatinine clearance from 10 to 21 mL/min in 24 hours and decreased the incidence of dialysis from 52% to 23% ($P < .05$).

These results generated a large randomized, controlled, multicenter study in which 504 patients were prospectively identified as having oliguric (urine output, <400 mL/day) or nonoliguric acute tubular necrosis and randomized to receive anaritide or placebo for 24 hours.[87] In patients with oliguric acute renal failure, anaritide infusion induced significantly greater dialysis-free survival than placebo did, 27% versus 8% ($P < .008$). However, in nonoliguric acute renal failure, anaritide actually appeared to worsen survival (48% versus 59% with placebo). Of note, anaritide induced a decrease in blood pressure and urine flow rate in nonoliguric patients, whereas in oliguric patients, blood pressure was less affected and the urine flow rate increased.

To further evaluate these findings, the study was repeated in a multicenter, randomized, double-blind, placebo-controlled trial of 222 patients with oliguric acute renal failure.[88] No differences were noted in dialysis requirement, dialysis-free survival, or 60-day mortality between anaritide and placebo. However, patients receiving anaritide had significantly more hypotension during infusion of the study drug.

These studies emphasize the difficulty of translating promise in animal studies to successful outcome in large clinical trials and also emphasize the importance of maintenance of renal perfusion pressure in acute renal failure, given the loss of renal autoregulation that occurs.[8]

PERIOPERATIVE ISCHEMIC AND NEPHROTOXIC INJURY

This section will review perioperative agents and events that may disrupt normal renal physiology. If the disruption is severe enough or occurs in susceptible individuals, it may induce ischemic or nephrotoxic renal injury.

Anesthetic Drugs

The choice of an anesthetic technique to preserve renal function during and after surgery is predicated on the preservation of RBF and perfusion pressure; suppression of vasoconstrictor, salt-retaining stress responses to surgical stimulation and postoperative pain; and avoidance or curtailment of nephrotoxic insults. No single anesthetic drug alone meets these criteria.

Regional Anesthesia
Spinal or epidural anesthesia (see Chapter 43) that achieves sympathetic blockade of the 4th through 10th thoracic segments is extremely effective in suppressing the sympathoadrenal stress response and release of catecholamines, renin, and AVP. During major surgery, RBF and GFR are preserved as long as adequate renal perfusion pressure is maintained.[89-91] Maintenance of adequate perfusion pressure implies careful titration of the block, especially in elderly patients with cardiovascular disease, and may necessitate a 25% to 50% increase in intraoperative fluid administration.[92] However, Gamulin and colleagues[93] found that the renal sympathetic blockade obtained by epidural anesthesia did not block increases in renal vascular resistance induced by infrarenal aortic cross-clamping, nor did it prevent postoperative decreases in creatinine clearance.

General Anesthesia
The overall effect on renal function of anesthetic drugs in common use (see Chapters 7, 10, and 11) has been well summarized by Priano.[30] All anesthetic techniques and agents tend to decrease GFR and intraoperative urine flow. Some drugs also decrease RBF, but the FF is usually increased, which implies that angiotensin-induced efferent arteriolar constriction limits the decrease in GFR. However, these effects are much less significant than those caused by surgical stress or aortic cross-clamping, and after emergence from anesthesia they usually resolve promptly. Any anesthetic technique that induces hypotension will result in decreased urine flow because of altered peritubular capillary hydrostatic gradients, even if renal autoregulation is preserved (as it generally is during anesthesia). Permanent injury seldom results unless the kidneys are abnormal to begin with or the hypovolemic insult is prolonged and exacerbated by nephrotoxic injury.

Halothane, enflurane, or isoflurane with nitrous oxide induces mild to moderate reductions in RBF and GFR, primarily as a result of their effects on the central circulation (myocardial depression, peripheral pooling).[94] These effects can be attenuated by previous hydration. High-dose opioid techniques using fentanyl or sufentanil do not depress myocardial contractility and have minimal effect on RBF and GFR. They are also considerably more effective in suppressing the release of catecholamines, angiotensin II, aldosterone, and AVP during surgery than volatile agents are. However, during CPB, both AVP and catecholamine levels rise markedly despite high-dose opioid anesthesia.[95] Intravenous agents such as thiopental and diazepam cause minor changes in renal function, about a 10% to 15% deviation from control. Ketamine increases RBF but decreases the urine flow rate, possibly through sympathetic activation; it preserves RBF during hemorrhagic hypovolemia.[96]

Nephrotoxicity of Volatile Anesthetics

The potential nephrotoxicity of volatile anesthetics (see Chapter 8) is due to their metabolic breakdown to free fluoride ions, which cause a tubular lesion that results in loss of concentrating ability and polyuric acute renal failure.[97] Toxicity is exacerbated by aminoglycosides or previous renal dysfunction. Peak fluoride levels less than 50 μm/L seldom induce injury, whereas levels over 150 μm/L are associated with a high incidence of polyuric acute renal failure.[98] Administration of methoxyflurane at more than one minimum alveolar concentration (MAC) for more than 2 hours is capable of generating a peak fluoride level greater than 100 μm/L, and for this reason methoxyflurane is no longer used. Enflurane is metabolized more rapidly, and most studies indicated that peak fluoride levels seldom rise above 25 μm/L. The antituberculotic agent isoniazid enhances fluoride production, but only isolated reports of fluoride-induced nephrotoxicity from enflurane have ever appeared. Isoflurane produces peak fluoride levels less than 4 m/L, and halothane is not metabolized to fluoride at all.[99]

The potential nephrotoxicity of sevoflurane remains controversial. Although its metabolism generates more fluoride than enflurane metabolism does, clinically significant fluoride-induced nephrotoxicity has not been detected. Compound A, a vinyl ether formed by the degradation of sevoflurane at low flow through carbon dioxide absorbents, is capable of inducing renal injury in rats. Although acute renal failure has not been reported in humans, Eger and coauthors reported evidence of transient renal injury (albuminuria, tubular enzymuria) in volunteers subjected to 8 hours of 1.25 MAC sevoflurane at a 2-L/min gas flow.[100] No changes were detected in urinary concentrating ability, serum creatinine, or BUN. Subsequently, Eger and colleagues[101] described a dose-response relationship between biochemical markers of glomerular and tubular injury (urinary albumin, α-glutathione-S-transferase) and compound A exposure expressed as parts per million per hour. They suggested that the threshold of renal injury is 80 to 168 ppm/hr based on their observation of altered biochemical markers with 1.25 MAC sevoflurane at 2 L/min for 4 hours, which was not seen after 2 hours and not at all with desflurane.

Other laboratories have disputed Eger and associates' findings. Bito and coworkers compared 6-hour patient exposure to low- and high-flow sevoflurane with low-flow isoflurane and found no differences in BUN, creatinine, or tubular enzymes for 3 days postoperatively.[102] Kharasch and colleagues[103] had similar results with the use of sevoflurane or isoflurane at 1 L/min in 73 patients undergoing procedures lasting longer than 2 hours, and they concluded that a moderate duration of low-flow sevoflurane anesthesia, even with the formation of compound A, is as safe as low-flow isoflurane anesthesia. Ebert and colleagues[104] attempted to duplicate the original 8-hour Eger sevoflurane study in volunteers at two sites with blinded laboratory analyses. Biochemical derangements were minimal and transient, and no significant changes were detected in BUN, creatinine, or creatinine clearance. Despite the similarity in experimental design, the mean level of compound A was about 25% lower and mean arterial pressure about 10% higher than in the Eger study, which may have accounted for the difference in results.

In summary, clinically significant renal injury with the use of low-flow sevoflurane anesthesia has not been reported in patients, even with moderate preexisting renal dysfunction. The relationship between compound A formation, biochemical injury, and clinically relevant renal dysfunction remains unclear and unproven. Nonetheless, it appears prudent to follow current FDA guidelines, which recommend a fresh gas flow of at least 2 L/min to inhibit compound A formation and its rebreathing and to enhance its washout.

Positive-Pressure Ventilation

Positive-pressure ventilation (see Chapter 75) and positive end-expiratory pressure (PEEP) decrease RBF, GFR, sodium excretion, and the urine flow rate.[105] The extent of depression of renal function depends on the mean airway pressure. Thus, the impact on the kidney is greater with inverse ratio ventilation than with intermittent mandatory ventilation (IMV) and greater with IMV than with spontaneous ventilation with PEEP (continuous positive airway pressure).

These changes are largely mediated by transmission of airway and intrapleural pressure to the intravascular space and lead to decreases in venous return, transmural (i.e., effective) cardiac filling pressure, and cardiac output. Transmission may actually be attenuated in acute lung injury because of poor lung compliance. High levels of mean airway pressure may compress the pulmonary arterial circulation, increase right ventricular afterload, and induce the intraventricular septum to shift into the left ventricle and decrease its filling and cardiac output.[106] Positive-pressure ventilation increases inferior vena cava pressure and renal venous pressure and may increase tubular sodium reabsorption by increases in peritubular capillary pressure.

The decrease in cardiac output and systemic arterial pressure results in a carotid and aortic baroreceptor-mediated increase in sympathetic nerve tone in the kidney with subsequent renal vasoconstriction, antidiuresis, and antinatriuresis. Volume receptors in the atria respond to decreased filling by reducing ANP secretion, which results in increased sympathetic tone, renin activation, and AVP activity.

Salt and water retention during airway pressure therapy was originally surmised to be due to an AVP effect,[107] but it is now thought that sympathetic responses are more important and that sodium retention is largely the result of decreased sodium delivery to the tubules. The renin-angiotensin-aldosterone system undoubtedly augments the renal responses to positive-pressure ventilation. Annat and associates[108] found that PEEP at 15 cm H_2O depressed cardiac output, RBF, GFR, and urine volume by 20% to 30% and was associated with increases in renin and aldosterone but not AVP. The impairment in renal function induced by airway pressure therapy can be prevented or reversed by preserving normal circulatory status, either by hydration[109] or by the use of dopamine.[110]

Induced Hypotension

During anesthesia with induced hypotension, a substantial reduction in GFR and the urine flow rate is common. However, when the duration of hypotension is less than 2 hours, no permanent impairment in renal function occurs, even in elderly patients.[111] Vasodilator agents used to induce hypotension differ in their effect on RBF. Administration of sodium nitroprusside decreases renal vascular resistance but tends to shunt blood flow away from the kidney. Moreover, its administration is associated with marked renin-angiotensin activation and catecholamine release, which results in rebound hypertension if the infusion is suddenly discontinued. Nitroglycerin decreases RBF less than sodium nitroprusside does.[112] The selective DA_1 dopaminergic agonist fenoldopam is capable of providing induced hypotension without any significant decrease in RBF.[113]

Aortic Cross-Clamping

The relative effects of suprarenal and infrarenal aortic cross-clamping (see Chapter 52) on renal function in patients undergoing major vascular surgery have been studied.[19] Regardless of the position of the aortic cross-clamp, RBF is decreased to 50% of normal during surgical preparation of the aorta, presumably because of direct compression or reflex spasm of the renal arteries. After release of the suprarenal cross-clamp, RBF increases above normal (reflex hyperemia), but the GFR remains depressed to a third of control for up to 2 hours. After 24 hours, the GFR is still only two thirds of control. Tubular functions (concentrating ability, sodium and water conservation) are markedly impaired, but urine flow is maintained. Myers and Moran[114] observed that these changes resemble an attenuated form of acute tubular necrosis. In the aforementioned study, all patients received mannitol pretreatment, which probably limited the tubular insult because oliguria was uncommon and recovery was relatively rapid. However, cross-clamp times longer than 50 minutes were associated with prolonged depression of the GFR and transient azotemia.[19]

Infrarenal aortic cross-clamping may also impair RBF and GFR by inducing decreases in cardiac output in response to increased systemic vascular resistance.[115] Atheromatous embolism of the renal arteries may be induced by cross-clamping or manipulation in areas of dense aortic plaque. Partial or complete cortical necrosis may occur but is usually irreversible.

Renal Protection during Aortic Cross-Clamping

Mannitol has been used for more than 40 years to provide renal protection during aortic cross-clamping.[116] Its protective effects have been clearly demonstrated in animal models of ischemic acute tubular necrosis,[117] but few prospective controlled human studies have been conducted. Low-dose dopamine has commonly been used during major vascular surgery. In a canine study of thoracic aortic cross-clamping, RBF, GFR, and urine flow remained impaired for a considerable time after cross-clamp release. This delay was not prevented by prophylactic dopamine.[72] In a human study of infrarenal cross-clamping, Paul and coworkers[118] compared diuretic therapy with a combination of mannitol and dopamine versus fluid loading with saline to a pulmonary artery occlusion pressure of 12 to 15 mm Hg. Although mannitol and dopamine substantially increased urine flow and sodium excretion during cross-clamping, they were no better than saline in attenuating residual GFR depression after cross-clamp release.

Cardiopulmonary Bypass

CPB (see Chapter 50) induces hypotension with nonpulsatile flow, which promotes renal vasoconstriction and decreased RBF. Norepinephrine levels increase progressively during bypass, and the renin-angiotensin system is activated. Acute renal failure has been associated with persistent elevation of plasma renin levels.[114] Thromboxane, released from activated platelets, and vascular elaboration of endothelin could add to renal vasoconstriction during extracorporeal circulation. Tubular enzymuria and microalbuminuria, an index of subclinical injury to the nephron, are consistently observed during CPB.[119] Despite these observations, acute renal failure occurs in less than 2% of all patients. Nonetheless, when it does occur after cardiac surgery, acute renal failure is associated with a forbidding mortality rate—60% to 90%.

Renal Protection during Cardiopulmonary Bypass

As yet, no evidence has been presented that pulsatile perfusion during CPB offers an advantage with respect to RBF, catecholamine release, or renal outcome. Although plasma renin activity is suppressed by pulsatile perfusion, microalbuminuria persists.[120] Badner and colleagues[121] found no difference in postoperative renal function in a group of patients with normal kidneys undergoing pulsatile or nonpulsatile CPB. Case series claiming that pulsatile CPB confers protection to patients with chronic renal insufficiency who are undergoing cardiac surgery do exist, but unfortunately they are neither randomized nor prospective.[122]

It has been observed in animal studies of CPB that RBF is dependent on renal perfusion pressure and that infusion of dopamine does not increase RBF during low-pressure states.[9] This observation suggests that autoregulation may be impaired during CPB. However, Hilberman and associates[123] found no relationship between low flow

(<50 mL/kg/min) or low mean arterial pressure (<50 mm Hg) and postoperative acute renal failure. Instead, the severity of postoperative renal dysfunction and its outcome correlated with the severity of cardiac dysfunction after CPB.[124]

Other important risk factors for postoperative renal dysfunction after cardiac surgery include the complexity of the surgery (e.g., combined procedures versus simple revascularization) and preoperative renal function. In a prospective review of more than 4000 cases at the Cleveland Clinic, Higgins and coworkers[125] observed that the risk of renal morbidity and mortality increases exponentially when the preoperative serum creatinine level is greater than 1.9 mg/dL.

There is little evidence that the "prophylactic" administration of low-dose dopamine has a protective role during CPB in patients with normal[126] or impaired renal function[127] who are undergoing cardiac surgery. Moreover, dopamine may induce tachycardia even in the low-dose range and is associated with a higher incidence of postoperative supraventricular and ventricular arrhythmias.[128]

Nephrotoxic Insults

Drug-Induced Nephrotoxicity

Nephrotoxic injury by drugs (e.g., aminoglycosides, cyclosporine, amphotericin B, cisplatin) or contrast dyes seldom occurs unless coexisting risk factors exist.[10] Such factors may be acute (shock, hypovolemia, congestive heart failure) or chronic (advanced age, diabetes, chronic renal insufficiency). The risk of nephrotoxicity increases exponentially with the number of risk factors and nephrotoxic combinations.

Nephrotoxic acute renal failure is usually nonoliguric, with loss of concentrating ability and slowly progressive azotemia. As the GFR declines, accumulation of renally excreted drugs exacerbates nephrotoxicity unless drug levels are carefully monitored and the dosage repeatedly adjusted. However, the prognosis for recovery is good if these agents are discontinued in time and no coexistent organ failure is present.

Aminoglycosides

Aminoglycosides (gentamicin, tobramycin, amikacin) are polycationic compounds that are filtered into the proximal tubule, where they bind to anionic brush border membrane phospholipids. Their nephrotoxicity is directly related to their polycationic status, so neomycin (six cationic sites) is more destructive than gentamicin (five sites) or streptomycin (three sites).[129] They are absorbed into intracellular lysosomes by endocytosis and thence released into the cytosol. Within the cell, they induce defects in lysosomes, plasma membranes, and mitochondria and, in particular, inhibit oxidative phosphorylation and the synthesis of high-energy phosphate compounds such as ATP.

Aminoglycoside-induced nephrotoxicity is directly related to sustained high trough serum levels, especially when associated with advanced age, preexisting renal disease, renal vasoconstrictive states (sepsis, hypovolemia, liver disease, congestive heart failure), adjuvant drug

therapy (loop diuretics, vancomycin, cephalosporins, NSAIDs, cyclosporine, amphotericin B), and electrolyte disorders (hypokalemia, hypomagnesemia, hypercalcemia, and metabolic acidosis).[130]

Prevention of aminoglycoside nephrotoxicity depends on maintenance of adequate hydration, avoidance or removal of the risk factors enumerated earlier, and careful monitoring of serum aminoglycoside levels. A daily 2-hour creatinine clearance measurement can also be helpful in the early detection of aminoglycoside-induced nephrotoxicity and appropriate dose adjustment for GFR. Once-daily administration of aminoglycosides to achieve a high therapeutic level with an adequate trough period for renal recovery may limit the occurrence of nephrotoxicity.[131] Low-dose dopamine increases the renal clearance of aminoglycosides, but it is not known whether this increased clearance protects against tubular injury.

Non-steroidal Anti-inflammatory Drugs

COX-1 is inhibited by NSAIDs such as indomethacin, meclofenamate, and ketorolac for about 8 to 24 hours. A single dose of aspirin causes irreversible acetylation of COX-1. In platelets, the impact lasts for the lifetime of these cells (7 to 10 days), but the kidney resynthesizes COX within 24 to 48 hours. The renal protective function of prostaglandins is "switched on" by injury, as illustrated by the fact that NSAIDs cause nephrotoxicity in ischemic, but not normal kidneys. During conditions of stress, impaired prostaglandin activity results in decreased RBF and GFR, increased renal vascular resistance, attenuated diuretic responsiveness, and hyperkalemia.

Adverse effects of NSAIDs and aspirin have been demonstrated in animal models of hemorrhage, endotoxemia, increased venous pressure, and low cardiac output and in humans with mild underlying renal dysfunction who also have congestive heart failure, ascites, or systemic lupus erythematosus.[132] However, in an individual patient, the risk of NSAIDs-induced nephrotoxicity is very much dependent on the milieu. Postoperative analgesia with a single agent such as ketorolac is extremely unlikely to cause injury in a relatively young, healthy, well-hydrated patient. The risk of nephrotoxic injury increases exponentially with the addition of concomitant nephrotoxins (e.g., contrast dye, aminoglycosides) in the presence of acute or chronic cardiovascular instability.

NSAIDs selective for COX-2 inhibitors appear to be less likely to cause gastric irritation and erosion. However, no evidence as yet indicates that they decrease the risk of nephrotoxic injury in comparison to nonselective COX inhibitors. Similar precautions regarding hydration and selection of low-risk patients should be taken.

Cyclosporine

Cyclosporine is a remarkably potent immunosuppressive agent and, together with steroids and azathioprine, is routinely used to prevent rejection after organ transplantation (see Chapter 56). Indeed, heart, lung, and liver transplantation increased exponentially after its release in 1981. It causes renal injury in part because it induces sympathetic hyperreactivity, hypertension, and renal vasoconstriction.

Preexisting renal dysfunction, hypovolemia, and other nephrotoxic insults exacerbate its nephrotoxic effects. Many transplant patients must tolerate a moderately elevated serum creatinine (1.5 to 2 mg/dL) to sustain adequate immunosuppression. A related calcineurin immunosuppressive agent, tacrolimus (FK-506), is somewhat less nephrotoxic than cyclosporine and has largely replaced it in liver transplantation. A number of alternative immunosuppressive agents (e.g., mycophenolate) have been developed in an effort to decrease or eliminate the cyclosporine requirement during induction.

In patients undergoing cadaveric renal transplantation, the calcium channel blocker diltiazem was added to the graft preservative solution, infused into the donor for 48 hours, and then given orally.[133] The incidence of transplant acute tubular necrosis decreased from 41% to 10%, and when acute renal failure did occur, the hemodialysis requirement was significantly less. Diltiazem impairs cyclosporine metabolism, so plasma cyclosporine levels are higher, with fewer episodes of early acute rejection, but it protects against cyclosporine nephrotoxicity.[134] The cyclosporine dosage may be reduced by 30% to achieve the same drug levels and thus represents a substantial cost savings to patients.

Radiocontrast Dyes

The nephrotoxicity of contrast dyes probably involves microvascular obstruction by crenated red cells, as well as direct tubular toxicity by release of free oxygen radicals. The risk is markedly increased in diabetic renal insufficiency, hypovolemia, congestive heart failure, and myeloma.[135] Radiocontrast dyes are hypertonic and cause an osmotic diuresis, which induces a false sense of security but exacerbates hypovolemia and renal damage. Azotemia commences 24 to 48 hours after exposure and peaks at 3 to 5 days. Surgery performed during this period greatly increases the risk of perioperative acute renal failure.

Prevention of nephrotoxicity depends on adequate hydration and deferral of elective surgical procedures until the effects of the dye have been evaluated and treated.[136] Nonionic, low-osmolar radiocontrast agents are less nephrotoxic, but they are expensive and offer an optimal cost-benefit ratio only when used in high-risk situations, such as diabetic nephropathy.[131]

A number of pharmacologic agents have possible roles in preventing or attenuating contrast nephropathy, but none replace hydration as first-line protection (see later). Intravenous mannitol has been used for many years but may exacerbate injury if it induces dehydration through excessive osmotic diuresis. Some evidence indicates that calcium channel blockers may be protective, but recent interest has focused on antioxidants and dopaminergic agonists.

N-Acetylcysteine and Fenoldopam

Tepel and coauthors reported that prophylactic administration of the antioxidant N-acetylcysteine (600 mg orally twice daily) attenuated renal injury in a study of 83 patients with chronic renal insufficiency (mean serum creatinine, 2.4 mg/dL) undergoing contrast radiography.[137] Only 2% of patients receiving N-acetylcysteine had an increase in serum creatinine of greater than 0.5 mg/dL versus 21% of patients receiving saline placebo, and mean serum creatinine concentrations actually decreased. However, in a subsequent study of 183 patients with less severe renal dysfunction (mean serum creatinine, 1.5 mg/dL), Briguori and colleagues found that N-acetylcysteine provided better protection than did saline alone only when a low dose of contrast dye was used.[138]

A number of retrospective reviews or case series have been published that attest to the benefit of prophylactic fenoldopam infusion (<0.1 µg/kg/min) in preventing or attenuating contrast nephropathy in high-risk patients. This benefit has not yet been confirmed by randomized prospective trials. In a double-blind randomized study of 45 patients, Tumlin and coworkers found that fenoldopam infusion prevented a contrast-induced decrease in RBF, but the study was underpowered to detect differences in renal outcome.[139]

A randomized prospective study was designed by Allaqaband and colleagues to compare N-acetylcysteine, fenoldopam, and placebo in 123 high-risk patients undergoing contrast radiography for cardiovascular procedures.[49] No difference was found in the incidence of increased serum creatinine (>0.5 mg/dL) in any of the groups, and the authors concluded that neither N-acetylcysteine nor fenoldopam offered any benefit over saline.

Pigment Nephropathy

Pigment nephropathy implies acute renal injury as a result of the nephrotoxic effect of the heme pigments myoglobin, hemoglobin, and bilirubin.

Rhabdomyolysis and Myoglobinemia

Muscle necrosis (rhabdomyolysis) occurs most commonly with direct trauma involving major crush or thermal injury. However, it also occurs with acute muscle ischemia induced by vascular disease or injury or by prolonged immobilization. Compartment syndromes exacerbate rhabdomyolysis. They are particularly likely to occur with major hemorrhage in an extremity or when vascular insufficiency coexists with tissue edema (e.g., femoral placement of an intra-aortic balloon after vein harvesting). Dramatic increases in metabolic rate (severe exercise, prolonged fever, status epilepticus or myoclonus), severe hypophosphatemia, or direct proteolysis (acute pancreatitis) can all precipitate rhabdomyolysis.[140]

Myoglobin, the oxygen-carrying heme pigment of muscle, is released into the bloodstream (myoglobinemia) and rapidly excreted by the glomerulus at a plasma threshold of 0.03 mg/dL. Delivery of myoglobin to the proximal tubule is greater in a well-muscled individual with normal GFR than in a cachectic patient with low GFR. At a urine pH of less than 5.6, myoglobin is transformed into ferrihematin, which precipitates in the proximal tubule.[141] Renal damage is facilitated by hypovolemia (i.e., low tubular flow) and acidic urine. Because of the associated hypercatabolic state, oliguria is associated with acute hyperkalemia, hypocalcemia, anion-gap metabolic acidosis, and rapid azotemia. Serum creatinine and BUN increase very rapidly (1.0 to 1.5 mg/dL/day and 20 to 30 mg/dL/day, respectively).

The most important aid to the diagnosis of rhabdomyolysis is a high index of suspicion. The affected muscle may be obviously ischemic or swollen, painful, and edematous. Urine myoglobin often tests positive without reddish urine. The serum is clear because of the low renal threshold for myoglobin excretion, whereas hemoglobinemia is associated with pink serum. Serial total creatinine phosphokinase (CPK) is a helpful guide to the severity of rhabdomyolysis (i.e., CPK-MM release).[142] Renal damage is much more likely when total CPK exceeds 10,000 U/L.

Prevention of acute nephrotoxic tubular necrosis is dependent on maintenance of high RBF and tubular flow. Urine flow should be kept between 100 and 150 mL/hr by osmotic diuresis with intravenous mannitol, 6.25 to 12.5 g every 6 hours, with or without intravenous furosemide, 10 to 20 mg as required.[143] Urine pH should be kept above 5.6 with intravenous sodium bicarbonate, 50 mEq intravenously, as required, or acetazolamide, 250 mg every 6 hours, or both. However, because no prospective data have confirmed the beneficial effect of urinary alkalinization, urine pH should not be increased at the expense of causing significant acid-base imbalance. Calcium should be given to treat hyperkalemia only.

Hemolysis and Hemoglobinemia

Acute intravascular hemolysis caused by mismatched blood transfusion (ABO incompatibility) is a direct and devastating renal insult. The renal damage is thought to be predominantly due to red blood cell stroma rather than free hemoglobin. Management is essentially the same as for rhabdomyolysis.

Jaundice and Bilirubinemia

A direct correlation has been found between the degree of preoperative obstructive jaundice and postoperative renal dysfunction.[144] When cholestasis causes conjugated bilirubin to increase above 8 mg/dL, bile salt excretion effectively ceases, and portal septicemia and renal damage ensue. This situation is analogous to hepatorenal syndrome and sepsis, in which circulating endotoxins induce renal vasoconstriction and damage (vasomotor nephropathy).

Administration of preoperative oral bile salts (e.g., sodium taurocholate) or intravenous mannitol may provide perioperative renal protection in patients with severe obstructive jaundice. In a prospective, randomized study in patients with obstructive jaundice undergoing surgery, Plusa and Clark[145] found no difference in renal outcome between these two regimens. However, mannitol provokes a brisk osmotic diuresis, and it is important to replace urinary losses appropriately. Diuresis-induced hypovolemia negates the protective effect of mannitol.[146]

Sepsis

Sepsis is the most common cause of new-onset acute renal failure in the postoperative period (see Chapter 74). Renal function may deteriorate progressively without defined episodes of hypotension. In addition, sepsis predisposes the kidney to further ischemic and nephrotoxic insults, such as concomitant aminoglycoside use.[147] Acute renal failure itself and hemodialysis perpetuate sepsis by activating leukocytes. Sepsis may induce renal damage by hypotension and vasomotor nephropathy and through the direct and indirect effects of endotoxin.

A reasonable amount of evidence suggests that renal autoregulation may be impaired in sepsis and that RBF and GFR decline pari passu with systemic vascular resistance and mean arterial pressure. Hypotension in turn sets off a cascade of neurohormonal responses (sympathoadrenal activity; renin-angiotensin, vasopressin, and thromboxane activation) that result in decreased RBF, GFR, sodium excretion, and urine flow. The severity of renal dysfunction appears to be directly related to the severity of sepsis and the degree of plasma renin activation.[148]

Renal dysfunction in sepsis is characterized as a vasomotor nephropathy, which implies renal vasoconstriction in the face of an increased total cardiac index. Renal vasoconstriction, mesangial cell contraction, a decreased ultrafiltration coefficient, and decreased GFR are induced by endotoxin and by compounds activated in sepsis.[149] These compounds include endothelin and eicosanoids such as thromboxane, PGF_2, and the leukotrienes C_4 and D_4. PGF_2, which mimics the action of thromboxane, is formed during leukostasis when arachidonic acid is oxidized by free oxygen radicals.

Endotoxin causes leukocyte arachidonic acid to undergo lipoxygenation to form leukotrienes; it also impairs their biliary elimination. In addition, experimental infusion of lipopolysaccharide (endotoxin) directly decreases RBF, GFR, and tubular concentrating ability and increases urinary loss of tubular enzymes. It causes sequestration of leukocytes in peritubular capillaries, induces endothelial lesions by releasing neutrophil-derived elastase (enhanced by reperfusion injury), and potentiates renal ischemia such that brief hemodynamic instability causes rapid loss of renal function. It also potentiates nephrotoxicity. The changes caused by endotoxin are mimicked by the cytokine tumor necrosis factor-α.

It has been estimated that nephrotoxic renal insufficiency will develop in about 10% to 26% of septic patients receiving aminoglycoside antibiotics.[130] Aminoglycoside nephrotoxicity is enhanced by the interaction of fever, renal vasoconstriction, hypovolemia, and endotoxin. In the presence of these and other risk factors (see earlier), the use of alternative non-nephrotoxic antibiotics should be considered to cover gram-negative infections, including penicillins (ticarcillin), cephalosporins (ceftazidime), carbapenems (imipenem), or monobactams (aztreonam).

Renal Protection in Septic Shock (see Chapter 74)

Anti-inflammatory Drugs

Cumming and colleagues[150] demonstrated a marked renal protective effect of a selective thromboxane synthetase inhibitor (U63557A) on laparotomy in a volume-loaded sheep peritonitis model. Administration of the selective inhibitor either before or 30 minutes after surgery prevented deterioration in creatinine clearance, urinary sodium excretion, and the urine flow rate. Beneficial effects have also been observed with aprotinin, perhaps through its anti-inflammatory action.[44] In contrast, nonselective COX inhibition by NSAIDs worsens renal function in sepsis by decreasing synthesis of the renal vasodilator prostacyclin.[151]

The use of pharmacologic doses of methylprednisolone in septic shock was discredited by two large multicenter studies showing no beneficial effect on outcome.[152,153] Moreover, patients who received steroids had significant increases in BUN but not in serum creatinine, thus suggesting a prerenal state induced by increased protein catabolism.[154] Other potentially adverse effects of high-dose steroids include impaired mitochondrial function, impaired leukocyte function, and inhibition of phospholipase A_2 resulting in decreased synthesis of intrarenal vasodilator prostaglandins.

Supranormal Oxygen Delivery

Over the last decade there has been considerable controversy in the concept of supranormal oxygen delivery to tissues to overcome the defect that exists in oxygen utilization by septic tissues.[155] This approach consists of inotropic support and blood transfusion to drive global oxygen delivery (Do_2) to one of three end points: to a Do_2 level consistently found in survivors (600 mL/min/m²), when global oxygen consumption (Vo_2) no longer increases with increasing Do_2 (consumption independence), or when blood lactate levels start to decline. The benefits of supranormal oxygen delivery on outcome have been disputed, and high-dose inotropic and vasopressor support may themselves have adverse consequences. Moreover, renal Do_2 and Vo_2 differ markedly from systemic indices. Renal Vo_2 is largely determined by tubular metabolic function, which is regulated by fluid and electrolyte changes. In a volume-loaded septic porcine model, inotropic support with dobutamine increased systemic Do_2 and Vo_2 but did not increase renal Do_2 and Vo_2.[25] Furthermore, decreased global renal Do_2 does not appear to cause tubular damage, possibly because tubular work and Vo_2 are decreased when the GFR declines.[156]

Dopaminergic Drugs

Low-dose dopamine (1 to 3 µg/kg/min) is frequently administered to septic patients in the belief that it confers renal protection through renal vasodilation or perhaps by inhibition of the Na^+-K^+–ATPase pump and decreases in renal tubular Vo_2.

It is also administered in combination with more potent pressors (dobutamine, epinephrine, and norepinephrine) in sepsis in the hope of enhancing hepatic, renal, and mesenteric perfusion. Some animal data support this practice. In a nonseptic dog study in which RBF was measured by thermodilution, the addition of low-dose dopamine to a norepinephrine infusion of 0.2 to 1.6 µg/kg/min increased RBF by 40% to 50%.[24] However, a subsequent study demonstrated that although low-dose dopamine increased RBF when added to an epinephrine infusion in healthy sheep, this benefit could not be found in an intraperitoneal sepsis model.[157] Low-dose dopamine can increase hepatic Do_2, but possibly at the expense of splanchnic oxygenation.

In patients with sepsis syndrome (signs of sepsis without hypotension), low-dose dopamine infusion doubled the urine flow rate and increased creatinine clearance by 60% without any change in systemic hemodynamics.[158] However, the renal response to dopamine decreased significantly after 48 hours of dopamine infusion, possibly

as a result of downregulation of renal dopaminergic receptors or diuresis-induced contraction of intravascular volume. In patients with established septic shock who required catecholamines for blood pressure support, low-dose dopamine did not alter systemic hemodynamics or renal function.

The prophylactic administration of low-dose dopamine in sepsis appears to have been laid to rest by a large prospective controlled study conducted by the Australian and New Zealand Intensive Care Society. They randomized 328 patients with signs of systemic inflammatory response syndrome and early renal dysfunction (oliguria or increasing serum creatinine) to dopamine, 2 µg/kg/min, or placebo. They found no differences in serum creatinine, dialysis requirement, intensive care unit or hospital length of stay, or overall mortality.[159]

The potential role of dopexamine in septic shock remains speculative. Most studies have examined its role in splanchnic and hepatic perfusion rather than in renal protection. In animal models of sepsis, dopexamine has improved splanchnic and hepatic Do_2, but its β_2-adrenergic activity in causing tachycardia and hypotension may limit its application in clinical sepsis. Smithies and associates[160] administered dopexamine to patients with sepsis syndrome, acute respiratory failure, and at least one other organ system failure. The cardiac index increased and gastric intramucosal pH (an index of splanchnic perfusion) improved significantly.

Norepinephrine

In patients with septic shock, profound hypotension, and oliguria, vasopressor therapy with norepinephrine may actually improve renal function by enhancing renal perfusion pressure. Desjars and colleagues[7] evaluated a group of septic patients who remained oliguric despite volume resuscitation and the use of dopamine in doses of up to 15 µg/kg/min. The addition of norepinephrine and reduction of dopamine to a low-dose level resulted in an improvement in mean arterial pressure from 50 to 70 mm Hg, a tripling of urine flow, and a doubling of creatinine clearance. Norepinephrine increased systemic vascular resistance with little change in the cardiac index or Do_2. Subsequent studies have confirmed that the use of norepinephrine to keep mean arterial pressure greater than 60 mm Hg results in improved cardiac function (increase in stroke volume and decrease in heart rate) and GFR without deleterious effects on the cardiac index, oxygen extraction, or Vo_2.[161]

Large doses of norepinephrine may be required to achieve these goals because in septic shock, the peripheral vasculature is notoriously refractory to norepinephrine-induced vasoconstriction as a result of massive inducible nitric oxide release as well as vasopressin deficiency (see the next section). Nonetheless, these findings strongly support the concept that renal autoregulation is impaired in sepsis and that maintenance of adequate renal perfusion pressure is an important component of renal protection.

Arginine Vasopressin

Patients in vasodilatory shock have inappropriately low plasma levels of AVP and marked vascular sensitivity to its exogenous administration at low doses.[162] Vasodilatory shock is defined as hypotension, an increased cardiac index, and low systemic vascular resistance refractory to pressors such as norepinephrine. Septic shock is its most common manifestation, but it is also characteristic of the contact activation syndrome induced by CPB or ventricular assist devices.[163]

Landry and coworkers[164] observed unusual sensitivity to the vasoconstrictor effects of infused AVP in patients with septic shock and profound hypotension despite catecholamine infusion. Infusion of AVP at doses of 2.4 U/hr, less than one tenth of those used in the treatment of bleeding esophageal varices, resulted in a dramatic increase in systolic blood pressure from 92 ± 4 to 146 ± 4 mm Hg (mean $\pm$ SEM, $P < .001$), and catecholamine infusions were able to be discontinued. In an associated report,[165] the authors observed that urine flow increased concomitantly in three of five patients, from an average of 30 to 110 mL/hr.

Plasma AVP levels were remarkably low (3.1 ± 1.0 pg/mL) and significantly lower than in a cohort of patients in cardiogenic shock who were also receiving catecholamines (22.7 ± 2.2 pg/mL, $P < .001$).[164] It has been postulated that this "AVP deficiency" may be the result of excessive baroreceptor-mediated AVP release from sustained hypotension. This theory is strongly supported by a canine study demonstrating almost complete depletion of radiolabeled AVP in the posterior pituitary after 1 hour of hemorrhagic shock (Fig. 20-21).[162]

A second mechanism for sensitivity to AVP in septic patients is explained by its effect on the potassium-ATP (K_{ATP}) channel.[162] Intracellular acidosis, lactic acid accumulation, and ATP depletion close K_{ATP} channels in the sarcolemma of vascular smooth muscle. This closing of channels traps potassium outside the cell and hyperpolarizes the membrane, which in turn closes the calcium channels essential for norepinephrine-induced vasoconstriction. AVP binds at the K_{ATP} channel and opens it, thereby reversing membrane hyperpolarization and restoring sensitivity to norepinephrine.

In summary, the beneficial effect of AVP on renal function in sepsis may in part be due to enhanced renal

perfusion pressure in the face of abnormal autoregulation, as well as the fact that AVP preferentially constricts the efferent arteriole, thereby improving FF and GFR.[40]

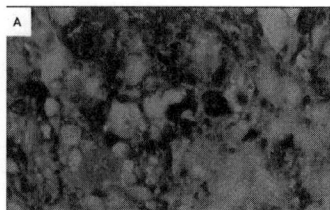

Figure 20–21 Baroreflex-induced arginine vasopressin (AVP) depletion in dogs. **A,** Section of the posterior pituitary gland (neurohypophysis) from a normal dog. The macrovesicles are stained with antivasopressin serum, a reaction indicative of replete stores of vasopressin. **B,** Section of the neurohypophysis from a dog after severe hemorrhagic hypotension (mean arterial pressure, <40 mm Hg) for 1 hour. The minimal staining with antivasopressin serum is indicative of profound baroreflex-induced depletion of AVP stores. (Reprinted, by permission, from Landry DW, Oliver JA: The pathogenesis of vasodilatory shock. N Engl J Med 345:588-595, 2001.)

KEY POINTS

1. The renal medulla receives less than 10% of RBF, and metabolically active structures in the juxtamedullary zone and medulla are at constant risk of hypoxia.

2. Increases in efferent arteriolar tone mediated by angiotensin, catecholamines, and vasopressin provide an important compensatory mechanism to maintain glomerular filtration pressure in the face of mild to moderate hypotension.

3. Over a wide range of blood pressure, renal autoregulation maintains GFR and RBF, but not urine flow, which is pressure dependent.

4. The kidney regulates a constant balance between vasoconstrictor, salt-retaining systems that protect against hypovolemia and hypotension and vasodilator, salt-excreting systems that protect against hypervolemia and hypertension.

5. The most metabolically active sites in the renal tubule are the proximal tubule and the medullary thick ascending limb, which play an important role in the pathogenesis of ischemic and nephrotoxic acute tubular necrosis, respectively.

6. Renal clearance estimates the virtual volume of plasma cleared of substance "x" per unit time, which allows us to estimate effective RPF and GFR, depending on how substance "x" is handled by the kidney.

7. A doubling of serum creatinine implies a halving of the GFR.

8. Serum creatinine does not increase above normal levels until the GFR is less than 50 mL/min; in cachectic individuals, it may still be in the normal range when the estimated GFR is between 20 and 30 mL/min.

9. ANP is released in response to increases in atrial volume and induces increases in urine flow and sodium excretion (natriuresis), which could be considered "endogenous renal protection."

10. Renal autoregulation is lost or impaired during acute renal failure, sepsis, and CPB, and vasoconstrictor drugs that maintain or restore renal perfusion pressure improve RBF.

REFERENCES

1. Tisher CC, Madsen KM: Anatomy of the kidney. In Brenner BM (ed): Brenner & Rector's The Kidney, 6th ed. Philadelphia, WB Saunders, 2000, pp 3-67.
2. Stanton BA, Koeppen BM: Elements of renal function. In Berne RM, Levy MN (eds): Physiology, 4th ed. St Louis, CV Mosby, 1998, pp 677-698.
3. Maddox DA, Brenner BM: Glomerular ultrafiltration. In Brenner BM (ed): Brenner & Rector's The Kidney, 6th ed. Philadelphia, WB Saunders, 2000, pp 319-374.
4. Thurau K, Boylan JW: Acute renal success: The unexpected logic of oliguria in acute renal failure. Am J Med 61:308-315, 1976.

5. Shipley RE, Study RS: Changes in renal blood flow, extraction of inulin, glomerular filtration rate, tissue pressure and urine flow with acute alterations of renal artery pressure. Am J Physiol 167:676-688, 1951.

6. Aukland K, Oien AH: Renal autoregulation: Models combining tubuloglomerular feedback and myogenic response. Am J Physiol 252:F768-F783, 1987.

7. Desjars PH, Pinaud M, Bugnon D, et al: Norepinephrine has no deleterious renal effects in human septic shock. Crit Care Med 17:426-429, 1989.

8. Kelleher SP, Robinette JB, Miller F, Conger JD: Effect of hemorrhagic reduction in blood pressure on recovery from acute renal failure. Kidney Int 31:725-730, 1987.

9. Mackay JH, Feerick AE, Woodson LC, et al: Increasing organ blood flow during cardiopulmonary bypass in pigs: Comparison of dopamine and perfusion pressure. Crit Care Med 23:1090-1098, 1995.

10. Brezis M, Rosen S: Hypoxia of the renal medulla—its implications for disease. N Engl J Med 332:647-655, 1995.

11. Kasiske BL, Keane WF: Laboratory assessment of renal disease: Clearance, urinalysis and renal biopsy. In Brenner BM (ed): Brenner & Rector's The Kidney, 6th ed. Philadelphia, WB Saunders, 2000, pp 1129-1170.

12. Tobias GJ, McLaughlin RF, Hopper J: Endogenous creatinine clearance: A valuable clinical test of glomerular filtration and a prognostic guide in chronic renal disease. N Engl J Med 266:317-323, 1962.

13. Sladen RN, Endo E, Harrison T: Two-hour versus 22-hour creatinine clearance in critically ill patients. Anesthesiology 67:1013-1016, 1987.

14. Shin B, Mackenzie C, Helrich M: Creatinine clearance for early detection of posttraumatic renal dysfunction. Anesthesiology 64:605-609, 1986.

15. Wesson LG, Lauler DP: Diurnal cycle of glomerular filtration rate and sodium and chloride excretion during responses to altered salt and water balance in man. J Clin Invest 40:1967-1977, 1961.

16. Kim KE, Onesti G, Ramirez O, et al: Creatinine clearance in renal disease. A reappraisal. BMJ 4:11-14, 1969.

17. Moran SM, Myers BD: Course of acute renal failure studied by a model of creatinine kinetics. Kidney Int 27:928-937, 1985.

18. Doolan PD, Alpen EL, Theil GB: A clinical appraisal of the plasma concentration and endogenous clearance of creatinine. Am J Med 32:65-81, 1962.

19. Myers BD, Miller DC, Mehigan JT, et al: Nature of the renal injury following total renal ischemia in man. J Clin Invest 73:329-341, 1984.

20. Cockroft DW, Gault MH: Prediction of creatinine clearance from serum creatinine. Nephron 16:31-41, 1976.

21. Robert S, Zarowitz BJ, Peterson EL, Dumler F: Predictability of creatinine clearance estimates in the critically ill. Crit Care Med 21:1487-1495, 1993.

22. Stanton BA, Koeppen BM: Control of body fluid osmolality and volume. In Berne RM, Levy MN (eds): Physiology, 4th ed. St Louis, CV Mosby, 1998, pp 715-743.

23. Bryan AG, Bolsin SN, Vianna PTG, Haloush H: Modification of the diuretic and natriuretic effects of a dopamine infusion by fluid loading in preoperative cardiac surgical patients. J Cardiothorac Vasc Anesth 9:158-163, 1995.

24. Schaer GL, Fink MP, Parrillo JE: Norepinephrine alone versus norepinephrine plus low-dose dopamine: Enhanced renal blood flow with combination pressor therapy. Crit Care Med 13:492-496, 1985.

25. Haywood GA, Tighe D, Moss R, et al: Goal directed therapy with dobutamine in a porcine model of septic shock: Effects on systemic and renal oxygen transport. Postgrad Med J 67(Suppl 1):S36, 1991.

26. Aronson S, Wiencek JG, Feinstein SB, et al: Assessment of renal blood flow with contrast ultrasonography. Anesth Analg 76:964, 1993.

27. Thorburn GD, Kopald HH, Herd JA, et al: Intrarenal distribution of nutrient blood flow determined by krypton-85 in the unanesthetized dog. Circ Res 13:290-307, 1963.

28. Hollenberg NK, Epstein M, Rosen SM, et al: Acute oliguric failure in man: Evidence for preferential renal cortical ischemia. Medicine (Baltimore) 47:455-474, 1968.

29. Aukland K: Methods for measuring renal blood flow: Total flow and regional distribution. Annu Rev Physiol 42:543-555, 1980.

30. Priano LL: Effects of anesthetic agents on renal function. In Barash PG (ed): Refresher Courses in Anesthesiology. Philadelphia, JB Lippincott, 1985, pp 143-156.

31. Schrier RW: Effects of the adrenergic nervous system and catecholamines on systemic and renal hemodynamics, sodium and water excretion and renin secretion. Kidney Int 6:291-306, 1974.

32. Levens NR, Peach MJ, Carey RM: Role of the intrarenal renin-angiotensin system in the control of renal function. Circ Res 48:157-167, 1981.

33. Ballerman BJ, Zeidel ML, Gunning ME, Brenner BM: Vasoactive peptides and the kidney. In Brenner BM, Rector FCJ (eds): The Kidney, 4th ed. Philadelphia, WB Saunders, 1991, pp 510-583.

34. Hricik D, Browning P, Kopelman R, et al: Captopril-induced functional renal insufficiency in patients with bilateral renal-artery stenoses or renal-artery stenosis in a solitary kidney. N Engl J Med 308:373-376, 1983.

35. Wynckel A, Ebikili B, Melin JP, et al: Long-term follow-up of acute renal failure caused by angiotensin converting enzyme inhibitors. Am J Hypertens 11:1080-1086, 1998.

36. Colson P, Ribstein J, Mimran A, et al: Effect of angiotensin converting enzyme inhibition on blood pressure and renal function during open heart surgery. Anesthesiology 72:23-27, 1990.

37. Genuth SM: The adrenal glands. In Berne RM, Levy MN (eds): Physiology, 4th ed. St Louis, CV Mosby, 1998, pp 930-964.

38. Baylis PH: Posterior pituitary function in health and disease. Clin Endocrinol Metab 12:747-770, 1983.

39. Bartter FC, Schwartz WB: The syndrome of inappropriate secretion of antidiuretic hormone. Am J Med 42:790-806, 1967.

40. Edwards RM, Trizna W, Kinter LB: Renal microvascular effects of vasopressin and vasopressin antagonists. Am J Physiol 256:F274-F278, 1989.

41. Levenson DJ, Simmons CEJ, Brenner BM: Arachidonic acid metabolites, prostaglandins and the kidney. Am J Med 72:354-374, 1982.

42. Johnston PA, Bernard DB, Perrin NS, et al: Prostaglandins mediate the vasodilatory effect of mannitol in the hypoperfused rat kidney. J Clin Invest 68:127-133, 1981.

43. Gerber JG, Olsen RD, Nies AS: Interrelationship between prostaglandins and renin release. Kidney Int 19:816-821, 1981.

44. Cumming AD: Acute renal failure and sepsis: Therapeutic approaches. Nephrol Dial Transplant 4:159-163, 1994.

45. Nasjletti A, Malik KU: Renal kinin-prostaglandin relationship: Implications for renal function. Kidney Int 19:860-868, 1981.

46. Gorfinkel HJ, Szidon JP, Hirsch LJ, et al: Renal performance in experimental cardiogenic shock. Am J Physiol 222:1260-1268, 1972.

47. de Bold AJ, Borenstein HB, Veress AT, Sonnenberg H: A rapid and potent natriuretic response to intravenous injection of atrial myocardial extract in rats. Life Sci 28:89-94, 1981.

48. Laragh J: Atrial natriuretic hormone, the renin-angiotensin axis, and blood-pressure electrolyte homeostasis. N Engl J Med 313:1330-1340, 1985.

49. Allaqaband S, Tumuluri R, Malik AM, et al: Prospective randomized study of N-acetylcysteine, fenoldopam, and saline for prevention of radiocontrast-induced nephropathy. Cathet Cardiovasc Interv 57:279-283, 2002.

50. Maack T, Camargo MJF, Kleinert HD, et al: Atrial natriuretic factor: Structure and functional properties. Kidney Int 27:607-615, 1985.

51. Shannon RP, Libby E, Elahi D, et al: Impact of acute reduction in chronically elevated left atrial pressure on sodium and water excretion. Ann Thorac Surg 46:430-437, 1988.

52. Goldberg L, Rajfer S: Dopamine receptors: Applications in clinical cardiology. Circulation 72:245-248, 1985.
53. Bello-Reuss E, Higashi Y, Kaneda Y: Dopamine decreases fluid reabsorption in the straight portions of the rabbit proximal tubule. Am J Physiol 242:F634-F640, 1982.
54. Olsen NV: Effects of dopamine on renal haemodynamics, tubular function, and sodium excretion in normal humans. Dan Med Bull 45:282-297, 1998.
55. Eklof AC: The natriuretic response to a dopamine DA1 agonist requires endogenous activation of dopamine DA2 receptors. Acta Physiol Scand 160:311-314, 1997.
56. Holtbäck U, Kruse MS, Brismar H, Aperia A: Intrarenal dopamine coordinates the effect of antinatriuretic and natriuretic factors. Acta Physiol Scand 168:215-218, 2000.
57. Kuchel O, Buu NT, Unger T: Dopamine sodium relationship: Is dopamine part of the endogenous natriuretic system? Contrib Nephrol 13:27, 1978.
58. Steudel W, Hurford WE, Zapol WM: Inhaled nitric oxide: Basic biology and clinical applications. Anesthesiology 91:1090-1121, 1999.
59. Ito S, Carretero OA, Abe K: Nitric oxide in the regulation of renal blood flow. New Horizons 3:615-623, 1995.
60. Lieberthal W: Biology of ischemic and toxic renal tubular cell injury: Role of nitric oxide and the inflammatory response. Curr Opin Nephrol Hypertens 7:289-295, 1998.
61. Landin L, Lorente JA, Renes E, et al: Inhibition of nitric oxide synthesis improves the vasoconstrictive effect of nora-drenaline in sepsis. Chest 106:250-256, 1994.
62. Goligorsky MS, Noiri E: Duality of nitric oxide in acute renal injury. Semin Nephrol 19:263-271, 1999.
63. Noiri E, Peresleni T, Miller F, Goligorsky MS: In vivo targeting of inducible NO synthase with oligodeoxynucleotides protects rat kidney against ischemia. J Clin Invest 97:2377-2383, 1996.
64. Fozard JR, Hannon JP: Adenosine receptor ligands: Potential as therapeutic agents in asthma and COPD. Pulm Pharmacol Ther 12:111-114, 1999.
65. Lee HT, Emala CW: Protective effects of renal ischemic preconditioning and adenosine pretreatment: Role of A(1) and A(3) receptors. Am J Physiol Renal Physiol 278:F380-F387, 2000.
66. Lee HT, Emala CW: Systemic adenosine given after ischemia protects renal function via A(2a) adenosine receptor activation. Am J Kidney Dis 38:610-618, 2001.
67. Armstrong DK, Dasta JF, Reilley TF, Tallman RDJ: Effect of haloperidol on dopamine-induced increase in renal blood flow. Drug Intell Clin Pharmacol 20:543-546, 1986.
68. Hughes A, Thom S, Martin G, et al: The action of a dopamine (DA1) receptor agonist, fenoldopam, in human vasculature in vivo and in vitro. Br J Clin Pharmacol 22:535-540, 1986.
69. Olsen NV, Olsen MH, Bonde J, et al: Dopamine natriuresis in salt-repleted, water-loaded humans: A dose-response study. Br J Clin Pharmacol 43:509-520, 1997.
70. Hilberman M, Maseda J, Stinson E, et al: The diuretic properties of dopamine in patients after open-heart operation. Anesthesiology 61:489-494, 1984.
71. MacGregor DA, Smith TE, Prielipp RC, et al: Pharmacokinetics of dopamine in healthy male subjects. Anesthesiology 92:338-346, 2000.
72. Pass L, Eberhart R, Brown J, et al: The effect of mannitol and dopamine on the renal response to thoracic aortic cross-clamping. J Thorac Cardiovasc Surg 95:608-612, 1988.
73. Ter Wee PM, Smit AJ, Rosman JB, et al: Effect of intravenous infusion of low-dose dopamine on renal function in normal individuals and in patients with renal disease. Am J Nephrol 6:42-46, 1986.
74. Swygert TH, Roberts LC, Valek TR, et al: Effect of intraoperative low-dose dopamine on renal function in liver transplant recipients. Anesthesiology 75:571-576, 1991.
75. Grundmann R, Kindler J, Meider G, et al: Dopamine treatment of human cadaver kidney graft recipients: A prospectively randomized trial. Lancet 2:827-828, 1980.
76. Olsen NV, Lund J, Jensen PF, et al: Dopamine, dobutamine, and dopexamine. A comparison of renal effects in unanesthetized human volunteers. Anesthesiology 79:685-694, 1993.
77. Ghosh S, Gray B, Oduro A, Latimer R: Dopexamine hydrochloride: Pharmacology and use in low cardiac output states. J Cardiothorac Vasc Anesth 5:382-389, 1991.
78. Murphy MB, Murray CB, Shorten GD: Fenoldopam—a selective peripheral dopamine-receptor agonist for the treatment of severe hypertension. N Engl J Med 345:1548-1557, 2001.
79. Singer I, Epstein M: Potential of dopamine A-1 agonists in the management of acute renal failure. Am J Kidney Dis 31:743-755, 1998.
80. Tobimatsu M, Konomi K, Saito S, Tsumagari T: Protective effect of prostaglandin E$_1$ on ischemia-induced acute renal failure in dogs. Surgery 98:45-52, 1985.
81. Neumayer HH, Gellert J, Luft FC: Calcium antagonists and renal protection. Ren Fail 15:353-358, 1993.
82. Diamond J, Cheung J, Fang L: Nifedipine-induced renal dysfunction. Am J Med 77:905-909, 1984.
83. Bauer J, Sunderrajan S, Reams G: Effects of calcium entry blockers on renin-angiotensin-aldosterone system, renal function and hemodynamics, salt and water excretion and body fluid composition. Am J Cardiol 56:62H-67H, 1985.
84. Conger JD, Falk SA, Hammond WS: Atrial natriuretic peptide and dopamine in established acute renal failure in the rat. Kidney Int 40:21-28, 1991.
85. Seki G, Suzuki K, Nonaka T, et al: Effects of atrial natriuretic peptide on glycerol induced acute renal failure in the rat. Jpn Heart J 33:383-393, 1992.
86. Rahman SN, Kim GE, Mathew AS, et al: Effects of atrial natriuretic peptide in clinical acute renal failure. Kidney Int 45:1731-1738, 1994.
87. Allgren RL, Marbury TC, Rahman SN, et al: Anaritide in acute tubular necrosis. N Engl J Med 336:828-834, 1997.
88. Lewis J, Salem MM, Chertow GM, et al: Atrial natriuretic factor in oliguric acute renal failure. Anaritide Acute Renal Failure Study Group. Am J Kidney Dis 36:767-774, 2000.
89. Kennedy W, Sawyer T, Gerbershagen H, et al: Simultaneous systemic cardiovascular and renal haemodynamic measurements during high spinal anaesthesia in normal man. Acta Anaesthesiol Scand 37:163-171, 1970.
90. Silvarjan M, Amory D, Lindbloom L, et al: Systemic and regional blood flow changes during spinal anesthesia in the rhesus monkey. Anesthesiology 43:78-88, 1975.
91. Ecoffey C, Edouard A, Pruszczynski W, et al: Effects of epidural anesthesia on catecholamines, renin activity and vasopressin changes induced by tilt in elderly men. Anesthesiology 62:294-297, 1985.
92. Lunn J, Dannemiller FJ, Stanley TH: Cardiovascular responses to clamping of the aorta during epidural and general anesthesia. Anesth Analg 58:372-376, 1979.
93. Gamulin Z, Forster A, Simonet F, et al: Effects of renal sympathetic blockade on renal hemodynamics in patients undergoing major aortic abdominal surgery. Anesthesiology 65:688-692, 1986.
94. Gelman S, Gowler KC, Smith LR: Regional blood flow during isoflurane and halothane anesthesia. Anesth Analg 63:557-565, 1984.
95. Stanley TH, Berman L, Green O, et al: Plasma catecholamine responses to fentanyl-oxygen anesthesia for coronary artery operation. Anesthesiology 53:250-253, 1980.
96. Priano LL: Alteration of renal hemodynamics by thiopental, diazepam and ketamine in conscious dogs. Anesth Analg 61:853-862, 1982.
97. Mazze RI, Trudell JR, Cousins MJ: Methoxyflurane metabolism and renal dysfunction: Clinical correlation in man. Anesthesiology 35:247, 1971.
98. Cousins MJ, Mazze RI: Methoxyflurane nephrotoxicity: A study of dose response in man. JAMA 225:1611-1616, 1973.
99. Mazze RI, Cousins MJ, Barr GA: Renal effects and metabolism of isoflurane in man. Anesthesiology 40:536-542, 1974.
100. Eger EI 2nd, Koblin DD, Bowland T, et al: Nephrotoxicity of sevoflurane versus desflurane anesthesia in volunteers. Anesth Analg 84:160-168, 1997.
101. Eger EI, Gong D, Koblin DD, et al: Dose-related biochemical markers of renal injury after sevoflurane versus desflurane anesthesia in volunteers. Anesth Analg 85:1154-1163, 1997.

102. Bito H, Ikeuchi Y, Ikeda K: Effects of low-flow sevoflurane anesthesia on renal function. Anesthesiology 86:1231-1237, 1997.

103. Kharasch ED, Frink EJJ, Zager R, et al: Assessment of low-flow sevoflurane and isoflurane effects on renal function using sensitive markers of tubular toxicity. Anesthesiology 86:1238-1253, 1997.

104. Ebert TJ, Frink EJ, Kharasch ED: Absence of biochemical evidence for renal and hepatic dysfunction after 8 hours of 1.25 minimum alveolar concentration sevoflurane anesthesia in volunteers. Anesthesiology 88:601-610, 1998.

105. Doherty D, Sladen RN: Effects of positive airway pressure on renal function. *In* Lumb PL (ed): Postoperative Mechanical Ventilation. Philadelphia, JP Lippincott, 1990, pp 369-386.

106. Jardin F, Forest JC, Boisante L, et al: Influence of positive end-expiratory pressure on left ventricular performance. N Engl J Med 304:387-392, 1981.

107. Sladen A, Laver MB, Pontoppidan H: Pulmonary complications and water retention in prolonged mechanical ventilation. N Engl J Med 279:448-453, 1968.

108. Annat G, Viale JP, Xuan BB, et al: Effect of PEEP ventilation on renal function, plasma renin, aldosterone, neurophysins and urinary ADH, and prostaglandins. Anesthesiology 58:136-141, 1983.

109. Venus B, Mathru M, Smith RA, et al: Renal function during application of positive end-expiratory pressure in swine: Effects of hydration. Anesthesiology 62:765-769, 1985.

110. Hemmer M, Suter PM: Treatment of cardiac and renal effects of PEEP with dopamine in patients with acute respiratory failure. Anesthesiology 50:399-403, 1979.

111. Thompson GE, Miller RD, Stevens WC, et al: Hypotensive anesthesia for total hip arthroplasty: A study of blood loss and organ function, brain, heart, liver and kidneys. Anesthesiology 48:91-96, 1978.

112. Colley PS, Silvarjan M: Regional blood flow in dogs during halothane anesthesia and controlled hypotension produced by nitroprusside or nitroglycerin. Anesth Analg 63:503-510, 1984.

113. Aronson S, Goldberg LI, Glock D, et al: Effects of fenoldopam on renal blood flow and systemic hemodynamics during isoflurane anesthesia. J Cardiothorac Vasc Anesth 5:29-32, 1991.

114. Myers BD, Moran SM: Hemodynamically mediated acute renal failure. N Engl J Med 314:97-105, 1986.

115. Gamulin Z, Forster A, Morel D, et al: Effects of infra-renal aortic cross-clamping on renal hemodynamics in humans. Anesthesiology 61:394-399, 1984.

116. Barry K, Cohen A, Knochel J, et al: Mannitol infusion. II. The prevention of acute functional renal failure during resection of an aneurysm of the abdominal aorta. N Engl J Med 264:967-971, 1961.

117. Burke TJ, Cronin RE, Duchin KL, et al: Ischemia and tubule obstruction during acute renal failure in dogs: Mannitol in protection. Am J Physiol 238:F305-F314, 1980.

118. Paul MD, Mazer CD, Byrick RJ, et al: Influence of mannitol and dopamine on renal function during elective infrarenal aortic cross-clamping in man. Am J Nephrol 6:427-434, 1986.

119. Ip-Yam PC, Murphy S, Baines M, et al: Renal function and proteinuria after cardiopulmonary bypass: The effects of temperature and mannitol. Anesth Analg 78:842-847, 1994.

120. Canivet JL, Larbuisson R, Damas P, et al: Plasma renin activity and urine beta 2-microglobulin during and after cardiopulmonary bypass: Pulsatile vs non-pulsatile perfusion. Eur Heart J 11:1079-1082, 1990.

121. Badner NH, Murkin JM, Lok P: Differences in pH management and pulsatile/nonpulsatile perfusion during cardiopulmonary bypass do not influence renal function. Anesth Analg 75:696-701, 1992.

122. Matsuda H, Hirose H, Nakano S, et al: Results of open heart surgery in patients with impaired renal function as creatinine clearance below 30 ml/min. The effects of pulsatile perfusion. J Cardiovasc Surg (Torino) 27:595-599, 1986.

123. Hilberman M, Myers B, Carrie G, et al: Acute renal failure following cardiac surgery. J Thorac Cardiovasc Surg 77:880-888, 1979.

124. Hilberman M, Derby GC, Spencer RJ, et al: Sequential pathophysiological changes characterizing the progression from renal dysfunction to acute renal failure following cardiac operation. J Thorac Cardiovasc Surg 79:838-844, 1980.

125. Higgins TL, Estafanous FG, Loop FD, et al: Stratification of morbidity and mortality outcome by preoperative risk factors in coronary artery bypass patients. A clinical severity score. JAMA 267:2344-2348, 1992.

126. Myles PS, Buckland MR, Schenk NJ, et al: Effect of "renal-dose" dopamine on renal function following cardiac surgery. Anaesth Intensive Care 21:56-61, 1993.

127. Costa P, Ottino GM, Matani A, et al: Low-dose dopamine during cardiopulmonary bypass in patients with renal dysfunction. J Cardiothorac Anesth 4:469-473, 1990.

128. Chiolero R, Borgeta A, Fisher A: Postoperative arrhythmias and risk factors after open heart surgery. Thorac Cardiovasc Surg 39:81-84, 1991.

129. Wardle N: Acute renal failure in the 1980s: The importance of septic shock and of endotoxemia. Nephron 30:193-200, 1982.

130. Zager RA: Endotoxemia, renal hypoperfusion, and fever: Interactive risk factors for aminoglycoside and sepsis-associated acute renal failure. Am J Kidney Dis 20:223-230, 1992.

131. Wetzels JF, Burke TJ, Schrier RW: Prevention and attenuation of acute renal failure. Curr Opin Nephrol Hypertens 1:133-140, 1992.

132. Clive D, Stoff J: Renal syndromes associated with nonsteroidal antiinflammatory drugs. N Engl J Med 310:563-572, 1984.

133. Kunzendorf U, Walz G, Brockmoeller J, et al: Effects of diltiazem upon metabolism and immunosuppressive action of cyclosporine in kidney graft recipients. Transplantation 52:280-284, 1991.

134. Neumayer HH, Kunzendorf U, Schreiber M: Protective effects of calcium antagonists in human renal transplantation. Kidney Int Suppl 36:87-93, 1992.

135. Parfrey PS, Griffiths SM, Barrett BJ, et al: Contrast material–induced renal failure in patients with diabetes mellitus, renal insufficiency or both. A prospective, controlled study. N Engl J Med 320:143, 1989.

136. Eisenberg RL, Bank WO, Hedgecock MW: Renal failure after major angiography can be avoided with hydration. Am J Radiol 136:859, 1981.

137. Tepel M, van der Giet M, Schwarzfeld C, et al: Prevention of radiographic-contrast-agent–induced reductions in renal function by acetylcysteine. N Engl J Med 343:180-184, 2000.

138. Briguori C, Manganelli F, Scarpato P, et al: Acetylcysteine and contrast agent–associated nephrotoxicity. J Am Coll Cardiol 40:298-303, 2002.

139. Tumlin JA, Wang A, Murray PT, Mathur VS: Fenoldopam mesylate blocks reductions in renal plasma flow after radio-contrast dye infusion: A pilot trial in the prevention of contrast nephropathy. Am Heart J 143:894-903, 2002.

140. Gabow PA, Kaehny WD, Kelleher SP: The spectrum of rhabdomyolysis. Medicine (Baltimore) 61:141, 1982.

141. Clyne DH, Kant KS, Pesce AJ, Pollack VE: Nephrotoxicity of low molecular weight serum proteins. Physicochemical interactions between myoglobin, hemoglobin, Bence-Jones protein and Tamm-Horsfall mucoprotein. Curr Probl Clin Biochem 9:299, 1979.

142. Ellinas PA, Rosner F: Rhabdomyolysis: Report of eleven cases. JAMA 84:617-624, 1992.

143. Ron D, Taitelman U, Michaelson M, et al: Prevention of acute renal failure in traumatic rhabdomyolysis. Arch Intern Med 144:277, 1984.

144. Wait RB, Kahng KU: Renal failure complicating obstructive jaundice. Am J Surg 157:256-263, 1989.

145. Plusa SM, Clark NW: Prevention of postoperative renal dysfunction in patients with obstructive jaundice: A comparison of mannitol-induced diuresis and oral sodium taurocholate. J R Coll Surg Edinb 36:303-305, 1991.

146. Gubern JM, Martinez-Rodenas F, Sitges-Serra A: Use of mannitol as a measure to prevent postoperative renal failure in patients with obstructive jaundice [letter]. Am J Surg 159:444-445, 1990; comment.

147. Zager RA: Sepsis-associated acute renal failure: Some potential pathogenetic and therapeutic insights. Nephrol Dial Transplant 4:164-167, 1994.

148. Cumming AD, Driedger AA, McDonald JW, et al: Vasoactive hormones in the renal response to systemic sepsis. Am J Kidney Dis 11:23-32, 1988.

149. Badr KF: Sepsis-associated renal vasoconstriction: Potential targets for future therapy. Am J Kidney Dis 20:207-213, 1992.

150. Cumming AD, McDonald JW, Lindsay RM, et al: The protective effect of thromboxane synthetase inhibition on renal function in systemic sepsis. Am J Kidney Dis 13:114-119, 1989.

151. Garella S, Matarese RA: Renal effects of prostaglandins and clinical adverse effects of nonsteroidal anti-inflammatory agents. Medicine (Baltimore) 63:165-181, 1984.

152. Bone RC, Fisher CJ, Clemmer TP, et al: A controlled clinical trial of high-dose methylprednisolone in the treatment of severe sepsis and septic shock. N Engl J Med 317:653-658, 1987.

153. Effect of high-dose glucocorticoid therapy on mortality in patients with clinical signs of systemic sepsis. The Veterans Administration Systemic Sepsis Cooperative Study Group. N Engl J Med 317:659-665, 1987.

154. Slotman GJ, Fisher CJJ, Bone RC, et al: Detrimental effects of high-dose methylprednisolone sodium succinate on serum concentrations of hepatic and renal function indicators in severe sepsis and septic shock. The Methylprednisolone Severe Sepsis Study Group. Crit Care Med 21:191-195, 1993.

155. Rudis MI, Basha MA, Zarowitz BJ: Is it time to reposition vasopressors and inotropes in sepsis? Crit Care Med 24:525-537, 1996.

156. Weber A, Schwieger IM, Poinsot O, et al: Sequential changes in renal oxygen consumption and sodium transport during hyperdynamic sepsis in sheep. Am J Physiol 262(Pt 2):F965, 1992.

157. Bersten AD, Rutten AJ: Renovascular interaction of epinephrine, dopamine, and intraperitoneal sepsis. Crit Care Med 23:537-544, 1995.

158. Lherm T, Troche G, Rossignol M, et al: Renal effects of low-dose dopamine in patients with sepsis syndrome or septic shock treated with catecholamines. Intensive Care Med 22:213-219, 1996.

159. Bellomo R, Chapman M, Finfer S, et al: Low-dose dopamine in patients with early renal dysfunction: A placebo-controlled randomised trial. Australian and New Zealand Intensive Care Society (ANZICS) Clinical Trials Group. Lancet 356:2139-2143, 2000.

160. Smithies M, Yee TH, Jackson L, et al: Protecting the gut and the liver in the critically ill: Effects of dopexamine. Crit Care Med 22:789-795, 1994.

161. Hesselvik JF, Brodin B: Low-dose norepinephrine in patients with septic shock and oliguria: Effects on afterload, urine flow and oxygen transport. Crit Care Med 17:179-180, 1989.

162. Landry DW, Oliver JA: The pathogenesis of vasodilatory shock. N Engl J Med 345:588-595, 2001.

163. Argenziano M, Choudri AF, Oz MC, et al: A prospective randomized trial of arginine vasopressin in the treatment of vasodilatory shock after left ventricular assist device placement. Circulation 96(9 Suppl):II-286-II-290, 1997.

164. Landry DW, Levin HR, Gallant EM, et al: Vasopressin deficiency contributes to the vasodilation of septic shock. Circulation 95:1122-1125, 1997.

165. Landry DW, Levin HR, Gallant EM, et al: Vasopressin pressor hypersensitivity in vasodilatory septic shock. Crit Care Med 25:1279-1282, 1997.

21 Cerebral Physiology and the Effects of Anesthetics and Techniques

Piyush M. Patel and John C. Drummond

Regulation of Cerebral Blood Flow 813
Chemical Regulation 814
Myogenic Regulation (Autoregulation) 817
Neurogenic Regulation 817
Viscosity Effects on Cerebral Blood Flow 817
Vasoactive Drugs 818
Age 820

Effects of Anesthetics on Cerebral Blood Flow and Cerebral Metabolic Rate 820
Intravenous Anesthetics 821
Inhaled Anesthetics 825
Muscle Relaxants 831

Other Effects of Anesthetics on Cerebral Physiology 832
Cerebrospinal Fluid Dynamics 832
Blood-Brain Barrier 832
Epileptogenesis 833

Cerebral Physiology in Pathologic States 833
Cerebral Ischemia—Pathophysiology 833
Brain Protection 837
Chronic Arterial Hypertension 842
Brain Tumors 842
Coma and Epilepsy 843

The effects of anesthetic drugs and techniques on cerebral physiology and, in particular, their effects on cerebral blood flow (CBF) and metabolism are reviewed in this chapter. The final section presents a brief discussion of pathophysiologic states, including cerebral ischemia, and cerebral protection. The chapter gives the most emphasis to information that is of immediate relevance to the rationale for the anesthetic and intensive care management of patients with intracranial pathology. Chapter 53 presents the clinical management of these patients in detail. Neurologic monitoring, including the effects of anesthetics on the electroencephalogram (EEG) and evoked responses, is reviewed in Chapter 38.

REGULATION OF CEREBRAL BLOOD FLOW

Anesthetics cause dose-related and reversible alterations in many aspects of cerebral physiology, including CBF, cerebral metabolic rate (CMR), and electrophysiologic function (EEG, evoked responses). The effects of anesthetic drugs and techniques have the potential to adversely affect the diseased brain and performance of the neurosurgical procedure and are therefore of clinical importance in patients with neurologic disease. However, in certain instances, the effects of general anesthesia on CBF and CMR can be manipulated to improve both the operative course and the clinical outcome of patients with neurologic disorders.

The adult human brain weighs approximately 1350 g and therefore represents about 2% of total-body weight. However, it receives 12% to 15% of cardiac output. This high flow rate is a reflection of the brain's high metabolic rate. At rest, the brain consumes oxygen at an average rate of approximately 3.5 mL of oxygen per 100 g of brain tissue per minute. Whole-brain O_2 consumption ($13.5 \times 3.5 = 47$ mL/min) represents about 20% of total-body oxygen utilization. Normal values for CBF,

Table 21-1   Normal cerebral physiologic values

CBF	
Global	45-55 mL/100 g/min
Cortical (mostly gray matter)	75-80 mL/100 g/min
Subcortical (mostly white matter)	~20 mL/100 g/min
$CMRO_2$	3-3.5 mL/100 g/min
CVR	1.5-2.1 mm Hg/100 g/min/mL
Cerebral venous Po_2	32-44 mm Hg
Cerebral venous So_2	55%-70%
ICP (supine)	8-12 mm Hg

CBF, cerebral blood flow; $CMRO_2$, cerebral metabolic rate of oxygen; CVR, cerebral vascular resistance; ICP, intracranial pressure.

Table 21-2   Factors influencing cerebral blood flow*

Factor	Comment
Chemical/Metabolic/Humoral	
Cerebral metabolic rate (CMR)	CMR influence assumes intact flow-metabolism coupling, the mechanism of which is not fully understood
Anesthetics	
Temperature	
Arousal/seizures	
$Paco_2$	
Pao_2	
Vasoactive drugs	
Anesthetics	
Vasodilators	
Vasopressors	
Myogenic	
Autoregulation/mean arterial pressure	The autoregulation mechanism is fragile, and in many pathologic states cerebral blood flow is regionally pressure passive
Rheologic	
Blood viscosity	
Neurogenic	
Extracranial sympathetic and parasympathetic pathways	Contribution and clinical significance poorly defined
Intra-axial pathways	

*See text for discussion.

CMR, and other physiologic variables are provided in Table 21-1.

Approximately 60% of the brain's energy consumption[1] is used to support electrophysiologic function. The depolarization-repolarization activity that occurs and is reflected in the EEG requires energy expenditure for the maintenance and restoration of ionic gradients and for the synthesis, transport, and reuptake of neurotransmitters. The remainder of the energy consumed by the brain is involved in cellular homeostatic activities. Local CBF and local CMR within the brain are very heterogeneous, and both are approximately four times greater in gray matter than white matter. The cell population of the brain is also heterogeneous in its oxygen requirements. Glial cells make up about half the brain's volume and require less energy than neurons. Besides providing a physically supportive latticework for the brain, glial cells are important in the reuptake of neurotransmitters and the delivery and removal of metabolic substrates and wastes.

The brain's substantial demand for substrate must be met by adequate delivery of oxygen and glucose. However, the space constraints imposed by the noncompliant cranium and meninges require that blood flow not be excessive. Not surprisingly, there are elaborate mechanisms for the regulation of CBF. These mechanisms, which include chemical, myogenic, and neurogenic factors, are listed in Table 21-2. The precise mechanisms of these effects are for the most part not well understood. However, a substantial volume of largely recent research indicates that modulation of the arginine–nitric oxide (NO)–cyclic guanosine monophosphate system[2,3] is central to the changes in cerebral vascular tone caused by several processes, including hypercapnia,[4,5] increased CMR,[6,7] volatile anesthetics,[8-10] and neurogenic mechanisms.[11-13]

Chemical Regulation

Several factors cause changes in the cerebral biochemical environment that result in adjustments in CBF, including changes in CMR, $Paco_2$, and Pao_2.

Cerebral Metabolic Rate

Increased neuronal activity results in increased local brain metabolism, and this increase in CMR is associated with a well-matched, proportional change in CBF.[14,15] Regional CBF and CMR measurements performed during maneuvers designed to activate specific brain regions provide evidence of the strict local "coupling" of CMR and CBF.[16-19] Although the precise mechanisms that mediate flow-metabolism coupling have not been defined, the available data implicate local by-products of metabolism (K^+, H^+, lactate, adenosine). Glutamate, released with increased neuronal activity, results in the synthesis and release of NO. NO is a potent cerebral vasodilator that plays an important role in flow and metabolism coupling.[6,7] More recent data have highlighted the role of glia in flow-metabolism coupling. Uptake of glutamate, released from neurons, by glia triggers increased glial metabolism and lactate production. Glial processes make contact with neurons and capillaries, and hence glia may serve as a conduit for the coupling of increased neuronal activity with increased glucose consumption and regional blood flow.[20] Nerves that innervate cerebral vessels release peptide neurotransmitters such as vasoactive intestinal peptide (VIP), neuropeptide Y, substance P, and calcitonin gene–related peptide. These neurotransmitters may also be potentially involved in neurovascular coupling. Flow and metabolism coupling within the brain is a complex physiologic process that is regulated not by a single mechanism, but by a combination of metabolic, glial, neural, and vascular factors.

CMR is influenced by several phenomena in the neurosurgical environment, including the functional state of the nervous system, anesthetics, and temperature.

FUNCTIONAL STATE. CMR decreases during sleep and increases during sensory stimulation, mental tasks, or arousal of any cause. During epileptic activity, CMR increases may be extreme, whereas in coma, CMR may be substantially reduced.

ANESTHETICS. The effect of individual anesthetics on CMR is presented in greater detail later in this chapter in the section "Effects of Anesthetics on Cerebral Blood Flow and Cerebral Metabolic Rate." In general, anesthetics suppress CMR, with ketamine and nitrous oxide (N_2O) being notable exceptions. It appears that the component of CMR on which they act is that associated with electrophysiologic function.[21] With several anesthetics, including barbiturates,[21] isoflurane,[22] sevoflurane,[23] desflurane,[24] propofol,[25] and etomidate,[26] increasing plasma concentrations cause progressive suppression of EEG activity and a concomitant reduction in CMR. However, increasing the plasma level beyond what is required to first achieve suppression of the EEG results in no further depression of CMR. The component of CMR required for maintenance of cellular integrity, the "housekeeping" component, is apparently unaltered by intravenous anesthetics (Fig. 21-1).

Values of the cerebral metabolic rate of oxygen ($CMRO_2$) observed when complete suppression of the EEG is achieved with different anesthetics are very similar. The inference that anesthetic-induced EEG suppression represents a single physiologic state no matter what anesthetic is used follows easily. However, there is evidence to the contrary. When barbiturates are administered to the point of EEG suppression, a uniform depression of CBF and CMR occurs throughout the brain. When suppression occurs during isoflurane administration, the relative reductions in CMR and CBF are greater in the neocortex than in other portions of the cerebrum.[27-29] Electrophysiologic responsiveness also varies. Cortical somatosensory evoked responses to median nerve stimulation can be recorded readily at doses of thiopental far in excess of those required to cause complete suppression of the EEG,[30] but they are difficult to elicit at concentrations of isoflurane associated with a burst suppression pattern, such as, 1.5 minimum alveolar concentration (MAC) (Fig. 21-2).[31] In addition, the EEG characteristics of the burst suppression states that occur just before complete suppression differ among anesthetics.[32] These differences may be of some relevance to discussions of differences in the "protective" potential of anesthetics that can produce EEG suppression because it is apparent that "burst suppression" does

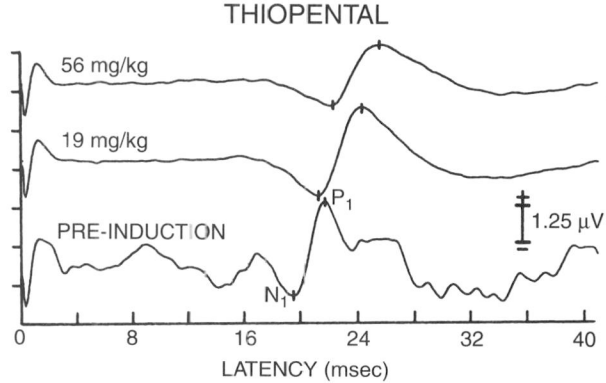

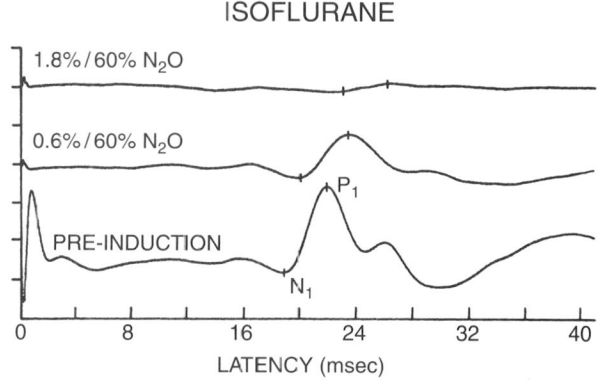

Figure 21-2 Cortical somatosensory evoked responses to median nerve stimulation in humans before induction and during anesthesia with thiopental and isoflurane/N_2O. In spite of an equivalent or greater degree of reduction in cerebral metabolic rate with thiopental, cortical evoked responses are better preserved[30] than during anesthesia with isoflurane,[31] which suggests that the electroencephalographic suppression achieved with different anesthetic agents should not be assumed to be equivalent electrophysiologic states. The cumulative thiopental doses and expired concentrations of isoflurane and N_2O are indicated.

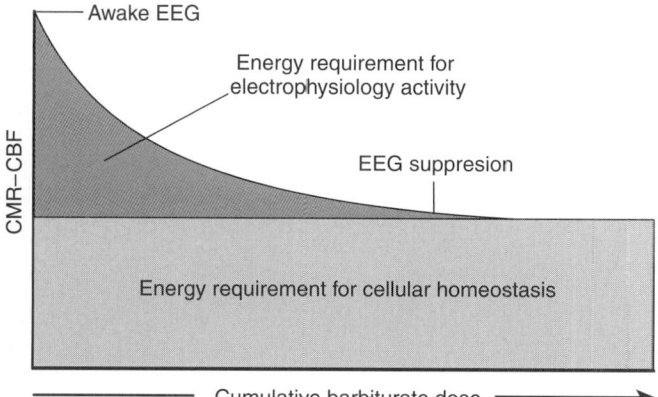

Figure 21-1 The interdependency[21] of cerebral electrophysiologic function and cerebral metabolic rate (CMR). Administration of various anesthetics,[21,22,26] including barbiturates, results in a dose-related reduction in the cerebral metabolic rate of oxygen ($CMRO_2$) and cerebral blood flow (CBF). The maximum reduction occurs with the dose that results in electrophysiologic silence. At this point, energy utilization associated with electrophysiologic activity has been reduced to zero, but energy utilization for cellular homeostasis persists unchanged. Additional barbiturate causes no further decrease in CBF or $CMRO_2$. EEG, electroencephalogram.

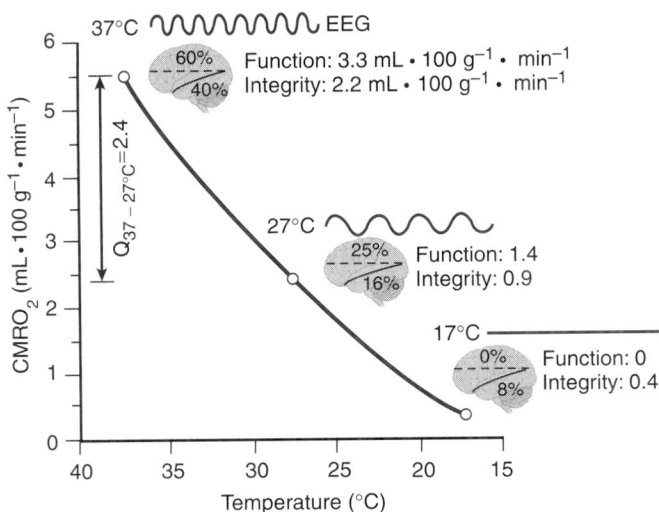

Figure 21-3 The effect of temperature reduction on the cerebral metabolic rate of oxygen (CMRO₂). Hypothermia reduces both of the components of cerebral metabolic activity identified in Figure 21-1: that associated with neuronal electrophysiologic activity ("Function") and that associated with maintenance of cellular homeostasis ("Integrity"). This effect is in contrast to anesthetics that alter only the functional component. The ratio of CMR at 37°C to that at 27°C, the Q_{10} ratio, is shown in the graph. EEG, electroencephalogram. (Adapted from Michenfelder JD: Anesthesia and the Brain: Clinical, Functional, Metabolic, and Vascular Correlates. New York, Churchill Livingstone, 1988.)

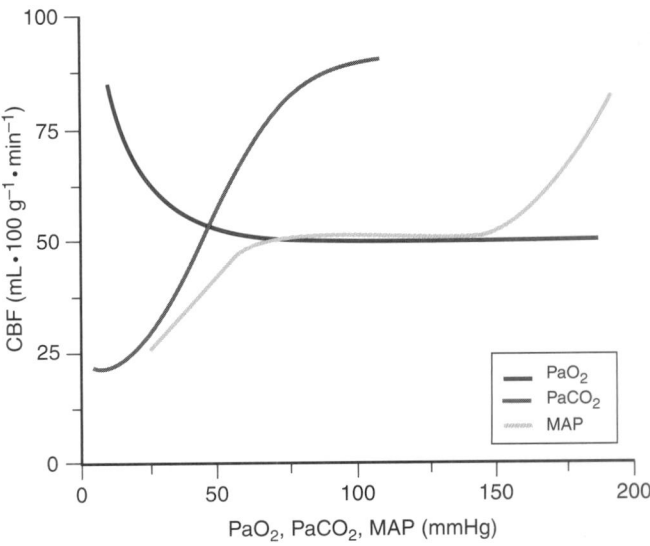

Figure 21-4 Changes in cerebral blood flow (CBF) caused by independent alterations in Paco₂, Pao₂, and mean arterial pressure (MAP).

not represent a uniform physiologic state, irrespective of the anesthetic used to produce it.

TEMPERATURE. The effects of hypothermia on both normal and ischemic brain have been reviewed in detail.[1,33,34] CMR decreases by 6% to 7%/°C of temperature reduction.[1] As is the case with some anesthetics, hypothermia can also cause complete suppression of the EEG (at about 18°C to 20°C). However, in contrast to anesthetics, temperature reduction beyond that at which EEG suppression first occurs does produce a further decrease in CMR (Fig. 21-3). This decrease occurs because although anesthetics reduce only the component of CMR associated with neuronal function, hypothermia causes decreases in the rate of energy utilization associated with both electrophysiologic function and the basal component associated with maintenance of cellular integrity. These decreases were once assumed to be proportional. However, mild hypothermia preferentially suppresses the basal component of CMR.[35,36] CMRO₂ at 18°C is less than 10% of normothermic control values, which probably accounts for the brain's tolerance of moderate periods of circulatory arrest at these and lower temperatures.

Hyperthermia has an opposite influence on cerebral physiology. Between 37°C and 42°C, CBF and CMR increase.[37] However, above 42°C a dramatic reduction in cerebral oxygen consumption occurs, an indication of a threshold for a toxic effect of hyperthermia that may occur as a result of protein (enzyme) degradation.

PaCO₂. CBF varies directly with Paco₂ (Fig. 21-4). The effect is greatest within the range of physiologic Paco₂ variation. CBF changes 1 to 2 mL/100 g/min for each 1–mm Hg change in Paco₂ around normal Paco₂ values.[38]

This response is attenuated below a Paco₂ of 25 mm Hg.[38] Under normal circumstances, CBF sensitivity to changes in Paco₂ ($\Delta CBF/\Delta Paco_2$) appears to be positively correlated with resting levels of CBF.[39] Accordingly, anesthetics that alter resting CBF cause changes in the CO₂ response of the cerebral circulation. The magnitude of the reduction in CBF by hypocapnia is greater when resting CBF is high (as might occur during anesthesia with volatile anesthetics). Conversely, when resting CBF is low, the magnitude of the hypocapnia-induced CBF reduction is decreased. Nonetheless, CO₂ responsiveness has been observed in normal brain during anesthesia with all of the numerous anesthetics that have been studied.

The changes in CBF caused by Paco₂ are apparently dependent on pH alterations in the extracellular fluid of the brain.[40] NO, especially NO of neuronal origin, is an important, though not exclusive mediator of CO₂-induced vasodilatation.[4,5,41-43] In particular, in primates, NO's relevance may be limited to the cerebral cortex.[5] In humans, NO inhibition significantly attenuates the hyperemic response to hypercapnia.[44] The vasodilator response to hypercapnia is also mediated in part by prostaglandins; administration of indomethacin reduces the vasodilator response by about 60%.[45] The changes in extracellular pH and CBF occur rapidly after Paco₂ adjustments because CO₂ diffuses freely across the cerebrovascular endothelium. Note that in contrast to respiratory acidosis, acute systemic metabolic acidosis has little immediate effect on CBF because the blood-brain barrier (BBB) excludes the hydrogen ion (H⁺) from the perivascular space. Although the CBF changes in response to alterations in Paco₂ occur rapidly, they are not sustained. In spite of the maintenance of increased arterial pH, CBF returns to normal over a period of 6 to 8 hours[46-48] because cerebrospinal fluid (CSF) pH gradually returns to normal as a result of the extrusion of bicarbonate. Consequently, a patient who has had a sustained period of hyperventilation or hypoventilation deserves special consideration. Acute normalization of $Paco_2$ will result in significant CSF acidosis (after hypocapnia) or alkalosis (after hypercapnia). The former will result in increased CBF with a concomitant increase in intracranial pressure (ICP) that will depend on the prevailing intracranial compliance. The latter conveys the theoretical risk of ischemia.

Pao_2. Changes in Pao_2 from 60 to over 300 mm Hg have little influence on CBF. Below a Pao_2 of 60 mm Hg, however, CBF increases rapidly (see Fig. 21-4). The mechanisms mediating the cerebral vasodilation during hypoxia are not fully understood but may include neurogenic effects initiated by peripheral or neuraxial chemoreceptors, as well as local humoral influences. At least part of the hyperemic response to hypoxia is mediated by NO of neuronal origin.[49] Hypoxia-induced hyperpolarization of vascular smooth muscle by the opening of adenosine triphosphate (ATP)-dependent K^+ channels also leads to vasodilation. Recent studies have indicated that the rostral ventrolateral medulla (RVM) serves as an oxygen sensor within the brain.[50] Stimulation of the RVM by hypoxia results in an increase in CBF (but not CMR), and lesions of the RVM suppress the magnitude of the CBF response to hypoxia. The response to hypoxia is synergistic with the hyperemia produced by hypercapnia and acidosis. At high Pao_2 values, CBF decreases modestly.[51] At 1 atm of oxygen, CBF is reduced by 12%.[52]

Myogenic Regulation (Autoregulation)

Autoregulation refers to the capacity of the cerebral circulation to adjust its resistance so that it can maintain CBF constant over a wide range of mean arterial pressure (MAP) values. In normal human subjects, the limits of autoregulation occur at MAP values of approximately 70 and 150 mm Hg (see Fig. 21-4). The lower limit of autoregulation (LLA) has been widely quoted as an MAP of 50 mm Hg. Although this number may be correct for some animal species, the available data argue that the LLA is considerably higher in humans.[53] Note that the units used on the x axis of "autoregulation curves" will influence the correct inflection points of the curve. When the x axis is "mean arterial pressure," the normal average LLA is not less than 70 mm Hg (with considerable interindividual variation).[54-58] However, cerebral perfusion pressure (CPP) is the ideal independent variable, but because ICP is not usually measured in normal subjects, CPP (MAP – ICP) is rarely available. Assuming a normal ICP in a supine subject of 10 to 15 mm Hg, an LLA of 70 expressed as MAP corresponds to an LLA of 55 to 60 mm Hg expressed as CPP.

Above and below the autoregulatory plateau, CBF is pressure dependent (pressure passive) and varies linearly with CPP. Autoregulation is influenced by various pathologic processes and, in addition, by the time course over which CPP changes occur. Even within the range over which autoregulation normally occurs, a rapid change in arterial pressure will result in a transient (3 to 4 minutes) alteration in CBF.[59]

The precise mechanism by which autoregulation is accomplished is not known. According to the myogenic hypothesis, changes in CPP lead to direct changes in the tone of vascular smooth muscle; this process appears to be passive. NO may participate in the vasodilation associated with hypotension in some species[60,61] but not, according to a single study, in primates.[62] Autonomic innervation of cerebral blood vessels may also contribute to autoregulation of blood flow (discussed in the next section).

Neurogenic Regulation

Considerable evidence has shown that the cerebral vasculature is extensively innervated.[63] The density of innervation declines with vessel size, and the greatest neurogenic influence appears to be exerted on larger cerebral arteries.[64] This innervation includes cholinergic (parasympathetic[65] and nonparasympathetic),[66-68] adrenergic (sympathetic[69] and nonsympathetic),[70] serotonergic,[71,72] and VIPergic[73] systems of extra- and intra-axial origin. It is certain that in animals there is an extracranial sympathetic influence through the superior cervical ganglion[69,74-77] and parasympathetic innervation through the sphenopalatine ganglion.[65] The intra-axial pathways are less well defined, although there is considerable evidence of innervation arising from several nuclei in animals, including the locus ceruleus,[70] the fastigial nucleus,[68] the dorsal raphe nucleus,[72] and the basal magnocellular nucleus of Meynert.[66,67] Evidence of the functional significance of neurogenic influences has been derived from studies of CBF autoregulation[74,76,78-80] and ischemic injury.[81,82] Hemorrhagic shock, a state with high sympathetic tone, results in a lower CBF at a given MAP than occurs when hypotension is produced with sympatholytic drugs, presumably because during shock, a sympathetically mediated vasoconstrictive effect shifts the lower end of the "autoregulatory" plateau (Fig. 21-5) to the right. It is not clear what the relative contributions of humoral and neural mechanisms are to this phenomenon; however, a neurogenic component is certainly operative in some species because sympathetic denervation increases CBF during hemorrhagic shock.[74,78,83] Activation of cerebral sympathetic innervation also shifts the upper limit of autoregulation to the right and offers some protection against hypertensive breakthrough of the BBB.[79,80] Experimental interventions that alter these neurogenic control pathways influence outcomes after standardized ischemic insults,[81,82] presumably through influences on vascular tone and therefore CBF. The nature and influence of such pathways in humans are not known, and at present, there are no clinical interventions designed to manipulate these pathways that are relevant to neurosurgical patients.[84]

Viscosity Effects on Cerebral Blood Flow

Blood viscosity can influence CBF. Hematocrit is the single most important determinant of blood viscosity.[85] In healthy subjects, variation of hematocrit within the normal range (33% to 45%) probably results in only trivial alteration in CBF. Beyond this range, changes are more substantial.[85,86] In anemia, cerebral vascular resistance is reduced and CBF increases. However, this increase in CBF may result not only from a reduction in viscosity but also

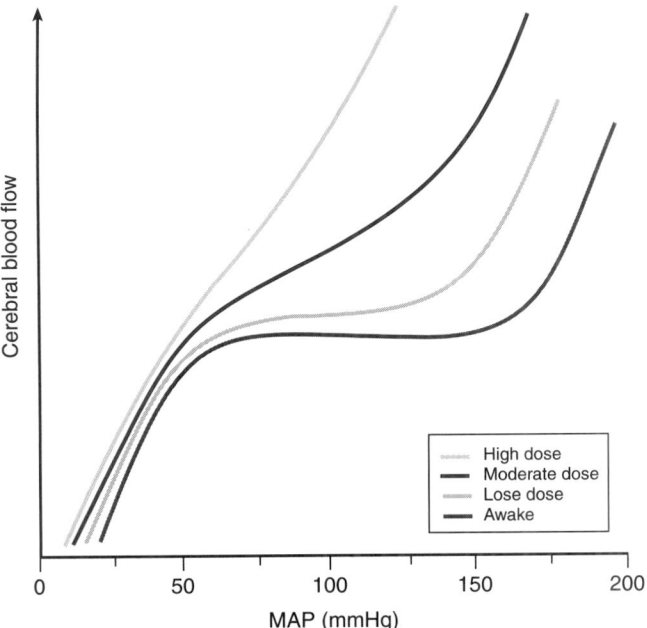

Figure 21–5 Schematic representation of the effect of increasing concentrations of a typical volatile anesthetic on autoregulation of cerebral blood flow. Dose-dependent cerebral vasodilation results in attenuation of autoregulatory capacity. Both the upper and lower thresholds are shifted to the left. MAP, mean arterial pressure.

in response to reduced oxygen-carrying capacity of blood.[87] The effect of a reduction in viscosity on CBF is more obvious in the setting of focal cerebral ischemia, when vasodilation in response to impaired oxygen delivery is probably already maximal. In this setting, the reduction in viscosity achieved by hemodilution results in increases in CBF in the ischemic territory.[88-91] The best available information suggests that in the setting of focal cerebral ischemia, a hematocrit of 30% to 34% will result in optimal oxygen delivery.[92,93] However, manipulation of viscosity in patients with acute ischemic stroke has not been shown to be of benefit in reducing the extent of cerebral injury.[94] Hence, viscosity is not a target of manipulation in patients at risk from cerebral ischemia, with the possible exception being those with hematocrit values in excess of 55%.

Vasoactive Drugs (also see Chapter 16)

A large number of drugs with intrinsic vascular effects are used in contemporary anesthetic practice, including both anesthetics and numerous vasoactive drugs used specifically for hemodynamic manipulation. This section will deal with the latter. The actions of anesthetics are discussed in a later section.

Systemic Vasodilators

Most drugs used to induce hypotension (including sodium nitroprusside, nitroglycerin, hydralazine, adenosine, and calcium channel blockers) also cause cerebral vasodilation. As a result, CBF either increases or is maintained at prehypotensive levels. In addition, CBF is maintained at a lower MAP when hypotension is induced

with a cerebral vasodilator rather than either hemorrhage or a noncerebral vasodilator such as the ganglionic blocker trimethaphan.[95] In contrast to direct vasodilators, the angiotensin-converting enzyme inhibitor enalapril does not have any significant impact on CBF.[96] Anesthetics that vasodilate the cerebral circulation simultaneously cause increases in cerebral blood volume (CBV) with the potential to increase ICP. The ICP effects of these drugs are empirically less dramatic when hypotension is induced slowly,[97] probably because of the more effective interplay of compensatory mechanisms (CSF and venous blood shifts) when changes occur more slowly.

Catecholamine Agonists/Antagonists

Numerous drugs with agonist and antagonist activity at catecholamine receptors (α_1, α_2, β, and dopamine) are in common use. The effects of these drugs on cerebral physiology are dependent on basal blood pressure, the magnitude of the systemic blood pressure changes that occur as a result of administration of the drug of interest, the status of the autoregulation mechanism, and the status of the BBB. A given drug may have direct effects on cerebral vascular smooth muscle or indirect effects, or both, that are mediated by the cerebral autoregulatory response to changes in systemic blood pressure. When autoregulation is preserved, increases in systemic pressure would be expected to increase CBF if basal blood pressure is either below or above the lower and upper limits of autoregulation, respectively. When basal pressure is within the normal autoregulation range, an increase in systemic pressure does not affect CBF significantly because the normal autoregulatory response to rising MAP entails cerebral vasoconstriction (an increase in cerebral vascular resistance) to maintain constant CBF. When autoregulation is defective, CBF will vary in direct relation to systemic pressure. The information in the following sections and in Table 21-3 emphasizes data obtained from investigations of pressor agents in intact preparations and gives greatest weight to results obtained in humans and higher primates.

α_1-Agonists

A frequently encountered clinical concern is that the administration of drugs with α_1-agonist effects (phenylephrine, norepinephrine) will lead to a reduction in CBF. Data derived from studies in both humans and nonhuman primates do not support this belief. Intracarotid infusion of norepinephrine in doses that raised MAP from 95 to 117 mm Hg and intravenous infusion that raised MAP from 95 to 142 mm Hg resulted in no change in CBF.[98] Intracarotid infusion of norepinephrine in baboons in a dose sufficient to increase MAP by 10% had no effect on CBF.[99] Administration of phenylephrine to patients maintained on cardiopulmonary bypass did not decrease CBF.[100] There are, however, some species differences with regard to the CBF response to α-agonists. α_1-Agonists also do not appear to cause cerebral vasoconstriction in rats,[101-104] but they do produce modest decreases in CBF in dogs and goats; this reduction in CBF can be blocked by α_1-antagonists.[105-108]

CBF increases have been attributed to norepinephrine. Such increases might occur if autoregulation were defective

Table 21–3 Best estimates of the influence of pure catecholamine receptor agonists and specific pressor substances on cerebral blood flow and cerebral metabolic rate*

Agonist	Cerebral Blood Flow	Cerebral Metabolic Rate
Pure		
α_1	0/–	0
α_2	–	0
β	+	+
β (BBB open)	+++	+++
Dopamine	++	0
Dopamine (high dose)	?–	?0
Mixed		
Norepinephrine	0/–	0/+
Norepinephrine (BBB open)	+	+
Epinephrine	+	+
Epinephrine (BBB open)	+++	+++

*Where species differences occurred, data from primates were given preference. See the text for a complete discussion.
BBB, blood-brain barrier.
+ indicates increase; – indicates decrease; the number of symbols indicates the magnitude of the effect; 0 indicates no effect.

or its limit exceeded. In some instances, the increases may be the result of BBB abnormalities. Some data suggest that β-mimetic drugs (norepinephrine has β_1-activity) cause activation of cerebral metabolism[109] with a parallel coupled increase in CBF, and this effect is likely to be most apparent when these drugs can gain greater access to the brain parenchyma through a defective BBB (see the next section on epinephrine).[99,102,110]

In summary, it seems likely that circulating α_1-agonists will have little direct influence on CBF in humans, with the exception that norepinephrine may cause vasodilation when the BBB is defective.

β-Agonists

β-Adrenergic receptor agonists, in small doses, have little direct effect on the cerebral vasculature. In larger doses and in association with physiologic stress, they can cause an increase in CMR with an accompanying increase in CBF.[111] The β_1-receptor is probably the mediator of these effects.[112] Olesen[98] observed no change in CBF in unanesthetized human volunteers in response to an intracarotid infusion of approximately 6 μg/min of epinephrine, a dose that caused no change in MAP. However, when King and colleagues[113] administered a larger dose of epinephrine, 37 μg/min intravenously (a dose sufficient to increase MAP from 91 to 109 mm Hg), CBF and $CMRO_2$ rose by 22% and 24%, respectively.

Evidence has shown that a BBB defect enhances the effect of β-agonists.[99,110,114] Intracarotid norepinephrine does not have an effect on CBF and CMR in normal baboons. However, when the BBB is disrupted by intracarotid injection of hypertonic urea, norepinephrine increased CBF and CMR.[99] Artru and associates demonstrated that epinephrine causes an elevation in $CMRO_2$ in dogs, but only when the BBB was made permeable.[110] Note that in neither of these studies were CBF/CMR changes observed without a BBB abnormality. These observations beg the interpretation that β-agonists will increase CBF and CMR only when the BBB is injured.

However, in the human study of King and coworkers (mentioned earlier), MAP was apparently not excessively high and CBF/CMR increases nonetheless occurred. Accordingly, it does not appear that BBB injury is a necessary condition in humans for the occurrence of β-mediated increases in CBF and CMR, although it will probably exaggerate the phenomenon.

β-Adrenergic Blockers

β-Blockers reduce or have no effect on CBF and CMR. In two investigations in humans, propranolol, 5 mg intravenously,[115] and labetalol, 0.75 mg/kg intravenously,[116] had no effect on CBF and CBF volume (CBFV), respectively. Dubois and associates observed modest reductions in CBF when labetalol was administered to craniotomy patients who became hypertensive during emergence from anesthesia.[117] Esmolol shortens seizures induced by electroconvulsive therapy (ECT), thus suggesting that it does cross the normal BBB.[118] Esmolol was reported in abstract form to have no effect on CBF and CMR as long as CPP was maintained.[119] Catecholamine levels at the time of administration of β-adrenergic blockers or the status of the BBB (or both) may influence the effect of these drugs. The database with respect to these possibilities is incomplete. However, data suggest that β-blockers are unlikely to have adverse effects on patients with intracranial pathology, other than effects secondary to changes in perfusion pressure.

Dopamine

Dopamine is widely used in the treatment of hemodynamic dysfunction. In addition, it is commonly used to augment the function of the normal cardiovascular system when elevation of MAP is desired as an adjunct to the treatment of focal cerebral ischemia, especially in the setting of vasospasm. Nonetheless, its effects on CBF and CMR have not been defined with certainty. Taken together, the available data[103,106,120-123] suggest that the predominant effect of dopamine in the normal cerebral vasculature, when administered in low doses, is probably slight vasodilation with minimal CMR change. Increased CMR in discrete regions of the brain, such as the choroid plexus and basal ganglia, has been reported. However, overall cortical blood flow is not influenced.[124] Vasoconstriction of the cerebral circulation is not observed even when dopamine is administered in doses up to 100 µg/kg/min. In that same investigation, the same doses of dobutamine were associated with CBF and CMR increases of 20% to 30%.[123]

α_2-Agonists

Interest in α_2-agonists is currently high because of their apparent analgesic and sedative effects. This class includes dexmedetomidine and clonidine, with the latter being a much less specific and less potent α_2-agonist. A number of investigations have demonstrated that dexmedetomidine decreases CBF with no effect on $CMRO_2$.[125-129] Dexmedetomidine-induced constriction of isolated cerebral vessels[130] and reversal of this effect with the simultaneous administration of an α_2-antagonist suggest that vasoconstriction is mediated by postsynaptic α_2-receptors.[131] In addition, α_2-agonists may act at a central site, such as the locus ceruleus,[70] and cause neurogenically mediated vasoconstriction.

Two investigations in human volunteers have confirmed the ability of dexmedetomidine to decrease CBF. Dexmedetomidine dose-dependently decreased middle cerebral artery (MCA) flow velocity, with the maximum reduction being approximately 25%.[132] In a more recent investigation, dexmedetomidine (1-µg/kg load and infusion at either 0.2 or 0.6 µg/kg/hr) decreased CBF by about 30%.[133] Although dexmedetomidine reduced MAP modestly, the reduction was not outside the normal limits of autoregulation. Of interest was the observation that the reduction in CBF was apparent even after the dexmedetomidine infusion had been discontinued for 30 minutes. The dose of dexmedetomidine that was administered resulted in significant sedation. Although it is possible that the reduction in CBF was associated with a reduction in CMR, the experimental studies cited earlier argue otherwise. These data provide reasonable evidence for the notion that dexmedetomidine is a cerebral vasoconstrictor. Accordingly, caution should be exercised in its use in patients in whom CBF is compromised.

Age (also see Chapters 60 and 62)

Aging, from childhood to late adulthood, is associated with a progressive reduction in CBF and $CMRO_2$.[134,135] This reduction may reflect the progressive neuronal loss that occurs with age.

EFFECTS OF ANESTHETICS ON CEREBRAL BLOOD FLOW AND CEREBRAL METABOLIC RATE

This section deals with the effect of anesthetics on CBF and CMR. It includes limited mention of influences on autoregulation, CO_2 responsiveness, and CBV. Discussions of effects on CSF dynamics, the BBB, and

epileptogenesis are presented in the later section "Cerebral Physiology in Pathologic States."

In neuroanesthesia, considerable emphasis is placed on the manner in which anesthetic drugs and techniques influence CBF. The rationale is twofold. First, delivery of energy substrates is dependent on CBF, and in the setting of ischemia, modest alterations in CBF can substantially influence neuronal outcome. Second, control and manipulation of CBF are central to the management of ICP because as CBF varies in response to vasoconstrictor-vasodilator influences (e.g., $Paco_2$ and volatile anesthetics), CBV varies linearly with it, albeit with some variation among anesthetics in the CBF-CBV ratio.[136] In normal brain, CBV is approximately 5 mL/100 g of brain tissue,[137] and over a $Paco_2$ range of approximately 25 to 70 mm Hg, CBV changes by about 0.049 mL/100 g for each 1-mm Hg change in $Paco_2$.[138,139] In an adult brain weighing about 1400 g, this can amount to a 20-mL change in total CBV for a $Paco_2$ range of 25 to 55 mm Hg.

Although CBV and CBF usually vary in parallel, exceptions do occur. CBV increases during cerebral ischemia,[140,141] and it may vary independently of CBF when MAP is the manipulated variable. Autoregulation normally serves to prevent MAP-related increases in CBV. In fact, as cerebral circulation constricts to maintain CBF constant in the face of rising MAP, CBV actually decreases.[142] When autoregulation is impaired or its upper limit ($\approx$150 mm Hg) is exceeded, CBF and CBV then increase in parallel as arterial pressure rises (see Fig. 21-4). Declining MAP results in a progressive increase in CBV as the cerebral circulation dilates to maintain constant flow, and exaggerated increases in CBV occur as MAP falls below the LLA.[142] In normal subjects, the initial increases in CBV do not result in significant elevation of ICP because there is latitude for compensatory adjustments by other intracranial compartments (e.g., translocation of venous blood and CSF to extracerebral vessels and the spinal CSF space, respectively). When intracranial compliance* is reduced, an increase in CBV can cause herniation or reduce CPP sufficiently to cause ischemia.

Several investigations on the effects of anesthetics on CBV in normal brain have been conducted.[144-146] In general, the effects observed confirm a parallel relationship between CBF and CBV. However, the relationship is not consistently 1:1,[136,147] and CBF-independent influences on CBV may occur. It is also an unexplored possibility that anesthetics may influence the venous side of the cerebral circulation. Although the intracranial veins are a largely passive compartment, some evidence indicates that in certain species, there is some active control of venous caliber by either neurogenic or humoral mechanisms.[75,77,148]

---

*Note a well-entrenched misuse of terminology.[143] The "compliance" curve that is commonly drawn to describe the intracranial pressure-volume relationship (Fig. 52-2) actually depicts the relationship $\Delta P/\Delta V$ (elastance) and not $\Delta V/\Delta P$ (compliance). What is here referred to as "reduced compliance" is more correctly described as "increased elastance." Not all disciplines, including most notably neurosurgery, have adopted the revised terminology. The authors have therefore left the misuse uncorrected herein.

At present, no evidence has shown that these direct effects have clinical significance. Nonetheless, the importance of blood volume on the venous side of the cerebral circulation should not be overlooked. Passive engorgement of these vessels as a result of the head-down posture, compression of the jugular venous system, or high intrathoracic pressure can have dramatic effects on ICP (see Fig. 53-4).

Intravenous Anesthetics (see Chapters 10 and 11)

The general pattern of the effect of intravenous anesthetics is one of parallel alterations in CMR and CBF. The vast majority of intravenous anesthetics cause a reduction in both. Ketamine, which causes an increase in CMR and CBF, is the exception. The effects of selected intravenous anesthetics on human CBF are compared in Figure 21-6.

It is probable that intravenous anesthetic–induced changes in CBF are largely the result of effects on CMR with parallel (coupled) changes in CBF. If this were the entire explanation, the CBF/CMR ratio would be the same for all anesthetics, but it is not. It is therefore likely that there are also direct effects on cerebral vascular smooth muscle (e.g., vasoconstriction, vasodilation, alteration of autoregulatory function) that make contributions to the net effect. For instance, although barbiturates are generally thought of as cerebral vasoconstrictors, some barbiturates actually cause relaxation of cerebral vascular smooth muscle in isolated vessel preparations.[161-163] However, a substantial reduction in CMR occurs in vivo, and the net effect at the point of EEG suppression is vasoconstriction and a substantial decrease in CBF.[21] It appears that in general, autoregulation and CO_2 responsiveness are preserved during administration of intravenous anesthetics.

Barbiturates

A dose-dependent reduction in CBF and CMR occurs with barbiturates. With the onset of anesthesia, CBF and $CMRO_2$ are reduced by about 30%.[164,165] When large doses of thiopental cause complete EEG suppression, CBF and CMR are reduced by about 50%.[21,149,166] Further increases in the dose of barbiturate have no additional effect on CMR.[21,167] These observations suggest that the major effect of nontoxic doses of depressant anesthetics is a reduction in the component of cerebral metabolism that is linked to electrical brain function (e.g., neurophysiologic activity), with only minimal effects on the second component, that related to cellular homeostasis (see Fig. 21-1).

Tolerance to the CBF/CMR effects of barbiturates may develop quickly.[168,169] In patients with severe head injury in whom "barbiturate coma" was maintained for 72 hours, the thiamylal blood concentration required to maintain EEG burst suppression was observed to be increased by the end of the first 24 hours and continued to increase over the next 48 hours.[170] During deep pentobarbital anesthesia, autoregulation is maintained to arterial pressures as low as 60 mm Hg.[171] CO_2 responsiveness also persists.[172]

Propofol

The effects of propofol (2,6-diisopropylphenol) on CBF and CMR appear to be quite similar to those of the barbiturates.

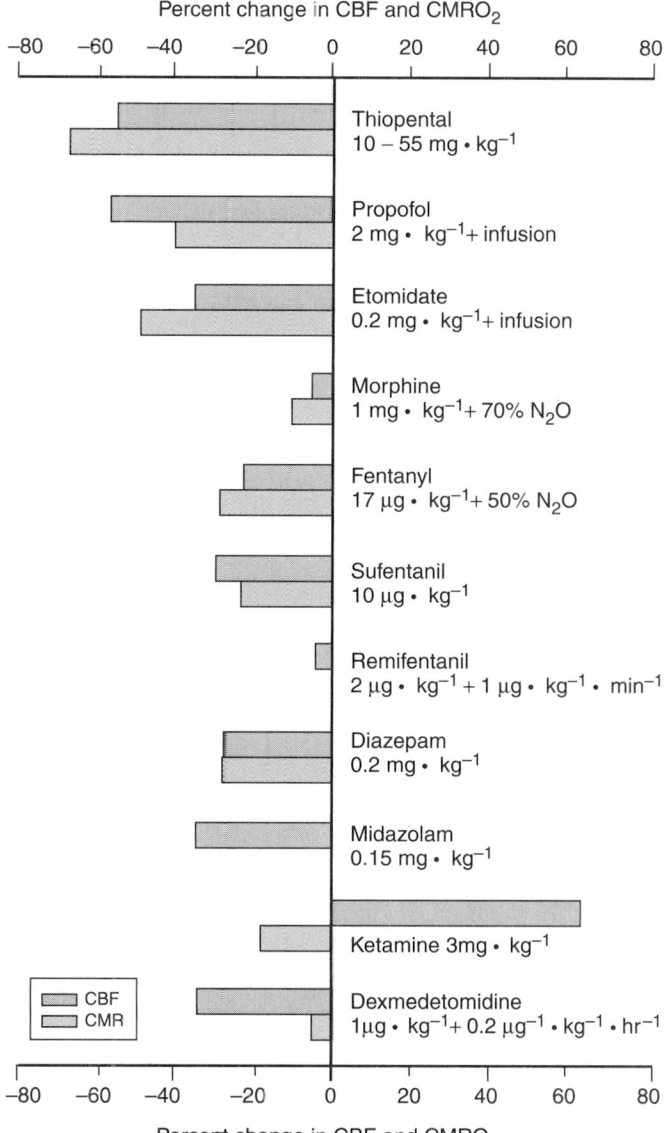

Figure 21–6 Changes in cerebral blood flow (CBF) and the cerebral metabolic rate of oxygen ($CMRO_2$) caused by intravenous anesthetic agents. The data are derived from human investigations and are presented as the percent change from unanesthetized control values. Dexmedetomidine CMR values were determined on a background of 0.5% isoflurane anesthesia. See the text for details. No data for the $CMRO_2$ effects of midazolam in humans are available. (Data from references 149-160.)

Three investigations in humans have revealed substantial reductions in both CBF and CMR after the administration of propofol.[150,173] Stephan and colleagues[150] administered propofol by bolus plus infusion (2 mg/kg and 0.2 mg/kg/min, respectively) and observed average CBF and CMR decreases of 51% and 36%, respectively. In patients undergoing lower extremity surgery with epidural anesthesia, infusion of 100 μg/kg/min of propofol resulted in a reduction in CBF of approximately 15% and a reduction in CMR of 18%.[174] Alkire and associates assessed cerebral glucose metabolism in volunteers by positron emission tomography (PET) before and during infusion of propofol to the point of unresponsiveness.[175]

The whole-brain metabolic rate decreased by 48% to 58%, with limited regional heterogeneity observed. A combination of propofol and fentanyl decreased subdural pressure in patients with intracranial tumors and decreased the arteriovenous oxygen saturation difference ($AVDO_2$) in comparison to isoflurane-fentanyl or sevoflurane-fentanyl anesthesia.[176] Ravussin and colleagues measured lumbar CSF pressure during induction of anesthesia by slow bolus administration of propofol (1.5 mg/kg over a 30-second period) in patients scheduled for craniotomy.[177] They observed maximal average reductions in lumbar CSF pressure and CPP of 32% and 10%, respectively. Collectively, these investigations in human subjects indicate that propofol effects reductions in CMR and secondarily decreases CBF, CBV, and ICP.

Both CO_2 responsiveness and autoregulation appear to be preserved during the administration of propofol in humans,[178,179] even when propofol is administered in doses that produce burst suppression of the EEG.[180] The magnitude of the reduction in CBF during hypocapnia is decreased during propofol administration. This effect is probably due to CMR suppression–induced cerebral vasoconstriction, thereby limiting further hypocapnia-mediated vasoconstriction. Seizures and opisthotonos have been reported to occur after propofol anesthesia.[181-185] However, systematic studies in both humans[186-188] and animals,[189,190] though identifying the occurrence of occasional dystonic and choreiform[186] movements, have failed to confirm the notion that propofol is proconvulsant. In fact, propofol appears to be anticonvulsant in animals (mice).[189,190] Furthermore, ECT seizures were shorter after induction with propofol than with methohexital,[191] which is more consistent with an anticonvulsant effect. In addition, propofol sedation has been widely used during "awake" resection of seizure foci and other intracranial lesions.[187,188,192] Although pronounced high-amplitude beta-frequency activity in the EEG has been observed,[193] there has not been an unexpected incidence of seizures.

Etomidate

The effects of etomidate on CBF and CMR are also superficially similar to those of barbiturates. Roughly parallel reductions in CBF and CMR occur in humans[151,194] and are in general accompanied by progressive suppression of the EEG.[195] Induction of anesthesia with either thiopental or etomidate resulted in a similar reduction in MCA flow velocity of about 27%.[196] The CBF/CMR changes are substantial. Renou and coworkers[151] gave approximately 0.2 mg/kg of etomidate to adults and observed mean reductions in CBF and CMR of 34% and 45%, respectively. In dogs, as is the case with barbiturates, no further reduction in CMR occurs when additional drug is administered beyond a dose sufficient to produce EEG suppression.[26] This latter phenomenon has not been demonstrated in humans. However, Bingham and colleagues[197] observed that etomidate lowered ICP when administered to severely head injured patients in whom EEG activity was well preserved, but it was ineffective when there was substantial antecedent EEG suppression. Canine data reviewed by Milde and colleagues[26] suggest that though substantial, the global CMR suppression

attainable with etomidate is slightly less profound than that achieved with isoflurane and barbiturates. These data are consistent with the observations of Davis and associates[198] that unlike barbiturates, which cause CMR suppression throughout the brain, the CMR suppression caused by etomidate is regionally variable and occurs predominantly in the forebrain structures.

Etomidate has been shown to be effective in reducing ICP without causing a reduction in CPP in patients with intracranial tumors[199] and head-injured patients.[200] However, etomidate administration has been shown to result in an exacerbation of brain tissue hypoxia and acidosis in patients in whom the MCA was temporarily occluded during surgery.[201] Additional concerns regarding the occurrence of adrenocortical suppression and renal injury caused by the propylene glycol vehicle[202] will probably preclude more than episodic use.

Reactivity to CO_2 is preserved in humans during etomidate administration.[151,195] Autoregulation has not been evaluated. Myoclonus and epileptogenesis are discussed in a later section.

Narcotics

Despite inconsistencies in the available information, it is likely that narcotics have relatively little effect on CBF and CMR in the normal, unstimulated nervous system.[203] When changes occur, the general pattern is one of modest reductions in both CBF and CMR. The inconsistencies in the literature probably arise largely because in many studies, the "control" states entailed paralysis and nominal sedation, often with nitrous oxide alone. In these studies, in which substantial reductions in CBF and CMR were frequently observed, the effect of the narcotic was probably a combination of the inherent effect of the drug plus a substantial component attributable to reduction in arousal. Comparable effects related to reduction of arousal may occur and be important clinically. However, they should be viewed as nonspecific effects of sedation or pain control, or both, rather than specific properties of narcotics. The following discussion emphasizes investigations in which control measurements were unlikely to have been markedly influenced by arousal phenomena.

MORPHINE. When morphine ($\approx$1 mg/kg) was administered as the sole agent in humans, Moyer and colleagues[204] observed no effect on global CBF and a 41% decrease in $CMRO_2$. The latter is a substantial reduction, and the absence of a simultaneous CBF adjustment is surprising. No other investigations of morphine alone in humans have been conducted. Jobes and coworkers gave morphine (1 and 3 mg/kg) with 70% N_2O to patients and observed no significant change in CBF or CMR.[152] The N_2O that was used might be expected to have caused a tendency toward increases in CBF and CMR. The relative absence of net changes in these variables from the awake control measurements suggests a small to moderate depressive effect of morphine on CBF and CMR at this large dose. Takeshita and associates[205] gave morphine, 3 mg/kg, to dogs sedated with 70% N_2O ($\approx$0.6 MAC). They observed reductions in global CBF and $CMRO_2$ of approximately 60% and 17%, respectively. These data cannot be completely reconciled, and the data of Jobes and colleagues[152] (presented earlier) are probably relevant to the most common clinical situations. Recall, however, that morphine can cause substantial histamine release in individual patients. Histamine is a cerebral vasodilator that will cause an increase in CBV and a CBF effect that will vary depending on the systemic blood pressure response.

Autoregulation was observed to be intact between MAP values of 60 and 120 mm Hg in human volunteers anesthetized with morphine, 2 mg/kg, and 70% N_2O.[206]

FENTANYL. Limited human data are available. Vernhiet and colleagues[153] measured CBF and $CMRO_2$ before and during anesthesia with 12 to 30 (mean, 16) µg/kg of fentanyl plus 50% N_2O in patients about to undergo cerebral angiography. Atropine and pancuronium were the only other drugs administered. Neither CBF nor $CMRO_2$ changed significantly from awake control values in their group of six subjects. However, one of the patients (an epileptic with a normal computed tomography [CT] scan) had dramatic and unexplained increases in both CBF and $CMRO_2$. For the remaining five, CBF and $CMRO_2$ decreased by 21% and 26%, respectively ($P < .05$). The data for fentanyl/N_2O presented in Figure 21-6 are derived from these five patients who received an average of 17 µg/kg of fentanyl. Murkin and coworkers measured CBF before and after induction of anesthesia with high-dose fentanyl, 100 µg/kg, and diazepam, 0.4 mg/kg.[207] CBF fell by 25%, although part of this effect may well have been the result of the benzodiazepine (see later) rather than fentanyl. Firestone and associates, using PET, observed a heterogeneous CBF response to 1.5 µg/kg of fentanyl in healthy volunteers. Increases occurred in the frontal, temporal, and cerebellar areas simultaneous with decreases in discreet areas associated with pain-related processing.[208] Additional data have been derived from animal experiments. McPherson and Traystman[209] administered fentanyl (25 µg/kg) to pentobarbital-anesthetized dogs and observed no effect on CBF and CMR. CO_2 responsiveness and autoregulation were unaffected, and the hyperemic CBF response to hypoxia also remained intact. Several investigations in lightly anesthetized animals[210-212] have demonstrated much larger fentanyl-induced reductions in CBF or CMR (or both) than those observed in humans.

These data taken together suggest that fentanyl will cause a moderate global reduction in CBF and CMR in the normal quiescent brain and will, like morphine, cause larger reductions when administered during arousal.

ALFENTANIL—CBF EFFECTS. McPherson and colleagues[213] administered alfentanil, 320 µg/kg, to pentobarbital-anesthetized dogs. They observed no changes in CBF, CMR, CO_2 responsiveness, autoregulation, or the CBF response to hypoxia. No studies of the CMR effects of alfentanil in humans have been performed. Schregel and coworkers administered 25 to 50 µg/kg of alfentanil to patients receiving 60% N_2O after induction of anesthesia with thiopental.[214] CBFV decreased transiently. A Doppler measure of MCA diameter was simultaneously unchanged, thus suggesting that the CBFV reduction was indicative of a decrease in CBF. Mayberg and colleagues also observed no changes in CBFV in response to 25 to 50 µg/kg of alfentanil given to patients during maintenance of anesthesia with isoflurane-N_2O.[215]

SUFENTANIL—CBF EFFECTS. Although some laboratory investigations have revealed apparent sufentanil-induced increases in CBF and CMR,[216] most investigations in both animals[211,217,218] and humans indicate that sufentanil causes, depending on the dose, either no change or reductions in CBF and CMR. Stephan and associates[154] measured CBF and $CMRO_2$ in patients before and after induction of anesthesia with 10 µg/kg of sufentanil. They observed a 29% reduction in CBF and a 22% reduction in $CMRO_2$. Murkin and colleagues, in a study involving the same dose of sufentanil and a similar design, made essentially identical observations.[219] Mayer and coworkers gave 0.5 µg/kg of sufentanil to volunteers and observed no change in CBF.[220] Weinstabl and colleagues observed reductions in CBFV when 1.0 and 2.0 µg/kg of sufentanil were given to intensive care unit (ICU) patients with increased ICP.[221] Neither Weinstabl and colleagues[221] nor Mayer and coworkers,[220] who administered sufentanil to healthy volunteers, observed changes in CBF velocity after 0.5 µg/kg of sufentanil.

SUFENTANIL—ICP EFFECTS. The data from the aforementioned studies lead to the anticipation of no change or a reduction in ICP as a result of the administration of either sufentanil or alfentanil. With respect to sufentanil, the bulk of the data derived from animals[215-218,222] and humans[221,223-226] have revealed no change in ICP after its administration. However, in some investigations in humans, sufentanil was associated with modest increases in neuraxis pressure.[227-229] Subsequent investigations appear to indicate that the ICP increases associated with sufentanil are at least in large part the consequence of a normal autoregulatory response to the sudden MAP reduction that can occur as a result of sufentanil administration.[230] The "message" for the clinician should probably be that sufentanil (and for that matter, fentanyl as well[225]) are best administered in a manner that does not produce a sudden reduction in MAP. MAP reduction will clearly reduce CPP and may increase ICP, each of which, when sufficiently extreme, may be deleterious. However, it should be noted that the ICP increases attributed to sufentanil have been small. Furthermore, four investigations[231-234] that compared conditions in the surgical field, including pressure under brain retractors,[231] identified no adverse influences attributable to sufentanil. Accordingly, sufentanil need not be viewed as contraindicated in any way, although it should be used with attention to its effect on MAP.

ALFENTANIL—ICP EFFECTS. Although fewer data are available, the general pattern is similar and the conclusions should be the same as for sufentanil (preceding paragraph).[227,235-238] Alfentanil was included with fentanyl and sufentanil in two of the investigations of conditions in the surgical field mentioned in connection with sufentanil.[231,232] No adverse effects were noted.

REMIFENTANIL. Investigations of moderate doses of remifentanil in patients have revealed minimal effects that are very similar to those of the other synthetic narcotics (with the exception of its substantially shorter duration of action). In patients undergoing craniotomy for supratentorial space-occupying lesions, 1 µg/kg of remifentanil caused no change in ICP.[239] In a second investigation in craniotomy patients, approximately 0.35 µg/kg/min of remifentanil resulted in CBF values comparable to those observed with moderately deep anesthesia with either isoflurane/N_2O or fentanyl/N_2O,[240] and CO_2 responsiveness was preserved. Greater doses of remifentanil may have more substantial effects. CBFV in the MCA decreased 30% in response to 5 μg/kg followed by 3 μg/kg/min of remifentanil at constant MAP in patients being anesthetized for bypass surgery.[241] A lower dose of 2 μg/kg followed by an infusion of 3 μg/kg/min, however, did not affect CBFV. Quantitatively similar observations were made after a large dose of sufentanil in patients undergoing cardiac anesthesia (see earlier).[154]

It should be noted that in the aforementioned studies, remifentanil was administered with other drugs that might influence cerebral hemodynamics. More recent studies in human volunteers have demonstrated that the infusion of low (sedative) doses of remifentanil can increase CBF. A PET study in human subjects to whom remifentanil, 0.05 and 0.15 μg/kg/min, was administered revealed increases in CBF in the prefrontal, inferior parietal, and supplementary motor cortices; reductions in CBF were observed in the cerebellum, superior temporal lobe, and midbrain gray matter.[242] The relative increase in CBF was greater with administration of the higher dose of remifentanil. Similar data were obtained by Lorenz and colleagues, who used magnetic resonance imaging for the determination of CBF.[243,244] The underlying mechanisms for the increases in CBF are not clear. However, the disinhibition produced by low-dose remifentanil infusion may have contributed. In aggregate, the available human data indicate that in low sedative doses, the administration of remifentanil alone can effect minor increases in CBF. With higher doses or with the concomitant administration of anesthetic adjuvants, CBF is either unaltered or modestly reduced.

Benzodiazepines

Benzodiazepines cause parallel reductions in CBF and CMR in humans and monkeys. CBF and $CMRO_2$ decreased by 25% when 15 mg of diazepam was given to head-injured patients.[155] Lorazepam administered to monkeys in doses sufficient to cause sedation reduced CBF by 24% and $CMRO_2$ by 21%.[245] The effects of midazolam on CBF (but not CMR) have also been studied in humans. Forster and associates observed a 30% to 34% reduction in CBF[156,246] after the administration of 0.15 mg/kg of midazolam to awake healthy human volunteers. Veselis and colleagues, using PET, observed a global reduction in CBF of 12% after a similar dose and noted that the decreases occurred preferentially in the brain regions associated with arousal, attention, and memory.[247] CO_2 responsiveness was preserved.[248]

The foregoing studies indicate that benzodiazepines should cause a moderate reduction in CBF in humans and suggest that the effect may be metabolically coupled. The extent of the maximal CBF/CMR reduction produced by benzodiazepines is probably intermediate between the decreases caused by narcotics (modest) and barbiturates (substantial).[21,249,250] It appears that benzodiazepines should be safe to administer to patients with intracranial hypertension, provided that respiratory depression and an associated increase in $Paco_2$ do not occur.

Flumazenil

Flumazenil is a highly specific, competitive benzodiazepine receptor antagonist. It had no effect on CBF when administered to unanesthetized human volunteers.[246,251] In two investigations in dogs with normal intracranial compliance,[249,252] flumazenil resulted in reversal of the CBF-, CMR-, and ICP-lowering effects of midazolam. Although Knudsen and coworkers[253] observed no change in either CBF or CMR when patients were aroused from midazolam anesthesia with flumazenil at the conclusion of craniotomy for resection of brain tumor, Chiolero and coauthors[254] reported severe increases in ICP when flumazenil was given to midazolam-sedated head-injured patients in whom ICP was poorly controlled before the administration of flumazenil. These latter observations are consistent with two animal investigations. In the investigation of Fleischer and coworkers mentioned earlier,[249] flumazenil not only reversed the CBF and CMR effects of midazolam but also caused a substantial, though short-lived, overshoot above premidazolam levels in both CBF (by 44% to 56%) and ICP (by 180% to 217%). CMR did not rise above control levels, thus indicating that the CBF increase was not metabolically coupled. A similar increase in CBF after flumazenil reversal of midazolam has also been observed in cats.[255] The CBF overshoot effect is unexplained but may be a neurogenically mediated arousal phenomenon.[256] Flumazenil should probably be avoided or used very cautiously to reverse benzodiazepine sedation in patients with impaired intracranial compliance.

Droperidol

No human investigations on the CBF/CMR effects of droperidol in isolation have been conducted. However, the information available from animal investigations and administration of drug combinations in humans[212,257-260] taken together suggests that droperidol is not a cerebral vasodilator and probably has little effect on CBF and CMR in humans. The occasional ICP increases that have been observed[258] probably reflect normal autoregulation-mediated vasodilation in response to an abrupt fall in MAP.

Ketamine

Among the intravenous anesthetics, ketamine is unique in its ability to cause increases in both CBF and CMR.[157,261-264] Animal studies indicate that the changes in CMR are regionally variable. In rats, substantial increases occur in limbic system structures simultaneous with modest changes or small decreases in cortical structures.[262,265] PET studies in humans have demonstrated that subanesthetic doses of ketamine (0.2 to 0.3 mg/kg) can increase global CMR by about 25%.[266] The greatest increase in CMR occurred in the frontal and anterior cingulate cortex. A relative reduction in CMR in the cerebellum was also observed. Commercially available formulations of ketamine contain both the (S)- and (R)-ketamine enantiomers. (S)-ketamine increases CMR substantially, whereas the (R)-ketamine enantiomer tends to decrease CMR, particularly in the temperomedial cortex and the cerebellum.[267] These changes in CMR are accompanied by corresponding changes in CBF.[268] Because autoregulation is maintained during ketamine anesthesia,[269] the observed effects of ketamine on cerebral hemodynamics indicate that ketamine increases CMR and secondarily increases CBF. CO_2 responsiveness is preserved.[270]

The anticipated ICP correlate of the increase in CBF has been confirmed to occur in humans.[270,271] However, anesthetics (diazepam, midazolam, isoflurane/N_2O, propofol) have been shown to blunt or eliminate the ICP or CBF increases associated with ketamine.[254,271-274] In fact, decreases in ICP have been reported in response to relatively large doses of ketamine (1.5 to 5 mg/kg) administered to propofol-sedated head-injured patients.[275] Accordingly, although ketamine is probably best avoided as the sole anesthetic in patients with impaired intracranial compliance, it may be reasonable to use it cautiously in patients who are simultaneously receiving the other drugs mentioned earlier.

Lidocaine

Lidocaine produces a dose-related reduction in $CMRO_2$ in experimental animals.[276] In dogs, 3 mg/kg lowered $CMRO_2$ by 10%, and 15 mg/kg reduced it by 27%. When very large doses (160 mg/kg) were given to dogs on cardiopulmonary bypass, the reduction in $CMRO_2$ was apparently greater than that seen with high-dose barbiturates.[166] This greater reduction in $CMRO_2$ with lidocaine may occur because the membrane-stabilizing effect of lidocaine also reduces the energy requirement for maintenance of membrane integrity. In unanesthetized human volunteers, Lam and coworkers observed CBF and CMR reductions of 24% and 20%, respectively, after the administration of 5 mg/kg of lidocaine over a 30-minute period followed by an infusion of 45 µg/kg/min.[277]

Bedford and colleagues[278] compared the effectiveness of bolus doses of thiopental (Pentothal), 3 mg/kg, and lidocaine, 1.5 mg/kg, in controlling the acute increase in ICP that occurred after the application of a pinhead holder or skin incision in craniotomy patients. The two regimens were equally effective in causing a reduction in ICP. However, the decrease in MAP was greater with thiopental. Accordingly, a bolus dose of lidocaine is a reasonable adjunct to the prevention or treatment of acute ICP elevation and has been recommended for use in the prevention of increases in ICP associated with endotracheal suctioning.[279] Note that large doses of lidocaine can produce seizures in humans and some experimental animals[280]; however, lidocaine-induced seizures have not been reported in anesthetized humans. Nonetheless, it seems appropriate to restrict lidocaine doses to amounts that achieve serum levels less than the seizure threshold (>5 to 10 µg/mL) in awake humans.[281] Viegas and Stoelting[282] reported peak serum concentrations of 6.6 to 8.5 µg/mL after a 2-mg/kg bolus of lidocaine. Bolus doses of 1.5 to 2.0 mg/kg therefore seem appropriate.

Inhaled Anesthetics

Volatile Anesthetics

The pattern of effects of volatile anesthetics on cerebral physiology is a striking departure from that observed with the intravenous agents, which generally cause parallel reductions in CMR and CBF. All volatile anesthetics, similar to intravenous sedative-hypnotic drugs, suppress cerebral metabolism in a dose-related manner.[22,283-287] Volatile anesthetics also possess intrinsic cerebral vasodilatory activity because of direct effects on vascular smooth muscle. The net effect of volatile anesthetics on CBF is therefore a balance between a reduction in CBF caused by CMR suppression and augmentation of CBF as a result of direct cerebral vasodilation. When administered in a dose of 0.5 MAC, the CMR suppression–induced reduction in CBF predominates, and net CBF decreases in comparison to the awake state. At 1.0 MAC, CBF remains unchanged; at this dose, CMR suppression and vasodilatory effects are in balance. Beyond 1.0 MAC, the vasodilatory activity predominates, and CBF increases significantly even though CMR is substantially reduced.

The increase in CBF produced by volatile anesthetics at doses greater than 1.0 MAC has been interpreted as evidence of uncoupling of flow and metabolism. However, considerable evidence indicates that coupling (CBF adjustments paralleling changes in CMR) persists during anesthesia with volatile anesthetics.[28,284,288-292] Accordingly, it is probably more accurate to say that the CBF/CMR ratio is altered (increased) by volatile anesthetics. This alteration is dose related, and under steady-state conditions, there is a positive correlation between MAC multiples and the $CBF/CMRO_2$ ratio[38,285,293,294]; that is, higher MAC levels cause greater "luxury" perfusion.

The important clinical consequences of administration of volatile anesthetics are derived from the increases that can occur in CBF and CBV and, consequently, ICP. Of the commonly used volatile anesthetics, the order of vasodilating potency is approximately halothane >> enflurane > desflurane ≈ isoflurane > sevoflurane.[29,287,291,295-298]

CBF EFFECTS. Volatile anesthetics possess intrinsic vasodilatory activity, and they not only modify cerebral autoregulation but also produce dose-dependent reductions in systemic blood pressure. Hence, their effects on CBF and CMR are best evaluated when arterial pressure is supported to a common level. In addition, the cerebrovascular effects of volatile anesthetics are modulated by the simultaneous administration of other central nervous system (CNS)-active drugs. It is therefore important to understand the control state (awake, sedated, or anesthetized) against which the CBF and CMR effects of volatile anesthetics are compared. The best information about the cerebrovascular effects of volatile anesthetics is obtained from studies in which a nonanesthetized awake control state is used.

Data on the cerebrovascular effects of halothane and enflurane are limited. Initial studies in humans demonstrated that administration of 1 MAC halothane significantly increased CBF in comparison to preanesthetic CBF values, even when systemic blood pressure was substantially reduced.[299] The same investigators subsequently showed that in humans, when MAP is maintained at 80 mm Hg, 1.1 MAC levels of halothane increased CBF by as much as 191% and decreased CMR by about 10%[295,299] (Fig. 21-7). When compared with awake values, 1.2 MAC enflurane also increased CBF and decreased CMR by 45% and 15%, respectively.[303] The dramatic increases in CBF with a simultaneous modest reduction in CMR attest to the cerebral vasodilatory properties of halothane and enflurane. Isoflurane, by contrast, does not increase CBF

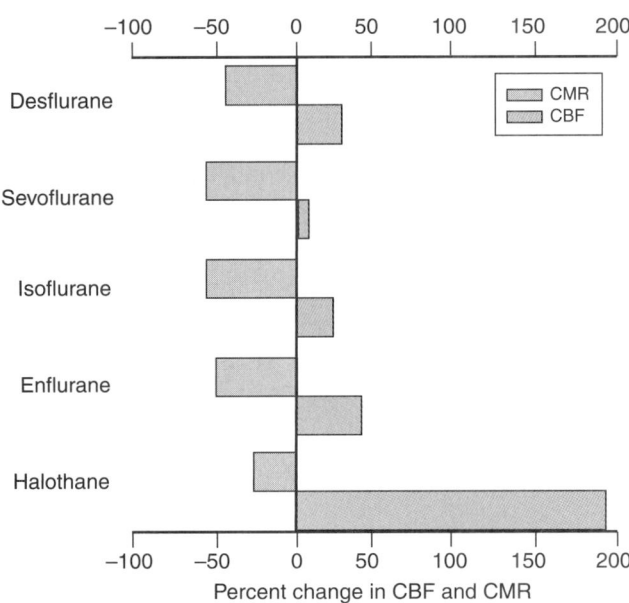

Figure 21–7 Estimated changes in cerebral blood flow (CBF) and the cerebral metabolic rate of oxygen (CMRO$_2$) caused by volatile anesthetics. The CBF data for halothane, enflurane, and isoflurane were obtained during 1.1 minimum alveolar concentration (MAC) anesthesia (with blood pressure support) in humans[295] and are expressed as the percent change from awake control values. The CMRO$_2$ data for halothane, enflurane, and isoflurane were obtained from cats[285,300] and are expressed as the percent change from N$_2$O-sedated control values. Data for sevoflurane were obtained during 1.1 MAC anesthesia in rabbits and are expressed as the percent change from a morphine/ N$_2$O-anesthetized control state.[287] CBF values were obtained in patients who received 1 MAC sevoflurane anesthesia.[301] Desflurane data were obtained in patients to whom 1 MAC desflurane was administered.[302]

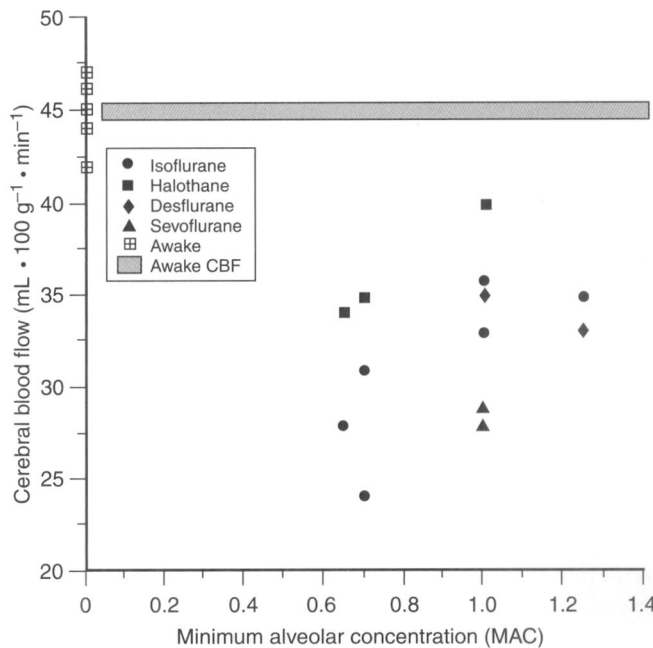

A

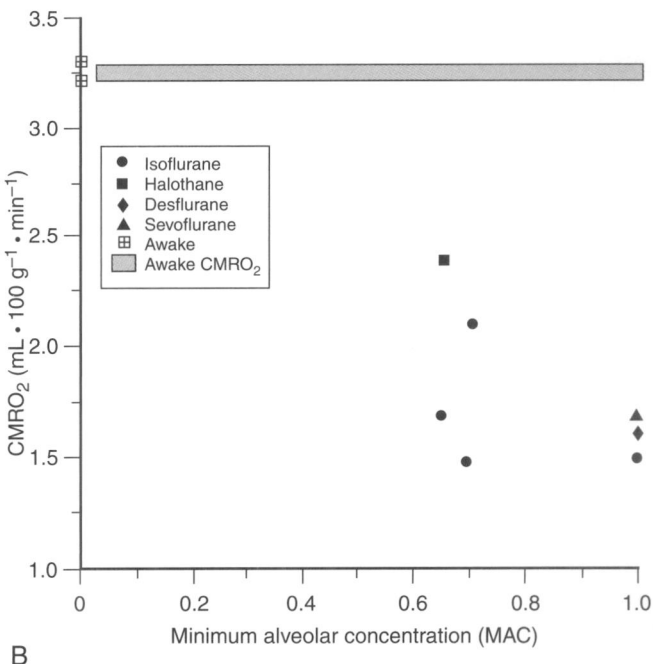

B

Figure 21–8 Effect of volatile anesthetics on cerebral blood flow (CBF) (**A**) and the cerebral metabolic rate of oxygen (CMRO$_2$) (**B**) in humans. The results are a composite of CBF and CMR values obtained from a number of separate investigations.[175,297,301,302,304-315] In these studies, Pa$_{CO_2}$ was maintained in the normocapnic range ($\approx$35 to 40 mm Hg) and mean arterial pressure was supported. In most of the investigations, CBF was measured by the inert gas technique. This technique measures primarily cortical CBF and, as such, might underestimate global CBF.

as much as halothane or enflurane does. Human studies have shown that in 1.1 MAC doses, isoflurane increases CBF by about 19% when systemic pressure is maintained within the normal range. CMR is reduced by about 45%.[292]

More recent investigations have shown that both sevoflurane and desflurane can significantly reduce CBF in humans in comparison to CBF values in awake nonanesthetized patients. In 1.0 MAC concentrations, sevoflurane[301] and desflurane[302] decreased CBF by 38% and 22% and CMR by 39% and 35%, respectively. These results, which suggest that the cerebral vasodilation produced by isoflurane is greater than that produced by sevoflurane and desflurane, were obtained with CBF measured by the inert gas technique. This technique measures CBF primarily within the cortex and may therefore have substantially underestimated global CBF. In addition, other investigations in humans, most using transcranial Doppler measurement of MCA flow velocity, indicate that the differences in the effects of isoflurane, desflurane (Fig. 21-8), and sevoflurane are, at best, modest.[291,298,316] It should be noted that a strictly quantitative comparison between these volatile anesthetics is not possible given the variations in blood pressure among study group patients. In addition, there is some discrepancy among studies in the literature regarding the magnitude of the effects of volatile anesthetics on CBF.

Much of this inconsistency may occur because of the interaction of regionally selective CBF methods with the heterogeneity within the cerebrum of the CBF effects of volatile anesthetics. See the later section "Distribution of CBF/CMR Changes."

CMR EFFECTS. All the volatile anesthetics cause reductions in CMR. The degree of $CMRO_2$ reduction that occurs at a given MAC level is less with halothane than with the other four agents (see Fig. 21-7). Sevoflurane's effect on $CMRO_2$ is very similar to that of isoflurane (see Fig. 21-7).[287] The available information, derived from separate investigations, suggests that desflurane causes slightly less suppression of $CMRO_2$ than isoflurane does, especially at concentrations above 1.0 MAC.[22,286] Although a direct comparison of the $CMRO_2$ effects of all the volatile anesthetics has not been performed in humans, collation of data from a number of investigations has shown that in 1.0 MAC doses, isoflurane, sevoflurane, and desflurane reduce $CMRO_2$ (AVDO$_2$ difference in arterial and jugular bulb blood samples) by 25%,[304] 38%,[301] and 22%,[317] respectively. PET studies in humans have also shown that halothane (0.9 MAC) and isoflurane (0.5 MAC) can decrease the cerebral metabolic rate of glucose (CMRg) by 40% and 46%, respectively.[175,318] The $CMRO_2$ reduction is dose related. With isoflurane (and almost certainly desflurane and sevoflurane as well), maximal reduction is attained simultaneously with the occurrence of EEG suppression.[22,286] This reduction occurs at clinically relevant concentrations (i.e., 1.5 to 2.0 MAC) in humans.[291,319] In dogs, administration of additional isoflurane up to 6.0% end-tidal volume results in no further reduction in CMR and no indication of metabolic toxicity.[22] Halothane presents a contrast to this pattern. Halothane concentrations in excess of 4.0 MAC are required to achieve EEG isoelectricity in dogs, and additional halothane causes a further reduction in $CMRO_2$ in concert with alterations in energy charge. The latter changes, which are reversible, suggest interference with oxidative phosphorylation.[283] These data indicate that unlike isoflurane, halothane can produce reversible toxicity when administered in very high concentrations.

The CBF and CMR dose-response relationships are somewhat alinear for volatile anesthetics. The initial appearance of an EEG pattern associated with the onset of anesthesia with halothane, enflurane, and isoflurane is accompanied by a precipitous decline in $CMRO_2$.[164] Thereafter, $CMRO_2$ declines in a slower dose-dependent manner. Other studies during anesthetic induction with halothane have observed marked increases in CBF before any alteration in CMR.[165] This finding suggests that the direct effect of a volatile anesthetic on smooth muscle may develop more rapidly than influences related to depression of CMR.

DISTRIBUTION OF CBF/CMR CHANGES. The regional distribution of anesthetic-induced changes in CBF and CMR differ markedly with halothane and isoflurane. Halothane produces relatively homogeneous changes throughout the brain. CBF is globally increased and CMR is globally depressed. The changes caused by isoflurane are more heterogeneous. CBF increases are greater in the subcortical areas and hindbrain structures than in the neocortex.[28,29,320] For CMR the converse is true, with a greater

reduction in the neocortex than the subcortex.[27] In humans, 1.0 MAC sevoflurane (Fig. 21-9) results in a reduction in CBF within the cortex and an increase in CBF within the cerebellum.[305] These effects of sevoflurane are similar to those produced by isoflurane.[29,305] Desflurane has not been submitted to similar local CBF studies. However, given the similarity of its effects on the

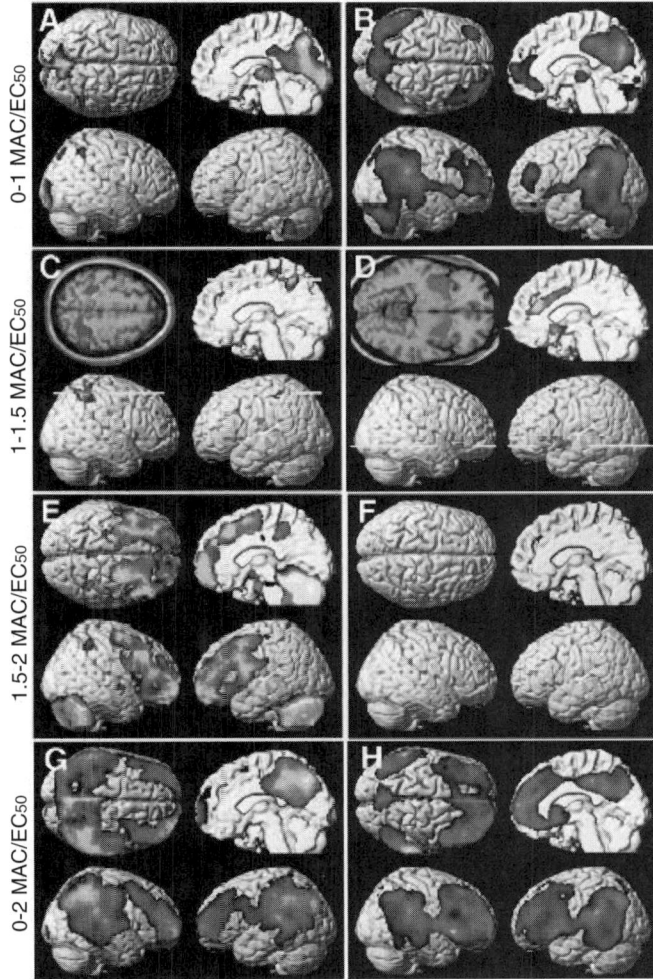

Figure 21–9 Dose-dependent redistribution of cerebral blood flow (CBF) in humans. Positron emission tomography (PET) scans demonstrate a dose-dependent reduction in CBF in both sevoflurane-anesthetized *(left)* and propofol-anesthetized subjects *(right)*. During sevoflurane anesthesia, an increase in concentration from 1.5 to 2.0 minimum alveolar concentration (MAC) leads to an increase in CBF within the subcortex, particularly in the cerebellum. A gradual reduction in mean arterial pressure (MAP) was observed with increasing concentrations of sevoflurane, and MAP was not supported. The CBF values would be expected to be considerably greater had blood pressure been maintained within the normal range. Therefore, the CBF values represented in the figure probably underestimate true CBF during sevoflurane anesthesia. In propofol-anesthetized subjects, CBF was uniformly decreased and redistribution of CBF was not observed. (Data from Kaisti K, Metsahonkala L, Teras M, et al: Effects of surgical levels of propofol and sevoflurane anesthesia on cerebral blood flow in healthy subjects studied with positron emission tomography. Anesthesiology 96:1358-1370, 2002.)

EEG (suggesting similar cortical CMR and CBF effects), the interim assumption of similar heterogeneity in CBF distribution seems reasonable. These distribution differences may explain certain apparent contradictions in reported CBF effects in the existing literature for isoflurane. Methods that can assess the entire cerebrum and measure true global CBF (microspheres, PET, autoradiography) will reveal greater increases in CBF than those that emphasize the cortical compartment (radioactive xenon techniques, transcranial Doppler, venous outflow). For instance, Eintrei and coauthors reported no increase in CBF when isoflurane was administered to patients undergoing craniotomy,[296] yet Adams,[321] Grosslight,[322] and Campkin[323] and their colleagues reported that administration of isoflurane to normocapnic subjects with intracranial pathology can result in increases in CSF pressure. The CBF methodology used by Eintrei and coworkers[296] measured cortical flow exclusively, and accordingly, the results of the three investigations are again consistent with a pattern of minimal vasodilation in the cortex and greater increases in CBF in the remainder of the brain.

CEREBRAL VASODILATION BY VOLATILE ANESTHETICS—CLINICAL IMPLICATIONS. The data presented thus far, in sum, indicate that isoflurane, desflurane, and sevoflurane may have a modest cerebral vasodilating effect in the human cortex when administered in doses of 1 MAC or less. In fact, as shown in Figure 21-8, administration of volatile anesthetics can effect net decreases in CBF. These data, however, should be interpreted with considerable caution because the critical variable that is of interest in the clinical sphere is CBV. Although there is a direct correlation between CBF and CBV, as noted earlier, the relationship is not strictly 1:1. The magnitude of the changes in CBV is significantly less than changes in CBF, and a modest reduction in CBF may not necessarily be accompanied by a reduction in CBV. This relationship is exemplified by clinical investigations in which a significant increase in ICP (and by extension, CBV) was observed in patients to whom isoflurane was administered in doses that would be expected to effect a reduction in CBF.[321,323] Although the induction of hypocapnia mitigated the increase in ICP in these studies, other investigations have revealed that hyperventilation may not be effective in blunting isoflurane-induced increases in ICP in patients with intracranial tumors.[322] In experimental investigations of cerebral injury, volatile anesthetics increased ICP significantly, and this rise in ICP was not ameliorated by hypocapnia.[324] Collectively, these data suggest that volatile anesthetics will have minimal effects on cerebral hemodynamics in patients with normal intracranial compliance. However, in patients with abnormal intracranial compliance, the potential for volatile anesthetic–induced increases in CBV and ICP exists. Accordingly, one should use discretion when administering volatile anesthetics in the setting of large mass lesions, unstable ICP, or sufficient derangement of cerebral physiology that CO_2 responsiveness and flow-metabolism coupling may be impaired in some or all of the brain. When they occur (a somnolent, vomiting patient with papilledema, a large mass, and compressed basal cisterns), the clinician may be well advised to use a predominantly

intravenous technique until such time as the cranium and dura are open and the effect of the anesthetic technique can be directly assessed. These events will be relatively rare in elective neurosurgery.

Situations in which there has been substantial antecedent lowering of CMR by drug administration or disease processes should also justify caution in the use of volatile anesthetics. If a volatile anesthetic has a substantial direct vasodilating effect on the cerebral vasculature that is normally offset by an opposing metabolically mediated vasoconstricting influence, it might be surmised that when a near-maximal reduction in CMR has occurred, introduction of the volatile anesthetic will have a predominantly vasodilating effect.[180,289] There are data to support this prediction. Murphy and coworkers[295] observed no increase in CBF (versus awake control measurements) during anesthesia with 0.6 and 1.1 MAC isoflurane (with blood pressure support), but at 1.6 MAC, CBF had increased by 100%. Maekawa and colleagues[27] measured CBF and local CMRg in rats both awake and during anesthesia with increasing concentrations of isoflurane. Isoflurane at 1 MAC resulted in an average CMRg decrease of 54% of the awake control value in five cortical areas and no change in average CBF. An additional 1.0 MAC (i.e., a total of 2.0 MAC) caused a further CMRg reduction of only 20% of the control value, and CBF simultaneously increased by 70% (Fig. 21-10). These data together suggest that isoflurane is a significant cerebral vasodilator when administered in concentrations at

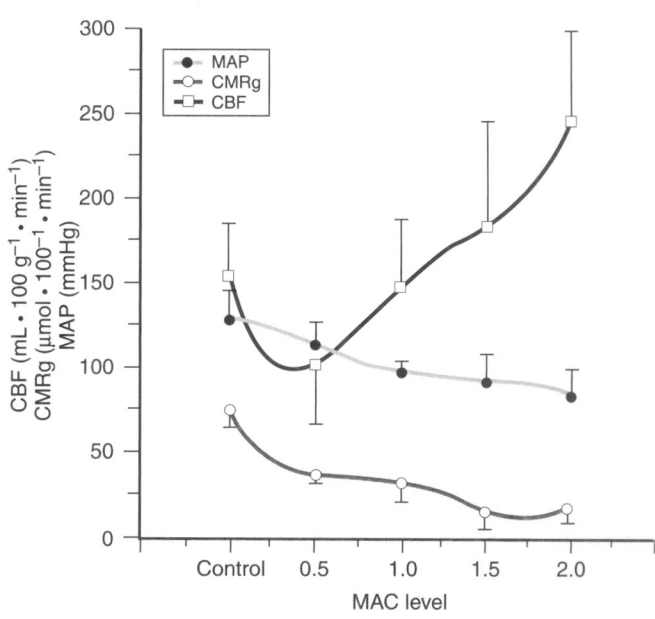

Figure 21–10 Relationship between changes in the cerebral metabolic rate for glucose (CMRg) and cerebral blood flow (CBF) in the motor-sensory cortex in rats during isoflurane anesthesia. Most of the CMR suppression caused by isoflurane had occurred by 1.0 minimum alveolar concentration (MAC), and in this concentration range CBF is not increased. Thereafter, additional isoflurane causes little further reduction in CMR, and cerebral vasodilation occurs. These data (±SD), from Maekawa and colleagues,[27] suggest the importance of metabolic coupling in determining the CBF effects of isoflurane.

and above those associated with near-maximal CMR suppression or, perhaps, when administered in situations where the component of CMR that is associated with electrophysiologic function is already suppressed by other drugs[180,289] or pathologic processes.

The net vasodilating effect of equi-MAC concentrations of isoflurane, desflurane, and sevoflurane is less in humans than that of halothane, and the former are probably therefore preferable if a volatile anesthetic is to be used in the setting of impaired intracranial compliance. That is not to say that halothane is contraindicated in these circumstances. It has clearly been demonstrated that when hypocapnia is established before the introduction of halothane, the increases in ICP that might otherwise occur in a normocapnic patient with poor intracranial compliance can be prevented or greatly attenuated.[325] Nonetheless, most clinicians will prefer isoflurane, desflurane, or sevoflurane because the margin for error is probably wider than with halothane.

TIME DEPENDENCE OF CBF EFFECTS. The effect of volatile anesthetics on CBF has been shown to be time dependent in animal investigations. After an initial increase, CBF falls substantially, with a steady state near pre–volatile anesthetic levels reached between 2½ and 5 hours after exposure.[46,320,326] The mechanism of this effect is not understood, and the phenomenon was not evident in humans studied during 3- or 6-hour exposure to halothane, isoflurane, desflurane, or sevoflurane.[291,327]

CEREBRAL BLOOD VOLUME. The extensive investigation of the influence of volatile anesthetics on CBF has been based primarily on the concern that cerebral vasodilation, produced by volatile anesthetics, might increase ICP. It should be noted, however, that it is CBV and not CBF per se that influences ICP. The vast majority of intracranial blood is within the cerebral venous circulation, and although there is a reasonable correlation between vasodilation-induced increases in CBF and CBV, the magnitude of CBF changes is considerably greater than the changes in CBV (Fig. 21-11). Hence, changes in CBF do not reliably predict changes in CBV and, by extension, in ICP. Nonetheless, the available data do indicate that CBV is considerably greater during isoflurane anesthesia than during propofol or pentobarbital anesthesia.[136] In addition, CBV responds to changes in Pa_{CO_2} by a reduction in CBV with hypocapnia and an increase in CBV with hypercapnia.[328] The magnitude of the change in CBV is, however, less than the change in CBF.

CO₂ RESPONSIVENESS AND AUTOREGULATION. CO_2 responsiveness is well maintained during anesthesia with all of the volatile anesthetics.[38,297,329-331] By contrast, autoregulation of CBF in response to rising arterial pressure is impaired. This impairment appears to be most apparent with anesthetics that cause the greatest cerebral vasodilation[285,295] and is dose related (see Fig. 21-5).[332,333] Sevoflurane may cause less impairment in autoregulation than other volatile anesthetics do. Recent studies surprisingly reported no change in CBFV in response to phenylephrine-induced MAP increases during anesthesia with 1.2 to 1.5 MAC sevoflurane[331,334,335] or in CBF during hemorrhagic hypotension.[336] The autoregulatory response to rising pressure is, however, rarely of significance in clinical neuroanesthesia. If anything, it is the

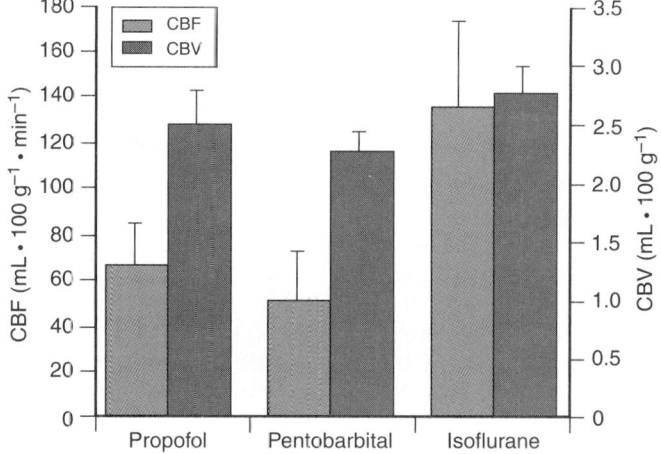

Figure 21–11 Effect of anesthetics on cerebral blood flow (CBF) and cerebral blood volume (CBV). When compared with isoflurane, propofol and pentobarbital effected substantial reductions in CBF. However, CBV reductions were more modest.[136] These data indicate that the magnitude of the effect of anesthetic agents on CBF is substantially greater than the effect on CBV. Hence, a reduction in CBF may not lead to equivalent reductions in CBV.

CBF response to falling pressure that is important, and as with all vasodilators, CBF is preserved to lower MAP during administration of volatile anesthetics with no evidence of differences among the various agents. Direct comparisons of CBF with isoflurane, desflurane, and sevoflurane during hypotension are not available.

EPILEPTOGENESIS. Enflurane is potentially epileptogenic in the clinical setting. Of particular relevance to neuroanesthesia is the observation that hypocapnia potentiates seizure-type discharges during enflurane anesthesia.[337] A 50% decrease in $CMRO_2$ was noted in human volunteers anesthetized with 3% enflurane, but with the onset of seizure activity, $CMRO_2$ returned to normal,[338] thus indicating preservation of flow-metabolism coupling. Note that there is no evidence that this type of EEG activity is deleterious when oxygen delivery is maintained during the event. However, because seizure activity can elevate brain metabolism by as much as 400%, the use of enflurane, especially in high doses and with hypocapnia, should probably be avoided in patients who are predisposed to seizures or have occlusive cerebrovascular disease.

The EEG-activating property of enflurane has been used intraoperatively to activate and identify seizure foci that are to be surgically resected, and in this situation, spike activity not present preoperatively has been observed to persist after surgery.[339] In addition, two reports have described seizures in the immediate postoperative period after enflurane anesthesia in both predisposed[340] and nonpredisposed individuals.[341] No apparent permanent sequelae have resulted from these events, and in fact, this association is not a rigorously proven one. At worst, such occurrences are extremely uncommon.

Isoflurane can cause EEG spiking and myoclonus, but in the experimental setting it has not been associated with the frank epileptoid activity induced by enflurane.

The clinical experience with isoflurane is very large, and unexplained "seizure-like activity" has been reported in only two patients. One incident occurred intraoperatively[342] and the other immediately postoperatively.[343] It therefore appears that epileptogenesis is not a clinical concern with isoflurane. In fact, isoflurane has been successfully used to control EEG seizure activity in refractory status epilepticus.[344]

Seizures have been reported to occur during induction of anesthesia with high concentrations of sevoflurane in children, including those without a recognized seizure diathesis.[345,346] In two healthy human subjects, EEG burst suppression with 2 MAC sevoflurane was accompanied by epileptiform discharges that were observed during EEG monitoring.[347] These discharges were associated with a significant increase in CBF, thus demonstrating that flow and metabolism coupling was preserved. In patients with temporal lobe epilepsy, the administration of 1.5 MAC sevoflurane elicited widespread paroxysmal interictal EEG activity. Of note was the observation that paroxysmal activity was not restricted to the ictal focus and that the administration of sevoflurane was not of any assistance in localization of the epileptogenic region of the brain.[348] The development of tonic-clonic movements indicative of seizure activity has also been reported in otherwise healthy patients on emergence from sevoflurane anesthesia.[349,350] In all of the reported cases of seizure activity associated with sevoflurane anesthesia, untoward sequelae have not been documented. These reports highlight sevoflurane's ability, albeit small, to evoke epileptiform activity, and accordingly, the use of sevoflurane in patients with epilepsy should be undertaken with appropriate caution.

Nitrous Oxide

The available data unequivocally indicate that N_2O can cause increases in CBF, CMR, and ICP. At least a portion of the CBF and CMR increases may be the result of a sympathoadrenal stimulating effect of N_2O.[351] The magnitude of the effect varies considerably depending on the presence or absence of other anesthetics (Fig. 21-12). When N_2O is administered alone, very substantial increases in CBF and ICP can occur. In sharp contrast, when N_2O is administered in combination with intravenous drugs, including barbiturates, benzodiazepines, narcotics, and propofol, its cerebral vasodilating effect is attenuated or even completely inhibited. The addition of N_2O to anesthesia induced with a volatile anesthetic will result in moderate CBF increases.

N_2O ADMINISTERED ALONE. The most dramatic reported increases in ICP or CBF in humans[354,355] and experimental animals[351,356,357] have occurred when N_2O was administered alone or with minimal background anesthesia. For instance, Henriksen and Jorgensen[354] recorded ICP before and during spontaneous breathing of 66% N_2O by patients with intracranial tumors. Mean ICP rose from 13 to 40 mm Hg. The CBF increases observed in humans are more modest than those observed in animals, but they are still substantial.[352] Whether these substantial increases represent the effects of N_2O per se or whether they reflect the nonspecific effects of "second-stage" arousal phenomena is not known.

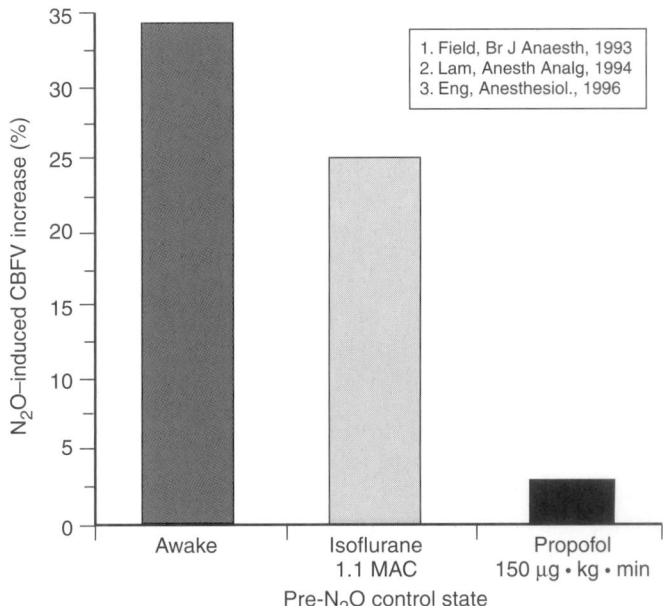

Figure 21–12 Mean percent increases in cerebral blood flow volume (CBFV) in the middle cerebral artery of normocapnic subjects exposed to 60% N_2O after control recording in three conditions: awake,[352] 1.1 minimum alveolar concentration (MAC) isoflurane,[290] and propofol, 150 μg/kg/min.[353]

N_2O ADMINISTERED WITH INTRAVENOUS ANESTHETICS. When N_2O is administered in conjunction with certain intravenous anesthetics, its CBF effect may be considerably reduced. Phirman and Shapiro[358] observed that a reproducible increase in ICP that had occurred in response to administration of 70% N_2O to a comatose patient was prevented by previous administration of a combination of pentothal and diazepam in spite of no change in baseline ICP. In an investigation of patients with intracranial tumors and poor intracranial compliance (mean preinduction ICP, 27 mm Hg),[359] 50% N_2O introduced during barbiturate anesthesia and after the induction of hypocapnia had a negligible effect on ICP. Jung and colleagues compared lumbar CSF pressure in patients with brain tumors during the administration of 0.7% isoflurane or 70% N_2O after induction of anesthesia with a barbiturate. Lumbar CSF pressure was modestly, but significantly greater with N_2O.[360] That the increase was less dramatic than those cited earlier for N_2O alone may reflect the presence of residual barbiturate. Benzodiazepines administered alone blunt the CBF response to N_2O in both animals and humans.[361,362] Narcotics appear to have a similar effect. Jobes and coauthors[152] reported that anesthesia with 1 mg/kg of morphine plus 70% N_2O resulted in no change in CBF from awake control values. Because of the very minor effect of morphine on CBF, these data suggest that N_2O did not cause substantial cerebral vasodilation. In a study using transcranial Doppler, Eng and associates observed no change in CBF velocity when N_2O was introduced in patients anesthetized with propofol.[353]

N_2O ADMINISTERED WITH VOLATILE ANESTHETICS. In most investigations, including several in humans, in which N_2O has been added to an anesthetic of 1.0 MAC or greater, substantial CBF increases have been recorded.[290,293,363-369] Algotsson and coworkers[370] examined the effect of an approximately equi-MAC substitution of N_2O for isoflurane. They compared CBF in patients anesthetized with 1.5 MAC isoflurane and 0.75 MAC isoflurane plus 65% N_2O. They observed 43% greater CBF with the latter, again consistent with a substantial vasodilating effect by N_2O in the presence of a volatile anesthetic. Similar observations were made by Lam and colleagues and Strebel and associates.[290,369] Several investigations confirm that CBF will be less with 1.0 MAC of isoflurane than with a 1.0 MAC combination achieved with 50% to 65% N_2O and isoflurane.[290,306,370]

The results of three investigations, including one in humans, indicate that this vasodilating effect of N_2O may be positively correlated with the concentration of inhaled anesthetic[365,366,369] and suggest that in general, the CBF increase caused by N_2O is exaggerated at higher concentrations of both halothane and isoflurane.

N_2O Effects on CMR. No uniform agreement regarding the effect of N_2O on CMR has not reached. Parallel changes in CBF and CMR,[351,356] CBF increases without an alteration in CMR,[368,371,372] and CMR alteration occurring without changes in CBF[373] have all been reported. This variability is doubtless the product of differences in species, methods, depth of background anesthesia, and interactions with simultaneously administered drugs. Few data derived from humans are available. Wollman and coauthors[373] reported that 70% N_2O caused a 15% reduction in $CMRO_2$ in human volunteers. However, both premedication and induction of anesthesia were accomplished with barbiturates, and the control group was nonconcurrent. Algotsson and coworkers[370] reported no difference in $CMRO_2$. From animal experimentation it appears likely that at least in some circumstances, N_2O causes increases in CMR. The "cleanest" investigation is that of Pelligrino and colleagues,[356] who measured cortical CBF and CMR in awake goats that received N_2O without premedication or other supplements. After 60 minutes of N_2O inhalation, cortical $CMRO_2$ was increased to 170% and global CBF to 143% of control values. The goats showed no evidence of an excitement stage. They became lethargic and experienced a fall in plasma epinephrine levels suggesting the absence of stress.

The CBF response to CO_2 is preserved during administration of N_2O.[366,368,373]

Clinical Implications. In spite of the inconsistencies that are evident, data indicate that the vasodilatory action of N_2O can be clinically significant in neurosurgical patients with reduced intracranial compliance.[354] However, it appears that N_2O-induced cerebral vasodilation can be considerably blunted by the simultaneous administration of intravenous anesthetics, although not all anesthetics have been evaluated and the dose-response relationships are not well defined. N_2O has been widely used in neurosurgery, and banishing it is inconsistent with the accumulated experience. Nonetheless, in circumstances wherein ICP is persistently elevated or the surgical field is persistently "tight," N_2O should be viewed as a potential contributing factor. In addition, the ability of N_2O to rapidly enter a closed gas space should be recalled, and it should be avoided or omitted when a closed intracranial gas space may exist.

Muscle Relaxants (see Chapter 13)

Nondepolarizing Relaxants

The only recognized effect of nondepolarizing relaxants on the cerebral vasculature occurs through the release of histamine. Histamine can result in a reduction in CPP because of the simultaneous increase in ICP (caused by cerebral vasodilation) and decrease in MAP.[374] It is not entirely clear, when the BBB is intact, whether histamine directly causes cerebral vasodilation or whether it is a secondary (autoregulatory) response to a reduction in MAP. d-Tubocurarine is the most potent histamine releaser among the available muscle relaxants. Metocurine, atracurium, and mivacurium also release histamine in lesser quantities.[375,376] This effect is likely to be clinically inconsequential[377] unless these agents are administered in the large doses necessary to achieve intubating conditions rapidly. Of this group of drugs, cisatracurium has the least histamine-releasing effect. No evidence of histamine release was seen after the administration of 0.15 mg/kg (three times the dose effective in 95% [ED_{95}] for twitch depression) of cisatracurium in neurosurgical ICU patients.[378]

Vecuronium, in relatively large doses of 0.1 to 0.14 mg/kg, had no significant effect on cerebral physiology in patients with brain tumors.[379,380] Pipecuronium and rocuronium have not been studied but should similarly be without direct effect, and no adverse events have been reported.

The indirect actions of relaxants may also have effects on cerebral physiology. Pancuronium given as a large bolus dose can cause an abrupt increase in arterial pressure. This increased arterial pressure might elevate ICP in the setting of impaired intracranial compliance and defective autoregulation; however, no significant clinical event has ever been reported. Muscle relaxation may reduce ICP because coughing and straining are prevented, and this results in lowering of central venous pressure with a concomitant reduction in cerebral venous outflow impedance.[381]

A metabolite of atracurium, laudanosine, may be epileptogenic. However, although large doses of atracurium caused an EEG arousal pattern in dogs, CBF, CMR, and ICP were unaltered.[382] In cats, the seizure threshold for lidocaine-induced seizures was not different during paralysis with atracurium, vecuronium, or pancuronium.[383] In rabbits, administration of laudanosine did not increase the severity of the epileptoid activity caused by direct application of cephalosporin to the cortical surface.[384] It appears highly unlikely that epileptogenesis will occur in humans with atracurium.[385,386]

In summary, vecuronium, pipecuronium, rocuronium, atracurium, mivacurium, cisatracurium, metocurine, and pancuronium (if acute elevation in MAP is prevented with the latter) are all reasonable drugs for use in patients with or at risk for intracranial hypertension. Doses of metocurine, atracurium, and mivacurium should be limited to ranges not associated with hypotension. Curare (for the diehards) is best administered slowly and in small divided doses to avoid substantial histamine release.

Succinylcholine

Succinylcholine can produce an increase in ICP in lightly anesthetized humans. Minton and colleagues[387] studied patients with intracranial tumors. Their subjects received morphine, 0.1 mg/kg, 1 hour before induction of anesthesia with thiopental, 6 mg/kg. The patients were ventilated by mask with 70% N_2O to maintain normocapnia and then received succinylcholine, 1 mg/kg. ICP increased from 15 ± 1 (SE) to a maximum of 20 ± 2 mm Hg after 1 to 3 minutes and returned to baseline in 8 to 10 minutes. The effect appears to be the result of cerebral activation (as evidenced by EEG changes and increases in CBF) caused by afferent activity from the muscle spindle apparatus.[388-390] Note, however, that correlation between the occurrence of visible muscle fasciculations and an increase in ICP is poor. As might be expected with what appears to be an arousal phenomenon, deep anesthesia has been observed to prevent succinylcholine-induced ICP increases in the dog.[388] In humans, the increase in ICP is also blocked by paralysis with vecuronium[387] and by "defasciculation" with metocurine, 0.03 mg/kg.[391] The efficacy of other defasciculating agents has not been examined in humans. However, defasciculation with pancuronium did not prevent increases in ICP in the dog.[389]

Although succinylcholine can produce increases in ICP, it need not be viewed as contraindicated in circumstances in which its use for rapid attainment of paralysis is otherwise seen as appropriate. Kovarik and coworkers observed no ICP change after the administration of succinylcholine, 1 mg/kg, to nonparalyzed, ventilated neurosurgical ICU patients, 6 of 10 of whom had sustained head injury.[392] Their observations are very relevant because it is in precisely this population of patients that the issue of the use of succinylcholine arises most frequently. Given that the ICP effect of succinylcholine may be an arousal phenomenon caused by increased afferent traffic from muscle spindles,[390] it is not unreasonable that disease processes that substantially blunt the level of consciousness might similarly blunt this response. As with many drugs, the concern should be not whether it is used but how it is used. If administered with proper attention to the control of carbon dioxide tension, blood pressure, and depth of anesthesia and after defasciculation, preferably with metocurine pending additional information, little hazard should attend its use.

OTHER EFFECTS OF ANESTHETICS ON CEREBRAL PHYSIOLOGY

Cerebrospinal Fluid Dynamics

Adult humans have approximately 150 mL of CSF, half within the cranium and half in the spinal CSF space.

CSF, which is formed in the choroid plexuses and to a lesser extent by transependymal diffusion from the brain's interstitium into the ventricular system, is replaced about three times per day.[393] It functions both as a cushion for the CNS and as an excretory pathway. Anesthetics have been shown to influence both the rate of formation and the rate of reabsorption of CSF. Table 21-4 provides nonquantitative information regarding the direction of influences of common anesthetics. All the information has been derived from animals[394-401] because these processes have not been examined in humans. They may be of relevance when a prolonged closed-cranium procedure is to be performed in a patient with poor intracranial compliance. The most deleterious potential combination of effects in the setting of poor intracranial compliance is increased CSF production and decreased reabsorption. In the dog, this pattern occurs with enflurane, which is perhaps another reason (in addition to the potential for epileptogenesis in the presence of cerebral injury and hypocapnia) for omission of enflurane in this circumstance.

The time course of these effects on CSF dynamics is slow. In clinical situations in which the CSF space is to be opened (most craniotomies) or in which a ventriculostomy is in place, they are probably of relatively little clinical importance.

Blood-Brain Barrier

In most of the body's capillary beds, fenestrations approximately 65 Å in diameter are found between endothelial cells. In the brain, with the exception of the choroid plexus, the pituitary, and the area postrema, tight junctions reduce this pore size to approximately 8 Å. As a result, large molecules and most ions are prevented from entering the brain's interstitium. There is little evidence that anesthetics alter the function of this "blood-brain barrier" in most circumstances. However, it has repeatedly been demonstrated that acute hypertension can breach the barrier[402-404] and that certain anesthetics facilitate this phenomenon.[405] Forster and colleagues[406] observed that extravasation of Evans blue into rabbit brain was greater when acute hypertension occurred during anesthesia with halothane than with thiopental. It is probable that this effect is the nonspecific result of cerebral vasodilation[407] rather than a specific effect of halothane. These results were obtained in the setting of extreme, abrupt hypertension in animals with an initially normal BBB. Evidence also indicates that anesthetics may influence the leakiness of an abnormal BBB at normotension. Smith and Marque[408] subjected dogs to 5 hours of anesthesia after a freeze lesion (which causes an opening in the BBB). Accumulation of

Table 21-4 Effects of anesthetics on the rate of cerebrospinal fluid secretion and absorption

	Halothane	Enflurane	Isoflurane	Desflurane	Fentanyl	Etomidate
Secretion	↓	↑	—	↑*	—	↓
Absorption	↓	↓	↑	—	↑	↑

Upward arrows indicate an increase in the rate of CSF absorption or secretion, and downward arrows indicate a decrease. The information is presented nonquantitatively, and effects may vary with dose. The data are derived from various investigations in animals.[394-401]
*Hypocapnia only.

cerebral water at 24 hours was less in animals anesthetized with pentobarbital or fentanyl-droperidol-N$_2$O than with halothane, enflurane, or isoflurane. To our knowledge, no peer-reviewed investigation has attempted a comparison of the effects of anesthetics on BBB function during anesthesia in normotensive humans.

Epileptogenesis

An extensive review of the convulsant and anticonvulsant effects of anesthetics and adjuvants is available.[409,410] Several commonly used anesthetics have some epileptogenic potential, particularly in predisposed individuals. A concern is that seizure activity may go unrecognized in an anesthetized and paralyzed patient and result in neuronal injury if substrate demand (CMR) exceeds supply for a prolonged period.[411] A second concern is that the epileptogenic effect will persist in the postanesthesia period and seizures will occur in less well controlled circumstances than exist in the operating room. In practice, it appears that spontaneous seizures during or after anesthesia have been extremely rare events. Nonetheless, in patients with processes that might predispose to seizures, it seems prudent to avoid the use of potentially epileptogenic agents in situations in which reasonable alternatives are available.

Enflurane and Sevoflurane
The epileptogenic properties of enflurane and sevoflurane are discussed in the earlier section on volatile anesthetics.

Methohexital
Myoclonic activity is sometimes observed with methohexital, and this drug has been used to activate seizure foci during cortical mapping.[412,413] One clinical report[414] describes the occurrence of seizures in two pediatric patients after induction doses of methohexital administered rectally in one and intramuscularly in the other. Both these patients had temporal lobe lesions and had previously had seizures. It appears that it is specifically patients with seizures of temporal lobe origin, typically of the psychomotor variety, who are at risk for activation of seizures by methohexital.[414,415] Recurrent spontaneous seizures after methohexital anesthesia for ECT have never been reported.

Ketamine
Ketamine can elicit seizures in patients with an epileptic diathesis.[416] Depth electrode recordings in epileptic patients revealed the occurrence of isolated subcortical seizure activity originating in the limbic and thalamic areas during ketamine anesthesia and demonstrated that this subcortical activation may not be reflected in surface EEG recordings.[417] The occurrence of seizures after ketamine anesthesia in neurologically normal subjects has also been reported on only two occasions,[418,419] and in one of these instances the seizure threshold may have been lowered by aminophylline.

Etomidate
Etomidate frequently produces myoclonus that is not associated with epileptiform activity on the EEG.[420] A single instance of severe, sustained myoclonus immediately after anesthesia with etomidate by infusion has been reported.[421] Etomidate has also been shown to precipitate generalized epileptic EEG activity in epileptic patients,[422] and its use in this population should probably be avoided. However, it has been used electively, in low doses, to activate seizure foci for the purposes of intraoperative EEG localization.[423] In our experience (unpublished), selective activation of a quiescent focus can be achieved with 0.1 mg/kg. Larger doses are more likely to lead to generalized activation.

Etomidate has also been noted to be associated with longer seizures in response to ECT than occur after methohexital or propofol. Remarkably, etomidate, in the dose range of 0.15 to 0.3 mg/kg, does not cause dose-related ECT seizure inhibition as is readily demonstrated with the other two agents.[424]

The preceding information not withstanding, no convincing reports have indicated that in normal subjects, epileptogenesis and the use of etomidate need to be restricted on this basis. In fact, etomidate has been used to control refractory status epilepticus.[425]

Narcotics
Seizures or limbic system hypermetabolism (or both) can be readily elicited in some animal species with narcotics.[211,426-429] Although an increase in CBF in deep brain structures associated with pain processing has been observed in human volunteers,[208] humans do not have a clinically apparent correlate of the hypermetabolism effect seen in animals. Several anecdotal reports, unaccompanied by EEG recordings, maintain that grand mal convulsions have occurred in patients who received both high[430] and low doses of fentanyl.[431,432] However, systematic investigations of EEG changes during the administration of relatively large doses of fentanyl, sufentanil, and alfentanil in humans have not documented neuroexcitatory activity,[433-435] and the "seizures" may have been an exaggerated rigidity phenomenon. The exception is the observation that alfentanil, 50 µg/kg, can augment temporal lobe spike activity in patients with temporal lobe epilepsy.[436] Note that untreated rigidity may itself also have important CNS consequences. An increase in ICP was observed when alfentanil-induced rigidity occurred in rats during controlled ventilation.[381] The effect probably arose because the associated increase in CVP caused cerebral venous congestion. In the absence of ventilatory support, both hypercapnia and hypoxemia may also occur.

Atracurium
See the discussion regarding the atracurium metabolite laudanosine in the section on nondepolarizing muscle relaxants.

CEREBRAL PHYSIOLOGY IN PATHOLOGIC STATES

Cerebral Ischemia—Pathophysiology

Critical CBF Thresholds
The brain has a high rate of energy utilization and very limited energy storage capacity. It is therefore extremely

vulnerable in the event of interruption of substrate (oxygen, glucose) supply. Under normal circumstances, global CBF is maintained at approximately 50 mL/100 g/min. In the face of a declining CBF and therefore declining oxygen supply, neuronal function deteriorates progressively rather than in an all-or-none fashion (Fig. 21-13). The brain has a substantial reserve below normal CBF levels, and it is not until CBF has fallen to approximately 22 mL/100 g/ min that EEG evidence of ischemia begins to appear. At a CBF level of approximately 15 mL/100 g/min, the cortical EEG is isoelectric. However, only when CBF is reduced to about 6 mL/100 g/ min are indications of potentially irreversible membrane failure (elevated extracellular potassium[437] and loss of the direct cortical response[441]) rapidly evident. As CBF decreases in the flow range between 15 and 10 mL/100 g/ min, a progressive deterioration in energy supply occurs that eventually leads, with a time course that may last hours[439,442] rather than minutes, to membrane failure and neuronal death. The brain regions falling within this CBF range (6 to 15 mL/100 g/ min) encompass brain tissue in which neuronal dysfunction is temporarily reversible but within which neuronal death will occur if flow is not restored; these brain regions are referred to as the ischemic penumbra.[431,443] Studies defining the progression to cerebral infarction within the penumbra have been performed principally in the cerebral cortex of baboons[437,438] and monkeys,[439] and the actual CBF levels at which the various decrements in function occur may vary with both the anesthetic[440,444] and species. However, in humans anesthetized with halothane and N$_2$O, the CBF threshold for the initial EEG change[445] is similar to that observed in the animal investigations.

Models of Cerebral Ischemia

Much has been made of the difference between complete cerebral ischemia, as occurs during cardiac arrest, and incomplete cerebral ischemia, as may occur during occlusion of a major cerebral vessel or severe hypotension. However, from the clinician's vantage, the important difference is that the residual blood flow during incomplete ischemia may result in enough oxygen delivery to allow for some generation of ATP and thereby stave off the catastrophic irreversible membrane failure that occurs within minutes during normothermic complete cerebral ischemia. This difference in the rate of failure of the energy supply[446,447] (Fig. 21-14) can result in a much greater apparent tolerance for focal or incomplete ischemia than for complete global ischemia (e.g., cardiac arrest). The difference is in reality a matter of severity rather than the actual initial pathophysiology of the insult, with the exception that limited residual perfusion may potentially be detrimental in the event of hyperglycemia. There is also a theoretical concern that low levels of residual flow will provide sufficient oxygen delivery to permit the formation of oxygen radicals. However, the observation that focal ischemia is better tolerated than complete global ischemia argues against major importance.

Energy Failure and Excitotoxicity

Energy failure is the central event that occurs during cerebral ischemia.[448] ATP is required for maintenance of the normal membrane ionic gradient, and energy failure rapidly ensues with membrane depolarization and influx of sodium and calcium into the neuron. Voltage-dependent

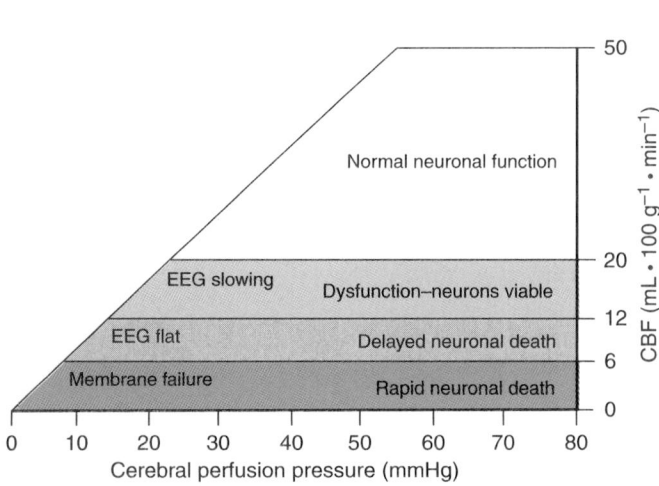

Figure 21–13 Relationships between cerebral perfusion, cerebral blood flow (CBF), the electroencephalogram (EEG), and the functional status/viability of neurons. Note that in the approximate CBF range of 6 to 12 mL/kg/min, the energy supply is insufficient to support electrophysiologic activity (i.e., EEG flat), but it can prevent complete membrane failure and neuronal death for extended periods. These areas are referred to as the ischemic penumbra.[437] The data are derived from studies in the cerebral cortex of barbiturate-anesthetized baboons[437,438] and unanesthetized monkeys.[439] The CBF and mean arterial pressure thresholds may vary with the anesthetic and species.[440]

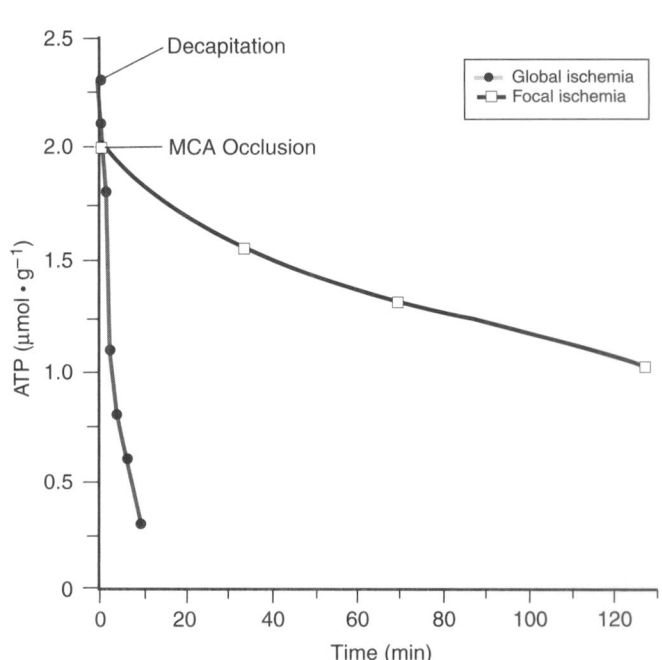

Figure 21–14 Comparison of the rates of failure of the energy supply (adenosine triphosphate [ATP]) in complete global ischemia (produced by decapitation in dogs[447]) and incomplete focal ischemia (middle cerebral artery occlusion [MCA] in monkeys[446]). In the presence of residual CBF, failure of the energy supply is substantially delayed.

calcium channels are then activated and calcium gains entry into the cytosol. Depolarization of presynaptic terminals also results in the release of massive quantities of excitatory neurotransmitters, particularly glutamate, into the synaptic cleft.[449] Activation of glutamatergic receptors, the N-methyl-D-aspartate (NMDA) and α-amino-3-hydroxy-5-methyl-4-isoxazopropionic acid (AMPA) receptors, adds to Na and Ca influx (Fig. 21-15). Initiation of cellular signaling by activation of metabotropic receptors leads to the release of stored Ca from endoplasmic reticulum by inositol triphosphate (IP₃). Ionic influx is

accompanied by influx of water, and neuronal swelling occurs rapidly after membrane depolarization. The injury that is initiated by excessive glutamate receptor activity is referred to as excitotoxicity.

Calcium is a ubiquitous second messenger in cells and is a cofactor required for the activation of a number of enzyme systems. The rapid, uncontrolled increase in cytosolic Ca levels initiates the activation of a number of cellular processes that contribute to injury. Cytoskeletal proteins such as actin are cleaved by activated proteases.[450] These enzymes also degrade a number of the protein

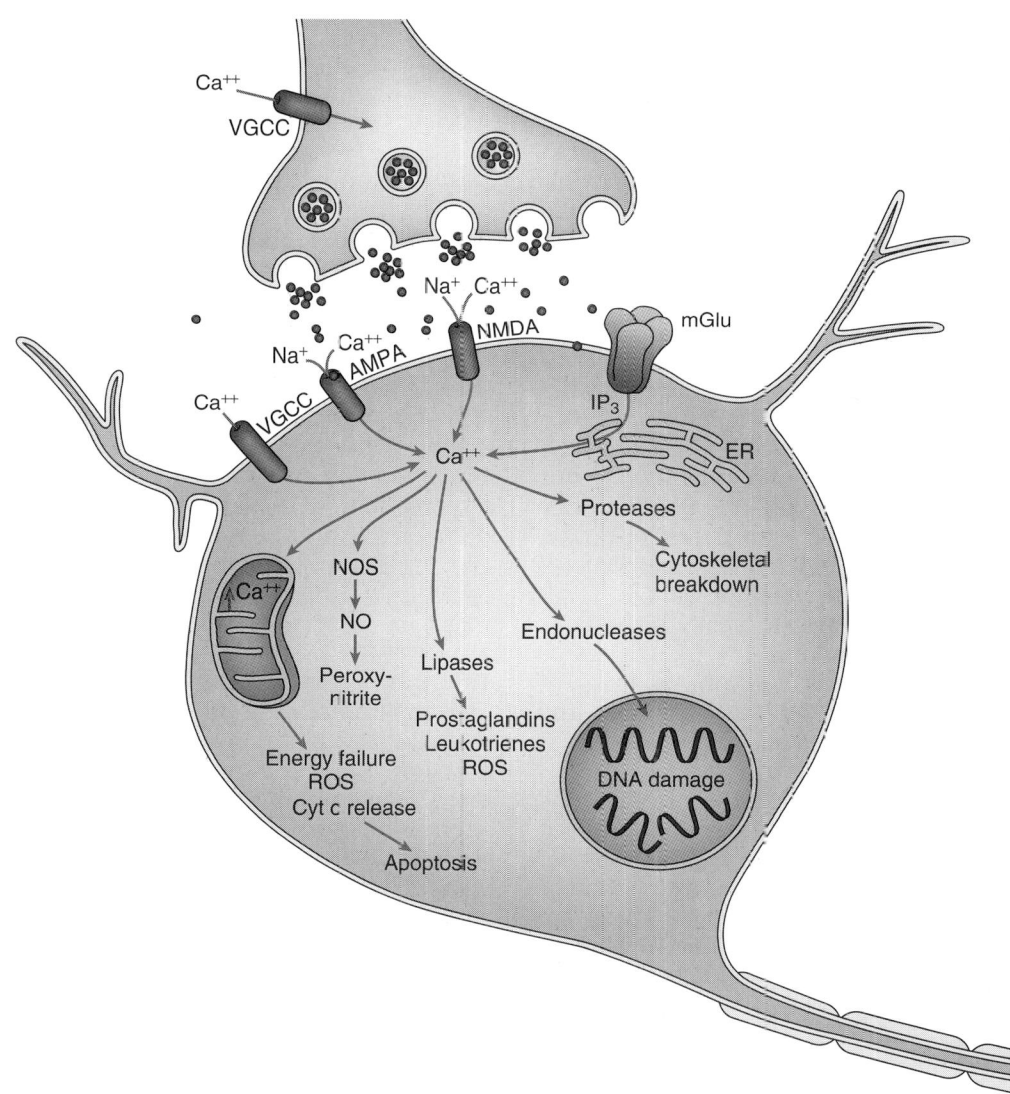

Figure 21–15 During ischemia, depletion of adenosine triphosphate leads to neuronal depolarization and the subsequent release of supranormal quantities of neurotransmitters, especially glutamate. Excessive stimulation of ligand-gated channels and the simultaneous opening of voltage-dependent Ca²⁺ channels permits rapid entry of Ca²⁺ into neurons. Stimulation of metabotropic glutamate receptors (mGlu) generates inositol triphosphate (IP₃), which causes release of Ca²⁺ from the endoplasmic reticulum (ER)/mitochondria. Activation of the α-amino-3-hydroxy-5-methyl-4-isoxazopropionic acid (AMPA)-gated subset of glutamate receptors also permits excessive entry of sodium (Na⁺). Excessive free Ca²⁺ results in the activation of numerous enzymes: protease activation causes breakdown of the cytoskeleton of the neuron; lipases damage plasma membrane lipids and release arachidonic acid, which is metabolized by cyclooxygenases and lipoxygenases to yield free radicals and other mediators of cell injury; activation of nitric oxide synthase (NOS) leads to release of nitric oxide (NO) and, in turn, the generation of peroxynitrite, a highly reactive free radical; and activated endonucleases damage DNA, thereby rendering the neuron susceptible to apoptosis. Injury to mitochondria leads to energy failure, free radical generation, and the release of cytochrome c (Cyt c) from mitochondria; the latter is one of the means by which neuronal apoptosis is initiated. NMDA, N-methyl-D-aspartate; ROS, reactive oxygen species; VGCC, voltage-gated calcium channels.

constituents of the neuron. Lipases attack cellular lipids and produce membrane damage. An important lipase, phospholipase A_2, releases fatty acids such as arachidonic acid from membranes.[451] Metabolism of arachidonic acid into prostaglandins and leukotrienes by cyclooxygenase and lipoxygenase is accompanied by generation of the superoxide free radical. The latter, in combination with other free radicals generated in response to mitochondrial injury, can lead to lipid peroxidation and membrane injury. Prostaglandins and leukotrienes also evoke an inflammatory response, and they are powerful chemotactic agents. Activation of platelets within cerebral microvessels, as well as the influx of white blood cells into damaged areas, aggravates ischemic injury by occluding the vasculature.

DNA damage is also an important event during ischemic neuronal injury. Generation of free radicals from arachidonic acid metabolism, from injured mitochondria, and from the production of peroxynitrite from NO leads to oxidative injury to DNA.[452] Activation of endonucleases also produces DNA strand breaks. Under normal circumstances, DNA injury results in the activation of poly-ADP ribose-polymerase (PARP), an enzyme that participates in DNA repair. With excessive DNA injury, PARP activity increases dramatically, and this increased activity can lead to depletion of nicotinamide adenine dinucleotide (NAD), a substrate of PARP.[452] NAD is also an important coenzyme in energy metabolism, and its depletion further exacerbates energy failure.

Lactate formation is an additional element of the pathophysiologic process. Lactic acid is formed as a result of the anaerobic glycolysis that takes place after failure of the supply of oxygen. The associated decline in pH contributes to deterioration of the intracellular environment. An increased preischemic serum glucose level may accelerate this process by providing additional substrate for anaerobic glycolysis.[453-456]

NO,[2,3,457] which has emerged as a probable mediator of CBF changes in many normal physiologic states (see the preceding sections), is also of relevance to the pathophysiology of ischemia. NO is, in fact, a weak free radical[457,458] that in turn leads to the generation of a more reactive species (peroxynitrite), and it is a "killer substance" used by macrophages.[2] In cerebral ischemia, NO is probably both friend and foe.[459] It is likely that during a period of focal ischemia, the vasodilating effect of NO (probably constitutively elaborated NO of endothelial origin) serves to augment collateral CBF.[460] However, in the postischemic phase, NO (probably inducible NO of neuronal origin) contributes to neuronal injury.[460]

Collectively, the simultaneous and unregulated activation of a number of cellular pathways overwhelms the reparative and restorative processes within the neuron and ultimately leads to neuronal death.

Nature of Neuronal Death

The neuronal death that occurs in response to these processes has been categorized as necrotic or apoptotic in nature. Necrotic death of neurons, mediated by excitotoxic injury, is characterized by rapid cellular swelling, condensation and pyknosis of the nucleus, and swelling of the mitochondria and endoplasmic reticulum. A characteristic of these necrotic neurons is the presence of an acidophilic cytoplasm.[461] Necrotic neuronal death results

in local infiltration of the brain by inflammatory cells. A consequence of this inflammation is a considerable amount of collateral damage.

Neuronal apoptosis, a form of cellular suicide, has also been demonstrated in a variety of models of cerebral ischemia. Apoptosis is characterized by condensation of chromatin, involution of the cell membrane, swelling of mitochondria, and cellular shrinkage. In the later stages of apoptosis, neurons fragment into several apoptotic bodies, which are then cleared from the brain.[461] The lack of a substantial inflammatory response to apoptotic death limits injury to the surrounding neurons that have survived the initial ischemic insult.

A number of biochemical pathways that lead to apoptosis have been described. Initiation of apoptosis by the release of cytochrome c from injured mitochondria has been studied the most (Fig. 21-16). Cytochrome c is restricted from the cytoplasm by the outer mitochondrial membrane.[462] When mitochondria are injured, pores within the outer membrane allow cytochrome c to be released into the cytoplasm, where it interacts with pro-caspase-9 and apoptosis-activating factor to produce an apoptosome.[463] Procaspase-9 undergoes activation by proteolytic cleavage. Activated caspase-9 then activates caspase-3. The latter serves as an executor of apoptosis by cleaving a number of protein substrates that are essential in DNA repair (such as PARP). Activation of caspase-3 can also occur by inflammatory signaling through activation of tumor necrosis factor-α (TNF-α) and caspase-8.[464] It should be noted that the neuronal injury that occurs in response to ischemia cannot easily be divided into necrosis or apoptosis. The nature of neuronal death probably encompasses a spectrum in which some neurons undergo necrosis or apoptosis whereas others undergo cell death that has features of both necrosis and apoptosis.

Timing of Neuronal Death (also see Chapter 79)

The traditional concept of ischemic injury was that neuronal death was restricted to the time of ischemia and during the early reperfusion period. However, more recent data indicate that postischemic neuronal injury is a dynamic process in which neurons continue to die for a long period after the initiating ischemic insult (Fig. 21-17).[465-467] This delayed neuronal death, which was first demonstrated in models of global cerebral ischemia, has been demonstrated during focal ischemia as well. The extent of delayed neuronal death depends on the severity of the ischemic insult. With severe ischemia, most neurons undergo rapid death. With more moderate insults, neurons that survive the initial insult undergo delayed death. This ongoing neuronal loss contributes to the gradual expansion of cerebral infarction after focal ischemia. In experimental studies, evidence of cerebral inflammation, which can theoretically contribute to further injury, has been demonstrated even 6 to 8 months after the primary ischemia.

The occurrence of delayed neuronal death has important implications for the evaluation of studies in which neuroprotective strategies are investigated. A wide variety of interventions have shown neuroprotective efficacy in studies in which the extent of injury is evaluated within 3 to 4 days after ischemia. However, this neuroprotective efficacy may not be sustained. Recent data indicate that

Figure 21–16 Cellular processes that lead to neuronal apoptosis. Cytochrome *c* (cyt c), which is normally restricted to the space between the inner and outer mitochondrial membranes, is released in response to mitochondrial injury. Cytochrome *c*, in combination with apoptosis activating factor (apaf), activates caspase-9 by proteolytic cleavage. Activated caspase-9 then leads to activation of caspase-3. This enzyme cleaves a number of substrates, including those necessary for DNA repair. Within the mitochondria, bax augments and bcl prevents the release of cytochrome *c*. Cytochrome *c* release can also be initiated by bid, a substance that is activated by caspase-8 through tumor necrosis factor-α (TNF) signaling. In addition, caspase-8 can directly activate caspase 3. Excessive activation of poly-ADP ribose-polymerase (PARP), an enzyme integral to DNA repair, depletes cellular stores of oxidized nicotinamide adenine dinucleotide (NAD^+). Depletion of NAD^+ further exacerbates the energy failure because it is central to energy metabolism. ATP, adenosine triphosphate.

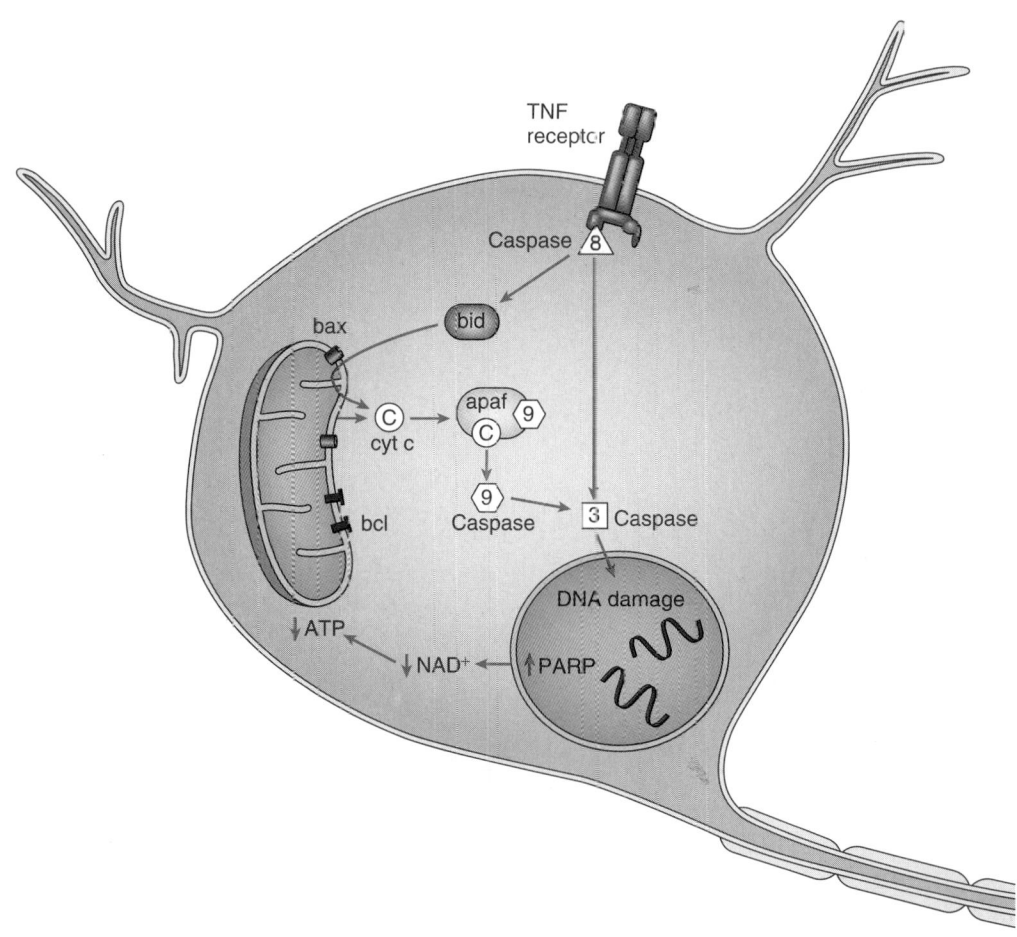

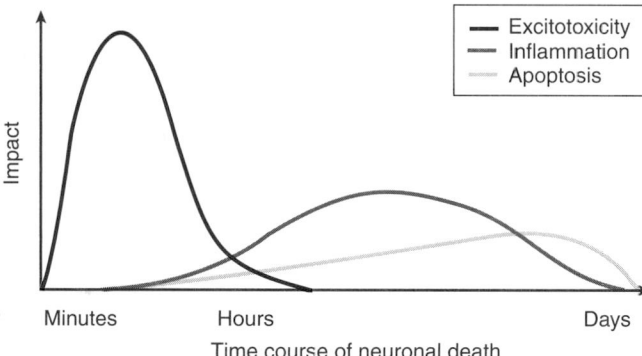

Figure 21–17 Time course of neuronal death. Excitotoxic (glutamate-mediated) injury results in neuronal death within the first few hours after the onset of ischemia. Brain tissue injury elicits an inflammatory response, an important process in removal of injured tissue and healing, that leads to a substantial amount of collateral damage. Inflammation-mediated neuronal death can continue for several days. Neuronal apoptosis can occur in injured neurons that survived the initial insult. Apoptotic neuronal death has been demonstrated to occur for many days after the initiating ischemic insult. It is now apparent that ischemic neuronal death is a dynamic process in which neurons continue to die for a long period. (Adapted from Dirnagl U, Iadecola C, Moskowitz MA: Pathobiology of ischaemic stroke: An integrated view. Trends Neurosci 22:391-397, 1999.)

cerebral infarction undergoes gradual expansion, and a reduction in injury attributed to a particular therapeutic intervention is no longer apparent when the injury is evaluated after a long postischemic recovery period.[465,466] Long-term (greater than 1 month) evaluation of the efficacy of a particular intervention is therefore important.

Brain Protection

The literature on cerebral ischemia and brain protection is vast, and a detailed discourse on this topic is beyond the scope of the present discussion. A number of excellent recent reviews on the subject are available.[461,463,467-471] The numerous brain protection strategies that have been studied in both the laboratory and the clinic can be classified according to the phase of this sequence that each addresses. They are listed in Table 21-5. The focus of the present discussion will be anesthetic-mediated neuroprotection.

Considerations Relevant to Complete Global Ischemia (Cardiac Arrest) (also see Chapter 78)

Maintenance of adequate perfusion pressure after cardiac arrest is of considerable importance. Hypotension developing after resuscitation from cardiac arrest may aggravate

Table 21–5 Clinical trials of drugs in acute stroke

Drugs to Improve Blood Flow	
Antithrombotic drugs (also see Stroke Prevention below)	Heparin
	Low-molecular-weight heparins
	Dalteparin
	Enoxaparin
	Nadroparin
	Tinzaparin
	Danaparoid (Org 10172; low-molecular-weight heparinoid)
Antiplatelet drugs (also see Stroke Prevention below)	Aspirin
	Abciximab
Fibrinogen-depleting drugs	Ancrod
	Defibrase
Drugs to improve capillary flow	Pentoxifylline
Thrombolytics	Prourokinase
	Streptokinase
	Tenecteplase
	Tissue plasminogen activator
	Urokinase

Drugs to Protect Brain Tissue (Neuroprotective Agents)	
Calcium channel blockers	Nimodipine
Calcium chelators	DP-b99
Free radical scavengers—antioxidants	Ebselen
	Tirilazad
GABA agonists	Clomethiazole
Glutamate antagonists	AMPA antagonists
	GYKI 52466
	NBQX
	YM90K
	ZK-200775 (MPQX)
	Kainate antagonist
	SYM 2081
	NMDA antagonists
	Competitive NMDA antagonists
	CGS 19755 (Selfotel)
	NMDA channel blockers
	Aptiganel (Cerestat)
	CP-101,606
	Dextrorphan
	Dextromethorphan
	Magnesium
	Memantine
	MK-801
	NPS 1506
	Remacemide
	Glycine site antagonists
	ACEA 1021
	GV150526
	Polyamine site antagonists
	Elprodil
	Ifenprodil
Growth factors	Fibroblast growth factor (bFGF)

Table 21–5 Clinical trials of drugs in acute stroke—cont'd

Leukocyte adhesion inhibitor	Anti-ICAM antibody (Enlimomab)
Nitric oxide inhibitor	Hu23F2G
Opioid antagonists	Lubeluzole
Phosphatidylcholine precursor	Naloxone
	Nalmefene
Serotonin agonist	Citicoline (CDP-choline)
Sodium channel blocker	Bay x 3072
Potassium channel opener	Fosphenytoin
	Lubeluzole
	619C89
Mechanism unknown or uncertain	Piracetam
	Lubeluzole

Stroke Prevention	
Anticoagulants	Low-molecular-weight heparins
	Dalteparin
	Enoxaparin
	Nadroparin
	Tinzaparin
	Danaparoid (Org 10172; low-molecular-weight heparinoid)
	Warfarin
Antihypertensive drugs	Candesartan cilexetil
	Eprosartan
	Nitrendipine
	Perindopril
Antiplatelet drugs	Aspirin
	Clopidogrel
	Dipyridamole
	Ticlopidine
	Triflusal
	GP IIa/IIIb inhibitors
	Lotrafiban
Estradiol	
Vitamins	

Please note that this is a list of *investigational* drugs that have been tested in animals or humans for treatment of stroke. Inclusion in this list does not mean that a drug is effective in stroke. Several drugs here have been shown to be ineffective in acute stroke trials.
AMPA, α-amino-3-hydroxy-5-methyl-4-isoxazopropionic acid; GABA, γ-aminobutyric acid; ICAM, intercellular adhesion molecule; NMDA, N-methyl-D-aspartate.

the microcirculatory and vasospastic processes occurring at this time and increase brain damage. A late phase of intracranial hypertension may occur and is due to the development of extensive cerebral edema, probably both vasogenic and cytotoxic in etiology, associated with brain necrosis. Attempts to control this type of intracranial hypertension with osmotherapy usually fail. ICP monitoring is not generally used because the patients in whom these delayed ICP increases develop have sustained massive tissue damage.

Both barbiturates and calcium channel blockers have been administered after cardiac arrest. The former are ineffective.[472-474] The calcium channel blocker nimodipine improved neurologic outcome when administered after complete global ischemia in a primate model,[475] but it was ineffective after complete global ischemia in the cat[476,477] and dog.[478] In a small cohort (51 patients) of cardiac arrest victims, nimodipine was shown to improve CBF but not neurologic outcome.[479] In a second trial involving approximately 150 cardiac arrest victims, no overall benefit in neurologic outcome was observed.[480] However, a subset of patients in whom initiation of advanced life support was delayed for more than 10 minutes demonstrated improved survival. This single study cannot serve as justification for the administration of nimodipine after cardiac arrest, especially in the face of the unequivocally negative results of the multicenter lidoflazine cardiac arrest study.[481] Once again, the important therapeutic objectives are maintenance of normocapnia and normotension, normalization of systemic pH, avoidance of hyperthermia, and prevention and treatment of seizures.

Induced mild hypothermia has recently been shown to be effective in reducing mortality and morbidity in patients who sustain a cardiac arrest.[482] Induction of mild hypothermia in the range of 32°C to 34°C for a period of about 24 hours improved neurologic outcome and survival 6 months after cardiac arrest when compared with the normothermic group. Mild hypothermia was induced without difficulty. Passive rewarming of patients was accomplished slowly over a period of 8 hours. The incidence of complications was similar to that in the control normothermic group. This important study is one of the first to demonstrate the feasibility and efficacy of induced hypothermia as a treatment to prevent injury from global ischemia. Undoubtedly, induced hypothermia will now be added to the armamentarium for the treatment of cerebral complications of cardiac arrest.

Considerations Relevant to Focal (Incomplete) Ischemia

Protection by Anesthetics

Before discussing individual drugs, it should be noted that a general theme that can be extracted from the protection-by-anesthetics literature, in particular for volatile anesthetics, is that anesthesia per se is protective. It appears that for undefined reasons, reducing the level of systemic stress associated with a standardized experimental insult results in an improved outcome.[483,484] In reviewing the protection-by-anesthetics literature, readers should be conscious of the possibility that the protective benefit ascribed to an intervention with an anesthetic may in fact be the product of exaggeration of the injury in a high-stress control state (e.g., N_2O "sedation").

BARBITURATES. The protective efficacy of barbiturates in focal cerebral ischemia has been reported numerous times in animals,[485-491] with only a single demonstration of effectiveness in humans.[492] The effect has been attributed principally to suppression of CMR. However, CBF redistribution effects and free radical scavenging[493] have been suggested to contribute, and there is evidence that CMR suppression is not the sole mechanism.[494-496] Suppression of CMR might logically be expected to be of benefit to brain regions in which oxygen delivery was

inadequate to meet normal demands but was sufficient to allow energy consumption by some ongoing electrophysiologic activity (i.e., in which the EEG was abnormal but not flat). Such regions are likely to be limited in size in the setting of focal ischemia, yet several of the animal investigations suggest a very substantial protective effect.[485,487-489] Review of these experiments reveals that the methods used to monitor and maintain temperature, though accepted at the time, were below the standards that have evolved from more recent understanding of the effects of both deliberate[497,498] and inadvertent[499] hypothermia. Unrecognized cerebral hypothermia may well have been a factor in some of the cited investigations, and it is therefore possible that the protective efficacy of barbiturates may have been overestimated. Although more recent publications involving suitable temperature control methods do in fact indicate a protective effect by barbiturates,[496,500,501] the magnitude of that effect was modest in comparison to the results of earlier studies. Barbiturate-induced EEG suppression in an already anesthetized patient may still be logical therapy when it can be applied before or early in the course of a period of temporary focal ischemia, such as temporary occlusion during aneurysm surgery. However, the judgment to institute such therapy should be made after consideration of the risk of the occlusive event, the patient's cardiovascular status, and the physician's willingness to accept the possible prolongation of arousal, as well as after objectively determining the probable magnitude of the protective effect.

Numerous investigations in animals and humans have failed to demonstrate any protective effect of barbiturates in the setting of global cerebral ischemia (e.g., cardiac arrest).[472,502]

Because CMR suppression has been the presumed mechanism of effect, barbiturates have traditionally been administered to produce a maximal reduction in CMR (which is nearly complete when EEG burst suppression has been achieved). However, data presented by Warner and colleagues[496] demonstrated that the same protective benefit (expressed as reduction in infarct volume) could be achieved with a third of the burst suppression dose.[496] This finding raises a clinically important issue. The various barbiturates (thiopental, thiamylal, methohexital, pentobarbital) have similar effects on CMR and have generally been assumed to have equal protective efficacy. However, if the mechanism of protection is a pharmacologic effect other than CMR reduction, is it reasonable to assume equivalence among the barbiturates? Recent data suggest that the neuroprotective efficacy of barbiturates is not similar. In a direct comparison of three clinically used barbiturates, methohexital and thiopental, but not pentobarbital, reduced injury in an animal model of focal ischemia.[503] These data suggest that mechanisms other than, or at least in addition to, metabolic suppression may contribute to the protective effect of barbiturates.

ISOFLURANE/VOLATILE ANESTHETICS. Isoflurane is also a potent suppressant of CMR in the cerebral cortex, and EEG evidence suggestive of a protective effect in humans[440] has been reported. In comparison to the awake or N_2O-fentanyl–anesthetized state, isoflurane has consistently been shown to be neuroprotective in models of hemispheric,[504] focal,[505] and nearly complete ischemia.[506,507] Of interest is the recent observation that isoflurane's neuroprotective efficacy is not sustained.[508] When injury is evaluated 2 days after ischemia, a robust reduction in injury is observed with isoflurane anesthesia. However, by 14 days, this reduction in injury was not apparent. These data indicate that neuronal injury continues well into the postischemic recovery period and that the neuroprotection that is evident shortly after ischemia may not persist for the long term. The neuroprotective effect of isoflurane is not substantially different from that of other volatile anesthetics.[484,491,498,500,501,509-514] Sevoflurane has been shown to reduce ischemic injury in animal models of focal[515] and hemispheric ischemia[516]; its efficacy is not different from that of halothane. Desflurane also reduces neuronal injury to the same extent that isoflurane does.[517] The available data therefore suggest that adequate anesthesia per se may have a protective effect[483,484] versus the awake state, but there does not appear to be any difference in neuroprotective efficacy among the volatile anesthetics.

PROPOFOL. EEG suppression can also be achieved with clinically feasible doses of propofol. Anecdotal information suggests that it is being used to provide "protection" during both aneurysm surgery[518] and carotid endarterectomy. In experimental models of cerebral ischemia, the extent of neurologic injury in propofol-anesthetized animals was similar to that in halothane-anesthetized animals.[519] Given the previous demonstration that halothane can reduce injury, these data provide indirect evidence of propofol's neuroprotective efficacy. In a more recent investigation, cerebral infarction was significantly reduced in propofol-anesthetized animals than in awake animals.[520] A direct comparison of propofol to pentobarbital has also demonstrated that cerebral injury after focal ischemia is similar in animals anesthetized with the two agents.[521] Collectively, these data are consistent with the premise that propofol can reduce ischemic cerebral injury, at least in the short term. Sustained neuroprotection with propofol has not been evaluated.

ETOMIDATE. Etomidate was proposed as early as 1988 as a potential protective drug in the setting of aneurysm surgery.[522] It too produces CMR suppression to an extent equivalent to the barbiturates, and like the barbiturates, etomidate is an agonist at the (inhibitory) type A γ-aminobutyric acid (GABA$_A$) receptor. At that time, no investigations of etomidate using histologic end points had been conducted. Subsequently, in a model of temporary forebrain ischemia, a very small protective effect, relative to anesthesia with 1.1 MAC halothane or isoflurane or anesthesia with thiopental, was demonstrated in the hippocampus, but no protective effects were seen in other brain regions, including the cortex, reticular nucleus of the thalamus, and the striatum.[523,524] In a later investigation using a model of temporary MCA occlusion,[501] the volume of injury was not reduced by etomidate relative to a 1.2 MAC halothane-anesthetized control group. In fact, the volume of injury with etomidate was significantly larger than in the control group. In patients subjected to temporary intracranial vessel occlusion, administration of etomidate results in greater tissue hypoxia and acidosis than equivalent desflurane anesthesia does. The aggravation of injury produced by etomidate (an imidazole) may be related to direct binding of NO[525] as a consequence of etomidate-induced hemolysis,[526] combined with direct inhibition of the NO synthase enzyme by etomidate.[527] Therefore, no scientific support exists for the current use[528] of etomidate for "cerebral protection."

Calcium Channel Blockers

It is now an established clinical practice to administer nimodipine orally (the intravenous preparation is not approved for clinical use in North America) for 21 days beginning as soon as possible after subarachnoid hemorrhage.[529] However, it has not yet become standard practice to administer nimodipine or any other calcium channel blocker routinely after neurologic stroke occurring in the operating room or any other environment. In spite of favorable results in small trials,[530,531] not all investigations in stroke victims have confirmed the benefits of nimodipine.[532] Those that did demonstrate beneficial effects saw them only in limited post hoc patient subsets, that is, those in whom therapy was initiated quickly.[530,531]

Other Drugs

A remarkable number of drugs have shown neuroprotective efficacy in animal studies. However, to date, large-scale randomized trials of a variety of drugs in patients with stroke have not demonstrated neuroprotection with any drug (see Table 21-5). With the exception of tissue plasminogen activator for thrombolysis and the calcium channel blockers nimodipine and nicardipine for the management of subarachnoid hemorrhage, pharmacologic neuroprotective drugs are not available for the treatment of patients with cerebral ischemia.

Cerebral Ischemia: Influence of Physiologic Variables

CEREBRAL PERFUSION PRESSURE. Measures designed to augment CBF (an important determinant of energy supply) are also important. In the "ischemic penumbra" (described earlier), small improvements in CBF have the potential to prolong neuronal survival substantially. Maintenance of a high normal CPP can augment collateral CBF[101] and has been shown to result in improvement in various neurophysiologic parameters, including neurologic function.[533-535] By contrast, hypotension can reduce CBF and exacerbate injury. Therefore, in patients with cerebral ischemia, hypotension should be treated promptly and normotension should be restored. The target MAP should be based on knowledge of a patient's preexisting blood pressure. In most patients, maintenance of MAP in the 70– to 80–mm Hg range should be adequate. Note, however, that augmentation of CPP in the high-normal range carries the inadequately explored risks of increased edema and hemorrhagic infarction if used as support during more than brief periods of ischemia, particularly when several hours has elapsed since the onset of ischemia.

CARBON DIOXIDE TENSION. Normocapnia should be maintained. Hypercapnia has the potential to cause an intracerebral steal phenomenon and may worsen intracellular pH. In spite of some support for the occurrence of a favorable so-called Robin Hood or inverse steal,[252,536] hypocapnia has not generally proved effective in either laboratory or clinical settings.[537-541] Pending further information, normocapnia remains the standard practice.

TEMPERATURE (also see Chapter 40). Hypothermia is firmly and justifiably established as the principal cerebral protective technique for circulatory arrest procedures. It unequivocally enhances cerebral tolerance for episodes of ischemia. For deep hypothermia, this effect has been presumed to be largely a function of reduction of CMR. Whereas pharmacologic agents, such as the barbiturates, reduce only that component of CMR associated with electrophysiologic "work" (about 60% of $CMRO_2$ in the awake state), hypothermia causes a reduction in both electrophysiologic energy consumption and energy utilization related to maintenance of cellular integrity, and mild hypothermia may preferentially suppress the latter.[35,36] Recently, there has been a surge of interest in mild hypothermia as a cerebral protective technique. A substantial number of laboratory studies have demonstrated that mild degrees of hypothermia (2°C to 4°C) during an episode of ischemia can confer substantial protection as measured histologically.[33,497,498,542-545] In addition, evidence from animal studies indicates that hypothermia initiated in the immediate postischemic period confers protective benefits.[499,546-549]

These recent observations regarding mild hypothermia have cast doubt on the notion that CMR suppression is the sole mediator of the cerebral protective effects of hypothermia. This doubt has arisen because the amount of CMR suppression associated with protective degrees of hypothermia is in some instances less than that associated with pharmacologic interventions that have been less clearly protective. Microdialysis investigations in the setting of cerebral ischemia have revealed that hypothermia has a very striking inhibitory effect on the release of various neurotransmitters[542] (recall the pathophysiologic "cascade" discussion earlier), and it may well be that the protective effects of hypothermia are far more dependent on influences on several steps in the biochemistry of ischemia (Table 21-6) than on suppression of CMR.[550]

Table 21–6   Possible mechanisms of cerebral protection by mild hypothermia*

Reduction of the cerebral metabolic rate
Decreased release of excitatory neurotransmitters
Inhibition of activation of protein kinase C (early)
Preservation of late postischemic enzyme function
Protein kinase C
Calcium-calmodulin kinase II
Ubiquitin
Reduction of free radical formation
Inhibition of DNA transcription
Inhibition of apoptosis
Inhibition of proinflammatory cytokines

*For details, see Maher J, Hachinski V: Hypothermia as a potential treatment for cerebral ischemia. Cerebrovasc Brain Metab Rev 5:277-300, 1993; and Colbourne F, Sutherland G, Corbett D: Postischemic hypothermia: A critical appraisal with implications for clinical treatment. Mol Neurobiol 14:171-201, 1997.)

On the strength of the animal investigations cited earlier, mild hypothermia (32°C to 34°C) is being used in some centers in anticipation of possible focal ischemic events (e.g., aneurysm surgery). A preliminary investigation of induced mild hypothermia as a neuroprotective strategy in patients undergoing cerebral aneurysm clipping demonstrated the feasibility of inducing mild hypothermia, and the initial results in a limited number of patients are encouraging.[551] The clinical trial is currently under way and should be completed within the next few years. A number of clinical trials of induced hypothermia in a limited number of stroke patients have been conducted. To date, these trials have demonstrated the feasibility of inducing hypothermia in the range of 33°C to 35°C,[552-555] even in patients who are not subjected to endotracheal intubation and mechanical ventilation.[556] Hypothermia was associated with improved ICP and CPP. However, complications are frequent, particularly thrombocytopenia, bradycardia, ventricular ectopy, hypotension, and infection. In addition, intractable increase in ICP can occur during rewarming, even if the elevation in temperature is gradual and accomplished over a period of several hours. These side effects attest to the need to conduct proper randomized trials to appropriately evaluate the efficacy of mild hypothermia in stroke patients. Such trials are currently under way.

The development of cerebral ischemia contributes to the pathophysiology of head injury.[557,558] Based on this evidence, induction of mild hypothermia has also been evaluated in head-injured patients. Although the initial small single-institution trials of mild hypothermia in head injury[559-562] were promising, the results of a large randomized clinical trial suggest that hypothermia may not necessarily be neuroprotective in the setting of head injury.[563] Methodologic concerns about that study have prompted a re-evaluation of hypothermia in head-injured patients, and trials are presently being conducted.

Hyperthermia has been shown to be deleterious to outcome after standardized ischemic events.[514,543,564,565] Hyperthermia before, during, and after ischemic events should be prevented or treated.

GLUCOSE. The withholding of glucose-containing solutions in situations in which cerebral ischemia may occur is now an established practice. This practice is based on numerous demonstrations in animal models of brain and spinal cord ischemia that elevation in plasma glucose before episodes of either complete or incomplete ischemia results in an aggravation of neurologic injury.[453-455,566-569] However, it should be noted that most investigations have involved adult animals and that there is less certainty regarding the adverse effects of hyperglycemia in immature subjects such as neonates.[570] Furthermore, it should be noted that only some[571,572] and not all[573-577] of the investigations in humans have provided confirmation of an independent effect of serum glucose on neurologic outcome. A recurrent theme in the discussion of these studies is that the elevation in glucose levels may be a result of the stress associated with a severe insult, either ischemic or traumatic, rather than its cause. In addition, the inevitable questions of whether and how quickly immediate insulin treatment of an elevated plasma glucose level reduces the risk to normoglycemic levels have not been examined thoroughly. It is our opinion that at this juncture, acute insulin administration (with its attendant risk of hypoglycemia) in patients with modest glucose elevation (e.g., 175 to 250 mg/dL) is not yet justified.

SEIZURES, pH. Normalization of systemic pH, prevention and treatment of seizures, which dramatically increase CMR, and control of ICP and CPP are all, though mundane and lacking the appeal of a pharmacologic silver bullet, important elements in brain protection and resuscitation.

INTRAVASCULAR VOLUME/HEMATOCRIT MANIPULATION. Although hemodilution has not proved effective in studies of human stroke, both laboratory and human data support the practice, and it is an established part of management of the ischemia associated with vasospasm. However, the data do not currently justify routine hemodilution (a hematocrit of 30% to 35% is the theoretical optimum) in patients in whom focal ischemia might occur in the operating room.[578] On the other hand, the potentially deleterious effects of hemoconcentration should help further suppress the out-of-date notion that neurosurgical patients should be "run dry." An increased hematocrit, because of viscosity effects, reduces CBF.[85] It is our unsubstantiated opinion that in anticipation of a procedure wherein incomplete ischemia might occur, such as carotid endarterectomy, a hematocrit in excess of 55% should be lowered by preoperative phlebotomy.

It is quite apparent from the discussion just presented that the efficacy of pharmacologic brain protection is, at best, limited. By contrast, the potential for exacerbation of preexisting cerebral injury, either ischemic or traumatic, is substantial. Accordingly, effort should be focused on maintenance of physiologic parameters (perfusion pressure, oxygenation, normocapnia, temperature management, control of hyperglycemia, and seizure prophylaxis) within the appropriate range and less on pharmacologic agents to reduce cerebral injury.

DEFERRING ELECTIVE PROCEDURES AFTER STROKE. The risks of extension of cerebral infarction in the event of subsequent anesthesia and surgery have not been studied systematically. In patients who have suffered a stroke, CBF undergoes marked changes. Areas of both high and low CBF occur, and stabilization of regional CBF and CMR is apparent after about 2 weeks.[579] Loss of normal vasomotor responses (CO_2 responsiveness, autoregulation) in the early postinsult period is very common,[580-582] and changes persist beyond 2 weeks in a small percentage of stroke victims.[581,582] BBB abnormalities, as reflected by accumulation of CT contrast or brain scan isotopes, are still present 4 weeks after the insult,[583] and histologic resolution of large infarcts is not complete for several months. The available information does not allow a definite statement regarding how long elective procedures should be deferred. A 6-week delay should give some assurance of the probable recovery of autoregulation, CO_2 responsiveness, and BBB integrity. However, the size and location of the infarction should be weighed. A small infarction in silent cortex may give wider latitudes than a large lesion that has resulted in a paresis that is still resolving. A recent prospective study suggested that in patients with nondisabling stroke, early carotid endarterectomy can be safely performed within 2 weeks of the stroke.[584] However, in patients with larger strokes, pending other information, it seems reasonable to defer elective surgery for at least 4 weeks after a cerebral vascular accident and preferably for 6 weeks from the point at which a stable postinsult neurologic state has been achieved.

Chronic Arterial Hypertension

A recurrent concern is that of acceptable levels of blood pressure reduction in chronically hypertensive patients. Firm guidelines have not been established. However, from the vantage of cerebral well-being, limiting elective MAP reduction to 30% to 35% of resting mean levels seems appropriate for both hypertensive and normotensive patients. It is reasonable that the same guidelines might apply in both populations because in chronic hypertension, both the upper and lower limits of autoregulation are shifted to the right with apparently little distortion.[54]

The rationale for a limit of 30% to 35% is as follows. It has been demonstrated that MAP reductions of 50% in nonanesthetized patients, both normotensive and hypertensive, will commonly produce reversible symptoms of cerebral hypoperfusion.[54,585,586] Although even greater reductions will probably be tolerated, provided that exposure is brief, the hematocrit is reasonable, and the cerebral vasculature is patent, we counsel against it. A reduction in MAP of this magnitude will result in the patient, normal or hypertensive, "falling off" the lower end of the autoregulatory plateau. It has been demonstrated that a reduction in MAP of 25% will bring both normotensive and hypertensive patients to the LLA.[54] As the reduction in MAP exceeds 25% of baseline, CBF values will be below normal, albeit in subjects free of occlusive vascular disease, but above the threshold for neurophysiologic dysfunction or injury (see Fig. 21-4). However, physiologic reserve is being encroached on, with little margin left for error or for other causes of impaired cerebral oxygen delivery (low hematocrit, unrecognized cerebrovascular disease).

It has been demonstrated in animals that treatment of chronic hypertension can restore the LLA to normal.[587,588] A similar phenomenon has been observed in humans by Strandgaard, although restoration was incomplete and failed to occur after as long as 12 months of treatment in some subjects.[54] It is an unexplored possibility that the extent of restoration of the LLA with antihypertensive therapy is agent dependent. Some may restore the LLA more effectively than others do. In particular, angiotensin-converting enzyme inhibitors have been shown to decrease the LLA acutely in both normotensive and hypertensive subjects.[55,589]

Intracranial Hypertension

Control of intracranial hypertension is discussed in detail in Chapter 53.

Brain Tumors

Few data are available regarding the physiology of intracranial tumors. Arbit and colleagues[590] measured CBF in cerebral tumors with laser-Doppler technology. In general, they found that tumors had lower CBF than normal brain did. Autoregulation was occasionally apparent, and CO_2 responsiveness was usually present. The investigation of Schregel and coworkers, who measured MCA velocity and vessel area in tumor patients, also revealed that CO_2 responsiveness was occasionally abnormal and that ipsilateral to the tumor, hyperventilation was sometimes associated with paradoxical increases in MCA flow velocity.[591] Animal experiments have shown that regional CBF and CBV are higher in the tumor region and that the response to hyperventilation (reduction in CBF and CBV) is preserved.[328] Measurement of regional CBF in the area of the tumor might also be a useful predictor of the grade of intracranial gliomas; both regional CBF and regional CBV are greater with higher-grade gliomas.[592] Considerable edema is often found in association with intracranial tumors. Bedford and coworkers[593] showed that the radiologic extent of the edema (which presumably represents the extent of abnormal vessel leakiness) correlated with the severity of the elevation in ICP that occurred in association with intubation-related hypertension. Empirically, the edema associated with tumors is improved by steroids,[594] and a reduction in tumor edema is accompanied by a reduction in regional CBF.[595] In patients with intracranial tumors,[596] BBB function is improved by the administration of dexamethasone over a time course as short as 6 hours. See Chapter 53 for a complete discussion.

Coma and Epilepsy

Coma, regardless of its etiology, is associated with reductions in brain metabolism. In the case of lesions occurring in the reticular activating system, the reduction in CMR probably represents a normal physiologic adjustment to reduced functional activity. During generalized seizure activity, CMR and CBF may increase dramatically.[411] The intensive motor and brain activity associated with generalized seizures leads to the development of systemic and cerebral acidosis, often accompanied by a reduction in arterial oxygenation, an increase in $Paco_2$, and peripheral lactic acidosis. If generalized seizure activity continues unabated, arterial hypotension ensues. With muscular relaxation and measures ensuring adequate oxygenation and ventilation, the systemic acidosis and hypotension can be avoided and the severity of cerebral acidosis diminished. During relatively brief episodes of continuous seizures, the brain seems able to meet the high metabolic demands.[411] However, even with effective ventilation and maintenance of perfusion pressure, when seizures continue for a prolonged period, they can lead to the development of irreversible neuronal damage.[597] Therapy aimed at interrupting the seizure and restoring a normal balance between cerebral metabolic demand and blood flow is indicated. Barbiturates, benzodiazepines, or other potent anticonvulsants are appropriate. Adequate ventilation, oxygenation, and maintenance of blood pressure are important adjunctive measures. Muscle relaxants must be viewed as purely symptomatic therapy because they do not alter the abnormal cerebral electrical activity.

The potentially injurious nature of seizures justifies attention to prevention. Practices vary. However, patients who have sustained a severe head injury or subarachnoid hemorrhage and any patient in whom a substantial cortical incision is planned are at risk, and prophylactic anticonvulsants should be considered.

KEY POINTS

1. The brain has a rapid metabolic rate, and it receives approximately 15% of the cardiac output. Under normal circumstances, CBF is approximately 50 mL/100 g/min. The gray matter receives 80% and the white matter receives 20% of this blood flow.

2. Approximately 60% of the brain's energy consumption is used to support electrophysiologic function. The remainder of the energy consumed by the brain is involved in cellular homeostatic activities.

3. CBF is tightly coupled to local cerebral metabolism. When cerebral activity in a particular region of the brain increases, a corresponding increase in blood flow to that region occurs. Conversely, suppression of cerebral metabolism leads to a reduction in blood flow.

4. CBF is autoregulated and maintained constant over a MAP range of 65 to 150 mm Hg. CBF is pressure passive when MAP is either below the lower limit or above the upper limit of autoregulation.

5. CBF is also under chemical regulation. It varies directly with arterial carbon dioxide tension ($Paco_2$) in the range of 25 to 70 mm Hg. With a reduction in Pao_2 to less than 60 mm Hg, CBF increases dramatically. Changes in temperature affect CBF primarily by suppression of cerebral metabolism.

6. Systemic vasodilators (nitroglycerin, nitroprusside, hydralazine, calcium channel blockers) vasodilate the cerebral circulation and can, depending on MAP, increase CBF. Vasopressors such as phenylephrine, norepinephrine, ephedrine, and dopamine do not have significant direct effects on cerebral circulation. Their effect on CBF is dependent on their effect on systemic blood pressure. When MAP is less than the lower limit of autoregulation, vasopressors increase systemic pressure and thereby increase CBF. If systemic pressure is within the limits of autoregulation, vasopressor-induced increases in systemic pressure have little effect on CBF.

7. All modern volatile anesthetics suppress CMR and, with the exception of halothane, can produce burst suppression of the EEG. At that level, CMR is reduced by about 60%. Volatile agents have dose-dependent effects on CBF. In sub-MAC doses, CBF is not significantly altered. Beyond 1 MAC doses, direct cerebral vasodilation results in an increase in CBF.

8. Barbiturates, etomidate, and propofol decrease CMR and can produce burst suppression of the EEG. At that level, CMR is reduced by about 60%. Flow and metabolism coupling is preserved, and therefore CBF is decreased. Opiates and benzodiazepines effect minor decreases in CBF and CMR, whereas ketamine

can increase CMR (with a corresponding increase in blood flow) significantly.

9. Brain stores of oxygen and substrates are limited, and the brain is exquisitely sensitive to reductions in CBF. Severe reductions in CBF (<10 mL/100 g/min) lead to rapid neuronal death. Ischemic injury is characterized by early excitotoxicity and delayed apoptosis.

10. Barbiturates, propofol, ketamine, and the volatile anesthetics have neuroprotective efficacy and can reduce ischemic cerebral injury. In the case of volatile anesthetics, the reduction in cerebral injury is transient, and long-term protection of neurons is not achieved. Etomidate administration is associated with regional reductions in CBF, which can exacerbate ischemic brain injury.

REFERENCES

1. Michenfelder JD: Anesthesia and the Brain: Clinical, Functional, Metabolic, and Vascular Correlates. New York, Churchill Livingstone, 1988.
2. Moncada S, Palmer RMJ, Higgs EA: Nitric oxide: Physiology, pathophysiology, and pharmacology. Pharmacol Rev 43:109-142, 1991.
3. Snyder SH, Bredt DS: Biological roles of nitric oxide. Sci Am 266:68-71, 74-77, 1992.
4. Wang Q, Pelligrino DA, Baughman VL, et al: The role of neuronal nitric oxide synthase in regulation of cerebral blood flow in normocapnia and hypercapnia in rats. J Cereb Blood Flow Metab 15:774-778, 1995.
5. McPherson RW, Kirsch JR, Ghaly RF, Traystman RJ: Effect of nitric oxide synthase inhibition on the cerebral vascular response to hypercapnia in primates. Stroke 26:682-687, 1995.
6. Ayata C, Ma J, Meng W, et al: L-NA–sensitive rCBF augmentation during vibrissal stimulation in type III nitric oxide synthase mutant mice. J Cereb Blood Flow Metab 16:539-541, 1996.
7. Cholet N, Seylaz J, Lacombe P, Bonvento G: Local uncoupling of the cerebrovascular and metabolic responses to somatosensory stimulation after neuronal nitric oxide synthase inhibition. J Cereb Blood Flow Metab 17:1191-1201, 1997.
8. McPherson RW, Kirsch JR, Traystman RJ: Effect of N-nitro-L-arginine on cerebral vasodilation by halothane and isoflurane [abstract]. Anesthesiology 77:A173, 1992.
9. Koenig HM, Pelligrino DA, Albrecht RF: Halothane vasodilatation and nitric oxide in rat pial vessels [abstract]. Anesthesiology 77:A751, 1992.
10. Koenig HM, Pelligrino DA, Wang Q, Albrecht RF: Role of nitric oxide and endothelium in rat pial vessel dilation response to isoflurane. Anesth Analg 79:886-891, 1994.
11. Iadecola C: Nitric oxide participates in the cerebrovasodilation elicited from cerebellar fastigial nucleus. Am J Physiol 263:R1156-R1161, 1992.
12. Raszkiewicz JL, Linville DG, Kerwin JF, et al: Nitric oxide synthase is critical in mediating basal forebrain regulation of cortical cerebral circulation. J Neurosci Res 33:129-135, 1992.
13. Kimura T, Yu J-G, Edvinsson L, Lee TJ-F: Cholinergic, nitric oxidergic innervation in cerebral arteries of the cat. Brain Res 773:117-124, 1997.
14. Lou HC, Edvinsson L, MacKenzie ET: The concept of coupling blood flow to brain function: Revision required? Ann Neurol 22:289-297, 1987.
15. Miyauchi Y, Sakabe T, Maekawa Y, et al: Responses of EEG, cerebral oxygen consumption and blood flow to peripheral nerve stimulation during thiopentone anaesthesia in the dog. Can Anaesth Soc J 32:491-498, 1985.
16. Cameron OG, Modell JG, Hichwa RD, et al: Changes in sensory-cognitive input: Effects on cerebral blood flow. J Cereb Blood Flow Metab 10:38-42, 1990.
17. Frostig RD, Lieke EE, Ts'o DY, Grinvald A: Cortical functional architecture and local coupling between neuronal activity and the microcirculation revealed by in vivo high-resolution optical imaging of intrinsic signals. Proc Natl Acad Sci U S A 87:6082-6086, 1990.
18. Perlmutter JS, Lich LL, Margenau W, Bucholz S: PET measured evoked cerebral blood flow responses in an awake monkey. J Cereb Blood Flow Metab 11:229-235, 1991.
19. Hyder F, Behar KL, Martin MA, et al: Dynamic magnetic resonance imaging of the rat brain during forepaw stimulation. J Cereb Blood Flow Metab 14:649-655, 1994.
20. Bonvento G, Lacombe P, Seylaz J: Effects of electrical stimulation of the dorsal raphe nucleus on local cerebral blood flow in the rat. J Cereb Blood Flow Metab 9:251-255, 1989.
21. Michenfelder J: The interdependency of cerebral function and metabolic effects following massive doses of thiopental in the dog. Anesthesiology 41:231-236, 1974.
22. Newberg LA, Milde JH, Michenfelder JD: The cerebral metabolic effects of isoflurane at and above concentrations that suppress cortical electrical activity. Anesthesiology 59:23-28, 1983.
23. Scheller MS, Tateishi A, Drummond JC, Zornow MH: The effects of sevoflurane on cerebral blood flow, cerebral metabolic rate for oxygen, intracranial pressure, and the electroencephalogram are similar to those of isoflurane in the rabbit. Anesthesiology 68:548-551, 1988.
24. Rampil IJ, Laster M, Dwyer RC, et al: No EEG evidence of acute tolerance to desflurane in swine. Anesthesiology 74:889-892, 1991.
25. Bruhn J, Bouillon T, Shafer S: Onset of propofol-induced burst suppression may be correctly detected as deepening of anaesthesia by approximate entropy but not by bispectral index. Br J Anaesth 87:505-507, 2002.
26. Milde LN, Milde JH, Michenfelder JD: Cerebral functional, metabolic and hemodynamic effects of etomidate in dogs. Anesthesiology 63:371-377, 1985.
27. Maekawa T, Tommasino C, Shapiro HM, et al: Local cerebral blood flow and glucose utilization during isoflurane anesthesia in the rat. Anesthesiology 65:144-151, 1986.
28. Hansen TD, Warner DS, Todd MM, et al: Distribution of cerebral blood flow during halothane versus isoflurane anesthesia in rats. Anesthesiology 69:332-337, 1988.
29. Reinstrup P, Ryding E, Algotsson L, et al: Distribution of cerebral blood flow during anesthesia with isoflurane or halothane in humans. Anesthesiology 82:359-366, 1995.
30. Drummond JC, Todd MM, U HS: The effect of high dose sodium thiopental on brain stem auditory and median nerve somatosensory evoked potentials in humans. Anesthesiology 63:249-254, 1985.
31. Peterson DO, Drummond JC, Todd MM: The effects of halothane, enflurane, isoflurane, and nitrous oxide on somatosensory evoked potentials in humans. Anesthesiology 65:35-40, 1986.
32. Akrawi WP, Drummond JC, Kalkman CJ, Patel PM: A comparison of the electrophysiologic characteristics of EEG burst-suppression as produced by isoflurane, thiopental, etomidate and propofol. J Neurosurg Anesthesiol 8:40-46, 1996.
33. Maher J, Hachinski V: Hypothermia as a potential treatment for cerebral ischemia. Cerebrovasc Brain Metab Rev 5:277-300, 1993.
34. Kataoka K, Mitani A, Yanese H, et al: Ischemic neuronal damage: How does mild hypothermia modulate it? Mol Clin Neuropathol 28:191-195, 1996.
35. Nemoto EM, Klementavicius R, Melick JA, Yonas H: Suppression of cerebral metabolic rate for oxygen ($CMRO_2$) by mild hypothermia compared with thiopental. J Neurosurg Anesthesiol 8:52-59, 1996.
36. Klementavicius R, Nemoto EM, Yonas H: The Q10 ratio basal cerebral metabolic rate for oxygen in rats. J Neurosurg 85:482-487, 1996.

37. Busija DW, Leffler CW, Pourcyrous M: Hyperthermia increases cerebral metabolic rate and blood flow in neonatal pigs. Am J Physiol 255:H343-H346, 1988.
38. Smith AL, Wollman H: Cerebral blood flow and metabolism: Effects of anesthetic drugs and techniques. Anesthesiology 36:378-400, 1972.
39. Sato M, Pawlik G, Heiss WD: Comparative studies of regional CNS blood flow autoregulation and responses to CO_2 in the cat. Stroke 15:91-97, 1984.
40. Koehler RC, Traystman RJ: Bicarbonate ion modulation of cerebral blood flow during hypoxia and hypercapnia. Am J Physiol 243:H33-H40, 1982.
41. Iadecola C, Zhang F: Nitric oxide–dependent and –independent components of cerebrovasodilation elicited by hypercapnia. Am J Physiol 266:R546-R552, 1994.
42. Iadecola C, Xu X: Nitro-L-arginine attenuates hypercapnic cerebrovasodilation without affecting cerebral metabolism. Am J Physiol 266:R518-R525, 1994.
43. Smith JJ, Lee JG, Hudetz AG, et al: The role of nitric oxide in the cerebrovascular response to hypercapnia. Anesth Analg 84:363-369, 1997.
44. Schmetterer L, Findl O, Strenn K, et al: Role of NO in the O_2 and CO_2 responsiveness of cerebral and ocular circulation in humans. Am J Physiol 273:R2005-R2012, 1997.
45. Heinert G, Nye P, Paterson D: Nitric oxide and prostaglandin pathways interact in the regulation of hypercapnic cerebral vasodilation. Acta Physiol Scand 166:183-193, 1999.
46. Albrecht RF, Miletich DJ, Madala LR: Normalization of cerebral blood flow during prolonged halothane anesthesia. Anesthesiology 58:26-31, 1983.
47. Raichle ME, Posner JB, Plum F: Cerebral blood flow during and after hyperventilation. Arch Neurol 23:394-403, 1970.
48. Plum F, Siesjo BK: Recent advances in CSF physiology. Anesthesiology 42:708-730, 1975.
49. Hudetz AG, Shen H, Kampine JP: Nitric oxide from neuronal NOS plays a critical role in cerebral capillary flow response to hypoxia. Am J Physiol 274:H982-H989, 1998.
50. Golanov E, Reis DJ: Oxygen sensitive neurons of the rostral ventrolateral medulla contribute to hypoxic cerebral vasodilation. J Physiol (Lond) 495:201-216, 1996.
51. Omae T, Ibayashi S, Kusuda K, et al: Effects of high atmospheric pressure and oxygen on middle cerebral blood flow velocity in humans measured by transcranial Doppler. Stroke 29:94-97, 1998.
52. Jacobson I, Harper AM, McDowall DG: The effects of oxygen at 1 and 2 atmospheres on the blood flow and oxygen uptake of the cerebral cortex. Surg Gynecol Obstet 119:737-742, 1964.
53. Drummond JC: The lower limit of autoregulation: Time to revise our thinking [letter]? Anesthesiology 86:1431-1433, 1997.
54. Strandgaard S: Autoregulation of cerebral blood flow in hypertensive patients. The modifying influence of prolonged antihypertensive treatment on the tolerance to acute, drug-induced hypotension. Circulation 53:720-727, 1976.
55. Waldemar G, Schmidt JF, Andersen AR, et al: Angiotensin converting enzyme inhibition and cerebral blood flow autoregulation in normotensive and hypertensive man. J Hypertens 7:229-235, 1989.
56. Larsen FS, Olsen KS, Hansen BA, et al: Transcranial Doppler is valid for determination of the lower limit of cerebral blood flow autoregulation. Stroke 25:1985-1988, 1994.
57. Olsen KS, Svenden LB, Larsen FS, Paulson OB: Effect of labetalol on cerebral blood flow, oxygen metabolism and autoregulation in healthy humans. Br J Anaesth 75:51-54, 1995.
58. Olsen KS, Svendsen LB, Larsen FS: Validation of transcranial near-infrared spectroscopy for evaluation of cerebral blood flow autoregulation. J Neurosurg Anesthesiol 8:280-285, 1996.
59. Greenfield JC, Rembert JC, Tindall GT: Transient changes in cerebral vascular resistance during the Valsalva maneuver in man. Stroke 15:76-79, 1984.
60. Toyoda K, Fujii K, Ibayashi S, et al: Role of nitric oxide in regulation of brain stem circulation during hypotension. J Cereb Blood Flow Metab 17:1089-1096, 1997.
61. Kobari M, Fukuuchi Y, Tomita M, et al: Role of nitric oxide in regulation of cerebral microvascular tone and autoregulation of cerebral blood flow in cats. Brain Res 667:255-262, 1994.
62. Thompson BG, Pluta RM, Girton ME, Oldfield EH: Nitric oxide mediation of chemoregulation but not autoregulation of cerebral blood flow in primates. J Neurosurg 84:71-78, 1996.
63. Branston NM: Neurogenic control of the cerebral circulation. Cerebrovasc Brain Metab Rev 7:338-349, 1995.
64. Dahl E: The innervation of the cerebral arteries. J Anat 115:53-63, 1973.
65. Hara H, Zhang Q-J, Kuroyanagi T, Kobayashi S: Parasympathetic cerebrovascular innervation: An anterograde tracing from the sphenopalatine ganglion in the rat. Neurosurgery 32:822-827, 1993.
66. Sato A, Sato Y: Cerebral cortical vasodilatation in response to stimulation of cholinergic fibres originating in the nucleus basalis of Meynert. J Auton Nerv Syst 30(Suppl):S137-S140, 1990.
67. Adachi T, Biesold D, Inanami O, Sato A: Stimulation of the nucleus basalis of Meynert and substantia innominata produces widespread increases in cerebral blood flow in the frontal, parietal and occipital cortices. Brain Res 514:163-166, 1990.
68. Iadecola C, Reis DJ: Continuous monitoring of cerebrocortical blood flow during stimulation of the cerebellar fastigial nucleus: A study by laser-Doppler flowmetry. J Cereb Blood Flow Metab 10:608-617, 1990.
69. Tuor UI: Local distribution of the effects of sympathetic stimulation on cerebral blood flow in the rat. Brain Res 529:224-231, 1990.
70. Reddy SVR, Yaksh TL, Anderson RE Jr, Sundt TM Jr: Effect in cat of locus coeruleus lesions on the response of cerebral blood flow and cardiac output to altered $PaCO_2$. Brain Res 365:278-288, 1985.
71. Edvinsson L, Dequeurce A, Duverger D, et al: Central serotonergic nerves project to the pial vessels of the brain. Nature 306:55-57, 1983.
72. Underwood MD, Bakalian MJ, Arango V, et al: Regulation of cortical blood flow by the dorsal raphe nucleus: Topographic organization of cerebrovascular regulatory regions. J Cereb Blood Flow Metab 12:664-673, 1992.
73. Hara H, Jansen I, Ekman R, et al: Acetylcholine and vasoactive intestinal peptide in cerebral blood vessels: Effect of extirpation of the sphenopalatine ganglion. J Cereb Blood Flow Metab 9:204-211, 1989.
74. Busija DW: Sympathetic nerves reduce cerebral blood flow during hypoxia in awake rabbits. Am J Physiol 247:H446-H451, 1984.
75. Auer LM, Edvinsson L, Johansson BB: Effect of sympathetic nerve stimulation and adrenoceptor blockade on pial arterial and venous calibre and on intracranial pressure in the cat. Acta Physiol Scand 119:213-217, 1983.
76. MacKenzie ET, McGeorge AD, Graham DI, et al: Effects of increasing arterial pressure on cerebral blood flow in the baboon, influence of the sympathetic nervous system. Pflugers Arch 378:189-195, 1979.
77. Bevan JA: Autonomic pharmacologist's guide to the cerebral circulation. Trends Pharmacol Sci 5:234-236, 1984.
78. Fitch W, MacKenzie ET, Harper AM: Effects of decreasing arterial blood pressure on cerebral blood flow in the baboon. Influence of the sympathetic nervous system. Circ Res 37:550-557, 1975.
79. Johansson BB, Auer LM: Neurogenic modification of the vulnerability of the blood-brain-barrier during acute hypertension in conscious rats. Acta Physiol Scand 117:507-511, 1983.
80. Tuor UI: Acute hypertension and sympathetic stimulation: Local heterogeneous changes in cerebral blood flow. Am J Physiol 263:H511-H518, 1992.
81. Reis DJ, Berger SB, Underwood MD, Khayata M: Electrical stimulation of cerebellar fastigial nucleus reduces ischemic infarction elicited by middle cerebral artery occlusion in rat. J Cereb Blood Flow Metab 11:810-818, 1991.

82. Koketsu N, Moskowitz MA, Kontos HA, et al: Chronic parasympathetic sectioning decreases regional cerebral blood flow during hemorrhagic hypotension and increases infarct size after middle cerebral artery occlusion in spontaneously hypertensive rats. J Cereb Blood Flow Metab 12:613-620, 1992.

83. Shibata M, Einhaus S, Schweitzer JB, et al: Cerebral blood flow decreased by adrenergic stimulation of cerebral vessels in anesthetized newborn pigs with traumatic brain injury. J Neurosurg 79:696-704, 1993.

84. MacFarlane R, Moskowitz MA, Sakas DE, et al: The role of neuroeffector mechanisms in cerebral hyperperfusion syndromes. J Neurosurg 75:845-855, 1991.

85. Harrison MG: Influence of haematocrit in the cerebral circulation. Cerebrovasc Brain Metab Rev 1:55-67, 1989.

86. Thomas DJ, Marshall J, Russell RW, et al: Effect of haematocrit on cerebral blood-flow in man. Lancet 2:941-943, 1977.

87. Cole DJ, Drummond JC, Patel PM, Marcantonio S: Effects of viscosity and oxygen content on cerebral blood flow in ischemic and normal rat brain. J Neurol Sci 124:15-20, 1994.

88. Cole DJ, Drummond JC, Shapiro HM, et al: The effect of hypervolemic-hemodilution with and without hypertension on cerebral blood flow following middle cerebral artery occlusion in the rat. Anesthesiology 71:580-585, 1989.

89. Korosue K, Ishida K, Matsuoka H, et al: Clinical, hemodynamic, and hemorrheological effects of isovolemic hemodilution in acute cerebral infarction. Neurosurgery 23:148-153, 1988.

90. Origitano TC, Wascher TM, Reichman H, Anderson DE: Sustained increased cerebral blood flow with prophylactic hypertensive hypervolemic hemodilution ("triple-H" therapy) after subarachnoid hemorrhage. Neurosurg 27:729-740, 1990.

91. Korosue K, Heros RC: Mechanism of cerebral blood flow augmentation by hemodilution in rabbits. Stroke 23:1487-1493, 1992.

92. Kee DB, Wood JH: Rheology of the cerebral circulation. Neurosurgery 15:125-131, 1984.

93. Lee SH, Heros RC, Mullan JC, Korosue K: Optimum degree of hemodilution for brain protection in a canine model of focal cerebral ischemia. J Neurosurg 80:469-475, 1994.

94. Aichner FT, Fazekas F, Brainin M, et al: Hypervolemic hemodilution in acute ischemic stroke: The Multicenter Austrian Hemodilution Stroke Trial (MAHST). Stroke 29:743-749, 1998.

95. Maekawa T, McDowall DG, Okuda Y: Brain-surface oxygen tension and cerebral cortical blood flow during hemorrhagic and drug-induced hypotension in the cat. Anesthesiology 51:313-320, 1979.

96. Akopov S, Simonian N: Comparison of isradipine and enalapril effects on regional carotid circulation in patients with hypertension with unilateral carotid artery stenosis. J Cardiovasc Pharmacol 30:562-570, 1997.

97. Marsh ML, Shapiro HM, Smith RW, Marshall LF: Changes in neurologic status and intracranial pressure associated with sodium nitroprusside administration. Anesthesiology 51:336-338, 1979.

98. Olesen J: The effect of intracarotid epinephrine, norepinephrine, and angiotensin on the regional cerebral blood flow in man. Neurology 22:978-987, 1972.

99. MacKenzie ET, McCulloch J, O'Keane M, et al: Cerebral circulation and norepinephrine: Relevance of the blood-brain barrier. Am J Physiol 231:483-488, 1976.

100. Rogers AT, Stump DA, Gravlee GP, et al: Response of cerebral blood flow to phenylephrine infusion during hypothermic cardiopulmonary bypass: Influence of Pa_{CO_2} management. Anesthesiology 69:547-551, 1988.

101. Drummond JC, Oh Y-S, Cole DJ, Shapiro HM: Phenylephrine-induced hypertension decreases the area of ischemia following middle cerebral artery occlusion in the rat. Stroke 20:1538-1544, 1989.

102. Berntman L, Dahlgren N, Siesjo BK: Influence of intravenously administered catecholamines on cerebral oxygen consumption and blood flow in the rat. Acta Physiol Scand 104:101-108, 1978.

103. Tuor UI, Edvinsson L, McCulloch J: Catecholamines and the relationship between cerebral blood flow and glucose use. Am J Physiol 251:H824-H833, 1986.

104. Sokrab TE, Johansson BB: Regional cerebral blood flow in acute hypertension induced by adrenaline, noradrenaline and phenylephrine in the conscious rat. Acta Physiol Scand 137:101-106, 1989.

105. Ekstrom-Jodal B, von Essen C, Haggendal E: Effects of noradrenaline on the cerebral blood flow in the dog. Acta Neurol Scand 50:11-26, 1974.

106. von Essen C: Effects of dopamine, noradrenaline and 5-hydroxytryptamine on the cerebral blood flow in the dog. J Pharm Pharmacol 24:668, 1972.

107. Oberdorster G, Lang R, Zimmer R: Direct effects of alpha- and beta-sympathomimetic amines on the cerebral circulation of the dog. Pflugers Arch 340:145-160, 1973.

108. Lluch S, Reimann C, Glick G: Evidence for the direct effect of adrenergic drugs on the cerebral vascular bed of the unanesthetized goat. Stroke 4:50-56, 1973.

109. Nemoto EM, Klementavicius R, Melick JA, Yonas H: Norepinephrine activation of basal cerebral metabolic rate for oxygen ($CMRO_2$) during hypothermia in rats. Anesth Analg 83:1262-1267, 1996.

110. Artru A, Nugent M, Michenfelder JD: Anesthetics affect the cerebral metabolic response to circulatory catecholamines. J Neurochem 36:1941-1946, 1981.

111. Bryan RM: Cerebral blood flow and energy metabolism during stress. Am J Physiol 259:H269-H280, 1990.

112. Sercombe R, Aubineau P, Edvinsson L, et al: Pharmacological evidence in vitro and in vivo for functional beta$_1$ receptors in the cerebral circulation. Pflugers Arch 368:241-244, 1977.

113. King BD, Sokoloff L, Wechsler RL: The effects of l-epinephrine and l-norepinephrine upon cerebral circulation and metabolism in man. J Clin Invest 31:273-279, 1951.

114. Abdul-Rahman A, Dahlgren N, Johansson BB, Siesjö BK: Increase in local cerebral blood flow induced by circulating adrenaline: Involvement of blood-brain barrier dysfunction. Acta Physiol Scand 107:227-232, 1979.

115. Madsen PL, Vorstrup S, Schmidt JF, Paulson OB: Effect of acute and prolonged treatment with propranolol on cerebral blood flow and cerebral oxygen metabolism in healthy volunteers. Eur J Clin Pharmacol 39:295-297, 1990.

116. Schroeder T, Schierbeck J, Howardy P, et al: Effect of labetalol on cerebral blood flow and middle cerebral arterial flow velocity in healthy volunteers. Neurol Res 13:10-12, 1991.

117. Dubois M, Caputy A, MacCosbe P, et al: Cerebral blood flow measurements during blood pressure control with intravenous labetalol following craniotomy. J Neurosurg Anesthesiol 4:176-181, 1992.

118. Howie MB, Black HA, Zvara D, et al: Esmolol reduces autonomic hypersensitivity and length of seizures induced by electroconvulsive therapy. Anesth Analg 71:384-388, 1990.

119. Bunegin L, Albin MS, Gelineau EF: Effect of esmolol on cerebral blood flow during intracranial hypertension and hemorrhagic hypovolemia [abstract]. Anesthesiology 67:A424, 1987.

120. von Essen C, Zervas NT, Brown DR, et al: Local cerebral blood flow in the dog during intravenous infusion of dopamine. Surg Neurol 13:181-188, 1980.

121. von Essen C: Effects of dopamine on the cerebral blood flow in the dog. Acta Neurol Scand 50:39-52, 1974.

122. Toda N: Dopamine vasodilates human cerebral artery. Experientia 39:1131-1132, 1983.

123. Bandres J, Yao L, Nemoto EM, et al: Effects of dobutamine and dopamine on whole brain blood flow and metabolism in unanesthetized monkeys. J Neurosurg Anesthesiol 4:250-256, 1992.

124. Townsend JB, Ziedonis DM, Bryan RM, et al: Choroid plexus blood flow: Evidence for dopaminergic influence. Brain Res 290:165-169, 1984.

125. Karlsson B, Forsman M, Roald OK, et al: Effect of dexmedetomidine, a selective and potent alpha2-agonist, on cerebral blood flow and oxygen consumption during halothane anesthesia in dogs. Anesth Analg 71:125-129, 1990.

126. James IM, Larbi E, Zaimis E: The effect of acute intravenous administration of clonidine on cerebral blood flow in man. Br J Pharmacol 39:198P-199P, 1970.

127. Kanawati IS, Yaksh TL, Anderson RE, Marsh RW: Effects of clonidine on cerebral blood flow and the response to arterial CO_2. J Cereb Blood Flow Metab 6:358-365, 1985.

128. Crosby G, Russo MA, Szabo MD, Davies KR: Subarachnoid clonidine reduces spinal cord blood flow and glucose utilization in conscious rats. Anesthesiology 73:1179-1185, 1990.

129. Lee H-W, Caldwell JE, Dodson B, et al: The effect of clonidine on cerebral blood flow velocity, carbon dioxide cerebral vasoreactivity, and response to increased arterial pressure in human volunteers. Anesthesiology 87:553-558, 1997.

130. Coughlan MG, Lee JG, Bosnjak ZJ, et al: Direct coronary and cerebral vascular responses to dexmedetomidine: Significance of endogenous nitric oxide synthesis. Anesthesiology 77:998-1006, 1992.

131. Busija DW, Leffler CW: Exogenous norepinephrine constricts cerebral arterioles via α_2-adrenoceptors in newborn pigs. J Cereb Blood Flow Metab 7:184-188, 1987.

132. Zornow MH, Maze M, Dyck JB, Shafer SL: Dexmedetomidine decreases cerebral blood flow velocity in humans. J Cereb Blood Flow Metab 13:350-353, 1993.

133. Prielipp RC, Wall MH, Tobin JR, et al: Dexmedetomidine-induced sedation in volunteers decreases regional and global cerebral blood flow. Anesth Analg 95:1052-1059, 2002.

134. Marchal G, Rioux P, Petit-Taboué M-C, et al: Regional cerebral oxygen consumption, blood flow, and blood volume in healthy human aging. Arch Neurol 49:1013-1020, 1992.

135. Meyer JS, Terayama Y, Takashima S: Cerebral circulation in the elderly. Cerebrovasc Brain Metabol Rev 5:122-146, 1993.

136. Todd MM, Weeks J: Comparative effects of propofol, pentobarbital, and isoflurane on cerebral blood flow and blood volume. J Neurosurg Anesthesiol 8:296-303, 1996.

137. Powers WJ, Raichle ME: Positron emission tomography and its application to the study of cerebrovascular disease in man. Stroke 16:361-365, 1985.

138. Greenberg JH, Alavi A, Reivich M, et al: Local cerebral blood volume response to carbon dioxide in man. Circ Res 43:324-331, 1978.

139. Grubb RL, Raichle ME, Eichling JO, Ter-Pogossian MM: The effects of changes in $Paco_2$ on cerebral blood volume, blood flow, and vascular mean transit time. Stroke 5:630-639, 1974.

140. Gibbs JM, Wise RJS, Leenders KL, Jones T: Evaluation of cerebral perfusion reserve in patients with carotid-artery occlusion. Lancet 1:310-314, 1984.

141. Montgomery EB, Grubb RL, Raichle ME: Cerebral hemodynamics and metabolism in postoperative cerebral vasospasm and treatment with hypertensive therapy. Ann Neurol 9:503-506, 1981.

142. Ferrari M, Wilson DA, Hanley DF, Traystman RJ: Effects of graded hypotension on cerebral blood flow, blood volume, and mean transit time in dogs. Am J Physiol 262:H1908-H1914, 1992.

143. Lanier WL, Warner DO: Intracranial elastance versus intracranial compliance: Terminology should agree with that of other disciplines [letter]. Anesthesiology 77:403-404, 1992.

144. Artru AA: Relationship between cerebral blood volume and CSF pressure during anesthesia with isoflurane or fentanyl in dogs. Anesthesiology 60:575-579, 1984.

145. Artru AA: Relationship between cerebral blood volume and CSF pressure during anesthesia with halothane or enflurane in dogs. Anesthesiology 58:533-539, 1983.

146. Archer DP, Labreque P, Tyler JL, et al: Cerebral blood volume is increased in dogs during administration of nitrous oxide or isoflurane. Anesthesiology 67:642-648, 1987.

147. Weeks JB, Todd MM, Warner DS, Katz J: The influence of halothane, isoflurane, and pentobarbital on cerebral plasma volume in hypocapnic and normocapnic rats. Anesthesiology 73:461-466, 1990.

148. Ulrich K, Kuschinsky W: In vivo effects of alpha-adrenoceptor agonists and antagonists on pial veins of cats. Stroke 16:880-884, 1985.

149. Pierce EC, Lambertsen CJ, Deutsch S, et al: Cerebral circulation and metabolism during thiopental anesthesia and hyperventilation in man. J Clin Invest 41:1664-1671, 1962.

150. Stephan H, Sonntag H, Schenk HD, Kohlhausen S: Effects of Disoprivan (propofol) on the circulation and oxygen consumption of the brain and CO_2 reactivity of brain vessels in the human [in German]. Anaesthesist 36:60-65, 1987.

151. Renou AM, Vernhiet J, Macrez P, et al: Cerebral blood flow and metabolism during etomidate anaesthesia in man. Br J Anaesth 50:1047-1050, 1978.

152. Jobes DR, Kennell EM, Bush GL, et al: Cerebral blood flow and metabolism during morphine–nitrous oxide anesthesia in man. Anesthesiology 47:16-18, 1977.

153. Vernhiet J, Macrez P, Renou AM, et al: Effets des fortes doses de morphinomimetiques (fentanyl et fentathienyl) sur la circulation cerebrale du sujet normal. Ann Anesth Franc 18:803-810, 1977.

154. Stephan H, Groger P, Weyland A, et al: The effect of sufentanil on cerebral blood flow, cerebral metabolism and the CO_2 reactivity of the cerebral vessels in man [in German]. Anaesthesist 40:153-160, 1991.

155. Cotev S, Shalit MN: Effects of diazepam on cerebral blood flow and oxygen uptake after head injury. Anesthesiology 43:117-122, 1975.

156. Forster A, Juge O, Morel D: Effects of midazolam on cerebral blood flow in human volunteers. Anesthesiology 56:453-455, 1982.

157. Takeshita H, Okuda Y, Sari A: The effects of ketamine on cerebral circulation and metabolism in man. Anesthesiology 36:69-75, 1972.

158. Paris A, Scholz J, von Knobelsdorff G, et al: The effect of remifentanil on cerebral blood flow velocity. Anesth Analg 87:569-573, 1998.

159. Kofke WA, Attaallah AF, Kuwabara H, et al: The neuropathologic effects in rats and neurometabolic effects in humans of large dose remifentanil. Anesth Analg 94:1229-1236, 2002.

160. Zornow MH, Fleischer JE, Scheller MS, et al: Dexmedetomidine, an alpha 2 adrenergic agonist, decreases cerebral blood flow in the isoflurane anesthetized dog. Anesth Analg 70:624-630, 1990.

161. Marin J, Lobato RD, Rico ML, et al: Effect of pentobarbital on the reactivity of isolated human cerebral arteries. J Neurosurg 54:521-524, 1981.

162. Ogura K, Takayasu M, Dacey RG: Differential effects of pentobarbital on intracerebral arterioles and venules of rats in vitro. Neurosurgery 28:537-541, 1991.

163. Moriyama S, Nakamura K, Hatano Y, et al: Responses to barbiturates of isolated dog cerebral and mesenteric arteries contracted with KCl and prostaglandin $F_{2\alpha}$. Acta Anaesthesiol Scand 34:523-529, 1990.

164. Stulken EH, Milde JH, Michenfelder JD, Tinker JH: The nonlinear responses of cerebrospinal metabolism to low concentrations of halothane, enflurane, isoflurane, and thiopental. Anesthesiology 46:28-34, 1977.

165. Albrecht RF, Miletich DJ, Rosenberg R, Zahed B: Cerebral blood flow and metabolic changes from induction to onset of anesthesia with halothane or pentobarbital. Anesthesiology 47:252-256, 1977.

166. Astrup J, Rosenorn J, Cold GE, et al: Minimum cerebral blood flow and metabolism during craniotomy. Effect of thiopental loading. Acta Anaesthesiol Scand 28:478-481, 1984.

167. Astrup J, Sørensen PM, Sørensen HR: Inhibition of cerebral oxygen and glucose consumption in the dog by hypothermia, pentobarbital, and lidocaine. Anesthesiology 55:263-268, 1981.

168. Altenburg BM, Michenfelder JD, Theye RA: Acute tolerance to thiopental in canine cerebral oxygen consumption studies. Anesthesiology 31:443-457, 1969.
169. Gronert GA, Michenfelder JD, Sharbrough FW, Milde JH: Canine cerebral metabolic tolerance during 24 hours of deep pentobarbital anesthesia. Anesthesiology 55:110-113, 1981.
170. Sawada Y, Sugimoto H, Kobayash H, et al: Acute tolerance to high-dose barbiturate treatment in patients with severe head injuries. Anesthesiology 56:53-54, 1982.
171. Reivich M: Regulation of the cerebral circulation. Clin Neurosurg 1:378-418, 1969.
172. Kassell NF, Hitchon PW, Gerk MK, et al: Influence of changes in arterial pco_2 on cerebral blood flow and metabolism during high-dose barbiturate therapy in dogs. J Neurosurg 54:615-619, 1981.
173. Vandesteene A, Trempont V, Engelman E, et al: Effect of propofol on cerebral blood flow and metabolism in man. Anaesthesia 43:42-43, 1988.
174. Oshmia T, Karasawa F, Satoh T: Effects of propofol on cerebral blood flow and the metabolic rate of oxygen in humans. Acta Anaesthesiol Scand 46:831-835, 2002.
175. Alkire MT, Haier RJ, Barker SJ, et al: Cerebral metabolism during propofol anesthesia in humans studied with positron emission tomography. Anesthesiology 82:393-403, 1995.
176. Petersen KD, Landsfeldt U, Cold GE, et al: Intracranial pressure and cerebral hemodynamics in patients with cerebral tumors. Anesthesiology 98:329-336, 2003.
177. Ravussin P, Guinard JP, Ralley F, Thorin D: Effect of propofol on cerebrospinal fluid pressure and cerebral perfusion pressure in patients undergoing craniotomy. Anaesthesia 43:37-41, 1988.
178. Fox J, Gelb AW, Enns J, et al: The responsiveness of cerebral blood flow to changes in arterial carbon dioxide is maintained during propofol–nitrous oxide anesthesia in humans. Anesthesiology 77:453-456, 1992.
179. Craen RA, Gelb AW, Murkin JM, Chong KY: Human cerebral autoregulation is maintained during propofol air/O_2 anesthesia [abstract]. J Neurosurg Anesthesiol 4:298, 1992.
180. Matta BF, Mayberg TS, Lam AM: Direct cerebrovasodilatory effects of halothane, isoflurane and desflurane during propofol-induced isoelectric electroencephalogram in humans. Anesthesiology 83:980-985, 1995.
181. Cameron AE: Opisthotonus again [letter]. Anaesthesia 42:1124, 1987.
182. Hopkins CS: Recurrent opisthotonus associated with anaesthesia [letter]. Anaesthesia 43:904, 1988.
183. Jones GW, Boykett MH, Klok M: Propofol, opisthotonus and epilepsy [letter]. Anaesthesia 43:905, 1988.
184. DeFriez CB, Wong HC: Seizures and opisthotonos after propofol anesthesia. Anesth Analg 75:630-632, 1992.
185. Bevan JC: Propofol-related convulsions. Can J Anaesth 40:805-809, 1993.
186. Borgeat A, Dessibourg C, Popovic V, et al: Propofol and spontaneous movements: An EEG study. Anesthesiology 74:24-27, 1991.
187. Cheng MA, Tempelhoff R, Silbergeld DL, et al: Large-dose propofol alone in adult epileptic patients: Electrocorticographic results. Anesth Analg 83:169-174, 1996.
188. Samra SK, Sneyd JR, Ross DA, Henry TR: Effects of propofol sedation on seizures and intracranially recorded epileptiform activity in patients with partial epilepsy. Anesthesiology 82:843-851, 1995.
189. Lowson S, Gent JP, Goodchild CS: Anticonvulsant properties of propofol and thiopentone: Comparison using two tests in laboratory mice. Br J Anaesth 64:59-63, 1990.
190. Lowson S, Gent JP, Goodchild CS: Convulsive thresholds in mice during the recovery phase from anaesthesia induced by propofol, thiopentone, methohexitone and etomidate. Br J Pharmacol 102:879-882, 1991.
191. Rampton AJ, Griffin RM, Stuart CS, et al: Comparison of methohexital and propofol for electroconvulsive therapy: Effects on hemodynamic responses and seizure duration. Anesthesiology 70:412-417, 1989.
192. Herrick IA, Craen RA, Gelb AW, et al: Propofol sedation during awake craniotomy for seizures: Patient-controlled administration versus neurolept analgesia. Anesth Analg 84:1280-1284, 1997.
193. Drummond JC, Iragui-Madoz VJ, Alksne JF, Kalkman CJ: Masking of epileptiform activity by propofol during seizure surgery. Anesthesiology 76:652-654, 1992.
194. Cold GE, Eskesen V, Eriksen H, et al: CBF and $CMRO_2$ during continuous etomidate infusion supplemented with N_2O and fentanyl in patients with supratentorial cerebral tumour. A dose-response study. Acta Anaesthesiol Scand 29:490-491, 1985.
195. Cold GE, Eskesen V, Eriksen H, Lyon BB: Changes in $CMRO_2$, EEG and concentration of etomidate in serum and brain tissue during craniotomy with continuous etomidate supplemented with N_2O and fentanyl. Acta Anaesthesiol Scand 30:159-163, 1986.
196. Kofke WA, Dong ML, Bloom M, et al: Transcranial Doppler ultrasonography with induction of anesthesia for neurosurgery. J Neurosurg Anesthesiol 6:89-97, 1994.
197. Bingham RM, Procaccio F, Prior PF, Hinds CJ: Cerebral electrical activity influences the effects of etomidate on cerebral perfusion pressure in traumatic coma. Br J Anaesth 57:843-848, 1985.
198. Davis DW, Mans AM, Biebuyck JF, Hawkins RA: Regional brain glucose utilization in rats during etomidate anesthesia. Anesthesiology 64:751-757, 1986.
199. Modica PA, Tempelhoff R: Intracranial pressure during induction of anaesthesia and tracheal intubation with etomidate-induced EEG burst suppression. Can J Anaesth 39:236-241, 1992.
200. Dearden NM, McDowall DG: Comparison of etomidate and althesin in the reduction of increased intracranial pressure after head injury. Br J Anaesth 57:361-368, 1985.
201. Hoffman WE, Charbel FT, Edelman G, et al: Comparison of the effect of etomidate and desflurane on brain tissue gases and pH during prolonged middle cerebral artery occlusion. Anesthesiology 88:1188-1194, 1998.
202. Levy ML, Aranda M, Zelman V, Giannotta SL: Propylene glycol toxicity following continuous etomidate infusion for the control of refractory cerebral edema. Neurosurgery 37:363-371, 1995.
203. Hoehner PJ, Whitson JT, Kirsch JR, Traystman RJ: Effect of intracarotid and intraventricular morphine on regional cerebral blood flow and metabolism in pentobarbital-anesthetized dogs. Anesth Analg 76:266-273, 1993.
204. Moyer JH, Pontius R, Morris G, Hershberger R: Effect of morphine and n-allylnormorphine on cerebral hemodynamics and oxygen metabolism. Circulation 15:379-384, 1957.
205. Takeshita H, Michenfelder JD, Theye RA: The effects of morphine and n-allylnormorphine on canine cerebral metabolism and circulation. Anesthesiology 37:605-612, 1972.
206. Jobes DR, Kennell E, Bitner R, et al: Effects of morphine–nitrous oxide anesthesia on cerebral autoregulation. Anesthesiology 42:30-34, 1975.
207. Murkin JM, Farrar JK, Tweed WA, et al: Relationship between cerebral blood flow and O_2 consumption during high-dose narcotic anesthesia for cardiac surgery [abstract]. Anesthesiology 63:A44, 1985.
208. Firestone LL, Gyulai F, Mintun M, et al: Human brain activity response to fentanyl imaged by positron emission tomography. Anesth Analg 82:1247-1251, 1996.
209. McPherson RW, Traystman RJ: Fentanyl and cerebral vascular responsivity in dogs. Anesthesiology 60:180-186, 1984.
210. Baughman VL, Hoffman WE, Albrecht RF, Miletich DJ: Cerebral vascular and metabolic effects of fentanyl and midazolam in young and aged rats. Anesthesiology 67:314-319, 1987.
211. Keykhah MM, Smith DS, Carlsson C, et al: Influence of sufentanil on cerebral metabolism and circulation in the rat. Anesthesiology 63:274-277, 1985.
212. Michenfelder JD, Theye RA: Effects of fentanyl, droperidol and Innovar on canine cerebral metabolism and blood flow. Br J Anaesth 43:630-636, 1971.

213. McPherson RW, Krempasanka E, Eimerl D, Traystman RJ: Effects of alfentanil on cerebral vascular reactivity in dogs. Br J Anaesth 57:1232-1238, 1985.
214. Schregel W, Schafermeyer H, Muller C, et al: The effect of halothane, alfentanil and propofol on blood flow velocity, blood vessel cross section and blood volume flow in the middle cerebral artery [in German]. Anaesthesist 41:21-26, 1992.
215. Mayberg TS, Lam AM, Eng CC, et al: The effect of alfentanil on cerebral blood flow velocity and intracranial pressure during isoflurane–nitrous oxide anesthesia in humans. Anesthesiology 78:288-294, 1993.
216. Milde LN, Milde JH, Gallagher WJ: Effects of sufentanil on cerebral circulation and metabolism in dogs. Anesth Analg 70:138-146, 1990.
217. Werner C, Hoffman WE, Baughman VL, et al: Effects of sufentanil on cerebral blood flow, cerebral blood flow velocity, and metabolism in dogs. Anesth Analg 72:177-181, 1991.
218. Bunegin L, Albin MS, Ernst PS, Garcia C: Cerebrovascular responses to sufentanil citrate in primates with and without intracranial hypertension [abstract]. Anesth Analg 70:S42, 1990.
219. Murkin JM, Farrar JK, Tweed WA: Sufentanil anaesthesia reduces cerebral blood flow and cerebral oxygen consumption [abstract]. Can J Anaesth 35:S131, 1988.
220. Mayer N, Weinstabl C, Podreka I, Spiss CK: Sufentanil does not increase cerebral blood flow in healthy human volunteers. Anesthesiology 73:240-243, 1990.
221. Weinstabl C, Mayer N, Spiss CK: Sufentanil decreases cerebral blood flow velocity in patients with elevated intracranial pressure. Eur J Anaesthesiol 9:481-484, 1992.
222. Sheehan PB, Zornow MH, Scheller MS, Peterson BM: The effects of fentanyl and sufentanil on intracranial pressure and cerebral blood flow in rabbits with an acute cryogenic brain injury. J Neurosurg Anesthesiol 4:261-267, 1992.
223. Weinstabl C, Mayer N, Richling B, et al: Effect of sufentanil on intracranial pressure in neurosurgical patients. Anaesthesia 46:837-840, 1991.
224. Werner C, Kochs E, Hoffman WE, et al: Sufentanil does not change cerebral hemodynamics and ICP in head injured patients [abstract]. J Neurosurg Anesthesiol 4:313, 1992.
225. Jamali S, Ravussin P, Archer D, et al: The effects of bolus administration of opioids on cerebrospinal fluid pressure in patients with supratentorial lesions. Anesth Analg 82:600-606, 1996.
226. Lauer KK, Connolly LA, Schmeling WT: Opioid sedation does not alter intracranial pressure in head injured patients. Can J Anaesth 44:929-933, 1997.
227. Marx W, Shah N, Long C, et al: Sufentanil, alfentanil, and fentanyl: Impact on cerebrospinal fluid pressure in patients with brain tumors. J Neurosurg Anesthesiol 1:3-7, 1989.
228. Sperry RJ, Bailey PL, Reichman MV, et al: Fentanyl and sufentanil increase intracranial pressure in head trauma patients. Anesthesiology 77:416-420, 1992.
229. Albanese J, Durbec O, Viviand X, et al: Sufentanil increases intracranial pressure in patients with head trauma. Anesthesiology 79:493-497, 1993.
230. Werner C, Kochs E, Bause H, et al: Effects of sufentanil on cerebral hemodynamics and intracranial pressure in patients with brain injury. Anesthesiology 83:721-726, 1995.
231. Herrick I, Gelb A, Manninen PH, et al: Effects of fentanyl, sufentanil, and alfentanil on brain retractor pressure. Anesth Analg 72:359-363, 1991.
232. From RP, Warner DS, Todd MM, Sokoll MD: Anesthesia for craniotomy: A double-blind comparison of alfentanil, fentanyl, and sufentanil. Anesthesiology 73:896-904, 1990.
233. Bristow A, Shalev D, Rice B, et al: Low-dose synthetic narcotic infusions for cerebral relaxation during craniotomies. Anesth Analg 66:413-416, 1987.
234. Shupak RC, Harp JR: Comparison between high-dose sufentanil-oxygen and high-dose fentanyl-oxygen for neuroanaesthesia. Br J Anaesth 57:375-381, 1985.
235. Jung R, Shah N, Reinsel R, et al: Cerebrospinal fluid pressure in patients with brain tumors: Impact of fentanyl versus alfentanil during nitrous oxide–oxygen anesthesia. Anesth Analg 71:419-422, 1990.
236. Moss E: Alfentanil increases intracranial pressure when intracranial compliance is low. Anaesthesia 47:134-136, 1992.
237. Markovitz BP, Duhaime A-C, Sutton L, et al: Effects of alfentanil on intracranial pressure in children undergoing ventriculoperitoneal shunt revision. Anesthesiology 76:71-76, 1992.
238. Souter MJ, Andrews PJD, Piper IR, Miller JD: Effects of alfentanil on cerebral haemodynamics in an experimental model of traumatic brain injury. Br J Anaesth 79:97-102, 1997.
239. Warner DS, Hindman BJ, Todd MM, et al: Intracranial pressure and hemodynamic effects of remifentanil versus alfentanil in patients undergoing supratentorial craniotomy. Anesth Analg 83:348-353, 1996.
240. Ostapkovich N, Baker KZ, Fogerty-Mack P, et al: Cerebral blood flow and CO_2 reactivity is similar during remifentanil/ N_2O and fentanyl/N_2O anesthesia. Anesthesiology 89:358-363, 1998.
241. Paris A, Scholz J, von Knobelsdorff G, et al: The effect of remifentanil on cerebral blood flow velocity. Anesth Analg 87:569-573, 1998.
242. Wagner K, Wiloch F, Kochs E, et al: Dose-dependent regional cerebral blood flow changes during remifentanil infusion in humans. Anesthesiology 94:732-739, 2001.
243. Lorenz I, Kolbitsch C, Hormann C, et al: The influence of nitrous oxide and remifentanil on cerebral hemodynamics in conscious human volunteers. Neuroimage 17:1056-1064, 2002.
244. Lorenz L, Kolbitsch C, Schocke M, et al: Low-dose remifentanil increases regional cerebral blood flow and regional cerebral blood volume, but decreases regional mean transit time and regional cerebrovascular resistance in volunteers. Br J Anaesth 85:199-204, 2000.
245. Rockoff MA, Naughton KVH, Shapiro HM, et al: Cerebral circulatory and metabolic responses to intravenously administered lorazepam. Anesthesiology 53:215-218, 1980.
246. Forster A, Juge O, Louis M, Nahory A: Effects of a specific benzodiazepine antagonist (RO 15-1788) on cerebral blood flow. Anesth Analg 66:309-313, 1987.
247. Veselis RA, Reinsel RA, Beattie BJ, et al: Midazolam changes cerebral blood flow in discrete brain regions: An $H_2^{15}O$ positron emission tomography study. Anesthesiology 87:1106-1117, 1997.
248. Forster A, Juge O, Morel D: Effects of midazolam on cerebral hemodynamics and cerebral vasomotor responsiveness to carbon dioxide. J Cereb Blood Flow Metab 3:246-249, 1983.
249. Fleischer JE, Milde JH, Moyer TP, Michenfelder JD: Cerebral effects of high-dose midazolam and subsequent reversal with RO 15-1788 in dogs. Anesthesiology 68:234-242, 1988.
250. Nugent M, Artru AA, Michenfelder JD: Cerebral metabolic, vascular and protective effects of midazolam maleate. Anesthesiology 56:172-176, 1982.
251. Wolf J, Friberg L, Jensen J, et al: The effect of the benzodiazepine antagonist flumazenil on regional cerebral blood flow in human volunteers. Br J Anaesth 34:628-631, 1990.
252. Artru AA: Flumazenil reversal of midazolam in dogs: Dose-related changes in cerebral blood flow, metabolism, EEG, and CSF pressure. J Neurosurg Anesthesiol 1:46-55, 1989.
253. Knudsen L, Cold GE, Holdgård HO, et al: Effects of flumazenil on cerebral blood flow and oxygen consumption after midazolam anaesthesia for craniotomy. Br J Anaesth 67:277-280, 1991.
254. Chiolero RL, Ravussin P, Anderes JP, et al: The effects of midazolam reversal by RO 15-1788 on cerebral perfusion pressure in patients with severe head injury. Intensive Care Med 14:196-200, 1988.
255. Kumano H, Shimomura T, Furuya H, et al: Effects of flumazenil during administration of midazolam on pial vessel diameter and regional cerebral blood flow in cats. Acta Anaesthesiol Scand 37:567-570, 1993.

256. Lanier WL, Albrecht RF, Iaizzo PA: Divergence of intracranial and central venous pressures in lightly anesthetized, tracheally intubated dogs that move in response to a noxious stimulus. Anesthesiology 84:605-613, 1996.

257. Sari A, Okuda Y, Takeshita H: The effects of Thalamonal on cerebral circulation and oxygen consumption in man. Br J Anaesth 44:330-334, 1972.

258. Misfeldt BB, Jorgensen PB, Spotoft H, Rønde F: The effects of droperidol and fentanyl on intracranial pressure and cerebral perfusion. Br J Anaesth 48:963-968, 1976.

259. Miller R, Tausk HC, Stark DCC: Effect of Innovar, fentanyl and droperidol on the cerebrospinal fluid pressure in neurosurgical patients. Can J Anaesth 22:502-508, 1975.

260. Fitch W, Barker J, Jennett WB, McDowall DG: The influence of neuroleptanalgesic drugs on cerebrospinal fluid pressure. Br J Anaesth 41:800-806, 1969.

261. Fukuda S, Murakawa T, Takeshita H, Toda N: Direct effects of ketamine on isolated canine cerebral and mesenteric arteries. Anesth Analg 62:553-558, 1983.

262. Cavazzuti M, Porro CA, Biral GP, et al: Ketamine effects on local cerebral blood flow and metabolism in the rat. J Cereb Blood Flow Metab 7:806-811, 1987.

263. Hougaard K, Hansen A, Brodersen P: The effect of ketamine on regional cerebral blood flow in man. Anesthesiology 41:562-567, 1974.

264. Strebel S, Kaufmann M, Maître L, Schaefer HG: Effects of ketamine on cerebral blood flow velocity in humans. Influence of pretreatment with midazolam or esmolol. Anaesthesia 50:223-228, 1995.

265. Crosby G, Crane AM, Sokoloff L: Local changes in cerebral glucose utilization during ketamine anesthesia. Anesthesiology 56:437-443, 1982.

266. Vollenweider FX, Leenders KL, Oye I, et al: Differential psychopathology and patterns of cerebral glucose utilisation produced by (S)- and (R)-ketamine in healthy volunteers using positron emission tomography (PET). Eur Neuropsychopharmacol 7:25-38, 1997.

267. Vollenweider FX, Leenders KL, Scharfetter C, et al: Metabolic hyperfrontality and psychopathology in the ketamine model of psychosis using positron emission tomography (PET) and [^{18}F] fluorodeoxyglucose (FDG). Eur Neuropsychopharmacol 7:9-24, 1997.

268. Holcomb HH, Lahti AC, Medoff DR, et al: Sequential regional cerebral blood flow brain scans using PET with H$_2$^{15}O demonstrate ketamine actions in CNS dynamically. Neuropsychopharmacology 25:165-172, 2001.

269. Schmidt A, Ryding E, Akeson J: Racemic ketamine does not abolish cerebrovascular autoregulation in the pig. Acta Anaesthesiol Scand 47:569-575, 2003.

270. Shapiro HM, Wyte SR, Harris AB: Ketamine anesthesia in patients with intracranial pathology. Br J Anaesth 44:1200-1204, 1972.

271. Belopavlovic M, Buchthal A: Modification of ketamine-induced intracranial hypertension in neurosurgical patients by pretreatment with midazolam. Acta Anaesthesiol Scand 26:458-462, 1982.

272. Mayberg TS, Lam AM, Matta BF, et al: Ketamine does not increase cerebral blood flow velocity or intracranial pressure during isoflurane/nitrous oxide anesthesia in patients undergoing craniotomy. Anesth Analg 81:84-89, 1995.

273. Akeson J, Bjorkman S, Messeter K, Rosén I: Low-dose midazolam antagonizes cerebral metabolic stimulation by ketamine in the pig. Acta Anaesthesiol Scand 37:525-531, 1993.

274. Sakai K, Cho S, Fukusaki M, et al: The effects of propofol with and without ketamine on human cerebral blood flow velocity and CO$_2$ response. Anesth Analg 90:377-382, 2000.

275. Albanése J, Arnaud S, Rey M, et al: Ketamine decreases intracranial pressure and electroencephalographic activity in traumatic brain injury patients during propofol sedation. Anesthesiology 87:1328-1334, 1997.

276. Sakabe T, Maekawa T, Ishikawa T, Takeshita H: The effects of lidocaine on canine cerebral metabolism and circulation related to the electroencephalogram. Anesthesiology 40:433-441, 1974.

277. Lam AM, Donlon E, Eng CC, et al: The effect of lidocaine on cerebral blood flow and metabolism during normocapnia and hypocapnia in humans [abstract]. Anesthesiology 79:A202, 1993.

278. Bedford RF, Persing JA, Pobereskin L, Butler A: Lidocaine or thiopental for rapid control of intracranial hypertension? Anesth Analg 59:435-437, 1980.

279. Donegan MF, Bedford RF: Intravenously administered lidocaine prevents intracranial hypertension during endotracheal suctioning. Anesthesiology 52:516-518, 1980.

280. Tommasino C, Maekawa T, Shapiro HM: Local cerebral blood flow during lidocaine-induced seizures in rats. Anesthesiology 64:771-777, 1986.

281. Stoelting RK: Pharmacology and Physiology in Anesthetic Practice. Philadelphia, JB Lippincott, 1987.

282. Viegas O, Stoelting RK: Lidocaine in arterial blood after laryngotracheal administration. Anesthesiology 43:491-493, 1975.

283. Michenfelder JD, Theye RA: In vivo toxic effects of halothane on canine cerebral metabolic pathways. Am J Physiol 229:1050-1055, 1975.

284. Michenfelder JD, Cucchiara RF: Canine cerebral oxygen consumption during enflurane anesthesia and its modification during induced seizures. Anesthesiology 40:575-580, 1974.

285. Todd MM, Drummond JC: A comparison of the cerebrovascular and metabolic effects of halothane and isoflurane in the cat. Anesthesiology 60:276-282, 1984.

286. Lutz LJ, Milde JH, Milde LN: The cerebral functional, metabolic, and hemodynamic effects of desflurane in dogs. Anesthesiology 73:125-131, 1990.

287. Scheller MS, Tateishi A, Drummond JC, Zornow MH: The effects of sevoflurane on cerebral blood flow, cerebral metabolic rate for oxygen, intracranial pressure, and the electroencephalogram are similar to those of isoflurane in the rabbit. Anesthesiology 68:548-551, 1988.

288. Kuramoto T, Oshita S, Takeshita H, Ishikawa T: Modification of the relationship between cerebral metabolism, blood flow and electroencephalogram by stimulation during anesthesia in the dog. Anesthesiology 51:211-217, 1979.

289. Drummond JC, Todd MM, Scheller MS, Shapiro HM: A comparison of the direct cerebral vasodilating potencies of halothane and isoflurane in the New Zealand white rabbit. Anesthesiology 65:462-467, 1986.

290. Lam AM, Mayberg TS, Eng CC, et al: Nitrous oxide–isoflurane anesthesia causes more cerebral vasodilation than an equipotent dose of isoflurane in humans. Anesth Analg 78:462-468, 1994.

291. Kuroda Y, Murakami M, Tsuruta J, et al: Blood flow velocity of middle cerebral artery during prolonged anesthesia with halothane, isoflurane, and sevoflurane in humans. Anesthesiology 87:527-532, 1997.

292. Lenz C, Rebel A, Klaus V, et al: Local cerebral blood flow, local cerebral glucose utilization, and flow-metabolism coupling during sevoflurane versus isoflurane anesthesia in rats. Anesthesiology 89:1480-1488, 1998.

293. Sakabe T, Kuramoto T, Kumagae S, Takeshita H: Cerebral responses to the addition of nitrous oxide to halothane in man. Br J Anaesth 48:957-962, 1976.

294. Heath KJ, Gupta S, Matta BF: The effects of sevoflurane on cerebral hemodynamics during propofol anesthesia. Anesth Analg 85:1284-1287, 1997.

295. Murphy FL, Kennell EM, Johnstone RE, et al: The effects of enflurane, isoflurane, and halothane on cerebral blood flow and metabolism in man [abstract]. Paper presented at the Annual Meeting of the American Society of Anesthesiologists, October 1974, pp 62-63.

296. Eintrei C, Leszniewski W, Carlsson C: Local application of ^{133}xenon for measurement of regional cerebral blood flow (rCBF) during halothane, enflurane, and isoflurane anesthesia in humans. Anesthesiology 63:391-394, 1985.

297. Ornstein E, Young WL, Ostapkovich N, et al: Comparative effects of desflurane and isoflurane on cerebral blood flow [abstract]. Anesthesiology 75:A209, 1991.

298. Johnson J, Sperry RJ, Lam A, Artru A: A phase III, randomized, open-label study to compare sevoflurane and isoflurane in neurosurgical patients. Anesth Analg 80:S214, 1995.

299. Wollman H, Alexander SC, Cohen PJ, et al: Cerebral circulation of man during halothane anesthesia. Anesthesiology 25:180-184, 1964.

300. Todd MM, Drummond JC, Shapiro HM: Comparative cerebrovascular and metabolic effects of halothane, enflurane, and isoflurane [abstract]. Anesthesiology 57:A332, 1982.

301. Mielck F, Stephan H, Weyland A, Sonntag H: Effects of one minimum alveolar anesthetic concentration sevoflurane on cerebral metabolism, blood flow, and CO_2 reactivity in cardiac patients. Anesth Analg 89:364-369, 1999.

302. Mielck F, Stephan H, Buhre W, et al: Effects of 1 MAC desflurane on cerebral metabolism, blood flow and carbon dioxide reactivity in humans. Br J Anaesth 81:155-160, 1998.

303. Sakabe T, Maekawa T, Fujii S, et al: Cerebral circulation and metabolism during enflurane anesthesia in humans. Anesthesiology 59:532-536, 1983.

304. Fraga M, Maceiras P, Rodino S, et al: The effects of isoflurane and desflurane on intracranial pressure, cerebral perfusion pressure, and cerebral arteriovenous oxygen content differences in normocapnic patients with supratentorial brain tumors. Anesthesiology 98:1085-1090, 2003.

305. Kaisti K, Metsahonkala L, Teras M, et al: Effects of surgical levels of propofol and sevoflurane anesthesia on cerebral blood flow in healthy subjects studied with positron emission tomography. Anesthesiology 96:1358-1370, 2002.

306. Reinstrup P, Ryding E, Algotsson L, et al: Regional cerebral blood flow (SPECT) during anaesthesia with isoflurane and nitrous oxide in humans. Br J Anaesth 78:407-411, 1997.

307. Bundgaard H, Oettingen G, Larsen K, et al: Effects of sevoflurane on intracranial pressure, cerebral blood flow and cerebral metabolism. Acta Anesthesiol Scand 42:621-627, 1998.

308. Madsen J, Cold G, Hansen E, Bardrum B: The effect of isoflurane on cerebral blood flow and metabolism in humans during craniotomy for small supratentorial cerebral tumors. Anesthesiology 66:332-336, 1987.

309. Ornstein E, Young W, Fleischer L, Ostapkovich N: Desflurane and isoflurane have similar effects on cerebral blood flow in patients with intracranial mass lesions. Anesthesiology 79:498-502, 1993.

310. Algotsson L, Messeter K, Nordstrom C, Ryding E: Cerebral blood flow and oxygen consumption during isoflurane and halothane anesthesia in man. Acta Anesthesiol Scand 32:15-20, 1988.

311. Kolbitsch C, Lorenz I, Hormann C, et al: Sevoflurane and nitrous oxide increase regional cerebral blood flow (rCBF) and regional cerebral blood volume (rCBV) in a drug-specific manner in human volunteers. Magn Reson Imaging 19:1253-1260, 2001.

312. Kolbitsch C, Lorenz I, Hormann C, et al: A subanesthetic concentration of sevoflurane increases regional cerebral blood flow and regional cerebral blood volume and decreases regional mean transit time and regional cerebrovascular resistance in volunteers. Anesth Analg 91:156-162, 2000.

313. Lorenz I, Hormann C, Luger T, et al: Influence of equianaesthetic concentrations of nitrous oxide and isoflurane on regional cerebral blood flow, regional cerebral blood volume, and regional mean transit time in human volunteers. Br J Anaesth 87:691-698, 2001.

314. Alkire M, Pomfrett CJ, Haier RJ, et al: Functional brain imaging during anesthesia in humans: Effects of halothane on global and regional cerebral glucose metabolism. Anesthesiology 90:701-709, 1999.

315. Young WL, Prohovnik I, Ornstein E, et al: The effect of arteriovenous malformation resection on cerebrovascular reactivity to carbon dioxide. Neurosurgery 27:257-267, 1990.

316. Ornstein E, Young WL, Fleischer LH, Ostapkovich N: Desflurane and isoflurane have similar effects on cerebral blood flow in patients with intracranial mass lesions. Anesthesiology 79:498-502, 1993.

317. Milde LN, Milde JH: Cerebral effects of sufentanil in dogs with reduced intracranial compliance. Anesth Analg 68:S196, 1989.

318. Alkire MT, Haier RJ, Shah NK, Anderson CT: Positron emission tomography study of regional cerebral metabolism in humans during isoflurane anesthesia. Anesthesiology 86:549-557, 1997.

319. Rampil IJ, Lockhart SH, Eger EI, et al: The electroencephalographic effects of desflurane in humans. Anesthesiology 74:434-439, 1991.

320. Boarini DJ, Kassell NF, Coester HC, et al: Comparison of systemic and cerebrovascular effects of isoflurane and halothane. Neurosurgery 15:400-409, 1984.

321. Adams RW, Cucchiara RF, Gronert GA, et al: Isoflurane and cerebrospinal fluid pressures in neurosurgical patients. Anesthesiology 54:97-99, 1981.

322. Grosslight K, Foster R, Colohan AR, Bedford RF: Isoflurane for neuroanesthesia: Risk factors for increases in intracranial pressure. Anesthesiology 63:533-536, 1985.

323. Campkin TV, Flinn RM: Isoflurane and cerebrospinal fluid pressure—a study in neurosurgical patients undergoing intracranial shunt procedures. Anaesthesia 44:50-54, 1989.

324. Scheller MS, Todd MM, Drummond JC: A comparison of the ICP effects of isoflurane and halothane after cryogenic brain injury in rabbits. Anesthesiology 67:507-512, 1987.

325. Adams RW, Gronert GA, Sundt TM, Michenfelder JD: Halothane, hypocapnia and cerebrospinal fluid pressure in neurosurgery. Anesthesiology 37:510-517, 1972.

326. Warner DS, Boarini DJ, Kassell NL: Cerebrovascular adaptation to prolonged halothane anesthesia is not related to cerebrospinal fluid pH. Anesthesiology 63:243-248, 1985.

327. Fleischer LH, Young WL, Ornstein E, Ostapkovich N: Cerebral blood flow in humans does not decline over time during isoflurane or desflurane anesthesia [abstract]. Anesthesiology 77:A167, 1992.

328. Cenic A, Craen R, Lee T, Gelb A: Cerebral blood volume and blood flow responses to hyperventilation in brain tumors during isoflurane or propofol anesthesia. Anesth Analg 94:661-666, 2002.

329. Madsen JB, Cold GE, Hansen ES, Bardrum B: Cerebral blood flow, cerebral metabolic rate of oxygen and relative CO_2-reactivity during craniotomy for supratentorial cerebral tumours in halothane anaesthesia. A dose-response study. Acta Anaesthesiol Scand 31:454-457, 1987.

330. Drummond JC, Todd MM: The response of the feline cerebral circulation to $Paco_2$ during anesthesia with isoflurane and halothane and during sedation with nitrous oxide. Anesthesiology 62:268-273, 1985.

331. Cho S, Fujigaki T, Uchiyama Y, et al: Effects of sevoflurane with and without nitrous oxide on human cerebral circulation. Anesthesiology 85:755-760, 1996.

332. Morita H, Bleyaert AL, Stezoski SW, Nemoto EM: The effect of halothane anesthesia on cerebral blood flow, autoregulation and cerebral metabolism of oxygen and glucose [abstract]. Paper presented at the Annual Meeting of the American Society of Anesthesiologists, October 1974, pp 63-64.

333. Strebel S, Lam AM, Matta B, et al: Dynamic and static cerebral autoregulation during isoflurane, desflurane, and propofol anesthesia. Anesthesiology 83:66-76, 1995.

334. Gupta S, Heath K, Matta BF: Effect of incremental doses of sevoflurane on cerebral pressure autoregulation in humans. Br J Anaesth 79:469-472, 1997.

335. Vavilala MS, Lee LA, Lee M, et al: Cerebral autoregulation in children during sevoflurane anaesthesia. Br J Anaesth 90:636-641, 2003.

336. Lu H, Werner C, Englehard K, et al: The effects of sevoflurane on cerebral blood flow autoregulation in rats. Anesth Analg 87:854-858, 1998.

337. Neigh JL, Garman JK, Harp JR: The electroencephalographic pattern during anesthesia with Enthrane. Anesthesiology 35:482-487, 1971.

338. Wollman H, Smith AL, Hoffman JC: Cerebral blood flow and oxygen consumption in man during electroencephalographic seizure patterns induced by anesthesia with Ethrane [abstract]. Fed Proc 28:356, 1967.

339. Fleming DC, Fitzpatrick J, Fariello RG, et al: Diagnostic activation of epileptogenic foci by enflurane. Anesthesiology 52:431-433, 1980.

340. Opitz A, Brecht S, Stenyel E: Enflurane anesthesia in epileptics [in German]. Anaesthesist 26:329-332, 1977.

341. Kruczek M, Albin MS, Wolf S, Bertoni JM: Postoperative seizure activity following enflurane anesthesia. Anesthesiology 53:175-176, 1980.

342. Hymes JA: Seizure activity during isoflurane anesthesia. Anesth Analg 64:367-368, 1985.

343. Harrison JL: Postoperative seizures after isoflurane anesthesia. Anesth Analg 65:1235-1236, 1986.

344. Kofke WA, Young RSK, Davis P, et al: Isoflurane for refractory status epilepticus: A clinical series. Anesthesiology 71:653-659, 1989.

345. Komatsu H, Taie S, Endo S, et al: Electrical seizures during sevoflurane anesthesia in two pediatric patients with epilepsy. Anesthesiology 81:1535-1537, 1994.

346. Haga S, Shima T, Momose K, et al: Anesthetic induction of children with high concentrations of sevoflurane [in Japanese]. Jpn J Anesthesiol 41:1951-1955, 1992.

347. Kaisti K, Jaaskelainen S, Rinne JO, et al: Epileptiform discharges during 2 MAC sevoflurane anesthesia in two healthy volunteers. Anesthesiology 91:1952-1955, 1999.

348. Hisada K, Morioka T, Fukui K, et al: Electrocorticographic activities in patients with temporal lobe epilepsy. J Neurosurg Anesthesiol 13:333-337, 2001.

349. Hilty CA, Drummond JC: Seizure-like activity on emergence from sevoflurane anesthesia. Anesthesiology 93:1357-1358, 2000.

350. Terasako K, Ishii S: Postoperative seizure-like activity following sevoflurane anesthesia. Anesth Analg 96:1239-1240, 2003.

351. Nakanishi O, Ishikawa T, Imamura Y, Hirakawa T: Inhibition of cerebral metabolic and circulatory responses to nitrous oxide by 6-hydroxydopamine in dogs. Can J Anaesth 44:1008-1013, 1997.

352. Field LM, Dorrance DE, Krzeminska EK, Barsoum LZ: Effect of nitrous oxide on cerebral blood flow in normal humans. Br J Anaesth 70:154-159, 1993.

353. Eng C, Lam AM, Mayberg TS, et al: The influence of propofol with and without nitrous oxide on cerebral blood flow velocity and CO$_2$ reactivity in humans. Anesthesiology 77:872-879, 1992.

354. Henriksen HT, Jorgensen PB: The effect of nitrous oxide on intracranial pressure in patients with intracranial disorders. Br J Anaesth 45:486-491, 1973.

355. Moss E, McDowall DG: I.C.P increases with 50% nitrous oxide in oxygen in severe head injuries during controlled ventilation. Br J Anaesth 51:757-761, 1979.

356. Pelligrino DA, Miletich DJ, Hoffman WE, Albrecht RA: Nitrous oxide markedly increases cerebral cortical metabolic rate and blood flow in the goat. Anesthesiology 60:405-412, 1984.

357. Theye RA, Michenfelder JD: The effects of nitrous oxide on canine cerebral metabolism. Anesthesiology 29:1119-1124, 1968.

358. Phirman JR, Shapiro HM: Modification of nitrous oxide–induced intracranial hypertension by prior induction of anesthesia. Anesthesiology 46:150-151, 1977.

359. Misfeldt BB, Jorgensen PL, Rishoj M: The effect of nitrous oxide and halothane upon the intracranial pressure in hypocapnic patients with intracranial disorders. Br J Anaesth 46:853-858, 1974.

360. Jung R, Reinsel R, Marx W, et al: Isoflurane and nitrous oxide: Comparative impact on cerebrospinal fluid pressure in patients with brain tumors. Anesth Analg 75:724-728, 1992.

361. Hoffman WE, Miletich DJ, Albrecht RF: The effects of midazolam on cerebral blood flow and oxygen consumption and its interaction with nitrous oxide. Anesth Analg 65:729-733, 1986.

362. Knudsen L, Cold GE, Holdgård HO, et al: The effects of midazolam on cerebral blood flow and oxygen consumption. Interaction with nitrous oxide in patients undergoing craniotomy for supratentorial tumors. Anaesthesia 45:1016-1019, 1990.

363. Manohar M, Parks C: Porcine regional brain and myocardial blood flows during halothane-O$_2$ and halothane–nitrous oxide anesthesia: Comparisons with equipotent isoflurane anesthesia. Am J Vet Res 45:465-473, 1984.

364. Manohar M, Parks CM: Porcine brain and myocardial perfusion during enflurane anesthesia without and with nitrous oxide. J Cardiovasc Pharmacol 6:1092-1101, 1984.

365. Manohar M, Parks C: Regional distribution of brain and myocardial perfusion in swine while awake and during 1.0 and 1.5 MAC isoflurane anaesthesia produced without or with 50% nitrous oxide. Cardiovasc Res 18:344-353, 1984.

366. Drummond JC, Scheller MS, Todd MM: The effect of nitrous oxide on cortical cerebral blood flow during anesthesia with halothane and isoflurane, with and without morphine, in the rabbit. Anesth Analg 66:1083-1089, 1987.

367. Todd MM: The effects of Paco$_2$ on the cerebrovascular response to nitrous oxide in the halothane-anesthetized rabbit. Anesth Analg 66:1090-1095, 1987.

368. Kaieda R, Todd MM, Warner DS: The effects of anesthetics and Paco$_2$ on the cerebrovascular, metabolic, and electroencephalographic responses to nitrous oxide in the rabbit. Anesth Analg 68:135-143, 1989.

369. Strebel S, Kaufmann M, Anselmi L, Schaefer HG: Nitrous oxide is a potent cerebrovasodilator in humans when added to isoflurane. Acta Anaesthesiol Scand 39:653-658, 1995.

370. Algotsson L, Messeter K, Rosén I, Holmin T: Effects of nitrous oxide on cerebral haemodynamics and metabolism during isoflurane anaesthesia in man. Acta Anaesthesiol Scand 36:46-52, 1992.

371. Baughman VL, Hoffman WE, Miletich DJ, Albrecht RF: Cerebrovascular and cerebral metabolic effects of N$_2$O in unrestrained rats. Anesthesiology 73:269-272, 1990.

372. Roald OK, Forsman M, Heier MS, Steen PA: Cerebral effects of nitrous oxide when added to low and high concentrations of isoflurane in the dog. Anesth Analg 72:75-79, 1991.

373. Wollman H, Alexander SC, Cohen PJ, et al: Cerebral circulation during general anesthesia and hyperventilation in man. Anesthesiology 26:329-334, 1965.

374. Tarkkanen L, Laitinen L, Johansson G: Effects of d-tubocurarine on intracranial pressure and thalamic electrical impedance. Anesthesiology 40:247-251, 1974.

375. Basta SJ, Savarese JJ, Ali HH, et al: Histamine-releasing potencies of atracurium, dimethyl tubocurarine and tubocurarine. Br J Anaesth 55:105S-106S, 1983.

376. Basta SJ: Clinical pharmacology of mivacurium chloride: A review. J Clin Anesth 4:153-163, 1992.

377. Rosa G, Orfei P, Sanfilippo M, et al: The effects of atracurium besylate (Tracrium) on intracranial pressure and cerebral perfusion pressure. Anesth Analg 65:381-384, 1986.

378. Schramm WM, Papousek A, Michalek-Sauberer A, et al: The cerebral and cardiovascular effects of cisatracurium and atracurium in neurosurgical patients. Anesth Analg 86:123-127, 1998.

379. Rosa G, Sanfilippo M, Vilardi V, et al: Effects of vecuronium bromide on intracranial pressure and cerebral perfusion pressure. Br J Anaesth 58:437-440, 1986.

380. Stirt JA, Maggio W, Haworth C, et al: Vecuronium: Effect on intracranial pressure and hemodynamics in neurosurgical patients. Anesthesiology 67:570-573, 1987.

381. Benthuysen JL, Kien ND, Quam DD: Intracranial pressure increases during alfentanil-induced rigidity. Anesthesiology 68:438-440, 1988.

382. Lanier WL, Milde JH, Michenfelder JD: The cerebral effects of pancuronium and atracurium in halothane-anesthetized dogs. Anesthesiology 63:589-597, 1985.

383. Lanier WL, Sharbrough FW, Michenfelder JD: Effects of atracurium, vecuronium or pancuronium pretreatment on lignocaine seizure thresholds in cats. Br J Anaesth 60:74-80, 1988.

384. Tateishi A, Zornow MH, Scheller MS, Canfell PC: Electroencephalographic effects of laudanosine in an animal model of epilepsy. Br J Anaesth 62:548-552, 1989.

385. Chapple DJ, Miller AA, Ward JB, Wheatley PL: Cardiovascular and neurological effects of laudanosine. Br J Anaesth 59:218-225, 1987.

386. Standaert FG: Magic bullets, science, and medicine. Anesthesiology 63:577-578, 1985.
387. Minton MD, Grosslight K, Stirt JA, Bedford RF: Increases in intracranial pressure from succinylcholine: Prevention by prior nondepolarizing blockade. Anesthesiology 65:165-169, 1986.
388. Lanier WL, Milde JH, Michenfelder JD: Cerebral stimulation following succinylcholine in dogs. Anesthesiology 64:551-559, 1986.
389. Lanier WL, Iaizzo PA, Milde JH: Cerebral function and muscle afferent activity following intravenous succinylcholine in dogs anesthetized with halothane: The effects of pretreatment with a defasciculating dose of pancuronium. Anesthesiology 71:87-95, 1989.
390. Lanier WL, Iaizzo PA, Milde JH, Sharbrough FW: The cerebral and systemic effects of movement in response to a noxious stimulus in lightly anesthetized dogs. Anesthesiology 80:392-401, 1994.
391. Stirt JA, Grosslight KR, Bedford RF, Vollmer D: "Defasciculation" with metocurine prevents succinylcholine-induced increases in intracranial pressure. Anesthesiology 67:50-53, 1987.
392. Kovarik DW, Mayberg TS, Lam AM, et al: Succinylcholine does not change intracranial pressure, cerebral blood flow velocity, or the electroencephalogram in patients with neurologic injury. Anesth Analg 78:469-473, 1994.
393. Cutler RWP, Spertell RB: Cerebrospinal fluid: A selective review. Ann Neurol 11:1-10, 1982.
394. Artru AA: Effects of halothane and fentanyl on the rate of CSF production in dogs. Anesth Analg 62:581-585, 1983.
395. Artru AA: Effects of halothane and fentanyl anesthesia on resistance to reabsorption of CSF. J Neurosurg 60:252-256, 1984.
396. Artru AA: Isoflurane does not increase the rate of CSF production in the dog. Anesthesiology 60:193-197, 1984.
397. Artru AA: Effects of enflurane and isoflurane on resistance to reabsorption of cerebrospinal fluid in dogs. Anesthesiology 61:529-533, 1984.
398. Artru AA, Nugent M, Michenfelder JD: Enflurane causes a prolonged and reversible increase in the rate of CSF production in the dog. Anesthesiology 57:255-260, 1982.
399. Maktabi MA, Elbokl FF, Faraci FM, Todd MM: Halothane decreases the rate of production of cerebrospinal fluid. Anesthesiology 78:72-82, 1993.
400. Artru AA: Rate of cerebrospinal fluid formation, resistance to reabsorption of cerebrospinal fluid, brain tissue water content, and electroencephalogram during desflurane anesthesia in dogs. J Neurosurg Anesthesiol 5:178-186, 1993.
401. Artru AA: Dose-related changes in the rate of cerebrospinal fluid formation and resistance to reabsorption of cerebrospinal fluid following administration of thiopental, midazolam, and etomidate in dogs. Anesthesiology 69:541-546, 1988.
402. Hatashita S, Hoff JT, Ishii S: Focal brain edema associated with acute arterial hypertension. J Neurosurg 64:643-649, 1986.
403. Sokrab T-EO, Johansson BB, Kalimo H, Olsson Y: A transient hypertensive opening of the blood-brain barrier can lead to brain damage. Acta Neuropathol 75:557-565, 1988.
404. Mayhan WG: Disruption of blood-brain barrier during acute hypertension in adult and aged rats. Am J Physiol 258:H1735-H1738, 1990.
405. Johansson BB, Linder L-E: Do nitrous oxide and lidocaine modify the blood-brain barrier in acute hypertension in the rat? Acta Anaesth Scand 24:65-68, 1980.
406. Forster A, Horn KV, Marshall LF, Shapiro HM: Anesthetic effects on blood-brain barrier function during acute arterial hypertension. Anesthesiology 49:26-30, 1978.
407. Johansson B: Blood-brain barrier dysfunction in acute arterial hypertension after papaverine-induced vasodilation. Acta Neurol Scand 50:573-580, 1974.
408. Smith AL, Marque JJ: Anesthetics and cerebral edema. Anesthesiology 45:64-72, 1976.
409. Modica PA, Tempelhoff R, White PF: Pro- and anticonvulsant effects of anesthetics (Part I). Anesth Analg 70:303-315, 1990.
410. Modica PA, Tempelhoff R, White PF: Pro- and anticonvulsant effects of anesthetics (Part II). Anesth Analg 70:433-444, 1990.
411. Kreisman NR, Magee JC, Brizzee BL: Relative hypoperfusion in rat cerebral cortex during recurrent seizures. J Cereb Blood Flow Metab 11:77-87, 1991.
412. Archer DP, McKenna JMA, Morin L, Ravussin P: Conscious-sedation analgesia during craniotomy for intractable epilepsy: A review of 354 consecutive cases. Can J Anaesth 35:338-344, 1988.
413. Ford EW, Morrell F, Whisler WW: Methohexital anesthesia in the surgical treatment of uncontrollable epilepsy. Anesth Analg 61:997-1001, 1982.
414. Rockoff MA, Goudsouzian NG: Seizures induced by methohexital. Anesthesiology 54:333-335, 1981.
415. Musella L, Wilder BJ, Schmidt RP: Electroencephalographic activation with intravenous methohexital in psychomotor epilepsy. Neurology 21:594-602, 1971.
416. Bennett DR, Madsen JA, Jordan WS, Wiser WC: Ketamine anesthesia in brain-damaged epileptics. Neurology 23:449-460, 1973.
417. Ferrer-Allado T, Brechner VL, Dymond A, et al: Ketamine-induced electroconvulsive phenomena in the human limbic and thalamic regions. Anesthesiology 38:333-344, 1973.
418. Steen P, Michenfelder JD: Neurotoxicity of anesthetics. Anesthesiology 50:437-453, 1979.
419. Hirshman CA, Krieger W, Littlejohn G, et al: Ketamine-aminophylline-induced decrease in seizure threshold. Anesthesiology 56:464-467, 1982.
420. Ghoneim MM, Yamada T: Etomidate: A clinical and electroencephalographic comparison with thiopental. Anesth Analg 56:478-485, 1977.
421. Laughlin TP, Newberg LA: Prolonged myoclonus after etomidate anesthesia. Anesth Analg 64:80-82, 1985.
422. Ebrahim ZY, DeBoer GE, Luders H, et al: Effect of etomidate on the electroencephalogram of patients with epilepsy. Anesth Analg 65:1004-1006, 1986.
423. Gancher S, Laxer KD, Krieger W: Activation of epileptogenic activity by etomidate. Anesthesiology 61:616-618, 1984.
424. Avramov MN, Husain MM, White PF: The comparative effects of methohexital, propofol, and etomidate for electroconvulsive therapy. Anesth Analg 81:596-602, 1995.
425. Yeoman P, Hutchinson A, Byrne A, et al: Etomidate infusions for the control of refractory status epilepticus. Intensive Care Med 15:255-259, 1989.
426. Maekawa T, Tommasino C, Shapiro HM: Local cerebral blood flow with fentanyl-induced seizures. J Cereb Blood Flow Metab 4:88-95, 1984.
427. DeCastro J, VanDeWater A, Wouters L, et al: Comparative study of cardiovascular neurological and metabolic side-effects of eight narcotics in dogs. Acta Anaesthesiol Belg 30:5-9, 1979.
428. Kofke WA, Garman RH, Tom WC, et al: Alfentanil-induced hypermetabolism, seizure, and histopathology in rat brain. Anesth Analg 75:953-964, 1992.
429. Kofke WA, Garman RH, Stiller RL, et al: Opioid neurotoxicity: Fentanyl dose-response effects in rats. Anesth Analg 83:1298-1306, 1996.
430. Rao TLK, Mummaneni N, El-Etr AA: Convulsions: An unusual response to intravenous fentanyl administration. Anesth Analg 61:1020-1021, 1982.
431. Safwat AM, Daniel D: Grand mal seizure after fentanyl administration [letter]. Anesthesiology 59:78, 1983.
432. Hoien A: Another case of grand mal seizure after fentanyl administration [letter]. Anesthesiology 60:387-388, 1984.
433. Murkin JM, Moldenhauer CC, Hug CC, Epstein CM: Absence of seizures during induction of anesthesia with high dose fentanyl. Anesth Analg 63:489-494, 1984.
434. Smith NT, Westover CJ, Quinn M, et al: An electroencephalographic comparison of alfentanil with other narcotics and with thiopental. J Clin Monit 1:236-244, 1985.
435. Smith NT, Dec-Silver H, Sanford TJ, et al: EEGs during high-dose fentanyl-, sufentanil-, or morphine-oxygen anesthesia. Anesth Analg 63:386-393, 1984.

436. Cascino GD, So EL, Sharbrough FW, et al: Alfentanil-induced epileptiform activity in patients with partial epilepsy. J Clin Neurophysiol 10:520-525, 1993.

437. Astrup J, Symon L, Branston NM, Lassen NA: Cortical evoked potential and extracellular K^+ and H^+ at critical levels of brain ischemia. Stroke 8:52-57, 1977.

438. Branston NM, Symon L, Crockard HA, Pasztor E: Relationship between the cortical evoked potential and local cortical blood flow following acute middle cerebral artery occlusion in the baboon. Exp Neurol 45:195-208, 1974.

439. Jones TH, Morawetz RB, Crowell RM, et al: Thresholds of focal cerebral ischemia in awake monkeys. J Neurosurg 54:773-782, 1981.

440. Michenfelder JD, Sundt TM, Fode N, Sharbrough FW: Isoflurane when compared to enflurane and halothane decreases the frequency of cerebral ischemia during carotid endarterectomy. Anesthesiology 67:336-340, 1987.

441. Carter LP, Yamagata S, Erspamer R: Time limits on reversible cortical ischemia. Neurosurgery 12:620-623, 1983.

442. Kaplan B, Brint S, Tanabe J, et al: Temporal thresholds for neocortical infarction in rats subjected to reversible focal cerebral ischemia. Stroke 22:1032-1039, 1991.

443. Hossmann KA: Viability thresholds and the penumbra of focal ischemia. Ann Neurol 36:557-365, 1994.

444. Perkins WJ, Lanier WL, Schroeder DR, et al: Critical regional cerebral blood flow determined using logistic regression analysis [abstract]. Anesthesiology 87:A173, 1997.

445. Sundt TM, Sharbrough FW, Piepgras DG, et al: Correlation of cerebral blood flow and electroencephalographic changes during carotid endarterectomy. Mayo Clin Proc 56:533-543, 1981.

446. Michenfelder JD, Sundt TM: Cerebral ATP and lactate levels in the squirrel monkey following occlusion of the middle cerebral artery. Stroke 2:319-326, 1971.

447. Michenfelder JD, Theye RA: The effects of anesthesia and hypothermia on canine cerebral ATP and lactate during anoxia produced by decapitation. Anesthesiology 33:430-439, 1970.

448. Siesjo BK: Pathophysiology and treatment of focal cerebral ischemia. Part I: Pathophysiology. J Neurosurg 77:169-184, 1992.

449. Benveniste H, Drejer J, Schousboe A, Diemer NH: Elevation of the extracellular concentrations of glutamate and aspartate in rat hippocampus during transient cerebral ischemia monitored by intracerebral microdialysis. J Neurochem 43:1369-1374, 1984.

450. Furukawa K, Fu W, Li Y, et al: The actin-severing protein gelsolin modulates calcium channel and NMDA receptor activities and vulnerability to excitotoxicity in hippocampal neurons. J Neurosci 17:8178-8186, 1997.

451. Chen ST, Hsu CY, Hogan EL, et al: Thromboxane, prostacyclin, and leukotrienes in cerebral ischemia. Neurology 36:466-470, 1986.

452. Pieper AA, Verma A, Zhang J, Snyder SH: Poly (ADP-ribose) polymerase, nitric oxide and cell death. Trends Pharmacol Sci 20:171-181, 1999.

453. Marsh WR, Anderson RE, Sundt TM: Effect of hyperglycemia on brain pH levels in areas of focal incomplete cerebral ischemia in monkeys. J Neurosurg 65:693-696, 1986.

454. Chopp M, Welch KMA, Tidwell CD, Helpern JA: Global cerebral ischemia and intracellular pH during hyperglycemia and hypoglycemia in cats. Stroke 19:1383-1387, 1988.

455. Smith M-L, vonHanwehr R, Seisjo BK: Changes in extra- and intracellular pH in the brain during and following ischemia in hyperglycemic and moderately hypoglycemic rats. J Cereb Blood Flow Metab 6:574-583, 1986.

456. Folbergrová J, Memezawa H, Smith M-L, Siesjö BK: Focal and perifocal changes in tissue energy state during middle cerebral artery occlusion in normo- and hyperglycemic rats. J Cereb Blood Flow Metab 12:25-33, 1992.

457. Dawson TM, Dawson VL, Snyder SH: A novel neuronal messenger molecule in brain: The free radical, nitric oxide. Ann Neurol 32:297-311, 1992.

458. Beckman JS: The double-edged role of nitric oxide in brain function and superoxide-mediated injury. J Dev Physiol 15:53-59, 1991.

459. Iadecola C: Bright and dark sides of nitric oxide in ischemic brain injury. Trends Neurosci 20:132-139, 1997.

460. Samdani AF, Dawson TM, Dawson VL: Nitric oxide synthase in models of focal ischemia. Stroke 28:1283-1288, 1997.

461. Lipton P: Ischemic cell death in brain neurons. Physiol Rev 79:1431-1568, 1999.

462. Fiskum G, Murphy AN, Beal MF: Mitochondria in neurodegeneration: Acute ischemia and chronic neurodegenerative diseases. J Cereb Blood Flow Metab 19:351-369, 1999.

463. Hou ST, MacManus JP: Molecular mechanisms of cerebral ischemia–induced neuronal death. Int Rev Cytol 221:93-148, 2002.

464. Velier JJ, Ellison JA, Kikly KK, et al: Caspase-8 and caspase-3 are expressed by different populations of cortical neurons undergoing delayed cell death after focal stroke in the rat. J Neurosci 19:5932-5941, 1999.

465. Kawaguchi M, Kimbro JR, Drummond JC, et al: Isoflurane delays but does not prevent cerebral infarction in rats subjected to focal ischemia. Anesthesiology 92:1335-1342, 2000.

466. Du C, Hu R, Csernansky C, et al: Very delayed infarction after mild focal cerebral ischemia: A role for apoptosis? J Cereb Blood Flow Metab 16:195-201, 1996.

467. Dirnagl U, Iadecola C, Moskowitz M: Pathobiology of ischaemic stroke: An integrated view. Trends Neurosci 22:391-397, 1999.

468. Zauner A, Daugherty WP, Bullock MR, Warner DS: Brain oxygenation and energy metabolism: Part I—biological function and pathophysiology. Neurosurgery 51:289-301, 2002.

469. Graham S, Chen J: Programmed cell death in cerebral ischemia. J Cereb Blood Flow Metab 21:99-109, 2001.

470. Chan PH: Reactive oxygen radicals in signaling and damage in the ischemic brain. J Cereb Blood Flow Metab 21:2-14, 2001.

471. Mattson MP, Duan W, Pedersen WA, Culmsee C: Neurodegenerative disorders and ischemic brain diseases. Apoptosis 6:69-81, 2001.

472. Abramson NA: Randomized clinical study of thiopental loading in comatose survivors of cardiac arrest. N Engl J Med 314:397-403, 1986.

473. Todd MM, Chadwich HC, Shapiro HM, et al: The neurologic effects of thiopental therapy following cardiac arrest in cats. Anesthesiology 57:76-86, 1982.

474. Gisvold SE, Safar P, Hendrickx HHL, et al: Thiopental treatment after global ischemia in pig-tailed monkeys. Anesthesiology 60:88-96, 1984.

475. Steen PA, Gisvold SE, Milde JH, et al: Nimodipine improves outcome when given after complete cerebral ischemia in primates. Anesthesiology 62:406-414, 1985.

476. Tateishi A, Fleischer JE, Drummond JC, et al: Nimodipine does not improve neurologic outcome after 14 minutes of cardiac arrest in cats. Stroke 20:1044-1050, 1989.

477. Tateishi A, Scheller MS, Drummond JC, et al: Failure of nimodipine to improve neurologic outcome after eighteen minutes of cardiac arrest in the cat. Resuscitation 211:191-206, 1991.

478. Steen PA, Newberg LA, Milde JH, Michenfelder JD: Cerebral blood flow and neurologic outcome when nimodipine is given after complete cerebral ischemia in the dog. J Cereb Blood Flow Metab 4:82-87, 1984.

479. Forsman M. Aarseth HP, Nordby HK, et al: Effects of nimodipine on cerebral blood flow and cerebrospinal fluid pressure after cardiac arrest: Correlation with neurologic outcome. Anesth Analg 68:436-443, 1989.

480. Roine RO, Kaste M, Kinnunen A, et al: Nimodipine after resuscitation from out-of-hospital ventricular fibrillation: A placebo-controlled, double-blind, randomized trial. JAMA 264:3171-3177, 1990.

481. Lidoflazine: Brain Resuscitation Clinical Trial II Study Group. A randomized clinical study of a calcium-entry blocker (Lidoflazine) in the treatment of comatose survivors of cardiac arrest. N Engl J Med 324:1225-1231, 1991.

482. Hypothermia after Cardiac Arrest Study Group: Mild therapeutic hypothermia to improve the neurologic outcome after cardiac arrest. N Engl J Med 346:549-556, 2002.

483. Hoffman WE, Cheng MA, Thomas C, et al: Clonidine decreases plasma catecholamines and improves outcome from incomplete ischemia in the rat. Anesth Analg 73:460-464, 1991.

484. Hoffman WE, Thomas C, Albrecht RF: The effect of halothane and isoflurane on neurologic outcome following incomplete cerebral ischemia in the rat. Anesth Analg 76:279-283, 1993.

485. Smith AL, Hoff JT, Nielsen SL, Larson CP: Barbiturate protection in acute focal cerebral ischemia. Stroke 5:1-7, 1974.

486. Hoff JT, Smith AL, Hankinson HL, Nielsen SL: Barbiturate protection from cerebral infarction in primates. Stroke 6:28-33, 1975.

487. Michenfelder JD, Milde JH, Sundt TM: Cerebral protection by barbiturate anesthesia. Use after middle cerebral artery occlusion in Java monkeys. Arch Neurol 33:345-350, 1976.

488. Lawner PM, Laurent JP, Simeone FA, Fink EA: Effect of extracranial-intracranial bypass and pentobarbital on acute stroke in dogs. J Neurosurg 56:92-96, 1982.

489. Selman WR, Spetzler RF, Roski RA, et al: Barbiturate coma in focal cerebral ischemia. Relationship of protection to timing of therapy. J Neurosurg 56:685-690, 1982.

490. Hoff JT, Nishimura M, Newfield P: Pentobarbital protection from cerebral infarction without suppression of edema. Stroke 13:623-628, 1982.

491. Nehls DG, Todd MM, Spetzler RF, et al: A comparison of the cerebral protective effects of isoflurane and barbiturates during temporary focal ischemia in primates. Anesthesiology 66:453-464, 1987.

492. Nussmeier NA, Arlund C, Slogoff S: Neuropsychiatric complications after cardiopulmonary bypass: Cerebral protection by a barbiturate. Anesthesiology 64:165-170, 1986.

493. Shapiro HM: Barbiturates in brain ischemia. Br J Anaesth 57:82-95, 1985.

494. Todd MM, Warner DS: A comfortable hypothesis re-evaluated: Cerebral metabolic rate depression and brain protection during ischemia [editorial]. Anesthesiology 76:161-164, 1992.

495. Nakashima K, Todd MM, Warner DS: The relation between cerebral metabolic rate and ischemic depolarization. Anesthesiology 82:1199-1208, 1995.

496. Warner DS, Takaoka S, Wu B, et al: Electroencephalographic burst suppression is not required to elicit maximal neuroprotection from pentobarbital in a rat model of focal cerebral ischemia. Anesthesiology 84:1475-1484, 1996.

497. Busto R, Dietrich WD, Globus MY-T, et al: Small differences in intraischemic brain temperature critically determine the extent of ischemic neuronal injury. J Cereb Blood Flow Metab 7:729-738, 1987.

498. Sano T, Drummond JC, Patel PM, et al: A comparison of the cerebral protective effects of isoflurane and mild hypothermia in a model of incomplete forebrain ischemia in the rat. Anesthesiology 76:221-228, 1992.

499. Buchan A, Pulsinelli WA: Hypothermia but not the N-methyl-D-aspartate antagonist, MK-801, attenuates neuronal damage in gerbils subjected to transient global ischemia. J Neurosci 10:311-316, 1990.

500. Warner DS, Zhou J, Ramani R, Todd MM: Reversible focal ischemia in the rat: Effects of halothane, isoflurane, and methohexital anesthesia. J Cereb Blood Flow Metab 11:794-802, 1991.

501. Drummond JC, Cole DJ, Patel PM, Reynolds LW: Focal cerebral ischemia during anesthesia with etomidate, isoflurane or thiopental: A comparison of the extent of cerebral injury. Neurosurgery 37:742-749, 1995.

502. Gisvold SE, Safar P, Hendrick HHL, et al: Thiopental treatment after global brain ischemia in pigtailed monkeys. Anesthesiology 60:88-96, 1984.

503. Cole DJ, Cross LM, Drummond JC, et al: Thiopentone and methohexital, but not pentobarbitone, reduce early focal cerebral ischemic injury in rats. Can J Anaesth 48:807-814, 2001.

504. Baughman VL, Hoffman WE, Miletich DJ, et al: Neurologic outcome in rats following incomplete cerebral ischemia during halothane, isoflurane or N₂O. Anesthesiology 69:192-198, 1988.

505. Soonthan-Brant V, Patel PM, Drummond JC, et al: Fentanyl does not increase brain injury after focal cerebral ischemia in rats. Anesth Analg 88:49-55, 1999.

506. Mackensen GB, Nellgard B, Kudo M, et al: Peri-ischemic cerebral blood flow (CBF) does not explain beneficial effects of isoflurane on outcome from near complete forebrain ischemia in rats. Anesthesiology 93:1102-1106, 2000.

507. Nellgard B, Mackensen GB, Pineda J, et al: Anesthetic effects on cerebral metabolic rate predict histologic outcome from near-complete forebrain ischemia in the rat. Anesthesiology 93:431-436, 2000.

508. Kawaguchi M, Kimbro JR, Drummond JC, et al: Effects of isoflurane on neuronal apoptosis in rats subjected to focal ischemia. J Neurosurg Anesthesiol 12:385, 2000.

509. Warner DS, Desphande JK, Wieloch T: The effect of isoflurane on neuronal necrosis following near-complete forebrain ischemia in the rat. Anesthesiology 64:19-23, 1986.

510. Baughman VL, Hoffman WE, Miletich DJ, et al: Neurologic outcome in rats following incomplete cerebral ischemia during halothane, isoflurane, or N₂O. Anesthesiology 69:192-198, 1988.

511. Milde LN, Milde JE, Lanier WL, et al: Comparison of the effects of isoflurane and thiopental on neurologic outcome and neuropathology after temporary focal cerebral ischemia in primates. Anesthesiology 69:905-913, 1988.

512. Gelb AW, Boisvert DP, Tang C, et al: Primate brain tolerance to temporary focal cerebral ischemia during isoflurane- or sodium nitroprusside-induced hypotension. Anesthesiology 70:678-683, 1989.

513. Ruta TS, Drummond JC, Cole DJ: A comparison of the area of histochemical dysfunction after focal cerebral ischaemia during anaesthesia with isoflurane and halothane in the rat. Can J Anaesth 38:129-135, 1991.

514. Warner DS, Todd MM, McFarlane C, et al: Sevoflurane and halothane reduce focal ischemic brain damage in the rat: Possible influence on thermoregulation. Anesthesiology 79:985-992, 1993.

515. Warner DS, McFarlane C, Todd MM, et al: Sevoflurane and halothane reduce focal ischemic brain damage in the rat. Anesthesiology 79:985-992, 1993.

516. Werner C, Mollenberg O, Kochs E, Schulte JE: Sevoflurane improves neurological outcome after incomplete cerebral ischaemia in rats. Br J Anaesth 75:756-760, 1995.

517. Engelhard K, Werner C, Reeker W, et al: Desflurane and isoflurane improve neurological outcome after incomplete cerebral ischaemia in rats. Br J Anaesth 83:415-421, 1999.

518. Ravussin P, deTribolet N: Total intravenous anesthesia with propofol for burst suppression in cerebral aneurysm surgery: Preliminary report of 42 patients. Neurosurgery 32:236-240, 1993.

519. Ridenour TR, Warner DS, Todd MM, Glonet TX: Comparative effects of propofol and halothane on outcome from temporary middle cerebral artery occlusion in the rat. Anesthesiology 76:807-812, 1992.

520. Gelb AW, Bayona NA, Wilson JX, Cechetto DF: Propofol anesthesia compared to awake reduces infarct size in rats. Anesthesiology 96:1183-1190, 2002.

521. Pittman JE, Sheng H, Pearlstein RD, et al: Comparison of the effects of propofol and pentobarbital on neurologic outcome and cerebral infarction size after temporary focal ischemia in the rat. Anesthesiology 87:1139-1144, 1997.

522. Batjer HH, Frankfurt AI, Purdy PD, et al: Use of etomidate, temporary arterial occlusion, and intraoperative angiography in surgical treatment of large and giant cerebral aneurysms. J Neurosurg 68:234-240, 1988.

523. Watson JC, Drummond JC, Patel PM, et al: An assessment of the cerebral protective effects of etomidate in a model of incomplete forebrain ischemia in the rat. Neurosurgery 30:540-544, 1992.

524. Sano T, Patel PM, Drummond JC, Cole DJ: A comparison of the cerebral protective effects of etomidate, thiopental and isoflurane in a model of forebrain ischemia in the rat. Anesth Analg 76:990-997, 1993.

525. McKay L, Drummond JC, Cole DJ, et al: Effect of nitric oxide on focal cerebral ischemic injury during etomidate or halothane anesthesia in rats [abstract]. Anesthesiology 85:A1181, 1996.

526. Nebauer AE, Doenicke A, Hoernecke R, et al: Does etomidate cause haemolysis? Br J Anaesth 69:58-60, 1992.

527. Wolff DJ, Datto GA, Samatovicz RA, Tempsick RA: Calmodulin-dependent nitric-oxide synthase. Mechanism of inhibition by imidazole and phenylimidazoles. J Biol Chem 268:9425-9429, 1993.

528. Samson D, Batjer HH, Bowman G, et al: A clinical study of the parameters and effects of temporary arterial occlusion in the management of intracranial aneurysms. Neurosurgery 34:22-28, discussion 28-29, 1994.

529. Pickard JD, Murray GD, Illingworth R, et al: Effect of oral nimodipine on cerebral infarction and outcome after subarachnoid haemorrhage: British Aneurysm Nimodipine Trial. BMJ 298:636-642, 1989.

530. Gelmers HJ, Gorter K, DeWeerdt CJ, Wiezer HJA: A controlled trial of nimodipine in acute ischemic stroke. N Engl J Med 318:203-207, 1988.

531. Rosenbaum D, Zabramski J, Frey J, et al: Early treatment of ischemic stroke with a calcium antagonist. Stroke 22:437-441, 1991.

532. Trust Study Group: Randomised, double-blind, placebo-controlled trial of nimodipine in acute stroke. Lancet 336:1205-1209, 1990.

533. Wise G, Sutter R, Burkholder J: The treatment of brain ischemia with vasopressor drugs. Stroke 3:135-140, 1972.

534. Cole DJ, Drummond JC, Osborne TN, Matsumura J: Hypertension and hemodilution during cerebral ischemia reduce brain injury and edema. Am J Physiol 259:H211-H217, 1990.

535. Young WL, Solomon RA, Pedley TA, et al: Direct cortical EEG monitoring during temporary vascular occlusion for cerebral aneurysm surgery. Anesthesiology 71:794-799, 1989.

536. Soloway M, Nadel W, Albin MS, White RJ: The effect of hyperventilation on subsequent cerebral infarction. Anesthesiology 29:975-980, 1968.

537. Waltz AG, Sundt TM, Michenfelder JD: Cerebral blood flow during carotid endarterectomy. Circulation 45:1091-1096, 1972.

538. Christensen MS, Paulson OB, Olesen J, et al: Cerebral apoplexy (stroke) treated with or without prolonged artificial hyperventilation: 1. Cerebral circulation, clinical course, and cause of death. Stroke 4:568-619, 1973.

539. Michenfelder JD, Sundt TM: The effect of $Paco_2$ on the metabolism of ischemic brain in squirrel monkeys. Anesthesiology 38:445-453, 1973.

540. Michenfelder JD, Milde JH: Failure of prolonged hypocapnia, hypothermia, or hypertension to favorably alter acute stroke in primates. Stroke 8:87-91, 1977.

541. Ruta TS, Drummond JC, Cole DJ: The effect of acute hypocapnia on local cerebral blood flow during middle cerebral artery occlusion in isoflurane anesthetized rats. Anesthesiology 78:134-140, 1993.

542. Busto R, Globus MY-T, Dietrich WD, et al: Effect of mild hypothermia on ischemia-induced release of neurotransmitters and free fatty acids in rat brain. Stroke 20:904-910, 1989.

543. Minamisawa H, Smith M-L, Siesjö BK: The effect of mild hyperthermia and hypothermia on brain damage following 5, 10, and 15 minutes of forebrain ischemia. Ann Neurol 28:26-33, 1990.

544. Welsh FA, Sims RE, Harris VA: Mild hypothermia prevents ischemic injury in gerbil hippocampus. J Cereb Blood Flow Metab 10:557-563, 1990.

545. Ridenour TR, Warner DS, Todd MM, McAllister AC: Mild hypothermia reduces infarct size resulting from temporary but not permanent focal ischemia in rats. Stroke 23:733-738, 1992.

546. Boris-Möller F, Smith M-L, Siesjö BK: Effects of hypothermia on ischemic brain damage: A comparison between preischemic and postischemia cooling. Neurosci Res Commun 5:87-94, 1989.

547. Busto R, Dietrich WD, Globus MY-T, Ginsberg MD: Post-ischemic moderate hypothermia inhibits CA1 hippocampal neuronal ischemic injury. Neurosci Lett 101:299-304, 1989.

548. Baker CJ, Onesti MT, Solomon RA: Reduction by delayed hypothermia of cerebral infarction following middle cerebral artery occlusion in the rat: A time-course study. J Neurosurg 77:438-444, 1992.

549. Coimbra C, Drake M, Boris-Moller F, Wieloch T: Long-lasting neuroprotective effect of postischemic hypothermia and treatment with an anti-inflammatory/antipyretic drug. Evidence for chronic encephalopathic processes after ischemia. Stroke 27:1578-1585, 1996.

550. Ginsberg MD, Sternau LL, Globus MY-T, et al: Therapeutic modulation of brain temperature: Relevance to ischemic brain injury. Cerebrovasc Brain Metab Rev 4:189-225, 1992.

551. Hindman BJ, Todd MM, Gelb AW, et al: Mild hypothermia as a protective therapy during intracranial aneurysm surgery: A randomized prospective pilot trial. Neurosurgery 44:23-32, discussion 32-33, 1999.

552. Steiner T, Friede T, Aschoff A, et al: Effect and feasibility of controlled rewarming after moderate hypothermia in stroke patients with malignant infarction of the middle cerebral artery. Stroke 32:2833-2835, 2001.

553. Georgiadis D, Schwarz S, Kollmar R, Schwab S: Endovascular cooling for moderate hypothermia in patients with acute stroke. Stroke 32:2550-2553, 2001.

554. Krieger DW, DeGeorgia MA, Abou-Chebl A, et al: Cooling for acute ischemic brain damage (COOL AID). Stroke 32:1847-1854, 2001.

555. Schwab S, Georgiadis D, Berrouschot J, et al: Feasibility and safety of moderate hypothermia after massive hemispheric infarction. Stroke 32:2033-2035, 2001.

556. Kammersgaard LP, Rasmussen BH, Jorgensen HS, et al: Feasibility and safety of inducing modest hypothermia in awake patients with acute stroke through surface cooling: A case-control study. Stroke 31:2251-2256, 2000.

557. Bouma GJ, Muizelaar JP, Choi SC, et al: Cerebral circulation and metabolism after severe traumatic brain injury: The elusive role of ischemia. J Neurosurg 75:685-693, 1991.

558. Graham DI, Ford I, Adams JH, et al: Ischaemic brain damage is still common in fatal non-missile head injury. J Neurol Neurosurg Psychiatry 52:346-350, 1989.

559. Marion DW, Obrist WD, Carlier PM, et al: The use of moderate therapeutic hypothermia for patients with severe head injuries: A preliminary report. J Neurosurg 79:354-362, 1993.

560. Shiozaki T, Sugimoto H, Taneda M, et al: Effect of mild hypothermia on uncontrollable intracranial hypertension after severe head injury. J Neurosurg 79:363-368, 1993.

561. Clifton GL, Allen S, Barrodale P, et al: A phase II study of moderate hypothermia in severe brain injury. J Neurotrauma 10:263-273, 1993.

562. Metz C, Holzschuh M, Bein T, et al: Moderate hypothermia in patients with severe head injury: Cerebral and extracerebral effects. J Neurosurg 85:533-541, 1996.

563. Clifton GL, Miller ET, Choi SC, et al: Lack of effect of induction of hypothermia after acute brain injury. N Engl J Med 344:556-563, 2001.

564. Kuroiwa T, Bonnekoh P, Hossmann KA: Prevention of postischemic hyperthermia prevents ischemic injury of CA1 neurons in gerbils. J Cereb Blood Flow Metab 10:550-556, 1990.

565. Baena RC, Busto R, Dietrich WD, et al: Hyperthermia delayed by 24 hours aggravates neuronal damage in rat hippocampus following global ischemia. Neurology 48:768-773, 1997.

566. Pulsinelli WA, Waldman S, Rawlinson D, Plum F: Moderate hyperglycemia augments ischemic brain damage: A neuropathologic study in the rat. Neurology 32:1239-1246, 1982.

567. Lanier WL, Stangland KJ, Scheithauer BW, et al: The effects of dextrose infusion and head position on neurologic outcome after complete cerebral ischemia in primates: Examination of a model. Anesthesiology 66:39-48, 1987.

568. Drummond JC, Moore SS: The influence of dextrose administration on neurologic outcome after temporary spinal cord ischemia in the rabbit. Anesthesiology 70:64-70, 1989.

569. Nakakimura K, Fleischer JE, Drummond JC, et al: Glucose administration prior to cardiac arrest significantly worsens neurologic outcome in cats. Anesthesiology 72:1005-1011, 1990.

570. Vannucci RC, Brucklacher RM, Vannucci SJ: The effect of hyperglycemia on cerebral metabolism during hypoxia-ischemia in the immature rat. J Cereb Blood Flow Metab 16:1026-1033, 1996.

571. Müllner M, Sterz F, Binder M, et al: Blood glucose concentration after cardiopulmonary resuscitation influences functional neurological recovery in human cardiac arrest survivors. J Cereb Blood Flow Metab 17:430-436, 1997.

572. Weir CJ, Murray GD, Dyker AG, Lees KR: Is hyperglycaemia an independent predictor of poor outcome after acute stroke? Results of a long term follow up study. BMJ 314:1303-1306, 1997.

573. Longstreth WT, Diehr P, Cobb LA, et al: Neurologic outcome and blood glucose levels during out-of-hospital cardiopulmonary resuscitation. Neurology 36:1186-1191, 1986.

574. Woo J, Lam CWK, Kay R, et al: The influence of hyperglycemia and diabetes mellitus on immediate and 3-month morbidity and mortality after acute stroke. Arch Neurol 47:1174-1177, 1990.

575. Frasco P, Croughwell N, Blumenthal J, et al: Association between blood glucose level during cardiopulmonary bypass and neuropsychiatric outcome [abstract]. Anesthesiology 75:A55, 1991.

576. Toni D, Sacchetti ML, Argentino C, et al: Does hyperglycaemia play a role on the outcome of acute ischaemic stroke patients? J Neurol 239:382-386, 1992.

577. Matchar DB, Divine GW, Heyman A, Feussner JR: The influence of hyperglycemia on outcome of cerebral infarction. Ann Intern Med 117:449-456, 1992.

578. Archer DP: The role of bloodletting in the prevention and treatment of asthenic apoplexy. J Neurosurg Anesthesiol 6:51-53, 1994.

579. Lenzi GL, Frackowiak RSJ, Jones T: Cerebral oxygen metabolism and blood flow in human cerebral ischemic infarction. J Cereb Blood Flow Metab 2:321-335, 1982.

580. Paulson OB: Regional cerebral blood flow in apoplexy due to occlusion of the middle cerebral artery. Neurology 20:63-77, 1970.

581. Agnoli A, Fieschi C, Bozzao L, et al: Autoregulation of cerebral blood flow. Studies during drug-induced hypertension in normal subjects and in patients with cerebral vascular diseases. Circulation 38:800-812, 1968.

582. Fieschi C, Agnoli A, Prencipe M, et al: Impairment of the regional vasomotor response of cerebral vessels to hypercarbia in vascular diseases. Eur Neurol 2:13-30, 1969.

583. Olsen TS: Regional cerebral blood flow after occlusion of the middle cerebral artery. Acta Neurol Scand 73:321-337, 1986.

584. Ballotta E, Da Giau G, Baracchini C, et al: Early versus delayed carotid endarterectomy after a non-disabling ischemic stroke: A prospective, randomized study. Surgery 131:287-293, 2002.

585. Finnerty FA, Witkin L, Fazekas JF: Cerebral hemodynamics during cerebral ischemia induced by acute hypotension. J Clin Invest 33:1227-1232, 1954.

586. Njemanze PC: Critical limits of pressure-flow relation in the human brain. Stroke 23:1743-1747, 1992.

587. Vorstrup S, Barry DI, Jarden JO, et al: Chronic antihypertensive treatment in the rat reverses hypertension-induced changes in cerebral blood flow autoregulation. Stroke 15:312-318, 1984.

588. Toyoda K, Fujii K, Ibayashi S, et al: Attenuation and recovery of brain stem autoregulation in spontaneously hypertensive rats. J Cereb Blood Flow Metab 18:305-310, 1998.

589. Paulson OB, Vorstrup S, Anderson AR, et al: Converting enzyme inhibition resets cerebral autoregulation at lower blood pressure. J Hypertens 3:S487-S488, 1985.

590. Arbit E, DiResta GR, Bedford RF, et al: Intraoperative measurement of cerebral and tumor blood flow with laser-Doppler flowmetry. Neurosurgery 24:166-170, 1989.

591. Schregel W, Geibler C, Winking M, et al: Transcranial Doppler monitoring during induction of anesthesia: Effects of propofol, thiopental, and hyperventilation in patients with large malignant brain tumors. J Neurosurg Anesthesiol 5:86-93, 1993.

592. Shin JH, Lee HK, Kwun BD, et al: Using relative cerebral blood flow and volume to evaluate the histopathologic grade of cerebral gliomas: Preliminary results. AJR Am J Roentgenol 179:783-789, 2002.

593. Bedford RF, Morris L, Jane JA: Intracranial hypertension during surgery for supratentorial tumor: Correlation with preoperative computed tomography scans. Anesth Analg 61:430-433, 1982.

594. Yeung WTI, Lee T-Y, Maestro RFD, et al: Effect of steroids on iopamidol blood-brain transfer constant and plasma volume in brain tumors measured with X-ray computed tomography. J Neuro-oncology 18:53-60, 1994.

595. Van Roost D, Hartmann A, Quade G: Changes of cerebral blood flow following dexamethasone treatment in brain tumour patients. Acta Neurochir (Wien) 143:37-43, 2001.

596. Jarden JO, Dhawan V, Moeller JR, et al: The time course of steroid action on blood-to-brain and blood-to-tumor transport of ^{82}Rb: A positron emission tomographic study. Ann Neurol 25:239-245, 1989.

597. Wasterlain CG: Mortality and morbidity from serial seizures: An experimental study. Epilepsia 15:155-176, 1974.

CHAPTER
22 Neuromuscular Physiology and Pharmacology

J. A. Jeevendra Martyn

Neuromuscular Transmission   860
Overview   860
Morphology   860
Quantal Theory   861

The Neuromuscular Junction   862
Formation of Neurotransmitter at
   Motor Nerve Endings   862
Nerve Action Potential   862
Synaptic Vesicles and Recycling   863
Process of Exocytosis   864
Acetylcholinesterase   864
Postjunctional Receptors   865
Synthesis and Stabilization of Postsynaptic
   Receptors   866
Basic Electrophysiology of
   Neurotransmission   866

**Drug Effects on Postjunctional
   Receptors   867**
Classic Actions of Nondepolarizing Muscle
   Relaxants   867

Classic Action of Depolarizing Muscle
   Relaxants   868
Nonclassic and Noncompetitive Actions of
   Neuromuscular Drugs   869
Desensitization Block   869
Channel Block   870
Phase II Block   870

**Biology of Prejunctional and
   Postjunctional Nicotinic
   Receptors   871**
Immature or Extrajunctional versus Mature or
   Junctional Isoforms   871
Myopathy of Critical Illness and Acetylcholine
   Receptors   873
Prejunctional Receptors   873

**Antagonism of Neuromuscular
   Block   875**
Mechanism of Antagonism   875
Classes of Drugs Used   875

The physiology of neuromuscular transmission could be analyzed and understood at the most simple level by using the classic model of nerve signaling to muscle through the acetylcholine receptor. The mammalian neuromuscular junction is the prototypical and most extensively studied synapse. Research has provided more detailed information on the processes that, within the classic scheme, can modify neurotransmission and response to drugs. One example of this is the role of qualitative or quantitative changes in acetylcholine receptors modifying neurotransmission and response to drugs.[1,2] In myasthenia gravis, for example, the decrease in acetylcholine receptors results in decreased efficiency of neurotransmission (and therefore muscle weakness)[3] and altered sensitivity to neuromuscular relaxants.[1,2] Another example is the importance of nerve-related (prejunctional) changes that alter neurotransmission and response to drugs.[1,4] At still another level is the evidence that muscle relaxants act in ways that are not encompassed by the classic scheme of unitary site of action. The observation that muscle relaxants can have prejunctional effects[5] or that some nondepolarizers can also have agonist-like stimulatory actions on the receptor[6] while others have effects not explainable by purely postsynaptic events[7] has provided new insights into some previously unexplained observations. Although this multifaceted action-response scheme makes the physiology and pharmacology of neurotransmission more complex, these added insights also bring experimentally derived knowledge much closer to clinical observations.

Crucial to the seminal concepts that have developed relative to the neurotransmitter acetylcholine and its receptor systems has been the introduction of powerful and contemporary techniques in molecular biology, immunology, and electrophysiology, as well as more elegant techniques for observations of neuromuscular junction in vivo.[8] These have augmented the more traditional pharmacologic, protein chemical, morphologic, and cytologic approaches.[9] Research has elucidated the manner in which the nerve ending regulates the synthesis and release of transmitter and the release of trophic factors, both of which control muscle function, and how these processes are influenced by exogenous and endogenous substances.[8-11] Research continues into how receptors are synthesized and anchored at the end plate, the role of the nerve terminal in the maturation process, and the synthesis and control of acetylcholinesterase, the enzyme that breaks down acetylcholine. Several reviews that provide detailed insights into these areas are available.[8-13]

NEUROMUSCULAR TRANSMISSION

Overview

Neuromuscular transmission occurs by a fairly simple and straightforward mechanism. The nerve synthesizes acetylcholine and stores it in small, uniformly sized packages called *vesicles*. Stimulation of the nerve causes these vesicles to migrate to the surface of the nerve, rupture, and discharge acetylcholine into the cleft separating nerve from muscle. Acetylcholine receptors in the end plate of the muscle respond by opening its channels for influx of sodium ions into the muscle to depolarize the muscle. The end-plate potential created is continued along the muscle membrane by the opening of the sodium channels present throughout the muscle membrane, initiating a contraction.[13] The acetylcholine immediately detaches from the receptor and is destroyed by acetylcholinesterase enzyme, which also is in the cleft. Drugs, notably depolarizing relaxants or carbachol (a synthetic analog of acetylcholine not destroyed by acetylcholinesterase), can also act on these receptors to mimic the effect of acetylcholine and cause depolarization of the end plate. These drugs are therefore called *agonists* of the receptor, because to a greater or lesser extent, at least initially, they stimulate the receptor. Nondepolarizing relaxants also act on the receptors, but they prevent acetylcholine from binding to the receptor and so prevent depolarization by agonists. Because these nondepolarizers prevent the action of agonists (e.g., acetylcholine, carbachol, succinylcholine), they are referred to as *antagonists* of the acetylcholine receptor. Other compounds, frequently called *reversal agents* or *antagonists of neuromuscular paralysis* (e.g., neostigmine), inhibit acetylcholinesterase enzyme and therefore impair the hydrolysis of acetylcholine. The increased accumulation of undegraded acetylcholine can effectively compete with nondepolarizing relaxants, displacing the latter from the receptor (i.e., law of mass action), antagonizing the effects of nondepolarizers.

Morphology

The neuromuscular junction is specialized on the nerve side and on the muscle side to transmit and receive chemical messages.[8-12] Each motor neuron runs without interruption from the ventral horn of the spinal cord to the neuromuscular junction as a large, myelinated axon. As it approaches the muscle, it branches repeatedly to contact many muscle cells, to gather them into a functional group known as a *motor unit*. The architecture of the nerve terminal is quite different from that of the rest of the axon. As the terminal reaches the muscle fiber, it loses its myelin to form a spray of terminal branches against the muscle surface and is covered by Schwann cells.[10] This arrangement conforms to the architecture on the synaptic area of muscle membrane (Fig. 22-1). The nerve is separated from the surface of the muscle by a gap of approximately 20 nm, called the *junctional cleft*. The nerve and muscle are held in tight alignment by protein filaments called basal lamina, which span the cleft between nerve and end plate. The muscle surface is heavily corrugated, with deep invaginations of the junctional cleft—the primary and secondary clefts—between the folds in the muscle membrane; the end plate's total surface area is very large. The depths of the folds also vary between muscle types and species. The human neuromuscular junctions, relative to muscle size, are smaller than those of the mouse, although the junctions are located on muscle fibers that are much larger. Human junctions have longer junctional foldings and deeper gutters.[11] The functional significance of these folds is unclear. The shoulders of the folds are densely populated with acetylcholine receptors, about 5 million of them in each junction. These receptors are sparse in the depths between the folds. Instead, these deep areas contain sodium channels.

The trophic function of the nerve is vital for the development and maintenance of adequate neuromuscular function. Before birth, each muscle cell commonly has contacts with several nerves and has several neuromuscular junctions.[14] At birth, all but one of the nerves retract, and a single end plate remains. Once formed, the nerve-muscle contact, especially the end plate, is durable. Even if the original nerve dies, the one replacing it innervates exactly the same region of the muscle. The nerve endings on fast muscles are larger and more complicated than those on slow muscles. The reason for this is unclear. These differences in the nerve endings on the muscle surfaces may play a role in the differences in the response to muscle relaxants of fast and slow muscles.

Because all the muscle cells in a unit are excited by a single neuron, stimulation of the nerve electrically or by an action potential originating from the ventral horn or by any agonist, including depolarizing relaxants (e.g., succinylcholine), causes all muscle cells in the motor unit to contract synchronously. The synchronous contraction of the cells in a motor unit is fasciculation and often is vigorous enough to be observed through the skin. Although most adult human muscles have only one neuromuscular junction per cell, an important exception is some of the cells in the extraocular muscles. The extraocular muscles are "tonic" muscles, and unlike other mammalian striated muscles, they are multiply innervated, with several neuromuscular junctions strung along the surface of each muscle cell.[15] These muscles contract and relax slowly, rather than quickly as other striated muscles do; they can maintain a steady contraction, or contracture, whose strength is proportional to the stimulus received.

Figure 22–1 Adult neuromuscular junction with the three cells that constitute the synapse: the motor neuron (i.e., nerve terminal), muscle fiber, and Schwann cell. The motor neuron from the ventral horn of the spinal cord innervates the muscle. Each fiber receives only one synapse. The motor nerve loses its myelin to terminate on the muscle fiber. The nerve terminal, covered by a Schwann cell, has vesicles clustered about the membrane thickenings, which are the active zones, toward its synaptic side and mitochondria and microtubules toward its other side. A synaptic gutter, made up of a primary and many secondary clefts, separates the nerve from the muscle. The muscle surface is corrugated, and dense areas on the shoulders of each fold contain acetylcholine receptors. The sodium channels are present at the clefts and throughout muscle membrane.

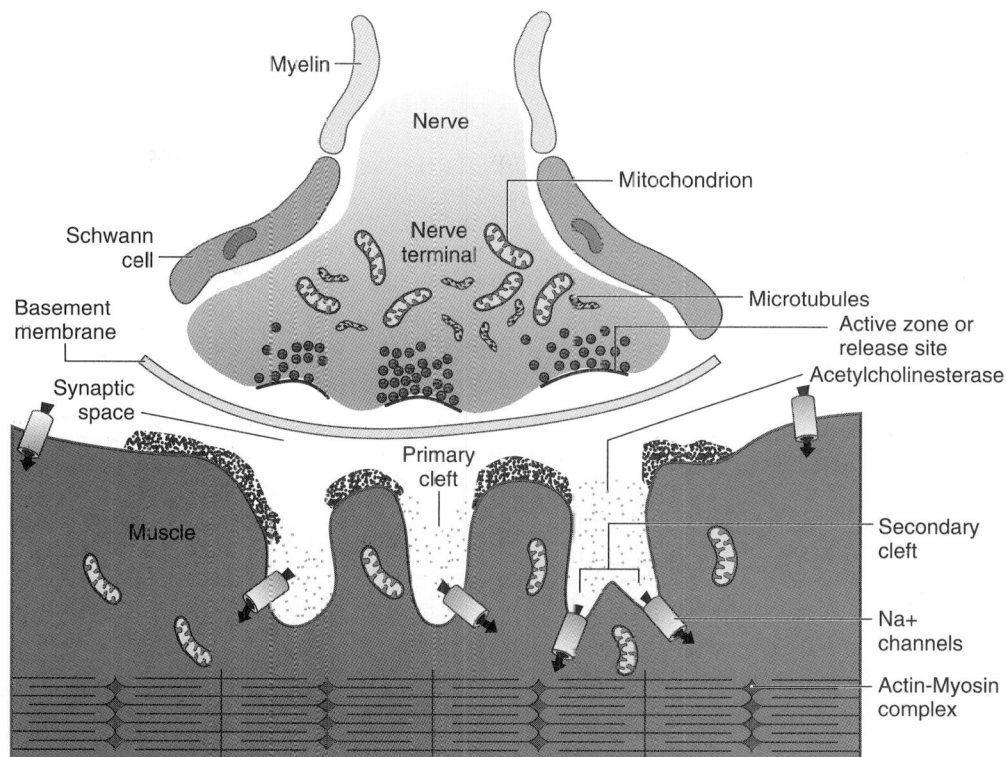

Physiologically, this specialization apparently holds the eye steadily in position. These muscles are important to an anesthetist because depolarizing relaxants affect them differently than they do most skeletal muscles. Instead of causing a brief contraction followed by paralysis, the drugs cause a long-lasting contracture response, which pulls the eye against the orbit and contributes to an increase in the pressure of the intraocular fluid[16] (see Chapter 65). The clinical significance of this has been questioned. Although many textbooks invoke the reported extrusion of intraocular content with succinylcholine, the basis for this seems to be anecdotal.[17]

The perijunctional zone is the area of muscle immediately beyond the junctional area, and it is critical to the function of the neuromuscular junction. The perijunctional zone contains a mixture of the receptors, which include a smaller density of acetylcholine receptors and high-density sodium channels (see Fig. 22-1). The admixture enhances the capacity of the perijunctional zone to respond to the depolarization (i.e., end-plate potential) produced by acetylcholine receptors and to transduce it into the wave of depolarization that travels along the muscle to initiate muscle contraction. The density of sodium channels in the perijunctional area is richer than in more distal parts of the muscle membrane.[18] The perijunctional zone is close enough to the nerve ending to be influenced by transmitter released from it. Moreover, special variants (i.e., isoforms) of receptors (see "Biology of Prejunctional and Postjunctional Nicotinic Receptors") and sodium channels can appear in this area at different stages of life and in response to abnormal decreases in nerve activity. Congenital abnormalities in the acetylcholine receptor[3] or the sodium channels (i.e., mutations)[19]

are also known. These variabilities seem to contribute to the differences in response to relaxants that are seen in patients with different pathologic conditions and ages.[1,20] Such qualitative differences may also play a role in altered muscle function (see "Myopathy of Critical Illness and Acetylcholine Receptors").

Quantal Theory

The contents of the nerve ending are not homogeneous. As shown in Figure 22-1, the vesicles are congregated in the portion toward the junctional surface, whereas the microtubules, mitochondria, and other support structures are located toward the opposite side. The vesicles containing transmitter are ordered in repeating clusters alongside small, thickened, electron-dense patches of membrane, referred to as *active zones* or *release sites*. This thickened area is a cross section of a band running across the width of the synaptic surface of the nerve ending, believed to be the structure to which vesicles attach (active zones) before they rupture into the junctional cleft (see "Process of Exocytosis"). High-resolution scanning electron micrographs reveal small protein particles arranged alongside the active zone between vesicles. These particles are believed to be special channels, the voltage-gated calcium channels, that allow calcium to enter the nerve and cause the release of vesicles.[21] The rapidity with which the neurotransmitter is released (200 μsec) suggests that the voltage-gated calcium channels are close to the release sites.

When observing the electrophysiologic activity of a skeletal muscle, small, spontaneous, depolarizing potentials at neuromuscular junctions can be seen. These potentials have only one-hundredth the amplitude of the evoked end-plate potential produced when the motor nerve is stimulated. Except for amplitude, these potentials resemble the end-plate potential in the time course and the manner in which they are affected by drugs. These small-amplitude potentials are called *miniature end-plate potentials* (MEPPs). Statistical analysis led to the conclusion that they are unitary responses; that is, there is a minimum size for the MEPP, and the sizes of all MEPPs are equal to or multiples of this minimum size. Because MEPPs are too big to be produced by a single molecule of acetylcholine, it was deduced that they are produced by uniformly sized packages, or *quanta*, of transmitter released from the nerve (in the absence of stimulation). The stimulus-evoked end-plate potential is the additive depolarization produced by the synchronous discharge of quanta from several hundred vesicles. The action potential that is propagated to the nerve ending allows entry of calcium into the nerve through voltage-gated calcium channels, and this causes vesicles to migrate to the active zone, fuse with the neural membrane, and discharge their acetylcholine into the junctional cleft.[21,22] Because the release sites are located immediately opposite the receptors on the postjunctional surface, little transmitter is wasted, and the response of the muscle is coupled directly with the signal from the nerve.

The alignment of the presynaptic receptor site is achieved by adhesion molecules or specific cell-surface proteins located on both sides of the synapse that grip each other across the synaptic cleft and hold the prejunctional and postjunctional synaptic apparatuses together.[23] One such protein implicated in synapse adhesion is neurexin, which binds to neuroligins on the postsynaptic membrane. The amount of acetylcholine released by each nerve impulse is large, at least 200 quanta of about 5000 molecules each, and the number of acetylcholine receptors activated by transmitter released by a nerve impulse also is large, about 500,000. The ions (mostly Na^+ and some Ca^{2+}) that flow through the channels of the activated receptors cause a maximum depolarization of the end plate, which causes an end-plate potential that is greater than the threshold for stimulation of the muscle. This is a very vigorous system. The signal is carried by more molecules of transmitter than are needed, and they evoke a response that is greater than needed. At the same time, only a small fraction of the available vesicles and receptors or channels are used to send each signal. Consequently, transmission has a substantial margin of safety, and at the same time, the system has substantial capacity in reserve.[24]

THE NEUROMUSCULAR JUNCTION

Formation of Neurotransmitter at Motor Nerve Endings

The axon of the motor nerve carries electrical signals from the spinal cord to the muscles and has all of the biochemical apparatus needed to transform the electrical signal into a chemical one. All the ion channels, enzymes, other proteins, macromolecules, and membrane components needed by the nerve ending to synthesize, store, and release acetylcholine and other trophic factors are made in the cell body and are transmitted to the nerve ending by axonal transport[10,25] (Fig. 22-2). The simple molecules choline and acetate are obtained from the environment of the nerve ending, the former by a special system that transports it from the extracellular fluid to the cytoplasm and the latter in the form of acetyl coenzyme A from mitochondria. The enzyme choline acetyltransferase brings about the reaction of choline and acetate to form acetylcholine, which is stored in cytoplasm until it is transported into vesicles, which are in a better position for release.

Nerve Action Potential

During a nerve action potential, sodium from outside flows across the membrane, and the resulting depolarizing voltage opens calcium channels, which allow entry of the calcium ions into the nerve and cause the release of acetylcholine. A nerve action potential is the normal activator that releases the transmitter acetylcholine. The number of quanta released by a stimulated nerve is greatly influenced by the concentration of ionized calcium in the extracellular fluid. If calcium is not present, depolarization of the nerve, even by electrical stimulation, will not produce release of transmitter. Doubling the extracellular calcium results in a 16-fold increase in the quantal content of an end-plate potential. The calcium current persists until the membrane potential is returned to normal by outward fluxes of potassium from inside the nerve cell. With the calcium channels on the nerve terminal are the potassium channels, including the voltage-gated and calcium-activated potassium channels, whose function is to limit calcium entry into nerve and therefore depolarization.[13] The calcium current can be prolonged by potassium channel blockers (e.g., 4-aminopyridine, tetraethylammonium), which slow or prevent potassium efflux out of the nerve. The increase in quantal content produced in this way can reach astounding proportions.[10,26] An effect of increasing the calcium in the nerve ending is also seen clinically as the so-called posttetanic potentiation, which occurs after a nerve of a patient paralyzed with a nondepolarizing relaxant is stimulated at high, tetanic frequencies. Calcium enters the nerve with every stimulus, but because it cannot be excreted as quickly as the nerve is stimulated, it accumulates during the tetanic period. Because the nerve ending contains more than the normal amount of calcium for some time after the tetanus, a stimulus applied to the nerve during this time causes the release of more than the normal amount of acetylcholine. The abnormally large amount of acetylcholine antagonizes the relaxant and causes the characteristic increase in the size of the twitch (see Chapters 30 and 39).

Calcium enters the nerve through specialized proteins called *calcium channels*.[13,25] Of the several types of calcium channels, two seem to be important for transmitter release, the P channels and the slower L channels. The P channels, probably the type responsible for the normal release of transmitter, are found only in nerve terminals.[10,27] In motor nerve endings, they are located immediately adjacent to the active zones (see Fig. 22-2).

Figure 22–2 The working of a chemical synapse, the motor nerve ending, including some of the apparatus for transmitter synthesis. The large, intracellular structures are mitochondria. Acetylcholine, synthesized from choline and acetate by acetylcoenzyme A, is transported into coated vesicles, which are moved to release sites. A presynaptic action potential, which triggers calcium influx through specialized proteins (Ca^{2+} channels), causes the vesicles to fuse with the membrane and discharge transmitter. Membrane from the vesicle is retracted from the nerve membrane and recycled. Each vesicle can undergo various degrees of release of contents— from incomplete to complete. The transmitter is inactivated by diffusion, catabolism, or reuptake. The *inset* provides a magnified view of a synaptic vesicle. Quanta of acetylcholine together with ATP

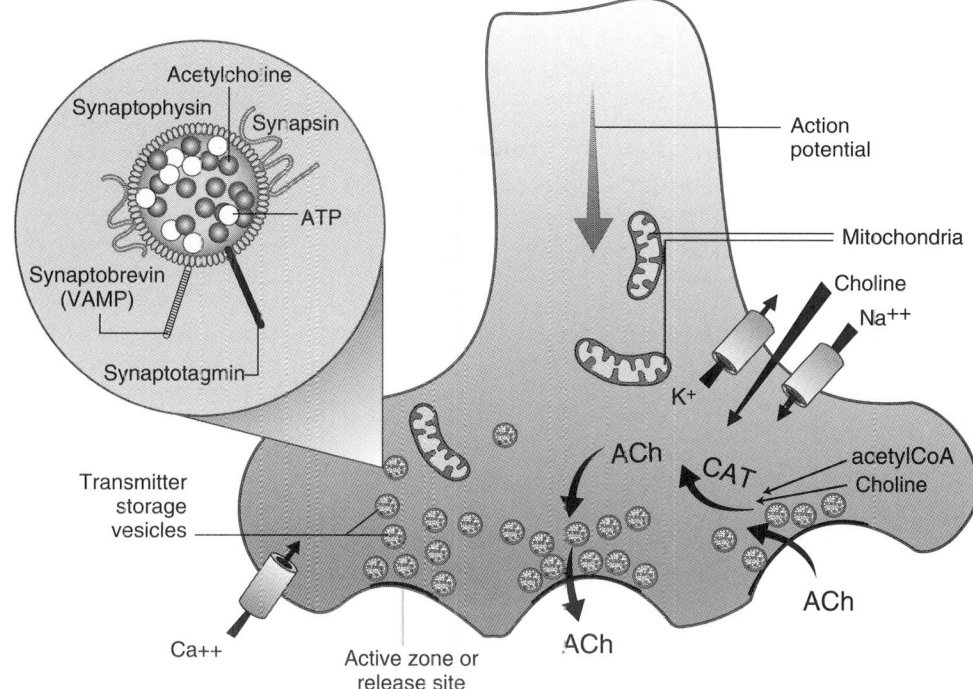

are stored in the vesicle and covered by vesicle membrane proteins. Synaptophysin is a vesicle membrane component glycoprotein. Synaptotagmin is the vesicle's calcium sensor. Phosphorylation of another membrane protein, synapsin, facilitates vesicular trafficking to the release site. Synaptobrevin (VAMP) is a SNARE protein involved in attaching the vesicle to the release site (see Fig. 22-3). ACh, acetylcholine; acetyl CoA, acetyl coenzyme A; CAT, choline acetyltransferase.

They are voltage-dependent; they are opened and closed by the changes in membrane voltage caused by the nerve action potential. Alterations in calcium entry into nerve ending can also alter release of transmitter. Eaton-Lambert myasthenic syndrome is an acquired autoimmune disease in which antibodies are directed against voltage-gated calcium channels at nerve endings.[4,28] In this syndrome, the decreased function of the calcium channel causes decreased release of transmitter, resulting in inadequate depolarization and muscle weakness. Patients with myasthenic syndrome exhibit increased sensitivity to depolarizing and nondepolarizing relaxants.[1]

Higher than normal concentrations of bivalent inorganic cations (e.g., magnesium, cadmium, manganese) can also block calcium entry through P channels and profoundly impair neuromuscular transmission. This is the mechanism for muscle weakness in the mother and fetus when magnesium sulfate is administered to treat preeclampsia. The P channels, however, are not affected by calcium entry–blocking drugs, such as verapamil, diltiazem, and nifedipine. These drugs have profound effects on the slower L channels present in the cardiovascular system. As a result, the L-type calcium channel blockers at therapeutic doses have no significant effect on the normal release of acetylcholine or on the strength of normal neuromuscular transmission. There have been a few reports, however, that calcium entry–blocking drugs may increase the block of neuromuscular transmission induced by nondepolarizing relaxants. The effect is small, and not all investigators have been able to observe it.

The explanation may lie in the fact that nerve endings also contain L-type calcium channels.

Synaptic Vesicles and Recycling

There seem to be two pools of vesicles that release acetylcholine, a readily releasable store and a reserve store, sometimes called VP2 and VP1, respectively.[25,29] The vesicles in the former are a bit smaller and are limited to an area very close to the nerve membrane, where they probably are bound to the active zones. These vesicles are the ones that ordinarily release transmitter. The release seems to occur when calcium ion enters the nerve through the P channels lined up on the sides of the active zones.[29] This calcium needs to move only a very short distance (i.e., a few atomic radii) to encounter a vesicle and to activate the proteins in the vesicle wall involved in a process known as docking[30] (see "Process of Exocytosis"). The activated protein seems to react with the nerve membrane to form a pore, through which the vesicle discharges its acetylcholine into the junctional cleft. Studies using fluorescent proteins have visualized how synaptic vesicles fuse with release sites and release their contents, which are then retrieved.[31] Some vesicles stay open briefly before retrieval and do not completely collapse into the surface membrane ("kiss and run"). Others stay open longer and probably do not completely collapse ("compensatory"). Still others completely collapse and are not retrieved until another stimulus is delivered ("stranded").[31]

Most vesicles in the nerve ending are the larger reserve (VPI) vesicles. These are firmly tethered to the cytoskeleton by many proteins, including actin, synapsin (an actin-binding protein), and spectrin.[32] From their position on the cytoskeleton, they may be moved to the readily releasable store to replace worn-out vesicles or to participate in transmission when the nerve is called on to work especially hard (e.g., when it is stimulated at very high frequencies or for a very long time). Under such strenuous circumstances, calcium may penetrate more deeply than normal into the nerve or may enter through L channels to activate calcium-dependent enzymes, which cause breakage of the synapsin links that hold the vesicles to the cytoskeleton, thereby allowing the vesicles to be moved to the release sites. Repeated stimulation requires the nerve ending to replenish its stores of vesicles filled with transmitter, a process known as mobilization. The term commonly is applied to the aggregate of all steps involved in maintaining the nerve ending's capacity to release transmitter—everything from the acquisition of choline and the synthesis of acetate to the movement of filled vesicles to the release sites. The uptake of choline and the activity of choline acetyltransferase, the enzyme that synthesizes acetylcholine, probably are the rate-limiting steps.[10,11,21-27]

Process of Exocytosis

The readily releasable pool of synaptic vesicles constitutes those vesicles readily available for release. During an action potential and calcium influx, neurotransmitter is released. Studies have shed some light on the inner workings by which the vesicle releases its contents. A conserved set of membrane proteins known as SNAREs (soluble *N*-ethylmaleimide-sensitive attachment protein receptors) are involved in the fusion, docking, and release of acetylcholine at the active zone. The whole process is called *exocytosis*. The SNAREs include the synaptic-vesicle protein synaptobrevin and the plasmalemma-associated proteins synataxin and synaptosome-associated protein of 25 kd (SNAP-25).[33] The current model for protein-mediated membrane fusions in exocytosis is as follows. Syntaxin and SNAP-25 are complexes attached to plasma membrane. After initial contact, the synaptobrevin on the vesicle forms a ternary complex with syntaxin/SNAP-25. Synaptotagmin is the protein on the vesicular membrane that acts as a calcium sensor and localizes the synaptic vesicles to synaptic zones rich in calcium channels, stabilizing the vesicles in the docked state.[34] The assembly of ternary complex forces the vesicle close to the underlying nerve terminal membrane (i.e., active zone), and the vesicle is then ready for release (Fig. 22-3). The vesicle can release part or all of its contents, some of which can be recycled to form new vesicles.[31] Botulinum toxin and tetanus neurotoxins, which selectively digest one or all of these three SNARE proteins, blocks exocytosis.[35] The result is muscle weakness or paralysis. These toxins in effect produce a partial or complete chemical denervation. Botulinum toxin is used therapeutically to treat spasticity or spasm in several neurologic and surgical diseases and cosmetically to correct wrinkles.

Acetylcholinesterase

The acetylcholine released from the nerve diffuses across the junctional cleft and reacts with specialized receptor proteins in the end plate to initiate muscle contraction. Transmitter molecules that do not react immediately with

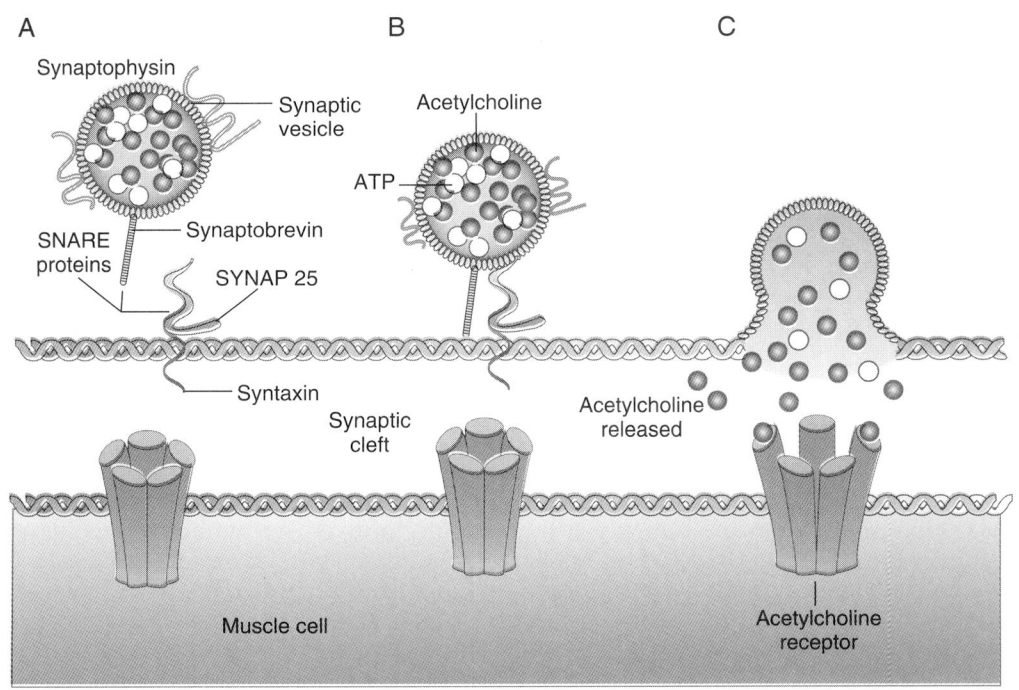

Figure 22–3 Model for protein-mediated membrane fusion and exocytosis. **A,** The release of acetylcholine from the vesicles is mediated by a series of proteins collectively called SNARE proteins. Synaptotagmin is the neuronal Ca^{2+} receptor detecting Ca^{2+} entry. Synaptobrevin (i.e., vesicle-associated membrane protein [VAMP]) is a filament-like protein on the vesicle. **B,** During depolarization and calcium entry, synaptobrevin on the vesicle unfolds and forms a ternary complex with syntaxin/SNAP-25. This process is facilitated by phosphorylation of synapsin, also present on the vesicle membrane. **C,** Assembly of the ternary complex forces the vesicle in close apposition to the nerve membrane at the active zone with release of its contents, acetylcholine. The fusion is disassembled, and the vesicle is recycled.

a receptor or those released after binding to the receptor are destroyed almost instantly by the acetylcholinesterase in the junctional cleft. Acetylcholinesterase at the junction is the asymmetric or A12 form protein made in the muscle, under the end plate. The acetylcholinesterase (enzyme classification 3.1.1.7) is a type-B carboxylesterase enzyme. There is a smaller concentration of it in the extrajunctional area. The enzyme is secreted from the muscle but remains attached to it by thin stalks of collagen fastened to the basement membrane.[12,25] Most of the molecules of acetylcholine released from the nerve initially pass between the enzymes to reach the postjunctional receptors, but as they are released from the receptors, they invariably encounter acetylcholinesterase and are destroyed. Under normal circumstances, a molecule of acetylcholine reacts with only one receptor before it is hydrolyzed. Acetylcholine is a potent messenger, but its actions are very short lived because it is destroyed in less than 1 millisecond after it is released.

There are congenital and acquired diseases related to altered activity of acetylcholinesterase enzyme. Congenital absence of the secreted enzyme (in knock-out mice), leads to impaired maintenance of motor neuronal system and organization of nerve terminal branches.[36] Many syndromes due to congenital abnormalities of cholinesterase enzymes have been described and result in neuromuscular disorders whose symptoms and signs usually resemble those of myasthenia.[37] Denervation decreases the acetylcholinesterases at the junctional and extrajunctional areas.[2] Other acquired diseases of cholinesterases are related to chronic inhibition of acetylcholinesterase by organophosphate pesticides or nerve gas (e.g., sarin) or to chronic pyridostigmine therapy given as prophylaxis against nerve gas poisoning.[38] Symptoms from chronic fatigue to muscle weakness have been attributed to chronic cholinesterase inhibition, underscoring the importance of acetylcholinesterase in normal and abnormal neuromuscular function.

Postjunctional Receptors

The similarity of the acetylcholine receptors among many species and the abundance of acetylcholine receptors from the *Torpedo* electric fish have greatly facilitated research in this area. The availability of the messenger ribonucleic acids (mRNAs) of humans and other species and of deoxyribonucleic acids (DNAs) has allowed the study of the receptor in artificial systems such as oocytes from frogs and mammalian cells that do not express the receptor, such as CCS or fibroblast cells. It is also possible by molecular techniques to mutate receptors to simulate pathologic states and then study receptor function in these artificial systems. By using these and related techniques, much has been learned about the synthesis, composition, and biologic function and the mechanisms that underlie physiologic and pharmacologic responses in the acetylcholine receptors.[1,7,39-41] It is evident that two isoforms of postjunctional receptors exist, a junctional or mature and an extrajunctional or immature receptor (see "Biology of Prejunctional and Postjunctional Nicotinic Receptors").[1,25] The differences between receptor subtypes, however, can be neglected in a general discussion of the role of receptors in neuromuscular transmission.

The acetylcholine receptors are synthesized in muscle cells and are anchored to the end-plate membrane by a special 43-kd protein known as rapsyn. This cytoplasmic protein is associated with acetylcholine receptor in a 1:1 ratio.[8] The receptors, formed of five subunit proteins, are arranged like the staves of a barrel into a cylindrical receptor with a central pore for ion channeling. The key features are sketched in Figure 22-4. The receptor protein has a molecular mass of about 250,000 daltons.

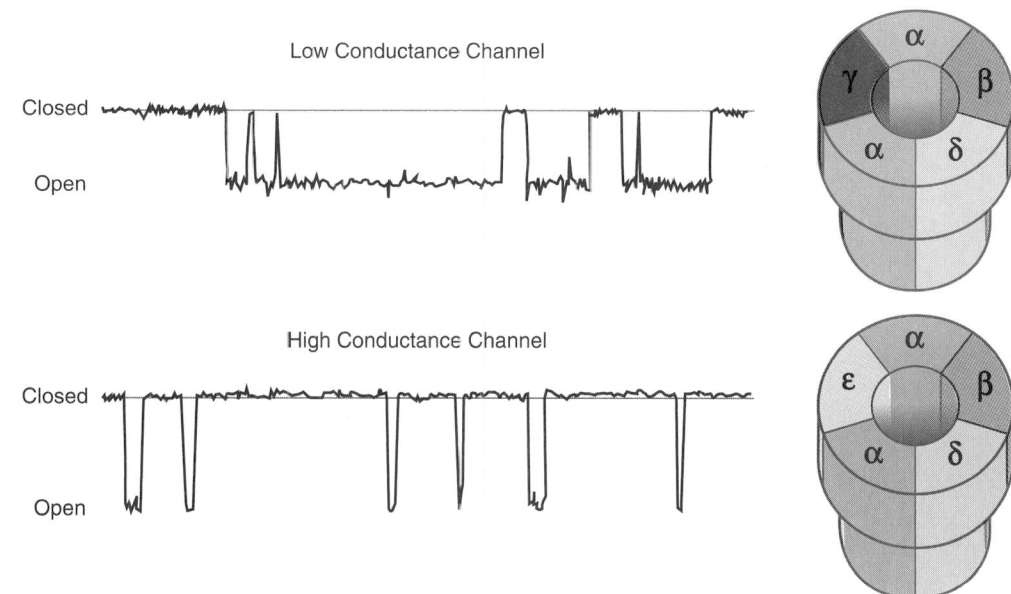

Figure 22–4 Sketch of acetylcholine receptor channels *(right)* and tracings of cell-patch records of receptor channel openings *(left)*. The mature, or junctional, receptor consists of two α-subunits and one each of β-, δ-, and ε-subunits. The immature, extrajunctional or fetal form consists of two α- and one each of β, δ, and γ-subunits. These subunits are arranged around the central cation channel. The immature isoform containing the γ-subunit shows long open times and low-amplitude channel currents. The mature isoform containing the ε-subunit shows shorter open times and high-amplitude channel currents. Substitution of the ε-subunit for the γ-subunit gives rise to the fast-gated, high-conductance channel type.

Each receptor has five subunits, which are designated α, β, δ, and ε or γ; there are two subunits of α and one of each of the others.[1,2] Each of the subunits consists of approximately 400 to 500 amino acids. The receptor protein complex passes entirely through the membrane and protrudes beyond the extracellular surface of the membrane and into the cytoplasm. The binding site for acetylcholine is on each of the α-subunits, and these are the sites of competition between the receptor agonists and antagonists. Agonists and antagonists are attracted to the binding site, and either may occupy the site, which is located near cysteine residues (unique to the α-chain) at amino acid positions 192-193 of the α-subunit.[42] Radiolabeled α-bungarotoxin from the cobra, used to quantitate the receptor, binds to heptapeptide region 189-199 of the α-subunit.[43]

Synthesis and Stabilization of Postsynaptic Receptors

Muscle tissue is formed from the mesoderm and initially appear as myoblasts. The myoblasts fuse to produce myotubes, which therefore have multiple nuclei. As the myotubes mature, the sarcomere, which is the contractile element of the muscle consisting of actin and myosin, develops. The protein, β-integrin, seems essential for myoblast fusion and sarcomere assembly.[44] Shortly after, the motor nerve axons grow into the developing muscle, and these axons bring in nerve-derived signals (i.e., growth factors), including agrin, that are key to maturation of the myotubes to muscle.[45] Agrin is a protein from the nerve that stimulates postsynaptic differentiation by activating muscle-specific kinase (MuSK), a tyrosine kinase expressed selectively in muscle. With signaling from

agrin, the acetylcholine receptors, which have been scattered throughout the muscle membrane, cluster at the area immediately beneath the nerve. Agrin together with other growth factors called neuregulins also induce the clustering of other critical muscle-derived proteins, including MUSK, rapsyn, and ERBB proteins, all of which are necessary for maturation and stabilization of the acetylcholine receptors at the junction (Fig. 22-5). Just before and shortly after birth, the immature, γ-subunit–containing acetylcholine receptors are converted to the mature, ε-subunit–containing receptors. Although the mechanism of this change is unclear, a neuregulin (growth factor) called ARIA (for acetylcholine receptor–inducing activity), which binds to one of the ERBB receptors, seems to play a role.[46]

Basic Electrophysiology of Neurotransmission

Progress in electrophysiologic techniques has moved at an equal pace with advances in molecular approaches to study the receptor. Patch-clamping is a technique in which a glass micropipette is used to probe the membrane surface until a single functional receptor is encompassed. The tip of the pipette is pressed into the lipid of the membrane, and the electronic apparatus is arranged to keep the membrane potential clamped (i.e., fixed) and to measure the current that flows through the channel of the receptor. The solution in the pipette can contain acetylcholine, tubocurarine, another drug, or a mixture of drugs. By application of these drugs to the receptor through the micropipette, electrical changes can be monitored.

Figure 22-6 illustrates the results of the classic depolarizing action of acetylcholine on end-plate receptors. Normally, the pore of the channel is closed by the

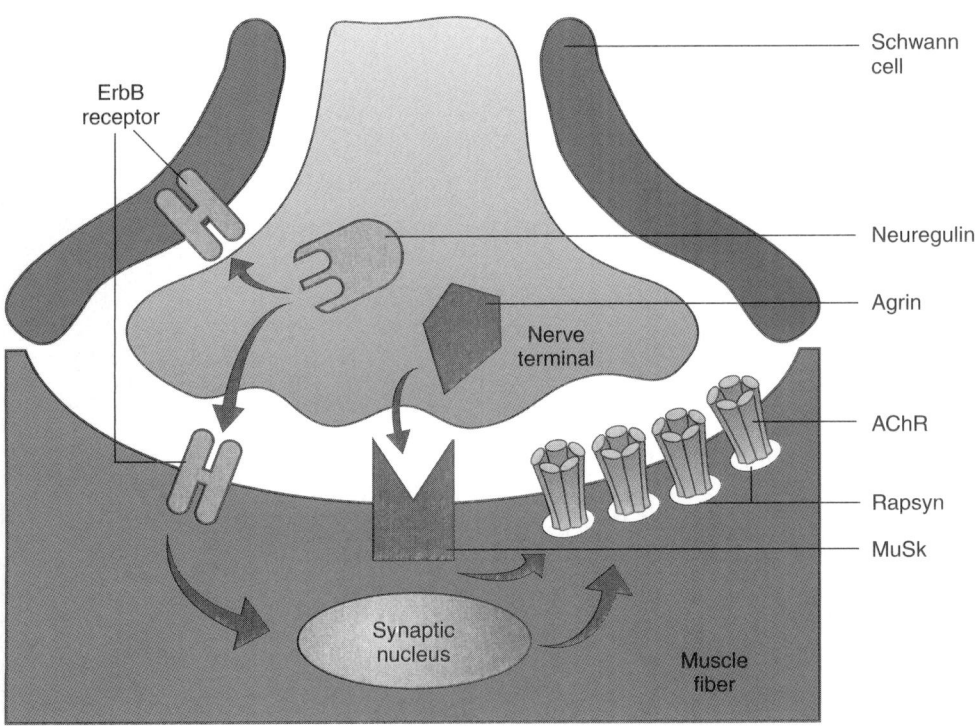

Figure 22–5 Diagram of agrin- and ARIA/neuregulin-dependent events during neuromuscular junction maturation. After establishment of a nerve on the muscle, growth factors, including agrin and ARIA (acetylcholine receptor–inducing activity), are released. Agrin interacting with its receptor MuSK (muscle-specific kinase) enhances the clustering of the synaptic proteins, including acetylcholine receptors (AChRs), rapsyn, and ERBB receptors. ARIA is the best candidate for involvement in the conversion of γ-subunit–containing immature receptor to ε-subunit–containing mature (innervated) receptor, which is synapse specific and therefore not inserted in the extrajunctional area.

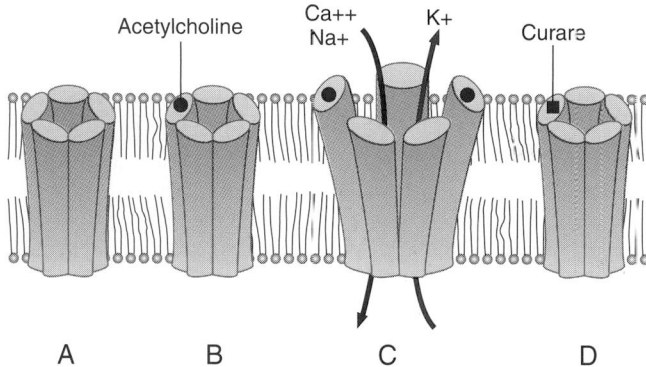

Figure 22–6 The actions of acetylcholine or curare on end-plate receptors. **A,** The ion channel is inactive and does not open in the absence of acetylcholine. **B,** Even the binding of one acetylcholine molecule *(filled circle)* to one of two binding sites does not open the channel. **C,** When acetylcholine binds to recognition sites of both α-subunits simultaneously *(filled circle)*, it triggers a conformation change that opens the channel and allows ions to flow across the membrane. **D,** The action of antagonists such as curare *(filled square)*. Acetylcholine is in competition with tubocurarine for the receptor's recognition site but may also react with acetylcholinesterase. Inhibiting the enzyme increases the lifetime of acetylcholine and the probability that it will react with a receptor. When one of the two binding (recognition) sites is occupied by curare, the receptor will not open, even if the other binding site is occupied by acetylcholine.

approximation of the cylinders (i.e., subunits). When an agonist occupies both α-subunit sites, the protein molecule undergoes a conformational change that forms a channel in the center through which ions can flow along a concentration gradient (see Fig. 22-6). When the channel is open, there is a flow of sodium and calcium from the outside of the cell to the inside and of potassium from the inside to the outside. The channel in the tube is large enough to accommodate many cations and electrically neutral molecules, but it excludes anions (e.g., chloride). The current carried by the ions depolarizes the adjacent membrane. The net current is depolarizing and creates the end-plate potential that stimulates the muscle to contract. In this instance, downward-going (i.e., depolarizing) rectangular pulses (see Fig. 22-4) can be recorded by the electrophysiologic technique described previously.

The pulse stops when the channel closes and one or both agonist molecules detach from the receptor. The current that passes through each open channel is minuscule, only a few picoamperes (about 10^4 ions/msec). However, each burst of acetylcholine from the nerve normally opens about 500,000 channels simultaneously, and the total current is more than adequate to produce depolarization of the end plate and contraction of muscle. The opening of a channel causes the conversion of chemical signals from a nerve to current flows to end-plate potentials, leading to muscle contraction. We are used to thinking of the end-plate potential as a graded event, which may be reduced in magnitude or extended in time by drugs, but in reality, the end-plate potential is the summation of many all-or-nothing events occurring simultaneously at myriad ion channels. It is these tiny events that are affected by drugs.

Receptors that do not have two molecules of agonists bound remain closed. Both α-subunits must be occupied simultaneously by agonist; if only one of them is occupied, the channel remains closed (see Fig. 22-6). This is the basis for the prevention of depolarization by antagonists. Drugs such as tubocurarine act by binding to either or both α-subunits, preventing acetylcholine from binding and opening the channel. This interaction between agonists and antagonists is competitive, and the outcome—transmission or block—depends on the relative concentrations and binding characteristics of the drugs involved (see "Drug Effects on Postjunctional Receptors").

Individual channels are also capable of a wide variety of conformations.[47,48] They may open or stay closed, affecting total current flow across the membrane, but they can do more. They may open for a longer or shorter time than normal, open or close more gradually than usual, open briefly and repeatedly (i.e., chatter), or pass fewer or more ions per opening than they usually do. Their function also is influenced by drugs, changes in the fluidity of the membrane, temperature, the electrolyte balance in the milieu, and other physical and chemical factors.[49] Receptor channels are dynamic structures that are capable of a wide variety of interactions with drugs and of entering a wide variety of current-passing states. All these influences on channel activity ultimately are reflected in the strength or weakness of neuromuscular transmission and the contraction of a muscle.

DRUG EFFECTS ON POSTJUNCTIONAL RECEPTORS

Classic Actions of Nondepolarizing Muscle Relaxants

Neurotransmission occurs when the action potential releases acetylcholine and binds to the receptor. All nondepolarizing relaxants impair or block neurotransmission by competitively preventing the binding of acetylcholine to its receptor. The final outcome (i.e., block or transmission) depends on the relative concentrations of the chemicals and their comparative affinities for the receptor. Figure 22-6 shows a system exposed to acetylcholine and tubocurarine. One receptor has attracted two acetylcholine molecules and opened its channel, where current will flow to depolarize that segment of membrane. Another has attracted one tubocurarine molecule; its channel will not open, and no current will flow, even if one acetylcholine molecule binds to the other site. The third receptor has acetylcholine on one α-subunit and nothing on the other. What will happen depends on which of the molecules binds. If acetylcholine binds, the channel will open, and the membrane will be depolarized; if tubocurarine binds, the channel will stay closed, and the membrane will not be depolarized. At other times, one or two tubocurarine molecules may attach to the receptor, in which case the receptor is not available to agonists; no current flow is recorded. In the presence of moderate concentrations of tubocurarine, the amount of current flowing through the entire end plate at any instant is reduced from normal, which results in a smaller end-plate potential and, if carried far enough, a block of neurotransmission or production of neuromuscular paralysis.

Normally, acetylcholinesterase enzyme destroys acetylcholine and removes it from the competition for a receptor, so that tubocurarine has a better chance of inhibiting transmission. If, however, an inhibitor of the acetylcholinesterase such as neostigmine is added, the cholinesterase cannot destroy acetylcholine. The concentration of agonist in the cleft remains high, and this high concentration shifts the competition between acetylcholine and tubocurarine in favor of the former, improving the chance of two acetylcholine molecules binding to a receptor even though tubocurarine is still in the environment. Cholinesterase inhibitors overcome the neuromuscular paralysis produced by nondepolarizing relaxants by this mechanism. The channel opens only when acetylcholine attaches to both recognition sites. A single molecule of antagonist, however, is adequate to prevent the depolarization of that receptor. This modifies the competition by biasing it strongly in favor of the antagonist. Mathematically, if the concentration of tubocurarine is doubled, the concentration of acetylcholine must be increased fourfold if acetylcholine is to remain competitive. Paralysis produced by high concentrations of antagonist is more difficult to reverse than those produced by low concentrations. After large doses of nondepolarizing relaxants, reversal drugs may be ineffective until the concentration of the relaxant in the perijunctional area decreases to a lower level by redistribution or elimination of the drug.

Classic Action of Depolarizing Muscle Relaxants

Depolarizing relaxants, at least initially, simulate the effect of acetylcholine and therefore can be considered agonists despite the fact that they block neurotransmission after initial stimulation. Structurally, succinylcholine is two molecules of acetylcholine bound together. It is therefore not surprising that it can mimic the effects of acetylcholine. Succinylcholine or decamethonium can bind to the receptor, open the channel, pass current, and depolarize the end plate. These agonists, similar to acetylcholine, attach only briefly; each opening of a channel is of very short duration, 1 millisecond or less. The response to acetylcholine, however, is over in milliseconds because of its rapid degradation by acetylcholinesterase, and the end plate resets to its resting state long before another nerve impulse arrives. In contrast, the depolarizing relaxants characteristically have a biphasic action on muscle—an initial contraction, followed by relaxation lasting minutes to hours. The depolarizing relaxants, because they are not susceptible to hydrolysis by acetylcholinesterase, are not eliminated from the junctional cleft until after they are eliminated from the plasma. The time required to clear the drug from the body is the principal determinant of how long the drug effect lasts. Whole-body clearance of the relaxant is very slow compared with acetylcholine, even when the plasma cholinesterase is normal. Because relaxant molecules are not cleared from the cleft quickly, they react repeatedly with receptors, attaching to one almost immediately after

separating from another, thereby repeatedly depolarizing the end plate and opening channels.

The quick shift from excitation of muscle contraction to blockade of transmission by depolarizing relaxants occurs because the end plate is continuously depolarized. This comes about because of the juxtaposition at the edge of the end plate on the muscle membrane—a different kind of ion channel, the sodium channel, that does not respond to chemicals but opens when exposed to a transmembrane voltage change. The sodium channel is also a cylindrical transmembrane protein through which sodium ions can flow. Two parts of its structure act as gates that allow or stop the flow of sodium ions.[50] Both gates must be open if sodium is to flow through the channel; the closing of either cuts off the flow. Because these two gates act sequentially, a sodium channel has three functional conformation states and can move progressively from one state to another (Fig. 22-7).

When the sodium channel is in its resting state, the lower gate (i.e., the time-dependent or inactivation gate) is open, but the upper gate (i.e., the voltage-dependent gate) is closed, and sodium ions cannot pass. When the molecule is subject to a sudden change in voltage by depolarization of the adjacent membrane, the top gate opens, and because the bottom (time-dependent) gate is still open, sodium flows through the channel. The voltage-dependent gate stays open as long as the molecule is subject to a depolarizing influence from the membrane around it; it will not close until the depolarization disappears. However, shortly after the voltage-dependent gate opens, the bottom gate closes and again cuts off the flow of ions. It cannot open again until the voltage-dependent gate closes. When the depolarization of the end plate stops, the voltage-dependent gate closes, the time-dependent one opens, and the sodium channel returns to its resting state. This whole process is short lived when depolarization occurs with acetylcholine. The initial response of a depolarizing muscle relaxant resembles that of acetylcholine, but because the relaxant is not hydrolyzed rapidly, depolarization of the end plate is not brief.

Depolarization of the end plate by the relaxant initially causes the voltage gate in adjacent sodium channels to open, causing a wave of depolarization to sweep along

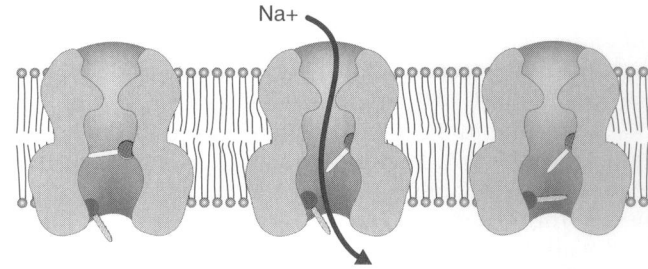

Figure 22–7 Sketch of sodium channel. The *bars* represent parts of the molecule that act as gates. The upper bar is voltage dependent; the lower bar is time dependent. The left side of the drawing represents the resting state. Once activated by a voltage change, the molecule and its gates progress as illustrated (*left to right*).

the muscle, producing muscle contraction. Shortly after the voltage-dependent gate opens, the time-dependent inactivation gate closes. Because the relaxant is not removed from the cleft, the end plate continues to be depolarized. Because the sodium channels immediately adjacent to the end plate are influenced by the depolarization of the end plate, their voltage-dependent gates stay open, and their inactivation gates stay closed. Because sodium cannot flow through a channel that has a closed inactivation gate, the perijunctional muscle membrane does not depolarize. When the flow of ions though the sodium channels in the perijunctional zone stops because the inactivation gates have closed, the channels downstream (beyond the perijunctional zone) are freed of depolarizing influence. In effect, the perijunctional zone becomes a buffer that shields the rest of the muscle from events at the end plate. Consequently, the muscle membrane is separated into three zones: the end plate, which is depolarized by succinylcholine; the perijunctional muscle membrane, in which the sodium channels are frozen in an inactivated state; and the rest of the muscle membrane, in which the sodium channels are in the resting state. Because a burst of acetylcholine from the nerve cannot overcome the inactivated sodium channels in the perijunctional zone, neuromuscular transmission is blocked. This phenomenon is also called *accommodation*. During accommodation, when the synapse is inexcitable through the nerve (transmitter), direct electrical stimulation of muscle causes muscle contraction because the sodium channels beyond the junctional area are in the resting excitable state.

The extraocular muscles contain tonic muscle, which is multiply innervated and chemically excitable along most of its surface.[15] Accommodation does not occur, and these muscles can undergo a sustained contracture in the presence of succinylcholine. The tension so developed forces the eye against the orbit and accounts for part of the increase in intraocular pressure produced by depolarizing relaxants. There is also evidence that the extraocular muscles contain a special type of receptor that does not become desensitized (discussed later) in the continued presence of acetylcholine or other agonists.[51]

Nonclassic and Noncompetitive Actions of Neuromuscular Drugs

Several drugs can interfere with the receptor, directly or through its lipid environment, to change transmission. These drugs react with the neuromuscular receptor to change its function and to impair transmission but do not act through the acetylcholine-binding site. These reactions cause drug-induced changes in the dynamics of the receptor, and instead of opening and closing sharply, the modified channels are sluggish. They open more slowly and stay open longer, or they close slowly and in several steps, or both. These effects on channels cause corresponding changes in the flow of ions and distortions of the end-plate potential. The clinical effect depends on the molecular events. For example, procaine, ketamine, inhaled anesthetics, or other drugs that dissolve in the membrane lipid may change the opening or closing characteristics of the channel.[52,53] If the channel

is prevented from opening, transmission is weakened. If, however, the channel is prevented from or slowed in closing, transmission may be enhanced. These drugs do not fit the classic model, and the impaired neuromuscular function is not antagonized by increasing perijunctional acetylcholine concentrations with cholinesterase inhibitors. Such drugs can be involved in two clinically important reactions receptor desensitization and channel blockade. The former occurs in the receptor molecule, and the latter occurs in the ion channel.

Desensitization Block

The acetylcholine receptor, because of its flexibility and the fluidity of the lipid around it, is capable of existing in a number of conformational states.[49,52-54] Because the resting receptor is free of agonist, its channel is closed. The second state exists when two molecules of agonists are bound to the α-subunit of the receptor, and the receptor has undergone the conformation change that opens the channel and allows ions to flow. These reactions are the bases of normal neuromuscular transmission. Some receptors that bind to agonists, however, do not undergo the conformation change to open the channel. Receptors in these states are called *desensitized* (i.e., they are not sensitive to the channel-opening actions of agonists). They bind agonists with exceptional avidity, but the binding does not result in the opening of the channel. The mechanisms by which desensitization occurs are not known. The receptor macromolecule, 1000 times larger by weight than most drugs or gases, provides many places at which the smaller molecules may act. The interface between lipid and receptor protein provides additional potential sites of reaction. Several different conformations of the protein are known, and because acetylcholine cannot cause the ion channel to open in any of them, they all are included in the functional term *desensitization*. Some evidence suggests that desensitization is accompanied by phosphorylation of a tyrosine unit in the receptor protein.[55,56]

Although agonists (e.g., succinylcholine) induce desensitization, the receptors are in a constant state of transition between resting and desensitized states whether agonists are present or not. Agonists do promote the transition to a desensitized state or, because they bind very tightly to desensitized receptors, trap a receptor in a desensitized state. Antagonists also bind tightly to desensitized receptors and can trap molecules in these states. This action of antagonists is not competitive with that of acetylcholine; it may be augmented by acetylcholine if the latter promotes the change to a desensitized state. Desensitization can lead to significant misinterpretations of data. Superficially, the preparation seems to be normal, but its responsiveness to agonists or antagonists is altered. One variety occurs very rapidly, within a few milliseconds after application of an agonist. This may explain the increased sensitivity to nondepolarizers after prior administration of succinylcholine. There also is the phenomenon caused by prolonged administration of depolarizing relaxants and known as *phase II block* (see "Phase II Block"). This frequently is referred to as a desensitization blockade but should not be, because desensitization of receptors is only one of many phenomena that contribute to the process.

Many other drugs used by anesthetists also promote the shift of receptors from a normal state to a desensitized state.[52-54] These drugs, some of which are listed in Table 22-1, can weaken neuromuscular transmission by reducing the margin of safety that normally exists at the neuromuscular junction, or they can cause an apparent increase in the capacity of nondepolarizing agents to block transmission. These actions are independent of the classic effects based on competitive inhibition of acetylcholine. The presence of desensitized receptors means that fewer receptor channels than usual are available to carry transmembrane current. The production of desensitized receptors decreases the efficacy of neuromuscular transmission. If many receptors are desensitized, insufficient normal ones are left to depolarize the motor end plate, and neuromuscular transmission will not occur. Even if only some receptors are desensitized, neuromuscular transmission will be impaired, and the system will be more susceptible to block by conventional antagonists such as tubocurarine or pancuronium.

Channel Block

Local anesthetics and calcium-entry blockers block the flow of sodium or calcium through their respective channels, explaining the term *channel-blocking drugs*. Similarly, a block to the flow of ions can occur at the acetylcholine receptor with concentrations of drugs used clinically and may contribute to some of the phenomena and drug interactions seen at the receptor. Two major types, closed channel and open channel block, can occur.[57,58] In a closed channel block, certain drugs can occupy the mouth of the channel, preventing ions from passing through the channel to depolarize the end plate. The process can take place even when the channel is not open. In an open channel block, a drug molecule enters a channel that has been opened by reaction with acetylcholine but does not necessarily penetrate all the way through. Open channel blockade is a use-dependent block, which means that molecules can enter the channel only when it is open. In open and closed channel blocks, the normal flow of ions through receptor is impaired, resulting in prevention of depolarization of the end plate and a weaker or blocked neuromuscular transmission. However, because the action is not at the acetylcholine recognition site, it is not a competitive antagonism of acetylcholine and is not relieved by anticholinesterases that increase concentrations of acetylcholine. Increasing the concentration of acetylcholine may cause the channels to open more often and thereby become more susceptible to blockade by use-dependent compounds. There is evidence that neostigmine and related cholinesterase inhibitors can act as channel-blocking drugs.[57]

Channel blockade is believed to play a role in some of the antibiotics, cocaine, quinidine, piperocaine, tricyclic antidepressants, naltrexone, naloxone, and histrionicotoxin-induced alterations in neuromuscular function. Muscle relaxants, in contrast, can bind to the acetylcholine recognition site of the receptor and occupy the channel. Pancuronium preferentially binds to the recognition site. Gallamine seems to act equally at the two sites. Tubocurarine is in between; at low doses, those that produce minimal blockage of transmission clinically, the drug is essentially a pure antagonist at the recognition site; at larger doses, it also enters and blocks channels. Decamethonium and succinylcholine as agonists can open channels and, as slender molecules, also enter and block them. Decamethonium and some other long, thin molecules can penetrate all the way through the open channel and enter the muscle cytoplasm. Whether prolonged administration of nondepolarizers, as in the intensive care situation, can result in entry of the relaxant, occupation of the channel, and entry of drug into the cytosol is unknown. This effect may partially explain the muscle weakness associated with relaxant therapy in the intensive care unit.

Phase II Block

Phase II block is a complex phenomenon that occurs slowly at junctions continuously exposed to depolarizing agents. The junction is depolarized by the initial application of a depolarizing relaxant, but then the membrane potential gradually recovers toward normal, even though the junction is still exposed to drug. Neuromuscular transmission usually remains blocked throughout the exposure. Several factors are involved. The repeated opening of channels allows a continuous efflux of potassium and influx of sodium, and the resulting abnormal electrolyte balance distorts the function of the junctional membrane. Calcium entering the muscle through the opened channels can cause disruption of receptors and sub–end-plate elements themselves. The activity of a sodium-potassium adenosine triphosphatase pump in the membrane increases with increasing intracellular sodium and, by pumping sodium out of the cell and

Table 22–1 Drugs that can cause or promote desensitization of nicotinic cholinergic receptors	
Volatile anesthetics	Acetylcholinesterase inhibitors
Halothane	Neostigmine
Methoxyflurane	Pyridostigmine
Isoflurane	Difluorophosphate (DFP)
Antibiotics	Local anesthetics
Polymyxin B	Dibucaine
Cocaine	Lidocaine
Alcohols	Prilocaine
Ethanol	Etidocaine
Butanol	Phenothiazines
Propanol	Chlorpromazine
Octanol	Trifluoperazine
Barbiturates	Prochlorperazine
Thiopental	Phencyclidine
Pentobarbital	Ca^{2+} channel blockers
Agonists	Verapamil
Acetylcholine	
Decamethonium	
Carbachol	
Succinylcholine	

potassium into it, works to restore the ionic balance and membrane potential toward normal. As long as the depolarizing drug is present, the receptor channels remain open, and ion flux through them remains high.[59]

Factors influencing the development phase II block include the duration of exposure to the drug, the particular drug used and its concentration, and even the type of muscle (i.e., fast or slow). Interactions with anesthetics and other agents also affect the process. All of these drugs may also have prejunctional effects on the rate and amount of transmitter release and mobilization. With so many variables involved in the interference with neuromuscular transmission, phase II block is a complex and ever-changing phenomenon. The reversal response of a phase II block produced by a depolarizing muscle relaxant to administration of cholinesterase inhibitors is difficult to predict. It is therefore best that reversal by cholinesterase inhibitors is not attempted, although the response to tetanus or train-of-four stimulation resembles that produced by nondepolarizers.

BIOLOGY OF PREJUNCTIONAL AND POSTJUNCTIONAL NICOTINIC RECEPTORS

Immature or Extrajunctional versus Mature or Junctional Isoforms

There are two variants of the postjunctional acetylcholine receptors. The acetylcholine receptor isoform present in the innervated, adult neuromuscular junction is referred to as the adult, mature, or junctional receptor. Another isoform is expressed when there is decreased activity in muscle, as seen in the fetus before innervation; after lower or upper motor neuron injury, burns, or sepsis; or after other events that cause increased muscle protein catabolism.[60,61] To contrast with the mature or junctional receptors, the other isoform is referred to as the immature, extrajunctional, or fetal form of acetylcholine receptor. Some evidence suggests that the immature isoform is not seen in muscle protein catabolism and wasting occurring with malnutrition.[61] The differences in the protein structure of the two isoforms cause significant qualitative variations among the responses of individual patients to relaxants and seem to be responsible for some of the anomalous results that are observed when administering relaxants to particular individuals. These qualitative differences in the isoforms can also cause variations in function of muscle (see "Myopathy of Critical Illness and Acetylcholine Receptors").[37]

In addition to their structural compositions, the two isoforms have other characteristics that are different.[1,8,50] At the molecular level, both types of receptors consists of five subunits (see Fig. 22-4). The mature junctional receptor is a pentamer of two α-subunits and one each of the β-, δ-, and ε-subunits. The immature receptor consists of two α-subunits and one each of β-, δ-, and γ-subunits; that is, in the immature receptor, the γ-subunit is present instead of the ε-subunit. The γ- and ε-subunits differ from each other very little in amino acid homology, but the

differences are great enough to affect the physiology and pharmacology of the receptor and its ion channel. Although the names junctional and extrajunctional imply that each is located in the junctional and extrajunctional areas, this is not strictly correct. Junctional receptors are always confined to the end plate (perijunctional) region of the muscle membrane. The immature, or extrajunctional, receptor may be expressed anywhere in the muscle membrane. Despite the name *extrajunctional*, they are not excluded from the end plate. During development and in certain pathologic states, the junctional and extrajunctional receptors can coexist in the perijunctional area of the muscle membrane (Fig. 22-8).

Quite unlike other cells, muscle cells are unusual in that they have many, usually hundreds of, nuclei per cell. Each of these nuclei has the genes to make both types of receptors. Multiple factors, including electrical activity, growth factor signaling (e.g., insulin, agrin, ARIA), and the presence or absence of innervation, control the expression of the two types of receptor isoforms.[8,10,25,46] This is most clearly seen in the developing embryo as the neuromuscular junction is formed. Before they are innervated, the muscle cells of a fetus synthesize only the immature receptors—hence the term *fetal isoform of receptor*. The synthesis is directed by nearly all the nuclei in the cell, and the receptors are expressed throughout the membrane of the muscle cell (see Fig. 22-8). As the fetus develops and the muscles become innervated, muscle cells begin to synthesize the mature isoform of receptors, which are inserted exclusively into the developing (future) end plate area. The nerve releases several growth factors that influence the synthetic apparatus of the nearby nuclei. First, nerve-supplied factors induce the subsynaptic nuclei to increase synthesis of the acetylcholine receptors. Next, the nerve-induced electrical activity results in repression of receptors in the extrajunctional area. The nerve-derived growth factors, including agrin and ARIA/neuregulin, cause the receptors to cluster in the subsynaptic area and prompt expression of the mature isoform[8,46] (see Fig. 22-5). In conditions associated with insulin resistance, there seems to be proliferation of acetylcholine receptors beyond the junctional area. Conditions in which insulin resistance (i.e., decreased growth factor signaling) has been observed include immobilization, burns, and denervation.[62-64] In these conditions, there is associated upregulation of the acetylcholine receptors and expression of the immature isoforms.[61,65,66]

Before innervation, acetylcholine receptors are present throughout the muscle membrane. After innervation, the acetylcholine receptors become more and more concentrated at the postsynaptic membrane and are virtually absent in the extrasynaptic area at birth. The innervation process progresses somewhat slowly during fetal life and matures during infancy and early childhood.[8,20,25] With time, the immature receptors diminish in concentration and disappear from the peripheral part of the muscle. In the active, adult, normal, innervated muscle, only the nuclei under and very near the end plate direct the synthesis of receptor; only the genes for expressing the mature receptors are active. The nuclei beyond the junctional area are not active, and therefore no receptors are expressed anywhere in the muscle cells beyond the

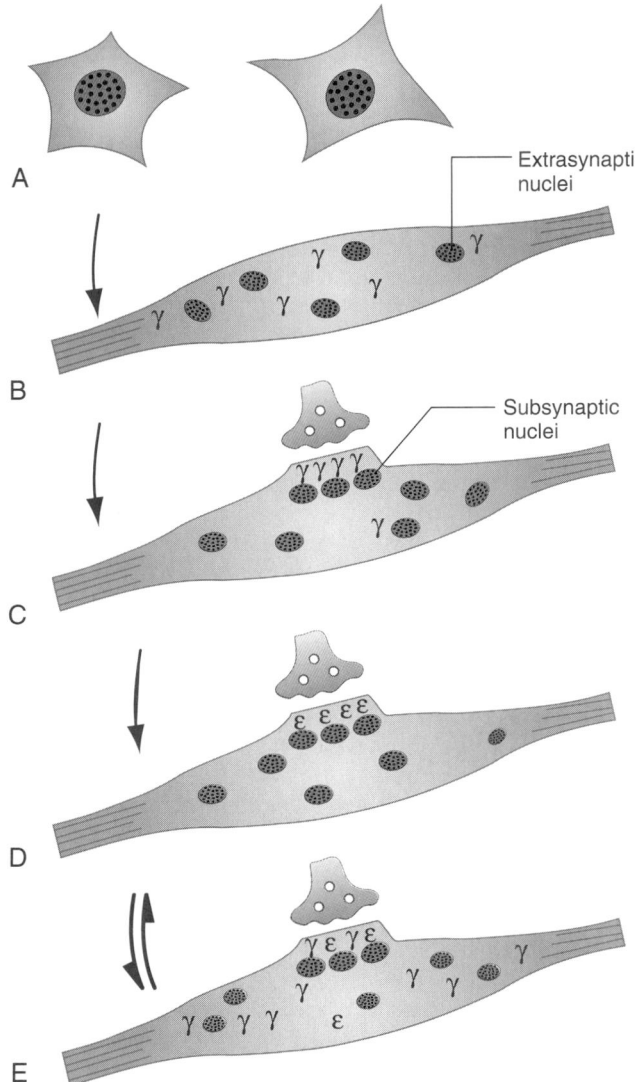

Figure 22–8 Distribution of acetylcholine receptors in developing adult, mature, and denervated muscle. **A** and **B,** In the early fetal stage, mononucleated myoblasts, derived from the mesoderm, fuse to form multinucleated myotubes. The γ-subunit–containing immature acetylcholine receptors are scattered throughout the muscle membrane. **C,** As the nerve makes contact with muscle, clustering of the receptors occurs at the synapse and is associated with some loss of extrasynaptic receptors. **D,** Maturation of the junction is said to occur when ε-subunit–containing receptors replace the γ-subunit–containing receptors. Even mature muscle is multinucleated, but it is devoid of extrasynaptic nuclei. **E,** Denervation or another pathologic state (e.g., burns, immobilization, chronic muscle relaxant therapy, sepsis) leads to re-expression of the γ-subunit receptor at the junctional and the extrajunctional areas. The latter changes are potentially reversible.

postsynaptic membrane of the newborn and that from a patient with myasthenia gravis are not too different. In patients with myasthenia gravis, the receptor numbers are usually decreased because of autoantibodies directed against the acetylcholine receptor.[3] It is not surprising therefore that neurotransmission is not as efficient in the newborn and patient with myasthenia gravis. A child is usually about 2 years old before nerve-muscle contacts are mature.

Proteins implicated in the linking of the mature receptors to the cytoskeleton include utrophin, α- and β-dystroglycan, and rapsyn. Several lines of evidence indicate that the clustering, expression, and stabilization of the mature receptors are triggered by at least three growth factors: agrin, ARIA, and calcitonin gene–related peptide.[8,11] Agrin is also released from the muscle, but muscle-derived agrin does not seem to be as important in the clustering and maturation of the receptor. ARIA is made in the nerve and seems to play a role in the maturation of vesicular arrangement and conversion of the γ to ε switch.[46,67] All of these growth factors interact with distinct membrane and cytosolic receptor proteins, causing phosphorylation, activation of nuclear (gene) transcriptional systems. Agrin signals through MuSK and ARIA through ERBB receptors (see Fig. 22-5). These receptors control qualitative and quantitative changes at the junction. Once begun, the process is very stable, and the nuclei in the junctional area continue to express mature receptors.

The extrajunctional receptors can reappear soon after upper and lower motor denervation and in certain pathologic states (e.g., burns, immobilization, chronic muscle relaxant therapy, loss of electrical activity). Stimulating a denervated muscle with an external electrical stimulus can prevent the appearance of the immature receptors. It has been suggested that the calcium that enters the muscle during activity is important to the suppression process.[68] In the pathologic states previously enumerated, if the process is severe and prolonged, extrajunctional receptors are inserted all over the surface of the muscle, including the perijunctional area (see Fig. 22-8). The junctional nuclei also continue to make mature receptors. The end plates consist of mature and immature receptors. The synthesis of immature receptors is initiated within hours of inactivity, but it takes several days for the whole muscle membrane to be fully covered with receptors. This upregulation of receptors has implications for the use of depolarizing and nondepolarizing relaxants.

The changes in subunit composition (γ versus ε) in the receptor confer certain changes in electrophysiologic (functional), pharmacologic, and metabolic characteristics.[1,25] The mature receptors are metabolically stable, with half-life approximating 2 weeks, whereas the immature receptor has a metabolic half-life of less than 24 hours. Immature receptors have a smaller single-channel conductance and a 2- to 10-fold longer mean channel open time than mature receptors (see Fig. 22-4). The changes in subunit composition may also alter the sensitivity or affinity, or both, of the receptor for specific ligands. Depolarizing or agonist drugs such as succinylcholine and acetylcholine depolarize immature receptors more easily, resulting in cation fluxes; one-tenth to one-hundredth

perijunctional area. Conversion of all of the γ-subunit– to ε-subunit–containing acetylcholine receptors in the perijunctional area continues to take place after birth. In the rat, it takes about 2 weeks.[8] In humans, this process takes longer. At birth, the postsynaptic membrane itself is also not as specialized; the newborn junction has simplified synaptic folds, a widened synaptic space, and reduced numbers of acetylcholine receptors. Morphologically, the doses, necessary for mature receptors, can effect depolarization.[69] Potency of nondepolarizers is also reduced, demonstrated as resistance to nondepolarizers documented in burns, denervation, and immobilization.[1,61,65,66] This resistance may be related to decreased affinity of the receptor to nondepolarizers and to the upregulation of receptors in the perijunctional area. Data suggest that some nondepolarizers may also cause a partial agonist response in immature receptors, explaining the decreased potency.[6] The altered sensitivities for cholinergic ligands may also result from changes in composition of the lipid membrane surrounding the receptor that is known to occur with some pathologic states.[49]

The sensitivity to muscle relaxants may occur in only certain parts of the body or certain muscles if only some muscles are affected by the diminution of nerve activity (e.g., after a stroke). The sensitivity to relaxants can begin to change between 24 and 72 hours after an injury or hospitalization. The most serious side effect with the use of succinylcholine in the presence of upregulated receptors in one or more muscle is hyperkalemia.[1,2,69] In these subjects, the receptors can be scattered over a large surface of the muscle. Immature receptors are especially sensitive to succinylcholine. The channels opened by the agonist allow potassium to escape from the muscle and enter the blood. If a large part of the muscle surface consists of upregulated (immature) receptor channels, each of which stays open for a longer time, the amount of potassium that moves from muscle to blood can be very large. The resulting hyperkalemia can cause dangerous disturbances in cardiac rhythm, including ventricular fibrillation. Moreover, it is difficult to prevent the hyperkalemia by the prior administration of nondepolarizers because extrajunctional receptors are not very sensitive to block by nondepolarizing relaxants.[1] Larger than normal doses of nondepolarizers may attenuate the increase in blood potassium but cannot completely prevent it. However, hyperkalemia and cardiac arrest can occur after succinylcholine administration, even in the absence of denervation states. This is seen in certain congenital muscle dystrophies, in which the muscle membrane is prone to damage by succinylcholine releasing potassium into the circulation.[69]

Myopathy of Critical Illness and Acetylcholine Receptors

Critical illnesses (see Chapters 75 and 76) such as sepsis, trauma, and burns induce functional and pharmacologic aberrations at the skeletal muscle, similar to that seen with upper or lower motor neuron injuries. The aberrant pharmacologic responses consist of a hyperkalemic response to succinylcholine and resistance to nondepolarizers.[1,2] The important functional change in muscle associated with critical illness is muscle weakness, resulting in hypoventilation, dependence on respirators, and decreased mobilization.[70,71] The pathognomic biochemical feature in all of these critical illnesses is the upregulation of acetylcholine receptors with expression of the immature (γ-subunit) isoform of receptors.[60-61,65-66]

The immature isoform has different electrophysiologic characteristics from those of the mature form, including prolonged open-channel time. In some clinical conditions, the presence of a prolonged open-channel time (due to congenital mutations in the receptor) is associated with muscle weakness.[37,72,73] These conditions present as progressive muscle weaknesses and impaired neuromuscular transmission without overt degeneration of the motor end plate. The receptor numbers typically are not significantly reduced. In all of these congenital conditions with prolonged open-channel time, there is delayed closure of the acetylcholine receptor ion channel. This leads to increased calcium load into the cytosol, progressive widening, and accumulation of debris in the synaptic cleft, resulting in reduced efficiency of released neurotransmitter and reduced safety factor. In the pathologic state of burns, sepsis, and trauma, in which muscle weakness is a concomitant finding, the expression of the immature isoform at the perijunctional membrane may have a role in muscle weakness. The presence of immature isoform can lead to prolonged open-channel time.[25] Whether these immature receptors play a role in the myopathy by this mechanism is unclear. The expression of the immature isoform may decrease the number of mature isoforms, a situation akin to myasthenia gravis, in which the mature receptor number at the junction is decreased.

In mice, deletion of the mature ϵ-subunit–containing receptors causes muscle weakness, despite the expression of immature receptors at the postjunctional membrane.[74] When there is de novo expression of immature isoforms of the receptor containing the γ-subunit, signaling through receptor tyrosine kinases or through growth factors (e.g., insulin) seems to be impaired.[62-64] Decreased signaling of growth factors such as agrin and ARIA may account for the dispersion of the acetylcholine receptors from the junctional area to areas throughout the muscle membrane with concomitant expression of the immature isoform of receptor, even in the junctional area.[75] These changes may play a role in the inefficient neurotransmission. The deficiency or absence of growth factor signaling (by means of insulin) leads to decreased anabolism of protein and enhanced muscle protein breakdown, including apoptosis, resulting in the loss of contractile elements. Apoptosis occurring in cardiac muscle contributes significantly to myocardial dysfunction.[76] The loss of muscle mass from apoptosis and decreased protein synthesis due to the decreased anabolic effect of insulin and other growth factors[77,78] may compound the skeletal muscle weakness related to ineffective neurotransmission related to expression of immature receptor. Signaling through receptor kinases and its effects on acetylcholine expression and apoptosis are intense areas of research by many groups. Correction of the altered signaling mechanism may reverse the expression of the immature to mature isoform, attenuate the loss of muscle mass due to apoptosis in muscle, and correct the muscle weakness associated with critical illness.

Prejunctional Receptors

Acetylcholine receptors exist as a variety of forms separate from that seen in muscle.[79] These receptors are expressed in peripheral neurons, autonomic and sensory ganglia, and in the central nervous system. There is also direct and indirect evidence for their existence in lymphocytes, fibroblasts, chondrocytes, macrophages, and granulocytes. Sixteen acetylcholine subunit genes have been cloned from vertebrates. They include various combinations of α-subunits (α_1 through α_9) and β-subunits (β_1 through β_4) and one each of γ-, δ-, and ϵ-subunits.

Prejunctional- or nerve terminal–associated cholinergic receptors have been demonstrated pharmacologically and by molecular biology techniques, but their form and functions are not well understood compared with those in the postjunctional area. Many drugs with an abundance of potential targets for drug action can affect the capacity of the nerve terminal to carry out its functions. The trophic function to maintain the nerve-muscle contact involves release and replenishment of acetylcholine together with trophic factors that require signaling through many receptors, of which the prejunctional nicotinic receptor is just one. Succinylcholine produces fasciculations that can be prevented by nondepolarizing relaxants. Because a fasciculation is, by definition, the simultaneous contraction of the multitude of muscle cells in a single motor unit and because only the nerve can synchronize all the muscles in its motor unit, it became apparent that succinylcholine must also act on nerve endings. Because nondepolarizing relaxants prevent fasciculation, it was concluded that they acted on the same prejunctional receptor. Since then, it has been shown many times that very small doses of cholinergic agonists (e.g., succinylcholine) and antagonists (e.g., curare) affect nicotinic receptors on the nerve ending, the former by depolarizing the ending and sometimes inducing repetitive firing of the nerve and the latter by preventing the action of agonists.[5]

Another clue to differences between prejunctional and postjunctional acetylcholine receptors was the finding that although both receptors can bind α-bungarotoxin, prejunctional binding was reversible, whereas postjunctional binding was not. Additional clues were found in the many demonstrations of quantitative differences in the reaction of prejunctional and postjunctional nicotinic receptors to cholinergic agonists and antagonists.[79,80] For instance, it was known that tubocurarine binds very poorly to the recognition sites of ganglionic nicotinic cholinoceptors and is not a competitive antagonist of acetylcholine at this site. Decamethonium is a selective inhibitor of the muscle receptor, and hexamethonium is a selective inhibitor of the nicotinic receptors in the autonomic ganglia.[79] Instead, D-tubocurarine and hexamethonium can block the opened channels of these receptors and owe their ability to block ganglionic transmission to this property. The functional characteristics of the prejunctional receptor channels may also be different. For example, the depolarization of motor nerve endings initiated by administration of acetylcholine can be prevented by tetrodotoxin, a specific blocker of sodium flux with no effect on the end plate.

Specific information on the molecular organization of the neuronal nicotinic receptors on motor neuron terminal is lacking, but work on other parts of the nervous system such as the brain and ganglia indicate that they are structurally quite different from those found on the

postjunctional muscle membrane.[79,80] Some of the subunit composition is similar, but other subunits do not resemble that of the postjunctional receptor. Of the 16 different nicotinic acetylcholine receptors gene product identified, only 11 (α_2 to α_9 and β_2 to β_4) are thought to contribute nicotinic receptors expressed in neurons. Most strikingly, nervous tissue does not contain genes for γ-, δ-, or ϵ-receptor subunits; it contains only the genes for the α- and β-subunits. The α- and β-subunit genes in nerve and muscle are not exactly the same; they are variants. Muscle contains only one gene for each of the subunits, which are called α_1 and α_1-subunit. In contrast, nervous tissue contains neither of these, but rather contains a number of related genes designated α_2 through α_9. To emphasize the distinction between neural and muscle nicotinic receptors, the former sometimes are designated *Nn* and the latter *Nm*. With so many different subunits available, there are many possible combinations, and it is not known which combinations are found in motor nerves. Their physiologic roles have also not been completely characterized. Expression of neuronal nicotinic acetylcholine receptors in vitro systems has confirmed that muscle relaxants and their metabolites can bind to these receptors.[81] Whether adverse effects observed during prolonged administration of relaxants could be attributed to interaction of relaxant with neuronal acetylcholine receptors is unclear.

The nicotinic receptor in the nerve ending of the neuromuscular junction may serve the function of regulator of transmitter release, as shown in other parts of the nervous system. The nicotinic receptor on the junctional surface of the nerve senses transmitter in the cleft and, by means of a positive-feedback system, causes the release of more transmitter. In other parts of the nervous system, this positive feedback is complemented by a negative-feedback system, which senses when the concentration of transmitter in the synaptic cleft has increased appropriately and shuts down the release system. Indirect evidence suggests that these receptors are muscarinic cholinergic receptors. Convincing data that motor nerve endings contain muscarinic receptors or a negative feedback system are not available for the motor neuron. The nerve ending is also known to bear several other receptors, such as opioid, adrenergic, dopamine, purine, and adenosine receptors and receptors for endogenous hormones, neuropeptides, and a variety of proteins. The physiologic roles of these receptors or the effects of anesthetics on them are unknown.

The motor nerves take up choline, synthesize acetylcholine, store it in vesicles, and move the vesicles into position to be released by a nerve action potential, a series of processes known collectively as *mobilization*. Muscle relaxants to a greater or lesser extent seem to influence this mobilization process by acting on the prejunctional nicotinic acetylcholine receptor. Tubocurarine and related muscle relaxants have a profound effect in decreasing the nerve's capacity to prepare more acetylcholine for release. Tubocurarine has no direct effect on the release process for acetylcholine; the amount of transmitter released is controlled by the availability of releasable acetylcholine and the amount of calcium that enters the nerve. Although it has frequently been observed that nondepolarizing relaxants do not diminish the transmitter released by a single nerve impulse or the first in a high-frequency train of impulses, they sharply decrease the release triggered by subsequent nerve pulses in the train. The most common manifestation of this is the so-called tetanic fade commonly seen after a nondepolarizing relaxant is administered. This effect is thought to result from inhibition of the process that replenishes releasable acetylcholine.[5]

ANTAGONISM OF NEUROMUSCULAR BLOCK

Mechanism of Antagonism

The nondepolarizing relaxants block (see Chapter 13) neuromuscular transmission predominantly by competitive antagonism of acetylcholine at the postjunctional receptor. The most straightforward way to overcome their effects is to increase the competitive position of acetylcholine. Two factors are important, the first of which is the concentration of acetylcholine. Increasing the number of molecules of acetylcholine in the junctional cleft changes the agonist-to-antagonist ratio and increases the probability that agonist molecules will occupy the recognition sites of the receptor. It also increases the probability that an unoccupied receptor will become occupied. Normally, only about 500,000 of the 5 million available receptors are activated by a single nerve impulse, and a large number of receptors is in "reserve" and could be occupied by an agonist. The second factor important to the competitive position of acetylcholine is the length of time acetylcholine is in the cleft. Acetylcholine must wait for the antagonist to dissociate spontaneously before it can compete for the freed site. The nondepolarizing relaxants bind to the receptor for slightly less than 1 millisecond, which is longer than the normal lifetime of acetylcholine. The destruction of acetylcholine normally takes place so quickly that most of it is destroyed before any significant number of antagonist molecules have dissociated from the receptor. Prolonging the time during which acetylcholine is in the junction allows time for the available acetylcholine to bind to receptor when the antagonist dissociates from the receptors.

Classes of Drugs Used

Three classes of drugs, potassium channel-blocking drugs, acetylcholinesterase inhibitors, and the γ-cyclodextrin derivatives, can be used clinically to reverse non–depolarizer-induced paralysis.[82,83] The best known of the potassium blocking drugs is 4-aminopyridine. Its actions are predominantly prejunctional; it impedes the efflux of potassium from the nerve ending. Because the efflux of potassium is the event that normally ends the action potential of the nerve ending, this action prolongs the depolarization of the nerve. Because the flux of calcium into the nerve continues for as long as the depolarization lasts, drugs of this class indirectly increase the flux of calcium into the nerve ending. The nerve releases more

acetylcholine and for a longer time than usual, conditions that are effective in antagonizing nondepolarizing relaxants. Because they act prejunctionally, these drugs can antagonize a block produced by certain antibiotics that act on the nerve ending, notably the polymyxins. Although 4-aminopyridine and drugs like it can be used clinically, their use is severely restricted because they are not specific. They affect the release of transmitters by all nerve endings, including motor nerves, autonomic nerves, and central nervous system components. Their use is accompanied by a variety of undesirable effects, and in practice, they are used only in special circumstances. A most serious side effect of potassium channel blockers is seizures.

The more commonly used antagonists of neuromuscular block (e.g., neostigmine, pyridostigmine, edrophonium) inhibit acetylcholinesterase by mechanisms that are similar but not identical.[82] Neostigmine and pyridostigmine are attracted by an electrostatic interaction between the positively charged nitrogen in the molecules and the negatively charged catalytic site of the enzyme. This produces a carbamylated enzyme, which is not capable of further action (i.e., the catalytic site is blocked and the enzyme is inhibited). Edrophonium has neither an ester nor a carbamate group, but it is attracted and bound to the catalytic site of the enzyme by the electrostatic attraction between the positively charged nitrogen in the drug and the negatively charged acetylcholinesterase site of the enzyme. Edrophonium also seems to have prejunctional effects, enhancing the release of acetylcholine from the nerve terminal. This effect is therefore useful when deep neuromuscular block needs reversal. Of the three commonly used anticholinesterases, edrophonium shows by far the greatest selectivity between acetylcholinesterase and butyrylcholinesterase, the serum esterase that hydrolyzes succinylcholine and mivacurium. It greatly favors the former enzyme and therefore seems to be the most desirable agent to reverse mivacurium. However, if the patient has normal serum esterase, pharmacokinetic factors are the principal determinants of the duration of blockade, and the activity of serum esterase or the lack of it plays only a minor role in the recovery. There is little reason to prefer one or another reversal drug on these grounds. Anticholinesterases are administered for prolonged periods in the treatment of myasthenia gravis[3] and as prophylaxis in cases of nerve gas poisoning.[38] Ironically, prolonged administration of cholinesterase inhibitors can also lead to a myasthenia-like state with muscle weakness.[84]

The cholinesterase inhibitors act preferentially at the neuromuscular junction and act at other synapses that use the same transmitter, including muscarinic receptors. An atropine-like drug should be administered with the cholinesterase inhibitor to counter the effects of the acetylcholine that accumulates in the muscarinic synapses of the gut, bronchi, and cardiovascular system. These three anticholinesterase inhibitors do not affect synapses in the central nervous system because all are quaternary ammonium ions, which do not easily penetrate the blood-brain barrier. A quaternary ammonium derivative of atropine, such as glycopyrrolate, which does not diffuse through the blood-brain barrier, frequently is used to limit the anticholinergic effects to the periphery. Other cholinesterase inhibitors, notably physostigmine and tacrine, are not quaternary ammonium compounds, and they have profound effects in the central nervous system. These may be antagonized by atropine but not by its quaternary ammonium analog derivatives. Unlike the other cholinesterase inhibitors, physostigmine and tacrine are also potent inhibitors of the enzyme phosphodiesterase, which plays an important role in the regulation of transmitter release at many synapses in the central nervous system. This action may be related to the reported efficacy of these two drugs in the treatment of Alzheimer's dementia.

Cholinesterase inhibitors also have actions at the postjunctional membrane independent of its effects on the enzyme. Several of these compounds contain methyl groups on a positively charged nitrogen, and they can act as agonists on the receptor channels, initiating ion flow and enhancing neuromuscular transmission. Neostigmine, physostigmine, and certain organophosphates can increase the frequency of MEPPs and increase the quantal content of end-plate potentials, but the importance of the increased transmitter release to reversal of neuromuscular blockade is not clear. Continuous exposure to the carbamate- or organophosphate-containing inhibitors causes degeneration of prejunctional and postjunctional structures, apparently because these structures accumulate toxic amounts of calcium. Calcium channel blockers such as verapamil prevent the neural actions of these drugs. All the drugs of this class also act in or on receptors to influence the kinetics of the open-close cycle and to block the ion channel.[57,58] The clinical significance of the drugs on reversal of nondepolarizers is not known.

A new approach to reversing residual neuromuscular block is by direct binding of the relaxant by means of chemical interaction. Antidote drugs that work by binding other drugs include protamine, citrate anticoagulation, lead or copper chelators, and RNA molecules recombinantly engineered to bind drugs. Cyclodextrins (i.e., small, cyclic polysaccharides) are one such compound synthesized from starch by bacteria as early as 1891. The γ-cyclodextrin derivative ORG25969 binds steroidal relaxants with very high affinity, resulting in inactive muscle relaxants. The kidney then removes these complexes. Preliminary studies show promising results.[83]

KEY POINTS

1. The neuromuscular junction provides a rich array of receptors and substrates for drug action. Several drugs used clinically have multiple sites of action. The muscle relaxants are not exceptions to the rule that most drugs have more than one site or mechanism of action. The major actions seem to occur by the mechanisms and at the sites described for decades: agonistic and antagonistic actions at postjunctional receptors for depolarizing and nondepolarizing relaxants, respectively. This description of neuromuscular drug action is a simplistic one. Neuromuscular transmission is impeded by nondepolarizers because they prevent access of acetylcholine to its recognition site on the postjunctional receptor.

2. If the concentration of nondepolarizer is increased, another, noncompetitive action—block of the ion channel—is superimposed. The paralysis is also potentiated by the prejunctional actions of the relaxant, preventing the release of acetylcholine. The latter can be documented as fade that occurs with increased frequency of stimulation. A more accurate description of the relaxant effects recognizes that the neuromuscular junction is a complex and dynamic system, in which the phenomena produced by drugs are composites of actions that vary with drug, dose, activity in the junction and muscle, time after administration, the presence of anesthetics or other drugs, and the age and condition of the patient.

3. Inhibition of the postjunctional acetylcholinesterase by anticholinesterases increases concentration of acetylcholine, which can compete and displace the nondepolarizer-reversing paralysis. These anticholinesterases also have other effects, including those on nerve terminals and on the receptor, by means of an allosteric mechanism. Cyclodextrins are reversal compounds that detoxify the effects of steroidal muscle relaxants only by directly binding to them.

4. Depolarizing compounds initially react with the acetylcholine recognition site and, like the transmitter, open ion channels and depolarize the end-plate membrane. Unlike the transmitter, they are not subject to hydrolysis by acetylcholinesterase and so remain in the junction. Soon after administration of the drug, some receptors are desensitized and, although occupied by an agonist, do not open to allow current to flow to depolarize the area.

5. If the depolarizing relaxant is applied in high concentration and allowed to remain at the junction for a long time, other effects occur. These include entry of the drug into the channel to obstruct it or to pass through it into the cytoplasm. Depolarizing relaxants also have effects on prejunctional structures, and the combination of prejunctional and postjunctional effects plus secondary ones on muscle and nerve homeostasis results in the complicated phenomenon known as *phase II blockade*.

6. Intense research in the area of neuromuscular transmission continues at a rapid pace. The newer observations on receptors, ion channels, membranes, and prejunctional functions reveal a much broader range of sites and mechanisms of action for agonists and antagonists.

7. Some of the other drugs used clinically (e.g., botulinum toxin) have effects on the nerve and therefore indirectly on muscle.[35] Nondepolarizing relaxants administered even for 12 hours or prolonged periods can have effects on postsynaptic receptor simulating denervation.[85,86] In recognizing these sites and mechanisms, we begin to bring our theoretical knowledge closer to explaining the phenomena observed when these drugs are administered to living humans.

8. Most recent work seems to be focused on the postjunctional membrane and the control of acetylcholine receptor expression in normal and diseased states. The presence or absence of the mature and immature isoforms seems to complicate matters further. In certain pathologic states (e.g., sepsis, burns, immobilization, chronic use of relaxants), upregulation of acetylcholine receptors occurs, usually with expression of the immature isoform. The altered functional and pharmacologic characteristics of these receptors results in increased sensitivity with hyperkalemia to succinylcholine and resistance to nondepolarizers.

9. An area of increasing attention is the control of the expression of mature versus immature receptors and the role of the immature isoform of the receptor in the muscle weakness associated with the diseases enumerated. The immature isoform expression is probably related to aberrant growth factor signaling. Mutations in the acetylcholine receptor, which result in prolonged open-channel time, similar to that seen with the immature receptor, even the presence of normal receptor numbers, can lead to a myasthenia-like state.[37] The weakness is usually related to the prolonged open-channel time. It is possible that the synaptic area expression of the immature receptor, which has a prolonged open-channel time, may simulate a myasthenia-like state.

10. Attenuated growth factor (e.g., insulin) signaling may also cause apoptosis in muscle. Loss of muscle mass due to apoptosis may compound the muscle weakness of critical illness related to expression of immature isoform receptors. In the future, it may be possible to manipulate the signaling mechanism to alter the expression of the receptor isoforms, attenuate apoptosis, and improve muscle function. Alternatively, these goals could be achieved by gene therapy.

REFERENCES

1. Martyn JAJ, White DA, Gronert GA, et al: Up-and-down regulation of skeletal muscle acetylcholine receptors. Anesthesiology 76:822, 1992.
2. Naguib M, Flood P, McArdle JJ, Brenner HR: Advances in neurobiology of the neuromuscular junction: Implications for the anesthesiologist. Anesthesiology 96:202, 2002.
3. Drachman DB: Myasthenia gravis. N Engl J Med 330:1797, 1994.
4. Vincent A, Dalton P, Clover L, et al: Antibodies to neuronal targets in neurological and psychiatric diseases. Ann N Y Acad Sci 992:48, 2003.
5. Bowman WC, Prior C, Marshall IG: Presynaptic receptors in the neuromuscular junction. Ann N Y Acad Sci 604:69, 1990.
6. Fletcher GH, Steinbach JH: Ability of depolarizing neuromuscular blocking drugs to act as partial agonists at fetal and adult mouse muscle nicotinic receptors. Mol Pharmacol 49:938, 1996.
7. Paul M, Kindler CH, Fokt RM, et al: Isobolographic analysis of non-depolarising muscle relaxant interactions at their receptor site. Eur J Pharmacol 438:35, 2002.
8. Sanes JR, Lichtman JW: Induction, assembly, maturation and maintenance of a postsynaptic apparatus. Nat Rev Neurosci 2:791, 2001.
9. Lukas RJ, Bencherif M: Heterogeneity and regulation of nicotinic acetylcholine receptors. Int Rev Neurobiol 34:25, 1992.
10. Kelly RB: The cell biology of the nerve terminal. Neuron 1:431, 1988.
11. Marques MJ, Conchello JA, Lichtman JW: From plaque to pretzel Fold formation and acetylcholine receptor loss at the developing neuromuscular junction. J Neurosci 20:3663, 2000.
12. Taylor P, Schumacher M, MacPhee-Quingley K, et al: The structure of acetylcholinesterase: Relationship to its function and cellular disposition. Trends Neurosci 10:93, 1987.
13. Catterall WA: Structure and functions of voltage-gated ion channels. Annu Rev Biochem 64:493, 1995.
14. Personius KE, Balice-Gordon RJ: Activity-dependent editing of neuromuscular synaptic connections. Brain Res Bull 53:513, 2000.
15. Buttner-Ennever JA, Horn AK: Oculomotor system: A dual innervation of the eye muscles from the abducens, trochlear, and oculomotor nuclei. Mov Disord 2:S2, 2002.
16. Durant NN, Katz RL: Suxamethonium. Br J Anaesth 54:195, 1982.
17. Vachon CA, Warner DO, Bacon DR: Succinylcholine and the open globe. Tracing the teaching. Anesthesiology 99:220, 2003.
18. Betz WJ, Caldwell JH, Kinnamon SC: Increased sodium conductance in the synaptic region of rat skeletal muscle fibers. J Physiol (Lond) 352:189, 1984.
19. Yu FH, Catterall WA: Overview of the voltage-gated sodium channel family. Genome Biol 4:207, 2003.
20. Goudsouzian NG, Standaert FG: The infant and the myoneural junction. Anesth Analg 65:1208, 1986.
21. Heuser JE, Reese TS: Structural changes after transmitter release at the frog neuromuscular junction. J Cell Biol 88:564, 1981.
22. Rash JE, Walrond JP, Morita M: Structural and functional correlates of synaptic transmission in the vertebrate neuromuscular junction. J Electron Microsc Tech 10:153, 1988.
23. Littleton JT, Sheng M: Neurobiology: Synapses unplugged. Nature 424:931, 2003.
24. Wood SJ, Slater CR: Safety factor at the neuromuscular junction. Prog Neurobiol 64:393, 2001.
25. Hall Z, Merlie JR: Synaptic structure and development: The neuromuscular junction. Cell 72:99-121, 1993.
26. Katz B, Miledi R: Estimates of quantal content during "chemical potentiation" of transmitter release. Proc R Soc Lond [Biol] 215:369, 1979.
27. Uchitel OD, Protti DA, Sanchez V, et al: P-type voltage dependent calcium channel mediates presynaptic calcium influx and transmitter release in mammalian synapses. Proc Natl Acad Sci U S A 89:3330, 1992.
28. Waterman S, Pinto A, Lang B, et al: The role of autoantibodies in Lambert-Eaton myasthenic syndrome. Ann N Y Acad Sci 84:596, 1998.
29. Südhof TC: The synaptic vesicle cycle revisited. Neuron 28:317, 2000.
30. Valtorta F, Jahn R, Fesce R, et al: Synaptophysin (p38) at the frog neuromuscular junction: Its incorporation into the axolemma and recycling after intense quantal secretion. J Cell Biol 107:2717, 1988.
31. Rizolli SO, Betz WJ. All change at the synapse. Nature 423:591, 2003.
32. Augustine GJ, Burns ME, DeBello WM, et al. Proteins involved in synaptic vesicle trafficking. J Physiol (Lond) 520:33, 1999.
33. Jahn R, Hanson PI: SNAREs line up in new environment. Nature 393:14, 1998.
34. Sugita S, Shin OH, Han W, et al: Synaptotagmins form a hierarchy of exocytotic Ca(2+) sensors with distinct Ca(2+) affinities. EMBO J 21:270, 2002.
35. Turton K, Chaddock JA, Acharya KR: Botulinum and tetanus neurotoxins: Structure, function and therapeutic utility. Trends Biochem Sci 27:552, 2002.

36. Heeroma JH, Plomp JJ, Roubos EW, Verhage M: Development of the mouse neuromuscular junction in the absence of regulated secretion. Neuroscience 120:733, 2003.

37. Engel AG, Ohno K, Sine SM: Congenital myasthenic syndromes: Progress over the past decade. Muscle Nerve 27:4, 2003.

38. Abraham RB, Rudick V, Weinbroum AA: Practical guidelines for acute care of victims of bioterrorism: Conventional injuries and concomitant nerve agent intoxication. Anesthesiology 97:989, 2002.

39. Gu Y, Forsayeth JR, Verall S: Assembly of the mammalian muscle acetylcholine receptor in transfected COS cells. J Cell Biol 114:799, 1991.

40. Changeux J-P, Edelstein SJ: On allosteric transitions and acetylcholine receptors. Trends Biochem 19:399, 1994.

41. Kopta C, Steinbach JH: Comparison of mammalian adult and fetal nicotinic acetylcholinic receptors stably expressed in fibroblasts. J Neurosci 14:3922, 1994.

42. Pedersen SE, Cohen JB: D-Tubocurarine binding sites are located at alpha-gamma and alpha-delta subunit interfaces of the nicotinic acetylcholine receptor. Proc Natl Acad Sci U S A 87:2785, 1990.

43. Griesmann GE, McCormick DJ, De Aizpurua HJ, et al: α-Bungarotoxin binds to human acetylcholine receptor α-subunit peptide 185-199. J Neurochem 54:1541, 1990.

44. Gullberg D: Cell biology: The molecules that make muscle. Nature 424:138, 2003.

45. Burden SJ: Building the vertebrate neuromuscular synapse. J Neurobiol 53:501, 2002.

46. Tansey MG, Chu GC, Merlie JP: ARIA/HRG regulates AChR epsilon subunit gene expression at the neuromuscular synapse via activation of phosphatidylinositol 3-kinase and Ras/MAPK pathway. J Cell Biol 134:46, 1996.

47. Barrantes FJ: Muscle end plate cholinoceptors. Pharmacol Ther 38:331, 1988.

48. McCarthy MP, Stroud RM: Conformational states of the nicotinic acetylcholine receptor from Torpedo californica induced by the binding of agonist, antagonist, and local anesthetics. Equilibrium measurements using tritium-hydrogen exchange. Biochemistry 28:40, 1989.

49. Karlin A, DiPaola M, Kao PN, Lobel P: Functional sites and transient states of the nicotinic acetylcholine receptor. In Hille B, Fambrough DM (eds): Proteins of Excitable Membranes. Society of General Physiologists. New York, Wiley Interscience, 1987, p 43.

50. Marban E, Yamagishi T, Tomaselli GF: Structure and function of voltage-gated sodium channels. J Physiol 508:647, 1998.

51. Dionne VE: Two types of nicotinic acetylcholine receptors at slow fibre end-plates of the garden snake. J Physiol 409:313, 1989.

52. Raines DE: Anesthesia and nonanesthetic volatile compounds have dissimilar activities on nicotinic acetylcholine receptor desensitization kinetics. Anesthesiology 84:663, 1996.

53. Sine SM: The nicotinic receptor ligand binding domain. J Neurobiol 53:431, 2002.

54. Gage PW, Hammill OP: Effects of anesthetics on ion channels in synapses. Int Rev Neurophysiol 25:3, 1981.

55. Swope SL, Qu Z, Huganir RL: Phosphorylation of nicotinic acetylcholine receptor by protein tyrosine kinases. Ann N Y Acad Sci 757:197, 1995.

56. Plested CP, Tang T, Spreadbury I, et al: AChR phosphorylation and indirect inhibition of AChR function in seronegative MG. Neurology 59:1682, 2002.

57. Albuquerque EX, Alkondon M, Pereira EF, et al: Properties of neuronal nicotinic acetylcholine receptors: Pharmacologic characterization and modulation of synaptic function. J Pharmacol Exp Ther 280:1117, 1997.

58. Maelicke A, Coban T, Storch A, et al: Allosteric modulation of Torpedo nicotinic acetylcholine receptor ion channel activity by noncompetitive agonists. J Receptor Signal Transduc Res 17:11, 1997.

59. Creese R, Head SD, Jenkinson DF: The role of the sodium pump during prolonged end-plate currents in guinea-pig diaphragm. J Physiol 384:377, 1987.

60. Martyn JAJ: Basic and clinical pharmacology of the acetylcholine receptor: Implications for the use of neuromuscular relaxants. Keio J Med 44:1, 1995.

61. Ibebunjo C, Martyn JAJ: Thermal injury induces greater resistance to D-tubocurarine in local than in distant muscles in the rat. Anesth Analg 91:1243-1249, 2000.

62. Ikezu T, Okamoto T, Yonezawa K, et al: Analysis of thermal injury-induced insulin resistance in rodents: Implication of post-receptor mechanism. J Biol Chem 272:25289-25295, 1997.

63. Hirose M, Kaneki M, Yasuhara S, et al: Immobilization depresses insulin signaling in skeletal muscle. Am J Physiol 279:E1235, 2000.

64. Hirose M, Kaneki M, Sugita H, et al: Long-term denervation impairs insulin receptor substrate (IRS)-1–mediated insulin signaling in skeletal muscle. Metabolism 50:216, 2001.

65. Ibebunjo C, Nosek MT, Itani M, Martyn JAJ: Mechanisms for the paradoxical resistance to D-tubocurarine during immobilization-induced muscle atrophy. J Pharmacol Exp Ther 87:443-451,1997.

66. Hogue C, Itani M, Martyn JAJ: Resistance to D-tubocurarine in lower motor neuron injury is related to increased acetylcholine receptors at the neuromuscular junction. Anesthesiology 73:703, 1990.

67. Missias AC, Chu GC, Klocke BJ, et al: Maturation of the acetylcholine receptor in skeletal muscle: Regulation of the AChR γ-to-ε switch. Dev Biol 179:223, 1996.

68. Cohen-Cory S: The developing synapse: Construction and modulation of synaptic structures and circuits. Science 298:770, 2002.

69. Gronert GA: Cardiac arrest after succinylcholine: Mortality greater with rhabdomyolysis than receptor upregulation. Anesthesiology 94:523, 2001.

70. Fletcher SN, Kennedy DD, Ghosh IR, et al: Persistent neuromuscular and neurophysiologic abnormalities in long-term survivors of prolonged critical illness. Crit Care Med 31:1012, 2003.

71. Herridge MS, Cheung AM, Tansey CM, et al: One-year outcomes in survivors of the acute respiratory distress syndrome. N Engl J Med 348:683, 2003.

72. Beeson D, Newland C, Croxen R, et al: Congenital myasthenic syndromes: Studies of the AChR and candidate genes. Ann N Y Acad Sci 841:181, 1998.

73. Gomez CM, Maselli RA, et al: Novel delta subunit mutation in slow-channel syndrome causes severe weakness by novel mechanisms. Ann Neurol 51:102, 2002.

74. Witzemann V, Schwartz H, Koenen M, et al: Acetylcholine receptor epsilon-subunit deletion causes muscle weakness and atrophy in juvenile and adult mice. Proc Nat Acad Sci U S A 93:13286, 1996.

75. Altiok N, Altiok S, Changeaux JP: Heregulin-stimulated acetylcholine receptor gene expression in muscle: Requirement for MAP kinase and evidence for a parallel inhibitory pathway independent of electrical activity. EMBO J 16:717, 1997.

76. Olivetti G, Abbi R, Quaini F, et al: Apoptosis in the failing human heart. N Engl J Med 336:1131, 1997.

77. Yasuhara S, Kanakubo E, Perez M-E, et al: Burn injury induces skeletal muscle apoptosis with activation of caspase pathways in rats. The Carl Moyer Award for the best scientific paper at the Annual Meeting of the American Burn Association 1999. J Burn Care Rehabil 20:462, 1999.

78. Yasuhara S, Perez M-E, Kanakubo E, et al: Skeletal muscle apoptosis following burns is associated with activation of pro-apoptotic signals. Am J Physiol 279:1114, 2000.

79. Lukas RJ, Changeux J-P, Novère NL, et al: International union of pharmacology. XX. Current status of the nomenclature for nicotinic acetylcholine receptors and their subunits. Pharmacol Rev 51:397, 1999.

80. Galzi JL, Changeux JP: Neuronal nicotinic receptors: Molecular organization and regulation. Neuropharmacology 34:563, 1995.

81. Chiodini F, Charpantier E, Muller D, et al: Blockade and activation of the human neuronal nicotinic acetylcholine receptors by atracurium and laudanosine. Anesthesiology 94:643, 2001.

82. Taylor P: Anticholinesterase agents. *In* Gilman AG, Goodna LS, Rall TW, Murad F (eds): Pharmacological Basis of Therapeutics, 9th ed. New York, Macmillan, 1996, p 161.

83. Bom A, Clark JK, Palin R: New approaches to reversal of neuromuscular block. Curr Opin Drug Discov Devel 5:793, 2002.

84. Richtsfeld M, Yasuhara S, Blobner M, Martyn JAJ: Chronic administration of pyridostigmine leads to a myasthenia-like with down-regulation of acetylcholine receptors. Young Investigator Award for abstract to be presented at ASCCA at the ASA Annual Meeting, San Francisco, CA, October 2003.

85. Fink H, Yasuhara S, Blobner M, Martyn JA: Up-regulation of acetylcholine receptors during subchronic infusion of pancuronium is caused by a post-transcriptional mechanism related to disuse. Crit Care Med 32:509, 2004.

86. Yanez P, Martyn JAJ: Prolonged D-tubocurarine infusion and/or immobilization causes upregulation of acetylcholine receptors and hyperkalemia to succinylcholine. Anesthesiology 84:384, 1996.

CHAPTER
23 Statistical Methods in Anesthesia

Stanley H. Rosenbaum

Introduction   881

Statistical Approaches   882

Types of Data   882

Descriptive Statistics   882

Normal Distribution   882
Measures of Central Tendency   883
Measures of Dispersion   883
Graphing the Data   884

Regression Analysis   884
Univariate versus Multivariate Regression   884

Hypothesis Testing   885
Power   885
Confidence Intervals   885

Study Design   886

Data Dredging and the Problem of
Multiple Comparisons   887

Choice of Tests   887
Nonparametric Statistics   887
Contingency Tables   888
Paired versus Unpaired Data   888
Two-Group versus Multiple-Group
Analysis   888

Bayesian Approach to
Probability   888

Evidence-Based Medicine   889

Conclusion   889

INTRODUCTION

The advance of scientific knowledge in the past half millennium has been closely related to the linkage between experimental results and mathematical assessment of empirical observations. It is the role of the branch of mathematics termed "statistics" to describe the results of experiments and analyze, as best as can be done mathematically, the causes and effects behind the experiments.

A serious problem for a clinician or clinical scientist who wishes to use statistical methodology is that it is a modern branch of mathematics, much of it developed in the past century. Its mathematical sophistication is often considerably beyond that of the university-level calculus that is the upper limit of conventional medical training. Furthermore, many statistical methods involve extremely long and tedious calculations that require computerized techniques to be practical. This drawback leads us to the quandary that although statistical methods are useful and often essential to the understanding of medical science, they may be subtle to comprehend and difficult to use.

It cannot be the role of a chapter in a book such as this to derive or even genuinely explain the mathematics behind statistical methods. Many accessible introductory texts give some of the reasoning and rough, cookbook approaches to practical usage (see the Selected Readings list). In real life, almost no one ever does any sort of statistical calculations beyond the most simple with paper and pencil. Application programs for statistical calculations are widely available for personal computers. Many of them are reasonably well documented and simple enough to use without much preparation.

The problem we have with these statistical programs for personal computers is that the assumptions behind the statistics remain subtle. It is very easy to use the wrong method or approach and still have the program generate an output that, though appearing to be correct, is simply wrong. The old computer adage of "garbage in, (statistically misleading) garbage out" is very easy to achieve with a computer package and a data file.

It is the goal of this chapter to provide some of the correct language for describing statistics and to suggest the proper methodology for the use of statistics in some standard situations. Some of the classic errors common in medical statistics will be indicated. Of course, readers must be familiar with whatever program they actually use.

STATISTICAL APPROACHES

Within the broad rubric of statistics, several distinct and valuable areas can be viewed separately. "Descriptive statistics" is the use of mathematical methods to describe or categorize a collection of data that result from a set of empirical observations. "Statistical testing" is the broad approach to the determination of conclusions from a set of observations. Within each of these categories are many separate techniques.

TYPES OF DATA

It must be remembered that behind every statistical methodology there are formal mathematical definitions and proofs. Although it may sometimes seem that a simple intuitive approach is sufficient to understand what is happening, mathematical statistics can be misleading and unforgiving. The mathematical proofs and calculations that are behind our statistical tables and computation programs make strict distinctions among the several types of data (Table 23-1).

One type of data, termed *interval* data, are simple *continuous* numerical measurements (e.g., 1.2, 33.4). Often, we describe *discrete* numerical measurements, such as counts or integral quantities in the same categorization. This approach is occasionally misleading: the claim that a "typical family has 2.3 children" is meaningful in a crude way, even though the quantification of children is obviously not a continuous numerical fraction. In practical use, both continuous and discrete data can be handled by techniques similar to those used for interval data.

The other major grouping of data is *categorical* data. One type of categorical data is *ordinal* data, which refers to the ordering or ranking of subjects (e.g., 1st, 3rd, 10th). It is important to be careful to resist the temptation to regard the number of the ranking as an interval number, that is, to confuse "first" with the number "1," and so on. Such grouping does not usually have much meaning in reality and is false to the mathematics if an attempt is then made to manipulate the number as though it were an interval value.

Another similar category is *binary* data (e.g., up versus down, greater versus lesser). The most general grouping is the simple *category* (e.g., red, green, blue; cancer, diabetes, ulcer). When using simple or binary categories it is incorrect to attach numbers to the groups and try to get numerical results—the mathematics are not appropriate and the results are not likely to mean much. Specific statistical techniques for categorical data are necessary.

Table 23–1 Types of data

Data Type	Examples
Interval	1.1, 22
Ordinal	1st, 3rd
Categorical—binary	Male/female, live/die
Categorical—multiple	Red, green, blue

DESCRIPTIVE STATISTICS

Our most general statistical goal is to describe our data set. The simplest method is to just present all the crude data. For small data sets, the actual measurements can be presented. For larger amounts of data, a graph or statistical plot of the data can be helpful. One can frequently see trends and groupings in a picture that are very difficult to describe numerically. It is often suggested that before any mathematical method is applied to data analysis, a graphic plot be produced. If the data do not look "right" to the naked eye, a wise statistical analyst will be very careful to avoid misleading results. The choice of the correct format for the statistical plot can be an art form, and special data manipulation computer programs can be useful to search for visual clues in a data set.

NORMAL DISTRIBUTION

Perhaps the most powerful numerical concept of mathematical statistics is the *normal distribution,* often called the "bell-shaped curve." The idea of a most likely central value with other values scattered evenly to both sides is a classic statistical concept with deep mathematical roots. It fits in nicely with our intuitive idea of a "true" value with measurements distributed randomly around that true value such that more values are close to the center than are distant.

Many typical data sets follow a normal distribution around a center point. This distribution, sometimes also called a gaussian distribution, is derived from the assumption that there is a center, "true" value and that deviations from the center are random and diminish in likelihood the farther the values get from the center.

The strict use of normal distribution implies very large amounts of continuous interval data. When, as is usual, our data set does not meet this criterion, approximations are needed. Fortunately, most computerized statistical programs can deal with this problem with good effect.

In general, the mathematical description of the placement of the values is termed the *distribution*. There are many, mostly uncommon distributions other than normal distribution. They yield different curves and have specific mathematical properties. Not all data sets, even if they look like a bell-shaped curve, are normal distributions. If the curve is too wide (i.e., many distant outlying points) or too narrow or uneven, the mathematics derived for normal distributions will not work well.

When data follow a normal distribution or, more generally, any specific mathematical distribution, the methods of *parametric* statistics can be used. The term parametric refers to the ability to describe the distribution with a specific set of values. Frequently, such is not possible, and *nonparametric* statistical methods are necessary. These methods make fewer mathematical assumptions about the distribution of the data, but they are more difficult and can be less robust in finding statistical distinctions. Conversely, if parametric statistical methods are applied to data that are not normally distributed, false or misleading results can be calculated. This type of error is common and can be prevented by using appropriate tests or checking the data for normality before applying tests that assume it.

In practical use, we often treat our data as though they follow a normal distribution. However, wise investigators will use the tests in their computer statistics packages to test for normality and recognize that if the data do not follow a normal distribution, other methods will be needed.

Measures of Central Tendency

In describing data, the first task is to give some indication of the approximate value, range, or size of what is being described. How this is done depends on the type of data involved (Table 23-2). For categorical or binary data, all that may be possible is to give the counts in each group. For categorical data with many groups, the most populous groups may be named and listed in order. For ordinal data, summary description may be difficult; often, first place or last place will be the most interesting.

The *median* is the center or middle data point if the data can be ordered from smallest to largest. This value would apply both to interval data and to ordinal types of categorical data. For interval data, many mathematical techniques can be applied. The simplest is the *mean*, or the simple average value of the numerical data, with each data point being counted equally. In a *weighted mean*, the individual points may be added in unequally, with some getting more credit (i.e., "weight") than others.

For interval data that can be analyzed mathematically, the data may be fitted to a curve, which means that a mathematical formula is computed that closely fits the measured data points, often by using a computer and sophisticated calculations. The relationship can be as simple as a straight line, or a complicated mathematical formula with exponentials, polynomials, or other functions included as may be needed. The various computed values in these formula would be the *parameters* of the curves. The data would thus be described by the parameters of the formula approximated to the observed data. For the simple case of a straight-line approximation to data, the parameters would be the slope and intercept of the line. For complex equations fitted to data, the parameters would be the various computed numbers that make up the equations.

The *mode* is the most common value in a set of data points. This concept can be misleading if the data are truly continuous because every data point would then probably be different (if only infinitesimally so) from every other point. Hence, to describe the mode of continuous data it makes the most sense to group the values into brief intervals. In this sense, the interval with the most points within it is the modal interval. The mode may also be a very misleading description of the central tendency of a data set because there may be no reason for the most common value to be anywhere near the middle.

Numerical data can be described by categorizing the values into *percentiles* or similar groups. The meaning here is that for the, say, 10th percentile, 10% of the data points are at or below that value. The 50th percentile corresponds to the median of the data set, and the 99th percentile is the value at or above 99% of the data points. Similarly, quartiles, quintiles, or other groups can be computed. With any method used to describe data, the choice of the description may subtly bias us in how we think about the result. In the simple data set [2, 2, 3, 7, 14], the mode = 2, the median = 3, and the mean = 5.6. Which, if any, of these representations is more accurate? The answer depends on how we want to use the data because no one representation is perfect.

Measures of Dispersion

Often we want to describe not only the values of our data but also how the data are spread out. For data that follow a normal distribution, the classic approach is to compute the *standard deviation* (SD) of the data. With this value, roughly 68% of the data fall within 1 SD of the mean and roughly 95% fall within 2 SD of the mean value. The larger the SD, the wider the "bell-shaped" curve, and the smaller the SD, the narrower the curve.

Another way of looking at this concept is to consider that if we were making measurements of an unknown value and our values were scattered in a random normal distribution around that value, it is likely that about 68% of the data points would be within 1 SD of the true value. Of course, this result is only the most probable outcome, and in any real set of randomly distributed data we could be unlucky and have very atypical points.

For data that do not follow a normal distribution, it can be difficult to describe the dispersion of the data set in a standard fashion. Often, just the *range* of the data, from lowest to highest, is given. Occasionally, the data may be so scattered, with very distant extremes, that the range is not as useful as reporting the 25th to 75th percentiles of the data.

Caution

Because it is so easy to use a computer package to calculate the SD, we must be particularly cautious about using it. Frequently, data do not fit nicely into the normal distribution with a symmetric bell shape and unbounded tails out in both directions. As an example, consider a population with widely dispersed ages, but with many children. It would be easy to get a mean value for the age of 10, with an SD of 15. Clearly, no values lie at the lower end of the distribution with ages of −5. In such situations, the SD has some merit in describing the spread of the data but is, by strict mathematics, being misapplied.

Standard Error of the Mean

Just as random numerical data can often be described by the SD, the means computed from multiple grouped determinations of the data set can be described by making

Table 23–2   Measures of central tendency
Mean ± standard deviation
Mode
Median
Percentiles

a computation very similar to the SD but applied not to the measured data but to the computed means. This computed quantity is termed the *standard error of the mean* (SEM). As more data sets are gathered, with each data point being a measurement of what is a "true," but unknown, value the means of the data sets will very probably get closer and closer to that true value. Hence, as more and more data are gathered, the SEM will get smaller and smaller. This concept is intuitively very reasonable—as we make more and more measurements of a value, we should be getting a mean value closer and closer to the "true" value, even if the data points themselves remain scattered.

The difference between SD and SEM is important. SD is used to describe the data, SEM is used for computations about the certainty of the mean of the data. Because our computer packages can as easily provide either of these values and SEM is a smaller value, one is tempted to describe the data by the SEM. Although this is not dishonest if clearly labeled, it can certainly be misleading. If you have a very large number of data points, the SEM will be very small, but widely dispersed data will have a large SD no matter how many points are measured.

Graphing the Data

All experienced statisticians will stress that before statistical calculations are applied to a new data set, the data be plotted in some graphic format. If the data are widely scattered, look asymmetric, or have a specific pattern, that information is useful in determining the statistical tools to be applied. Furthermore, noting the presence of extreme outlying points may be a clue to mathematical or experimental errors.

REGRESSION ANALYSIS

Data may often fit a mathematical formula, which may be a straight line (e.g., a linear relationship) or just about any sort of continuous mathematical formula. In *regression analysis,* we use the power of the computer program to determine the mathematical formula that best fits the data. To do this we have to provide the program with the type of curve to use, for example, a straight line, quadratic equation, or exponential curve. The program will then provide us with the parameters within the selected equation that best fit the data points.

The art of regression is complex. The first problem is to pick the appropriate mathematical relationship to fit the data. Graphing the data is obviously very useful for this. There are also some mathematical subtleties in how to best fit the data to the curve, but by far the most common method is a *least-squares* approach that minimizes the square of the distance of each data point from the proposed curve. Although this methodology is about 2 centuries old, it clearly benefits from the use of modern computerized calculations, without which it would be practically unusable.

The computer program for regression analysis will provide the parameters of the fitted equation, such as the slope and y intercept for a straight line, and also some information about how well these parameters fit the data. The user has to be cautious in using the fitted equation if the agreement is poor because almost any jumble of data can be fitted to some equation, albeit with terrible agreement. It is fair to stress that the human eye has real power to judge trends, so if a graph of the data does not look like it fits the curve, the wise will be very skeptical of the result.

Univariate versus Multivariate Regression

In fitting data in a regression analysis, the first step is to choose the variables that will be used as independent variables. In *univariate* analysis, only one variable is used for the data fit, and the data are plotted and the computations performed by using that one variable to describe the data. As an example, the weights of a group of subjects may be compared with their heights. However, in the real world, many possible variables can almost always be used to determine an outcome. In *multivariate* analysis, more than one variable is used to describe the observed results. In the weight example, the subjects' weights might be analyzed by using heights, ages, and gender. Note that in this multivariate example, the outcome is a continuous interval variable, but is determined by a collection of interval variables (age, height) and a categorical variable (gender). The precise mathematical techniques that are used for multivariable analysis will depend on the nature of the variable used; in general, a mixed group of variables makes the most sense with real-world data.

On first approaching analysis of a data set, a simple univariate analysis may help in understanding the relationships involved. However, the data analyst must be cautioned that subtle relationships can be missed with only univariate analysis if the relevant variable is not used. As an example, heart rate may correlate with the dosage of pain medicine in an injured patient, but the causal relationship for both is likely to depend on the degree of pain.

With multivariate regression analysis, many potential pitfalls can readily be encountered with computerized calculations. One critical category of problems derives from the relationships that the various variables may have with one another, which is often described by indicating how *independent* these variables are in relation to one another. For an independent variable, the values of one variable do not tell what the values of the other would be. In the example of weight versus age and height, we would expect age and height to be independent in adults. Mathematically, it would be determined that age and height are *uncorrelated*. However, in children, age and height are correlated, so weight could be expressed as a function of weight versus age or weight versus height. In this last case, a multivariate analysis that focused on independent variables might just produce the result that weight is a function of height and throw out the relationship between weight and age. Hence, when many variables are involved, caution must be applied so that experimentally important relationships are not missed because they do not add mathematically to the results. Sophisticated statistical computer packages will look for these sorts of problems. Identification of significant correlation among the different variables would suggest that some information may be lost if only independent variables are reported. If a simpler statistical program is used, it would be wise to perform multivariate analyses with some of the variables left out to see whether other possible relevant relationships appear.

Another type of problem that can be misleading with multivariable relationships occurs in the situation in which the computer program produces a variable that correlates only weakly with the data, but does so with high reliability. This situation would be expressed in linear analysis as a result with a small correlation coefficient but a very good "P value" (more about "P" later). The fact that the correlation is not probably a statistical fluke does not offer much to the experimental analysis if the correlation is poor—the data are not well explained by the relationship. Here, the confusion comes from the fact that although the correlation is weak and does not explain much, the calculation shows very high confidence in the presence of this weak correlation.

HYPOTHESIS TESTING

A very common use of statistical techniques is to test a question, called the *hypothesis*. Also often termed *significance testing*, this approach yields the valuable concept of the "P value." It is this P value that is often used to summarize the statistical strength of the data analysis in supporting or rejecting the hypothesis. If we were comparing groups, we often describe the test as a comparison of the *null hypothesis*, which states that there is no difference between two groups of data, and the *alternative hypothesis*, which states that there is a difference. If we were analyzing a single grouping of data and performing a comparison of two descriptions of the data, such as determining whether the mean value of the group as calculated from the data is different from 0, the two hypotheses would be "mean = 0" versus "mean = measured value $\neq 0$."

The P value is computed from the observed data as the probability of obtaining this data set if in reality the null hypothesis were true. It is important to note that this calculation assumes the null hypothesis and is not the same as saying that P is the probability that the alternative hypothesis is true. If in reality the null hypothesis is true, it would be unlikely that we observe something else in our data. In actual experimental situations, all data have some randomness, so we can never be certain that our observation is not just chance and bad luck.

In hypothesis testing we choose a *level of significance*, termed the *alpha* value, and declare that if P is less than alpha, the result is statistically significant and accepted as true. If P is not less than alpha, we reject the hypothesis (equivalent to accepting the null hypothesis). Remember the logical sequence: we choose alpha in advance, then compute P from the data. If P is less than alpha, we agree to accept the hypothesis and we reject the null hypothesis. The P value is the chance that the null hypothesis was true but, through our bad luck, the data came out as observed anyhow. Typically, we set alpha equal to .05 and

want P less than that. For that P value, it would mean that the chance of the data coming out this way was less than a probability of 5% (P = .05) if the null hypothesis were in fact true.

Choosing the level of significance is an arbitrary decision. We might want to be very sure that we did not erroneously reject the null hypothesis and set alpha at .01. It is common in biomedical studies to pick an alpha value of .05. Also be aware that a very small P value may lead us to reject the null hypothesis but may not give us much information about the exact nature of the alternative. As an example, tossing a coin and getting six heads in a row might lead us to reject the null hypothesis that the coin is a fair coin, but it is not enough information to convince us that the coin always comes up heads. We calculate the P value from the data assuming the null hypothesis and use a small value of P to allow us to reject the null hypothesis, yet that does not fully characterize the alternative hypothesis.

Power

It should seem intuitively obvious that the ability of a statistical test to make a valid determination depends on the amount of data available. With only a few observations or data points, we cannot be as certain about a conclusion as if we had large amounts of data. If our goal were determining the fairness of a coin, tossing it twice would not convince us of much; tossing it a thousand times, however, would give us a good idea about its nature. In statistical hypothesis testing, the *power* of a study is a description of the ability of the study to detect a true difference. A statistical hypothesis test may fail to achieve significance (fail to get P < alpha) if either the data truly do not reflect a difference or if there are so few data points that the mathematics yields a poor P value. We define a *beta error* as the probability of falsely accepting the null hypothesis (calculated by assuming that the alternative hypothesis is true), and the *power = 1 − beta*. For the power to be good, that is, the beta value to be small, we want our study to have enough data points so that if a difference is observed between the null and alternative hypotheses, we can accept it with reliability.

A sample size calculation is often performed before an experiment is undertaken to determine how much data would be necessary to have a reasonable chance of observing what is guessed to be the observed result. Standard computer programs are available that will compute the number of data points necessary when the alpha and power values are provided and some estimate is made of the likely observed effect. It is important to be cautious about any study that is interpreted as "negative," that is, reports no significant difference between the study groups. It may be that no difference truly exists, but it may also be that the sample size was too small to determine a difference with statistical significance.

Confidence Intervals

It is becoming more common in reporting statistical measurements to use *confidence intervals* as a description of the statistical determination. A range of values may be given such that it is determined with some likelihood (often picked at 95%) that the true values lie within that range. For expressing simple results, the confidence interval is equivalent to providing a mean ± SD. This method becomes particularly useful for describing results when we want to describe "no difference" in correct statistical fashion. Here, the proper description would be that the true difference lies in an interval less than "x" with the given statistical confidence.

In sum, for hypothesis testing we want the following:
- Null hypothesis—e.g., mean = measure value "m"
- Alternative hypothesis—e.g., mean = 0
- Alpha value (chosen in advance)—e.g., alpha = .05
- Power (chosen in advance in conjunction with a sample size calculation so that we have enough data points)—e.g., power = 0.8
- P value—computed for data

We can say that we have a significant difference between the null and alternative hypotheses if *P* is less than alpha. If we are describing a value, we can give it as a confidence interval, and if we are saying that there is "no difference," we can describe it as a difference (if any) in the interval less than some computed value.

STUDY DESIGN

The essence of scientific study is generally some numerical determination of a result. It is this numerical analysis that we approach with our statistical calculations. However, without a careful design of the study in the way that the numerical data are generated, formal statistical analysis of the numbers will yield scant benefits and may even be very misleading. In the typical study we are usually attempting to either characterize some variable (e.g., mean or trend) or make a choice to accept or reject among various hypotheses. No matter what the question is in our minds, we must always be careful that the results genuinely answer the question and that we are not misleading ourselves with inappropriate conclusions.

Scientific studies may be *observational* studies in which we gather data without performing any specific intervention affecting the assignment of groups or effects on group members. Because in an observational study we have to take what we find as data, we are always very subject to other unrecognized factors that may distort our interpretation or limit our ability to ask questions about our data.

In an *interventional* study, we pick the group members, determine what is being done to them, and attempt to look out for and eliminate potential confusion before the data are collected. A *clinical trial* is a typical interventional study in which different therapies are compared.

In the design of a scientific study one major fear is a statistical *bias,* which is a systematic effect in the study that produces an error in our interpretation of the results. When considering the various possible study designs, we need to beware of the potential biases that may creep in. A *selection bias* occurs when we are comparing groups with respect to some variable, but do not realize that the groups are different in other (but important) ways.

Because groups of subjects may differ in multiple ways, our assignment of subjects into groups may result, either from misdirected choice or just random "bad luck," in groups that are not fairly comparable. So although we think that our results are determined by the variable under study, it may really be that some other factor misleads us in our conclusion. As an example, consider a study that is comparing surgical and medical treatment of some illness and ends up with a grouping in which a higher proportion of men than women are undergoing surgical therapy. Any conclusion from this study about surgery versus medical therapy is biased and might be truly just reflecting a difference in the results of therapy on men versus women.

A *confounding bias* occurs when multiple variables are intimately intertwined so that although we may assume that the variable under study is important, the truth is that the confounding variable is more important. As an example, consider a study attempting to determine the effects of obesity on longevity. Because diabetes mellitus is very closely correlated to obesity, a result that purported to be about obesity might easily be more accurate about diabetes. When variables do not correlate with each other so that changes in one do not go along with changes in the other, we call them (in a rough nonmathematical sense) *independent* variables. Variables that are correlated with each other are not independent.

A *measurement* bias occurs if the methods used for making measurements when comparing different groups have different scales or sensitivities. As an example, consider attempting to get a history of chest pain in groups of patients with and without known coronary artery disease. Patients who know that they have heart disease might be imagined to remember brief pain more thoroughly than healthy patients do, or perhaps they might deny pain more in their wish to believe that they are healthy—here the art of the experimenter is to predict and avoid such biases.

In a *blinded* study (more properly called a *masked* study), measurement bias may be avoided if the person performing the measurement does not know which group is being measured so that subtle bias in approaching or determining the data can be avoided. As an example, consider an active drug being compared with an inactive placebo. A researcher who knew which patient was taking the active drug might be more diligent in pursuing benefits or side effects. In a *double-blind* clinical study, neither the patients nor the experimenters obtaining the data should know which subjects are in which group to avoid subtle measurement bias.

Observational studies may be categorized as case, case-control, or cohort studies. In a simple *case study*, an individual case or group of cases is reported. Such reports may demonstrate the existence of some observation or effect, provide the presumably typical character of the observation, and suggest a therapy or natural history. These types of studies do not have the nature of a proof because it is always a possibility that some other hidden effect is producing the observation or that the observed characteristics are atypical in some fashion. Nevertheless, often "seeing is believing," so much of what is reported in medicine is in the form of case observations.

The distinction between cohort and case-control studies is important, but often misinterpreted. In both categories, groups of subjects are compared, usually in regard to the effects of some intervention. In a *case-control* study, the factor separating the groups is determined *after* the intervention. Typically, a comparison is made of some outcome in one group, the case group, versus a similar group that does not have the outcome and functions as the control group. Because the groups are separated after the intervention, selection biases or unappreciated confounding variables can mislead the investigators. As an example, consider a study investigating the effects of hypertension on surgical mortality. If the groups are divided into patients with and without perioperative cardiac events, it may well be that one group will be different from the other. However, such a result may be misleading; perhaps it is really the renal disease that is associated with the hypertension that is significant (a confounding bias). Alternatively, perhaps patients with hypertension are sent to surgery by their physicians only when they have worse surgical problems, so the groups are not fairly compared (a selection bias).

In a cohort study, the study group is monitored before the intervention occurs. The group is assembled to be as similar as possible and then monitored forward in time. Such studies are useful for describing the natural history of disease and may be helpful in suggesting etiologies. However, as with the other observational studies, selection and confounding bias may occur and lead to misleading results.

A case-control study is sometimes termed a *retrospective* study because the analysis can only be done after the subjects complete the study (so that it can be determined to which group they belong). In this sense, a cohort study is a *prospective* study inasmuch as the data must be gathered before the intervention. Unfortunately, these terms may be misused because obviously, a case-control study can be planned in advance ("prospectively"). In addition, no matter how truly prospective a study is, once the data are gathered, the analyses are performed after the fact ("retrospectively"). These terms are best avoided.

After considering the nature of observational trials we can see the strength of the interventional clinical trial, where the investigators determine the membership of the groups to be compared in advance and attempt to make the groups as alike as possible. In a *randomized clinical trial,* the subjects are assigned by chance to the groups so that if there are some fluctuations in the subjects or some subtle selection bias, the effect will be the same in each group (and presumably cancel out in the result). Such a study is necessarily prospective in nature.

Randomized clinical trials are the idealized standard in medical research because they give the best chance to minimize biases. However, the effort and expense in setting up a clinical trial may be very considerable. Recognize that such a trial requires patients to be enrolled before the medical intervention is performed. Patients give up choice of the therapy that they receive and allow their therapy to be randomly selected among various options. Such trials (even if they involve standard therapies) require full ethical board clearance and explicit patient consent.

Even with the best clinical trial methodology, potential difficulties include dealing with subtle selection biases regarding who is entered into the trial. Studies that are actively watched by investigators and their highly motivated associates may result in atypical practices that cannot be generalized into standard clinical practice. The patients in clinical trials are themselves mostly motivated by the search for personal benefit and cannot be depended on to follow protocols strictly or to stay with a program that does not appear to be successful to them.

DATA DREDGING AND THE PROBLEM OF MULTIPLE COMPARISONS

In all our statistical interpretations regarding the acceptance of data-determined conclusions, we always recognize that there is the random chance of a highly unlikely statistical result being misinterpreted as the typical true conclusion. A coin tossed six times and coming up all heads might lead us to conclude the coin was not fairly balanced, yet that will happen every $2^6 = 64$ times that it is attempted even with an entirely fair coin. When we pick an alpha value of .05, we are roughly saying that about 5% of the time we will accept misleading random errors as though they were true. This is roughly equivalent to recognizing that for every 20 experiments we do, perhaps 1 will be wrongly accepted as true based solely on bad luck and random chance. If we analyze a large set of data in many ways, some random results may appear statistically significant just based on this sort of chance. This is the error of *"data dredging."*

In a similar manner, if a very large number of independent comparisons are made between two groups of subjects and we accept an error rate of 5%, we might get a false, but statistically "significant" result about once for every 20 comparisons made. This is the error of *"multiple comparisons."* Mathematical methods are available to correct for these errors—what is most relevant for the consumer of the statistical analysis is to recognize the presence of the error and look for the correction.

CHOICE OF TESTS

Nonparametric Statistics

When calculating the random distribution of some variable it is easy to visualize the values as clustered around some center value in the well-known bell-shaped (termed "normal") distribution. However, as noted earlier, not all data have such a nice distribution. Data that are not in interval format, such as nominal data (e.g., red, black; male, female) or ordinal data (first, third), cannot be described by mathematical distributions with parameters such as the mean or SD. Such a situation calls for nonparametric statistics. Nonparametric statistical methods are typically used for the analysis of nominal or ordinal data. Data that are distributed in a very atypical skewed fashion (a "non-normal" distribution) will not be properly handled by analyses that have the mathematical assumptions of normality; such data will need nonparametric analysis.

The first step in considering the choice of a statistical test is to decide whether statistical methods that assume a normal distribution are appropriate or whether nonparametric methods are needed (Table 23-3). A test for normality is included in typical statistical computer packages.

Contingency Tables

A very common nonparametric statistical problem is the analysis of a table of data in which each cell in the table is a count in a particular category. The question is to determine whether the groups are statistically different from one another. As an example, consider the question of men versus women and their political affiliation, Republican versus Democrat, in which a 2×2 table is generated. If additional political groups are added, say Green and Undeclared, we then have a 2×4 table. If we wished to analyze these data to determine whether men and women differ in political affiliation or whether Democrats versus Greens differ in gender distribution, we would apply nonparametric statistical methods appropriate to a contingency table.

Paired versus Unpaired Data

If statistical methods are applied to analyze data from multiple groups and each individual data point comes from a separate and distinct source, the mathematics behind the statistics assumes an independence and randomness that would not be the same if the sources are highly related. As an example, consider a study of blood pressure in two groups of subjects, one treated with medication and the other untreated. Because blood pressure measurements can be widely scattered in distribution, depending on the subjects' previous medical condition, a small drug effect might be difficult to notice. However, if the same individuals were studied before and after therapy, the wide initial variations might cancel out and small effects would be noticed. In this latter study, the data points can be paired, one in each group, to detect these small effects. A study in which the data can be paired can be very sensitive in picking out small changes. Conversely, the erroneous use of paired statistics might suggest a statistically significant result when one does not exist.

Two-Group versus Multiple-Group Analysis

In a simple statistical analysis we may be characterizing one group of data or comparing that group with a standard value. It is slightly more intricate to compare two groups when we want to characterize each group and determine whether the groups are statistically different. Much more concern must be applied to the situation when we have three or more groups. In this case of multiple groups, two distinct types of questions can be asked. First, we might wish to know whether the groups are significantly different or whether they are all the same (with any numerical differences attributed solely to random fluctuations). Second, if we do conclude that the groups are statistically not all the same, we might want to know which groups are different from one another—that is, are they all distinct or are just one or a few different whereas the rest are similar to each other.

In summary, three questions should be asked when choosing between tests (see Table 23-3):
1. One group, two groups, or many groups?
2. Paired or unpaired groups?
3. Parametric (interval data following a normal distribution) or nonparametric methods?

BAYESIAN APPROACH TO PROBABILITY

The commonsense meaning of the term "probability" can readily become confusing within the mathematical morass of formal statistics. In practice, we commonly use and interchange two definitions for probability. In the *frequentist* approach, we view the probability of an occurrence as the fraction of occasions that the selected event would occur if the trial were repeated many times. So we say that the probability of a fair coin coming up heads is .5 because if we toss it many times, we would get about 50% heads.

However, in many real-life situations we cannot repeat the trials many times to get a frequency of occurrence for an event. In the *subjectivist* approach, we assign a probability to an event based on our best guess or opinion. Such subjective assessments are very similar to what we do in medicine when we make an interpretation based on opinion and experience. This approach is often termed *bayesian* statistics because of a mathematical

Table 23–3	Choice of tests		
Comparison Goal	**Normally Distributed (Parametric) Interval Data**	**Nonparametric Interval Data**	**Categorical Data**
Describe group	Mean ± SD	Median, mode, percentile	Counts and proportions
Compare group with value	*t*-Test	Wilcoxon	Chi-square
Compare two groups	Unpaired *t*-test	Mann-Whitney	Chi-square, Fisher
Two paired groups	Paired *t*-test	Wilcoxon	McNemar
Three or more groups	ANOVA	Kruskal-Wallis	Chi-square
Multiple matched groups	Repeated-measures ANOVA	Friedman	—
Regression	Linear regression	Nonparametric regression	Logistic regression

ANOVA, analysis of variance; SD, standard deviation.

formula, Baye's equation, that is used to manipulate subjective probabilities.

The powerful practical insight that comes from bayesian statistics lies in the requirement that we start statistical calculations with an initial probability of an event. This very much matches the real-life situation, in which any test or prediction depends on the patient under study. It is generally medically unwise to consider a diagnosis for a patient unless we take the patient's own characteristics into account. It is obvious to any clinician that an abnormal cardiogram suggesting myocardial ischemia would not mean the same thing in a healthy 30-year-old as it would in his obese hypertensive grandfather. In a similar argument, a negative exercise stress test does not give us great confidence that a very high-risk patient is free of cardiac disease (because the chance of disease is so high and stress tests are notorious for missing disease in some patients).

In medical situations, bayesian statistics are mostly used for the interpretation of diagnostic or predictive data. The term "bayesian" is often an indication that the patients' or population's a priori chances of disease should be considered when applying a predictive test.

When using diagnostic or predictive tests, the concepts of sensitivity and specificity are very useful because they are not dependent on the population. *Sensitivity* is, roughly, the ability of the test to pick up the disease, and *specificity* indicates the ability of the test to avoid false alarms. To use these terms we define four possible situations:

True positive (TP): The patient has disease and the test is positive.

False positive (FP): The patient does not have disease and the test is positive.

True negative (TN): The patient does not have disease and the test is negative.

False negative (FN): The patient has disease and the test is negative.

By definition,

$$\text{Sensitivity} = TP/(TP + FN)$$

$$\text{Specificity} = TN/(TN + FP)$$

The ideal test has a sensitivity of 1, which indicates that the test picks up all the patients with the disease, and a specificity of 1, which indicates that the test never falsely claims that a healthy patient is diseased.

It is also sometimes useful to define the following:

$$\text{Positive predictive value (PPV)} = TP/(TP + FP)$$

$$\text{Negative predictive value (NPV)} = TN/(TN + FN)$$

Remember that although the sensitivity and specificity of a test do not depend on the characteristics of the population, they certainly do depend on the quality of the test. However, PPV and NPV are dependent on the tested population—this situation is where our comment about "bayesian" is relevant. (Although it is not the goal of this chapter to prove these claims, the reader may be convinced by considering what happens to sensitivity, specificity, PPV, and NPV in situations in which the test is applied to a population in whom the disease is absent so that only TN and FP are nonzero: PPV is vanishingly small and NPV approaches 1. Similarly, for a population with almost all patients having disease, PPV goes to 1 and NPV vanishes.)

The bayesian insight can now be stated that we apply diagnostic or predictive tests only to populations of subjects who are somewhat likely to test positive, but not "excessively" so. If we test subjects who are very likely to test positive, a positive test is confirmatory and a negative may be more likely to be a false-negative than a true-negative result. Similarly, if the tested population is very unlikely to have the specified disease, a negative test is only confirmatory and a positive test is more likely to be a false-positive than a true result.

EVIDENCE-BASED MEDICINE

Making judgments in science is an intricate process. Our decisions are formed by theoretical reasoning, extrapolation from empirical data, traditional conventions, and, often, local authorities. Most modern philosophers of science recognize that the old view of the scientific method as a totally unbiased approach to the interpretation of raw data is naive. All the data we collect in any experiment is created, selected, and interpreted within the context of our theory-based view of the world. Furthermore, more than one theoretical explanation can generally be given for any one set of data. All this being the case, it must still be stressed that modern medicine has passed from the era when "practice" and "art" were sufficient justification for medical decision making. *Evidence-based medicine* is the fashionable term for the approach to medical decision making in which careful use is made of the applicable experimental scientific data. Controlled clinical trials and large-scale observational studies are important methods for this approach. A *meta-analysis* is a report of data that combines results from multiple similar studies to create a statistically more powerful study with many more data points and a better opportunity to come to a statistically significant conclusion.

The practicing clinician has many sources that analyze empirical evidence and provide guidance for medical decisions. Governmental groups and private medical organizations have produced many guidelines and clinical practice documents that assess the quality of available evidence and make suggestions. To give further guidance, these suggestions may also be ranked by confidence. The most reliable data backed by well-established theories would give recommendations with the greatest weight. Reports that are backed by weaker data such as uncontrolled studies give recommendations with less confidence in the evidence.

CONCLUSION

Clinicians use statistical methodology both to analyze their own data and to assess the value of others' scientific reports. Because data analysis is generally the application of one of a number of commercial computer packages, each with its own menus, formatting, and subtle caveats, the most valuable suggestion to the budding statistician is to know the program, read the manual, and plot the data. The human visual system is well adapted to see groups and trends—if the conclusions do not look like they fit the data, caution and skepticism are prudent.

When assessing the value of a scientific report, a careful clinician reads the "methods" section and asks the questions suggested earlier: Are the subjects selected to minimize bias? Are the statistical methods appropriate? Is the study large enough to be statistically powerful? Are the conclusions warranted by the evidence? Can the conclusions from this study be extended to cover more general cases or do they apply only to the limited situation under study?

Finally, despite the best statistical approaches and the most careful experimental procedures, a wise clinician recognizes that even some apparently well done experiments can yield erroneous conclusions. A study that produces an important clinical conclusion, especially one that seems to change tradition or violate previous theoretical understanding, bears confirmation by another group using different patients in a different setting. Healthy skepticism is the basis of good statistics and good science.

KEY POINTS

1. Always plot your data. Significant trends should be visible to the eye.
2. Know your statistics program well enough to be sure that it is calculating what you want.
3. Interval data should not be treated like categorical data—the mathematics is different.
4. Many statistical methods assume that the data are distributed "normally," that is, in a symmetric bell-shaped curve; these methods can be misleading if the data are not normally distributed.
5. SD is used to describe the spread of data, and SEM is used to compare data sets.
6. Multivariate regression, which relates the outcome variable to more than one other factor, requires more data but will probably pick up correlations that may be missed if only univariate regression is used.
7. When using multivariate regression, if two variables correlate closely with each other, the statistical package may miss reporting one as correlating with the outcome.
8. In hypothesis testing, a negative result may indicate no real difference or may just mean that the study

was underpowered to pick up a true, but small difference.
9. A *P* value is the probability that the observed result will occur, assuming no true difference between the tested hypotheses, which is not the same as the probability of the difference being true.
10. A bayesian approach to diagnostic testing recognizes the fact that the value of a test depends on the patient population: if the test is almost always truly positive in the population, false-negative results will outnumber true-negative ones and make the test less useful. This is also the situation if the test is almost always truly negative, in which case false positives cause the confusion.
11. Selection biases make many real-life clinical studies difficult to interpret. Randomized clinical trials are the best way to minimize this problem.
12. Beware of the error of "data dredging." Applying too many tests to insufficient data will probably find something that, misleadingly, seems significant.

SELECTED READINGS

Standard Statistical Computer Packages

Instat, GraphPad Software, San Diego, California.
A simple, very user-friendly program with good built-in help.

JMP, SAS Institute, Cary, North Carolina.
The SAS group's simple stand-alone program. Though relatively simple when compared with the full SAS program, its completeness leads to some complexity for the beginner.

SPSS, SPSS Inc, Chicago, Illinois.
A full featured, expensive, and very powerful program that is accessible to the nonprofessional statistics user. The help files are usable and exhaustive.

SAS, SAS Institute, Cary, North Carolina.
Expensive, very complex, very powerful. This standard package of programs is the one most commonly used by professional biomedical statisticians. Not for the amateur.

Selected Introductory Statistics Texts

Altman D: Practical Statistics for Medical Research. Boca Raton, Florida, CRC Press, 1990.
Well organized and complete. A good course textbook.

Dawson B: Basic & Clinical Biostatistics. New York, McGraw-Hill, 2000.
Suitable for self-study, fairly complete.

Feinstein A: Clinical Epidemiology. Philadelphia, WB Saunders, 1985.
Enormously insightful about the structure and problems of clinical research.

Glantz S: Primer of Biostatistics. New York, McGraw-Hill, 2001.
Very clear, very popular; also has a very simple-to-use statistics program that may be purchased with the book.

Anesthesia Management

CHAPTER
24 Risk of Anesthesia

Lee A. Fleisher

Issues Related to Study Design   894
Types of Studies   894
Problems Inherent in Studying
Anesthesia-Related Risk   896

Mortality Related to Anesthesia   897
Surgery without Anesthesia   897
Early Studies of Anesthesia-Related
Mortality   897
Anesthesia-Related Mortality Studies
after 1980   899
Perioperative Mortality in Outpatient
Surgery   902
Analysis of Intraoperative Cardiac Arrests   903
Use of Computer Analysis   904
Other Approaches to Discern the Root Cause of
Morbidity and Mortality   904
Issues Associated with Anesthesia-Related
Mortality   905

Risks Related to the Patient   906

Special Patient Groups   909
Obstetrics   909
Pediatrics   912
Geriatrics   914

**Risks Directly Related to the
Anesthetic Drug   914**

Risks Related to Surgery   915

**Risks Related to Location of Surgery
and Postoperative Monitoring   915**

**Risks Related to the Anesthesia
Provider   917**

Risks to the Anesthesiologist   918

Improving Anesthesia Safety   919

**Future Directions in Perioperative
Risk   920**

Summary   920

Much attention has been focused on the risks of anesthesia—surgery-related risks to the patient and occupational risks to the anesthesiologist. From the patient's perspective, it is important to provide an accurate assessment of the probability of complications and to study perioperative morbidity and mortality as a means of quality assurance to improve outcome. Numerous studies have attempted to define the probability of morbidity and mortality, with wide variability of results. Risk indices have been developed to identify patients who have a higher probability of developing complications, and it has become evident that individual genetic makeup can affect outcome. In all of these areas, as well as in clinical discussions with patients, the key issue is what risk are we attempting to define.

For the risk of anesthesia, there are multiple factors that enter into the equation. A myopic perspective could include only the morbidity and mortality that occurs intraoperatively. From a quality-assurance perspective, any death within 48 hours after use of an anesthetic is evaluated for potential relevancy. Other investigators have evaluated 30-day morbidity and mortality as part of their estimation of anesthesia-related and surgery-related risks. With respect to ambulatory surgery, 30-day outcomes may be too long, and complications within the first 7 days may be relevant. For patients with cardiac disease, myocardial infarction or cardiac enzyme release in the perioperative period can have implications for months to years.[1,2] It is important to define the time perspective when evaluating the studies (Table 24-1).

It is also important to differentiate the potential risk that is solely attributable to administration of anesthesia from the risks that anesthesia may modify. From a quality-assurance perspective, a patient with coronary artery disease who has a perioperative myocardial infarction would have the primary cause of morbidity assigned to the disease, but administration of perioperative β-blockers might have prevented the adverse outcome. Anesthesiologists must view perioperative organ protection as part of their goals to provide the highest quality of care and reduce perioperative risk.[3] Another example is the use of regional anesthesia to reduce graft thrombosis for patients undergoing infrainguinal arterial reconstruction.[4-6] One outcome that has benefited from regional anesthesia is graft thrombosis and the need for reoperation or amputation. However, the benefit from regional anesthesia was found in only two studies; the third study had a much lower rate of graft thrombosis, suggesting that the benefit may manifest only

Table 24–1 Time perspective of anesthetic morbidity and mortality studies

Study	Year	Time Perspective
Beecher and Todd[21]	1954	All deaths on the surgical services
Dornette and Orth[43]	1956	Deaths in the operating room or after failure to regain consciousness
Clifton and Hotten[47]	1963	Any death under, attributable to, or without return of consciousness after anesthesia
Harrison[51]	1978	Death within 24 hours
Marx et al.[35]	1973	Death within 5 days
Hovi-Viander[53]	1980	Death within 3 days
Lunn and Mushin[64]	1982	Death within 6 days
Tiret and Hatton[61]	1986	Complications within 24 hours
Mangano et al.[93]	1996	Death within 2 years

Adapted from Derrington MC, Smith G: A review of studies of anaesthetic risk, morbidity and mortality. Br J Anaesth 59:827, 1987.

if the rate of complication is sufficiently large. Assessment of risk therefore depends on the rate of complications.

Traditionally, anesthesiologists and investigators have focused on issues of death and major morbidity such as myocardial infarction, pneumonia, and renal failure. It is becoming increasingly important to include outcomes that affect economic issues, quality of life, and satisfaction for the patient (Table 24-2). For example, nausea and vomiting that delays or prevents discharge to home is important from the perspective of economics and quality of life. Readmission to the hospital after outpatient surgery is an important component of outcome studies.[7] Overall satisfaction with care is increasingly included as an outcome.[8-10] Further research is required to assess the influence of anesthesia care for nonmorbid outcomes and the importance of these outcomes from a patient-oriented perspective.

Many studies have also looked at what some investigators describe as *surrogate end points*.[11] For example, nausea and vomiting that do not require treatment or do not delay discharge do not have the same impact as episodes that do affect these outcomes. Myocardial ischemia on the electrocardiogram is another example of a surrogate outcome that may not lead directly to overt morbidity.[12] In determining the risk of anesthesia, it is important to define the outcome of greatest significance.

Perioperative risk is multifactorial and depends on the interaction of anesthesia-, patient-, and surgery-specific

factors (Fig. 24-1). With respect to anesthesia, the effects of the agents and the skills of the practitioner are important. Similarly, the surgeon's skills and the surgical procedure itself affect perioperative risk. From the patient's perspective, the question remains whether coexisting disease raises the probability of complications to a level such that the benefit of the surgery is outweighed by the risk. Anesthesiologists frequently have focused on perioperative risk, but the patient is most concerned with management of the disease process. As the specialty focuses on its role in the 21st century, it is important to acknowledge the patient's perspective and desire to undergo procedures that prolong life or improve quality of life. Increasing the ability of the anesthesiologist to affect the decision-making process and the overall risk is the future challenge.

Given these various goals, perspectives, and influences, this chapter attempts to define the current state of knowledge in this area. With the increasing interest in evidence-based medicine, it is important to define what is known and not known. Because it would be unethical to compare operations performed with the use of an "ideal anesthetic" with those using a less ideal or no anesthetic, virtually all studies looking at the factors that contribute to perioperative mortality involve evaluations of large cohorts of patients. However, since the 1990s there have been several well-designed, randomized clinical trials to evaluate different anesthesia regimens, which has advanced the field. This chapter also reviews the literature, with an emphasis on the strength of the evidence for the conclusions.

Table 24–2 Examples of common outcome measures

Outcome	Example
Mortality	
Morbidity	
Major	Myocardial infarction
	Pneumonia
	Pulmonary embolism
Minor	Nausea
	Vomiting
	Readmission
Patient satisfaction	
Quality of life	

ISSUES RELATED TO STUDY DESIGN

Types of Studies

To interpret the literature, it is important to understand the strengths and limitations of the various study designs. *Prospective cohort studies* involve the identification of a group of subjects who are monitored over time for the occurrence of an outcome of interest. The goal is to identify patients who develop the outcome. For studies of perioperative mortality, individual cases can be reviewed to determine the cause of mortality.

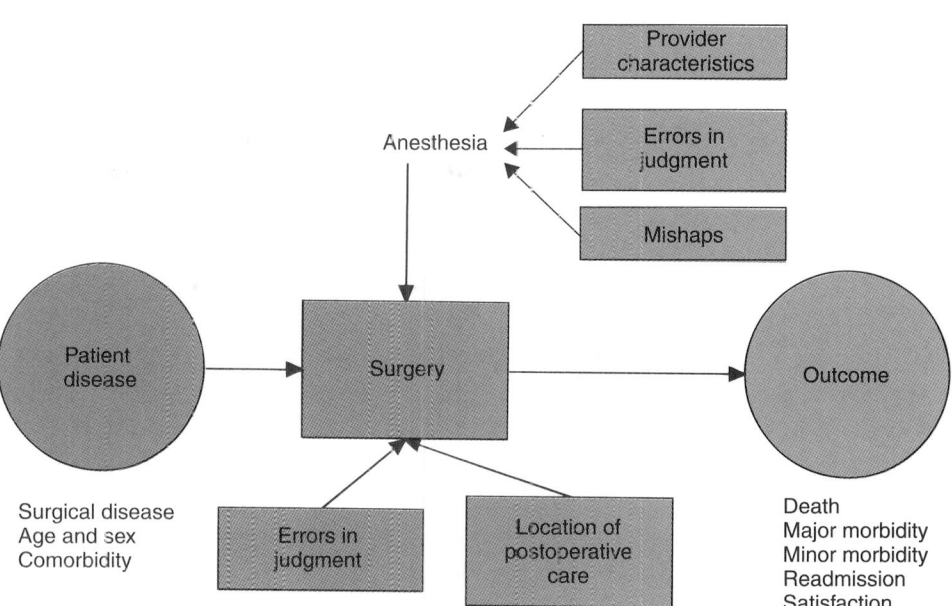

Figure 24–1 Representation of the influences of various components on poor perioperative outcomes. Surgical, anesthetic, and patient characteristics all contribute to outcome. Anesthesia-related contributions can include issues of judgment and mishaps, as well as characteristics of the provider. The surgical procedure itself affects outcome, as does the location of intraoperative and postoperative care.

Alternatively, data on all patients in the cohort can be obtained, and factors that are associated with the development of morbidity or mortality can be discerned. An example of a prospective cohort study identifying factors associated with perioperative cardiac morbidity and mortality is that of Goldman and colleagues,[13] which led to the development of the Cardiac Risk Index.

Another example of a prospective cohort study is one in which patients with a known disease are studied for the development of predefined outcomes. Such studies provide the natural history of the disease. For example, studies of patients who have sustained a myocardial infarction could be important in determining the optimal time between the infarct and surgery.[14-16]

Although prospective cohort studies have important value in identifying risk factors for the outcome of interest, there are significant limitations. The selection of the cohort of interest can significantly affect the results obtained. The larger the cohort, the more the results can be generalized. A second bias is that many patients may be lost to follow-up. In perioperative studies, this may not be an important issue for short-term outcomes. The importance of a risk factor depends on the completeness of the data. For example, if the presence of severe angina were not included in the database, it could not be considered as a risk factor, and other factors may appear to be more important.[13]

A specific example of a prospective cohort study is the *randomized clinical trial.* Randomized clinical trials represent the gold standard for evidence of causation. They have defined inclusion and exclusion criteria, treatment protocols, and outcomes of interest. They are usually single- or double-blinded (to patient and physician) studies and are designed to test the effect of a new drug or intervention. They rarely are used as a means of identifying risk, but they may be used to determine whether a risk factor is truly linked by a causal relationship or is simply an association. For example, hypothermia in the perioperative period has been associated with an increased

incidence of perioperative ischemia, a surrogate marker for morbidity.[17] In a randomized clinical trial, the use of forced-air warming to maintain normothermia was associated with a significantly lower incidence of perioperative morbid cardiac events.[18] Randomized clinical trials directed at interventions that reduce the frequency of a given risk factor in the population are frequently performed after the results of a prospective cohort study to confirm the findings of an association between poor outcome and that factor.

Randomized clinical trials derive their strength from an evidence-based perspective because of their high degree of internal validity; the randomization scheme and use of placebo (or accepted alternative treatments) provide strong evidence that the results are related to the intervention. Importantly, these trials have a lower degree of external validity because the intervention may not behave in the same manner when it is diffused in a more heterogeneous population in whom treatment is not defined.

Retrospective studies involve identification of patients who have sustained an outcome and definition of risk factors associated with the outcome. An example of a retrospective design is a *case-control study.* Case-control studies identify patients with the outcome of interest. Frequently, these patients are included as part of a prospective cohort study. The prevalence of a risk factor in the patients with the outcome (i.e., cases) is compared with the prevalence of the risk factor in matched controls to maximize the efficiency and power of the results. The ratio of cases to controls can be varied, yielding greater power with an increasing number of controls.

Case-control studies are subject to several biases. The exact definitions of cases and controls can influence the analysis. Frequently, patients are matched for age and gender, but other factors may play an important role. It is critical that the exposure precedes the outcome, and a dose-response gradient further confirms the relationship.

Problems Inherent in Studying Anesthesia-Related Risk

Several issues related to studying anesthesia-related risk can affect the findings. For example, multiple definitions of perioperative mortality exist. In particular, the time frame in which a death can be attributed to the surgery and delivery of anesthesia varies. Because in-hospital stays have shortened, many events related to surgery may occur after discharge. This is particularly the case with ambulatory or short-stay surgery, for which recovery from anesthesia occurs at home. As we continue to monitor our patients for safety, it will be important to extend follow-up care beyond the traditional hospital setting, and many recent studies have included such an approach.

A major problem in any study of risk is the actual rate of complications in the population of interest. There are multiple sources of data for studying perioperative risk. Although some of the original studies used data from only one or a small group of institutions, such approaches may not be practical in the current era. As demonstrated throughout this chapter, most individuals believe that risk related to anesthesia has decreased over time, although this premise has been questioned.[19] For example, the rate of anesthesia-related mortality described in the Confidential Enquiry into Perioperative Deaths (CEPOD) of 1987 was 1 in 185,000 patients, compared with the 1 in 2680 cases reported by Beecher and Todd about 30 years earlier.[20,21] Considering the current rate, any study would have to be enormous to detect anesthesia-related mortality. Such a study would require information from a large number of sites or data covering multiple years from a single institution.[22] Considering concerns in the United States regarding confidentiality and legal liability, a multicenter study of risk in unselected patients would be difficult to undertake. Such problems may not be inherent in other countries.

Another issue is the effect of the act of studying outcome. As in any study of risk, the actual rate of complication decreases as a result of increased observation. This is frequently observed as a lower than expected rate of complications in the placebo arm of a randomized, controlled trial.

An alternative approach is to identify bad outcomes and study them for patterns of errors. For example, Cheney and colleagues[23] developed the American Society of Anesthesiologists (ASA) Closed Claims Study (ACCS). By obtaining the records of major events that led to legal litigation, they were able to identify factors that contributed to bad outcomes. With this methodology, selected morbidities that lead to litigation can be identified. The limitation of this methodology is that the actual rates of complications are not known; only the number of closed legal claims is identified. Cases that do not result in litigation are not included in the database.

Several attempts have been made to establish large epidemiologic databases. One example of such an approach has been the work of Mangano and the Multicenter Study of Perioperative Ischemia group with regard to cardiac surgery. This group used their database to evaluate issues such as the rate and importance of atrial fibrillation after cardiac surgery and the use of aspirin.[24,25] Other approaches include the development of cardiac surgery databases by the Society of Thoracic Surgeons, the U.S. Veterans Administration, and the New England Collaborative Project.[26-30] These databases are used to define risk factors for poor outcome, to benchmark local to national complication rates, and as educational tools. Such databases include little or no information regarding anesthesia practice. They include a predominance of patients from academic or major medical centers, whereas smaller or community hospitals may have very different patterns of care. Although these databases may provide extremely important information to improve care, the ability to generalize results to the nonacademic centers is unknown.

This final issue of the institutional site of the surgery may have other implications related to the pattern of care at a particular hospital. Although studies frequently categorize risk as related to anesthesia, surgery, or patient disease, postoperative care may have a profound impact on risk. For example, the risk of pulmonary embolism may be related to nursing care and the frequency of patient ambulation after surgery.[31] The presence of an intensivist who makes daily rounds and higher nurse staffing ratios may also affect outcome.[32-34] Variations in the total care provided by a hospital, including the anesthesiologists and surgeons, may significantly affect outcomes.

One advance in determining local complication rates is the development of hospital information systems. The use of computer databases in the assessment of risk began with Marx and colleagues[35] in the 1970s. These information systems now are almost a requirement of survival for the hospital. The ability to query these systems will make large-scale studies of institutional risk much less burdensome in the future. Reich and coworkers[36] used one such system to identify intraoperative hemodynamic abnormalities, including pulmonary hypertension, hypotension during cardiopulmonary bypass, and pulmonary diastolic hypertension after cardiopulmonary bypass, as independent predictors of mortality, stroke, and perioperative myocardial infarction beyond the effects of other preoperative risk factors.

When extremely large sample sizes are needed, administrative databases may be among the most cost-effective approaches to this issue. Examples of administrative databases include Medicare claims files, private insurance company claims, and hospital electronic records. These databases include a small number of data points for an extremely large number of subjects. For example, the Medicare database includes financial data, disease codes (International Classification of Diseases, 9th revision [ICD-9]), and procedure codes (Current Procedural Terminology [CPT]) for each patient. It also includes information regarding location of care and provider type. The Medicare claims file is being extensively used to provide benchmarks for rates of mortality and major complications after coronary bypass surgery.[37] Hospitals can compare their rates with those of neighboring and competing hospitals and may use these data as markers for quality of hospital care.[38,39] Silber and colleagues[40] took an alternative approach to the use of Medicare databases and evaluated perioperative factors that influence failure to rescue. *Failure to rescue* is the concept whereby the actual rate of complications associated with death is studied rather than the overall death and complication rate.[40] The underlying assumption is that higher quality of care results in a lower rate of fatal outcomes, even among patients who sustain complications.

MORTALITY RELATED TO ANESTHESIA

The first report of the delivery of anesthesia (ether) for an operative procedure was in 1846. Only 2 years later, there was a report of a death attributable to anesthesia.[41] In that report, Hannah Greener died on induction with chloroform. Since that time, there have been numerous investigations into the cause of anesthesia-related death. The first formal investigation of anesthesia-related deaths was published by John Snow in 1858.[42] Snow analyzed 50 cases of death during chloroform anesthesia. At that time, mortality occurred principally in healthy patients undergoing minor procedures, suggesting that anesthesia was the principal cause of mortality. Subsequent studies reported deaths of patients with significant comorbidities undergoing major surgical procedures; in these cases, the cause of mortality was frequently multifactorial.

Surgery without Anesthesia

Surgical procedures were carried out before the introduction of anesthetics. The key to success was the speed of the procedure, with successful amputations lasting only 30 seconds. Strong assistants and restraints were frequently required. Alternatively, decreased cerebral perfusion by means of bilateral carotid compression was used to decrease sensation during the procedure. Surgical procedures were associated with significant risk of death and, at a minimum, were associated with severe pain. The development of anesthesia has been heralded as one of the great advances of modern medicine because it allowed surgery to advance.

Early Studies of Anesthesia-Related Mortality

One of the earliest systematic approaches to anesthesia-related risk[21,35,43-53] occurred in 1935, when Ruth[54] helped establish the first anesthesia study commission to analyze perioperative deaths. The commissioners relied on voluntary submission of cases and determined the cause of death by majority vote. Both of these methodologies were deemed inadequate in subsequent years (Table 24-3).

From a pragmatic standpoint, determining the cause of anesthesia-related mortality is important if information from the analysis can be used to improve subsequent care. This concept was best voiced by Sir Robert MacIntosh in 1948.[55] He stated that many anesthesia-related deaths were preventable and that improved education was the best means to avoid unnecessary mortality. He went so far as to suggest that all development of new drugs be halted for 5 years to direct more attention to training young anesthetists. He attempted to focus attention on postoperative care, suggesting that more deaths occurred after patients were returned to the ward than intraoperatively. His final comments were related to the need to establish a formal inquiry mechanism for determining the cause of any death, because such an analysis could lead to improved practice. In many ways, the CEPOD was the culmination of such a philosophy.[20]

A major advance in the analysis of anesthesia-related risk was the 1954 report by Beecher and Todd[21] of anesthesia-related deaths at 10 institutions. Their study included 599,548 anesthesia procedures. The cause of mortality was determined at the local institution by consensus of a surgeon and the chief anesthetist of the institution. Each death was characterized as having one primary cause and could have multiple secondary causes. The overall chance of mortality from any cause was 1 per 75 cases. Anesthesia was the primary cause of mortality in 1 of 2680 procedures, and it was a primary or contributory cause of mortality in 1 of 1560 procedures. Surgical error

Table 24–3   Estimates of the incidence of mortality related to anesthesia before 1980

Study	Year	Number of Anesthetics	Primary Cause	Primary and Associated Cause
Beecher and Todd[21]	1954	599,548	1:2680	1:1560
Dornette and Orth[43]	1956	63,105	1:2427	1:1343
Schapira et al.[44]	1960	22,177	1:1232	1:821
Phillips et al.[45]	1960	—	1:7692	1:2500
Dripps et al.[46]	1961	33,224	1:852	1:415
Clifton and Hotton[47]	1963	205,640	1:6048	1:3955
Memery[48]	1965	114,866	1:3145	1:1082
Gebbie[49]	1966	129,336	—	1:6158
Minuck[50]	1967	121,786	1:6766	1:3291
Marx et al.[35]	1973	34,145	—	1:1265
Bodlander[52]	1975	211,130	1:14,075	1:1703
Harrison[51]	1978	240,483	—	1:4537
Hovi-Viander[53]	1980	338,934	1:5059	1:1412

From Ross AF, Tinker JH: Anesthesia risk. In Miller RD (ed): Anesthesia, 3rd ed. New York, Churchill Livingstone, 1990.

in diagnosis, judgment, or technique was the primary cause of death in 1 of 420 cases, and patient disease was the primary cause in 1 of 95 cases. The authors placed these figures in the perspective of treating other causes of mortality:

> Data are present to show that death from anesthesia is of sufficient magnitude to constitute a public health problem. Anesthesia kills several times as many citizens each year out of the total population of the country as does poliomyelitis. Consideration of the millions of dollars rightly spent in attacking poliomyelitis and the next to nothing, comparatively, spent in anesthesia research makes clear an urgent need.

Dornette and Orth[43] reported on deaths occurring in the operating room at their institution during a 12-year period from 1943 through 1954. During this period, 95 patients died on the operating table, 12 patients suffered an intraoperative cardiac arrest and died postoperatively, and 1 patient died in the recovery room. This resulted in a total of 108 deaths in 63,105 anesthesia procedures. In 19 cases, the death was judged to be the result of the operation. In 13 patients, preexisting disease was judged to be the cause of death. The patient's condition plus the operation was a cause of death in 29 instances. Anesthesia was the primary cause of death in 26 cases (2 of which were the result of an overdose of local anesthetic administered by a surgeon) and a partial cause in an additional 21 patients. The rate of mortality totally attributable to anesthesia was 1 in 2427 cases, and the rate of mortality totally or partially attributable to anesthesia was 1 in 1343 cases.

Dripps and colleagues[46] at the University of Pennsylvania surveyed their experience during the 10-year period from 1947 through 1957. They identified 1285 operative deaths (i.e., death within 30 days) in approximately 120,000 anesthesia procedures, for a gross mortality rate of 1.1%. This definition includes late deaths, in contrast to many studies that have focused on the intraoperative period or the first 48 postoperative hours. After review of the hospital records, the investigators determined whether anesthesia was definitely or possibly contributory to each death. Among patients who underwent spinal anesthesia, mortality definitely related to anesthesia occurred in 1 of 1560 procedures, and mortality definitely or possibly related to anesthesia occurred in 1 of 780 procedures. Among those who underwent general anesthesia, mortality was definitely related to anesthesia in 1 of 536 cases and definitely or possibly related in 1 of 259 cases. Mortality was correlated with physical status with the use of the ASA Physical Status Classification scoring system. The higher mortality figures compared with other reports may be related to the higher physical acuity at this hospital. Importantly, deaths attributable to anesthesia did not occur among any of the 16,000 patients with ASA class I physical status.

Dripps and colleagues[46] compared their data with those of Beecher and Todd.[21] The principal intraoperative complications were hypotension and hypoxia. Virtually all patients who had spinal anesthesia had intraoperative complications, but postoperative complications were rare in this group. The investigators believed that anesthesia-related mortality had improved since the start of the study, mainly because of improvements in cardiac resuscitation, more rational transfusion therapy, standard use of recovery rooms, and efficient use of mechanical ventilators.

There were a number of reports from individual hospitals or a small group of hospitals during the subsequent 2 decades.[49] The Baltimore Anesthesia Study Committee[45] reviewed 1024 deaths occurring on the day of or the day after a surgical procedure to determine the potential contribution of anesthesia. This short period of observation (48 hours) contrasts with the 30-day period used by Dripps and coworkers.[46] For each case reviewed, the committee determined whether anesthesia was the principal cause or one of several contributing factors. In 196 cases (19.2%), the committee voted that anesthesia management contributed to the death of the patient. Anesthesia was the principal cause of death in approximately one third of cases (64 of 196), with one half of those being related to improper management of the anesthetic. The researchers estimated the rate of operative mortality rate as 4 in 10,000 operations using these data and applying rates of surgery from the National Health Survey. In more than 50% of all cases studied, death occurred in the patient's room, leading the investigators to emphasize the need for routine use of postanesthesia care areas. In an attempt to educate practitioners and prevent duplication of preventable causes of death, each of the perioperative deaths was discussed.

Schapira and coworkers[44] reported on mortality occurring within 24 hours after surgery between the years 1952 and 1956 at Montefiore Hospital in New York. They ascribed 27 deaths to anesthesia, including 18 in which anesthesia was a primary cause and 9 in which it was contributory. The overall prevalence of death partially or totally attributable to anesthesia was 1 in 1232 procedures.

Clifton and Hotton[47] reported 162 deaths associated with anesthesia in 205,640 operations performed at the Royal Prince Alfred Hospital in Sydney, Australia, between 1952 and 1962. They calculated that the incidence of mortality totally attributable to anesthesia was 1 in 3955, that attributable to surgery was 1 in 2311, and that attributable to patient disease was 1 in 1996 procedures. One cause of postoperative mortality was respiratory insufficiency. The researchers argued that many of these complications would have been prevented by the use of a recovery unit. The potential safety advantages of a postanesthesia care unit (PACU) constituted a general theme in reports from the 1960s.

Dinnick[56] reported 600 deaths associated with anesthesia as part of a series of investigations sponsored by the Association of Anaesthetists in London. This represents the second report from this group since a committee was established to collect clinical data in 1949. The first report included a review of 1000 fatalities and concluded that "in the majority of the reports there were departures from accepted practice." The initial report, published in 1956, found that regurgitation or vomiting was the main factor for death, whereas the second report, published in 1964, found that low blood volume was more important. Underventilation was the second most common finding, accounting for 25% of the cases.

Bodlander[52] provided a follow-up report of anesthesia-related mortality at the Royal Prince Alfred Hospital for the years 1963 to 1972. The incidence of mortality totally attributed to anesthesia decreased to 1 in 1702 cases, whereas anesthesia contributed to mortality in 1 in 502 cases, compared with 1 in 1208 for the years 1952 to 1962. The reduction in anesthesia-related deaths was attributed to an increase in the number of qualified staff and the degree of supervision.

Marx and colleagues[35] evaluated the incidence of death within 7 days after surgery among 34,145 consecutive patients at the Bronx Municipal Hospital Center between 1965 and 1969. A total of 645 patients died, and a death report form was constructed based on that developed by a committee of the New York Academy of Medicine. The deaths were then analyzed in relation to perioperative data available from a computer system. The patient's preexisting disease was considered to be the primary cause of death in 83% of cases, operation in 10%, and anesthesia in only 4% (1 of 1265 cases). Although mortality rose progressively with age, physical status correlated best with the incidence of mortality.

Marx and colleagues[35] also determined the relationship between type of anesthesia and mortality. Regional anesthesia was associated with the lowest incidence of death, local anesthesia with the highest; the incidence for general anesthesia was intermediate. Although this relationship was significantly different between groups, the difference appeared to be related to patient risk factors, a finding supported by a study by Cohen and colleagues.[51a]

Farrow and coworkers[57,58] studied hospital mortality after 108,878 anesthesia procedures in Cardiff, Wales, between 1972 and 1977. The crude mortality rate was 2.2 per 100 patients. Mortality was greatest among patients older than 65 years. The mortality rate also increased with the severity of disease and the need for emergent operations.

Harrison[51] evaluated mortality associated with 240,483 anesthesia procedures performed between 1967 and 1976 at Groote Schuur Hospital in Cape Town, South Africa. Data were collected prospectively, beginning in 1956. Anesthesia was the cause of death or major contributory factor in 0.22 cases per 1000 procedures, compared with 0.33 per 1000 operations in the previous 10 years. Anesthesia contributed to 2.2% of all of the deaths associated with surgery. The most common causes of anesthesia-related mortality, in order of frequency, were hypovolemia, respiratory inadequacy after neuromuscular blockade, complications of tracheal intubation, and inadequate postoperative care. Although the improvement in anesthesia-related mortality could not be directly attributed to specific improvements in care, four specific changes did occur: continuing improvement in routine monitoring, an increase in the ratio of consultants to registrars (British system residents), a decrease in the case load per anesthesiologist, and the introduction of recovery rooms and intensive care units (ICUs).

Studies before 1980 demonstrated steady improvements in anesthesia-related mortality. Studies performed throughout the world focused on identifying the causative factors for perioperative mortality. Several general themes emerged. Anesthesia represents a small but significant cause of perioperative mortality, perioperative respiratory complications represent a major complication, and elucidation of the causes of perioperative mortality and education about these causes should lead to improved outcomes.

Anesthesia-Related Mortality Studies after 1980

Whereas studies conducted before 1980 typically focused on one institution or a small group of institutions, studies since then have frequently been performed on a national basis. Improvements in anesthesia-related and overall mortality have made the analysis of a single institution inadequate because of the small sample size. For example, Holland[59] reported the deaths occurring within 24 hours after an anesthesia procedure in New South Wales, Australia. A committee of six anesthesiologists, three surgeons, an obstetrician, a general practitioner, and a medical administrator was established in 1960 and reviewed all such cases except during a 3-year period between mid-1980 and mid-1983. Four categories were established to define the relationship of anesthesia to operative morbidity and mortality (Table 24-4). Between 1960 and 1985, information was obtainable on 92% to 96% of all cases. Twenty-five percent of the 5262 deaths in that period were deemed attributable in whole or in part to the anesthesia procedure. The incidence of anesthesia-attributable deaths decreased from 1 in 5500 procedures performed in 1960 to 1 in 10,250 in 1970 and then to 1 in 26,000 in 1984 (Table 24-5). Based on these estimates, the investigators asserted that it was at least five times safer to undergo anesthesia in 1984 compared with 1960, particularly for healthy individuals. A subsequent follow-up report stated that factors under the control of the anesthesiologist caused or contributed to perioperative mortality at a rate of 1 in 20,000 operations.[60]

Table 24–4   Edwards classification of the relationship of anesthesia to operative morbidity and mortality*

Category	Definition
I	When it is reasonably certain that the event or death was caused by the anesthetic agent or technique of administration or in other ways coming directly within the anesthetist's province
II	Similar to type I cases, but ones in which there is some element of doubt about whether the agent or technique was entirely responsible for the result
III	Cases in which the patient's adverse event or death was caused by the anesthetic and the surgical technique
IV	Events entirely referable to surgical technique

From Holland R: Anaesthetic mortality in New South Wales. Br J Anaesth 59:834, 1987.

Table 24–5   Estimated risk of mortality in New South Wales, Australia

Year	No. of Deaths	Estimated Anesthetics	Deaths per Anesthesia
1960	55	300,000	1:5500
1970	39	400,000	1:10,250
1984	24	550,000	1:26,000

From Holland R: Anaesthetic mortality in New South Wales. Br J Anaesth 59:834, 1987.

Table 24–6   Incidence of complications partially or totally related to anesthesia

Complications	Partially Related	Totally Related	Total*
All complications	1:1887	1:1215	1:739
Death	1:3810	1:13,207	1:1957
Death and coma	1:3415	1:7924	1:2387

*Total number of anesthetics: 198,103.
From Tiret L, Desmonts JM, Hatton F, Vourc'h G: Complications associated with anaesthesia—A prospective survey in France. Can Anaesth Soc J 33:336-344, 1986.

The latter study demonstrated a preponderance of male over female patients (1.7:1). The reason for this finding is unclear, although it confirms other reports. Importantly, 64% of the deaths were deemed inevitable, suggesting that only one third were preventable.

The New South Wales Committee determined the primary error in management that led to each perioperative death. The most frequent primary cause was inadequate preparation of the patient, followed by a wrong choice of anesthetic drug. From the committee's standpoint, a wrong choice of agent included administering a renally excreted agent to a patient with chronic renal failure. The third most common error was inadequate crisis management during the initial decade of the study, but this cause was much less important during the period from 1983 through 1985. Inadequate postoperative management was the second most common cause of problems during the final years of the study.

The New South Wales study of anesthesia-related mortality evaluated the contribution of the anesthetist on perioperative mortality. Four groups of providers were identified: specialists, nonspecialists, CRNAs, and residents. The absolute number of anesthesia-related deaths decreased in all groups but was most pronounced for the nonspecialists. During the period from 1960 through 1969, the resident medical officer frequently provided anesthesia. During this same period, it was found that residents contributed significantly to the mortality observed among "good-risk" patients, which led to a phasing out of the resident medical officer as a member of the anesthesia work force.

Under the direction of the French Ministry of Health, Tiret and colleagues[61] carried out a prospective survey of complications associated with anesthesia in France between 1978 and 1982 from a representative sample of 198,103 anesthesia procedures chosen at random from hospitals throughout the country. The sample included a survey of 460 public and private hospitals. The investigators evaluated the occurrence of death or coma within 24 hours after surgery. The opinions of the participating anesthesiologist and that of the National Committee of Assessors were determined, and the latter was accepted if there was disagreement. In the group studied, 268 patients had major complications, 67 patients died, and 16 patients had persistent coma. Death was totally related to anesthesia for 1 in 13,207 procedures and partially related for 1 in 3810 (Table 24-6). Sixty-two percent of the coma cases were deemed totally attributable to

anesthesia, with the remainder being partially attributable to anesthesia. The French survey confirmed previous findings that major complications occurred more frequently in older patients, those undergoing emergency operations, and those with more extensive comorbidities as measured by the ASA physical status classification.

One of the most important findings of the survey was that postanesthesia respiratory depression was the largest cause of death and coma that were totally attributable to anesthesia (Table 24-7). Almost all of the patients who had respiratory depression leading to a major complication had received narcotics and muscle relaxants that had not been reversed. They also reported a high incidence of anaphylactoid shock, which the investigators contended was caused primarily by the use of Althesin and succinylcholine. There was no category of drug overdose, which might have been a more appropriate label for some of these cases.

The study by Tiret and colleagues[61] had the advantage of collecting data prospectively, allowing more accurate estimation of overall mortality than many of the other studies completed. A major limitation of the study was that only deaths occurring within 24 hours after surgery were included, ignoring late deaths that were the direct result of intraoperative complications.

Tikkanen and Hovi-Viander[62] studied death associated with anesthesia and surgery in Finland and compared the results in 1986 with those collected in 1975. Mortality related to anesthesia decreased during the 9-year period; the incidence of anesthesia-related mortality was 0.15 per 10,000 procedures in 1986.

Lunn and colleagues[63-65] published two reports on anesthesia-related surgical mortality in the United Kingdom. When a death occurred in a hospital within 6 days after surgery, a questionnaire was sent to the patient's anesthetist and surgeon. For 59.3% of the 4034 reported deaths, both the surgeon and the anesthetist returned the forms. The replies were reviewed anonymously by two assessors, and differences of opinion were determined by arbitration. After review, further details were obtained if the reply indicated that anesthesia was at least partly responsible for the death. The second report was based on an analysis of 197 reports of death within 6 days after anesthesia during 1981. In this report, 43% of the deaths were found by the assessors to have

Table 24–7   Causes of death or coma totally attributable to anesthesia in French survey

Problem	No. of Complications	No. of Deaths	No. of Comas
Equipment failure	5	1	1
Intubation complication	16	1	1
Aspiration gastric contents	27	4	2
Postoperative respiratory depression	28	7	5
Anaphylactoid shock	31	1	1
Cardiac arrest	17	1	—

From Tiret L, Desmonts JM, Hatton F, Vourc'h G: Complications associated with anaesthesia—A prospective survey in France. Can Anaesth Soc J 33:336-344, 1986.

nothing to do with anesthesia, 41% were partly attributable to anesthesia, and 16% were totally attributable to anesthesia. Of the 32 cases for which death was totally attributable to anesthesia, most were caused by faulty anesthesia technique or postoperative respiratory failure.

The pioneering work of Lunn and others led to the development of the CEPOD, which assessed almost 1 million cases of anesthesia during a 1-year period in 1987 in three large regions of the United Kingdom.[20,66] Unique to this study was the establishment of "crown privilege" by the government to allow total confidentiality:

The Secretary of State is satisfied that the disclosure of documents about individual cases prepared for the Enquiry into Perioperative Deaths would be against the public interest and would undermine the whole basis of a confidential study. The data or information sent to the Confidential Enquiry into Perioperative Deaths is therefore protected from subpoena...

Deaths occurring within 30 days after surgery were included in the study. There were 4034 deaths in an estimated 485,850 operations, resulting in a crude mortality rate of 0.7% to 0.8%. Surgery contributed totally or partially in 30% of all cases. Progression of the presenting disease contributed to death in 67.5% of the cases, and progress of an intercurrent disease was relevant in 44.3%. Anesthesia was considered the sole cause of death in only three individuals, for a rate of 1 in 185,000 cases, and anesthesia was contributory in 410 deaths, for a rate of 7 in 10,000 cases (Table 24-8).

There are several potential causes for the improvement in mortality between the CEPOD study and previous studies, including cases from the same group. One explanation is that improvement in care led to improvement in outcome. Many of the deaths that would previously have been classified as "anesthesia totally contributory" were later classified as "anesthesia partially contributory."

An important aspect of the CEPOD study was that it established anesthesia- and surgery-related factors that contributed to mortality. The five most common causes of death are shown in Table 24-9. Of the 410 perioperative deaths, there were 9 cases of aspiration or vomiting and 18 cases of cardiac arrest. A large proportion of elderly women had fractures of the femoral neck. The death rate was inversely related to the seniority of the operating surgeon and to preoperative preparation. The operating surgeon was a consultant in only 19% of the orthopedic cases, compared with 47% overall.

The CEPOD study also provided important information regarding anesthesia practice. Patients were seen preoperatively in more than 80% of the cases but postoperatively in less than 50%. Although the electrocardiogram was monitored in 97% of cases, core temperature was assessed in only 7%. Muscle relaxants were used in more than 50% of the cases, but a nerve stimulator was used in only 14%.

The assessors concluded that avoidable factors were present in about 20% of the perioperative deaths. Contributing factors for anesthesiologists and surgeons

Table 24–8   Death totally attributable to each component of risk in the Confidential Enquiry into Perioperative Deaths

Component	Mortality Rate Contribution
Patient	1:870
Operation	1:2860
Anesthetic	1:185,056

Adapted from Buck N, Devlin HB, Lunn JL: Report of a Confidential Enquiry into Perioperative Deaths, Nuffield Provincial Hospitals Trust. London, The King's Fund Publishing House, 1987.

Table 24–9   Most common clinical causes of death in the Confidential Enquiry into Perioperative Deaths

Cause of Death	Percent of Total
Bronchopneumonia	13.5
Congestive heart failure	10.8
Myocardial infarction	8.4
Pulmonary embolism	7.8
Respiratory failure	6.5

Adapted from Buck N, Devlin HB, Lunn JL: Report of a Confidential Enquiry into Perioperative Deaths, Nuffield Provincial Hospitals Trust. London, The King's Fund Publishing House, 1987.

tended to be failure to act appropriately with existing knowledge (rather than lack of knowledge), equipment malfunction, and fatigue. However, the researchers suggested that inadequate supervision was a problem and that no operation on a patient with an ASA physical status of class IV or V should be performed without direct consultation with the appropriate anesthesia or surgical authority (Table 24-10).

Several large national studies have been published since the CEPOD. Pedersen and colleagues[67] performed a series of studies in the late 1980s in Denmark to look at factors attributable to anesthesia that led to serious morbidity or mortality. They performed a prospective study of 7306 anesthesia procedures. In a method similar to that used in earlier studies, three anesthetists reviewed the records of complications and determined whether the cause was attributable to anesthesia (no distinction was made between totally and partially contributing factors). Complications attributable to anesthesia occurred in 43 patients (1 of 170), and 3 patients (1 of 2500) died. Complications in the 43 patients, in order of incidence, included cardiovascular collapse in 16 (37%), severe postoperative headache after regional anesthesia in 9 (21%), and awareness under anesthesia in 8 (19%). The researchers determined that 37% of the anesthesia-related morbidity was preventable. The three deaths occurred in severely ill patients (ASA physical status class III or greater), and two of these deaths were judged to be preventable.

Cohen and coworkers[51a] developed a methodology for studying anesthesia outcome in four teaching hospitals in Canada. They developed a new anesthesia record to serve as a data collection instrument. Research nurses reviewed all inpatient records within 72 hours after surgery, conducted interviews of the patients using a standardized instrument, and conducted a telephone survey of most of the outpatients. Assessment of the contribution of anesthesia to each complication was determined using the classification of the New South Wales Committee on Anaesthesia Mortality (see Table 24-4). In a total of 6914 anesthesia procedures in adults, there were no deaths directly attributable to anesthesia.

Lagasse[19] reviewed perioperative deaths (i.e., deaths occurring within 2 days after surgery) at a suburban university hospital network between 1992 and 1994 and an urban university hospital network between 1995 and 1999. There were a total of 347 deaths in 184,472 cases. Anesthesia-related mortality (i.e., death to which error by an anesthesia practitioner contributed) occurred in 1 of every 12,641 procedures in the suburban setting and in 1 of 13,322 procedures in the urban setting. Mortality increased with increasing ASA physical status (Fig. 24-2). In reviewing data over the previous decade, the investigators estimated that the anesthesia-related mortality rate had remained stable at approximately 1 death per 13,000 procedures, with wide variation making it impossible to detect trends in anesthesia safety.

Perioperative Mortality in Outpatient Surgery

Warner and colleagues[181] at the Mayo Clinic studied major morbidity and mortality occurring within 1 month after ambulatory surgery in 38,598 patients (see Chapter 68). Four patients died, two of myocardial infarction and two in an automobile accident (Fig. 24-3). The two deaths from myocardial infarction occurred at least 1 week after surgery and were not directly attributable to anesthesia. Considering the rate of mortality directly related to anesthesia described in the CEPOD study, no deaths would be expected in a study of this size.

Fleisher and colleagues[68] performed a claims analysis of patients undergoing 16 different surgical procedures in a nationally representative (5%) sample of Medicare beneficiaries for the years 1994 through 1999. A total of 564,267 procedures were studied, with 360,780 in an outpatient hospital, 175,288 in an ambulatory surgery center (ASC), and 28,199 in an office. On the day of surgery, no deaths occurred in the office, but 4 occurred in the ASC (2.3 per 100,000), and 9 occurred in the outpatient

Table 24–10 Grade of physician according to time of operation in the Confidential Enquiry into Perioperative Deaths

Grade	Anesthetist		Surgeon	
	Day*	Night†	Day*	Night†
Consultant	50	25	45	34
Others	50	75	55	66

*Day represents Monday through Friday, 9 AM to 7 PM.
†Night represents Monday through Friday, 7 PM to 9 AM, and Saturday and Sunday.
Adapted from Buck N, Devlin HB, Lunn JL: Report of a Confidential Enquiry into Perioperative Deaths, Nuffield Provincial Hospitals Trust. London, The King's Fund Publishing House, 1987.

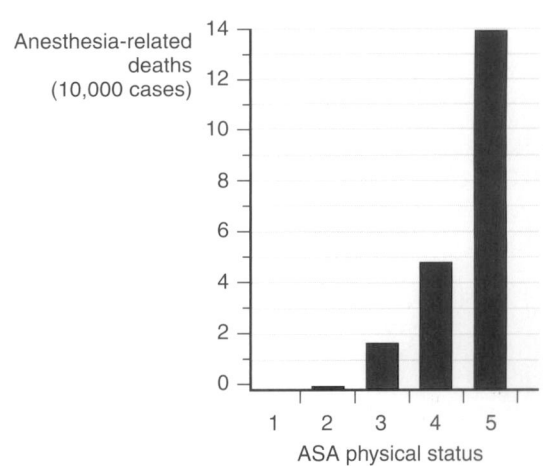

Figure 24–2 Relationship between the American Society of Anesthesiologists (ASA) physical status classification and perioperative mortality (within 2 days of surgery) related to anesthesia provided in urban and suburban institutions. (Adapted from Lagasse RS: Anesthesia safety: Model or myth? A review of the published literature and analysis of current original data. Anesthesiology 97:1609, 2002.)

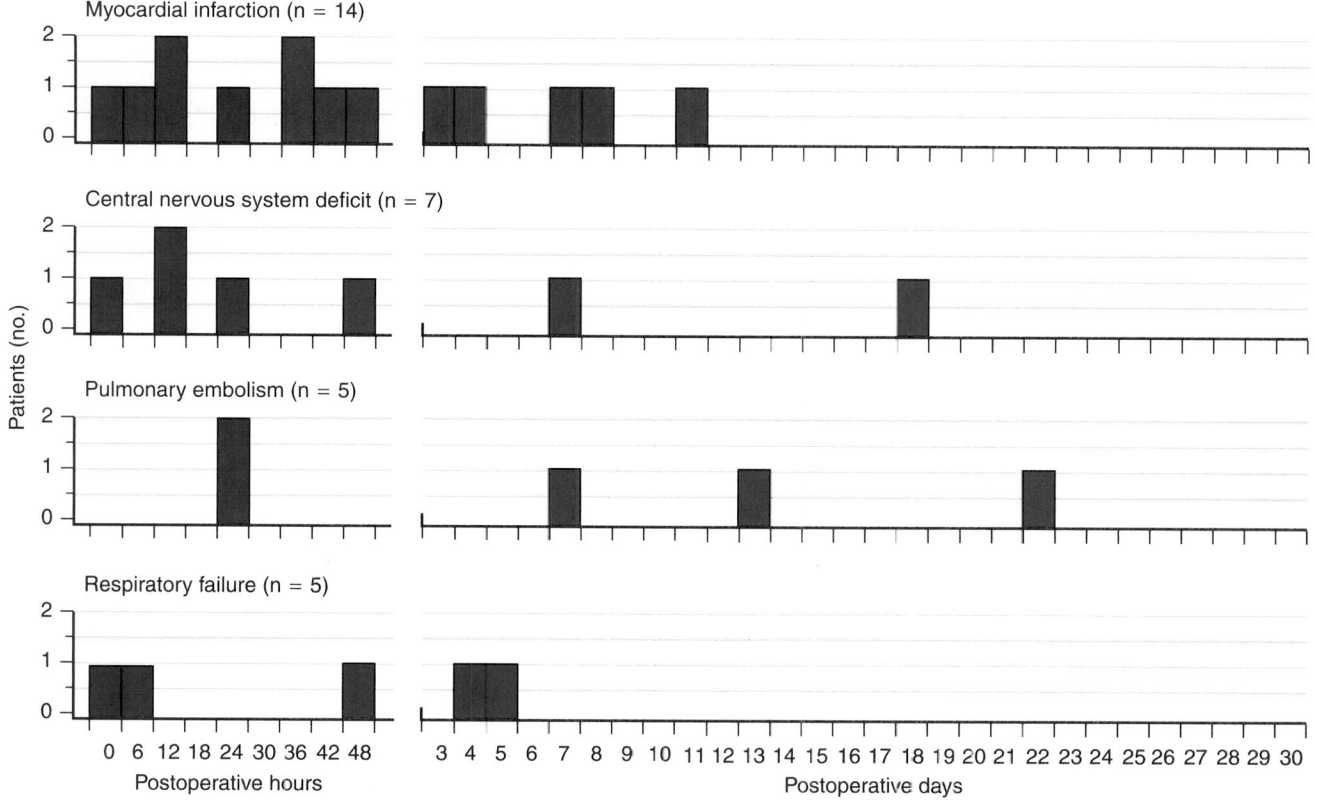

Figure 24–3 Timing of perioperative events in patients undergoing ambulatory surgery. Many of the events occur within the first 48 hours and probably are related to the stress of surgery. A subset of events occurring after this period may be related to background event rates. The overall rate of morbidity was lower than expected for a similar cohort of age-matched nonsurgical patients. (From Warner MA, Shields SE, Chute CG: Major morbidity and mortality within 1 month of ambulatory surgery and anesthesia. JAMA 270:1437, 1993.)

hospital (2.5 per 100,000). The 7-day mortality rate was 35 per 100,000 in the office setting, 25 per 100,000 in the ASC, and 50 per 100,000 in the outpatient hospital. The rate of admission to an inpatient hospital within 7 days was 9.08 per 1000 in the office, 8.41 per 1000 in the ASC, and 21 per 1000 in the outpatient hospital. This was one of the first attempts to assess the rates of mortality in a diverse group of outpatient surgery locations.

Analysis of Intraoperative Cardiac Arrests

Rather than studying perioperative mortality associated with anesthesia, several studies have evaluated intraoperative fatal and nonfatal cardiac arrests[22,69-77] (Table 24-11). In this situation, there are sufficient numbers of complications to perform an analysis at a single institution. Keenan and Boyan[78] studied the incidence and causes of cardiac arrest related to anesthesia at the Medical College of Virginia during a 15-year period. There were a total of 27 cardiac arrests during 163,240 procedures, for an incidence of 1.7 per 10,000 cases. Fourteen patients died, for an incidence of 0.9 per 10,000 cases. Pediatric patients had a threefold higher risk of arrest than adults did; emergency cases had a sixfold greater risk. Specific errors in anesthesia management could be identified in 75% of cases, most commonly inadequate ventilation and absolute overdose of an inhaled anesthetic. The time of

day did not appear to influence the rate of anesthesia-related cardiac arrest. From an educational perspective, the investigators identified progressive bradycardia preceding all but one arrest, suggesting that early identification and treatment may prevent complications.

Olsson and Hallen[79] studied the incidence of intraoperative cardiac arrests at the Karolinska Hospital in Stockholm, Sweden, from 1967 to 1984. A total of 170 arrests occurred in 250,543 anesthesia procedures performed. Sixty patients died, resulting in a mortality rate of 2.4 per 10,000 procedures. After elimination of cases of inevitable death (e.g., rupture of a cerebral aneurysm, trauma), the rate of mortality caused by anesthesia was 0.3 deaths per 10,000 procedures. The most common causes of anesthesia-related cardiac arrest were inadequate ventilation (27 patients), asystole after succinylcholine (23 patients), and postinduction hypotension (14 patients). The incidence of cardiac arrest increased with increasing severity of comorbid disease, as assessed by the ASA physical status classification. In evaluating the incidence of intraoperative cardiac arrest over time, there was a considerable decline between 1967 and 1984, coincident with the increased number of anesthesia specialists employed at the clinic.

Biboulet and colleagues[77] studied fatal and nonfatal cardiac arrests encountered during anesthesia and during the first 12 postoperative hours in the PACU or ICU in

Table 24–11   Cardiac arrest series when the denominator is more than 40,000 anesthetics

Study	Years	Total No. of Anesthetics	Rate of Arrest
Hanks and Papper[69]	1947-1950	49,728	1:2162
Ehrenhaft et al.[70]	1942-1951	71,000	1:2840
Bonica[71]	1945-1952	90,000	1:6000
Blades[72]	1948-1952	42,636	1:21,318
Hewlett et al.[73]	1950-1954	56,033	1:2061
Briggs et al.[74]	1945-1954	103,777	1:1038
Keenan and Boyan[78]	1969-1978	107,257	1:6704 (P)
Cohen et al.[76]	1975-1983	112,721	1:1427 (C)
Tiret et al.[61]	1978-1982	198,103	1:3358 (C)
Tiret et al.[61]	1978-1982	198,103	1:11,653 (P)
Keenan and Boyan[78]	1979-1988*	134,677	1:9620 (P)
Newland et al.[22]	1989-1999	72,959	1:14,493 (P)
Newland et al.[22]	1989-1999	72,959	1:7299 (C)

C, contributory cause; P, primary cause.
*Since pulse oximetry was introduced in 1984, no "preventable respiratory" cardiac arrests have occurred.
Adapted from Brown DL: Anesthesia risk: A historical perspective. *In* Brown DL (ed): Risk and Outcome in Anesthesia, 2nd ed. Philadelphia, JB Lippincott, 1992.

a single hospital in France. Eleven cardiac arrests related to anesthesia were identified among 101,769 anesthesia procedures (1.1 per 10,000). The mortality rate related to anesthesia was 0.6 per 10,000 cases. The major causes of death were anesthetic overdose, hypovolemia, and hypoxemia; 10 of the 11 cases had at least one human error, and all were classified as avoidable.

Newland and colleagues[22] reported anesthesia-related cardiac arrests from 72,959 procedures over a 10-year period in a teaching hospital in the United States. They judged that 15 cardiac arrests of a total of 144 were related to anesthesia (0.69 per 10,000 procedures), and in an additional 10 cases, anesthesia was considered contributory, for a total rate of 1.37 per 10,000 procedures (95% CI: 0.52-2.22). The risk of death related to anesthesia-attributable perioperative cardiac arrest was 0.55 per 10,000 procedures. Most of the arrests were related to medication administration, airway management, or technical problems of central venous access.

Cardiac arrests may be related to quality of care. The ability to resuscitate patients from an intraoperative cardiac arrest may reflect the skills of the care providers. Additional research is required to determine the validity of such an approach.

Use of Computer Analysis

Use of computer databases has enhanced the ability of investigators to identify perioperative complications. In one of the earliest computer analyses of postanesthesia deaths, Marx and colleagues[35] identified 645 individuals who died within 7 days after surgery from a total cohort of 34,145 consecutive surgical patients. The rate of mortality related to anesthesia was 1 in 1265 cases; in 1 in 1707 cases, death was related to postoperative management. The investigators deemed two thirds of all of the deaths to be preventable. Sanborn and colleagues[80] used a computer anesthesia record to identify intraoperative

incidents with high sensitivity and specificity. They were able to demonstrate that perioperative deaths occurred more frequently in patients who sustained an intraoperative incident than those who did not.

Other Approaches to Discern the Root Cause of Morbidity and Mortality

The accumulating data clearly demonstrate that risk directly attributable to anesthesia has declined over time. The cause for this reduction in mortality is unclear. Numerous factors have been implicated in the improved outcome, including new monitoring modalities, new anesthetic drugs, and changes in the anesthesia workforce. However, it is difficult to document reduced risk related to any one factor (issues related to manpower are addressed later). Although using newer monitoring modalities, particularly pulse oximetry, would be expected to improve outcomes, no randomized trial has been able to document such a conclusion.[81] This limitation supports the need for continued monitoring of complications and their root cause with studies such as the ACCS.

Studies similar to the CEPOD have not been performed in the United States, most likely because of the legal system, and information related to perioperative mortality must be obtained from other sources. The Professional Liability Committee of the ASA conducted a nationwide survey of closed insurance claims for major anesthesia mishaps. In the ACCS, fatal and nonfatal outcomes were reviewed. Among the fatal events, unexpected cardiac arrest during spinal anesthesia was observed in 14 healthy patients from the initial 900 claims.[82] The cases were analyzed in detail to identify patterns of management that might have led to the event. Two patterns were identified: oversedation leading to respiratory insufficiency and inappropriate resuscitation of high spinal sympathetic blockade.

Tinker and coworkers[83] queried the ACCS to determine the role of monitoring devices in the prevention of anesthesia mishaps. They reviewed 1097 anesthesia-related claims and determined that 31.5% of the negative outcomes could have been prevented by the use of additional monitors, primarily pulse oximetry and capnography. Injuries that were deemed preventable with additional monitoring resulted in dramatically more severe injury and cost of settlement than did those judged nonpreventable with additional monitoring. In almost 90% (305 of 346) of the preventable cases, at least one clinical sign of abnormality was identified by the existing monitors.

Caplan and colleagues[84] reviewed the ACCS for respiratory events (Table 24-12). These claims represented the single largest class of injury (34%), with death or brain damage occurring in 85% of cases. They identified inadequate ventilation, esophageal intubation, and difficult tracheal intubation as the primary causes of respiratory events. Most of the outcomes were thought by the investigators to be preventable with better monitoring (Fig. 24-4). Although no randomized trial has demonstrated the value of pulse oximetry or capnography, an analysis of claims supports the value of such monitoring. This analysis also formed part of the basis for the ASA Task Force on Management of the Difficult Airway guidelines and algorithm.[85]

Cooper and colleagues[86-89] approached the problem of sample size for determining perioperative morbidity by identifying "critical incidences," which were defined as those that were preventable but could lead to undesirable outcomes. This definition included events that led to no or only transient effects for the patient. The investigation involved collecting data on anesthesia-related human errors and equipment failures from anesthesiologists, residents, and nurse anesthetists. In a series of reports, the authors identified frequent incidences, such as disconnections in breathing circuits, and causes of discovery of errors, such as intraoperative relief. They confirmed that equipment failure was a small cause of anesthesia mishaps (4%), whereas human error was dominant. They suggested that future studies of anesthesia-related mortality and morbidity should classify events according to a strategy for prevention rather than outcome alone.

Buffington and coworkers[90] studied the ability of attendees of an anesthesia meeting to identify five faults intentionally created in a standard anesthesia machine. A survey was distributed, and the answer sheets were scored with respect to the number of correct answers. Only 3.4% of the respondents found all five faults. The average number of faults detected was 2.2. The professional background of the participants did not influence the ability to find the faults; distributions were similar between physicians and CRNAs. There was a small improvement in fault-finding ability among those with more than 10 years of experience. Studies such as these highlight the problem of the practitioner's ability to identify conditions that may lead to anesthesia mishaps. Whether improved technology or education can reduce some basal level of mishaps is unknown.

Issues Associated with Anesthesia-Related Mortality

Most of the studies have focused on in-hospital and short-term mortality, but perioperative complications may be the events that directly lead to death. For example, a perioperative stroke or myocardial infarction may lead to death after the period of analysis. Even small myocardial infarctions or unstable angina during the perioperative period has been associated with worse long-term survival in several studies.[2,91,92] Should these "late" deaths be attributed to anesthesia complications for the purpose of such analyses? Results from several studies add to the dilemma. For example, Mangano and colleagues[93] performed a randomized clinical trial in which 7 days of perioperative β-blockade was compared with placebo in high-risk patients undergoing noncardiac surgery. They reported significantly improved survival at 6 months, which remained significant during the 2 years of follow-up. In a subsequent report regarding this trial, Wallace and coworkers[94] demonstrated that the improved survival in the group receiving β-blockade was associated with a significantly lower incidence of perioperative myocardial ischemia but no difference in perioperative cardiac events. The authors of the original study suggested that atenolol resulted in better plaque stabilization during the perioperative period, resulting in improved long-term survival. If the hyperdynamic perioperative state is not well controlled, this theory suggests that more plaques become destabilized and progress to acute occlusion and sudden death. If atenolol is not used and patients die within 6 months of surgery, should this be attributed to an error in anesthesia and perioperative management? Part of the answer relies on the strength of this study to support the conclusion that routine use of atenolol does result in improved long-term survival. However, work by Poldermans and colleagues[3] demonstrated a reduction in perioperative morbidity and mortality in high-risk vascular patients given perioperative β-blockade, supporting its use in this subset of patients.

The potential effects of anesthesia on long-term survival were suggested in an abstract by Weldon and colleagues.[95] They demonstrated that deeper maintenance levels of anesthesia, as assessed by a bispectral index (BIS) monitor, were associated with higher 1-year postoperative

Table 24–12 Distribution of adverse respiratory events in the American Society of Anesthesiologists Closed Claims Study

Event	No. of Cases	Percent of 522 Respiratory Claims
Inadequate ventilation	196	38
Esophageal intubation	94	18
Difficult tracheal intubation	87	17
Inadequate inspired oxygen concentration	11	2

From Caplan RA, Ward RJ, Posner K, Cheney FW: Unexpected cardiac arrest during spinal anesthesia: A closed claims analysis of predisposing factors. Anesthesiology 68:5, 1988.

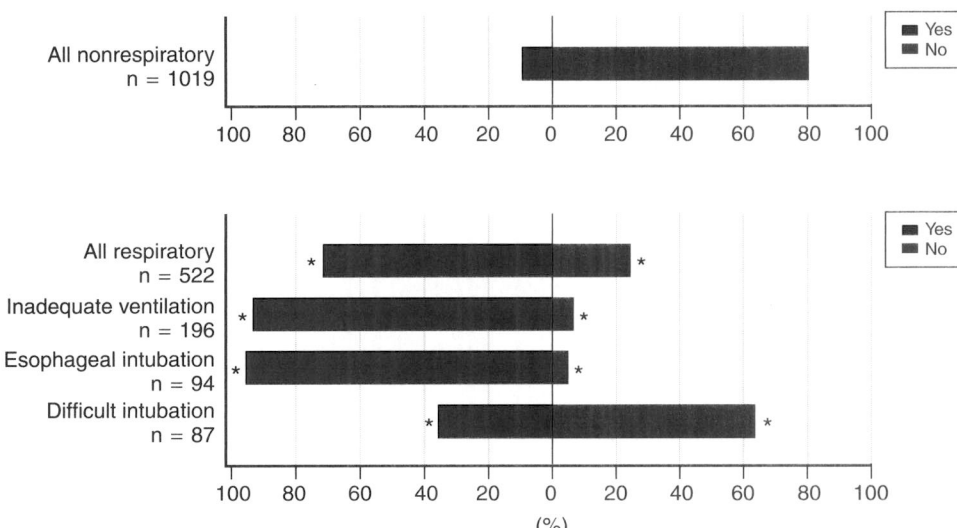

Figure 24–4 Relationship between adverse events in the American Society of Anesthesiologists (ASA) Closed Claims Study and preventable complications. Preventable events related to respiratory complications were significantly more common than those related to all nonrespiratory complications. Of the respiratory complications, difficult intubation had the least number of preventable complications (P < 0.05 compared with nonrespiratory claims). (From Caplan RA, Posner KL, Ward RJ, Cheney FW: Adverse respiratory events in anesthesia: A closed claims analysis. Anesthesiology 72:828, 1990.)

death rates for patients 40 years and older undergoing major, noncardiac surgery. Further work is required to determine whether these results reflect a true pathophysiologic link between perioperative management and long-term outcome or a simple statistical association.

RISKS RELATED TO THE PATIENT

Perioperative morbidity and mortality increase with increasing patient comorbidity. The original ASA physical status scoring system was proposed in 1941 and included six categories.[96] It was intended to standardize terminology and allow statistical analysis of outcomes between sites.[97] The original classification avoided the inclusion of surgical variables and was restricted to preoperative patient characteristics. It was revised in 1961 by Dripps and colleagues[46] to five categories, which were then adopted by the ASA.

The simplest example of such a relationship is the incidence of mortality correlated with ASA physical status. In their original study of perioperative mortality, Dripps and coworkers[46] demonstrated that mortality increased as severity of comorbid disease increased, as assessed by the ASA physical status classification. Several investigators have re-evaluated the relationship between operative mortality and ASA physical status classification. The studies by Pedersen[67] and Tiret[61] and their colleagues demonstrated such relationships. Vacanti and coworkers[98] also demonstrated the relationship between increasing mortality and decreasing physical status in 68,388 cases.

In Canada, Cohen and colleagues[51a] analyzed 100,000 anesthesia procedures and determined mortality within 7 days of operation using governmental vital statistics mortality data between the years 1975 and 1984. They established a computer database for each procedure that included age, preoperative conditions, ASA physical status, anesthesia technique, monitors, and other factors. The overall 7-day mortality rate was 71.04 deaths per 10,000 procedures. The mortality rate increased with advanced age, and it showed a marked increase among those older

than 80 years. Rates were low for normal, healthy individuals and for those undergoing minor procedures. The investigators developed a multiple logistic regression model to determine the independent predictors of mortality. Significant risk markers for increasing mortality were advanced age, male gender, increasing physical status score, major or intermediate surgery, emergency procedure, having a complication in the operating room, narcotic anesthesia techniques, and having received only one or two anesthetic drugs (Table 24-13).

In an attempt to look at each of the categories of contributing factors independently, Cohen's group[51a] constructed receiver-operator characteristic curves. There was no increment in prediction of mortality beyond that based on characteristics of the patient plus surgery. Plots including "other" or anesthesia-related factors showed almost complete overlap with curves including only patient- and surgery-specific factors.

One of the limitations of the ASA physical status classification is that ranking is a subjective measure conferred by the practitioner rather than an objective measure determined by the presence of specific disease states. Owens and coworkers[99] evaluated this hypothesis by asking 255 anesthesiologists to classify 10 hypothetical patients. In six of the cases, there was general agreement among the practitioners about classification of the patient; in the other four cases, there was divergence of opinion. The key finding of this study was that the ASA physical status classification is "useful but suffers from a lack of scientific precision."[99]

Rather than evaluating the risk of overall mortality, many studies have attempted to define the patient characteristics associated with morbidity and mortality related to a particular organ system. In evaluating the risk directly related to the patient's condition, it is important to understand the limitations of the methodology. All such studies evaluate the predictive value of a clinical or laboratory risk factor for a defined perioperative complication. In this approach, a cohort of individuals of interest is defined. In the optimal state, the study is performed prospectively, and the outcome of interest is assessed in a rigorous,

Table 24–13   Risk factors associated with increased odds of dying within 7 days for all cases

Variable	All Procedures: Relative Odds of Dying within 7 Days	95% Confidence Limits
Patient Related		
Age (yr)		
60-79/<60	2.32	1.70, 3.17
80+/<60	3.29	2.18, 4.96
Sex (F/M)	0.77	0.59, 1.00
Physical status score (3-5/1-2)	10.65	7.59, 14.85
Surgery Related		
Major/minor	3.82	2.50, 5.93
Intermediate/minor	1.76	1.24, 2.5
Length of anesthesia (≤2 hr/<2 hr)	1.08	0.77, 1.50
Emergency/elective	4.44	3.38, 5.83
Other Factors		
Year of operation (1975-1979/1980-1984)	1.75	1.32, 2.31
Had a complication in the operating or recovery room (yes/no)	1.42	1.06, 1.89
Anesthesia Related*		
Experience of anesthetist (>600 procedures for ≥8 yr/ <600 procedures for <8 yr)	1.06	0.82, 1.37
Inhalation with narcotic/inhalation alone	0.76	0.51, 1.15
Narcotic alone/inhalation alone	1.41	1.01, 2.00
Narcotic with inhalation/inhalation alone	0.79	0.47, 1.32
Spinal/inhalation alone	0.53	0.29, 0.98
No. of anesthetic drugs (1-2/3+)	2.94	2.20, 3.84

*All cases performed with the five most frequently used anesthetic techniques.
Adapted from Cohen MM, Duncan PG, Tate RB: Does anesthesia contribute to operative mortality? JAMA 260:2861, 1988.

blinded fashion. Unfortunately, many of the studies focus on selected patients and include a retrospective design, methods that greatly limit their generalizability and validity. For example, many studies evaluating risk factors in vascular surgery patients include only patients who are referred for diagnostic testing rather than a consecutive series of patients.

Many studies have adopted the approach of defining a cohort of individuals, determining their clinical and laboratory risk factors, and using multivariate modeling to determine the factors associated with increased risk. Frequently, perioperative risk is used to define intraoperative and postoperative complications. A major limitation in the use of multivariate modeling for this purpose is the assumption that the intraoperative period is a "black box" and that care is not modified by knowledge of the risk factor (Fig. 24-5). However, anesthesiologists do modify their intraoperative care of high-risk patients in an attempt to reduce the risk. Changes in medical care over time and better knowledge about high-risk patients should result in reduction of risk related to specified clinical factors. For this reason, many of the indices developed previously may no longer have clinical validity.

In designing a multivariate risk index for perioperative morbidity and mortality, only factors that are included in the analysis and in the patient population of interest can be included in the final model. For example, if the

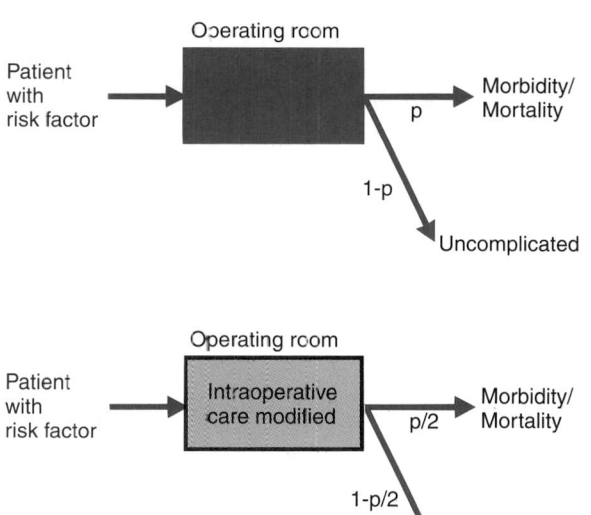

Figure 24–5 The concept of the *black box* for risk indices. In developing a risk index, patients with a specific risk factor enter the operating room and have a complication at a rate *p*. If the anesthesiologist is aware of the importance of the risk factor and can modify care to reduce such risk (*p/2*), the risk factor may no longer be significant. If the risk factor is ignored, complications may again occur in such patients.

population studied represents a unique referral bias, some risk factors may be overrepresented, and others may not be present in sufficient quantity to study. An example is unstable angina in the original Cardiac Risk Index developed by Goldman and colleagues.[13] Because patients with unstable angina present only for emergency surgery, that risk factor is rarely represented in many indices.

There are numerous specific disease states that increase perioperative risk. Cardiovascular disease is the most extensively studied, with the goal of identifying patients at greatest risk for fatal and nonfatal myocardial infarction. One of the earliest attempts to define cardiac risk was performed by Goldman and colleagues[13] at the Massachusetts General Hospital. They studied 1001 patients older than 45 years who were undergoing noncardiac surgery, excluding patients who underwent transurethral resection of the prostate under spinal anesthesia. Using multivariate logistic regression, they demonstrated nine clinical factors associated with increased morbidity and mortality. Each of these risk factors was associated with a given weight in the logistic regression equation, which was converted into points in the index. An increasing number of points was associated with increasing perioperative cardiac morbidity or mortality.

There have been several attempts to validate the Goldman Cardiac Risk Index. Zeldin[100] prospectively determined the Cardiac Risk Index for 1140 surgical patients and reported that the overall accuracy of the index was as high as in the original study, although the rate of complications in the highest-risk group was less than originally reported. Larsen and coworkers[101] also found that the Cardiac Risk Index demonstrated good accuracy in 2609 consecutive unselected patients older than 40 years. Domaingue and colleagues[102] studied patients undergoing various vascular surgery procedures and reported a higher probability of major cardiac complications than that reported by Goldman and coworkers[13]; however, they also demonstrated a higher rate of complications with increasing cardiac risk class. The validity of the Cardiac Risk Index is more controversial for vascular surgery patients. Jeffrey and colleagues[103] evaluated the rate of cardiac complications in 99 patients undergoing elective abdominal aortic surgery and demonstrated a similar pattern of increased overall complication rates with increasing cardiac risk. A higher percentage (7%) of patients in the lowest category in their study sustained a cardiac complication. White and colleagues[104] demonstrated the value of the Goldman Cardiac Risk Index for long-term survival after vascular surgery. Several other studies were unable to demonstrate any relationship between the Cardiac Risk Index and perioperative cardiac complications, with a high incidence of complications found in patients with a Cardiac Risk Index of I or II.[105,106] When the ASA physical status classification was compared with the Goldman Cardiac Risk Index in a cohort of 16,277 patients undergoing noncardiac surgery,[107] both indices demonstrated predictive value, although the objective Goldman Cardiac Risk Index had little increased value over the more subjective ASA physical status classification.

Other investigators have attempted to develop risk indices. Detsky and coworkers[108] studied a cohort of individuals who were referred to an internal medicine service for preoperative evaluation. Many of the factors identified by Goldman[13] were confirmed or slightly modified in the Detsky index, and angina was added to the risk factors. The researchers advocated the calculation of a pretest probability of complication based on the type of surgery, after which the Detsky Modified Risk Index is applied with the use of a nomogram. In this manner, the overall probability of complications can be determined as a function of the surgical procedure and of patient disease. The Detsky index was advocated as the starting point for risk stratification in the American College of Physicians Guideline on preoperative evaluation.[109] In an attempt to update the original index, Lee and colleagues[110] at the Brigham and Women's Hospital studied 4315 patients 50 years or older who were undergoing elective major noncardiac procedures in a tertiary-care teaching hospital. Six independent predictors of complications were identified and included in a Revised Cardiac Risk Index: high-risk type of surgery, history of ischemic heart disease, history of congestive heart failure, history of cerebrovascular disease, preoperative treatment with insulin, and preoperative serum creatinine level higher than 2.0 mg/dL. The rate of major cardiac complications increased with the number of risk factors.

Numerous risk indices developed for cardiac surgery have been developed.[111-116] The goal has been to identify patients who are at greatest risk for adverse perioperative outcomes, not specifically anesthesia-related risk. Many of these indices focus on anatomic considerations for perioperative risk. They are extremely useful in risk adjustment to assess rates of mortality. For example, the State of New York annually publishes data on mortality rates associated with coronary bypass grafting by surgeon and by hospital.[117-119] For comparison of rates across institutions, risk figures must be adjusted so that institutions that perform predominantly high-risk surgery are not penalized.

Patients undergoing vascular surgery represent a cohort with very high perioperative complication rates.[120] Clinical risk indices and noninvasive diagnostic testing have been used to identify patients with the highest rates of perioperative mortality and major morbidity. Numerous studies demonstrated that the presence of a reversible defect on thallium imaging and new regional wall motion abnormalities on dobutamine echocardiography predicts those with a high perioperative risk.[121-130] As use of these technologies spread, the tests lost much of their predictive value because they were used in lower-risk patients.[131,132] Subsequent studies demonstrated that the tests should be applied only to patients who are at moderate or high risk and identified a group of clinical characteristics that define the group for whom the test can have optimal predictive characteristics. Eagle and colleagues[133] determined the value of clinical risk factors for predicting perioperative cardiac events and the additive value of noninvasive testing based on the preoperative risk profile. Five clinical predictors were identified: age older than 70 years, diabetes mellitus, angina, ventricular ectopic activity being treated, and Q waves on an electrocardiogram. Among patients undergoing major vascular surgery, an increasing number of clinical variables was associated with an increasing perioperative risk. The presence of thallium redistribution after dipyridamole infusion further identified a high-risk cohort among patients with one or two clinical risk factors. A subsequent multi-institutional report used a Bayesian approach to define the additive value of these risk factors and thallium markers to identify patients at high risk for complications.[134]

Vanzetto and coworkers[135] performed a prospective evaluation in which an expanded number of clinical variables was identified in a cohort of patients undergoing major vascular surgery. Cardiovascular morbidity and mortality was determined prospectively in this population. An increasing number of clinical variables was associated with increasing perioperative risk. Most importantly, dipyridamole thallium imaging was performed only in the subset of patients with two or more clinical variables, and the results of the test were not made available to the clinicians caring for the patients. In this well-performed study, the presence of thallium redistribution identified a cohort with an incrementally greater perioperative risk compared with those with negative scan results and a similar number of clinical variables.

Similar to the work with dipyridamole thallium imaging, dobutamine stress echocardiography can be further quantified. The presence of wall motion abnormalities at a slow heart rate is the best predictor of increased perioperative risk; large areas of defect are of secondary importance.[130] Boersma and colleagues[136] assessed the value of dobutamine stress echocardiography with respect to the extent of wall motion abnormalities and use of β-adrenergic blockers during surgery (see Chapter 27). They assigned one point for each of the following characteristics: age older than 70 years, current angina, myocardial infarction, congestive heart failure, prior cerebrovascular accident, diabetes mellitus, and renal failure. As the total of number of clinical risk factors increases, perioperative cardiac event rates also increase. Dobutamine stress echocardiography was performed only for patients with a significant number of risk factors, and patients who demonstrated new wall motion abnormalities had higher event rates than those with the same clinical risk score but without new wall motion abnormalities.

As part of their study of anesthesia-related mortality, Pedersen and colleagues[67] evaluated the occurrence of cardiovascular and pulmonary complications. For a total of 7306 anesthesia procedures, they reported a 6.3% incidence of intraoperative or postoperative cardiovascular complications and a 4.8% incidence of intraoperative or postoperative pulmonary complications. Acute myocardial infarction occurred in 0.16% of the patients. The investigators evaluated a number of characteristics, including gender, age, presence of ischemic heart disease, duration of anesthesia, and type of surgery, and assessed their relationship to cardiovascular and pulmonary complications and overall mortality in the hospital (Table 24-14). Cardiopulmonary complications were associated with advanced age (>70 years), preoperative signs of ischemic heart disease with recent myocardial infarction, chronic heart failure, chronic lung disease, and abdominal surgery, particularly of an emergency nature. They observed

that the use of pancuronium was associated with worse perioperative outcome, a finding reminiscent of the curare-related deaths of the 1940s and 1950s.

Numerous studies have evaluated the importance of single variables such as hypertension on perioperative risk. Goldman and Caldera[137] evaluated a cohort of patients undergoing noncardiac surgery with general anesthesia. Hypertension did not denote a group with increased perioperative risk, although the number of patients with diastolic blood pressure greater than 110 mm Hg was insufficient to draw any conclusions. This study highlighted the problems related to generalization of results, because many subsequent researchers have suggested that surgery be delayed for patients with a diastolic blood pressure greater than 110 mm Hg. In one of the few studies to demonstrate a relationship, Hollenberg and coworkers[138] identified hypertension and the presence of left ventricular hypertrophy as predictors of perioperative ischemia, but they did not consider their independent relationship with perioperative major morbidity.

Examples of a prospective cohort study to identify the risk of a particular clinical factor include studies of the rate of perioperative reinfarction in patients who sustained a previous myocardial infarction. Traditionally, risk assessment for noncardiac surgery was based on the time interval between the myocardial infarction and surgery. Multiple studies have demonstrated an increased incidence of reinfarction if the myocardial infarction occurred within 6 months of surgery.[14-16] With improvements in perioperative care, this difference has decreased.

The previous example of assessing risk illustrates the issue of changes in management over time. The importance of the intervening time interval may no longer be valid in the current era of thrombolytics, angioplasty, and risk stratification after acute myocardial infarction. Although many patients with myocardial infarction continue to have myocardium at risk for subsequent ischemia and infarction, in others, the critical area of coronary stenosis is totally occluded or widely patent. For example, the use of percutaneous transluminal coronary angioplasty (PTCA) is associated with a reduced incidence of death or reinfarction within 6 months.[139] Patients should be evaluated from the perspective of their risk for ongoing ischemia. In their guidelines for perioperative evaluation of noncardiac surgery, the American Heart Association/American College of Cardiology Task Force on Assessment of Diagnostic and Therapeutic Cardiovascular Procedures [140] proposed that patients who have had a myocardial infarction within less than 30 days should be considered the group at highest risk; after that period, risk stratification is based on disease severity and exercise tolerance.

SPECIAL PATIENT GROUPS

Obstetrics

Maternal mortality is rare, and the anesthesia-related component of maternal delivery represents only a small fraction of all maternal deaths, making the study of this

Table 24–14   Factors associated with increased perioperative complications

Risk Factors	No. of Anesthetics (n = 7306)*	Cardiovascular Complications %	(odds ratio)	Pulmonary Complications %	(odds ratio)	Mortality in Hospital %	(odds ratio)
Sex							
Female	4587	4.9		3.7		0.7	
Male	2634	8.8[†]	(1.8)	6.6[†]	(1.8)	2.2[†]	(3.2)
Age (yr)							
<50	3965	2.6		2.3		0.3	
50-90	2043	8.2		6.7		1.8	
70-79	886	14.3[†]		8.9		2.9[†]	
≥80	293	16.7[†]		10.2[†]		5.8[†]	
Ischemic heart disease	103	29.1[†]	(6.5)	8.7	(1.9)	2.9	(2.5)
Myocardial infarction							
>1 yr	125	20.8[†]		7.7		4.0[†]	
≤1 yr	26	38.5[†]		10.4[†]		7.7[†]	
Chronic heart failure	199	35.2[†]		15.1[†]	(3.8)	9.0[†]	(9.9)
Hypertension	380	11.8[†]	(2.1)	7.1[†]	(1.6)	1.3	(1.1)
Hypertension (SBP ≤90 mm Hg)	127	16.5[†]	(2.5)	17.3[†]	(4.0)	9.4[†]	(9.8)
Chronic obstructive lung disease	201	12.4[†]	(2.1)	12.4	(3.0)	5.0[†]	(4.7)
Renal failure	153	14.4[†]	(2.2)	11.8[†]	(2.4)	5.9[†]	(5.2)
Diabetes mellitus	141	9.2	(1.5)	7.1	(1.5)	2.1[†]	(1.8)
Neurologic disease	34	5.9	(1.0)	8.8[†]	(1.9)	2.9	(2.4)
Cancer	1257	7.0	(1.1)	5.5	(1.2)	1.1	(1.0)
Cancer (abdominal)	242	19.8[†]	(3.2)	19.4[†]	(4.3)	5.0[†]	(5.4)
Emergency surgery	2454	7.4[†]	(1.3)	6.3[†]	(3.0)	2.8[†]	(3.2)
Duration of anesthesia (min)							
<30	1774	1.2		0.6		0.1	
30-179	4621	6.8		4.5		1.3	
180-299	470	17.9[†]		13.4[†]		3.2[†]	
≥300	162	20.4[†]		30.2[†]		4.9[†]	
Minor surgery	4916	3.2		1.8		0.3	
Major surgery	2113	13.0[†]	(4.1)	10.6	(5.8)	3.1[†]	(4.9)
Total		6.3		4.8		1.2	

*The analysis shows the maximum number of patients in the various groups.
[†]P < .05 indicates a statistically significant higher rate of complications and mortality compared with the rest of the total incidence.
SBP, systolic blood pressure.
From Pedersen T: Complications and death following anaesthesia: A prospective study with special reference to the influence of patient-, anaesthesia-, and surgery-related risk factors. Dan Med Bull 41:319, 1994.

problem difficult or impossible in any one institution (see Chapter 58). A series of studies was performed between 1974 and 1985 to determine the rate of complications in the United States and England. One of the first reports was for the period of 1974 to 1978. Kaunitz and colleagues[141] reported an anesthesia-related death rate of 0.6 per 100,000 births using data from all 50 states. Endler and coworkers[142] studied births in Michigan between 1972 and 1984 and reported 15 maternal deaths in which anesthesia was the primary cause and 4 deaths in which anesthesia was contributory. This resulted in a rate of 0.82 anesthesia-related deaths per 100,000 live births. Eleven of the 15 deaths were associated with cesarean section. Obesity and emergency surgery were risk factors in many patients. Complications related to regional anesthesia were problems during the early part of the study, whereas failure to secure a patent airway was the primary cause of mortality in later years. There were no anesthesia-related maternal deaths in the final 2 years of the study. The incidence of anesthesia-related death was markedly higher among black women, which the investigators suggested might have been related to an inability to detect cyanosis. Rochat and colleagues[143] studied 19 areas of the United States between 1980 and 1985 and reported 0.98 anesthesia-related deaths per 100,000 live births. They observed that maternal mortality did not decrease over the time of the study.

The Confidential Enquiry into Maternal Deaths in England and Wales has been assessing maternal deaths since 1952.[144] Records of all maternal deaths are sent to a district medical officer, who sends an inquiry form to all health practitioners involved in the care of those patients. These forms are evaluated by a senior obstetrician and an anesthesia assessor. Morgan[144] reported the maternal deaths from anesthesia between 1952 and 1981 (Table 24-15). The total maternal mortality rate decreased

Table 24–15 Maternal mortality figures obtained from the Confidential Enquiry into Maternal Deaths in England and Wales

Years	Maternal Mortality per 1000 Total Births	Number of Deaths from Anesthesia	Percentage of True Maternal Deaths from Anesthesia	Percentage with Avoidable Factors*
1952-1954	0.53	49	4.5	—
1955-1957	0.43	31	3.6	77
1958-1960	0.33	30	4.0	80
1961-1963	0.26	28	4.0	50
1964-1966	0.20	50	8.7	48
1967-1969	0.16	50	10.9	68
1970-1972	0.13	37	10.4	76
1973-1975	0.11	31	13.2	90
1976-1978	0.11	30	13.2	93
1979-1981	0.11	22	12.2	100

From Morgan M: Anaesthetic contribution to maternal mortality. Br J Anaesth 59:842, 1987.

over time, and the percentage of deaths related to anesthesia increased, although the absolute number of deaths from anesthesia decreased. During the early years of the study, endotracheal intubation was rarely performed during obstetric anesthesia. Later reports advocated the use of endotracheal intubation after thiopentone-suxamethonium, and technical difficulties with intubation were identified. The other major finding of this study was that the experience of the anesthetist in obstetric anesthesia was the most important factor in anesthesia-related maternal mortality.

Several studies have attempted to define the cause of anesthesia-related maternal deaths. Insights into the cause of maternal mortality can also be elicited from the ACCS. In 1991, Chadwick and colleagues[145] published a report of closed malpractice claims related to 190 obstetric cases, representing 127 cesarean sections and 63 vaginal deliveries. The most frequent complications were maternal death and brain damage in the newborn. There were 15 maternal deaths among patients who had regional anesthesia and 26 among patients who had general anesthesia. Because the absolute number of patients who underwent each type of anesthesia was unknown, the risk attributable to

anesthesia could not be determined, unlike the subsequent report from Hawkins and coworkers.[148]

Hawkins and coworkers[148] obtained data from the ongoing National Pregnancy Mortality Surveillance System of the Centers for Disease Control and Prevention (CDC). Using state data on births and fetal deaths from 1979 through 1990, three obstetric anesthesiologists reviewed the records to determine the possible risk related to anesthesia. A total of 129 women died of anesthesia-related causes during the study period, most (82%) during cesarean section, and the incidence decreased over time (Table 24-16). The decreased mortality rate appeared to be related to increased use of regional anesthesia. The primary cause of mortality was related to the type of anesthesia. For general anesthesia, 73% of the deaths were related to airway problems. Unlike the Confidential Enquiry into Maternal Deaths in England, the United States study lacked the extensive detail for each event, and the absolute cause of mortality therefore remained somewhat in doubt. In particular, the researchers acknowledge that general anesthesia may be used more often for patients with a higher acuity of disease, which may account for the higher mortality rate

Table 24–16 Numbers, case-fatality rates, and risk ratios of anesthesia-related deaths during cesarean section delivery by type of anesthesia in the United States, 1979-1984 and 1985-1990

Population	Number of Deaths		Case-Fatality Rate		Risk Ratio	
	1979-1984	1985-1990	1979-1984	1985-1990	1979-1984	1985-1990
General	33	32	20.0* (95% CI 17.7,22.7)	32.3* (95% CI 25.9,49.3)	2.3 (95% CI 1.9,2.9)	16.7 (95% CI 12.9, 21.8)
Regional	19	9	8.6† (95% CI 1.8,9.4)	1.9† (95% CI 1.8,2.0)	Referent	Referent

*Per million general anesthetics for cesarean section.
†Per million regional anesthetics for cesarean section.
CI, confidence interval.
Adapted from Hawkins JL, Gibbs CP, Orleans M, et al: Obstetric anesthesia work force survey, 1981 versus 1992. Anesthesiology 87:135, 1997.

associated with its use. The availability of national databases should allow accurate tracking of mortality to ensure that appropriate quality-assurance and quality-improvement systems are in place.

Panchal and colleagues[146] conducted a retrospective case-control study using patients' records from a state-maintained anonymous database of all nonfederal Maryland hospitals that performed deliveries between 1984 and 1997 (Fig. 24-6). Variables studied included patient demographics and ICD-9 (Clinical Modification) diagnosis and procedure codes. Of the 822,591 hospital admissions for delivery during the 14-year study period, there were 135 maternal deaths. The most common diagnoses associated with mortality during hospital admission for delivery were preeclampsia or eclampsia (22.2%); postpartum hemorrhage or obstetric shock (22.2%); pulmonary complications (14%); blood clot or amniotic embolism, or both (8.1%); and anesthesia-related complications (5.2%).

Gibbs and coworkers[147] surveyed 1200 hospitals in 1981 and sent questionnaires to the chiefs of anesthesia and obstetrics. Anesthesiologists were available for obstetric anesthesia in only 21% of all hospitals and at night and on the weekends in only 15%. Hospitals with fewer than 500 deliveries per year had the most striking deficiencies in anesthesia personnel. Even for cases in which general anesthesia was provided for cesarean section, an anesthesiologist was involved in the care only 44% of the time, whereas hospitals with greater than 1500 deliveries per year had an anesthesiologist present 85% of the time. The researchers did not evaluate the relationship between outcome and staffing models. The survey was performed again in 1992.[148] Compared with 1981, the researchers found a marked increase in the availability of labor analgesia and a decrease in the use of general anesthesia. In more than one half of the anesthesia procedures for cesarean section, care was provided by nurse anesthetists without medical direction by an anesthesiologist. How these trends in staffing have affected maternal mortality requires further evaluation.

Pediatrics

There are few studies of anesthesia-related risk in the pediatric population (see Chapter 60). Two themes emerge from these studies: Very young infants are at increased risk, and anesthesia-related risk is reduced in centers with specialized pediatric anesthesia facilities. In the report by Beecher and Todd,[21] there was a "disproportionate number" of anesthesia-related deaths of children younger than 10 years.

Graff and colleagues[149] from the Baltimore Anesthesia Study Committee reported 335 operative deaths in the pediatric age group. Of these, 58 were thought to be primarily or partially attributable to anesthesia. The percentage of operative deaths attributable to anesthesia was relatively constant among age groups at 16.6% to 21.7%. The estimated anesthesia-associated mortality rate was 3.3 deaths per 10,000 operations for those younger than 15 years, compared with 0.6 for those between 15 and 24 years old and 11.7 for those older than 64 years. More than one half of the patients were categorized as ASA physical status class I or II, suggesting that most deaths occurred in children with good anesthesia risk. Most deaths occurred during tonsillectomy, which probably reflects the fact that tonsillectomy is the most common operation in this age group. The investigators attempted to determine the phase of the operation that was associated with highest risk. Improper management of the anesthetic accounted for approximately one half of the cases. Respiratory complications (e.g., underventilation, aspiration of vomitus or blood) were apparent in 82% of the anesthesia-related deaths. The investigators suggested that female patients are at a better operative risk than male patients in all age groups.

Tiret and colleagues[150] published a study of pediatric anesthesia risk in 1988. They prospectively studied major anesthesia-related complications in pediatric patients in 440 hospitals in France between 1978 and 1982. There were 27 major complications in 40,240 cases, which included 12 cardiac arrests and 1 death. The incidence of major complications and that of cardiac arrests were

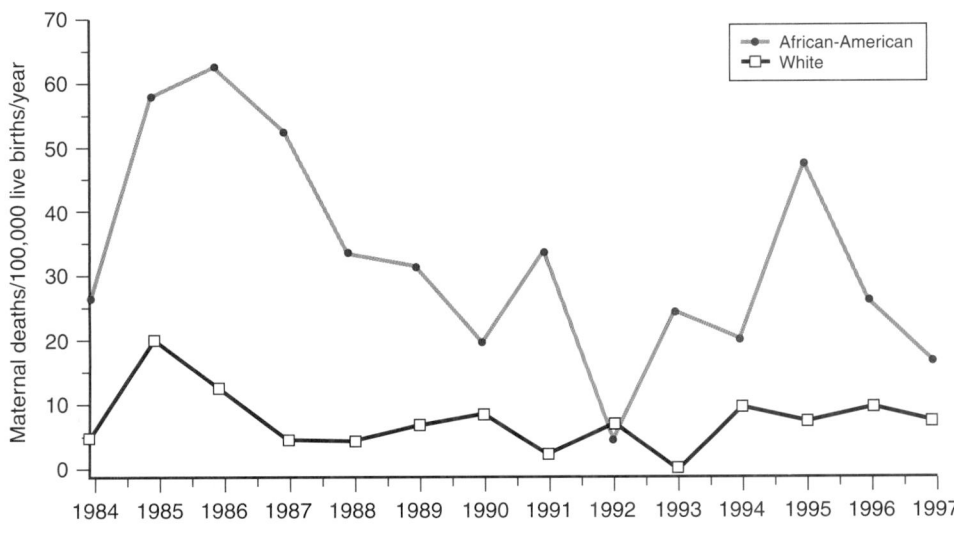

Figure 24–6 Delivery mortality ratios by race in Maryland, from 1984 to 1997, using discharge summaries. (From Panchal S, Arria AM, Labhsetwar SA: Maternal mortality during hospital admission for delivery: A retrospective analysis using a state-maintained database. Anesth Analg 93:134, 2001.)

Table 24-17 Incidence of complications per 1000 anesthetics for infants and children compared with results for adults

	All Complications	Cardiac Arrests	Deaths
Infants <1 yr	4.3*	1.9	ns
Children 1-14 yr	0.5	0.2	0.03
Total 0-14 yr	0.7*	0.3	0.02*
Adults ≥15 yr	1.5	0.7	0.4

*$P < .001$; ns = not significant.
From Tiret L, Desmonts JM, Hatton F, Vourc'h G: Complications associated with anaesthesia—A prospective survey in France. Can Anaesth Soc J 33:336, 1986.

significantly higher for infants than for older children. The rate of cardiac arrests related to anesthesia was highest among infants (19 per 10,000) and lowest among children (2.1 per 10,000) (Table 24-17). Most complications in infants involved the respiratory system, predominantly airway problems and aspiration. Older children experienced respiratory and cardiac complications, which occurred most frequently during induction and recovery.

Cohen and colleagues[151] studied 29,220 anesthesia procedures at the Winnipeg Children's Hospital. Data were collected from mid-1982 to 1987 and stored in a databank. Data on patients' coexisting medical conditions and postoperative follow-up were obtained within 72 hours. Complications included death, cardiac arrest, drug incident, airway obstruction, and minor complications such

as nausea and vomiting, arrhythmias, and sore throat. Neonates underwent a higher percentage of major vascular or cardiac and intra-abdominal procedures, and older children had a higher incidence of extremity procedures. Intraoperative cardiac arrest occurred most frequently in patients younger than 1 year of age (4 in 2901 procedures) compared with older children. Postoperatively, minor events such as nausea and vomiting were more common in older children, whereas respiratory events were more common in infants and younger children (Table 24-18). Compared with adult patients, children experienced different complications, which frequently extended well into the postoperative period. In a comparison of 2-year periods between 1982 and 1987, the rates of intraoperative events were found to be stable, and the rate of postoperative complications decreased. The researchers suggested that identification of these problems could lead to changes in management that result in improved outcomes.

In 1994, the Pediatric Perioperative Cardiac Arrest (POCA) Registry[152] was formed to determine the clinical factors and outcomes associated with cardiac arrest in anesthetized children. For institutions in the registry, standardized data from each cardiac arrest in an anesthetized child 18 years or younger are submitted. A total of 289 cardiac arrests occurred in the 63 institutions in the database during the first 4 years of the registry, of which 150 were judged to be related to anesthesia (1.4 per 10,000 anesthesia procedures), with a 26% mortality rate. Medication-related causes and cardiovascular causes of cardiac arrest were most common (Fig. 24-7). Anesthesia-related cardiac arrest occurred most often in patients younger than 1 year of age and in patients with severe underlying disease. The goal of the registry is similar to that of the closed claims studies—to identify

Table 24-18 Summary of perioperative events by age group*

Event	<1 Month (n = 361)	1–12 Months (n = 2544)	1–5 Years (n = 13,484)	6–10 Years (n = 7184)	11+ Years (n = 5647)
Any intraoperative event	14.96	7.31	7.10	12.22	9.69
Any recovery-room event	16.61	7.23	12.20	14.88	15.23
Any postoperative event					
Minor event†	13.57	10.30	20.32	31.49	32.44
Major event‡	23.82	7.51	3.26	3.37	3.33
Any event§					
Among patients seen	48.89	25.92	37.50	50.52	51.33
Among all patients	41.55	23.47	33.16	45.04	45.78

*All figures are given as the percentage of events per total anesthetics.
†Includes nausea and vomiting, sore throat, muscle pain, headache, dental conditions, positional conditions, conditions involving extremities, eye conditions, croup, temperature, behavioral problem, thrombophlebitis, arterial line problem, awareness, and "other" problems.
‡Includes "other respiratory" conditions, cardiovascular disorders, nerve palsy, hepatic disorders, renal disorders, seizures, surgical complications, and death.
§Percentage of total anesthetics in which there was at least one event in the intraoperative, recovery-room, or later postoperative period.
Adapted from Cohen MM, Cameron CB, Duncan PG: Pediatric anesthesia morbidity and mortality in the perioperative period. Anesth Analg 70:160, 1990.

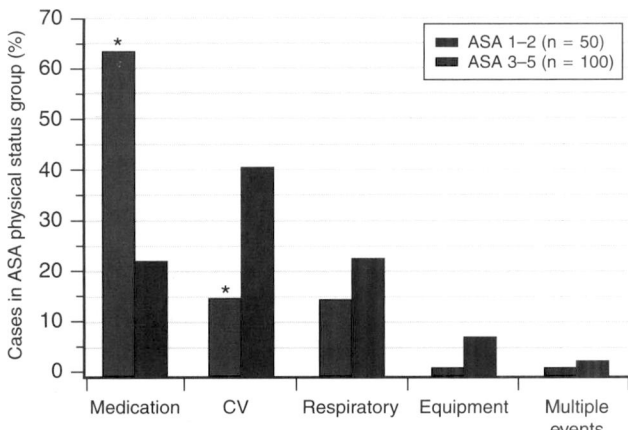

Figure 24–7 Causes of perioperative cardiac arrests in the pediatric population in the Pediatric Perioperative Cardiac Arrest Registry. Medication-related and cardiovascular (CV) causes of cardiac arrest were most common. (Adapted from Morray JP, Geiduschek JM, Ramamoorthy C, et al: Anesthesia-related cardiac arrest in children: Initial findings of the Pediatric Perioperative Cardiac Arrest [POCA] Registry. Anesthesiology 93:6, 2000.)

the causes in this unique population and thereby identify preventive strategies.

Geriatrics

Numerous studies have documented the importance of advanced age to perioperative risk (see Chapter 62). In many of the original studies on factors associated with perioperative mortality, the highest rates of death after surgery occurred among the youngest and the oldest patients. Age was implicated as one of the factors in the risk indices developed by Goldman, Detsky, and Pedersen. Age is predominantly analyzed as a dichotomous variable, with many studies focusing on age greater than 70 years.

One of the issues regarding the mortality rate in the geriatric population is the definition of this group. Multiple definitions have been used for advanced age, including patients older than 65, 70, 80, or 90 years. Denney and Denson[153] evaluated risk of surgery in patients older than 90 years. They suggested that the prevailing philosophy in 1972—that surgery might not be appropriate in this cohort considering the high perioperative risk—was without objective supporting data. They reported 272 patients undergoing 301 operations at the University of Southern California Medical Center and found, contrary to their expectation, that the risk was more than justified in at least 70% of the nonagenarians. They reported that serious bowel obstruction was the only underlying comorbidity associated with a prohibitive perioperative mortality rate (63%).

Djokovic and Hedley-Whyte[154] studied outcome after surgery in 500 patients older than 80 years at the Harvard Medical System. They found that mortality was predicted by ASA physical status classification, with greater comorbidity associated with increasing risk. Myocardial infarction was the leading cause of postoperative death. Patients without significant comorbidities (ASA class I)

had a mortality rate of less than 1%. The data suggest that surgery is safe in this cohort and that risk is not a function of age but of coexisting disease.

Del Guercio and Cohn[155] investigated the value of preoperative invasive monitoring in obtaining hemodynamic and cardiopulmonary variables for predicting operative risk in the elderly. A total of 148 consecutive patients older than 65 years were studied preoperatively in an ICU. Only 13.5% had normal physiologic measurements. Advanced and uncorrectable functional deficits were found in 63% of patients, and all of those who underwent the planned operation died. This further supports the contention that coexisting disease, not age, is the risk.

The elderly patient presents a difficult issue for the anesthesiologist. Atherosclerosis increases with advancing age, and the heart muscle itself ages. Further preoperative evaluation in the elderly usually focuses on the identification of comorbidity. Based on the accumulating evidence, it is these factors that influence perioperative risk.

RISKS DIRECTLY RELATED TO THE ANESTHETIC DRUG

Numerous studies have evaluated the influence of choice of anesthesia on outcome, a question that is discussed throughout this book. From a global perspective, there does not appear to be one best anesthesia technique. In a multivariate analysis by Cohen and coworkers[51a] of 100,000 anesthesia procedures performed in Canada, the choice of drug did not provide any additional prognostic information for predicting mortality beyond that of patient disease and the surgical procedure. In univariant analysis, monitored anesthesia care did appear to be associated with worse outcomes, but this was attributable to its use for sicker patients (see Table 24-13).

One question that has plagued the anesthesia literature is the issue of inherent toxicity of the anesthetics. There are important distinctions between undesirable side effects of anesthesia and true toxicity. In the initial reports of the mid-20th century, there was much concern about curare toxicity. Recent discussions of anesthetic toxicity have focused on halothane and sevoflurane. The issues for halothane were fulminant hepatic necrosis and death. The issue for sevoflurane was whether its metabolite, compound A, was nephrotoxic. After several case reports of hepatic necrosis after halothane anesthesia, a retrospective study of 856,500 anesthesia procedures at 34 institutions was undertaken.[156-158] In all but nine cases, hepatic necrosis could be explained by other causes. Of the remaining nine cases, only seven received halothane. Halothane could be associated with hepatitis and hepatic failure, but the incidence was very low.

Despite concern about the renal toxicity of sevoflurane (see Chapter 8), the overall safety of this drug has been sufficiently established for the U.S. Food and Drug Administration to allow its continued sale in the United States. Some laboratory studies have supported the contention that sevoflurane reacts with soda lime to form compound A and that this metabolite can lead to renal toxicity.[159,160] However, clinical studies have been unable to confirm this potentially detrimental effect.[161,162]

Numerous studies have attempted to define the "safest" anesthetic for high-risk patients. In the late 1980s, there was particular concern that isoflurane caused coronary steal in patients with coronary stenosis and collaterals and that this could result in myocardial ischemia.[163,164] A series of studies was conducted to evaluate the rate of perioperative cardiac morbidity and mortality in patients undergoing coronary artery bypass grafting to determine the importance of the agent used for general anesthesia.[165-169] All of these studies demonstrated no difference in outcome, supporting the contention that there is no one safest anesthesia technique.

A series of randomized trials demonstrated improved outcome with regional rather than general anesthesia.[5,6,170-174] For lower extremity and pelvic surgery, regional anesthesia was associated with a lower incidence of graft thrombosis and deep vein thrombosis, as well as decreased bleeding. For vascular surgery patients, the primary finding was a lower incidence of graft thrombosis and need for reoperation in patients undergoing infrainguinal bypass surgery; however, the largest of these studies was unable to demonstrate any difference in outcome based on anesthesia technique.[5,6,173] The rate of this complication was low in the total cohort in the largest trial, making it impossible to detect any difference based on technique.

Rodgers and coworkers[175] published a large meta-analysis of regional versus general anesthesia. Neuraxial blockade was found to reduce postoperative mortality and other serious complications. The size of some of these benefits remained uncertain.

RISKS RELATED TO SURGERY

The surgical procedure itself significantly influences perioperative risk. In virtually every study performed, emergency surgery is associated with additional risk. For example, in the study of Goldman and colleagues,[13] emergency surgery was associated with the second highest weight (i.e., number of points), after active signs of congestive heart failure. In the same study, intrathoracic and abdominal procedures were determined to have a higher risk.

In some cases, the risk related to surgery is a function of the underlying disease processes and the stress related to the surgical procedure. Cardiovascular surgery is associated with the highest risk of any procedure. The risks related to cardiac surgery are reviewed in Chapter 50. Vascular surgery is among the highest-risk group of the noncardiac procedures. Although aortic reconstructive surgery has traditionally been considered the procedure with highest risk, infrainguinal procedures have shown a similar rate of cardiac morbidity in several studies.[176,177] In an attempt to analyze the causes for the high complication rate on a relatively peripheral procedure, L'Italien and coworkers[177] demonstrated that the extent of coronary artery disease is higher among patients undergoing infrainguinal procedures and most likely accounts for the excess morbidity and mortality.

Ashton and colleagues[178] evaluated perioperative morbidity and mortality in a cohort of patients at a Veterans Hospital. Although vascular surgery was among the highest-risk procedures, amputation was associated with the highest in-hospital cardiac complication rate within this subgroup. This finding most likely represents the more severe nature of the cardiovascular disease in these patients and the prolonged hospitalization needed to facilitate recuperation. As in the study by Goldman and colleagues,[13] intra-abdominal, thoracic, and orthopedic procedures were associated with increased risk. In another report, Ashton[178a] evaluated the rate of perioperative myocardial infarction in patients undergoing transurethral resection of the prostate. Despite the high incidence of coronary artery disease in this population, the incidence of perioperative myocardial infarction was only 1%.

Numerous studies have evaluated the perioperative complication rate related to superficial procedures. Backer and coworkers[179] evaluated the rate of perioperative myocardial reinfarction in patients undergoing ophthalmologic surgery. They demonstrated that the rate of perioperative cardiac morbidity after ophthalmologic surgery was extremely low, even in patients with recent myocardial infarction. Virtually all studies have confirmed that ophthalmologic surgery is very safe under anesthesia.[180] Warner and colleagues[181] studied patients undergoing ambulatory surgery and reported no anesthesia-related deaths in more than 45,000 cases.

Eagle and colleagues[182] evaluated the contribution of coronary artery disease and its treatment on perioperative cardiac morbidity and mortality by surgical procedure. They evaluated patients enrolled in the Coronary Artery Surgery Study who had documented coronary artery disease and who received medical therapy or coronary revascularization and then underwent noncardiac surgery during the subsequent 10-year period. The rates of perioperative myocardial infarction and death were determined, and the surgical procedures were divided into three broad categories. Major vascular surgery was associated with the highest risk, with a combined morbidity and mortality of greater than 10%. Procedures associated with a combined complication rate of 1% to 5% included intra-abdominal, thoracic, and head and neck operations. In all of these cases, patients who had previously undergone coronary artery bypass grafting had a significantly lower combined morbidity and mortality rate than those in the medically treated group. Low-risk procedures included breast, skin, urologic, and orthopedic surgery. These broad groups of surgical procedures were the basis for the definitions of surgical risk published in the guidelines on perioperative cardiovascular evaluation for noncardiac surgery by the American Heart Association/American College of Cardiology Task Force on Assessment of Diagnostic and Therapeutic Cardiovascular Procedures[140] (Table 24-19).

RISKS RELATED TO LOCATION OF SURGERY AND POSTOPERATIVE MONITORING

Perioperative risk varies among hospitals for major procedures such as coronary artery bypass grafting and

Table 24–19 Cardiac risk stratification for noncardiac surgical procedures

Cardiac Risk*	Surgical Procedures
High (often >5%)	Emergent major operations, particularly in the elderly
	Aortic and other major vascular surgery
	Peripheral vascular surgery
	Anticipated prolonged surgical procedures associated with large fluid shifts and/or blood loss
Intermediate (usually <5%)	Carotid endarterectomy
	Head and neck surgery
	Intraperitoneal and intrathoracic surgery
	Orthopedic surgery
	Prostate surgery
Low† (usually <1%)	Endoscopic procedures
	Superficial procedure
	Cataract surgery
	Breast surgery

*Cardiac risk is the combined incidence of cardiac death and nonfatal myocardial infarction.
†Low-risk cases usually do not require further preoperative cardiac testing.
Adapted from Eagle K, Brundage B, Chaitman B, et al: Guidelines for perioperative cardiovascular evaluation of the noncardiac surgery. A report of the American Heart Association/American College of Cardiology Task Force on Assessment of Diagnostic and Therapeutic Cardiovascular Procedures. Circulation 93:1278, 1996.

abdominal aortic aneurysm repair[183,184] (see Chapters 50 and 52). Multiple studies have documented a relationship between surgical volume and mortality. Although surgical skill most certainly plays a role in the rate of complications and mortality, local factors may also play an important role. For example, low surgical volume may lead to less skilled anesthesia and postoperative care. The influence of each of these factors on overall morbidity and mortality is unknown.

Although the value of postoperative monitoring and care in an ICU has never been documented in a randomized clinical trial, many investigators have suggested that such care is one of the primary reasons for improved morbidity and mortality in recent years. For patients undergoing major vascular surgery, several investigators have suggested that more intense postoperative monitoring could obviate the need for preoperative cardiac testing and revascularization.[185,186] One potential value of risk assessment is the identification of patients who could benefit from referral to centers with more extensive perioperative resources. Patients with a low probability of perioperative morbidity and mortality could have surgery performed locally, and individuals at higher risk could receive benefit from transfer to a larger center.

It is estimated that 60% of all surgical procedures are performed on an outpatient basis, and this percentage is increasing annually. Review of the literature to determine the safety of this shift from the inpatient to the outpatient arena reveals a striking lack of good evidence to document such safety. Warner and coworkers[181] studied the safety of surgery on an ambulatory basis in 38,598 patients. They documented only 33 episodes of major morbidity or mortality within 1 month after surgery. Major morbidity included 14 myocardial infarctions, 7 central nervous system deficits, 5 pulmonary embolisms, and 5 cases of respiratory failure (see Fig. 24-3). When adjusted for age and gender, these rates of major morbidity

and mortality were lower than those expected in the nonsurgical population. However, Olmstead County, Minnesota, the site of Warner's study, represented a unique population with high standards for health care. Facilities were immediately available to care for any unexpected emergency or admission. The study was performed during an era in which the patients were primarily healthy individuals undergoing peripheral or superficial procedures.

The type and extent of surgical procedures performed in an outpatient setting is constantly changing, and procedures associated with greater perioperative risk are increasingly performed on an outpatient basis. The value of overnight observation in a hospital setting as opposed to immediate discharge home has been studied for a number of surgical procedures. One of the first procedures advocated to be performed on an ambulatory basis was tonsillectomy. In 1968, a case series of 40,000 outpatient tonsillectomies was reported with no deaths.[187a] Details on patient selection and length of postoperative monitoring were vague. Based on insurance company and state mandates, performance of tonsillectomy on an outpatient basis became routine.[187] Beginning in the mid-1980s and continuing in the 1990s, a number of articles evaluated the risk of early discharge. For example, Carithers and colleagues[188] at Ohio State University analyzed 3000 tonsillectomies and argued that early discharge might be hazardous and economically unwarranted. The rate of readmission for active bleeding between 5 and 24 hours after surgery was reported to be between 0.2% and 0.5%.[189-193] Although the absolute rate of readmission is low, it represents a substantial risk for children. Whether the benefits of early discharge outweigh the risks is a decision society will have to make.

Another procedure being performed on an outpatient basis is mastectomy. An analysis of Medicare claims demonstrated that the rate of outpatient mastectomy increased from only two procedures reported to Medicare in 1986 to 10.8% of the mastectomies performed in this population in 1995.[194] The investigators compared the rate of readmission within 7 days after surgery for those who had the procedure on an inpatient basis with those treated on an outpatient basis, adjusting for severity of disease. Simple mastectomies performed on an outpatient basis had a significantly higher rate of readmission compared with 1-day stays, with an adjusted odds ratio of 1.84. There were 33.8 readmissions per 1000 cases for the outpatient surgeries, compared with 24.2 readmissions for the 1-day length of stay surgeries. Compared with the group treated on an outpatient basis, there were significantly lower rates of readmission after 1-day stays for infection (4.1 versus 1.8 per 1000 cases), nausea and vomiting (1.1 versus 0 per 1000 cases), and pulmonary embolism or deep vein thrombosis (1.1 versus 0 per 1000 cases). Similarly, modified radical mastectomies performed on an outpatient basis had a significantly higher rate of readmission compared with 1-day stays, with an adjusted odds ratio of 1.72. The researchers suggested that patients who have the procedure on an outpatient basis may wait longer at home until seeking medical care and therefore may present with more advanced symptoms.

There is increasing interest in performing surgery and providing anesthesia in office-based settings. There are no good data to determine the safety of such practices, although there have been a flurry of high-profile cases in which patients have died in plastic surgery and dental offices. Anesthesia and sedation are frequently provided by individuals other than anesthesiologists or nurse anesthetists in these settings, and there are reports of office nurses or even clerical help administering anesthetic agents.

There has been an attempt to quantify the incidence of complications in an office-based setting. The American Association for Ambulatory Plastic Surgery Facilities (AAAPSF) mailed a survey to their members to determine the incidence of complications occurring in office facilities.[195] The overall response rate was 57%. The findings showed that 0.47% of patients had at least one complication, including bleeding, hypertension, infection, and hypotension, and 1 of 57,000 patients died. Assuming that these are very minor procedures performed only on healthy individuals, a rate of mortality that is three times the current estimate for anesthesia-related complications is a concern. Further research and quality-assurance mechanisms need to be in place before this practice is generalized. One of the problems inherent in an office-based setting is the inability to perform quality-assurance reviews. For example, few surgeons or anesthesiologists would be willing to allow their "competitors" to review their complication rate unless mandated to perform such a review.

The problems in evaluating the risk of outpatient surgery include the lack of any large database compiled from a diverse group of settings and the lack of uniform standards for quality assurance. Although the Joint Committee for the Accreditation of Hospitals accredits ASCs, as do two other organizations, accreditation is still not widespread and remains optional. Although ambulatory care centers have led the way in performing appropriate follow-up of their patients at home, such follow-up is not uniformly complete. As of 1998, only three states had established regulations for office-based settings, and these regulations vary greatly. The implications of the lack of regulation are unclear, but issues related to emergency plans and resuscitation equipment may be left to the discretion of the local personnel, potentially placing patients at risk.

The decision to perform a procedure in an ambulatory setting is based on the surgeon's preference and the insurance company's mandates. Frequently, a case series by a surgeon or review by an insurance company demonstrates that otherwise healthy individuals can undergo a given procedure safely in an outpatient setting. The need for subsequent medical attention or use of resources at home is not necessarily taken into account. This may lead to insurance company mandates that the procedure be performed in all patients in an ambulatory setting. The generalization from healthy individuals to patients with comorbid disease may not be justified in the absence of data to demonstrate its safety. As an advocate for the patient, the anesthesiologist should continue to evaluate the safety of such practices and determine when the risks of ambulatory surgery outweigh any potential benefits. It is also important to determine whether the insurance companies are in essence transferring the risk of undergoing surgery from the medical system to the patient.

RISKS RELATED TO THE ANESTHESIA PROVIDER

The added risk associated with the provider of anesthesia is an emotionally charged issue, particularly in the United States. Over the history of the specialty, various individuals have provided anesthesia, including anesthesiologists, general medical officers, residents, and CRNAs.

The importance of the anesthesiologist to outcome is best illustrated by the work of Slogoff and Keats.[196] They studied the association of perioperative myocardial ischemia and cardiac morbidity in patients undergoing coronary artery bypass grafting. They found that perioperative myocardial infarction occurred significantly more frequently in patients with ischemia before the bypass operation. They then reported the rate of ischemia and infarction by anesthesiologist (identified by number). Anesthesiologist no. 7 had a significantly higher rate of complications than the average for the rest of the group. Operator technique or experience may affect risk. This observation parallels similar findings that surgical volume (and presumably experience) is associated with outcome.

Several studies have attempted to evaluate the complication rates and risks associated with various care provider models. Bechtoldt,[197] as a member of the North Carolina Anesthesia Study Committee, evaluated 900 perioperative deaths from an estimated 2 million anesthesia procedures performed in North Carolina between 1969 and 1976. Data were obtained from the medical examiner's report, the routine death certificate, and a questionnaire completed by the person who administered the anesthetic.

The committee concluded that 90 of these deaths were related to anesthesia. About one half of the anesthesia-related deaths occurred in the operating room, including 19 that occurred on induction. With information attained from a survey of hospitals, they then determined the relationship between mortality and anesthesia provider based on the total number of procedures administered by each group (Fig. 24-8). The lowest rate of anesthesia-related deaths (1 per 28,166 procedures) occurred in patients who received anesthesia from an anesthesia care team (physician anesthesiologist and CRNA), and the highest rate (1 per 11,432 procedures) was associated with anesthesia administered by a dentist (1 per 11,432); the rate for the nurse anesthetist–only cohort was intermediate (1 per 20,723). The large number of cases in which the care provider was unknown and the reliance on hospital estimates of the number of cases performed by each group made interpretation difficult.

The Stanford Center for Health Care Research[198] also evaluated the impact of provider on outcome of care. They prospectively collected data from 8593 patients undergoing 15 surgical procedures over a 10-month period (May 1973 through February 1974). Using a risk-adjustment methodology, the actual patient outcome was compared with that predicted by the patient's health status and operative procedure. The investigators reported that death plus severe morbidity was 11% higher than predicted for patients who received their care in a nurse anesthetist–only setting, 3% lower than predicted for physician-only care, and 20% lower than predicted for an anesthesia care team environment. Because of the small sample size, these findings did not reach statistical significance between the groups.

The differences in outcome among anesthesia providers are extremely difficult to study from a methodologic standpoint. The impact of specific provider types may be greatest in specific situations. For example, there may be no difference in outcome for healthy individuals, particularly if no complications occur. In contrast, patients with significant comorbidities and those who sustain perioperative complications may benefit from having providers with specific skill sets. One way to study such issues is to evaluate the rate of survival after complications. Silber and colleagues[199] at the University of Pennsylvania advocated such an approach. They studied the medical records of 5972 surgical patients randomly selected from 531 hospitals. They evaluated patient and hospital characteristics, including the number and type of physicians, board-certification status, and ratio of care providers. The 30-day mortality rate correlated with patient characteristics. Failure to rescue (i.e., prevent death) after an adverse event was inversely associated with the proportion of board-certified anesthesiologists on staff in each facility. Improved perioperative survival was significantly associated with the presence of an increased number of board-certified anesthesiologists.

As a follow-up to this study, Silber and colleagues[200] compared the outcomes of surgical patients for whom anesthesia care was or was not personally performed or medically directed by an anesthesiologist. Medicare claims records were analyzed for all elderly patients in Pennsylvania who underwent general surgical or orthopedic procedures between 1991 and 1994. The 30-day mortality rate and the mortality rate after complications (i.e., failure to rescue) were lower when anesthesiologists directed anesthesia care, even after adjustment for patient and hospital characteristics.

Silber and colleagues[201] employed similar methodology to determine the importance of board certification in perioperative risk. Adjusted odds ratios for death (1.13; 95% CI: 1.00-1.26; $P < .04$) and for failure to rescue (1.13; 95% CI: 1.01-1.27; $P < .04$) were greater when care was delivered by noncertified, midcareer anesthesiologists.

The marked increase in the number of anesthesiologists has been paralleled by a dramatic decrease in malpractice insurance premiums for anesthesiologists.[202] Because these premiums are based on the number and severity of claims, these data suggest that anesthesia is getting safer. The issue remains unresolved, and further research into the importance of anesthesia provider to outcome is required.

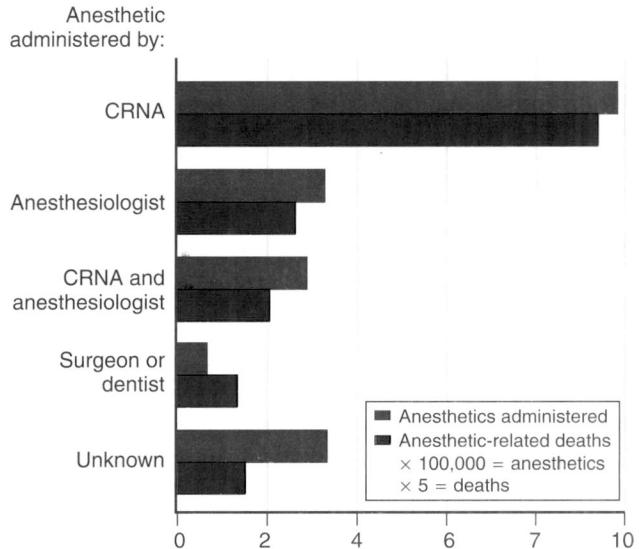

Figure 24–8 Relationship between anesthesia provider and anesthesia-related deaths in North Carolina. The number of cases performed by each group was estimated from a survey of hospitals. The certified registered nurse anesthetist (CRNA) and the anesthesiologist care team were associated with the best outcomes, whereas the surgeon or dentist practicing anesthesia was associated with the worst. (From Bechtoldt AA: Committee on anesthesia study. Anesthetic-related deaths: 1969-1976. N C Med J 42:253, 1981.)

RISKS TO THE ANESTHESIOLOGIST

Several potential risks to the anesthesiologist are related to the provision of care (see Chapter 88), including the medicolegal risk, the risk of an allergic reaction, and the risk of a needlestick injury and transmission of disease from the patient to the practitioner. The medicolegal risks are described in Chapter 89.

It is becoming increasing apparent that anesthesiologists are at risk for latex allergy, which can lead to a life-threatening reaction. Many anesthesiologists realize that they are sensitized to latex and apply appropriate precautions. The problem is that many sensitized individuals are asymptomatic. Brown and coworkers[203] studied 168 eligible anesthesiologists and nurse anesthetists working in the anesthesia department of The Johns Hopkins Hospital. The prevalence of latex allergy with clinical symptoms was 2.4% and that of latex sensitization without clinical symptoms was 10.1%. The prevalence of irritant or contact dermatitis was 24%. These data suggest that latex is an important problem to the anesthesiologist and that there is a need to transform the hospital to a latex-free environment.

There has always been concern that anesthesiologists are at risk for contracting a disease from a patient. In the past, the risk was primarily hepatitis, but the human immunodeficiency virus (HIV) is a greater concern today. In a review of the literature, Berry and Greene[204] reported that at least 20 different pathogens have been transmitted through accidental needlestick injuries.

Among anesthesia personnel in several studies conducted in the United States, hepatitis B seropositivity ranged from 12.7% to 48.6%, a rate at least four times greater than that in the general population.[205-207] The risk of hepatitis B infection after a percutaneous exposure to antigen-positive blood is estimated to be 27% to 43%.[208] The development of the hepatitis B vaccine has substantially reduced this risk. Hepatitis C virus has been identified as a major cause of post-transfusion hepatitis. There have been several reports of occupationally acquired hepatitis in health care workers.[209] Because up to 50% of infected individuals develop signs of chronic liver infection, this represents a potentially serious problem.

Among the greatest fears of the health care worker is HIV infection. The risk of acquiring HIV is approximately 0.4% from a single percutaneous exposure to blood or bloody fluid from an HIV-infected patient.[210] There has been at least one case report of an anesthesiologist who was infected with HIV from a needlestick injury during insertion of a central venous catheter into an HIV-positive patient.[211]

Several strategies have been developed to reduce the transmission of communicable diseases (see Chapter 88). Although anesthesiologists traditionally think of the risk to the patient, they must now include the risk to themselves. The widespread adoption of universal precautions should reduce the rate of infection; however, anesthesiologists have not accepted these recommendations widely. In a study of nine hospitals, 59% of the contaminated percutaneous injuries were preventable.[212] In a theoretical model of risk of HIV infection, it was estimated that the 30-year occupational risk was 0.10% to 0.22% in low-prevalence areas and 8.26% to 13% in high-prevalence areas.[213] The researchers suggested that double-gloving practices may lead to reduced risk.

IMPROVING ANESTHESIA SAFETY

Over the past several decades, there have been major initiatives to improve the safety of anesthesia. In 1984,

Cooper, Kitz, and Ellison hosted the first International Symposium on Preventable Anesthesia Mortality and Morbidity in Boston. Approximately 50 anesthesiologists from around the world attended the meeting and, after much debate, established a series of definitions of outcome, morbidity, and mortality (Table 24-20). These meetings have been held every 2 years since the first symposium. The Anesthesia Patient Safety Foundation was established as a result of the Boston meeting. The society has been active in publishing widely circulated newsletters and awarding annual grants. Similar societies have been established in countries outside the United States, and a National Patient Safety Foundation has been created on the same model.

Starting with the ACCS, there has been much interest in establishing guidelines for best and safest practice. Practice policies or guidelines are summations by clinicians of the available evidence about the benefits and risks of particular treatment plans. Guidelines are a method of codifying recommendations regarding the use of a given technology. Several types of recommendations fall into the general category of a practice parameter. A *standard* implies that a therapy or practice should be performed for patients with a particular condition. Standards are approved only if an assessment of the probabilities and utilities of the group indicate that the decision to choose the treatment or a strategy would be virtually unanimous. If a particular therapy or strategy is considered a standard, it is a cost-effective measure for those for whom it is being recommended. Standards are intended to be applied rigidly. The ASA has established Standards for Intraoperative Monitoring, which were developed from safety guidelines adopted by the Harvard University hospital system. Guidelines are intended to be more flexible than standards, but they should be followed in most cases. Depending on the patient, the setting, and other factors, guidelines can and should be

---

Table 24–20 Proposed definitions from the 1994 International Symposium on Preventable Anesthesia Morbidity and Mortality

Outcome
 Normal
 Abandoned procedure
 Morbidity
 Death
Morbidity
 An unplanned, unwanted, undesirable consequence of
  anesthesia
Mortality
 Death that occurs before recovery from effects of a drug
  or drugs given to facilitate a procedure
 Death that occurs during an attempt to relieve the pain
  of a condition
 Death that results from an incident that occurs while the
  drugs are effective

Adapted from Pierce EC Jr: The 34th Rovenstine Lecture: 40 years behind the mask: Safety revisited. Anesthesiology 84:965, 1996.

tailored to fit individual needs. Like standards, guidelines should be cost-effective methods. A number of specific guidelines have been adopted by the ASA for diverse issues such as the difficult airway,[214] use of the pulmonary artery catheter,[215] and use of blood components.[216] The goal is to define the evidence on which optimal practice can be based.

There is much interest in the use of anesthesia simulators to train and test individuals and their ability to react to simulated crises.[217-221] Standardized scenarios have been developed for making comparisons among individuals.[222,223] Further research is required to determine how best to use this technology in anesthesia training and in recertification.

FUTURE DIRECTIONS IN PERIOPERATIVE RISK

The impact of genetics on perioperative risk has been well known since the elucidation of the inheritance pattern of malignant hyperthermia. With malignant hyperthermia, there is a clear link between the autosomal dominant disease and an adverse outcome after administration of an anesthetic.[226] There is increasing interest in evaluating the impact of genetic polymorphism on overall perioperative outcome, even if the link to anesthesia is less well defined. For example, apolipoprotein E4 has been shown to modulate neurologic injury and recovery after a variety of acute ischemic insults, including coronary artery bypass grafting.[227] Polymorphism of the glycoprotein GPIIIa constituent of the platelet integrin receptor has also been correlated with postoperative cognitive decline.

SUMMARY

The risks related to anesthesia have dramatically decreased over the past several decades. It is clear that death totally attributable to anesthesia is rare. Patient disease and the type and perhaps the location of surgical procedures have a greater effect on overall outcome. With these changes in risk, the anesthesiologist must now focus on nonmorbid outcomes, and there must be continued vigilance to maintain the high standards of hospital-based anesthesia in nonhospital settings.

KEY POINTS

1. Perioperative risk is multifactorial and depends on the interaction of anesthesia-, surgery-, and patient-specific factors.
2. Anesthesia-related (and surgery-related) risk includes morbidity and mortality within 30 days, although shorter periods may be relevant depending on the extent of surgery.
3. Anesthesia and the actions of anesthesiologists may completely or partially cause perioperative morbidity

and mortality, but the actions of the anesthesiologist may also decrease or modify risk related to patient disease.
4. In the literature on anesthesia-related risk, the rates of morbidity and mortality depend on the wide variety of definitions found.
5. Studies of anesthesia-related risk have found that postanesthesia respiratory depression is the largest cause of death and coma totally attributable to anesthesia; this finding prompted the development of postanesthesia care units.
6. Research into anesthesia-related cardiac arrests has found them to be attributable to medication administration, airway management, and technical problems of central venous access.
7. Multivariate modeling using logistic regression equations can be used to determine factors associated with increased risk in the cohort and in individuals and has been used to develop risk indices such as the Cardiac Risk Index.
8. Surveys of maternal mortality suggest that the absolute rate of complications by anesthesia type has not decreased but that the increased use of regional anesthesia has led to improvements in outcome.
9. Medication-related and cardiovascular causes of cardiac arrest were the most common causes in the Pediatric Perioperative Cardiac Arrest registry.
10. With increases in outpatient surgery, increased surveillance is required to ensure that appropriate procedures are performed in appropriate locations.

REFERENCES

1. Mangano DT, Browner WS, Hollenberg M, et al: Long-term cardiac prognosis following noncardiac surgery. The Study of Perioperative Ischemia Research Group. JAMA 268:233, 1992.
2. Kim LJ, Martinez EA, Faraday N, et al: Cardiac troponin I predicts short-term mortality in vascular surgery patients. Circulation 106:2366, 2002.
3. Poldermans D, Boersma E, Bax JJ, et al: The effect of bisoprolol on perioperative mortality and myocardial infarction in high-risk patients undergoing vascular surgery. Dutch Echocardiographic Cardiac Risk Evaluation Applying Stress Echocardiography Study Group. N Engl J Med 341:1789, 1999.
4. Christopherson R, Beattie C, Frank SM, et al: Perioperative morbidity in patients randomized to epidural or general anesthesia for lower extremity vascular surgery. Perioperative Ischemia Randomized Anesthesia Trial Study Group. Anesthesiology 79:422, 1993.
5. Bode RH, Jr, Lewis KP, Zarich SW, et al: Cardiac outcome after peripheral vascular surgery. Comparison of general and regional anesthesia. Anesthesiology 84:3, 1996.
6. Tuman KJ, McCarthy RJ, March RJ, et al: Effects of epidural anesthesia and analgesia on coagulation and outcome after major vascular surgery. Anesth Analg 73:696, 1991.
7. Twersky R, Fishman D, Homel P: What happens after discharge? Return hospital visits after ambulatory surgery. Anesth Analg 84:319, 1997.
8. Cohn LH, Rosborough D, Fernandez J: Reducing costs and length of stay and improving efficiency and quality of care in cardiac surgery. Ann Thorac Surg 64(Suppl 6):S58, 1997.

9. Fleisher LA, Metzger SE, Lam J, Harris A: Perioperative cost-finding analysis of the routine use of intraoperative forced-air warming during general anesthesia. Anesthesiology 88:1357, 1998.

10. Klafta JM, Roizen MF: Current understanding of patients' attitudes toward and preparation for anesthesia: A review. Anesth Analg 83:1314, 1996.

11. Fisher DM: Surrogate end points. Are they meaningful [editorial]? Anesthesiology 81:795, 1994.

12. Fleisher LA: ...but, is suppression of postoperative ST segment depression an important outcome [editorial]? Anesth Analg 84:709, 1997.

13. Goldman L, Caldera DL, Nussbaum SR, et al: Multifactorial index of cardiac risk in noncardiac surgical procedures. N Engl J Med 297:845, 1977.

14. Tarhan S, Moffitt EA, Taylor WF, Giuliani ER: Myocardial infarction after general anesthesia. JAMA 220:1451, 1972.

15. Rao TLK, Jacobs KH, El-Etr AA: Reinfarction following anesthesia in patients with myocardial infarction. Anesthesiology 59:499, 1983.

16. Shah KB, Kleinman BS, Sami H, et al: Reevaluation of perioperative myocardial infarction in patients with prior myocardial infarction undergoing noncardiac operations. Anesth Analg 71:231, 1990.

17. Frank SM, Beattie C, Christopherson R, et al: Unintentional hypothermia is associated with postoperative myocardial ischemia. The Perioperative Ischemia Randomized Anesthesia Trial Study Group. Anesthesiology 78:468, 1993.

18. Frank SM, Fleisher LA, Breslow MJ, et al: Perioperative maintenance of normothermia reduces the incidence of morbid cardiac events. A randomized clinical trial. JAMA 277:1127, 1997.

19. Lagasse RS: Anesthesia safety: Model or myth? A review of the published literature and analysis of current original data. Anesthesiology 97:1609, 2002.

20. Buck N, Devlin HB, Lunn JL: Report of a Confidential Enquiry into Perioperative Deaths. Nuffield Provincial Hospitals Trust. London, The King's Fund Publishing House, 1987.

21. Beecher HK, Todd DP: A study of deaths associated with anesthesia and surgery. Ann Surg 140:2, 1954.

22. Newland MC, Ellis SJ, Lydiatt CA, et al: Anesthetic-related cardiac arrest and its mortality: A report covering 72,959 anesthetics over 10 years from a US teaching hospital. Anesthesiology 97:108, 2002.

23. Cheney FW, Posner K, Caplan RA, Ward RJ: Standard of care and anesthesia liability. JAMA 261:1599, 1989.

24. Mathew JP, Parks R, Savino JS, et al: Atrial fibrillation following coronary artery bypass graft surgery: Predictors, outcomes, and resource utilization. Multicenter Study of Perioperative Ischemia Research Group. JAMA 276:300, 1996.

25. Mangano DT: Aspirin and mortality from coronary bypass surgery. N Engl J Med 347:1309, 2002.

26. Nugent WC: Clinical applications of risk-assessment protocols in the management of individual patients. Ann Thorac Surg 64(Suppl 6):S68, 1997.

27. Grover FL, Shroyer AL, Edwards FH, et al: Data quality review program: The Society of Thoracic Surgeons Adult Cardiac National Database. Ann Thorac Surg 62:1229, 1996.

28. Grover FL, Shroyer AL, Hammermeister KE: Calculating risk and outcome: The Veterans Affairs database. Ann Thorac Surg 62(Suppl 5):S6, 1996.

29. Clark RE: The development of The Society of Thoracic Surgeons voluntary national database system: Genesis, issues, growth, and status. Best Pract Benchmarking Healthc 1:62, 1996.

30. Clark RE: The STS Cardiac Surgery National Database: An update. Ann Thorac Surg 59:1376, 1995.

31. Todd CJ, Freeman CJ, Camilleri-Ferrante C, et al: Differences in mortality after fracture of hip: The East Anglian audit. BMJ 310:904, 1995.

32. Pronovost PJ, Jenckes MW, Dorman T, et al: Organizational characteristics of intensive care units related to outcomes of abdominal aortic surgery. JAMA 281:1310, 1999.

33. Pronovost PJ, Angus DC, Dorman T, et al: Physician staffing patterns and clinical outcomes in critically ill patients: A systematic review. JAMA 288:2151, 2002.

34. Aiken LH, Clarke SP, Sloane DM, et al: Hospital nurse staffing and patient mortality, nurse burnout, and job dissatisfaction. JAMA 288:1987, 2002.

35. Marx GF, Mateo CV, Orkin LR: Computer analysis of postanesthetic deaths. Anesthesiology 39:54, 1973.

36. Reich DL, Bodian CA, Krol M, et al: Intraoperative hemodynamic predictors of mortality, stroke, and myocardial infarction after coronary artery bypass surgery. Anesth Analg 89:814, 1999.

37. Ghali WA, Ash AS, Hall RE, Moskowitz MA: Statewide quality improvement initiatives and mortality after cardiac surgery. JAMA 277:379, 1997.

38. Mukamel DB, Mushlin AI: Quality of care information makes a difference: An analysis of market share and price changes after publication of the New York State Cardiac Surgery Mortality Reports. Med Care 36:945, 1998.

39. Hannan EL, Racz MJ, Jollis JG, Peterson ED: Using Medicare claims data to assess provider quality for CABG surgery: Does it work well enough? Health Serv Res 31:659, 1997.

40. Silber JH, Williams SV, Krakauer H, Schwartz JS: Hospital and patient characteristics associated with death after surgery. A study of adverse occurrence and failure to rescue. Med Care 30:615, 1992.

41. Beecher HK: The first anesthesia death with some remarks suggested by it on the fields of the laboratory and clinic in the appraisal of new anesthetic agents. Anesthesiology 2:443, 1941.

42. Snow J: On chloroform and other anesthetics. London, John Churchill, 1858.

43. Dornette WHL, Orth OS: Death in the operating room. Anesth Analg 35:545, 1956.

44. Schapira M, Kepes ER, Hurwitt ES: An analysis of deaths in the operating room and within 24 hours of surgery. Anesth Analg 39:149, 1960.

45. Phillips OC, Frazier TM, Graff TD, DeKornfeld TJ: The Baltimore anesthesia study committee; review of 1,024 postoperative deaths. JAMA 174:2015, 1960.

46. Dripps RD, Lamont A, Eckenhoff JE: The role of anesthesia in surgical mortality. JAMA 178:261, 1961.

47. Clifton BS, Hotten WIT: Deaths associated with anaesthesia. Br J Anaesth 35:250, 1963.

48. Memery HN: Anesthesia mortality in private practice. JAMA 194:127, 1965.

49. Gebbie D: Anaesthesia and death. Can Anaesth Soc J 13:390, 1966.

50. Minuck M: Death in the operating room. Can Anaesth Soc J 13:390, 1967.

51. Harrison GG: Death attributable to anaesthesia: A 10-year survey (1967-1976). Br J Anaesth 50:1041, 1978.

51a. Cohen MM, Duncan PG, Tate RB: Does anesthesia contribute to operative mortality? JAMA 260:2859, 1988.

52. Bodlander FMS: Deaths associated with anaesthesia. Br J Anaesth 47:36, 1975.

53. Hovi-Viander M: Death associated with anaesthesia in Finland. Br J Anaesth 52:483, 1980.

54. Ruth HS: Anesthesia study commissions. JAMA 127:514, 1945.

55. Macintosh RR: Deaths under anaesthetics. Br J Anaesth 21:107, 1948.

56. Dinnick OP: Deaths associated with anaesthesia. Anaesthesia 19:536, 1964.

57. Farrow SC, Fowkes FG, Lunn JN, et al: Epidemiology in anaesthesia: A method for predicting hospital mortality. Eur J Anaesthesiol 1:77, 1984.

58. Farrow SC, Fowkes FGR, Lunn JN, et al: Epidemiology in anaesthesia. II. Factors affecting mortality in hospital. Br J Anaesth 54:811, 1982.

59. Holland R: Anaesthetic mortality in New South Wales. Br J Anaesth 59:834, 1987.

60. Warden JC, Horan BF: Deaths attributed to anaesthesia in New South Wales, 1984-1990. Anaesth Intensive Care 24:66, 1996.

61. Tiret L, Desmonts JM, Hatton F, Vourc'h G: Complications associated with anaesthesia—A prospective survey in France. Can Anaesth Soc J 33:336, 1986.

62. Tikkanen J, Hovi-Viander M: Death associated with anaesthesia and surgery in Finland in 1986 compared to 1975. Acta Anaesthesiol Scand 39:262, 1995.

63. Lunn JN: The study on anaesthetic-related mortality. Anaesthesia 35:617, 1980.

64. Lunn JN, Mushin WW: Mortality associated with anesthesia. Anaesthesia 37:856, 1982.

65. Lunn JN, Hunter AR, Scott DB: Anaesthesia-related surgical mortality. Anaesthesia 38:1090, 1983.

66. Lunn JN, Devlin HB: Lessons from the Confidential Enquiry into Perioperative Deaths in three NHS regions. Lancet 2:1384, 1987.

67. Pedersen T, Eliasen K, Henriksen E: A prospective study of mortality associated with anaesthesia and surgery: Risk indicators of mortality in hospital. Acta Anaesthesiol Scand 34:176, 1990.

68. Fleisher LA, Pasternak LR, Herbert R, Anderson GF: Inpatient admission and death after outpatient surgery in elderly patients: Importance of the patient, system and location of care. Arch Surg 2004.

69. Hanks EC, Papper EM: Cardiac resuscitation. N Y State J Med 51:1801, 1951.

70. Ehrenhaft JL, Eastwood DW, Morris LE: Analysis of twenty-seven cases of acute cardiac arrest. J Thorac Surg 22:592, 1951.

71. Bonica JJ: Cardiac arrest. Northwest Med 52:719, 1953.

72. Blades B: Cardiac arrest. JAMA 155:709, 1954.

73. Hewlett TH, Gilpatrick CW, Bowers WF: Cardiac arrest. Surg Gynecol Obstet 102:607, 1956.

74. Briggs BD, Sheldon DB, Beecher HK: Cardiac arrest. A study of a thirty-year period of operating room deaths at Massachusetts General Hospital, 1925-1954. JAMA 160:1439, 1956.

75. Keenan RL, Boyan CP: Decreasing frequency of anesthetic cardiac arrest. J Clin Anesth 3:354, 1991.

76. Cohen MM, Duncan PG, Pope WDB, Wolkenstein C: A survey of 112,000 anaesthetics at one teaching hospital (1975-83). Can Anaesth Soc J 33:22, 1986.

77. Biboulet P, Aubas P, Dubourdieu J, et al: Fatal and non-fatal cardiac arrests related to anesthesia. Can J Anaesth 48:326, 2001.

78. Keenan RL, Boyan CP: Cardiac arrest due to anesthesia. JAMA 253:2373, 1985.

79. Olsson GL, Hallen B: Cardiac arrest during anaesthesia. A computer-aided study in 250,543 anaesthetics. Acta Anaesthesiol Scand 32:653, 1988.

80. Sanborn KV, Castro J, Kuroda M, Thys DM: Detection of intraoperative incidents by electronic scanning of computerized anesthesia records. Comparison with voluntary reporting. Anesthesiology 85:977, 1996.

81. Moller JT, Svennild I, Johannessen NW, et al: Perioperative monitoring with pulse oximetry and late postoperative cognitive dysfunction. Br J Anaesth 71:340, 1993.

82. Caplan RA, Ward RJ, Posner K, Cheney FW: Unexpected cardiac arrest during spinal anesthesia: A closed claims analysis of predisposing factors. Anesthesiology 68:5, 1988.

83. Tinker JH, Dull DL, Caplan RA, et al: Role of monitoring devices in prevention of anesthetic mishaps: A closed claims analysis. Anesthesiology 71:541, 1989.

84. Caplan RA, Posner KL, Ward RJ, Cheney FW: Adverse respiratory events in anesthesia: A closed claims analysis. Anesthesiology 72:828, 1990.

85. Practice guidelines for management of the difficult airway. A report by the American Society of Anesthesiologists Task Force on Management of the Difficult Airway. Anesthesiology 78:597, 1993.

86. Cooper JB: Toward prevention of anesthetic mishaps. Int Anesthesiol Clin 22:167, 1984.

87. Cooper JB, Newbower RS, Kitz RJ: An analysis of major errors and equipment failures in anesthesia management: Considerations for prevention and detection. Anesthesiology 60:34, 1984.

88. Newbower RS, Cooper JB, Long CD: Learning from anesthesia mishaps: Analysis of critical incidents in anesthesia helps reduce patient risk. QRB Qual Rev Bull 7:10, 1981.

89. Cooper JB, Newbower RS, Long CD, McPeek B: Preventable anesthesia mishaps: A study of human factors. Anesthesiology 49:399, 1978.

90. Buffington CW, Ramanathan S, Turndorf H: Detection of anesthesia machine faults. Anesth Analg 63:79, 1984.

91. Yeager RA, Moneta GL, Edwards JM, et al: Late survival after perioperative myocardial infarction complicating vascular surgery. J Vasc Surg 20:598, 1994.

92. Lopez-Jimenez F, Goldman L, Sacks DB, et al: Prognostic value of cardiac troponin T after noncardiac surgery: 6-month follow-up data. J Am Coll Cardiol 29:1241, 1997.

93. Mangano DT, Layug EL, Wallace A, Tateo I: Effect of atenolol on mortality and cardiovascular morbidity after noncardiac surgery. Multicenter Study of Perioperative Ischemia Research Group. N Engl J Med 335:1713, 1996.

94. Wallace A, Layug B, Tateo I, et al: Prophylactic atenolol reduces postoperative myocardial ischemia. McSPI Research Group. Anesthesiology 88:7, 1998.

95. Weldon BC, Mahla ME, Van dea MT, Monk TG: Advancing age and deeper intraoperative anesthetic levels are associated with higher first year death rates. Anesthesiology 97:A1, 2002.

96. Saklad M: Grading of patients for surgical procedures. Anesthesiology 62:206, 1941.

97. Keats AS: The ASA classification of physical status: A recapitulation. Anesthesiology 49:233, 1978.

98. Vancanti CJ, VanHouten RJ, Hill RC: A statistical analysis of the relationship of physical status to postoperative mortality in 68,388 cases. Anesth Analg 49:564, 1970.

99. Owens WD, Felts JA, Spitznagel J: ASA physical status classifications. Anesthesiology 49:239, 1978.

100. Zeldin RA: Assessing cardiac risk in patients who undergo noncardiac surgical procedures. Can J Surg 27:402, 1984.

101. Larsen SF, Olesen KH, Jacobsen E, et al: Prediction of cardiac risk in non-cardiac surgery. Eur Heart J 8:179, 1987.

102. Domaingue CM, Davies MJ, Cronin KD: Cardiovascular risk factors in patients for vascular surgery. Anaesth Intensive Care 10:324, 1982.

103. Jeffrey CC, Kunsman J, Cullen DJ, Brewster DC: A prospective evaluation of cardiac risk index. Anesthesiology 58:462, 1983.

104. White GH, Advani SM, Williams RA, Wilson SE: Cardiac risk index as a predictor of long-term survival after repair of abdominal aortic aneurysm. Am J Surg 156:103, 1988.

105. McEnroe CS, O'Donnell TF, Yeager A, et al: Comparison of ejection fraction and Goldman risk factor analysis to dipyridamole-thallium imaging 201 studies in the evaluation of cardiac morbidity after aortic aneurysm surgery. J Vasc Surg 11:497, 1990.

106. Lette J, Waters D, Lassonde J, et al: Postoperative myocardial infarction and cardiac death. Predictive value of dipyridamole-thallium imaging and five clinical scoring systems based on multifactorial analysis. Ann Surg 211:84, 1990.

107. Prause G, Ratzenhofer-Comenda B, Pierer G, et al: Can ASA grade or Goldman's cardiac risk index predict peri-operative mortality? A study of 16,227 patients. Anaesthesia 52:203, 1997.

108. Detsky A, Abrams H, McLaughlin J, et al: Predicting cardiac complications in patients undergoing non-cardiac surgery. J Gen Intern Med 1:211, 1986.

109. Palda VA, Detsky AS: Perioperative assessment and management of risk from coronary artery disease. Ann Intern Med 127:313, 1997.

110. Lee TH, Marcantonio ER, Mangione CM, et al: Derivation and prospective validation of a simple index for prediction of cardiac risk of major noncardiac surgery. Circulation 100:1043, 1999.

111. Magovern JA, Sakert T, Magovern GJ, et al: A model that predicts morbidity and mortality after coronary artery bypass graft surgery. J Am Coll Cardiol 28:1147, 1996.

112. Newman MF, Wolman R, Kanchuger M, et al: Multicenter preoperative stroke risk index for patients undergoing coronary artery bypass graft surgery. Multicenter Study of Perioperative Ischemia (McSPI) Research Group. Circulation 94(Suppl 9):II74, 1996.

113. Jones RH, Hannan EL, Hammermeister KE, et al: Identification of preoperative variables needed for risk adjustment of short-term mortality after coronary artery bypass graft surgery. The Working Group Panel on the Cooperative CABG Database Project. J Am Coll Cardiol 28:1478, 1996.

114. Weightman WM, Gibbs NM, Sheminant MR, et al: Risk prediction in coronary artery surgery: A comparison of four risk scores. Med J Aust 166:408, 1997.

115. Higgins TL, Estafanous FG, Loop FD, et al: ICU admission score for predicting morbidity and mortality risk after coronary artery bypass grafting. Ann Thorac Surg 64:1050, 1997.

116. Iezzoni LI, Ash AS, Shwartz M, et al: Predicting in-hospital deaths from coronary artery bypass graft surgery. Do different severity measures give different predictions? Med Care 36:28, 1998.

117. Hannan EL, Kilburn H Jr, O'Donnell JF, et al: Adult open heart surgery in New York State: An analysis of risk factors and hospital mortality rates. JAMA 264:2768, 1990.

118. Hannan EL, Kumar D, Racz M, et al: New York State's Cardiac Surgery Reporting System: Four years later. Ann Thorac Surg 58:1852, 1994.

119. Hannan EL, Kilburn H Jr, Racz M, et al: Improving the outcomes of coronary artery bypass surgery in New York State. JAMA 271:761, 1994.

120. Hertzer NR, Bevan EG, Young JR, et al: Coronary artery disease in peripheral vascular patients: A classification of 1000 coronary angiograms and results of surgical management. Ann Surg 199:223, 1984.

121. Boucher CA, Brewster DC, Darling RC, et al: Determination of cardiac risk by dipyridamole-thallium imaging before peripheral vascular surgery. N Engl J Med 312:389, 1985.

122. Cutler BS, Leppo JA: Dipyridamole thallium 201 scintigraphy to detect coronary artery disease before abdominal aortic surgery. J Vasc Surg 5:91, 1987.

123. Eagle KA, Singer DE, Brewster DC, et al: Dipyridamole-thallium scanning in patients undergoing vascular surgery. Optimizing preoperative evaluation of cardiac risk. JAMA 257:2185, 1987.

124. Elliott BM, Robison JG, Zellner JL, Hendrix GH: Dobutamine-201Tl imaging. Assessing cardiac risks associated with vascular surgery. Circulation 84(Suppl 5):III54, 1991.

125. Lane RT, Sawada SG, Segar DS, et al: Dobutamine stress echocardiography for assessment of cardiac risk before noncardiac surgery. Am J Cardiol 68:976, 1991.

126. Langan Er, Youkey JR, Franklin DP, et al: Dobutamine stress echocardiography for cardiac risk assessment before aortic surgery. J Vasc Surg 18:905, 1993.

127. Lette J, Waters D, Lapointe J, et al: Usefulness of the severity and extent of reversible perfusion defects during thallium-dipyridamole imaging for cardiac risk assessment before noncardiac surgery. Am J Cardiol 64:276, 1989.

128. Poldermans D, Fioretti PM, Forster T, et al: Dobutamine stress echocardiography for assessment of perioperative cardiac risk in patients undergoing major vascular surgery. Circulation 87:1506, 1993; see comments.

129. Poldermans D, Fioretti PM, Boersma E, et al: Dobutamine-atropine stress echocardiography and clinical data for predicting late cardiac events in patients with suspected coronary artery disease. Am J Med 97:119, 1994.

130. Poldermans D, Arnese M, Fioretti PM, et al: Improved cardiac risk stratification in major vascular surgery with dobutamine-atropine stress echocardiography. J Am Coll Cardiol 26:648, 1995.

131. Baron JF, Mundler O, Bertrand M, et al: Dipyridamole-thallium scintigraphy and gated radionuclide angiography to assess cardiac risk before abdominal aortic surgery. N Engl J Med 330:663, 1994.

132. Mangano DT, London MJ, Tubau JF, et al: Dipyridamole thallium-201 scintigraphy as a preoperative screening test. A reexamination of its predictive potential. Study of Perioperative Ischemia Research Group. Circulation 84:493, 1991.

133. Eagle KA, Coley CM, Newell JB, et al: Combining clinical and thallium data optimizes preoperative assessment of cardiac risk before major vascular surgery. Ann Int Med 110:859, 1989.

134. L'Italien GJ, Paul SD, Hendel RC, et al: Development and validation of a Bayesian model for perioperative cardiac risk assessment in a cohort of 1081 vascular surgical candidates. J Am Coll Cardiol 27:779, 1996.

135. Vanzetto G, Machecourt J, Blendea D, et al: Additive value of thallium single-photon emission computed tomography myocardial imaging for prediction of perioperative events in clinically selected high cardiac risk patients having abdominal aortic surgery. Am J Cardiol 77:143, 1996.

136. Boersma E, Poldermans D, Bax JJ, et al: Predictors of cardiac events after major vascular surgery: Role of clinical characteristics, dobutamine echocardiography, and beta-blocker therapy. JAMA 285:1865, 2001.

137. Goldman L, Caldera DL: Risks of general anesthesia and elective operation in the hypertensive patient. Anesthesiology 50:285, 1979.

138. Hollenberg M, Mangano DT, Browner WS, et al: Predictors of postoperative myocardial ischemia in patients undergoing noncardiac surgery. The Study of Perioperative Ischemia Research. JAMA 268:205, 1992.

139. Stone GW, Grines CL, Browne KF, et al: Predictors of in-hospital and 6-month outcome after acute myocardial infarction in the reperfusion era: The Primary Angioplasty in Myocardial Infarction (PAMI) Trial. J Am Coll Cardiol 25:370, 1995.

140. Eagle K, Brundage B, Chaitman B, et al: Guidelines for perioperative cardiovascular evaluation of the noncardiac surgery. A report of the American Heart Association/American College of Cardiology Task Force on Assessment of Diagnostic and Therapeutic Cardiovascular Procedures. Circulation 93:1273, 1996.

141. Kaunitz AM, Hughes JM, Grimes DA, et al: Causes of maternal mortality in the United States. Obstet Gynecol 65:605, 1985.

142. Endler GC, Mariona FG, Sokol RJ, Stevenson LB: Anesthesia-related maternal mortality in Michigan, 1972 to 1984. Am J Obstet Gynecol 159:187, 1988.

143. Rochat RW, Koonin LM, Atrash HK, Jewett JF: Maternal mortality in the United States: Report from the Maternal Mortality Collaborative. Obstet Gynecol 72:91, 1988.

144. Morgan M: Anaesthetic contribution to maternal mortality. Br J Anaesth 59:842, 1987.

145. Chadwick HS, Posner K, Caplan RA, et al: A comparison of obstetric and nonobstetric anesthesia malpractice claims. Anesthesiology 74:242, 1991.

146. Panchal S, Arria AM, Labhsetwar SA: Maternal mortality during hospital admission for delivery: A retrospective analysis using a state-maintained database. Anesth Analg 93:134, 2001.

147. Gibbs CP, Krischer J, Peckham BM, et al: Obstetric anesthesia: A national survey. Anesthesiology 65:298, 1986.

148. Hawkins JL, Gibbs CP, Orleans M, et al: Obstetric anesthesia work force survey, 1981 versus 1992. Anesthesiology 87:135, 1997.

149. Graff TD, Phillips OC, Benson DW, Kelley G: Baltimore Anesthesia Study Committee: Factors in pediatric anesthesia mortality. Anesth Analg 43:407, 1964.

150. Tiret L, Nivoche Y, Hatton F, et al: Complications related to anaesthesia in infants and children. A prospective survey of 40,240 anaesthetics. Br J Anaesth 61:263, 1988.

151. Cohen MM, Cameron CB, Duncan PG: Pediatric anesthesia morbidity and mortality in the perioperative period. Anesth Analg 70:160, 1990.

152. Morray JP, Geiduschek JM, Ramamoorthy C, et al: Anesthesia-related cardiac arrest in children: Initial findings of the Pediatric Perioperative Cardiac Arrest (POCA) Registry. Anesthesiology 93:6, 2000.

153. Denney JL, Denson JS: Risk of surgery in patients over 90. Geriatrics 27:115, 1972.

154. Djokovic JL, Hedley-Whyte J: Prediction of outcome of surgery and anesthesia in patients over 80. JAMA 242:2301, 1979.

155. Del Guercio LR, Cohn JD: Monitoring operative risk in the elderly. JAMA 243:1350, 1980.
156. DeBacker LJ, Longnecker DS: Prospective and retrospective searches for liver necrosis following halothane anesthesia. Serum enzyme study and case report. JAMA 195:157, 1966.
157. Aach R: Halothane and liver failure. JAMA 211:2145, 1970.
158. Subcommittee of the National Halothane Study of the Committee on Anesthesia, National Academy of Sciences-National Research Council: Summary of the National Halothane Study: Possible association between halothane anesthesia and postoperative hepatic necrosis. JAMA 197:775, 1966.
159. Nishiyama T, Aibiki M, Hanaoka K: Inorganic fluoride kinetics and renal tubular function after sevoflurane anesthesia in chronic renal failure patients receiving hemodialysis. Anesth Analg 83:574, 1996.
160. Levine MF, Sarner J, Lerman J, et al: Plasma inorganic fluoride concentrations after sevoflurane anesthesia in children. Anesthesiology 84:348, 1996.
161. Rooke GA, Ebert T, Muzi M, Kharasch ED: The hemodynamic and renal effects of sevoflurane and isoflurane in patients with coronary artery disease and chronic hypertension. Sevoflurane Ischemia Study Group. Anesth Analg 82:1159, 1996.
162. Conzen PF, Nuscheler M, Melotte A, et al: Renal function and serum fluoride concentrations in patients with stable renal insufficiency after anesthesia with sevoflurane or enflurane. Anesth Analg 81:569, 1995.
163. Buffington CW, Romson JL, Levine A, et al: Isoflurane induces coronary steal in a canine model of chronic coronary occlusion. Anesthesiology 66:280, 1987.
164. Becker LC: Is isoflurane dangerous for the patient with coronary artery disease [editorial]? Anesthesiology 66:259, 1987.
165. Slogoff S, Keats AS: Randomized trial of primary anesthetic agents on outcome of coronary artery bypass operations. Anesthesiology 70:179, 1989.
166. Slogoff S, Keats AS, Dear WE, et al: Steal-prone coronary anatomy and myocardial ischemia associated with four primary anesthetic agents in humans. Anesth Analg 72:22, 1991.
167. Leung JM, Hollenberg M, O'Kelly BF, et al: Effects of steal-prone anatomy on intraoperative myocardial ischemia. The SPI Research Group. J Am Coll Cardiol 20:1205, 1992.
168. Leung JM, Goehner P, O'Kelly BF, et al: Isoflurane anesthesia and myocardial ischemia: Comparative risk versus sufentanil anesthesia in patients undergoing coronary artery bypass graft surgery. The SPI Research Group. Anesthesiology 74:838, 1991.
169. Inoue K, Reichelt W, el-Banayosy A, et al: Does isoflurane lead to a higher incidence of myocardial infarction and perioperative death than enflurane in coronary artery surgery? A clinical study of 1178 patients. Anesth Analg 71:469, 1990.
170. Hjelmstedt A, Sahlstedt B, Maripuu E: Comparative influences of epidural and general anaesthesia on deep venous thrombosis and pulmonary embolism after total hip replacement. Acta Chir Scand 147:125, 1981.
171. Rivers SP, Scher LA, Sheehan E, Veith FJ: Epidural versus general anesthesia for infrainguinal arterial reconstruction. J Vasc Surg 14:764, 1991.
172. Shir Y, Frank SM, Brendler CB, Raja SN: Postoperative morbidity is similar in patients anesthetized with epidural and general anesthesia for radical prostatectomy. Urology 44:232, 1994.
173. Christopherson R, Glavan NJ, Norris EJ, et al: Control of blood pressure and heart rate in patients randomized to epidural or general anesthesia for lower extremity vascular surgery. Perioperative Ischemia Randomized Anesthesia Trial (PIRAT) Study Group. J Clin Anesth 8:578, 1996.
174. Norman JG, Fink GW: The effects of epidural anesthesia on the neuroendocrine response to major surgical stress: A randomized prospective trial. Am Surg 63:75, 1997.
175. Rodgers A, Walker N, Schug S, et al: Reduction of postoperative mortality and morbidity with epidural or spinal anaesthesia: Results from overview of randomized trials. BMJ 321:1493, 2000.
176. Krupski WC, Layug EL, Reilly LM, et al: Comparison of cardiac morbidity between aortic and infrainguinal operations. Study of Perioperative Ischemia (SPI) Research Group. J Vasc Surg 15:354, 1992.
177. L'Italien GL, Cambria RP, Cutler BS, et al: Comparative early and late cardiac morbidity among patients requiring different vascular surgery procedures. J Vasc Surg 21:935, 1995.
178. Ashton CM, Petersen NJ, Wray NP, et al: The incidence of perioperative myocardial infarction in men undergoing noncardiac surgery. Ann Intern Med 118:504, 1993.
178a. Ashton CM, Thomas J, Wray NP, et al: The frequency and significance of ECG changes after transurethral prostate resection. J Am Geriatr Soc 39:575,1991.
179. Backer CL, Tinker JH, Robertson DM, Vlietstra RE: Myocardial reinfarction following local anesthesia for ophthalmic surgery. Anesth Analg 59:257, 1980.
180. Schein OD, Katz J, Bass EB, et al: The value of routine preoperative medical testing before cataract surgery. Study of Medical Testing for Cataract Surgery. N Engl J Med 342:168, 2000.
181. Warner MA, Shields SE, Chute CG: Major morbidity and mortality within 1 month of ambulatory surgery and anesthesia. JAMA 270:1437, 1993.
182. Eagle KA, Rihal CS, Mickel MC, et al: Cardiac risk of non-cardiac surgery: Influence of coronary disease and type of surgery in 3368 operations. CASS Investigators and University of Michigan Heart Care Program. Coronary Artery Surgery Study. Circulation 96:1882, 1997.
183. Kantonen I, Lepantalo M, Salenius JP, et al: Mortality in abdominal aortic aneurysm surgery: The effect of hospital volume, patient mix and surgeon's case load. Eur J Vasc Endovasc Surg 14:375, 1997.
184. Luft HS, Bunker JP, Enthoven AC: Should operations be regionalized? The empirical relation between surgical volume and mortality. N Engl J Med 301:1364, 1979.
185. Rosenfeld BA, Breslow MJ, Dorman T: Postoperative management strategies may obviate the need for most preoperative cardiac testing [letter]. Anesthesiology 84:1266, 1996.
186. D'Angelo AJ, Puppala D, Farber A, et al: Is preoperative cardiac evaluation for abdominal aortic aneurysm repair necessary? J Vasc Surg 25:152, 1997.
187. Raymond CA: Study questions, safety, economic benefits of outpatient tonsil/adenoid surgery [news]. JAMA 256:311, 1986.
187a. Chiang TM, Sukis AE, Ross DE: Tonsillectomy performed on an outpatient basis: report of a series of 40,000 cases without a death. Arch Otolaryngol 88:307, 1968.
188. Carithers JS, Gebhart DE, Williams JA: Postoperative risks of pediatric tonsilloadenoidectomy. Laryngoscope 97:422, 1987.
189. Mitchell RB, Pereira KD, Friedman NR, Lazar RH: Outpatient adenotonsillectomy. Is it safe in children younger than 3 years? Arch Otolaryngol Head Neck Surg 123:681, 1997.
190. Gabalski EC, Mattucci KF, Setzen M, Moleski P: Ambulatory tonsillectomy and adenoidectomy. Laryngoscope 106:77, 1996.
191. Gerber ME, O'Connor DM, Adler E, Myer CM 3rd: Selected risk factors in pediatric adenotonsillectomy. Arch Otolaryngol Head Neck Surg 122:811, 1996.
192. Schloss MD, Tan AK, Schloss B, Tewfik TL: Outpatient tonsillectomy and adenoidectomy: Complications and recommendations. Int J Pediatr Otorhinolaryngol 30:115, 1994.
193. Truy E, Merad F, Robin P, et al: Failures in outpatient tonsillectomy policy in children: A retrospective study in 311 children. Int J Pediatr Otorhinolaryngol 29:33, 1994.
194. Warren JL, Riley GF, Potosky AL, et al: Trends and outcomes of outpatient mastectomy in elderly women. J Natl Cancer Inst 90:833, 1998.
195. Morello DC, Colon GA, Fredricks S, et al: Patient safety in accredited office surgical facilities. Plast Reconstr Surg 99:1496, 1997.
196. Slogoff S, Keats AS: Does perioperative myocardial ischemia lead to postoperative myocardial infarction? Anesthesiology 62:107, 1985.

197. Bechtoldt AA: Committee on anesthesia study. Anesthetic-related deaths: 1969-1976. N C Med J 42:253, 1981.
198. Forrest WH: Outcome: The effect of the provider. *In* Hirsh RA, Forrest WH (eds): Health Care Delivery in Anesthesia. Philadelphia, George F. Stickley, 1980, p 137.
199. Silber JH, Williams SV, Krakauer H, Schwartz JS: Hospital and patient characteristics associated with death after surgery: A study of adverse occurrence and failure to rescue. Med Care 30:615, 1992.
200. Silber JH, Kennedy SK, Even-Shoshan O, et al: Anesthesiologist direction and patient outcomes. Anesthesiology 93:152, 2000.
201. Silber JH, Kennedy SK, Even-Shoshan O, et al: Anesthesiologist board certification and patient outcomes. Anesthesiology 96:1044, 2002.
202. Abenstein JP, Warner MA: Anesthesia providers, patient outcomes and costs. Anesth Analg 82:1273, 1996.
203. Brown RH, Schauble JF, Hamilton RG: Prevalence of latex allergy among anesthesiologists: Identification of sensitized but asymptomatic individuals. Anesthesiology 89:292, 1998; see comments.
204. Berry AJ, Greene ES: The risk of needlestick injuries and needlestick-transmitted diseases in the practice of anesthesiology. Anesthesiology 77:1007, 1992.
205. Denes AE, Smith JL, Maynard JE, et al: Hepatitis B infection in physicians. Results of a nationwide seroepidemiologic survey. JAMA 239:210, 1978.
206. Berry AJ, Isaacson IJ, Hunt D, Kane MA: The prevalence of hepatitis B viral markers in anesthesia personnel. Anesthesiology 60:6, 1984.
207. Berry AJ, Isaacson IJ, Kane MA, et al: A multicenter study of the prevalence of hepatitis B viral serologic markers in anesthesia personnel. Anesth Analg 63:738, 1984.
208. Henderson DK: HIV-1 in the Health Care Setting. *In* Mandell GL, Douglas RG, Bennett JE (eds): Principles and Practice of Infectious Disease, 3rd ed. New York, Churchill Livingstone, 1990, p 2221.
209. Kiyosawa K, Sodeyama T, Tanaka E, et al: Hepatitis C in hospital employees with needlestick injuries. Ann Intern Med 115:367, 1991.
210. Marcus R: CDC Cooperative Needlestick Surveillance Group: Surveillance on health care workers exposed to blood from patients infected with the human immunodeficiency virus. N Engl J Med 319:1118, 1988.
211. Busby J: Through the valley of many shadows: HIV infected physicians. Tex Med 87:36, 1991.
212. Greene ES, Berry AJ, Arnold WP 3rd, Jagger J: Percutaneous injuries in anesthesia personnel. Anesth Analg 83:273, 1996.
213. Buergler JM, Kim R, Thisted RA, et al: Risk of human immunodeficiency virus in surgeons, anesthesiologists, and medical students. Anesth Analg 75:118, 1992; see comments.
214. Practice guidelines for management of the difficult airway. A report by the American Society of Anesthesiologists Task Force on Management of the Difficult Airway. Anesthesiology 78:597, 1993.
215. Practice guidelines for pulmonary artery catheterization. A report by the American Society of Anesthesiologists Task Force on Pulmonary Artery Catheterization. Anesthesiology 78:380, 1993.
216. Practice guidelines for blood component therapy. A report by the American Society of Anesthesiologists Task Force on Blood Component Therapy. Anesthesiology 84:732, 1996.
217. Holzman RS, Cooper JB, Gaba DM, et al: Anesthesia crisis resource management: Real-life simulation training in operating room crises. J Clin Anesth 7:675, 1995.
218. Howard SK, Gaba DM, Fish KJ, et al: Anesthesia crisis resource management training: Teaching anesthesiologists to handle critical incidents. Aviat Space Environ Med 63:763, 1992.
219. Schwid HA, O'Donnell D: Anesthesiologists' management of simulated critical incidents. Anesthesiology 76:495, 1992.
220. Popp HJ, Schecke T, Rau G, et al: An interactive computer simulator of the circulation for knowledge acquisition in cardio-anesthesia. Int J Clin Monit Comput 8:151, 1991.
221. Gaba DM, DeAnda A: A comprehensive anesthesia simulation environment: Recreating the operating room for research and training. Anesthesiology 69:387, 1988.
222. Devitt JH, Kurrek MM, Cohen MM, et al: Testing the raters: Inter-rater reliability of standardized anaesthesia simulator performance. Can J Anaesth 44:924, 1997.
223. Devitt JH, Kurrek MM, Cohen MM, et al: Testing internal consistency and construct validity during evaluation of performance in a patient simulator. Anesth Analg 86:1160, 1998.
224. Pedersen T: Complications and death following anaesthesia: A prospective study with special reference to the influence of patient-, anaesthesia-, and surgery-related risk factors. Dan Med Bull 41 319, 1994.
225. Pierce EC Jr: The 34th Rovenstine Lecture: 40 years behind the mask: Safety revisited. Anesthesiology 84:965, 1996.
226. Tordiff BE, Newman MF, Saunders AM, et al: Preliminary report of a genetic basis for cognitive decline after cardiac operations. The Neurologic Outcome Research Group of the Duke Heart Center. Ann Thorac Surg 64:715, 1997.
227. Hopkins PM: Malignant hyperthermia: advances in clinical management and diagnosis. Br J Anaesth 85:118, 2000.

CHAPTER
25 Preoperative Evaluation

Michael F. Roizen

Rationale   927

The Changing Nature of Preoperative
  Evaluation   932

Uncovering Patient Factors
  That Increase the Risk of
  Anesthesia   932
  The History   933
  The Physical Examination   938

Detecting Disease: History, Physical
  Examination, and Chart Review
  Versus Laboratory Tests   939
  Laboratory Tests Are Ineffective
    Screening Devices   940
  The 2002 ASA Preoperative Testing
    Advisory   940
  Patient Risk   944
  Medicolegal Liability   944
  Operating Room Schedules   946

Preoperative and Preprocedure
  Testing   946
  The Low Predictive Value of an "Abnormal"
    Laboratory Test Result   947
  A Simplified Benefit-Risk Analysis
    of Testing   949
  Lead-Time and Length-Time Biases   950
  Laboratory Test Abnormalities in Asymptomatic
    Populations   950

Implementing Accuracy and
  Efficiency in Preoperative
  Evaluation   962
  The Danger of Underordering Tests   972

Errors Made by Physicians When
  Ordering Tests   972

Information Management in
  Preoperative and Preprocedure
  Evaluation and Outcome
  Enhancement   973
  Informatics and the Preoperative
    Evaluation   973
  Improving Patient Satisfaction with
    the Preoperative Evaluation   981

Gaining the Resources and Consensus
  to Initiate and Maintain an
  Anesthesia Preoperative and
  Preprocedure Clinic   981
  Developmental and Organizational
    Changes   982
  The Necessity for Teamwork   982
  The Economic Concerns and Benefits of
    Developing a PPAC   984
  The Strategic Need to Market the
    PPAC   985
  Renovation of Facilities   987
  Daily Operations and Procedures of
    the PPAC   987
  The Anesthesia Medical Consultation   988
  Perioperative Quality Assurance
    Indicators   988
  Cost-Effectiveness of the PPAC   988
  The Evolution of Anesthesiology   990

Summary   990

RATIONALE

The ultimate goals of preoperative and preprocedure medical assessment of patients who are to undergo anesthesia care are to reduce the morbidity of surgery, to increase the quality but decrease the cost of perioperative care, and to return the patient to desirable functioning as quickly as possible. We include preprocedure in this assessment period because anesthesia care increasingly involves rendering the patient more comfortable during procedures that do not involve classic surgery. Traditionally, these goals have been facilitated by a preoperative meeting between the patient and the anesthesiologist. The meeting now has six specific purposes:

1. To obtain pertinent information about the patient's medical history and physical and mental conditions, in

order to determine which tests and consultations are needed

2. Guided by patient choices and the risk factors uncovered by the medical history, to choose the care plans to be followed
3. To obtain informed consent
4. To educate the patient about anesthesia, perioperative care, and pain treatments in the hope of reducing anxiety and facilitating recovery
5. To make perioperative care more efficient and less expensive
6. To utilize the operative experience to motivate the patient to more optimal health and thereby improve perioperative and/or long-term outcome

Reducing the patient's anxiety and obtaining informed consent are discussed in other chapters. Most data indicate that recovery occurs more quickly when the anesthesiologist allays the patient's concerns, informs the patient about what is to come, and plans postoperative pain therapy with the patient[1-5] (also see Chapter 72). The next three functions of preoperative evaluation are closely related: the acquisition of a pertinent medical history, including information about physical and medical conditions.

No. 6 in this list—improving outcome by using interventions in a preoperative and preprocedure assessment clinic—perioperative and long-term outcome changes with aspirin, β-adrenergic receptor blocking agents, cholesterol management drugs, diet, exercise, immunization, smoking cessation, and other interventions instituted in a clinic or by a primary care physician that use the operative experience to motivate more optimal health for daily life—is relatively new: Can you change therapy now and into the immediate postoperative period and alter the perioperative outcome and/or long-term outcome? Rolled into this new function are three other questions:

Do you have enough time to initiate such that that change will make a positive outcome difference to the patient?
Do you have the time to motivate the patient to accept such?
Can you motivate the patient to initiate such?

These four questions affect the decisions about testing, consultation, and discussion of care plans with the patient and lead to patient education, setting expectations for the patient's postoperative pain therapy and recovery plan, and cost reduction, and possibly leading to a high quality of life long-term. This may impose an additional important function (some would say opportunity for the specialty and individual physician; some would say burden for the anesthesiologist) as perioperative physician motivating the patient. This function derives from the judgment and continuing data that show that a patient in optimal shape for daily living has a better perioperative and long-term outcome than one not in such shape. However, this function also requires the preoperative or preprocedure interview to be conducted earlier (days, not hours, prior to surgery) to have maximum effectiveness and places the perioperative physician into the mainstream of medical care. As medicine has evolved, perhaps nowhere has the mutation demanded of physicians been greater than in perioperative care.

Thus, major functions of preoperative and preprocedure evaluation—optimizing patient health before surgery and/or planning the most appropriate perioperative management—improve perioperative and long-term outcome—reduce perioperative costs. Data supporting this claim are substantial, but indirect; studies of perioperative morbidity over five decades repeatedly show that preoperative patient conditions and perioperative optimization of care are significant predictors of postoperative morbidity.[6-70] Specifically, less severe manifestations of adverse preoperative conditions are associated with lower perioperative morbidity and mortality (Table 25-1 and Fig. 25-1).

These data strongly imply (some would say *prove*) that preoperative treatment or alteration of such conditions and habits such as congestive heart failure, diabetes, cardiovascular demand reduction, blood vessel inflammation, physical inactivity, and smoking, to name only a few, can reduce the severity of disease, improve patient quality of life and functioning, and thus reduce perioperative morbidity and mortality. Moreover such changes have been shown to improve longer-term quality of life

Table 25–1   Mortality risk for elective surgery, determined for various degrees of coexisting disease

Preoperative Condition	Overall Clinical Assessment of Patient				
	Good	Minor Impairment	Major Impairment	Poor	Moribund*
Impairment of general health by disease requiring surgery	1.9	1.4	4.9	21.5	52.6
Ischemic heart disease	1.1	1.6	4.3	40.1	56.3
Chronic lower respiratory tract infection	2.0	0.9	3.7	19.8	66.7
Cardiac failure	5.3	4.1	7.5	20.8	28.6
Obesity	0.3	0.3	2.2	14.6	50.0
Impaired renal function	1.4	2.8	4.4	22.5	50.0
Diabetes	1.3	1.6	5.8	14.9	—
No preoperative condition	0.2	0.7	3.5	16.1	50.0

*Mortality figures for this group were based on small numbers for each condition.
Modified from Fowkes FGR, Lunn JN, Farrow SC, et al: Epidemiology in anaesthesia. III: Mortality risk in patients with coexisting physical disease. Br J Anaesth 54:819, 1982.

Hospital Mortality
Age (yr)

Preoperative disease
and surgery

	<50	50-69	≥70

Chronic heart failure — <50: 0.1% / 0.5%; 50-69: 0.4% / 2%; ≥70: 0.8% / 4%

Renal failure — <50: 0.2% / 1%; 50-69: 0.9% / 2%; ≥70: 2% / 9%

Abdominal surgery — <50: 0.3% / 2%; 50-69: 1% / 6%; ≥70: 3% / 12%

Chronic heart failure and renal failure — <50: 0.7% / 3%; 50-69: 3% / 13%; ≥70: 6% / 24%

Chronic heart failure and abdominal surgery — <50: 0.9% / 4%; 50-69: 4% / 17%; ≥70: 7% / 30%

Renal failure and abdominal surgery — <50: 2% / 8%; 50-69: 2% / 32%; ≥70: 16% / 50%

Chronic heart failure, renal failure, and abdominal surgery — <50: 6% / 26%; 50-69: 22% / 60%; ≥70: 37% / 76%

Figure 25–1 Estimated risk of hospital mortality in relation to age, preoperative disease, and surgery. Elective surgery, *top triangles*; emergency surgery, *bottom triangles*. (From Pedersen T, Eliasen K, Henriksen E: A prospective study of mortality associated with anaesthesia and surgery: Risk indicators of mortality in hospital. Acta Anaesthesiol Scand 34:176, 1990.)

and outcome. For this to occur, preoperative and preprocedure assessment must be accomplished far enough in advance to give the physician a "second opinion" that guides therapy and consultations toward optimizing the preoperative health status of the patient. This step obliges the preoperative evaluator to take a thorough history and to determine the extent of consultation with the primary care physician that is needed to judge optimal health and the potential for improvement of preoperative status.

Preoperative consultations may initiate additional risk-modification tactics, such as reducing tachycardia[5] or the stress on plaque,[31-42] controlling hypertension,[51-53] perioperative cessation of smoking,[54-57] nutritional fortification,[60,61] immunization,[62] reducing inflammation in blood vessels,[43-48] and stamina/strength training,[63-70] and in this way may improve perioperative outcome. Preoperative evaluation produces other benefits as well. Patient education about perioperative care expectations can radically reduce the length of stay and costs (Table 25-2) and, as previously mentioned, substantially improve quality of life.

Can this process of preoperative assessment be accomplished in isolation by a primary care physician or internist? Although much of the process probably could be, a condition considered "optimal for daily life" (e.g., some degree of prerenal azotemia in the patient with congestive heart failure) may not be "optimal preoperative status" (at which time vasodilation may cause hypotension or permanent renal impairment or both). Furthermore, the process of preoperative evaluation and risk factor modification requires a broad knowledge of the *content* of scientific perioperative care and a deep understanding of the *context* in which that knowledge is applied. Understanding the context—the environmental, sociological, ethical, and team concepts and the economic influences—of perioperative care is almost as important as the technical knowledge upon which the practice of perioperative care rests. Thus, compulsive attention to the effects of planned perioperative maneuvers on patient physiology would be desirable—perhaps even necessary—if the benefit of such preplanning is deemed worth the cost. Furthermore, the perioperative time presents a more meaningful period to

Table 25–2 The benefits of combining changes in pain therapy with preoperative education of the patient regarding perioperative expectations, as shown for three clinical pathways*

	Clinical Pathways		
	#1 ("Standard") (n = 117)	#2 (n = 142)	#3 (n = 46)
Operating room time (h)	4.9 ± 1.2	3.7 ± 0.4	3.7 ± 0.4
Blood loss (mL)	1,948 ± 740	1,240 ± 527	1,147 ± 510
Length of stay (days)	4.6 ± 1.2	1.7 ± 0.6	1.12 ± 0.3
Hospital cost	$21,870	$14,206	$12,886
Satisfaction with pain therapy (% of patients)	86.7%	94%	97.5%
Overall satisfaction (% of patients)	90%	90.5%	92%
Readmission rate	2.4%	2%	0?%

*Preoperative education of the surgical patient about perioperative expectations, coupled with changes in pain therapy, can radically reduce the length of stay and costs without loss of patient satisfaction. Pathway #1 = data collected before preoperative education and changes in pain therapy; pathway #2 = data collected after education and the first change in pain therapy; pathway #3 = data collected after education and further refinement in pain therapy.
Modified from Worwag E, Chodak GFW: Overnight hospitalization after radical prostatectomy: The impact of two clinical pathways on patient satisfaction, length of hospitalization, and morbidity. Anesth Analg 87:62, 1998, with permission.

many patients that allows motivation to make changes in therapy or behavior that many patients do not make at less meaningful times.

Preoperative evaluation by a physician is not inexpensive. However, later sections of this chapter show how preoperative planning can be much less expensive than current practices because of the ability to order tests selectively and to use education and information tools to increase efficiency, to shorten the length of stay, to reduce the rate of cancellations, and to increase patient satisfaction. In addition, preoperative assessment can uncover hidden conditions that could cause problems both during and after surgery. In this way, the anesthesiologist is able to anticipate problems and plan therapy intended to prevent or minimize the effects of such problems.[5,18,31-70]

A study at the University of Florida found that preanesthetic evaluations provided information leading to changes in care plans for more than 15% of all healthy patients (i.e., American Society of Anesthesiologists [ASA] physical status I and II patients), and for 20% of all patients in general.[24] Care plans were changed because of information from observation and history: the most common conditions causing changes were gastric reflux, insulin-dependent diabetes mellitus, asthma, and suspected difficult intubation (Table 25-3). However, the data did not indicate that these changes improved patient outcome. Nevertheless, practitioners seem to believe that the discovery of these conditions calls for a change in plans, which is usually implemented in a way that delays operating room (OR) schedules and increases costs. Examples of last-minute changes are administration of an H_2-blocker 1 to 2 hours before, a β-blocker 1 hour before, and an oral antacid immediately before entry to the OR; the obtaining of equipment to measure blood glucose levels; the obtaining of a history of the patient's diabetic course and treatment from the primary care doctor as well as from the patient; the performance of fiberoptic laryngoscopy; or additional skilled help. Thus, even if preoperative evaluation were not to alter outcome to any great degree,

its ability to reduce costs by reducing laboratory tests and delays in obtaining equipment or treatments perceived to be beneficial (and medicolegally required) would be substantial and would warrant its use.

Data from Stanford,[25,26] the University of Chicago,[5,67-69] the University of South Florida,[27] the University of Rochester,[28] the University of Massachusetts,[29] and community hospitals in London, Ontario,[30] and in Australia[68,69] and elsewhere[39-48] confirm these cost and outcome advantages. Furthermore, a negative history and physical examination can lead to decreased resource utilization for healthy patients[23] and for those with comorbid conditions but without risk factors requiring high intensity care.[74] In addition, preoperative evaluation gives practitioners confidence that they will not be surprised by unexpected patient conditions and gives patients confidence that the health care system is responding to their individual conditions and is focused on their well-being in the perioperative period and beyond.

In the beginning, the preoperative assessment described above relied only on accurate history-taking and physical examination. In the 1960s, multiphasic screening laboratory tests were added to the process. This chapter evaluates the goals of preoperative medical assessment and the *relative* importance of history-taking, physical examination, and laboratory testing regarding the improvement of perioperative outcome but then goes beyond these knowledge-based steps.

Beginning with the first edition of *Anesthesia* in 1981, I have attempted to describe not only current practices but also the need for innovative change. In the first edition (before the use of diagnosis-related groups [DRGs] to establish fees, and before that cost-based push to reduce testing), I discussed the lack of benefit from nonselective laboratory testing. In the second edition (1986), I described how cost-benefit and benefit-risk analyses again pointed to the need to reduce the amount of laboratory testing. The third edition (1991) also came to a nontraditional conclusion: we needed to change the way we usually

Table 25-3   Medical problems discovered on preanesthetic evaluation that could prompt a change in patient management

History Point	Concern/Area to Evaluate	Anesthesia Plans That May Require Extra Time
Airway perceived as difficult to intubate	Head, eyes, ears, nose, throat: airway; prior anesthesia outcomes	Obtain fiberoptic equipment; obtain skilled help
Asthma	Pulmonary disease	Optimize therapy; use bronchodilators; possibly extubate during deep anesthesia
Diabetes, insulin-dependent	Endocrine, metabolic, diabetes	Discuss insulin management with patient and primary care doctor; monitor blood glucose intraoperatively; determine presence of autonomic neuropathy and plan management appropriately, such as administration of metoclopramide and PACU or ICU stay
Drug abuse	Social history	Consider HIV testing; prescribe medications to avoid withdrawal symptoms in perioperative period
Gastroesophageal reflux or hiatus hernia	Gastrointestinal disease: hiatus hernia	Administer H_2 antagonists or oral antacids and use rapid-sequence induction of anesthesia; or use awake intubation techniques and obtain appropriate equipment
Heart disease: valve disease, risk of subacute bacterial endocarditis	Antibiotic prophylaxis	Arrange for antibiotic administration 1 h prior to surgery
Malignant hyperthermia history, family history, or suspected potential history	Prior anesthetic/surgical history	Obtain clean anesthesia machine; use appropriate technique and precautions; have agents to treat malignant hyperthermia available
Monoamine oxidase inhibitors	CNS: psychiatric/medication	Discontinue therapy preoperatively if patient is not suicidal; plan for perioperative pain therapy
Pacemaker or automatic implantable cardiac defibrillator	Cardiovascular disease: electrocardiogram	Evaluate cause of pacemaker implementation; obtain repolarizing equipment or magnet; use electrocautery with altered position; use bipolar electrocautery
Peripheral motor neuropathy	CNS disease: neurologic deficit	Avoid depolarizing muscle relaxants
Pregnancy or uncertain pregnancy status	Genitourinary: pregnancy	Monitor fetal heart rate; use oral antacids; adjust induction of anesthesia; determine status of pregnancy
Pulmonary tuberculosis	Pulmonary disease: tuberculosis	Use disposable breathing circuit or clean equipment; ensure adequate treatment of patient prior to surgery
Renal insufficiency	Genitourinary disease	Monitor fluid status intraoperatively

CNS, central nervous system; HIV, human immunodificiency virus; ICU, intensive care unit; PACU, postanesthetic care unit.
The database format presented is one maintained at the University of Chicago, but it is modeled after one described by the University of Florida and is modified from data from Gibby GL, Gravenstein JS, Layon AJ, Jackson KI: How often does the preoperative interview change anesthetic management? [abstract]. Anesthesiology 77:A1134,1992.

perform preoperative evaluation. The fourth edition of this chapter again suggested a major break with current practice: unless we instituted a system of performing careful preoperative evaluations on all patients, we were in danger of doing too little assessment and even too little testing. In some areas of the United States, the pendulum may have swung too far to the "no-test" and "cursory-assessment" side.

Not surprisingly, in the fifth edition (1999), this chapter accentuated the need to develop consensus in making a preoperative clinic effective for all and to implement an effective electronic information system ("informatics") process. It also emphasized the dramatic benefits of instituting a functional preoperative clinic that has gone

through the stages of efficient patient evaluation, appropriate test selection, and effective prerequisite education of the patient and that is organized in such a way that patient satisfaction is increased. The importance and benefits of adding *patient education* to these processes was also highlighted, as were the information services that make the process more efficient for all caregivers as well as for the patient. I now emphasize the metamorphosis of preoperative evaluation into a period that can motivate a higher quality of life and thereby improve long-term as well as immediate outcome.

I believe that just as the practice of anesthesia has changed during the past decade, the practice of preoperative evaluation also needs to change to ensure that the best cost-benefit and benefit-risk goals are attained. Specifically, data indicate that we can produce optimal cost-benefit and benefit-risk strategies for perioperative care only when we reduce testing to that indicated by history-taking and when we institute effective patient education informed by appropriate choices for pain therapy. Outcome can be improved, patient satisfaction increased, and hospital stays shortened appropriately when the patient is educated intensively about pain therapy and recovery in the preoperative clinic. In this way, cardiovascular stress reduction, inflammation treatment, diet, physical activity, and tobacco habits can be changed to improve outcome.

The difficulty is that we must obtain a thorough history far enough in advance to allow us to perform selected tests and to implement the necessary therapies and motivational strategies without disrupting surgical schedules and the patient's perioperative care plans. This must also be done far enough in advance to give the patient and his or her significant others time to plan for the options that have been selected.

THE CHANGING NATURE OF PREOPERATIVE EVALUATION

Preoperative evaluation strives to answer three questions: Is the patient in optimal health? Can, or should, the patient's physical or mental condition be improved before surgery? Does the patient have any health problems or use any medications that could unexpectedly influence perioperative events? Such an evaluation must include the long-accepted standard practices: review of hospital chart(s) and prior anesthesia records, consultation with the primary care physician, history-taking, physical examination, evaluation of laboratory tests obtained, ordering of additional laboratory tests, and discussion of perioperative anesthesia plans (including alternatives for intraoperative and postoperative analgesia) with the patient in a way that provides accurate information and reduces patient anxiety. However, the practice of medicine has changed. The cost-conscious and outcome-focused environment of the 2000s has made it difficult for anesthesiologists to achieve these goals using the style of the 1980s and earlier.

For example, the increased need to minimize costs means fewer or no preoperative hospital days for the patient. More than 65% of all operations are performed on an outpatient basis, almost 10% in the surgeon's office, and another 20% to 30% as morning admissions. Unfortunately, the increasing age of patients often means a greater likelihood of concurrent disease. Unlike the old days, when the entire evening before surgery could be spent learning about the medically complex patient, anesthesiologists are now being asked to perform preoperative evaluation as they "run" from case to case. They are being asked to deliver more for less and at the same time to meet the continuing demand of administrators and surgeons to shorten turnover times. In such time-pressured situations, the anesthesiologist may be justifiably uncomfortable about the adequacy and comprehensiveness of his or her preoperative evaluation. Did I remember to ask the patient whether he or she had a drink during the past 72 hours, or whether he or she has ever had a problem with drinking?

(These are currently the two most sensitive and specific questions to ask when trying to determine the likelihood of alcoholism.[75,76]) Did I forget to ask other questions—for example, whether any family members had hepatitis?

It is very difficult to make an adequate preoperative evaluation in 5 to 15 minutes, and it is impossible to change any therapy or optimize any care that requires more than 10 minutes without increasing costs and inconveniencing all concerned. Furthermore, the pressure to proceed, even when there may be increased or unknown risk, is much greater when time is short than when such evaluations are done in advance. Frequently, old records are not available.[77,78] Also, the pressure to proceed quickly probably makes the consent process less informed and the discussion of anxiety relief and preoperative pain therapy plans less thorough. Also, the patient and significant others have little or no time to "digest" information about what to expect regarding the perioperative care plan.

Do we need to change our system? Clearly, a change is needed if preoperative assessment is to be adequate, and more so if anesthesiology as a specialty is to continue to lead the movement fostering patient safety, optimizing perioperative outcome, and motivating a higher quality of life with fewer health care costs. To perform these assessments efficiently, the anesthesiologist needs to know about the patient, to educate the patient, and to motivate the patient.

Preoperative evaluation is intrinsically valuable, and interacting with the patient in this way is an enjoyable and productive part of the practice of anesthesia and can continue to make anesthesia a specialty integral to and valuable for the health of the nation and of the individual patient. Also, for the practical-minded, inadequate preoperative assessment is now one of the top three causes of lawsuits against anesthesiologists. Nevertheless, in the current atmosphere, there is not enough time to assess the patient preoperatively using traditional methods. Before suggesting solutions to this problem, this chapter will evaluate the importance of preoperative assessment, as well as the conditions that may be sought and determined from such assessment.

UNCOVERING PATIENT FACTORS THAT INCREASE THE RISK OF ANESTHESIA

This chapter provides information the anesthesiologist needs to know to ensure that his or her patient is asymptomatic from the standpoint of anesthetic risk. The management of patients found to be symptomatic is discussed in Chapter 27. Ensuring that the patient is asymptomatic requires knowledge of the patient factors that increase the perioperative risk of anesthesia, because it is those factors that must be eliminated.

Major surgery usually represents a tremendous assault on the human organism. The body has an elaborate defense mechanism that alerts it to, and helps it escape from, trauma. The job of the anesthesiologist is *not* simply to put the patient to sleep and to wake him or her when surgery is over, but to maintain homeostasis during the assault of surgery and to provide pain relief to blunt the effects after the assault. To do this, the anesthesiologist must interfere with the stress response induced by pain, anticipate periods when the stress response will not be present, plan for the rare situations in which the patient's medical problems may occur acutely, and, at the same time, manage any chronic medical conditions.

Even when the stress of surgery is not felt consciously, it evokes a complex physiologic response. Much of this response is meant to allow the body to escape trauma. For example, blood flow is diverted from the kidney and liver to the heart and head, and blood pressure rises. Thus, the system most needed to be in a "good" state of health, the cardiovascular system, has first priority.[9,18-22] Elaborate and simple tests and history-taking processes have evolved to evaluate the cardiovascular system, especially in aged patients or patients with comorbid disease.[58,59,79-81] We will evaluate the process of history-taking first.

The History

Unfortunately, illnesses in systems other than the cardiovascular have an effect on perioperative risk. The following is a list of relatively common conditions we ensure are not present before assuming that the patient is asymptomatic.[24,82,83] Chapters 24 and 27 discuss the increased risk posed by the problems discovered, and Chapter 27 describes optimization of the patient's physical condition, anticipation of potential problems, and possible therapies for the problems, and deals with managing drug regimens prior to procedures and surgery. The evaluation process that follows represents our initial screening procedure for disease. Although the process attempts to be relatively inclusive, it cannot cover all possible conditions that might be encountered when dealing with surgical patients.

First Areas of Concern and the Rule of Threes

The rule of threes indicates that three aspects of acute history, three aspects of chronic history, and three aspects of physical examination make a difference to perioperative outcome. The three aspects of acute history are:
1. Exercise tolerance
2. History of present illness and its treatments
3. When the patient last visited with her or his primary care physician

The three aspects of chronic history are:
1. Medications and causes for their use and allergies
2. Social history including drug, alcohol, and tobacco use and cessation
3. Family history and history of prior illnesses and operations

The three aspects of physical examination are:
1. Airway
2. Cardiovascular
3. Lung, plus those aspects specific to the patient's condition or planned procedure, such as a sensory nerve examination if a regional block is planned (more about physical examination later).

Included first in the history are general items, such as whether the patient has received recent medical care, or whether the patient has received recent medical care, or

has taken medication, or has allergies. (See Table 25-2 for an example of how such information is obtained from a patient when the institution does not use a computerized medical record.) Questions also are asked about prior exposure to anesthetics and subsequent problems:

When did you last have anesthesia?
Do you have any problems with anesthesia? Have any of your family members had any problems with anesthesia?
Do you have allergies?
What are you allergic to?
Have you had any blood tests in the last 6 months?
Have you had a chest x-ray in the last 2 months?
Have you had an electrocardiogram (ECG) in the last 2 months?
Has your stool been checked for blood or have you had a colonoscopy, etc., in the last year?
Have you been a patient in a hospital, an emergency department, or an outpatient surgery center in the last 2 years? If so, why? What part of the hospital (for example, critical care unit)? How long were you there?
Do you take any medications?
What medications do you take?
Do you take any medications not prescribed by your doctor, that you purchase through the internet or from a shelf at a drugstore, health food store, or grocery store?
Do you take any supplements or vitamins or minerals? (These can interact substantially with perioperative medications.)[84-87]

Also included in this category of questions are items about artificial devices (e.g., hearing aids, false eyes) and use of alcohol:

Do you wear contact lenses?
Do you currently use eye drops prescribed by a doctor?
When did you have an alcoholic drink?
Have you ever had a drinking problem?

Because patients tend to give socially acceptable answers on sensitive subjects (Trigg DJ et al, unpublished data),[88] when probing in these types of areas a checklist or computer-aided history may be more valid than an interview. Sensitive subjects include risk factors for use of illegal drugs and for human immunodeficiency virus (HIV) infection. Nevertheless, the personal interview is essential for in-depth questioning.

Cardiovascular Disease

Most important is to determine the patient's cardiovascular reserve.[58,59,65-70,79-81] To do this, you can ask about the maximum amount the patient can walk or the greatest number of floors she or he can climb without the need to stop, or you can determine an ejection fraction from prior testing or the patient's record during stress testing. The ability to do 4 metabolic equivalents (METs) of exercise,[58-59,65] the equivalent of walking 5 city blocks or climbing two flights of stairs at a reasonable rate without having to stop (Table 25-4) correlates in multiple studies with better perioperative outcome[58,59,65-70,78-81]

We try to ensure that the patient does not have the following cardiovascular conditions: congestive heart failure, cardiomyopathies, ischemic heart disease (stable or unstable), valvular or subvalvular heart disease, hypertension (diastolic or systolic[37]), disturbances in cardiac rhythm, pericarditis, arteritis, or other manifestations of atherosclerosis.

Table 25–4 Estimated energy requirements for various activities*

Metabolic Equivalents (METs)	Activity
1 MET	Can you take care of yourself?
	Can you eat, dress, and use the toilet?
	Can you walk indoors around the house?
	Can you walk a block or two on level ground at 2 to 3 mph (3.2 to 4.8 km/h)?
4 METs	Can you climb a flight of stairs or walk up a hill?
	Can you walk on level ground at 4 mph (6.4 km/h)?
	Can you run a short distance?
	Can you do heavy work around the house such as scrubbing floors or moving heavy furniture?
	Can you participate in moderate recreational activities such as golfing, bowling, dancing, doubles tennis, or throwing a baseball or football?
10 METs	Can you participate in strenuous sports such as swimming, singles tennis, football, basketball, or skiing?

*Adapted from the Duke Activity Status Index and the American Heart Association Exercise Standards.
From Eagle KA, Berger PB, Calkins H, et al: ACC/AHA guideline update for perioperative cardiovascular evaluation for noncardiac surgery—executive summary: A report of the American College of Cardiology/American Heart Association Task Force on Practice Guidelines (Committee to Update the 1996 Guidelines on Perioperative Cardiovascular Evaluation for Noncardiac Surgery). J Am Coll Cardiol 39:542, 2002.

These conditions require further evaluation to make sure that optimal treatment has been achieved before surgery (see Chapter 27). In the outcome studies described previously, congestive heart failure incurred the highest risk.[6-22]

Questions should not be limited to the cardiovascular system. For example, to search for alcoholic cardiomyopathy, the following inquiries are made:
Have you had a drink in the last 72 hours?
Have you ever had a problem with drinking?

As mentioned previously, these two questions are the most sensitive and specific questions to ask when trying to determine the possibility of alcoholism.[75,76]

Exercise tolerance should also be checked—for example, the patient's ability to walk up stairs, play sports, and perform chores (mowing lawns, making beds, vacuuming), without becoming short of breath.

Typical questions regarding the cardiovascular system include the following:
What is the most vigorous activity you've done in the last 3 weeks?
How far have you walked in the last week without stopping?
Can you walk a block without stopping? When did you last do so?
Can you walk 4 blocks without stopping? When did you last do so?
Have you ever awakened and felt short of breath?
Do you become short of breath after climbing a flight of stairs or after walking a short distance?
When did you last climb a flight of stairs?
Are you able to walk up stairs at the same rate as 5 years ago?
Can you climb 2 flights of stairs without stopping? When did you last do so?
Have you ever had a heart attack, or have you ever been treated for a possible heart attack?
Do you have heart problems such as skipped heart beats, angina, or chest pain?
Have you been told that you have a heart murmur or rheumatic fever?

Have you ever been told that you have mitral valve prolapse?
Have you ever had heart or lung surgery?
Do your ankles ever swell?
Are you ever short of breath? When?
Do you ever have chest pains, angina, chest heaviness, or chest tightness?
Do you ever have indigestion that does *not* occur after overeating?
Have you ever been told by your doctor to exercise or diet to control high blood pressure?
Have you ever been a patient in a critical care unit (cardiac care unit, intensive coronary care unit)?
Have you passed out or nearly passed out in the last year? Why?[89]
Do you sleep with more than one pillow at night? (This question is useful only for men and women over age 60, as 50% of younger women sleep with two pillows [Trigg DJ et al, unpublished data][88].)
Do you currently take water pills or diuretics?
Do you take medication for high blood pressure or medication to prevent high blood pressure?
Do you currently take potassium pills or powder?
Do you currently take anticoagulants or blood-thinning medicine?
Have you ever been told to take, or have you ever been given, antibiotics before routine dental work?

Sometimes these questions are asked in a different order, so that the patient is not startled or confused by them, as if they were a "pop quiz." To avoid surprising or confusing the patient, questions are asked in a "set." For instance, all questions related to medication are asked at the same time.

Respiratory and Airway Problems
Because airway problems cause substantial risk, the most important consideration regarding the respiratory system is securing the airway (also see Chapters 17 and 42). Therefore, evidence of airway obstruction and restriction

of neck and jaw movement is sought. The end result of exposure to toxins (whether environmental or related to smoking) is also sought: emphysema, bronchitis, and chronic infections. We try to ensure that asthma is not present and that other conditions, such as obesity, have not progressed to the point of limiting respiratory function or causing sleep apnea.[90-94]

The personal interview (no matter when performed) is usually quite efficient in revealing the condition of the airway, respiratory reserve, and the possible need for laboratory evaluation, such as pulmonary function testing with bronchodilators or blood gas analysis or both. Questioning the partner (if present) of those who snore or who have daytime somnolence can alert one to the probability of sleep apnea. While the presence of undiagnosed sleep apnea increases postoperative risk, we do not yet know appropriate interventions or benefit-risk strategies to gain more definitive diagnosis of such in a preoperative meeting. It is probable, although there are no data confirming this, that preoperative screening for sleep apnea in obese men over age 50 and in women over age 60 who snore and have daytime somnolence will prove to provide an outcome benefit.

The personal interview may also be the best time to educate the patient and family members about the time needed for cessation of smoking (and other use of tobacco products) in order to be beneficial (see Chapter 27).[54-57]

Questions that usually elicit information about the general condition of the mouth and airway and possible reactions to anesthesia include the following:

Do you wear dentures, a crown, a partial, or a bridge?

Are any of your teeth loose, cracked, chipped, or capped?

Have you ever had anesthesia?

Have you or any blood relative ever had any problems with anesthesia? (This question not only helps reveal possible airway problems but also elicits information about some rarer diseases, such as malignant hyperthermia, glucose-6-phosphate dehydrogenase [G6PD] deficiency, acute porphyria, allergies, sickle cell disease, neurologic disorders, and hiatus hernia. It usually also elicits concerns about postoperative nausea and vomiting and thus provides an opportunity to reassure the patient, to plan the choice of anesthetic, to ask female patients about their last menstrual period, and to use preanesthetic suggestion, for those physicians believing in the value of this practice.)

Can you open your mouth fully?

Do your joints ever click, pop, or hurt?

Have you ever been treated for a problem of the jaw joint (that is, a temporomandibular joint [TMJ] problem)?

Have you ever been hoarse for more than 1 month?

Do you snore, or do others say you snore? (This question proved to be the best predictor of difficult intubation when our computer-based health history was compared with outcome studies[48] but was not very specific [four of five patients who answered yes to this question did not have a difficult intubation].)

Do you ever fall asleep in the daytime? Have you ever had a near-miss car accident because you almost fell asleep in the daytime? Was this not after a period of intentional sleep deprivation? How often?

Have you gained weight recently? (A 10% weight gain increases the number of apneic episodes by 30%.[95])

Have you ever had cancer?

Have you ever had, or been treated for, arthritis?

Do you have neck stiffness or problems moving your head?

Have you ever been told you had diphtheria? (Diphtheria can cause narrowing of the airway.)

The following questions search for lung disease:

Have you ever had pneumonia? When?

Have you ever undergone lung surgery?

Do you have shortness of breath, wheezing, chest pain, bronchitis, asthma, or emphysema?

Do you cough regularly or frequently?

Do you cough up mucus (sputum or phlegm)?

In the last 4 weeks, have you had a fever, chills, cold, or flu?

Do you smoke or have you ever smoked? When did you stop?

Do you use spit or chew tobacco?

Have you ever smoked half a pack or more of cigarettes a day on a regular basis?

Have you ever smoked a pipe or cigars on a regular basis?

Hepatic and Gastrointestinal Disease

Past and present hepatic disease increases the risk of certain surgical procedures (see Chapter 27), sometimes contributes to abnormal clotting and pharmacokinetics, and may present medicolegal concerns (e.g., in the case of postanesthetic jaundice). Hepatic disease also increases the risk of surgery for nonhepatic problems (see Chapter 27).

Gastrointestinal diseases may increase the potential for aspiration of gastric contents. For example, the gastroparesis of ulcer disease is often accompanied by solid food in the stomach, and inflammatory bowel disease may be accompanied by arthritis in the neck. Gastrointestinal disease also increases the potential for dehydration, electrolyte disturbances, and anemia. The presence of gastrointestinal or hepatic disease can give clues about possible endocrine, pulmonary or cardiac disease (e.g., gastritis in the alcoholic patient could indicate alcoholic cardiomyopathy).

Questions that screen for gastrointestinal or hepatic disease include the following:

Have you ever been diagnosed as having a hiatus hernia?

Have you ever had hepatitis, yellow jaundice, liver disease, or malaria?

Have you ever had gallstones or gallbladder disease?

Are your stools ever bloody or black and tarry?

Have you seen bright red blood on your stool or on toilet tissue after wiping?

Have your bowel habits changed this year?

Do you often have diarrhea?

Have you ever vomited blood or material that looks like coffee grounds in the last 6 months?

Do you have frequent nausea or vomiting?

Have you lost weight this year without trying?

Has your appetite for food changed in the last year?

Are you eating the same foods you ate a year ago?

Have you had heartburn within the last month?

Are you now being treated, or have you been treated, for ulcer disease?

Are you currently taking antacids such as Tagamet (cimetidine), Zantac (ranitidine), Pepcid (famotidine), Prilosec (omeprazole), AcipHex (rabeprazole), or Axid (nizatidine)?

Patient's Name _____ Age _____ Sex _____

Planned Operation _____ Date of Surgery _____

Surgeon _____ Primary Doctor _____ Here before: ☐ Yes ☐ No

Cardiologist? _____ When last seen _____ Is your cardiologist at this institution? ☐ Yes ☐ No

Your height _____ Your weight: _____ Your weight at age 21: _____

1. Please list **ALL OPERATIONS** (and approximate dates)

a. _____ d. _____

b. _____ e. _____

c. _____ f. _____

2. Please list any **ALLERGIES** to medicines, latex or other (and your reaction to it)

a. _____ c. _____

b. _____ d. _____

3. Please list **ALL MEDICATIONS** you have taken in the last month (include OVER THE COUNTER drugs, inhalers, herbals, dietary supplements, vitamins, and aspirin)

Name of Drug	**Dose & Frequency**	**Name of Drug**	**Dose & Frequency**
a.		f.	
b.		g.	
c.		h.	
d.		i.	
e.		j.	

(Please check YES or NO and circle specific problems)   YES   NO

4. Have you taken steroids (prednisone or cortisone) in the last year? ☐ ☐

5. Have you ever smoked? (quantify in _____ packs/day for _____ years) ☐ ☐

     Do you still smoke? ☐ ☐

     Do you drink alcohol? (if so, when was your last drink? _____) ☐ ☐

       If so, have you ever had a problem drinking? ☐ ☐

     Do you use any illegal drugs? ☐ ☐

6. Can you walk up TWO flights of stairs without stopping? ☐ ☐

7. When did you last walk up two flights of stairs _____ or walk 6 blocks without stopping _____ ?

8. Have you had any problems with your heart? **(circle)** (chest pain or pressure, heart attacks, abnormal EKG, skipped beats, heart murmur, palpitation, heart failure {fluid in the lungs}, require antibiotics before routine dental care) ☐ ☐

9. Do you have or have you ever had high blood pressure? ☐ ☐

10. Have you had any problems with your lungs or your chest? **(circle)** (shortness of breath, emphysema, bronchitis, asthma, TB, abnormal chest x-ray) ☐ ☐

11. Are you ill or were you recently ill with a cold, fever, chills, flu or productive cough? ☐ ☐

     Describe recent changes

12. Have you or anyone in your family had serious bleeding problems? **(circle)** (prolonged bleeding from nosebleed, gums, tooth extractions, or surgery) ☐ ☐

13. Have you had any problems with your blood (anemia, leukemia, sickle cell disease, blood clots, transfusions)? If yes, when ☐ ☐

14. Have you ever had problems with your: **(circle)** ☐ ☐

     Liver (cirrhosis, hepatitis, jaundice)? ☐ ☐

     Kidney (stones, failure, dialysis)? ☐ ☐

     Digestive system (frequent heartburn, hiatus hernia, stomach ulcer)? ☐ ☐

     Back, neck or jaws (TMJ, rheumatoid arthritis)? ☐ ☐

Figure 25–2 Preoperative and Preprocedure Assessment Clinic (PPAC) Form 4: Patient preoperative and preprocedure history.

(Continued)

(Please check YES or NO and circle specific problems)   YES   NO

15.   Have you ever had: **(circle)**

      Seizures, epilepsy, or fits?

      Stroke, facial, leg or arm weakness, difficulty speaking?

      Cramping pain in your legs with walking?

      Problems with hearing, vision or memory?

16.   Have you ever been treated for cancer with chemotherapy or radiation therapy? **(circle)**

17.   Women: could you possibly (even remotely) be pregnant?

      Last menstrual period began:

18.   Have you ever had problems with anesthesia or surgery? **(circle)** (severe nausea or vomiting,

      malignant hyperthermia (in blood relatives or self), prolonged drowsiness, anxiety, breathing

      difficulties)

19.   Do you have any chipped or loose teeth, dentures, caps, bridgework, braces, problems

      opening your mouth, swallowing or choking? **(circle)**

20.   Do your physical abilities limit your daily activities?

21.   Do you snore?

22.   Please list any medical illnesses not noted above:

_____

_____

23.   Additional comments/questions for nurse or anesthesiologist

_____

_____

_____

Figure 25–2—cont'd

Bleeding Problems

Bleeding can occur because of a hereditary deficiency of clotting factors or because of abnormal platelet or vascular function caused by disease or drugs. The following questions search for such abnormalities:

Have you ever had a blood problem such as anemia or leukemia?

Have you ever had a problem with blood clotting?

Have you ever had a serious bleeding problem?

Have you received a blood transfusion since 1979?

Do you use any medications such as aspirin or vitamins such as vitamin E or supplements such as ginseng or garlic known to affect blood clotting? How much? How often? When did you last use such?

These questions are often asked in two ways, as patients seem to need time to recall such events. For example:

Has a family member or blood relative ever had a serious bleeding problem?

Have you ever had prolonged or unusual bleeding from cuts, nosebleeds, minor bruises, tooth extractions, or surgery?

Have you ever had excessive bleeding that required blood transfusion?

Renal Disease

Renal disease can contribute to bleeding because of a functional platelet deficit associated with renal impairment (see Chapter 27). In addition, renal insufficiency can increase risk because it produces anemia (prior to, or in the absence of, optimal erythropoietin therapy, which might be considered preoperatively to decrease transfusion need and to improve functional recovery (see Chapter 27), electrolyte disturbances, peripheral neuropathy, and abnormalities in drug metabolism and excretion. The following questions search for renal disease:

Have you ever had any kidney problem?

Have you ever had kidney failure, dialysis, or more than two kidney infections?

Have you ever had kidney stones?

Are you undergoing dialysis for kidney problems?

Have you had changes in bowel or bladder function in the last year?

Has your appetite for food changed in the last year? (Voluntary avoidance of foods having a high protein content is a subtle sign of renal disease.)

Endocrine Disturbances

Endocrine disturbances and the end-organ effects of diabetes or thyroid, parathyroid, pituitary, adrenal (and carcinoid) disease can increase perioperative risk substantially. For instance, morbidity and mortality increase 5- to 10-fold because of the nephropathy and autonomic insufficiency of diabetes (see Chapter 27). The following questions help ensure the patient does not have endocrine-related diseases:

Do you wake up at night to urinate? How often?

Have you ever been told that you have diabetes or sugar diabetes?

Do you take, or have you taken steroids, cortisone, muscle-building supplements or steroids, or DHEAs or adrenocorticotropic hormone (ACTH) in the last year?

Do you perspire (sweat) much more than others or a great deal every now and then?

How often do you have headaches?

Does your face flush or get red every now and then, even when you are not exercising?

The last three questions attempt to rule out the hazardous perioperative situation of undiscovered pheochromocytoma or carcinoid syndromes. Both conditions can now be well managed if known about in advance (see Chapter 27). Both, however, incur a mortality rate as high as 10% if undiscovered prior to operation.

The following questions search for symptoms of thyroid and parathyroid disease:

Have you ever taken medicine (e.g., Synthroid [levothyroxine]) or had radioactive iodine (^{131}I) for thyroid disease?

Do you consistently like the room warmer or colder than your spouse does?

Do you have muscle cramps or spasms in your legs more than three times a year?

Neurologic Disease

Physical examination can add significantly to one's impressions and can reduce the necessity for some questions, particularly regarding neurologic disease. Nevertheless, to exclude neurologic disease, the following questions are usually asked:

Have you ever had a seizure, convulsion, fit, stroke, or paralysis?

Have you ever been diagnosed as having a tremor?

Have you ever had migraine headaches?

Have you ever had nerve injury, multiple sclerosis, or any other disorder of the nervous system?

Have you ever had numbness, tingling, or "pins-and-needles" in your arm or leg that has lasted more than 2 hours?

Have you taken antidepressant, sedative, tranquilizing, or antiseizure medications in the last year? Do you take SAM-e (adenosyl methionine) or St. John's Wort because of feeling blue? (I might add, if the patient is a woman over age 45 years, Do you take any medications for hot flashes or for peri- or postmenopausal symptoms?[84-87]).

Musculoskeletal Disease

Because arthritis affects the ease of securing the airway, I usually ask about potential musculoskeletal system disease during the search for airway and lung disease. A brief review could include the following questions:

Have you ever had low back pain?

Have you been working at your usual job or doing your normal activities in the last week?

Have you taken pain pills or had pain shots in the last 6 months?

Sensitive Areas of Concern

One area not yet discussed concerns more difficult-to-manage subjects, such as the possibility of pregnancy, and the possibility of pregnancy in a minor, asymptomatic hemoglobinopathies when intense counseling and consultation service are not available, illicit drug use, and the potential for acquired immunodeficiency syndrome (AIDS).

I believe that such matters should be handled in concert with hospital or facility policy.[96] However, because this kind of information can affect perioperative risk and plans, my usual procedure is to search for clues in the history. If one has taken the time to gain the patient's confidence so that the patient understands that these questions are being asked in order to provide better care, success is possible. If one tries to approach these sensitive areas in the 5 to 15 minutes usually allotted, the process is awkward at best and usually does not succeed. In fact, patients seem to answer these questions more reliably on a checklist paper-and-pencil form or on a computer-based health history (Trigg DJ et al, unpublished data).[71,88]

Under optimal conditions, the questions that can be asked include the following:

Within the last 2 years, have you taken nonprescription drugs, such as cocaine, crack, heroin, or LSD?

Have you been exposed to the body fluids (blood, semen, urine, or saliva) of anyone likely to have the AIDS virus?

Are you in any of the groups at high risk for AIDS (homosexuals, bisexuals, hemophiliacs, and those who have had sex with a prostitute within the last 18 years)?

Would you like to undergo a test to find out whether you have been exposed to the AIDS virus?

From an institutional point of view, in the future AIDS testing will be an especially important consideration.

The Physical Examination

The physical examination looks for the same conditions sought by the history. However, the Rule of Threes indicates the three aspects of the physical examination (airway, cardiovascular, and lung) that may augment, or be better than, the history for detecting the presence of undiagnosed disease or a condition that may affect perioperative outcome; other aspects to be explored include those specific to the patient's condition or planned procedure, such as a sensory nerve examination if a regional block is planned.

The physical examination consists of the following processes:

- Determination of arterial blood pressure in both arms, and in at least one arm 2 minutes after the patient assumes the upright position after lying down.
- Examination of the pulses and of the chest for heaves, thrusts, pulsations, murmurs, and gallops (third and fourth heart sounds). (Some believe that obtaining ankle blood pressure is useful in assessing the risk for cardiovascular disease,[97,98] but this process is not routine.)
- Examination of the carotid and jugular pulses. (I have found that patients expect to be partially undressed for this exam and consider the examiner unprofessional if he or she does not auscultate blood pressure sounds using a bell or diaphragm held to the skin.)
- Examination of the chest and auscultation of the bases of the heart for subtle rales suggestive of congestive heart failure, or for rhonchi, wheezes, and other sounds indicative of lung disease. (Although history-taking may detect these symptoms that point to lung disease as accurately as auscultation, the patient expects a "good" physician to auscultate his or her lungs preoperatively. Thus, this part of the physical examination also helps increase patient confidence.)

- Observation of the patient's walk for signs of neurologic disease and to assess back mobility and general health.
- Examination of the eyes for abnormal movement and, along with the skin, for signs of jaundice, cyanosis, nutritional abnormalities, and dehydration.
- The fingers are checked for clubbing.
- Examination of the airway and mouth for neck mobility, tongue size, oral lesions, and ease of intubation (see Chapter 42).
- Functional evaluation of cardiovascular risk by observing vigor and stamina in walking. (I frequently take the pulse of the patient and myself prior to and after climbing two flights of stairs with the patient, while we talk about other subjects. My own pulse change acts as a control, alerting me when to be concerned about the patient's exercise capacity: if the patient's pulse rate exceeds an increase of 40 beats per minute after climbing two flights [twice my usual pulse change], I worry that the patient cannot do much more than 4 METs of activity [see Table 25-4].)
- Examination of the legs for bruising, edema, clubbing, mobility, sensation, and adequacy of hair growth (or skin texture) as signs of circulatory competence.

Although these portions of the history-taking and physical examination are routine, they are usually not recorded. Because the Health Care Financing Administration (HCFA) has insisted on recording of procedures as proof of their performance, it is advisable to use information system processes to document what has been done (see later).

DETECTING DISEASE: HISTORY, PHYSICAL EXAMINATION, AND CHART REVIEW VERSUS LABORATORY TESTS

Because more than 80% of patients receiving anesthesia are either outpatients or "come-and-stay" patients (i.e., patients admitted to the hospital after surgery), patients cannot be evaluated preoperatively as they were during the 1970s. A new system had to be devised. The resulting set of questions is extensive, consisting of more than 100 items.

I believe that use of a written or automated questionnaire to ask the screening questions, if coupled with a personal interview to pursue positive answers, does not decrease the accuracy or perceived personalization of the care given (see later) (Trigg DJ et al, unpublished data),[71,88,99-102]. Therefore, I began using this combination for inpatients as well (this process is described later in the chapter), especially for "come-and-stay" patients. My task is to explore in depth any positive results from the history-taking and to spend the rest of the time discussing issues that the patient is concerned about, as well as educating the patient about postoperative recovery pain and other plans and motivating him or her to adopt medications or lifestyle changes that have been shown to beneficially affect perioperative outcome.

Furthermore, storing the history and physical information electronically and securely (described later in this chapter) allows the anesthesiologist who is providing care to assess the patient's data the day or night before surgery. Most anesthesiologists have developed ways of putting the classic pattern (chart review; history-taking; physical examination; and discussion of risks, alternative anesthetic plans, and postoperative pain therapies) together so that all of these questions are part of a compassionate flow of thought that helps the patient recall information. A rigid, specific order for questioning is usually unnecessary.

The anesthesiologist must remember that older male patients tend to deny symptoms, often seeing disease as a sign of frailty. Some patients believe that their symptoms indicate a life-threatening disease and therefore resist seeking medical help (and answering questions) until help is imperative. Seeing a physician who has adopted beneficial lifestyle changes motivates the patient to do so.[103,104] Despite such obstacles to obtaining pertinent information, seeing the patient before surgery does give the anesthesiologist one strong advantage: patients are usually willing and eager to share information. Surgery is usually a major event for both men and women; no patient really views any surgery as "minor." Thus, the preoperative interview can elicit vital information and is a powerful time to motivate patients to choose healthy options such as adhering to blood pressure normalization therapy, stopping smoking, and initiating a program of regular walking ands strength training. The trick is to work with the surgeons to have appointments scheduled far enough in advance to make the lifestyle and drug programs meaningful in perioperative as well as long term outcomes.

Some investigators have suggested that anesthesiologists forget the history and just use laboratory tests to screen for disease. A review of the literature strongly suggests otherwise: the history (whether obtained personally, by questionnaire, or by telephone interview by person or computer screening device), and the investigation of positive answers in an in-person interview is many times more effective in screening for disease than the use of laboratory tests alone. Also, the combination of history and personal interview can be a much less expensive process and avoids the medicolegal problems and inefficiency associated with excessive laboratory testing. Furthermore, testing is not a great personal motivator; even using abnormal test results to motivate compliance is only a small fraction as effective as is human-to-human interaction.[105]

The data presented below lead us to believe that the combination of history-taking (from personal interview or questionnaire supplemented by personal interview) and physical examination is the best tool for optimal evaluation of patients and optimal selection of laboratory tests (i.e., selection of only those tests that have a greater chance of benefiting rather than harming the patient).

The primary problem with ordering batteries of laboratory tests for all patients is that laboratory tests are not very good screening devices for disease. In addition, the subsequent "extra" tests that physicians order as a follow-up of supposedly abnormal results are costly. More important is the fact that nonindicated tests often represent additional risk for the patient, increase medicolegal risk for the physician, and render ORs in outpatient centers and hospitals inefficient.

Laboratory Tests Are Ineffective Screening Devices

In general, results of preoperative laboratory testing have been regarded as supplements to the patient's health history and physical examination. Collectively, this information has been the primary source of patient data available to the anesthesiologist. In the perioperative management of the patient, the anesthesiologist may alter the care of the patient based on preoperative laboratory test results. If a preoperative test suggests a change in the care of an individual such that the health of the patient is improved or a potential problem is avoided, then that test has been beneficial to the patient. *Other preoperative tests, the results of which are normal and merely borderline, may only distract the physician*; the results of these tests create no benefit but rather inconvenience, or worse, harm, through distraction. Furthermore, if a preoperative test suggests a change in the care of an individual so that the health of the patient suffers or a problem arises, that test decreases the overall quality of medical care and is harmful to the patient. One common example is a situation in which abnormal results on a chest radiograph obtained for a 40-year-old man solely because he is scheduled for surgery leads to a computed tomographic needle biopsy that produces normal results but also a pneumothorax. This sequence shows how a "benign" test can result in harm. Thus, testing can incur a risk-benefit ratio that is higher than 1.

On the whole, not much benefit appears to result from unindicated routine laboratory testing. Leonard and co-workers[106] reported that biochemical screening tests had no significant value in the preoperative screening of pediatric patients expected to be hospitalized for less than one week. When Korvin and associates[107] reviewed biochemical tests given routinely to 1,000 patients on hospital admission, none of the tests produced a new diagnosis that was unequivocally beneficial to the patient. In an ambitious, controlled trial of multiphasic screening of 1,500 patients, Olsen and co-workers[108] found no difference in morbidity between control groups and groups subjected to screening tests. Durbridge and colleagues[109] compared 1,500 patients randomly assigned to undergo or not undergo screening tests on admission. With respect to length of hospital stay or patient outcome, no benefit resulted from the 8,363 extra tests performed for the group undergoing screening tests. Narr et al.[23,110] found that more than 3,000 patients classified as American Society of Anesthesiologists (ASA) I or II failed to benefit from laboratory testing, and that absence of tests in over 1,000 ASA I patients (average age, 21.4 years) did not adversely affect medical care.

Many studies have compared the yield from indicated (warranted based on history or risk group) versus unindicated (unwarranted) preoperative testing[111-131] (Table 25-5) (Apfelbaum JL et al, unpublished data). Few unindicated tests have yielded beneficial changes in perioperative care: at most, only 16 of more than 16,000 patients who had unindicated preoperative tests benefited from such testing. Furthermore, this figure represents the most optimistic interpretation, because four patients in the study conducted by Kaplan et colleagues.[111] received no benefit, and in another study,[116] the benefit of treating asymptomatic

anemia in seven patients prior to non–blood-loss surgery was not clear.

The 2002 ASA Preoperative Testing Advisory

In 2002, the ASA published a guide for preoperative preparation of the patient prior to operative and nonoperative procedures.[78] This publication followed an Internal Health Organization review of preoperative testing and a Medicare statement on preoperative testing. The fact that it was an "advisory" rather than a guideline highlights the point that the data are not robust enough to state recommendations with absolute certainty. Five findings from the ASA Advisory that are echoed in the other reviews bear emphasis:

1. No test, but rather a physician review stating that "this patient is in optimal shape for daily living" is usual for patients undergoing minimally invasive surgery.
2. Evaluation should occur prior to the day of surgery if the patient is not absolutely healthy or the procedure is other than "minimally invasive"(that is, testing was at least partially to be selected based on the invasiveness of the procedure).
3. Certain tests were found to be usual for the most invasive type of surgery.
4. About 17% of anesthesiologists obtained pregnancy testing routinely for all women in the potentially pregnant calendar ages of 11 to 55 years, irrespective of the patient's statement that "there is no way I could potentially be pregnant."

We will review these findings in turn.

The ASA Advisory's statement that it is appropriate that no test but a physician review saying "this patient is in optimal shape for daily living" for patients undergoing minimally invasive surgery is based on the data presented above buttressed by two randomized controlled studies of minimally invasive procedures.

In the first and largest study, Schein and colleagues[132] randomly allocated over 19,000 patients at nine centers scheduled to undergo cataract extraction with or without lens implantation to be tested routinely or tested only when indicated. No difference in outcome, hospitalization rate, or any measure of morbidity, mortality, cost, or satisfaction occurred between the "test routinely" and "test only when indicated" groups. The accompanying editorial reiterated the point (I am biased, because I wrote it) that each patient was seen by and under the care of a primary care physician who had already done sufficient testing and management to be able to state that each patient was in optimal shape for daily living.[133]

In a similar but smaller subsequent study of slightly over 1,000 patients, Lira and colleagues[134] found the same result: patients who are in ideal shape for daily living as judged by a physician need no additional testing prior to a minimally invasive surgical procedure. Those findings and the results of earlier studies indicate that it is appropriate to segregate patients by invasiveness of procedure to help select tests. A regimen for such segregation by invasiveness of procedure is suggested in Table 25-6. It is significant that the data and schemata listed in this table require that the patient's condition be judged optimal for daily living. Does this mean that patients should be routinely

Table 25–5 Reported yields (abnormal, significantly abnormal, changes in care) for unindicated versus indicated laboratory testing

Study (Population, n)	Total No. of Tests	Percentage of all Tests Abnormal	Unindicated Tests (No. [1%])	Percentage of Abnormal Results Acted on (%)	No. of Unindicated/ Indicated Results That Change Management	No. of Unindicated/ Indicated Potential Benefits	Used to Define Abnormal
Kaplan et al[111] (1985) (elect. surg., 1,000)	2,785	3.45	1,828 (65.6)	—	0/—	4/—	Action limits
Narr et al[110] (1991) (elect. surg., 3,782)	18,910	0.87	—	28.5	47 total	10 total	Substantially abnormal
McKee and Scott[112] (1987) (elect. surg., 397)	794*	2.14	—	0	0 total	13 total	Reference range
Turnbull and Buck[113] (1987) (cholecystectomy, 1,010)	3,646*	2.30†	—	8.3	7 total	4/6	Reference range
Johnson et al[114] (1988) (ambul. surg., 212)	424*	24.06†	—	0.98	1 total	0/13	Reference range
Muskett and McGreevy[115] (1986) (consec. surg.,§ 200)	1,007*	38.63†	—	18.5	5/71‡	0/—	—
O'Connor and Drasner[116] (1990) (elect. surg.,‖ 486)	937	12.9†	—	15.7	24/—	7/—	Clinically significant
Hackmann et al[117] (1991) (day surg.,‖ 2,649)	2,649	0.53	2,605 (98.3)	7.1	0/1	0/1	Hb < 10 g/dL
Roy et al[118] (1991) (elect. surg.,‖ 2,000)	2,000	0.55	—	27.3	3 total	3 total	Hb < 10 g/dL
Nigam et al[119] (1990) (tonsillectomy,‖ 250)	250	0.80	—	0	0/0	0/2	Hb ≤ 10 g/dL
Baron et al[120] (1992) (elect. surg.,‖ 1,863)	1,863	1.13	—	0	0/0	—	30% > Hct ?50%
Rohrer et al[121] (1988) (elect. surg., 282)	1,119	5.90	514 (45.9)	—	3/0000	0/21	Reference range
Lawrence and Kroenke[122] (1988) (orthop. surg.,¶ 200)	200	17.00†	180 (90.0)	29.4	6/4	0/3	Lawrence and Kroenke[87]
Apfelbaum et al**,†† (elect. surg., 1,746)	21,318	16.1	10,899 (51.1)	18.4	13/121	1/91	Action limits
Asaf et al[123]	719	25.3*	719 (100)	0	0/—	7/—	Reference range
Johnson and Mortimer[124]	773	10*	773 (100)	3	2/—	0/—	Reference range
Alsomait et al[125]	14,000	14.1*	90 (90.8)	0	0/0	0/0	Reference range

*Electrocardiographic (ECG) and/or chest radiographic results excluded.
†Urinalysis results included.
‡ECG and chest radiographic results included.
§A high medical risk population at a Veterans Affairs Medical Center Hospital.
‖Pediatric population (<18y).
¶Clean-wound, nonprosthetic knee procedures.
**Includes author of this manuscript.
††Apfelbaum JL et al (unpublished data).
This table was coauthored with Dr. Raj Kim.

Table 25–6 Types of surgical procedures for which anesthesia may be administered

Type	General Definition	Specific Examples
A	*Minimally invasive* procedures that have little potential to disrupt normal physiology and are associated with only rare periprocedure morbidity related to the anesthetic; these procedures rarely require blood administration, invasive monitoring, and/or postoperative management in a critical care setting	Cataract extraction, diagnostic arthroscopy, postpartum interval tubal ligation
B	*Moderately invasive* procedures that have a modest or intermediate potential to disrupt normal physiology; these procedures may require blood administration, invasive monitoring, or postoperative management in a critical care setting	Carotid endarterectomy, transurethral resection of the prostate, and laparoscopic cholecystectomy
C	*Highly invasive* procedures that typically produce significant disruption of normal physiology; these procedures commonly require blood administration, invasive monitoring, or postoperative management in a critical care setting	Total hip replacement, open aortic valve replacement, and posterior fossa craniotomy for aneurysm

started on aspirin, β-adrenergic receptor blocking agents, statins, physical activity (walking and strength exercises), immune boosting and immunization therapy preprocedure? It did not, in the studies by Schein and Lira and associates, but it may, in the future (see later).

The segregation of patients based on the degree of invasiveness of the planned surgery as well as on the patient's condition brings up certain issues: when to perform a preoperative evaluation in order to determine the condition of the patient, and what to do if you disagree with the primary care physician about the patient's status as optimal for daily living. The judgment about invasiveness depends not just on the CPT (Current Procedural Terminology) code of the American Medical Association (AMA) but also on the surgeon—a laparoscopic cholecystectomy can be minimally invasive in a gifted surgeon's hands, is moderately invasive in most, and is highly invasive in some. The classification of surgical procedures outlined in Table 25-6 is based on the anesthesiologist's evaluation or judgment of usual invasiveness. Such preoperative evaluation almost certainly must of necessity occur prior to the day of surgery if the patient is not absolutely healthy or the procedure is other than "minimally invasive"(that is, testing is at least partially to be selected based on the invasiveness of the procedure).

As to disagreement with the primary care physician's evaluation, or if there is no primary care evaluation, the dialogue of the Advisory committee was and is clear: the final arbitrator of perioperative evaluation is the anesthesiologist providing anesthesia care for the patient. We will review the other two unexpected findings from the Advisory—about tests for highly invasive procedures and pregnancy tests later in this chapter. Let us now review why laboratory tests do not have more benefit for the perioperative patient.

Although laboratory tests can aid in ensuring that a patient's preoperative condition is optimal once a disease is suspected or diagnosed, such tests have several shortcomings as screening devices for the discovery of unknown disease. First, they frequently fail to uncover pathologic conditions. Second, they detect abnormalities the discovery of which does not necessarily improve patient care or outcome. Also, laboratory tests are inefficient in screening for asymptomatic diseases. Finally, most abnormalities discovered on preoperative screening, or even on admission screening for nonsurgical purposes, are not recorded (other than on the laboratory report) or pursued appropriately.

By itself, the detection of abnormalities does not justify testing, because most abnormalities in asymptomatic patients do not reflect the presence of disease. For tests reported as continuous results, the distribution of results in a population of patient is gaussian (i.e., normal). The values defining "abnormal" are set arbitrarily, so that test results exceeding those of the highest 2.5% of healthy individuals, or falling below those of the lowest 2.5% of healthy individuals, are said to be abnormal. Test results between these two extremes are "within the reference range." Therefore, 5% of test results from patients without disease will be "outside the hospital reference range." If one were to order 100 hemoglobin determinations for a sample of healthy patients, 5% of the results would be expected to be "abnormal." Ordering multiple preoperative tests increases the chances of at least one abnormal result.

Assuming that results of tests are independent of one another, the more tests ordered, the higher the likelihood of an abnormal result. For example, if two tests are ordered for a patient without disease, the chance of both being normal is 0.95 × 0.95 or 0.90. For 20 tests, the chance that all would be normal would be only 36%. The chance that at least one result will be abnormal is 64%. Thus, if one uses more than 13 tests to screen patients before surgery, one should expect at least one abnormal test result.

AIDS testing provides another example. More than 92% of the population at low risk for HIV infection who have positive (abnormal) results on two enzyme-linked immunosorbent assays (ELISAs) and one Western blot test in reality do not have HIV infection.[130] Therefore, it is not surprising that the benefit from nonselective testing is so low or that so few abnormal results arising from unwarranted tests are acted on (Table 25-5). Mammography is another example. If both mammograms and breast examinations were performed yearly starting when women are 40 years old, by age 50 over 49 percent would have had a false-positive test on examination, and over 20 percent a breast biopsy for benign disease.[135]

Even for the very elderly, a patient group at higher risk for morbidity and mortality during surgery, the ultimate benefit of routine laboratory screening is doubtful. Domoto and colleagues[136] examined the yield and benefit of a battery of 19 screening laboratory tests performed routinely in 70 functionally intact elderly patients (average age, 82.6 years) who resided at a chronic care facility. The 70 patients underwent 3,905 screening tests. "New abnormal" results occurred in 5 of the 19 screening tests. Most of these "new abnormalities" were only minimally outside the normal range. Only four discoveries (0.1 percent of all tests ordered) led to a change in patient management, none of which, these workers concluded, benefited any patient in any important way.

Wolf-Klein and associates[137] retrospectively studied the results of annual laboratory screening of a population of 500 institutionalized and ambulatory elderly patients (average age, 80 years). From the 15,000 tests performed, 756 new abnormalities were discovered, 690 of which were ignored. Sixty-six of the new abnormalities were evaluated; the result was 20 new diagnoses, 12 of which were treated. Two patients of the 500 ultimately may have benefited from eradication of asymptomatic bacteriuria (although eradication of this condition has not been shown to improve the quality of life or to extend life[138]).

Studies show that the history and physical examination are the best ways to screen for disease. Delahunt and Turnbull[139] evaluated 803 patients who were assessed preoperatively for varicose vein stripping or inguinal herniorrhaphy. A total of 1,972 tests produced only 63 abnormalities not indicated by history or physical findings. Furthermore, in no instance did the discovery of these abnormalities influence patient management.

Another study retrospectively evaluated 690 admissions for elective pediatric surgical procedures.[140] Bates and colleagues[141] found that at least 40% of repeat tests carried out in a large teaching hospital were redundant. The history and physical examination indicated the probability of abnormalities in all 12 patients in whom an abnormality was detected by laboratory testing. Clinical diagnosis, and not laboratory testing, was the apparent basis for any change in operative plans.

Narr and co-workers[23] at the Mayo Clinic found no harm from omitting *all* laboratory testing for ASA I patients. The sample size of this study was large enough to indicate that more harm than benefit would probably occur by testing ASA I patients. One exception should be noted: the median age of these patients was 21.4 years, making the conclusion about testing of ASA I patients over 40 years of age unclear. Narr and colleagues have acted on their data: no tests are now obtained on ASA I patients undergoing surgery at the Mayo Clinic. Review of a sampling of such patients' records and outcome indicates the validity of such an approach, and others have reported cost savings and operating efficiency resulting from this practice.[110,142]

Several studies have compared groups of hospitalized patients undergoing routine laboratory screening tests (to supplement the history and physical examination) with groups not undergoing routine screening tests. Wood and Hoekelman[143] found that abnormal results from the history, physical examination, or laboratory examination changed the preoperative clinical course for 28 of 1,924 children: surgery was postponed for all 28 children. For only 3 of these children did laboratory tests indicate an abnormality not suggested by the history or physical examination. Thus, the history and physical examination dictated the appropriate laboratory testing for all but 3 of 1,924 patients.

A more specific conclusion is also possible. The abnormalities discovered in these three patients were found on chest radiographs. (These children were part of a study comparing perioperative outcome at two hospitals, one that required chest radiograph as a screening test for elective surgery in children and one that did not.) There were no differences noted in anesthetic or perioperative complications between the two groups. Therefore, Wood and Hoekelman recommended that chest radiographs not be obtained routinely for apparently healthy children.

Even in a referral population, history and physical examination determine more than 90% of the clinical course when a patient is referred for consultation about cardiovascular, neurologic, or respiratory disease.[144] Other studies also have demonstrated that the history and physical examination accurately indicate all areas in which subsequent laboratory testing proves beneficial to patients. For example, Rabkin and Horne[145,146] examined the records of 165 patients having a "new" abnormality on the ECG that was "surgically significant" (i.e., a change from a previous tracing that represents a condition possibly affecting perioperative management or outcome). In only two instances were anesthetic or surgical plans altered by the discovery of "new abnormalities" found on the ECG but not indicated by history. Thus, even for these 165 patients, for whom the benefits of a laboratory test should have been maximal because abnormalities were detected before surgery, the history or physical examination determined case management most of the time. Furthermore, in one of the two instances of altered case management (a patient who had atrial fibrillation), physical examination should have indicated the need for an ECG. A history or physical examination was not available for the other patient.

Table 25-5 shows that patients who benefit from testing have risk factors, symptoms, or other conditions in their history that call for testing. In our own study (Apfelbaum JL et al, unpublished data), in patients who were symptomatic with risk factors for disease or who only had risk factors for disease, 606 (5.8%) of 10,419 test results were significantly abnormal. Of these, 124 tests (1.2%) affected care. Of these patients, 6 tests resulted in harm (6 in 10,419, or 0.06%), whereas 91 patients (91 in 10,419, or 0.9%) benefited from a change in care. In contrast, for asymptomatic patients who had no risk factors for disease, only 121 (1.1%) of the 10,899 test results were significantly abnormal. Of these, 10 tests (0.01%) affected care. During the study, every change in care that benefited or harmed a patient stemmed from a single test result. Therefore, the 13 "care-affecting" tests represented 13 "care-affected" patients. Of these 13 patients, 5 (in 10,899, or 0.05%) asymptomatic patients were harmed, whereas only one (in 10,899 test results, or 0.009%) of the patients benefited from a change in care. Neither harm nor benefit was thought to result from the other seven changes in care. These results confirm the studies of the more than 20,000 patients of Schein and Lira (discussed previously) who also did not benefit from laboratory testing once their physicians had determined that they were in optimal shape for daily living.[132,134]

In summary, the studies cited point to the lack of benefit from routine laboratory tests as a method of assessing patients preoperatively. Many of these laboratory tests have been shown to be superfluous to patient care management. History and physical examination are considered the most effective ways of screening for disease. Laboratory tests can be used to screen for disease when the patient has appropriate risk factors and when such tests have proved effective. However, the better use of such tests is to confirm clinical diagnoses or to optimize the patient's condition prior to surgery.

Patient Risk

Unnecessary testing may lead physicians to pursue and treat borderline and false-positive laboratory abnormalities. This observation does not imply that all standard screening tests should be discontinued. Some are beneficial, such as the mammogram for all women over 40 or 50 years of age,[108,109,135] the test for occult blood or colonoscopy in stool for all people over 40 years of age,[126,127,129] and the Papanicolaou (Pap) smear for sexually active females.[126,127,129] However, few studies have examined whether increased testing and the follow-up on false-positive test results adversely affect patients. In one study addressing this issue, Roizen and associates[82] retrospectively examined the adverse effects of chest radiographs on patients. For 606 patients, 386 additional chest radiographs were ordered without indication of need. Among those 386 patients, the discovery of only one abnormality (an elevated hemidiaphragm probably caused by phrenic nerve palsy) may have resulted in improved care for that patient. On the other hand, the existence of lung shadows on chest radiographs of three patients led to three sets of invasive tests, including one thoracotomy, but no discovery of disease. These procedures caused considerable morbidity, including one pneumothorax and 4 months of disability, for these three patients.

Tape and Muslin[149] found a similar result when examining the benefits and risks of chest radiographs obtained preoperatively in Rochester, New York. Of 341 patients admitted for vascular surgery, nine had radiographic findings that led to clinical action. Specifically, three patients (two with congestive heart failure and one with pulmonary fibrosis) may have benefited from the findings. However, all three patients were known by history to have the disease shown on chest radiographs. In addition, six patients were subjected to a potentially detrimental clinical response. Two had a false diagnosis of tuberculosis, with subsequent therapy for one patient; two others had false diagnosis of nodules; and the last two had falsely normal chest radiographic readings. All the beneficial effects attributed to preoperative chest radiographs accrued to patients who had an obvious clinical history of pulmonary or cardiac disease. Orkin[150] has further explained the basis of the risk of testing asymptomatic patients.

Similarly, in another study, even though few patients benefited by preoperative testing that was warranted by history or risk factors (91 of 1,746), even fewer were harmed by such testing (one patient) (Apfelbaum JL et al, unpublished data). In contrast, testing of asymptomatic patients was more risky than beneficial to patient health. Specifically, 1 in every 2,000 preoperative tests (1 in 300 patients) led to patient harm because of the pursuit of abnormalities indicated by those tests; 1 in 10,000 tests (1 in 1,746 patients) led to benefit (Apfelbaum JL et al, unpublished data).

In another study, Turnbull and Buck[113] examined the charts of 2,570 patients undergoing cholecystectomy to determine the value of preoperative tests. With four possible exceptions, history and physical examinations successfully indicated the need for all tests that ultimately benefited the patients. For those four patients, it is doubtful that any benefit actually occurred as a result of preoperative tests. Among them was one patient who had emphysema detected only by chest radiograph; this patient had preoperative physiotherapy without subsequent postoperative complications. Two patients had unsuspected hypokalemia (potassium levels of 3.2 and 3.4 mEq/L in blood) and received treatment prior to operation. Current data in the literature indicate that no harm occurs to patients undergoing surgery with this degree of hypokalemia and that severe harm may be caused by treating such patients with oral or intravenous administration of potassium (Table 25-7).[151-155] The fourth patient possibly benefiting from preoperative testing had an asymptomatic hemoglobin concentration of 9.9 g/dL and was given a blood transfusion prior to cholecystectomy. Because cholecystectomy is not normally associated with major blood loss, one might conclude that this patient also received no benefit from preoperative laboratory testing and its pursuit but was exposed to the risk of transfusion. Thus, it is not clear that any patient in this study benefited from preoperative screening tests given without indication for need by history or physical examination.

In another study, only two patients (who had eradication of asymptomatic bacteriuria) benefited from the 9,720 screening tests that were given.[156] At least one patient was seriously harmed from pursuit and treatment of abnormalities on screening tests. In this patient, atrial fibrillation and congestive heart failure developed after institution of thyroid therapy (for borderline low thyroxine levels) and free thyroxine index tests. It is unclear whether these investigators examined other patients for potential harm arising from the pursuit and treatment of abnormalities on screening tests.

To determine benefits and risks, screening mammography has been evaluated in a real-life practice setting.[135] Although yearly screening was beneficial, over 20% of the women who did not have disease were subjected to a breast biopsy. Furthermore, more than 49% of these "normal" women would have been subjected to a breast biopsy if each had had a yearly mammogram and clinical breast exam. Thus, even when benefits exceed risk, there is substantial risk in routine testing.

Medicolegal Liability

"Extra testing"—testing not warranted by findings on a medical history—does not provide medicolegal protection

Table 25–7   Risk of potassium supplementation*

| | Route of Administration | | | |
	Oral	IV	Oral and IV	All Routes
Patients (no.)	1,910	2,192	819	921
Death	3 (0.2%)	3 (0.15%)	1 (0.1%)	7 (0.14%)
Life-threatening reaction or death	6 (0.3%)	7 (0.35%)	14 (1.7%)	28 (0.57%)
Hyperkalemia	74 (3.9%)	34 (1.6%)	71 (8.7%)	179 (3.6%)
Other side effects	53 (2.8%)	18 (0.8%)	33 (4.0%)	283 (5.7%)

*One in 200 patients given potassium supplementation dies or has a life-threatening reaction.
Data from Lawson DH: Adverse reactions to potassium chloride. Q J Med 43:433, 1974; and Lawson DH, Hutcheon AW, Jick H: Life-threatening drug reactions amongst medical inpatients. Scot Med J 24:127, 1979.

against liability (also see Chapter 89). Studies show that 30% to 95% of all unexpected abnormalities found on preoperative laboratory tests are not noted on the chart before surgery[111,122,137,143,145,146,157-167] (Table 25-8). This lack of notation occurs not only at university medical centers but at community hospitals as well.

Moreover, the failure to pursue an abnormality appropriately poses a greater risk of medicolegal liability than does failure to detect that abnormality.[167] In this way, extra testing increases the medicolegal risk to physicians. In addition, the HCFA is attempting to make failure to pursue abnormalities grounds for charging physicians

Table 25–8   Unrecorded abnormalities on preoperative tests

Series	Type Test	Unexpected Abnormalities (n)	Unexpected Abnormalities Noted on Chart Preoperatively* (%)
Lorenzi and Cohen[†]	PT/PTT	20	5
Rabkin and Horne[145,146]	ECG	157	31
Kaplan et al[111]	CBC/PTT Glucose/SMA 6	12[‡]	17
Robbins and Rose[157]	PT	23	39
Wood and Hoekelman[143]	Hematocrit	15[‡]	27
Parkerson[158,159,§]	Multiple	343	38
	Multiple; >10% abnormal	63?	60
Williamson et al[160,§]	Urinalysis	164	17
	FBS	63	32
	Hemoglobin	32	16
Huntley et al[161,§]	Multiple	343	67
Daughaday et al[162]	Multiple	167	60
Epstein et al[163]	T_4	111	60
Wheeler et al[164]	Hemoglobin	258	71
Kelley and Mamlin[165,§]	Multiple	852	64-85
Wolf-Klein et al[137,§]	Multiple	756	7-73(avg. 50)
Lawrence and Kroenke[122]	Urinalysis	180	29
Umbach et al[166]	Chest radiographs	116	59
Narr et al[110]	Multiple	160	40
O'Connor and Drasner[116]	Hemoglobin and urinalysis	97	51

*Recording of an unexpected abnormality on the patient's chart, either preoperatively or at any time other than on the laboratory test report printout.
[†]Personal communication.
[‡]Abnormalities potentially significant to perioperative management.
[§]Test not obtained preoperatively.
CBC, complete blood count; ECG, electrocardiogram; FBS, fasting blood sugar; PT, prothrombin time; PTT, partial thromboplastin time; SMA 6, simultaneous multichannel analyses of sodium, potassium, chloride, bicarbonate, urea nitrogen, and creatinine levels in blood; T_4, thyroxine.

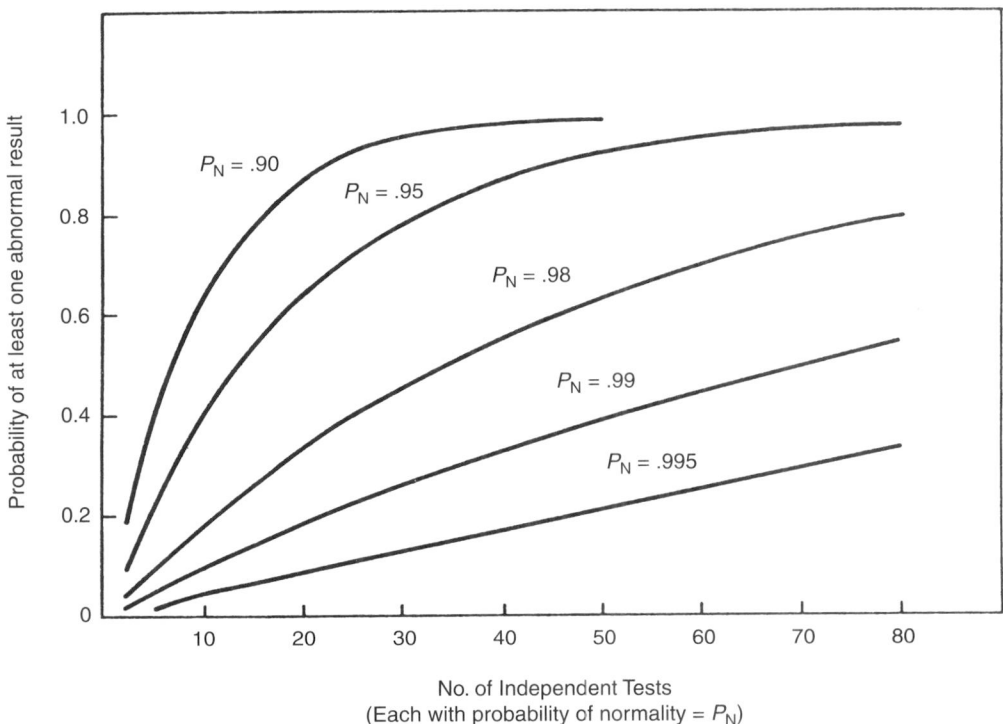

Figure 25–3 Probability of at least one abnormal result on multiple independent trials of tests, each with a probability (P_N) of a normal result, for selected values of P_N. (From Berwick DM: Screening in health fairs. A critical review of benefits, risks, and costs. JAMA 254:1492, 1985.)

with inadequate practice. However, such lack of attention to unexpected abnormalities is a completely reasonable response; the data discussed previously[168] (Fig. 25-3) indicate that most unexpected abnormalities in asymptomatic patients occur in patients who are actually healthy.

Furthermore, pursuit of unexpected abnormalities in asymptomatic patients is more likely to harm than benefit such patients. It is logical that pursuit of unindicated testing poses liability, as the tests were not warranted, and the statistics of testing theory as well as data in the literature indicate that the pursuit of such abnormalities is more likely to cause harm than to prove beneficial. Thus, the problems associated with nonselective batteries of tests include both direct and indirect risks to patients and society (Table 25-9).

Operating Room Schedules

According to hospital administrators in the United States, surgeons say they order preoperative tests to satisfy anesthesiologists: surgeons find it easier just to order all the tests and let the anesthesiologist sort them out (also see Chapter 86) . Surgeons also believe that it is much more efficient to order batteries of tests than to have an anesthesiologist, who sees the patient the night before or the morning of surgery, obtain the tests on an emergency basis. This line of reasoning overlooks the fact that abnormalities arising from tests performed in the battery fashion are usually not discovered until the night before or the morning of surgery, if at all. Then, the discovery of abnormal results delays or postpones OR schedules, as effort and time are wasted to obtain consultant review of false-positive or slightly abnormal results. Also, data show clear cost reductions from delegating test selection to anesthesiologists,[26-30] as well as other benefits from educational practices that are discussed later in this chapter.[5,31-40,54-72,169]

PREOPERATIVE AND PREPROCEDURE TESTING

Most hospitals, many anesthesia departments, many outpatient surgical centers, and now many office-based operatories have rather arbitrary rules and recommendations regarding tests that should be performed before elective surgery. With good intentions, anesthesiologists tried to follow those rules, and problems began. The inexpensive

Table 25–9 Consequences of using nonselective batteries of preoperative tests

	Consequences
Direct risks to patients	*False-positive* results (i.e., an erroneous "abnormality" on a radiograph or electrocardiogram) may initiate follow-up activities that are harmful to the patient. *False-negative* results encourage the overlooking of true problems or instill a false sense of security.
Indirect risk to patients	Diverts physician's attention to nonvital issues.
Cost to society	Reduces resources available to care for others.
Cost to physicians	Failure to pursue abnormalities increases medicolegal risks.

multiphasic screening batteries of tests subsequently developed by the Kaiser Hospitals and Health Plan seemed to be the answer to this confusing and arbitrary process.[170] Physicians believed they could now order inexpensive batteries of tests and thus efficiently screen for disease. However, physicians were still trying to determine which tests to order before surgery, and what to do with the unexpectedly abnormal result on the morning of surgery. Kaiser found that this system of preoperative multiphasic screening was not practical.[171] The system produced so many false-positive and false-negative results that the subsequent harm vastly outweighed any possible benefit. Nevertheless, the notion of "the more testing, the better" is still with us.

The Low Predictive Value of an "Abnormal" Laboratory Test Result

Understanding what constitutes an "abnormal" laboratory test result requires an appreciation of the way "normal" values are determined. A normal range is based on the typical distribution of the gaussian curve.[172] For example, assuming a gaussian distribution and hemoglobin values of 13.5 to 16.7 g/dL ("reference range") for healthy men, one can expect 5% of "normal" men to have a test result outside that range.

Of prime importance in preoperative evaluation is knowing the percentage of abnormal laboratory test values that truly indicates disease. If the anesthetic management of a patient is altered because of a test abnormality, that abnormality should indicate a condition (1) that poses a significant risk of preoperative morbidity that can be lessened by preoperative treatment, (2) that cannot be discovered through history-taking and physical examination, and (3) that is sufficiently prevalent in the population to justify the risk of performing the follow-up test. To be cost-efficient, the test should be sufficiently "sensitive" (have "positivity in disease") and sufficiently "specific" (have "negativity in health"). That is, test results should be positive if the patient has disease and negative if the patient is healthy.[172-174] In fact, what a clinician really wants to know is what a positive or negative test means for the individual patient in front of him or her. The values representing the predictive ability of a positive or negative test ("positive predictive values" and "negative predictive values") depend on the pretest population probability.[172-174]

We shall now consider the significance of false-positive and false-negative results and the prevalence of disease in the test population in relation to abnormal laboratory test results. (I am indebted to Drs. Jorgen Hilden and Anders Hald, whose comments have helped make this section clearer.) For example, patients with pneumonia would have the notation "pneumonia" (or some significant abnormality) written as the diagnosis on their chest radiograph reports. Let us assume that the specificity of a test (its negativity in health) is 98.3%; that is, 983 of 1,000 people who actually do not have asymptomatic pneumonia will have a comment such as "without evidence of pneumonia" or "normal" written on their chest radiograph reports. Next, let us assume that 0.5% of the asymptomatic population under age 40 who are about to undergo routine elective surgery has pneumonia. Given the preceding assumptions, what is the likelihood that a person whose chest radiograph report reads "pneumonia" would actually have pneumonia?

If we test 100,000 asymptomatic persons, and 0.5% are assumed to be diseased, this means that 500 people would have undetected pneumonia. If the sensitivity of chest radiographs to pneumonia is assumed to be 75%, 375 of these people would have abnormal radiographs. Then, if specificity is assumed to be 98.3%, 97,809 of the 99,500 healthy people would have normal results on chest radiographs. This means that 1,691 (1.7%) would have abnormal radiographic results. Thus, of 2,066 patients having a diagnosis of pneumonia based on chest radiographs, 1,691 (82%) of the results would be falsely positive. Therefore, it is entirely possible that 82% of the chest radiographs indicating "infiltrate compatible with pneumonia" in otherwise asymptomatic persons would actually be radiographs of totally healthy people. Expressed in another way, when the above assumptions discussed are applied, the likelihood that an asymptomatic person would actually have pneumonia when the chest radiograph contains that notation is only 18%; that is, for this patient group, the predictive value of a positive test (the "positive predictive value") is only 18%.

Only patients with abnormal test results who actually have disease ("true positives") benefit from laboratory testing. Let us assume that 2.2% of the chest radiographs in the under-age-40 population are positive, and that, for each true positive, perioperative mortality decreases by 50%. If we use the 82% false-positive rate derived previously, the number of patients benefiting per 1,000 radiographs is 3.9 (true positives per 1,000 = all positives − false positives; i.e., [2.2% × 1,000] − [82% percent − 2.2 percent × 1,000] = 3.9 patients). Therefore, a reduction in operative mortality of 50%, or 1 per 20,000 (i.e., 3.9 − 0.5 × 0.0005), gives 0.000095 fewer deaths per 1,000 operations when preoperative chest radiographs are obtained.

Hilden and Hald (personal communication) question whether this is a logical calculation. For example, one study analyzed outcomes for asymptomatic patients.[175] The death rate for this group was 1 in 10,000. Of these deaths, more than 90% were caused by avoidable problems unrelated to unknown diseases. Therefore, at most, fewer than 10% of the deaths of asymptomatic individuals could be attributed to preoperative conditions, and probably fewer than 10% of those deaths (<1% of the total, or 1 in 1,000,000) would be related to pneumonia. Thus, the intuitive value is similar to what we have estimated. Furthermore, from an examination of the data in Tables 25-5 and 25-10, it is evident that few chest radiographs in the under-40 asymptomatic population led to benefit. In addition, the harm from these tests has not yet been considered.

Translating this figure into the present value for years of life saved per 1,000 chest radiographs yields the following: 0.000095 fewer deaths per 1,000 operations × 22.62 years saved per life saved = 0.0022 years of life (22.62 is the present value of 60 more years of life for a 20-year-old, per Neuhauser[172]). At the University of Chicago, the 0.0022 years of life saved would cost $78,000 (an anteroposterior and lateral chest radiograph cost $78, not including fees for consultations, repeated radiographs, or other laboratory tests or procedures). Therefore, each year of life saved by

Table 25–10 Screening chest radiographs: Incidence of abnormal test results, the discovery of which may change management of anesthesia

Age(y)	Series	Patients Examined (n)	Abnormalities*(%)	New Abnormalities† (%)
0-14	Farnsworth et al[176]	350	8.9	0.3
0-18	Brill et al[177]	1,000	1.9	0.7
0-19	Sagel et al[178]	521	0	0
0-19	Sane et al[179]	1,500	5.4	2.2
0-19	Wood and Hoekelman	749	4.7	1.2
1-20	Rees et al[180]	46	0	0
20-29	Sagel et al[178]	894	1	—
21-30	Rees et al[180]	62	3	—
≤30	Loder[181]	437	10.1	0.2
≤30	Hubbell et al[182]	12	0	0
≤30	Maigaard et al[183]	1,256	≤4.5	0
0-39	Umbach et al[166]	305	3.0	—
30-39	Sagel et al[178]	942	2.3	—
≤40	Catchlove et al[184]	29	0	0
≤40	Collen et al[170]	15,978	2.1	—
≤40	Sagel et al[178]	2,357	1.3	1.3
≤40	McKee and Scott[112,‡]	26	7.7	3.9
≤40	Combined[112,176-179,181-183,§]	6,787	4.0	0.8
40-49	Sagel et al[178]	928	7.1	
<40	Velanovich[185]	—	3.1	—
40-49	Umbach et al[166]	290	6.2	—
40-59	Collen et al[170]	21,489	7.4	—
41-50	Hubbell et al[182]	28	17.9	0
41-50	Rees et al[180]	119	19	—
41-50	McKee and Scott[112,‡]	53	17	0
30-69	Loder[181]	515	≤6.0	—
31-40	Rees et al[180]	93	13	—
31-40	Hubbell et al[182]	22	22.5	4.5
40-60	Velanovich[185]	NA	23.9	—
≥40	Sagel et al[178]	3,689	23.9	6.0
≥40	Catchlove et al[184]	50	0	0
≥40	Thomsen et al[186]	1,823	2.3	0.2
50-59	Umbach et al[166]	247	10.9	—
50-59	Sagel et al[178]	733	20.3	—
51-60	Hubbell et al[182]	87	36.8	4.4
51-60	Rees et al[180]	121	40.0	—
51-60	McKee and Scott[112,‡]	85	40.0	0
>55	Gupta et al[187,‡]	346	5.5	0.9
60-69	Umbach et al[166]	202	13.3	—
60-69	Sagel et al[178]	977	29.7	—
61-70	Boghosian and Mooradian[188]	78	≤49	—
>60	Boghosian and Mooradian[188]			
	Without risk factor‡	44	34.0	—
	With risk factors	92	62.0	—
>60	Collen et al[170]	7,196	19.2	—
>60	Hubbell et al[182]	145	44.1	4.8‖
>60	McKee and Scott[112,‡]	163	44.2	1.9
>60	Velanovich[185]	NA	31.9	—
61-70	Rees et al[180]	134	43.3	—
61-70	Hubbell et al[182]	94	36.2	5.4
>65	Sewell et al[189]	28	21	—
≥69	Loder[181]	48	≤72.9	—
≥?70	Wolf-Klein et al[137]	500	1.9	—
≥70	Sagel et al[178]	832	41.7	—
≥70	Törnebrandt and Fletcher[180]	100	37	8.1?
≥70	Boghosian and Mooradian[188]			
	Without risk factors‡	58	≤59	—
	With risk factors	45	≤64	—

(Continued)

Table 25–10   Screening chest radiographs: Incidence of abnormal test results, the discovery of which may change management of anesthesia—Cont'd

Age (y)	Series	Patients Examined (*n*)	Abnormalities*(%)	New Abnormalities† (%)
≥71	Levinstein et al[156]	121	84.4	0.9
70-79	Umbach et al[166]	110	27.2	—
71-80	Rees et al[180]	76	61.8	—
71-80	Hubbell et al[182]	28	57.1	0
>80	Umbach et al[166]	21	33.3	—
>80	Hubbell et al[182]	23	60.9	8.7
20-89	Fink et al[191]	127	46	—
74-97	Domoto et al[136]	69	72.5	33
>81	Rees et al[180]	16	68.8	—
?0-?90	Wiencek et al[192]	403	≤25.1	2.4
0-90	Delahunt and Turnbull[139]	860	—	0
24-90	Tape and Mushlin[149,¶]	318	33	0
0-?90	Petterson and Janower[193]	1,530	9.8	1.3
0-?90	Turnbull and Buck[113,¶]	691	5.5	—
0-?90	Royal College[134]	3,052	3.8	—
0-?90	Rucker et al[195,‡]	371	0.3	—
0-?90	Blery et al[128]	2,765	0.7	0.1
0-90+	Weibman et al[196,¶]	734	5.0	—
0-90+	Muskett and McGreevy[115]	119	29.4	5.0
0-90+	Gagner and Chiasson[197]	1,000	7.4	—

*These data constitute an edited summary of the data presented by various articles, edited to select abnormalities that might change management of anesthesia.

†Abnormalities not already known or suspected by history or physical examination.

‡Patients were asymptomatic.

§Combined studies in younger-than-40 population excluding two studies, those by Rees et al[180] and Collen et al.[170]

‖0% changed treatment.

¶Tape and Mushlin[149] studied vascular surgery patients; Turnbull and Buck,[113] cholecystectomy patients; and Weibman and colleagues,[196] cancer patients.

obtaining chest radiographs costs about $35,500,000 (78,000 divided by 0.0022).

However, just as there are other costs (e.g., pursuing some false-positive chest shadows will result in computed tomographic needle biopsies and lobectomies in totally healthy patients[109-112]), there are other benefits (e.g., treatment of some patients having solitary nodules or mediastinal masses may prolong life). Let us arbitrarily assume that these costs and benefits are equal. One is forced to conclude that screening for an asymptomatic disease having a low prevalence rate is a very expensive and possibly risky procedure.

A Simplified Benefit-Risk Analysis of Testing

The above analysis is only a cost-benefit and not a benefit-risk analysis and therefore disregards the possible harm of unwarranted testing, which in fact does incur risk (Fig. 25-4). Let us assume that the chest radiograph in the under-age-40 population has a sensitivity of 75% and a specificity of 95% (these values are better than the best in the literature for readings referenced by a single radiologist). Let us also assume that the prevalence of disease detectable by the test is 0.5%, that the benefit from true positives is 20 in 100 (better than the best in

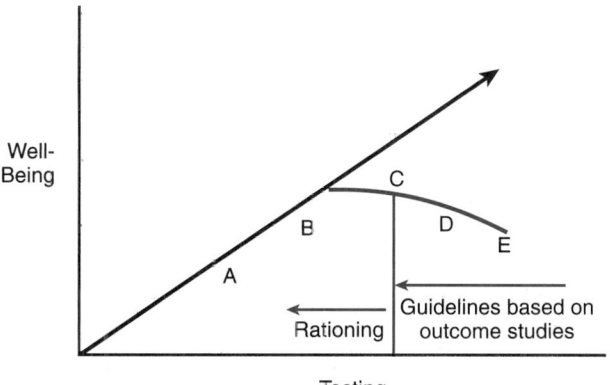

Figure 25–4 Theory and actuality of what happens to well-being as testing increases. The straight line represents the common theory that "the more testing, the better"; that is, that well-being increases with testing. The A-to-E curve shows what actually happens as testing increases. At a certain point (point C), more harm than good may result. Therefore, point C represents the optimal point in the well-being versus testing relationship. The goal of using guidelines is to direct resources from point E to point C (to reduce testing and to increase well-being). Unless health-care providers allocate health resources in a cost-efficient manner, governmental restrictions will move testing from point C to point A—that is, will ration testing that improves well-being.

Table 25–11   Hypothetic benefit-risk analyses for two tests, under three circumstances

Test:	Chest Radiograph	Electrocardiogram	
Patient:	<40-Year-Old Asymptomatic Patient (%)	30-Year-Old-Asymptomatic Man, to Search for MI	47-Year-Old Asymptomatic Man, to Search for MI and Conduction Disturbance
Sensitivity of test	75	33%	50%
Specificity of test	95	90%	90%
Prevalence of disease detectable by test	0.5	~2.1%	~15%
Benefit from true-positives	20	20%	20%
Harm rate for false-positives	6	6%	6%
Benefit per 1,000 patients			
Predicted true-positives	3.8	7	75
Benefited patients	0.8	1.4	15
Harm per 1,000 patients			
Predicted false-positives	4.9	97.9	85
Harmed patients	3	5.9	5.1
Conclusion:	Harm greater than benefit: do not test!		Benefit greater than harm: test!

MI, myocardial infarction.

the literature)[110-125] (see Table 25-6) (Apfelbaum JL et al, unpublished data), and that harm from false-positive results is 6 in 100 (see previous discussion)[82,149] (Apfelbaum JL et al, unpublished data). For the asymptomatic under-age-40 population, the result would be harm to three individuals and benefit to only 0.8 individuals per 1,000 chest radiographs (Table 25-11). Similar analyses are possible for other tests and situations (see Table 25-11).

Lead-Time and Length-Time Biases

Two important concepts related to the reported benefits and risks of screening tests deserve consideration: lead-time and length-time biases.[198] These two factors can indicate an apparent benefit of testing when there is none. Let us examine screening for lung cancer in smokers and screening for breast cancer. In a Czechoslovakian trial of screening of smokers, men at high risk were randomly assigned to either chest radiography twice a year or no screening.[199] No difference in mortality from lung cancer occurred. However, the 5-year survival rate from the time of diagnosis was 23% for the screened group and 0% for the control group. Thus this apparent improvement was entirely owing to earlier diagnosis ("lead-time bias"). In fact, mortality from lung cancer was actually higher in the screened group, indicating that the real effect of screening and subsequent intervention was negative.

Black and Welch[198] reviewed the only other trial of screening strategies using diagnostic radiology evaluated in a randomized trial. In the first (and to date, only) randomized trial of mammographic screening—the Malmö mammographic screening trial[200]—the benefits of this test also seem to disappear. Women over 45 years of age were randomly assigned to either regular mammography or no screening. Although survival from the time of diagnosis was 80% higher for the screened group, no difference

existed in mortality from the time of randomization. Thus, the apparent increase in the survival rate for screened patients was entirely owing to lead-time bias (earlier diagnosis) and length-time bias (less severe cases diagnosed) associated with screening test detection, and not to any benefit from the screening strategy itself.

Before one concludes that no tests should occur preoperatively, let us remember that detection of subclinical conditions in high-risk groups and optimization of therapy for clinical conditions can result in less perioperative morbidity, fewer changes in perioperative plans, and better informed discussions of risk with the patient and significant others. In fact, more recent tests of mammography have also shown this lead-time bias but have shown a survival benefit as well: about two thirds of the benefit of screening mammograms in the over-age-40 population was due to lead time and one third to a real survival advantage.[201]

Laboratory Test Abnormalities in Asymptomatic Populations

Does Surgical Procedure Influence Laboratory Test Choice and Requirements?

A decade ago the answer to these two questions was no. Today, as we indicated above, the answer is yes. Some operations incur such low rates of morbidity and mortality that a test is not indicated unless it is necessary for "routine" preventive care of the patient. Examples would be diagnostic knee arthroscopy and cataract extraction. Table 25-6 divides procedures into three types. Type A procedures are minimally invasive operations that produce little tissue trauma and minimal blood loss. I believe that *no* laboratory testing is indicated for these operations, based on preoperative status alone (such a division was proposed in the ASA Advisory for Preanesthesia Evaluation discussed earlier). That assumes that the patient is seen and followed by a primary care physician and judged to be in optimal health for daily living by that physician. Obviously, some laboratory testing may be required for patients undergoing such procedures, in order to provide preventive care or to optimize such patients' medical condition if they are not already in optimal health for daily living (even a haircut can pose a risk for someone in severe congestive heart failure). On the other hand, type B and C procedures are progressively more risky and invasive. For these procedures, it becomes increasingly important to optimize any adverse conditions (even the less severe ones) that exist preoperatively. Therefore, type B and C procedures often require more preoperative testing. There are insufficient data to be able to state there is a definitive benefit to additional preoperative screening for type B procedures, but in the absence of such data, most physicians err on the side of caution and obtain the same data that are appropriate for type C procedures.

Chest Radiographs

What abnormalities on chest radiographs can influence management of anesthesia? Certainly it may be important to know about the existence of the following conditions before proceeding to anesthesia and surgery: tracheal deviation or compression; mediastinal masses; pulmonary nodules; a solitary lung mass; aortic aneurysm; pulmonary edema; pneumonia; atelectasis; new fractures of the vertebrae, ribs, and clavicles; dextrocardia; and cardiomegaly. However, a chest radiograph probably would not detect the degree of chronic lung disease requiring a change in anesthetic technique any better than would the history or physical examination.

Table 25-10[112,113,149,156,166,170,176-197] shows the prevalence of conditions that a chest radiograph might detect. These data show that abnormalities are rare in the asymptomatic individual. In fact, the risks associated with chest radiographs probably exceed their possible benefit if the patient is asymptomatic and less than 75 years of age. This analysis is predicated on maximizing benefit to all patients as a general group, because one cannot say which individual patients will benefit and which will be harmed. Thus, chest radiographs are not warranted for any asymptomatic patient who is less than 75 years of age and free of risk factors. In fact, this conclusion may apply to those older than 75 years of age as well.

Electrocardiograms

The incidence of ECG abnormalities has been determined by studies of patients (Hsu J et al, unpublished data)[113,114,170,171,202-208] and epidemiologic surveys of healthy people.[183] The abnormalities on the ECG that have the potential to alter management of anesthesia are as follows: atrial flutter or fibrillation; first-, second-, and third-degree atrioventricular block; changes in ST segment suggesting myocardial ischemia or recent pulmonary embolism; premature ventricular and atrial contractions, especially those that are frequent (i.e., greater than 3 per minute); left or right ventricular hypertrophy; short PR interval; Wolff-Parkinson-White syndrome; myocardial infarction; prolonged QT segment (this has special importance and gained prominence as a cause of perioperative morbidity and mortality); and tall peaked T waves. What is the incidence of finding these abnormalities on the 12-lead preoperative screening ECG but not on a standard monitor lead 1 or an MCL_5 lead applied immediately before induction of anesthesia in the OR?

Before answering that question, some qualifiers apply. First, few of the studies on the incidence of ECG abnormalities (Apfelbaum JL et al, unpublished data)[78,79,167] excluded patients having histories or physical examinations indicating cardiac problems. Second, the studies do not distinguish those findings evident on monitoring leads from findings evident on only 6- or 12-lead ECGs[112-114,128,136,145,146,156,170,183,185-210] (Table 25-12).

Table 25–12   Percentage of patients having abnormalities determined by screening electrocardiograms[*]

Age (y)	Sex	Series	Patients Examined (n)	Total Abnormalities[†](%)	Specific Abnormalities			
					LVH	MI	ST Changes	AV Block
16-19	M	Ostrander et al[204]	216	20.3	17.8	0.0	0.9	1.4
16-19	F	Ostrander et al[204]	24	5.9	1.3	0.0	4.2	0.4
20-29	M	Ostrander et al[204]	452	14.0	7.1	0.2	6.0	0.7
20-29	F	Ostrander et al[204]	577	11.3	0.2	0.2	9.9	1.0
20-29	M	Collen et al[170]	3,000	9.6	—	—	—	—
30-39	F	Collen et al[170]	4,000[‡]	9.3	—	—	—	—
>30	Either	Maigaard et al[183]	1,256	>4.5	—	0.1	—	—
30-39	M	Ostrander et al[204]	676	—	3.0	0.0	6.9	1.3
30-39	F	Ostrander et al[204]	699	—	0.4	0.1	11.6	1.6
30-39	M	Collen et al[170]	4,000[‡]	12.1	—	—	—	—
30-39	F	Collen et al[170]	5,000[‡]	11.7	—	—	—	—
35-44	M	Kannel et al[203,205]	—	—	2.9	—	—	—
35-44	F	Kannel et al[203,205]	—	—	0.9	—	—	—
<40	Either	Blery et al[128]	2,256	0.6	—	—	—	—
<40	Either	Apfelbaum et al[206,§,‖]	510	0	—	—	—	—
<40	Either	McKee and Scott[112,§]	23	13 (0)	—	—	—	—

(Continued)

Table 25–12 Percentage of patients having abnormalities determined by screening electrocardiograms*—Cont'd

Age (y)	Sex	Series	Patients Examined (n)	Total Abnormalities[†] (%)	Specific Abnormalities			
					LVH	MI	ST Changes	AV Block
<40	Either	Gold et al[209]	94	37	—	—	—	—
<40	Either	Velanovich[185]	NA	15.8	—	—	—	—
>40	Either	Johnson et al[114]	212	66	2.8	13.2	23.1	2.8
40-49	M	Ostrander et al[204]	468	24*	4.1	1.7	16.1	1.5
40-49	F	Ostrander et al[204]	474	21[‡]	0.6	0.8	17.2	0.6
40-49	M	Collen et al[170]	4,000[‡]	17.6	—	—	—	—
40-49	F	Collen et al[170]	5,000[‡]	15.6	—	—	—	—
40-49	Either	Gold et al[209]	260	36	—	—	—	—
41-50	Either	McKee and Scott[112,§]	53	1.9 (0)	—	—	—	—
<45	?	Moorman et al[207,§]	275	0.4	—	—	—	—
45-54	M	Kannel et al[203,205]	—	—	4.8	—	—	—
45-54	F	Kannel et al[203,205]	—	—	3.6	—	—	—
40-60	Either	Velanovich[185]	NA	47.5	—	—	—	—
>45	?	Morman et al[207,§]	500	1.4	—	—	—	—
>50	Either	Yipintsoi et al[202]	424[§]	14.4[§]	—	—	—	—
50-59	M	Ostrander et al[204]	330	30[‡]	3.3	5.1	20.8	1.2
50-59	F	Ostrander et al[204]	327	40[‡]	3.4	0.9	32.4	2.1
50-59	M	Collen et al[170]	5,000[‡]	24.9	—	—	—	—
50-59	F	Collen et al[170]	6,000[‡]	20.7	—	—	—	—
50-59	Either	Gold et al[209]	163	44	—	—	—	—
51-60	Either	McKee and Scott[112,§]	84	23.8 (0)	—	—	—	—
55-64	M	Kannel et al[203,205]	—	—	10.1	—	—	—
55-64	F	Kannel et al[203,205]	—	—	4.1	—	—	—
<60	Either	Rabkin and Horne[145,146]	309	13.5	2.5	1.6	11.0	1.0
>60	Either	Rabkin and Horne[145,146]	503	24.4	2.2	1.9	13.0	0.6
			—	42.3	—	—	—	—
>60	Either	McKee and Scott[112,§]	163	(1.3)	—	—	—	—
>60	Either	Gold et al[209]	134	62	—	—	—	—
>60	Either	Velanovich[185]	—	61.5	—	—	—	—
>65	Either	Seymour et al[208]	222	52.7	—	—	—	—
60-69	M	Ostrander et al[204]	177	—	8.4	9.0	37.1	4.5
60-69	F	Ostrander et al[204]	196	—	10.2	6.1	42.4	4.1
60-69	M	Collen et al[170]	2,000[‡]	35.1	—	—	—	—
60-69	F	Collen et al[170]	3,000[‡]	29.7	—	—	—	—
65-74	M	Kannel et al[203,205]	—	—	7.1	—	—	—
65-74	F	Kannel et al[203,205]	—	—	9.6	—	—	—
>?70	Either	Wolf-Klein et al[137]	500	11.9	—	—	—	—
>70	M	Collen et al[170]	1,000[‡]	52.2	—	—	—	—
>70	F	Collen et al[170]	1,000[‡]	41.2	—	—	—	—
≥71	Either	Levinstein et al[156]	121	24.4	0.7	13.8	6.3	3.6
70-79	M	Ostrander et al[204]	100	—	7.9	9.9	46.5	7.9
70-79	F	Ostrander et al[204]	119	—	11.8	2.5	43.8	6.7
74-97	Either	Domoto et al[136]	69	27.5	—	—	—	—
>80	M	Ostrander et al[204]	26	—	11.5	7.7	46.2	19.2
>80	F	Ostrander et al[204]	43	—	16.3	4.7	58.2	9.3
0-?90	Either	Blery et al[128,§]	2,256	0.6 (0.3)	—	—	—	—
0-?90	Either	Turnbull and Buck[113]	632	14.6	Combined: 0.67			
0-?90	Either	Muskett and McGreevy[115]	145	1.3	—			—

*All studies are 12-lead studies, except for that of Collen et al[170] which is a 6-lead study.

[†]These data constitute an edited summary of data given in several series, edited to select abnormalities that might change management of anesthesia. *Numbers in parentheses indicate abnormalities judged retrospectively by the authors of the paper to be significant to perioperative management.*

[‡]Values are approximations that represent "best-guess" numbers from data not explicitly stated in the reports.

[§]Patients were asymptomatic.

‖Apfelbaum JL et al, unpublished data (patients were asymptomatic).

AV, atrioventricular; LVH, left ventricular hypertrophy; MI, myocardial infarction.

Table 25-13   Patients found to have a new abnormality on an ECG and on previous ECG*

| | New Abnormality with a previously | | | |
	Normal ECG		Abnormal ECG	
Age(y)	<60	≥60	<60	≥60
No. of patients/total no.	18/180	42/192	24/129	81/310
% new abnormalities	10	21.9	18.6	26
Abnormality				
T wave	11 (6.1%)	18 (9.4%)	10 (7.8%)	19 (6.1%)
ST segment	7 (3.9%)	9 (4.7%)	6 (4.7%)	20 (6.4%)
Arrhythmias				
SVT or PVC	3 (1.7%)	7 (3.6%)		8 (2.6%)
Others, including PAC	3 (1.7%)	6 (3.1%)	1 (0.8%)	1 (0.3%)
QRS duration		8 (4.2%)	2 (1.6%)	14 (4.5%)
LVH	3 (1.7%)	4 (2.1%)	5 (3.9%)	7 (2.3%)
Q wave	4 (2.2%)	3 (1.6%)	1 (0.8%)	7 (2.3%)
Ventricular conduction defects	5 (2.6%)	1 (0.8%)	7 (2.3%)	7 (2.3%)
AV block	2 (1.0%)	3 (2.3%)	1 (0.3%)	

*Numbers in parentheses are percentage of patients; two-thirds of patients had a previous ECG within 2 years of their new ECG.
AV, atrioventricular; ECG, electrocardiogram; LVH, left ventricular hypertrophy; PAC, premature atrial contractions; PVC, premature ventricular contractions; SVT, supraventricular tachycardia.
Data from Rabkin and Horne.[145,146]

The data in Table 25-13 and elsewhere[210,211] show that abnormalities on the ECG are relatively common and increase exponentially with age. Averaging all those data indicates that the incidence of abnormal preoperative electrocardiographic results will exceed 10% at 40 years of age and will be 25% by 60 years of age. These estimates pool abnormalities for both sexes. Clearly, the studies that looked for abnormalities on the ECG after first ensuring that the patient was asymptomatic[112,202,128] found a much lower incidence of significant abnormalities. McKee and Scott[112] found no abnormalities significant to perioperative care for 160 individuals who had no cardiac symptoms and were under 60 years of age, and only two abnormalities for 163 patients over 60 years of age. Moorman and colleagues[207] reported that only 1 of 275 asymptomatic patients 45 years of age or less had abnormalities on preoperative ECGs. In the study by Blery and co-workers,[128] only 0.6% of 2,256 patients under age 40 who had no cardiac or pulmonary symptoms had an abnormality on preoperative ECGs. Our group found no abnormalities on ECG that were significant to, or altered, perioperative care for 510 patients judged to be asymptomatic on the basis of results from a video questionnaire[206] (Apfelbaum JL et al, unpublished data). This study is discussed later in this chapter.

How useful is it to repeat ECGs if the patient has had an ECG within the past 2 years? Rabkin and Horne[145,146] addressed this question. "New abnormalities" on a subsequent ECG occur with significant frequency—approximately 25% to 50% as frequently as all abnormalities occurring on the previous ECG (see Table 25-13). Thus, one would be justified in obtaining screening ECGs prior to elective surgery for all patients over 40 years of age, even those who have recently had an ECG if it is more than 5 months old or was abnormal. (See Table 25-11 for an analysis of the risk versus benefit of obtaining an ECG for asymptomatic patients.)

Some physicians have questioned even that conclusion. Goldberger and O'Konski[176] believe that the most important potential benefit of the preoperative ECG is detection of previously unrecognized myocardial infarction. This risk increases with age. However, even for the highest-risk group, men 75 years of age or older, the estimated incidence of unrecognized Q-wave infarction within the preceding 6 months is relatively small (< 0.5%). Goldberger and O'Konski concluded that the risk from obtaining a preoperative ECG and subsequent reactions probably exceeds its benefit if patients are asymptomatic, do not have important risk factors for coronary disease, and are under 45 (men) or 55 (women) years of age. If we use the data in Table 25-12 and apply the benefit-risk analysis described in the section on chest radiographs, ECGs are indicated for asymptomatic patients of average risk (no special family history of premature arterial aging diseases such as stroke, heart attack, or peripheral vascular disease prior to age 40) undergoing type B or C procedures who are over 40 (men) or 50 (women) years of age.

These estimates do not account for the differences in physiologic age that exist between patients of the same calendar age. I believe that these differences are important. Although I also believe that physiologic age ("RealAge"*) should be the factor used to determine the need for testing, this hypothesis has not been widely tested. We know that conditions such as normal blood pressure, regular vigorous exercise, the absence of exposure

---

*The term was coined by Dr. Michael Roizen,[212] who is a scientific advisor to RealAge, Inc., and has an equity interest in that company. He is the author of several books published by HarperCollins, including "RealAge: Are You as Young as You Can Be?" (a #1 New York Times Bestseller, and #1 in four other countries), "The RealAge Diet," "Cooking the RealAge Way," and "The RealAge Makeover: Looking Younger, Living Longer."

Hemoglobin, Hematocrit, and White Blood Cell Counts

The classic references on hemoglobin, hematocrit, and white blood cell counts, and the inferences they allow, have stood the test of time. We describe them now, so that the reader will understand the rationale for decisions and practices used today.

In 1964, Wasserman and Gilbert[214] reported that of 28 patients with uncontrolled polycythemia (hemoglobin >16 g/dL) who underwent major surgery, 22 (79%) had complications and 10 (36%) died. This group was compared with 53 patients who had controlled polycythemia (hemoglobin <16 g/dL) and major surgery; 15 (28%) had complications, and 3 (5%) died. In both groups, most of the complications were related to polycythemia (e.g., hemorrhage or thrombosis). Other data confirm that polycythemia is an independent risk factor for cardiovascular mortality.[215] Admittedly, the study of Wasserman and Gilbert had deficiencies: it was a retrospective study, no time frame was given, and "minor" surgery was excluded. Also, the study did not explain why polycythemia was controlled preoperatively for some patients but not for others. Nevertheless, knowledge and pretreatment of polycythemia decreased perioperative morbidity and mortality, but there is little or no data on what levels are appropriate to treat. Most physicians arbitrarily rely on the limited data of Wasserman and Gilbert[214] and do not treat unless the hemoglobin level is greater than 16 mg/dL.

Not even such weak evidence exists for treatment of normovolemic anemia. Rothstein[216] concluded that hemoglobin of 9 g/dL is adequate for patients over 3 months of age but should exceed 10 g/dL for younger patients (see Chapters 47 and 48). As emphasized by Roy and colleagues,[118] the age of the patient at the time of discovery of anemia often points to its cause. Anemia in the neonatal period is often attributable to recent blood loss, isoimmunization, congenital hemolytic anemia, or congenital infection. Anemia first detected 3 to 6 months after birth suggests a congenital disorder of hemoglobin synthesis or structure. Therefore, assays of hemoglobin concentration in the first 6 months may represent the first opportunity for analysis. This use of the perioperative period for screening (or case finding) necessitates a proactive procedure for referring the patient and parents for counseling and/or treatment (ideally integrated through an automated information [informatics] system linking preoperative clinic and primary care physicians). Thus, preoperative evaluation can add to a patient's prior medical database.

This point—that preoperative evaluations and documentation of data from the history are often not complete—was reiterated by Hackmann and colleagues[117] in their study of the prevalence of anemia. They reported that several patients whose anemia was not properly suspected had conditions (Hirschsprung's disease, pyloric stenosis, or history of anemia accompanying juvenile rheumatoid arthritis) that should have alerted the anesthesiologist. Similarly, it was difficult to find a perioperative benefit in search for even common hemoglobinopathies (see later) in asymptomatic individuals.[217] These investigators also emphasized the importance of obtaining a thorough history.

Should asymptomatic anemia be treated prior to non–blood-loss surgery, as O'Connor and Drasner[116] and others have done? Does this practice produce more benefit than harm? Does iron therapy at this early age contribute to late ischemic heart disease? Is this the function of preoperative testing—to spot chronic conditions? Although there are no definite answers to these questions, I agree with O'Connor and Drasner that these practices are indicated if one sets up the preoperative assessment to function in that role. This means that the anesthesiologist and the clinic would constitute second-opinion consultants to the primary care physician. It would also require that the preoperative assessment be performed sufficiently early (at least 1 week before surgery) and be vested with enough authority to postpone surgery in a timely enough fashion to avoid any decrease in OR efficiency.

If the preoperative assessment is not done in advance or is not vested with sufficient authority, perhaps asymptomatic anemia prior to non–blood-loss surgery should not be treated preoperatively. This seems to be confirmed by studies showing that patients survive anesthesia and type-A surgery when hemoglobin levels are above 8.0 g/dL.[218,219] No data confirm the hypothesis that preoperative treatment of moderate or mild normovolemic anemia in such patients decreases perioperative morbidity or mortality. Similarly, no data exist regarding the possible harm from abnormal white blood cell counts found preoperatively. Therefore, the following ranges of "surgically acceptable values" are arbitrary: for hematocrit, 29% to 57% for men and 27% to 54% for women; for white blood cell count, 2,400 to 16,000/mm^3 for both men and women. When values fall outside these ranges, I recommend seeking an alternative diagnosis before instituting anesthesia or surgery.[219]

How many healthy patients have this degree of abnormality in hematocrit or white blood cell count? No such patient was found in either study of the 223 and 2,010 patients judged healthy by history (i.e., history indicated no need for tests).[111,206] Table 25-14 provides the only other available data, which are limited. If we assume that 10% of all abnormalities are outside the "surgically acceptable" range (see Table 25-14), and if we apply the benefit-risk analysis described in the section on chest radiographs, we would conclude that either preoperative hematocrit or hemoglobin levels should be determined for all female surgical patients and for all male surgical patients over 64 years of age who are undergoing type B or C surgical procedures. Red cell antigen screening would be warranted for all patients undergoing procedures involving possible blood loss of more than 2 U/70 kg body weight (type B and C surgical procedures).[221,222] White blood cell counts appear to be rarely, if ever, justified for asymptomatic patients.

Table 25–14 Abnormalities discovered by screening hemoglobin tests and WBC counts

Age (y)	Sex	Series	Patients Examined (n)	Hemoglobin Abnormalities (%)	WBC Count Abnormalities (%)
<1	Either	Roy et al[118]	257	1.1	
<1	Either	Hackmann et al[117]	269	2.6	
1-5	Either	Roy et al[118]	1,113	0.7	
3-12	Either	Nigam et al[119]	250	0.8	
5-18	Either	Roy et al[118]	630	0	
<18	Either	Hackmann et al[117]	2,649	0.5	
<18	Either	Baron et al[120]	1,863	1.1	
<18	Either	O'Connor and Drasner[116]	468	11.9	2.7
1-19	Either	Hackmann et al[117]	2,380	0.3	
<19	Either	Wood and Hoekelman[143]	1,924	0.8	
<40	M	Collen et al[170]	6,941	1.9	2.6
<40	F	Collen et al[170]	9,037	12.6	2.6
≥18	Either	Parkerson[159]	392	18.8	10.7
>19	Either	Johnson et al[114]	212	2.4*	0
32-90	Either	Johnson and Mortimer[124]	100*	12	7
<40	Either	McKee and Scott[112*]	96*	0	0
<40	Either	Velanovich[185]	—†	12	
40-59	M	Collen et al[170]	11,832	3.1	2.2
40-59	F	Collen et al[170]	9,657	10.1	2.2
41-50	Either	McKee and Scott[112*]	53*	5.7	?
40-60	Either	Velanovich[185]	—†	15.5	
51-60	Either	McKee and Scott[112*]	85*	0	0
≥60	M	Collen et al[170]	4,062	5.6	1.7
≥60	F	Collen et al[170]	3,134	5.5	1.7
>60	Either	McKee and Scott[112*]	163*	6.1	?
>60	Either	Velanovich[185]	—†	31.6	
>?70	Either	Wolf-Klein et al[137]	551	33.2	17.4
>71	Either	Levinstein et al[156]	121	27.8	4.0
74-97	Either	Domoto et al[136]	70	11.4	4.3
Unspecified	Either	Turnbull and Buck[113]	1,005*	0.7	0.1
Unspecified	Either	Muskett and McGreevy[115]	199	60.8	34.8
				9.0‡	5.1‡
Unspecified	Either	Kaplan et al[111*]	293	0‡	0‡
Unspecified	Either	Gold and Wolfersberger[223*]	3,375	0.33	
Unspecified	Either	Carmalt et al[220]	278	30.4§	
Unspecified	Either	Huntley et al[161]	119	23	
Unspecified	Either	Williamson et al[160]	982	3.2	
Unspecified	Either	Blery et al[128*]	1,728	1.1	

*Patients were asymptomatic.
†A total of 520 patients were examined, but no age distribution was presented.
‡Abnormalities significant to perioperative management.
§Carmalt and co-workers[220] found that 24.5% were new abnormalities. Two patients had hemoglobin values of less than 8 g/dL, 17 had values of 8 to 10 g/dL, and 21 had values of 10 to 12 g/dL.

Blood Chemistries, Urinalysis, and Clotting Studies

What blood chemistries would have to be abnormal, and how abnormal would they have to be, to justify changing one's perioperative management? Abnormal hepatic or renal function might change the choice and dose of anesthetic or adjuvant drugs. Approximately 1 in 700 supposedly healthy patients actually harbors hepatitis, and 1 in 3 of those patients will become jaundiced.[224,225] However, our group found no asymptomatic patient who denied exposure to hepatitis who then became jaundiced after uneventful surgery[206] (Roizen MF, unpublished data for more than 11,500 patients in a prospective study of the "HealthQuiz" [discussed later]; Hsu J et al, unpublished data). These data suggest that either the screening history suffices or the incidence of asymptomatic hepatitis is decreasing.

Data from the National Veterans Affairs Surgical Risk Study[61] found that the albumin level was an important predictor of perioperative morbidity and mortality in every surgical specialty. Therefore, one could argue for determining, and I believe it is appropriate to determine, albumin levels preoperatively for all patients about to undergo class C procedures.

Table 25-15* presents the available data regarding abnormalities found on screening blood chemistries. Unexpected abnormalities are reported for 2% to 10% of patients screened, and these abnormalities lead to many additional tests that usually (approximately 80%) have no significance for the patient. In fact, as described in the section on laboratory tests as ineffective screening devices, if 20 chemistry tests are ordered for a healthy individual, there is a 64% chance that results of at least one test will be abnormal (see Fig. 25-3). Unexpected abnormalities that are significant arise in 2% to 5% percent of patients studied. Of these abnormalities, approximately 70% percent are related to blood glucose[226] and blood urea nitrogen (BUN) levels. Note that the screen for diabetes may soon shift from random determinations of blood glucose levels to determination of the concentration of glycosylated hemoglobin (Hb A_{1c}). The 9 to 20 additional tests on the screening simultaneous multi-channel analysis (SMA) of 12 to 20 variables lead to very few important discoveries affecting anesthesia. In fact, the false-positive rate is so high (i.e., 96.5% for the test for calcium) that the value representing cost versus benefit for most of these tests (even when the tests are free) is negative, as is the value representing benefit versus risk. Examination of the data reported by Berwick[168] in Table 25-15 helps clarify the difficulty of screening. More than 75% of the abnormalities (see the line in Table 25-15 in which $n = 76,519$) were not even outside the range that caused the laboratories at these health screening fairs to notify the patient or physician of an abnormal value (see the line in Table 25-15 in which $n = 86,006$), let alone be judged significant to the patient's health.

It appears that only blood glucose (or its successor Hb A_{1c}), albumin, and BUN assays are indicated before type B and C procedures. Even then, BUN is indicated only for patients over 65 years of age, and glucose (or Hb A_{1c}) only for individuals over 75 years of age. No blood chemistry tests are warranted for patients less than 65 years of age. Furthermore, because the antibody test for hepatitis A and C are useful after infection has occurred, the medicolegal risk posed by postanesthetic jaundice should be even less.

Abnormalities are common on urinalysis[†] (Table 25-16) (Apfelbaum JL, et al, unpublished data). The quality of urinalysis results obtained by dipstick technique has been variable at best.[236] In addition, these abnormal results usually do not lead to beneficial changes in management. Most of the results that do lead to beneficial changes could have been obtained by history or determination of BUN and glucose (or Hb A_{1c}) levels, tests that are already recommended for all patients over 65 and 75 years of age, respectively. Thus, urinalysis, although initially inexpensive, becomes an expensive test to justify on a benefit-cost or benefit-risk basis.

Although partial thromboplastin time (PTT) and pro-thrombin time (PT) are useful tests for screening patients who have a history of bleeding, their value as screening tests for asymptomatic patients has never been shown* (Table 25-17). Virtually no asymptomatic patient in the literature has had unequivocal benefit from clotting function studies performed preoperatively (see Table 25-17). Most patients show symptoms or have a medication history suggesting the possible need for clotting function tests. Suchman and Mushlin[242] and Macpherson[243] reviewed the data, as we did,[82] and came to the same conclusion: preoperative clotting function testing for asymptomatic patients who have no risk factors for coagulopathy is incapable of predicting perioperative bleeding. No information is gained from either an abnormal or a normal result on clotting studies in low-risk patients. Figure 25-5 presents an algorithm that can be used to segregate high- and low-risk patients.[244]

One patient deserves special comment: the patient taking aspirin or aspirin-containing compounds. Aspirin at a dose of 3 to 10 mg/kg of body weight daily does not seem to pose a risk of bleeding, and is even beneficial enough for some groups to begin instituting it in preoperative clinics.[43,44] But this practice is just now going from banned to advocated due to early evidence of benefit to patient outcome.

Because the pharmacokinetics of aspirin change when more than 2 g/70 kg of body weight is consumed daily, a patient should be evaluated if he or she is on large doses of aspirin (more than six 325-mg tablets a day) and has not discontinued aspirin consumption sufficiently early to ensure that there is no appreciable level of acetylsalicylic acid in the blood for 24 hours before surgery. (This is the period in which acetylsalicylic acid would have to be absent for the generation of the approximately 50,000 new platelets/mm^3 needed for normal platelet aggregation.) The patient should also be evaluated if surgical hemostasis cannot be ensured or if a regional procedure into a closed space is planned. Nonsteroidal anti-inflammatory drugs (NSAIDs) present similar problems.[245] (For further explanation of these situations, see the section in Chapter 27 regarding interruption of a drug regimen prior to surgery.)

Tests for HIV, Pregnancy, Hemoglobinopathies, Malignant Hyperthermia, Magnesium Deficiency, and Low Albumin Levels

Tests for HIV infection and pregnancy and screening for hemoglobinopathy and malignant hyperthermia raise ethical questions that may require close attention to institutional policy and the immediate availability of counseling services. Moreover, all of these tests have risks. The physician may therefore decide to limit testing to only "at-risk" populations (e.g., for pregnancy testing, only female patients who believe they may be pregnant). As noted previously, the ASA Practice Advisory survey of members found that 17% of all members obtained a

---

*See references 110-113, 128, 136-139, 156, 159, 168, 170, 206, 220, 224-234.
†See references 113-116, 122, 136, 137, 141, 142, 156, 160, 161, 168, 170, 185, 223, 235, 236.

*See references 110, 111, 115, 121, 123-125, 128, 134, 156, 157, 237-242.

Table 25–15 Screening blood chemistries: Percentage of patients having abnormalities

Age (y)	Series	Patients Examined (n)	BUN	Cr	Glucose	AST or SGOT	Uric Acid	Cholesterol	Albumin	Total Protein	Ca²⁺	VDRL	ALK PTAse	Bilirubin	K⁺	Phosphate
0-65	Narr et al[110]	3,782	—	—	1.9	0.3	—	—	—	—	—	—	—	—	0.2	—
10-54	Schemel[225]	7,620	—	—	—	0.144	—	—	—	—	—	—	—	—	—	—
12-90	Alsumait et al[125]	1000	—	1.6	8.2	—	—	—	—	—	—	—	—	—	4.0	—
15-85	Carmalt et al[220,*]	296	1.4	1.0	2.0	0	—	0.3	0	—	0.3	—	0	0	0.3	—
>18	Parkerson[159]	397	—	1.2	15.8	2.8	7.9	6.1	—	—	2.0	—	—	1.2	6.6	—
>18	Schneiderman et al[227]	547	—	9.3	—	1.3	—	—	—	—	—	—	9.7	3.7	—	—
>18	[Bryan data][228,229]	623	1.1	—	5.0	—	4.5	—	1.4	2.4	1.0	—	—	—	4.0	—
>25	Peery[230,*]	1,771	18	—	21	3.1	36	30	0.5	0.5	—	—	1.3	—	3.6	—
32-90	Johnson and Mortimer[124]	100	17	14	8	—	—	—	—	—	—	—	—	—	6	—
<40	McKee and Scott[112,†]	96	0	—	—	—	—	—	—	—	—	—	—	—	0	—
40-59	Collen et al[170]	21,489	—	1.4	5.6	4.6	4.8	2.7	0.3	4.4	1.3	1.9	—	—	—	—
41-50	McKee and Scott[112,†]	53	0	—	—	—	—	—	—	—	—	—	—	—	0	—
>40	Collen et al[170]	15,978	—	0.8	4.6	3.6	3.4	1.7	0.4	3.5	1.4	0.8	—	—	—	—
51-60	McKee and Scott[112,†]	85	0	—	—	—	—	—	—	—	—	—	—	—	0	—
>60	Collen et al[170]	7,196	—	2.7	8.3	4.5	6.0	3.0	0.4	3.9	1.5	2.3	—	—	—	—
>60	McKee and Scott[112,†]	163	2.5	—	—	—	—	—	—	—	—	—	—	—	0	—
>70	Wolf-Klein et al[137]	500	24.6	14.5	24.6	9.4	7.7	13.8	20.4	9.9	7.2	—	23.2	1.7	5.4	—
>71	Levinstein et al[156]	121	36	10.8	29.0	0.8	7.2	6.9	27.8	19.2	5.6	—	19.0	0.7	3.0	—
74-97	Dunlop et al[136]	70	30	—	26.5	9.2	8.6	17.2	0	2.1	1.0	—	9.2	2.1	—	1.0
All	Wataneeyawech and Kelly[224]	6,540	—	—	—	0.234	—	—	—	—	—	—	—	—	—	—

(Continued)

957

Table 25–15 Screening blood chemistries: Percentage of patients having abnormalities—cont'd

Age (y)	Series	Patients Examined (n)	BUN	Cr	Glucose	AST or SGOT	Uric Acid	Cholesterol	Albumin	Total Protein	Ca²⁺	VDRL	ALK PTAse	Bilirubin	K⁺	Phosphate
All	Bryan et al[228]	2,846	1.4	—	5.6	—	—	—	1.4	0.7	0.3	—	—	—	0.3	—
All	Friedman et al[231]	8,446	3.4	3.3	5.9	2.7	2.7	3.8	1.5	2.5	5.4	—	3.9	2.4	1.4	—
All	Delahunt and Turnbull[139],†	332	0	0	—	—	—	—	—	—	—	—	—	—	0.3	—
All	Young and Drake[233],*	390	6.4	3.7	7.5	—	—	—	—	—	2.0	—	—	—	0	—
All	Berwick[168]	86,006‡	0.7	0.3	1.2	0.5	1.2	0.8	0.02	0.09	0.5	—	0.7	0.3	1.8	—
All	Berwick[168]	76,519	1.6	1.3	3.5	2.5	2.9	5.1	1.5	1.2	2.8	—	2.6	4.0	3.2	—
All	Boonstra and Jackson[233],*	12,000	—	—	—	—	—	—	—	—	5.0*	—	—	—	—	—
All	Apfelbaum et al[206],§	1,784‖	2.0	1.8	3.4	1.8	—	—	0.3	1.3	1.0	—	1.3	—	2.6¶	0.3
All	Apfelbaum et al[206],§	Variable (asymptom.)‡	0.3	0.3	0.1	0.2	—	—	0.2	0.3	0.7	—	0.6	—	1.8¶	—
All	Whitehead[234]	2,871	3.4	—	10.0	1.8	9.2	9.3	2.9	—	9.2	—	8.3	6.0	4.7	—
All	Turnbull and Buck[113],†	995	0.1	0.2	0.7	—	—	—	—	—	—	—	—	—	1.4	—
All	Blery et al[128],†	~2,800	0.1	0.1	0.1	—	—	—	—	—	—	—	—	—	0.5	—

*A high percentage of these findings were analyzed in more depth and were found to be clinically unimportant.
†Patients were asymptomatic.
‡Significantly abnormal (outside action limits).[111]
§Also, Apfelbaum JL et al, unpublished data.
‖Symptomatic or asymptomatic patients.
¶Pertains to all abnormalities for all electrolytes measured, not just K⁺.

ALK PTAse, alkaline phosphatase; AST, aspartate aminotransferase; BUN, blood urea nitrogen; Ca²⁺, calcium; Cr, creatinine; K⁺, potassium; SGOT, serum glutamicoxaloacetic transminase; VDRL, serologic test for syphilis, developed by the Venereal Disease Research Laboratory.

Table 25–16   Abnormalities discovered by screening urinalysis

Age (y)	Sex	Series	Patients Examined (n)	Abnormalities (%)	Significant Abnormalities (%)
<18	Either	O'Connor and Drasner[116]	453	15	0.4
<19	Either	Wood and Hoekelman[142]	1,859	1.7	0.5
Unspecified	Either	Huntley et al[161]	119	61	—
5-12	F	Cardiff-Oxford[235]	16,800	1.8	—
15-?	Either	Lawrence and Kroenke[122]	180	15	<1.6
Unspecified	Either	Gold and Wolfersberger[223]	3,375	2.7	—
Unspecified	Either	Williamson et al[160]	982	16.7	—
Unspecified	Either	Collen et al[170]	44,663	14.6	—
Unspecified	Either	Muskett and McGreevy[115]	144	22.4	—
Unspecified	Either	Berwick[168]	235	2.6	—
Unspecified	Either	Turnbull and Buck[113,*]	995	4.3	—
>19	Either	Johnson et al[114]	212	39	<1.9 (?0)
>?70	Either	Wolf-Klein et al[137]	550	12.9	—
≥71	Either	Levinstein et al[156]	121	25.8[†]	—
74-97	Either	Domoto et al[136]	70	9.2	—

*Patients were asymptomatic.
†Was only 1.4% when a dipstick technique was used.

pregnancy test for all women in the potentially child-bearing age range (variously described, with ranges that extend from 11 to 60 calendar years of age). Magnesium testing is a special concern.

Testing of asymptomatic patients for AIDS is unlikely to be the most effective way of uncovering the disease. One program screening for HIV in asymptomatic individuals was able to produce an "acceptably low false-positive rate" by diagnosing HIV infection after only one sample of blood produced positive results on three different tests, and after the second sample of blood had been used for verification.[130] Thus, for pregnancy, hemoglobinopathies, and HIV infection, the history is still the best tool for identifying those who should be tested or those who are at risk of the condition.

In the past, no screening test has existed for susceptibility to malignant hyperthermia syndrome (MHS) other than a personal or family history of the condition (also see Chapter 27). Several new tests are available; none uses genetic testing, but one is expected to be available shortly. Despite previous studies suggesting a single localization of this disorder to chromosome 19q, Levitt and colleagues[246] and other groups have observed evidence for significant genetic heterogeneity in MHS. Nevertheless, they found seven MHS families in which the identified genetic aberrations appear linked to chromosome 17q11.2-24. Because the gene encoding the adult muscle sodium channel a-subunit (SCN4A) has also been localized to this region of the long arm of chromosome 17,

this area may be the site of a primary defect in MHS. However, because the specific site cannot yet be identified, linkage analysis for MHS coupled with polymerase chain amplification might be used in the future to screen for MHS in high-risk patients.

It is still too early to predict the usefulness of these tests as a screening procedure for MHS or for other genetic diseases such as diabetes. Other screening tests for MHS have not been reliable enough to use for any but "at-risk" individuals (e.g., children with a history of myopathies who are undergoing surgery for strabismus, patients having a family history of problems with anesthesia, and patients with a history of abnormal (red) appearance, thermoregulation, and reactions to minor stresses) (Fig. 25-6) (also see Chapter 27).

Magnesium (Mg) deficiency represents another special situation. Putatively it is much more common than other ion deficiencies, and Mg treatment has been advocated as extremely beneficial.[247] However, because no data appear to link preoperative treatment of Mg deficiency with benefit, screening with tests appears superfluous. Let us expand on this concept.

Hypomagnesemia is a prevalent laboratory finding in hospitalized patients (11% to 16%; Table 25-18). The total serum level of Mg represents the protein-bound (physiologically inactive) Mg, as well as the ionized (physiologically active) Mg. (Total serum Mg constitutes less than 1% of total body Mg, there being no constant ratio between the two values.)

Table 25–17 Percentage of patients having coagulation abnormalities, as determined by screening prothrombin time, partial thromboplastin time, platelet count, or bleeding time tests

Age (y)	Series	Patients Examined (n)	Percentage with Abnormalities of				Percentage with Surgically Significant Abnormalities of			
			PT	PTT	PLT CNT	BT	PT	PTT	PLT CNT	BT
?<18	Asaf et al[123]	416	32.4 (121/373)	17.6 (61/346)			0 (0/416)			
20-90	Robbins and Rose[157]	1,025		14 (143/1,025)			0 (0/1,025)			
Unspecified	Baranetsky and Weinstein[237]	2,600	0.2 (5/2,600)				0 (0/2,600)			
Unspecified	Barber et al[238]	1,941 (including 141 with risk factors)				6 (110/1,941)*			22.2 (43/1,941)*	
		1,800				1.5 (27/1,800)*			0.19 (2/1,800)*	
20-90	Blery et al[128]	~2,900	0.1 (4/2,931)	0.1 (4/2,914)	0.3 (10/3,546)		0 (0/2,931)	0 (0/2,914)	0.03 (1/3,576)	
12-90	Alsumait et al[125]	1000	1.4 (14/1000)	1.2 (12/1000)	1.1 (11/1000)	0.4 (17/3,845)	0 (0/1000)	0 (0/1000)	0 (0/1000)	0 (0/3,845)
20.25-65	Narr et al[110]	3,782			1.2 (40/3,782)				0 (0/3,782)	
0-93	Lorenzi and Cohen (personal communication)	578	3.5(20/578)				0 (0/578)			
>18	Kalpan et al[111]	154					0 (0/154)			
>18	Macpherson et al[239]	1,109	1.8 (12/668)	2.8 (29/1,008)	10.1 (108/1,022)		0 (0/668)	0 (0/1,008)	0 (0/1,022)	
>18	Rohrer et al[121] With risk factors	282	0.6 (1/159)	6.3 (10/159)	8.2 (20/117)	7.4 (14/170)	0.6 (1/154)	71.4 (73/159)	22.6 (73/117)	? (0/154)
	Asymptomatic		0.8 (1/123)	2.4 (3/123)	8.0 (13/103)	3.8 (4/105)	0 (0/123)	0 (0/123)	0 (0/103)	0 (0/105)
32-90	Johnson and Mortimer[124]	100			6 (6/100)				0 (0/100)	
>71	Levinstein et al[156]	121			4.0					
Unspecified	Turnbull and Buck[113]	1,005	0 (0/213)	1.5 (3/210)	0 (0/1,005)		0 (0/123)	0 (0/210)	0 (0/1,005)	
Unspecified	Bushnick et al[240]	640	0.8 (5/591)	0.3 (2/640)						
Unspecified	Eisenberg et al[241]	750					0 (0/750)			
Unspecified	Muskett and McGreevy[115]	200	3.9 (5/128)	3.9 (5/126)			0 (0/128)	0 (0/126)		
Unspecified	Suchman and Mushlin[242] With known risk factors	1,004		10.4 (104/1,004)				4.6 (46/1,004)		
	Without known risk factors	11,334	13.3 (243/1,927)					0.71† (13/1,827)		

*Number in parenthesis represents number of patients.

†An abnormal PTT was not more likely to predict hemorrhage than was a normal PTT and was not helpful in preoperative management.

BT, bleeding time; PLT CNT, platelet count; PT, prothrombin time; PTT, partial thromboplastin time.

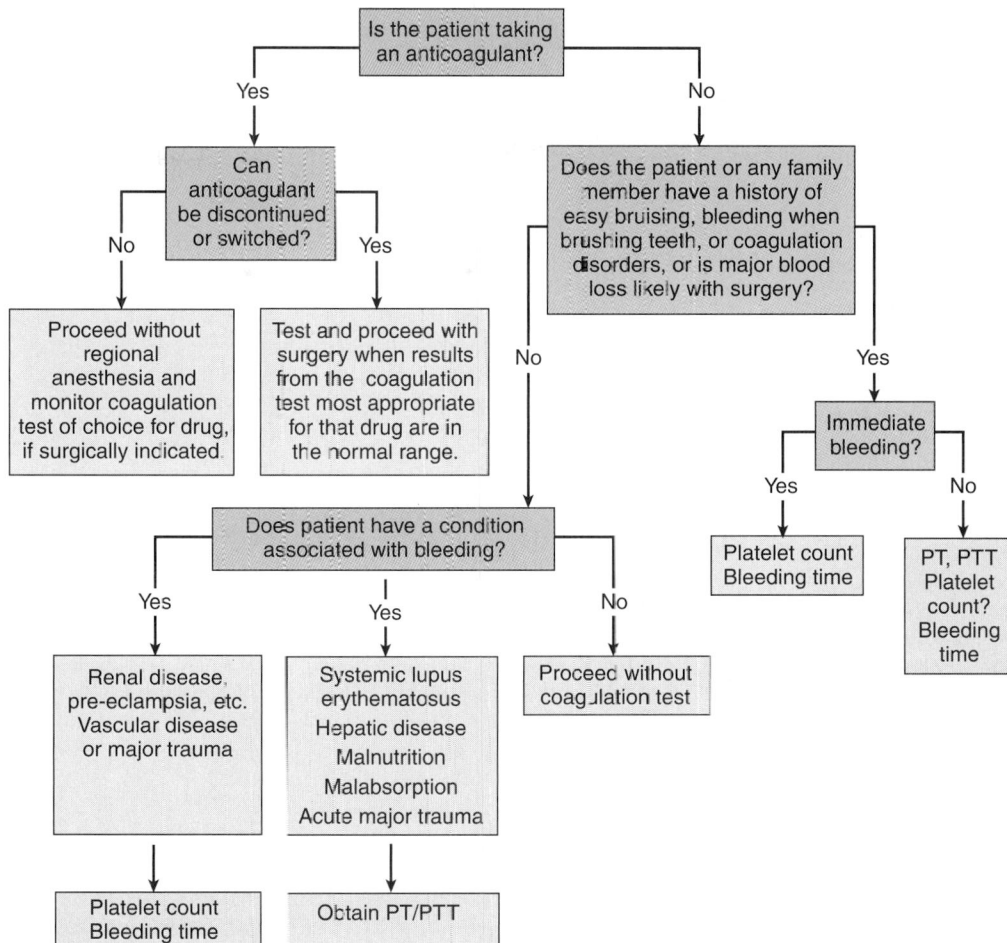

Figure 25–5 Procedure for determining whether coagulation tests are needed. PT, prothrombin time; PTT, partial thromboplastin time. (Redrawn and modified from Roizen MF, Hurd MJ: Preoperative patient evaluation. *In* Rogers MC (ed): Current Practice in Anesthesiology, 2nd ed. St. Louis, Mosby–Year Book, 1990, p 14.)

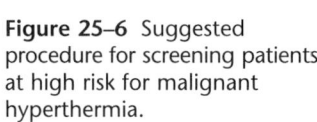

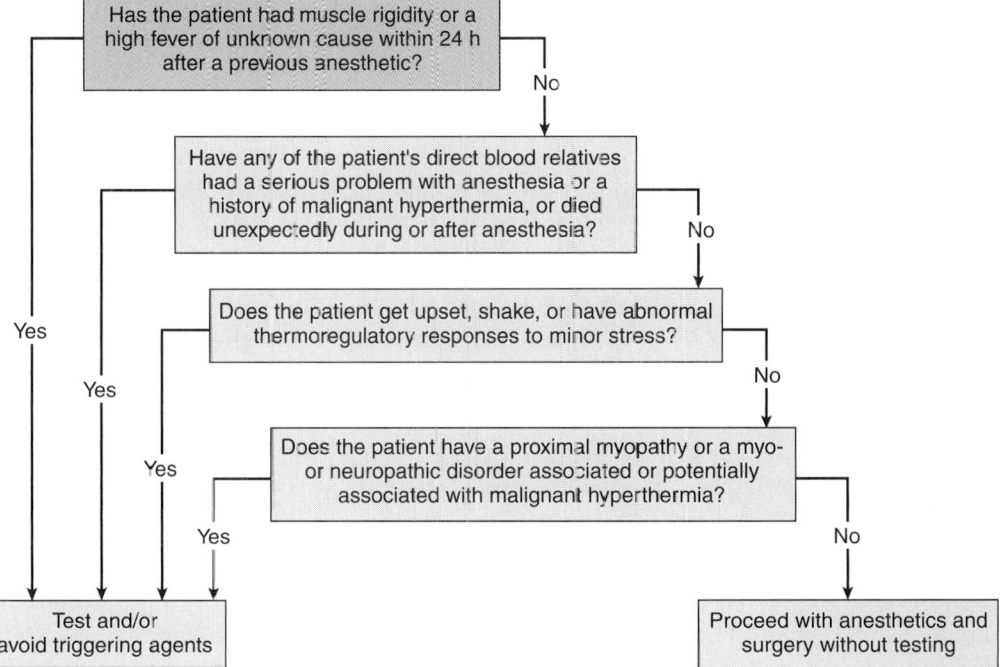

Figure 25–6 Suggested procedure for screening patients at high risk for malignant hyperthermia.

Table 25–18 Prevalence of hypomagnesemia among hospitalized patients

	Wong et al[247]	Whang and Ryder[254]	Lum[255]	Reinhart and Desbiens[250]	Chernow et al[256]
Setting	LA County/USC Medical Center	Urban primary care hospital	VAMC	Community referral hospital	Mass. Gen. Hosp.
Patient selection criteria	Random; hospitalized patients	Random; hospitalized patients	Acute medical/ surgical patients	Consecutive medical ICU patients	Postoperative ICU patients*
No. of subjects	621	1,033†	353	102	193
Hypomagnesemia					
Definition	<1.2 mEq/L	<0.74 mmol/L	<0.72 mmol/L	<1.4 mEq/L	<1.5 mEq/L
Prevalence‡	11.0%	47.1%	26.1%	20%	61%
Technique for measuring serum Mg	ACA, or AAS on a Perkin Elmer 560 B	ACA	ACA III	AAS	AAS (Varian 1275)

*Undergoing major abdominal, thoracic, or vascular procedures.
†The number of test results, not the number of patients.
‡Refers to test results, not patients, i.e., the number of abnormal test results ÷ the number of test results.
AAS, atomic absorption spectrophotometry; ACA, Du Pont Automatic Clinical Analyzer; ICU, intensive care unit; LA, Los Angeles; Mass. Gen. Hosp., Massachusetts General Hospital, Boston; USC, University of Southern California, Los Angeles; VAMC, Veterans Affairs Merical Center.
Courtesy of Dr. Allan Jo and colleagues.

Fanning and colleagues[248] showed that intravenous administration of Mg for 4 days after coronary artery bypass grafting decreased the incidence and severity of atrial fibrillation. Specifically, 14 patients in the control group had 42 episodes of fibrillation, 2 of whom required cardioversion. In contrast, 7 patients in the Mg-treated group had 12 episodes of atrial fibrillation, and none required cardioversion. In a similar study, intraoperative administration of Mg after cardiopulmonary bypass decreased the frequency of postoperative ventricular arrhythmias (8 of 50 [16%] in the Mg-treated group versus 17 of 50 [34%] in the placebo-treated group, $P < 0.04$).[249]

Some investigators believe that serum Mg should be measured routinely in hospitalized patients because of the high prevalence of hypomagnesemia coupled with the difficulty of diagnosing hypomagnesemia on clinical grounds alone.[247,250] One investigator argues that common sense dictates that nonessential surgery be deferred until Mg depletion has been corrected, again with no data to support such an assertion.[251] I could not find any data indicating better perioperative outcome in patients not undergoing cardiovascular surgery because of routine detection and correction of hypomagnesemia. The benefit of decreased frequency of cardiac dysrhythmias after cardiac surgery[248,249] occurred with or without preoperative hypomagnesemia. If one is going to use magnesium empirically, one probably should have a measure of renal function and should monitor magnesium levels (or reflexes in the awake patient), but no data indicate that such levels should be routinely determined before surgery.

The National Veterans Affairs Surgical Risk Study found that albumin levels were an important predictor of outcome after surgery.[61,222] Furthermore, changes in this level after enteral nutrition have been important predictors

of perioperative outcome in malnourished or otherwise very sick patients (see Chapter 27). It may therefore be time to add this laboratory test for patients undergoing surgical class C procedures, and for patients who have a physiologic age (RealAge) of over 85 who are undergoing surgical class B procedures.

Even sophisticated laboratory tests have not been better in controlled trials than the history and physical examination in estimating the risk from a diagnosis. This lack of benefit from laboratory testing has applied to diagnoses as relatively amenable to laboratory diagnosis as the differential diagnosis of systolic murmurs,[252] assessment of nutritional status,[253] and diagnosis of cardiac and gastrointestinal disease.[89]

IMPLEMENTING ACCURACY AND EFFICIENCY IN PREOPERATIVE EVALUATION

The ability of preoperative evaluation of even healthy patients (ASA physical status I or II) to detect important symptoms and medical history makes its benefit greater than its risk. Furthermore, preoperative evaluation done in advance is ultimately cost-efficient, as it minimizes expensive delays on the day of surgery. (Table 25-19 shows the laboratory tests recommended for asymptomatic patients by various investigators and institutions.) In addition, such assessment can be used to limit the amount of testing to only that warranted by symptoms or risk-grouping (Table 25-20). The protocol described in Table 25-20 (and the algorithms derived from it [see Figs. 25-7 to 25-13]) do have certain requirements if the patient's preoperative condition is to be optimized. A careful history and physical examination must be performed using The Rule of Threes discussed previously. Also, any condition indicating the existence of one of the disease entities presented in Table 25-20 must be searched for, and that condition must be specifically tested for in patients undergoing type B or C surgical procedures. This protocol clearly places the burden of accuracy on the history-taker. Furthermore, use of the protocol does require that a system be in place so that the physician performing the assessment views the test results and communicates the readiness of the patient for surgery, or the need for further testing/consultation, to the primary care physician, surgeon, and scheduling system. *This step places an additional burden on the preoperative assessor: he or she must determine what degree of consultation with the primary care physician and surgeon is necessary to judge optimal health for perioperative care.*

Two possible objections by the assessor immediately come to mind:

1. Why can't the primary care physician do the evaluation and send it to me?
2. It's a time-consuming process for which I get no compensation.

In their simplest forms, the answers to these objections are:

1. The primary care physician is not specifically trained in preoperative assessment.
2. Ultimately, preoperative evaluation is very cost-effective for the institution, the health care payors, and the patients. It is justifiable to compensate the anesthesiologist for preoperative assessment at the same rate as for OR time.

First Objection
Although the primary care physician can render a patient's condition optimal for daily living, he or she does not have the anesthesiologist's depth of understanding of the physiologic changes caused by surgery or the requirements that must be met to facilitate class B and C surgical procedures and to optimize perioperative outcome. An example of this is the induction by the primary care physician of some degree of prerenal azotemia for the patient with congestive heart failure. Even though prerenal azotemia may make the patient more comfortable for the conditions of daily living, it predisposes the patient to hypovolemic disaster during surgery. Unfortunately, careful attention to optimizing the perioperative condition is highly desirable but is not compatible with the current state of knowledge and functioning of primary care physicians. Such knowledge is more available and of better quality than in prior decades,[263-265] and many reports have highlighted the importance of this aspect of care.[9,266-268] Nevertheless, the training, knowledge, and ability of primary care physicians are still very deficient in this aspect of consultation.

In addition, the preoperative meeting of anesthesiologist and patient should serve other important functions:
• Informing the patient about treatment options
• Educating the patient about anesthesia, perioperative care, and pain treatment in the hope of reducing anxiety and facilitating recovery[5]

The meeting may serve another important function:
• Motivating (by using the perioperative experience) the patient to achieving more optimal health and thereby improve perioperative and/or long-term outcome.

At this time, none of these functions is performed adequately by most primary care physicians, and there is no one better trained to do so than the anesthesiologist.

Second Objection
It is cost-efficient for both the institution and the health care provider to have the anesthesiologist perform preoperative assessments, *provided a system is set up to make the process cost-efficient.* In the OR, the anesthesia service earns revenue only when a patient is undergoing surgery. Thus, the goals of the hospital in producing a cost-efficient OR environment and the goals of the anesthesia department are closely aligned. Long turnover times, unused OR time, and delays in the OR schedule have many disadvantages. They waste the resources of the anesthesia department, reduce the cost-efficiency of hospitals, impede teaching, frustrate surgeons, and decrease harmonious teamwork among health care providers. Such inefficiencies make the hospital, surgical center, and office-based operatory less competitive when fees are determined on the basis of "capitated-care" (payment of fixed fees), a diagnosis-related group (DRG), or an ambulatory care group (ACG).

Because many countries, and especially the United States, are undergoing multiple transitions in the way care is paid for, it is important to note that in all systems efficiency in OR utilization and transition to functional recovery postoperatively or post-procedurally is valuable for all systems. Therefore, it is optimal to facilitate smooth transfer of the patient into the OR. In addition, if preoperative assessment by an anesthesiologist were supplemented by informatics systems linking primary care provider, surgeon, OR, and perioperative care site, more cost-efficiencies could be obtained. For example, a history would not be obtained by the internist, surgeon, surgical resident, anesthesiologist, anesthesia resident, and three teams of nurses—all with imperfect information transfer between them, much duplication of laboratory services, and many delays. Thus, even though the rules for payment have changed, those who live in a capitated care environment will find it cost-efficient to have a system that facilitates preoperative assessment sufficiently early to minimize OR delays, reduce unwarranted testing, facilitate relief of patient anxiety, and speed recovery. Part of the job of the anesthesiologist and of anesthesia societies is to ensure that the value of these services is remunerated appropriately.

For the anesthesiologist, several effective systems could be instituted. Supported by consultation 1 week or more before surgery, or by some other second-opinion mechanisms encouraged by appropriate CPT codes and fee schedules, such systems *could* pay for themselves (Fig. 25-14). Initiating such a system is not easy, but failure to do so will make the anesthesiologist and his or her practice site less efficient and more costly, less marketable and desirable to patients; and a continuing source of frustration to surgeons, OR administrators, and anesthesiologists.

Table 25–19   Recommended test guidelines for asymptomatic patients

Age	Roizen[257] (1994) (Simplified) 1	Roizen[257] (1994) 2		Roizen[83] (1990) 3 ♂	♀	Roizen[258] (1986) 4 ♂	♀	Roizen[259] (1981) 5 ♂	♀	Eiseman[260]* (1989) 6	Velanovich[261] (1991) 7
<6 mo				None	Hb or Hct	None	Hct or Hb	?SGOT ?BUN ?Gluc	Hb or Hct SGOT ?BUN ?Gluc	CBC Elect BUN/Gluc Urin Protime PTT PLT Cnt CXR ECG FOBT	
6 mo 2 y	Hb or HCT	♂ None	♀ Hb or HCT ?Preg test								
6 y											
18 y 30 y											ECG
40 y	Hct ECG	Hct ECG		BUN Gluc ECG	Hb or Hct BUN/ Gluc ECG	BUN/ Gluc ECG	Hct or Hb BUN/ Gluc ECG	?SGOT BUN/ Gluc ECG	Hb or Hct ?SGOT BUN/ Gluc ECG		Hct BUN/Gluc/Creat Tot Prot/Alb/ Lymph Cnt CXR ECG
50 y		Hct ECG									
60 y				Hb or Hct BUN/Gluc CXR ECG		Hb or Hct BUN/Gluc CXR ECG		Hb or Hct BUN/Gluc CXR ECG ?SGOT			
65 y	Hct ECG BUN/Gluc	Hct BUN ECG									
70 y											
75 y and over		Hct BUN/Gluc ECG									

*Recommendations of the American College of Surgeons.
†Recommendations of the Mayo Clinic, Rochester, Minn.
‡Personal communication with JV Roth (Albert Einstein Hospital, NY).
§Personal communication with SL Kaplan (Westfall Surgery Center, Rochester, NY).
Alb, albumin; BUN/Gluc, blood urea nitrogen and glucose; CBC, complete blood count; Creat, creatinine; ECG, electrocardiogram; Elect, electrolytes; CXR, chest radiograph; FOBT, fecal occult blood test; Gluc, glucose; Hb, hemoglobin; Hct, hematocrit; Lymph Cnt, lymphocyte count; PLT Cnt, platelet count; Preg, pregnancy; Protime, prothrombin time; PTT, partial thromboplastin time; SGOT, serum gluatamic-oxaloacetic transaminase; Tot Prot, total protein; Urin, urinalysis.

Table 25–19   Recommended test guidelines for asymptomatic patients—cont'd

Larson[262] (1992)	Blery et al[128] (1986)		McKee and Scott[112] (1987)		Narr et al[110,†] (1991)	Macpherson et al[239] (1990)		Albert Einstein Hospital[‡] (1993)	Westfall Surgical Center[§]
8	**9**		**10**		**11**	**12**		**13**	**14**
CBC Urin	Minor surg None	Major surg Hct or Hb	None		None	Minor surg None	Major surg CBC	None	None
								CBC	
	ECG	Hct or Hb ECG	CBC		ECG Creat/Gluc	BUN ECG	CBC BUN ECG	CBC ECG	ECG
CBC Urin Elect BUN Creat Gluc CXR ECG			CBC ECG						
			Minor surg CBC ECG	Major surg CBC BUN Elect ECG CXR	CBC Creat/Gluc ECG CXR	BUN ECG CXR	C3C BUN ECG	CBC BUN CXR Elect Gluc	
	BUN Creat Elect ECG	Hct BUN/Creat Elect ECG							

Table 25–20 Preoperative and Preprocedure Assessment Clinic (PPAC) simplified strategy for preoperative and preprocedure testing based on co-morbid conditions (Form 3)

	CBC w/plt	T/S & ALB	β-hCG	PT/PTT	Elec	BUN/Cr	Glu	AST/Alkp	ECG	CXR	UA
Disease-based indications											
Alcohol abuse	x			x				x	x		
Adrenal cortical disease	x				x		x				
Anemia	x										
Cancer, except skin, without known metastases	x									x	
Diabetes					x	x	x		x		
Hematologic (significant)abnormalities	x	x		x							
Exposure to hepatitis								x			
Hepatic disease				x		x		x			
Malignancy with chemotherapy	x			x*		x		x	±	x	
Malnutrition	x	x		±	x						
Morbid obesity						x	x		x		
Peripheral vascular disease or stroke	x				x	x	x				
Personal or family history of bleeding	x			x				±			
Poor exercise tolerance or "Real Age" over 64	x					x	x				
Possibly pregnant			x								
Pulmonary disease	x								±	x†	
Renal disease	x				x	x			x		
Rheumatoid arthritis	x								x	x†	
Sleep apnea	x								x		
Smoking >40 pk-yr	x								x	x†	
Suspected UTI or prosthesis insertion											x
Systemic Lupus						x			x	x†	
Therapy-based indications											
Radiation therapy	x								x	x	
Use of anticoagulants	x			x							
Use of digoxin and diuretics					x	x			x		
Use of statins								x	x		
Use of steroids					x	x	x				
Procedure-based indications											
Procedure with significant blood loss	x	x									
Procedure with radiograhic dye						x					
Class C procedure	x	x			x	x					

†For leukemias only.
‡For active, acute process only.
*Class C Procedures typically disrupt normal physiology and commonly require blood transfusions, invasive monitoring, and/or postoperative ICU care. CBC w/plt, complete blood count with platelets; T/S, type & screen; ALB, albumin; β-hCG, pregnancy test; PT/PTT, prothrombin time/INR/partial thromboplastin time; Elec, electrolytes; BUN/Cr, blood urea nitrogen/creatinine; Glu, glucose; AST/AlkP, aspartate transaminase/alkaline phosphatase; ECG, electrocardiogram; CXR, chest x-ray; UA, urinalysis; ±, consider. All tests are valid for 6 months unless condition has changed, with the exception of abnormal prior ECG and β-hCG for pregnancy.
Data from Roizen,[89] Kaplan et al,[111] and Biery et al.[128]

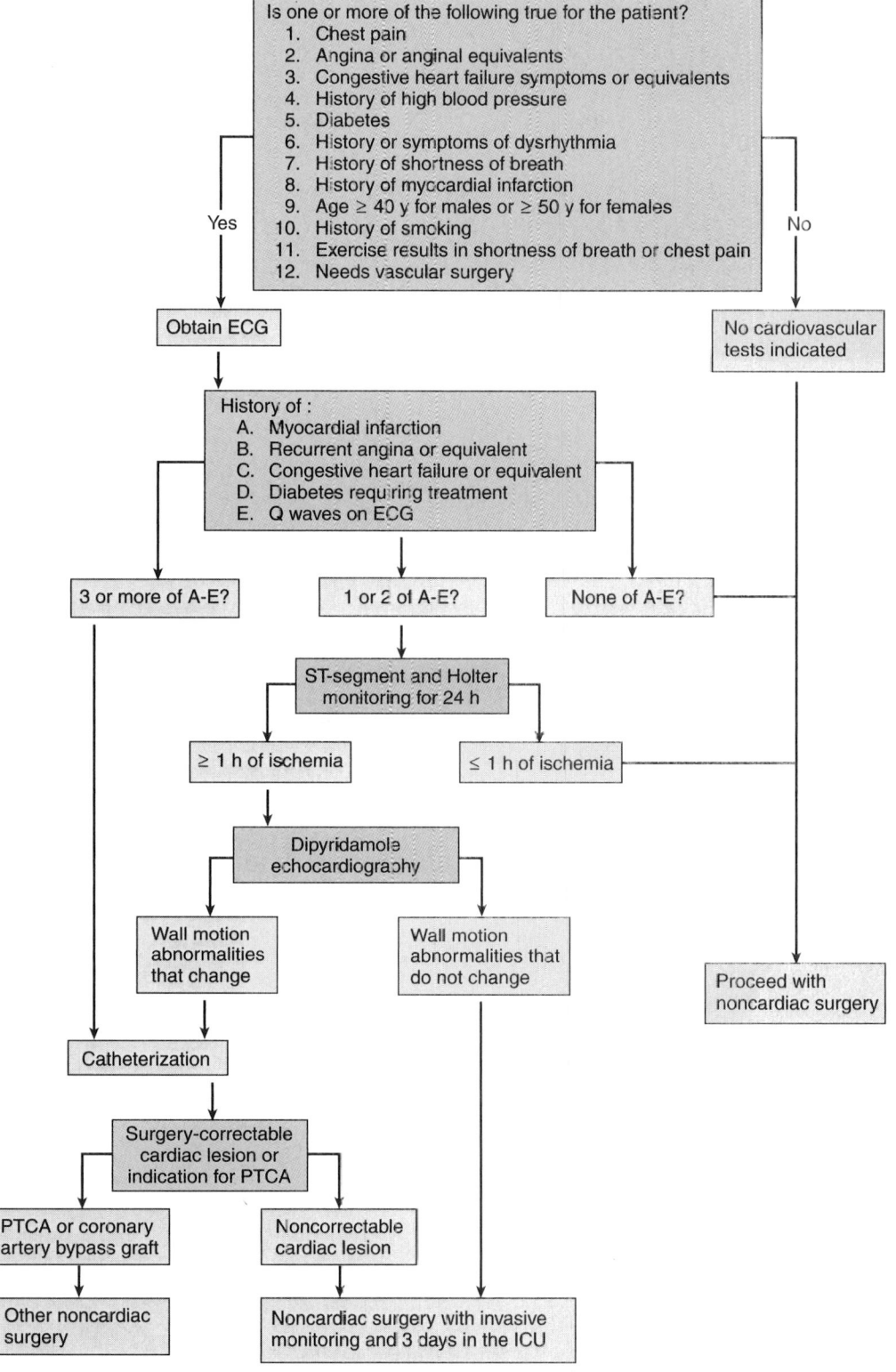

Figure 25–7 Evaluating cardiovascular risk for patients undergoing noncardiac surgery: the procedure for determining which cardiovascular laboratory tests are necessary. The history is used to segregate patients into groups for testing and/or invasive monitoring. ECG, electrocardiogram; ICU, intensive care unit; PTCA, percutaneous transluminal coronary angioplasty.

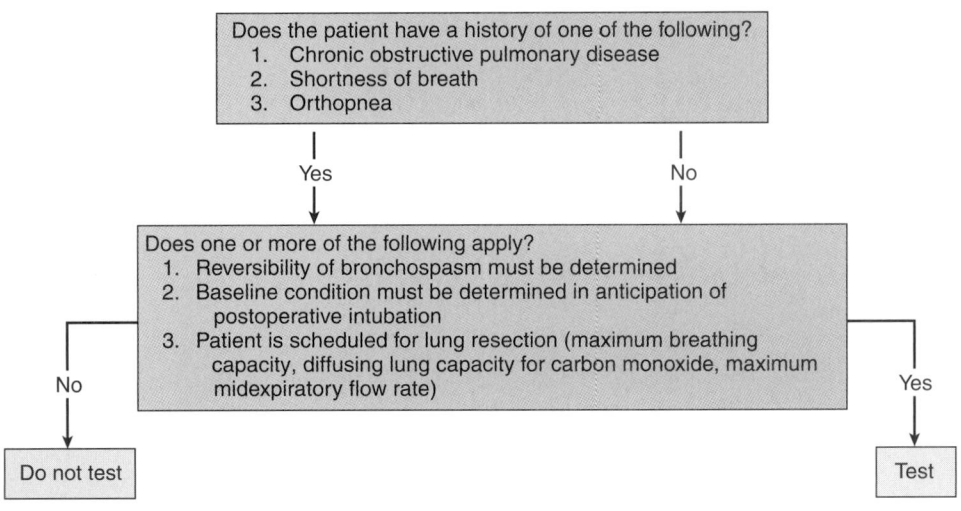

Figure 25–8 Procedure for determining when pulmonary function tests are warranted.

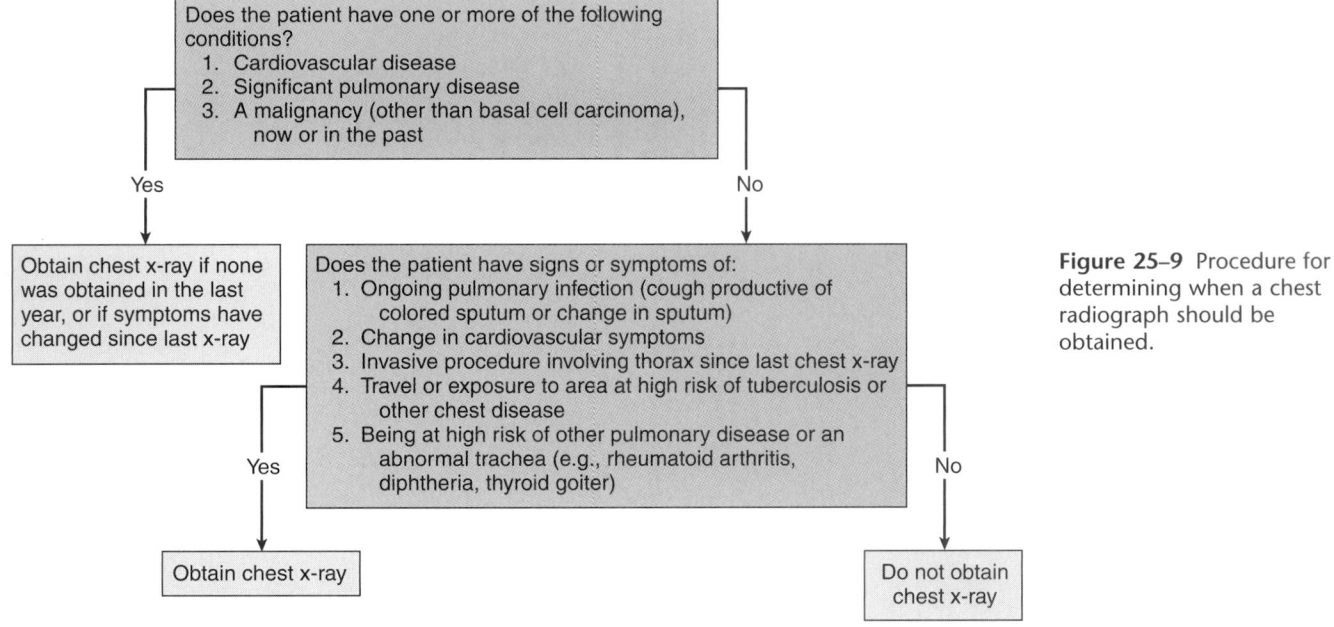

Figure 25–9 Procedure for determining when a chest radiograph should be obtained.

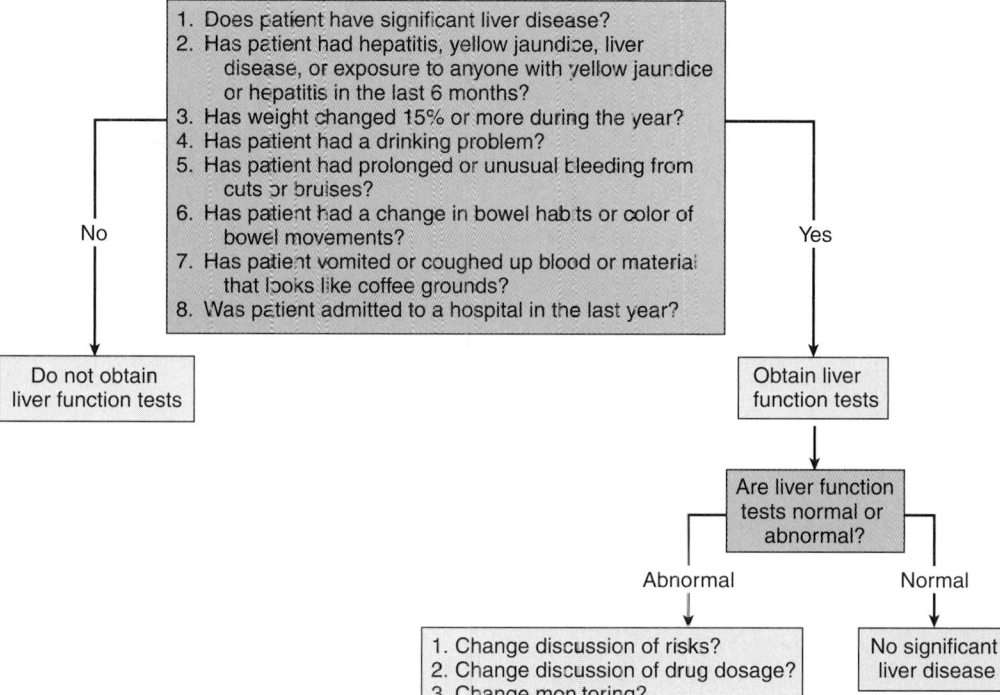

Figure 25–10 Procedure for soliciting the signs and symptoms of significant liver disease that warrant the performance of liver function tests.

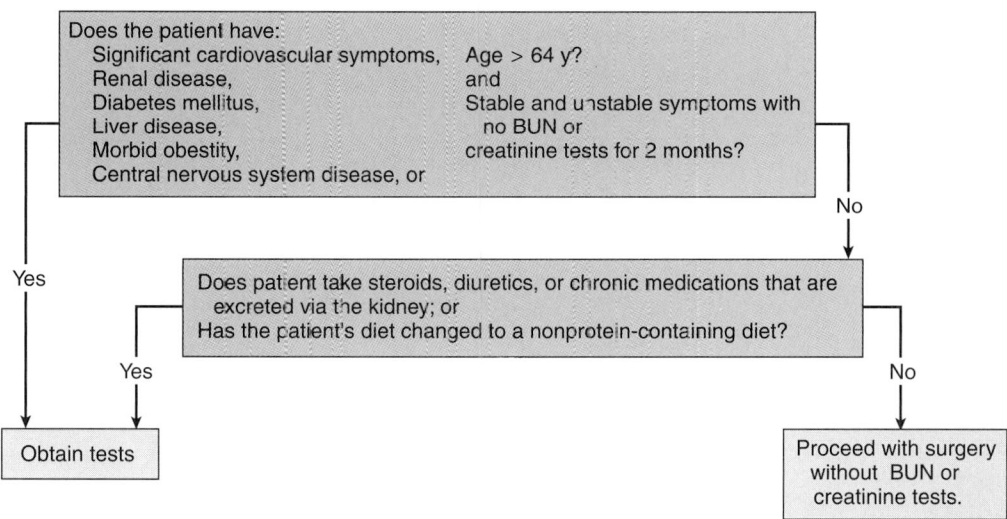

Figure 25–11 Procedure for determining when blood urea nitrogen (BUN) or creatinine levels should be obtained.

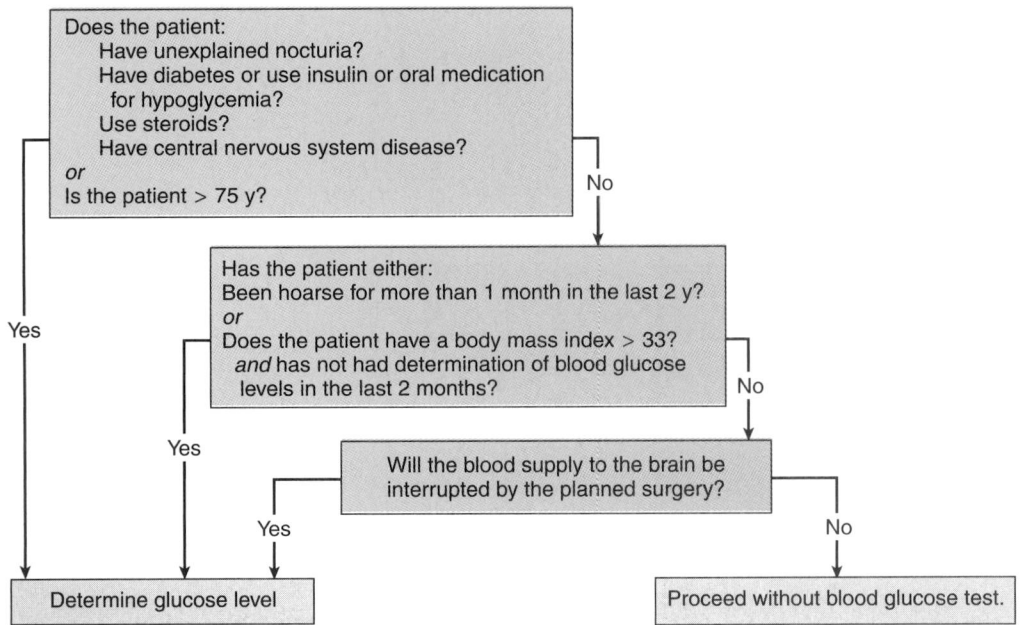

Figure 25–12 Procedure for determining when blood glucose levels should be obtained.

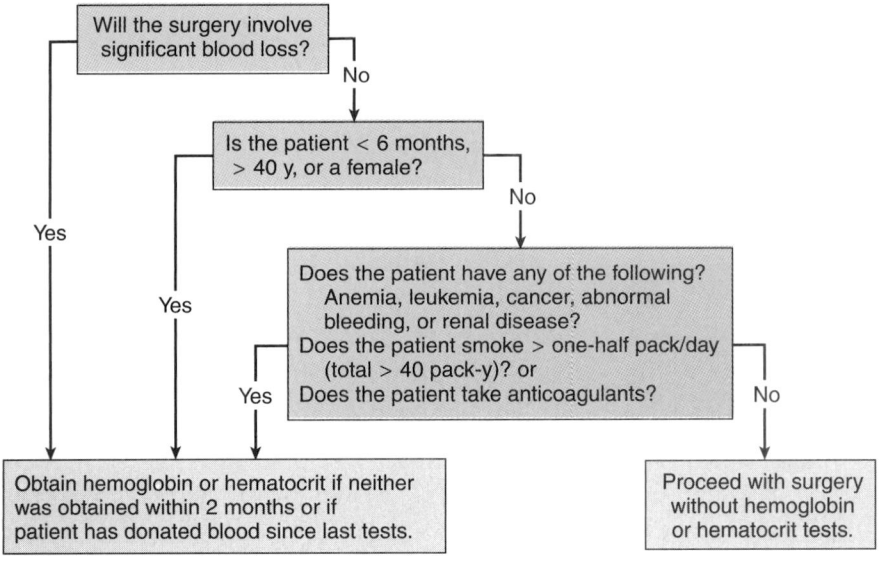

Figure 25–13 Procedure for determining when hemoglobin levels or a hematocrit should be obtained.

MED-HIST #:

PATIENT NAME:

PHYSICIAN:

DATE OF SERVICE _____/_____/_____

ANESTHESIOLOGIST _____

DIAGNOSIS _____   ICD-9 _____

REFERRING M.D. _____

LOCATION:

- 11. [ ] OFFICE or CLINIC
  12. [ ] PAIN CLINIC
  13. [ ] ICU
  14. [ ] OTHER_____
  15. [ ] INPATIENT FLOOR_____

- 20. [ ] HealthQuiz (interpretation of information stored in a computer)   99090

  OFFICE CONSULTATION (new or established patient)

  21. [ ] PROBLEM FOCUSED (15 min)   99241
  22. [ ] EXPANDED PROBLEM FOCUSED (15-30 min)   99242

- 23. [ ] DETAILED, MORE THAN 1 SYSTEM (30-40 min)   99243
  24. [ ] COMPREHENSIVE, MODERATELY COMPLEX   99244
          MEDICAL DECISION-MAKING (40-60 min)
  25. [ ] COMPREHENSIVE, COMPLEX MEDICAL DECISION-MAKING   99245

  INPATIENT CONSULTATION (new or established patient)

  31. [ ] PROBLEM FOCUSED (20 min)   99251
  32. [ ] EXPANDED PROBLEM FOCUSED (20-40 min)   99252
  33. [ ] DETAILED, MORE THAN 1 SYSTEM (40-55 min)   99253
  34. [ ] COMPREHENSIVE, MODERATELY COMPLEX MEDICAL   99254
          DECISION-MAKING (55-80 min)
  35. [ ] COMPREHENSIVE, COMPLEX MEDICAL   99255
          DECISION-MAKING (80-110 min)

  SPECIAL SERVICES: TELEPHONE CALLS WITH PATIENT OR PHYSICIANS

  41. [ ] BRIEF   99371
  42. [ ] INTERMEDIATE   99372
  43. [ ] LENGTHY   99373
  44. [ ] GROUP CONFERENCES WITH A TEAM OF M.D.'s (first 30 min)   99361

  OFFICE VISITS, NEW PATIENT

  51. [ ] PROBLEM FOCUSED (10 min)   99201
  52. [ ] EXPANDED PROBLEM FOCUSED (20 min)   99202

- 53. [ ] DETAILED, MORE THAN 1 SYSTEM (30 min)   99203
          DECISION-MAKING (45 min)
  55. [ ] COMPREHENSIVE, COMPLEX MEDICAL DECISION-MAKING (60 min)   99205

  CRITICAL CARE SERVICES

  61. [ ] CRITICAL CARE (first hour)
  62. [ ] CRITICAL CARE (each additional 30 min)
          Number of additional 30-min periods _____

•Indicates most common choices

Figure 25–14 Billing form used to report preoperative second opinion or consultation activities to payers.

The Danger of Underordering Tests

Inadequate preoperative evaluation leads to the missing of potential problems or to delays in the OR schedule for at least 15% of even healthy (ASA I) patients.[24] In addition, trying to reduce testing without such a system of assessment in place may not be beneficial. Since 1979, physicians at three university practices were found to decrease the ordering of unwarranted tests almost 1.5 times as fast as they decreased the ordering of indicated tests (19.6% and 12.9%, respectively).[269] This would be good if the benefit from decreasing unjustified tests outweighed the benefit of ordering the truly useful ones. However, the possible benefit from a justified test is probably more than 1.5 times the possible benefit from not ordering an unjustified test, at least regarding preoperative tests. Therefore, the net changes that have occurred in preoperative test selection since 1979 may not be beneficial. One is forced to conclude that a better system for obtaining the warranted tests and for eliminating the unwarranted tests may be a necessary supplement to education and to standard endorsements for the reduction of costs and errors if selective application of laboratory tests is to be beneficial.[269] This process calls for the use of information systems and an evaluative clinic. The need for an information system and clinic to make the idea work is accentuated by data on the errors made when selecting tests without the availability of an information system.

Errors Made by Physicians When Ordering Tests

Selecting tests when there are no information systems to help has one major problem: it is a difficult procedure for physicians to complete successfully. *Even when physicians agree to use specific, agreed-upon criteria based on history and physical examination to order tests selectively and thereby reduce routine testing, they still make a surprising number of mistakes when ordering tests.* Approximately 30% to 40% of patients who *should* have certain tests (based on agreed-upon criteria such as those in Table 25-20) do not get such tests, and 20% to 40% of patients who should *not* have certain tests are nevertheless subjected to them. For instance, Blery and co-workers[128] examined 3,866 surgical patients in France. Even after medical personnel had been educated regarding which criteria indicated a need for which tests, 30% of the tests were ordered without need; another 22% of tests should have been ordered but were not. Thus, surgeons and anesthesiologists not only increased costs but also failed to obtain possibly valuable information.

These mistakes occur mainly because integrating the history, physical examination, and indications for laboratory tests is not an easy process. Even when criteria for testing have been previously agreed upon by surgeons and anesthesiologists, the number of variables one must remember makes arriving at correct conclusions a complex task. As an example, let us consider how many mistakes are made regarding one commonly used preoperative test, the chest radiograph.

Charpak and co-workers[270] examined the value of preoperative screening chest radiographs for 3,849 patients.

Surgeons and anesthesiologists agreed that any of the following findings on history or physical examination would warrant ordering a chest radiograph: any lung or cardiovascular disease; any malignant disease; current smoking by patients over 50 years of age; major surgical emergencies; immunodepression; and, for immigrants, absence of prior health examination. Surgeons made their decisions regarding ordering of chest radiographs after seeing the patient. Even with this agreement on criteria, of 1,426 chest radiographs that should have been ordered for this group of 3,849 patients, 271 were ordered but not warranted, and 596 were not ordered but should have been. Although clinical judgment may account for some of these discrepancies, most of these lapses appear simply to be errors. If so many errors occurred for a single test, even more errors would be likely if patients were subjected to multiple testing.

Data from studies performed by our group confirm this rate of error.[269] We tested the hypothesis that for the period 1979 through 1988, physicians voluntarily and substantially reduced the ordering of preoperative tests not justified by history and physical examination. Reviewing 2,093 medical records from every other year of that period (and studying four operations at each of three cities), we investigated the indications for, and the performance of, preoperative tests. During this period, the incidence of unwarranted laboratory tests obtained preoperatively decreased from 32.2% to 25.8%. This decrease was irregular and varied from operation to operation, from test to test, and from city to city.

Furthermore, an unexpected 12% decrease (from 92.9% to 80.9%) in the ordering of *indicated* preoperative tests occurred. Overall, 66.9% of tests obtained preoperatively in 1979 were not warranted, decreasing to 60.1% in 1987. If the possible benefit of ordering only appropriate tests outweighed the possible harm of not ordering a needed test, the net result would still be a benefit to society. Unfortunately, however, the possible benefit of performing a needed test is probably more than twice the possible harm of performing an unnecessary test.

We concluded that the pressures to order tests more optimally and to do assessments more quickly have not been accompanied by changes in practice patterns that ultimately benefit the patient. In order for the net benefit to accrue to the patient, a better *information* system is needed for obtaining the truly necessary tests and for not ordering the unwarranted ones. On the other hand, punitive measures to reduce testing may save money but may impair health care. This may be the approach the HCFA is attempting, which now requires the use of diagnosis-related codes (International Classification of Diseases, edition 9 [ICD-9]) for reimbursement of testing.

Can physicians do better at preoperative evaluation than a 5- to 15-minute history-taking prior to induction of anesthesia for outpatient or "come-and-stay" patients (those to be admitted after surgery)? They can, and should, for their patients' sake and their own. The British have reached the same conclusion.[271] A change in the system of obtaining patient histories and ordering tests has been advocated even for internists.[272-274]

Just as the need for a more effective *theoretical* system of preoperative evaluation became evident, the study just described reinforced our belief that the actual *information* system used for ordering tests also needed to change, in order to improve the efficiency of the process.

INFORMATION MANAGEMENT IN PREOPERATIVE AND PREPROCEDURE EVALUATION AND OUTCOME ENHANCEMENT

Being unaware of previously occurring in-hospital and perioperative events can lead to perioperative disaster in a subsequent surgical procedure. For example, an unanticipated difficult airway or allergic reaction that occurred earlier but is not known can (and has) contributed to disasters in subsequent anesthesia care. Avoiding such disasters would seem to be a solvable problem in an age of records, paper or otherwise. Yet anyone who has practiced in a large modern-day American hospital (university or community) knows that past charts are often not available. Even when the patient is seen in a surgeon's office or perioperative clinic, the transfer of records and consent forms can be a weak link in the chain of communication. Enter the information age and the promise of making the chain perfect.

Informatics and the Preoperative Evaluation

Because we currently practice in an environment called the "Information Age," how is it possible that we still have trouble obtaining the information we need? As our health care institutions switch to electronically stored patient records, theoretically this problem should vanish. However, these institutions and a variety of vendors that now offer programs for automating the preoperative assessment frequently fail to provide operational solutions. These "turnkey" products are often isolated implementations of paper records. Such preoperative systems have not achieved wide acceptance, despite their introduction more than 3 decades ago.[275,276] However, planned with the overall goals of the preoperative evaluation in mind, information systems can be used successfully to improve patient care and the efficiency of the overall system.

Such a system requires an accurate and complete database storing the patient's current health status and past anesthesia and surgical experiences. The sources for the data may be varied and have been collected at disparate locations and times. The ideal database should include the history of the current surgical problem plus past medical, social, and surgical histories. It should also include review of organ systems, current physical examinations and perioperative plans, and notes on discussions with the patient and significant others. This database can also be used when providing ancillary services such as laboratory tests and consultations. Once the perioperative plan has been formulated, a record can be clearly communicated to the patient, the surgeon, and the anesthesiologist's colleagues. Finally, by establishing an accurate baseline status, the information that has been acquired can be used to initiate quality assurance procedures.

This section provides an introduction to the use of information systems and identifies important issues for the clinician who is considering implementing such a system.

Collection of Data

Traditionally, the physician obtained the information he or she needed by talking with the patient, scanning the available paper chart, consulting other physicians, and collecting reports from laboratories or consultants. These data were then recorded in a note. The information was often incomplete at the time the note was written (missing lab data or uncompleted consultation). Thus, the note that may have needed to be updated often wasn't.

To standardize the format and help the physician obtain important information, many facilities use forms that range from simple headings placed on a page to detailed checklists (see Fig. 25-2 for a checklist our group now sends to surgeons and proceduralists to be completed by the patient prior to seeing an anesthesiologist). As physician contact time has become more limited, ancillary personnel have been recruited to help acquire and assemble the required data. Patients are also being asked to spend more time completing checklists or questionnaires that cover many points in their history. Compared with the current procedure, automation should be able to improve many of these processes. For example, the use of electronic information systems (informatics) can reduce or eliminate the redundant entry of information in a record, a situation that frequently creates discrepancies in that record.

The expense of obtaining these histories increases because we often rely on professionals to obtain the routine history rather than focus on the details that are abnormal or important to the planned care. The process could be less expensive if patients completed the screening process themselves. There are many ways the patient could do this. When patients are given a clear reason for their input and a clear and simple format for answering questions, the patient-completed questionnaire can be an accurate and powerful tool.[6,276]

One of the first systems used for this purpose was the HealthQuiz.* Developed in 1987, this system consisted of a laptop device that had a simple liquid crystal display and three buttons; the patient pressed a "yes," "no," or "not sure" button to answer health-related questions. The HealthQuiz was a simple system, not unlike many of the small electronic games becoming popular at the time, and it was readily accepted by patients. Its program consisted of a branching algorithm made up of 254 items. The wording of each question was carefully prepared and validated so that consistent answers were given whether the patient was responding to a human or to the computer or was later asked the same question again. The initial questions were standard health history items

---

*The author developed this video preoperative health questionnaire at the University of Chicago to help ameliorate the problem of inefficient preoperative assessments and test selection methods. Consequently, the University of Chicago owns the rights to commercialize the product. Both the University of Chicago and Johns Hopkins University may benefit from commercialization of this technology and the applications described herein (see www.Healthquiz.com for further explanation).

pertinent to anesthesia care and were based on health maintenance guidelines.[59,66] Subsequently, a variety of questionnaires were developed for general medicine, pediatrics, and preventive health.

Although compact and easy to use, the HealthQuiz required the use of a dedicated unit for producing the questionnaire. In 1993, the rapid expansion of the Internet into health care and even the patient's home prompted the development of a networked version of the system, the HealthQuiz Plus 2, which could be accessed from any computer by means of an Internet browser. This concept has been extended, and now the patient can

complete the questionnaire from any touch-tone phone. The system also allows on-line viewing of the report and the ability to hone in on questions, suggested laboratory tests, or risk assessments to examine the underlying questions, answers, and logic.

Data are also available at the point of care and are easily transferred to other medical information systems. For example, justification of laboratory tests by the assignment of diagnosis-related codes (ICD-9) is produced for each test suggested, and this information can be given to the laboratory to aid in reimbursement (Figs. 25-15 and 25-16). Such procedures supersede the old but still often

---

```
ANESTHESIA AND CRITICAL CARE RESEARCH FOUNDATION
PATIENT SUMMARY REPORT v.2.1  (c) 1992, 1993


70-year old ASIAN FEMALE  ID # 1839751
```

SYMPTOMS REVIEW		
PULM	Hx pneumonia	DOB: 09/15/22
GI	Hx hiatus hernia	DATE: 08/02/93
CV	?? palpitations	HT: 153.0 cm
CV	?? Hx murmur or rheumatic fever	WT: 69.0 kg
CV	1 Flight DOE	BMI: 29.47
CV	?? Ankle swelling	BP: 150 /85
CV	High blood pressure	HR: 84 /min
CV	Stairs w/o SOB	HQASA: 2.50
CV	Grocery exercise w/o SOB	VALIDITY: GOOD
PSH	S/P hysterectomy	

ALLERGIES

Non-drug allergies

SUGGESTED LABS

BUN/CREAT   ECG

ICD-9:   ICD-9:

MEDICATIONS

Acetaminophen
Antacid meds
Pain meds
Antihypertensives
Hormone replacement

PERTINENT ANESTHESIA CARE ITEMS		TOBACCO/ETOH/IVDA
Loose/chipped teeth	Previous anesthesia	Quit smoking >8 mo
Hx snoring	Caps or bridge	

Figure 25–15 The HealthQuiz Plus 2 computer device uses the patient's answers to its questionnaire to produce this summary of the patient's health history and suggested laboratory tests, annotated with International Classification of Diseases, ninth edition (ICD-9) codes. BMI, body mass index; BP, blood pressure; BUN, blood urea nitrogen; CREAT, creatinine; CV, cardiovascular; DOB, date of birth; DOE, dyspnea on exertion; ECG, electrocardiogram; GI, gastrointestinal; HQASA1-5, Health Quiz ASA status square; HR, heart rate; HT, height; Hx, history; IVDA, intravenous drug abuse; PSH, past surgical history; PULM, pulmonary; SOB, shortness of breath; S/P, status post; WT, weight.

ANESTHESIA AND CRITICAL CARE RESEARCH FOUNDATION
TEST RATIONALE REPORT v.2.1 (c) 1992, 1993

70-year old   ASIAN   FEMALE   ID# 1839751   8/02/93

Listed below is the rationale for each laboratory test suggested for the patient. Please consult the Preoperative
Test Selection Software Manual for a complete description, with reference to clinical practice guidelines and
the best medical evidence available.

RATIONALE FOR DETERMINING BUN/CREATININE LEVELS:

1   If the answer to Q 577 ("Do you have high blood pressure?") is YES or NOT SURE:

Hypertensive patients often have abnormal renal function. In fact, one of the goals of treating
hypertension is to prevent renal dysfunction.

2   If the answer to Q 617 ("Do you currently take any medication for high blood pressure?") is YES or NOT
SURE:

Hypertensive patients often have abnormal renal function. In fact, one of the goals of treating hypertension is
to prevent renal dysfunction.

RATIONALE FOR OBTAINING AN ECG:

1   If the answer to Q 529 ("Have you been told you have a heart murmur or rheumatic fever?") is YES or NOT
SURE:

Although heart murmurs and rheumatic fever do not necessarily produce abnormalities on ECG, when
abnormalities are found on ECG, they can often be a help in diagnosing left atrial or ventricular enlargement
from either volume or pressure overload. ICD-9 _____

2   If the answer to Q 561 ("Do you become short of breath after climbing one flight of stairs or after walking a
short distance?") is YES:

HealthQuiz outcome studies show that patients who have a history of dyspnea after climbing one flight of
stairs or walking one block are at higher risk of ECG abnormalities. ICD-9 _____

3   If the answer to Q 577 ("Do you have high blood pressure?") is YES or NOT SURE:

One of the adverse concomitants of hypertension is left ventricular hypertrophy. Although the sensitivity of
the ECG for the detection of left ventricular hypertrophy is debated, the ECG costs less than an
echocardiogram for the detection of hypertrophy. In the absence of echocardiography and in the presence of
high blood pressure, an ECG may be used as an initial screening test. ICD-9 _____

4   If the answer to Q 617 ("Do you currently take any medicine to control high blood pressure?") is YES or
NOT SURE:

One of the adverse concomitants of hypertension is left ventricular hypertrophy. Although the sensitivity of
the ECG in detecting left hypertrophy is debated, the ECG costs less than an echocardiogram for the detection
of hypertrophy. In the absence of echocardiography and the presence of high blood pressure, an ECG may
be used as an initial screening test. ICD-9 _____

Figure 25–16   Example of the summary sheet that gives the physician the rationale for each of the tests suggested for the patient. This sheet is generated by the HealthQuiz computer device, which uses the patient's answers to the HealthQuiz questionnaire, plus 480 algorithms programmed into the device, to make its decisions; it also provides International Classification of Diseases, ninth edition (ICD-9) codes for each choice. ECG, electrocardiogram.

used paper-and-pencil check-off lists (Figs. 25-17 and 25-18), and even newer ones that are able to be scanned, as shown in Figure 25-2. However, this system has not been adopted by many institutions because of the cost to use it (approximately one dollar per patient) and the difficulty of integrating the system into the practice setting.

Although the value of the preoperative evaluation has been discussed, efforts to improve efficiency cause anesthesiologists to consider whether some patients may be assessed just as effectively immediately before surgery. To be successful, this plan should accomplish three key goals:

1. Gain information about the planned procedure.
2. Determine the patient's current health status.
3. Allow the patient to obtain information about his or her planned anesthetic before surgery.

Optimally the evaluation should be done far enough in advance to allow motivating the patient to adopt healthier behaviors, such as regular physical activity and smoking cessation, and to institute therapies such as aspirin, β-adrenergic receptor blocking drugs, statins, and others that will facilitate better perioperative and long-term outcomes. Tools such as the patient-completed health history, along with accessibility to previous information on perioperative care and other available data, can provide the second leg of the triad with minimal provider resources, identifying patients who need to come to the clinic for additional evaluation. Finally, on-line educational resources, perhaps in association with a brief call from the anesthesiologist, can complete the process of discussing the anesthesia plan with the patient. This plan would allow patients to present on the day of surgery yet minimize the potential for the discovery of unplanned conditions that would delay care, disrupt the OR schedule, or, worse, lead to adverse events.

Physician, hospital, and health system methods for data gathering that include radiology reports, laboratory test reports, and prior operative notes and anesthetic records are now becoming more widespread. They may use not only standard computer terminals but also hand-held devices. These systems are able to decrease redundant data entries by communicating with other data sources, such as hospital billing systems (for demographic data), patient-completed questionnaires, internet educational and reference resources such as e-pocrates, data from other providers, and order entry for such items as added β-adrenergic receptor blocking agents, smoking cessation aids, statins, aspirin, and even walking prescriptions. Such processes allow more than one provider to record information for the evaluation and to effectively communicate that information to the anesthesiologist or other care-givers at different times or locations.

The provider systems are still evolving. Ease of use and ease of data entry are very important for acceptance by physicians, who seem to have a very short tolerance time for clumsy system performance. Also, because typing on a computer can interfere with the physician-patient interaction, a conscious effort must be made to move away from the computer and address the patient directly, so that he or she does not "feel like a number."

Laboratory systems, pharmacies, and administrative billing systems have led the way in providing on-line data systems. These data may be integrated into the collection process if suitable computer interfaces can be constructed. More problematic is the incorporation of older records, as well as notes or other nondigital data from outside sources.

SKR 2# M.D. Checklist for Ordering Preoperative Laboratory Tests^{TM}

(Check indication if positive: Only one positive indication is needed per item.)

Patient Name: _____

Scheduled Operation: _____

TESTS TO BE OBTAINED	INDICATION FOR ORDERING TEST
Hgb/HCT	_____Potentially bloody operation (blood to be cross-matched preoperatively)
	_____Known anemia
	_____Bleeding disorder
	_____Hematologic malignancy
	_____Patient undergoing radiation or chemotherapy
	_____Chronic renal failure
	_____Severe chronic disease
	_____Other (specify):_____
WBCs (Differential will be obtained automatically if WBC or Hgb is abnormal.)	_____Infection
	_____Disease of WBCs
	_____Patient undergoing radiation or chemotherapy
	_____Immunosuppressive therapy or steroid therapy
	_____Hypersplenism
	_____Aplastic anemia
_____ Check here if you wish differential in any case.	_____Collagen vascular disease
	_____Other (specify): _____
	_____
	_____
PT/PTT	_____Known or suspected coagulation abnormality
	_____Anticoagulant therapy or anticipated therapy
	_____Hemorrhage or anemia
	_____Thrombosis
	_____Liver disease
	_____Malabsorption or poor nutrition
	_____Other (specify): _____
	_____
	_____

Continued

Figure 25–17 Sample checklist for determining which preoperative laboratory tests should be obtained. CPK, creatine phosphokinase; ECG, electrocardiogram; HCT, hematocrit; Hgb, hemoglobin; PT, prothrombin time; PTT, partial thromboplastin time; SIADH, syndrome of inappropriate antidiuretic hormone secretion; SMA 6 and SMA 12, simultaneous multichannel analyses of 6 and 12 blood components, respectively; WBCs, white blood cells.

PLATELETS

_____Known platelet abnormality
_____Hemorrhage or purpura
_____Leukemia
_____Patient undergoing radiation or
          chemotherapy
_____Hypersplenism
_____Some anemias (aplastic, autoimmune,
          myelophthisic, pernicious)
_____Transplant rejection
_____Other

SMA 6

_____Age 60 yr or older
_____Use of diuretics
_____Renal disease
_____Other fluid or electrolyte abnormality
          (diarrhea, SIADH, diabetes insipidus, severe
          liver disease, malabsorption, fever)
_____Other (specify):_____
_____

SMA 12

_____Age 60 yr or older
_____Diabetes mellitus
_____Hypoglycemia
_____Pancreatic disease
_____Pituitary disease
_____Adrenal disease, steroid therapy
_____Liver disease or exposure to hepatitis
_____Patient undergoing radiation or
          chemotherapy
_____Parathyroid disease

ECG

_____Age 40 yr or older
_____Known or suspected cardiac abnormality
_____Other (specify):_____
_____

OTHER TESTS DESIRED
(specify indication):

_____Urinalysis
_____Rapid plasma reagin [syphilis screening
          test]
_____CPK isoenzymes

OTHERS

_____
_____
_____

(Test name and indication):

_____
_____
_____

Figure 25–17 Cont'd.

Collation of Data: The Perioperative Database

Databases consist of an "engine" and an interface. The engine is the computer program that actually stores and retrieves information. Many commercial engines such as Dbase, Sybase, and Access, as well as proprietary programs written by vendors, are available. Although a full discussion of the different engines is beyond the scope of this chapter, several questions that must be addressed when evaluating any database system are discussed here.

First, these systems range from intensely complex, requiring a full-time programmer available for maintenance and modifications, to relatively user-friendly, perhaps maintainable by a physician who has some background in database management. When selecting a system, the potential buyer must consider the resources required for maintenance.

Second, these systems vary in their ability to exchange information with other database systems, such as a hospital-based information system. I believe that ease of exchange, both now and in the future, should be considered in the selection of a system. Third, the hardware that

implements the system also warrants some consideration, although to a lesser degree than the previous two criteria. Today, processor speed and storage on desktop systems are making the selection of hardware a less critical issue than before.

Finally, thoughtful design of the interface system is very important, because this feature determines the everyday ease and usefulness of the system. Many installed medical information systems (estimated at 30% in 2004, down from 45% in 1999) have not been successful, even though they are technologically sound. A large portion of these failures is due to nonacceptance by users.

Clinicians want to be able to easily specify how they get information in and out of the system (the interface), and to be able to modify that interface without being charged for each change in format of a report. Programs such as Access include so-called "drag-and-drop" formats that allow the user to easily create new input and report forms. Other systems may require programming assistance or, in the case of a proprietary system, a more formal process with the vendor in order to change the system.

The hardware systems that run these programs have become more affordable and accessible, and many of these systems can run on personal computers. However, the clinic environment is much more demanding than the office environment. The physician working in an office can tolerate a certain amount of instability and downtime on a computer, but these conditions cannot be allowed in a clinic without considerable consequences. For example, if a paper record is unavailable for one or two cases, the cases may be delayed for 20 minutes. If the server or network is unavailable, 15 ORs will be delayed for 20 minutes each.

Information systems in a clinic environment should have adequate backup in order to meet the clinical demands of being available 24 hours a day. The cost of having adequate backup and supporting personnel must be included in any planned installation. Maintenance costs for information systems can be as high as 70% of a system's total cost over the its life span. Security concerns and documenting conformance with the HIPAA make the use of a personal computer use more difficult, even as distributed databases become more useable and more desirable (given equal security systems, it is more time-consuming and more difficult to hack into 4,000 computers than one central database).

Integration of Information

If an electronic information system only collects information and duplicates the current paper system, the cost-benefit advantage is likely to be marginal. Furthermore, it is highly unlikely that merely automating the collection of data will produce significant time savings for those involved. The benefits become clear when data are analyzed and disseminated.

The first benefit concerns the reporting of data to facilitate evaluation, discussion, and subsequent care of the patient. By necessity, the paper record had to report data in the order it was recorded. Reexamination of the paper report may show that simple electronic reformatting of the displayed information, allowing key points to be emphasized, is beneficial. If the reports are available on-line, they no longer need a linear presentation. Only the

---

SKR Preoperative Patient Questionnaire™

Patient Name: _____

Age: _____

	Yes	No	Don't Know
1. Do you currently take any of the following medications?			
a. Aspirin (Excedrin, Anacin, Bufferin, Alka-Seltzer)	_____	_____	_____
b. Anticoagulants (blood-thinning medicine)	_____	_____	_____
c. Quinidine or diltiazem, verapamil, nifedipine, propranolol or Inderal (heart rhythm medicines)	_____	_____	_____
d. Diuretics (water pills)	_____	_____	_____
e. Antihypertensive drugs (blood pressure pills)	_____	_____	_____
f. Digitalis (heart pills)	_____	_____	_____
g. Immunosuppressive drugs (e.g., cyclosporine, cyclophosphamide, azathioprine, 6-mercaptopurine)	_____	_____	_____
h. Steroids (e. g., prednisone, prednisolone)	_____	_____	_____
2. Have you ever been treated for cancer with chemotherapy or radiation (x-ray) therapy?	_____	_____	_____
3. Do you currently have any problems with your:			
a. Liver (e.g., cirrhosis, hepatitis, yellow jaundice, malaria)	_____	_____	_____
b. Kidneys (e.g., stones, infection, failure, dialysis)	_____	_____	_____
c. Spleen	_____	_____	_____
d. Blood (e.g., anemia, leukemia, sickle cell disease)	_____	_____	_____
4. Have you or anyone in your family ever had a serious bleeding problem?	_____	_____	_____
5. Have you ever had prolonged or unusual bleeding from nosebleeds, tooth extractions, cuts or surgery (e.g., tonsillectomy, hernia, hysterectomy)?	_____	_____	_____
6. Do you bleed from your teeth or gums when you brush your teeth?	_____	_____	_____
7. Are your stools sometimes bloody or black and tarry?	_____	_____	_____
8. Have you vomited blood and material that looks like coffee grounds?	_____	_____	_____
9. Have you received a blood transfusion within the last 6 mo?	_____	_____	_____

Continued

Figure 25–18 Sample patient questionnaire for determining which preoperative laboratory tests should be obtained.

10. Have you recently had fever, chills, cold, or flu?   _____ _____ _____

11. Have you ever been told you have sugar diabetes?   _____ _____ _____

12. Do you wake up to urinate more than once a night?   _____ _____ _____

13. Do you have muscle cramps or spasms?   _____ _____ _____

14. Do you have problems with your lungs and chest (e.g., chest pain, skipped heart beats, high blood pressure)?   _____ _____ _____

15. Do you have problems with your lungs or chest (e.g., smoke one pack or more per day, shortness of breath, chest pain, emphysema, asthma, bronchitis)?   _____ _____ _____

16. Have you recently been exposed to anyone with hepatitis (yellow jaundice)?   _____ _____ _____

17. Are you pregnant?   _____ _____ _____

18. Is there any possibility that you are pregnant?   _____ _____ _____

19. Do you have a cough, or do you cough frequently?   _____ _____ _____

20. Do you cough up sputum?   _____ _____ _____

21. When you cough up sputum, have you noticed a change in the color or consistency or type of the sputum?   _____ _____ _____

22. Do you have epilepsy, fits, or seizures?   _____ _____ _____

23. Do you have neck or back problems?   _____ _____ _____

24. Have you or any blood relative had problems related to an operation?   _____ _____ _____

25. Have you lost weight recently?   _____ _____ _____

26. Are you scheduled to have an operation?   _____ _____ _____
    If so, which one?_____

27. What medicines do you take?
    a. _____   d. _____
    b. _____   e. _____
    c. _____   f. _____

Others:_____   _____

_____   _____

Figure 25–18 Cont'd.

key points may be initially presented, with additional details available through a mechanism that allows the user to select a statement or fact on the screen and to obtain additional details or information.

The computer can provide reference material on unfamiliar conditions or drugs—sometimes even automatically, as in the case of warnings about possible drug interactions. Also, when an institution wants to guide and track use of its resources, the computer can suggest preferred clinical pathways. The system may actually do an initial analysis of the data, based on algorithms, to assist in clinical decision-making. The ASA and other standard-setting organizations, including the committee advising the state of Maine, recognize the importance of clinical judgment and the interaction between patient and physician (Fig. 25-19).

Such systems have the advantages of always posing a comprehensive set of questions to the patient and of not forcing the clinician to compromise comprehensiveness because of time constraints. Beers and colleagues[277] showed that such a system did a better job of obtaining accurate and complete patient histories than time-pressed clinicians. Computer-assisted analysis of data will expand as methods are developed for computers to use all the data they have accumulated.

Research can be another opportunity for benefit.[278-280] However, as an initial warning, it should be emphasized that these systems build large data sets rapidly, and the temptation to search the data for a correlation is both strong and misguided. Correlations found in this manner are often misleading and, only if supported by logic, may at best provide the basis for asking more formal questions. Pursuit of these questions, in a prospective fashion, can be rewarding. Fleisher and colleagues[281] used such a system to determine that the risk for similar Medicare patients undergoing similar operations was substantially

STATEMENT ON ROUTINE PREOPERATIVE LABORATORY AND DIAGNOSTIC SCREENING

(Approved by House of Delegates on October 14, 1987 and last amended on October 13, 1993)

Preanesthetic laboratory and diagnostic testing is often essential; however, no routine* laboratory or diagnostic screening† test is necessary for the preanesthetic evaluation of patients. Appropriate indications for ordering tests include the identification of specific clinical indicators or risk factors (e.g. age, pre-existing disease, magnitude of the surgical procedure). Anesthesiologists, anesthesiology departments or health care facilities should develop appropriate guidelines for preanesthetic screening tests in selected populations after considering the probable contribution of each test to patient outcome. Individual anesthesiologists should order test(s) when, in their judgment, the results may influence decisions regarding risks and management of the anesthesia and surgery. Legal requirements for laboratory testing where they exist should be observed. The results of tests relevant to anesthetic management should be reviewed prior to initiation of the anesthetic. Relevant abnormalities should be noted and action taken, if appropriate.

*Routine refers to a policy of performing a test or tests without regard to clinical indications in an individual patient.

†Screening means efforts to detect disease in unselected populations of asymptomatic patients.

A

BASIC STANDARDS FOR PREANESTHESIA CARE
(Approved by House of Delegates on October 14, 1987)

These standards apply to all patients who receive anesthesia or monitored anesthesia care. Under unusual circumstances, e.g. extreme emergencies, these standards may be modified. When this is the case, the circumstances shall be documented in the patient's record.

Standard I: An anesthesiologist shall be responsible for determining the medical status of the patient, developing a plan of anesthesia care, and acquainting the patient or the responsible adult with the proposed plan.

The development of an appropriate plan of anesthesia care is based upon:

1. Reviewing the medical record.

2. Interviewing and examining the patient to:

   a. Discuss the medical history, previous anesthetic experiences.

   b. Assess those aspects of the physical condition that might affect decisions regarding perioperative risk and management.

3. Obtaining and/or reviewing tests and consultations necessary to the conduct of anesthesia.

4. Determining the appropriate prescription of preoperative medications as necessary to the conduct of anesthesia.

B The responsible anesthesiologist shall verify that the above has been properly performed and documented in the patient's record.

Figure 25–19 Two standards published by the American Society of Anesthesiologists (ASA) in the ASA Directory of Members 1998. (A) Statement on routine preoperative laboratory and diagnostic screening. The routine use of laboratory or diagnostic screening tests is not an essential part of the preanesthetic evaluation of patients. (B) Basic standards for preanesthesia care. The history, physical examination, and chart review are essential when obtaining tests as part of preanesthesia care. (From American Society of Anesthesiologists The ASA Directory of Members, 1998. Park Ridge, IL. American Society of Anesthesiologists, 1998.)

higher in a surgeon's office than in a hospital outpatient surgical center. In the future, the ability to connect pre-operative data with outcomes captured electronically will only increase the usefulness of these databases as tools.

Through improved coding and billing, the use of pre-operative databases has been shown to improve economies and cost recovery.[26,27,280] These improvements in cost-recovery mechanisms, along with improvements in laboratory utilization and reimbursement for medically indicated ICD-9–coded test ordering, may justify the cost of implementing a system in the context of a preoperative clinic (see later).

Dissemination of Information
One of the main reasons for instituting an electronic record is to ensure availability of the collected and analyzed data on the day of surgery. At one institution, 20% of manually completed forms were being lost in the process. This loss

would happen most frequently when either the date or location of surgery was changed after the preoperative visit. Also, many practitioners work at multiple sites, within the same institution, at different surgeons' offices or ambulatory care centers, or across the city or even across state lines. The ability to review information for any patient at any site the night before surgery allows the anesthesiologist to better plan and prepare for the next day's cases, and to call the patient, with substantial knowledge about that patient. This process enhances both patient care and efficiency of the ORs.

Institutions vary in the frequency with which patients return, but having the basic information for a patient from a previous procedure can be time-saving for subsequent elective operations. It can even be life-saving in the event of an urgent procedure for which old records are unavailable and the patient cannot provide a history.

Every discussion of information systems must consider security and confidentiality. The same access that is necessary for efficient dissemination of information can have negative effects on patient trust and a significant legal, financial, and criminal impact if improperly used. It is crucial that the system has both controlled access and accurate logging of use to minimize the opportunity for inappropriate use and to identify abuse. Users of the system must be informed of the significant and strictly applied penalties for improper use of the records. This area requires that expert assistance, both technical and legal, should be obtained by anyone who is implementing an information system containing patient data.

Improving Patient Satisfaction with the Preoperative Evaluation

Our group uses the information system to increase patient satisfaction with preoperative evaluation in several ways (Foss JF, personal communication). For example, the most important factor in decreasing patient satisfaction was delay in seeing a physician. Therefore, we use the system to decrease this time interval.

The University of Chicago system logs the arrival time of the patient at the clinic. After the patient has completed his or her self-administered questionnaire on health matters, the system uses those answers to determine the risk status of that patient. A "triage nurse" then uses that risk status, definitions of the three levels of surgery (minimally invasive surgery, surgery of moderate intensity, or major surgery), and the functional age of the patient (i.e., his or her physiologic age [RealAge], not chronologic age) to determine what level of visit with the anesthesiologist is required. A comprehensive visit takes 20 minutes or more and assesses the patient who has an ASA status of 2.0 or higher, *or* is undergoing major surgery, *or* has a biologic age over 65. The next category, the visit of intermediate intensity, takes 15 to 25 minutes. These patients have an ASA status of 1.5 to 2, *or* are undergoing type B surgery, *or* have a biologic age of 61 to 65. Finally, the "expedited visit" takes 5 to 10 minutes and evaluates the patient who has an ASA status of 2 or less, *and* is undergoing minimally invasive surgery, *and* has a biologic age of less than 61.

Once the appropriate level of visit has been determined, the patient is made ready to see the anesthesiologist. He or she is placed in an examination room and dressed to the waist in a hospital gown. Blood pressure, heart rate, height, and weight are recorded, and a self-entered history is completed by the patient.

The patient's status is entered into the computer system, and the times to each room are tracked on the local area networked computer system. A red light signals when an "expedited patient" is ready to be seen. The anesthesiologist will often excuse himself or herself from the comprehensive-visit patient and see the expedited patient immediately. (Comprehensive-visit patients seem not to object to the interruption, as they understand that they require, and will receive, extra physician time.) The total time for patients is not reduced, but the delay until the patient first sees the physician is decreased.

Another way to use an information system to improve patient satisfaction is to ask patients to complete a self-administered questionnaire after surgery. The questionnaire, given by phone or, if in-hospital, by computer or paper and pencil, can assess the patient's satisfaction with the anesthesia service's performance and pain therapy. Feedback for such results has improved performance in the University of Chicago system by physicians in satisfying patients' pain relief requirements.

Information systems are not a replacement for good care, nor is it likely that they will decrease the time spent with patients. However, if carefully designed and implemented, information systems can enhance the acquisition and management of data, so that physicians can spend more of the time they do have with patients in attending to their care. Although such systems can decrease the risks of caring for a patient by providing a complete working database, they are also capable of introducing new risks regarding confidentiality of data and dependence on availability of the system. No matter how much automation, education, or informatics you decide to employ, the factor most important in achieving success is marshalling the resources and consensus of department members and users (surgeons, obstetricians, radiologists, administrators) to institute such a considerable undertaking.

GAINING THE RESOURCES AND CONSENSUS TO INITIATE AND MAINTAIN AN ANESTHESIA PREOPERATIVE AND PREPROCEDURE CLINIC

The anesthesiologist is the specialist most knowledgeable in evaluating and managing operative medical complexities as they relate to anesthesia and surgery. "The assessment of, consultation for and preparation of patients for anesthesia," is part of the American Board of Anesthesiology's definition of the practice of anesthesiology.*

As changes in the health care system decrease reimbursement and the length of stay in the hospital, more

---

*Booklet of Information. Raleigh, North Carolina, American Board of Anesthesiology, pg. 2, 2002.

and more surgical patients are entering the hospital on an outpatient basis or as same-day admissions. Same-day admissions present the anesthesiologist with a formidable challenge from both an organizational and a clinical perspective. The amount of time available to evaluate even medically complex patients has decreased. This fact and the consequent need to redefine and expand the traditional practice of anesthesia, especially outside the operating room, have been accepted as necessary among anesthesiologists in both academic and community practices.[282,283]

The preoperative evaluation is often the first encounter a patient has with anesthesia and health system- or hospital-based services. Examination facilities, personalized services, and organizational efficiency during the evaluation often influence a patient's perception of the quality of health care at an institution. As previously mentioned, our group has found that the rapidity with which a physician sees the patient is *the* most important factor in determining patient satisfaction with the preoperative process (Foss JF et al, personal communication).

The establishment of a centralized anesthesia preoperative evaluation clinic (APEC) or what I call a "Preoperative And Preprocedure Assessment Clinic" (PPAC)[25,26,284-290] can be a positive investment for the anesthesia group and the hospital, as it becomes a recognized center for decreasing perioperative costs, improving the efficiency of clinical services, implementing clinical pathways that educate and increase market share, and increasing patient and surgeon satisfaction with perioperative and periprocedure services.

Developmental and Organizational Changes

The goal of the APEC, or PPAC (I have used these terms interchangeably, although I now prefer PPAC), is to provide a comprehensive anesthesia service for physicians and their presurgical and preprocedure patients. One centralized location provides all anesthesia consultations, physical examinations, laboratory and electrocardiographic services, educational resources, and hospital registrations and insurance authorizations. Modifying the existing clinical practice to provide cost-effective preoperative evaluation can be approached by a variety of methods, educational tools, and uses of data (Table 25-21).

Certain advantages do accrue when a PPAC is established, but implementation may require stages of change and growth. (I advocate taking incremental steps up the organizational ladder to efficiency: improvement of preoperative testing, implementation of education about perioperative care, and then implementation of education about expectations on pain therapy.) Instituting such a clinic requires a commitment from more than the anesthesia department. Without the support of surgical services and without administrative, financial, and emotional commitment, the PPAC will not realize its full potential and may even incur extra costs rather than savings. However, with such commitment, the health system will increase the quality of care and will decrease costs. Nevertheless, logical as it is, such commitment will not come easily.

The development of the PPAC represents a collaboration between hospital administration and the departments of anesthesia, surgery, gynecology, and nursing. Table 25-22 lists the operational goals for a PPAC.

A timeline for the development of a PPAC should be defined for hospital administration in a business plan. The plan should clearly describe not only reasonable and sustainable goals but also the financial, political, and emotional support necessary for success of the PPAC. The plan should also include analysis of the existing method of providing preoperative evaluation, recommended changes, developmental strategies, descriptions of PPAC management and organizational imperatives, and evaluation of financial risk.

The development of a PPAC begins with a departmental commitment to improve the current system. Even the simplest of changes can enhance the quality of patient care. For example, having a patient complete an anesthesia medical questionnaire in the surgeon's office and then having that information transmitted to the anesthesiologist for review several days before surgery would greatly increase the anesthesiologist's awareness of the patient's medical status.

I advise regularly sending (every 3 months) NPO guidelines, a letter about the clinic and its policies, and a set of forms reminding them of its functioning (Figs. 25-20 to 25-22 and Table 25-20; also see Fig. 25-2) to all surgeons and proceduralists. The information could then be made available to the surgeon, OR, and anesthesiologists the day before the anticipated surgery. This practice could reduce the delays and cancellations that occur when unexpected medical problems are present or unresolved at the scheduled time of surgery.

The Necessity for Teamwork

The PPAC is an integrated partnership having visible alliances with the departments of anesthesia and nursing, and often surgery and obstetrics, but always with the hospital or health system administration. Frequently the existing system of preoperative assessment is beleaguered by the need for change in many of the time-honored traditions, structures, and processes.

Table 25–21 Key areas to consider in promoting cost-effective preoperative preparation

1. Physician education and modification of physician practice (e.g., learn the cost of each diagnostic test ordered preoperatively, plan length of stay with pain therapy practitioners)
2. Practice guidelines
3. Clinical pathways (requires interdepartmental teamwork)
4. Information sharing (e.g., in areas of evaluative protocols and avoiding duplication of services)
5. Economic analysis (e.g., cost-identification, effectiveness, cost-benefit studies)
6. Medical resource management (e.g., in the efficiency and effectiveness of the preoperative process)
7. Education about, and reassessment of, perioperative satisfaction and plans for perioperative pain therapy
8. Outcomes measurement and management

Table 25–22   Operational goals for a preoperative and preprocedure assessment clinic (PPAC)

1. To improve the client's perception of the preoperative evaluation experience by increasing personalized patient care, comfort, and convenience
2. To provide a centralized site for preoperative evaluation
3. To institute an anesthesia scheduling system for timely patient access and flow
4. To ensure the presence of an anesthesiologist on site when patients are present
5. To appoint a medical director of the PPAC to coordinate all activities
6. To ensure the availability of medical records and surgical notes at the time of the preoperative evaluation
7. To decrease logistical shuffling of patients to multiple hospital service areas
8. To integrate and coordinate services through on-site facilities for admitting/registration, insurance authorization, laboratory tests, and electrocardiographic studies
9. To improve the education of patients and families about the elements of their surgical procedure and the proposed anesthesia care, including postoperative pain control options
10. To educate patients about what to expect regarding postoperative feeding and discharge needs
11. To ensure and coordinate cost-effective ordering of preoperative laboratory and diagnostic studies
12. To provide an anesthesia medical consultation service for evaluation of medically complex inpatients and outpatients
13. To decrease the number of cancellations and delays in the operative procedures on the day of surgery
14. To enlist the skills of a nurse practitioner to assist in preoperative evaluations and patient/family education
15. To develop protocols, policies, and clinical pathways
16. To perform quality assurance reviews
17. To maximize efficiency in operating room function and turnover time by coordinating all preoperative information at one location (the anesthesia preoperative evaluation clinic [APEC])
18. To enhance patient and surgeon satisfaction

Figure 25–20 Example of letter to colleagues and their staffs in other specialties about policies of the Preoperative and Preprocedure Assessment Clinic (PPAC).

Date *(issued every three months)*

Dear Surgical and Proceduralist Colleagues *(in this day of medical staff mail merge, I advocate personalizing this letter)*:

Many of you have asked for requirements and/or guidelines as to which patients need to be seen in the Preoperative and Preprocedure Assessment Clinic (PPAC) prior to surgery. Our goals are to better identify those patients who are likely to benefit from a before-day-of-procedure consultation with an anesthesiologist and to help you prepare those who will not be seen until the day-of-procedure.

Many patients who are undergoing minor procedures and are generally healthy are inconvenienced by a PPAC visit. Additionally, there is no evidence to suggest that they are benefited by being seen ahead of time. We do have limited resources and hope to use them appropriately for the best outcome for all our patients. However, many who do not need to be seen may still wish to be seen. We do not want to limit that.

In an effort to better serve patients who are scheduled for anesthesia services we are enclosing several documents that may be of assistance. You will find:

a) Referral guidelines, PPAC Form 1 *(Figure 25-21)*
b) Healthy Patient Testing guidelines, PPAC Form 2 *(Figure 25-22)*
c) Testing Grid for Patients with Co-Morbid Conditions guidelines, PPAC Form 3 *(Table 25-20)*
d) Patient history form to be completed by the patient prior to the PPAC appointment or the visit with the anesthesiologist on the day of the procedure, PPAC Form 4 *(Figure 25-2)*
e) NPO guidelines *(not included in this chapter)*.

These, like all processes in medicine are always works in progress that we will attempt to improve. We need your feedback and will greatly appreciate any suggestions for improvement. You can reach us at *(phone number)*.

Sincerely,

Name
Medical Director, Preoperative and Preprocedure Assessment Clinic

Encls.

Patients who are healthy without any medical problems do not need to have an appointment in the Preoperative and Preprocedure Assessment Clinic (PPAC).

For patients NOT seen in the PPAC:

1. Please follow the testing guidelines in PPAC Forms 2 and 3 *(see Figures 25-22 and Table 25-20).*

2. Please ensure correct NP status. See attached OR policy form.

3. Please be sure patients are instructed to take perioperative medications appropriately. See PPAC Form 4 *(see Figure 25-2)*

4. You may find PPAC Form 4 helpful in deciding which patients may benefit from a PPAC evaluation.

5. PPAC Form 4 should be given to all patients to complete and bring either to their PPAC appointment or to their anesthesiologist on the day of their procedure.

6. Please be sure all pertinent medical information from outside our system (diagnostic tests, especially blood work, cardiac stress texts, echocardiograms, catheterizations, PFTs, consultation, etc.) are available on the day of the procedure. Usually patients with such tests should be seen in the PPAC.

7. "Clearance letters/notes" are rarely sufficient to design a safe anesthetic. A letter summarizing the patient's medical problems and condition, preferably indicating that these are optimized, along with the actual diagnostic tests are necessary.

   If sufficient and appropriate evaluation and preparation are not available on the day of the procedure for those patients with chronic medical conditions who you choose NOT to send to the PPAC it may be necessary to delay or postpone surgery until adequate information or optimization is achieved. We especially encourage you to utilize the PPAC for complex patients or those undergoing major procedure (Class C on PPAC Form 2 [Figure 25-22]).

If you have any questions or comments please contact Dr. *(name)* at *(phone number or e-mail address).*

Figure 25–21 Preoperative and Preprocedure Assessment Clinic (PPAC) referral guidelines (Form 1).

Figure 25-23 shows the fundamental goals that the PPAC strives to accomplish. These goals recognize and encourage clinical responsibility in the portioning of services and, most important, in the sharing of financial costs and savings in the PPAC enterprise. That is, because the department that bears the cost of making the PPAC function is not always the department that enjoys the subsequent savings, transfers of funds are necessary to make the system really work fairly for all concerned. These transfers, plus agreement on the incentives and goals, should be considered *before* institution of the PPAC.

To encourage the referral of patients to the PPAC by surgeons, anesthesiologists can identify the clinical (and perhaps marketing) advantages. Interviewing surgeons regarding their concerns and problems with preoperative assessment helps identify the changes that will be necessary. Likewise, administrators can be interviewed regarding their desires for efficiency of patient care, for increased patient education and satisfaction, and for marketing advantages. Such a process marks the anesthesiologist as an active partner and a resource for improving perioperative care.

In addition to the primary mandate of patient safety, our surgical colleagues are also concerned with avoiding cancellations and OR delays, and with reducing costs and improving patient satisfaction through education, in order to facilitate marketing. To enhance the anesthesiologist's commitment to the PPAC and to increase the patient referral base, an "informal assurance" may be given that if the patient is deemed appropriate and remains medically stable, the patient's care will proceed to surgery without cancellation or delay. This process requires that the entire anesthesia group support the PPAC program and protocols, and means that not all physicians can give consultations in the PPAC. It also means that this position requires an experienced clinician.

The Economic Concerns and Benefits of Developing a PPAC

What are the costs and benefits of a PPAC, and who ultimately supports it financially? This question is pertinent because the costs of a PPAC are borne by one group but the benefits accrue to another. One of the basic principles

These guidelines are to be used for HEALTHY patients. PPAC Form 3 (Table 25-20), **A SIMPLIFIED STRATEGY FOR PREOPERATIVE AND PREPROCEDURE TESTING BASED UPON CO-MORBID CONDITIONS,** *can be used to determine diagnostic tests for patients with medical problems.*

1. For patients of any age undergoing **Class A procedures,** which are defined as minimally invasive (e.g., cataracts under MAC, diagnostic arthroscopy, breast biopsy), we do not require or recommend ANY routine lab tests. However, tests may be indicated based on medical problems. **Healthy** patients require no tests. *One exception is to obtain a baseline creatinine level in any patient undergoing a procedure that includes injection of contrast dye.*

2. For **Class B procedures** (moderately invasive, in which blood loss or major hemodynamic changes are rare) testing is primarily indicated for patients with medical problems. **Therefore, healthy patients of any age do not require laboratory tests for Class B procedures.** *One exception is to obtain a baseline creatinine in any patient undergoing a procedure that includes injection of contrast dye.* However, you may elect to do an ECG based strictly on age (men ≥ 40 and women ≥ 50). Be aware, however, that CMS (Medicare and Medicaid) will not pay for a "routine preoperative ECG". You must be able to select an appropriate diagnosis and ICD-9 code (pallor, dizziness, HTN, obesity, lipid disorder, are frequently used) and be supported by a diagnosis that is documented on your H&P. CBC, electrolytes, BUN, creatinine, LFTs, PT/PTT are done only if patients have medical conditions that support a need for these tests, see PPSC Form 2.

3. For **Class C procedures** (typically disrupt normal physiology, commonly require blood transfusions, invasive monitoring and/or postoperative ICU care) we definitely recommend CBC w/platelets, electrolytes, BUN and creatinine. Other tests (e.g. PT/PTT, LFTs) are indicated based on comorbid conditions, see PPSC Form 2. ECG is the same as indication for Class B procedures but we encourage you to find an "acceptable" diagnosis to allow an ECG in men ≥ 40 and women ≥ 50, based on likelihood of finding an abnormality that may affect perioperative or periprocedure care and likelihood of a risk factor—hypertension, obesity, diabetes, smoking, lipid abnormality, CRP abnormality, lack of exercise, etc.

4. We do not recommend "routine" pregnancy tests prior to the day of surgery. However, one needs to do a careful history and order pregnancy tests as indicated.

5. Generally, tests one within 6 months are acceptable (unless major abnormalities are present or the patient's condition has changed, which necessitate more recent labs), with the exception of ECGs that need to be repeated after 3 months if abnormal.

If you have further questions, *Dr. Name* can be reached at *Number or email*

Figure 25–22 Preoperative and Preprocedure Assessment Clinic (PPAC) testing guidelines for the healthy (Form 2).

of economic analysis of a new venture is that comparison and choices must be made between the existing use of resources and the proposed alternative.

Any financial support given to a PPAC by a hospital will be based on price, quality, and value. Therefore, a cost analysis of the current system of preoperative evaluation will describe the problems, effectiveness, and cost of the traditional system, and the subsequent surgical effectiveness of the new system. This document is more effective if it is comprehensive and focuses on opportunities for improvement.

The strategic alliance and partnership with hospital/health system administration and the departments of nursing and surgery (obstetrics, gynecology, and radiology) toward the common goals of improvement in quality, cost reductions, and reduced length of stay through educational programs requires that the financial support and gains of the PPAC be delegated responsibly and fairly. For example, the facility and professional staff and the maintenance, equipment, registration, and phlebotomy personnel associated with the PPAC would incur cost to the hospital/health system administration. Nursing and educational resources will be supported through the department of nursing or anesthesia cost center. Similarly, benefits from reductions in length of stay and reduced OR times and cancellations should be shared among the parties.

The PPAC staff can be cross-trained to provide services to other areas of the OR during periods of reduced patient volume. This sharing of resources would decrease PPAC costs and increase PPAC "profits." An anesthesiologist would serve as medical director of the PPAC. Table 25-23 lists the sequential elements of a PPAC business plan.

The Strategic Need to Market the PPAC

The concept of public relations and marketing of the PPAC may be unfamiliar to the anesthesiologist.

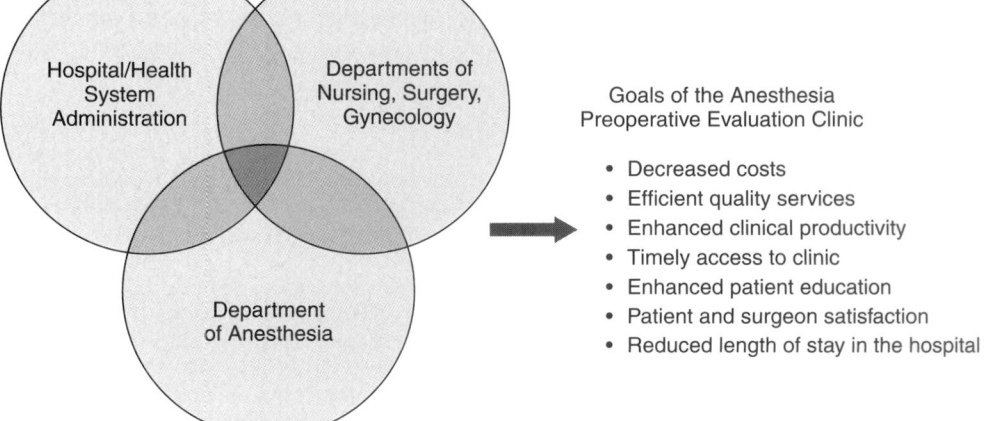

Figure 25–23 The anesthesia preoperative evaluation clinic is a constructive partnership working toward the achievement of common goals. The sharing of resources and budgetary costs is apportioned.

Hospital/Health System Administration

Departments of Nursing, Surgery, Gynecology

Department of Anesthesia

Goals of the Anesthesia Preoperative Evaluation Clinic

- Decreased costs
- Efficient quality services
- Enhanced clinical productivity
- Timely access to clinic
- Enhanced patient education
- Patient and surgeon satisfaction
- Reduced length of stay in the hospital

Table 25–23   Outline of a business plan for a preoperative and preprocedure assessment clinic (PPAC)

The business plan for a PPAC provides or describes the following items:

I. An Executive Summary
A one-paragraph summary of the PPAC program

II. Description of the PPAC
The objective or mission of the PPAC (see Fig. 25-20)
The names of the proposed PPAC medical director, department chair
The location within the hospital designated for the PPAC (define an area, even if currently occupied)
The development stage (is there an existing preoperative program?)
The services of the PPAC (see operational goals, Table 25-23)
Anesthesiology specialty information (i.e., anesthesiologists are the experts in operating room medicine and preoperative evaluation)

III. Analysis of General Factors Affecting Viability of the PPAC
Volume and medical condition of preoperative patients (present a graph for past years)
Anticipated growth trends
Vulnerability to economic factors (e.g., fee-for-service is decreasing, managed care is increasing, hospitals need to decrease costs)
Technological factors (e.g., anesthesia and surgical procedures are becoming increasingly more complex)
Regulatory issues (the PPAC conforms to all local, state, and federal policies)
Financial considerations

IV. Definition of Target Markets
All outpatient and same-day admissions (i.e., increased smooth flow of the healthy patient through the health care system and educational processes, often starting in the surgical office)
The medically complex patient undergoing anesthesia and surgery

V. Discussion of Factors Relating to Competition
The competitive position of the PPAC (the anesthesiologist is the operating room and preoperative medicine expert)
Barriers to entry (primary care physicians/consultants believe they have sufficient specialty knowledge to clear patients for anesthesia and surgery)
Future competition

VI. Description of Effective Marketing Strategies
Increased visibility, which increases viability of the PPAC
Use of hospital/health system news media to explain who anesthesiologists are and what they do
Formation of strategic partnerships with the departments of nursing, surgery, and gynecology, and with the hospital/health system administration
Informal assurance that cases will be facilitated by anesthesia if seen in the PPAC
Presentations at surgical, medical, gynecologic, pediatric, and administrative grand rounds and conferences

VII. Description of Operational Aspects of the PPAC
Facilities (e.g., examination rooms, phlebotomy/ECG room)
Equipment and supplies
Variable labor requirements (e.g., nurse practitioner, anesthesiologist)
Daily anticipated operations and flow
Quality assurance and utilization review (see Table 25-24)
Management information systems

VIII. Description of Management and Organization of the PPAC
The clinical and administrative director
Inclusion of the department of nursing and of the hospital administration
Organization management (presented in a flow chart)

IX. Description of the Developmental Goals of the PPAC
Short-term goals (changes in clinical practice)
Long-term goals (e.g., renovation of facilities)
A time line (demonstrates a developmental plan)
The growth strategy (projection of 6-month, 1-year, and 5-year goals)
Evaluation of risk (as long as patients have surgical needs, risk is minimal)

X. Discussion of Financial Matters
Income statement (consider a facility fee, anesthesia medical consultation charge, projected hospital/health system cost savings, and market share enrichment)
Variable expenditures (i.e., PPAC personnel and resources: 90% of expenditures, facility housekeeping and supplies)
Balance sheet

Increased visibility of the anesthesiologist in a PPAC increases awareness of the clinical expertise of the anesthesiologist and his or her role in developing clinical pathways, preoperative outcome enhancing therapies such as β-adrenergic blocking agents, statins, and aspirin, and pain therapy that decrease the patient's length of stay. For example, at one of the author's institutions, preoperative evaluation and postoperative pain therapy groups are linked (i.e., provided by the same team of physicians, a subgroup of a department) in order to facilitate patient education and rapid discharge. The result has been superior satisfaction on the part of patients and other health care providers.

Hospital/health system publications, presentations at medical, surgical, and gynecologic grand rounds (and administrative grand rounds, if such exist at your institution), and personal communication with physicians increase the awareness of surgeons, hospitals, and health systems regarding the direct influence of the PPAC and anesthesiologist on cost-effective preoperative patient management. Many hospitals have an office of planning and development or a media center that can participate in marketing and educational strategies to promote the PPAC and its policies and educational programs.

Renovation of Facilities

The centralization and modernization of preoperative evaluation procedures represented by a PPAC are long-term investments in the proper facilities and benefit the patient, anesthesia group, and hospital. Focusing all services into one area produces a center that is visible and efficient. Table 25-24 lists the facilities that constitute the APEC at Stanford University Hospital and the University of Chicago.

Table 25–24 Facilities of the anesthesia preoperative evaluation clinic (APEC) at Stanford University Hospital and the University of Chicago*

The APEC at Stanford University consists of the following facilities (information for the University of Chicago is shown in brackets):
1. Five combination office and examination rooms [10]
2. A patient and family education room (preoperative teaching) [1]
3. A patient-centered media and video room [0]
4. A phlebotomy and electrocardiography room [8 are set up for this]
5. An on-site office for the APEC medical director [1]
6. A registration and reception area [1]
7. On-site restroom facilities [2]
8. A large, comfortable patient lounge [1]
9. An area for admitting and financial services [yes]
10. Approximately 2,200 square feet for facilities [2,600]
11. Conference room and shared chart and computer support room [University of Chicago only]

*All areas are accessible to wheelchairs.

Daily Operations and Procedures of the PPAC

The daily operations of the PPAC will vary according to patient volume, severity of the patient's medical conditions, availability of the facility, and employee resources. However, we are able to suggest a general operational structure that represents several PPACs currently in existence.

A PPAC facility can serve 40 to 60 patients a day. The full-time PPAC requires availability of assessment from 8 AM to 6 PM Monday through Friday. The average time needed from check-in to discharge of ASA I patients is 40 minutes; of ASA II patients, 60 minutes; and of ASA III or IV patients, 80 minutes. Approximately one third of that time is spent with a clinician. If fewer than 25 patients are seen daily, a half-day clinic may be appropriate. In this instance, physicians might rotate to the OR after 5-hour stints, because work in the PPAC is intense.

To allow patients to be evaluated in a timely and efficient manner, the PPAC appointment schedule and scheduling system is made available to the surgical specialty clinics. The surgeon's specific OR reservation can be linked to the requirement that a patient must also have a PPAC appointment. This practice not only facilitates anesthesia appointments but also encourages the delivery of patient-centered care.

Previously, most patients ("drop-ins") would come to the PPAC in large numbers in the mid-afternoon and would consequently experience long waits for anesthesia evaluation. Although this situation has been greatly improved by scheduling of appointments, some flexibility regarding "drop-ins" helps accommodate patients requiring urgent surgical decisions and patients from outside the hospital area.

After registration, the patient is processed through hospital/health system admissions, utilization review, and financial services, located in the PPAC. These processes are coordinated with the patient's completion of a preoperative questionnaire[291] (see Fig. 25-2) that seeks information about pertinent medical history, previous surgeries, and medications. These processing services and completion of the questionnaire are scheduled with the goal of maximizing efficient use of physician time. The patient's medical history record is available at the time of the PPAC appointment because the medical records department has received, by electronic communication and 24 to 72 hours earlier, a list of the patient's scheduled appointments for that day.

The anesthesia evaluator interviews and examines the patient and obtains (via facsimile, secure e-mail, internet available secure databases, or phone) whatever outside medical information is needed to complete the assessment. At one site (the University of Chicago), all this information is directly entered into a patient database. Appropriate laboratory, diagnostic, and ECG requirements are determined and obtained on-site in the PPAC. The centralization of services is a significant convenience for patients, who no longer need to visit several hospital sites to complete preoperative requirements. ECGs are evaluated before the patient leaves the PPAC. All laboratory tests are reviewed at the end of the clinic day.

A perioperative educator (usually a nurse) provides individualized education for the patient and family in the preoperative teaching center located in the PPAC. Preoperative education increases the patient's understanding of what to expect regarding postoperative pain therapy and, by decreasing anxiety and fear, achieves its goal of increasing patient comfort. Additionally, preoperative patient education reduces pain and the length of stay in the phase II recovery area and inpatient facilities, and sets the expectations regarding recovery and the needs of the patient on discharge from the hospital. The educational program is organized with the help of the specific surgical service and the office of hospital/health system planning in order to provide patients with videotapes and descriptions of expectations and plans.

Previously, each surgical service had a nurse educator who provided perioperative education for patients. The PPAC program reduced use of this hospital resource significantly and currently coordinates all education through the centralized PPAC location. The preoperative teaching center has a variety of anatomic models, brochures, charts, prostheses, specific videotapes made for this process, and other items to help patients understand their proposed anesthetic, surgical, and perioperative management. Some items can even focus on preventive long-term care (such as cessation of smoking, exercise programs, control of blood pressure, and medications). The anesthesia perioperative database program generates pharmacy orders as well as written instructions for the patient and significant others (see later). These instructions specify where to go, when to be there, which medications to take, and what to expect in the perioperative period.

The staff telephones patients on the afternoon or evening before surgery to confirm arrival time, to reinforce instructions, and to answer any questions. This contact by telephone helps to avoid delays and cancellations on the day of surgery.

The Anesthesia Medical Consultation

The PPAC provides an important service—the anesthesia medical consultation. This is not simply a routine preoperative examination but a conference requested by a primary care physician or surgeon who seeks advice on the suitability of the patient for anesthesia in light of the patient's medical condition. Obtaining these consultations 6 or more days before the planned day of surgery has many advantages. It facilitates the planning of intraoperative anesthesia and monitoring requirements, the obtaining of outside consultations and additional testing, and preparation for perioperative pain therapy and discharge. Although this system seems formidable, it was assembled in small steps by a team. The members of the team have agreed in advance not only to develop the plan but also who has responsibility for each aspect of the plan.

An anesthesia medical consultation increases the awareness of surgeons and patients regarding the expertise of the anesthesiologist in perioperative medicine. This process has led to a greater role for the anesthesiologist in perioperative medicine (see The Evolution of Anesthesiology section). This consultation may initiate diagnostic and/or therapeutic actions for a specific medical problem, including referral of the patient to a specialist such as a cardiologist, for help in evaluating and managing a specific concern.

The expertise of the anesthesiologist is evident when he or she is involved in the decision-making process regarding consultations. Fischer[25] reported a 73% reduction in unnecessary consultations with medical specialists when the anesthesiologist was involved in the consultation decision process, an obvious system cost saving.

Regarding billings, PPAC consultations are first coded using the CPT of the AMA. A professional fee is then submitted, and reimbursement is requested. Although routine visits (those usual in the past) are not billed for, the educational/evaluation process that differs from the past is billed for, and any savings that accrue from reduced length of stay are shared in order to fund the clinic.

Perioperative Quality Assurance Indicators

A database system will allow entry and analysis of quality assurance indicators for the PPAC. System problems that cause costly surgical delays or cancellations, together with practices requiring improvement or enhancement, are easily identifiable. Figure 25-24 summarizes data from the previous section on preoperative informatics to suggest a database format that allows evaluation of quality assurance indicators for the PPAC.

Cost-Effectiveness of the PPAC

The responsibilities of the anesthesiologist are unique in the preoperative process. He or she is the final clinical pathway or "gatekeeper" for the patient entering the OR and for the facilitation of postoperative pain therapy. As such, the PPAC anesthesiologist is a central figure in the review and implementation of practice guidelines[5,292-294] and clinical pathways. He or she also participates in sharing of information (such as patient evaluation protocols and consultations), efforts to avoid duplication of services, studies on identification of costs and benefits, and the evaluation of the management of medical resources and measurements of outcome.

Because the anesthesiologist is the specialist best able to evaluate intraoperative medical complexities as they relate to anesthesia and surgery, he or she is also best qualified to define and coordinate the appropriate preoperative studies needed for optimal intraoperative management of the patient.

Diagnostic Studies and the PPAC

Using guidelines plus clinical judgment seems to be more cost-effective than using only clinical judgment or batteries of tests. These guidelines are provided to surgeons for review and are based primarily on the patient's age, medical status, proposed surgical procedure, and judgment of the clinician.

Four recent studies reported a reduction in testing and hospital costs when preoperative diagnostic testing was

```
┌─────────────────────────────────┐                    PREOP PROGRAM
│                                 │          QUALITY & SERVICE INDICATOR FORM
│                                 │
│                                 │
│                                 │          Today's Date: _____
│                                 │
│                                 │          Date of Surgery: _____
│         (Addressograph)         │
└─────────────────────────────────┘
```

Anesthesia Evaluator: _____   Referring Clinic: _____

- Scheduled Appointment: ☐ Yes ☐ No

- Arrived ±30 Minutes of Appt. Time: ☐ Yes ☐ No

- Patient Triaged Out: ☐ Yes ☐ No

- Patient Chart Available: ☐ Yes ☐ No ☐ Ordered

- Time First Seen in Preop Clinic: _____ (military time)

- Time in Preop Program < 90 Minutes: ☐ Yes ☐ No

    If No, cause of delay in Preop Program:

    ☐ No Chart

    ☐ Outside Records/Tests Did Not Arrive With Patient

    Time to Find Old/Recent: ☐ ECG ☐ Chest X-Ray ☐ MUGA ☐ PFT's
                              ☐ ECHO ☐ Stress Test ☐ Lab Work

    ☐ Complex History, No H&P, Start From the Beginning for History

    ☐ Lab Order Problems/Changes   ☐ Call Resident

    ☐ Wait to Clear Patient's ECG

    ☐ Consult With Medical Director

    ☐ Medical Director Not Available, Find Appropriate Person

    ☐ Contact Outside Source for Additional Information

    ☐ Patient Arrived After 5:00 P.M.

    ☐ Patient Had Surgery Recently, Chart Not Available, Start All Over With Information

    ☐ Clinical Complication That Could Postpone or Cancel Surgery

    ☐ Language Barrier w/Interpreter   ☐ Language Barrier w/NO Interpreter

    ☐ Physical Disabilities

    ☐ Teaching

    ☐ Nursing Assessment Forms

    ☐ Solved Problems Unrelated to Anesthesia; explain: _____

    ☐ Cardiac Surgical Team Not Available

```
┌───────────────────────────┐
│        EVALUATOR          │
│      (military time)      │
│                           │
│  TIME IN: _____   │
│  TIME OUT: _____   │
│  PT. LEVEL: _____   │
│                           │
│  TEACH:  Yes( )  No( )    │
│                           │
│          TOTAL            │
│  VISIT TIME IN: _____   │
│  VISIT TIME OUT: _____   │
└───────────────────────────┘
```

Comments: _____

Figure 25–24 A quality assurance form used by an anesthesia preoperative evaluation clinic to assess the quality and efficiency of its service. ECG, electrocardiogram; ECHO, echocardiogram; H&P, history and physical examination; MUGA, multiple uptake gated analysis; PFT's, pulmonary function tests.

coordinated through the anesthesiologist in the PPAC. The reductions in testing and in average hospital costs per patient were, respectively, 55.1 percent and $112.09,[25] 28.6 percent and $20.89,[289] 55 percent and $137.[27] Roizen and associates[291] reported a $100 decrease in costs per patient.

The PPAC and Delays and Cancellations in the Surgery Schedule

Day-of-surgery delays and cancellations, OR downtime, and loss of hospital revenue decrease when an unstable medical condition is determined *before* the day of surgery (see also Chapter 86). Several authors have reported

Table 25–25 Decrease in surgical cancellations for patients evaluated in the anesthesia preoperative evaluation clinic (APEC)

Investigator	Decrease in Surgical Cancellations
Fischer[25]	88%
Pollard et al[26]	20%
Boothe[289]	60%
Macarthur et al[285]	5 times lower

decreased day-of-surgery cancellations when patients were referred to a PPAC prior to the day of surgery (Table 25-25). The anesthesiologist becomes the primary physician identified with preoperative cost containment and improved quality of perioperative patient care. Furthermore, educating the patient about what to expect regarding postoperative pain therapy and feeding decreases his or her length of stay in the hospital.

Incentives for Cost Reductions

The contribution of the anesthesiologist to cost savings for the hospital or health system is often not obvious and is frequently difficult to quantify. However, the PPAC provides several areas of identifiable cost reductions to the hospital or health system for which the anesthesiologist is directly responsible.

A contractual agreement negotiated with the hospital or health system can recognize that the anesthesia department influences hospital or health care system costs. Fischer[25] reported a one-year hospital cost reduction of $1.01 million spent for unnecessary preoperative testing, and Starsnic and colleagues[289] reported a 1-year cost reduction of $643,056 when preoperative diagnostic studies were coordinated through the PPAC.

The Evolution of Anesthesiology

Health care is in an active state of transformation and reform. The next decade will be a transition-rich environment for consolidations, affiliations, and improving quality of care. The anesthesiologist-directed preoperative evaluation clinic represents a successful partnership between hospital and physician and a framework for growth in our specialty and improvement in outcome for patients.

Anesthesiologists are being asked to provide optimal, efficient patient care within the limitation of finite resources. Current dynamic changes in the field of anesthesiology require a fundamental reassessment and restructuring of the manner in which clinical anesthesia care is provided.

The anesthesia preoperative assessment is a medical evaluation of the patient's current condition, integrated with the anesthesiologist's unique knowledge of the potential clinical and operative events that may occur. Is it time to use this resource to improve patient outcome? Clear data now indicate the outcome benefits (and cost savings to the patient and to society) of instituting the following measures:

1. β-Adrenergic receptor blockade for 2 weeks for all patients over 60 years of age without contraindications who are scheduled for type B and C procedures (see Chapter 27)
2. Statins for 2 weeks for all patients not already receiving such who are scheduled for type B and C procedures
3. Aspirin for all patients over 40 years of age who are scheduled for type B and C procedures that do not involve a closed space lesion, plastic surgery, or retinal surgery (although retinal surgery has shown outcome benefits from perioperative aspirin in at least one study)
4. Physical activity regimen and smoking cessation programs for all patients who are scheduled for type B and C procedures.[31-72]

Will anesthesiology adopt these changes and be a more vibrant specialty in the future, or will these changes become the responsibility of the primary care physician, making preoperative evaluation part of another specialty? And will acceptance or abandonment of such changes determine the viability of the specialty of anesthesiology and its value to society in the future?

I believe the answers are obvious! You, the reader of this chapter, have the ability to make anesthesiology a specialty of the future or a dinosaur of the past. The expanding role of the anesthesiologist beyond the OR has redefined our specialty for the hospital, our colleagues, and the community regarding our clinical expertise, effectiveness, and contribution to quality patient care.

A successful anesthesia PPAC provides the foundation for preparation of the patient for surgery. It results in considerable advantages for the anesthesiologist, improves the quality of care and value for our patients, and provides visible hospital leadership in responding to rapidly changing health care demands.

SUMMARY

Our primary goal has to be efficient delivery of quality care. Patients undergoing surgery move through a continuum of medical care to which the primary care physician, internist, anesthesiologist, and surgeon contribute in a partnership that ensures the best outcome possible. No aspects of medicine require greater cooperation than the performance of surgery and the perioperative care of a patient. For the anesthesiologist, this responsibility starts in a preoperative and preprocedure assessment. The importance of integrating practice is even greater because of the increasing life span of our population. As the number of elderly patients increases, so does the need for preoperative consultation to plan for comorbidities and multiple drug regimens, knowledge of which is crucial to successful patient management.

At a time when medical information is encyclopedic, it is difficult for even the most conscientious anesthesiologist to keep abreast of medical issues relevant to perioperative patient management. Thus, the proposed PPAC facilitates those most sought-after goals: improved quality of care and reduced costs. We physicians can demonstrate to our constituency—the patients—and to their watchdog—the government—that the present system of preoperative evaluation can be changed to increase efficiency, to reduce costs substantially, and to improve the quality of care. At the same time, anesthesiologists can lessen their own anxiety about performing the very best evaluation possible.

KEY POINTS

1. The ultimate goals of preoperative and pre-procedure medical assessment of patients who are receiving anesthesia care are to reduce the morbidity of surgery, to increase the quality but decrease the cost of perioperative care, and to return the patient to desirable functioning as quickly as possible.
2. The basis for preoperative and preprocedure evaluation are data demonstrating that patient conditions and perioperative optimization of care are significant predictors of postoperative morbidity.
3. Preoperative and preprocedure evaluation offer an opportunity to motivate a patient to achieve a higher quality of life and thereby improve long-term as well as immediate outcome.
4. The three areas of acute history that impact perioperative evaluation are exercise tolerance, history of present illness, and when the patient last visited with her/his primary care physician.
5. The three aspects of chronic history that impact perioperative evaluation are medications and reasons for their use, and allergies; social history, including drug, alcohol, and tobacco use and cessation; and family history and history of prior illness.
6. The three aspects of the physical examination are airway, cardiovascular and pulmonary evaluation.
7. In general, not much benefit appears to arise from unindicated routine laboratory testing, and testing should be reserved for those for whom the results may lead to improved care or avoidance of a potential problem.
8. In 2002 the ASA, because of a lack of conclusive data to produce an evidence-based guideline, produced a preoperative testing advisory, which outlined the available studies and provided details regarding consultants' opinions on the value of different diagnostic tests.
9. The extent of a surgical procedure influences the need for routine testing; low-risk procedures require no or minimal diagnostic testing.
10. Informatics may be critical to the efficient and effective preoperative evaluation by ensuring accurate transfer of information to the anesthesia team.

Acknowledgments

The author gratefully acknowledges the contributions of Drs. Joseph Foss and Stephen Fischer in the 5th Edition of this chapter; of Dr. Terrance Winn in the revisions of this chapter in this edition; of Dr. Raj Kim, who coauthored the analysis of benefit versus risk for laboratory tests and Table 25-4; and of Dr. Allan Jo, who provided the summary of testing for, and treatment of, magnesium deficiency.

REFERENCES

1. Egbert LD, Battit GE, Turndorf H, Beecher HK: The value of the preoperative visit by an anesthetist. A study of doctor-patient rapport. JAMA 185:553, 1963.
2. Egbert LD, Battit GE, Welch CE, Bartlett MK: Reduction of postoperative pain by encouragement and instruction of patients. A study of doctor-patient rapport. N Engl J Med 270:825, 1964.
3. Wolfer JA, Davis CE: Assessment of surgical patients' preoperative emotional condition and postoperative welfare. Nurs Res 19:402, 1970.
4. Anderson EA: Preoperative preparation for cardiac surgery facilitates recovery, reduces psychological distress, and reduces the incidence of acute postoperative hypertension. J Consult Clin Psychol 55:513, 1987.
5. Worwag E, Chodak GFW: Overnight hospitalization after radical prostatectomy: The impact of two clinical pathways on patient satisfaction, length of hospitalization, and morbidity. Anesth Analg 87:62, 1998.
6. Vacanti CJ, Van Houten RJ, Hill RC: A statistical analysis of the relationship of physical status to postoperative mortality in 68,388 cases. Anesth Analg 49:564, 1970.
7. Lewin I, Lerner AG, Green SH, et al: Physical class and physiologic status in the prediction of operative mortality in the aged sick. Ann Surg 174:217, 1971.
8. Silber JH, Williams SV, Krakauer H, Schwartz JS: Hospital and patient characteristics associated with death after surgery. A study of adverse occurrence and failure to rescue. Med Care 30:615, 1992.
9. Goldman L, Caldera DL, Nussbaum SR, et al: Multifactorial index of cardiac risk in noncardiac surgical procedures. N Engl J Med 297:845, 1977.
10. Keats AS: The ASA classification of physical status—a recapitulation. Anesthesiology 49:233, 1978.
11. Olsson GL, Hallén B: Cardiac arrest during anaesthesia. A computer-aided study in 250 543 anaesthetics. Acta Anaesthesiol Scand 32:653, 1988.
12. Bechtoldt AA Jr: Committee on Anaesthesia Study. Anesthetic-related deaths: 1969-1976. NC Med J 42:253, 1981.
13. Rehder K: Clinical evaluation of isoflurane. Complications during and after anaesthesia. Can J Anaesth 29, suppl:S44, 1982.
14. Cohen MM, Duncan PG: Physical status score and trends in anesthetic complications. J Clin Epidemiol 41:83, 1988.
15. Farrow SC, Fowkes FGR, Lunn JN, et al: Epidemiology in anaesthesia. I: Factors affecting mortality in hospital. Br J Anaesth 54:811, 1982.
16. Fowkes FGR, Lunn JN, Farrow SC, et al: Epidemiology in anaesthesia. III: Mortality risk in patients with coexisting physical disease. Br J Anaesth 54:819, 1982.
17. Tiret L, Hatton F, Desmonts JM, Vourc'h G: Prediction of outcome of anaesthesia in patients over 40 years: A multifactorial risk index. Stat Med 7:947, 1988.
18. Cohen MM, Duncan PG, Tate RB: Does anesthesia contribute to operative mortality? JAMA 260:2859, 1988.
19. Lunn JN, Farrow SC, Fowkes FGR, et al: Epidemiology in anaesthesia. I: Anaesthetic practice over 20 years. Br J Anaesth 54:803, 1982.
20. Hosking MP, Warner MA, Lobdell CM, et al: Outcomes of surgery in patients 90 years of age or older. JAMA 261:1909, 1989.
21. Duncan PG, Cohen MM, Tweed WA, et al: The Canadian four-centre study of anaesthetic outcomes: III. Are anaesthetic complications predictable in day surgical practice? Can J Anaesth 39:440, 1992.
22. Pedersen T, Eliasen K, Henriksen E: A prospective study of mortality associated with anaesthesia and surgery: Risk indicators of mortality in hospital. Acta Anaesthesiol Scand 34:176, 1990.
23. Narr BJ, Hansen TR, Warner MA: Preoperative laboratory screening in healthy Mayo patients: Cost-effective elimination of tests and unchanged outcomes. Mayo Clin Proc 66:155, 1991.

24. Gibby GL, Gravenstein JS, Layon AJ, Jackson KI: How often does the preoperative interview change anesthetic management? [abstract]. Anesthesiology 77:A1134, 1992.

25. Fischer SP: Development and effectiveness of an anesthesia preoperative evaluation clinic in a teaching hospital. Anesthesiology 85:196, 1996.

26. Pollard JB, Zboray AL, Mazze RI: Economic benefits attributed to opening a preoperative evaluation clinic for outpatients. Anesth Analg 83:407, 1996.

27. Fu ES, Scharf JE, Glodek J: Preoperative testing: A comparison between HealthQuiz recommendations and routine ordering. Am J Anesthesiol 24:237, 1997.

28. Vogt AW, Henson LC: Unindicated preoperative testing: ASA physical status and financial implications. J Clin Anesth 9:437, 1997.

29. Nardella A, Pechet L, Snyder LM: Continuous improvement, quality control, and cost containment in clinical laboratory testing. Effects of establishing and implementing guidelines for preoperative tests. Arch Pathol Lab Med 119:518, 1995.

30. Larocque BJ, Maykut RJ: Implementation of guidelines for preoperative laboratory investigations in patients scheduled to undergo elective surgery. Clin J Surg 37:397, 1994.

31. Stone JG, Foëx P, Sear JW, et al: Myocardial ischemia in untreated hypertensive patients: effect of a single small oral dose of beta-adrenergic blocking agent. Anesthesiology 68:495, 1988.

32. Slogoff S, Keats AS: Does chronic treatment with calcium entry blocking drugs reduce perioperative myocardial ischemia? Anesthesiology 68:676, 1988.

33. Roizen MF: Should we all have a sympathectomy at birth? Or at least perioperatively? Anesthesiology 68:482, 1988.

34. Pasternack PF, Grossi EA, Baumann FG, et al: Beta blockade to decrease silent myocardial ischemia during peripheral vascular surgery. Am J Surg 158:113, 1989.

35. Mangano DT, Layug EL, Wallace A, et al: Effect of atenolol on mortality and cardiovascular morbidity after noncardiac surgery. Multicenter Study of Perioperative Ischemia Research Group (McSPI). N Engl J Med 335:1713, 1996.

36. Poldermans D, Boersma E, Bax JJ, Thomson IR, et al: The effect of bisoprolol on perioperative mortality and myocardial infarction in high-risk patients undergoing vascular surgery. Dutch Echocardiographic Cardiac Risk Evaluation Applying Stress Echocardiography Study Group. N Engl J Med 341:1789, 1999.

37. Auerbach AD, Goldman L: Beta-blockers and reduction of cardiac events in noncardiac surgery: Scientific review. JAMA 287:1435, 2002.

38. Boersma E, Poldermans D, Bax JJ, et al: Predictors of cardiac events after major vascular surgery: Role of clinical characteristics, dobutamine echocardiography, and beta-blocker therapy. JAMA:1865, 2001.

39. Urban MK, Markowitz SM, Gorden MA, et al: Postoperative prophylactic administration of beta-adrenergic blockers in patients at risk for myocardial ischemia. Anesth Analg 90:1257, 2000.

40. VanDenKerkhof EG, Milne B, Parlow JL: Knowledge and practice regarding prophylactic perioperative beta blockade in patients undergoing noncardiac surgery: A survey of Canadian anesthesiologists. Anesth Analg 96:1558, 2003.

41. Wallace A, Layug B, Tateo I, et al: Prophylactic atenolol reduces postoperative myocardial ischemia. McSPI Research Group [see comments]. Anesthesiology 88:7, 1998.

42. Zaugg M, Tagliente T, Lucchinetti E, et al: Beneficial effects from beta-adrenergic blockade in elderly patients undergoing noncardiac surgery. Anesthesiology 91:1674, 1999.

43. Mangano DT: Aspirin and mortality from coronary bypass surgery. N Engl J Med 347:1309, 2002.

44. Neilipovitz DT, Bryson GL, Nichol G: The effect of perioperative aspirin therapy in peripheral vascular surgery: A decision analysis. Anesth Analg 93:573, 2001.

45. Durazzo AE, Machado FW, et al: Reduction in cardiovascular events after vascular surgery with atorvastatin. A randomized trial. J Vascular Surg 39:967, 2004.

46. Eagle KA, Berger PB, Calkins H, et al: ACC/AHA guideline update for perioperative cardiovascular evaluation for noncardiac surgery—executive summary: A report of the American College of Cardiology/American Heart Association Task Force on Practice Guidelines (Committee to Update the 1996 Guidelines on Perioperative Cardiovascular Evaluation for Noncardiac Surgery). J Am Coll Cardiol 39:542, 2002.

47. Nass CM, Allen JK, et al: Secondary prevention of coronary artery disease in patients undergoing elective surgery for peripheral arterial disease. VASC Med 6:35, 2001.

48. Poldermans, Bax JJ, Kertai MD, et al: Statins are associated with a reduced incidence of perioperative mortality in patients undergoing major noncardiac vascular surgery. Circulation 107:1848, 2003.

49. Shojania KG, Duncan BW, McDonald KM, Wachter RM: Safe but sound patient safety meets evidence based medicine. JAMA 508, 2002.

50. Stevens RD, Burri H, Tramer MR: Pharmacologic myocardial protection in patients undergoing noncardiac surgery: A quantitative systematic review. Anesth Analg 97:623, 2003.

51. Stamler J, Stamler R, Neaton JD: Blood pressure, systolic and diastolic, and cardiovascular risks. US population data. Arch Intern Med 153:598, 1993.

52. SHEP Cooperative Research Group: Prevention of stroke by antihypertensive drug treatment in older persons with isolated systolic hypertension. Final results of systolic hypertension in the elderly program (SHEP). JAMA 265:3255, 1991.

53. The fifth report of the Joint National Committee on detection, evaluation, and treatment of high blood pressure. Ann Intern Med 153:154, 1993.

54. Skolnick ET, Vomvolakis MA, Buck KA, et al: Exposure to environmental tobacco smoke and the risk of adverse respiratory events in children receiving general anesthesia. Anesthesiology 88:1144, 1998.

55. Warner MA, Offerd KP, Warner ME, et al: Role of preoperative cessation of smoking and other factors in postoperative pulmonary complications: A blinded prospective study of coronary artery bypass patients. Mayo Clin Proc 64:609, 1989.

56. Fiore MC, Jorenby DE, Schensky AE, et al: Smoking status as the new vital sign: Effect of assessment and intervention in patients who smoke. Mayo Clin Proc 70:209, 1995.

57. Munday IT, Desai PM, Marshall CA, et al: The effectiveness of pre-operative advice to stop smoking: A prospective controlled trial. Anaesthesia 48:816, 1993.

58. Reilly DF, McNeely MJ, Doerner D, et al: Self-reported exercise tolerance and the risk of serious perioperative complications. Arch Intern Med 159:2185, 1999.

59. Smith TP, Kinasewitz GT, Tucker WY, et al: Exercise capacity as a predictor of post-thoracotomy morbidity. Am Rev Respir Dis 129:730, 1984.

60. Starker PM, Group FE, Askanazi J, et al: Serum albumin levels as an index of nutritional support. Surgery 91:194, 1982.

61. Khuri SF, Daley J, Henderson W, et al: Risk adjustment of the postoperative mortality rate for the comparative assessment of the quality of surgical care: Results of the National Veterans Affairs Surgical Risk Study. J Am Coll Surg 185:315, 1997.

62. Brownstein AB, Roizen MF: A compelling rationale for using preoperative visits to complete adult immunizations. J Clin Anesth 10:338, 1998.

63. Tinetti ME, Williams CS: Falls, injuries due to falls, and the risk of admission to a nursing home. N Engl J Med 337:1279, 1997.

64. Kujala UM, Kaprio J, Sarna S, Koskenvuo M: Relationship of leisure-time physical activity and mortality. The Finnish twin cohort. JAMA 279:440, 1998.

65. Sgura FA, Kopecky SL, Grill JP, Gibbons RJ: Supine exercise capacity identifies patients at low risk for perioperative cardiovascular events and predicts long-term survival. Am J Med 108:334, 2000.

66. Gulati M, Pandey DK, Arnsdorf MF, et al: Exercise capacity and the risk of death in women—The St. James Women Take Heart Project. Circulation 108:1554, 2003.

67. Myers J, Prakash M, Froelicher V, et al: Exercise capacity and mortality among men referred for exercise testing. N Engl J Med 346:793, 2002.

68. Gilbey HJ, Ackland TR, Wang AW, et al: Exercise improves early functional recovery after total hip arthroplasty. Clin Orthopaed Related Res 408:193, 2003.

69. Wang AW, Gilbey HJ, Ackland TR: Perioperative exercise programs improve early return of ambulatory function after total hip arthroplasty. Am J Phys Med Rehabil 81:801, 2002.

70. Debigare R, Maltais F, Whittom F, et al: Feasibility and efficacy of home exercise training before lung volume reduction. J Cardiopulm Rehabil 19:235, 1999.

71. Apfelbaum J, Roizen MF, Robinson D, et al: How frequently do asymptomatic patients benefit from the pursuit of abnormalities in their preoperative test results [abstract]? Anesthesiology 73:A1254, 1990.

72. Moller AM, Pedersen T, Villebro N, Norgaard P: Impact of lifestyle on perioperative smoking cessation and postoperative complication rate. Prev Med 36:704, 2003.

73. Kirsh EJ, Worwag EM, Sinner M, Chodak GW: Using outcome data and patient satisfaction surveys to develop policies regarding minimum length of hospitalization after radical prostatectomy. Urology 56:101, 2000.

74. Charlson ME, MacKenzie CR, Gold JP: Preoperative autonomic function abnormalities in patients with diabetes mellitus and patients with hypertension. J Am Coll Surg 179:1, 1994.

75. Cyr M, Wartman SA: The effectiveness of routine screening questions in the detection of alcoholism. JAMA 259:51, 1988.

76. Adams WL, Barry KL, Fleming MF: Screening for problem drinking in older primary care patients. JAMA 276:1964, 1996.

77. Gibby GL, Schwab WK: Availability of records in an outpatient preanesthetic evaluation clinic. J Clin Monit Comput 14:385, 1998.

78. Practice Advisory for Preoperative Evaluation: A report by the American Society of Anesthesiologists Task Force on Preanesthetic Evaluation. Anesthesiology 96:485, 2000. (www.asahq.org/practice/preeval.pdf)

79. Cahalin L, Pappagianopoulos P, Prevost S, et al: The relationship of the 6-min walk test to maximal oxygen consumption in transplant candidates with end-stage lung disease. Chest 108:452, 1995.

80. Older P, Smith R, Courtney P, Hone R: Preoperative evaluation of cardiac failure and ischemia in elderly patients by cardiopulmonary exercise testing. Chest 104:701, 1993.

81. Older P, Hall A: The role of cardiopulmonary exercise testing for preoperative evaluation of the elderly. In Wassserman K (ed): Exercise Gas Exchange in Heart Disease. Armonk, New York, Futura Publishing, 1996, p 287.

82. Roizen MF, Kaplan EB, Schreider BD, et al: The relative roles of the history and physical examination, and laboratory testing in preoperative evaluation for outpatient surgery: The "Starling" curve in preoperative laboratory testing. Anesthesiol Clin North Am 5:15, 1987.

83. Roizen MF: Preoperative evaluation. In Miller RD (ed): Anesthesia, vol 1, 3rd ed. New York, Churchill Livingstone, 1990, p 743.

84. Roizen MF: Is a patient's history of food supplement use simply supplementary? J Clin Anesth 10:89, 1998.

85. Ang-Lee MK, Moss J, Yuan CS: Herbal medicines and perioperative care. JAMA 11:208, 2001.

86. Flanagan K: Preoperative assessment: Safety considerations for patients taking herbal products. J PeriAnesthes Nurs 16:19, 2001.

87. Markowitz JS, Donovan JL, DeVane CL, et al: Effect of St. John's wort on drug metabolism by induction of cytochrome P450 3A4 enzyme. JAMA 290:500, 2003.

88. Lutner RE, Roizen MF, Stocking CB, et al: The automated interview versus the personal interview. Do patient responses to preoperative health questions differ? Anesthesiology 75:394, 1991.

89. Mitchell TL, Tornelli JL, Fisher TD, et al: Yield of the screening review of systems: A study on a general medical service. J Gen Intern Med 7:393, 1992.

90. Benumof JL: Obstructive sleep apnea in the adult obese patient: Implications for airway management. J Clin Anesth 13:144, 2001.

91. Nieto FJ, Young TB, Lind BK, et al: Association of sleep-disordered breathing, sleep apnea, and hypertension in a large community based study. JAMA 283:1829, 2000.

92. Mooe T, Franklin KA, Holmstrom K, et al: Sleep-disordered breathing and coronary artery disease. Long-term prognosis. Am J Respir Crit Care Med 164:1910, 2001.

93. Ostermeier AM, Roizen MF, Hautkappe M, et al: Three sudden postoperative respiratory arrests associated with epidural opioids in patients with sleep apnea. Anesth Analg 85:452-460, 1997.

94. Gottlieb DJ, Whitney CW, Bonekat WH, et al: Relation of sleepiness to respiratory disturbance index. The sleep heart health study. Am J Respir Crit Care Med 159:502, 1999.

95. Peppard PE, Young T, Palta M, et al: Longitudinal study of moderate weight change and sleep-disordered breathing. JAMA 284:3015, 2000.

96. Epstein B: Controversies in outpatient anesthesia. In White PF (ed): Outpatient Anesthesia. New York, Churchill Livingstone, 1990, p 473.

97. Leng GC, Fowkes FGR, Lee AJ, et al: Use of ankle brachial pressure index to predict cardiovascular events and death: A cohort study. BMJ 313:1440, 1996.

98. Kuller LH, Shemanski L, Psaty BM, et al: Subclinical disease as an independent risk factor for cardiovascular disease. Circulation 92:720, 1995.

99. Roizen MF, Coalson D, Hayward RSA, et al: Can patients use an automated questionnaire to define their current health status? Med Care 30(suppl):MS74, 1992.

100. Badner NH, Craen RA, Paul TL, Doyle JA: Anaesthesia preadmission assessment: A new approach through use of a screening questionnaire. Can J Anaesth 45:87, 1998.

101. Essin DJ, Dishakjian R, deCiutiis VL, et al: Development and assessment of a computer-based preanesthetic patient evaluation system for obstetrical anesthesia. J Clin Monit 14:95, 1998.

102. Kobak KA, Taylor LV, Dottl SL, et al: A computer-administered telephone interview to identify mental disorders. JAMA 278:905, 1997.

103. Roizen MF: The RealAge Makeover: Looking Younger, Living Longer! New York, HarperCollins, 2004.

104. Hash RB, Munna RK, Vogel RL, Bason JJ: Does physician weight affect perception of health advice? Prev Med 36:41, 2003.

105. O'Malley PG, Feuerstein IM, Taylor AJ: Impact of electron beam tomography, with or without case management, on motivation, behavioral change, and cardiovascular risk profile: A randomized controlled trial. JAMA 289:2215, 2003.

106. Leonard JV, Clayton BE, Colley JRT: Use of biochemical profile in Children's Hospital: Results of two controlled trials. BMJ 2:662, 1975.

107. Korvin CC, Pearce RH, Stanley J: Admissions screening: Clinical benefits. Ann Intern Med 83:197, 1975.

108. Olsen DM, Kane RL, Proctor PH: A controlled trial of multiphasic screening. N Engl J Med 294:925, 1976.

109. Durbridge TC, Edwards F, Edwards RG, Atkinson M: Evaluation of benefits of screening tests done immediately on admission to hospital. Clin Chem 22:968, 1976.

110. Narr BJ, Hansen TR, Warner MA: Preoperative laboratory screening in healthy Mayo patients: Cost-effective elimination of tests and unchanged outcomes. Mayo Clin Proc 66:155, 1991.

111. Kaplan EB, Sheiner LB, Boeckmann AJ, et al: The usefulness of preoperative laboratory screening. JAMA 253:3576, 1985.

112. McKee RF, Scott EM: The value of routine preoperative investigations. Ann R Coll Surg Engl 69:160, 1987.

113. Turnbull JM, Buck C: The value of preoperative screening investigations in otherwise healthy individuals. Arch Intern Med 147:1101, 1987.

114. Johnson H Jr, Knee-Ioli S, Butler TA, et al: Are routine preoperative laboratory screening tests necessary to evaluate ambulatory surgical patients? Surgery 104:639, 1988.

115. Muskett AD, McGreevy JM: Rational preoperative evaluation. Postgrad Med J 62:925, 1986.

116. O'Connor ME, Drasner K: Preoperative laboratory testing of children undergoing elective surgery. Anesth Analg 70:176, 1990.

117. Hackmann T, Seward DJ, Sheps SB: Anemia in pediatric day-surgery patients: Prevalence and detection. Anesthesiology 75:27, 1991.

118. Roy WL, Lerman J, McIntyre BG: Is preoperative haemoglobin testing justified in children undergoing minor elective surgery? Can J Anaesth 38:700, 1991.

119. Nigam A, Ahmed K, Drake-Lee AB: The value of preoperative estimation of haemoglobin in children undergoing tonsillectomy. Clin Otolaryngol 15:549, 1990.

120. Baron MJ, Gunter J, White P: Is the pediatric preoperative hematocrit determination necessary? South Med J 85:1187, 1992.

121. Rohrer MJ, Michelotti MC, Nahrwold DL: A prospective evaluation of the efficacy of preoperative coagulation testing. Ann Surg 208:554, 1988.

122. Lawrence VA, Kroenke K: The unproven utility of preoperative urinalysis. Clinical use. Arch Intern Med 148:1370, 1988.

123. Asaf T, Reuveni H, Yermiahu T, et al: The need for routine pre-operative coagulation screening tests (prothrombin time PT/partial thromboplastin time PTT) for healthy children undergoing elective tonsillectomy and/or adenoidectomy. Int J Pediatr Otorhinolaryngol 61:217, 2001.

124. Johnson RK, Mortimer AJ: Routine pre-operative blood testing: is it necessary? Anaesthesia 57:914, 2002.

125. Alsumait BM, Alhumood SA, Ivanova T, et al: A prospective evaluation of preoperative screening laboratory tests in general surgical patients. Med Princ Pract 11:42, 2002.

126. Sox HC Jr (ed): Common Diagnostic Tests: Use and Interpretation, 2nd ed. Philadelphia, American College of Physicians, 1990.

127. Hayward RSA, Steinberg EP, Ford DE, et al: Preventive care guidelines: 1991. In Eddy DM (ed): Common Screening Tests. Philadelphia, American College of Physicians, 1991.

128. Blery C, Szatan M, Fourgeaux B, et al: Evaluation of a protocol for selective ordering of preoperative tests. Lancet 1:139, 1986.

129. Hayward RSA, Steinberg EP, Ford DE, et al: Preventive care guidelines: 1991. Ann Intern Med 114:758, 1991.

130. Burke DS, Brundage JF, Redfield RR, et al: Measurement of the false positive rate in a screening program for human immunodeficiency virus infections. N Engl J Med 319:961, 1988.

131. Houry S, Georgeac C, Hay JM, et al: A prospective multicenter evaluation of preoperative hemostatic screening tests. The French Associations for Surgical Research. Am J Surg 170:19, 1995.

132. Schein OD, Katz J, Bass EB, et al: The value of routine preoperative medical testing before cataract surgery. N Engl J Med 342:168, 2000.

133. Roizen MF: More preoperative assessment by physicians and less by laboratory tests [editorial]. N Engl J Med 342:204, 2000.

134. Lira RPC, Nascimento MA, Moreira-Filho DC, et al: Are routine preoperative medical tests needed with cataract surgery? Pan Am J Public Health 10:13, 2001.

135. Elmore JG, Barton MB, Moceri VM, et al: Ten-year risk of false positive screening mammograms and clinical breast examinations. N Engl J Med 338:1089, 1998.

136. Domoto K, Ben R, Wei JY, et al: Yield of routine annual laboratory screening in the institutionalized elderly. Am J Public Health 75:243, 1985.

137. Wolf-Klein GP, Holt T, Silverstone FA, et al: Efficacy of routine annual studies in the care of elderly patients. J Am Geriatr Soc 33:325, 1985.

138. Abrutyn E, Mossey J, Berlin JA, et al: Does asymptomatic bacteriuria predict mortality and does antimicrobial treatment reduce mortality in elderly ambulatory women? Ann Intern Med 120:827, 1994.

139. Delahunt B, Turnbull PRG: How cost-effective are routine preoperative investigations? N Z Med J 92:431, 1980.

140. Rosselló PJ, Ramos Cruz A, Mayol PM: Routine laboratory tests for elective surgery in pediatric patients: Are they necessary? Bol Assoc Med P R 72:614, 1980.

141. Bates DW, Boyle DL, Rittenberg E, et al: What proportion of common diagnostic tests appear redundant? Am J Med 104:361, 1998.

142. Van Klei WA, Moons KGA, et al: Effect of outpatient preoperative evaluation on cancellation of surgery and length of hospital stay. Anesth Analg 94:644, 2002.

143. Wood RA, Hoekelman RA: Value of the chest x-ray as a screening test for elective surgery in children. Pediatrics 67:447, 1981.

144. Sandler G: Costs of unnecessary tests. Br J Med 2:21, 1979.

145. Rabkin SW, Horne JM: Preoperative electrocardiography: Its cost-effectiveness in detecting abnormalities when a previous tracing exists. Can Med Assoc J 121:301, 1979.

146. Rabkin SW, Horne JM: Preoperative electrocardiography: Effect of new abnormalities on clinical decisions. Can Med Assoc J 128:146, 1983.

147. Salzmann P, Kerlikowske K, Phillips K: Cost-effectiveness of extending screening mammography guidelines to include women 40 to 49 years of age. Ann Intern Med 127:955, 1997.

148. Bar L, Yen MF, Vitak B, et al: Mammography service screening and mortality in breast cancer patients: 20-year follow-up before and after introduction of screening. Lancet 361:1405, 2003.

149. Tape TG, Mushlin AI: How useful are routine chest x-rays of preoperative patients at risk for postoperative chest disease? J Gen Intern Med 3:15, 1988.

150. Orkin FK: Practice standards: The Midas touch or the emperor's new clothes? Anesthesiology 70:567, 1989.

151. Hirsh IA, Tomlinson DL, Slogoff S, Keats AS: The overstated risk of preoperative hypokalemia. Anesth Analg 67:131, 1988.

152. Vitez TS, Soper LE, Wong KC, Soper P: Chronic hypokalemia and intraoperative dysrhythmias. Anesthesiology 63:130, 1985.

153. Harrrington JT, Isner JM, Kassirerr JP: Our national obsession with potassium. Am J Med 73:155, 1982.

154. Lawson DH: Adverse reactions to potassium chloride. Q J Med 43:433, 1974.

155. Lawson DH, Hutcheon AW, Jick H: Life threatening drug reactions amongst medical in-patients. Scot Med J 24:127, 1979.

156. Levinstein MR, Ouslander JG, Rubenstein LZ, Forsythe SB: Yield of routine annual laboratory tests in a skilled nursing home population. JAMA 258:1909, 1987.

157. Robbins JA, Rose SD: Partial thromboplastin time as a screening test. Ann Intern Med 90:796, 1979.

158. Parkerson GR Jr: Cost analysis of laboratory tests in ambulatory primary care. J Fam Pract 7:1001, 1978.

159. Parkerson GR Jr: Determinants of physician recognition and follow-up of abnormal laboratory values. J Fam Pract 7:341, 1978.

160. Williamson JW, Alexander M, Miller GE: Continuing education and patient care research. Physician response to screening test results. JAMA 201:938, 1967.

161. Huntley RR, Steinhauser R, White KL, et al: The quality of medical care: Techniques and investigation in the outpatient clinic. J Chronic Dis 14:630, 1961.

162. Daughaday WH, Erickson MM, White W, et al: Evaluation of routine 12-channel chemical profiles on patients admitted to a university general hospital. In Benson ES, Strandjord PE (eds): Multiple Laboratory Screening. San Diego, Academic Press, 1969, p 181.

163. Epstein KA, Schneiderman LJ, Bush JW, Zettner A: The "abnormal" screening serum thyroxine (T4): Analysis of physician response, outcome, cost and health effectiveness. J Chronic Dis 34:175, 1981.

164. Wheeler LA, Brecher G, Sheiner LB: Clinical laboratory use in the evaluation of anemia. JAMA 238:2709, 1977.

165. Kelley CR, Mamlin JJ: Ambulatory medical care quality. Determination by diagnostic outcome. JAMA 227:1155, 1974.

166. Umbach GE, Zubek S, Deck H-J, et al: The value of preoperative chest x-rays in gynecological patients. Arch Gynecol Obstet 243:179, 1988.

167. Robertson WM: Medical Malpractice: A Preventive Approach. Seattle, University of Washington Press, 1985.

168. Berwick DM: Screening in health fairs. A critical review of benefits, risks, and costs. JAMA 254:1492, 1985.

169. Singh NA: A randomized controlled trial of progressive resistance training in depressed elders. J Gerontol 52:M27, 1997.

170. Collen MF, Feldman R, Siegelaub AB, Crawford D: Dollar cost per positive test for automated multiphasic screening. N Engl J Med 283:459, 1970.

171. Collen MF (ed): Multiphasic Health Testing Services. New York, John Wiley & Sons, 1978.

172. Neuhauser D: Cost-effective clinical decision making. Pediatrics 60:756, 1977.

172a. Robbins JA, Mushlin AI: Preoperative Evaluation of the healthy patient. Med Clin North Am 63:1145, 1979.

173. Pauker SG, Kopelman RI: Interpreting hoofbeats: Can Bayes help clear the haze? N Engl J Med 327:1009, 1992.

174. Coley CM, Barry MJ, Fleming C, Mulley AG: Early detection of prostate cancer. Part I: Prior probability and effectiveness of tests. Ann Intern Med 126:394, 1997.

175. Tinker JH, Dull DL, Caplan RA, et al: Role of monitoring devices in prevention of anesthetic mishaps: A closed claims analysis. Anesthesiology 71:541, 1989.

176. Farnsworth PB, Steiner E, Klein RM, SanFilippo JA: The value of routine preoperative chest roentgenograms in infants and children. JAMA 244:582, 1980.

177. Brill PW, Ewing ML, Dunn AA: The value (?) of routine chest radiography in children and adolescents. Pediatrics 52:125, 1973.

178. Sagel SS, Evens RG, Forrest JV, Bramson RT: Efficacy of routine screening and lateral chest radiographs in a hospital-based population. N Engl J Med 29:1001, 1974.

179. Sane SM, Worsing RA Jr, Wiens CW, Sharma RK: Value of preoperative chest x-ray examinations in children. Pediatrics 60:669, 1977.

180. Rees AM, Roberts CJ, Bligh AS, Evans KT: Routine preoperative chest radiography in non-cardiopulmonary surgery. BMJ 1:1333, 1976.

181. Loder RE: Routine pre-operative chest radiography. 1977 compared with 1955 at Peterborough District General Hospital. Anaesthesia 33:972, 1978.

182. Hubbell FA, Greenfield S, Tyler JL, et al: The impact of routine admission chest x-ray films on patient care. N Engl J Med 312:209, 1985.

183. Maigaard S, Elkjaer P, Stefansson T: Vaerdien af preoperative rutinerøntgenundersøgelse af thorax og ekg.[English abstract: Value of routine preoperative radiographic examination of the thorax and ECG.] Ugeskr Laeger 140:769, 1978.

184. Catchlove BR, Wilson RM, Spring S, Hall J: Routine investigations in elective surgical patients. Their use and cost effectiveness in a teaching hospital. Med J Aust 2:107, 1979.

185. Velanovich V: Preoperative laboratory screening based on age, gender, and concomitant medical diseases. Surgery 115:56, 1994.

186. Thomsen HS, Gottlieb J, Madsen JK, et al: Rutinemaessig røntgenundersøgelse af thorax inden kirurgiske indgreg i universel anaestesi. [English abstract: Routine radiographic examination of the thorax prior to surgical intervention under general anesthesia.] Ugeskr Laeger 140:765, 1978.

187. Gupta SD, Gibbons FJ, Sen I: Routine chest radiography in the elderly. Age Ageing 14:11, 1985.

188. Boghosian SG, Mooradian AD: Usefulness of routine preoperative chest roentgenograms in elderly patients. J Am Geriatr Soc 35:142, 1987.

189. Sewell JMA, Spooner LLR, Dixon AK, Rubenstein D: Screening investigations in the elderly. Age Ageing 10:165, 1981.

190. Törnebrandt K, Fletcher R: Pre-operative chest x-rays in elderly patients. Anaesthesia 37:901, 1982.

191. Fink DJ, Fang M, Wyle FA: Routine chest x-ray films in a Veterans Hospital. JAMA 245:1056, 1981.

192. Wiencek RG, Weaver DW, Bouwman DL, Sachs RJ: Usefulness of selective preoperative chest x-ray films. A prospective study. Am Surg 53:396, 1987.

193. Petterson SR, Janower ML: Is the routine preoperative chest film of value? Appl Radiol 6:70, 1977.

194. Royal College of Radiologists Working Party on the Effective Use of Diagnostic Radiology: Preoperative chest radiology. National study by the Royal College of Radiologists. Lancet 2:83, 1979.

195. Rucker L, Frye EB, Staten MA: Usefulness of screening chest roentgenograms in preoperative patients. JAMA 250:3209, 1983.

196. Weibman MD, Shah NK, Bedford RF: Influence of preoperative chest x-rays on the perioperative management of cancer patients [abstract]. Anesthesiology 67:A332, 1987.

197. Gagner M, Chiasson A: Preoperative chest x-ray films in elective surgery: A valid screening tool. Can J Surg 33:271, 1990.

198. Black WC, Welch HG: Advances in diagnostic imaging and overestimations of disease prevalence and the benefits of therapy. N Engl J Med 328:1237, 1993.

199. Kubik A, Parkin DM, Khlat M, et al: Lack of benefit from semi-annual screening for cancer of the lung: Follow-up report of a randomized controlled trial on a population of high-risk males in Czechoslovakia. Int J Cancer 45:26, 1990.

200. Andersson I, Aspergren K, Janzon L, et al: Mammographic screening and mortality from breast cancer: The Malmö mammographic screening trial. BMJ 297:943, 1988.

201. Tabar L, Yen MF, Vitak B, et al: Mammography service screening and mortality in breast cancer patients: 20-year follow-up before and after introduction of screening. Lancet 361:1405, 2003.

202. Yipintsoi T, Vasinanukorn P, Sanguanchua P: Is routine pre-operative electrocardiogram necessary? J Med Assoc Thai 72:16, 1989.

203. Gordon T, Kannel WB: The Framingham Massachusetts study twenty years later. In Kessler II, Levin ML (eds): The Community as an Epidemiologic Laboratory: A Casebook of Community Studies. Baltimore, Johns Hopkins Press, 1970, p 123.

204. Ostrander LD Jr, Brandt RL, Kjelsberg MO, Epstein FH: Electrocardiographic findings among the adult population of a total natural community, Tecumseh, Michigan. Circulation 31:888, 1965.

205. Kannel WB, McGee D, Gordon T: A general cardiovascular risk profile: The Framingham study. Am J Cardiol 38:46, 1976.

206. Apfelbaum J, Robinson D, Murray WJ, et al: An automated method to validate preoperative test selection: First results of a multicenter study [abstract]. Anesthesiology 71:A928, 1989.

207. Moorman JR, Hlatky MA, Eddy DM, et al: The yield of the routine admission electrocardiogram. A study in a general medical service. Ann Intern Med 103:590, 1985.

208. Seymour DG, Pringle R, MacLennan WJ: The role of the routine pre-operative electrocardiogram in the elderly surgical patient. Age Ageing 12:97, 1983.

209. Gold BS, Young ML, Kinman JL, et al: The utility of preoperative electrocardiograms in the ambulatory surgery patient. Arch Intern Med 152:301, 1992.

210. Sox HC Jr, Garber AM, Littenberg B: The resting electrocardiogram as a screening test. A clinical analysis. Ann Intern Med 111:489, 1989.

211. Goldberger AL, O'Konski M: Utility of the routine electrocardiogram before surgery and on general hospital admission. Critical review and new guidelines. Ann Intern Med 105:552, 1986.

212. Roizen MF: RealAge: Are You As Young As You Can Be? New York, HarperCollins, 1999.

213. Stamler J, Stamler R, Neaton JD, et al: Low risk-factor profile and long-term cardiovascular and non-cardiovascular mortality and life expectancy: findings for 5 large cohorts of young adults and middle-aged men and women. JAMA 282:2012, 1999.

214. Wasserman LR, Gilbert HS: Surgical bleeding in polycythemia vera. Ann N Y Acad Sci 115:122, 1964.

215. Erikssen G, Thaulow E, Sandvik L, et al: Haematocrit: A predictor of cardiovascular mortality? J Intern Med 234:493, 1993.

216. Rothstein P: What hemoglobin level is adequate in pediatric anesthesia? Anesthesiol Update 1:2, 1978.

217. Pemberton PL, Down JF, Porter JB, Bromley LM: A retrospective observational study of pre-operative sickle cell screening. Anaesthesia 57:334, 2002.

218. Weiskopf RB, Viele MK, Feiner J, et al: Human cardiovascular and metabolic response to acute, severe isovolemic anemia. JAMA 279:217, 1998.

219. Carson JL, Duff A, Berlin JA, et al: Perioperative blood transfusion and postoperative mortality. JAMA 279:199, 1998.

220. Carmalt MHB, Freeman P, Stephens AJH, Whitehead TP: Value of routine multiple blood tests in patients attending the general practitioner. BMJ 1:620, 1970.

221. Moore SB, Reisner RK, Offord KP: Morning admission for a same-day surgical procedure: Resolution of a blood bank problem. Mayo Clin Proc 64:406, 1989.

222. Daley J, Khuri SF, Henderson W, et al: Risk adjustment of the postoperative morbidity rate for the comparative assessment of the quality of surgical care: Results of the National Veterans Affairs Surgical Risk Study. J Am Coll Surg 185:328, 1997.

223. Gold BD, Wolfersberger WH: Findings from routine urinalysis and hematocrit on ambulatory oral and maxillofacial surgery patients. J Oral Surg 38:677, 1980.

224. Wataneeyawech M, Kelly KA Jr: Hepatic diseases unsuspected before surgery. N Y State J Med 75:1278, 1975.

225. Schemel WH: Unexpected hepatic dysfunction found by multiple laboratory screening. Anesth Analg 55:810, 1976.

226. Singer DE, Samet JH, Coley CM, Nathan DM: Screening for diabetes mellitus. Ann Intern Med 109:639, 1988.

227. Schneiderman LJ, DeSalvo L, Baylor S, Wolf PL: The "abnormal" screening laboratory results. Its effect on physician and patient. Arch Intern Med 129:88, 1972.

228. Bryan DJ, Wearne JL, Viau A, et al: Profile of admission chemical data by multichannel automation: An evaluative experiment. Clin Chem 12:137, 1966.

229. Schoen I: Clinical chemistry. A retrospective look at routine screening. Calif Med 108:430, 1968.

230. Peery TM: The role of the laboratory in health evaluation, Interim Report No. 77, from the 1964 Technicon International Symposium, New York, NY, as quoted in Schoen I: Clinical chemistry, a retrospective look at routine screening. Calif Med 108:430, 1968.

231. Friedman GD, Goldberg M, Ahuja JN, et al: Biochemical screening tests. Effect of panel size on medical care. Arch Intern Med 129:91, 1972.

232. Young DM, Drake TGH: Unsolicited laboratory information, presented to the College of American Pathologists, Chicago, 18 Oct 1965, as quoted in Schoen I: Clinical chemistry, a retrospective look at routine screening. Calif Med 108:430, 1968.

233. Boonstra CE, Jackson CE: The clinical value of routine serum calcium analysis. Ann Intern Med 57:963, 1962.

234. Whitehead TP: Multiple analyses and their use in the investigation of patients. Adv Clin Chem 14:389, 1971.

235. Cardiff-Oxford Bacteriuria Study Group: Sequelae of covert bacteriuria in schoolgirls. A four-year follow-up study. Lancet 1:889, 1978.

236. Challand GS: Is ward biochemical testing cheap and easy? Intensive Care World 4:9, 1987.

237. Baranetsky NG, Weinstein P: Partial thromboplastin time for screening. Ann Intern Med 91:498, 1979.

238. Barber A, Green D, Galluzzo T, Ts'ao C-H: The bleeding time as a preoperative screening test. Am J Med 78:761, 1985.

239. Macpherson DS, Snow R, Lofgren RP: Preoperative screening: value of previous tests. Ann Intern Med 113:969, 1990.

240. Bushnick JB, Eisenberg JM, Kinman J, et al: Pursuit of abnormal coagulation screening tests generates modest hidden preoperative costs. J Gen Intern Med 4:493, 1989.

241. Eisenberg JM, Clarke JR, Sussman SA: Prothrombin and partial thromboplastin times as preoperative screening tests. Arch Surg 117:48, 1982.

242. Suchman AL, Mushlin AI: How well does the activated partial thromboplastin time predict postoperative hemorrhage? JAMA 256:750, 1986.

243. Macpherson DS: Preoperative laboratory testing: should any tests be "routine" before surgery? Med Clin North Am 77:289, 1993.

244. Roizen MF, Hurd MJ: Preoperative patient evaluation. *In* Rogers MC (ed): Current Practice in Anesthesiology, 2nd ed. St. Louis, Mosby–Year Book, 1990, p 14.

245. Souter AJ, Fredman B, White PF: Controversies in the perioperative use of nonsterodial [sic] antiinflammatory drugs. Anesth Analg 79:1178, 1994.

246. Levitt RC: Prospects for the diagnosis of malignant hyperthermia susceptibility using molecular genetic approaches. Anesthesiology 76:1039, 1992.

247. Wong ET, Rude RK, Singer FR, Shaw ST Jr: A high prevalence of hypomagnesemia and hypermagnesemia in hospitalized patients. Am J Clin Pathol 79:348, 1983.

248. Fanning WJ, Thomas CS Jr, Roach A, et al: Prophylaxis in atrial fibrillation with magnesium sulfate after coronary bypass grafting. Ann Thorac Surg 52:529, 1991.

249. England MR, Gordon G, Salem M, Chernow B: Magnesium administration and dysrhythmias after cardiac surgery. A placebo-controlled, double-blind, randomized trial. JAMA 268:2395, 1992.

250. Reinhart RA, Desbiens NA: Hypomagnesemia in patients entering the ICU. Crit Care Med 13:506, 1985.

251. Gambling DR, Birmingham CL, Jenkins LC: Magnesium and the anaesthetist. Can J Anaesth 35:644, 1988.

252. Lembo NJ, Dell'Italia LJ, Crawford MH, O'Rourke RA: Bedside diagnosis of systolic murmurs. N Engl J Med 318:1572, 1988.

253. Baker JP, Detsky AS, Wesson DE, et al: Nutritional assessment. A comparison of clinical judgment and objective measurements. N Engl J Med 306:969, 1982.

254. Whang R, Ryder KW: Frequency of hypomagnesemia and hypermagnesemia. Requested vs routine. JAMA 263:3063, 1990.

255. Lum G: Hypomagnesemia in acute and chronic care patient populations. Am J Clin Pathol 97:827, 1992.

256. Chernow B, Bamberger S, Stoiko M, et al: Hypomagnesemia in patients in postoperative intensive care. Chest 95:391, 1989.

257. Roizen MF: Preoperative evaluation. *In* Miller RD (ed): Anesthesia, vol 1, 4th ed. New York, Churchill Livingstone, 1994, p 827.

258. Roizen MF: Routine preoperative evaluation. *In* Miller RD (ed): Anesthesia. vol 1, 2nd ed. New York, Churchill Livingstone, 1986, p 225.

259. Roizen MF: Routine preoperative evaluation. *In* Miller RD (ed): Anesthesia, vol. 1. New York, Churchill Livingstone, 1981, p 3.

260. Eiseman B: Necessary preoperative tests. *In* Wilmore DW, Brennan MF, Harken AH, et al (eds): Medicine: Care of the Surgical Patient, American College of Surgeons, vol 2. New York, Scientific American, 1989, p 1.

261. Velanovich V: The value of routine preoperative laboratory testing in predicting postoperative complications: A multivariate analysis. Surgery 109:236, 1991.

262. Larson CP Jr: Evaluation of the patient and preoperative preparation. *In* Barash PG, Cullen BF, Stoelting RK (eds): Clinical Anesthesia, 2nd ed. Philadelphia, Lippincott, 1992, p 545.

263. Roizen MF: The preoperative cardiology consult: What the cardiologist should know about anesthesia. *In* Parmley WW, Chatterjee K (eds): Cardiology, vol. 2 (Cardiovascular Disease). Philadelphia, Lippincott, 1993, p 1.

264. Preoperative and Perioperative Care. *In* Medical Knowledge Self-Assessment Program 13, Primary Care Medicine.

Philadelphia, American College of Physicians, 2003, pp 131-140.

265. Mukherjee D. Eagle KA: Perioperative cardiac assessment for noncardiac surgery: Eight steps to the best possible outcome. Circulation 107:2771, 2003.

266. Mangano DT, Browner WS, Hollenberg M, et al: Long-term cardiac prognosis following noncardiac surgery. JAMA 268:233, 1992.

267. Hollenberg M, Mangano DT, Browner WS, et al: Predictors of postoperative myocardial ischemia in patients undergoing noncardiac surgery. JAMA 268:205, 1992.

268. Charlson ME, MacKenzie CR, Ales K, et al: Surveillance for postoperative myocardial infarction after noncardiac operations. Surg Gynecol Obstet 167:407, 1988.

269. Macario A, Roizen MF, Thisted RA, et al: Reassessment of preoperative laboratory testing has changed the test-ordering patterns of physicians. Surg Gynecol Obstet 75:539, 1992.

270. Charpak Y, Blery C, Chastang C, et al: Usefulness of selectively ordered preoperative tests. Med Care 26:95, 1988.

271. Curran J, Chmielewski AT, White JB, Jennings AM: Practice of preoperative assessment by anaesthetists. BMJ 291:391, 1985.

272. Mancuso CA: Impact of New Guidelines on Physicians' Ordering of Preoperative Tests. J Gen Intern Med 14:166, 1999.

273. Tierney WM, McDonald CJ, Hui SL, Martin DK: Computer predictions of abnormal test results. Effects on outpatient testing. JAMA 259:1194, 1988.

274. Tierney WM, Miller ME, Overhage JM, McDonald CJ: Physician inpatient order writing on microcomputer workstations. Effects on resource utilization. JAMA 269:379, 1993.

275. Chodoff P, Gianaris CD: A nurse-computer assisted preoperative anesthesia management system. Comput Biomed Res 6:371, 1973.

276. Tompkins BM, Tompkins WJ, Loder E, Noonan AF: A computer-assisted preanesthesia interview: value of a computer-generated summary of patient's historical information in the preanesthesia visit. Anesth Analg 59:3, 1980.

277. Beers RA, O'Leary CE, Franklin PD: Comparing the history-taking methods used during a preanesthetic visit: The HealthQuiz versus the written questionnaire. Anesth Analg 86:134, 1998.

278. Forrest WJ, Bellville JW: The use of computers in clinical trials. Br J Anaesth 39:311, 1967.

279. Galla SJ, Schwarzbach R, Buccigrossi R: A computer program for analysis of anesthetic records. Anesthesiology 30:565, 1969.

280. Gibby GL, Paulus DA, Sirota DJ, et al: Computerized pre-anesthetic evaluation results in additional abstracted comorbidity diagnoses. J Clin Monit 13:35, 1997.

281. Fleisher L: Access and use of health care vary by type of Medicaid managed care program. Find Brief 6:1, 2003.

282. Saidman LJ: The 33rd Rovenstine Lecture. What I have learned from 9 years and 9,000 papers. Anesthesiology 83:191, 1995.

283. Longnecker D: Planning the future of anesthesiology. Anesthesiology 84:495, 1996.

284. Burk N, Mazzei W: The need for an anesthesia preoperative evaluation center [abstract]. Anesth Analg 70:S44, 1990.

285. Macarthur AJ, Macarthur C, Bevan JC: Preoperative assessment clinic reduces day surgery cancellations [abstract]. Anesthesiology 75:A1109, 1991.

286. Conway JB, Goldberg J, Chung F: Preadmission anaesthesia consultation clinic. Can J Anaesth 39:1051, 1992.

287. Finegan BA: Preadmission and outpatient consultation clinics. Can J Anaesth 39:1009, 1992.

288. Boothe P: Changing the admission process for elective surgery: An economic analysis. Can J Anaesth 42:391, 1995.

289. Starsnic MA, Guarnieri DM, Norris MC: Efficacy and financial benefit of an anesthesiologist-directed university preadmission evaluation clinic. J Clin Anesth 9:299, 1997.

290. Fischer SP, Cost-effective preoperative evaluation and testing. Chest 1159(suppl):96S-100S, 1999.

291. Roizen MF, Kaplan EB, Sheiner LB, et al: Elimination of unnecessary laboratory tests by preoperative questionnaire [abstract]. Anesthesiology 61:A455, 1984.

292. Eddy DM: Resolving conflicts in practice policies. JAMA 264:389, 1990.

293. Ginsburg WH: When does a guideline become a standard? The new American Society of Anesthesiologists guidelines give us a clue. Ann Emerg Med 22:121, 1993.

294. Roizen MF, Fleisher LA: Medical guidelines by other societies: Should we ignore or influence them? Anesth Analg 82:679, 1996.

CHAPTER
26 Pulmonary Function Testing

Thomas J. Gal

Clinical Spirometry   999
Vital Capacity   999
Time-Expired Spirogram   1000
Maximum Breathing Capacity   1002
Respiratory Muscle Strength   1002

**Physiologic Determinants of
Maximum Flow Rates   1002**
Flow-Volume Relationships   1003
Airway Compression and Flow
    Limitation   1004
Sites and Mechanisms of Decreased Air Flow
    in Disease   1004

**Measurement of Airway
Obstruction   1005**
Airway Resistance   1005
Forced Expiratory Maneuvers   1006

Flow-Volume Loops   1007
Defining Normal Values   1009

Tests of Gas Exchange Function   1010
Alveolar-Arterial Oxygen Tension
    Difference   1010
Multiple-Breath Nitrogen Washout   1010
Diffusing Capacity of the Lung   1010

**Pulmonary Function Testing in
Surgical Patients   1011**

**Evaluation of the Patient for Lung
Resection   1012**
Indications and Criteria   1012
Exercise Capacity   1013

**Preoperative Measures to Improve
Lung Function   1014**

Pulmonary function testing continues to play a role in traditional preoperative evaluation of patients undergoing major surgery. Although it is simple and risk free, such testing is often performed in a reflex fashion without real indications because of limited physiologic and clinical insight on the part of many practicing physicians. As a result, these practitioners are often uncomfortable interpreting test data and are unsure about what the data mean or what was actually measured.

Such preoperative screening is aimed at identifying individuals with abnormal lung function not so much to detect unrecognized disease as to quantitate its severity in the hope of reducing the risk of postoperative ventilatory impairment and other respiratory complications. The subjective information provided by the medical history and the findings on physical examination seldom identify the actual abnormalities of respiratory function, and the findings are often poor indicators of the severity of disease. In contrast, pulmonary function testing provides objective, standardized measurements for assessing the presence and severity of respiratory dysfunction. These measurements also enable the clinician to monitor the progression of any impairment and to document the response to therapy (e.g., bronchodilators). The tests fall into two major groups: those that detect abnormalities of

gas exchange and those related to the mechanical ventilatory function of the lungs and chest wall. This discussion deals principally with the latter group.

The cornerstone of all pulmonary function testing is clinical spirometry. There are numerous other tests, including some that purport to indicate abnormalities of gas exchange. This chapter reviews the measurement techniques and interprets the physiologic basis and significance of many of these tests. The aim is to provide a better understanding of the defects identified by each testing scheme. Such information does not merely serve to impress a board examiner or a colleague; it also enhances the anesthesiologist's role as a consultant in the rational perioperative management of the cases evaluated. Management considerations include the risk of postoperative morbidity, resectability of lung tissue, and management of the anesthetic.

CLINICAL SPIROMETRY

Vital Capacity

The most common measurement of lung function is the vital capacity (VC). John Hutchinson is given the credit for inventing the spirometer and for coining the term *vital capacity* in the mid-19th century.[1] The VC is the largest volume measured after an individual inspires deeply and maximally to total lung capacity (TLC) and then exhales completely to residual volume (RV) into a spirometer. The maneuver is performed without concern for rapidity of effort. Normal values for VC are lower in supine subjects than in sitting ones and vary directly with height and inversely with age. In general, a given VC is suspected of being abnormal if it falls below 80% of the predicted value. Patients with abnormally low values for VC are said to have restrictive disease. The decreased VC associated with restrictive disease may result from lung pathology such as pneumonia, atelectasis, or pulmonary fibrosis. It may also occur with a loss of distensible lung tissue (e.g., after surgical excision). Decreased VC is also seen in the absence of lung disease. In this case, muscle weakness, abdominal swelling, or pain may prevent the patient from obtaining a full inspiration or a maximum expiratory effort.

Time-Expired Spirogram

After a maximum inspiratory effort, a subject exhales as forcefully and rapidly as possible, and the volume of gas is called the *forced vital capacity* (FVC). The exhaled volume is recorded with respect to time. The rate of airflow during this rapid, forceful exhalation indirectly reflects the flow resistance properties of the airways. When airway obstruction occurs, the FVC tends to be less than the standard VC because airways reach flow limitation early and air trapping occurs. In healthy subjects, the two maneuvers usually result in almost equal measured volumes. Because the FVC maneuver is an artificial one, patients must be instructed carefully, and they often require practice attempts before performing the test adequately. Generally, three acceptable tracings are required for analysis. These FVC maneuvers must be characterized by an initial full inspiration to TLC, followed by an abrupt onset of exhalation and continued maximum effort throughout exhalation to RV. The exhalation should take at least 4 seconds and should not be interrupted by coughing, glottic closure, or any mechanical obstruction.[2]

The FVC is reduced by the same conditions that reduce VC. To identify airway obstruction, flow rates are determined by calculation of the volume exhaled during certain time intervals. Most commonly measured is the volume exhaled in the first second, called the *forced expiratory volume in 1 second* (FEV$_1$). The FEV$_1$ can be expressed as the absolute volume in liters, and typical values for various patient groups are listed in Table 26-1. The FEV$_1$ provides an even better perspective on the degree of airway obstruction when it is expressed as a percentage of the FVC (FEV$_1$/FVC).

For the purposes of reporting and calculating values, the largest observed FVC and FEV$_1$ from any of the three acceptable spirograms are used, even if they are not obtained from the same curve.[2] Normal, healthy subjects can exhale 75% to 80% of FVC in the first second; the remaining volume is exhaled in two or three additional seconds (Fig. 26-1). Diseases such as asthma and bronchitis,

Table 26–1 Clinical ranges for 1-second forced expiratory volume (FEV$_1$)	
Clinical Range (L)	**Patient Group**
3.0-4.5	Normal adult
1.5-2.5	Mild-to-moderate obstruction
<1.0	Qualifies as handicapped
0.8	Disability
0.5	Severe emphysema

which obstruct the airway, reduce expiratory flow rates and therefore reduce FEV$_1$ and FEV$_1$/FVC. An obstructive defect is essentially characterized by a disproportionate decrease in the airflow rate relative to the actual volume exhaled (i.e., FVC) and indicates airway narrowing and flow limitation during expiration. Values for FEV$_1$/FVC that are lower than 70% reflect mild obstruction, those lower than 60% suggest moderate obstruction, and those lower than 50% indicate severe obstruction. Because the FEV$_1$/FVC represents a ratio, it is important to realize that identical percentage values may not indicate equivalent degrees of lung dysfunction. For example, a patient with an FEV$_1$ of 1.5 L and an FVC of 3.0 L does not have the same degree of impairment as a similar-sized patient with an FEV$_1$ of 0.75 L and an FVC of 1.5 L, although both have an FEV$_1$/FVC ratio of 50%.

Restrictive diseases are not usually associated with airway obstruction but do cause decreases in FVC. Although the absolute volume of FEV$_1$ may be reduced on a similar

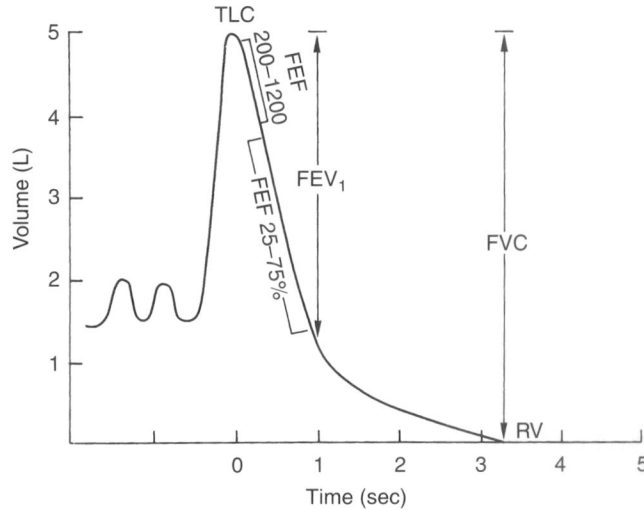

Figure 26-1   Forced vital capacity (FVC) maneuver in a subject with a normal lung. Exhaled volume is plotted against time as the subject expires forcefully, rapidly, and completely to residual volume (RV) after a maximum deep inspiration to total lung capacity (TLC). FEV$_1$, forced expired volume in 1 second; FEF$_{200-1200}$, forced expiratory flow between 200 and 1200 mL of expired volume; FEF$_{25\%-75\%}$, forced expiratory flow over the midportion of vital capacity (i.e., from 25% to 75% of expired volume).

basis, the FEV$_1$ expressed as a percentage of FVC is usually normal (e.g., FEV$_1$/FVC = 70%). The essential physiologic characteristic of a restrictive defect is a reduction in total lung volume (i.e., TLC). However, the presence of such a defect is usually implied when FVC is reduced and the ratio of FEV$_1$/FVC is normal or increased. The impacts of various mechanical abnormalities on VC and these dynamic lung volumes are summarized in Table 26-2.

The maximum flow rate during an FVC maneuver occurs in the initial 0.1 second and is called the *peak flow rate* (measured in liters per second or liters per minute). Peak flow can be estimated by drawing a tangent to the steepest part of the FVC spirogram, but this method is subject to large errors. More commonly, maximum flow is measured as the average flow during the liter of gas expired after the initial 200 mL during an FVC maneuver (see Fig. 26-1). This is usually designated as *forced expiratory flow between 200 and 1200 mL of FVC* (FEF$_{200-1200}$); however, the term *maximum expiratory flow rate* has also been used. This flow is slightly lower than the true peak flow, which can be measured conveniently with a hand-held flow meter (Fig. 26-2) or more accurately with a pneumotachygraph. Peak flow is markedly affected by obstruction of large airways and is particularly responsive to bronchodilator therapy. Because repeat measurements are convenient to obtain, the peak flow rate can be used to monitor therapeutic responses in patients with acute asthma. Normal values in healthy men younger than 40 years are typically 500 L/min or more. Values less than 200 L/min in surgical candidates suggest impaired cough efficiency and a strong likelihood of postoperative complications.[3] The test is much less unpleasant and exhausting for patients than the FVC maneuver; it therefore provides a valuable tool to identify gross pulmonary disability at the bedside.

Although peak flow is largely a function of the caliber of the airways, it also greatly depends on expiratory muscle strength and on the patient's effort and coordination. As a result, the measurement can be variable. In contrast, high degrees of effort are not required to achieve maximum expiratory flow at intermediate and low lung volumes during forced expiration. Flow is often measured over the middle half of the FVC (i.e., between 25% and 75% of the expired volume). This parameter, formerly called the *maximum midexpiratory flow,* is now referred to as the *forced midexpiratory flow* (FEF$_{25\%-75\%}$). Because the flow does not include the initial, highly effort-dependent portion of forced expiration, FEF$_{25\%-75\%}$ is often referred to as *effort independent.* This designation is not entirely appropriate, because FEF$_{25\%-75\%}$ can be decreased by marked reductions in expiratory effort and by a submaximal inspiration before the maneuver. The latter artificially

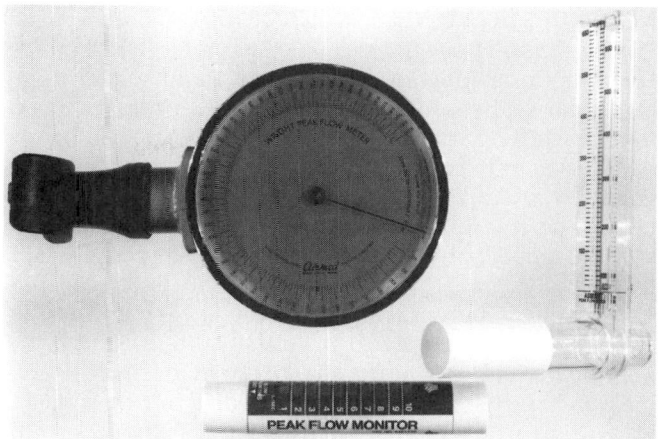

Figure 26–2 Three hand-held peak flow meters. The classic Wright meter (Air Med Limited, Harlow, England) and the Assess peak flow meter (Health Scan Products, Cedar Grove, NJ) quantitate the peak flow rate. The smaller peak flow monitor (Biotrine Corporation, Woburn, MA) allows the patient to tape over the holes before blowing. If the flow rate indicated by the first uncovered hole is reached, a hornlike sound is produced by a metal, reedlike device within the tube.

reduces the FVC and, along with it, the FEF$_{25\%-75\%}$. The same flow rates may also decrease with truly maximum effort, compared with slightly submaximal effort.[4,5] This phenomenon, called *negative effort dependence,* appears to be an artifact of measuring volume changes at the mouth rather than actual changes in thoracic gas volume, which differ in terms of the dynamic airway compression that occurs with truly maximum effort.

The FEF$_{25\%-75\%}$ is a highly variable spirometric index, largely because of its dependence on the absolute volume of FVC and on changes in expiratory time with various degrees of airway obstruction. Values for FEF$_{25\%-75\%}$ in healthy young men average 4.5 to 5.0 L/sec, but because of wide variations even in normal subjects, the predicted limits of normal may be as low as 2 L/sec. The measurement has often been proposed as a sensitive indicator of early obstruction in the small distal airways. However, patients undergoing spirometry for suspected airway obstruction almost always had normal values for FEF$_{25\%-75\%}$ when FEV$_1$/FEV was 75% or greater.[6] One exception may occur in patients with restrictive ventilatory defects, in whom the FEF$_{25\%-75\%}$ may be markedly reduced and the FEV$_1$/FVC normal. However, lung volumes, as reflected by the TLC, the FVC, and the absolute volume of FEV$_1$, are all reduced, and the FEF$_{25\%-75\%}$ does not appear to be any more sensitive than FEV$_1$ in detecting mild abnormalities of lung dysfunction.

Table 26–2 Forced vital capacity (FVC) and 1-second forced expiratory volumes (FEV$_1$) in disease states

Disease States	FVC	FEV$_1$	FEV$_1$/FVC
Airway obstruction (asthma, bronchitis)	Normal	Decreased	Decreased
Stiff lungs (pneumonia, pulmonary edema, pulmonary fibrosis)	Decreased	Decreased	Normal
Respiratory muscle weakness (myasthenia gravis, myopathies)	Decreased	Decreased	Normal

Maximum Breathing Capacity

Dynamic lung function is routinely evaluated in many pulmonary function laboratories by measuring the maximum breathing capacity or, more specifically, the *maximum voluntary ventilation* (MVV). This is the largest volume that can be breathed per minute by voluntary effort, and it is an estimate of the peak ventilation available to meet physiologic demands. The patient is instructed to breathe as hard and fast as possible for 12 seconds. The measured volume is extrapolated to 1 minute and is expressed in units of liters per minute. Because high rates of airflow are required for the MVV, the measurement is significantly affected by changes in airway resistance. MVV is usually reduced in patients with obstructive airway disease and correlates reasonably well with FEV_1 measured in liters (MVV $\cong$ FEV_1 × 35). Discrepancies between the measured MVV and that predicted by FEV_1 often indicate inconsistent or submaximal inspiratory effort.[7] The MVV as a comprehensive test of ventilatory function is also altered by factors other than airway obstruction, including the elastic properties of the lung and chest wall, respiratory muscle strength, learning, coordination, and motivation. In healthy male adults, MVV averages 150 to 175 L/min. This extremely high level of ventilatory effort cannot be maintained for much longer than 1 minute. However, approximately 80% of the MVV can be sustained by healthy subjects for as long as 15 minutes and up to 60% for even longer periods. Abnormally low values (<80% of predicted) do not identify specific defects but do indicate gross impairment in respiratory function. The unique value of the test for the surgical candidate may lie in its dependence on intangible variables, such as cooperation, motivation, and stamina.

Respiratory Muscle Strength

All measurements of pulmonary function that require patient effort (e.g., FVC, FEV_1 peak flow, MVV) are influenced by the strength of the respiratory muscles. The latter can be specifically evaluated by measurement of maximum static respiratory pressures. The pressures are generated against an occluded airway during a maximum forced inspiratory or expiratory effort and are usually measured with aneroid gauges.[8] *Maximum static inspiratory pressure* (PImax) is measured when inspiratory muscles are at their optimal length near RV (Fig. 26-3). Similarly, *maximum static expiratory pressure* (PEmax) is measured when expiratory muscles are optimally stretched after a full inspiration to near TLC. In young adult men, the PImax is about –125 cm H_2O, and the PEmax is about +200 cm H_2O.

The pressure measured at the mouth includes that generated by the respiratory muscles and a portion of that resulting from the elastic recoil of the respiratory system. The latter is essentially zero at functional residual capacity (FRC). Pressures measured at FRC are less than at the extremes of lung volume (see Fig. 26-3), but unlike the other values, they reflect solely the pressures developed by the respiratory muscles.

A PImax of –25 cm H_2O or less indicates severe inability to take a deep breath, whereas a PEmax of less than

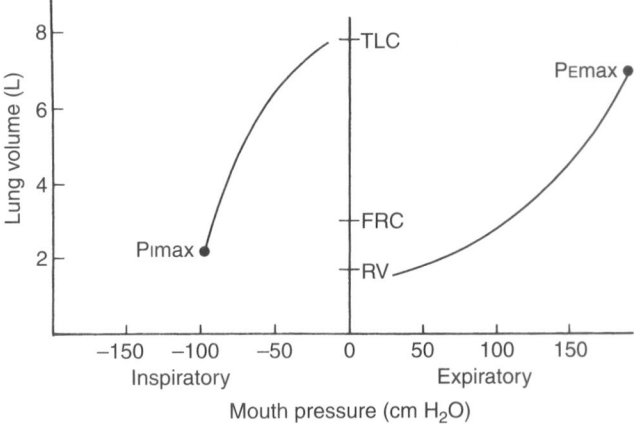

Figure 26–3 Normal values for maximum static inspiratory pressure (PImax) and expiratory pressure (PEmax), measured at the mouth, are plotted as a function of lung volume from residual volume (RV) to total lung capacity (TLC). FRC, functional residual capacity.

+40 cm H_2O suggests severely impaired coughing ability. Although these pressures are not measured routinely in all pulmonary function laboratories, they are particularly useful in the evaluation of patients with neuromuscular disorders. For these patterns, the VC has long been used to indicate the severity of respiratory muscle weakness and to predict respiratory failure. Measurements of respiratory muscle strength can more readily identify patients in whom respiratory muscle weakness is the prime cause of hypercapnic respiratory failure.[9]

PHYSIOLOGIC DETERMINANTS OF MAXIMUM FLOW RATES

The maximum flow rates that can be achieved during pulmonary function testing maneuvers depend on three factors, each of which is highly influenced by the volume of the lung at the time. Foremost is the degree of effort, or the driving pressure generated by muscle contraction. The expiratory effort reflected by PEmax is maximum at high lung volumes near TLC and decreases as lung volume decreases (see Fig. 26-3). Conversely, PImax is achieved at low lung volumes near RV and diminishes at higher lung volumes.

A second important determinant of maximum flow is the elastic *recoil pressure of the lung* (PL). At all lung volumes from RV to TLC, the lung has a tendency to recoil inward (Fig. 26-4). The PL therefore is greatest at TLC (25 to 30 cm H_2O) and lowest at RV (2 to 3 cm H_2O). The PL is opposed by the outward *recoil pressure of the chest wall* (Pcw), except at very high lung volumes. The *recoil pressure of the respiratory system* (Prs) is the algebraic sum of PL + Pcw. PL and Pcw are equal and opposite at a certain point (i.e., Prs = 0). This volume is the FRC that is the respiratory system's normal resting volume.

A third factor, which opposes the two driving pressures, is the resistance to flow provided by the airways. This *airway resistance* (Raw) is determined by the size of the airways. Because airways are largest at high lung volumes

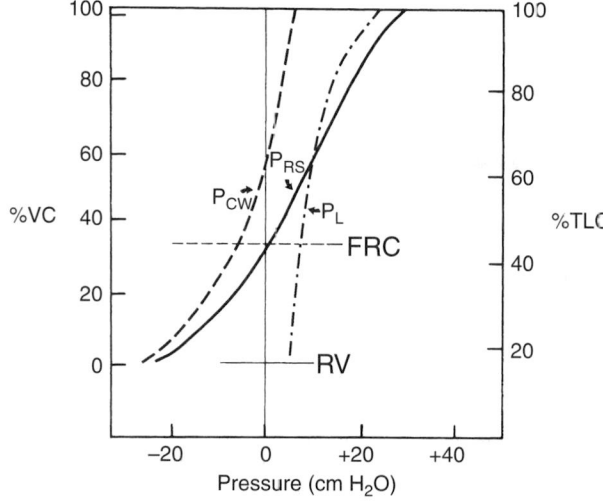

Figure 26–4 Elastic recoil pressures for the lung (P_L), chest wall (P_{CW}), and total respiratory system (P_{RS}) are plotted as a function of lung volume. FRC, functional residual capacity; RV, residual volume; TLC, total lung capacity; VC, vital capacity.

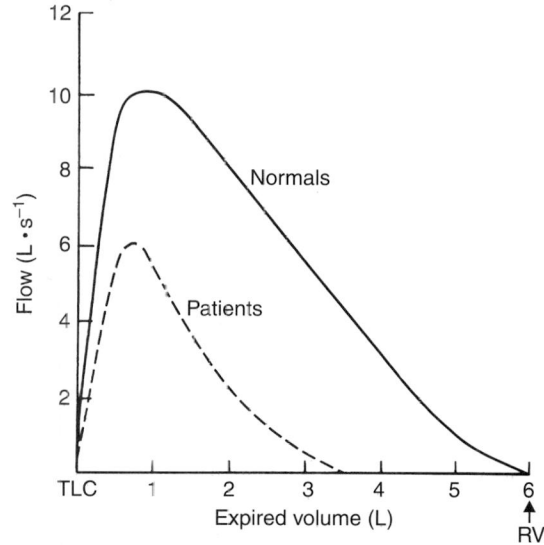

Figure 26–6 Idealized maximum expiratory flow-volume curves for normal subjects are contrasted with those typically seen for patients with obstructive airway disease. Expiratory flow is plotted as a function of lung volume during maximum expiration from total lung capacity (TLC) to residual volume (RV).

and smallest at RV, Raw is greatest at RV and least at TLC (Fig. 26-5A). The inverse relationship between Raw and lung volume is not linear. The reciprocal of Raw, *airway conductance* (Gaw), which is linearly related to lung volume (see Fig. 26-5B), is often used to identify bronchoconstriction or bronchodilation.

Flow-Volume Relationships

Because all determinants of maximum flow depend on lung volume, a useful format for assessing the flow-resistive properties of the airways is to plot flow as a function of volume during the FVC maneuver. At the beginning of the forced expiration, the rate of flow quickly rises to a maximum or peak value at a lung volume very near to

TLC. As expiration continues, lung volume decreases, airways narrow, resistance increases, and flow rates progressively decrease. The impact of obstructive airway disease on such flow rates is emphasized in Figure 26-6. In patients with airway obstruction, flows are reduced over the full range of lung volume, from TLC to RV.

The influence of expiratory effort on the flow-volume curves is important. An individual can inscribe different flow-volume curves with different efforts, although each may have the same FVC. At large lung volumes close to TLC, air flow rises with increasing effort, as shown by curve A of Figure 26-7. With decreasing effort, curves B and C exhibit decreased flows in this high range of lung volume,

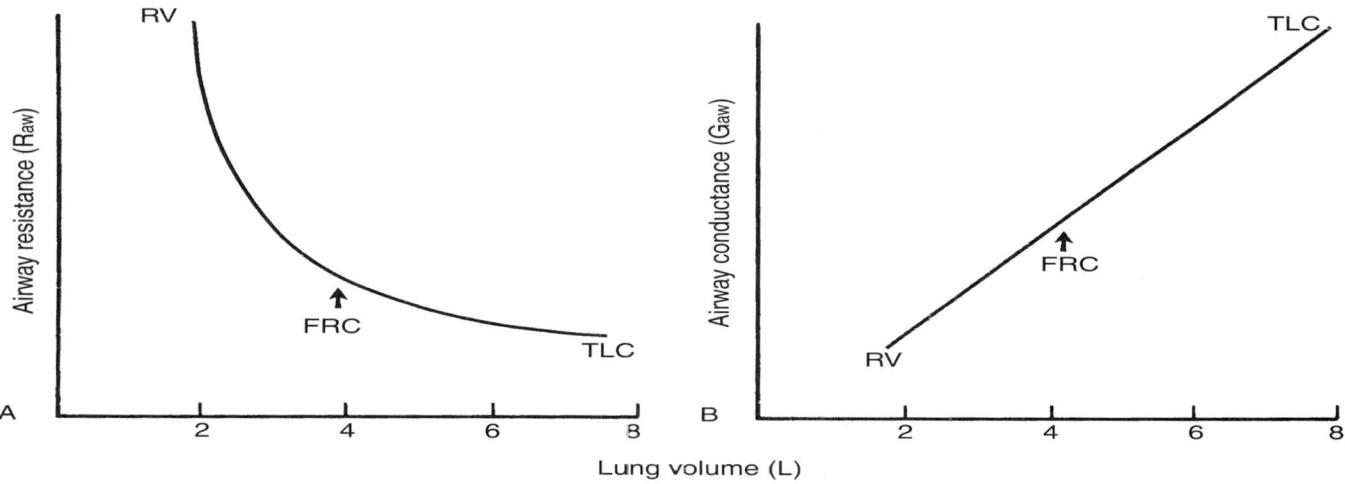

Figure 26–5 The hyperbolic relationship of airway resistance (Raw) to lung volume (**A**) is contrasted with the linear relationship (**B**) of its reciprocal airway conductance (Gaw). FRC, functional residual capacity; RV, residual volume; TLC, total lung capacity.

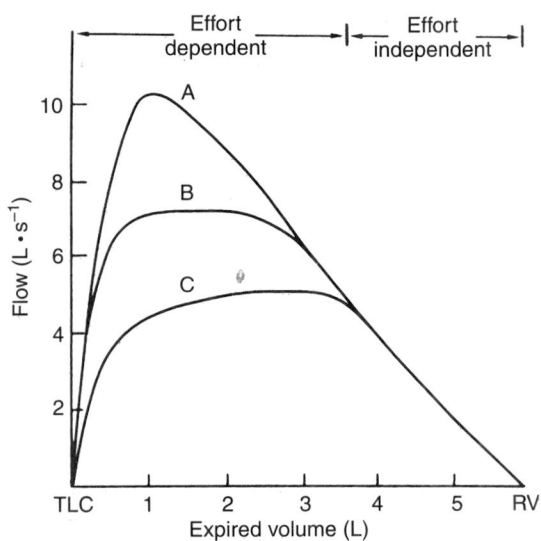

Figure 26–7 Forced expiratory flow-volume curves for a normal subject. The exhalation from total lung capacity (TLC) to residual volume (RV) was performed at three levels of effort: maximum (curve A), intermediate (curve B), and minimal (curve C).

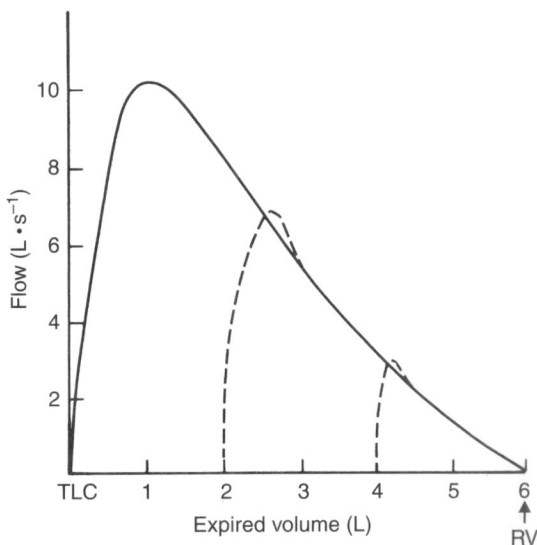

Figure 26–8 Forced expiratory flow-volume curves inscribed during maximum maneuvers performed by beginning at total lung capacity (TLC) and at 2 and 4 L below TLC. RV, residual volume.

but all three curves merge at a point and continue together to RV. At these intermediate and low lung volumes, only moderate effort is needed to produce maximum flow. Because increased expiratory effort has little effect on increasing these flows, there is little difference between the three curves, and this portion of the curve is referred to as *effort independent*. At this point, flow is largely a function of the other two variables (P_L and R_{aw}). Exaggerated effort may decrease these flows, as with $FEF_{25\%-75\%}$.[4,5]

The rate of airflow during forced expiration is influenced by the effort expanded and by the lung volume at which the expiratory maneuver is begun. True maximum flows occur only when expiration is begun at or near TLC. When forced expirations are begun with maximum effort from volume below TLC (Fig. 26-8), peak flow is not as high, but flows quickly conform to the same performance envelope as if the maneuvers were begun at TLC. Even some healthy subjects can exhibit a decreased FEV_1/FVC ratio on the normal volume-time spirogram when the forced expirations are started from such submaximal volumes. Therein lies some of the advantage of a flow-volume plot compared with the volume-time tracing with conventional spirometry.

Airway Compression and Flow Limitation

The failure of increasing effort to further augment flow over the lower two thirds of the VC results from dynamic compression of the airways. This has been described in a model of flow limitation called the *equal pressure point* (EPP) concept. The pressure head, which moves air from the alveoli to the mouth, is provided by the *alveolar pressure* (P_{ALV}). At any given lung volume, alveolar pressure is the sum of *lung elastic recoil pressure* (P_L) and *pleural pressure* (P_{PL}). At any lung volume when there is no flow, such as at end inspiration (Fig. 26-9A), P_{PL} is subatmospheric and counterbalances P_L. The sum (P_{ALV}) is zero, as are

pressures at the mouth and through the remaining airways. During forced expiration (see Fig. 26-9B), P_{PL} rises above atmospheric pressure (i.e., becomes positive), and the increased P_{ALV} again is the sum of P_L and P_{PL}. Pressure is dissipated along the airway to overcome resistance to flow and finally reaches zero at the mouth. At some point along the airway, the intraluminal pressure falls to a level that equals the surrounding P_{PL}. This site is the EPP. Toward the mouth (i.e., downstream), the lateral pressure within the airway lumen is less than the compressing P_{PL}, and the airways tend to collapse. After maximum flow is reached, further increases in P_{PL} from extra effort do not affect airflow in the upstream segment (i.e., from EPP toward the alveoli), because the driving pressure along this portion of the airway is equal to P_L. Therein lies the origin of the term *effort independent*. The increased P_{PL} produces more compression of the downstream airways (i.e., from EPP to mouth). Increasing effort produces more and more airway compression but fails to increase flow.

The principal value of this dynamic airway compression is in the production of an effective cough. Even though maximum flows may not be reached, the compressed downstream airway develops an increased linear velocity of airflow, which maximizes the removal of secretions along airway walls. At intermediate lung volumes, EPPs lie in segmental bronchi, but they may move farther upstream toward the alveoli at lower lung volumes. The dynamic compression involves primarily the lobar and mainstem bronchi and the intrathoracic trachea. Coughing is therefore most effective in removing material from these relatively large airways.

Sites and Mechanisms of Decreased Air Flow in Disease

Abnormal expiratory flow rates may be seen in many disease states and may result from alterations in any of the

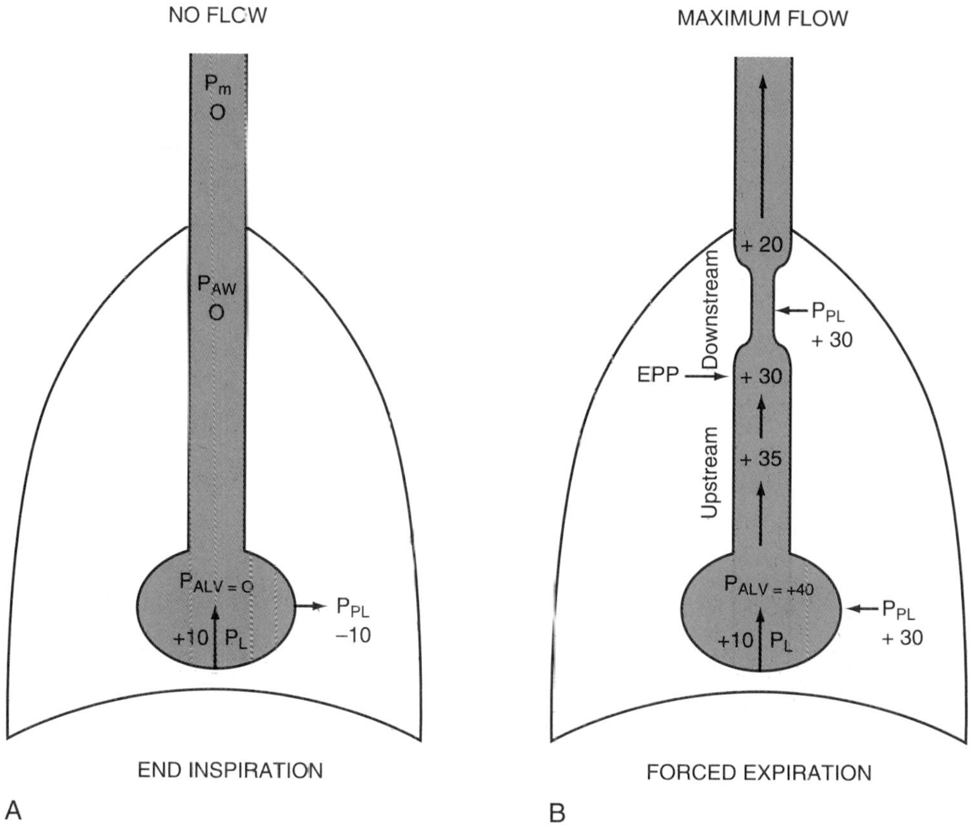

Figure 26–9 A model depicting the equal pressure point (EPP) concept of expiratory flow limitation. P_{ALV}, alveolar pressure; P_{AW}, intraluminal airway pressure; P_{PL}, pleural pressure; P_m, mouth pressure.

three major determinants of flow (i.e., P_{Emax}, P_L, and Raw), as seen in Table 26-3. For example, patients with neuromuscular disease who may exhibit decreased expiratory flows include those with myasthenia gravis, muscular dystrophy, Guillain-Barré syndrome, and spinal cord transection. Decreased ability to generate expiratory effort is the principal cause of low expiratory flows in these patients, who seldom exhibit increases in Raw or decreases in P_L. Other categories of restrictive disease, such as musculoskeletal deformities (e.g., kyphoscoliosis, ankylosing spondylitis, interstitial lung disease), are often associated with near-normal muscle strength. In these situations, expiratory flows may be slightly increased because of an increased P_L associated with

reductions in lung volume. Reduced lung volumes associated with long-term neuromuscular disease also may be associated with increases in P_L, which may result in more normal expiratory flow rates.

The classic example of decreased expiratory flow associated with decreased lung recoil (P_L) is emphysema. In this disease, expiratory muscle strength is usually adequate, and lung distention tends to increase airway size, such that Raw is also usually normal. Conversely, in patients with bronchitis and asthma, airway narrowing is prominent. In these two variants of obstructive lung disease, the major factor reducing flow is increased Raw. Early changes in these obstructive lung diseases may be confined to the smaller peripheral airways. Narrowing in these airways may reduce expiratory flows at middle and low lung volumes, but it does not appreciably affect measurements in Raw or the other determinants of airflow.

MEASUREMENT OF AIRWAY OBSTRUCTION

Airway Resistance

Of the standard techniques used to evaluate airway obstruction, Raw measurements appear to be the most direct. The technique is rapid and noninvasive and requires merely that a subject pant once or twice per second through a mouthpiece and with a noseclip in place. During normal breathing, a major fraction of the resistance

Table 26–3 Mechanisms for decreased expiratory flow rates

Disease	Physiologic Variables		
	P_{Emax}	Raw	P_L
Neuromuscular weakness	↓	N	N
Emphysema	N	N	↓
Asthma, bronchitis	N	↑	N
Peripheral airway disease	N	N	N

N, normal; P_{Emax}, maximum static expiratory pressure; Raw, airway resistance; P_L, lung elastic recoil pressure; ↑, increased; ↓, decreased.

to airflow resides in the nose, pharynx, and larynx and can mask changes taking place in the lungs. The use of a mouthpiece bypasses the nose to minimize the effects of the upper airway on the measurement. The panting maneuver is used to keep the larynx dilated and to reduce its influence on the total resistance to airflow. The measurements of Raw require the subject to sit in a constant-volume body plethysmograph ("body box"), which also permits recording of the thoracic gas volume and thereby provides an accurate appraisal of the effects of lung volume on Raw. Lung volume is estimated by use of Boyle's law to relate changes in box pressure and mouth pressure, and Raw is calculated from changes in box pressure and flow.[10] The subjects initially pant against a closed mouthpiece, usually at end expiration. Thoracic gas volume (i.e., FRC) is calculated from the relationship of box pressure to mouth pressure (Fig. 26-10). The shutter in the mouthpiece is then opened, and continued panting inscribes the relationship between box pressure and flow at the mouth to derive Raw. The upper limit of normal Raw is usually considered to be 2 cm H_2O in 1 second. To eliminate passive changes in Raw as a result of differences in lung volume, the reciprocal of Raw, Gaw, is calculated (see Fig. 26-5). The Gaw is usually divided by the lung volume at which the measurement is made (usually FRC) to obtain specific Gaw. The coefficient of variation (standard deviation/mean × 100) in normal baseline values for a single subject is usually small (<10%). Specific Gaw is a

highly reproducible measurement that can identify changes in the caliber of the intrapulmonary airways. However, a considerable portion of normal airway resistance resides in the upper airways and can be significantly increased with head flexion, which reduces the caliber of the hypopharynx.[11,12] It is important that patients position themselves as erectly as possible when using the mouthpiece in the body box.

Forced Expiratory Maneuvers

Despite the specificity and sensitivity of Raw measurements, airway obstruction is more commonly evaluated by measurements of maximum forced expiration. The indices obtained from forced expiration, unlike Raw, are determined by a complex interrelationship of flow-resistive properties of intrathoracic airways and elastic recoil of the lung. The simplest of such measurements is the peak expiratory flow, which is conveniently measured with a variable orifice flow meter. The peak flow occurs early in a forced expiration, when flow limitation has not occurred in the airways; flow therefore depends greatly on effort and on the subject's cooperation. However, because variation for the measurement in the same subject is surprisingly low, peak expiratory flow is a fairly reproducible test of airway function.

Another extensively used indirect measure of airway dimensions is the FEV_1. During the first 25% of an FVC

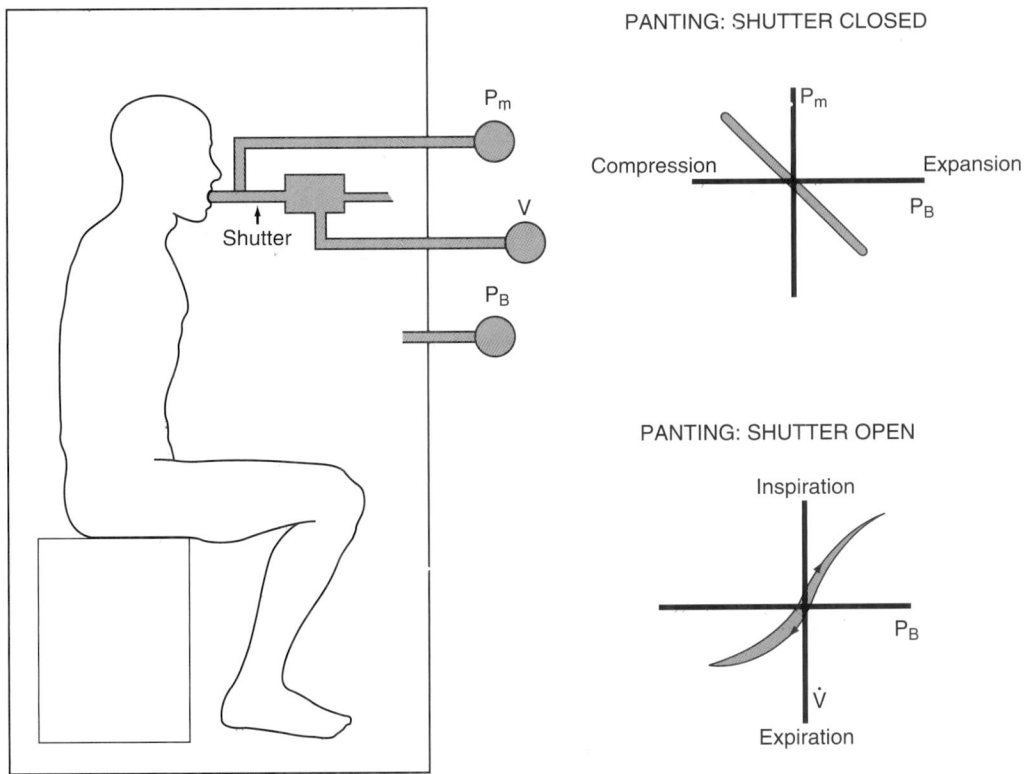

Figure 26–10 Diagram of the constant-volume body plethysmograph used to measure airway resistance and lung volume. When a subject pants against an obstructed mouthpiece (shutter closed), box pressure (P_B) is plotted against mouth pressure (P_m). Changes in P_B are converted to changes in lung volume by calibration of the box with known volumes of added gas and observation of P_B changes. As the subject pants through the open mouthpiece, flow (V) replaces P_m on the plot, and airway resistance is computed from the relationship between P_B and V.

maneuver, flow reflects dimensions of the airways between the alveoli and the mouth and is effort dependent. Although the physiologic parameters governing the remaining flow are complex, FEV_1, like peak flow, is simple and reproducible and therefore is a useful index of airway function. The measurement is subject to day-to-day variability, which is greater in patients with obstructive airway disease than in normal patients.[13] These changes in FEV_1 must exceed 15% to signify bronchodilation or constriction. An even greater potential variability applies to measurements of $FEF_{25\%-75\%}$. It is also necessary to account for the possibilities of negative effort dependence and, more importantly, the changes in FVC that may occur. For example, in patients with bronchodilation, FVC may increase but may produce a misleading decrease in $FEF_{25\%-75\%}$.[14] The measurement therefore should be adjusted to the same absolute lung volume (i.e., the same segment of FVC below TLC) (Fig. 26-11).

Traditionally, the response to bronchodilators is expressed as the percentage of change in FEV_1 from a baseline value. Healthy normal subjects and those with very mild obstruction typically exhibit a minimal increase in FEV_1 (<5%). Likewise, patients with severe baseline obstruction respond poorly because of accompanying secretions and airway edema. The most dramatic improvement occurs in patients with moderate obstruction; in these patients, the response to bronchodilators follows a bell-shaped distribution.[15] Because of the variability of response patterns, reliance on FEV_1 changes may underestimate the efficacy of bronchodilator therapy. The spirometric *inspiratory capacity* (IC), which reflects the degree of lung hyperinflation as a result of airway obstruction, has been suggested as a more useful alternative.[16]

Additional assessment of the flow-resistive properties of the airways can be obtained from maximum expiratory flow-volume (MEFV) curves, which illustrate the relationship between airflow and lung volume during an FVC maneuver (see Fig. 26-6). A typical response when bronchoconstriction is induced consists of diminished flows throughout the sole MEFV curve envelope (Fig. 26-12). Ventilatory flows and FVC usually decrease, and RV increases. Expiratory flows must be measured at the same reference lung volume. This is usually at a fixed percentage of the baseline or normal FVC and requires that all curves be superimposed at TLC.

In normal subjects, full inflation to TLC may remove the bronchoconstriction induced by mechanical stimuli or drugs, whereas in asthmatics, an increase in bronchomotor tone may accompany the same deep inspiration. To overcome these variable effects of a full inspiration on bronchial tone, flows can be measured with partial expiratory flow-volume curves. In this case, the maximum forced expiration is started at or slightly above the middle of the FVC (Fig. 26-13). In all cases, the partial expiratory flow-volume curve is followed by a full inhalation to TLC and a maximum forced exhalation to RV to obtain a reference MEFV curve. Flows are usually measured between 20% and 40% of the VC above the RV. Because partial expiratory flow-volume curves are unaffected by changes in upper airway resistance, they are sensitive to the change in the intrapulmonary airways

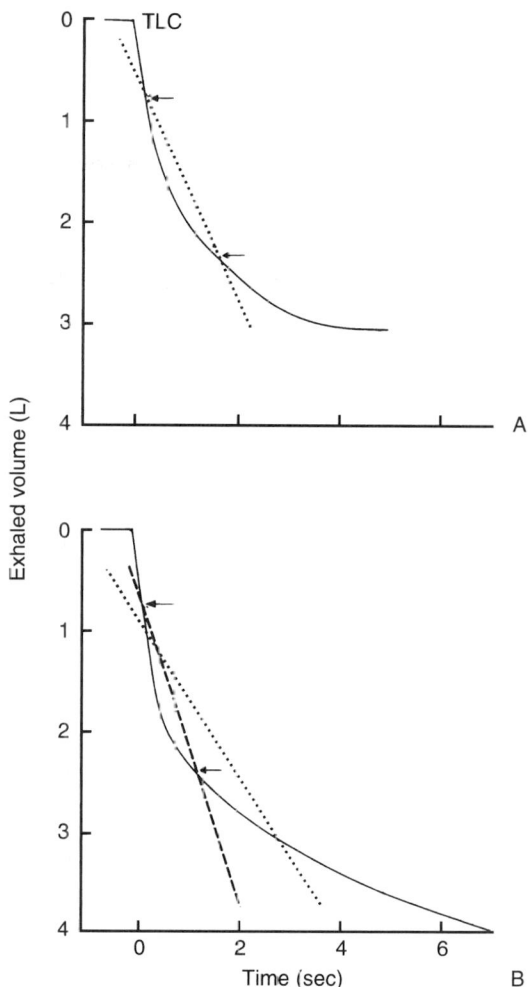

Figure 26–11 Forced expiratory spirograms before (**A**) and after (**B**) bronchodilator therapy. Notice that the forced vital capacity (FVC) is increased in **B**, but flow over its midportion ($FEF_{25\%-75\%}$) is decreased unless adjusted to the same volume (i.e., the portion of the FVC below total lung capacity [TLC]). The artifact results from the increased FVC as a result of bronchodilation. If $FEF_{25\%-75\%}$ is measured over the same volume segment as in **A**, the value increases.

and have been suggested as a useful alternative to Raw for detecting bronchoconstrictor and bronchodilator responses.

Flow-Volume Loops

The finding of reduced peak flow, MVV, and FEV_1 without additional clinical evidence of chronic obstructive lung disease may indicate the presence of an obstructing lesion of the upper airway, larynx, or trachea. In some cases, this obstruction may be suspected by a careful history and physical examination, but in many instances, it may stimulate diffuse airway obstruction and may suggest a marked degree of lung dysfunction. The latter is most likely to occur in patients who are to undergo head and neck surgery and may present for operative procedures

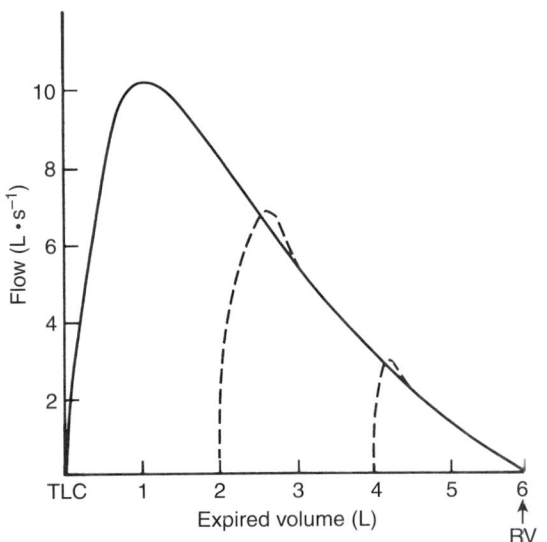

Figure 26–12 Maximum expiratory flow-volume curves before *(solid line)* and after *(broken lines)* induced bronchoconstriction. Flow is plotted against expired volume, which is expressed in liters (L), from total lung capacity (TLC) to residual volume (RV).

fully to TLC and then perform an FVC maneuver. This is followed immediately by a maximum inspiration as quickly as possible back to TLC (Fig. 26-14). Expiratory flow decreases over the latter half of the exhaled volume, despite the sustained expiratory effort indicated by the high positive P_{PL}. During maximum inspiration, airways do not undergo compression. Rather, with increasing inspiratory effort, airways become distended by the subatmospheric (negative) P_{PL}, and flow is increased. The entire inspiratory portion of the loop and the expiratory curve near TLC depend highly on effort. The ratio of expiratory flow to inspiratory flow at 50% of VC (i.e., mid-VC ratio) is normally about 1.0. This ratio is particularly useful in identifying upper airway obstruction, in which case inspiratory flow tends to be reduced more than expiratory flow, and the mid-VC ratio is increased (>1).

Flow-volume loops aid in detecting upper airway obstruction and may help to localize the site and identify the nature of the obstruction. Several characteristic patterns have been described. Perhaps the most common lesion is a fixed obstruction, such as a benign stricture resulting from tracheostomy or tracheal intubation. A tumor or mass such as a goiter may produce a similar picture, as would breathing through a fixed external resistance. No significant change in airway diameter occurs during inspiration or expiration. As a result, expiratory flows show a plateau of constant flow over the effort-dependent portion of the VC. Inspiratory flows show a similar plateau (Fig. 26-15A). Because both are reduced by nearly the same extent, the mid-VC ratio remains approximately 1.0.

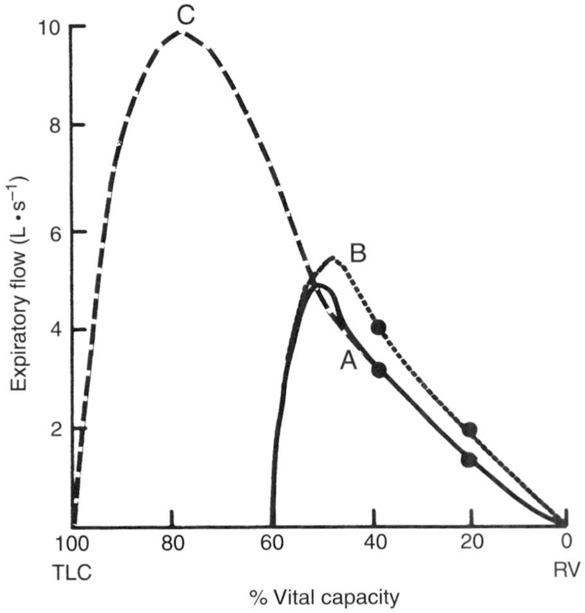

related to these lesions. Flow-volume loops provide a graphic analysis of flow at various lung volumes and have been used to discriminate among patients with upper obstructive lung lesions. Flow and volume are plotted simultaneously on an XY recorder as subjects inhale

Figure 26–13 Partial expiratory flow-volume curves before (A) and after (B) bronchodilator treatment. Forced expiration is begun just above midpoint of vital capacity (VC). Flows are quantitated at 20% and 40% of VC above residual volume (RV). A reference maximum expiratory curve (C) is also inscribed by beginning exhalation from total lung capacity (TLC).

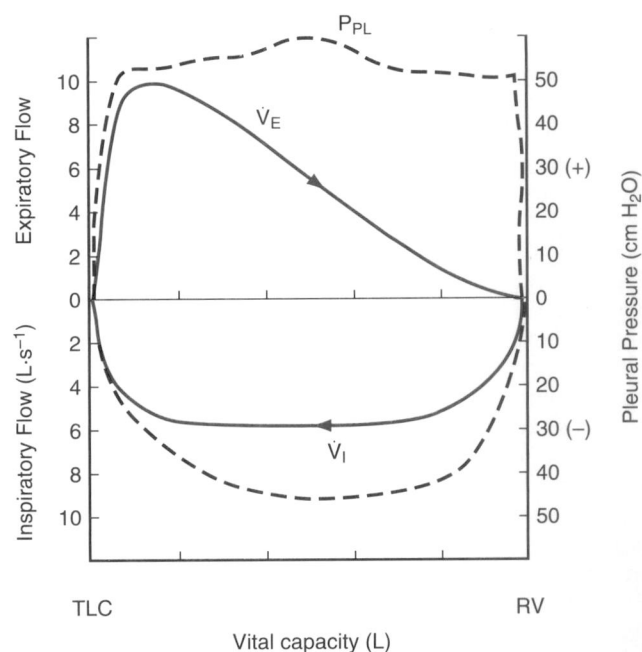

Figure 26–14 Schematic representation of a maximum inspiratory ($\dot{V}_I$) and expiratory ($\dot{V}_E$) flow-volume loop in a normal subject. The pleural pressure (P_{PL}) associated with the maximum effort is plotted as a function of lung volume from total lung capacity (TLC) to residual volume (RV). $\dot{V}_I$ and $\dot{V}_E$ at the midpoint (50%) of vital capacity are indicated by *arrows.*

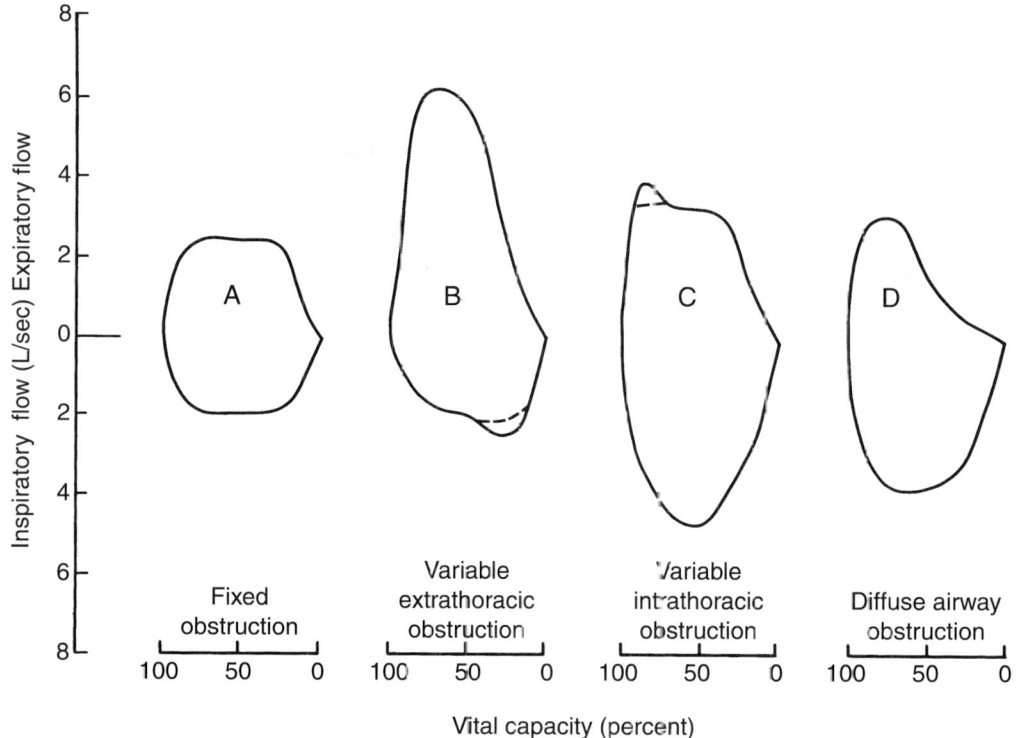

Figure 26–15 Maximum inspiratory and expiratory flow-volume curves (i.e., flow-volume loops) in four types of airway obstruction.

A lesion whose influence varies with the phase of respiration is called a *variable obstruction*. To understand the impact of such lesions on flow, it is necessary to characterize the behavior of the three basic partitions of the airway (Table 26-4).

Variable extrathoracic obstructions (see Fig. 26-15B) are most commonly associated with vocal cord paralysis, which is usually accompanied by inspiratory stridor. A similar pattern may be seen with marked pharyngeal muscle weakness in curarized volunteers[17] and in patients with chronic neuromuscular disorders.[18] The flow pattern occasionally has been identified in patients with severe obstructive sleep apnea. During forced inspiration, the negative transmural pressure inside the airway tends to collapse the airway with increasing effort and therefore reduces inspiratory flow. During expiration, the

positive pressure within the upper airway tends to decrease the obstruction, and expiratory flow is reduced far less and may even be normal. The mid-VC ratio of expiratory to inspiratory flow is often greater than 2.0.

The other form of variable obstruction occurs intrathoracically and is usually caused by tumors of the trachea or major bronchi. During forced expiration, the high P_{PL}s decrease airway diameter and may increase the obstruction. A plateau flow usually occurs during expiration when the compressed airway lumen assumes its minimal size at the area of the lesion (see Fig. 26-15C). During inspiration, lowering of P_{PL} surrounding the airway tends to decrease the obstruction, and the inspiratory portion of the flow-volume loop may be normal. The mid-VC ratio of expiratory flow is low, as in the case of diffuse airway obstruction (see Fig. 26-15D). However, the shapes of the curves differ. Figure 26-15D, an example of diffuse or distal airway obstruction, exhibits abnormal decreased flow in the segment near the RV. Figure 26-15C demonstrates normal flow in this area.

The physiologic diagnosis of upper airway obstruction is sometimes difficult in patients with diffuse airway obstruction (e.g., chronic bronchitis, asthma). These conditions themselves produce significant abnormalities of the flow-volume loop (see Fig. 26-15D), and flow-volume loops identify upper airway obstruction best in the absence of significant generalized airway disease.

Defining Normal Values

One important aspect of pulmonary function testing is defining what is normal and what indicates the presence of respiratory disease. Results are commonly interpreted in relation to reference values to determine whether they

Table 26–4 Airway partitioning and behavior
Upper (Extrathoracic)
Surrounding soft tissue unsupporting
Collapses during inspiration
Expands during expiration
Intrathoracic
Outer surface exposed to pleural pressure
Expands during inspiration
Collapses during expiration
Distal (Pulmonary)
Intimately related to lung tissue
Collapses as expiration proceeds

lie within a certain normal range. One statistically acceptable approach is to define as abnormal the lowest 5% of the reference population. For most tests, results from large numbers of normal patients have been used to generate regression equations based on age, gender, race, and most importantly, height. Although a number of clinical laboratories designate values of FVC and FEV_1 less than 80% of predicted as abnormal, this arbitrary standard has no statistical basis and should be avoided.

Assuming a gaussian distribution, the 95% confidence limits can be derived as 1.65 times the coefficient of variation. The latter is the quotient of the standard deviation and the mean. For FVC and FEV_1, coefficients of variation are 12% to 13% in large groups of normal subjects.[19] A value of 1.65 times these variations indicates that a measurement must be about 21% lower than the mean to be considered abnormal. Because the coefficient of variation for $FEF_{25\%-75\%}$ is about 25% in similar populations, values must be 40% below the population mean before they are truly considered abnormal.

TESTS OF GAS EXCHANGE FUNCTION

Alveolar-Arterial Oxygen Tension Difference

Abnormally high *alveolar-arterial oxygen tension gradients* (P_{AO_2}–P_{aO_2}) during room air breathing are common in asymptomatic smokers and in patients with minimal signs of chronic bronchitis. Although the P_{AO_2}–P_{aO_2} appears to be a sensitive means of detecting regional ventilation-perfusion ($\dot{V}/\dot{Q}$) inequalities, the test is not widely used for screening purposes because of the difficulty in measuring alveolar oxygen tension (P_{AO_2}), which must be estimated from the alveolar air equation. The oxygen tension of the warmed and humidified inspired gas in the trachea is represented as P_{IO_2}. The gas in the alveoli also contains carbon dioxide. As a rule, less carbon dioxide is produced than oxygen consumed. The ratio of carbon dioxide production to oxygen consumption is the *respiratory exchange ratio* (R), which is usually assumed to be 0.8. A simple calculation of P_{AO_2} for bedside use may be derived by dividing the arterial carbon dioxide tension (P_{aCO_2}) by R or by multiplying the carbon dioxide value by 1.25 and then subtracting the value from P_{IO_2}. The alveolar gas equation may be written as follows:

$$P_{AO_2} = P_{IO_2} - P_{aCO_2}/R$$

The normal P_{AO_2}–P_{aO_2} in subjects breathing room air averages 8 mm Hg in young persons and increases linearly with age. By the eighth decade, typical values may reach 25 mm Hg. This widening of the P_{AO_2}–P_{aO_2} with age and in disease states results solely from decreases of P_{aO_2}, not P_{AO_2}.

The simple bedside measurement of room air arterial O_2 tension (P_{aO_2}) provides a useful estimate of lung function. A value of less than 60 mm Hg indicates significant if not advanced lung disease, unless drug-induced hypoventilation is responsible. The P_{aO_2} has also been used in conjunction with the *peak expiratory flow rate* (PEFR) for the differentiation of dyspnea of cardiac versus pulmonary origin. This *dyspnea differentiation index* (DDI) is PEFR × P_{aO_2}/1000.[20] Patients with pulmonary dyspnea typically have lower PEFR values and a lower DDI than cardiac patients with dyspnea.

Multiple-Breath Nitrogen Washout

Measurements of the uneven distribution of ventilation are also sensitive to mild airway obstruction. If the resident nitrogen in the lung is washed out by breathing 100% oxygen, the concentration of nitrogen decreases as cumulative expired volume decreases. If the distribution of ventilation is normal and uniform, the lung appears to behave as a single compartment that produces a relatively fast, single-exponential washout curve for nitrogen (Fig. 26-16). In the abnormal patient with lung disease and nonuniform ventilation, the curve deviates from the single exponential and appears to contain more than one ventilatory compartment. Different lung units have their nitrogen diluted at different rates. The fast, well-ventilated alveoli cause a rapid decrease in expired nitrogen, whereas slow, poorly ventilated areas produce a prolonged tail on the washout curve. Unequal time constants throughout the lung may explain the phenomena. Although multiple-breath nitrogen washout appears to be a sensitive test, appropriate analysis of the curve is tedious and requires computer analysis to be practical as a screening test.

Diffusing Capacity of the Lung

The role of diffusion in producing abnormalities in gas exchange is of little importance and for practical purposes can be ignored under resting conditions. Limitation of diffusion consists of an oxygen gradient between alveolar and end-capillary oxygen tensions. This value is normally zero. Only if cardiac output is increased and the fraction of inspired oxygen is decreased does

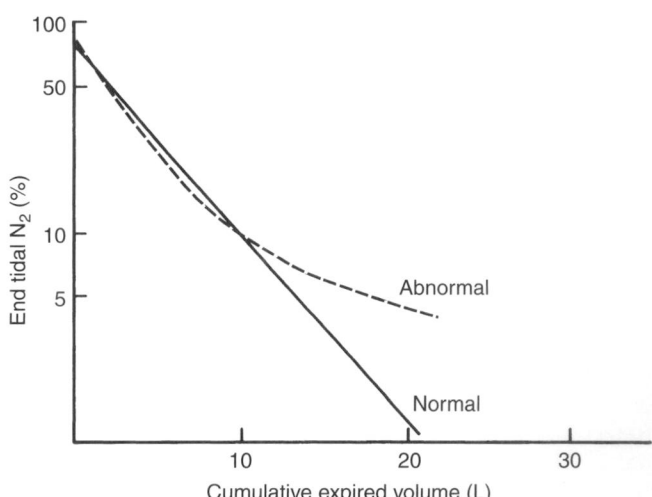

Figure 26–16 Schematic representation of multiple-breath nitrogen washout curves in a young, healthy nonsmoker (Normal) and in an asymptomatic smoker (Abnormal). Expired nitrogen concentration is plotted on a logarithmic scale against cumulative expired volume during pure oxygen breathing.

such a gradient develop. Examples of such situations are high levels of exercise and breathing at altitudes above 10,000 feet.

Diffusing capacity of the lungs (DL) is defined as the rate at which a gas enters the blood divided by its driving pressure. The latter term is the gradient between alveolar and end-capillary tensions. DL is expressed in units of milliliters per minute per millimeter of mercury.

In addition to driving pressure, DL is determined by the thickness of the alveolar-capillary membrane. DL is influenced by the number of capillaries in the alveolar wall, which determines the area of the alveolar-capillary membrane surface. Measurement of DL provides information about the amount of functioning capillaries in contact with ventilated air spaces. The number of functioning capillaries may be reduced in certain pulmonary vascular and parenchymal disease states. The brief inhalation of nontoxic low concentrations of carbon monoxide (CO) has become standard in most pulmonary function laboratories for this purpose.

CO has several features that make the gas useful for measuring DL. It has 200 times the affinity for hemoglobin as oxygen does and therefore does not build up rapidly in plasma. CO concentration is low in the blood under normal conditions, and pulmonary capillary tension can be assumed to be zero. Of the techniques using CO, the rebreathing method is least influenced by changes in $\dot{V}/\dot{Q}$ distributions.

To measure the CO diffusing capacity of the lungs (DLCO), three values must be obtained: the milliliters of CO transferred from alveoli to blood per minute, the mean alveolar CO tension (PACO), and the pulmonary capillary CO tension (PCCO):

$$DLCO = \frac{CO\ mL/min/mmHg}{PACO - PCCO}$$

Of the several techniques for estimating DLCO, the most widely employed is the single-breath test. In the single-breath method, the patient inspires a dilute mixture of CO and holds the breath for 10 seconds. During this period, CO leaves alveolar gas to enter the blood in proportion to the diffusing capacity. The number of milliliters of CO transferred is calculated from the percentage of CO in alveolar gas at the beginning and at the end of the breath-hold by infrared analysis. To do this, the FRC must be calculated from the helium dilution and then added to the inspiratory volume. The PCCO is essentially zero and can be ignored.

The single-breath method requires very little patient cooperation and is relatively simple to perform because it requires no blood samples. It is relatively insensitive to the backpressure of CO in the blood and is only mildly affected by $\dot{V}/\dot{Q}$ inequalities. Disadvantages include the extensive mathematical computations and the requirement for 1.3 L or greater inspired volume with a breath-hold. The latter may not be feasible in the dyspneic patient or in the exercising subject.

Normal values of DLCO range from 20 to 30 mL/min/mm Hg and depend on lung size. The use of helium enables determination of total alveolar volume (VA). Dividing DLCO by VA normalizes for lung volume.

Decreases in DLCO are caused by emphysema, lung resection, pulmonary emboli, and anemia, all of which effectively decrease surface area by reducing capillary blood volume. Other diseases, such as pulmonary fibrosis, sarcoidosis, and alveolar proteinosis, increase alveolar wall thickness, which also decreases DLCO. Increased DLCO is rarely of much clinical concern. Many conditions that increase pulmonary blood volume result in an increased DLCO, including the supine position, exercise, obesity, and left-to-right intracardiac shunts.

PULMONARY FUNCTION TESTING IN SURGICAL PATIENTS

Significant postoperative changes in pulmonary function in many surgical patients include phenomena such as reduced lung volumes, rapid and shallow breathing, and impaired gas exchange. These alterations in pulmonary function may occur as a result of the anesthetic, the surgical procedure, the associated body position, or the medications administered immediately after surgery. These changes, which occur in normal patients, may be more severe in patients undergoing surgery who have compromised pulmonary function and therefore may produce significant postoperative pulmonary complications. Such complications usually include bronchospasm, bronchitis with purulent sputum, disabling cough pneumonia, and respiratory failure, as indicated by altered blood gas values. Preexisting lung dysfunction is the major factor associated with postoperative pulmonary problems. Also important are incisional site and size, as well as possible surgical trauma to lung tissue. Both considerations render the patient who is to undergo thoracic surgery a prime candidate for evaluation.

Prevailing opinion suggests that preoperative pulmonary function testing provides the clinician with important information regarding the potential for postoperative respiratory morbidity. If pulmonary function data are of value, which patients are candidates for such testing? Although no general agreement exists about which patients should be tested, the prime candidates are those in whom there is a reasonable expectation of abnormal pulmonary function. This broad list was outlined by Tisi[21] (Table 26-5).

Table 26–5 Factors prompting preoperative pulmonary evaluation: Tisi guidelines

Age >70
Morbid obesity
Thoracic surgery
Upper abdominal surgery
History of smoking, cough
Any pulmonary disease

From Tisi GM: Preoperative evaluation of pulmonary function: Validity, indications, and benefits. Am Rev Respir Dis 119:293, 1979.

Conflicting data abound regarding these rather broad criteria. The American College of Chest Physicians has proposed a more stringent set of guidelines (Table 26-6). Adherence to these stricter guidelines has been recommended as a means of decreasing unnecessary and costly spirometric testing.[22]

Initial identification of most of these patients is accomplished by history, physical examination, and chest radiographic studies. The chest x-ray film is a particularly valuable clinical marker for clinically severe disease, especially if it identifies lung hyperinflation, which has been associated with a 33% rate of significant postoperative pulmonary complications.[23]

Which pulmonary function studies are appropriate for preoperative evaluation? The objective of testing in the preoperative setting is not to detect mild, early lung disease but to predict the likelihood of pulmonary complications. The physician must ask whether the test results alter perioperative management or sufficiently affect risk estimates such that planned surgery is altered or even postponed. Other factors, such as the cost of testing and even the risk of testing, must also be considered. No single test appears to be the best predictor of risk, probably because none assesses all of the factors that are important regardless of whether complications may occur. The optimal scheme for evaluating patients preoperatively is by means of arterial blood gas analysis and the FEV_1, FVC, FEV_1/FVC, peak flow, and $FEF_{25\%-75\%}$, which can be obtained from a single spirometric study. Abnormalities on such spirometric tests seem to correlate with the incidence of postoperative pulmonary complications.

Although the evaluation of preoperative pulmonary function is largely aimed at predicting the risk of postoperative complications, the identification of abnormal lung function, particularly obstructive airway disease, is also important to reduce intraoperative morbidity. A reduced FEV_1/FVC, for example, documents the existence of airway obstruction and suggests the likelihood of increased airway reactivity. The site and the nature of many surgical procedures often provide very little latitude for choosing between regional and general anesthesia. In patients with airway obstruction and heightened airway reactivity, airway instrumentation (e.g., laryngoscopy, tracheal intubation) is fraught with the hazard of provoking reflex bronchoconstriction, particularly under light planes of anesthesia. In many patients with obstructive airway disease, the deeper levels of inhaled anesthesia required to blunt such airway reflexes are difficult to achieve because of poor $\dot{V}/\dot{Q}$ matching and, if achieved, the levels are poorly tolerated by the cardiovascular system. To minimize airway responses, it is important to other prophylactic measures, which may include anticholinergics and β-agonists inhaled as aerosols before surgery and intravenous opioids and lidocaine administered before airway instrumentation.

Patients with abnormally low FEV_1 values before surgery are likely to experience severe hypercapnia if they are allowed to breathe spontaneously under general anesthesia.[24] The magnitude of the carbon dioxide increase is directly related to the degree of reduction in FEV_1 and develops largely because the rapid, shallow breathing pattern characteristic of anesthetized patients worsens $\dot{V}/\dot{Q}$ matching. It is essential to control ventilation in these patients. With controlled ventilation, low respiratory rates (<10 breaths/min) are desirable to minimize $\dot{V}/\dot{Q}$ mismatch, which arises largely because of the prolonged time required to move air in and out of the obstructed airways. Because of this obstruction, low inspiratory flow rates have long been advocated to lessen peak airway pressure and to presumably minimize barotrauma and circulatory disturbances. However, evidence suggests the opposite. In patients with chronic obstructive pulmonary disease who were ventilated with customary tidal volumes (10 mL/kg), respiratory system resistance decreased as inspiratory flow rates were increased from 0.25 to 1.5 L/s.[25] The investigators postulated that this effect was caused by decreases in thoracic tissue resistance or was a reflection of improvement in time-constant inequalities or in the viscoelastic behavior of the respiratory system, or both. Other studies have shown that a high inspiratory flow rate in such patients produced improved gas exchange and was not complicated by barotrauma or circulatory depression.[26,27] An important consequence of the increased inspiratory flow rate was a reduced inspiratory time, which allowed increased time for exhalation. Increased expiratory time provides more complete emptying of alveoli, which must occur through high-resistance airways. With a shorter expiratory time, which inevitably occurs with the increased inspiratory time needed with a lower inspiratory flow, alveoli are not allowed to empty completely, and they receive less gas volume at the same distending pressures during inspiration.

Table 26–6 Factors prompting preoperative pulmonary function testing: American College of Physicians Guidelines

Lung resection
Smoking history, dyspnea
Cardiac surgery
Upper abdominal surgery
Lower abdominal surgery
Uncharacterized pulmonary symptoms

From Hnatiuk OW, Dillard TA, Torrington KG: Adherence to established guidelines for preoperative pulmonary function. Chest 107:1294, 1995.

EVALUATION OF THE PATIENT FOR LUNG RESECTION

Indications and Criteria

Resection of lung disease results in a greater impairment in postoperative lung function than does most other types of surgery (see Chapter 49). Lung resection in patients with pulmonary dysfunction is associated with a high risk of postoperative complications, even the possibility of death. These patients require a more extensive pulmonary evaluation, particularly if removal of an entire lung is anticipated. A major aim of the evaluation is to decide whether the removal of lung tissue can be tolerated without compromising pulmonary function to a degree that the patient dies from pulmonary insufficiency or is severely disabled. The long-term ability to withstand such lung resection is related to the amount and functional status of the lung parenchyma removed and, more importantly, to the function of the remaining lung tissue. Removal of lung from an already compromised patient may be followed by inadequate gas exchange, pulmonary hypertension, and incapacitating dyspnea. The role of the anesthesiologist is to be aware of these risks, but the decision about whether a patient can tolerate the proposed resection with acceptable risk rests with the surgeon and pulmonologist.

Although much of the literature in this area emphasizes long-term disability of the pneumonectomy patient, the immediate impact on pulmonary function may be as great in patients undergoing lobectomy because of surgical trauma to the remaining tissue of the same lung. Results of pulmonary function studies must be viewed in light of the patient's age, the status of the cardiovascular system, and the patient's cooperation and motivation. Data on pneumonectomy patients collectively indicate that removal of the entire lung is likely to be tolerated if the preoperative pulmonary function meets the following criteria: (1) FEV_1 greater than 2 L and FEV_1/FVC ratio of at least 50%, (2) MVV greater than 50% of predicted, and (3) RV/TLC ratio less than 50%.

If any of these criteria is not met, more sophisticated split-function pulmonary testing is indicated to estimate the relative functional contribution of each lung. If, for example, the lung to be removed contributes less to ventilatory function than the other lung does, low spirometric values are not as ominous. Usually, split-function pulmonary testing consists of xenon radiospirometry to assess ventilation and macroaggregates of iodine or technetium to scan perfusion. The relative contribution of each lung to total ventilation or perfusion can be used to predict postoperative pulmonary function. A predicted postoperative FEV_1 of at least 800 mL should be required before pneumonectomy is performed. The risk of significant resting carbon dioxide retention and resting dyspnea appears to be high with FEV_1 values less than this. If surgery is still contemplated in the face of a low predicted FEV_1 value, an invasive study is recommended. The pulmonary artery of the lung to be removed can be subjected to occlusion by a balloon. If pulmonary hypertension (mean pulmonary arterial pressure >35 mm Hg) and arterial hypoxemia (Pao_2 <45 mm Hg) do not occur, it can be assumed that the remaining lung may be able to accommodate the entire cardiac output. Such a patient may be allowed to undergo surgery despite failure to fulfill the mechanical ventilatory criterion. The indications for performing this invasive procedure are not agreed on universally, but many physicians still heed the advice of Olsen and colleagues that balloon occlusion, if feasible, should be performed when the less invasive studies are inconclusive.

Exercise Capacity

There has been an increased emphasis on preoperative evaluation of exercise capacity before lung resection since the late 1990s. This assessment is important because it considers cardiopulmonary interactions. Qualitative estimates of cardiopulmonary reserve can be derived from the medical history, physical examination, and arterial blood gas measurements. Additional qualitative estimates of exercise capacity may be symptom limited (e.g., dyspnea). The best example of such testing is stair climbing. The ability to climb three flights of stairs (one flight = 20 six-inch-high steps) at the patient's own pace without stopping is associated with decreased morbidity and mortality. In contrast, an inability to climb two flights identifies a high risk. Many such patients also exhibit a significant (>4%) decrease in oxygen saturation when pulse oximetry is used.[28]

A more quantitative estimate of cardiopulmonary function can be obtained by measuring the maximum oxygen uptake during exercise. Continued observations have suggested that a patient's maximum oxygen uptake ($\dot{V}o_2$max) during exercise is an accurate preoperative means of identifying patients who are likely to experience post-thoracotomy morbidity.[29] The $\dot{V}o_2$max is essentially a measure of physical fitness and therefore reflects the ability to survive the stresses of the perioperative period and beyond. During exercise, the lung must accommodate the increased ventilation and blood flow, much as the remaining lung does after pneumonectomy. Patients with $\dot{V}o_2$max values of 20 mL/kg/min or more had minimal morbidity.[29] Those with a $\dot{V}o_2$max of 15 mL/min or less had increased cardiopulmonary complications, whereas those whose $\dot{V}o_2$max was less than 10 mL/kg/min appeared to have an unacceptably high risk and a mortality rate greater than 30% in the short term. Insight into these $\dot{V}o_2$max values is provided by evidence that a two-flight stair climb (20 steps/min) without dyspnea approximates a $\dot{V}o_2$max of 16 mL/kg/min. Standardized laboratory measurement of exercise $\dot{V}o_2$max has become the gold standard for assessing cardiorespiratory function and predicting outcome in patients undergoing lung resection.

Another simple test that requires little equipment and correlates well with $\dot{V}o_2$max is the 6-minute walk test. Its popularity has led to the establishment of standardization guidelines.[30] A patient who is able to walk 180 feet in 1 minute (2 mph) has a 6-minute walk distance of 1080 feet, which corresponds approximately to a $\dot{V}o_2$max of 12 mL/kg/min. Distances of less than 2000 feet for the 6-minute walk test indicate a $\dot{V}o_2$max of less than 15 mL/kg/min.[28]

Increasing evidence suggests that resting pulmonary function, as reflected by spirometric testing, does not accurately predict exercise performance in patients with more severe lung disease.[31] Cardiopulmonary exercise testing may be necessary to evaluate the degree of impairment. Exercise testing has become attractive because it reflects gas exchange, ventilation, tissue oxygenation, and cardiac output. If cardiac output is increased, blood flow to the pulmonary vascular bed increases, as occurs when flow is diverted to the remaining lung tissue after resection. Patients who otherwise might have been considered inoperable on the basis of low FEV_1 values may be considered to be operative candidates because of their performance and high $\dot{V}o_2$max during exercise. Conversely, patients with marked reductions in exercise $\dot{V}_{O_2}max$ before surgery appear to be at high risk for postoperative morbidity, regardless of how well they performed on routine and split-function pulmonary testing.

PREOPERATIVE MEASURES TO IMPROVE LUNG FUNCTION

Aside from assessing operability in candidates for lung resection, the major goal of identifying preoperative pulmonary dysfunction is to alter outcome by reducing the morbidity and mortality associated with postoperative pulmonary complications (see Chapters 25 and 27). The assumption is that patients identified as having abnormal function may benefit from therapeutic measures to improve lung function, thereby reducing the likelihood of postoperative complications. Numerous applications of such therapy to poor-risk patients have decreased postoperative complications to levels approaching those found in patients with normal function.

Ideally, a comprehensive rehabilitation regimen of exercise, nutrition, education, and, most importantly, physiotherapy can improve the functional capacity of patients with significant lung disease.[32] However, such extensive therapy is not practical preoperatively, and limited therapy usually is carried out for 48 to 72 hours before surgery. It is equally important that some of the measures be continued after surgery. The treatment regimen is aimed largely at four modalities: (1) smoking cessation, (2) mobilization of secretions, (3) therapy for bronchospasm, and (4) improved motivation and stamina. Although it is generally assumed that smoking cessation is followed by a decrease in the volume of airway secretions and in airway reactivity and by improved mucociliary transport, these beneficial effects take 2 to 4 weeks to manifest. The shorter-term effects (48 to 72 hours) may instead be increased secretions and hyperactive airways. The major benefit from discontinuing smoking in the immediate preoperative period appears to be the decrease in carboxyhemoglobin content and better oxygen availability to the tissues.[33] There is additional evidence that the sensitive upper airway reflexes of smokers are reduced by abstinence. It is therefore reasonable to expect the adverse events so common during the induction of anesthesia (i.e., cough, breath-holding, and laryngospasm) to be reduced.[34]

The removal of secretions is an important component of preoperative preparation, because their persistence increases the likelihood of infection and increased airway reactivity. Antibiotic therapy for patients with chronic bronchitis may be helpful, but the secretions are best loosened by adequate hydration systematically and by heating of aerosol therapy agents. The use of mucolytic agents and oral expectorants is at best of questionable benefit and is fraught with the hazards of increased airway irritability and other side effects, such as gastrointestinal irritation. Mucociliary clearance is impaired in such patients, and cough is ineffective because of an inability to generate sufficient airflow rates. Mechanical measures must be used to dislodge secretions and move them into the more proximal airways, where cough can more readily remove secretions. Such therapy is limited to percussion and vibration combined with postural drainage.

Reactive airways and reversible airflow obstruction are common features, especially in patients presenting for thoracic surgery. The use of medications to establish and sustain normal airway function is important in the perioperative period. β_2-Sympathomimetic aerosols are the mainstays for treatment and prevention of bronchospasm. The use of the quaternary anticholinergic compound ipratropium may also be helpful, particularly if tachycardia is a concern with β_2-sympathetic drugs. Theophylline is often added to this regimen; however, there is considerable concern regarding the toxicity and limited efficacy of intravenous theophylline when it is administered in the setting of acute disease.

Patients should be prepared for thoracotomy by improving motivation and stamina. Education and practice with incentive spirometry devices are important in the maintenance of postoperative lung volume and coughing efficacy. Such preparation and continued postoperative use appears to be far more effective than intermittent positive-pressure breathing therapy.

Use of the preparatory respiratory care maneuvers ultimately benefits the patient and contributes to reducing the incidence and severity of postoperative respiratory complications. The question remains, however, whether such an improved outcome is reflected in pulmonary function on spirometric testing. It may be unreasonable to expect a dramatic reversal in airflow obstruction and improved blood gas values with such a brief (48 to 72 hours) regimen. Gracey and colleagues[35] evaluated pulmonary function before surgery in patients with chronic obstructive pulmonary disease on such a standardized regimen. Although this therapy produced statistically significant changes in several test results of pulmonary function, the functional significance of the changes was doubtful. Nevertheless, the incidence of complications in these patients was dramatically reduced, as has been shown in numerous other studies. There are no definitive data that can identify whether this reduced complication rate results specifically from the preparation regimen, the use of specific agents or techniques, or the increased attention paid to patients in whom airway obstruction or other pulmonary dysfunction is identified.

It appears reasonably well established that patients whose clinical history and physical examination suggest the presence of pulmonary disease are at increased risk if spirometric results are abnormal. It is unclear exactly what should be done for such patients other than an abbreviated regimen of preoperative preparation and concern intraoperatively for control of airway reactivity. Equally uncertain is which test best predicts risk and what further testing is appropriate for patients with abnormal spirometric results. Nevertheless, in patients who are about to undergo pulmonary resection, exercise testing seems to provide the best predictive insight.

KEY POINTS

1. The primary goal of preoperative pulmonary function testing is not to detect lung disease but to quantitate its severity.

2. Chest radiography is a valuable indicator for severe disease, especially in patients with lung hyperinflation.

3. The FEV_1, which is customarily used as an index of airway obstruction, provides a better perspective of the degree of obstruction when it is expressed as a percentage of FVC (i.e., FEV_1/FVC).

4. Patients with abnormally low FEV_1 values are likely to experience severe hypercapnia if allowed to breathe spontaneously under general anesthesia.

5. MVV, the most comprehensive test of ventilatory function, is significantly affected by airway obstruction. It is also affected by lung and chest wall elasticity, respiratory muscle strength, coordination, and motivation.

6. The maximum flow rates achievable during pulmonary function testing maneuvers depend on three factors, all of which are related to lung volume: effort or driving pressure, elastic recoil pressure of the lung, and flow resistance of the airways.

7. The upper (extrathoracic) airway, because of the surrounding soft tissue, collapses during inspiration and expands during expiration. The intrathoracic airway responds to pleural pressure changes and therefore expands during inspiration and collapses during expiration.

8. The DDI is equal to $PEFR \times Pao_2/1000$.[20] Patients with pulmonary dyspnea typically have lower PEFR values and a lower DDI than cardiac patients with dyspnea.

9. Evaluation of patients for thoracic surgery is aimed at deciding whether removal of a lung can be tolerated without causing pulmonary insufficiency or severe disability.

10. Ability to climb three flights of stairs without stopping is associated with decreased morbidity and mortality after lung resection.

REFERENCES

1. Hess D: History of pulmonary function testing. Respir Care 34:427, 1989.
2. American Thoracic Society: Standardization of spirometry: Update. Am J Respir Crit Care Med 152:1107, 1995.
3. Stein M, Koota GM, Simon M, et al: Pulmonary evaluation of surgical patients. JAMA 181:765, 1962.
4. Suratt PM, Hooe DM, Owens DA, et al: Effect of maximal versus submaximal expiratory effort on spirometric values. Respiration 42:233, 1981.
5. Krowka MJ, Enright PL, Rodarte JR, et al: Effect of effort on measurement of forced expiratory volume in one second. Am Rev Respir Dis 136:829, 1987.
6. Gelb AF, Williams AJ, Zamel N: Spirometry: FEV_1 vs FEF 25-75 percent. Chest 84:473, 1983.
7. Dillard TA, Oleh HW, McCumber TR: Maximum voluntary ventilation: Spirometric determinants in chronic obstructive

8. Black LF, Hyatt RE: Maximal respiratory pressures: Normal values and relationship to age and sex. Am Rev Respir Dis 103:641, 1971.
9. Braun NMT, Arora NS, Rochester DF: Respiratory muscle and pulmonary function in polymyositis and other proximal myopathies. Thorax 38:616, 1983.
10. Dubois AB, Botelho SY, Comroe JH: A new method for measuring airway resistance in man using a body plethysmograph: Values in normal subject and in patients with respiratory disease. J Clin Invest 35:327, 1956.
11. Suratt PM, Gal TJ, Hooe DM: Effect of head flexion on airway resistance measured in a body plethysmograph. Br J Dis Chest 75:204, 1981.
12. Siistro G, Stanescu D, Dooms G, et al: Head position modifies upper airway resistance in men. J Appl Physiol 64:1285, 1988.
13. Rozas CJ, Goldman AL: Daily spirometric variability: Normal subjects and subjects with chronic bronchitis with and without airflow obstruction. Arch Intern Med 142:1287, 1982.
14. Cockroft DW, Berscheid BA: Volume adjustment of maximum mid-expiratory flow: Importance of changes in total lung capacity. Chest 78:585, 1980.
15. Enright PL, Lebowitz MD, Cockroft DW: Physiologic measures: Pulmonary function tests. Asthma outcome. Am J Respir Crit Care Med 149:59, 1994.
16. O'Donnell D: Assessment of bronchodilator efficacy in symptomatic COPD. Is spirometry useful? Chest 117(Suppl 2):42S, 2000.
17. Gal TJ, Arora NS: Respiratory mechanics in supine subjects during progressive partial curarization. J Appl Physiol 52:57, 1982.
18. Vincken WG, Elleker MG, Cusio MG: Flow-volume loop changes reflecting respiratory muscle weakness in chronic neuromuscular disorders. Am J Med 83:673, 1987.
19. Pennock BE, Rogers RM, McCaffree DR: Changes in measured spirometric indices: What is significant? Chest 80:97, 1981.
20. Ailani RK, Ravakhah K, DiGiovine B, et al: Dyspnea differentiation index. A new method for rapid separation of cardiac vs. pulmonary dyspnea. Chest 116:1100, 1999.
21. Tisi GM: Preoperative evaluation of pulmonary function: Validity, indications, and benefits. Am Rev Respir Dis 119:293, 1979.
22. Hnatiuk OW, Dillard TA, Torrington KG: Adherence to established guidelines for preoperative pulmonary function. Chest 107:1294, 1995.
23. Kroenke K, Lawrence VA, Theroux JF, et al: Postoperative complications after thoracic and major abdominal surgery in patients with and without obstructive lung disease. Chest 104:1445, 1993.
24. Pietak S, Weenig CS, Hickey RF, et al: Anesthetic effects on ventilation in patients with chronic obstructive disease. Anesthesiology 42:160, 1975.
25. Tantucci C, Coreil C, Chasse M, et al: Flow resistance in patients with chronic obstructive pulmonary disease in acute respiratory failure. Am Rev Respir Dis 144:384, 1991.
26. Connors AF, McAferee D, Gray BA: Effect of inspiratory flow rate on gas exchange during mechanical ventilation. Am Rev Respir Dis 124:537, 1981.
27. Tuxen DV, Lane S: The effects of ventilatory pattern on hyperinflation, airway pressures, and circulation in mechanical ventilation of patients with severe airflow obstruction. Am Rev Respir Dis 136:872, 1987.
28. Ninan M, Summers KE, Landranau RJ, et al: Standardized exercise oximetry predicts post pneumonectomy outcome. Ann Thorac Surg 64:328, 1997.
29. Walsh GL, Morice RC, Putnam JB, et al: Resection of lung cancer is justified in high-risk patients selected by oxygen consumption. Ann Thorac Surg 58:704, 1994.

30. ATS Statement: Guidelines for the six minute walk test. Am J Respir Crit Care Med 166:111, 2002.

31. Ortega F, Montemayor T, Sanchez A, et al: Role of cardiopulmonary exercise testing and the criteria used to determine disability in patients with severe chronic obstructive disease. Am J Respir Crit Care Med 150:747, 1994.

32. Kesten S: Pulmonary rehabilitation and surgery for end-stage lung disease. Clin Chest Med 18:174, 1997.

33. Erskine RJ, Murphy PJ, Langton JA: Sensitivity of upper airway reflexes in cigarette smokers: Effect of abstinence. Br J Anaesth 73:298, 1994.

34. Dennis A, Curran J, Sheriff J, et al: Effects of passive and active smoking on induction of anaesthesia. Br J Anaesth 73:450, 1994.

35. Gracey DR, Divertie MB, Didier EP: Preoperative pulmonary preparation of patients with chronic obstructive pulmonary disease: A prospective study. Chest 76:123, 1979.

27 Anesthetic Implications of Concurrent Diseases

Michael F. Roizen and Lee A. Fleisher

Role of the Primary Care Physician or Consultant   1018

Diseases Involving the Endocrine System and Disorders of Nutrition   1019
Pancreatic Disorders   1019
Disorders of Nutrition, Including Obesity   1027
Hyperalimentation (Total Parenteral or Enteral Nutrition)   1034
Adrenocortical Malfunction   1035
Adrenal Medullary Sympathetic Hormone Excess: Pheochromocytoma   1042
Hypofunction or Aberration in Function of the Sympathetic Nervous System (Dysautonomia)   1044
Thyroid Dysfunction   1045
Disorders of Calcium Metabolism   1048
Pituitary Abnormalities   1051

Diseases Involving the Cardiovascular System   1053
Hypertension   1053
Ischemic Heart Disease   1060
Valvular Heart Disease   1077
Cardiac Conduction Disturbances   1083

Disorders of the Respiratory and Immune Systems   1085
General Preoperative and Preprocedure Considerations   1085
Specific Diseases   1089

Diseases of the Central Nervous System, Neuromuscular Diseases, and Psychiatric Disorders   1093
Coma   1094
Epileptic Seizures   1094
Infectious Diseases of the Central Nervous System, Degenerative Disorders of the Central Nervous System, and Headache   1095
Back Pain, Neck Pain, and Spinal Canal Syndromes   1096
Demyelinating Diseases   1096
Metabolic Diseases   1096
Neuromuscular Disorders   1098
Down Syndrome   1099
Preoperative Prediction of Increased Intracranial Pressure during Neurosurgery   1099
Mental Disorders   1100

Renal Disease, Infectious Diseases, and Electrolyte Disorders   1100
Renal Disease   1100
Infectious Disease   1103
Electrolyte Disorders   1104

Gastrointestinal and Liver Diseases   1107
Gastrointestinal Disease   1107
Liver Disease   1110

Hematologic Disorders and Oncologic Disease   1111
Hematologic Disorders   1111
Oncologic Disease   1117

Patients Given Drug Therapy for Chronic and Acute Medical Conditions   1118
Pharmacologic Processes in the Sympathetic Nervous System   1119
Antihypertensive Drugs   1119
Mood-Altering Drugs   1122
Sympathomimetic Drugs   1124
Other Drugs   1124
Interrupting a Drug Regimen before Surgery   1125

This chapter reviews conditions requiring special preoperative and preprocedure evaluation and/or intraoperative or procedure management, or postprocedure care. Patients undergoing surgery move through a continuum of medical care to which a primary care physician, an internist or pediatrician, an anesthesiologist, and a surgeon, radiologist, or obstetrician-gynecologist contribute to ensure the best outcome possible. No aspect of medical care requires greater cooperation among physicians than does performance of a surgical operation or complex procedure involving multiple specialists and the perioperative care of a patient. The importance of integrating physicians' expertise is even greater within the context of the increasing life span of our population.[1] As the number of the elderly and the very old (those older than 85 years) grows, so does the need of surgical patients for preoperative consultation to help plan for comorbidity and multiple drug regimens, knowledge of which is crucial to successful patient management. At a time when medical information is encyclopedic, it is difficult, if not impossible for even the most conscientious anesthesiologist to keep abreast of the medical issues relevant to every aspect of perioperative or periprocedure patient management. This chapter reviews such issues.

As with "healthy" patients (also see Chapter 25), it is the history and physical examination that most accurately predict not only the associated risks but also the likelihood that a monitoring technique or change in therapy will be beneficial or necessary for survival. This chapter emphasizes instances in which specific information should be sought in history taking, physical examination, or laboratory evaluation. Although controlled studies designed to confirm that optimizing a patient's preoperative or preprocedure physical condition would result in lower morbidity have not been performed for most diseases, it is logical to assume that such is the case. Studies showing the benefits of optimizing specific preprocedure conditions are highlighted. The fact that such preventive measures would cost less than treating the morbidity that would otherwise occur is an important consideration in a cost-conscious environment.

Recent data indicate that minimally invasive procedures such as cataract extraction, magnetic resonance imaging (MRI), or diagnostic arthroscopy (see Table 25-6 in Chapter 25), performed in conjunction with the best current anesthetic practices, pose no greater risk than daily living does and thus might not be considered an opportunity for special evaluation. Nonetheless, preanesthetic and preprocedure evaluations were found to provide information that led to changes in health care plans for more than 15% of all American Society of Anesthesiologists (ASA) class I and II patients (and for >20% of all patients in general) at the University of Florida (Gibby GL et al., personal communication). Although these changes in care plans were attributable to data found by history taking and observation (the most common being gastric reflux, diabetes mellitus requiring insulin, asthma, and suspected difficult intubation), no data show that patient outcome was improved by such changes. Nevertheless, logic caused practitioners to alter plans for such patients in ways that would delay operating room schedules and increase costs. Examples would

be administering a β-adrenergic blocking drug, aspirin, or a statin (or any combination) the night before rather than delaying surgery to do so on the morning of surgery; administering a histamine type 2 (H_2) antagonist 1 to 2 hours before and an oral antacid immediately before entry into the operating room; ensuring the availability of equipment to measure blood glucose levels; obtaining a history of the patient's diabetic course and treatment from the primary care doctor, as well as from the patient; and performing a fiberoptic laryngoscopic examination or procuring additional skilled attention. Thus, even if preoperative and preprocedure evaluation might not alter the outcome in an important way, its ability to decrease cost by reducing unwarranted laboratory testing and delays in obtaining treatment and equipment perceived to be beneficial (and medicolegally required) would be substantial and would warrant its use.

Examples of determining the costs of such benefits can be found in Chapter 25 or in this chapter in the section on preoperative and preprocedure preparation of patients with cardiovascular disease. The following conditions are discussed in this chapter:

1. Diseases involving the endocrine system and disorders of nutrition
2. Diseases involving the cardiovascular system
3. Disorders of the respiratory and immune system
4. Diseases of the central nervous system (CNS), neuromuscular diseases, and mental disorders
5. Diseases involving the kidney, infectious diseases, and disorders of electrolytes
6. Diseases involving the gastrointestinal (GI) tract or the liver
7. Diseases involving hematopoiesis and various forms of cancer
8. Diseases of aging or those that occur more commonly in the aged, as well as chronic and acute medical conditions requiring drug therapy (also see Chapter 62).

ROLE OF THE PRIMARY CARE PHYSICIAN OR CONSULTANT

The role of the primary care physician or consultant is not to select or suggest anesthetic or surgical methods but rather to optimize the patient's preoperative and preprocedure status regarding conditions that increase the morbidity and mortality associated with surgery.

Quotations and a table in a *Medical Knowledge Self-Assessment Program* published by the leading organization representing internists, the American College of Physicians, highlight this role for the consultant:[2]

Consultation practice is an important component of virtually every internist's professional activity and in some specialties accounts for up to 50% of patient care time. Effective interaction with colleagues in other specialties requires a thorough grounding in the language and science of these other disciplines as well as an awareness of basic guidelines for consultation [Table 27-1]. ... The consulting internists' role in perioperative care is focused on the elucidation of medical factors that

Table 27–1   Guidelines for consultation practice

1. Complete a prompt, thorough, generalist-oriented evaluation.
2. Respond specifically to the question(s) posed.
3. Indicate clearly the perioperative importance of any observations and recommendations outside the area of initial concern.
4. Provide focused, detailed, and precise diagnostic and therapeutic guidance.
5. Emphasize verbal communication with the anesthesiologist and surgeon, particularly to resolve complex issues.
6. Avoid chart notations that unnecessarily create or exacerbate regulatory or medicolegal risk.
7. Use frequent follow-up visits in difficult cases to monitor clinical status and compliance with recommendations.

From American College of Physicians: Medical consultation. *In* Medical Knowledge Self-Assessment Program IX, Part C, Book 4. Philadelphia, American College of Physicians, 1992, p 939.

may increase the risks of anesthesia and surgery. ... Selecting the anesthetic technique for a given patient, procedure, surgeon, and anesthetist is highly individualized and remains the responsibility of the anesthesiologist rather than the internist.

Optimizing a patient's preoperative and preprocedure condition is a cooperative venture between the anesthesiologist and the internist, pediatrician, surgeon, or family physician. If the primary care physician cannot affirm that the patient is in the very best physical state attainable (for that patient) by that physician and his or her consultants, the anesthesiologist and physician should do what is necessary to optimize that condition. Failure to consult with the primary care physician preoperatively or before a complex procedure is as risky as not checking the oxygen in the spare tanks. In fact, statements that describe the preoperative and preprocedure physical condition of the patient (e.g., "This patient is in optimum shape" and "I believe the mitral stenosis is more severe than the slight degree of mitral insufficiency") are much more useful to the anesthesiologist than statements that suggest overall clearance ("cleared for surgery") or perioperative procedures ("prevent hypoxia and hypotension").

Primary care physicians can prepare and treat a patient to provide optimal conditions for daily life. However, they do not have the depth of understanding of the anesthesiologist regarding the physiologic changes brought on by surgery and the manipulations in function that must be made to facilitate surgery and procedures and optimize perioperative and periprocedure outcomes. One example would be the induction of some degree of prerenal azotemia in a patient with congestive heart failure (CHF) by the primary care physician. The volume depletion associated with prerenal azotemia may make a cardiac patient more comfortable in daily life but would predispose that patient to hypovolemic disaster during and after surgery and complex procedures. Thus, even though it would be desirable for the primary care physician to start the process of preparing the patient for the

needs of surgery or complex procedures, this activity would not be compatible with the current state of knowledge or functioning of the vast majority of primary care physicians. Although such education is more readily available and of better quality than in previous decades[3-7] and although Fleisher, Goldman, Charlson, and their coworkers and even cardiologic organizations have provided considerable data regarding the importance of this aspect of care,[7-10] the training, knowledge, and ability of primary care physicians are still very deficient in this aspect of consultation. Without understanding the physiologic changes that occur perioperatively, it is difficult to prescribe the appropriate therapy. It is therefore part of the anesthesiologist's job to instruct the patient's consultants about the type of information needed from the preoperative and preprocedure consultation.

DISEASES INVOLVING THE ENDOCRINE SYSTEM AND DISORDERS OF NUTRITION

Pancreatic Disorders

Preoperative and Preprocedure Diabetes Mellitus
This section makes nine major points regarding diabetes:

1. Diabetes itself may not be as important to perioperative outcome as its end-organ effects are (see point 3 for exceptions). Although the presence of diabetes has long been assumed to increase perioperative risk, results from epidemiologic studies may not support this assumption in patients not requiring management in the intensive care unit (ICU). These studies segregated the effects of diabetes per se on the organ system from the effects of the complications of diabetes (e.g., cardiac, nervous system, renal, and vascular disease) and the effects of old age and the accelerated aging that diabetes causes. Surgical mortality rates in the diabetic population are on average five times higher than rates in the nondiabetic population.[11,12] However, in epidemiologic studies in which diabetes itself was segregated from the complications of diabetes (including cardiac and vascular disease) and old age, this finding was questioned.[12,13] Similarly, if diabetics undergoing major vascular surgery are compared with nondiabetics matched for the type of surgery, age, sex, weight, and complicating diseases, there is no difference in the mortality rate or the number of postoperative complications.[13] Even in patients requiring ICU management, long-standing diabetes does not appear to be as important an issue as the end-organ dysfunction that exists and the degree of glucose control in the perioperative/periprocedure and ICU periods.[14-16]

2. Because diabetes represents at least two disease processes, its perioperative management may differ between these.

3. The Diabetes Control and Complication Trial for type 1 diabetics, the U.K. Prospective Diabetes Study for type 2 diabetics, and the Kumamoto studies all show that chronic tight control of blood sugar and blood pressure (BP) along with physical activity

results in a major delay in microvascular complications and perhaps indefinite postponement in type 2 diabetic patients.[17,18] However, current debate centers on the benefit associated with tight control in the perioperative period and on the benefit-risk ratio. Evidence indicates that tight control of blood glucose might be of benefit for pregnant diabetics (and their future offspring)[19] (also see Chapter 58), for diabetics undergoing cardiopulmonary bypass (also see Chapters 50 and 51), for those with (global) CNS ischemia[20] (also see Chapter 53), and for patients requiring postoperative or postprocedure care in an ICU. Little evidence indicates that tight control is of substantial benefit to any other group; the benefit-risk ratio of tight control has not been examined for any other group of patients.[14-16]

4. Different regimens permit almost any degree of perioperative control of blood glucose levels, but the tighter the control desired, the more frequently blood glucose levels must be monitored. Three treatment regimens are outlined later.

5. The major risk factors for diabetics undergoing surgery are the end-organ diseases associated with diabetes: cardiovascular dysfunction, renal insufficiency, joint collagen tissue abnormalities (limitation in neck extension,[21] poor wound healing), inadequate granulocyte production, and neuropathies.[11,13-16,22,23] Thus, a major focus of the anesthesiologist should be the preoperative and preprocedure evaluation and treatment of these diseases to ensure optimal preoperative and preprocedure conditions.

6. Regional anesthesia may be indicated to facilitate some procedures. The following considerations should be kept in mind regarding the use of regional anesthesia for diabetic patients. Local anesthetic requirements are lower and the risk of nerve injury is higher in diabetic patients.[24,25] In addition, combining local anesthetics with epinephrine may pose an even greater risk of ischemic or edematous nerve injury (or both) in diabetics.

7. Nosocomial infection rates are probably decreased with outpatient surgery; the frequency of complications may be decreased in diabetics most at risk by either tight control of blood glucose or intense postoperative care, or both.

8. The number of people known to be diabetic is enormous and progressively increasing in the United States and the world. This growth has been fueled by the rise in type 2 diabetes caused by weight gain in the adult population.

9. Both forms of diabetes cause accelerated aging. Thus, the risks involved in caring for someone with diabetes is similar to those for someone much older, that is, someone who has a much higher physiologic age (or "RealAge"[26,27]).

Non–insulin-dependent (type 2) diabetics account for more than 90% of the over 18 million diabetics in the United States,[28] but a diagnosis has been made in only 60%. The medical cost for these patients was over $150 billion in 2002 and has increased at more than 10% per year since 1996. At the current rate of growth, there will be 250 million diabetics in the world in 2010. These individuals tend to be elderly, overweight, and relatively resistant to ketoacidosis and susceptible to the development of a hyperglycemic-hyperosmolar nonketotic state. The diagnosis of diabetes is made with a fasting blood glucose level greater than 125 mg/dL (7.0 mmol/L), and impaired glucose tolerance is diagnosed if the fasting level is below 125 mg/dL (7.0 mmol/L) but greater than 110 (6.1). Plasma insulin levels are normal or elevated in type 2 diabetics but are relatively low for the level of blood glucose. This hyperinsulinemia by itself is postulated to cause accelerated cardiovascular disease.[29]

Insulin originates in the pancreas. Pancreatic islets are composed of at least three cells: alpha cells, which secrete glucagon; beta cells, which secrete insulin; and delta cells, which contain secretory granules. Insulin is first synthesized as proinsulin, converted to insulin by proteolytic cleavage, and then packaged into granules within the beta cells. A large quantity of insulin, normally about 200 U, is stored in the pancreas; continued synthesis is stimulated by glucose. A basal, steady-state release of insulin is provided by the beta granules, in addition to release controlled by stimuli external to the beta cell. Basal insulin secretion continues in the fasted state and is crucial to inhibition of catabolism and ketoacidosis. Glucose and fructose are the primary regulators of insulin release. Other stimulators of insulin release include amino acids, glucagon, GI hormones (gastrin, secretin, cholecystokinin-pancreozymin, and enteroglucagon), and acetylcholine. Epinephrine and norepinephrine inhibit insulin release by stimulating α-adrenergic receptors and stimulate insulin release at β-adrenergic receptors.

Diabetes mellitus is a heterogeneous group of disorders that have the common feature of a relative or absolute lack of insulin. The disease is characterized by a multitude of hormone-induced metabolic abnormalities, by a diffuse microvascular lesion, and by long-term end-organ complications. Diabetes can be divided into two very different diseases that share these end-organ abnormalities. Type 1 diabetes is associated with autoimmune diseases and has a concordance rate of 40% to 50% (i.e., if one of a pair of monozygotic twins had diabetes, the likelihood that the other twin would have diabetes is 40% to 50%). In type 1 diabetes, the patient is insulin deficient and susceptible to ketoacidosis if insulin is withheld. In type 2, the concordance rate is 100% (i.e., genetic material is both necessary and sufficient for the development of type 2 diabetes). These patients are not susceptible to the development of ketoacidosis in the absence of insulin, and they have peripheral insulin resistance. Gestational diabetes develops in more than 2% of all pregnancies and increases the risk for type 2 diabetes to 17% to 63% within 15 years.

Type 1 and type 2 diabetes differ in other ways as well. Contrary to a long-standing belief, patient age does not allow a firm distinction between type 1 and type 2 diabetes; type 1 diabetes can develop in an older person. A diabetes-producing variant of Coxsackie B4 virus has been isolated from the pancreas of a patient who died of diabetic ketoacidosis (type 1 diabetes). This virus was also recovered from mice bred to be diabetes prone after inoculation of the virus had produced hyperglycemia and pancreatic beta cell necrosis coincident with rising antibody titers.[30] Thus, the intrinsic genetic "vulnerability" in insulin-dependent type 1 diabetes mellitus may consist of a diminished capacity of beta cells to survive exposure to potentially damaging extrinsic agents. Type 1 diabetes is associated with a 15% prevalence of other autoimmune diseases, including Graves' disease, Hashimoto's thyroiditis, Addison's disease, and myasthenia gravis.

Currently, therapy for type 2 diabetes usually begins with exercise and dietary management. A diet rich in fiber with less saturated fat and daily physical activity for 30 minutes are often associated with normalization of fasting blood glucose levels and delay of glucose intolerance in more than 50% of subjects.[31] The next stage of therapy is the use of oral hypoglycemic medications to stimulate the release of insulin by pancreatic beta cells and improve tissue responsiveness to insulin by reversing the postbinding abnormality. The common orally administered drugs are tolazamide (Tolinase), tolbutamide (Orinase), and the newer sulfonylureas glyburide (Micronase), glipizide (Glucotrol), and glimepiride. These last drugs have a longer blood glucose–lowering effect that persists for 24 hours or more and fewer drug-drug interactions. Oral hypoglycemic drugs may produce hypoglycemia for as long as 50 hours after intake (chlorpropamide [Diabinese] has the longest half-life). Other drugs include metformin, which decreases hepatic glucose output and may increase peripheral responsiveness to glucose (and is associated with lactic acidosis if the patient becomes dehydrated); acarbose, which decreases glucose absorption; and the thiazolidinediones (rosiglitazone and pioglitazone), which increase peripheral responsiveness to insulin.[32] Troglitazone, another drug of this latter class, has been taken off the market because of 61 cases of acute renal failure after its use. Increasingly, physicians advocating tight control of blood sugar levels are giving insulin to "maturity-onset" insulin-dependent diabetic patients twice a day or even more frequently.[33,34]

Insulin-dependent diabetics tend to be young, nonobese, and susceptible to the development of ketoacidosis. Plasma insulin levels are low or nonmeasurable, and therapy requires insulin replacement. Patients with insulin-dependent diabetes experience an increase in their insulin requirements in the postmidnight hours, which may result in early-morning hyperglycemia (dawn phenomenon). This accelerated glucose production and impaired glucose utilization are due to nocturnal surges in secretion of growth hormone (GH).[35] Normal patients and diabetics taking insulin have steady-state levels of insulin in their blood. (Unfortunately, traditional values for insulin pharmacokinetics are derived from studies designed as though the diabetic received only one shot of insulin in a lifetime.) Absorption of insulin is highly variable and dependent on the type and species of insulin, the site of administration, and subcutaneous blood flow. Nevertheless, attainment of a steady state is dependent on periodic administration of the preparations received by the patient. Thus, it seems logical to perioperatively continue the combinations of preparations that the patient had been receiving chronically after examining the patient's blood glucose monitoring logbook for the degree of control. (In our clinical experience, erratic control can foreshadow perioperative hypoglycemia.)

Acute complications in diabetic patients include hypoglycemia and diabetic ketoacidosis, as well as hyperglycemic, hyperosmolar, nonketotic coma. Diabetic patients are also subject to a series of long-term complications that lead to considerable morbidity and premature mortality, including cataracts, neuropathies, retinopathy, and angiopathy involving peripheral and myocardial vessels. The leading cause of the blindness associated with renal failure in the United States is diabetes. Many of these complications will bring the diabetic patient to surgery. The evidence that hyperglycemia itself accelerates these complications or that tight control of blood sugar levels decreases the rapidity of the progression of microangiopathic disease is becoming more definitive.[17,18,36,37]

Glucose itself may be toxic because high levels can promote nonenzymatic glycosylation reactions leading to the formation of abnormal proteins that may decrease elastance and wound-healing tensile strength.[38] The decrease in elastance is responsible for the stiff joint syndrome and for the fixation of the atlanto-occipital joint that makes intubation difficult.[21,39,40] Furthermore, elevations in glucose may increase the production of macroglobulins by the liver, thereby increasing blood viscosity, and may promote intracellular swelling by favoring the production of nondiffusible, large molecules (e.g., sorbitol). Newer drug therapies (e.g., aldose reductase inhibitors) aim to decrease intracellular swelling by inhibiting the formation of such large molecules.

Studies on the long-term outcome of type 1 and type 2 diabetics indicate that tight control of blood glucose and blood sugar substantially prevents such complications (Table 27-2).[17,18]

Perioperative management of a diabetic patient may affect the surgical outcome. Physicians advocating tight control of blood glucose levels point to the evidence of increased wound-healing tensile strength and decreased wound infections in animal models of diabetes (type 1) under tight control and the development of infections, renal failure, other serious complications, and death in patients requiring intensive care.[14-16,41]

Infections account for two thirds of postoperative complications and about 20% of perioperative deaths in diabetic patients. Experimental data suggest that many factors can make a diabetic patient vulnerable to infection. Many alterations in leukocyte function have been demonstrated in hyperglycemic diabetics, including decreased chemotaxis and impaired phagocytic activity of granulocytes, as well as reduced intracellular killing of pneumococci and staphylococci.[42,43] When diabetic patients are treated aggressively and blood glucose levels are kept below 270 mg/dL, the phagocytic function of granulocytes is improved and intracellular killing of bacteria is restored to nearly normal levels.[44]

Diabetic patients have been thought to experience more infections in clean wounds than nondiabetics do. In a review of 23,649 surgical patients, the rate of wound infection in clean incisions was 10.7% for diabetics versus 1.8% for nondiabetics.[45] However, when age is accounted for, the incidence of wound infection in diabetic surgical patients does not differ significantly from that in nondiabetic patients. In addition, hyperglycemia may worsen the neurologic outcome after intraoperative cerebral ischemia.

Table 27–2   Tight control of blood glucose levels reduces chronic complications in type 1 diabetic patients

Measure and Results	Type 1 Diabetic Patients	
	Group Undergoing Intensive Control of Blood Glucose	*Control Group*
Measurement of blood glucose levels	≥4/day	1/day
Insulin injections	≥3/day, or an insulin pump was used	1-2/day
Diet	Special diet	Usual diabetic diet
Physician office visits	1-4/mo	Once every 3 mo
Results after 6 yr		
Diabetic retinopathy	70% less than control	
Treatment needed for retinopathy	50% less than control	
Significant nephropathy	50% less than control	
Neuropathy	60% less than control	

Modified from Reichard P, Nilsson BY, Rosenqvist U: The effect of long-term intensified insulin treatment on the development of microvascular complications of diabetes mellitus. N Engl J Med 329:304-309, 1993.

Blood glucose levels may affect neurologic recovery after a global ischemic event. In a study of 430 consecutive patients resuscitated after out-of-hospital cardiac arrest, mean blood glucose levels were higher in patients who never awakened (341 ± 13 mg/dL) than in those who did awaken (262 ± 7 mg/dL).[46] Among patients who awakened, those with persistent neurologic deficits had higher mean glucose levels (286 ± 15 mg/dL) than did patients without deficits (251 ± 7 mg/dL). These results are consistent with the finding that hyperglycemia during a stroke is associated with poorer short- and long-term neurologic outcomes. Although several questions remain, the likelihood that blood glucose is a determinant of brain damage after global ischemia is supported by the vast majority of animal studies after *global* CNS ischemia[20] and by most, but not all studies after *focal* CNS ischemia.[20] The preponderance of data after CNS ischemia indicates that levels of glucose higher than 150 or 250 mg/dL have an adverse effect on CNS recovery. Until better data are available, many will argue that a diabetic patient about to undergo surgery in which hypotension or reduced cerebral blood flow may occur should have a blood glucose level below 200 mg/dL during a period of cerebral ischemia. Some special situations may also influence how tightly one should manage a patient's glucose level, such as surgery requiring cardiopulmonary bypass, surgery in pregnant patients, and emergency surgery in patients with diabetic ketoacidosis or hyperosmolar nonketotic coma.

Diabetics undergoing coronary artery bypass graft (CABG) surgery in 1980 had a perioperative mortality rate of 5% versus 1.5% for nondiabetics.[47] In this study and in most other studies of diabetic patients undergoing CABG surgery, important additional risk factors or confounding variables were not considered, including the incidence and extent of hypertension, ventricular dysfunction, and CHF or the severity of coronary artery disease.

The aforementioned study of 340 diabetics and 2522 nondiabetics undergoing CABG surgery in 1980 demonstrated only a moderate increase in operative mortality for diabetics (1.8% versus 0.6%).[47] In the postbypass phase, patients with diabetes were found to require inotropic therapy and intra-aortic balloon pump support five times more frequently than nondiabetics did. This increased need for therapy in diabetics is due to several possible factors. Diabetics with angina have more extensive coronary artery disease than nondiabetic patients do. They are also more likely to have hypertension, cardiomegaly, diffuse hypokinesis, and previous myocardial infarction (MI). Insulin-dependent diabetics with coronary artery disease, impaired stress responses, and autonomic nerve dysfunction appear to have stiffer ventricles with a greater elevation in left ventricular end-diastolic pressure than matched nondiabetic controls do.[48-50] During cardiopulmonary bypass, hypothermia and stress reactions decrease the response to insulin and result in marked hyperglycemia (even when the perfusate and intravenous solutions do not contain glucose). Administration of washed cells has been advocated for small individuals because acid citrate dextrose– or adenine-supplemented blood can result in significant hyperglycemia. These changes are exaggerated in diabetic patients, and administration of insulin may have little effect until rewarming is achieved. In a number of recently reported cases, inotropic agents were ineffective in maintaining cardiac contractility, although filling pressures, sinus rhythm, serum electrolytes, and arterial blood gases (ABGs) were adequate. Blood sugar levels were elevated in each case. After intravenous infusion of insulin, effective myocardial contractions returned and allowed easy and rapid weaning from bypass. The effect of glucose levels on neurologic outcome during cardiopulmonary bypass is both unclear and controversial.

Many diabetics requiring emergency surgery for trauma or infection have significant metabolic decompensation, including ketoacidosis. Frequently, little time is available for stabilization of the patient, but even a few hours may be sufficient for correction of any fluid and electrolyte disturbances that are potentially life threatening. It is futile to delay surgery in an attempt to eliminate ketoacidosis completely if the underlying surgical condition will lead to further metabolic deterioration. The likelihood of intraoperative cardiac arrhythmias and hypotension resulting from ketoacidosis will be reduced if volume depletion and hypokalemia are at least partially treated.

Insulin therapy is initiated with a 10-U intravenous bolus of regular insulin, followed by continuous insulin infusion. The rate of infusion is determined most easily if one divides the last serum glucose value by 150 (or 100 if the patient is receiving steroids, has an infection, or is considerably overweight). The actual amount of insulin administered is less important than regular monitoring of glucose, potassium, and pH. Because the number of insulin-binding sites is limited, the maximum rate of glucose decline is fairly constant and averages 75 to 100 mg/dL/hr, regardless of the dose of insulin.[51] During the first 1 to 2 hours of fluid resuscitation, the glucose level may fall more precipitously. When serum glucose reaches 250 mg/dL, the intravenous fluid should include 5% dextrose.

The volume of fluid required for therapy varies with the overall deficit; it ranges from 3 to 5 L and may be as high as 10 L. Despite losses of water in excess of losses of solute, sodium levels are generally normal or reduced. Factitious hyponatremia caused by hyperglycemia or hypertriglyceridemia may result in this seeming contradiction. The plasma sodium concentration decreases by about 1.6 mEq/L for every 100-mg/dL increase in plasma glucose above normal. Initially, normal saline is infused at a rate of 250 to 1000 mL/hr, depending on the degree of volume depletion and cardiac status. Some measure of left ventricular volume should be monitored in diabetics who have a history of myocardial dysfunction. About a third of the estimated fluid deficit is corrected during the first 6 to 8 hours and the remaining two thirds over the next 24 hours.

The degree of acidosis is determined by measurement of ABGs and detection of an increased anion gap:

$$Na^+ - (Cl^- + HCO_3^-)$$

Acidosis with an increased anion gap (≥16 mEq/L) in an acutely ill diabetic may be caused by ketones in ketoacidosis, lactic acid in lactic acidosis, increased organic acids from renal insufficiency, or all three problems. In ketoacidosis, plasma levels of acetoacetate, β-hydroxybutyrate, and acetone are increased. Plasma and urinary ketones are measured semiquantitatively with Ketostix and Acetest tablets. The role of bicarbonate therapy in diabetic ketoacidosis is controversial. Myocardial function and respiration are known to be depressed at a blood pH below 7.0 to 7.10, yet rapid correction of acidosis with bicarbonate therapy may result in alterations in CNS function and structure. These alterations may be caused by (1) paradoxical development of cerebrospinal fluid and CNS acidosis from rapid conversion of bicarbonate to carbon dioxide and diffusion of the acid across the blood-brain barrier, (2) altered CNS oxygenation with decreased cerebral blood flow, and (3) the development of unfavorable osmotic gradients. After treatment with fluids and insulin, β-hydroxybutyrate levels decrease rapidly, whereas acetoacetate levels may remain stable or even increase before declining. Plasma acetone levels remain elevated for 24 to 42 hours, long after blood glucose, β-hydroxybutyrate, and acetoacetate levels have returned to normal; the result is continuing ketonuria.[51] Persistent ketosis with a serum bicarbonate level less than 20 mEq/L in the presence of a normal glucose concentration is an indication of the continued need for intracellular glucose and insulin for reversal of lipolysis.

The most important electrolyte disturbance in diabetic ketoacidosis is depletion of total-body potassium. Deficits range from 3 to 10 mEq/kg body weight. Serum potassium levels decline rapidly and reach a nadir within 2 to 4 hours after the start of intravenous insulin administration. Aggressive replacement therapy is required. The potassium administered moves into the intracellular space with insulin as the acidosis is corrected. Potassium is also excreted in urine because of the increased delivery of sodium to the distal renal tubules that accompanies volume expansion. Phosphorus deficiency in ketoacidosis as a result of tissue catabolism, impaired cellular uptake, and increased urinary losses may give rise to significant muscular weakness and organ dysfunction. The average phosphorus deficit is approximately 1 mmol/kg body weight. Replacement is needed if the plasma concentration falls below 1.0 mg/dL.[51]

Glucotoxicity

Chronic tight control of blood glucose has been motivated by a theoretical concern about five potential glucotoxicities, plus the results from three major randomized outcome studies involving diabetic patients.[17,18]

Glucose itself may be toxic because high levels can promote nonenzymatic glycosylation reactions that lead to the formation of abnormal proteins. These proteins may decrease elastance, which is responsible for the stiff joint syndrome (and difficult intubation secondary to fixation of the atlanto-occipital joint), as well as decrease wound-healing tensile strength. Furthermore, elevations in glucose may increase macroglobulin production by the liver (which would increase blood viscosity) and promote intracellular swelling by favoring the production of nondiffusible, large molecules (such as sorbitol). Some drug therapies (e.g., aldose reductase inhibitors) endeavor to decrease intracellular swelling by inhibiting the formation of such large molecules.

Glycemia also disrupts autoregulation. Glucose-induced vasodilation prevents target organs from protecting against increases in systemic BP. A glycosylated hemoglobin level of 8.1% is the threshold at which the risk of microalbuminuria increases logarithmically. A person with type 1 diabetes who has microalbuminuria greater than 29 mg/day has an 80% chance of experiencing renal insufficiency. The threshold for glycemic toxicity differs for various vascular beds. For example, the threshold for retinopathy is a glycosylated hemoglobin value of 8.5% to 9.0% (12.5 mmol/L or 225 mg/dL), and that for cardiovascular disease is an average blood glucose value of 5.4 mmol/L (96 mg/dL). Thus, different degrees of hyperglycemia may be required before different vascular beds are damaged, or certain degrees of glycemia are associated with other risk factors for vascular disease. Another view is that perhaps severe hyperglycemia and microalbuminuria are simply concomitant effects of a common underlying cause. For instance, diabetics in whom microalbuminuria develops are more resistant to insulin, insulin resistance is associated with microalbuminuria in first-degree relatives of type 2 diabetics, and persons who are normoglycemic but subsequently have clinical diabetes are at risk for atherogenesis before the onset of disease.

Tight control retards all these glucotoxicities and may have other benefits in retarding the severity of diabetes itself.[17,18,52]

Thus, management of intraoperative glucose might be influenced by specific situations, such as the type of operation, pregnancy,[53,54] and the expected global CNS insult; the bias of the patient's primary care physician; or the type of diabetes. Type 1 diabetic patients definitely need insulin and might be considered candidates for tight control of blood glucose levels. Type 2 diabetic patients have insulin, and current data indicate they do not benefit from tight perioperative control unless they need intensive care.[14-16,55]

The key to managing blood glucose levels perioperatively in diabetic patients is to set clear goals and then monitor blood glucose levels frequently enough to adjust therapy to achieve these goals. Three regimens that afford various degrees of perioperative control of blood glucose levels are discussed in the following sections.

Classic "Non–Tight Control" Regimen

Aim: To prevent hypoglycemia, ketoacidosis, and hyperosmolar states.

Protocol:

1. On the day before surgery, the patient should be given nothing by mouth (NPO) after midnight; a 13-oz glass of clear orange juice should be at the bedside or in the car for emergency use.
2. At 6 AM on the day of surgery, infuse a solution of intravenous fluids containing 5% dextrose through plastic cannulas at a rate of 125 mL/hr/70 kg body weight.
3. After starting the intravenous infusion, give half the usual morning insulin dose (and the usual type of insulin) subcutaneously.
4. Continue 5% dextrose solutions through the operative period and give at least 125 mL/hr/70 kg body weight.
5. In the recovery room, monitor blood glucose concentrations and treat on a sliding scale.

Such a regimen has been found to meet its goals.[56]

"Tight Control" Regimen 1

Aim: To keep plasma glucose levels at 79 to 120 mg/dL. Maintenance of such levels may improve wound healing and prevent wound infections, improve neurologic outcome after global or focal CNS ischemic insults, or improve weaning from cardiopulmonary bypass.

Protocol:

1. On the evening before surgery, determine the preprandial blood glucose level.
2. Through a plastic cannula, begin an intravenous infusion of 5% dextrose in water at a rate of 50 mL/hr/ 70 kg body weight.
3. "Piggyback" an infusion of regular insulin (50 U in 250 mL or 0.9% sodium chloride) to the dextrose infusion with an infusion pump (Fig. 27-1). Before attaching this piggyback line to the dextrose infusion, flush the line with 60 mL of infusion mixture and discard the flushing solution. This approach saturates insulin-binding sites on the tubing.[57]
4. Set the infusion rate by using the following equation: Insulin (U/hr) = plasma glucose (mg/dL)/150.

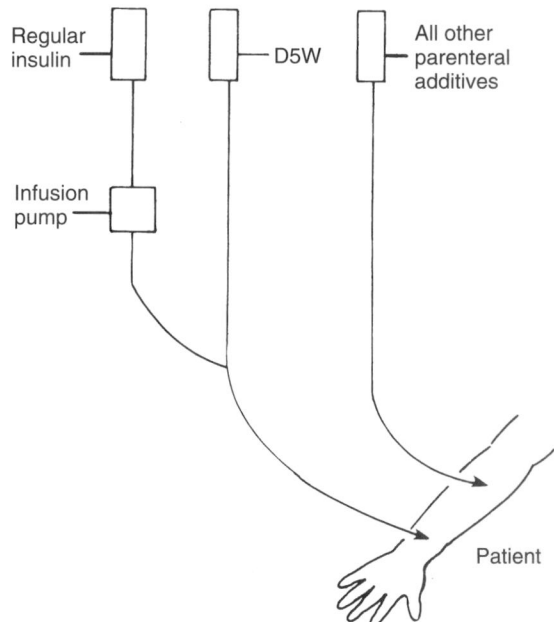

Figure 27–1 Arrangement of intravenous lines for infusion of regular insulin in a regimen tightly controlling blood glucose levels in diabetic patients undergoing surgery. D5W, 5% dextrose in water.

(*Note:* The denominator should be 100 if the patient is taking corticosteroids, e.g., 10 mg of prednisolone a day or its equivalent, not to include inhaled steroids.)

5. Repeat blood glucose measurements every 4 hours as needed, and adjust insulin appropriately to obtain blood glucose levels of 100 to 200 mg/dL.
6. On the day of surgery, intraoperative fluids and electrolytes are managed by continued administration of non–dextrose-containing solutions, as described in steps 3 and 4.
7. Determine the plasma glucose level at the start of surgery and every 1 to 2 hours for the rest of the 24-hour period. Adjust the insulin dosage appropriately.

Although we have not found it necessary to treat hypoglycemia (i.e., blood glucose levels <50 mg/dL), we have been prepared to do so with 15 mL of 50% dextrose in water. In such circumstances, the insulin infusion would be terminated. This regimen has been found to accomplish its objectives, with the exception of such tight goals for blood glucose, even in very "brittle" diabetics (i.e., those extremely resistant to treatment) given high doses of steroids.[58]

"Tight Control" Regimen 2

Aim: Same as for Tight Control Regimen 1.

Protocol:

1. Obtain a "feedback mechanical pancreas" and set the controls for the desired plasma glucose regimen.
2. Institute two appropriate intravenous lines.

This last regimen may well supersede all others if the cost of a mechanical pancreas can be reduced and if control of hyperglycemia is shown to make a meaningful difference perioperatively; it has *superseded* all others in many ICUs, and for good reason (Table 27-3).[14-16]

Table 27–3 Therapy for 1548 postsurgical diabetics in the Leuven intensive care unit study*

Glucose Therapy (mg/dL)	Intensive Rx (80-110)	Conventional Rx (180-200)
Death in the ICU	4.6%	8.0%
After 5 days in the ICU	10.6%	20.2%
1st 5 ICU days	1.7%	1.8%
All deaths	7.2%	10.9%
>14 days in the ICU	11.4%	15.7%
>14 days ventilated	7.5%	11.9%
Rx dialysis	4.8%	8.2%
Polyneuropathy	28.7%	51.9%

*Decreased complication rates and improved survival were observed in the group treated by tight control.

Diabetes and Accelerated Physiologic Aging

Adverse perioperative outcomes have repeatedly and substantially correlated with the age of the patient,[7,9,12,26,27,59-61] and diabetes does cause physiologic aging. When one translates the results of the Diabetes Control and Complications Trials into age-induced physiologic changes, a type 1 diabetic who has poor control of blood sugar ages approximately 1.75 years physiologically for every chronologic year of the disease and 1.25 years if blood sugar has been controlled tightly.[26] A type 2 diabetic ages about 1.5 years for every chronologic year of the disease and about 1.06 years with tight control of blood sugar and BP.[18,26,27,31] Thus, when providing care for a diabetic patient, one must consider the associated risks to be those of a person who is much older physiologically. That is, a diabetic's physiologic age ("RealAge") is considerably higher than that person's calendar age just by virtue of having the disease.[1]

The increased prevalence of obesity and lack of physical exercise seem to be major contributors to the increased prevalence of type 2 diabetes. As with type 1 diabetes, tight control of blood sugar, increased physical activity, and reduction in weight appear to reduce the accelerated aging associated with type 2 diabetes and even to substantially delay appearance of the disease. Although such a reduction in aging should reduce the perioperative risk for diabetic patients, no controlled trials have confirmed this theory.

Other Conditions Associated with Diabetes

Diabetes is associated with microangiopathy (in retinal and renal vessels), peripheral neuropathy, autonomic dysfunction, and infection. Diabetics are often treated with angiotensin-converting enzyme (ACE) inhibitors, even in the absence of gross hypertension, in an effort to prevent the effects of disordered autoregulation, including renal failure.[17,18,62]

Before surgery, assessment and optimization of treatment of the potential and potent end-organ effects of diabetes are at least as important as assessment of the diabetic's current overall metabolic status. Information about a diabetic patient that might merit special attention before surgery includes the therapeutic, dietary, and exercise or physical activity regimens; adequacy of glucose control; previous surgical and anesthetic responses; and presence of the end-organ effects of diabetes. In our experience, many diabetic patients pay extreme attention to glucose control. expect each physician to ask about it, and are annoyed (and probably rightly so) if the physicians treating them in the perioperative period are not at least as concerned about the glucose level as the patients have had to be. Thus, if just to avoid making the patient angry (and, we believe, for more value than that), the anesthesiologist should inquire in some depth about the diabetic's control of blood glucose levels. Basic laboratory examinations might include determination of fasting blood sugar levels, electrolytes, and blood urea nitrogen (BUN) or creatinine levels, as well as an electrocardiogram (ECG). Scheduling the operative procedure early in the day avoids prolonging the catabolic state and minimizes the risk of preoperative hypoglycemia.

If one is to believe the few studies we have, the presence of autonomic neuropathy makes the operative period more hazardous and the postoperative period crucial to survival. Evidence of autonomic neuropathy might be routinely sought before surgery. Patients with diabetic autonomic neuropathy are at increased risk for gastroparesis (and consequent aspiration) and for intraoperative and postoperative cardiorespiratory arrest. Data indicate that diabetics who exhibit signs of autonomic neuropathy, such as early satiety, lack of sweating, lack of pulse rate change with inspiration or orthostatic maneuvers, and impotence, have a very high incidence of painless myocardial ischemia[50,57-59,63,64] and gastroparesis. Some investigators have successfully used 10 mg of metoclopramide preoperatively to facilitate gastric emptying of solids (Fig. 27-2). Interference with respiration or sinus automaticity by pneumonia or by anesthetics, pain medications, or sedative drugs appears to be the precipitating cause in most cases of sudden cardiorespiratory arrest.[1] Measuring the degree of sinus arrhythmia or beat-to-beat variability provides a simple, accurate test for significant autonomic neuropathy. The difference between the maximum and minimum heart rate on deep inspiration is normally 15 beats/min but was found to be 5 beats/min or less in all patients who sustained cardiorespiratory arrest.[63]

Other characteristics of patients with autonomic neuropathy include postural hypotension with a decrease in BP of more than 30 mm Hg, resting tachycardia, nocturnal diarrhea, and dense peripheral neuropathy. Diabetics with significant autonomic neuropathy may have impaired respiratory responses to hypoxia and are particularly susceptible to the action of drugs that have depressant effects. These patients may warrant very close, continuous cardiac and respiratory monitoring for 24 to 72 hours postoperatively, although such logical treatment has not been tested in a rigorous, controlled trial.[23] In the absence of autonomic neuropathy, we would favor outpatient surgery for a diabetic (Table 27-4).

Anticipated Newer Treatments for Diabetes

At least four major changes in care for diabetic patients have made it to the clinical trial stage:

- Implanted (like a pacemaker) glucose analyzer with electronic transmission to a surface (watch) monitor

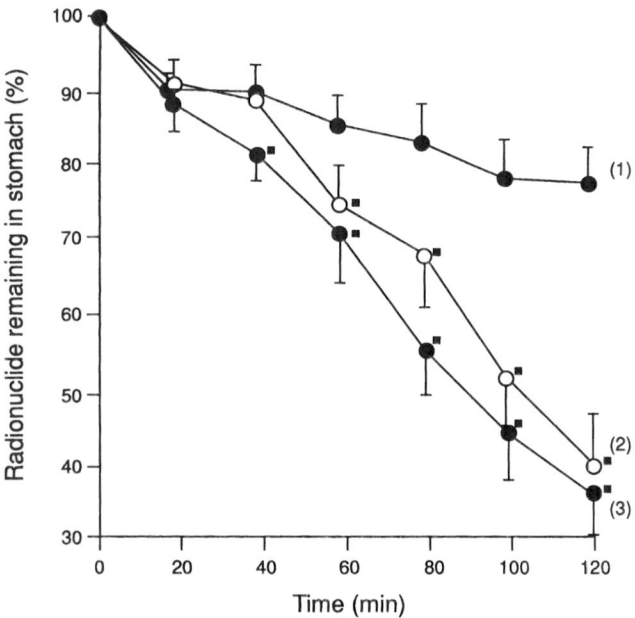

Figure 27–2 Gastric emptying time (mean ± SD) of a solid test meal in three groups of patients: diabetics (line 1), diabetics given metoclopramide (10 mg intravenously) 1.5 hours before the test meal (line 2), and nondiabetics (line 3). (From Wright RA, Clemente R, Wathen R: Diabetic gastroparesis: An abnormality of gastric emptying of solids. Am J Med Sci 289:240, 1985.)

- A glucagon-like peptide receptor antagonist such as GIP-1
- New islet transplantation medication that makes islet cell transplants much more successful and rejection medication less hazardous
- Medications such as INGAP peptide, which may cause regrowth of normally functioning islet cells (without needing transplantation)

Table 27–4 Should a diabetic be an outpatient or a morning admittance patient?

Outpatient If	Morning Admittance Patient If
Can evaluate history in advance	Cannot evaluate history
End-organ disease does not require monitoring	End-organ disease requires invasive monitoring
Prehydration is available or is unnecessary	Needs careful prehydration
No CNS ischemia or planned cardiopulmonary bypass	CNS ischemia is present or cardiopulmonary bypass is planned
Not pregnant	Pregnant
Patient or vested home "mate" can determine blood glucose level	Patient cannot determine blood glucose level
Has vested home "mate"	No vested individual
Can take temperature or look for "red" wound	Cannot take temperature or look for "red" wound
Plan higher admit rate (no data)	Social care network is unsuitable

You can imagine how some of these treatments may radically change the therapies used in the perioperative period. If regrowth of islets becomes common, type 1 diabetes could all but disappear; if implanted minute-to-minute glucose reading is possible, tight control may be much easier and more expected.

Current Focus for Diabetes Perioperatively

Perhaps as important as arranging for tight control in a diabetic needing intensive care is keeping in mind that diabetic patients have an increased incidence of atherosclerosis and all its complications. These patients are particularly susceptible to episodes of painless myocardial ischemia and cardiovascular instability.[65-67] In fact, over 80% of the ischemic episodes that occur in both patients who have myocardial ischemia and those who are diabetic are "silent." However, a 65-year-old diabetic is as likely to die of a cardiovascular event in the next several years as a person who has just had a heart attack (Table 27-5).[68] These data dramatically illustrate the increased risk of cardiovascular disease in diabetics who do not have symptoms. As with other endocrinopathies, the cardiovascular system should be a focus for the anesthetist's attention in diabetic patients.

Insulinoma and Other Causes of Hypoglycemia

Hypoglycemia in persons not treated for diabetes is rare. Hypoglycemia in nondiabetics can be caused by such diverse entities as pancreatic islet cell adenoma or carcinoma, large hepatoma, large sarcoma, alcohol ingestion, use of β-adrenergic receptor blocking drugs, haloperidol, hypopituitarism, adrenal insufficiency, altered physiology after gastric or gastric bypass surgery, hereditary fructose intolerance, antidiabetic drug ingestion, galactosemia, or autoimmune hypoglycemia.[69] The last four entities cause postprandial reactive hypoglycemia. Because restriction of oral intake prevents severe hypoglycemia, the practice of keeping the patient NPO and infusing small amounts of a solution containing 5% dextrose greatly lessens the possibility of perioperative postprandial reactive hypoglycemia. The other causes of hypoglycemia can cause serious problems during the perioperative period.[70]

Symptoms of hypoglycemia fall into two groups: adrenergic excess (tachycardia, palpitations, tremulousness, or diaphoresis) and neuroglycopenia (headache, confusion, mental sluggishness, seizures, or coma). All these symptoms may be masked by anesthesia, so blood glucose levels should be determined frequently in such patients to ensure that hypoglycemia is not present. Because manipulation of an insulinoma can result in massive insulin release, this tumor should probably be operated on only at centers equipped with a mechanical pancreas; new data may indicate that the somatostatin analog octreotide will make such operations much less risky in all settings.[71,72]

Muir and colleagues[71] managed 38 patients undergoing resection of insulinoma. Every 15 minutes these investigators determined the plasma glucose concentration in these patients, in whom a mechanical pancreas produced no increase in plasma glucose. Although 9 of the 38 patients became significantly hypoglycemic (i.e., plasma glucose concentrations <50 mg/dL), only 4 of 253 measurements taken before resection showed a decrease in glucose of

Table 27–5   Seven-year risk of cardiovascular events in nondiabetics and type 2 diabetics without previous myocardial infarctions*

	Nondiabetics		Type 2 Diabetics without Previous MI (*n* = 890)
	Without Previous MI (n = 1304)	*With Previous MI (n = 69)*	
Fatal or nonfatal MIs, per 100 person-years	0.5	3.0	3.2
Death from cardiovascular causes, per 100 person-years	0.3	2.6	2.5

*The 7-year risk for cardiovascular events in type 2 diabetes who have *not* had a previous myocardial infarction (MI) is the same as for nondiabetics who *have* had a previous MI. Values are adjusted for age and sex (median age at start, approximately 58 years). Adapted from Haffner SM, Lehto S, Rönnemaa T, et al: Mortality from coronary heart disease in subjects with type 2 diabetes and in nondiabetic subjects with and without prior myocardial infarction. N Engl J Med 339:229, 1998, with permission.

more than 20 mg/dL in any 15-minute period. Muir and associates[71] believe that intermittent sampling of plasma glucose (every 15 minutes) may be satisfactory as long as the plasma glucose concentration is kept at 60 mg/dL or above. In this series, the absence or presence of hyperglycemic rebound after tumor resection was not of predictive value in determining the completeness of insulinoma resection. Other causes of hypoglycemia do not involve the release of insulin in such vast quantities (or at all); therefore, less frequent (every 1 to 2 hours) intraoperative blood glucose determinations and continuous dextrose infusion appear to be sufficient.

Perioperative use of the somatostatin analog octreotide, which suppresses insulin release from such tumors, appears to make the perioperative period a logarithm safer in anecdotal experience. Whether all tumors respond to this drug similarly and thus radically reduce the hazard from resection of insulinoma remains to be determined.[72]

Disorders of Nutrition, Including Obesity

Hyperlipoproteinemia, Hyperlipidemia, and Hypolipidemia

Hyperlipidemia may result from obesity, estrogen or corticoid therapy, uremia, diabetes, hypothyroidism, acromegaly, alcohol ingestion, liver disease, inborn errors of metabolism, or pregnancy. Hyperlipidemia may cause premature coronary or peripheral vascular disease or pancreatitis.[73] Most cholesterol is carried in serum by low-density lipoprotein (LDL), whereas approximately 30% of total serum cholesterol is carried by high-density lipoprotein (HDL). Increased LDL cholesterol, a form of hyperlipidemia, appears to be associated with premature atherosclerosis, as is decreased HDL cholesterol. HDL cholesterol is carried in roughly equivalent amounts on two types of HDL: on a less dense HDL_2 subfraction that is negatively associated with coronary artery disease and on a more dense HDL_3 subfraction that is unrelated to coronary artery disease.

In regard to the production of atherosclerosis, LDL is distinguished from HDL by associating L with "lousy" and H with "healthy." That is, the oxidized form of LDL constitutes a risk factor for atherosclerosis, whereas HDL is believed to carry dangerous cholesterol away from the periphery, to be metabolized by the liver, and is therefore protective. Levels of HDL are 25% higher in women than men; low levels of HDL in women are associated with premature atherosclerosis. Cigarette smoking lowers HDL levels, whereas regular exercise (particularly strenuous exercise, but even nonstrenuous exercise) and a small daily intake of alcohol raise HDL levels. However, alcohol increases HDL_3, the HDL subfraction thought to be inert with respect to coronary artery disease; octogenarians have high levels of HDL.

Data showing that coronary events can be reduced by treating individuals with even normal levels of LDL cholesterol with the "statins"—drugs that raise HDL and lower LDL cholesterol levels—resulted from a decade of rapid progress in preventing reinfarction in high-risk patients.[74-78] Secondary prevention efforts were successful when these high-risk patients stopped smoking, reduced their BP, controlled stress, increased physical activity, and used aspirin, folate, β-blocking drugs, angiotensin inhibitors, diet, and other drugs to reduce their levels of LDL and increase their levels of HDL.[79,80]

Although controlling the diet remains a major treatment modality for all types of hyperlipidemia,[79,81] the drugs fenofibrate and gemfibrozil, which are used to treat hypertriglyceridemia, can cause myopathy, especially in patients with hepatic or renal disease; clofibrate is also associated with an increased incidence of gallstones. Cholestyramine binds bile acids, as well as oral anticoagulants, digitalis drugs, and thyroid hormones. Nicotinic acid causes peripheral vasodilation and should probably not be continued through the morning of surgery. Probucol (Lorelco) decreases the synthesis of apoprotein A-I; its use is associated on rare occasion with fetid perspiration or prolongation of the QT interval (or both) and sudden death in animals.

The West of Scotland Coronary Prevention Study and its congeners produced convincing evidence that drugs in the "statin" class (3-hydroxy-3-methylglutaryl–coenzyme A [HMG-CoA] reductase inhibitors) prevent the morbidity and mortality related to arterial aging and vascular disease, as well as their consequences, such as coronary arterial disease, stroke, and peripheral vascular insufficiency.[75,76]

Table 27–6 Acute coronary events in patients with average cholesterol levels who were given lovastatin: results from the Air Force/Texas coronary atherosclerosis prevention study

	Lovastatin Group (20-40 mg/day)	Placebo Group	P Value
No. of patients	3304	3301	NS
% men	85%	85%	NS
Age (mean ± SD, yr)			
Men	58 ± 7	58 ± 7	NS
Women	62 ± 5	63 ± 5	NS
First acute major coronary events	116	183	<.001
Unstable angina	60	87	.02
Myocardial infarction	57	95	.002
Revascularization	106	157	.001
Coronary events	163	215	.006

Abstracted from Downs JR, Clearfield M, Weis S, et al: Primary prevention of acute coronary events with lovastatin in men and women with average cholesterol levels. Results of AFCAPS/TexCAPS. JAMA 279:1615, 1998, with permission.

Thus, the statins—lovastatin (Mevacor), pravastatin (Pravachol), simvastatin, fluvastatin, atorvastatin (Lipitor), and rosuvastatin (Crestor)—are mainstays of therapy.

However, the report of Downs and coworkers[75] from the Air Force/Texas Coronary Atherosclerosis Prevention Study went further. It showed a 37% reduction in the risk of first acute major coronary events in patients who had not only no risk factors for coronary artery aging but also normal (average) LDL cholesterol levels (Table 27-6). In this study lovastatin did not alter mortality rates, but that had been true for many early short-term trials with the statins. Although much of the effect of the statins has been attributed to their lipid-lowering effects, statins have also been shown to modify endothelial function, inflammatory responses, plaque stability, and thrombogenicity.[80] The report of Downs and colleagues broadened the use of statins, and they remain mainstays of therapy for hyperlipidemia. Statins are drugs that block HMG-CoA reductase, the rate-limiting enzyme of cholesterol synthesis. Their use is occasionally accompanied by liver dysfunction, CNS dysfunction, and severe depression not related to the high cost of each drug and its cogeners. Recent data indicate that statins provide the substantial benefit of reversing inflammation in arteries, as evidenced by their ability to decrease highly specific C-reactive protein (hs-CRP) and pull cholesterol from plaques.[79,82,83]

Hypolipidemic conditions are rare diseases often associated with neuropathy, anemia, and renal failure. Although anesthetic experience with hypolipidemic conditions has been limited, some specific recommendations can be made: continuation of caloric intake and intravenous administration of protein hydrolysates and glucose throughout the perioperative period.

Obesity*

No randomized controlled trials give irrefutable evidence that preoperative evaluation of obese patients, even before bariatric surgery, makes a significant difference in

patient mortality. However, much evidence indicates that such evaluations, as for other patients, makes the perioperative period more efficient, reduces provider and patient anxiety, and sets appropriate expectations that lead to increased patient satisfaction with pain therapy and the entire perioperative experience. We believe that such an assessment can also spot important variations in airway, pulmonary, cardiovascular, metabolic, and nervous system physiology that lead to improved provider preparedness, patient outcome, and the feeling of both about the quality of the perioperative care. Such may be an important element of surgery in the obese, especially for bariatric surgery. Moreover, motivating and ensuring prophylaxis for deep vein thrombosis can be an important determinant of the acute outcome inasmuch as pulmonary emboli are the greatest cause of perioperative 30-day mortality. Importantly, any contribution that the anesthesiologist can make toward evaluating the psychological attitude and preparation of the patient (for example, the patient stopped exercising 3 weeks ago) is usually most welcomed and important to the surgeon. For it is the psychological readiness of each patient and that patient's commitment to outcome after this operation that appear to determine its long-term worth for that patient.

Obesity in society and in an individual may not be of recent origin, but the rapid increase in treatments involving successful surgery for obesity without huge morbidity is. Recently, the rate and number of obese persons in all societies have been increasing with epidemic speed. In fact, obesity may be increasing even faster than surgery for it is. For example, in the United States, more than 50% of adults weigh more than 20% above what is considered the optimum body weight for their height—a recent increase from 30%.[84] Furthermore, this increase occurred in just 18 years. One measure of obesity is body mass index (BMI), for which a value above 31 kg/m² represents morbid obesity and its risks and a value above 27 for women and 28 for men corresponds to weight 25% above ideal (Table 27-7). The pathophysiologic consequences of obesity involve every major organ system.[85] Many of the metabolic, hormonal, and physiologic changes associated with obesity (e.g., insulin resistance, decreased number of

---

*Much of this section of the chapter is modified from Beers and Roizen, in press, with permission.

Table 27–7   Obesity as a function of body mass index*

| Height‡ | | Average Weight (Men and Women)† | | | | | | |
| | | 19-34 yr | | | ≥35 yr | | | |
ft/in	cm	lb	Average kg	Average BMI	lb	Average kg	Average BMI	BMI 20% > Ideal
5'0"	152.4	97-128	51.1	22.0	108-138	55.9	24.1	27.5
5'1"	154.9	101-132	53.0	22.0	111-143	57.7	24.8	27.5
5'2"	157.5	104-137	54.7	22.0	115-148	59.5	23.9	27.5
5'3"	160.0	107-141	56.4	22.0	119-152	61.5	24.0	27.5
5'4"	162.6	111-146	58.4	22.0	122-157	63.4	24.0	27.5
5'5"	165.1	114-150	60.0	22.0	126-162	65.5	24.0	27.5
5'6"	167.6	118-155	62.0	22.0	130-167	67.5	24.0	27.5
5'7"	170.2	121-160	63.9	22.0	134-172	69.5	24.0	27.5
5'8"	172.7	125-164	65.7	22.0	138-178	71.5	24.0	27.5
5'9"	175.3	129-169	67.7	22.0	142-183	73.8	24.0	27.5
5'10"	177.8	132-174	69.6	22.0	146-188	75.9	24.0	27.5
5'11"	180.3	136-179	71.6	22.0	151-194	78.4	24.1	27.5
6'0"	182.9	140-184	73.7	22.0	155-199	80.4	24.0	27.5
6'1"	185.4	144-189	75.7	22.0	159-205	82.7	24.0	27.5
6'2"	188.0	148-195	77.9	22.0	164-210	85.0	24.0	27.5
6'3"	190.5	152-200	80.0	22.0	168-216	87.2	24.0	27.5

*Body mass index (BMI) = weight (in kilograms) ÷ height^2 (in meters).
†Without clothes.
‡Without shoes.
Data from Roizen MF: Preoperative Test Selection Program Software Manual of Version 2.15L. Pleasanton, CA, Nellcor, 1994.

insulin receptors, and subsequent diabetes mellitus) can be induced by overfeeding normal subjects and can be reversed by weight reduction. Despite obesity being the condition that is increasing most in both percentage and numerical terms, few studies have examined the nonsurgical perioperative factors that make a difference in morbidity after bariatric operations. In fact, surgery is almost always reserved for patients with medical complications of obesity rather than just obesity per se. This stance is controversial because many patients consider obesity without overt medical complications to be a major cause of an adverse quality of life. However, but in terms of outcome, it is obesity's complications that cause most of its aging effects.[85] Obesity itself, its complications, and its treatment have significance for the anesthesiologist. A person who is 30% overweight has a 40% increased chance of dying of heart disease and a 50% increased chance of dying of a stroke. Obesity is also associated with higher resource utilization (more perioperative days in the hospital) and greater perioperative morbidity and mortality, such as deep vein thrombosis and its consequences, most often as a result of inactivity.[86,87]

Although many conditions associated with obesity (diabetes, hyperlipidemia, cholelithiasis, gastroesophageal reflux disease, cirrhosis, degenerative joint and disk disease, venous stasis and thrombotic/embolic disease, sleep disorders, and emotional and altered body image disorders) contribute to chronic morbidity in the obese, the main concerns for the anesthesiologist have been the same for over 3 decades—derangements of the cardiopulmonary system.[88,89]

In obese patients, gas exchange may be impaired not only by altered cardiopulmonary mechanisms but also by

management of a difficult airway, loss of functional residual capacity (FRC), and ensuing rapid desaturation when anesthesia is induced; by a propensity for desaturation in the recumbent (as opposed to the upright) position and the potential need to induce anesthesia and recovery in such patients in the upright position; by a propensity for and the presence of sleep apnea, chronic respiratory insufficiency, pulmonary hypertension, and a predisposition to deep vein thrombosis and its consequences; and by a need for active participation to overcome uncomfortableness and motivate ambulation in the postoperative period.

Obstruction of the airway by the abundant soft tissue in the upper airway frequently produces hypoxemia and hypercapnia, and obesity significantly increases the risk of difficult tracheal intubation.[90,91] FRC decreases because the weight of the torso and abdomen makes diaphragmatic excursions more difficult and more position dependent, a problem made worse by mechanical ventilation. For many obese patients, this process causes FRC to be less than closing volume and decreases the time of safe apnea before hypoxia occurs (Amalraj S, personal communication) (Fig. 27-3). Furthermore, obese patients have increased volume and acidity of gastric juices preoperatively (Fig. 27-4), perhaps indicating the wisdom of premedicating such patients with cimetidine, ranitidine, Bicitra, or metoclopramide. (The simplest, least expensive, scientifically tested regimen appears to be administration of cimetidine the night and morning before surgery [Fig. 27-5] [Amalraj S, personal communication]). Others would conclude that awake intubation is indicated, but a preference for this technique must be balanced by the realization that most episodes of gastroesophageal reflux and the greatest

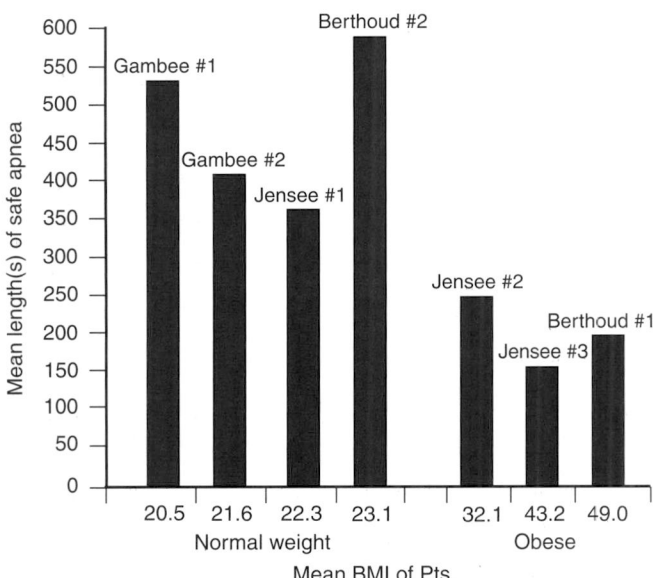

Figure 27–3 Duration of safe apnea before hemoglobin desaturation in obese and normal-weight patients (90% oxygen saturation), as reported by various studies. BMI, body mass index. (Amalraj S, personal communication.)

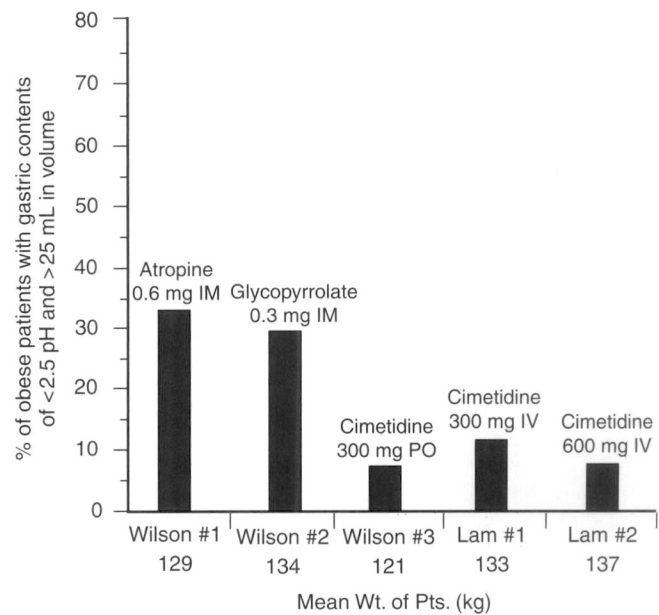

Figure 27–5 Effect of drugs on the risk of pulmonary aspiration in obese patients, as reported by various studies. (Amalraj S, personal communication.)

potential for pulmonary aspiration occur from and during "bucking" on an endotracheal tube.[92,93] Obesity is also a significant risk factor for postoperative hypoxemia,[94] a situation partially remedied by placing the patient in the semirecumbent (rather than the supine) position for the first 48 to 72 hours of recovery.[95]

Morbid obesity (BMI >30 kg/m²) is the most common and a major risk factor for obstructive sleep apnea (OSA).[96] An increase in BMI by about two units (e.g., from 27 to 29) increases the likelihood of coexisting OSA by a factor of 4.[97] OSA in the obese generally improves after weight reduction.[98] Whereas the prevalence of OSA in the

general U.S. population is 2% in women and 4% in men,[96] it is 3% to 25% and 40% to 78% in morbidly obese women and men, respectively.[97-101] Sleep apnea in obese patients is usually obstructive and a consequence of both airway narrowing from abundant peripharyngeal adipose tissue and an abnormal decrease in upper airway muscle tone during rapid eye movement (REM) sleep.[96]

The presence and severity of OSA in obese patients cannot be reliably predicted by BMI, neck circumference, pulmonary function tests, daytime room-air ABGs, or questionnaires to detect and quantify sleep-related complaints (or any combination of these factors).[102-106] In the United States, sleep apnea is undiagnosed in 80% to 90% of sufferers.[97,107] Consequently, preoperative patients with this condition frequently have suggestive symptoms, but no previous evaluation. (Bariatric surgery may be a better option than chronic tracheostomy in patients with OSA, and the need for tracheostomy is frequently listed as an indication for such bariatric surgery.)

The definitive diagnostic test for OSA is polysomnography. The presence of sleep apnea is defined as 5 or more apneic events (cessation of airflow lasting 10 seconds or longer despite continued respiratory effort) per hour or 15 or more hypopneic events (decrease in airflow of more than 50% lasting 10 seconds or longer) per hour during a 7-hour sleep study.[108] The apneic-hypopneic index is the total number of apneic or hypopneic events (or both) per hour during sleep; the severity of OSA is directly related to the magnitude of this index.[96] Hypopneic and apneic events are associated with arousal from REM sleep and oxyhemoglobin desaturation. Daytime somnolence is a frequent complaint because sleep is fragmented such that the patient cannot sustain adequate intervals of REM sleep. Concomitant with apneic/hypopneic events, sympathetic nervous system activation occurs in response to hypoxemia.

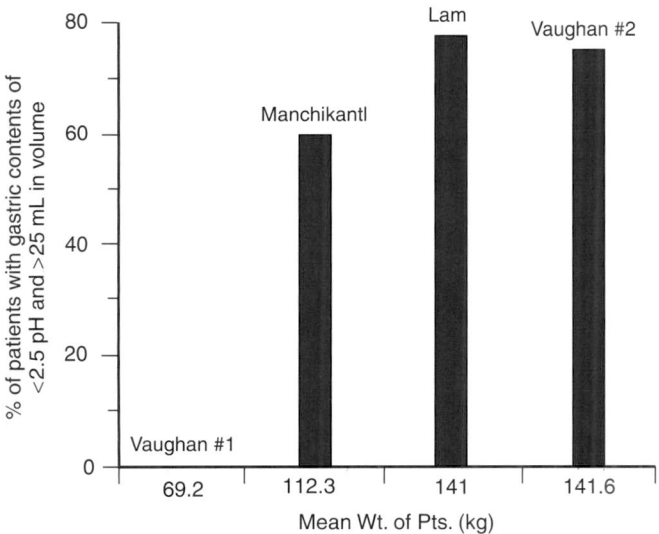

Figure 27–4 Relationship between weight and risk factors for pulmonary aspiration, as reported by four studies. (Amalraj S, personal communication.)

This finding may explain the strong association between OSA and systemic hypertension.[109]

Detection of OSA in obese patients presenting for bariatric surgery may be important for two reasons. First, patients with OSA are more sensitive to the consequences of the depressant effects of hypnotics and opioids on airway muscle tone and respiration.[110] Postoperative parenteral or neuraxial opioid administration to obese patients with OSA carries the potential for fatal or near-fatal respiratory misadventure.[111,112] More intense postoperative nursing care and monitoring may be indicated when symptoms or signs of sleep apnea exist and either systemic or neuraxial opioids are necessary for postoperative pain control.[111] Second, OSA is associated with difficulty performing laryngoscopy[113,114] and difficult mask ventilation.[115] In addition, obese patients have reduced oxygen stores because of their diminished expiratory reserve volume.[116,117] The combination of these factors sets the stage for airway catastrophe. Because a large percentage of obese patients have sleep apnea, identification of those who probably do *not* have the condition may be more appropriate; in fact, some experts recommend presuming that *all* morbidly obese patients presenting for bariatric surgery have OSA. Thus, they recommend that all preoperative patients scheduled for bariatric surgery be trained in the use of continuous positive airway pressure (CPAP) or bilevel positive airway pressure (BiPAP).[118]

In the absence of previous polysomnographic testing, the presence and severity of OSA in a preoperative bariatric surgical patient are most conveniently assessed by the history. Useful information can often be elicited from the patient's roommate or sleeping partner. Historical information presumptive of sleep apnea includes habitual snoring, interrupted breathing during sleep (apneic spells followed by short gasps, grunts, or resuscitative snorting), impaired daytime performance, morning headache, and irritability.[96] Systemic hypertension[107,109] and increased neck circumference (>40 to 42 cm at the cricoid cartilage)[108,119] are consistent with the presumptive diagnosis of OSA. Other abnormalities associated with OSA that are detected by physical examination are somnolence and physical signs of difficult mask airway or difficult intubation (e.g., Mallampati class III or IV, hypognathia, decreased thyromental distance).[110,112,114]

Polysomnographic testing might be indicated in morbidly obese preoperative patients who habitually snore and report daytime somnolence or have observed periods of interrupted breathing during sleep (or both).[96] However, morbid obesity and symptoms of OSA per se are not indications for preoperative pulmonary function testing and room-air blood gas analysis. In the absence of uncharacterized symptoms or signs of pulmonary disease, these tests have neither predictive value nor utility in optimizing the postoperative management or outcome of bariatric surgery patients.[111,120-122]

Obesity per se is not a common cause of chronic respiratory insufficiency.[123] Clinically significant impairment in gas exchange and pulmonary function are more common when chronic obstructive pulmonary disease (COPD) and obesity coexist. The two conditions together cause greater impairment in gas exchange than expected from simple summation of the impairment caused by each pathophysiologic process.[124] As in all patients, the presence of concomitant pulmonary system disease may be detected by a smoking history and symptoms or signs such as coughing, wheezing, or dyspnea on exertion.

In obese patients, chronic daytime hypoxemia is a better predictor of pulmonary hypertension and cor pulmonale than the presence and severity of OSA are.[125-127] Room-air pulse oximetry may be a useful, noninvasive means to screen patients for daytime hypoxemia, particularly if measured and compared in both the upright and supine positions. A *supine* room-air Spo_2 of less than 96% may merit further investigation (e.g., pulmonary function tests, room-air ABGs, chest radiographs, and echocardiography). An elevated hematocrit may also be a clue to chronic hypoxemia.

A syndrome characterized by chronic daytime hypoventilation, dubbed the obesity-hypoventilation syndrome (OHS), can develop in a subgroup of obese patients.[123] OHS is also associated with chronic daytime hypoxemia (Po_2 <65 mm Hg), conveniently detected during the preoperative visit by routine measurement of room-air pulse oximetry. Sustained hypercapnia (Pco_2 >45 mm Hg) in an obese patient without significant obstructive pulmonary disease is diagnostic for this syndrome. These patients are typically extremely obese (BMI >40 kg/m^2), and the likelihood of OHS increases strongly as BMI increases.[128] The precise underlying pathophysiology of OHS is unclear and probably multifactorial; however, chronic alveolar hypoventilation may be attributed to the compressive effect of extreme adiposity on the thoracic cage and diaphragm.[106,123] Most obese patients with OHS also have OSA; nevertheless, obese patients with OSA do not commonly have OHS.[106,123] Patients on the "severe" end of the OHS spectrum who have signs and symptoms of cor pulmonale are termed "pickwickian."[106] In one study of obese patients with OSA but without airflow obstruction, 56 of 58 patients with chronic daytime hypoxemia were proved by testing to have OHS.[127]

The reason to be wary of and to try to diagnose whether obesity coexists with either OHS *or* COPD is that such a combination often causes chronic daytime hypoxemia. Chronic daytime hypoxemia leads to pulmonary hypertension, right ventricular hypertrophy, or right ventricular failure (or any combination of these sequelae). These conditions (pickwickian) are associated with increased perioperative morbidity and mortality, and assessment of these patients may require extensive testing to guide preoperative medical optimization and postoperative management.[106,109,110,129]

Prevalent ECG findings in obese patients are low QRS voltage, left ventricular hypertrophy or strain, left atrial abnormality, and T-wave flattening in the inferior and lateral leads.[130] ECG evidence in the obese of right ventricular hypertrophy or strain, right axis deviation, right bundle branch block, or P pulmonale is not common in the absence of pulmonary hypertension and cor pulmonale.

Morbid obesity with minimal or no coexisting pulmonary conditions (e.g., no OHS or COPD) will be referred to as "simple" obesity. In simple obesity, the pathophysiology of mild alterations in daytime gas exchange and pulmonary function may also result from compression and restriction of the chest wall and diaphragm by excess adipose tissue.[131] Typically, in the obese, the expiratory reserve volume (ERV) and FRC are most affected and reduced to 60% and 80% of normal, respectively. If ERV decreases below closing volume, airway closure occurs during normal tidal breathing, and dependent alveoli are relatively or completely underventilated. Daytime hypoxemia results if the shunt and ventilation-perfusion mismatch are of sufficient magnitude. After massive weight loss, morbidly obese patients demonstrate marked improvement in Pao_2 and the alveolar-arterial oxygen gradient, and variables reflecting oxygenation improve to an extent directly proportional to the increase in ERV.[132,133]

Whereas vital capacity in simple obesity is reduced to 90% of control, it is reduced to 60% of normal in OHS.[134] The additional reduction in lung volume seen in OHS may be sufficient to cause marked increases in distal airway resistance. Airway resistance, increased by 133% in simple obesity, is increased by 650% in OHS.[134] In comparison to simple obesity, forced expiratory volume in 1 second (FEV_1) and the maximum expiratory flow rate and maximum voluntary ventilation are reduced by 40%[134] in OHS. Accompanying these physiologic changes are the mechanical disadvantages of an overstretched diaphragm. In combination, these factors may lead to chronic respiratory muscle fatigue and the chronic hypoventilation characteristic of OHS.[106] In addition, the reduced lung volume associated with OHS may further impair ventilation-perfusion matching and cause decreases in Pao_2 and increases in the A-a gradient greater than those of simple obesity. However, most of the reduction in Pao_2 in OHS patients is postulated as being due to alveolar hypoxia from hypercapnia.[106]

Especially in patients with OHS, the supine position further reduces lung volume and increases distal airway resistance.[116,131] Ferretti and associates[99] found that orthopnea in obese patients may be attributable to these physiologic causes. During the preoperative assessment, the extent of dyspnea that the patient experiences in the supine position may yield useful information.

In the perioperative setting, the reduction in chest wall and diaphragmatic muscle tone after induction of general anesthesia and skeletal muscle relaxation further impairs oxygenation. In simple obesity, the net effect may reduce ERV and FRC to less than 50% of preinduction values, thereby excluding even more alveoli from effective gas exchange.[131] In addition, reduction of ERV and FRC predisposes to atelectasis and limits effective clearance of secretions in the postoperative period.

ERV is the primary source of oxygen reserve during apnea. Therefore, in an obese patient, preoxygenation is less effective, and after apnea, the time to hemoglobin desaturation below 90% is reduced.[135,136] In an obese, anesthetized, relaxed patient, the combination of a reduced "apneic oxygenation reserve" and the likelihood of difficulty with positive-pressure mask ventilation amplifies the potential for a hypoxemic misadventure.[137,138] Elective awake tracheal intubation may be the safest approach if a patient scheduled for bariatric surgery has signs indicating a potential for difficult intubation, such as poor visualization of the posterior pharyngeal wall.[139] Positioning the patient with a roll under the scapulas and an occipital rest and asking the patient to fully extend at the atlanto-occipital joint before induction may facilitate awake or conventional laryngoscopy and intubation.

After major open abdominal surgery and without postoperative oxygen supplementation, even normal patients experience hypoxemia (Spo_2 <90%) that persists several days and is most prevalent and severe on the night of the second postoperative day.[140] On the first postoperative day after open bariatric surgery, 75% of obese patients had a Pao_2 less than 60 mm Hg; Pao_2 averaged 14 mm Hg less than preoperative baseline measurements.[141] Although some improvement was seen, oxygenation remained significantly less than baseline during the subsequent postoperative days. These facts emphasize the importance of obtaining a preoperative assessment of baseline oxygenation (by pulse oximetry) and preparing for specific treatments should preoperative values minus 14 mm Hg be hazardous.

More extensive pulmonary function tests and preoperative treatment of any treatable abnormality (e.g., infectious and bronchospastic components of pulmonary disease) may be indicated for obese patients who smoke or have pulmonary symptoms (e.g., chronic cough, sputum production, wheezing, shortness of breath at rest or on minor exertion). Such evaluation may be indicated even for laparoscopic bariatric surgery. Although laparoscopic bariatric surgery may have fewer adverse effects on postoperative pulmonary gas exchange and require less postoperative analgesia, there is always the potential that the surgeon will need to convert to an "open" procedure. However, if an open procedure is likely and the obesity is severe, ABGs might also be analyzed to quantitate the degree of hypoventilation and aid in assessing the most appropriate time to extubate the trachea.

Postoperative continuous oxygen supplementation and maintenance of the semirecumbent or upright posture[142] might be a prudent strategy for all bariatric surgery patients. However, oxygen therapy alone may not be adequate, as determined by coexisting OSA, COPD, or OHS; postoperative opioid analgesic needs; and preexisting hypoxemia or orthopnea. If a need for opioid analgesics is anticipated in obese patients with OSA, OHS, COPD, the baseline Spo_2 is less than 96%, or a history of orthopnea is elicited, postoperative CPAP or BiPAP therapy might be useful.

Nasal CPAP, a treatment of OSA since 1981, acts by "splinting" the airway during inspiration.[143] Given a patient compliance rate of 50% to 80%, it may be prudent to question whether the patient will accept this nocturnal therapy.[143] In normal-weight patients undergoing major abdominal surgery, nasal CPAP plus supplemental oxygen was not shown to decrease hypoxemic events the first postoperative night.[144] However, in surgical patients with OSA, postoperative nasal CPAP therapy has been shown to prevent episodic apneic events associated with fluctuations in BP.[145]

BiPAP, a more recent refinement of respiratory therapy, combines CPAP with additional inspiratory pressure support. Prophylactic BiPAP (12 cm H_2O inspiratory pressure, 4 cm H_2O expiratory pressure) during the first 24 to 48 hours after bariatric surgery significantly improved forced vital capacity (FVC), FEV_1, and oxygenation as reflected by continuous SpO_2 monitoring.[146,147] The improvement in lung volume persisted for several days and led to quicker recovery to baseline spirometric volumes; however, the complication rate and length of postoperative stay were not shown to be altered by this therapy.

It is unclear whether it is appropriate to delay bariatric surgery for aggressive optimization of airway status and oxygenation with CPAP or BiPAP therapy. Rennotte and colleagues[148] did not observe any major postoperative respiratory complications in 14 patients treated with nasal CPAP for up to 3 weeks before surgery, but without a prospective control group, it could not be determined whether complications would have occurred without such preparation. Two to three weeks may be necessary to not only maximize medical benefits but also allow sufficient time for patients unfamiliar with CPAP or BiPAP therapy to acclimate to nocturnal use of the device. Three weeks of nightly CPAP treatment before bariatric surgery improved the left ventricular ejection fraction and afterload in obese patients with coexisting heart failure.[149] Eight weeks of preoperative nasal CPAP therapy may be required to treat hypertension secondary to OSA.[150] After surgery, treatment should be applied as early as possible after extubation.[129]

Cardiopulmonary Evaluation of Obese Patients

EVALUATION AND PREVENTION OF VENOUS STASIS AND THROMBOEMBOLISM. Although assessment of venous status might seem strange as the first priority on cardiovascular evaluation, its importance and prominence become obvious when one looks at mortality data. Venous emboli that enter the pulmonary circulation are the major source of pulmonary dysfunction leading to the 1% to 2% 30-day mortality rate. Most mortality in the 30-day perioperative period after bariatric surgery is due to pulmonary embolism (this cause of mortality is three or more times more frequent than anastomotic leak with subsequent sepsis). Various drug regimens to decrease the thrombotic tendency have been attempted, but there is no agreement. The use of low-molecular-weight heparin might limit postoperative pain therapy options, and preoperative administration of aspirin and subsequent warfarin (Coumadin) to an international normalized ratio (INR) of 2.3 might be the current treatment of choice. The use of warfarin, a vitamin K antagonist, can be problematic postoperatively inasmuch as most patients after Roux-en-Y gastrojejunostomy malabsorb fat and fat-soluble substances, including vitamin K. This malabsorption makes the dose of warfarin difficult to control, and daily adjustment will often be required for at least a few weeks. Nevertheless, preoperative evaluation for venous stasis is difficult; many surgeons insist on preoperative exercise for at least an hour of walking or bicycle exercise 3 days a week for 6 weeks and the absence of leg symptoms (pain, soreness, or redness). Other surgeons or groups require 30 minutes of walking each day (see later for psychological factors that determine success). Factors that decrease the risk for venous stasis in multiple patients include preoperative exercise and antithrombotic drug and perhaps stocking prophylaxis, nonpolycythemic hematocrit, increased cardiac output, and early ambulation. Thus, evaluation of exercise status and drug therapy, absence of preexisting venous disease or signs or symptoms of venous disease, optimal hydration, and perioperative drug therapy all aimed at early ambulation might be the goals of this area of evaluation and prophylaxis. However, whatever is done, it should be remembered that this area is the major determinant of perioperative survival.

CARDIOVASCULAR EVALUATION OF OBESE PATIENTS. Cardiac output must increase approximately 0.01 L/min to perfuse each kilogram of adipose tissue. As a result, obese patients often have hypertension, which can cause cardiomegaly and left ventricular failure. Care should be taken to use a BP cuff of correct size when quantitating the degree of hypertension present.

The obese may have limited cardiac reserve and poor tolerance for stress induced by hypotension, hypertension, tachycardia, or fluid overload associated with the preoperative and preprocedure period. Massively obese patients with carbon dioxide retention are called pickwickian, alveolar hypoventilation being the hallmark of this condition. Other components of the pickwickian syndrome are somnolence, hypoxemia, failure of the right side of the heart, and secondary polycythemia. Many of these patients have right ventricular failure (also see Chapter 32 for monitoring considerations). Thus, preoperative and preprocedure assessment should include not only history taking and physical examination with an emphasis on drug therapy and cardiopulmonary problems, but also an ECG examination looking specifically for left or right ventricular hypertrophy, ischemia, and conduction defects.

Obese persons may metabolize lipophilic drugs to a greater degree (and for longer periods) than their thin counterparts. More fluorine is produced from enflurane given to obese patients than to thin ones. One would assume that responses to drugs stored in fat (e.g., narcotics, barbiturates, volatile anesthetics) would be prolonged in the obese. There is no evidence, however, that use of the more soluble anesthetics delays recovery time in obese subjects. The dose requirements of pharmacologic drugs used for analgesia and airway management are also altered by significant overweight status (BMI >27.5). Increased body fat increases the volume of distribution of sufentanil and slows its elimination. In one study, the elimination half-life of sufentanil was 208 minutes for eight obese patients (mean weight, 94 kg) versus 135 minutes for eight controls (mean weight, 70 kg).[151] Similarly, muscle relaxants that depend on hepatic blood flow for elimination (i.e., pancuronium, vecuronium, and rocuronium) appear to have dosage requirements that are directly proportional to body surface area, as well as longer twitch recovery times. The 25% to 75% twitch recovery time for vecuronium was 38.4 minutes for obese patients (mean weight, 93 kg) versus 17.6 minutes for nonobese patients (mean weight, 61 kg).[152]

The anesthesiologist should also be aware of conditions caused by remedies other than bariatric surgery used to treat obesity.[153] Drastic dieting can produce acidosis, hypokalemia, and hyperuricemia; protein hydrolysate liquid diets are associated with intractable ventricular arrhythmias.[154] These problems seem to have disappeared as diets have changed from hydrolyzed collagen fasts to the currently used very-low-calorie diet.

Drug treatment of obesity also has implications for the anesthesiologist. Amphetamines (and probably mazindol) given *acutely* increase anesthetic requirements; by contrast, amphetamines administered *chronically* decrease anesthetic requirements (see the section on chronic drug therapy). Amphetamines may interfere with the action of vasoactive drugs given to treat hypotension or hypertension.

Because many obese patients have tried drug therapies, the anesthesiologist should consider asking questions about the use of adjuvants. If such drugs have been used, the anesthesiologist might consider auscultation and echocardiography to search for mitral valve regurgitant lesions because some dietary aids of the past (notably "phen-fen") have been associated with these conditions. Other dietary herbs are also known to cause liver dysfunction, so searching for the use of these adjuvants may be important. Fenfluramine (a drug that inhibits the serotonergic system) by itself may decrease both anesthetic requirements and BP.

Psychiatric Considerations
Psychological evaluation is crucial for patient success after bariatric surgery. The year after surgery is not easy, let alone the week after. The patient must be sapient and engaged and must be able to have the discipline to keep a food diary. The evaluation of the anesthesiologist can provide valuable clues—has the patient been walking daily, for example. The patient needs to be emotionally stable. Choices that the anesthesiologist can uncover that correlate with failure are street drug abuse, unaddressed major psychiatric disorders/illness, compulsive eating disorder, and the diagnosis of fibromyalgia or chronic fatigue syndrome. If such are searched for and found on preoperative evaluation, communication among all, including the surgeon, can spare the health care team much frustration and save the patient much distress.

Musculoskeletal Concerns, Evaluation for Positioning, and Other Issues
Other features of obesity are of prognostic and perioperative importance to the anesthesiologist as well. Because of excessive and extensive subcutaneous fat and large size of the extremities, proper positioning of the patient, placement of monitoring devices, and establishment of intravenous sites are more difficult to accomplish, and BP (and the choice of cuff size) is less easy to ascertain than for patients of normal weight.

Preoperative consideration of the positioning of obese patients may eliminate some postoperative problems. In a retrospective study, Warner and colleagues[155] found that patients whose BMI was greater than 38 kg/m² had a 29% incidence of postoperative ulnar neuropathy versus a 1% incidence in controls. Upper brachial plexus root injury may result from extreme rotation of the head and cervical spine to the opposite side.[156] Lower root injury may result from hyperabduction of the arm on the same side as the injury. Preoperatively, one may assess sites vulnerable to pressure injury. Intraoperatively, pressure

point checks and repositioning periodically make good sense.

Preoperative evaluation of the deep venous system of the legs is difficult in the obese. (Even more sponges and instruments are left in the obese.) Routine prophylaxis for deep venous thrombosis is commonly initiated preoperatively, a prudent practice given that obesity is a major risk factor for sudden postoperative death from massive pulmonary thromboembolism. Anticoagulant prophylaxis is likely to be ordered by the surgeon, and such therapy must be considered if a central neuraxial catheter is to be inserted and used for postoperative analgesia. Furthermore, the incidence of wound infection, deep vein thrombosis, and pulmonary embolism is increased; the latter two should probably be guarded against with subcutaneous heparin and early ambulation. Thus, a knowledge of or discussion with the specific surgeon of preferences for postoperative prophylaxis of deep vein thrombosis and its consequences and preparation of the patient for this plan may be an important aspect of the preoperative meeting of the anesthesiologist and patient.

Anorexia Nervosa, Bulimia, and Starvation
Many endocrine and metabolic abnormalities occur in patients with anorexia nervosa, a condition characterized by starvation to the point of 40% loss of normal weight, hyperactivity, and a psychiatrically distorted body image. Many anorectic patients exhibit impulsive behavior, including suicide attempts, and intravenous drug use is much more common than in the general population. Acidosis, hypokalemia, hypocalcemia, hypomagnesemia, hypothermia, diabetes insipidus, and severe endocrine abnormalities mimicking panhypopituitarism need attention before anesthesia and surgery. Similar problems occur in bulimia (bulimorexia), a condition that may affect as many as 50% of female college students[157] and is even unintentionally present in many elderly.[158] As in severe protein deficiency (kwashiorkor), anorexia nervosa and bulimia may be accompanied by ECG alterations, including a prolonged QT interval, atrioventricular (AV) block, and other arrhythmias; sensitivity to epinephrine; and cardiomyopathy.[157,159] Total depletion of body potassium makes the addition of potassium to glucose solutions useful; however, fluid administration can precipitate pulmonary edema in these patients. Esophagitis, pancreatitis, and aspiration pneumonia are more frequent in these patients, as is delayed gastric emptying. Thus, invasive monitoring (radial artery and pulmonary artery catheterization) may be indicated for anorectic, bulimic, and malnurtured patients requiring emergency surgery. Elective surgery should probably be delayed until the abnormalities are treated.

Hyperalimentation (Total Parenteral or Enteral Nutrition) (also see Chapter 77)

Hyperalimentation (i.e., total parenteral nutrition [TPN]) consists of concentrating hypertonic glucose calories in the normal daily fluid requirements. The solutions contain protein hydrolysates, soybean emulsions (i.e., Intralipid), or synthetic amino acids. The major benefits of TPN or enteral nutrition have been fewer complications postoperatively and shorter hospital stays for patients scheduled to have no oral feeding for 7 days or who were malnourished preoperatively.[160,161] Starker and colleagues[162] found that the response to TPN, as monitored by serum albumin levels, predicted the postoperative outcome.[163] The group demonstrating a rise in serum albumin with TPN had diuresis, weight loss, and fewer complications (1 of 15 patients) than did the group that gained weight and had a decrease in serum albumin (8 of 16 patients had 15 complications) (Fig. 27-6). These data are echoed by those in the Veterans Administration (VA) studies, which reported that the serum albumin level was one of the most powerful predictors of perioperative outcome.[160,161]

The major complications of hyperalimentation are sepsis and metabolic abnormalities. The central lines used for TPN require application with an absolutely aseptic technique and should not be used routinely as an intravenous route for drug administration. Major metabolic complications of TPN relate to deficiencies and the development of hyperosmolar states. Complications of hypertonic dextrose can develop if the patient has insufficient insulin (diabetes mellitus) to metabolize the sugar or if insulin resistance occurs (e.g., because of uremia, burns, or sepsis).[160]

A gradual decrease in the infusion rate of TPN prevents the hypoglycemia that can occur on abrupt discontinuance. Thus, the infusion rate of TPN should be decreased the night before anesthesia and surgery or be continued throughout the operation at its current rate. The main reason for slowing or discontinuing TPN before anesthesia is to avoid intraoperative hyperosmolarity secondary to accidental rapid infusion of the solution or hypoglycemia

if the infusion is discontinued because of the high levels of endogenous insulin and lower levels of glucose present in the usual crystalloid solutions.[160] Hypophosphatemia is a particularly serious complication that results from the administration of phosphate-free or phosphate-depleted solutions for hyperalimentation. The low serum phosphate level causes a shift of the oxygen dissociation curve to the left. The resulting low 2,3-diphosphoglycerate and adenosine triphosphatase levels mean that cardiac output must increase for oxygen delivery to remain the same. Hypophosphatemia of less than 1.0 mg/dL of blood may cause hemolytic anemia, cardiac failure, tachypnea, neurologic symptoms, seizures, and death. In addition, long-term TPN is associated with deficiencies in trace metals such as copper (refractory anemia), zinc (impaired wound healing), and magnesium.

For these reasons, we have adopted the following practices.[160] Infusion of TPN or enteral nutrition is reduced beginning the night before surgery, and a 5% or 10% dextrose solution is substituted preoperatively. If serum glucose phosphate and potassium concentrations (measured preoperatively) are abnormal, they are restored to within normal limits. Strict asepsis is maintained. Conversely, we often continue infusing the TPN solution by using a pump system or enteral nutrition, strictly maintaining its normal rate and asepsis, administering all fluids through a different intravenous site, and performing a rapid-sequence induction of anesthesia (for those who received enteral nutrition).

Adrenocortical Malfunction*

Three major classes of hormones—androgens, glucocorticoids, and mineralocorticoids—are secreted by the adrenal cortex.[163,154] For each class, an excess or a deficiency of hormone produces a characteristic clinical syndrome. The widespread use of steroids can also make the adrenal cortex unable to respond normally to the demands placed on it by surgical trauma and subsequent healing.[165-174] The increase in unindicated (scanning) computed tomographic (CT) abdominal imaging procedures has meant that many adrenal masses have unfortunately been discovered only incidentally.[175-178] Several points relative to adrenal cortical management deserve attention:

Controlled comparisons of perioperative management for patients who have disorders of adrenal function are lacking, although we use steroids more and more commonly, with the results of some controlled trials available for specific uses.[163,179] However, a review of the possible pathophysiologic changes in the adrenal cortex and techniques for their management should enable us to improve the perioperative care of patients with adrenal abnormalities.

Physiologic Properties of Adrenocortical Hormones
Androgens
Androstenedione and dehydroepiandrosterone, weak androgens arising from the adrenal cortex,[180] constitute major sources of androgen in women (and have gained

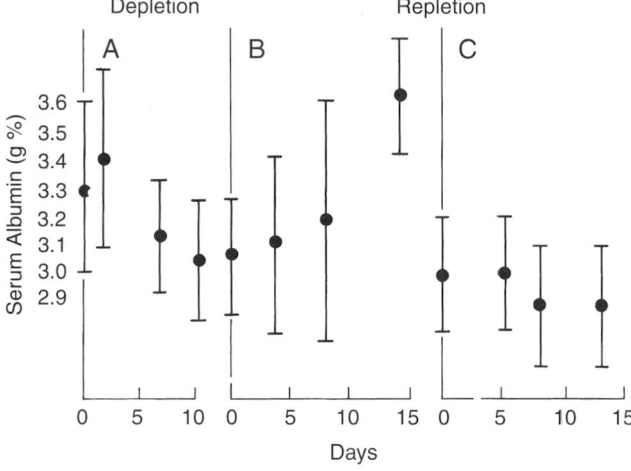

Figure 27–6 A-C, The response to hyperalimentation (repletion), as measured by variation in serum albumin levels, predicted the outcome of surgery. Patients who responded (**B**) to nutritional support with increased albumin levels had a significantly better outcome than did those whose albumin level did not increase (**C**). See the text for a more complete explanation. (Adapted from Starker PM, Group FE, Askanazi J, et al: Serum albumin levels as an index of nutritional support. Surgery 91:194, 1982.)

---

*Much of this section of the chapter is modified from Lampe and Roizen,[163] with permission.

prominence for their use or abuse by baseball players seeking to hit more home runs). Excess secretion of androgen causes masculinization, pseudopuberty, or female pseudohermaphroditism. With some tumors, androgen is converted to an estrogenic substance, in which case feminization results.[180] No special anesthetic evaluation is needed for such patients. Some congenital enzyme defects that cause androgen abnormalities also result in glucocorticoid and mineralocorticoid abnormalities that should be evaluated before surgery.[180] Most of these patients are treated with exogenous glucocorticoids and mineralocorticoids and consequently require supplementation of these hormones perioperatively (see later).

Glucocorticoids

The principal glucocorticoid, cortisol, is an essential regulator of carbohydrate, protein, lipid, and nucleic acid metabolism. Cortisol is believed to exert its biologic effects through a sequence of steps initiated by binding of hormone to stereospecific intracellular cytoplasmic receptors. This bound complex stimulates nuclear transcription of specific mRNAs. These mRNAs are then translated to give rise to proteins that mediate the ultimate effects of hormones.

Most cortisol is bound to corticosterone-binding globulin (CBG, transcortin). It is the relatively small amounts of unbound cortisol that enter cells to induce actions or to be metabolized. Conditions that induce changes in the amount of CBG include liver disease and nephrotic syndrome, both of which result in decreased circulating levels of CBG, and estrogen administration and pregnancy, which result in increased CBG production. Total serum cortisol levels may become elevated or depressed under conditions that alter the amount of bound cortisol, and yet the unbound, active form of cortisol is present in normal amounts. The most accurate measure of cortisol activity is the level of urinary cortisol—that is, the amount of unbound, active cortisol filtered by the kidney.

The serum half-life of cortisol is 80 to 110 minutes.[171] However, because cortisol acts through intracellular receptors, pharmacokinetic data based on serum levels are not good indicators of cortisol activity. After a single dose of glucocorticoid, serum glucose is elevated for 12 to 24 hours; improvement in pulmonary function in patients with bronchial asthma can still be measured 24 hours after glucocorticoid administration.[171] Treatment schedules for glucocorticoid replacement are therefore based not on the measured serum half-life but on the well-documented prolonged end-organ effect of these steroids. Hospitalized patients requiring chronic glucocorticoid replacement therapy are usually treated twice daily, with a slightly higher dose given in the morning than in the evening to simulate the normal diurnal variation in cortisol levels.[163] For patients who require parenteral "steroid coverage" during and after surgery (see later paragraphs), administration of glucocorticoid every 12 hours is appropriate.[169,170] The relative potencies of glucocorticoids are listed in Table 27-8. Cortisol is inactivated primarily in the liver and is excreted as 17-hydroxycorticosteroid. Cortisol is also filtered and excreted unchanged into urine.

The synthetic glucocorticoids vary in their binding specificity in a dose-related manner. When given in supraphysiologic doses (more than 30 mg/day), cortisol and cortisone bind to mineralocorticoid receptor sites and cause salt and water retention and loss of potassium and hydrogen ions.[171] When these steroids are administered in maintenance doses of 30 mg/day or less, patients require a specific mineralocorticoid for electrolyte and volume homeostasis.[171] Many other steroids do not bind to mineralocorticoid receptors, even at high doses, and have no mineralocorticoid effect[171] (see Table 27-8).

Secretion of glucocorticoids is regulated by pituitary adrenocorticotropic hormone (ACTH). ACTH is synthesized from a precursor molecule (pro-opiomelanocortin) that is metabolized to form an endorphin (β-lipotropin) and ACTH. Episodic secretion of ACTH has a diurnal rhythm that is normally greatest during the early morning hours in men, later in women, and is regulated at least in part by light-dark cycles. Its secretion is stimulated by release of corticotropin-releasing factor (CRF) from the hypothalamus. (An abnormality in the diurnal rhythm of corticoid secretion has been implicated as a cause of so-called jet lag.) Cortisol and other glucocorticoids exert negative feedback at both the pituitary and hypothalamic levels to inhibit the secretion of ACTH and CRF. If one destroys the CRF- or ACTH-producing cells, the adrenal takes more than 30 days to atrophy to the point where acute administration of exogenous ACTH will cause almost no adrenal responsiveness.

Mineralocorticoids

Aldosterone, the major mineralocorticoid secreted in humans, comes from the zona glomerulosa of the adrenal cortex and causes reabsorption of sodium and secretion of potassium and hydrogen ions, thereby contributing to electrolyte and volume homeostasis.[181] This action is most prominent in the distal renal tubule but also occurs in the salivary and sweat glands. The major regulator of aldosterone secretion is the renin-angiotensin system. Juxtaglomerular cells in the cuff of the renal arterioles are sensitive to decreased renal perfusion pressure or volume

Table 27–8 Relative potency and equivalent doses for commonly used glucocorticoids

Steroids	Relative Glucocorticoid Potency	Equivalent Glucocorticoid Dose (mg)
Short Acting		
Cortisol (hydrocortisone)	1.0	20.0
Cortisone	0.8	25.0
Prednisone	4.0	5.0
Prednisolone	4.0	5.0
Methylprednisolone	5.0	4.0
Intermediate Acting		
Triamcinolone	5.0	4.0
Long Acting		
Betamethasone	25.0	0.60
Dexamethasone	30.0	0.75

Data from Axelrod L: Glucocorticoid therapy. Medicine (Baltimore) 55:39, 1976.

and, consequently, secrete renin.[181] Renin splits the precursor angiotensinogen (from the liver) into angiotensin I, which is further converted by a converting enzyme, primarily in the lung, to angiotensin II. Angiotensin II binds to specific receptors to increase mineralocorticoid secretion, which is also stimulated by an increased potassium concentration and, to a lesser degree, by ACTH.[181]

Adrenocortical Hormone Excess

Glucocorticoid Excess

Glucocorticoid excess (Cushing's syndrome) resulting from either endogenous oversecretion or chronic treatment with higher than physiologic-dose glucocorticoids produces a moon-faced plethoric individual with a centripetal distribution of fat (truncal obesity and skinny extremities), thin skin, easy bruising, and striae. Muscle wasting is common, but the heart and diaphragm are usually spared. A test for this syndrome is to ask the patient to get up from a chair without using the hands. An inability to do so indicates proximal muscle weakness consistent with Cushing's syndrome. These patients often have osteopenia as a result of decreased formation of bone matrix and impaired absorption of calcium. Fluid retention and hypertension (because of increases in renin substrate and vascular reactivity caused by glucocorticoid) are common. Such patients may also have hyperglycemia and even diabetes mellitus from inhibition of peripheral use of glucose, as well as anti-insulin action and concomitant stimulation of gluconeogenesis (Table 27-9).

The most common cause of Cushing's syndrome is the administration of glucocorticoids for such conditions as arthritis, asthma, and allergies.[163] In these conditions, the adrenal glands atrophy and cannot respond to stressful situations (e.g., the preoperative and preprocedure period) by secreting more steroid. Thus, additional glucocorticoids may be required perioperatively (see the later section "Patients Taking Steroids for Other Reasons"). Spontaneous Cushing's syndrome may be caused by pituitary production of ACTH (65% to 75% of all spontaneous cases), which is usually associated with pituitary microadenoma, or by nonendocrine ectopic ACTH production (principally by tumors of the lung, pancreas, or thymus).[182] Ten percent to 20% of cases of spontaneous Cushing's syndrome are caused by an ACTH-independent process, either an adrenal adenoma or carcinoma.

Special preoperative and preprocedure considerations for patients with Cushing's syndrome include regulating diabetes and hypertension and ensuring that intravascular fluid volume and electrolyte concentrations are normal. Ectopic ACTH production may cause marked hypokalemic alkalosis.[163] Treatment with the aldosterone antagonist spironolactone will stop the potassium loss and help mobilize excess fluid. Because of the high incidence of severe osteopenia and the risk of fractures, meticulous attention must be paid to positioning of the patient.[163] In addition, glucocorticoids are lympholytic and immunosuppressive and thus increase the patient's susceptibility to infection.[183] The tensile strength of healing wounds decreases in the presence of glucocorticoids, an effect that is at least partially reversed by the topical administration of vitamin A.[184]

Specific considerations pertain to the surgical approach for each cause of Cushing's syndrome. For example, nearly three fourths of cases of spontaneous Cushing's disease result from a pituitary adenoma that secretes ACTH. Our perioperative treatment of patients who have Cushing's disease and a pituitary microadenoma differs from that of patients who have a pituitary adenoma associated with amenorrhea and galactorrhea. A patient with Cushing's disease is inclined to bleed more easily and (on the basis of anecdotal evidence) tends to have higher central venous pressure (CVP). Thus, during transsphenoidal tumor resection in such patients, we routinely monitor CVP and maintain it in the low end of the normal range. In other cases of transsphenoidal resection of microadenoma, such monitoring is needed only infrequently.

Ten percent to 15% of patients with Cushing's syndrome exhibit adrenal overproduction of glucocorticoids from an adrenal adenoma or carcinoma.[163] If either unilateral or bilateral adrenal resection is planned, we normally begin administering glucocorticoids at the start of resectioning of the tumor. Despite the absence of definitive studies, we normally give 100 mg of hydrocortisone hemisuccinate or hydrocortisone phosphate every 24 hours intravenously. We reduce this amount over a period of 3 to 6 days until a maintenance dose is reached. Beginning on day 3, the surgeons that we have worked with most also give a mineralocorticoid, 9α-fluorocortisol (0.05 to 0.1 mg/day). In certain patients, both steroids may require several adjustments. This therapy continues if the patient has undergone bilateral resection. For a patient who has undergone unilateral adrenal resection, therapy is individualized according to the status of the remaining adrenal gland. The incidence of pneumothorax in open adrenal resection approaches 20%; the diagnosis of pneumothorax

Table 27–9 Clinical features of hyperadrenalism (Cushing's syndrome) and hypoadrenalism

Cushing's Syndrome	Hypoadrenalism
Central obesity	Weight loss
Proximal muscle weakness	Weakness, fatigue, lethargy
Osteopenia at a young age and back pain	Muscle and joint pain
Hypertension	Postural hypotension and dizziness
Headache	Headache
Psychiatric disorders	Anorexia, nausea, abdominal pain, constipation, diarrhea
Purple stria	
Spontaneous ecchymoses	
Plethoric facies	
Hyperpigmentation	Hyperpigmentation
Hirsutism	
Acne	
Hypokalemic alkalosis	Hyperkalemia, hyponatremia
Glucose intolerance	Occasional hypoglycemia
Kidney stones	Hypercalcemia
Polyuria	Prerenal azotemia
Menstrual disorders	
Increased leukocyte count	

is sought and treatment is begun before the wound is closed.

Bilateral adrenalectomy in patients with Cushing's syndrome is associated with a high incidence of postoperative complications and a perioperative mortality rate of 5% to 10%; it often results in permanent mineralocorticoid and glucocorticoid deficiency. Ten percent of patients with Cushing's syndrome who undergo adrenalectomy have an undiagnosed pituitary tumor. After reduction of high levels of cortisol by adrenalectomy, the pituitary tumor enlarges. These pituitary tumors are potentially invasive and may produce large amounts of ACTH and melanocyte-stimulating hormone, thereby increasing pigmentation.

Adrenal tumors are at least 85% incidentalomas—that is, discovered incidentally during screening (and largely unindicated) CT scans. Nonfunctioning adrenal adenomas are found in up to 10% of patients on autopsy.[178] Functioning adenomas are generally treated surgically; often, the contralateral gland resumes functioning after several months. Frequently, however, the effects of carcinomas are not cured by surgery. In such cases, administration of inhibitors of steroid synthesis, such as metyrapone or mitotane (o,p'-DDD[2,2-bis(2-chlorophenyl-4-chlorophenyl)-1,1-dichloroethane]), may ameliorate some symptoms but may not improve survival. These drugs and the aldosterone antagonist spironolactone may aid in reducing symptoms in the case of ectopic ACTH secretion if the primary tumor proves unresectable. Patients given these adrenal suppressants are also prescribed chronic glucocorticoid replacement therapy (i.e., the goal of therapy is complete adrenal suppression). These patients should be considered to have suppressed adrenal function, and glucocorticoid replacement should be increased perioperatively.

Mineralocorticoid Excess

Excess mineralocorticoid activity (common with glucocorticoid excess because most glucocorticoids have some mineralocorticoid properties) leads to potassium depletion, sodium retention, muscle weakness, hypertension, tetany, polyuria, inability to concentrate urine, and hypokalemic alkalosis.[185] These symptoms constitute primary hyperaldosteronism, or Conn's syndrome (a cause of low-renin hypertension because renin secretion is inhibited by the effects of the high levels of aldosterone).

Primary hyperaldosteronism is present in 0.5% to 1% of hypertensive patients who have no other known cause of hypertension.[185] Primary hyperaldosteronism most often results from unilateral adenoma, although 25% to 40% of patients have been found to have bilateral adrenal hyperplasia. Intravascular fluid volume, electrolyte concentrations, and renal function should be restored to within normal limits preoperatively by administering the aldosterone antagonist spironolactone. The effects of spironolactone are slow in onset and increase for 1 to 2 weeks.[185] A patient who has a serum potassium level of 2.9 mEq/L may have a total-body potassium deficit of as little as 40 mEq or as much as 400 mEq. Frequently, at least 24 hours is required to restore potassium equilibrium.[186-188] A normal serum potassium level does not necessarily imply correction of a total-body deficit of potassium.

In addition, patients with Conn's syndrome have a high incidence of hypertension and ischemic heart disease; hemodynamic monitoring should be appropriate for the degree of cardiovascular impairment.[189] A retrospective anecdotal study indicated that the intraoperative hemodynamic status was more stable when BP and electrolytes were controlled preoperatively with spironolactone than when other antihypertensive drugs were used.[164] However, the efficacy of optimizing the perioperative status of patients who have disorders of glucocorticoid or mineralocorticoid secretion has not been clearly established. We have assumed that gradual restoration of a normal condition is good medicine and that it would decrease perioperative morbidity and mortality.

Adrenocortical Hormone Deficiency

Glucocorticoid Deficiency

Withdrawal of steroids or suppression of synthesis by steroid therapy is the leading cause of underproduction of corticosteroids.[163] Management of this type of glucocorticoid deficiency is discussed in the later section "Patients Taking Steroids for Other Reasons." Other causes of adrenocortical insufficiency include defects in ACTH secretion and destruction of the adrenal gland by autoimmune disease, tuberculosis, hemorrhage, or cancer; some forms of congenital adrenal hyperplasia (see previous discussion); and administration of cytotoxic drugs.

Primary adrenal insufficiency (Addison's disease) is associated with local destruction of all zones of the adrenal cortex and results in both glucocorticoid and mineralocorticoid deficiency if the insufficiency is bilateral; common symptoms and signs are listed in Table 27-9. Autoimmune disease is the most common cause of primary (nonexogenous) bilateral ACTH deficiency in the United States, whereas tuberculosis is the most common cause worldwide. Tuberculosis is associated with decreased adrenal function but large adrenal glands, as is also common in sarcoidosis, histoplasmosis, amyloidosis, metastatic malignancy, and adrenal hemorrhage. Destruction or partial destruction by trauma and by human immunodeficiency virus (HIV) and other infections such as cytomegalovirus, mycobacteria, and fungi is being recognized more frequently.

An increasingly common cause of adrenal insufficiency associated with large adrenal glands is heparin-induced thrombocytopenia, which might be considered in every patient who has received heparin and has hypotension.

Autoimmune destruction of the adrenals may be associated with other autoimmune disorders, such as some forms of type 1 diabetes and Hashimoto's thyroiditis. Enzymatic defects in cortisol synthesis also cause glucocorticoid insufficiency, compensatory elevations in ACTH, and congenital adrenal hyperplasia.[180] Because adrenal insufficiency usually develops slowly, such patients are subject to marked pigmentation (from excess ACTH trying to stimulate an unproductive adrenal gland) and cardiopenia (apparently secondary to chronic hypotension).[163]

Secondary adrenal insufficiency occurs when ACTH secretion is deficient, often because of a pituitary or hypothalamic tumor. Treatment of pituitary tumors by surgery or radiation may result in hypopituitarism and subsequent adrenal failure.[163]

If unstressed, glucocorticoid-deficient patients usually have no perioperative problems. However, acute adrenal crisis (addisonian crisis) can occur when even a minor stress is present (e.g., upper respiratory infection).[163,167,190] Preparation of such a patient for anesthesia and surgery should include treatment of hypovolemia, hyperkalemia, and hyponatremia.[173] Because these patients cannot respond to stressful situations, it was traditionally recommended that they be given a stress dose of glucocorticoids (about 200 mg hydrocortisone/70 kg body weight/day) perioperatively. However, Symreng and colleagues[169] gave 25 mg of hydrocortisone phosphate intravenously to adults at the start of the operative procedure, followed by 100 mg intravenously over the next 24 hours. Because using the minimum drug dose that would produce an appropriate effect is desirable, this latter regimen seems attractive. Such a regimen has proved to be as successful as a regimen using maximum doses (about 300 mg hydrocortisone per 70 kg body weight per day—see the later section "Patients Taking Steroids for Other Reasons"). Thus, we now recommend giving 100 mg of hydrocortisone phosphate intravenously every 24 hours.[169,170]

Mineralocorticoid Deficiency

Hypoaldosteronism, a less common condition,[191] can be congenital or can occur after unilateral adrenalectomy or prolonged administration of heparin. In addition, it can also be a consequence of long-standing diabetes and renal failure. Nonsteroidal inhibitors of prostaglandin synthesis may also inhibit renin release and exacerbate this condition in patients who have renal insufficiency.[191] Plasma renin activity is below normal and fails to increase appropriately in response to sodium restriction or diuretic drugs. Most symptoms are caused by hyperkalemic acidosis rather than hypovolemia; in fact, some patients are hypertensive. These patients can have severe hyperkalemia, hyponatremia, and myocardial conduction defects.[191] These defects can be treated successfully by administering mineralocorticoids (9α-fluorocortisol, 0.05 to 0.1 mg/day) preoperatively.[191] Doses must be carefully titrated and monitored to avoid an increase in hypertension.

Patients Taking Steroids for Other Reasons

Perioperative Stress and the Need for Corticoid Supplementation

Many experimental studies and other reports (mostly anecdotal) concerning the adrenal responses of normal patients to the perioperative period, as well as the responses of patients taking steroids for other diseases, indicate the following:

1. Perioperative stress is related to the degree of trauma and the depth of anesthesia. Deep general or regional anesthesia causes the usual intraoperative glucocorticoid surge to be postponed to the postoperative period.[192]
2. A few patients who have suppressed adrenal function will have perioperative cardiovascular problems if they do not receive supplemental steroids perioperatively.[166-174]
3. Although, on occasion, a patient who chronically takes steroids becomes hypotensive perioperatively, only rarely has this event been documented sufficiently to

implicate glucocorticoid or mineralocorticoid deficiency as the cause.[166-174]
4. Acute adrenal insufficiency occurs only rarely but can be life threatening.[166-174]
5. There is little risk in giving these patients steroid coverage equivalent to 100 mg of hydrocortisone hemisuccinate perioperatively.[163,169,170]

In a well-controlled study of glucocorticoid replacement in primates, the investigators clearly defined the life-threatening events that can be associated with inadequate perioperative corticosteroid replacement.[170] This study further defined the physiologic and hemodynamic consequences of inadequate cortisol replacement; an alternative dose regimen is suggested that has stood the test of a decade and has altered management methods to possibly improve patient safety. In this study, adrenalectomized primates and sham-operated controls were maintained on physiologic doses of steroids for 4 months. The animals were then randomly allocated to groups that received subphysiologic (one tenth the normal cortisol production), physiologic, or supraphysiologic (10 times the normal cortisol production) doses of cortisol for 4 days preceding abdominal surgery (cholecystectomy). Hemodynamic variables were measured by means of arterial and pulmonary artery catheters. The animals were maintained on their randomized dosage schedules during and after surgery. The group given subphysiologic doses of steroid perioperatively had a significant increase in postoperative mortality. Death rates for the physiologic and supraphysiologic replacement groups were the same and did not differ from the rate for sham-operated controls. Death in the subphysiologic replacement group was related to severe hypotension associated with a significant decrease in systemic vascular resistance and a reduced left ventricular stroke work index. Filling pressures of the heart were unchanged when compared with those in control animals. There was no evidence of hypovolemia or severe CHF. Despite the low systemic vascular resistance, the animals did not become tachycardic. All these responses are compatible with the previously documented interaction of glucocorticoids and catecholamines and thus suggest that glucocorticoids mediate catecholamine-induced increases in cardiac contractility and maintenance of vascular tone.

The investigators used a sensitive measure of wound healing involving hydroxyproline accumulation. All treatment groups, including the group given supraphysiologic doses of glucocorticoids, had the same capacity for wound healing. Furthermore, perioperative administration of supraphysiologic doses of corticosteroids produced no adverse metabolic consequences.

This well-conducted study confirms several long-standing intuitive impressions concerning patients who have inadequate adrenal function as a result of either underlying disease or administration of exogenous steroids. Inadequate replacement of corticosteroids perioperatively can lead to addisonian crisis and death. Administration of supraphysiologic doses of steroids for a short time perioperatively caused no discernible complications. However, at least theoretical negative consequences can occur when large doses of steroids are given (see later). It is clear that inadequate corticosteroid coverage can cause death. What is not so clear is what dose of steroid should be recommended for replacement therapy. The authors of the previously discussed study on monkeys were reluctant to recommend simple physiologic steroid replacement doses for human patients perioperatively.[170] We agree that a prospective, randomized double-blind trial in patients receiving physiologic doses of steroids is needed before current recommendations are modified.[169,170] In any case, we never supplement perioperatively with a dose lower than what the patient has already been receiving.[171]

Which patients definitely need supplementation? If in doubt, how can a patient's need for glucocorticoid supplementation be determined? Because the risk is low, we normally provide supplementation for any patient who has received steroids within a year.[165,166,169-174,180-182,184] Data indicate that topical application of steroids (even without the use of occlusive dressings) can suppress normal adrenal responses for as long as 9 months to 1 year[165,171] (Table 27-10).

How can one determine when adrenal responsiveness has returned to normal? The morning plasma cortisol level does not reveal whether the adrenal cortex has recovered sufficiently to ensure that cortisol secretion will increase adequately to meet the demands of stress. Inducing hypoglycemia with insulin has been advocated as a sensitive test of pituitary-adrenal competence but is impractical and probably a more dangerous practice than simply administering glucocorticoids. If the plasma cortisol concentration is measured during acute stress, a value of more than 25 µg/dL assuredly (and a value >15 µg/dL probably) indicates normal pituitary-adrenal responsiveness. In another test of pituitary-adrenal sufficiency, the baseline plasma cortisol level is determined. Then, 250 µg of synthetic ACTH (cosyntropin) is given, and plasma cortisol is measured 30 to 60 minutes later.[172] An increase in plasma cortisol of 6 to 20 µg/dL or more is normal.[193] A normal response indicates recovery of pituitary-adrenal axis function. A lesser response usually indicates pituitary-adrenal insufficiency, possibly requiring perioperative supplementation with steroids.

Typically, laboratory data defining pituitary-adrenal adequacy are not available before surgery. However, rather than delay surgery or test most patients, we assume that any patient who has taken steroids at any time during the preceding year has suppressed pituitary-adrenal function and will require perioperative supplementation.

Under perioperative conditions, the adrenal glands secrete 116 to 185 mg of cortisol daily. Under maximum stress, they may secrete 200 to 500 mg/day. Good correlation exists between the severity and duration of the operation and the response of the adrenal gland. "Major surgery" would be represented by procedures such as colectomy and "minor surgery" by procedures such as herniorrhaphy. In one study of 20 patients during major surgery, the mean maximal concentration of cortisol in plasma was 47 µg/dL (range, 22 to 75 µg/dL). Values remained above 26 µg/dL for a maximum of 72 hours after surgery. During minor surgery, the mean maximal concentration of cortisol in plasma was 28 µg/dL (range, 10 to 44 µg/dL).

Although the precise amount required has not been established, we usually intravenously administer the maximum amount of glucocorticoid that the body manufactures in response to maximal stress (i.e., approximately 200 mg/day of hydrocortisone phosphate/70 kg body weight).[169,170,192] For minor surgical procedures, we usually give hydrocortisone phosphate intravenously, 100 mg/day/70 kg body weight. Unless infection or some other perioperative complication develops, we decrease this dose by approximately 25% per day until oral intake can be resumed. At this point, the usual maintenance dose of glucocorticoids can be administered.

Risks of Supplementation

Rare complications of perioperative steroid supplementation include aggravation of hypertension, fluid retention, inducement of stress ulcers, and psychiatric disturbances. Although data are not available to assess the incidence of the following risks, two common complications of short-term perioperative supplementation with glucocorticoids are described in the literature: abnormal wound healing and an increased rate of infections.[166,169-174,181-185] This evidence is inconclusive, however, because it relates to acute glucocorticoid administration and not to chronic administration of glucocorticoids with increased doses at times of stress. Ehrlich and Hunt[184] found that moderate to large doses of steroids exert their morphologic effects best within 3 days of injury. They postulated that inhibition of the early inflammatory process by steroids after wounding was responsible for the delay in healing. Vitamin A was found to be somewhat protective against delayed healing, presumably because of its effect on

Table 27–10   Recovery of hypothalamic-pituitary adrenal function after withdrawal of steroids

Recovery Time (mo)	Plasma 17-Hydroxycorticoid Values	Plasma ACTH Values	Adrenal Response to Exogenous ACTH	Response to Metyrapone
1	Low*	Low	Low	Low
2-5	Low	High†	Low	Low
6-9	Normal	Normal	Low	Low
>9	Normal	Normal	Normal	Normal

*Various subjective manifestations of mild adrenal insufficiency occur during this stage.
†The diurnal rhythm of plasma concentrations is qualitatively normal during this stage.
ACTH, adrenocorticotropic hormone.
Data from Graber AL, Ney RI, Nicholson WE, et al: Natural history of pituitary-adrenal recovery following long-term suppression with corticosteroids. J Clin Endocrinol Metab 25:11, 1965.

stabilizing lysosomes.[184] In contrast to these studies that suggest a deleterious effect of perioperative glucocorticoid administration on wound healing in rats, a study involving primates suggests that high doses of glucocorticoids, administered perioperatively, do not impair sensitive measures of wound healing.[170] Other data provide no better insight into these problems.[166,169-174,181,182,184] These data are not conclusive regarding a short-term increase in supplementation. However, an overall assessment of these results suggests that short-term perioperative supplementation with steroids has a small, but definite deleterious effect on wound healing that is perhaps partially reversed by topical administration of vitamin A.

Information regarding the risk of infection from perioperative glucocorticoid supplementation is also unclear. Winstone and Brooke[194] reported 4 cases of septicemia in 18 surgical patients given perioperative glucocorticoid supplementation. No similar complications occurred in 17 others who were also taking glucocorticoids but who were not given perioperative supplementation. In other studies, no increased risk of serious infections was reported.[163] Data indicate that the risk of infection in a patient chronically taking steroids is real, but these data are inadequate to conclude that perioperative supplementation with steroids increases that risk.

Adrenal Cortex Function in the Elderly
(also see Chapter 62)
Production of androgens by the adrenal gland progressively decreases with age.[195] This decrease in androgen activity has no known implications for anesthesia. Plasma levels of cortisol are unaffected by increasing age. Levels of CBG are also unaffected by age, which suggests that a normal fraction of free cortisol (1% to 5%) is present in elderly patients. Several investigators have noted a progressively impaired ability of aged patients to metabolize and excrete glucocorticoids. In normal individuals, the quantity of 17-hydroxycorticosteroids excreted is reduced by half by the seventh decade. This decreased excretion undoubtedly reflects the reduced renal function that occurs with aging. When excretion of cortisol metabolites is expressed as a function of creatinine clearance, the age difference disappears. Further reductions in cortisol clearance may be due to impaired hepatic metabolism of circulating cortisol.

The rate of secretion of cortisol is 30% lower in the elderly. This reduced secretion is an appropriate compensatory mechanism for maintaining a normal level of cortisol in the face of decreased hepatic and renal clearance of cortisol. It is important to the anesthesiologist that the reduced cortisol production can be overcome during periods of stress and that the elderly display an entirely normal adrenal response to the administration of ACTH and to stresses such as hypoglycemia.

Both underproduction and overproduction of glucocorticoids are generally considered diseases of younger individuals. The highest incidence of Cushing's disease of either pituitary or adrenal origin occurs during the third decade of life. The most common cause of spontaneous Cushing's disease is benign pituitary adenoma.[182] However, in patients older than 60 years in whom Cushing's disease develops, the most likely cause is adrenal carcinoma

or ectopic ACTH production from tumors usually located in the lung, pancreas, or thymus.

Effect of Etomidate on Adrenal Function
(also see Chapter 10)
Even a single dose of etomidate for induction of anesthesia suppresses adrenal function.[196] The clinical significance of adrenal suppression by etomidate is unknown, but there is justifiable concern over the continued use of etomidate without steroid supplementation.

Etomidate is an imidazole sedative-hypnotic that induces rapid loss of consciousness with minimal cardiovascular depression, even in compromised patients. Etomidate has been administered in two clinical settings—as a bolus for induction of anesthesia and as a continuous infusion for prolonged sedation in the ICU setting. The pattern of adrenal suppression appears to be related to dose and time and is associated with narcotic coadministration; it differs with the duration of administration and the absence of narcotic coadministration.[196]

In rats and humans, etomidate inhibits two essential adrenocortical enzymes, 11β-hydroxylase and cholesterol side chain cleavage enzyme.[196] We believe that it is important to clarify the difference between the adrenal suppression caused by etomidate and the stated goal of several anesthesiologists to provide stress-free anesthesia. It appears that providing a level of anesthesia that prevents grimacing, sweating, extreme elevations in BP and heart rate, and an outpouring of the neurohumoral mediators of stress is evidence that we have adequately depressed CNS function and protected our patients from some of the unwanted side effects of surgery. This goal is different from etomidate's inhibition of peripheral adrenocortical enzymes that occurs as an unwanted side effect of the drug when it is administered in combination with narcotics.

Thus, it has been documented that adrenal reserve is compromised for at least 24 hours after a single induction dose of etomidate in most patients.[197] Should hypotension or electrolyte abnormalities associated with adrenal insufficiency (hyponatremia and hyperkalemia) occur in a patient who has recently received etomidate, we agree with previous suggestions[196] that corticosteroids should be administered in stress doses (e.g., cortisol, 100 mg/day) and be tapered as noted in the earlier section "Patients Taking Steroids for Other Reasons."

Adrenal Incidentaloma
Adrenal tumors are found in as many as 10% of autopsies, and the increased use of imaging techniques brings many of these tumors to clinical attention before death. Previously, size was used as a discriminator: tumors larger than 6 cm were surgically removed because of the high probability of malignancy. Those smaller than 3 cm were monitored, and those 3 to 6 cm were investigated.

Recent data from three large series[175-178] and success from laparoscopic removal[198,199] have called for a re-evaluation. The three series found a significant number of adrenal carcinomas and pheochromocytomas (approximately 3% of each), an occasional aldosteronoma (approximately 1%), and a not insignificant number of metastases from as yet undiscovered primary tumors (approximately 10%). These data may indicate the need for a more aggressive approach to adrenal incidentalomas that are smaller than 6 cm.

Adrenal Medullary Sympathetic Hormone Excess: Pheochromocytoma

Less than 0.1% of all cases of hypertension are caused by pheochromocytomas, or catecholamine-producing tumors derived from chromaffin tissue.[200] Nevertheless, these tumors are clearly important to the anesthetist inasmuch as 25% to 50% of hospital deaths in patients with pheochromocytoma occur during induction of anesthesia or during operative procedures for other causes.[201] Though usually found in the adrenal medulla, these vascular tumors can occur anywhere, such as in the right atrium, the spleen, the broad ligament of the ovary, or the organs of Zuckerkandl at the bifurcation of the aorta.[202] Malignant spread, which occurs in less than 15% of pheochromocytomas, usually proceeds to venous and lymphatic channels with a predisposition for the liver. This tumor is occasionally familial or part of the pluriglandular-neoplastic syndrome known as multiple endocrine adenoma type IIa or type IIb and is manifested as an autosomal dominant trait. Type IIa consists of medullary carcinoma of the thyroid, parathyroid adenoma or hyperplasia, and pheochromocytoma. What used to be called type IIb is now often called pheochromocytoma in association with phakomatoses such as von Recklinghausen's neurofibromatosis and von Hippel-Lindau disease and cerebellar hemangioblastoma. Often, bilateral tumors are found in the familial form. Localization of tumors can be achieved by MRI or CT scans, metaiodobenzylguanidine (MIBG) nuclear scanning, ultrasonography, or intravenous pyelography studies (in decreasing order of combined sensitivity and specificity).

Symptoms and signs that may be solicited preoperatively and preprocedurely and that are suggestive of pheochromocytoma are excessive sweating; headache; hypertension; orthostatic hypotension; previous hypertensive or arrhythmic response to induction of anesthesia or to abdominal examination; paroxysmal attacks of sweating, headache, tachycardia, and hypertension; glucose intolerance; polycythemia; weight loss; and psychological abnormalities. In fact, the occurrence of combined symptoms of paroxysmal headache, sweating, and hypertension is probably a more sensitive and specific indicator than any one biochemical test for pheochromocytoma[200,202-205] (Table 27-11). Despite more than 2000 articles in the literature about pheochromocytoma, little is known about what factors in care affect perioperative morbidity.[206-209]

Although no controlled, randomized, prospective clinical studies have investigated the value of preoperative and preprocedure use of adrenergic receptor blocking drugs, the use of such drugs is generally recommended before surgery. These drugs probably reduce the complications of hypertensive crisis, the wide BP fluctuations during manipulation of the tumor (especially until venous drainage is obliterated), and the myocardial dysfunction that occurs perioperatively. A reduction in mortality associated with resection of pheochromocytoma (from 40% to 60% to the current 0% to 6%) occurred when α-adrenergic receptor blockade was introduced as preoperative and preprocedure preparatory therapy for such patients[205-211] (Table 27-12).

α-Adrenergic receptor blockade with prazosin or phenoxybenzamine restores plasma volume by counteracting the vasoconstrictive effects of high levels of catecholamines. This re-expansion of fluid volume is often followed by a decrease in hematocrit. Because some patients may be very sensitive to the effects of phenoxybenzamine, it should initially be given in doses of 20 to 30 mg/70 kg orally once or twice a day. Most patients usually require 60 to 250 mg/day. The efficacy of therapy should be judged by the reduction in symptoms (especially sweating) and stabilization of BP. For patients who have carbohydrate intolerance because of inhibition of insulin release mediated by α-adrenergic receptor stimulation, α-adrenergic receptor blockade may reduce fasting blood sugar levels. For patients who exhibit ST-T changes on ECG, long-term preoperative and preprocedure α-adrenergic receptor blockade (1 to 6 months) has produced ECG and clinical resolution of catecholamine-induced myocarditis.[206-212]

Table 27–11 Characteristics of tests for pheochromocytoma

Test/Symptoms	Sensitivity (%)	Specificity (%)	Likelihood Ratio Positive Result*	Likelihood Ratio Negative Result†
Vanillylmandelic acid excretion	81	97	27.0	0.20
Catecholamine excretion	82	95	16.4	0.19
Metanephrine excretion	83	95	16.6	0.18
Abdominal computed tomography scan	92	80	4.6	0.10
Concurrent paroxysmal hypertension, headache, sweating, and tachycardia‡	90	95	18.0	0.10

*The ratio representing the likelihood of a positive result is obtained by dividing the sensitivity by 1 and then subtracting the specificity.
†The ratio representing the likelihood of a negative result is obtained by subtracting the sensitivity from 1 and then dividing by the specificity.
‡Data for concurrent paroxysmal symptoms are best estimates from available data.
Modified from Pauker SG, Kopelman RI: Interpreting hoofbeats: Can Bayes help clear the haze? N Engl J Med 327:1009, 1992.

Table 27–12 Perioperative mortality associated with resectioning of pheochromocytoma*

Year of Series	Study	Mortality (%)	Patients in Series (N)
1951	Apgar (review)	45/0	91
1951	Apgar	33.0	12
1963	Stackpole	13.0	100
Earlier than 1960	Mayo Clinic	0.0-26.0	101 (?)
Later than 1960	Mayo Clinic	2.9 (?)	44 (?)
Earlier than 1967	Modlin (without α-blockade)	18.0	17
Later than 1967	Modlin (with α-blockade)	2.0	41
1976-1993	Scott	3.0	33
1976-1993	Roizen	0.0	56
1974-1994	Lucon	2.0	50

*Data were abstracted from studies discussed in Roizen and colleagues[208] and include more recent patient information.

β-Adrenergic receptor blockade with propranolol is suggested for patients who have persistent arrhythmias or tachycardia[206-212] because these conditions can be precipitated or aggravated by α-adrenergic receptor blockade. β-Adrenergic receptor blockade should not be used without concomitant α-adrenergic receptor blockade lest the vasoconstrictive effects of the latter go unopposed and thereby increase the risk of dangerous hypertension.

The optimal duration of preoperative therapy with phenoxybenzamine has not been studied. Most patients require 10 to 14 days, as judged by the time needed to stabilize BP and ameliorate symptoms. On the basis of our experience, this is a minimal period of time.[207,208,212] Because the tumor spreads slowly, little is lost by waiting until medical therapy has optimized the patient's preoperative condition. Accordingly, we recommend using the following criteria:

1. No in-hospital BP reading higher than 165/90 mm Hg should be evident for 48 hours before surgery. We often measure arterial BP every minute for 1 hour in a stressful environment (our postanesthesia care unit). If no BP reading is greater than 165/90, this criterion is considered satisfied.
2. Orthostatic hypotension should be present, but BP on standing should not be lower than 80/45 mm Hg.
3. The ECG should be free of ST-T changes that are not permanent.
4. No more than one premature ventricular contraction (PVC) should occur every 5 minutes.

Other drugs, including prazosin, calcium channel blocking drugs, clonidine, and magnesium, have also been used to achieve suitable degrees of α-adrenergic blockade before surgery.

Although specific anesthetic drugs have been recommended, we believe that optimal preoperative preparation, gentle induction of anesthesia, and good communication between the surgeon and anesthesiologist are most important. Virtually all anesthetic drugs and techniques (including isoflurane, sevoflurane, sufentanil, remifentanil, fentanyl, and regional anesthesia) have been used with success. In fact, all drugs studied are associated with a high rate of transient intraoperative arrhythmias[207] (Table 27-13). We have avoided halothane because it sensitizes the myocardium and may increase arrhythmogenic

Table 27–13 Incidence of perioperative complications in a randomized study of patients undergoing resectioning of pheochromocytoma under one of four anesthetic techniques

	Anesthetic*			
	Enflurane (6)	Halothane (6)	Droperidol and Fentanyl (7)	Regional (5)
Ventricular tachycardia				
Needing no treatment	5	5	6	5
Needing treatment	0	1	1	0
Vasodilator needed				
Intraoperatively	6	6	7	5
Postoperatively	0	1†	1†	0
Vasopressor needed				
Intraoperatively	0	1	1	0
Postoperatively	0	0	0	0
Myocardial infarction‡	0	0	0	0
Renal failure‡	0	0	0	0
Congestive heart failure‡	0	1	1	1
Stroke‡	0	0	0	0
Death‡	0	0	0	0

*Number of patients shown in parentheses.
†Not all the abnormally secreting tumor tissue was removed from the patient.
‡Occurring postoperatively.
Data from Roizen MF, Horrigan RW, Koike M, et al: A prospective randomized trial of four anesthetic techniques for resection of pheochromocytoma [abstract]. Anesthesiology 57:A43, 1982.

frequency, as well as desflurane because it may precipitate non-neurogenic catecholamine release. No good data indicate that these biases are appropriate.

Because of ease of use, we prefer to give phenylephrine hydrochloride (Neo-Synephrine) or dopamine for hypotension and nitroprusside for hypertension. Phentolamine (Regitine) has too long an onset and duration of action. Occasionally (five times in >80 pheochromocytoma resections), we have used a β-adrenergic blocking agent (esmolol is now the preferred agent) for severe tachycardia without hypertension or volume depletion. Painful or stressful events such as intubation often cause an exaggerated stress response in less than perfectly anesthetized patients who have pheochromocytoma. This response is caused by release of catecholamines from nerve endings that are "loaded" by the reuptake process. Such stresses may cause catecholamine levels of 200 to 2000 pg/mL in normal patients. For a patient with pheochromocytoma, even simple stress can lead to blood catecholamine levels of 2000 to 20,000 pg/mL. However, infarction of a tumor, with release of products onto peritoneal surfaces, or surgical pressure causing release of products can result in blood levels of 200,000 to 1,000,000 pg/mL—a situation that should be anticipated and avoided (ask for a temporary stay of surgery, if at all possible, while the rate of nitroprusside infusion is increased). Once the venous supply is secured and if intravascular volume is normal (as measured by pulmonary wedge pressure), normal BP usually results. However, some patients become hypotensive and occasionally require massive infusions of catecholamines. On rare occasion, patients remain hypertensive intraoperatively. Postoperatively, about 50% remain hypertensive for 1 to 3 days—and initially have markedly elevated but declining plasma catecholamine levels—at which time all but 25% become normotensive. It is important to interview other family members and perhaps advise them to inform their future anesthetist about the potential for such familial disease.

Hypofunction or Aberration in Function of the Sympathetic Nervous System (Dysautonomia)

Disorders of the sympathetic nervous system include Shy-Drager syndrome, Riley-Day syndrome, Lesch-Nyhan syndrome, Gill's familial dysautonomia, diabetic dysautonomia, and the dysautonomia of spinal cord transection.

Although individuals can function well without an adrenal medulla, a deficient peripheral sympathetic nervous system occurring late in life poses major problems for many facets of life[213-223]; nevertheless, perioperative sympathectomy or its equivalent has been recommended by some.[224-238] A primary function of the sympathetic nervous system appears to be regulation of BP and intravascular fluid volume during changing of body position. Common features of all the syndromes of hypofunctioning of the sympathetic nervous system are orthostatic hypotension and decreased beat-to-beat variability in heart rate. These conditions can be caused by deficient intravascular volume, deficient baroreceptor function (as also occurs in carotid artery disease[239]), abnormalities in CNS function (as in Wernicke or Shy-Drager syndrome), deficient neuronal stores of norepinephrine (as in idiopathic orthostatic

hypotension[214] and diabetes[19]), or deficient release of norepinephrine (as in traumatic spinal cord injury[213]). These patients may have an increased number of available adrenergic receptors (a compensatory response) and an exaggerated response to sympathomimetic drugs.[240] In addition to other abnormalities, such as retention of urine or feces and deficient heat exchange, hypofunctioning of the sympathetic nervous system is often accompanied by renal amyloidosis. Thus, electrolyte and intravascular fluid volume status should be evaluated preoperatively. Because many of these patients have cardiac abnormalities, intravascular fluid volume might be assessed preoperatively with a Swan-Ganz catheter or transesophageal echocardiography rather than measurement of CVP (also see Chapters 32 and 33).

Inasmuch as functioning of the sympathetic nervous system is not predictable in these patients, we generally use slow, gentle induction of anesthesia and treat sympathetic excess or deficiency by infusing, with careful titration, drugs that directly constrict (phenylephrine) or dilate (nitroprusside) blood vessels or that stimulate (isoproterenol) or depress (esmolol) the heart rate. We prefer these drugs to agonists or antagonists, which may indirectly release catecholamines. A 20% perioperative mortality rate for 2600 patients with spinal cord transection has been reported,[221] thus indicating that such patients are difficult to manage and deserve particularly close attention.

After reviewing 300 patients with spinal cord injuries, Kendrick and coworkers[241] concluded that autonomic hyperreflexia syndrome does not develop if the lesion is below spinal dermatome T7. If the lesion is above that level (splanchnic outflow), 60% to 70% of patients experience extreme vascular instability. The trigger to this instability, or a *mass reflex* involving noradrenergic and motor hypertonus,[215] can be a cutaneous, proprioceptive, or visceral stimulus (a full bladder is a common initiator). The sensation enters the spinal cord and causes a spinal reflex, which in normal persons is inhibited from above. Sudden increases in BP are sensed in the pressure receptors of the aorta and carotid sinus. The resulting vagal hyperactivity produces bradycardia, ventricular ectopia, or various degrees of heart block. Reflex vasodilation may occur above the level of the lesion and result in flushing of the head and neck.

Depending on the length of time since spinal cord transection, other abnormalities may occur. Acutely (i.e., <3 weeks from the time of spinal injury), retention of urine and feces is common and, by elevating the diaphragm, may impair respiration. Disimpaction of the intestine alleviates this respiratory problem. Hyperesthesia is present above the lesion; reflexes and flaccid paralysis are present below the lesion. The intermediate period (3 days to 6 months) is marked by a hyperkalemic response to depolarizing drugs.[220] The chronic phase is characterized by a return of muscle tone, a positive Babinski sign, and frequently, the occurrence of hyperreflexia syndromes (e.g., mass reflex, see earlier).

Thus, in addition to meticulous attention to perioperative intravascular volume and electrolyte status, the anesthesiologist should know—by history taking, physical examination, and laboratory data—the status of the patient's myocardial conduction (as revealed by ECG), the status of renal functioning (by noting the ratio of creatinine to BUN), and the condition of the respiratory muscles (by determining the ratio of FEV_1 to FVC) (also see Chapter 26). The anesthesiologist may also obtain a chest radiograph if atelectasis or pneumonia is suspected on the basis of history taking or physical examination. Temperature control, the presence of bone fractures or decubitus ulcers, and normal functioning of the urination and defecation systems must be assessed. Confirmation of the latter prevents postoperative pneumonia or atelectasis caused by high positioning of the diaphragm.

Thyroid Dysfunction

The major thyroid hormones are thyroxine (T_4), a prohormone product of the thyroid gland, and the more potent 3,5,3-triiodothyronine (T_3), a product of both the thyroid and extrathyroidal enzymatic deiodination of T_4. Under normal circumstances, approximately 85% of T_3 is produced outside the thyroid gland. Production of thyroid secretions is maintained by secretion of thyroid-stimulating hormone (TSH) in the pituitary, which in turn is regulated by secretion of thyrotropin-releasing hormone (TRH) in the hypothalamus. Secretion of TSH and TRH appears to be negatively regulated by T_4 and T_3. Many believe that all effects of thyroid hormones are mediated by T_3 and that T_4 functions as a prohormone.

Thyroid hormones create their effects through several mechanisms. Binding of T_3 to high-affinity nuclear receptors (TR_α and TR_β) and subsequent activation of DNA-directed mRNA synthesis may account for the anabolic growth and developmental effects, plus some caloriogenic effect, of thyroid hormones. Patients with the syndrome of thyroid hormone resistance have point mutations in TR_β. Thyroid hormone is also responsible for an increased concentration of adrenergic receptors, which may account for many of its cardiovascular effects.

Because T_3 has a greater biologic effect than T_4 does, one would expect the diagnosis of thyroid disorders to be based on levels of T_3. However, this is not usually the case. The diagnosis of thyroid disease is confirmed by one of several biochemical measurements: levels of free T_4 or total serum concentrations of T_4 and the "free T_4 estimate." This estimate is obtained by multiplying total T_4 (free and bound) by the thyroid-binding ratio (formerly called resin T_3 uptake) (Table 27-14). Free T_4 can be accurately

measured by many laboratories. Direct measurement of free T_4 obviates the need to account for changes in binding protein synthesis and affinity caused by other conditions. The T_3-binding ratio measures the extra quantity of serum protein-binding sites. This measurement is necessary because thyroxine-binding globulin (TBG) is abnormally high during pregnancy, hepatic disease, and estrogen therapy (all of which would elevate the total T_4 level) (Table 27-15). Reliable interpretation of measurements of the total hormone concentration in serum necessitates data on the percentage of bound hormone. The thyroid hormone–binding ratio test provides this information. In this test, ^{131}I-labeled T_3 is added to a patient's serum and allowed to reach an equilibrium binding state. A resin is then added that binds the remaining radioactive T_3. Resin uptake is greater if the patient has fewer TBG-binding sites. In normal patients, resin T_3 uptake (the thyroid hormone–binding ratio) is 25% to 35%. When serum TBG is elevated, the thyroid hormone–binding ratio is diminished (see Table 27-14). When serum TBG is diminished, as in nephrotic syndrome, in conditions in which glucocorticoids are increased, or in chronic liver disease, the thyroid hormone–binding ratio is increased.

The free T_4 estimate and the free T_3 estimate are frequently used as measures of a patient's serum T_4 and T_3 hormone concentration. To obtain these estimates, the concentration of total serum T_4 or total serum T_3 is multiplied by the measured thyroid hormone–binding ratio.

Table 27-15 Factors influencing serum levels of thyroxine-binding globulin

Conditions Increasing Serum Levels	Conditions Decreasing Serum Levels
Use of oral contraceptives	Testosterone
Pregnancy	Use of corticosteroids
Use of estrogen	Severe illness
Infectious hepatitis	Cirrhosis
Chronic active hepatitis	Nephrotic syndrome
Neonatal state	Inherited conditions
Acute intermittent porphyria	?Phenytoin
Inherited conditions	

Table 27-14 Biochemical measurements of thyroid function that account for variation in production of thyroid-binding globulin

	Examples of Normal Thyroid Status					
	FT_4E	=	T_4	×	THBR	TSH
Normal	0.19 (0.12-0.25)	=	0.6 (0.4-0.9)	×	31% (25%-35%)	0.2 (0.2-0.8)
During use of oral contraceptives	0.19	=	1.3	×	15%	0.3
During use of corticosteroids	0.18	=	0.3	×	60%	0.3

FT_4E is the free T_4 (thyroxine) estimate. It is usually obtained by multiplying the total T_4 concentration (the free amount and the amount bound to protein) by the thyroid hormone–binding ratio (THBR, formerly called the resin T3 uptake). THBR is a measure of the bound thyroid hormone–binding protein. TSH is the thyroid-stimulating hormone secreted by the pituitary in the negative feedback loop. (TSH increases when FT_4E is low in hypothyroidism.)

Values of these two indices are normal in the event of a primary alteration in binding, but not in secretion of thyroid hormone.

Hyperthyroidism can be diagnosed by measuring levels of TSH after administration of TRH. Although administering TRH normally increases TSH levels in blood, even a small increase in the T_4 or T_3 level in blood abolishes this response. Thus, a subnormal or absent serum TSH response to TRH is a very sensitive indicator of hyperthyroidism.[242] In one group of disorders involving hyperthyroidism, serum TSH levels are elevated in the presence of elevated levels of free thyroid hormone.

Measurement of the α-subunit of TSH has been helpful in identifying the rare patients who have a pituitary neoplasm and who usually have increased α-subunit concentrations. Some patients are clinically euthyroid in the presence of elevated levels of total T_4 in serum. Certain drugs, notably gallbladder dyes, propranolol, glucocorticoids, and amiodarone, block the conversion of T_4 to T_3, thereby elevating T_4 levels. Severe illness also slows this conversion. Levels of TSH are often high in situations in which the rate of conversion is decreased. In hyperthyroidism, cardiac function and responses to stress are abnormal; return of normal cardiac function parallels the return of TSH levels to normal.

Hyperthyroidism

Although hyperthyroidism is usually caused by the multinodular diffuse enlargement in Graves' disease (also associated with disorders of the skin or eyes, or both), it can also occur with pregnancy,[243] thyroiditis (with or without neck pain), thyroid adenoma, choriocarcinoma, or TSH-secreting pituitary adenoma.[244] Five percent of women have thyrotoxic effects 3 to 6 months postpartum and tend to have recurrences with subsequent pregnancies. Major manifestations of hyperthyroidism are weight loss, diarrhea, warm moist skin, weakness of large muscle groups, menstrual abnormalities, osteopenia, nervousness, jitteriness, intolerance to heat, tachycardia, cardiac arrhythmias, mitral valve prolapse,[245] and heart failure. When the thyroid is functioning abnormally, the entity most threatened is the cardiovascular system. When diarrhea is severe, dehydration should be corrected preoperatively. Mild anemia, thrombocytopenia, increased serum alkaline phosphatase, hypercalcemia, muscle wasting, and bone loss frequently occur in hyperthyroidism. Muscle disease usually involves the proximal muscle groups; it has not been reported to cause respiratory muscle paralysis. In the apathetic form of hyperthyroidism (seen most commonly in persons older than 60 years), cardiac effects dominate the clinical picture.[246] Signs and symptoms include weight loss, anorexia, and cardiac effects such as tachycardia, irregular heart rhythm, atrial fibrillation (in 10%), heart failure, and occasionally, papillary muscle dysfunction.[245,246]

Although β-adrenergic receptor blockade can control the heart rate, its use is fraught with hazard in a patient already experiencing CHF. However, a decreasing heart rate may improve heart-pumping function. Thus, hyperthyroid patients who have fast ventricular rates, who are in CHF, and who require emergency surgery are given esmolol guided by changes in pulmonary artery wedge

pressure and their condition. If slowing the heart rate with a small dose of esmolol (50 µg/kg) does not aggravate heart failure, we administer more esmolol. We believe that we should aim to avoid imposing surgery on any patient whose thyroid function is clinically abnormal. Therefore, we believe that only "life or death" emergency surgery should preclude making the patient pharmacologically euthyroid, a process that can take 2 to 6 weeks. Antithyroid medications include propylthiouracil or methimazole, both of which decrease the synthesis of T_4 and may enhance remission by reducing TSH receptor antibody levels (the primary pathologic mechanism in Grave's disease). Propylthiouracil also decreases the conversion of T_4 into the more potent T_3. However, the literature indicates a trend toward preoperative preparation with propranolol and iodides alone.[247] This approach is quicker (i.e., 7 to 14 days versus 2 to 6 weeks); it shrinks the thyroid gland, as does the more traditional approach; it decreases conversion of the prohormone T_4 into the more potent T_3; and it treats symptoms but may not correct abnormalities in left ventricular function.[248] Regardless of the approach, antithyroid drugs should be administered chronically and on the morning of surgery. If emergency surgery is necessary before the euthyroid state is achieved, if subclinical hyperthyroidism progresses without adequate treatment,[249] or if hyperthyroidism gets out of control during surgery, intravenous administration of esmolol, 50 to 500 µg/kg, could be titrated to restore a normal heart rate (assuming the absence of CHF) (see earlier). In addition, intravascular fluid volume and electrolyte balance should be restored. However, administering propranolol or esmolol does not invariably prevent "thyroid storm."[250]

No controlled study has demonstrated clinical advantages of any anesthetic drug over another for surgical patients who are hyperthyroid. A review of cases performed at the University of California, San Francisco, from 1968 to 1982 revealed that virtually all anesthetic drugs and techniques[251] have been used without adverse effects even being remotely attributable to the drug or technique. Furthermore, although some investigators have recommended that anticholinergic drugs (especially atropine) be avoided inasmuch as they interfere with the sweating mechanism and cause tachycardia, atropine has been given as a test for the adequacy of antithyroid treatment. Because patients are now subjected to operative procedures only when euthyroid, the traditional "steal" of a heavily premedicated hyperthyroid patient (so commonly found in the iodine-deficient locales surrounding the Lahey, Mayo, and Cleveland Clinics) in the operating room has vanished.

A patient with a large goiter and an obstructed airway can be handled in the same way as any other patient with problematic airway management. Preoperative medication should avoid excessive sedation, and an airway should be established, often with the patient awake. A firm armored endotracheal tube is preferable and should be passed beyond the point of extrinsic compression. It is most useful to examine CT scans of the neck preoperatively to determine the extent of compression. Maintenance of anesthesia usually presents little difficulty. Postoperatively, extubation should be performed under optimal circumstances for reintubation in the event that the tracheal rings have been weakened and the trachea collapses.

Of the many possible postoperative complications (nerve injuries, bleeding, and metabolic abnormalities), "thyroid storm" (discussed later), bilateral recurrent nerve trauma, and hypocalcemic tetany are the most feared. Bilateral recurrent laryngeal nerve injury (by trauma or edema) causes stridor and laryngeal obstruction as a result of unopposed adduction of the vocal cords and closure of the glottic aperture. Immediate endotracheal intubation is required, usually followed by tracheostomy to ensure an adequate airway. This rare complication occurred only once in more than 30,000 thyroid operations at the Lahey Clinic. Unilateral recurrent nerve injury often goes unnoticed because of compensatory overadduction of the uninvolved cord. However, we often test vocal cord function before and after this surgery by asking the patient to say "e" or "moon." Unilateral nerve injury is characterized by hoarseness and bilateral nerve injury by aphonia. Selective injury to the adductor fibers of both recurrent laryngeal nerves leaves the abductor muscles relatively unopposed, and pulmonary aspiration is a risk. Selective injury to the abductor fibers leaves the adductor muscles relatively unopposed, and airway obstruction can occur. Bullous glottic edema, an additional cause of postoperative respiratory compromise, has no specific cause or known preventive measure.

The intimate involvement of the parathyroid gland with the thyroid gland can result in inadvertent hypocalcemia during surgery for thyroid disease. Complications relating to hypocalcemia are discussed in the later section "Hypocalcemia."

Because postoperative hematoma can compromise the airway, neck and wound dressings are placed in a crossing fashion (rather than vertically or horizontally) and should be examined for evidence of bleeding before a patient is discharged from the recovery room.

Thyroid Storm

"Thyroid storm" is the name for the clinical diagnosis of a life-threatening illness in a patient whose hyperthyroidism has been severely exacerbated by illness or surgery. Thyroid storm is characterized by hyperpyrexia, tachycardia, and striking alterations in consciousness.[251] It can thus be manifested very similarly to malignant hyperthermia, pheochromocytoma, or neuroleptic malignant syndrome.[210] No laboratory tests are diagnostic of thyroid storm, and the precipitating (nonthyroidal) cause is the major determinant of survival. Therapy can include blocking the synthesis of thyroid hormones by administering antithyroid drugs, blocking the release of preformed hormone with iodine, meticulous attention to hydration and supportive therapy, and correcting the precipitating cause. Blocking the sympathetic nervous system with reserpine, guanethidine, or α- and β-receptor antagonists may be exceedingly hazardous and requires skillful management and constant monitoring of the critically ill patient.

Thyroid dysfunction, either hyperthyroidism or hypothyroidism, develops in more than 10% of patients treated with the antiarrhythmic agent amiodarone.[252] Approximately 35% of the drug's weight is iodine, and

a 200-mg tablet releases about 20 times the optimal daily dose of iodine. This iodine can lead to reduced synthesis of T_4 or increased synthesis. In addition, amiodarone inhibits the conversion of T_4 into the more potent T_3.

Patients receiving amiodarone might be considered to be in need of special attention preoperatively and may even require special attention to anesthesia, not just because of the arrhythmia that led to such therapy but also to ensure that no perioperative dysfunction or surprises occur because of unsuspected thyroid hyperfunction or hypofunction.[253] Many patients with amiodarone-induced thyrotoxicosis receive steroids for a period of time, another area of questioning that might be triggered by the use of amiodarone in a preoperative patient.

Hypothyroidism

Hypothyroidism is a common disease that occurs in 5% of a large population in Great Britain, in 3% to 6% of a healthy older population in Massachusetts, and in 4.5% of a medical clinic population in Switzerland. The apathy and lethargy that often accompany hypothyroidism frequently delay its diagnosis, so the perioperative period may be the first opportunity to spot many such hypothyroid patients. However, hypothyroidism is usually subclinical, serum concentrations of thyroid hormones are in the normal range, and only serum TSH levels are elevated.[254,255] The normal range of TSH is 0.3 to 4.5 mU/L, and TSH values of 5 to 15 mU/L are characteristic of this entity.[255] In such cases, hypothyroidism may have little or no perioperative significance. However, a retrospective study of 59 mildly hypothyroid patients found that more hypothyroid patients than control subjects required prolonged postoperative intubation (9 of 59 versus 4 of 59) and had significant electrolyte imbalances (3 of 59 versus 1 of 59) and bleeding complications (4 of 59 versus 0 of 59).[256] Because only a small number of charts were examined, these differences did not reach statistical significance. In another study, overt hypothyroidism later developed in a high percentage of patients with a history of subclinical hypothyroidism.[257] Thus, a previous history of subclinical hypothyroidism may indicate the need to search for and be concerned about the possibility of overt hypothyroidism.

In the less frequent occurrences of overt hypothyroidism, the relative lack of thyroid hormone results in slow mental functioning, slow movement, dry skin, arthralgias, carpal tunnel syndrome, periorbital edema, intolerance to cold, depression of the ventilatory responses to hypoxia and hypercapnia,[258] impaired clearance of free water with or without hyponatremia, "hung-up reflexes," slow gastric emptying, sleep apnea,[259] and bradycardia. In extreme cases, cardiomegaly, heart failure, and pericardial pleural effusions are manifested as fatigue, dyspnea, and orthopnea.[260] Hypothyroidism is often associated with amyloidosis, which may produce an enlarged tongue, abnormalities of the cardiac conduction system, and renal disease. Hypothyroidism decreases the anesthetic requirement slightly.[261] The tongue may be enlarged in a hypothyroid patient even in the absence of amyloidosis, and such enlargement may hamper endotracheal intubation.

A rising TSH level is a most sensitive indicator of failing thyroid function. Ideal preoperative and preprocedure management of hypothyroidism consists of restoring normal thyroid status: we routinely administer the normal dose of levothyroxine the morning of surgery, even though these drugs have long half-lives (1.4 to 10 days). (Levothyroxin is the preferred therapy because it allows the controlling enzyme systems to regulate TSH secretion as well as conversion to T_3.)[262] Reduced GI absorption of levothyroxine may occur with the coadministration of cholestyramine or aluminum hydroxide, iron, a high-bran meal, or sucralfate or colestipol. For patients in myxedema coma requiring emergency surgery, liothyronine can be given intravenously (with fear of precipitating myocardial ischemia, however) while supportive therapy is undertaken to restore normal intravascular fluid volume, body temperature, cardiac function, respiratory function, and electrolyte balance.

Treating hypothyroid patients with symptomatic coronary artery disease poses special problems and may require compromises in the general practice of preoperatively restoring euthyroidism with drugs.[260] Although both levothyroxine and esmolol may be given, adequate amelioration of both ischemic heart disease and hypothyroidism may be difficult to achieve. The need for thyroid therapy must be balanced against the risk of aggravating the anginal symptoms. One review suggested early consideration of coronary artery revascularization.[263] It advocated initiating thyroid replacement therapy in the ICU soon after the patient's arrival from the operating room and myocardial revascularization surgery. However, several deaths from arrhythmia and CHF, as well as cardiogenic shock with infarction, have occurred while patients who were not given thyroid therapy were awaiting surgery. Thus, true emergency coronary artery revascularization should be considered in patients with both severe coronary artery disease and significant hypothyroidism.

In hypothyroidism, respiratory control mechanisms do not function normally.[258] However, the response to hypoxia and hypercapnia and the clearance of free water become normal with thyroid replacement therapy.[258,260] Drug metabolism is anecdotally reported to be slowed, and awakening times from sedatives are reported to be prolonged during hypothyroidism. However, few formal studies and none in humans of the pharmacokinetics and pharmacodynamics of sedatives or anesthetic drugs have been published.[264] These concerns disappear when thyroid function is normalized preoperatively. Addison's disease (with its relative steroid deficiency) is more common in hypothyroidism, and some endocrinologists routinely treat noniatrogenic hypothyroid patients with stress doses of steroids perioperatively because both conditions are commonly caused by autoimmune responses. The possibility that this steroid deficiency exists should be considered if the patient becomes hypotensive perioperatively. Body heat mechanisms are inadequate in hypothyroid patients, so temperature should be monitored and maintained, especially in patients requiring emergency surgery. Because of an increased incidence of myasthenia gravis in hypothyroid patients, it may be advisable to use a peripheral nerve stimulator to guide administration of muscle relaxants (see Chapter 39).

Thyroid Nodules and Carcinoma

More than 90% of thyroid nodules are benign, yet identifying malignancy in a solitary thyroid nodule is a difficult and important procedure. Male patients and patients with previous radiation therapy to the head and neck have an increased likelihood of malignant disease in their nodules. Often, needle biopsy and scanning are sufficient for the diagnosis, but occasionally, excisional biopsy is needed. Papillary carcinoma accounts for more than 70% of all thyroid carcinomas. Simple excision of lymph node metastases appears to be as efficacious for patient survival as radical neck procedures. Follicular carcinoma accounts for about 15% of thyroid carcinomas, is more aggressive, and has a less favorable prognosis.

Medullary carcinoma, the most aggressive form of thyroid carcinoma, is associated with a familial incidence of pheochromocytoma, as are parathyroid adenomas. For this reason, a history might be obtained from patients who have a surgical scar in the thyroid region so that the possibility of occult pheochromocytoma can be ruled out.

Disorders of Calcium Metabolism

The three substances that regulate serum concentrations of calcium, phosphorus, and magnesium—parathyroid hormone (parathyrin, PTH), calcitonin, and vitamin D—act on bone, kidney, and gut. Calcium excess in blood is due to either malignancy or hyperparathyroidism in over 90% of patients. PTH stimulates bone resorption and inhibits renal excretion of calcium, two conditions that lead to hypercalcemia. Calcitonin can be considered an antagonist to PTH. Through its metabolites, vitamin D aids in the absorption of calcium, phosphate, and magnesium from the gut and facilitates the bone resorptive effects of PTH.[265]

Hyperparathyroidism and Hypercalcemia

Primary hyperparathyroidism occurs in about 0.1% of the population, most commonly begins in the third to fifth decades of life, and occurs two to three times more frequently in women than men. Primary hyperparathyroidism usually results from enlargement of a single gland, commonly an adenoma and very rarely a carcinoma. Hypercalcemia almost always develops.

Calcium is the chief mineral component of the body; it provides structure to the skeleton and performs key roles in neural transmission, intracellular signaling, blood coagulation, and neuromuscular functioning. Ninety-nine percent of the 1000 g of calcium present in the average human body is stored in bone. The normal total serum calcium level is 8.6 to 10.4 mg/dL, as measured in most laboratories. Fifty percent to 60% is bound to plasma proteins or is complexed with phosphate or citrate. The value is dependent on the albumin level, with a decline of 0.8 mg/dL for each 1 g/dL drop in albumin. Calcium binding to albumin is pH dependent: binding decreases with acidic pH and increases with alkaline pH. It should be noted that serum calcium and not ionized calcium decreases with decreases in albumin levels. Although ionized calcium is the clinically significant fraction, the cost and technical difficulties of stabilizing the electrodes used for measurement have limited the available assays.

Nevertheless, PTH and vitamin D_3 work to keep the level stable within 0.1 mg/dL in any individual.

Many of the prominent symptoms of hyperparathyroidism are a result of the hypercalcemia that accompanies it. Regardless of the cause, hypercalcemia can produce any of a number of symptoms, the most prominent involving the renal, skeletal, neuromuscular, and GI systems— anorexia, vomiting, constipation, polyuria, polydipsia, lethargy, confusion, formation of renal calculi, pancreatitis, bone pain, and psychiatric abnormalities. Free intracellular calcium initiates or regulates muscle contraction, release of neurotransmitters, secretion of hormones, enzyme action, and energy metabolism.

Nephrolithiasis occurs in 60% to 70% of patients with hyperparathyroidism. Sustained hypercalcemia can result in tubular and glomerular disorders, including proximal (type II) renal tubular acidosis. Polyuria and polydipsia are common complaints.

Skeletal disorders related to hyperparathyroidism are osteitis fibrosa cystica and simple diffuse osteopenia. The rate of bone turnover is five times higher in patients with hyperparathyroidism than in normal controls. Patients may have a history of frequent fractures or complain of bone pain, the latter especially in the anterior margin of the tibia.

Because free intracellular calcium initiates or regulates muscle contraction, neurotransmitter release, hormone secretion, enzyme action, and energy metabolism, abnormalities in these end organs are often symptoms of hyperparathyroidism. Patients may experience profound muscle weakness, especially in proximal muscle groups, as well as muscle atrophy. Depression, psychomotor retardation, and memory impairment may occur. Lethargy and confusion are frequent complaints.

Peptic ulcer disease is more common in these patients than in the rest of the population. Production of gastrin and gastric acid is increased. Anorexia, vomiting, and constipation may also be present.

Approximately a third of all hypercalcemic patients are hypertensive, but the hypertension usually resolves with successful treatment of the primary disease. Neither hypertension nor minimally invasive surgery seems to alter the perioperative risk of surgery in such patients in comparison to the usual hypertensives.[266,267] Even octogenarians with asymptomatic hyperparathyroidism can be operated on without mortality and with morbidity no different from that in younger individuals, thus encouraging the use of parathyroidectomy as preventive care therapy.[268,269] Long-standing hypercalcemia can lead to calcifications in the myocardium, blood vessels, brain, and kidneys. Cerebral calcifications may cause seizures, whereas renal calcifications lead to polyuria that is unresponsive to vasopressin.

The most useful confirmatory test for hyperparathyroidism is a radioimmunoassay for PTH. In fact, some surgeons monitor PTH levels intraoperatively to determine whether they have resected the causative adenoma.[270] In hyperparathyroid patients, hormone levels are abnormal for a given level of calcium. The level of inorganic phosphorus in serum is usually low, but it may be within normal limits. Alkaline phosphatase is elevated if considerable skeletal involvement is present.

Glucocorticoid administration reduces the level of calcium in blood in many other conditions that cause hypercalcemia, but not usually in primary hyperparathyroidism. In sarcoidosis, multiple myeloma, vitamin D intoxication, and some malignant diseases, all of which can cause hypercalcemia, administration of glucocorticoids may lower serum calcium levels through an effect on GI absorption. This effect occurs to a lesser degree in primary hyperparathyroidism.

Hypercalcemia may also occur as a consequence of secondary hyperparathyroidism in patients who have chronic renal disease. When phosphate excretion decreases as a result of a lower nephron mass, serum calcium levels fall because of deposition of calcium and phosphate in bone. Secretion of PTH subsequently increases, which causes the fraction of phosphate excreted by each nephron to increase. Eventually, the chronic intermittent hypocalcemia of chronic renal failure leads to chronically high levels of serum PTH and hyperplasia of the parathyroid glands.

What should be done for asymptomatic patients with primary hyperparathyroidism? This question has become the subject of a major controversy, for which no definitive answer exists. *Symptomatic* primary hyperparathyroidism is usually treated surgically, as is hyperparathyroidism in young patients or those with azotemia, bone demineralization, or chronic total calcium elevations greater than 12 mg/dL. If the patient refuses surgery or if other illnesses make surgery inadvisable, medical management can be difficult. This difficulty occurs when hyperfunctioning parathyroid glands secrete more hormone as the serum calcium concentration is lowered—as though the calcium set point for feedback regulation of PTH secretion had been raised.

Patients with moderate hypercalcemia who have normal renal and cardiovascular function present no special preoperative and preprocedure problems. The ECG can be examined preoperatively and intraoperatively for shortened PR or QT intervals (Fig. 27-7). Because severe hypercalcemia can result in hypovolemia, normal

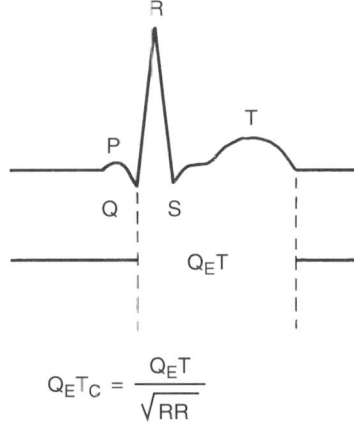

$$Q_ET_C = \frac{Q_ET}{\sqrt{RR}}$$

Figure 27–7 Measurement of the QTc interval (properly termed Q_ET_C to indicate that it begins with the start of the Q wave, lasts throughout the QT interval, ends with the end of the T wave, and is corrected for heart rate). RR is the RR interval in seconds. (From Hensel P, Roizen MF: Patients with disorders of parathyroid function. Anesthesiol Clin North Am 5:287, 1987.)

intravascular volume and electrolyte status should be restored before commencement of anesthesia and surgery.

Management of hypercalcemia can include increasing urinary calcium excretion by means of hydration and diuresis. Restoration of intravascular volume, augmentation and excretion of urinary sodium, and administration of diuretics (furosemide is commonly used) generally increase urinary calcium excretion substantially. Complications of these interventions include hypomagnesemia and hypokalemia.

In emergency situations, vigorous expansion of intravascular volume usually reduces serum calcium to a safe level (<14 mg/dL); administration of furosemide is also often helpful in these situations. Phosphate should be given to correct hypophosphatemia because it decreases calcium uptake into bone, increases calcium excretion, and stimulates breakdown of bone. Hydration and diuresis, accompanied by phosphate repletion, suffice in the management of most hypercalcemic patients. Other measures decrease reabsorption of bone and include pamidronate sodium (90 mg intravenously), salmon calcitonin (100 to 400 U), and plicamycin.

Calcitonin lowers serum calcium levels through direct inhibition of bone resorption. It can decrease serum calcium levels within minutes after intravenous administration. Side effects include urticaria and nausea.

It is especially important to know whether the hypercalcemia has been chronic because serious cardiac, renal, or CNS abnormalities may have resulted.

Hypocalcemia

Hypocalcemia (caused by hypoalbuminemia, hypoparathyroidism, hypomagnesemia, or chronic renal disease) is not usually accompanied by a clinically evident cardiovascular disorder. The most common cause of hypocalcemia is hypoalbuminemia. In true hypocalcemia (i.e., when the free calcium concentration is low), myocardial contractility is affected. That is, myocardial contractility varies directly with levels of blood ionized calcium, although contractility decreased only 20% when ionized calcium levels changed from 1.68 to 1.34 mmol/L.[271] The clinical signs of hypocalcemia are clumsiness; convulsions; laryngeal stridor; depression; muscle stiffness; paresthesia (oral and perioral); parkinsonism; tetany; Chvostek's sign; dry, scaly skin, brittle nails, and coarse hair; low serum concentrations of calcium; prolonged QT intervals; soft tissue calcifications; and Trousseau's sign.

Hypocalcemia delays ventricular repolarization, hence increasing the QTc interval (normal, 0.35 to 0.44 second). With electrical systole prolonged, the ventricles may fail to respond to the next electrical impulse from the sinoatrial node and a 2:1 heart block results. Prolongation of the QT interval is a moderately reliable ECG sign of hypocalcemia, not for the population as a whole, but for the individual patient.[272] Thus, monitoring the QT interval as corrected for the heart rate (Fig. 27-7) is a useful, but not always accurate means of monitoring hypocalcemia in any individual patient. CHF may also occur with hypocalcemia, but this is rare. Because CHF in patients with coexisting heart disease is reduced in severity when calcium and magnesium ion levels are restored to normal, these levels might be normal before surgery in a patient

with impaired exercise tolerance or signs of cardiovascular dysfunction.[265,271] Sudden decreases in blood levels of ionized calcium (as with chelation therapy) can result in severe hypotension.

Patients with hypocalcemia may have seizures. They may be focal, jacksonian, petit mal, or grand mal in appearance, indistinguishable from such seizures in the absence of hypocalcemia. Patients may also have a type of seizure called cerebral tetany, which consists of generalized tetany followed by tonic spasms. Therapy with standard anticonvulsants is ineffective and may even exacerbate these seizures (by an anti–vitamin D effect). In long-standing hypoparathyroidism, calcifications may appear above the sella; these calcifications represent deposits of calcium in and around small blood vessels of the basal ganglia. They may be associated with a variety of extrapyramidal syndromes.

The most common cause of *acquired hypoparathyroidism* is surgery on the thyroid or parathyroid glands. Other causes include autoimmune disorders, therapy with iodine 131, hemosiderosis, neoplasia, and granulomatous disease. *Idiopathic hypoparathyroidism* has been divided into three categories: an isolated persistent neonatal form, branchial dysembryogenesis, and autoimmune candidiasis related to multiple endocrine deficiency.

Pseudohypoparathyroidism and *pseudopseudohypoparathyroidism* are rare hereditary disorders characterized by short stature, obesity, rounded face, and shortened metacarpals. Patients with pseudohypoparathyroidism have hypocalcemia and hyperphosphatemia despite high serum levels of PTH. These patients have a deficient end-organ response to PTH because of abnormalities in G protein function.

Because treatment of hypoparathyroidism is not surgical, hypoparathyroid patients who come to the operating room are those who require surgery for an unrelated condition. Their calcium, phosphate, and magnesium levels should be measured both preoperatively and postoperatively. Patients with symptomatic hypocalcemia might be treated with intravenous calcium gluconate before surgery. Initially, 10 to 20 mL of 10% calcium gluconate may be given at a rate of 5 mL/min. The effect on serum calcium levels is of short duration, but a continuous infusion with 10 mL/min of 10% calcium gluconate in 500 mL of solution over a period of 6 hours helps keep serum calcium at adequate levels.

The objective of therapy is to bring the symptoms under control before surgery and anesthesia. For patients with chronic hypoparathyroidism, the objective is to keep the serum calcium level in the lower half of the normal range. A preoperative and preprocedure ECG is useful for maintaining the QTc interval. The preoperative and preprocedure QTc value may be used as a guide to the serum calcium level if rapid laboratory assessment is not possible. Changes in the calcium level may alter the duration of muscle relaxation, so such alterations might be monitored by using a twitch monitor in these (as well as all other) patients.[273]

The intimate involvement of the parathyroid gland with the thyroid gland can result in unintentional hypocalcemia during surgery for diseases of either organ. Because of the affinity of their bones for calcium, this relationship is crucial in patients with advanced osteitis.

Internal redistribution of magnesium or calcium ions, or both, may occur (into "hungry bones") after parathyroidectomy and cause either hypomagnesemia or hypocalcemia, or both. Because the tendency to tetany increases with alkalosis, hyperventilation is usually assiduously avoided. The most prominent manifestations of acute hypocalcemia are distal paresthesias and muscle spasm (tetany). Potentially fatal complications of severe hypocalcemia include laryngeal spasm and hypocalcemic seizures. The clinical sequelae of magnesium deficiency include cardiac arrhythmias (principally ventricular tachyarrhythmias), hypocalcemic tetany, and neuromuscular irritability independent of hypocalcemia (tremors, twitching, asterixis, and seizures).

In addition to monitoring total serum calcium or ionized calcium postoperatively, one can test for the Chvostek and Trousseau signs. (Note that serum calcium and not ionized calcium is dependent on the albumin level, with a decline of about 0.8 mg/dL for each 1 g/dL drop in serum albumin level.) Because the Chvostek sign can be elicited in 10% to 15% of patients who are not hypocalcemic, an attempt should be made to elicit it preoperatively to ensure that its appearance is meaningful. The Chvostek sign is a contracture of the facial muscles produced by tapping the ipsilateral facial nerves at the angle of the jaw. The Trousseau sign is elicited by applying a BP cuff at a level slightly above the systolic level for a few minutes. The resulting carpopedal spasm, with contractions of the fingers and an inability to open the hand, stems from the increased muscle irritability in hypocalcemic states, aggravated by ischemia produced by the BP cuff.

Osteoporosis

Fifty percent of women older than 65 years sustain an osteoporotic fracture. (Because men are living longer, osteoporosis will probably become an increasing problem for them too, and recent reports indicate a 15% per decade hip fracture rate for men older than 65 years.) Osteoporosis is the thinning of bone that causes low bone mass and thus weakening of this living tissue to the point of breakage. Known risk factors include age, relative lifetime estrogen deficiency (late menarche, amenorrhea, early menopause, nulliparity), deficiency of dietary calcium, tobacco use, increased aerobic exercise in combination with decreased weight-bearing exercise, decreased weight-bearing exercise by itself, use of soft drinks, and Asian or white ancestry. Although therapy for osteoporosis (use of biphosphates, bone mineral depositors, weight-bearing exercises, calcium, vitamin D, estrogen, and now designer estrogens that may be useful for men, such as Evista) does not have major known implications for anesthesia care, bone fractures in such patients have occurred on movement to and from an operating table. Thus, the precautions mentioned earlier for hyperparathyroid patients relative to self-positioning and careful positioning may be useful.

Pituitary Abnormalities

Anterior Pituitary Hypersecretion

The anterior pituitary gland consists of five identifiable types of secretory cells (and the hormones that they secrete): somatotrophs (GH), corticotrophs (ACTH), lactotrophs (prolactin), gonadotrophs (luteinizing hormone [LH] and follicle-stimulating hormone [FSH]), and thyrotrophs (TSH). Secretion of these pituitary hormones is largely regulated by a negative-feedback loop by hypothalamic regulatory hormones and by signals that originate from the target site of pituitary action. Six hypothalamic hormones have been characterized: dopamine, the prolactin-inhibiting hormone; somatostatin, the GH release–inhibiting hormone; GH-releasing hormone (GHRH); corticotropin-releasing hormone (CRH); gonadotropin-releasing hormone (GnRH or LHRH); and TRH. Most pituitary tumors (>60%) are hypersecretory and are classified according to the excess production of a specific anterior pituitary hormone.

The three most common disorders of pituitary hypersecretion are those related to excesses of prolactin (amenorrhea, galactorrhea, and infertility), ACTH (Cushing's syndrome), or GH (acromegaly). In addition to knowing the pathophysiologic processes of the disease involved, the anesthesiologist must determine whether the patient recently underwent air pneumoencephalography. If so, nitrous oxide should not be used; this practice lessens the risk of intracranial hypertension from gas collection. CT or MRI of the sella has largely replaced neuroencephalography, but the latter is still performed.

Acromegaly is a syndrome that consists of characteristic facies, weakness, enlargement of the hands (often to the point of rendering the usual oximeter probes difficult to use) and feet, thickening of the tongue (often to the point of making endotracheal intubation difficult), and enlargement of the nose and mandible with spreading of the teeth (often to the point of requiring larger than normal laryngoscopic blades).[274,275] The patient may even appear myxedematous. Other findings include abnormal glucose tolerance and osteoporosis. The most specific test for acromegaly is measurement of GH before and after glucose administration. The typical acromegalic has very elevated fasting levels of GH (usually above 10 g/mL), and the levels do not change appreciably after the oral administration of glucose. In the normal state, glucose markedly suppresses the GH level. A few patients with active acromegaly have normal levels of fasting GH, and GH levels are not suppressed by glucose. In addition, elevated plasma insulin-like growth factor type I (IGF-I), also known as somatomedin C, is pathognomonic of GH excess. The drug L-dopa, which normally causes an elevation of GH in normal subjects, either has no effect or lowers GH levels in acromegalics. More than 99% of cases of acromegaly are attributable to pituitary adenoma. Thus, the primary treatment of acromegaly is transsphenoidal surgery. If the pituitary tumor is not totally removed, patients are often offered external pituitary irradiation. In the case of suprasellar extension, conventional transfrontal hypophysectomy is often performed. The dopaminergic agonist bromocriptine can lower GH levels, but the long-term follow-up with this drug is not favorable. Octreotide, a long-acting analog of somatostatin, now given in depot form about once a month, produces effective palliation in 50% of patients.

The effects of excessive GH stem from both direct actions of the hormone on tissue and stimulation of the production of somatomedins. Excessive GH often results in retention of sodium and potassium, inhibition of the peripheral action of insulin (which can result in diabetes mellitus), and premature atherosclerosis (often associated with cardiomegaly). Exertional dyspnea may be related to either heart failure or respiratory insufficiency as a result of kyphoscoliosis. Cardiac arrhythmias are common. We do not yet know the incidence of these problems in elderly men now being treated with or receiving GH (recombinant) for the possible improvement of functional status. Preoperative and preprocedure evaluation of a patient who has acromegaly or who is receiving GH might begin by determining whether significant cardiac, hypertensive, pulmonary, or diabetic problems exist. If so, preoperative and preprocedure evaluation should proceed along the lines described in the sections discussing those topics. In addition, difficulty with endotracheal intubation should be anticipated in an acromegalic patient; lateral neck films or CT scans of the neck and direct or indirect visualization can identify patients with subglottic stenosis or an enlarged tongue, mandibles, epiglottis, or vocal cords.[275,276] If placement of an arterial line is necessary, a brachial or femoral site may be preferable to a radial site.[277]

Prolactin has been one of the most interesting markers to identify patients with pituitary tumors. Elevated prolactin levels are often, but not invariably associated with galactorrhea. Females commonly present with amenorrhea, and males present with impotence. Optimal therapy for prolactin-secreting tumors is now believed to be the dopamine agonist bromocriptine or cabergoline. These drugs, which are extremely effective in controlling the prolactin level and restoring gonadotropin function, are used when fertility is desired. When normal menses, contraception, and skeletal integrity are desired, birth control pills are the treatment.[278] Side effects of bromocriptine include orthostatic hypotension, gastroparesis (possible increased risk of aspiration), constipation, and nasal congestion (possible need for oral intubation).[278] With large prolactin-secreting tumors (macroadenomas), loss of other pituitary function is common, and evaluation of thyroid and adrenocortical status is indicated. Preoperative and preprocedure preparation of patients with Cushing's syndrome is discussed in the section on ACTH excess.

Anterior Pituitary Hypofunction

Anterior pituitary hypofunction results in deficiency of one or more of the following hormones: GH, TSH, ACTH, prolactin, or gonadotropin. Preoperative and preprocedure preparation of patients who are chronically deficient in ACTH and TSH is discussed earlier. No special preoperative and preprocedure preparation is required for a patient deficient in prolactin or gonadotropin; deficiency in GH, however, can result in atrophy of cardiac muscle, a condition that may necessitate preoperative and preprocedure cardiac evaluation. Nonetheless, anesthetic problems have not been documented in patients with isolated GH deficiency. Acute deficiencies are another matter.

Acute pituitary deficiency is often caused by bleeding into a pituitary tumor. In surgical specimens of resected adenomas, as many as 25% show evidence of hemorrhage.

These patients often present with acute headache, visual loss, nausea or vomiting, ocular palsy, disturbances of consciousness, fever, vertigo, or hemiparesis. In such patients, rapid transsphenoidal decompression should be accompanied by consideration of replacement therapy, including glucocorticoids and treatment of increased intracranial pressure.

Obstetric anesthesiologists are often aware of these pituitary failure problems: Sheehan's syndrome is the clinical manifestation of pituitary infarction associated with hypotension after or during obstetric hemorrhage. Conditions that strongly suggest this diagnosis are failure to start postpartum lactation, increasing fatigue, cold intolerance, and especially hypotension unresponsive to volume replacement and pressors.

Posterior Pituitary Hormone Excess and Deficiency

Secretion of vasopressin, or antidiuretic hormone (ADH), is enhanced by increased serum osmolality or the presence of hypotension. Inappropriate secretion of vasopressin, without relation to serum osmolality, results in hyponatremia and fluid retention. This inappropriate secretion can result from a variety of CNS lesions; from drugs such as nicotine, narcotics, chlorpropamide, clofibrate, vincristine, vinblastine, and cyclophosphamide; and from pulmonary infections, hypothyroidism, adrenal insufficiency, and ectopic production from tumors. Preoperative and preprocedure management of a surgical patient with inappropriate secretion of vasopressin includes appropriate treatment of the causative disorders and restriction of water. Occasionally, drugs that inhibit the renal response to ADH (e.g., lithium or demeclocycline) should be administered preoperatively to restore normal intravascular volume and electrolyte status.

Most of the clinical features associated with the syndrome of inappropriate antidiuretic hormone (SIADH) secretion are related to hyponatremia and the resulting brain edema; these features include weight gain, weakness, lethargy, mental confusion, obtundation, and disordered reflexes and may culminate in convulsions and coma. This form of edema rarely leads to hypertension.

SIADH should be suspected in any patient with hyponatremia who excretes urine that is hypertonic relative to plasma. The following laboratory findings further support the diagnosis:
1. Urinary sodium >20 mEq/L
2. Low serum levels of BUN, creatinine, uric acid, and albumin
3. Serum sodium <130 mEq/L
4. Plasma osmolality <270 mOsm/L
5. Urine hypertonic relative to plasma

Noting the response to water loading is a useful way of evaluating patients with hyponatremia. Patients with SIADH are unable to excrete dilute urine even after water loading. Assay of ADH in blood can confirm the diagnosis. Too vigorous treatment of chronic hyponatremia can result in disabling demyelination.[279,280] The increase in serum sodium should not be greater than 1 mEq/L/hr[279,280] (see the discussion of hyponatremia in the later section "Electrolyte Disorders").

Patients with mild to moderate symptoms of water intoxication can be treated with restriction of fluid intake to about 500 to 1000 mL/day. Patients with severe water intoxication and CNS symptoms may need vigorous treatment consisting of intravenous administration of 200 to 300 mL of 5% saline solution over a period of several hours, followed by fluid restriction.

Treatment should be directed at the underlying problem. If SIADH is drug induced, use of the drug should be withdrawn. Inflammation should be treated with appropriate measures, and neoplasms should be managed with surgical resection, irradiation, or chemotherapy, whichever is indicated.

No drugs are available that can suppress release of ADH from the neurohypophysis or from a tumor. Dilantin and narcotic antagonists such as naloxone and butorphanol have some inhibiting effect on physiologic ADH release but are clinically ineffective in patients with SIADH. Drugs that block the effect of ADH on renal tubules include lithium, which is rarely used because its toxicity often outweighs its benefits, and demethylchlortetracycline in doses of 900 to 1200 mg/day. The latter drug interferes with the ability of the renal tubules to concentrate urine, thereby causing excretion of isotonic or hypotonic urine and lessening the hyponatremia. Demethylchlortetracycline can be used in ambulatory patients with SIADH when it is difficult to restrict fluids.

When a patient with SIADH comes to the operating room for any surgical procedure, fluids are managed by measuring central volume status by CVP, pulmonary artery lines, or the cross-sectional left ventricular area at end-diastole on transesophageal echocardiography and by frequent assays of urine osmolarity, plasma osmolarity, and serum sodium, including the period immediately after surgery. Despite the common impression that SIADH is frequently seen in elderly patients in the postoperative period, studies have shown that the patient's age and the type of anesthetic used have no bearing on the postoperative development of SIADH. It is not unusual to see many patients in the neurosurgical ICU suffering from this syndrome. The diagnosis is usually one of exclusion. Patients with SIADH generally require only fluid restriction; very rarely is hypertonic saline needed.

Lack of ADH, which results in diabetes insipidus, is caused by pituitary disease, brain tumors, infiltrative diseases such as sarcoidosis, head trauma (including trauma after neurosurgery), or lack of a renal response to ADH. The last can occur as a result of such diverse causes as hypokalemia, hypercalcemia, sickle cell anemia, obstructive uropathy, and renal insufficiency. Preoperative or preprocedure treatment of diabetes insipidus consists of restoring normal intravascular volume by replacing urinary losses, administering desmopressin nasally, and giving daily fluid requirements intravenously.

Perioperative management of patients with diabetes insipidus is based on the extent of the ADH deficiency. Management of a patient with complete diabetes insipidus and a total lack of ADH does not usually present any major problem as long as the side effects of the drug are avoided and the presence of the condition is known before surgery. Just before surgery, the patient is given the usual dose of DDAVP (desmopressin acetate) intranasally or an intravenous bolus of 100 mU of aqueous vasopressin, followed by constant infusion of 100 to 200 mU/hr.[281]

The dose is usually adjusted to permit the daily breakthrough polyuria that avoids the iatrogenic syndrome of SIADH. We have found it useful to continue that dosing regimen perioperatively in all ambulatory patients who can take fluid orally in the postoperative period. All the intravenous fluids given intraoperatively should be isotonic to reduce the risk of water depletion and hypernatremia. Plasma osmolality should be measured every hour, both intraoperatively and immediately after surgery. If plasma osmolality rises well above 290 mOsm/L, hypotonic fluids can be administered; the rate of the intraoperative vasopressin infusion can be increased to more than 200 mU/hr.

For patients who have a partial deficiency of ADH, it is not necessary to use aqueous vasopressin perioperatively unless plasma osmolality rises above 290 mOsm/L. Nonosmotic stimuli (e.g., volume depletion) and the stress of surgery usually cause the release of large quantities of ADH perioperatively. Consequently, these patients require only frequent monitoring of plasma osmolality during this period.

Because of side effects, the dose of vasopressin should be limited to that necessary for control of diuresis.[282] The oxytoxic and coronary artery–constricting properties of vasopressin make this limit especially applicable to patients who are pregnant or have coronary artery disease.[282]

Another problem for anesthesiologists is the care of patients who come to the operating room with a vasopressin drip for the treatment of bleeding from esophageal varices. This treatment is less common since the advent of laser therapy for varices. However, when vasopressin is given, the vasoconstrictive effect of vasopressin on the splanchnic vasculature is used to decrease bleeding. Such patients are often volume depleted and may have concomitant coronary artery disease. Because vasopressin has been shown to markedly decrease oxygen availability, primarily as a result of decreased stroke volume and heart rate, monitoring of tissue oxygen delivery may be useful. In 1982, Nikolic and Singh[283] described a patient with a history of angina pectoris who received a combination of cimetidine and vasopressin for esophageal varices. Bradyarrhythmias and AV block occurred and necessitated placement of a pacemaker. On two occasions, discontinuation of either of these drugs alleviated the symptoms. This effect indicates that the combination of cimetidine and vasopressin could be deleterious to the heart because of the combined negative inotropic and arrhythmogenic effects of the two drugs.

DISEASES INVOLVING THE CARDIOVASCULAR SYSTEM

Hypertension (also see Chapter 24)

Analysis of the perioperative treatment of hypertension is important because of the prevalence of the condition (30% of the general population in the United States), the great risk in perioperative care of a hypertensive patient, and the high cost of unnecessary delays in surgery. The controversy centers around two issues. Does inadequate control of hypertension result in complications that could be prevented with some control? How much control of BP is needed and for how long? That is, does overzealous control just create unnecessary postponements of elective surgery or, worse, predispose the patient to exaggerated adverse drug reactions and greater hemodynamic instability than not so zealous control does?

Because of the controversy regarding the appropriateness of preoperative treatment of hypertension, the original articles that stimulated this controversy will be evaluated. Smithwick and Thompson[284] and Brown[285] reported overall mortality rates of 2.5% to 3.6%, respectively, for hypertensive patients undergoing sympathectomy between 1935 and 1947. These values were five or six times higher than those for normotensive patients undergoing similar operations. Obviously, these patients were not randomly assigned to treatment or nontreatment groups, and no attempt was made to ensure that end-organ disease was equivalent in the two groups. In 1929, Sprague[286] analyzed the records of 75 patients with hypertensive cardiac disease and found that 24 (32%) died during or shortly after operations involving general anesthesia.

In the early 20th century, severely ill patients did not do well perioperatively; however, whether *preoperative* treatment would have improved the surgical outcome is unknown. The evolution of drug therapy for hypertension was hampered in the late 1950s and early 1960s by the publication of case reports of severe hypotension and bradycardia in patients given antihypertensive drugs before surgery. Tailoring of the anesthetic dose to the patient's condition and the realization that sympatholytic antihypertensive drugs decrease anesthetic requirements[287] caused such case reports to disappear from the literature.

A more recent prospective controlled double-blind study by the VA provided a rationale for lifelong treatment of hypertension: such treatment decreased the incidence of stroke, CHF, and progression to renal insufficiency and accelerated (malignant) hypertension[288,289] (Table 27-16). Many other studies have confirmed the beneficial effect of treating hypertension, even in patients with diastolic pressures of 90 to 104 mm Hg.[290-292] One study has indicated caution when adding diuretics to the therapeutic limits in treating a patient with an abnormal ECG whose BP does not decrease after administration of the usual doses of diuretic drugs (see the later section "Hypokalemia").[293] There is also controversy regarding the use of calcium channel blockers in patients with coronary artery disease.

Table 27–16 Effect on morbidity of treating hypertension (average diastolic blood pressure, 90-114 mm Hg)

	Control Group	Treatment Group
5-yr morbidity	55%	18%
Death	19/194	8/186
Terminating CHF	5	0
Terminating stroke	6	0
All CHF	11	0
All strokes	20	5

CHF, congestive heart failure.
Data from Veterans Administration Cooperative Study Group on Antihypertensive Agents: Effects of treatment on morbidity in hypertension: Results in patients with diastolic blood pressure averaging 90 through 114 mm Hg. JAMA 213:1143, 1970.

For several short-acting dihydropyridine calcium channel blockers, a meta-analysis of first-line therapy for hypertension suggested the possibility of harm.[294] A meta-analysis of drugs used in stable angina demonstrated significantly worse outcomes in patients taking nifedipine versus β-blockers.[295] However, other analyses suggest that nifedipine is safe in patients with cardiovascular disease, particularly if the long-acting formulation is used.[296,297]

Substantial benefit has also been shown for treatment of isolated systolic hypertension (systolic BP >160 mm Hg and diastolic BP <90 mm Hg) in the elderly[298] (Table 27-17) and in diabetics.[299] However, overvigorous treatment of hypertension can result in a "J curve" for morbidity, especially in patients with coronary artery stenosis (i.e., if BP is reduced too much, morbidity starts to increase again)[291,300] (Fig. 27-8), although these findings are controversial.[301] Other studies in experimental models of hypertension and in humans indicate even more than prophylactic benefit: treatment results in regression of cardiac hypertrophy and autonomic nerve alterations of hypertension. U.S. government statistics reveal significant decreases (>50%) in the death rate from stroke from 1969 to 1992 and a 40% overall decrease in age-adjusted cardiovascular mortality. Deaths related to hypertensive cardiovascular disease and to MI have decreased dramatically since 1974, and this decrease accounts for most of the decline in cardiovascular death in this time period.

Table 27–17 Effect of treating isolated systolic hypertension on morbidity*

	Morbidity (Events, *n*)		
	Active Treatment Group (n = 2365)	Placebo Group (n = 2371)	Relative Risk
Deaths	213	242	0.87
Strokes	96	149	0.63
Transient ischemic attacks	62	82	0.75
Myocardial infarction	50	74	0.67
Coronary artery bypass graft	30	47	0.63
Angioplasty	19	22	0.86
Left ventricular failure	48	102	0.46

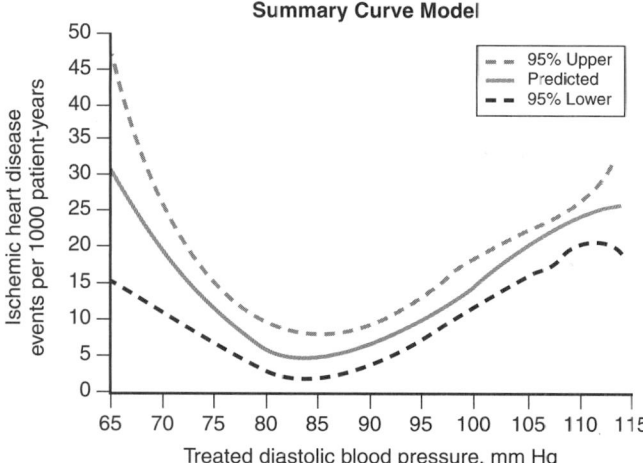

Figure 27–8 Studies that stratified cardiac events by treated diastolic blood pressure levels. Ischemic Heart Disease Events is a combination of morbidity and mortality. The summary curve was calculated by using a systematic decrease of 10 mm Hg in diastolic blood pressure levels. Surrounding *dashed curves* show the 95% confidence intervals. (Redrawn from Farnett L, Mulrow CD, Linn WD, et al: The J-curve phenomenon and the treatment of hypertension. Is there a point beyond which pressure reduction is dangerous? JAMA 265:489, 1991.)

This decrease (at least in localized communities) correlates with successful control of hypertension. This strong evidence from the VA studies and from epidemiologic data have led to the belief that all patients with a diastolic BP above 90 mm Hg should be treated, regardless of age. Although the median BP in the United States is 129/86 mm Hg, the ideal BP for the prevention of arterial aging is 115/76 mm Hg.[26,27] Furthermore, as the Framingham studies have shown, we gain approximately 20 mm Hg in systolic BP and 10 mm Hg in diastolic BP as we age from 30 to 65. This finding is important because every 10–mm Hg increase in systolic BP and every 8–mm Hg increase in diastolic BP age the arteries the equivalent of 4 years. Therefore, preventing these increases would make the average 65-year-old person only 52 years old physiologically.[26] If 115/76 mm Hg is the ideal, why, then, do we accept 130 or even 140/85 or 90 mm Hg before treatment? Arterial aging could be greatly mitigated if we advocated a more aggressive approach to treating BP that exceeds 115/76 mm Hg.

The Framingham data also indicate that one should prevent elevations in both systolic and diastolic BP.[291] In fact, investigations of the Framingham study show that there is nothing to suggest a greater impact of diastolic BP on aging of the arteries.

However, the question is whether elective surgery should be postponed and patient and physician schedules disrupted so that treatment can be instituted and stabilized, even for systolic hypertension alone. Several schools of thought exist, the two oldest represented by studies conducted by Prys-Roberts and colleagues[302] in 1971 and by Goldman and Calder[303] in 1979. Several other studies (Bedford and Feinstein,[304] Asiddao et al.,[305] Stone et al.,[225,308] Flacke et al.,[227] Ghignone et al.,[228]

Tuman et al.,[232] Ellis et al.,[306] Charlson et al.,[8] Mangano et al.,[226,307] Wolfsthal,[309] Pasternack et al.[310]) have also been cited. Weksler and colleagues[311] investigated the issue of preoperative hypertension in a study using a randomized design, but the results may be very limited. Only one study has directly assessed the relationship between cardiovascular disease and preoperative isolated systolic hypertension. In a multicenter study of patients undergoing CABG surgery, the presence of isolated systolic hypertension has been associated with a 30% increased incidence of perioperative cardiovascular complications when compared with normotensive individuals, but no study has addressed the importance of isolated systolic hypertension in noncardiac surgery.[312] Unfortunately, each of these studies has deficiencies that prevent the establishment of a definitive answer to this question. However, we now believe that the weight of evidence from these studies taken together compels an answer.

Critical Analysis of the Data of Prys-Roberts and Colleagues

Followers of Prys-Roberts and colleagues[302] believe that preoperative treatment of hypertension lowers the incidence of perioperative morbidity and mortality. This study compared three groups: a control group consisting of seven elderly normotensive patients with an average mean arterial BP of 89.5 mm Hg, a group of seven hypertensive patients whose high BP was not treated preoperatively (four were being treated not for high BP but for its complications) and who had an average mean arterial BP of 129.5 mm Hg, and a group of 15 hypertensive patients whose high BP was treated preoperatively and who had an average mean arterial BP of 129.9 mm Hg. The same doses of thiopental and halothane were given to all groups of patients, and measurements were made of absolute change in mean arterial BP, cardiac arrhythmias, and ECG evidence of ischemia. Patients with untreated hypertension had the greatest absolute fall in BP and the highest percentage of arrhythmias and ischemia.

Several flaws in study design create serious doubt whether the relationship between preoperative treatment of hypertension and perioperative morbidity has been evaluated objectively in this investigation. First, the wisdom of administering the same dose of anesthetic to both groups of patients should be questioned. If the anesthetic dose had been titrated to the anesthetic needs of the patient, would the results have been different? Second, BP did not differ between the treated and untreated groups. In addition, at least four of the seven hypertensive patients who were not treated for high BP were "sicker" than any of the hypertensive patients who were treated. Why some patients were treated for hypertension and others were not was not explained; selection definitely did not occur on a random basis. Finally, it was not stated whether surgery was similar for all groups.

This study does indicate that patients who are sick preoperatively have more problems perioperatively than healthy patients do. This has been shown many times (see Fowkes and colleagues[12] and Cohen and Duncan[313] for reviews). However, from these data, the efficacy of preoperative treatment of hypertension cannot be established. This study and others by the same group nonetheless provide useful data regarding the hemodynamic consequences of anesthesia when a standard technique is used on patients who have untreated hypertension.

Critical Analysis of the Data of Goldman and Caldera

The school of thought represented by Goldman and Caldera[303] advocates that preoperative treatment of hypertension does not affect the outcome. Goldman and Caldera state that their study is a prospective one. However, the only prospective aspect of their study appears to be that patients were examined preoperatively. These investigators compared surgical outcomes in three groups: sick hypertensive patients whose high BP was treated preoperatively; less sick hypertensive patients whose high BP was "undertreated" preoperatively; and less sick, only moderately hypertensive patients who received no treatment preoperatively. No difference in outcome between the groups was found.

This study has several flaws in design. Patients were not randomly assigned regarding preoperative treatment, undertreatment, or nontreatment of hypertension. In addition, sicker patients were allocated to the treated hypertensive group (Table 27-18), thus biasing the study results toward favoring nontreatment of hypertension.

Other flaws concern statistical methods. Only 117 hypertensive patients were studied, and only 34 of the 117 patients who were hypertensive at surgery had a diastolic BP of at least 100 mm Hg (see Table 27-16). If the rate of morbid complications was assumed to be 20% in the untreated group and if treatment was assumed to reduce morbidity by 50%, then by power analysis,[314] Goldman and Caldera[303] would have had to compare approximately 237 patients to have an 80% chance of finding a difference at a confidence level of 0.05. If a lower rate of morbidity in the untreated group (e.g., 15%) and a lesser reduction in the rate of morbidity (e.g., 33%) were assumed, substantially more patients would have to be studied to be 80% sure that no difference occurred, even at the 0.05 confidence level. For example, if the rate of morbid complications was assumed to be 15% in the untreated group and if treatment was assumed to reduce morbidity by 33%, 764 patients would have had to be studied in each group to be 80% certain that no difference occurred, the confidence level being 0.05. These major flaws in study design make it impossible to ascertain whether preoperative treatment of hypertension decreased perioperative morbidity.

Critical Analysis of the Data of Bedford and Feinstein and the Data of Wolfsthal

Bedford and Feinstein[304] and Wolfsthal[309] and their supporters believe that BP instability is the condition most frequently predicting morbid perioperative complications. In the Bedford-Feinstein study, the responses of three groups to rapid-sequence induction were compared prospectively. Patients were allocated to groups based on the initial admitting room BP and the average presurgical in-hospital BP: group I (30 patients) had a BP of less than 140/90 mm Hg during and after admission (normal BP group), group II (12 patients) had a BP of greater than 140/90 mm Hg on admission but less than 140/90 mm Hg during hospitalization (labile BP group), and group III (8 patients) had a BP greater than 140/90 mm Hg during and after admission (hypertensive BP group). Whether any of the patients in the labile or hypertensive BP groups were receiving therapy for hypertension, had end-organ complications of hypertension (e.g., ischemic heart disease), or were told that they were hypertensive was not stated. Patients were given standard (i.e., not tailored to the patient's condition) premedication (morphine, diazepam, and atropine) and standard rapid-sequence induction (thiopental, 3 to 4 mg/kg intravenously; succinylcholine, 1.5 mg/kg intravenously). After intubation, the heart rate and BP increased significantly in all three groups. The increase was greatest in the labile BP group, which had an increase from a mean BP of 102 ± 5 to 152 ± 4 mm Hg. Eight of 12 patients in that group required additional thiopental or vasodilating drugs (or both) to normalize BP, and transient ST-segment depression in lead II occurred in 2 of 12. No patient in either of the other two groups required similar treatment or had ST-segment changes seen on ECG.

Thus, this study does indicate that patients with labile BP may require more careful titration of anesthetic drugs than those whose BP is either normal or high but stable. However, we do not know whether the results would have been different if the anesthetic had been titrated to the anesthetic needs of the individual patient. Nor do we know whether the groups had equivalent baseline end-organ disease. We do not even know how many patients were being treated for hypertension. Similar deficiencies[7] are present in retrospective analyses of the effect of hypertension on perioperative hemodynamic lability (Wolfsthal[309]) and perioperative outcomes (Mangano studies[307] and Charlson and associates[8,315-317]). Although such deficiencies mean that we do not know whether preoperative treatment

Table 27–18 Analysis of treatment groups used by Goldman and Caldera[303] to evaluate the effectiveness of preoperative treatment of hypertension in surgical patients

| Preoperatively Hypertensive Patients | n | Preoperatively | | | |
		Diastolic BP >99 mm Hg (n)	BUN >30 mg/dL (n)	Angina or CHF (%)	TIAs (%)
Treated successfully*	79	0	8	47	13
Treated unsuccessfully	40	34	13	40	18
Not treated	77		1	26	4

lessened the perioperative risk for these particular hypertensive patients, the deficiencies do not decrease the importance of preoperative hypertension as a marker predicting increased perioperative cardiovascular and renal risk.

Critical Analysis of the Data of Asiddao and Colleagues

The study conducted by Asiddao and colleagues[305] is cited by those advocating preoperative treatment of hypertension. In this study, records of 166 cases of unilateral carotid endarterectomy were reviewed to investigate the association of preoperative and intraoperative factors with perioperative complications. Asiddao and coworkers found that postoperative hypertension (i.e., systolic BP >200 mm Hg or diastolic BP >110 mm Hg) and transient postoperative neurologic deficits occurred more commonly in the 21 patients with poor preoperative control of BP (BP >170/95 mm Hg) (52% and 23.8%, respectively) than in the 79 patients with adequate BP control (BP <170/95 mm Hg) (35% and 2.5%, respectively) or in the 66 normotensive patients (17% and 1.5%, respectively). No statistically significant difference was found between the groups regarding permanent neurologic sequelae of surgery or the rate of myocardial ischemia.

The study by Asiddao and associates[305] does not tell us whether postoperative hypertension caused the transient neurologic deficits or whether these deficits resulted in a compensation of postoperative hypertension. We also do not know whether the three groups were equivalent in end-organ manifestations of preoperative disease. Nor does the study tell us why BP was not controlled preoperatively in some patients or whether preoperative normalization of BP would have reduced the rate of postoperative complications. This study does tell us that patients who have high BP before surgery are likely to have high BP after surgery.

Critical Analysis of the Data of Stone and Associates

Stone and associates[225,308] gave one of a variety of β-adrenergic blocking drugs or placebo as preoperative medication to a group of mildly hypertensive patients, and knowing to which group the patients were assigned, the investigators then looked for ischemic episodes. They observed a significantly greater incidence of brief ischemic episodes during induction and emergence in the untreated patients than in patients given a β-adrenergic blocking drug as premedication (Table 27-19). Although on the surface the results seem to clearly establish the efficacy of β-blocking drugs in reducing perioperative ischemic episodes in patients who are mildly hypertensive preoperatively, two limitations might temper our enthusiasm. First, there seems to be a problem with randomization. Even though characteristics of the groups are not statistically different, they are numerically different. One therefore wonders whether bias was introduced by the fact that the control group underwent more vascular operations and had more preexisting coronary artery disease than the treatment groups did. Second, the observers' awareness of which patients belonged to which treatment group could introduce insidious and subtle differences in management, such as provision of inadequate anesthesia, a closer search for myocardial ischemia, or

Table 27–19 Myocardial ischemia and sympathectomy in "mildly" hypertensive patients[225,308]

	Control Group	Mildly Hypertensive Patients Receiving a β-Adrenergic Receptor Blocking Drug Immediately Preoperatively
Development of myocardial ischemia	11	2
No evidence of myocardial ischemia	28	87

Data from Stone JG, Foëx P, Sear JW, et al: Myocardial ischemia in untreated hypertensive patients. Effect of a single small oral dose of a beta-adrenergic blocking agent. Anesthesiology 68:495, 1988.

more lengthy sampling of ECG strips from the control group. Although one wishes that a double-blind study could be performed in such a situation and perhaps it is possible to do so, the effect on heart rate induced by β-adrenergic blockade may make such a study difficult. Stone and coworkers[225] clearly note the limitations of their study and should be congratulated for not extrapolating or expanding their conclusions beyond that allowed by the data.

Some may comment that the tachycardia that was allowed to occur was severe and therefore indicative of inadequate anesthesia and that the authors have merely demonstrated that β-adrenergic blockade takes the place of a skillful anesthesiologist. We hesitate to come to that conclusion because we believe that these investigators really tried to provide the best anesthesia care possible. We doubt that even the subtle bias of an unblinded study could have caused this degree of inadequate anesthesia, but one must consider that possibility. Nevertheless, this study and several other published papers[226-228,232,306,309] demonstrating that clonidine or other techniques depress sympathetic nervous system responses during anesthesia all imply that modifying the response of the sympathetic nervous system, whether on the α-adrenergic side with clonidine, on the β-adrenergic side with one of the β-adrenergic blocking drugs used by Stone and colleagues,[225] with deep general anesthesia,[230] or with regional anesthesia,[229] may be all that is needed preoperatively in a mildly hypertensive patient. Data from the Multicenter Study of Perioperative Ischemia (McSPI) research group (see review in the next section) substantiates this point of view.[226]

Critical Analysis of the Data of the McSPI Group

Mangano and coworkers in the McSPI group[226] evaluated patients at risk for coronary artery disease who were undergoing noncardiac surgery. Those meeting the inclusion criteria listed in Table 27-20 were randomly assigned to receive atenolol or placebo for 7 days, as outlined in Table 27-21. Although no difference in morbidity occurred in the first 2 weeks, atenolol produced significantly higher survival rates at 1 and 2 years (Table 27-22). The difference was so great that administering atenolol was

Table 27–20   Eligibility criteria used by the McSPI group for treatment with atenolol on the morning of surgery and for the subsequent 2 weeks

Surgery and anesthesia	Patient scheduled for elective noncardiac surgery requiring general anesthesia
Cardiac risks	Patient at risk for coronary artery disease, as indicated by the presence of at least 2 of the following: Age ≥65 yr Typical angina Atypical angina with a positive stress test Hypertension Smoking (current) Total cholesterol >240 mg/dL Diabetes
Other criteria	No current congestive heart failure, bronchospasm, 3rd-degree heart block

Abstracted from Mangano DT, Layug EL, Wallace A, et al: Effect of atenolol on mortality and cardiovascular morbidity after noncardiac surgery. N Engl J Med 335:1713, 1996.

Table 27–22   Benefits of administration of atenolol for 1 week in patients at risk for coronary artery disease who were undergoing noncardiac surgery: the McSPI study

	Placebo Group (n = 101)	Atenolol Group (n = 99)	P Value
6-mo survival rate	92%	100%	.001
1-yr survival rate	86%	97%	.005
2-yr survival rate	79%	91%	.019

From Mangano DT, Layug EL, Wallace A, et al: Effect of atenolol on mortality and cardiovascular morbidity after noncardiac surgery. N Engl J Med 335:1713, 1996, with permission.

the equivalent of making the average 69-year-old man 3.7 years younger physiologically than the same patient not given atenolol.[26] Even though these data did not pertain solely to hypertensive patients (about 65% did relate to such patients), the results speak clearly about the benefit of controlling BP and "hemodynamic stress" in similar patients. Thus, we believe that the weight of evidence provides a clear answer to our question. The long-lasting benefit from even short-duration therapy indicates that

Table 27–21   Protocol for administration of atenolol in patients at risk for coronary artery disease who were undergoing noncardiac surgery: the McSPI study

Patient criteria	Heart rate ≥55 beats/min Systolic blood pressure (BP) ≥100 mm Hg Absence of congestive heart failure Absence of 3rd-degree heart block Absence of bronchospasm
Protocol	(1) 5 mg of atenolol IV preoperatively over 5-min period. If criteria continue to be met, another 5 mg of atenolol IV over 5-min period (2) Repeat #1 immediately after surgery (3) On postoperative day 1 and for all days until discharge up through day 7, same drug regimen as in #1 and #2 every 12 hr or once orally (50 mg if heart rate >55 beats/min but no higher than 65 beats/min and systolic BP >100 mm Hg, or 100 mg if heart rate >65 beats/min and systolic BP >100 mm Hg)

Modified from Mangano DT, Layug EL, Wallace A, et al: Effect of atenolol on mortality and cardiovascular morbidity after noncardiac surgery. N Engl J Med 335:1713, 1996, with permission.

prevention of plaque disruption may be the mechanism of benefit.[318]

Critical Analysis of the Study by Weksler and Colleagues

Weksler and colleagues[311] studied 989 chronically treated hypertensive patients who underwent noncardiac surgery with a diastolic BP between 110 and 130 mm Hg and who had no previous MI, unstable or severe angina pectoris, renal failure, pregnancy-induced hypertension, left ventricular hypertrophy, previous coronary revascularization, aortic stenosis, preoperative dysrhythmias, conduction defects, or stroke.[311] The control group had their surgery postponed and they remained in the hospital for BP control, and the study patients received 10 mg of nifedipine intranasally. The observed patients did not have any statistically significant differences in postoperative complications, which suggested that this subset of patients without significant cardiovascular comorbidity can proceed with surgery despite elevated BP on the day of surgery. The ability to generalize these findings is limited because of the absence of neurologic or cardiovascular complications in either group, thus suggesting that this was a very low-risk population and not the population that presents the greatest diagnostic dilemma. Study participants were limited to "well-controlled" hypertensives who were severely hypertensive only on the day of surgery and may not apply to chronically "poorly controlled" hypertensives.

Recommendations

Although preoperative systolic BP has been found to be a significant predictor of postoperative morbidity,[225,260, 282-290,292-298,300-309,311,315-317,319-322] no data definitively establish whether preoperative treatment of hypertension reduces perioperative risk. Until a definitive study is performed (and that would unfortunately be extremely difficult to do), we recommend letting the weight of evidence guide preoperative treatment of a patient with hypertension. Such treatment would be based on three general beliefs: (1) The patient should be educated regarding the importance of lifelong treatment of hypertension,[226,288,289,291-299,301,323,324] even isolated systolic hypertension. (2) Perioperative hemodynamic fluctuations occur less frequently in treated than in untreated hypertensive patients (as demonstrated by Prys-Roberts and colleagues[302] and confirmed by Goldman and Caldera,[303] Mangano and associates,[307] and Wolfsthal[309]). (3) Hemodynamic fluctuations have some relationship to morbidity. The data of Stone and coworkers,[225] the McSPI group,[226] Pasternack and colleagues,[310] and Weksler and associates[311] imply that rapid correction of BP or prevention of increases in heart rate may be all that is needed. However, data from animals that had declining renal function with acute reductions in arterial BP accentuate the risks of such reductions.[325] Even though other epidemiologic data confirm these risks,[300,301] the hazards of BP fluctuations and acute hypertension may be serious in an untreated hypertensive subject.[326] Modern drug therapy for hypertension appears to reduce these risks but does so for many with a decrement in quality of life that causes many patients to avoid such medications.[327] Specific racial differences need to be considered before treatment (African-Americans respond less well to β-adrenergic receptor blocking drugs and ACE inhibitors but as well to calcium channel antagonists as whites do).[328]

In addition to deciding whether a hypertensive patient needs treatment and ensuring that none of the complications of antihypertensive drugs are present, preoperative management should include a search for end-organ damage secondary to hypertension—that is, changes in the CNS and coronary arteries, myocardium, aorta, carotid arteries, kidneys, and peripheral blood vessels. This type of injury may affect perioperative management. For example, the presence of renal disease may alter the choice and dosage of anesthetic drugs. Similarly, recent myocardial ischemia may warrant a delay in elective surgery. Knowing the location of myocardial ischemia would indicate which ECG lead should be monitored intraoperatively (also see Chapter 34). In addition, to guide intraoperative regulation of BP and to judge the effects of therapy, we obtain multiple BP readings in both arms while the patient is in various positions. We do this even if these readings are obtained in the preoperative holding area, in the preprocedure evaluation clinic (see Chapter 25), or in the operating room rather than on a ward the night before surgery. It is possible that patients admitted the morning of surgery do not receive as good care, but the difference in outcome is small. We try to minimize that difference by being especially careful.

We use such preoperative data to determine the individualized range of values that we consider tolerable by a particular patient during and after surgery. That is, if BP is 180/100 mm Hg and the heart rate is 96 beats/min on admission with no signs or symptoms of myocardial ischemia, we feel confident that the patient can tolerate these levels during surgery. If during the night BP decreases to 80/50 mm Hg and the heart rate to 48 beats/min and the patient does not wake with signs of a new cerebral deficit, we believe that the patient can safely tolerate such levels during anesthesia. Therefore, on the basis of preoperative data, we derive an individualized set of values for each patient. We then try to keep cardiovascular variables within that range and, in fact, plan before

induction what therapies to use to accomplish that goal (e.g., administration of more/less anesthesia, nitroglycerin or nitroprusside/dopamine, dobutamine, phenylephrine, propranolol/isoproterenol, or atropine) (Fig. 27-9). We believe that this type of planning is especially important for a patient with suspected cardiovascular disease and relatively unimportant for a totally healthy patient. We do not know for certain that keeping cardiovascular variables within an individualized range of acceptable values improves the surgical outcome, but we do believe that such a plan reduces morbidity. For example, in several studies, major intraoperative deviations in BP or heart rate, or both, from the preoperative level have correlated with the occurrence of myocardial ischemia.[302-305,316,317,320-322,329,330]

Preoperative Administration of all Antihypertensive Drugs

We routinely administer all antihypertensive drugs preoperatively, except ACE inhibitors or angiotensin II antagonists (AIIAs). For these, we convert to intravenous preparations, which we administer after establishing hemodynamic stability. Coriat and colleagues[331] found that ACE inhibitors were associated with hypotension in 100% of patients during induction versus about 20% in whom ACE inhibitors were withheld on the morning of surgery.

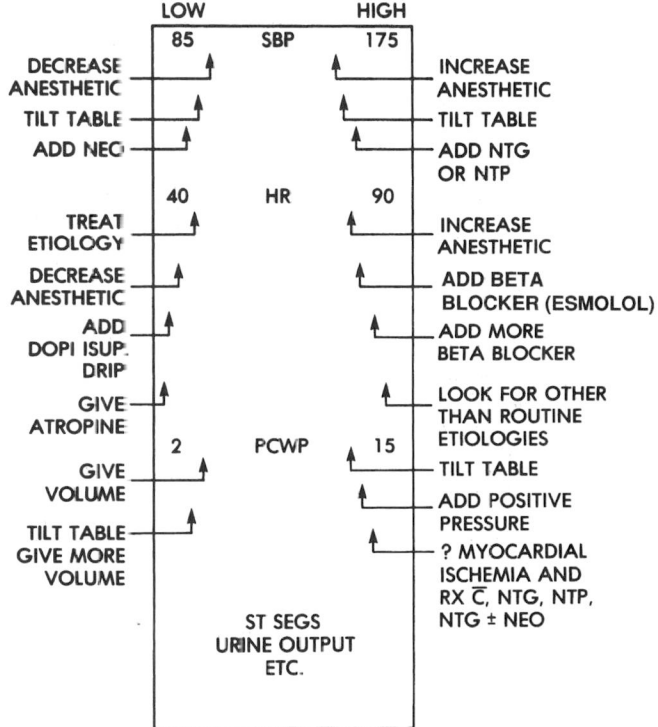

Figure 27–9 Window of acceptable values for cardiovascular variables during and after surgery. This hypothetic range of "safe" cardiovascular values for one patient illustrates possible therapies that might be used if actual perioperative values approached the high or low end of that range. The range of safe values, variables treated, and therapies are tailored to the patient and surgical situation. DOPI ISUP, dopamine or Isuprel; HR, heart rate; NEO, Neo-Synephrine; NTG, nitroglycerin; NTP, nitroprusside; PCWP, pulmonary capillary wedge pressure; SBP, systemic blood pressure.

Bertrand and colleagues performed a prospective randomized study in which it was demonstrated that more severe hypotensive episodes requiring vasoconstrictor treatment occur after induction of general anesthesia in patients chronically treated with an AIIA and receiving this drug on the morning before surgery than in those in whom AIIAs were discontinued on the day before surgery.[332] If these drugs were continued, vasopressin is the drug of choice for refractory hypotension. Although the long-term adverse effects of withholding therapy on the morning of surgery were not assessed, we withhold therapy until either oral fluid is able to be consumed (ambulatory patients) or we can convert to intravenously or nasogastrically administered alternatives (patients who remain NPO postoperatively). We even administer the patient's chronic diuretics on the morning of surgery because the major effect of diuretics after 1 week of therapy is arteriolar vasodilation and assessment of urine output may be inaccurate if the diuretic is abruptly discontinued on the morning of surgery.

Ischemic Heart Disease

Identifying Ischemic Heart Disease

Any of the following conditions may indicate the presence of ischemic heart disease: a history of viselike chest pain, with or without radiation to the inner aspect of the arm or neck; dyspnea on exertion, on exposure to cold, with defecation, or after eating (especially postmenopausal women who do not take estrogen); orthopnea; paroxysmal nocturnal dyspnea; nocturnal coughing; nocturia; previous or current peripheral or pulmonary edema; history of MI; family history of coronary artery disease; diagnosis of MI by ECG or elevated levels of enzymes; and cardiomegaly. Other patients who should be suspected of having ischemic heart disease include those who have diabetes, hypertension (especially if they are cigarette smokers or hyperlipemic),[31,32,333] left ventricular hypertrophy on ECG or echocardiogram,[77,78,334,335] peripheral vascular disease (Lichtor JL and colleagues, personal communication),[335-342] carotid bruits,[339-345] asymptomatic carotid artery occlusion,[339,340] or unexplained tachycardia or fatigue.

The more difficult question to answer is how common ischemic heart disease is in asymptomatic patients or those with a normal ECG but predisposing conditions. The history appears to be the best indicator of coronary artery disease. Tomatis and coworkers[336] recorded coronary angiograms for "nearly all patients" who presented for aortoiliac reconstruction or resection of an abdominal aortic aneurysm. Of those with normal ECG results and histories not suggestive of coronary artery disease, 38% had stenosis of at least 50% in one or more coronary arteries, and 14% had stenosis of at least 75% in one or more coronary arteries. The percentages of patients with stenosis were the same for asymptomatic patients with abnormal ECG findings. However, a normal ECG result was not sensitive in ruling out significant stenosis when vascular disease was present: 44% of patients with normal ECGs and peripheral vascular disease had stenosis of at least 50% in one or more coronary arteries, and 30% had stenosis of at least 75%.

Hertzer and associates[337,338] found angina and a history of myocardial disease to be reliable indicators of coronary artery disease. These investigators studied 1000 patients with peripheral vascular disease. Of the 500 patients with normal ECG results and no history of myocardial disease, 37% had narrowing of at least 70% in one or more coronary arteries. By contrast, of those suspected of having coronary artery disease because of history or ECG results (or both), 78% had narrowing of this same degree. In addition, patients who currently had angina had a 66% incidence of either severe correctable or severe inoperable coronary artery disease, whereas those who had peripheral vascular disease but no angina had an incidence of only 22.5%. For women, knowing the estrogen status appears to be crucial to interpreting other aspects of their cardiovascular history.[346] Thus, in addition to the symptoms just listed that are sought by routine questioning,[347] information about age, smoking, history of diabetes, cholesterol level, exercise tolerance, and estrogen status can all help predict the likelihood of coronary artery disease.

Are these data from 20 and 30 years ago still valid today? We believe so. Even though the average age of the typical surgical patient in the United States is now about 10 years higher than it was 25 years ago (Lichtor JL and colleagues, personal communication), the physiologic age (i.e., the RealAge) of the patients now being operated on is probably similar to that of patients 20 years ago.[26,27] Therefore, although the age-adjusted mortality rates for coronary artery disease have decreased by approximately 45% and the age-adjusted mortality rate for all in-hospital surgical procedures has fallen by over 45%, aging of the surgical population has caused us to face the same risks that we faced 2 decades ago.

Although over 80% of all episodes of myocardial ischemia are "silent,"[348,349] patients with myocardial ischemia are *not* "silent." For example, even though the episodes of myocardial ischemia may have been silent, for all 165 patients studied by Rabkin and Horne[347,350] who had ECG evidence of coronary artery disease, the patient's history gave an indication of the risk of coronary artery disease. This has also been the finding of our own studies[347,351] and several others when physiologic age of 75 years or older has been added to the factors in a clinical history that would indicate myocardial ischemia. These indicators consist of the following: chest pain, typical or atypical; dyspnea on exertion or exposure to cold, with defecation, or after eating; nocturnal coughing; nocturia; previous or current peripheral or pulmonary edema; history of MI; a family history (especially sibling history) of coronary artery disease; cardiomegaly; abnormal ECG results; diabetes, hypertension; hyperlipemia; left ventricular hypertrophy; peripheral vascular disease; cigarette smoking; carotid artery bruits; peripheral vascular surgery; and unexplained tachycardia.

Several studies of asymptomatic carotid artery disease have shown very high perioperative mortality rates and life risk from associated ischemic heart disease.[339,343-345] Barnes and Marszalek[340] found perioperative mortality rates of 18.2% and 15%, respectively, for patients with an asymptomatic carotid bruit or occlusive disease but a rate of only 2.1% for patients undergoing similar peripheral vascular procedures who did not have a carotid bruit.

Table 27–23   Carotid artery bruits and the risk of stroke in elective surgery

Study	Incidence of Stroke in Patients	
	With Bruits	*Without Bruits*
Ropper et al.[343]	1/104	4/631
Of those having vascular surgery	1/37	4/130
Barnes et al.[339]	5/85*	0/364
Perioperative deaths	10.6%	0.3%
Reed et al.[345]		
CABG surgery; 54 strokes	13/54†	4/54†

*All patients included in this study were undergoing vascular surgery. These 85 patients also had either a bruit or significant carotid artery obstruction, or both.

†Case-control study. These investigators examined the incidence of carotid bruit in patients who had strokes after CABG surgery. CABG, coronary artery bypass graft.

Although the existence of asymptomatic carotid bruits did not predict the site of stroke or greatly influence the incidence of perioperative stroke,[282-284] it did predict mortality from ischemic heart disease (Table 27-23). Another point of view is found in the retrospective case-controlled review of strokes after CABG surgery.[345] In that review, strokes after CABG surgery were 3.9 times more likely to occur if a carotid bruit was present preoperatively than if such were not present. The group was too small to determine whether the site of the bruit predicted the site of the stroke. As little as 15% percent of patients with triple-vessel coronary artery disease have abnormal resting ECGs.[335] Transient ischemic attacks (TIAs) are even more predictive. The 5% to 6% annual mortality rate after TIAs in a 60-year-old individual is due mainly to MI; this rate is similar to the 4% annual mortality rate for a 60-year-old with stable angina pectoris.[352]

The important point to remember is that the history is the best indicator of coronary artery disease. In most series, the sensitivity and specificity of the history in indicating coronary artery disease range from 80% to 91% (Lichtor JL and colleagues, personal communication).[333,335-337,345,350,351,353,354] The history has higher sensitivity and specificity than most tests in indicating such disease (also see Chapter 25 for the definition of sensitivity and specificity). However, one test is gaining in popularity because it has been demonstrated to be easy to perform and to accurately predict perioperative morbidity.

One Easy Noninvasive Test and Two Easy Measures—But *Does* Preoperative Treatment Improve Outcome?

Fowkes and colleagues[77,355,356] are testing a simple-to-measure index that would predict the degree of subclinical arterial aging that exists and the likelihood of subsequent cardiovascular events and death: the ratio of systolic BP in the posterior tibial artery of the ankle (as measured by Doppler) to systolic BP in the brachial artery (as measured by cuff). This index has predicted 8- and 10-year cardiovascular mortality in nonoperated patients: the incidence of cardiovascular death was 85% higher in those with an index of less than 0.7. The index is made even more powerful when combined with other historical factors. Patients who had an index of less than 0.9, were hypertensive, and currently smoked had a 43.8% risk of cardiovascular events in the next 5 years, as opposed to the 15.6% risk for those who had identical conditions but an index of 1.0 or higher.

Older's exercise index ("aerobic threshold") seems to have the same goal[357,358]—to predict the degree of subclinical arterial aging. The RealAge system attempts to do the same thing with its measurements but uses a much broader range of modifiable factors.[26,27]

However, the key payoff would be the demonstration that using such tests would motivate patients to modify health-related habits, which in turn would improve their index values. This result would then have to be correlated with beneficial effects on perioperative cardiovascular events. (Examples of changes in health-related habits include food choices, smoking and smoke inhalation, increased physical activity, consumption of antioxidants, use of aspirin, use of β-blocking drugs, use of statins, weight reduction, BP control, anti-inflammatory treatments, and flossing of teeth.) Although an increasing body of data[26,27,342,359,360] seem to predict that such changes would occur, they have not yet been confirmed. Such a study would be incredibly difficult to execute successfully, but would any study be more worthwhile?

Perioperative Morbidity

The presence of coronary artery disease, its severity, the time of the most recent myocardial tissue death, the arteries affected, ventricular function and reserve, and the complications and treatment of the disease are important information to the anesthesiologist. These variables influence the manner in which anesthesia is given and, in fact, may determine whether anesthesia and surgery should be postponed.

Previous Myocardial Infarction

Numerous epidemiologic studies[189,322,323,361-370] (Table 27-24) (but none in the last 9 years) have shown that if a previous MI and subsequent surgery are separated by less than 6 months, the perioperative reinfarction rate is 5% to 86% (1.5 to 10 times higher than the value when previous MI and subsequent surgery are separated by more than 6 months), and the mortality rate is 23% to 86%. After 6 months, the perioperative reinfarction rate seems to stabilize at 2% to 6%. An investigation by Schoeppel and colleagues[368] in which a small number of patients were studied produced a 0% mortality rate in the first year after infarction but a perioperative reinfarction rate of 16.7% and a mortality rate of 67% in patients experiencing perioperative reinfarction. Because the incidence and timing of perioperative reinfarction in the study by Schoeppel and coworkers differ so much from those variables in the other studies listed in Table 27-24, we have placed little emphasis on that study. However, for all 12 of the studies listed in Table 27-24, the overall reinfarction rates are similar.[189,315-317,320-323,351,353,354,361-371] These data do not include patients who underwent immediate

Table 27–24 Incidence of perioperative myocardial infarction or mortality in patients with previous myocardial infarction

Time from MI Operation (mo)	Arkins et al[361] 1963: Mort	Topkins and Artusio[362] 1959-1963		Fraser et al[363] 1960-1964 Mort	Tarhan et al[364] 1967-1970		Sapala et al[365] 1970-1974		Steen et al[366] 1970		von Knorring[370] 1981	
		Reinf	*Mort*		*Reinf*	*Mort*	*Reinf*	*Mort*	*Reinf*	*Mort*	*Reinf*	*Mort*
0-3	40% (11/27)	54.5%	*	38% (19/38)	37% (3/8)	*	86% (6/7)	86% (6/7)	27% (2/18)		25%	*
4-6	*	(12/22)	*	*	16% (3/19)	*			11% (2/18)		(4/16)	
7-12	*	25.0% (9/36)	*	*	5% (2/42)	*					18% (2/11)	*
13-18	*	22.4%	*	*	4% (1/27)	*						
19-24	*	(11/49)	*	*	4% (1/21)	*	5.7% (9/159)	1.9% (3/159)	5.4%		11%	
25-36	*	5.9% (3/51)	*	*	5%	*			(30/544)		(10/89)	*
>36	*	1.0% (5/493)	*	*	(11/232)							
Unknown	*	42.8% (3/7)	*	*	5.6% (7/73)	*					22% (9/41)	*
Total patients with MI	*	6.5% (43/658)	4.7% (31/658)	*	6.6% (28/422)	3% (15/422)	9% (15/166)	5.4% (9/166)	6.1% (36/587)	4.2% (25/587)	15.9% (25/157)	4% (7/157)

*Mortality was not stated.
MI, myocardial infarction: Mort, mortality: Reinf, reinfarction.

angiography, clot dissolution therapy, angioplasty, or stent therapy.

The study conducted by Rao and associates[189] deserves special comment because it proposes to show a vast decrease in the perioperative reinfarction rate with the use of modern monitoring techniques. Rates of perioperative reinfarction and mortality were compared in two groups of patients who had previous MIs and were operated on at two different time periods: 364 patients between 1973 and 1976 and 733 patients between 1976 and 1982. Rao and coworkers attribute the reduction in the overall perioperative reinfarction rate (from 7.7% to 1.9%) and in each time period (i.e., from 36% to 5.8% when surgery occurs within 3 months of a previous MI) to invasive monitoring and rapid treatment of cardiovascular variables when values deviated from normal. These two practices apply to both the intraoperative period and the first 72 postoperative hours. (The 72-hour period may be critical because virtually all 12 studies and others showed that reinfarction was most likely to occur 24 to 96 hours after surgery[189,322,323,361-378] [Table 27-25].) Most of the reduction in the perioperative reinfarction rate applied to patients older than 65 years. (MI makes the physiologic age or risk of death equivalent to that of someone 3 to 17 years older, depending on the location of the infarction and the decrease in left ventricular ejection fraction.[26,27])

An editorial evaluating the study by Rao and colleagues stated that the use of historical controls may have biased the conclusions. Moreover, a different patient mix, improved skills of the surgeon and anesthetist, and other unidentified or unmeasured changes over time may have contributed to the reduction in the reinfarction rate.

Despite the evidence of an increased risk for surgery in patients with a recent MI, Rivers and associates demonstrated relatively low cardiac morbidity (20%) in a cohort of 30 patients requiring urgent or emergency vascular procedures in the first 6 weeks after an MI.[377] Four postoperative deaths (three cardiac related) and two nonfatal reinfarctions occurred. Cardiac complications did not correlate with age, interval from MI to surgery within the initial 6 weeks, type of anesthesia, or complexity of the operation.

Normalization of hemodynamics by pulmonary artery catheter monitoring and 3 days in an ICU also appears to reduce perioperative morbidity in vascular surgery patients, a group at high risk for postoperative cardiac morbidity. In a randomized controlled trial, Berlauk and coworkers[378] examined that intervention scheme, which was similar to the one investigated by Rao and associates,[189] for patients undergoing vein graft bypass for limb salvage from 1986 to 1990. Forty-five patients were randomly assigned to group 1 (i.e., pulmonary artery catheterization performed ≥12 hours before surgery, followed by treatment for hemodynamic optimization). The 44 other patients were randomly assigned to either group 2 (23 patients; i.e., pulmonary artery catheterization within 3 hours of surgery, followed by a shorter treatment for

Table 27–24 Incidence of perioperative myocardial infarction or mortality in patients with previous myocardial infarction—cont'd

Goldman et al[367] 1975-1976		Eerola et al[327] 1970-1974		Schoeppel et al[368] 1980		Rao et al[190] 1973-1976		Rao et al[190] 1976-1982		Shah et al[371] 1983-1986	
Reinf	Mort	Reinf	Mort	Reinf	Mort	Reinf	Mort	Reinf	Mort	Reinf	Mort
4.5% (1/22)	23% (5/22)	8% (1/12)	8% (1/12)	0% (0/1)	0% (0/1)	30% (4/11)	*	5.8% (3/52)	*	4.3% (1/23)	
	5.9% (1/12)	5.9% (1/17)	0% (0/1)	0% (0/8)	0% (0/8)	26% (8/3)	*	2.3% (2/36)	*	0% (0/18)	
						5% (6/127)	*	1.0% (1/104)	*		
0% (0/13)						5% (6/114)		1.6% (4/258)	*		
	8% (1/13)			0% (0/10)	0% (0/10)					5.7% (10/74)	
		4.9% (4/82)	12% (1/82)				*		*		
3.3% (2/66)	3.3% (2/66)					5% (4/81)		1.7% (4/235)			
				0% (0/26)	0% (0/26)						
	8.9% (9/109)			5.7% (3/53)	3.8% (2/53)	7.7% (28/364)	4.1% (15/364)	1.9% (14/733)	0.7% (5/733)	4.7% (13/275)	1.1% (3/275)

hemodynamic optimization) or to group 3 (21 control patients; i.e., no preoperative catheterization or hemodynamic optimization, no treatment guided by CVP monitoring, and minimal or no stay in the ICU).

Berlauk and colleagues reported that patients undergoing less intensive treatment (group 3) were significantly more likely to have intraoperative complications (tachycardia, hypotension, arrhythmia) than were patients in group 1. The overall incidence of postoperative complications (renal failure, CHF, MI, graft thrombosis, death) was 18% for group 1, 13% for group 2, and 43% for group 3. Half the complications in group 3 were attributable to early graft thrombosis and accounted for most of the difference in complication rates. The authors conjectured that the increased incidence of thrombosis was due to poor cardiac output. No significant difference in mortality existed between groups. Although Berlauk and coauthors reported a higher incidence of postoperative cardiac morbidity in the control group, this conclusion is difficult to follow because discrepancies exist between their calculations and data provided elsewhere in the paper. For example, their Table 5 reports three postoperative cardiac complications in group 1, two in group 2, and five in group 3. However, their Table 4 says that only three patients in group 3 (numbers 1, 7, and 8) experienced these complications. Simple explanations for these discrepancies may exist but were not evident to us or to the Task Force on Pulmonary Artery Catheterization of the ASA.[379]

This study had other deficiencies that preclude definitive advice on ways of reducing morbidity in patients with

Table 27–25 When do myocardial infarctions occur after vascular surgery?

Investigators	Year Published	Examined Prospectively	Postoperative				
			Day 0	Day 1	Day 2	Day 3	Day 4
Plumlee and Boettner[372]	1972	No	11/24	3/24	1/24	2/24	
Tarban et al[364]	1972	No		14/71	8/71	22/71	13/71
Rao et al[190]	1983	No		8/28	7/28	10/28	3/28
		No		3/14	4/14	7/14	
Becker and Underwood[373]	1987	?	11/28	6/28	9/28	0/28	1/28
Total (4 studies)			22	34	29	41	17

a previous MI: the outcome did not differ significantly between the groups undergoing "normalization" of hemodynamics more than 12 hours before surgery versus less than 3 hours before surgery. Furthermore, the rationale for group assignments in this study is unclear. Rather than randomly assign the 89 patients to three groups of equal size, the investigators created two randomly selected groups and then subdivided the second group into a separate randomization that created imbalanced sample sizes. Group assignments may not have been truly random because of significant preoperative differences between groups regarding the incidence of angina and CHF and hemodynamic indices. Berlauk and colleagues[378] explained that *"although the randomization sequence was performed at the beginning of the study, actual patient entry into the study was finalized the evening before surgery. Bias of the chief surgical resident, who determined the operating room schedule, may account for the lack of patients with angina. ..."* Furthermore, the role of pulmonary artery catheterization and hemodynamic optimization by aggressive management in reducing perioperative morbidity in a patient with a previous MI is unclear.[380,381] Sandham and colleagues performed a randomized trial comparing goal-directed therapy guided by a pulmonary artery catheter with standard care without the use of a pulmonary artery catheter. The subjects were 1994 high-risk (ASA class III or IV) patients 60 years or older who were scheduled for urgent or elective major surgery, followed by stay in an ICU. They observed no difference in outcomes, further questioning the value of the routine use of pulmonary artery catheters as a means of reducing perioperative morbidity and mortality. Other workers have pointed out that certain surgical procedures (e.g., ophthalmic operations) have low perioperative reinfarction rates[366-368,380] whereas others (e.g., vascular operations[367,374-378,382-387]) have high reinfarction rates. The study by Rao and colleagues[189] does confirm that the perioperative reinfarction rate is higher in the first 6 months after a previous MI. Postponement of surgery for patients who have had an MI less than 6 months earlier should reduce the mortality associated with anesthesia. Again, however, we are lacking data analyzing whether such risk changes with preoperative segregation by clinical criteria or provocative testing. The guidelines promulgated by the American College of Cardiology and the American Heart Association seem to indicate a liberalization of surgery to 6 weeks after infarction in "low-risk patients."[10] The rationale for this liberalization relates to changes in management of MI in the nonoperative setting (i.e., thrombolytics, percutaneous coronary interventions) and its influence on the natural history of coronary artery disease. The less severe the coronary artery disease, the more similar the patient's anticipated survival curve to that of patients who do not have coronary artery disease[388] and, probably, the less the perioperative risk.[378,389,390] Waiting 6 weeks will allow the myocardium to heal and reduce the risk of arrhythmias and rupture of ventricular aneurysms.

Preoperative Testing: Analyses of Benefit versus Risk and Cost

Treadmill exercise testing, bicycle ergometry, dipyridamole-thallium imaging, dobutamine stress echocardiography,

Table 27–26   Adverse cardiac events after abnormal preoperative tests: relative risks (combined) and costs of tests

Test	Studies (N)	RR (95% CI)	Cost (U.S. $)
DTS	11	6.3 (3.0-13.1)	1200-1400
RNV	5	3.8 (1.5-9.4)	500-600
AECG	6	3.7 (2.0-7.1)	300-550
DSE	3	19.0 (5.9-60.8)	1000-1200

AECG, ambulatory electrocardiography; CI, confidence interval; DSE, dobutamine stress echocardiography; DTS, dipyridamole-thallium scintigraphy; RNV, estimation of ejection fraction by radionuclide ventriculography; RR, relative risk.

preoperative Holter monitoring, noninvasive imaging, the ankle-brachial pressure index (see the earlier section "One Easy Noninvasive Test . . ."), and cardiac catheterization also add information to the history and thereby increase our knowledge about the likelihood of cardiac disease and perioperative cardiac function.[353,374-376,383-387,391] Mantha and coworkers[387] performed a meta-analysis to determine which preoperative noninvasive test was most predictive of the risk of an adverse cardiovascular outcome after vascular surgery. They concluded that the presence of wall motion abnormalities during dobutamine stress echocardiography was both predictive and most cost-effective (Table 27-26 and Fig. 27-10). Similarly, Shaw and colleagues[391b] performed a meta-analysis of studies available through 1994 on dipyridamole-thallium imaging and dobutamine stress echocardiography before major vascular surgery and demonstrated that the prognostic value of noninvasive stress imaging abnormalities for perioperative ischemic events is comparable between available techniques but that the accuracy varies with the prevalence of coronary artery disease.

ECG criteria for myocardial ischemia during or after exercise consist of at least 1 mm of J-point depression with downsloping or horizontal ST segments; slowly upsloping ST-segment depression, defined as 2 mm of ST depression measured 80 milliseconds from the J point; and ST-segment elevation[345] (Fig. 27-11). Other responses to treadmill testing that are predictive of severe multivessel or left main stem coronary artery disease include ST-segment depression exceeding 2.5 mm, serious ventricular arrhythmias at low heart rates or early (first 3 minutes) onset of ischemic ST-segment depression, or prolonged duration of the ischemic ST-segment depression in the post-test recovery period (>8 minutes).[353]

Non-ECG responses to treadmill testing that predict severe coronary artery disease include low achieved heart rates (≤120 beats/min), systolic hypotension (decrease of >10 mm Hg) in the absence of hypovolemia or antihypertensive medications, rise in diastolic BP to higher than 110 mm Hg, and an inability to exercise beyond 3 minutes. The treadmill test responses predictive of severe multivessel or left main stem coronary artery disease (or both) are listed in Table 27-27. Clearly, however, the response to the test must be interpreted in light of the patient's history and with the knowledge that it is more predictive for men than women[353] (Table 27-28).

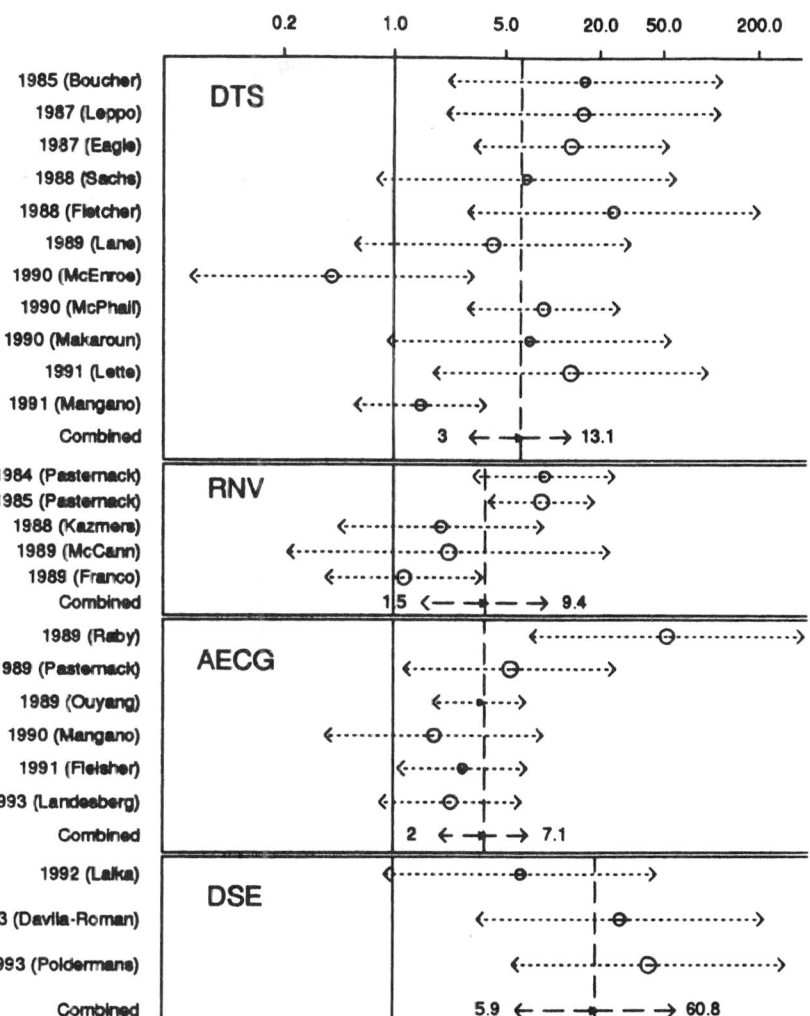

Figure 27–10 Relative risks and confidence intervals resulting from the use of four preoperative tests to predict adverse outcomes after vascular surgery, as reported by various studies. Names at the left refer to the first author of studies reviewed by Mantha and colleagues.[387] *Broken vertical lines* represent combined relative risks, as assessed by each test. AECG, ambulatory electrocardiography; DSE, dobutamine stress echocardiography; DTS, dipyridamole-thallium scintigraphy; RNV, estimate of ejection fraction by radionuclide ventriculography. (Adapted from Mantha S, Roizen MF, Barnard J, et al: Relative effectiveness of preoperative noninvasive cardiac evaluation tests on predicting adverse cardiac outcomes following vascular surgery: A meta-analysis. Anesth Analg 79:422, 1994.)

ECG Patterns Indicative of Myocardial Ischemia

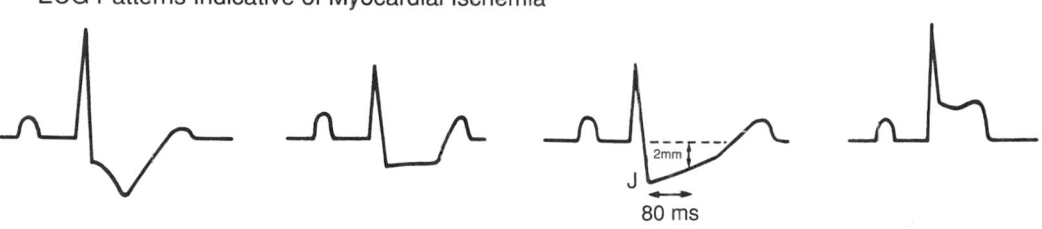

ECG Patterns Not Indicative of Myocardial Ischemia

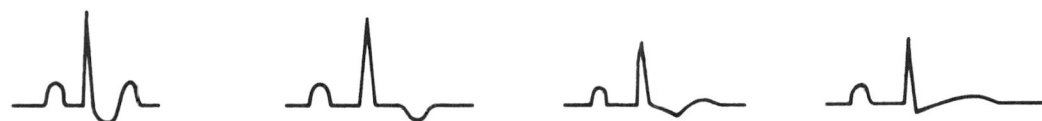

Figure 27–11 Electrocardiographic (ECG) criteria for myocardial ischemia consist of 1 mm or more of J-point depression with downsloping or horizontal ST segments; slowly upsloping ST-segment depression, defined as 2 mm of ST depression measured 80 milliseconds from the J point; and ST-segment elevation. Whereas ST-segment depression indicates nontransmural ischemia, ST-segment elevation often connotes more severe degrees of ischemia reflecting transmural injury. The structure of the ST-segment slope is predictive of the severity of coronary disease shown angiographically, with downsloping ST depression indicating severe two- and three-vessel coronary artery disease more often than either horizontal or slowly upsloping ST depression does and ST-segment elevation indicating high-grade, usually proximal arterial obstruction in patients without previous myocardial infarction. (Reproduced with permission from Goldschlager N: Use of the treadmill test in the diagnosis of coronary artery disease in patients with chest pain. Ann Intern Med 97:383, 1982.)

Table 27–27 Treadmill test responses predictive of severe multivessel and/or left main coronary artery disease

Electrocardiographic responses
  ST-segment response
    Downsloping
    Elevation
  ST-segment depression exceeding 2.5 mm
  Serious ventricular arrhythmias occurring at low heart
    rates (120-130 beats/min)
  Early onset (first 3 min) of ischemic ST-segment
    depression of elevation
  Prolonged duration in the post-test recovery period
    (≥8 min) of ischemic ST-segment depression
Nonelectrocardiographic criteria
  Low achieved heart rate (≤120 beats/min)
  Hypotension* (≥10–mm Hg fall in systolic blood pressure)
  Rise in diastolic blood pressure (≥110-120 mm Hg)
  Low achieved rate-pressure product (≤15,000)
  Inability to exercise beyond 3 min

*In the absence of antihypertensive medications or hypovolemia of any cause.
Modified from Goldschlager N: Use of the treadmill test in the diagnosis of coronary artery disease in patients with chest pain. Ann Intern Med 97:383, 1982.

An inability to increase the heart rate (cardiac risk index [CRI]) above 90 beats/min after supine bicycle exercise for 2 minutes at 50 rpm has been shown to predict perioperative MI with 80% sensitivity. This test is claimed by its investigators to have better sensitivity (80%) with a small sacrifice in specificity (53%) than the Goldman CRI (sensitivity, 60%; specificity, 64%). This same group recommended this test for geriatric patients at low risk (according to the Goldman CRI) to identify the "false-negatives" of the Goldman CRI or for geriatric patients at risk for perioperative MI. Limitations of this test, however, are recognized in patients with impaired joint mobility, dementia, muscle weakness, claudication, or exertional angina.[376] Ejection fractions greater than 50% (and normal left ventricular size on plain chest radiographs) predict good perioperative cardiac function and survival.[390,391]

For dipyridamole-thallium scanning, patients received dipyridamole (0.56 mg/kg) intravenously over a 4-minute period while their heart rate, BP, and ECG were monitored. After an additional 2 minutes, when the effect of dipyridamole was considered maximal, 2 mCi of thallium 201 was administered intravenously. Five minutes after the administration of thallium, initial images were taken for 8 consecutive minutes. Delayed images were obtained 3 hours later. Anterior, 45-degree, and 70-degree left anterior oblique projections were taken each time. Dipyridamole causes vasodilation and an increase in coronary blood flow. Because stenotic vessels cannot dilate normally, areas of myocardium supplied by them will take up less thallium during scanning than will areas supplied by normal vessels and will show up as filling defects on immediate images. On late images, after the vasodilation has resolved, thallium is redistributed to these previously underperfused areas.

Dipyridamole infusion resulted in an increase in heart rate of 17 beats/min, a decrease in systolic BP of 17 mm Hg, and chest pain in 30% of patients, which was reversible with 125 mg of aminophylline intravenously. ECGs were examined for ischemic changes, defined as 1-mm or more horizontal or downsloping ST-segment depression. Myocardial regions on initial and delayed images were graded as being normal, as showing fixed deficits (without redistribution), or as showing one or more segments with thallium redistribution (with or without evidence of fixed deficits). Initial studies[383,384,392] (reviewed by Mantha and colleagues[387]) have shown this test to be valuable in further stratifying high risk, as assessed by five clinical factors (CHF, diabetes mellitus, history of ventricular ectopy, angina, and history of MI). Of patients with thallium redistribution, 45% had a perioperative MI, whereas 7% of patients without redistribution had a perioperative MI ($P = .001$). Dipyridamole-thallium scanning has been suggested to be valuable in stratifying patients with intermediate risk, as assessed by five clinical factors (Q waves on resting ECG, history of ventricular ectopy, diabetes, age >70 years, and angina) that were identified by logistic regression on several clinical findings and Goldman CRIs and Dripp classes. Fletcher and colleagues[392] found the test superior to clinical assessment in identifying high-risk patients for further angiographic study, prophylactic CABG surgery, or intensive intraoperative and

Table 27–28 Electrocardiographic response of angiographically demonstrated coronary artery disease to treadmill exercise

Clinical Characteristics	Prevalence of Coronary Artery Disease (%)	Predictive Accuracy of a Positive Test (%)	Predictive Accuracy of a Negative Test (%)
Asymptomatic	5	10-20	95-100
Noncardiac chest pain	10-25	45-50	80-85
Cardiac chest pain			
Atypical, or probable, angina	50-70	80-85	65-70
Typical, or definite, angina	85-95	95-100	50-55

Modified from Goldschlager N: Use of the treadmill test in the diagnosis of coronary artery disease in patients with chest pain. Ann Intern Med 97:383, 1982.

postoperative management. Dipyridamole-thallium scanning may reveal redistribution when coronary narrowing is only 40% to 60%. This process may aid in the management of higher-risk patients by initiating invasive monitoring, with prompt medication for hemodynamic changes. These actions may have artificially decreased the incidence of perioperative MI in the studies of thallium scanning cited. Because the results of thallium scans in all these studies were made known to the caretakers, patients with positive scans may have received more invasive monitoring, as well as coronary angiography, angioplasty, medications, and CABG surgery. The discriminating capacity of this test may improve with further classification of redistribution segments by size and number and by additional projections (see Fig. 27-10 and Table 27-26). Additionally, both increased lung uptake and left ventricular cavity dilation are indicative of ventricular dysfunction with ischemia. Several investigative groups have demonstrated that delineation of "low" and "high" risk thallium scans (larger area of defect, increased lung uptake, and left ventricular cavity dilation) markedly improved the test's predictive value.[393] This study indicates that patients with "high" risk thallium scans have a particularly increased risk for perioperative morbidity and long-term mortality and might be segregated for high-intensity therapy.

Twenty-four– to 48-hour Holter monitoring of intermediate-risk patients has been shown to be effective in detecting asymptomatic ischemia and has an excellent negative predictive value and a fair positive predictive value for postoperative cardiac complications (see Fig. 27-10 and Table 27-26). Preoperative ischemia increases the risk for intraoperative ischemia threefold to fourfold. Raby and colleagues[385] studied 176 vascular surgery patients who were asymptomatic for ischemic cardiac disease and found preoperative ischemia on Holter monitoring to be an independent factor with high correlation for significant postoperative cardiac complications (e.g., infarction, unstable angina, and ischemic pulmonary edema). In this series, 24- to 48-hour Holter monitoring detected two of three patients with positive stress test results and four patients with postoperative cardiac complications who did not have a history suggestive of ischemic heart disease. With an overall sensitivity of 92%, specificity of 88%, positive predictive value of 38%, and negative predictive value of 99%, Holter monitoring may be the test of choice for evaluating intermediate-risk patients who have no suggestive history or for patients who are unable to undergo an exercise stress test. Importantly, other investigators have demonstrated the value of silent ambulatory ECG monitoring, although the negative predictive values have not been as high as originally reported. Fleisher and colleagues[7] demonstrated a similar predictive value of dipyridamole-thallium imaging and ambulatory ECG monitoring; however, the quantity of silent ischemia could not be used to identify patients at greatest risk who might benefit from further testing and coronary revascularization. Limitations of this method are seen in patients with left bundle branch block, left ventricular hypertrophy, strain, and ST-T changes with digoxin because of the difficulties in analyzing ST-segment changes.

Studies of visual interpretation of the coronary angiogram suggest that the physiologic effects of most coronary artery obstruction cannot be determined accurately by conventional angiographic approaches.

Dobutamine stress echocardiography has also been tested for its ability to predict adverse cardiac outcome in patients undergoing vascular surgery.[387,394-397] For this test, an abnormal result or a positive result consists of new regional wall motion abnormalities or worsening of existing regional wall motion abnormalities on echocardiography during infusion of dobutamine. A negative result consists of the absence of any change on echocardiography during dobutamine infusion. This test has high predictive value for adverse cardiac events (although the findings of Mantha and coworkers[387] are limited to only three studies of dobutamine stress echocardiography for this purpose). The relative risk (95% confidence interval [CI]) of an adverse outcome predicted by the test was 19 (5.9 to 60.8) (see Fig. 27-10 and Table 27-26), which suggests that this test is very "effective." It is interesting to note that unlike the other studies, the study of Mantha and colleagues[387] found that the predictive value increased over the time period that the test was available. Boersma and associates[397b] assessed the value of dobutamine stress echocardiography with respect to the extent of wall motion abnormalities and the ability of preoperative β-blocker treatment to attenuate risk in patients undergoing major aortic surgery. They assigned 1 point for each of the following characteristics: age older than 70 years, current angina, MI, CHF, previous cerebrovascular disease, diabetes mellitus, and renal failure. As the total number of clinical risk factors increases, perioperative cardiac event rates also increase.

Studies have concentrated on the identification and stratification of risk in the intermediate-risk group of patients who would benefit most from a preoperative cardiac workup and risk assessment. Goldman and colleagues[367] prospectively studied 1001 patients older than 40 years undergoing a broad variety of emergency and elective surgery. Multiple regression analysis of the data showed that nine factors independently correlated with the development of life-threatening or fatal cardiac complications: (1) the presence of an S_3 gallop, jugular vein distention or CHF; (2) a history of MI in the preceding 6 months; (3) a cardiac rhythm other than sinus; (4) the occurrence of more than five PVCs per minute; (5) performance of intraperitoneal, intrathoracic, or aortic surgery; (6) patient age older than 70 years; (7) significant valvular aortic stenosis; (8) emergency surgery; and (9) poor general medical condition. On the basis of this study, the investigators developed a method of computing a CRI (Table 27-29). This study suggests that the history and physical examination account for 29 of 53 points in assessing the cardiac risk of the general surgical population and that the initial history and physical examination permit selection of intermediate-risk patients for further evaluation. Eagle and colleagues[383] studied 200 vascular surgery patients, a population with a high incidence of cardiovascular disease, and by logistic regression, found the following to be independent risk factors: Q waves on resting ECG, history of ventricular ectopy, diabetes, age older than 70 years, angina, and CHF.

Similarly, Poldermans and associates studied a vascular surgery population with dobutamine stress echocardiography.[399] Clinical variables identify 33% of patients at very low risk for perioperative complications of vascular surgery, in whom further testing is redundant. In all other candidates, dobutamine-atropine stress echocardiography is a powerful tool that identifies patients at intermediate risk and a small group at very high risk. Again, multiple regression studies suggest that initial clinical evaluation suffices for selecting patients for further evaluation.

One of the most recent clinical risk indices was developed by investigators at the Brigham and Women's Hospital, who studied 4315 patients aged 50 years who were undergoing elective major noncardiac procedures in a tertiary care teaching hospital.[400] Six independent predictors of complications were identified and included in a revised CRI: high-risk type of surgery, history of ischemic heart disease, history of CHF, history of cerebrovascular disease, preoperative treatment with insulin,

Table 27–30 Simplified revised cardiac risk index

Factors That Make a Difference in Outcome
High-risk surgery
History of ischemic heart disease
History of congestive heart failure
History of cerebrovascular disease
Preoperative treatment with insulin
Preoperative serum creatinine level greater than 2.0 mg/dL

Rates of major cardiac complications if you had zero, one, two, or three of these factors were 0.4% to 0.5%, 0.9% to 1.3%, 4% to 7%, and 9% to 11%, respectively, after elective major noncardiac surgery. See the text for details.
From Lee TH, Marcantonio ER, Mangione CM, et al: Derivation and prospective validation of a simple index for prediction of cardiac risk of major noncardiac surgery. Circulation 100:1043-1049, 1999.

and preoperative serum creatinine level greater than 2.0 mg/dL (Table 27-30). (Rates of major cardiac complication with zero, one, two, or three of these factors were 0.5%, 1.3%, 4%, and 9%, respectively, in the derivation cohort and 0.4%, 0.9%, 7%, and 11%, respectively, in 1422 patients in the validation cohort.)

The Cleveland Clinic group has established a clinical severity scoring system to characterize risk before coronary artery bypass surgery[401] (Table 27-31 and Fig. 27-12). This system predicts cardiovascular morbidity and gives stratification points for the risk of an adverse cardiovascular outcome in patients with preoperative renal insufficiency, diabetes, age, anemia, COPD, mitral valve insufficiency, aortic valve stenosis, cerebrovascular disease, and surgery performed on an emergency basis—many factors found by Goldman and colleagues to affect outcome adversely. Therefore, diseases that impinge on the cardiovascular system, such as renal insufficiency and diabetes, have important effects in predicting cardiovascular morbidity. What is the role of preoperative or preprocedure treatment of these conditions?

The American College of Cardiology/American Heart Association Task Force on Perioperative Cardiovascular Evaluation for Noncardiac Surgery used data such as those just presented, combined with expert opinion, to propose a series of algorithms for preoperative evaluation of such patients (Tables 27-32 to 27-34, Fig. 27-13).[10] They did this because of the importance of a surgical event to a patient's long-term prognosis and because surgery may present the first opportunity for long-term evaluation, risk management, and motivation of the patient. First, the clinician must evaluate the urgency of the surgery and the appropriateness of a formal preoperative assessment. Next, it should be determined whether the patient has undergone a previous coronary revascularization procedure or coronary evaluation. Patients with unstable coronary syndromes should be identified and appropriate treatment instituted. Finally, the decision to undergo further testing depends on the interaction of clinical risk factors, surgery-specific risk, and functional capacity. *High clinical risk markers* include acute coronary syndromes and severe valvular disease. *Intermediate predictors* of increased risk are factors that have been associated with higher

Table 27–29 Computation of the cardiac risk index*†

Criteria	Points
1. History	
a. Age >70 yr	5
b. MI in previous 6 mo	10
2. Physical examination	
a. S_3 gallop or JVD	11
b. Important VAS	3
3. Electrocardiogram	
a. Rhythm other than sinus of PACs on last preoperative ECG	7
b. >5 PVCs/min documented at any time before surgery	7
4. General status	
Po_2 <60 or Pco_2 >50 mm Hg, K <3.0 or HCO_3 <20 mEq/L, BUN >50 or Cr >3.0 mg/dL, abnormal AST, signs of chronic liver disease, or patient bedridden from noncardiac causes	3
5. Surgery	
a. Intraperitoneal, intrathoracic, or aortic surgery	3
b. Emergency surgery	4
Total possible points	**53**

*To calculate a score, the number of points from all factors that the patient possesses are summed.
†Patients are further segregated into class I (0 to 5 points), with a risk of 1% to 7% for major complications; class II (6 to 12 points), risk of 7% to 11%; class III (13 to 25 points), risk of 14% to 38%; and class IV (≥26 points, risk of 30% to 100%.
AST, aspartate transaminase; BUN, blood urea nitrogen; Cr, creatinine; ECG, electrocardiogram; HCO_3, bicarbonate; JVD, jugular vein distention; K, potassium; MI, myocardial infarction; PACs, premature atrial contractions; Pco_2, partial pressure of carbon dioxide; Po_2, partial pressure oxygen; PVCs, premature ventricular contractions; VAS, valvular aortic stenosis.
Modified from Goldman L, Caldera DL, Nussbaum SR, et al: Multifactorial index of cardiac risk in noncardiac surgical procedures. N Engl J Med 297:845, 1977. Risk calculations from Goldman et al.,[367] Detsky et al.,[375] and Jeffrey et al.[398]

Table 27–31 Use of preoperative factors to predict risk of adverse outcome after coronary artery bypass graft surgery: clinical severity scoring system of the Cleveland Clinic

Preoperative Factors	Score	Morbidity Odds Ratio
Surgery performed on an emergency basis	6	9.0
Serum creatinine levels		
141-167 µmol/L (1.6-1.8 mg/dL)	1	
≥168 µmol/L (≥1.9 mg/dL)	4	2.8
Severe left ventricular dysfunction	3	2.1
Reoperation	3	2.5
Operative mitral valve insufficiency	3	2.6
Age		
65-74 yr	1	1.5
≥75 yr	2	1.9
Previous vascular surgery	2	1.4
Chronic obstructive pulmonary disease	2	1.5
Anemia (hematocrit ≤34%)	2	1.6
Operative aortic valve stenosis	1	1.5
Weight ≤65 kg	1	1.5
Diabetes, taking oral or insulin therapy	1	1.5
Cerebrovascular disease	1	1.4

Modified from Higgins TL, Estafanous FG, Loop FD, et al: Stratification of morbidity and mortality outcome by preoperative risk factors in coronary artery bypass patients. A clinical severity score. JAMA 267:2344, 1992.

perioperative risk in multiple studies. The guidelines currently consider mild angina pectoris, previous MI, compensated or previous CHF, chronic renal insufficiency, and diabetes mellitus as intermediate risk factors. *Minor predictors* of risk are those associated with coronary artery disease, but their relationship with perioperative cardiac complications is less well established. These predictors include advanced age, an abnormal ECG, rhythm other than sinus, low functional capacity, history of stroke, and uncontrolled systemic hypertension, with low functional status being most important. For patients at intermediate clinical risk, both exercise tolerance and the extent of the

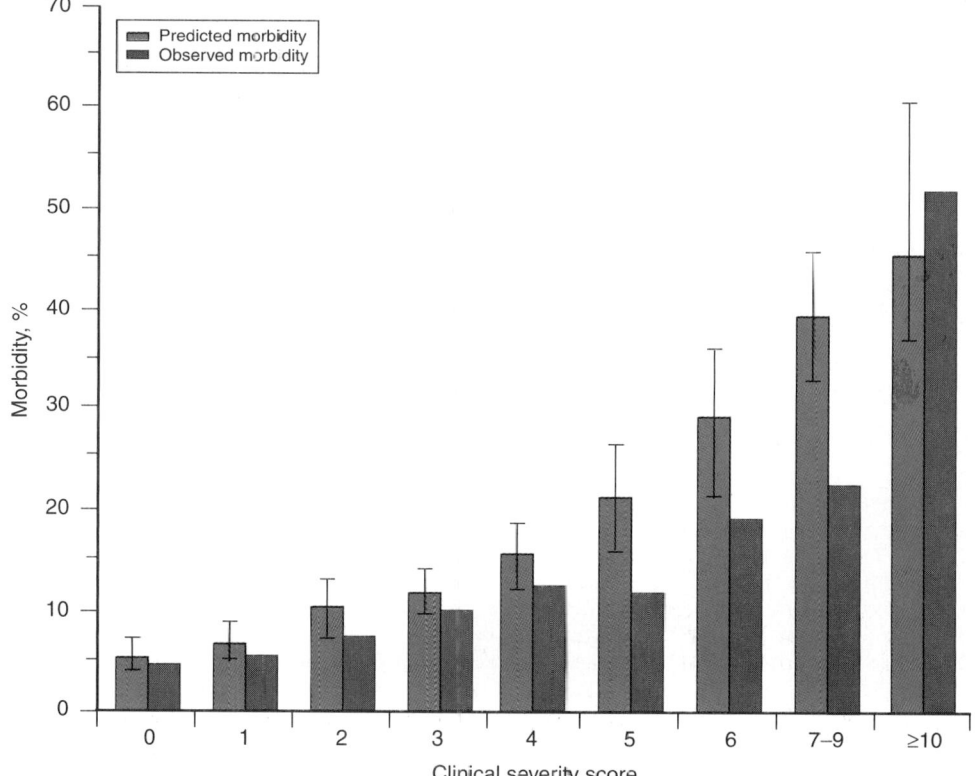

Figure 27–12 The observed morbidity after coronary artery bypass surgery versus the morbidity predicted by a clinical severity scoring system that evaluated various pertinent preoperative conditions. Morbidity was lower than the predicted 99.4% confidence interval at scores 2, 5, 6, and 7 to 9. The model may not be validated prospectively because of changes in clinical management that could result in complications. The *vertical lines* at top of the *bars* indicate confidence intervals. (Redrawn from Higgins TL, Estafanous FG, Loop FD, et al: Stratification of morbidity and mortality outcome by preoperative risk factors in coronary artery bypass patients. A clinical severity score. JAMA 267:2344, 1992.)

Table 27–32 Clinical predictors of increased perioperative cardiovascular risk (myocardial infarction, congestive heart failure, death)

Degree	Clinical Predictors

Major	Unstable coronary syndromes
	  Recent myocardial infarction* with evidence of ischemic risk, as determined by clinical symptoms or noninvasive study
	  Unstable or severe† angina (Canadian class III or IV)‡
	Decompensated congestive heart failure
	Significant arrhythmias
	  High-grade atrioventricular block
	  Symptomatic ventricular arrhythmias in the presence of underlying heart disease
	  Supraventricular arrhythmias with uncontrolled ventricular rate
	  Severe valvular disease

Intermediate	Mild angina pectoris (Canadian class I or II) Previous myocardial infarction, as determined by history or pathologic Q waves Compensated or previous congestive heart failure Diabetes mellitus
Minor	Advanced age Abnormal electrocardiogram (left ventricular hypertrophy, left bundle branch block, ST-T abnormalities) Rhythm other than sinus (e.g., atrial fibrillation) Low functional capacity (e.g., inability to climb one flight of stairs with a bag of groceries) History of stroke Uncontrolled systemic hypertension

*The American College of Cardiology National Database Library defines recent myocardial infarction as one that occurred more than 7 days but less than 31 days ago.
†May include stable angina in patients who are unusually sedentary.
‡Campeau L: Grading of angina pectoris. Circulation 54:522-523, 1976.
From Eagle KA, Berger PB, et al: ACC/AHA guideline update for perioperative cardiovascular evaluation for noncardiac surgery—executive summary: A report of the American College of Cardiology/American Heart Association Task Force on Practice Guidelines (Committee to Update the 1996 Guidelines on Perioperative Cardiovascular Evaluation for Noncardiac Surgery). J Am Coll Cardiol 39:542-553, 2002, with permission.

Table 27–33 Estimated energy requirements for various activities*

Metabolic Equivalents (METs)	Activity
1 MET	Can you take care of yourself? Can you eat, dress, and use the toilet? Can you walk indoors around the house? Can you walk a block or two on level ground at 2 to 3 mph (3.2 to 4.8 km/hr)?
4 METs	Can you climb a flight of stairs or walk up a hill? Can you walk on level ground at 4 mph (6.4 km/hr)? Can you run a short distance? Can you do heavy work around the house such as scrubbing floors or moving heavy furniture? Can you participate in moderate recreational activities such as golfing, bowling, dancing, doubles tennis, or throwing a baseball or football?
10 METs	Can you participate in strenuous sports such as swimming, singles tennis, football, basketball, or skiing?

*Adapted from the Duke Activity Status Index and the American Heart Association Exercise Standards.
From Eagle KA, Berger PB, et al: ACC/AHA guideline update for perioperative cardiovascular evaluation for noncardiac surgery—executive summary: A report of the American College of Cardiology/American Heart Association Task Force on Practice Guidelines (Committee to Update the 1996 Guidelines on Perioperative Cardiovascular Evaluation for Noncardiac Surgery). J Am Coll Cardiol 39:542-553, 2002, with permission.

Table 27–34   Stratification of cardiac risk for noncardiac surgical procedures

Cardiac Risk*	Noncardiac Surgical Procedure
High reported cardiac risk (often >5%)	Emergency major operations, particularly in the elderly Aortic and other major vascular procedures Peripheral vascular procedures Anticipated prolonged surgical procedures associated with large fluid shifts and/or blood loss
Intermediate reported cardiac risk (generally <5%)	Carotid endarterectomy Head and neck procedures Intraperitoneal and intrathoracic procedures Orthopedic surgery Prostate surgery
Low reported cardiac risk[†] (generally <1%)	Endoscopic procedures Superficial procedures Cataract surgery Breast surgery

*Combined incidence of cardiac death and nonfatal myocardial infarction.
[†]These procedures generally do not require further preoperative cardiac testing.
From Eagle KA, Berger PB, et al: ACC/AHA guideline update for perioperative cardiovascular evaluation for noncardiac surgery—executive summary: A report of the American College of Cardiology/American Heart Association Task Force on Practice Guidelines (Committee to Update the 1996 Guidelines on Perioperative Cardiovascular Evaluation for Noncardiac Surgery). J Am Coll Cardiol 39:542-553, 2002, with permission.

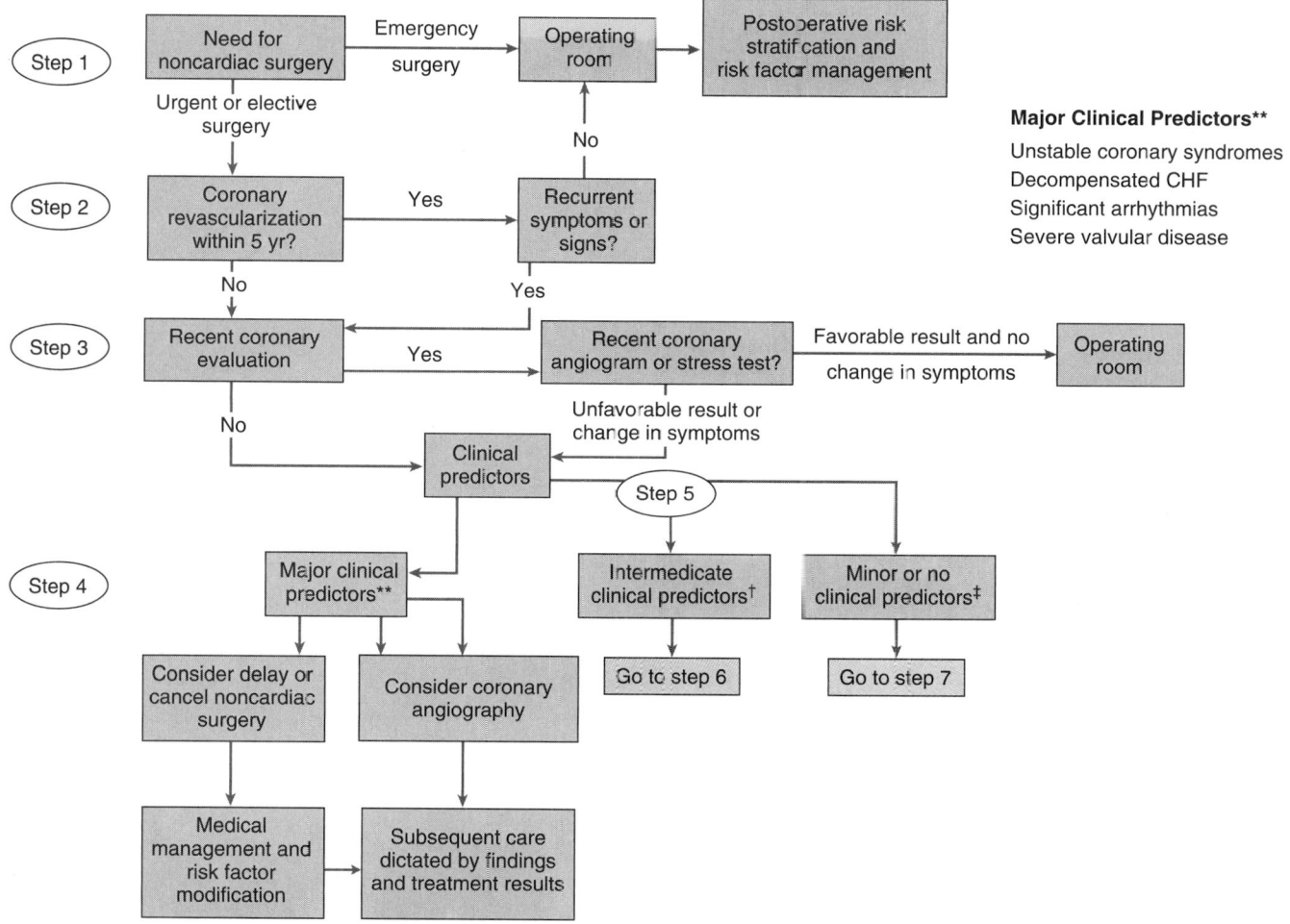

Figure 27–13 Coronary risk assessment. Risk stratification strategies for determining a patient's candidacy for preoperative noninvasive testing before elective surgery. CHF, congestive heart failure; ECG, electrocardiogram; MET, metabolic equivalent; MI, myocardial infarction. (Redrawn from Eagle KA, Berger PB, et al: ACC/AHA guideline update for perioperative cardiovascular

(Continued)

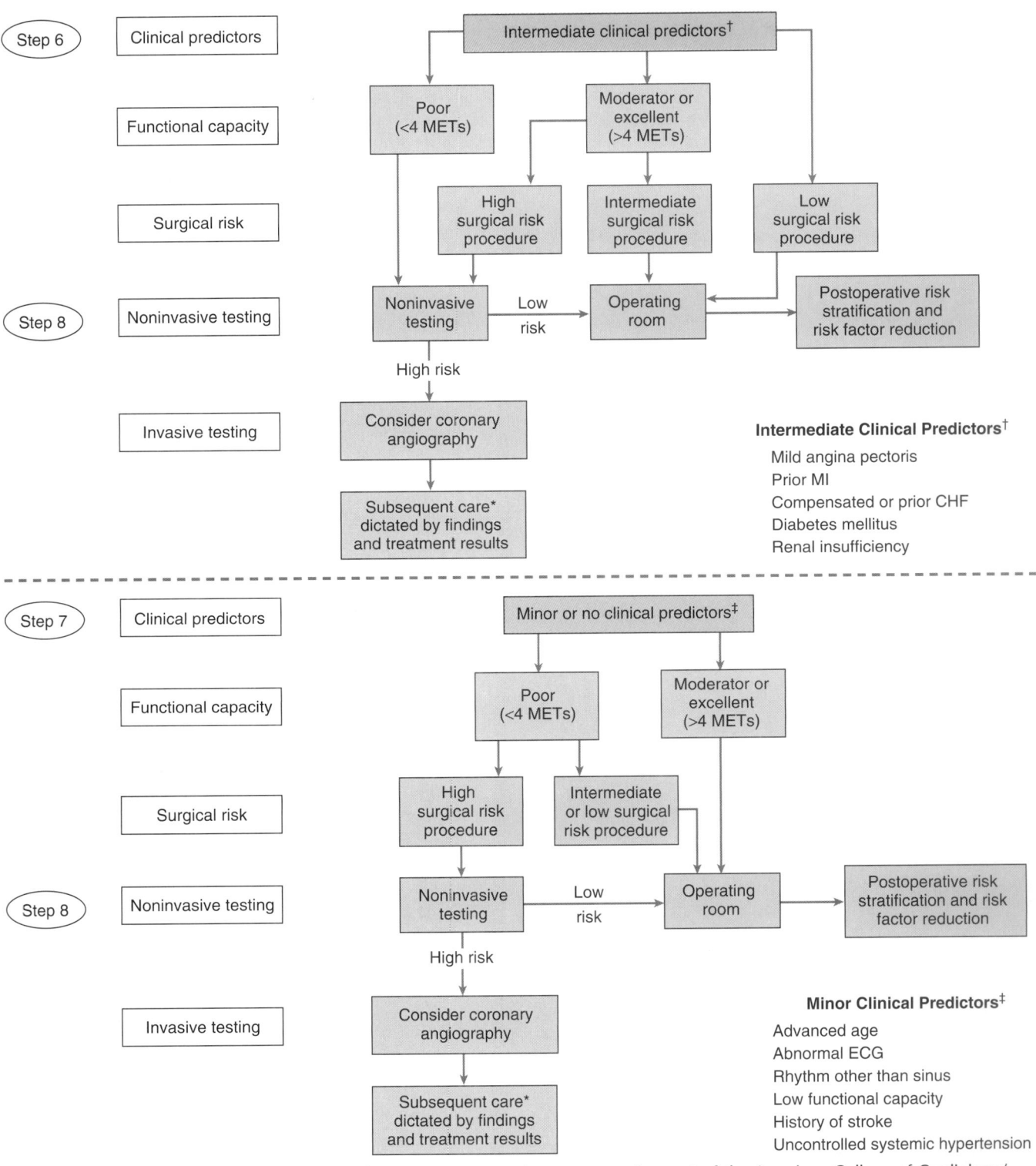

Figure 27–13—cont'd evaluation for noncardiac surgery—executive summary: A report of the American College of Cardiology/American Heart Association Task Force on Practice Guidelines [Committee to Update the 1996 Guidelines on Perioperative Cardiovascular Evaluation for Noncardiac Surgery]. J Am Coll Cardiol 39:542-553, 2002.)

surgery are taken into account in regard to the need for further testing. The importance of exercise capacity was shown by Reilley and colleagues[401b] (see Chapter 25 for more information on this aspect of preoperative and preprocedure evaluation). Patients who could not walk four

blocks and climb two flights of stairs were considered to have poor exercise tolerance and were found to have twice as many perioperative cardiovascular complications as those with better functional status. The likelihood of a serious complication occurring was inversely related to the number of blocks that could be walked or flights of stairs that could be climbed. Importantly, no preoperative cardiovascular testing should be performed if the results will not change perioperative management.

Since publication of the algorithm in 1996, several studies have suggested that this stepwise approach to the assessment of coronary artery disease is both efficacious and cost-effective.[402,403] Licker and colleagues compared the data of two consecutive 4-year periods (1993 to 1996 [control period] versus 1997 to 2000 [intervention period]). Implementation of the American College of Cardiology/American Heart Association guidelines[10] was associated with increased use of preoperative stress myocardial imaging (44.3% versus 20.6%; $P < .05$) and coronary revascularization (7.7% versus 0.8%; $P < 0.05$). During the intervention period, there was a significant decrease in the incidence of cardiac complications (from 11.3% to 4.5%) and an increase in event-free survival at 1 year after surgery (from 91.3% to 98.2%). Froehlich and colleagues[402] compared 102 historical control patients with 94 patients after implementation of the guideline and 104 patients late after implementation of the guideline. Both resource utilization and cost were reduced after implementation of the guideline, and the effect was sustained for 2 years.

Thus, the major signposts of perioperative myocardial function that we can obtain before surgery are the risk factors for arterial aging and a history of ischemic pain (and its relationship to exercise), CHF, diabetes, and renal insufficiency. The value of this information is slightly enhanced by a 6-minute walk test; determination of the ankle-brachial pressure index; ECG and non-ECG responses to bicycle or treadmill exercise; determination of the ejection fraction; and the use of ECG, radionuclide imaging, radionuclide imaging after dipyridamole, wall motion changes during dobutamine infusion, or angiography.[307,315-317,353,374-376,383-387,391-400,402-404]

Relationship to Previous Coronary Artery Bypass Graft or to Percutaneous Transluminal Coronary Artery Angioplasty

Much of the information on which altered perioperative anesthetic management of ischemic heart disease is based is derived from studies of patients undergoing aortic and CABG procedures. Although CABG relieves angina and increases exercise tolerance (as did many placebo operations and medications before it),[405] improved survival occurs only in patients with significant left main coronary artery disease[386,406] and those with mild to moderate impairment in left ventricular function.[407] However, a potential additional benefit of CABG surgery or percutaneous transluminal coronary angioplasty (PTCA) with or without stents has been documented. Reduced perioperative morbidity during subsequent noncardiac surgical procedures may be an additional benefit of surviving CABG surgery or PTCA.[10,337,338,389,407-409] Eagle and colleagues reported on a long-term analysis of patients entered into the Coronary Arteries Surgery Study (CASS).[410] They studied patients assigned to medical or surgical treatment of coronary artery disease for over 10 years who subsequently underwent 3368 noncardiac operations in the years after assignment of coronary treatment. The rate of perioperative MI and death was stratified by the type of surgical procedure. Specifically, low-risk surgeries such as skin, breast, urologic, and minor orthopedic procedures were associated with a total morbidity and mortality of less than 1% regardless of coronary treatment type, and previous revascularization did not affect the outcome. Intermediate-risk surgery such as abdominal, thoracic, and carotid endarterectomy was associated with a combined morbidity and mortality of 1% to 5%, with a small but significant improvement in outcome noted in patients who had previously undergone revascularization. The most significant improvement in outcome was seen in patients undergoing major vascular surgery such as abdominal or lower extremity revascularization. In this cohort, mortality after noncardiac surgery was reduced by two thirds in patients who had received bypasses or had revascularization with PTCA (with or without stents). However, this observational study did not randomize patients and was undertaken in the 1970s and 1980s, before significant advances in medical, surgical, and percutaneous coronary strategies.

To provide definitive data for this hypothesis, a randomized controlled study would be necessary; such a trial is currently ongoing.[411] Importantly, CABG surgery may simply constitute a "survival test." That is, it may cause reinfarction or death, or both, in patients who would have sustained an MI or who would have died after noncardiac surgery.[389] This conclusion appears to be likely because patients who do poorly during and after CABG surgery are those with poor left ventricular function and increased left ventricular end-diastolic pressure.[409] Patients with these same cardiovascular conditions also have increased perioperative risk after noncardiac surgery.[315,317,337,338,367,374-376,383-387,390,392] Therefore, one proposal to decrease perioperative risk in patients severely disabled with angina (or ischemic heart disease) is to study the coronary arteries and perform PTCA (with or without stenting) or CABG, if indicated, before their noncardiac surgery.

Hertzer and associates[337,338] did just this. Knowing that survival after vascular surgery depends mainly on preserving myocardial function, these investigators obtained coronary angiograms and proposed CABG surgery (when appropriate) for 1001 consecutive patients needing peripheral vascular surgery (regardless of the degree of suspicion of coronary artery disease before angiography). CABG was believed to be indicated in 251 patients, 226 of whom underwent CABG, with 12 (5.31%) operative deaths; of these patients, 130 subsequently underwent peripheral vascular procedures, with only 1 death.

Do these figures imply that mortality was decreased or increased by the CABG procedure? Did some patients not undergo their initially indicated vascular procedure because of the morbidity associated with CABG? (The report did not indicate why 26 patients who initially were scheduled for peripheral vascular procedures did not undergo these procedures after CABG.) The long-term prognosis for Hertzer's patients was better in those who underwent CABG before their noncardiac surgery than in those who did not: the 5-year cardiac survival rate was 82.5% versus 74%. In fact, in the CASS series, previous CABG surgery or PTCA (versus medical therapy) reduced the risk to that of someone 4 years younger (Fig. 27-14).

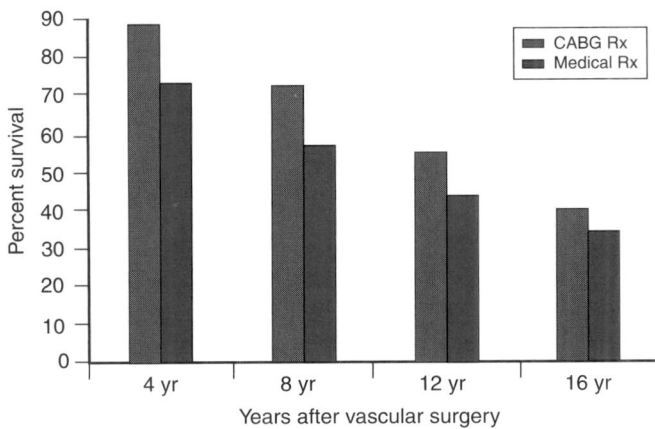

Figure 27–14 Long-term survival of 1834 patients with peripheral vascular disease who were enrolled in the Coronary Artery Surgery Study (CASS) registry. Survival rates are shown for those undergoing coronary artery bypass grafting (CABG) versus medical therapy before their vascular surgery. (Redrawn from Rihal CS, Eagle KA, Mickel MC, et al: Surgical therapy for coronary artery disease among patients with combined coronary artery disease and peripheral vascular disease. Circulation 91:46, 1995.)

This risk reduction was equivalent to that found by the McSPI group for β-adrenergic receptor blocking therapy on the day of surgery and 7 subsequent days.[226,412]

Are these therapies additive? We do not have an answer. Again, the work of Hertzer and associates describes a nonrandomized series.[337,338] Huber and colleagues[409] try to make the point that vascular surgery after PTCA is safer than vascular surgery without PTCA, but their series had a rate of serious complications (failed PTCA, MI, death) from PTCA of more than 10%. Posner and coworkers used an administrative data set of patients who underwent PTCA and noncardiac surgery in Washington state.[413] They matched coronary disease patients undergoing noncardiac surgery with and without previous percutaneous coronary interventions (PCI) and looked at cardiac complications. In this nonrandomized design, they noted a significantly lower rate of 30-day cardiac complications in patients who underwent PTCA at least 90 days before the noncardiac surgery. Importantly, PCI within 90 days of noncardiac surgery did not improve outcome. Although the explanation for these results is unknown, they may support the notion that PTCA performed "to get the patient through surgery" may not improve their perioperative outcome because cardiac complications may not occur in patients with stable or asymptomatic coronary stenosis and because PTCA (before embedding drugs into stents or radiation therapy) may actually destabilize some coronary plaques. Patients with destabilized plaques are subject to morbidity early in the increased coagulant phase of the hours, days, or weeks after noncardiac surgery.

PTCA with coronary stenting poses several special issues. Kaluza and coauthors reported on the outcome of 40 patients who underwent prophylactic coronary stent placement less than 6 weeks before major noncardiac surgery requiring general anesthesia.[414] The time between stenting and surgery appeared to be the main determinant of outcome, and the authors recommend that a minimum of 2 weeks and preferably 4 weeks elapse before elective surgery. Wilson and colleagues reported on 207 patients who underwent noncardiac surgery within 2 months of stent placement.[6] A total of 8 patients died or suffered an MI, all of whom were among the 168 patients undergoing surgery within 6 weeks after stent placement. No events occurred in the 39 patients who underwent surgery 7 to 9 weeks after stent placement. These authors suggest that whenever possible, noncardiac surgery should be delayed more than 6 weeks after stent placement, by which time stents are generally endothelialized and a course of antiplatelet therapy to prevent stent thrombosis has been completed.

Therefore, the hypothesis that CABG or PTCA decreases morbidity and mortality in patients undergoing subsequent noncardiac surgery remains a hypothesis. (Although previous CABG or PTCA reduces the risk of subsequent noncardiac surgery, does the combination of revascularization and noncardiac surgery lead to a better outcome than just the noncardiac surgery alone?) In the absence of randomized data, decision analysis models can be used to address the issue.[415-417] Such models assume that patients with significant coronary artery disease would undergo CABG surgery before noncardiac surgery. The models found that the optimal decision was sensitive to local morbidity and mortality rates within the clinically observed range. These models suggest that preoperative testing for the purpose of coronary revascularization is not the optimal strategy if perioperative morbidity and mortality are low. If long-term survival is included in the models, coronary revascularization may lead to an improved overall outcome and be a cost-effective intervention,[417] particularly in patients with significant left main or three-vessel coronary stenosis (or both). Landesberg and colleagues demonstrated that long-term survival after major vascular surgery is significantly improved if patients with moderate to severe ischemia on preoperative dipyridamole-thallium imaging undergo selective coronary revascularization.[418]

Summary of Preoperative and Intraoperative Factors that Correlate with Perioperative Morbidity

Summarizing a large number of studies, we list the following preoperative findings as conditions that correlate with perioperative morbidity and that can be corrected before surgery:

1. Recent MI[190,327,361-371]
2. Severe CHF (i.e., sufficiently severe to produce rales, an S_3 gallop, or distention of the jugular vein)*
3. Severe angina (see Table 27-35 for classification of the severity of angina)[367,374,386,390,399,400,413-417,419]
4. Heart rhythm other than sinus[365,367,374-376]
5. Premature atrial contractions[367]
6. More than five PVCs per minute (though unconfirmed in later studies)[365,367]
7. Chronic renal insufficiency;
8. BUN levels higher than 50 mg/dL or potassium levels below 3.0 mEq/L[367,399-401]

---

*See references 190, 307, 315, 317, 365, 367, 374-379, 381-386, 390, 399-401, 410, 413-417, 419.

Table 27–35 Classification of angina by the New York Heart Association and the Canadian Cardiovascular Society

NYHA	CCS
I. Ordinary physical activity such as walking or climbing stairs does not cause angina. Angina with strenuous or rapid prolonged exertion at work or recreation or with sexual relations	I. Ordinary physical activity such as walking and climbing stairs does not cause angina. Angina with strenuous or rapid or prolonged exertion at work or recreation
II. Slight limitation of ordinary activity. Walking or climbing stairs rapidly, walking uphill, and walking or stair climbing after meals or in the cold, in wind, under emotional stress, or only for a few hours after awakening. Walking more than two blocks on the level or more than one flight of stairs at a normal pace and under normal conditions	II. Slight limitation of ordinary activity. Walking or climbing stairs rapidly, walking uphill, and walking or stair climbing after meals or in cold, in wind, when under emotional stress, or only for a few hours after awakening. Walking more than two blocks on the level and climbing more than one flight of ordinary stairs at a normal pace and under normal conditions
III. Marked limitation of ordinary physical activity. Walking one or two blocks on the level and climbing one flight of stairs under normal conditions and at a normal pace "Comfortable at rest"	III. Marked limitation of ordinary physical activity. Walking one to two blocks on the level and climbing more than one flight under normal conditions
IV. Inability to carry out any physical activity without discomfort—anginal syndrome may be present at rest	IV. Inability to carry out any physical activity without discomfort— anginal syndrome *may be* present at rest

Preoperative factors that correlate with perioperative risk but cannot be altered include (1) old physiologic or chronologic age (perioperative risk increases with age),[*] (2) significant aortic stenosis,[367,401,422] (3) emergency surgery,[190,313,361,367,374-376,390,401] (4) cardiomegaly,[317,367,374-376,390,401] (5) history of CHF,[†] (6) angina (or a history of angina or ischemia) on ECG,[190,307,353,365,367,374-379,381-386,390] (7) abnormal ST-segment or inverted or flat T waves on ECG,[8,367,374,376] abnormal QRS complex on ECG,[367] and (8) a significant mitral regurgitant murmur.[367,401]

---

[*]See references 26, 27, 313, 367, 374-378, 387, 399, 402, 410, 420, 421.
[†]See references 190, 315, 317, 365, 367, 374-379, 381-386, 390, 392, 401.

Significant intraoperative factors that correlate with perioperative risk and that may be avoided or altered are as follows: (1) unnecessary use of vasopressors,[423,424] (2) unintentional hypotension[316,328,366,367] (this point is controversial, however, because some investigators have found that unintentional hypotension does not correlate with perioperative morbidity[421,424]), (3) hypothermia,[425] (4) too low or too high a hematocrit,[426,427] and (5) lengthy operations.[334,361,366,367]

Significant intraoperative factors that correlate with perioperative morbidity and probably cannot be avoided are (1) emergency surgery and (2) thoracic or intraperitoneal surgery or above-the-knee amputations.[334,365-367, 374-379,381-390,392,401,420]

Although the evidence for these factors is fairly substantial, virtually no data are derived from prospective randomized studies indicating that treatment of the aforementioned conditions reduces perioperative risk in patients with ischemic heart disease. Nevertheless, all logic dictates that such treatment does reduce risk. Thus, the goal in giving anesthesia to patients with ischemic heart disease is to achieve the best preoperative condition obtainable by treating conditions that correlate with perioperative risk. The next step is to intraoperatively monitor for conditions that correlate with perioperative risk and, by careful attention to detail, avoid circumstances that lead to perioperative risk. Although local anesthesia may reduce perioperative risk,[365,380] epidemiologic studies do not indicate any significant differences in perioperative morbidity in patients with ischemic heart disease who are given local anesthesia as opposed to general anesthesia.

Preoperative and Preprocedure Evaluation

Preoperative evaluation of a patient with ischemic heart disease should include a review of the clinical course of any previous MIs and a review of studies made subsequent to those events. Because patients most likely to benefit are those who have severe coronary artery disease (i.e., multivessel left main stem coronary artery disease) and ejection fractions of 21% to 50%, some strategies have been devised to limit routine exercise testing, dipyridamole-thallium scanning, Holter monitoring, dobutamine stress echocardiography, and angiographic testing to only these patients (Figs. 27-15 to 27-17).[10,393,410,414-416,428] That these studies have been or are being performed implies something about the patient's cardiac function.

The preoperative evaluation should also include a review of the results of exercise studies, Holter monitoring, other noninvasive tests such as dobutamine stress echocardiography, and coronary angiography to determine which ECG lead to monitor for ischemia. Although in theory, the ECG lead that first indicates ischemia or best represents the stenosed artery on exercise should be the first to reveal ischemia in the operating room, no study has confirmed this assumption. If no exercise or coronary angiographic study has been performed, precordial lead V_5 is preferred.[8,307,429,430]

Preoperative and Preprocedure Therapy

The only known way to increase oxygen supply to the myocardium of patients with coronary artery stenosis

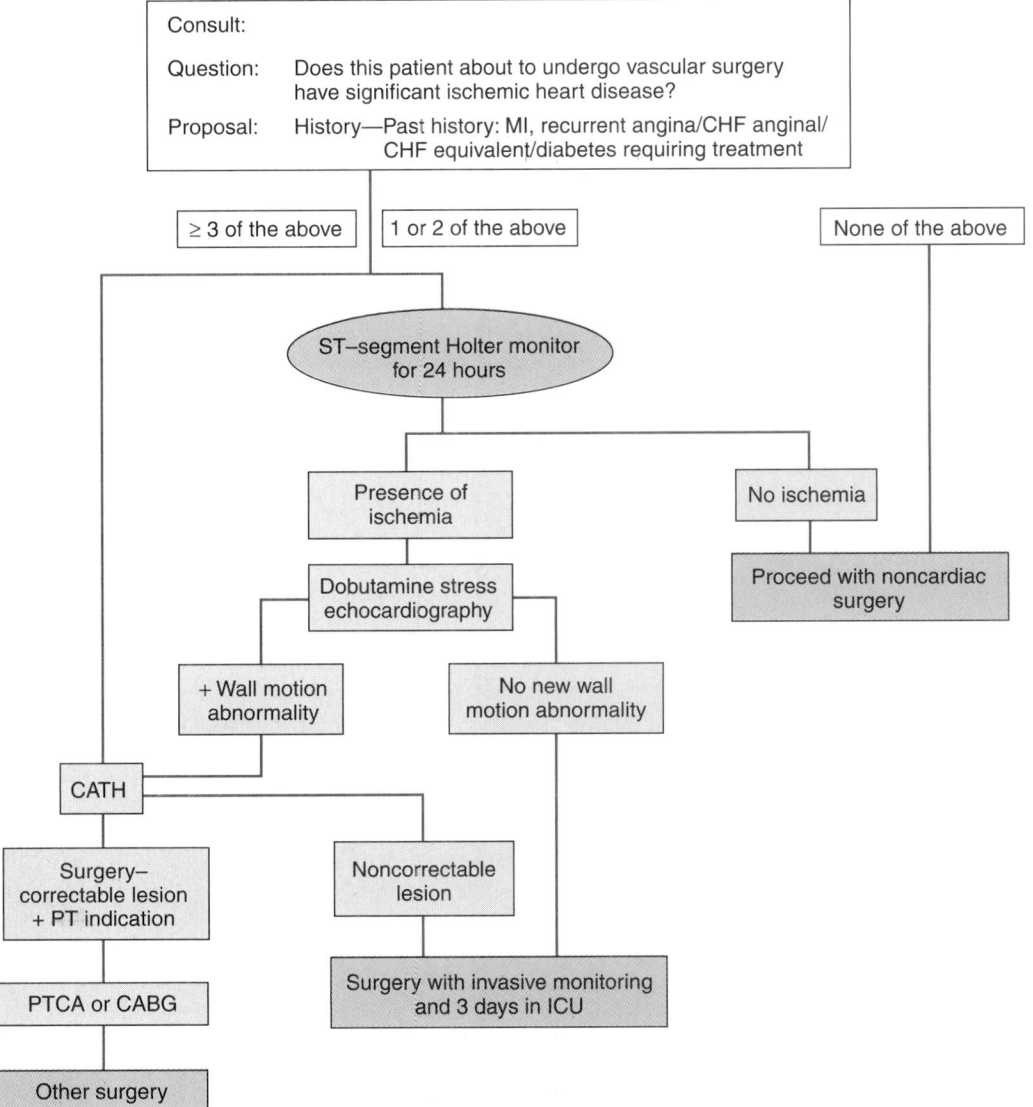

Figure 27–15 Assessment of cardiac risk in a patient about to undergo vascular surgery. If the clinical index is high, coronary arteriography (CATH) is recommended, with subsequent coronary artery bypass grafting (CABG) or percutaneous transluminal coronary angioplasty (PTCA) for those with correctable lesions and patient (PT) consent. An equivocal history is followed by Holter monitoring and, if Holter monitoring is abnormal, by dobutamine stress echocardiography. CHF, congestive heart failure; ICU, intensive care unit; MI, myocardial infarction. (See the text and data of Fig. 27-9 for analyses by Mantha and colleagues.[387])

is to maintain diastolic BP, hemoglobin concentration[401,431,432] (Fig. 27-18), and oxygen saturation. The main goal of anesthesia practice for these patients has been to decrease the determinants of myocardial oxygen demand, heart rate, ventricular wall tension, and contractile performance.[308,310,382,431-433] Thus, medical management designed to preserve all viable myocardial tissue may include the following:

1. Administration of β-adrenergic receptor blocking drugs (propranolol, atenolol, esmolol, or metoprolol) to decrease contractility and the heart rate.
2. Vasodilation (with nitroglycerin or its "long-acting" analogs nitroprusside, hydralazine, or prazosin) to decrease ventricular wall tension.[225-228,306,308,310] The use of Swan-Ganz catheters[379,434] and transesophageal echocardiography for this type of patient is described

in Chapters 32 and 33, and the intraoperative management of patients with ischemic heart disease is discussed in further detail in Chapter 50 and in recent guidelines.[10]

3. β-Blocker therapy. Multiple studies have now evaluated the benefit of perioperative pharmacologic therapy, including β-blockers, calcium channel blockers, and α2-agonists.[435-437] Keeping cardiovascular variables within an acceptable range and the rate-pressure product below the threshold for angina appears to be an appropriate objective.[190,226,310,329,330,433,438] Specifically, prophylactic use of β-adrenergic blocking agents has been suggested as level I evidence for the prevention of perioperative cardiac morbidity in high-risk patients.[439-445]

4. Aspirin, statins, exercise, and diet. These choices seem to be indicated in many patients, as reviewed in

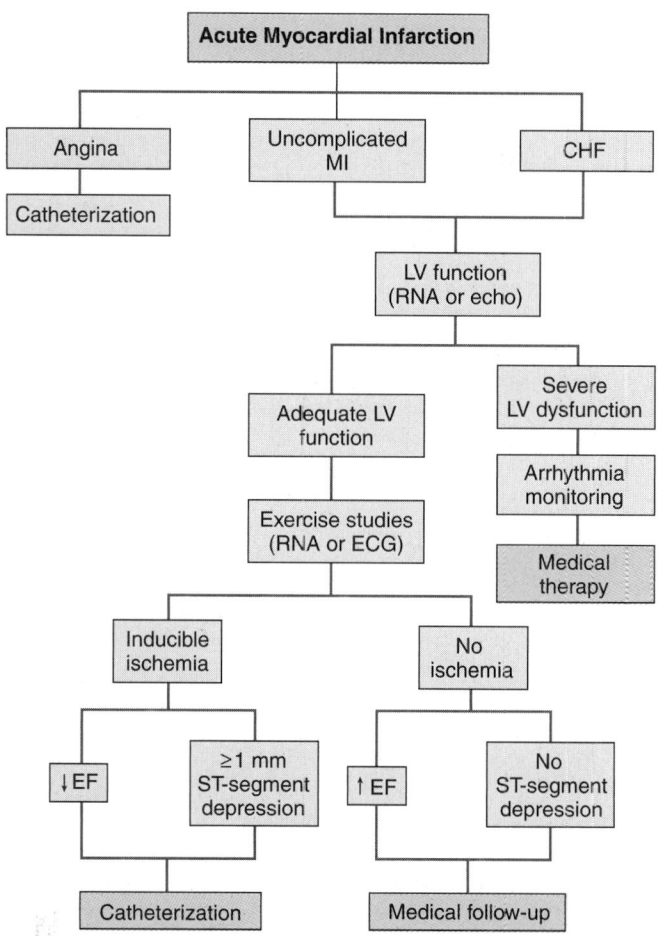

Figure 27–16 Strategy for identifying patients who should undergo cardiac catheterization after acute myocardial infarction (MI). This strategy is based on clinical assessment, evaluation of left ventricular (LV) function by radionuclide angiography (RNA) or echocardiography (Echo), analysis of arrhythmias, and stress testing. CHF, overt congestive heart failure; ECG, electrocardiogram; EF, ejection fraction. (Redrawn from Epstein SE, Palmeri ST, Patterson RE: Evaluation of patients after acute myocardial infarction. Indications for cardiac catheterization and surgical intervention. N Engl J Med 307:1487, 1982.)

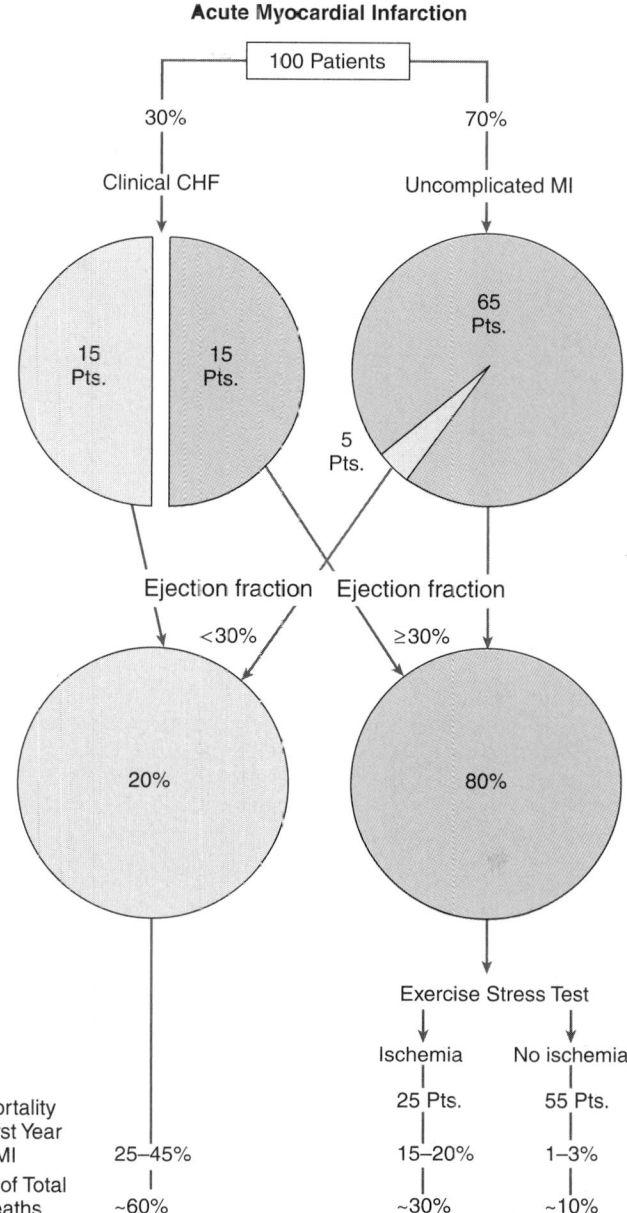

Figure 27–17 First-year mortality rates for patients with acute myocardial infarction (MI) according to subgroup. *Pink areas* represent patients with ejection fractions of more than 30%; *gray areas* represent patients with ejection fractions of less than 30%. (The percentages are, by necessity, rough approximations.) CHF, overt congestive heart failure. (Redrawn from Epstein SE, Palmeri ST, Patterson RE: Evaluation of patients after acute myocardial infarction. Indications for cardiac catheterization and surgical intervention. N Engl J Med 307:1487, 1982.)

Chapter 25 under "Chronic Drug Therapy."[5] Briefly, we believe that drugs given chronically (e.g., antihypertensive medications and some ACE inhibitors) should be continued through the morning of surgery (see earlier). The topic of chronic drug therapy is discussed in more detail in the last section of this chapter. In high-risk patients undergoing major surgery, specifically those with known ischemic heart disease undergoing major vascular, abdominal, and thoracic surgery, perioperative β-blocker therapy should be continued.

Valvular Heart Disease

Major alterations in the preoperative management of patients with valvular heart disease have been made regarding the use of anticoagulant therapy and are now based on the causes of disease. Preoperative and intraoperative management of patients with valvular heart disease is discussed in Chapter 50; nevertheless, a few important points concerning preoperative care are emphasized here. Of prime importance is realizing that stenotic lesions are managed in a fashion exactly opposite that for regurgitant lesions. Therefore, the type of lesion that exists should be determined preoperatively. Although the causes of various forms of valvular heart disease have not

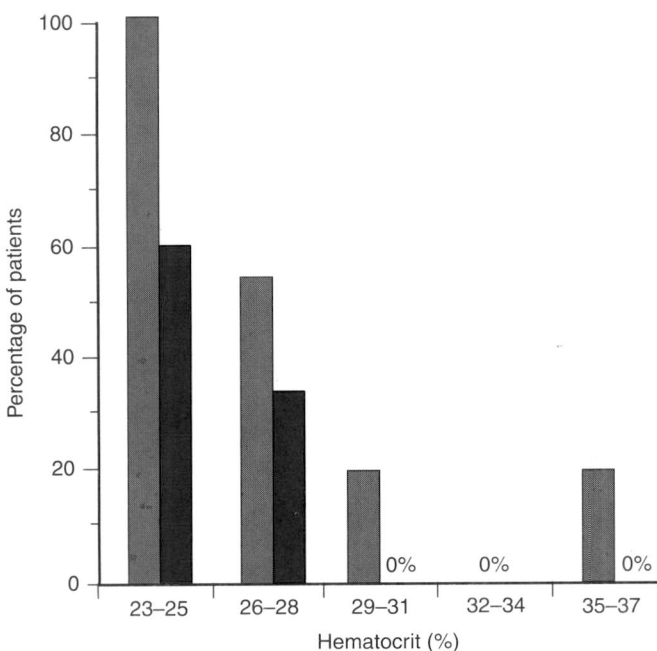

Figure 27–18 Relationship of postoperative myocardial ischemia *(black bars)* and morbid cardiac events *(red bars)* to hematocrit for 27 high-risk patients undergoing infrainguinal arterial bypass. (Data from Nelson AH, Fleisher LA, Rosenbaum SH: The relationship between postoperative anemia and cardiac morbidity in high risk vascular patients in the ICU. Crit Care Med 21:860, 1993.)

changed, the relative frequency has. Rheumatic valvulitis is much less common today than it was in the 1970s, and syphilitic aortitis has all but disappeared. Now common are congenital bicuspid aortic stenosis, mitral valve prolapse, hypertrophic cardiomyopathy (also called asymmetric septal hypertrophy or subvalvular aortic stenosis), and mitral valve insufficiency as a result of calcification and drug therapy.

The prognosis and, presumably, the perioperative risk for patients with valvular heart disease depend on the stage of the disease.[398,422] Although stenotic lesions progress faster than regurgitant lesions do, regurgitant lesions secondary to infective endocarditis, rupture of the chordae tendineae, or ischemic heart disease can be rapidly fatal. Left ventricular dysfunction is common in the late stage of valvular heart disease. Once again, the history and physical examination appear to be the most sensitive and specific indicators of disease and disease stage[446,447] (Table 27-36).

Preoperative maintenance of drug therapy can be crucial; for example, a patient with aortic stenosis can deteriorate rapidly with the onset of atrial fibrillation or flutter because the atrial contribution to left ventricular filling can be critical in maintaining cardiac output. One of the most serious complications of valvular heart surgery and valvular heart disease before surgery is cardiac arrhythmia. Conduction disorders and chronic therapy with antiarrhythmic and inotropic drugs are discussed elsewhere in this chapter. The reader is referred elsewhere

Table 27–36 Bedside diagnosis of systolic murmurs: sensitivity, specificity, and predictive value of diagnostic maneuvers

Maneuver	Response	Murmur	Sensitivity (%)	Specificity (%)	Predictive Value Positive (%)	Negative (%)
Inspiration	Increase	Right sided	100	88	67	100
Expiration	Decrease	Right sided	100	88	67	100
Müller maneuver	Increase	Right sided	15	92	33	81
Valsalva maneuver	Increase	Hypertrophic cardiomyopathy	65	96	81	92
Squatting to standing	Increase	Hypertrophic cardiomyopathy	95	84	59	98
Standing to squatting	Decrease	Hypertrophic cardiomyopathy	95	85	61	99
Leg elevation	Decrease	Hypertrophic cardiomyopathy	85	91	71	96
Handgrip	Decrease	Hypertrophic cardiomyopathy	85	75	46	95
Handgrip	Increase	Mitral regurgitation and ventricular septal defect	68	92	84	81
Transient arterial occlusion	Increase	Mitral regurgitation and ventricular septal defect	78	100	100	87
Amyl nitrite inhalation	Decrease	Mitral regurgitation and ventricular septal defect	80	90	85	87

Modified from Lembo NJ, Dell'Italia LJ, Crawford MH, O'Rourke RA: Bedside diagnosis of systolic murmurs. N Engl J Med 318:1572, 1988.

in this book (Chapter 51) or to other sources[448,449] for discussion of the management of a child with congenital heart disease who is undergoing noncardiac surgery.

Mitral Valve Prolapse

Mitral valve prolapse, perhaps the most frequent valvular abnormality, occurs in 5% to 17% of otherwise healthy people. It is associated with atrioseptal secundum defects,[450,451] thoracic skeletal abnormalities (as a result of the time of development of these structures), and for unknown reasons, migraine anxiety neurosis and autonomic dysfunction. Hereditary transmission has been proposed to occur through autosomal dominance with reduced expressivity in humans. Mitral valve prolapse is also associated with von Willebrand's syndrome and polycystic kidney disease, and the presence of one condition might call forth a search (by at least history and physical examination) for the other.

Mitral valve prolapse is either asymptomatic or is manifested as palpitations, dyspnea, atypical chest pain, dizziness, syncope, or sudden death. Supraventricular arrhythmias (associated with AV bypass tracts and the pre-excitation syndrome) occur in more than 50% of patients with mitral valve prolapse. Ventricular arrhythmias (usually in surgery) occur in 45% of such patients, bradyarrhythmias in 25%, and sudden death in 1.4%.[450,451] The frequent occurrence of transient cerebral ischemia has resulted in the chronic use of aspirin or anticoagulants in patients with mitral valve prolapse, and the potential for endocarditis has led to the recommendation for prophylaxis with antibiotics before known bacteremic events[450-453] and the avoidance of head-up positions and decreased afterload in such patients.

Preoperative Antibiotic Prophylaxis for Endocarditis

Patients who have any form of valvular heart disease, as well as those with intracardiac (ventricular septal or atrial septal defects) or intravascular shunts, should be protected against endocarditis at the time of a known bacteremic event. Endocarditis has occurred in a sufficiently significant number of patients with hypertrophic cardiomyopathy (subvalvular aortic stenosis, asymmetric septal hypertrophy) and mitral valve prolapse to warrant the inclusion of these two conditions in the prophylaxis regimen.

Is endotracheal intubation a bacteremic event? Bacteremia occurs after the following events at these rates: dental extraction, 30% to 80%; brushing of teeth, 20% to 24%; use of oral irrigation devices, 20% to 24%; barium enema, 11%; transurethral prostate resection, 10% to 57%; upper gastrointestinal endoscopy, 8%; nasotracheal intubation, 16% (4 of 25 patients); and orotracheal intubation, 0% (0 of 25 patients).[454,455] Thus, although bacteremia from orotracheal intubation is rare, we believe that prophylaxis should be given to patients with valvular heart disease before instituting instrumentation of the gallbladder, GI tract, oropharynx, or genitourinary tract. The choice of antibiotic for prophylaxis should be aimed at the most commonly occurring (i.e., most numerous) pathogen[456] (Table 27-37). Note that these prophylactic regimens should be altered to prevent sepsis after specific surgical procedures[457] (Table 27-38). Guidelines of the

American Heart Association state that all antimicrobial prophylaxis should be started 30 minutes to 1 hour rather than 24 hours before a known bacteremic event so that therapeutic levels are achieved without superinfecting the patient with unusual pathogens.[456,457]

Cardiac Valve Prostheses and Anticoagulant Therapy and Prophylaxis for Deep Venous Thrombosis

In patients with prosthetic valves, the risk of increased bleeding during a procedure in a patient receiving antithrombotic therapy has to be weighed against the increased risk of thromboembolism caused by stopping the therapy. Common practice in patients undergoing noncardiac surgery with a mechanical prosthetic valve in place is for cessation of anticoagulant therapy 3 days before surgery. This time frame allows the INR to fall to less than 1.5 times normal. The oral anticoagulants can then be resumed on postoperative day 1. Using a similar protocol, Katholi and colleagues found no perioperative episodes of thromboembolism or hemorrhage in 25 patients.[458] An alternative approach in patients at high risk for thromboembolism is conversion to heparin during the perioperative period. The heparin can then be discontinued 4 to 6 hours before surgery and resumed shortly thereafter. Current prosthetic valves may have a lower incidence, and the risk of heparin may outweigh the benefit in the perioperative setting. According to the American Heart Association/American College of Cardiology guidelines, heparin can usually be reserved for those who have had a recent thrombus or embolus (arbitrarily within 1 year), those with demonstrated thrombotic problems when previously off therapy, those with a Björk-Shiley valve, and those with more than three risk factors (atrial fibrillation, previous thromboembolism, hypercoagulable condition, and mechanical prosthesis).[459] A lower threshold for recommending heparin should be considered in patients with mechanical valves in the mitral position, in whom a single risk factor would be sufficient evidence of high risk. Subcutaneous low-molecular-weight heparin offers an alternative outpatient approach.[460] It is appropriate for a surgeon and cardiologist to discuss the optimal perioperative management for such a patient.

Regional anesthetic techniques might be avoided, although this issue is controversial.[461-476] Many practitioners do not hesitate to use regional anesthesia in the face of prophylaxis for deep venous thrombosis.[465,468,470,472] However, epidural hematoma has been associated with anticoagulant therapy in many reports. Large retrospective reviews of outcome after epidural or spinal anesthesia, or both, during or shortly before initiation of anticoagulant therapy with heparin have not reported neurologic dysfunction related to hematoma formation in any patient.[465-468] This paucity of damaging epidemiologic evidence, though reassuring, does not reduce the need for frequent evaluation of neurologic function and search for back pain in the perioperative period after regional anesthesia in any patient receiving any clotting function inhibitor, including aspirin.[473-476] The risk of regional anesthesia concurrent with prophylaxis for deep venous thrombosis with heparin is greater with the use of low-molecular-weight heparin. (Heparin-induced

Table 27–37 Endocarditis prophylaxis: recommended antibiotic regimens*

	Dosage for Adults	Dosage for Children (in No Case to Exceed Adult Dose)
Dental and Upper Respiratory Procedures Likely to Produce Bacteremia (i.e., Tonsilloadenoidectomy, Bronchoscopy, Nasal Intubation, Nasogastric Tube Placement)		
Oral		
Amoxicillin	3 g 1 hr before procedure and 1.5 g 6 hr later	50 mg/kg
Amoxicillin, penicillin allergy:		
Erythromycin ethylsuccinate	800 mg	20 mg/kg 1 hr before procedure and 10 mg/kg 6 hr later
or		
Erythromycin stearate	1 g PO 2 hr before procedure and half the initial dose 6 hr later	
or		
Clindamycin	300 mg orally 1 hr before procedure and 150 mg 6 hr after initial dose	10 mg/kg and 5 mg/kg 6 hr later
Parenteral		
Ampicillin	2 g IM or IV 30 min before procedure	50 mg/kg IM or IV 30 min before procedure
Penicillin allergy: clindamycin	300 mg IV 30 min before procedure	10 mg/kg IV 30 min before procedure
Gastrointestinal and Genitourinary Procedures (i.e., GI or GU Surgery or Instrumentation or Surgery Involving a Tissue Possibly Contaminated with GI or GU Organisms)		
Parenteral		
Ampicillin	2 g IM or IV 30 min before procedure	50 mg/kg IM or IV 30 min before procedure
Plus gentamicin	1.5 mg/kg (not to exceed 80 mg) IM or IV 30 min before procedure	2.0 mg/kg IM or IV 30 min before procedure
Plus amoxicillin	1.5 g PO 6 hr after ampicillin and gentamicin or repeat ampicillin and gentamicin after initial dose	50 mg/kg
Penicillin, amoxicillin allergy: vancomycin	1 g IV infused slowly over 1-hr period before procedure	20 mg/kg IV infused slowly over 1-hr period beginning 1 hr before procedure
Plus gentamicin	1.5 mg/kg (not to exceed 80 mg) IM or IV 30 min before procedure	2.0 mg/kg IM or IV 30 min before procedure
Oral		
Amoxicillin	3 g 1 hr before procedure and 1.5 g 6 hr after initial dose	50 mg/kg 1 hr before procedure and 25 mg/kg 6 hr after initial dose

*The frequently used cephalosporins are not recommended. A single dose of the parenteral drugs is probably adequate because bacteremias after most oral cavity and diagnostic procedures are of short duration. However, one or two follow-up doses may be given at 8- to 12-hour intervals in selected patients, such as hospitalized patients judged to be at higher risk.

Table 27–38 Prevention of wound infection and sepsis in surgical patients

Nature of Operation	Probable Pathogens	Recommended Drugs	Adult Dosage before Surgery*
Clean			
Cardiac			
Prosthetic valve, coronary artery bypass graft, and other open heart surgery	*Staphylococcus epidermidis, Staphylococcus aureus,* enteric gram-negative bacilli	Cefazolin or vancomycin†	1 g IV 1 g IV
Vascular			
Arterial surgery involving the abdominal aorta, a prosthesis, or a groin incision	*S. aureus, S. epidermidis,* enteric gram-negative bacilli	Cefazolin or vancomycin†	1 g IV 1 g IV
Lower-extremity amputation for ischemia	*S. aureus, S. epidermidis,* enteric gram-negative bacilli, clostridia	Cefazolin or vancomycin†	1 g IV 1 g IV

(continued)

Table 27-38   Prevention of wound infection and sepsis in surgical patients—cont'd

Nature of Operation	Probable Pathogens	Recommended Drugs	Adult Dosage before Surgery*
Neurosurgery			
Craniotomy	S. aureus, S. epidermidis	Cefazolin or	1 g IV
		vancomycin†	1 g IV
Orthopedic			
Total joint replacement,	S. aureus, S. epidermidis	Cefazolin or	1 g IV
internal fixation of fractures		vancomycin†	1 g IV
Ocular	S. aureus, S. epidermidis,	Gentamicin or tobramycin	Multiple drops
	streptococci, enteric	or neomycin-gramicidin-	topically over 2-24 hr
	gram-negative bacilli,	polymyxin B	
	Pseudomonas	Cefazolin	100 mg SC at end of procedure
Clean-Contaminated			
Head and neck			
Entering oral cavity	S. aureus, streptococci, oral	Cefazolin	1 g IV
or pharynx	anaerobes	or clindamycin	600 mg IV
Gastroduodenal	Enteric gram-negative bacilli,	High risk, gastric bypass,	1 g IV
	gram-positive cocci	or percutaneous	
		endoscopic gastrostomy	
		only: cefazolin	
Biliary tract	Enteric gram-negative bacilli,	High risk only: cefazolin	1 g IV
	enterococci, clostridia		
Colorectal	Enteric gram-negative bacilli,	Oral neomycin plus	
	anaerobes	erythromycin base‡	
		Parenteral: cefoxitin	1 g IV
		or cefotetan	
Appendectomy	Enteric gram-negative bacilli,	Cefoxitin or cefotetan	1 g IV
	anaerobes		
Vaginal or abdominal	Enteric gram-negative bacilli,	Cefazolin	1 g IV
hysterectomy	anaerobes, group B		
	streptococci, enterococci		
Cesarean section	Same as for hysterectomy	High risk only: cefazolin	1 g IV after cord clamping
Abortion§	Same as for hysterectomy	Aqueous penicillin G	1 million U IV
		or doxycycline	300 mg PO§
Dirty‖			
Ruptured viscus	Enteric gram-negative bacilli,	Cefoxitin or	1 g IV q6h
	anaerobes, enterococci	cefotetan,	1 g IV q12h
		with or without	
		gentamicin;	1.5 mg/kg IV q8h
		or clindamycin	600 mg IV q6h
		and gentamicin	1.5 mg/kg IV q8h
Traumatic wound¶	S. aureus, group A	Cefazolin	1 g IV q6h
	streptococci, clostridia		

*Parenteral prophylactic antimicrobial drugs for clean and clean-contaminated surgery can be given as a single intravenous dose just before surgery. Cefazolin can also be given intramuscularly. For prolonged operations, additional intraoperative doses should be given every 4 to 8 hours for the duration of the procedure.

†For hospitals in which methicillin-resistant S. aureus and S. epidermidis frequently cause wound infection or for patients allergic to penicillins or cephalosporins. Rapid intravenous administration may cause hypotension, which could be especially dangerous during induction of anesthesia.

‡After appropriate diet and catharsis, 1 g of each at 1, 2, and 11 PM the day before surgery. An alternative is oral lavage solution (Golytely, Med Lett Drug Ther 27:39, 1985) from 1 to 6 PM (4 to 6 hours) until rectal effluent is clear, followed by neomycin, 2 g, and metronidazole, 2 g orally at 7 and 11 PM (Wolff et al., Arch Surg 123:895, 1988).

§Aqueous penicillin G or doxycycline is recommended for first-trimester abortion in patients considered to be at high risk for pelvic infection, including those with previous pelvic inflammatory disease, previous gonorrhea, or multiple sex partners. The dosage of doxycycline should be divided into 100 mg 1 hour before abortion and 200 mg ½ hour after. For midtrimester abortion, cefazolin, 1 g IV, is recommended.

‖For "dirty" surgery, therapy should usually be continued for 5 to 10 days.

¶For bite wounds in which probable pathogens may also include oral anaerobes, Eikenella corrodens (human), and Pasteurella multocida (dog and cat) (Weber and Hansen, Infect Dis Clin North Am 5:663, 1991), some Medical Letter consultants recommend the use of amoxicillin-clavulanate (Augmentin) or ampicillin-sulbactam (Unasyn).

Modified from Antimicrobial prophylaxis in surgery. Med Lett Drugs Ther Guidelines 20:27, 2004.

thrombocytopenia has been treated successfully with intravenous immunoglobulin.[470]) The American Society of Regional Anesthesia and Pain Management has issued a consensus statement on the use of regional anesthesia in anticoagulated patients.[477] They suggest that the decision to perform spinal or epidural anesthesia/analgesia and the timing of catheter removal in a patient receiving antithrombotic therapy should be made on an individual basis, with the small, though definite risk of spinal hematoma weighed against the benefits of regional anesthesia for a specific patient.

Deep venous thrombosis is so common in postoperative patients that almost 1% of postsurgical patients die of fatal pulmonary embolism[478] (Table 27-39). Because of this high mortality risk, prophylaxis against deep venous thrombosis has attained widespread acceptance; thus, prophylaxis often begins with 5000 U of heparin given subcutaneously 2 hours before surgery.[478-480] Other trials

Table 27–39   Incidence of deep venous thrombosis and fatal pulmonary embolism and recommended prophylaxis

| Type of Surgery | Incidence of | | | Recommended Prophylaxis |
	Deep Venous Thrombosis (%)	Proximal Deep Venous Thrombosis (%)	Fatal Pulmonary Embolism (%)	
General				
Age >40 yr	10	<1	0.1	
Age >60 yr	10-40	3-15	0.8	
Malignancy	50-60			
				Low-dose heparin with or without compression stockings
Thoracic	30			*or*
Vascular				External pneumatic compression
Aortic repair	26			
Peripheral	12			
Urologic				
Open prostatectomy	40			
TURP	10			
Other urologic	30-40			
Major gynecologic				
With malignancy	40			
Without malignancy	10-20			
Neurosurgery				
Craniotomy	20-80			External pneumatic compression
Laminectomy	4-25		1.5-3.0	
Orthopedic				Low-dose heparin and external pneumatic compression
				or
Total-hip replacement	40-80	10-20	1.0-5.0	Warfarin
Hip fracture	48-75		1.0-5.0	*or*
Tibial fracture	45			Adjusted-dose heparin
				or
				Low-molecular-weight heparin
Total knee	60-70	20	1.0-5.0	External pneumatic compression
				or
				Warfarin
				or
Head, neck, chest wall	11			Low-dose heparin
Medical				
Acute myocardial infarction	30	6		Ambulation
Stroke	60-75			*or*
Acute spine injury	60-100			Low-dose heparin
Other bed bound	26			

TURP, transurethral resection of the prostate.

have shown equal effect with external pneumatic compression.[479,481] Persuading surgeons to use this technique may provide greater assurance in using regional anesthesia. Such an option, however, is not available for patients with a prosthetic valve.

Another problem that can arise is managing a pregnant patient with a prosthetic valve during delivery. It is recommended that warfarin be replaced by subcutaneous heparin during the peripartum period. During labor and delivery, elective induction is advocated with discontinuance of all anticoagulant therapy, as indicated for the particular valve prosthesis (discussed earlier).[482]

Auscultation of the prosthetic valve should be performed preoperatively to verify normal functioning[483] (Fig. 27-19). Abnormalities in such sounds warrant preoperative consultation and verification of functioning.

Cardiac Conduction Disturbances

Cardiac Arrhythmias (also see Chapters 34 and 35)

Bradyarrhythmias, especially if profound or associated with dizziness or syncope, are generally managed with pacemakers. However, on rare occasion, chronic bifascicular block (right bundle branch block with a left anterior or posterior hemiblock or a left bundle branch block with combined left anterior and posterior hemiblocks), even when only a first-degree heart block is present, progresses to complete heart block and sudden perioperative death. Such progression is rare, however. In six studies, less than 2% of the approximately 266 patients with bifascicular block progressed to complete heart block perioperatively.[484-489]

On the other hand, these patients have a high 5-year mortality rate (160 of 554 patients, or 29%). Most of the deaths were related to tachyarrhythmias or MI—events not usually preventable by traditional pacemakers.[490] Thus, the presence of a bifascicular block on ECG should make the anesthesiologist more worried about associated coronary artery disease or left ventricular dysfunction. Nevertheless, these patients rarely have complete heart block perioperatively. Therefore, prophylactic preoperative insertion of temporary pacing wires for bifascicular block does not seem warranted. However, a central route can be established in advance in the event that a temporary pacemaker needs to be inserted (most operating rooms do not rely on transthoracic pacing, although such might be attempted if available).[491] The actual pacemaker equipment and appropriate personnel should be immediately available and tested regularly because symptomatic heart block does occur perioperatively in more than 1% of patients.[484-488] One study appears to have confirmed this rate of at least 1% for patients undergoing cardiac surgery.[492] One percent of patients who had no preoperative insertion of a pacing pulmonary artery catheter subsequently required pacing before cardiopulmonary bypass. By contrast, 19% of patients who had such a catheter in place underwent cardiac pacing before cardiopulmonary bypass. Predictors of the need for pacing included previous symptomatic bradyarrhythmia, a history of transient complete AV block, and aortic valve disease.

More than five PVCs per minute on preoperative examination correlate with perioperative cardiac morbidity.[367,375,376,390] To the classic criteria for treating PVCs

Prosthesis type	Mitral Prosthesis	Acoustic Characteristics	Aortic Prosthesis	Acoustic Characteristics
Ball Valves	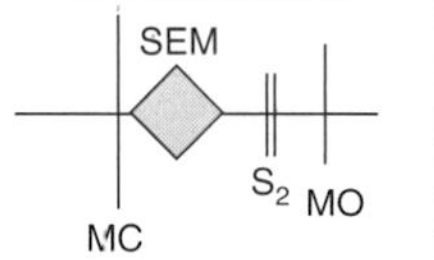 SEM / S₂ MO / MC	1) A_2–MO Interval 0.07–0.11 sec. 2) MV > MC 3) II-III/VI Systolic ejection murmer (SEM) 4) No diastolic murmur	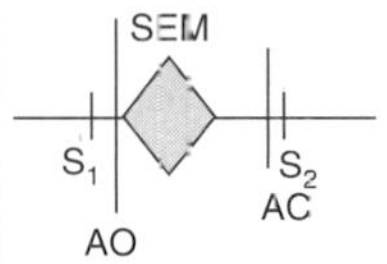 SEM / S₁ S₂ AC / AO	1) S_1–AO Interval 0.07 sec. 2) AO > AC 3) II/VI harsh SEM 4) No diastolic murmur
Disc Valves	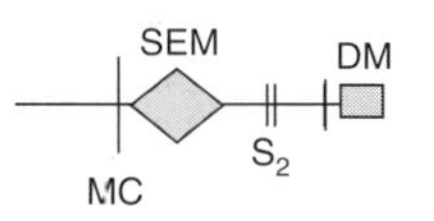 SEM DM / S₂ / MC	1) A_2–MO Interval 0.05–0.09 sec. 2) MO is rarely heard 3) II/VI is usually heard 4) II-III/VI diastolic rumble is usually heard	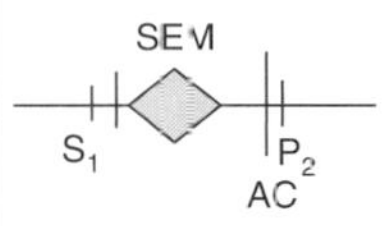 SEM / S₁ P₂ AC	1) S_1–AO Interval 0.04 sec. 2) AO is uncommonly heard AC is usually heard 3) II/VI SEM is usually heard 4) Occasional diastolic murmur
Porcine Valves	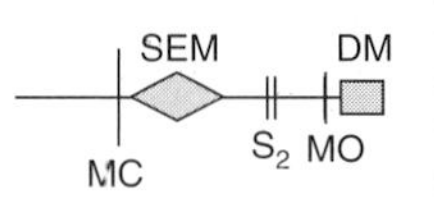 SEM DM / S₂ MO / MC	1) A_2–MO Interval 0.01 sec. 2) MO is audible 50% 3) I-II/VI apical SEM 50% 4) Diastolic rumble $1/2$–$2/3$	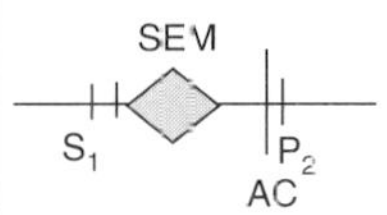 SEM / S₁ P₂ AC	1) S_1–AO Interval 0.03–0.08 sec. 2) AO is uncommonly heard AC is usually heard 3) II/VI SEM in most 4) No diastolic murmur
Bileaflet Valve (St. Jude)			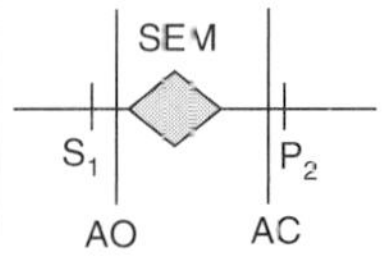 SEM / S₁ P₂ / AO AC	1) AO and AC commonly heard 2) A soft SEM is common

Figure 27–19 Summary of the normal acoustic characteristics of valve prostheses according to type and location. A_2, aortic second sound; AC, aortic valve closure sound; AO, aortic valve opening sound; DM, diastolic murmur; MC, mitral valve closure sound; MO, mitral valve opening sound; P_2, pulmonary second sound; S_1, first heart sound; S_2, second heart sound; SEM, systolic ejection murmur. (Redrawn from Smith ND, Raizada V, Abrams J: Auscultation of the normally functioning prosthetic valve. Ann Intern Med 95:594, 1981.)

(the presence of R-on-T couplets, the occurrence of more than three PVCs per minute, and multifocality of PVCs) must be added frequent (>10/hr over a 24-hour period) and repetitive ventricular beats. Electrophysiologic and programmed ventricular stimulation studies are being used to indicate and guide treatment for patients with ischemic heart disease or recurrent arrhythmias and for survivors of out-of-hospital cardiac arrest.[493] Although such patients are often treated with antiarrhythmic therapy, attention to their underlying condition should be a focus of our preoperative management. Chronic antiarrhythmic therapy is discussed in the last section of this chapter. Torsades de pointes is an arrhythmia characterized by episodes of alternating electrical polarity such that the major vector of the QRS complex seems to alternate around an isoelectric line. The hallmark enabling differential diagnosis from ventricular tachycardia is the unusual response of this arrhythmia to commonly used antiarrhythmic drugs. That is, the use of drugs that prolong the QT interval (e.g., quinidine, procainamide, disopyramide, some of the antihistamines, and the antipsychotic phenothiazines) may well make the arrhythmia more frequent or of longer duration. Reports of the sudden occurrence of torsades de pointes during surgery have been rare in the anesthesia literature. Immediate therapy consists of the administration of magnesium or electrical cardioversion, followed by overdrive cardiac pacing or the administration of β-adrenergic agonists and discontinuation of drugs that prolong the QT interval.

Premature atrial contractions and cardiac rhythm other than sinus also correlate with perioperative cardiac morbidity.[367,375] These arrhythmias may be more a marker of poor cardiovascular reserve than a specific cause of perioperative cardiac complications.

Pre-excitation syndrome is the name for supraventricular tachycardias associated with AV bypass tracts.[494] Successful treatment, which is predicated on an understanding of the clinical and electrophysiologic manifestations of the syndrome, consists of either catheter ablation techniques[490] or surgery using preoperative and intraoperative techniques that avoid release of sympathetic substances and other vasoactive substances and therefore tachyarrhythmias.[495-497] Anesthesia for electrophysiologic procedures is discussed in Chapters 50 and 68.

Pacemakers (Control of Arrhythmias)

The types of pacemakers available and the indications for their use have changed significantly since 1980. More than 90% of pacemakers are inserted for the treatment of bradyarrhythmias occurring either after tachycardia (bradytachy syndrome) or by themselves (i.e., in sick sinus syndrome or AV conduction disorders). Physiologic pacing is an attempt to increase the patient's hemodynamic response to increased metabolic demands. An increase in heart rate provides greater augmentation of cardiac output than maintenance of AV synchrony does. The rate of pacemaker insertion has also declined by more than 50% since 1980; in 1984 a publication by the American College of Cardiology and the American Heart Association of indications for pacemaker insertion codified these changes in practice patterns. The most common pacemaker for this type of dysfunction is the ventricular R-wave–inhibited (demand) type (VVI) (letter codes are described later and in Table 27-40). More complex pacemakers are presently being used to provide better cardiac output in stressful situations and decrease myocardial wall stress[498] or to treat ventricular or supraventricular tachyarrhythmias. Lithium batteries now give a pacemaker a 5- to 10-year life span. Programmable pacemakers are adjustable for sensitivity and rate. Currently available atrial pacemakers fired by an outside radiofrequency source permit termination of reentrant or pre-excitation atrial arrhythmias; similarly, ventricular pacemakers can be used to terminate supraventricular tachycardia and recurrent ventricular tachycardia.[499] Thus, in addition to learning about the patient's underlying disease, current condition, and drug therapy, the anesthesiologist must learn, preoperatively, the following information about any implanted pacemaker[499]:

1. The indication for placement of the pacemaker and the default rhythm (i.e., what rhythm occurs if the pacemaker does not capture).
2. The type of pacemaker (demand, fixed, or radiofrequency), the chamber paced, and the chamber sensed. Pacemakers have traditionally been given a five-letter code (see Table 27-40). However, most pacemakers implanted since 1980 have codes consisting of only the first three letters. The *first* letter indicates the chamber paced (i.e., V = ventricle, A = atrium, D = dual or both). The *second* letter indicates the chamber sensed (i.e., V = ventricle, A = atrium, D = dual, O = none). The *third* letter indicates the sensing pattern (i.e., O = no sensing, fixed mode; I = inhibited, demand pacer; T = triggered, meaning that the sensing of an electrical impulse triggers a pacemaker spike; D = dual, i.e., both T and I). For example, a VOO pacemaker paces the ventricle, does not sense, and is in a fixed mode.

Table 27–40 The North American Society for Pacing and Electrophysiology/British Pacing and Electrophysiology Group (NSAPE/BPEG) generic (NBG)* five-letter code for pacemaker systems

First Letter: Chamber Paced	Second Letter: Chamber Sensed	Third Letter: Mode of Response	Fourth Letter (If Used): Programmable Features	Fifth Letter (If Used): Arrhythmia Treatment
A = atrium	A = atrium	T = triggered	P = programmable (single)	O = none
V = ventricle	V = ventricle	I = inhibited	M = multiprogrammable	P = pacing (antitachyarrhythmia)
D = dual	D = dual	D = dual (T & I)	O = not programmable	S = shock
O = none	O = none	O = not applicable	R = rate modulated	D = dual (P & S)

*N, NSAPE; B, BPEG; G, generic.

Note: Positions I to III are used exclusively for antibradyarrhythmia function.

In other words, it is a fixed-rate ventricular pacemaker. A VVI pacemaker paces the ventricle, senses the ventricle, and is inhibited. It is a ventricular-inhibited demand pacemaker. A DVI pacemaker paces both the atrium and ventricle, senses only the ventricle, and is inhibited. Thus, it is a sequential AV demand pacemaker that fires when it does not sense intrinsic ventricular activity. Rate-modulated pacemakers increase the heart rate in response to increased demand. They have special sensors and are placed in patients who may have abnormal sinus node function. These pacemakers have an R in the fourth position of the pacemaker letter code[498] (e.g., VVIR; see Table 27-40). A DDDCP pacemaker has multiprogrammable "physiologic" dual-chamber pacing with telemetry and antitachyarrhythmia-pacing capability. An OOOPS is a simple, programmable cardioverter, defibrillator, or cardioverter-defibrillator. It cannot be overemphasized that no generic code can describe every antiarrhythmic device in a comprehensive and unambiguous fashion. It seems to us that it is beneficial to consult with an electrophysiologist/cardiologist before anesthetizing any patient who has a pacemaker.

3. How to detect deterioration in battery function (increased rate or decreased rate).

4. How to change the mode or fire the pacemaker if it is of the radiofrequency type. (These procedures should not only be learned by anesthesiologists but also be demonstrated to them. In addition, the magnet or programming device [or both] should be in or near the operating room at the time of surgery.)

5. The current rate and sensitivity settings of the pacemaker.

6. Whether the pacemaker is currently functioning and how well.

Because demand pacemakers can sense electrocautery, which sometimes inhibits pacemaker firing, asystole can occur in a pacemaker-dependent patient. A review of the causes of interference has recently been published.[500] Most pacemakers can be converted to a fixed rate, and the anesthesiologist can take the following precautions: (1) have the cardiologist demonstrate how such conversion is done and (2) have the necessary magnet or programming device, or both, available in the operating room. In addition, the ground plate should be as far from the pulse generator and lead as possible, a bipolar form of electrocautery should be used, and if possible, some measure of blood flow should be monitored (i.e., Doppler detector, pulse oximetry unaffected by electrocautery, or intra-arterial line). The rationale for the last measure is that electrocautery temporarily affects the accuracy of ECG results; because asystole could occur during this period, a measure of blood flow is necessary. Currently, at least eight manufacturers produce a total of more than 80 types of pacemakers, with a variety of default programs. A default program is the secondary program (i.e., the generator circuit) to which the primary program will revert if it senses problems in the initial circuit. Because default programs differ, pacemaker malfunction will be manifested differently depending on the brand and model. Thus, it is necessary to learn before surgery how problems will be manifested with each pacemaker during surgery.[499]

The most common cause of temporary pacemaker malfunction is lack of contact between the electrode wire and the endocardium. Pacemaker spikes continue to exist on the ECG oscilloscope, even when no myocardial contractions propel blood. This situation has occurred with muscular exertion, blunt trauma, cardioversion, and positive-pressure ventilation.[501] Treatment consists of advancing the electrode until it captures, administering isoproterenol (if that worked in the past), external pacing, or failing that, cardiopulmonary resuscitation.

During the preoperative examination, the anesthesiologist can also assess progression of underlying disease (e.g., CHF, electrolyte disorders, and the condition of all systems related to the underlying disease). Antiarrhythmic therapy and its implications are discussed in the last section of this chapter.

DISORDERS OF THE RESPIRATORY AND IMMUNE SYSTEMS

General Preoperative and Preprocedure Considerations

Although little may seem to have changed in the preoperative preparation of patients with respiratory disease, this impression is not true. Major changes in drug therapy have occurred, and appreciation has increased regarding the effects of smoking and sleep apnea on perioperative and chronic care.[502-515] (Preoperative and preprocedure identification and perioperative care of patients with sleep apnea are discussed in the earlier section on obesity.)

The main purpose of preoperative testing is to identify patients at risk for perioperative complications and to institute appropriate perioperative therapy. Preoperative assessment can also establish baseline function and the feasibility of surgical intervention. Whereas numerous investigators have used pulmonary function tests to define inoperability or high-risk versus low-risk groups for pulmonary complications, few have been able to demonstrate that the performance of any specific preoperative or intraoperative measure reliably decreases perioperative pulmonary morbidity or mortality. Because routine preoperative pulmonary testing and care are discussed extensively in Chapters 26 and 75, the current discussion is limited to an assessment of the effectiveness of this type of care.

In fact, few randomized prospective studies indicate an outcome benefit of preoperative preparation; a larger cohort has implied a benefit of intraoperative and postoperative pain therapy techniques[516-518] (usually planned preoperatively; see Chapter 25). Stein and Cassara[519] randomly allocated 48 patients to undergo preoperative therapy (cessation of smoking, administration of antibiotics for purulent sputum, and use of bronchodilating drugs, postural drainage, chest physiotherapy, and ultrasonic nebulizer) or no preoperative therapy. The no-treatment group had a mortality of 16% and morbidity of 60%, as opposed to 0% and 20%, respectively, for the treatment group. In addition, the treatment group spent an average of 12 postoperative days in the hospital as compared with 24 days for the 21 survivors in the no-treatment group.

Collins and colleagues[520] prospectively examined the benefits of preoperative antibiotics, perioperative chest physiotherapy and therapy with bronchodilating drugs, and routine postoperative analgesia (morphine) on postoperative respiratory complications in patients with COPD. Of these therapies, only preoperative treatment with antibiotics had a beneficial effect.

Warner and coworkers[521] collected data retrospectively about smoking history and prospectively (concurrently) about pulmonary complications for 200 patients undergoing CABG surgery. These investigators documented that 8 weeks or more of smoking cessation was associated with a 66% reduction in postoperative pulmonary complications. Smokers who stopped for less than 8 weeks actually had an increase (from 33% for current smokers to 57.1% for recent quitters) in the rate of one or more of the six complications surveyed: purulent sputum with pyrexia; need for respiratory therapy care; bronchospasm requiring therapy; pleural effusion or pneumothorax (or both) necessitating drainage; segmental pulmonary collapse, as confirmed by radiography; or pneumonia necessitating antibiotic therapy. Others have found that both shorter and longer periods of cessation of smoking were needed before achieving cardiovascular[522-524] and hematologic benefit.[525] Of note, Bluman and associates[526] performed a retrospective chart review of 410 patients undergoing noncardiac surgery at a VA hospital. Current smoking was associated with a nearly sixfold increase in risk for a postoperative pulmonary complication. Reduction in smoking within 1 month of surgery was not associated with a decreased risk of postoperative pulmonary complications. Nakagawa and coauthors also reported higher pulmonary complication rates in patients undergoing pulmonary surgery who quit within 4 weeks of surgery than in current smokers or those who had stopped smoking for more than 4 weeks.[527] The fact that anesthesiologists rarely see their patients 4 weeks or more before surgery presents a dilemma: if one is unable to advise the patient to stop smoking 8 weeks or more before surgery, is it preferable for the patient to continue smoking? Perhaps these data will further support the implementation of preoperative and preprocedure assessment clinics in which anesthesiologists are able to advise and counsel patients about risk reduction. When Skolnick and coworkers[515] studied 602 children prospectively, exposure to passive smoking (as measured by urinary cotinine, the major metabolite of nicotine) correlated directly with airway complications. Children with the least exposure to passive smoke had the fewest complications.

Celli and associates[528] performed a randomized prospective controlled trial of intermittent positive-pressure breathing (IPPB) versus incentive spirometry and deep-breathing exercises in 81 patients undergoing abdominal surgery. The groups exposed to a respiratory therapist (regardless of the treatment given) had more than a 50% lower incidence of clinical complications (30% to 33% versus 88%) and shorter hospital stays than the control group did. Thus, this third prospective study indicates that outcome improves when there is any concern about lung function on the part of someone knowledgeable in maneuvers designed to clear lung secretions.

Bartlett and coworkers[529] randomly assigned 150 patients undergoing extensive laparotomy to one of two groups.

One group received preoperative instruction in and postoperative use (10 times per hour) of incentive spirometry. The other group received similar medical care but no incentive spirometry. Only 7 of 75 patients using incentive spirometry had postoperative pulmonary complications, as opposed to 19 of 75 in the control group. However, other studies have not shown a benefit for specific treatments or have been too contaminated with bias to have a clear result emerge. Lyager and colleagues[530] randomly assigned 103 patients undergoing biliary or gastric surgery to receive either incentive spirometry with preoperative and postoperative chest physiotherapy or only preoperative and postoperative chest physiotherapy. No difference in the postoperative course or pulmonary complications was found between the two groups. Other studies have shown a specific benefit (i.e., above that provided by routine care) for chest physiotherapy and IPPB. These studies are usually poorly controlled, not randomized, or retrospective in design (or any combination of the three); these deficiencies probably substantially bias the results toward finding a benefit in reducing postoperative pulmonary complications.[531-534] Although randomized prospective studies showed no benefit or actual harm from chest physiotherapy and IPPB on the resolution of pneumonia[535,536] or postoperative pulmonary complications,[520,528,533,536-539] the four studies cited earlier[519,520,528,529] and numerous retrospective studies[521,531-533] strongly suggest that preoperative evaluation and treatment of patients with pulmonary disease actually decrease perioperative respiratory complications, even if only by causing a change in anesthetic techniques.[516]

Recent meta-analyses have suggested a benefit of anesthetic and pain management with respect to respiratory outcomes. Rodgers and colleagues reviewed 141 trials involving 9559 patients who had been randomized to receive neuraxial blockade or general anesthesia. Overall mortality was significantly lower in the neuraxial blockade group (2.1% versus 3.1%). The relative risk of pneumonia in the neuraxial group was 0.61 (CI, 0.48 to 0.81), and the relative risk of respiratory depression was 0.41 (CI, 0.23 to 0.73).

Not all studies demonstrate beneficial effects of pretreatment. In afebrile outpatient ASA I and II children with no lung disease or findings who underwent noncavitary, nonairway surgery for under 3 hours, neither albuterol nor ipratropium premedication decreased adverse events.[540]

Evaluation of dyspnea is especially useful and thus warrants discussion here (for a review of the specific pulmonary function tests that identify high-risk groups, see Chapter 26). Boushy and coworkers[539] found that grades of preoperative dyspnea correlated with postoperative survival. (Grades of respiratory dyspnea are provided in Table 27-41.) Mittman[541] demonstrated an increased risk of death after thoracic surgery from 8% in patients without dyspnea to 56% in patients who were dyspneic. Similarly, Reichel[542] found that no patients died after pneumonectomy if they were able to complete a preoperative treadmill test for 4 minutes at the rate of 2 mph on level ground. Other studies have found that the history and physical examination of an asthmatic subject can also predict the need for hospitalization.[504,543] Wong and

Table 27–41 Grade of dyspnea caused by respiratory problems (assessed in terms of walking on the level at a normal pace)

Category	Description
0	No dyspnea while walking on the level at a normal pace
I	"I am able to walk as far as I like, provided I take my time."
II	Specific (street) block limitation ("I have to stop for a while after one or two blocks.")
III	Dyspnea on mild exertion ("I have to stop and rest while going from the kitchen to the bathroom.")
IV	Dyspnea at rest

Modified from Boushy SF, Billing DM, North LB, et al: Clinical course related to preoperative pulmonary function in patients with bronchogenic carcinoma. Chest 59:383, 1971.

colleagues[544] found that the risk index (Table 27-42) correlated with postoperative pulmonary complications. Other than dyspnea, what preoperative conditions make postoperative respiratory complications more likely[534,544-546] (see Chapter 74)?

Table 27–42 Classification of risk of pulmonary complications for thoracic and abdominal procedures

Category	Points*
I. Expiratory spirogram	
A. Normal (% FVC + % FEV_1/FVC >150)	0
B. % FVC + % FEV_1/FVC = 100-150	1
C. % FVC + % FEV_1/FVC < 100	2
D. Preoperative FVC < 20 mL/kg	3
E. Postbronchodilator FEV_1/FVC < 50%	3
II. Cardiovascular system	
A. Normal	0
B. Controlled hypertension, myocardial infarction without sequelae for more than 2 yr	0
C. Dyspnea on exertion, orthopnea, paroxysmal nocturnal dyspnea, dependent edema, congestive heart failure, angina	1
III. Nervous system	
A. Normal	0
B. Confusion, obtundation, agitation, spasticity, discoordination, bulbar malfunction	1
C. Significant muscular weakness	1
IV. Arterial blood gases	
A. Acceptable	0
B. $Paco_2$ >50 mm Hg or Pao_2 <60 mm Hg on room air	1
C. Metabolic pH abnormality >7.50 or <7.30	1
V. Postoperative ambulation	
A. Expected ambulation (minimum, sitting at bedside) within 36 hr	0
B. Expected complete bed confinement for ≥36 hr	1

Arozullah and associates developed the first validated multifactorial risk index for postoperative respiratory failure, defined as mechanical ventilation for more than 48 hours after surgery or reintubation and mechanical ventilation after postoperative extubation.[547] In a prospective cohort study of 181,000 male veterans as part of The National Veterans Administration Surgical Quality Improvement Program, seven factors independently predicted risk (Table 27-43). With increasing numbers of risk factors present, the rate of complications increased from 0.5% (class 1) to 26.6% (class 4). Arozullah and colleagues subsequently developed a risk index for postoperative pneumonia by using data on 160,805 patients undergoing major noncardiac surgery and validated the index by using data on an additional 155,266 patients.[548] Patients were divided into five risk classes by using risk index scores (Table 27-44). Pneumonia rates were 0.2% in those with 0 to 15 risk points, 1.2% in those with 16 to 25 risk points, 4.0% in those with 26 to 40 risk points, 9.4% in those with 41 to 55 risk points, and 15.3% in those with more than 55 risk points.

From our perspective, the important information and conditions to search for during the history taking and physical examination are as follows:
1. Dyspnea (see Table 27-41).
2. Coughing and production of sputum. Sputum, if present, should be Gram-stained and cultured, and appropriate antibiotic treatment should be instituted.

Table 27–43 Preoperative predictors of postoperative respiratory failure

Variable	Odds Ratio (95% Confidence Interval)
Type of surgery	
Abdominal aortic aneurysm	14.3 (12.0-16.9)
Thoracic	8.14 (7.17-9.25)
Neurosurgery, upper abdominal, or peripheral vascular	4.21 (3.80-4.67)
Neck	3.10 (2.40-4.01)
Other surgery*	1.00 (reference)
Emergency surgery	3.12 (2.83-3.43)
Albumin <0.30 g/L	2.53 (2.28-2.80)
Blood urea nitrogen >0.30 mg/dL	2.29 (2.04-2.56)
Partially or fully dependent status	1.92 (1.74-2.11)
History of COPD	1.81 (1.66-1.98)
Age (yr)	
≥70	1.91 (1.71-2.13)
60-69	1.51 (1.36-1.69)
<60	1.00 (reference)

*Other surgeries include ophthalmologic, ear, nose, mouth, lower abdominal, extremity, dermatologic, spine, and back surgery.
COPD, chronic obstructive pulmonary disease.
From Arozullah AM, Daley J, Henderson WG, et al: Multifactorial risk index for predicting postoperative respiratory failure in men after major noncardiac surgery. The National Veterans Administration Surgical Quality Improvement Program. Ann Surg 232:242-253, 2000, with permission.

Table 27–44 Postoperative pneumonia risk index

	Preoperative Risk Factor Point Value
Type of surgery	
Abdominal aortic aneurysm repair	15
Thoracic	14
Upper abdominal	10
Neck	8
Neurosurgery	8
Vascular	3
Age	
80 yr	17
70-79 yr	13
60-69 yr	9
50-59 yr	4
Functional status	
Totally dependent	10
Partially dependent	6
Weight loss >10% in past 6 mo	7
History of chronic obstructive pulmonary disease	5
General anesthesia	4
Impaired sensorium	4
History of cerebrovascular accident	4
Blood urea nitrogen level	
<2.86 mmol/L (0.8 mg/dL)	4
7.85-10.7 mmol/L (22-30 mg/dL)	2
≥10.7 mmol/L (≥30 mg/dL)	3
Transfusion >4 U	3
Emergency surgery	3
Steroid use for chronic condition	3
Current smoker within 1 yr	3
Alcohol intake >2 drinks/day in past 2 wk	2

From Arozullah AM, Khuri SF, Henderson WG, et al: Development and validation of a multifactorial risk index for predicting postoperative pneumonia after major noncardiac surgery. Ann Intern Med 135:847-857, 2001, with permission.

3. Recent respiratory infection. Viral respiratory infections affect respiratory function by giving rise to increased airflow obstruction that may persist for as long as 5 weeks.[549,550] These infections also adversely affect the respiratory mechanisms responding to bacteria. However, whether the incidence of complications in normal children is lessened by waiting 5 weeks until the symptoms of respiratory infection have disappeared is open to question.[551-556] Elwood and colleagues recently studied afebrile outpatient tertiary care children (aged 2 months to 18 years, N = 109) without lung disease or findings who underwent noncavitary, nonairway surgery for under 3 hours and did not find any association between adverse events and either upper respiratory tract infection (URI) within 6 weeks (n = 76) or URI within 7 days (n = 21).[540] Therefore, the risk and benefits of delaying surgery must be balanced in patients with URI if they are afebrile.
4. Hemoptysis.

5. Wheezing and previous use of bronchodilating drugs and corticosteroids (systemic or inhaled). Wheezing often suggests potentially reversible airway obstruction but is a notoriously poor indicator of the degree of obstruction. In addition, not all wheezing is caused by bronchospasm. Cardiac and other pulmonary causes must be differentiated from asthma.[557] Drug therapy for asthma should be ascertained and optimized if possible.[558] Asthmatics have a fourfold increase in perioperative respiratory complications. Holleman and Simel[504] found that auscultated audible wheezing on nonforced expiration (along with a 70-pack-year history of smoking and patient sensation of wheezing) was a reliable sign of severe airflow limitation.
6. Pulmonary complications from previous surgery. Prolonged endotracheal intubation after surgery can be required by many conditions, most notably respiratory and neuromuscular disorders.
7. A history of smoking. The incidence of respiratory complications is higher in tobacco smokers than nonsmokers.[521,531,532,559,560]
8. Age, general history of the patient, and any other significant physical findings. Although other disease conditions probably increase a patient's respiratory risk, the documentation on this hypothesis is barely adequate.[544] Old age definitely increases respiratory and cardiac risk,[521,530,547,548,559,561,562] although it is less important in ambulatory surgery.[563] In a multivariate analysis, McAlister and colleagues reported that age older than 65 years was associated with an odds ratio of 1.8 for pulmonary complications.[560] Cardiovascular history and examination are obviously important in themselves but are also especially helpful in revealing signs of pulmonary hypertension, such as right ventricular lift (i.e., lift over the lower part of the sternum), fixed and widely split second heart sound, and S_4 gallop at the left sternal border.
9. Breathing frequency and form. Pursed lips, cyanosis, and the use of accessory muscles should be noted. Vocal cord dysfunction occurs commonly from both psychosocial illness and an attempt to increase end-expiratory pressure.[564]
10. Body habitus:
    a. Abnormalities of the chest wall, trauma, kyphoscoliosis with restrictive lung disease. Development of a barrel chest is a late manifestation of obstructive lung disease.
    b. Obesity. There is controversy regarding the influence of obesity on postoperative pulmonary complications. In an analysis of 12 studies conducted between 1968 and 2000, obesity was associated with a relative risk of 1.3 for postoperative pulmonary complications, but this risk was not clinically significant.[565] However, a weight 30% over ideal doubles the incidence of respiratory complications according to one author (Amalraj S, personal communication).[90-95,106-108,110-114,535,559]
    c. OSA is associated with increased pulmonary complications, primarily hypercapnia and hypoxia,[110-112,118,566] as well as a threefold increased rate of unplanned ICU stay.

11. Adequacy of the upper airway, presence of tracheal deviation, ease of facemask application, ease of endotracheal intubation.
    a. McAlister and coauthors reported that a maximal laryngeal height of 4 cm or less was associated with an odds ratio of 2.0 for pulmonary complications after nonthoracic surgery.[560]
12. Presence of rales, rhonchi, wheezing (especially on nonforced expiration), diaphragmatic excursion, and air movement and the ratio of expiratory to inspiratory time.[504]
13. Site of proposed surgery. Upper abdominal surgery increases the incidence of perioperative pulmonary complications.[516,519,532,544,545,567]
14. Surgery performed on an emergency basis. Wong and colleagues[544] found that surgery performed on an emergency basis increased the risk of perioperative pneumonia 13-fold in patients with severe COPD.

Chapters 25 and 26 review the value of chest radiographs and pulmonary function tests in identifying patients with preoperative pulmonary disease, as well as which tests should be ordered and for whom. A recent study suggests that clinical evaluation is more accurate than abnormal spirometry. Warner and colleagues used a matched control design to study smokers undergoing abdominal surgery and found no significant differences in the incidence of prolonged intubation, pneumonia, or prolonged ICU stay in those with abnormal findings on spirometry.[568] Any patient who will require postoperative ventricular support should be considered for preoperative testing. Although we have yet to find the ideal pulmonary function test that guarantees success or that predicts a poor outcome that could be improved by therapy, the following conditions are relatively good predictors of complications associated with resection of a lung: a maximum breathing capacity of less than 40 or 50 L/min/70 kg, an FEV_1/FVC ratio of less than 40% of predicted, an FEV_1 of less than 1.2 L, or a maximum midexpiratory flow rate of less than 50 L/min.[531,534,541-545,569-571]

To these conditions is now added the diffusing capacity of the lung for carbon monoxide (D_{LCO}).[391,570,571] D_{LCO} decreases with fixed obstructive lung disease (i.e., emphysema) but remains normal in bronchospastic disease. In one study, when preoperative D_{LCO} was less than 60% of predicted, the mortality rate was 25% and the pulmonary morbidity rate was 45%, whereas a D_{LCO} of 100% or greater of predicted was associated with a 0% mortality rate and a 11% pulmonary morbidity rate. A subsequent study confirmed these findings.[571] Although we have always tried to reduce laboratory studies, they may prove useful in a patient with COPD who requires pulmonary surgery. Further analysis is necessary to determine whether the finding of a normal D_{LCO} may allow expansion of the usual spirometric criteria to permit successful pulmonary resection in patients who are currently excluded as candidates for such operations. We conduct such tests on any patient with dyspnea of grade II or higher or any patient who shows significant abnormalities or risk on the first 13 factors listed earlier. Wong and coworkers[544] found that the Shapiro score (see Table 27-42) and ASA physical status independently predicted adverse outcomes after surgery in patients with severe obstructive

pulmonary disease. Although this score depends heavily on abnormal pulmonary function test results for grading risk, abnormalities in the cardiovascular, neuromuscular, and central nervous systems, plus restrictions in ambulation, can also increase the risk score. A Shapiro score of 5 points or more was associated with a 17-fold higher risk of perioperative death and a 14-fold higher risk of postoperative bronchospasm after nonthoracic surgery.[544]

Despite the lack of definitive data establishing the efficacy of preoperative pulmonary testing and therapy, we recommend the following approach:
1. Eradicate acute infections and suppress chronic infections by using appropriate diagnostic measures and antibiotic treatment.
2. Relieve bronchospasm by using inhaled corticosteroids and bronchodilating drugs and document such relief with measurements of FEV_1 (also see Chapters 26 and 75).
3. In patients with bronchial asthma, consider the administration of corticosteroids beginning at least 48 hours before surgery in patients with a significant history of bronchospastic disease to achieve the maximal effect at the time of surgery. No randomized data support such an approach, but studies have not shown an increase in the risk of respiratory infection or wound complications.[572,573]
4. Institute measures to improve sputum clearance and familiarize the patient with respiratory therapy equipment (incentive spirometry) and postural drainage maneuvers. Initiate practice coughing and deep-breathing exercises (also see Chapters 26 and 75).
5. Treat uncompensated right ventricular heart failure with digoxin, diuretics, oxygen, and drugs that decrease pulmonary vascular resistance (e.g., hydralazine).[574]
6. The use of low-dose heparin prophylactically to decrease the incidence of venous thrombosis (and pulmonary emboli) has been the standard.[478-480,575] More recently, the use of low-molecular-weight heparin and intermittent compression stockings has become standard for high-risk patients.[576,577]
7. Identify and treat suspected or diagnosed sleep apnea with CPAP or BiPAP or other measures as indicated earlier (in the section "Obesity").
8. Encourage reduction or cessation of smoking at least 4 weeks and preferably 8 weeks or more before surgery.[521] Although the debate about cessation of smoking includes more than pulmonary risk, cardiovascular, hematologic, and aspiration risk has also not been shown to be responsive to short-term cessation.[521-525] Perhaps the benefit of using a major life event, an operation, to promote cessation of smoking is worth the increased short-term risk that encouraging cessation within a day or two of surgery would entail; the latter hypothesis remains to be tested. Even young people who smoke only a half to a pack of cigarettes per day exhibit abnormalities in respiratory function.[578] Avoiding passive smoking also appears beneficial.[515]

Specific Diseases

Pulmonary Vascular Diseases
Pulmonary vascular diseases include pulmonary hypertension secondary to heart disease (postcapillary disorders),

parenchymal lung disease (pulmonary precapillary disorders), pulmonary embolism, and cor pulmonale from COPD.[579] Optimal preoperative management of these conditions requires treatment of the underlying disease.[579,580] Because pulmonary embolism can be particularly difficult to diagnose, it is crucial to be especially alert to the possibility of this disease. The clinical findings of pulmonary emboli are not always present or specific for the diagnosis. The history may include tachypnea, dyspnea, palpitations, syncope, chest pain, or hemoptysis. Physical examination can reveal a pleural rub, wheezing, rales, a fixed and split second heart sound, right ventricular lift, or evidence of venous thrombosis, none of which is present in most patients. If the ECG shows an S_1-Q_3 pattern, spiral CT or lung perfusion scans can be obtained to rule out the diagnosis of pulmonary emboli. A high degree of suspicion is necessary to warrant angiography, and anticoagulation or fibrinolytic therapy. If possible, the reactivity of the pulmonary vasculature should be determined, for it may be enhanced or decreased by such drugs as nifedipine, hydralazine, nitroglycerin, prazosin, tolazoline, phentolamine, and nitric oxide. Monitoring of pulmonary artery pressure is often required; preoperative measures should be undertaken to ensure that the patient is not exposed to conditions that elevate pulmonary vascular resistance (i.e., hypoxia, hypercapnia, acidosis, lung hyperinflation, hypothermia)[581] or that decrease blood volume (prolonged restriction of fluid intake) or systemic vascular resistance.

Infectious Diseases of the Lung

Preoperative evaluation and treatment should follow the basic guidelines outlined in the introduction to this section; treatment of the underlying disease should be completed before all but emergency surgery is performed. It bears repeating that viral respiratory infections do affect respiratory function by giving rise to increased airflow obstruction (especially in the small airways) that may persist for at least 5 weeks. Viral respiratory infections also adversely affect the respiratory mechanisms that defend against bacteria. Within 5 weeks of an upper respiratory infection, children may have an increased incidence of perioperative respiratory tract complications after intubation.[551-556] It appears appropriate to delay surgery that requires tracheal intubation for all children (and possibly all adults) for 5 weeks after an upper respiratory infection.[551-556] However, in afebrile outpatient ASA I and II children with no lung disease or findings who underwent noncavitary, nonairway surgery lasting less than 3 hours, Elwood and coauthors reported that there was no association between either recent URI or active URI and desaturation, wheeze, cough, stridor, or laryngospasm causing desaturation.[540]

Even though elective surgery should be postponed whenever infectious diseases of the lung are present, patients undergoing emergency surgery often have nosocomial infections and immunocompromised systems. The predominant pathogens for nosocomial pneumonia are gram-negative bacilli, *Staphylococcus aureus, Haemophilus influenzae,* anaerobes, and pneumococci. Furthermore, tuberculosis has been increasing since 1985, probably because of reactivation in patients infected with HIV. Tuberculosis leads to chronic pulmonary and systemic symptoms. Affected patients may have malaise, headache, fever, hemoptysis, and extrapulmonary diseases affecting the skin, cervical lymph nodes, kidneys, pericardium, and meninges. Active disease is treated with isoniazid and rifampin for 9 months. Therapy should probably be started before surgery; for patients coming from countries with a high incidence of resistance to isoniazid, initial therapy might include more than two drugs. Administration of treatment before these emergency patients (many of whom have adult respiratory distress syndrome) are brought to the operating room might include initiation of anti-infective therapy, optimization of fluid status and gas exchange, and therapy for the underlying pathophysiologic process.[580-585]

Chronic Obstructive Pulmonary Disease

Treatment of COPD (reactive airways) may include the use of β-adrenergic drugs, parasympatholytic agents (especially for exercise-induced asthma), systemic or inhaled corticosteroids, and leukotriene antagonists.[502-514,586] An estimated 5% of the population has bronchospasm. Some investigators recommend using inhaled bronchodilators as first-line drugs and reducing the dose of inhaled steroids, such as beclomethasone dipropionate, budesonide, mometasone, or fluticasone, which are inactivated after absorption. However, in large doses, these "inhaled" steroids can suppress adrenal function, and supplemental systemic corticosteroids may be needed at times of stress (see earlier discussion under the section on adrenocortical malfunction). Preoperative assessment must include gaining knowledge of drug regimens and their effects and education of the patient regarding proper use of an inhaler (Table 27-45) because these drugs can interact dangerously with anesthetics (see the last section of this chapter) or can be used inappropriately and therefore produce side effects without maximum benefit.[502-514] No known interaction between the inhaled anticholinergic ipratropium bromide and muscle relaxants has been reported. Patients can feel fine at rest but must be tested by exercise or spirometry to document the degree of

---

Table 27–45 Procedures for correct use of a metered-dose inhaler

Remove the cap and hold the inhaler upright.

Shake the inhaler.

Tilt the head back slightly and exhale steadily to functional residual capacity.

Position the inhaler by using a spacer between the actuator and the mouth.

Press down on the inhaler while taking a slow, deep breath (3 to 5 seconds).

Hold the full inspiration for at least 5 and up to 10 seconds, if possible, to allow the medication to reach deeply into the lungs.

Repeat inhalations as directed. Waiting 1 minute after inhalation of the bronchodilator may permit subsequent inhalations to penetrate more deeply into the lungs and is necessary to ensure proper dose delivery.

Rinse the mouth and expectorate after using the inhaler.

current bronchospasm. Furthermore, a symptomatic response to bronchodilators in an asymptomatic patient may not predict whether the patient responds to bronchodilator therapy. An estimated 10% of asthmatic patients exhibit sensitivity to aspirin and may react not only to compounds containing aspirin but also to tartrazine, yellow dye No. 5, indomethacin, other nonsteroidal anti-inflammatory drugs, and aminopyrine.[587]

COPD takes several forms. Bronchial asthma, which occurs in 3% to 5% of the population, is characterized by reversible airway obstruction. When airway obstruction is partially reversible (by steroids or adrenergic mediators), it is often accompanied by chronic bronchitis. Some of the drugs may improve aspects of lung function other than bronchial muscle tone.[554] The majority of patients with a history of chronic cough and production of sputum on most days for 3 months a year for at least 2 years have chronic bronchitis. These patients are (or almost always have been) smokers, although environmental and occupational or genetic predisposition may contribute to hypertrophy of the mucous glands in the major airways, to hyperplasia of the goblet cells, and to edema and inflammation of the airways. They will have a decreased DLCO, whereas patients with pure bronchospasm will have a normal DLCO. Hyperinflation of the air spaces, abnormal dilation, and destruction of acinar units distal to the terminal bronchiole define emphysema. The destruction of alveolar membranes is believed to be related to an imbalance favoring destructive proteases (the most important of which are neutrophil derived) over protective circulating antiproteases (the most important of which is α_1-antitrypsin). Cigarette smoking increases the protease-antiprotease ratio. The destruction of alveolar structures limits expiratory airflow by decreasing both elastic lung recoil and radial lung traction, and the loss of alveolar capillary blood volume results in decreased DLCO. Cystic fibrosis is characterized by dilatation and hypertrophy of the bronchial glands, mucous plugging of the peripheral airways, and often, bronchitis, bronchiectasis, and bronchiolectasis. For all these conditions, the measures recommended earlier in this section, as well as appropriate hydration to allow for mobilization of secretions, should be followed.

Interstitial and Immune Lung Diseases
Included in this heterogeneous group of diseases are the hypersensitivity lung diseases, environmental exposure diseases, inorganic dust diseases, radiation-induced lung disease, sarcoidosis, collagen vascular disorders (systemic lupus erythematosus, polymyositis, dermatomyositis, Sjögren's syndrome, rheumatoid arthritis, systemic sclerosis), Goodpasture's syndrome, idiopathic pulmonary hemosiderosis, Wegener's granulomatosis, and the autoimmune diseases.[588] CT scans localize pulmonary inflammation and have become the primary decision-making tool in diagnosing infiltrative lung disease.[589,590] Many of these disorders affect not only the lungs but also the blood vessels, the conduction system of the heart, the myocardium, the joints (including those of the upper airway and larynx), and the renal, hepatic, and central nervous systems as well. The reader is referred to a textbook of internal medicine to aid in understanding the pathophysiologic

processes and full preoperative assessment of these conditions. Therapy for these conditions includes the use of anti-inflammatory drugs, corticosteroids, and immunosuppressive therapies.

Neoplasms
Solitary nodules are tumors that are less than 6 cm in diameter, surrounded by lung parenchyma, and not associated with adenopathy or pleural effusion. The cure rate for bronchogenic carcinoma manifested as a solitary nodule is 50%—much better than the "cure" rate for other manifestations.[591] (It should be remembered that tuberculosis can mimic cancer so closely that surgery has even been performed.) Blood studies, including calcium and alkaline phosphatase levels, and liver function studies help confirm that the neoplasm has not disseminated. If these studies and the history and physical examination show no abnormal findings, it is unlikely that bone, brain, or hepatic MRI or CT scanning techniques will indicate metastasis. Surgery need not await the results of these tests because few patients not found to have metastatic disease by simple blood tests, history, and physical examination will prove to have such disease detected by these scans. Survival depends on the stage of the tumor and the age of the patient.[592]

Surgical resection is the primary therapy for non–small cell carcinomas (e.g., adenocarcinoma, squamous cell carcinoma, and large cell carcinoma). These carcinomas account for 75% of all lung carcinomas, 12% of all malignant tumors, and 20% of all cancer deaths in the United States.[593] Success of surgery can be predicted by the stage of the tumor. The most widely accepted staging system for these carcinomas is the tumor-node-metastasis (TNM) classification. In this system, T1 lesions are smaller than 3 cm in diameter, T2 lesions are larger than 3 cm, T3 lesions invade the chest call mediastinum or diaphragm, and T4 lesions invade the heart or great vessels. The designation N0 indicates no lymph node involvement; N1, tracheobronchial or hilar lymph node involvement; and N3, contralateral or supraclavicular lymph node involvement. M0 connotes no metastases, and M1, systemic metastases.

Patients in stage I who have small primary tumors (T1N0M0) usually undergo lobectomy and have a 5-year survival rate of 50%. Surgical procedures that spare the pulmonary parenchyma—wedge resection or bronchial sleeve resection—are reserved for patients with COPD and heart disease, although thoracoscopic resection may radically improve localization and tolerance of procedures. Patients in stage II (T1N1M0 or T2N1M0) also undergo total resection and have a 5-year survival rate of 30%. Patients in stage IIIa (T3N0M0 or T1 or T2N2M0) undergo resection for cure but currently have a 5-year survival rate of only 17%.[592] Postresection radiotherapy has not been demonstrated to improve survival as yet, and mass screening programs do not lead to a better prognosis (see Chapter 25 sections on lead and length time biases). Diagnostic typing and staging often involve percutaneous transthoracic aspiration, which is associated with a 30% incidence of pneumothorax.[592]

The combination of chemotherapy and radiation therapy is the current treatment of choice for small cell carcinomas of the lung.[594] Oat cell (small cell) carcinoma of the lung and bronchial adenomas are known for their secretion of endocrinologically active substances, such as ACTH-like hormones. Squamous cell cancers in the superior pulmonary sulcus produce Horner's syndrome, as well as characteristic pain in areas served by the eighth cervical nerves and first and second thoracic nerves. These tumors are now treated with preoperative radiation; surgical resection leads to an almost 30% "cure" rate.

Anaphylaxis, Anaphylactoid Responses, and Allergic Disorders Other than Those Related to Lung Diseases and Asthma

Anaphylactic and Anaphylactoid Reactions

Anaphylaxis is a severe life-threatening allergic reaction. *Allergic* applies to immunologically mediated reactions, as opposed to those caused by pharmacologic idiosyncrasy, by direct toxicity or drug overdosage, or by drug interaction.[590,595,596] Anaphylaxis is the typical immediate hypersensitivity reaction (type I). Such reactions are produced by immunoglobulin E (IgE)-mediated release of pharmacologically active substances. These mediators in turn produce specific end-organ responses in the skin (urticaria), the respiratory system (bronchospasm and upper airway edema), and the cardiovascular system (vasodilation, changes in inotropy, and increased capillary permeability). Vasodilation occurs at the level of the capillary and postcapillary venule and leads to erythema, edema, and smooth muscle contraction. This clinical syndrome is called *anaphylaxis*. By contrast, *anaphylactoid reaction* denotes an identical or very similar clinical response that is not mediated by IgE or (usually) an antigen-antibody process.[597]

In anaphylactic reactions, an injected substance can serve as the allergen itself. Low-molecular-weight agents are believed to act as haptens that form immunologic conjugates with host proteins. The offending substance, whether hapten or not, may be the parent compound, a nonenzymatically generated product, or a metabolic product formed in the patient's body. When an allergen binds immunospecific IgE antibodies on the surface of mast cells and basophils, histamine and eosinophilic chemotactic factors of anaphylaxis (ECF-A) are released from storage granules in a calcium- and energy-dependent process.[595] Other chemical mediators are rapidly synthesized and subsequently released in response to cellular activation. These mediators include slow-reacting substance of anaphylaxis (SRS-A), which is a combination of three leukotrienes; other leukotrienes[598]; kinins; platelet-activating factors; adenosine; chemotactic factors; heparin; tryptase; chymase; and prostaglandins, including the potent bronchoconstrictor prostaglandin D_2, eosinophil growth and activating factors, mast cell growth factors, and proinflammatory and other factors that contribute to the IgE isotype switch.

The end-organ effects of the mediators produce the clinical syndrome of anaphylaxis. Usually, a first wave of symptoms, including vasodilation and a feeling of impending doom, is quickly followed by a second wave as the cascade of mediators amplifies the reactions. In a sensitized patient, onset of the signs and symptoms caused by these mediators is usually immediate but may be delayed 2 to 15 minutes or, in rare instances, as long as

2.5 hours after the parenteral injection of antigen.[598,599] After oral administration, manifestations may occur at unpredictable times.

Mast cell proliferation, together with severe progressive inflammation, contributes to the worsening of symptoms that occurs even after an allergen load is no longer present. The antigen present in cells and lymphocytes, as well as activated mast cells, starts to make cytokines. These proinflammatory cytokines recruit more inflammatory cells, which promotes tissue edema and mediates a second wave of mast cell degranulation. This second wave can promote recurrence of severe symptoms 6 to 8 hours later and necessitates, some believe, at least 8 hours of continued ICU-like observation.

In addition, there are multiple effector processes by which biologically active mediators can be generated to produce an anaphylactoid reaction. Activation of the blood coagulation and fibrinolytic systems, the kinin-generating sequence, or the complement cascade can produce the same inflammatory substances that result in an anaphylactic reaction. The two mechanisms known to activate the complement system are called classical and alternative. The classical pathway can be initiated through IgG or IgM (transfusion reactions) or plasmin. The alternative pathway can be activated by lipopolysaccharides (endotoxin), drugs (Althesin[597]), radiographic contrast media,[600] membranes (nylon tricot membranes for bubble oxygenators[601]), cellophane membranes of dialyzers,[602] vascular graft material,[603] latex or latex-containing products,[604,605] and perfluorocarbon artificial blood. The most common agents that are responsible for intraoperative anaphylaxis are muscle relaxants.[606] However, latex accounts for a significant number of these reactions, and the incidence of intraoperative anaphylaxis caused by latex is increasing. It is now probably the second most important cause of intraoperative anaphylaxis. In addition, histamine can be liberated independent of immunologic reactions.[607] Mast cells and basophils release histamine in response to chemicals or drugs. Most narcotics can release histamine[607] and produce an anaphylactoid reaction, as can radiographic contrast media,[600] *d*-tubocurarine,[608] and thiopental. What makes some patients susceptible to release of histamine in response to drugs is unknown, but hereditary and environmental factors may play a role.

Intravenous contrast material is probably the most frequently used agent that causes anaphylactoid reactions. Because diagnostic (skin and other) tests are helpful only in IgE-mediated reactions, pretesting is not useful for contrast reactions. Pretreatment with diphenhydramine, cimetidine (or ranitidine), and corticosteroids has been reported to be useful in preventing or ameliorating anaphylactoid reactions to intravenous contrast material[600,609] and perhaps to narcotics and chymopapain.[610,611] Unfortunately, very large doses of steroids (1 g of methylprednisolone intravenously) may be necessary to obtain a beneficial effect.[612] The efficacy of large-dose steroid therapy has not been confirmed. Other common substances associated with anaphylactic or anaphylactoid reactions that might merit preoperative therapy include antibiotics, volume expanders, and blood products[595,613,614] (Table 27-46). The anesthesiologist should be prepared preoperatively to treat an anaphylactic or anaphylactoid response.

Table 27–46   Incidence of anaphylactic or anaphylactoid reactions to some common agents

Agent	Incidence
Plasma protein	
Plasma protein derivative	0.019
Human serum albumin	0.011
Dextran 60/75	0.069
Dextran 40	0.007
Starch	
Hydroxyethyl starch	0.085
Penicillin	0.002*
Chymopapain	0.3-1.5

*Fatal reactions.
Data modified from Ring and Messner,[613] Levy and colleagues,[595] and Moss and coworkers.[610]

In some cases, a patient with a history of an anaphylactic or anaphylactoid reaction must receive a substance suspected of producing such a reaction (e.g., iodinated contrast material). In addition, some patients have a higher than average likelihood of having a reaction, thus warranting well-planned pretreatment and therapy for possible anaphylactic and anaphylactoid reactions.[595]

Minimizing Risks Preoperatively

Although virtually all evidence on this subject is merely anecdotal, enough consistent thought recurs through the literature to justify proposing an optimal approach to these problems. First, predisposing factors should be sought; patients with a history of atopy or allergic rhinitis should be suspected as being at risk. Because anaphylactic and anaphylactoid reactions to contrast media occur 5 to 10 times more frequently in patients with a previously suspected reaction, consideration should be given to the administration of both H_1 and H_2 receptor antagonists for 16 to 24 hours before exposing these patients to a suspected allergen. H_1 receptor antagonists appear to require this much time to act on the receptor. Volume status should be optimized,[595] and perhaps large doses of steroids (2 g of hydrocortisone) should also be administered before exposing patients to agents associated with a high incidence of anaphylactic or anaphylactoid reactions.[612,613,615] Older patients and patients taking β-adrenergic blocking drugs present special problems; they are at higher risk of having complications from both pretreatment (especially vigorous hydration) and therapy for anaphylactic reactions and are less responsive to treatment regimens.[616] One approach is to avoid drugs likely to trigger anaphylactic or anaphylactoid reactions or alter the treatment protocol for this group. Drawing blood for later analysis, especially of tryptase, can be useful in clarifying the diagnosis.[617]

With the increasing incidence of latex hypersensitivity, attempts have been made to make much of the operating room environment latex free; however, costs and preferences have resulted in the continued use of latex-containing gloves in many hospitals. In allergic patients, care should be taken to ensure that no latex-containing products are present in the operating room.

Primary Immunodeficiency Diseases

Primary immunodeficiency diseases are usually manifested early in life as recurrent infections. Along with survival achieved with antibiotic and antibody treatment have come new prominent features: cancer and allergic and autoimmune disorders. Hereditary angioneurotic edema is an autosomal dominant genetic disease characterized by episodes of angioneurotic edema involving the subcutaneous tissues and submucosa of the GI tract and airway and often manifested as abdominal pain. These patients have a functionally impotent inhibitor or deficiency of an inhibitor to complement component C1. Treatment of an acute attack is supportive because epinephrine, antihistamines, and corticosteroids often fail to work. Plasma transfusions have been reported to resolve attacks or make them worse (theoretically by supplying either C1 esterase inhibitor or previously depleted complement components). The severity of attacks can be prevented or decreased by drugs that are either plasmin inhibitors (e.g., ε-aminocaproic acid [EACA] and tranexamic acid) or androgens (e.g., danazol). Because trauma can precipitate acute attacks, prophylactic therapy with danazol, intravenous EACA, plasma, or all three is recommended before elective surgery. Reports have also described the successful use of a partially purified C1 esterase inhibitor in two patients.[618,619]

Most of the 1 in 700 persons who have selective IgA deficiency (i.e., <5 mg/dL) have repeated serious infections or connective tissue disorders.[620] These infections commonly involve the respiratory tract (e.g., sinusitis, otitis) or GI tract (manifested as diarrhea or malabsorption, or both). If the patient has rheumatoid arthritis, Sjögren's syndrome or systemic lupus erythematosus, the anesthetist should consider the possibility of isolated IgA deficiency. However, patients with this disorder can be otherwise healthy. Because antibodies to IgA may develop in these patients if previously exposed to IgA (as might occur from a previous blood transfusion), subsequent blood transfusions can cause anaphylaxis, even when they contain washed erythrocytes. Transfusions should therefore consist of blood donated by another IgA-deficient patient.

Many immunomodulators are now being given to augment cancer treatments[621]; no interactions between these modulators, no effects on the incidence of immune reactions during anesthesia, and no interactions with anesthetic effects have been reported except those regarding immune-suppressing drugs (see the last section of this chapter).

DISEASES OF THE CENTRAL NERVOUS SYSTEM, NEUROMUSCULAR DISEASES, AND PSYCHIATRIC DISORDERS

Taking the history and performing the physical examination suggested in Chapter 25 should help identify almost all significant neurologic or mental disease. Information gathered from the history that would warrant further investigation includes a previous need for postoperative ventilation in a patient without inordinate lung disease, which would indicate the possibility of metabolic neurologic disorders such as porphyria, alcoholic myopathy, other myopathies, neuropathies, and neuromuscular disorders such as myasthenia gravis. Other historical information warranting further investigation would be the use of drugs such as steroids; guanidine; anticonvulsant, anticoagulant, and antiplatelet drugs; lithium; tricyclic antidepressant drugs; phenothiazines; and butyrophenones.

Although preoperative treatment of most neurologic disorders has not been reported to lessen perioperative morbidity, knowledge of the pathophysiologic characteristics of these disorders is important in planning intraoperative and postoperative management. Thus, preoperative knowledge about these disorders and their associated conditions (e.g., cardiac arrhythmias with Duchenne's muscular dystrophy or respiratory and cardiac muscle weakness in dermatomyositis) may reduce perioperative morbidity. A primary goal of neurologic evaluation is to determine the site of the lesion in the nervous system. Such localization to one of four levels (supratentorial compartment, posterior fossa, spinal cord, peripheral nervous system) is essential for accurate diagnosis and appropriate management. (Disorders accompanied by increased intracranial pressure and cerebrovascular disorders are discussed in Chapter 53.)

Coma

Little is known about specific anesthetic or perioperative or periprocedural choices that alter outcome for a comatose patient, but as for all other conditions, it is imperative to know the cause of the coma so that drugs can be avoided that might worsen the condition or that might not be metabolized because of organ dysfunction. First, the patient should be observed. Yawning, swallowing, or licking of the lips implies a "light" coma with major brainstem function intact. If consciousness is depressed but respiration, pupillary reactivity to light, and eye movements are normal and no focal motor signs are present, metabolic depression is likely. Abnormal pupillary responses may indicate hypoxia, hypothermia, local eye disease, or drug intoxication with belladonna alkaloids, narcotics, benzodiazepines, or glutethimide; pupillary responses may also be abnormal, however, after the use of eye drops. Other metabolic causes of coma include uremia, hypoglycemia, hepatic coma, alcohol ingestion, hypophosphatemia, myxedema, and hyperosmolar nonketotic coma. Except in extreme emergencies, such as uncontrolled bleeding or a perforated viscus, care should be taken to render the patient as metabolically normal as possible before surgery. This practice and documenting the findings on the chart preoperatively lessen any confusion regarding the cause of intraoperative and postoperative problems. However, too rapid correction of uremia or hyperosmolar nonketotic coma can lead to cerebral edema, a shift of water into the brain as a result of a reverse osmotic effect caused by the dysequilibrium of urea concentration.

The physical examination can be extremely helpful preoperatively in assessing the prognosis.[622-626] Arms flexed at the elbow (i.e., decorticate posture) imply bilateral hemisphere dysfunction but an intact brainstem, whereas extension of the legs and arms (bilateral decerebrate posture)

implies bilateral damage to structures at the upper brainstem or deep hemisphere level. Seizures are often seen in patients with uremia and other metabolic encephalopathies. Hyperreflexia and upward-pointing toes suggest a structural CNS lesion or uremia, hypoglycemia, or hepatic coma; hyporeflexia and downward-pointing toes with no hemiplegia generally indicate no structural CNS lesion.

Epileptic Seizures

Epileptic seizures result from paroxysmal neuronal discharges of abnormally excitable neurons. Six percent to 10% of individuals younger than 70 years will experience a seizure at some time during their lifetime. Fifty percent to 70% of patients with one seizure will never have another. However, 70% of people with two seizures will have an epileptic focus, be candidates for antiseizure medications, and be subject to withdrawal seizures after anesthesia if such medications are not continued.[627] A seizure is the term for the clinical event defined as a paroxysmal alteration in neurologic function caused by a synchronous, rhythmic depolarization of brain cortical neurons. Epilepsy is the condition manifested by recurrent, unprovoked seizures. Sometimes syncopal episodes can be mistaken for seizures, especially when interviews are compressed in the short time frame of a preoperative visit. We believe that each patient who gives a history of recent undiagnosed syncope or seizure should be seen by a specialist in this field before proceeding with anesthesia because anesthesia can provoke these conditions (see later).[628] Twenty-five percent of patients with a seizure have a normal electroencephalogram (EEG) when interictal. Thus, a negative EEG does not indicate that someone with a seizure will not have a withdrawal seizure when emerging from anesthesia. Seizures can be generalized (arising from deep midline structures in the brainstem or thalamus, usually without an aura or focal features during the seizure), partial focal motor, or sensory seizures (the initial discharge comes from a focal unilateral area of the brain, often preceded by an aura). As with cerebrovascular accidents and coma, knowing the origin may be crucial to understanding the pathophysiologic processes of the disease and to managing the intraoperative and postoperative course.

Epileptic seizures can arise from discontinuation of sedative-hypnotic drugs or alcohol, use of narcotics, uremia, traumatic injury, neoplasms, infection, congenital malformation, birth injury, drug use (e.g., amphetamines, cocaine), hypercalcemia or hypocalcemia, blood in the ventricle or hypoxia, and vascular disease and vascular accidents. Thirty percent of epileptic seizures have no known cause. Most partial seizures are caused by structural brain abnormalities (secondary to tumor, trauma, stroke, infection, and other causes).

An epileptic patient requires no special anesthetic management other than that for the underlying disease. Most authorities believe that anticonvulsant medications should be given in the therapeutic range[627-629] and continued through the morning of surgery, even in pregnant women; they should also be given postoperatively, even in mothers who plan to breast-feed, according to guidelines published by the American Academy of Neurology.

Many of the epileptic drugs, including phenytoin, carbamazepine, and phenobarbiturate, alter the hepatic metabolism of many drugs and induce cytochrome P450 enzyme activity. Drug-drug interactions are much less problematic with the newer epileptic drugs such as gabapentin and topirimate.[627] Appropriate treatment of status epilepticus may include general anesthesia.[629] In one controlled trial, phenobarbital was more rapidly effective in controlling status epilepticus than was diazepam followed by phenytoin.[629] The frequency of side effects and required tracheal intubation was similar for both regimens. High concentrations of enflurane (especially with hyperventilation) can be associated with EEG evidence of epileptic activity and tonic-clonic movements.[630] These seizures, however, do not appear to have serious sequelae. Enflurane anesthesia does not seem to increase seizure activity in patients with a history of convulsive disorders, and it even suppresses seizures induced by electroshock, pentylenetetrazole, strychnine, picrotoxin, or bemegride.[631] Thus, other than the use of current drug therapy and heeding precautions taken for the underlying disease, no known changes in perioperative management seem to be indicated.

Infectious Diseases of the Central Nervous System, Degenerative Disorders of the Central Nervous System, and Headache

Many degenerative CNS disorders have been traced to slowly developing viral diseases or even the presence of certain proteins or viral particles ("prions"). No special perioperative anesthetic considerations appear to apply for infectious disorders of the CNS other than those for increased intracranial pressure and avoiding occupational exposure and transmission of disease to health care workers (also see Chapter 53). The appropriate prophylactic measures to take if one comes in contact with meningococcal disease or other infectious CNS diseases are still not well established. The use of *H. influenzae* type b vaccine has made meningitis an adult disease.[632]

Parkinson's disease is a degenerative disorder of the CNS that may or may not be caused by a virus. Clinically, Parkinson's disease, chronic manganese intoxication, phenothiazine or butyrophenone toxicity, Wilson's disease, Huntington's chorea, traumatic boxing injury, the effects of street drug toxins such as methylphenyltetrahydropyridine (MPTP), and carbon monoxide encephalopathy all have similar initial features: bradykinesia, muscular rigidity, and tremor. The substantia nigra and nerve terminals in the striatum (caudate nucleus and putamen) degenerate, and the clinical signs presumably result from decreased production (by at least 70% to 80%) of dopamine in the neurons of the basal ganglia leading to the putamen and caudate nucleus. The effects of this dopaminergic deficiency may be compounded by the unopposed effects of cholinergic neurons bordering the basal ganglia. The resulting clinical syndrome (parkinsonism) includes tremor, rigidity, akinesia, and postural instability. This syndrome can be spotted easily during the stair or even hall walk that we recommend as part of the basic physical examination evaluation (see Chapter 25).

Newer therapies have been developed to arrest or even reverse the progression of this disease. Therapy is directed

at (1) increasing the neuronal release of dopamine or the receptor's response to dopamine, (2) stimulating the receptor directly with bromocriptine and lergotrile, (3) implanting dopaminergic tissue, or (4) decreasing cholinergic activity. New therapies using the monoamine oxidase inhibitor deprenyl or adrenal medullary transplants to slow the progression of disease appear promising,[633,634] and even treatment with high-dose coenzyme Q10 appears strikingly beneficial.[27] Experience with deprenyl in the perioperative milieu is insufficient to make proscriptions about its use. Anticholinergic agents have been the initial drugs of choice because they decrease tremor more than muscle rigidity. Dopamine does not pass the blood-brain barrier, so its precursor L-dopa (levodopa) is used. Unfortunately, L-dopa is decarboxylated to dopamine in the periphery and can cause nausea, vomiting, and arrhythmia. These side effects are diminished by the administration of α-methylhydrazine (carbidopa), a decarboxylase inhibitor that does not pass the blood-brain barrier. Refractoriness to L-dopa develops, and it is now debated whether the drug should be used only when symptoms cannot be controlled with other anticholinergic medications. "Drug holidays" have been suggested as one means of restoring the effectiveness of these compounds, but cessation of such therapy may result in a marked deterioration of function and a need for hospitalization. Therapy for Parkinson's disease should be initiated before surgery and be continued through the morning of surgery; such treatment seems to decrease drooling, the potential for aspiration, and ventilatory weakness.[635-637] Reinstituting therapy promptly after surgery is crucial,[628,633-638] as is avoiding drugs such as the phenothiazines and butyrophenones (droperidol), which inhibit the release of dopamine (and perhaps alfentanil) or compete with dopamine at the receptor.[635] Carbidopa/levodopa in low doses (20 to 200 mg nightly versus the usual 60 to 600 mg/day for Parkinson's disease) is commonly used in the non-parkinsonian restless leg syndrome of the elderly (present in 2% to 5% of individuals older than 60 years). This drug too should be given the night before and the night immediately after surgery. Clozapine (a benzodiazepine) does not appear to worsen the movement disorders of Parkinson's disease and has been used postoperatively to stop levodopa-induced hallucinations.

Dementia, a progressive decline in intellectual function, can be caused by treatable infections (e.g., syphilis, cryptococcosis, coccidioidomycosis, Lyme disease, tuberculosis), depression (a trial of antidepressants is indicated in most patients), side effects of medications (digitalis has slowed brain function more than the heart rate), myxedema, vitamin B_{12} deficiency, chronic drug or alcohol intoxication, metabolic causes (liver and renal failure), neoplasms, partially treatable infections (HIV), untreatable infections (Creutzfeldt-Jakob syndrome), or decreased acetylcholine in the cerebral cortex (Alzheimer's disease). This last condition occurs in more than 0.5% of Americans.[625,639-641] Although these patients are often given cholinergic agonists, controlled trials of these drugs have not as yet shown major significant benefits.[639,640,642] Gingko has been advocated and has improved subjective symptoms in 37% of patients versus 23% of those given placebo. Although later controlled trials have failed to confirm its benefits in early Alzheimer's or in healthy elderly individuals, gingko is still popular. However, the prevalence of Alzheimer's disease and the desperation of the patients and their families have now widened such therapies. Cholinergic medications have been shown to improve functioning in patients with Alzheimer's disease.[643] These families often desire surgery, but the interactions of these drugs and therapies with perioperative analgesic and anesthetic drug therapies are not well established. Most reversible dementias are either drug-induced delirium or depression.[639,640,644] At present, early results with stimulation at "threshold testing" are promising and seem to stimulate dendritic regrowth and may reverse some or much of the cognitive decline. Such computer programs and games are in early testing. Creutzfeldt-Jakob disease has been transmitted inadvertently by surgical instruments and corneal transplants; the causative virus or protein particle is not inactivated by heat, disinfectants, or formaldehyde.

More than 90% of patients with chronic recurring headaches are categorized as having migraine, tension, or cluster headaches. The mechanism of tension or cluster headaches may not differ qualitatively from that for migraine headaches; all may be manifestations of labile vasomotor regulation.[645] A headache is said to be migraine if it is characterized by four of the following five "POUNDing" conditions: if it is *P*ulsating, if it lasts *O*ne day or more, if it is *U*nilateral, if there is *N*ausea, and if it *D*isturbs daily activities.[646]

Treatment of cluster and migraine headaches centers on the use of serotonin drugs such as sumatriptan or ergotamine and its derivatives.[645-647] Other drugs that may be effective are propranolol, calcium channel inhibitors, cyproheptadine, prednisone, antihistamines, tricyclic antidepressants, phenytoin, and diuretic drugs, as well as biofeedback. Giant cell arteritis, glaucoma, and all the meningitides, including Lyme disease, are other causes of headache that might benefit from treatment before surgery.[648] No other special treatment is indicated preoperatively for a patient who has a well-delineated cause for the headaches. Acute migraine attacks can sometimes be terminated by ergotamine tartrate aerosol or by injection of sumatriptan or dihydroergotamine mesylate intravenously; general anesthesia has also been used. We normally continue all prophylactic headache medicine, except aspirin (because of the potential for bleeding), through the morning of surgery.

Back Pain, Neck Pain, and Spinal Canal Syndromes

Acute spinal cord injury is discussed earlier in the section on autonomic dysfunction. Although it is a common problem, little is written about the anesthetic management of syndromes related to herniated disks, spondylosis (usually of advancing age), and the congenital narrowing of the cervical and lumbar canal that gives rise to symptoms of nerve root compression.[649,650] One report stresses the importance of the vascular component in the mechanism of damage to the spinal cord and, hence, the theoretical desirability of slight hypertension perioperatively.[651] Another report suggests the use of awake intubation, a fiberoptic bronchoscope, and evoked potential monitoring.[649] Preoperative management of a patient about to

undergo chemonucleolysis is discussed earlier in the section on anaphylaxis. Other than the commonsense approach of seeking neurologic consultation or, if necessary, using awake positioning of patients in a comfortable position before emergency root decompression procedures, no special procedures appear to be necessary.

Demyelinating Diseases

Demyelinating diseases constitute a diffuse group of diseases ranging from those with uncertain cause (e.g., multiple sclerosis, where genetic, epidemiologic, and immunologic factors are probably all involved and interferon-beta appears to be a promising treatment[652]) to those that follow infection, vaccination (e.g., Guillain-Barré syndrome), or antimetabolite treatment of cancer. Therefore, demyelinating diseases can have very diverse symptoms. Apparently, there is a risk of relapse of these diseases immediately after surgery.[653] Because relapse may occur as a result of rapid electrolyte changes in the perioperative period, such changes might be avoided. In addition, perioperative administration of steroids has been advocated as a protective measure.[279] Multiple sclerosis and demyelinating diseases in general are the most common cause of nontraumatic disability in young adults. The age-adjusted survival rate is 80% of that of unaffected individuals, or put another way, the average patient with multiple sclerosis ages 1.2 years for every year that they have the disease. However, the variability of the disease makes this average rate of aging almost meaningless. Thus far, no mode of treatment has been shown to alter most of these disease processes, although ACTH, steroids, interferon-beta, glatiramer acetate (Copaxone), and plasmapheresis may ameliorate or abbreviate a relapse, even alter disease progression, especially progression of multiple sclerosis and (if started within 2 weeks of onset) Guillain-Barré syndrome.[654] Such an effect is consonant with the hypothesis of an immunologic disorder being the cause of these diseases.

Sleep apnea may be considered a demyelinating or degenerative CNS disease or a peripheral disease of obesity, depending on its etiology. Both types (central and peripheral etiologies) appear to be increasingly common and are present in more than 5% of elderly African-Americans. Because sleep apnea poses many problems for postoperative pain control, we now recommend using only nonsteroidal anti-inflammatory drugs for pain relief if we cannot monitor these patients in a second-stage recovery unit.[655-657] Preprocedure and preoperative identification of patients and therapy for sleep apnea are discussed in the earlier section "Obesity."

Metabolic Diseases

Included in the category of metabolic diseases is nervous system dysfunction secondary to porphyrias, alcoholism, uremia, hepatic failure, and vitamin B_{12} deficiency. The periodic paralysis that can accompany thyroid disease is discussed under "Neuromuscular Disorders" (see later).

Alcoholism or heavy alcohol intake is associated with acute alcoholic hepatitis (also see Chapter 55), the activity of which declines as alcohol is withdrawn; with myopathy and cardiomyopathy, which can be severe; and with withdrawal syndromes. The best questions to ask in seeking a history of alcohol intake are "Have you ever had a drinking problem?" and "Have you had a drink in the last 24 hours?" These questions have higher sensitivity and specificity than many other longer series of questions about alcoholism[658] (see Chapter 25). Within 6 to 8 hours of withdrawal, the patient may become tremulous, a state that usually subsides within days or weeks. Alcoholic hallucinosis and withdrawal seizures generally occur within 24 to 36 hours. These seizures are generalized grand mal attacks; when focal seizures occur, other causes should be sought. Delirium tremens usually appears within 72 hours of withdrawal and is often preceded by tremulousness, hallucinations, or seizures. These three symptoms, combined with perceptual distortions, insomnia, psychomotor disturbances, autonomic hyperactivity, and in a large percentage of cases, another potentially fatal illness (e.g., bowel infarction or subdural hematoma), are components of delirium tremens. This syndrome is now treated with benzodiazepines. Nutritional disorders of alcoholism include alcoholic hypoglycemia and hypothermia, alcoholic polyneuropathy, Wernicke-Korsakoff syndrome, and cerebellar degeneration. In alcoholic patients (i.e., those who drink at least two six packs of beer or 1 pint of whiskey per day or the equivalent), emergency surgery and anesthesia (despite alcoholic hepatitis) are not associated with worsening abnormalities in liver enzymes. In addition, about 20% of alcoholic patients also have COPD. A patient who has a history of alcohol abuse therefore warrants careful examination of many systems for quantification of preoperative physical status.

Although hepatic failure can lead to coma with high-output cardiac failure, unlike uremia, it does not lead to chronic polyneuropathy. Uremic polyneuropathy is a distal symmetric sensorimotor polyneuropathy that may be improved by dialysis. The use of depolarizing muscle relaxants in patients with polyneuropathies has been questioned (also see Chapter 13). We believe that patients who have a neuropathy associated with uremia should not be given succinylcholine because of a possible exaggerated hyperkalemic response.

Pernicious anemia caused by vitamin B_{12} deficiency may result in subacute combined degeneration of the spinal cord; the signs are similar to those of chronic nitrous oxide toxicity. Both pernicious anemia and nitrous oxide toxicity are associated with peripheral neuropathy and disorders of the pyramidal tract and posterior column (which governs fine motor skills and the sense of body position). Combined-system disease can also occur without anemia, as can nitrous oxide toxicity in dentists and nitrous oxide abusers. Patients with B_{12} deficiency and anemia, if treated with folate, improve hematologically but progress to dementia and severe neuropathy. It may thus be prudent to give an intramuscular injection of 100 μg of vitamin B_{12} or 800 μg orally before giving folate to a patient who has signs of combined-system degeneration.[659]

The porphyrias are a constellation of metabolic diseases that result from an autosomally inherited lack of

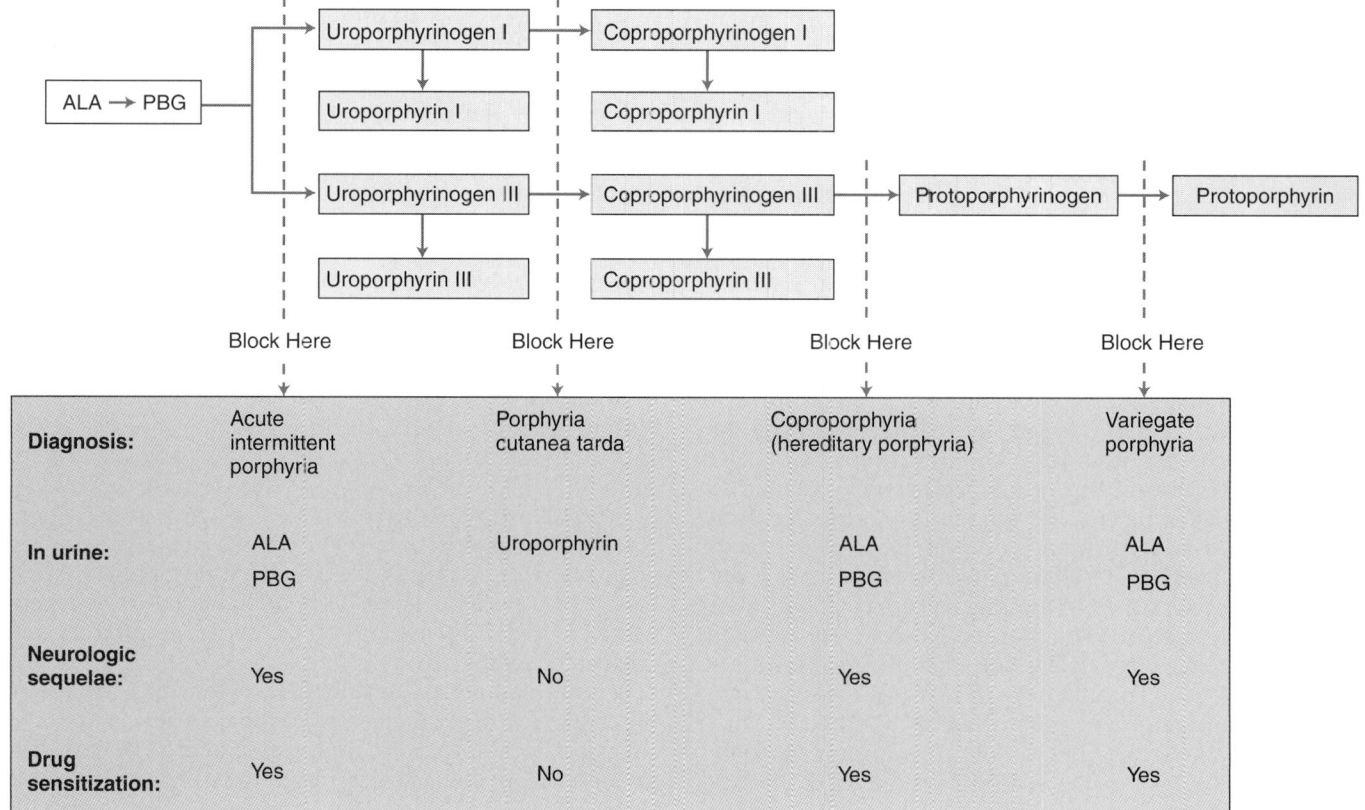

Figure 27–20 Schematic depiction of the functional enzyme deficits that occur in some of the porphyrias. ALA, aminolevulinic acid; PBG, porphobilinogen.

functional enzymes active in the synthesis of hemoglobin. Figure 27-20 schematically depicts the abnormalities that result from these enzyme deficits. It is important to note that type 1, 3, and 4 porphyrias can cause life-threatening neurologic abnormalities. These conditions are characterized by the presence of aminolevulinic acid (ALA) or porphobilinogen (or both) in urine; these substances do not occur in porphyria cutanea tarda, a disease that does not incur neurologic sequelae.[660] In acute intermittent porphyria, the typical pattern consists of acute attacks of colicky pain, nausea, vomiting, severe constipation, psychiatric disorders, and lesions of the lower motor neuron that can progress to bulbar paralysis. Certain drugs can induce the enzyme ALA synthetase and thereby exacerbate the disease process.[661-663] These sensitizing drugs include barbiturates, meprobamate, chlordiazepoxide, glutethimide, diazepam, hydroxydione, phenytoin, imipramine, pentazocine, birth control pills, ethyl alcohol, sulfonamides, griseofulvin, and ergotamine preparations. Patients often have attacks during infection, fasting, or menstruation. Administration of glucose suppresses ALA synthetase activity and prevents or ablates acute attacks. Drugs used in anesthetic management that are reported to be safe for patients with porphyria include neostigmine (Prostigmin), atropine, gallamine, succinylcholine, *d*-tubocurarine, pancuronium, nitrous oxide, procaine, propofol, propanidid, etomidate, meperidine, fentanyl, morphine, droperidol, promazine, promethazine, and chlorpromazine.[661-663] Although ketamine has been used, postoperative psychoses attributable to the disease may be difficult to distinguish from those possibly caused by ketamine. In addition, although ketamine and etomidate are reported to be safe in humans, they seem to be porphyrinogenic in rats. Propofol has been used without provoking porphyria in at least two susceptible patients.[661,662]

Neuromuscular Disorders

Neuromuscular disorders consist of conditions affecting any major component of the motor unit: motor neuron, peripheral nerve, neuromuscular junction, and muscle. Neuropathies may involve all components of the nerve, thereby producing sensory, motor, and autonomic dysfunction, or only one component. Myopathies may involve only the proximal or distal muscles, or both.

Myasthenia gravis (also see Chapter 13) is a disorder of the muscular system caused by partial blockade or destruction of nicotinic acetylcholine receptors by IgG antibodies. This syndrome is characterized by fluctuating ophthalmoplegia, ptosis, and bulbar, respiratory, or limb weakness and is confirmed by a beneficial response to cholinergic drugs.[664,665] These patients often have other autoimmune diseases, including rheumatoid arthritis and hypothyroidism. Thirty-three percent of patients with myasthenia gravis have bulbar symptoms (and are therefore subject to problems with disposal of secretions) at initial evaluation, and more than 60% of people with myasthenia gravis will have bulbar symptoms at some time during their life. This symptom should not be confused with respiratory muscle weakness, which occurs much less commonly.

The severity of the disease correlates with the ability of antibodies to decrease the number of available acetylcholine receptors.[664] Treatment of myasthenia is usually begun with anticholinesterase drugs, but in moderate and severe disease, treatment progresses to steroids and thymectomy.[664,665] Immunosuppressive drugs and plasmapheresis are initiated if the more conservative measures fail, and intravenous immunoglobulin, a rapid-onset therapy, is reserved for acute exacerbations and myasthenic crises.[664,665]

One major problem for the anesthesiologist involves the use of muscle relaxants and their reversal.[666] Because much of the care of myasthenia gravis patients involves tailoring the amount of anticholinesterase medication to the maximal muscle strength of the patient, derangement of the course of the patient during surgery could necessitate reassessment of the drug dosage. For that reason, several researchers recommend withholding all anticholinergic drugs for 6 hours before surgery and reinstituting medication postoperatively with extreme caution because the sensitivity of these patients to such drugs may have changed. In addition, there has been some concern that anticholinergic drugs may lead to a high incidence of bowel anastomotic leaks in patients who have undergone bowel anastomosis. Small doses of succinylcholine can be used to facilitate endotracheal intubation; tiny doses of nondepolarizing drugs can be used for intraoperative relaxation not achieved by regional anesthesia or volatile anesthetics. Controlled ventilation is usually required for at least 24 to 48 hours postoperatively.[665-667] This practice is especially important in cases involving myasthenia gravis of more than 6 years' duration, chronic obstructive lung disease, daily pyridostigmine requirement of 750 mg in association with significant bulbar weakness, and vital capacity of less than 40 mL/kg.[667]

Lambert-Eaton syndrome (myasthenic syndrome) is characterized by proximal limb muscle weakness and is associated with antibodies directed against the voltage-gated calcium channels in presynaptic nerve terminals. Strength or reflexes may increase with repetitive effort. Affected patients have decreased release of acetylcholine at the neuromuscular junction. Guanidine therapy enhances the release of acetylcholine from nerve terminals and improves strength. Men who have this syndrome generally have small cell carcinoma of the lung or other malignancy, whereas women often have malignancy, sarcoidosis, thyroiditis, or a collagen-related vascular disease. In addition, these patients have increased sensitivity to both depolarizing and nondepolarizing muscle relaxants.[668] Lambert-Eaton syndrome is also associated with an autonomic nervous system defect manifested by gastroparesis, orthostatic hypotension, and urinary retention.

Dermatomyositis and polymyositis are characterized by proximal limb muscle weakness with dysphagia. These conditions are associated with malignancy or collagen-related vascular disease and often involve respiratory and cardiac muscle.

Periodic paralysis is another disease in which sensitivity to muscle relaxants increases. Periodic weakness starts in childhood or adolescence and is precipitated by rest after exercise, sleep, cold, surgery, or pregnancy. Hypokalemic and hyperkalemic forms exist and are associated with cardiac arrhythmias. Like thyrotoxic periodic paralysis, these hypokalemic and hyperkalemic forms usually spare the respiratory muscles. Anesthetic management consists of minimizing stress and maintaining normal fluid and electrolyte status and body temperature.[668-671]

Muscular dystrophy patients now survive into their late twenties or early thirties. Complicating their disease are respiratory infections, kyphoscoliosis, muscle contractions, and cardiac abnormalities. Duchenne's muscular dystrophy, the most common of the muscular dystrophies, is a sex-linked recessive disease involving the Xp21 locus.[672] It occurs after 2 years of age, at which time patients experience a rapid progression of muscle disease that leads to incapacity in their teens. Cardiac involvement is common when the disease affects the proximal and pelvic muscles, and respiratory failure is a frequent cause of death. Limb-girdle muscular dystrophy is not as severe as Duchenne's muscular dystrophy; it occurs later in life, has cardiac involvement, and is transmitted as an autosomal recessive trait. Facioscapulohumeral muscular dystrophy (FSHMD) is a disease of autosomal dominant inheritance that has a mild clinical form in adolescence. Patients with FSHMD have a normal life span without an increased risk of cardiac complications; however, postoperative respiratory deaths have been recorded. Myotonic dystrophy is a disease in which continued active contraction of muscles persists after voluntary effort or stimulation has ceased. This autosomally dominant inherited disease begins at 20 to 40 years of age and is associated with cardiomyopathy, baldness, testicular atrophy, cataracts, intellectual and emotional abnormalities, and premature death in the 50- to 60-year-old range. The facial, sternocleidomastoid, distal, and pharyngeal muscles become weak and atrophy. Because the disease involves the muscles themselves and not their innervation, conduction anesthesia cannot produce adequate relaxation of tonic muscles. Gastric dilation has also been reported to be a problem, as has malignant hyperthermia. As with the other forms of muscular dystrophy, most problems in myotonic dystrophy arise from cardiac arrhythmias and inadequacy of the respiratory muscles.[672] For all the forms of muscular dystrophy, as for all the neuropathies (discussed earlier), there have been problems related to exaggerated serum potassium release after the administration of depolarizing muscle relaxants (also see Chapter 13).

Malignant hyperthermia (also see Chapter 29) in the patient or in a relative of the patient merits careful history taking and at least consideration of performing a test for susceptibility to the condition (see Chapter 25). Prophylaxis with intravenous dantrolene sodium (Dantrium) may also be warranted (also see Chapter 29). In some cases, malignant hyperthermia has been associated with recognizable musculoskeletal abnormalities such as strabismus, ptosis, myotonic dystrophy, hernias, kyphoscoliosis, muscular dystrophy, central core disease, and marfanoid syndrome. Appropriate preparation for a patient with previous masseter spasm, or trismus, is a matter of considerable debate. We prepare for malignant hyperthermia (i.e., we ensure a contaminant-free machine, use nontriggering agents, and have a malignant hyperthermia cart in the room) but do not routinely perform muscle biopsy or prescribe dantrolene prophylaxis.[673,674] Malignant hyperthermia occurs most frequently in children and adolescents, the incidence

being 1 in 14,000 administrations of anesthetic. The incidence increases to 1 in 2500 patients requiring squint surgery. Questions to ask parents during the preoperative evaluation include the following: "Does your child become rigid when upset?" and "Does your child sweat profusely when upset?" However, the sensitivity and specificity of such questions in predicting malignant hyperthermia have not been confirmed. The hope is to soon have a genetic screening test to detect most forms of malignant hyperthermia, but as yet such a test remains an unrealized promise. The reader is referred to Chapters 25 and 29 for a complete discussion of the screening procedure to use.

Down Syndrome

Down syndrome (trisomy 21) occurs once in 1000 live births. It is associated with congenital cardiac lesions such as endocardial cushion defects (40%), ventricular septal defects (27%), patent ductus arteriosus (12%), and tetralogy of Fallot (8%), and prophylactic antibiotics should be used before predictable bacteremic events. Down syndrome is also associated with upper respiratory infections, with atlanto-occipital instability (in about 15% of patients,[675-678] in whom it is asymptomatic in most cases, but it is recommended that all patients be treated as though they have atlanto-occipital instability) and laxity of other joints, with thyroid hypofunction (50%), with an increased incidence of subglottic stenosis, and with enlargement of the tongue (or a decreased oral cavity size for a normal-sized tongue).[677,679] No abnormal responses to anesthetics or anesthetic adjuvants have been substantiated. A reported sensitivity to atropine has been disproved, although administration of atropine to any patient given digoxin for atrial fibrillation should be done with extreme care.[679] Examination for the conditions associated with Down syndrome should precede surgery.

Preoperative Prediction of Increased Intracranial Pressure during Neurosurgery

Symptoms and signs of increased intracranial pressure include morning headache or headache made worse by coughing, nausea, vomiting, disturbances in consciousness, history of large tumors, tumors involving the brainstem, neck rigidity, and papilledema. Patients with these signs, large ventricles (as seen on radiography or images of the brain), or edema surrounding supratentorial tumors should be considered at risk for intraoperative intracranial hypertension. These patients may benefit from preoperative treatment or anesthetic management that assumes this possibility[680] (also see Chapter 53).

Other preoperative considerations for patients with neurologic disease that can cause intracranial hypertension are the associated hypoventilation and hypoxia in patients who have severe hemiplegia and the presence of subarachnoid bleeding or other forms of intracranial hemorrhage (especially likely in women given heparin who have two or more cerebral infarcts on CT scan). Many strokes or TIAs have a possible cardiac origin (59 of 184 patients).[681,682] The drugs used to prevent cerebral arterial spasm—calcium channel blockers—are discussed in the last section of this chapter.

Mental Disorders

Perhaps the most important preoperative consideration for patients with mental disorders, in addition to developing rapport, is understanding their specific drug therapy and its effects and side effects. More than 15% of all adult patients undergoing surgery are taking one of these therapies or have recently been taking one of these therapies. Lithium, tricyclic antidepressants, selective serotonin reuptake inhibitors, other antidepressants that defy classification such as bupropion, phenothiazines, butyrophenones, and monoamine oxidase inhibitors are used in these patients.[683] These drugs have potent effects and side effects that are discussed in the last section of this chapter.

RENAL DISEASE, INFECTIOUS DISEASES, AND ELECTROLYTE DISORDERS

One may ask why preoperative preparation of a patient with renal disease is discussed in the same section as preoperative preparation of a patient with an infectious disease. Although it is commonly recommended that no surgery except emergency or curative (e.g., drainage of an abscess) operations be performed in patients with infectious disease, it has become evident that renal insufficiency can be caused by antimicrobial drugs[684] and that sepsis, not shock, is probably the leading cause of acute postoperative renal failure.[685] The anesthesiologist has an important role to play in preventing the onset and consequences of renal failure and its initiators.[686,687] The linking of renal failure to electrolyte disorders is more obvious: the kidney is the primary organ for regulating body osmolality and fluid volume and has a major role in excretion of the end products of metabolism. In performing these functions, the kidney becomes intimately involved in the excretion of electrolytes.

A patient with renal insufficiency whose own kidneys are still functioning is distinct not only from a patient with end-stage renal disease whose renal functions are provided by dialysis but also from a patient who has a transplanted kidney. These three groups of patients require very different preoperative preparation. In addition, acute changes in renal function present quite a different problem than do chronic alterations in function.[686,687] Certain renal diseases require different preoperative preparation than others, but generally, renal disease of any origin presents the same preoperative problems (also see Chapters 20, 37, and 54).

Renal Disease

Causes and Systemic Effects of Renal Disorders
Nephrotic syndrome may develop in patients with glomerular diseases without disturbing tubular function. The soundness of tubular function is an important consideration because tubular dysfunction with attendant uremia presents quite different problems than glomerular disease with only nephrotic syndrome does. This is not to minimize the adverse effects of glomerular disease; nephrotic syndrome consists of massive proteinuria and consequent hypoalbuminemia. The resulting reduction in plasma oncotic pressure diminishes plasma volume and calls forth compensatory mechanisms that result in retention of sodium and water. As a result, a common clinical finding in nephrotic syndrome is edema. Thus, patients with nephrotic syndrome may have excess total-body water and decreased intravascular volume. In addition, diuretics are often given in an attempt to decrease edema. Although serum creatinine and creatinine clearance have limitations as indices of the glomerular filtration rate (GFR) (inulin clearance is still the gold standard), these measurements are, for now, the most readily available to the anesthesiologist.[687] Plasma creatinine levels reflect endogenous muscle catabolism and dietary intake, as well as urinary excretion. Urinary excretion depends on both filtration and secretion by the kidney. Drugs that are commonly used in the preoperative and perioperative periods can distort this measure of glomerular filtration: cimetidine and trimethoprim interfere with secretion by increasing plasma creatinine and decreasing creatinine clearance without altering filtration.[687] It should also be remembered that the commonly used methods for measuring creatinine have a 95% confidence limit of more than 20% for a GFR greater than 30 mL/min. Thus, a normal creatinine level of 1.3 mg/dL might give a measured value ranging from 1.0 to 1.5 mg/dL.[687]

Furthermore, in patients with nephrotic syndrome in whom renal tubular function has been preserved, hypovolemia appears to be a significant cause of deteriorating tubular renal function.[687-691] Consequently, we advocate the same intense preoperative, intraoperative, and postoperative fluid management for patients with nephrotic syndrome as we do for patients with diminished tubular function. Admittedly, no randomized study has shown that close control of intravascular volume status in these groups of patients preserves renal tubular function (or any other measure of perioperative morbidity) to a greater degree than less rigid control does.

Uremia, the end result of renal tubular failure (i.e., failure of the concentrating, diluting, acidifying, and filtering functions), is manifested in many ways. Changes occur in the cardiovascular, immunologic, hematologic, neuromuscular, pulmonary, and endocrine systems, as well as in bone. These alterations are ascribed either to the toxic end products of protein metabolism or to an imbalance in functioning of the kidney. As the number of functioning nephrons diminishes, the still-functioning nephrons attempt to increase some solute and body composition preservation functions at the expense of other functions, such as excretion of phosphate. The accumulation of phosphate increases parathormone levels, which in turn produces osteodystrophy. Osteodystrophy can be managed by (1) restriction of dietary phosphate, (2) the use of gels (e.g., aluminum hydroxide or carbonate) that bind with intestinal phosphate, (3) calcium supplementation, or (4) parathyroidectomy.[692]

Certain alterations in patients with uremia, such as neuropathy, are most logically attributed to an accumulation of toxic metabolites. Peripheral neuropathy is most often sensory and involves the lower extremities, but it may also be motor; peripheral neuropathies are often improved with hemodialysis and can be dramatically reversed with transplantation. The use of depolarizing muscle relaxants in patients with peripheral neuropathy is controversial and is discussed in the section on neuropathies. Tubular function is commonly assessed by acidifying and concentrating capabilities.[693] Although such tests are crude, these capabilities are usually readily assessed by measuring urine pH and specific gravity. Better assessment of renal blood flow, for the purpose of improving renal blood flow and its distribution, is promised by the use of contrast ultrasound in the operating room.[694] Along with the altered volume status and cardiac complications in uremic patients, autonomic neuropathy may contribute to hypotension during anesthesia. Atherosclerosis is often accelerated in uremic patients; hypertension, with its attendant consequences, is very common.

Cardiac failure (especially episodic failure) frequently occurs in uremic patients because of the presence of many adverse conditions: anemia with increasing myocardial work, hypertension, atherosclerosis, and altered volume status. Pericarditis can manifested by pericardial rub alone or by pain (with or without hemorrhage). Cardiac tamponade should be ruled out on the basis of clinical features and by echocardiography if this diagnosis is seriously suspected preoperatively. In addition, cardiac tamponade should be treated or planned for preoperatively.

If anemia is present, its severity generally parallels the degree of uremia; chronically uremic patients seem to adapt well to anemia. No hard data have substantiated the need to give a preoperative blood transfusion to a chronically uremic patient, even when the preoperative hematocrit is as low as 16 or 18 vol%. Even in nonuremic patients in an ICU, a recent randomized trial was unable to demonstrate improved outcome with a liberal transfusion strategy.[695] One of the major historical reasons for not transfusing blood in patients with end-stage renal disease has been disproved: data show that the more blood transfusions a transplant recipient receives before transplantation, the greater the chance that the transplant will function successfully.[696] This immunosuppressive effect of transfusions is now routinely used in transplantation. However, the development of recombinant human erythropoietin may obviate the need for transfusions in chronically uremic patients in the future. Administration of recombinant human erythropoietin to patients in chronic and progressive renal failure resulted in an average increase in hematocrit of 10% above baseline within 3 weeks, with no serious side effects.[697] Balancing of the immunosuppressive use of blood transfusions versus the benefits of erythropoietin and the risks of transfusion remains to be determined. In uremic patients, coagulation and platelet adhesiveness may be abnormal and factor III activity decreased. Even uremic patients not given corticosteroids or immunosuppressive drugs may demonstrate abnormal immunity, perhaps meriting increased attention regarding procedures that lessen patient cross-contamination.

Uremic patients exhibit a wide variety of metabolic and endocrinologic disorders in addition to hyperparathyroidism,[692] including impaired carbohydrate tolerance, insulin resistance, type IV hyperlipoproteinemia,

autonomic insufficiency, hyperkalemia, and anion-gap acidosis (caused by an inability of the kidneys to reabsorb filtered bicarbonate and excrete sufficient ammonium into urine).[698] Furthermore, the excretion and pharmacokinetics of drugs are different in uremic patients than in normal patients. In addition, complications of hemodialysis include hepatitis B (and persistent hepatitis B antigenemia), nutritional deficiencies, electrolyte and fluid imbalances, and mental disorders. Because these conditions can lead to serious perioperative morbidity, they should be evaluated before surgery. No data, however, have substantiated the hypothesis that preoperative optimization of these metabolic and endocrinologic disorders reduces perioperative risk in uremic patients.

As with uremic patients, preoperative optimization of volume status is paramount in patients with kidney stones.[699] Seventy-five percent of all kidney stones are composed of calcium oxalate. Patients with these stones often take diuretic drugs, avoid calcium-rich foods, or restrict salt intake. Prevention of dehydration by institution of intravenous fluid therapy along with restricted oral intake of protein may be as important for these patients as it is for patients with struvite or uric acid stones. Struvite stones often result from urinary infection. Uric acid stones can be prevented by treatment with allopurinol, by preoperative hydration, or by alkalization of urine. Acidosis may contribute to stone formation. Again, optimal intravascular volume status is important in preventing stones and preserving renal function. More thorough discussion of renal function and physiology is provided in Chapter 20. Chapter 54 deals with the complexities of managing patients for renal surgery and other urologic procedures.

Creatinine clearance in conjunction with free water clearance appears to be the most accurate way of quantifying, for pharmacokinetic purposes, the degree of decreased renal function[700,701] (also see Chapter 37). For a patient with stable renal function, creatinine clearance, which is a rough estimate of GFR, can be approximated by noting the serum creatinine level: a doubling of the creatinine level represents a halving of GFR. Thus, a patient with a stable serum creatinine level of 2 mg/dL would have a GFR of approximately 60 mL/min. A stable serum creatinine level of 4 mg/dL would accompany a GFR of approximately 30 mL/min, and a stable serum creatinine level of 8 mg/dL would accompany a GFR of 15 mL/min or less. When pregnancy and considerable edema are not present and the serum creatinine level is stable, the following formulas can be used to estimate creatinine clearance and free water clearance.[700,702,703]

$$\text{Creatinine clearance} = \frac{[140 - \text{Age(yr)}] \times \text{Body weight (kg)}}{72 \times \text{Serum creatinine (mg/dL)}}$$

$$\text{Free water clearance} = \text{Urine flow (mL/hr)}$$
$$- \left[\frac{\text{Urine osmolality (mOsm/L)} \times \text{Urine flow (mL/hr)}}{\text{Plasma osmolality (mOsm/L)}} \right]$$

Note that renal function must be stable. Unstable renal function is often associated with changes in serum creatinine levels that lag by several days. Although knowing the serum creatinine level is more useful than knowing the BUN level, the latter provides some information, as discussed in the next section.

Free water clearance is a measure of renal concentrating ability and is normally –25 to +100 mL/hr; it becomes more positive in renal insufficiency states. It may also become more positive in patients who have a head injury or high blood alcohol levels or in those undergoing aggressive fluid infusion or administration of diuretics.[701]

Patients with Insufficient but Functioning Kidneys

One of the greatest challenges for the anesthesiologist is presented by patients with insufficient renal function whose renal function must be preserved during surgery. Additionally, the presence of chronic renal failure is associated with higher rates of perioperative cardiac morbidity, which may warrant further evaluation for the presence of occult coronary artery disease.[704] The many uremic symptoms and great perioperative morbidity associated with uremia can probably be avoided by attention to detail in the preoperative and perioperative management of patients with insufficient, but still functioning kidneys.[685-692]

First, studies demonstrate that acute postoperative renal failure is associated with an extremely high mortality rate.[399-401,403,410,705] There are multiple risk factors for the development of perioperative renal dysfunction. The most important risk factors include preexisting renal disease, heart surgery involving cardiopulmonary bypass or aortic surgery involving cross-clamping of the thoracic or abdominal aorta, and ongoing sepsis. In a systematic review of 28 studies by Novis and colleagues, preoperative renal risk factors such as increased serum creatinine, increased BUN, and preoperative renal dysfunction were repeatedly found to predict postoperative renal dysfunction.[702] Mangano and coworkers performed a prospective cohort study of 2222 patients with or without concurrent vascular surgery.[705] They identified five independent preoperative predictors of renal dysfunction: age 70 to 79 years (relative risk [RR], 1.6; 95% CI, 1.1 to 2.3) or age 80 to 95 years (RR, 3.5; CI, 1.9 to 6.3), CHF (RR, 1.8; CI, 1.3 to 2.6), previous myocardial revascularization (RR, 1.8; CI, 1.2 to 2.7), type 1 diabetes mellitus (RR, 1.8; CI, 1.1 to 3.0) or preoperative serum glucose levels exceeding 16.6 mmol/L (RR, 3.7; CI, 1.7 to 7.8), and preoperative serum creatinine levels of 124 to 177 μmol/L (RR, 2.3; CI, 1.6 to 3.4).

Moreover, acute perioperative renal failure is most likely to occur in patients who have renal insufficiency before surgery, are older than 60 years, and have preoperative left ventricular dysfunction.[706] Proper hydration before surgery probably decreases the mortality after acute renal failure induced by radiocontrast agents.[690-692] Clues regarding the presence of hypovolemia or hypervolemia should be sought from the history and physical examination (e.g., weight loss or gain, thirst, edema, orthostatic hypotension and tachycardia, flat neck veins, dry mucous membranes, decreased skin turgor). In seriously ill patients, insertion of a pulmonary arterial catheter will permit more precise monitoring of intravascular fluid volume. Other causes of deterioration in function in chronic renal insufficiency are low cardiac output or low renal blood flow (in prerenal azotemia, whether because of cardiac failure or because of fluid depletion from diuretic drugs,

BUN often increases disproportionately to increases in creatinine), urinary tract infection, use of nephrotoxic drugs, hypercalcemia, and hyperuricemia. These conditions and drugs should be avoided; if any of these conditions exist, they should be treated preoperatively.

To preserve normal renal function, infusion of saline, mannitol, furosemide, or low-dose dopamine has been recommended.[707-713] However, these therapies should be initiated with caution because saline infusions and mannitol can lead to fluid overload and myocardial damage; in addition, diuretic drugs given intraoperatively can produce postoperative hypovolemia, which worsens renal function. Very high concentrations of mannitol may also cause acute renal failure.[714] A meta-analysis of 58 trials involving the use of dopamine for renal protection/treatment, only 17 of which were randomized, was unable to demonstrate any benefit from the use of low-dose dopamine.[715] Maintenance of normal intravascular fluid volume can be guided by pulmonary capillary wedge pressure and has prevented impairment of renal function after abdominal aortic reconstruction, even when urinary volumes were low.[716] Fenoldopam is a dopamine analog that causes natriuresis and increases renal blood flow and urine output.[717] Several small studies have reported renoprotective effects of fenoldopam in patients undergoing cardiopulmonary bypass and infrarenal aortic aneurysm repair.[718-720]

Anesthetic drugs have been studied in patients with renal insufficiency. In a randomized trial, general anesthesia with desflurane or isoflurane did not exacerbate renal insufficiency.[721] Despite concern that sevoflurane leads to the production of compound A, which impairs renal functioning, a randomized trial of low-flow sevoflurane versus low-flow isoflurane anesthesia in patients with stable renal insufficiency did not demonstrate any difference in any measured renal function parameter.[722]

Patients Undergoing Dialysis

Patients with chronic (and at times acute) renal failure require renal replacement therapy, including conventional intermittent hemodialysis, peritoneal dialysis, and continuous renal replacement therapy (CRRT). CRRT includes a wide variety of techniques whose perioperative management has recently been reviewed[723] (Table 27-47). Although the primary indication for CRRT is acute renal failure, it can also be used for fluid clearance, correction of electrolyte abnormalities, and management of metabolic acidosis. It can be used in surgical patients without significant hemodynamic abnormalities. These patients may return to the operating room and their assessment and management may be complicated by the underlying disease and the use of systemic anticoagulation to prevent filter and circuit clotting. In patients undergoing intermittent treatment with hemodialysis or peritoneal dialysis, the procedure is discontinued before entering the operating room. For CRRT, the anesthesiologist must determine the appropriateness of discontinuing the therapy. With short procedures, the therapy can almost always be stopped and the arterial and venous ends of the circuit connected and run in the bypass mode. CRRT can also be used to manage fluids during surgery by changing the dialysate. If CRRT is continued, its effect on drug dosing

Table 27-47   Characteristics of renal replacement therapy

Renal Replacement Therapy	Blood Pump	Replacement Fluid (RF)/ Dialysate (D)	Intraoperative Use
Conventional intermittent hemodialysis	Yes	D	No
Peritoneal dialysis	No	D	No
Slow continuous ultrafiltration	Yes/no	None	Yes
Continuous arteriovenous hemodialysis	No	D	No
Continuous arteriovenous hemodiafiltration	No	RF, D	No
Continuous venovenous hemofiltration	Yes	RF	Yes
Continuous venovenous hemodialysis	Yes	D	Yes
Continuous venovenous hemodiafiltration	Yes	RF, D	Yes

From Petroni KC, Cohen NH: Continuous renal replacement therapy: Anesthetic implications. Anesth Analg 94:1288-1297, 2002, with permission.

must be recognized. In addition to effects on renal elimination of drugs, there are effects from changes in protein binding and volume of distribution, as well as drug removal effects from membrane permeability, membrane surface area, the ultrafiltration rate, and the dialysate flow rate.

Because a patient undergoing dialysis has already lost natural renal functioning, the emphasis in preoperative assessment shifts toward protecting other organ systems and optimally maintaining vascular access sites for cannulation. Usually, this does not require invasive monitoring. Emphasis is placed on intravascular fluid volume and electrolyte status, which can be ascertained by knowing when the patient last underwent dialysis, how much weight was normally gained or lost with dialysis, whether the fluid loss was peritoneal or intravascular, and what electrolyte composition the blood was dialyzed against. Although preoperative dialysis may benefit patients who have hyperkalemia, hypercalcemia, acidosis, neuropathy, and fluid overload, the resulting dysequilibrium between fluid and electrolytes can cause problems. Because hypovolemia induced by dialysis can lead to intraoperative hypotension, we try to avoid weight and fluid reduction in patients undergoing preoperative dialysis. In addition, hypopnea has been found to occur during and after dialysis when the dialysate contained acetate.[724] Avoiding an acetate bathing solution may prevent this cause of hypoventilation.

Patients Who Have Received a Renal Transplant

More than 140,000 patients have received renal transplants (versus 300,000 currently undergoing dialysis in the United States). Approximately 60% are still alive, although a third must undergo dialysis (approximately 50,000 patients are now awaiting transplantation).[725] The advantages, in addition to increased survival, include improvement of the anemia, endocrine and sexual function, and fatigue that inhibit employment and enjoyment for dialysis patients. The disadvantages are the cost and risks of the transplant operation and the chronic use of immunosuppressants. When these patients have subsequent surgery, the status of their renal function must be determined (i.e., whether they have normal renal function, insufficient but still functioning kidneys, or end-stage renal disease requiring hemodialysis). Descriptions of side effects

from immunosuppressive drugs should also be sought. The drugs used preoperatively and intraoperatively to prevent acute rejection themselves have serious side effects that encourage close monitoring of blood glucose and cardiovascular function.[696,726,727] Because renal transplantation greatly increases the risk of infection, it is very important to avoid invasive monitoring and prevent patient cross-contamination.

Drugs in Renal Failure

Patients with renal azotemia have a threefold or higher risk of an adverse drug reaction than those with normal renal function do.[728-733] The risk is increased by two conditions. (1) *Excessive pharmacologic effects* result from high levels of a drug or its metabolite (e.g., the metabolite of meperidine) in blood because of physiologic changes in target tissues induced by the uremic state. An example would be excessive sedation in a uremic patient with standard blood levels of sedative-hypnotic drugs. (2) *Excessive administration of electrolytes with drugs* also increases the risk of an adverse drug reaction. For example, penicillin standardly has 1.7 mEq of potassium per 1 million U.[728-733] Administration of standard doses of drugs that depend on renal excretion for their elimination can result in drug accumulation and enhanced pharmacologic effect. Bennett and associates[728] and Gibson[731] have provided dosing guidelines for many drugs used by anesthesiologists for patients with and without renal failure. For example, patients with end-stage renal disease required significantly higher propofol doses to achieve the clinical end point of hypnosis than patients with normal renal function did.[732]

Infectious Disease

Because it is commonly recommended that no surgery except emergency or essential surgery (e.g., drainage of an abscess) be performed when an acute infectious disease is present and because renal insufficiency can be caused by antimicrobial drugs,[684,689,690] renal function and organ damage from renal insufficiency should be assessed preoperatively when infectious disease is present. Prophylactic administration of antibiotics (see Tables 27-37 and 27-38) helps prevent sepsis from bacteremic interventions.[734,735]

If therapeutic levels of an antibiotic are given and a reduction in fever occurs (presumably because of decreased levels of released interleukin-2), spinal anesthesia might be considered by the anesthesiologist (using benefit-risk judgments) when an acute infectious disease is present.[736]

Sepsis is a leading cause of postoperative morbidity,[685,686,690,691] probably through a decrease in systemic vascular resistance related to activation of the complement system and other mediators. Thus, attention to the effects of antibiotic drugs must be supplemented by attention to intravascular volume status.[688-691,737,738] The degree of impairment of the infected organ and its effect on anesthesia should be assessed. For instance, endocarditis merits examination of volume status; antibiotic and other drug therapy and side effects[739]; myocardial function; and renal, pulmonary, neurologic, and hepatic function—organ systems that can be affected by endocarditis.

Although all surgery except emergency or essential operations is proscribed when an acute infectious disease is present[549-561,567-571,740] (also see the section on upper respiratory infections in the pulmonary section of this chapter), many such diseases (e.g., influenza and pneumococcal pneumonia) are becoming less frequent because of successful immunization recommendations and programs.[741,742] Whether the preoperative clinic can or should be used to increase the use of preventive vaccines is currently being studied, but it is unclear whether vaccination in the 48 hours before surgery is effective or risky.[743] Furthermore, even though acute infections are less common, surgery in patients with chronic viral diseases such as hepatitis and HIV is more frequent. Many of these patients may also harbor opportunistic infections such as tuberculosis or may have other systemic problems. Whether anesthesia or surgery, or both, exacerbates these infections or their systemic manifestations is not clear.[744]

At least two other considerations merit preoperative consideration: patient isolation to prevent contamination of the patient and health care providers. Both concerns are real and are the focus of at least several published volumes. Nosocomial infection is a major source of postsurgical morbidity.[745-751] Acquired immunodeficiency syndrome (AIDS)[752] and many forms of hepatitis (A, B, and C) appear to be due to viral infections but require direct contact with blood or body fluids. Screening for specific viruses or for the chronic end-organ effects of these viruses[753-755] is now being done to reduce the risk of infection to both recipients and health care personnel during blood transfusions. The usual precautions appear to be largely effective,[756] but the risk is considerable if these precautions are not followed meticulously.[757]

Electrolyte Disorders (also see Chapters 37, 41, and 46)

Disorders of calcium, magnesium, and phosphate balance were discussed in the section on diseases involving the endocrine system and disorders of nutrition.

Hyponatremia and Hypernatremia

Electrolyte disorders are usually detected by determining the levels of electrolytes in serum. These concentrations reflect the balance between water and electrolytes. The osmolality of all body fluids is normally maintained within the narrow physiologic range of 285 to 290 mOsm/kg H_2O by integration of three key processes: thirst, release of ADH, and responsiveness of the medullary collecting ducts to ADH. Because of the permeability of biologic membranes, intracellular osmolality and extracellular osmolality are almost always equal and can be estimated by the following formula:

$$2[Na^+](mEq/L) + \frac{[Glucose](mg/dL)}{18} + \frac{[BUN](mg/dL)}{2.8} = mOsm/kg$$

This formula will become easier to calculate when we convert fully to the Système International d'Unités (metric system) because millimoles (mmol) can be substituted for mg/(factor) in the above formula to read

$$2[Na^+] + [Glucose] + [BUN] = mOsm/kg$$

with concentrations expressed in millimoles per liter (mmol/L). Although secretion of ADH is tightly controlled by osmotic stimuli at 285 to 290 mOsm/kg, the osmotic threshold for thirst is high (300 mOsm/kg), thus making this sign an important guide to volume deficiency.

Hyponatremia is perhaps the third most common fluid-electrolyte abnormality in hospitalized patients. (Magnesium deficiency occurs in as many as 25% [see Chapter 25] and potassium deficiency, discussed later in this section, in as many as 10%.) Hyponatremia can occur

---

Table 27–48 Types and causes of hypotonic hyponatremia*

Hypovolemic
Gastrointestinal losses
    Vomiting
    Diarrhea
Skin losses
Third-space losses
Lung losses
Renal losses
    Diuretics
    Renal damage
    Urinary tract obstruction
Adrenal insufficiency
Isovolemic
Syndrome of inappropriate secretion of antidiuretic hormone
Renal failure
Water intoxication
Hypokalemia
Dysfunctional osmostat
Hypervolemic
Congestive heart failure
Nephrosis
Liver dysfunction

*Serum osmolality less than 280 mOsm/L.

in isotonic, hypertonic, or hypotonic forms. For example, isotonic hyponatremia can develop in protein or liquid accumulation states such as myeloma. Hypertonic hyponatremia can be present with hyperglycemia or with infusions of glycine (as in the transurethral resection of the prostate [TURP] syndrome[758]). Hypotonic hyponatremia is the largest classification and is subdivided according to the status of the extracellular fluid into hypovolemic, isovolumic, or hypervolemic hypotonic hyponatremia. All three types require that excretion of renal water be impaired despite continued intake of dilute fluid. Common causes of *hypovolemic* hypotonic hyponatremia (see Table 27-48) are GI losses[759] (vomiting, diarrhea), third-space losses (diuretics or salt-wasting nephropathy), or adrenal insufficiency. *Hypervolemic* hypotonic hyponatremic states complicate severe cardiac failure,[760] cirrhosis, nephrotic syndrome, or renal failure and are characterized by retention of sodium with disproportionately larger amounts of water.

The more common *isovolumic* hypotonic hyponatremia is caused by retention of water without sodium. Because edema is not usually clinically apparent, such patients appear isovolumic. Edema is most often caused by SIADH, which in turn may be caused by CNS or pulmonary tumors or dysfunction. Secretion of ADH increases with age, thus rendering the elderly more prone to hyponatremia. Drugs that potentiate the secretion of ADH (tricyclic antidepressants and vincristine) or its effects on the medullary collecting duct system in the kidney (nonsteroidal anti-inflammatory drugs and chlorpropamide) or that have similar effects (oxytocin) may be more likely to cause hyponatremia in the elderly. To establish the diagnosis of SIADH, the physician should determine that the patient is free of renal and cardiac dysfunction, has normal adrenal and thyroid function, and is normovolemic. Urine osmolality would then be found to exceed 100 mOsm/kg, serum osmolality would be low, and urine sodium excretion would be higher than 20 mEq/L (20 mOsm/L).

Disturbances in serum sodium therefore reflect alterations in glucose metabolism, renal function, or accumulation of body water. The last can be affected by disturbances in thirst, release of ADH, and renal function. Thus, hyponatremia reflects a relative excess of free water and can occur when total-body sodium increases (as in edematous disorders), when total-body sodium is normal (as in excess of free water because of SIADH), or when total-body sodium decreases (as occurs with too aggressive use of diuretic drugs). Definition of the cause defines the treatment. For instance, water restriction is the mainstay of therapy for SIADH. Administration of demeclocycline is another option that corrects SIADH by inducing a reversible nephrogenic diabetes insipidus. The anesthesiologist is faced with the question of what levels of electrolytes require treatment before anesthesia. Although slowly developing hyponatremia usually produces few symptoms, the patient may be lethargic and apathetic. Chronic hyponatremia is better tolerated than acute hyponatremia because of mechanisms regulating intracellular fluid volume that alleviate brain edema; the loss of other solutes from cells decreases the osmotic movement of water into cells. Nonetheless, severe chronic hyponatremia (i.e., serum sodium levels <123 mEq/L) can

cause brain edema.[761,762] By contrast, acute hyponatremia may be manifested by severe symptoms requiring emergency treatment: profound cerebral edema with obtundation, coma, convulsions, and disordered reflexes and thermoregulatory control.[761,762] Depending on the cause and relative total sodium and water content, treatment can range from administration of hypertonic saline or mannitol (with or without diuretic drugs) to restriction of fluids or administration of other drugs.[280,761,762] Because neurologic damage may develop if the serum sodium concentration is increased too rapidly, the rate of increase should not exceed 1 mEq/L/hr.[279,280,762] After the serum sodium concentration has reached 125 mEq/L, therapy may consist of water restriction; more rapid correction may result in CNS demyelination.[279,280,762] In hyponatremic patients who have excess total-body water secondary to SIADH, serum levels can be corrected by giving furosemide, 1 mg/kg, and hypertonic saline to replace the loss of electrolytes in urine.[279,761,762] The diagnosis of SIADH is discussed earlier in this chapter (see the section "Pituitary Abnormalities").

Neither acute nor chronic hyponatremia necessitates the restoration of serum sodium to normal levels; brain swelling usually disappears at a serum sodium level of 130 mEq/L. This leaves us with the question of what levels of serum sodium make anesthesia more risky. Because no data exist to answer this question, to allow for some error in caring for patients, we have arbitrarily chosen a flexible concentration of 131 mEq/L as the lower sodium limit for elective surgery. A discussion of intraoperative hyponatremia in patients undergoing transurethral prostatectomy[758] can be found in Chapter 54.

Hypernatremia occurs much less commonly than hyponatremia. It is often iatrogenic in origin (e.g., it can be caused by failure to provide sufficient free water to a patient who is unconscious or who has had a recent stroke-induced deficit of the thirst mechanism) and can occur in the presence of low, normal, or excess total-body sodium. The primary symptoms of hypernatremia relate to brain cell shrinking. Because too rapid correction of hypernatremia can lead to cerebral edema and convulsions, correction should be made gradually. Again, with no data to support this stance, we believe that all patients undergoing surgery should have serum sodium concentrations of less than 150 mEq/L before anesthesia.

Hypokalemia and Hyperkalemia

Hypokalemia and hyperkalemia are also discussed in Chapters 25, 37, 41, and 46. The relationship between the measured potassium concentration in serum and total-body potassium stores can best be described with a scattergram.[186,763] Only 2% of total-body potassium is stored in plasma (4200 mEq in cells and 60 mEq in extracellular fluid). In normal persons, 75% of the 50 to 60 mEq/L of total-body potassium is stored in skeletal muscle, 6% in red blood cells, and 5% in the liver. Thus, a 20% to 25% change in potassium levels in plasma could represent a change in total-body potassium of 1000 mEq or more if the change were chronic or as little as 10 to 20 mEq if the change were acute.

As with serum sodium levels,[761,762] acute changes in serum potassium levels appear to be less well tolerated than chronic changes. Chronic changes are relatively well tolerated because of the equilibration of serum and intracellular stores that takes place over time to return the resting membrane potential of excitable cells to nearly normal levels.

Hyperkalemia can result from factitious elevation of potassium (as in red blood cell hemolysis); excessive exogenous potassium from sources such as salt substitutes or, in large amounts, bananas; cellular shifts in potassium (as a result of metabolic acidosis, tissue and muscle damage after burns, use of depolarizing muscle relaxants, or intense catabolism of protein); and decreased renal excretion (as occurs in renal failure, renal insufficiency with trauma, and therapy with potassium-sparing diuretic drugs, especially when combined with ACE inhibitors or mineralocorticoid deficiency).[763-769] Factitious hyperkalemia can occur when a tourniquet is left on too long or even by simple fist clenching.[770]

The major danger in anesthetizing patients who have disorders in potassium balance appears to be abnormal cardiac function—that is, both electrical disturbance[764-767] and poor cardiac contractility.[765,766] Hyperkalemia lowers the resting membrane potential of excitable cardiac cells and decreases the duration of the myocardial action potential and upstroke velocity. This decreased rate of ventricular depolarization, plus the beginning of repolarization in some areas of the myocardium while other areas are still undergoing depolarization, produces a progressively widening QRS complex that merges with the T wave into a sine wave on the ECG.

Above a potassium level of 6.7 mEq/L, the degree of hyperkalemia and the duration of the QRS complex correlate well.[764] This correlation is even better than the correlation between the serum potassium level and T-wave changes. Nevertheless, the earliest manifestations of hyperkalemia are narrowing and peaking of the T wave. Though not diagnostic of hyperkalemia, T waves are almost invariably peaked and narrow when serum potassium levels are 7 to 9 mEq/L. When serum potassium levels exceed 7 mEq/L, atrial conduction disturbances appear, as manifested by a decrease in P-wave amplitude and an increase in the PR interval. Supraventricular tachycardia, atrial fibrillation, PVCs, ventricular tachycardia, ventricular fibrillation, or sinus arrest may all occur.

The ECG and cardiac alterations associated with hyperkalemia are potentiated by low serum levels of calcium and sodium. Intravenous administration of saline, bicarbonate, glucose with insulin (1 U/2 g glucose), and calcium can reverse these changes by shifting some extracellular potassium into the cell.

β-Adrenergic stimuli also cause redistribution of potassium into the cell. Indeed, the plasma potassium concentration measured in samples immediately before surgery is usually 0.2 to 0.8 mEq/L lower than that measured during the less stressful period 1 to 3 days before surgery.[771] β-Adrenergic receptor blocking drugs such as propranolol can be used to prevent such an effect preoperatively. A β-adrenergic receptor stimulating agent (20 mg of nebulized albuterol for a 70-kg patient) can be used to treat hyperkalemia when it occurs; it decreases potassium levels 1.0 mEq/L within 30 minutes, and its effect lasts 2 hours.[772] Although nebulized β₂-agonists effectively

lower plasma potassium concentrations by stimulating sodium- and potassium-dependent adenosine triphosphatase, this therapy should be used as an adjunct to rather than a substitute for more established measures. Kayexalate (sodium polystyrene sulfonate) enemas can be given to bind potassium in the gut in exchange for sodium. Dialysis against a hypokalemic solution will also decrease serum potassium levels. However, in a hyperkalemic patient, hypoventilation can be dangerous during anesthesia[654,658,773,774] because each 0.1 change in pH can produce a 0.4- to 1.5-mEq/L change in serum potassium levels in the opposite direction. For example, if pH decreases from 7.4 to 7.3, serum potassium levels could increase from 5.5 to 6.5 mEq/L.[767]

Hypokalemia can be caused by inadequate intake of potassium, excessive GI loss (through diarrhea, vomiting, nasopharyngeal suctioning, chronic use of laxatives, or ingestion of cation exchange resins, as in certain wines), excessive renal loss (because of use of diuretic drugs, renal tubular acidosis, chronic chloride deficiency, metabolic alkalosis, mineralocorticoid excess, excessive ingestion of licorice, use of antibiotics, ureterosigmoidostomy, and diabetic ketoacidosis), and shifts of potassium from extracellular to intracellular compartments (as occur in alkalosis, insulin administration, β-adrenergic agonist administration or stress, barium poisoning, and periodic paralysis). As with hyperkalemia, knowledge of the cause of potassium deficiency and the appropriate preoperative evaluation and treatment of that cause may be as important as treatment of the deficiency itself. Also like hyperkalemia, hypokalemia may reflect small or vast changes in total-body potassium. Acute hypokalemia may be much less well tolerated than chronic hypokalemia. The major worrisome manifestations of hypokalemia pertain to the circulatory system, both the cardiac and peripheral components. In addition, chronic hypokalemia results in muscle weakness, hypoperistalsis, and nephropathy.

Cardiovascular manifestations of hypokalemia include autonomic neuropathy, which results in orthostatic hypotension and decreased sympathetic reserve; impaired myocardial contractility; and electrical conduction abnormalities, which can result in sinus tachycardia, atrial and ventricular arrhythmias, and disturbances in intraventricular conduction that can progress to ventricular fibrillation. That these are real concerns for a hypokalemic patient has been shown far too often.[764-766,772,775-777] In addition to arrhythmias, the ECG shows widening of the QRS complex, ST-segment abnormalities, progressive diminution of the T-wave amplitude, and progressive increase in the U-wave amplitude.[778] Surawicz[764] found these changes to be invariably present when serum potassium levels decreased to below 2.3 mEq/L. Although U waves are not specific for hypokalemia, they are sensitive indicators of the condition. Replenishing the total-body potassium deficit for a depletion reflected by a serum deficit of 1 mEq/L (e.g., from 3.3 to 4.3 mEq/L) may require 1000 mEq of potassium. Even if this amount could be given instantaneously (and it should not be replenished at a rate exceeding 250 mEq/day), it would take 24 to 48 hours to equilibrate in all tissues.[187,188] Potassium-depleted myocardium is unusually sensitive to digoxin, calcium, and most important, potassium.

Rapid potassium infusion in a hypokalemic patient can produce arrhythmias as severe as those produced by hypokalemia itself.[188,779-781] One potential strategy to prevent hypokalemia from anxiety and stress includes premedication with clonidine.[782]

Thus, the decision to proceed with surgery and anesthesia in the face of acute or chronic depletions or excesses of potassium depends on many factors.[783-790] One must know the cause and treatment of the underlying condition creating the electrolyte imbalance and the effect of that imbalance on perioperative risk and physiologic processes. The urgency of the operation, the degree of electrolyte abnormality, the medications given, the acid-base balance, and the suddenness or persistence of the electrolyte disturbance are all considerations. For example, one small study of patients undergoing vascular access procedures with preoperative potassium levels of greater than 6 mmol/L demonstrated no adverse outcomes.[788] Similarly, in a cohort study in which 38 patients had a preoperative potassium level over 5.5 mEq/L, there were no dysrhythmias or major morbidity associated with the use of succinylcholine.[789]

Retrospective epidemiologic studies attribute significant risk to the administration of potassium (even chronic oral administration).[784,785] In one study, 1910 of 16,048 consecutive hospitalized patients were given oral potassium supplements. Of these 1910 patients, hyperkalemia contributed to death in 7, and the incidence of complications of potassium therapy was 1 in 250. Armed with such data, many internists do not prescribe oral potassium therapy for patients given diuretic drugs. Yet these patients frequently become moderately hypokalemic.[791,792] Modest hypokalemia occurs in 10% to 50% of patients given diuretic drugs. Should surgery be delayed to subject such patients to the risks of potassium therapy?

Three studies investigated whether modest hypokalemia was a problem by prospectively seeking arrhythmias on the ECGs of patients who had various preoperative levels of potassium.[786,787,790] No difference in the incidence of arrhythmias occurred in 25 normokalemic (K > 3.4 mEq/L) patients, 25 moderately hypokalemic (K = 3 to 3.4 mEq/L) patients, and 10 severely hypokalemic (K < 2.9 mEq/L) patients.[786] Wahr and coauthors studied 2402 patients undergoing elective coronary artery bypass grafting and reported that a serum potassium level less than 3.5 mmol/L was a predictor of serious perioperative arrhythmia (odds ratio [OR], 2.2; 95% CI, 1.2 to 4.0), intraoperative arrhythmia (OR, 2.0; 95% CI, 1.0 to 3.6), and postoperative atrial fibrillation/flutter (OR, 1.7; 95% CI, 1.0 to 2.7).[790] The inability of the eye to pick up these changes—or even the inability of Holter recordings for short periods[793] (which seem to not have been obtained in this study)—points to the need for confirming studies.

Other studies indicate that modest hypokalemia can have severe consequences.[792,794,795] Holland and coworkers[795] treated 21 patients with 50 mg of hydrochlorothiazide twice a day for 4 weeks. These patients had a history of becoming hypokalemic during diuretic therapy; none of them had cardiac disease or was taking other medication. Before and after diuretic therapy, 24-hour ambulatory ECGs were recorded. This study is also subject to the limitations of Holter monitoring.[793] Ventricular ectopy,

including complex ventricular ectopy (multifocal PVCs, ventricular couplets, ventricular tachycardia), developed in 7 of the 21 patients (33%). Potassium repletion decreased the number of ectopic ventricular beats per patient from 71.2 to 5.4/hr. Apparently, some patients are sensitive to even minor potassium depletion. In the Multiple Risk Factor Intervention Trial involving 361,662 patients, more than 2000 of whom were treated for hypertension with diuretics, the reduction in serum potassium after diuretic therapy was greater in those with PVCs.[792] Although we recommend that hypokalemic patients be given potassium supplements, the merit of this practice is unclear.

Our personal criteria for preoperative potassium therapy are as follows. As a rule, all patients undergoing elective surgery should have normal serum potassium levels. However, we do not recommend delaying surgery if the serum potassium level is above 2.8 mEq/L or below 5.9 mEq/L, if the cause of the potassium imbalance is known, and if the patient is in otherwise optimal condition. This range of safe potassium levels is arbitrary and has changed from 3.3 in 1979, to 3.1 in 1986, to 2.9 in 1990 on the lower side and from 5.6 in 1979, to 5.7 in 1986, to 5.9 in 1990 on the upper side as more data have become available on the safety of preoperative hypokalemia and the dangers of replacing potassium in a hospital environment[784,785] (see Table 25-5 in Chapter 25). We subject all patients with end-stage renal failure to dialysis (using the same arbitrary safe range) before all surgical procedures except truly emergency ones (as in instances of imminent exsanguination). In studies on dogs in 1978, Tanifuji and Eger[796] determined the relationships between electrolyte status and anesthetic requirements that may require intraoperative consideration: hyponatremia and hypo-osmolality decreased the minimum alveolar concentration (MAC), hypernatremia increased MAC, and hyperkalemia did not affect the anesthetic requirement.

GASTROINTESTINAL AND LIVER DISEASES

The reader should also see the discussion of porphyrias in the section on neurologic disease, the discussion of nutritional deficiencies in the section on disorders of nutrition, and pediatric disorders such as transesophageal fistula in Chapters 60 and 77.

Gastrointestinal Disease

Preoperative Search for Diverse Associated Disorders in Gastrointestinal Disease

Although preoperative preparation of the GI tract is usually the responsibility of the surgeon and although the GI tract frequently does not need to be extensively evaluated by the anesthesiologist, GI disease can and often does cause derangements in many or all other systems. Such disturbances can affect the safety of anesthesia for the patient. Thus, the anesthesiologist may need to not only optimize the patient's condition through extensive preoperative preparation but also have knowledge of disease processes and their effects to guide the patient smoothly through the perioperative period. The major advances of correcting fluid and electrolyte disorders and optimizing nutritional status before surgery now allow surgery to be performed in patients with GI disease previously deemed to be at too great a risk and may have lessened the risk for others.[159-162,797,798] Still, in patients with GI disease, thorough assessment of intravascular fluid volume and electrolyte concentrations and nutrition is essential, including an evaluation of the supervening side effects of these therapies (e.g., hypophosphatemia from parenteral nutrition, hyperkalemia or cardiac arrhythmias from too vigorous treatment of hypokalemia, and CHF from too rapid or too vigorous treatment of hypovolemia).

In addition to the vast alterations in fluids, electrolytes, and nutrition that can occur with such diverse GI diseases as neoplasms and pancreatitis, patients with GI disorders can have gastroesophageal reflux disease,[799] bowel obstruction, vomiting, or hypersecretion of acid. These effects may merit rapid induction of anesthesia with the application of cricoid pressure or awake endotracheal intubation, preoperative nasogastric suctioning, or preoperative use of histamine receptor blocking agents (also see Chapter 42). Clotting abnormalities may need to be corrected because fat-soluble vitamin K (often malabsorbed) is necessary for the synthesis of factors V, VII, IX, and X in the liver (also see Chapter 55). Liver disease is often associated with GI disease and, if severe enough, can also result in a deficiency of clotting factors synthesized by the liver.

Other factors should be remembered in any preoperative evaluation of a patient with GI disease. First, closed spaces containing gas expand by absorbing nitrous oxide. Such expansion can lead to ischemic injury or GI viscus rupture, or both.[800] Second, GI surgery predisposes the patient to sepsis; sepsis and decreased peripheral vascular resistance can lead to massive fluid requirements, cardiac failure, and renal insufficiency. Recently, the wound infection rate has been declining. This decrease may be attributable to the use of better technique, more appropriate prophylactic use of antibiotics, better nutrition, less invasive (laparoscopic and endoscopic) surgery, or surgical resection of even solid tumors.[457,800-804] Third, patients with GI disease may have many other associated disorders not directly related to the GI tract. For example, they may be anemic from deficiencies in iron, intrinsic factor, folate, or vitamin B_{12}. They may also manifest neurologic changes from combined-system disease. Respiration may be impaired because of heavy cigarette smoking, peritonitis, abscess, pulmonary obstruction, previous incisions, aspiration, or pulmonary embolism (as occurs with ulcerative colitis or with thrombophlebitis in the bedridden).[805] These patients may also have hepatitis, cholangitis, side effects from antibiotic drugs or other medications, massive bleeding with anemia and shock, or psychological derangements.

Because GI disease can be accompanied by so many diverse associated disorders, the clinician must clearly search for other system involvement and preoperatively assess and treat such disorders appropriately. Discussion of two specific diseases, ulcerative colitis and carcinoid tumor, will highlight the importance of involvement of other systems in GI disease.

Ulcerative Colitis and Carcinoid Tumors as Examples of Gastrointestinal Disease Affecting Other Systems

Patients with ulcerative colitis often have psychological problems. They may also have phlebitis; deficiencies in iron, folate, or vitamin B_{12}; anemia; or clotting disorders caused by malabsorption. They may be malnourished or dehydrated or have electrolyte abnormalities. In addition, ulcerative colitis can be accompanied by massive bleeding, bowel obstruction or perforation or toxic megacolon causing respiratory compromise, hepatitis, arthritis, iritis, spondylitis, or diabetes secondary to pancreatitis.

The site of origin of carcinoid tumors in more than 75% of patients is the GI tract.[806] Within the GI tract, carcinoid tumors have been documented to occur from the esophagus to the rectum. The most frequent site is the appendix, but carcinoids in this location rarely, if ever, metastasize or produce carcinoid syndrome. Tumors arising in the ileocecal region have the highest incidence of metastases. Carcinoid tumors originating from other sites than the GI tract, such as the head and neck, lung, gonads, thymus, breast, and urinary tract, have also been reported. Cardiac involvement, though frequently reported, is usually limited to right-sided valvular and myocardial plaque formation.[807]

Not all patients with carcinoid tumors have symptoms attributable to secretion of hormone by the tumor. Some can, however, and unexpected carcinoid can be manifested during surgery by hypersecretion of gastric fluid.[808] The most comprehensive series in the literature indicates that only 7% of patients have carcinoid syndrome, which typically consists of flushing, diarrhea, and valvular heart disease. Of those with the syndrome, approximately 74% have cutaneous flushing; 68%, intestinal hypermotility; 41%, cardiac symptoms; and 18%, wheezing. Factors influencing symptoms include the location of the tumor and the specific hormones produced and secreted. Although it is generally believed that if patients do not exhibit carcinoid syndrome, the tumors are not producing serotonin (5-hydroxytryptamine [5-HT]), but such may not be the case. Approximately 50% of patients with carcinoid tumors of the GI tract demonstrate evidence of 5-HT production as manifested by elevated urinary levels of 5-hydroxyindoleacetic acid (5-HIAA), a metabolic product of 5-HT. Carcinoid syndrome is usually associated with ileal carcinoid tumors that have metastasized to the liver. Presumably, the liver clears mediators released from the tumor. Impairment of this clearing ability by the metastatic tumor results in carcinoid syndrome.

Most patients with carcinoid tumors and increased urinary 5-HIAA have typical carcinoid tumors originating from the midgut (ileum or jejunum). These patients excrete only small amounts of 5-hydroxytryptophan (5-HTP). Patients with atypical carcinoid tumors that originate in the foregut (bronchus, stomach, and pancreas) excrete large amounts of 5-HT and 5-HTP, as well as moderately higher amounts of 5-HIAA.

Although it is generally agreed that 5-HT is responsible for the diarrhea experienced by patients with carcinoid tumors, other neurohumoral agents may contribute to the flushing and hypotension,[806] including dopamine, histamine, and some of the neuropeptides such as substance P, neurotensin, vasoactive intestinal peptide, and somatostatin.

The net physiologic effect of circulating 5-HT represents a composite of both direct action (mediated by 5-HT receptors) and indirect action (mediated through modulation of adrenergic neurotransmission). The existence of several subtypes of 5-HT receptors may account for the different effects of 5-HT on various serotonin-sensitive tissue beds. Indirect actions are effected through alterations in catecholamine release and depend on the level of circulating 5-HT.

5-HT has little, if any direct effect on the heart. With elevated levels, however, positive chronotropic and inotropic myocardial effects may occur, mediated by the release of noradrenaline (norepinephrine). Effects of serotonin on the vasculature include both vasoconstriction and vasodilation.

Alterations in GI function attributed to 5-HT include increased motility and net intestinal secretion of water, sodium chloride, and potassium. 5-HT reportedly causes bronchoconstriction in many animals, but rarely in humans. Asthmatics are a possible exception. Carcinoid tumors are frequently manifested as diarrhea with fluid and electrolyte abnormalities. Because these tumors secrete vasoactive substances, patients can exhibit hypotension or hypertension along with the flush associated with release of vasoactive substances. Vasoactive substances can be released from the tumor by any number of substances, including catecholamines. Until the 1990s, management of this tumor was a real challenge for the anesthesiologist. Thus, anesthesiologists of that era had to tread a fine line between avoiding substances known to release 5-HT (e.g., d-tubocurarine and morphine) and inducing anesthesia so light that painful stimuli activate a sympathetic stress response.[809,810] The anesthesiologist also needed to be ready and able to treat hypotension, decreased peripheral vascular resistance, bronchospasm, and hypertension. α-Adrenergic receptor blockade with the phenothiazines, butyrophenones, or phenoxybenzamine and β-adrenergic receptor blockade with propranolol have been advocated to prevent catecholamine-mediated release of vasoactive substances. These practices, however, can lead to hypotension. Nevertheless, that difficulty in managing carcinoid syndrome seemed to change with the availability of a somatostatin analog. In fact, somatostatin is now such a powerful inhibitor of the release of peptides from carcinoid tumors and an inhibitor of the peptic effects on receptor cells that it is the therapy of choice for preoperative, intraoperative, and postoperative management of carcinoid symptoms and crises.[806,809] However, the ease of management of most patients[806,809-814] should not lull the anesthesiologist into being unprepared—in fact, somatostatin has caused problems of its own and has failed to prevent severe hypotension and bronchospasm.[815,816]

In patients with severe hypotension that is not treatable with somatostatin, the drug of choice is either angiotensin or vasopressin. (Angiotensin is not commercially available in the United States but is an approved drug that is available by contacting Novartis.) However, the vasoactive substances released by carcinoid tumors cause fibrosis of the heart valves that often results in pulmonic stenosis or tricuspid insufficiency. To increase cardiac output in a patient with tricuspid insufficiency, the anesthesiologist should avoid drugs or situations that increase pulmonary vascular resistance (e.g., angiotensin, vasopressin, acidosis, hypercapnia, hypothermia) (also see Chapters 50 and 51). In addition, the production of large amounts of 5-HT (equal to 200 mg/day of 5-HIAA) can lead to the development of niacin deficiency with pellagra (as occurs with diarrhea, dermatitis, and dementia).

Acute elevation of plasma kinin activity in carcinoid patients has been postulated for many years as the explanation for the symptoms of carcinoid syndrome. Physiologic effects of kinins are known to include vasodilation of smaller resistance vessels and stimulation of the release of histamine from mast cells. The latter action potentiates their own vasodilating properties and further reduces systolic and diastolic BP. In addition, increases in vascular permeability may lead to edema. Kinins are not known to affect the myocardium directly.

Steroids have been effective in treating the symptoms of bronchial carcinoid tumors. Although prophylactic preoperative administration and intraoperative therapeutic use have been described, controlled studies of beneficial effects are lacking. Aprotinin, like steroids, inhibits the kallikrein cascade. This drug is believed to be capable of blocking the proteinase activity of kallikrein, and some reports have described a dramatic clinical response.

A subset of patients with symptoms of carcinoid syndrome excrete histamine at increased levels in their urine. Histamine causes vasodilation of small blood vessels, which leads to flushing and decreased total peripheral resistance. Histamine is known to cause bronchoconstriction, particularly in patients with bronchial asthma and other pulmonary diseases. Its role in carcinoid bronchospasm, if any, is uncertain. Histamine receptor blocking drugs have been used with some success in alleviating the flushing associated with carcinoid syndrome. H2 antagonism alone was found to be just as effective as combination therapy in preventing symptoms; pure H1 antagonism, however, was ineffective. These therapies have been relegated to a second-line defense since the use of somatostatin.

Catecholamines aggravate the symptoms of carcinoid syndrome, presumably by stimulating release of hormone by the tumor. The mechanism by which this release occurs remains obscure. Adrenergic receptors have not been demonstrated in carcinoid tumors, nor do these tumors usually have neural innervation. Perhaps adrenergic stimuli work through their mechanical effects on the gut and vessels to stimulate the release of tumor products. Treatment of patients with carcinoid tumors by means of α- and β-adrenergic antagonists has been beneficial in ameliorating flushing in some instances but ineffective in others.

The results of prospective studies on somatostatin to ameliorate the symptoms of carcinoid syndrome have been dramatic. In several case reports involving a total of 46 patients, all but 2 had rapid, dramatic improvement in flushing.[806-809,811-814] Similar results have been obtained in patients with diarrhea. Somatostatin appears to be a major advancement in the treatment of carcinoid syndrome.

It might logically be concluded that preoperative preparation of a patient with carcinoid syndrome would be similar to that for a patient with pheochromocytoma: titration of adrenergic, histaminic, and serotonergic receptor blocking drugs to maximum effect while monitoring intravascular volume status and adding somatostatin before surgery. Although this approach is logical, preoperative symptoms do not correlate with perioperative symptoms, and only the last two therapeutic options (optimization of intravascular fluid status and administration of somatostatin) are most effective.

Bronchospasm with or without flushing also develops in many patients when vasoactive substances are released. Thus, a patient with carcinoid tumor may be well or may be severely incapacitated by pulmonary, neurologic, nutritional, fluid, electrolytic, or cardiovascular disturbances.[806,809] Therefore, although the GI system in itself may not require extensive preoperative preparation, GI disease can cause disturbances in any or all other systems that require extensive preoperative preparation to optimize the patient's condition plus preoperative knowledge of physiology and the effects of diseases to guide patients through the perioperative period smoothly. In addition, the anesthesiologist's understanding of the nature of the surgery probably aids in determining the system involvement caused by the GI disorder.

Another preoperative consideration is that patients with GI diseases (perhaps even more so than those with other diseases) have had to endure the psychosocial trauma of having to live with their disease for long periods or the necessity of facing such a prospect.[817] They need emotional support and holistic kindnesses as much as, if not more than others, without sacrificing scientific rigor in the treatment of their condition. Obtaining relevant psychological data while gathering medical information, sitting (not standing) while taking the history, and empathizing with the patient about how difficult it must be to accomplish tasks with this disease (stressing accomplishments, we have found) legitimize the physician's interests in and support of the patient's pain and other psychosocial issues. The time spent sitting and talking with the patient also allows the anesthesiologist to discuss options for pain therapy with the patient, why systemic morphine might be avoided in a patient with a fresh bowel anastomosis,[818] and other issues that show the anesthesiologist to be both a competent physician and particularly concerned with that patient's well-being. In addition to an appreciation of the organic effects of their disease, attention to emotional support of these patients perioperatively presents opportunities to use one's full skills as a physician to bring about healing.

Liver Disease

What are the risks of giving anesthesia to patients with acute liver disease who require emergency surgery? What are the risks of giving anesthesia to patients with chronic impairment of liver function? What can be done to minimize these risks? Although one might think that the experiences gained from providing anesthesia for liver transplantation would answer many of these questions, there is a substantial difference between optimizing cardiovascular function to meet the needs of a new liver (e.g., supply of nutrients) and maintaining liver function in a diseased liver. Because hepatic function and physiology are discussed in Chapter 55, we will mention only that the liver performs many functions: it synthesizes substances

(e.g., proteins, clotting factors), detoxifies the body of both drugs and the products of normal human metabolism, excretes waste products, and stores and supplies energy. Tests of liver function assess synthesis (cholesterol levels, prothrombin time [PT], albumin levels), cellular integrity (aspartate aminotransferase [AST], alanine aminotransferase [ALT], lactate dehydrogenase, alkaline phosphatase), the liver's ability to detoxify the body (e.g., ammonia, direct bilirubin, or lidocaine levels), and the liver's ability to excrete certain substances (sulfobromophthalein retention, total bilirubin levels).

In examining the effects of anesthesia (with or without surgery) on liver function and measures to reduce risk in patients with preexisting liver disease, investigators have often looked at one or more of the aforementioned tests or, more commonly, at major end points of morbidity (jaundice) or mortality. The evidence can be summarized as follows: the last data we have (too old now, but it is the last data we have) indicate that without anesthesia or surgery, approximately 1 in 700 to 800 patients who are otherwise healthy and scheduled for surgery will have abnormal preoperative results of liver function tests; of these patients, jaundice will develop in 1 in 3 (also see Chapter 25 for these studies).[819,820] In our preliminary study, *every* patient with abnormal liver function tests has been symptomatic preoperatively.[351] Therefore, the risk may be less than described (see Chapter 25).[821]

All anesthetics tested (general, narcotic–nitrous oxide, and regional) have caused transient abnormalities in liver function test results. These abnormalities were magnified by upper intra-abdominal surgery and occurred regardless of preexisting liver disease.[773,822-829] Patients whose preoperative liver function tests are abnormal will obviously have a higher incidence of abnormal results on postoperative liver function tests.[773,822-824,826,827] Lacking in the literature are investigations that studied patients with compromised hepatic function to determine how to decrease the risk of surgery and anesthesia. Also lacking are comparisons of outcome after various perioperative strategies for managing different causes of hepatic dysfunction (i.e., viral [or even one virus versus another virus], toxic, or drug induced). In addition to preexisting hepatic disease and the operative site, hypokalemia, hypotension, sepsis, and the need for blood transfusion all contribute to postoperative hepatic dysfunction. Thus, anesthesia and surgery probably exacerbate hepatic disease and thereby clearly increase morbidity and mortality.[773,822-823,826,827] Only one study, on alcoholic liver disease, has implied otherwise.[773]

The main goal of the anesthesiologist is to avoid making the hepatic disease (with perhaps its metabolic and CNS toxicity) worse and increasing the chance of renal failure, coma, and death.[830] Studies of portal hypertension have shown that mortality can be 50% when preoperative serum albumin concentrations are lower than 3 g/dL, preoperative serum bilirubin levels are greater than 3 mg/dL, and ascites and encephalopathy are present; mortality can be even higher when the PT is grossly abnormal. By contrast, mortality decreases to 10% when preoperative serum albumin levels are 3 to 3.5 g/dL, preoperative serum bilirubin levels are 2 to 3 mg/dL, PT is normal, and encephalopathy is absent. The risks of anesthetizing a patient with chronic liver disease not requiring a portacaval shunt are detailed only sporadically but appear to be greater than those associated with anesthetizing a healthy patient.[819-834]

In the late 1970s and 1980s it was debated whether halothane should be given to patients with hepatitis or biliary tract disease. The National Halothane Study did not find halothane to cause massive hepatic necrosis—or any other hepatic abnormality—more frequently than any other anesthetic[699] and, in fact, demonstrated its safety in biliary tract surgery. Prospective studies have been contradictory at best regarding whether repeat exposure to halothane within a short time elevates liver enzyme levels to a greater degree than other anesthetics do.[835-838] Because the incidence of hepatitis attributable only to halothane would be very low, very large groups would have to be studied. The incidence of postoperative jaundice and hepatitis not attributable to halothane is much greater than the incidence of hepatitis attributable only to halothane, and the absence of differentiating pathologic features makes halothane-induced hepatitis difficult to exclude as a possibility. Newer tests imply an immunologic basis to the continuation of either hepatitis or liver dysfunction after the initial mechanism (e.g., if hypoxia begets the injury, the immune mechanism continues it) and are supported by resolution of a prolonged case of halothane hepatitis after treatment.[839] Although other cases that have resolved after steroid therapy have been presented, those cases did not, in fact, have a long enough period before the beginning of their resolution when the disease was stable to conclude that steroids made a difference and that this was not the natural course of the disease. One case is inconclusive but certainly implies that a controlled trial should be instituted. This subject is perhaps even more important now that several forms of viral hepatitis (acute and chronic) are treatable; left untreated, hepatitis C evolves to chronic type C hepatitis in 50% of patients and to cirrhosis in 20% of those in whom chronic hepatitis develops. Treatment with interferon-alfa (leukocyte) appears to reduce the risk of these consequences substantially.[753,754]

More sensitive tests of hepatocellular dysfunction after anesthesia and surgery, such as glutathione-S-transferase, reveal impairment more frequently.[840] One is left to conclude that both metabolic and immunologic mechanisms can contribute to hepatocellular dysfunction after anesthesia and surgery. Are these related to anesthesia or surgery? Internists almost always point to anesthesia and must be educated to shed light on their bias, although this need is less with better diagnostic tests[753,755] and with the possibility of treatment of some forms of hepatitis.[753,754]

Thus, the strong bias of internists makes anesthetic-induced hepatitis ("halothane hepatitis") a popular diagnosis despite the higher incidence of viral and drug hepatitis.[773,838-853] Another factor producing possible bias is the fact that animal models of halothane hepatitis incorporate liver hypoxia or pretreatment with polyvinyl chlorides, conditions that can themselves adversely affect liver function. No irrefutable evidence has implicated halothane as being better or worse than any other anesthetic for patients with preexisting liver disease. However, should liver disease worsen postoperatively, the tendency is to blame halothane (even when it has not

been in the operating room for 20 years). Anesthesia is certainly less likely than hypoxia, trauma, viral hepatitis, drug-induced hepatitis, or sepsis to cause serious hepatic injury.[819,852] No one has yet determined whether a time limit exists within which repeat exposure to an anesthetic is more dangerous than exposure to various anesthetics or after which repeat anesthesia is as safe as a first exposure to an anesthetic. The common consistent feature of many forms of chronic liver disease is a vulnerability to decreased oxygen delivery to the hepatic artery. This vulnerability occurs because of increased resistance to portal vein blood flow. Many stimuli, including surgical palpation, appear to decrease oxygen delivery to the hepatic artery. Thus, anesthesia and surgery may affect hepatic well-being after surgery in a patient with an already compromised liver.

What should physicians do to avoid contracting hepatitis or giving it to patients? It is cost-effective for anesthesia personnel to receive the appropriate vaccines and take appropriate precautions.[821,853-856] What should a physician with hepatitis B do to prevent infecting patients? That subject is discussed in detail elsewhere.[857]

Liver disease severe enough to affect hepatic synthesis can impair the detoxification of many drugs,[839,840,852,858-861] including muscle relaxants[858-861] (also see Chapter 13), and can disturb coagulation (also see Chapter 48) but may or may not affect anesthetic requirements greatly.[862,863] Administration of fresh frozen plasma may be needed to correct coagulation disorders.

HEMATOLOGIC DISORDERS AND ONCOLOGIC DISEASE

Hematologic Disorders

Anemia and Polycythemia
Chapter 25 discusses the evidence that normovolemic anemia or polycythemia increases perioperative morbidity. The results indicate that knowledge and pretreatment of polycythemia might decrease perioperative morbidity and mortality.

Except for patients with ischemic heart disease (see later), no such evidence exists for normovolemic anemia (this topic is also reviewed in Chapter 25).[431,432] Thus, there are no specific preoperative routines for anemia itself, except regarding patients who have or are likely to have ischemic heart disease (as determined by risk factors).[864-869] For these patients, hematocrits above or below 29% to 34% were found in two separate studies to be associated with increased episodes of myocardial ischemia after vascular surgery[431,432] (see Fig. 27-18). For patients at risk for current ischemic heart disease, data indicate that transfusion to a hematocrit level of 29% to 34% may be appropriate (also, see the earlier section on cardiovascular diseases). It should be remembered that anemia is a reduction in circulatory erythrocyte mass below the range of values considered normal for persons of the same sex at the same location (age older than 6 months, race, and ethnic background do not explain anemia). Each erythrocyte lives for approximately 120 days; therefore, replacement of 15 to 20 mL of senescent cells needs to be accomplished in the absence of diseases that destroy or cause loss of blood cells. Moreover, the symptoms of anemia—headache, weakness, exertional dyspnea, and loss of endurance—do not provide much information about the severity, rapidity of onset, and cardiorespiratory effects of the underlying cause of the anemia.

Furthermore, because anemia can be a hallmark of many other diseases possibly affecting perioperative anesthetic management, the preoperative presence of anemia requires a search for and treatment of the underlying cause. For instance, anemia could indicate renal insufficiency or a drug reaction, both of which could alter anesthetic management. For this reason, the cause of anemia should be known preoperatively. Similarly, polycythemia can be a primary disease (e.g., polycythemia vera), or it can be secondary to smoking, the use of diuretic drugs, chronic use of androgens, hypoxia, or other forms of chronic lung/heart disease. Phlebotomies are quite effective for patients with mild polycythemia. Cerebral blood flow improves when the hematocrit is kept below 45%.[866,867] No prospective controlled study has been performed on humans regarding a possible decrease in perioperative morbidity or wound healing[431,432,864-869] from perioperative treatment of anemia or polycythemia. The time of most danger to the patient may be the early recovery room period, during which time oxygen delivery to the lungs is perhaps at its worst[431,432] (also see Chapters 71 and 74). When religious convictions prohibit blood transfusion and the patient is anemic or may become anemic, therapeutic options include autotransfusion with the salvaged or removed blood always connected to (or in contact with) the patient and the use of blood substitutes. Although perfluorocarbons have fallen into disrepute because of effects on reticuloendothelial function, other substitutes, including hemoglobin-based substitutes, may become available, and synthetic erythropoietin will find greater use in preoperative prophylaxis and preoperative predeposit blood programs.[811,870] This subject is discussed in greater detail in Chapters 47 and 48.

Erythropoietin is one of the substances necessary for normal production of red blood cells. Production and secretion of erythropoietin from the peritubular cells of the kidney are stimulated by tissue hypoxia. Signal transduction of this hypoxic stimulus depends on a heme-containing oxygen-sensing protein that mediates changes in the stability of messenger RNA from chromosome 7 in erythropoietin-producing cells. Erythropoietin triggers quiescent, early erythroid progenitor cells into cycle by acting like a mitogen and facilitating differentiation into late committed erythroid progenitor cells. In normoxic individuals, synthesis of erythropoietin is not stimulated until the concentration of hemoglobin falls below 10.5 g/dL. In severe anemia, erythropoietin levels can increase more than 1000-fold. Iron, folic acid, and vitamin B_{12} are also needed for normal maturation of erythrocytes. Several forms of anemia present special situations, such as sickle cell anemia, hereditary spherocytosis, and the autoimmune hemolytic anemias.

Sickle Cell Anemia and Related Hemoglobinopathies

The sickle cell syndromes constitute a family of hemoglobinopathies caused by abnormal genetic transformation of amino acids in the heme portion of the hemoglobin molecule.[871] The sickle cell syndromes arise from a mutation in the β-globin gene that changes the sixth amino acid from valine to glutamic acid. A major pathologic feature of sickle cell disease is the aggregation of irreversibly sickled cells in blood vessels. The molecular basis of sickling is the aggregation of deoxygenated hemoglobin B molecules along their longitudinal axis.[871] This abnormal aggregation distorts the cell membrane and thereby produces a sickle shape. Irreversibly sickled cells become dehydrated and rigid and can cause tissue infarcts by impeding blood flow and oxygen to tissues.[871-875] Some have challenged this hypothesis, with several studies showing enhanced adhesion of sickled erythrocytes to vascular endothelium.[876] Some other abnormal hemoglobins interact with hemoglobin S to various degrees and give rise to symptomatic disease in patients heterozygous for hemoglobin S and one of the other hemoglobins such as the hemoglobin of thalassemia (hemoglobin C).

Three tenths of 1% of the African American population in the United States has sickle cell–thalassemia disease (hemoglobin SC); these patients also have end-organ disease and symptoms suggestive of organ infarction. For these patients, perioperative considerations should be similar to those for patients with sickle cell disease (hemoglobin SS), discussed later.

Whereas 8% to 10% of African Americans have the sickle cell trait (hemoglobin AS), 0.2% are homozygous for sickle cell hemoglobin and have sickle cell anemia. Sickle cell trait is a heterozygous condition in which the individual has one βS globin gene and one βA globin gene, which results in the production of both hemoglobin S and hemoglobin A, with a predominance of hemoglobin A. Sickle cell trait should not be considered a disease because hemoglobin AS cells begin to sickle only when the oxygen saturation of hemoglobin is below 20%. No difference has been found between normal persons (those with hemoglobin AA) and those with hemoglobin AS regarding survival rates or the incidence of severe disease, with one exception: patients with hemoglobin AS have a 50% increase in pulmonary infarction. However, single case reports of a perioperative death and a perioperative brain infarct in two patients with hemoglobin AS disease do exist,[875,877] and a report of death believed to be due to aortocaval compression during general anesthesia that resulted in a sickling crisis does exist.[878] Frequent measurement of oxygen saturation (pulse oximetry) in multiple areas of the body is recommended, including the ear and toe in pregnant patients.[878] A retrospective review of exercise in military recruits showed that soldiers with sickle cell trait had a higher risk of sudden death after extreme exertion during basic training than did black soldiers with only hemoglobin A—32 per 100,000 versus 1 per 1,000,000.[879] Although this magnitude of increase may not seem great, the vasoactive responses of the perioperative period can be similar to those of moderate to extreme exertion.

The pathologic end-organ damage that occurs in sickle cell states is attributable to three processes: the sickling or adhesion (or both) of cells in blood vessels, which causes infarcts and subsequent tissue destruction secondary to tissue ischemia; hemolytic crisis secondary to hemolysis;

and aplastic crises that occur with bone marrow exhaustion, which can rapidly result in severe anemia. Logic dictates that patients currently in crisis not undergo surgery except for extreme emergencies, and then only after an exchange transfusion.[873,875-880]

Because sickling is increased with lowered oxygen tensions, acidosis, hypothermia, and the presence of more desaturated hemoglobin S, current therapy includes keeping the patient warm and well hydrated, giving supplemental oxygen, maintaining high cardiac output, and not creating areas of stasis with pressure or tourniquets. Meticulous attention to these practices in periods when we do not usually pay most careful attention (i.e., waiting in the preinduction area) or when gas exchange may be most unmatched to the cardiovascular-metabolic demands (early postoperative period) may be important in lessening morbidity. Even following these measures routinely, with no special emphasis placed on the periods described, succeeded in reducing mortality to 1% in several series of patients with sickle cell syndromes.[877-831] Retrospective review of patient charts led the authors of those studies to conclude that at most, a 0.5% mortality rate could be attributed to the interaction between sickle cell anemia and anesthetics.

Can this rate be decreased?[872,881-883] Several investigators have advocated using partial exchange transfusions perioperatively. In children with sickle cell anemia and acute lung syndromes, partial exchange transfusion improved clinical symptoms and blood oxygenation. In addition, serum bilirubin levels decreased in patients with acute liver injury. Clinical improvement of pneumococcal meningitis and cessation of hematuria in papillary necrosis also accompanied exchange transfusion.[872,884] The goal of exchange transfusion is to increase the concentration of hemoglobin A to 40% and the hematocrit to 35%. The 40% figure is an arbitrary one because no controlled studies have established the threshold ratio of hemoglobin A to S that would render blood unable to sickle in vivo. To achieve the 40% ratio in a 70-kg adult, about 4 U of washed erythrocytes would have to be exchanged; the system is inexpensive but efficient.

The possible decrease in preoperative morbidity after partial exchange transfusion has not been compared with the risks of exchange, except in two studies[874,885] in which the risks of exchange were found to exceed the benefits. In the first study, a retrospective review of 82 surgical procedures performed between 1978 and 1986 in 60 patients, no advantage was noted for preoperative exchange transfusion, as measured by a decrease in postoperative complications.[835] (However, only the sickest may have received exchange because patients were not randomly allocated to exchange or nonexchange groups.) A slight increase in postoperative atelectasis requiring treatment was seen in patients given preoperative transfusions. More than 50% of the patients given transfusions had a postoperative complication. Patients who began with a hematocrit of more than 36% had a lower rate of complications.[885] In the second study, a randomized comparison of aggressive versus conservative transfusion practices in 551 patients (604 operations), perioperative sickling complications were *not* different between groups, and transfusion-related complications were substantially less in the conservative group.[874] Therefore, our recommendation is to pay meticulous attention to preventing conditions that increase sickling or that cause infection and to limit exchange transfusion to crisis situations. Perhaps giving higher concentrations of enriched oxygen to patients undergoing laparoscopic procedures should also become routine. Induction of hyponatremia has been shown to abort acute sickle cell crisis; however, this treatment has not gained widespread acceptance. Other conditions are common in sickle cell syndromes: pulmonary dysfunction with increased shunting, renal insufficiency, gallstones, small MIs, priapism, stroke, aseptic necrosis of bones and joints, ischemic ulcers, retinal detachment from neovascularization, and complications of repeated transfusions.

Recently, bone marrow transplantation with low-risk regimens that produce hematopoietic chimerism seem promising.[886] This regimen may make all other older therapies irrelevant if it is as successful as it now seems to be.

In thalassemia, globin structures are normal, but because of gene deletion, the rate of synthesis of either the α- or β-chains of hemoglobin (α- and β-thalassemia, respectively) decreases.[887-889] Two copies of the gene that codes for the α-globin chain are located on chromosome 16. Deletion of all four of these genes causes cell death in utero, and three deletions cause severe chronic hemolysis and a shortened life span. "α-Thalassemia-1 (trait)" occurs when two genes have been deleted and mild anemia results; "α-thalassemia-2 (silent)" occurs when the two genes have been deleted but no mild anemia or microcytosis results. In α-thalassemia trait, the hemoglobin A_2 level is normal. β-Thalassemia is associated with an excess of α-chains, which denature developing erythrocytes, thereby leading to their premature death in marrow or to shortened survival in the circulation. An elevated hemoglobin A_2 level is the hallmark of β-thalassemia trait, a common cause of mild anemia and microcytosis. Bone marrow transplantation and pharmacologic manipulation of hemoglobin F synthesis are being tried in these hemoglobinopathies, as is direct gene replacement therapy. These therapies seem to be promising in even reversing liver failure from previous iron overload.[890] These syndromes are common in Southeast Asia, India, and the Middle East and in people of African descent.

In thalassemia, facial deformity from erythropoietin-stimulated ineffective erythropoiesis (ineffective because of a genetic inability to produce useful hemoglobin) has been reported to make endotracheal intubation difficult.[887,888] This one case report[888] has not been amplified, and there are no reports of this complication in patients with sickle cell anemia. However, the anemia associated with these syndromes often produces a compensatory hyperplasia of the erythroid marrow, which in turn is associated with severe skeletal abnormalities.[887-889]

Cytoskeletal Anemias (Hereditary Spherocytosis and Elliptocytosis), Enzyme-Deficient Anemias, and Autoimmune Hemolytic Anemias

Congenital abnormalities of the erythrocyte membrane are becoming better understood. In elliptocytosis and hereditary spherocytosis, the membrane is more permeable to cations and more susceptible to lipid loss when cell energy is depleted than is the membrane of a normal red blood cell. Both hereditary spherocytosis (present in 1 in 5000 people) and hereditary elliptocytosis are inherited as autosomal dominant traits. In both disorders, defects in the membrane are thought to result from a mutation of spectrin, a structural protein of the membrane cytoskeleton.[891] Although the therapeutic role of splenectomy in these diseases is not fully defined, in severe disease, splenectomy is known to improve the shortened life span of the red blood cell 100% (from 20 to 30 days to 40 to 70 days). Because splenectomy predisposes the patient to gram-positive septicemia (particularly pneumococcal), perhaps patients should be given pneumococcal vaccine preoperatively before predictable bacteremic events. No specific problems related to anesthesia have been reported for these disorders.

Glucose-6-phosphate dehydrogenase (G6PD) deficiency (a gender-linked recessive trait) is also reported to occur in approximately 8% of African-American men.[892] Young cells have normal activity, but older cells are grossly deficient when compared with normal cells. A deficiency in G6PD results in hemolysis of the erythrocyte and the formation of Heinz bodies. Red cell hemolysis can also occur with intercurrent infections or after the administration of drugs that produce substances requiring G6PD for detoxification (e.g., methemoglobin, glutathione, and hydrogen peroxide). Drugs to be avoided are sulfa drugs, quinidine, prilocaine, lidocaine, antimalarial drugs, antipyretic drugs, non-narcotic analgesics, vitamin K analogs, and perhaps sodium nitroprusside.

The autoimmune hemolytic anemias include cold antibody anemia, warm antibody anemia (idiopathic), and drug-induced anemia.[893-895] Cold antibody hemolytic anemias are mediated by IgM or IgG antibodies, which at room temperature and below cause red blood cells to clump. When these patients are given blood transfusions, the cells and all fluid infusions must be warm, and body temperature must be meticulously maintained at 37°C if hemolysis is to be prevented. Warm antibody (or "idiopathic") hemolytic anemia is a difficult management problem characterized by chronic anemia, the presence of antibodies active against red blood cells, a positive Coombs test, and difficulty in crossmatching blood. For patients undergoing elective surgery, autologous transfusions, predeposit of blood with or without erythropoietin stimulation,[870] and blood from rare Rh-negative red blood cell donors or the patient's first-degree relatives (or both) can be used. In emergency situations, the possibility of autotransfusion, splenectomy, or corticosteroid treatment should be discussed with a hematologist knowledgeable in this area.

Drug-induced anemias have three mechanisms. In receptor-type hemolysis, a drug (e.g., penicillin) binds to the membrane of the red blood cell, and the complex stimulates the formation of an antibody against the complex. In "innocent bystander" hemolysis, a drug (e.g., quinidine, sulfonamide) binds to a plasma protein, thereby stimulating an antibody (IgM) that cross-reacts with an erythrocyte. In autoimmune hemolysis, the drug stimulates the production of an antibody (IgG) that cross-reacts with the erythrocyte. Drug-induced hemolytic anemias generally cease when therapy with the drug ends. In emergency situations, the least incompatible cells available should be used for blood transfusion.

Granulocytopenia

Granulocyte mechanisms have undergone experimental elaboration in the last decade, partly because of the molecular biologic revolution: in addition to erythropoietin (discussed earlier), more than 14 hemolymphopoietic growth factors or cytokines have been characterized biochemically and cloned genetically. These growth factors interact with cell-surface receptors to produce their major actions[896] (Table 27-49). The use of the colony-stimulating factors has permitted more intense oncologic treatment. The few reports related to their perioperative effects detail

Table 27-49   Major effects of hemolymphopoietic growth factors/cytokines

Cytokine	Other Names	Biologic Effects
Erythropoietin		Erythrocyte production
Interleukin-3 (IL-3)	Multicolony-stimulating factor Stem cell activating factor Persisting cell-stimulating factor Hemopoietin-2	Stimulates proliferation and differentiation of granulocyte, macrophage, eosinophil, mast cell, megakaryocyte, T- and B-cell lineages, and early myeloid stem cells. Interacts with erythropoietin to stimulate erythroid colony formation, stimulates proliferation of AML blasts, and stimulates histamine release by mast cells
Granulocyte colony-stimulating factor (G-CSF)	Differentiation factor MGI-2	Stimulates granulocyte lineage proliferation and differentiation. Acts on early myeloid stem cells, especially in association with other factors; synergizes with IL-3 to stimulate megakaryocyte colony formation. Increases neutrophil phagocytes and antibody-dependent cell-mediated cytotoxicity. Releases neutrophils from bone marrow and is chemotactic for neutrophils and monocytes. Enhances phagocytosis and antibody-dependent cell-mediated cytotoxicity and oxidative metabolism of neutrophils. Stimulates monocyte killing of *Mycobacterium avium-intracellulare* and *Candida* species, tumoricidal activity of monocytes, antibody-dependent cell-mediated cytotoxicity, and expression of cell-surface proteins

(continued)

Table 27–49 Major effects of hemolymphopoietic growth factors/cytokines—cont'd

Cytokine	Other Names	Biologic Effects
Granulocyte-macrophage colony-stimulating factor (GM-CSF)		Stimulates granulocyte, macrophage, and megakaryocyte proliferation and differentiation, early myeloid stem cells, and—in the presence of erythropoietin—erythropoiesis. Enhances cytotoxic and phagocytic activity of neutrophils against bacteria, yeast, parasites, and antibody-coated tumor cells. Increases surface expression of neutrophil adhesion proteins and enhances eosinophil cytotoxicity, macrophage phagocytosis, and basophil histamine release. Amplifies IL-2–stimulated T-cell proliferation and stimulates B-cell lines to proliferate
Colony-stimulating factor-1	Macrophage colony-stimulating factor	Stimulates predominantly macrophage-monocyte proliferation and differentiation with lesser effects on granulocytes. Acts synergistically with other factors on earlier myeloid stem cells. Stimulates macrophage phagocytosis, killing, migration, antitumor activity, and metabolism. Stimulates secretion of plasminogen activator, G-CSF, interferon, IL-3, or tumor necrosis factor by peritoneal macrophages
Interleukin-1 (α and β)	Endogenous pyrogen Hemopoietin-1 Osteoclast-activating factor Lymphocyte-activating factor	Induces synthesis of acute-phase proteins by hepatocytes. Activates resting T cells, cofactor for T- and B-cell proliferation. Chemotactic for monocytes and neutrophils. Induces production of growth factors, including G-CSF, GM-CSF, IL-6, CSF-1, IL-3, and interferon by many cells. Radioprotective in mice
Interleukin-2	T-cell growth factor	Growth factor for T cells, activates cytotoxic T lymphocytes, promotes synthesis of other cytokines, enhances natural killer cell function
Interleukin-4	B-cell stimulating factor-1 B-cell differentiation factor (BCDF) IgG induction factor	Enhances antibody production (IgG and IgE) and upregulates class II MHC molecules and Fc receptors on B cells. Costimulant with anti-IgM antibodies for induction of DNA synthesis in resting B cells. Stimulates growth of activated T cells. In the presence of IL-3, enhances mast cell growth, with G-CSF enhances granulocytes of GM colony formation, and with erythropoietin and/or IL-1 stimulates erythroid and megakaryocyte colony formation
Interleukin-5	Eosinophil differentiation factor (EDF) T-cell replacing factor (TRF) B-cell growth factor-II (BCGF-II) B-cell differentiation factor (BCDF)	Enhances antibody production (IgA). Promotes proliferation and IgG secretion by B-cell lines and induces hapten-specific IgG secretion in vitro by in vivo primed B cells. Promotes differentiation by normal B cells. Stimulates eosinophil production and differentiation (GM-CSF and IL-3 act synergistically with IL-5 to stimulate eosinophil proliferation and differentiation). Enhances synthesis of IL-2 receptors
Interleukin-6	B-cell stimulating factor-2 (BSF-2) Interferon-B₂ T-cell activation factor Hybridoma growth factor	B-cell differentiation and IgG secretion. T cells activated to cytotoxicity. Synergizes with IL-3 on early marrow myeloid stem cells and stimulates proliferation and differentiation of granulocytes, macrophages, eosinophils, mast cells, and megakaryocytes, as well as platelet production (may be a thrombopoietin)
Interleukin-7	Lymphopoietin-1	Stimulates pre–B-cell production. Stimulates T-cell proliferation
Interleukin-8*	Neutrophil-activating factor T-cell chemotactic factor	Inflammatory mediator; stimulates activation of neutrophils
Interleukin-9		Stimulates erythroid colony formation and proliferation of a megakaryocyte cell line
Interleukin-10	Cytokine synthesis–inhibiting factor	Inhibits cytokine production by T_H1 cells
Interleukin-11		Stimulates B-cell, megakaryocyte, and mast cell lineages
C-Kit ligand	Mast cell factor Stem cell factor Hemolymphopoietic growth factor-1	Acts on relatively early stem cells synergistically with other cytokines. Stimulates pre-B cells

*Not considered a true growth factor, but included here for completeness.

AML, acute myeloblastic leukemia; MHC, major histocompatibility complex; T_H1, first of the thymus-derived cells.

Modified from Quesenberg PJ, Schafer AI, Schreiber AD, et al: Hematology. In American College of Physicians: Medical Knowledge Self-Assessment. Philadelphia, American College of Physicians, 1991, p 374.

the adverse consequences that such therapies can have on gas exchange when adverse immunologic effects occur.[897]

In patients who have fewer than 500 granulocytes per milliliter of blood and established sepsis, the use of growth factor and granulocyte transfusion has been shown to prolong life.[898-900] Although bone marrow transplantation is being used increasingly, complications usually occur after transplantation, not on harvesting of cells (at which time the anesthesiologist who is not involved in critical care is most frequently involved). Abnormal results on pulmonary function testing before bone marrow transplantation seem to predict complications after transplantation, but not so strongly as to preclude transplantation.[901]

Platelet Disorders

Although *inherited* platelet disorders are rare, *acquired* disorders are quite common and affect at least 20% of all patients in medical and surgical ICUs, with infections and drug therapies being the leading causes.[902] Both acquired and inherited platelet conditions cause skin and mucosal bleeding, whereas defects in plasma coagulation produce deep tissue bleeding or delayed bleeding.[903] Perioperative treatment of inherited platelet disorders (e.g., Glanzmann's thrombasthenia, Bernard-Soulier syndrome, Hermansky-Pudlak syndrome) consists of platelet transfusions. EACA has recently been used successfully (experimentally, 1 g/70 kg four times daily) to decrease perioperative bleeding in thrombocytopenic patients. The much more common acquired disorders may respond to one of several therapies. Immune thrombocytopenias, such as those associated with lupus erythematosus, idiopathic thrombocytopenic purpura, uremia, hemolytic-uremic syndrome, platelet transfusions, heparin, and thrombocytosis, may respond to steroids, splenectomy, platelet pheresis, eradication of *Helicobacter pylori,* or alkylating agents or may require platelet transfusions, plasma exchange, whole blood exchange, or transfusion; sometimes these disorders do not respond to anything.[470,903-906] Traditionally, splenectomy is performed when steroid therapy fails or reaches a dosage that poses unacceptable risks of toxicity. Newer agents such as anti-D immune globulin and rituximab may induce desirable remissions in idiopathic thrombocytopenic purpura without splenectomy.

Thrombotic thrombocytopenic purpura is a rare disorder of unknown cause. Despite various therapies, this disorder carries a very high mortality rate. However, the introduction of plasmapheresis has improved response rates dramatically in patients with this disease. One uncontrolled study implies that the benefit lies not only in improvement of the hematologic picture but also in prevention of adult respiratory distress syndrome, a leading cause of death in these patients.[906] In that study, early institution of plasmapheresis improved oxygenation.

By far the largest number of platelet abnormalities consists of drug-related defects in the aggregation and release of platelets. Aspirin irreversibly acetylates platelet cyclooxygenase, the enzyme that converts arachidonic acid to prostaglandin endoperoxidases. Because cyclooxygenase is not regenerated in the circulation within the life span of the platelet and because this enzyme is essential for the aggregation of platelets, one aspirin may affect platelet function for a week. All other drugs that inhibit platelet function (e.g., vitamin E, indomethacin, sulfinpyrazone, dipyridamole, tricyclic antidepressant drugs, phenothiazines, furosemide, steroids) do not inhibit cyclooxygenase function irreversibly; these drugs disturb platelet function for only 24 to 48 hours. If emergency surgery is needed before the customary 8-day period for platelet regeneration after aspirin therapy or if the 2-day period for other drugs has not elapsed, administration of 2 to 5 U of platelet concentrates will return platelet function in a 70-kg adult to an adequate level and platelet-induced clotting dysfunction to normal.[903,907] Only 30,000 to 50,000 normally functioning platelets/mL are needed for normal clotting. Because low-dose aspirin therapy (<650 mg/day) allows aspirin to be gone from the body 24 hours after the last dose and because the body makes 70,000 platelets/mL blood per day, a 48-hour period after the last aspirin in minidose therapy should be sufficient time for platelet aggregation to become normal. This may be the time period that must pass to avoid platelet transfusions and their associated risks. One platelet transfusion will increase the platelet count from 4000 to 20,000/mL blood; the platelet half-life is about 8 hours.[903,907] Although designer aspirin that affects only one part of the cyclooxygenase tree may soon be available, the form that is most likely to be used may cause clotting disturbances (without the GI effects, however) that are equal to those caused by the currently available form of aspirin.

Heparin-induced thrombocytopenia can develop within hours on re-exposure to heparin in a previously sensitized patient. Lepirudin and argatroban are new direct thrombin inhibitors effective in therapy for heparin-induced thrombocytopenia.[908]

Major risk factors for thrombosis include factor V Leiden and prothrombin 20210A mutations, elevated plasma homocysteine, and the antiphosphoid antibody syndrome.[909,910] Clinicians facing these challenging patients might seek expert local consultation for help with management.

Hemophilia and Related Clotting Disorders

Abnormalities in blood coagulation as a result of defects in plasma coagulation factor are either inherited or acquired. Inherited disorders include X-linked hemophilia A (a defect in factor VIII activity), von Willebrand's diseases (defect in the von Willebrand component of factor VIII), hemophilia B (a sex-linked deficiency of factor IX activity), and other less common disorders. The sex-linked origin of some of these disorders means that hemophilia occurs almost exclusively in the male offspring of female carriers; men do not transmit the disease to their male offspring.

In elective surgery, levels of the deficient coagulation factor should be assayed 48 hours before surgery and the level restored to 40% of normal before surgery. One unit of factor concentrate per kilogram of body weight normally increases the factor concentration by 2%. Thus, in an individual essentially devoid of activity, administration of 20 U/kg body weight would be required as an initial dose. Because the half-life is 6 to 10 hours for factor VIII and 8 to 16 hours for factor IX, approximately 1.5 U/hr/kg of factor VIII or 1.5 U/2 hr/kg of factor IX should be given. Additional administration of factors VIII and IX should be guided by the activity of the clotting factors for about 6 to 10 days postoperatively.[911-913]

These factors are available in various preparations: the newer genetically engineered von Willebrand factor, cryoprecipitate, which contains 20 U/mL, is obtained from regular donors (the risk of hepatitis being 1:200 for 5-mL lots) or from fresh frozen plasma (which contains 1 U/mL). Some risk of transmitting hepatitis and AIDS accompanies transfusion but, with better testing, much less than formerly.[914-918] Current screening of blood for AST or ALT levels is believed to result in a much lower risk of hepatitis C and even AIDS from transfusion. Theoretically, antigenic testing for HIV should further decrease the risk of transmission by blood products. Heat treatment is also reported to reduce the risk substantially. Factor IX, but not factor VIII is contained in prothrombin complex concentrates; however, these concentrates may contain activated clotting factors, which can lead to disseminated intravascular coagulation (DIC) and a high risk of hepatitis. In addition, although EACA or tranexamic acid (0.5 mg/kg) is sometimes administered as a fibrinolytic inhibitor, these substances carry with them a significant risk of DIC. Additional hazards of modern therapy include acute and chronic hepatitis, AIDS, hypersensitivity reactions, psychic trauma, chronic pain with narcotic addiction, and inhibition of factors, especially VIII.

An antibody that inactivates factor VIII or IX (fresh frozen plasma fails to increase clotting factor activity after incubation with the patient's plasma) develops in approximately 10% of patients with either hemophilia A or B. These acquired anticoagulants are usually composed of IgG, are poorly removed by plasmapheresis, and are variably responsive to immunosuppressive drugs. The use of prothrombin complex concentrates can be lifesaving but carries the risk of DIC and hepatitis.

Vitamin K deficiency is discussed in the section on liver disease. To review, vitamin K–dependent clotting factors (II, VII, IX, and X) require vitamin K for the postsynthetic addition of γ-carboxyl groups to glutamate residues; administration of vitamin K or fresh frozen plasma can correct these deficiencies.

Patients who come to the operating room after having received many units of blood (as in massive GI bleeding) may have deficient clotting. This impaired clotting is initially caused by depletion of platelets, which occurs after approximately 10 to 15 U of blood has been given, and later, by depletion of coagulation factors[919,920] (see Chapter 47). Treatment of these deficiencies can be corrected with platelet concentrates—each concentrate is normally suspended in 50 mL of fresh plasma; thus, coagulation factors are also replaced.

Urokinase, streptokinase, and tissue plasminogen activator (t-PA) have been used to treat pulmonary embolism, deep venous thrombosis, stroke, and arterial occlusive disease. These drugs accelerate the lysis of thrombi and emboli, in contrast to heparin, which may prevent, but not dissolve a thrombus. Bleeding complications associated with these fibrinolytic agents are the result of dissolution of hemostatic plugs and can be quickly reversed by discontinuing the medication and replenishing plasma fibrinogen with cryoprecipitate or plasma. However, cryoprecipitate and plasma are seldom needed preoperatively because the fibrinolytic activity of urokinase and streptokinase usually dissipates within 1 hour of discontinuing their administration. Nonetheless, insufficient data have accumulated to prescribe the ideal preoperative preparation and intraoperative management of hemostasis in patients recently treated with urokinase, streptokinase, or t-PA. Postponing surgery for three half-lives of the drug (increases in plasmin activity in blood can be assayed for ≥ 4 to 8 hours) may not be possible, and meticulous observation of the operative field for hemostasis may not suffice.[921,922] The process may be even more complex in a vascular or cardiac patient who requires heparin administration intraoperatively. To correct fibrinogen deficiency in these patients, some clinicians administer fibrinogen before surgery and EACA at heparin administration. We usually delay or avoid giving EACA until heparin is administered in an effort to minimize the risk of thrombosis.

Desmopressin is now being tried in operations associated with high blood loss as a routine measure to decrease bleeding and transfusion requirements. Desmopressin therapy began as treatment of platelet dysfunction in von Willebrand's disease but has since expanded to routine use in patients undergoing cardiovascular surgery and frequent use in other high–blood loss operations. This increased use was prompted by the finding that desmopressin decreases bleeding and transfusion requirements.[923] Whether the side effects of desmopressin exceed the benefits remains to be determined and will probably influence how routine its administration becomes.

The problem of patients taking oral anticoagulants is discussed in the cardiovascular section of this chapter.[462-475, 478-481] Regional anesthetic techniques might be avoided in patients given anticoagulant drugs.[462-475,478-481] Whether these regional techniques should also be avoided in patients treated prophylactically with low-dose subcutaneous heparin has not been studied. The effects of heparin sulfate can be reversed by titrating protamine with the activated clotting time used as a guide. Our group usually gives approximately 1 mg of protamine per 3 to 4 mg of heparin administered within the last 8 hours. Pharmacologic research is searching for specific molecular subtypes of heparin that have different anticoagulant potencies, binding affinities for antithrombin III, antithrombotic effects, and platelet aggregating effects (see the pulmonary section in this chapter on prophylaxis for deep venous thrombosis). The search is for a "new" heparin preparation that will block thrombosis without causing clinical bleeding (see earlier). Such a development might change our ways of monitoring clotting function. As of now, the new heparins appear to increase the risk of epidural hematoma. Determining the bleeding time, platelet count, partial thromboplastin time, and PT will identify almost all problems in patients with a suspected clotting or bleeding disorder (also see Chapter 47). As explained in Chapter 25, these screening tests should probably not be obtained for asymptomatic patients.

Oncologic Disease

Patients with malignant tumors may be otherwise healthy or may be desperately ill with nutritional, neurologic, metabolic, endocrinologic, electrolyte, cardiac, pulmonary, renal, hepatic, hematologic, or pharmacologic disabilities. Thus, determining the other disabilities accompanying malignant tumors requires evaluation of all systems. Abnormalities frequently accompanying such tumors include hypercalcemia either by direct bone invasion or by ectopic elaboration of parathyroid hormone or other bone-dissolving substance, uric acid nephropathy, hyponatremia (especially with small cell, or oat cell, carcinoma of the lung), nausea, vomiting, anorexia and cachexia, fever, tumor-induced hypoglycemia, intracranial metastases (10% to 20% of all cancers), peripheral nerve or spinal cord disorders, meningeal carcinomatosis, toxic neuropathies secondary to anticancer therapy, and paraneoplastic neurologic syndromes (dermatomyositis, Eaton-Lambert syndrome, myopathics, and distal neuropathies).

Many patients with malignant tumors are given large doses of analgesics and should be kept comfortable during the perioperative period. Avoiding drug dependence is of no practical importance in terminally ill patients.[924,925] Marijuana (tetrahydrocannabinol) depresses the CNS vomiting center and may be more effective than the phenothiazines or butyrophenones in suppressing the nausea associated with cancer and its therapy; marijuana decreases anesthetic requirements 15% to 30%.[926] Immunomodulators, stimulating factors or cytokines, gene identification,[927,928] and drugs for treating side effects (e.g., midazolam or ondansetron) have given new hope for safer, more effective therapy with fewer limiting side effects. The effect of ondansetron in preventing vomiting and the effect of midazolam in preventing "memory-stimulated vomiting" have been important additions.

The toxicity of cancer chemotherapy is related to the drugs used and the dose. For radiation therapy, damage occurs when the following doses are exceeded: lungs, 1500 rad; kidneys, 2400 rad; heart, 3000 rad; spinal cord, 4000 rad; intestine, 5500 rad; brain, 6000 rad; and bone, 7500 rad. The toxicities of biologic and immunomodulating therapies are related to the change in immune function that they cause.[621,896,897,899] Alkylating agents cause bone marrow depression, including thrombocytopenia, as well as alopecia, hemorrhagic cystitis, nausea, and vomiting. The alkylating agents, including cyclophosphamide and mechlorethamine, can act as anticholinesterase and prolong neuromuscular blockade.[929] The antineoplastic alkaloid vincristine produces peripheral neuropathy and SIADH, and vinblastine produces myelotoxicity. Cisplatin is also associated with peripheral neuropathy and severe nausea. Nitrosoureas can produce severe hepatic and renal damage, as well as bone marrow toxicity, myalgia, and paresthesia. Folic acid analogs such as methotrexate have been linked to bone marrow depression, ulcerative stomatitis, pulmonary interstitial infiltrates, GI toxicity, and occasionally, severe liver dysfunction. Fluorouracil and floxuridine, both pyrimidine analogs, cause bone marrow toxicity, megaloblastic anemia, nervous system dysfunction, and hepatic and GI alterations. Purine analogs (mercaptopurine, thioguanine) have bone marrow depression as their primary toxic effect. Anthracycline antibiotics (doxorubicin, daunorubicin, mithramycin, mitomycin C, bleomycin) can all cause pulmonary infiltrates; cardiomyopathy (especially doxorubicin and daunorubicin); myelotoxicity; and GI, hepatic, and renal disturbances.

The wisdom of anesthetizing patients given bleomycin has been questioned. A retrospective study by Goldiner and coauthors[930] reported postoperative deaths in five consecutive patients given bleomycin. All five patients died of postoperative respiratory failure. Using the same anesthetic technique, Goldiner and coworkers[930] then anesthetized 12 patients, limited the inspired oxygen concentration to 22% to 25% perioperatively, and replaced much of the blood loss with colloids rather than crystalloids. None of the 12 patients died. These investigators postulated that bleomycin caused epithelial cell edema that progressed to necrosis of type I alveolar cells, fluid leakage into the alveolar space, and the formation of "hyaline membranes" similar to that associated with oxygen toxicity.[931] Goldiner and colleagues[930] believe that this pathophysiologic similarity indicates a possible synergistic relationship between oxygen and bleomycin. However, LaMantia and coworkers[932] retrospectively analyzed the changes in 16 patients undergoing surgery after bleomycin therapy. Thirteen patients were given oxygen at inspired concentrations of 37% to 45%. No instances of postoperative respiratory failure occurred. Animal data do not support this effect of bleomycin in altering the toxicity of hyperoxia.[933] Thus, data are currently available to support all practices regarding oxygen administration to patients given bleomycin. We prefer to keep inspired oxygen concentrations at the lowest level that provides adequate tissue oxygenation. When in doubt about side effects in patients undergoing cancer chemotherapy, our practice is to seek advice from two experts.

PATIENTS GIVEN DRUG THERAPY FOR CHRONIC AND ACUTE MEDICAL CONDITIONS

A steadily increasing number of potent drugs are being used to treat disease, and the average hospitalized patient receives more than 10 drugs. Many drugs have side effects that might make anesthesia more risky or patient management more difficult. Knowing the pharmacologic properties and potential side effects of commonly used drugs helps the anesthesiologist avoid pitfalls during anesthesia and surgery.

The first step in avoiding these pitfalls is to obtain a drug history from the patient, including vitamins, herbs, and supplements.[26,934] Then, for every drug, medicine, and over-the-counter preparation that the patient is using, the anesthesiologist should know the name, classification of drug, diseases and conditions for which it is prescribed, and common side effects. Having this knowledge before surgery helps the anesthesiologist avoid making mistakes that might turn minor side effects into life-threatening situations. If necessary, the anesthesiologist should return to the patient's bedside to search for signs or symptoms of these effects. Unnecessary drugs should be discontinued for at least three and preferably five half-lives of the drugs. This period should be longer if metabolites of the drug have activity and longer half-lives. For essential or beneficial drugs, the optimal dose should be determined in consultation with the treating physician; the optimal dose is that maximizing the ratio of therapeutic value to the risk of drug toxicity. Side effects should be sought and either corrected preoperatively or at least planned for in anesthetic management. For instance, if a patient is made hypokalemic with diuretic drugs, hypokalemia might be corrected before surgery; an even better approach would be to avoid hyperventilation during surgery (see the earlier section on hypokalemia). This line of reasoning and planning is best done at least 1 week before surgery. Ideally, the surgeon, internist, primary care practitioner, and anesthesiologist should communicate regarding these topics well in advance of surgery. Understanding the side effects of chronic drug therapy that affect the sympathetic nervous system requires some knowledge of the basic pharmacologic characteristics of the sympathetic nervous system.[811,812]

Pharmacologic Processes in the Sympathetic Nervous System

The autonomic nervous system is discussed in detail in Chapter 16. Although that review is comprehensive, it is important to remember several points related to the pharmacology of the sympathetic nervous system when considering chronic drug therapy.

Norepinephrine, dopamine, and epinephrine exert their physiologic effect by interacting with an appropriate receptor at the target tissue. The primary receptor acts through intermediary messenger systems (including cyclic 3′,5′-adenosine monophosphate [cAMP] or G-stimulatory or G-inhibitory proteins, or both) or can change the conformation (and hence the affinity for ligands) of bordering or neighboring receptors. These bordering or neighboring receptor effects may account for many of the multitude of effects associated with catecholamines. The three major types of catecholamine receptors are α-adrenergic, β-adrenergic, and dopaminergic. These receptors are subdivided as follows:

α_1-*Receptor:* Stimulation constricts vascular smooth muscle and thus increases peripheral vascular resistance.

α_2-*Receptor:* Stimulation inhibits the release of norepinephrine itself (constituting negative feedback to the sympathetic neuron). These receptors are largely presynaptic, although postsynaptic vasoconstricting α_2-receptors exist on blood vessels.

β_1-*Receptor:* Stimulation increases the heart rate and the strength of cardiac contractions.

β_2-*Receptor:* Stimulation causes dilation of smooth muscles of the blood vessels and airway, relaxation of uterine smooth muscle, and a variety of endocrine effects, including secretion of renin.

β_3-*Receptor:* Stimulation results in greater release of norepinephrine from the sympathetic neuron (constituting positive feedback to the sympathetic neuron).

DA_1-*receptor:* Stimulation causes dilation of vascular smooth muscle, notably in renal and mesenteric blood vessels.

DA_2-*receptor:* Stimulation inhibits the release of norepinephrine (presynaptic) and may also inhibit, through its ganglionic actions, the release of acetylcholine. The class of dopamine receptors involved in locomotion, inhibition of intestinal motility (antagonism of which accounts for the increase in gastric emptying by metoclopramide), and vomiting is not known. These different effects may be caused by slight differences in receptor conformations.

The action of sympathomimetic substances is terminated through an unusual process: the nerve ending uses an active reuptake system to recapture most of the norepinephrine from the target tissue (see Chapter 16). Obviously, blockage of this system permits more norepinephrine to remain free to produce physiologic effects. In addition to this reuptake system, two enzymes transform catecholamines metabolically: monoamine oxidase (MAO) and catechol-O-methyltransferase (COMT) (see Chapter 16).

Antihypertensive Drugs

Many antihypertensive drugs and almost all mind-altering drugs affect sympathetic neuronal storage, uptake, metabolism, or release of neurotransmitters. For instance, the antihypertensive drug reserpine depletes the granules of norepinephrine, epinephrine, and dopamine in both the brainstem and periphery. Depletion of transmitters in sympathetic nerve endings renders drugs such as ephedrine and metaraminol ineffective because these drugs act primarily by releasing catecholamines (Fig. 27-21). Guanethidine and guanadrel deplete granular norepinephrine and affect only the peripheral sympathetic system. In amounts used clinically, reserpine decreases MAC by 20% to 30%, whereas guanethidine has no effect on anesthetic requirements.[287] In addition to causing a lack of response to indirect-acting vasopressors, reserpine can cause denervation supersensitivity and hyperresponsiveness (with

Figure 27–21 Antihypotensive drugs such as metaraminol (Aramine), tyramine, and ephedrine create their effect by releasing catecholamines from the granules of the nerve terminal. Therefore, when treatment with drugs such as methyldopa, reserpine, or guanethidine depletes the store of norepinephrine (NE) in the granules, little NE remains for release, and the antihypotensive drugs have been rendered ineffective.

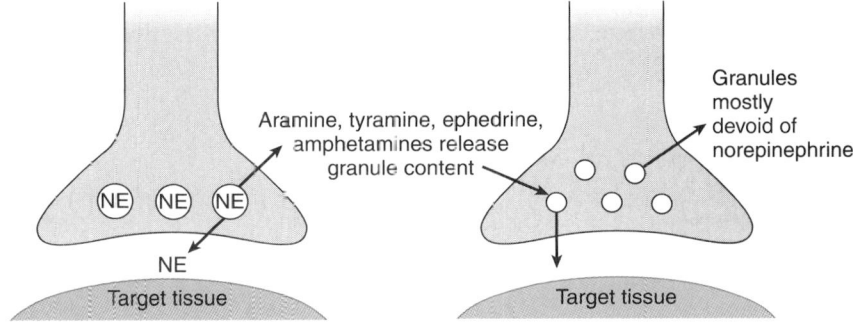

hypertension or tachycardia, or both) to the usual doses of direct-acting sympathetic amines, such as phenylephrine (Neo-Synephrine), isoproterenol, norepinephrine, epinephrine, and dopamine.[933,935-938] Thus, in patients who have been treated with drugs that alter sympathetic neurotransmitter release, uptake, metabolism, or receptor function, some problems may occur: hypotension, hypertension, and bradycardia should be treated by titrating doses of direct-acting vasoconstrictors such as phenylephrine, vasodilators such as nitroprusside, or chronotropic drugs such as atropine, isoproterenol, or dopamine.

Another group of antihypertensive drugs consists of "false neurotransmitters." False neurotransmitters replace norepinephrine in the granules at the nerve ending. α-Methyldopa (Aldomet) becomes α-methyldopamine, which is further metabolized to α-methyl norepinephrine (Fig. 27-22). In some nerve endings and for some receptors, α-methyldopamine or α-methylnorepinephrine is more potent than dopamine or norepinephrine as dopaminergic or α-adrenergic receptor stimulants. However, at most nerve endings, the false neurotransmitters are less potent stimulants; this lower degree of stimulation is one means by which their antihypertensive action is produced. Alternatively, α-methyldopa may act by stimulating the brainstem sympathetic nervous system. When this system antagonizes the peripheral sympathetic nervous system, the activity of the latter decreases and BP is reduced. Through its central effect, α-methyldopa decreases anesthetic requirements 20% to 40%.[287]

In addition to altering the response to exogenously administered vasopressors, these neurotransmitter-depleting drugs can also produce side effects: psychic depression, nightmares, drowsiness, nasal stuffiness, diarrhea, bradycardia, and orthostatic hypotension with impotence (reserpine).[938,939] Guanethidine and guanadrel can cause orthostatic hypotension, bradycardia, asthma, diarrhea, and inhibition of ejaculation. α-Methyldopa is associated with drowsiness, orthostatic hypotension, bradycardia, diarrhea, acute or chronic hepatitis, cirrhosis, and autoimmune hemolytic anemia (i.e., a positive Coombs test result).[938] Because of these side effects, ACE inhibitors (captopril, enalapril, lisinopril, enalaprilat, and

ramipril) and angiotensin II receptor blockers are being used increasingly as first-line drugs and appear to improve the quality of life of patients taking antihypertensive drugs.[324] One of the angiotensin II receptor blockers—valsartan—when combined with a diuretic, actually increases libido in both men and women while decreasing BP. However, ACE inhibitors and angiotensin II receptor blockers may be associated with more peripheral vasodilation and hypotension on induction of anesthesia than sympatholytics are.[940] Added to this group are the ACE receptor blocking agents. These last two classes of drugs are associated with such severe hypotension with standard anesthetic induction that we discontinue or at least consider discontinuing the use of these drugs preoperatively (see earlier).[331]

Catecholamine or sympathetic receptor blocking drugs affect the three major types of catecholamine receptors: α-adrenergic, β-adrenergic, and dopaminergic. The existence of subdivisions (e.g., β_1 and β_2) suggested the possibility that some drugs would be found to affect only one set of receptors. For example, terbutaline is used more frequently than isoproterenol because terbutaline is said to exert a preferential effect on β_2-receptors (i.e., dilation of bronchial smooth muscle), thereby avoiding the cardiac stimulation produced by drugs that stimulate β_1-receptors. In fact, the selectivity is dose related. At a certain dose, a direct β_2-receptor stimulating drug will affect only those receptors but, at a higher dose, will stimulate both β_1- and β_2-receptors. The effect of a given dose varies with each patient. A certain dose may stimulate β_1- and β_2-receptors in one patient but neither receptor in another patient. More and more selective blocking drugs are being developed in hope of widening the margin between β_1- and β_2- and α-adrenergic effects. Ultimately, however, even more selectivity is desired. It would be advantageous to be able to decrease the heart rate without changing myocardial contractility or to increase contractility without changing the heart rate. Such is the goal of much drug research and the development of dobutamine. However, to date, all such selectivity appears to be dose related, even for dobutamine.[941]

Metoprolol (Lopressor) and atenolol (Tenormin) (both β_1-adrenergic receptor blocking drugs) and propranolol, betaxolol, timolol, esmolol, pindolol, oxprenolol, acebutolol, carteolol, penbutolol, and nadolol are widely available β-adrenergic receptor blocking drugs used for chronic therapy in the United States. Because nadolol has poor lipid solubility, it has a long elimination half-life (17 to 24 hours) and does not cross the blood-brain barrier readily. Although selective β-adrenergic receptor blocking drugs should be more appropriate in patients with increased airway resistance or diabetes, this advantage is apparent only when low doses are used. The use of β-adrenergic receptor blocking drugs has become widespread because these drugs treat everything from angina and hypertension to priapism and stage fright. These drugs appear to decrease morbidity and mortality in patients who have initially survived MI[236,942,943] and to increase perioperative survival (see the earlier section on cardiovascular disease and Chapter 25).[226,310,318]

Propranolol is the current standard for β-adrenergic receptor blocking drugs. Smulyan and colleagues[944] studied

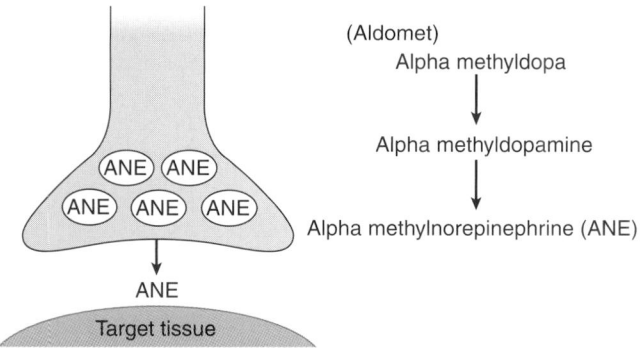

Figure 27–22 In the granules of the nerve terminal, α-methyldopa (Aldomet) is converted enzymatically to α-methyldopamine by the same enzyme that converts dopa to dopamine. α-Methyldopamine is converted to α-methylnorepinephrine by the same enzyme that converts dopamine to norepinephrine.

the problems of long-term propranolol hydrochloride therapy in adult patients who must undergo abdominal surgery. Because these patients cannot take oral medications postoperatively for many days, they must be protected against perioperative sympathetic stimulation and the propranolol withdrawal syndrome. A continuous intravenous infusion of propranolol (3 mg/hr, regardless of the patient's weight) given postoperatively accomplished these goals: postoperative serum propranolol levels and β-adrenergic receptor blockade returned to their "usual" preoperative levels. The hypotensive and bradycardic effects of propranolol and general anesthesia appear to be additive.[945] Because of its shorter half-life (3 to 10 minutes), esmolol has replaced propranolol in critical care (including anesthesia) settings because errors in therapy or side effects, such as increased airway resistance, vanish much more quickly than if propranolol were administered.[946] Propranolol does not affect anesthetic requirements,[947] and one would expect the same lack of effect from other "pure" β-adrenergic receptor blocking drugs. The regimen for atenolol was presented earlier (see Tables 27-20 and 27-21).

α-Adrenergic receptor blocking drugs include phentolamine, prazosin, terazosin, doxazosin, phenoxybenzamine, the phenothiazines, and the butyrophenones (e.g., droperidol). Dopaminergic receptor antagonists include the antischizophrenic drugs (phenothiazines and butyrophenones) and metoclopramide. The receptor blocking drugs inhibit the action of sympathomimetic drugs at the receptor in a dose-related fashion. Thus, propranolol lowers BP by blocking the tendency of norepinephrine and epinephrine to increase the rate and force of contractions of the heart (and perhaps their tendency to increase the secretion of renin as well). To overcome this blockade, one need only provide more β-receptor stimulating drug. Thus, high doses of vasopressors may be needed to increase BP in a patient given large doses of propranolol.

When administration of β-adrenergic receptor blocking drugs is terminated, sympathetic stimulation often increases, as though the body had responded to the presence of these drugs by increasing sympathetic neuron activity. Thus, propranolol and nadolol (to name just two) withdrawal can be accompanied by a hyper–β-adrenergic condition that increases myocardial oxygen demands. Administering propranolol or metoprolol can cause bradycardia, CHF, fatigue, dizziness, depression, psychoses, bronchospasm, and Peyronie's disease.[938,939] Side effects of dopaminergic receptor blocking drugs are discussed later in this chapter. Prazosin (Minipress), terazosin, and oxazocin are α₁-adrenergic receptor blocking drugs used to treat hypertension, ischemic cardiomyopathy, receding hairlines, and benign prostatic hypertrophy because they dilate both veins and arteries and reduce sphincter tone. These drugs are associated with vertigo, palpitations, depression, dizziness, weakness, and anticholinergic effects.

Brainstem sympathomimetic drugs stimulate α-adrenergic receptors in the brainstem. Clonidine (Catapres), a drug with a half-life of 12 to 24 hours, guanabenz, and guanfacine (Tenex) are α₂-adrenergic receptor stimulants. Presumably, α₂-adrenergic agonists, including clonidine, guanabenz, and guanfacine, chronically lower BP through the central brainstem adrenergic stimulation referred to previously. They may also be used chronically to treat opiate,

cocaine, food, and tobacco withdrawal. Occasionally, withdrawal from clonidine can precipitate a sudden hypertensive crisis, analogous to that occurring on withdrawal from propranolol, and cause a hyper–β-adrenergic condition. The degree of hypertensive crisis after clonidine withdrawal is now being debated. (Although intravenous clonidine is not yet available in the United States, a skin patch of clonidine has been approved and is being used preoperatively to ablate sympathomimetic responses perioperatively.) Tricyclic antidepressant drugs and presumably phenothiazines and the butyrophenones interfere with the action of clonidine. Although administration of a butyrophenone (e.g., droperidol) to a patient taking clonidine, guanabenz, or guanfacine chronically could theoretically precipitate a hypertensive crisis, none has been reported. Clonidine administration can be accompanied by drowsiness, dry mouth, orthostatic hypotension, bradycardia, and impotence. Acute clonidine or dexmedetomidine administration decreases anesthetic requirements by 40% to 60%; chronic administration decreases requirements by 10% to 20%.[227,228,306,948] Because of the relative safety of these drugs and their ability to decrease anesthetic requirements, block narcotic-induced muscle rigidity, and provide pain relief, their popularity preoperatively is increasing.[227,228,306,948-954]

Three other classes of antihypertensive drugs affect the sympathetic nervous system indirectly: diuretics, arteriolar dilators, and slow (calcium) channel blocking agents. Thiazide diuretic drugs are associated with hypochloremic alkalosis, hypokalemia, hyperglycemia, hyperuricemia, and hypercalcemia. The potassium-sparing diuretic drug spironolactone is associated with hyperkalemia, hyponatremia, gynecomastia, and impotence. All diuretic drugs can cause dehydration. The thiazide diuretics and furosemide appear to prolong neuromuscular blockade.[955] The arteriolar dilator hydralazine can cause a lupus-like condition (usually with renal involvement), nasal congestion, headache, dizziness, CHF, angina, and GI disturbances. Such a syndrome is nonexistent with the other direct vasodilator on the U.S. market, minoxidil.

The slow-channel calcium ion antagonists ("calcium channel blocking drugs") inhibit the transmembrane influx of calcium ions into cardiac and vascular smooth muscle. Such inhibition reduces the heart rate (negative chronotropy); depresses contractility (negative inotropy); decreases conduction velocity (negative dromotropy); and dilates coronary, cerebral, and systemic arterioles[956] (Fig. 27-23). Verapamil, diltiazem, and nifedipine all produce such effects, but to varying degrees and apparently by similar, but different mechanisms.[956,957] These mechanisms relate to the three different classes of calcium channel antagonists that they represent: the phenylalkylamines, the benzothiazepines, and the dihydropyridines, respectively.[956,957] Nifedipine is the most potent of the three as a smooth muscle dilator, whereas verapamil and diltiazem have negative dromotropic and inotropic effects and vasodilating properties. Diltiazem has weak vasodilating properties when compared with nifedipine and has less AV conduction effect than verapamil does. Thus, verapamil and diltiazem can increase the PR interval and produce AV block. In fact, reflex activation of the sympathetic nervous system may be necessary during the

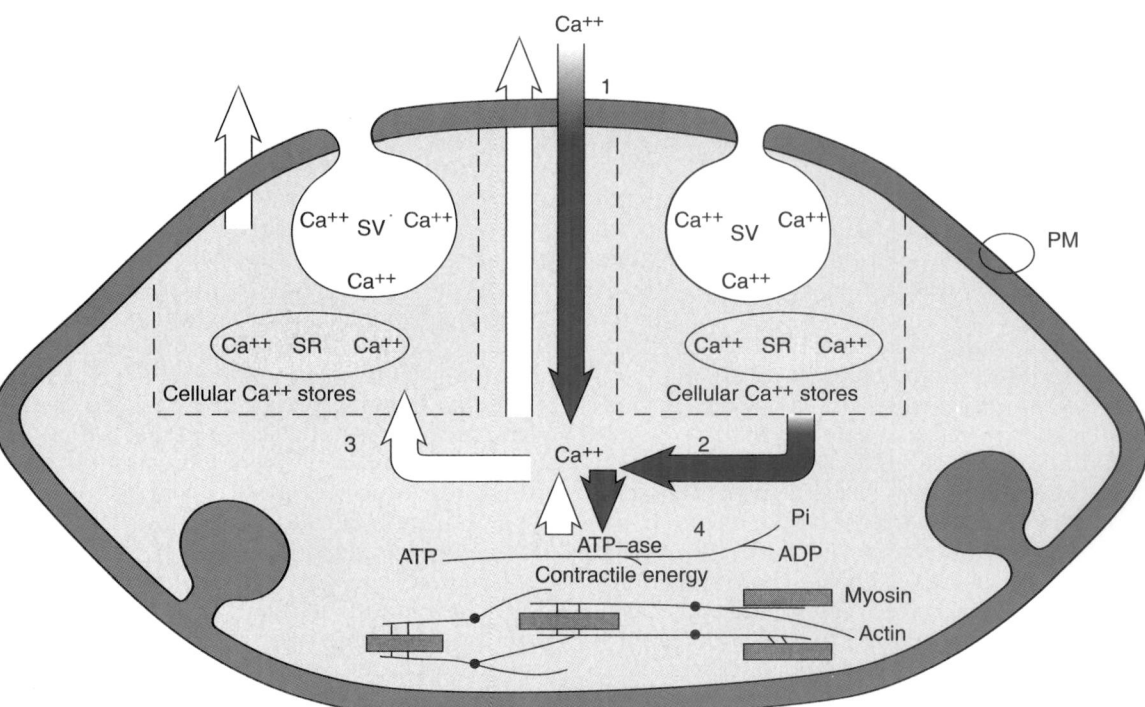

Figure 27–23 Schematic drawing of a smooth muscle cell showing calcium flux and possible sites of interference by halothane and nifedipine. The concentration of calcium (Ca^{2+}) in the cytoplasm increases (*red arrows*) because of entry through the plasma membrane (PM) and release from surface vesicles (SV) or the sacroplasmic reticulum (SR). When the concentration of cytoplasmic Ca^{2+} is sufficiently high, adenosine triphosphate (ATP) is activated. Splitting of ATP by adenosine triphosphatase (ATPase) into phosphatidylinositol (Pi) and adenosine diphosphate (ADP) provides the interaction and contraction of actin filaments and myosin particles constituting muscle fibers. The concentration of cytoplasmic Ca^{2+} decreases (*white arrows*) with the return of Ca^{2+} to cellular stores and the extracellular transport of Ca^{2+}. Both halothane and nifedipine probably (1) inhibit the entry of Ca^{2+} and (2) may also interfere with cytoplasmic Ca^{2+} flux by reducing the release of Ca^{2+} by the SR, by (3) reducing storage and reuptake, or by (4) blocking ATPase or the contractile mechanism (or both). (Redrawn from Tosone SR, Reves JG, Kissin I, et al: Hemodynamic responses to nifedipine in dogs anesthetized with halothane. Anesth Analg 62:903, 1983.)

administration of diltiazem, and especially during verapamil therapy, to maintain normal conduction. Clearly, verapamil and diltiazem must be titrated very carefully when a patient is already taking a β-adrenergic receptor blocking drug or when adding β-blocking drugs to a patient already taking verapamil or diltiazem. Although the increased death rate in patients taking calcium channel blocking drugs as antihypertensive treatment (versus other agents) has cast doubt on their utility, calcium channel blocking drugs are still widely prescribed.

The use of calcium channel blocking drugs has several important implications for anesthetic management.[956,958-968] First, the effects of inhaled and narcotic anesthetics and nifedipine in decreasing systemic vascular resistance, BP, and contractility may be additive.[956,959-962] Similarly, verapamil and anesthetics (inhaled anesthetics, nitrous oxide, and narcotics) increase AV conduction times and additively decrease BP, systemic vascular resistance, and contractility.[960-962,965,968] Second, verapamil and presumably the other calcium channel blocking drugs have been found to decrease anesthetic requirements by 25%.[958] These drugs can produce neuromuscular blockade, potentiate both depolarizing and nondepolarizing neuromuscular blocking drugs, and in at least one type of myopathy (Duchenne's muscular dystrophy), even precipitate respiratory failure.[963,964,966] Finally, because

slow-channel activation of calcium is necessary to cause spasms of cerebral and coronary vessels, bronchoconstriction, and normal platelet aggregation, these drugs may have a role in treating ischemia of the nervous system, bronchoconstriction, and unwanted clotting disorders perioperatively.[963] All three drugs are highly protein bound and may displace or be displaced by other drugs that are also highly protein bound (e.g., lidocaine, bupivacaine, diazepam, disopyramide, and propranolol). Adverse consequences can be minimized by titrating the inhaled or narcotic drug to the hemodynamic and anesthetic effects. By monitoring for side effects, the anesthetist can prevent side effects from becoming serious (S. Slogoff and coworkers, personal communication). Hemodynamic, but not electrophysiologic changes can usually be reversed by administering calcium.[967] Reversal of the electrophysiologic effects may occur if "industrial" doses of β-adrenergic agonists are given.

Mood-Altering Drugs

Mood-altering drugs are the most frequently prescribed medications in the United States. They include monoamine oxidase inhibitors (MAOIs), selective serotonin reuptake inhibitors (SSRIs), phenothiazines, tricyclic antidepressant drugs, other antidepressants that fail previous drug category classification such as bupropion, and drugs of abuse such as cocaine. MAOIs, which include isocarboxazid (Marplan), phenelzine (Nardil), pargyline (Eutonyl), tranylcypromine (Parnate), and deprenyl, bind irreversibly to the enzyme MAO, thereby increasing intraneuronal levels of amine neurotransmitters (serotonin, norepinephrine, dopamine, epinephrine, octopamine). This increase is associated with an antidepressant effect, an antihypertensive effect, an antinarcoleptic effect, elevation of liver enzymes, and delayed onset of Parkinson's disease (deprenyl).[633] Because two forms of the enzyme (MAO-A and MAO-B) are selective in vitro for substrate (MAO-A is selective for serotonin, dopamine, and norepinephrine; MAO-B for tyramine and phenylethylamine), presumably MAOIs selective for MAO-A or MAO-B would have different effects.[969] This is not known for certain inasmuch as deprenyl (selegiline [Eldepryl]), an MAO-B–selective drug, improves a dopamine deficiency state, parkinsonism.[633]

Interactions between MAOIs and a variety of foods and drugs containing indirect-acting sympathomimetic substances such as ephedrine or tyramine (found especially in aged cheeses) can occur for as long as 2 weeks after the last dose of MAOI is given. The most serious effects of this interaction are convulsions and hyperpyrexic coma (particularly after narcotics).

Anesthetic management of a patient given an MAOI can be chaotic; for this reason it is widely accepted practice to discontinue MAOIs at least 2 to 3 weeks before any planned operation.[970-980] An alternative point of view has been expressed regarding severely psychotic patients or emergency surgery.[969,981-983] Clearly, the risk of discontinuing MAOIs must be weighed against the risk of suicidal tendencies in some patients deprived of MAOIs. There are no reported experiences of interactions between narcotics and deprenyl, so judgments about possible worsening of Parkinson's disease and continuing MAOIs have no basis in data. It should be noted that severe reactions have occurred when too short an interval existed between the administration of MAOIs and tricyclic antidepressants.[849] Emergency surgery on patients given MAOIs can be punctuated by hemodynamic instability. A regional block can be attempted as treatment of postoperative pain to avoid having to give narcotics. Cases of hyperpyrexic coma after the administration of most narcotics have been reported in humans, and animal studies document a 10% to 50% incidence of hyperpyrexic coma in animals pretreated with MAOIs and then given a variety of narcotics.[970-980] These reactions appear to be treated best by therapy supporting vital functions.

Alternative drugs for the treatment of severe depression include the tricyclic antidepressant drugs: amitriptyline (Elavil, Endep), imipramine (Tofranil, Presamine), desipramine (Norpramin), doxepin (Adapin, Sinequan), nortriptyline (Aventyl), fluoxetine (Prozac), trazodone (Desyrel), and bupropion (Wellbutrin).[975] Tricyclic antidepressant drugs also block the reuptake of neurotransmitters and cause their acute release. Given chronically, these drugs decrease stores of noradrenergic catecholamines. Tricyclic antidepressant drugs also produce side effects similar to those of atropine (dry mouth, tachycardia, delirium, urinary retention) and can cause changes on the ECG (changes in the T wave, prolongation of the QRS complex, bundle branch block or other conduction abnormalities, or PVCs). Although arrhythmias induced by tricyclic antidepressants have been treated successfully with physostigmine, bradycardia has sometimes occurred.[975] Drug interactions with tricyclic antidepressants include those related to blockade of the reuptake of norepinephrine (such as interference with the action of guanethidine) and fatal arrhythmias after halothane and pancuronium.[984-986] Such interactions, though predictable for a population of patients, may not alter a patient's threshold for arrhythmias. The newer antidepressants (the SSRIs) can also have serious side effects. Fluoxetine, a tricyclic that also has an SSRI effect, causes nausea, vomiting, headaches, nervousness, and possibly paranoia and ideas of suicide more commonly than the other tricyclics do,[975] but it is less likely to cause anticholinergic effects or orthostatic hypotension. Bupropion may cause nausea, vomiting, seizures, agitation, tremor, excitement, and increased motor activity, but only rarely causes anticholinergic effects or orthostatic hypotension. Switching between drugs for depression can cause hyperpyrexia and coma. Thus, switching before surgery should not be requested casually.[975]

The effectiveness of phenothiazines and butyrophenones in schizophrenia suggests a dopamine receptor blocking action. In addition, these drugs possess varying degrees of parasympathetic stimulation and ability to block α-adrenergic receptors. The phenothiazines include chlorpromazine (Thorazine, Chlor-PZ), promazine (Sparine), triflupromazine (Vesprin), fluphenazine (Prolixin), trifluoperazine, prochlorperazine (Compazine), and many others. The butyrophenones include droperidol and haloperidol (Haldol). Both the phenothiazines and butyrophenones produce sedation, depression, and antihistaminic, antiemetic, and hypothermic responses. They are also associated with cholestatic jaundice, impotence, dystonia, and photosensitivity. Other side effects associated with phenothiazines include orthostatic hypotension (partly as a result of α-adrenergic blockade) and ECG abnormalities such as prolongation of the QT or PR intervals, blunting of T waves, depression of the ST segment, and on rare occasion, PVCs and torsades de pointes.[975,985,986] Although few data are available on the antidepressant drugs selective for serotonin (the SSRIs), occasional case reports of severe hypotension and cardiac arrest with severe bradycardia have been presented in abstract form.

Several important drug interactions are noteworthy for the phenothiazine derivatives. The effects of CNS depressants (especially narcotics and barbiturates) are enhanced by the concomitant administration of phenothiazines. In addition, the CNS seizure threshold is lowered by the administration of phenothiazines, which should be avoided in patients who are epileptic or withdrawing from any drug that depresses the CNS. The antihypertensive effects of guanethidine and guanadrel are blocked by tricyclic antidepressant drugs and the phenothiazines.[938] Lithium carbonate is used to treat manic depression, but it is more effective in preventing mania than relieving depression. In excitable cells, lithium mimics sodium and decreases the release of neurotransmitters both centrally and peripherally. Lithium prolongs neuromuscular blockade[987] and may decrease anesthetic requirements because it blocks brainstem release of norepinephrine, epinephrine, and dopamine.

Psychoactive drugs such as amphetamines (including methamphetamines and their smokable derivative in crystal form known as "ice") and cocaine acutely release norepinephrine, epinephrine, and dopamine and block their reuptake. Taken chronically, they deplete the nerve endings of these neurotransmitters.

Drugs that appear to increase central α-adrenergic release increase anesthetic requirements, whereas drugs that appear to decrease central α-adrenergic release decrease anesthetic requirements. (This may not be the mechanism by which they alter anesthetic requirements, but it is a convenient way of remembering the alteration.) Drugs that affect only the β-adrenergic receptors do not alter anesthetic requirements.[227,228,287,947,948,988,989]

Sympathomimetic Drugs (also see Chapter 16)

Many antiasthmatic drugs (bronchodilators) such as terbutaline, aminophylline, and theophylline are sympathomimetic drugs that can interact with volatile anesthetics to cause cardiac arrhythmias. Halothane (and to some degree most other volatile anesthetics) sensitizes the myocardium to exogenous catecholamines.[990-993] Sensitization means that the minimum dose of exogenous epinephrine administered intravenously that is needed to produce PVCs would be lower in patients anesthetized with halothane than in awake patients.

How much epinephrine is safe to give when halothane is the anesthetic? Katz and Bigger[990] reported that the administration of 0.15 mL/kg of a 1:100,000 epinephrine solution per 10-minute period (not to exceed 0.45 mL/kg of a 1:100,000 solution per hour) was safe. Several studies have shown that lidocaine given with epinephrine affords extra protection and that enflurane and isoflurane are less sensitizing than halothane.[991-993] Because halothane is a potent bronchodilator,[994] it may be the best choice for anesthetizing patients with asthma.[995] However, such may not be the case; many asthmatic patients are already taking exogenous catecholamines such as xanthines as chronic bronchodilator therapy.

Xanthines are effective bronchodilators because they produce β-adrenergic stimulation in two ways: they cause release of norepinephrine[996,997] and also inhibit the breakdown of cAMP,[998] the mediator of many of the actions of β-adrenergic receptor agonists.[545] Phosphodiesterase catalyzes the breakdown of cAMP. Thus, inhibition of phosphodiesterase by theophylline increases the concentration of cAMP. Marcus and associates[996] and Westfall and Flemming[997] showed that at least 40% of the inotropic effects of aminophylline are due to its ability to release norepinephrine directly. Experimentally, aminophylline decreases the threshold for ventricular fibrillation.[999]

Plasma theophylline levels of 5 mg/L are needed to reduce abnormally high airway resistance. No further beneficial effects are obtained when levels exceed 20 mg/L; instead, toxic effects appear.[1000] Theophylline (aminophylline is a combination of 85% theophylline and 15% ethylenediamine) is metabolized largely by the liver, with less than 10% being excreted unchanged in urine. The average half-life is 4.4 ± 1.15 hours in adults, and clearance is 1.2 mL/min/kg.[1000] Significant liver disease or pulmonary edema can decrease clearance of the drug by half and by a third, respectively.[1001] Cigarette smokers clear aminophylline more rapidly than nonsmokers do.[1002]

An interaction between aminophylline and halothane appears to be a frequent, predictable occurrence: of 16 dogs anesthetized with 1% halothane and given high-dose bolus injections of aminophylline, 12 had ventricular arrhythmias and 8 had ventricular tachycardia or fibrillation.[1003-1005] Thus, it is advisable to wait three drug half-lives after the last dose of aminophylline is given (i.e., approximately 13 hours in normal individuals) before using halothane to anesthetize an asthmatic patient. Using another anesthetic that is a bronchodilator[994] but is less likely to predispose the patient to catecholamine-induced arrhythmias[991-993] (e.g., enflurane or isoflurane or sevoflurane) or using inhaled or systemic steroids started several days in advance might be alternatives in patients requiring aminophylline or other exogenous sympathomimetic drugs before or during surgery.[1006]

Other Drugs

Drugs other than those discussed earlier in this chapter have implications for anesthetic management. The therapies that have been discussed include anticoagulants and fibrinolytics (in the hematologic section), endocrinologic preparations excluding birth control pills but including corticosteroids (in the section on endocrinologic disease), antihypertensive drugs (earlier in this section and in the section on cardiovascular diseases), anticonvulsant drugs (in the section on neurologic disorders), and cancer chemotherapeutic agents (in the section on oncology).

Antiarrhythmic Drugs

Antiarrhythmic drugs include local anesthetics (lidocaine, procaine), anticonvulsant (phenytoin) or antihypertensive (propranolol) drugs, calcium channel blocking drugs, or primary antiarrhythmic drugs. These drugs are classified into five major categories: local anesthetics that alter phase 0 and phase 4 depolarization (quinidine, procainamide, and flecainide), local anesthetics that affect only phase 4 depolarization (lidocaine, tocainide, phenytoin, encainide), β-adrenergic receptor antagonists, antiadrenergic drugs (bretylium, disopyramide, amiodarone), and calcium entry blockers. These drugs are discussed elsewhere in this chapter and in Chapter 16. A useful reference with suggestions about drug therapy for cardiac arrhythmias and monitoring of side effects was published by the *Medical Letter on Drugs and Therapeutics*.[1007] A lack of adverse reports does not indicate that all these drugs should be continued through the time of surgery; pharmacokinetic studies have not yet determined whether anesthesia (or anesthesia with specific agents) alters the volume of distribution or clearance of these drugs to an extent sufficient to warrant changing the dosage or dosage schedule in the perioperative period. The dearth of reports on this subject may be due to a lack of significant drug interaction or to a lack of awareness that untoward events could be caused by such an interaction.

The pharmacologic characteristics of the various antiarrhythmic drugs can affect anesthetic management.

Disopyramide is similar to quinidine and procainamide in its antiarrhythmic effectiveness. Disopyramide is excreted mainly by the kidneys, but hepatic disease increases its half-life. This drug often produces anticholinergic effects, including tachycardia, urinary retention, and psychosis. Hepatitis has also been reported to have occurred after its use.[1007] Little is known of the interaction of bretylium with anesthetics. Because bretylium blocks the release of catecholamines, chronic therapy with this drug has been associated with hypersensitivity to vasopressors.[1007] Quinidine is dependent on the kidneys for excretion, can produce vagolytic effects that can decrease AV block, and is associated with blood dyscrasias and GI disturbances.[1007] Most of the antiarrhythmic drugs enhance nondepolarizing neuromuscular blockade. Reports have confirmed this enhancement for quinidine, phenytoin, lidocaine, procainamide, and propranolol.[1008-1016] Amiodarone, an antiadrenergic drug used to treat recurrent supraventricular and ventricular tachycardia, causes thyroid dysfunction as a result of the large amount of iodine in its structure (see the section on thyroid disorders earlier in this chapter), as well as peripheral neuropathy, and has been associated with hypertension, bradyarrhythmias, and reduced cardiac output during anesthesia.[1017] The drug has a half-life of 29 days, and pharmacologic effects persist for over 45 days after its discontinuance.[1018] No data document such an effect for depolarizing muscle relaxants.

Antibiotics

Many antibacterial agents are nephrotoxic or neurotoxic (or both), and many prolong neuromuscular blockade (also see Chapter 13).[1010-1016] The only antibiotics devoid of neuromuscular effects appear to be penicillin G and the cephalosporins.[1015] Most enzyme-inducing drugs do not increase the metabolism of enflurane or isoflurane. However, isoniazid appears to induce the microsomal enzymes responsible for the metabolism of at least enflurane, thereby increasing the possibility of fluorine-associated renal damage after enflurane.[1019] Appropriate antibiotic prophylaxis for surgery (see Tables 27-37 and 27-38) requires a knowledge of the probability of infection for that type of surgical procedure and, if the incidence of infection warrants, the use of a drug regimen directed against the most likely infecting organisms.[457]

Digitalis

Digitalis preparations have a limited margin of safety, and the risk of toxicity increases with hypokalemia.[1020] Although there is good rationale for administering digoxin prophylactically before surgery,[574,1021] we generally avoid doing so because potassium concentrations can fluctuate widely during anesthesia as a result of fluid shifts, ventilatory acid-base derangements, and adjuvant treatments[734,770-772] and because intraoperative arrhythmias caused by digitalis toxicity may be difficult to differentiate from those having other sources. Digitalis intoxication can be manifested by such diverse cardiac arrhythmias as junctional escape rhythm, PVCs, ventricular bigeminy or trigeminy, junctional tachycardia, paroxysmal atrial tachycardia with or without block, sinus arrest, sinus exit block, Mobitz type I or II blocks, or

ventricular tachycardia.[1020] However, anesthetics appear to protect against digitalis toxicity, at least in animal studies.[1022-1025] A titrated cardioversion technique using at first 10- and then 20-, 30-, 40-, 50-, 75-, 100-, 150-, and 200-J doses resulted in safe cardioversion in the presence of digitalis and propofol or midazolam hypnosis.[1026] For patients in atrial fibrillation, the ventricular response should guide the choice of dose of digitalis.

Medications for Glaucoma (also see Chapter 65)

Medications for glaucoma include two organophosphates: echothiophate and isoflurophate. These drugs inhibit serum cholinesterase, which is responsible for the hydrolysis and inactivation of succinylcholine and ester-type local anesthetics such as procaine, chloroprocaine, and tetracaine.[1027-1029] These ester-type local anesthetics should be avoided in patients treated with eye drops containing organophosphate. Table 27-50 lists other medications related to anesthesia and their side effects (from the National Registry for Drug-Induced Ocular Side Effects, Oregon Health Sciences University, 3181 SW Sam Jackson Park Road, Portland, OR 97201; 503-279-8456).

Magnesium, Cimetidine, and Oral Contraceptives

Magnesium is given to treat eclampsia; it can cause neuromuscular blockade by itself and potentiates neuromuscular blockade by both nondepolarizing and depolarizing muscle relaxants.[1030,1031] Cimetidine reduces hepatic blood flow and inhibits enzymatic degradation of drugs by the liver. Thus, higher blood levels and prolonged elimination half-lives may result when drugs that are metabolized by the liver (e.g., lidocaine, procaine, some narcotics, and propranolol) are given to patients taking cimetidine chronically or acutely.[1032,1033] The risk of postoperative venous thrombosis increases when oral contraceptives are used preoperatively.[1034,1035] Although some authorities recommend changing from oral contraceptives to topical methods of birth control 2 to 4 weeks before surgery,[1036] no controlled study has determined whether birth control pills should be discontinued before surgery or the resulting incidence of pregnancy. Other authorities recommend preventing venous thromboembolism by using low-dose heparin, guided by a determination of efficacy and cost-effectiveness.[478-480] Because estrogens greatly decrease the incidence of cardiovascular disease and osteoporosis, their use in the elderly is being encouraged.[346] Thus, the uncertainty surrounding prophylaxis for heart disease (created by the dilemma of long-term benefit versus the short-term risk of thromboembolism) needs better data for resolution.

Interrupting a Drug Regimen before Surgery

If a drug is needed for treatment preoperatively, it should be continued through surgery. We provide patients and other professionals with a detailed list (Table 27-51) that we supply through our preanesthesia and preprocedure assessment clinic. It must often be specifically requested because many patients and nurses perceive the NPO directive to include drugs.[1037,1038] The only exception to this general rule of not altering preoperative drug therapy might pertain to (1) MAOIs, (2) anticoagulants and fibrinolytic

Table 27–50   Common ophthalmologic drugs and their anesthetically important interactions

Drug (Trade Name)	Toxicities and Specific Treatments
Glaucoma: Primary goal is to reduce IOP by	
Miotics and epinephrine: increase outflow of aqueous humor	
β-Blockade and carbonic anhydrase inhibitors: reduce production of aqueous humor	
Osmotic drugs: transiently decrease volume	
Miotics	
Parasympathomimetics	
Pilocarpine (Adsorbocarpine, Isopto Carpine, Pilocar, Pilocel)	
Carbachol	
Acetylcholinesterase inhibitors	*Tox:* Hypersalivation, sweating, N/V, bradycardia, hypotension, bronchospasm, CNS effects, coma, respiratory arrest, death
Physostigmine	
Demecarium	*Rx:* Atropine, pralidoxime (Protopam)
Isoflurophate (Floropryl)	*Ix:* Succinylcholine—prolonged apnea (drugs must be discontinued 4 wk before)
Echothiophate (Echodide, Phospholine)	
Epinephrine (Epitrate, Murocoll, Mytrate, Epifrin, Glaucon, Epinal, Eppy)	*Tox:* (rare) Tachycardia, PVCs, HTN, headache, tremors
	Ix: Avoid drugs that sensitize to catecholamines, e.g., halothane
β-Blockers	*Tox:* J-blockade with bradycardia, exacerbation of asthma, CNS depression, lethargy, confusion
Timolol (Timoptic)	
Betaxolol (Betoptic [? β₁ selective])	Synergy noted with systemic drugs
Levobunolol (Betagan)	
Carbonic anhydrase inhibitors	*Tox:* Anorexia, GI disturbances, "general miserable feeling" and malaise, paresthesias, diuresis, hypokalemia (transient), renal colic and calculi, hyperuricemia, thrombocytopenia, aplastic anemia, acute respiratory failure in patients with COPD
Acetazolamide (Diamox)	
Dichlorphenamide (Daranide, Oratrol)	
Ethoxzolamide (Cardrase, Ethamide)	
Methazolamide (Neptazane)	
Osmotic drugs	*Tox:* Dehydration, hyperglycemia, nonketotic hyperosmolar coma (rare). Fatalities with mannitol secondary to CHF or intracranial bleeding
Glycerin (Glyrol, Osmoglyn)	
Isosorbide (Ismotic)	
Urea (Urevert, Ureaphil)	Urea may cause thrombosis
Mannitol (Osmitrol)	
Intraocular acetylcholine (Miochol)	*Tox:* Hypotension, bradycardia
	Rx: Atropine
Mydriatics and cycloplegics: Provide pupillary dilatation and paralysis of accommodation	
Anticholinergics block muscarinic receptors; paralyzing in iris	
α-Adrenergics contract the dilator of the iris	
Anticholinergics	*Tox:* Dry mouth, flushing, thirst, tachycardia, seizure, hyperactivity, transient psychosis, rare coma, and death
Atropine (Atropisol, Bufopto, Isopto Atropine)	
Cyclopentolate, alone (Cyclogyl) or with phenylephrine-homatropine (Cyclomydril)	*Rx:* Physostigmine
Scopolamine tropicamide (Homatrocel, Isopto Homatropine, Isopto Hyoscine, Murocoll #19, Mydriacyl)	
α-Adrenergics	*Tox:* Tachycardia, HTN, PVCs, myocardial ischemia, agitation
Phenylephrine (Efricel, Mydfrin, Neo-Synephrine)	
Hydroxyamphetamine (Paredrine)	

CHF, congestive heart failure; CNS, central nervous system; COPD, chronic obstructive pulmonary disease; GI, gastrointestinal; HTN, hypertension; IOP, intraocular pressure; Ix, interaction; N/V, nausea and vomiting; PVCs, premature ventricular contractions; Rx, treatment; Tox, toxicity.

drugs (e.g., clopidogrel [Plavix]) if surgical hemostasis is needed, (3) nicotinic acid, (4) dosage adjustments for insulin and corticosteroids, (5) ACE inhibitors and receptor antagonists (angiotensin II receptor blocking drugs), and (6) drugs for erectile dysfunction (i.e., sildenafil [Viagra], vardenafil [Levitra], tadalafil [Cialis], or similar drugs). These recommendations require that the anesthesiologist be aware of the pharmacologic characteristics, interactions,

and anesthetic implications of drugs described earlier in this chapter.[331,1039,1040]

When in doubt about a disease or a drug, we consult the following textbooks: *Harrison's Principles of Internal Medicine; Anesthesia and Uncommon Diseases: Pathophysiologic and Clinical Correlations; Anesthesia and Co-Existing Disease; Essence of Anesthesia Practice; Anesthetic Implications of Congenital Anomalies in Children; Pharmacology and*

Table 27–51 Preoperative and preprocedure medication instruction guidelines (PPAC Form 5)

Instruct patients to take the following medications with a small sip of water EVEN IF OTHERWISE NPO:
Antihypertensive medications—Continue on the day of the operation or procedure
Diuretics—Continue on the day of the operation or procedure
Cardiac medications (e.g., digoxin)—Continue on the day of the procedure
Antidepressant, antianxiety, and psychiatric medications—Continue on the day of the operation or procedure
Thyroid medications—Continue on the day of the operation or procedure
Birth control pills—Continue on the day of the operation or procedure
Eye drops—Continue on the day of the operation or procedure
Heartburn or reflux medications (e.g., Prilosec, Zantac)—Continue on the day of the operation or procedure
Narcotic pain medications—Continue on the day of the operation or procedure
Antiseizure medications—Continue on the day of the operation or procedure
Asthma medications—Continue on the day of the operation or procedure
Steroids (oral and inhaled)—Continue on the day of the operation or procedure
Statins (e.g., Zocor, Lipitor)—Continue on the day of the operation or procedure
Aspirin—Usually continue; discontinue 7 days before plastic surgery and surgery on the retina
COX-2 inhibitors—Continue on the day of the operation or procedure unless the surgeon specifies (usually concerned about bone healing)
NSAIDs—Usually continue; discontinue 48 hr before plastic surgery and surgery on the retina
Vitamins, iron, Premarin—Discontinue on the day of the operation or procedure
Topical medications (e.g. creams and ointments)—Discontinue on the day of the operation or procedure
Oral hypoglycemic drugs—Discontinue on the day of the operation or procedure
Insulin—For all patients, discontinue all regular or combination (70/30 preparations) insulin on the day of the operation or procedure. Type 2 diabetics should discontinue *all* insulins of any type. Type 1 diabetics should take a small amount (usually $\frac{1}{3}$) of their usual AM long-acting insulin (e.g., Lente or NPH) on the day of the operation or procedure. Type 1 diabetics should not take any short-acting insulin such as regular insulin on the day of the procedure. Patients with an insulin pump should continue their basal rate *only*.
Viagra, Levitra, Cialis or similar drugs—Discontinue 36 hr before surgery
Warfarin (Coumadin)—Discontinue 4 days before surgery except for patients undergoing cataract surgery without a bulbar block
Plavix (clopidogrel)—Discontinue 7 days before surgery except for vascular patients or those undergoing cataract surgery
Herbals and nonvitamin supplements—Discontinue 7 days before surgery
MAOIs—Patients taking these antidepressant medications need an anesthesia consultation before surgery (preferably 3 wk before surgery)

COX, cyclooxygenase; MAOIs, monoamine oxidase inhibitors; NPO, nothing by mouth; NSAIDs, nonsteroidal anti-inflammatory drugs.

Physiology in Anesthetic Practice; and *Goodman and Gilman's The Pharmacologic Basis of Therapeutics.* It is then wise to consult two experts on the drug or disease and determine who is best able to care for the patient. The expert who is best qualified should be observed while attending to the patient, not only preoperatively and intraoperatively but also postoperatively. It is important to remember that few prospective controlled studies have shown that any preoperative technique, treatment, or management decreases perioperative risk. However, common sense and foreknowledge of potential pitfalls, as well as diligence in avoiding those pitfalls, should reduce avoidable perioperative complications.

KEY POINTS

1. The history and physical examination most accurately predicts the risks and the likelihood of changes in monitoring or therapy.
2. For diabetic patients, end-organ dysfunction and the degree of glucose control in the perioperative and periprocedural periods are the critical issues with regard to risk.
3. The key to managing blood glucose levels in diabetic patients perioperatively is to set clear goals and then monitor blood glucose levels frequently enough to adjust therapy to achieve these goals.
4. Obesity is associated with multiple comorbidities, including diabetes, hyperlipidemia, and chololithiasis, but the primary concern is derangements of the cardiopulmonary system.
5. Obstructive sleep apnea is important to recognize because of the increased sensitivity to and the consequence of depressing the effects of hypnotics and opioids on airway muscle tone and respiration, as well as the difficulty with laryngoscopy and mask ventilation.
6. Although no controlled, randomized prospective clinical studies have been performed to evaluate the use of adrenogenic receptor blocking drugs in patients undergoing pheochromocytoma, the preoperative use of such drugs is generally recommended before surgery.

7. For patients with hypertension, we recommend the routine administration of all drugs preoperatively except angiotensin-converting enzyme inhibitors and angiotensin II antagonists.
8. Evaluation of a patient with cardiovascular disease depends on the clinical risk factors, extent of surgery, and exercise tolerance.
9. In patients with pulmonary disease, the following should be assessed: dyspnea, coughing and production of sputum, recent respiratory infection, hemoptysis, wheezing, previous pulmonary complications, smoking history, and physical findings.
10. In patients with pulmonary disease, several strategies, including cessation of smoking 8 weeks or more before surgery, have been suggested.
11. Risk factors for perioperative renal dysfunction include advanced age, congestive heart failure, previous myocardial revascularization, diabetes, and elevated baseline creatinine.
12. The main concern for a patient with renal disease is making it worse and thereby increasing the chance of renal failure, coma, and death.
13. Mild perioperative anemia may be significant only in patients with ischemic heart disease.
14. Careful management of chronic drug administration can include questions about the effects and side effects of alternative as well as prescription drugs.

REFERENCES

1. Wei JY: Age and the cardiovascular system. N Engl J Med 327:1735, 1992.
2. Medical consultation. *In* Medical Knowledge Self-Assessment Program IX, Part C, Book 4. Philadelphia, American College of Physicians, 1992, p 939.
3. Hamilton WK: Do let the blood pressure drop and do use myocardial depressants! Anesthesiology 45:273, 1976.
4. Roizen M: The preoperative cardiology consult: What the cardiologist should know about anesthesia. *In* Parmley W, Chatterjee K (eds): Cardiology. Philadelphia, JB Lippincott, 1993, p 1.
5. Gluck R, Munoz E, Wise L: Preoperative and postoperative medical evaluation of surgical patients. Am J Surg 155:730, 1988.
6. Wilson SH, Fasseas P, Orford JL, et al: Clinical outcome of patients undergoing non-cardiac surgery in the two months following coronary stenting. J Am Coll Cardiol 42:234-240, 2003.
7. Fleisher LA, Eagle KA: Clinical practice. Lowering cardiac risk in noncardiac surgery. N Engl J Med 345:1677, 2001.
8. Charlson ME, MacKenzie CR, Ales K, et al: Surveillance for postoperative myocardial infarction after noncardiac operations. Surg Gynecol Obstet 167:407, 1988.
9. Goldman L, Caldera DL, Nussbaum SR, et al: Multifactorial index of cardiac risk in noncardiac surgical procedures. N Engl J Med 297:845, 1977.
10. Eagle KA, Berger PB, Calkins H, et al: ACC/AHA guideline update for perioperative cardiovascular evaluation for noncardiac surgery—executive summary: A report of the American College of Cardiology/American Heart Association Task Force on Practice Guidelines (Committee to Update the 1996 Guidelines on Perioperative Cardiovascular Evaluation for Noncardiac Surgery). J Am Coll Cardiol 39:542-553, 2002.
11. Walsh DB, Eckhauser FE, Ramsburgh SR, et al: Risk associated with diabetes mellitus in patients undergoing gall-bladder surgery. Surgery 91:254, 1982.
12. Fowkes, FGR, Lunn JN, Farrow SC, et al: Epidemiology in anesthesia. III. Mortality risk in patients with coexisting physical disease. Br J Anaesth 54:819, 1982.
13. Hjortrup A, Rasmussen BF, Kehlet H: Morbidity in diabetic and nondiabetic patients after major vascular surgery. BMJ 287:1107, 1983.
14. Van den Berghe G, Wouters P, Weekers F, et al: Intensive insulin therapy in critically ill patients. N Engl J Med 345:1359-1367, 2001.
15. Finney SJ, Zekveld C, Elia A, Evans TW: Glucose control and mortality in critically ill patients. JAMA 290:2041-2047, 2003.
16. Krinsley JS: Association between hyperglycemia and increased hospital mortality in a heterogeneous population of critically ill patients. Mayo Clin Proc 78:1471-1478, 2003.
17. The Diabetes Control and Complications Trial (DCCT)/ Epidemiology of Diabetes Interventions and Complications Research Group: Retinopathy and nephropathy in patients with type I diabetes four years after a trial of intensive therapy. N Engl J Med 342:381-389, 2000.
18. UK Prospective Diabetes Study Group: Tight blood pressure control and risk of macrovascular and microvascular complications in type II diabetes. BMJ 317:703-713, 1998.
19. Kenepp NB, Shelley WC, Gabbe SG, et al: Fetal and neonatal hazards of maternal hydration with 5% dextrose before cesarean section. Lancet 1:1150, 1982.
20. Wass CT, Lanier WL: Glucose modulation of ischemic brain injury: Review and clinical recommendations. Mayo Clin Proc 71:801-812, 1996.
21. Reissell E, Orko R, Maunuksela E-L, Lindgren L: Predictability of difficult laryngoscopy in patients with long-term diabetes mellitus. Anaesthesia 45:1024, 1990.
22. Burgos LG, Ebert TJ, Asiddao C, et al: Increased intraoperative cardiovascular morbidity in diabetes with autonomic neuropathy. Anesthesiology 70:591, 1989.
23. Charlson ME, MacKenzie CR, Gold JP: Preoperative autonomic function abnormalities in patients with diabetes mellitus and patients with hypertension. J Am Coll Surg 179:1, 1994.
24. Kalichman MW, Calcutt NA: Local anesthetic–induced conduction block and nerve fiber injury in streptozotocin-diabetic rats. Anesthesiology 77:941, 1992.
25. Eastwood DW: Anterior spinal artery syndrome after epidural anesthesia in a pregnant diabetic patient with scleredema. Anesth Analg 73:90, 1991.
26. Roizen MF: RealAge: Are You As Young As You Can Be? New York, HarperCollins, 1999.
27. Roizen MF: The RealAge Makeover: Take Years off Your Looks and Add Them to Your Life! New York, HarperCollins, 2004.
28. Narayan KM, Boyle JP, Thompson TJ, et al: Lifetime risk for diabetes mellitus in the United States. JAMA 290:1884-1890, 2003.
29. Wingard DL, Barrett-Connor EL, Ferrara A: Is insulin really a heart disease risk factor? Diabetes Care 18:1299, 1995.
30. Yoon J-W, Austin M, Onodera T, et al: Virus-induced diabetes mellitus. N Engl J Med 300:1173, 1979.
31. Tuomilehto J, Lindstrom J, Eriksson JG, et al: Finnish Diabetes Prevention Study Group. Prevention of type 2 diabetes mellitus by changes in lifestyle among subjects with impaired glucose tolerance. N Engl J Med 344:1343-1350, 2001.
32. Inzucchi SE, Maggs DG, Spollett GR, et al: Efficacy and metabolic effects of metformin and troglitazone in type II diabetes mellitus. N Engl J Med 338:867, 1998.
33. Hayward RA, Manning WG, Kaplan SH, et al: Starting insulin therapy in patients with type 2 diabetes. Effectiveness, complications, and resource utilization. JAMA 278:1663, 1997.
34. Coldwell JA: Controlling type 2 diabetes. Are the benefits worth the costs? JAMA 278:1700, 1997.
35. Campbell PJ, Bolli GB, Cryer PE, et al: Pathogenesis of the dawn phenomenon in patients with insulin-dependent diabetes mellitus. N Engl J Med 312:1473, 1985.
36. Stern MP, Rosenthal M, Haffner SM: A new concept of impaired glucose tolerance: Relation to cardiovascular risk. Atherosclerosis 5:311, 1985.

37. Brenner BM: Hemodynamically mediated glomerular injury and the progressive nature of kidney disease. Kidney Int 23:647, 1983.

38. Gottrup F, Andreassen TT: Healing of incisional wounds in stomach and duodenum: The influence of experimental diabetes. J Surg Res 31:61-68, 1981.

39. Grgic A, Rosenbloom AL, Weber FT, et al: Joint contracture— common manifestation of childhood diabetes mellitus. J Pediatr 88:584, 1976.

40. Salzarulo HH, Taylor LA: Diabetic "stiff joint syndrome" as a cause of difficult endotracheal intubation. Anesthesiology 64:366, 1986.

41. Goodson WH III, Hunt TK: Studies of wound healing in experimental diabetes mellitus. J Surg Res 22:221, 1977.

42. Bagdade JD: Phagocytic and microbiological function in diabetes mellitus. Acta Endocrinol (Copenh) 83(Suppl 205): 27, 1976.

43. Nolan CM, Beaty HN, Bagdade JD: Further characterization of the impaired bactericidal function of granulocytes in patients with poorly controlled diabetes. Diabetes 27:889, 1978.

44. McMurry JF: Wound healing with diabetes mellitus. Better glucose control for better wound healing in diabetics. Surg Clin North Am 64:769, 1984.

45. Cruse PJ, Foord R: A 5-year prospective study of 23,649 surgical wounds. Arch Surg 107:206, 1973.

46. Longstreth WT, Inui TS: High blood glucose level on hospital admission and poor neurological recovery after cardiac arrest. Ann Neurol 15:59, 1984.

47. Johnson WD, Pedraza PM, Kayser KL: Coronary artery surgery in diabetics: 261 consecutive patients followed four to seven years. Am Heart J 104:823-827, 1982.

48. Borow KM, Jaspan JB, Williams KA, et al: Myocardial mechanics in young adult patients with diabetes mellitus: Effects of altered load, inotropic state and dynamic exercise. J Am Coll Cardiol 15:1508, 1990.

49. Croughwell N, Lyth M, Quill TJ, et al: Diabetic patients have abnormal cerebral autoregulation during cardiopulmonary bypass. Circulation 82(Suppl IV):IV-407, 1990.

50. Tsueda K, Huang KC, Dumont SW, et al: Cardiac sympathetic tone in anaesthetized diabetics. Can J Anaesth 38:20, 1991.

51. Kitabchi AE, Wall BM: Diabetic ketoacidosis. Med Clin North Am 79:9, 1995.

52. The Diabetes Control and Complications Trial Research Group: Effect of intensive therapy on residual β-cell function in patients with type 1 diabetes in the Diabetes Control and Complications Trial. A randomized, controlled trial. Ann Intern Med 128:517, 1998.

53. Ramanathan S, Khoo P, Arismendy J: Perioperative maternal and neonatal acid-base status and glucose metabolism in patients with insulin-dependent diabetes mellitus. Anesth Analg 73:105, 1991.

54. Kenepp NB, Shelley WC, Gabbe SG, et al: Fetal and neonatal hazards of maternal hydration with 5 percent dextrose before cesarean section. Lancet 1:1150, 1982.

55. Daykin AP: Anesthetic and surgical stress in the diabetic patient: Carbohydrate homeostasis. Int Anesthesiol Clin 26:206, 1988.

56. Walts LF, Miller J, Davidson MB, Brown J: Perioperative management of diabetes mellitus. Anesthesiology 55:104-109, 1981.

57. Peterson L, Caldwell J, Hoffman J: Insulin adsorbance to polyvinyl chloride surfaces with implications for constant-infusion therapy. Diabetes 25:72, 1976.

58. Meyer EJ, Lorenzi M, Bohannon NV, et al: Diabetic management by insulin infusion during major surgery. Am J Surg 137:323, 1979.

59. Farrow SC, Fowkes FGR, Lunn JN, et al: Epidemiology in anaesthesia. II: Factors affecting mortality in hospital. Br J Anaesth 54:811, 1982.

60. Glaser RB: Morbidity and mortality from major vascular surgery. In Roizen MF (ed): Anesthesia for Vascular Surgery. New York, Churchill Livingstone, 1990, p 8.

61. Khuri SF, Daley J, Henderson W, et al: Risk adjustment of the postoperative mortality rate for the comparative assessment of the quality of surgical care: Results of the National Veterans Affairs Surgical Risk Study. J Am Coll Surg 185:315, 1997.

62. Ravid M, Brosh D, Levi Z, et al: Use of enalapril to attenuate decline in renal function in normotensive, normoalbuminuric patients with type 2 diabetes mellitus. A randomized, controlled trial. Ann Intern Med 128:982, 1998.

63. Page MM, Watkins PJ: Cardiorespiratory arrest and diabetic autonomic neuropathy. Lancet 1:14, 1978.

64. Thomas AN, Pollard BJ: Renal transplantation and diabetic autonomic neuropathy. Can J Anaesth 36:590, 1989.

65. Heino A: Operative and postoperative nonsurgical complications in diabetic patients undergoing renal transplantation. Scand J Urol Nephrol 22:53, 1988.

66. Hirsch IB, McGill JB, Cryer PE, White PF: Perioperative management of surgical patients with diabetes mellitus. Anesthesiology 74:346, 1991.

67. Eldridge AJ, Sear JW: Peri-operative management of diabetic patients. Any changes for the better since 1985? Anaesthesia 51:45, 1996.

68. Haffner SM, Lehto S, Rönnemaa T, et al: Mortality from coronary heart disease in subjects with type 2 diabetes and in nondiabetic subjects with and without prior myocardial infarction. N Engl J Med 339:229, 1998.

69. Service J: Hypoglycemias. J Clin Endocrinol Metab 76:269, 1993.

70. Schreider BD, Uitvlugt A, Roizen MF: Anesthesia for patients with insulinoma and other causes of hypoglycemia. Anesthesiol Clin North Am 5:357, 1987.

71. Muir JJ, Endres SM, Offord K, et al: Glucose management in patients undergoing operation for insulinoma removal. Anesthesiology 59:371, 1983.

72. Reubi J-C, Laissue JA: Multiple actions of somatostatin in neoplastic disease. Trends Pharmacol Sci 16:110, 1995.

73. Schaefer EJ, Levy RI: Pathogenesis and management of lipoprotein disorders. N Engl J Med 312:1300, 1985.

74. Larsen ML, Illingworth DR: Drug treatment of dyslipoproteinemia. Med Clin North Am 78:225, 1994.

75. Downs JR, Clearfield M, Weis S, et al: Primary prevention of acute coronary events with lovastatin in men and women with average cholesterol levels. Results of AFCAPS/TexCAPS. JAMA 279:1615, 1998.

76. Shepherd J, Cobbe SM, Ford I, et al: Prevention of coronary heart disease with pravastatin in men with hypercholesterolemia. N Engl J Med 333:1301, 1995.

77. Fowkes FGR, Price JF, Leng GC: Targeting subclinical atherosclerosis. BMJ 316:1764, 1998.

78. Grundy SM, Balady GJ, Criqui MH, et al: Primary prevention of coronary heart disease: Guidance from Framingham. A statement for healthcare professionals from the AHA Task Force on Risk Reduction. Circulation 97:1876, 1998.

79. Campbell NC, Thain J, Deans HG, et al: Secondary prevention in coronary heart disease: Baseline survey of provision in general practice. BMJ 316:1430, 1998.

80. von der Weijden T, Grol R: Preventing recurrent coronary heart disease. We need to attend more to implementing evidence based medicine. BMJ 316:1400-1401, 1998.

81. Knopp RH, Walden CE, Retzlaff BM, et al: Long-term cholesterol-lowering effects of 4 fat-restricted diets in hypercholesterolemic and combined hyperlipidemic men. The dietary alternatives study. JAMA 278:1509, 1997.

82. Rosenson RS, Tangney CC: Antiatherothrombotic properties of statins. Implications for cardiovascular event reduction. JAMA 279:1643, 1998.

83. Nissen SE, Tuzcu EM, Schoenhagen P, et al: Effect of intensive compared with moderate lipid-lowering therapy on progression of coronary atherosclerosis. A randomized clinical trial. JAMA 291:1071-1080, 2004.

84. Flegal KM, Carroll MD, Ogden CL, Johnson CL: Prevalence and trends in obesity among US adults, 1999-2000. JAMA 288:1723-1727, 2002.

85. Fontaine KR, Redden DT, Wang C, et al: Years of useful life lost due to obesity. JAMA 289:187-193, 2003.

86. Andres R: Effect of obesity on total mortality. Int J Obesity 4:381, 1980.

87. Quesenberry CP Jr, Caan B, Jacobson A: Obesity, health services use, and health care costs among members of a health maintenance organization. Arch Intern Med 158:466, 1998.

88. Fox GS, Whalley DG, Bevan DR: Anaesthesia for the morbidly obese. Experience with 110 patients. Br J Anaesth 53:811, 1983.

89. Taylor RR, Kelly TM, Elliott CG, et al: Hypoxemia after gastric bypass surgery for morbid obesity. Arch Surg 120:1298, 1985.

90. Wilson SL, Mantena NR, Halverson JD: Effects of atropine, glycopyrrolate, and cimetidine on gastric secretions in morbidly obese patients. Anesth Analg 60:37, 1981.

91. Rocke DA, Murray WB, Rout CC, Gouws E: Relative risk analysis of factors associated with difficult intubation in obstetric anesthesia. Anesthesiology 77:67, 1992.

92. Illing L, Duncan PG, Yip R: Gastroesophageal reflux during anaesthesia. Can J Anaesth 39:466, 1992.

93. Hardy J-F, Lepage Y, Bonneville-Chouinard N: Occurrence of gastroesophageal reflux on induction of anaesthesia does not correlate with the volume of gastric contents. Can J Anaesth 37:502, 1990.

94. Hudes ET, Marans HJ, Hirano GM, et al: Recovery room oxygenation: A comparison of nasal catheters and 40 percent oxygen masks. Can J Anaesth 36:20, 1989.

95. Vaughan RW, Bauer S, Wise L: Effect of position (semirecumbent versus supine) on postoperative oxygenation in markedly obese subjects. Anesth Analg 55:37, 1976.

96. Strollo PJ, Rogers RM: Obstructive sleep apnea. N Engl J Med 334:99-104, 1996.

97. Young T, Palta M, Dempsey J, et al: The occurrence of sleep-disordered breathing among middle-aged adults. N Engl J Med 328:1230-1235, 1993.

98. Rajala R, Partinen M, Sane T, et al: Obstructive sleep apnoea syndrome in morbidly obese patients. J Intern Med 230:125-129, 1991.

99. Ferretti A, Giampiccolo P, Cavalli A, et al: Expiratory flow limitation and orthopnea in massively obese subjects. Chest 119:1401-1408, 2001.

100. Resta O, Foschino-Barbaro MP, Legari G, et al: Sleep-related breathing disorders, loud snoring and excessive daytime sleepiness in obese subjects. Int J Obes Relat Metab Disord 25:669-675, 2001.

101. Vgontzas AN, Tan TL, Bixler EO, et al: Sleep apnea and sleep disruption in obese patients. Arch Intern Med 154:1705-1711, 1994.

102. van Boxem TJ, de Groot GH: Prevalence and severity of sleep disordered breathing in a group of morbidly obese patients. Neth J Med 54:202-206, 1999.

103. Herer B, Roche N, Carton N, et al: Value of clinical, functional, and oximetric data for the prediction of obstructive sleep apnea in obese patients. Chest 116:1537-1544, 1999.

104. van Kralingen KW, de Kanter W, de Groot GH, et al: Assessment of sleep complaints and sleep-disordered breathing in a consecutive series of obese patients. Respiration 66:312-316, 1999.

105. Serafini FM, MacDowell Anderson W, et al: Clinical predictors of sleep apnea in patients undergoing bariatric surgery. Obes Surg 11:28-31, 2001.

106. Koenig SM: Pulmonary complications of obesity. Am J Med Sci 321:249-279, 2001.

107. Silverberg DS, Iaina A, Oksenberg A. Treating obstructive sleep apnea improves essential hypertension and quality of life. Am Fam Physician 65:229-236, 2002.

108. Benumof JL: Obstructive sleep apnea in the adult obese patient: Implications for airway management. J Clin Anesth 13:144-156, 2001.

109. Peppard PE, Young T, Palta M, Skatrud J. Prospective study of the association between sleep-disordered breathing and hypertension. N Engl J Med 342:1378-1384, 2000.

110. Dhonneur G, Combes X, Leroux B, Duvaldestin P: Postoperative obstructive apnea. Anesth Analg 89:762-767, 1999.

111. Boushra NN: Anaesthetic management of patients with sleep apnoea syndrome. Can J Anaesth 43:599-616, 1996.

112. Ostermeier AM, Roizen MF, Hautkappe M, et al: Three sudden respiratory events associated with epidural opioids in patients with sleep apnea. Anesth Analg 85:452-460, 1997.

113. Hiremath AS, Hillman DR, James AL, et al: Relationship between difficult tracheal intubation and obstructive sleep apnoea. Br J Anaesth 80:606-611, 1998.

114. Siyam M, Benhamou D: Difficult endotracheal intubation in patients with sleep apnea syndrome. Anesth Analg 95:1098-1102, 2002.

115. Langeron O, Masso E, Huraux C, et al: Prediction of difficult mask ventilation. Anesthesiology 92:1229-1236, 2000.

116. Biring MS, Lewis MI, Liu JT, Mohsenifar Z: Pulmonary physiologic changes of morbid obesity. Am J Med Sci 318:293-297, 1999.

117. Rochester DF: Obesity and pulmonary function. *In* Alpert MA, Alexander JK (eds): The Heart and Lung in Obesity. Armonk, NY, Futura, 1998, pp 108-132.

118. Ebeo CT, Benotti PN, Byrd RP, et al: The effect of bi-level positive airway pressure on postoperative pulmonary function following gastric surgery for obesity. Respir Med 96:672-676, 2002.

119. Riley RW, Powell NB, Guilleminault C, et al: Obstructive sleep apnea surgery: Risk management and complications. Otolaryngol Head Neck Surg 117:648-652, 1997.

120. Hnatiuk OW, Dillard TA, Torrington KG: Adherence to established guidelines for preoperative pulmonary testing. Chest 107:1294-1297, 1995.

121. Roche N, Herer B, Roig C, Huchon G: Prospective testing of two models based on clinical and oximetric variables for prediction of obstructive sleep apnea. Chest 121:747-752, 2002.

122. Crapo RO, Kelly TM, Elliott CG, Jones SB: Spirometry as a preoperative screening test in morbidly obese patients. Surgery 99:763-768, 1986.

123. Kessler R, Chaouat A, Schinkewitch P, et al: The obesity-hypoventilation syndrome revisited. A prospective study of 34 consecutive cases. Chest 120:369-376, 2001.

124. Chaouat A, Weitzenblum E, Krieger J: Association of chronic obstructive pulmonary disease and sleep apnea syndrome. Am J Respir Crit Care Med 151:82-86, 1995.

125. Blankfield RP, Hudgel DW, Tapolyai AA, Zyzanski SJ: Bilateral leg edema, obesity, pulmonary hypertension, and obstructive sleep apnea. Arch Intern Med 160:2357-2362, 2000.

126. Bradley TD, Rutherford R, Grossman RF, et al: Role of daytime hypoxemia in the pathogenesis of right heart failure in the obstructive sleep apnea syndrome. Am Rev Respir Dis 131:835-839, 1985.

127. Al-Mobeireek AF, Al-Kassimi FA, Al-Majed SA, et al: Clinical profile of sleep apnea syndrome. Saudi Med J 21:180-183, 2000.

128. Akashiba T, Kawahara S, Kosaka N, et al: Determinants of chronic hypercapnia in Japanese men with obstructive sleep apnea syndrome. Chest 121:415-421, 2002.

129. Tung A, Rock P: Perioperative concerns in sleep apnea. Curr Opin Anaesthesiol 14:671-678, 2000.

130. Alpert MA, Terry BE, Cohen MV, et al: The electrocardiogram in morbid obesity. Am J Cardiol 85:908-910, 2000.

131. Pelosi P, Croci M, Ravagnan I, et al: Respiratory system mechanics in sedated, paralyzed, morbidly obese patients. J Appl Physiol 82:811-818, 1997.

132. Vaughan RW, Cork RC, Hollander D: The effect of massive weight loss on arterial oxygenation and pulmonary function tests. Anesthesiology 54:325-328, 1981.

133. Hakala K, Maasilta P, Sovijarvi AR: Upright body position and weight loss improve respiratory mechanics and daytime oxygenation in obese patients with obstructive sleep apnea. Clin Physiol 20:50-55, 2000.

134. Rochester DF: Obesity and pulmonary function. *In* Alpert MA, Alexander JK (eds): The Heart and Lung in Obesity. Armonk, NY, Futura, 1998, pp 108-132.

135. Berthoud MC, Peacock JE, Reilly CS: Effectiveness of preoxygenation in morbidly obese patients. Br J Anaesth 67:464-466, 1991.

136. Jense HG, Dubin SA, Silverstein PI, O'Leary-Escolas U: Effect of obesity on safe duration of apnea in anesthetized humans. Anest Analg 72:89-93, 1991.

137. Rose DK, Cohen MM: The airway: Problems and predictions in 18,500 patients. Can J Anaesth 41:372-383, 1994.

138. Brodsky JB, Lemmens HJM, Brock-Utne JG, et al: Morbid obesity and tracheal intubation. Anesth Analg 94:732-736, 2002.

139. Voyagis GS, Kyriakis KP, Dimitriou V, Vrettou I: Value of oropharyngeal Mallampati classification in predicting difficult laryngoscopy among obese patients. Eur J Anaesthesiol 15:330-334, 1998.

140. Rosenberg J, Ullstad T, Rasmussen J, et al: Time course of postoperative hypoxemia. Eur J Surg 160:137-143, 1994.

141. Taylor RR, Kelly TM, Elliott CG, et al: Hypoxemia after gastric bypass surgery for morbid obesity. Arch Surg 120:1298-1302, 1985.

142. Vaughan RW, Bauer S, Wise L: Effect of position on postoperative oxygenation in markedly obese subjects. Anesth Analg 55:37-41, 1976.

143. Loadsman JA, Hillman DR: Anaesthesia and sleep apnoea. Br J Anaesth 86:254-266, 2001.

144. Drummond GB, Stedul K, Kingshott R, et al: Automatic CPAP compared with conventional treatment for episodic hypoxemia and sleep disturbance after major abdominal surgery. Anesthesiology 96:817-826, 2002.

145. Reeder MK, Goldman MD, Loh L, et al: Postoperative obstructive sleep apnoea. Hemodynamic effects of treatment with nasal CPAP. Anaesthesia 46:849-853, 1991.

146. Ebeo CT, Benotti PN, Byrd RP, et al: The effect of bi-level positive airway pressure on postoperative pulmonary function following gastric surgery for obesity. Respir Med 96:672-676, 2002.

147. Joris JL, Sottiaux TM, Chiche JD, et al: The effect of bilevel positive airway pressure nasal ventilation on the postoperative pulmonary restrictive syndrome in obese patients undergoing gastroplasty. Chest 111:665-670, 1997.

148. Rennotte MT, Baele P, Aubert G, Rodenstein DO: Nasal continuous positive airway pressure in the perioperative management of patients with obstructive sleep apnea submitted to surgery. Chest 107:367-374, 1995.

149. Tkacova R, Rankin F, Fitzgerald FS, et al: Effects of continuous positive airway pressure on obstructive sleep apnea and left ventricular afterload in patients with heart failure. Circulation 98:2269-2275, 1998.

150. Wilcox I, Grunstein RR, Hedner JA, et al: Effect of nasal continuous positive airway pressure during sleep on 24-hour blood pressure in obstructive sleep apnea. Sleep 16:539-544, 1993.

151. Schwartz AE, Matteo RS, Orstein E, et al: Pharmacokinetics of sufentanil in obese patients. Anesth Analg 73:790, 1991.

152. Weinstein JA, Matteo RS, Orstein E, et al: Pharmacodynamics of vecuronium and atracurium in the obese surgical patient. Anesth Analg 67:1149, 1988.

153. Rosenbaum M, Leibel RL, Hirsch J: Obesity. N Engl J Med 337:396, 1997.

154. Sours HE, Frattali VP, Brand CD, et al: Sudden death associated with very low calorie weight reduction regimens. Am J Clin Nutr 34:453, 1981.

155. Warner MA, Warner ME, Martin JT: Ulnar neuropathy: Incidence, outcome, and risk factors in sedated and anesthetized patients. Anesthesiology 81:1332-1340, 1994.

156. Sawyer RJ, Richmond MN, Hickey JD, Jarratt JA: Peripheral nerve injuries associated with anaesthesia. Anaesthesia 55:980-991, 2000.

157. Goldbloom DS, Kennedy SH, Kaplan AS, et al: Anorexia nervosa and bulimia nervosa. Can Med Assoc J 140:1149, 1989.

158. Donini LM, Savina C, Cannella C: Eating habits and appetite control in the elderly: The anorexia of aging. Int Psychogeriatr 15:73-87, 2003.

159. Arnold DE, Rose RJ, Stoddard P: Intraoperative cardiac dysrhythmias in a patient with bulimic anorexia nervosa. Anesthesiology 67:1003, 1987.

160. Veterans Administration Total Parenteral Nutrition Cooperative Study Group: Perioperative total parenteral nutrition in surgical patients. N Engl J Med 325:525, 1991.

161. Nicholas JM, Cornelius MW, Tchorz KM, et al: A two institution experience with 226 endoscopically placed jejunal feeding tubes in critically ill surgical patients. Am J Surg 186:583-590, 2003.

162. Starker PM, La Sala PA, Askanazi J, et al: The responses to TPN, a form of nutritional assessment. Ann Surg 198:720, 1983.

163. Lampe GH, Roizen MF: Anesthesia for patients with abnormal function of the adrenal cortex. Anesthesiol Clin North Am 5:245, 1987.

164. Hanowell ST, Hittner KC, Kim YD, et al: Anesthetic management of primary aldosteronism. Anesthesiol Rev 9:36, 1982.

165. Rabinowitz IN, Watson W, Farber EM: Topical steroid depression of the hypothalamic-pituitary-adrenal axis in psoriasis vulgaris. Dermatologica 154:321, 1977.

166. Knudsen L, Christiansen LA, Lorentzen JE: Hypotension during and after operation in glucocorticoid-treated patients. Br J Anaesth 53:295, 1981.

167. Cassinello Ogea C, Giron Nombiela JA, Ruiz Tramazaygues J, et al: Severe perioperative hypotension after nephrectomy with adrenalectomy [in Spanish]. Rev Esp Anestesiol Reanim 49:213-217, 2002.

168. Pleym H, Spigset O, Kharasch ED, Dale O: Gender differences in drug effects: Implications for anesthesiologists. Acta Anaesth Scand 47:241-259, 2003.

169. Symreng T, Karlberg BE, Kågedal B, et al: Physiological cortisol substitution of long-term steroid-treated patients undergoing major surgery. Br J Anaesth 53:949, 1981.

170. Udelsman R, Ramp J, Gallucci WT, et al: Adaptation during surgical stress: A reevaluation of the role of glucocorticoids. J Clin Invest 77:1377, 1986.

171. Axelrod L: Glucocorticoid therapy. Medicine (Baltimore) 55:39, 1976.

172. Graber AL, Ney RI, Nicholson WE, et al: Natural history of pituitary-adrenal recovery following long-term suppression with corticosteroids. J Clin Endocrinol Metab 25:11, 1965.

173. Ackerman GL, Nolsn CM: Adrenocortical responsiveness after alternate-day corticosteroid therapy. N Engl J Med 278:405-409, 1968.

174. Streck WF, Lockwood DH: Pituitary adrenal recovery following short-term suppression with corticosteroids. Am J Med 66:910, 1979.

175. Cook DM, Loriaux DL: The incidental adrenal mass. Am J Med 101:88, 1996.

176. Linos DA, Stylopoulos N, Raptis SA: Adrenaloma: A call for more aggressive management. World J Surg 20:788, 1996.

177. Mantero F, Masini AM, Opocher G, et al: Adrenal incidentaloma: An overview of hormonal data from the National Italian Study Group. Horm Res 47:284, 1997.

178. Cook DM: Adrenal mass. Endocrinol Metab Clin North Am 26:829-852, 1997.

179. Volk T, Schmutzler M, Engelhardt L, et al: Effects of different steroid treatment on reperfusion-associated production of reactive oxygen species and arrhythmias during coronary surgery. Acta Anaesthesiol Scand 47:667-674, 2003.

180. Derksen J, Negesser SK, Meinders AE, et al: Identification of virilizing adrenal tumors in hirsute women. N Engl J Med 331:968-973, 1994.

181. Hollenberg NK, Williams GH: Hypertension, the adrenal and the kidney: Lessons from pharmacologic interruption of the renin-angiotensin system. Adv Intern Med 25:327, 1980.

182. Tyrrell JB, Brooks RM, Fitzgerald PA, et al: Cushing's disease. Selective trans-sphenoidal resection of pituitary microadenomas. N Engl J Med 298:753-758, 1978.

183. Dale DC, Fauci AS, Wolff SM: Alternate-day prednisone. Leukocyte kinetics and susceptibility to infections. N Engl J Med 291:1154, 1974.

184. Ehrlich HP, Hunt TK: Effects of cortisone and vitamin A on wound healing. Ann Surg 167:324-328, 1968.

185. Young WF Jr: Pheochromocytoma and primary hyperaldosteronism: Diagnostic approaches. Metab Clin North Am 26:801-827, 1997.

186. Jasani BM, Edmonds CJ: Kinetics of potassium distribution in man using isotope dilution and whole-body counting. Metabolism 20:1099, 1971.

187. Johnson JE, Hartsuck JM, Zollinger RM Jr, et al: Radiopotassium equilibrium in total body potassium: Studies using ^{43}K and ^{42}K. Metabolism 18:663, 1969.

188. Surawicz B, Chlebus H, Mazzoleni A: Hemodynamic and electrocardiographic effects of hyperpotassemia: Differences in response to slow and rapid increases in concentration of plasma K. Am Heart J 73:647, 1967.

189. Rao TLK, Jacobs KH, El-Etr AA: Reinfarction following anesthesia in patients with myocardial infarction. Anesthesiology 59:499, 1983.

190. Oh SH, Patterson R: Surgery in corticosteroid-dependent asthmatics. J Allergy Clin Immunol 53:345-351, 1974.

191. Schambelan M, Sebastian A: Hyporeninemic hypoaldosteronism. Adv Intern Med 24:385, 1979.

192. Oyama T, Taniguchi K, Jin T, et al: Effects of anaesthesia and surgery on plasma aldosterone concentration and renin activity in man. Br J Anaesth 51:747, 1979.

193. Nieman LK, Oldfield EH, Wesley R, et al: A simplified morning corticotrophin-releasing hormone stimulation test for the differential diagnosis of adrenocorticotrophin-dependent Cushing's syndrome. J Clin Endocrinol Metab 77:1308, 1993.

194. Winstone NE, Brooke BN: Effects of steroid treatment on patients undergoing operation. Lancet 1:973, 1961.

195. Migeon C, Keller A, Lawrence B, Shepard T: DHA and androsterone levels in human plasma. Effect of age and sex: Day-to-day and diurnal variations. J Clin Endocrinol Metab 17:1051, 1957.

196. Wagner RL, White PF, Kan PB, et al: Inhibition of adrenal steroidogenesis by the anesthetic etomidate. N Engl J Med 310:1415, 1984.

197. Zurick AM, Sigurdsson H, Koehler LS, et al: Magnitude and time course of perioperative adrenal suppression with single dose etomidate in male adult cardiac surgical patients [abstract]. Anesthesiology 65:A248, 1986.

198. Gagner M, Breton G, Pharand D, Pomp A: Is laparoscopic adrenalectomy indicated for pheochromocytomas? Surgery 120:1076, 1996.

199. Linos DA, Stylopoulos N, Boukis M, et al: Anterior, posterior, or laparoscopic approach for the management of adrenal diseases? Am J Surg 173:120, 1997.

200. Bravo EL: Evolving concepts in the pathophysiology, diagnosis and treatment of pheochromocytoma. Endocr Rev 15:356, 1994.

201. St John Sutton MG, Sheps SG, Lie JT: Prevalence of clinically unsuspected pheochromocytoma: Review of a 50-year autopsy series. Mayo Clin Proc 56:354, 1981.

202. Brown IE, Milshteyn M, Kleinman B, et al: Case 3-2002 pheochromocytoma presenting as a right intra-atrial mass. J Cardiothorac Vasc Anesth 16:370-373, 2002.

203. Witteles RM, Kaplan EL, Roizen MF: Sensitivity of diagnostic and localization tests for pheochromocytoma in clinical practice. Arch Intern Med 160:2521-2524, 2000.

204. Pauker SG, Kopelman RI: Interpreting hoofbeats: Can Bayes help clear the haze? N Engl J Med 327:1009, 1992.

205. Lucon AM, Pereira MAA, Mendonça BB, et al: Pheochromocytoma: Study of 50 cases. J Urol 157:1208, 1997.

206. Desmonts JM, le Houelleur J, Remond P, et al: Anaesthetic management of patients with pheochromocytoma: A review of 102 cases. Br J Anaesth 49:991, 1977.

207. Roizen MF, Horrigan RW, Koike M, et al: A prospective randomized trial of four anesthetic techniques for resection of pheochromocytoma [abstract]. Anesthesiology 57:A43, 1982.

208. Roizen MF, Hunt TK, Beaupre PN, et al: The effect of alpha-adrenergic blockade on cardiac performance and tissue oxygen delivery during excision of pheochromocytoma. Surgery 94:941, 1983.

209. Witteles RM, Kaplan EL, Roizen MF: Safe and cost-effective preoperative preparation of patients with pheochromocytoma. Anesth Analg 91:302-304, 2000.

210. Allen GC, Rosenberg H: Pheochromocytoma presenting as acute malignant hyperthermia—a diagnostic challenge. Can J Anaesth 37:593, 1990.

211. Zakowski M, Kaufman B, Berguson P, et al: Esmolol use during resection of pheochromocytoma: Report of three cases. Anesthesiology 70:875, 1989.

212. Roizen MF, Schreider BD, Hassan SZ: Anesthetic for patients with pheochromocytoma. Anesthesiol Clin North Am 5:269, 1987.

213. Goldstein DS, Holmes C, Cannon RO III, et al: Sympathetic cardioneuropathy in dysautonomias. N Engl J Med 336:696, 1997.

214. Ziegler MG, Lake CR, Kopin IJ: The sympathetic nervous system defect in primary orthostatic hypotension. N Engl J Med 296:293, 1977.

215. Naftchi NE, Wooten GF, Lowman EW, et al: Relationship between serum dopamine-β-hydroxylase activity, catecholamine metabolism, and hemodynamic changes during paroxysmal hypertension in quadriplegia. Circ Res 35:850, 1974.

216. Cohen CA: Anesthetic management of a patient with the Shy-Drager syndrome. Anesthesiology 35:95, 1971.

217. McCaughey TJ: Familial dysautonomia as an anaesthetic hazard. Can J Anaesth 12:558, 1965.

218. Meridy HW, Creighton RE: General anaesthesia in eight patients with familial dysautonomia. Can J Anaesth 18:563, 1971.

219. Stowe DF, Bernstein JS, Madsen KE, et al: Autonomic hyperreflexia in spinal cord injured patients during extracorporeal shock wave lithotripsy. Anesth Analg 68:788, 1989.

220. Gronert GA, Theye RA: Pathophysiology of hyperkalemia induced by succinylcholine. Anesthesiology 43:89, 1975.

221. Jousse AT, Wynne-Jones M, Breithaupt DJ: A follow-up study of life expectancy and mortality in traumatic transverse myelitis. Can Med Assoc J 98:770, 1968.

222. Bevan DR: Shy-Drager syndrome. A review and a description of the anaesthetic management. Anaesthesia 34:866, 1979.

223. Malan MD, Crago RR: Anaesthetic considerations in idiopathic orthostatic hypotension and the Shy-Drager syndrome. Can J Anaesth 26:322, 1979.

224. Roizen MF: Should we all have a sympathectomy at birth? Or at least preoperatively? Anesthesiology 68:482, 1988.

225. Stone JG, Foëx P, Sear JW, et al: Myocardial ischemia in untreated hypertensive patients. Effect of a single small oral dose of a beta-adrenergic blocking agent. Anesthesiology 68:495, 1988.

226. Mangano DT, Layug EL, Wallace A, et al: Effect of atenolol on mortality and cardiovascular morbidity after noncardiac surgery. N Engl J Med 335:1713, 1996.

227. Flacke JW, Bloor BC, Flacke WE, et al: Reduced narcotic requirement by clonidine with improved hemodynamic and adrenergic stability in patients undergoing coronary bypass surgery. Anesthesiology 67:11, 1987.

228. Ghignone M, Calvillo O, Quintin L: Anesthesia and hypertension: The effect of clonidine on perioperative hemodynamics and isoflurane requirements. Anesthesiology 67:3, 1987.

229. Yeager MP, Glass DD, Neff RK, Brinck-Johnsen T: Epidural anesthesia and analgesia in high-risk surgical patients. Anesthesiology 66:729, 1987.

230. Roizen MF, Lampe GH, Benefiel DJ, et al: Is increased operative stress associated with worse outcome [abstract]. Anesthesiology 67:A1, 1987.

231. Fleisher LA, Rosenbaum SH, Nelson AH, Barash PG: The predictive value of preoperative silent ischemia for postoperative ischemic cardiac events in vascular and nonvascular surgery patients. Am Heart J 122:980, 1991.

232. Tuman KJ, McCarthy RJ, Spiess BD, et al: Effect of pulmonary artery catheterization on outcome in patients

undergoing coronary artery surgery. Anesthesiology 70:199, 1989.

233. Anand KJS, Hickey PR: Halothane-morphine compared with high-dose sufentanil for anesthesia and postoperative analgesia in neonatal cardiac surgery. JAMA 326:1, 1992.

234. Bland JHL, Lowenstein E: Halothane-induced decrease in experimental myocardial ischemia in the non-failing canine heart. Anesthesiology 45:287, 1976.

235. Klassen GA, Bramwell RS, Bromage PR, Zborowska-Sluis DT: Effect of acute sympathectomy by epidural anesthesia on the canine coronary circulation. Anesthesiology 52:8, 1980.

236. Norris RM, Clarke ED, Sammel NL, et al: Protective effect of propranolol in threatened myocardial infarction. Lancet 2:907, 1978.

237. Levine JD, Dardick SJ, Roizen MF, et al: The contribution of sensory afferents and sympathetic efferents to joint injury in experimental arthritis. J Neurosci 6:3423, 1986.

238. Feigl EO: The paradox of adrenergic coronary vasoconstriction. Circulation 76:737, 1987.

239. Wade JG, Larson CP, Hickey RF, et al: Carotid endarterectomy and carotid chemoreceptor and baroreceptor function in man. N Engl J Med 282:823, 1970.

240. Hui KKP, Conolly ME: Increased numbers of beta receptors in orthostatic hypotension due to autonomic dysfunction. N Engl J Med 304:1473, 1981.

241. Kendrick WW, Scott JW, Jousse AT, et al: Reflex sweating and hypertension in traumatic transverse myelitis. Treat Serv Bull (Ottawa) 8:437, 1953.

242. Woeber KA: Update on the management of hyperthyroidism and hypothyroidism. Arch Intern Med 160:1067-1071, 2000.

243. Amino N, Mori H, Iwatani Y, et al: High prevalence of transient postpartum thyrotoxicosis and hypothyroidism. N Engl J Med 306:849, 1982.

244. Farling PA. Thyroid disease. Br J Anaesth 85:15-28, 2000.

245. Channick BJ, Adlin EV, Marks AD, et al: Hyperthyroidism and mitral-valve prolapse. N Engl J Med 305:497, 1981.

246. Forfar JC, Miller HC, Toft AD: Occult thyrotoxicosis: A correctable cause of "idiopathic" atrial fibrillation. Am J Cardiol 44:9, 1979.

247. Feek CM, Sawers JSA, Irvine WJ, et al: Combination of potassium iodide and propranolol in preparation of patients with Graves' disease for thyroid surgery. N Engl J Med 302:883, 1980.

248. Forfar JC, Muir AL, Sawers SA, Toft AD: Abnormal left ventricular function in hyperthyroidism: Evidence for a possible reversible cardiomyopathy. N Engl J Med 307:1165, 1982.

249. Tenerz Å, Forberg R, Jansson R: Is a more active attitude warranted in patients with subclinical thyrotoxicosis? J Intern Med 228:229, 1990.

250. Eriksson M, Rubenfeld S, Garber AJ, et al: Propranolol does not prevent thyroid storm. N Engl J Med 296:263, 1977.

251. Roizen MF, Becker CE: Thyroid storm: A review of cases at University of California, San Francisco. Calif Med 115:5, 1971.

252. Loh KC: Amiodarone-induced thyroid disorders: A clinical review. Postgrad Med J 76:133-140, 2000.

253. Williams M, Lo Gerfo P: Thyroidectomy using local anesthesia in critically ill patients with amiodarone-induced thyrotoxicosis: A review and description of the technique. Thyroid 12:523-525, 2002.

254. Murkin JM: Anesthesia and hypothyroidism: A review of thyroxine physiology, pharmacology, and anesthetic implications. Anesth Analg 61:371, 1982.

255. Sawin CT, Castelli WP, Hershman JM, et al: The aging thyroid: Thyroid deficiency in the Framingham Study. Arch Intern Med 145:1386, 1985.

256. Weinberg AD, Brennan MD, Gorman CA, et al: Outcome of anesthesia and surgery in hypothyroid patients. Arch Intern Med 143:893, 1983.

257. Vanderpump MPJ, Tunbridge WMG, French JM, et al: The incidence of thyroid disorders in the community: A twenty-year follow-up of the Wickham Survey. Clin Endocrinol 43:55, 1995.

258. Zwillich CW, Pierson DJ, Hofeldt FD, et al: Ventilatory control in myxedema and hypothyroidism. N Engl J Med 292:662, 1975.

259. Hattori H, Hattori C, Yonekura A, Nishimura T: Two cases of sleep apnea syndrome caused by primary hypothyroidism. Acta Otolaryngol Suppl 550:59-64, 2003.

260. Bough EW, Crowley WF, Ridgway EC, et al: Myocardial function in hypothyroidism. Relation to disease severity and response to treatment. Arch Intern Med 138:1476, 1978.

261. Babad AA, Eger EI II: The effects of hyperthyroidism and hypothyroidism on halothane and oxygen requirements in dogs. Anesthesiology 29:1087, 1968.

262. Karga HJ, Papapetrou PD, Karpathios SE, et al: L-thyroxine therapy attenuates the decline in serum triiodothyronine in nonthyroidal illness induced by hysterectomy. Metabolism 52:1307-1312, 2003.

263. Levine HD: Compromise therapy in the patient with angina pectoris and hypothyroidism: A clinical assessment. Am J Med 69:411, 1980.

264. McMurphy RM, Hodgson DS, Bruyette DS, Fingland RB: Cardiovascular effects of 1.0, 1.5, and 2.0 minimum alveolar concentrations of isoflurane in experimentally induced hypothyroidism in dogs. Vet Surg 25:171-178, 1996.

265. Hensel P, Roizen MF: Patients with disorders of parathyroid function. Anesthesiol Clin North Am 5:287, 1987.

266. Lind L, Ljunghall S: Blood pressure reaction during the intraoperative and early postoperative periods in patients with primary hyperparathyroidism. Expl Clin Endocrinol 102:409-413, 1994.

267. Gallagher SF, Denham DW, Murr MM, Norman JG: The impact of minimally invasive parathyroidectomy on the way endocrinologists treat primary hyperparathyroidism. Surgery 134:910-917, 2000.

268. Kebebew E, Duh QY, Clark OH: Parathyroidectomy for primary hyperparathyroidism in octogenarians and nonagenarians: A plea for early surgical referral. Arch Surg 138:867-871, 2003.

269. Mihai R, Farndon JR: Parathyroid disease and calcium metabolism. Br J Anaesth 85:29-43, 2000.

270. Kao PC, van Heerden JA, Taylor RL: Intraoperative monitoring of parathyroid procedures by a 15-minute parathyroid hormone immunochemiluminometric assay. Mayo Clin Proc 69:532, 1994.

271. Lang RM, Fellner SK, Neumann A, et al: Left ventricular contractility varies directly with blood ionized calcium. Ann Intern Med 108:524, 1988.

272. Rumancik WM, Denlinger JK, Nahrwold ML, et al: The QT interval and serum ionized calcium. JAMA 240:366, 1978.

273. Munir MA, Jaffar M, Arshad M, et al: Reduced duration of muscle relaxation with rocuronium in a normocalcemic hyperparathyroid patient. Can J Anaesth 50:558-561, 2003.

274. Melmed S, Ho K, Klibanski A, et al: Clinical review 75: Recent advances in pathogenesis, diagnosis, and management of acromegaly. J Clin Endocrinol Metab 80:3395, 1995.

275. Schmitt H, Buchfelder M, Radespiel-Troger M, Fahlbusch R: Difficult intubation in acromegalic patients: Incidence and predictability. Anesthesiology 93:110-114, 2000.

276. Dougherty TB, Cronau LH Jr: Anesthetic implications for surgical patients with endocrine tumors. Int Anesthesiol Clin 36:31-44, 1998.

277. Campkin TV: Radial artery cannulation: Potential hazard in patients with acromegaly. Anaesthesia 35:1008, 1980.

278. Molitch EM: Diagnosis and treatment of prolactinomas. Adv Intern Med 44:117-153, 1999.

279. Rojiani AM, Prineas JW, Cho ES: Protective effect of steroids on electrolyte-induced demyelination. J Neuropathol Exp Neurol 46:495, 1987.

280. Ayus JC, Krothapalli RK, Arieff AI: Changing concepts in the treatment of severe symptomatic hyponatremia: Rapid correction and possible relation to central pontine myelinolysis. Am J Med 78:897, 1985.

281. Robertson GL: Diabetes insipidus. Endocrinol Metab Clin North Am 24:549, 1995.

282. Corliss RJ, McKenna DH, Sialers S, et al: Systemic and coronary hemodynamic effects of vasopressin. Am J Med Sci 256:293, 1968.

283. Nikolic G, Singh JB: Cimetidine, vasopressin and chronotropic incompetence. Med J Aust 2:435, 1982.

284. Smithwick RH, Thompson JE: Splanchnicectomy for essential hypertension. JAMA 152:1501, 1953.

285. Brown BR: Anesthesia and essential hypertension. In Hershey SG (ed): ASA Refresher Courses in Anesthesiology, vol 7. Philadelphia, JB Lippincott, 1979, p 41.

286. Sprague HB: The heart in surgery. An analysis of results of surgery on cardiac patients during the past ten years at the Massachusetts General Hospital. Surg Gynecol Obstet 49:54, 1929.

287. Miller RD, Way WL, Eger EI II: The effects of alpha-methyldopa, reserpine, and guanethidine on minimum alveolar anesthetic requirement (MAC). Anesthesiology 29:1153, 1968.

288. Veterans Administration Study on Antihypertensive Agents: Effects of treatment on morbidity in hypertension. JAMA 202:1028, 1967.

289. Veterans Administration Cooperative Study Group on Antihypertensive Agents: Effects of treatment on morbidity in hypertension: Results in patients with diastolic blood pressure averaging 90 through 114 mm Hg. JAMA 213:1143, 1970.

290. Moser M, Hebert P, Hennekens CH: An overview of the meta-analyses of the hypertension treatment trials. Arch Intern Med 151:1277, 1991.

291. Kannel WB: Blood pressure as a cardiovascular risk factor. Prevention and treatment. JAMA 275:1571, 1996.

292. Hypertension Detection and Follow-up Program Cooperative Group: The effect of treatment on mortality in "mild" hypertension. N Engl J Med 307:976, 1982.

293. Multiple Risk Factor Intervention Trial Research Group: Multiple risk factor intervention trial. Risk factor changes and mortality results. JAMA 248:1465, 1982.

294. Psaty BM, Smith NL, Siscovick DS, et al: Health outcomes associated with antihypertensive therapies used as first-line agents. A systematic review and meta-analysis. JAMA 277:739-745, 1997.

295. Heidenreich PA, McDonald KM, Hastie T: Meta-analysis of trials comparing beta-blockers, calcium antagonists, and nitrates for stable angina. JAMA 281:1927-1936, 1999.

296. Jollis, JG, Simpson RJ Jr, Chowdhury MK, et al: Calcium channel blockers and mortality in elderly patients with myocardial infarction. Arch Intern Med 159:2341-2348, 1999.

297. Opie, LH, Yusuf S, Kubler W: Current status of safety and efficacy of calcium channel blockers in cardiovascular diseases: A critical analysis based on 100 studies. Prog Cardiovasc Dis 43:171-196, 2000.

298. SHEP Cooperative Study Group: Prevention of stroke by antihypertensive drug treatment in older persons with isolated systolic hypertension. Final results of the Systolic Hypertension in the Elderly Program (SHEP). JAMA 265:3255, 1991.

299. Curb JD, Pressel SL, Cutler JA, et al: Effect of diuretic-based antihypertensive treatment on cardiovascular disease risk in older diabetic patients with isolated systolic hypertension. JAMA 276:1886, 1996.

300. Farnett L, Mulrow CD, Linn WD, et al: The J-curve phenomenon and the treatment of hypertension. Is there a point beyond which pressure reduction is dangerous? JAMA 265:489, 1991.

301. Hasebe N, Kido S, Ido A, et al: Reverse J-curve relation between diastolic blood pressure and severity of coronary artery lesion in hypertensive patients with angina pectoris. Hypertens Res 25:381-387, 2002.

302. Prys-Roberts C, Meloche R, Foëx P: Studies of anesthesia in relation to hypertension. I: Cardiovascular responses of treated and untreated patients. Br J Anaesth 43:122, 1971.

303. Goldman L, Caldera DL: Risks of general anesthesia and elective operation in the hypertensive patient. Anesthesiology 50:285, 1979.

304. Bedford RF, Feinstein B: Hospital admission blood pressure: A predictor for hypertension following endotracheal intubation. Anesth Analg 59:367, 1980.

305. Asiddao CB, Donegan JH, Whitesell RC, et al: Factors associated with perioperative complications during carotid endarterectomy. Anesth Analg 61:631, 1982.

306. Ellis JE, Drijvers G, Shah MN, et al: Topical clonidine fails to reduce postoperative stress response after noncardiac surgery. Anesth Analg 74:S85, 1992.

307. Mangano DT, Browner WS, Hollenberg M, et al: Association of perioperative myocardial ischemia with cardiac morbidity and mortality in men undergoing noncardiac surgery. N Engl J Med 323:1781, 1990.

308. Stone JG, Foëx P, Sear JW, et al: Risk of myocardial ischemia during anesthesia in treated and untreated hypertensive patients. Br J Anaesth 61:675, 1988.

309. Wolfsthal SD: The clinical characteristics and perioperative blood pressure lability in hypertensive patients referred for preoperative medical evaluation [abstract]. Clin Res 37:8034A, 1989.

310. Pasternack PF, Grossi EA, Baumann FG, et al: Beta blockade to decrease silent myocardial ischemia during peripheral vascular surgery. Am J Surg 158:113, 1989.

311. Weksler N, Klein M, Szendro G, et al: The dilemma of immediate preoperative hypertension: To treat and operate, or to postpone surgery? J Clin Anesth 15:179-183, 2003.

312. Aronson S, Boisvert D, Lapp W: Isolated systolic hypertension is associated with adverse outcomes from coronary artery bypass grafting surgery. Anesth Analg 94:1079-1084, 2002.

313. Cohen MM, Duncan PG: Physical Status Score and trends in anesthetic complications. J Clin Epidemiol 41:83, 1988.

314. Fleiss JL: Statistical Methods for Rates and Proportions. New York, John Wiley & Sons, 1973, p 178.

315. Charlson ME, MacKenzie R, Gold JP, et al: Postoperative renal dysfunction can be predicted. Surg Gynecol Obstet 169:303, 1989.

316. Charlson ME, MacKenzie CR, Gold JP, et al: Preoperative characteristics predicting intraoperative hypotension and hypertension among hypertensives and diabetics undergoing noncardiac surgery. Ann Surg 212:66, 1990.

317. Charlson ME, MacKenzie CR, Gold JP, et al: Risk for postoperative congestive heart failure. Surg Gynecol Obstet 172:95, 1991.

318. Burke AP, Farb A, Malcom GT, et al: Coronary risk factors and plaque morphology in men with coronary disease who died suddenly. N Engl J Med 336:1276, 1997.

319. Ayobe MH, Tarazi RC: Reversal of changes in myocardial β-receptors and inotropic responsiveness with regression of cardiac hypertrophy in renal hypertensive rats (RHR). Circ Res 54:125, 1984.

320. Schneider AJL, Knoke JD, Zollinger RM Jr, et al: Morbidity prediction using pre- and intraoperative data. Anesthesiology 51:4, 1979.

321. Eerola M, Eerola R, Kaukinen S, et al: Risk factors in surgical patients with verified preoperative myocardial infarction. Acta Anaesthesiol Scand 24:219, 1980.

322. Mauney FM, Ebert PA, Sabiston DC: Postoperative myocardial infarction: A study of predisposing factors, diagnosis and mortality in a high risk group of surgical patients. Ann Surg 172:497, 1970.

323. Garraway WM, Whisnant JP: The changing pattern of hypertension and the declining incidence of stroke. JAMA 258:214, 1987.

324. Rutan GH, Kuller LH, Neaton JD, et al: Mortality associated with diastolic hypertension and isolated systolic hypertension among men screened for the Multiple Risk Intervention Trial. Circulation 77:504, 1988.

325. Okuda S, Onoyama K, Motomura K, et al: Effect of acute reduction in blood pressure on renal function of rats with diseased kidneys. Nephron 45:311, 1987.

326. Mayhan WG, Faraci FM, Heistad DD: Disruption of the blood-brain barrier in cerebrum and brain stem during acute hypertension. Am J Physiol 251:H1171, 1986.

327. Croog SH, Levine S, Testa MA, et al: The effects of antihypertensive therapy on the quality of life. N Engl J Med 314:1657, 1986.

328. Materson BJ, Reda DJ, Cushman WC, et al: Single-drug therapy for hypertension in men. A comparison of six antihypertensive agents with placebo. N Engl J Med 328:914, 1993.

329. Slogoff S, Keats AS: Does perioperative myocardial ischemia lead to postoperative myocardial infarction? Anesthesiology 62:107, 1985.

330. Slogoff S, Keats AS: Further observations on perioperative myocardial ischemia. Anesthesiology 65:539, 1986.

331. Coriat P, Richer C, Douraki T, et al: Influence of chronic angiotensin-converting enzyme inhibition in anesthetic induction. Anesthesiology 81:299, 1994.

332. Bertrand M, Godet G, Meersschaert K, et al: Should the angiotensin II antagonists be discontinued before surgery? Anesth Analg 92:26-30, 2001.

333. Kuller LH, Shemanski L, Psaty BM, et al: Subclinical disease as an independent risk factor for cardiovascular disease. Circulation 92:720, 1995.

334. Lichtor JL, Roizen MF, Lane B, Thisted R: Change in mortality rate for surgical procedures 1979 to 1994. Personal communication.

335. Benchimol A, Harris CL, Desser KB, et al: Resting electrocardiogram in major coronary artery disease. JAMA 224:1489, 1973.

336. Tomatis LA, Fierens EE, Verbrugge GP: Evaluation of surgical risk in peripheral vascular disease by coronary angiography: A series of 100 cases. Surgery 71:429, 1972.

337. Hertzer NR, Beven EG, Young JR, et al: Coronary artery disease in peripheral vascular patients. A classification of 1000 angiograms and results of surgical management. Ann Surg 199:223, 1984.

338. Hertzer NR, Young JR, Beven EG, et al: Late results of coronary bypass in patients with infrarenal aortic aneurysms. The Cleveland Clinic Study. Ann Surg 205:360, 1987.

339. Barnes RW, Liebman PR, Marszalek PB, et al: The natural history of asymptomatic carotid disease in patients undergoing cardiovascular surgery. Surgery 90:1075, 1981.

340. Barnes RW, Marszalek PB: Asymptomatic carotid disease in the cardiovascular surgical patient: Is prophylactic endarterectomy necessary? Stroke 12:497, 1981.

341. Operating to prevent stroke [editorial]. Lancet 337:1255, 1991.

342. Markus RA, Mack WJ, Azen SP, Hodis HN: Influence of lifestyle modification on atherosclerotic progression determined by ultrasonographic change in the common carotid intima-media thickness. Am J Clin Nutr 65:1000, 1997.

343. Ropper AH, Wechsler LR, Wilson LS: Carotid bruit and the risk of stroke in elective surgery. N Engl J Med 307:1388, 1982.

344. Heyman A, Wilkinson WE, Heyden S, et al: Risk of stroke in asymptomatic persons with cervical arterial bruits. A population study in Evans County, Georgia. N Engl J Med 302:838, 1980.

345. Reed GL, Singer DE, Picard EH, DeSanctis RW: Stroke following coronary-artery bypass surgery: A case-control estimate of the risk from carotid bruits. N Engl J Med 319:1246, 1988.

346. Morise AP, Dalal JN, Duval RD: Value of a simple measure of estrogen status for improving the diagnosis of coronary artery disease in women. Am J Med 94:491, 1993.

347. Roizen MF: Preoperative Test Selection Program Software Manual of Version 2.15L. Pleasanton, CA, Nellcor, 1994.

348. Deanfield JE, Maseri A, Selwyn AP, et al: Myocardial ischaemia during daily life in patients with stable angina: Its relation to symptoms and heart rate changes. Lancet 1:753-758, 1983.

349. McCann RL, Clements FM: Silent myocardial ischemia in patients undergoing peripheral vascular surgery: Incidence and association with perioperative cardiac morbidity and mortality. J Vasc Surg 9:583, 1989.

350. Rabkin SE, Horne JM: Preoperative electrocardiography: Effect of new abnormalities on clinical decisions. Can Med Assoc J 128:146, 1983.

351. Apfelbaum J, Robinson D, Murray WJ, et al: An automated method to validate preoperative test selection: First results of a multicenter study [abstract]. Anesthesiology 71:A928, 1989.

352. Biller J, Saver JL: Transient ischemic attacks—populations and prognosis. Mayo Clin Proc 69:493, 1994.

353. Goldschlager N: Use of the treadmill test in the diagnosis of coronary artery disease in patients with chest pain. Ann Intern Med 97:383, 1982.

354. Weiner DA, Ryan TJ, McCabe CH, et al: Exercise stress testing. Correlations among history of angina, ST-segment response and prevalence of coronary-artery disease in the Coronary Artery Surgery Study (CASS). N Engl J Med 301:230, 1979.

355. Leng GC, Fowkes FGR, Lee AJ, et al: Use of ankle brachial pressure index to predict cardiovascular events and death: A cohort study. BMJ 313:1440, 1996.

356. Kornitzer M, Dramaix M, Sobolski J, et al: Ankle/arm pressure index in asymptomatic middle-aged males: An independent predictor of ten-year coronary heart disease mortality. Angiology 46:211, 1995.

357. Older P, Smith R, Courtney P, Hone R: Preoperative evaluation of cardiac failure and ischemia in elderly patients by cardiopulmonary exercise testing. Chest 104:701, 1993.

358. Older P, Hall H: The role of cardiopulmonary exercise testing for preoperative evaluation of the elderly. In Wasserman K (ed): Exercise Gas Exchange in Heart Disease. Armonk, NY, Futura, 1996, p 421.

359. Russell LB, Carson JL, Taylor WC, et al: Modeling all-cause mortality: Projections of the impact of smoking cessation based on the NHEFS. Am J Public Health 88:630, 1998.

360. Vita AJ, Terry RB, Hubert HB, Fries JF: Aging, health risks, and cumulative disability. N Engl J Med 338:1035, 1998.

361. Arkins R, Smessaert AA, Hicks RG: Mortality and morbidity in surgical patients with coronary artery disease. JAMA 190:485, 1964.

362. Topkins MJ, Artusio JF: Myocardial infarction and surgery: A five year study. Anesth Analg 43:715, 1964.

363. Fraser JG, Ramachandran PR, Davis HS: Anesthesia and recent myocardial infarction. JAMA 199:318, 1972.

364. Tarhan S, Moffitt EA, Taylor WF, et al: Myocardial infarction after general anesthesia. JAMA 199:318, 1972.

365. Sapala JA, Ponka JL, Duvernow WFC: Operative and nonoperative risks in the cardiac patient. J Am Geriatr Soc 23:529, 1975.

366. Steen PA, Tinker JH, Tarhan S: Myocardial reinfarction after anesthesia and surgery. JAMA 239:2566, 1976.

367. Goldman L, Caldera DL, Southwick FS, et al: Cardiac risk factors and complications in noncardiac surgery. Medicine (Baltimore) 57:357, 1978.

368. Schoeppel SL, Wilkinson C, Waters J, et al: Effects of myocardial infarction on perioperative cardiac complications. Anesth Analg 62:493, 1983.

369. Knapp RB, Topkins MJ, Artusio JF Jr: The cerebrovascular accident and coronary occlusion in anesthesia. JAMA 182:332, 1962.

370. von Knorring J: Postoperative myocardial infarction: A prospective study in a risk group of surgical patients. Surgery 90:55, 1981.

371. Shah KB, Kleinman BS, Sami H, et al: Reevaluation of perioperative myocardial infarction in patients with prior myocardial infarction undergoing noncardiac operations. Anesth Analg 71:231, 1990.

372. Plumlee JE, Boettner RB: Myocardial infarction during and following anesthesia and operation. South Med J 65:886, 1972.

373. Becker RC, Underwood DA: Myocardial infarction in patients undergoing noncardiac surgery. Cleve Clin J Med 54:25, 1987.

374. Eagle KA, Boucher CA: Cardiac risk of noncardiac surgery. N Engl J Med 321:1330, 1989.

375. Detsky AS, Abrams HB, McLaughlin JR, et al: Predicting cardiac complications in patients undergoing non-cardiac surgery. J Gen Intern Med 1:211, 1986.

376. Gerson MC, Hurst JM, Hertzberg VS, et al: Cardiac prognosis in noncardiac surgery. Ann Intern Med 103:832, 1985.

377. Rivers SP, Scher LA, Gupta SK, Veith FJ: Safety of peripheral vascular surgery after recent acute myocardial infarction. J Vasc Surg 11:70-75, discussion 76, 1990.

378. Berlauk JF, Abrams JH, Gilmour IJ, et al: Preoperative optimization of cardiovascular hemodynamics improves outcome in peripheral vascular surgery: A prospective, randomized clinical trial. Ann Surg 214:289, 1991.

379. American Society of Anesthesiologists Task Force on Pulmonary Artery Catheterization: Practice guidelines for pulmonary catheterization. A report by the American Society of Anesthesiologists Task Force on Pulmonary Artery Catheterization. Anesthesiology 78:380, 1993.

380. Backer CL, Tinker JH, Robertson DM, et al: Myocardial reinfarction following local anesthesia for ophthalmic surgery. Anesth Analg 59:257, 1980.

381. Wolf GL, Lynch S, Berlin I: Intra-ocular surgery with general anesthesia. Arch Ophthalmol 93:323, 1975.

382. Roizen MF: Anesthesia goals for surgery to relieve or prevent visceral ischemia. In Roizen MF (ed): Anesthesia for Vascular Surgery. New York, Churchill Livingstone, 1990, p 171.

383. Eagle KA, Coley CM, Newell JB, et al: Combining clinical and thallium data optimizes preoperative assessment of cardiac risk before major vascular surgery. Ann Intern Med 110:859, 1989.

384. Boucher CA, Brewster DC, Darling RC, et al: Determination of cardiac risk by dipyridamole-thallium imaging before peripheral vascular surgery. N Engl J Med 312:389, 1985.

385. Raby KE, Goldman L, Creager MA, et al: Correlation between preoperative ischemia and major cardiac events after peripheral vascular surgery. N Engl J Med 321:1296, 1989.

386. Lette J, Waters D, Lapointe J, et al: Usefulness of the severity and extent of reversible perfusion defects during thallium-dipyridamole imaging for cardiac risk assessment before noncardiac surgery. Am J Cardiol 64:276, 1989.

387. Mantha S, Roizen MF, Barnard J, et al: Relative effectiveness of preoperative noninvasive cardiac evaluation tests on predicting adverse cardiac outcomes following vascular surgery: A meta-analysis. Anesth Analg 79:422, 1994.

388. Bruschke AVG, Proudfit WL, Sones FM: Progress study of 590 consecutive nonsurgical cases of coronary disease followed 5-9 years. Circulation 47:1147, 1973.

389. Mahar LJ, Steen PA, Tinker JH, et al: Perioperative myocardial infarction in patients with coronary artery disease with and without aorta-coronary bypass grafts. J Thorac Cardiovasc Surg 76:533, 1978.

390. Kennedy JW, Kaiser GC, Fisher LD, et al: Clinical and angiographic predictors of operative mortality from the Collaborative Study in Coronary Artery Surgery (CASS). Circulation 63:793, 1981.

391. Mangano DT, Hedgcock MW, Wisneski JA: Noninvasive prediction of ventricular dysfunction: Coronary artery disease [abstract]. Anesthesiology 57:A21, 1982.

391b. Shaw LJ, Eagle KA, Gersh BJ, Miller DD: Meta-analysis of intravenous dipyridamole-thallium-201 imaging (1985 to 1994) and dobutamine echocardiography (1991 to 1994) for risk stratification before vascular surgery. J Am Coll Cardiol 27:787-798, 1996.

392. Fletcher JP, Antico VF, Gruenwald S, Kershaw LZ: Dipyridamole-thallium scan for screening of coronary artery disease prior to vascular surgery. J Cardiovasc Surg 29:666, 1988.

393. Fleisher LA, Rosenbaum SH, Nelson AH, et al: Preoperative dipyridamole thallium imaging and ambulatory electrocardiographic monitoring as a predictor of perioperative cardiac events and long-term outcome. Anesthesiology 83:906-917, 1995.

394. Lane RT, Sawada SG, Segar DS, et al: Dobutamine stress echocardiography for assessment of cardiac risk before noncardiac surgery. Am J Cardiol 68:976, 1991.

395. Lalka SG, Sawada SG, Dalsing MC, et al: Dobutamine stress echocardiography as a predictor of cardiac events associated with aortic surgery. J Vasc Surg 15:831, 1992.

396. Dávila-Román VG, Waggoner AD, Sicard GA, et al: Dobutamine stress echocardiography predicts surgical outcome in patients with aortic aneurysm and peripheral vascular disease. J Am Coll Cardiol 21:957, 1993.

397. Poldermans D, Fioretti PM, Forster T, et al: Dobutamine stress echocardiography for assessment of perioperative cardiac risk in patients undergoing major vascular surgery. Circulation 87:1506, 1993.

397b. Boersma E, Poldermans D, Bax JJ, et al: Predictors of cardiac events after major vascular surgery: Role of clinical characteristics, dobutamine echocardiography, and beta-blocker therapy. JAMA 285:1865-1873, 2001.

398. Jeffrey CC, Kunsman J, Cullen DJ, Brewster DC: A prospective evaluation of cardiac risk index. Anesthesiology 58:462, 1984.

399. Poldermans D, Arnese M, Fioretti PM, et al: Improved cardiac risk stratification in major vascular surgery with dobutamine-atropine stress echocardiography. J Am Coll Cardiol 26:648-653, 1995.

400. Lee TH, Marcantonio ER, Mangione CM, et al: Derivation and prospective validation of a simple index for prediction of cardiac risk of major noncardiac surgery. Circulation 100:1043-1049, 1999.

401. Higgins TL, Estafanous FG, Loop FD, et al: Stratification of morbidity and mortality outcome by preoperative risk factors in coronary artery bypass patients. A clinical severity score. JAMA 267:2344, 1992.

401b. Reilly DF, McNeely MJ, Doerner D, et al: Self-reported exercise tolerance and the risk of serious perioperative complications. Arch Intern Med 159:2185-2192, 1999.

402. Froehlich JB, Karavite D, Russman PL, et al: American College of Cardiology/American Heart Association preoperative assessment guidelines reduce resource utilization before aortic surgery. J Vasc Surg 36:758-763, 2002.

403. Licker M, Khatchatourian G, Schweizer A, et al: The impact of a cardioprotective protocol on the incidence of cardiac complications after aortic abdominal surgery. Anesth Analg 95:1525-1533, 2002.

404. Bittner V, Weiner DH, Yusuf S, et al: Prediction of mortality and morbidity with a 6-minute walk test in patients with left ventricular dysfunction. JAMA 270:1702, 1993.

405. Benson H, McCallie DP: Angina pectoris and the placebo effect. N Engl J Med 300:1424, 1979.

406. Takaro T, Hultgren HN, Lipton MJ, et al: The VA cooperative randomized study of surgery for coronary arterial occlusive disease. II: Subgroup with significant left main lesions. Circulation 54:(Suppl 3)III-107, 1976.

407. Reed RC, Murphy ML, Hultgren HN, et al: Survival of men treated for chronic stable angina pectoris. A cooperative randomized study. J Thorac Cardiovasc Surg 75:1, 1978.

408. Crawford ES, Morris GC, Howell JF, et al: Operative risk in patients with previous coronary artery bypass. Ann Thorac Surg 26:215, 1978.

409. Huber KC, Evans MA, Bresnahan JF, et al: Outcome of noncardiac operations in patients with severe coronary artery disease successfully treated preoperatively with coronary angioplasty. Mayo Clin Proc 67:15, 1992.

410. Eagle KA, Rihal CS, Mickel MC, et al: Cardiac risk of noncardiac surgery: Influence of coronary disease and type of surgery in 3368 operations. CASS Investigators and University of Michigan Heart Care Program. Coronary Artery Surgery Study. Circulation 96:1882-1887, 1997.

411. McFalls EO, Ward HB, Krupski WC, et al: Prophylactic coronary artery revascularization for elective vascular surgery: Study design. Veterans Affairs Cooperative Study Group on Coronary Artery Revascularization Prophylaxis for Elective Vascular Surgery. Control Clin Trials 20:297-308, 1999.

412. Rihal CS, Eagle KA, Mickel MC, et al: Surgical therapy for coronary artery disease among patients with combined coronary artery and peripheral vascular disease. Circulation 91:46, 1995.

413. Posner KL, Van Norman GA, Chan V: Adverse cardiac outcomes after noncardiac surgery in patients with prior percutaneous transluminal coronary angioplasty. Anesth Analg 89:553-560, 1999.

414. Kaluza GL, Joseph J, Lee JR, et al: Catastrophic outcomes of noncardiac surgery soon after coronary stenting. J Am Coll Cardiol 35:1288-1294, 2000.

415. Fleisher LA, Skolnick ED, Halroyd KJ, Lehmann HP: Coronary artery revascularization before abdominal aortic aneurysm surgery: A decision analytic approach. Anesth Analg 79:661-669, 1994.

416. Mason JJ, Owens DK, Harris RA, et al: The role of coronary angiography and coronary revascularization before noncardiac surgery. JAMA 273:1919-1925, 1995.

417. Glance LG: Selective preoperative cardiac screening improves five-year survival in patients undergoing major vascular surgery: A cost-effectiveness analysis. J Cardiothorac Vasc Anesth 13:265-271, 1999.

418. Landesberg G, Mosseri M, Wolf YG, et al: Preoperative thallium scanning, selective coronary revascularization, and long-term survival after major vascular surgery. Circulation 108:177-183, 2003.

419. Hultgren HN, Pfeifer JF, Angell WW, et al: Unstable angina: Comparison of medical and surgical management. Am J Cardiol 39:734, 1977.

420. Santos AL, Gelperin A: Surgical mortality in the elderly. J Am Geriatr Soc 23:42, 1975.

421. Driscoll AC, Hobika JH, Etsten BE, et al: Clinically unrecognized myocardial infarction following surgery. N Engl J Med 264:633, 1961.

422. O'Keefe JH, Shub C, Rettke SR: Risk of noncardiac surgical procedures in patients with aortic stenosis. Mayo Clin Proc 64:400, 1989.

423. Smith JS, Roizen MF, Cahalan MK, Benefiel DJ: Does anesthetic technique make a difference? Augmentation of systolic blood pressure during carotid endarterectomy: Effects of phenylephrine versus light anesthesia and of isoflurane versus halothane on the incidence of myocardial ischemia. Anesthesiology 69:846, 1988.

424. Riles TS, Kopelman I, Imparato AM: Myocardial infarction following carotid endarterectomy: A review of 683 operations. Surgery 85:249, 1979.

425. Frank SM, Fleisher LA, Breslow MJ, et al: Perioperative maintenance of normothermia reduces the incidence of morbid cardiac events: A randomized clinical trial. JAMA 277:1127, 1997.

426. Erikssen G, Thaulow E, Sandvik L, et al: Haematocrit: A predictor of cardiovascular mortality? J Intern Med 234:493, 1993.

427. Nelson AH, Fleisher LA, Rosenbaum SH: Relationship between postoperative anemia and cardiac morbidity in high-risk vascular patients in the intensive care unit. Crit Care Med 21:860, 1993.

428. Fleisher LA, Skolnick ED, Holyrod KJ, Lehmann HP: Coronary artery revascularization before abdominal aortic aneurysm surgery: A decision analytic approach. Anesth Analg 79:661, 1994.

429. Roy WL, Edelist G, Gilbert B: Myocardial ischemia during non-cardiac surgical procedures in patients with coronary-artery disease. Anesthesiology 54:393, 1979.

430. Kaplan JA, King SB: The precordial electrocardiographic lead (V_5) in patients who have coronary-artery disease. Anesthesiology 45:570, 1976.

431. Christopherson R, Frank S, Norris E, et al: Low postoperative hematocrit is associated with cardiac ischemia in high-risk patients [abstract]. Anesthesiology 75(Suppl 3A):A99, 1991.

432. Nelson AH, Fleisher LA, Rosenbaum SH: The relationship between postoperative anemia and cardiac morbidity in high risk vascular patients in the ICU. Crit Care Med 21:860, 1993.

433. Roizen MF, Beaupre PN, Alpert RA, et al: Monitoring with two-dimensional transesophageal echocardiography. J Vasc Surg 1:300, 1984.

434. Naylor CD, Sibbald WJ, Sprung CL, et al: Pulmonary artery catheterization: Can there be an integrated strategy for guideline development and research promotion? JAMA 269:2407, 1993.

435. Nishina K, Mikawa K, Uesugi T, et al: Efficacy of clonidine for prevention of perioperative myocardial ischemia: A critical appraisal and meta-analysis of the literature. Anesthesiology 96:323-329, 2002.

436. Stevens RD, Burri H, Tramer MR: Pharmacologic myocardial protection in patients undergoing noncardiac surgery: A quantitative systematic review. Anesth Analg 97:623-633, 2003.

437. Wijeysundera DN, Beattie WS: Calcium channel blockers for reducing cardiac morbidity after noncardiac surgery: A meta-analysis. Anesth Analg 97:634-641, 2003.

438. Rehman A, Zalos G, Andrews NP, et al: Blood pressure changes during transient myocardial ischemia: Insights into mechanisms. J Am Coll Cardiol 30:1249, 1997.

439. Heidenreich PA, McDonald KM, Hastie T, et al: Meta-analysis of trials comparing beta-blockers, calcium antagonists, and nitrates for stable angina. JAMA 281: 1927-1936, 1999.

440. Shojania KG, Duncan BW, McDonald KM, Wachter RM: Safe but sound: Patient safety meets evidence-based medicine. JAMA 288:508-513, 2002.

441. Chenoweth DE, Cooper SW, Hugli TE, et al: Complement activation during cardiopulmonary bypass. N Engl J Med 304:497, 1981.

442. Auerbach AD, Goldman L: β-Blockers and reduction of cardiac events in noncardiac surgery: Clinical applications. JAMA 287:1445-1447, 2002.

443. Auerbach AD, Goldman L: β-Blockers and reduction of cardiac events in noncardiac surgery: Scientific review. JAMA 287:1435-1444, 2002.

444. Leape LL, Berwick DM, Bater DW: What practices will most improve safety? Evidence-based medicine meets patient safety. JAMA 288:501-507, 2002.

445. Palda VA, Detsky AS: Perioperative assessment and management of risk from coronary artery disease. Ann Intern Med 127:313-328, 1997.

446. Lembo NJ, Dell'Italia LJ, Crawford MH, O'Rourke RA: Bedside diagnosis of systolic murmurs. N Engl J Med 318:1572, 1988.

447. Etchells E, Bell C, Robb K: Does this patient have an abnormal systolic murmur? JAMA 277:564, 1997.

448. Hollinger I: Diseases of the cardiovascular system. In Katz R, Steward D (eds): Anesthesia and Uncommon Pediatric Diseases. Philadelphia, WB Saunders, 1993, p 93.

449. Noonan JA: Association of congenital heart disease with syndromes or other defects. Pediatr Clin North Am 25:797, 1978.

450. Devereux RB: Recent developments in the diagnosis and management of mitral valve prolapse. Curr Opin Cardiol 10:107, 1995.

451. Bor DH, Himmelstein DU: Endocarditis prophylaxis for patients with mitral valve prolapse: A quantitative analysis. Am J Med 76:711, 1984.

452. Bartels C, Bechtel J, Hossmann V, Horsch S: Cardiac risk stratification for high-risk vascular surgery. Circulation 95:2473-2475, 1997.

453. Clemens JD, Horwitz RI, Jaffe CC, et al: A controlled evaluation of the risk of bacterial endocarditis in persons with mitral-valve prolapse. N Engl J Med 307:776, 1982.

454. Berry FA, Blanketbaker WL, Ball CG: A comparison of bacteremia occurring with nasotracheal and orotracheal intubation. Anesth Analg 52:873, 1973.

455. Shull HJ, Greene BM, Allen SD, et al: Bacteremia with upper gastrointestinal endoscopy. Ann Intern Med 83:212, 1975.

456. Dajani AS, Bisno AL, Chung KJ, et al: Prevention of bacterial endocarditis. Recommendations by the American Heart Association. JAMA 264:2919, 1990.

457. Antimicrobial prophylaxis in surgery. Med Lett Drugs Ther Guidelines 20:27, 2004.

458. Katholi RE, Nolan SP, McGuire LB: Living with prosthetic heart valves. Subsequent noncardiac operations and the risk of thromboembolism or hemorrhage. Am Heart J 92:162-167, 1976.

459. Bonow RO, Carabello B, et al: Guidelines for the management of patients with valvular heart disease: Executive summary. A report of the American College of Cardiology/American Heart Association Task Force on Practice Guidelines (Committee on Management of Patients with Valvular Heart Disease). Circulation 98:1949-1984, 1998.

460. Ezekowitz MD: Anticoagulation management of valve replacement patients. J Heart Valve Dis 11(Suppl 1):S56-S60, 2002.

461. Edelson RN, Chernik NL, Posner JB: Spinal subdural hematomas complicating lumbar puncture. Arch Neurol 31:134, 1974.

462. Reddy NB, Rao TLK: Regional anesthesia for vascular surgery of the lower extremities: Considerations regarding anticoagulation. In Roizen MF (ed): Anesthesia for Vascular Surgery. New York, Churchill Livingstone, 1990, p 367.

463. Brem SS, Hafler DA, Van Uitert RL, et al: Spinal subarachnoid hematoma: A hazard of lumbar puncture resulting in reversible paraplegia. N Engl J Med 303:1020, 1981.

464. Owens EL, Kasten GW, Hessel EA II: Spinal subarachnoid hematoma after lumbar puncture and heparinization: A case report, review of the literature, and discussion of anesthetic implications. Anesth Analg 65:1201, 1986.

465. Rao TLK, El-Etr AA: Anticoagulation following placement of epidural and subarachnoid catheters: An evaluation of neurologic sequelae. Anesthesiology 55:618, 1981.

466. Bargon HC, LaRaja RD, Rossi G, Atkinson D: Continuous epidural analgesia in the heparinized vascular surgical patient: A retrospective review of 912 patients. J Vasc Surg 6:144, 1987.

467. Onishchuk JL, Carlsson C: Epidural hematoma associated with epidural anesthesia: Complications of anticoagulant therapy. Anesthesiology 77:1221, 1992.

468. Odoom JA, Sih IL: Epidural analgesia and anticoagulant therapy: Experience with one thousand cases of continuous epidurals. Anaesthesia 38:254, 1983.

469. Locke GE, Giorgio AJ, Biggers SL Jr, et al: Acute spinal epidural hematoma secondary to aspirin-induced prolonged bleeding. Surg Neurol 5:293, 1976.

470. Frame JN, Mulvey KP, Phares JC, Anderson MJ: Correction of severe heparin-associated thrombocytopenia with intravenous immunoglobulin. Ann Intern Med 111:946, 1989.

471. Tekkok IH, Cataltepe O, Tahta K, Bertan V: Extradural haematoma after continuous extradural anaesthesia. Br J Anaesth 67:112, 1991.

472. Waldman SD, Feldstein GS, Waldman HJ, et al: Caudal administration of morphine sulphate in anticoagulated and thrombocytopenic patients. Anesth Analg 66:267, 1987.

473. Horlocker TT, Wedel DJ, Offord KP: Does preoperative antiplatelet therapy increase the risk of hemorrhagic complications associated with regional anesthesia? Anesth Analg 70:631, 1990.

474. Macdonald R: Aspirin and extradural blocks. Br J Anaesth 66:1, 1991.

475. Amrein PC, Ellman L, Harris WH: Aspirin-induced prolongation of bleeding and perioperative blood loss. JAMA 245:1825, 1981.

476. Vandermeulen EP, Van Aken H, Vermylen J: Anticoagulants and spinal-epidural anesthesia. Anesth Analg 79:1165, 1994.

477. Horlocker TT, Wedel DJ, Benzon H, et al: Regional anesthesia in the anticoagulated patient: Defining the risks (the second ASRA Consensus Conference on Neuraxial Anesthesia and Anticoagulation). Reg Anesth Pain Med 28:172-197, 2003.

478. International Multicentre Trial: Prevention of fatal postoperative pulmonary embolism by low doses of heparin. Lancet 2:45, 1975.

479. Consensus Conference: Prevention of venous thrombosis and pulmonary embolism. JAMA 256:744, 1988.

480. Collins R, Scrimgeour A, Yusuf S, Peto R: Reduction in fatal pulmonary embolism and venous thrombosis by perioperative administration of subcutaneous heparin. N Engl J Med 318:1162, 1988.

481. Gallus A, Raman K, Darby T: Venous thrombosis after elective hip replacement—the influence of preventive intermittent calf compression and on surgical technique. Br J Surg 70:17, 1983.

482. Lutz DJ, Noller KL, Spittell JA Jr, et al: Pregnancy and its complications following cardiac valve prostheses. Am J Obstet Gynecol 131:460, 1978.

483. Smith ND, Raizada V, Abrams J: Auscultation of the normally functioning prosthetic valve. Ann Intern Med 95:594, 1981.

484. Pastore JO, Yurchak PM, Janis KM, et al: The risk of advanced heart block in surgical patients with right bundle branch block and left axis deviation. Circulation 57:677, 1978.

485. Berg GR, Kotler MN: The significance of bilateral bundle branch block in the preoperative patient. A retrospective electrocardiographic and clinical study in 30 patients. Chest 59:62, 1971.

486. Rooney S-M, Goldiner PL, Muss E: Relationship of right bundle-branch block and marked left axis deviation to complete heart block during general anesthesia. Anesthesiology 44:64, 1976.

487. Kunstadt D, Punja M, Cagin N, et al: Bifascicular block: A clinical and electrophysiologic study. Am Heart J 86:173, 1973.

488. Venkataraman K, Madias JE, Hood WB Jr: Indications for prophylactic preoperative insertion of pacemakers in patients with right bundle branch block and left anterior hemiblock. Chest 68:501, 1975.

489. Gauss A, Hübner C, Radermacher P, et al: Perioperative risk of bradyarrhythmias in patients with asymptomatic chronic bifascicular block or left bundle branch block. Does an additional first-degree atrioventricular block make any difference? Anesthesiology 88:679, 1998.

490. Ruskin JN: Catheter ablation for supraventricular tachycardia. N Engl J Med 324:1660, 1991.

491. Kelly JS, Royster RL: Noninvasive transcutaneous cardiac pacing. Anesth Analg 69:229, 1989.

492. Risk SC, Brandon D, D'Ambra MN, et al: Indications for the use of pacing pulmonary artery catheters in cardiac surgery. J Cardiothorac Vasc Anesth 6:275, 1992.

493. Ruskin JN, DiMarco JP, Garan H: Out-of-hospital cardiac arrest. Electrophysiologic observations and selection of long-term antiarrhythmic therapy. N Engl J Med 303:607, 1980.

494. Prystowsky EN: Diagnosis and management of the pre-excitation syndromes. Curr Probl Cardiol 13:225, 1988.

495. McAnulty JH, Rahimtoola SH, Murphy E, et al: Natural history of "high-risk" bundle-branch block. Final report of a prospective study. N Engl J Med 307:137, 1982.

496. Rose MR, Koski G: Anesthesia in patients with Wolff-Parkinson-White syndrome [abstract]. Anesthesiology 69:A146, 1988.

497. Sadowski AR, Moyers JR: Anesthetic management of the Wolff-Parkinson-White syndrome. Anesthesiology 51:553, 1979.

498. Furman S: Rate-modulated pacing. Circulation 82:1081, 1990.

499. Shapiro WA, Roizen MF, Singleton MA, et al: Intraoperative pacemaker complications. Anesthesiology 63:319, 1985.

500. Rozner MA: Review of electrical interference in implanted cardiac devices. Pacing Clin Electrophysiol 26(4 Pt 1): 923-925, 2003.

501. Thiagarajah S, Azar I, Agres M, et al: Pacemaker malfunction associated with positive-pressure ventilation. Anesthesiology 58:565, 1983.

502. Anthonisen NR, Connet JE, Kiley JP, et al: Effect of smoking intervention and the use of an inhaled anticholinergic bronchodilator on the rate of decline of FEV_1. The Lung Health Study. JAMA 272:1497, 1994.

503. European Respiratory Society: Optimal assessment and management of chronic obstructive pulmonary disease (COPD). Eur Respir J 8:1398, 1995.

504. Holleman DR Jr, Simel DL: Does the clinical examination predict airflow limitation? JAMA 273:313, 1995.

505. Lacasse Y, Guyatt GH, Goldstein RS: The components of a respiratory rehabilitation program: A systematic overview. Chest 111:1077, 1997.

506. Saint S, Bent S, Vittinghoff E, Grady D: Antibiotics in chronic obstructive pulmonary disease exacerbations. A meta-analysis. JAMA 273:957, 1995.

507. Thompson WH, Nielson CP, Carvalho P, et al: Controlled trial of oral prednisone in outpatients with acute COPD exacerbations. Am J Respir Crit Care Med 154:407, 1996.

508. NAEP Expert Panel Report 2: Guidelines for the diagnosis and management of asthma. Public Health Service. US Department of Health and Human Services Publication No. 97-4051A, May 1997 (http://www.nhlbi.nih.gov/nhlbi/nhlbi.htm).

509. Cockcroft DW: Management of acute severe asthma. Ann Allergy Asthma Immunol 75:83, 1995.

510. Tinkelman DG, Reed CE, Nelson HS, Offord KP: Aerosol beclomethasone dipropionate compared with theophylline as primary treatment of chronic, mild to moderately severe asthma in children. Pediatrics 92:64, 1993.

511. Dompeling E, van Schayck CP, van Grunsven PM, et al: Slowing the deterioration of asthma and chronic obstructive pulmonary disease observed during bronchodilator therapy by adding inhaled corticosteroids. A 4-year prospective study. Ann Intern Med 118:770, 1993.

512. Calligaro KD, Azurin DJ, Dougherty MJ, et al: Pulmonary risk factors of elective abdominal aortic surgery. J Vasc Surg 18:914, 1993.

513. Homer CJ: Asthma disease management. N Engl J Med 337:1461, 1997.

514. Sur S, Hunt LW, Crotty TB, Gleich GJ: Sudden-onset fatal asthma. Mayo Clin Proc 69:495, 1994.

515. Skolnick ET, Vomvolakis MA, Buck KA, et al: Exposure to environmental tobacco smoke and the risk of adverse respiratory events in children receiving general anesthesia. Anesthesiology 88:1144, 1998.

516. Ballantyne JC, Carr DB, deFerranti S, et al: Comparative effects of postoperative analgesic therapies upon respiratory function: Meta-analysis of initial randomized control trials. Anesth Analg 86:598, 1998.

517. Rodgers A, Walker N, Schug S, et al: Reduction of postoperative mortality and morbidity with epidural or spinal anaesthesia: Results from overview of randomised trials. BMJ 321:1493, 2000.

518. Wu CL, Caldwell MD: Effect of post-operative analgesia on patient morbidity. Best Pract Res Clin Anaesthesiol 16:549-563, 2002.

519. Stein M, Cassara EL: Preoperative pulmonary evaluation and therapy for surgery patients. JAMA 211:787, 1970.

520. Collins CD, Darke CS, Knowelden J: Chest complications after upper abdominal surgery: Their anticipation and prevention. BMJ 1:401, 1968.

521. Warner MA, Offord KP, Warner ME, et al: Role of preoperative cessation of smoking and other factors in postoperative pulmonary complications: A blinded prospective study of coronary artery bypass patients. Mayo Clin Proc 64:609, 1989.

522. Robinson K, Conroy RM, Mulcahy R: When does the risk of acute coronary heart disease in ex-smokers fall to that in non-smokers? A retrospective study of patients admitted to hospital with a first episode of myocardial infarction or unstable angina. Br Heart J 62:16, 1989.

523. Rosenberg L, Kaufman D, Helmrich S, Shapiro S: The risk of myocardial infarction after quitting smoking in men under 55 years of age. N Engl J Med 313:1511, 1985.

524. Gordon T, Kannell WB, McGee D: Death and coronary attacks in men after giving up smoking: A report from the Framingham Study. Lancet 2:1345, 1974.

525. Ernst E, Matrai A: Abstention from chronic cigarette smoking normalizes blood rheology. Atherosclerosis 64:75, 1987.

526. Bluman LG, Mosca L, Newman N, Simon DG: Preoperative smoking habits and postoperative pulmonary complications. Chest 113:883-889, 1998.

527. Nakagawa M, Tanaka H, Tsukuma H, Kishi Y: Relationship between the duration of the preoperative smoke-free period and the incidence of postoperative pulmonary complications after pulmonary surgery. Chest 120:705-710, 2001.

528. Celli BR, Rodriguez KS, Snider GL: A controlled trial of intermittent positive pressure breathing, incentive

529. spirometry, and deep breathing exercises in preventing pulmonary complications after abdominal surgery. Am Rev Respir Dis 130:12, 1984.

529. Bartlett RH, Brennan ML, Gazzaniga AB, et al: Studies on the pathogenesis and prevention of postoperative pulmonary complications. Surg Gynecol Obstet 137:925, 1973.

530. Lyager S, Wernberg M, Rajani N, et al: Can postoperative pulmonary conditions be improved by treatment with the Bartlett-Edwards incentive spirometer after upper abdominal surgery? Acta Anaesthesiol Scand 23:312, 1979.

531. Tisi GM: Preoperative evaluation of pulmonary function validity, indications, benefits. Am Rev Respir Dis 119:293, 1979.

532. Hedley-Whyte J, Burgess GE, Feeley TW, et al: Critical analysis of preventive measures. In Applied Physiology of Respiratory Care. Boston, Little, Brown, 1976, p 119.

533. Pontoppidan H: Mechanical aids to lung expansion in nonintubated surgical patients. Am Rev Respir Dis 122:109, 1980.

534. Celli BR: What is the value of preoperative pulmonary function testing? Med Clin North Am 77:309, 1993.

535. Graham WGB, Bradley DA: Efficacy of chest physiotherapy in the resolution of pneumonia. N Engl J Med 299:624, 1978.

536. Connors AF Jr, Hammon WE, Martin RJ, et al: Chest physical therapy. The immediate effect on oxygenation in acutely ill patients. Chest 78:559, 1980.

537. Cottrell JE, Siker ES: Preoperative intermittent positive-pressure breathing therapy in patients with chronic obstructive lung disease: Effect on postoperative pulmonary complications. Anesth Analg 52:258, 1973.

538. Forthman HJ, Shepard A: Postoperative pulmonary complications. South Med J 62:1198, 1969.

539. Boushy SF, Billing DM, North LB, et al: Clinical course related to preoperative pulmonary function in patients with bronchogenic carcinoma. Chest 59:383, 1971.

540. Elwood T, Morris W, Martin LD, et al: Bronchodilator premedication does not decrease respiratory adverse events in pediatric general anesthesia. Can J Anaesth 50:277-284, 2003.

541. Mittman C: Assessment of operative risk in thoracic surgery. Am Rev Respir Dis 84:197, 1961.

542. Reichel J: Assessment of operative risk of pneumonectomy. Chest 62:570, 1972.

543. Fischl MA, Pitchenik A, Gardner LB: An index predicting relapse and need for hospitalization in patients with acute bronchial asthma. N Engl J Med 305:783, 1981.

544. Wong DH, Weber EC, Schell MJ, et al: Factors associated with postoperative pulmonary complications in patients with severe COPD. Anesth Analg 80:276, 1995.

545. Wiener-Kronish JP, Matthay MA: Preoperative evaluation. In Murray J, Nadel J (eds): Textbook of Respiratory Medicine. Philadelphia, WB Saunders, 1988, p 683.

546. Roukema JA, Carol EJ, Prins JG: The prevention of pulmonary complications after upper abdominal surgery in patients with non-compromised pulmonary status. Arch Surg 123:30, 1988.

547. Arozullah AM, Daley J, Henderson WG, Khuri SF: Multifactorial risk index for predicting postoperative respiratory failure in men after major noncardiac surgery. The National Veterans Administration Surgical Quality Improvement Program. Ann Surg 232:242-253, 2000.

548. Arozullah AM, Khuri SF, Henderson WG, et al: Development and validation of a multifactorial risk index for predicting postoperative pneumonia after major noncardiac surgery. Ann Intern Med 135:847-857, 2001.

549. Hall WJ, Douglas RG, Hyde RW, et al: Pulmonary mechanics after uncomplicated influenza A infection. Am Rev Respir Dis 113:141, 1976.

550. Green GM, Jakab GJ, Low RB, et al: Defense mechanisms of the respiratory membrane. Am Rev Respir Dis 115:479, 1977.

551. Tait AR, Knight PR: The effects of general anesthesia on upper respiratory tract infections in children. Anesthesiology 67:930, 1987.

552. DeSoto H, Patel RI, Soliman IE, Hannallah RS: Changes in oxygen saturation following general anesthesia in children with upper respiratory infection signs and symptoms undergoing otolaryngological procedures. Anesthesiology 68:276, 1988.

553. Fennelly ME, Hall GM: Anaesthesia and upper respiratory tract infections—a non-existent hazard? Br J Anaesth 64:535, 1990.

554. Cohen MM, Cameron CB: Should you cancel the operation when a child has an upper respiratory tract infection? Anesth Analg 72:282, 1991.

555. Jacoby DB, Hirshman CA: General anesthesia in patients with viral respiratory infections: An unsound sleep? Anesthesiology 74:969, 1991.

556. Kinouchi K, Tanigami H, Tashiro C, et al: Duration of apnea in anesthetized infants and children required for desaturation of hemoglobin to 95%. The influence of upper respiratory infection. Anesthesiology 77:1105, 1992.

557. Fishman AP: Cardiac asthma—a fresh look at an old wheeze. N Engl J Med 320:1346, 1989.

558. Dunlap NE, Fulmer JD: Corticosteroid therapy in asthma. Clin Chest Med 5:669-683, 1984.

559. Latimer RG, Dickman M, Day WC, et al: Ventilatory patterns and pulmonary complications after upper abdominal surgery determined by preoperative and postoperative computerized spirometry and blood gas analysis. Am J Surg 122:622, 1971.

560. McAlister FA, Khan NA, Straus SE, et al: Accuracy of the preoperative assessment in predicting pulmonary risk after nonthoracic surgery. Am J Respir Crit Care Med 167:741-744, 2003.

561. Tarhan S, Moffitt EA, Sessler AD, et al: Risk of anesthesia and surgery in patients with chronic bronchitis and chronic obstructive pulmonary disease. Surgery 74:720, 1973.

562. Pereira ED, Fernandes AL, da Silva Arcao M, et al: Prospective assessment of the risk of postoperative pulmonary complications in patients submitted to upper abdominal surgery. Sao Paulo Med J 117:151-160, 1999.

563. Chung F, Mezei G, Tong D, et al: Pre-existing medical conditions as predictors of adverse events in day-case surgery. Br J Anaesth 83:262-270, 1999.

564. Newman KB, Mason UG 3rd, Schmaling KB: Clinical features of vocal cord dysfunction. Am J Respir Crit Care Med 152:1382, 1995.

565. Smetana GW: Preoperative pulmonary assessment of the older adult. Clin Geriatr Med 19:35-55, 2003.

566. Gupta RM, Parvizi J, Hanssen AD, Gay PC: Postoperative complications in patients with obstructive sleep apnea syndrome undergoing hip or knee replacement: A case-control study. Mayo Clin Proc 76:897-905, 2001.

567. Knudson J: Duration of hypoxemia after uncomplicated upper abdominal and thoraco-abdominal operations. Anaesthesia 25:372, 1970.

568. Warner DO, Warner MA, Offord KP, et al: Airway obstruction and perioperative complications in smokers undergoing abdominal surgery. Anesthesiology 90:372-379, 1999.

569. Boysen PG, Block AJ, Moulder PV: Relationship between preoperative pulmonary function tests and complications after thoracotomy. Surg Gynecol Obstet 152:813, 1981.

570. Furguson MK, Little L, Rizzo L, et al: Diffusing capacity predicts morbidity and mortality after pulmonary resection. J Thorac Cardiovasc Surg 96:894, 1988.

571. Markos J, Mullan BP, Hillman DR, et al: Preoperative assessment as a predictor of mortality and morbidity after lung resection. Am Rev Respir Dis 139:902, 1989.

572. Pien LC, Grammer LC, Patterson R: Minimal complications in a surgical population with severe asthma receiving prophylactic corticosteroids. J Allergy Clin Immunol 82:696-700, 1988.

573. Kabalin CS, Yarnold PR, Grammer LC: Low complication rate of corticosteroid-treated asthmatics undergoing surgical procedures. Arch Intern Med 155:1379-1384, 1995.

574. Selzer A, Walter RM: Adequacy of preoperative digitalis therapy in controlling ventricular rate in postoperative atrial fibrillation. Circulation 34:119, 1966.

575. Ginsberg JS: Management of venous thromboembolism. N Engl J Med 335:1816, 1996.

576. Geerts WH, Heit JA, Clagett GP, et al: Prevention of venous thromboembolism. Chest 119(1 Suppl):132S-175S, 2001.

577. O'Donnell M, Weitz JI: Thromboprophylaxis in surgical patients. Can J Surg 46:129-135, 2003.

578. Neiwoehner DE, Kleinerman J, Rice DB: Pathologic changes in the peripheral airways of young cigarette smokers. N Engl J Med 291:755, 1974.

579. Matthay RA, Niederman MS, Wiedemann HP: Cardiovascular pulmonary interaction in chronic obstructive pulmonary disease with special reference to pathogenesis and management of cor pulmonale. Med Clin North Am 74:571, 1990.

580. Dorinsky PM, Gadek JE: Mechanisms of non-pulmonary organ failure in ARDS. Chest 96:885, 1989.

581. Domino KB, Wetstein L, Glasser SA, et al: Influence of mixed venous oxygen tension ($P\bar{v}o_2$) on blood flow to atelectatic lung. Anesthesiology 59:428, 1983.

582. Combs DL, O'Brien RJ, Geiter LJ: USPHS tuberculosis short-course chemotherapy trial 21: Effectiveness, toxicity, and acceptability. The report of final results. Ann Intern Med 112:397, 1990.

583. Niederman MS, Craven DE, Fein AM, Schultz DE: Pneumonia in the critically ill hospitalized patient. Chest 97:170, 1990.

584. Murray JF, Mills J: Pulmonary infectious complications of human immunodeficiency virus infection: Parts 1 and 2. Am Rev Respir Dis 5:1356, 1582, 1990.

585. Skerrett SJ, Niederman MS, Fein AM: Respiratory infections and acute lung injury in systemic illness. Clin Chest Med 10:469, 1989.

586. Barnes PJ: A new approach to the treatment of asthma. N Engl J Med 321:1517, 1989.

587. Settipane GA, Dudupakkam RK: Aspirin intolerance. III: Subtypes, familial occurrence and cross reactivity with tartrazine. J Allergy Clin Immunol 56:215, 1975.

588. Crystal RG, Bitterman PB, Rennard SI, et al: Interstitial lung disease of unknown cause: Disorders characterized by chronic inflammation of the lower respiratory tract. N Engl J Med 310:154, 1984.

589. Mathieson JR, Mayo JR, Staples CA, Müller NL: Chronic diffuse infiltrative lung disease: Comparison of diagnostic accuracy of CT and chest radiography. Radiology 171:111, 1989.

590. Cooper JAD (ed): Drug-induced pulmonary disease. Clin Chest Med 11:1, 1990.

591. Williams DE, Pairolero PC, Davis CS, et al: Survival of patients surgically treated for stage I lung cancer. J Thorac Cardiovasc Surg 82:70, 1981.

592. Woodring JH: Lung cancer. Radiol Clin North Am 28:489, 1990.

593. Cancer Statistics for the United States. www.cdc.gov/nchs/products/pubs/pubd/hus/trendtables.htm 200.

594. Aisner J: Extensive-disease small-cell lung cancer: The thrill of victory the agony of defeat. J Clin Oncol 14:658, 1996.

595. Levy JH, Roizen MF, Morris JM: Anaphylactic and anaphylactoid reactions: A review. Spine 11:282, 1986.

596. Kemp SF, Lockey RF, Wolf BL, Lieberman P: Anaphylaxis. A review of 266 cases. Arch Intern Med 155:1749, 1995.

597. Watkins J: Anaphylactoid reactions to I.V. substances. Br J Anaesth 51:51, 1979.

598. Smith PL, Kagey-Sobotka A, Bleecker ER, et al: Physiologic manifestations of human anaphylaxis. J Clin Invest 66:1072, 1980.

599. Delage C, Irey NS: Anaphylactic deaths: A clinicopathologic study of 43 cases. J Forensic Sci 17:525, 1972.

600. Bettman MA: Radiographic contrast agents—a perspective. N Engl J Med 317:891, 1987.

601. Chenoweth DE, Cooper SW, Hugli TE, et al: Complement activation during cardiopulmonary bypass. N Engl J Med 304:497, 1981.

602. Craddock PR, Fehr J, Brigham KL, et al: Complement and leukocyte-mediated pulmonary dysfunction in hemodialysis. N Engl J Med 296:769, 1977.

603. Roizen MF, Rodgers GM, Valone FH, et al: Anaphylactoid reactions to vascular graft material presenting with vasodilation and subsequent disseminated intravascular coagulation. Anesthesiology 71:331, 1989.

604. Swanson MC, Bubak ME, Hunt LW, et al: Quantification of occupational latex aeroallergens in a medical center. J Allergy Clin Immunol 94:445, 1994.

605. Mertes PM, Laxenaire MC: Allergic reactions occurring during anaesthesia. Eur J Anaesthesiol 19:240-262, 2002.

606. Lieberman P: Anaphylactic reactions during surgical and medical procedures. J Allergy Clin Immunol 110(2 Suppl): S64-S69, 2002.

607. Rosow CE, Moss J, Philbin DM, et al: Histamine release during morphine and fentanyl anesthesia. Anesthesiology 56:93, 1982.

608. Moss J, Rosow CE, Savarese JJ, et al: Role of histamine in the hypotensive action of d-tubocurarine in humans. Anesthesiology 55:19, 1981.

609. Millbern SM, Bell SD: Prevention of anaphylaxis to contrast media. Anesthesiology 50:56, 1979.

610. Moss J, McDermott DJ, Thisted RA, et al: Anaphylactic/anaphylactoid reactions in response to Chymodiactin (chymopapain). Anesth Analg 63:253, 1984.

611. Philbin DM, Moss J, Akins CW, et al: The use of H$_1$ and H$_2$ histamine antagonists with morphine anesthesia: A double-blind study. Anesthesiology 55:292, 1981.

612. Halevy S, Altura BT, Altura BM: Pathophysiological basis for the use of steroids in the treatment of shock and trauma. Klin Wochenschr 60:1021, 1982.

613. Ring J, Messmer K: Incidence and severity of anaphylactoid reactions to colloid volume substitutes. Lancet 1:466, 1977.

614. Milner LV, Butcher K: Transfusion reactions reported after transfusion of red blood cells and of whole blood. Transfusion 18:493, 1978.

615. Barach EM, Nowak RM, Lee TG, et al: Epinephrine for treatment of anaphylactic shock. JAMA 251:2118, 1984.

616. Toogood JH: Risk of anaphylaxis in patients receiving beta-blocker drugs. J Allergy Clin Immunol 81:1, 1988.

617. Van Arsdel PP Jr, Larson EB: Diagnostic tests for patients with suspected allergic disease. Ann Intern Med 110:304 1989.

618. Del Pizzo A: Hereditary angioneurotic edema. Anesthesiol Rev 5:41, 1978.

619. Hosea SW, Santaella ML, Brown EJ, et al: Long-term therapy of hereditary angioedema with danazol. Ann Intern Med 93:809, 1982.

620. Oxelius V-A, Laurell A-B, Lindquist B, et al: IgG subclasses in selective IgA deficiency. Importance of IgG2-IgA deficiency. N Engl J Med 304:1476, 1981.

621. Fauci AS, Rosenberg SA, Sherwin SA, et al: Immunomodulators in clinical medicine. Ann Intern Med 106:421, 1987.

622. Levy DE, Caronna JJ, Singer BH, et al: Predicting outcome from hypoxic-ischemic coma. JAMA 253:1420, 1985.

623. Plum F, Posner JB: The Diagnosis of Stupor and Coma. 3rd ed. Philadelphia, FA Davis, 1980.

624. Lowenstein DH, Massa SM, Rowbotham MC, et al: Acute neurologic and psychiatric complications associated with cocaine abuse. Am J Med 83:841, 1987.

625. Barry PP, Moskowitz MA: The diagnosis of reversible dementia in the elderly, a critical review. Arch Intern Med 148:1914, 1988.

626. Boguosslavsky J, Meineberg O: Eye-movement disorders in brain-stem and cerebellar stoke. Arch Neurol 44:141, 1987.

627. Drugs for epilepsy. Med Lett Drugs Ther 45:57-64, 2003.

628. Roberts R: Differential diagnosis of sleep disorders, non-epileptic attacks and epileptic attacks. Curr Opin Neurol 11:135-9, 1998.

629. Shaner DM, McCurdy SA, Herring MO, et al: Treatment of status epilepticus: A prospective comparison of diazepam and phenytoin versus phenobarbital and optional phenytoin. Neurology 38:202, 1988.

630. Joas TA, Stevens WC, Eger EI II: Electroencephalographic seizure activity in dogs during anesthesia. Br J Anaesth 43:739, 1971.

631. Opitz A, Brechts B, Stenzel E: Enflurane anaesthesia for epileptic patients. Anaesthesist 26:329, 1977.

632. Schuchat A, Robinson K, Wenger JD, et al: Bacterial meningitis in the United States in 1995. N Engl J Med 337:970, 1997.

633. Parkinson Study Group: Impact of deprenyl and tocopherol treatment on Parkinson's disease in DATATOP patients requiring levodopa. Ann Neurol 39:37, 1996.

634. Goetz CG, Olanow CW, Koller WC, et al: Multicenter study of autologous adrenal medullary transplantation to the corpus striatum in patients with advanced Parkinson's disease. N Engl J Med 320:337, 1989.

635. Mets B: Acute dystonia after alfentanil in untreated Parkinson's disease. Anesth Analg 72:557, 1991.

636. Muzzi DA, Black S, Cucchiara RF: The lack of effect of succinylcholine on serum potassium in patients with Parkinson's disease. Anesthesiology 71:322, 1989.

637. Ngai SH: Parkinsonism, levodopa, and anesthesia. Anesthesiology 37:344, 1972.

638. Wiklund RA, Ngai SH: Rigidity and pulmonary edema after Innovar in a patient on levodopa therapy: Report of a case. Anesthesiology 35:545-547, 1971.

639. Skoog I, Nilsson J, Palmertz B, et al: A population-based study of dementia in 85-year-olds. N Engl J Med 328:153, 1993.

640. Petersen RC, Smith GE, Waring SC, et al: Mild cognitive impairment: Clinical characterization and outcome. Arch Neurol 56:303-308, 1999.

641. Ross GW, Abbott RD, Petrovitch H, et al: Frequency and characteristics of silent dementia among elderly Japanese-American men. The Honolulu-Asia Aging Study. JAMA 277:800, 1997.

642. Snowdon DA, Greiner LH, Mortimer JA, et al: Brain infarction and the clinical expression of Alzheimer disease. The Nun Study. JAMA 277:813, 1997.

643. Drugs for Alzheimer's disease. Med Lett Drugs Ther 43:53, 2001.

644. Hemmelgarn B, Suissa S, Huang A, et al: Benzodiazepine use and the risk of motor vehicle crash in the elderly. JAMA 278:27, 1997.

645. Mozkowitz MA: Basic mechanisms in vascular headache. Neurol Clin 8:801, 1990.

646. Michel P, Henry P, Letenneur L, et al: Diagnostic screen for assessment of IHS criteria for migraine by general practitioners. Cephalalgia 12:54, 1993.

647. MacIntyre PD, Bhargava B, Hogg KJ, et al: Effect of subcutaneous sumatriptan, a selective 5HT-1 agonist, on the systemic, pulmonary, and coronary circulation. Circulation 87:401, 1993.

648. Shadick NA, Phillips CB, Logigian EL, et al: The long-term clinical outcomes of Lyme disease. A population-based retrospective cohort study. Ann Intern Med 121:560, 1994.

649. Ovassapian A, Land P, Schafer MF, et al: Anesthetic management for surgical corrections of severe flexion deformity of the cervical spine. Anesthesiology 58:370, 1983.

650. Dahm LS, Dickson JH, Harrison GH: Perioperative and anesthetic management in the patient with scoliosis. Anesthesiol Rev 9:13, 1982.

651. Ferguson RJ, Caplan LR: Cervical spondylitic myelopathy. Neurol Clin 3:373, 1985.

652. Rudick RA, Cohen JA, Weinstock-Guttman B, et al: Management of multiple sclerosis. N Engl J Med 337:1604, 1997.

653. Basket PJF, Armstrong R: Anaesthetic problems in multiple sclerosis: Are certain agents contraindicated? Anaesthesia 25:397, 1970.

654. McKhann GM, Griffin JW, Cornblath DR, et al: Plasmapheresis and Guillain-Barré syndrome: Analysis of prognostic factors and the effect of plasmapheresis. Ann Neurol 23:347, 1988.

655. Ancoli-Israel S, Klauber MR, Stepnowsky C, et al: Sleep-disordered breathing in African-American elderly. Am J Respir Crit Care Med 152:1946, 1995.

656. Ostermeier AM, Roizen MF, Hautkappe M, et al: Three sudden postoperative respiratory arrests associated with

epidural opioids in patients with sleep apnea. Anesth Analg 85:452, 1997.

657. Aldrich MS: Narcolepsy. N Engl J Med 323:389, 1990.

658. Cyr MG, Wartman SA: The effectiveness of routine screening questions in the detection of alcoholism. JAMA 259:51, 1988.

659. Toh B-H, van Driel IR, Gleeson PA: Pernicious anemia. N Engl J Med 337:1441, 1997.

660. Jensen NF, Fiddler DS, Striepe V: Anesthetic considerations in porphyrias. Anesth Analg 80:591, 1995.

661. Kantor G, Rolbin SH: Acute intermittent porphyria and caesarean delivery. Can J Anaesth 39:282, 1992.

662. Meissner PN, Harrison GG, Hift RJ: Propofol as an I.V. anaesthetic induction agent in variegate porphyria. Br J Anaesth 66:60, 1991.

663. McNeill MJ, Bennet A: Use of regional anaesthesia in a patient with acute porphyria. Br J Anaesth 64:371, 1990.

664. Massey JM: Treatment of acquired myasthenia gravis. Neurology 48:S46-S51, 1997.

665. d'Empaire G, Hoaglin DC, Perlo VP, et al: Effect of prethymectomy plasma exchange on postoperative respiratory function in myasthenia gravis. J Thorac Cardiovasc Surg 89:592, 1985.

666. Eisenkraft JB, Book WJ, Mann SM, et al: Resistance to succinylcholine in myasthenia gravis: A dose response study. Anesthesiology 69:760, 1988.

667. Eisenkraft JB, Papatestas AE, Kahn CH, et al: Predicting the need for postoperative mechanical ventilation in myasthenia gravis. Anesthesiology 65:79, 1986.

668. Small S, Ali HH, Lennon VA, et al: Anesthesia for unsuspected Lambert-Eaton myasthenic syndrome with autoantibodies and occult small cell lung carcinoma. Anesthesiology 76:142, 1992.

669. Lema G, Urzua J, Moran S, Canessa R: Successful anesthetic management of a patient with hypokalemic familial periodic paralysis undergoing cardiac surgery. Anesthesiology 74:373, 1991.

670. Ashwood EM, Russell WJ, Burrow DD: Hyperkalaemic periodic paralysis. Anaesthesia 47:579, 1992.

671. Gutmann DH, Fischbeck KH: Molecular biology of Duchenne and Becker's muscular dystrophy: Clinical applications. Ann Neurol 26:189, 1989.

672. Smith CL, Bush GH: Anesthesia and progressive muscular dystrophy. Br J Anaesth 57:1113, 1985.

673. Schwartz L, Rockoff MA, Koka BV: Masseter spasm with anesthesia: Incidence and implications. Anesthesiology 61:772, 1984.

674. Rosenberg H: Trismus is not trivial, editorial. Anesthesiology 67:453, 1987.

675. Pueschel SM, Scola FH: Atlantoaxial instability in individuals with Down syndrome: Epidemiologic, radiographic, and clinical studies. Pediatrics 80:55, 1987.

676. Morray JP, MacGillivray R, Duker G: Increased perioperative risk following repair of congenital heart disease in Down's syndrome. Anesthesiology 65:221, 1986.

677. Roizen NJ, Patterson D: Down's syndrome Lancet 361:1281-1289, 2003.

678. Freeman SB, Taft LF, Dopoley KJ, et al: Population-based study of congenital heart defects in Down syndrome. Am J Med Genet 80:213-217, 1998.

679. Kobel M, Creighton RE, Steward DJ: Anaesthetic considerations in Down's syndrome: Experience with 100 patients and a review of the literature. Can J Anaesth 29:593, 1982.

680. Bedford RF, Morris L, Jane JA: Intracranial hypertension during surgery for supratentorial tumor: Correlation with preoperative computed tomography scans. Anesth Analg 61:430, 1982.

681. Ramirez-Lassepas M, Quinones MR: Heparin therapy for stroke: Hemorrhagic complications and risk factors for intracerebral hemorrhage. Neurology 34:114, 1984.

682. Rem JA, Hachinski VC, Boughner DR, Barnett HJ: Value of cardiac monitoring and echocardiography in TIA and stroke patients. Stroke 16:950, 1985.

683. Drugs for psychiatric disorders. Treatment guideline. Med Lett Drugs Ther 11:69-76, 2003.

684. Appel GB, Neu HC: The nephrotoxicity of antimicrobial agents. N Engl J Med 296:663, 722, 784, 1977.

685. Fischer RP, Polk HC Jr: Changing etiologic patterns of renal insufficiency in surgical patients [editorial]. Surg Gynecol Obstet 140:85, 1975.

686. Better OS, Stein JH: Early management of shock and prophylaxis of acute renal failure in traumatic rhabdomyolysis. N Engl J Med 322:825, 1990.

687. Levey AS, Perrone RD, Madias NE: Serum creatinine and renal function. Annu Rev Med 39:465, 1988.

688. Byrick RJ, Rose DK: Pathophysiology and prevention of acute renal failure: The role of the anaesthetist. Can J Anaesth 37:457, 1990.

689. Berns AS: Nephrotoxicity of contrast media. Kidney Int 36:730, 1989.

690. Myers BD, Moran SM: Hemodynamically mediated acute renal failure. N Engl J Med 314:97, 1986.

691. Shusterman N, Strom BL, Murray TG, et al: Risk factors and outcome of hospital-acquired acute renal failure: A clinical epidemiologic study. Am J Med 83:65, 1987.

692. Bernard DB: Extrarenal complications of the nephrotic syndrome [clinical conference]. Kidney Int 33:1184, 1988.

693. Thadhani R, Pascual M, Bonventre JV: Acute renal failure. N Engl J Med 334:1448, 1996.

694. Aronson S, Thisthelwaite RJ, Walker R, et al: Safety and feasibility of renal blood flow determination during surgery with perfusion ultrasonography. Anesth Analg 80:353, 1995.

695. Hebert PC, Wells G, Blajchman MA, et al: A multicenter, randomized, controlled clinical trial of transfusion requirements in critical care. Transfusion Requirements in Critical Care Investigators, Canadian Critical Care Trials Group. N Engl J Med 340:409-417, 1999.

696. Rao KV, Anderson RC, O'Brien TJ: Factors contributing for improved graft survival in recipients of kidney transplants. Kidney Int 24:210, 1983.

697. Eschbach JW, Kelly MR, Haley NR, et al: Treatment of the anemia of progressive renal failure with recombinant human erythropoietin. N Engl J Med 321:158, 1989.

698. Burke GR, Gulyassy PF: Surgery in the patient with renal disease and related electrolyte disorders. Med Clin North Am 63:1191, 1979.

699. Coe FL, Parks JH, Asplin JR: The pathogenesis and treatment of kidney stones. N Engl J Med 327:1141, 1992.

700. Kellen M, Aronson S, Roizen MF, et al: Predictive and diagnostic tests of renal failure: A review. Anesth Analg 78:134, 1994.

701. Shin B, Mackenzie CF, Helrich M: Creatinine clearance for early detection of posttraumatic renal dysfunction. Anesthesiology 64:605, 1986.

702. Novis BK, Roizen MF, Aronson S, Thisted RA: Association of preoperative risk factors with postoperative acute renal failure. Anesth Analg 78:143, 1994.

703. Rowe JW, Andres R, Tobin JD, et al: The effect of age on creatinine clearance in men: A cross-sectional and longitudinal study. J Gerontol 31:155, 1976.

704. Lee TH, Marcantonio ER, Mangione CM, et al: Derivation and prospective validation of a simple index for prediction of cardiac risk of major noncardiac surgery. Circulation 100:1043-1049, 1999.

705. Mangano CM, Diamondstone LS, Ramsay JG, et al: Renal dysfunction after myocardial revascularization: Risk factors, adverse outcomes, and hospital resource utilization. The Multicenter Study of Perioperative Ischemia Research Group. Ann Intern Med 128:194-203, 1998.

706. Koning HM, Koning AJ, Leusink JA: Serious acute renal failure following open heart surgery. Thorac Cardiovasc Surg 33:283, 1985.

707. Kleinknecht D, Ganeval D, Gonzalez-Duque LA, et al: Furosemide in acute oliguric renal failure: A controlled trial. Nephron 17:51, 1976.

708. Flancbaum L, Choban PS, Dasta JF: Quantitative effects of low-dose dopamine on urine output in oliguric surgical intensive care unit patients. Crit Care Med 22:61, 1994.

709. Hanley MJ, Davidson K: Prior mannitol and furosemide infusion in a model of ischemic acute renal failure. Am J Physiol 241:F556, 1981.

710. Davis RF, Lappas DG, Kirklin JK, et al: Acute oliguria after cardiopulmonary bypass: Renal functional improvement with low-dose dopamine infusion. Crit Care Med 10:852, 1982.

711. Polson RJ, Park GR, Lindop MJ, et al: The prevention of renal impairment in patients undergoing orthotopic liver grafting by infusion of low dose dopamine. Anaesthesia 42:15, 1987.

712. Paul MD, Mazer CD, Byrick RJ, et al: Influence of mannitol and dopamine on renal function during elective infrarenal aortic clamping in man. Am J Nephrol 6:427, 1986.

713. Crowley K, Clarkson K, Hannon V, et al: Diuretics after transurethral prostatectomy: A double-blind controlled trial comparing furosemide and mannitol. Br J Anaesth 65:337, 1990.

714. Dorman, HR, Sondheimer JH, Cadnapaphornchai P: Mannitol-induced acute renal failure. Medicine (Baltimore) 69:153-159, 1990.

715. Kellum JA, Decker J: Use of dopamine in acute renal failure: A meta-analysis. Crit Care Med 29:1526-1531, 2001.

716. Alpert RA, Roizen MF, Hamilton WK, et al: Intraoperative urinary output does not predict postoperative renal function in patients undergoing abdominal aortic revascularization. Surgery 95:707, 1984.

717. Murphy MB, McCoy CE, Wever RR, et al: Augmentation of renal blood flow and sodium excretion in hypertensive patients during blood pressure reduction by intravenous administration of the dopamine1 agonist fenoldopam. Circulation 76:1312-1318, 1987.

718. Halpenny M, Lakshmi S, O'Donnell A, et al: The effects of fenoldopam on coronary conduit blood flow after coronary artery bypass graft surgery. J Cardiothorac Vasc Anesth 15:72-76, 2001.

719. Halpenny M, Rushe C, Breen P, et al: The effects of fenoldopam on renal function in patients undergoing elective aortic surgery. Eur J Anaesthesiol 19:32-39, 2002.

720. Caimmi PP, Pagani L, Micalizzi E, et al: Fenoldopam for renal protection in patients undergoing cardiopulmonary bypass. J Cardiothorac Vasc Anesth 17:491-494, 2003.

721. Litz RJ, Hubler M, Lorenz W, et al: Renal responses to desflurane and isoflurane in patients with renal insufficiency. Anesthesiology 97:1133-1136, 2002.

722. Conzen PF, Kharasch ED, Czerner SF, et al: Low-flow sevoflurane compared with low-flow isoflurane anesthesia in patients with stable renal insufficiency. Anesthesiology 97:578-584, 2002.

723. Petroni KC, Cohen NH: Continuous renal replacement therapy: Anesthetic implications. Anesth Analg 94:1288-1297, 2002.

724. Dolan MJ, Whipp BJ, Davidson WD, et al: Hypopnea associated with acetate hemodialysis: Carbon dioxide–flow–dependent ventilation. N Engl J Med 305:72, 1981.

725. Renal Data System: USRDS 2001 Annual Data Report: Atlas of End Stage Renal Disease in the United States. Bethesda, MD, National Institute of Diabetes and Digestive and Kidney Diseases, 2001.

726. Roth S, Kuperberg JP: Adverse responses following intraoperative administration of Orthoclone OKT3. Anesth Analg 62:822, 1989.

727. Myers BD, Sibley R, Newton L, et al: The long-term course of cyclosporine-associated chronic nephropathy. Kidney Int 33:590, 1988.

728. Bennett WM, Aronoff GR, Morrison G, et al: Drug prescribing in renal failure: Dosing guidelines for adults. Am J Kidney Dis 3:155, 1983.

729. Rubin AL, Stenzel KH, Reidenberg MM: Symposium on drug action and metabolism in renal failure. Am J Med 62:459, 1977.

730. Bennett WM, Aronoff GR, Golper TA, et al: Drug Prescribing in Renal Failure. Dosing Guidelines for Adults. 2nd ed. Philadelphia, American College of Physicians, 1991.

731. Gibson TP: Renal disease and drug metabolism: An overview. Am J Kidney Dis 8:7, 1986.

732. Goyal P, Puri GD, Pandey CK, Srivastva S: Evaluation of induction doses of propofol: Comparison between endstage renal disease and normal renal function patients. Anaesth Intensive Care 30:584-587, 2002.

733. Dawling S, Crome P: Clinical pharmacokinetic considerations in the elderly: An update. Clin Pharmacokinet 17:236, 1989.

734. Keighley MRB: Antibiotics in biliary disease: The relative importance of antibiotic concentrations in the bile and serum. Gut 17:495, 1976.

735. Platt R, Zaleznik DF, Hopkins CC, et al: Perioperative antibiotic prophylaxis for herniorrhaphy and breast surgery. N Engl J Med 322:153, 1990.

736. Chestnut DH: Spinal anesthesia in the febrile patient. Anesthesiology 76:667, 1992.

737. Rackow EC, Astiz ME: Pathophysiology and treatment of septic shock. JAMA 266:548, 1991.

738. Knaus WA, Wagner DP: Multiple systems organ failure: Epidemiology and prognosis. Crit Care Clin 5:522, 1989.

739. The choice of antibacterial drugs. Med Lett Drugs Ther 46:13, 2004.

740. Shapiro BA, Kacmarek RM, Cane RD, et al: Clinical Application of Respiratory Care. 4th ed. St Louis, Mosby–Year Book, 1991.

741. Shapiro ED, Berg AT, Austrian R, et al: The protective efficacy of polyvalent pneumococcal polysaccharide vaccine. N Engl J Med 325:1453, 1991.

742. Gardner P, Schaffner W: Immunization of adults. N Engl J Med 328:1252, 1993.

743. Brownstein AB, Roizen MF: A compelling rationale for using preoperative visits to complete adult immunizations. J Clin Anesth 10:338, 1998.

744. Schwartz D, Schwartz T, Cooper E, Pullerits J: Anaesthesia and the child with HIV infection. Can J Anaesth 38:626, 1991.

745. Platt R, Polk BF, Murdock B, et al: Mortality associated with nosocomial urinary-tract infection. N Engl J Med 307:637, 1982.

746. Albert RK, Condie F: Hand-washing patterns in medical intensive-care units. N Engl J Med 304:1465, 1981.

747. Farber BF, Kaiser DL, Wenzel RP: Relation between surgical volume and incidence of postoperative wound infection. N Engl J Med 305:200, 1981.

748. Gross PA, Neu HC, Aswapokee P, et al: Deaths from nosocomial infections: Experience in a university hospital and a community hospital. Am J Med 68:219, 1980.

749. Bryan CS, Reynolds KL: Bacteremic nosocomial pneumonia: Analysis of 172 episodes from a single metropolitan area. Am Rev Respir Dis 129:668, 1984.

750. Maki DG, Botticelli JT, Le Roy ML, Thielke TS: Prospective study of replacing administration sets for intravenous therapy at 48- vs 72-hour intervals: 72 hours is safe and cost-effective. JAMA 258:1771, 1987.

751. Maki DG, Ringer M: Evaluation of dressing regimens for prevention of infection with peripheral intravenous catheters: Gauze, a transparent polyurethane dressing, and an iodophor-transparent dressing. JAMA 258:2396, 1987.

752. Popovic M, Sarngadharan MG, Read E, et al: Detection isolation, and continuous production of cytopathic retroviruses (HTLV-III) from patients with AIDS and pre-AIDS. Science 224:497, 1984.

753. Sharara AI, Hunt CM, Hamilton JD: Hepatitis C. Ann Intern Med 125:658, 1996.

754. Hoffnagle JH, Di Bisceglie AM: The treatment of chronic viral hepatitis. N Engl J Med 336:347, 1997.

755. Dodd RY: The risk of transfusion-transmitted infection. N Engl J Med 327:419, 1992.

756. Dworsky ME, Welch K, Cassady G, et al: Occupational risk for primary cytomegalovirus infection among pediatric health-care workers. N Engl J Med 309:950, 1983.

757. Buergler JM, Kim R, Thisted RA, et al: The risk of human immunodeficiency virus in surgeons, anesthesiologists, and medical students. Anesth Analg 75:118, 1992.

758. Jensen V: The TURP syndrome. Can J Anaesth 38:90, 1991.

759. Ostia JR: The binge-purge syndrome: A common albeit unappreciated cause of acid-base and fluid electrolyte disturbances. South Med J 80:58, 1987.

760. Schrier RW: Pathogenesis of sodium and water retention in high-output and low-output cardiac failure, nephrotic syndrome, cirrhosis, and pregnancy (Pts 1 and 2). N Engl J Med 319:1065, 1127, 1988.

761. Arieff AI, Llacki F, Massry SG: Neurologic manifestations and morbidity of hyponatremia: Correlation with brain water and electrolytes. Medicine (Baltimore) 55:121, 1976.

762. Sterns RH: Severe symptomatic hyponatremia: Treatment and outcome. Ann Intern Med 107:656, 1987.

763. Muldowney FP, Williams RT: Clinical disturbances in serum sodium and potassium in relation to alteration in total exchangeable sodium, exchangeable potassium and total body water. Am J Med 35:768, 1963.

764. Surawicz B: Relationship between electrocardiogram and electrolytes. Am Heart J 73:814, 1967.

765. Sack D, Kim ND, Harrison CE Jr: Contractility and subcellular calcium metabolism in chronic potassium deficiency. Am J Physiol 226:756, 1974.

766. Wong KC, Vitez TS: Electrolyte imbalance. Semin Anesth 2:161, 1983.

767. Goggin MJ, Joekes AM: Gas exchange in renal failure. I: Dangers of hyperkalaemia during anaesthesia. BMJ 2:244, 1971.

768. Busch EH, Ventura HO, Lavie CJ: Heparin-induced hyperkalemia. South Med J 80:1450, 1987.

769. Rimmer JM, Horn JF, Gennari FJ: Hyperkalemia as a complication of drug therapy. Arch Intern Med 147:867, 1987.

770. Don BR, Sebastian A, Cheitlin M, et al: Pseudohyperkalemia caused by fist clenching during phlebotomy. N Engl J Med 322:1290, 1990.

771. Kharasch ED, Bowdle TA: Hypokalemia before induction of anesthesia and prevention by β_2 adrenoceptor antagonism. Anesth Analg 72:216, 1991.

772. Allon M, Dunlay R, Copkney C: Nebulised albuterol for acute hyperkalemia in patients on hemodialysis. Ann Intern Med 110:426, 1989.

773. Zinn SE, Fairley HB, Glenn JD: Liver function in patients with mild alcoholic hepatitis, after enflurane, nitrous oxide–narcotic, and spinal anesthesia. Anesth Analg 64:487, 1985.

774. Ellefson RD: Porphyrinogens, porphyrins, and the porphyrias. Mayo Clin Proc 57:454, 1982.

775. Edwards R, Winnie AP, Ramamurthy S: Acute hypocapneic hypokalemia: An iatrogenic anesthetic complication. Anesth Analg 56:786, 1977.

776. Lawson NW, Butler GH, Rat CT: Alkalosis and cardiac arrhythmias. Anesth Analg 52:951, 1973.

777. Adrogué HJ, Madias NE: Management of life-threatening acid-base disorders. First of two parts. N Engl J Med 338:26, 1998.

778. Aldinger KA, Samaan NA: Hypokalemia with hypercalcemia. Prevalence and significance in treatment. Ann Intern Med 87:571, 1977.

779. Wong KC, Kawamura R, Hodges MR, et al: Acute intravenous administration of potassium chloride to furosemide pretreated dogs. Can J Anaesth 24:203, 1977.

780. Kawamura R, Wong KC, Hodges MR: Intravenous potassium chloride in hypokalemic dogs pretreated with digoxin. Anesth Analg 57:108, 1978.

781. Kunin AS, Surawicz B, Sims EAH: Decrease in serum potassium concentrations and appearance of cardiac arrhythmias during infusion of potassium with glucose in potassium-depleted patients. N Engl J Med 266:228, 1962.

782. Hahm TS, Cho HS, Lee KH, et al: Clonidine premedication prevents preoperative hypokalemia. J Clin Anesth 14:6-9, 2002.

783. Wilkinson PL, Ham J, Miller RD: Preoperative hyperkalemia and elective surgery. In Wilkinson PL, Ham J, Miller RD (eds): Clinical Anesthesia. Case Selections from the University of California, San Francisco. St Louis, CV Mosby, 1980, p 54.

784. Lawson DH: Adverse reactions to potassium chloride. Q J Med 43:433, 1974.

785. Lawson DH, Hutcheon AW, Jick H: Life threatening drug reactions amongst medical in-patients. Scott Med J 24:127, 1979.

786. Vitez TS, Soper LE, Wong KC, Soper P: Chronic hypokalemia and intraoperative dysrhythmias. Anesthesiology 63:130, 1985.

787. Hirsch IA, Tomlinson DL, Slogoff S, Keats AS: The overstated risk of preoperative hypokalemia. Anesth Analg 67:131, 1988.

788. Olson RP, Schow AJ, McCann R, et al: Absence of adverse outcomes in hyperkalemic patients undergoing vascular access surgery. Can J Anaesth 50:553-557, 2003.

789. Schow AJ, Lubarsky DA, Olson RP, Gan TJ: Can succinylcholine be used safely in hyperkalemic patients? Anesth Analg 95:19-122, 2002.

790. Wahr JA, Parks R, Boisvert D, et al: Preoperative serum potassium levels and perioperative outcomes in cardiac surgery patients. Multicenter Study of Perioperative Ischemia Research Group. JAMA 281:2203-2210, 1999.

791. Dyckner T, Wester PO: Ventricular extrasystoles and intracellular electrolytes before and after potassium and magnesium infusions in patients on diuretic treatment. Am Heart J 97:12, 1979.

792. Cohen JD, Neaton JD, Prineas RJ, Daniels KA: Diuretics, serum potassium and ventricular arrhythmias in the multiple risk factor intervention. Am J Cardiol 60:548, 1987.

793. Morganroth J, Michelson EL, Horowitz LN, et al: Limitations of routine long-term electrocardiographic monitoring to assess ventricular ectopic frequency. Circulation 58:408, 1978.

794. Duke M: Thiazide-induced hypokalemia: Association with acute myocardial infarction and ventricular fibrillation. JAMA 239:43, 1978.

795. Holland OB, Nixon JV, Kuhnert L: Diuretic-induced ventricular ectopic activity. Am J Med 70:762, 1981.

796. Tanifuji Y, Eger EI II: Brain sodium, potassium and osmolality: Effect on anesthetic requirement. Anesth Analg 57:404, 1978.

797. Kornbluth A, Sachar DB: Ulcerative colitis practice guidelines in adults. American College of Gastroenterology, Practice Parameters Committee. Am J Gastroenterol 92:204, 1997.

798. Lindor KD, Fleming CR, Ilstrup DM: Preoperative nutritional status and other factors that influence surgical outcome in patients with Crohn's disease. Mayo Clin Proc 60:393, 1985.

799. Kahrilas PJ: Gastroesophageal reflux disease. JAMA 276:983, 1996.

800. Eger EI II, Saidman LJ: Hazards of nitrous oxide anesthesia in bowel obstruction and pneumothorax. Anesthesiology 26:61, 1965.

801. Antimicrobial prophylaxis. Med Lett Drugs Ther 43:92-97, 2001.

802. Jain NK, Larson DE, Schroeder KW, et al: Antibiotic prophylaxis for percutaneous endoscopic gastrostomy. Ann Intern Med 107:824, 1987.

803. Gorbach SL: Antimicrobial prophylaxis for appendectomy and colorectal surgery. Rev Infect Dis 13(Suppl 10):S815, 1991.

804. Peterson WJ: Peptic ulcer—an infectious disease? West J Med 152:167, 1990.

805. Ross AHM, Smith MA, Anderson JR, et al: Late mortality after surgery for peptic ulcer. N Engl J Med 307:519, 1982.

806. Longnecker M, Roizen MF: Patients with carcinoid syndrome. Anesthesiol Clin North Am 5:313, 1987.

807. Botero M, Fuchs R, Paulus DA, Lind DS: Carcinoid heart disease: A case report and literature review. J Clin Anesth 14:57-63, 2002.

808. Pandharipande PP, Reichard PS, Vallee MF: High gastric output as a perioperative sign of carcinoid syndrome. Anesthesiology 96:755-756, 2002.

809. Veall GRQ, Peacock JE, Bax NDS, Reilly CS: Review of the anaesthetic management of 21 patients undergoing laparotomy for carcinoid syndrome. Br J Anaesth 72:335, 1994.

810. Philbin DM, Coggins CH: Plasma antidiuretic hormone levels in cardiac surgical patients during morphine and halothane anesthesia. Anesthesiology 49:95, 1978.

811. Marsh HM, Martin JK Jr, Kvols LK, et al: Carcinoid crisis during anesthesia: Successful treatment with a somatostatin analogue. Anesthesiology 66:89, 1987.

812. Watson JT, Badner NH, Ali MJ: The prophylactic use of octreotide in a patient with ovarian carcinoid and valvular heart disease. Can J Anaesth 37:798, 1990.

813. McCrirrick A, Hickman J: Octreotide for carcinoid syndrome. Can J Anaesth 38:339, 1991.

814. Quinlivan JK, Roberts WA: Intraoperative octreotide for refractory carcinoid-induced bronchospasm. Anesth Analg 78:400, 1994.

815. Dilger JA, Rho EH, Que FG, Sprung J: Octreotide-induced bradycardia and heart block during surgical resection of a carcinoid tumor. Anesth Analg 98:318-320, 2004.

816. Zimmer C, Kienbaum P, Wiesemes R, Peters J: Somatostatin does not prevent serotonin release and flushing during chemoembolization of carcinoid liver metastases. Anesthesiology 98:1007-1011, 2003.

817. Drossman DA, McKee DC, Sandler RS, et al: Psychosocial factors in the irritable bowel syndrome. A multivariate study of patients and non-patients with irritable bowel syndrome. Gastroenterology 95:701, 1988.

818. Aitkenhead AR, Robinson S: Influence of morphine and pethidine on the incidence of anastomotic dehiscence after colonic surgery. Br J Anaesth 63:230P, 1989.

819. Wataneeyawech M, Kelly KA Jr: Hepatic diseases, unsuspected before surgery. N Y State J Med 75:1278, 1975.

820. Schemel WH: Unexpected hepatic dysfunction found by multiple laboratory screening. Anesth Analg 55:810, 1976.

821. Lentschener C, Ozier Y: What anaesthetists need to know about viral hepatitis. Acta Anaesthesiol Scand 47:794-803, 2003.

822. Baden JM, Serra M, Fujinaga M, Mazze RI: Halothane metabolism in cirrhotic rats. Anesthesiology 67:660, 1987.

823. Harville DD, Summerskill WH: Surgery in acute hepatitis— cause and effects. JAMA 184:257, 1963.

824. Viegas O, Stoelting RK: LDH_5 changes after cholecystectomy and hysterectomy in patients receiving halothane, enflurane or fentanyl. Anesthesiology 51:556, 1979.

825. Smith AA, Volpitto PP, Gramling ZW, et al: Chloroform, halothane and regional anesthesia: A comparative study. Anesth Analg 52:1, 1973.

826. Ronk W: Liver function chemistries after enflurane and narcotic-N_2O anesthesia. AANA J 46:507-511, 1978.

827. The National Halothane Study, Bunker JP, Forrest WH, Mosteller F, et al (eds): A Study of the Possible Association between Halothane Anesthesia and Postoperative Hepatic Necrosis. Washington, DC, US Government Printing Office, 1969.

828. Shingu K, Eger EI II, Johnson BH, et al: Effect of oxygen concentration, hyperthermia, and choice of vendor on anesthetic-induced hepatic injury in rats. Anesth Analg 62:146, 1983.

829. La Mont JT: Postoperative jaundice. Surg Clin North Am 54:637, 1974.

830. Black PM: Predicting the outcome from hypoxic-ischemic coma: Medical and ethical implications. JAMA 254:1215, 1985.

831. Resnick RH, Iber FL, Ishihara AM, et al: A controlled study of the therapeutic portacaval shunt. Gastroenterology 67:843, 1974.

832. Green J, Beyar R, Sideman S, et al: The "jaundiced heart": A possible explanation for postoperative shock in obstructive jaundice. Surgery 100:14, 1986.

833. Aranha GV, Sontag SJ, Greenlee HB: Cholecystectomy in cirrhotic patients: A formidable operation. Am J Surg 143:55, 1982.

834. Metcalf AMT, Dozois RR, Wolff BG, Beart RW Jr: The surgical risk of colectomy in patients with cirrhosis. Dis Colon Rectum 30:529, 1987.

835. Wright R, Eade OE, Chisholm M, et al: Controlled prospective study of the effect on liver function of multiple exposures to halothane. Lancet 6:817, 1975.

836. Trowell J, Peto R, Smith AC: Controlled trial of repeated halothane anaesthetics in patients with carcinoma of the uterine cervix treated with radium. Lancet 1:821, 1975.

837. Allen PJ, Downing JW: A prospective study of hepatocellular function after repeated exposures to halothane or enflurane in women undergoing radium therapy for cervical cancer. Br J Anaesth 49:1035, 1977.

838. Fee JPH, Black GW, Dundee JW, et al: A prospective study of liver enzyme and other changes following repeat administration of halothane and enflurane. Br J Anaesth 51:1133, 1979.

839. Moore DH, Benson GD: Prolonged halothane hepatitis: Prompt resolution of severe lesion with corticosteroid therapy. Dig Dis Sci 31:1269, 1986.

840. Hussey AJ, Howie J, Allan LG, et al: Impaired hepatocellular integrity during general anaesthesia, as assessed by measurement of plasma glutathione S-transferase. Clin Chim Acta 161:19, 1986.

841. Dykes MHM: Is halothane hepatitis chronic active hepatitis [editorial]? Anesthesiology 46:233, 1977.

842. Bréchot C, Nalpas B, Couroucé A-M, et al: Evidence that hepatitis B virus has a role in liver-cell carcinoma in alcoholic liver disease. N Engl J Med 306:1384, 1982.

843. Sipes I, Brown B: An animal model of hepatotoxicity associated with halothane anesthesia. Anesthesiology 45:622, 1976.

844. Klatskin G, Kimberg DV: Recurrent hepatitis attributable to halothane sensitization in an anesthetist. N Engl J Med 280:515, 1969.

845. Douglas HJ, Eger EI II, Biava CG, et al: Hepatic necrosis associated with viral infection after enflurane anesthesia. N Engl J Med 296:553, 1977.

846. Gall EA: Report of the pathology panel: National Halothane Study. Anesthesiology 29:233-248, 1968.

847. Stoelting RK, Blitt CD, Cohen PJ, Merin RG: Hepatic dysfunction after isoflurane anesthesia. Anesth Analg 66:147, 1987.

848. Malnick SD, Mahlab K, Borchardt J, et al: Acute cholestatic hepatitis after exposure to isoflurane. Ann Pharmacother 36:261-263, 2002.

849. Plummer JL, Hall PM, Jenner M, et al: Effect of treatment with phenobarbitone or isoniazid on hepatotoxicity due to prolonged subanesthetic halothane inhalation. Pharmacol Toxicol 62:74, 1988.

850. Hubbard AK, Roth TP, Gandolfi AJ, et al: Halothane hepatitis patients generate an antibody response toward a covalently bound metabolite of halothane. Anesthesiology 68:791, 1988.

851. Farrell G, Prendergast D, Murray M: Halothane hepatitis: Detection of constitutional susceptibility factor. N Engl J Med 313:1310, 1985.

852. Lewis JH, Zimmerman HJ, Ishak KG, Mullick FG: Enflurane hepatotoxicity: A clinicopathologic study of 24 cases. Ann Intern Med 98:984, 1983.

853. Stevens CE, Taylor PE, Rubinstein P, et al: Safety of the hepatitis B vaccine. N Engl J Med 312:375, 1985.

854. Berry AJ, Isaacson IJ, Hunt D, et al: The prevalence of hepatitis B viral markers in anesthesia personnel. Anesthesiology 60:6, 1984.

855. Mulley AG, Silverstein MD, Dienstag JL: Indications for use of hepatitis B vaccine, based on cost-effectiveness analysis. N Engl J Med 307:644, 1982.

856. Cody SH, Nainan OV, Garfein RS, et al: Hepatitis C virus transmission from an anesthesiologist to a patient. Arch Internal Med 162:345-350, 2002.

857. Naulty JS, Reves JG, Tobey RR, et al: Hepatitis and operating room personnel: An approach to diagnosis and management. Anesth Analg 56:360, 1977.

858. Duvaldestin P, Agoston S, Henzel D, et al: Pancuronium pharmacokinetics in patients with liver cirrhosis. Br J Anaesth 50:1131, 1978.

859. Orko R, Ailia A, Rosenberg PH: Effect of biliary obstruction on muscle relaxation with vecuronium. Eur J Anaesthesiol 5:9, 1988.

860. Arden JR, Lynam DP, Castagnoli KP, et al: Vecuronium in alcoholic liver disease: A pharmacokinetic and pharmacodynamic analysis. Anesthesiology 68:771, 1988.

861. Parker CJR, Hunter JM: Pharmacokinetics of atracurium and laudanosine in patients with hepatic cirrhosis. Br J Anaesth 62:177, 1989.

862. Swerdlow BN, Holley FO, Maitre PO, Stanski DR: Chronic alcohol intake does not change thiopental anesthetic requirement, pharmacokinetics, or pharmacodynamics. Anesthesiology 72:455, 1990.

863. Johnston RE, Kulp RA, Smith TC: Effects of acute and chronic ethanol administration on isoflurane requirement in mice. Anesth Analg 54:277, 1975.

864. Audet A-M, Goodnough LT: Practice strategies for elective red blood cell transfusion. American College of Physicians. Ann Intern Med 116:403, 1992.

865. Welch HG, Meehan KR, Goodnough LT: Prudent strategies for elective red blood cell transfusion. Ann Intern Med 116:393, 1992.

866. Thomas DJ, Du Boulay GH, Marshall J, et al: Effect of hematocrit on cerebral blood flow in man. Lancet 2:941, 1977.

867. Thomas DJ: Whole blood viscosity and cerebral blood flow [editorial]. Stroke 13:285, 1982.

868. Crystal GJ, Rooney MW, Salem MR: Myocardial blood flow and oxygen consumption during isovolumic hemodilution alone and in combination with adenosine-induced controlled hypotension. Anesth Analg 67:539, 1988.

869. Heughan C, Grislis G, Hunt TK: The effect of anemia on wound healing. Ann Surg 179:163, 1974.

870. Goodnough LT, Rudnick S, Price TH, et al: Increased preoperative collection of autologous blood with recombinant human erythropoietin therapy. N Engl J Med 321:1163, 1989.

871. Bunn HF: Pathogenesis and treatment of a sickle cell disease. N Engl J Med 337:762, 1997.

872. Adams RJ, McKie VC, Hsu L, et al: Prevention of a first stroke by transfusions in children with sickle cell anemia and abnormal results on transcranial Doppler ultrasonography. N Engl J Med 339:5, 1998.

873. Platt OS, Thorington BD, Brambella DJ, et al: Pain in sickle cell disease: Rates and risk factors. N Engl J Med 325:11, 1991.

874. Vichinsky EP, Haberkern CM, Neumayr L, et al: A comparison of conservative and aggressive transfusion regimens in the perioperative management of sickle cell disease. N Engl J Med 333:206, 1995.

875. Dalal FY, Schmidt GB, Bennett EJ, et al: Sickle-cell trait, a report of a postoperative neurological complication. Br J Anaesth 46:387, 1974.

876. Turhan A, Weiss LA, Mohandas N, et al: Primary role for adherent leukocytes in sickle cell vascular occlusion: A new paradigm. Proc Natl Acad Sci U S A 99:3047-3051, 2002.

877. Oduro KA, Searle JF: Anaesthesia in sickle-cell states: A plea for simplicity. BMJ 4:596, 1972.

878. Dunn A, Davies A, Eckert G, et al: Intraoperative death during caesarean section in a patient with sickle-cell trait. Can J Anaesth 34:67, 1987.

879. Kark JA, Posey DM, Schumaeker IIR, Ruehle CJ: Sickle cell trait as a risk factor for sudden death in physical training. N Engl J Med 317:781, 1987.

880. Homi J, Reynolds J, Skinner A, et al: General anesthesia in sickle-cell disease. BMJ 1:1599, 1979.

881. Bischoff RJ, Williamson A III, Dalali MJ, et al: Assessment of the use of transfusion therapy perioperatively in patients with sickle cell hemoglobinopathies. Ann Surg 207:434, 1988.

882. Morrison JC, Wiser WL: The use of prophylactic partial exchange transfusion in pregnancies associated with sickle cell hemoglobinopathy. Obstet Gynecol 48:516, 1976.

883. Morrison JC, Whybrew WD, Bucovaz ET: Use of partial exchange transfusion preoperatively in patients with sickle cell hemoglobinopathies. Am J Obstet Gynecol 132:59, 1978.

884. Lanzkowsky P, Shende A, Karayalcin G, et al: Partial exchange transfusion in sickle cell anemia: Use in children with serious complications. Am J Dis Child 132:1206, 1978.

885. Tuck SM, James CE, Brewster EM, et al: Prophylactic blood transfusion in maternal sickle cell syndromes. Br J Obstet Gynaecol 94:121, 1987.

886. Krishnamurti L, Blazar BR, Wagner JE: Bone marrow transplantation without myeloablation for sickle cell disease. N Engl J Med 344:68, 2001.

887. Beutler E: The common anemias. JAMA 259:2433, 1988.

888. Orr D: Difficult intubation: A hazard in thalassemia. A case report. Br J Anaesth 39:585, 1967.

889. Pootrakul P, Hungsprenges S, Fucharoen S, et al: Relation between erythropoiesis and bone metabolism in thalassemia. N Engl J Med 304:1470-1473, 1981.

890. Muretto P, Angelucci E, Lucarelli G: Reversibility of cirrhosis in patients cured of thalassemia by bone marrow transplantation. Ann Intern Med 136:667-672, 2002.

891. Lux SE, Wolfe LC: Inherited disorders of the red cell membrane skeleton. Pediatr Clin North Am 27:463, 1980.

892. Beutler E: Glucose-6-phosphate dehydrogenase deficiency. N Engl J Med 324:169, 1991.

893. Engelfriet CP, Overbeeke MA, van der Berne AE: Autoimmune hemolytic anemia. Semin Hematol 29:3, 1992.

894. Schilling RF: Is nitrous oxide a dangerous anesthetic for vitamin B_{12}–deficient subjects? JAMA 255:1605, 1986.

895. Beebe DS, Bergen L, Palahniuk RJ: Anesthesia utilizing plasmapheresis and forced air warming in a patient with severe cold agglutinin hemolytic anemia. Anesth Analg 76:1144, 1993.

896. Quesenberg PJ, Schafer AI, Schreiber AD, et al: Hematology. *In* American College of Physicians: Medical Knowledge Self-Assessment. Philadelphia, American College of Physicians, 1991, p 374.

897. Tobias JD, Furman WL: Anesthetic considerations in patients receiving colony-stimulating factors (G-CSF and GM-CSF). Anesthesiology 75:536, 1991.

898. Alavi JB, Root RK, Djerassi I, et al: A randomized clinical trial of granulocyte transfusion for infection in acute leukemia. N Engl J Med 296:706, 1977.

899. Gabrilove JL, Jakubowski A, Scher H, et al: Effect of granulocyte colony stimulating factor on neutropenia and associated morbidity due to chemotherapy for transitional-cell carcinoma of the urothelium. N Engl J Med 318:1414, 1988.

900. Quie PG: The white cells: Use of granulocyte transfusions. Rev Infect Dis 9:189, 1987.

901. Crawford SW, Fisher L: Predictive value of pulmonary function tests before marrow transplantation. Chest 101:1257, 1992.

902. McCrae KR, Bussel JB, Mannucci PM, et al: Platelets: An update on diagnosis and management of thrombocytopenic disorders. Hematology (Am Soc Hematol Educ Program) 282-305, 2001.

903. Petrovitch CT: The bleeding patient. *In* Roizen MF (ed): Anesthesia for Vascular Surgery. New York, Churchill Livingstone, 1990, p 465.

904. Kelton JG: Management of the pregnant patient with idiopathic thrombocytopenic purpura. Ann Intern Med 99:796, 1983.

905. King DJ, Kelton JG: Heparin-associated thrombocytopenia. Ann Intern Med 100:535, 1984.

906. Douzinas EE, Markakis K, Karabinis A, et al: Early plasmapheresis in patients with thrombotic thrombocytopenic purpura. Crit Care Med 20:57, 1992.

907. Majerus PW, Miletich JP: Relationships between platelets and coagulation factors in hemostasis. Annu Rev Med 29:41, 1978.

908. Lewis BE, Wallis DE, Berkowitz MD, et al: Argatroban anticoagulant therapy in patients with heparin-induced thrombocytopenia. Circulation 103:1838-1843, 2001.

909. Bauer KA : The thrombophilias: Well-defined risk factors with uncertain therapeutic implications. Ann Intern Med 135:367-373, 2001.

910. Levine JS, Branch DW, Rauch J: The antiphospholipid syndrome. N Engl J Med 346:752-763, 2002.

911. Evans BE: Dental treatment for hemophiliacs: Evaluation of dental program (1975-1976) at the Mount Sinai Hospital International Hemophilia Training Center. Mt Sinai J Med 44:409, 1977.

912. Zauber NP, Levin J: Factor IX levels in patients with hemophilia B (Christmas disease) following transfusion with concentrates of factor IX or fresh frozen plasma (FFP). Medicine (Baltimore) 56:213, 1977.

913. Brettler DB, Levine PH: Factor concentrates for treatment of hemophilia: Which one to choose? Blood 73:2067, 1989.

914. Curran JW, Lawrence DN, Jaffe H, et al: Acquired immunodeficiency syndrome (AIDS) associated with transfusions. N Engl J Med 310:69, 1984.

915. Safety of therapeutic products used for hemophilia patients. MMWR Morb Mortal Wkly Rep 37:441, 1988.

916. Briere RO: Serum ALT levels: Effect of sex, race, and obesity on unit rejection rate. Transfusion 28:392, 1988.

917. Sloand EM, Pitt E, Klein HG: Safety of the blood supply. JAMA 274:1368, 1995.

918. Preparation of von Willebrand's factor. Med Lett Drugs Ther 35:51, 1993.

919. Miller RD: Complications of massive blood transfusions. Anesthesiology 39:82, 1973.

920. Sherman LA: Alterations in hemostasis during massive transfusion. *In* Nusbacher J (ed): Massive Transfusion. Washington, DC, American Association of Blood Banks, 1978, p 51.

921. Lee KF, Manchell J, Rankin JS, et al: Immediate versus delayed coronary grafting after streptokinase treatment: Postoperative blood loss and clinical results. J Thorac Cardiovasc Surg 95:216, 1988.

922. Dickman CA, Shedd SA, Spetzler RF, et al: Spinal epidural hematoma associated with epidural anesthesia: Complications of systemic heparinization in patients receiving peripheral vascular thrombolytic therapy. Anesthesiology 72:947, 1990.

923. Czer LS, Bateman TM, Gary RJ, et al: Treatment of severe platelet dysfunction and hemorrhage after cardiopulmonary bypass: Reduction in blood product usage with desmopressin. J Am Coll Cardiol 9:1139, 1987.

924. Marks RM, Sachar EJ: Undertreatment of medical inpatients with narcotic analgesics. Ann Intern Med 78:173, 1973.

925. Brigden ML, Barnett JB: A practical approach to improving pain control in cancer patients. West J Med 146:580, 1987.

926. Vitez TS, Way WL, Miller RD, et al: Effect of delta-9-tetrahydrocannabinol on cyclopropane MAC in the rat. Anesthesiology 38:525, 1973.

927. Drugs of choice for cancer chemotherapy. Med Lett Drugs Ther 39:21, 1997.

928. Bishop JM: Molecular themes in oncogenesis. Cell 64:235, 1991.

929. Chung F: Cancer, chemotherapy, and anesthesia. Can J Anaesth 29:364, 1982.

930. Goldiner P, Carlon GC, Cvitkovic E, et al: Factors influencing postoperative morbidity and mortality in patients treated with bleomycin. BMJ 1:1664, 1978.

931. Singer MM, Wright F, Stanley LK, et al: Oxygen toxicity in man: A prospective study in patients after open-heart surgery. N Engl J Med 283:1473, 1970.

932. LaMantia KR, Glick JH, Marshall BE: Supplemental oxygen does not cause respiratory failure in bleomycin-treated surgical patients. Anesthesiology 60:65, 1984.

933. Matalon S, Harper WV, Nickerson PA, Olszowka J: Intravenous bleomycin does not alter the toxic effects of hyperoxia in rabbits. Anesthesiology 64:614, 1986.

934. Roizen MF: Is a patient's history of food supplement use simply supplementary? J Clin Anesth 10:89, 1998.

935. Weiner N, Taylor P: Neurohumoral transmission and the autonomic nervous system. *In* Gilman AG, Goodman LS, Rall TW, et al (eds): Goodman and Gilman's The Pharmacological Basis of Therapeutics, 7th ed. New York, Macmillan, 1985, p 66.

936. Lake CR, Chernow B, Feuerstein G, et al: The sympathetic nervous system in man: Its evaluation and the measurement of plasma NE. *In* Ziegler MG, Lake CR (eds): Norepinephrine. Baltimore, Williams & Wilkins, 1984, p 1.

937. Burn JH, Rand MJ: Actions of sympathomimetic amines on animals treated with reserpine. J Physiol (Lond) 144:314, 1958.

938. Drugs for hypertension. Med Lett Drugs Ther 37:45, 1995.

939. Drugs that cause psychiatric symptoms. Med Lett Drugs Ther 35:65, 1993.

940. Woodside J Jr, Garner L, Bedford RF, et al: Captopril reduces the dose requirement for sodium nitroprusside induced hypotension. Anesthesiology 60:413, 1984.

941. Sethna DH, Gray RJ, Moffitt EA, et al: Dobutamine and cardiac oxygen balance in patients following myocardial revascularization. Anesth Analg 61:917, 1982.

942. The Norwegian Multicenter Study Group: Timolol-induced reduction in mortality and reinfarction in patients surviving acute myocardial infarction. N Engl J Med 304:801, 1981.

943. Frishman WH, Furberg CD, Friedewald WT: β-Adrenergic blockade for survivors of acute myocardial infarction. N Engl J Med 310:830, 1984.

944. Smulyan H, Weinberg SE, Howanitz PJ: Continuous propranolol infusion following abdominal surgery. JAMA 247:2539, 1982.

945. Slogoff S, Keats AS, Hibbs CW, et al: Failure of general anesthesia to potentiate propranolol activity. Anesthesiology 47:504, 1977.

946. Gold MR, Dec GW, Cocca-Spofford DC, Thompson BT: Esmolol and ventilatory function in cardiac patients with COPD. Chest 100:1215, 1991.

947. Tanifuji Y, Eger EI II: Effect of isoproterenol and propranolol on halothane MAC in dogs. Anesth Analg 55:383, 1976.

948. Bloor BC, Flacke WE: Reduction in halothane anesthetic requirement by clonidine, an alpha-adrenergic agonist. Anesth Analg 61:741, 1982.

949. Weinger MB, Segal IS, Maze M: Dexmedetomidine, acting through central alpha-2 adrenoceptors, prevents opiate-induced muscle rigidity in the rat. Anesthesiology 71:242, 1989.

950. Ghignone M, Noe C, Calvillo O, Quintin L: Anesthesia for ophthalmic surgery in the elderly: The effects of clonidine on intraocular pressure, perioperative hemodynamics, and anesthetic requirement. Anesthesiology 68:707, 1988.

951. Engelman E, Lipszyc M, Gilbart E, et al: Effects of clonidine on anesthetic drug requirements and hemodynamic response during aortic surgery. Anesthesiology 71:178, 1989.

952. Maze M, Tranquilli W: Alpha-2 adrenoreceptor agonists: Defining the role in clinical anesthesia. Anesthesiology 74:581, 1991.

953. Segal IS, Jarvis DJ, Duncan SR, et al: Clinical efficacy of oral-transdermal clonidine combinations during the perioperative period. Anesthesiology 74:220, 1991.

954. Muzi M, Goff DR, Kampine JP, et al: Clonidine reduces sympathetic activity but maintains baroreflex responses in normotensive humans. Anesthesiology 77:864, 1992.

955. Miller RD, Sohn YJ, Matteo RS: Enhancement of d-tubocurarine neuromuscular blockade by diuretics in man. Anesthesiology 45:442, 1976.

956. Katz AM: Cardiac ion channels. N Engl J Med 328:1244, 1993.

957. Millard RW, Grupp G, Grupp IL, et al: Chronotropic, inotropic, and vasodilator actions of diltiazem, nifedipine, and verapamil. Circ Res 52(Suppl I):I-29, 1983.

958. Maze M, Mason DM: Verapamil decreases the MAC for halothane in dogs. Anesth Analg 62:274, 1983.

959. Reves JG, Kissin I, Lell WA, et al: Calcium entry blockers: Uses and implications for anesthesiologists. Anesthesiology 57:504, 1982.

960. Hysing ES, Chelly JE, Doursout M-F: Cardiovascular effects of and interaction between calcium blocking drugs and anesthetics in chronically instrumented dogs. III: Nicardipine and isoflurane. Anesthesiology 65:385, 1986.

961. Merin RG, Chelly JE, Hysing ES, et al: Cardiovascular effects of and interaction between calcium blocking drugs and anesthetics in chronically instrumented dogs. IV: Chronically administered oral verapamil and halothane, enflurane, and isoflurane. Anesthesiology 66:140, 1987.

962. Kapur PA, Matarazzo DA, Fung DM, Sullivan KB: The cardiovascular and adrenergic actions of verapamil or diltiazem in combination with propranolol during

halothane anesthesia in the dog. Anesthesiology 66:122, 1987.

963. Dale J, Landmark KH, Myhre E: The effects of nifedipine, a calcium antagonist, on platelet function. Am Heart J 105:103, 1983.

964. Zalman F, Perloff JK, Durant NN, et al: Acute respiratory failure following intravenous verapamil in Duchenne's muscular dystrophy. Am Heart J 105:510, 1983.

965. Zimpfer M, Fitzal S, Tonzcar L: Verapamil as a hypotensive agent during neuroleptanaesthesia. Br J Anaesth 53:885, 1981.

966. Durant NN, Nguyen N, Katz RL: Potentiation of neuromuscular blockade by verapamil. Anesthesiology 60:298, 1984.

967. Nugent M, Tinker JH, Moyer TP: Verapamil worsens rate of development and hemodynamic effects of acute hyperkalemia in halothane anesthetized dogs: Effects of calcium therapy. Anesthesiology 60:435, 1984.

968. Lalka SG, Rhodes RS, Lina AA, et al: Effect of calcium entry and β blockade during infrarenal aortic clamping. J Surg Res 46:246, 1989.

969. Michaels I, Serrins M, Shier NQ, Barash PG: Anesthesia for cardiac surgery in patients receiving monoamine oxidase inhibitors. Anesth Analg 63:1014, 1984.

970. Evans-Prosser CDG: The use of pethidine and morphine in the presence of monamine oxidase inhibitors. Br J Anaesth 40:279, 1968.

971. Campbell GD: Dangers of monamine oxidase inhibitors. BMJ 1:750, 1963.

972. Rogers KJ, Thornton JA: The interaction between monamine oxidase inhibitors and narcotic analgesics in mice. Br J Pharmacol 36:470, 1969.

973. Sjoqvist F: Psychotropic drugs. 2. Interaction between monamine oxidase (MAO) inhibitors and other substances. Proc R Soc Med 58:967, 1965.

974. Monamine oxidase inhibitors for depression. Med Lett Drugs Ther 31:11, 1989.

975. Drugs for psychiatric disorders. Med Lett Drugs Ther 33:43, 1991.

976. Roizen MF: Monoamine oxidase inhibitors: Are we condemned to relive history, or is history no longer relevant? J Clin Anesth 2:293, 1990.

977. Noble WH, Baker A: MAO inhibitors and coronary artery surgery: A patient death. Can J Anaesth 39:1061, 1992.

978. Wells DG, Bjorksten AR: Monoamine oxidase inhibitors revisited. Can J Anaesth 36:64, 1989.

979. Hirshman CA, Linderman KS: Anesthesia and monoamine oxidase inhibitors. JAMA 261:3407, 1989.

980. Stack CG, Rogers P, Linter SPK: Monoamine oxidase inhibitors and anaesthesia: A review. Br J Anaesth 60:222, 1988.

981. El-Ganzouri AR, Ivankovich AD, Braverman B, McCarthy R: Monoamine oxidase inhibitors: Should they be discontinued preoperatively? Anesth Analg 64:592, 1985.

982. Ebrahim ZY, O'Hara JF, Borden L, Tetzlaff J: Monoamine oxidase inhibitors and elective surgery. Cleve Clin J Med 60:129, 1993.

983. Clarke AG: MAOI's and Anaesthesia. Can J Anaesth 43:641, 1996.

984. Edwards RE, Miller RD, Roizen MF, et al: Cardiac effects of imipramine and pancuronium during halothane and enflurane anesthesia. Anesthesiology 50:421, 1979.

985. Veith RC, Raskind MA, Caldwell JH, et al: Cardiovascular effects of tricyclic antidepressants in depressed patients with chronic heart disease. N Engl J Med 306:954, 1982.

986. Richelson E, El-Fakahany E: Changes in the sensitivity of receptors for neurotransmitters and the actions of some psychotherapeutic drugs. Mayo Clin Proc 57:576, 1982.

987. Martin BA, Kramer PM: Clinical significance of the interaction between lithium and a neuromuscular blocker. Am J Psychiatry 139:1326, 1982.

988. Johnston RR, Way WL, Miller RD: Alteration of anesthetic requirements by amphetamine. Anesthesiology 36:357, 1972.

989. Stoelting RK, Creasser CW, Martz RC: Effect of cocaine administration on halothane MAC in dogs. Anesth Analg 54:422, 1975.

990. Katz RL, Bigger JT: Cardiac arrhythmias during anesthesia and operation. Anesthesiology 33:193, 1970.

991. Joas TA, Stevens WC: Comparison of the arrhythmic doses of epinephrine during Forane, halothane and enflurane anesthesia in dogs. Anesthesiology 35:48, 1971.

992. Johnston RR, Eger EI II, Wilson C: A comparative interaction of epinephrine with enflurane, isoflurane and halothane in man. Anesth Analg 55:709, 1976.

993. Horrigan RW, Eger EI II, Wilson CB: Epinephrine-induced arrhythmias during enflurane anesthesia in man: A nonlinear dose-response relationship and dose-dependent protection from lidocaine. Anesth Analg 57:547, 1978.

994. Hirshman CA, Bergman NA: Halothane and enflurane protect against bronchospasm in an asthma dog model. Anesth Analg 57:629, 1978.

995. Shnider SM, Papper EM: Anesthesia for the asthmatic patient. Anesthesiology 22:886, 1961.

996. Marcus ML, Skelton CL, Graver LE, et al: Effects of theophylline on myocardial mechanics. Am J Physiol 222:1361, 1972.

997. Westfall DP, Flemming WW: Sensitivity changes in the dog heart to norepinephrine, calcium and aminophylline resulting from pretreatment with reserpine. J Pharmacol Exp Ther 159:98, 1968.

998. Rall TW, West TC: The potentiation of cardiac inotropic responses to norepinephrine by theophylline. J Pharmacol Exp Ther 139:269, 1963.

999. Horwitz LN, Spear JF, Moore EN, et al: Effect of aminophylline on the threshold for initiating ventricular fibrillation during respiratory failure. Am J Cardiol 35:376, 1975.

1000. Mitenko PA, Ogilvie RI: Pharmacokinetics of intravenous theophylline. Clin Pharmacol Ther 14:509, 1973.

1001. Piafsky KM, Ogilvie RI: Dosage of theophylline in bronchial asthma. N Engl J Med 292:1218, 1975.

1002. Hunt SN, Jusko WJ, Yurchak AM: Effect of smoking on theophylline disposition. Clin Pharmacol Ther 19:546, 1975.

1003. Takaori M, Loehning RW: Ventricular arrhythmias induced by aminophylline during halothane anaesthesia in dogs. Can J Anaesth 14:79, 1967.

1004. Takaori M, Loehning RW: Ventricular arrhythmias during halothane anaesthesia: Effect of isoproterenol, aminophylline, and ephedrine. Can J Anaesth 12:275, 1965.

1005. Roizen MF, Stevens WC: Multiform ventricular tachycardia due to the interaction of aminophylline and halothane. Anesth Analg 57:738, 1978.

1006. Stirt JA, Berger JM, Sullivan SF: Lack of arrhythmogenicity of isoflurane following administration of aminophylline in dogs. Anesth Analg 62:568, 1983.

1007. Drugs for cardiac arrhythmias. Med Lett Drugs Ther 38:75, 1996.

1008. Harrah MD, Way WL, Katzung BG: The interaction of d-tubocurarine with antiarrhythmic drugs. Anesthesiology 33:406, 1970.

1009. Telivuo L, Katz RL: The effects of modern intravenous local anesthetics on respiration during partial neuromuscular block in man. Anaesthesia 25:30, 1970.

1010. Miller RD, Way WL, Katzung BG: The potentiation of neuromuscular blocking agents by quinidine. Anesthesiology 28:1036, 1967.

1011. Pittinger CB, Eryasa Y, Adamson R: Antibiotic-induced paralysis. Anesth Analg 49:487, 1970.

1012. Singh YN, Harvey AL, Marshall IG: Antibiotic-induced paralysis of the mouse phrenic nerve–hemidiaphragm preparation, and reversibility by calcium and by neostigmine. Anesthesiology 48:418, 1978.

1013. Pittinger CB, Adamson R: Antibiotic blockade of neuromuscular function. Annu Rev Pharmacol 12:169, 1972.

1014. Becker LD, Miller RD: Clindamycin enhances a non-depolarizing neuromuscular blockade. Anesthesiology 45:84, 1976.

1015. Snavely SR, Hodges GR: The neurotoxicity of antibacterial agents. Ann Intern Med 101:92, 1984.

1016. McIndewar IC, Marshall RJ: Interactions between the neuromuscular blocking drug Org NC45 and some anaesthetic, analgesic and antimicrobial agents. Br J Anaesth 53:785, 1981.
1017. Navalgund AA, Alifimoff JK, Jakymec AJ, Bleyaert AL: Amiodarone-induced sinus arrest successfully treated with ephedrine and isoproterenol. Anesth Analg 65:414, 1986.
1018. Kannan R, Nademane K, Hendrickson JA, et al: Amiodarone kinetics after oral doses. Clin Pharmacol Ther 31:438, 1982.
1019. Rice SA, Sbordone L, Mazzo RI: Metabolism by rat hepatic microsomes of fluorinated ether anesthetics following isoniazid administration. Anesthesiology 53:489, 1980.
1020. Beller GA, Smith TW, Abelmann WH, et al: Digitalis intoxication. N Engl J Med 284:989, 1971.
1021. Ritchie AJ, Danton M, Gibbons JRP: Prophylactic digitalisation in pulmonary surgery. Thorax 47:41, 1992.
1022. Morrow DH: Anesthesia and digitalis toxicity. VI. Effect of barbiturates and halothane on digoxin toxicity. Anesth Analg 49:305, 1970.
1023. Pratila MG, Pratilas V: Anesthetic agents and cardiac electromechanical activity. Anesthesiology 49:338, 1978.
1024. Logic JR, Morrow DH: The effect of halothane on ventricular automaticity. Anesthesiology 36:107, 1972.
1025. Ivankovich AD, Miletich DJ, Grossman RK, et al: The effect of enflurane, isoflurane, fluroxene, methoxyflurane and diethyl ether on ouabain tolerance in the dog. Anesth Analg 55:360, 1976.
1026. Ali N, Dais K, Banks T, Sheikh M: Titrated electrical cardioversion in patients on digoxin. Clin Cardiol 5:417, 1982.
1027. Adverse systemic effects from ophthalmic drugs. Med Lett Drugs Ther 24:53, 1982.
1028. The Medical Letter Handbook of Adverse Drug Interactions, 2003.
1029. Pantuck EJ, Pantuck CB: Cholinesterases and anticholinesterases. In Katz RL (ed): Muscle Relaxants. Amsterdam, Excerpta Medica, 1975, p 143.
1030. Ghonelm MM, Long JP: The interaction between magnesium and other neuromuscular blocking agents. Anesthesiology 32:23, 1970.
1031. Del Castillo J, Engback L: The nature of neuromuscular block produced by magnesium. J Physiol (Lond) 124:370, 1954.
1032. Feely J, Wilkinson GR, McAllister CB, et al: Increased toxicity and reduced clearance of lidocaine by cimetidine. Ann Intern Med 96:592, 1982.
1033. Lam AM, Parkin JA: Cimetidine and prolonged post-operative somnolence. Can J Anaesth 28:450, 1981.
1034. Vessey MD, Doll R, Fairbairn AS, et al: Postoperative thromboembolism and the use of oral contraceptives. BMJ 3:123, 1970.
1035. Greene GR, Sartwell PE: Oral contraceptive use in patients with thromboembolism following surgery, trauma, or infection. Am J Public Health 62:680, 1972.
1036. Interruption of a drug regimen before anesthesia. Med Lett Drugs Ther 16:19, 1974.
1037. Wyld R, Nimmo WS: Do patients fasting before and after surgery receive their prescribed drug treatment? BMJ 296:744, 1988.
1038. Lesar TS, Briceland LL, Delcoure K, et al: Medication prescribing errors in a teaching hospital. JAMA 263:2329, 1990.
1039. Hassey MJ: Drug interactions in anaesthesia. Br J Anaesth 59:112, 1987.
1040. Update: Drugs in breast milk. Med Lett Drugs Ther 21:21, 1979.

CHAPTER
28 Patient Positioning

Ronald J. Faust, Roy F. Cucchiara, and Perry S. Bechtle

American Society of Anesthesiologists
    Closed Claims Data and Practice
    Advisories   1151

Pathophysiologic Considerations   1152
    Cardiovascular Considerations   1152
    Pulmonary Considerations   1152
    Neurologic Considerations   1153

Positions   1158
    Supine Position   1158

Lithotomy Position   1158
Lateral Position   1159
Lateral Oblique Position   1160
Trendelenburg Position   1162
Prone Position   1162
Positions for Orthopedic
    Surgery   1163
Position for Shoulder
    Surgery   1163
Sitting Position   1164

Like much else in anesthesia, positioning is expected to be always perfect, and any complications that arise as a result of it are met with surprise and concern. The goal of positioning is to facilitate the performance of the surgical procedure by the surgeon while ensuring that the position is physiologically safe for the anesthetized patient. In most practices, the surgeon and anesthesiologist work together to put the anesthetized patient into as ideal a position as safely as possible after induction of anesthesia. The importance of positioning is underscored by the fact that nerve damage is the second most common type of anesthetic complication represented in the American Society of Anesthesiologists (ASA) Closed Claims Database. However, there is a paucity of data confirming that positioning interventions affect outcome.

AMERICAN SOCIETY OF ANESTHESIOLOGISTS CLOSED CLAIMS DATA AND PRACTICE ADVISORIES

Two analyses of nerve injury cases from the ASA Closed Claims Database have been published, the most recent in 1999.[1] This database is derived from case summaries from the closed claims files of professional liability insurance companies. Of all anesthesia claims, death (32%), nerve damage (16%), and brain damage (12%) were the types most frequently settled. Six hundred seventy (16%) of 4183 total claims closed between 1970 and 1995 involved nerve injury claims. Table 28-1 summarizes the distribution of the most frequent injuries by gender. Although female claimants predominated in non-nerve damage claims, the distribution between genders was equal for nerve damage cases. Most nerve injuries occurred in adults; less than 1% of closed claims for nerve injury cases involved children.

Ulnar neuropathies predominated (28%) in the 670 nerve injury cases, followed by brachial plexus, lumbosacral nerve root, and spinal cord injuries in the ASA Closed Claims Database (Table 28-2). Ulnar neuropathies were far more common in male than female patients.

Some of the nerve injury cases are not related to positioning. An increasing incidence of spinal cord injuries in the database was observed for claims for injury occurring in the 1990s.[1] This trend may be related to increasing injuries from neuraxial blocks in anticoagulated patients, the introduction of low-molecular-weight heparin, and more blocks performed for chronic pain management. The ASA Closed Claims Database also includes reports on two patients who sustained cervical cord injuries when they fell off the operating room table!

In 1999, the ASA Task Force on Prevention of Perioperative Peripheral Neuropathies approved a practice advisory for the prevention of perioperative peripheral neuropathies.[2] The Task Force's report is called a *practice advisory* because this type of document is not supported by scientific literature to the same degree as standards or guidelines. The Task Force reviewed 509 positioning studies and found that only 6 demonstrated scientifically proven relationships between interventions and outcomes. Because there was so little objective information, the Task Force did not rely completely on the literature but built a consensus after obtaining consultant opinion from a body of anesthesiologists and other specialists with experience in patient positioning. The summary of the Task Force's advisory is reprinted in Table 28-3.

V1

Table 28–1 Distribution of the most common ASA Closed Claims Database Injuries by Gender and Age

Claim	Male (%)	Female (%)	Median Age (yr)	Age Range (yr)	Persons <16 Years Old (%)
Non-nerve damage (n = 3513)	38	61	39	0-94	11
All nerve damage (n = 670)	50*	49*	44*	1-86	1*
Ulnar (n = 190)	75*	23*	50*	20-82	0*
Brachial plexus (n = 137)	40	58	41†	1-80	1*
Lumbosacral root (n = 105)	29†	71†	37	20-83	0*
Spinal cord (n = 84)	52†	48†	54*	2-86	5†
All other nerves (n = 154)	42	58	40	5-81	2*

*$P \leq 0.01$ versus non-nerve damage claims.
†$P \leq 0.05$ versus non-nerve damage claims.
From Cheney FW, Domino KB, Caplan RA, et al: Nerve injury associated with anesthesia. Anesthesiology 90:1064, 1999.

PATHOPHYSIOLOGIC CONSIDERATIONS

Cardiovascular Considerations

It is one of the wonders of evolution and physiologic regulation that dinosaurs, giraffes, and humans have been able to assume postures in which the head is higher than the heart while perfusion to the brain is maintained. Physiologic mechanisms of changing vascular resistance and cardiac output allow the cardiovascular system to maintain adequate flow to the central nervous system despite position changes.

A complex system of local mechanisms (i.e., autoregulation) and reflexes in the venous and the arterial systems maintain blood pressure and blood flow during changes in position. Although these local mechanisms and reflexes work in concert, anesthesia can blunt the response of each element of the system, thereby altering the final response in either direction. The venous and atrial reflexes are served by mechanosensitive afferent nerves that respond to stretching of the great veins and heart chambers. These nerves tend to inhibit sympathetic outflow

Table 28–2 Distribution of claims for nerve injury

Nerve	Number of Claims	Percent of Total (n = 670)
Ulnar	190	28
Brachial plexus	137	20
Lumbosacral nerve root	105	16
Spinal cord	84	13
Sciatic	34	5
Median	28	4
Radial	18	3
Femoral	15	2
Other single nerves	43	6
Multiple nerves	16	2
Total	670	100

From Cheney FW, Domino KB, Caplan RA, et al: Nerve injury associated with anesthesia. Anesthesiology 90:1064, 1999.

when central blood volume is elevated. Arterial baroreflexes are also served by mechanosensitive afferent nerves located in the aortic arch and carotid arteries. They respond to stretch and tend to inhibit sympathetic outflow and activate the parasympathetic system when activated by a rise in arterial pressure. Conversely, a fall in pressure usually evokes sympathetic vasoconstriction and vagal withdrawal.

In the upright position, there is a considerable increase in transmural vascular pressure in the lower extremities because of the hydrostatic effects of the columns of blood. This increase is limited by increased pressure in the tissue surrounding the vessels, which is caused by muscle tone and contraction required to maintain the erect position and by venous valves. Even with this compensation, 0.5 to 1.0 L of blood can pool in the lower extremities, central venous pressure can fall to very low values, and cardiac output is reduced by about 20% in the upright position. Cardiac output tends to increase immediately on assumption of the supine position. Venous blood from the lower body returns to the central circulation and stroke volume increases. If contractility and arterial tone remained constant, arterial pressure would rise. Baroreceptor afferent impulses from the great veins, heart, and aortic receptors travel through the vagus nerve and from the carotid sinus through the glossopharyngeal nerve to the medulla. Increased efferent parasympathetic and decreased efferent sympathetic activity change the parasympathetic-sympathetic balance, decreasing heart rate, stroke volume, and contractility and reducing sympathetic vasoconstrictor activity. The result is that blood pressure remains relatively constant.

Pulmonary Considerations

During spontaneous ventilation, the rib cage and the diaphragm contribute to thoracic expansion. The abdomen also expands with inspiration to accommodate caudad motion of the diaphragm. In the supine position, abdominal expansion during inspiration is lessened and rib cage expansion is exaggerated compared with upright postures. In upright positions, the weight of the abdominal contents pulls the diaphragm caudad and helps to maintain

Table 28–3 Consensus Findings of the ASA Task Force on Prevention of Perioperative Peripheral Neuropathies

Preoperative Assessment
When judged appropriate, it is helpful to ascertain that patients can comfortably tolerate the anticipated operative position.

Upper Extremity Positioning
Arm abduction should be limited to 90 degrees in supine patients; patients who are positioned prone may comfortably tolerate arm abduction greater than 90 degrees.
Arms should be positioned to decrease pressure on the postcondylar groove of the humerus (i.e., ulnar groove). When arms are tucked at the side, a neutral forearm position is recommended. When arms are abducted on armboards, supination or a neutral forearm position is acceptable.
Prolonged pressure on the radial nerve in the spiral groove of the humerus should be avoided.
Extension of the elbow beyond a comfortable range may stretch the median nerve.

Lower Extremity Positioning
Lithotomy positions that stretch the hamstring muscle group beyond a comfortable range may stretch the sciatic nerve.
Prolonged pressure on the peroneal nerve at the fibular head should be avoided.
Neither extension nor flexion of the hip increases the risk of femoral neuropathy.

Protective Padding
Padded armboards may decrease the risk of upper extremity neuropathy.
The use of chest rolls in laterally positioned patients may decrease the risk of upper extremity neuropathies.
Padding at the elbow and at the fibular head may decrease the risk of upper and lower extremity neuropathies, respectively.

Equipment
Properly functioning automated blood pressure cuffs on the upper arms do not affect the risk of upper extremity neuropathies.
Shoulder braces in steep head-down positions may increase the risk of brachial plexus neuropathies.

Postoperative Assessment
A simple postoperative assessment of extremity nerve function may lead to early recognition of peripheral neuropathies.

Documentation
Charting specific positioning actions during the care of patients may result in improvements of care by (1) helping practitioners focus attention on relevant aspects of patient positioning and by (2) providing information that continuous improvement processes can lead to refinements in patient care.

From ASA Task Force on Prevention of Perioperative Peripheral Neuropathies: Practice advisory for the prevention of perioperative peripheral neuropathies. Anesthesiology 92:1168-1182, 2000.

functional residual capacity. In recumbent positions, the abdominal contents tend to displace the diaphragm cephalad, causing a decrease in functional residual capacity (by approximately 0.5 L in adults). While supine, dependent regions of the diaphragm move preferentially with breathing, such that preferential ventilation of dependent lung regions is favored. This aids in matching ventilation to perfusion because the dependent portions of the lung are also preferentially perfused. With the induction of anesthesia, the functional residual capacity further decreases in supine subjects (by approximately 0.5 L). The classic teaching is that this decrease in lung volume is caused by a cephalad shift of the diaphragm.[3] However, later studies show that the net end-expiratory position of the diaphragm does not shift significantly during anesthesia and paralysis, although its shape does change.[4-6] An inward motion of the rib cage and, under some conditions, increases in intrathoracic blood volume cause most of the decreases in functional residual capacity associated with anesthesia. Similar changes probably occur in other recumbent positions. These changes in thoracic configuration are associated with atelectasis in dependent lung areas, which significantly impairs gas exchange.

Neurologic Considerations

Anatomically, many of the body's muscles exert their force on tendons that glide around bony tubercles or through tendonous retinacula. This enables the muscles to exert their actions around joints whether the joints are extended or flexed. Some nerves follow similar anatomic courses. Although excessive flexion or extension can produce predictable problems in patients' nerves and muscles through excessive pressure and stretch, other mechanisms can also lead to positioning injuries.

Dylewsky and McAlpine[7] described four axonal reactions to injury. *Transient ischemic nerve blocks* occur with no structural nerve damage and last only minutes. *Neurapraxia* recovery takes 4 to 6 weeks and results from demyelination of peripheral fibers of the nerve trunk. *Axonotmesis* describes a complete disruption of the axons within an intact nerve sheath; recovery depends on regeneration of the distal nerve at 1 mm per day, but complete recovery is unlikely. *Neurotmesis* involves complete nerve disruption; surgical repair can produce only partial functional recovery at best.

Five in vivo mechanisms for perioperative peripheral neuropathies are stretch, compression, generalized ischemia, metabolic derangement, and surgical section.[7,8] As little as 10% to 15% elongation of a peripheral nerve is sufficient to cause changes in vital physiologic processes in a peripheral nerve.[9] Adverse affects of stretch and compression on nerves can be very subtle. Prielipp and coworkers[10] have demonstrated that when awake male volunteers are monitored with somatosensory evoked potentials (SSEP), half perceive no symptoms when pressure sufficient to cause SSEP changes is applied externally to the ulnar nerve. Caplan has likened this to "silent" myocardial ischemia, but also pointed out that there may be a certain threshold of pressure or duration of compression required to produce clinical symptoms.[11]

Metabolic diseases play a role in perioperative neuropathies such as diabetes, and nutritional problems such as pernicious anemia and alcoholic neuritis are common in surgical patients. Arteriosclerosis, drug, or heavy metal exposure and infectious diseases such as polio also can cause neuropathies. Perioperative cigarette smoking is associated with an increased incidence of postoperative neuropathies, presumably because of the vasoconstrictive effects of nicotine.[12]

Upper Extremity Nerve Injury During Anesthesia
Brachial Plexus

Brachial plexus injuries occur primarily in cardiothoracic procedures requiring median sternotomy. Shoulder braces used for head-down procedures have also been implicated as a cause of postoperative brachial plexus neuropathy, and this complication has also been described after some prone procedures.

Mechanisms for brachial plexus injury during median sternotomy include stretch or compression of the plexus during sternal separation, direct trauma from fractured 1st ribs, stretching related to internal mammary dissection, and trauma or hematoma related to internal jugular vein cannulation. Brachial plexus injuries constitute 20% of claims for nerve injury in the ASA Closed Claims Database (see Table 28-2).[1] A prospective study of patients undergoing open heart surgery found the incidence of these injuries to be as high as 4.9%.[7] Lower parts of the plexus are most often involved, producing painless motor deficits that usually resolve over 6 to 8 weeks.

Shoulder braces placed close to the neck of patients undergoing noncardiothoracic procedures in a steep head-down (Trendelenburg) position may put pressure directly on the upper roots and trunks of the brachial plexus. Braces placed more laterally may put excessive traction on the brachial plexus by displacing the shoulder inferiorly. Coppieters and coworkers[9] studied the effect of the brachial plexus tension test (BPTT), a clinical equivalent of straight leg raising in the upper extremity, in asymptomatic male volunteers. Their results led them to strongly discourage the use of shoulder braces in positioning patients for surgery. Nonsliding mattresses were recommended when shoulder braces were thought absolutely required for a steep head-down tilt.

The prone position has also been implicated in brachial plexus injuries. Although theoretical advantages may support tucking the arms at the side in prone patients or turning the head to the side of an arm abducted up, no data support this idea. Brachial plexus injuries in prone patients are rare.

Ulnar Neuropathy

Ulnar neuropathy was formerly attributed to intraoperative compression or stretching because of the nerve's vulnerable position at the elbow where it passes around the medial epicondyle of the humerus and under the retinaculum of the cubital tunnel (Fig. 28-1). The anatomic boundaries of the cubital tunnel are the floor (i.e., medial ligament of the elbow) and the roof (i.e., arcuate ligament, which extends from the medial epicondyle of the humerus to the medial aspect of the olecranon process of the ulna). The ulnar nerve then passes posteromedially to the tubercle of the coronoid process of the ulna; the arterial supply of the nerve in this area, the posterior recurrent ulnar artery, is very superficial. Anatomically, the tubercle of the coronoid process is 1.5 times larger in men and boys, who also are more likely to have a thicker cubital tunnel retinaculum. Women and girls have a much thicker layer of subcutaneous fat between the skin and the ulnar nerve at the cubital tunnel and the medial aspect of the coronoid process.[13]

An exhaustive retrospective study of the Mayo Clinic database for perioperative ulnar neuropathies occurring

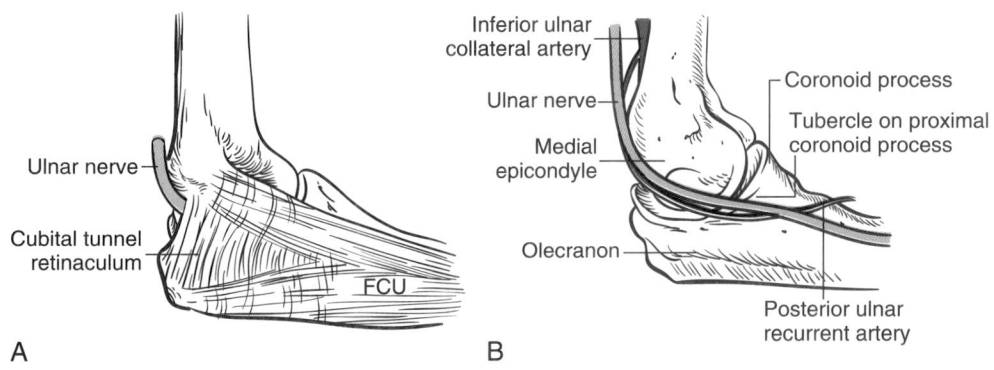

Figure 28–1 A, The retinaculum of the cubital tunnel is depicted distinct from the aponeurosis of the flexor carpi ulnaris (FCU) with which its distal margin blends. **B,** The ulnar nerve and its primary blood supply in the proximal forearm, the posterior ulnar recurrent artery, are superficial as they pass posteromedially to the tubercle of the coronoid process. (Adapted from Warner MA: Perioperative neuropathies. Mayo Clinic Proc 73:569, 571, 1998.)

over a 35-year period (1957-1991) was reported in 1994.[14] Ulnar neuropathies lasting longer than 3 months were identified in 414 of 1,129,692 consecutive patients (1 per 2729 patients) undergoing procedures requiring anesthesia or monitored anesthesia care. Seventy percent of the patients developing ulnar neuropathy were male. Almost half of the deficits were sensory only, and 80% of these patients regained complete sensation in 1 year. Only 35% of patients with mixed sensory and motor deficits recovered completely in 1 year.

Warner and coworkers[14] concluded that perioperative ulnar neuropathies might not be related to patient positioning for several reasons. Symptoms were not observed for more than 24 hours after the procedure in 57% of patients. Many of the neuropathies occurred in patients who did not receive general anesthesia. Bilateral ulnar neuropathies occurred in 9%. There were strong associations with several patient characteristics: male gender, very obese or very thin body habitus, and prolonged hospitalization (>14 days).

Two prospective studies further strengthened the suspicion that the injury associated with postoperative ulnar neuropathy does not usually occur intraoperatively. In the first, 1502 surgical patients were carefully assessed for neurologic signs and symptoms before and after surgery.[15] Warner and coworkers[15] found that seven patients (1 in 215) developed ulnar neuropathy perioperatively, but that none of the 7 was symptomatic within the first 2 postoperative days. The median onset of symptoms was the fourth postoperative day. Six of seven of the patients were men. In another prospective study of medical patients requiring no surgical procedures, 2 of 986 patients developed ulnar neuropathy.[16] It has become accepted that postoperative ulnar nerve palsy can occur without any apparent cause, even when positioning and padding of the patient's arms has been carefully done perioperatively. Postoperative ulnar nerve palsy is not always a preventable complication.[17]

Other Upper Extremity Nerve Injuries

The *radial nerve* may be injured where it wraps laterally around the middle of the humerus or laterally in its groove at the elbow. More muscular patients may be at higher risk because of limitations of extension of the elbow caused by hypertrophied biceps muscles and inflexible tendons. This may put the median or the anterior interosseous nerve on a greater stretch intraoperatively.[18] Transient *median nerve* carpal tunnel symptoms were identified in 27 of 1502 patients followed prospectively by Warner and coworkers[15] during the perioperative period. The *anterior interosseous nerve* contains no sensory fibers, but loss of it produces weakness of the thumb and index finger and a characteristic square pinch rather than an "O" on opposition of the thumb and index finger. Specific sensory and motor deficiencies caused by upper and lower extremity neuropathies are listed in Table 28-4.

Lower Extremity Neuropathies

A large, retrospective study found motor neuropathies persisting more than 3 months in 55 patients among those undergoing 198,461 procedures in the lithotomy position, which is an incidence of 1 in 3608.[19] Forty-three of the 55 neuropathies involved the common peroneal nerve. Motor function of the affected nerve recovered in 43% of the patients within 1 year. Three risk factors were strongly associated with increased risk of developing a neuropathy in the lithotomy position: prolonged surgery (>3 hours), very thin body habitus, and recent cigarette smoking.

Lithotomy Position Injuries

Warner and coworkers[20] also prospectively studied lower extremity neuropathies in 991 lithotomy patients. Fifteen patients (1.5%) developed neuropathies. The obturator, lateral femoral cutaneous, sciatic, and peroneal nerves were involved in five, four, three, and three patients, respectively. Fourteen of 15 patients presented with paresthesias; the symptoms resolved within 6 months in all but 1 patient. Prolonged positioning in the lithotomy position (>2 hours) and the extremes of body weight were found to contribute to an increased risk for lower extremity neuropathies after surgery in the lithotomy position in this prospective study.

Transient neurologic symptoms, also referred to as transient radicular irritation, can manifest as severe pain radiating down both legs after spinal anesthesia with lidocaine. The lithotomy position is associated with more frequent occurrences of this problem.[21]

Specific Nerve Injuries

The *common peroneal nerve* passes around the head of the fibula laterally, where it can be injured by compression by leg holders used to position patients in a lithotomy position (Fig. 28-2). The *sciatic nerve* can be stretched by hyperflexion of the hip and extension of the knee in patients in a lithotomy position.

The *femoral nerve* can be injured by compression by abdominal wall retractors. The *obturator nerve* passes through the pelvis and is occasionally injured by surgical retractors placed deep below the pelvic brim. Excessive flexion can also injure the obturator nerve.

The *lateral femoral cutaneous nerve* is sensory only. Excessive flexion of the hip on the abdomen may occasionally cause compression leading to temporary neuropathies.

Evaluation and Treatment of Perioperative Neuropathies

Warner has recommended early neurology consultation for patients with motor neuropathies; electromyographic (EMG) studies can be helpful to determine the location of the lesion and may provide information on the potential reversibility of any nerve deficit.[8] In contrast, sensory neuropathies often are transient, and initial reassurance might be all that is necessary.[8,22] Since anesthesiologists often will be unable to provide long-term surveillance of patients who develop sensory deficits, it seems prudent to seek neurology consultation for sensory deficits lasting more than 5 days.

Eye Complications

Eye complications are frustratingly common in patients who have undergone procedures in the prone position and

Table 28–4   Motor and sensory defects caused by perioperative peripheral neuropathies

Nerve	Motor Deficit	Sensory Deficit
Axillary	Loss of arm abduction by deltoid muscle	Deficit affects "arm-patch" area of the lateral shoulder.
Musculocutaneous	Loss of elbow flexion by biceps brachii (injury below the elbow yields sensory injury only)	Radial aspect of the volar forearm is affected.
Ulnar	A weak hand results from loss of function of many intrinsic hand muscles. Injuries at or above the elbow may produce weakness in the flexor digitorum profundus to ring and small fingers. Imbalance between interossei weakness (low ulnar nerve palsy) and digital flexor weakness (high ulnar nerve palsy) causes different degrees of ring and little finger "clawing."	The little finger and the ulnar (medial) half of the hand and ring finger are affected. The autonomous zone of sensory loss is the ulnar-palmar aspect of the little finger.
Radial	Loss of wrist and metaphalangeal joint extension results in wristdrop and fingerdrop. Lesions in the axilla also cause loss of elbow extension by the triceps brachii.	Radial aspect of the dorsal forearm is affected, continuing to the dorsum of the hand, thumb, and index and long fingers. The autonomous zone of sensory loss is in the region of the anatomic snuff box.
Median	Injury in the distal forearm (low median nerve palsy) results in impaired thumb opposition, abduction, and profound thenar atrophy. Lesions at or above the elbow (high median nerve palsy) may produce weakness in finger flexion and wrist flexion	Deficit affects the distal palm and palmar surfaces of the thumb and the index, long, and half of the ring fingers. The sole sensory innervation to the fingertips of the index and long fingers is affected. The autonomous zone is in the radial-palmar aspect of the index finger.
Anterior interosseous	Deficit causes loss of flexor pollicis longus and flexor digitorum profundus function of the index and possibly middle fingers. This results in an inability to form an "OK" sign. Loss of pronator quadratus function results in some weakness of pronation.	None
Femoral	Deficit causes loss of extension of the lower limb by the iliopsoas and quadriceps and gives rise to the purely sensory saphenous nerve (below).	Anterior surface of the thigh to the knee is affected.
Saphenous		Medial surfaces of the knee, leg, and foot are affected.
Obturator	Deficit impairs adduction of the thigh.	Medial surface of the thigh is affected.
Sciatic	Deficit impairs hamstring function in knee flexion and all motor function below the knee. Incomplete lesions typically affect the peroneal division preferentially	Sensory components of the tibial and common peroneal nerves are affected.
Tibial	Deficit impairs plantar flexion of the foot by the gastrocnemius and soleus muscles and inversion by the posterior tibialis, and causes loss of toe flexion by flexor hallucis longus and flexor digitorum.	Sole of the heel and foot is affected.
Sural		Lateral surface of foot is affected.
Common peroneal	Footdrop results from impaired ankle dorsiflexion. Deficit causes loss of eversion and toe extension.	Lateral surface of the leg and the dorsal surface of the foot are affected.
Lateral femoral cutaneous		Upper anterolateral thigh is affected.

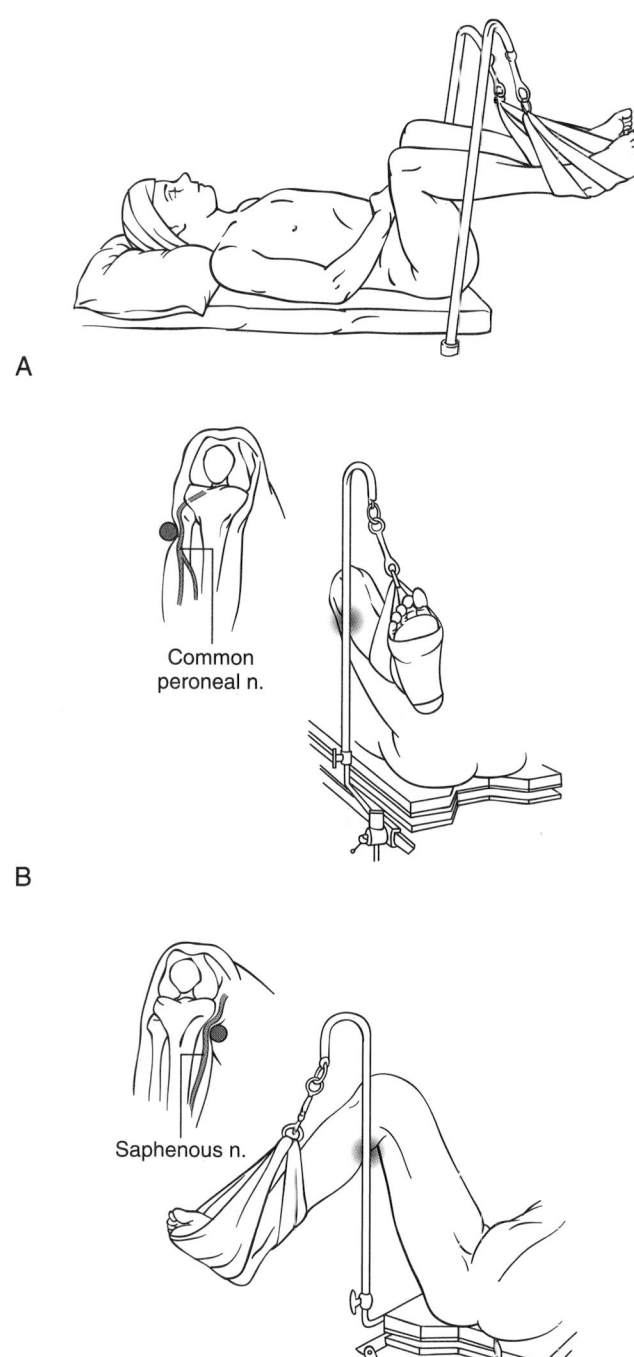

Figure 28–2 A, Lithotomy position, showing leg placement. **B** and **C,** Positioning is poor because the unpadded lithotomy leg holder can compress the common peroneal nerve laterally or the saphenous nerve medially. (Adapted from Martin JT: Lithotomy positions. Anesth Analg 1992;75:275 and from Smith BE: Obstetrics. *In* Martin JT, Warner MA [eds]: Positioning in Anesthesia and Surgery, 3rd ed. Philadelphia, WB Saunders, 1997, pp 47-70.)

are at risk in other positions as well. Eye complications constitute 3% of all claims in the ASA Closed Claims Database but have a higher frequency of payment than that for claims for other conditions. Figure 28-3 portrays a number of mechanisms leading to perioperative visual loss.

Corneal abrasions are most common, often involving the "down eye" in patients who were positioned prone with their heads turned to the side. One study put the prevalence at 0.17% for prone patients and found taping just after induction of anesthesia to be more effective than ophthalmic ointment used intraoperatively.[23] Although direct trauma can occur to the cornea, swelling of the dependent eye may be the mechanism causing the down eye to open slightly, allowing a slit-shaped area of cornea to dry. The patient with a corneal abrasion complains of eye pain and a foreign body sensation on awakening from anesthesia. Corneal abrasions usually heal quickly; the affected eye can be patched and antibiotic ointment applied to prevent bacterial infection that could lead to a corneal ulcer.

Pressure on the eyes should always be avoided. Small increases in pressure may occlude venous flow in the retina. If the pressure is slightly higher, arterial flow can be impaired and contribute to ischemia of the retina or optic nerve. Retinal artery occlusion usually manifests as a painless, monocular blindness with a pale edematous retina and a cherry-red spot at the fovea.

Ischemic optic neuropathy (ION) has been recognized as a serious complication of hemorrhage in cardiovascular, spinal, and other types of surgery, leading to blindness in one or both eyes postoperatively.[24,25] The association between blood loss, hypotension, and blindness was mentioned by Hippocrates. ION is caused by infarction or ischemia of the anterior or posterior parts of the optic nerve. The blood supply to the posterior optic nerve is a watershed zone where delicate connections exist between the small arterial branches of the central retinal artery and outer pial vessels from branches of the ophthalmic artery.[24]

Many patients with ION do not have atherosclerosis and other cardiovascular risk factors; the complication has been reported in patients as young as 13 years.[25] In an extensive review in patients undergoing cardiopulmonary bypass, ION was diagnosed in 17 of 27,915 patients (0.06%).[26] Four cases occurred in 501,342 anesthetics (0.0008%) not involving cardiopulmonary bypass at the same institution.[27] None of these involved spinal surgery, but three cases of ION involving spinal surgery occurred at this institution in the first 4 years after the review.

The ASA Professional Liability Committee established a Registry for Postoperative Visual Loss (POVL Registry) in 1999 to collect data on this problem (www. ASAclosedclaims.org) (see Chapter 82). In the first 4 years, 79 cases were collected. In contrast to the literature cited earlier, 67% of the ASA POVL Registry cases involved prone spinal procedures, and 81% were caused by ION. The median age of the reported cases was 49; the age range was 19 to 73.

Other factors such as stretch and compression of the optic nerve due to orbital swelling in the prone patient may be involved in ION. Significant swelling often occurs in the orbits after prolonged procedures done in the

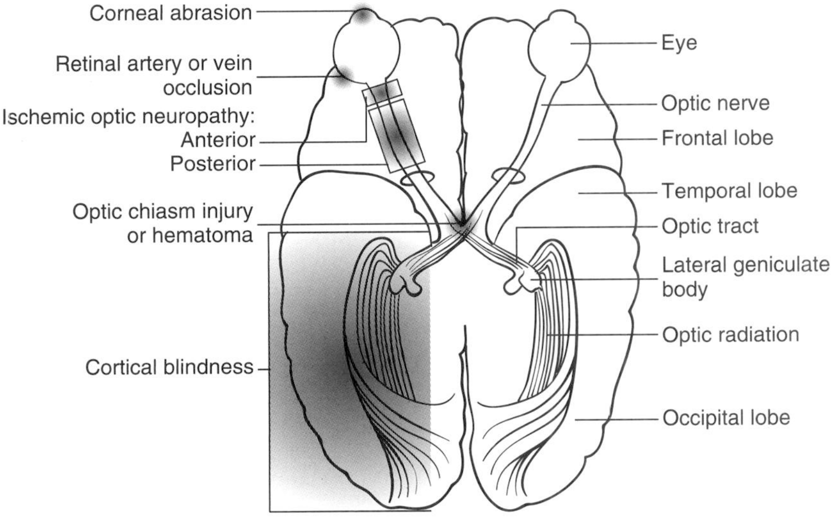

Corneal abrasion ————

Retinal artery or vein occlusion ————

Ischemic optic neuropathy:
Anterior ————
Posterior ————

Optic chiasm injury or hematoma ————

Cortical blindness ————

———— Eye

———— Optic nerve

———— Frontal lobe

———— Temporal lobe

———— Optic tract

———— Lateral geniculate body

———— Optic radiation

———— Occipital lobe

Figure 28–3 Causes of perioperative eye complications are depicted. Corneal abrasions are most common. Swelling or pressure can lead to retinal vein or artery occlusion. Ischemic optic neuropathy is caused by infarction of the optic nerve. Injuries to the optic chiasm can occur during pituitary surgery, and cortical blindness can occur after some cardiac and neurosurgical procedures. (Adapted from Williams EL, Hart WM, Tempelhoff R: Postoperative ischemic optic neuropathy. Anesth Analg 80:1018-1029, 1995.)

prone position; this swelling could affect circulation in the orbit posterior to the globe or cause stretching of the ophthalmic nerves.

Cortical blindness from hemorrhagic or embolic infarctions of the occipital lobe also occurs in the perioperative period, most commonly in patients after cardiac and neurosurgical procedures (see Fig. 28-3). Injuries or bleeding in the optic chiasm can lead to blindness after pituitary surgery.

POSITIONS

Supine Position

The supine position is the most commonly used position for surgical procedures. Because it is probably also the most commonly used position for natural sleep, it might be considered to be risk free. However, as shown in the ASA Closed Claims Database, ulnar neuropathies are the most common perioperative nerve injury, and most are associated with surgical procedures done in this position.[1]

Positioning of the upper extremities in a supine patient has been addressed. Pressure on the ulnar groove and the spiral groove of the humerus where the radial nerve passes must be avoided, but is there an ideal position for the arms? The ASA Practice Advisory recommended that arm abduction should be limited to 90 degrees and that the forearm and hand be supinated or kept in neutral position (not pronated) when an armboard is used (see Table 28-3).[2] Supination of the forearm was also recommended by Coppieters and colleagues[9] after their studies involving the brachial plexus tension test and by Prielipp and coworkers,[10] who used a computerized pressure sensing mat to determine positions that resulted in the least pressure over the ulnar groove.[9,10] Although the ASA Practice Advisory consensus was that padding at the elbow "may decrease" the risk of upper extremity neuropathy, it was pointed out that there were no data to prove this.[2] In 27% of the 190 patients with ulnar nerve injuries

in the ASA Closed Claims Database, elbow padding was specifically mentioned.[1] Inappropriate use of padding (too tight) may increase the risk of perioperative neuropathy.

It is necessary in some cases to tuck one or both arms by a patient's side to improve surgical access. In obese patients, it can be quite difficult to tuck the patient's upper extremity by his or her abdomen and hips without risking excessive pressure on the hand or forearm. This practice has led to compartment syndromes in the hand and forearm that required surgical release in some patients. Difficulties can be compounded if an intravenous line infiltrates in an arm that is tucked beside the body. Neuromuscular blockade monitoring is also hampered when there is no access to an upper extremity.

Lithotomy Position

The lithotomy position is used frequently in gynecologic and urologic surgery. The simultaneous elevation of the legs while the person is in the supine position provides the advantages of reducing torsion on the pelvis and lower back. Translocation of the vascular volume is promoted centrally. However, the areas that support the weight of the legs provide points of potential nerve and muscle injury (see Fig. 28-2). The goal is to suspend or support the legs so that they are flexed at the hips perpendicular to the torso and spread far enough apart to allow appropriate access to the perineum and abdomen. Sometimes, less flexion of the hips is required. There are several devices to support the legs, with vertical bars common to all of them. The support from the bars may be by built-in concave metal supports or by straps (Figs. 28-2 and 28-4). Both of these positions usually require additional padding.

There is risk of injury to the peroneal nerve if it is compressed between the head of the fibula and the bar or the support structures. Pressure over the medial tibial condyle may result in saphenous nerve injury (see Fig. 28-2). More common nerve injuries associated with the lithotomy position are discussed in "Lower Extremity Neuropathies."

V1

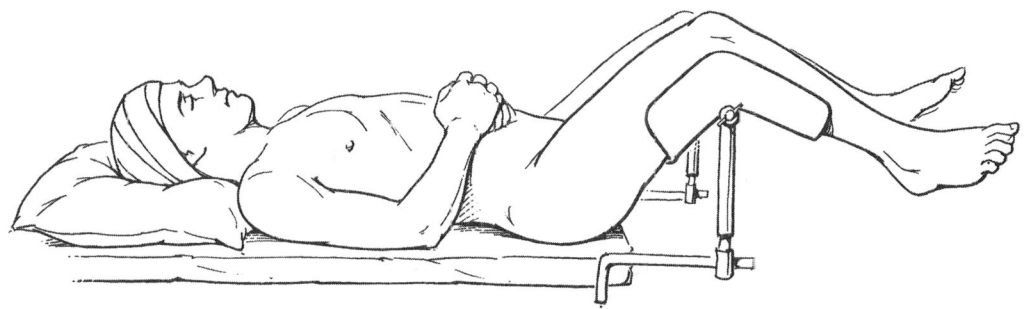

Figure 28–4 Lithotomy position with less hip flexion for endoscopic procedures such as transurethral resection of the prostate. (Adapted Martin JT. Lithotomy positions. *In* Martin JT, Warner MA [eds]: Positioning in Anesthesia and Surgery, 3rd ed. Philadelphia, WB Saunders, 1997, p 50.)

Lower extremity compartment syndrome is a recognized complication of the lithotomy position. A review of 572,498 surgical procedures done between 1989 and 1999 at the Mayo Clinic found 13 cases of compartment syndrome requiring fasciotomy.[28] The complication was not limited to the lithotomy position (1 per 8720), occurring almost as frequently in the lateral position (1 per 9711) and in some supine patients (1 per 92,441). Surgical procedures in which compartment syndromes developed were longer (7.2 hours) on average than the mean length of procedures for all patents (2.7 hours) during the study period.

A devastating injury in this position, which is fortunately uncommon, is hand and finger injury. As the foot of the bed is being rolled to a vertical position, care must be taken that the fingers are not caught in the gap and crushed (Fig. 28-5). Compartment syndrome of the hand can occur if it is compressed between the buttocks and the operating table. In the lithotomy position, pooling of the preparation solution under the buttocks and lower back can result in a chemical burn; it is wise to remove all drapes in this area after preparation so that puddles of residual solution can be removed.

Lateral Position

Thoracotomy and total-hip arthroplasty patients are usually placed in the lateral position. The arm is placed perpendicular to the torso on a pillow or on an overarm rest to support its weight (Fig. 28-6); the arm is often taped in this position. Care must be taken that the tape does not impinge on the ulnar nerve at the elbow or on the radial

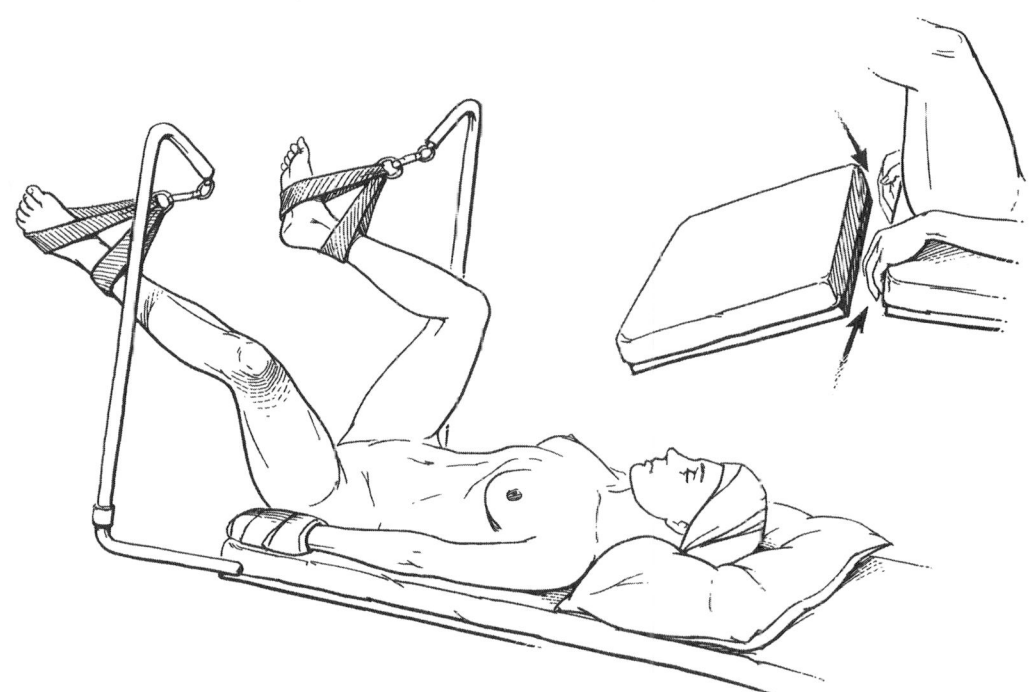

Figure 28–5 Lithotomy position with straps instead of stirrups for leg support. *Inset* shows the risk to the fingers when the lower portion of the operating table is lowered. (Adapted from Martin JT: Lithotomy positions. *In* Martin JT, Warner MA [eds]: Positioning in Anesthesia and Surgery, 3rd ed. Philadelphia, WB Saunders, 1997, p 67.)

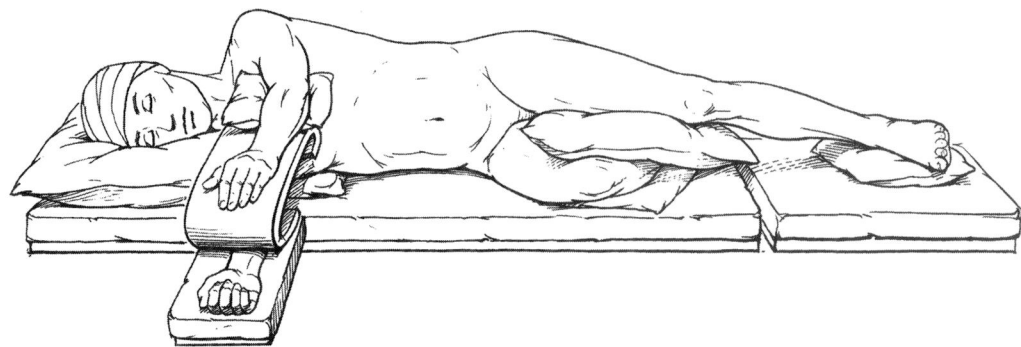

Figure 28–6 The lateral position, showing the upper arm rest in position; axillary roll, which supports the chest to free the axilla; and one type of leg positioning. (Adapted from Day LJ: Unusual positions: Orthopedics: Surgical aspects. *In* Martin JT [ed]: Positioning in Anesthesia and Surgery, 2nd ed. Philadelphia, WB Saunders, 1987, p 226.)

nerve as it wraps around the radial groove in the upper third of the humerus. For some thoracotomy procedures, a higher chest exposure is needed, and the arm is placed above the shoulder plane. Special care must be taken to avoid plexus injury in these situations (Fig. 28-7). Tension on the brachial plexus can be reduced by bringing the arm into a more anterior plane with the body. The lower area of the chest is generally supported with an axillary roll, which often is a 1-L bag of intravenous fluid wrapped in a towel. This places the weight of the chest on the rib cage and prevents the shoulder and axilla from being compressed; compression of the axilla can lead to brachial plexus injury in the down arm. Palpation of the arterial pulse in the down arm is sometimes used as a measure of the adequacy of decompression. However, because the axillary brachial plexus can be substantially compressed well before pulses are lost, this method is probably insufficient evidence of safety. If the peripheral

arm pulse is absent, substantial compression must have already occurred, and the patient and chest roll should be repositioned.

Rhabdomyolysis much like that in a crush injury, arterial insufficiency resulting in below-the-knee amputation, massive swelling of the thigh, and renal failure associated with myoglobinuria have been reported.[29] Use of the pulse oximeter to detect excessive pressure on the femoral triangle has been suggested.[30]

Lateral Oblique Position

The lateral oblique position (i.e., the three-quarters prone position) is used primarily for exposure of the posterior fossa in neurosurgery but may be used for other procedures on the back and upper neck. In this position, the torso is rotated from supine to lateral (Fig. 28-8). The upper leg is brought forward and flexed slightly, and

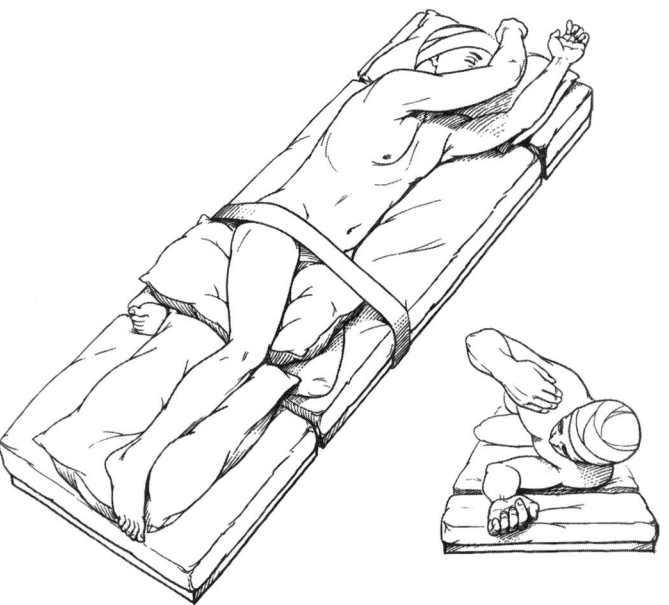

Figure 28–7 The lateral decubitus position for thoracotomy, showing a more headward position of the arms to facilitate surgical exposure. (Adapted from Lawson NW, Meyer DJ: Lateral positions. *In* Martin JT, Warner MA [eds]: Positioning in Anesthesia and Surgery, 3rd ed. Philadelphia, WB Saunders, 1997, p 134.)

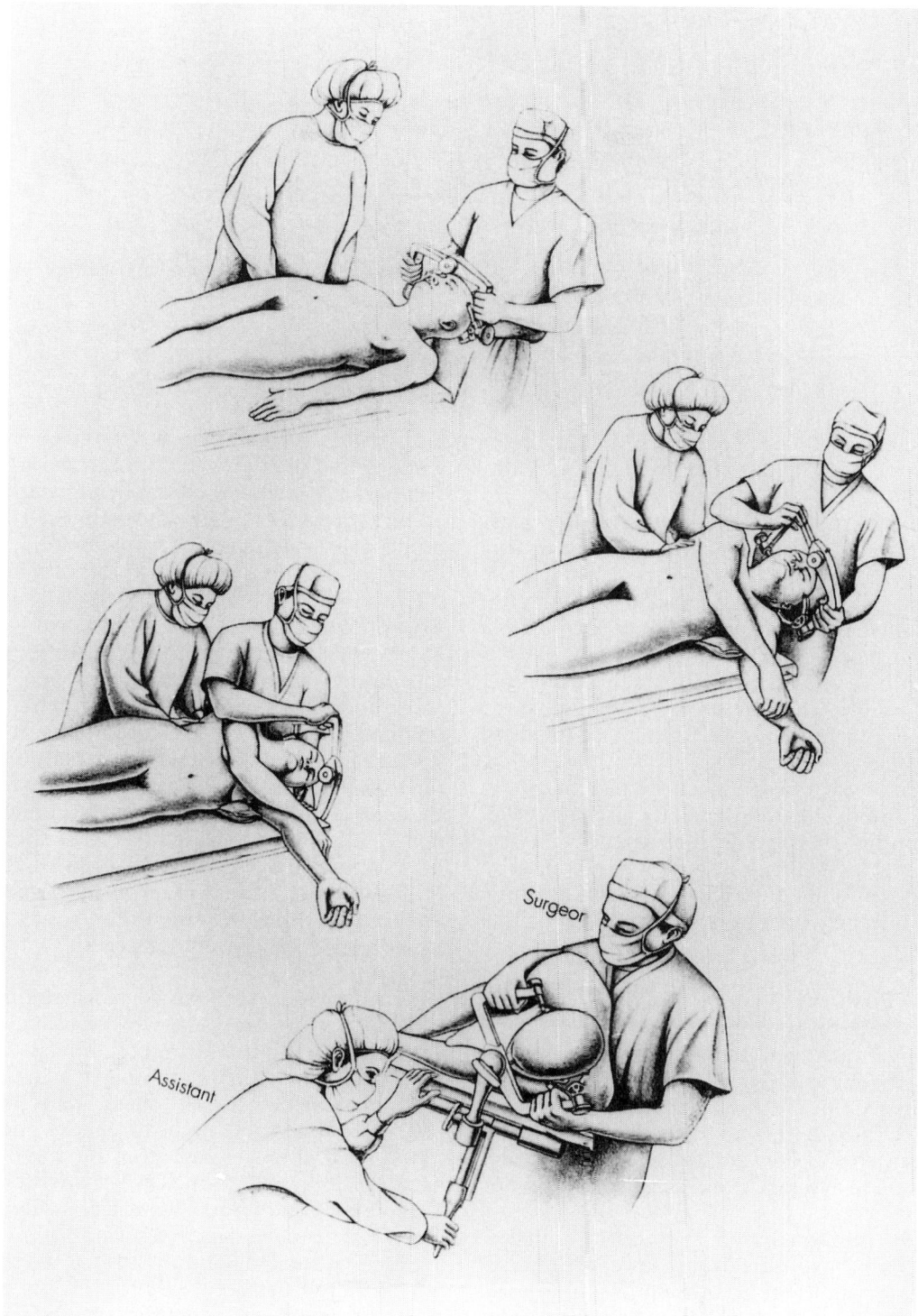

Figure 28–8 Movement of the patient from the supine to the lateral oblique position. (From Tew JM, Scodary DJ: Surgical positioning. *In* Apuzzo MJ [ed]: Brain Surgery: Complication Avoidance and Management. New York, Churchill Livingstone, 1993, p 1609.)

the lower leg is left straight. The head-holder pins may be placed before or after the patient is turned. An axillary roll is placed under the chest to support the weight of the body and to prevent the down axilla from being compressed. This is done at an angle, slightly higher posteriorly and slightly more caudad anteriorly. It should be possible to get part of a hand in the space between the chest wall and the axilla. The lower shoulder is brought to the forward edge of the bed or just slightly over it (Fig. 28-9). The patient is then rotated to the three-quarters prone position so that the occipital or lateral occipital skull is accessible to the surgeon. The upper arm is placed downward

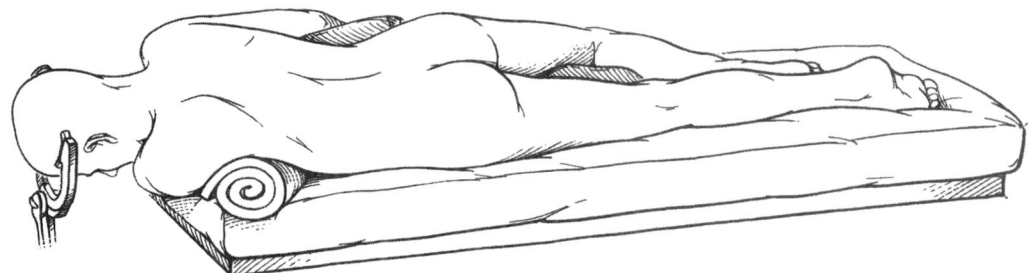

Figure 28–9 The lateral oblique (three-fourths prone) position. The axillary roll is placed under the chest, and the lower shoulder is brought forward to the edge of the bed or just slightly over the edge.

near the side wherever it falls comfortably. The upper shoulder must not be so high that it interferes with surgical access.

For the park bench position, the lower arm is placed posteriorly and parallel to the torso of a patient in the lateral oblique position. This position places considerable weight on the head of the humerus and acromion, and these areas should be padded carefully without excess bulk. Attention must be paid to the lower breast to prevent pressure on the nipple and areola. Extreme flexion of the head may compromise cervical spinal cord perfusion; quadriplegia can occur in the prone position despite this precaution.[31]

There are several difficulties in placing a patient in the lateral oblique position, and it is more difficult than lateral or prone positioning. Pressure on the dependent axilla and its contents and breast tissue are appropriate concerns, but there are no real guidelines for how much pressure is acceptable. Clinical experience must ultimately be the guide.

Trendelenburg Position

The Trendelenburg (head-down) modification of the supine position places the head down, often with the knees flexed, so that the patient does not slide headward on the table. The risks of shoulder braces to the brachial plexus were discussed earlier, and they are strongly discouraged.[2] When they cannot be avoided, nonsliding mattresses are recommended.

The head-down position moves the viscera cephalad and is used to improve exposure during lower abdominal surgery, to increase venous return after spinal anesthesia, or to increase central blood volume to facilitate jugular or subclavian cannulation. This position increases central venous pressure, intracranial and intraocular pressure, myocardial work, and pulmonary venous pressure and decreases pulmonary compliance and functional residual capacity.[32] Nevertheless, in a study in morbidly obese patients undergoing laparoscopy, the head-down position was shown to result in few changes in respiratory mechanics.[33] Endotracheal intubation is usually necessary to protect the airway and prevent pulmonary aspiration. There is one case report of a patient who had a cerebral hemorrhage during such a procedure and emerged with a significant neurologic deficit.[34] Clinical swelling of the

face, eyelids, conjunctiva, and tongue has been observed, along with a plethoric color of venous stasis in the head and neck. Lingual and buccal nerve neuropathy can also occur.[35] In patients with substantial swelling, it may be prudent to delay removal of the endotracheal tube until airway swelling has resolved.

Prone Position

The prone position is commonly used to provide surgical access to the posterior spine, lower extremities, and posterior fossa of the skull. Before induction of anesthesia, the cervical range of motion the patient can achieve comfortably (laterally and in flexion and extension) should be assessed along with the range of motion of the shoulders. Older patients and those with shoulder problems often cannot move their arms up to 90 degrees, and it is impossible to put their arms out on armboards after the patients are prone; the arms are then tucked at their sides intraoperatively, preventing access to intravenous and arterial lines.

Turning the head to the side is safe for most patients as long as pressure on the down eye is avoided; this offers fair access to the airway and endotracheal tube. Turning the neck can be difficult or impossible in the older patient with an arthritic neck. For them, foam pillows are available that support the forehead, cheeks, and chin but have cutouts for the eyes, mouth, and nose (Jackson Table Headrest Pillow, Orthopedic Systems, Inc., Union City, CA). One device (Prone View, Oceanside, CA) props the face in a foam pillow above a mirror so that the exact position of the eyes and mouth can be seen. The horseshoe headrest has been used for this purpose, but it supports the head on only the cheeks and forehead, is unstable during operating table adjustments, and makes it difficult to keep pressure off the eyes. In patients with known cervical problems, the head is often positioned in a pinion head holder so that the neck can be kept in neutral position, excessive flexion and extension are avoided, the neck is stable throughout the surgical procedure, and access to the airway is facilitated.

Inattentive positioning of a prone female's breasts can lead to postoperative tenderness and possibly to tissue injury. Extremely large breasts can lead to some instability of the thorax of a woman in the prone position. Although lateral displacement of the breasts is possible, common practice is to position them medially. Like most other aspects of positioning, no controlled studies can be found. Martin wrote, "However, an informal, nonstatistical, chaperoned interrogation of female patients and nursing personnel who represented a variety of body habitus indicated that lateralizing traction on breasts was painful to most women, whereas medial and cephalad compression was not."[36]

Chest rolls support the thorax and extend down to the hips. Their primary purpose is to prevent increased abdominal pressure in the prone patient, allowing room for diaphragmatic excursion. In addition to causing increased pulmonary pressures for mechanically ventilated patients, increased pressure in the abdominal cavity can also be transmitted to veins in the epidural space, leading to increased bleeding in the surgical fields. In obese patients, it is easier to use special tables and frames (e.g., Jackson table, Relton frame) that allow more space for the abdomen to hang down.

Lumbar flexion is frequently used to facilitate surgical exposure in that level of the spine. This can be produced by flexion of the table or by attachments that allow the patient to be placed in a kneeling position with some weight supported on the knees and shins. Table flexion usually causes the patient to move down on the table, and the position of the head, face, and arms must be carefully checked while these adjustments are being made.

The clinical impression is that hypotension occurs more often in prone patients than in those in any other surgical position. Hypotension probably is caused by venous pooling in the legs.

Positions for Orthopedic Surgery

Femoral neck fractures and midfemoral fractures needing open reduction and internal fixation require different positions because of the need for surgical access and for roentgenographic and fluoroscopic guidance (Figs. 28-10 and 28-11). The lateral decubitus position typically is used for total-hip arthroplasty (see Chapter 61). The down hip and leg are at risk during total-hip arthroplasty in the lateral decubitus position.

The orthopedic fracture table consists of a body section to support the head and thorax, a sacral plate for the pelvis with a perineal post, and adjustable footplates. The most important features of the table are the ability to maintain traction on a lower extremity and to obtain surgical and fluoroscopic access. Because the patients requiring this table are often in pain, anesthesia is usually induced before the patient is moved to the table. If regional anesthesia is used, the fracture side should be placed up to decrease the pain until the anesthetic takes affect. After the patient has been transferred, the upper extremity on the fracture side should be placed so that it does not interfere with surgical access to the fracture; placing it across the chest directly or over an armboard is effective. Complications from this position include brachial plexus injury, lower extremity compartment syndrome, and pudendal nerve injury related to the perineal post.

Position for Shoulder Surgery

The use of the "beach chair," "barber's chair," or semirecumbent position is increasing in popularity in parallel with surgical procedures on the shoulder. The key element of the position is that it provides anterior and posterior access to the shoulder, with the upper extremity freely mobile. Extreme rotation of the head away from the operative side can result in stretching of the brachial plexus during surgical manipulation. Figure 28-12 shows one method of securing the endotracheal tube and head to prevent movement and accidental extubation. The surgical field is clearly higher than the heart, so air embolism is a risk. An impressive complication of shoulder arthroscopy

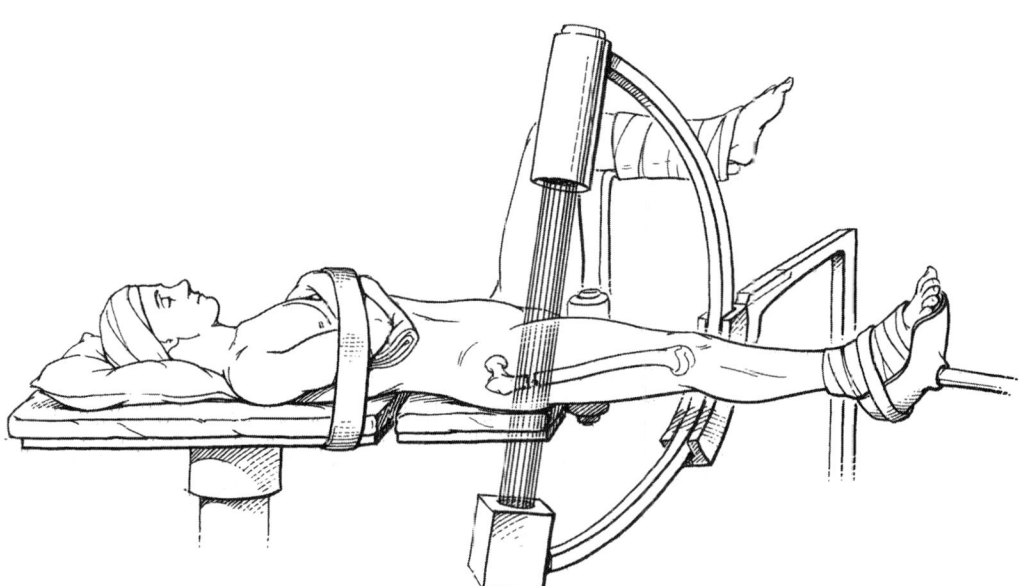

Figure 28–10 Femoral neck fractures can be managed in the supine position on the fracture table. (Adapted from Martin JT: Lithotomy positions. *In* Martin JT, Warner MA [eds]: Positioning in Anesthesia and Surgery, 3rd ed. Philadelphia, WB Saunders, 1997, p 54.)

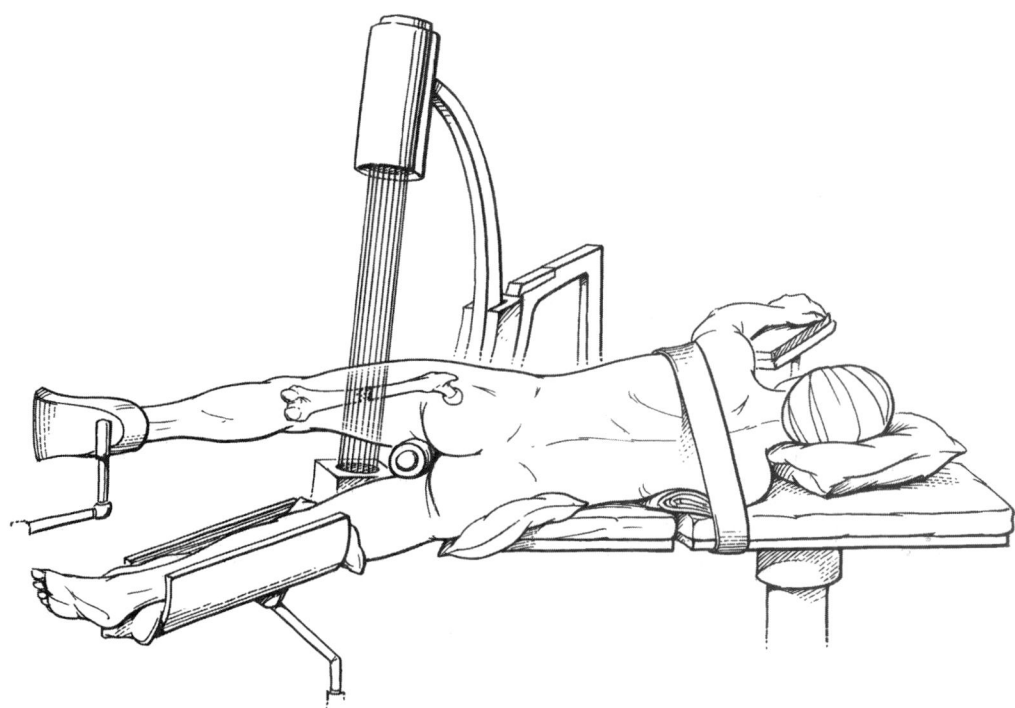

Figure 28–11 For midfemoral fractures, the patient is placed on the fracture table in the lateral position with the legs spaced and positioned to allow roentgenography at an angle in several planes. (Adapted from Day LJ: Unusual positions: Orthopedics: Surgical aspects. *In* Martin JT [ed]: Positioning in Anesthesia and Surgery, 2nd ed. Philadelphia, WB Saunders, 1987, p 229.)

is rapid, progressive, and complete airway obstruction, caused by extravasation of the fluid used during the visualization out of the capsule and into the tissues of the neck.[37]

Sitting Position

The sitting position is said to offer some surgical advantages for posterior cervical procedures and posterior fossa craniotomies. Surgeons may weigh these advantages differently, but most can agree that ease of surgical exposure, amount of blood pooling in the operative field, and operative position of the surgeon are different among the sitting, lateral, and prone positions. Access to the endotracheal tube, reduction of facial swelling, and better cardiovascular stability are notable advantages of the sitting position in anesthetic management. Risks of posterior fossa craniectomy in the sitting position include venous air embolism, paradoxical air embolism to the arterial circulation, hypotension, vascular instability resulting from brainstem

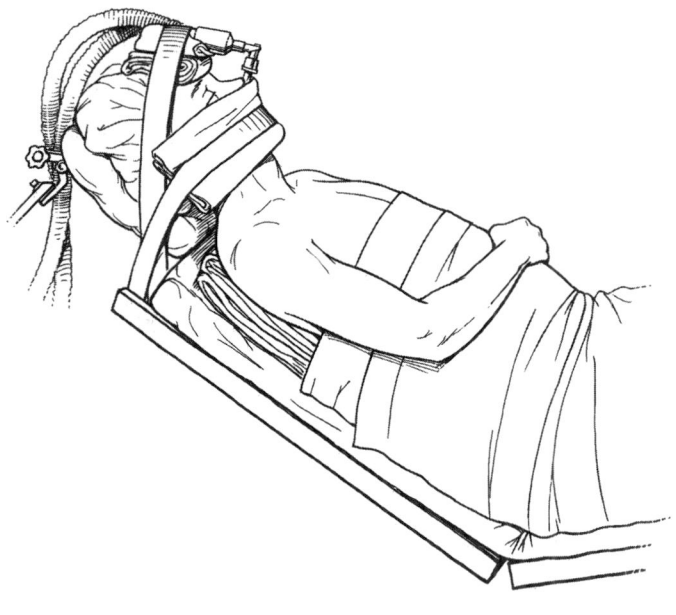

Figure 28–12 Lateral view of the upright shoulder position. The endotracheal tube and head are secured to prevent movement and accidental extubation.

manipulation, specific cranial nerve stimulation, airway obstruction, position-related brainstem ischemia, and macroglossia. These are not unique to the sitting position and may occur in other positions. Management should be directed at the prevention, early detection, and treatment of these problems.

There is much concern about the use of the sitting position, although there is a large body of information about its safety. Several large published series show a favorable safety record for operations using the sitting or prone positions.[38-40] A study by Black and colleagues[38] put the problem into perspective, and the results are consistent with those of other studies. These authors retrospectively reviewed 579 posterior fossa craniectomies (333 sitting and 246 horizontal) performed concurrently from 1981 through 1984. Intraoperatively, the incidence of hypotension did not differ between the two groups from induction of anesthesia to incision or from incision to closure. About 20% of the patients in each group became hypotensive during each of these periods; all responded to vasopressors or fluids, or both. The incidence of venous air embolism in patients monitored by Doppler ultrasound was significantly greater in the sitting position (45%) than in the horizontal position (12%). Sitting patients required transfusion less often than prone patients, and the transfused volume was lower.[38] No prospective, randomized comparison of the sitting and prone positions has been performed.

Several details should be considered when a patient is placed into a sitting or semirecumbent position (Fig. 28-13). Strict attention to detail should be paid to the flexion of the neck to prevent excessive flexion of the neck in sitting and other positions to prevent spinal cord eschemia, obstruction of carotid and vertebral arteries, and embolic or thrombotic stroke.[41] The decision about what constitutes excessive neck flexion is difficult; clinical experience and preanesthetic evaluation of range of motion may be most helpful. Warner[42] recommended avoidance of any position that would place the head and neck at the extreme limit of a range of motion. In general, the physician should be able to place two fingers between the chin and the sternum when positioning is complete.

In the sitting position, the arms tend to hang by the side. When muscle relaxants are used, the downward force caused by the weight of the arms is sufficient to stretch the brachial plexus beneath the clavicle and compress the neuromuscular bundle to the upper extremity, causing arm paralysis or weakness. Blankets are usually placed under the elbow and forearm to support the weight of the arm so that there is no downward stretch on the arm, and the arm is pushed up slightly, giving the appearance of a slight shoulder shrug.

The hips are often flexed because position tends to place the buttocks at an angle to support the weight of the body and because it is thought to aid venous return. The hips should be at the break in the table, with the lumbar area against the back of the table. If the patient "slouches" lower, the cervical operating field may be too low to clear the top of the table and the torso and thighs may not be in a stable position on the operating table. The legs must not be outstretched, however, because this places considerable tension on the sciatic nerve and can result in postoperative weakness. Bending the legs at the knees removes this tension, and placing an artificial fat pad under the buttocks and the sciatic notch of the pelvis may reduce the chances of pressure ischemia of the sciatic nerve. Venous return may be aided and thromboembolism may be prevented by the use of alternative

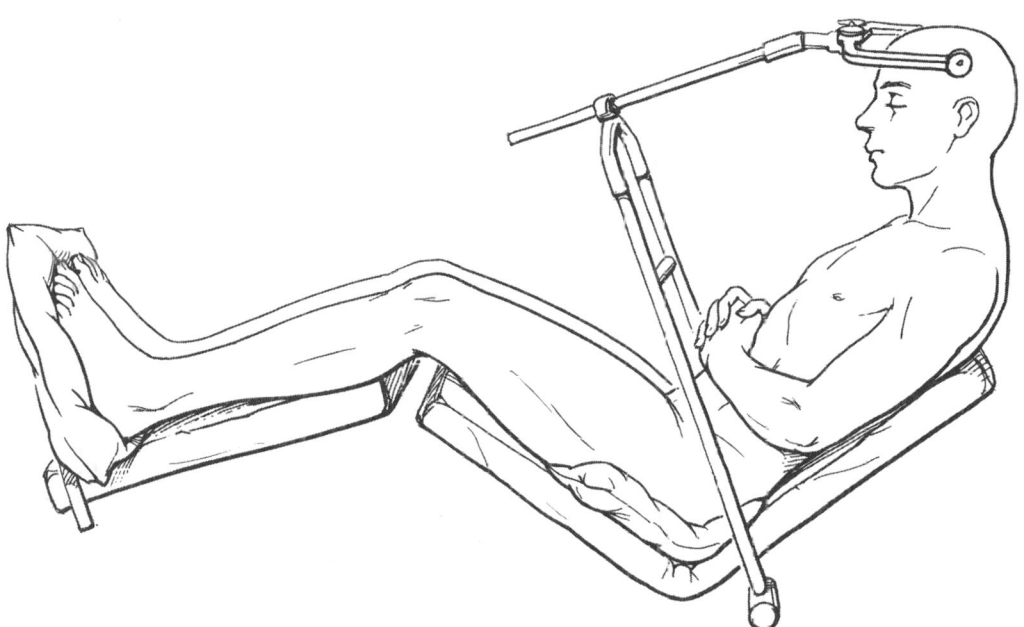

Figure 28–13 The patient is in a semi-sitting position with the knees flexed slightly. The headrest support is fastened to the upper part of the table so that the head can be lowered without changing the relationship of the pinion head holder to the torso. The arms must be supported (not shown) so that the weight of the arm does not stretch the brachial plexus. The buttock area is padded. (Adapted from Martin JT: The head-elevated positions: Anesthesiologic considerations. *In* Martin JT [ed]: Positioning in Anesthesia and Surgery, 2nd ed. Philadelphia, WB Saunders, 1987, p 81.)

inflatable leg wraps (e.g., sequential thromboembolic disease stockings).

REFERENCES

1. Cheney FW, Domino KB, Caplan RA, et al: Nerve injury associated with anesthesia. Anesthesiology 90:1062-1069, 1999.
2. ASA Task Force on Prevention of Perioperative Peripheral Neuropathies: Practice advisory for the prevention of perioperative peripheral neuropathies. Anesthesiology 92:1168-1182, 2000.
3. Froese AB, Bryan AC: Effects of anesthesia and paralysis on diaphragmatic mechanics in man. Anesthesiology 41:242-255, 1974.
4. Kleinman BS, Frey K, VanDrunen M, et al: Motion of the diaphragm in patients with chronic obstructive pulmonary disease while spontaneously breathing versus during positive pressure breathing after anesthesia and neuromuscular blockade. Anesthesiology 97:298-305, 2002.
5. Krayer S, Rehder K, Vettermann J, et al: Position and motion of the human diaphragm during anesthesia-paralysis. Anesthesiology 70:891-898, 1989.
6. Warner DO, Warner MA, Ritman EL: Human chest wall function while awake and during halothane anesthesia. I. Quiet breathing. Anesthesiology 82:6-19, 1995.
7. Dylewsky W, McAlpine FS: Peripheral nervous system. In Martin JT, Warner MA (eds): Positioning in Anesthesia and Surgery, 3rd ed. Philadelphia, WB Saunders, 1997.
8. Warner MA: Perioperative neuropathies. Mayo Clinic Proc 73:567-574, 1998.
9. Coppieters MW, Van De Velde M, Stappaerts KH: Positioning in anesthesiology. Anesthesiology 97:75-81, 2002.
10. Preilipp RC, Morell RC, Walker FO, et al: Ulnar nerve pressure. Anesthesiology 91:345-354, 1999.
11. Caplan RA: Will we ever understand perioperative neuropathy? A fresh approach offers hope and insight. Anesthesiology 91:335-336, 1999.
12. Warner MA, Martin JT, Schroeder DR, et al: Lower-extremity motor neuropathy associated with surgery performed on patients in a lithotomy position. Anesthesiology 81:6-12, 1994.
13. Contreras MG, Warner MA, Charboneau WJ, et al: The anatomy of the ulnar nerve at the elbow: Potential relationship of acute ulnar neuropathy to gender differences. Clin Anat 11:372-378, 1998.
14. Warner MA, Warner ME, Martin JT: Ulnar neuropathy: Incidence, outcome, and risk factors in sedated or anesthetized patients. Anesthesiology 81:1332-1340, 1994.
15. Warner MA, Warner DO, Matsumoto JY, et al: Ulnar neuropathy in surgical patients. Anesthesiology 90:54-59, 1999.
16. Warner MA, Warner DO, Harper CM, et al: Ulnar neuropathy in medical patients. Anesthesiology 92:613-615, 2000.
17. Stoelting RK: Postoperative ulnar nerve palsy—Is it a preventable complication? Anesth Analg 76:7-9, 1993.
18. Contreras MG, Warner MA, Carmicheal SW, et al: Perioperative anterior interosseous neuropathy. Anesthesiology 96:243-245, 2002.
19. Warner MA, Martin JT, Schroeder DR, et al: Lower-extremity motor neuropathy associated with surgery performed on patients in a lithotomy position. Anesthesiology 81:6-12, 1994.
20. Warner MA, Warner DO, Harper CM, et al: Lower extremity neuropathies associated with lithotomy positions. Anesthesiology 93:938-942, 2000.
21. Pollock JE, Neal JM, Stephenson CA, et al: Prospective study of the incidence of transient radicular irritation in patients undergoing spinal anesthesia. Anesthesiology 84:1361-1367, 1996.
22. Warner MA: Perioperative neuropathies in the lower extremities. In Faust RJ (ed): Anesthesiology Review, 3rd ed. New York, Churchill Livingstone, 2002.
23. Cucchiara RF, Black S: Corneal abrasion during anesthesia surgery. Anesthesiology 69:978-979, 1988.
24. Williams EL, Hart WM, Tempelhoff R: Postoperative ischemic optic neuropathy. Anesth Analg 80:1018-1029, 1995.
25. Brown RH, Schauble JF, Miller NR: Anemia and hypotension as contributors to perioperative loss of vision. Anesthesiology 80:222-226, 1994.
26. Nuttall GA, Garrity JA, Dearani JA, et al: Risk factors for ischemic optic neuropathy after cardiopulmonary bypass: A matched case/control study. Anesth Analg 93:1410-1416, 2001.
27. Warner ME, Warner, MA, Garrity JA, et al: The frequency of perioperative vision loss. Anesth Analg 93:1417-1421, 2001.
28. Warner ME, LaMaster LM, Thoeming AK, et al: Compartment syndrome in surgical patients. Anesthesiology 94:705-708, 2001.
29. Lachiewicz PF, Latimer HA: Rhabdomyolysis following total hip arthroplasty. J Bone Joint Surg Br 73:576-579, 1991.
30. Smith JW, Pellicci PM, Sharrock N, et al: Complications after total hip replacement: The contralateral limb. J Bone Joint Surg Am 71:528-535, 1991.
31. Deem S, Shapiro HM, Marshall LF: Quadriplegia in a patient with cervical spondylosis after thoracolumbar surgery in the prone position. Anesthesiology 75:527-528, 1991.
32. Wilcox S, Vandam LD: Alas, poor Trendelenburg and his position! A critique of its uses and effectiveness. Anesth Analg 67:574-578, 1998.
33. Sprung J, Whalley DG, Falcone T, et al: The impact of morbid obesity, pneumoperitoneum, and posture on respiratory system mechanics and oxygenation during laparoscopy. Anesth Analg 94:1345-1350, 2002.

34. Oliver SB, Cucchiara RF, Warner MA, et al: Unexpected focal neurologic deficit on emergence from anesthesia: A report of three cases. Anesthesiology 67:823-826, 1987.
35. Winter R, Munro M: Lingual and buccal nerve neuropathy in a patient in the prone position: A case report. Anesthesiology 71:452-454, 1989.
36. Martin JT: The prone position: Anesthesiologic considerations. In Martin JT (ed): Positioning in Anesthesia and Surgery, 2nd ed. Philadelphia, WB Saunders, 1987.
37. Hynson JM, Tung A, Guevara JE, et al: Complete airway obstruction during arthroscopic shoulder surgery. Anesth Analg 76:875-878, 1993.
38. Black S, Ockert DB, Oliver WC, et al: Outcome following posterior fossa craniectomy in patients in the sitting or horizontal position. Anesthesiology 69:49-56, 1988.
39. Young ML, Smith DS, Murtagh F, et al: Comparison of surgical and anesthetic complications in neurosurgical patients experiencing venous air embolism in the sitting position. Neurosurgery 18:157-161, 1986.
40. Duke DA, Lynch JJ, Harner SG, et al: Venous air embolism in sitting and supine patients undergoing vestibular schwannoma resection. Neurosurgery 42:1282-1286, 1998.
41. Gravenstein N, Grundy BL, Lobato EB: The central nervous system. In Martin JT, Warner MA (eds): Positioning in Anesthesia and Surgery, 3rd ed. Philadelphia, WB Saunders, 1997.
42. Warner MA: Positioning of the head and neck. In Martin JT, Warner MA (eds): Positioning in Anesthesia and Surgery, 3rd ed. Philadelphia, WB Saunders, 1997.

29 Malignant Hyperthermia

Gerald A. Gronert, Isaac N. Pessah, Sheila M. Muldoon, and Timothy J. Tautz

History   1170

**Pathophysiology and Molecular
    Biology   1170**
Molecular Events in Excitation-Contraction
    Coupling   1171
Ryanodine Receptor   1173
Factors Other Than Ryanodine Receptor
    Abnormalities   1174

Genetics   1174
Distribution of *RYR1* Mutations   1174
Inheritance and Penetrance of Malignant
    Hyperthermia   1176
Discordance in Malignant Hyperthermia
    Testing   1176
Functional Changes in *RYR1* Associated with
    Malignant Hyperthermia Mutations   1176

Dantrolene   1177

**Specific Organ and Tissue
    Abnormalities   1178**
Skeletal Muscle   1178
Heart   1179

Sympathetic Nervous System   1180
Miscellaneous Abnormalities   1180

Clinical Syndromes   1180
Trismus-Masseter Spasm   1180
Sudden, Unexpected Pediatric Cardiac
    Arrest   1181
Rhabdomyolysis   1181

**Triggering of Malignant
    Hyperthermia   1182**
Anesthetic Triggering   1182
Awake Triggering: Exercise and Heat
    Stroke   1182

Diagnosis   1183

Association with Other Disorders   1183

Treatment   1184

**Anesthesia for Susceptible
    Patients   1184**

Evaluation of Susceptibility   1185

Summary   1186

Malignant hyperthermia (MH), an eerie and erratic metabolic mayhem, is a clinical syndrome that in its classic form occurs during anesthesia with a potent volatile agent such as halothane and the depolarizing muscle relaxant succinylcholine, producing rapidly increasing temperature (by as much as 1°C/5 min) and extreme acidosis. The effects result from loss of control of intracellular calcium levels and compensatory acute, uncontrolled increases in skeletal muscle metabolism that may proceed to severe rhabdomyolysis. Initially, the mortality rate was 70%; earlier diagnosis and use of dantrolene have reduced it to less than 5%. MH now occurs in muted forms because of diminished use of succinylcholine, diagnostic awareness, early detection through end-expired carbon dioxide, use of less potent triggers, and use of drugs that attenuate

its onset. Wilson and colleagues[1] first used the term *malignant hyperthermia* in print in 1966. A Danish survey[2] indicates an incidence of fulminant MH of one case per 250,000 anesthetics. However, considering only potent anesthetics and succinylcholine, one case of fulminant MH occurred per 62,000 anesthetics. The incidence of suspected MH was one case per 16,000 anesthetics or one case per 4,200 anesthetics involving potent volatile agents in combination with succinylcholine.

Public education and communication are provided by a layman's organization, Malignant Hyperthermia Association of the United States (MHAUS, 11 E. State Street, P.O. Box 1069, Sherburne, New York 13460-1069; telephone: 1-607-674-7901; fax: 1-607-674-7910; email: mhaus@norwich.net; web site: www.mhaus.org) and by a medical professional's 24-hour, 7-day telephone service for emergency consultation, the MH Hotline (1-800-MHHYPER, or 1-800-644-9737). The professional subsidiary of MHAUS, the North American MH Registry, collates findings from biopsy centers in Canada and the United States and provides access to specific patient data through the Hotline or its Director, Dr. Barbara Brandom (North American MH Registry of MHAUS, Room 7449, Department of Anesthesiology, Children's Hospital, University of Pittsburgh, 3705 Fifth Avenue at DeSoto St., Pittsburgh, Pennsylvania, 15213-2583; telephone: 1-888-274-7899; fax: 1-412-692-8658; email: bwb@pitt.edu).

Of the three forms of the ryanodine receptor, RYR1, RYR2, and RYR3, only mutations in RYR1 have been linked to MH. The genetics of MH and the related abnormal function of RYR1 are being investigated at the molecular biologic level, with the porcine model providing intricate detail. Equivalent parallels in humans are limited by scarcer material for scientific study and the difficulty in identifying underlying sources of abnormal responses, complicated by the fact that phenotypes vary within a genotype (i.e., discordance between genetic results and MH testing by contracture studies). Dantrolene remains essential in therapy, although its mechanism of action is elusive. Standardization of in vitro MH muscle contracture testing with two slightly different protocols, the European (contracture test [IVCT]) and the North American (caffeine-halothane contracture test [CHCT]), has resulted in sufficiently large databases to confirm sensitivity and specificity. Diagnostic challenges occur with intra-anesthetic changes that mimic MH, particularly in its earlier manifestations.

HISTORY

Between 1915 and 1925, one family experienced three anesthetic-induced MH deaths featuring rigidity and hyperthermia and was puzzled for decades regarding the cause of these deaths. Susceptibility was eventually confirmed in three descendants.[3] In 1929, Ombrédanne[4] described anesthesia-induced postoperative hyperthermia and pallor in children with significant mortality (i.e., Ombrédanne's syndrome) but did not detect familial relationships. Critical worldwide insight into MH began in 1960, when Denborough and Lovell[5] described a 21-year-old Australian with an open leg fracture who was more anxious about anesthesia than about surgery because 10 of his relatives had died during or after anesthesia. Lovell initially anesthetized him with the then-new agent halothane, halted it when signs of MH appeared, and subsequently used spinal anesthesia. Further evaluations of affected families came from George Locher in Wausau, Wisconsin, in conjunction with Beverly Britt in Toronto, Canada. Direct skeletal muscle involvement rather than central loss of temperature control was established by recognition of increased muscle metabolism or muscle rigidity early in the syndrome, low-threshold contracture responses,[6] and elevated values for creatine kinase (CK).

Swine inbred for muscle development (e.g., Landrace, Pietrain, Poland China) provide an excellent animal model. The single-point mutation producing porcine MH is probably caused by the random occurrence of the altered *RYR1* allele, followed by deliberate inbreeding for desirable traits. International sharing of breeding stock accounts for its worldwide spread. Affected swine are detected by testing for the ubiquitous Arg615Cys mutation. The experimental model evolved from earlier reports describing unsuitable pork[7]; the stresses of the abattoir result in accelerated metabolism and rapid deterioration of the muscle, resulting in pale, soft, exudative pork.[8] Its incidence increased with breeding patterns designed to produce rapid growth rate, superior muscling, and hybrid vigor, although the drawback is a link with stress susceptibility. This increased incidence led to the term *porcine stress syndrome*.[9] Any stresses, such as separation, shipping, weaning, fighting, coitus, or preparation for slaughter, can lead to increased metabolism, acidosis, rigidity, fever, and death.

In 1966, Hall and coworkers[10] reported MH induced by halothane and succinylcholine in stress-susceptible swine. The human and porcine forms are virtually identical in comparisons of the clinical and laboratory changes of anesthesia-induced MH.[11] In 1975, Harrison[12] described the efficacy of dantrolene in preventing and treating porcine MH, which was confirmed in humans by a multihospital evaluation of dantrolene used to treat unanticipated anesthetic-induced episodes.[13] MH in swine is a manifestation of a generalized susceptibility to stress. Stress-induced awake triggering is common in MH-susceptible swine but uncommon in MH-susceptible humans.

MH presents several paradoxes. Anesthetics are inconsistent in their ability to trigger MH and are frequently ineffective in triggering episodes in affected humans[14]; this may be related to delay of the response by various depressants and nondepolarizing muscle relaxants.[15] Conversely, "safe" anesthetics, which are more appropriately described as those less likely to trigger MH, can still be associated with apparent MH episodes; these have always responded appropriately to dantrolene.[16] Susceptible individuals appear normal in regard to structure and function until they are stressed, complicating detection of the condition. Detection requires an anesthetic challenge, an invasive and destructive muscle biopsy with contracture responses to caffeine or halothane, or genetic investigation for causative mutations.

PATHOPHYSIOLOGY AND MOLECULAR BIOLOGY

MH is a myopathy, usually subclinical, that features an acute loss of control of intracellular calcium ions (Ca^{2+}). Normal muscle contraction is initiated at the neuromuscular junction (i.e., the motor end plate). Acetylcholine is released from the terminals of motor neurons and diffuses a short distance to the postsynaptic membrane, where binding to nicotinic cholinergic receptors triggers a wave of depolarization referred to as an *excitatory postsynaptic potential* (EPSP) that leads to action potentials that propagate to transverse tubules (T tubules). The T tubules act as conduits to bring action potentials deep within the myofibrils, where their excitatory signal is transduced to the junctional face of sarcoplasmic reticulum (SR) within the muscle cells to initiate release of Ca^{2+} stored within the SR terminal cisternae. In skeletal muscle, the release of SR Ca^{2+} is an essential step for contraction. The whole process, from T-tubule depolarization to release of SR Ca^{2+}, is called excitation-contraction (EC) coupling. Knowledge of the molecular events contributing to EC coupling is essential to understanding the cause of MH.

Skeletal EC coupling begins deep within the T-tubule membrane at high-density, voltage-gated L-type Ca^{2+} channels, historically labeled *dihydropyridine receptors* (DHPRs). The DHPR possesses an integral membrane voltage sensor whose function is to respond to T-tubule depolarization and initiate long-range conformational changes within the Ca^{2+} channel complex. Voltage-dependent activation of DHPR opens an integral Ca^{2+}-selective conductance path that permits entry of small amounts of Ca^{2+} into the muscle cell. The entry of Ca^{2+} into the skeletal myotube is not necessary for engaging skeletal-type EC coupling. Rather, one of the DHPR subunits (α_{1S}-subunit) provides physical links between DHPRs within T tubules and Ca^{2+} release channels within junctional SR. Skeletal muscle expresses a specific type of Ca^{2+} release channel called the *skeletal isoform*, or RYR1. Skeletal EC coupling is the result of physical coupling between α_{1S}-subunits and RYR1 at specialized "triadic" regions where the T-tubule membrane comes in close apposition to junctional SR and does not depend on the influx of Ca^{2+}. After EC coupling is initiated, the free, ionized, unbound intracellular Ca^{2+} concentration within the relaxed muscle cell increases from 10^{-7} M to about 5×10^{-5} M. The increase in Ca^{2+} removes the troponin inhibition from the contractile proteins, resulting in muscle contraction. Intracellular Ca^{2+} pumps (i.e., sarcoplasmic/endoplasmic reticulum Ca^{2+}-ATPase [SERCA] pumps) rapidly reaccumulate Ca^{2+} back into the SR, and relaxation occurs when the concentration is restored to less than mechanical threshold. Contraction and relaxation require adenosine triphosphate (ATP); both are energy-related processes that consume ATP (Fig. 29-1).

Clinical and laboratory data for swine and humans indicate decreased control of intracellular Ca^{2+}, resulting in a release of free, unbound, ionized Ca^{2+} from storage sites that normally maintain muscle relaxation. Aerobic and anaerobic forms of metabolism increase to provide added ATP to drive the Ca^{2+} pumps that maintain Ca^{2+} homeostasis in SR and mitochondria and across the sarcolemma in extracellular fluid. Virtually all of these reactions are exothermic (i.e., they produce heat). Rigidity occurs when unbound myofibrillar Ca^{2+} approaches the contractile threshold. Dantrolene is therapeutic because it reduces Ca^{2+} release from the SR without altering Ca^{2+} reuptake.

Molecular Events in Excitation-Contraction Coupling

Understanding the mechanisms underlying MH requires a more detailed description of the process of EC coupling, the process by which skeletal muscle transforms a chemical signal in the form of a neurotransmitter at the surface

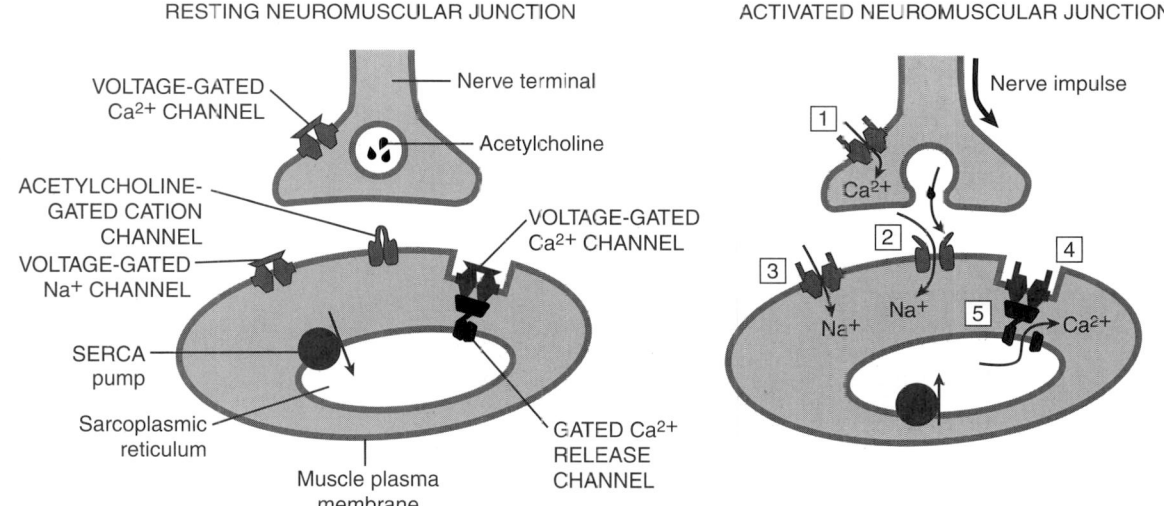

Figure 29–1 The key ion channels involved in neuromuscular transmission and excitation contraction coupling. Nerve impulses arriving at the nerve terminal activate voltage-gated Ca^{2+} channels (1). The resulting increase in cytoplasmic Ca^{2+} concentration is essential in exocytosis of acetylcholine. Binding of acetylcholine to postsynaptic nicotinic cholinergic receptors activates an integral nonselective cation channel, which depolarizes the sarcolemmal membrane (2). Depolarizing the sarcolemma to threshold activates voltage-gated Na^+ channels (3), which propagate action potential impulses deep into the muscle through the transverse tubule system. Within the transverse tubule system, L-type voltage-gated Ca^{2+} channels sense membrane depolarization and undergo a conformational change (4). A physical link between the α_1-subunit and the ryanodine receptor is thought to transfer the signal to sarcoplasmic reticulum to induce the release of stored Ca^{2+} (5). (Adapted from Alberts B, Bray D, Lewis J, et al: Molecular Biology of the Cell, 3rd ed. New York, Garland Press, 1994.)

of the fiber into muscle contraction.[17-19] Figure 29-1 depicts a neuromuscular junction in which an efferent motor neuron synapses with muscle fibers to form a motor end plate. Membrane depolarization at the nerve terminal activates voltage-dependent Ca^{2+} channels on the presynaptic membrane. Most members of the family of voltage-dependent Ca^{2+} channels are composed of five subunits: α_1, α_2, β, γ, and δ. Although subunits α_2, β, γ, and δ contribute important membrane targeting and modulatory functions, it is the larger α_1-subunit that performs essential functions of voltage sensing and conduction of Ca^{2+}. Specifically, it is the N-type channel (i.e., $Ca_V2.1$ in International Union of Pharmacology nomenclature, α_{1A} in alternate nomenclature) that is primarily responsible for depolarized induced Ca^{2+} entry into motor nerve terminals. Rise of cytosolic Ca^{2+} concentrations within the nerve terminals initiates a process of vesicle migration and fusion that leads to exocytosis of acetylcholine stored within the synaptic vesicles. Simultaneous release of thousands of quanta of acetylcholine results in EPSPs. Acetylcholine binds to nicotinic acetylcholine receptors, which are nonselective cation channels, and activates inward current (primarily carried by sodium ions), thereby depolarizing the muscle cells. When EPSPs sum to threshold, action potentials are propagated from the sarcolemma to the T tubule. Acetylcholinesterase in the synaptic cleft catalyzes rapid breakdown of acetylcholine; rapid removal from the cleft enables the motor unit to be ready for another stimulus within a few milliseconds.

Within the T-tubule membrane of skeletal muscle, a highly homologous relative of the N-type channels, the L-type voltage-gated Ca^{2+} channel ($Ca_V1.1$ or α_{1S}), or DHPR, is enriched within the T-tubule membrane. Three chemical classes of drugs used for controlling cardiovascular function—dihydropyridines, phenylalkylamines, and benzothiazepines—are also capable of blocking DHPRs by direct interaction with α_1-subunits. In skeletal muscle, it is α_{1S}-DHPR that participates in EC coupling. Unique to skeletal muscle is the highly ordered arrangement of α_{1S}-DHPRs into linear arrays of clustered tetrads. Electron microscopic and immunocytochemical analyses indicate that each α_{1S}-DHPR tetrad is close to (superimposed above) a single RYR1 within the junctional face of SR terminal cisternae (Fig. 29-2). Because each functional RYR1 channel is composed of a tetramer of four identical subunits, each α_{1S}-DHPR overlies a single RYR1 subunit. The relative restrictions imposed by the dimensions of α_{1S}-DHPR tetrads and RYR1 tetramers permit only alternate RYR1 channels to pair with α_{1S}-DHPR tetrads. In common with other voltage-gated ion channels, each α_{1S}-DHPR possesses a stretch of amphipathic amino acids within the fourth α-helix (S4) of each of four transmembrane domains that functions as a voltage sensor within the T-tubule membrane. Membrane depolarization induces a discrete movement of charge within the S4 segment of the α_{1S}-DHPR. A mechanical signal, thought to be in the form of a conformational transition, is transmitted to the cytoplasmic loop between repeats II and III of the α_{1S}-DHPR. Significant evidence exists for a direct physical coupling between the II-III loop of α_{1S}-DHPR and multiple noncontiguous regions within the large, hydrophilic cytoplasmic domain of RYR1. Such physical links transmit essential signals across the narrow gap of the triadic junction that activate RYR1 and release Ca^{2+} from SR. This conformational coupling model is consistent with the nature of skeletal muscle EC coupling,

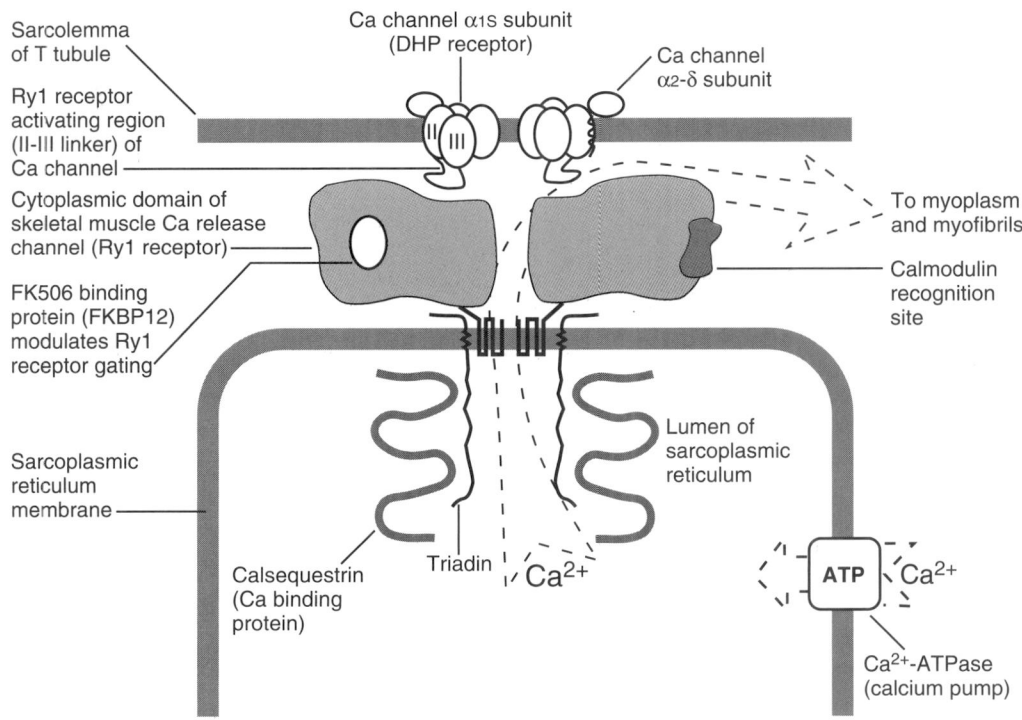

Figure 29–2 Schematic representation of the triad junction of skeletal muscle shows the junctional foot protein (ryanodine receptor [RyR1]) and its associated proteins. In skeletal muscle, the α_{1S}-subunit of the dihydropyridine receptor (DHPR) participates in excitation-contraction coupling. These physical links transmit essential signals across the narrow gap of the triadic junction that activate RyR1 and release Ca^{2+} from the sarcoplasmic reticulum. (Adapted from Pessah IN, Lynch C III, Gronert GA: Complex pharmacology of malignant hyperthermia. Anesthesiology 84:1275, 1996.)

which is independent of extracellular Ca^{2+}. However, after the initial signal activates Ca^{2+} release from SR, Ca^{2+}-induced Ca^{2+} release appears to play a role in regulating the temporal and quantitative characteristics of RYR1 activation. RYR1 also sends a retrograde signal to α_{1S}-DHPR, enhancing its Ca^{2+} entry function. However, unlike Ca^{2+} entry mediated by α_{1S}-DHPR, which is essential for cardiac EC coupling, Ca^{2+} entry through α_{1S}-DHPR is neither essential nor needed for engaging skeletal type EC coupling. Bidirectional signaling between α_{1S}-DHPR and RYR1 in skeletal muscle appears to represent a fundamental mechanism involving conformational coupling between sarcoplasmic/endoplasmic reticulum Ca^{2+} release channels and voltage- or store-operated Ca^{2+} entry (SOC) channels within the surface membrane in a variety of mammalian cells.

After release into the sarcoplasm, Ca^{2+} is rapidly removed through active transport by SERCA pumps located on junctional and longitudinal SR. Calsequestrin inside the lumen of SR binds to Ca^{2+} and further enhances Ca^{2+} loading within SR. Cytosolic Ca^{2+} is typically brought back to basal nanomolar concentration within 30 msec of muscle contraction. The rapid removal of cytosolic Ca^{2+} is essential for normal muscle relaxation and requires rapid termination of Ca^{2+} efflux from SR. Aberrant termination of RYR1 activity has emerged as a key underlying mechanism in MH susceptibility.

Ryanodine Receptor

The toxic plant alkaloid ryanodine was first purified and characterized from the powdered stem wood and roots of *Ryania speciosa Vahl* by Rogers and coworkers in 1948. The alkaloid produces profound rigidity in skeletal muscle.[17,19,20] Isolation of 9,21-dehydroryanodine from *Ryania* facilitated the synthesis of radiolabeled ryanodine ([³H]ryanodine) and permitted direct studies aimed at understanding the mechanism of this muscle poison. The availability of [³H]ryanodine led to identification of the RYR receptor, which is synonymous with the junctional foot protein and possesses Ca^{2+}-release channel activity. RYRs bind [³H]ryanodine with selectivity, and the high-affinity binding interaction is sensitive to the conformational state of the channel (see Fig. 29-2). High-affinity and low-affinity ryanodine binding sites appear to be located within a 76-kd tryptic fragment from the carboxyl terminus of RYR1 of rabbit skeletal muscle (Fig. 29-3). MacLennan's group[19] reports that the hydrophobic segments within residues 3985-4362 are thought to form the M_1 through M_4 transmembrane domains, enabling RYR1 to span the SR membrane four times. The M_1 through M_4 domains of RYR1 have high sequence homology to the analogous domains of inositol triphosphate receptors, suggesting a possible role in forming the sarcoplasmic/endoplasmic reticulum Ca^{2+} channel pore.

Skeletal (RYR1), cardiac (RYR2), and brain (RYR3) isoforms are encoded by three genes located on human chromosomes 19q13.1, 1q42.1-q43, and 15q14-q15, respectively. Based on sedimentation analysis and channel reconstitution studies in bilayer lipid membranes, each functional RYR consists of four identical subunits. Multiple isoforms of RYR are coexpressed in many cell types.

Coexpression of different RYR isoforms in HEK293 cells has revealed that RYR2 is capable of physically interacting with RYR3 and RYR1, but that RYR1 does not interact with RYR3.[20] Whether formation of mixed oligomeric RYRs extends beyond heterologous expression models such as HEK293 cells to mammalian tissue in situ has not been determined.

Complementary DNA (cDNA) sequence analysis reveals that each RYR protomer is composed of 5032 to 5037, 4968 to 4976, and 4872 amino residues with calculated molecular masses of 564 to 565, 565, and 552 kd for the RYR1, RYR2, and RYR3 isoforms, respectively. Typically, a sequence homology of 66% to 70% is observed between any two conspecific isoforms. RYR receptors are also highly conserved in the same tissue among different species (>95% sequence homology of RYR1 found in mammalian skeletal muscle of human, pig, and rabbit). The tetrameric organization of the RYR1 from skeletal muscle has been corroborated by electron microscopy of cryosections of purified RYR1 protein. Three-dimensional reconstruction of RYR1 cryosections has revealed the quatrefoil appearance of each homo-oligomer, with four radial channels on the cytoplasmic face that may converge into a single, common transmembrane pore on the luminal face. Evidence of direct coupling of α_{1S}DHPR and RYR1 has been demonstrated by expressing chimeric $\alpha_{1S/C}$-DHPR cDNAs in dysgenic myotubes that lack constitutive expression of α_{1S}-DHPR. Such studies have provided compelling evidence that the cytoplasmic region between repeats II and III (i.e., cytosolic II-III loop) contains a stretch of 46 amino acids (L720 to Q765) that is essential for engaging bidirectional signaling with RYR1, even in the presence of drastic alterations of sequence surrounding residues L720 to L765.[19,21,22]

In addition to α_{1S}DHPR, RYR1 has been shown to interact with and be modulated by several intracellular accessory proteins. Calmodulin interacts directly with RYR1 of skeletal muscle, with a stoichiometry of two to three calmodulin molecules per subunit. The calmodulin sites with greatest affinity have been localized to the foot region of RYR1 (see Fig 29-2). Through a mechanism independent of kinase activity, calmodulin enhances channel activity at low cytoplasmic Ca^{2+}, whereas it inhibits channel activity at optimal Ca^{2+} (10 to 100 nM). Calsequestrin, the major Ca^{2+} binding protein within the SR lumen, links indirectly to a luminal domain of RYR1. The conformational change in RYR1 also conveys information to the SR lumen through calsequestrin and may be essential in regulating the Ca^{2+} release process. Functional interactions between RYR1 and calsequestrin may play an important role in regulating excitability of the Ca^{2+} channel in response to different filling states of SR. Triadin, a 95-kd, highly basic glycoprotein, was initially suggested to couple RYR1 and the α_1-subunit of DHPR; however, amino acid analysis of triadin indicates only a single pass through the SR membrane, which contradicts its hypothesized role in coupling. The extremely high density of basic residues in the luminal terminus of triadin may be critical in interacting with the acidic moiety of RYR1. The linkage between RYR1 and triadin is thought to provide an anchorage site for calsequestrin within the SR lumen.

FKBP12, the major T-cell immunophilin, tightly associates with RYR1 in skeletal muscle with a stoichiometry of four molecules per channel oligomer. The site on RYR1 that recognizes FKBP12 is distinct from that which binds calmodulin (see Fig. 29-2). Binding of FKBP12 appears to stabilize the closed conformation of the Ca^{2+} channel complex and its full conductance transitions. The immunosuppressant FK506 promotes dissociation of FKBP12 from RYR1 by competing with a common binding site essential for protein-protein interaction of the heterocomplex. The resulting FKBP12-deficient channel conducts current with multiple subconductance states. In the presence of channel activators such as Ca^{2+} and caffeine, activity of the FKBP12-deficient channel is further enhanced by increasing the mean open time and open probability. Association of FKBP12 to RYR1 may promote cooperativity among subunits. Dissociation of FKBP12 with FK506 increases maximal binding capacity of [^{3}H]ryanodine with lowered binding affinity, suggesting loss of negative allosteric interaction between high-affinity and low-affinity [^{3}H]ryanodine binding sites. The association of FKBP12 with the RYR1 complex may be involved in promoting cooperativity between neighboring channels. The "coupled gating" behavior of multiple channels has been reported in measurements with multiple channels reconstituted in membrane lipid bilayer by use of recombinant RYR1 (coexpressed with FKBP12) and native SR. Introduction of FK506 dissociates FKBP12 from the recombinant RYR1 complex and eliminates the coupled gating behavior of multiple channels. The cooperativity between neighboring RYR1 channels may contribute significantly to the robust release of Ca^{2+} from SR during EC coupling.

Homer proteins form an adapter system that regulates coupling of group 1 metabotropic glutamate receptors with intracellular inositol triphosphate receptors and is modified by neuronal activity. Homer proteins physically associate with RYR1 and regulate gating responses to Ca^{2+}, depolarization, and caffeine. The EVH1 domain appears to mediate the actions of Homer on RYR1 function.[23] Dyspedic myotubes expressing RYR1 with a point mutation of a putative Homer-binding domain exhibit significantly reduced amplitude in their responses to potassium ion (K^+) depolarization compared with cells expressing wild-type protein. Homer therefore appears to be a direct modulator of increased Ca^{2+} release and EC coupling in skeletal myotubes.

Two novel proteins (60 kd and 90 kd), whose function is unknown, are also associated with the RYR1 complex. One possesses kinase activity, and the other is the substrate of this kinase. Another 150/160-kd protein also is associated with RYR1. Phosphorylation of the 150/160-kd protein by casein II kinase inhibits RYR1 channel activity.

Factors Other Than Ryanodine Receptor Abnormalities

Other cellular processes affect MH episodes. The pathophysiology of MH may be affected by various inherited abnormalities, especially in heterogeneic humans, or by secondary changes prompted by the altered RYR1. These processes include changes involving inositol triphosphate, lipase and fatty acids, and catecholamines; oxidation-reduction activity; ionic reactivity; and the mechanical threshold of muscle.

GENETICS

Mutations in *RYR1* occur in at least 50% of susceptible subjects and almost all families with central core disease (CCD). More than 30 missense mutations[24] and one deletion[25] have been associated with a positive contracture test (CHCT or IVCT) result or clinical MH, or both. Genetic heterogeneity in MH is documented by five other loci (17q21-24, 1q32, 3q13, 7q21-24, and 5 p), designated as malignant hyperthermia susceptibility (MHS) 2 through 6, respectively. The only known gene other than *RYR1* is the one coding for the α_{1S}-subunit of DHPR, *CACNL1A3*, in MHS3. Two causative mutations in this gene are linked to less than 1% of MHS families worldwide.[26] For practical purposes, the *RYR1* gene remains the target for genetic analysis.

Distribution of *RYR1* Mutations

Multiple mutations that segregate with MHS are dispersed throughout the *RYR1* gene, and many silent polymorphisms are present in the coding region.[27] Some of these have been found in patients with CCD, and in others, the *RYR1* mutation is associated with CCD and MH phenotypes (Fig. 29-3). All reported mutations lead to an amino acid change or, in one case, a deletion, and all are putatively functional.[24,25] Until recently, it was thought that most *RYR1* mutations were clustered between amino acid residues 35 and 614 (MH/CCD region 1) and amino acid residues 2163 and 2458 (MH/CCD region 2) in the myoplasmic foot region of the protein, but a third hotspot is in the carboxyl-terminal transmembrane loop of the receptor, where MHS/CCD region 3 mutations may cluster.[28] The first mutation found in this region (Ile4898Thr) was identified in a large Mexican family with a severe and highly penetrant form of CCD, but no evidence of clinical MH was found despite exposure of 18 members to triggering anesthetics. Subsequently, 14 more mutations associated with CCD have been identified in this region, but many are private, found only in the index case and his or her family. However, mutations causing MH exist in this region. In one large Maori family, the mutation Thr4826Ile was found in five probands who experienced clinical episodes of MH and in 130 members diagnosed by IVCT.[29]

Regional differences in the frequencies of common MHS mutations are observed across Europe. The G341R mutation (Table 29-1) is present in about 6% of Irish, English, and French families but is rare in Northern Europe. The Arg614Cys mutation is more common in German families but less frequent in other European families. G2434R, the most prevalent mutation in the United Kingdom, accounting for 17.5% of MHS families, has a low frequency in continental Europe.[26] Frequencies of *RYR1* gene mutations detected in North Americans vary significantly from those found in Europe.[25] The Arg614Cys and Val2168Met mutations, common in Germany and

RYR1: gene structure and mutational spots

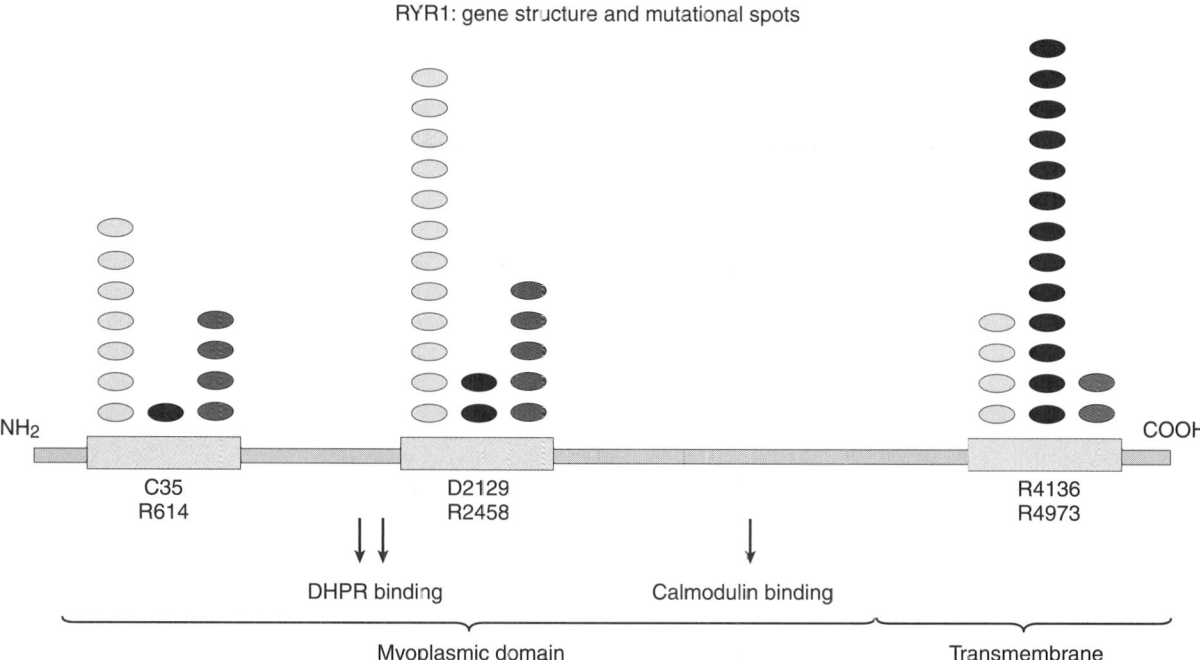

Figure 29–3 Ryanodine receptor 1 gene *(RYR1)* structure and mutational hot spots. Amino- and carboxyl-terminal domains are indicated as NH$_2$ and COOH, respectively. Myoplasmic and transmembrane domains are shown at the bottom and *arrows* indicate dihydropyridine receptor (DHPR) and calmodulin binding sites. Red boxes indicate mutational hot spots with amino acid numbers below. The ovals above represent mutations associated with malignant hyperthermia (gray), central core disease (black), or both (red). (Courtesy of N. Sambuughin, Barrow Neurological Institute, Phoenix, AZ.)

Table 29–1 Findings of the North American malignant hyperthermia mutation panel, 2002

Exon	Mutation*	RYR1 Amino Acid Change	No. of Families in North America[†]	Estimated Incidence in Europe	Phenotype
6	C487T	R163C	2	2-7%	MHS, CCD
9	G742A	G248R	2 (1+1)	2%	MHS
11	G1021A	G341R	1	6-17%	MHS
17	C1840T	R614C	6 (4+2)	4-45%	MHS
39	C6487T	R2163C	2	4%	MHS
39	G6488A	R2163H	0	1%	MHS, CCD
39	G6502A	V2168M	1	8%	MHS, CCD
40	C6617T	T2206M	2	One family	MHS
44	Deletion	ΔG2347	2	0%	MHS
44	G7048A	A2350T	1	0%	MHS
45	G7303A	G2434R	9 (5+4)	4-10%	MHS
45	G7307T	R2435H	1	2.5%	MHS, CCD
46	G7361A	R2454H	4	One family	MHS
46	C7372	R2458C	0	4%	MHS
46	G7373A	R2458H	0	4%	MHS
101	G14582A	A4861H	0	Multiple families	CCD
102	T14693C	I4898T	0	Multiple families	MHS, CCD

*Criteria for the 17 mutations: (1) they occur in more than one family in North America or Europe, and (2) previously tested sequence variant shows that it is not a polymorphism.
[†]Data collaboration of the Uniformed Services University of the Health Sciences, Thomas Jefferson University, Wake Forest University, University of California, Davis, and Barrow Neurological Institute, + indicates those also found in Canada (e.g., for exon 45, four families with the mutation G2434R were found in Canada).
CCD, central core disease; MHS, malignant hyperthermia susceptibility.

Switzerland, are rare in North America. Moreover, the G341Arg mutation, common in Ireland, England, and France, was not detected in the first 73 North American MH-susceptible patients screened for causative mutations. The mutation common to Europe and North America is G2434Arg, occurring in 4% to 7% of European and 5.5% of North American families. Overall, the mutations identified in North Americans accounted for 22% of the screened population, similar to studies in Germany and Italy.[25] In Europe, IVCT data and *RYR1* mutations correlate well for the response to caffeine but not to halothane. In North America, all patients identified with a causative *RYR1* mutation were highly positive for the halothane response in the CHCT, but less so for caffeine. This variation may be caused by differences in the method of delivery and the concentration of halothane used in the IVCT and CHCT (see "Evaluation of Susceptibility"). Genetic screening in European and North American studies targeted only regions 1 and 2, the original two hot spots in the gene, accounting for about one fourth of the coding region of the *RYR1* gene. The absence of *RYR1* mutations in the rest of the screened population may be explained by mutations located outside these two regions or by involvement of other genes.

Inheritance and Penetrance of Malignant Hyperthermia

No longer can the inheritance of human MH be considered solely autosomal dominant with variable penetrance, because more than one genetic locus has been identified in some families. Six nonconsanguineous families harbor at least two genes causing MH.[30] MHS homozygotes are common in affected pigs but rare in human populations. MHS homozygous humans appear clinically normal but exhibit stronger responses to IVCT and CHCT than do heterozygous individuals.[31] They do not exhibit signs or symptoms of CCD.

Discordance in Malignant Hyperthermia Testing

Discordance has confounded linkage analysis worldwide. Examples include IVCT-tested normal (MHN) patients carrying an *RYR1* mutation or an IVCT-tested positive (MHS) patient who does not carry the familial *RYR1* mutation. Several explanations are possible: inexact thresholds for the IVCT or CHCT leading to errors in determining MHN or MHS; variable penetrance; and other unknown genes or modifier genes. Robinson and associates demonstrated by the transmission disequilibrium test (TDT) that loci on chromosomes 5 and 7 and, to a lesser extent, loci on chromosomes 1 and 7 influence susceptibility to MH.[32] A number of families have two *RYR1* mutations on separate haplotypes.[30] Because of discordance, it is not possible to exclude MH on the basis of genetic testing alone.[33]

European Guidelines for Screening

In 2000, the European MH group[33] formulated guidelines for *RYR1* mutation screening with linkage data to other loci for some MH families, but the investigators emphasized the vital role for the IVCT in the diagnosis of MH.

These guidelines have reduced the number of relatives requiring contracture testing without increasing risk[26,34] and include the following:
1. Confirmation of MHS in a family member (preferably a proband) by IVCT before genetic testing.
2. Use of 15 *RYR1* mutations characterized by in vitro functional assays for the genetic protocol.
3. If a causative mutation is detected in a first-degree relative, MHS is confirmed, and IVCT is omitted.
4. If a familial mutation is not detected, IVCT is necessary.

Future Genetic Testing in North America

In contrast to European genetic efforts, only a small number of MH susceptible families have been extensively investigated by North American phenotyping, linkage analysis, and screening of specific genes. Collaborative protocols over the past 5 years between MH biopsy centers and molecular biologists have screened 140-160 unrelated MHS subjects for mutations in the RYR1 gene (see "Distribution of RYR1 Mutations"). In September 2002, MHAUS sponsored a meeting of molecular geneticists and MH experts to examine expanded screening in North America. They achieved consensus on several points:
1. Genetic testing limitations include low sensitivity due to diversity of the mutations and genes.
2. The *RYR1* gene is the primary focus for genetic testing, but further studies are required for more complete understanding of the relationship between mutations and susceptibility.
3. Guidelines for referral and education are needed to establish clinical testing in a Clinical Laboratories Improvement Act (CLIA)–certified laboratory.
4. A North American MH *RYR1* Mutation Panel was established and agreed on a table of mutations (see Table 29-1).

Functional Changes in *RYR1* Associated with Malignant Hyperthermia Mutations

Altered SR Ca^{2+} channel gating kinetics appear to underlie the uncontrolled skeletal muscle metabolism associated with administration of halogenated anesthetics or depolarizing agents. The sustained elevation of the Ca^{2+} level in the sarcoplasm results in abusive stimulation of aerobic and glycolytic metabolism, which accounts for combined acidosis, rigidity, altered permeability, and hyperkalemia. Although studies using Ca^{2+}-selective microelectrodes have indicated that MH-affected muscle has a higher level of resting Ca^{2+}, the findings have not been confirmed by radiometric fluorescent Ca^{2+} dyes. Study of the chronologic relationship of the biochemical and clinical development of porcine MH demonstrates that the increase in intracellular Ca^{2+} concentration precedes the increase in expired carbon dioxide and the classic first sign, tachycardia.[35]

Extensive study of the porcine model has defined the biochemical and functional changes in SR Ca^{2+} transport and RYR1 function underlying MH. The validity of the single-point porcine *RYR1* mutation[36] for defining MH malfunction is affirmed by use of the fluorescent calcium indicator indo-1 to determine the concentration of Ca^{2+} in myoblastic cells transfected with wild-type or mutated *RYR1* complementary DNA. The cells expressing the porcine *RYR1* mutation showed higher sensitivity to caffeine. Clinical doses of halothane resulted in a rapid increase of intracellular Ca^{2+} concentration in cells expressing the mutated RYR1, whereas no changes in intracellular Ca^{2+} concentration were observed in cells expressing the wild-type receptor. These results provide definitive evidence that a single amino acid mutation, Arg615Cys, in RYR1 causes porcine MH.[17-19]

Although active SR Ca^{2+} accumulation appears to be normal in MH-affected pig muscle, significant abnormalities in the process of Ca^{2+} release have been documented in several types of in vitro bioassays. In skinned muscle fiber preparations, the rate and the extent of Ca^{2+} release from SR were higher in fibers with MH abnormalities. These results in skinned fibers correlate well with those obtained from isolated SR membrane preparations enriched in RYR1 protein. Although initial studies revealed a difference in the Ca^{2+} threshold for activation for SR Ca^{2+} release, later studies using rapid-quench methods found no apparent difference in the sensitivity of SR Ca^{2+} release with respect to Ca^{2+}. O'Brien and Li[37] developed a microassay that revealed functional differences in Ca^{2+} transport in SR membranes isolated from normal or from MHS pigs. They found that SR from MHS swine had normal maximal Ca^{2+}-ATPase pumping but that the activity of RYR1 after addition of a bolus of Ca^{2+} was 50% greater in heterozygotes and 100% greater in homozygotes for the mutation. Hypersensitivity to receptor agonists, such as caffeine, and an associated hyposensitivity to inhibition with magnesium (Mg^{2+}) was also demonstrated. There has been some controversy about whether changes exist in the sensitivity of MH-affected muscles to inhibition by Mg^{2+} compared with normal fibers. Owen and colleagues[38] demonstrated that fibers from pigs heterozygous or homozygous for the *RYR1* MH allele needed only a smaller reduction in the free concentration of Mg^{2+} to induce Ca^{2+} release from SR. Dantrolene counteracted the effect of reduced Mg^{2+} inhibition in MH-affected muscle. The abnormal responsiveness of MH-affected muscle to various stimuli may result from the reduced ability of myoplasmic Mg^{2+} to inhibit Ca^{2+} release from SR.

Reconstitution of channels isolated from MHS pigs studied in bilayer lipid membranes has revealed significantly reduced sensitivity to inactivating concentrations of Ca^{2+}, whereas the sensitivity of channels to activating Ca^{2+} remains unchanged. The Ca^{2+} channels from MHS pigs exhibit a significantly higher open probability compared with wild-type channels across a broad range of Ca^{2+} concentrations (7 µM to 10 µM) on the cytoplasmic face when measured at pH 6.8. Whether Ca^{2+} channels reconstituted in bilayer lipid membranes from pigs with MH susceptibility exhibit an altered response to inhibition by Mg^{2+} remains controversial. In porcine MH, Mg^{2+} inhibition of RYR1 channels was not altered, whereas there is a threefold lower potency for Mg^{2+} inhibition of MH-affected Ca^{2+} channels. Similar findings were seen in human MHS skinned fibers.[39] The underlying cause of these various porcine experimental results is unclear, but

the concentration of monovalent ions in measuring channel activity might have influenced the inhibitory potency of Mg^{2+}. Channels isolated from pigs heterozygous for the MH mutation suggest that the heterozygous porcine population of Ca^{2+} release channels contains heterotetramers with properties distinct from those of MH homozygote or normal channels. The data also imply that the population of Ca^{2+} release channels in humans with MHS who are heterozygous for a dominant mutation in this protein also contains heterotetrameric channels. In contrast to Ca^{2+} uptake and release studies with isolated SR, single-channel measurements have failed to reveal an altered sensitivity of channels to activation by caffeine.

Radioligand-receptor binding studies with nanomolar concentrations of [³H]ryanodine have determined differences between SR isolated from normal humans and pigs and those with MH susceptibility. [³H]Ryanodine binding assays represent a sensitive means of assessing functional anomalies regulating the channel pore by use of a simple tube assay. This is possible because [³H]ryanodine binds to a conformationally sensitive site within or near the channel pore. Mickelson and coworkers[17] first demonstrated that the binding of [³H]ryanodine to MH homozygotic porcine heavy SR exhibited an altered Ca^{2+} dependence at the low-affinity (inhibitory) Ca^{2+} site and a lower affinity for ryanodine compared with normal porcine SR. However, the maximum capacity of SR to bind [³H]ryanodine was the same in both tissues, indicating an altered structure or function, or both, of the receptor rather than a change in expression associated with the disease. Studies performed with RYR1 isolated from human biopsies revealed a higher affinity for [³H]ryanodine and a higher sensitivity to activation by caffeine with MHS preparations. Surprisingly, it was the activation, not the inactivation, of the binding of [³H]ryanodine by Ca^{2+} that was abnormal in human MH SR.

DANTROLENE

Dantrolene is the drug of choice for preventing and reversing the symptoms of MH. Dantrolene sodium is a hydantoin derivative (1-[[[5-(4-nitrophenyl)-2-furanyl]methylene]imino]-2,4-imidazolidinedione) that relaxes but does not totally paralyze skeletal muscle. These properties of dantrolene have been closely correlated with its ability to reduce Ca^{2+} efflux from SR in vitro. Dantrolene (20 µM) counteracts the effect of reduced Mg^{2+} inhibition in MH-affected muscle.[38] Caffeine contractures induced after K^+ conditioning of porcine skeletal muscle were found to render muscles refractory to brief electrical stimulation, but there was still an enhancement of contracture tension elicited by subsequent direct caffeine stimulation of SR calcium release. This enhanced sensitivity to caffeine was inhibited by dantrolene (20 µM) and its water-soluble analog azumolene (150 µM).

Preparations of skeletal SR membrane vesicles have been used to examine the ability of dantrolene to alter Ca^{2+} fluxes. Dantrolene (10 to 90 µM) was shown to inhibit SR Ca^{2+} release, especially when assayed in the presence of caffeine and adenine nucleotide. Later, depolarization-induced

Ca^{2+} release, measured from triadic vesicles by use of a stopped-flow apparatus and fura-2, was shown to be inhibited by dantrolene.[40] However, the exact mechanism by which dantrolene induces muscle relaxation is unclear, and some results have been conflicting. For example, halothane-activated RYR1 from frog skeletal muscle was unaffected by concentrations of dantrolene as high as 100 μM, whereas single-channel studies with porcine and human RYR1 revealed a biphasic action of dantrolene: channel activation at low (0.5 to 2 nM) concentrations and channel inhibition at a higher (5 μM) concentration. Species variability may in part account for this difference.

Experiments of radioligand-receptor binding performed with [3H]ryanodine have shown that under certain assay conditions, micromolar concentrations of dantrolene or its water-soluble derivative azumolene could inhibit the binding of ryanodine to its conformationally sensitive site. In this respect, doxorubicin-stimulated binding was much more inhibited by dantrolene than by caffeine or Ca^{2+}-stimulated binding. These results are in agreement with Ca^{2+} transport studies with skeletal SR, in which azumolene was shown to block doxorubicin-induced Ca^{2+} release. However, a later investigation found little pharmacologic overlap between the modulation of [3H]ryanodine and [3H]dantrolene binding sites in porcine skeletal muscle. For example, the binding of [3H]dantrolene was insensitive to ryanodine and Ca^{2+} and adenine nucleotides. Experiments performed with [3H]dantrolene have revealed that specific binding sites for the drug colocalize to junctional SR membranes with [3H]ryanodine binding sites. [3H]Dantrolene binding sites were not detected in T-tubule membranes or sarcolemmal membranes.

The idea that dantrolene suppresses SR Ca^{2+} release as a result of direct interactions with RYR1 has been somewhat controversial. Significant progress has been made to positively identify the location of dantrolene binding sites within the EC coupling machinery. Paul-Pletzer and associates[41] demonstrated that [3H]azidodantrolene, a pharmacologically active, photoaffinity analog of dantrolene, specifically labels the amino terminus of RYR1. The [3H]azidodantrolene binding site was localized to the 1400–amino acid residue fragment of RYR1 cleaved by *n*-calpain, a tissue-specific isoform of this Ca^{2+} and thiol-activated protease. More detailed analysis further localized the [3H]azidodantrolene binding site to a single domain containing the core sequence corresponding to amino acid residues 590 through 609 of RYR1.[42] Evidence of the specificity of the [3H]azidodantrolene photoaffinity-labeling procedure was provided based on the observation that a monoclonal antibody that recognizes the 172-kd, *n*-calpain–cleaved, amino-terminal fragment inhibited [3H]azidodantrolene photolabeling of RYR1 in SR in a concentration-dependent manner. Ikemoto and coworkers[43,44] proposed that this very region of the RYR1 structure (DP1 domain) participates in interdomain interactions that stabilize the closure of the Ca^{2+} channel state. Based on this model, one possible mechanism by which dantrolene inhibits release of SR Ca^{2+} is by directly binding to the DP1 region and stabilizing the interdomain interaction of DP1.[42] How dantrolene binding to the DP1 domain stabilizes rather than destabilizes interdomain interactions remains a mystery.

SPECIFIC ORGAN AND TISSUE ABNORMALITIES

Skeletal Muscle

Affected human muscle frequently has no histologic defect or else has protean nonspecific pathology so variable that none can be directly attributed to MH. These include central cores, internal nuclei, target fibers, supercontracted fibrils, and marked variation in fiber diameter.[45]

Metabolism, Enzymatic Considerations, Heat Production, Contractures, and Fiber Type

Affected muscle is close to loss of control of intracellular Ca^{2+}. With that, aerobic (oxygen consumption [$\dot{V}O_2$]) and glycolytic metabolism increase dramatically. There is an approximately threefold increase in $\dot{V}O_2$ and a 15- to 20-fold increase in blood lactate level, with related acid-base imbalances. The earliest changes appear as an increase in muscle intracellular Ca^{2+} concentration[35] and in the venous effluent from skeletal muscle, as decreases in pH or partial pressure of oxygen (PO_2), or as increases in PCO_2, lactate, potassium, or temperature.[46] These changes occur before the increases in heart rate, temperature, and circulating catecholamine levels. The most sensitive early sign during anesthesia is an increase in expired carbon dioxide (during constant ventilation), but it can be misleading (see "Diagnosis"). Heat production during acute MH derives from aerobic metabolism, glycolysis, neutralization of hydrogen ions, and hydrolysis of high-energy phosphate compounds involved in ion transport and in the contraction-relaxation process.[47] Precise calculations of the expended energy are difficult because of unsteady metabolic and circulatory states, variable and uncontrolled heat loss, and production of heat by neutralization of acid.

Muscle rigidity in MH is a contracture, similar to a muscle cramp, that is nonpropagated, prolonged, and sometimes irreversible. Contractures are used in tissue baths in the laboratory to study various aspects of MH. The lack of consistent correlation of fiber type or fiber proteins with abnormal function underscores the difficulties in analyzing this disorder; stress is necessary to detect the abnormality. The altered RYR1 protein is expressed in fast and slow fibers.

Calcium

The SR is the intracellular organelle primarily responsible for control of intracellular Ca^{2+} transients, and mitochondria serve a secondary reserve function in binding Ca^{2+}. When intracellular Ca^{2+} levels increase beyond the capabilities of the SR, mitochondria aid in binding. The mitochondrion provides the greatest supply of ATP through aerobic metabolism; only secondarily does it bind and store Ca^{2+}. There is evidence of muscle mitochondrial binding and accumulation of Ca^{2+} during acute episodes of porcine MH.[48] Mitochondrial deficiencies do not explain the diminished aerobic responses in MH. $\dot{V}O_2$ consistently increases about threefold during MH, in contrast to the 10-fold increase possible during severe exercise. In view of the serious acid-base imbalances and depletion of muscle energy stores, this increase seems paradoxically low.

Perhaps $\dot{V}o_2$ and ATP production by mitochondria is limited during MH by several factors, including ATP translocation, mitochondrial Ca^{2+} binding, intracellular acid-base status, and electrolyte aberrations.

Ca^{2+} antagonists are associated with hyperkalemia and potentially increased mortality in vivo when used in conjunction with dantrolene.[49] They do not prevent or effectively treat MH in susceptible pigs.[50,51] In addition to the risk of hyperkalemia with Ca^{2+} antagonists and dantrolene, there is the added hazard that the hyperkalemia could trigger MH in susceptible skeletal muscle.[52]

Electrophysiologic Measurements

The Ca^{2+}-control abnormalities of MH are reflected in altered electrophysiology. Multiple-pulse stimulation of porcine muscle (i.e., six pulses with 5-msec spacing) demonstrated an increase in tension and an increased rate of rise of tension in susceptible pigs; this difference was accentuated after dantrolene was given, and the susceptible pig muscle recovered much more effectively from the effects of dantrolene than did that of the normal animals.[53] This confirms abnormally increased Ca^{2+} transients through intracellular organelles. Similar differences in humans were inaccurate by MH testing,[54] although one study suggests better precision.[55] During slaughter, affected swine are found to have a lower (and rapidly declining) resting membrane potential than that of normal swine.[56,57] This may contribute to the rapid decline of muscle pH and energy stores because this is prevented or attenuated by curarization and ventilation to maintain oxygenation.[56] Halothane lowers mechanical threshold in susceptible and normal muscle, predisposing susceptible muscle toward the development of a contracture.[58]

Channelopathies

One of the considerations regarding MH and disorders of EC coupling is the existence of channelopathies, disorders of the voltage-gated ion channels that control fluxes of ions across membranes.[18] These channels are ion-conducting proteins with a membrane-spanning pore, gates, and voltage sensors, equipping them for passage of sodium, calcium, and chloride ions. Chloride channels provide 75% to 80% of membrane conductance at rest, contributing to the fast repolarization phase of the action potential. These channels are present in the surface and inner membranes of all excitable and most nonexcitable cells. There are naturally occurring mutations that alter their function with specific pathologic consequences. Abnormalities relating to skeletal muscle pathology include those of the sodium channel (i.e., hyperkalemic periodic paralysis, paramyotonia congenita, and some others, known collectively as potassium-aggravated myotonias), potassium channel (i.e., myokymias such as episodic ataxia), calcium channel (i.e., DHPR mutations causing hypokalemic periodic paralysis or dysgenic muscle in mice), and the chloride channel (i.e., myotonia congenita in humans, mice, and goats). The RYR1 is not a voltage-gated channel.

Implications of Findings in Skeletal Muscle

The single-point mutation of RYR1 in all susceptible swine is the major cause of porcine MH,[36] and other abnormalities are secondary or occur in parallel. Inositol trisphosphate is a major physiologic second messenger mobilizing Ca^{2+} from endoplasmic reticulum, but it does not seem to be involved in MH because it lacks the surface membrane interactions possessed by the RYR1 for SR.[17,19,20] Altered lipase, fatty acids, and triglycerides may play a more important role.[59] Free radical peroxidation probably occurs during porcine MH as an adaptive response to sustained stress that contributes to abnormal calcium homeostasis and fatty acid metabolism.[60] Volatile anesthetics and succinylcholine represent a stress for skeletal muscle because they perturb membranes and disturb Ca^{2+} homeostasis. In general, normal muscle can withstand and compensate for these stresses. In susceptible muscle, the membrane perturbation induced by halothane or the depolarization induced by succinylcholine may cause an earlier Ca^{2+} release that strikingly stimulates greater Ca^{2+} release. Coupled with the lower mechanical threshold, an early MH response may result.[58] Although MH-susceptible muscle may briefly tolerate these stresses, a cascading cycle of increasing metabolism, temperature, and acidosis eventually results. Skeletal muscle, about 40% of body weight, represents a sleeping giant in regard to metabolism, and once aroused, it dominates whole-body responses. MH-affected muscle may always be closer to loss of control than normal muscle. Normal muscle can respond abnormally with extremely prolonged effort, such as the overstraining disease or capture myopathy of wild animals after prolonged chase.[61]

Heart

Myocardial function is severely altered in human and porcine MH. Tachycardia and arrhythmias are followed by hypotension, decreased cardiac output, and eventual cardiac arrest. Porcine data suggest that these alterations are secondary; increased myocardial oxygen consumption during MH is related to β-agonist stimulation of sympathetic activation without the lactate production or potassium efflux that suggests a primary MH response.[62] Porcine MH myocardium does not respond abnormally to exaggerated concentrations of calcium, digoxin, potassium, or carbon dioxide.[52] Overall, the heart appears to be affected primarily by the tremendous, potentially ischemic demands placed on it by exaggerated whole-body metabolism.[63]

Central Nervous System

Central nervous system involvement during fulminant human MH appears to result from increased temperature, acidosis, hyperkalemia, hypoxia, and hypo-osmolality related to fluid shifts as factors in acute cerebral edema. The extreme picture includes coma, areflexia, and fixed, dilated pupils. Recovery varies and is related to the duration and severity of the MH episode. Severe fever (to 42.5°C [108.5°F]) may result in a virtually flat electroencephalogram and coma, but recovery is still possible.[64]

MH is not a central nervous system disorder, as demonstrated by the fact that a tourniquet-isolated limb remains flaccid during the whole-body rigidity of an acute episode.[65] Cerebral oxygen consumption and lactate production are not increased in swine during MH episodes.[66]

Kochs and colleagues[67] observed early profound electroencephalographic depression during porcine MH and improvement with dantrolene, which they interpreted as primary brain involvement. Hofer and coworkers[68] contradicted this opinion by correlating alteration of electroencephalographic and cerebral metabolites with beginning whole-body MH episodes.

Sympathetic Nervous System

Activation of the sympathetic nervous system occurs early during MH. Fight, fright, or flight can initiate an MH episode in susceptible swine without anesthetic agents.[9] This is rarely observed in humans (see "Awake Triggering: Exercise and Heat Stroke"). During MH, circulating levels of epinephrine and norepinephrine increase markedly (e.g., from less than 1 ng/mL to 30 ng/mL). Sympathetic responses appear to be secondary in porcine MH, although the physiologic effects of sympathetic excitation can magnify the changes of an MH episode. For example, metabolic responses precede altered sympathetic activity[46]; the MH response is unaltered despite acute sympathetic denervation (total spinal anesthesia)[69]; infusion of norepinephrine to blood levels greater than those associated with MH does not trigger MH[70,71]; and norepinephrine does not potentiate halothane-induced porcine MH, although triggering is delayed when blood flow to muscle is reduced.[71] β-Agonist effects result in pronounced myocardial stimulation.[62] Administration of α-agonists and β-agonists does not result in increased metabolism in susceptible porcine muscle.[70,72]

Sympathetic antagonists may protect from or ameliorate episodes of MH by lowering body temperature and modifying acid-base changes.[73] The β-antagonists appear to increase heat loss and potentially increase muscle perfusion. β-Antagonists attenuate metabolism and fever during MH but do not improve survival.[73] They block myocardial stimulation of porcine MH, but this stimulation is secondary to β-agonist effects without evidence for myocardial MH.[62] There is no direct evidence that the sympathetic nervous system initiates MH.[46]

Miscellaneous Abnormalities

Disseminated intravascular coagulation is caused by the release of tissue thromboplastin during fever, acidosis, hypoxia, hypoperfusion, and gross alterations in membrane permeability.[46] Porcine MH erythrocytes show greater fragility and peroxidation.[74] Lymphocytes reflect MH mutations and constitute a means for MH testing.[75,76] These findings directly support the alteration of porcine tissue other than skeletal muscle by MH.

Liver from normal swine transplanted into MH-susceptible swine remains normal, and liver from swine homozygous for MH that is transplanted into normal swine functions as normal.[77] Pulmonary changes during MH appear to be secondary to systemic manifestations. These include tachypnea, hyperventilation, $\dot{V}$ and $\dot{Q}$ abnormalities, increased blood and expired carbon dioxide, decreased blood Po_2, and ultimately, pulmonary edema. The increase in whole-body carbon dioxide stores during MH is better reflected by measurements of expired carbon dioxide or venous carbon dioxide than arterial measurements. Renal function during active MH is altered indirectly; oliguria and anuria result from shock, ischemia, cardiac failure, myoglobinuria, and myoglobinemia.

CLINICAL SYNDROMES

Fulminant MH is rare. The usually muted onset is quickly detected by increased levels of expired carbon dioxide, developing tachycardia, or muscle rigidity. Onset can be acute and rapid if anesthesia includes a potent inhaled anesthetic or succinylcholine. It can be delayed and may not be overt until the patient is in the recovery room. Once initiated, the course of MH can be rapid. When clinical signs, such as increased expired carbon dioxide, muscle rigidity, tachycardia, and fever, suggest MH, the association is not strong unless more than one abnormal sign is observed. A single adverse sign usually does not indicate MH.

Volatile anesthetics and succinylcholine cause affected subjects to undergo a striking increase in aerobic and anaerobic metabolism, resulting in intense production of heat, carbon dioxide, and lactate and an associated respiratory and metabolic acidosis.[11,46] These reactions markedly alter whole-body acid-base balance and temperature because of skeletal muscle bulk (40%) and are magnified as temperature increases. Whole-body rigidity occurs in almost all pigs and in most humans. Temperature may exceed 43°C (109.4°F), $Paco_2$ may exceed 100 mm Hg, and pHa may be less than 7.00. Associated with this increased permeability of muscle are increased serum levels of potassium, ionized calcium, CK (although MH-related changes do not differ overall from CK changes observed during surgery[78]), myoglobin, and serum sodium.[46] Later, serum potassium and calcium levels decrease; muscle edema may occur. Sympathetic hyperactivity (e.g., tachycardia, sweating, hypertension) occurs early as a sign of increased metabolism. With metabolic exhaustion, cellular permeability increases with whole-body edema, including acute cerebral edema. As MH progresses, disseminated intravascular coagulation and cardiac or renal failure may develop. MH is a disorder of increased metabolism; it need not involve increased temperature, for example, if heat loss is greater than production or if cardiac output plummets early. The clinical MH syndrome can occur as a final common pathway in situations that may not involve susceptibility to MH, as various disorders may mimic MH (Table 29-2).[79-84]

Trismus-Masseter Spasm

Trismus-masseter spasm is defined as jaw muscle rigidity in association with limb muscle flaccidity after administration of succinylcholine. It is a unique property of jaw muscle in normal people. Masseter and lateral pterygoid muscles contain slow tonic fibers that can respond to depolarizers with a contracture.[85,86] This is manifested clinically on exposure to succinylcholine as an increase in jaw muscle tone, well defined by van der Spek and associates.[87] When this increase in jaw muscle tone becomes exaggerated, prolonged, and tight ("jaws of steel"),

Table 29–2   Mimics of malignant hyperthermia

Disorder	Reference
Alcohol therapy for limb arteriovenous malformation	81
Contrast dye	144
Cystinosis	145
Diabetic coma	80
Drug toxicity or abuse	46
Environmental heat gain more than loss	64
Equipment malfunction, increased carbon dioxide	114
Exercise hyperthermia	106-111,146
Freeman-Sheldon syndrome	151
Heat stroke	109-113
Hyperthyroidism	79
Hypokalemic periodic paralysis	83
Intracranial free blood	82
Muscular dystrophies (Duchenne, Becker)	84
Myotonias	18
Neuroleptic malignant syndrome	116
Osteogenesis imperfecta	147
Pheochromocytoma	148
Prader-Willi syndrome	149
Rhabdomyolysis	46,90-92
Sepsis	46
Ventilation problems	114
Wolf-Hirschhorn syndrome	150

the likelihood of MH increases greatly. There is a spectrum of normal responses: a tight jaw that becomes a rigid jaw and then a very rigid jaw (Fig. 29-4). Somewhere in the area of the declining curve is the boundary for the MH population; the difficulty is in defining it. Trismus may still occur after pretreatment with a defasciculating dose of a nondepolarizing relaxant. If there is rigidity of other muscles in addition to trismus, the association with MH is absolute; anesthesia should be halted as soon as

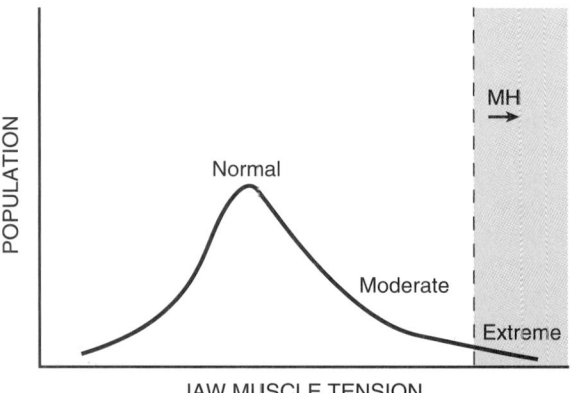

Figure 29–4 Succinylcholine usually increases jaw muscle tone slightly. In some patients, this increase is moderate, and in very few, the effect is extreme (i.e., "jaws of steel"). As much as 50% of this latter group may be susceptible to malignant hyperthermia (MH). Somewhere in the area of the declining curve is the boundary for the MH population.

possible and treatment of MH begun. The following discussion considers trismus without rigidity of other muscles.

After trismus occurs, proper monitoring should include end-expired carbon dioxide, examination for pigmenturia, and arterial or venous blood sampling for CK, acid-base status, and electrolyte levels, particularly potassium. The initial degree of tightness of the jaw and its duration suggest the gravity of the response. For patients with jaws of steel, the procedure should be halted, especially if the condition persists for more than several minutes. If the jaw is slightly resistant to opening, the anesthesiologist may continue anesthesia during proper monitoring. If the jaw is modestly tight and distinctly a problem, there are two choices: halt the procedure or continue with nontriggering agents. Any suggestion of MH should prompt MH therapy, including the use of dantrolene. The patient with a fever may have an exaggerated response to succinylcholine's effect in increasing jaw muscle tension. Patients who experience trismus should undergo testing for MH susceptibility. Trismus occurring after use of nondepolarizing muscle relaxants is not apparently related to MH or to hyperkalemia.[88]

Sudden, Unexpected Pediatric Cardiac Arrest

MH rarely begins as an abrupt cardiac arrest after the use of succinylcholine. In the absence of upregulation of nicotinic skeletal muscle acetylcholine receptors,[89] this reflects an occult myopathy that responds to succinylcholine with abrupt massive rhabdomyolysis and an associated acute rapid massive hyperkalemia.[90-92] It is devastating to caregivers and family because an apparently healthy child can scarcely be resuscitated because of the difficulties in aiding redistribution of potassium to diminish hyperkalemic levels. Heroic efforts, including cardiopulmonary bypass, can be successful.[93] These cases may respond acutely to calcium because it aids in counteracting hyperkalemia by reestablishing the ionic membrane balance in the heart and to dantrolene because of its effect in stabilizing muscle membrane permeability. Myopathic muscle continually suffers marked stress, and dantrolene may help to relieve that by attenuating calcium fluxes until more ATP is generated. Because of potential cerebral ischemia, glucose should be administered with caution. Succinylcholine continues to be valuable, because a nondepolarizing relaxant has not yet matched its advantages, but there should be precise indications for its use in young children.

Rhabdomyolysis

Rhabdomyolysis may occur during an MH episode or trismus, but milder forms occur more often than realized. In a study of 11 normal children, those given succinylcholine had a serum myoglobin level of 1187±615 ng/mL, in contrast to 30±9 ng/mL in those not given succinylcholine.[94] Myoglobinuria with rhabdomyolysis can occur in various muscle disorders and without exposure to succinylcholine.[92] Because of the virtual identity of myoglobin and hemoglobin, myoglobinuria can be misdiagnosed as hemolysis during MH. Any unusual anesthetic incident—muscle response, arrhythmia, trismus, or fever—should prompt examination of urine color and plasma electrolytes, especially potassium.

TRIGGERING OF MALIGNANT HYPERTHERMIA

Acute episodes of MH depend on three variables: a genetic (perhaps rarely acquired) predisposition, the absence of inhibiting factors, and the presence of a sufficiently potent anesthetic or nonanesthetic trigger.

Anesthetic Triggering

Anesthetic drugs that trigger MH include halothane, enflurane, isoflurane, desflurane, sevoflurane, and succinylcholine. Desflurane and sevoflurane are less potent triggers, producing a more gradual onset of MH.[95,96] The onset may be explosive if succinylcholine is used.[46] Inbred, susceptible swine are identified during an inhalation induction with a potent volatile anesthetic; they develop pronounced hind limb rigidity within 5 minutes.[46] Prior exercise even an hour before induction of anesthesia increases the severity and hastens the onset of these attacks in swine.[46] Mild hypothermia, depressants such as barbiturates and tranquilizers, and nondepolarizing relaxants delay the onset of MH.[15,97,98]

Susceptible humans respond less predictably than swine to these triggers. Many affected humans have previously tolerated potent triggers without visible difficulty.[14] This unpredictability may in part be related to the delaying effects described earlier, as well as to a brief anesthetic. Some patients have experienced MH episodes during anesthesia that did not involve recognized triggering agents; fortunately, all have responded appropriately to dantrolene. The mechanism of anesthetic triggering in humans is unsolved.

Succinylcholine has several variant responses that can occur singly or in combination. The first is a muscle contracture, also observed in muscle that is myotonic or denervated.[89] The second is a change in muscle membrane permeability without contracture, resulting in the release of CK and myoglobin from muscle. Even in normal patients, succinylcholine releases CK and myoglobin from muscle in small amounts. This action is exaggerated in the presence of halothane and attenuated by curare[46]; myoglobin release can be fairly marked even in the absence of obviously discolored urine.[94] The third response is an increase in metabolism, as in MH, which is usually associated with muscle contracture and increased membrane permeability.[46]

Nitrous oxide has been proposed as a weak trigger of human MH.[46] This is most unlikely because it has been used repeatedly and safely as the basic anesthetic in MH-susceptible humans and swine. Hyperbaric nitrous oxide does not produce MH in susceptible swine, even in concentrations causing apnea.[99]

Nondepolarizing muscle relaxants block the effects of succinylcholine in triggering MH. They attenuate the effects of volatile anesthetics.[15,97] D-Tubocurarine has been incriminated as an MH trigger because it produced fever in two susceptible children.[46] D-Tubocurarine results in greater lactate production in susceptible pigs exposed to environmental stress,[46] but it has not been shown to be a trigger; it does produce a contracture in denervated muscle, suggesting that it may have a mild depolarizing action that is not generally apparent.[100] Reversal of a nondepolarizing neuromuscular blockade does not trigger MH.

Episodes of MH have been reported during various operative procedures, with general or regional anesthesia, and in extremes of ages. Prior fever or succinylcholine-induced trismus should not be ignored, even if the patient survived without obvious mishap.[101] The youngest probable case of MH involved succinylcholine-related muscle rigidity in utero just before birth.[102] Presumably, the fetus inherited the paternal susceptibility that was triggered by maternal anesthesia.

Prolonged propofol infusions in pediatric intensive care are associated with complications that may mimic MH reactions.[103,104] Propofol is not an MH trigger, and its effects on membranes of MH-affected skeletal muscle are stabilizing and opposite to those of volatile triggers.[105]

Awake Triggering: Exercise and Heat Stroke

Porcine environmental stress such as exercise, heat stress, anoxia, apprehension, and excitement triggers MH (see "History").[46,72] These responses are related to muscle movement or to increased temperature. Susceptible swine in vitro or in vivo react to carbachol or heat (41°C to 42°C) with abnormally increased oxygen consumption and lactate production, but not to α-sympathetic or β-sympathetic agonists, or both.[72] Abnormal responses can be blocked or delayed by nondepolarizing relaxants.[15,46,56,97] However, mechanisms in porcine awake MH may not relate to human awake MH.

Epidemiologic studies reveal that exercise-induced symptoms occur more frequently in MHS patients,[106] including exercise-induced rhabdomyolysis.[107,108] A novel mutation with an Arg401Cys substitution in the amino terminus occurred in three cases of exercise-induced rhabdomyolysis.[108] There was a stress-induced hyperthermic death of a 12-year-old boy. He had an MH episode during sevoflurane anesthesia and was treated successfully with dantrolene.[109] Eight months later, after a football game in the setting of an ambient temperature of 80°F (26.7°C), he complained of weakness, tingling in his extremities, and muscle stiffness. He was hot, diaphoretic, and hyperventilating. Seizures and respiratory arrest occurred; jaw rigidity prevented endotracheal intubation. Ventricular fibrillation occurred, and cardiopulmonary resuscitation was begun. In the hospital, his rectal temperature was 108°F (42.2°C), pH was 6.76, and potassium level was 8.8 mEq/L. Despite dantrolene, resuscitation was unsuccessful. Autopsy revealed normal cardiac anatomy and no explanatory pathology. Analysis of DNA in the boy (postmortem) and his father revealed an altered *RYR1* gene sequence of C487T, with a substitution of arginine for cysteine 163. Other reports relate heat stroke, sudden and unexpected death, unusual stress and fatigue, or myalgias to possible awake MH episodes.[110-113] Stresses include exercise and environmental exposure to volatile vapors. Despite these rare exceptions, susceptible patients with no history of prior problems may live their everyday lives normally.

DIAGNOSIS

MH is a disorder of increased metabolism, and early signs may be subtle (see "Clinical Syndromes"). These must be distinguished from other disorders with similar signs (see Table 29-2). Postoperative fever alone seldom represents MH.

When the diagnosis is obvious (i.e., fulminant MH or succinylcholine-induced rigidity with rapid metabolic changes), there is marked hypermetabolism and heat production, and there may be little time left for specific therapy to prevent death or irreversible sequelae. If end-tidal carbon dioxide increases and ventilation is then increased to maintain normal end-tidal values, diagnosis of MH may be delayed.[114] A clinical grading scale aids in establishing the likelihood of MH in specific problem cases. It is based on weighted scores for muscle tone, muscle breakdown, acid-base parameters, temperature, tachycardia or other arrhythmias, and response to dantrolene. This scale is hampered if clinical laboratory evaluation has been minimal.[115]

In general, MH is not expected to occur when nontriggers are administered (see "Anesthesia for Susceptible Patients"). When volatile anesthetics or succinylcholine is used, MH should be suspected if there is increased end-expired carbon dioxide, undue tachycardia, tachypnea, arrhythmias, mottling of the skin, cyanosis, increased temperature, muscle rigidity, sweating, or unstable blood pressure. If any of these occur, signs of increased metabolism, acidosis, or hyperkalemia must be sought. Analysis of arterial blood gases demonstrates metabolic acidosis and may show respiratory acidosis if the patient is unable to increase ventilation as metabolism increases. Central venous oxygen and carbon dioxide levels change more markedly than do those in arterial blood; therefore, end-expired carbon dioxide or venous carbon dioxide levels more accurately reflect whole-body stores. Venous carbon dioxide, unless the blood drains an area of increased metabolic activity, should have PCO_2 levels only about 5 mm Hg greater than that of expected or measured $PaCO_2$. In small children, particularly without oral food or fluid for a prolonged period, base deficit may be 5 mEq/L because of their smaller energy stores. Any patient who is suspected of having an MH episode should be reported to the North American Registry using the rare disease protocol (AMRA) available from the MHAUS web site.

ASSOCIATION WITH OTHER DISORDERS

The King-Denborough syndrome, characterized by short stature, musculoskeletal abnormalities, and mental retardation, is associated with susceptibility to MH, as is CCD. CCD was present in the family of Denborough's original patient[5] and discovered during later evaluations. Duchenne dystrophy is an X-linked myopathy; the associated deterioration of muscle membranes can result in a clinical MH episode on exposure to membrane perturbors such as MH triggers despite normal contracture testing results.[84] Patients with Duchenne dystrophy can respond to anesthesia with sudden, acute, difficult-to-resuscitate cardiac arrest or sudden, acute rhabdomyolysis, even without the use of succinylcholine.[84,90-92] Patients with any occult myopathy, even without exposure to succinylcholine, may experience these potentially and rapidly disastrous anesthetic events.[90-92]

Neuroleptic malignant syndrome[116] (NMS) is an uncommon condition caused by central effects of drugs with dopamine antagonist properties, including antipsychotics (e.g., haloperidol), and by drugs used for sedation or as antiemetics (e.g., Compazine, metoclopramide, droperidol). In affected patients, these drugs may cause a reaction involving a range of symptoms culminating in fulminant MH–like hypermetabolism. The onset ranges from hours to days after beginning drug treatment. There are three key clinical components of NMS. First, the patient usually experiences an impairment of motor function with generalized rigidity, akinesia, or extrapyramidal disturbances, or some combination of these conditions. Second, deterioration in mental status occurs, producing coma, stupor, or delirium. Third, hyperpyrexia develops, with deterioration and lability of other "vegetative" functions, resulting in diaphoresis, dehydration, fluctuations in blood pressure and heart rate, and tachypnea. Duration averages 7 to 10 days, with gradual recovery that parallels the slow metabolism of the triggering drugs.

NMS patients may experience predictable complications of hypermetabolism, including rhabdomyolysis, renal failure, disseminated intravascular coagulation, thromboembolism, and sudden cardiac arrest. Treatment involves discontinuation of the drugs and symptomatic control of temperature, acid-base balance, intravenous fluid balance, and muscle tone. Specific pharmacotherapy is empirical. Clinical reports support consideration of benzodiazepines, dopamine agonists, and dantrolene. Dantrolene aids in therapy because it lowers muscle heat production and therefore body temperature, and it eases rigidity without the need for tracheal intubation. In refractory cases and patients with prominent catatonic features, electroconvulsive therapy has helped. Succinylcholine, usually part of such therapy, may risk hyperkalemia in patients with muscle necrosis. Although often similar in presentation, NMS and MH result from different pathophysiology. Unlike MH, dopamine antagonists trigger NMS in the brain; it may respond to centrally acting agents, electroconvulsive therapy, and neuromuscular blockers. MH triggers appear safe in NMS patients and their families. Some NMS patients have had positive MH muscle biopsy results, but their significance is unclear.

The relationship of isolated CK elevations and MH susceptibility remains unclear. Some have had positive contracture testing, and others with a long-standing benign course have received triggers uneventfully.[117] Less convincing is a direct association of MH with other disorders: crib death, or sudden infant death syndrome; Smith-Lemli-Opitz syndrome[118]; and Charcot-Marie-Tooth syndrome.[119] Exercise and heat stroke are discussed under "Awake Triggering: Exercise and Heat Stroke." Succinylcholine induces contractures in myotonic muscle, which could be confused with MH. Myotonic goats develop brief rigidity after succinylcholine administration but, even with the concomitant use of halothane, show no evidence of MH. In myotonia, there appears to be rigidity in the absence of serious metabolic abnormalities; infrequent positive biopsy results appear to be related to non-MH factors.

TREATMENT

Discontinuation of the trigger may be adequate treatment for acute MH if the onset is slow or if exposure was brief. Dantrolene, the therapeutic mainstay, is packaged in 20-mg bottles with sodium hydroxide for a pH of 9 to 10 (otherwise it will not dissolve) and mannitol (converts the hypotonic solution to isotonic). Dantrolene must be dissolved in sterile water rather than solutions because the extra molecules lead to a salting-out effect and greater difficulty in dissolving it. It may be heated to hasten solution.[120] In a large adult, as many as 10 bottles may be required. Dantrolene's cardiac effects are complex and include interactions with calcium antagonists (see "Calcium"). Dantrolene has a half-life of at least 10 hours in children and adults.[121,122] It does not paralyze; peak effects include moderate muscle weakness with adequate strength for deep breathing and coughing. Weakness is accentuated in myopathic patients. Aside from cholestasis during long-term (>3 weeks) therapy, dantrolene has no serious side effects.

Acute therapy for MH can be summarized as follows:
1. Discontinue all anesthetic agents and hyperventilate with 100% oxygen. Normal ventilation is that required to remove metabolic carbon dioxide. With increased aerobic metabolism, normal ventilation must increase. However, carbon dioxide production is also increased because of neutralization of fixed acid by bicarbonate; hyperventilation removes this additional carbon dioxide.
2. Repeat administration of dantrolene (2 mg/kg, every 5 minutes to a total dose of 10 mg/kg, if needed, although doses to 29 mg/kg have been used).[123]
3. Administer bicarbonate (2 to 4 mEq/kg). Continued efflux of lactate from skeletal muscle may result in recurrent acidosis[124] because lactate, being ionized, slowly crosses the muscle cell membrane to extracellular fluid.
4. Control fever by iced fluids, surface cooling, cooling of body cavities with sterile iced fluids, and a heat exchanger with a pump oxygenator.[93] The clinician must not become so preoccupied with cooling and other busy work that he or she neglects the prime factor in therapy: intravenous administration of dantrolene. Cooling should be halted at 38°C to 39°C to prevent inadvertent hypothermia.
5. Monitor urinary output to prevent shock to kidneys or acute tubular necrosis and to examine for myoglobinuria.
6. Further therapy is guided by blood gases, electrolytes, temperature, arrhythmia, muscle tone, and urinary output.
7. Analyze electrolytes; CK concentrations; liver profile; levels of blood urea nitrogen, lactate, and glucose;

coagulation studies (e.g., INR, platelet count, prothrombin time, fibrinogen, fibrin-split or degradation products); and serum hemoglobin and myoglobin and urine hemoglobin and myoglobin.

The clinical course determines further therapy and studies. Dantrolene should probably be repeated at least every 10 to 15 hours (its half-life) for several doses.[121,122] Recrudescence of MH can approach 50%, usually within 6.5 hours.[123] Treatment of hyperkalemia should be slow. The plasma K+ level must be serially monitored because it may be an important factor in treatment (e.g., persistently elevated K+ level may prevent defibrillation).[93] The most effective way to lower serum potassium is reversal of MH by effective doses of dantrolene. Calcium administration is indicated only for related arrhythmias or for poor cardiac function. However, when indicated, calcium and cardiac glycosides may be safely used because their administration to the susceptible pig does not trigger MH.[52] They can be lifesaving during persistent hyperkalemia.[90-92]

Permanent neurologic sequelae, such as coma or paralysis, may occur in advanced cases, probably from inadequate cerebral oxygenation and perfusion for the increased metabolism and because of the fever, acidosis, hypo-osmolality with fluid shifts, and potassium release. Even satisfactory care during anesthesia may not prevent neurologic complications. Measurements of intracranial pressure may help in the evaluation of cerebral edema. Disseminated intravascular coagulation or consumptive coagulopathy may be caused by hemolysis, release of tissue thromboplastins, overt tissue damage, or shock. The best treatment is adequate therapy for MH to prevent stagnation of peripheral blood flow and to lower temperature.

Among the ineffective therapeutic adjuncts are calcium antagonists and sympathetic antagonists. Calcium antagonists do not increase porcine survival.[50,51] They may interact with dantrolene to produce hyperkalemia, which can result in retriggering MH[52] or in myocardial depression.[49] Magnesium reduces the increase in intracellular calcium during porcine MH but does not prevent the increase in metabolism. Although it may play a role in MH mechanisms (see "Pathophysiology and Molecular Biology"),[38] its therapeutic value appears to be minimal.

Early diagnosis and treatment of MH are essential. Complications are difficult to treat and may lead to serious and permanent sequelae. Retriggering may occur as dantrolene is redistributed or metabolized. The physician should contact the MH Hotline to verify treatment and report the case using an AMRA form.

ANESTHESIA FOR SUSCEPTIBLE PATIENTS

Anesthesia should consist of nitrous oxide, barbiturates, etomidate, propofol, opiates, tranquilizers, or nondepolarizing muscle relaxants. Potent volatile agents and succinylcholine must be avoided, even in the presence of dantrolene. Some human patients have experienced a hypermetabolic state despite these precautions, but they have always responded favorably to intravenous dantrolene. Preoperative dantrolene is not needed because the use of nontriggering agents is almost always associated with uneventful anesthesia. If used, 1 to 2 mg/kg should be given intravenously just before induction to avoid the side effects of lengthy pretreatment. In obstetric cases, it is best given after the cord is clamped to avoid the problems of a floppy child, because cord blood levels may approach 65% of maternal levels.[125] Regional anesthesia is safe and may be preferred. Amide anesthetics had been considered dangerous in susceptible patients because they induce or worsen contractures in vitro as a result of their effect in increasing calcium efflux from the SR. However, these effects require millimolar concentrations, far greater than plasma values achieved in clinical use. Porcine and human studies demonstrated the lack of danger of amide anesthetics. Intravenous lidocaine was used as long ago as 1970 to treat acute MH without harm and with apparently good results.[6]

Anesthetic machines may be "cleansed" of potent volatile agents by removal or sealing of the vaporizers, change of soda lime, perhaps replacement of the fresh gas outlet hose, and use of a disposable circle with a flow of 10 L/min for 5 minutes. After flow is reduced, the volatile agent's concentration may again increase. A gas analyzer demonstrates a continuous volatile vapor concentration. This is important because some new machines require a constant high flow to minimize volatile agent concentrations.[126]

The anesthesiologist should confidently discuss the anesthetic care with the patient, assuring him or her that all will be done to avoid difficulties with MH and that the appropriate drugs, knowledge, and skills are immediately at hand if any problems occur. Many of these patients have undergone procedures uneventfully, such as dental analgesia and obstetric anesthesia, before the diagnosis of susceptibility was made. The patient can enter the therapeutic environment in a reassured, relaxed, and comfortable state. Outpatient procedures are feasible in most environments; the time of discharge depends on usual outpatient criteria. Any facility using MH triggers on an inpatient or outpatient basis should have dantrolene immediately available.

Several species, such as pigs, dogs, cats, and horses, have suffered MH episodes.[46] A canine colony inbred for MH has the canine *RYR1* gene.[127] Cosgrove and colleagues[128] examined contractures in greyhounds in conjunction with a triggering anesthetic challenge; all findings were normal. Continuing study of the capture myopathy of wild animals, more recently in feral deer, suggests that this is "overstraining" during the chase of normal animals rather than a genetic disorder similar to MH.[129]

EVALUATION OF SUSCEPTIBILITY

Evaluation includes a history and physical examination for the detection of subclinical abnormality. A genealogy with specific information about anesthetic exposure and agents can estimate the likelihood of exposure to triggering agents. Blood CK values, when determined in a resting, fasting state without recent trauma, reflect muscle membrane stability. When CK level is elevated in a close relative of a person with known MH susceptibility, the relative may be considered to have MH susceptibility

without contracture testing. If the CK level is normal on several occasions, there is no predictive value, and contracture studies are necessary. The patient must travel to the test center for surgical biopsy to ensure viability and accurate results.

Muscle biopsy contracture studies, performed at about 30 centers around the world, use exposures to halothane, caffeine, halothane plus caffeine, and ryanodine.[33] 4-Chloro-*m*-cresol may add to precision.[130] There is a crisis in the United States, with only six test centers (December 2003), in part because of medical care limitations. This is inappropriate considering geography and population. Contracture responses are sometimes positive in patients with myopathies that bear no direct relationship to MH and therefore may not indicate susceptibility. Dantrolene must be avoided before the biopsy, because it masks the response to contracture-producing drugs. After a patient is diagnosed with MHS, DNA testing for mutations should follow. When one is detected, other relatives with that mutation are considered to have MHS without the need for the invasive contracture test, and they need not travel to a testing center (see "Genetics").

For the student of anesthesia, susceptible individuals have a lower threshold to contracture-producing drugs. The muscle specimen must be viable (i.e., twitch when stimulated electrically) because the contracture threshold may vary if the fiber is deteriorating. Bath kinetics are stable with the use of experienced laboratories, and variations in temperature have less effect than anticipated on contracture thresholds.[131]

Advice should be given to the susceptible patient. Precautions are necessary in regard to general anesthesia, and triggers include all potent volatile agents and succinylcholine. Awake episodes are uncommon, and if not experienced before the diagnosis, they are an unlikely problem. Military personnel may have restrictions because of the necessary avoidance of combat trauma and the possible mandatory use of triggers, and soldiers with MH susceptibility may be less desirable because some authorities believe that they may fatigue sooner with harsh military conditioning because of their subclinical myopathy.

The predictive value (i.e., percentage of positive results that are true positives) or efficiency (i.e., percentage of all results that are true, whether positive or negative) of contracture testing in determining susceptibility cannot be estimated. False-positive results resulting from cautious interpretation or decreased specificity are masked because the patient will never be exposed to triggering agents. European and North American contracture protocols have yielded sufficient multicenter data to confirm acceptable test results.[132,133] Separation of control patients from MH patients was based on purely clinical information using the clinical grading scale.[115] Both protocols have 97% to 99% sensitivity (i.e., frequency of positive results in the patients with clinically established MH) and acceptable (78% to 94%) specificity (i.e., frequency of negative results in low-risk controls). Threshold values attempt to provide 100% sensitivity to detect all MHS patients; this restriction limits specificity.

The North American testing protocol (CHCT) uses incremental caffeine concentrations of 0.5, 1, 2, 4, 8, and 32 mM and uses 3% halothane as a bolus application.

It yields two diagnoses: normal (MHN) or abnormal (MHS). The European testing protocol (IVCT) uses additional steps in its increments: caffeine concentrations of 0.5, 1, 1.5, 2, 3, 4, and 32 mM, and halothane in concentrations of 0.5%, 1%, 2%, and sometimes 3%. Greater fractionation of caffeine and halothane increments in the European protocol results in lower diagnostic thresholds (i.e., 0.2 g for both drugs).[132] The lesser fractionation of increments in the North American protocol leads to greater thresholds (0.3 g) for caffeine and a relatively large gray area for halothane of about 0.5 to 0.8 g.[133] Interpretation of IVCT yields three diagnoses: MHS, for which halothane and caffeine results are abnormal; MHN, for which both results are normal; and equivocal (MHE), for which only one result is abnormal. Fewer MHE diagnoses and better genetic correlations exist when contractures are markedly abnormal instead of near threshold; this may lessen discordance.[134,135]

What is needed in MH testing is an accurate, noninvasive or nondestructive measure of susceptibility that has no overlap between the ranges of normal and susceptible responses. A promising innovative in vivo human application involves physiologically based microdialysis infusion of caffeine or halothane into muscle of MH-susceptible patients, triggering exaggerated localized changes in acid-base balance.[136,137] White blood cells express MH mutations and provide a substrate for genetic analysis.[75,76,138,139] Nuclear magnetic resonance has promise;[140] the difficulty is to standardize a stress, such as forearm ischemia, that can differentiate susceptible tissue from normal. Although early ultrasound results were encouraging, study results for skeletal muscle were inaccurate in humans with MH susceptibility.[141] Adnet and coworkers[142] examined masseter muscle in a skinned fiber in vitro preparation in attempts to explain its propensity for contracture. They observed greater sensitivity to Ca^{2+} and caffeine than that in quadriceps muscle. Their findings were contradicted in a contracture study of masseter biopsy specimens taken during major craniofacial cancer surgery.[143] These responded similarly to quadriceps.

SUMMARY

MH is a subclinical myopathy featuring an eerie and erratic metabolic mayhem that is unmasked on exposure to potent volatile anesthetics or succinylcholine. Skeletal muscle acutely and unexpectedly increases its oxygen consumption and lactate production, resulting in greater heat production, respiratory and metabolic acidosis, muscle rigidity, sympathetic stimulation, and increased cellular permeability. MH-susceptible skeletal muscle differs from normal muscle in that it is always closer to loss of control of Ca^{2+} concentration within the muscle fiber, and it can involve a generalized alteration in cellular or subcellular membrane permeability. This is an EC coupling defect resulting from an alteration in the receptor encoded by *RYR1*. It is a homozygous, single-point mutation of *RYR1* in swine and a heterozygous disorder in humans, in whom there may also be a modification of RYR1 protein function by interacting structures, membranes, or enzymes; MH may occur as a final common path phenomenon. Diagnosis rests on extraordinary temperature, acid-base alterations,

and muscle aberrations. Specific treatment is the action of dantrolene on muscle Ca^{2+} movements; symptomatic treatment is by reversal of acid-base and temperature changes. Evaluation of affected families is guided by measurements of circulating CK, analysis of drug-induced muscle contractures (by European IVCT and North American CHCT protocols), and genetic testing of DNA samples. General or regional anesthesia is safe for patients susceptible to MH, provided that care is taken to specially prepare the anesthesia machine and to avoid all potent volatile anesthetics and succinylcholine if a general technique is chosen.

Research on MH has yielded insights into the physiology of metabolism and into the molecular biology of genetic muscle disorders. Remaining challenges include identification of all genetic mutations responsible for human MH, elucidation of the mechanism that links exposure to the subsequent loss of Ca^{2+} control, development of noninvasive and nondestructive testing for susceptibility, and determination of the mode of action of dantrolene.

KEY POINTS

1. MH is an anesthetic-related disorder of increased metabolism of skeletal muscle. It is an inherited condition and occurs in swine and humans.

2. Skeletal muscle accounts for approximately 40% of body weight; its increased metabolism therefore has a profound effect on whole-body metabolism.

3. Signs of MH, including tachycardia, increased expired carbon dioxide, muscle rigidity, and increased temperature, are related to increased metabolism.

4. Function of the ryanodine receptor of skeletal muscle is abnormal in MH, causing barely controlled calcium concentration within the cell.

5. Added loss of control of intracellular calcium leads to marked metabolic stimulation within the cell to provide extra ATP to drive the calcium pumps that restore calcium to its reservoirs (e.g., SR, mitochondrion, extracellular fluid).

6. Dantrolene markedly attenuates loss of calcium from SR, restoring metabolism to normal, with reversal of the signs of metabolic stimulation.

7. MH is inherited; one mutation accounts for all porcine MH, and more than 30 mutations account for human MH.

8. Evaluation of persons susceptible to MH includes contracture of a skeletal muscle biopsy specimen with halothane or caffeine, estimation of muscle permeability by measurement of plasma CK level, and evaluation of DNA to identify mutations. Only DNA testing is needed to evaluate swine MH.

9. Future MH goals include advancement of genetic evaluations in North American and European medical programs and finances that are stronger for supporting genetic studies, identification of the mode of action of dantrolene, determination of the immediate cause of MH triggering, and development of effective, nondestructive tests for MH susceptibility.

REFERENCES

1. Wilson RD, Nichols RJ Jr, Dent TE, et al: Disturbances of the oxidative-phosphorylation mechanism as a possible etiological factor in sudden unexplained hyperthermia occurring during anesthesia. Anesthesiology 27:231, 1966.
2. Ording H: Investigation of malignant hyperthermia susceptibility in Denmark. Dan Med Bull 43:111, 1996.
3. Harrison GG, Issacs H: Malignant hyperthermia: An historical vignette. Anaesthesia 47:54, 1992.
4. Ombrédanne L: De l'influence de l'anesthésique employé dans la ganèse des accidents post-opératoires de pâleur-hyperthermie observés chez les nourrissons. Rev Med Française 10:617, 1929.
5. Denborough MA, Lovell RRH: Anaesthetic deaths in a family. Lancet 2:45, 1960.
6. Kalow W, Britt BA, Terreau ME, et al: Metabolic error of muscle metabolism after recovery from malignant hyperthermia. Lancet 2:89, 1970.
7. Herter M, Wilsdorf G: Die Bedeutung des Schweines für die Fleischversorgung, vol 270. Berlin, Arbeiten der Deutscher Landwirtschaft-Gesellschaft, 1914.
8. Briskey EJ: Etiological status and associated studies of pale, soft, exudative porcine musculature. Adv Food Res 13:89, 1964.
9. Topel DG, Bicknell EJ, Preston KS, et al: Porcine stress syndrome. Mod Vet Pract 49:40, 1968.
10. Hall LW, Woolf N, Bradley JWP, et al: Unusual reaction to suxamethonium chloride. Br Med J 2:1305, 1966.
11. Berman MC, Harrison GG, Bull AB, et al: Changes underlying halothane-induced malignant hyperpyrexia in Landrace pigs. Nature 225:653, 1970.
12. Harrison GG: Control of the malignant hyperpyrexic syndrome in MHS swine by dantrolene sodium. Br J Anaesth 47:62, 1975.
13. Kolb ME, Horne ML, Martz R: Dantrolene in human malignant hyperthermia: A multicenter study. Anesthesiology 56:254, 1982.
14. Bendixen D, Skovgaard LT, Ording H: Analysis of anaesthesia in patients susceptible to malignant hyperthermia before diagnostic in vitro contracture test. Acta Anaesth Scand 41:480, 1997.
15. Gronert GA, Milde JH: Variations in onset of porcine malignant hyperthermia. Anesth Analg 60:499, 1981.
16. Pollock N, Hodges M, Sendall J: Prolonged malignant hyperthermia in the absence of triggering agents. Anaesth Intensive Care 20:520, 1992.
17. Berchtold MW, Brinkmeier H, Muntener M: Calcium ion in skeletal muscle: Its crucial role for muscle function, plasticity, and disease. Physiol Rev 80:1215, 2000.
18. Kleopa K, Barchi RL: Genetic disorders of neuromuscular ion channels. Muscle Nerve 26:299, 2002
19. Du GG, Sandhu B, Khanna VK, et al: Topology of the Ca^{2+} release channel of skeletal muscle sarcoplasmic reticulum (R_YR1). Proc Natl Acad Sci 99:16725, 2002.
20. Xiao B, Masumiya H, Jiang D, et al: Isoform-dependent formation of heteromeric Ca^{2+} release channels (ryanodine receptors). J Biol Chem 277:41778, 2002.
21. Grabner M, Dirksen RT, Suda N, et al: The II-III loop of the skeletal muscle dihydropyridine receptor is responsible for the bi-directional coupling with the ryanodine receptor. J Biol Chem 274:21913, 1999.
22. Wilkens CM, Kasielke N, Flucher BE, et al: Excitation-contraction coupling is unaffected by drastic alteration of the sequence surrounding residues L720-L764 of the alpha(1S) II-III loop, Proc Natl Acad Sci U S A 98:5892, 2001.
23. Feng W, Tu J, Yang T, et al: Homer regulates gain of ryanodine receptor type 1 channel complex. J Biol Chem 277:44722, 2002.
24. McWilliams S, Nelson T, Sudo RT, et al: Novel skeletal muscle ryanodine receptor mutation in a large Brazilian family with malignant hyperthermia. Clin Genet 62:80, 2002.
25. Sambuughin N, Sei Y, Gallagher KL, et al: North American malignant hyperthermia population—Screening of the ryanodine receptor gene and identification of novel mutations. Anesthesiology 95:594, 2001.
26. Robinson RL, Brooks C, Brown SL, et al: RYR1 mutations causing central core disease are associated with more severe malignant hyperthermia in vitro contracture test phenotypes. Hum Mutation 20:88, 2002.
27. McCarthy TV, Quane KA, Lynch PJ: Ryanodine receptor mutations in malignant hyperthermia and central core disease. Hum Mutat 15:410, 2000.
28. Lynch PJ, McCarthy T: Molecular aspects of malignant hyperthermia and central core disease. Channelopathies 3:55, 2000.
29. Brown RL, Pollock NA, Couchman KG, et al: A novel ryanodine receptor mutation and genotype-phenotype correlation in a large malignant hyperthermia New Zealand Maori pedigree. Hum Mol Genet 9:1515, 2000.
30. Monnier N, Krivosic-Horber R, Payen J-F, et al: Presence of two different genetic traits in malignant hyperthermia families: Implication for genetic analysis, diagnosis, and incidence of malignant hyperthermia susceptibility. Anesthesiology 97:1067, 2002.
31. Fletcher JE, Tripolitis L, Hubert M, et al: Genotype and phenotype relationships for mutations in the ryanodine receptor in patients referred for diagnosis of malignant hyperthermia. Br J Anaesth 75:307, 1995.
32. Robinson R, Hopkins P, Carsana A, et al: Several interacting genes influence the malignant hyperthermia genotype. Hum Genet 112:217, 2003.
33. Urwyler A, Deufel T, McCarthy T, et al: Guidelines for molecular genetic detection of susceptibility to malignant hyperthermia. Br J Anaesth 86:283, 2001.
34. Rueffert H, Olthoff D, Deutrich C, et al: Mutation screening in the ryanodine receptor 1 gene (RYR1) in patients susceptible to malignant hyperthermia who show definite IVCT results: Identification of three novel mutations. Acta Anaesth Scand 46:692, 2002.
35. Ryan JF, Lopez JR, Sanchez VB, et al: Myoplasmic calcium changes precede metabolic and clinical signs of porcine malignant hyperthermia. Anesth Analg 79:1007, 1994.
36. Fujii J, Otsu K, Zorzato F, et al: Identification of a mutation in porcine ryanodine receptor associated with malignant hyperthermia. Science 253:448, 1991.
37. O'Brien PJ, Li G: Rapid, simple and sensitive microassay for skeletal muscle homogenates in the functional assessment of the Ca^{2+}-release channel of sarcoplasmic reticulum: Application to diagnosis of susceptibility to malignant hyperthermia. Mol Cell Biochem 167:61, 1997.
38. Owen VJ, Taske NL, Lamb GD: Reduced Mg^{2+} inhibition of Ca^{2+} release in muscle fibers of pigs susceptible to malignant hyperthermia. Am J Physiol 272:C203, 1997.
39. Duke AM, Hopkins PM, Steele DS: Effects of Mg^{2+} and SR luminal Ca^{2+} on caffeine-induced Ca^{2+} release in skeletal muscle from humans susceptible to malignant hyperthermia. J Physiology 544:85, 2002.
40. Yamaguchi N, Igami K, Kasai M: Kinetics of depolarization-induced calcium release from skeletal muscle triads in vitro. J Biochem 121:432, 1997.
41. Paul-Pletzer K, Palnitkar SS, Jimenez LS, et al: The skeletal muscle ryanodine receptor identified as a molecular target of [3H]azidodantrolene by photoaffinity labeling. Biochemistry 40:531, 2001.
42. Paul-Pletzer K, Yamamoto T, Bhat MB, et al: Identification of a dantrolene-binding sequence on the skeletal muscle ryanodine receptor. J Biol Chem 277:34918, 2002.
43. Ikemoto N, Yamamoto T: Postulated role of inter-domain interaction within the ryanodine receptor in Ca^{2+} channel. Trends Cardiovasc Med 10:310, 2000.
44. Yamamoto T, Ikemoto N: Spectroscopic monitoring of local conformational changes during the intramolecular domain-domain interaction of the ryanodine receptor. Biochemistry 41:1492, 2002.
45. Monnier N, Romero NB, Lerale J: Familial and sporadic forms of central core disease are associated with mutations in the C-terminal domain of the skeletal muscle ryanodine receptor. Hum Mol Gen 10:2581, 2001.
46. Gronert GA: Malignant hyperthermia. Anesthesiology 53:395, 1980.

47. Hall GM, Bendall JR, Lucke JN, et al: Porcine malignant hyperthermia. II. Heat production. Br J Anaesth 48:305, 1976.
48. Stadhouders AM, Viering WAL, Verburg MP, et al: In vivo induced malignant hyperthermia in pigs. III. Localization of calcium in skeletal muscle mitochondria by means of electron microscopy and microprobe analysis. Acta Anaesthesiol Scand 28:14, 1984.
49. Saltzman LS, Kates RA, Corke BC, et al: Hyperkalemia and cardiovascular collapse after verapamil and dantrolene administration in swine. Anesth Analg 63:272, 1984.
50. Harrison GG, Wright IG, Morrell DF: The effects of calcium channel blocking drugs on halothane initiation of malignant hyperthermia in MHS swine and on the established syndrome. Anaesth Intensive Care 16:197, 1988.
51. Gallant EM, Foldes FF, Rempel WE, et al: Verapamil is not a therapeutic adjunct to dantrolene in porcine malignant hyperthermia. Anesth Analg 64:601, 1985.
52. Gronert GA, Ahern CP, Milde JH, et al: Effect of CO_2, calcium, digoxin, and potassium on cardiac and skeletal muscle metabolism in malignant hyperthermia susceptible swine. Anesthesiology 64:24, 1986.
53. Quinlan JG, Iaizzo PA, Gronert GA, et al: Use of dantrolene plus multiple pulses to detect stress-susceptible porcine muscles. J Appl Physiol 60:1313, 1986.
54. Quinlan JG, Wedel DJ, Iaizzo PA: Multiple-pulse stimulation and dantrolene in malignant hyperthermia. Muscle Nerve 13:904, 1990.
55. Hoyer A, Veeser M, Albrecht Y: Repetitive stimulation differentiates distinctly malignant hyperthermia-susceptible (MHS) from non-susceptible (MHN) human muscles in vitro. Anesthesiology 95:A1017, 2001.
56. Bendall JR: The effect of pre-treatment of pigs with curare on the postmortem rate of pH fall and onset of rigor mortis in the musculature. J Sci Food Agric 17:333, 1966.
57. Schmidt GR, Goldspink G, Roberts T, et al: Electromyography and resting membrane potential in longissimus muscle of stress-susceptible and stress-resistant pigs. J Anim Sci 34:379, 1972.
58. Gallant EM, Gronert GA, Taylor SR: Cellular membrane potential and contractile threshold in mammalian skeletal muscle susceptible to malignant hyperthermia. Neurosci Lett 28:181, 1982.
59. Wieland SJ, Gong Q-H, Fletcher JE, et al: Altered sodium current response to intracellular fatty acids in halothane-sensitive skeletal muscle. Am J Physiol 271:C347, 1996.
60. Duthie GG, Arthur JR: Free radicals and calcium homeostasis: Relevance to MH? Free Radic Biol Med 14:435, 1993.
61. Martucci RW, Jessup DA, Gronert GA, et al: Blood gases and catecholamine levels in capture stressed desert bighorn sheep. J Wildl Dis 28:250, 1992.
62. Gronert GA, Theye RA, Milde JH, et al: Catecholamine stimulation of myocardial oxygen consumption in porcine malignant hyperthermia. Anesthesiology 49:330, 1978.
63. Roewer N, Dziadzka A, Greim CA, et al: Cardiovascular and metabolic responses to anesthetic-induced malignant hyperthermia in swine. Anesthesiology 83:141, 1995.
64. Cabral R, Prior PF, Scott DF, et al: Reversible profound depression of cerebral electrical activity in hyperthermia. Electroencephalogr Clin Neurophysiol 42:697, 1977.
65. Satnick JH: Hyperthermia under anesthesia with regional muscle flaccidity. Anesthesiology 30:472, 1969.
66. Artru AA, Gronert GA: Cerebral metabolism during porcine malignant hyperthermia. Anesthesiology 53:121, 1980.
67. Kochs E, Hoffman WE, am Esch JS: Improvement of brain electrical activity during treatment of porcine malignant hyperthermia with dantrolene. Br J Anaesth 71:881, 1993.
68. Hofer RE, Wedel DJ, Sharbrough FW: The effects of malignant hyperthermia on cerebral metabolites and the electroencephalogram in Pietrain swine. Anesthesiology 79:A435, 1993.
69. Gronert GA, Milde JH, Theye RA: Role of sympathetic activity in porcine malignant hyperthermia. Anesthesiology 47:411, 1977.
70. Gronert GA, White DA: Failure of norepinephrine to initiate porcine malignant hyperthermia. Pflugers Arch 411:226, 1988.
71. Maccani RM, Wedel DJ, Hofer RE: Norepinephrine does not potentiate porcine malignant hyperthermia. Anesth Analg 82:790, 1996.
72. Gronert GA, Milde JH, Taylor SR: Porcine muscle responses to carbachol, α- and β-adrenoceptor agonists, halothane or hyperthermia. J Physiol (Lond) 307:319, 1980.
73. Lister D, Hall GM, Lucke JN: Porcine malignant hyperthermia. III. Adrenergic blockade. Br J Anaesth 48:831, 1976.
74. Cooper P, Meddings JB: Erythrocyte membrane fluidity in malignant hyperthermia. Biochim Biophys Acta 1069:151, 1991.
75. Sei Y, Gallagher KL, Basile AS: Skeletal muscle type ryanodine receptor is involved in calcium signaling in human B lymphocytes. J Biol Chem 274:5995, 1999.
76. Girard T, Cavagna D, Padovan E, et al: B-lymphocytes from malignant hyperthermia susceptible patients have an increased sensitivity to skeletal muscle ryanodine receptor activators. J Biol Chem 276:48077, 2001.
77. Carr RJ, Belani KG, Iaizzo PA, et al: Porcine malignant hyperthermia and liver transplantation: Further insight into systemic pathophysiology. Anesth Analg 80:S68, 1995.
78. Antognini JF: Creatine kinase alterations after acute malignant hyperthermia episodes and common surgical procedures. Anesth Analg 81:1039, 1995.
79. Nishiyama K, Kitahara A, Natsume H, et al: Malignant hyperthermia in a patient with Graves' disease during subtotal thyroidectomy. Endocr J 48:227, 2001.
80. Wappler F, Roewer N, Kochling A, et al: Fulminant malignant hyperthermia associated with ketoacidotic coma. Intensive Care Med 22:809, 1996.
81. Behnia R: Systemic effects of absolute alcohol embolization in a patient with a congenital arteriovenous malformation of the lower extremity. Anesth Analg 80:415, 1995.
82. Kitanaka C, Inoh Y, Toyoda T, et al: Malignant brain stem hyperthermia caused by brain stem hemorrhage. Stroke 25:518, 1994.
83. Lambert C, Blanloeil Y, Krivosic-Horber R, et al: Malignant hyperthermia in a patient with hypokalemic periodic paralysis. Anesth Analg 79:1012, 1994.
84. Gronert GA, Fowler W, Cardinet GH III, et al: Absence of malignant hyperthermia contractures in Becker-Duchenne dystrophy at age 2. Muscle Nerve 15:52, 1992.
85. Butler-Browne GS, Eriksson P-O, Laurent C, et al: Adult human masseter muscle fibers express myosin isozymes characteristic of development. Muscle Nerve 11:610, 1988.
86. Morgan DL, Proske U: Vertebrate slow muscle: Its structure, pattern of innervation, and mechanical properties. Physiol Rev 64:103, 1984.
87. van der Spek AFL, Reynolds PI, Fang WB, et al: Changes in resistance to mouth opening induced by depolarizing and non-depolarizing neuromuscular relaxants. Br J Anaesth 64:21, 1990.
88. Albrecht A, Wedel DJ, Gronert GA: Masseter muscle rigidity and non-depolarizing neuromuscular blocking agents. Mayo Clin Proc 72:329, 1997.
89. Martyn JAJ, White DA, Gronert GA, et al: Up-and-down regulation of skeletal muscle acetylcholine receptors: Effects on neuromuscular blockers. Anesthesiology 76:822, 1992.
90. Larach MG, Rosenberg H, Gronert GA, et al: Hyperkalemic cardiac arrest during anesthesia in infants and children with occult myopathy. Clin Pediatr (Phila) 36:9, 1997.
91. Schulte-Sasse U, Eberlein HJ, Schmucker I: Sollte die Verwendung von Succinylcholin in der Kinderanästhesie neu überdacht werden? Anaesthol Reanimat 18:13, 1993.
92. Gronert GA: Cardiac arrest after succinylcholine: Mortality greater with rhabdomyolysis than receptor upregulation. Anesthesiology 94:523, 2001.
93. Lee G, Antognini JF, Gronert GA: Complete recovery after prolonged resuscitation and cardiopulmonary bypass for hyperkalemic cardiac arrest. Anesth Analg 79:172, 1994.
94. Brustowicz RM, Moncorge C, Koka BV: Metabolic responses to tourniquet release in children. Anesthesiology 67:792, 1987.
95. Allen GC, Brubaker CL: Human malignant hyperthermia associated with desflurane anesthesia: The onset of MH. Anesth Analg 86:1328, 1998.

96. Shulman M, Braverman B, Ivankovich AD, Gronert GA: Sevoflurane triggers malignant hyperthermia in swine. Anesthesiology 54:259, 1981.

97. Hall GM, Lucke JN, Lister D: Porcine malignant hyperthermia. IV. Neuromuscular blockade. Br J Anaesth 48:1135, 1976.

98. Iaizzo PA, Kehler CH, Carr RJ, et al: Prior hypothermia attenuates malignant hyperthermia in susceptible swine. Anesth Analg 82:803, 1996.

99. Gronert GA: Hyperbaric nitrous oxide and malignant hyperpyrexia. Br J Anaesth 53:1238, 1981.

100. McIntyre AR, King RE, Dunn AI: Electrical activity of denervated mammalian skeletal muscle as influenced by D-tubocurarine. J Neurophysiol 8:297, 1945.

101. Lips FJ, Newland M, Dutton G: Malignant hyperthermia triggered by cyclopropane during cesarean section. Anesthesiology 56:144, 1982.

102. Sewall K, Flowerdew RMM, Bromberger P: Severe muscular rigidity at birth: Malignant hyperthermia syndrome? Can Anaesth Soc J 27:279, 1980.

103. Cannon ML, Glazier SS, Bauman LA: Metabolic acidosis, rhabdomyolysis, and cardiovascular collapse after prolonged propofol infusion. J Neurosurg 95:1053, 2001.

104. Kelly DF: Editorial: Propofol-infusion syndrome. J Neurosurg 95:925, 2001.

105. Fruen BR, Mickelson JR, Roghair TJ, et al: Effects of propofol on Ca^{2+} regulation by malignant hyperthermia-susceptible muscle membranes. Anesthesiology 82:1274, 1995.

106. Wappler F, Fiege M, Antz M, et al: Hemodynamic and metabolic alterations in response to graded exercise in a patient susceptible to malignant hyperthermia. Anesthesiology 92:268, 2000.

107. Wappler F, Fiege M, Steinfath M, et al: Evidence for susceptibility to malignant hyperthermia in patients with exercise-induced rhabdomyolysis. Anesthesiology 94:95, 2001.

108. Davis M, Brown R, Dickson A, et al: Malignant hyperthermia associated with exercise-induced rhabdomyolysis or congenital abnormalities and a novel RYR1 mutation in New Zealand and Australian pedigrees. Br J Anaesth 88:508, 2002.

109. Tobin JR, Jason DR, Nelson TE, et al: Malignant hyperthermia and apparent heat stroke (Correspondence). JAMA 286:168, 2001.

110. Ogletree JW, Antognini JF, Gronert GA: Postexercise muscle cramping associated with positive malignant hyperthermia contracture testing. Am J Sports Med 24:49, 1996.

111. Ryan JF, Tedeschi LG: Sudden unexplained death in a patient with a family history of malignant hyperthermia. J Clin Anesth 9:66, 1997.

112. Anetseder M, Hartung E, Klepper S, et al: Gasoline vapors induce severe rhabdomyolysis. Neurology 44:2393, 1994.

113. Denborough MA, Hopkinson KC, Banney DG: Firefighting and malignant hyperthermia. Br Med J 296:1442, 1988.

114. Karan SM, Crowl F, Muldoon SM: Malignant hyperthermia masked by capnographic monitoring. Anesth Analg 78:590, 1994.

115. Larach MG, Localio AR, Allen GC, et al: A clinical grading scale to predict malignant hyperthermia susceptibility. Anesthesiology 80:771, 1994.

116. Caroff SN, Rosenberg H, Mann SC: Neuroleptic malignant syndrome in the critical care unit. Crit Care Med 30:2609, 2002.

117. Reijneveld JC, Notermans NC, Linssen WHJP, et al: Benign prognosis in idiopathic hyper-CK-emia. Muscle Nerve 23:575, 2000.

118. Haji-Michael PG, Hatch DL: Smith-Lemli-Opitz syndrome and malignant hyperthermia. Anesth Analg 83:200, 1996.

119. Ducart A, Adnet P, Renaud B, et al: Malignant hyperthermia during sevoflurane anesthesia. Anesth Analg 80:609, 1995.

120. Mitchell LW, Leighton BL: Warmed diluent speeds dantrolene reconstitution. Can J Anaesth 50:127, 2003.

121. Lerman J, McLeod ME, Strong HA: Pharmacokinetics of intravenous dantrolene in children. Anesthesiology 70:625, 1989.

122. Flewellen EH, Nelson TE, Jones WP, et al: Dantrolene dose response in awake man: Implications for management of malignant hyperthermia. Anesthesiology 59:275, 1983.

123. Brandom BW, Larach MG, North American MH Registry: Reassessment of the safety and efficacy of dantrolene. Anesthesiology 97:A1199, 2002.

124. Gronert GA, Ahern CP, Milde JH: Treatment of porcine malignant hyperthermia: Lactate gradient from muscle to blood. Can J Anaesth 33:729, 1986.

125. Shime J, Gare D, Andrews J, et al: Dantrolene in pregnancy: Lack of adverse effects on the fetus and newborn infant. Am J Obstet Gynecol 159:831, 1988.

126. Schönell LHB, Sims C, Bulsara M: Preparing a new generation anaesthetic machine for patients susceptible to malignant hyperthermia. Anaesth Intens Care 31:58, 2003.

127. Roberts MC, Mickelson JR, Patterson EE, et al: Autosomal dominant canine malignant hyperthermia is caused by a mutation in the gene encoding the skeletal muscle calcium release channel (RYR1). Anesthesiology 95:716, 2001.

128. Cosgrove SB, Eisele PH, Martucci RW, et al: Evaluation of Greyhound susceptibility to malignant hyperthermia using halothane-succinylcholine anesthesia and caffeine-halothane contractures. Lab Anim Sci 42:482, 1992.

129. Antognini JF, Eisele PH, Gronert GA: Evaluation for malignant hyperthermia susceptibility in black-tailed deer. J Wildlife Dis 32:678, 1996.

130. Wappler F, Anetseder M, Baur CP, et al: Multicentre evaluation of in vitro contracture testing with bolus administration of 4-chloro-m-cresol for diagnosis of malignant hyperthermia susceptibility. European J Anaesth 20:528, 2003.

131. Antognini JF, Gronert GA: Effect of temperature variation (22C-44C) on halothane and caffeine contracture testing in humans. Acta Anaesthesiol Scand 41:639, 1997.

132. Ording H, Brancadoro V, Cozzolino S, et al: In vitro contracture test for diagnosis of malignant hyperthermia following the protocol of the European MH group: Results of testing patients surviving fulminant MH and unrelated low-risk subjects. Acta Anaesthesiol Scand 41:955, 1997.

133. Allen GC, Larach MH, Kunselman AR: The sensitivity and specificity of the caffeine halothane contracture test: A report from the North American malignant hyperthermia registry. Anesthesiology 88:579, 1998.

134. Islander G, Ording H, Bendixen D, et al: Reproducibility of in vitro contracture test results in patients tested for malignant hyperthermia susceptibility. Acta Anaesth Scand 46:1144, 2002.

135. Robinson RL, Anetseder MJ, Brancadoro V, et al: Recent advances in the diagnosis of malignant hyperthermia susceptibility: How confident can we be of genetic testing? European J Human Genet 11:342, 2003.

136. Anetseder M, Hager M, Müller CR, et al: Diagnosis of susceptibility to malignant hyperthermia by use of a metabolic test. Lancet 359:1579-1580, 2002; 362:494, 2003.

137. Anetseder M, Hager M, Müller R, et al: Provocative metabolic testing for malignant hyperthermia by intramuscular caffeine and halothane application in humans. Anesthesiology 97:A432, 2002.

138. Kraev N, Loke JCP, Kraev A, et al: Protocol for the sequence analysis of ryanodine receptor subtype 1 gene transcripts from human leukocytes. Anesthesiology 99:289, 2003.

139. Loke JCP, Kraev N, Sharma P, et al: Detection of a novel ryanodine receptor subtype 1 mutation (R328W) in a malignant hyperthermia family by sequencing of a leukocyte transcript. Anesthesiology 99:297, 2003.

140. Bendahan D, Kozak-Ribbens G, Confort-Gouny S, et al: Definition of a diagnostic score of malignant hyperthermia using P-31 magnetic resonance spectroscopy [in French]. Ann Fr Anesth Reanim 15:583, 1996.

141. Antognini JF, Anderson M, Cronan M, et al: Ultrasonography: Not useful in detecting susceptibility to malignant hyperthermia. J Ultrasound Med 13:371, 1994.

142. Adnet PJ, Reyford H, Tavernier BM, et al: In vitro human masseter muscle hypersensitivity: A possible explanation for increase in muscle tone. J Appl Physiol 80:1547, 1996.

143. Melton AT, Antognini JF, Gronert GA: Caffeine- or halothane-induced contractures of masseter muscle are similar to those of vastus muscle in normal humans. Acta Anaesth Scand 43:764, 1999.

144. Mozley PD: Malignant hyperthermia following intravenous iodinated contrast media. Diagn Gynecol Obstet 3:81, 1981.

145. Purday JP, Montgomery CJ, Blackstock D: Intraoperative hyperthermia in a paediatric patient with cystinosis. Paediatr Anaesth 5:389, 1995.

146. Scully RE (ed): Case records of the Mass. General Hospital. N Engl J Med 331:259, 1994.

147. Peluso A, Cerullo M: Malignant hyperthermia susceptibility in patients with osteogenesis imperfecta. Paediatr Anaesth 5:398, 1995.

148. Allen GC, Rosenberg H: Phaeochromocytoma presenting as acute malignant hyperthermia: A diagnostic challenge. Can J Anaesth 37:595, 1990.

149. Arakura K, Narita M, Nisimura C, et al: Malignant hyperthermia in a child with Prader-Willi syndrome. Anesth Resuscitation 32(Suppl):53, 1996.

150. Ginsburg R, Purcell-Jones GMH: Malignant hyperthermia in the Wolf-Hirschhorn syndrome. Anaesthesia 43:386, 1988.

151. Jones R, Dolcourt J: Muscle rigidity following halothane anesthesia in two patients with Freeman-Sheldon syndrome. Anesthesiology 77:599, 1992.

CHAPTER
30 Fundamental Principles of Monitoring Instrumentation

James F. Szocik, Steven J. Barker, and Kevin K. Tremper

Introduction   1191

Basic Principles   1192
Nature of Physics and Measurement   1192
Accuracy   1193
Signal Processing   1193

Pressure Measurement   1196
Principles of Pressure (Mass, Force,
    and Energy)   1196
Static Pressure Measurement
    (Manometer)   1198
Dynamic Pressure Measurement
    (Transducer)   1199
Signal-Processed Pressure Measurement
    (Noninvasive Blood Pressure Monitor)   1201

Flow Measurement   1202
Principles of Flow   1202
Mass/Volume Flow Meters (Urometer,
    Volumeter, Dilutional Measurements)   1203
Velocity/Flow Measurements
    (Venturi, Pitot, Doppler)   1203
Balance-of-Pressure Flow Meters
    (Bourdon Tube, Thorpe Tube)   1204
Vane Spirometer Flow Meters
    (Wright Spirometer)   1205
Summary of Flow Measurement   1205

Measurement Using Sound   1205
Principles of Sound   1205

Passive Sound Examination
    (Stethoscope)   1206
Active Sound Examination (Percussion,
    Echo, Doppler)   1206

Measurement Using Electricity   1208
Principles of Electricity   1208
Passive Electrical Examination
    (Electrocardiograph,
    Electroencephalograph)   1210
Active Electrical Examination
    (Somatosensory Evoked Potentials   1211

Measurement Using Light   1212
Principles of Light   1212
Light as a Multifunctional Tool:
    Beer-Lambert Law   1212
Light Absorbance Monitors (Capnometer,
    Anesthetic Analyzer)   1213
Pulse Oximeters   1213
Raman Scattering   1215

Temperature Measurement   1216
Principles of Temperature   1216
Temperature Monitors (Thermometer,
    Thermistor, Thermocouple,
    Thermopile, Liquid Crystal)   1216

Appendices   1218

INTRODUCTION

Patient monitoring has been a key aspect of anesthesiology since its beginnings as a medical specialty. As anesthesiology has grown more sophisticated and complex, so have the monitors and the data that they produce. The anesthesiologist's senses of sight, hearing, and touch, at first expanded with the stethoscope, sphygmomanometer, and electrocardiograph, are now supplemented by the pulse oximeter, expired gas analyzer, evoked potential monitor, and transesophageal echocardiograph, to name a few. The complexity of some of these devices can be intimidating, and we are tempted to regard them as incomprehensible "black boxes" that provide us with clinical data. However, to do so would be to shirk an important part of our clinical responsibility. We must be able to not only understand and interpret the data from our monitors but also anticipate and recognize errors associated with their use. We cannot accomplish this goal without understanding how these devices work.

The purpose of this chapter is to provide an understanding of the scientific principles underlying the design and function of our most commonly used monitors. An introduction defining some concepts of basic physics is followed by more detailed descriptions of the principles. The text and figures explain these principles predominantly in a qualitative manner. For those desiring a more quantitative explanation, the relevant equations are provided in the appendices to this chapter.

BASIC PRINCIPLES

Nature of Physics and Measurement

What is monitoring? The verb *monitor* (derived from the Latin *monere*, "to warn") means to check systematically or to keep watch over. In the context of anesthesiology, monitoring means using both our senses and electronic devices to repeatedly or continuously measure important variables in an anesthetized patient.

Physics is the science of matter and energy and interactions between the two; that is, it is the study of everything in the physical universe. Physics encompasses everything from the motions and inner workings of the atom to those of galaxies. Physics is quantitative, and mathematics is the language of physics. In fact, Isaac Newton invented "the calculus" as a tool for expressing and studying the laws of physics. Our monitors are also quantitative. Before we can discuss and understand the complexity of modern anesthetic monitors, we must quantitatively define what we are attempting to measure.

We measure and monitor mass and energy: how much of a substance is present and in what energy state. Much of what we desire to monitor is outside the range of human physical senses. Therefore, we must make measurements in this insensible realm with devices that enhance or extend our senses. Just as the senses have limitations and can be "fooled" under certain circumstances (Fig. 30-1), our physiologic monitors are limited by their design and can also be fooled under some conditions. Intelligent users of these devices must understand their basic design assumptions to predict when they are likely to produce erroneous data.

As we make measurements of mass, space, time, and other physical variables, we often encounter confusion between the terms *units* and *dimensions*. A dimension describes the measure by which a physical variable is expressed quantitatively. For example, length (l) is the dimension used to describe distance, height, or width. Units are specific ways of measuring a given dimension: meters, feet, furlongs, and light-years are all units of length. In basic mechanics, all dimensions can be expressed in terms of the three *fundamental dimensions* of mass (m), length (l), and time (t). In problems of energy transport, an additional dimension of temperature or heat content must be added. In electricity and magnetism, the dimension of charge is also required.

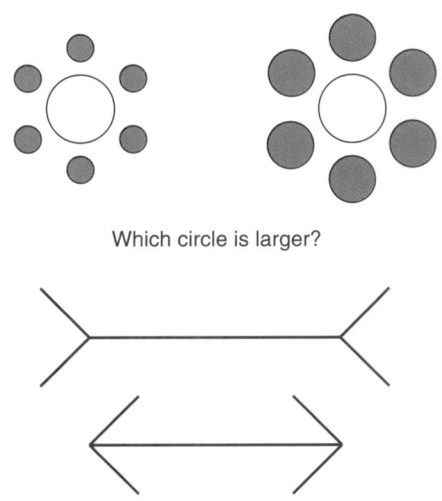

Which circle is larger?

Which line is longer?

Figure 30–1 Optical illusions. We perceive the circles to be different sizes because we infer the size by relative dimensions. The closeness of the smaller circles makes the inner circle appear smaller, and vice versa. The lines appear to be different sizes because we use straight-line perspective to estimate size and distance. This illusion reportedly does not work in cultures where straight lines are not used. Therefore, our internal perceptions lead us to err in estimating size and length. In the same way, the internal programming of our monitors can lead us to misinterpret results.

As stated earlier, *units* are specific ways of measuring a particular dimension. Although there are many units of mass, length, and time, the scientific community has standardized to the *Systeme International d'Unites*, or SI units: length in meters, mass in kilograms, time in seconds. To understand how all quantities in basic mechanics can be expressed in terms of mass (m), length (l), and time (t), we must introduce one (and *only* one) equation: Newton's second law of motion, the basis of all classic physics:

$$F = ma \tag{1}$$

Stated in English, force equals mass times acceleration. Force and acceleration are *vectors;* that is, they have both magnitude and direction. Mass is a *scalar;* it has only magnitude. From this simple equation we can see that the dimensions of force must be the dimensions of mass times those of acceleration. Acceleration is the rate of change in velocity, and velocity is the rate of change in distance. Thus, velocity has dimensions of length divided by time, l/t, and acceleration has dimensions of l/t/t, or l/t^2. The SI units of acceleration are meters per second per second, or m/sec². Because the SI unit of mass is the kilogram, Equation 1 tells us that the unit of *force* must be kg-m/s² (kilogram-meters per second squared). This unit is called the *newton,* after Sir Isaac, so 1 N = 1 kg-m/s².

Other dimensions and units can be derived in the same way. For example, kinetic energy is proportional to mass times velocity squared (mv²), so its dimensions are m(l/t)², and its SI unit is kg-m²/sec². Because "kilogram-meter squared per second squared" is quite a mouthful, we define this unit of energy as the *joule*. The term *power* refers to the time derivative of energy, that is, the change in energy per unit time. The unit of power is thus the joule per second, which we call the *watt*. One watt equals 1 J/sec. Throughout physics, there are many other "practical units" that can always be related to SI units. For example, we are all familiar with *horsepower* as a unit of the power of an engine. One horsepower equals 746 W.

Measurement is the determination of a physical quantity (e.g., mass, length, time, energy, and any of their derivatives). Measuring depends on a physical interaction. If a mass or energy does not interact with anything, it cannot be perceived to exist. As we have stated, physics uses the second, meter, and kilogram to measure time, space, and matter. How do we define the size of these standard units? Historically, the second was defined as a fraction (1/60 of 1/60 of 1/24) of a day. However, because of tidal forces on the earth, the days are becoming longer, and the second is now defined as the interval required for 9,192,631,770 vibrations of the cesium 133 atom measured via an atomic beam clock. The meter was originally one ten millionth of the distance from the North Pole to the Equator. In 1960, the meter was redefined to be 1,650,763.73 wavelengths of orange-red light from a krypton 86 lamp. Today, the meter is defined as the distance that light travels in a vacuum during a time of 1/299,792,458 second because time can be measured with better accuracy and precision than the wavelengths of a krypton lamp. The gram was originally defined as the weight of the volume of pure water at 4°C that occupies a cube that is one hundredth of a meter on all sides. Today, the kilogram is defined as a unit of mass based on a physical standard (a platinum-iridium cylinder).

Temperature is related to the energy per unit mass of a substance in the form of motion on an atomic level. When an object of higher temperature is brought into contact with one of lower temperature, thermal energy, or *heat*, spontaneously passes from the "hot" to the "cold" object until the two reach equilibrium at a temperature between the two original temperatures. In gases, temperature is a quantitative measure of the kinetic energy of molecular motion per unit mass. In 1742, Celsius proposed a temperature scale of *degrees* with the freezing point of water used as 0°C and the boiling point of water at 1-atm pressure used as 100°C. A temperature of absolute zero is defined as the point at which the molecules in a substance are in their lowest possible energy state. This condition occurs at −273.15°C or, in SI units, 0° Kelvin (K).

Physical measurements can be either continuous or discrete. That is, we can measure a distance of 3.1416 m, but we cannot measure out 3.1416 eggs. We consider most numerically defined quantities to be continuous. However, when we measure very tiny quantities (wavelengths of light, energies of photons, masses of atoms), we find that our measurements are not continuous; they change in small jumps, or *quanta*. Continuous measurement is thus an illusion, but a practical one for most purposes.

Accuracy

All measurements have errors. Error is usually determined by the comparison of a measurement to a "gold standard" of that measure. Unfortunately, all measurements, even the so-called gold standards, are subject to errors with respect to reproducibility. From a clinician's perspective, we can depend on a physiologic measurement only if it is accurate to the degree required for clinical decision making. For example, systemic blood pressure can be measured in several ways. We can listen to Korotkoff sounds by the use of a sphygmomanometer cuff and stethoscope; we can rely on an oscillometric automated noninvasive blood pressure device, or if we need continuous measurement, we may place an arterial cannula.[1] Unfortunately, each of these techniques provides a slightly different arterial blood pressure value, and each has different sources of error. Our choice of method may be determined by accuracy or by our needs for the frequency of the data and the ease of retrieving these data. An automatic oscillometric device is usually chosen over manual auscultatory measurements for ease of acquisition and reproducibility. Two people taking auscultatory blood pressure measurements may hear the Korotkoff sounds at slightly different points and record different blood pressures. The required accuracy of a clinical monitor is determined by the smallest change in the measured variable that could affect a clinical decision. The requirements for "absolute accuracy" (is the measured value correct?) may be different from the requirements for "relative accuracy" (does the measured value follow trends?).

For example, a pulse oximeter estimates arterial hemoglobin oxygen saturation by measuring light absorbance. The pulse oximeter saturation estimate, Spo_2, is compared with the hemoglobin saturation determined from analysis of an arterial blood sample by a laboratory co-oximeter, Sao_2. Some errors are associated with arterial blood sampling and in vitro analysis of the sample by the co-oximeter. Nevertheless, the co-oximeter is considered to be the gold standard in this comparison of methods.

The pulse oximeter's saturation value can be compared with that of the co-oximeter by the determination of *bias* and *precision* (Fig. 30-2). Bias is the average difference between simultaneous values from the two methods, or the systematic error. If a pulse oximeter reads an average of 5% higher than the co-oximeter does, it has a bias of 5%, and we can adjust for that systematic error by recalibrating the device. Precision is the standard deviation of the difference between the two measurements, and it quantifies the random error, or "scatter." A higher value for precision indicates a larger random error. (This statistic may be more appropriately called "imprecision.") If the random error is too large, the device may not be clinically useful. We can adjust for systematic error (bias) by recalibration, but there is no way to adjust for random error.[2]

Signal Processing

Some physiologic values are constant over time, whereas others vary. When a measured value changes over time, it constitutes a signal. Many physiologic processes generate signals that cannot be perceived by our senses or are too small to measure directly. We must process and amplify these signals, a situation that introduces new problems. The first step in processing is to convert the raw physiologic variable (e.g., pressure, temperature, velocity) into

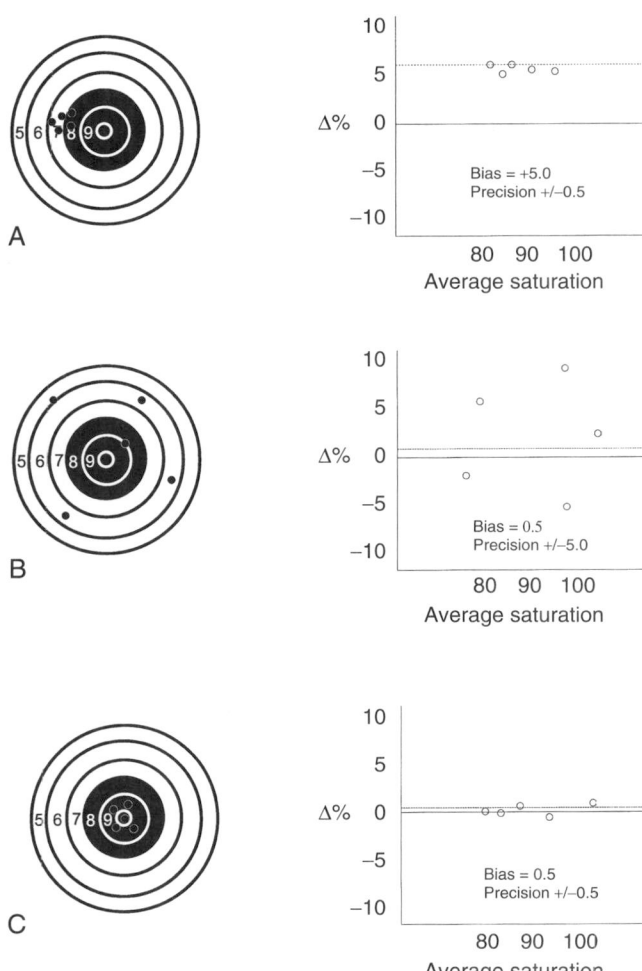

Figure 30–2 Accuracy and precision. The bias plot is a way to compare two different methods of measuring the same variable. Examples are plotted above on the right for saturation values, blood analysis versus pulse oximetry. It is a plot of the difference between the two measurements being compared versus the average of those two measurements. If one method constantly measures slightly higher than the other by a consistent value, it has a positive bias. If it has only slight variation around that bias, it is said to have very low random error (or precision, which equals the standard deviation of the differences) (**A**). **B**, The values are randomly scattered such that the average difference is near zero, but the precision value is very large. This large random error makes the device unusable because calibration will not improve this random error. **C**, The optimal device, that is, a bias near zero and a very small precision (standard deviation of the differences). No amount of calibrating or "sighting in" could cause **B** to become more accurate because the error is randomly scattered.

another form of energy, usually electrical. This conversion is accomplished by a *transducer* (Fig. 30-3). For example, a pressure transducer converts pressure (force/area) into an electrical signal, which can then be amplified and processed. The processed output is usually transmitted to a display device.

When an analog signal (e.g., voltage versus time) is amplified, both the background noise and the desired signal are amplified (Fig. 30-4). Various techniques can be used to enhance the signal-to-noise ratio. For instance,

most pulse oximeters assume that a patient's pulse rate is between 30 and 300 beats per minute. Therefore, the instrument filters out any pulsations that occur at frequencies below 30 or above 300 (see the section on alternating current, capacitors, and impedance). In some cases, a desired signal can be repeated and summated, and the accompanying random noise becomes a smaller fraction of the signal. Evoked potentials are an excellent example of this process. The evoked response signal for a single stimulus is actually much smaller than the random noise, but this signal is nearly identical after each stimulus. Therefore, by summing the potentials after many stimuli, we reinforce the evoked response signal but not the noise (Fig. 30-5).

Finally, the waveform of any periodic signal can be represented by a summation of sinusoidal waves, called a "Fourier series" (Fig. 30-6).[3] The component sine waves can be described by their frequency and amplitude (or power, which is proportional to the square of the amplitude). Thus, a waveform originally expressed as amplitude versus time is *transformed* into a plot of power versus frequency (Fig. 30-7). The resulting plot, called the "power spectrum," is a common form for displaying and interpreting some types of waveform data, such as the electroencephalogram (see Chapter 38).

When we monitor a patient, we measure physical quantities in a physiologic setting, and these measurements are subject to error and uncertainty. Our task as anesthesiologists is to understand both the physiologic and the physical limitations of these measurements, judge the potential for error, and make clinical decisions in the face of these uncertainties.

A new form of signal analysis has entered the realm of anesthesiology. Our recording of vital signs and patient data, first begun a century ago by Harvey Cushing,[4] is a primitive form of signal analysis. To quote Dr. Cushing[5]:

> In all serious or questionable cases the patient's pulse and blood-pressure, their usual rate and level having been previously taken under normal ward conditions, should be followed throughout the entire procedure, and the observations recorded on a plotted chart. Only in this way can we gain any idea of physiological disturbances—whether given manipulations are leading to shock, whether there is a fall of blood-pressure from loss of blood, whether the slowed pulse is due to compression, and so on.

The signal, whether an observed pupillary sign, palpated pulse, transduced pressure, or auscultated breath sound, was integrated by the anesthetist, interpreted (is this real or is it artifact?), and charted (data storage). Modern data recorders use the same principles. Additionally, data storage has become much more complex. Not only must the signal be transduced, but it must also be recorded, either in raw or in processed form (Fig. 30-8). This point is important because it introduces new possibilities in monitoring (trends, signals, feedback to user) and new pitfalls. Imagine an anesthesia record that would alert you to future potential physiologic issues from currently monitored data and predictive algorithms, that is, an intelligent anesthesia record. New problems are introduced

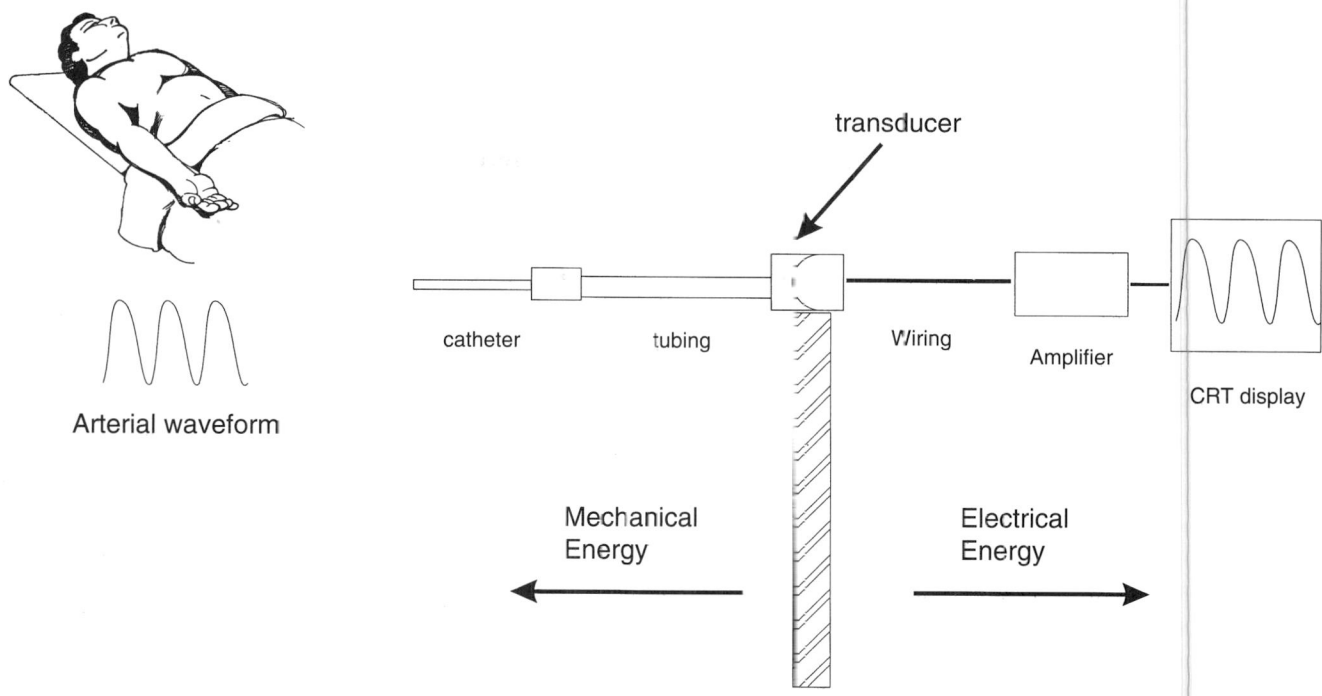

Figure 30–3 Transducer. A transducer changes a signal from one form of energy to another. A common transducer in anesthesia changes mechanical energy, such as an arterial pulse, into electrical energy. Microphones and speakers are also examples of transducers.

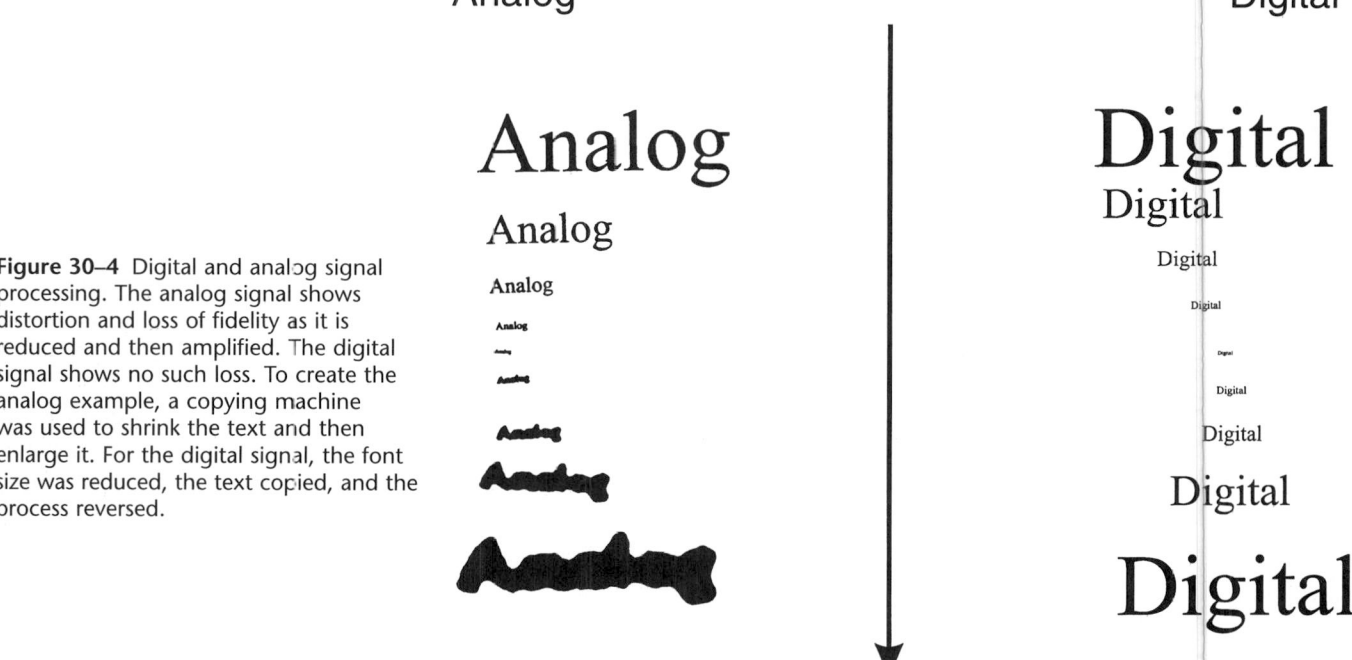

Figure 30–4 Digital and analog signal processing. The analog signal shows distortion and loss of fidelity as it is reduced and then amplified. The digital signal shows no such loss. To create the analog example, a copying machine was used to shrink the text and then enlarge it. For the digital signal, the font size was reduced, the text copied, and the process reversed.

signal and noise   pure noise

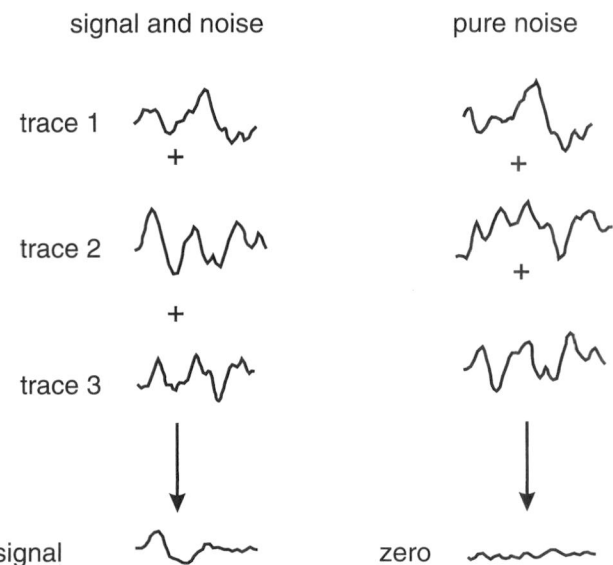

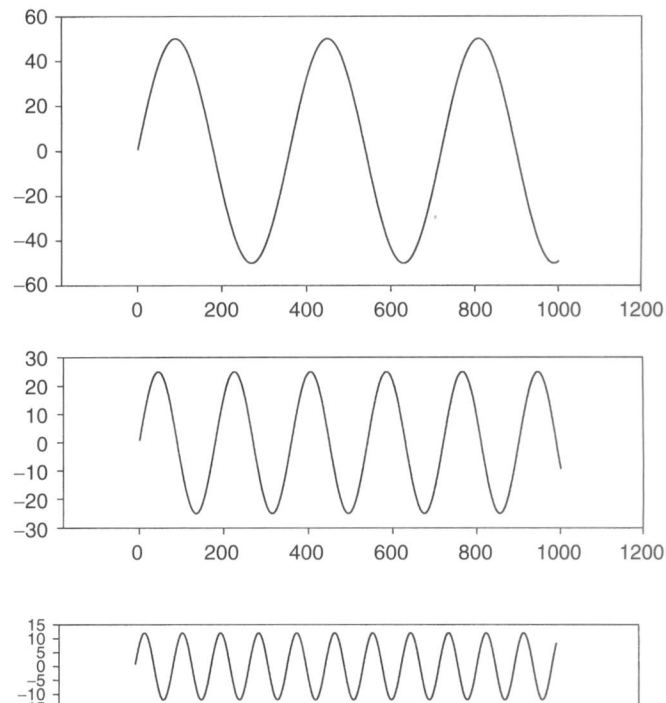

Figure 30–5 Somatosensory evoked potentials. A background signal can be separated from random noise by repeatedly adding the signals. The noise (random) is equally likely to be positive or negative; hence, adding positive and negative yields zero with multiple summations.

by such technology: security, potential loss of data (loss of not only a single chart or data point, but of all the charts), and erroneous signal processing.

PRESSURE MEASUREMENT

Principles of Pressure (Mass, Force, and Energy)

Many of our monitors are based on fundamental principles of the mechanics of solids and fluids, usually a derivation of F = ma. We discuss a few of these principles in this section and provide common examples of each.

Many of our monitors measure force, which is related to mass and acceleration as described by Equation 1, Newton's second law. The force may be generated by gravity, a beating heart, a compressed gas, or a contracting muscle. When we weigh a patient, we are determining the force exerted by gravity at the earth's surface on the patient's mass (m). This gravitational force (F_g) is related to mass by the formula

$$F_g = mg \qquad (2)$$

where g, the gravitational constant for acceleration, equals 9.8 N/kg (Fig. 30-9). Many anesthetic monitors measure pressure, which is force divided by the area of the surface on which that force is exerted. Pressure thus has dimensions of force/area, and its SI unit is the newton/meter^2, which is called the *pascal*. Because the pascal is a very small unit of pressure, we usually choose to use *kilopascal*, which equals 1000 Pa.

As noted earlier, kinetic energy is proportional to mass times velocity squared and is measured in kg-m^2/sec^2, or joules.

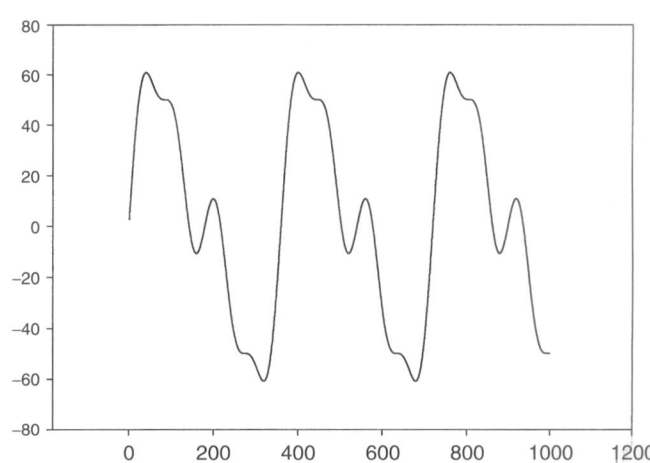

Figure 30–6 Fourier series. This pseudoarterial waveform was generated by adding the three sine waves with the following characteristics: y = 50 sin x, y = 25 sin 2x, y = 12 sin 4x.

If a force (F) acts on a mass (m) over a distance (d), we define *work* as the product of the force and distance: W = Fd. It can be shown from Equation 1 (using a little calculus; see Appendix 1 at the end of this chapter) that the work performed on a mass equals the change in its kinetic energy:

$$W = Fd = \Delta \tfrac{1}{2}(mv^2) \qquad (3)$$

Work has dimensions of force times distance and SI units of newton-meters. Because work and energy change are equivalent, 1 N-m must equal 1 kg-m^2/sec^2 = 1 joule (J). This equivalence of units can be verified by Equation 1.

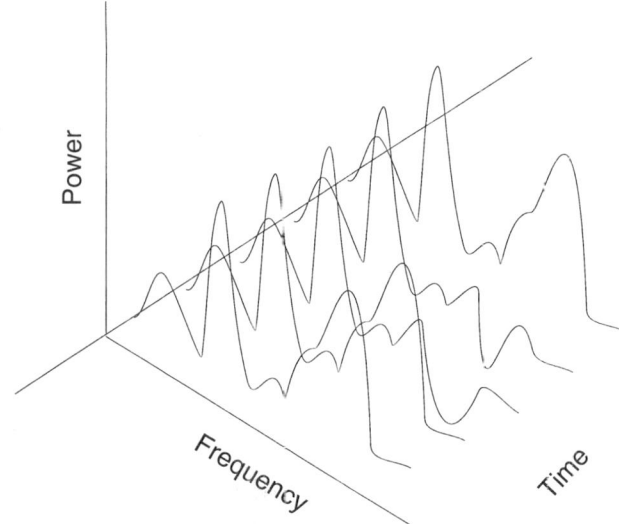

Figure 30–7 Spectral arrays. A compressed spectral array can display the frequency on the *x* axis and power on the *y* axis. A number of these arrays can be aligned with time as a third axis to give an indication of changes in power over time.

The relationship of work and energy leads to the concept of *potential energy*. If we lift mass (m) by a height (z) above the floor and let it fall, the force of gravity (F_g = mg) acts on the mass through the distance (z), thus doing work:

$$W = Fd = mgz \qquad (4)$$

At the end of its fall, the mass has a kinetic energy equal to the work performed, mgz (Equation 3). Therefore, we say that when the mass is raised to the height z above the floor, we have given it a potential energy equal to mgz. A 1-kg mass lifted 1 m off the floor has a potential energy of 9.8 J. This potential energy can be converted into the kinetic energy of motion simply by letting the mass fall. Potential energy can be stored in many other forms besides height (called "gravitational potential"), for example, a compressed spring, gas at high pressure in a tank, or the electrical potential of a battery (Fig. 30-10).

Energy is related to matter in one additional way through Einstein's famous equation $E = mc^2$. That is to say, matter and energy are the same "stuff." In the absolute sense, usually reserved for thermonuclear weapons, atomic reactors, and the sun, matter can be converted into energy,

Figure 30–8 Advanced signal processing. After a signal has been transduced (see Fig. 30-3) and initially processed (see Figs. 30-4 to 30-7), it can then be further analyzed, converted into data streams for transfer and storage, encoded for security, and linked to other signals for presentation to the user as information.

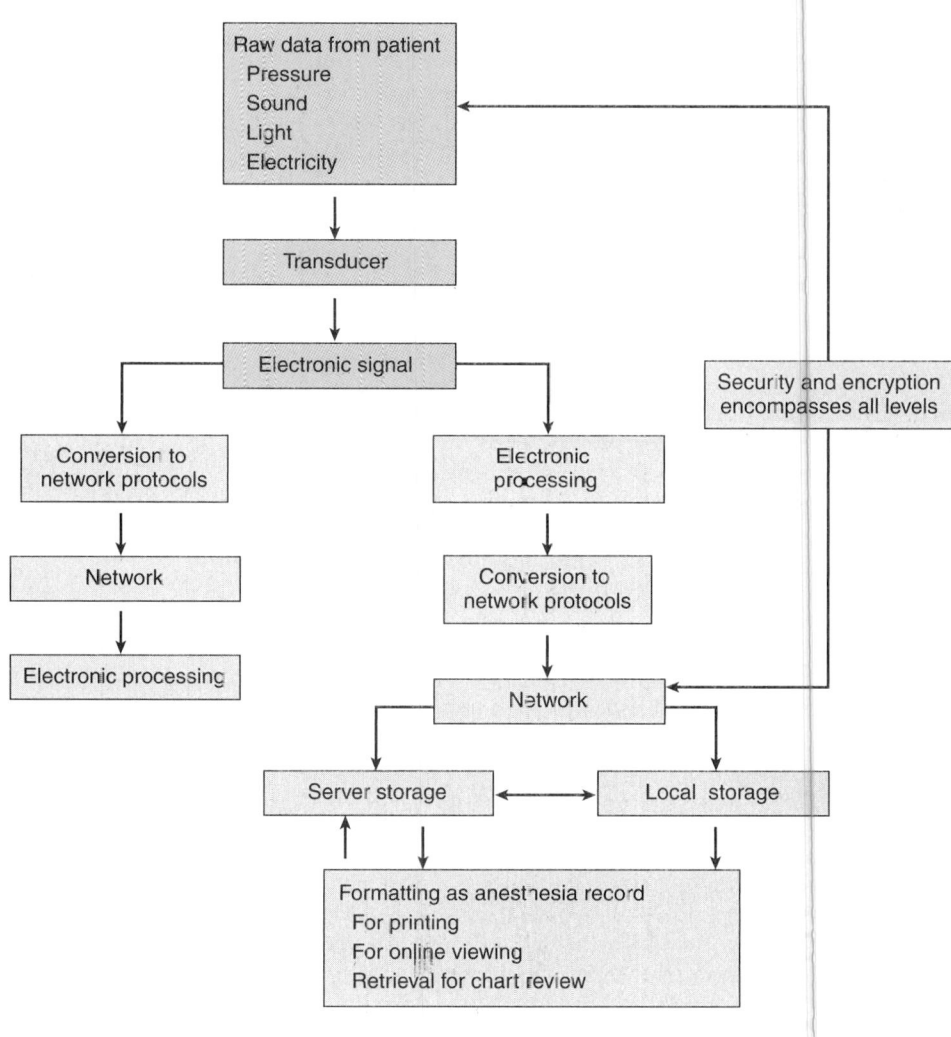

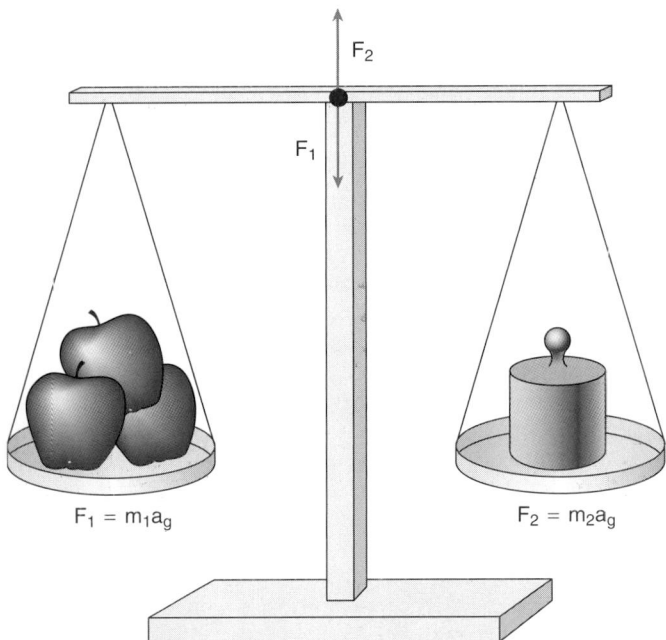

Figure 30–9 Balance. A scale is in balance when the forces are equal and in opposite directions. The force of gravity on the unknown mass of fruit is balanced by the known standard masses on the opposite side of the balance. $F_1 = F_2$, and hence $m_1 a_g = m_2 a_g$; because $a_g = a_g$, $m_1 = m_2$. a_g, acceleration caused by gravity.

and vice versa. If a 1-kg mass were completely converted to energy by means of $E = mc^2$, it would yield 8.987×10^{16} J (Table 30-1).

We have already defined power as the rate of change in energy per unit time. With the additional relationship between work and energy (Equation 3), it is clear that power is also the "rate of work," or the amount of work performed per unit time. Thus, the unit of power (1 W = 1 J/sec) can also be expressed as the newton-meter/second.

Static Pressure Measurement (Manometer)

We have defined pressure as the force acting on a surface per unit area. A *fluid* is defined as matter that continuously deforms (changes shape) as long as any stress (surface force) is applied to it. Fluids are subdivided into liquids, which are relatively incompressible, and gases, which are compressible.

Pressure exists and can be measured everywhere within a fluid, even when it is not in contact with a rigid surface. Although the SI unit of pressure is the pascal (or newton per meter squared), in medicine we more commonly use units such as millimeters of mercury (mm Hg) and centimeters of water (cm H_2O). How does a unit of length become a unit of pressure? This is the principle of the liquid manometer, the oldest method of pressure measurement. The manometer *balances* the pressure to be measured against the pressure exerted by a vertical column of liquid of known density, for example, mercury and water. The density of a fluid is its mass per unit volume, which has SI units of kilograms per cubic meter

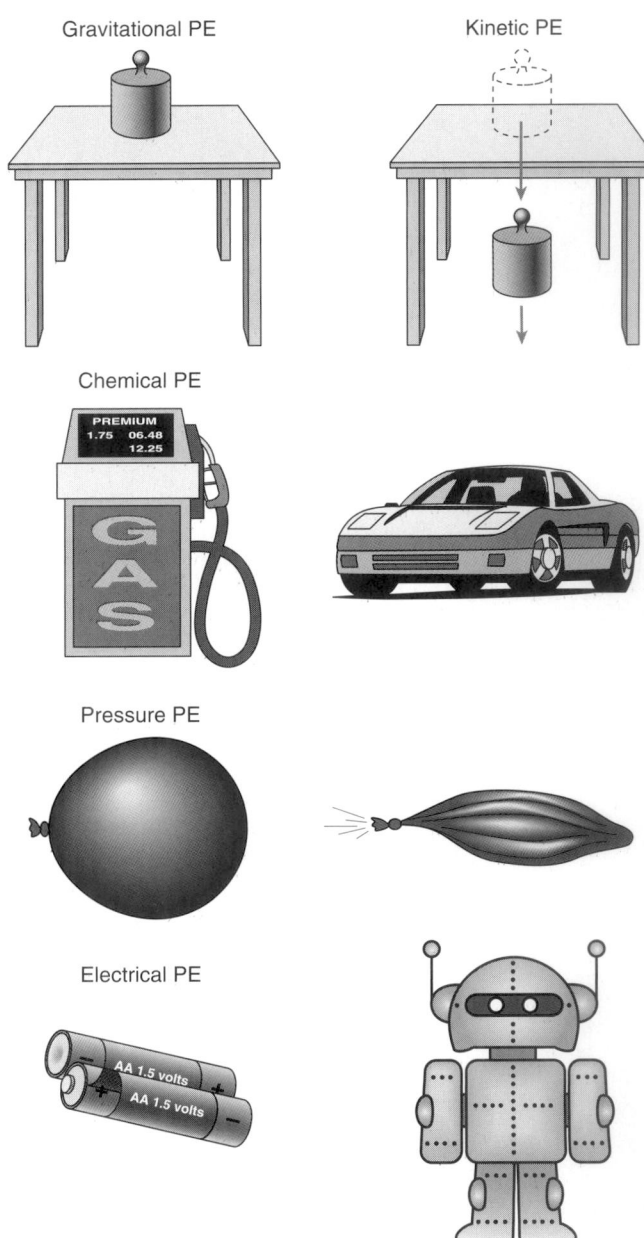

Figure 30–10 Potential energy and kinetic energy. Potential energy is stored energy that can be released or converted into kinetic energy, the energy of motion. Energy can be stored as gravitational, chemical, electrical, and other forms of potential energy.

(kg/m^3) or, commonly, grams per milliliter. The pressure exerted by a liquid column of height (z) and density (ρ) is simply ρgz (see Appendix 2 for derivation). If the manometer liquid is mercury, which has a density of 13,600 kg/m^3, the manometer pressure in pascals is

$$P \text{ (Pa)} = 13,600 \times 9.8 \times z \text{ (m)} = 1.333 \times 10^5 \times z \text{ (m)}$$

Because these large numbers are rather awkward, we express p in kilopascals (kPa) and z in millimeters of mercury (mm Hg):

$$P \text{ (kPa)} = 0.1333z \text{ (mm Hg)}$$

Table 30–1 Comparison of energy levels of common and uncommon events

Event	Energy
1-kg mass falling 1 m on Earth	9.8 J
Heartbeat	10 J (at rest, 60 beats/min, 10 W)
Internal defibrillation for ventricular fibrillation	30 J
Maximal output of a surface defibrillator	360 J
1 kcal	4186 J
Car battery	$1.8 \text{ MJ} = 1.8 \times 10^6 \text{ J}$
Kilogram of fat	$3.8 \times 10^7 \text{ J}$
Ton of TNT	$4.2 \times 10^9 \text{ J}$
Atomic bomb (Hiroshima)	15 kilotons = $15 \times 10^3 \times 4.2 \times 10^9 \text{ J} = 6.3 \times 10^{14} \text{ J}$
Hydrogen bomb	1 megaton = $4.2 \times 10^{15} \text{ J}$
1 kg converted completely to energy	$8.987 \times 10^{16} \text{ J}$
The sun (4.2×10^9 kg matter/sec)	3.8×10^{26} J/sec

Modified from Hecht E: Physics: Algebra/Trig. Pacific Grove, CA, Brooks/Cole, 1994.

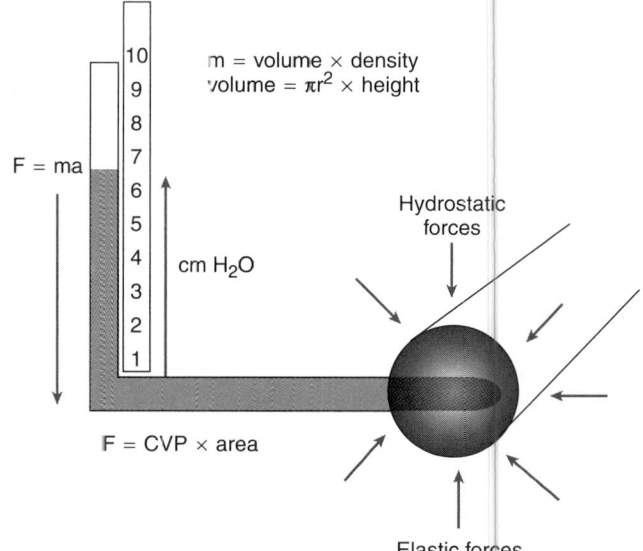

Figure 30–11 Manometer. A water manometer uses a balance of forces. In this case, downward pressure of the fluid, as determined by its density and height, balances the upward pressure of the central venous system caused by hydrostatic and elastic recoil forces.

A useful reference for the various pressure units in use today is the pressure of the earth's atmosphere at sea level, called "one atmosphere" or 1 atm:

$$1 \text{ atm} = 101.3 \text{ kPa}$$
$$= 760 \text{ mm Hg}$$
$$= 14.7 \text{ pounds/square inch (psi)}$$
$$= 988 \text{ cm H}_2\text{O}$$

For slowly changing pressures, a water or mercury manometer is simple and dependable (Fig 30–11). The manometer cannot respond quickly to rapid changes in pressure because of its inertia; that is, the mass of the liquid column resists rapid changes in height. If a fluid-filled catheter is connected to a patient, the height of the fluid in the manometer determines the mean pressure at the tip of the catheter. If the pressure measured is central venous pressure, we can use these data to infer right ventricular preload. Because this manometer is in direct continuity with the patient's circulation, the manometer fluid must be compatible with blood; that is, it must be iso-osmolar, as well as nontoxic.

Dynamic Pressure Measurement (Transducer)

Accurate measurement of a rapidly changing pressure, such as arterial blood pressure, is more difficult and complex. There are many characteristics of the pressure-versus-time waveform that we might wish to determine. Systolic, diastolic, and mean arterial pressure is given by the maximum, minimum, and average pressure values during the cardiac cycle (Fig. 30–12). In addition, we can measure the maximum upward slope of the waveform

during systole, which is related to the speed of ventricular ejection. An abnormally rapid downslope after aortic valve closure (indicated by the dicrotic notch) suggests possible aortic insufficiency. Thus, the details of the pressure-time waveform, as well as its maxima and minima, are potentially important to the clinician.

A modern pressure transducer is a device that changes either electrical resistance or capacitance in response to changes in pressure on a solid-state device. The variable transducer resistance is placed in an electrical circuit involving three known resistances (Wheatstone bridge; see Appendix 3), and the change in resistance is converted into electrical voltage. The moving part of the

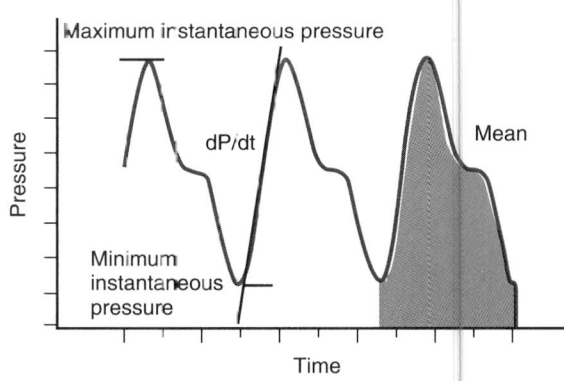

Figure 30–12 Arterial waveform. Systolic pressure is defined as the instantaneous maximal pressure; diastolic, the instantaneous minimal pressure; and mean, the average pressure over a cycle. dP/dT refers to the upstroke of the arterial pressure, that is, the rate of pressure generation. Mean pressure is estimated as diastolic plus one third the pulse pressure (systolic − diastolic) when only systolic and diastolic pressure is known.

transducer itself is very small and has little mass. However, it is not clinically or commercially practical to place the transducer in contact with arterial blood, so we use a liquid-filled tube to connect the intra-arterial catheter to the pressure transducer. This system of a fluctuating driving pressure (i.e., the arterial pressure being measured), a liquid-filled tube, and a pressure transducer is mechanically equivalent to the mass-spring harmonic oscillator shown in Figure 30-13. The mass (m) represents the mass of the fluid in the tubing. The spring represents the elasticity of the tubing. The damper, shown schematically as a piston moving in oil, represents the friction generated by the fluid moving to and fro in the tubing.

A more commonly encountered harmonic oscillator is that of a car driving down a bumpy dirt road (see Fig. 30-13). In this case, the oscillating driving pressure is provided by the bumps in the road, which force the car wheel to oscillate up and down. The car springs are analogous to the compliance of the arterial pressure tubing, and the car's shock absorbers, which oppose motion of the wheel in either direction, are analogous to the friction of the fluid moving back and forth in the fluid-filled tube. Depending on the frequency of the bumps (i.e., driving pressure frequency), the system can either suppress the bumpy road or may initiate dramatically increased oscillations. The frequency of the driving force that causes maximal amplification of the signal is called the natural

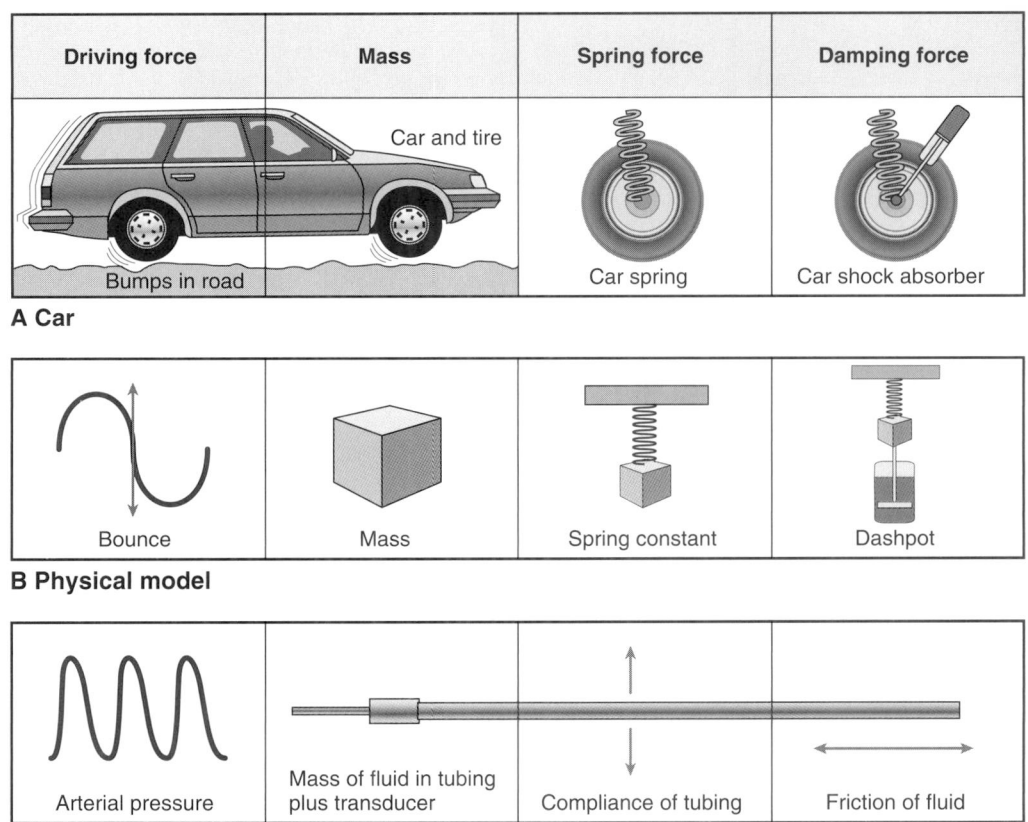

Figure 30–13 A to **C,** Damping and resonance. Pressure measured in an invasive arterial catheter can actually overshoot or amplify the real blood pressure. This phenomenon is referred to as the dynamic frequency response of the fluid-filled arterial line and transducer system. The phenomenon has a physical model that can generate an equation to predict the output pressure response, depending on the frequency of the input pressure and several physical parameters of the system. In the physical model on the *right,* driving pressure (arterial blood pressure) acts on a mass (the fluid within the arterial pressure tubing) by pushing it up and down against a spring, which stores energy (the compliant pressure tubing), and on a dash pot, which opposes motion in either direction (the resistance of the fluid as it moves to and fro within the pressure tubing). Depending on the input frequency, the output may undergo amplification as it reaches a specific frequency, known as the resonant frequency of the system. On the *left* side of the figure is a common phenomenon noted when a car drives along a bumpy dirt road. In this situation, the driving force is the bumps in the road, which act on the tire. The car spring is equivalent to compliance to the pressure tubing, and the shock absorber corresponds to the resistance of fluid moving back and forth in the arterial line. The mass of the fluid is analogous to the mass of the front of the car. You may have experienced the phenomenon: when you reach a certain speed as you are driving along a bumpy road, the front of the car starts to oscillate with increasing amplitude. If you speed up or slow down, this phenomenon disappears. The car bounces highest when you have reached the resonant frequency of this harmonic oscillator. See Appendix 4 for a detailed mathematical description of this process.

resonant frequency (Fig. 30-14). The degree of amplification is directly related to the mass and inversely related to the amount of friction present; for large amounts of friction, attenuation rather than amplification occurs (see Appendix 4).

To visualize this concept intuitively, hang a weight on the end of a rubber band while holding the upper end of the band in your hand. If you move your hand up and down slowly, the weight follows your hand movements almost exactly. As you increase the frequency of your hand oscillations, the weight begins to "lag" behind your hand, and the amplitude of the weight movement begins to increase. As you approach the natural frequency of this simple system, you will observe the phenomenon of "resonance" when the amplitude of the weight motion becomes very large. If you try different rubber bands and weights, you will find that stiffer bands or smaller weights yield higher natural frequencies. The same is true of our fluid-coupled pressure transducer system. Stiffer (i.e., less compliant) tubing or a shorter length of tubing (less mass) produces higher natural frequencies in this system; that is, it requires a much higher pulse rate before amplification.

To minimize the potential of amplification of the real arterial pressure, the system should have very noncompliant (i.e., stiff) tubing and the total mass of liquid in the system should also be minimized, which can be accomplished by having small-diameter tubing and as short a length as possible. In most clinical systems, the natural resonant frequency is 10 to 15 Hz, which is much higher than the primary frequency of the arterial waveform (the heart rate is 60 to 120 beats/min or 1 to 2 Hz). Unfortunately, the arterial waveform is not a sine wave, but is the more complex shape shown in Figure 30-6 and is made up of a summation of sine waves, a Fourier series. The higher-frequency components of the arterial waveform (higher harmonics) are the ones that are closer to the natural frequency and are therefore amplified. This is

why we see a "whip" in the waveform when the peak systolic pressure and the initial upstroke are amplified significantly above the true systolic pressure, even if the heart rate itself is not in the range of the resonant frequency. In theory, mean arterial pressure should be the same because this amplification of systolic pressure also produces a reduction in diastolic pressure (see Appendix 4).

These fast-responding pressure transducers are often used to measure both central venous pressure and pulmonary artery pressure. As such, they have a frequency response much greater than necessary to faithfully reproduce the actual signal. However, the clinical meaning and interpretation of measurements from pulmonary artery catheters have been under scrutiny for years.[6] A recent study[7] has shown no definitive benefit in patient outcomes from the use of pulmonary artery catheters. These "problems" with pulmonary artery catheters are not the result of physical flaws in the catheter or the transducer, but reside within the meaning of the information that we extract from the data.

Signal-Processed Pressure Measurement (Noninvasive Blood Pressure Monitor)

Systolic pressure can be estimated by noting return of the flow pulse after occlusion of the artery by a cuff. The return of flow can be detected by (1) simple palpation of the radial artery, (2) recording with a Doppler device over the radial artery, or (3) the use of a pulse oximeter. Most anesthesiologists are familiar with the loss of pulse oximeter signal when the noninvasive blood pressure monitor is cycling.

The automated noninvasive blood pressure monitoring devices used in most operating rooms make use of a more sophisticated application of this principle. These devices monitor the oscillating signal generated in the cuff by the arterial pressure changes. The cuff first inflates to above systolic pressure, at which point the signal and oscillations are abolished. Then the cuff slowly deflates in a stepwise fashion. The pressure at which the signal first appears is interpreted as the systolic pressure. The signal increases in amplitude as the cuff pressure decreases. The point at which the signal is at maximal amplitude is interpreted as mean arterial pressure. As cuff pressure decreases further, the oscillations drop off rapidly. Diastolic pressure is mathematically inferred from the systolic and mean values (Fig. 30-15).[8] Errors can be introduced in the same manner as for manual auscultation of Korotkoff sounds: too small or too large a cuff requires a higher or a lower pressure to occlude arterial flow, and stiff atherosclerotic arteries are resistant to compression. External compression caused by patient motion or the surgeon leaning on the noninvasive blood pressure monitoring cuff can cause oscillations in cuff pressure that are not related to arterial pressure and may result in an erroneous reading, most commonly a high diastolic pressure.

Mercury sphygmomanometers are being phased out of use in some countries and hospitals, which leads to questions regarding the accuracy and precision of alternative devices such as the aforementioned noninvasive automated blood pressure monitors and aneroid sphygmomanometers.[9,10]

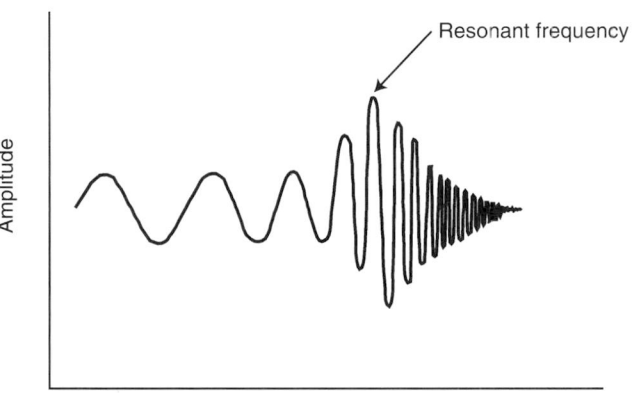

Figure 30–14 Amplitude and frequency. As the frequency increases, the amplification can increase to a maximum, and then the signal becomes attenuated. (Adapted from Sykes MK, Vickers MD, Hull CJ: Principles of Measurement and Monitoring in Anaesthesia and Intensive Care, 3rd ed. Oxford, Blackwell, 1991.)

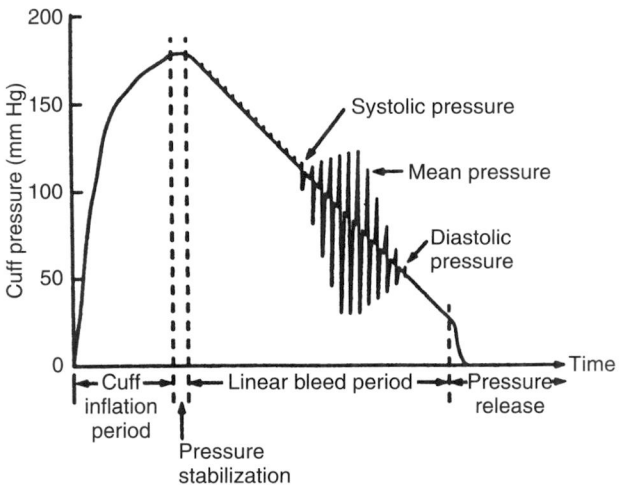

Figure 30–15 Noninvasive blood pressure measurement. Using the signal from the arterial pulse, oscillometric blood pressure measurements are obtained by determining the point at which the signal is first detected, its maximal amplitude, and the signal decay rate.[8] (Adapted from Ehrenwerth J, Eisenkraft J: Anesthesia Equipment: Principles and Applications. St Louis, Mosby–Year Book, 1993.)

FLOW MEASUREMENT

Principles of Flow

Pressure in fluids can be thought of as a form of potential energy, as described earlier. Kinetic energy in fluids is expressed in terms of *flow*, the bulk movement of fluid with a given direction and speed. We must carefully distinguish between fluid *flow* and fluid *velocity*, which are often confused. Flow ($\dot{Q}$) refers to the volume of fluid passing a particular location per unit of time; its SI units are meter cubed per second, but it is more commonly measured in milliliters per second or liters per minute. Fluid velocity (U) is simply the speed of the fluid at a particular point in space, measured in meters per second. By analogy, imagine a multilane freeway: the speed (velocity) of individual cars may vary depending on the lane; the flow is the number of cars passing a point per minute. The potential energy of pressure can be converted into the kinetic energy of flow; for example, the hydrostatic pressure generated by gravity acting on a vertical column of liquid can be transformed into flow by opening a valve at the bottom of the column. Pressure and flow can also change independently. With the human

circulatory system used as an example, a healthy young trauma patient can have relatively high blood pressure but low blood flow (hypovolemic shock) with high systemic resistance. On the other hand, a septic patient can have very low blood pressure accompanied by high blood flow (high-output septic shock). The total mechanical energy of a moving fluid is the sum of the kinetic (flow) energy and the potential (pressure) energy (Table 30-2) .

A pressure gradient exerts a force on the fluid, and the fluid tends to accelerate in the direction of *decreasing* pressure. Pressure gradient is only one of the forces that commonly act on fluids; other forces include gravity (discussed earlier) and viscous force or friction. If these other forces are negligible and the fluid is incompressible (i.e., a liquid with constant density), the equation of motion (F = ma) can be integrated to yield

$$P + \tfrac{1}{2}\rho U^2 = P_0 \qquad (5)$$

where P is pressure, ρ is fluid density, U is the magnitude of the fluid velocity, and P_0 is a constant called the *stagnation pressure* (see Appendix 5). This form of the *Bernoulli equation* tells us that as velocity increases in a frictionless flow, pressure decreases and vice versa. This concept resolves the common misconception that pressure always decreases in the direction of flow. For example, in the flow inside a tube (a pipe or a large vein) of gradually increasing diameter, fluid velocity (U) decreases in the downstream direction as the diameter and cross-sectional area of the tube increase. As U decreases, Equation 5 tells us that P actually increases in the direction of flow. This example again shows the relationship of potential and kinetic energy in fluids: as the kinetic energy of this tube flow decreases (U^2 falls) in the flow direction, the potential energy increases (P rises) by an equal amount. The total energy remains constant because we have assumed no friction.

Flow can be determined by knowing the average velocity of the fluid across the tube. In laminar flow, Figure 30-16A, the velocity profile is distributed such that the highest velocity is in the center and the fluid at the edges is virtually stationary. In turbulent flow, the velocity profile is "flattened" (Fig. 30-16B). Some monitors measure flow directly, but most measure flow indirectly, by either pressure or velocity measurements.

The Bernoulli equation applies to a specific subset of flow parameters as listed earlier. Many flows important to anesthesiologists do not follow the Bernoulli equation. Most commonly, the flow that we desire to measure is not laminar but turbulent. The transition from laminar

Table 30–2	Comparison of hydrodynamic and electrical energy commonly encountered	
Water	**Electricity**	**Energy**
Squirt gun	Static electric spark	High pressure, low flow, low energy
Garden hose	House current	Moderate pressure, moderate flow, moderate energy
	Car battery	Low pressure, moderate flow, moderate energy
River flood		Low pressure, huge flow, huge energy
Fire hose	High-tension wires	High pressure, high flow
	Lightning	High pressure, high flow

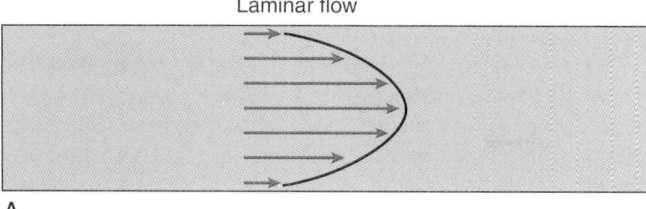

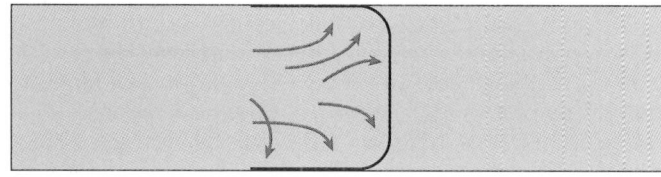

Figure 30–16 Laminar and turbulent flow. In a smooth-walled tube at low flow rates (i.e., small pressure gradients), the flow rate is laminar; that is, flow moves smoothly in concentric circles, with the centermost area having the greatest flow velocity and the area nearest the wall of the tube being virtually stationary. As the flow rate (and pressure gradient) increases, the flow transitions from laminar to turbulent. Instead of a neatly ordered flow, the velocities are more randomly distributed, energy is dissipated as heat, and the energy needed for a given flow rate increases. Many factors govern this transition, including size of the tube, viscosity of the fluid, flow rate, and pressure gradient. These factors are combined in determination of the Reynolds number (see Appendix 5).

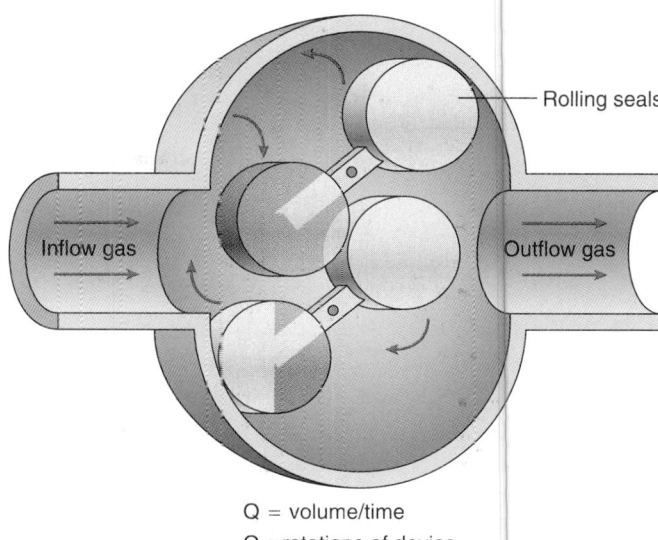

$$Q = \text{volume/time}$$
$$Q \propto \text{rotations of device}$$

Figure 30–17 Volumeter. Flow can be described as volume over time. This design of flow meter allows gas to pass only in little aliquots, each of which turns a counter to measure the amount flowing past. When divided by time, this method results in flow measurement. (Adapted from Ehrenwerth J, Eisenkraft J: Anesthesia Equipment: Principles and Applications. St Louis, Mosby–Year Book, 1993.)

to turbulent flow depends on the type of fluid and the shape of the flow. The fluid factors are summarized in the Reynolds number:

$$Re = \rho UD/\mu \qquad (6)$$

where ρ is the density of the fluid, U is the mean flow velocity, D is the diameter of the tube, and μ is the viscosity of the fluid. Thus, as the average speed of flow increases, the flow becomes more turbulent. In straight tubes, the change from laminar to turbulent flow occurs at an Re value greater than 2100 (see Appendix 5). Many flow meters require laminar flow for their measured values (pressure or velocity) to be accurately transformed into a flow measurement (e.g., Pitot tube; see later).

Mass/Volume Flow Meters (Urometer, Volumeter, Dilutional Measurements)

We can actually measure the mass or volume of fluid flowing per unit time by catching fluid in a container and either weighing it or measuring its volume. The common urometer for measuring urine volume is an example. The volumeter used in North American Drager anesthesia machines also measures aliquots of volume integrated over time to measure tidal and minute volume (Fig. 30-17).[11]

Both volume and mass flow can be measured by dilutional techniques. If some measurable indicator (a bolus of dye, a thermal pulse, oxygen consumption, carbon dioxide production) is injected into a flow and its concentration is

measured downstream, the volume flow ($\dot{Q}$) can be calculated by integration. The most common medical application is determination of cardiac output by the pulmonary artery thermodilution method (see Appendix 6). Errors associated with these methods involve using the wrong injectate volume (too small a volume resulting in too large a flow) or an error in temperature measurement (see the section on temperature).

"Continuous" cardiac output using an electric heating coil to warm the blood removes errors associated with fluid injectate techniques but introduces the need to average the smaller signal over a longer time base. Additionally, there is an upper limit to warming the blood, so signal quality is reduced in febrile patients.[12] The mass flow of carbon dioxide or oxygen can be used to measure cardiac output by the Fick equation and modifications (see Appendix 6). By using these variables, a change in metabolic rate can lead to errors in measurement.

Velocity/Flow Measurements (Venturi, Pitot, Doppler)

A Venturi tube is one with a very gradual contraction and expansion in the tube, in contrast to the sudden contraction of an orifice flow meter (Fig. 30-18) . Because the contraction is smooth and gradual, the Bernoulli equation (Equation 5) applies to this geometry. If we measure the pressure difference between the widest and the narrowest parts of the Venturi tube, we can solve the Bernoulli equation for velocity (see Appendix 5). The Venturi tube derives fluid velocity (U) from the pressure difference, not volume flow ($\dot{Q}$). In laminar flow, fluid velocity is proportional to flow. The Venturi tube is used in many industrial applications and is also used on some aircraft to measure speed.

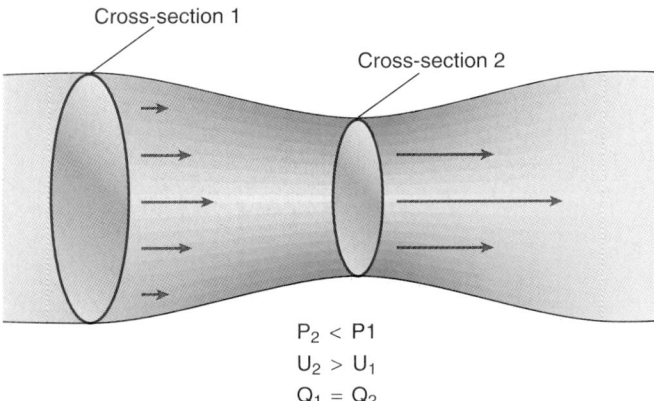

Figure 30–18 Venturi tube. By measuring the pressure difference between two points in a laminar flow, the average flow velocity can be determined because the mass flow must be the same (see Appendix 5).

A Pitot tube is a cylindric tube whose open end is pointed directly into the flow, that is, "upstream" (Fig. 30-19). The pressure measured in the Pitot tube is the *stagnation pressure*, given earlier by Equation 5. If we also measure the static pressure (p) (the p_1 side port in the figure) and we know the fluid density ρ, we can easily solve Equation 5 for the fluid velocity (U). Note again that the Pitot tube derives velocity (U), not volume flow ($\dot{Q}$). The Pitot tube is simple and reliable and is almost universally used on aircraft to measure their speed. In anesthesia, the Pitot tube is used in Datex Ultima monitors. To measure gas flow in two directions, the Datex monitor incorporates two Pitot tubes, one facing in each direction. Additionally, the monitor samples gas composition to correct for the density and viscosity of the gas mixture.

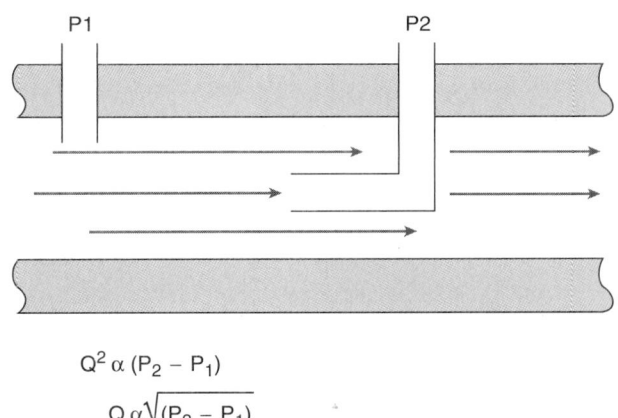

Figure 30–19 Pitot tube. As flows increase, wall pressure decreases as a result of the Bernoulli principle. The Pitot tube measures the difference in pressure from the middle of the flow to the wall and converts this difference to a flow measurement (see Appendix 5). (Adapted from Ehrenwerth J, Eisenkraft J: Anesthesia Equipment: Principles and Applications. St Louis, Mosby–Year Book, 1993.)

Balance-of-Pressure Flow Meters (Bourdon Tube, Thorpe Tube)

If flow in a tube passes through a sudden restriction such as an orifice, the volume flow ($\dot{Q}$) is proportional to the area of the orifice and the square root of the pressure drop through the orifice. (The Bernoulli Equation 5 does not apply to this flow geometry.) This is the principle of all orifice flow meters, including the floating bobbin rotameter of an anesthesia machine (see Appendix 5).

The most common flow meter seen by anesthesiologists is the rotameter on the anesthesia machine (Fig. 30-20). This variable-orifice flow meter uses a balance of forces to determine pressure change. When the flow meter valve is opened, the flow of gases through the annular orifice between the bobbin and the tapered glass tube provides a force to raise the bobbin. As the bobbin rises, the area of the annular gap between the bobbin and the tube increases as a result of the taper of the tube. As the area of this gap (orifice) increases, the pressure change across the bobbin decreases because the pressure change across an orifice is inversely proportional to the square of the orifice area. The bobbin ceases its upward motion at an equilibrium point when the downward force of gravity is balanced by the upward pressure forces. Thus, the height of the bobbin in the tube is proportional to the gas flow. Although this flow meter is simple in principle, its application becomes more complex when the flow in the tube changes from laminar to turbulent as velocity and diameter increase. For mathematical derivations, see Appendix 5.

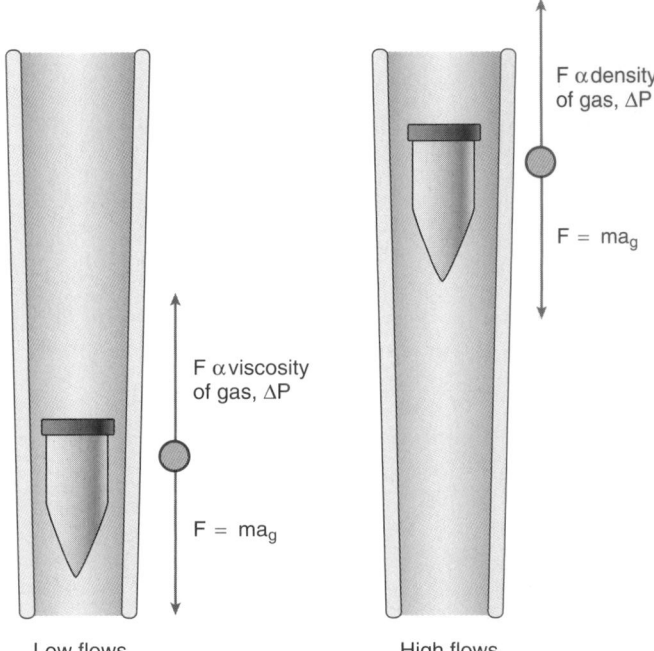

Figure 30–20 Thorpe tube flow meter. At low flows, the viscosity of gas predominates (acts like a tube), and the flows balance when the gravitational attraction equals the pressure gradient across the equivalent orifice. At higher flows, density takes over, and the balance is the same, except for the formula determining pressure (acts like an orifice) (see Appendix 5).

Another flow meter (Bourdon tube, Fig. 30-21) keeps the orifice constant and allows the pressure to vary. As flow ($\dot{Q}$) increases, the gradient of P_1 to P_2 increases and causes the flattened metal tube to uncoil and move the pointer.

Vane Spirometer Flow Meters (Wright Spirometer)

Vanes or propellers placed in a confined flow turn at a rate proportional to the volume flow if there is no friction in the propeller bearings. Various vane spirometers (Fig. 30-22) (e.g., Wright spirometer) work by this principle. These devices tend to be less accurate at both very high and low flow rates because of frictional forces.

Summary of Flow Measurement

Certain problems are associated with every method of measuring flow. Because not all gases are pure with a known, constant density, flow meters based on the Bernoulli Equation 5 are subject to errors. Furthermore, any device inserted into a fluid flow can disturb the flow by its presence. For example, a rotating vane spirometer may reduce the gas flow at high flow rates because of friction. Several methods of flow or fluid velocity measurement are dependent on a pressure measurement (Pitot tube, Venturi tube, orifice flow meter); hence, the flow measurement is no more accurate than the pressure measurement.

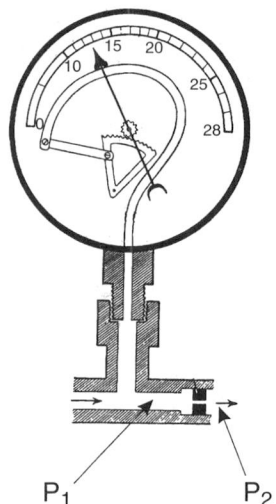

$$Q \propto P_1 - P_2 \propto \text{resistance} \propto r^4$$

Figure 30–21 Bourdon tube flow meter. Unlike the Thorpe tube, which has constant pressure but a variable orifice, the Bourdon tube has a constant orifice but variable pressure. The tube uncoils under the high backpressure. This drawback makes it unsuitable for use in low-pressure respiratory systems. However, it receives much use in portable oxygen tanks. Of note, if the orifice is increased in radius, the flow meter will under-read actual flow. If dirty (i.e., decreased radius), the flow will be overestimated. (From Mushin WW, Jones PL: Physics for the Anaesthetist, 4th ed. Oxford, Blackwell, 1987.)

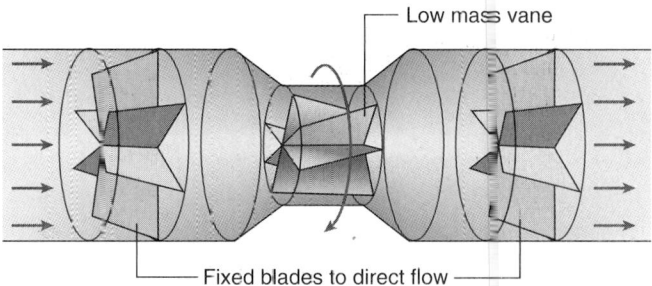

$$Q \propto \text{momentum (mV)}$$

Figure 30–22 Vane spirometer. Moving gases contain kinetic energy, which can be sampled by a rotating "windmill" in the gas stream.[13] (Adapted from Ehrenwerth J, Eisenkraft J: Anesthesia Equipment: Principles and Application. St Louis, Mosby–Year Book, 1993.)

MEASUREMENT USING SOUND

Principles of Sound

Sound waves are small fluctuations in pressure, density, and velocity that can propagate through matter of any form: solid, liquid, or gas. Unlike electromagnetic waves such as light (see the section on light), sound cannot propagate through a vacuum. Sound is called a *longitudinal wave* because the motion of the particles occurs in the same direction as wave propagation. In contrast, waves on the surface of the ocean are *transverse waves* because the motion of the particles is mainly perpendicular to the direction of wave propagation (Fig. 30-23).

In 1842, Christian Johann Doppler first described the apparent change in pitch of a sound that occurred when either the source of the sound or the listener was moving.[14] This Doppler effect now has several applications in patient monitoring, including precordial and esophageal Doppler ultrasound monitoring of local blood velocities or cardiac output.

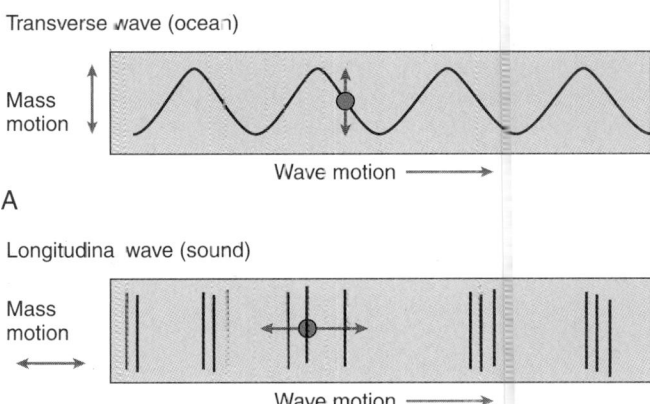

Figure 30–23 Transverse (**A**) and longitudinal (**B**) waves. In transverse waves (e.g., ocean waves), the particles move perpendicular to the motion of the wave. In longitudinal waves (e.g., sound waves), the particles move back and forth in the direction of the wave. The actual matter in either wave does not move much. The energy transfers without mass transfer.

When a sound source is moving toward the listener, the apparent pitch increases, and vice versa. The amount of frequency shift depends on whether the listener or the sound source is moving (Fig. 30-24; see Appendix 7). Because changes in the frequency of sine waves can be measured precisely, the Doppler principle provides a very accurate method of measuring the velocity of moving sound reflectors. At the high frequencies often used ($\geq$5 MHz), objects as small as red corpuscles can scatter enough sound for detection.

Sound has been used for many years in medical diagnosis and monitoring. It can be used as a diagnostic method in two ways: passive and active. In a passive examination, the sounds generated by the patient are studied. The basic examination of this type uses the stethoscope. In an "active" examination, acoustic energy is transmitted into the patient, and the resulting interaction of this energy with the patient is analyzed for information. Both types of examination use the same physics principles.

Passive Sound Examination (Stethoscope)

Vibrations, such as those caused by the closing and opening of heart valves or air moving through the respiratory passages, travel through the body as sound waves. Sound is generally conducted better and more rapidly in liquids than in gases. Thus, bronchial breath sounds are heard better when the bronchi are surrounded by lung consolidation. When sound waves reach a sudden change in density, some of the energy is reflected.

Some simple facts about sound waves can facilitate an understanding of the reflection and scattering process in the body. First, all sound waves can be represented as a summation of sinusoidal waves of various frequencies and amplitudes. This process of Fourier or power spectral analysis has been discussed earlier in this chapter. A note from a musical instrument thus consists of a sine wave at the "fundamental frequency" plus many "harmonics." The fundamental is the frequency that describes the pitch of the tone: middle C is standardized at 256 Hz, for example. Harmonics are sine waves at frequencies that are multiples of the fundamental frequency.

Fortunately for our ears, all of these many frequencies propagate at the same speed, the speed of sound (called "a"). For ideal gases, the speed of sound is proportional to the square root of temperature. The speed of sound in air at room temperature is 344 m/sec, or 1129 ft/sec or

770 miles/hr (mph). At an altitude of 13,000 m (40,000 ft), where the standard temperature is –57°C, the speed of sound is only 295 m/sec, or 661 mph. The speed of sound is much higher in liquids than gases. For example, the speed of sound through water at 15°C is 1450 m/sec. This value approximates the speed of sound through most of the solid parts of the body. In solids, the speed of sound varies greatly, with a range of 54 m/sec in rubber to 6000 m/sec in granite. Reflection of sound occurs at interfaces where the product of the tissue density and the speed of sound ($\rho \times a$) changes suddenly. Larger changes in this "acoustic impedance" result in greater reflection and less transmission. In the human body, the largest changes in acoustic impedance occur at gas-tissue boundaries: the lungs and the gastrointestinal tract. Reflection of sound thus makes it difficult to auscultate heart tones through an air-filled, emphysematous chest. For the same reason, a transthoracic echocardiograph provides less detail than the transesophageal technique does; in the former case, the lungs are in the way.

The first attempts to gather information about the inside of the patient by using sound involved placing one's ear directly on the patient. Although this procedure had many limitations, it led to development of the modern stethoscope, which is based on the physical principles of sound transmission. The stethoscope uses a large diaphragm to transmit and concentrate the sound energy. The bell acts as both an amplifier and a low-pass filter to transmit low-frequency diastolic rumbles. The physics of stethoscopy were described in depth by Rappaport and Sprague.[15]

In a simple stethoscopic examination, errors are introduced by "signal processing," that is, lack of appropriate knowledge on the part of the listener. Because it is a nonpowered, nontechnologic device (the energy levels come from the phenomena themselves), an esophageal or precordial stethoscope has additional value in being a continuous monitor during power outages. Physical limits to the technique include air space disease (in itself an informational finding), inability to place the monitor appropriately, and lack of quantifiable data.

Active Sound Examination (Percussion, Echo, Doppler)

The earliest "active" acoustic diagnostic technique was percussion of the chest wall. A skilled clinician can use

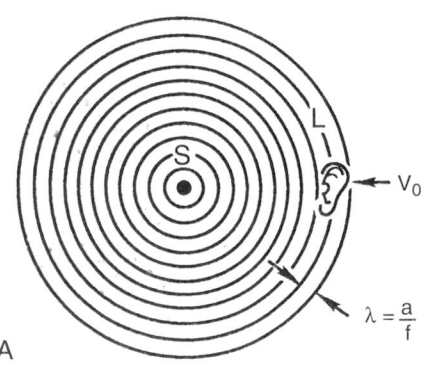 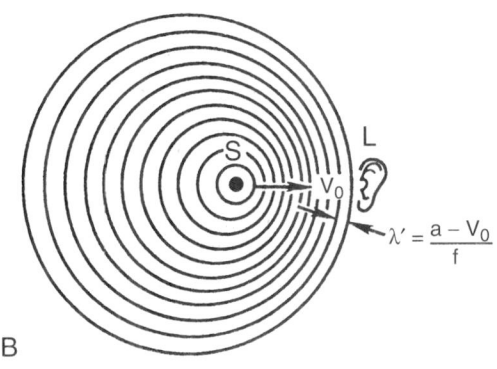

Figure 30–24 Doppler effect. **A,** When a listener is moving toward a stationary sound source, the frequency increases because the listener traverses more waves per unit time than a stationary listener does. **B,** When a sound source is moving toward a stationary listener, the wave fronts "stack up," thereby causing an apparent increased frequency.

$$\lambda = \frac{a}{f}$$

$$\lambda' = \frac{a - V_0}{f}$$

this method to detect consolidation of the lungs, pleural effusion, and a few other chest pathologies. Though based on transmission and reflection of sound, percussion is purely qualitative and is unable to accurately localize pathologic changes. Modern ultrasound improves on percussion by using shorter-wavelength sound waves and quantitative detection of their reflections (echoes).

The resolution of an examination is limited by the wavelength of the sound used (Fig. 30-25). Using ultrasound at frequencies in the megahertz (10^6 cycles/sec) range allows resolution of much smaller objects. The wavelength of 1.0-MHz sound waves in solid tissue is about 1.5 mm, whereas the wavelength of a 256-Hz tone (middle C) in tissue is 5.7 m.

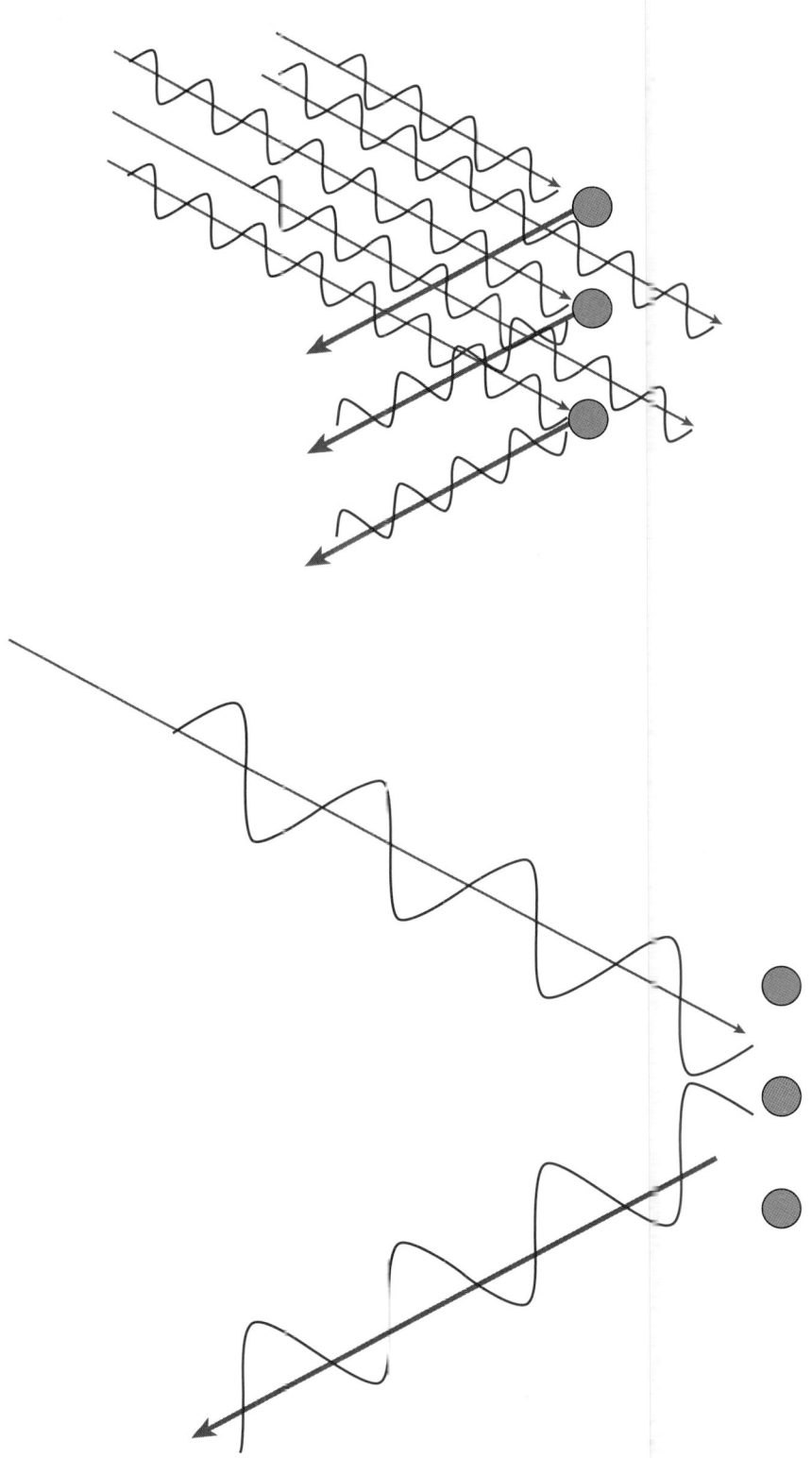

Figure 30–25 Wave size and resolution. Wave reflection depends on the relative size of waves and objects. For small objects, small waves are needed for good reflection and resolution. **A,** The object size is large relative to the wave size, which results in good spatial resolution. **B,** The object size is small relative to the wavelength, which leads to poor resolution of the objects. This principle applies to light waves also. Hence, electron microscopes can resolve smaller objects than light microscopes can because the wavelengths used are smaller. Imagine running an unsharpened pencil over a fine (1-mm grid) or coarse (1-cm grid) screen. The pencil sticks in the larger holes while passing over the smaller ones. Sharpening the pencil to a point improves the resolution.

With the use of esophageal transducers, echocardiography has become a popular intraoperative monitoring technique.[16,17] Sound waves in the 2- to 10-MHz range are transmitted toward the heart in short bursts or pulses. After each pulse, the transducer passively listens to the reflected echoes from various tissues. The ability to place the transducer in the esophagus is advantageous because sound does not then have to pass through air spaces or bone on its way to and from the heart. The speed of sound through the heart and surrounding soft tissues is a nearly constant 1540 m/sec. Thus, the elapsed time between transmission of the pulse and receipt of the echo provides the distance to the reflecting structure. The sound beam from the transducer is projected in a narrow "searchlight" pattern, so the exact direction of reflecting structures is also known.

The Doppler effect is used in echocardiography to determine the presence and degree of valvular regurgitation by converting the Doppler shift of sound waves reflected from erythrocytes into a color display (see Appendix 7; also see Chapter 33). Cardiac output has been estimated from descending thoracic aortic blood velocity by using a Doppler technique. These devices estimate the blood flow in the descending aorta and ignore flow to the head and arms. They calibrate descending aortic flow to cardiac output by assuming a constant proportional relationship between the two flows.

MEASUREMENT USING ELECTRICITY

Principles of Electricity

Most of our monitors and other anesthesiology apparatus use the basic principles of electricity and magnetism. Nearly all of our transducers use some form of electrical energy as their output, and the subsequent data processing and display are entirely electrical. We review some of the principles in this section by using examples from medical equipment.

Static Electricity

Electricity is a manifestation of a property called *charge* that is inherent in matter. The charge can be negative, positive, or neutral. Static electricity involves charges at rest: like charges repel one another, whereas opposite charges attract. What we usually mean by the word "electricity" involves the flow of charges, or the electrical *current*. Current flows in one direction in "direct-current" (DC) electronic devices and alternates back and forth in "alternating-current" (AC) devices.

The SI unit of charge is the *coulomb*, and the smallest quantum of charge is the charge of an electron, which is equal but opposite the charge of a proton. An *electrostatic* force is exerted between two charged objects and is directly proportional to the product of the two charges and inversely proportional to the square of the distance between them:

$$F = k \times q_1 \times q_2/r^2 \text{—Coulomb's law} \qquad (7)$$

This force is attractive when the charges are of opposite sign and repulsive when they are of the same sign.

In a Nobel Prize–winning experiment, Robert Millikan determined the charge of an electron by suspending charged oil drops between two horizontal charged plates such that the electrostatic force balanced the gravitational force and the drops were held in midair (Fig. 30-26). Approximately 20 years later, his son, Glen Allen Millikan, developed one of the earliest infrared ear oximeters, the forerunner of the pulse oximeter (see the section on the pulse oximeter).

Direct Current

Just as mechanical energy may be stored as potential energy, electrical energy can be stored as a *potential difference*. A common analogy is to compare electrical potential difference with water pressure (Fig. 30-27, see Table 30-2). The potential difference (V) between points A and B is defined as the work required to move a unit charge from A to B (see the discussion of the relationship of work and energy, earlier in this chapter). The SI unit of potential difference is the *volt*; hence, the term voltage is often used for potential difference. Charges can move easily through *conductors*, but they do not move well through *insulators*, also called *dielectrics*. If a potential (V) exists between A and B and these two points are connected by a conductor, charges will flow between them and produce a current (I).

The SI unit of current is the coulomb per second, called the *ampere*. If A and B are separated by an insulator, no current will flow until the potential difference becomes so great that a breakdown of the insulator occurs. For example, if A and B are separated by dry air, no current will flow until the potential difference reaches 3000 V/mm. At this potential gradient, air suddenly becomes a conductor, and a current flows in the form of a visible (and audible) spark. To generate a spark between two electrodes 1 cm apart, one must create a potential difference of 30,000 V. Lightning is a larger manifestation of the same phenomenon.

A battery is a chemical cell that produces a constant potential difference between two electrodes, which is called *electromotive force* (EMF). The battery can provide a continuous source of electrons, or current, to flow through

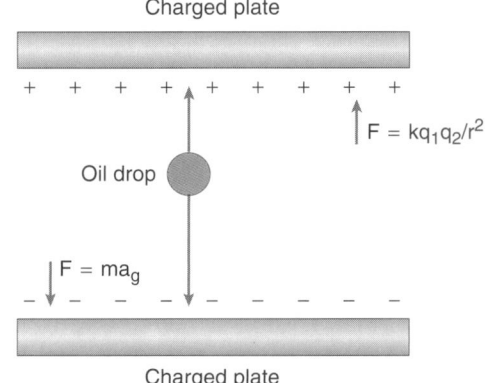

Figure 30–26 Electric force. The quantity of charge on an electron was determined by balancing the electric force on an oil drop against the gravitational force on the same drop. $F_1 = kq_1q_2/r^2 = F_2 = m_1a_g$.

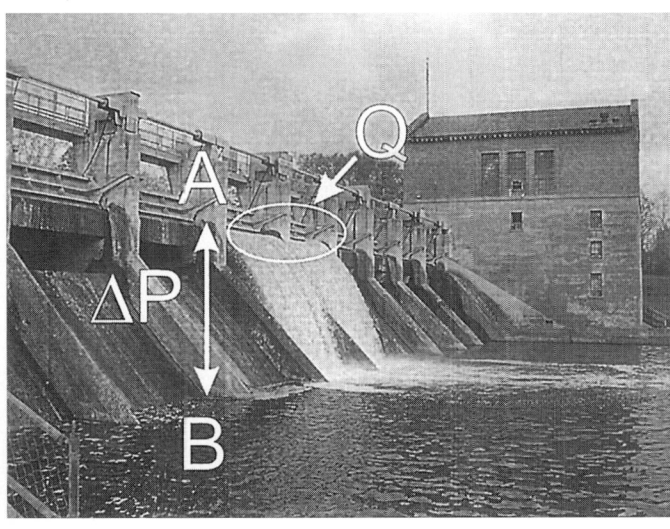
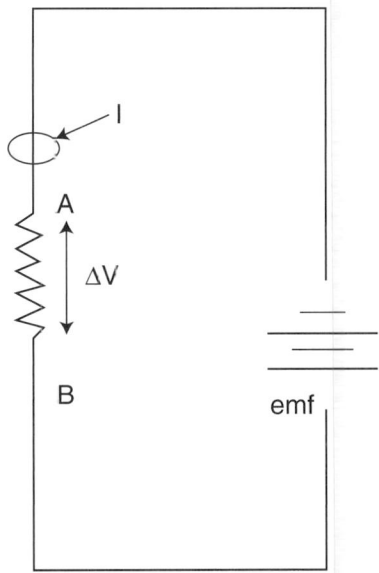

Figure 30–27 Water and electricity. The pressure drop over the dam (A to B) is analogous to the voltage drop over the resistance (A to B) (e.g., light bulb). The amount of flow (width of water) (Q) is analogous to the current (I). Both falling water and electrical potential can do work, as evidenced by the use of dams to generate electricity and electricity to pump water.

any conducting circuit connected between its electrodes. Flow of electricity is opposed by *resistance,* analogous to resistance in water pipes. In most materials, resistance (R) is related to voltage (V) and current flow (I) in the following manner:

$$V = IR\text{—Ohm's law} \qquad (8)$$

This relationship is called Ohm's law, and materials that follow this behavior are called ohmic materials. This example is analogous to hemodynamic flow, in which the pressure drop (mean arterial pressure – central venous pressure) equals cardiac output times systemic vascular resistance.

$$\Delta P = CO \times SVR \qquad (9)$$

The power (i.e., rate of work, see discussion earlier in this chapter) required to drive an electric current is the product of voltage and current: P = VI. By combining this formula with Ohm's law (V = IR), we have $P = I^2R = V^2/R$. Thus, if we double the current through a fixed resistance (R), we use four times the original power. This power loss in resistors is dissipated as heat, which is the reason why nearly all electrical devices become warm during use.

A *capacitor* is a device that stores charge (Q) in direct proportion to the potential difference (V) between its two electrodes: Q = CV. The proportionality constant (C) is called *capacitance,* which is measured in SI units of *farads.* When a capacitor is connected to a battery, current flows until the capacitor is charged to the point that the potential across the capacitor equals the EMF of the battery: V = Q/C = EMF (Fig. 30-28). When we push the "charge" button of a defibrillator, this kind of circuit is activated to charge a capacitor to the desired level. As shown in Figure 30-28B, time is required to charge a capacitor.

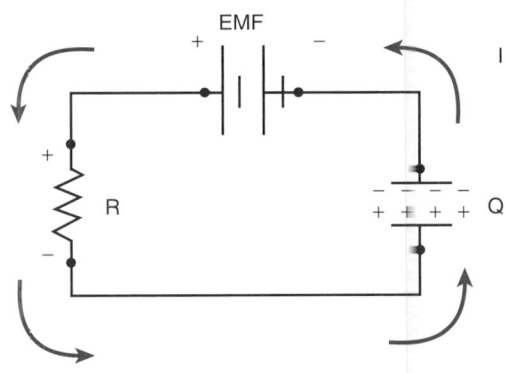

DC current, charge and voltage vs. time

A

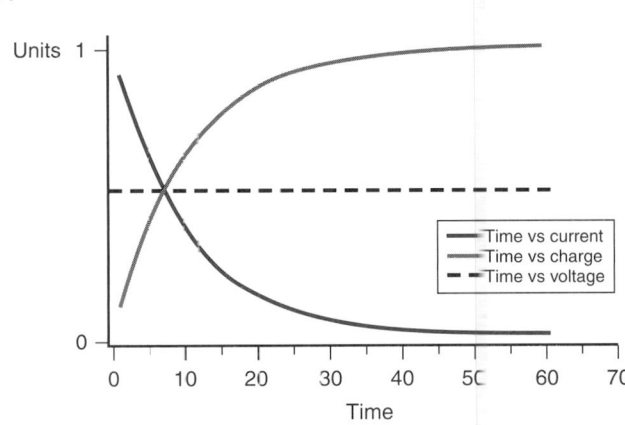

B

Figure 30–28 Resistance and capacitance in a direct-current circuit. **A,** Under direct current, the resistance impedes flow, with a voltage drop developing across the resistance. The capacitor allows current to flow until the charge builds on the capacitor (**B**). Under direct current, the voltage is constant over time, and the current flow decreases as the charge on the capacitor increases. This type of circuit is used to charge a defibrillator.

For a large capacitor, more time is required. Hence, it takes longer to charge a defibrillator to 200 J than to 50 J.

Alternating Current

In an AC circuit, the current and the voltage fluctuate rapidly (Fig. 30-29). There are many important differences between AC and DC power. The voltage in common AC house power fluctuates sinusoidally at a frequency of 60 Hz (50 Hz in Europe). We characterize the amplitude of such a fluctuating voltage by calculating its root mean square (RMS), that is, the square root of the time average of V^2. Thus, for AC house power, $V_{RMS} = 115$ V (230 V in Europe). Current in an AC system is also constantly changing and is likewise measured as an RMS value.

AC circuits have three forms of *impedance:* resistance (R), capacitance (C), and *inductance* (L). An inductor is a circuit element whose impedance increases with the frequency (f) of the current fluctuations ($R = 2\pi i f L$). Conversely, the impedance of a capacitor decreases with increasing frequency ($R = 1/2\pi i f C$). Inductors thus tend to block high frequencies, whereas capacitors tend to block low frequencies (Fig. 30-30). This principle is used in stereo systems to direct the signal to either the woofer (low-frequency) speaker or the tweeter (high-frequency) speaker. In medical

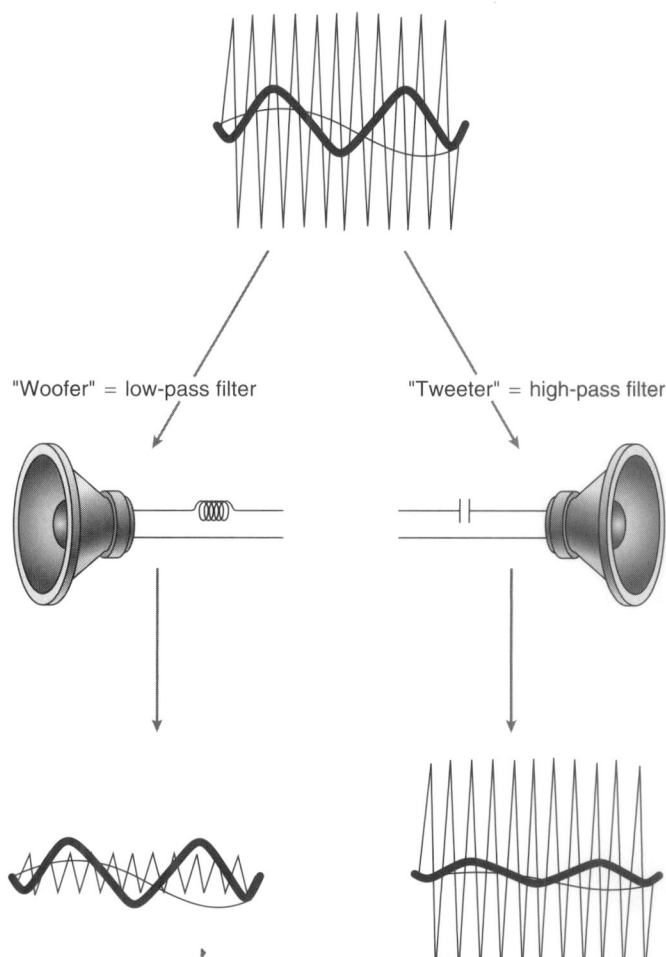

"Woofer" = low-pass filter

"Tweeter" = high-pass filter

Figure 30–30 Woofer and tweeter. Stereo speakers use resistors to act as impedance to the high-frequency components of sound, and only the bass frequencies are allowed to pass to the woofer speaker. Capacitors are used as a high-pass filter to allow only the high frequencies to get to the tweeter. The 60-Hz interference from electrical appliances can be decreased by a similar process. (From Hecht E: Physics: Algebra/Trig. Pacific Grove, CA, Brooks/Cole, 1994.)

instruments, inductance and capacitance circuits can be used to "filter" the signal, for example, decreasing the amount of 60-Hz interference from AC wiring.

Passive Electrical Examination (Electrocardiograph, Electroencephalograph)

Electrocardiograph

Now that some of the basics of electricity have been described, we can discuss the electrocardiograph (ECG) and the electroencephalograph (EEG), where the sources of EMF are the heart and the brain. Electrical potentials on biologic surfaces are too small to observe directly and must be amplified and processed before display. ECG potentials on the skin are in the 1-mV range, and EEG potentials are near 0.1 mV.

Figure 30-31 illustrates why electrical potentials on biologic surfaces are so small. The heart generates an electrical

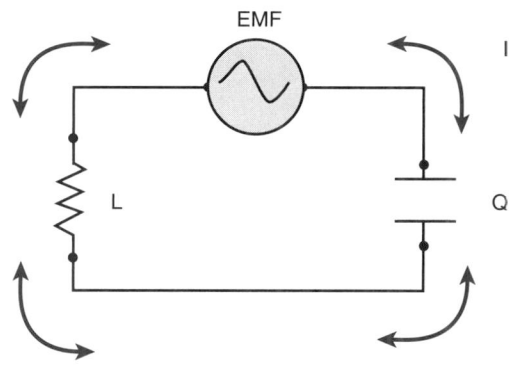

AC current, charge and voltage vs. time

A

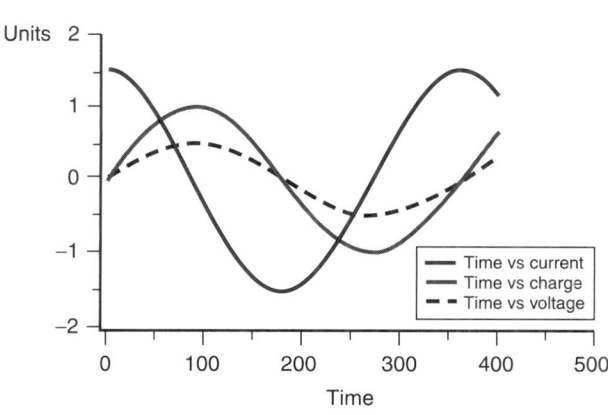

B

Figure 30–29 Resistance and capacitance in an alternating-current (AC) circuit. In an AC circuit (**A**), unlike a direct-current circuit, the capacitor does not block current flow. The capacitor and resistance act to shift the phase of the AC current. Current changes lag behind voltage changes (**B**).

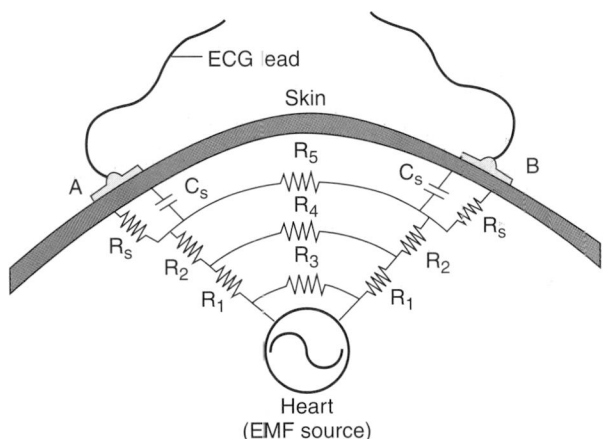

Figure 30–31 Why electrocardiographic potentials are so small. Multiple resistances and capacitances in the body decrease the potential and distort the waveform before the electromotive force reaches the surface.

signal as a result of the synchronous depolarization and repolarization of multiple cells. The electrical potentials generated by the heart are measured by two skin electrodes, A and B. As the figure shows, there are multiple effective resistances and capacitances in the tissues between the EMF source and the measuring electrodes. These impedances lower the magnitude of the voltage signal at the skin. The "shunt" resistors R_3, R_4, and R_5 combined with the "series" resistors R_1, R_2, and R_3 form what is called a *voltage divider network*. Lower values of shunt resistance or higher values of series resistance result in smaller voltages at the skin. The capacitance of the skin (C_s) also acts to attenuate the low-frequency components and distort the waveform. Skin resistance, which may be a megaohm (10^6 ohms) for dry skin, can be reduced to a few hundred ohms by conductive gels.

If a DC voltage is applied between two body surface electrodes, current flows through the tissues between them. Although the electrical current in metals consists entirely of electron flow, in tissues, both positive and negative ions migrate. Negative ions tend to accumulate at the positive electrode (the anode), and positive ions accumulate at the negative electrode (the cathode). This collection of anions and cations near each electrode creates its own EMF, and this force opposes the EMF that set up the original current. The current therefore decreases, so the effective impedance between the electrodes increases. This phenomenon, called *polarization of electrodes,* has two harmful effects. First, the increased impedance from polarization can attenuate the ECG signal for several seconds after defibrillation or DC cardioversion. Such attenuation could be misinterpreted as a lack of electrical activity and result in inappropriate administration of a second shock. The second consequence of prolonged application of DC voltage is accumulation of a local concentration of toxic ions near electrode sites, a condition that can cause burns or tissue necrosis. A partial solution to the problem is the use of a nonpolarizable electrode, such as a silver and silver chloride combination. This electrode can act as a source of, or "sink," for both anions and cations, thereby minimizing the accumulation

of ions. Most disposable ECG electrodes now use such materials. Even these electrodes, however, are nonpolarizable for only a limited time, and the application of prolonged DC voltage between any tissue electrodes must be avoided.

Electroencephalograph

Similar problems complicate measurements of the EEG, but in this case, the signal is only one tenth the amplitude: 100 μV versus 1 mV for the ECG. The spontaneous surface EEG provides eight or more channels of amplitude (surface voltage)-versus-time data, which is of limited use for monitoring in the operating room. For rapid interpretation and diagnosis, the amplitude-versus-time data are usually transformed into plots of amplitude versus frequency. This process of power spectral analysis has been discussed in the section on signal processing. The EEG power spectrum facilitates rapid diagnosis of hemisphere asymmetries and changes in frequency content that accompany either deep anesthesia or cerebral hypoxia. "Bispectral density" is a newer method of analyzing the EEG that determines levels of correlation between various frequency components in the power spectrum. This type of analysis may provide improved determination of the depth of anesthesia in some settings.

Active Electrical Examination (Somatosensory Evoked Potentials)

A muscle twitch is elicited by generating a 0.2- to 0.3-msec pulse of current to depolarize a motor nerve. This motor nerve then conducts the impulse to the muscle, where a twitch is generated. We can understand the "in-use" failings of this device by following the path of the signal. Clearly, we must start with an adequate power source (no power = no twitch). Aside from intrinsic mechanical failure, if the coupling of the electrodes to the patient is poor, that is, if the electrodes are dry or good skin contact is not made, or both, the circuit has high resistance, very little current will flow (see earlier discussion and Equation 8), and a diminished twitch is generated. In summary, the simplest way to be certain that this monitor is functioning properly is to perform both a positive (see the desired response, i.e., thumb twitch, before the chosen drug is given) control and a negative control (see the twitch disappear in response to administered drug) (see Chapter 39).

Evoked potential (evoked response) monitors can determine the status of multiple parts of the sensory nervous system by measuring the central nervous system response to a discrete sensory stimulus. The stimulus can be auditory, optical, or peripheral sensory. The amplitude of the evoked response measured at the skin can be very small—5 μV in the case of some cortical potentials. This very small signal is in a "sea" of spontaneous EEG (100-μV amplitude) signals. We therefore resort to a signal enhancement technique called "ensemble averaging." Rather than trying to measure the response to a single stimulus, we average the responses from hundreds (or thousands) of stimuli. Because the evoked responses occur consistently at the same time after the stimulus, this averaging process reinforces the signal from the evoked response, and the random "noise" cancels itself. In this way, we commonly measure signals whose amplitude is perhaps 1/20th the amplitude of the background noise (see Fig. 30-5).

MEASUREMENT USING LIGHT

Principles of Light

What we commonly refer to as light is electromagnetic radiation in the visible range. Every substance with a temperature above absolute zero emits electromagnetic radiation. This radiation is characterized by a frequency and wavelength that are related by the speed of light: frequency = speed of light ÷ wave length. (c = speed of light = 3×10^8 m/sec or 186,400 miles/sec or 7.5 times around the earth's circumference in 1 second.) High energies are associated with high frequencies and short wavelengths, such as those of gamma rays and x-rays. As wavelength increases to the micron range, ultraviolet radiation proceeds to visible light, and at larger wavelengths, infrared is then followed by microwaves and radio waves with wavelengths in the kilometer range.

Electromagnetic waves and sound waves have some important differences. The particles in motion in sound waves are in the same direction as the propagation (longitudinal waves), whereas electromagnetic waves are perpendicular to the direction of propagation (transverse waves). Sound waves can propagate only through matter, whereas electromagnetic waves propagate through a vacuum without attenuation. The speed of light is about 1 million times faster than the speed of sound in air. If an observer is moving relative to a sound source, measurement of the speed of sound depends on the observer's own motion, but the speed of light is the same to any observer and any frame of reference. This statement is a basic premise of Einstein's special theory of relativity. At the high-frequency end of the electromagnetic spectrum are two forms of ionizing radiation: x-rays and gamma rays. These high-frequency waves are capable of knocking electrons out of their orbits and can thereby cause cell injury and death or ontogenesis. Gamma rays are commonly emitted by decaying radioactive nuclei.

Visible light and infrared light demonstrate several properties common to all electromagnetic radiation. Light represents a form of energy that when passing through matter, may be reflected, transmitted, or absorbed. Although light itself cannot be stored, it can be converted into some other form of energy such as electricity, chemical energy, and heat. In addition, light can be generated from other forms of energy, including heat (incandescent), electrical (gas discharge), and chemical (photoluminescent) energy.

Light as a Multifunctional Tool: Beer-Lambert Law

When light passes through matter, it is transmitted, absorbed, or reflected. The relative absorption or reflection of light is used in several monitoring devices to estimate the concentrations of dissolved substances, for example, carbon dioxide in respiratory gas and hemoglobin in plasma. The field of absorption spectrophotometry is based on the Beer-Lambert law, which states that if a known intensity of light illuminates a chamber of known dimensions, the concentration of the dissolved substance can be determined if the incident and transmitted light intensity is measured:

$$I_t = I_i e^{-dC\alpha} \tag{10}$$

Solved for C,

$$C = 1/d\alpha \ \ln I_i/I_t \tag{11}$$

where C is the concentration of the dissolved substance, d is the path length of the light a, and α is an absorption constant for the substance C at the wavelength used. I_i and I_t are the incident and transient light intensity, respectively. The unknown concentration (C) is inversely proportional to the path length (d) of light and directly proportional to the log of the ratio of incident light to transmitted light intensity (Fig. 30-32). Red light and infrared light are generally used because the constituents of interest to anesthesiologists (anesthetic agents, CO_2, hemoglobin) absorb light in that range. It is also fortunate that red and infrared light can penetrate tissue and may therefore be used to measure the concentration of hemoglobin species in living tissue (see the section on

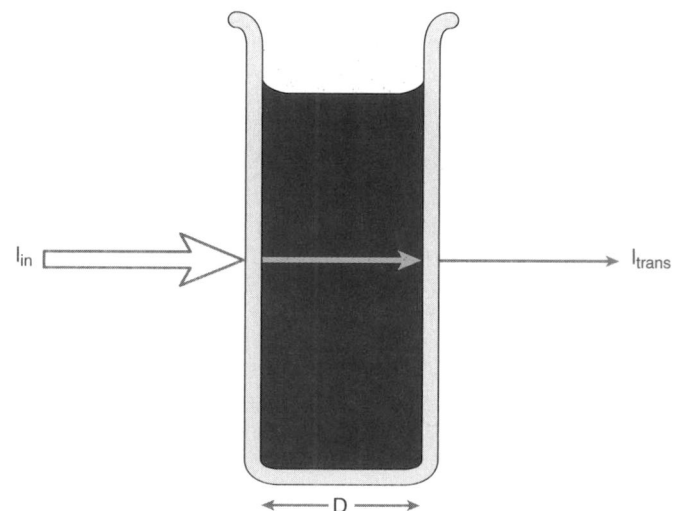

I_{trans}	= $I_{in}e^{-(D \times C \times a_\lambda)}$
I_{trans}	= intensity of light transmitted
I_{in}	= intensity of incident light
D	= distance light is transmitted through the liquid
C	= concentration of solute (oxyhemoglobin)
a_λ	= extinction coefficient of the solute (a constant)

Figure 30–32 Cuvette. Light entering the cuvette is reflected and absorbed. The concentration of substances absorbing and reflecting light can be determined by measuring the amount of light entering and exiting the system.

pulse oximeters). Infrared light is absorbed by small molecules only if they have bonds and are asymmetric. Therefore, nitrogen, oxygen, and helium cannot be measured by infrared light. Another limitation of infrared light is that it is absorbed by ordinary glass; therefore, the measurement chambers for these devices must be made of sapphire, which is permeable to red and infrared light.

Light Absorbance Monitors (Capnometer, Anesthetic Analyzer)

Capnographs and anesthetic analyzers both use the Beer law by analyzing constituents of the respiratory gas stream. The physical design of most capnometers is divided into two categories: mainstream and sidestream. In mainstream capnometers, the light absorption chamber is placed directly in the airway, and the light source shines throughout the chamber, with CO_2 being measured during inspiration and expiration directly. Advantages of this technique are a very fast response time and no problems with clogging of the sampling tubes, which is a disadvantage of sidestream capnometers. Disadvantages include the necessity of having a potentially heavy, expensive infrared measurement device placed directly in the endotracheal tube and the unavailability of devices that can measure both anesthetic agents and CO_2. The most commonly used devices in the operating room are sidestream capnometers. A small capillary sampling tube is attached to the airway, and samples are aspirated at 200 to 300 mL/min into the measurement chamber, which is within the monitor. The advantages of this method are just the opposite of the disadvantages of the mainstream capnometers, that is, the sampling tube is lightweight, and the device can be used to measure carbon dioxide and anesthetic agents. Disadvantages relate mostly to the delayed response time and potential clogging of the aspiration tubing.[18]

Agent analyzers and capnography function by the same physical principles, but with different wavelengths of light being used (Fig. 30-33). The mixture of gases can interfere with each other, so compensations are built into current devices.

Pulse Oximeters

Oximeters are devices that use light absorbance measurements to determine the concentration of various species of hemoglobin. One of the first in vivo oximeters was a noninvasive monitor used in aviation research during World War II. This device transilluminated tissue (the earlobe) with the light of two wavelengths. One wavelength was sensitive to changes in oxyhemoglobin, and the other was not. In effect, the earlobe acted as a test tube containing the suspended hemoglobin. For a review of the development of pulse oximetry, the reader is referred to an article by Severinghaus and Astrup.[19]

Before specific engineering problems are discussed, we need to define what we wish to measure. Adult blood usually contains four species of hemoglobin: oxyhemoglobin (HbO_2), reduced hemoglobin (Hb), methemoglobin (metHb), and carboxyhemoglobin (COHb). Each of these hemoglobin species has a different light absorption profile.

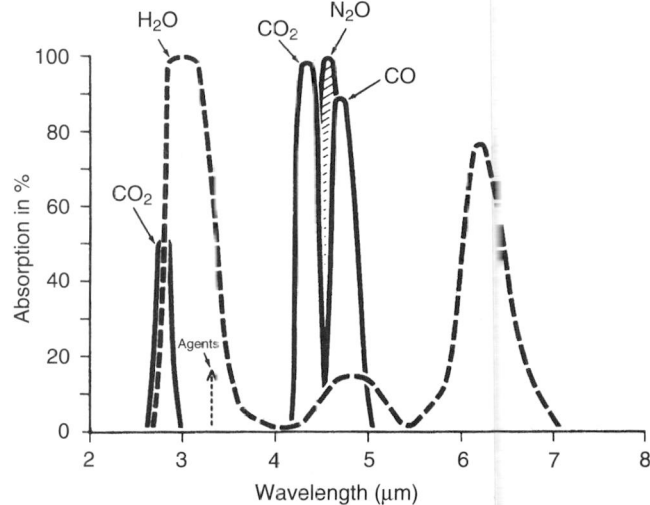

Figure 30–33 Absorption spectra of some gases and materials important to anesthesia. Note that absorption is not constant over wavelengths. Therefore, it is important to choose the proper wavelength to measure. In addition, when multiple substances are present, it is still possible to measure their concentrations, provided that enough wavelengths are available. (The solution becomes one of multiple equations with multiple unknowns.) (From Gravenstein JS, Paulus DA, Hayes TJ: Capnography in Clinical Practice. Boston, Butterworths, 1989.)

Figure 30-34 illustrates the different absorption constants for each hemoglobin species over a range of light from red to infrared. Except in pathologic conditions, metHb and COHb occur in low concentrations. Fractional hemoglobin saturation ($O_2Hb\%$) is defined as the ratio of HbO_2 to total hemoglobin:

$$O_2Hb\% = HbO_2/(HbO_2 + Hb + metHb + COHb)$$

Measuring this quantity requires four wavelengths of light and produces four simultaneous Beer-Lambert equations to solve for the four hemoglobin species. Because metHb and COHb do not contribute to oxygen transport, *functional saturation* is defined as the ratio of HbO_2 to HbO_2 plus reduced hemoglobin:

$$Sao_2 = HbO_2/(HbO_2 + Hb)$$

Although functional saturation depends explicitly on only HbO_2 and Hb, four light wavelengths are still required to measure it in the presence of significant concentrations of COHb and metHb.[20,21] If the concentrations of metHb and COHb are both zero, $O_2Hb\%$ and Sao_2 become identical.

The pulse oximeter performs substantial signal processing of optically transduced physiologic data. Although the principle governing pulse oximetry is straightforward, application of this principle to produce a clinically useful device involves significant engineering problems.[20,22] The remainder of this section describes the physical and physiologic problems of pulse oximeter design and the engineering solutions to these problems. The discussion is divided into basic design and management of signal artifacts.

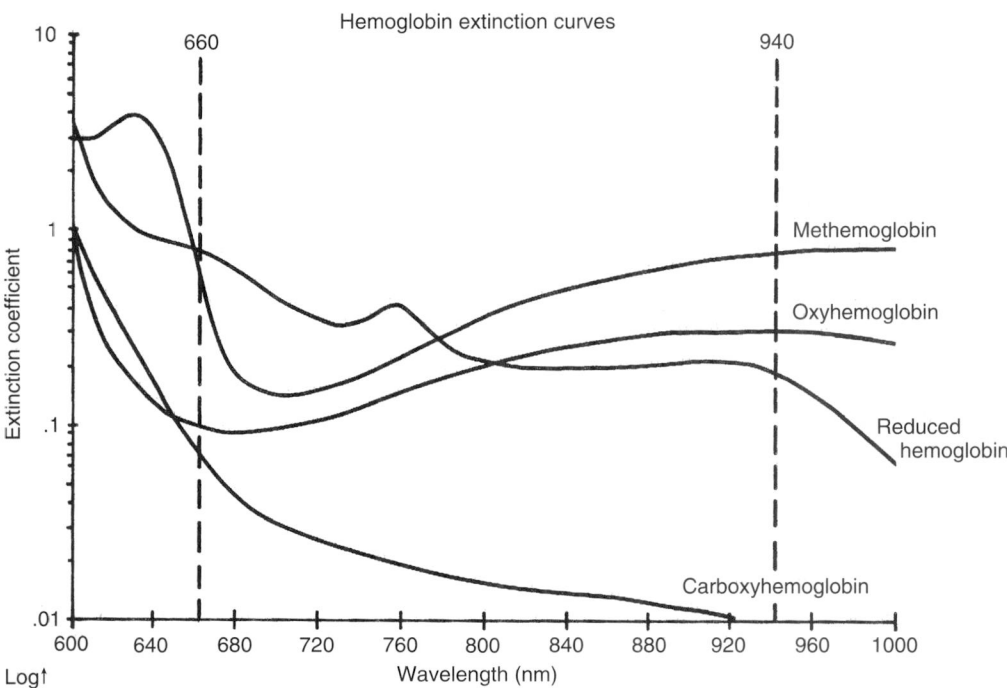

Figure 30–34 Hemoglobin extinction curves. Pulse oximetry uses the wavelengths of 660 and 940 nm because they are available in solid-state emitters (not all wavelengths are able to be emitted from diodes). Unfortunately, HbCO and HbO$_2$ absorb equally at 660 nm. Therefore, HbCO and HbO$_2$ both read as Sao$_2$ to a conventional pulse oximeter. In addition, Hbmet and reduced Hb share absorption at 660 nm and interfere with correct Sao$_2$ measurement. (Courtesy of Susan Manson, Biox/Ohmeda, Boulder, Colorado, 1986.)

Basic Design of Pulse Oximeters

Noninvasive in vivo oximeters measure red and infrared light transmitted through and reflected by a tissue bed. Accurate estimation of Sao$_2$ by this method entails several technical problems. First, there are many light absorbers in the transmitted light path other than arterial hemoglobin (e.g., skin, soft tissue, and venous and capillary blood). The pulse oximeter accounts for the effects of absorption of light by tissue and venous blood by assuming that only arterial blood pulsates. Figure 30-35 schematically illustrates the series of absorbers in a typical sample of living tissue. At the top of the figure is the AC component, which represents absorption of light by the pulsating arterial blood. The DC (baseline) component represents absorption of light by the tissue bed, including venous, capillary, and nonpulsatile arterial blood. Pulsatile expansion of the arteriolar bed increases the light path length (Equations 10 and 11), thereby increasing absorbency. Pulse oximeters use only two wavelengths of light: 660 nm (red light) and 940 nm (near-infrared light). The pulse oximeter first determines the AC component of absorbance at each wavelength and then divides this value by the corresponding DC component to obtain a "pulse-added" absorbance, which is independent of the incident light intensity. The oximeter then calculates the ratio (R) of the two pulse-added absorbances (one for each wavelength)[20]:

$$R = (AC\ 660/DC\ 660)/(AC\ 940/DC\ 940) \quad (12)$$

Finally, the value of R is related to the displayed saturation estimate Spo$_2$ by a "look-up table" programmed into the oximeter's software. The tables used in all commercial pulse oximeters are based on experimental studies in healthy human volunteers. Although each manufacturer's exact calibration curve is proprietary, these curves are very similar. For instance, when the ratio of red-to-infrared pulse-added absorbance is 1.0, the displayed Spo$_2$ is approximately 85%. This fact has clinical implications, which are discussed in the next section.

Signal Artifact Management

Probably the most difficult engineering problem in pulse oximetry is identification of the fluctuating absorbance pattern of arterial blood in a sea of electromagnetic and other artifacts. Artifacts have three major sources: ambient light, low perfusion (weak pulse, low AC-to-DC signal ratio), and motion (high AC-to-DC signal ratio). All these sources of artifacts produce a low signal-to-noise ratio.

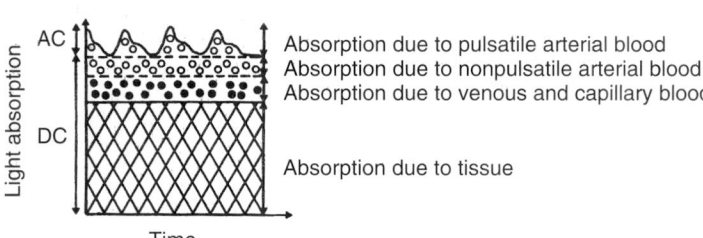

Figure 30–35 Pulse oximetry signals. A primary difficulty with pulse oximetry is that the pulsatile signal is small in comparison to the total absorbance of the ear or finger being examined. Pulsatile flow is needed to determine Sao$_2$. (Adapted from Ohmeda Pulse Oximeter Model 3700 Service Manual.)

The photodiodes used in the sensor to detect light cannot differentiate one wavelength of light from another. Therefore, the detector does not know whether the light received originates from the red light-emitting diode (LED), the infrared LED, or the room lights. This problem is solved in most pulse oximeters by alternating the red and infrared LED sources. The red LED is turned on first, and the photodiode detector produces a current resulting from the red LED plus the room lights. Next, the red LED is turned off and the infrared LED is turned on. The photodiode signal then represents the infrared LED plus the room lights. Finally, both LEDs are turned off, and the photodiode generates a signal from the room lights alone. This sequence is repeated hundreds of times per second. In this way, the oximeter attempts to eliminate light interference even in a quickly changing background of room light.[19] Some sources of fluctuating light can cause problems despite this clever design. Artifact from ambient light can be minimized simply by covering the sensor with an opaque shield.

Another engineering problem is that of a low AC-to-DC signal ratio, or low perfusion. When a small pulsatile absorbance signal is detected, the pulse oximeter amplifies the signal and estimates saturation from the ratio of the amplified absorbances. In this way, the pulse oximeter can estimate saturation values of SpO_2 for a wide range of patients who generate different amplitudes for pulsatile absorbance. Unfortunately, as with a radio receiver, when a weak signal is amplified, the background noise, or "static," is also amplified. At the highest amplifications (which can be up to a million times), some pulse oximeters may analyze this noise signal and generate an SpO_2 value from it. Because the noise is usually equal in the red and the infrared signals, the ratio of the two is often near unity (1.0), which yields a displayed saturation of approximately 85%. This problem could be demonstrated in early pulse oximeters by placing a piece of paper in the sensor between the photodiode and the LED. Many early models amplified the background noise while searching for a pulse until they eventually displayed a pulse and saturation value derived from the noise. To prevent this type of artifact, manufacturers have now incorporated minimum values for the signal-to-noise ratio, below which the device displays no value for SpO_2. Some oximeters also display a low–signal strength error message; in addition, many display a plethysmographic wave for visual identification of noise.

Patient motion (high AC-to-DC signal ratio) may be the most difficult artifact to eliminate. Engineers have tried several approaches to this problem, beginning with increasing the signal-averaging time. If the device averages its measurements over a longer period, the effect of an intermittent artifact is usually less. However, this longer averaging period also slows the response time to any acute change in SaO_2. Most pulse oximeters now allow the user to select one of several time-averaging modes. In addition, the designer can use sophisticated algorithms to identify and reject spurious signals.

One innovation aimed at reducing motion artifact is based on the premise that motion causes pulsations of venous blood within the tissue bed. Conventional pulse oximetry cannot distinguish these venous pulsations from those of arterial blood; hence, large errors or loss of signal can result. In the new signal-processing algorithm developed by Masimo, the oximeter actually computes a venous "noise reference signal," which is common to both light wavelengths. The noise reference is then subtracted from the total signal, and a "true" arterial signal is left. Tests in human volunteers as well as preliminary clinical studies indicate that this new technology represents an improvement in pulse oximeter performance in low signal-to-noise ratio situations.[23,24]

Over the past decade, other in vivo oximeters have been developed to measure light reflected by living tissue in an attempt to determine tissue hemoglobin saturation in specific organs. Using reflected rather than transmitted light adds complexity because the path length of the light through the tissue may be tortuous and make calibration difficult. Nevertheless, a signal reflected from living tissue may produce useful information regarding the average saturation of the hemoglobin within the tissue illuminated by the reflectance oximeter.[25] For example, a cerebral oximeter may be able to measure mean brain hemoglobin saturation, which reflects the intracerebral balance between venous and arterial blood, as well as the oxygenation of both.

Raman Scattering

As stated earlier, light of a specific energy can be absorbed by or emitted from a substance, depending on its allowable levels of vibrational, rotational, and electronic energy. Another absorption and re-emission phenomenon of light scattering occurs in a very small percentage of interactions. In this process, called Raman scattering, light in the visible and ultraviolet range is absorbed by molecules of a substance, thereby producing unstable vibrational or rotational energy states. Because these excited states are unstable, some of the absorbed energy is immediately re-emitted, thereby allowing the molecule to relax into a stable state. This Raman scattering signal occurs very infrequently; therefore, most photons pass through the gas sample without taking part in this particular absorption–re-emission phenomenon. If the intensity of the transmitted light is sufficiently great, the Raman-scattered signal can be measured and used to identify the molecules within the gas sample. Because the signal is scattered light, it is emitted in all directions relative to the incident beam.[18,26] The Raman light is of low intensity, so it is best to measure it at right angles to the high-intensity exciting beam.

An advantage of Raman scattering over gas analysis based on absorption of infrared light is that a spectrum of Raman scattering lines can be used to identify all types of molecules in the gas phase (e.g., O_2 and N_2). Because it involves only vibrational and rotational energy states, Raman scattering cannot be used to identify single atoms. As discussed earlier, infrared absorption can be used to analyze molecules with a dipole moment and therefore cannot be used to identify oxygen or nitrogen. A disadvantage of Raman scattering as a clinical tool is the requirement for a very high-intensity laser light source to produce the small Raman-scattered signal.[18,26]

TEMPERATURE MEASUREMENT (also see Chapter 40)

Principles of Temperature

Moving matter contains energy. Even stationary objects are moving at the atomic level. This kinetic energy of molecules and atoms is described as temperature. When all atomic motion ceases, the substance is said to be at absolute zero. This state provides a reference point for all temperature measurements. Heat has been defined as a form of internal kinetic energy that flows between two contacting bodies at different temperatures.

The amount of heat required to raise the temperature of 1 g of a given substance by 1°C is called the *specific heat* of that substance. The calorie, a common heat unit, is the amount of heat required to raise the temperature of 1 g of water from 14.5°C to 15.5°C. One calorie is equal to 4.184 J. When we refer to calories in terms of the calories in the food that we eat or the calories that we expend while exercising, we are actually referring to kilocalories, or thousands of calories. The total amount of heat energy in an object thus depends on its specific heat, its temperature, and its mass. For example, although a cup of 60°C coffee is much "hotter" than a 30°C swimming pool, the coffee contains much less total thermal energy than the pool does. The same is true for potential energy stored as pressure potential or electrical potential. A small container at high pressure may have less potential energy than a larger container at lower pressure.

Temperature Monitors (Thermometer, Thermistor, Thermocouple, Thermopile, Liquid Crystal)

Three general techniques can be used for measuring temperature: those based on expansion of a material as the temperature of the material increases, those based on changes in electrical properties with temperature, and those based on optical properties of a material. As heat is added to most substances (gases, liquids, or solids), motion of the molecules increases, and the volume of the material expands at constant pressure. Depending on the material, this expansion can be calibrated linearly to changes in temperature. Liquids are most commonly used, specifically, mercury, because its effective range extends from its freezing point of −39°C to approximately 250°C.[27] Mercury thermometers have two general disadvantages. They require 2 to 3 minutes for complete thermal equilibration (mercury has a high specific heat). In addition, they are enclosed in a glass tube, which may break and injure the patient.[28] Thermometers based on the expansion of gas (Bourdon tube) or metal (bimetallic strip) are frequently used as thermostats because they respond slowly to transient changes in temperature.

Electrical techniques for measuring temperature can be subdivided into three categories: resistance thermometers, thermistors, and thermocouples. Resistance thermometers operate on the principle that the electrical resistance of metals increases with temperature. These devices most frequently use a platinum wire as the temperature-sensitive resistor, a battery, and a galvanometer to measure current, which can be calibrated to temperature. The platinum wire is incorporated into a Wheatstone bridge circuit, which accurately measures very small changes in resistance (Fig. 30-36).

When compared with a platinum thermometer, a thermistor is a semiconductor that displays the opposite behavior with regard to electrical resistance. Specifically, as the thermistor is heated, its resistance decreases. Thermistors, being solid-state devices, can be manufactured as extremely small devices and therefore have a fast response to change in temperature (i.e., little heat is needed to increase their temperature). Most of the temperature probes used in anesthesia, from the ones at the end of Swan-Ganz catheters to esophageal probes, are thermistors.

Physical problems with thermistors are few: broken wires lead to high resistance and improper interpretation of temperature. More common are poor probe placement and misinterpretation of the value, such as placing the esophageal probe in the oral pharynx and measuring airway temperature, not core temperature. The optical properties of materials can be used to measure temperature in two ways: (1) the infrared emission of a body can be measured by using a device known as a thermopile and the emission then converted to temperature, and (2) a liquid crystal "matrix" can be placed in direct contact with the desired zone and an optical change can be observed (a change in color). The most commonly encountered example of infrared temperature measurement involves the tympanic membrane temperature monitor used in pediatrics and on hospital wards.[29] The infrared detector produces an electrical signal that is proportional to the fourth power of the difference in absolute temperatures of the objects. The following formula describes the specifics: $Q_{1,2} = K (T_1^4 - T_2^4)$, where $Q_{1,2}$ is net heat transfer (W/cm²),

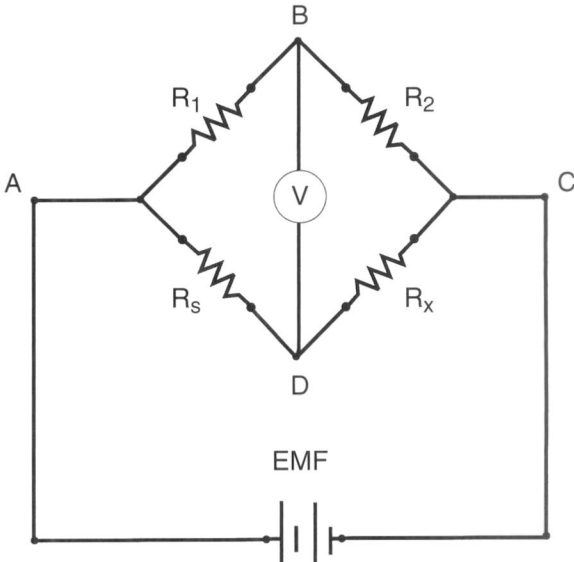

Figure 30–36 Wheatstone bridge. A Wheatstone bridge is an electronic circuit designed so that an unknown resistance can be calculated by knowing two sets of variables: (1) the voltage drop across the bridge and (2) the other resistances in the circuit (see Appendix 3).

K is the Stefan-Boltzmann constant, and T_1 and T_2 are the absolute temperatures of the two objects (°K). In theory, this method of measuring the core temperature should be accurate. However, in practice, improper placement and lack of calibration, but not cerumen, contribute to real-world errors.[30-32] Additionally, the probe is rather large for intraoperative use.

Liquid crystal measures of temperature (commonly found in "mood rings") are often used for skin temperature monitoring. Just as the molecules in a liquid crystal watch display change their optical properties with a small electric current (becoming polarized and dark), the molecules in a liquid crystal temperature device change their optical properties with temperature (resulting in a rainbow of colors). The crystal matrix is sensitive to pressure as well as temperature. (By touching a broken LCD display panel, one can note the visual rainbow of changing colors.) The reported clinical accuracy of liquid crystal devices varies.[33,34] In conclusion, new monitors are being developed almost continuously, but new physical principles are revealed only rarely. Physics as a science is trying to simplify and render the universe in absolute terms. The terms and principles outlined here will be referred to multiple times in subsequent chapters.

KEY POINTS

1. Accuracy and precision are different. Accuracy is how close a value is to the true value. Precision is how repeatable the measurements are. An inaccurate, but precise monitor can be re-calibrated to be accurate, but an imprecise monitor cannot be improved.
2. Invasive pressure monitors are affected by damping and resonance. Damping leads to distortion, signal loss, and lowering of peak values. Resonance can lead to amplification and overestimation of the peak value.
3. Flow measurements are one of the most difficult to obtain and usually involve indirect measures. (For example, a temperature change or pressure drop is measured and a flow value is derived. A small error in the initial measurement leads to a much larger error in the derived flow value.)
4. Pulse oximetry combines analysis of optical plethysmography and absorption analysis with empirical data to produce an estimate of Sao_2.
5. Wavelength and frequency are related to the speed of the wave by the following formula: speed = wavelength × frequency. Shorter wavelengths improve the resolution of both light and ultrasound measurements.
6. Filtering can improve the signal display, but it can also result in smoothing and loss of information.
7. A signal can be extracted from noise by repeated measurements because the noise is random over time but the signal is not.
8. Electrical signals can be converted from analog to digital. Conversion can introduce some artifacts but can allow for greater storage and analysis capabilities.

REFERENCES

1. DeGowin EL, DeGowin RL: Bedside Diagnostic Examination, 5th ed. New York, Macmillan, 1987.
2. Bland JM, Altman DG: Statistical methods for assessing agreement between two methods of clinical measurement. Lancet 1:307-310, 1986.
3. Sykes MK, Vickers MD, Hull CJ: Ultrasound. In Principles of Measurement and Monitoring in Anaesthesia and Intensive Care, 3rd ed. Oxford, Blackwell, 1991.
4. Beecher HK: The first anesthetic records (Cushing and Codman). Surg Gynecol Obstet 71:689-692, 1940.
5. Cushing H: Technical methods of performing certain cranial operations. Surg Gynecol Obstet 6:237-246, 1908.
6. Connors AF Jr, Speroff T, Dawson NV, et al: The effectiveness of right heart catheterization in the initial care of critically ill patients. JAMA 276:889-897, 1996.
7. Sandham JD, Hull RD, Brant RF, et al: A randomized, controlled trial of the use of pulmonary-artery catheters in high-risk surgical patients. N Engl J Med 348:5-14, 2003.
8. Quill TJ: Blood pressure monitoring. In Ehrenwerth J (ed): Anesthesia Equipment Principles and Applications. St Louis, Mosby–Year Book, 1993, p 274.
9. O'Brien E: Has conventional sphygmomanometry ended with the banning of mercury? Blood Press Monit 7:37-40, 2002.
10. Ireland J: In praise of mercury sphygmomanometers. Electronic readings of blood pressure seem to be higher than readings obtained with mercury sphygmomanometers. BMJ 322:1249, 2001.
11. Cicman JH, Gotzon J, Himmelwright C, et al: Operating Principles of Narkomed Anesthesia Systems, 2nd ed. Telford, PA, WE Andrews, 1998.
12. Q2 CCO/SvO2 Monitoring System Operating Manual [computer program]. North Chicago, Abbott Laboratories, 1998.
13. Szocik JF, Tremper K, Barker SJ: Fundamental principles of monitoring and instrumentation. In Miller RD (ed): Anesthesia, vol 1, 5th ed. San Francisco, Churchill Livingstone, 2000, pp 1053-1086.
14. Resnick R, Halliday D: Physics for Students of Science and Engineering. New York, John Wiley & Sons, 1960.
15. Rappaport MB, Sprague H: physiologic and physical laws that govern auscultation, and their clinical application. Am Heart J 21:257, 1941.
16. Cahalan MK, Litt L, Botvinick EH, Schiller NB: Advances in noninvasive cardiovascular imaging: Implications for the anesthesiologist. Anesthesiology 66:356-372, 1987.
17. Clements FM, de Bruijn NP: Perioperative evaluation of regional wall motion by transesophageal two-dimensional echocardiography. Anesth Analg 66:249-261, 1987.
18. Gravenstein JS, Paulus JS, Hayes TJ: Capnography in Clinical Practice. Boston, Butterworths, 1989.
19. Severinghaus JW, Astrup PB: History of blood gas analysis. Int Anesthesiol Clin 25:1-224, 1987.
20. Tremper KK, Barker SJ: Pulse oximetry. Anesthesiology Jan 70:98-108, 1989.
21. Barker SJ, Tremper KK, Hyatt J: Effects of methemoglobinemia on pulse oximetry and mixed venous oximetry. Anesthesiology 70:112-117, 1989.
22. Pologe JA: Pulse oximetry: Technical aspects of machine design. Int Anesthesiol Clin 25:137-153, 1987.
23. Dumas C, Wahr JA, Tremper KK: Clinical evaluation of a prototype motion artifact resistant pulse oximeter in the recovery room. Anesth Analg 83:269-272, 1996.
24. Barker SJ, Shah NK: The effects of motion on the performance of pulse oximeters in volunteers (revised publication). Anesthesiology 86:101-108, 1997.
25. Wahr JA, Tremper KK, Samra S, Delpy DT: Near-infrared spectroscopy: Theory and applications. J Cardiothorac Vasc Anesth 10:406-418, 1996.
26. Westenskow DR, Smith KW, Coleman DL, et al: Clinical evaluation of a Raman scattering multiple gas analyzer for the operating room. Anesthesiology 70:350-355, 1989.

27. Budavari S, O'Neil MJ, Smith A, Heckelman P: The Merck Index, 11th ed. Rahway, NJ, Merck, 1989.
28. Moxham JP, Lee PK: Broken glass mercury thermometer: A difficult airway foreign body. Otolaryngol Head Neck Surg 127:339-341, 2002.
29. Shinozaki T, Deane R, Perkins FM: Infrared tympanic thermometer: Evaluation of a new clinical thermometer. Crit Care Med 16:148-150, 1988.
30. Pransky SM: The impact of technique and conditions of the tympanic membrane upon infrared tympanic thermometry. Clin Pediatr (Phila) 30(4 Suppl):50-52, discussion 60, 1991.
31. Terndrup TE, Rajk J: Impact of operator technique and device on infrared emission detection tympanic thermometry. J Emerg Med 10:683-687, 1992.
32. Chamberlain JM, Terndrup TE: New light on ear thermometer readings. Contemp Pediatr 11:66-76, 1994.
33. Vaughn MS, Cork RC, Vaughn RW: Inaccuracy of liquid crystal thermometry to identify core temperature trends in postoperative adults. Anesth Analg 61:284-287, 1982.
34. Ikeda T, Sessler DI, Marder D, Xiong J: Influence of thermoregulatory vasomotion and ambient temperature variation on the accuracy of core-temperature estimates by cutaneous liquid-crystal thermometers. Anesthesiology 86:603-612, 1997.

APPENDIX 1

Distance versus Time under Constant Acceleration: Equivalence of Potential and Kinetic Energy

Velocity **v** is the rate at which distance is changing; that is, it is the time derivative of distance:

$$\mathbf{v} = d\mathbf{x}/dt \tag{1}$$

The variable **v** is written in boldface type to indicate that it is a vector: it has both magnitude and direction. Distance **x** is a vector pointing from the origin to the present location of the particle or object; it is called the "position vector." Time (t) is a scalar; it has magnitude but no direction and is therefore written in plain type.

Acceleration (**a**) is the time rate of change of velocity. Thus, it is the time derivative of the velocity vector, or the second derivative of distance with respect to time.

$$\mathbf{a} = d\mathbf{v}/dt = (d/dt)(d\mathbf{x}/dt) = d^2\mathbf{x}/dt^2 \tag{2}$$

If an object starts with zero velocity (**v** = 0) at time zero (t = 0) and then accelerates with constant acceleration (**a**), its velocity at time t will be simply **v** = **a**t. To calculate the distance traveled by the object between time t = 0 and time t, we must divide the time interval 0 to t into a series of very small intervals, each of time length dt. The distance traveled during the interval dt is simply the velocity at that time multiplied by the time interval:

$$d\mathbf{x} = \mathbf{v}dt = (\mathbf{a}t)dt \tag{3}$$

In the second step, we have substituted the constant acceleration relationship **v** = **a**t from above. Now to compute the total distance traveled, we must sum the distance from all of the small dt time intervals that occur between 0 and t.

$$\mathbf{x} = \Sigma(\mathbf{a}t)dt \tag{4}$$

If we allow the length of the time interval dt to approach zero, the summation process becomes the *integral* with respect to time from time zero to time t.

$$x = \int vdt = \int (at)dt = \frac{1}{2}at^2 \tag{5}$$

Thus, an object starting from rest at t = 0 and moving with constant acceleration (**a**) will move a distance $\frac{1}{2}\mathbf{a}t^2$ in time t. If this is a falling object (in a vacuum, where there is no air resistance), a = g = 9.8 m/sec², and the distance formula becomes

$$\mathbf{x} = \frac{1}{2}gt^2 = (4.9)t^2 \tag{6}$$

In the first second the object falls 4.9 m; at the end of 2 seconds, it has fallen 19.6 m; after 3 seconds, 44.1 m; and so on. The kinetic energy (KE) of a moving object is

$$KE = \frac{1}{2}mv^2 \tag{7}$$

where m is the mass of the object and v is the magnitude of its velocity (also called *speed*). Note that v used in this sense is in plain type, not boldface. Consider again the falling object that started at position x = 0 at time t = 0 and falls a distance h:

$$h = \tfrac{1}{2}gt^2, \text{ or}$$

$$t = \sqrt{(2h/g)} \tag{8}$$

Because velocity v = at = gt, we have by substitution from Equation 8

$$V = gt = g\sqrt{(2h/g)} = \sqrt{(2gh)} \tag{9}$$

The kinetic energy is given by

$$KE = \tfrac{1}{2}mv^2 = \tfrac{1}{2}m(2gh) = mgh \tag{10}$$

Now let us consider the *work* required to lift the fallen object back to its original height of h. Recall that work is defined as the force exerted times the distance over which the force acts: W = Fd. The force of gravity acting on our object is F_g = mg, so the work required to lift it the distance (h) back to x = 0 is

$$W = Fd = (mg)d = mgh \tag{11}$$

Thus, the work required to restore the object equals the kinetic energy possessed by the object at the bottom of its fall, KE = W = mgh. When we lift the object from x = h back to x = 0, we have increased its *potential energy* (PE) by the amount mgh. This potential energy can be converted to kinetic energy by allowing the object to fall the distance h. This type of potential energy, called *gravitational potential*, has a value that clearly depends on where we locate the origin of our coordinates, x = 0. However, it is the *change* in potential energy, not its absolute value, that the potential energy/kinetic energy balances:

$$\Delta KE = -\Delta PE \tag{12}$$

The change in kinetic energy is equal to and of opposite sign to the change in potential energy.

APPENDIX 2

Physics of Hydrostatic Pressure

A liquid manometer is a simple and reliable means of monitoring pressures that do not change rapidly. It simply uses the weight of a measured vertical column of liquid to balance the pressure exerted against the bottom of the column. We have defined weight as the force exerted by gravity on a mass (m) F_g = mg. To determine the weight of a column of liquid of known dimensions (the manometer in Fig. 30-11), we must first know the density (mass per unit volume) of the liquid. Density has dimensions of m/l^3, and the SI units are kilograms per cubic meter (kg/m^3). Because liquids are almost incompressible, their density is little influenced by pressure (but affected by temperature). The density of water at room temperature is 997.8 kg/m^3, or 1.0 g/cm^3.

The pressure (p) exerted by the bottom of the vertical column of liquid in a manometer (see Fig. 30-11) is determined as follows. If the cross-sectional area of the liquid cylinder is A and the height of the cylinder is z, its volume is V = Az. If the liquid has a density of ρ, the mass of the column is

$$m = \rho V = \rho Az \tag{1}$$

and its weight is

$$W = mg = \rho Azg \tag{2}$$

The liquid column exerts a force equal to its weight on its base, whose surface area is A, thus creating the following pressure on the surface:

$$p = \text{Force/Area} = \rho Azg/A = \rho gz \tag{3}$$

The pressure exerted by the manometer is therefore independent of its cross-sectional area (A); it depends on only the density of the working fluid and the vertical height of the column. If we know the liquid density, measurement of the column height (z) allows us to calculate the pressure (p). For example, if the working fluid is mercury (e.g., sphygmomanometers), the density is 13,680 kg/m³ (13.68 g/cm³, or 13.68 times the density of water). The relationship of pressure to height of the column is then

$$p = \rho gz = (13,600 \text{ kg/m}^3)(9.8 \text{ N/kg})(z)$$

$$p \text{ [N/m}^2] = 133,300(z) \tag{4}$$

The unit of pressure newton/meter² (N/m²) is called the pascal (Pa). Because a pascal is a small unit of pressure, we usually use kilopascals (10³ Pa) or kPa. If we express p in kPa and z in millimeters of mercury (rather than meters), Equation 4 becomes

$$p \text{ [kPa]} = 0.1333(z) \text{ [mm]} \tag{5}$$

APPENDIX 3

Wheatstone Bridge

The Wheatstone bridge is a network of four resistors connected as shown in Figure 30-36, with a battery or direct-current voltage source (electromotive force) connected between A and C and a voltmeter (V) connected between B and D. The bridge is said to be "balanced" when the voltmeter reads zero potential difference between points B and D. From Ohm's law (V = IR), it is easy to show that balance occurs when $R_x = R_s \times (R_2/R_1)$. If R_s is an adjustable standard resistor and R_1 and R_2 are fixed known resistors, the balanced bridge provides a very precise means of determining R_x, the unknown resistance. This principle has many applications in biomedical engineering, including strain gauge pressure transducer measurements. In this case, the transducer itself is the unknown resistance R_x.

APPENDIX 4

Amplification Artifact of a Fluid Tube/Transducer Pressure Wave

The amplification artifact of a fluid tube/transducer pressure waveform can be calculated if a few properties of the system are known. The most relevant part of this solution is the response amplitude, which is plotted against the driving frequency (f) in Figure 30-14. This figure shows some important properties of fluid-coupled transducers and other harmonic oscillators. One of these properties is the existence of a resonant frequency, f_0, which is defined as follows:

$$f_0 = \frac{1}{2}\pi\sqrt{k/m}$$

Remember, m is the mass of the system and k is the elasticity, or spring constant.

As we increase the amount of damping (i.e., friction; c is the friction constant), we observe a decrease in the peak amplitude at resonance, and the frequency at which the peak occurs decreases slightly. The damping coefficient (z) is defined as follows:

$$z = c/\sqrt{2km}$$

Even though the arterial pressure waveform is not actually sinusoidal, Figure 30-14 shows the most important characteristics of the pressure transducer response. Any combination of catheter, tubing, and transducer can be characterized by two quantities: a resonant frequency (f_0) and a damping coefficient (z). Gardner measured these quantities for many transducer and tubing systems and found that most systems have resonant frequencies of 10 to 20 cycles/sec or hertz (Hz) and damping coefficients of 0.2 to 0.3. For clinical systems, the maximum amplification factor (the ratio of transducer output to input waveform amplitude) at resonance is near 2.5.

If the resonant frequency is 10 Hz (600 cycles/min), one might conclude that amplification plays little role in the clinical range of pulse rates, which are 5 to 10 times smaller. However, the arterial pressure waveform is not a sine wave. It can be represented as a summation of sine waves (a Fourier series) with frequencies up to many times the pulse rate. It is these higher harmonic frequencies that are amplified most and that yield the spiked appearance of a poorly processed arterial waveform. Depending on the shape of the actual arterial pressure wave, this distortion can introduce a 20% to 40% "overshoot" error in systolic blood pressure readings. Even worse, this error is dependent on the pulse rate, so an error determined for a particular patient at the beginning of administration of an anesthetic may not remain constant.

From this discussion we can easily predict how to optimize the performance of a pressure transducer system. First, the resonant frequency (f_0) should be as high as possible. Therefore, the value for k in Equation 1 should be large (i.e., the spring should be "stiff"), and the value for m should be small (i.e., the cannula and pressure tubing should be as stiff and inelastic as possible). To minimize the mass of the moving fluid, the tubing should be short in length and small in diameter. Judging from plots of amplitude versus frequency/resonant frequency at different damping coefficients, the optimal damping coefficient would be 0.4 to 0.5. One should also carefully eliminate air bubbles from the system because they add elasticity and friction, thereby lowering the resonant frequency. In a clinical system, one can determine the approximate f_0 and z of a transducer system if graphic output is available. If the high-pressure flush is turned on and then quickly off at a high chart speed (50 mm/sec), the tracing oscillates through several cycles at a frequency near f_0. The damping coefficient can be found by determining the ratio of amplitudes of successive peaks on the tracing. This is a practical example of how fundamental principles of mechanics can be used to predict and optimize the performance of monitoring systems. These concepts of mechanics will recur in later sections of this chapter.

APPENDIX 5

Flow Meters, Bernoulli's Principle, Laminar and Turbulent Flow

The equations governing the motion of fluids are expressions of Newton's second law, F = ma. Forces associated with fluids fall into three major categories: (1) gravity, (2) pressure, and (3) friction. In the example using manometers, the gravitational force per unit volume of fluid is simply ρg, acting in the vertical direction. Pressure forces are actually the result of differences in pressure from one point to another and are expressed mathematically as the negative of the pressure gradient. (A pressure gradient is a vector in the direction of the maximal rate of pressure increase, with magnitude equal to the pressure derivative in that direction.) Friction is proportional to viscosity, the physical property of a fluid that relates shear stress to rate of strain.

$$P_0 = p + \tfrac{1}{2}\rho U^2 + \rho gz \tag{1}$$

Equation 1 shows the relationship between velocity and pressure of a fluid in a flow that meets the conditions described. For flows in tubes, the manometer technique provides an easy method of measuring mean pressure. Therefore, the simplest flow meters apply a combination of these two principles to a tube of changing cross-sectional diameter. For example, the Venturi flow meter shown in Figure 30-18 consists of a tube of varying cross-sectional area that has two ports for measurement of pressure. The Bernoulli equation for points 1 and 2 in the figure becomes

$$P_1 + \tfrac{1}{2}\rho U_1^2 = P_2 + \tfrac{1}{2}\rho U_2^2 \tag{2}$$

Here, the gravity terms have canceled out because the tube is horizontal, but these terms are usually negligible for gas flows in any direction.

The volume of the fluid flow (Q) (also called flux) at both locations must be the same because no fluid is entering or leaving through the tube walls. The dimensions and SI units for the volume of fluid flow are l^3/t and m^3/sec, respectively. This volume is determined at each cross section of the tube by multiplying the average velocity (U) by the cross-sectional area (A):

$$Q = U_1 A_1 = U_2 A_2 \tag{3}$$

Assuming that A_1, A_2, P_1, and P_2 are known, we now have two equations for the two unknowns U_1 and U_2. Solving these for the velocity U_1 produces

$$U_1 = \sqrt{\left[2(P_1 - P_2)/\rho(1 - A_1^2/A_2^2)\right]} \qquad (4)$$

To find the volume of the flow (Q), we merely multiply this result by A_1. Note that velocity is proportional to the square root of the pressure drop or that the pressure change varies as velocity squared. For a given U_1, or the magnitude of flow velocity, the pressure drop varies as the square of the ratio of the areas, or the fourth power of the ratio of the diameters. If we choose an A_2 greater than A_1, Equation 4 implies that P_2 is greater than P_1. In this case, the pressure increases in the direction of flow, a change that initially seems contrary to intuition.

The bobbin flow meters (also called variable-orifice flow meters) in anesthesia machines use a similar principle. These devices consist of a slightly tapered vertical tube and a bobbin or ball that fits inside the tube (see Fig. 30-20). The cross-sectional area of the ring-shaped gap between the bobbin and the tube wall is proportional to the height of the bobbin. Because changes in the cross-sectional area of flow are abrupt rather than gradual (as in Fig. 30-20), the Bernoulli equation does not accurately describe this type of flow. The flow above the bobbin (i.e., downstream) is highly turbulent, and turbulence is a condition that dissipates kinetic energy into heat. However, introduction of the empirical constant C_d enables one to use the same formulation as in Equation 4:

$$Q = C_d A\sqrt{\left[2(P_1 - P_2)\right]/\rho} \qquad (5)$$

and

$$P_1 - P_2 = (\tfrac{1}{2}\rho Q^2)/(C_d^2 A^2) \qquad (6)$$

where C_d is a dimensionless constant called the discharge coefficient. This constant varies with the shape of the orifice and with the value for another dimensionless parameter, the Reynolds number (Re). The Reynolds number, the overall ratio of inertial forces to viscous forces in a particular flow, is determined as follows:

$$Re = \rho UL/\mu \qquad (7)$$

where U is mean flow velocity, L is a characteristic length for the flow (in our flow meter, L is the diameter of the tube), and μ is the viscosity of the fluid. The dimension for viscosity is M/LT. The value for the Reynolds number is important to any fluid flow because it determines some of the most important characteristics of the flow. For example, the transition from laminar, or "smooth," flow to turbulent flow is determined by the shape of the flow and the Reynolds number. Flow in a long, straight, smooth-walled tube becomes turbulent at an Re value of approximately 2100. On the other hand, flow through an abrupt orifice, such as that of the flow meter in Figure 30-20, becomes turbulent at an Re value of less than 100.

Returning now to the function of the flow meter, one can see that as gas flows upward through the tapered tube, the bobbin begins to rise. As the bobbin rises, the cross-sectional area of the orifice (A) increases because of the taper of the tube; therefore, the drop in pressure ($P_1 - P_2$) decreases. The bobbin reaches an equilibrium position for a given volume of flow (Q) when the pressure lifting the bobbin is exactly equal to the weight of the bobbin. In this type of flow meter, the pressure difference is fixed by the bobbin weight, and the area of the orifice varies with the volume of the flow, hence the name variable-orifice flow meter. Equations 5 and 6 show that calibration of these flow meters depends on both the density and the viscosity of the gas: density (ρ) appears explicitly, and viscosity (μ) appears in the dependence of C_d on the Reynolds number. If we use the wrong gas in a particular flow meter, Equations 5 and 6 and the viscosity and density of the new gas enable us to predict the change in calibration.

APPENDIX 6

Measurement of Cardiac Output by the Thermal Dilution and Mass Flow Technique

A commonly used method of measuring blood flow is dilutional calculation, that is, dye or thermal dilution. These methods are simply mass or energy balances that determine the volume of fluid that has been diluted by adding a volume of dye or a given thermal energy. If you have a bucket of water at room temperature (25°C) and you want to determine the volume of water in the bucket, you could add a known volume of water at a known temperature. If 100 mL of water at 35°C is added to the bucket and the final temperature is 27°C, the unknown volume can be calculated by balancing the heat energy associated with the dilutional process, assuming that no heat is lost to the environment. This dilutional process can be used to measure blood flow by completing this same heat balance measured over time. Thermodilution cardiac output measurements can have significant error as a result of the many assumptions associated with the technique, such as rapid injection of the thermodilution injectate; accurate temperature and volume of the injected fluid; constant known heat capacity of blood, which in reality is a function of the hematocrit value; little heat loss to the lung; and so on.

Thermistor probes are most commonly used for clinical monitoring of patient temperature because they are inexpensive, small, and flexible. For these reasons, the thermistor probe is also used to measure cardiac output determined by the thermodilution technique. Computation of cardiac output performed in this manner is, in effect, a heat balance for the right side of the heart. (Heat balance is a method of accounting for all heat in a process or change involving transfer of heat.) The technique consists of quick injection of a known volume of a sterile solution (usually 10 mL of 5% dextrose in water) into the right side of the heart while a sensor notes the temperature of the blood in the pulmonary artery. It is assumed that the cold injected solution equilibrates thermally with the blood as it perfuses the pulmonary artery but that the solution does not acquire heat from other tissues. The following equation is the solution of this heat balance:

$$CO = \left[\rho_i C_i V_i (T_b - T_i)(60 C_r)\right] / \left[(\rho_b C_b) \int_0^\infty T_b(t) dt\right]$$

where CO is cardiac output (L/min); ρ_i and ρ_b are the densities of the injectate and blood, respectively; C_i and C_b are the heat capacities of the injectate and blood, respectively; V_i is the volume of the injectate; T_b and T_i are the temperature of the blood and the injectate, respectively; Cr is a computational constant that corrects for the rising temperature of the injectate; and the integration is the area under the thermodilution curve. Because the injectate warms as it is injected through the catheter before mixing with the blood, the correction factor Cr is applied to the equation.

The same principle of balance used for temperature determination of cardiac output can be applied to O_2 or CO_2 balance as well. Classically, oxygen balance is used as described by Fick. Measurement of oxygen consumption and content is cumbersome, and a modification of the Fick equation using CO_2 production is also used. NICO is a new partial rebreathing method using the following equation:

$$Q = \dot{V}co_2 / (C\bar{v}co_2 - Caco_2)$$

Cardiac output (Q) is simply the expired CO_2 divided by the arterial-venous difference in CO_2. Assuming that Q does not change, the equations for CO_2 elimination must be the same with or without rebreathing, where N indicates normal breathing and R indicates rebreathing. By rearranging the equations, cardiac output is the ratio of the change in elimination of CO_2 divided by the change in arterial CO_2 content. Arterial CO_2 content is derived from the slope of P_{ETCO_2}.

$$Q = \dot{V}co_{2N}/(C\bar{v}co_{2N} - Caco_{2N}) = \dot{V}co_{2R}/(C\bar{v}co_{2R} - Caco_{2R}) = \frac{\Delta \dot{V}co_2}{\Delta Caco_2}$$

Therefore, we can see that potential errors are induced by violations of the following assumptions: (1) change in Q during the measurement period, (2) change in metabolic rate and hence production of CO_2, and (3) change in ventilation.

As a trend analysis, patients with chronic obstructive lung disease, in which the absolute value of $Paco_2$ is widely different from P_{ETCO_2}, may have an absolute error in Q determination by this method, but the relative changes should track.

APPENDIX

Ultrasound

The simplest sound wave to represent mathematically is a sinusoidal wave propagating in one dimension:

$$p' = p_0 \sin\left[(2\pi/\lambda)(x - at)\right] \tag{1}$$

where p′ is the pressure fluctuation, λ is the wavelength (distance between waves), x is the coordinate in the direction of propagation, and a is the speed of propagation, or the speed of sound.

The amplitude of a sound wave is measured by the root mean square value of the pressure fluctuations. This value is called the sound pressure level (SPL). Because the range of SPL values is often very wide, a logarithmic scale is used:

$$SPL = 20 \log (p*/P_0) \tag{2}$$

where p* is the root mean square pressure fluctuation and P_0 is a reference pressure chosen as the lowest sound pressure detectable by the human ear. This pressure representing the threshold of hearing is 2×10^{-8} kPa at a sound frequency of 2 kHz (2000 cycles/sec). The units in this SPL scale are called decibels. Thus, a sound pressure of 2×10^{-8} kPa corresponds to an SPL of zero decibels (0 dB), the lowest audible sound level [($p*/P_0 = 1$; log (1) = 0)]. Quiet conversation has an SPL of approximately 40 to 50 dB, or a pressure 10 to 300 times that of the threshold of hearing.

When sound waves encounter a sudden change in the properties of the conducting medium, some of the sound is transmitted through the new medium, and some of it is reflected, or "scattered," in many directions. Although the mathematics of this process are complex, one conclusion is readily apparent: the greater the mismatch in density and compressibility between the two media, the more sound that is reflected. The quantity that best determines the degree of reflection at an interface between two media is the ratio (R) of the products of density (ρ) and the speed of sound (a) through the two media:

$$R = (\rho_1 a_1)/(\rho_2 a_2) \tag{3}$$

We can easily see that the greatest acoustic mismatch in the body occurs between solid tissues and the lungs. Both the density and the speed of sound are much lower in the air-filled lungs than in solid tissues. Therefore, ultrasonography cannot "look" through the lungs at tissues or organs on the other side. The second greatest mismatch occurs between soft tissues and bone, the latter having a much higher ρa than the former. In 1842, Christian Johann Doppler first described the apparent change in pitch of a sound that occurred when either the source of the sound or the listener was moving. This Doppler effect now has several applications in patient monitoring, including precordial and esophageal Doppler ultrasound devices that measure local blood velocities or cardiac output. If a sound source radiating a frequency (f) is stationary and the listener is moving (see Fig. 30-24A), the wavelength of the waves can be determined by the equation

$$\lambda = a/f \tag{4}$$

because the time between wave fronts is 1/f and the waves are moving at the speed of sound (a). If the listener moves toward the source at speed V_0, the velocity of the listener relative to the moving wave fronts is $(a + V_0)$. The number of wave fronts that the listener encounters per unit time is therefore

$$f' = \text{Velocity/Distance between waves} = (a + V_0)/\lambda \tag{5}$$

Because the sound frequency for a stationary listener is $f = a/\lambda$ (Equation 4), the frequency f' heard by the moving listener becomes

$$f' = (a + V_0)/\lambda = f + (V_0/\lambda) = f + (V_0 f/a) = f[1 + (V_0/a)] \tag{6}$$

The apparent frequency of the listener is thus increased by the factor $[1 + (V_0/a)]$. A listener moving toward the source at half the speed of sound hears a frequency 1.5 times that of a stationary listener.

Now consider a stationary listener and a source moving at speed V_0, as shown in Figure 30-24B. The wave fronts are no longer concentric circles; they are more closely spaced in the direction that the source is moving. If the frequency of the sound emitted at the source is f, the source moves a distance V_0/f during each vibration. The wavelength in the direction of motion is thus shortened by V_0/f and becomes $1 = (a - V_0)/f$. The waves themselves are traveling at speed a, so the frequency heard by the stationary listener is

$$f' = a/\lambda' = af/(a - V_0) = f[1/(1 - V_0/a)] \tag{7}$$

Now, if the source is moving at half the speed of sound toward the listener, the apparent frequency doubles. Compare this situation with the preceding one in which the listener is moving and the apparent frequency increases by only 50%. Doppler ultrasound systems combine the two situations shown in Figure 30-24. The initial acoustic source is a stationary transducer, and the sound from this device is scattered from a moving target (e.g., red blood cells). The scattered sound then returns to a stationary listener: the receiving transducer. In effect, the target is a moving listener hearing a stationary source; the target then reradiates the sound as a moving source toward a stationary listener. The frequency heard by the receiving transducer is obtained by combining Equations 6 and 7:

$$f' = f\left[\frac{1 + V/a}{1 - V/a}\right]$$

In this example we have assumed that the target is moving toward the ultrasound transducers at speed V. If the target is moving at half the speed of sound, the observed frequency is increased by a factor of 3! Because changes in the frequency of sine waves can be measured precisely, the Doppler principle provides a very accurate method of measuring the velocity of moving sound reflectors. At the high frequencies often used (≥ 5 MHz), objects as small as red corpuscles can scatter enough sound for detection.

Ultrasound imaging is exceptionally complex. For simplicity's sake, recall the submarine movies wherein the sonar operator calls out "range 2000 yards, bearing 36 degrees." These two parameters are critical in describing some of the math of ultrasound.

The first factor to consider is the maximal range of the ultrasound, which is described by the following relationship:

$$r_{max} = cT/2$$

That is, the maximal range equals the speed of sound in tissue (≈ 1540 m/sec) multiplied by the time T between pulses divided by 2. A further limitation is the fact that the energy dissipates in the tissue. (You need to tap harder when percussing to detect deeper structures). For deeper penetration into tissues, one requires higher energies and slower pulse rates. Wavelength and frequency are related in the following manner:

$$\lambda = c/f$$

where f is the frequency, λ is the wavelength, and c is the speed of sound.

Next we need to consider both the axial resolution (is the enemy destroyer 2000 yards distant, or 2005?) and the annular resolution (is the bearing 36 or 38 degrees?). Sound in tissue spreads out in a bandwidth around a fundamental frequency. So to determine the necessary bandwidth for an axial resolution of 2 mm, the following rough approximation holds:

$$B = 2c/\Delta r$$

where Δr is the axial resolution. Therefore we need a bandwidth of 1 54 MHz to get an axial resolution of 2 mm.

For annular resolution ($\Delta\theta$), remember that the beam spreads out the further it goes from the source. Without deriving the mathematics, two factors determine annular resolution, the frequency and the aperture. Aperture size is limited to a size that will fit into or onto a human. Remember that a 1-degree error at a 1-cm range will increase at a 10-cm range: circumference = $2\pi r$: $1/360 \times 2 \times \pi \times 1 = 0.17$ mm; thus, at 10 cm, circumference = 1.7 mm.

CHAPTER
31 Measuring Depth of Anesthesia

Donald R. Stanski and Steven L. Shafer

Definitions of Anesthetic Depth   1227
Historical Definitions   1227
A Modern Definition of the
    Anesthetic State   1230

Memory and Awareness   1236
Recall, Conscious or Explicit Memory   1237
Detection of Auditory Input, Unconscious or
    Implicit Memory   1238
Implications of Explicit,
    Intraoperative Recall   1238

**Hypnotics, Analgesics, and
Anesthetic Depth   1239**
Inhaled Anesthetics   1239

Intravenously Administered (Nonopioid)
    Anesthetics   1243
Opioids   1246

**Electrophysiologic
Monitoring   1249**
Spontaneous Electroencephalogram   1249
Bispectral Electroencephalographic
    Monitoring   1250
Other Measures of Anesthetic
    Depth   1257

Summary   1258

Anesthesiologists appear to define the state of "anesthesia" the same way that Justice Potter Stewart, without disclosing his research, defined pornography in 1964: "I know it when I see it." This definition is inadequate to quantitatively measure the anesthetic state. Anesthesiologists proffer multiple and sometimes inconsistent views on quantitative measures of the anesthetic state. Fortunately, an integrated, quantitative concept of the anesthetic state can now be built on the incremental knowledge developed since the introduction of anesthesia over a century ago.

The chapter is divided into three general sections. The first section discusses two related topics: the evolving definitions of depth of anesthesia and the problem of recall (memory) and awareness. The history of attempts to define "depth of anesthesia" make one realize that our knowledge of the specific attributes of the drugs used in clinical practice has to be incorporated into our understanding of anesthetic depth.

The second section of this chapter involves basic pharmacologic concepts relevant to the scientific investigation of depth of anesthesia. This brief review, which includes an overview examining the interaction of two anesthetic drugs, prepares the reader for the third section, which discusses specific drugs and clinical situations in two subsections. The first subsection discusses clinical measures of anesthetic depth that derive directly from the patient. Each discussion begins with a review of the scientific approaches available to quantitate the relationship of

drug dose or plasma concentration to the resulting drug effects. This fundamental anesthetic clinical pharmacology is needed to then integrate the different drugs into the clinical administration of an anesthetic and subsequently interpret the drug interactions relative to the fundamental "depth of anesthesia." The second subsection discusses electrophysiologic approaches to assessing depth of anesthesia. These approaches represent the application of technology to the issue of quantitation of anesthetic drug effect and depth of anesthesia. Depth of anesthesia is the interaction of two drug effects fundamental to clinical anesthesia. One drug effect involves the hypnotic component, which creates unconsciousness. The second drug effect involves the analgesic component, which decreases the body's reflex response to noxious stimuli. The interaction of these two components allows anesthesia to be delivered to patients in a safe and effective manner over a broad range of clinical situations.

DEFINITIONS OF ANESTHETIC DEPTH

Historical Definitions

The word "anesthesia" was first used by the Greek philosopher Dioscorides in the first century of the current era to describe the narcotic effect of the plant mandragora.

The word reappeared in the 1771 *Encyclopaedia Britannica,* where it was defined as a "privation of the senses."[1] After the introduction of ether anesthesia by Morton in 1846, Oliver Wendell Holmes coined the word to describe the new phenomenon that made surgical procedures possible.

Plomley,[2] in 1847, was the first to attempt to define depth of anesthesia. He described three stages: intoxication, excitement (both conscious and unconscious), and the deeper levels of narcosis. In that same year, John Snow[3] described "five degrees of narcotism" for ether anesthesia. The first three stages encompassed induction of anesthesia, and the last two represented surgical anesthesia. Eleven years later, Snow[4] turned his attention to chloroform. Snow's excellent characterizations of ether and chloroform anesthesia described the following signs: conjunctival reflex; regular, deep, automatic breathing; movement of the eyeballs; and inhibition of the intercostal muscles. Many of these clinical signs were later "rediscovered."[5] Because oxygen was not readily available until the early 1900s, Snow and his successors tried to minimize the use of deep anesthesia to decrease morbidity and mortality.

The early 1900s saw the introduction of premedication with sedatives or opioids. In addition, anesthetics with more rapid onset, such as nitrous oxide and ethylene, became available. Therefore, the anesthetic excitement phase could be traversed more rapidly with the use of preanesthetic medication and rapid-onset inhaled anesthetics. In 1937, Guedel published his classic description of the clinical signs of ether anesthesia.[6] He used clear physical signs involving somatic muscle tone, respiratory patterns, and ocular signs (Fig. 31-1) to define four stages. The first stage, analgesia, is characterized by slow, regular breathing with the diaphragm and intercostal muscles and the presence of the lid reflex. The subject experiences complete amnesia, analgesia, and sedation. In the second

stage (delirium), the subject experiences excitement, unconsciousness, and a dream state with uninhibited activity. Ventilation is irregular and unpredictable. Reflex dilatation of the pupils occurs, the lid reflex is intact, and the risk of clinically important reflex activity (e.g., vomiting, laryngospasm, or arrhythmias) increases. The third stage (surgical anesthesia) consists of four progressive planes. Plane 1 is characterized by slight somatic relaxation, regular periodic breathing, and active ocular muscles. During plane 2, breathing changes, inhalation becomes briefer than exhalation, and a slight pause separates inhalation and exhalation. The eyes become immobile. In plane 3, the abdominal muscles are completely relaxed, and diaphragmatic breathing is very prominent. The eyelid reflex is absent. In plane 4, the intercostal muscles are completely paralyzed, and paradoxical rib cage movement occurs. Breathing is irregular, and the pupils are dilated. In Guedel's fourth stage (respiratory paralysis), muscles become flaccid, and the eyes widely dilate. Cardiovascular and respiratory arrest occurs, as does cardiovascular collapse.

In 1954, Artusio[7] expanded Guedel's description of ether analgesia (stage 1) into three planes. In plane 1, the patient has no amnesia or analgesia. In plane 2, the patient has total amnesia and partial analgesia. In plane 3, the patient has complete analgesia and amnesia, but is comfortable and responsive to verbal stimulation; there is little depression of reflexes. The clinical signs of depth of anesthesia defined by Guedel and others had significant practical utility for the administration of ether, cyclopropane, and chloroform anesthesia. The success of using clinical signs to assess ether anesthetic depth arises partly from the established hypnotic and analgesic effects that ether provides, which differ from those of the current inhaled anesthetics used in modern anesthetic practice.

Beginning in 1942, small doses of the muscle relaxant *d*-tubocurarine were used with the deep levels of ether

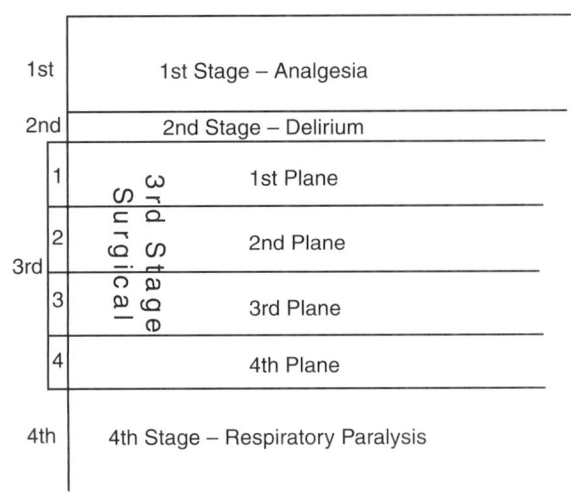

Showing division of anesthesia into four stages and the division of the third or surgical stage into four planes.

A

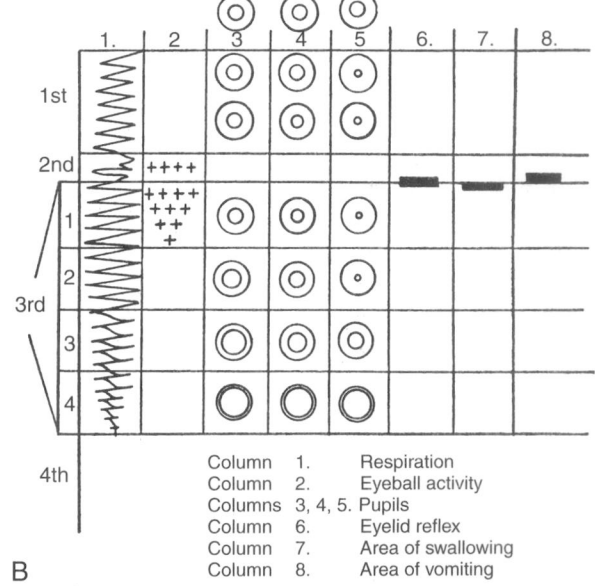

Column 1. Respiration
Column 2. Eyeball activity
Columns 3, 4, 5. Pupils
Column 6. Eyelid reflex
Column 7. Area of swallowing
Column 8. Area of vomiting

B

Figure 31–1 Guedel's classic text described the stages and planes of ether anesthesia (**A**) and then related them to clinical signs or relevant reflexes (**B**). (From Guedel AE: Inhalational Anesthesia: A Fundamental Guide. New York, Macmillan, 1937.)

anesthesia that produced plane 2 or 3 of Guedel's stage III. Respiration was assisted when necessary. Over time, the dose of *d*-tubocurarine began to increase as fully controlled ventilation became commonplace. Anesthesiologists soon realized that they could combine controlled ventilation and large doses of muscle relaxants with low concentrations of inhaled anesthetics to reduce the risk of toxicity (cardiovascular and respiratory depression) and increase the speed of emergence from anesthesia. However, the use of muscle relaxants eliminated two valuable types of clinical signs of depth of anesthesia: the rate and volume of respiration and the degree of muscle relaxation induced by the anesthetic.[7] Seven of the nine components of Guedel's classification system involved skeletal muscle activity. When muscle relaxants are used with ether anesthesia, only pupil size and lacrimation are left as clinical signs. These signs are inadequate to judge anesthetic depth clinically.[8] A 1945 editorial in the *Lancet* discussed the clinical problems that muscle relaxants would create,[9] and descriptions of patient awareness during surgery later began to appear in the literature.[10]

In 1957, Woodbridge[11] examined the diverse use of anesthetic drugs at that time. He defined anesthesia as having four components: (1) sensory blockade of afferent nerve impulses; (2) motor blockade of efferent impulses; (3) reflex blockade of the respiratory, cardiovascular, or gastrointestinal tract; and (4) mental block, sleep, or unconsciousness. Different drugs could be used to achieve each effect. However, Woodbridge made no effort to define methods of assessing each of these components.

In a 1987 editorial, Prys-Roberts[12] contributed to the concept of depth of anesthesia by redefining which elements are truly relevant to anesthesia. He began by observing that depth of anesthesia is difficult to define because anesthetists have approached the issue in terms of the drugs available to them rather than the patient's needs during surgery. Prys-Roberts believed that the noxious stimulation of surgery induces a variety of reflex responses that may be independently modified to the benefit of the patient. One important premise is that pain is the conscious perception of noxious stimuli. Thus, he defined anesthesia as a state in which the patient neither perceives nor recalls noxious stimuli as a result of drug-induced unconsciousness. The loss of consciousness is considered a threshold or all-or-none (quantal) phenomenon. By this definition, there can be no degrees of anesthesia or any variable depth of anesthesia. Prys-Roberts defined

anesthesia in terms of the drugs producing unconsciousness and modification of noxious stimuli, and he classified them by pharmacologic properties of the drugs and not by their ability to produce components of the state of anesthesia.

Prys-Roberts focused his concepts on the body's response to noxious stimuli, which he defined as factors causing potential or actual cell damage: mechanical, chemical, thermal, or radiation induced. Figure 31-2 shows the somatic and autonomic responses to noxious stimuli. In this scheme, one reads from left to right and from top to bottom to see the order in which reflex responses are suppressed by anesthetic drugs. For example, somatic responses include both sensory and motor activity. Sensory input obtained through the central nervous system (CNS) can originate from somatic or visceral tissue. The subject must be conscious to perceive pain. Low concentrations of inhaled or intravenously administered anesthetics can eliminate recall of pain, but they allow a motor response. The motor response to noxious stimuli is typically an all-or-none reflex withdrawal of the stimulated part. Eger and colleagues[13] used this movement response as a clinical end point in developing the concept of minimum alveolar concentration (MAC).

The response of the respiratory system is part of the autonomic response described by Prys-Roberts. The motor response to noxious stimuli can involve an increase in tidal volume or the frequency of breathing. This ventilatory response may occur even if there is no somatic motor response to surgical stimulation. A higher concentration is required to suppress the breathing response than to suppress the somatic response to noxious stimuli.

Prys-Roberts divided autonomic responses into three categories. The hemodynamic response consists of autonomic responses to noxious stimuli, namely, increased sympathoadrenal activity that elevates arterial blood pressure and the heart rate. The sudomotor response consists of sweating. Release of hormones is an extremely difficult response to eliminate completely.

Prys-Roberts considered pain relief, muscle relaxation, and suppression of autonomic activity to be discrete pharmacologic events. These events may be engendered by specific drugs. Some drugs can produce all these end points; others can achieve only one or two. The only feature common to most anesthetics is suppression of sensory perception and production of unconsciousness. He considered inclusion of muscle relaxation in the definition of

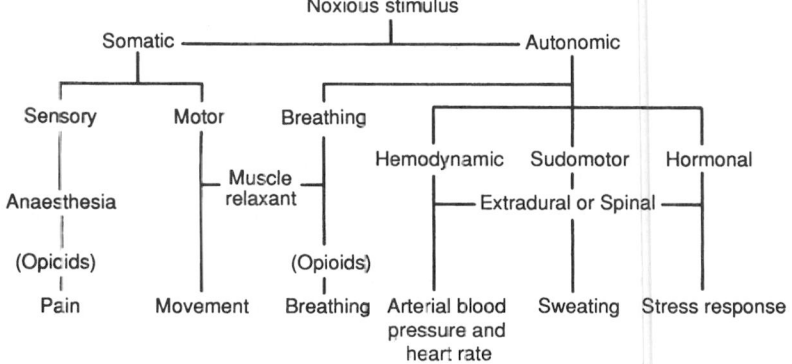

Figure 31–2 Depth of anesthesia can be defined by suppression of the relevant clinical responses to noxious stimuli, as proposed by Prys-Roberts. (Modified from Prys-Roberts C: Anaesthesia: A practical or impossible construct [editorial]? Br J Anaesth 59:1341, 1987.)

the anesthetic state illogical and confusing. Although muscle relaxation is necessary for laryngoscopy and surgical access, it is neither a component of anesthesia nor an alternative to adequate anesthesia.

Kissin,[14] in a 1993 editorial, expanded, refined, and further contributed to the definition of anesthesia. He began by indicating that a wide spectrum of pharmacologic actions by different drugs can be used to create the general anesthetic state. These pharmacologic actions include analgesia, anxiolysis, amnesia, unconsciousness, and suppression of somatic motor, cardiovascular, and hormonal responses to the stimulation of surgery. Kissin stated that the spectrum of effects that constitute the state of general anesthesia should not be regarded as several components of anesthesia resulting from one anesthetic action but, instead, should be considered as separate pharmacologic actions, even if the anesthesia is produced by one drug. Kissin then reviewed a series of investigative studies and concepts that supported his hypothesis:

1. Several groups of drugs (benzodiazepines, opioids, α_2-agonists) that induce anesthesia by acting on specific receptors can have their anesthetic effects reversed by the administration of a specific receptor antagonist.

2. There is growing understanding that the molecular mechanisms of general anesthesia are more specific than was suggested by the previous unitary hypothesis of anesthesia.

3. The rank order of effects for two important goals of anesthesia (hypnotic effect and blockade of somatic motor response to noxious stimuli) can be different for different classes of anesthetics. Opioids induce blockade of the movement response to noxious stimulation before hypnosis occurs. For intravenous anesthetics, the opposite occurs.

4. When studies of anesthetic interactions are undertaken, the type of interaction (synergism, antagonism, summation) for one component of anesthesia may differ from that of another component.

5. Classic theories of anesthesia, based on the unitary nonspecific mechanisms of anesthetic action, suggest that one anesthetic may be freely replaceable by another and that the anesthetic effects of combinations of anesthetics should be additive. Many combinations of anesthetic drugs prove to be supra-additive for the hypnotic effects, a finding suggesting that the mechanisms of hypnotic action of different components of a combination are different.

If one understands general anesthesia as a spectrum of separate pharmacologic actions that vary according to the goals of anesthesia, certain conclusions can be made regarding the measurement of anesthetic potency and depth of anesthesia. Kissin stated that "Diversity of pharmacological actions that in combination provide anesthesia make[s] it almost impossible to determine the potency of different actions with one measure."[14]

A Modern Definition of the Anesthetic State

What Is Anesthesia?

The sine qua non of the anesthetized state is unconsciousness, the lack of conscious processing of thoughts. The crux of the difficulty in defining "anesthetic depth" is that unconsciousness cannot be measured directly. What can be measured is response to stimulation. Does the patient move when his name is called? Does the response to incision suggest conscious perception? Does the heart rate or blood pressure go up in response to surgical manipulation? Does the patient remember events, conversations, or pain? As observed by Prys-Roberts (see Fig. 31-2), anesthesia is nonresponsiveness, broadly defined. The "depth" of anesthesia is determined by the stimulus applied, the response measured, and the drug concentration at the site of action that blunts responsiveness.

As defined elsewhere in this chapter, the state of consciousness can also be inferred, though not directly measured, by analysis of electroencephalographic (EEG) information. Such analysis can be done by using either spectral-based techniques such as the "bispectral (BIS) index" or evoked potentials such as auditory evoked potentials. These indices do not directly measure unconsciousness or unresponsiveness. However, through extensive validation it is clear that these measures are predictive of the likelihood of response, provided that the anesthetic state has been induced with the drugs used to calibrate the electrophysiologic measure.

Nonresponsiveness can be introduced by deep sleep, an unusually boring chapter, or 2% isoflurane. What distinguishes the nonresponsiveness of the anesthetic state from the nonresponsiveness of normal sleep is the differential in stimulus that can penetrate the state of nonresponsiveness and rouse the brain to conscious perception. The hypnotic drugs used in anesthesia (propofol, thiopental, inhaled anesthetics, ketamine) are each capable of producing such profound CNS depression that even the most painful surgical stimulus cannot rouse patients from a state of nearly total nonresponsiveness. However, if the surgical stimulus can be attenuated before reaching the cortical level, less drug is required to maintain the state of nonresponsiveness.

Attenuation of surgical stimulation is the function of analgesic drugs (e.g., opioids) and local anesthetics. The interaction between analgesics and hypnotics is thus fundamental to understanding and defining anesthetic depth. Table 31-1 indicates the components of defining depth of anesthesia used in the remainder of this chapter.

Extending ideas proposed by Glass in 1998,[15] consciousness can thus be perceived as a balance within the cortex between depression and excitation (Fig. 31-3, upper right). The cortex is primarily depressed by hypnotics, although opioids and nitrous oxide also have sedating

---

Table 31–1 Components needed to define depth of anesthesia

Afferent stimulus
Efferent response
Equilibrated concentrations of analgesic components
Equilibrated concentrations of hypnotic components
Equilibrated concentrations of other relevant drugs
    (e.g., β-blockers, muscle relaxants, local anesthetics)
Interaction surface relating drug concentrations to the
    probability of a given response to a given stimulus

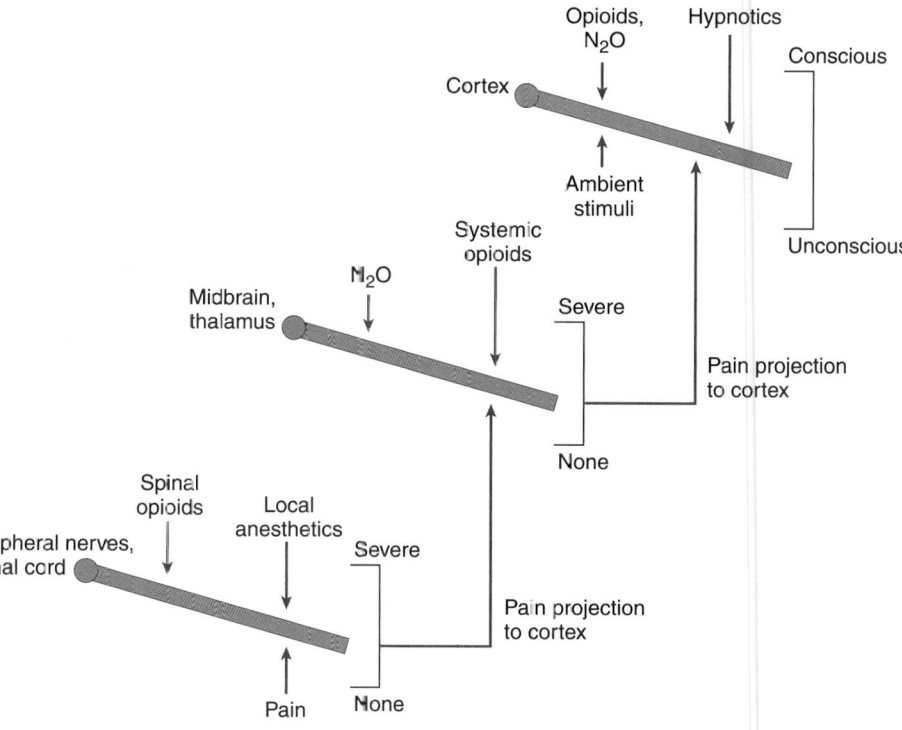

Figure 31–3 Stylized view of the interaction between hypnotics, which depress consciousness, and analgesics, which suppress noxious stimuli.

properties that depress the cortex. Cortical depression promotes unconsciousness. These effects are opposed by both ambient stimulation (e.g., music, a hard cold mattress) and the excitatory effects of pain projected from the thalamus and midbrain on the cortex.

Figure 31-3 also shows the influence of opioids, nitrous oxide, and local anesthetics in preventing noxious stimulation from reaching the cortex. Systemic opioids act primarily on the midbrain and thalamus,[16] whereas neuraxial opioids act on the spinal cord. Local anesthetics act either at the spinal cord (for neuraxial blocks) or on peripheral nerves (e.g., nerve blocks and local infiltration). Nitrous oxide exerts some of its analgesic effects through spinal mechanisms,[17,18] as well as midbrain mechanisms,[19] but for simplicity we will lump it together with opioids at the midbrain. The net effect of analgesic and local anesthetics is to attenuate the transmission of painful sensation to the cortex, thereby reducing the amount of hypnotic required to obtain a state of nonresponsiveness.

The Pharmacologic View of the Anesthetic State
Figure 31-4 reduces the model in Figure 31-3 to a highly simplified pharmacologic view. The subcortical actions in Figure 31-3 have been compressed to a single site of action, the midbrain. Similarly, Figure 31-4 compresses all analgesics, including nitrous oxide, local anesthetics, and opioids, to just "opioids." Finally, Figure 31-4 equates "unconsciousness," which is clearly cortical, with "nonresponsiveness," which involves both cortical and subcortical structures. The result is a simplified pharmacologic structure that may provide insight into the interaction between analgesics and hypnotics on consciousness and responsiveness.

In Figure 31-4, painful stimuli arrive in the midbrain. Opioids attenuate the response. The magnitude of the

stimulus affects both the magnitude of the output and the apparent potency of the opioids. Another way of saying this is that it takes more opioid to attenuate an intensely painful stimulus than a modestly painful stimulus. This has been repeatedly demonstrated, as shown in Figure 31-5.[20] Pharmacologically, the effect of opioids on attenuating the pain signal at the midbrain can be expressed by using a standard sigmoid Emax pharmacodynamic equation:

$$\text{Pain out} = \text{Pain in} \cdot \left(1 - \frac{\text{Opioid}^{\gamma}}{\text{Opioid}^{\gamma} + (\text{Opioid}_{50} \cdot \text{Pain in})^{\gamma}}\right)$$

in which "pain in" is the afferent painful stimulus entering the midbrain, "pain out" is the efferent painful stimulus transmitted to the cortex, "opioid" is the opioid concentration in the midbrain, "opioid$_{50}$" is the equilibrated opioid concentration associated with 50% attenuation of the "pain in" for an afferent pain intensity of 1, and γ is the steepness of the opioid concentration-versus-response relationship. Opioid$_{50}$ is multiplied by "pain in" to reflect the decreased potency of opioids in attenuating severe pain, as shown in Figure 31-5.

In Figure 31-4 the output of the midbrain is projected to the cortex, where the CNS-arousing characteristics of pain are balanced by the CNS-depressant effects of hypnotics. The pharmacologic expression of this relationship would be

$$\frac{\text{Probability of}}{\text{nonresponsiveness}} = 1 - \frac{\text{Hypnotic}^{\eta}}{\text{Hypnotic}^{\eta} + (\text{Hypnotic}_{50} \cdot \text{Stimulus in})^{\eta}}$$

where "stimulus in" is the "pain out" projecting from the midbrain plus the ambient stimulation, "hypnotic" is the concentration of the sedative-hypnotic in the cortex, "hypnotic$_{50}$" is the concentration associated with

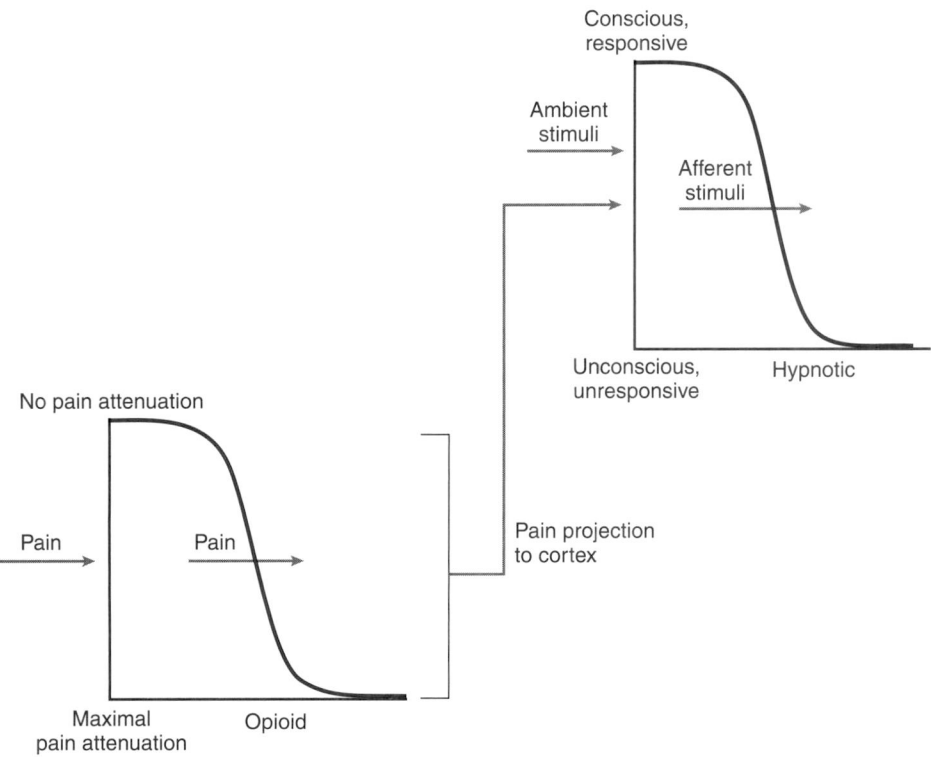

Figure 31–4 Pharmacologic interpretation of the interaction between hypnotics and analgesics.

a 50% probability of nonresponsiveness when the "stimulus in" equals 1, and η is the steepness of the hypnotic concentration–versus–probability of nonresponsiveness relationship.

If we integrate these cascading models of drug effect, we get a response surface as shown in Figure 31-6. The x and y axes of Figure 31-6 are the equilibrated concentrations of opioid and hypnotic, respectively, The z axis of Figure 31-6

is the probability of nonresponsiveness. This surface has the fundamental properties of the opioid-hypnotic relationship. Near the origin for drug concentrations, labeled "1" on the surface, there is no chance of nonresponsiveness, probably because the patient is wide awake. In fact, the floor of the figure indicates that a minimum amount

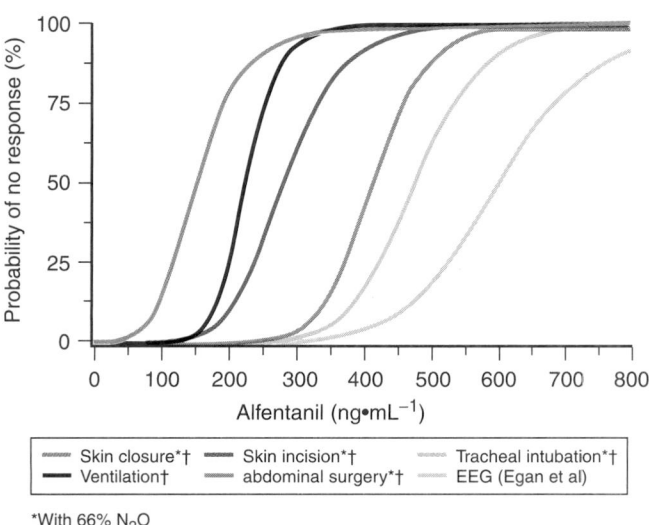

*With 66% N_2O
†Ausems et al

Figure 31–5 The effect of increasingly painful stimulation on the opioid concentration-versus-response relationship.[20] As pain intensity increases, the apparent potency of the opioids decreases.

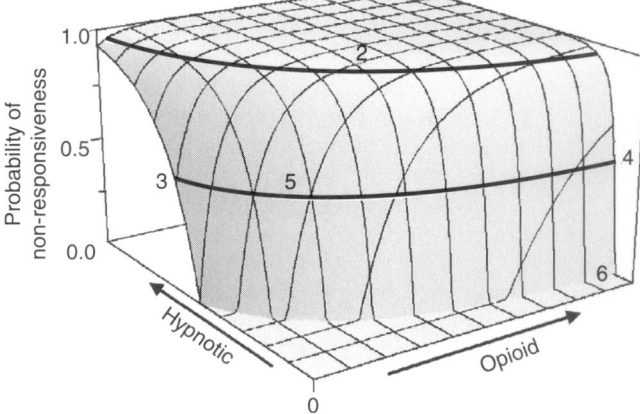

Figure 31–6 Relationship between opioid and hypnotic drug concentrations and the probability of nonresponsiveness. 1, No chance of nonresponsiveness; 2, no chance of response; 3, hypnotic concentration-versus-response relationship in the absence of opioids; 4, hypnotic concentration-versus-response relationship in the presence of large doses of opioids; 5, area of maximum synergy between opioids and hypnotics; 6, in the absence of hypnotics, even profound levels of opioids cannot suppress the response; *red line* in the middle of the surface, the 50% isobole; *red curve* at the top of the surface, 95% isobole.

of drug must be given before the patient has any chance of nonresponsiveness. On the other side of the surface, labeled "2," enough opioid and hypnotic are present to ensure virtually no chance of response. The red line in the middle of the surface is the 50% isobole. This line shows the opioid and hypnotic concentrations associated with a 50% probability of responsiveness. It extends from the curve for the hypnotic concentration-versus-response relationship in the absence of opioids on the far left, labeled "3," to the hypnotic concentration-versus-response relationship in the presence of large quantities of opioids on the right, labeled "4." The relationship between hypnotics and opioids is highly synergistic in that when the drugs are used in combination (for example, at the point labeled "5"), it takes far less of either drug than would be the case were the opioids or hypnotics used alone. Notice how some hypnotic is required to achieve the anesthetized state. In the absence of a hypnotic, even profound levels of opioids are unable to produce a state of nonresponsiveness, as can be seen at point "6" on the surface.[21-24] However, a modest amount of opioid profoundly reduces the concentration of hypnotic necessary for nonresponsiveness, as seen at point "5." Beyond this point, additional opioid has only modest effect in further reducing the hypnotic dose required for drug effect. The corollary is that large doses of hypnotic are required in the absence of an opioid.[25-27] The red curve at the top of the surface is the 95% isobole. This curve defines the opioid and hypnotic combinations associated with a 95% probability of nonresponsiveness. Because the surface is very steep, once there is a modest probability of nonresponsiveness, a modest increase in drug concentration is all that is required to move from a 50% chance of nonresponsiveness to a 95% chance of nonresponsiveness.

Figure 31-6 is intentionally left unitless to illustrate that a very simple model of the anesthetic state, as shown in Figure 31-3, generates a pharmacologic response surface that is very much like those seen in virtually all drug interaction trials.[28]

The ability of inhaled anesthetics to induce immobility in response to noxious stimulation is mediated by the spinal cord, not the cortex.[29-31] We also know that intravenous opioids primarily work at the level of the midbrain. Experimentally, the interaction between inhaled anesthetics and opioids in preventing movement response to noxious stimulation looks very close to Figure 31-6. Thus, it seems logical that downward projections from the midbrain to the spinal cord[32] are responsible for the MAC-sparing properties of opioids. As such, a pharmacologic model of the effect of opioids on MAC would resemble Figure 31-4 with a few changes to reflect opioids attenuating the signal at the dorsal horn and the response end point (movement) mediated by the spinal cord rather than the cortex.

Experimental Characterization of the Anesthetic State

To quantify anesthetic depth, we must be rigorous about the definition of the z axis in Figure 31-6, nonresponsiveness. Consider a complex matrix of stimuli and responses, as shown in Figure 31-7. Stimuli can be roughly divided into benign and noxious. Benign stimuli are not physically painful. Thus, responses to benign stimuli are readily suppressed by hypnotics alone, with minimal need for analgesic drugs. Noxious stimuli are physically painful, and thus responses to noxious stimuli are more readily suppressed in the presence of analgesics. Among the noxious stimuli, skin incision appears somewhat in the middle; it is more stimulating than electrical pain, but much less stimulating than laryngoscopy. Figure 31-7 presents the noxious stimuli in approximately increasing order.

Responses can be categorized as verbal, purposeful movement, involuntary movement, ventilation, hemodynamic response, sudomotor response, the formation of implicit and explicit memories, and EEG responses, as shown in Figure 31-7. The responses also tend to follow a rank order in that loss of verbal response precedes loss of purposeful movement, which precedes loss of involuntary movement. Opioids tend to ablate hemodynamic response

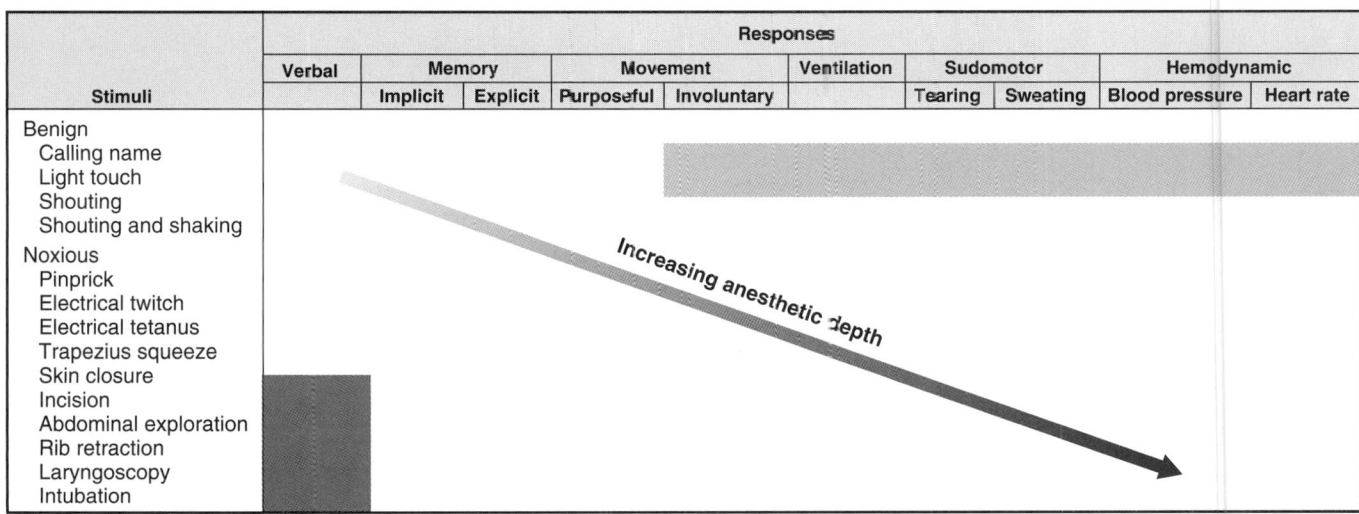

Stimuli	Responses									
	Verbal	Memory		Movement		Ventilation	Sudomotor		Hemodynamic	
		Implicit	Explicit	Purposeful	Involuntary		Tearing	Sweating	Blood pressure	Heart rate
Benign Calling name Light touch Shouting Shouting and shaking **Noxious** Pinprick Electrical twitch Electrical tetanus Trapezius squeeze Skin closure Incision Abdominal exploration Rib retraction Laryngoscopy Intubation					Increasing anesthetic depth					

Figure 31-7 Matrix of relevant stimuli and responses. Stimuli are in approximately increasing order of noxiousness. Responses are in approximately increasing order of difficulty of suppression. As the cells progress from left to right and from top to bottom, increasingly larger doses of anesthetic are required to suppress a given response to a given stimulus.

before movement, whereas hypnotics tend to ablate movement response before hemodynamic response.[33] Given this tendency, we would anticipate that the interaction surfaces between opioids and hypnotics for hemodynamic response and movement response would have several intersections. Frequently, the responses are grouped. For example, the responses that suggest conscious perception, such as verbal, voluntary movement, and memory, might be grouped together. Responses that are autonomic in nature, such as hemodynamic and sudomotor response, are logically grouped together.

For simplicity we will consider complete nonresponsiveness to be a lack of any of these responses. If we were interested only in consciousness, we might not include involuntary movement, ventilation response, hemodynamic response, or sudomotor response in our list of important responses because they can still occur in the absence of any conscious perception.

Figure 31-7 shows a matrix of stimuli and responses with 140 cells. Not all the cells are clinically relevant. For example, one rarely has involuntary movements, hyperventilates, or has autonomic responses to hearing one's name called, although beauty pageants and Internal Revenue Service visits are notable counterexamples. On the converse side, anesthesia should never be so inadequate that patients scream on incision. Thus, some cells in Figure 31-7 have been removed as being clinically uninteresting, which leaves 122 cells to define anesthetic depth. If we wanted to fully characterize the ability of isoflurane and fentanyl to create a state of nonresponsiveness for each of the listed responses to any of the listed stimuli, we would need to characterize the response surface (Fig. 31-6) for each clinically relevant cell! With so many choices of stimuli and interactions, it is not surprising that anesthesiologists cannot agree on a simple definition of anesthetic depth. Fortunately, it is not really necessary to characterize the response to every stimulus. If we characterize the response to a benign stimulus, such as shaking and

shouting, and several noxious stimuli, such as electrical tetanus, incision, laryngoscopy, and intubation, we will have captured the clinically relevant range of benign and noxious stimulation.

To this we must add the matrix of hypnotics versus opioids. Commonly used hypnotics include the anesthetic gases halothane, isoflurane, sevoflurane, and desflurane and the intravenous hypnotics propofol, thiopental, etomidate, and midazolam. Commonly used opioids include fentanyl, alfentanil, sufentanil, remifentanil, morphine, meperidine, hydromorphone, methadone, and (in Europe) tramadol and piritramide. With 8 hypnotics and 10 opioids, there are 80 combinations. Eighty combinations times 122 interactions yields 9760 combinations of opioids, hypnotics, stimuli, and responses. To this we must then add the influence of age, disease, genetics, and other factors. Clearly, it is impossible to create response surfaces to characterize how opioids and hypnotics produce a state of nonresponsiveness for all possible combinations of drugs, patients, stimuli, and responses.

Fortunately, there are powerful generalizations that provide both clinical insight and tractable experimental design. The most important is that for any stimulus-response pair, depth of anesthesia is the probability of nonresponse. More generally, *depth of anesthesia is the probability of nonresponse to stimulation, calibrated against the strength of the stimulus, the difficulty of suppressing the response, and the drug-induced probability of nonresponsiveness.* Anesthetic depth ranges from a 100% probability of an easily suppressed response (verbal answer) to a mild stimulus (e.g., calling one's name) and readily suppressed responses (e.g., verbal answer) to a 100% probability of nonresponse to profoundly noxious stimuli (e.g., intubation) and responses that are difficult to suppress (e.g., tachycardia). Table 31-1 lists the components needed to define anesthetic depth.

Figure 31-8 integrates the role of anesthetic drugs in the stimulus-response relationship. It shows three stimuli of

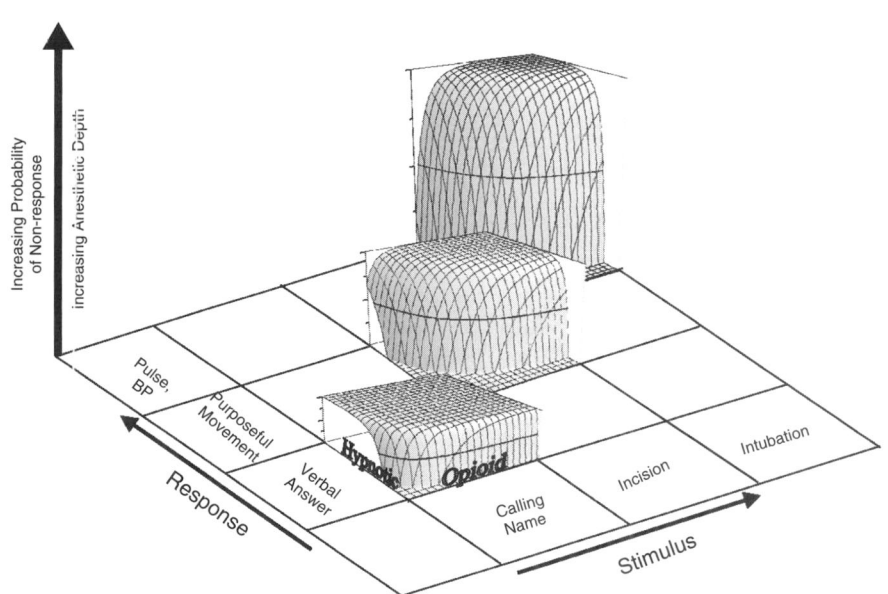

Figure 31–8 The role of opioid and hypnotics in the stimulus-response relationship for three stimuli of increasing intensity and three increasingly difficult responses to suppress. Each cell would have its own opioid-hypnotic interaction surface, and three are displayed. The vertical axis is the probability of nonresponse. Verbal nonresponsiveness to name calling is readily suppressed, even at light levels of anesthesia. In contrast, profound levels of anesthesia are required to suppress the hemodynamic response to intubation.

increasing intensity: name calling, incision, and intubation. It also shows three different responses to stimuli that are increasingly difficult to suppress: verbal, movement, and hemodynamic response. Within three of the cells are representative opioid-hypnotic interactions. As seen in the cells, verbal response to name calling is readily suppressed by hypnotics, with only modest effect from opioids. Movement to incision requires more hypnotic and opioid to suppress. Additionally, the "z" probability axis has been stretched vertically to indicate that a 100% chance of nonresponse to incision is a more profound level of drug effect than is a 100% chance of nonresponse to name calling. Suppressing the most difficult response, hypertension and tachycardia, to the most profound stimulus, intubation, requires even more opioid and hypnotic. Additionally, the probability axis is further elongated vertically, thus indicating that suppression of the hemodynamic response to intubation requires a more profound drug effect than does suppressing movement to incision. The distant response surface in Figure 31-8 demonstrates a profound anesthetic depth based on the stimulus, the response, and the drug-induced probability of nonresponse. As demonstrated in Figure 31-8, anesthetic depth ranges from a 100% chance of a verbal response to a verbal command (wide awake, no drug) to enough opioid and hypnotic to provide a 100% chance of no hemodynamic response to intubation.

For the inhaled anesthetics, MAC creates a unifying principle. Although each inhaled anesthetic has some pharmacologic peculiarities, in general, they have parallel dose-response curves across drugs (e.g., isoflurane versus sevoflurane versus desflurane) and across stimuli-response pairs (MAC$_{awake}$,[34,35] MAC, MAC$_{BAR}$[36,37] [MAC of anesthetic necessary to prevent the β-adrenergic response to skin incision]). Thus, by knowing the relative values of MAC, one can infer the relative values of the other stimulus-response relationships. There is less similarity among the intravenous hypnotics. Fortunately, only propofol and midazolam are commonly used to induce and maintain the anesthetic state, which limits the number of clinically interesting intravenous anesthetic combinations.

Despite conflicting reports of pharmacologic idiosyncrasies with each member of the fentanyl series, fentanyl, alfentanil, sufentanil, and remifentanil appear to differ mainly in potency, with otherwise parallel concentration-versus-response relationships. Morphine, meperidine, hydromorphone, and methadone appear to differ in both potency and intrinsic efficacy, with slightly lower maximal analgesic effect than noted with the fentanyl series of opioids. These latter four also have their own pharmacologic quirks, particularly meperidine.

Nitrous oxide is not only the oldest of the anesthetic drugs still in common use but remains one of the least well understood. It has properties of hypnotics, with an identifiable MAC of about 1 atm,[38] and is a modestly potent analgesic as well. Although the interaction of nitrous oxide with opioids,[39] inhaled anesthetics,[40,41] and propofol[42,43] has been characterized, no studies have gathered enough data to generate the response surfaces needed to fully understand the interactions of this nearly ubiquitous anesthetic drug.

Fundamental Relationships That Characterize the Anesthetic State

Based on the simplifying assumptions, we need to understand a limited number of prototypic drug combinations: isoflurane-fentanyl, isoflurane–nitrous oxide, nitrous oxide–fentanyl, propofol-fentanyl, propofol–nitrous oxide, midazolam–nitrous oxide, and midazolam-fentanyl. For each of these combinations, characterization of the response surface for a handful of stimuli and responses would allow understanding of current clinical practice and provide for definition of the full range of anesthetic depth:

1. Loss of response to shouting and shaking
   a. Any response is considered (i.e., "MAC$_{awake}$")
2. Loss of response to electrical tetanus
   a. Verbal response or purposeful movement
   b. Any autonomic (hemodynamic or sudomotor) response
   c. Any memory response
3. Loss of response to an intermediate stimulus (incision, trapezius muscle squeeze)
   a. Purposeful movement (i.e., "MAC")
   b. Any autonomic (hemodynamic or sudomotor) response (i.e., "MAC$_{BAR}$")
   c. Any memory response
4. Loss of response to laryngoscopy/intubation
   a. Purposeful movement
   b. Any autonomic (hemodynamic or sudomotor) response
   c. Any memory response
5. The unstimulated concentration–versus–EEG response relationship

We now have a matrix of just 11 stimulus-versus-response relationships. Multiplication by our seven prototypic drug combinations yields 77 response surfaces, from which we can infer the rest of the surfaces through scaling based on MAC for inhaled drugs and C$_{50}$ (plasma concentration that results in 50% drug effect) for intravenous drugs and the relative rankings of stimuli and responses. Moreover, the combinations range from light anesthesia, with modest stimulation and easily attenuated responses found in the upper right corner of Figure 31-7, to deep anesthesia, with profound stimuli and very difficult to ablate responses found in the lower right corner of Figure 31-7.

Figure 31-9 shows examples of response surfaces for a modest stimulus on the left (withdrawal in response to electrical tetanus) and a profound stimulus on the right (movement in response to intubation). These interaction surfaces are based on the same model as the interaction surface shown in Figure 31-6; they differ only in the intensity of the afferent painful signal. We find the same pattern when we examine real data. The left image in Figure 31-10 shows the response surface for MAC reduction of isoflurane by fentanyl.[23] The right image of Figure 31-10 shows the interaction of propofol with alfentanil on blunting all responses to intubation.[24] The shapes of these curves are not exactly like the shapes derived from our hypnotic-opioid interaction model because (1) the investigators were interested only in characterizing the interaction at the level of a 50% response and thus did not gather enough data to characterize the upper and lower edges of either curve and (2) the mathematical function used was multiple logistic regression, which has several

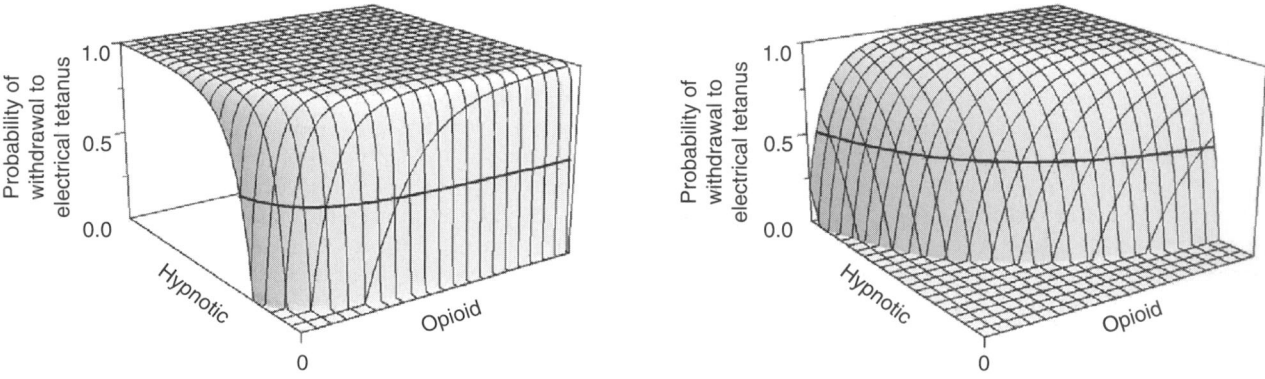

Figure 31–9 Examples of response surfaces for a modest stimulus on the *left* (withdrawal to electrical tetanus) and a profound stimulus on the *right* (movement response to intubation), based on the model shown in Figure 31-6 with differing intensity of the afferent painful signal. The figure on the *left* shows a relatively mild stimulus-response combination, whereas the figure on the *right* shows a profoundly noxious stimulus-response combination.

shortcomings as a model of drug interaction. Nevertheless, the figures demonstrate the intrinsic synergy between opioids and hypnotics in producing unresponsiveness, as well as the tendency for more profoundly noxious stimulation (e.g., intubation) to generate more synergy between the analgesic and hypnotic components of anesthesia.

Given our broad definition of anesthetic depth as providing nonresponsiveness to a wide range of stimuli and response pairs (Figure 31-7), one might wonder what drugs constitute anesthetics. For example, one can envision an anesthetic consisting of β-blockers to blunt the hemodynamic response, trimethaphan to prevent tearing, a ventilator to control respiration, duct tape to prevent movement, and scopolamine to prevent memory. There is no chance of any response to any stimulation, so (1) is the patient deeply anesthetized? and (2) are β-blockers, trimethaphan, ventilators, muscle relaxants, scopolamine, and duct tape anesthetics?

The answer to both questions is "yes." For the first question, if the proposed technique could truly provide a 100% chance of nonresponse (and we haven't tried this personally), it would be clinically indistinguishable from a conventional hypnotic-opioid technique that produced a similar state of nonresponsiveness. However, because scopolamine is a sedative and not usually associated with loss of consciousness, we would require a priori evidence that the scopolamine dose reliably produced unconsciousness and not just amnesia of the surgery. Our answer to the second question is "yes, duct tape is an anesthetic." This reductio ad absurdum demonstrates the ambiguity in the word "anesthetic" as a noun referring to a class of drugs. Drugs are defined by their actions. Because the creation of a state of nonresponsiveness ("anesthesia") involves so many drug actions, the term "anesthetic" should not be used to suggest a particular drug class. In particular, "anesthetics" should not be used to describe drugs that suppress consciousness because they are more accurately termed "hypnotics."

MEMORY AND AWARENESS

Before the introduction of anesthesia in 1846, surgical operations were uncommon. Robertson[44] unearthed two

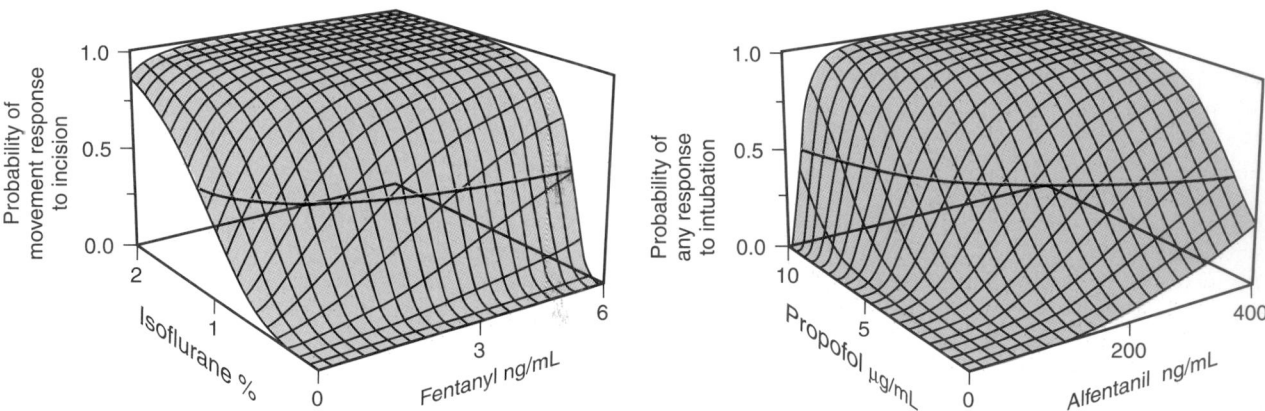

Figure 31–10 The *left image* shows the response surface for minimum alveolar concentration reduction of isoflurane by fentanyl.[23] The *right image* shows the interaction of propofol with alfentanil on blunting all responses to intubation.[24] Both figures demonstrate the intrinsic synergy between opioids and hypnotics in producing unresponsiveness.

descriptions of the torture suffered by victims of surgical operations performed before the introduction of anesthesia. In spite of the introduction of surgical anesthesia, however, the vivid descriptions of pain during surgery have not been eliminated completely. Reports of awareness, recall, and memory under anesthesia still occur in clinical practice.

Vickers[45] described two degrees of inadequate depth of anesthesia. The first degree involves recall or retention of memory of an event that occurred while under anesthesia. Conscious or explicit memory refers to intentional or conscious recollection of previous experiences as assessed by tests of recall or recognition. The second degree of inadequate anesthesia involves responsiveness to auditory input, also called "wakefulness." Wakefulness has been described as the responding of a patient to a verbal command during or after surgery without recall of the stimulus. Unconscious or implicit memory refers to changes in performance or behavior that are produced by previous experience on tests that do not require any intentional or conscious recollection of those experiences.[46]

Recall, Conscious or Explicit Memory

In some clinical situations, the risk of intraoperative recall is high. Bogetz and Katz[47] examined the incidence of recall in 51 patients who underwent surgical procedures after major trauma. Thirty-seven patients with stable hemodynamic status were able to receive drugs for induction and maintenance of anesthesia. In this group, four had intraoperative recall. Two of the four patients considered this awareness their worst hospital experience. Fourteen of the 51 subjects were so severely injured and hemodynamically unstable that no anesthetic was administered for at least 20 minutes of surgery. Six of 14 of these patients (43%) recalled events from their surgery. Two of the latter subjects considered this intraoperative awareness the worst aspect of their hospital experience. A more recent study by Lubke and coworkers could not find evidence of explicit memory in a series of minor and major trauma patients.[48] The difference between these two studies, one in 1984 and the second in 1999, may reflect better resuscitation of trauma patients, which would increase the tolerance of anesthetic drugs. Lubke and colleagues' patients had a mean BIS index value of 54, thus suggesting adequate hypnosis.

The most comprehensive prospective study to date on intraoperative recall has been reported by Sandin and coauthors, who found that 18 patients out of 11,785 (0.15%) had awareness under general anesthesia.[49] The incidence of awareness was 0.18% in procedures that used neuromuscular blocking drugs and 0.10% in the absence of these drugs. They interviewed patients on three different occasions: in the recovery room, when recall was detected in only 39%; again at 1 to 3 days, when recall was detected in 33%; and finally at 7 to 14 days, when the final cases were detected. They demonstrated the need for multiple attempts to detect awareness by using a structured interview technique because of the risk of underreporting from single interviews. Finally, Sandin and associates, in an analysis of individual cases, suggested that a reduced incidence of recall of intraoperative events

would not be achieved by monitoring of end-tidal anesthetic gas concentrations or by more frequent use of benzodiazepines.

Ghoneim recently reviewed cases of recall in different anesthetic situations.[50] The incidence of awareness in a nonobstetric and noncardiac surgical population approximates 0.2%. A higher incidence is reported for obstetric general anesthesia, 0.4%. The incidence in cardiac surgery ranges from 1.1% to 1.5%. Finally, as indicated earlier, major trauma cases can have a range of awareness from 11% to 43%.

Intraoperative awareness or recall has occurred with high-dose opioid anesthesia. In one case report, the patient had intraoperative awareness and hypertensive crises when fentanyl (96 µg/kg) and diazepam (0.28 mg/kg) were administered after preanesthetic medication with morphine and scopolamine.[51] Previous case reports using high-dose opioid anesthesia had not documented a significant hemodynamic response associated with intraoperative awareness.[52,53] Two clinical signs possibly predicting the occurrence of recall are movement and autonomic response. The use of muscle relaxants can eliminate the movement response, which leaves only autonomic activity as a measure of intraoperative awareness. To circumvent the problem of complete muscle paralysis, Tunstall[54,55] proposed using the isolated forearm technique to allow the possibility of movement during and after the administration of muscle relaxants. This procedure involves the application of a tourniquet to an extremity before the administration of muscle relaxants. Because the muscles do not receive the relaxant, the extremity is not paralyzed and can be monitored for movement.

This technique has been used to study the relationship of purposeful muscle movement to intraoperative recall. Schultetus and colleagues[56] used the isolated arm technique to compare the incidence of movement and recall in patients given ketamine, thiopental, or a combination of the two induction drugs for cesarean section. For 11 of 24 subjects given thiopental (2 mg/kg) or the combination of ketamine (0.5 mg/kg) and thiopental (2 mg/kg), movement occurred in the isolated arm. Four of the 24 patients had dreams, whereas 3 of the 24 had intraoperative recall. In 12 subjects given only ketamine (1 mg/kg), 1 had a movement response, and none had recall.

Russell[57,58] showed that the incidence of movement with the isolated arm technique can vary markedly with the choice of anesthetic. The incidence of intraoperative movement was 44% after nitrous oxide and fentanyl anesthesia, but it was only 7% after a continuous infusion of etomidate with fentanyl. The high incidence of wakefulness (as judged by movement) in the nitrous oxide–fentanyl group caused the investigators to terminate the study. Although the incidence of purposeful movement in the isolated arm was high, the incidence of actual intraoperative recall was low (only one subject).

Other investigators have not been able to correlate other clinical signs of light anesthesia or postoperative recall to the isolated arm movement response.[59-61] Moreover, the effects of ischemia from prolonged inflation of the tourniquet at pressures higher than arterial blood pressure on this methodology are unknown. Abouleish and Taylor[62] could not correlate movement, size of pupils, or changes in blood pressure with awareness or dreams in patients given morphine (0.2 mg/kg) and diazepam (0.1 mg/kg) after cesarean section. The foregoing studies suggest that the occurrence of purposeful movement in an isolated extremity is not a good predictor of intraoperative recall.

Detection of Auditory Input, Unconscious or Implicit Memory

Although the patient may not overtly recall a stimulus or an event, auditory input can register in the brain during apparently adequate surgical anesthesia. Auditory and verbal input must be "meaningful" for it to register in the patient's memory. Frequently, hypnosis or other cues may be needed to elicit recall.

Levinson[63] performed the classic study of detection of meaningful auditory input under anesthesia. Ten volunteers undergoing dental surgery were given thiopental followed by nitrous oxide and diethyl ether. Monitoring the EEG for an irregular slow-wave–high-voltage pattern allowed the anesthetist to maintain a similar depth of anesthesia in all patients. This EEG pattern was considered equivalent to moderate to deep ether anesthesia. During surgery, the anesthetist provided verbal stimulation to the patient in the form of an intraoperative crisis by verbally stating that cyanosis was present and then treated appropriately. All 10 patients had no spontaneous recall of the simulated intraoperative crisis. Under hypnosis, however, four patients could remember the frightening words in exact detail. An additional four remembered someone speaking to them. All eight became anxious and either emerged spontaneously from their hypnotic trance or refused to continue exploring the event. One subject had activation of the EEG pattern when the intraoperative crisis occurred, but no recall of the event.

Blacher[64] described his efforts to duplicate Levinson's experiment by using noxious, threatening verbal stimuli and hypnosis for subsequent recall. He reported similar findings, but he did not complete the project because he considered it too inhumane. Benign verbal stimuli did not produce significant evidence of auditory recall. He postulated that a noxious or crisis event was required. Bennett and coworkers[65] randomly assigned 33 subjects to receive either no intraoperative verbal stimuli or a personalized, but nonthreatening instruction to pull on their ear during a postoperative interview. Anesthesia was maintained with nitrous oxide, halothane, or enflurane. All subjects given the intraoperative suggestion did not recall the event. The incidence of pulling on the ear during the postoperative interview was significantly higher in patients given the intraoperative message than in those not given the message. This and other studies[66,67] suggest that unconscious memory may occur during general anesthesia, as shown by the effect of intraoperative suggestion on postoperative behavior. Other studies with similar methodology, however, demonstrate no unconscious memory.[68-70]

In a volunteer study examining the effect of subanesthetic concentrations of nitrous oxide and isoflurane on memory and responsiveness, Dwyer and colleagues[71] demonstrated that memory was decreased by increasing concentrations of each anesthetic. Both conscious and unconscious memories of the information presented during anesthetic administration were prevented by 0.45 MAC isoflurane, but they were not completely prevented by 0.6 MAC nitrous oxide. Although this volunteer study had significant methodologic rigor, it did not address the impact that surgical stimulation could have on anesthetic concentrations required to prevent conscious and unconscious memory. The stimuli in this study involved only verbal and visual input, stimuli less intense than surgical manipulation.

Veselis and colleagues[72] used the best current clinical pharmacology methodology to characterize the pharmacodynamics of anesthetic drugs used during sedation when the patient is still awake and cooperative, but amnestic. The authors evaluated the effects of midazolam, propofol, thiopental, and fentanyl on volunteer participants' memory of words and pictures at equisedative plasma concentrations. Controlling for sedation was essential in this research because sedation itself can produce amnesia resulting from inattention to the stimuli presented for later recall. Equi-sedative concentrations were as follows: midazolam, 64.5 ng/mL; propofol, 0.7 µg/mL; thiopental, 2.9 µg/mL; and fentanyl, 0.9 ng/mL. The plasma concentrations of drugs that result in 50% of maximal effect (Cp_{50}) for loss of memory to words were 56 ng/mL for midazolam, 0.62 µg/mL for propofol, 4.5 µg/mL for thiopental, and 3.2 ng/mL for fentanyl. Large effects on memory were produced only by propofol and midazolam. Thiopental had mild memory effects, whereas fentanyl had none. These findings have relevance for examining the choice of drug for sedation, but they cannot be translated into an anesthetic situation with general anesthesia, surgical stimulation, and prevention of intraoperative recall. Although certain drugs used in anesthesia have very specific effects in combating recall (e.g., scopolamine, benzodiazepines), we still do not know whether routine use of these drugs will guarantee lack of intraoperative recall.[73]

Implications of Explicit, Intraoperative Recall

Limited information is available on the postoperative consequences of intraoperative recall. Blacher[74] described a traumatic post–cardiac surgery neurosis involving anxiety and irritability, repeated nightmares, preoccupation with death, and a reluctance to discuss these symptoms. He attributed this postoperative state to patients' being awake and paralyzed during open heart surgery. These patients responded favorably to assurances that their postoperative difficulties may have been caused by awareness during surgery.

Ghoneim and Block[75] reviewed the consequences of intraoperative or explicit recall. The two most frequent complaints were an ability to hear events during surgery and the sensation of weakness/paralysis, with some patients experiencing pain. Patients particularly recall conversations that are of a negative nature concerning themselves or their medical condition. The most frequently reported postoperative effects were sleep disturbances, dreams, nightmares, flashbacks, and daytime anxiety. For many patients, the experience of awareness may not leave prolonged aftereffects; in some, however, a post-traumatic stress disorder marked by repetitive nightmares, anxiety, irritability, a preoccupation with death, and a concern with sanity can develop. It is unclear why a post-traumatic distress syndrome develops in some patients and not in others.

Lennmarken and associates[76] provided follow-up information on the intraoperative awareness patients prospectively identified by Sandin and colleagues.[49] Nine of the 18 patients with documented explicit recall of surgery were interviewed 2 years later. Four of the nine were still severely disabled because of psychiatric/psychological sequelae and fulfilled the clinical criteria for post-traumatic stress disorder. All these victims had been offered and received therapy for the intraoperative awareness immediately after it was identified. This study suggests a need for longer-term follow-up of patients who experience awareness during surgery.

Ghoneim has summarized the large body of investigation attempting to understand the role of implicit memory for events during anesthesia.[77] Implicit memory while under anesthesia refers to changes in performance or behavior that can be produced by previous experience or tests that do not require any intentional or conscious recall of these experiences. These investigations have studied the indirect memory of patients and responses to behavioral and therapeutic suggestions made under anesthesia. At very light levels of anesthesia, it can be demonstrated that memory and implicit recall can occur, whereas deeper levels of anesthesia eliminate the ability to detect any implicit recall or memory. There is no good, consistent evidence that verbal therapeutic suggestions given during anesthesia, which would involve implicit memory, can meaningfully alter postoperative performance (i.e., pain management, prevention of side effects). Ghoneim concludes that implicit memory after anesthesia has proved to be an elusive phenomenon.

HYPNOTICS, ANALGESICS, AND ANESTHETIC DEPTH

Inhaled Anesthetics

Movement Response and the MAC Concept

The purposeful movement of a body part in response to noxious perioperative stimuli has been extensively used as a clinical sign of anesthesia. Using this movement to quantitate anesthetic response induced by potent inhaled anesthetics, Eger and Merkel and their colleagues[13,78] defined MAC as the minimum alveolar concentration of inhaled anesthetic required to prevent 50% of subjects from responding to a painful stimulus with "gross purposeful movement." Readers are referred to excellent review articles that document development of the MAC concept and its many applications in anesthesia.[79,80] The MAC concept has four basic components: (1) an all-or-none (quantal) movement response must occur after the application of a supramaximal noxious stimulus; (2) end-tidal concentrations of anesthetic in the alveoli, considered an equilibrated sample site, are used as an indication of the concentration of anesthetic in the brain; (3) appropriate mathematical quantitation of the relationship between the alveolar concentration of anesthetic and the quantal response is used to estimate

MAC; and (4) MAC can be quantitated for altered physiologic and pharmacologic states.

For determination of MAC in humans, the standard noxious stimulus has been the initial surgical skin incision.[13] Skin incision represents a reproducible form of supramaximal surgical stimulation. There has been no systematic examination of other perioperative surgical stimuli (e.g., peritoneal traction) representing more profound surgical manipulation than skin incision or endotracheal intubation. For determination of MAC in animals, the standard stimulus has been the application of a surgical clamp to the base of the tail. After examining other noxious stimuli in dogs, Eger and colleagues[13] concluded that tail clamping represented the most noxious stimulation that was clinically reproducible and not excessively traumatic. The MAC concept has been expanded by evaluating other clinical end points and defined stimuli. Stoelting and associates[31] determined the MAC of anesthetic that would allow opening of the eyes on verbal command during emergence from anesthesia ("MAC$_{awake}$"). This stimulation is less intense than surgical skin incision, and response occurs at lower concentrations of anesthetic than is the case with movement to skin incision. Generally, MAC$_{awake}$ values are a third to a fourth the MAC values for surgical incision. Yakaitis and coworkers[82] determined the MAC of inhaled anesthetic that would inhibit movement and coughing during endotracheal intubation ("MAC$_{intubation}$"). Intubation is significantly more stimulating than skin incision, and higher concentrations of inhaled anesthetic are required to eliminate the movement response. Finally, Roizen and associates[83] investigated the MAC of anesthetic necessary to prevent an adrenergic response to skin incision ("MAC$_{BAR}$"), as measured by the concentration of catecholamine in venous blood. When one examines the values for (1) MAC$_{awake}$, (2) MAC$_{skin incision}$, (3) MAC$_{intubation}$, and (4) MAC$_{BAR}$, one sees a family of concentration-versus-response curves that characterize the hypnotic effects of inhaled anesthetics relative to defined clinical stimuli.

Zbinden and colleagues[84] undertook a comprehensive examination of the effects of different noxious stimuli on the purposeful movement response with isoflurane. Twenty-six healthy surgical patients were administered isoflurane only with adequate inspired/end-tidal equilibration. Multiple noxious stimuli were applied at varying end-tidal isoflurane concentrations. From the resulting data, the authors were able to define a family of concentration-versus-response curves for different noxious stimuli, as displayed in Figure 31-11. The end-tidal isoflurane concentrations that resulted in a 50% probability of no movement response to different stimuli were as follows: verbal responsiveness, 0.37%; trapezius muscle squeeze, 0.84%; laryngoscopy, 1.0%; 50-Hz electrical tetanus, 1.03%; skin incision, 1.16%; and laryngoscopy with intubation, 1.76%. This study demonstrates how varying clinical stimuli require different isoflurane concentrations to prevent a clinical response and can be used to define a concentration-versus-response relationship for the hypnotic effects of isoflurane.

A second component of the MAC concept involves use of the alveolar concentration of an anesthetic as an indication of drug concentration. Because the concentration

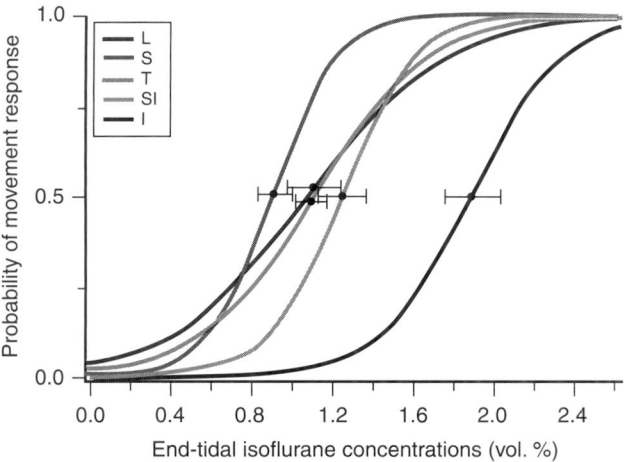

Figure 31–11 Logistic regression analysis of the end-tidal isoflurane concentration relative to the predicted probability of no movement response for different noxious stimuli. *Bars* indicate the 95% confidence bounds to the end-tidal concentration with a 50% probability of response. I, laryngoscopy/intubation; L, laryngoscopy; S, trapezius muscle squeeze; SI, skin incision; T, tetanic nerve stimulation. (Redrawn with modification from Zbinden AM, Maggiorini M, Petersen-Felix S, et al: Anesthetic depth defined using multiple noxious stimuli during isoflurane/oxygen anesthesia. I. Motor reactions. Anesthesiology 80:253, 1994.)

of gas is defined as a percentage of 1 atm at sea level, it is independent of barometric pressure and elevation. Additionally, partial pressures of inhaled anesthetics at equilibrium should be similar in all body parts, such as the alveolus, blood, and brain. Thus, the measured end-tidal partial pressure of inhaled anesthetic (representative of the alveolar concentration) is in direct proportion to the underlying concentration in the brain. Because cerebral blood perfusion is large, it is possible to achieve an

equilibration among end-tidal, alveolar, arterial, and brain anesthetic partial pressures within 15 minutes of exposure to a constant end-tidal anesthetic concentration. Eger and Bahlman[85] quantitated the difference between arterial and end-tidal partial pressures of halothane. If the difference between the inspired and end-tidal partial pressures was less than 10%, the difference between end-tidal and arterial concentrations would be minimal.

A third component of the MAC concept involves the use of appropriate mathematical approaches to quantitate the relationship between dose and response. The original MAC concept of Eger and colleagues[13] used a "bracketing approach" in humans and animals. In an individual patient, a fixed end-tidal concentration of anesthetic was achieved, and the response to a single skin incision was observed. Depending on the patient's response or lack of response, the next patient received a higher or lower concentration. A single measurement was obtained per patient. Patients were studied over a range of end-tidal concentrations. They were placed in groups of four; the subject having the lowest end-tidal (alveolar) concentration of anesthetic was the first to be studied. For each group, the percentage of patients moving in response to stimulation was plotted against the average end-tidal concentration for that group. A visual line of "best fit" through these points yielded the concentration at which 50% of patients would respond (i.e., the MAC). An example of such analysis is presented in Figure 31-12, which uses the concentration-versus-response data gathered for halothane alone, for halothane with morphine premedication, and for halothane with 70% nitrous oxide. Both morphine premedication and 70% nitrous oxide decreased the MAC value for halothane.[86]

In animal studies, it was possible to manipulate the end-tidal concentration of anesthetic and apply the tail clamp stimuli on multiple occasions. A MAC value can be obtained for each animal by sequentially increasing or decreasing the end-tidal concentrations to bracket the value between movement and no movement. De Jong and Eger[87]

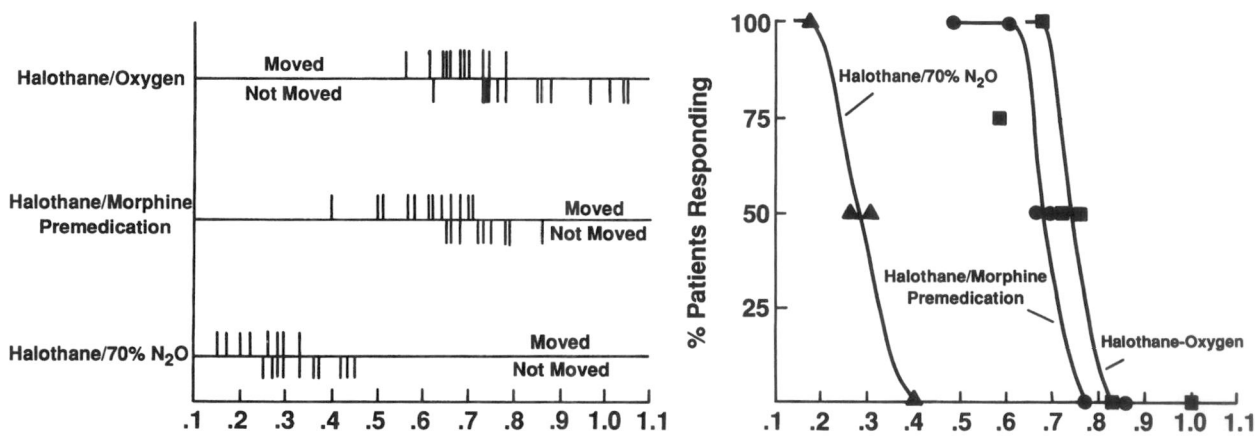

Alveolar Concentration of Halothane

Figure 31–12 Minimal alveolar concentration necessary to prevent movement in 50% of subjects receiving a noxious stimulus for halothane combined with (1) oxygen, (2) oxygen and morphine premedication (0.15 mg/kg intramuscularly), and (3) 70% nitrous oxide. The anesthetic requirement for halothane is greatly decreased by nitrous oxide and less so by premedication with morphine. (Modified from Saidman LJ, Eger EI II: Effect of nitrous oxide and of narcotic premedication on the alveolar concentration of halothane required for anesthesia. Anesthesiology 25:302, 1964.)

extended the analysis of MAC data by using more appropriate mathematical/statistical techniques to quantitate the relationship between alveolar anesthetic concentration and response/no response data. Nonlinear logistic regression analysis was used to estimate the probability of no movement at any given end-tidal concentration.[88] The logistic regression analysis produced values for MAC comparable to those produced by the bracketing technique. Logistic regression allowed estimation of the variance associated with the estimate of MAC. It was also possible to extrapolate the probability of movement from 50% to any given probability within the curve. Thus evolved the concept of end-tidal partial pressure of inhaled anesthetic that inhibited response in 95% of patients. Investigators have examined the relationship between $MAC_{skin\ incision}$ and a more noxious stimulus, $MAC_{intubation}$,[82] or a less noxious stimulus, MAC_{awake}.[34] When different inhaled anesthetics are compared, the ratio of $MAC_{skin\ incision}$ to $MAC_{intubation}$ or MAC_{awake} is relatively constant. When the possible relationship between synergism and antagonism of four different potent inhaled anesthetics was examined relative to nitrous oxide, no evidence of a relationship could be demonstrated.[89]

A fourth feature of MAC is that it has served as a sensitive tool to determine the interaction of other anesthetics and CNS drugs with the inhaled anesthetics. Other drugs used in anesthesia decrease anesthetic requirements, as measured by a reduction in MAC. In addition, numerous altered physiologic states (e.g., aging) change the requirements for inhaled anesthetics. Table 31-2 summarizes the results of studies regarding factors that affect MAC.

Much of the previous research on MAC assumed that the lack of movement response with inhaled anesthetics was due to anesthetic effects on the central, cortical brain tissues. This assumption has been challenged. In 1993, Rampil and colleagues demonstrated that the spinal cord represents a major site of action for inhaled anesthetics.[29] Their studies showed that the MAC of isoflurane in rodents was identical in value for intact animals and rodents that were decorticate or decerebrate, a finding suggesting that the main ability of inhaled anesthetics in preventing purposeful movement occurs at the spinal cord level.[29,30] Antognini and Schwartz also drew the same conclusions from experiments whereby they determined MAC in the goat by having the animal's brain isolated from the remainder of the body through a complex cardiopulmonary bypass procedure.[31] These investigators demonstrated that the MAC value for the goat was approximately twice as large when only the brain was exposed to isoflurane as opposed to both the brain and the spinal cord. These series of studies demonstrate that the response to purposeful movement is achieved by inhaled anesthetics at subcortical anatomic levels, on the spinal cord. Eger and associates proposed that volatile anesthetics cause a lack of movement response to noxious stimuli by action in the spinal cord and create a hypnotic/amnestic loss of consciousness at a supraspinal, cortical site of action.[90]

Other Clinical Responses
Responses other than purposeful movement have been investigated as possible clinical measures of the depth of anesthesia: the rate and volume of ventilation in

Table 31–2 Factors that affect the minimum alveolar concentration

Effect on MAC	Factors (Study Subjects)
Decrease	Hypothermia (animals)
	Severe hypotension (animals)
	Age (humans)
	Opioids, ketamine (humans, animals)
	Chronic administration of amphetamine (animals)
	Reserpine, α-methyldopa (animals)
	Cholinesterase inhibitors (animals)
	Intravenous local anesthetics (humans, animals)
	Pregnancy (animals)
	Hypoxemia (Pao_2 <40 mm Hg) (animals)
	Anemia (animals)
	α_2-Agonists (animals, humans)
Increase	Hyperthermia (animals)
	Hyperthyroidism (animals)
	Alcoholism (humans)
	Acute administration of dextroamphetamine (animals)
No effect	Duration of anesthesia (humans, animals)
	Sex (human, animals)
	Metabolic acid-base status (animals)
	Hypercapnia and hypocapnia (humans, animals)
	Isovolemic anemia (animals)
	Hypertension (animals)

Adapted from Quasha AL, Eger EI II, Tinker JH: Determination and applications of MAC. Anesthesiology 53:315, 1980.

spontaneously breathing subjects, eye movement, the diameter and reactivity of pupils to light, heart rate, arterial blood pressure, and autonomic signs such as sweating. It has not been possible, however, to use these clinical signs to generate uniform measures of depth of anesthesia for inhaled anesthetics. Although some clinical signs do correlate with depth of anesthesia for certain inhaled anesthetics, the same cannot be said for other inhaled anesthetics.[91]

Zbinden and colleagues[92] systematically examined the interaction of isoflurane concentrations with the hemodynamic response to different noxious stimuli. In 26 healthy surgical patients receiving different equilibrated end-tidal concentrations of isoflurane, the following noxious stimuli were applied, several of them on multiple occasions: trapezius muscle squeeze, 50-Hz electrical tetanus, laryngoscopy, laryngoscopy with intubation, and skin incision. With continuous recording of intra-arterial hemodynamics, acute increases in heart rate and systolic blood pressure were noted and related to the isoflurane concentration and the presence or absence of purposeful movement. Table 31-3 presents the absolute increase in systolic blood pressure and heart rate at the isoflurane end-tidal

Table 31–3   Hemodynamic response to defined noxious stimuli under isoflurane anesthesia

Stimulus	End-Tidal Concentration That Suppresses Movement in 50% of Patients (ET$_{50}$) (Percent atm)	Change in Systolic Blood Pressure for Patients at ET$_{50}$ (mm Hg)	Change in Heart Rate for Patients at ET$_{50}$ (Beats/min)
Trapezius muscle squeeze	0.90	9	5
Electrical tetanus	1.10	15	15
Laryngoscopy	1.07	23	17
Skin incision	1.24	34	35
Laryngoscopy and intubation	1.87	53	36

Adapted from Zbinden AM, Petersen-Felix S, Thomson DA: Anesthetic depth defined using multiple noxious stimuli during isoflurane/oxygen anesthesia. II. Hemodynamic responses. Anesthesiology 80:261, 1994.

concentration that had a 50% probability of no purposeful movement for that specific stimulus. Different noxious stimuli result in different degrees of hemodynamic response. There is a relative rank order of the degree of hemodynamic response, with laryngoscopy and intubation being the most intense stimuli. Multiple regression analysis demonstrated that the type of stimulation had the highest influence on the increase in blood pressure, with the isoflurane concentration being the least important. Figure 31-13 presents the baseline systolic blood pressure and subsequent increase in systolic pressure at a measured isoflurane concentration for subjects receiving a skin incision. The shaded areas represent the linear regression relationship of isoflurane concentration versus prestimulus and poststimulus systolic blood pressure. Increasing the isoflurane concentration did not prevent the increase in systolic blood pressure, even at very high end-tidal concentrations. Rather, increasing the isoflurane concentration only decreased the prestimulation systolic pressure such that the noxious stimuli returned systolic pressure closer to the normal, awake values. Similar results were found with the other noxious stimuli on both heart rate and systolic blood pressure response, with the degree

of hemodynamic response being determined by the nature of the noxious stimuli.

The clinical implications of these data relative to judging the anesthetic depth of inhaled anesthetics from the hemodynamic response are significant. When used as a sole agent, even at high concentrations isoflurane is unable to suppress hemodynamic responses to noxious stimuli. Instead, the hemodynamic control seen with high isoflurane concentrations occurs as a result of a decrease in the prestimulation hemodynamic baseline value. Thus, although hemodynamic responses are the most commonly used clinical measures to judge the inhaled anesthetic depth of anesthesia, the scientific basis for this is certainly not obvious. This study is important evidence that isoflurane is providing hypnotic anesthetic effects with minimal analgesic effect, as judged by the profound hemodynamic responses that occurred with noxious stimuli. In clinical practice, additional anesthetic drugs are commonly used with inhaled anesthetics. Daniel and colleagues[37] examined how fentanyl (0 to 3 μg/kg) and 60% nitrous oxide alter the heart rate, mean arterial blood pressure, and catecholamine response (components of MAC$_{BAR}$) during desflurane and isoflurane anesthesia.

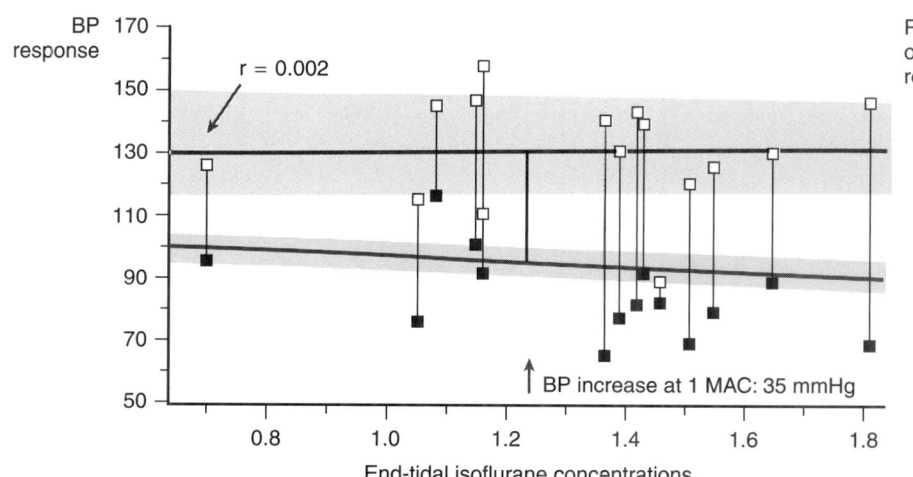

Figure 31–13 Response of systolic blood pressure (BP, mm Hg) to skin incision as a function of end-tidal isoflurane concentration. *Filled squares,* systolic blood pressure before stimulation; *open squares,* systolic blood pressure after stimulation; *lower oblique line,* regression line to systolic blood pressure before stimulation (r = −.46); *upper line,* regression line to systolic blood pressure after skin incision (r = .0002); *shaded area,* 95% confidence interval for regression lines; *vertical arrow,* median effective isoflurane concentration for the motor response of the stimulation pattern. (Redrawn from Zbinden AM, Petersen-Felix S, Thomson DA: Anesthetic depth defined using multiple noxious stimuli during isoflurane/oxygen anesthesia. II. Hemodynamic responses. Anesthesiology 80:261, 1994.)

Fentanyl, 1.5 µg/kg, reduced MAC_{BAR} for desflurane from 1.3 to 0.4 MAC and for isoflurane from 1.3 to 0.55 MAC. Increasing the fentanyl dose to 3 µg/kg did not cause further change in the MAC_{BAR} values for both inhaled anesthetics. Figure 31-14 shows an interaction surface for fentanyl and isoflurane based on modifying the model reported by McEwan to increase the C_{50} in the absence of fentanyl by 1.3 and adjusting the isoflurane C_{50} in the presence of an effect-site fentanyl concentration of 1.36 ng/mL (corresponding to a 1.5-mg/kg bolus) to 0.4 MAC. The black arrow shows the reduction in MAC_{BAR} demonstrated by Daniel. It is clear from the figure that additional opioid would not be expected to yield further significant reductions in MAC_{BAR}. This study suggests that the addition of analgesic components, such as nitrous oxide and fentanyl, can prevent the sympathetic stimulation and hemodynamic responses seen with noxious surgical stimuli when inhaled anesthetics are used.

Intravenously Administered (Nonopioid) Anesthetics

Traditionally, these intravenous anesthetics were used solely for induction of anesthesia as a single intravenous bolus. Only with the clinical introduction of propofol have these agents been infused for maintenance of anesthesia, in which case assessment of the depth of anesthesia becomes more relevant.

Assessing Depth during Induction of Anesthesia

Induction of anesthesia often consists of a rapid intravenous bolus injection of a hypnotic (e.g., propofol, thiopental, etomidate). Plasma concentrations peak within a half to 1 minute and decline rapidly on redistribution of the drug. The rapidly changing plasma concentrations cause a corresponding fluctuation in the degree of CNS depression. The depth of anesthesia increases rapidly (causing loss of consciousness), peaks, and then decreases as plasma concentrations decline. CNS depression lags behind the plasma concentration and is manifested as hysteresis on curves plotting effect against plasma concentration. The non–steady-state conditions produced by rapid administration of a drug make assessment of the relationship of plasma concentration and depth of anesthesia difficult, if not impossible, during bolus intravenous administration.

Clinical end points useful in assessing the depth of anesthesia during induction include loss of verbal responsiveness, loss of eyelid reflex, and loss of corneal reflex. Typical stimulation occurring during induction of anesthesia includes laryngoscopy and intubation, which constitute profoundly noxious stimuli. Frequently, response to these two procedures cannot be eliminated completely with just the intravenously administered hypnotic. In one study, administration of thiopental (6 mg/kg) was followed by an average increase in systolic blood pressure of 53 mm Hg on laryngoscopy and intubation.[93] In another study, administration of thiamylal (4 mg/kg) was followed by an increase in mean arterial blood pressure from 92 mm Hg (control) to 136 mm Hg on laryngoscopy.[94] Because most intravenous hypnotics do not provide significant analgesia, the hemodynamic response to major noxious stimuli is great, even when large doses are given. Thus, assessment of the depth of anesthesia with the use of clinically relevant noxious stimuli such as laryngoscopy and intubation requires the concurrent administration of other analgesic drugs (opioids or nitrous oxide) to provide reasonable and clinically acceptable hemodynamic control.

Most research on estimating the depth of anesthesia induced by intravenous anesthetics has focused on the relationship between dose and response. For example, Brett and Fisher[95] reported that the dose of thiopental associated with a 50% probability of no movement in response to a firm squeeze of the trapezius muscle was 3 to 7 mg/kg for adults and more than 7 mg/kg for infants 1 to 11 months of age. It is possible that a larger initial volume of distribution or a more rapid redistribution (both pharmacokinetic mechanisms) in infants accounts for the difference in dose requirement. It is also possible that brain sensitivity to thiopental differs for infants and adults. Dose-response studies cannot differentiate between these two very different mechanisms.

Dose-response studies can have meaningful scientific and clinical value if they are performed with multiple measures of drug effect, concomitant variables, and appropriate statistical data analysis. Avram and associates[96] demonstrated this point by successfully examining the thiopental induction dose requirement using an EEG end point (3 to 5 seconds of isoelectric signal), clinical end points (dropping of a syringe), and measurement of multiple covariates (age, gender, lean body mass, cardiac output). Avram's group[95] concluded that age and either lean or total body weight are the most important predictors of thiopental dose requirement, with gender and cardiac output being less important. Jacobs and Reves[97] provided editorial comment on this article and used

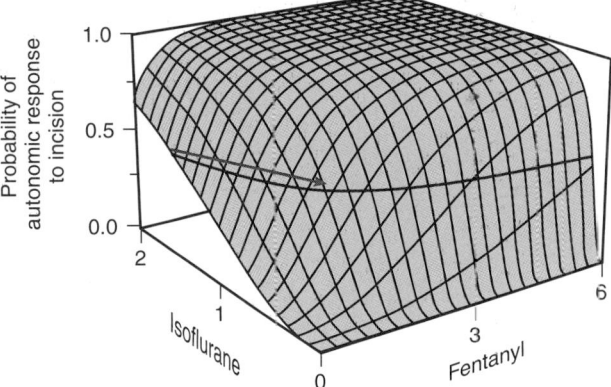

Figure 31–14 Interaction surface for fentanyl and isoflurane reflecting suppression of the autonomic response. The surface is based on the isoflurane interaction reported by McEwan and colleagues,[23] but modified to increase the C_{50} of isoflurane in the absence of fentanyl by 1.3 and adjusting the isoflurane C_{50} in the presence of an effect-site fentanyl concentration of 1.36 (corresponding to a 1.5-mg/kg bolus) to 0.4 MAC, as reported by Daniel.[37] The *black arrow* shows the reduction in MAC_{BAR} demonstrated by Daniel and associates.[37]

computer simulations to confirm and extend the findings of the study by Avram and colleagues.

Assessing Depth during Maintenance of Anesthesia

Becker[98] presented one of the first studies to quantitate the relationship between plasma concentrations of an intravenous anesthetic (in this case, thiopental) and clinical measures of depth of anesthesia. First studying patients anesthetized with 67% nitrous oxide and thiopental, Becker found that the corneal reflex and movement response to a firm squeeze of the trapezius muscle correlated highly with the movement response to surgical stimulation (cervical dilation or skin incision). He then related the plasma concentration of thiopental to three clinical signs (loss of eyelid reflex, loss of corneal reflex, and absence of movement in response to squeezing the trapezius muscle) in another group of patients given thiopental/oxygen anesthesia. Anesthesia was induced with thiopental, 2 to 2.5 mg/kg, followed by an intravenous infusion of 1 to 1.5 mg/kg/min. Patients were observed for the three clinical signs. Arterial blood samples drawn at these clinical end points were analyzed for both total plasma concentration and free (or unbound) plasma concentrations of thiopental. Plasma levels of thiopental gathered under these pseudo–steady-state conditions, especially free or unbound plasma levels, are believed to be accurate predictors of brain levels of the drug and are therefore good indicators of the depth of anesthesia. The eyelid reflex was lost at significantly lower levels of thiopental than the corneal reflex or movement response was. Similar plasma concentrations of thiopental were needed for loss of the corneal reflex and for loss of the movement response to squeeze of the trapezius muscle, both of which had been found to correlate highly with loss of movement in response

to skin incision. Becker did not report hemodynamic responses to the corneal or trapezius stimuli. For the patients given 67% nitrous oxide, the plasma concentrations of thiopental necessary to achieve the same surgical end points were as much as 71% lower than those in patients given only thiopental.

Hung and colleagues[99] proposed a conceptual approach to examining intravenous anesthetic pharmacodynamics that involved clinical measures. A computer-driven infusion pump using a pharmacokinetic model of thiopental disposition was used to rapidly achieve and then maintain constant thiopental plasma concentrations in 26 surgical patients. A low (10 to 40 µg/mL) and then high (40 to 90 µg/mL) constant thiopental plasma concentration was achieved and then maintained for 10 minutes. After allowing 5 minutes for blood-brain equilibration, the following sequential clinical stimuli were applied to the patients at 1-minute intervals: verbal command, 50-Hz electrical tetanus, trapezius muscle squeeze, laryngoscopy, and laryngoscopy followed by intubation. Purposeful movement response was used as the measure of clinical response. Logistic regression was used to relate the measured constant thiopental plasma concentration to the presence or absence of movement and to estimate the Cp_{50} value. Figure 31-15 displays the thiopental plasma concentration versus response/no response in the data, along with the logistic regression characterization. Prevention of movement during intubation required significantly higher thiopental concentrations (78.8 µg/mL) relative to laryngoscopy (50.7 µg/mL), trapezius muscle squeeze (39.8 µg/mL), electrical tetanus (30.3 µg/mL), and verbal responsiveness (15.6 µg/mL). These data confirm the utility of purposeful movement as a measure of the depth of anesthesia for intravenous anesthetics and demonstrate that

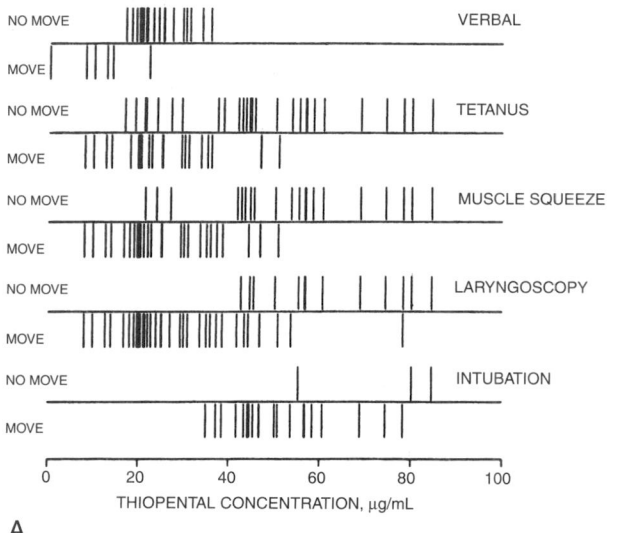

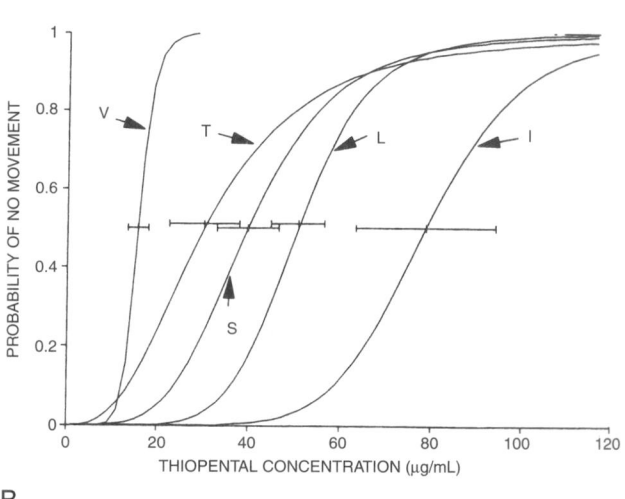

A

B

Figure 31–15 A, Move/no move versus serum thiopental concentration for five different clinical stimuli. Each *bar* indicates the serum thiopental concentration and response to stimuli applied to an individual patient. **B,** Predicted probability of no movement versus serum thiopental concentrations obtained by using logistic regression of the data indicated in **A.** The *bars* indicate the 95% confidence bounds of the estimate of serum thiopental concentration that produces a 50% probability of no movement response. I, laryngoscopy/intubation; L, laryngoscopy; S, trapezius muscle squeeze; T, tetanic nerve stimulation; V, verbal. (From Hung OR, Varvel JR, Shafer SL, et al: Thiopental pharmacodynamics. II. Quantitation of clinical and electroencephalographic depth of anesthesia. Anesthesiology 77:237, 1992.)

different noxious stimuli can be statistically separated with this methodology. The conceptual approach developed by Hung and coworkers[99] can be used to examine how altered physiologic states and diseases change the intravenous anesthetic requirement.

Kazama and colleagues[26] examined the pharmacodynamics of propofol alone and then of propofol with fentanyl by using the defined noxious stimuli/movement responses that Hung and associates[99] used for thiopental and the hemodynamic methodology developed by Zbinden and colleagues[92] for isoflurane. Kazama and coworkers found propofol Cp_{50} values for the following defined stimuli: loss of verbal responsiveness, 4.4 µg/mL; electrical tetanus, 9.3 µg/mL; laryngoscopy, 9.8 µg/mL; skin incision, 10.0 µg/mL; and intubation, 17.4 µg/mL. With the addition of a steady-state fentanyl plasma concentration of 1 or 3 ng/mL, there was only a minimal decrease in the propofol Cp_{50} for loss of verbal responsiveness: 11% for 1 ng/mL and 17% for 3 ng/mL. For the other, more intense noxious stimuli (tetanus, laryngoscopy, skin incision, and intubation), a much greater decrease in propofol Cp_{50} occurred. Fentanyl, 1 ng/mL, decreased Cp_{50} values 31% to 34%, whereas fentanyl, 3 ng/mL, decreased Cp_{50} values 50% to 55%. Further increases in fentanyl plasma concentrations did not lead to additional decreases in propofol Cp_{50} values. Kazama and colleagues found that the systolic blood pressure response to propofol alone was profound, similar to what Zbinden and coauthors[92] described. The addition of fentanyl to propofol attenuated the systolic blood pressure increases in a dose-dependent manner. The conceptual methodology used by Kazama and associates allows for characterization of anesthetic depth with multiple, defined noxious stimuli. The combination of the hypnotic anesthetic propofol with the analgesic effects of fentanyl allows a clinically successful anesthetic to be given to patients with quantitative methodology.

Quantitation of the clinical depth of anesthesia for the combination of an opioid and an intravenous anesthetic was reported by Vuyk and colleagues.[100] The pharmacodynamic methodology developed by Ausems and coworkers[39] was used to examine the interaction of a constant plasma concentration of propofol (in place of nitrous oxide) as alfentanil was titrated to clinical responses. Propofol had a significant interaction with alfentanil, thus decreasing the total dose of alfentanil and the alfentanil plasma concentrations needed for adequate anesthesia. Table 31-4 indicates how the total dose of alfentanil needed decreased from 22.8 mg with 66% nitrous oxide to 10.3 mg with a steady-state propofol plasma concentration of 4 µg/mL. The mechanism of this decreased dose requirement was a marked potentiation of alfentanil such that alfentanil plasma concentrations needed to achieve the same degree of pharmacologic effect were two to four times lower with propofol.

In a subsequent study, Vuyk and coworkers used this same methodology, but they randomized the surgical subjects to receive a range of constant propofol blood concentrations.[24] With blood propofol concentrations increasing from 2 to 10 µg/mL, the alfentanil Cp_{50} decreased from 170 to 25 ng/mL for laryngoscopy, from 280 to

Table 31–4 Interaction of propofol and nitrous oxide with alfentanil in lower abdominal surgery

Event	Alfentanil Cp_{50} (ng/mL) in Conjunction with	
	Propofol	Nitrous Oxide
Steady-state propofol or nitrous oxide concentration	4.0 ± 0.6 µg/mL (range, 3.2-4.9)	66%
Intubation	92 ± 20*	429 ± 42*
Skin incision	55 ± 16*	101 ± 16*
Intra-abdominal dissection	66 ± 38†	206 ± 65†
Total alfentanil dose (mg)	10.3 ± 6.1†	22.8 ± 6.4†

*±SE.
†±SD.
Modified from Vuyk J, Lim T, Engbers FHM, et al: Pharmacodynamics of alfentanil as a supplement to propofol or nitrous oxide for lower abdominal surgery in female patients. Anesthesiology 78:1036, 1993.

23 ng/mL for intubation, from 259 to 9 ng/mL for opening of the peritoneum, and from 209 to 16 ng/mL for the intra-abdominal surgical stimulus. With plasma alfentanil concentrations increasing from 10 to 150 ng/mL, the Cp_{50} for propofol to regaining of consciousness decreased from 3.8 to 0.8 µg/mL. This study confirms the profound, synergistic interaction of propofol with alfentanil. Vuyk and colleagues used computer simulations of their data to suggest that the optimal blood propofol and plasma alfentanil concentrations that allow the most rapid recovery from intraoperative anesthesia occur at a propofol concentration of 3.5 µg/mL and an alfentanil concentration of 85 ng/mL. An editorial[101] comment on this study provided more general guidelines for using the quantitative interaction of propofol and alfentanil to design dosing regimens for total intravenous anesthesia.

In clinical practice, intravenously administered anesthetic drugs are frequently combined with other drugs that provide additional analgesia (opioids, nitrous oxide, potent inhaled anesthetics). As indicated earlier, large intravenously administered doses of thiopental or propofol are less than effective in eliminating the hemodynamic response to relevant clinical stimuli such as laryngoscopy and intubation.[26,93,94] Fentanyl decreases the anesthetic requirement for thiopental or propofol by providing antinociceptive effects that the intravenous hypnotics do not provide.[26,102] Clinically, the hemodynamic response to laryngoscopy, intubation, or skin incision is most commonly used to assess depth of anesthesia. The use of muscle relaxants to ease endotracheal intubation precludes use of the movement response. Because laryngoscopy and intubation are single events, if clinical depth is inadequate (e.g., in the event of a profound hemodynamic response), additional intravenous anesthetics, opioids, or maintenance anesthetic drugs are rapidly administered. When precise hemodynamic control becomes important (as in coronary artery disease), larger doses of opioids are used instead of intravenously administered anesthetics.

Opioids

Opioid analgesics are extensively used for premedication, as a supplement to regional and general anesthesia, as the primary anesthetic agent, and as an analgesic for postoperative pain (see Chapter 72). The analgesia produced by these drugs through specific receptor systems within the CNS decreases autonomic, endocrine, and somatic responses to noxious stimulation. Although opioids have been used as sole anesthetics, they create incomplete hypnotic effects at very large doses. Opioids need to be combined with hypnotic drugs to induce the anesthetic state.

Opioids as Complete Anesthetics

In 1947, Neff and colleagues[103] used meperidine as an intravenous supplement to nitrous oxide/oxygen anesthesia in what is now known as a "balanced anesthesia" technique. The later use of opioids as complete anesthetics coincided with the development of cardiac surgery and intensive care during the 1970s. Providing anesthesia for patients with severe valvular or congenital heart disease without causing cardiovascular collapse was problematic before the use of opioids. These early cardiac surgery patients were extremely ill and had little or no circulatory reserve. During the late 1960s, Lowenstein and associates[104] noted the hemodynamic stability of patients undergoing mechanical ventilation who were given frequently large doses of intravenous morphine to suppress respiration in intensive care units. This observation encouraged Lowenstein and coworkers to become the first to administer morphine (0.5 to 3.0 mg/kg) as the only anesthetic drug. The resulting cardiovascular stability in acutely ill patients with acquired valvular heart disease was impressive. As cardiac surgery advanced in methodology, patients with ischemic heart disease began to undergo surgical anesthesia. Unfortunately, morphine anesthesia was less satisfactory for these patients, in whom hypertension, tachycardia, and awareness during surgery developed, in contrast to patients with valvular heart disease.[104]

In 1978, Stanley and Webster[105] introduced the concept of high-dose fentanyl for cardiac anesthesia. This technique minimized the undesirable effects of morphine on induction (hypotension) and provided better hemodynamic stability in patients with good ventricular function and ischemic heart disease. As clinical experience with fentanyl increased, however, investigators found that even increasingly large doses of fentanyl could not always produce complete unresponsiveness, as defined in Figure 31-8, for the most potent stimuli and difficult-to-suppress responses.[106] This discovery raised the important issue of whether opioids are "complete anesthetics" or are, as suggested in Figure 31-3, only potent analgesics and weak hypnotics.

Human and animal studies show that opioids are not complete anesthetics. Wynands and colleagues[21] used moderate to large doses of fentanyl (50 to 150 μg/kg) only, with no other anesthetic drugs (no hypnotic component), and measured plasma concentrations at defined surgical stimuli (intubation, skin incision, sternotomy, aortic root dissection) in patients with good ventricular function who were undergoing coronary surgery. Figure 31-16 shows the relationship among drug concentrations, stimulation,

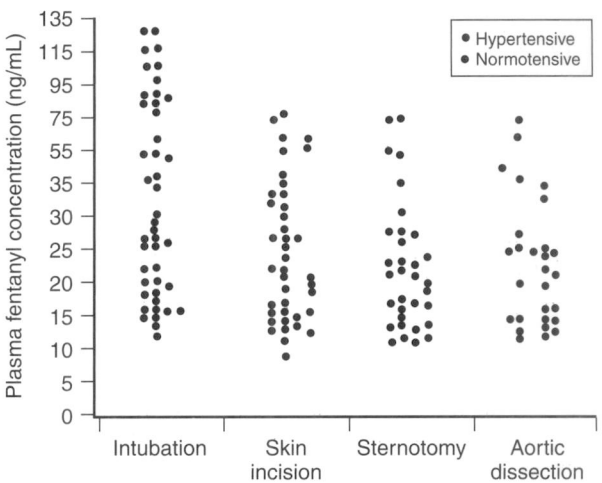

Figure 31–16 Plasma concentration of fentanyl at the time of certain clinical stimuli, along with the presence or absence of hypertension. During sternotomy and aortic dissection, even high plasma concentrations of fentanyl (>15 ng/mL) do not always prevent hypertension. (Redrawn with modification from Wynands JE, Wong P, Townsend GE, et al: Narcotic requirements for intravenous anesthesia. Anesth Analg 63:101, 1984.)

and hemodynamic response. In approximately 20% of patients, extremely high plasma concentrations of fentanyl (15 ng/mL) did not eliminate hemodynamic responses, defined as a 20% increase in systolic blood pressure. These results have been confirmed by Hynynen and colleagues[107] and Philbin and coworkers.[108] Using more precise methodology than previous investigators, Thompson and associates[109] have shown that distinct concentration-response relationships exist for fentanyl and sufentanil when used in moderate to high doses for cardiac surgery with concurrent isoflurane for hypnosis and hemodynamic control as the clinical end point.

The investigations conducted by Murphy and Hug[110] in measuring the depth of opioid anesthesia in animals (dogs) also address the issue of whether opioids are complete anesthetics. These investigators examined the ability of fentanyl to decrease enflurane MAC. They first anesthetized the dog with enflurane and determined MAC. Several infusions of fentanyl at progressively higher rates were used to obtain a constant steady-state plasma concentration of fentanyl in each animal. After each increase in infusion rate, enflurane MAC was determined again. Measurement of opioid concentrations in blood samples ensured that several different steady-state plasma concentrations of fentanyl were obtained in each animal. Murphy and Hug found that even high plasma concentrations of fentanyl (20 ng/mL) did not decrease enflurane MAC beyond 60% to 70% of its initial value (Fig. 31-17). That is, there was a ceiling to the enflurane-sparing effect. Morphine, sufentanil, and alfentanil also decrease enflurane MAC and have a similar ceiling effect in dogs.[111-113]

McEwan and colleagues undertook similar studies in humans and characterized the decrease in isoflurane MAC with varying constant fentanyl plasma concentrations achieved with a computer-driven infusion pump.[23] Movement response to initial skin incision was examined

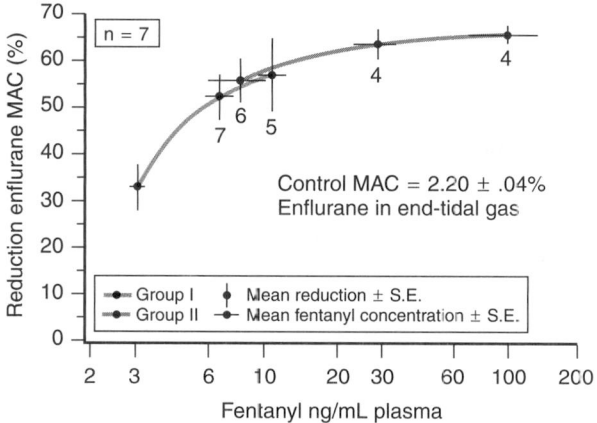

Figure 31–17 Percent reduction in enflurane minimum alveolar concentration (MAC) as a function of plasma concentrations of fentanyl. Each *point* represents the mean concentration (±SEM) for fentanyl in plasma and the average percent (±SEM) reduction in enflurane MAC. Numbers of dogs below the *vertical standard error bars* indicate the numbers per data point. (Redrawn from Murphy MR, Hug CC Jr: The anesthetic potency of fentanyl in terms of its reduction of enflurane MAC. Anesthesiology 57:485, 1982.)

relative to end-tidal isoflurane concentrations. McEwan and coworkers[23] found very similar results in humans to those observed by Hug and colleagues in dogs. Isoflurane MAC decreased 39% at a steady-state fentanyl plasma concentration of 1 ng/mL and 63% at a fentanyl plasma concentration of 3 ng/mL. Increasing fentanyl plasma concentrations to more than 3 ng/mL produced minimal further reduction in isoflurane MAC. The maximal MAC reduction was 82% at a steady-state fentanyl plasma concentration of 10.6 ng/mL. Similar MAC reduction results have been obtained with other inhaled anesthetics (desflurane, sevoflurane) and other opioids (alfentanil, sufentanil, remifentanil).[114,115]

Comparable results are found when other end points of inhaled anesthetics and opioid interactions are examined, including MAC$_{awake}$ and MAC$_{BAR}$;[36,37,116,117] a ceiling effect of the opioid occurs at defined steady-state plasma concentrations.

Clinical Signs of Inadequate Anesthesia and Plasma Concentration of Opioids

Ausems and colleagues[118] used pharmacodynamic modeling concepts to relate clinical signs of inadequate opioid anesthesia to plasma concentrations of the drug. In their study paradigm, patients were premedicated with a benzodiazepine, anesthesia was induced with alfentanil (150 μg/kg), and the trachea was intubated with the aid of succinylcholine. Anesthesia was maintained with 70% nitrous oxide and a variable-rate infusion of alfentanil. The infusion was titrated to the following clinical end points: (1) increased systemic arterial blood pressure greater than 15 mm Hg higher than the patient's normal value; (2) heart rate exceeding 90 beats/min in the absence of hypovolemia; (3) somatic responses such as body movements (minimal muscle paralysis allowed physical movement), swallowing, coughing, grimacing, or opening of the

eyes; and (4) autonomic signs of inadequate anesthesia (e.g., lacrimation, flushing, or sweating). If any clinical signs occurred, the infusion rate was increased 25 to 50 μg/kg/hr, and a small bolus dose (7 μg/kg) was given. Good hemodynamic control was possible in all subjects. If no clinical signs occurred, however, the infusion rate was decreased at regular 15-minute intervals.

Table 31-5 shows the incidence of response to intraoperative noxious stimuli in 37 patients; three different types of surgical procedures are represented. Although hypertension was the most common clinical response, the other three clinical measures occurred a significant number of times. The authors could not predict which patients would have somatic responses, tachycardia, or hypertension. Measurement of plasma concentrations made it possible to describe the concentration-versus-response relationship for different perioperative stimuli. Figure 31-18A shows the relationship between the plasma concentration of alfentanil and response/no response for three clinical end points: intubation, skin incision, and skin closure. Regarding elimination of the response to noxious stimulation, intubation required significantly higher plasma concentrations of alfentanil than skin incision did, and skin closure required significantly lower concentrations than skin incision did.

Table 31–5 Response of 37 patients to noxious intraoperative stimulation during anesthesia with alfentanil and nitrous oxide*

	Surgical Procedure		
	Breast	Lower Abdominal	Upper Abdominal
No. of patients	12	14	11
Hemodynamic responses			
Hypertension	4 (1-7)	4 (1-7)	5 (1-7)
Tachycardia	0 (0-1)	1 (0-4)	3 (1-7)
Somatic responses			
Body movement, swallowing, coughing, grimacing, eye opening	2 (0-4)	5 (0-9)	2 (0-6)
Other autonomic signs of inadequate anesthesia			
Lacrimation, flushing, sweating	0 (0-1)	0 (0-3)	1 (0-2)

*Data are presented as the median number of response episodes per patient. Numbers in parentheses represent the range of number of episodes among the patients in each group. Hypertension is an increase in systemic arterial systolic blood pressure of more than 15 mm Hg above the patient's normal value; tachycardia is a heart rate higher than 90 beats per minute in the absence of hypovolemia.

Data from Ausems ME, Hug CC Jr, Stanski DR, et al: Plasma concentrations of alfentanil required to supplement nitrous oxide anesthesia for general surgery. Anesthesiology 65:362, 1986.

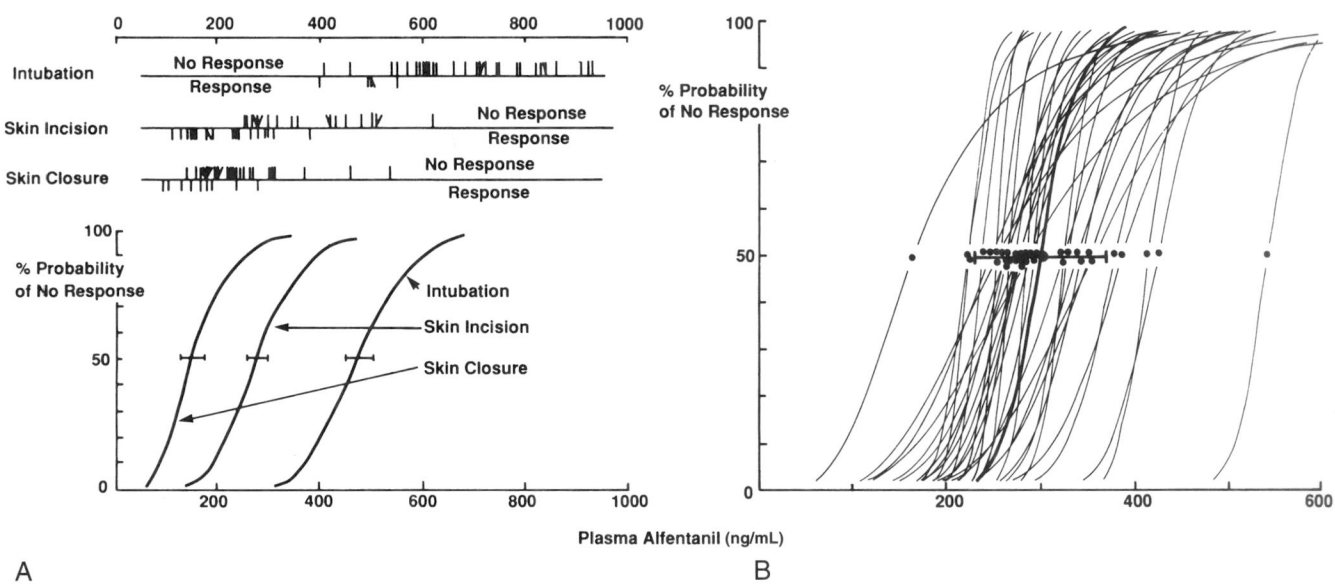

Figure 31–18 A, Relationship between the plasma concentration of alfentanil and response/no response at three specific events of short duration. The quantal data are characterized by logistic regression in the *lower panel,* ±SE for the Cp_{50}, which is the alfentanil plasma concentration associated with a 50% probability of no response. (From Ausems ME, Hug CC Jr, Stanski DR, et al: Plasma concentrations of alfentanil required to supplement nitrous oxide anesthesia for general surgery. Anesthesiology 65:362, 1986.) **B,** Plasma concentration of alfentanil versus the probability of no response for each of 34 patients during the intra-abdominal phase of lower abdominal surgery. *Dots* represent the Cp_{50} values, and the *heavy dark line* represents the average response of the 34 patients. (From Ausems ME, Vuyk J, Hug CC Jr, et al: Comparison of computer-assisted infusion versus intermittent bolus administration of alfentanil as a supplement to nitrous oxide for lower abdominal surgery. Anesthesiology 68:851, 1988.)

The use of logistic regression made it possible to define Cp_{50} values for these clinical events (Table 31-6). Plasma concentrations of alfentanil were varied in the individual subject during surgery to obtain multiple response/no response data points, after which a curve plotting plasma concentration against response was constructed for each

subject (Fig. 31-18B).[118] Especially noteworthy are the steep slope of the individual curves and the moderate pharmacodynamic variability among individuals. Table 31-6 demonstrates that upper abdominal surgery required significantly higher plasma concentrations of alfentanil than lower abdominal or breast surgery did.

The foregoing pharmacodynamic modeling concept has been used to examine the alfentanil dose requirement, pharmacokinetics, and pharmacodynamics in patients with heavy alcohol consumption. Lemmens and colleagues[119] showed that moderate consumers of alcohol (20 to 40 g/day) have an increased requirement for alfentanil because of decreased CNS sensitivity to this opioid. The Cp_{50} of alfentanil in patients with alcohol consumption was 522 ± 104 ng/mL versus 208 ± 26 ng/mL in a control group. This finding suggests that there may be cross-tolerance between opioids and ethanol. Lemmens and coworkers[120] also defined the role of plasma protein binding in determining the clinical effects of alfentanil anesthesia. By examining the alfentanil plasma concentration–versus–clinical response relationship, both total bound and free, and the degree of alfentanil plasma protein binding, they found a significant negative correlation ($r = .67$) between Cp_{50} (total drug) and the free fraction of alfentanil. These data suggest that 45% of the variability in alfentanil CNS response, as estimated by the Cp_{50}, could be explained by variability in the plasma protein binding of alfentanil.

Remifentanil is a newer opioid that is related to the fentanyl family of short-acting, 4-aniliopiperidine derivatives; however, it is unique in having ester linkages that are susceptible to hydrolysis by nonspecific blood and tissue esterases, thereby resulting in very rapid metabolism.

Table 31–6 Cp_{50} values for perioperative events and intraoperative manipulation associated with three types of surgical procedures during alfentanil anesthesia

Event	Cp_{50} (ng/mL)
Single events	
Intubation	475 ± 28*
Skin incision	279 ± 20
Skin closure	150 ± 23
Spontaneous ventilation	233 ± 13
Intraoperative manipulation	
Breast surgery	270 ± 63†
Lower abdominal	309 ± 44
Upper abdominal	412 ± 35
Spontaneous ventilation	233 ± 13

*Standard error of the estimated value for the parameter.
†Values are presented as mean ± SD.
Cp_{50}, plasma concentration of a drug producing a 50% chance of suppressing a response to a given stimulus.
Data from Ausems ME, Vuyk J, Hug CC Jr, et al: Comparison of computer-assisted infusion versus intermittent bolus administration of alfentanil as a supplement to nitrous oxide for lower abdominal surgery. Anesthesiology 68:851, 1988.

Egan and colleagues[121] described the comparative clinical pharmacology of remifentanil and alfentanil. Both opioids have a similar small volume of distribution because of limited tissue solubility; however, remifentanil has significantly higher metabolic clearance, 2.9 L/minute versus 0.36 L/minute for alfentanil. Remifentanil has a similar rate of blood-brain equilibration, with a $t_{1/2} k_{eC}$ value of 1.6 minutes versus 0.96 minute for alfentanil. Remifentanil, however, is significantly more potent than alfentanil, with an EEG Cp_{50} value of 19.9 ng/mL versus 375.9 ng/mL for alfentanil. Minto and colleagues[122,123] quantitated the population pharmacokinetics and dynamics of this opioid by using simulation techniques to develop dosing guidelines. Drover and colleagues[124] applied the opioid anesthetic depth concepts developed by Ausems and associates[39] to define therapeutic plasma concentrations of remifentanil in surgical patients.

The rapid blood-brain equilibration of alfentanil and remifentanil means that a given plasma concentration has a close relationship to the CNS concentration and hence to drug effect.[125] Drugs with a slower rate of blood-brain equilibration (e.g., fentanyl, sufentanil, morphine) would be less amenable to the type of pharmacodynamic analysis of the plasma concentration–versus–clinical effect relationship used by Ausems and coworkers.[39] Glass and colleagues[126] applied the fundamental concepts proposed by Ausems and coworkers[39] to fentanyl by using a computer-driven infusion pump to obtain constant fentanyl plasma concentrations from induction of anesthesia to skin incision. Because of the long equilibration delay between plasma and the effect site in the CNS ($t_{1/2} k_{e0}$ of 4.7 minutes), a significant period of time was allowed between establishing the constant plasma concentration and application of the noxious stimuli. Only fentanyl and 70% nitrous oxide were used, no premedication or induction sedative was given, and fentanyl plasma concentrations were also measured. After skin incision, patients were observed for purposeful somatic movement. The fentanyl plasma concentration that had a 50% probability of no movement (Cp_{50}) with 70% nitrous oxide was 3.26 ng/mL.

The approach to opioid administration presented by Ausems and colleagues[39] provides useful insight into clinical assessment of the analgesic component of depth of anesthesia. Overdosage with opioids cannot be judged intraoperatively. Only at the end of anesthesia, when spontaneous ventilation should occur, does one know whether administration of opioids has been excessive. To prevent overdosage, Ausems and coworkers[39] proposed using a viable rate of infusion in which one titrates plasma concentrations to clinical effect to find the lowest possible effective rate of opioid administration. To achieve this end point, one must look for clinical signs of inadequate anesthesia. Once the infusion rate just causing inadequate anesthesia has been determined, one increases the rate slightly, thus providing adequate anesthesia. The steep slope of the concentration-versus-response curve for alfentanil (see Fig. 31-18B) demonstrates that a small increase in plasma concentration of the drug rapidly converts inadequate anesthesia (100% probability of response to stimuli) to adequate anesthesia. Because of moderate variability in the pharmacokinetics of alfentanil, this process of titrating the dose (infusion rate) against clinical effect and

pharmacodynamics is necessary for each patient. This concept is most applicable to alfentanil, which has rapid blood-brain equilibration,[125] and it is ideal with remifentanil, which has extremely rapid and predictable pharmacokinetics along with rapid blood-brain equilibration.[121] Intermittent intravenous bolus administration of opioids is not as efficient as variable-rate infusion when titrating plasma concentrations of opioids to clinical effect.[118]

ELECTROPHYSIOLOGIC MONITORING

Spontaneous Electroencephalogram

The realization that anesthetic drugs alter the EEG dates back to the discovery that the brain produces electrical activity (see Chapter 38).[127] In 1875, Caton[128] used chloroform to convince himself that the electrical oscillations from the brain were indeed biologic in origin. During the 1920s and 1930s, when electronic amplifiers allowed recording of these small voltages through the skull, Berger[129] measured the influence of chloroform on the EEG. In 1937, Gibbs and coauthors[130] reported that anesthetics changed EEG activity from low-voltage fast waves to high-voltage slow waves and postulated that the EEG could be used to measure the effects of anesthesia. In 1952, Faulconer[131] demonstrated with ether that the depth of anesthesia, based on recognition of EEG patterns, correlated with the arterial concentration of ether. He also demonstrated that the presence of nitrous oxide lowered the arterial concentration of ether necessary to produce a given EEG effect.

The EEG can be considered a measure of the depth of anesthesia for several reasons. It represents cortical electrical activity derived from summated excitatory and inhibitory postsynaptic activity, which is controlled and paced by subcortical thalamic nuclei. This electrical activity has direct physiologic correlates relevant to the depth of anesthesia. Cerebral blood flow and cerebral metabolism are related to the degree of EEG activity.[132] Anesthetic drugs affect both cerebral physiology and EEG patterns. The EEG is a noninvasive indicator of cerebral function when the patient is unconscious and unresponsive. Although recording of the raw EEG involves accumulating a large amount of information and EEG tracings, new computer analysis techniques can summarize and distill the EEG into a condensed, descriptive format (the "processed" EEG).[133,134] Rampil[135] reviewed the value of the processed EEG in the clinical practice of anesthesia.

Inadequate anesthesia generally causes EEG activation. Peripheral noxious stimuli reach the brain through afferent systems that pass through the ascending reticular activating systems of the brainstem. These systems regulate corticocerebral function and thus affect the underlying EEG pattern. Noxious stimuli can cause three types of changes in the EEG: (1) desynchronization with the appearance of 20- to 60-Hz fast rhythms (EEG activation), (2) the appearance of 6- to 10-Hz spindles, and (3) bursts of 1- to 3-Hz slow waves.[136] These patterns vary with individual anesthetics and with the nature of the stimulation.[137] For example, during light levels of thiopental anesthesia in dogs (steady-state plasma concentrations of 15 to 27 µg/mL), supramaximal stimulation of the sciatic nerve caused EEG activation and increased cerebral metabolic oxygen requirements and blood flow by 15%.[138] During deep levels of thiopental anesthesia (37 to 49 µg/mL), stimulation produced no change in these variables. A distinct threshold concentration of thiopental seems to block the response to noxious stimuli during anesthesia in animals.

The EEG is a valuable tool because it reflects cerebral physiology, it is a continuous and noninvasive measure, and it changes markedly on administration of anesthetic drugs.[139] However, early studies concluded that the EEG was not a meaningful measure of the depth of anesthesia. Galla and colleagues[140] examined raw EEG signals for 43 patients and correlated EEG patterns with clinical signs of anesthesia. A discrepancy seemed to exist between the clinical signs and EEG patterns, especially during induction and emergence. During induction, clinical signs indicated that the patients were more lightly anesthetized than the EEG patterns suggested, whereas on emergence, clinical signs indicated greater anesthetic depth. Levy[141] investigated processed EEG signals during induction and before bypass in patients undergoing cardiac surgery who were given potent inhaled anesthetics and opioids. He examined a series of univariate descriptors, including median frequency (the frequency below which 50% of the EEG power is located) and spectral edge (the frequency below which 95% of the EEG power is located). He concluded that the multimodal EEG activity observed in 64% of cases precluded the use of single univariate parameters to describe the anesthetic state. Berezowskyj and coworkers[142] had similar findings with the use of power spectral analysis in patients given nitrous oxide, opioid, and halothane for anesthesia. Clinical assessment of the depth of anesthesia did not correlate well with EEG patterns.

Two studies attempted to correlate univariate EEG parameters to the clinical end point of awakening from anesthesia. Drummond and colleagues[143] examined five numeric descriptors derived from the processed EEG during imminent arousal (spontaneous movement, coughing, or eye opening) from isoflurane/nitrous oxide anesthesia. These authors determined the threshold value for each parameter that best served to predict imminent arousal. Although several parameters (median frequency, spectral edge 90% frequency, total power, and frequency band ratio) predicted imminent arousal with sensitivities of 90% and specificities of 82% to 90%, none of the EEG descriptors could serve as a completely reliable, sole predictor of imminent arousal. Long and coworkers[144] undertook a similar analysis using either isoflurane or fentanyl anesthesia. For isoflurane anesthesia, these investigators found that awakening was always presaged by an abrupt decrease in power in the 1- to 4-Hz frequency range (decrease in delta power). During emergence from fentanyl/nitrous oxide anesthesia, obvious change in the overall EEG power spectrum was noted; however, the same numeric EEG descriptors that were predictive of awakening from isoflurane also occurred during emergence from fentanyl. These two studies concluded that consistent trends in the EEG can be expected to occur with changing depth of anesthesia, with the available EEG descriptors providing potentially useful trend information regarding the changing depth of anesthesia. However, the sensitivity and specificity of the available parameters are such that none can serve as the sole indicator of anesthetic depth.

Dwyer and colleagues[145] examined the power spectrum of the EEG in surgical patients receiving 0.6 to 1.4 MAC isoflurane-only anesthesia with skin incision. A second group of volunteers received 0.15 to 0.45 MAC isoflurane with memory testing. Different time-dependent EEG frequency parameters (e.g., spectral edge, median frequency) were examined relative to the clinical measures. The authors found that isoflurane caused some decrease in EEG activity. However, no difference in EEG parameters was found between subjects who moved and those who did not move with skin incision. In volunteers receiving low-dose isoflurane, memory of the information presented did not correlate with values of any EEG parameter. The authors concluded that the examined EEG parameters did not predict depth of anesthesia as defined by response to surgical skin incision, response to verbal command, or development of memory.

The previously described clinical research attempting to relate EEG effects to clinical anesthetic depth has resulted in inconclusive findings. When single anesthetic drugs are examined under defined conditions, it has been possible to demonstrate unambiguous relationships between EEG parameters and anesthetic drug concentrations and to use pharmacokinetic and pharmacodynamic modeling concepts to link drug concentrations to EEG drug effects.[146] Different EEG waveform data analysis approaches have been used to define different univariate EEG parameters as measures of anesthetic drug effect. The most powerful application has been to further understand the fundamental clinical pharmacology of the anesthetic drugs. By using a statistical approach called "semilinear canonic correlation," drug-specific EEG measures have been identified for opioids,[147] midazolam,[148] and propofol[149] and have proved robust when prospectively tested.[150]

Application of the EEG to measure clinical depth of anesthesia failed previously for several reasons: a lack of understanding of the effects of interactions of several concurrently administered anesthetic drugs on the EEG, no standard approach to choosing an optimal EEG parameter, and finally, no clear definition of a "gold standard" for measurement and assessment of the clinical depth of anesthesia. Attempts to apply the MAC concept of inhaled anesthetics (i.e., movement responses to skin incision) have been inconclusive, as reflected in the previously discussed studies because the spinal-versus-cortical mechanisms of purposeful movement were not understood until recently.[29-31]

Bispectral Electroencephalographic Monitoring

In the 1990s, Aspect Medical Systems, a medical device company in Natick, Massachusetts, undertook an integrated research effort to develop the EEG as a measure of anesthetic depth.* The Aspect EEG monitor quantitates the anesthetic effects on the brain, specifically, the hypnotic component of anesthesia. The device presents

---

*Dr. Stanski, coauthor of this chapter, is a member of the board of directors of Aspect Medical Systems.

a continuous EEG parameter, the bispectral (BIS) index, which ranges from an awake, no-drug-effect value of 95 to 100 to zero with no detectable EEG activity. Successful development of the Aspect BIS EEG monitoring system can be identified with the following concepts:

1. The simultaneous use of multiple EEG signal–processing approaches captured incremental information that was not captured with traditional approaches based on a single signal-processing approach, such as fast Fourier transformation.
2. Multiple clinically relevant measures (movement, hemodynamics, drug concentrations, consciousness, recall) in patients and volunteers were gathered with concurrent EEG data.
3. Advanced multivariate statistical data analysis was used to correlate the components of the multiple EEG signal–processing approaches with the clinical data to create the univariate BIS parameter.
4. Prospective clinical evaluation of the BIS index was performed at multiple institutions under varying anesthetic and surgical conditions.
5. The BIS index was recognized as measuring the hypnotic components of the anesthetic and was relatively insensitive to the analgesic (e.g., opioid) components of an anesthetic.
6. Prospective clinical trials demonstrated that BIS monitoring could improve the outcome of an anesthetic regimen.
7. Simple hardware and sensors were developed and are commercially available to facilitate high-quality signal capture despite the noisy electrical environment of the operating room.

Bispectral Electroencephalographic Signal Processing

Bispectral EEG signal processing has been reviewed by Rampil[151] and by Sigl and Chamoun.[152] To date, most EEG signal processing has involved a form of spectral analysis, which examines the EEG signal during a small slice of time (epoch) as a function of frequency. The frequency analysis decomposes the EEG signal into a series of sine waves by Fourier analysis. Each sine wave is described with an amplitude, frequency, and phase angle. The sine wave amplitude is half the peak-to-peak voltage, the frequency is the number of cycles per second, and the phase angle describes the time offset of the sine wave relative to the start of the epoch. The output of the Fourier analysis is a histogram showing the frequency, amplitudes, and phase of the sine waves that taken together, create the EEG signal. Fourier analysis assumes that the signal pattern is constant during the epoch. Thus, it poorly handles signals that abruptly change during an epoch, such as burst suppression. Traditional spectral analysis ignores the phase data and assumes that the frequency constituents are uncorrelated (linear).

In contrast, BIS analysis assumes that frequencies may be correlated and uses the phase information to look for evidence of phase coupling among frequency bands, termed "bicoherence." The meaning of EEG phase relationships is not yet clear; however, the general notion is that an awake brain has multiple signal generators, working independently, and hence displays little synchronization.

As the brain falls asleep, fewer independent signal generators are active, and thus the resulting EEG is more likely to reflect coupling (bicoherence) between signal generators. In addition, BIS analysis has several useful properties that promote noise suppression beyond what is possible with conventional spectral analysis.[151] Thus, BIS analysis provides additional information about the EEG signal than is captured by traditional spectral analysis approaches that consider only frequency and amplitude.

Developing the Bispectral (BIS) Index

The BIS index is a complex, proprietary EEG parameter that has been under development since 1987 by Aspect Medical Systems. In 1996, the U.S. Food and Drug Administration approved the commercially available version as a monitor of anesthetic effect on the brain. Figure 31-19 displays the conceptual process whereby Aspect took EEG and clinical data from approximately 1500 subjects and 5000 hours of EEG signal gathered under a broad range of anesthetic regimens. The EEG was processed by first removing high- and low-frequency artifacts, electrocardiographic signals, pacemaker spikes, eye blinks, wandering baseline, and alternating current interference. The EEG data were then analyzed by three different approaches: Fourier, BIS, and time domain analysis (Fig. 31-20). Time domain analysis was used to characterize burst suppression and isoelectricity. The EEG was smoothed across the power spectrum and bispectrum by using a moving average. The analysis then examined the degree of beta or high frequency (14 to 30 Hz), the amount of low-frequency synchronization, and the presence of fully or nearly suppressed periods (i.e., isoelectric signal).

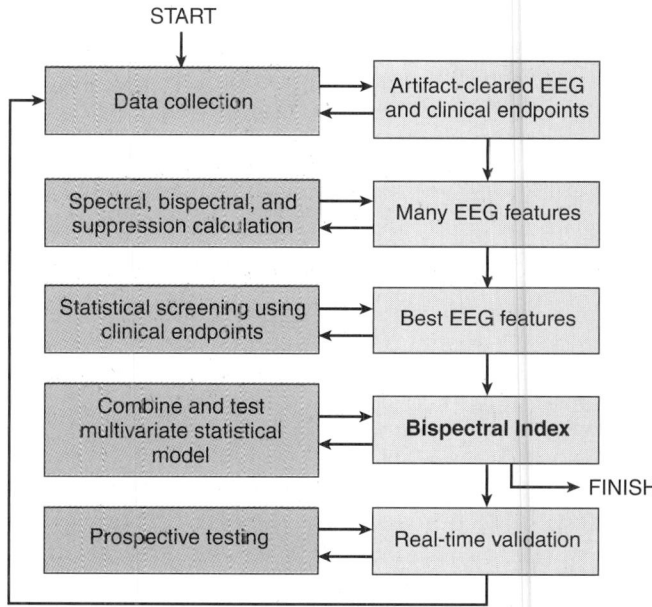

Figure 31–19 Key steps used during development of the bispectral algorithm. Statistical modeling was used to identify the best features of the electroencephalogram for recognition of clinical end points. The circular path notes that the process was iterative. (Redrawn from Kelley SD: Monitoring Level of Consciousness during Anesthesia and Sedation. Natick, MA, Aspect Medical Systems, 2003.)

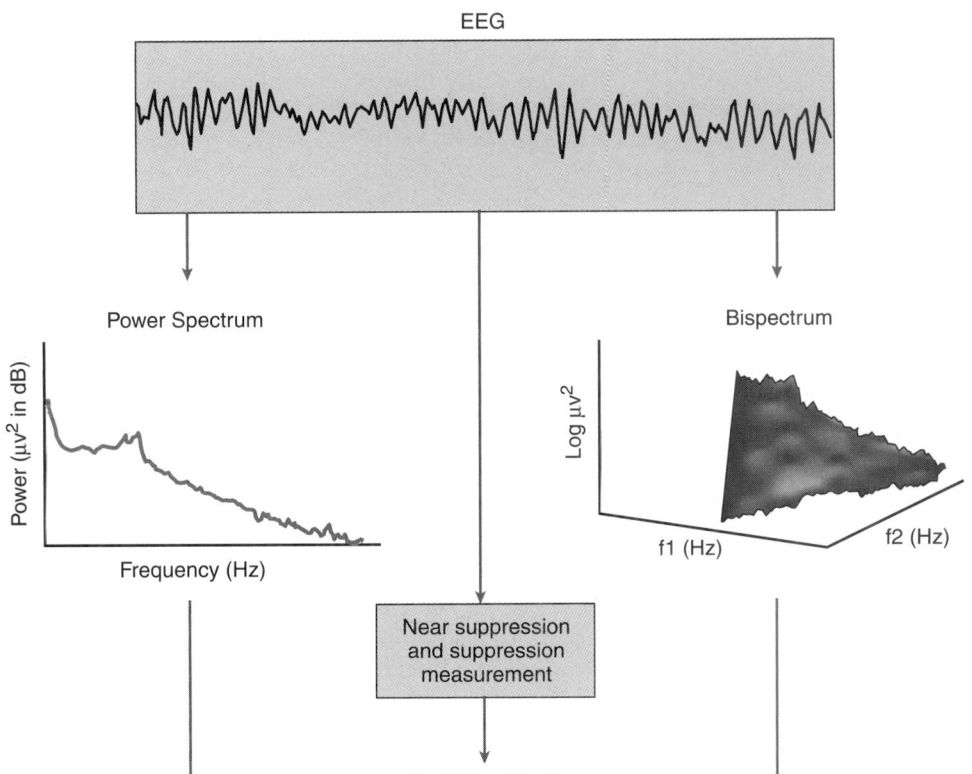

EEG

Power Spectrum

Bispectrum

Figure 31–20 Schematic diagram of signal processing paths integral to generating a single bispectral (BIS) index value. After digitization and artifact rejection, original electroencephalographic (EEG) epochs undergo three primary paths of analysis—power spectral analysis, BIS analysis, and time-based analysis for suppression/near suppression—to look for key EEG features. The BIS algorithm, based on statistical modeling, combines the contributions of each of the identified features to generate the scaled BIS index. (Redrawn from Kelley SD: Monitoring Level of Consciousness during Anesthesia and Sedation. Natick, MA, Aspect Medical Systems, 2003.)

The algorithm to determine final calculation of the BIS value (0 to 100) involved performing a multivariate statistical analysis, similar to semilinear canonic correlation,[147] on the aforementioned EEG data relative to a clinical database that was gathered from multiple different clinical studies over the past 15 years. As prototype versions of the BIS index were developed over a period of several years, subsequent clinical testing was used to improve and refine the algorithms and components of the EEG parameter. The BIS algorithm was adapted to handle burst suppression EEG, to minimize the initial activation of the EEG seen with some anesthetic drugs, and to optimally use the components of Fourier analysis and bispectrum analysis. Thus, the BIS index is a complex parameter composed of a combination of time domain, frequency domain, and higher-order spectral subparameters derived from clinical data that measure the hypnotic component of an anesthetic.[151] The BIS parameter has been and remains a work in progress. Over the past decade the BIS parameter has been modified based on new data about the EEG response to novel anesthetic drugs and drug combinations, as well as to incorporate new signal collection and noise rejection technology.

Clinical Development and Validation of the Bispectral Index

The initial studies with early versions of the BIS algorithm in the early 1990s attempted to correlate the BIS index to predict movement in response to skin incision with the use of isoflurane/oxygen,[152] propofol/nitrous oxide[153] or propofol/alfentanil anesthesia.[154] In the first major clinical evaluation of the BIS technology, a large,

multicenter study by Sebel and colleagues[155] randomized 300 patients into two groups. Both groups received an anesthetic regimen designed so that approximately half of all patients would move at skin incision. In the control group, the BIS index was passively recorded and not used for titration. In the BIS-titrated group, drug concentrations were increased to produce a BIS value less than 60. In the control group, the BIS index was a mean of 66 ± 19 (standard deviation [SD]) with a 43% movement rate. In the BIS-adjusted group, the BIS index was lower, a mean of 51 ± 19 (SD) with a significantly lower movement rate of 13%. In this multicenter trial, some centers used primarily opioids with nitrous oxide, whereas others used propofol or isoflurane as the primary anesthetic. The study also found that reliability of the BIS index was strongly influenced by anesthetic technique. When hypnotic drugs such as propofol or isoflurane are used as the primary anesthetic, changes in the BIS index correlate with the probability of a movement response to skin incision. When opioid analgesics are used at higher doses, the correlation to patient movement became much less significant. This information, when linked to the understanding that purposeful movement to skin incision reflects the spinal action of anesthetics instead of their cortical effects, provided fundamental understanding of how development of the BIS algorithm had to be focused on the hypnotic components of anesthesia, specifically, the clinical measures of consciousness and memory. A subsequent series of studies described in the following paragraphs provided the data and clinical understanding to create the current algorithm to calculate the BIS index.

Glass and coworkers[156] designed a study to examine the relationship among BIS index, measured drug concentrations, and increasing levels of sedation when the anesthetic drugs propofol, midazolam, isoflurane, and alfentanil were given to volunteers in a controlled manner. Data from this study were used to further optimize the BIS algorithm. Seventy-two volunteers received a single drug at four or five defined, increasing target plasma concentrations that ultimately created an unconscious subject. The BIS index, arterial drug or end-tidal concentrations, and subjective sedation and memory scores were measured. The BIS index was significantly correlated to measured drug concentrations, as well as clinical measures of sedation. None of the alfentanil patients lost consciousness and had minimal change in the BIS index, a finding confirming that the BIS index is not sensitive to low concentrations of opioid analgesics. Fifty percent and 95% of the volunteers were unconscious at BIS values of 67 and 50, respectively.

Liu and colleagues[157] demonstrated in 26 surgical subjects that the BIS index accurately tracked the degree of clinical sedation with intermediate (4 mg) to large (20 mg) doses of midazolam given during regional anesthesia. Response to a loud voice (observer assessment of alertness/sedation [OAA/S] score of 3) corresponded to a BIS index of 87 ± 6 (SD) and a 40% probability of recall. A deeper end point, lack of response to mild prodding (OAA/S score of 2) corresponded to a BIS value of 81 ± 8 (SD) and resulted in complete lack of recall. When midazolam created an unresponsive subject, the mean BIS index was 69.2 ± 13.9 (SD). Similar results were found by these investigators for propofol when given under regional anesthesia.[158] Katoh and coworkers[159] had similar results with low, sedating doses of sevoflurane and also with higher, anesthetic concentrations in 69 surgical patients. Both the BIS index and end-tidal sevoflurane concentrations were correlated to clinical sedation scores

of the patients. The BIS index decreased almost linearly from a median value of 95 to 45 with an end-tidal sevoflurane concentration increasing from 0.2% to 1.4%. Sevoflurane concentrations greater than 1.4% produced a limited further reduction in the BIS index. Flaishon and colleagues[160] examined the behavior of the BIS index when surgical patients were given a single intravenous bolus of propofol, 2 mg/kg, or thiopental, 4 mg/kg, with concurrent muscle relaxants. The isolated arm technique was used to identify loss and then return of consciousness. No patient with a BIS index of less than 58 was conscious; a BIS index of less than 65 signified a less than 5% probability of return of consciousness within 50 seconds.

Kearse and associates[161] undertook a more detailed examination of memory and response to command during propofol/nitrous oxide sedation with BIS monitoring. These investigators found a strong association between the BIS index and response to command, whether the command consisted simply of a uniform voice asking a volunteer to move a hand or foot or incorporated graded and then varied stimuli. The relationship between the BIS index and responsiveness scores remained consistent over time and with increases or decreases in propofol concentrations. No subject was responsive when the BIS index was less than 57.

Johansen and Sebel[162] have reviewed the historical clinical development and current applications of BIS monitoring in clinical anesthesia.

Interpreting the Bispectral Index

Figure 31-21 displays the numerical value of the BIS index, from 0 to 100 relative to clinical end points, and the underlying EEG signal. BIS values of 0 represent an isoelectric EEG, whereas values of 100 represent an awake CNS. After administration of a hypnotic drug, the BIS index decreases from an awake value of 100 as the patient's

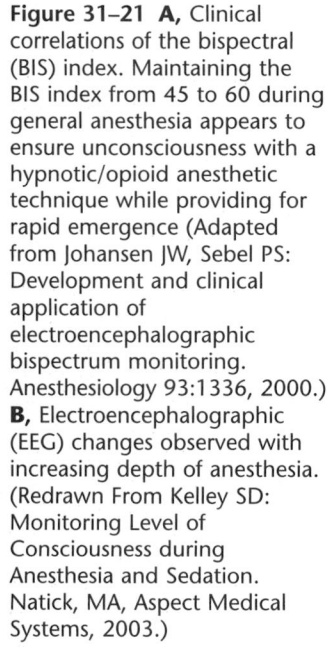
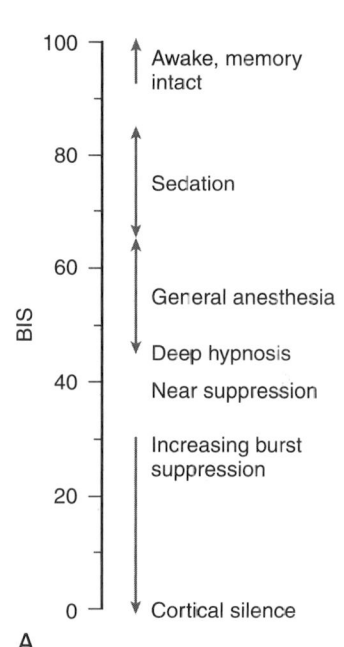
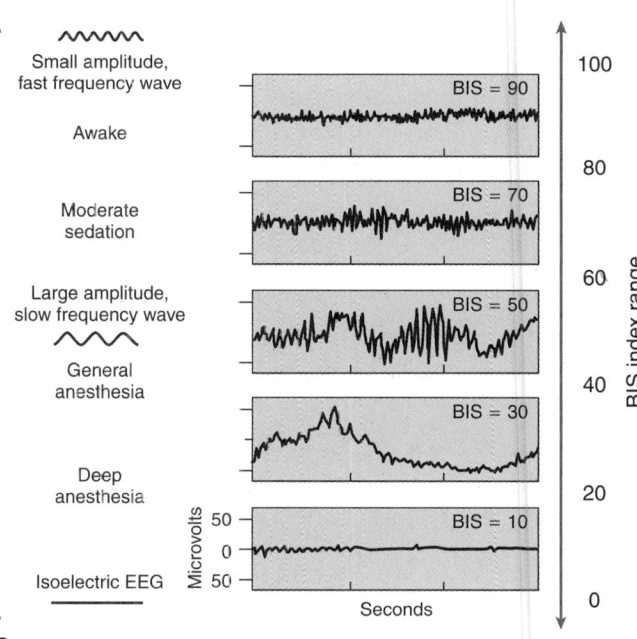

Figure 31–21 A, Clinical correlations of the bispectral (BIS) index. Maintaining the BIS index from 45 to 60 during general anesthesia appears to ensure unconsciousness with a hypnotic/opioid anesthetic technique while providing for rapid emergence (Adapted from Johansen JW, Sebel PS: Development and clinical application of electroencephalographic bispectrum monitoring. Anesthesiology 93:1336, 2000.) **B,** Electroencephalographic (EEG) changes observed with increasing depth of anesthesia. (Redrawn From Kelley SD: Monitoring Level of Consciousness during Anesthesia and Sedation. Natick, MA, Aspect Medical Systems, 2003.)

level of consciousness undergoes a series of transitions. At a BIS index of 60, the probability of consciousness is low. A BIS index of less than 40 represents deep hypnosis and an EEG approaching isoelectricity. BIS values of 40 to 60 reflect adequate hypnotic effect for general anesthesia with reasonably rapid recovery to consciousness. Loss of consciousness will tend to occur at BIS values between 70 and 80. Like all electrophysiologic measures, one must correlate the individual clinical state to the BIS value in each patient to adjust for variability between patients. Figure 31-22 displays the current understanding of the relationship between the BIS value and the probability of response to either voice or explicit memory recall. The curve for memory impairment is to the left of the curve for verbal responsiveness.

A limited number of studies examined the relationship of the BIS index to direct measures of brain function. Alkire[163] studied the correlation between the cerebral metabolic rate, as measured by positron emission tomography, and the BIS index during propofol and isoflurane anesthesia. Volunteers served as their own controls. After baseline measurements, volunteers received increasing amounts of propofol or isoflurane until they were unconscious (BIS values of 30 to 50). This study demonstrated a linear relationship between decreasing BIS index and a reduction in cerebral metabolic rate, thus indicating a physiologic link of the quantitated EEG and cerebral metabolism under the influence of hypnotic drugs.

Ludbrook and colleagues[164] examined the relationship between propofol brain concentrations, as estimated by simultaneous arterial/jugular bulb venous blood sampling during propofol induction of anesthesia, and cerebral blood flow and BIS measurements. Although significant inter-subject variability was seen, calculated propofol brain concentrations and BIS values were closely correlated.

The relationship between noxious stimuli, opioid response, and the BIS index has been determined. Early studies had demonstrated that low concentrations of

opioids did not change the BIS response during propofol or inhaled anesthetics.[155,156] Iselin-Chaves and coworkers[165] performed a volunteer study that examined sedation score and the presence/absence of recall during stepped increases of propofol and propofol with alfentanil (50 or 100 ng/mL). The BIS index, sedation, and memory function were highly correlated, and the BIS value was not affected by the low alfentanil concentration.

Guignard and associates[166] extended this understanding by examining the response of the BIS index to the interaction of noxious stimuli (laryngoscopy/tracheal intubation) during propofol administration with and without remifentanil in surgical patients. Computer-controlled infusion of propofol was used to achieve a constant target effect-site concentration of 4 μg/mL. Hemodynamics, movement response, and the BIS index were measured during tracheal intubation. With only propofol at a target effect-site concentration of 4 μg/mL, the BIS index decreased to a mean of approximately 45. Intubation resulted in a significant increase in BIS values to a mean of 70. When computer-controlled infusion of remifentanil was added to achieve target effect-site concentrations of 2 to 16 ng/mL, the interaction of remifentanil on BIS values was obvious. Before intubation, these remifentanil concentrations did not change the BIS values during propofol hypnosis. Progressively increasing concentrations of remifentanil blunted the increase in BIS index after intubation. Remifentanil target effect-site concentrations of 8 and 16 ng/mL resulted in a minimal increase in the BIS index, hemodynamic stability, and no purposeful movement. This study demonstrated that significant noxious stimuli given with only a hypnotic present (e.g., propofol, inhaled anesthetics) will result in significant hemodynamic response with an increase in BIS index values. The addition of adequate opioid analgesia results in hemodynamic control and less or no change in the BIS value.

Ropcke and colleagues[167] demonstrated similar EEG activation and increase in BIS values when desflurane only (no opioids) was given to surgical patients during intra-abdominal surgery. They demonstrated that in unstimulated patients before the initiation of surgery, a desflurane end-tidal concentration of 2.2% was needed to achieve a mean BIS value of 50. The desflurane end-tidal concentration needed to achieve a BIS value of 50 increased to 6.8% during intra-abdominal noxious surgical stimulation. The authors did not examine how opioid analgesia would change the response observed with desflurane. These two studies indicate that with inadequate analgesia (opioid) during significant noxious surgical stimuli, one can expect the BIS index to increase. Low concentrations of opioid in the presence of a hypnotic drug with no noxious stimuli present will not change the BIS value. Higher doses/concentrations of opioids can result in EEG slowing and a decrease in the BIS index, either alone or with hypnotic anesthetic drugs present.

Two studies suggest that nitrous oxide given in concentrations of up to 70% have minimal effect on the BIS index. Rampil and coworkers[168] demonstrated in volunteers that although nitrous oxide concentrations up to 50% did alter the spectral content of the EEG, there were minimal changes in the BIS index. The subjects did not exhibit

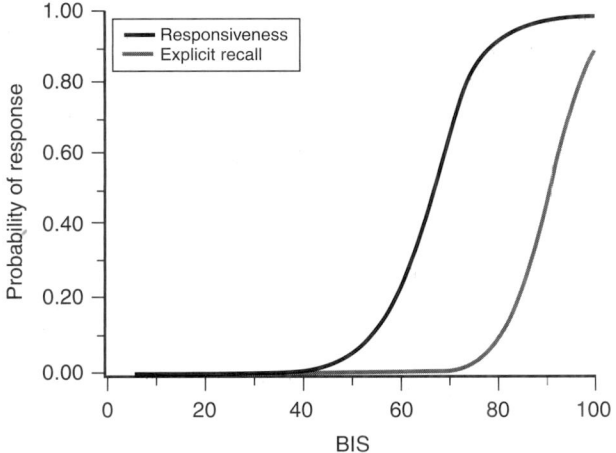

Figure 31–22 The reduction in verbal responsiveness to command (*red line*) and memory (*black line*) with decreased bispectral (BIS) index values. BIS values less than 60 are associated with a very low probability of awareness. (Redrawn from Kelley SD: Monitoring Level of Consciousness during Anesthesia and Sedation. Natick, MA, Aspect Medical Systems, 2003.)

any signs of CNS depression at these concentrations. Coste and colleagues[169] examined the interaction of propofol used to induce anesthesia, orotracheal intubation, and the BIS index. Anesthesia was induced in surgical patients with a computer-driven infusion pump that achieved a target propofol effect-site concentration of 4 μg/mL. Propofol decreased the BIS index to 57 to 60. The addition of 60% to 70% nitrous oxide in a second group of patients did not result in any change in the BIS value. Clinically, fewer patients experienced a movement response in the nitrous oxide group, whereas the hemodynamic response to orotracheal intubation was not different between the two groups. These studies suggest that nitrous oxide in concentrations of 50% to 70% results in a degree of analgesia with minimal impact on the BIS index when hypnotic drugs are used concurrently.

Katoh and coworkers[170] examined the effects of increasing age on the relationship of sevoflurane sedation relative to the BIS index. They studied 96 surgical patients 18 to 85 years of age. The patients were sedated at sevoflurane end-tidal concentrations ranging from 0.4% to 0.9%, and verbal responsiveness to loud name calling (OAA/S score of 3) or mild prodding (OAA/S score of 2) was determined. The BIS index was linearly related to end-tidal sevoflurane concentrations. Sevoflurane end-tidal concentrations of 0.4% to 0.5% produced BIS values of 80 to 95, whereas sevoflurane end-tidal concentrations of 0.8% to 0.9% produced BIS values of 60 to 80. The authors found that MAC_{awake} was age related, with the elderly having a significantly lower value than younger patients did. The relationship of the probability of no response to verbal command versus the BIS index was not age related. These data suggest that the BIS index can be used to adjust for the aged-related change in sevoflurane potency. Similar studies will be needed to examine the age independence of BIS values at deeper clinical end points of hypnotic drug effect.

Several other factors that will be encountered in clinical anesthesia care can interact with the BIS index. The moderate changes in body temperature that occur during cardiopulmonary bypass can change the EEG signal and hence the BIS index. Mathew and colleagues[171] showed that in patients undergoing cardiopulmonary bypass with constant effect-site concentrations of fentanyl and midazolam, hypothermia decreased the BIS index by 1.12 units per degree Celsius decline in temperature. Body temperature ranged from approximately 32°C to 37°C in this clinical study. In healthy volunteers, mild core hyperthermia (increase of 2°C) did not alter the BIS index.[172]

Infusion of esmolol can also alter the BIS index. Johansen[173] has shown in surgical patients that during a stable propofol/alfentanil anesthetic (propofol target effect-site concentration of 5.5 μg/mL, alfentanil effect-site concentration of 50 or 150 ng/mL), a 30-minute infusion of esmolol (1-mg/kg bolus, 250 μg/kg/min) decreased the BIS index from 37 ± 6 (SD) to 22 ± 6 (SD). Discontinuation of esmolol reversed these changes. Menigaux and associates[174] demonstrated that when esmolol was given during induction with propofol only, the BIS index was not different from that of the control group (propofol, no esmolol) before intubation. BIS values were approximately 45 before intubation. With intubation,

the BIS value increased in the control group to approximately 60, whereas the BIS value in the esmolol group was unchanged. These two studies indicate that there is a complex interaction of β-adrenoreceptor blockade during anesthesia with relevant noxious stimuli and measurement of the hypnotic component with the BIS index. β-Adrenoreceptor blockade both alters the EEG arousal response to noxious stimuli when inadequate analgesia is present and can decrease the BIS index during adequate clinical anesthesia.

Epidural anesthesia can also decrease the amount of hypnotic anesthetic needed for sedation. Hodgson and Liu[175] have shown that the end-tidal concentration of sevoflurane needed to achieve a BIS index of 50 was 0.59% in patients receiving a lidocaine epidural for surgical procedures whereas a sevoflurane end-tidal concentration of 0.92% was needed to achieve a BIS index of 50 in patients receiving general anesthesia or general anesthesia with an intravenous infusion of lidocaine to match the plasma concentrations achieved during the epidural anesthetic. This study demonstrates that the deafferentation induced by regional anesthesia results in supraspinal effects that change hypnotic anesthetic requirements.

The dissociative anesthetic ketamine can create excitatory effects on the EEG. Ketamine doses that create unresponsiveness (0.25 to 0.5 mg/kg) did not change the BIS index.[176] When ketamine is used with other hypnotics that decrease the BIS index, such as propofol, an additive interaction occurs on the pharmacodynamic end points that is not reflected in the BIS index.[177] Thus, the BIS index may not have clinical utility when used with ketamine alone or with other anesthetic drugs.

Bispectral Index and Clinical Utility/Outcome

Several studies have examined the clinical and economic outcome benefits of BIS monitoring in routine surgery. Gan and colleagues[178] studied 302 subjects receiving a propofol/alfentanil/nitrous oxide anesthetic regimen in four different institutions. Half the subjects were randomized to a "standard practice" whereby the propofol and alfentanil were titrated to provide a stable anesthetic with the fastest possible recovery. The BIS index was recorded in this group but was not displayed to the practitioner. The remaining subjects received "standard practice plus BIS monitoring." In this group, propofol infusions were titrated to achieve a target BIS value between 45 and 60 during surgery and 60 to 75 during the final 15 minutes of the anesthetic regimen. Patients in the BIS group required significantly lower normalized propofol infusion rates (134 versus 116 μg/kg/min), were extubated significantly sooner (11.2 versus 7.3 minutes), had a higher percentage of patients oriented on arrival in the recovery room (43% versus 23%), and had more rapid discharge from the recovery room. This study demonstrated that titrating propofol with BIS monitoring during balanced anesthesia decreased propofol use and significantly improved recovery with no difference in intraoperative conditions.

Song and colleagues[179] presented similar findings with inhaled anesthetics. Sixty surgical patients were randomized to receive desflurane or sevoflurane with 65% nitrous oxide and low doses of fentanyl. Half the patients were randomized to standard practice in which the inhaled anesthetic was titrated according to clinical end points and judgment. The second group had the volatile anesthetic titrated to a BIS value of 60. During the maintenance period, BIS values were significantly lower in the standard-treatment group (mean, 42), a finding suggesting deeper anesthesia than in the BIS-titrated group with a mean of 60. Volatile anesthetic use in the BIS-titrated group was 30% to 38% lower than in the control group. Similarly, times to verbal responsiveness were 30% to 55% shorter in the BIS-titrated group. This study demonstrated that titrating desflurane and sevoflurane with the use of BIS monitoring decreased utilization of the drugs and contributed to faster emergence from anesthesia.

Three clinical trials have been undertaken to examine the value of BIS monitoring relative to intraoperative awareness. The B-Aware trial is an Australian prospective, randomized, double-blind multicenter trial involving patients at high risk of awareness (cesarean section, high-risk cardiac surgery, trauma surgery, or rigid bronchoscopy).[180] Patients were assessed for awareness at 2 to 6 hours, 24 to 36 hours, and 30 days. An independent, blinded committee assessed each report of awareness. BIS-guided anesthesia reduced the risk of awareness by 82% ($n = 1227$, 2 patients) in comparison to the control group ($n = 1238$, 11 patients).

The AIM study was a prospective multicentered study of 19,576 patients undergoing general anesthesia at seven geographically dispersed institutions in the United States.[181] All patients were interviewed postoperatively and 1 week after surgery with a structured interview technique. A total of 25 cases (0.13%) of awareness were identified, and they occurred at a fairly consistent rate in the seven different institutions. High-risk procedures such as cardiac surgery had a higher incidence (0.95%) than lower-risk orthopedic procedures did (0.1%). These findings are similar to previous reports of the incidence of awareness from Australia and Sweden. Awareness is a ubiquitous phenomenon with an incidence between 1 and 2 cases per 1000 anesthetics.

The SAFE-II study is Swedish awareness follow-up evaluation of 5100 patients who underwent BIS monitoring during surgery.[182] The use of BIS monitoring was associated with a significantly reduced incidence of awareness (78% reduction) when compared with historical controls from the same hospitals and investigators.[49] These three studies demonstrate that awareness occurs in current clinical practice and that routine BIS monitoring can significantly reduce this risk to patients.

The relationship of anesthetic management to patient morbidity and mortality has generally focused on the immediate perioperative time period, that is, the hours to days surrounding surgery and anesthesia. Information on the effects of anesthetic management on long-term postoperative mortality rates is limited. Weldon and coauthors[183] reported that deep maintenance anesthetic levels are associated with higher 1-year postoperative death rates in patients 40 years and older undergoing major, noncardiac surgery. These investigators monitored the BIS index in 907 patients undergoing general anesthesia for major elective surgery (excluding cardiac and intracranial procedures) lasting at least 2 hours. The anesthetic technique was not controlled, and the anesthesiologist was blind to the BIS values. The percentage of time that the BIS index was less than 40, between 40 and 60, or greater than 60 was measured during the maintenance phase of the anesthetic. The authors examined the incidence of death at 1 year in the group. Mortality was significantly higher if the BIS index was less than 40 in patients older than 40 years. Increasing age and lower BIS values were both independently associated with higher mortality rates. Lennmarken and colleagues[184] confirmed these finding with a retrospective analysis of a previously published study examining the incidence of awareness using BIS monitoring. The authors found in the cohort of 5077 consecutive subjects monitored with the BIS index that a low BIS value increased the risk of 1-year mortality. Monk and coworkers examined 1-year postoperative mortality in a large Medicare hospital database linking hospitals that used BIS monitoring.[185] This retrospective analysis also suggested that hospitals that routinely use BIS monitoring have decreased 1-year postoperative mortality.

Clinical Use of the Bispectral Index

The previously described development of the BIS index and its application to patient care monitoring represent the first scientifically validated and commercially supported monitor of anesthetic drug effect on the CNS. The BIS index primarily measures the effects of hypnotics on the EEG. The synergistic interaction of opioids with volatile or intravenous hypnotics on clinical end points (hemodynamics, movement responses) is more profound than reflected by the EEG. As a result, the BIS index is most accurate when used with anesthetics consisting of a low or moderate dose of opioid analgesic and a hypnotic drug (volatile inhaled anesthetic, intravenous anesthetic) titrated to the BIS response. Low opioid doses enable the BIS index to accurately reflect the pharmacodynamics of the hypnotic drugs on the CNS. High-dose opioids yield significant synergy with the hypnotic drugs, as demonstrated by Glass and colleagues,[114,115] such that minimal amounts of hypnotic drug are required to obtain adequate anesthesia. Because the reduced hypnotic dose in high-dose opioid techniques results in less profound hypnotic EEG drug effect, the BIS response is less reliable with a high-dose opioid technique.

Clinical use of BIS monitoring involves separating the hypnotic and analgesic components of an anesthetic regimen. The concept entails titration of the hypnotic drug (e.g., isoflurane, desflurane, sevoflurane, propofol, midazolam) to lower the BIS value to 40 to 60 (see Fig. 31-21). This range appears to be the therapeutic window associated with a high probability of unconsciousness. A small to moderate amount of analgesic drug (opioid) is also given with the hypnotic drug. The anesthesiologist then evaluates the clinical and BIS responses to the surgical procedure over time. During times of intense surgical stimulation, if the BIS index increases and the patient exhibits movement and hemodynamic responses, the anesthesiologist should respond by increasing the hypnotic component to lower the BIS value to the 40 to 60 range. If the BIS value is in the 40 to 60 range and movement and hemodynamic responses continue, incremental opioid should be added to increase the analgesic component of the anesthetic until movement and hemodynamics are controlled. As the end of the anesthetic regimen approaches, the hypnotic component should be decreased to allow the BIS index to increase.

BIS monitoring provides an important new dimension to the ability to adjust the components of an anesthetic in a logical manner. Figure 31-23 presents a tabular summary of the algorithm that will allow maximal utility of the BIS index during anesthesia.

Other Measures of Anesthetic Depth

Evoked Responses

Sensory or nerve stimulation produces a low-amplitude signal, or evoked response, within the CNS. This evoked response can be separated by means of special computer signal–averaging techniques from the underlying, spontaneous EEG. The ability to evoke a response is a measure of the functional integrity of the sensory receptors and the pathways between the sensory receptor and neural generator of peaks in the evoked response waveform. Evoked responses are used primarily to monitor the functional integrity of the neural structures, to identify neural structures, and to diagnose neurophysiologic conditions. Because evoked responses are sensitive to anesthetic drugs, they have been investigated as possible measures of anesthetic drug effect and depth of anesthesia.[139] The sensory stimulation most commonly used in recording of evoked responses is somatosensory (electrical) stimulation of peripheral nerves, auditory stimulation using clicks at the auditory canal, visual stimulation using flashing lights, or electrical stimulation of tooth pulp.

Recording of evoked responses involves recording EEG epochs synchronized to the repetitive sensory stimuli.

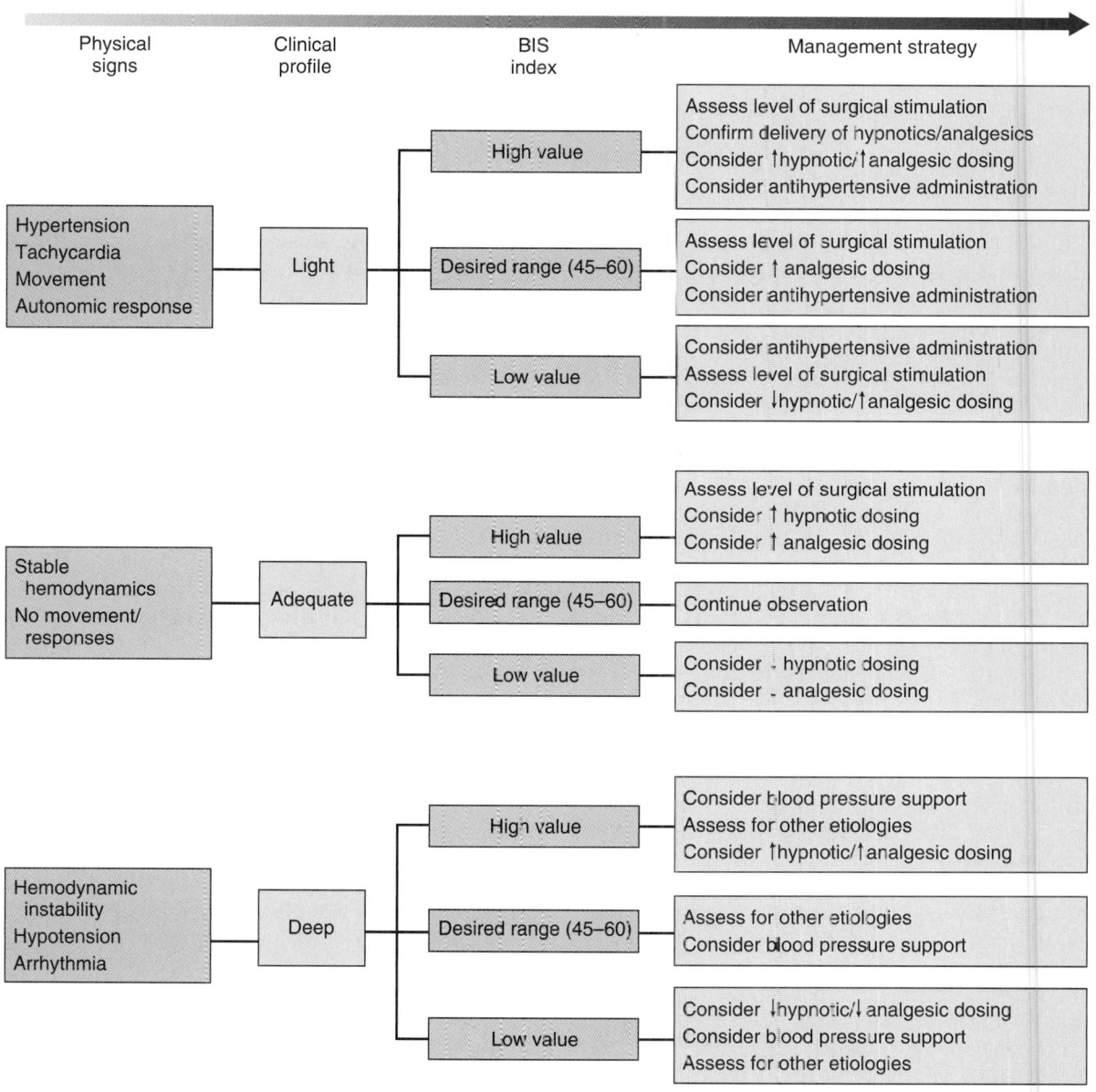

Figure 31-23 Strategy for titrating hypnotic and opioid based on integration of the bispectral (BIS) index value with observed clinical response. (Redrawn from Kelley SD: Monitoring Level of Consciousness during Anesthesia and Sedation. Natick, MA, Aspect Medical Systems, 2003.)

Computer techniques for processing EEG signals extract the evoked potential from the underlying EEG. Typically, the algorithm requires 100 to 1000 stimuli to extract the evoked potential from the underlying EEG signal. Therefore, the evoked response represents a time-versus-voltage relationship that can be quantitated by measuring the poststimulus latency and interpeak amplitudes in the waveform. Evoked response methodology has been reviewed by Grundy.[186,187]

Many investigations have been performed with evoked potentials, with special emphasis on midlatency auditory evoked potentials (MLAEPs).[188-195] MLAEPs have been shown to be significantly affected by anesthetic hypnotic drugs in a graded, reversible, and nonspecific manner. Specifically, the amplitudes (microvolts) and the latency (milliseconds) of the waves Pa and Nb have been examined. Hypnotic anesthetic drugs decrease the amplitudes and increase the latencies of these two waves. Opioids in clinically relevant concentrations produce minimal changes in MLAEPs.[196]

Iselin-Chaves and colleagues[197] compared the MLAEP and BIS index in volunteers receiving stepped increases in propofol concentrations or propofol and alfentanil while recording clinical sedation scores. They found that both the BIS and MLAEP patterns showed significant changes with increasing levels of sedation, with the Pa and Nb waves decreasing in amplitude and increasing in latency. The BIS index correlated better with clinical sedation scores relative to the MLAEPs; however, MLAEPs showed the best correlation with plasma drug concentrations. The addition of 100 ng/mL alfentanil did not affect the relationship between MLAEP and loss of consciousness.

MLAEPs have inconveniences that to date have limited their clinical use.[197] These limitations include (1) considerable time needed to produce a response, 0.5 to 5 minutes; (2) complex setup, with MLAEPs typically requiring more than 5 minutes of patient preparation; (3) need for intact hearing; and (4) lack of a univariate parameter calibrated to the anesthetic state. Mantzaridis and Kenny addressed some of these limitations by introducing a new MLAEP parameter, the auditory evoked potential (AEP) index, based on a proprietary algorithm.[198] The AEP simplifies interpretation of the MLAEP waveforms, but it still requires significant time for the signal-averaging process. Jensen and coworkers developed a new adaptive method for extracting the MLAEP from the EEG signal that involves an autoregressive model with an exogenous input (ARX) to allow extraction of the AEP signal within 15 to 25 sweeps of 110-msec duration; the process results in only a 6-second delay.[199] This concept has been incorporated into a commercially available device that calculates the A-Line ARX Index (AAI) from the fast-extracted MLAEP waveform analysis (A-Line Monitor, Danmeter A/S, Odense, Denmark). The AAI, like the BIS index, ranges from 100 (awake) to 0 (deep hypnotic effect). This variable represents the only commercially available device analogous to the BIS monitor, but it uses AEPs. Struys and colleagues[200] compared this autoregressive modeling with exogenous input of MLAEPs to the BIS index in patients receiving propofol. Target effect-site concentrations were achieved and progressively increased in steps with clinical measurement of the level of sedation (OAA/S scores) and defined noxious stimuli. Both the BIS index and the AAI were accurate indicators of the level of sedation and loss of consciousness. With clinical stimuli, greater variability was seen with the AAI than with the BIS index. The BIS index correlated best with propofol effect-site concentrations. Neither methodology predicted reaction to noxious stimuli. Hemodynamic variables were poor indicators of the hypnotic state.

One recent study compared the AAI with the BIS index in surgical patients undergoing transitions from wakefulness to unconsciousness.[201] The authors concluded that the BIS index and AAI were superior to hemodynamic variables and classic single-parameter EEG variables (i.e., median frequency). The BIS index provided better discrimination between unconscious and awake states than the AAI index did.

SUMMARY

Horace Well's demonstration of nitrous oxide at Massachusetts General Hospital in 1846 was declared a "humbug" because an inadequate nitrous oxide dose failed to fully blunt the patient's perception of pain from a dental extraction. Ever since, anesthesiologists have struggled with varying definitions of this triad—stimulus, response, and anesthetic drug—in an effort to find a common definition of anesthetic depth. The definition of "depth of anesthesia" has constantly changed over the past 160 years as the drugs used to administer anesthesia evolved and the fundamental knowledge of anesthetic drug effects increased.

In this edition of *Anesthesia* we have defined anesthetic depth as the probability of nonresponse to stimulation, calibrated against the strength of the stimulus, the difficulty of suppressing the response, and the drug-induced probability of nonresponsiveness at defined drug effect-site concentrations. This definition requires that multiple different stimuli and responses be measured at well-defined drug concentrations. No specific individual stimulus and response measurement will capture depth of anesthesia in a clinically or scientifically meaningful manner. Thus, the anesthesiologist must understand a complex matrix of stimuli, responses, and anesthetic drugs, including their pharmacodynamic (and generally synergistic) interactions. This definition captures the nature of current routine clinical care whereby anesthesiologists observe a series of stimuli from talking to the patient preoperatively to skin incision to intubation. They also observe a range of responses ranging from verbal response to movement to tachycardia and hypertension, and they calibrate these observations of stimuli and responses against the anesthetic drugs used to reduce the probability of response by constantly adjusting the administered dose to achieve the desired anesthetic depth.

In our definition of "depth of anesthesia" we define the need for two components to induce the anesthetic state: hypnosis created with drugs such as propofol or the inhaled anesthetics and analgesia created with the opioids or nitrous oxide. We demonstrate the scientific evidence that profound degrees of hypnosis in the absence of analgesia will not prevent the hemodynamic responses to profoundly noxious stimuli. In addition, profound degrees of analgesia do not guarantee unconsciousness. However, the combination of hypnosis and analgesia suppresses the hemodynamic response to noxious stimuli and guarantees unconsciousness. The synergy between hypnotics and analgesics is used every day by every anesthesiologist in clinical practice. We also demonstrate that this concept can be captured with a three-dimensional interaction surface (hypnotic concentration on the y axis, analgesic concentration on the x axis, probability of nonresponsiveness to defined stimuli on the z axis) that can be accurately estimated with available clinical data for currently used anesthetic drugs.

The BIS index is presently the most extensively validated measure of "depth of anesthesia." This monitor correlates well with the effects of hypnotics (particularly propofol, thiopental, and inhaled anesthetic gases) on memory, sedation, and consciousness. The BIS index does not measure the intrinsic brain state. It measures hypnotic drug effect. Nevertheless, titration guided by the BIS index appears to decrease the incidence of intraoperative awareness, currently estimated at 0.2% in healthy patients undergoing general anesthesia. An electrophysiologic measure of analgesia parallel to the BIS index and hypnotic assessment is not currently available.

There is considerable room for the development of additional technology and pharmacologic insight into measures of the depth of anesthesia. The opioid/hypnotic concentration–versus–response surface relationship has not been characterized for many stimulus-response pairs. There are many additional drug interactions that might be profitably characterized (e.g., opioids versus α_2-adrenergic agonists), as well as higher-dimensional drug interactions (e.g., three-drug interaction surfaces[28]). There are cells in the stimulus-response matrix for which only poor EEG predictors (e.g., movement with opioid/nitrous oxide anesthesia, ketamine) are available. Certain important responses are poorly understood (e.g., inflammatory, humeral, neurophysiologic, and psychological responses). Our definition of anesthetic depth and measurement of anesthetic depth will expand as the matrix of stimuli, responses, and the drugs that influence the probability of nonresponse expands with new research and new knowledge.

KEY POINTS

1. The definition of "depth of anesthesia" has constantly evolved since the first demonstration of clinical anesthesia in the 1840s. The changing definitions have revolved around the available drugs used to provide anesthesia and the body of knowledge on their effects in humans.

2. Anesthesia is not a single pharmacologic process. It is a complex interaction of multiple stimuli, diverse responses, and the drug-induced probability of nonresponsiveness to the stimuli.

3. Anesthesia can be defined by its hypnotic (unconsciousness) and analgesic (pain relief) components. The hypnotic component can be induced by intravenous and inhaled anesthetics, whereas the analgesic component can be induced by opioids and local anesthetics. Some drugs, such as ether, nitrous oxide, and ketamine, provide both hypnotic and analgesic components to some degree.

4. Hypnotics, when given alone, will allow significant hemodynamic response to intense noxious stimuli. Opioids, when given alone, do not guarantee consistent unconsciousness or lack of movement response to intense noxious stimuli. A combination of the two can result in predictable unconsciousness and lack of hemodynamic response to intense noxious stimuli.

5. The interaction of the hypnotic and analgesic components can be characterized by a three-dimensional surface with hypnotic concentration on the y axis, analgesic concentration on the x axis, and probability of nonresponse on the z axis.

6. Characterization of the three-dimensional surface requires precise stimuli to be applied and specific responses to be measured at defined effect-site concentrations of the hypnotic and analgesic.

7. The specific stimuli-response pairs used to define anesthetic depth range from easily suppressed responses to mild stimulation, such as the verbal response to a verbal command, to difficult-to-suppress responses to intense stimuli, such as the hemodynamic response to intubation.

8. The interaction of hypnotics and analgesics is generally synergistic.

9. Current clinical anesthesia involves the physician carefully observing the clinical response to defined stimuli and then adjusting the hypnotic or analgesic dosage, or both, by using their synergistic interaction to achieve the clinical goals of hemodynamic control, lack of awareness, and rapid, safe induction and emergence.

10. The hypnotic effects of the intravenous and inhaled anesthetics can be measured with the bispectral index, an empirically derived EEG measure that has extensive clinical calibration.

11. The bispectral index is an empirically derived measure of hypnotic drug effect, including hypnotic-induced sedation, amnesia, loss of consciousness, and reduced cerebral metabolic rate.

12. A consequence of inadequate anesthetic depth is intraoperative awareness. The incidence of awareness in healthy patients is approximately 0.2% and can increase to 1.0% to 1.5% in higher-risk patient populations. Emerging evidence is indicating that intraoperative monitoring of the hypnotic component of an anesthetic can significantly decrease the risk of awareness.

REFERENCES

1. White DC: Anaesthesia: A privation of the senses. An historical introduction and some definitions. *In* Rosen M, Lunn JN (eds): Consciousness, Awareness, and Pain in General Anaesthesia. London, Butterworths, 1987, p 1.
2. Plomley F: Operations upon the eye [letter]. Lancet 1:134, 1847.
3. Snow J: On the Inhalation of the Vapors of Ether in Surgical Operations: Containing a Description of the Various Stages of Etherization, and a Statement of the Result of Nearly Eighty Operations in Which Ether Has Been Employed in St. George's and University College Hospitals. London, John Churchill, 1847. Reproduced by Lea & Febiger, Philadelphia, 1959.
4. Snow J: On Chloroform and Other Anesthetics. London, John Churchill, 1858.
5. Gillespie NA: The signs of anaesthesia. Anesth Analg 22:275, 1943.
6. Guedel AE: Inhalational Anesthesia: A Fundamental Guide. New York, Macmillan, 1937.
7. Artusio JF Jr: Di-ethyl ether analgesia: A detailed description of the first stage of ether analgesia in man. J Pharmacol Exp Ther 111:343, 1954.
8. Tomas DW, Runciman WB: Monitoring depth of anesthesia. Anaesth Intensive Care 16:69, 1988.
9. Curare in anaesthesia [editorial]. Lancet 2:81, 1945.
10. Winterbottom EH: Insufficient anaesthesia [letter]. BMJ 1:247, 1950.
11. Woodbridge PD: Changing concepts concerning depth of anesthesia. Anesthesiology 18:536, 1957.
12. Prys-Roberts C: Anaesthesia: A practical or impossible construct [editorial]? Br J Anaesth 59:1341, 1987.
13. Eger EL II, Saidman LJ, Brandstater B: Minimum alveolar anesthetic concentration: A standard of anesthetic potency. Anesthesiology 26:756, 1965.
14. Kissin I: General anesthetic action: An obsolete notion? Anesth Analg 76:215, 1993.
15. Glass PS: Anesthetic drug interactions: An insight into general anesthesia—its mechanism and dosing strategies. Anesthesiology 88:5-6, 1998.
16. Bencherif B, Fuchs PN, Sheth R, et al: Pain activation of human supraspinal opioid pathways as demonstrated by [^{11}C]-carfentanil and positron emission tomography (PET). Pain 99:589-598, 2002.
17. Fukuhara N, Ishikawa T, Kinoshita H, et al: Central noradrenergic mediation of nitrous oxide–induced analgesia in rats. Can J Anaesth 45:1123-1129, 1998.
18. Quock RM, Best JA, Chen DC, et al: Mediation of nitrous oxide analgesia in mice by spinal and supraspinal kappa-opioid receptors. Eur J Pharmacol 175:97-100, 1990.
19. Fang F, Guo TZ, Davies MF, Maze M: Opiate receptors in the periaqueductal gray mediate analgesic effect of nitrous oxide in rats. Eur J Pharmacol 336:137-141, 1997.
20. Egan TD, Muir KT, Hermann DJ, et al: The electroencephalogram (EEG) and clinical measure of opioid potency: Defining the EEG–clinical potency relationship ("fingerprint") with application to remifentanil. Int J Pharm Med 15:1-9, 2001.
21. Wynands JE, Wong P, Townsend GE, et al: Narcotic requirements for intravenous anesthesia. Anesth Analg 63:101, 1984.
22. Sebel PS, Glass PS, Fletcher JE, et al: Reduction of the MAC of desflurane with fentanyl. Anesthesiology 76:52-59, 1992.
23. McEwan AI, Smith C, Dyar O, et al: Isoflurane minimum alveolar concentration reduction by fentanyl. Anesthesiology 78:864, 1993.
24. Vuyk J, Lim T, Engbers FHM, et al: The pharmacodynamic interaction of propofol and alfentanil during lower abdominal surgery in women. Anesthesiology 83:8, 1995.
25. Smith C, McEwan AI, Jhaveri R, et al: The interaction of fentanyl on the Cp_{50} of propofol for loss of consciousness and skin incision. Anesthesiology 81:820-828, 1994.
26. Kazama T, Ikeda K, Morita K: Reduction by fentanyl of the Cp_{50} values of propofol and hemodynamic responses to various noxious stimuli. Anesthesiology 87:213, 1997.
27. Kazama T, Ikeda K, Morita K, et al: Propofol concentration required for endotracheal intubation with a laryngoscope or fiberscope and its interaction with fentanyl. Anesth Analg 86:872-879, 1998.
28. Minto CF, Schnider TW, Short TG, et al: Response surface model for anesthetic drug interactions. Anesthesiology 92:1603-1816, 2000.
29. Rampil IJ, Mason P, Singh H: Anesthetic potency (MAC) is independent of forebrain structures in the rat. Anesthesiology 78:707, 1993.
30. Rampil IJ: Anesthetic potency is not altered after hypothermic spinal cord transactions in rats. Anesthesiology 80:606, 1994.
31. Antognini JF, Schwartz K: Exaggerated anesthetic requirements in the preferentially anesthetized brain. Anesthesiology 79:1244, 1993.
32. Fields HL, Anderson SD: Evidence that raphe-spinal neurons mediate opiate and midbrain stimulation-produced analgesias. Pain 5:333-349, 1978.
33. Kazama T, Ikeda K, Morita K: The pharmacodynamic interaction between propofol and fentanyl with respect to the suppression of somatic or hemodynamic responses to skin incision, peritoneum incision, and abdominal wall retraction. Anesthesiology 89:894-906, 1998.
34. Stoelting RK, Longnecker DE, Eger EI II: Minimum alveolar concentrations in man on awakening from methoxyflurane, halothane, ether and fluroxene anesthesia: MAC awake. Anesthesiology 33:5-9, 1970.
35. Eger EI II: Age, minimum alveolar anesthetic concentration, and minimum alveolar anesthetic concentration-awake. Anesth Analg 93:947-953, 2001.
36. Roizen MF, Horrigan RW, Frazer BM: Anesthetic doses blocking adrenergic (stress) and cardiovascular responses to incision—MAC BAR. Anesthesiology 54:390-398, 1981.
37. Daniel M, Weiskopf RB, Noorani M, Eger EI II: Fentanyl augments the blockade of the sympathetic response to incision (MAC-BAR) produced by desflurane and isoflurane: Desflurane and isoflurane MAC-BAR without and with fentanyl. Anesthesiology 88:43-49, 1998.
38. Hornbein TF, Eger EI II, Winter PM, et al: The minimum alveolar concentration of nitrous oxide in man. Anesth Analg 61:553-556, 1982.
39. Ausems ME, Hug CC Jr, Stanski DR, et al: Plasma concentrations of alfentanil required to supplement nitrous oxide anesthesia for general surgery. Anesthesiology 65:362, 1986.
40. Ghouri AF, White PF: Effect of fentanyl and nitrous oxide on the desflurane anesthetic requirement. Anesth Analg 72:377-381, 1991.
41. Rampil IJ, Lockhart SH, Zwass MS, et al: Clinical characteristics of desflurane in surgical patients: Minimum alveolar concentration. Anesthesiology 74:429-433, 1991.
42. Stuart PC, Stott SM, Millar A, et al: Cp_{50} of propofol with and without nitrous oxide 67%. Br J Anaesth 84:638-639, 2000.
43. Ichinohe T, Aida H, Kaneko Y: Interaction of nitrous oxide and propofol to reduce hypertensive response to stimulation. Can J Anaesth 47:699-704, 2000.
44. Robertson HR: Without benefit of anesthesia: George Wilson's amputation and Fanny Burney's mastectomy. Ann R Coll Physicians Surg Can 22:27, 1989.
45. Vickers MD: Detecting consciousness by clinical means. *In* Rosen M, Lund NJ (eds): Consciousness, Awareness, and Pain in General Anesthesia. London, Butterworths, 1987, p 12.
46. Schacter DL: Implicit knowledge: New perspectives on unconscious processes. Proc Natl Acad Sci U S A 89:11113, 1992.
47. Bogetz MS, Katz JA: Recall of surgery for major trauma. Anesthesiology 61:6, 1984.
48. Lubke GH, Kerssens C, Phaf H, et al: Dependence of explicit and implicit memory on hypnotic state in trauma patients. Anesthesiology 90:670, 1999.
49. Sandin RH, Enlund G, Samuelsson P, et al: Awareness during anaesthesia: A prospective case study. Lancet 355:707, 2000.
50. Ghoneim MM: Awareness during anesthesia. Anesthesiology 92:597, 2000.

51. Mark JB, Greenberg LM: Intraoperative awareness and hypertensive crisis during high-dose fentanyl-diazepam-oxygen anesthesia. Anesth Analg 62:698, 1983.

52. Mummaneni N, Rao TLK, Montoya A: Awareness and recall with high-dose fentanyl-oxygen anesthesia. Anesth Analg 59:948, 1980.

53. Hilgenberg JC: Intraoperative awareness during high dose fentanyl-oxygen anaesthesia. Anesthesiology 54:341, 1981.

54. Tunstall ME: Detecting wakefulness during general anaesthesia for caesarean section. BMJ 1:1321, 1977.

55. Tunstall ME: The reduction of amnesic wakefulness during caesarean section. Anaesthesia 34:316, 1979.

56. Schultetus RR, Hill CR, Dharmaraj CM, et al: Wakefulness during cesarean section after anesthetic induction with ketamine, thiopental, or ketamine and thiopental combined. Anesth Analg 65:723, 1986.

57. Russell IF: Balanced anesthesia: Does it anesthetize [letter]? Anesth Analg 64:941, 1985.

58. Russell IF: Comparison of wakefulness with two anaesthetic regimens: Total I.V. balanced anaesthesia. Br J Anaesth 58:965, 1986.

59. Breckenridge J, Aitkenhead AR: Isolated forearm technique for detection of wakefulness during general anaesthesia [abstract]. Br J Anaesth 53:665P, 1981.

60. Bogod DG, Orton JK, Yau HM, et al: Detecting awareness during general anesthetic caesarean section: An evaluation of two methods. Anaesthesia 45:279, 1990.

61. Russell IF: Midazolam-alfentanil: An anesthetic? An investigation using the isolated forearm technique. Br J Anaesth 70:42, 1993.

62. Abouleish E, Taylor FH: Effect of morphine-diazepam on signs of anesthesia, awareness, and dreams of patients under NO for cesarean section. Anesth Analg 55:702, 1976.

63. Levinson BW: States of awareness during general anaesthesia: Preliminary communication. Br J Anaesth 37:544, 1965.

64. Blacher RS: Awareness during surgery [editorial]. Anesthesiology 61:1, 1984.

65. Bennett HL, Davis HS, Giannini JA: Non-verbal response to intraoperative conversation. Br J Anaesth 57:174, 1985.

66. Block RI, Ghoneim MM, Sum Ping ST, et al: Human learning during general anesthesia and surgery. Br J Anaesth 66:170, 1991.

67. McLintock TT, Aitken H, Downie CF, et al: Postoperative analgesic requirements in patients exposed to positive intraoperative suggestions. BMJ 301:788, 1990.

68. Woo R, Seltzer JL, Marr A: The lack of response to suggestion under controlled surgical anesthesia. Acta Anaesthesiol Scand 31:567, 1987.

69. Eich E, Reeves JL, Katz RL: Anesthesia, amnesia, and memory/awareness distinction. Anesth Analg 64:1143, 1985.

70. Block RI, Ghoneim MM, Sum Ping ST, et al: Efficacy of therapeutic suggestions for improved postoperative recovery presented during general anesthesia. Anesthesiology 75:746, 1991.

71. Dwyer R, Bennett HL, Eger EI, et al: Effects of isoflurane and nitrous oxide in subanesthetic concentrations on memory and responsiveness in volunteers. Anesthesiology 77:888, 1992.

72. Veselis RA, Reinsel RA, Feschenko VA, et al: The comparative amnestic effects of midazolam, propofol, thiopental and fentanyl at equisedative concentrations. Anesthesiology 87:49, 1997.

73. Pandit SK, Heisterkamp DV, Cohen PJ: Further studies on the anti-recall effect of lorazepam: A dose-time-effect relationship. Anesthesiology 45:495, 1976.

74. Blacher RS: On awakening paralyzed during surgery: A syndrome of traumatic neurosis. JAMA 234:67, 1975.

75. Ghoneim MM, Block RI: Learning and memory during general anesthesia, an update. Anesthesiology 87:387, 1997.

76. Lennmarken C, Bildfors K, Enlund G, et al: Victims of awareness. Acta Anaesthesiol Scand 46:229, 2002.

77. Ghoneim MM: Implicit memory for events during anesthesia. In Ghoneim MM (ed): Awareness during Anesthesia. Oxford, Butterworth-Heineman, 2001.

78. Merkel G, Eger EI II: A comparative study of halothane and halopropane anesthesia: Including the method for determining equipotency. Anesthesiology 24:346, 1963.

79. Quasha AL, Eger EI II, Tinker JH: Determination and applications of MAC. Anesthesiology 53:315, 1980.

80. Cullen DJ: Drugs and anesthetic depth. In Smith NT, Miller RD, Corbascio AN (eds): Drug Interactions in Anesthesia. Philadelphia, Lea & Febiger, 1981, p 287.

81. Stoelting RK, Longnecker DE, Eger EI II: Minimum alveolar concentrations in man on awakening from methoxyflurane, halothane, ether and fluroxene anesthesia: MAC awake. Anesthesiology 33:5, 1970.

82. Yakaitis RW, Blitt CD, Angiulo JP: End-tidal halothane concentration for endotracheal intubation. Anesthesiology 47:386, 1977.

83. Roizen MF, Horrigan RW, Frazer BM: Anesthetic doses blocking adrenergic (stress) and cardiovascular responses to incision: MAC BAR. Anesthesiology 54:390, 1981.

84. Zbinden AM, Maggiorini M, Petersen-Felix S, et al: Anesthetic depth defined using multiple noxious stimuli during isoflurane/oxygen anesthesia. I. Motor reactions. Anesthesiology 80:253, 1994.

85. Eger EI II, Bahlman SH: Is the end-tidal anesthetic partial pressure an accurate measure of the arterial anesthetic partial pressure? Anesthesiology 35:301, 1971.

86. Saidman LJ, Eger EI II: Effect of nitrous oxide and of narcotic premedication on the alveolar concentration of halothane required for anesthesia. Anesthesiology 25:302, 1964.

87. de Jong RH, Eger EI II: MAC expanded: AD_{50} and AD_{95} values of common inhalation anesthetics in man. Anesthesiology 42:384, 1975.

88. Waud DR: On biological assays involving quantal responses. J Pharmacol Exp Ther 183:577, 1972.

89. Torri G, Damia G, Fabiani ML: Effect of nitrous oxide on the anaesthetic requirement of enflurane. Br J Anaesth 46:468, 1974.

90. Eger EI, Koblin D, Harris RA, et al. Hypothesis: Inhaled anesthetics produce immobility and amnesia by different mechanisms at different sites. Anesth Analg 84:915, 1997.

91. Cullen DJ, Eger EI II, Stevens WC, et al: Clinical signs of anesthesia. Anesthesiology 36:21, 1972.

92. Zbinden AM, Petersen-Felix S, Thomson DA: Anesthetic depth defined using multiple noxious stimuli during isoflurane/oxygen anesthesia. II. Hemodynamic responses. Anesthesiology 80:261, 1994.

93. King BD, Harris LC Jr, Greifenstein FE, et al: Reflex circulatory responses to direct laryngoscopy and tracheal intubation performed during general anesthesia. Anesthesiology 12:556, 1951.

94. Stoelting RK: Circulatory changes during direct laryngoscopy and tracheal intubation: Influence of duration of laryngoscopy with or without prior lidocaine. Anesthesiology 47:381, 1977.

95. Brett CM, Fisher DM: Thiopental dose-response relations in unpremedicated infants, children, and adults. Anesth Analg 66:1024, 1987.

96. Avram MJ, Sanghvi R, Henthorn TK, et al: Determinants of thiopental induction dose requirements. Anesth Analg 76:10, 1993.

97. Jacobs JR, Reves JG: Effect site equilibration time is a determinant of induction dose requirement. Anesth Analg 76:1, 1993.

98. Becker KE Jr: Plasma levels of thiopental necessary for anesthesia. Anesthesiology 49:192, 1978.

99. Hung OR, Varvel JR, Shafer SL, et al: Thiopental pharmacodynamics. II. Quantitation of clinical and electroencephalographic depth of anesthesia. Anesthesiology 77:237, 1992.

100. Vuyk J, Lim T, Engbers FHM, et al: Pharmacodynamics of alfentanil as a supplement to propofol or nitrous oxide for lower abdominal surgery in female patients. Anesthesiology 78:1036, 1993.

101. Stanski DR, Shafer SL: Quantifying anesthetic drug interaction: Implications for drug dosing. Anesthesiology 83:1, 1995.

102. Tammisto T, Aromaa U, Korttila K: The role of thiopental and fentanyl in the production of balanced anaesthesia. Acta Anaesthesiol Scand 24:31, 1980.

103. Neff W, Mayer EC, de la Luz Percales M: Nitrous oxide and oxygen anesthesia with curare relaxation. Calif Med 66:67, 1947.

104. Lowenstein E, Hallowell P, Levine FH, et al: Cardiovascular response to large doses of intravenous morphine in man. N Engl J Med 281:1389, 1969.

105. Stanley TH, Webster LR: Anesthetic requirements and cardiovascular effects of fentanyl-oxygen and fentanyl-diazepam-oxygen anesthesia in man. Anesth Analg 57:411, 1978.

106. Waller JL, Hug CC Jr, Nagle DM, et al: Hemodynamic changes during fentanyl-oxygen anesthesia for aortocoronary bypass operation. Anesthesiology 55:212, 1981.

107. Hynynen M, Takkunen O, Salmenpera M, et al: Continuous infusion of fentanyl or alfentanil for coronary artery surgery: Plasma opiate concentrations, haemodynamics and postoperative course. Br J Anaesth 58:1252, 1986.

108. Philbin DM, Rosow CE, Schneider RC, et al: Fentanyl and sufentanil anesthesia revisited: How much is enough? Anesthesiology 73:5, 1990.

109. Thompson IR, Henderson BT, Singh K, et al: Concentration-response relationships for fentanyl and sufentanil in patients undergoing coronary artery bypass grafting. Anesthesiology 89:852, 1998.

110. Murphy MR, Hug CC Jr: The anesthetic potency of fentanyl in terms of its reduction of enflurane MAC. Anesthesiology 57:485, 1982.

111. Hall RI, Murphy MR, Hug CC Jr: The enflurane sparing effect of sufentanil in dogs. Anesthesiology 67:518, 1987.

112. Hall RI, Szlam F, Hug CC Jr: The enflurane-sparing effect of alfentanil in dogs. Anesth Analg 66:1287, 1987.

113. Murphy MR, Hug CC Jr: The enflurane sparing effect of morphine, butorphanol, and nalbuphine. Anesthesiology 57:489, 1982.

114. Glass PSA: Anesthetic drug interactions: An insight into general anesthesia—its mechanisms and dosing strategies. Anesthesiology 88:5, 1998.

115. Glass PSA, Gan TJ, Howell S, et al: Drug interactions: Volatile anesthetics and opiates. J Clin Anesth 9:18S, 1997.

116. Katoh T, Kobayashi S, Suzuke A, et al: The effect of fentanyl on sevoflurane requirements for somatic and sympathetic responses to surgical incision. Anesthesiology 90:398, 1999.

117. Katoh T, Ikeda K: The effect of fentanyl on sevoflurane requirements for loss of consciousness and skin incision. Anesthesiology 88:18, 1998.

118. Ausems ME, Vuyk J, Hug CC Jr, et al: Comparison of computer-assisted infusion versus intermittent bolus administration of alfentanil as a supplement to nitrous oxide for lower abdominal surgery. Anesthesiology 68:851, 1988.

119. Lemmens HJM, Bovill JG, Hennis PJ, et al: Alcohol consumption alters the pharmacodynamics of alfentanil. Anesthesiology 71:669, 1989.

120. Lemmens HJM, Burm AGL, Bovill JG, et al: Pharmacodynamics of alfentanil: The role of protein binding. Anesthesiology 76:65, 1992.

121. Egan TD, Minto CF, Hermann DJ, et al: Remifentanil vs alfentanil, comparative pharmacokinetics and pharmacodynamics in healthy adult male volunteers. Anesthesiology 84:821, 1996.

122. Minto CF, Schnider TW, Egan TD, et al: Influence of age and gender on the pharmacokinetics and pharmacodynamics of remifentanil. I. Model development. Anesthesiology 86:10, 1997.

123. Minto CF, Schnider TW, Shafer SL: Pharmacokinetics and pharmacodynamics of remifentanil. II. Model development. Anesthesiology 86:24, 1997.

124. Drover DR, Lemmens HJM: Population pharmacodynamics and pharmacokinetics of remifentanil as a supplement to nitrous oxide anesthesia for elective abdominal surgery. Anesthesiology 89:869, 1998.

125. Scott JC, Ponganis KV, Stanski DR: EEG quantitation of narcotic effect: The comparative pharmacodynamics of fentanyl and alfentanil. Anesthesiology 62:234, 1985.

126. Glass PS, Doherty M, Jacobs JR, et al: Plasma concentration of fentanyl, with 70% nitrous oxide, to prevent movement at skin incision. Anesthesiology 78:842, 1993.

127. Brazier MAB: The effect of drugs on the electroencephalogram of man. Clin Pharmacol Ther 5:102, 1964.

128. Caton R: The electrical currents of the brain [abstract]. BMJ 2:278, 1875.

129. Berger H: Uber das Elektrenkaphalogramm des Menschen. Arch Psychiatry 101:452, 1933.

130. Gibbs FA, Gibbs EL, Lennox WG: Effect on the electroencephalogram of certain drugs which influence nervous activity. Arch Intern Med 60:154, 1937.

131. Faulconer A Jr: Correlation of concentrations of ether in arterial blood with electro-encephalographic patterns occurring during ether-oxygen and during nitrous oxide, oxygen and ether anesthesia of human surgical patients. Anesthesiology 13:361, 1952.

132. Kuramoto T, Oshita S, Takeshita H, et al: Modification of the relationship between cerebral metabolism, blood flow, and electroencephalogram by stimulation during anesthesia in the dog. Anesthesiology 51:211, 1979.

133. Levy WJ, Shapiro HM, Maruchak G, et al: Automated EEG processing for intraoperative monitoring: A comparison of techniques. Anesthesiology 53:223, 1980.

134. Gregory TK, Pettus DC: An electroencephalographic processing algorithm specifically intended for analysis of cerebral electrical activity. J Clin Monit 2:190, 1986.

135. Rampil IJ: What every neuroanesthesiologist should know about electroencephalograms and computerized monitors. Anesthesiol Clin North Am 10:683, 1992.

136. Prior PF: The EEG and detection of responsiveness during anaesthesia and coma. In Rosen M, Lunn JN (eds): Consciousness, Awareness, and Pain in General Anaesthesia. London, Butterworths, 1987, p 34.

137. Bimar J, Bellville JW: Arousal reactions during anesthesia in man. Anesthesiology 47:449, 1977.

138. Miyauchi Y, Sakabe T, Maekawa T, et al: Responses of EEG, cerebral oxygen consumption and blood flow to peripheral nerve stimulation during thiopentone anaesthesia in the dog. Can Anaesth Soc J 32:491, 1985.

139. Clark DL, Rosner BS: Neurophysiologic effects of general anesthetics. I. The electroencephalogram and sensory evoked responses in man. Anesthesiology 38:564, 1973.

140. Galla SJ, Rocco AG, Vandam LD: Evaluation of the traditional signs and stages of anesthesia: An electroencephalographic and clinical study. Anesthesiology 19:328, 1958.

141. Levy WJ: Intraoperative EEG patterns: Implications for EEG monitoring. Anesthesiology 60:430, 1984.

142. Berezowskyj JL, McEwen JA, Anderson GB, et al: A study of anaesthesia depth by power spectral analysis of the electroencephalogram (EEG). Can Anaesth Soc J 23:1, 1976.

143. Drummond JC, Brann CA, Perkins DE, et al: A comparison of median frequency, spectral edge frequency, a frequency band power ratio, total power and dominance shift in the determination of depth of anesthesia. Acta Anaesthesiol Scand 35:693, 1991.

144. Long CW, Shah NK, Loughlin C, et al: A comparison of EEG determinants of near awakening from isoflurane and fentanyl anesthesia. Anesth Analg 69:169, 1989.

145. Dwyer RC, Rampil IJ, Eger EI, et al: The electroencephalogram does not predict depth of isoflurane anesthesia. Anesthesiology 81:403, 1994.

146. Stanski DR: Pharmacodynamic modeling of anesthetic EEG drug effects. Annu Rev Pharmacol Toxicol 32:421, 1992.

147. Gregg K, Varvel JR, Shafer SL: Application of semilinear canonical correlation to the measurement of opioid drug effect. J Pharmacokinet Biopharm 20:611, 1992.

148. Schnider TW, Minto CF, Fiset P, et al: Semilinear canonical correlation applied to the measurement of the electroencephalographic effects of midazolam and flumazenil reversal. Anesthesiology 84:510, 1996.

149. Schnider, TW, Minto CF, Shafer SL, et al: The influence of age on propofol pharmacodynamics. Anesthesiology 90:1502, 1999.

150. Gambús PL, Gregg KM, Shafer SL: Validation of the alfentanil canonical univariate parameter as a measure of opioid effect on the electroencephalogram. Anesthesiology 83:747-756, 1995.

151. Rampil IJ: A primer for EEG signal processing in anesthesia. Anesthesiology 89:980, 1998.

152. Sigl JC, Chamoun NG: An introduction to bispectral analysis for the electroencephalogram. J Clin Monit 10:392, 1994.

153. Kearse LA Jr, Manberg P, Chamoun N, et al: Bispectral analysis of the electroencephalogram correlates with patient movement to skin incision during propofol/nitrous oxide anesthesia. Anesthesiology 81:1365, 1994.

154. Vernon JM, Lang E, Sebel PS, Manberg P: Prediction of movement using bi-spectral EEG during propofol/alfentanil or isoflurane/alfentanil anesthesia. Anesth Analg 80:780, 1995.

155. Sebel PS, Lang E, Rampil IJ, et al: A multicenter study of bispectral electroencephalogram analysis for monitoring anesthetic effect. Anesth Analg 84:891, 1997.

156. Glass PS, Bloom M, Kearse L, et al: Bispectral analysis measures sedation and memory effects of propofol, midazolam, isoflurane and alfentanil in healthy volunteers. Anesthesiology 86:836, 1997.

157. Liu J, Singh H, White PF: Electroencephalogram bispectral analysis predicts the depth of midazolam-induced sedation. Anesthesiology 84:64, 1996.

158. Liu, J, Singh H, White PF: Electroencephalographic bispectral index correlates with intraoperative recall and depth of propofol-induced sedation. Anesth Analg 84:185, 1997.

159. Katoh T, Suzuki A, Ikeda K: Electroencephalographic derivatives as a tool for predicting the depth of sedation and anesthesia induced by sevoflurane. Anesthesiology 88:642, 1998.

160. Flaishon R, Windsor A, Sigl J, et al: Recovery of consciousness after thiopental or propofol: Bispectral index and the isolated forearm technique. Anesthesiology 86:613, 1997.

161. Kearse LA, Rosow C, Zaslavsky A, et al: Bispectral analysis of the electroencephalogram predicts conscious processing of information during propofol sedation and hypnosis. Anesthesiology 88:25, 1998.

162. Johansen JW, Sebel PS: Development and clinical application of electroencephalographic bispectrum monitoring. Anesthesiology 93:1336, 2000.

163. Alkire M: Quantitative EEG correlations with brain glucose metabolic rate during anesthesia in volunteers. Anesthesiology 89:323, 1998.

164. Ludbrook GL, Visco D, Lam AM: Propofol: Relation between brain concentrations, electroencephalogram, middle cerebral blood flow velocity and cerebral oxygen extraction during induction of anesthesia. Anesthesiology 97:1363, 2002.

165. Iselin-Chaves IA, Flaishon R, Sebel PS, et al: The effect of the interaction of propofol and alfentanil on recall, loss of consciousness and the bispectral index. Anesth Analg 87:949, 1998.

166. Guignard B, Menigaux C, Dupont X, et al: The effect of remifentanil on the bispectral index change and hemodynamic response after orotracheal intubation. Anesth Analg 90:161, 2000.

167. Ropcke H, Rehberg B, Koennen-Bergmann M, et al: Surgical stimulation shifts EEG concentration-response relationship with desflurane. Anesthesiology 94:390, 2001.

168. Rampil IJ, Kim JS, Lenhardt R, et al: Bispectral EEG index during nitrous oxide administration. Anesthesiology 89:671, 1998.

169. Coste C, Guignard B, Menigaux C, Chauvin M: Nitrous oxide prevents movement during orotracheal intubation without affecting BIS value. Anesth Analg 91:130, 2000.

170. Katoh T, Bito H, Sato S: Influence of age on hypnotic requirement, bispectral index, and 95% spectral edge frequency associated with sedation by sevoflurane. Anesthesiology 92:55, 2000.

171. Mathew JP, Weathersax KJ, East CJ, et al: Bispectral analysis during cardiopulmonary bypass: The effect of hypothermia on the hypnotic state. J Clin Anesth 13:301, 2001.

172. Lopez M, Ozaki M, Sessler D, et al: Mild core hyperthermia does not alter the electroencephalographic responses during epidural-enflurane anesthesia in humans. J Clin Anesth 5:425, 1993.

173. Johansen JW: Esmolol promotes electroencephalographic burst suppression during propofol/alfentanil anesthesia. Anesth Analg 93:1526, 2001.

174. Menigaux C, Guignard B, Adam F, et al: Esmolol prevents movement and attenuates the BIS response to orotracheal intubation. Br J Anaesth 89:857, 2002.

175. Hodgson PS, Liu SS: Epidural lidocaine decreases sevoflurane requirement for adequate depth of anesthesia as measured by the bispectral index monitor. Anesthesiology 94:799, 2001.

176. Morioka N, Ozaki M, Matsukawa T, et al: Ketamine causes a paradoxical increase in the bispectral index. Anesthesiology 87:A502, 1997.

177. Sakai T, Singh WD, Kudo T, et al: The effect of ketamine on clinical endpoints of hypnosis and EEG variables during propofol infusion. Acta Anaesthiol Scand 43:212, 1999.

178. Gan TJ, Glass PS, Windsor A, et al: Bispectral index monitoring allows faster emergence and improved recovery from propofol, alfentanil and nitrous oxide anesthesia. Anesthesiology 87:808, 1997.

179. Song D, Joshi GP, White PF: Titration of volatile anesthetics using bi-spectral index facilitates recovery after ambulatory anesthesia. Anesthesiology 87:842, 1997.

180. Myles PS, Leslie K, McNeil J, Chan MTV, and the B-Aware Trial Group: Bispectral index monitoring to prevent awareness during anaesthesia: The B-Aware Randomized Controlled Trial. Lancet 363:1747-1757, 2004.

181. Sebel PS, Bowdle A, Ghoneim M, et al: The incidence of awareness during anesthesia: A multicenter US study. Anesthesiology 99:A-360, 2003.

182. Lennmarken C, Ekman A, Sandin R: Incidence of awareness using BIS-monitoring. Anesth Analg 96:S133, 2003.

183. Weldon BC, Mahla ME, van der Aa M, et al: Advancing age and deeper intraoperative anesthetic levels are associated with higher first year death rates. Anesthesiology 97:A-1097, 2002.

184. Lennmarken C, Lindholm MJ, Greenwald SC, et al: Confirmation that low intraoperative BIS levels predict increased risk of post-operative mortality. Anesthesiology 99:A-303, 2003.

185. Monk T, Sigl J, Weldon BC: Intraoperative BIS utilization is associated with reduced one-year post-operative mortality. Anesthesiology 99:A-1361, 2003.

186. Grundy BL: Evoked potential monitoring. In Blitt ED (ed): Monitoring in Anesthesia and Critical Care Medicine. New York, Churchill Livingstone, 1985, p 345.

187. Grundy BL: Intraoperative monitoring of sensory-evoked potentials. Anesthesiology 58:72, 1983.

188. Thornton C, Catley DM, Jordan C, et al: Enflurane anaesthesia causes graded changes in the brainstem and early cortical auditory evoked response in man. Br J Anaesth 55:479, 1983.

189. Thornton C, Heneghan CPH, James MFM, et al: Effects of halothane or enflurane with controlled ventilation on auditory evoked potentials. Br J Anaesth 56:315, 1984.

190. Thornton C, Heneghan CPH, Navaratnarajah M, et al: Effect of etomidate on the auditory evoked response in man. Br J Anaesth 57:554, 1985.

191. Thornton C, Heneghan CPH, Navaratnarajah M, et al: Selective effect of Althesin on the auditory evoked response in man. Br J Anaesth 58:422, 1986.

192. Heneghan CPH, Thornton C, Navaratnarajah M, et al: Effect of isoflurane on the auditory evoked response in man. Br J Anaesth 59:277, 1987.

193. Thornton C, Konieczko K, Jones JG, et al: Effect of surgical stimulation on the auditory evoked response. Br J Anaesth 60:372, 1988.

194. Thornton C, Barrowcliffe MP, Konieczko KM, et al: The auditory evoked response as an indicator of awareness. Br J Anaesth 63:113, 1989.

195. Newton DEF, Thornton C, Konieczko K, et al: Auditory evoked response and awareness: A study in volunteers at sub-MAC concentrations of isoflurane. Br J Anaesth 69:122, 1992.

196. Schwender D, Rimkus T, Haessler R, et al: Effect of increasing doses of alfentanil, fentanyl and morphine on mid-latency auditory evoked potentials. Br J Anaesth 71:622, 1993.

197. Iselin-Chaves IA, Moalem HE, Gan TG, et al: Changes in the auditory evoked potentials and the bispectral index following propofol or propofol and alfentanil. Anesthesiology 92:1300, 2000.

198. Mantzaridis H, Kenny GH: Auditory evoked potential index: A quantitative measure of changes in auditory evoked potentials during general anesthesia. Anaesthesia 52:1030, 1997.

199. Jensen EW, Nygaard M, Hennenberg SW: On-line analysis of middle latency auditory evoked potentials (MLAEP) for monitoring depth of anesthesia in laboratory rats. Med Eng Phys 20:722, 1998.

200. Struys MMRF, Jensen EW, Smith W, et al: Performance of the ARX-derived auditory evoked potential index as an indicator of anesthetic depth. Anesthesiology 96:803, 2002.

201. Schmidt GN, Bischoff P, Standl T, et al: ARX-derived auditory evoked potential index and bispectral index during the induction of anesthesia with propofol and remifentanil. Anesth Analg 97:139, 2003.

CHAPTER
32 Cardiovascular Monitoring

Jonathan B. Mark and Thomas F. Slaughter

Introduction to Cardiovascular Monitoring: Extending the Physical Examination 1266
Stethoscopy 1266
Heart Rate Monitoring 1267
Pulse Rate Monitoring 1268

Arterial Blood Pressure Monitoring 1268
Indirect Measurement of Arterial Blood Pressure 1269
Direct Measurement of Arterial Blood Pressure 1272

Central Venous Pressure Monitoring 1286
Central Venous Cannulation 1286
Complications of Central Venous Pressure Monitoring 1293
Physiologic Considerations for Central Venous Pressure Monitoring: Diastolic Pressure-Volume Relationships and Transmural Pressure 1296
Normal Central Venous Pressure Waveforms 1297
Abnormal Central Venous Pressure Waveforms 1298

Pulmonary Artery Catheter Monitoring 1301
Pulmonary Artery Catheterization 1301
Complications of Pulmonary Artery Catheter Monitoring 1304
Physiologic Considerations for Pulmonary Artery Catheter Monitoring: Prediction of Left Ventricular Filling Pressure 1307
Normal Pulmonary Artery and Wedge Pressure Waveforms 1309
Left Atrial Pressure, Pulmonary Artery Wedge Pressure, and Pulmonary Capillary Pressure 1310
Abnormal Pulmonary Artery and Wedge Pressure Waveforms 1311
Use of Central Vascular Pressures to Estimate Left Ventricular Preload 1318
Predicting Left Ventricular End-Diastolic Pressure 1320

Pulmonary Artery Catheterization and Outcome Controversies 1323
Pulmonary Artery Catheterization: Indications 1325
Additional Features of Pulmonary Artery Catheters 1325
Cardiac Preload Assessment beyond the Pulmonary Artery Catheter: Systolic Pressure Variation and Other Dynamic Indicators 1326

Cardiac Output Monitoring 1327
Thermodilution Cardiac Output Monitoring 1328
Continuous Thermodilution Cardiac Output Monitoring 1330
Fick Cardiac Output Measurement 1331

Continuous Mixed Venous Oximetry Pulmonary Artery Catheters 1331

Right Ventricular Ejection Fraction Pulmonary Artery Catheters 1332

Pulmonary Artery Catheter–Derived Hemodynamic Variables 1333

Non–Pulmonary Artery Catheter–Based Methods for Cardiac Output and Perfusion Monitoring 1334
Ultrasound-Based Methods for Cardiac Output Monitoring 1334
Bioimpedance Cardiac Output Monitoring 1336
Partial CO_2 Rebreathing Fick Cardiac Output Monitoring 1337
Lithium Dilution Cardiac Output Monitoring 1337
Pulse Contour Cardiac Output Monitoring 1338
Other Techniques for Circulatory and Perfusion Monitoring 1338

Coagulation Monitoring 1338
Functional Measures of Coagulation 1339
Heparin Concentration Measurement 1340
Viscoelastic Measures of Coagulation 1341
Platelet Function Monitors 1342

INTRODUCTION TO CARDIOVASCULAR MONITORING: EXTENDING THE PHYSICAL EXAMINATION

Although some might consider electronic devices the only cardiovascular monitors, the fundamental basis for circulatory monitoring remains in the eyes, hands, and ears of the anesthesiologist. In many ways, the anesthesiologist's senses capture more information than even the most sophisticated electronic monitors. Combined with knowledge, experience, and sound clinical judgment, the physician's senses offer an integrated, panoramic view of the patient's condition, made even more valuable by an understanding of the clinical context present. Whereas instruments accurately and monotonously collect volumes of quantitative data, the clinician integrates, evaluates, and interprets the data and, in so doing, provides the most important aspect of patient monitoring.[1] Just as inspection, palpation, and auscultation are the cornerstones for standard physical examination of the cardiovascular system, these procedures are fundamental elements of perioperative cardiovascular monitoring. However, they must be adapted and focused on the unique requirements of surgical and critically ill patients, and their limitations must be recognized.

Many standard physical means of assessing the circulation are used throughout an operation. For many healthy patients undergoing minor procedures, these physical signs may provide a considerable fraction of the total cardiovascular monitoring. When the operation becomes more complex or the patient comes to surgery with more advanced or unstable cardiovascular disease, the extent of supplemental electronic monitoring grows accordingly. However, careful physical assessment still provides the clinician with an all-important backup system to confirm or refute information derived from other monitoring devices. The most obvious, perhaps trivial example is a patient whose electrocardiogram (ECG) shows asystole. Detection of a normal pulse by direct palpation focuses the anesthesiologist on correcting the monitoring artifact rather than initiating cardiopulmonary resuscitation. The clinical examination provides redundant monitoring for patient safety; the heart rate is monitored continuously by the ECG and confirmed when required by intermittent palpation of the pulse.

Early advances in cardiovascular assessment beyond the methods of basic physical examination were not readily accepted into medical practice. Around 1900, the introduction of sphygmomanometry to measure blood pressure was criticized because it would weaken clinical acuity by blunting the senses and acute perceptions of the clinician. Even stethoscopy had its critics, simply on the basis that it placed the physician at greater distance from the patient.[2] Today, these concerns appear foolish considering our patient care responsibilities in unusual environments such as magnetic resonance scanners, where remote monitoring is required. Nonetheless, there can be little doubt that increased reliance on electronic monitoring devices has diminished our fundamental clinical skills of physical assessment.

Palpation of the pulse and its rate and character should not be forgotten in the perioperative setting. Unique constraints in the operating room may dictate which pulses are accessible for monitoring. An anesthetist standing at the patient's head during induction of anesthesia can easily palpate the carotid artery, the superficial temporal artery anterior to the ear, or the facial artery at the mandible. When only an arm is accessible, the axillary, brachial, radial, and ulnar pulses may be examined. Even procedures necessitating that the anesthetist be positioned near the patient's feet permit palpation of femoral, popliteal, dorsalis pedis, and posterior tibial pulses. Many of these vessels also serve as suitable sites for sampling arterial blood or direct arterial cannulation for pressure monitoring. Perhaps most important, one should consider the unique opportunities for pulse monitoring during surgery rather than just the constraints of this environment. During cardiac surgery, the beating heart may be observed directly, and palpation of the ascending aorta by the surgeon provides a useful estimate of aortic blood pressure. In fact, the surgeon's evaluation of any arterial pulse within the surgical field should be considered whenever severe hemodynamic instability develops.

Clinical evaluation of venous pressure during anesthesia is technically difficult because of unusual patient positions, positive-pressure mechanical ventilation, and lack of access to observe the neck veins. However, early recognition of venous obstruction in an extremity or the head and neck may have important clinical consequences. Not only might this observation herald hemodynamic problems for the patient, but communicating these observations to the operating surgeon should also allow timely correction of associated technical problems.

Given that the cardiovascular system is responsible for the transport of substrates and by-products to and from all organ systems, monitoring end-organ function reflects the adequacy of performance of the cardiovascular system. Inspection of mucous membranes, skin color, and skin turgor can reveal pertinent clues about hydration, oxygenation, and perfusion. Additional simple clinical techniques include empirical estimation of fluid deficits and measurement of intraoperative blood loss. Decreased urine output may indicate hypovolemia or reduced cardiac output, and altered mental status may be a sign of inadequate cerebral perfusion. Unfortunately, preexisting end-organ dysfunction may confound interpretation of these simple physical signs and measurements. Furthermore, drugs may alter organ function directly. For example, general anesthesia makes it impossible to monitor mental status or sensory or motor function by physical examination, and diuretic therapy obviates monitoring urine output as an indicator of overall systemic perfusion. As a result, simple clinical assessment of end-organ function is of limited value in many anesthetized or critically ill patients, so additional cardiovascular monitoring techniques are required.

Stethoscopy

Although Laennec is credited with introducing the stethoscope into general medical practice in 1818, nearly a century elapsed before Harvey Cushing proposed in 1908 that the stethoscope be used as a routine continuous cardiopulmonary monitoring device during surgery.[3] Today, intraoperative monitoring with either a precordial or an esophageal stethoscope has become a fundamental extension of the physical examination for all anesthetized patients.[4,5]

Stethoscopy provides a simple and reliable means of listening to heart and breath sounds continuously throughout an operation. The most common equipment used for precordial stethoscopy consists of a heavy metal bell or accumulator attached to a length of rubber or plastic extension tubing and a custom-molded monaural plastic earpiece. Electronically amplified stethoscopes have been designed in an attempt to improve the quality and clarity of heart and breath sounds, and wireless systems using radio-transmitted signals allow continuous monitoring without the anesthetist being tethered to the patient by the stethoscope extension tubing.[6-8] However, stethoscopes with these electronic modifications have not supplanted the standard inexpensive mechanical device in everyday practice.

Though minimally invasive and practical only for a patient who is undergoing general endotracheal anesthesia, the esophageal stethoscope provides monitoring benefits not available with its precordial cousin. Clear breath sounds and distinct heart sounds are audible in most patients with the stethoscope tip positioned 28 to 30 cm from the incisors.[9] Esophageal temperature can be measured with a thermistor incorporated in the tip of the stethoscope. Specially configured stethoscopes permit transesophageal ECG recording, which may be useful in diagnosing atrial arrhythmias, right ventricular ischemia, or posterior left ventricular ischemia.[10,11] The esophageal stethoscope may also be a valuable therapeutic tool for treating intraoperative sinus bradycardia or junctional rhythm. For this special application, transesophageal atrial pacing can be accomplished with a stethoscope equipped with bipolar pacing electrodes on its outer surface.[12,13] Although use of the esophageal stethoscope is generally without significant risk, it has been associated with occasional complications, including hypoxemia from unintended tracheobronchial placement or compression of the membranous posterior portion of the trachea in small infants, loss down the esophagus, detachment of the acoustic cuff, and distortion of surgical anatomy in the neck.[14-16] Placement of the esophageal stethoscope may also cause pharyngeal or esophageal trauma and interfere with nasogastric tube positioning or transesophageal echocardiography.

Despite the apparent value of the precordial or esophageal stethoscope for basic monitoring of patient safety, its widespread application in clinical practice has diminished in recent years.[15,17] This decline may be driven by the routine use of pulse oximetry, capnography, and other electronic safety monitors that have become ubiquitous and even required by law in some locations. As a practical matter, clinicians may not recognize the loss of heart or breath sounds as readily as might be expected because of reliance on more modern electronic devices or the distractions and noise pollution inherent in the operating room. These practice patterns appear to be borne out by the 1993 Australian Incident Monitoring Study, which noted that a stethoscope was used in only 5% of the 1256 critical incidents reported. Furthermore, it was the first monitor to detect the morbid incident—cardiac arrest—in only one instance.[17]

The current role of intraoperative stethoscopy may be summarized as follows:

1. A stethoscope should be immediately available in all locations where anesthesia is administered. Its role in diagnosing important respiratory problems (e.g., bronchospasm) probably exceeds its value as a continuous circulatory monitor.
2. Monitors such as the oximeter, capnograph, and ECG detect untoward incidents more often than the stethoscope does, in part because it is difficult to concentrate continuously on listening to both heart and breath sounds while providing anesthesia care.
3. The stethoscope thus remains a valuable additional safety monitor, but only as a supplement to standard disconnect alarms, pulse oximetry, capnography, and direct observation of the patient.
4. Use of the stethoscope as a continuous monitor has become limited to special applications (e.g., pediatric anesthesia) and to institutions with insufficient resources to purchase electronic monitors.

Heart Rate Monitoring

The simplest and least invasive form of cardiac monitoring remains measurement of the heart rate. As a circulatory vital sign, the heart rate provides an important guide to the patient's baseline condition and the influence of anesthetics and surgical stimuli. The ability to estimate the heart rate quickly with a "finger on the pulse" is a skill as important as this expression is common. However, under most circumstances in modern anesthesia practice, electronic monitoring devices are used to provide a continuous, numeric display of the heart rate.

Although any monitor that senses the period of the cardiac cycle can be used to determine the heart rate, the most common technique applied in the operating room is the ECG. Current monitors use multiple ECG leads to sense cardiac electrical activity.[18] This redundancy aids in detection of the R wave and improves the accuracy of heart rate measurement. As a result, a single noisy lead, or one in which the R waves are of very low amplitude, will not prevent the monitor from calculating the heart rate accurately.

ECG measurement of the heart rate begins with accurate detection of the R wave and measurement of the R-R interval. The digital value displayed for the heart rate is generated from an algorithm designed to count and average a certain number of beats and then display a number that is updated every 5 to 15 seconds.[19] As a result, transient changes in heart rate may have little impact on the displayed digital value. For example, consider an episode of complete heart block that interrupts slow sinus rhythm. Depending on the algorithm used by the monitor, the digital value for heart rate may show only a slight reduction from the baseline value. In this instance, the heart rate of 49 beats/min displayed by the monitor fails to alert the clinician to the dangerous transient bradyarrhythmia (Fig. 32-1). Although the monitor could update the digital value for the heart rate after each beat calculated from the R-R interval, numbers would then be flashing on the display screen, changing with each heartbeat, because of the normal physiologic beat-to-beat variability in heart rate. Instead, the displayed digital value

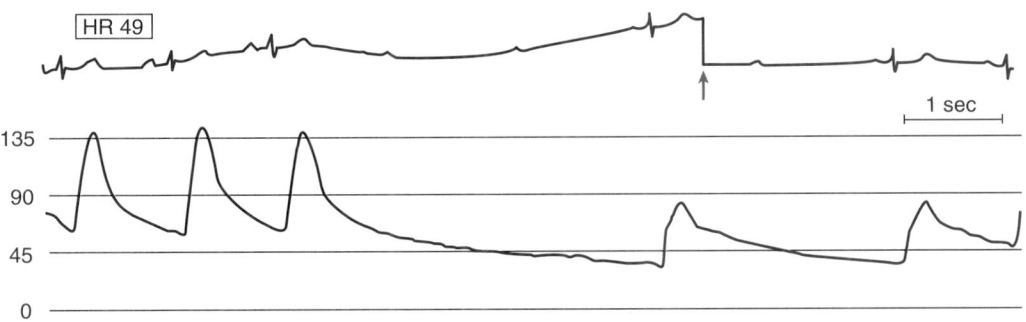

Figure 32–1 Digital heart rate (HR) displays may fail to warn of dangerous bradyarrhythmias. Direct observation of the electrocardiogram (ECG) and the arterial blood pressure traces reveals complete heart block and a 4-second period of asystole, whereas the digital display reports an HR of 49 beats/min. Note that the ECG filter *(arrow)* corrects the baseline drift so that the trace remains on the recording screen. (From Mark JB: Atlas of Cardiovascular Monitoring. New York, Churchill Livingstone, 1998, Fig. 13-2.)

for the heart rate is derived by the monitor by using a moving average filter that gives greater weight to the most recent values in deriving the average value for the display.

Occasionally, the clinician must check electrode attachment, increase ECG signal gain, or select alternative ECG leads to facilitate heart rate monitoring. Some monitors allow manual adjustment of the threshold or sensitivity for R-wave detection. Despite these measures, the monitor may display inaccurate heart rates when patient movement or other electrical interference distorts the ECG trace. In the operating room, such interference frequently occurs when the electrosurgical unit is in use. The ECG trace should always be visually inspected to confirm the numeric value for the heart rate displayed on the monitor. Spurious values are recognized quickly, and the true heart rate can be estimated from the ECG waveform tracing. In addition, the arterial pressure waveform or the pulse oximeter plethysmograph should be used to confirm the pulse rate in these instances.

Electrical interference in the ECG trace may arise from sources other than the electrosurgical unit. Power line noise appears as a 60-Hz artifact and may be eliminated by selecting narrower-bandpass ECG filters, including a 60-Hz notch filter. Other artifacts result from muscle twitching and fasciculations, as well as various medical devices, including lithotripsy machines, cardiopulmonary bypass equipment, and fluid warmers.[20] Paced rhythms often produce problems with ECG measurement of the heart rate. When tall pacing spikes are present, the monitor may misinterpret these high-amplitude signals as R waves and miscalculate the heart rate. Tall T waves may produce the same artifact when the monitor mistakenly counts these T waves as R waves. These problems may be lessened by decreasing ECG gain, adjusting R-wave detection sensitivity, or changing the ECG lead to one with a smaller pacing spike or T-wave amplitude.

Pulse Rate Monitoring

The distinction between heart rate and pulse rate centers on whether a given electrical depolarization and systolic contraction of the heart (heart rate) generates a palpable peripheral arterial pulsation (pulse rate). Pulse deficit describes the extent to which the pulse rate is less than the heart rate. Such deficit is typically seen in patients with atrial fibrillation, in which short R-R intervals compromise cardiac filling during diastole and result in a reduced stroke volume and imperceptible arterial pulse. The most extreme example of a pulse deficit is electrical-mechanical dissociation or pulseless electrical activity, seen in patients with cardiac tamponade, extreme hypovolemia, and other conditions in which cardiac contraction does not generate a palpable peripheral pulse.

Most monitors report the heart rate and pulse rate separately. The former is measured from the ECG trace, and the latter is determined from a selectable pulse source. The pulse oximeter plethysmograph trace provides a suitable pulse measurement source for most patients except those with severe arterial occlusive disease or marked peripheral vasoconstriction. In addition to indicating the pulse rate, this waveform may also provide supplementary diagnostic clues to cardiovascular function.[21] Other pulse rate sources include automatic noninvasive blood pressure devices, which determine the pulse rate from the pressure oscillations detected by the surrounding cuff, and invasive monitoring of the direct arterial pressure waveform.

Pulse rate monitoring and heart rate monitoring complement one another. Although monitoring both may seem redundant, such redundancy is intentional and being applied to modern computerized monitoring algorithms to reduce measurement errors and false alarms. In the end, however, as with all numeric information displayed on the bedside monitor, the clinician must scrutinize the analog ECG tracing and other waveforms to ensure the veracity of the digital values displayed by the bedside monitor.

ARTERIAL BLOOD PRESSURE MONITORING

Like the heart rate, blood pressure is a fundamental cardiovascular vital sign that describes the force driving tissue perfusion. Arterial blood pressure is the most important determinant of left ventricular afterload and, therefore, the workload of the heart. Consequently, frequent measurement of arterial blood pressure is a critical part of monitoring anesthetized or seriously ill patients. The importance of monitoring this vital sign is underscored by the fact that standards for basic anesthetic monitoring mandate measurement of arterial blood pressure at least every 5 minutes in all anesthetized patients.[4]

Techniques for measuring blood pressure fall into two major categories: indirect Riva-Rocci cuff devices and direct arterial cannulation and pressure transduction. These methods differ most notably in terms of the physical signal being monitored and the level of invasiveness of their application. Although direct arterial blood pressure measurement is the reference standard against which other methods are compared, even this technique can yield spurious results. As a result, blood pressures measured in clinical practice with different techniques often yield significantly different values.[22,23]

Indirect Measurement of Arterial Blood Pressure

Manual Intermittent Techniques

Most indirect methods of blood pressure measurement rely on a sphygmomanometer similar to the one first described by Riva-Rocci in 1896.[24] This apparatus included an arm-encircling inflatable elastic cuff, a rubber bulb to inflate the cuff, and a mercury manometer to measure cuff pressure.[25] Riva-Rocci described the measurement of systolic arterial blood pressure by determining the pressure at which the palpated radial arterial pulse disappeared as the cuff was inflated. The scientific rigor and attention to detail of Riva-Rocci's work are chronicled in a translation celebrating his original publications.[25]

A commonly used variation of the Riva-Rocci method is termed the return-to-flow technique. Whereas the Riva-Rocci technique recorded the pressure at which the pulse completely disappeared during cuff inflation, the return-to-flow method records the pressure at which the pulse reappears during cuff deflation. With this technique, systolic blood pressure can be estimated without a stethoscope by using only a cuff and manometer. When the patient has a finger pulse oximeter or indwelling arterial catheter in the ipsilateral arm, return to flow can be detected by reappearance of the plethysmographic or arterial pressure waveforms. Although return-to-flow methods provide a simple, rapid estimation of systolic blood pressure, they do not allow measurement of diastolic blood pressure.

To measure both systolic and diastolic arterial pressure, the most widely used intermittent manual method is the auscultatory technique, originally described by Korotkoff in 1905.[26,27] Using a sphygmomanometer, cuff, and stethoscope, Korotkoff measured blood pressure by auscultation of the sounds generated by arterial blood flow. These sounds are a complex series of audible frequencies produced by turbulent flow, instability of the arterial wall, and shock wave formation as external occluding pressure on the artery is reduced.[28] The pressure at which the first Korotkoff sound is heard is generally accepted as systolic pressure (phase I). The sound character progressively changes (phases II and III), becomes muffled (phase IV), and is finally absent (phase V). Diastolic pressure is recorded at phase IV or V. However, phase V may never occur in certain pathophysiologic states such as aortic regurgitation.[29]

A fundamental shortcoming of the auscultatory method of blood pressure measurement is its reliance on blood flow to generate Korotkoff sounds. Pathologic or iatrogenic causes of decreased peripheral blood flow, such as cardiogenic shock or high-dose vasopressor infusion, can attenuate or obliterate sound generation and result in significant underestimation of blood pressure.[30] In contrast, low compliance of the tissues underlying the cuff, as encountered in a shivering patient, will require an excessively high cuff-occluding pressure and produce "pseudohypertension."[28] Patients with severe calcific arteriosclerosis have relatively noncompressible arteries, which is another circumstance wherein cuff blood pressures will overestimate the true intra-arterial blood pressure.[31]

Other common sources of error during intermittent manual blood pressure measurement include selection of an inappropriate cuff size and excessively rapid cuff deflation. The width of the blood pressure cuff should be 20% greater than arm diameter, and the cuff should be applied snugly after any residual air has been squeezed out. The pneumatic bladder inside the cuff should span at least half the circumference of the arm and be centered over the artery. Although too large a cuff will generally work well and produce little error, the use of cuffs that are too narrow will result in overestimation of blood pressure (Fig. 32-2).[32,33] The cuff deflation rate is another important variable that influences manual blood pressure measurement. The decrease in cuff pressure should proceed slowly enough for the Korotkoff sounds to be detected and properly assigned to the current pressure in the cuff. Failure to identify the initial Korotkoff sounds will result in a falsely low measurement of blood pressure. A deflation rate of 3 mm Hg/sec limits this source of error, and coupling the deflation rate to the heart rate—2 mm Hg/beat—has been found to improve accuracy further.[34]

Automated Intermittent Techniques

Many limitations of manual intermittent blood pressure measurement have been overcome by automated noninvasive blood pressure (NIBP) devices, which are now used widely in medical care. By applying a single algorithm or

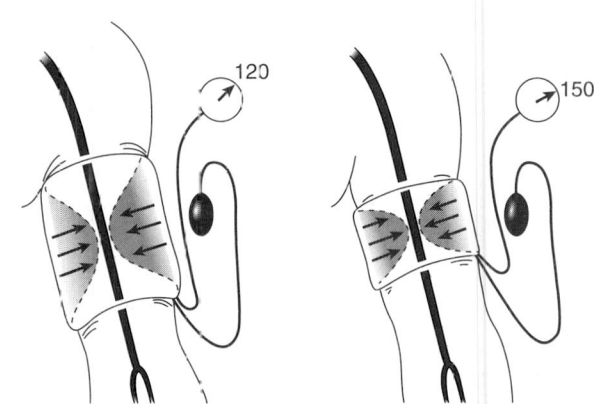

Figure 32–2 Effect of cuff size on manual blood pressure measurement. An inappropriately small blood pressure cuff yields erroneously high values for blood pressure because the pressure within the cuff is incompletely transmitted to the underlying artery.

method of data interpretation, NIBP devices provide values for systolic, diastolic, and mean arterial pressure. In addition, automated NIBP devices provide audible alarms and can transfer data to a computerized information system. However, the greatest advantage of automated NIBP devices over manual methods of blood pressure measurement is that they provide frequent, regular pressure measurements and free the operator to perform other vital clinical duties.

Most automated NIBP devices are based on oscillometry, a technique first described by von Recklinghausen in 1931.[35] In this method, variations in cuff pressure resulting from arterial pulsations during cuff deflation are sensed by the monitor and used to determine arterial blood pressure values. The pressure at which the peak amplitude of arterial pulsations occurs corresponds closely to directly measured mean arterial pressure (MAP),[36,37] and values for systolic and diastolic pressure are derived from proprietary formulas that examine the rate of change of the pressure pulsations. Systolic pressure is identified as the pressure at which pulsations are increasing and are at 25% to 50% of maximum. Diastolic pressure is the most difficult value to determine by oscillometry and is commonly recorded when the pulse amplitude has declined from the peak value by 80% (Fig. 32-3).[28]

Although oscillometry is used primarily in automated NIBP measurement, the same principles may be applied to determine blood pressure manually with a standard cuff and aneroid manometer. If the cuff is deflated slowly until the needle on the aneroid gauge begins to flicker or oscillate, the corresponding pressure value provides a close estimate of systolic blood pressure. The primary advantage of this technique is that it can be performed quickly, with only one hand on the inflation bulb and pressure relief valve.

In clinical practice, oscillometric automated NIBP measurement has focused largely on pressures measured from the upper part of the arm. Although the cuff sizes recommended for NIBP measurement have followed the guidelines used for manual auscultatory techniques, when standard cuff sizes are used in critically ill patients, the pressure values recorded underestimate true intra-arterial pressure, thus suggesting that smaller cuffs might be preferred for more accurate measurements in this setting.[38] On the other hand, if a patient's surgical procedure or medical condition requires that the cuff be applied to the calf, ankle, or thigh, an appropriately sized cuff must be used. Several investigators have proposed using neonatal-sized cuffs placed around the finger or thumb of an adult patient.[39-41] Although these alternatives may be applied in certain circumstances, their overall accuracy has not been widely validated and may not conform to accepted industry standards.[42]

Other techniques have been described for automated intermittent NIBP measurement. One method uses the Doppler principle to determine blood flow distal to an inflatable cuff,[43] a second involves photo-oscillometry to

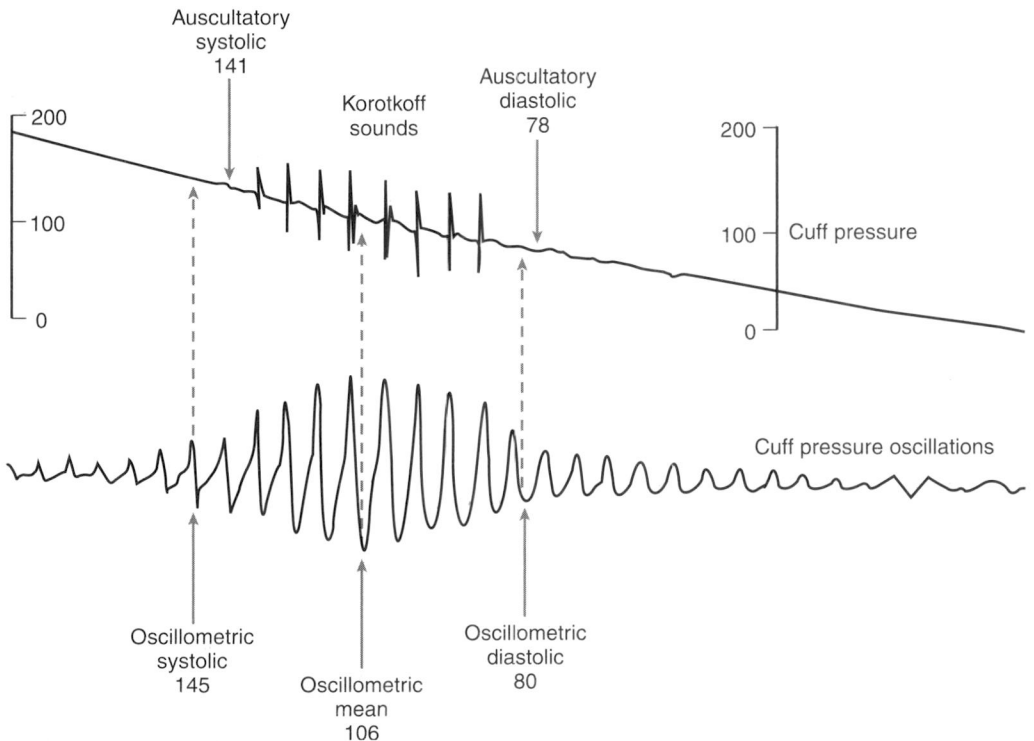

Figure 32–3 Comparison of blood pressure measurements by Korotkoff sounds and oscillometry. Oscillometric systolic blood pressure is recorded at the point where cuff pressure oscillations begin to increase, mean pressure corresponds to the point of maximal oscillations, and diastolic pressure is measured when the oscillations become attenuated. Note the correspondence between these measurements and the Korotkoff sounds that determine auscultatory systolic and diastolic pressure. (Redrawn from Geddes LA: Cardiovascular Devices and Their Applications. New York John Wiley, 1984, Fig 34-2. Reprinted by permission of John Wiley & Sons, Inc.)

detect brachial artery movement,[44] and another senses motion of the arterial wall.[45] Although these methods have been found to measure blood pressure with reasonable accuracy under some clinical circumstances, they all require additional sensing transducers, and their accuracy in critically ill patients is uncertain. Consequently, none has supplanted the standard oscillometric technique.

Even though automated NIBP measurements have been shown to closely approximate directly measured arterial pressure in controlled clinical settings,[22,33,37,46] numerous investigations underscore the disagreement that often exists when direct and indirect pressure measurements are compared, particularly when techniques are compared under changing hemodynamic conditions.[23,47-49] Standards for performance of automated NIBP devices have been advanced by the American Association for the Advancement of Medical Instrumentation (AAMI) and the British Hypertension Society. AAMI standards require that a monitor record blood pressure to within 5 ± 8 mm Hg (mean $\pm$ standard deviation [SD]) prediction error with respect to the reference method.[44] However, the clinical performance of an NIBP monitor should be evaluated by other criteria, including the number of outlier values, duration of discrepancies, magnitude of individual errors, and performance under variable clinical conditions.[44]

Complications of Noninvasive Blood Pressure Measurement

Even though automated blood pressure measurement techniques are considered noninvasive and relatively safe, complications have been reported (Table 32-1), including pain, petechiae and ecchymoses, limb edema, venous stasis and thrombophlebitis, peripheral neuropathy, and even compartment syndrome.[44,50-52] These morbid events occur more often after prolonged periods of excessively frequent cuff inflation/deflation cycling and are due to trauma or impaired distal limb perfusion. Other factors that may contribute include cuff misplacement across a joint or repeated attempts to determine blood pressure in the presence of an artifact-producing condition such as involuntary muscle tremors.[53] Caution should be exercised when using these monitors in patients with depressed consciousness, preexisting peripheral neuropathies, arterial or venous insufficiency, or irregular cardiac rhythms[50] or in those receiving anticoagulant or thrombolytic therapy.[54]

Automated Continuous Techniques

Advances in microprocessor and servomechanical control technology have enabled noninvasive techniques to

Table 32–1	Complications of noninvasive blood pressure measurement
Pain
Petechiae and ecchymoses
Limb edema
Venous stasis and thrombophlebitis
Peripheral neuropathy
Compartment syndrome

provide a reasonable representation of the arterial pressure waveform and a nearly continuous assessment of blood pressure without resorting to direct arterial cannulation. One such device measures finger blood pressure with an arterial volume-clamp method, designed and first reported by Penaz in 1973.[55] The device consists of a small cuff secured around the middle phalanx of a finger or the base of the thumb. The inflatable, flexible cuff contains an infrared photoplethysmograph linked through a servo-controlled mechanism housed within a small box strapped to the wrist. The plethysmograph continually measures the diameter of the digital arteries by transillumination. To begin monitoring, a "locking" calibration procedure is performed by varying cuff pressure to establish the vessel size at which oscillometric pressure variation is maximal, which corresponds to MAP. An electromechanical feedback loop is then established, and the external pressure applied to the cuff is varied continuously to keep the measured vessel size constant at the set point. Cuff pressure tracks arterial pressure throughout the cardiac cycle and is displayed on the monitor screen as a continuous waveform.[56-60]

Although several clinical investigators have demonstrated reasonable accuracy of finger blood pressure as a surrogate for intra-arterial pressure measurements,[61] a number of factors have precluded more widespread application of this technology. By definition, finger blood pressure monitoring records distal arterial pressure, which tends to be lower than brachial arterial pressure in elderly patients with atherosclerosis and higher than brachial pressure in young patients because of peripheral pulse wave amplification. Spasm of the finger arteries prevents accurate measurement in 5% of patients,[60] and some studies have noted substantial measurement errors in anesthetized and critically ill patients.[62-64] Unlike direct invasive arterial blood pressure monitoring, the finger pressure technique does not provide access for often-needed blood sampling. Because the "transducer" recording blood pressure with this method is the finger, the vertical height of the finger becomes an important determinant of the pressure recorded, just as transducer height is important with direct arterial pressure measurement. Finally, the potential for circulatory impairment of the distal end of the finger as a result of the constantly inflated cuff has been a cause for concern.[65]

Other automatic and continuous techniques have been used to measure blood pressure noninvasively. One such device reconstructs an arterial pressure waveform from measurements of arterial wall displacement after oscillometric calibration, but changes in arterial compliance appear to compromise the clinical performance of this instrument.[66] Another device uses pulse transit time as recorded from dual pulse oximeter probes placed on the ear and finger after oscillometric calibration from the contralateral arm, but it too has performed poorly in clinical settings, with indirectly monitored blood pressure changing in the opposite direction from direct intra-arterial pressure more than 30% of the time.[67] A third noninvasive method uses arterial tonometry, a variation of applanation tonometry in which a superficial artery (usually the radial) is compressed and partially flattened against the underlying bone.[68,69] This flattened arterial surface serves as a "transducer" for intravascular pressure acting perpendicularly against the vessel wall. An array of piezoelectric crystals positioned on the skin overlying this flattened portion of artery sense arterial pressure changes and translate them into a continuous arterial pressure waveform. The device is calibrated at intervals by cuff oscillometry from the upper part of the arm. Despite some reports of good clinical performance of this device,[69,70] it has limitations in pediatric patients[71] and those receiving vasodilating drugs.[44] In view of the ongoing limitations of all these technologies, it remains unclear whether any noninvasive technique will reduce the need for direct arterial pressure monitoring or whether these methods will replace automated intermittent oscillometry as the standard NIBP monitoring method in anesthesia and critical care.

Direct Measurement of Arterial Blood Pressure

Arterial cannulation with continuous pressure transduction and waveform display remains the accepted reference standard for blood pressure monitoring despite the fact that it is more costly, has the potential for more complications, and requires more technical expertise to initiate and maintain than noninvasive monitoring does. There are a number of reasons why clinicians should use this form of invasive pressure monitoring (Table 32-2). First and foremost, direct arterial pressure should be used when moment-to-moment blood pressure changes are anticipated and rapid detection of them is considered to be vital. Familiar examples include cardiac surgery with cardiopulmonary bypass, deliberate induced hypotension, vascular surgery with major arterial clamping, and anticipated need for infusion of vasoactive drugs. These conditions typically apply to patients with severe preexisting cardiovascular disease or hemodynamic instability or when the planned operative procedure is likely to cause large, sudden cardiovascular changes, rapid blood loss, or large fluid shifts. The Australian Incident Monitoring Study of 1993 confirmed the superiority of direct arterial pressure monitoring over indirect monitoring techniques for the early detection of intraoperative hypotension.[72]

In addition to continuous pressure monitoring, arterial catheterization provides reliable vascular access and obviates the need for multiple arterial or venous punctures for frequent blood sampling. Because of a variety of patient-related conditions, NIBP measurement may be inaccurate or prove technically impossible in some individuals, such as those with morbid obesity, burned extremities, or shock.[30] In these cases, direct arterial pressure monitoring

Table 32–2 Indications for arterial cannulation
Continuous, real-time blood pressure monitoring
Planned pharmacologic or mechanical cardiovascular manipulation
Repeated blood sampling
Failure of indirect arterial blood pressure measurement
Supplementary diagnostic information from the arterial waveform

may be the only method for blood pressure measurement and continual circulatory assessment.

Perhaps the most underemphasized value of direct arterial pressure monitoring is that arterial pressure waveform analysis may provide many important diagnostic clues to the patient's condition. More than a half century ago, Eather and colleagues emphasized these diagnostic insights in a paper that first introduced and advocated direct monitoring of "arterial pressure and pressure pulse contours" in anesthetized patients.[73] Some of these diagnostic insights are readily apparent and commonly sought, such as identification of the arterial dicrotic notch to guide proper timing for intra-aortic balloon counterpulsation, whereas others are more subtle, such as recognition of excessive variation in systolic blood pressure as a sign of hypovolemia.[74]

Percutaneous Radial Artery Cannulation

The radial artery is the most common site for invasive blood pressure monitoring in anesthesia and critical care because it is technically easy to cannulate and complications are uncommon, in part owing to the good collateral circulation of the hand.[75] For example, Slogoff and coauthors described 1700 cardiovascular surgical patients who underwent radial artery cannulation without ischemic complications despite evidence of radial artery occlusion after decannulation in more than 25% of patients.[76] Before attempting radial artery cannulation, many clinicians assess the adequacy of collateral flow to the hand by performing a modified Allen test. This bedside examination, originally described by E. V. Allen in 1929, provided a technique to assess arterial stenosis in the hands of patients with thromboangiitis obliterans.[77] To perform the Allen test, the examiner compresses the radial and ulnar arteries and asks the patient to make a tight fist to exsanguinate the palm. The patient then opens the fist while avoiding hyperextension of the wrist or fingers, and as occlusion of the ulnar artery is released, the color of the open palm is observed. Normally, the palm will have a striking flush in several seconds; severely reduced ulnar collateral flow is present when the palm remains pale for more than 10 seconds.

Although the Allen test is often used to identify patients at high risk for ischemic complications from radial artery catheterization, the predictive value of this test has been questioned. Many reports of permanent ischemic sequelae note that a normal Allen test result was present before catheterization.[78-81] In contrast, there are many descriptions of uncomplicated radial artery catheterization despite the presence of an abnormal Allen test before the procedure.[76,82,83] Although most patients show radial artery dominance with respect to overall hand perfusion, total radial artery occlusion does not appear to compromise distal perfusion.[84] Furthermore, Allen test results bear little relation to distal blood flow, as measured by fluorescein dye injection[85] or photoplethysmography.[86] Although it is obviously of great importance that the clinician minimize the chance of significant distal ischemia from arterial pressure monitoring, it appears that the Allen test cannot be relied on to avoid this adverse outcome.

Consistent, successful radial artery cannulation should be easily achievable with attention to a number of

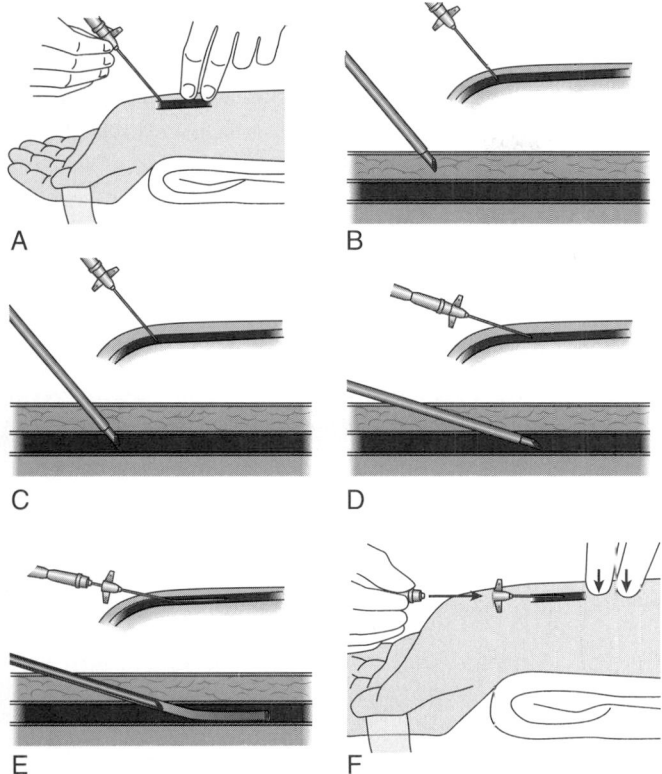

Figure 32–4 Percutaneous radial artery cannulation. **A,** The wrist is positioned and the artery identified by palpation. **B,** The catheter-over-needle assembly is introduced through the skin and advanced toward the artery. **C,** Entry of the needle tip into the artery is identified by the flash of arterial blood in the needle hub reservoir. **D,** The needle-catheter assembly is advanced at a lower angle to ensure entry of the catheter tip into the vessel. **E,** If blood flow continues into the needle reservoir, the catheter is advanced gently over the needle into the artery. **F,** The catheter is attached to pressure monitoring tubing while maintaining proximal occlusive pressure on the artery.

procedural details (Fig. 32-4). The wrist and hand are immobilized in mild dorsiflexion and secured with the wrist resting across a soft pad, folded towel, or stack of sponges. Excessive dorsiflexion of the wrist should be avoided because of the possibility of attenuating the pulse and injuring the median nerve from excessive stretch. The course of the radial artery proximal to the wrist is identified by gentle palpation, the skin is prepared with alcohol or povidone-iodine (Betadine), and a local anesthetic is injected intradermally and subcutaneously alongside the artery with a 25- or 26-gauge needle. Generous local anesthetic infiltration not only ensures that the procedure will be pain free but may also reduce vessel spasm at the time of arterial puncture. A small nick is placed in the skin at the intended puncture site with a No. 11 surgical blade or large hypodermic needle to prevent "burring" of the catheter tip as it passes through tough skin.

Next, the arterial catheter is checked for frictionless movement over the needle. The sterile plastic casing surrounding the catheter should be removed and inserted into the needle hub to serve as a reservoir for the blood

that pulses out when the artery is entered, or alternatively, a small syringe with the plunger removed should be used as a blood reservoir. Although a 20-gauge Teflon catheter is most commonly used for radial artery cannulation, the size (20- or 18-gauge) and composition (Teflon or polypropylene) of the catheter seem to have little influence on the frequency of complications.[76] The catheter is advanced toward the palpated artery at a comfortable angle, generally 30 to 45 degrees, and successful entry of the needle tip into the artery is confirmed by the "flash" of arterial blood flow into the needle hub and reservoir.

Because the needle protrudes slightly beyond the tip of the catheter, the needle tip is the only portion of the needle-catheter assembly that may have entered the arterial lumen when the flash of blood is first identified. To thread the catheter into the artery, the catheter angle should be reduced and the needle-catheter assembly advanced several millimeters (see Fig. 32-4). If blood continues to flow into the needle reservoir, it is certain that the needle and catheter are both within the lumen of the radial artery, and the catheter alone can now be advanced gently into the artery.

Failure to recognize that the needle is the leading edge of the needle-catheter assembly is responsible for most technical failures by inexperienced operators who try to advance the catheter into the radial artery when only the needle tip has entered the lumen. The catheter then "fails to thread" because its tip has not yet entered the radial artery. One should never try to advance the catheter unless blood is flowing into the collecting reservoir, thereby confirming that the catheter tip is within the arterial lumen. Once the catheter is fully advanced into the vessel lumen, the radial artery is occluded by applying proximal pressure, the needle is removed, the monitoring system pressure tubing is fastened to the catheter, an appropriate sterile dressing is applied, and the apparatus is securely taped or sutured to the wrist.

Some clinicians choose the "transfixion" technique for arterial cannulation, in which the front and back walls of the artery are punctured intentionally, the needle is removed from the catheter, and the catheter is withdrawn into the vessel lumen. Although it is unnecessary to place an additional hole in the back wall of the radial artery for successful cannulation, the technique per se does not appear to influence the incidence of postcannulation arterial thrombosis.[83,87,88]

If the needle punctures the back wall of the artery, it is not a grievous error as long as the operator recognizes it by observing that blood no longer enters the needle reservoir. Either the needle tip alone or both the needle and the catheter tips have pierced the back wall of the artery, and one can often determine which has occurred. At this point, one should not withdraw the entire needle-catheter assembly; rather, the needle alone should be retracted several millimeters into the catheter, thereby making the catheter tip the "leading edge." If arterial blood flow reappears in the collection reservoir, the catheter tip should be within the vessel lumen, and the catheter now may be advanced fully. Alternatively, if retraction of the needle into the catheter fails to restore blood flow into the collection reservoir, the catheter is pulled back slowly until pulsatile blood flow reappears, and then the catheter is advanced into the artery. The key point is for the operator to note at all times whether the needle tip or the catheter tip is the leading edge of the assembly.

When one is unsuccessful in threading the catheter into the artery, a sterile guidewire may be passed through the catheter into the artery to aid insertion. Many arterial cannulation kits have integrated needle-guidewire-catheter assemblies for this purpose. When these devices are used, the needle tip is introduced into the artery, the wire is inserted through the needle once arterial flow is detected, and the catheter is then inserted over the guidewire. Although some authors have suggested that guidewire-based techniques will improve arterial cannulation success rates in some patients,[89] it appears that success is more a function of operator experience and personal preference.[90]

Alternative Arterial Pressure Monitoring Sites

If the radial arteries are unsuitable for pressure monitoring, several alternative cannulation sites are available. The *ulnar artery* is cannulated by using a technique much like that described for the radial artery. Even in circumstances in which previous attempts to cannulate the ipsilateral radial artery have failed, the ulnar artery may be cannulated safely.[76] However, adequacy of collateral flow from the radial artery to the hand should be established before this procedure with a modified Allen test in which one releases radial artery occlusion, maintains ulnar artery compression, and observes restoration of flow to the hand.

Although the *brachial artery* does not have the anatomic benefit of the collateral circulation present in the hand, clinical trials have confirmed the safety of this cannulation site.[91,92] Bazaral and coauthors reported the use of more than 3000 brachial artery catheters in patients undergoing cardiac surgery over a 3-year period, with only one patient requiring a postoperative thrombectomy and no untoward sequelae.[93] A slightly longer catheter is preferred for the brachial site because of the need for the catheter to traverse the elbow joint. Other peripheral arteries occasionally chosen for pressure monitoring include the *dorsalis pedis, posterior tibial,* and *superficial temporal* arteries. The dorsalis pedis and posterior tibial arteries form the same collateral circulation to the foot that the radial and ulnar arteries provide to the hand. However, this anatomic safety feature is more theoretical than real in older adults because of the high incidence of lower extremity vascular disease in many of these same patients who require direct arterial pressure monitoring. Consequently, successful clinical experience using these smaller peripheral arteries for pressure monitoring has been reported predominantly in children.[94]

The *axillary artery* provides another site for long-term pressure monitoring. Advantages include patient comfort and mobility and access to a central arterial pressure waveform, and complications appear to be infrequent.[95,96] A wire-guided catheterization technique and a longer indwelling catheter may improve the success rate of axillary cannulation. If the axillary approach is chosen, the left side is preferred because its tip will lie distal to the aortic arch and great vessels. Clinicians should be aware,

however, that the risk of cerebral embolization is increased whenever more centrally located arterial catheters are used.

The *femoral artery* is the largest artery commonly selected for pressure monitoring, and it appears to have a safety record comparable to that of other sites.[97-99] As with axillary artery pressure monitoring, the femoral artery waveform more closely resembles aortic pressure than do waveforms recorded from peripheral sites. When compared with radial artery catheterization, the risk of distal ischemia after femoral artery cannulation may be reduced because of the large diameter of the artery, but atherosclerotic plaque embolization is more likely during initial guidewire and catheter placement. Although some investigators have shown an increase in infectious complications with femoral artery catheters,[96,100] others have not shown an increased risk.[98,99,101] Catheterization of the femoral artery is best achieved with a guidewire technique. The operator must be careful to puncture the femoral artery below the inguinal ligament, thereby limiting the risk of arterial injury causing uncontained hemorrhage into the pelvis or peritoneum, a potentially catastrophic complication.[102,103]

Complications of Direct Arterial Pressure Monitoring

The widespread application of invasive arterial pressure monitoring in anesthesia and intensive care is related, no doubt, to the extremely good safety record of this technique. Large clinical investigations confirm the low incidence of long-term complications after radial artery cannulation, in particular, the small risk of distal ischemia, which is probably less than 0.1%.[75,76] Although vascular complications from radial artery cannulation are rare, a number of factors have been identified that may increase the risk, including vasospastic arterial disease, previous arterial injury, thrombocytosis, protracted shock, high-dose vasopressor administration, prolonged cannulation, and infection.[78,104,105]

The Australian Incident Monitoring Study provides some noteworthy observational data on the incidence and types of complications of blood pressure monitoring.[72,106] Of 2000 untoward clinical events reported in this investigation, only 13 were related to peripheral arterial cannulation, fewer than the number associated with central venous or peripheral venous cannulation (18 and 33 incidents, respectively). Five of these 13 cases involved equipment faults or misassembly, in 3 cases the arterial line was mistaken for an intravenous line and used for drug injection, in 3 cases the arterial line was either disrupted or kinked, in 1 case a fragment of guidewire broke off inside the patient, and in only 1 instance did transient vasospasm follow radial artery cannulation.[106] A second report from this study, which focused entirely on blood pressure monitoring, noted that direct pressure monitoring failed or gave misleading results in 10 instances, including 5 in which there was either incorrect calibration, incorrect interpretation of the pressure display, or unrecognized subclavian artery stenosis.[72]

Certain clinically relevant conclusions can be drawn from these data. First, it is striking that many, if not most, of the complications from direct arterial pressure monitoring can be attributed to equipment misuse. This serves to highlight the importance of proper operator knowledge,

Table 32–3 Complications of direct arterial pressure monitoring

Distal ischemia, pseudoaneurysm, arteriovenous fistula
Hemorrhage
Arterial embolization
Infection
Peripheral neuropathy
Misinterpretation of data
Misuse of equipment

training, and experience in ensuring patient safety. Second, it is vital to have a system for the manual determination of blood pressure readily available at all times. The clinician should have a low threshold for measuring blood pressure manually from a different extremity, particularly when the results of invasive pressure monitoring do not match the patient's general clinical appearance.

Serious complications, though rare, do occur after arterial cannulation (Table 32-3). Reports describe pseudoaneurysm and arteriovenous fistula formation,[107] retained guidewire requiring surgical extraction,[108] fatal hemorrhage after difficult femoral artery cannulation,[102] and upper extremity compartment syndrome after brachial artery cannulation.[109] In almost all cases, however, there were technical problems during catheter placement or confounding medical problems such as shock or coagulopathy. Infectious complications are increasingly rare now that disposable transducers have replaced reusable ones. Because retrograde arterial embolism is possible whenever forceful flushing of a peripheral arterial catheter is performed,[110] special care should be exercised whenever more centrally located arterial catheters are used, including those in the superficial temporal artery or axillary artery or when monitoring from the central lumen of an intra-aortic balloon pump in the descending aorta.

Technical Aspects of Direct Blood Pressure Measurement

Direct measurement of arterial blood pressure requires that the pressure waveform from the cannulated artery be reproduced accurately on the bedside monitor. Not surprisingly, the displayed pressure signal is influenced significantly by the measuring system, including the arterial catheter, extension tubing, stopcocks, flush devices, transducer, amplifier, and recorder.[51,111-113] Consequently, it is important to understand how the monitoring system may influence the contour of the pressure waveform and the measured values for blood pressure.

The direct blood pressure monitoring systems used in the operating room and intensive care units are described as underdamped second-order dynamic systems.[111,113-119] These fluid-filled, catheter-transducer monitoring systems may be modeled after simple mass-spring systems. Intuitively, when the mass at the end of a spring is displaced and then released, a characteristic simple harmonic motion is observed. Clinical blood pressure monitoring systems exhibit similar physical behavior that depends on three characteristic physical properties: elasticity, mass, and friction. These three properties determine the

system operating characteristics, termed the *frequency response* or *dynamic response,* which in turn is characterized by two important system parameters, *natural frequency* (f_n, ω) and *damping coefficient* (ζ, Z, α, D). The natural frequency of the monitoring system quantifies how rapidly the system oscillates, and the damping coefficient quantifies the frictional forces that act on the system and determine how rapidly it comes to rest. Both parameters may be estimated or measured at the bedside, and they dramatically influence the appearance of the recorded pressure waveform.

Natural Frequency, Damping Coefficient, and Dynamic Response of Pressure Monitoring Systems

The arterial blood pressure waveform is a periodic complex wave that can be reproduced by Fourier analysis, which recreates the original complex pressure wave by summing a series of simpler sine waves of different amplitudes and frequencies.[113,120] The original pressure wave has a characteristic periodicity termed the *fundamental frequency,* which is equal to the pulse rate. Although the pulse rate is reported in beats per minute, fundamental frequency is reported in cycles per second or Hertz (Hz). For example, a pulse rate of 60 beats/min equals 1 beat/sec or 1 cycle/sec or 1 Hz.

The sine waves that sum to produce the complex wave have frequencies that are multiples or harmonics of the fundamental frequency. A crude arterial waveform that displays a systolic upstroke, systolic peak, dicrotic notch, and so forth can be reconstructed with reasonable accuracy from two sine waves, the fundamental frequency and the second harmonic (Fig. 32-5). If the original arterial pressure waveform contains high-frequency components such as a steep systolic upstroke, higher-frequency sine waves (and more harmonics) are needed to provide a faithful reconstruction of the original pressure waveform. As a general rule, 6 to 10 harmonics are required to provide

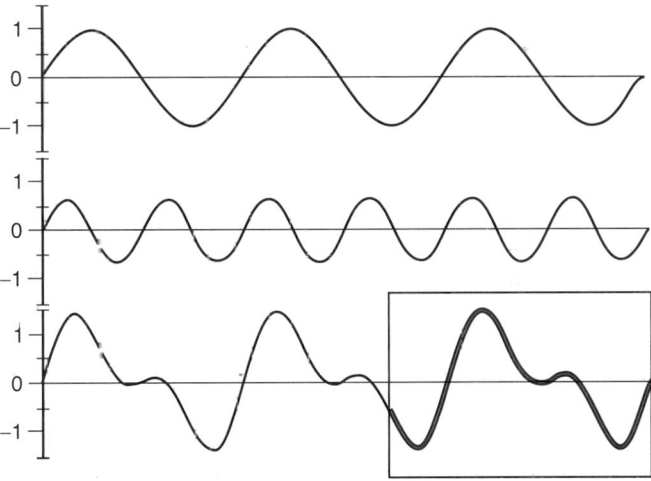

Figure 32–5 Arterial blood pressure waveform produced by the summation of sine waves. The fundamental wave *(top)* added to 63% of the second harmonic wave *(middle)* results in a pressure wave *(bottom)* that resembles an arterial blood pressure waveform *(box).* (Redrawn from Mark JB: Atlas of Cardiovascular Monitoring. New York, Churchill Livingstone, 1998, Fig. 9-1.)

distortion-free reproduction of most arterial pressure waveforms.[120,121] Hence, accurate blood pressure measurement in a patient with a pulse rate of 120 beats/min (2 cycles/sec or 2 Hz) requires a monitoring system dynamic response of 12 to 20 Hz. However, the faster the heart rate and the steeper the systolic pressure upstroke, the greater the dynamic response demands on the monitoring system.

If the monitoring system has a natural frequency that is too low, frequencies in the monitored pressure waveform will approach the natural frequency of the measurement system. As a result, the system will resonate, and pressure waveforms recorded on the monitor will be exaggerated or amplified versions of true intra-arterial pressure (Fig. 32-6). This phenomenon is the familiar arterial pressure waveform that displays overshoot, ringing, or resonance, and the systolic blood pressure recorded overestimates intra-arterial pressure. Tachycardia and steep systolic pressure upstrokes present the greatest challenge for clinical monitoring systems because the higher-frequency content of these waveforms more likely approaches the resonant frequency of the measurement system.

In addition to a sufficiently high natural frequency, the bedside monitoring system must also have an appropriate damping coefficient. An overdamped arterial pressure waveform is recognized by its slurred upstroke, absent dicrotic notch, and loss of fine detail. Severely overdamped pressure waves display a falsely narrowed pulse pressure, although MAP may remain reasonably accurate (Fig. 32-7). In contrast, underdamped pressure waveforms display systolic pressure overshoot and contain additional artifacts produced by the measurement

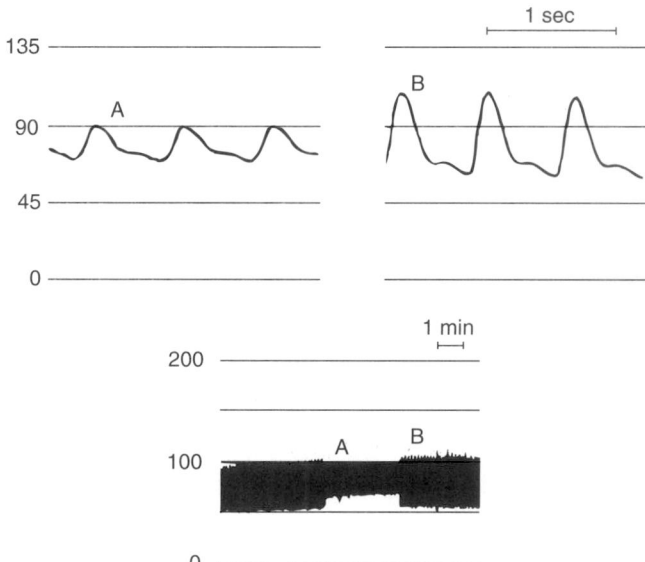

Figure 32–7 Overdamped arterial pressure waveform. The overdamped pressure waveform (*A*) shows a diminished pulse pressure when compared with the normal waveform (*B*). The slow-speed recording below demonstrates a 3-minute period of damped arterial pressure. Despite the damped pressure waveform, mean arterial pressure remains unchanged during this period. (Redrawn from Mark JB: Atlas of Cardiovascular Monitoring. New York, Churchill Livingstone, 1998, Fig. 9-3.)

system that are not part of the original intravascular pressure wave (see Fig. 32-6). It is a mistake to attach physiologic significance to these small artifactual waves that result from an underdamped monitoring system that continues to ring or oscillate abnormally in response to the input pressure signal.

Most catheter-tubing transducer systems are underdamped but have an acceptable natural frequency that exceeds 12 Hz. If the system's natural frequency is lower than 7.5 Hz, the pressure waveform is often distorted, and no amount of damping adjustment can restore the monitored waveform to adequately resemble the original waveform.[51,111] If, on the other hand, the natural frequency can be increased sufficiently (e.g., 24 Hz), damping will have minimal effect on the monitored waveform, and faithful reproduction of intravascular pressure is achieved more easily (Figs. 32-8 and 32-9). In other words, the lower the natural frequency of the monitoring system, the more narrow the range of damping coefficients that can be tolerated to ensure faithful reproduction of the pressure wave or adequate dynamic response. For example, if the monitoring system's natural frequency is 10 Hz, the damping coefficient must be between 0.45 and 0.6 for accurate pressure waveform monitoring. If the damping coefficient is too low, the monitoring system will be underdamped, resonate, and display factitiously elevated systolic blood pressure. In contrast, if the damping coefficient is too high, the system will be overdamped, systolic pressure will be falsely decreased, and fine detail in the pressure trace will be lost.

From these considerations, it follows that a pressure monitoring system will have optimal dynamic response

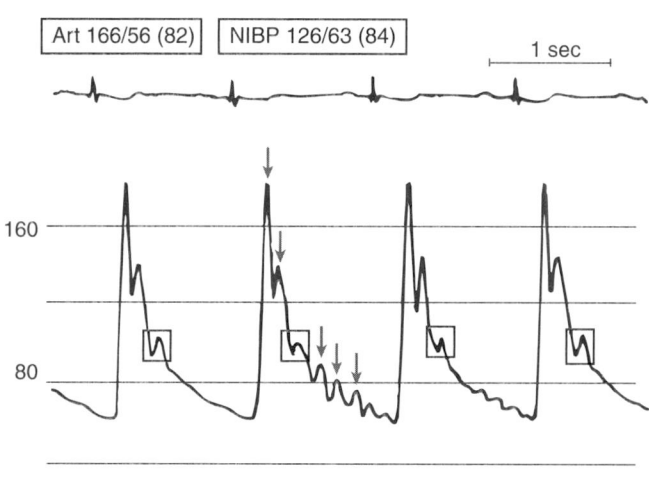

Art 166/56 (82) | NIBP 126/63 (84)

Figure 32–6 Underdamped arterial pressure waveform. Systolic pressure overshoot and additional small, nonphysiologic pressure waves *(arrows)* distort the waveform and make it hard to discern the dicrotic notch *(boxes)*. Digital values displayed for direct arterial blood pressure (ART 166/56, mean of 82 mm Hg) and noninvasive blood pressure (NIBP 126/63, mean of 84 mm Hg) show the differences in pressure measurement that arise because of an underdamped arterial pressure waveform. (Redrawn from Mark JB: Atlas of Cardiovascular Monitoring. New York, Churchill Livingstone, 1998, Fig. 9-4.)

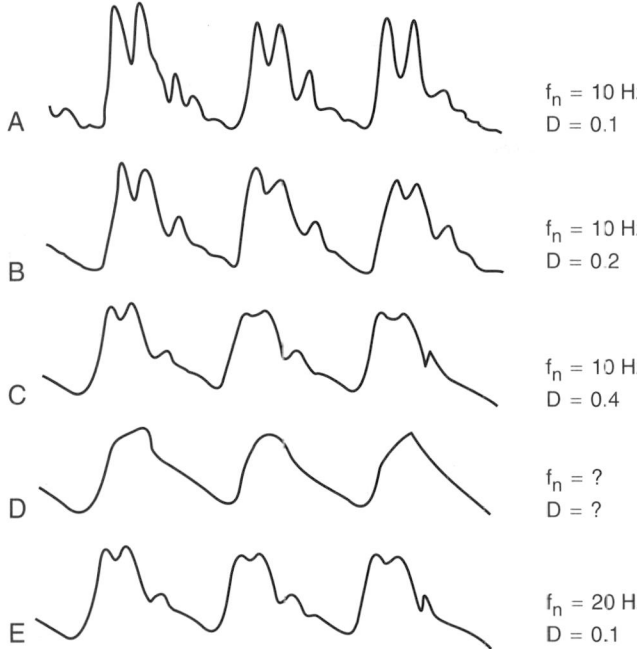

Figure 32–8 Interaction between damping coefficient (D) and natural frequency (f_n) in pressure waveform recordings. **A,** An underdamped pressure waveform (f_n = 10 Hz, D = 0.1) displays small artifactual waves and systolic pressure overshoot. **B,** A small increase in D (0.2) diminishes these artifacts. **C,** Critical damping (D = 0.4) provides an accurate pressure waveform, even though f_n remains low. **D,** Overdamping results in loss of fine detail and precludes determination of f_n or D. **E,** Increased f_n (20 Hz) allows a low D (0.1) to have minimal impact on waveform morphology. Notice the similarities between waveforms **C** and **E.** (Redrawn from Mark JB: Atlas of Cardiovascular Monitoring. New York, Churchill Livingstone, 1998, Fig. 9-7.)

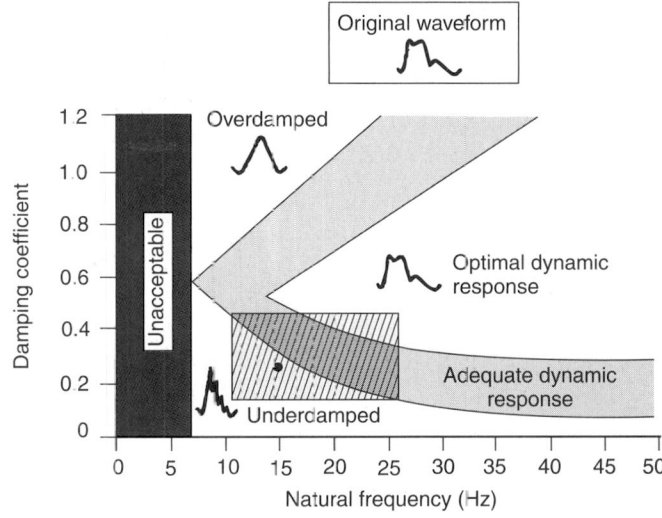

Figure 32–9 Interaction between damping coefficient and natural frequency. Depending on these two system parameters, catheter tubing-transducer systems fall into one of five different dynamic response ranges. Systems with an optimal dynamic response will faithfully record the most demanding pressure waveforms, whereas those with an adequate dynamic response will accurately record most pressure waveforms seen in clinical practice. Overdamped and underdamped systems introduce artifacts characteristic of these technical limitations. Systems with a natural frequency of less than 7 Hz are considered unacceptable. The *rectangular crosshatched box* indicates the ranges of damping coefficients and natural frequencies commonly encountered in clinical pressure measurement systems. The point within the box shows the mean values of 30 such systems recorded by Schwid.[122] (Redrawn from Mark JB: Atlas of Cardiovascular Monitoring. New York, Churchill Livingstone, 1998, Figs. 9-6, 9-8, and 9-11.)

if its natural frequency is as high as possible. In theory, this is achieved best by using short lengths of stiff pressure tubing and limiting the number of stopcocks and other monitoring system appliances.[112] Standard intravenous extension tubing should never be used because it is too compliant. Blood clots and air bubbles often trapped and concealed in stopcocks and other connection points system will have similar adverse influences on the dynamic response of the system.

Because typical clinical blood pressure monitoring systems are underdamped and display some degree of systolic pressure overshoot, it is tempting to try to increase the damping in the system by introducing a small air bubble into the monitoring tubing line, but this should not be done. Aside from the obvious risk of arterial air embolism and the potential for retrograde flushing of the air bubble into the cerebral circulation,[110] the air bubble will not improve the dynamic response of the system because any increase in system damping is always accompanied by a decrease in its natural frequency. Somewhat paradoxically, resonance in the system may increase and systolic pressure overshoot may be even greater because of the reduced natural frequency of the monitoring system. In this example (Fig. 32-10), a 0.1-mL air bubble markedly dampens the system but lowers the natural frequency and causes an artifactual 25–mm Hg increase in systolic pressure.

As an alternative to placing air bubbles in the monitoring system, devices can be added to increase damping without lowering the natural frequency (see Fig. 32-8). These devices improve impedance matching, which eliminates wave reflections and prevents resonance in the monitoring system.[111,115,119] Although some have advocated the use of these devices in monitoring systems,[111] others have highlighted the limitations of these devices, including an inability to adjust or tune the monitoring system to provide the most accurate in vivo pressure recordings.[44,119]

Even though limiting the pressure monitoring system to short extension tubing will optimize the system's dynamic response, clinical circumstances often require longer extension tubing, stopcocks for blood drawing, and other in-line sampling and flush devices. Thus, it becomes important to be able to assess the amount of distortion existing in the monitoring system in clinical use. Although one cannot accurately predict the total system's natural frequency or damping coefficient from knowledge of the values for individual system components,[112] the *fast-flush test* provides a convenient bedside method for determining these vital system performance parameters. This test can be performed without additional equipment beyond the normal monitors and recorders, and it assesses the dynamic response of the entire monitoring system, from catheter tip to transducer. Furthermore, it

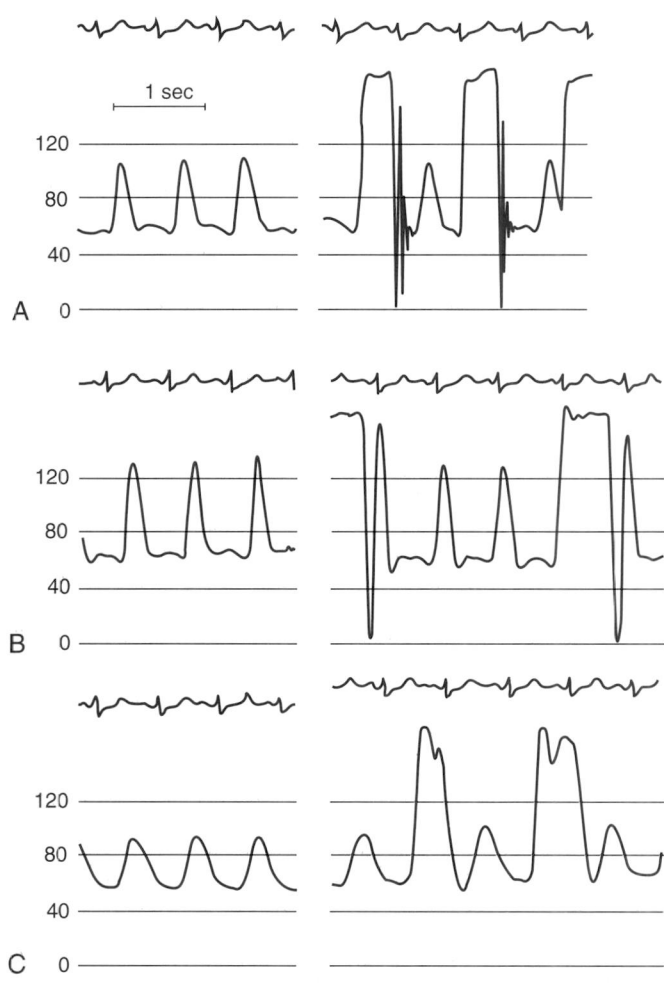

Figure 32–10 Effect of small air bubbles within arterial pressure monitoring systems. Arterial pressure waveforms are displayed along with superimposed fast flush square-wave artifacts. **A,** The original monitoring system has an adequate dynamic response (natural frequency, 17 Hz; damping coefficient, 0.2). **B,** A small 0.1-mL air bubble added to the monitoring system produces a paradoxical increase in arterial blood pressure. Note the decreased natural frequency of the system. **C,** A larger 0.5-mL air bubble further degrades the dynamic response and produces spurious arterial hypotension. (Redrawn from Mark JB: Atlas of Cardiovascular Monitoring. New York, Churchill Livingstone, 1998, Fig. 9-14.)

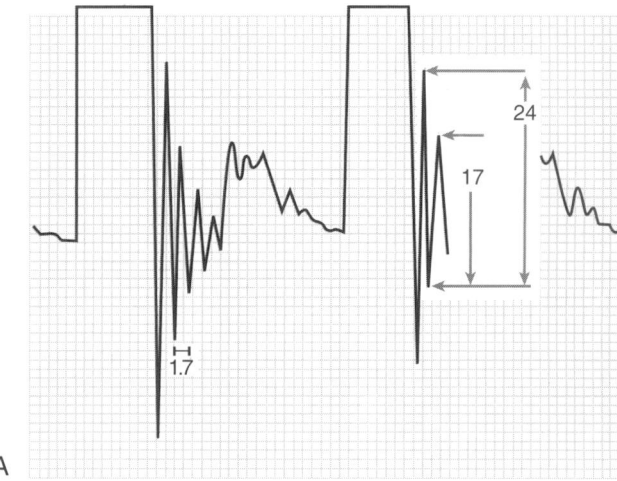

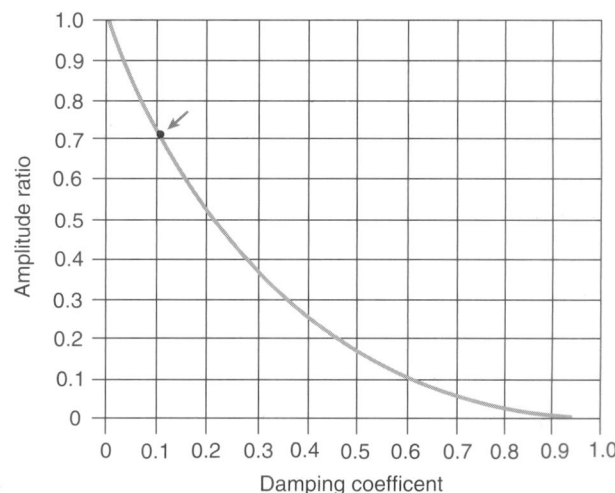

Figure 32–11 Clinical measurement of natural frequency and damping coefficient. **A,** Two square-wave fast-flush artifacts interrupt an arterial pressure waveform recorded on standard 1-mm grid paper at a speed of 25 mm/sec. Natural frequency is determined by measuring the period of one cycle of adjacent oscillation peaks (1.7 mm). The damping coefficient is determined by measuring the heights of adjacent oscillation peaks (17 and 24 mm). From these measurements, a natural frequency of 14.7 Hz and an amplitude ratio of 0.71 may be calculated. See the text for greater detail. **B,** Relationship between the amplitude ratio and the damping coefficient. The amplitude ratio determined in the fast-flush test in **A** corresponds to a damping coefficient of 0.11. (Redrawn from Mark JB: Atlas of Cardiovascular Monitoring. New York, Churchill Livingstone, 1998, Figs. 9-9 and 9-10.)

yields results that are essentially identical to those from standard laboratory square-wave testing.[111,114,116,117]

To perform this test, the fast-flush valve is opened briefly several times, and the resulting flush artifact is examined. The monitoring system's natural frequency is related to the time period or distance between two successive oscillation cycles. An example is illustrated in Figure 32-11, where the distance between two cycles is 1.7 mm at a recorder speed of 25 mm/sec (standard ECG speed). Natural frequency is then easily calculated: 1 cycle/1.7 mm × 25 mm/sec = 14.7 cycles/sec or 14.7 Hz. Note that the distance between successive oscillation cycles (i.e., cycles 1 to 2, 2 to 3) should be identical because this is a fundamental characteristic of the measurement system—its natural frequency. Furthermore, the tighter the oscillation cycles, the higher

the natural frequency. To measure natural frequency most accurately, a fast recording speed should be chosen (e.g., 50 mm/sec), several flush cycles should be examined, and an average value calculated.

The damping coefficient is determined from the flush artifact by measuring the amplitudes of successive oscillation cycles. The amplitude ratio thus derived indicates how quickly the measuring system comes to rest. A low amplitude ratio corresponds to a high damping coefficient, or a system that comes to rest quickly. Conversely, a high amplitude ratio corresponds to a low damping coefficient, or a system that tends to resonate. The damping coefficient can be calculated mathematically, but it is usually determined graphically from the measured amplitude ratio.[111,118] In this example, the amplitudes of two successive oscillation cycles are 24 and 17 mm, respectively, for an amplitude ratio of 17/24 or 0.71, which corresponds to a damping coefficient of 0.11 when using the graphic solution shown (see Fig 32-11). As in the case for measuring natural frequency, any two adjacent peaks may be used to determine the amplitude ratio because the ratio of successive peaks should be relatively constant. Again, this is a fundamental characteristic of the measurement system—the damping coefficient. Note that the monitoring system illustrated here has an adequate natural frequency of approximately 15 Hz but is notably underdamped, with a damping coefficient of 0.11. Consequently, this catheter-tubing-transducer system falls into the underdamped region illustrated in Figure 32-9, and one would expect to find systolic pressure overshoot in such a system.

Although the technical requirements for accurate blood pressure measurement are well known, these conditions are often unmet in routine clinical practice. Schwid examined the frequency response of 30 radial artery catheter-transducer systems used in routine intensive care monitoring.[122] Mean values (± SD) for natural frequency (14.7 ± 3.7 Hz) and damping coefficient (0.24 ± 0.07) were worse than values typically reported for measurements made under laboratory conditions, instead falling in the underdamped response region reported by Gardner.[111] Furthermore, the range of frequency responses (10.2 to 25.3 Hz) and damping coefficients (0.15 to 0.44) measured in this setting suggests that distortion of the arterial waveform is common in clinical practice, with systolic arterial pressure overshoot resulting from a relatively underdamped system being the most common problem. Figure 32-9 shows these data from Schwid[122] in the format suggested by Gardner[111] and graphically highlights this situation.

Several practical points for direct blood pressure monitoring in daily clinical practice emerge from these technical considerations. First, in an attempt to optimize the dynamic response of the monitoring system, one should try to keep the catheter-tubing-transducer system as simple as possible by using the minimum length of tubing and number of stopcocks required for patient care purposes. Second, one should know how the natural frequency and damping coefficient might be calculated with the fast-flush method. One practical application is that this testing allows the clinician to distinguish true hypotension from an artifact resulting from an excessively damped system caused by a large air bubble or blood clot in the catheter or tubing (see Fig. 32-10). A third relates to the clinical interpretation of systolic arterial blood pressure values. Because of the dynamic response limitations of most clinical pressure monitoring systems, direct measurement of systolic arterial pressure often exceeds indirect noninvasive measurement, simply because of underdamping and resonance (see Fig. 32-6).

Pressure Monitoring System Components

Arterial pressure monitoring systems have a number of components, beginning with the intra-arterial catheter and including extension tubing, stopcocks, in-line blood sampling set, pressure transducer, continuous-flush device, and electronic cable connecting the bedside monitor and waveform display screen. The stopcocks in the system provide sites for blood sampling and allow the transducer to be exposed to atmospheric pressure to establish a zero reference value. Newer systems include needleless blood sampling ports and in-line aspiration systems. These components permit blood drawing without the use of sharp needles and allow the aspirated waste blood to be returned to the patient within a convenient closed system. Modifications such as these are intended to reduce the risk of needle injury and blood exposure to health care workers, as well as decrease waste of the patient's blood during sampling. However, these additional features may degrade the dynamic response of the monitoring system and further exacerbate systolic arterial pressure overshoot.[123]

The flush device provides a continuous, slow (1 to 3 mL/hr) infusion of saline to purge the monitoring system and prevent thrombus formation within the arterial catheter. Historically, a dilute concentration of heparin (1 to 2 U/mL saline) has been added to this flush solution to further reduce the incidence of thrombosis,[124] but this practice increases the risk of heparin-induced thrombocytopenia and is not needed for routine practice.[125,126]

The flush device not only ensures continuous slow flushing of the line and catheter but also includes a spring-loaded valve that allows periodic, high-pressure flushing to purge the extension line of blood after an arterial sample has been taken. Despite the presence of both slow- and fast-flush systems, pressure monitoring systems appear to undergo a slow degradation in dynamic response over time, with a decrease in natural frequency and increase in damping coefficient.[127] The dynamic response can be restored, however, with periodic "manual" flushing of the system.

Transducer Setup: Zeroing, Calibrating, and Leveling

Before initiating patient monitoring, the pressure transducer must be zeroed, calibrated, and leveled to the appropriate position on the patient. The initial step in this process is to expose the transducer to atmospheric pressure by opening the adjacent stopcock to air, pressing the zero pressure button on the monitor, and thereby establishing the zero pressure reference value. The transducer now has a reference—ambient atmospheric pressure—against which all intravascular pressures are measured. This process underscores the fact that all pressures displayed on the monitor are referenced to atmospheric pressure, outside the body. Although clinicians generally refer to "zeroing the transducer," the transducer is actually exposed to atmospheric pressure through an open stopcock affixed to the transducer. To be precise, it is this air-fluid interface at the level of the stopcock that is the zero pressure locus. This point must be aligned with a specific position on the patient to ensure the correct transducer level.

When a significant change in pressure occurs, the zero reference value should be rechecked before initiating therapy. Opening the stopcock and exposing the transducer to atmospheric pressure can accomplish this quickly. The monitor should be inspected to ensure that the pressure trace overlies the zero pressure line on the display screen and the digital pressure value equals zero. Note that checking the zero value is different from establishing the zero reference, which is done at the beginning of the monitoring procedure.[128] If the stopcock is exposed to atmospheric pressure and pressure is not equal to zero, baseline drift of the transducer's electrical circuit may have occurred. Such transducer drift is caused by problems with membrane dome coupling to the electronic pressure transducing elements, as well as other technical problems with the transducer, the attached electrical cable, or the monitor itself.[51,129,130] These technical problems appear to be uncommon now that high-quality disposable transducers are widely available,[131] but they may be insidious, which underscores the importance of confirming "unexpected" arterial pressure values by checking them against a cuff pressure measurement.[132]

Historically, calibration of the transducer was the next step after the zeroing procedure. Calibration is an adjustment in system gain to ensure the proper response to a known reference pressure value. Traditionally, this has been performed by using a mercury manometer as the standard.[51] Currently, however, disposable pressure transducers meet or exceed the accuracy standards established by the AAMI and the American National Standards Institute.[131] Transducer calibration at the bedside thus appears to be unnecessary. By avoiding daily calibration, the attendant serious risks of arterial air embolism and infection may be reduced. In general, if a pressure transducer or monitoring cable is faulty, the initial zero value cannot be established, and the monitoring system must be changed. On rare occasion, despite successful zeroing the recorded pressure values appear erroneous, and a malfunctioning pressure transducer, cable, or monitor must be suspected and replaced.[129,130,132,133]

The final step in transducer setup is leveling the pressure monitoring zero point to the appropriate position on the patient. In general, zeroing and leveling the transducer are accomplished at the same time, before initiating patient monitoring. However, these are two distinct procedures. Zeroing exposes the transducer to ambient atmospheric pressure through an open stopcock. Leveling assigns this zero reference point to a specific position on the patient's body.

In a supine patient, pressure transducers are leveled most often to the midchest position in the midaxillary line,[51] a site chosen because it is easy to estimate by eye and provides a reasonable approximation for the midpoint of the heart in the chest. Although precise location for the zero reference level is important for all pressure monitoring, it is critical for measurement of cardiac filling pressures. An error of 10 mm Hg in arterial blood pressure measurement is generally of minor clinical importance, but the same error in central venous pressure (CVP) or pulmonary artery wedge pressure (PAWP) may have major diagnostic implications.

Despite the common practice of aligning pressure transducers at the midchest level, more accurate pressure monitoring will be achieved if the transducer is aligned approximately 5 cm below the sternal border in the fourth intercostal space.[134] Rather than align the transducer at the "midchamber" or midheart level, this preferred location

aligns the transducers with the upper-most blood levels in the cardiac chambers and thereby eliminates the confounding effect of hydrostatic pressure on the measurement of pressure in the cardiac chambers. Courtois and associates have shown that errors in measurement of left ventricular filling pressure of up to 7 mm Hg occur when transducers are leveled to the midchest rather than the top of the left ventricle.[134] Because many critically ill or anesthetized patients have direct arterial pressure measured along with other direct intravascular cardiac filling pressures, it seems prudent to use the same zero reference level for all direct pressure measurements.

In some circumstances, the clinician may choose to level the arterial pressure transducer at a different position on the body. During neurosurgical operations performed with the patient in a seated position, the pressure transducer is often aligned with the patient's ear to approximate the level of the circle of Willis and better estimate cerebral perfusion pressure. The transducer should not need to be rezeroed by pushing the zero pressure button on the monitor because only the reference level has been altered. In fact, if zero is rechecked, it should be unchanged, regardless of transducer location, because atmospheric pressure changes little over the few inches of height alteration being considered in this situation. Arterial blood pressure now recorded at the level of the head will be lower than that recorded at the heart, the difference being precisely equal to the hydrostatic pressure difference between the head and the heart (Fig. 32-12).[128]

Frequently, pressure transducers are attached to an intravenous pole, and patient position is altered by adjusting the height of the operating room table or intensive care bed. Raising the patient above the transducer will produce spuriously high pressures, whereas lowering the patient below the transducer will produce spuriously low pressures. Again, the error introduced is exactly equal to the hydrostatic pressure difference between the patient and transducer. Although these leveling artifacts are generally small relative to the magnitude of arterial blood pressure, they are of critical importance when measuring CVP or pulmonary artery pressure (PAP). Taping pressure transducers directly to the patient can obviate these leveling artifacts. Common major mistakes in pressure monitoring include failure to establish zero, failure to recheck the zero value for transducer drift, and failure to relevel the transducer appropriately after changes in patient position.[51]

Proper interpretation of blood pressure measurements from a patient in the lateral decubitus position requires an understanding of the distinction between zeroing and leveling pressure transducers and the differences between noninvasive and invasive blood pressure measurement (Fig. 32-13). While the patient is supine, blood pressure is 120/80 mm Hg in both arms, as measured by noninvasive cuffs and direct indwelling radial artery catheters. The patient is now placed in the right lateral decubitus position, the left arm is 20 cm above the heart, and the right arm is 20 cm below the heart. The invasive blood pressure transducers remain at the same level in the midthoracic position. Blood pressure measured in the left arm by cuff will be lower, 105/65 mm Hg, because the left arm is 20 cm above the level of the heart, whereas blood

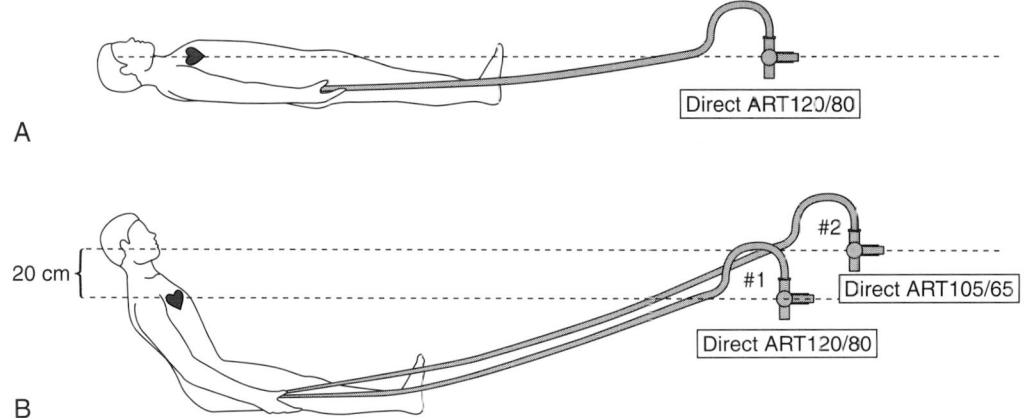

Figure 32–12 Effect of pressure transducer level on measurement of blood pressure. **A,** In a supine patient, the same arterial blood pressure (ART) is measured at the level of the heart or the brain. **B,** With the patient in the sitting position, blood pressure recorded from a transducer that remains at heart level (#1) will be unchanged, but blood pressure recorded from a transducer adjusted to the level of the brain (#2) will be lower by an amount equal to the hydrostatic pressure difference between these two transducer positions (20 cm H_2O or approximately 15 mm Hg). (Redrawn from Mark JB: Atlas of Cardiovascular Monitoring. New York, Churchill Livingstone, 1998, Fig. 9-19.)

pressure measured in the right arm by cuff will be higher, 135/95 mm Hg. However, blood pressure measured from either the left or right radial catheters will remain unchanged, 120/80 mm Hg, because the reference level for the pressure transducers remains fixed at the mid-chest position. Indeed, if the arterial pressure transducers were attached to the arms, the zero reference levels for the transducers would have changed as the patient assumed the lateral position, and pressures recorded from right and left radial artery catheters would equal those recorded by the ipsilateral noninvasive cuffs.

Normal Arterial Pressure Waveforms

Direct arterial pressure monitoring in anesthetized patients began more than 50 years ago.[73] In that early era, arterial pulse waveform analysis was noted to provide useful diagnostic information, but somewhat surprisingly, modern physicians pay little attention to the morphology and detail of the arterial pressure waveform. O'Rourke and Gallagher attribute this change in practice to the reliance on cuff sphygmomanometry, which provides "numbers which came to be linked in a simplistic way to cardiac strength (systolic pressure) and arteriolar

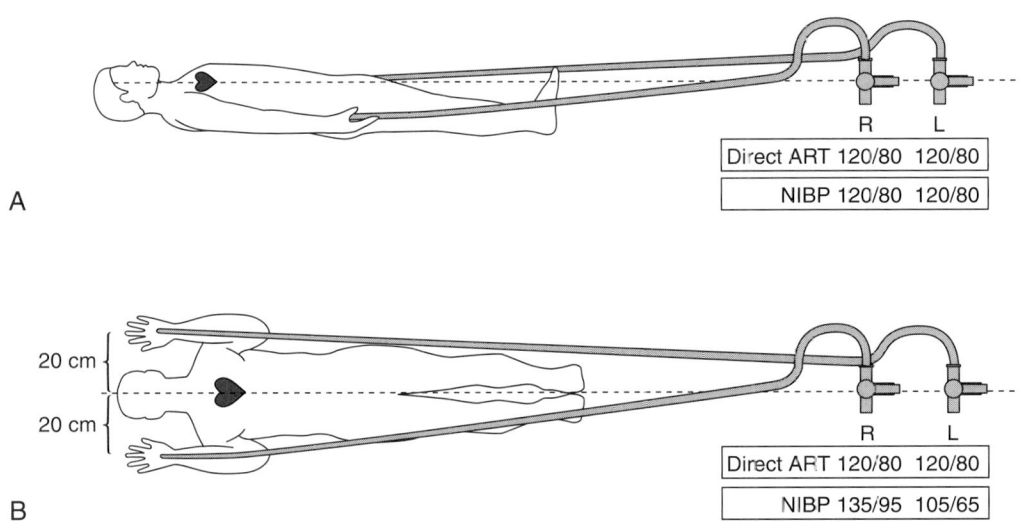

Figure 32–13 Effect of patient position on the relationship between direct arterial blood pressure (ART) and indirect noninvasive blood pressure (NIBP) measurements. **A,** In a supine patient, pressures measured from the right (R) or left (L) arms by either technique will be the same. **B,** In the right lateral decubitus position, ART recorded directly from the right and left radial arteries will remain unchanged as long as the respective pressure transducers remain at heart level. However, NIBP will be higher in the dependent right arm and lower in the nondependent left arm. Differences in NIBP are determined by the positions of the arms above and below the level of the heart and are equal to the hydrostatic pressure differences between the level of the heart and the respective arm. A 20-cm difference in height produces a 15–mm Hg difference in pressure. (Redrawn from Mark JB: Atlas of Cardiovascular Monitoring. New York, Churchill Livingstone, 1998, Fig. 9-22.)

tone (diastolic pressure). Pseudoscience had arrived with (these) numbers.... Even when monitored directly in operating theatres and critical care areas, anesthetists and intensivists show little interest in the waveform and base their judgments on values of systolic, diastolic and mean pressure."[135]

Because clinicians today benefit from the widespread availability of high-resolution, multicolored monitor displays, renewed interest in waveform analysis should expand clinical monitoring capabilities.[74] Appreciation of the diagnostic clues provided by the direct arterial pressure waveform requires full understanding of normal waveform components, their relationship to the cardiac cycle, and differences in waveforms recorded from different sites in the body.

The systemic arterial pressure waveform results from ejection of blood from the left ventricle into the aorta during systole, followed by peripheral arterial runoff of this stroke volume during diastole (Fig. 32-14). The systolic components follow the ECG R wave and consist of a steep pressure upstroke, peak, and decline and correspond to the period of left ventricular systolic ejection. The downslope of the arterial pressure waveform is interrupted by the dicrotic notch, then continues its decline during diastole after the ECG T wave, and reaches its nadir at end-diastole. The dicrotic notch recorded directly from the central aorta is termed the incisura (from the Latin, "a cutting into"). The incisura is sharply defined and is undoubtedly related to aortic valve closure.[136] In contrast, the peripheral arterial waveform generally displays a later, smoother dicrotic notch that only approximates the timing of aortic valve closure and depends more on properties of the arterial wall.[137] Note that the systolic upstroke

of the radial artery pressure trace does not appear for 120 to 180 milliseconds after inscription of the ECG R wave (see Fig. 32-14). This interval reflects the sum of times required for spread of electrical depolarization through the ventricular myocardium, isovolumic left ventricular contraction, opening of the aortic valve, left ventricular ejection, transmission of the aortic pressure wave to the radial artery, and finally, transmission of the pressure signal from the arterial catheter to the pressure transducer.

The bedside monitor displays numeric values for the systolic peak and end-diastolic nadir pressures. Measurement of mean pressure is more complicated and depends on the algorithm used by the monitor.[138] In simplest terms, MAP is equal to the area beneath the arterial pressure curve divided by the beat period and averaged over a series of consecutive heartbeats. Although MAP is often estimated as diastolic pressure plus one third times pulse pressure, this estimation can be misleading. At equivalent heart rates, narrow or thin arterial pressure waveforms spend more time at lower pressures, thereby resulting in low MAP, whereas wide or full arterial pressure waveforms spend more time at higher pressures, thereby resulting in higher MAP.

One of the most important features of the arterial pressure waveform is the phenomenon of *distal pulse amplification*. Pressure waveforms recorded simultaneously from different arterial sites will have different morphologies because of the physical characteristics of the vascular tree, namely, impedance and harmonic resonance (Fig. 32-15).[44,135,139,140] As the arterial pressure wave travels from the central aorta to the periphery, several characteristic changes occur. The arterial upstroke becomes steeper, the systolic peak becomes higher, the dicrotic notch appears later, the diastolic wave becomes more prominent, and end-diastolic pressure becomes lower. Thus, when compared with central aortic pressure, peripheral arterial waveforms have higher systolic pressure, lower diastolic

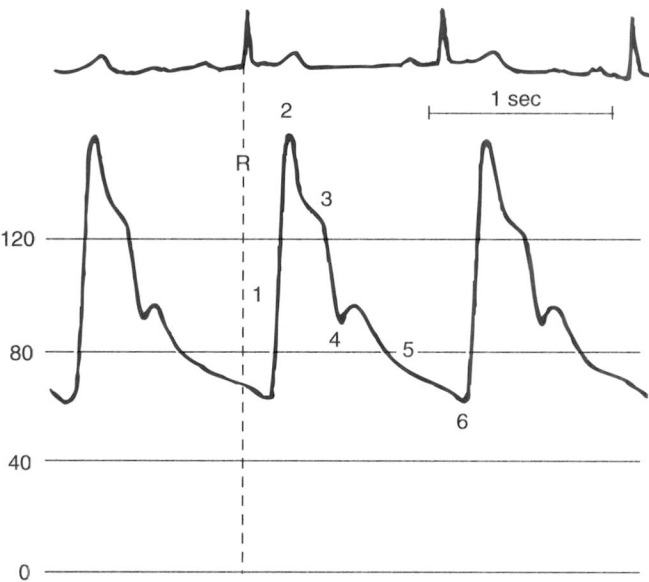

Figure 32–14 Normal arterial blood pressure waveform and its relationship to the electrocardiographic R wave. 1, Systolic upstroke; 2, systolic peak pressure; 3, systolic decline; 4, dicrotic notch; 5, diastolic runoff; 6, end-diastolic pressure. (Redrawn from Mark JB: Atlas of Cardiovascular Monitoring. New York, Churchill Livingstone, 1998, Fig. 8-1.)

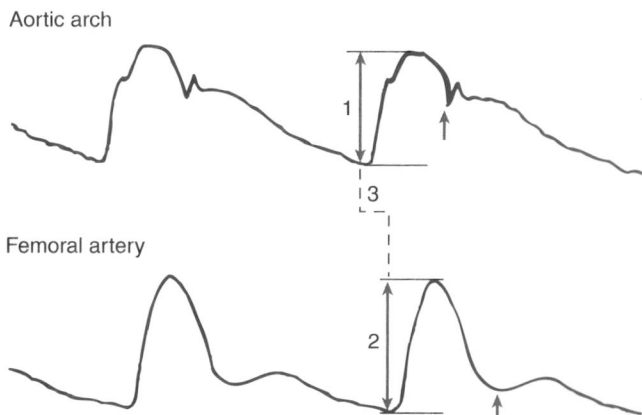

Figure 32–15 Distal pulse wave amplification of the arterial pressure waveform. When compared with pressure in the aortic arch, the more peripherally recorded femoral artery pressure waveform demonstrates a wider pulse pressure (compare 1 and 2), a delayed upstroke (3), a delayed, slurred dicrotic notch (compare short *arrows*), and a more prominent diastolic wave. (Redrawn from Mark JB: Atlas of Cardiovascular Monitoring. New York, Churchill Livingstone, 1998, Fig. 8-4.)

pressure, and wider pulse pressure. Furthermore, there is a delay in arrival of the pressure pulse at peripheral sites, so the systolic pressure upstroke begins approximately 60 milliseconds later in the radial artery than in the aorta. Despite morphologic and temporal differences between peripheral and central arterial waveforms, MAP in the aorta is just slightly greater than that in the radial artery.

Pressure wave reflection is the predominant factor that influences the shape of the arterial pressure waveform as it travels peripherally.[135,139,141-143] As blood flows from the aorta to the radial artery, mean pressure decreases only slightly because of little resistance to flow in the major conducting arteries. At the arteriolar level, mean blood pressure falls markedly as a result of the dramatic increase in vascular resistance at this site. This high resistance to flow diminishes pressure pulsations in small downstream vessels but acts to augment upstream arterial pressure pulses because of pressure wave reflection.[144] These intrinsic vascular phenomena determine the shape of the arterial pulse wave recorded from different sites in the body, in both health and disease. For example, elderly patients have reduced arterial distensibility, which results in early return of reflected pressure waves, increased pulse pressure, a late systolic pressure peak, and disappearance of the diastolic pressure wave (Fig. 32-16).

From these considerations, it becomes evident that the morphology of the arterial waveform and the precise values of systolic and diastolic blood pressure vary throughout the body under normal conditions in otherwise healthy individuals. Perhaps of even greater importance, the relationship between central and peripheral arterial pressure varies with age and is altered by various physiologic changes, pathologic conditions, and pharmacologic interventions.

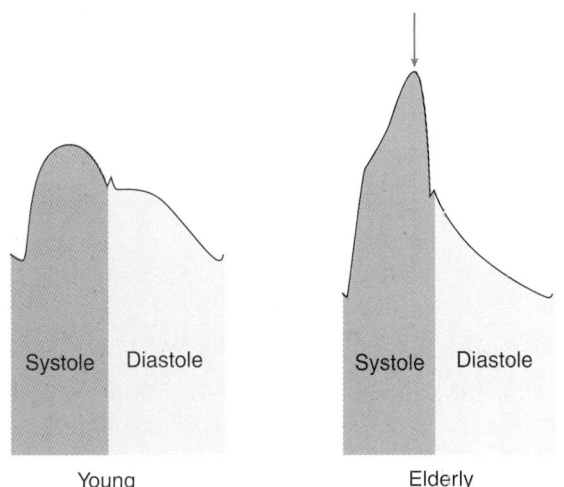

Figure 32–16 Impact of pressure wave reflection on arterial pressure waveforms. In elderly individuals with reduced arterial distensibility, early return of reflected waves increases pulse pressure, produces a late systolic pressure peak *(arrow)*, and attenuates the diastolic pressure wave. Myocardial oxygen balance is more tenuous in the elderly because these changes in blood pressure increase myocardial oxygen demand during systole and reduce myocardial oxygen supply during diastole.

Arterial Blood Pressure Gradients

In addition to the normal physiologic phenomena that exert subtle influences on the arterial pressure waveform, a number of pathophysiologic conditions cause exaggerated arterial pressure gradients in the body. Frank and coworkers demonstrated that 21% of patients undergoing peripheral vascular surgery had a blood pressure difference between the two arms that exceeded 20 mm Hg.[145] In view of the prevalence of this problem, when blood pressure is lower in one arm than the other or when the pulses are weaker on one side, one should never insert an arterial catheter on the side with the weaker pulse because determination of blood pressure from this site will probably underestimate true aortic pressure. In addition to atherosclerosis, other pathologic conditions such as arterial dissection or embolism preclude accurate pressure monitoring from the affected sites.

Unusual patient positions during surgery may produce regional arterial compression, and surgical retraction, particularly during cardiothoracic operations, can produce local vascular compression.[146,147] The nature of the operative procedure is always an important determinant of the appropriate site for arterial pressure monitoring. Operations requiring placement of a descending thoracic aortic cross-clamp may interrupt arterial flow to the left subclavian artery and its tributaries in the left arm, as well as branches of the aorta beyond the clamp. In these cases, blood pressure monitored from the right arm best estimates aortic root pressure and carotid arterial pressure and is used to guide anesthetic management. In addition, pressure may be monitored simultaneously from a femoral artery in an attempt to estimate perfusion pressure to vital organs distal to the aortic cross-clamp.

Various pathophysiologic disturbances may produce generalized arterial pressure gradients in the body and should be considered when choosing a site for arterial pressure monitoring. Large differences in peripheral and central arterial pressure may be seen in patients with shock. Femoral artery systolic pressure may exceed radial artery systolic pressure by more than 50 mm Hg in septic patients who require vasopressor infusions, an observation that has significant therapeutic implications for the management of critically ill patients.[148] Other vasoactive drugs, anesthetics (particularly neuraxial block), and changes in patient temperature produce pressure gradients that alter the relationship between central and peripheral arterial pressure measurements.[44] During hypothermia, thermoregulatory vasoconstriction causes radial arterial systolic pressure to exceed femoral artery systolic pressure, whereas during rewarming, vasodilation reverses this gradient and causes radial artery pressure to underestimate femoral artery pressure.[149]

A similar pressure gradient phenomenon has been described in cardiac surgical patients undergoing cardiopulmonary bypass (Fig. 32-17). Shortly after initiation of cardiopulmonary bypass, mean radial artery pressure is lower than mean femoral artery pressure, and this difference seems to persist during the bypass procedure.[150,151] Furthermore, in the initial minutes after bypass, radial arterial pressure continues to be lower than central aortic pressure, often by more than 20 mm Hg.[152-158] In most patients, these pressure differences persist after bypass for

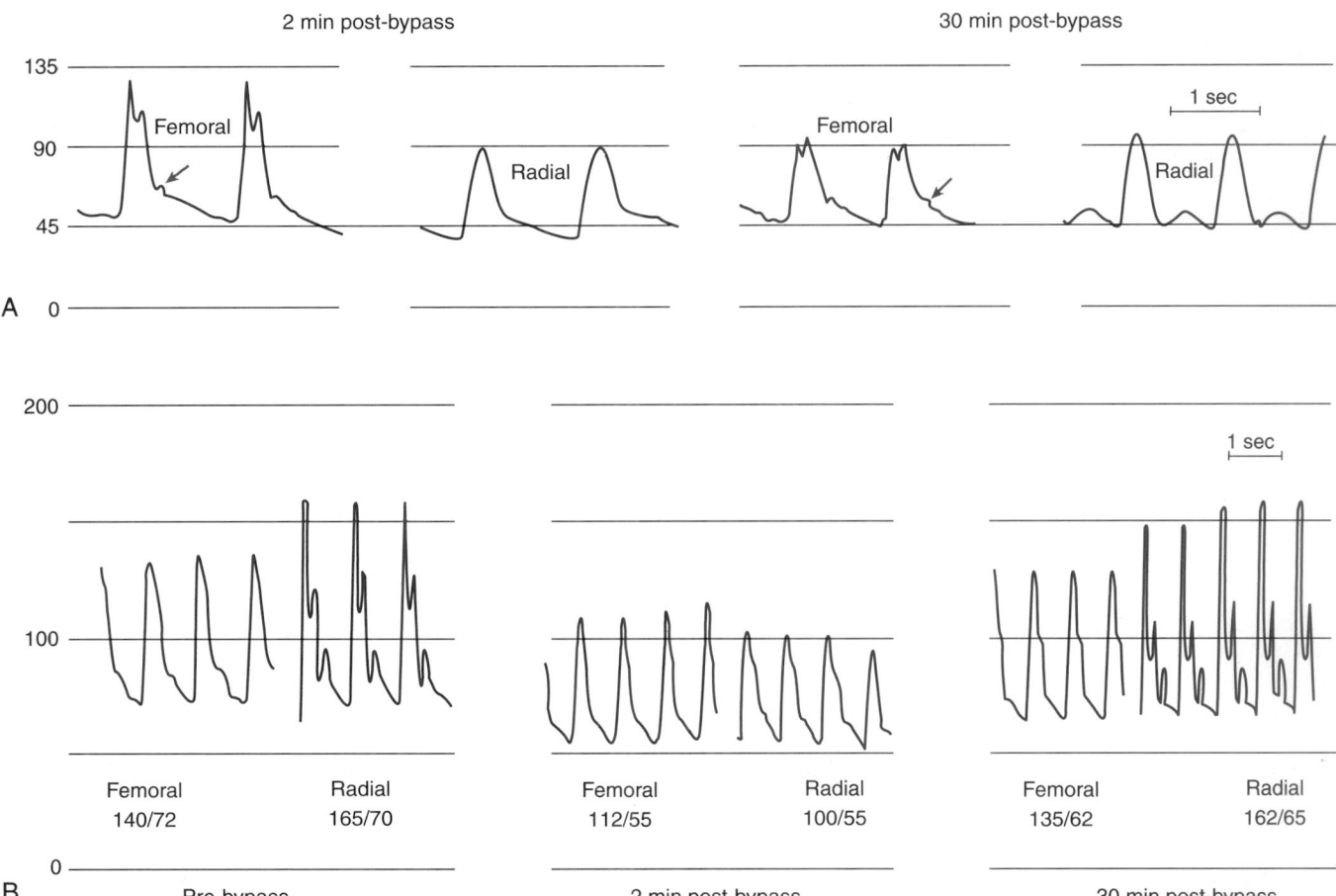

Figure 32–17 Arterial pressure gradients after cardiopulmonary bypass. **A,** Femoral and radial artery pressure traces recorded 2 minutes after bypass, when radial artery pressure underestimates the more centrally measured femoral artery pressure, and 30 minutes after bypass, when radial and femoral arterial pressures have been equalized and radial pressure has assumed a more typical morphology. Note that the dicrotic notch *(arrows)* is visible in the femoral pressure trace after bypass, but not initially in the radial pressure trace. **B,** Femoral and radial artery pressure traces recorded before cardiopulmonary bypass, 2 minutes after bypass, and 30 minutes after bypass. Note the changing relationship between femoral and radial artery pressure measurements at these different times.

only several minutes and resolve within an hour, but occasionally these pressure gradients are still present during the postoperative period. Although acute hemodilution alone does not appear to explain this phenomenon,[159] a number of etiologies have been proposed, including vasodilation and decreased resistance in the forearm and hand vasculature during rewarming on bypass,[152,154-157] radial artery vasoconstriction after aortic cross-clamping,[160] or decreased arterial elasticity.[161] At present, however, the complete mechanism remains unresolved.[158]

Abnormal Arterial Pressure Waveforms (also see Chapter 50)

Detailed examination of the morphologic features of individual arterial pressure waveforms can provide important diagnostic clues to a variety of pathologic conditions (Table 32-4). *Aortic stenosis* produces a fixed obstruction to left ventricular ejection that results in reduced stroke volume and an arterial pressure waveform that rises slowly (*pulsus tardus*) and peaks late in systole (Fig. 32-18). A distinct shoulder, termed the *anacrotic notch,* often distorts the pressure upstroke.[162] In addition, the dicrotic

Table 32–4 Arterial blood pressure waveform abnormalities

Condition	Characteristics
Aortic stenosis	Pulsus parvus (narrow pulse pressure) Pulsus tardus (delayed upstroke)
Aortic regurgitation	Bisferiens pulse (double peak) Wide pulse pressure
Hypertrophic cardiomyopathy	Spike and dome (midsystolic obstruction)
Systolic left ventricular failure	Pulsus alternans (alternating pulse pressure amplitude)
Cardiac tamponade	Pulsus paradoxus (exaggerated decrease in systolic blood pressure during spontaneous inspiration)

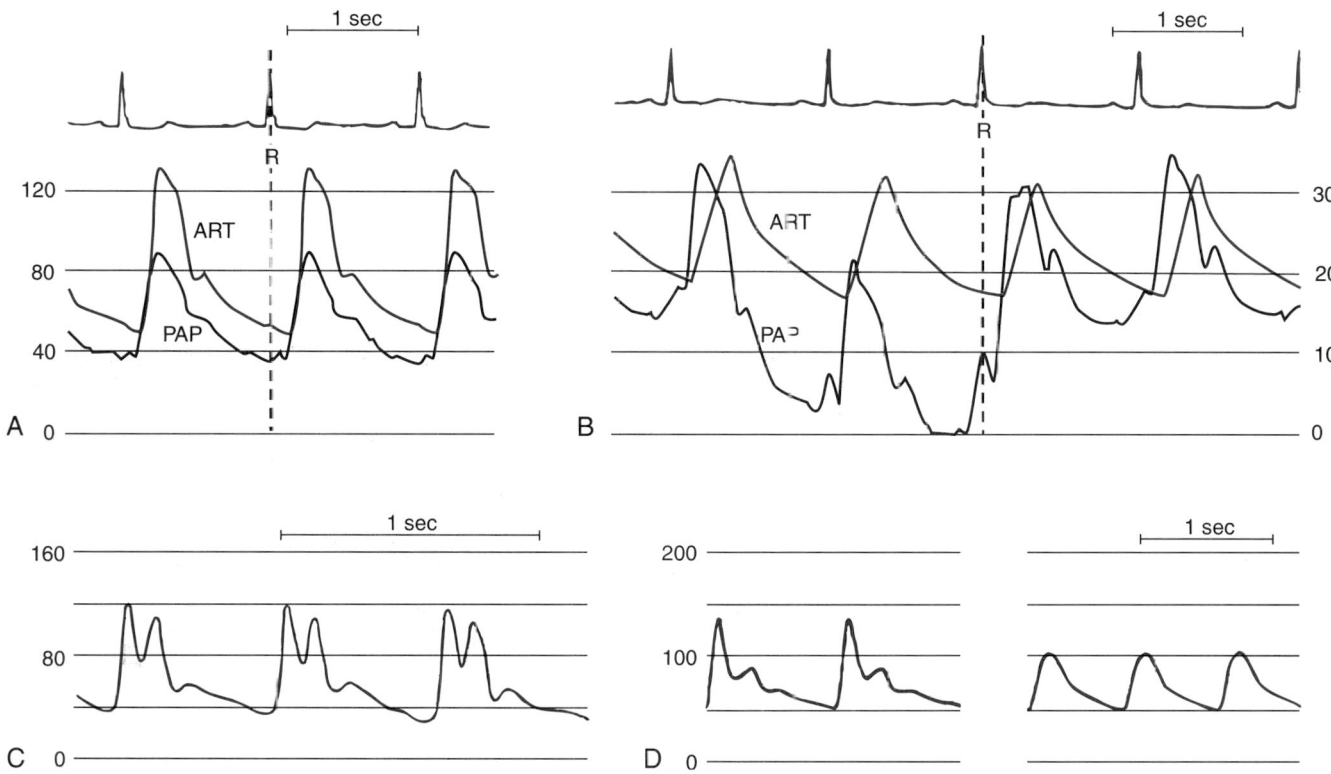

Figure 32–18 Influence of pathologic conditions on arterial pressure (ART) waveform morphology. **A,** Normal ART and pulmonary artery pressure (PAP) waveform morphologies demonstrating the similar timing of these waveforms relative to the electrocardiographic R wave. **B,** In aortic stenosis, the ART waveform is distorted and has a slurred upstroke and delayed systolic peak. These changes are particularly striking in comparison to the normal PAP waveform. Note the beat-to-beat respiratory variation in the PAP waveform. See the text for greater detail. For **A** and **B,** the ART scale is on the *left* and the PAP scale is on the *right*. **C,** Aortic regurgitation produces a bisferiens pulse and a wide pulse pressure. See the text for greater detail. **D,** An arterial pressure waveform in a patient with hypertrophic cardiomyopathy shows a peculiar "spike-and-dome" configuration. The pressure waveform assumes a more normal morphology after surgical correction of this condition. (Redrawn from Mark JB: Atlas of Cardiovascular Monitoring. New York, Churchill Livingstone, 1998, Figs. 3-3, 17-21, and 17-24.)

notch may not be discernible and the arterial pressure is small in amplitude *(pulsus parvus)*. All these features make the arterial pressure waveform appear overdamped, in contrast to the normal arterial pressure waveform, which has a sharp upstroke and distinct dicrotic notch.

In *aortic regurgitation,* the arterial pressure wave displays a sharp rise, wide pulse pressure, and low diastolic pressure as a result of runoff of blood into the left ventricle and the periphery during diastole. Because of the large stroke volume ejected from the left ventricle in this condition, the arterial pressure pulse may have two systolic peaks *(bisferiens pulse)* (see Fig. 32-18). These two peaks represent separate percussion and tidal waves, with the former resulting from left ventricular ejection and the latter arising from the periphery as a reflected wave.[162] The bisferiens pulse is also described in patients with mixed aortic regurgitation and stenosis and in those with hypertrophic cardiomyopathy, although the physiologic basis is different in the latter condition. In *hypertrophic cardiomyopathy,* the arterial pressure waveform assumes a peculiar bifid shape termed a "spike-and-dome" configuration. After an initial sharp pressure upstroke that results from rapid left ventricular ejection in early systole, arterial pressure falls rapidly as dynamic left ventricular outflow obstruction develops during midsystole, and a late

systolic reflected wave follows, thereby creating the characteristic double-peaked waveform (see Fig. 32-18).[162,163]

Observation of arterial waveform patterns over consecutive heartbeats provides an additional set of diagnostic clues. *Pulsus alternans* is recognized by the alternating beats of larger and smaller pulse pressures (Fig. 32-19). In general, it is considered to be a sign of severe left ventricular systolic dysfunction, often noted in patients with advanced aortic stenosis. It may be seen occasionally during general anesthesia, presumably as a consequence of the anesthetic-induced reduction in sympathetic nervous system activity in patients with underlying impairment in left ventricular contractility.[164] Pulsus alternans should be distinguished from the bigeminal pulse that arises from a bigeminal rhythm, usually ventricular bigeminy. Both abnormalities create an alternating pulse pressure in the arterial pressure waveform, but the rhythm is regular in pulsus alternans.

Pulsus paradoxus is an exaggerated inspiratory fall in systolic arterial pressure that exceeds 10 to 12 mm Hg during quiet breathing (see Fig. 32-19).[162,165,166] The term may be confusing because a small inspiratory reduction in blood pressure is a normal phenomenon, and pulsus paradoxus is not truly paradoxical, but rather an exaggeration of this normal inspiratory decline in blood pressure.

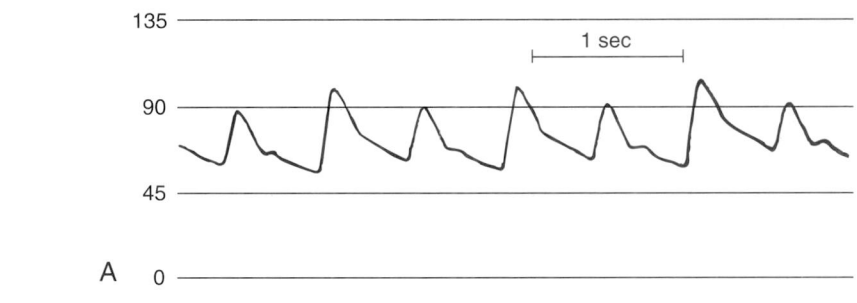

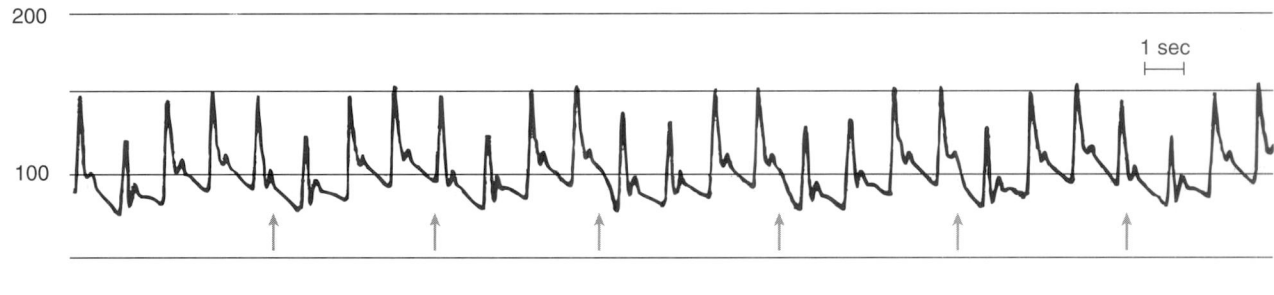

Figure 32–19 Beat-to-beat variability in arterial pressure waveform morphologies. **A,** Pulsus alternans. **B,** Pulsus paradoxus. The marked decline in systolic arterial pressure and pulse pressure during spontaneous inspiration *(arrows)* is characteristic of this condition. (Redrawn from Mark JB: Atlas of Cardiovascular Monitoring. New York, Churchill Livingstone, 1998, Fig. 18-10.)

Pulsus paradoxus is a characteristic, almost universal finding in cardiac tamponade and occurs in many patients with pericardial constriction. It is said to occur in patients with airway obstruction, bronchospasm, dyspnea, or any condition characterized by large swings in intrathoracic pressure. However, in cardiac tamponade, the pulse pressure and left ventricular stroke volume decrease during inspiration, in contrast to the blood pressure changes observed in patients with forced breathing patterns and exaggerated changes in intrathoracic pressure in which pulse pressure is relatively unchanged.[167]

The arterial pressure waveform provides diagnostic clues in other more unusual physiologic states. Proper timing of *intra-aortic balloon counterpulsation* mandates detailed interpretation of the arterial waveform (Fig. 32-20).[168] Even during nonpulsatile *cardiopulmonary bypass,* the minor variations in blood pressure created by the arterial roller head allow calculation and confirmation of the adequacy of systemic blood flow (see Fig. 32-20).[169]

CENTRAL VENOUS PRESSURE MONITORING

Indirect assessment of CVP through physical examination of the neck veins is a fundamental aspect of cardiovascular assessment, but one that has many shortcomings. One real anatomic limitation to the physical assessment of jugular venous pulsations results from the presence of competent venous valves that exist in the internal jugular veins of most individuals. These valves are located approximately 0.5 to 2.0 cm above the junction of the

internal jugular and subclavian veins bilaterally and withstand backpressures of 50 to 100 cm H_2O.[170-173] When CVP is increased, these valves are either incompetent or absent, particularly in patients with chronic severe tricuspid valve regurgitation.[173] In addition, the jugular veins may be impossible to identify in 20% of patients, and the bedside diagnosis of low, normal, or high CVP is often inaccurate, particularly in critically ill patients.[174-176] These general problems are compounded in the perioperative period, when visualization of the neck veins is further obscured and acute, large changes in CVP occur in many patients. As a result, direct measurement of CVP is performed frequently in hemodynamically unstable patients and those undergoing major operations.

Central Venous Cannulation

Cannulation of a large central vein is the standard clinical method for monitoring CVP and is also performed for a number of additional therapeutic interventions, such as providing secure vascular access for the administration of vasoactive drugs or to initiate rapid fluid resuscitation. Frequently, the central venous location is the only site available for intravenous access of any kind. Patients at risk for venous air emboli may have central venous catheters placed for aspiration of entrained air. Central venous access is required to initiate transvenous cardiac pacing, temporary hemodialysis, or pulmonary artery catheterization for more comprehensive cardiac monitoring (Table 32-5).

In certain patients, such as those with ischemic heart disease, the cardiovascular consequences of pain or anxiety

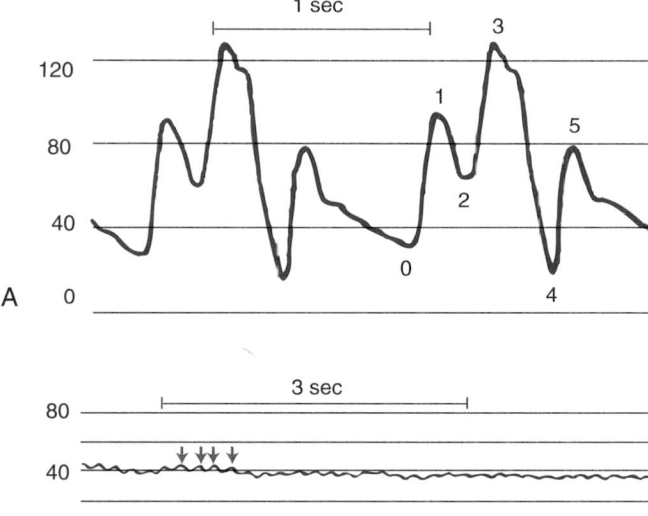

Figure 32–20 Unusual arterial pressure waveforms. **A,** Intra-aortic balloon counterpulsation with a 1:2 balloon-assist ratio produces a characteristic change in the arterial pressure waveform. Four cardiac cycles are shown, two with balloon assistance and two without. 0, Unassisted end-diastolic pressure; 1, unassisted systolic pressure; 2, dicrotic notch; 3, assisted or augmented diastolic pressure; 4, end-diastolic or presystolic dip; 5, assisted systolic pressure. Effective afterload reduction by the intra-aortic balloon is demonstrated by the presystolic dip pressure (4) lower than the unassisted end-diastolic pressure (0) and the assisted systolic pressure peak (5) lower than the unassisted systolic pressure peak (1). **B,** Arterial pressure waveform during cardio-pulmonary bypass. Small phasic pressure variations *(arrows)* result from the mechanical action of the bypass roller pump. The bypass pump flow rate may be estimated by measuring these pulsations. Nineteen pulsations are recorded in a 3-second time interval. In this case, the pump configured with $^3/_8$-inch tubing has an effective stroke volume of 27 mL. The pump flow rate may be calculated as follows: (19 pulsations/3 seconds) × (1 pump revolution/2 pulsations) × (27 mL/revolution) × (60 sec/min) = 5130 mL/min. This calculated pump flow rate should equal the flow rate displayed on the pump console (i.e., 5.2 L/min). (Redrawn from Mark JB: Atlas of Cardiovascular Monitoring. New York, Churchill Livingstone, 1998, Figs. 20-3 and 19-8.)

Table 32–5   Indications for central venous cannulation
Central venous pressure monitoring
Pulmonary artery catheterization and monitoring
Transvenous cardiac pacing
Temporary hemodialysis
Drug administration
Concentrated vasoactive drugs
Hyperalimentation
Chemotherapy
Drugs irritating to peripheral veins
Prolonged antibiotic therapy (e.g., endocarditis)
Rapid infusion of fluids (through large cannulas)
Trauma
Major surgery
Aspiration of air emboli
Inadequate peripheral intravenous access
Sampling site for repeated blood testing

during central venous or arterial cannulation may produce untoward hemodynamic changes.[177] Although some authors advocate postponing central venous catheterization until general anesthesia is established,[178] this option is not practical in critically ill patients in intensive care or in surgical patients who will not receive general anesthesia. Furthermore, pain-free vascular cannulation before induction of anesthesia is easily achieved through the use of adequate local anesthesia, intravenous sedatives, and careful patient observation.[179,180] In the end, the decision to perform central venous cannulation before or after induction of anesthesia is guided most often by individual patient and physician preferences or institutional practices. One should consider abandoning attempts at preoperative central venous cannulation in any patient who becomes overly sedated or uncooperative during the procedure, proceed with anesthetic induction and tracheal intubation as planned, and then gain central vascular access under more controlled circumstances.

Right Internal Jugular Vein Cannulation (also see CD Rom)

Many different techniques for internal jugular vein cannulation have been described, although the "central" approach described by Daily and colleagues is among the most popular and is described with minor modifications here.[181] Careful positioning will make the patient comfortable, improve identification of surface landmarks, and increase the likelihood of successful venipuncture. The patient is placed in the supine position with the head turned slightly to the left to expose the right side of the neck and keep the chin from interfering with the procedure. Pillows that cause the neck to be flexed should be removed, but forceful neck extension or extreme leftward rotation of the head should be avoided because this may alter cervical vascular anatomy, cause the internal jugular vein to overlie the carotid artery, and increase the risk of puncture of the carotid artery.[182]

Anatomic landmarks, including the sternal notch, clavicle, and sternocleidomastoid muscle, should be assessed before preparation and draping for the sterile procedure because these landmarks are better appreciated before they are covered by the sterile drape (Fig. 32-21). The carotid artery should be palpated and its course determined; it lies lateral to the trachea, usually under the more medial sternal head of the sternocleidomastoid muscle. The internal jugular vein lies in the groove between the sternal and clavicular heads of the sternocleidomastoid muscle, lateral and slightly anterior to the carotid artery. In many patients, venous pulsations from the internal jugular vein are observed directly within this groove and further identify the approximate site for venipuncture.

The patient should be calm, sedated, receiving supplemental oxygen if necessary, and monitored with an ECG, blood pressure monitor, and pulse oximeter. Because of the frequency and serious morbidity of infectious complications from central venous catheterization, strict aseptic technique is required. Formal guidelines to reduce these complications have been published by the Centers for Disease Control and Prevention and provide prudent recommendations that should be followed during all but the most emergent catheterizations.[183,184]

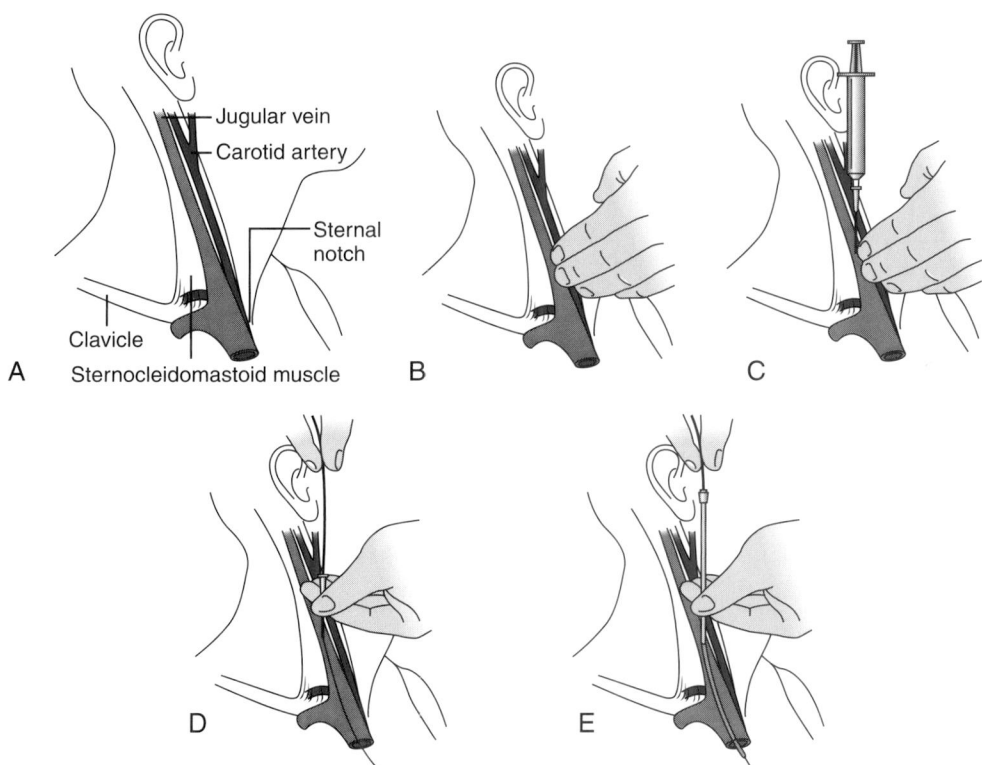

Figure 32–21 Technique for central venous cannulation of the right internal jugular vein. **A,** Important surface landmarks are identified. **B,** The course of the internal carotid artery is palpated. **C,** The internal jugular vein is punctured at the apex of the triangle formed by the two heads of the sternocleidomastoid muscle, with the needle tip directed toward the ipsilateral nipple. **D,** A guidewire is introduced through the thin-walled needle into the vein. **E,** The central venous cannula is inserted over the guidewire while making sure that the proximal end of the guidewire protrudes beyond the catheter and is controlled by the operator.

Good aseptic technique begins with hand washing before the procedure. A mask, cap, sterile gloves, and gown should always be used, even when placing the catheter in the operating room. The skin is cleansed widely from earlobe to clavicle to sternal notch with an appropriate antiseptic. Recent evidence suggests that 2% chlorhexidine may be preferred over the more widely used 10% povidone-iodine solution.[183,185] A meta-analysis showed a 50% reduction in bloodstream infection when chlorhexidine was used for skin disinfection rather than povidone-iodine.[186] The aseptic preparation is completed with the application of a large sterile drape that provides maximal barrier precautions.

Under these sterile conditions, the relevant anatomy is again identified, particularly the course of the carotid artery in the neck. An assistant then places the patient in a slight head-down (Trendelenburg) position to increase the diameter of the jugular vein in the neck. This step is occasionally omitted in a hypervolemic, dyspneic patient. The intended venipuncture site is anesthetized by subcutaneous infiltration of a local anesthetic solution (typically 1% lidocaine) with a 25- or 26-gauge needle. The local anesthetic wheal should be generous enough to allow pain-free suturing of the catheter insertion point at the end of the procedure.

With the fingers of the left hand gently resting on the carotid artery pulse as a valuable anatomic landmark, venipuncture then proceeds with a 22-gauge, 1½-inch

(3.8-cm) finger needle mounted on a 5-mL syringe (see Fig. 32-21). The needle is inserted at the apex of the triangle formed by the two heads of the sternocleidomastoid muscle, at an angle of approximately 30 degrees from the plane of the skin, and directed at the ipsilateral nipple. Gentle aspiration will identify the jugular vein when dark venous blood enters the syringe. Even though use of the small finder needle is an extra step in this procedure, it presumably increases the margin of safety[187] because unintentional puncture of the carotid artery with this small needle is less likely to result in significant bleeding and hematoma formation. Although blood may have been aspirated earlier during injection of the local anesthetic, the color of the blood may not be appreciated when it mixes with the local anesthetic solution, thereby making it difficult to distinguish venous from arterial blood. Thus, it is important that the finder needle be attached to an empty syringe during this step.

If blood is not aspirated as the finder needle is advanced and then withdrawn, additional needle passes may locate the internal jugular vein by fanning laterally in a small arc from the point where the needle enters the skin. As long as the carotid artery remains palpable medially, exploring in an orderly fashion with the finder needle directed slightly more laterally will often identify the vein with little risk of carotid artery puncture. If the vein is not located after several needle passes, the finder needle is withdrawn completely and checked for patency, the anatomy is reassessed, and the puncture may then proceed with the needle entering the skin several millimeters closer to the palpated carotid pulse but still directed in a sagittal or slightly lateral direction. One should resist the temptation to explore with a medial or leftward direction of the finder needle when this technique is being used because such exploration will increase the likelihood of unintentional carotid artery puncture.

After the internal jugular vein is located with the finder needle, the needle is gently withdrawn while the skin and surface anatomy remain fixed by the left hand. The vein is then punctured with an 18-gauge, 2½-inch (6.4 cm) thin-walled needle attached to a 5-mL syringe directed along the same track used by the finder needle while keeping in mind the location and depth of the identified internal jugular vein. It is common for the lumen of the jugular vein to be compressed as this larger thin-walled needle is advanced, and as a result, the needle pierces both front and back walls almost simultaneously.[188,189] Accordingly, the thin-walled needle should be inserted only slightly beyond the expected depth of the vein and then slowly withdrawn while maintaining gentle aspiration on the syringe. Frequently, venous entry of the needle is recognized during needle withdrawal by the sudden return of free-flowing venous blood.

Once successful venipuncture is confirmed by free aspiration of dark venous blood into the 5-mL syringe, the hub of the thin-walled needle is fixed with the fingers of the left hand, the syringe is detached, and venous blood should be observed to drip from the needle hub. A guidewire (generally 0.032 or 0.035 inch) is inserted through the needle by using either the J-shaped tip or the soft, flexible straight end. The wire should advance easily into the vein with little resistance. The ECG is monitored continuously to detect arrhythmias, which are common if the wire tip contacts the walls of the right atrium or ventricle.[190] From this point in the procedure, it is critical that the clinician maintain control over the guidewire and pay attention to its depth of insertion and continued sterility.

The puncture site is enlarged with a No. 11 scalpel blade to the size required for the intended catheter. A firm, tapered-tip vessel dilator may be inserted to dilate the subcutaneous tissues around the guidewire and allow a larger catheter to pass more smoothly. (When an introducer sheath is to be used for internal jugular vein cannulation, the dilator and sheath form one unit, and this separate dilation step is usually omitted.) The vessel dilator is removed, and the central venous catheter is inserted over the guidewire while traction on the skin is maintained. Again, the clinician must be attentive to the guidewire and ensure that a sufficient length protrudes from the catheter hub so that the wire may be extracted easily. The catheter is inserted to an appropriate depth that will place the tip in the superior vena cava, above its junction with the right atrium. This depth is typically 15 to 18 cm if the catheter is placed with the technique described.

Finally, the guidewire is withdrawn, the catheter is attached by a Luer-Lock connector to the monitoring or infusion tubing and sutured in place, and sterile gauze or transparent dressing is applied. Antibiotic ointment should not be applied to the insertion site because of the possibility of increasing the risk of catheter colonization with multidrug-resistant bacteria or *Candida*.[183,184,191]

Central venous catheters placed in the operating room are generally used for the duration of the surgical procedure without first confirming the location of the catheter tip radiographically. Before monitoring or infusion commences, aspiration of blood should confirm the intravenous location of each lumen of a multilumen catheter and remove any residual air from the catheter-tubing system. After surgery, however, the position of the catheter tip must always be confirmed radiographically. Catheter tips located within the heart or below the pericardial reflection on the superior vena cava increase the risk of cardiac perforation and fatal cardiac tamponade. Ideally, the catheter tip should lie within the superior vena cava, parallel to the vessel walls, and be positioned *below* the inferior border of the clavicles and *above* the level of the third rib, the T4 to T5 interspace, the azygos vein, the tracheal carina, or the takeoff of the right main stem bronchus.[192,193] Using fresh human cadavers, Albrecht and colleagues recently confirmed that the tracheal carina was always above the pericardial reflection on the superior vena cava, thus suggesting that catheter tips should always be located superior to this radiographic landmark.[194]

Choosing the Method, Catheter, and Site for Central Venous Cannulation

Since its introduction into clinical practice in the late 1960s,[181,195,196] percutaneous venipuncture of the right internal jugular vein has been the method preferred by anesthesiologists for central venous cannulation.[197] Reasons for this preference include the consistent, predictable anatomic location of the internal jugular vein; readily identified, palpable surface landmarks; and a short, straight course to the superior vena cava, which facilitates right heart catheterization. An internal jugular vein catheter is more accessible intraoperatively to the anesthesiologist, who is most often working at the patient's head, and perhaps of greatest importance, vascular cannulation is highly successful, generally reported in the 90% to 99% range.[197-199]

Numerous techniques have been described for percutaneous internal jugular vein cannulation.[200-202] Although it is unlikely that one single method will lead to the greatest success rate in the hands of all clinicians, it appears that certain techniques may result in a higher incidence of unintentional carotid artery puncture.[201] It seems prudent, therefore, to determine the location of the carotid pulse before attempted jugular vein cannulation and to continue to palpate the pulse gently during the initial steps of venipuncture while being careful to avoid excessive pressure that may compress the jugular vein. A right-handed operator easily does this, but continued palpation of the carotid artery during jugular venipuncture is awkward when a left-handed individual is performing the procedure. In this instance, it is best to evaluate the course of the carotid artery before, but not during the venipuncture.

Other adjunctive measures should be considered in an attempt to reduce complications during central venous cannulation, particularly the frequency of carotid arterial puncture during attempted internal jugular cannulation. Many individuals substitute a 2-inch, 18-gauge intravenous catheter for the 18-gauge thin-walled needle for venipuncture and guidewire placement. Although this catheter can be advanced completely into the vein, it becomes kinked more easily than a needle, thereby making it more difficult to recognize pulsatile arterial blood flow from unintentional arterial puncture. To confirm the intravenous location of this catheter, several things may be done. The color of the aspirated blood is examined, and it may be compared with a simultaneously obtained arterial sample or even sent for blood gas analysis. A more practical, quicker, and simpler method is to transduce the pressure from the 18-gauge catheter[203] or attach a sterile intravenous extension tubing set to create a simple vertical fluid manometer to estimate the pressure and distinguish arterial from venous catheterization.[204] Continuous pressure transduction of the thin-walled needle has been advocated as an even better method to detect arterial puncture and prevent arterial cannulation because the needle will not kink and thereby provide a misleading pressure waveform.[199,205] Although none of these measures are foolproof, they may provide a margin of safety and reduce the serious complications resulting from unintentional cannulation of the carotid artery with a large-bore catheter.

Widespread adoption of guidewire-based vascular cannulation methods has undoubtedly increased the safety of central venous cannulation. These techniques, originally described by Seldinger,[206] allow initial vascular puncture with a smaller-gauge needle, followed by guidewire placement and subsequent vessel dilation and cannulation with a large-bore catheter.[207] This method has virtually replaced the "catheter through the needle" method, which requires vascular puncture with a needle larger than the catheter and results in more complications from cannulation site hemorrhage and shearing of the catheter if it is withdrawn inappropriately through the insertion needle. Some central venous catheter insertion kits contain a modified syringe that allows the guidewire to be placed directly through the syringe plunger without disconnecting the syringe from the thin-walled needle. However, when this technique is used, one of the most valuable signs of unintentional arterial puncture is virtually impossible to recognize—namely, the pulsatile return of bright red blood through the thin-walled needle. Failure to recognize this sign may lead to erroneous arterial placement of a central venous catheter.[208]

Central venous catheters come in a variety of lengths, gauges, compositions, and lumen numbers.[209,210] These features vary according to the purpose of catheterization, whether for CVP monitoring or other therapeutic needs and whether intended for short- or long-term use. It is therefore critical that the physician choose the best catheter for any given application and thereby reduce risk to the patient caused by improper catheter selection. Although multilumen catheters are very popular because they allow simultaneous continuous pressure monitoring and fluid or drug infusion, their use has been associated with a greater risk of infection than has the use of single-lumen catheters.[184] Furthermore, multilumen catheters may have a greater propensity than single-lumen catheters to cause vascular perforation because more septations and stiffer plastic are required in the manufacturing process of a multilumen catheter.[209] A popular alternative

method for multilumen central venous access involves the use of a sidearm introducer sheath attached to a series of stopcocks for multiple drug infusions, with a single-lumen catheter inserted through the hemostasis valve used for simultaneous continuous CVP monitoring. Although the use of these larger introducer sheaths is not free from complications, they allow rapid placement of a pacing wire or pulmonary artery catheter for more intensive monitoring without the need for additional central venipunctures or catheter exchanges over a guidewire.

In patients at risk for major intraoperative blood loss and hemodynamic instability, two central venous catheters are frequently inserted. Some physicians advocate double cannulation of the same central vein (usually the right internal jugular) with two catheters in close proximity. In this technique, a guidewire is introduced into the internal jugular vein by the standard method. Then, before catheter placement, a second jugular venipuncture is performed, approximately 1 to 2 cm cephalad or caudad, and a second guidewire is introduced into the vein. Placing appropriate catheters over each guidewire and securing them at the skin in normal fashion completes the procedure. Limited evidence suggests that the incidence of major complications with this double-cannulation technique is no greater than with single central venous catheterization, although arrhythmias may be more common because of unintentional intracardiac placement of the guidewires.[211] However, it is not clear whether this approach is safer than central venous cannulation in two separate central veins. Serious reported complications of the double-cannulation technique include facial vein avulsion, catheter entanglement, and catheter fracture.[211-213] Double central venous cannulation must be reserved for patients whose needs for venous access and hemodynamic monitoring cannot be met through single cannulation.

Selecting the best site for safe and effective central venous cannulation ultimately requires that the physician consider the purpose of catheterization (pressure monitoring versus drug or fluid infusion), the patient's underlying medical condition, the intended operation, and the skill and experience of the physician performing the procedure. In patients with severe bleeding diatheses, it is best to choose a puncture site where bleeding from the vein or adjacent artery is easily detected and controlled with local compression. In this instance, an external jugular approach would be preferred over infraclavicular subclavian catheterization. Patients with severe emphysema or other patients who would be severely compromised by pneumothorax would be better candidates for right internal jugular cannulation than subclavian cannulation because of the higher risk of pneumothorax with the latter approach. If transvenous cardiac pacing were required in an emergency situation, catheterization of the right internal jugular vein is recommended because it provides the most direct course to the right ventricle. Trauma patients with their necks immobilized in a hard cervical collar are best resuscitated with the use of femoral or subclavian cannulas; the latter may be placed even more safely if the risk of pneumothorax is obviated by previous placement of thoracostomy tubes. The physician must recognize that the length of catheter inserted to position the catheter tip properly in the superior vena cava will vary according to the puncture site, being slightly (3 to 5 cm) greater when the left internal or external jugular veins are chosen versus the right internal jugular vein.[214] Finally, a physician's personal experience undoubtedly plays a significant role in determining the safest site for central venous cannulation, particularly when the procedure is performed under urgent or emergency circumstances.

Ultrasound-Guided Central Venous Cannulation

To increase the success and decrease the complications of central venous cannulation, different ultrasound-guided techniques have been described for cannulating the internal jugular vein,[215-218] subclavian vein,[219-222] and femoral vein.[223] Some methods use devices incorporated into the sterile field that provide real-time, two-dimensional ultrasound images of the pertinent vascular anatomy, particularly the relationship between the target vein and its adjacent artery. Alternatively, when a diagnostic echocardiograph machine is already available in the operating room, a standard short-focus surface transducer can be used to image the vascular anatomy (Fig. 32-22). Intraoperative transesophageal echocardiography has been advocated to guide central venous catheterization for congenital heart surgery.[224] Finally, Doppler-based nonimaging techniques provide a real-time, audible Doppler signal to guide venous cannulation based on distinguishing the continuous audible hum of the vein from the pulsatile signal of the artery.

In general, these ultrasound-guided techniques appear to have several advantages. Invariably, with ultrasound assistance, fewer needle passes are required for successful venous cannulation. In addition, most investigators have shown that ultrasound guidance reduces the time required for catheterization, increases overall success rates, and results in fewer complications.[225,226] In one of the largest controlled trials, Denys and coworkers used dedicated two-dimensional real-time imaging to cannulate the internal jugular vein in more than 900 patients and found that

ultrasound-guided cannulation was successful in all patients and reduced the risk of carotid artery puncture (1.7% versus 8.3%), brachial plexus irritation (0.4% versus 1.7%), and hematoma (0.2% versus 3.3%) when compared with landmark-guided techniques.[216]

Most published studies support the use of ultrasound guidance during central venous cannulation, and a recent report from the Agency for Healthcare Research and Quality advocates more widespread adoption of this practice.[226] Nonetheless, many of these procedures are still performed with landmark-based techniques because of the relatively high success rate and low morbidity of this procedure when performed by experienced individuals, the additional cost and perceived inconvenience of acquiring and using an ultrasound device, and concern that reliance on ultrasound-guided catheterization will prevent trainees from acquiring adequate skills for landmark-based central venous cannulation.

Notwithstanding these concerns, ultrasound studies have disclosed several important anatomic and technical insights that should lead to improved central venous cannulation in all patients, regardless of the technique used. The large central veins are readily distinguished from their accompanying arteries by their lack of pulsatility, marked enlargement during a Valsalva maneuver, and easy compressibility with the ultrasound probe. This provides several lessons for landmark-based venipuncture. When the internal jugular vein is not located easily with the finder needle, the clinician can increase the venous target size markedly by asking the patient to perform a Valsalva maneuver. In contrast, jugular venipuncture will be much more difficult if the vein is compressed during overzealous attempts to palpate and localize the carotid artery. Ultrasound imaging has demonstrated that both the subclavian[219] and internal jugular[216] veins are actually compressed, before vessel entry, by the cannulating needle as it advances. This observation explains the common clinical finding that venipuncture is recognized as often during needle withdrawal as during needle advancement. Furthermore, ultrasonography demonstrates that in a significant number of patients, the internal jugular vein lies directly over the carotid artery,[227,228] thereby increasing the risk of carotid artery puncture unless the needle is directed more laterally or lower in the neck where the internal jugular vein assumes a more lateral location.[215] Ultrasound-guided techniques may be particularly useful for increasing the success rate and decreasing complications when less experienced individuals and trainees perform central venous cannulation.[216,219] Perhaps of greatest importance, ultrasound-guided central venous cannulation provides a method to salvage the procedure when landmark-based methods are unsuccessful, thus making its use particularly attractive in high-risk patients in whom the clinician anticipates difficulty with vascular access.[216,218,219]

Alternative Central Venous Cannulation Sites

Left Internal Jugular Vein

Left internal jugular vein cannulation may be accomplished with a technique similar to the one described earlier for the right internal jugular vein, although several anatomic details make the left side less attractive than the right.

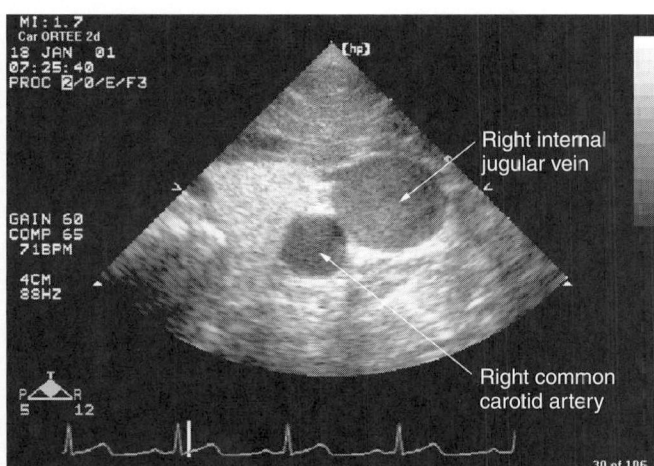

Figure 32–22 Transverse-plane ultrasound image showing the right internal jugular vein and its typical anatomic position anterior and lateral to the right common carotid artery.

The cupola of the pleura is higher on the left, which theoretically increases the risk of pneumothorax. The thoracic duct may be injured during venipuncture because it enters the venous system at the junction of the left internal jugular and subclavian veins.[229] The left internal jugular vein is often smaller than the right and demonstrates a greater degree of overlap of the adjacent carotid artery during head rotation. Catheters inserted from the left side of the patient must traverse the innominate (i.e., left brachiocephalic) vein and enter the superior vena cava perpendicularly, and their distal tips may impinge on the right lateral wall of the superior vena cava, thereby increasing the risk of vascular injury. (This anatomic disadvantage pertains to all left-sided catheterization sites and highlights the need for radiographic confirmation of proper catheter location.) In addition, because clinicians cannulate the left internal jugular vein much less often than the right, it is not surprising that cannulation of the left internal jugular vein is more difficult, more time consuming, and associated with more complications than right internal jugular cannulation is.[182,230]

Subclavian Vein

The subclavian vein is an important site for central venous cannulation and is particularly popular among surgeons and other physicians who place central venous catheters for emergency volume resuscitation and long-term intravenous therapy rather than for shorter-term monitoring purposes.[222,231,232] Advantages of subclavian venous cannulation include a lower risk of infection than with internal jugular or femoral sites,[183,184,233,234] ease of insertion in trauma patients who may be immobilized in a cervical collar, and increased patient comfort, especially for long-term intravenous therapy such as hyperalimentation and chemotherapy.

The most common technique used for subclavian vein cannulation is the infraclavicular approach.[232] The patient is placed in a slight head-down position with the arms fully adducted, the head is turned slightly away from the side of venipuncture, and a small bedroll is placed between the shoulder blades to fully expose the infraclavicular area. The skin is punctured 2 to 3 cm caudad to the midpoint of the clavicle, far enough from its inferior edge to avoid downward angulation of the needle as it is inserted just beneath the posterior surface of the clavicle. The needle tip is directed toward the suprasternal notch, which may be constantly identified by the fingers of the operator's other hand. If the subclavian vein is not entered in the first pass, the needle may be withdrawn and a second pass attempted in a slightly more cephalad direction while ensuring that the needle continues to hug the undersurface of the clavicle as it is advanced. Once the subclavian vein is punctured, catheterization proceeds in a manner similar to that described for jugular vein catheterization.

Several important technical details must be followed to ensure successful subclavian vein cannulation and avoid complications, particularly pneumothorax. Venipuncture generally proceeds without first identifying the vein with a smaller-gauge finder needle because the depth of the subclavian vein is often beyond the reach of the standard $1\frac{1}{2}$-inch, 22-gauge needle. A thin-walled needle is preferred over an 18-gauge catheter for venipuncture and guidewire placement because the 18-gauge catheter is easily kinked as it courses under the clavicle. Of greatest importance, however, the clinician should resist the temptation to make multiple needle thrusts if the subclavian vein is not punctured on the second or third attempt. It is clear that complications from this procedure, particularly the incidence of pneumothorax and subclavian artery puncture, are directly related to the number of attempts and are more common when venipuncture is unsuccessful.[222,232,234] Bilateral attempts at subclavian venipuncture should rarely be undertaken because of the potential serious morbidity of bilateral pneumothorax. Perhaps even more than in the case of internal jugular vein cannulation, the safety of subclavian venipuncture rests in the experience of the operator. In more practiced hands, the incidence of complications should be lower, with pneumothorax developing in less than 2% and arterial puncture in less than 5% of cases.[222,232]

External Jugular Vein

Both the right and left external jugular veins provide a safe alternative to internal jugular or subclavian vein cannulation. Because the external jugular veins are superficial, they allow central venous cannulation with essentially no risk of pneumothorax or unintended arterial puncture. In most instances, it is best to use an 18-gauge catheter rather than the thin-walled needle to introduce the guidewire because of the tortuous course of the external jugular vein and the frequent need to manipulate the guidewire repeatedly to direct it into the superior vena cava. A J-tipped guidewire should always be used because it may be advanced under the clavicle into the central circulation more successfully than a straight-tipped wire.[235,236] When the guidewire does not advance as desired and appears to be moving peripherally into the subclavian vein, abducting the ipsilateral shoulder beyond 90 degrees before advancing the wire may facilitate central venous passage. Alternatively, the patient's ipsilateral arm is placed at the side, and an assistant applies mild caudad traction on the shoulder to straighten the course of the external jugular vein while the wire is advanced. Essentially the only factors that preclude use of the external jugular veins for CVP monitoring are an inability to visualize and cannulate the vessel in the neck and advance the catheter into the central circulation. Unfortunately, these problems occur in approximately 20% of patients, thus limiting more widespread application of this technique.[203,237]

Femoral Vein

Femoral vein cannulation provides a useful site for CVP monitoring when the more common jugular and subclavian sites are not accessible, as in patients with burns, trauma, or surgical procedures that involve the head, neck, and upper part of the thorax or during cardiopulmonary resuscitation. Use of the femoral vein obviates many of the common complications of central venous catheterization, particularly pneumothorax and carotid or subclavian artery injury. Femoral venipuncture is performed below the inguinal ligament just medial to the palpated femoral arterial pulse in a manner similar to that used for femoral artery cannulation. Either a long (40 to 70 cm) catheter is positioned under ECG guidance in the inferior vena cava close to the cavoatrial junction,[238] or a shorter (15 to 20 cm) catheter is inserted from the femoral vein into the common iliac vein.[239] Both techniques provide intra-abdominal venous pressure measurements that agree closely with simultaneously obtained superior vena cava CVP values when these pressures are measured in mechanically ventilated, critically ill adults.[238,239] However, it is unclear whether intra-abdominal venous pressure will reflect intrathoracic CVP in spontaneously breathing patients, those who are not supine, or individuals with marked elevations in intrathoracic or intra-abdominal pressure. Disadvantages of the femoral venous route include an increased risk of thromboembolic and infectious complications.[183,233,234] In addition, femoral arterial or venous injury during attempted cannulation may result in intra-abdominal hemorrhage.

Axillary and Other Peripheral Veins

In patients with extensive, severe burn injuries, the axillary region is often spared and provides a useful site for either arterial or venous pressure monitoring.[240] Standard 20-cm CVP catheters placed in the axillary veins, approximately 1 cm medial to the palpated axillary artery, will allow measurement of pressure from the superior vena cava. Even more distal pressures measured from peripheral veins in the hand and forearm may provide a reasonably accurate estimate of CVP in selected surgical patients.[241] Modified volumetric infusion pumps can measure in-line peripheral venous pressure without the need for additional transducers and monitoring equipment.[242] Although this method of measuring CVP incurs no risk beyond that associated with placing any standard peripheral intravenous catheter, it has not been widely validated and cannot replace central venous cannulation in most circumstances.

Peripherally inserted central venous catheters (PICCs) have become a popular alternative to centrally inserted catheters in patients requiring long-term intravenous therapy. Advantages of PICCs include bedside placement under local anesthesia, extremely low risk of major insertion-related complications, and safe placement by nonphysicians (i.e., registered nurses and physician assistants). This technique may be particularly cost-effective because it eliminates the need for a minor operative procedure in patients who require a Hickman or Broviac central venous catheter.[243] Venous access for a PICC is obtained through an antecubital vein, preferably the basilic vein, which is generally more successfully catheterized than the cephalic vein because the latter is more tortuous, particularly at the clavipectoral fascia. Early reports described only modest success positioning PICCs in an appropriate central location, as well as a considerable risk of venous thrombosis,[244-246] but improvements in catheter design and insertion technique now result in successful placement and few complications in most patients.[243] Most PICCs placed for long-term therapeutic indications (chemotherapy or parenteral nutrition) are very flexible, nonthrombogenic silicone catheters. Less commonly, a standard polyurethane 40-cm intravenous catheter is inserted peripherally and advanced to a central location for short-term infusion of

vasoactive drugs or monitoring of CVP or PAP. When these standard long venous catheters are inserted from an antecubital vein, the catheter tip may advance into the heart as the arm is abducted, thereby increasing the risk of cardiac perforation or arrhythmias.[247,248] Whenever a PICC line is in place, the clinician should exercise caution when placing any additional central venous catheters because of the risk of shearing the PICC line within the central venous circulation.

Complications of Central Venous Pressure Monitoring

Complications of central venous cannulation have been recognized since this technique was introduced into clinical practice nearly 50 years ago. Overall, more than 15% of patients undergoing central venous catheterization suffer complications.[234]

Although serious immediate complications are infrequent when these procedures are performed by well-trained, experienced clinicians, infectious complications remain common, and this procedure continues to result in significant morbidity and mortality. Complications are often divided into mechanical, thromboembolic, and infectious etiologies (Table 32-6).

Mechanical Complications of Central Venous Catheterization

The incidence of complications depends on a number of factors, including the catheter insertion site and the patient's medical condition. Large retrospective and observational studies provide the best estimates of the most frequent complications. In general, *unintended arterial puncture*

Table 32–6   Complications of central venous pressure monitoring

Mechanical
  Vascular injury
    Arterial
    Venous
    Cardiac tamponade
  Respiratory compromise
    Airway compression from hematoma
    Pneumothorax
  Nerve injury
  Arrhythmias
Thromboembolic
  Venous thrombosis
  Pulmonary embolism
  Arterial thrombosis and embolism
  Catheter or guidewire embolism
Infectious
  Insertion site infection
  Catheter infection
  Bloodstream infection
  Endocarditis
Misinterpretation of data
Misuse of equipment

is the most common immediate mechanical complication. Shah and coauthors reported more than 6000 central venous catheterizations over a 5-year period, with more than 95% performed through the internal jugular vein.[249] In this series, the most common complication was carotid artery puncture, which occurred in 120 patients (1.9%) but did not result in any serious morbidity. Authors of other large studies report a somewhat higher incidence of arterial puncture during central venous catheterization ranging from approximately 3% to 15%.[198,199,222,234] In all likelihood, the frequency of arterial puncture with a small-gauge finding needle is even higher than these estimates. Though usually benign, on rare occasion, arterial puncture with even small-gauge needles may lead to serious complications such as arterial thromboembolism.[250]

If arterial puncture with a small needle occurs during central venous cannulation, the needle should be removed and external pressure applied for several minutes to prevent hematoma formation. In the event of unintentional cannulation of the carotid artery with a large-gauge catheter, the preferred clinical management is less certain. In the large series of Shah and coworkers, arterial cannulation with a 7.5-French introducer sheath occurred in four patients.[249] The sheath was removed immediately when its intra-arterial location was recognized by the high-pressure backflow of blood, and external compression was applied for 5 minutes. No hematoma formation requiring further treatment occurred in any patient. In contrast to this report, others describe hematoma formation after removal of the catheter from the artery, with a significant risk of airway compromise that may require urgent tracheal intubation and surgical exploration for hematoma evacuation or arterial repair.[106,198] When unintentional carotid artery cannulation occurs, it can usually be managed conservatively by removing the catheter, applying local compression to the puncture site, and monitoring the patient's airway and neurologic status. A vascular surgeon should be consulted promptly to help manage the complication. Under no circumstances should prolonged cannulation of the carotid artery be tolerated because arteritis, thrombus formation, and cerebral embolization may result.[251]

Vascular injuries from central venous catheterization have a range of clinical consequences. The most common minor complications are localized hematoma or injury to the venous valves.[171] More serious complications include vascular perforation into the pleural space or mediastinum resulting in hydrothorax, hemothorax, hydromediastinum, hemomediastinum, and chylothorax.[229,252-255] Other catastrophic rare vascular injuries have been reported, including aortic perforation[256] and avulsion of the facial vein.[212] Delayed vascular complications after central venous catheterization are uncommon but should be considered as potential consequences of this procedure. A number of these complications have been described in the literature, including aortoatrial fistula, venobronchial fistula, carotid artery–internal jugular vein fistula, and pseudoaneurysm formation.[257-260]

The most important life-threatening vascular complication of central venous catheterization is *cardiac tamponade* resulting from perforation of the intrapericardial superior vena cava, right atrium, or right ventricle and the resulting hemopericardium or unintentional pericardial instillation of intravenous fluid.[261,262] This injury was the single most common fatal complication of central venous cannulation among 3533 cases reported in the American Society of Anesthesiologists Closed Claims Project in 1996.[263,264] An update from the same project in 2002 revealed that vascular injury remains the most common complication of central venous catheterization, although since 1990, there has been a reduction in the fraction of fatal injuries attributed to cardiac tamponade.[265] Most reports document the avoidable nature of this catastrophic event and highlight that patients are predisposed to this complication when central venous catheter tips are malpositioned within the heart chambers or abutting the wall of the superior vena cava at a steep angle, recognized radiographically as a gentle curvature of the catheter tip within the superior vena cava.[266] These observations emphasize that radiographic confirmation of proper catheter tip location is mandatory, regardless of whether the catheter is inserted from a central or peripheral site. In fact, many early reports of catheter-related cardiovascular perforation suggest that peripheral catheters may present unusually high risk for this complication because arm abduction may cause the catheter tip to advance into a dangerous location within the heart.[247,267] When cardiac tamponade is caused by catheter-induced cardiac perforation, symptoms develop suddenly, so the physician must have a high index of suspicion if severe hypotension occurs in any patient with a central venous catheter in place. Cardiac arrhythmias may provide an early clue to the intracardiac location of the catheter tip.[248,268] Occasionally, both posteroanterior and lateral chest radiographs and injection of radiopaque contrast are required to locate the catheter tip precisely.[269]

Pneumothorax is often cited as the most common complication of subclavian central venous cannulation, although it appears that unintended arterial puncture occurs more often than pneumothorax, even with the subclavian site of venipuncture.[106,222] Mansfield and colleagues reported a 1.5% incidence of pneumothorax and a 3.7% incidence of subclavian arterial puncture in 821 patients who underwent attempted subclavian venous cannulation.[222] Pneumothorax occurs even less frequently with the internal jugular approach. Shah and coauthors reported a 0.5% incidence of pneumothorax in their series of nearly 6000 internal jugular catheterizations.[249] This is probably a conservative overestimate because most patients in this series underwent median sternotomy for cardiac surgery, a procedure that may have caused the pneumothorax in many of these patients. Small pneumothoraces may be managed by radiographic observation, with or without needle aspiration, assuming that the patient remains clinically stable. Tube thoracostomy is the best treatment of larger pneumothoraces or pneumothorax in a patient receiving positive-pressure mechanical ventilation or scheduled for major surgery. The physician must always be prepared for the possibility of tension pneumothorax and its adverse hemodynamic sequelae. In addition to pneumothorax, other respiratory tract injuries have been reported to occur with central venous catheterization, including subcutaneous and mediastinal emphysema, tracheal perforation, and rupture of an endotracheal tube cuff.[270]

Nerve injury is another potential complication of central venous cannulation. Damage may occur to the brachial plexus, stellate ganglion, phrenic nerve,[271] or vocal cords.[271,272] Chronic pain syndromes have been attributed to this procedure as well.[273]

Thromboembolic Complications of Central Venous Catheterization

Catheter-related thrombosis is a significant risk associated with central venous catheterization, and it occurs in as many as 15% of patients in medical intensive care units.[234] Subclavian catheters appear to have the lowest risk of this complication. Venous thrombosis may impair venous drainage or lead to superior vena cava syndrome or pulmonary thromboembolism.[274] The absolute risk and clinical importance of catheter-related thrombosis remain poorly defined.[234]

In addition to thromboembolism, other reported embolic complications of central venous catheterization include catheter, guidewire, and air embolism.[213,275-279] Invariably, these complications are the result of misuse of equipment, thereby highlighting the need for proper education and training of nurses and physicians responsible for the use of these devices.

Infectious Complications of Central Venous Catheterization

By far, the most common major late complication of central venous cannulation is *infection*. Bloodstream infections occur in approximately 5% of patients with standard central venous catheters and lead to an estimated 150,000 to 250,000 cases of catheter-related bacteremia or fungemia annually.[183,280] Given that the crude mortality associated with nosocomial bloodstream infections is nearly 35% and the cost of these infections can exceed $50,000 per episode, most simple efforts to reduce this complication appear to be both cost-effective and lifesaving.[183,280,281]

As previously noted, the starting point for prevention of infection is meticulous attention to aseptic technique.[202] When more long-term central venous cannulation is anticipated, the subclavian site is preferred because use of the jugular or femoral veins carries a higher risk of infection.[183,184,233,234,280] Multilumen catheters are associated with higher risk than single-lumen catheters are, although the added clinical functionality of such catheters often mandates their use.[282] The type of catheter inserted influences the rate of catheter colonization and subsequent bloodstream infection. Catheters are made from materials such as silicone, polyvinyl chloride, Teflon, and polyurethane. Furthermore, catheters of the same material may be manufactured differently, which influences their surfaces and the frequency of bacterial adherence to the surface.[283]

One recent improvement in catheter design has been incorporation of an antimicrobial treatment onto the catheter surface. Combinations of chlorhexidine and silver sulfadiazine or minocycline and rifampin have been shown to reduce rates of catheter colonization and bloodstream infection.[183,234,280,281] Other catheter modifications include the use of a silver-impregnated subcutaneous cuff with catheters intended for long-term use.[191]

When patients require central venous catheterization for more than 3 to 4 days, some clinicians recommend catheter replacement at a new site, others suggest exchanging the catheter over a guidewire, and still others believe that catheters should not be changed unless there are signs of infection or other clinical indications.[282,284,285] A systematic review of the literature from 1997 suggested that guidewire exchange of central venous catheters might be associated with a greater risk of infection but fewer mechanical complications than occur with placement of the catheter at a new site.[286] Current guidelines from the Centers for Disease Control and Prevention do not support routine catheter site changes or scheduled changes over a guidewire and provide other detailed recommendations for catheter management to reduce the risk of infectious complications.[183]

Other Complications of Central Venous Catheterization

Other miscellaneous adverse sequelae of central venous cannulation have been reported (see Table 32-6). Although their incidence is not clearly known, most appear to be uncommon. All physicians performing these procedures should recognize them, however, to limit the morbidity of central venous cannulation, particularly because many of these complications result from *operator error*.[106,264,287]

The use of *guidewires*, *vessel dilators*, and *large-bore catheters* carries certain additional risks that mandate meticulous attention to technique. The proximal tip of the guidewire must remain under the physician's control at all times to avoid inserting the wire too far into the heart and thus causing arrhythmias or heart block or potentially losing the guidewire within the circulation.[268,275] By design, vessel dilators are stiffer than central venous catheters and may cause significant trauma if inserted forcefully or further than necessary to dilate the subcutaneous tissue track from the skin to the vein.[264,288] Large-bore introducer sheaths and multilumen catheters have become popular because of their clinical usefulness, yet their size may increase the risk of cannulation-associated trauma, hemorrhage from unrecognized line disconnections, and major venous air embolism. Not only may air be entrained during initial cannulation,[277] but improperly connected large-bore cannulas may also pose an additional risk because of the large site for air entry directly into the central venous circulation.[276,278,279]

Unusual complications of central venous cannulation continue to be reported as new catheter modifications are designed, such as the antiseptic catheter surface treatment with chlorhexidine. Although more than 2.5 million of these catheters have been used in the United States without incident, rare but severe anaphylactoid reactions have been reported in Japanese patients.[289,290] A double-lumen 15.5-French catheter has been designed for use in immunocompromised patients to provide long-term central venous access and an introducer lumen to accommodate a standard pulmonary artery catheter for hemodynamic monitoring. It remains to be seen whether this type of extremely large catheter will create more problems than it solves.[291]

Although many complications of CVP monitoring relate to equipment misuse, the frequency of complications caused by data misinterpretation remains unknown. It is extremely likely, however, that clinicians misinterpret CVP measurements and have suboptimal understanding of CVP monitoring, just as has been demonstrated repeatedly for pulmonary artery catheter monitoring (see discussion to follow). Safe and effective use of CVP monitoring requires a detailed understanding of cardiovascular physiology, normal CVP waveforms, and common pathologic changes in these measurements.

Physiologic Considerations for Central Venous Pressure Monitoring: Diastolic Pressure-Volume Relationships and Transmural Pressure

Cardiac filling pressures are monitored to estimate cardiac filling volumes, which in turn determine the stroke output of the left and right ventricles. According to the Frank-Starling principle, the force of cardiac contraction is directly proportional to end-diastolic muscle fiber length at any given level of intrinsic contractility or inotropy. This muscle fiber length or preload is proportional to end-diastolic chamber volume. Even though it would be ideal to monitor cardiac chamber volumes continuously in critically ill patients, this goal remains elusive in clinical practice.

When a cardiac filling pressure is measured as a surrogate for estimating cardiac volume, one must not assume that these two variables always change in direct proportion or even in the same direction. In fact, the diastolic pressure-volume relationship in cardiac muscle is not linear, but rather curvilinear, with a progressively steeper slope at higher volumes (Fig. 32-23).[292,293] This diastolic

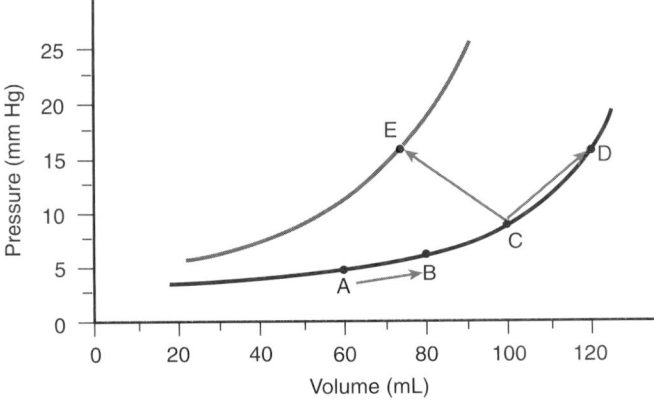

Figure 32–23 Ventricular diastolic pressure-volume relationship. Along the flat portion of the curve, a 20-mL increase in ventricular volume causes a small increase in ventricular pressure (A to B). In contrast, the same increase in volume along the steep portion of the ventricular filling curve causes a marked increase in filling pressure (C to D). Another problem associated with the use of filling pressure as a surrogate for filling volume arises when shifts in the pressure-volume relationship occur. At point C, ventricular volume is 100 mL and ventricular pressure is 8 mm Hg. An increase in filling pressure to 15 mm Hg may accompany either increased volume (D) or decreased volume (E). The latter occurs when ventricular compliance changes and shifts the ventricular diastolic pressure-volume relationship up and to the left. (Redrawn from Mark JB: Atlas of Cardiovascular Monitoring. New York, Churchill Livingstone, 1998, Fig. 15-2.)

pressure-volume relationship is one limb of a pressure-volume loop that describes the relationship between pressure and volume for the left or right ventricle during an entire cardiac cycle. When a ventricle is operating along the flat portion of its diastolic filling curve, a significant increase in filling volume or preload results in a small increase in filling pressure. In contrast, the same increase in filling volume causes a significant increase in filling pressure when the ventricle is operating on the steep portion of its curve.[294] An even more confusing situation arises when the diastolic pressure-volume relationship of the ventricle changes, for example, with the onset of myocardial ischemia. Rather than moving along the same diastolic pressure-volume curve, the ventricle now shifts to a different, steeper curve where somewhat paradoxically, an increase in filling pressure may accompany a decrease in filling volume.[295] As a result, one cannot assume that a given measured change in cardiac filling pressure reflects a proportional change in ventricular preload, and on occasion, diastolic pressure and volume can change in opposite directions.[295,296]

The relationship between ventricular volume and filling pressure depends on the portion of the pressure-volume curve over which the patient's heart is operating and the shape or slope of the curve. Commonly termed ventricular compliance, this change in pressure for a given change in volume ($\Delta P/\Delta V$) is actually the reciprocal of compliance and is more accurately termed ventricular elastance, distensibility, or stiffness.[297,298] A patient with an abnormally stiff ventricle will have a greater change in end-diastolic pressure for any given change in end-diastolic volume, and the converse is true for a patient with an abnormally compliant ventricle. By definition, diastolic dysfunction is present when ventricular pressure is abnormally elevated for any given ventricular volume.

The ventricular diastolic pressure-volume relationship is influenced by the intrinsic properties of the ventricle, such as the passive mechanical characteristics of cardiac muscle, chamber geometry, and relaxation. In addition, external forces exerted by the pericardium, the adjacent ventricle, the coronary vasculature, and pleural pressure will further influence ventricular pressure-volume relationships.[299-302] One should not equate cardiac filling pressures with filling volumes when patients are functioning over wide ranges of their diastolic pressure-volume curve or under conditions in which diastolic stiffness is abnormal or changing rapidly.

In general, all intravascular pressures measured in clinical practice are referenced to ambient atmospheric pressure. (Indeed, the first step in pressure transducer setup is to zero the transducer by exposing it to atmospheric pressure and assigning this pressure a value of zero by pressing the zero pressure button on the attached monitor. See "Technical Aspects of Direct Blood Pressure Monitoring.") Thus, a cardiac filling pressure of 10 mm Hg is 10 mm Hg higher than ambient atmospheric pressure. Does this pressure value accurately represent the distending force across the cardiac chamber wall at end-diastole?

To answer this question, one needs to consider transmural pressure. The cardiac chambers are all contained within the pericardium and thorax. Changes in pressure in the structures surrounding the heart will influence pressures recorded within the heart. Transmural pressure is the difference between chamber pressure and juxtacardiac or pericardial pressure. This transmural pressure determines ventricular preload, end-diastolic volume, or fiber length.[131,177] The same measured filling pressure, referenced to atmospheric pressure can be associated with markedly different transmural pressures and chamber volumes, depending on whether juxtacardiac pressure is high or low. Although juxtacardiac pressure can be ignored under some circumstances, marked alterations in pleural and pericardial pressure occur commonly and must be considered when any cardiac filling pressure is interpreted. Transmural pressure is always the pressure of physiologic interest. Because juxtacardiac pressure is not measured routinely, one always must consider that the measured central vascular pressure, referenced to ambient atmospheric pressure, may be a poor estimate of transmural pressure.[294,303]

Cardiac filling pressures are measured directly from a number of sites in the vascular system. CVP monitoring is the least invasive method, followed by PAP monitoring and left atrial pressure monitoring. Proper interpretation of all cardiac filling pressures requires knowledge of normal values for these pressures, as well as pressures in the cardiac chambers and great vessels and other measured and derived hemodynamic variables (Table 32-7).

Normal Central Venous Pressure Waveforms

Strictly speaking, CVP is the pressure at the junction of the venae cavae and right atrium and reflects the driving force for filling the right atrium and ventricle. Because the large

veins of the thorax, abdomen, and proximal ends of the extremities form a compliant reservoir for a sizable percentage of the total blood volume, CVP is highly dependent on the intravascular blood volume and intrinsic vascular tone of these capacitance vessels. In other words, CVP or right atrial pressure reflects the appropriateness of the blood volume to the capacity of the venous system.[304] In addition to providing a measure of the circulating blood volume, CVP reflects the functional capacity of the right ventricle. Based on the Frank-Starling mechanism, higher right heart filling pressures are required to maintain ventricular stroke output when right ventricular contractility is impaired. Thus, in clinical practice, CVP monitoring is used for assessment of blood volume and right heart function.[305] Normal CVP in an awake, spontaneously breathing patient ranges between 1 and 7 mm Hg.

Normal mechanical events of the cardiac cycle are responsible for the sequence of waves seen in a typical CVP trace. The CVP waveform consists of five phasic events, three peaks (a, c, v) and two descents (x, y) (Table 32-8, Fig. 32-24).[306-308] The most prominent wave is the *a wave* of atrial contraction, which occurs at end-diastole after the ECG P wave. The a wave increases atrial pressure and provides the "atrial kick" to fill the right ventricle through the open tricuspid valve. Atrial pressure decreases after the a wave as the atrium relaxes. This smooth decline in pressure is interrupted by the c wave. This wave is a transient increase in atrial pressure produced by isovolumic ventricular contraction which closes the tricuspid valve and displaces it toward the atrium. The c wave always follows the ECG R wave because it is generated during the onset of ventricular systole. (Note that the c wave observed in a jugular venous pressure trace might have a slightly more complex origin. This wave has been attributed to early systolic pressure transmission from the adjacent carotid artery and may be termed a carotid impact wave.[309] Because jugular venous pressure also reflects right atrial pressure, however, this c wave probably represents both arterial [carotid impact] and venous [tricuspid motion] origins.)

Atrial pressure continues its decline during ventricular systole because of continued atrial relaxation and

Table 32–7   Normal cardiovascular pressures

Pressure	Average (mm Hg)	Range (mm Hg)
Right Atrium		
a wave	6	2-7
v wave	5	2-7
Mean	3	1-5
Right Ventricle		
Peak systolic	25	15-30
End-diastolic	6	1-7
Pulmonary Artery		
Peak systolic	25	15-30
End-diastolic	9	4-12
Mean	15	9-19
Pulmonary Artery Wedge		
Mean	9	4-12
Left Atrium		
a wave	10	4-16
v wave	12	6-21
Mean	8	2-12
Left Ventricle		
Peak systolic	130	90-140
End-diastolic	8	5-12
Central Aorta		
Peak systolic	130	90-140
End-diastolic	70	60-90
Mean	90	70-105

Table 32–8   Central venous pressure waveform components

Waveform Component	Phase of Cardiac Cycle	Mechanical Event
a wave	End-diastole	Atrial contraction
c wave	Early systole	Isovolumic ventricular contraction, tricuspid motion toward the right atrium
v wave	Late systole	Systolic filling of the atrium
h wave	Mid to late diastole	Diastolic plateau
x descent	Midsystole	Atrial relaxation, descent of the base, systolic collapse
y descent	Early diastole	Early ventricular filling, diastolic collapse

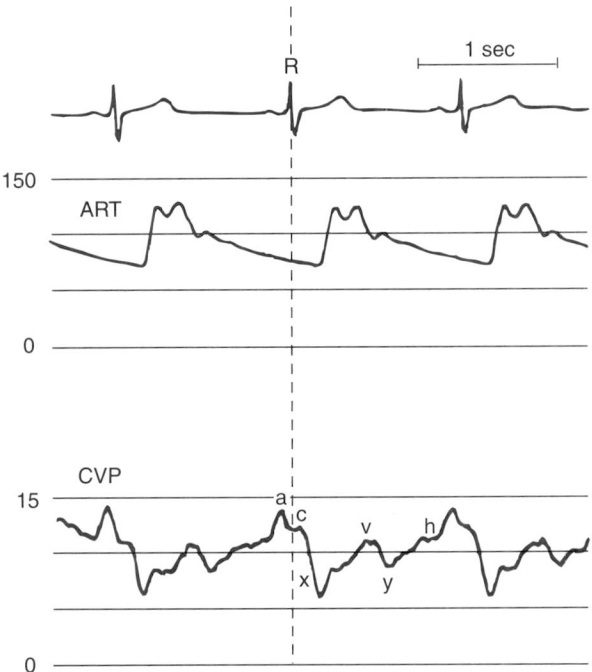

Figure 32–24 Normal central venous pressure (CVP) waveform. The diastolic components (y descent, end-diastolic a wave) and the systolic components (c wave, x descent, end-systolic v wave) are all clearly delineated. A mid-diastolic plateau wave, the h wave, is also seen because the heart rate is slow. Identification of the waveform is aided by timing the relationship between individual waveform components and the electrocardiographic R wave. Timing of the waveform with the arterial pressure (ART) trace is more confusing because of the relative delay in systolic arterial pressure upstroke. (Redrawn from Mark JB: Atlas of Cardiovascular Monitoring. New York, Churchill Livingstone, 1998, Fig. 2-5.)

changes in atrial geometry produced by ventricular contraction and ejection. This is the *x descent* or systolic collapse in atrial pressure. The x descent can be divided into two portions, x and x′, corresponding to the segments before and after the c wave. The last atrial pressure peak is the *v wave*, which is caused by venous filling of the atrium during late systole while the tricuspid valve remains closed. The v wave usually peaks just after the ECG T wave. Atrial pressure then decreases, thereby inscribing the *y descent* or diastolic collapse, as the tricuspid valve opens and blood flows from the atrium to the ventricle. (A final component of the CVP waveform, the *h wave*, occasionally appears as a pressure plateau in mid to late diastole. The h wave is not normally seen unless the heart rate is slow and venous pressure is elevated.[309,310]) In summary, the normal venous waveform components may be remembered as follows: the a wave results from atrial contraction; the c wave from tricuspid valve closure and isovolumic right ventricular contraction; and the v wave from ventricular ejection, which drives venous filling of the atrium.

Thus, in relation to the cardiac cycle and ventricular mechanical actions, the CVP waveform can be considered to have three systolic components (c wave, x descent, v wave) and two diastolic components (y descent, a wave). By recalling the mechanical actions that generate the pressure peaks and troughs, it is easy to identify these

waveform components properly by aligning the CVP waveform and the ECG trace and using the ECG R wave to mark end-diastole and the onset of systole. When the radial artery pressure trace is used for CVP waveform timing instead of the ECG, confusion may arise because the arterial pressure upstroke occurs nearly 200 milliseconds after the ECG R wave (see Fig. 32-24). This normal physiologic delay reflects the times required for the spread of electrical depolarization through the ventricle ($\approx$60 milliseconds), isovolumic left ventricular contraction ($\approx$60 milliseconds), transmission of the increase in aortic pressure to the radial artery ($\approx$50 milliseconds), and transmission of the increase in radial artery pressure through fluid-filled tubing to the transducer ($\approx$10 milliseconds).[113,136]

The normal CVP peaks are designated systolic (c, v) or diastolic (a) according to the phase of the cardiac cycle in which the wave begins. However, one generally identifies these waves not by their onset or upstroke but rather by the location of their peaks. For instance, the a wave generally begins and peaks in end-diastole, but the peak may appear delayed to coincide with the ECG R wave, especially in a patient with a short PR interval. In this instance, the a and c waves merge, and this composite wave is termed an a-c wave. Designation of the CVP v wave as a systolic event may be even more confusing. Although ascent of the v wave begins during late systole, the peak of the v wave occurs during isovolumic ventricular relaxation, immediately before opening of the atrioventricular valve and the y descent. Consequently, the most precise description would be that the v wave begins in late systole but peaks during isovolumic ventricular relaxation, the earliest portion of diastole. For clinical purposes, it is simplest to consider the v wave to be a systolic wave.

Although three distinct CVP peaks (a, c, v) and two troughs (x, y) are discernible in the normal venous pressure trace, heart rate changes and conduction abnormalities alter this pattern. A short ECG PR interval causes fusion of the a and c waves, and tachycardia reduces the length of diastole and the duration of the y descent, which causes the v and a waves to merge. In contrast, bradycardia causes each wave to become more distinct, with separate x and x′ descents visible and a more prominent h wave. Although in some circumstances other pathologic waves may be evident in the CVP trace, one should resist the temptation to assign physiologic significance to each small pressure peak because many will arise as artifacts of fluid-filled tubing-transducer monitoring systems. Instead, search for the expected waveform components, including the waveforms that are characteristic of the pathologic conditions suspected.

Abnormal Central Venous Pressure Waveforms

Various pathophysiologic conditions may be diagnosed or confirmed by examination of the CVP waveform (Table 32-9). One of the most common applications is the rapid diagnosis of cardiac arrhythmias.[311] In *atrial fibrillation* (Fig. 32-25), the a wave disappears and the c wave becomes more prominent because atrial volume is greater at end-diastole and the onset of systole owing to the absence of effective atrial contraction. Occasionally, atrial fibrillation or flutter waves may be seen in the CVP trace,

Table 32–9 Central venous pressure waveform abnormalities

Condition	Characteristics
Atrial fibrillation	Loss of a wave
	Prominent c wave
Atrioventricular dissociation	Cannon a wave
Tricuspid regurgitation	Tall systolic c-v wave
	Loss of x descent
Tricuspid stenosis	Tall a wave
	Attenuation of y descent
Right ventricular ischemia	Tall a and v waves
	Steep x and y descents
	M or W configuration
Pericardial constriction	Tall a and v waves
	Steep x and y descents
	M or W configuration
Cardiac tamponade	Dominant x descent
	Attenuated y descent
Respiratory variation during spontaneous or positive-pressure ventilation	Measure pressures at end-expiration

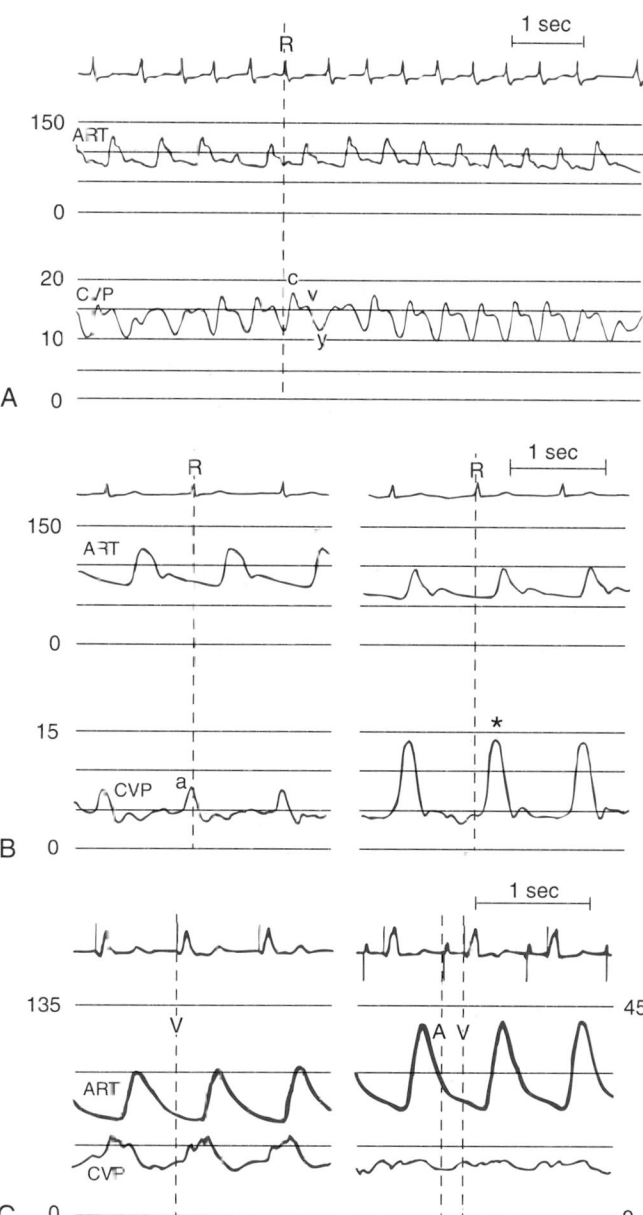

Figure 32–25 Central venous pressure (CVP) changes caused by cardiac arrhythmias. **A,** Atrial fibrillation. Note the absence of the a wave, a prominent c wave, and a preserved v wave and y descent. This arrhythmia also causes variation in the electrocardiographic (ECG) R-R interval and left ventricular stroke volume, which can be seen in the ECG and arterial pressure (ART) traces. **B,** Isorhythmic atrioventricular dissociation. In contrast to the normal end-diastolic a wave in the CVP trace (left panel), an early systolic cannon wave is inscribed (asterisk, right panel). The reduced ventricular filling accompanying this arrhythmia causes decreased arterial blood pressure. **C,** Ventricular pacing. Systolic cannon waves are evident in the CVP trace during ventricular pacing (left panel). Atrioventricular sequential pacing restores the normal venous waveform and increases arterial blood pressure (right panel). The ART scale is shown on the left, the CVP scale on the right. (Redrawn from Mark JB: Atlas of Cardiovascular Monitoring. New York, Churchill Livingstone, 1998, Figs. 14-1, 14-5, and 14-16.)

when the ventricular rate is slow. Isorhythmic *atrioventricular dissociation* or *junctional (nodal) rhythm* (see Fig. 32-25) alters the normal sequence of atrial contraction before ventricular contraction. Instead, atrial contraction now occurs during ventricular systole, when the tricuspid valve is closed, thereby inscribing a tall cannon a wave in the CVP waveform. Absence of normal atrioventricular synchrony during ventricular pacing (see Fig. 32-25) can be identified in a similar fashion by searching for cannon waves in the venous pressure trace. In these instances, CVP helps diagnosis the cause of arterial hypotension: loss of the normal end-diastolic atrial kick may not be as evident in the ECG trace as it is in the CVP waveform.

Right-sided valvular heart diseases alter the CVP waveform in different ways.[312] *Tricuspid regurgitation* (Fig. 32-26) produces abnormal systolic filling of the right atrium through the incompetent valve. A broad, tall systolic c-v wave is inscribed that begins in early systole and obliterates the systolic x descent in atrial pressure. The CVP trace is said to be ventricularized because it resembles right ventricular pressure. Note that this regurgitant wave differs in onset, duration, and magnitude from a normal CVP v wave caused by end-systolic atrial filling from the venae cavae. In patients with tricuspid regurgitation, right ventricular end-diastolic pressure is overestimated by the numeric display on the bedside monitor, which reports a single mean value for CVP. Instead, right ventricular end-diastolic pressure is estimated best by measuring the CVP value at the time of the ECG R wave, before the regurgitant systolic wave (see Fig. 32-26). Unlike tricuspid regurgitation, *tricuspid stenosis* (see Fig. 32-26) is a diastolic defect in atrial emptying and ventricular filling. Mean CVP is elevated, and a pressure gradient exists throughout diastole between the right atrium and ventricle. The a wave is unusually prominent and the y descent is attenuated because of the impaired diastolic egress of blood from the atrium. Other conditions that

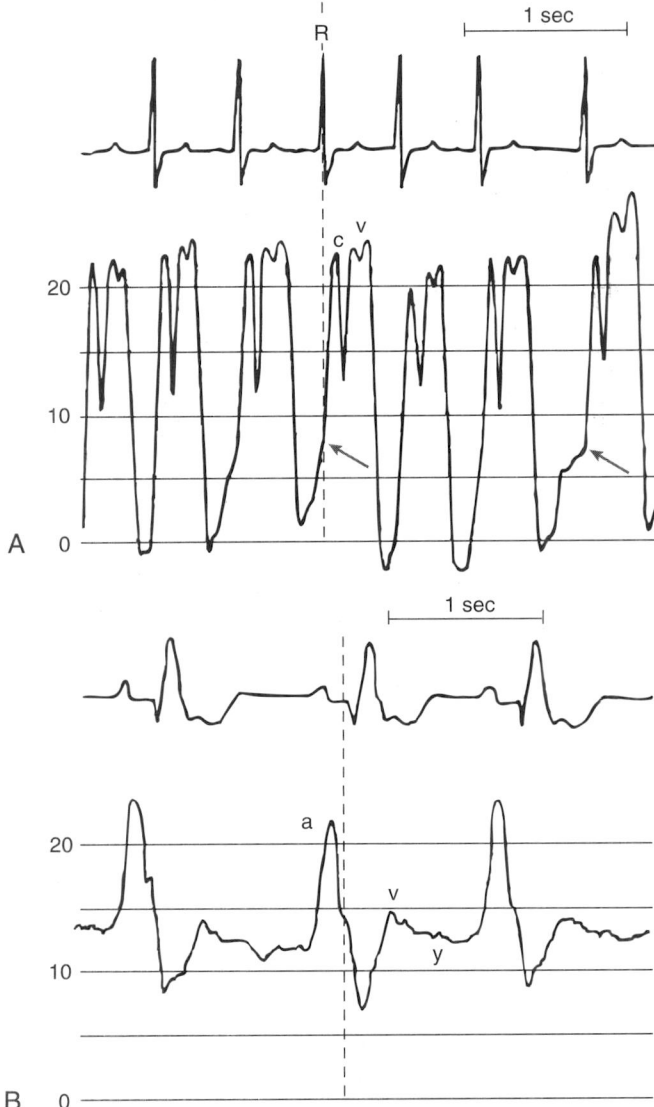

blood volume and right ventricular preload. As noted earlier, for this purpose, transmural CVP is always the pressure of physiologic interest. In clinical practice, however, we measure and record pressures referenced to ambient atmospheric pressure. Consequently, accurate interpretation of CVP requires the physician to consider alterations in intrathoracic or juxtacardiac pressure that occur during the respiratory cycle.[294,303] During spontaneous breathing (Fig. 32-27), inspiration causes a decrease in pleural and juxtacardiac pressure that is transmitted, in part, to the right atrium and lowers CVP. This same decrease in pleural pressure will influence other measured central vascular pressures in similar fashion. Note a subtle, but critically important observation about the measurement of central vascular pressures. Although CVP measured relative to atmospheric pressure decreases during the inspiratory phase of spontaneous ventilation, transmural CVP, the difference between right atrial pressure and juxtacardiac pressure, may actually increase slightly as more blood is drawn into the right atrium. The opposite pattern is observed during positive-pressure ventilation, in which inspiration increases intrathoracic pressure, raises the measured CVP, but decreases transmural CVP because the elevated intrathoracic pressure reduces venous return. In clinical practice, transmural pressures are rarely measured because of difficulty assessing juxtacardiac or intrathoracic pressure.

Figure 32–26 Central venous pressure (CVP) changes in tricuspid valve disease. **A,** Tricuspid regurgitation increases mean CVP, and the waveform displays a tall systolic c-v wave that obliterates the x descent. In this example, the a wave is not seen because of atrial fibrillation. Right ventricular end-diastolic pressure is estimated best at the time of the electrocardiographic R wave (arrows) and is lower than mean CVP. **B,** Tricuspid stenosis increases mean CVP, the diastolic y descent is attenuated, and the end-diastolic a wave is prominent. (Redrawn from Mark JB: Atlas of Cardiovascular Monitoring. New York, Churchill Livingstone, 1998, Figs. 17-3 and 17-15.)

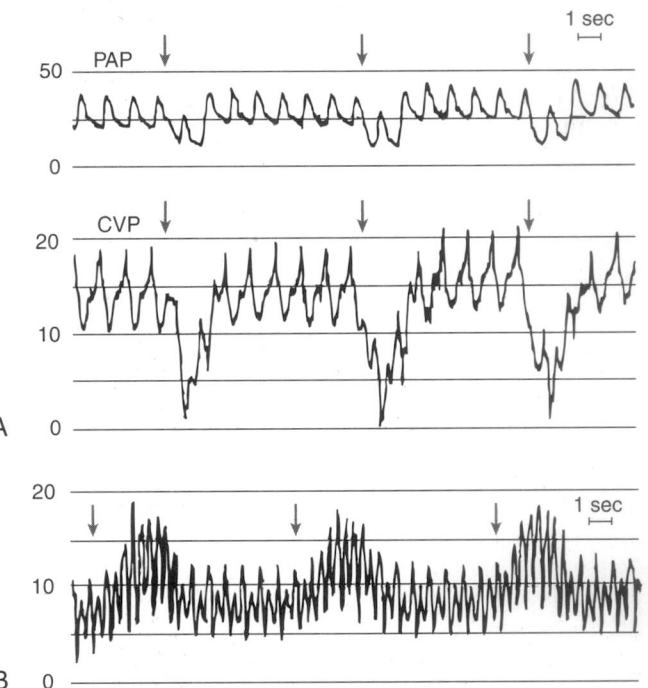

Figure 32–27 Respiratory influences on the measurement of central venous pressure (CVP). **A,** During spontaneous ventilation, the onset of inspiration (arrows) causes a reduction in intrathoracic pressure that is transmitted to both the CVP and the pulmonary artery pressure (PAP) waveforms. CVP should be recorded at end-expiration (mean CVP, 14 mm Hg). **B,** During positive-pressure ventilation, the onset of inspiration (arrows) causes an increase in intrathoracic pressure. CVP is still recorded at end-expiration (mean CVP, 8 mm Hg). (Redrawn from Mark JB: Atlas of Cardiovascular Monitoring. New York, Churchill Livingstone, 1998, Figs. 16-1 and 16-2.)

reduce right ventricular compliance, such as right ventricular ischemia, pulmonary hypertension, or pulmonic valve stenosis, may produce a prominent end-diastolic a wave in the CVP trace but do not attenuate the early diastolic y descent. CVP waveform morphology changes in other characteristic ways in the presence of pericardial diseases and right ventricular infarction. These patterns are interpreted best in conjunction with PAP monitoring, which is discussed in the next section.

Perhaps the most important application of CVP monitoring is to provide an estimate of the adequacy of circulating

Instead, end-expiratory values for cardiac filling pressure should be recorded in all patients to provide the best estimate of transmural pressure. At the end of expiration, intrathoracic and juxtacardiac pressures approach atmospheric pressure, whether the patient is breathing spontaneously or receiving positive-pressure mechanical ventilation (see Fig. 32-27). Proper pressure values can be determined by visual inspection of the CVP waveform on a calibrated monitor screen or paper recording. Under most circumstances, transmural CVP and the end-expiratory value for CVP will be close to one another. This facilitates comparison of CVP values (and other cardiac filling pressures) obtained from the same patient under varying patterns of ventilation, a common situation in anesthesia and critical care.

Not only can individual CVP waveforms provide unique diagnostic clues about the circulation, but trends in CVP during anesthesia and surgery are also useful in estimating fluid or blood loss and guiding replacement therapy. It is important to remember that the range in normal values is considerable and that small changes in CVP may reflect significant changes in circulating blood volume and right ventricular preload. Additional useful information may be derived from examining how a fluid bolus simultaneously alters CVP and other variables of clinical interest such as blood pressure, urine output, and so forth.

PULMONARY ARTERY CATHETER MONITORING

In 1970, Swan, Ganz, and colleagues introduced pulmonary artery catheterization into clinical practice for hemodynamic assessment of patients with acute myocardial infarction.[313-317] These catheters allowed accurate measurement of important cardiovascular physiologic variables at the bedside, and their popularity soared over the next 2 decades as they were used in an increasing number of critically ill and surgical patients. By the middle 1990s, estimated annual pulmonary artery catheter (PAC) sales in the United States approached 2 million catheters, with an estimated cost associated with their use in excess of $2 billion each year.[318]

The PAC provides measurements of several hemodynamic variables that many clinicians, including experts in intensive care, cannot accurately predict from standard clinical signs and symptoms.[319,320] However, despite this evidence that PACs provide cardiovascular measurements that supplement or correct clinical observations, it remains uncertain whether PAC monitoring leads to improved patient outcome.[321-325] Before considering this issue, we will review techniques for catheterization, complications associated with PAC use, the physiologic basis for PAC monitoring, interpretation of normal and pathologic PAC waveforms, and the relationship between PAC-derived measures of left ventricular filling pressure and left ventricular preload.

Pulmonary Artery Catheterization (also see CD ROM)

PACs can be placed from any of the central venous cannulation sites described earlier, but the right internal jugular vein is preferred because it provides the most direct route to the right heart chambers and thereby usually leads to successful catheterization. The procedure is conducted as already described for central venous cannulation, until the step where the venous catheter is to be inserted. At this point, a slightly larger skin nick is made to accommodate the large-bore (7.5 to 9.0 French) introducer sheath. This introducer has a hemostasis valve at its outer end, through which the PAC will be inserted, and a sidearm extension that allows continuous central venous access for fluid and drug administration. A tapered-tip, stiff dilator stylet is placed into the introducer sheath to facilitate passage of this large cannula over the guidewire from the skin, through the subcutaneous tissues, into the vein. Utmost care must be exercised when introducing this large dilator-cannula assembly by advancing it only to the depth required to enter the vein and then threading the introducer cannula completely into the vein over the guidewire and dilator. Finally, the guidewire and dilator are removed, the sidearm extension is secured to an intravenous infusion set with a Luer-Lock connector, and the introducer sheath is sutured in place.

The standard PAC has a 7.0-, 7.5-, or 8.0-French circumference and is 110 cm in length, with these distances marked at 10-cm intervals. It contains four separate internal lumens. One leads to the distal port at the catheter tip and is used for PAP monitoring. The second leads to a proximal port, located approximately 30 cm from the catheter tip, and is intended for CVP monitoring and fluid and drug administration. The third lumen leads to a balloon near the catheter tip, and the fourth contains fine wires leading to a temperature thermistor, just proximal to the balloon. This thermistor is used to monitor pulmonary artery blood temperature as part of the thermodilution method for cardiac output monitoring (see later).

The final steps in placing a PAC require the aid of a skilled assistant to help prepare the catheter and attach it properly to pressure monitoring transducers. The physician performing the catheterization removes the PAC from its package and inserts it through a sterile plastic sheath while being careful to not damage the balloon in this process.[326] This sheath or sleeve covers a length of the PAC residing outside the patient and thereby allows minor manipulations in PAC position during the monitoring period while attempting to maintain catheter sterility. The assistant then attaches the distal and proximal port hubs to the pressure monitoring system that will allow these waveforms to be displayed on the bedside monitor. These ports are flushed to ensure proper function and expel the air from these catheter lumens. The balloon is inflated with a 1.5-mL volume-limited syringe packaged with the PAC, and the balloon is tested by filling it completely with 1.5 mL of air to make certain that there are no leaks and that the balloon inflates symmetrically without obstructing the opening of the distal end of the lumen.[327]

The balloon should always be inflated with air, not liquid. The air-filled balloon at the tip of the catheter serves to carry the catheter forward with blood flow through the right heart chambers and helps "float" the catheter to its proper position in the pulmonary artery, much like the spinnaker on a sailboat is driven by the trailing wind.

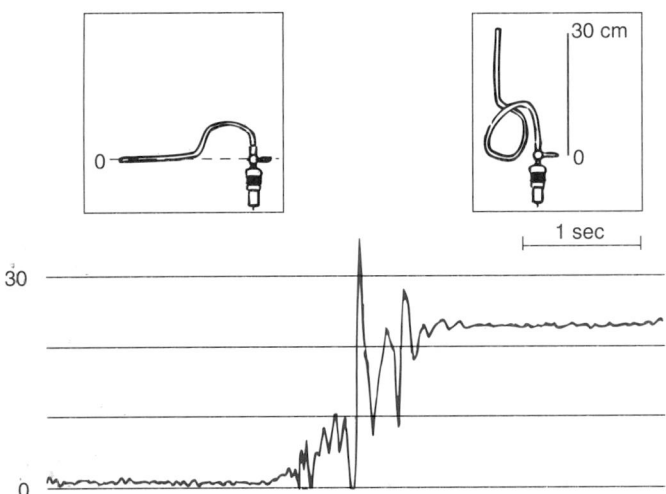

Figure 32–28 Bedside testing of the pulmonary artery catheter–pressure transducer system. With the tip of the catheter held at the level of the transducer and the heart, a pressure of 0 mm Hg is recorded. The catheter tip is raised to create a 30-cm vertical fluid column, and the resulting pressure display should equal 22 mm Hg (equivalent to 30 cm H_2O). (Redrawn from Mark JB: Atlas of Cardiovascular Monitoring. New York, Churchill Livingstone, 1998, Fig. 3-4.)

Some authors have suggested that the balloon may be inflated with sterile saline to aid catheter passage when difficulties such as severe tricuspid valve regurgitation are present.[328] However, this practice is dangerous and may increase the risk of pulmonary artery rupture. To reduce the risk of unintentional balloon inflation with liquid, the special balloon inflation syringe should remain attached to the PAC at all times.[329]

A simple maneuver should now be performed to check for proper assembly and function of the PAC monitoring system.[330,331] When the tip of the PAC is held near heart level, the recorded pressure should be 0 mm Hg, thereby confirming that the transducer was correctly adjusted to the level of the heart at the beginning of the procedure. The catheter tip is then raised up straight to create a 30-cm-tall vertical fluid column, which should produce a pressure of 22 mm Hg (equivalent to 30 cm H_2O), on the bedside monitor (Fig. 32-28). This quick, simple step ensures that the pressure recorded from the distal end of the lumen during PAC flotation is correct because it checks the integrity of the entire monitoring system from the tip of the catheter to the waveform display on the screen.

The PAC is inserted through the hemostasis valve of the introducer to a depth of 20 cm, or approximately 5 cm beyond the tip of the introducer sheath. A characteristic CVP waveform must be identified to confirm that the PAC tip is in the vena cava or right atrium. The gentle curvature of the PAC should be oriented to point just leftward of the sagittal plane (the 11-o'clock position as viewed from the patient's head). This orientation will facilitate catheter passage through the anteromedially located tricuspid valve. The balloon is inflated, and the catheter is advanced into the right atrium, through the tricuspid valve into the right ventricle, through the pulmonic valve into the pulmonary artery, and finally into the wedge position. Characteristic waveforms from each of these locations confirm proper catheter passage and placement (Fig. 32-29).

After PAWP is measured, the balloon is deflated, and the PAP waveform should reappear for continuous monitoring. Wedge pressure may be obtained periodically as needed by reinflating the balloon with 1.5 mL of air to allow the catheter to float distally until pulmonary artery occlusion again occurs. The clinician must recognize that the PAC tip advances to a smaller pulmonary artery each time that the balloon is inflated to measure wedge pressure. Similarly, the PAC should return to its monitoring position in the proximal portion of the pulmonary artery after the balloon is deflated. In some patients, the PAC may migrate distally even without balloon inflation. This problem is more common during cardiopulmonary bypass because of the repeated cardiac manipulations and temperature changes that alter the stiffness of the catheter.[332] Consequently, proper catheter position must be ensured throughout the monitoring period by frequent observation of the PAP waveform. If a PAWP trace appears without balloon inflation or with only partial

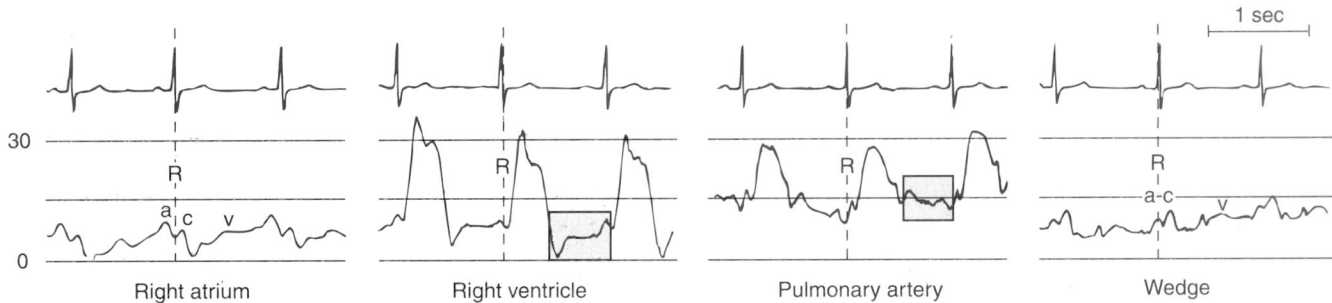

Figure 32–29 Characteristic waveforms recorded during passage of a pulmonary artery catheter. Right atrial pressure resembles a central venous pressure waveform and displays a, c, and v waves. Right ventricular pressure shows a higher systolic pressure than seen in the right atrium, although the end-diastolic pressures are equal in these two chambers. Pulmonary artery pressure shows a diastolic step-up when compared with ventricular pressure. Note also that right ventricular pressure increases during diastole whereas pulmonary artery pressure decreases during diastole (shaded boxes). Pulmonary artery wedge pressure has a morphology similar to that of right atrial pressure, although the a-c and v waves appear later in the cardiac cycle relative to the electrocardiogram. (Redrawn from Mark JB: Atlas of Cardiovascular Monitoring. New York, Churchill Livingstone, 1998, Fig. 3-1.)

balloon inflation, the balloon should be deflated and the catheter withdrawn several centimeters to reduce the risk of pulmonary vascular injury. Although the external protective sleeve covering the PAC is intended to maintain sterility during these minor adjustments in catheter position, the sleeve does not preclude contamination. Therefore, PACs should be manipulated only as necessary to maintain a proper safe location.[333]

Additional Guidelines for Pulmonary Artery Catheter Placement

From a right internal jugular vein puncture site, the right atrium should be reached when the PAC is inserted 20 to 25 cm, the right ventricle at 30 to 35 cm, the pulmonary artery at 40 to 45 cm, and the wedge position at 45 to 55 cm. When other sites are chosen for catheter placement, additional distance is required, typically an additional 5 to 10 cm from the left internal jugular and left and right external jugular veins, an additional 15 cm from the femoral veins, and an additional 30 to 35 cm from the antecubital veins.[331] These distances serve only as a rough guide, and waveform morphology must always be verified from the monitor display and catheter position confirmed with a chest radiograph. The tip of the PAC should be within 2 cm of the cardiac silhouette on a standard anteroposterior chest film.[334]

Keeping in mind these typical distances helps avoid complications caused by unintended catheter loops and knots within the heart. If a right ventricular waveform is not observed after inserting the catheter 40 cm, coiling in the right atrium is likely. Similarly, if a pulmonary artery waveform is not observed after inserting the catheter 50 cm, coiling in the right ventricle has probably occurred. The balloon should be deflated, the catheter withdrawn to 20 cm, and the PAC floating sequence repeated.

Although the right internal jugular vein is the primary site for pulmonary artery catheterization, failure to achieve venous cannulation or other medical and surgical considerations may require the use of alternative sites. For cardiac surgery, the left internal jugular vein is often the second choice because use of the subclavian veins poses a problem unique to this setting. After sternotomy and sternal retraction, a PAC inserted by the subclavian route may be compressed and kinked under the clavicle, thus making it impossible to withdraw or advance the catheter should this be required during the course of surgery.[335]

Regardless of the intended surgical procedure, whenever one plans to insert a PAC through the left internal jugular, subclavian, and particularly the external jugular veins, the more tortuous course of these vessels may make it difficult to advance the large-bore introducer sheath fully into the vessel. This is not a problem as long as the introducer cannula is withdrawn slightly to maintain a position in the vein that allows unimpeded intravenous infusion and free aspiration of venous blood. Often, the introducer cannula needs to remain in this partially inserted position while the PAC is introduced through its hemostasis valve. Because the PAC has a more flexible, smaller tip than the introducer does, the PAC might advance easily and completely into the central vein and right atrium. The PAC balloon may then be inflated and the procedure completed in normal fashion.

With the PAC in proper position, the introducer sheath can usually be fully guided into the central vein and sutured in place because the PAC has served, in essence, as a more effective "guidewire." Occasionally, the introducer sheath must remain partially or completely withdrawn to avoid acute angulation and kinking of the PAC as it leaves the sheath and enters the central vein.[335-337]

After successful venous cannulation, when attempts to advance the PAC to the right ventricle prove difficult, the physician should consider whether this difficulty is due to abnormal venous anatomy. The most common abnormality of the systemic veins is *persistence of the left superior vena cava*, which is present in approximately 0.1% to 0.2% of the general population and 2% to 9% of patients with other forms of congenital heart disease.[338-343] A persistent left superior vena cava descends along the left mediastinum and empties into the coronary sinus, which is dilated as a consequence of the abnormal venous drainage pattern. Occasionally, the condition is recognized radiographically by an abnormal appearance of the left side of the mediastinum and cardiac border or an abnormal pulsation of the left internal jugular vein. However, because of the lack of physiologic consequences of this abnormal venous anatomy, virtually all cases are asymptomatic and discovered incidentally at the time of attempted central venous or pulmonary artery catheterization. In patients with this anomaly, PAC placement may be difficult or impossible as a result of the tortuous course that the catheter must follow from the vena cava through the coronary sinus to reach the right heart chambers. Because a normal right superior vena cava is present in most of these patients, the anomaly is recognized only when attempted PAC placement proceeds from a left-sided vein. More rarely, difficult PAC placement is encountered during attempted right-sided venous cannulation because the right superior vena cava is absent as well. In these cases, the right internal jugular vein joins the persistent left superior vena cava by a bridging innominate vein. A rare form of atrial septal defect termed unroofed coronary sinus may also be encountered in patients with these venous abnormalities. This congenital defect provides a site for coronary sinus–left atrial communication, with the potential for a PAC to enter the left atrium and systemic circulation through this defect.[343] With any of these venous anomalies, PAC advancement into the coronary sinus may disclose an unexpected pressure waveform, coronary sinus pressure. This waveform has characteristics of both the downstream right atrial pressure and an indirectly transmitted, dampened left ventricular pressure waveform. Recognition requires that the physician have a clear appreciation for the expected waveforms encountered by the PAC as right heart catheterization proceeds.

A few additional points might aid successful positioning of the PAC. The air-filled balloon tends to float to nondependent regions as it passes through the heart into the pulmonary vasculature. Consequently, positioning a patient head down will aid flotation past the tricuspid valve, and tilting the patient onto the right side and head-up positioning will aid flotation out of the right ventricle and may reduce the frequency of malignant ventricular arrhythmias during catheterization.[344]

Because of gravitational and anatomic factors, most catheters float to the right pulmonary artery.[345,346] Thus, to catheterize the left pulmonary artery selectively, the patient should be positioned with the right side down.[347] Deep inspiration during spontaneous ventilation will increase venous return and right ventricular output transiently and may facilitate catheter flotation in a patient with low cardiac output. On occasion, a catheter may be floated to proper position when stiffened by injecting, through the distal lumen, 10 to 20 mL of the iced solution prepared for measurement of cardiac output. Finally, a catheter that is initially difficult to place may be positioned easily when hemodynamic conditions change, as commonly occurs after induction of general anesthesia and initiation of positive-pressure ventilation.

Complications of Pulmonary Artery Catheter Monitoring

The use of PACs has been associated with various adverse effects that may be divided into complications that occur during initial attempts to gain venous access, those occurring during pulmonary artery catheterization, late complications associated with catheter residence in the body, and adverse consequences associated with misuse of equipment and misinterpretation of data. For the most part, problems during attempts to gain central venous access are similar for PAP or CVP monitoring (see Table 32-6). However, catheterization of the right heart chambers beyond the cavoatrial junction may cause complications uniquely associated with PACs and rarely, if ever, seen with CVP monitoring alone (Table 32-10).

Although many PAC-related complications have been described over the past 25 years, their incidence is not clearly known because they are described, for the most part, in isolated case reports or small case series.[348] When all adverse effects are considered, including self-limited arrhythmias observed during catheter insertion, it appears that minor complications occur in more than 50% of catheterized patients.[318] However, of greater clinical relevance, major morbidity specifically attributable to PAC use is uncommon.[349,350] Based on an exhaustive review of the literature that included 860 publications in

Table 32–10   Complications of pulmonary artery catheter monitoring

Catheterization
    Arrhythmias, ventricular fibrillation
    Right bundle branch block, complete heart block
Catheter residence
    Mechanical, catheter knots
    Thromboembolism
    Pulmonary infarction
    Infection, endocarditis
    Endocardial damage, cardiac valve injury
    Pulmonary artery rupture
    Pulmonary artery pseudoaneurysm
Misinterpretation of data
Misuse of equipment

its 1993 report and another 90 newer studies in its 2003 update, the American Society of Anesthesiologists Task Force on Pulmonary Artery Catheterization has emphasized that the reported incidence of complications from PAC monitoring varies widely in the medical literature.[318] The task force suggested that serious complications caused specifically by pulmonary artery catheterization occur in 0.1% to 0.5% of PAC-monitored surgical patients. Two large prospective observational studies of more than 5000 patients each provide good support for this contention. In 1984, Shah and coauthors reported the use of PACs in 6245 patients undergoing cardiac and noncardiac operations.[249] Quite remarkably, only 10 patients (0.16%) had serious complications resulting in morbidity and only 1 patient (0.016%) died as a result of pulmonary artery catheterization. A 1998 European report of PAC use in 5306 patients undergoing cardiac operations confirmed a similar low incidence of major morbidity, with injury to the right ventricle or pulmonary artery occurring in only 4 patients (0.07%).[351] Finally, only 1 of the 2000 adverse events reported in the Australian Incident Monitoring Study of 1993 involved the use of a PAC, in contrast to 64 other adverse events involving access to the arterial or venous systems.[106] Although these large studies suggest that the incidence of serious complications attributable to use of the PAC is low, the frequency of complications in a particular clinical setting or patient group remains unknown. However, clinicians who use PACs must be familiar with all the potential complications associated with catheter use in an attempt to avoid these problems or recognize them early and treat them successfully.

Arrhythmias (also see Chapter 34) are the primary complication observed during pulmonary artery catheterization. In fact, self-limited atrial or ventricular arrhythmias are so common during PAC passage through the heart that most clinicians do not consider this a complication, but rather a confirmation that the PAC is traversing the cardiac chambers en route to the pulmonary artery. Shah and colleagues observed transient premature ventricular contractions in 68% and atrial dysrhythmias in 1.3% of their catheterized patients.[249] Of greater clinical significance, persistent ventricular arrhythmias requiring treatment occurred in only 3.1% of patients, none of whom suffered prolonged hemodynamic instability. Although the balloon-tipped PAC is less arrhythmogenic when it strikes the endocardium than a standard intravenous catheter or transvenous pacing wire is,[352] PACs have been reported to induce sustained atrial fibrillation, ventricular tachycardia, and ventricular fibrillation.[344,351-353]

As uncommon as these malignant arrhythmias may be, the physician must always consider this risk when placing a PAC and recognize that certain patients may be at increased risk. For example, in a patient with critical aortic stenosis scheduled for valve replacement, one may choose to avoid use of a PAC or delay flotation of the catheter until the heart is exposed and cardiopulmonary bypass support is immediately available. In general, the risk of *ventricular fibrillation* is greatest in patients with myocardial ischemia, particularly those with acute right ventricular ischemia.[354] In a study of 2821 patients who underwent pulmonary artery catheterization in the coronary care unit, ventricular fibrillation developed in 25 of 2327 (1.1%)

patients with acute myocardial infarction versus 0 of 494 (0%) without infarction, and the risk was greatest (4.2%) in the subset of patients in whom right ventricular infarction was diagnosed.[354]

Prophylactic use of intravenous lidocaine before pulmonary artery catheterization has not been shown to consistently reduce the incidence of ventricular arrhythmias.[355,356] When ventricular tachycardia or frequent ventricular premature beats occur during the catheterization procedure, the balloon should be deflated and the catheter withdrawn to the right atrium. This terminates the arrhythmia in nearly all cases, and the pulmonary artery may be catheterized by standard procedures once the arrhythmia has ceased. A more difficult clinical question arises when hemodynamically significant arrhythmias develop later in the monitoring period, after the PAC has been in place for hours or days. Although it is unlikely that the PAC is responsible for these new arrhythmias, the position of the catheter tip should always be checked by observation of the pressure waveform and chest radiograph. A catheter tip that is malpositioned within the right ventricle is significantly more arrhythmogenic than a catheter tip, cushioned by the inflated balloon, that is floating through the heart during initial catheterization. Once proper PAC position is confirmed and other causes of ventricular arrhythmia such as myocardial ischemia are excluded, several clues may point toward the PAC as being the cause of the rhythm disturbance, including left bundle branch block morphology of the ventricular premature beats, their resistance to medical therapy, and their response to withdrawal of the catheter into the right atrium.[352]

As the PAC passes through the right ventricle and strikes the interventricular septum, transient *right bundle branch block* occurs in up to 5% of patients.[357-359] This complication presumably results from the minor trauma of catheter passage through the heart. It occurs less frequently with balloon-tipped catheters than with standard stiff cardiac catheters, which are known to cause right or left bundle branch block, depending on which ventricular chamber is catheterized.[358,360] Right bundle branch block is of no real clinical consequence except in patients with preexisting left bundle branch block, in whom complete heart block may be precipitated. Despite this theoretical concern, *complete heart block* from pulmonary artery catheterization is uncommon. Shah and coworkers catheterized 113 patients with preexisting left bundle branch block, and complete heart block developed in only 1 patient (0.9%).[249] In a different population of 47 high-risk patients with left bundle branch block, many of whom had acute myocardial infarction or heart failure, Morris and associates inserted 82 PACs without a single episode of complete heart block during the catheterization or for 24 hours thereafter.[357] Prophylactic placement of a transvenous ventricular pacing wire is not necessary in patients with preexisting left bundle branch block who require PAC monitoring. Instead, transcutaneous pacing equipment, an external pulse generator, and a temporary transvenous pacing wire or pacing PAC should be readily available to treat heart block and severe bradycardia. It is important for the anesthesiologist to recognize that the onset of heart block from pulmonary artery catheterization may be delayed and only fully manifested after the administration of anesthetic drugs. For example, incomplete right bundle branch block after PAC insertion has been reported to progress to complete right bundle branch block and bradycardia after induction of anesthesia.[359]

Various *mechanical problems* with PACs or introducer sheaths have been reported, and a physician who is familiar with these potential problems should be able to avoid most of them. In the setting of cardiac surgery, PACs may be damaged by surgical instruments or become entrapped by sutures or the cannulas used for these operations.[249,361-367] Whenever the surgical procedure involves the right heart structures, it is prudent to ensure free movement of the PAC before chest closure.

Sternal retraction during cardiac surgery poses another mechanical problem with PACs, particularly when they are inserted through the external jugular or subclavian routes. The PAC may kink as it exits the introducer sheath and makes an acute angle between the sheath and vessel wall.[335-337] Withdrawing the introducer sheath slightly or limiting the amount of surgical retraction may resolve this problem. These mechanical difficulties should be suspected whenever there is a damped appearance of the monitored pressure traces or difficulty infusing fluid or withdrawing blood through one of the catheter lumens.

Although gross structural defects in the PAC should be recognized by inspection before catheter insertion, more subtle manufacturing problems may escape detection. Some of these, such as interluminal communications between the PAP, CVP, and balloon inflation lumens, may be suspected only when information derived from the catheters is inconsistent with other clinical data.[326,327,358,369]

PACs may dislodge temporary transvenous pacing wires, become entangled with other cardiac catheters, or form *knots* within the heart.[370-372] Arnaout and coauthors reported a PAC knot around the tricuspid valve chordae tendineae that resulted in severe tricuspid valve regurgitation after catheter removal.[370] Catheter knots should be suspected when difficulty is encountered during withdrawal of a PAC, and the diagnosis may be confirmed by chest radiography. Knots may be untied in vivo by radiologists with the use of intravascular snares and fluoroscopic guidance.[373] If the knot has already been drawn tight, removal under direct surgical exposure of the venous cannulation site may be required.[374] These problems are more likely when the PAC is inserted an excessive distance and the catheter loops or coils within the cardiac chambers, thus emphasizing the importance of prevention.

The use of PACs has been associated with thrombocytopenia,[375] and the catheter may serve as a nidus for intravascular thrombosis.[376] Although the incidence of *thromboembolic* complications is increased in patients who require PAC monitoring for longer periods, thrombi have been noted to be attached to a PAC within 1 to 2 hours of their insertion.[377,378] When drugs such as aprotinin and ε-aminocaproic acid are used to reduce perioperative bleeding, the risk of thrombus formation on the PAC may be even greater.[379,380] Although heparin bonding of the external surface has unquestionably reduced the thrombogenicity of PACs, it does not entirely eliminate this complication.[378,380,381] This predisposition to intravascular thrombosis in patients with PAC monitoring arises in part from the prosthetic catheter itself and in part from the subclinical endothelial injury produced by the catheter. Through autopsy examination of 32 patients who died with PACs in place, Connors and colleagues demonstrated that venous thrombi, fibrin strands, mural ecchymoses, or intimal petechiae were evident in 90% of patients.[382]

Although minor venous thrombi and pulmonary ischemic lesions are fairly common in patients with PAC monitoring, major pulmonary embolism arising from the use of a PAC is a rare occurrence.[376,383,384] Rather than thromboembolism, the most common cause of *pulmonary infarction* in patients with PACs is occlusion of pulmonary blood flow by a malpositioned catheter that occludes a branch of the pulmonary artery.[383] The radiographic hallmark of this condition is a wedge-shaped infiltrate radiating from the tip of a peripherally located PAC. This iatrogenic complication may be prevented by diligent monitoring of the PAP waveform recorded from the catheter tip to allow early recognition of a catheter that has migrated distally, wedged within a small pulmonary artery, and obstructed distal blood flow.

PAC-related *infection* occurs more commonly in patients who require monitoring for more than 3 days and those with preexisting sepsis.[385] Using sophisticated microbiologic techniques in 297 critically ill medical and surgical patients, Mermel and associates demonstrated a 22% incidence of local infection of the introducer sheath, but a low 0.7% incidence of bacteremia caused by the PAC.[386] Although PACs may be colonized from multiple sources, the patient's skin is the most important source of organisms, and it is the introducer sheath rather than the PAC itself that is usually the infected device. In view of these findings, it is not surprising that scheduled changes of PACs do not reduce the risk of bloodstream infection, particularly when the catheter is changed over a guidewire through the original venipuncture site.[387] If clinical factors mandate changing the PAC, placement through a new vascular access site will reduce the risk of infection in comparison to guidewire-assisted exchange. However, cannulation at a new puncture site carries a greater risk of mechanical complications, and these risks and benefits must be balanced in each individual patient.[387]

The most serious infection related to PACs is *endocarditis*. The pulmonic and tricuspid valves are the most likely sites, but right atrial endocarditis has also been reported.[388,389] Although these catastrophic infections appear to be rare, they represent part of the continuum of endocardial damage, thrombosis, and infection that has been documented to be associated with the use of PACs.[389] Immunocompromised, debilitated, and bacteremic patients may be at particular risk for these complications.

In addition to predisposing the patient to endocarditis, PACs may damage the right heart endocardium and the tricuspid and pulmonic valves.[382,389-391] Rowley and coworkers performed autopsies on 55 previously catheterized patients and found that 53% had right-sided *endocardial lesions*.[389] Although both severe *tricuspid regurgitation* and severe *pulmonic regurgitation* have been

reported,[370,390,391] these conditions are rare complications of PAC use. In general, the anatomic redundancy in valvular tissue appears to prevent clinically important valvular regurgitation in patients who have PACs in place. Using color flow Doppler echocardiography, Sherman and colleagues demonstrated that placement of a PAC caused a slight increase in the magnitude of tricuspid regurgitation, but in no instance did the PAC lead to severe right-sided valvular insufficiency.[392]

Perhaps the most life-threatening complication of pulmonary artery catheterization is one that is uncommon and often avoidable through meticulous attention to insertion and monitoring techniques. *Pulmonary artery rupture* occurs in approximately 0.02% to 0.2% of catheterized patients and appears to be a fatal complication in nearly 50% of cases.[249,393-396] Although it may occur in a variety of monitoring situations, many reported cases have involved patients undergoing heart surgery requiring cardiopulmonary bypass.[395-398] Several patient factors common to this clinical setting have been proposed to increase the risk of this complication, including hypothermia, anticoagulation, advanced age, and pulmonary hypertension.[398-400] The latter may predispose patients to arterial injury during balloon inflation as a result of the increased gradient between the proximal arterial and distal wedge pressures or because pulmonary hypertension distends the pulmonary vasculature and causes the PAC to wedge in a distal, less compliant vessel. Both factors may result in eccentric balloon inflation that could drive the exposed catheter tip into the vessel wall.[401,402] However, whether preexisting pulmonary hypertension increases the risk of pulmonary artery rupture during PAC monitoring remains unproven.

Several mechanisms for pulmonary artery injury have been proposed and investigated. Hardy and associates, studying cadaveric specimens, determined that the pressure required to rupture the pulmonary artery in patients older than 60 years was well within the range of pressures normally exerted during balloon inflation, thus suggesting that a balloon forcefully inflated in a pulmonary artery smaller than the balloon diameter may rupture the vessel wall.[400] Other proposed mechanisms for pulmonary artery rupture include chronic erosion by a catheter tip abutting the vessel wall or eccentric balloon inflation that forces the uncushioned catheter tip through the vessel wall.[399,403] Regardless of the precise mechanism by which pulmonary arterial injury occurs in an individual patient, case reports highlight that this complication often results from suboptimal catheter insertion and monitoring techniques. These procedural errors include unnecessary catheter manipulation, excessive insertion distances predisposing to catheter tips becoming lodged in distal small pulmonary arteries, unrecognized persistent wedge pressure, prolonged balloon inflation, or improper balloon inflation with liquid rather than air.[329,395,399,402,403] It is critical that the clinician recognize artifactual "overwedged" pressure recordings that indicate a peripheral location of the PAC tip or impaction against the vessel wall and correct this problem immediately by withdrawing the catheter into the proximal part of the pulmonary artery (see later).

The hallmark of catheter-induced pulmonary artery rupture is hemoptysis, which may cause life-threatening exsanguination or hypoxemia. Less commonly, this complication is manifested as occult hypotension or respiratory compromise. If the visceral pleura fails to contain the bleeding, free rupture into the pleural space produces a large hemothorax. When time allows, a chest radiograph helps make the diagnosis by revealing the hemothorax or a new infiltrate near the tip of a distally positioned PAC. This infiltrate may be confused with catheter-related pulmonary infarction, but its pattern of resolution and other clinical signs and symptoms help distinguish these diagnoses.[394] In confusing cases, the diagnosis may be made by performing a wedge angiogram, in which radiopaque dye injected through the wedged PAC will extravasate into the pulmonary parenchyma and thus identify the site of arterial disruption.[399]

Treatment focuses on stabilizing cardiorespiratory performance, maintaining adequate gas exchange, and arresting the hemorrhage. Specific therapeutic steps are highly individualized; they depend on the setting in which the complication occurs and may be quite different when pulmonary artery rupture is suspected in a debilitated patient in the intensive care unit versus a relatively fit patient undergoing cardiopulmonary bypass. The first priority is ensuring adequate pulmonary ventilation, which may require endobronchial intubation with either a single- or double-lumen endotracheal tube to allow selective unilateral lung ventilation and protect the unaffected lung.[404] Positive end-expiratory pressure (PEEP) applied to the affected lung may help control hemorrhage.[398] Anticoagulation, if present, should be reversed unless the patient must remain on cardiopulmonary bypass. Bronchoscopy is performed for tracheobronchial toilet and to localize the site of bleeding. Other maneuvers may be performed at the bedside to provide temporary control of hemorrhage. A bronchial blocker may be guided into the involved bronchus to tamponade the bleeding and prevent continued contamination of the uninvolved lung.[393] Management of the PAC itself in these circumstances is more controversial. Some authors recommend removing the catheter,[394] but others suggest leaving the PAC in place to monitor PAP and guide antihypertensive therapy targeted at lowering this pressure and reducing bleeding.[395] Others have suggested that the PAC balloon may be carefully reinflated and the catheter floated into the involved pulmonary artery to occlude the bleeding arterial segment as a temporizing measure.[393] Although these conservative medical treatments may be effective in some cases, many patients will require definitive surgical therapy, such as oversewing the involved pulmonary artery or resecting the involved segment, lobe, or lung[393,394,398,399]

Patients who have this complication and are managed with conservative medical therapy alone are at risk for *pseudoaneurysm* formation and secondary hemorrhage.[393,398,402,405,406] Because of these delayed risks and the high mortality associated with rebleeding, some authors have recommended follow-up pulmonary angiography and coil embolization or elective surgical resection in patients who were initially managed medically.[393,396,398,405,407]

A more insidious complication of PAC monitoring and perhaps the most common serious adverse effect from the use of this technology is *misinterpretation of data* leading to inappropriate, harmful therapy.[408-411] Although it is not clear what role this factor plays in creating complications in an individual patient, there is reason to believe that there are widespread knowledge deficits among practitioners who use PACs in clinical care. In 1990, Iberti and coauthors reported the results of a 31-question multiple-choice examination that tested knowledge of the PAC.[412] The test was administered to 496 resident and staff physicians in the medicine, surgery, and anesthesiology departments of 13 North American medical centers. The authors found a poor overall level of knowledge of PACs, as evidenced by a mean test score of only 67% correct answers, and they concluded, "there is reason to be concerned about the effective use of the PAC." Although higher scores were achieved by individuals with more training and more experience inserting PACs and using catheter-derived information in patient management, none of these factors ensured a high level of knowledge. Similarly disappointing results were subsequently obtained when this examination was administered to 216 critical care nurses,[413] 535 European intensive care physicians,[414] and 1095 members of the U.S. Society of Critical Care Medicine.[415] The authors of these reports seemed particularly concerned that PAWP measurement was performed incorrectly by 30% to 50% of the clinicians in these studies. Other authors have also noted the large interobserver variability in interpretation of PAC pressure tracings,[416] and more recent reports continue to document the inability of practicing cardiovascular anesthesiologists to measure wedge pressure accurately[417] and the failure of brief educational programs to improve this critical diagnostic skill.[418] Taken together, these observations highlight the fact that effective use of PACs requires a great deal of expertise and clinical experience, and even measuring the most fundamental PAC-derived variable, namely, wedge pressure, may prove to be a complicated exercise.[419-421] With these issues in mind, the physiologic basis for PAC monitoring will be reviewed, followed by a description of normal and pathologic PAC waveforms, with an emphasis of the physiologic mechanisms that produce them.

Physiologic Considerations for Pulmonary Artery Catheter Monitoring: Prediction of Left Ventricular Filling Pressure

Pulmonary artery catheterization is performed in critically ill patients to measure a range of hemodynamic variables, including cardiac output, mixed venous oxygen saturation, and most importantly, pulmonary artery diastolic and wedge pressures. These pressure measurements are used to estimate left ventricular filling pressure and help guide fluid and vasoactive drug administration when clinical signs, symptoms, or other monitored variables are thought to be inadequate or unreliable.

When a PAC floats to the wedge position, the inflated balloon at its tip isolates the distal pressure monitoring orifice from upstream PAP. Blood flow ceases between the catheter tip and a junction point where pulmonary veins draining the occluded pulmonary vascular region join other veins in which blood still flows toward the left atrium (Fig. 32-30). A continuous static column of blood now connects the wedged PAC tip to this junction point

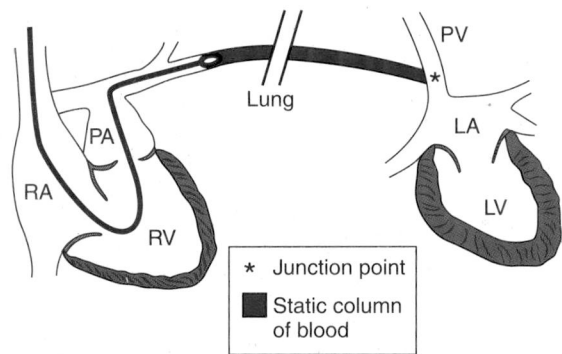

Figure 32–30 Pulmonary artery wedge pressure measurement creates a static column of blood connecting the catheter tip to a junction point where flow resumes in the pulmonary veins (PV) near the left atrium (LA). LV, left ventricle; PA, pulmonary artery; RA, right atrium; RV, right ventricle. (Redrawn from Mark JB: Atlas of Cardiovascular Monitoring. New York, Churchill Livingstone, 1998, Fig. 4-1.)

in the pulmonary veins near the left atrium. Thus, wedging the PAC functionally extends the catheter tip to measure the pressure at the point at which blood flow resumes on the venous side of the pulmonary circuit.[422] Because resistance to flow in the large pulmonary veins is negligible, PAWP provides an accurate, indirect measurement of both pulmonary venous pressure and left atrial pressure.[120,423]

Pulmonary artery diastolic pressure is often used as an alternative to wedge pressure as an estimate of left ventricular filling pressure. Under normal circumstances, resistance to pulmonary blood flow is low, and the pressure in the pulmonary artery at the end of diastole equilibrates with downstream pressure in the pulmonary veins and left atrium.[424-427] From a monitoring standpoint, pulmonary artery diastolic pressure has the added

advantage of being available for continuous monitoring, in contrast to wedge pressure, which can be measured only intermittently when the PAC balloon is inflated.

For pulmonary artery diastolic or wedge pressure to be a valid estimate of left ventricular filling pressure, a continuous, static column of blood must connect the tip of the wedged catheter and the draining pulmonary venous radicle. At the microcirculatory level, this connecting channel consists of thin pulmonary capillaries, which are subject to extramural compressive forces exerted by the surrounding alveoli. West and colleagues described a physiologic model of the pulmonary vasculature consisting of three zones that are based on the gravitationally determined relationships between PAP, pulmonary venous pressure, and alveolar pressure.[428] This lung zone model provides useful insight into conditions when the PAC may not provide accurate estimates of left ventricular filling pressure.

In lung physiologic zones 1 and 2, alveolar pressure can exceed pulmonary venous pressure (zone 2) or both PAP and pulmonary venous pressure (zone 1) (Fig. 32-31). A PAC positioned in these lung zones will be influenced by alveolar pressure, and the resultant pressure will bear little relationship to the downstream pulmonary venous pressure or left ventricular filling pressure. Under these circumstances, alveolar or airway pressure is being monitored rather than the intended vascular pressure in the left atrium or ventricle. Fortunately, in most clinical settings in which a PAC is used, patients are supine, which favors the creation of zone 3 conditions, and radiographic studies confirm that PAC tips lie below the level of the left atrium under these clinical conditions.[346] However, when patients are placed in the lateral or semi-upright position, considerable nondependent portions of their lungs may exhibit zone 2 behavior. In general, zones 1 and 2 become more extensive when left atrial pressure is low, when the PAC tip is located vertically

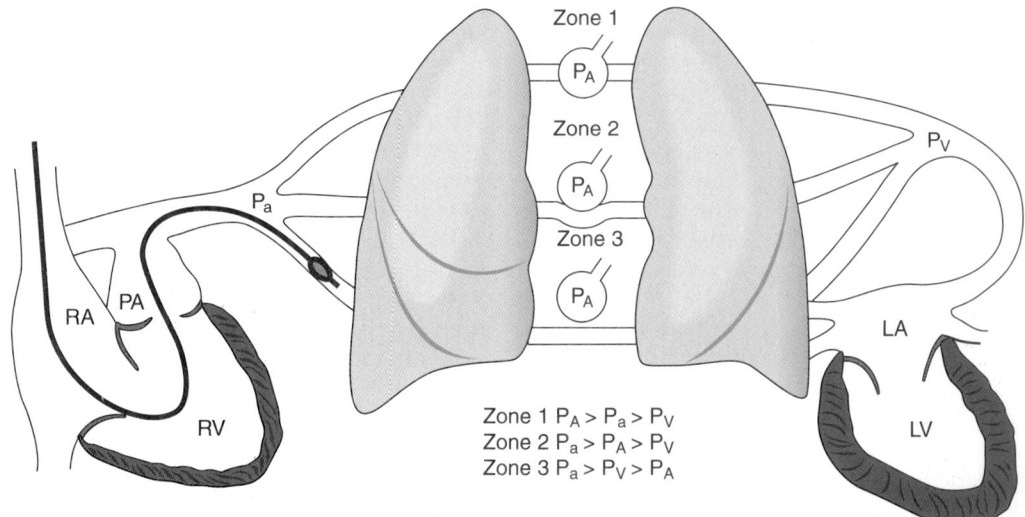

Zone 1 $P_A > P_a > P_V$
Zone 2 $P_a > P_A > P_V$
Zone 3 $P_a > P_V > P_A$

Figure 32–31 The pulmonary artery catheter tip must be wedged in lung zone 3 to provide an accurate measure of pulmonary venous (P_v) or left atrial (LA) pressure. When alveolar pressure (P_A) rises above P_v in lung zone 2 or above pulmonary arterial pressure (P_a) in lung zone 1, wedge pressure will reflect alveolar pressure rather than intravascular pressure. LV, left ventricle; PA, pulmonary artery; RA, right atrium; RV, right ventricle. (Redrawn from Mark JB: Atlas of Cardiovascular Monitoring. New York, Churchill Livingstone, 1998, Fig. 6-10.)

above the left atrium, or when alveolar pressure is high. Catheters that are wedged outside zone 3 may be suspected when the normal phasic wedge pressure a and v waves are absent, when wedge pressure varies markedly with the respiratory cycle, and when mean wedge pressure exceeds pulmonary artery diastolic pressure because this should never occur unless tall a or v waves are present in the wedge pressure trace.[120]

Normal Pulmonary Artery and Wedge Pressure Waveforms

As the flow-directed, balloon-tipped PAC is floated from a central vein to its proper position in the pulmonary artery, characteristic pressure waveforms are recorded (see Fig. 32-29). When the catheter tip reaches the superior vena cava or right atrium, a CVP waveform should be observed with its a, c, and v waves and low mean pressure value (see Table 32-7). At this point, the PAC balloon is inflated, and the catheter is advanced until it crosses the tricuspid valve to record right ventricular pressure. This waveform is recognized by the sudden increase in systolic pressure, the wide pulse pressure, and the low diastolic pressure that approximates CVP. The PAC next enters the right ventricular outflow tract and floats across the pulmonic valve into the main pulmonary artery. Often, this passage is heralded by arrhythmias, especially premature ventricular beats, as the balloon-tipped catheter strikes the right ventricular infundibulum. PAP is characterized by the step-up in diastolic pressure recorded as the catheter crosses the pulmonic valve. In the absence of pulmonic valve stenosis, pulmonary artery systolic pressure closely approximates right ventricular systolic pressure, but pulmonary artery diastolic pressure generally exceeds right ventricular diastolic pressure.

On occasion, it may be difficult to distinguish right ventricular pressure from PAP, particularly if only the numeric values for these pressures are examined. However, careful observation of the pressure waveforms, with a focus on the diastolic pressure contours, will allow these pressure waveforms to be distinguished. PAP decreases steadily during diastole as blood flows from the pulmonary artery toward the left atrium. In contrast, right ventricular pressure increases steadily during diastole as blood flows into the right ventricle through the open tricuspid valve (see Fig. 32-29).[331]

Under normal conditions, the PAP upstroke slightly precedes the radial artery pressure upstroke (Fig. 32-32) because of the longer duration of left ventricular isovolumic contraction, as well as the transmission time of the central aortic pressure upstroke to the downstream radial artery recording site. Although the PAP upstroke precedes the radial artery pressure upstroke by 50 milliseconds, peak PAP precedes peak radial artery pressure by only 10 milliseconds.[429] As a practical matter, the pulmonary and systemic arterial pressure waveforms appear to overlap on the bedside monitor, with these pressures rising, peaking, and falling at approximately the same points in time (see Fig. 32-32). Understanding these temporal relationships is critically important if one is to properly interpret abnormal pulmonary artery and wedge pressure waveforms, particularly when tall v waves are present in these traces (see later).

The PAC, with balloon inflated, finally reaches the wedge position. As noted earlier, wedge pressure is an indirect measurement of pulmonary venous pressure and left atrial pressure and should therefore resemble these pressure waveforms. Consequently, the PAWP waveform may be identified as a venous pressure trace that displays characteristic a and v waves and x and y descents. However, because of the pulmonary vascular bed interposed between the PAC tip and the left atrium, wedge pressure is a delayed representation of left atrial pressure.[423,430] On average, 160 milliseconds is required for the left atrial pressure pulse to traverse the pulmonary veins, capillaries, arterioles, and arteries. As a consequence of this delay, the wedge pressure a wave appears to follow the ECG R wave in early ventricular systole (see Fig. 32-32). However, the a wave is an end-diastolic pressure event produced by left atrial contraction. Recognition of

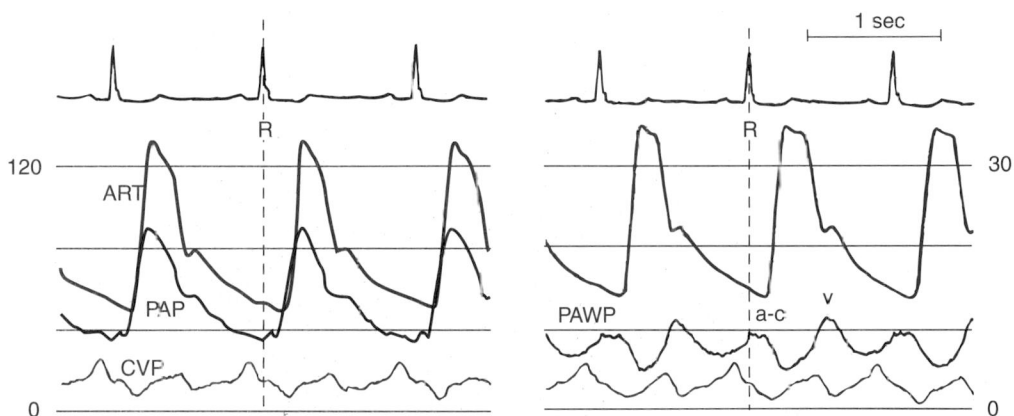

Figure 32–32 Temporal relationships between normal systemic arterial pressure (ART), pulmonary artery pressure (PAP), central venous pressure (CVP), and pulmonary artery wedge pressure (PAWP). Note that the PAWP a-c and v waves appear to occur later in the cardiac cycle than do their counterparts on the right side of the heart seen in the CVP trace. The ART scale is on the *left,* and the PAP, CVP, and PAWP scales are on the right. (Redrawn from Mark JB: Atlas of Cardiovascular Monitoring. New York, Churchill Livingstone, 1998, Fig. 3-3.)

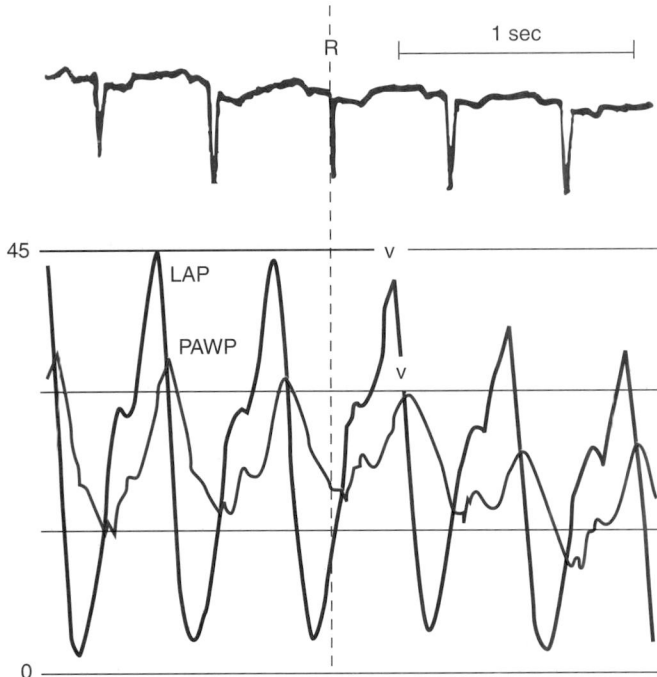

Figure 32–33 Pulmonary artery wedge pressure (PAWP) is a damped, delayed reflection of left atrial pressure (LAP). The tall regurgitant v waves (v) caused by severe mitral regurgitation are seen clearly in the LAP trace but appear delayed and smaller in magnitude in the PAWP trace. (Redrawn from Mark JB: Atlas of Cardiovascular Monitoring. New York, Churchill Livingstone, 1998, Fig. 4-4.)

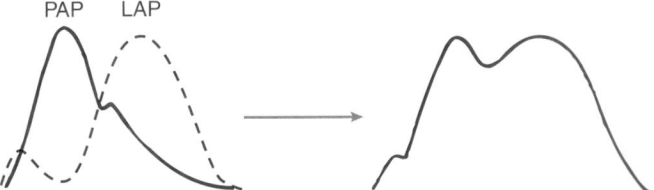

Figure 32–34 Tall left atrial pressure (LAP) a and v waves transmitted in a retrograde direction through the pulmonary vasculature distort the antegrade pulmonary artery pressure (PAP) waveform. The LAP a wave distorts systolic upstroke, and the v wave distorts the dicrotic notch. (Redrawn from Mark JB: Atlas of Cardiovascular Monitoring. New York, Churchill Livingstone, 1998, Fig. 4-10.)

this intrinsic time delay in phasic wedge pressure waves must be appreciated for proper interpretation of waveforms.

Not only is wedge pressure a delayed representation of left atrial pressure, but it is also a damped reflection of phasic atrial pressure waves. The amount of damping is variable, but when left atrial pressure waves are prominent, the pressure peaks may be significantly underestimated by the wedge trace (Fig. 32-33). Even though the wedge pressure waveform will always appear to be a damped, delayed version of left atrial pressure, the mean pressure recorded from these two sites should be similar under most circumstances.

To recognize prominent a or v waves in the wedge pressure trace, it is not always necessary to inflate the PAC balloon and obtain a wedge position (Fig. 32-34). Because the wedge pressure records pressure waves transmitted in retrograde fashion from the left atrium, these waves will normally sum with antegrade PAP waves produced by right ventricular ejection. The PAP trace thus becomes a composite wave reflecting both retrograde and antegrade components. Tall left atrial a or v waves will distort the normal PAP waveform appearance, with the a wave inscribed at the onset of systolic upstroke and the v wave distorting the dicrotic notch (see Fig. 32-34).[423,431] Once these waves are identified by wedging the PAC and comparing the pulmonary artery and wedge pressure traces, it is convenient and perhaps more prudent to "follow" the wedge pressure a and v waves in the unwedged

pulmonary artery pressure trace without repeatedly inflating the balloon to measure wedge pressure.

In summary, PAWP measured with a balloon-tipped PAC provides a delayed, damped estimate of left atrial pressure by measuring the pressure where flow resumes at a pulmonary venous junction point near the left atrium. Mean wedge pressure will always be lower than mean PAP; otherwise, blood would not flow in an antegrade direction. The wedge pressure waveform should display small a and v waves that should be identifiable if the pressure trace is displayed with sufficient gain and resolution on the monitor screen.

Left Atrial Pressure, Pulmonary Artery Wedge Pressure, and Pulmonary Capillary Pressure

Direct *left atrial pressure* monitoring is usually restricted to patients undergoing cardiac surgery. The most common technique for monitoring left atrial pressure involves catheterization of the left atrium with a thin catheter introduced through the right superior pulmonary vein and secured with a purse-string suture. The catheter is brought out through the skin beneath the xiphoid process and attached to a closed pressure monitoring tubing-transducer system. Because left atrial monitoring is discontinued in the postoperative period simply by withdrawing the left atrial catheter through the skin, trans-septal methods for monitoring left atrial pressure during surgery have been proposed to reduce the risk of bleeding after catheter removal.[432,433] Left atrial pressure measurement has also been performed for diagnostic cardiac catheterization by a retrograde arterial approach, trans-septal venous catheterization, and even percutaneous direct left atrial puncture from a right paravertebral insertion site.[434]

Today, direct left atrial pressure monitoring has largely been supplanted by PAC monitoring. This has occurred, no doubt, because the PAC simultaneously provides an estimation of left ventricular filling pressure as well as additional useful monitoring information, including CVP and cardiac output. Although some authors have shown modest discrepancies between left atrial pressure and PAWP in the period immediately after cardiopulmonary bypass, wedge pressure generally provides an excellent estimate of left atrial pressure in postoperative cardiac surgical patients.[426,435,436] However, a host of pathophysiologic conditions can alter the relationships between pulmonary artery diastolic, wedge, and left atrial pressure, and these conditions must be recognized to avoid misinterpretation of the data provided by these monitors (see later).

Direct left atrial pressure monitoring continues to be particularly useful in pediatric patients undergoing complex congenital heart surgery because of the difficulty of using some of the standard percutaneous techniques in this patient population. Gold and coauthors reported the use of more than 6000 transthoracic left atrial and right atrial pressure monitoring catheters, with complications from left-sided monitoring occurring in only 0.68% of 2393 catheters.[437] However, direct access to the left heart chambers always carries the risk of air and particulate embolization to the systemic circulation and thus requires close attention to proper management by the entire team of caregivers to ensure that line patency is maintained and flushing is performed with care.

The most common complication of direct left atrial pressure monitoring actually results from catheter removal. Because of the risk of bleeding from the cardiac site of catheter entry, the left atrial catheter must be removed before the mediastinal portion of the chest drains, and if the catheter cannot be withdrawn through the skin, surgical re-exploration is needed. Other rare complications of left atrial pressure monitoring include entrapment of the catheter in mechanical aortic or mitral valve prostheses,[437,438] fistula formation between the right superior pulmonary vein and the right main stem bronchus,[439] and unrecognized retained catheter fragments that serve as a source of systemic embolization.[440]

Normal left atrial pressure waveforms resemble CVP or right atrial pressure waveforms, although there are a few subtle morphologic distinctions. Because atrial depolarization originates in the sinoatrial node located at the junction of the superior vena cava and the right atrium, the right-sided a wave appears slightly earlier than the left-sided a wave (Fig. 32-35). Although the a wave is the most prominent pressure peak in a normal CVP trace, the v wave is often taller than the a wave in a normal left

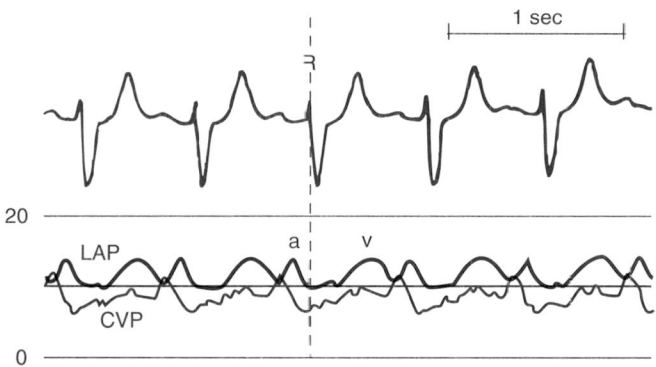

Figure 32–35 Normal temporal relationships between the electrocardiographic, central venous pressure (CVP), and left atrial pressure (LAP) traces. The LAP and CVP waveforms have nearly identical morphologies, although the CVP a wave slightly precedes the LAP a wave. (Redrawn from Mark JB: Atlas of Cardiovascular Monitoring. New York, Churchill Livingstone, 1998, Fig. 2-9.)

atrial pressure waveform, thus suggesting that right atrial contraction is generally more forceful than left atrial contraction and that the left atrium is less distensible than the right atrium during passive systolic filling.[136] Finally, the interval between right atrial contraction and right ventricular contraction is longer by approximately 40 milliseconds than the interval between left atrial contraction and left ventricular contraction.[136] Consequently, a and c waves are seen more often as separate waves in a right atrial pressure trace than in a left atrial pressure trace. In normal left atrial pressure waveforms, the a and c waves merge into a composite a-c wave, although most clinicians simply describe this pressure peak as the a wave. Similarly, the PAWP waveform generally displays only a and v waves because the wedge pressure c wave is obscured further as a result of the damping effect of the lung vasculature on the transmitted left atrial pressure waves.

The terms *pulmonary artery wedge pressure* and *pulmonary artery occlusion pressure* are used interchangeably and refer to the same measurement obtained from the tip of a PAC after balloon inflation and flotation to the wedged position. As already discussed, this pressure provides an indirect estimate of mean left atrial pressure. In contrast, the hydrostatic pressure in the pulmonary capillaries that drives edema formation according to the Starling equation is a different pressure that must exceed left atrial pressure to maintain antegrade blood flow through the lungs. This *pulmonary capillary pressure* must not be confused with wedge pressure or left atrial pressure, nor should these terms be used interchangeably.[441] Continued use of the phrase "pulmonary capillary wedge pressure" rather than pulmonary artery wedge pressure or occlusion pressure has perpetuated misconceptions about these measurements. Although the magnitude of the difference between pulmonary capillary pressure and wedge pressure is generally small, it can increase markedly when resistance to flow in the pulmonary veins is elevated.[442] In most situations, the major component of pulmonary vascular resistance (PVR) occurs at the precapillary, pulmonary arteriolar level. However, rare conditions such as pulmonary veno-occlusive disease may cause a marked increase in postcapillary resistance to flow within the pulmonary veins. A similar situation arises in other conditions that disproportionately increase pulmonary venous resistance, such as central nervous system injury, acute lung injury, hypovolemic shock, endotoxemia, and norepinephrine infusion.[441,443] Under these conditions, measurement of wedge pressure will underestimate pulmonary capillary pressure substantially and thereby underestimate the risk of hydrostatic pulmonary edema. Although pulmonary capillary pressure can be measured at the bedside by analyzing the decay in the PAP trace after inflation of the PAC balloon, these techniques have not been widely adopted in clinical practice.[444-449] To avoid confusion, the phrase "pulmonary capillary wedge pressure" should be abandoned because it is imprecise and misleading.

Abnormal Pulmonary Artery and Wedge Pressure Waveforms

PAC monitoring is subject to the same technical artifacts inherent in all invasive pressure monitoring techniques,

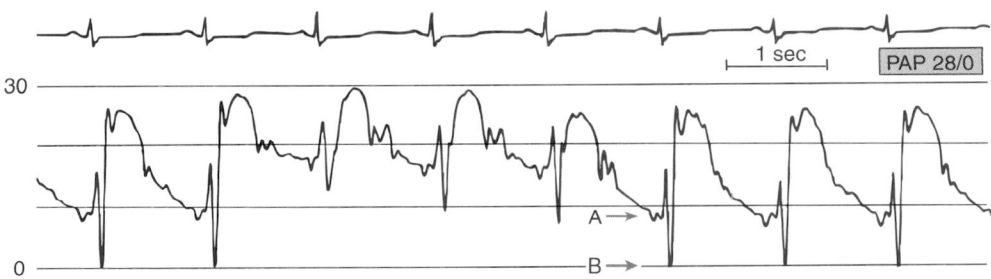

Figure 32–36 Artifactual pressure peaks and troughs in the pulmonary artery pressure (PAP) waveform caused by catheter motion. The correct value for pulmonary artery end-diastolic pressure is 8 mm Hg (A), although the monitor digital display erroneously reports the PAP as 28/0 mm Hg (B). (Redrawn from Mark JB: Atlas of Cardiovascular Monitoring. New York, Churchill Livingstone, 1998, Fig. 5-6.)

as well as some additional problems unique to this method.[403,450-452] Because the PAC is longer than other intravascular catheters, greater attention must be paid to ensure that the lumens are free from clot or air bubbles that will distort the pressure waveforms. In addition, the PAC passes through the heart and is subject to pressure-recording artifacts resulting from cardiac-induced catheter motion. These artifactual pressure spikes may be distinguished from the underlying physiologic pressure waveform by their unique morphology and timing.

The most common prominent pressure artifact observed in a PAC trace is a sharp pressure spike seen immediately after the ECG R wave at onset of systole (Fig. 32-36).[450,453] At this point in the cardiac cycle, tricuspid valve closure, right ventricular contraction, and ejection set the PAC in motion and inscribe a motion artifact in the pressure waveform. Note that this pressure artifact appears at the same time as the CVP c wave and may produce a factitiously low pressure or a pressure peak. If the bedside monitor detects this artifactual pressure nadir inappropriately, it may be erroneously designated as the pulmonary artery diastolic pressure (see Fig. 32-36). Repositioning the PAC by advancing or withdrawing it a few centimeters often ameliorates the problem.

Another common artifact in PAC pressure measurement occurs when attempts to inflate the balloon cause the catheter tip to become obstructed and thus fail to measure intravascular pressure. This phenomenon is generally termed *overwedging* and is usually caused by distal catheter migration and eccentric balloon inflation that forces the catheter tip against the wall of the pulmonary artery.

Rather than recording intravascular pressure, the catheter now records the gradually rising pressure produced by the continuous flush system as it builds up pressure against the obstructed distal opening (Fig. 32-37). Note that overwedged pressure is devoid of pulsatile detail, is much higher than pulmonary diastolic pressure, and continuously rises toward the flush pressure level. These observations all suggest that this cannot be an accurate measurement of PAWP.

As emphasized earlier, each PAC balloon inflation allows the catheter tip to migrate distally several centimeters to reach the wedge position. This flotation process generally occurs over several cardiac cycles. When a wedge pressure tracing appears during partial balloon inflation, it suggests that the PAC is located inappropriately in a smaller, distal branch of the pulmonary artery. The catheter should be withdrawn before overwedging results in vascular injury or pulmonary infarction. A distally positioned catheter may overwedge itself without balloon inflation. This problem must be recognized immediately by observing the waveform, and the PAC must be withdrawn until a normal PAP tracing is restored.

Pathophysiologic conditions involving the left-sided cardiac chambers or valves produce characteristic changes in the pulmonary artery and wedge pressure waveforms (Table 32-11).[454] One of the most widely recognized abnormalities is the tall v wave of *mitral regurgitation* (Fig. 32-38). Unlike a normal wedge pressure v wave produced by late systolic pulmonary venous inflow, which fills the left atrium while the mitral valve is closed, the prominent v wave of mitral regurgitation begins in

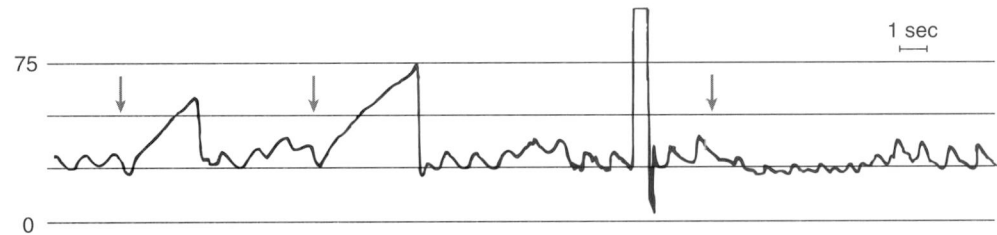

Figure 32–37 Overwedging of the pulmonary artery (PA) catheter causes artifactual waveform recordings. The first two attempts to inflate the PA catheter balloon *(first two arrows)* produce a nonpulsatile, increasing pressure caused by an occluded catheter tip. After the catheter is withdrawn slightly, balloon inflation allows proper wedge pressure measurement *(third arrow)*. Before the third attempt at balloon inflation, the PA pressure lumen is flushed. Flushing restores the appropriate pulsatile pressure detailed to the PA and wedge pressure waveforms on the right side of the trace. (Redrawn from Mark JB: Atlas of Cardiovascular Monitoring. New York, Churchill Livingstone, 1998, Fig. 5-7.)

Table 32–11 Pulmonary artery wedge pressure waveform abnormalities

Condition	Characteristics
Mitral regurgitation	Tall regurgitant c-v wave
	Obliteration of x descent
Ventricular septal defect	Tall antegrade v wave
Mitral stenosis	Tall a wave
	Attenuation of y descent
Myocardial ischemia	Tall a waves
	Tall v waves

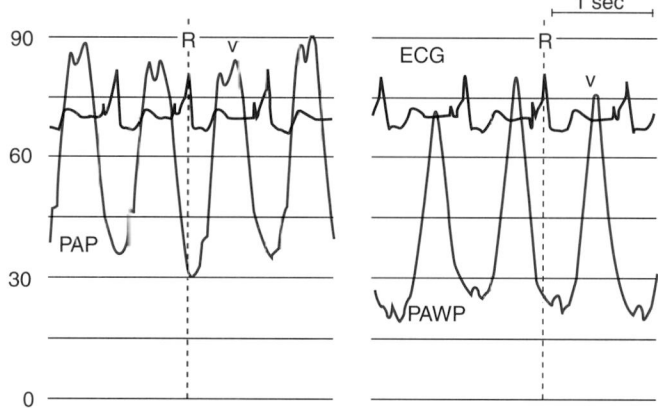

Figure 32–39 Severe mitral regurgitation. A tall systolic v wave (v) is inscribed in the pulmonary artery wedge pressure (PAWP) trace and also distorts the pulmonary artery pressure (PAP) trace, thus giving it a bifid appearance. The electrocardiogram (ECG) is abnormal because of ventricular pacing. Left ventricular end-diastolic pressure is estimated best by measuring PAWP at the time of the electrocardiographic R wave, before onset of the regurgitant v wave. Note that mean PAWP exceeds left ventricular end-diastolic pressure in this condition. (Redrawn from Mark JB: Atlas of Cardiovascular Monitoring. New York, Churchill Livingstone, 1998, Fig. 17-11.)

early systole and might be more precisely designated a regurgitant c-v wave. Mitral regurgitation causes fusion of the c and v waves and obliteration of the systolic x descent because the isovolumic phase of left ventricular systole is eliminated as a result of the retrograde ejection of blood into the left atrium.[312] Because the prominent v wave of mitral regurgitation is generated during ventricular systole, mean wedge pressure overestimates left ventricular filling pressure, just as measurement of mean CVP in patients with severe tricuspid regurgitation overestimates right ventricular filling pressure (see Fig. 32-26). In patients with severe mitral regurgitation, left ventricular end-diastolic pressure is estimated best by measuring wedge pressure before onset of the regurgitant v wave (Figs. 32-38 and 32-39). Although mean wedge pressure exceeds left ventricular end-diastolic pressure in patients with severe mitral regurgitation, mean wedge pressure remains a good approximation of mean left atrial pressure. Consequently, the regurgitant v wave contributes to left atrial hypertension and the subsequent risk of hydrostatic pulmonary edema.

When large v waves are present in the wedge pressure trace, it is critically important to recognize them and be able to distinguish the wedge pressure waveform from the unwedged PAP waveform. At first glance, a wedge trace with a tall systolic v wave resembles a typical unwedged PAP trace, but closer observation reveals a number of discriminating morphologic details. The PAP upstroke is

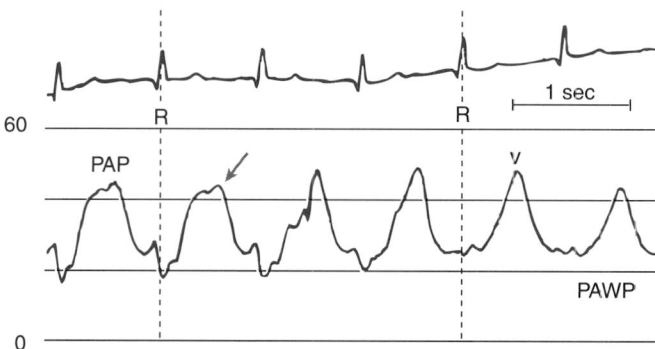

Figure 32–38 Mitral regurgitation. A tall regurgitant v wave (v) is seen in the pulmonary artery wedge pressure (PAWP) trace and may also be noted in the unwedged pulmonary artery pressure (PAP) waveform (arrow). (Redrawn from Mark JB: Atlas of Cardiovascular Monitoring. New York, Churchill Livingstone, 1998, Fig. 17-5.)

steeper and slightly precedes the systemic arterial pressure upstroke, whereas a wedge tracing with a prominent v wave has a more gradual upstroke that begins after the radial artery pressure upstroke. Although the PAP peak occurs at about the same time as the systemic arterial pressure peak and the ECG T wave, the wedge pressure v wave reaches its peak later in the cardiac cycle, after the ECG T wave (see Figs. 32-38 and 32-39).[312,429] This so-called rightward shift in the PAP waveform should be recognized by careful scrutiny and comparison of the ECG systemic arterial, pulmonary artery, and wedge pressure traces. Another feature that distinguishes pulmonary artery and wedge pressure traces in patients with severe mitral regurgitation is the unusual morphology of the pulmonary artery waveform itself. The prominent regurgitant v wave distorts the pulmonary artery waveform by giving it a bifid appearance in systole and obscuring the normal end-systolic dicrotic notch (see Figs. 32-38 and 32-39). This is most evident in patients with the tallest wedge pressure v waves.[431,455] By recognizing these subtle, but important diagnostic details, a clinician may monitor the wedge pressure v wave by observing the unwedged PAP trace and obviate the need for repeated balloon inflation. Of greater importance, one can avoid the disastrous situation in which a PAC migrates distally and becomes wedged unintentionally without balloon inflation and the clinician, not recognizing the wedge tracing, attempts to inflate the balloon and ruptures the pulmonary artery.

Although some clinicians use the height of the wedge pressure v wave as an indicator of the severity of mitral regurgitation, this practice is fraught with problems and has some fundamental physiologic limitations.[456-460] Because wedge pressure is a damped reflection of left atrial pressure, there may be some instances in which a prominent left atrial pressure v wave is not transmitted to the wedge pressure trace.[461] More important, the wedge pressure v wave is a pressure surrogate for a volume event, namely, regurgitant systolic filling across the incompetent mitral valve.

A closer look at the left atrial pressure-volume relationships helps explain the apparently paradoxical coexistence of severe mitral regurgitation and a normal PAWP trace.[457,462] Three factors determine whether mitral regurgitation produces a prominent v wave in the left atrial or wedge pressure traces: left atrial volume (often termed the patient's "volume status"), left atrial compliance, and regurgitant volume (Fig. 32-40). Given that the left atrial pressure-volume relationship is curvilinear, the same volume of regurgitation will result in a variable increment in systolic pressure, depending on the preexisting atrial volume at the onset of systole. Similarly, the shape of the left atrial pressure-volume curve, which reflects atrial stiffness or compliance, will determine the height of the pressure wave for any given regurgitant volume. Accordingly, patients with acute mitral regurgitation tend to have tall wedge pressure v waves because they have smaller, stiffer left atria than do patients with chronic valvular regurgitation. Although the total regurgitant volume of blood entering the left atrium will influence the height of the v wave, this is clearly not the only determinant of v wave magnitude. Therefore, it is not surprising that wedge pressure v waves are neither sensitive nor specific indicators of the severity of mitral regurgitation.[457-460] Prominent wedge pressure v waves may exist in the absence of mitral regurgitation when left atrial pressure is high, as might occur when the left atrium is compressed.[463] Tall v waves are also seen commonly in patients with hypervolemia, congestive heart failure, and ventricular septal defects.[457] Note that the giant v waves observed in patients with *ventricular septal defects* are not caused by retrograde flow, but rather by excessive antegrade systolic flow into the left atrium from the left-to-right shunt, which increases pulmonary blood flow and systolic atrial filling through the pulmonary veins.[456]

In contrast to mitral regurgitation, which distorts the systolic portion of the wedge pressure waveform, *mitral stenosis* alters the morphology of the diastolic portions of this waveform. In this condition, the holodiastolic pressure gradient across the mitral valve results in an increased mean wedge pressure, a slurred early diastolic y descent, and a tall end-diastolic a wave. Similar hemodynamic abnormalities are seen in patients with left atrial myxoma or whenever there is obstruction to mitral flow. Diseases that increase left ventricular stiffness (e.g., left ventricular infarction, pericardial constriction, aortic stenosis, and systemic hypertension) produce changes in wedge pressure that resemble in part those seen in mitral stenosis. In these conditions, mean wedge pressure is increased and the trace displays a prominent a wave, but the y descent remains steep because of the absence of obstruction to flow across the mitral valve during diastole. Because patients with advanced mitral stenosis often have coexisting atrial fibrillation, the a wave will not be present in many of these cases, although the other hemodynamic features persist (Fig. 32-41).[312]

Myocardial ischemia is accompanied by a number of physiologic abnormalities that are detectable with the PAC. Ischemia impairs left ventricular relaxation and thereby results in diastolic dysfunction. This pattern of ischemia is particularly characteristic of the demand ischemia associated with tachycardia or induced by rapid atrial pacing.[295,464-469] Impaired ventricular relaxation results in a stiffer, less compliant left ventricle in diastole, which leads to increased left ventricular end-diastolic pressure. Not only does this, in turn, increase left atrial and wedge pressure, but the morphology of these waveforms changes as well, with the phasic a and v wave components becoming more prominent as diastolic filling pressure increases.[467,470-476] Although myocardial ischemia will often be detectable as a rise in pulmonary artery diastolic, mean, or systolic pressure, these changes are generally less striking than the accompanying change in wedge pressure and the new appearance of tall a and v waves (Fig. 32-42). In patients with left ventricular ischemia, the tall wedge pressure a wave is produced by

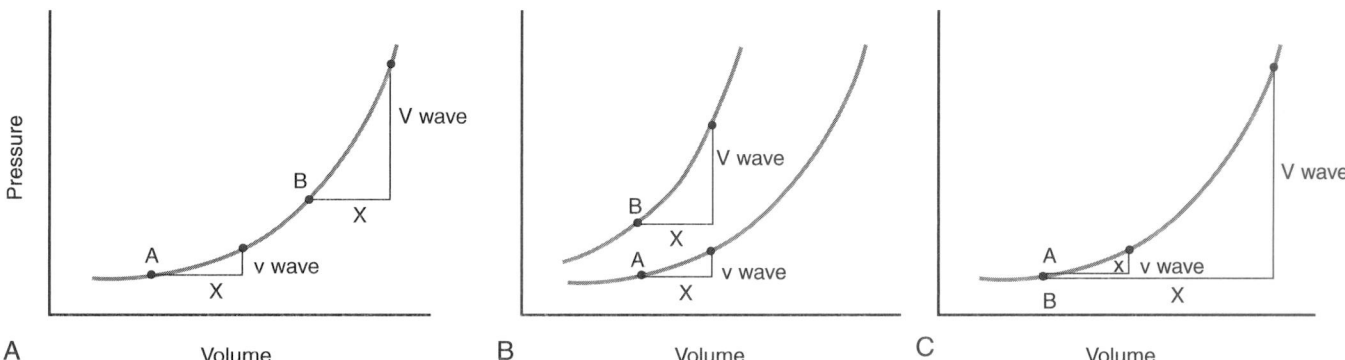

Figure 32–40 Height of the v wave as an indicator of the severity of mitral regurgitation. Left atrial pressure-volume curves describe the three factors that determine the height of the v wave. **A,** Influence of left atrial volume. For the same regurgitant volume (x), the left atrial v wave will be taller if baseline atrial volume is greater (point B versus point A). **B,** Influence of left atrial compliance. For the same regurgitant volume (x), the left atrial v wave will be taller if baseline atrial compliance is reduced (point B versus point A). **C,** Influence of regurgitant volume. Beginning at the same baseline left atrial volume (points A and B), if regurgitant volume increases (X versus x), the left atrial pressure v wave will increase (V versus v). (Redrawn from Mark JB: Atlas of Cardiovascular Monitoring. New York, Churchill Livingstone, 1998, Fig. 17-13.)

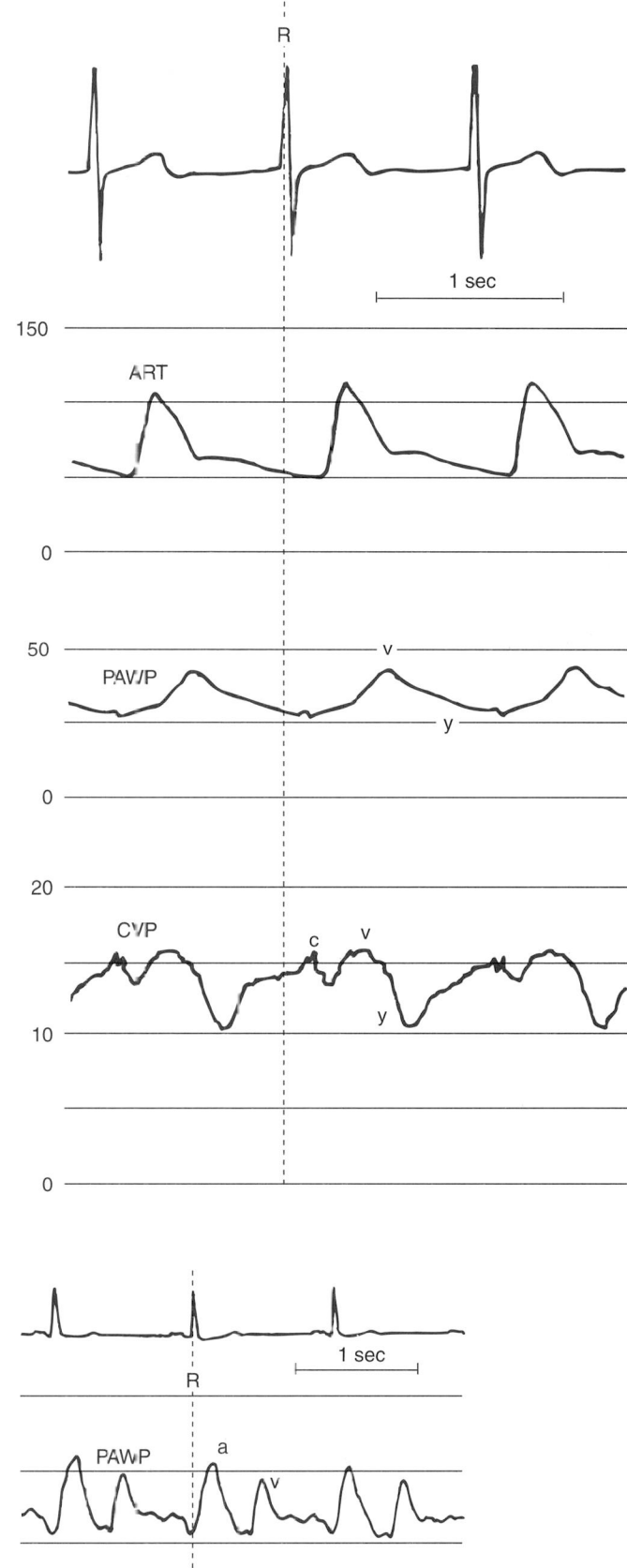

Figure 32–41 Mitral stenosis. Mean pulmonary artery wedge pressure (PAWP) is increased (35 mm Hg), and the diastolic y descent is markedly attenuated. Compare the slope of the y descent in the PAWP trace with the y descent in the central venous pressure (CVP) trace. In addition, compare this PAWP y descent with the PAWP y descent in mitral regurgitation (see Figs. 32-38 and 32-39). Because of atrial fibrillation, a waves are not seen in the PAWP or CVP traces. ART, arterial blood pressure. (Redrawn from Mark JB: Atlas of Cardiovascular Monitoring. New York, Churchill Livingstone, 1998, Fig. 17-19.)

Figure 32–42 Myocardial ischemia. Pulmonary artery pressure (PAP) is relatively normal and mean pulmonary artery wedge pressure (PAWP) is only slightly elevated (15 mm Hg). However, PAWP morphology is markedly abnormal, with tall a waves (21 mm Hg) resulting from the diastolic dysfunction seen in this condition. (Redrawn from Mark JB: Atlas of Cardiovascular Monitoring. New York, Churchill Livingstone, 1998, Fig. 12-4.)

end-diastolic atrial contraction into a stiff, incompletely relaxed left ventricle and underscores the fact that the atrial kick provides a greater than normal contribution to ventricular filling under these conditions.[425,474,477] Although the diastolic dysfunction accompanying myocardial ischemia leads to an increase in left ventricular end-diastolic pressure, this pressure elevation often coexists with decreased left ventricular end-diastolic volume or preload.[295] The dissociation between filling pressure and filling volume in this condition must be appreciated to avoid diagnostic and therapeutic errors.

Myocardial ischemia produces a characteristic pattern of left ventricular systolic dysfunction in addition to the diastolic abnormalities noted earlier. Systolic dysfunction is the hallmark of supply ischemia caused by a sudden reduction or cessation of coronary blood flow to a region of the myocardium.[466,478] With severe systolic dysfunction, changes in global left ventricular contractile performance may be detected with hemodynamic monitoring. As the ejection fraction falls and left ventricular end-diastolic volume and pressure rise, hemodynamic monitoring will show systemic arterial hypotension and elevated pulmonary diastolic and wedge pressure. This hemodynamic pattern is uncommon during anesthesia and surgery and suggests severe systolic myocardial dysfunction.[479-481] A more common hemodynamic manifestation of myocardial ischemia occurs when left ventricular geometry is distorted or when the region of ischemic myocardium underlies a papillary muscle.[482] Acute mitral valve regurgitation may result, not because of any inherent abnormality of the mitral valve leaflets, but rather because of critical alterations in the supporting structures of the mitral valve, including the mitral annulus, chordae tendineae, papillary muscles, and underlying left ventricular myocardium.[482,483] This form of mitral regurgitation is often termed "papillary muscle ischemia" or "functional mitral regurgitation." As noted earlier, PAC monitoring is particularly well suited to detect this event by revealing the onset of new regurgitant v waves in the pulmonary artery or wedge pressure trace (see Figs. 32-38 and 32-39).

Whether the PAC should be used in high-risk patients as a supplemental monitor for detection of myocardial ischemia remains uncertain.[484-487] However, if physicians choose this form of monitoring, they should have a clear understanding of the mechanism by which ischemia alters pulmonary artery and wedge pressure and an appreciation for the anticipated pressure waveform changes. None of the current methods of detecting perioperative myocardial ischemia is perfectly sensitive or specific. Although patients with left ventricular ischemia are likely to have higher mean wedge pressure than those without ischemia, these differences are small and may be difficult to detect clinically.[476] Furthermore, clear quantitative threshold values for mean wedge pressure or a and v wave peak pressures that are diagnostic of ischemia have not been identified, perhaps because of the wide variation in the normal range of these pressures. Consequently, when a PAC is used to diagnose myocardial ischemia, the best approach is to integrate the PAC data with other monitored values and use changes in pulmonary artery or wedge pressure as parts of the diagnostic puzzle.[467,488]

Right ventricular ischemia produces characteristic hemodynamic patterns that may be recognized with PAC monitoring. Just as left ventricular ischemia increases PAWP, right ventricular ischemia increases CVP, and this is one of the few situations in which CVP may be higher than wedge pressure. In addition, CVP waveform morphology changes in a characteristic manner and displays a prominent a wave resulting from right ventricular diastolic dysfunction and a prominent v wave resulting from ischemia-induced tricuspid regurgitation.[11,306,467,489,490] The CVP waveform in this condition is described as having an M or W configuration, which refers to the tall a and v waves and steep x and y descents. Severe *pulmonary artery hypertension* may also result in secondary right ventricular ischemia and dysfunction and increased CVP, but this condition is distinguished from primary right ventricular dysfunction in that PAP and the calculated PVR are not increased in the latter condition.

The CVP waveform in right ventricular infarction shares many morphologic features with that recorded from patients with *restrictive cardiomyopathy* or *pericardial constriction*, including elevated mean pressure, prominent a and v waves, and steep x and y descents.[489,491] The pathophysiologic feature common to these conditions is impaired right ventricular diastolic compliance and is often termed "restrictive physiology." In pericardial constriction, this arises from the restraining effect of the diseased pericardium, whereas in restrictive cardiomyopathy and right ventricular infarction, diastolic dysfunction impairs ventricular relaxation and increases intrinsic ventricular stiffness. Pericardial constriction, also termed constrictive pericarditis or pericardial restriction, limits cardiac filling because of the rigid, often calcified pericardial shell. Impaired venous return decreases end-diastolic volume, stroke volume, and cardiac output. Despite reduced cardiac volumes, cardiac filling pressures are markedly elevated and equal in all four chambers of the heart at end-diastole (Fig. 32-43). Although PAC monitoring reveals this pressure equalization, the characteristic M or W configuration is more apparent in the CVP trace than in the PAWP trace, most likely because of the damping effect of the pulmonary vasculature on the left-sided filling pressure as recorded by the PAC.[167,492-494]

Another hemodynamic hallmark of pericardial constriction is observed in the right and left ventricular pressure traces. These traces demonstrate rapid, but short-lived early diastolic ventricular filling, which produces a diastolic "dip-and-plateau" pattern or "square root sign" (Fig. 32-44).[166,495] In some cases, particularly when the heart rate is slow, a similar waveform pattern may be noted in the CVP trace: a steep y descent (the diastolic dip) produced by rapid early diastolic flow from the atrium to the ventricle, followed by a mid-diastolic h wave (the plateau) from the interruption in flow imposed by the restrictive pericardial shell (see Figs. 32-43 and Fig. 32-44).

Like pericardial constriction, *cardiac tamponade* impairs cardiac filling, but in the case of tamponade, a compressive pericardial fluid collection produces this effect. This filling defect results in a marked increase in CVP and reduced cardiac diastolic volume, stroke volume, and cardiac output. Despite many similar hemodynamic features, tamponade and constriction may be distinguished by the

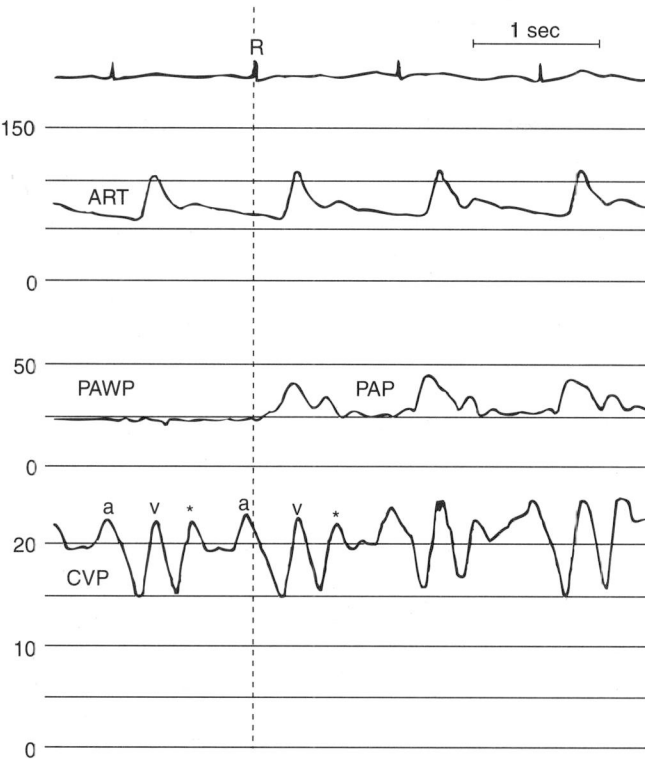

Figure 32–43 Pericardial constriction. This condition causes elevation and equalization of diastolic filling pressures in the pulmonary artery pressure (PAP), pulmonary artery wedge pressure (PAWP), and central venous pressure (CVP) traces. The CVP waveform reveals tall a and v waves with steep x and y descents and a mid-diastolic plateau wave *(asterisk)* or h wave. ART, arterial blood pressure. (Redrawn from Mark JB: Atlas of Cardiovascular Monitoring. New York, Churchill Livingstone, 1998, Fig. 18-1.)

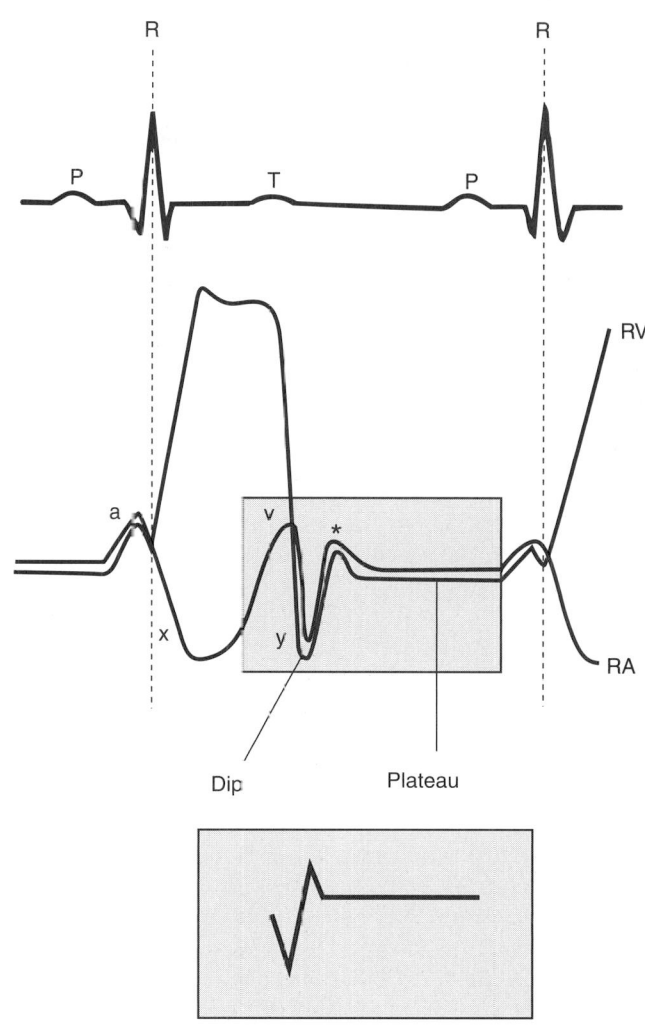

Figure 32–44 Pericardial constriction. The diastolic filling abnormality in this condition inscribes a "dip-and-plateau pattern" or "square root sign" in both the right ventricular (RV) and right atrial (RA) pressure traces. (Redrawn from Mark JB: Atlas of Cardiovascular Monitoring. New York, Churchill Livingstone, 1998, Fig. 18-3.)

different CVP waveforms seen in these two conditions. In tamponade, the venous pressure waveform appears more monophasic and is dominated by the systolic x pressure descent. The diastolic y pressure descent is attenuated or absent because early diastolic flow from the right atrium to the right ventricle is impaired by the surrounding compressive pericardial fluid collection (Fig. 32-45).[166,167,489,492,496-498] Clearly, other clinical and hemodynamic clues help distinguish these diagnoses, such as the presence of pulsus paradoxus, which is an almost invariable finding in cardiac tamponade (see Fig. 32-19).[499] CVP traces in pericardial constriction and cardiac tamponade thus have many similarities, but also important distinguishing features. As a general rule, the CVP waveform in pericardial constriction has prominent x and y descents or a predominant y descent, whereas in cardiac tamponade, the venous pressure waveform shows attenuation or obliteration of the y descent. Coexisting abnormalities such as tachycardia, arrhythmias, and atrial contractile failure may complicate interpretation of these waveforms. On occasion, localized pericardial constriction may simulate valvular stenosis, and hypovolemia may lower cardiac filling pressures to within the normal range and confound the diagnosis. In some instances, patients may show features of more than one condition, such as seen in patients with effusive-constrictive

pericarditis who have constriction of the heart by the visceral pericardium in addition to a pericardial effusion that compresses the heart.[500]

Probably the single most important waveform abnormality or interpretive problem in PAC monitoring is discerning the correct pressure measurement in patients receiving *positive-pressure mechanical ventilation* or those who have labored spontaneous respiration. When any pulmonary artery or wedge pressure recording is used to estimate ventricular preload, the physician must consider the confounding effects of changes in intrathoracic pressure that occur during the respiratory cycle. Just as in the case of CVP monitoring, transmural cardiac filling pressures are estimated best when end-expiratory pressure values are recorded (see the earlier section "Physiologic Considerations for Central Venous Pressure Monitoring: Diastolic Pressure-Volume Relationships and Transmural Pressure"). During positive-pressure mechanical ventilation,

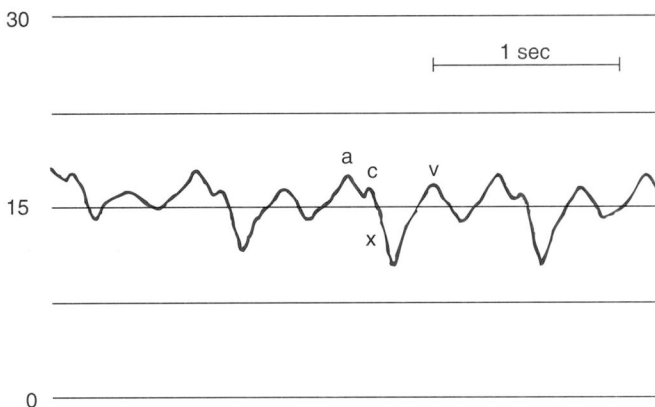

Figure 32–45 Cardiac tamponade. The central venous pressure waveform shows an increased mean pressure (16 mm Hg) and attenuation of the y descent. Compare with Figures 32-43 and 32-44. (Redrawn from Mark JB: Atlas of Cardiovascular Monitoring. New York, Churchill Livingstone, 1998, Fig. 18-5.)

Transduced PAWP	20	20	20
Transmural PAWP	25	10	25
LV compliance	Normal	Normal	Stiff
LV volume	Increased	Normal (or reduced)	Normal (or reduced)

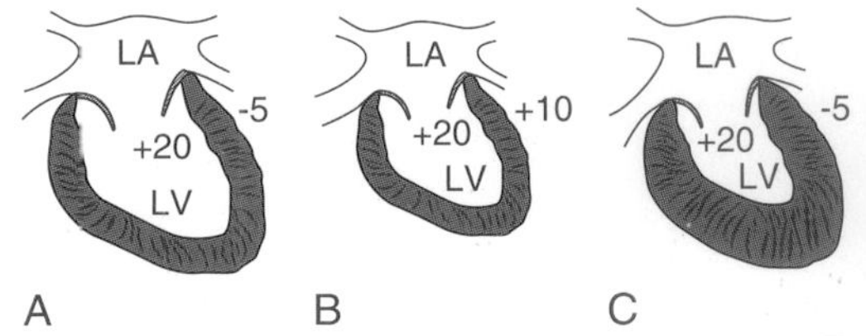

Figure 32–47 Influence of juxtacardiac pressure and ventricular compliance on left ventricular (LV) preload. There are three interpretations of an increased transduced pulmonary artery wedge pressure (PAWP, 20 mm Hg). **A,** Juxtacardiac pressure (−5 mm Hg) and LV compliance are normal, transmural PAWP is increased (25 mm Hg), and LV volume is increased. **B,** Juxtacardiac pressure is increased (+10 mm Hg), LV compliance is normal, transmural PAWP is decreased (10 mm Hg), and LV volume is normal or decreased. **C,** Juxtacardiac pressure is normal, LV compliance is decreased, transmural PAWP is increased (25 mm Hg), and LV volume is normal or decreased. LA, left atrium. (Redrawn from Mark JB: Atlas of Cardiovascular Monitoring. New York, Churchill Livingstone, 1998, Fig. 15-8.)

inspiration increases pulmonary artery and wedge pressure. By measuring these pressures at end-expiration, the confounding effect of this inspiratory increase in intrathoracic pressure is obviated (Fig. 32-46).[303] Forceful inspiration during spontaneous ventilation has the opposite effect, but again, measurement of these pressures at end-expiration eliminates this confounding factor (see Fig. 32-27). Bedside monitors are designed with algorithms that aim to identify and report the numeric values for end-expiratory pressures.[501-504] Unfortunately, these algorithms are notoriously inaccurate. The most reliable method for measuring central vascular pressures at end-expiration is examination of the waveforms on a calibrated monitor screen or paper recording.[504,505]

Use of Central Vascular Pressures to Estimate Left Ventricular Preload

Accurate, clinically meaningful interpretation of PAC-derived cardiac filling pressures requires a detailed understanding of the underlying physiologic principles, particularly the relationship between left ventricular filling pressure and preload. Although measurements such as pulmonary artery diastolic pressure and wedge pressure are used often as measures of left ventricular filling, many factors influence the relationship between filling

pressure and chamber volume. For example, consider how one might interpret measurement of a PAWP of 20 mm Hg (Fig. 32-47). This pressure is somewhat higher than the normal value, but depending on how this measured wedge pressure is interpreted, different treatments would be indicated. Proper interpretation of this filling pressure depends on two factors, juxtacardiac pressure and ventricular compliance. The most common interpretation of a wedge pressure of 20 mm Hg assumes that juxtacardiac pressure and ventricular compliance are normal and leads to the diagnosis of hypervolemia, with increased left ventricular end-diastolic volume causing the increased PAWP. One arrives at a different interpretation of this wedge pressure if juxtacardiac pressure is increased for any reason, including cardiac tamponade, pericardial constriction, or positive-pressure inspiration. Under these conditions, the same elevated filling pressure may be associated with normal or reduced left ventricular end-diastolic volume.

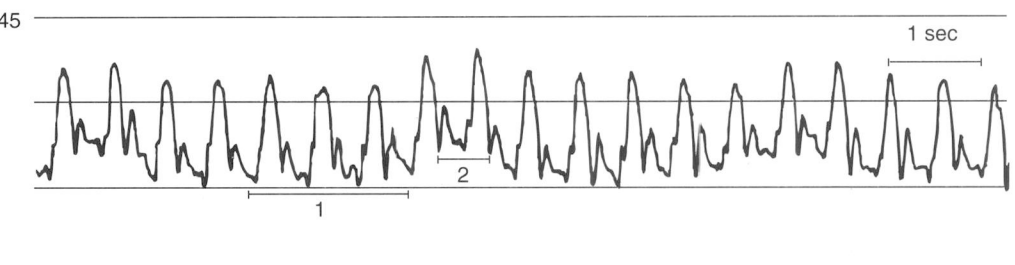

Figure 32–46 Influence of positive-pressure mechanical ventilation on pulmonary artery pressure. Pulmonary artery pressure should be measured at end-expiration (#1, 15 mm Hg) to obviate the artifact caused by positive-pressure inspiration (#2, 22 mm Hg). Compare with Figure 32-27. (Redrawn from Mark JB: Atlas of Cardiovascular Monitoring. New York, Churchill Livingstone, 1998, Fig. 16-3.)

Finally, a wedge pressure of 20 mm Hg has a third interpretation if ventricular compliance is decreased, such as might occur with diastolic dysfunction from myocardial ischemia, hypertrophy, or cardiomyopathy. Under these conditions, as in the case of increased juxtacardiac pressure, left ventricular volume may be normal or reduced despite elevated wedge pressure (see Fig. 32-47).

Deciding whether any given central vascular pressure is ideal for a particular patient may be a clinical challenge. When wedge pressure is extremely high or low, it is easy to recognize that this value must be adjusted to avoid pulmonary edema or improve cardiac output. However, things are rarely so clear-cut in critically ill patients, and the target value for optimal wedge pressure is uncertain and often decided empirically. Under these circumstances, a rapid fluid challenge may be a useful method to determine whether the PAWP value is optimal for the patient in any particular clinical setting. An intravenous bolus of crystalloid or colloid solution (250 to 500 mL) is given rapidly over a period of 15 minutes, and the change in wedge pressure is measured along with other pertinent hemodynamic variables. If the baseline wedge pressure is high or if a severe pulmonary capillary injury is present, a reduced volume may be used. Small increases in wedge pressure after the fluid challenge (e.g., less than 3 mm Hg) suggest that the ventricle is operating on the flat portion of its diastolic filling curve, whereas large increases in wedge pressure (e.g., 7 mm Hg or greater) suggest that the steep portion of the curve has been reached and that little further increase in stroke volume and cardiac output can be achieved without a substantial risk of producing hydrostatic pulmonary edema.[120,504]

As difficult as it may be to decide whether the wedge pressure is optimal for a particular patient, even greater uncertainty confronts a physician who uses CVP to determine whether cardiac preload is adequate or optimal. Clinicians have recognized for years that in many patients, CVP may be misleading[506-509] because of a number of anatomic and physiologic reasons.[294] The diastolic pressure-volume curves for the left and right ventricles are different, even in healthy individuals, with the left ventricle being stiffer or less compliant. Although investigators have shown that changes in CVP, pulmonary artery diastolic pressure, and wedge pressure all occur in the same direction,[510] the more important question is whether small changes in CVP are clinically detectable given that these small changes are often accompanied by much larger changes in PAWP, simply for the reason that the right and left ventricles have different diastolic pressure-volume relationships.[511]

The use of CVP to estimate left ventricular preload is associated with additional interpretive problems because of the fact that the right and left ventricles share a common septal wall and are both contained within the pericardium. Ventricular interdependence and pericardial constraint couple changes in right and left ventricular function such that a primary change in right ventricular filling may produce a secondary change in left ventricular filling by altering its diastolic pressure-volume relationship.[293,294,296,302,512] For example, acute pulmonary artery hypertension increases right ventricular end-diastolic volume and pressure, shifts the ventricular septum leftward, and increases left ventricular end-diastolic pressure while simultaneously decreasing left ventricular end-diastolic volume because of a shift in the left ventricular pressure-volume relationship to a steeper, stiffer curve.

Finally, numerous additional anatomic, physiologic, and pathophysiologic factors may alter the relationship between CVP and left ventricular preload (Fig. 32-48).[294] The further upstream from the left ventricle one records

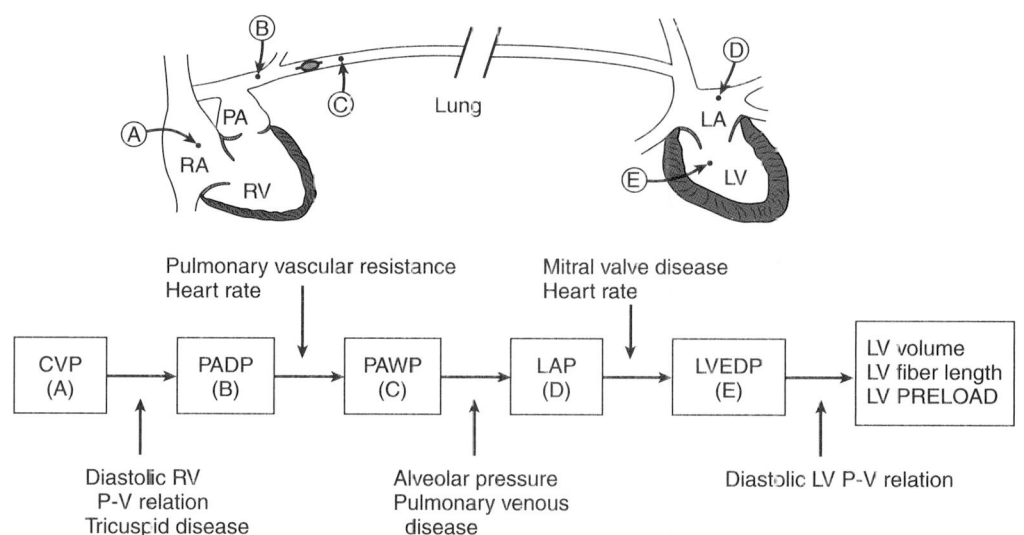

Figure 32–48 Anatomic and physiologic factors that influence the relationships between various measures of left ventricular (LV) filling and true LV preload. The further upstream filling pressure is measured, the more confounding factors may influence the relationship between this measurement and LV preload. CVP, central venous pressure; LA, left atrium; LAP, left atrial pressure; LVEDP, left ventricular end-diastolic pressure; PA, pulmonary artery; PADP, pulmonary artery diastolic pressure; PAWP, pulmonary artery wedge pressure; P-V, pressure-volume; RA, right atrium; RV, right ventricle. (Redrawn from Mark JB: Atlas of Cardiovascular Monitoring. New York, Churchill Livingstone, 1998, Fig. 15-5.)

the "filling pressure," the greater the number of these factors that may conspire to alter the relationship between the monitored pressure and left ventricular preload. In view of these considerations, it should be no surprise that reliance on CVP to estimate left ventricular preload is often misleading in critically ill patients. Furthermore, these same anatomic and physiologic factors may influence the relationship between pulmonary artery diastolic pressure, wedge pressure, left atrial pressure, and left ventricular end-diastolic pressure as measure of ventricular filling.

Predicting Left Ventricular End-Diastolic Pressure

Measurement of PAWP has two somewhat distinct purposes.[513] The first reason to measure wedge pressure is that it serves as an estimate for pulmonary capillary pressure. As such, wedge pressure offers a measure of the hydrostatic filtration pressure within the pulmonary capillaries that largely controls the formation of pulmonary edema. For this purpose, mean PAWP should be measured and reported. Although wedge pressure and capillary pressure are not identical, changes in PAWP generally mirror changes in pulmonary capillary pressure.

The second purpose for measuring wedge pressure is to estimate filling of the left ventricle. In this instance, the end-diastolic wedge pressure after atrial contraction best predicts left ventricular end-diastolic filling pressure or preload.[504] Left ventricular end-diastolic pressure is measured at the Z-point, identified on the left ventricular pressure trace as the point at which the slope of the ventricular pressure upstroke changes, approximately 50 milliseconds after the ECG Q wave and generally coinciding with the ECG R wave (Fig. 32-49).[136] Left ventricular end-diastolic pressure is a phasic pressure measured at end-diastole, not a mean diastolic pressure in the left ventricle. Although PAWP is generally reported as mean pressure, an end-diastolic component of wedge pressure can also be identified in its phasic pressure trace. In the presence of normal sinus rhythm, atrial contraction provides this end-diastolic mechanical event. Thus, measurement of the wedge pressure a wave peak provides a more accurate estimate of left ventricular end-diastolic pressure than that provided by mean wedge pressure (see Fig. 32-49).

The important distinction is that average or mean wedge pressure should be recorded to estimate pulmonary capillary pressure, the hydrostatic pressure in the lung, whereas the end-diastolic wedge pressure recorded after the a wave estimates left ventricular end-diastolic pressure or preload. As summarized eloquently by Mitchell and coworkers more than 40 years ago, "While the ventricular end diastolic pressure may be considered to be the hemodynamic 'stimulus' which determines the force of ventricular contraction, the mean atrial (or wedge) pressure may be considered the hemodynamic 'price' which the organism must pay for this stimulus to be provided."[514]

Pressure tracings from two patients, one with aortic stenosis and one with mitral regurgitation, help illustrate this important point (Fig. 32-50). Left ventricular end-diastolic pressure is elevated (25 mm Hg) in both patients and is well approximated by the left atrial (or wedge)

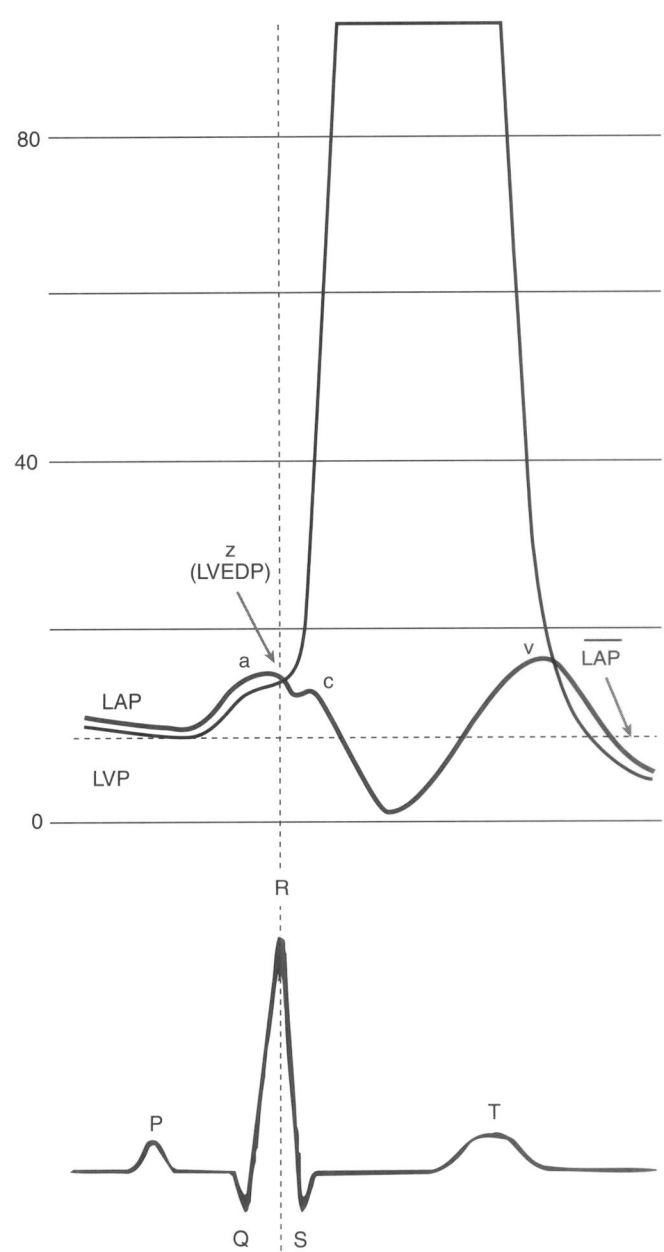

Figure 32–49 Relationship between left atrial pressure (LAP) and left ventricular end-diastolic pressure (LVEDP). LVEDP is measured at the Z-point on the left ventricular pressure (LVP) trace at the time of the electrocardiographic R wave. Mean LAP (9 mm Hg) underestimates LVEDP (15 mm Hg), but the LAP a wave pressure peak closely estimates LVEDP.[514] (Redrawn from Mark JB: Atlas of Cardiovascular Monitoring. New York, Churchill Livingstone, 1998, Fig. 6-1.)

pressure a wave peak. In both patients, this pressure provides the best single pressure estimate for left ventricular preload. Although both patients have the same left ventricular diastolic pressure, mean left atrial (or wedge) pressure is much higher in the patient with mitral regurgitation (30 mm Hg) than in the patient with aortic stenosis (15 mm Hg). The patient with aortic stenosis produces an end-diastolic pressure of 25 mm Hg with a strong left atrial contraction, as evidenced by the tall left atrial a wave.

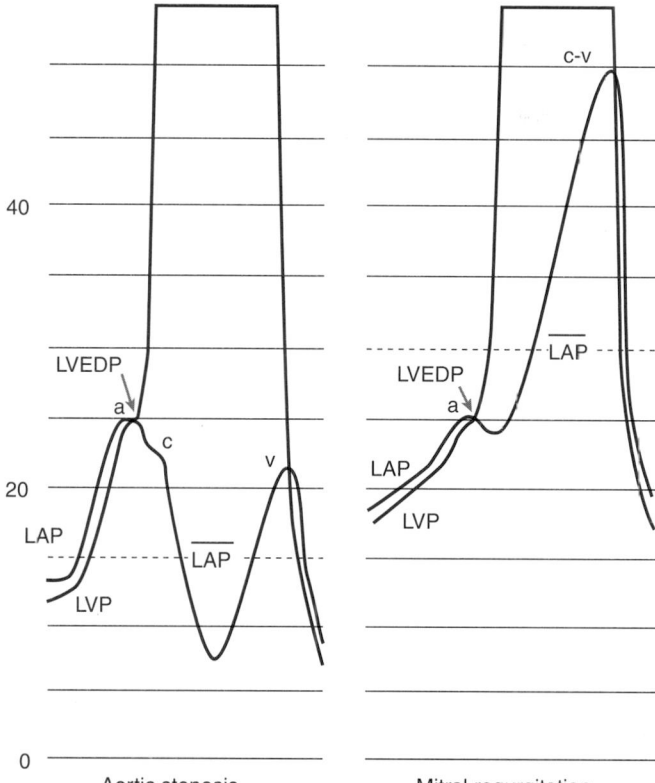

Figure 32–50 Relationship between left atrial pressure (LAP) and left ventricular end-diastolic pressure (LVEDP) in aortic stenosis and mitral regurgitation. LVEDP is elevated in both conditions (25 mm Hg), but mean LAP ($\overline{\text{LAP}}$) remains low in aortic stenosis (15 mm Hg) but high in mitral regurgitation (30 mm Hg) because of the regurgitant c-v wave inscribed during systole. LVP, left ventricular pressure. (Redrawn from Mark JB: Atlas of Cardiovascular Monitoring. New York, Churchill Livingstone, 1998, Fig. 6-2.)

This effective booster pump mechanism provides the necessary end-diastolic pressure with an acceptable mean left atrial pressure that does not place the patient at risk for pulmonary edema. In contrast, the patient with mitral regurgitation has a very high mean left atrial pressure (30 mm Hg) caused by the tall regurgitant c-v wave. Clearly, mean wedge pressure does not equal end-diastolic wedge pressure. This distinction is important, and it is often overlooked in daily clinical practice because of our emphasis on a single numeric value for wedge pressure.

PAC Underestimation of Left Ventricular End-Diastolic Pressure

When a PAC is used to estimate left ventricular filling pressure, in a number of situations this pressure is either underestimated (Table 32-12) or overestimated (Table 32-13) by the pulmonary artery diastolic or wedge pressure measurements.[513] Left ventricular *diastolic dysfunction* leading to decreased ventricular compliance is the most common cause of underestimation of left ventricular end-diastolic pressure.[515] The atrial contribution to left ventricular end-diastolic volume and pressure is normally less than 20%, but with diastolic dysfunction, this atrial contribution may approach 50%.[474,477] Under these conditions, the wedge pressure a wave will be unusually prominent and will provide a close estimate of left ventricular end-diastolic pressure, whereas mean wedge pressure will underestimate left ventricular filling (see Fig. 32-42).[425] In patients with *aortic regurgitation,* abnormal diastolic left ventricular filling occurs from the aorta as soon as left ventricular pressure falls below aortic pressure and continues after left atrial contraction and closure of the mitral valve. Left ventricular diastolic pressure continues to rise until end-diastolic pressure is reached at the onset of mechanical systole, which reestablishes antegrade flow from the left ventricle to the aorta. Because mitral valve closure occurs before end-diastole, mean PAWP and the wedge pressure a wave both underestimate left ventricular end-diastolic pressure.[425]

In the presence of *pulmonic regurgitation,* diastolic flow from the proximal portion of the pulmonary artery becomes bidirectional, antegrade toward the left atrium and retrograde into the right ventricle. When right ventricular diastolic pressure is lower than left atrial pressure, pulmonary artery diastolic flow seeks the lower-pressure pathway toward the right ventricle, and pulmonary artery diastolic pressure will underestimate PAWP, left atrial pressure, and left ventricular end-diastolic pressure.[513]

When PVR is normal, there is no pressure gradient across the pulmonary vascular bed at the end of diastole, and pulmonary artery diastolic pressure equilibrates with the downstream left atrial pressure. However, when right ventricular systole is delayed because of *right bundle branch block,* PAP continues to fall with the x or

Table 32–12 Underestimation of left ventricular end-diastolic pressure

Condition	Site of Discrepancy	Cause of Discrepancy
Diastolic dysfunction	Mean LAP < LVEDP	Increased end-diastolic a wave
Aortic regurgitation	LAP a wave < LVEDP	Mitral valve closure before end-diastole
Pulmonic regurgitation	PADP < LVEDP	Bidirectional runoff for pulmonary artery flow
Right bundle branch block	PADP < LVEDP	Delayed pulmonic valve opening
Postpneumonectomy	PAWP < LAP or LVEDP	Obstruction of pulmonary blood flow

LAP, left atrial pressure; LVEDP, left ventricular end-diastolic pressure; PADP, pulmonary artery diastolic pressure; PAWP, pulmonary artery wedge pressure.

Modified from Mark JB: Predicting left ventricular end-diastolic pressure. *In* Mark JB (ed): Atlas of Cardiovascular Monitoring. New York, Churchill Livingstone, 1998, p 59.

systolic descent in left atrial pressure. Under such conditions, pulmonary artery diastolic pressure will underestimate left ventricular end-diastolic pressure by as much as 7 mm Hg.[516]

A final condition in which PAC measurements underestimate left ventricular end-diastolic pressure is different from the pathophysiologic states just noted because in this condition, the process of measuring wedge pressure changes pulmonary blood flow and thereby influences left heart filling. Under normal conditions, inflation of the PAC balloon to measure wedge pressure interrupts antegrade blood flow through a small section of the lung and has no measurable effect on total pulmonary blood flow or left heart filling. However, after *pneumonectomy* and possibly other conditions that markedly decrease the pulmonary vascular bed, balloon inflation may occlude a significant portion of the remaining pulmonary vascular cross-sectional area. Mechanical obstruction of pulmonary blood flow results and causes increased CVP and decreased left atrial pressure, cardiac output, and systemic blood pressure.[517,518] Therefore, because PAC balloon inflation and measurement of wedge pressure lead to obstruction of pulmonary blood flow, the measured wedge pressure underestimates the left atrial and left ventricular end-diastolic pressures that existed before balloon inflation. This artifact should be suspected in the appropriate clinical setting, when a sudden reduction in systemic arterial pressure occurs coincident with PAC balloon inflation.

PAC Overestimation of Left Ventricular End-Diastolic Pressure

Respiratory influences on the pulmonary artery and wedge pressure traces are the most common cause of overestimation of left ventricular end-diastolic pressure (Table 32-13). In this regard, mechanical ventilation with *PEEP* poses a particular problem because it may create zone 1 or zone 2 lung conditions and cause PAWP to be influenced by alveolar pressure.[519] Formulas have been derived to adjust for the effects of PEEP on wedge pressure measurement. In general, mechanical ventilation with PEEP increases wedge pressure by an amount less than half the value of PEEP applied (i.e., 10 cm H_2O PEEP will raise

wedge pressure less than 5 cm H_2O or 4 mm Hg).[120,520] However, the ratio of chest wall compliance to lung compliance has a significant impact on the relationship between the level of PEEP and its effect on PAWP, and simple mathematical methods to adjust for this effect are not entirely reliable.[120,512,521,522] Alternative methods to correct for PEEP, such as measuring pleural pressure with an esophageal balloon, are cumbersome and not generally used. Prolonged discontinuation of PEEP before measuring wedge pressure is to be discouraged. Not only will circulatory dynamics change dramatically because of rebound central hypervolemia caused by translocation of blood from the periphery, but respiratory gas exchange may also deteriorate and be slow to recover.[120] As an alternative, Pinsky and colleagues found that transient airway disconnection for 2 to 3 seconds in patients receiving mechanical ventilation with PEEP allowed measurement of nadir wedge pressure, which proved to be a better and safer way to estimate left ventricular filling pressure at higher levels of PEEP.[522] When wedge pressure measurement did not change after abrupt airway disconnection, the on-PEEP wedge pressure measurement accurately reflected left ventricular filling pressure. However, when wedge pressure decreased after airway disconnection, the nadir wedge pressure reached within 3 seconds provided a more accurate measurement. Fortunately, most patients who require high levels of PEEP may not manifest these artifactual wedge pressure measurement problems. Studying patients with adult respiratory distress syndrome, Teboul and associates found that PAWP closely estimates left ventricular end-diastolic pressure at all levels of PEEP up to 20 cm H_2O.[523] This relative microvascular "protection" from the effects of PEEP presumably occurred because of the marked increase in lung stiffness that is seen in this condition.

When the pulmonary vasculature is normal, pulmonary blood flow ceases at end-diastole, and pulmonary artery diastolic pressure equals left atrial pressure.[524] However, if PVR increases, equilibration of PAP with downstream pressure does not occur. Under these conditions, the pulmonary vascular bed begins to resemble the systemic vasculature, where a large pressure gradient between systemic arterial pressure and right atrial pressure persists at end-diastole.

Table 32-13   Overestimation of left ventricular end-diastolic pressure

Condition	Site of Discrepancy	Cause of Discrepancy
Positive end-expiratory pressure	Mean PAWP > mean LAP	Creation of lung zone 1 or 2 or pericardial pressure changes
Pulmonary arterial hypertension	PADP > mean PAWP	Increased pulmonary vascular resistance
Pulmonary veno-occlusive disease	Mean PAWP > mean LAP	Obstruction to flow in large pulmonary veins
Mitral stenosis	Mean LAP > LVEDP	Obstruction to flow across the mitral valve
Mitral regurgitation	Mean LAP > LVEDP	Retrograde systolic v wave raises mean atrial pressure
Ventricular septal defect	Mean LAP > LVEDP	Antegrade systolic v wave raises mean atrial pressure
Tachycardia	PADP > mean LAP > LVEDP	Short diastole creates pulmonary vascular and mitral valve gradients

LAP, left atrial pressure; LVEDP, left ventricular end-diastolic pressure; PADP, pulmonary artery diastolic pressure; PAWP, pulmonary artery wedge pressure.
Modified from Mark JB: Predicting left ventricular end-diastolic pressure. *In* Mark JB (ed): Atlas of Cardiovascular Monitoring. New York, Churchill Livingstone, 1998, p 59.

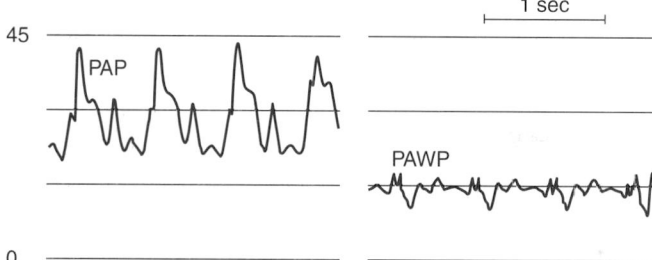

Figure 32–51 Pulmonary hypertension. The increased gradient across the pulmonary vasculature causes pulmonary artery diastolic pressure to exceed pulmonary artery wedge pressure (PAWP). PAP, pulmonary artery pressure. (Redrawn from Mark JB: Atlas of Cardiovascular Monitoring. New York, Churchill Livingstone, 1998, Fig. 6-11.)

Therefore, in the presence of *pulmonary arterial hypertension* caused by elevated PVR, pulmonary artery diastolic pressure overestimates wedge pressure, left atrial pressure, and left ventricular end-diastolic pressure (Fig. 32-51).

In contrast to the precapillary pulmonary vasoconstriction that exists in patients with pulmonary arterial hypertension, postcapillary obstruction to flow in the pulmonary veins may occur in the rare condition *pulmonary veno-occlusive disease*. Patients with this condition have normal left atrial pressure, but some disagreement exists regarding whether these patients have normal or elevated PAC-derived wedge pressure measurements.[120,441,525,526] In part, these different observations may relate to whether the PAC has been wedged successfully because the wedge position may be difficult to obtain in these patients or, in some instances, the measured wedge pressure may be recorded from a totally occluded vascular channel. The most important factor, however, is whether the patient has predominantly small-vein occlusion or large-vein occlusion. Obstruction to flow in the small pulmonary veins narrows the static column of blood connecting the wedged PAC tip with the flowing column in the larger pulmonary veins. Given that the partial obstruction involves only the static column, wedge pressure will measure normal pulmonary venous and left atrial pressure because there is no pressure drop across this partially obstructed vascular segment in the absence of flow. Conversely, large-vein obstruction creates a pressure gradient across the large veins as blood flows in them toward the left atrium. In this instance, wedge pressure will detect an increased pulmonary venous pressure and overestimate left atrial and ventricular diastolic pressure.[120,441,525,526] This model of pulmonary vein obstruction is consistent with the observations of Zidulka and Hakim, who measured wedge pressure in both large and small pulmonary arteries.[422] Other conditions may mimic the hemodynamic features of pulmonary veno-occlusive disease, including mediastinal fibrosis and intrathoracic or atrial tumors that obstruct pulmonary venous flow near the left atrium.

Mitral stenosis obstructs blood flow between the left atrium and left ventricle, and consequently, left atrial pressure will exceed left ventricular pressure throughout diastole. Furthermore, all upstream pressures recorded by the PAC will overestimate left ventricular end-diastolic

pressure as a result of the valvular obstruction.[527] Because the pressure gradient across the mitral valve is directly related to the flow across it, pulmonary artery diastolic and wedge pressures will overestimate left ventricular filling pressures even more when transmitral flow is increased by tachycardia or elevated cardiac output.

Left atrial pressure is increased in *mitral regurgitation* because of the abnormal leakage of blood across the incompetent valve during systole, and left ventricular end-diastolic pressure is better approximated by measuring wedge pressure before onset of the regurgitant c-v wave (see Figs. 32-38 and Fig. 32-39).[458] In contrast to patients with mitral stenosis, in whom left atrial pressure exceeds left ventricular pressure throughout diastole, a patient with mitral regurgitation has appropriate diastolic equilibration of atrial and ventricular pressures. The problem in mitral regurgitation is choosing the appropriate end-diastolic, pre–v wave pressure to use as an estimate of left ventricular end-diastolic pressure. Mean PAWP will overestimate left ventricular end-diastolic pressure in any patient whose wedge pressure displays tall systolic v waves, including those with *ventricular septal defect* and left ventricular failure.[456,457]

When *tachycardia* develops, the duration of diastole is shortened, and there is less time for egress of blood from the pulmonary vasculature to the left atrium and from the left atrium to the left ventricle. At both the mitral valve and pulmonary vascular levels, pressure gradients develop as the duration of diastole progressively decreases during tachycardia.[424,514,528] Consequently, pulmonary artery diastolic pressure overestimates mean PAWP, which in turn overestimates left ventricular end-diastolic pressure. Patients in atrial fibrillation will have more complete equilibration of pulmonary artery diastolic pressure and left ventricular end-diastolic pressure during longer R-R intervals. Consequently, these beats should be chosen to provide the best estimate of left ventricular end-diastolic pressure and preload.

In summary, there are many circumstances in which pulmonary artery diastolic or wedge pressure may underestimate or overestimate left ventricular end-diastolic pressure and thereby provide a misleading estimate of ventricular filling or preload. Some conditions are relatively common, whereas others are extremely rare, and frequently, several conditions coexist, further complicating the measurement problem. For example, a patient with mitral stenosis resulting in pulmonary hypertension in whom tachycardia develops has three reasons for the PAC-derived data to be in error and lead to a pulmonary artery diastolic pressure that markedly overestimates left ventricular end-diastolic pressure. Major clinical errors would result if the high pulmonary artery diastolic pressure is presumed to indicate increased left ventricular preload in a patient with these conditions.

Pulmonary Artery Catheterization and Outcome Controversies

Pulmonary artery catheterization has evoked more controversy than any other widely adopted cardiovascular monitoring practice because it is an expensive, invasive technique that is widely used but still not rigorously proven to improve patient outcome. The PAC controversy has been fueled in part by strongly worded editorials written by prominent physicians debating whether PAC use should be suspended pending better scientific proof of the efficacy of this monitoring practice.[529-534] The titles of these editorials convey the emotional nature of these issues—"Use and abuse of the balloon tip pulmonary artery (Swan-Ganz) catheter: Are patients getting their money's worth?";[535] "Swan song for the Swan-Ganz catheter?"[531]; and perhaps most provocative, "Death by pulmonary artery flow–directed catheter."[534] Although similar controversies surround the use of other widely adopted, high-tech clinical monitoring techniques, such as electronic fetal monitoring,[536-538] physicians who use PACs must appreciate the ongoing uncertainties surrounding PAC monitoring and be fully informed of the evidence that must guide patient selection.[539]

In 2003, the American Society of Anesthesiologists published an updated practice guideline for pulmonary artery catheterization that provided a current exhaustive review of the scientific evidence for the clinical effectiveness of PAC monitoring.[318] The inconsistent findings of the many studies in the literature were striking, with evidence both supporting[540-545] and refuting[323,324,546-552] the benefits of this technique. Many early studies reported small numbers of patients, which limited their validity and wider applicability, and larger more recent trials continue to have mixed results and limitations in study design. One of the earliest observational studies involving more than 1000 general surgical patients reported lower perioperative mortality and myocardial reinfarction rates in patients monitored with PACs versus historical controls,[553] but other large studies have not found a similar outcome benefit. One reason for these divergent results may be that clinical trials have focused on different populations, such as patients with acute myocardial infarction,[554,555] those undergoing cardiac surgery,[556,557] and critically ill patients with a variety of medical and surgical diseases.[322,558] Despite the large numbers of patients in some of these reports, many experts have questioned these studies because they were observational in design rather than randomized controlled trials.[318,349,559,560] Nonetheless, several of these studies have raised serious concern among physicians because they suggested that not only was the PAC ineffective, but patients who received PAC monitoring also suffered increased morbidity and mortality when compared with patients who did not receive such monitoring.[322,554,555]

Perhaps the most provocative of all these PAC outcome studies is one published in 1996, in which Connors and colleagues examined the association between PAC use during the first 24 hours of intensive care and subsequent survival.[322] This prospective cohort study included 5735 patients in five teaching hospitals as part of a larger 9000-patient study entitled "The study to understand prognoses and preferences for outcomes and risks of treatments (SUPPORT)."[561-564] The patients in this study were desperately ill; entry into the study required a predicted 6-month mortality rate in excess of 50%. Patients who underwent PAC monitoring were judged to be sicker by every measurement recorded, but the authors used case-matching analyses and applied a propensity score to adjust for these confounding medical covariates. To the extent that these statistical adjustments were successful, the results of the study were very worrisome. PAC-monitored patients had increased mortality, increased length of hospital stay, and increased cost. Moreover, no subgroup of patients appeared to benefit from PAC monitoring. Publication of this study was accompanied by a strongly worded editorial calling for a moratorium on PAC use or a randomized controlled trial to define its efficacy.[529]

The controversies surrounding PAC use have helped identify several key issues that remain unanswered but are intimately related to the basic question of PAC monitoring and patient outcome.

PAC Monitoring Outcome: Variable Skill, Knowledge, and Treatment Plans

Tremendous variability in the level of skill, knowledge, and confidence is found in nurses and physicians who use PACs.[412-415,417,418] Furthermore, experienced clinicians often choose different therapies when presented with the same PAC-derived hemodynamic data.[409-411] Some experts believe that failure to control for these factors has been responsible for the poor performance of the PAC in many of the clinical trials reported in the literature.[325,559,563,565] As noted by Fowler and Cook, "A [research study] design choice not to standardize treatment but to replicate day-to-day care in ICUs around the world may reflect the reality that there is nothing standard about 'standard practice,' and there is no proven 'best practice.'"[566] Consequently, because many studies have not provided an explicit description of the level of knowledge of the practitioners or how the PAC was used to guide care, the results of these studies have been called into question.[318,325]

PAC Monitoring Outcome: Variable Practice

The use of PACs varies widely between individual physicians, institutions, and geographic locations.[375,558,567,568] As in other parts of modern medicine, this begs the question regarding whether the PAC is overused in some settings or perhaps underused in others. Some authors have suggested that PAC use has been driven in part by the variation in regional medical care payment structures or the local mechanism for physician reimbursement.[349,567]

PAC Monitoring Outcome: Learning Bias

Learning bias may be another important factor that confounds determination of PAC effectiveness.[325,349] This phenomenon is well recognized in clinical medicine. In brief, it suggests that we now take better care of patients in general because we have learned such a great deal about cardiovascular pathophysiology and patterns of disease by using PACs that we now apply this knowledge effectively in the care of patients who do not have PAC monitoring.

PAC Monitoring Outcome: Early Intervention

Early use of PAC monitoring in the care of general surgical patients,[569,570] trauma patients,[544] cardiac surgical patients,[571] or elderly high-risk patients[541] has been emphasized by some authors as a requirement for improvement in clinical outcome. The studies of Shoemaker and coworkers in particular have underscored the importance of early monitoring and treatment to optimize tissue perfusion before irreversible organ damage occurs.[535,569,570] A recent randomized trial in emergency room patients with severe sepsis or septic shock showed reduced morbidity and mortality in those receiving early treatment guided by a special mixed venous oxygen–sensing CVP catheter.[572,573] Although this study used a modified CVP catheter rather than a PAC, it confirms a benefit to early intervention guided by specific hemodynamic parameters.

PAC Monitoring Outcome: Goal-Directed Therapy

The role of PAC monitoring in improving patient outcome is inextricably tied to the therapies that it guides. As several authors have noted, "if there is no good treatment for the pathophysiologic state that is identified, there is no expectation of therapeutic benefit from the diagnostic procedure."[334,349] This may be one of the key issues in our current conundrum, namely, our inability to effectively treat many serious illnesses, such as sepsis, even when the cardiovascular problems are clearly identified through PAC monitoring.

In terms of PAC-guided therapies, one of the most controversial is one in which the physician measures hemodynamic variables with the catheter and then attempts to increase oxygen delivery to some predetermined goal. This treatment algorithm has been termed "maximizing oxygen delivery," "goal-oriented therapy," or "supraphysiologic goal-driven treatment." In essence, these therapies involve PAC monitoring to guide fluid and inotropic drug administration, with various supranormal circulatory goals as end points: oxygen delivery greater than 600 mL/min/m^2, oxygen consumption greater than 170 mL/min/m^2, or cardiac index higher than 4.5 L/min/m^2. Although some investigations have shown an outcome benefit with this therapeutic approach,[545,569,571,574-578] others have shown either no effect of such therapy[579] or even increased mortality.[580] The uncertain efficacy of this therapeutic approach has been cited as a significant reason why PAC monitoring has not proved effective.[322,559] A complete consideration of this treatment strategy is beyond the scope of this discussion, but it remains an extremely controversial aspect of PAC monitoring.[581,582] Although most experts agree that PACs allow more accurate titration of traditional therapy in critically ill patients, some of the most "aggressive" therapies that it guides remain unproven.[583]

Pulmonary Artery Catheterization: Indications

The practice guidelines and consensus statements that have been generated over the past several years best summarize the current indications for PAC monitoring.[318,559,584-536] The most recent of these practice guidelines is the American Society of Anesthesiologists practice guideline published in 2003.[318] The guideline task force considered PAC monitoring to be appropriate or necessary, or both, in selected surgical patients undergoing procedures associated with a high risk of complications from hemodynamic changes (e.g. cardiac surgery) or in those with advanced cardiopulmonary diseases who would be at increased risk for adverse perioperative events because of their preoperative medical condition. Furthermore, the characteristics of the practice setting should be considered, including the proficiency and experience of clinicians who would be using perioperative PAC monitoring. In other words, three interdependent variables should help a physician determine when PAC monitoring is indicated: the patient, the surgical procedure, and the practice setting.

Many high-risk patients undergo low-risk operations that have little physiologic impact, and these individuals should not receive PAC monitoring. One example would be a patient with advanced ischemic cardiomyopathy who needs lower extremity amputation that could be performed with a regional anesthesia technique. In contrast, a relatively low-risk patient undergoing a very high-risk procedure may benefit from perioperative PAC monitoring. An example might be a patient with stable ischemic heart disease scheduled to undergo extensive abdominal cancer surgery. Finally, the third factor that determines whether PAC monitoring is appropriate relates to the individual practice setting.[318] Keats has termed this feature "the role of environment in the outcome of operation," by which he meant all the important unmeasurable aspects of each clinical setting, including among other things, surgical skills and experience.[587] Clearly, all physicians and nurses using the PAC must have the requisite knowledge and skills to use it safely and effectively. However, there is something that at the present time still defies objective assessment, and a short postgraduate educational program alone seems to be ineffective in improving PAC interpretation skills.[418]

To provide better scientific evidence to define appropriate indications for PAC monitoring, well-designed randomized clinical trials are required.[318,559,588-593] Such trials remain difficult to perform because of problems in gaining informed consent from critically ill patients, difficulty ensuring that physicians remain committed to trial guidelines, and obstacles encountered in patient selection bias and crossover from non-PAC monitoring to PAC monitoring.[549,588,589,594] The National Institutes of Health has recently undertaken large multicenter trials focused on PAC use in patients with acute respiratory distress syndrome and severe congestive heart failure.[321,595] Although these trials will help answer clinically important questions in these patient cohorts, they will have limited applicability for perioperative patients.

In 2003, Sandham and coauthors published the largest prospective randomized clinical trial to date focusing on the use of PACs in high-risk elderly surgical patients.[324,596] Nearly 2000 patients were randomized to receive goal-directed therapy guided by a PAC or standard care without a PAC. PAC monitoring did not lead to any benefit in terms of morbidity or mortality, and the PAC-monitored group had a higher rate of pulmonary embolism. The authors found that it was difficult to achieve the "supra-normal" physiologic goals desired in the PAC-treated group, a finding that was consistent with other trials. Perhaps of greatest importance, the authors demonstrated the ability to perform a well-controlled randomized clinical trial, considered to be a significant milestone in our search to determine the appropriate role of PAC monitoring in clinical practice.[596]

Additional Features of Pulmonary Artery Catheters

The popularity of PAC monitoring relates in large part to the fact that these catheters are multipurpose and provide a wide range of supplementary features for therapeutic and diagnostic applications. In addition to the standard lumens that allow measurement of PAP and CVP, catheters may have an additional venous infusion lumen opening either 20 or 30 cm from the catheter tip. Special PACs are available that allow temporary endocardial pacing or intracardiac ECG recording. One such catheter has five small electrodes embedded in its outer wall, two located approximately 20 cm from the catheter tip and three located approximately 30 cm from the catheter tip. Combinations of these electrodes allow bipolar endocardial ventricular, atrial, or atrioventricular pacing.[597] Other pacing PACs do not have the pacing electrodes permanently attached but instead have a special lumen that opens in the right ventricle, through which a thin bipolar wire may be introduced for endocardial ventricular pacing.[598] Another type of pacing PAC has special atrial and ventricular lumens that accommodate two separate wires to allow atrioventricular sequential pacing.[599] Although successful endocardial pacing is achieved in most patients with these catheters, reliable catheter positioning is more problematic than with standard PACs. Patient movement or PAC balloon inflation to measure wedge pressure may alter the position of the catheter or dislodge the wires within the heart and thereby interrupt pacing.

Cardiac Preload Assessment beyond the Pulmonary Artery Catheter: Systolic Pressure Variation and Other Dynamic Indicators

The starting point for resuscitation of a patient with circulatory failure is intravascular volume expansion to optimize cardiac preload. Goal-directed resuscitation is predicated on the availability of monitored information that accurately indicates whether specific hemodynamic goals are being achieved, including a measure of cardiac preload such as CVP or PAWP. As noted in the earlier discussion of CVP and PAC monitoring, use of these filling pressure surrogates for ventricular preload is subject to a number of confounding variables that complicate their interpretation. Moreover, these cardiac filling pressures are static indicators of preload: they may be in the low, normal, or high range, but not necessarily "optimal" for a given patient in a particular clinical setting.

Rather than these traditional static markers of cardiac filling, newer dynamic markers of volume responsiveness have been described that may provide more useful information for determining the appropriate end points for fluid resuscitation.[600] The variations in arterial blood pressure observed during positive-pressure mechanical ventilation are the most widely studied of these dynamic indicators of cardiac preload. These changes in blood pressure are readily observed on the bedside monitor in patients who are undergoing direct arterial blood pressure monitoring, and they result from changes in intrathoracic pressure and lung volume that occur during the respiratory cycle.[601-604]

During positive-pressure inspiration, increasing lung volume compresses and displaces the pulmonary venous reservoir and propels it into the left heart chambers, thereby increasing left ventricular preload. Simultaneously, the increase in intrathoracic pressure reduces left ventricular afterload. The increase in left ventricular preload and decrease in afterload produce an increase in left ventricular stroke volume and an increase in systemic arterial pressure. In most patients, the preload effects are more important, but in patients with severe left ventricular systolic failure, the reduction in afterload plays an important role in increasing left ventricular ejection. At the same time that left heart filling is increasing during early inspiration, the rising intrathoracic pressure causes a decrease in systemic venous return and right ventricular preload. The increased lung volume may also increase PVR slightly and thereby increase right ventricular afterload. These effects combine to reduce right ventricular ejection during inspiration.

Toward the end of inspiration or during early expiration, the reduced right ventricular stroke volume that occurred during inspiration crosses the pulmonary vascular bed and leads to reduced left ventricular filling. As a result, left ventricular stroke volume falls, and systemic arterial blood pressure decreases. This cyclic variation in systemic arterial pressure may be measured and quantified as the *systolic pressure variation (SPV)*.[303]

SPV is often subdivided into inspiratory and expiratory components by measuring the increase (Δ Up) and decrease (Δ Down) in systolic pressure in relation to the end-expiratory, apneic baseline pressure (Fig. 32-52). In a mechanically ventilated patient, the normal SPV is 7 to 10 mm Hg, with Δ Up being 2 to 4 mm Hg and Δ Down

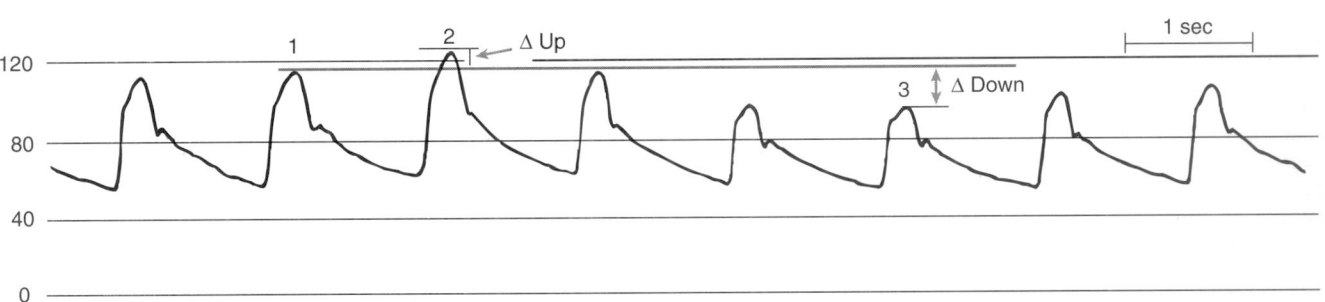

Figure 32–52 Systolic pressure variation. When compared with systolic blood pressure recorded at end-expiration (1), a small increase occurs during positive-pressure inspiration (2, Δ Up), followed by a decrease (3, Δ Down). Normally, the total variation in systolic pressure does not exceed 10 mm Hg. In this instance, the large Δ Down indicates hypovolemia even though systolic arterial pressure and the heart rate are relatively normal. (Redrawn from Mark JB: Atlas of Cardiovascular Monitoring. New York, Churchill Livingstone, 1998, Fig. 16-16.)

being 5 to 6 mm Hg.[605] The greatest clinical use of SPV has been in the early diagnosis of hypovolemia.[601,606-608] Both in experimental animals and patients, hypovolemia causes a dramatic increase in SPV, particularly Δ Down. Some authors have suggested that the increase in SPV and Δ Down may herald hypovolemia, even in patients in whom arterial blood pressure is maintained near normal levels by compensatory arterial vasoconstriction.[601,609]

In a heterogeneous group of intensive care patients, Marik demonstrated that a large SPV (>15 mm Hg) was highly predictive of a low PAWP (<10 mm Hg).[610] Using echocardiography to measure the left ventricular cross-sectional area as a surrogate for preload, Coriat and colleagues found Δ Down to be a better predictor of preload than wedge pressure was.[605]

Other uses of SVP focus on changes in the Δ Up portion of the arterial pressure trace. Just as Δ Down may reveal changes in cardiac preload, the Δ Up portion of the arterial pressure trace may provide clues to the afterload dependence of the left ventricle. Preliminary evidence suggests that a marked increase in Δ Up during positive-pressure inspiration occurs when the increased pleural pressure reduces transmural left ventricular pressure sufficiently that left ventricular stroke output increases in the failing, afterload-dependent left ventricle.[602-604,611]

As a dynamic indicator of cardiac preload, SPV and Δ Down provide valuable clinical information beyond that provide by static preload indicators such as CVP or wedge pressure. It appears that the magnitude of blood pressure variation accurately predicts patients who will subsequently respond to a volume challenge by increasing stroke volume and cardiac output. Using receiver-operator curve analysis, Tavernier and coworkers showed that the magnitude of Δ Down was a far better indicator of volume responsiveness than PAWP or echocardiographically derived left ventricular end-diastolic area was.[612]

Although most monitoring trials to date have examined SPV and Δ Down as indicators of preload, other closely related variables have also been found to be useful clinical measures of volume responsiveness. Some authors have suggested that rather than measure absolute SPV, focusing on Δ Down as a percentage of the systolic pressure during apnea will provide a more accurate measure of volume status, particularly in patients with large changes in blood pressure or significant arterial hypotension.[613] Another dynamic marker of preload based on arterial waveform analysis has been the pulse pressure variation (PPV), defined as the maximal difference in arterial pulse pressure measured over the course of the positive-pressure respiratory cycle divided by the average of the maximal and minimal pulse pressures.[609,614,615] Normal PPV should not exceed 13%.[609] Finally, new pulse contour methods for measurement of cardiac output (see later) allow on-line measurement of variations in left ventricular stroke volume, so-called *stroke volume variation (SVV)*.[609,616] Like the other related dynamic indicators of cardiac preload, the normal SVV is approximately 10%, and greater variability accurately predicts a positive response to a fluid challenge.[609,516]

Despite rapidly accumulating evidence for the value of SPV and its related measures as accurate predictors of cardiac preload, these measures have not found widespread clinical adoption for a number of reasons. The original description of this method required transient interruption of mechanical ventilation to identify an apneic baseline for measurement of Δ Down and Δ Up.[605] More recently, Schwid and Rooke have shown that use of the end-expiratory value for systolic blood pressure serves as an alternative suitable baseline that does not require a change in the pattern of ventilation.[617] Although an automated method for continual computation and display of SPV by the bedside monitor is not widely available, computer-derived measurements appear to be accurate and could be incorporated into newer monitoring devices.[618,619]

Finally, a large number of clinical factors preclude wider application of this technique. Although cyclic changes in systemic arterial pressure are often observed during spontaneous ventilation, using SPV to predict hypovolemia has been well validated only in patients receiving positive-pressure mechanical ventilation. Among other things, the tidal volume and changes in intrathoracic pressure during spontaneous ventilation are too variable from breath to breath for accurate interpretation of these respiratory-circulatory interactions.[605] The magnitude of the SPV observed in any patient will be influenced by positive-pressure ventilatory parameters, including tidal volume and peak inspiratory pressure. Values will be further confounded by the presence of arrhythmias, changes in chest wall and lung compliance, the addition of PEEP, and other pulmonary pathology.[619] As a final point, the physiologic basis for SPV is not entirely related to the changes in left ventricular preload described earlier,[620] and some studies have suggested that SPV is not as accurate as other more traditional measures (left ventricular area or wedge pressure) during severe hemorrhagic hypovolemia.[621]

CARDIAC OUTPUT MONITORING

Aside from its pressure monitoring capabilities, undoubtedly the most important feature of the PAC is its ability to measure cardiac output by the thermodilution method. Cardiac output is the total blood flow generated by the heart, and in a normal adult at rest, it ranges from 4.0 to 6.5 L/min (Table 32-14). To the extent that the body

Table 32–14   Normal hemodynamic values

	Average	Range
Cardiac output (L/min)	5.0	4.0-6.5
Stroke volume (mL)	75	60-90
Systemic vascular resistance (Wood units)	15	10-20
(Dynes · sec · cm^{-5})	1200	800-1600
Pulmonary vascular resistance (Wood units)	1	0.5-3
(Dynes · sec · cm^{-5})	80	40-180
Arterial oxygen content (mL/dL)	18	16-20
Mixed venous oxygen content (mL/dL)	14	13-15
Arteriovenous oxygen difference (mL/dL)	4	3-5
Oxygen consumption (mL/min)	225	200-250

regulates cardiac output to meet tissue metabolic requirements, measurement of cardiac output provides a global assessment of the circulation, including the neurohumoral influences on it. Cardiac output measurements are usually combined with other hemodynamic measurements (heart rate, arterial blood pressure, CVP, PAP, and wedge pressure) to allow calculation of additional important circulatory variables such as systemic vascular resistance (SVR) and PVR. Thus, the PAC provides a large fraction of the data that the critical care physician or anesthesiologist uses for comprehensive cardiovascular assessment.

Three factors have driven efforts to measure cardiac output in clinical practice. The first is the recognition that in many critically ill patients, low cardiac output leads to significant morbidity and mortality.[622,623] Second, clinical assessment of cardiac output is often inaccurate, and in particular, many gravely ill patients with severely decreased cardiac output have normal systemic arterial blood pressure, which can be clinically misleading.[622,624] Third, newer techniques for measurement of cardiac output are less invasive than PAC monitoring and thus might provide benefit to many patients without the attendant risks of invasive monitoring.[624-626]

Notwithstanding many of these considerations, the optimal cardiac output in a given clinical setting remains uncertain.[627] As noted earlier, goal-directed therapies often target specific cardiac output values or hemodynamic values related to cardiac output, and these therapeutic approaches have not gained wide acceptance because of the inconsistent results of clinical trials. A wide variety of techniques are currently available for measuring cardiac output and other blood flow variables, and the advantages and disadvantages of each method must be appreciated for proper clinical application.

Thermodilution Cardiac Output Monitoring

The thermodilution technique has become the de facto clinical standard for measuring cardiac output because of its ease of implementation and the long clinical experience using it in various settings. It is a variant of the *indicator dilution* method, in which a known amount of a tracer substance is injected into the bloodstream and its concentration change measured over time at a downstream site. As its name implies, the thermodilution method uses a thermal indicator.

The fundamental physical basis for the indicator dilution methods is given by the Stewart-Hamilton equation, named after the two investigators who were instrumental in the development of this technique.[628,629] Its most generalized form is given in Equation 1.

$$\dot{Q} = \frac{I}{\int_0^\infty C_I dt} \qquad (1)$$

where $\dot{Q}$ = cardiac output
I = amount of indicator

$\int_0^\infty C_I dt$ = integral of indicator concentration over time

Historically, various nontoxic dyes (Coomassie blue, Evans blue, indocyanine green) and radioactive tracers have been injected into both peripheral and central venous sites and their downstream concentrations analyzed, but these techniques were largely limited to cardiac catheterization laboratories and experimental studies.[630-633] The dye dilution methods have not maintained widespread clinical popularity because they require continuous withdrawal of arterial blood to plot the dye concentration curve, and the most common indicator, indocyanine green, can gradually build up with repeated injections. However, this method has been used to diagnose intracardiac shunts by observing the altered shape of the dye dilution curve that is produced by the abnormal recirculation of dye under these conditions.

Two developments have had a significant impact on the routine measurement of cardiac output in clinical practice. The first was the introduction of thermal indicators by Fegler,[634] and the second was the incorporation of a temperature-measuring thermistor in the tip of a PAC.[635-637] Several unique features of the thermodilution cardiac output monitoring technique have led to its widespread popularity and rapid clinical acceptance. It can be performed quickly and repeatedly, the measurement does not require advanced diagnostic or technical skills, and it uses a nontoxic, nonaccumulating, and nonrecirculating indicator.

When a thermal indicator is used to measure cardiac output, the Stewart-Hamilton equation must be modified (Equation 2).

$$\dot{Q} = \frac{(T_B - T_I) \cdot K}{\int_0^\infty \Delta T_B(t) dt} \qquad (2)$$

where $\dot{Q}$ = cardiac output (L/min)
T_B = blood temperature
T_I = injectate temperature
K = computational constant

$\int_0^\infty \Delta T_B(t) dt$ = integral of temperature change over time

Blood temperature is measured continuously by the thermistor at the tip of the PAC, and injectate temperature is measured by a second thermistor at the injectate port.[638] The computation constant (K) is provided in each PAC package insert, and it must be entered manually into the cardiac output computer before measurement of cardiac output. This constant is actually the product of three constants, V_I, K_1, and K_2, which are defined as follows.[639-641]

V_I = volume of injectate
K_1 = density factor (product of the injectate's specific heat and specific gravity, divided by the product of the blood's specific heat and specific gravity)
K_2 = computation constant (catheter dead space, heat exchange in transit, injection time, conversion factor for units of L/min)

These constants adjust for the amount of thermal signal that will be introduced with each injection, as influenced by the physical characteristics of the catheter (i.e., size and composition) and the intended injectate that will be used. Typically, normal saline or 5% dextrose solutions are used, and the minor differences in their physical characteristics have minimal influence (<2%) on cardiac output measurement.[640,642] The last factor in the thermodilution equation, the integral of temperature change over time, is equal to the area under the thermodilution curve and is calculated electronically by the cardiac output computer.

To perform a thermodilution cardiac output measurement, a fixed volume of iced or room-temperature fluid is injected as a bolus into the proximal CVP lumen of the PAC, and the resulting change in pulmonary artery blood temperature is recorded by the thermistor at the catheter tip. As in all other forms of cardiovascular monitoring, it is important to have a real-time display of the thermodilution curve resulting from each cardiac output measurement.[454,643] Such display allows the clinician to discern artifacts that would invalidate the cardiac output measurement, such as unstable blood temperature, recirculation, or incomplete indicator injection. Usually, a series of three cardiac output measurements performed in rapid succession are averaged to provide a more reliable result. Stetz and associates reviewed 14 clinical studies that compared thermodilution cardiac output with other methods, such as Fick or dye dilution, to determine the reproducibility of the thermodilution technique.[644] These authors found that when single injections were used to determine cardiac output, a difference between sequential cardiac output measurements of 22% was required to suggest a clinically significant change. In contrast, when three injections were averaged to determine the thermodilution measurement, a change greater than 13% indicated a clinically significant change in cardiac output.

When carefully performed, thermodilution cardiac output measurements appear to provide results that are within 5% to 10% of other reference methods.[636,640,645,646] Few complications are directly attributable to the technique itself, although tachyarrhythmias and bradyarrhythmias related to injection of the indicator have been reported.[637,647]

Sources of Error in Thermodilution Cardiac Output Monitoring

Several important technical issues and potential sources of error must be considered for proper interpretation of thermodilution cardiac output measurements (Table 32-15).[639-641] The thermodilution technique measures right ventricular output and pulmonary artery blood flow. In the face of *intracardiac* or *extracardiac shunts*, right ventricular and left ventricular output will not be equal.

Table 32–15 Factors influencing accuracy of thermodilution cardiac output measurement

Intracardiac or extracardiac shunts
Tricuspid or pulmonic valve regurgitation
Inadequate delivery of thermal indicator
    Central venous injection site within the catheter
      introducer sheath
    Warming of iced injectate
Thermistor malfunction from fibrin or clot
Pulmonary artery blood temperature fluctuations
    After cardiopulmonary bypass
    Rapid intravenous fluid administration
Respiratory cycle influences

In patients with left-to-right shunts, early recirculation of the thermal indicator can be seen to distort the downslope of the thermodilution curve.[641] Although mathematical solutions can be used to determine the shunt fraction based on further analysis of the distorted thermodilution curves caused by shunts, these solutions are not available on bedside cardiac output computers.[641]

Patients with *tricuspid* or *pulmonic valve regurgitation* pose additional problems for measurement of cardiac output by the thermodilution technique because of recirculation of the indicator across the incompetent valve. In patients with severe tricuspid regurgitation, the thermodilution curves have an abnormally prolonged decay time, and the measured cardiac output may be inaccurate.[454,639,641,648,649] Unfortunately, there is no simple method to correct for this problem. In the presence of significant tricuspid regurgitation, cardiac output is usually underestimated by the thermodilution method, but it may be overestimated, depending on the severity of valvular regurgitation and the magnitude of the cardiac output.[650]

Other technical problems with thermodilution cardiac output measurement are caused by *inadequate delivery of the thermal indicator,* which can occur when the proximal CVP injectate port is not fully within the right atrium but rather contained within the introducer sheath.[651] In this case, the thermal bolus will not be delivered properly, and an abnormal cardiac output curve will be produced.[652,653] This problem should be recognized when one has difficulty making the bolus injection in a patient whose PAC is inserted a relatively short distance, such as 40 cm from the insertion site. When an iced injectate is used, mishandling of syringes can warm the solution and reduce the thermal indicator administered. In addition, fibrin or blood clot on the PAC tip may lead to temperature-sensing *thermistor malfunction* and result in spurious cardiac output values.

Because this measurement method is a thermal-based technique, in many circumstances an unrecognized *fluctuation in blood temperature* may influence the cardiac output measurement. In most patients, pulmonary artery blood temperature falls rapidly in the initial minutes *after cardiopulmonary bypass,* when the rewarmed body core redistributes the heat gained at the end of bypass. As a result of this progressive decline in central core and pulmonary artery blood temperature, the thermal baseline is unstable. Thermodilution cardiac output measurements made in the minutes after bypass are notoriously unreliable and most often lead to marked underestimation of true cardiac output.[654] Other inaccuracies in thermodilution cardiac output measurement occur when pulmonary artery blood temperature changes because of *rapid fluid infusion* through a peripheral intravenous site, through the PAC introducer sheath, or through one of the proximal PAC ports.[655,656] Either overestimation or underestimation of cardiac output occurs, depending on the timing of the additional fluid bolus.

The clinician can understand and predict all these measurement artifacts by recalling the Stewart-Hamilton equation and recognizing that cardiac output is inversely proportional to the area under the thermodilution curve. Any factor that causes a factitious reduction in this area will result in an erroneous increase in measured cardiac output. For example, if the constant entered in the cardiac output computer was the value for a 10-mL injectate but only a 5-mL injectate was used, the injected thermal indicator would be half the intended amount. As a result, the area under the thermodilution curve would be approximately half the expected value, and the computed cardiac output would overestimate true cardiac output by a factor of 2.

The choice of iced (0°C) or room-temperature injectate has been examined in detail to determine the preferred method for accurate measurement of cardiac output. Although the size of the thermal bolus (and hence the signal-to-noise ratio) is increased when an iced injectate is used, this indicator is more time consuming, expensive, and cumbersome to prepare than a room-temperature injectate. In addition, if the injection port thermistor becomes disconnected during the use of iced injectate, the injectate temperature will be measured erroneously as room temperature and result in artifactually decreased cardiac output values because the $T_B - T_I$ term will be too small. However, several groups have demonstrated equivalent accuracy in cardiac output determinations when iced and room-temperature injectates are compared, so it appears that room-temperature injectate is preferred for almost all clinical applications.[657,658] In adults, an injectate volume of 10 mL should be used, particularly with room-temperature solutions, because the measurements will be more accurate than those using smaller 3- or 5-mL volumes.[658] In children, an injectate volume of 0.15 mL/kg is recommended.[641]

One of the more controversial issues in standard bolus thermodilution cardiac output monitoring is the proper timing of measurement in relation to the *respiratory cycle,* particularly in patients receiving positive-pressure mechanical ventilation. By the nature of its measurement and mathematical expression, cardiac output is reported as flow per minute, even though it is measured by a thermodilution curve that is generated over several seconds and based on a small number of heartbeats. The cardiac output computer usually measures the first 60% to 70% of this curve and then extrapolates the downslope exponential to the baseline temperature.[639,655] Because the stroke output of the right ventricle varies as much as 50% during the respiratory cycle, the limited "sampling" of right ventricular stroke volumes measured with the bolus thermodilution technique may lead to widely variable measurements of cardiac output, depending on the point during the respiratory cycle when the measurements are performed.[659,660] Although the reproducibility of consecutive measurements improves markedly when the bolus injections are synchronized to the same phase of the respiratory cycle,[661,662] accurate measurement of average cardiac output is achieved more reliably by making multiple injections during the different phases of the respiratory cycle and then averaging the results.[639,641,660,663] Because the pattern of variation in pulmonary blood flow during respiration depends on many factors, including the pattern of ventilation (spontaneous or positive pressure), respiratory rate, tidal volume, airway pressure, and so forth, there is no simple way to know whether timing measurements at end-expiration will always provide the highest, lowest, or an intermediate value for cardiac output.[639,660,661] In the end, the clinician is faced with

a tradeoff—accuracy versus reproducibility. Recent studies of continuous cardiac output (COO) monitoring techniques highlight these issues.

Continuous Thermodilution Cardiac Output Monitoring

Newer technologies applied to PAC monitoring allow nearly continuous CCO monitoring with the use of either warm[664-671] or cold[672] thermal indicators. The warm thermal technique is the one now widely accepted in clinical practice. In brief, this method involves the release of small quantities of heat from a 10-cm thermal filament incorporated into the right ventricular portion of a PAC approximately 15 to 25 cm from the catheter tip.[667,673] Commercially available CCO monitors use proprietary stochastic identification algorithms to analyze the thermal signal measured by the thermistor at the tip of the catheter. The heating filament is cycled on and off in a pseudorandom binary sequence, and cardiac output is derived from cross-correlation of the measured pulmonary artery temperature and the known sequence of heating filament activation. A basic assumption inherent in this technique is that the cardiac output remains constant during the interval analyzed for measurement.[674]

Typically, the displayed value for cardiac output is updated every 30 to 60 seconds and represents the average value for the cardiac output measured over the previous 3 to 6 minutes.[675] In a laboratory investigation examining how CCO measurements respond to unstable hemodynamic conditions such as hemorrhage and fluid resuscitation, Siegel and colleagues showed that CCO changes were markedly slower than those detected by ultrasonic flow probe, blood pressure, or mixed venous oxygen saturation.[674] In view of these inherent time delays, current warm thermal PAC CCO methods should not be considered continuous, real-time monitors, but rather techniques that provide continual, frequently updated cardiac output values.

In general, CCO methods appear to have good agreement with standard bolus thermodilution cardiac output measurements or electromagnetic flow probe techniques.[668,669,676] In a small, multicenter study, Mihm and associates found that CCO provided a clinically reliable measurement in a group of 47 intensive care unit patients.[665] The device performed well in patients with a wide range of cardiac outputs (1.6 to 10.6 L/min) and core temperatures (33.2°C to 39.8°C), and the method showed no deterioration in performance over the 72-hour monitoring period. In general, PAC-based CCO monitoring appears to be more reproducible or precise than standard bolus thermodilution techniques, although this may simply be a function of the fact that the continuous methods display a time-weighted, average cardiac output value as opposed to a single instantaneous measurement.[664,665,677,678]

Warm thermal CCO PACs have been fairly rapidly and widely accepted into clinical practice for a number of practical reasons. Although these catheters are more expensive than standard PACs, bolus injections for measurement of cardiac output are obviated, thereby potentially reducing nursing efforts and the risk of fluid overload or infection. However, like cold bolus thermodilution techniques, warm thermal CCO has certain methodologic pitfalls that must be recognized and avoided. As already emphasized, CCO monitors have an inherent 5- to 15-minute delay in responding to abrupt changes in cardiac output, and the magnitude of this delay depends on the type of physiologic perturbation, as well as the CCO computer monitor algorithm.[673,674] Although modifications of CCO algorithms have provided a "STAT Mode" rapid response time, acute changes in cardiac output are still detected more slowly by CCO monitoring than by other methods such as direct arterial pressure or mixed venous oximetry.[664,674] Claims that CCO monitoring provides the best early warning of important circulatory changes remain anecdotal at present.[671,679]

Because the CCO PAC measures a cardiac output value that is an average derived over the previous several minutes, the beat-to-beat variations in stroke volume that occur during a single respiratory cycle are all equally represented in the derived average value for cardiac output. In contrast, bolus thermodilution measurements will show quite different cardiac output values, depending on the phase of respiration during which they are recorded (see earlier discussion). Thus, the CCO-averaging algorithm obviates this physiologic effect that confounds bolus thermodilution cardiac output techniques. As a result, cardiac output measured by the CCO method may provide a more accurate measurement of average cardiac output for patients receiving positive-pressure mechanical ventilation. Although electronic smoothing or filtering is standard for all hemodynamic values displayed on the bedside monitor, such as heart rate, blood pressure, and so forth, the delay inherent in warm thermal CCO monitoring is much longer—minutes rather than seconds. In effect, the CCO technique involves a fundamental tradeoff between rapid response time and overall accuracy of measurement. The standards for these performance characteristics have not been defined but must balance the response time against the stability of the displayed value and its immunity from thermal noise.[678]

In summary, the CCO PAC monitoring technique is more reproducible and precise than bolus thermodilution cardiac output measurement, but the time delays inherent in the CCO technique require the clinician to rely on other monitored variables to detect acute circulatory changes. Because an external system for cold fluid injection is not required, the CCO technique requires less nursing time and may result in fewer measurement errors, less risk of fluid overload, and less risk of infection. The CCO computer and catheter require a significant amount of time to warm up and may work poorly in an environment with a great deal of thermal noise or rapid hemodynamic changes, such as the cardiac operating room.

Fick Cardiac Output Measurement

The Fick method for determination of cardiac output is a form of the indicator dilution technique in which exogenous indicators are not required, but instead, transported oxygen serves this purpose. This method was first proposed in 1870 by the German physiologist Adolph Fick, who described a means to determine blood flow by measuring overall oxygen uptake and content in blood.[680,681]

The Fick equation relates cardiac output to oxygen consumption and blood oxygen content and is recognizable as a special form of the generalized indicator dilution equation.

$$\dot{Q} = \frac{\dot{V}o_2}{(Cao_2 - C\bar{v}o_2) \cdot 10} \qquad (3)$$

where
$\dot{Q}$ = cardiac output (L/min)
$\dot{V}o_2$ = oxygen consumption (mL O_2/min)
Cao_2 = oxygen content of arterial blood (mL O_2/100 mL blood)
$C\bar{v}o_2$ = oxygen content of mixed venous blood (mL O_2/100 mL blood)

Multiplying the denominator by 10 converts deciliters to liters (10 dL = 1L).

The denominator of the Fick equation is the arteriovenous oxygen content difference. This difference is calculated from the arterial and mixed venous oxygen contents.
Cao_2 = hemoglobin concentration (g/dL) × 1.36 mL O_2/g hemoglobin × arterial hemoglobin saturation (%)
$C\bar{v}o_2$ = hemoglobin concentration (g/dL) × 1.36 mL O_2/g hemoglobin × venous hemoglobin saturation (%)

In general, the contribution of dissolved oxygen is ignored in these calculations because it is small (0.003 × the arterial or mixed venous partial pressure of oxygen).

To calculate cardiac output by the Fick method, arterial and mixed venous blood must be drawn for blood gas analysis. The latter requires pulmonary artery catheterization to collect a true mixed venous sample. In addition, oxygen consumption must be measured; traditionally, this measurement required collection of the patient's exhaled air over a period of several minutes with cumbersome equipment. In an attempt to simplify and automate the Fick technique, newer approaches have used pulse oximetry, pulmonary artery oximetry, and on-line respiratory gas analysis or indirect calorimetry to measure oxygen consumption.[582-684] Although clinicians sometimes estimate the Fick cardiac output by assuming a constant basal value for oxygen consumption of approximately 200 to 250 mL/min, this approach is likely to be inaccurate in critically ill patients.[643] Normal values for all these variables are given in Table 32-14.

CONTINUOUS MIXED VENOUS OXIMETRY PULMONARY ARTERY CATHETERS

Although the formal Fick cardiac output method is not applied widely in clinical practice, the physiologic relationships described by the Fick equation form the basis for another PAC-based monitoring technique termed continuous mixed venous oximetry. Rearrangement of the Fick equation reveals the four determinants of mixed venous hemoglobin saturation ($S\bar{v}o_2$):

$$S\bar{v}o_2 = Sao_2 - \frac{\dot{V}o_2}{\dot{Q} \cdot 1.36 \cdot Hgb} \qquad (4)$$

where
$S\bar{v}o_2$ = mixed venous hemoglobin saturation (%)
Sao_2 = arterial hemoglobin saturation (%)

$\dot{V}O_2$ = oxygen consumption (mL O_2/min)
$\dot{Q}$ = cardiac output
Hgb = hemoglobin concentration (g/dL)

To the extent that arterial hemoglobin saturation, oxygen consumption, and hemoglobin concentration remain stable, mixed venous hemoglobin saturation may be used as an indirect indicator of cardiac output. For example, when cardiac output falls, tissue oxygen extraction increases and the mixed venous blood will become more desaturated. However, as noted in this equation, mixed venous hemoglobin saturation also varies directly with arterial hemoglobin saturation and hemoglobin concentration and varies inversely with oxygen consumption. When any of these other variables change significantly, one cannot assume that a change in mixed venous hemoglobin saturation results solely from a change in cardiac output. Although these considerations may confound the use of mixed venous hemoglobin saturation as an indicator of cardiac output, monitoring this variable provides more comprehensive information about the balance of oxygen delivery and consumption by the body—not just cardiac output, but also the adequacy of cardiac output.[675]

Although mixed venous hemoglobin saturation may be determined by intermittent blood sampling from the pulmonary artery, a specially designed PAC can provide this information reliably and continuously. Fiberoptic bundles incorporated into the PAC determine the hemoglobin saturation in pulmonary artery blood based on the principles of reflectance oximetry and the use of either a two- or three-wavelength system. A special computer connected to this PAC displays mixed venous hemoglobin saturation continuously. In addition, these continuous mixed venous oximetry PACs allow standard thermodilution cardiac output measurements or are combined with warm thermal CCO capability, thereby providing both continual cardiac output and venous oximetry data.

Technical problems with continuous mixed venous oximetry are generally limited to improper positioning of the PAC tip against the vessel wall or inaccurate calibration.[671,675] Multi-wavelength fiberoptic technology and reflection intensity algorithms help reduce wall artifacts caused by spurious reflections from a PAC thrombus or the pulmonary arterial walls. These catheters are calibrated at the bedside before use but may also be calibrated in vivo from a pulmonary artery blood gas sample if the mixed venous saturation values are questionable.[685]

Most clinical trials comparing PAC-derived continuous venous oximetry values with laboratory analysis of pulmonary artery blood samples have show good agreement with little bias between techniques.[671] Despite the apparent accuracy of this technique, there are significant questions about the clinical value of this additional monitoring. Although normal values of mixed venous hemoglobin saturation are well known, the appropriate therapeutic target value for any individual patient remains uncertain.[671] Clearly, low values of mixed venous hemoglobin saturation indicate an overall inadequacy of oxygen delivery relative to total-body oxygen consumption. However, many critically ill patients with normal or high values for mixed venous hemoglobin saturation have regionally inadequate blood flow and tissue oxygen delivery that is not detected by global measurements such as mixed venous oximetry.

The continuous mixed venous oximetry PAC may be used to measure thermodilution cardiac output and arterial and mixed venous oxygen content values and thereby calculate oxygen consumption by rearrangement of the Fick equation. However, values of oxygen consumption derived from these measurements generally underestimate direct oxygen consumption measured by mass spectrometry, metabolic cart, or water-sealed spirometry.[581] Oxygen delivery may also be calculated from these PAC-derived values.

$$\dot{D}O_2 = \dot{Q} \cdot CaO_2 \tag{5}$$

where
$\dot{D}O_2$ = oxygen delivery
$\dot{Q}$ = cardiac output (dL/min)
CaO_2 = oxygen content of arterial blood (mL O_2/100 mL blood)

Many physicians have used these derived measures of oxygen consumption and oxygen delivery to guide treatment of critically ill patients. Unfortunately, as noted in the earlier discussions of pulmonary artery catheterization, this "goal-oriented therapy" has not been shown to result in improved patient outcomes in most instances. Few clinical trials have directly assessed the value of oximetry PAC monitoring versus standard PAC monitoring. A small 226-patient trial comparing CVP, PAC, and oximetry PAC monitoring for cardiac surgery failed to show any benefits for the oximetry PAC and noted increased costs associated with this technique.[549] More recently, in a large Veterans Affairs observational trial of 3265 cardiac surgical patients, 49% of the patients received continuous mixed venous oximetry PACs, and use of this catheter was associated with increased cost but no better outcome than observed in the standard PAC group.[686]

In summary, continuous mixed venous oximetry remains an appealing, widely used monitoring technology because of the ability of this technique to provide continuous information about the global oxygen supply-and-demand balance in the body. These catheters are more expensive than standard PACs, and clinical studies to date have not yet defined appropriate clinical indications for their use.[559,671,675,686]

RIGHT VENTRICULAR EJECTION FRACTION PULMONARY ARTERY CATHETERS

Although cardiovascular monitoring has focused predominantly on left ventricular performance, in some instances, right ventricular dysfunction may be the more important factor limiting the circulation.[687-690] Patient populations at increased risk for right ventricular dysfunction include those with chronic obstructive pulmonary disease, adult respiratory distress syndrome, pulmonary hypertension, and right ventricular ischemia and infarction.[691]

Standard techniques are available for monitoring right ventricular performance in patients with acute myocardial infarction involving the right ventricle. ECG monitoring using the V_4R lead has proved to be a sensitive and specific indicator of right ventricular ischemia and infarction.[692-694] PAC monitoring in patients with right ventricular infarction often reveals the characteristic hemodynamic patterns described earlier.[489,490,691,695] However, accurate evaluation of right ventricular performance in patients with other causes of right ventricular dysfunction has proved more complicated. In patients with severe respiratory failure, the confounding effects of mechanical ventilation with high levels of PEEP have made interpretation of cardiac filling pressures difficult and, in some cases, misleading.[675,696-699]

In intraoperative and critical care environments, measurement of the right ventricular ejection fraction (RVEF) with a specially designed PAC offers another method for evaluating right ventricular function. This method uses a standard PAC equipped with a rapid-response thermistor that detects and quantifies the small changes in pulmonary artery blood temperature that occur with each heartbeat.[700,701] The thermistor measures these temperature changes after bolus administration of an iced or room-temperature injectate, and the cardiac output computer measures the residual fraction of thermal signal after each heartbeat to determine the RVEF as 1 minus this average residual fraction.[701] Clearly, all factors that confound standard thermodilution cardiac output measurement will also interfere with accurate determination of RVEF. In addition, because the temperature changes measured by the RVEF PAC are small, beat-to-beat changes, the method will not work if the ECG R waves cannot be detected accurately, the R-R interval is short as a result of tachycardia, or the cardiac rhythm is irregular.[675] Comparison of PAC-based RVEF measurements with angiographic or nuclear techniques has yielded mixed results in terms of accuracy, but this may reflect, in part, the absence of a widely accepted reference standard for this measurement.[701-703]

Intraoperative use of the RVEF PAC has focused primarily on detection of right ventricular dysfunction in patients with coronary artery disease undergoing surgical revascularization. Reduced RVEF has been noted after cardiopulmonary bypass, particularly in patients with preexisting right coronary artery obstruction.[704-706] Anecdotally, an acute reduction in RVEF from its normal value of approximately 40% may provide an early sign of right ventricular ischemia.[707] However, RVEF is an extremely load-dependent measurement of right ventricular performance, and the clinician must keep this fact in mind to interpret this measurement properly.[675,697,698]

Clinical use of the RVEF PAC appears to have found its greatest application to date in critically ill patients, especially those with respiratory failure.[675,697-699,708] In these applications, the measurement of greatest interest has been right ventricular end-diastolic volume, which is derived mathematically from RVEF.

$$RVEDV = \frac{SV}{RVEF} \tag{6}$$

where RVEDV = right ventricular end-diastolic volume
SV   = stroke volume
RVEF = right ventricular ejection fraction

Right ventricular end-diastolic volume appears to correlate better with cardiac output than do standard preload

measurements such as CVP or PAWP.[675,698,699] These findings are not surprising given all the interpretive problems associated with monitoring of cardiac filling pressure previously discussed. Furthermore, the better correlation between right ventricular end-diastolic volume and cardiac output may result from the mathematical coupling of measurements because both are derivatives of stroke volume determined with the PAC. As in the case of standard PAC monitoring, however, the benefit of RVEF PAC monitoring in terms of patient outcome remains unproven.[559]

PULMONARY ARTERY CATHETER–DERIVED HEMODYNAMIC VARIABLES

The cardiovascular system is often modeled as an electrical circuit, with the relationship between cardiac output, blood pressure, and resistance to flow related in a manner similar to Ohm's law. The electrical version of this relationship is familiar as Equation 7.

$$V = I \cdot R \tag{7}$$

where V = voltage
I = current
R = resistance

The analogous formulas for determining SVR and PVR rearrange Ohm's law and replace voltage with blood pressure and current with blood flow.

$$SVR = \frac{MAP - CVP}{CO} \cdot (80) \tag{8}$$

$$PVR = \frac{MPAP - PAWP}{CO} \cdot (80) \tag{9}$$

where SVR = systemic vascular resistance
PVR = pulmonary vascular resistance
MAP = mean arterial pressure (mm Hg)
CVP = mean central venous pressure (mm Hg)
MPAP = mean pulmonary artery pressure (mm Hg)
PAWP = mean pulmonary artery wedge pressure (mm Hg)
CO   = cardiac output (L/min)

Multiplying by 80 corrects SVR and PVR values from Wood units (mm Hg/L/min) to standard metric units (dynes · sec · cm^{-5}).

Normal values for SVR and PVR are given in Table 32-14. Note that these calculations of SVR and PVR are based on a hydraulic fluid model that assumes continuous, laminar flow through a series of rigid pipes.[709,710] These calculations also use atrial pressure as the downstream pressure for systemic or pulmonary flow, with CVP used for right atrial pressure in the SVR calculation and PAWP used for left atrial pressure in the PVR calculation. Alternative methods to calculate resistance ignore the effect of these downstream pressures. For the systemic circulation, total resistance may be calculated from mean arterial pressure and cardiac output alone, and for the pulmonary circulation, total pulmonary resistance describes the ratio of mean pulmonary artery pressure and cardiac output.

All these resistance formulas oversimplify the behavior of the cardiovascular system. A more physiologic model of the systemic circulation considers the vasculature to be a series of collapsible vessels with intrinsic tone. This model, also called the vascular waterfall, describes a critical closing pressure in the downstream end of the circuit that exceeds right atrial pressure and serves to limit flow—an effective downstream pressure that is higher than the right atrial pressure used in the SVR formula. Detailed consideration of these issues is beyond the scope of this discussion and is available in other sources.[711,712] The important issue for clinicians is that therapy focused on the fine adjustment of SVR may be very misleading and should be avoided.

Additional problems arise when considering the pulmonary vasculature and using the formulas just presented as a measure of resistance to flow through the lung. The pulmonary vasculature is more compliant than the systemic vasculature, and marked increases in pulmonary blood flow may not produce any significant increase in PAP. In addition, flow usually ceases at end-diastole in the low-resistance pulmonary circuit.[443,713] Thus, changes in PVR may result from intrinsic alterations in pulmonary vascular tone (constriction or dilation), vascular recruitment, or rheologic dynamics.[710,713,714] For the pulmonary circuit, a better approach to evaluating changes in PVR may be to examine the end-diastolic gradient between pulmonary artery diastolic and wedge pressure (see Fig. 32-51).[714] Alternatively, more complex calculations of impedance rather than resistance will better describe these vascular properties of the pulmonary circuit.[715]

Another set of common calculations derived from standard hemodynamic variables adjusts these measurements for the patient's body surface area (BSA) in an attempt to normalize these measurements for patients of different size. BSA is generally determined from standard nomograms based on height and weight. The most commonly indexed variables are the cardiac index (cardiac index = cardiac output/BSA) and stroke volume index (stroke volume index = stroke volume/BSA). On occasion, SVR and PVR are indexed as well. Note, however, that indexed resistances are higher than nonindexed values because the cardiac index term is in the denominator of these equations. The appropriate formulas are SVR index = SVR × BSA and PVR index = PVR × BSA.

In theory, normalizing hemodynamic values through "indexing" should help clinicians determine appropriate normal physiologic ranges to assist in guiding therapy. Unfortunately, there is little evidence that these additional calculations provide valid normalizing adjustments. BSA is a biometric measurement with an obscure relationship to blood flow, and it does not adjust for variations between individuals based on age, sex, body habitus, or metabolic rate.[716] Although it is important to be aware of a patient's size and medical history when interpreting and treating changes in any of the measured or calculated hemodynamic variables, it is not appropriate to target therapy solely at achieving normal indexed values.

NON–PULMONARY ARTERY CATHETER–BASED METHODS FOR CARDIAC OUTPUT AND PERFUSION MONITORING

Ultrasound-Based Methods for Cardiac Output Monitoring

The popularity and safety of diagnostic Doppler echocardiography in clinical medicine have driven the application of these techniques for measurement of cardiac output. All of the ultrasound-based methods for cardiac output monitoring use the Doppler principle. When ultrasound waves strike moving objects, these waves are reflected back to their source at a different frequency, termed the Doppler shift frequency, that is directly related to the velocity of the moving objects and the angle at which the ultrasound beam strikes these objects. For blood flow measurements, the red blood cells flowing through a major artery serve as the moving objects targeted by the ultrasound beam. The Doppler equation describes these relationships (Equation 10). To measure blood flow velocity, this equation is rearranged to solve for velocity (Equation 11).

$$f = \frac{2f_0 \cdot v \cdot \cos\theta}{c} \tag{10}$$

$$v = \frac{f \cdot c}{2f_0 \cdot \cos\theta} \tag{11}$$

where
  f = Doppler shift frequency
  v = velocity of red blood cell targets
  f_0 = transmitted ultrasound beam frequency
  θ = angle between the ultrasound beam and the vector of red blood cell flow
  c = velocity of ultrasound in blood (approximately 1570 m/sec)

In general, measurement of blood flow velocity requires just a single measurement, the Doppler shift frequency, because the velocity of ultrasound in blood and the transmitted ultrasound frequency are known, and cosine θ is assumed to equal 1 as long as the angle of insonation is small. This assumption requires that the ultrasound beam be oriented as much as possible in a direction that is parallel to blood flow. For example, for angles less than 20 degrees, cosine θ will be greater than 0.94, thereby introducing an error of less than 6% in the cardiac output calculation.

Once the Doppler shift frequency is measured and blood flow velocity is calculated, stroke volume can be determined from Equation 12.

$$SV = v \cdot ET \cdot CSA \tag{12}$$

where
  SV = stroke volume (mL)
  v   = spatial average velocity of blood flow (cm/sec)
  ET = systolic ejection time (sec)
  CSA = cross-sectional area of the vessel (cm²)

Finally, cardiac output is derived as the product of stroke volume and heart rate.

One Doppler method that has been described for determination of cardiac output uses a PAC equipped with three 1-mm ultrasound transducers mounted on the front and rear surfaces of the catheter tip.[717-719] The theoretical advantages of *PAC Doppler cardiac output* monitoring are that the technique determines a space-averaged measurement of blood flow velocity in the pulmonary artery and an instantaneous measurement of vessel diameter throughout the cardiac cycle, thereby providing a form of CCO monitoring.[719,720] However, the modest accuracy of the technique and its requirement for pulmonary artery catheterization have limited clinical acceptance.

The Doppler principle has also been applied to measure cutaneous blood flow by *laser Doppler velocimetry*.[721] Because this method detects only changes in skin blood flow rather than absolute cardiac output, its use is confined mainly to determining the adequacy of graft tissue flow after microvascular anastomosis of major tissue flaps.

Several different ultrasound-based methods are used to measure cardiac output, each with slightly different equipment and measuring blood flow from a different site in the body. One method involves the use of an ultrasound probe mounted on the tip of an endotracheal tube to measure *transtracheal Doppler cardiac output* by insonation of aortic blood flow.[722,723] This method used pulsed-wave Doppler ultrasound to measure the flow velocity in the ascending aorta. The aortic cross-sectional area was determined by range-gating the Doppler signal in small 1-mm increments to measure aortic diameter and then calculating the aortic cross-sectional area, assuming the aorta to be a circular vessel.[723] Although early reports suggested that this method tracked directional changes in cardiac output accurately, Hausen and coauthors reported very poor performance of the device in the postoperative setting, with transtracheal Doppler measurements markedly underestimating thermodilution cardiac output values.[724] Practical considerations have also been unfavorable, including marked operator dependency for success because of a difficult user interface and poor signal stability.[725] This method required tracheal intubation and patient sedation, which further limited its applicability. When the Doppler signal is inadequate, the endotracheal tube cuff needed to be deflated and the tube repositioned, thus placing the patient at risk for pulmonary aspiration.[724] As a result of these considerations, transtracheal Doppler cardiac output measurement has not been widely accepted in clinical practice.

Esophageal Doppler Cardiac Output Monitoring

Other clinical methods to measure cardiac output with Doppler ultrasound have focused on less invasive approaches than the transtracheal or PAC techniques. One method was developed to measure blood flow velocity in the distal aortic arch with an ultrasound transducer applied to the suprasternal notch.[726] Further refinements of the technique used continuous-wave Doppler to measure the systolic velocity integral and estimate stroke volume in the ascending aorta.[727] By the 1980s, successful noninvasive measurement of cardiac output was reported involving the use of commercially available equipment to determine velocities in the ascending aorta with continuous-wave Doppler and the aortic cross-sectional area with A-mode pulsed echocardiography.[728-730] Although these *suprasternal Doppler cardiac output* techniques showed reasonable agreement with thermodilution methods, they were relatively labor intensive, required a fair degree of experience and expertise, and could not be accomplished in a significant number of critically ill medical and surgical patients.[728,730,731] Because they provided only intermittent measurements at best, clinical acceptance of this method was limited.

The evolution of Doppler techniques into practical clinical monitoring tools required an ultrasound transducer that could be positioned and left in place for continuous monitoring without the need for repeated adjustments or time-consuming measurements by the physician. Such a transducer was incorporated into the tip of a standard esophageal stethoscope to allow continuous monitoring of cardiac output by interrogating the blood flow profile in the descending thoracic aorta. This technique, *esophageal Doppler cardiac output* monitoring, is one of the more widely applied methods for noninvasive or minimally invasive monitoring of cardiac output.[626] In brief, the Doppler probe is inserted into the esophagus to a depth of approximately 35 cm from the incisors in a tracheally intubated patient. Probe position is adjusted to optimize the audible Doppler flow sound from the descending aorta. In most patients, optimal probe tip position is at the T5-6 vertebral interspace or the third sternocostal junction because the esophagus and the descending aorta lie in close proximity and run essentially parallel to one another at this location.[732-734] The ultrasound transducer is mounted at a fixed angle that is known by the cardiac output computer and used to correct the resulting Doppler shift frequency to provide an accurate velocity measurement (see earlier discussion).

The esophageal Doppler monitoring method interrogates blood flow in the descending thoracic aorta and therefore measures only a fraction of total cardiac output. Consequently, the esophageal Doppler probe must be "calibrated" by some method. Most early investigators performed this initial calibration with a suprasternal Doppler measurement of cardiac output in the ascending aorta.[729,735-739] In some instances, ascending aortic diameter was also measured by A-mode ultrasound,[729,735] whereas later versions of these monitors used a nomogram to estimate aortic diameter based on the patient's age, sex, height, and weight.[736-739]

The initial studies comparing cardiac output measured with the esophageal Doppler device with other methods showed variable performance of the new technique.[740,741] Although several investigators demonstrated accurate tracking of changes in cardiac output measured by thermodilution, there were significant differences in absolute cardiac output between methods, with the Doppler technique both underestimating and overestimating simultaneous thermodilution values.[729,736] Other investigations were even less favorable, thus suggesting that the esophageal Doppler method could not be relied on as a trend monitor.[738,739,742] It appeared that the suprasternal Doppler measurements and the aortic diameter measurements were often in error and did not provide suitable initial calibration of the esophageal Doppler probe. Furthermore, these initial calibration methods were cumbersome and time consuming and required significant operator expertise.

In recent years, the esophageal Doppler method for cardiac output monitoring has seen renewed enthusiasm, not so much as an accurate measure of absolute cardiac output, but as an estimate for systemic blood flow.[626,743] Singer and colleagues have popularized this technique in the United Kingdom by applying it to the care of critically ill patients and using newer features of the Doppler technique to discern additional hemodynamic information.[744-747] Improvements in instrument design have made it more informative to the clinician and much simpler to use. Current devices provide a clear visual display of the spectral Doppler waveform and calculate and display additional hemodynamic variables, including the peak blood flow velocity, flow acceleration, and the heart rate–corrected flow time. Some studies have shown that these additional measures provide useful information about left ventricular preload, contractility, and SVR.[626,744-749] Esophageal Doppler monitoring provides a continuous, beat-to-beat waveform that is proportional to left ventricular stroke volume. One of the more important values of the monitor may be that it focuses clinical attention on optimizing stroke volume rather than total cardiac output. Indeed, in critically ill patients, complications may be predicted better by low stroke volume than by low cardiac output.[750]

The newer esophageal Doppler monitoring devices are simpler to operate because they do not require the cumbersome calibration procedures demanded by earlier devices. The emphasis in developing these devices has been more toward providing a continuous measure of aortic blood flow rather than total cardiac output.[751,752] For the Doppler technique to provide accurate trending information, however, several assumptions must still remain valid. First, the angle between the esophageal Doppler probe and the descending aorta must be known and remain constant throughout the monitoring period. Second, the aortic cross-sectional area must remain constant. Third, the descending aortic flow must remain a constant proportion of the total cardiac output.[753]

The esophageal Doppler monitoring technique has a number of attributes that have aided its clinical acceptance. The technique is easy to use, minimally invasive, and inherently safe. It has been used successfully for days in tracheally intubated patients or sedated patients in the intensive care unit.[734] This monitoring can be initiated rapidly, usually within 5 minutes, and can be applied when pulmonary artery catheterization cannot be accomplished or is contraindicated.[754] It appears that limited experience is needed for clinical success—as few as 10 to 12 cases for accurate application of the technique.[734] A recent review of 25 clinical trials comparing esophageal Doppler cardiac output measurement with PAC thermodilution measurement noted that the Doppler cardiac output values correlated well with thermodilution measurements, showed minimal overall bias and good tracking of directional changes in thermodilution cardiac output, and had low intraobserver and interobserver measurement variability.[734]

The main limitation of esophageal Doppler cardiac output monitoring remains its accuracy as an absolute measure of cardiac output. In an attempt to address this problem, the latest modifications of these devices have focused on direct measurement of aortic diameter. These newer monitors use esophageal Doppler probes containing two ultrasound transducers. One is used to measure aortic blood flow by pulsed-wave Doppler, and the second measures aortic diameter simultaneously at the flow site by M-mode echocardiography.[732,733] These monitors display both the Doppler and the M-mode waveforms to promote user confidence in the quality of these signals. The advantage of the added aortic imaging data is that assumptions regarding aortic diameter are not needed and, instead, are replaced by continual aortic measurements. Whether these newer monitors will provide more accurate cardiac output values than possible with the simpler Doppler technologies remains uncertain.

Other limitations of the esophageal Doppler technique must also be appreciated by the physician to avoid pitfalls in interpretation of data. First and foremost, as emphasized earlier, the technique provides only an estimate of total cardiac output. Furthermore, for changes in cardiac output to be properly detected, the previously mentioned assumptions regarding descending aortic blood flow must remain valid. The technique is likely to be inaccurate in patients with aortic valve stenosis or regurgitation or those with thoracic aortic disease. Moreover, a fundamental assumption that descending aortic blood flow is approximately 70% of total cardiac output is not valid in the presence of conditions that redistribute blood flow, such as pregnancy, aortic cross-clamping, and after cardiopulmonary bypass.[729,734,737] The esophageal Doppler technique is not easily applied in non–tracheally intubated patients, and it cannot be used in individuals with esophageal pathology. Finally, like all ultrasound techniques, the acoustic window to acquire the Doppler signal may not be adequate in some individuals, thereby precluding use of this method.

The current clinical role for esophageal Doppler cardiac output monitoring is not to serve as a replacement for the PAC, but rather as an additional circulatory monitor in higher-risk patients who do not warrant invasive monitoring.[626,755] The popularity of this technique in the United Kingdom may reflect in part the much more restricted use of PACs in that country versus the United States. Preliminary studies have suggested that perioperative esophageal Doppler-guided volume resuscitation of moderate-risk surgical patients reduces perioperative morbidity and shortens the hospital stay.[756,757] If these results can be duplicated in other settings and with larger groups of patients, this technique may find a role as a more routine monitor in patients who are at increased risk for perioperative circulatory complications.

Bioimpedance Cardiac Output Monitoring

An interest in studying cardiovascular function during space flight initially prompted investigations of impedance plethysmography as a noninvasive method of determining cardiac output. The technique of *bioimpedance cardiac output* monitoring was first described by Kubicek and colleagues and is based on the changes in electrical impedance of the thoracic cavity that occur with the ejection of blood during cardiac systole.[758] Their original formula relates these bioimpedance measurements to stroke volume.

$$SV = \frac{\rho L^2}{Zo^2} \cdot VET \cdot max \frac{dZ}{dt} \qquad (13)$$

where SV   = stroke volume
 ρ = specific resistivity of blood
 L   = thoracic length
 Zo^2 = basal thoracic impedance
 VET   = ventricular ejection time

$max \frac{dZ}{dt}$ = maximum rate of change in impedance during systolic upstroke

Cardiac output is computed from the product of the derived stroke volume and heart rate. Over the years, this formula for deriving stroke volume has been modified based on refined models of the behavior of thoracic resistivity.[626,759,760]

Various devices have been marketed commercially that measure cardiac output by the bioimpedance method. Each requires the application of disposable electrodes to the skin surface along the sides of the neck and lateral aspect of the lower part of the thorax. Impedance measurements are made by applying a continuous small electrical current across the chest. Patient height, weight, and gender are entered into the monitor by the operator to allow calculation of the volume of the thoracic cavity. Bioimpedance cardiac output is computed for each cardiac cycle and continuously displayed as an average value over several heartbeats.

Validation studies comparing bioimpedance cardiac output measurement with other methods have produced inconsistent results.[626,739,740,760-766] Although many studies suggest that the bioimpedance method is accurate in healthy volunteers, its reliability deteriorates in critically ill patients, including those with sepsis, increased lung water, aortic regurgitation, and electronic cardiac pacing.[760,761,766] Because the bioimpedance method is an indirect measure of cardiac output with a complex mathematical derivation, it is not surprising that this monitoring method has not proved to be as reliable as some other techniques.

Recent reports of animal studies and small clinical trials have described changes in signal-processing techniques that have improved the accuracy of thoracic bioimpedance measurements.[767-770] In an attempt to further improve signal quality, an alternative approach to bioimpedance monitoring uses a specially designed endotracheal tube to measure electrical impedance changes in the ascending aorta.[771] Despite these refinements, bioimpedance cardiac output monitoring has not found broad clinical acceptance to date.

Partial CO$_2$ Rebreathing Fick Cardiac Output Monitoring

Another method of cardiac output monitoring that does not require pulmonary artery catheterization is the *partial CO$_2$ rebreathing Fick technique*.[772-774] Because of the difficulty encountered in measuring oxygen consumption or mixed venous hemoglobin saturation with the standard Fick method, this technique is based on a restatement of the Fick Equation for carbon dioxide elimination rather than oxygen uptake.

$$\dot{Q} = \frac{\dot{V}CO_2}{(C\bar{v}CO_2 - CaCO_2)} \qquad (14)$$

where $\dot{Q}$ = cardiac output
 $\dot{V}CO_2$ = rate of carbon dioxide elimination
 $C\bar{v}CO_2$ = carbon dioxide content of mixed venous blood
 $CaCO_2$ = carbon dioxide content of arterial blood

This method uses the change in CO$_2$ production and end-tidal CO$_2$ concentration in response to a brief, sudden change in minute ventilation.[775,776] With a specially designed breathing system and monitoring computer, this measurement is easily performed in any tracheally intubated patient. Every 3 minutes, a computer-controlled pneumatic valve intermittently increases dead space for a 50-second period, thereby causing partial rebreathing of exhaled gases. Changes in CO$_2$ production and end-tidal CO$_2$ in response to the rebreathing are used to calculate cardiac output by a differential version of the Fick equation for carbon dioxide. The attractive features of this method are that it is entirely noninvasive, it can be performed every few minutes, and the brief episodes of rebreathing pose no substantial risk to most patients, with end-tidal CO$_2$ values increasing by less than 3 mm Hg. However, as currently designed, accurate measurements with this technique require tracheal intubation for precise measurement of exhaled gases. Furthermore, changing patterns of ventilation may have an unpredictable influence on the measurement. As with all Fick-based techniques, the partial CO$_2$ rebreathing method measures pulmonary capillary blood flow as an indicator of total cardiac output and thus requires correction for pulmonary shunting.

The initial clinical trials suggest reasonably good agreement between the partial rebreathing CO$_2$ cardiac output method and other techniques such as thermodilution. However, as with most of these newer monitoring methods, the clinical trials are small and mainly focused on specific patient groups, particularly coronary artery bypass patients.[773,774] At present, the clinical role for this technique is focused mainly on short-term intraoperative applications or uncomplicated mechanically ventilated postoperative patients.

Lithium Dilution Cardiac Output Monitoring

The *lithium dilution* technique is another cardiac output monitoring method that derives its fundamental basis from indicator dilution principles.[777-779] In brief, after an intravenous bolus injection of a small dose of lithium chloride, an ion-selective electrode attached to a peripheral arterial catheter measures the lithium dilution curve, from which cardiac output is derived. Preliminary investigations suggest that this technique is accurate when compared with standard thermodilution methods or electromagnetic flowmetry.[780,781] As originally described, the technique required a central venous catheter for lithium injection, but recent studies indicate comparable accuracy with peripheral intravenous bolus administration of the lithium indicator.[782-784] Thus, the technique seems to provide a method for accurate measurement of cardiac output in a wide variety of critically ill patients who have only peripheral intravenous and arterial catheters.

Pulse Contour Cardiac Output Monitoring

In an attempt to provide continuous measurement of cardiac output, a number of techniques have focused on analysis of the arterial pulse pressure waveform. These methods, generally termed *pulse contour cardiac output,* determine cardiac output from computerized analysis of the pressure waveform recorded at various sites, including the aorta,[785] radial artery,[786] and even a finger in a noninvasive technique.[787,788] All these methods determine stroke volume and cardiac output from analysis of the arterial pressure pulse.[789] Although early studies comparing these techniques showed fairly poor agreement with other cardiac output measurements, more recent clinical trials in cardiac surgical patients have shown that the pulse contour methods provide an acceptable level of accuracy.[790-795] Two pulse contour methods are clinically available that differ in regard to the site of arterial pressure monitoring and the initial calibration technique. One method uses transpulmonary thermodilution calibration and requires femoral arterial catheterization,[796] which may limit its applicability in some centers. The other uses lithium dilution calibration and arterial pulse wave analysis from radial or brachial measurement sites.[797]

These pulse contour methods are based on solid physical principles, offer the potential for continuous beat-to-beat monitoring, and are calibrated with sound methods. Both systems use transpulmonary measurement of an indicator (either cold or lithium), thereby eliminating the confounding effects of the respiratory cycle encountered during standard PAC thermodilution cardiac output measurements. However, these techniques involve substantial computations and are based on physiologic models that may not always apply clinically. A number of issues remain with the pulse contour technique, including the nonlinearity of aortic compliance, the relationship between peripheral and aortic pressure, and the expected clinical problems encountered with the recording of arterial pressure waveforms, including resonance and damping.[789]

The clinical role of all these alternative methods for monitoring cardiac output remains in evolution. Advocates of flow monitoring argue that early preemptive therapy guided by these devices is more likely to improve patient outcome than delayed therapy is in critically ill patients who already have evidence of end-organ failure. In the acute care setting, noninvasive cardiac output monitoring methods that are easily applied during surgery or on initial arrival at the emergency department or intensive care unit may have a unique role in providing a bridge to more comprehensive, invasive monitoring with a PAC.

Other Techniques for Circulatory and Perfusion Monitoring

Other methods for detecting adequacy of the circulating blood volume or end-organ perfusion have focused on measurement of circulating blood volume. The *double indicator dilution* method is one technique for assessment of blood volume at the bedside. With the use of equipment for transpulmonary thermodilution measurement of cardiac output, cold indocyanine green dye is injected intravenously, and the dye dilution and cold dilution curves are recorded with an arterial catheter inserted in the femoral artery and positioned in the descending aorta. The dye serves as an intravascular marker, whereas the cold diffuses and is convected into the extravascular space. The monitoring computer derives the intrathoracic blood volume from these measurements.[798] Early investigations suggested that intrathoracic blood volume is a better measure of cardiac preload than traditional measurements such as CVP or PAWP are.[798-803]

Pulse dye densitometry is another method that may provide a bedside indication of the circulating blood volume that was previously measured only with complex radioactive isotope techniques. This method involves the intravenous injection of indocyanine green dye and detection of the dye with a peripheral pulse dye densitometer that uses two-wavelength light absorption, similar to a pulse oximeter.[804-807]

Other monitoring techniques aimed at detecting inadequate tissue blood flow have focused on the splanchnic circulation as a site that may provide an early indication of hypoperfusion. *Gastric tonometry* is a recently automated technique that allows measurement of gastric intramucosal P_{CO_2} and calculation of intramucosal pH with a semicontinuous air tonometer.[808-810] Some investigations have already noted the superiority of this end-organ monitor as an indicator of the adequacy of tissue perfusion and a predictor of perioperative complications or death.[756,810,811] Unfortunately, it is not known whether therapy directed at correcting such splanchnic hypoperfusion will confer clinical benefit.[812,813] These nontraditional cardiovascular monitoring techniques, such as measurement of intrathoracic blood volume and gastric intramucosal pH, offer new variables for cardiovascular monitoring that may augment or even supplant some current monitors.

COAGULATION MONITORING
(also see Chapters 47 and 50)

In contrast to hemodynamic monitoring, assessment of perioperative coagulation remains, at present, entirely an ex vivo process. Traditionally, coagulation monitoring in surgical patients has focused on preoperative testing to identify those at increased risk for perioperative bleeding and intraoperative monitoring of heparin therapy during cardiac and vascular surgery. More recently, the availability of increasingly sensitive and specific point-of-care coagulation monitors has provided an opportunity to guide the administration of blood components and hemostatic drugs more specifically, without the delays inherent in standard laboratory testing.

Monitoring heparin anticoagulation during cardiac and vascular surgery is widely recognized as essential for the safe performance of these operations. Heparin is a biopharmaceutical derived from bovine lung or porcine intestinal mucosa and is composed of a heterogeneous mixture of compounds with diverse anticoagulant activities.[814]

Consequently, variability in heparin activity and pharmacodynamic response is well documented. Various patient-specific factors also affect the pharmacodynamic response to heparin, including age, intravascular volume, and plasma/membrane concentrations of antithrombin III, heparin cofactor II, platelet factor 4, and other heparin-binding proteins.[814] Not surprisingly, therefore, patients exhibit widely different anticoagulant responses to the same standard dose of heparin.[815] Finally, heparin anticoagulation monitoring must be performed if only to prevent the rare, but potentially lethal complication resulting from failure to administer heparin as intended before cardiopulmonary bypass or arterial clamping.[816]

The ideal test of perioperative coagulation would be simple to perform, accurate, reproducible, diagnostically specific, and cost-effective. Although no single monitoring device available to date has all these ideal operating characteristics, many provide useful information to guide patient management. Particularly when combinations of these devices are used, they provide valuable diagnostic insight into the mechanism of a patient's perioperative coagulopathy. The importance of integrated monitoring described earlier for hemodynamic assessment is equally applicable to coagulation monitoring.

The commercially available point-of-care coagulation monitors used in the perioperative setting may be divided into four categories: functional measures of coagulation or assays that measure the intrinsic ability of the blood to clot, monitors of heparin concentration, viscoelastic measures of coagulation, and platelet function analyzers (Table 32-16).

Functional Measures of Coagulation

The activated coagulation time (ACT), described by Hattersley in 1966,[817] is a version of the Lee-White whole blood clotting time that is modified to include an initiator for contact activation of the coagulation system. This activator, frequently diatomaceous earth, is used to accelerate clot formation and reduce the time to completion of the assay.

Hattersley's original assay required manual mixing of a blood sample with the contact activator, followed by repeated visual assessment of the tube to determine the time to visible clot formation. More recent commercial ACT monitors simplify testing by automating clot detection. One of the more widely available ACT monitors uses a glass test tube that contains a small magnet at the bottom (Hemochron; International Technidyne, Inc., Edison, NJ). After adding a sample of blood, the tube is placed into the analyzer, where a constant temperature of 37°C is maintained, and the tube is rotated slowly while the magnet maintains contact with a proximity detection switch. As fibrin clot forms, the magnet becomes enmeshed and is pulled away from the detection switch, thereby triggering an alarm and providing an end time for the ACT measurement. Another ACT device uses a "plumb bob" flag assembly that is raised and dropped repeatedly through the sample vial containing blood and contact activator (Hepcon and ACT II; Medtronic Blood Management, Parker, CO). As clot forms, the rate of descent of the flag through blood slows and triggers an optical detector and alarms to signify the end time for the ACT.

Because each patient's baseline ACT measurement serves as a control for subsequent determinations, the method selected for ACT testing might appear to be unimportant. However, drugs used in the perioperative period, such as the antifibrinolytic drug aprotinin, may dramatically alter the times measured with different ACT monitoring systems. Aprotinin inhibits contact activation by celite (diatomaceous earth)[818] and produces an artifactual elevation of the celite ACT. If this interaction is not considered, an insufficient dose of heparin may be administered. Kaolin, an alternative contact activator, should be used to measure ACT in patients receiving aprotinin because it will bind the aprotinin and remove it from plasma.[818] It is not clear whether excess concentrations of aprotinin will overwhelm the kaolin-binding capacity and thereby affect the kaolin-activated ACT.

The ACT in normal individuals is approximately 107 ± 13 seconds (mean ± SD).[817] However, the time at which a patient's "baseline" ACT is measured can influence the result. After surgical incision, the baseline ACT decreases by more than 2 SD in patients undergoing cardiac surgery, perhaps because of release of tissue factor after tissue injury.[819] Heparin clearly prolongs the ACT because this test measures the clotting potential of the intrinsic and common pathways of coagulation. In addition to prolongation of the ACT by heparin, a prolonged ACT signifies an impaired ability of the blood sample to generate clot, for whatever reason. However, the ACT is relatively resistant to platelet dysfunction and is affected only by severe thrombocytopenia and platelet inhibitors such as prostacyclin or monoclonal antibodies directed against glycoprotein IIb/IIIa surface receptors.[820-822]

ACT testing is probably the most widely used perioperative coagulation monitor because of its simplicity, low cost, and ability to monitor anticoagulation when large doses of heparin are used as required for cardiac surgical procedures. However, certain limitations are associated with this method of monitoring. The ACT is relatively insensitive to low concentrations of heparin, and ACT measurements are not particularly reproducible.[823] These deficiencies are especially important when ACT monitoring is used to verify heparin neutralization with protamine. ACT monitoring may also be influenced by

Table 32–16 Point-of-care coagulation monitors

Functional measures of coagulation
   Activated coagulation time (ACT)
   Heparin management test (HMT)
   High-dose thrombin time (HiTT)
   Prothrombin time (PT)
   Activated partial thromboplastin time (aPTT)
Monitors of heparin concentration
   Protamine titration
   Ion-selective electrodes
Viscoelastic measures of coagulation
   Thromboelastograph (TEG)
   Sonoclot
Platelet function analyzers

phospholipid-bound microparticles extruded from the platelet surface during activation. These platelet microparticles artifactually shorten the ACT, even in the presence of residual heparin.[824] In addition to artifactually low ACT values, high ACT values longer than 600 seconds do not represent a linear dose-response relationship to high-dose heparin administration.[823] Furthermore, both hypothermia and hemodilution prolong the time to ACT clot formation. In some instances, these artifactual effects on measurement of the ACT may lead to false assumptions regarding the extent of anticoagulation. Reproducibility of the ACT may be improved by averaging duplicate ACT determinations.[825] ACT tubes containing either heparinase or protamine have been used in conjunction with unmodified ACT tubes to improve the sensitivity for detecting low heparin concentrations in blood.[826]

The heparin management test (HMT) (Pharmanetics, Morrisville, NC) offers promise as a solution to several problems associated with ACT monitoring during cardiac surgery. This method exploits recent advances in dry reagent chemistry for analysis of coagulation. The HMT uses a microprocessor-controlled analyzer and disposable test cards to provide a rapid, reproducible measure of functional anticoagulation in heparin-containing whole blood. A reaction chamber within each test card contains paramagnetic iron oxide beads and the dry chemical reagents necessary to activate coagulation in the blood sample.[827] After a drop of blood is added to the card, capillary action draws a small portion of this blood sample into the reaction chamber. An oscillating magnetic field is applied to the solution of blood, chemical reactants, and beads. A light beam passes through the test chamber and detects oscillations in the amplitude of transmitted light coincident with bead movement. As clot formation occurs, the beads become enmeshed within the clot, thereby reducing the amplitude of light oscillations to trigger the end time for the HMT measurement. The minute sample of blood drawn into the test chamber and the sensitivity of the clot detection method used in this system minimize confounding effects from hypothermia and hemodilution. Preliminary evaluation of this monitor during cardiac surgery suggests that the HMT may provide a more accurate and more reproducible measure of heparin activity than the ACT does.[828,829] Recently, the HMT has been incorporated into an array of tests performed on a single analyzer platform, the Rapidpoint Coag (Bayer Diagnostics, Tarrytown, NY). The HMT is performed in series with the heparin titration test (HTT) and the protamine response time (PRT) to acquire patient-specific recommendations for subsequent dosing of heparin and protamine, respectively. In addition, the Rapidpoint Coag analyzer has been used in concert with the ecarin clotting time (ECT) to monitor dosing of the specific thrombin inhibitor bivalirudin.[830]

A third measure of heparin anticoagulation, also used primarily during cardiac surgery, is the high-dose thrombin time (HiTT) (International Technidyne, Edison, NJ). The HiTT assay contains high reagent concentrations of thrombin to cleave fibrinogen directly and generate a fibrin clot. In the presence of these excess thrombin concentrations, clot formation occurs independently of plasma coagulation factors other than fibrinogen. As a result, the HiTT is prolonged by heparin (or other thrombin inhibitors), extreme degrees of hypofibrinogenemia or dysfibrinogenemia, and high concentrations of fibrin split products.[831,832] During most surgical procedures requiring heparin administration, HiTT prolongation will correlate with the heparin anticoagulant effect. The major limitation to more widespread use of the HiTT assay has been the limited shelf life of the thrombin reagent, which must be mixed just before performing the test.

Preoperative laboratory-based coagulation testing remains common practice in patients with a preexisting coagulopathy and those scheduled to undergo surgical procedures commonly associated with postoperative coagulopathy, such as cardiac or hepatic surgery. Most often, the prothrombin time (PT) and activated partial thromboplastin time (aPTT) are measured to provide baseline reference values for the patient, although the dose-response curves for these assays limit their usefulness when high-dose heparin anticoagulation is used. As point-of-care coagulation monitors that measure PT and aPTT become increasingly available, it is important to recognize that the test results from these monitors will not necessarily mirror the results reported by the hospital-based laboratory. Results from point-of-care coagulation monitoring may differ from laboratory testing because reagent sensitivities vary considerably from manufacturer to manufacturer and from one lot of reagent to another. In addition, laboratory-based testing relies on plasma samples, as opposed to whole blood samples commonly used in point-of-care testing.[833] Indeed, some of the delay inherent in laboratory-based testing results from the time required to process the plasma sample from the patient's whole blood. Because values obtained with point-of-care monitors are unlikely to agree with laboratory-based testing, their successful use in clinical practice will often require that baseline reference values be determined for each individual patient.

Heparin Concentration Measurement

Protamine titration is at present the most widely used method for determining heparin concentration in the perioperative setting. Protamine is a strongly basic polycationic protein that directly inhibits heparin in a stoichiometric manner. In other words, 1 mg of protamine will inhibit 1 mg (approximately 100 U) of heparin. This reaction forms the basis for the protamine titration method of measurement of heparin concentration. As increasing concentrations of protamine are added to a sample of heparin-containing blood, the time to clot formation decreases until the point at which the protamine concentration exceeds the heparin concentration in the blood sample, and then the time to clot formation increases. If a series of blood samples with incremental doses of protamine are analyzed, the sample in which the protamine and heparin concentrations are most closely matched will be the first one to generate a clot. Thus, by using protamine titration methodology, it is possible to estimate the heparin concentration present in a given sample of blood.[834]

Assuming that the heparin-protamine titration curve of an individual patient remains constant throughout the operative period, it is possible to use the protamine titration method to estimate the dose of heparin required to achieve a desired plasma heparin concentration. In a similar manner, determination of the heparin concentration at the conclusion of surgery allows a more precise estimate of the amount of protamine required to neutralize the circulating heparin. More precise administration of heparin and protamine may have a number of clinical advantages. Some investigations have suggested that thrombin activity during cardiopulmonary bypass may be reduced when stable heparin concentrations are maintained.[835] More effective thrombin inhibition during bypass should benefit patients by decreasing consumption of coagulation factors and thereby reducing postoperative bleeding.[836,837] Although protamine titration was initially performed manually, automated methods are currently available (Hepcon HMS; Medtronic Blood Management, Parker, CO). These monitors use cassettes of four to six protamine-containing vials to perform the titration assay. Different measurement cassettes are chosen, depending on the expected range of heparin concentration.

Protamine titration methodology is relatively sensitive to low concentrations of heparin and is limited only by the range of protamine concentrations provided for testing. For this reason, protamine titration has proved particularly useful for verifying heparin neutralization after protamine administration. This method for determining heparin concentration is relatively resistant to the influences of hypothermia and hemodilution. Furthermore, heparin concentration monitoring by protamine titration is not altered during aprotinin therapy, in contrast to celite ACT measurements. The major limitation of heparin concentration monitoring is failure to assess functional coagulation or the intrinsic clotting potential of the blood. To use an extreme example, consider a patient with a homozygous deficiency of antithrombin III. Although functional measures of coagulation, such as the ACT, would clearly identify these patients by failure to achieve the desired prolongation of the ACT after heparin administration, measures of heparin concentration alone would demonstrate the expected blood heparin level but would fail to identify the lack of anticoagulant effect.

Preliminary reports have described another method for measuring heparin concentration in whole blood with electrochemical sensors. These heparin sensors use a polyvinyl chloride membrane impregnated with triiododecylmethylammonium chloride (TDMAC) to produce an electric potential in response to heparin, which correlates well with laboratory-based measures of heparin concentration.[838] The heparin sensor offers several advantages over protamine titration methods for determination of the heparin concentration. First, the heparin sensor is not dependent on clot formation, which allows determination of heparin concentrations in patients with underlying coagulopathies, as well as in blood samples containing anticoagulants in addition to heparin, such as citrate or ethylenediaminetetraacetic acid (EDTA). In addition, the heparin sensor produces a linear response over a greater heparin concentration range than current protamine titration methods do. Rather than reporting

heparin concentration discontinuously, as necessitated by protamine titration cartridges, heparin concentrations determined with ion-selective membranes are reported over a continuous range. Despite the apparent advantages of these electrochemical sensors, their accuracy may be altered by high plasma concentrations of salicylate, nitrate, iodide, or bromide.[839] The clinical usefulness of these ion-selective electrodes awaits further development of these sensors into commercially applicable forms.

Viscoelastic Measures of Coagulation

Initially developed in the 1940s, viscoelastic measures of coagulation have undergone a resurgence in popularity. The unique aspect of viscoelastic monitors lies in their ability to measure the entire spectrum of clot formation from early fibrin strand generation through clot retraction and eventual fibrinolysis. The thromboelastograph (TEG) (Haemoscope, Niles, IL), developed by Hartert in 1948,[840] uses a small 0.35-mL blood sample placed into a disposable cuvette within the instrument. The cuvette is maintained at a temperature of 37°C and continuously rotates around an axis of approximately 5 degrees. A metal piston attached by a torsion wire to an electronic recorder is lowered into the blood within the cuvette. As clot formation occurs, the piston becomes enmeshed within the clot, and rotation of the cuvette is transferred to the piston and electronic recorder.

Although variables derived from the TEG tracing do not coincide directly with laboratory-based tests of coagulation, the TEG is capable of detecting characteristic abnormalities in clot formation and fibrinolysis.[841] Various parameters that describe the characteristics of clot formation and lysis are inscribed by the TEG recorder. The R value (reaction time) measures the time to initial clot formation (normal, 7.5 to 15 minutes). It is considered to be comparable to the whole blood clotting time and may be accelerated by adding celite to the TEG sample cuvette. The R value is prolonged by a deficiency of one or more plasma coagulation factors. Maximum amplitude (MA) provides a measure of clot strength and may be decreased by either qualitative or quantitative platelet dysfunction or decreased fibrinogen concentration. Normal MA is 50 to 60 mm. The alpha angle and K (BiKoatugulierung or coagulation) values measure the rate of clot formation and may be prolonged by any factor slowing clot generation, such as plasma coagulation factor deficiency or heparin anticoagulation (Figs. 32-53 and 32-54).

The Sonoclot (Sienco, Inc., Wheat Ridge, CO) provides an alternative viscoelastic measure of coagulation. When compared with TEG, the Sonoclot immerses a rapidly vibrating probe into a 0.4-mL sample of blood. As clot formation occurs, impedance to probe movement through the blood increases and generates an altered electrical signal and characteristic clot "signature." The Sonoclot may be used to derive the ACT, as well as provide information regarding clot strength and clot lysis.[842]

Both the TEG and Sonoclot generate characteristic diagrams by translating the mechanical resistance encountered by the sensor as it moves through the clotting blood sample. Measurements derived from these diagrams

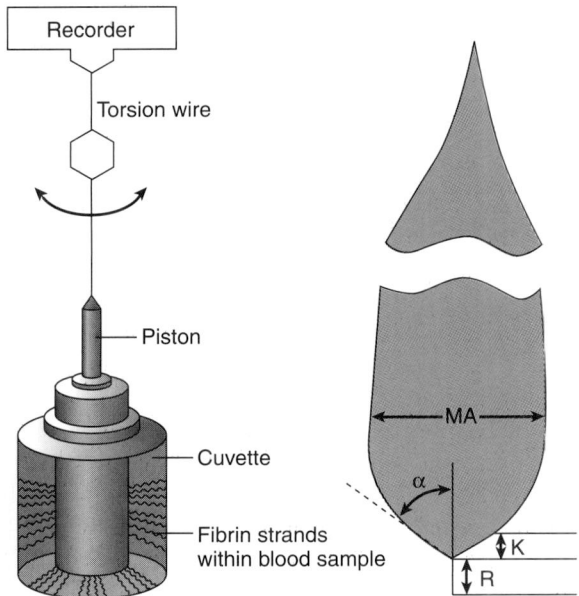

Figure 32–53 The functional components of the thromboelastograph consist of a rotating cuvette, a suspended piston attached to a torsion wire, and a recorder. As the blood sample clots, rotation of the cuvette is transferred to the torsion wire and translated by the recorder as a characteristic tracing. Quantitative parameters derived from the thromboelastograph trace are the reaction time (R), the BiKoatugulierung value or coagulation time (K), the alpha angle (α), and maximum amplitude (MA). See the text for greater detail. (Redrawn from Tuman K, Speiss B, McCarthy R, et al: Effects of progressive blood loss on coagulation as measured by thromboelastography. Anesth Analg 66:856, 1987.)

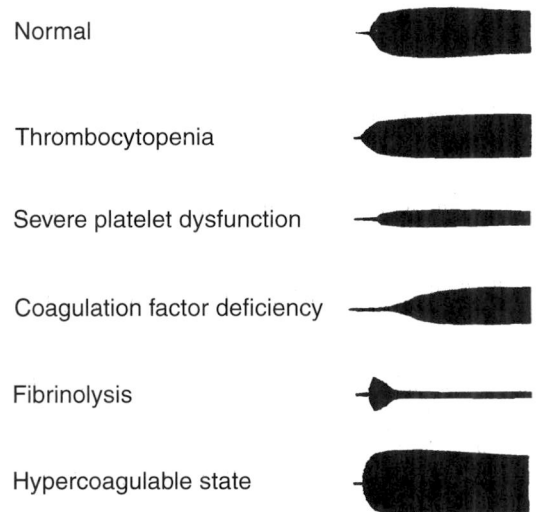

Figure 32–54 Characteristic thromboelastograph tracings.

have been related to more traditional measures of coagulation such as the ACT.[843] In addition, abnormal patterns have been associated with deficiencies in coagulation factors and functional platelet abnormalities.[844,845] One of the more common applications of the TEG analyzer is the real-time detection of excessive fibrinolysis during liver transplantation. The TEG may also be used to differentiate surgical bleeding from coagulopathy after cardiac surgery.[846,847] More widespread application of viscoelastic coagulation monitoring has been hindered by the lack of specificity associated with abnormal findings and the qualitative nature of assay interpretation. Recent computerization and automation of these instruments have improved reproducibility of the measurements and made the results more quantitative. Further modifications of viscoelastic measurement techniques, such as the addition of heparinase to TEG samples to allow monitoring during cardiopulmonary bypass, may lead to novel applications in the perioperative setting.[848]

Platelet Function Monitors

Despite tremendous advances in point-of-care monitoring of plasma coagulation, bedside assessment of platelet function has remained problematic. Although platelet function influences many point-of-care coagulation monitoring methods currently in use, these platelet-mediated effects are often nonspecific and unpredictable. The ACT is influenced only by profound platelet dysfunction,[820] and even though the TEG and Sonoclot are capable of detecting platelet abnormalities, their sensitivity and specificity are limited in terms of defining platelet dysfunction in the context of a complex perioperative coagulopathy. The standard method for identifying qualitative platelet dysfunction is laboratory-based optical aggregometry performed with specific platelet agonists in platelet-rich plasma. Unfortunately, this form of testing is technically demanding and cannot be performed at the bedside. Furthermore, alteration of platelet function by the method of sample preparation may affect the results.[849] Flow cytometry using fluorescent-labeled antibodies provides a sensitive method for quantitating platelet activation and platelet surface receptor availability. A further advantage of this form of platelet function analysis is the ability to use whole blood, thereby minimizing the potential for blood sampling and processing artifacts. However, as with platelet aggregation studies, flow cytometry requires substantial technical expertise and laboratory-based support.

Several platelet function assays specifically designed for use at the bedside have entered clinical trials. The HemoSTATUS (Medtronic Blood Systems, Parker, CO) platelet function test exploits the ability of platelet-activating factor (PAF) to accelerate clot formation of a kaolin-activated ACT. HemoSTATUS testing is performed on the Medtronic HMS coagulation analyzer by using a six-channel kaolin ACT cartridge preloaded with serially increasing concentrations of PAF. A clot ratio is determined for each individual patient assay based on the ratio of the PAF-accelerated ACT to the standard ACT. An individual patient's clot ratio is compared with a maximal clot ratio derived from normal volunteers to provide a relative measure of the patient's platelet function. In the presence of platelet dysfunction, higher concentrations of PAF are required to achieve a comparable PAF-activated ACT. When the HemoSTATUS monitor has been used after cardiac surgery, investigators demonstrated a relationship between platelet dysfunction and postoperative bleeding.[850] Furthermore, the maximal clot ratio as determined by HemoSTATUS has been demonstrated to improve after the administration of either desmopressin (DDAVP) or platelet concentrates. Other investigators, however, have failed to identify a relationship between platelet dysfunction as measured by HemoSTATUS and postoperative bleeding.[851,852]

Currently undergoing clinical trials, the Rapid Platelet Function Analyzer (RPFA; Accumetrix, San Diego, CA) is an automated turbidimetric whole blood assay of platelet function that assesses the ability of activated platelets to bind fibrinogen-coated polystyrene beads.[853] On addition of the test blood, thrombin receptor–activating peptide directly activates platelets within the sample, thereby stimulating expression of glycoprotein IIb/IIIa platelet surface receptors. As activated platelets bind and aggregate fibrinogen-coated beads, light transmission through the sample increases to generate a measurable signal. Although the RPFA is simple to operate and provides a rapid bedside measure of platelet function, a baseline reference measurement is required for each patient to calculate the extent of subsequent changes in platelet function, and the potential for application of this methodology in the perioperative setting remains unclear.

Plateletworks, a diagnostic assay of platelet aggregation, is performed with the Ichor hematology analyzer (Helena Laboratories, Beaumont, TX). The Plateletworks assay uses a hemocytometer to perform automated platelet counts on whole blood samples collected in the presence and absence of platelet-stimulating agonists such as collagen or adenosine diphosphate. The difference in platelet counts before and after addition of the agonist provides a direct measure of platelet aggregation and is reported as percent aggregation. Although applicability of the Plateletworks assay to the perioperative setting remains to be determined, preliminary investigations have demonstrated reasonable correlations between cell counts performed with the Ichor hematology analyzer and traditional laboratory-based instruments.[854] In addition, the Plateletworks assay has proved effective in identifying platelet dysfunction in the setting of glycoprotein IIb/IIIa antagonists and appears to correlate relatively well with laboratory-based measures of platelet aggregation.[855,856]

The PFA-100 (Platelet Function Analyzer; Dade International Inc, Miami) is unique among both laboratory-based and point-of-care platelet function monitors in that it incorporates high-shear conditions to simulate primary hemostasis after injury to a small vessel. Citrate-containing blood added to a disposable test cartridge is aspirated through a 200-μm capillary and then forced through a 150-mm aperture in a membrane containing collagen and either adenosine diphosphate or epinephrine.[857] Exposure of platelets within the blood sample to activating agents within the membrane under high-shear conditions stimulates platelet adherence and aggregation. As the platelet plug forms, blood flow through the aperture decreases and the time to aperture occlusion is displayed as the "closure time."

Although clinical trials with this instrument remain in progress, preliminary findings have demonstrated that the PFA-100 detects both congenital and acquired disorders of platelet function with a high degree of sensitivity and specificity.[858,859] Furthermore, the PFA-100 has proved effective as a measure of platelet function during cardiopulmonary bypass in adults, with preliminary data suggesting potential to identify postoperative coagulopathies.[846,860]

The Hemodyne Hemostasis Analyzer (Hemodyne, Richmond, VA), currently in clinical trials, specifically measures the force developed between platelets during clot formation and subsequent retraction. Using a sample of whole blood, the Hemodyne analyzer provides measures of platelet contractile force, the force produced by platelets during clot retraction, and clot elastic modulus, a measure of clot rigidity.[861] In preliminary investigations, platelet contractile force was reduced after cardiopulmonary bypass and modestly correlated with perioperative blood loss.[862]

Advances in our understanding of hemostasis and thrombosis at the molecular level have directly contributed to recent biotechnologic innovations in the assessment of perioperative hemostasis. Further advances in point-of-care coagulation monitoring offer the opportunity for clinicians to make more informed decisions about transfusion therapy and hemostatic drug administration to minimize bleeding in the perioperative setting.

KEY POINTS

1. Although a stethoscope should be present in every anesthetizing location, continuous stethoscopy is an insensitive method for early detection of untoward hemodynamic events.

2. Most automated noninvasive blood pressure measuring devices use an oscillometric measurement technique and rarely cause complications. Caution should be exercised in patients who cannot complain of arm pain, those with irregular rhythms that force repeated cuff inflation, and individuals receiving anticoagulant therapy.

3. Direct arterial pressure monitoring should be widely used in operative patients with severe cardiovascular diseases or those undergoing major surgical procedures that involve significant blood loss or fluid shifts.

4. The Allen test for palmar arch collateral arterial flow is not a reliable method to predict complications from radial artery cannulation. Despite the absence of anatomic collateral flow at the elbow, brachial artery catheterization for perioperative blood pressure monitoring is a safe alternative to radial or femoral arterial catheterization.

5. The accuracy of a directly recorded arterial pressure waveform is determined by the natural frequency and damping coefficient of the pressure monitoring system. The optimal dynamic response of the system

will be achieved when the natural frequency is high, thereby allowing accurate pressure recording across a wide range of damping coefficients.

6. Rather than the common placement at the midaxillary line, the preferred position for alignment (or "leveling") of external pressure transducers is approximately 5 cm posterior to the sternomanubrial junction. When using external transducers and fluid-filled monitoring systems, this transducer location will eliminate confounding hydrostatic pressure measurement artifacts.

7. Because of wave reflection and other physical phenomena, the arterial blood pressure recorded from peripheral sites has a wider pulse pressure than central aortic pressure does.

8. Methods to reduce mechanical complications from central venous catheters include the use of ultrasound vessel localization, venous pressure measurement before the insertion of large catheters, and radiographic confirmation that the catheter tip lies outside the pericardium and parallel to the walls of the superior vena cava.

9. Of the many complications of central venous and pulmonary artery catheters, catheter misuse and data misinterpretation are among the most common.

10. Pulmonary artery wedge pressure is a delayed and damped reflection of left atrial pressure. Wedge pressure provides a close estimate of pulmonary capillary pressure in many cases, but it may underestimate capillary pressure when postcapillary pulmonary vascular resistance is increased, as in patients with sepsis.

11. The use of central venous, pulmonary artery diastolic, or pulmonary artery wedge pressure as an estimate of left ventricular preload is subject to many confounding factors, including changes in diastolic ventricular compliance and juxtacardiac pressure.

12. Most randomized prospective clinical trials have failed to show that pulmonary artery catheter monitoring results in improved patient outcome. Reasons cited for these results include misinterpretation of catheter-derived data and failure of hemodynamic therapies that are guided by specific hemodynamic indices.

13. Systolic pressure variation, the change in systolic arterial blood pressure measured during a positive-pressure mechanical ventilation cycle, provides an accurate measure of left ventricular preload that is more reliable than central venous or pulmonary artery pressure measurements.

14. Thermodilution cardiac output monitoring, the most widely used clinical technique, is subject to thermal errors introduced by rapid intravenous fluid administration, positive-pressure mechanical ventilation, and tricuspid valve regurgitation.

15. Mixed venous hemoglobin saturation is inversely proportional to cardiac output, but is also dependent on arterial hemoglobin saturation, hemoglobin concentration, and oxygen consumption.

16. Newer methods of cardiac output monitoring, including esophageal Doppler and pulse contour analysis, allow beat-to-beat estimation of left ventricular stroke volume and measurement of other cardiovascular variables.

17. The activated coagulation time is the most widely used method for point-of-care coagulation testing and titration of intraoperative heparin therapy. Alternative coagulation tests assess blood heparin concentration, platelet function, or viscoelastic properties of the coagulation system.

REFERENCES

1. Gravenstein JS: Monitoring with our good senses. J Clin Monit Comput 14:451-453, 1998.
2. Vandam LD: The senses as monitors. *In* Blitt CD (ed): Monitoring in Anesthesia and Critical Care Medicine. New York, Churchill Livingstone, 1985, pp 5-24.
3. McIntyre JWR: Stethoscopy during anaesthesia. Can J Anaesth 44:535-342, 1997.
4. American Society of Anesthesiologists: Standards for Basic Anesthetic Monitoring, ASA Standards, Guidelines and Statements. Park Ridge, IL, American Society of Anesthesiologists, 1993, p 5.
5. Blitt CD: Precordial and esophageal stethoscopes. *In* Blitt CD (ed): Monitoring in Anesthesia and Critical Care Medicine. New York, Churchill Livingstone, 1985, pp 25-27
6. Barthram CN, Taylor L: The oesophageal and precordial stethoscope transducer as a monitoring and teaching aid. Anaesthesia 49:713-714, 1994.
7. Biro P: Electrically amplified precordial stethoscope. J Clin Monit 10:410-412, 1994.
8. Philip JH, Raemer DB: An electronic stethoscope is judged better than conventional stethoscopes for anesthesia monitoring. J Clin Monit 2:151-154, 1986.
9. Manecke GR, Poppers PJ: Esophageal stethoscope placement depth: Its effect on heart and lung sound monitoring during general anesthesia. Anesth Analg 86:1276-1279, 1998.
10. Kates RA, Zaidan JR, Kaplan JA: Esophageal lead for intraoperative electrocardiographic monitoring. Anesth Analg 61:781-785, 1982.
11. Trager MA, Feinberg BI, Kaplan JA: Right ventricular ischemia diagnosed by an esophageal electrocardiogram and right atrial pressure tracing. J Cardiothorac Anesth 1:123-125, 1987.
12. Pattison CZ, Atlee JL III, Matthews EL, et al: Atrial pacing thresholds measured in anesthetized patients with the use of an esophageal stethoscope modified for pacing. Anesthesiology 74:854-859, 1991.
13. Smith I, Monk TG, White PF: Comparison of transesophageal atrial pacing with anticholinergic drugs for the treatment of intraoperative bradycardia. Anesth Analg 78:245-252, 1994.
14. Cooper JO, Cullen BF: Observer reliability in detecting surreptitious random occlusions of the monaural esophageal stethoscope. J Clin Monit 6:271-275, 1990.
15. Prielipp RC, Kelly JS, Roy RC: Use of esophageal or precordial stethoscopes by anesthesia providers: Are we listening to our patients? J Clin Anesth 7:367-372, 1995.
16. Reitan JA, Barash PG: Noninvasive monitoring. *In* Saidman LJ, Smith NT (eds): Monitoring in Anesthesia, 2nd ed. Boston, Butterworth, 1984, pp 117-192.
17. Klepper ID, Webb RK, Van Der Walt JH, et al: The stethoscope: Applications and limitations—an analysis of 2000 incident reports. Anaesth Intensive Care 21:575-578, 1993.
18. Weinfurt PT: Electrocardiographic monitoring: An overview. J Clin Monit 6:132-138, 1990.

19. Block FE: What is heart rate, anyway? J Clin Monit 10:366-370, 1994.
20. Mark JB: Monitoring heart rate. *In* Mark JB (ed): Atlas of Cardiovascular Monitoring. New York, Churchill Livingstone, 1998, pp 205-217.
21. Murray WB, Foster PA: The peripheral pulse wave: Information overlooked. J Clin Monit 12:365-377, 1996.
22. Davis RF: Clinical comparison of automated auscultatory and oscillometric and catheter-transducer measurements of arterial pressure. J Clin Monit 1:114-119, 1985.
23. Bruner JMR, Krenis LJ, Kunsman JM, Sherman AP: Comparison of direct and indirect methods of measuring arterial blood pressure. Med Instrum 15:11-21, 97-101, 182-188, 1981.
24. Riva-Rocci S: Un nuovo sfigmomanometro. Gaz Med Torino 47:981, 1896.
25. Zanchetti A, Mancia G: The centenary of blood pressure measurement: A tribute to Scipione Riva-Rocci. J Hypertens 14:1-12, 1996.
26. Korotkoff NS: On the subject of methods of determining blood pressure. Bull Imp Med Acad St Petersburg 11:365, 1905.
27. Shevchenko YL, Tsitlik JE: 90th anniversary of the development by Nikolai S. Korotkoff of the auscultatory method of measuring blood pressure. Circulation 94:116-118, 1996.
28. Gorback MS: Considerations in the interpretation of systemic pressure monitoring. *In* Lumb PD, Bryan-Brown CW (eds): Complications in Critical Care Medicine. Chicago, Year Book, 1988, p 296.
29. Goldstein S, Killip T: Comparison of direct and indirect arterial pressures in aortic regurgitation. N Engl J Med 267:1121, 1962.
30. Cohn JN: Blood pressure measurement in shock. Mechanism of inaccuracy in auscultatory and palpatory methods. JAMA 199:972-976, 1967.
31. Messerli FH, Ventura HO, Amodeo C: Osler's maneuver and pseudohypertension. N Engl J Med 312:1548-1551, 1985.
32. Iyriboz Y, Hearon CM, Edwards K: Agreement between large and small cuffs in sphygmomanometry: A quantitative assessment. J Clin Monit 10:127-133, 1994.
33. Ramsey M: Blood pressure monitoring: Automated oscillometric devices. J Clin Monit 7:56-67, 1991.
34. Yong PG, Geddes LA: The effect of cuff pressure deflation rate on accuracy in indirect measurement of blood pressure with the auscultatory method. J Clin Monit 3:155-159, 1987.
35. von Recklinghausen H: Neue Wege zur Blutdruckmessung. Berlin, Springer-Verlag, 1931.
36. Posey JA, Geddes LA, Williams H, Moore AG: The meaning of the point of maximum oscillations in cuff pressure in the indirect measurement of blood pressure. Part 1. Cardiovasc Res Ctr Bull 8:15-25, 1969.
37. Yelderman M, Ream AK: Indirect measurement of mean blood pressure in the anesthetized patient. Anesthesiology 50:253-256, 1979.
38. Bur A, Hirschl MM, Herkner H, et al: Accuracy of oscillometric blood pressure measurement according to the relation between cuff size and upper-arm circumference in critically ill patients. Crit Care Med 28:371-376, 2000.
39. Green DW: Use of a neonatal noninvasive blood pressure module on adult patients. Anaesthesia 51:1129-1132, 1996.
40. Khan SQ, Wardlaw JM, Davenport R, et al: Use of a neonatal blood pressure cuff to monitor blood pressure in the adult finger—comparison with a standard adult arm cuff. J Clin Monit 14:233-238, 1998.
41. Lyew MA, Jamieson JW: Blood pressure measurement using oscillometric finger cuffs in children and young adults. Anaesthesia 49:895-899, 1994.
42. O'Brien E, Atkins W: Blood pressure measurement using oscillometric finger cuffs. Anaesthesia 50:743-744, 1995.
43. Kazamias TM, Gander MP, Franklin DL: Blood pressure measurement with Doppler ultrasonic flowmeter. J Appl Physiol 30:585-588, 1971.
44. Weiss BM, Pasch T: Measurement of systemic arterial pressure. Curr Opin Anaesthesiol 10:459-466, 1997.
45. Zahed B, Sadove MS, Hatano S: Comparison of automated Doppler ultrasound and Korotkoff measurements of blood pressure. Anesth Analg 50:699, 1971.
46. Borow KM, Newburger JW: Noninvasive estimation of central aortic pressure using the oscillometric method for analyzing systemic artery pulsatile blood flow: Comparative study of indirect systolic, diastolic, and mean brachial artery pressure with simultaneous direct ascending aortic pressure measurements. Am Heart J 103:879-886, 1982.
47. Van Bergen FH, Weatherhead DS, Treloar AE, et al: Comparison of indirect and direct methods of measuring arterial blood pressure. Circulation 10:481-490, 1954.
48. Nystrom E, Reid KH, Bennett R, et al: A comparison of two automated indirect arterial blood pressure meters: With recordings from a radial arterial catheter in anesthetized surgical patients. Anesthesiology 62:526-530, 1985.
49. Gravlee GP, Brockschmidt JK: Accuracy of four indirect methods of blood pressure measurement, with hemodynamic correlations. J Clin Monit 6:284-298, 1990.
50. Sutin KM, Longaker MT, Wahlander S, et al: Acute biceps compartment syndrome associated with the use of a noninvasive blood pressure monitor. Anesth Analg 83:1345-1346, 1996.
51. Gardner RM, Hollingsworth KW: Optimizing the electrocardiogram and pressure monitoring. Crit Care Med 14:651-658, 1986.
52. Bickler PE, Schapera A, Bainton CR: Acute radial nerve injury from use of an automatic blood pressure monitor. Anesthesiology 73:186-188, 1990.
53. Celoria G, Dawson JA, Teres D: Compartment syndrome in a patient monitored with an automated blood pressure cuff. J Clin Monit 3:139, 1987.
54. Alford JW, Palumbo MA, Barnum MJ: Compartment syndrome of the arm: A complication of noninvasive blood pressure monitoring during thrombolytic therapy for myocardial infarction. J Clin Monit Comput 17:163-166, 2002.
55. Penaz J: Photoelectric measurement of blood pressure, volume, and flow in the finger. Paper presented at the 10th International Conference on Medical and Biological Engineering, 1973, p 104.
56. Boehmer RD: Continuous, real-time, non-invasive monitor of blood pressure: Penaz methodology applied to the finger. J Clin Monit 3:282, 1987.
57. Hirschl MM, Binder M, Herkner H, et al: Accuracy and reliability of noninvasive continuous finger blood pressure measurement in critically ill patients. Crit Care Med 24:1684-1689, 1996.
58. Kurki T, Smith NT, Head N, et al: Noninvasive continuous blood pressure measurement from the finger: Optimal measurement conditions and factors affecting reliability. J Clin Monit 3:6-13, 1987.
59. Molhoek GP, Wesseling KH, Settels JJM: Evaluation of the Penaz servoplethysmomanometer for continuous, noninvasive measurement of finger blood pressure. Basic Res Cardiol 79:598, 1984.
60. Smith NT, Wesseling KH, de Wit B: Evaluation of two prototype devices producing noninvasive, pulsatile, calibrated blood pressure measurement from a finger. J Clin Monit 1:17-29, 1985.
61. Bos WJW, van Goudoever J, van Montfrans GA, et al: Reconstruction of brachial artery pressure from noninvasive finger pressure measurements. Circulation 94:1870-1875, 1996.
62. Gibbs NM, Larach DR, Derr JA: The accuracy of Finapress noninvasive mean arterial pressure measurements in anesthetized patients. Anesthesiology 74:647-652, 1991.
63. Bardoczky GI, Levarlet M, Engelman E, et al: Continuous noninvasive blood pressure monitoring during thoracic surgery. J Cardiothorac Vasc Anesth 6:51-54, 1992.
64. Pace NL, East TD: Simultaneous comparison of intraarterial, oscillometric, and Finapres monitoring during anesthesia. Anesth Analg 73:213-220, 1991.
65. Gravenstein JS, Paulus DA, Feldman J, McLaughlin G: Tissue hypoxia distal to a Penaz finger blood pressure cuff. J Clin Monit 1:120-125, 1985.
66. de Jong JR, Tepaske R, Scheffer G-J, et al: Noninvasive continuous blood pressure measurement: A clinical evaluation of the Cortronic APM 770. J Clin Monit 9:18-24, 1993.

67. Young CC, Mark JB, White W, et al: A clinical evaluation of continuous noninvasive blood pressure monitoring: Accuracy and tracking capabilities. J Clin Monit 11:245-252, 1995.

68. Weiss BM, Spahn DR, Rahmig H, et al: Radial artery tonometry: Moderately accurate but unpredictable technique of continuous non-invasive arterial pressure measurement. Br J Anaesth 76:405-411, 1996.

69. Kemmotsu O, Ueda M, Otsuka H, et al: Arterial tonometry for noninvasive, continuous blood pressure monitoring during anesthesia. Anesthesiology 75:333-340, 1991.

70. Kemmotsu O, Ueda M, Otsuka H, et al: Blood pressure measurement by arterial tonometry in controlled hypotension. Anesth Analg 73:54-58, 1991.

71. Kemmotsu O, Ohno M, Takita K, et al: Noninvasive, continuous blood pressure measurement by arterial tonometry during anesthesia in children. Anesthesiology 81:1162-1168, 1994.

72. Cockings JGL, Webb RK, Klepper ID, et al: Blood pressure monitoring—applications and limitations: An analysis of 2000 incident reports. Anaesth Intens Care 21:565-569, 1993.

73. Eather KF, Peterson LH, Dripps RD: Studies of the circulation of anesthetized patients by a new method for recording arterial pressure and pressure pulse contours. Anesthesiology 10:125-132, 1949.

74. Mark JB: Atlas of Cardiovascular Monitoring. New York, Churchill Livingstone, 1998.

75. Mandel MA, Dauchot PJ: Radial artery cannulation in 1000 patients. Precautions and complications. J Hand Surg 2:482-485, 1977.

76. Slogoff S, Keats AS, Arlund C: On the safety of radial artery cannulation. Anesthesiology 59:42-47, 1983.

77. Allen EV: Thromboangiitis obliterans: Methods of diagnosis of chronic obstructive lesions distal to the wrist with illustrative cases. Am J Med Sci 178:237, 1929.

78. Mangano DT, Hickey RF: Ischemic injury following uncomplicated radial artery catheterization. Anesth Analg 58:55-57, 1979.

79. Baker RJ, Chunprapaph B, Nyhus LM: Severe ischaemia of the hand following radial artery catheterization. Surgery 80:449-457, 1976.

80. Thompson SR, Hirschberg A: Allen's test re-examined. Crit Care Med 16:915, 1988.

81. Wilkins RG: Radial artery cannulation and ischaemic damage: A review. Anaesthesia 40:896-899, 1985.

82. Bedford RF, Wollman H: Complications of percutaneous radial artery cannulation: An objective prospective study in man. Anesthesiology 38:228-236, 1973.

83. Davis FM, Stewart JM: Radial artery cannulation. A prospective study in patients undergoing cardiothoracic surgery. Br J Anaesth 52:42-47, 1980.

84. Husum B, Palm T: Arterial dominance in the hand. Br J Anaesth 50:913-916, 1978.

85. McGregor AD: The Allen test—an investigation of its accuracy by fluorescein angiography. J Hand Surg [Br] 12:82-85, 1987.

86. Stead SW, Stirt JA: Assessment of digital blood flow and palmar collateral circulation. Int J Clin Monit Comput 2:29, 1985.

87. Cederholm I, Sorensen J, Carlsson C: Thrombosis following percutaneous radial artery cannulation. Acta Anaesthesiol Scand 30:227-230, 1986.

88. Jones RM, Hill AB, Nahrwold ML: The effect of method of radial artery cannulation on post-cannulation blood flow and thrombus formation. Anesthesiology 55:76, 1981.

89. Mangar D, Thrush DN, Connell GR, Downs JB: Direct or modified Seldinger guide wire–directed technique for arterial catheter insertion. Anesth Analg 76:714-717, 1993.

90. Gerber DR, Zeifman WE, Khouli HI, et al: Comparison of wire-guided and nonwire-guided radial artery catheters. Chest 109:761-764, 1996.

91. Barnes RW, Foster EJ, Jansen GA: Safety of brachial arterial catheterization as monitors in the intensive care unit—prospective evaluation with the Doppler ultrasonic velocity detector. Anesthesiology 44:260-264, 1976.

92. Moran KT, Halpin DP, Zide RS, et al: Long-term brachial artery catheterization: Ischemic complications. J Vasc Surg 8:76-78, 1988.

93. Bazaral MG, Welch M, Golding LAR, Badhwar K: Comparison of brachial and radial arterial pressure monitoring in patients undergoing coronary artery bypass surgery. Anesthesiology 73:38-45, 1990.

94. Randel SN, Tsang BH, Wung JT: Experience with percutaneous indwelling peripheral arterial catheterization in neonates. Am J Dis Child 141:848-851, 1987.

95. Brown M, Gordon LH, Brown OW: Intravascular monitoring via the axillary artery. Anaesth Intensive Care 13:38-40, 1985.

96. Gurman GM, Kriemerman S: Cannulation of big arteries in critically ill patients. Crit Care Med 13:217-220, 1985.

97. Ersoz CJ, Hedden M, Lain L: Prolonged femoral arterial catheterization for intensive care. Anesth Analg 49:160-164, 1973.

98. Russell JA, Joel M, Hudson RJ, et al: Prospective evaluation of radial and femoral artery catheterization sites in critically ill adults. Crit Care Med 11:936-939, 1983.

99. Thomas F, Burke JP, Parker J, et al: The risk of infection related to radial vs femoral sites for arterial catheterization. Crit Care Med 11:807-812, 1983.

100. Singh S, Nelson N, Acosta I, et al: Catheter colonization and bacteremia with pulmonary and arterial catheters. Crit Care Med 10:736-739, 1982.

101. Frezza EE, Mezghebe H: Indications and complications of arterial catheter use in surgical or medical intensive care units: Analysis of 4932 patients. Am Surg 64:127-131, 1998.

102. Muralidhar K: Complication of femoral arterial pressure monitoring. J Cardiothorac Vasc Anesth 12:128-129, 1998.

103. Sim EKW, Beynen FA, Danielson GK: Intraperitoneal hemorrhage following femoral artery cannulation for intraoperative monitoring: An unusual complication. J Clin Monit 9:295-296, 1993.

104. Rehfeldt KH, Sanders MS: Digital gangrene after radial artery catheterization in a patient with thrombocytosis. Anesth Analg 90:45-46, 2000.

105. Rose SH: Ischemic complications of radial artery cannulation: An association with a calcinosis, Raynaud's phenomenon, esophageal dysmotility, sclerodactyly, and telangiectasia variant of scleroderma. Anesthesiology 78:587-589, 1993.

106. Singleton RJ, Webb RK, Ludbrook GL, Fox AL: Problems associated with vascular access: An analysis of 2000 incident reports. Anaesth Intensive Care 21:664-669, 1993.

107. Coulter TD, Wiedemann HP: Complications of hemodynamic monitoring. Clin Chest Med 20:249-267, 1999.

108. Garey C, Sprung J, Thomas P: Unusual complication of arterial catheterization. Anesth Analg 76:668, 1993.

109. Horlocker TT, Bishop AT: Compartment syndrome of the forearm and hand after brachial artery cannulation. Anesth Analg 81:1092-1094, 1995.

110. Lowenstein E, Little JW, Lo HH: Prevention of cerebral embolization from flushing radial-artery cannulas. N Engl J Med 285:1414-1415, 1971.

111. Gardner RM: Direct blood pressure measurement—dynamic response requirements. Anesthesiology 54:227-236, 1981.

112. Heimann PA, Murray WB: Construction and use of catheter-manometer systems. J Clin Monit 9:45-53, 1993.

113. Shinozaki T, Deane RS, Mazuzan JE: The dynamic responses of liquid-filled catheter systems for direct measurements of blood pressure. Anesthesiology 53:498-504, 1980.

114. Kleinman B, Powell S, Kumar P, Gardner RM: The fast flush test measures the dynamic response of the entire blood pressure monitoring system. Anesthesiology 77:1215-1220, 1992.

115. Kleinman B: Understanding natural frequency and damping and how they relate to the measurement of blood pressure. J Clin Monit 5:137-147, 1989.

116. Kleinman B, Powell S, Gardner RM: Equivalence of fast flush and square wave testing of blood pressure monitoring systems. J Clin Monit 12:149-154, 1996.

117. Kleinman B, Frey K, Stevens R: The fast flush test—is the clinical comparison equivalent to its in vitro simulation? J Clin Monit Comput 14:485-489, 1998.

118. Geddes LA, Bourland JD: Technical note: Estimation of the damping coefficient of fluid-filled, catheter-transducer pressure-measuring systems. J Clin Eng 13:59-62, 1988.

119. Hipkins SF, Rutten AJ, Runciman WB: Experimental analysis of catheter-manometer systems in vitro and in vivo. Anesthesiology 71:893-906, 1989.

120. O'Quin R, Marini JJ: Pulmonary artery occlusion pressure: Clinical physiology, measurement, and interpretation. Am Rev Respir Dis 128:319-326, 1983.

121. Geddes LA: Handbook of Blood Pressure Measurement. Clifton, NJ, Humana Press, 1991.

122. Schwid HA: Frequency response evaluation of radial artery catheter-manometer systems: Sinusoidal frequency analysis versus flush method. J Clin Monit 4:181-185, 1988.

123. Woda RP, Dzwonczyk R, Buyama C, et al: On the dynamic performance of the Abbott Safeset blood-conserving arterial line system. J Clin Monit 15:215-221, 1999.

124. Wiedemann HP, Matthay MA, Matthay RA: Cardiovascular-pulmonary monitoring in the intensive care unit (Part 1). Chest 85:537-549, 1984.

125. Heeger PS, Backstrom JT: Heparin flushes and thrombocytopenia. Ann Intern Med 105:143, 1985.

126. Slaughter TF, Greenberg CS: Heparin-associated thrombocytopenia and thrombosis. Implications for perioperative management. Anesthesiology 87:667-675, 1997.

127. Promonet C, Anglade D, Menaouar A, et al: Time-dependent pressure distortion in a catheter-transducer system. Anesthesiology 92:208-218, 2000.

128. Mark JB: Technical requirements for direct blood pressure measurement. In Mark JB (ed): Atlas of Cardiovascular Monitoring. New York, Churchill Livingstone, 1998, pp 99-126.

129. Meyer RM, Kimovec MA, Hefner GG: Cable-testing device fails to indicate that hypertension is artifactual. J Clin Monit 9:54-59, 1993.

130. McDermott M, Dearlove OR: Nasogastric contents short-circuit pressure transducer. Anaesthesia 52:719, 1997.

131. Gardner RM: Accuracy and reliability of disposable pressure transducers coupled with modern pressure monitors. Crit Care Med 24:879-882, 1996.

132. Skidmore K, Chen J, Litt L: Arterial catheter pressure cable corrosion leading to artifactual diagnosis of hypotension. Anesth Analg 95:1192-1195, 2002.

133. Barbieri LT, Kaplan JA: Artifactual hypotension secondary to intraoperative transducer failure. Anesth Analg 62:112-114, 1983.

134. Courtois M, Fattal PG, Kovacs SJ, et al: Anatomically and physiologically based reference level for measurement of intracardiac pressures. Circulation 92:1994-2000, 1995.

135. O'Rourke MF, Gallagher DE: Pulse wave analysis. J Hypertens Suppl 14:S147-S157, 1996.

136. Braunwald E, Fishman AP, Cournand A: Time relationship of dynamic events in the cardiac chambers, pulmonary artery and aorta in man. Circ Res 4:100-107, 1956.

137. Schwid HA, Taylor LA, Smith NT: Computer model analysis of the radial artery pressure waveform. J Clin Monit 3:220-228, 1987.

138. Ream AK: Mean blood pressure algorithms. J Clin Monit 1:138-144, 1985.

139. O'Rourke MF, Yaginuma T: Wave reflections and the arterial pulse. Arch Intern Med 144:366-371, 1984.

140. Abrams JH, Cerra F, Holcroft JW: Cardiopulmonary monitoring. In Wilmore DW, Brennan MF, Harken AH, et al (eds): Care of the Surgical Patient. New York, Scientific American Medicine, 1989, pp 1-27.

141. Hettrick DA, Warltier DC: Ventriculoarterial coupling. In Warltier DC (ed): Ventricular Function. Baltimore, Williams & Wilkins, 1995, pp 153-180.

142. Murgo JP, Westerhof N, Giolma JP, Altobelli SA: Aortic input impedance in normal man: Relationship to pressure wave forms. Circulation 62:105-116, 1980.

143. Murgo JP, Westerhof N, Giolma JP, Altobelli SA: Manipulation of ascending aortic pressure and flow wave reflections with the Valsalva maneuver: Relationship to input impedance. Circulation 63:122-132, 1981.

144. Franklin SS, Weber MA: Measuring hypertensive cardiovascular risk: The vascular overload concept. Am Heart J 128:793-803, 1994.

145. Frank SM, Norris EJ, Christopherson R, Beattie C: Right- and left-arm blood pressure discrepancies in vascular surgery patients. Anesthesiology 75:457-463, 1991.

146. Kinzer JB, Lichtenthal PR, Wade LD: Loss of radial artery pressure trace during internal mammary artery dissection for coronary artery bypass graft surgery. Anesth Analg 64:1134-1136, 1985.

147. Mark JB: Arterial blood pressure. Direct vs. indirect measurement. In Mark JB (ed): Atlas of Cardiovascular Monitoring. New York, Churchill Livingstone, 1998, pp 81-89.

148. Dorman T, Breslow MJ, Lipsett PA, et al: Radial artery pressure monitoring underestimates central arterial pressure during vasopressor therapy in critically ill surgical patients. Crit Care Med 26:1646-1649, 1998.

149. Urzua J, Sessler DI, Meneses G, et al: Thermoregulatory vasoconstriction increases the difference between femoral and radial arterial pressures. J Clin Monit 10:229-236, 1994.

150. Chauhan S, Saxena N, Mehrotra S, et al: Femoral artery pressures are more reliable than radial artery pressures on initiation of cardiopulmonary bypass. J Cardiothorac Vasc Anesth 14:274-276, 2000.

151. Rich GF, Lubanski RE, McLoughlin TM: Differences between aortic and radial artery pressure associated with cardiopulmonary bypass. Anesthesiology 77:63-66, 1992.

152. Stern DH, Gerson JI, Allen FB, Parker FB: Can we trust the direct radial artery pressure immediately following cardiopulmonary bypass? Anesthesiology 62:557-561, 1985.

153. Mohr R, Lavee J, Goor DA: Inaccuracy of radial artery pressure measurement after cardiac operations. J Thorac Cardiovasc Surg 94:286-290, 1987.

154. Gravlee GP, Wong AB, Adkins TG, et al: A comparison of radial, brachial, and aortic pressures after cardiopulmonary bypass. J Cardiothorac Anesth 3:20-26, 1989.

155. Pauca AL, Hudspeth AS, Wallenhaupt SL, et al: Radial artery–to-aorta pressure difference after discontinuation of cardiopulmonary bypass. Anesthesiology 70:935-941, 1989.

156. Urzua J: Aortic-to–radial arterial pressure gradient after bypass. Anesthesiology 73:191, 1990.

157. Maruyama K, Horiguchi R, Hashimoto H, et al: Effect of combined infusion of nitroglycerin and nicardipine on femoral-to-radial arterial pressure gradient after cardiopulmonary bypass. Anesth Analg 70:428-432, 1990.

158. Hynson JM, Katz JA, Mangano DT: On the accuracy of intra-arterial pressure measurement: The pressure gradient effect. Crit Care Med 26:1623-1624, 1998.

159. Urzua J, Nunez G, Lema G, et al: Hemodilution does not alter the aortic-to-femoral arterial pressure difference in dogs. J Clin Monit Comput 15:429-433, 1999.

160. Baba T, Goto T, Yoshitake A, Shibata Y: Radial artery diameter decreases with increased femoral to radial arterial pressure gradient during cardiopulmonary bypass. Anesth Analg 85:252-258, 1997.

161. Kanazawa M, Fukuyama H, Kinefuchi Y, et al: Relationship between aortic-to–radial arterial pressure gradient after cardiopulmonary bypass and changes in arterial elasticity. Anesthesiology 99:48-53, 2003.

162. Braunwald E: The physical examination. In Braunwald E (ed): Heart Disease. A Textbook of Cardiovascular Medicine, 4th ed. Philadelphia, WB Saunders, 1992, pp 13-42.

163. Wynne J, Braunwald E: The cardiomyopathies and myocarditides: Toxic, chemical, and physical damage to the heart. In Braunwald E (ed): Heart Disease. A Textbook of Cardiovascular Medicine, 4th ed. Philadelphia, WB Saunders, 1992, pp 1398-1450

164. Freeman AB, Steinbrook RA: Recurrence of pulsus alternans after fentanyl injection in a patient with aortic stenosis and congestive heart failure. Can Anaesth Soc J 32:654-657, 1985.

165. McGregor M: Pulsus paradoxus. N Engl J Med 301:480-482, 1979.

166. Shabetai R, Fowler NO, Guntheroth WG: The hemodynamics of cardiac tamponade and constrictive pericarditis. Am J Cardiol 26:480-489, 1970.

167. Mark JB: Pericardial constriction and cardiac tamponade. *In* Mark JB (ed): Atlas of Cardiovascular Monitoring. New York, Churchill Livingstone, 1998, pp 313-326.

168. Mark JB: Intraaortic balloon counterpulsation. *In* Mark JB (ed): Atlas of Cardiovascular Monitoring. New York, Churchill Livingstone, 1998, pp 343-355.

169. Mark JB: Hemodynamic observations during cardiopulmonary bypass. *In* Mark JB (ed): Atlas of Cardiovascular Monitoring. New York, Churchill Livingstone, 1998, pp 327-341.

170. Dresser LP, McKiney WM: Anatomic and pathophysiologic studies of the human internal jugular valve. Am J Surg 154:220-224, 1987.

171. Imai M, Hanaoka Y, Kemmotsu O: Valve injury: A new complication of internal jugular vein cannulation. Anesth Analg 78:1041-1046, 1994.

172. Sum-Ping ST: Internal jugular valves: Competent or incompetent. Anesth Analg 78:1039-1040, 1994.

173. Fisher J, Vaghaiwalla F, Tsitlik J, et al: Determinants and clinical significance of jugular venous valve competence. Circulation 65:188-196, 1982.

174. McGee SR: Physical examination of venous pressure: A critical review. Am Heart J 136:10-18, 1998.

175. Cook DJ: Clinical assessment of central venous pressure in the critically ill. Am J Med Sci 299:175-178, 1990.

176. Cook DJ, Simel DL: Does this patient have abnormal central venous pressure? JAMA 275:630-634, 1996.

177. Lunn JK, Stanley TH, Webster LR, Bidwai AV: Arterial blood-pressure and pulse-rate responses to pulmonary and radial arterial catheterization prior to cardiac and major vascular operations. Anesthesiology 51:265-269, 1979.

178. Dzelzkalns R, Stanley TH: Placement of the pulmonary arterial catheter before anesthesia for cardiac surgery: A stressful, painful, unnecessary crutch. J Clin Monit 1:197-200, 1985.

179. Streisand JB, Clark NJ, Pace NL: Placement of the pulmonary arterial catheter before anesthesia for cardiac surgery: Safe, intelligent, and appropriate use of invasive hemodynamic monitoring. J Clin Monit 1:193-196, 1985.

180. Waller JL, Zaidan JR, Kaplan JA, Bauman DI: Hemodynamic responses to preoperative vascular cannulation in patients with coronary artery disease. Anesthesiology 56:219-221, 1982.

181. Daily PO, Griepp RB, Shumway NE: Percutaneous internal jugular vein cannulation. Arch Surg 101:534-536, 1970.

182. Sulek CA, Gravenstein N, Blackshear RH, Weiss L: Head rotation during internal jugular vein cannulation and the risk of carotid artery puncture. Anesth Analg 82:125-128, 1996.

183. O'Grady NP, Alexander M, Dellinger EP, et al: Guidelines for prevention of intravascular catheter–related infections. MMWR Morb Mortal Wkly Rep 51:1-29, 2002.

184. American Society of Anesthesiologists: Recommendations for Infection Control for the Practice of Anesthesiology, 2nd ed. Park Ridge, IL, American Society of Anesthesiologists, 1998, pp 15-19.

185. Prielipp RC, Sherertz RJ: Skin: The first battlefield. Anesth Analg 97:933-935, 2003.

186. Chaiyakunapruk N, Veenstra DL, Lipsky BA, Saint S: Chlorhexidine compared with povidone-iodine solution for vascular catheter-site care: A meta-analysis. Ann Intern Med 136:792-801, 2002.

187. Civetta JM, Gabel JC, Gemer M: Internal-jugular-vein puncture with a margin of safety. Anesthesiology 36:622-623, 1972.

188. Ellison N, Jobes DR, Troianos CA: Internal jugular vein cannulation. Anesth Analg 78:198, 1994.

189. Mangar D, Turnage WS, Mohamed SA: Is the internal jugular vein cannulated during insertion or withdrawal of the needle during central venous cannulation. Anesth Analg 76:1375, 1993.

190. Royster RL, Johnston WE, Gravelee GP: Arrhythmias during venous cannulation prior to pulmonary artery catheter insertion. Anesth Analg 64:1214-1216, 1985.

191. Maki DG, Cobb L, Garman JK, et al: An attachable silver-impregnated cuff for prevention of infection with central venous catheters: A prospective randomized multicenter trial. Am J Med 85:307-314, 1988.

192. Caruso LJ, Gravenstein N, Layon AJ, et al: A better landmark for positioning a central venous catheter. J Clin Monit Comput 17:331-334, 2002.

193. Kapadia CB, Heard SO, Yeston NS: Delayed recognition of vascular complications caused by central venous catheters. J Clin Monit 4:267-271, 1988.

194. Albrecht K, Nave J, Breitmeier D, et al: Applied anatomy of the superior vena cava—the carina as a landmark to guide central venous catheter placement. Br J Anaesth 92:75-77, 2004.

195. English IC, Frew RM, Pigott JF, Zaki M: Percutaneous catheterisation of the internal jugular vein 1969 [classical article]. Anaesthesia 50:1071-1076, 1995.

196. Jernigan WR, Gardner WC, Mahr MM, Milburn JL: The internal jugular vein for access to the central venous system. JAMA 218:97-98, 1971.

197. Sanford TJ: Internal jugular vein cannulation versus subclavian vein cannulation. An anesthesiologist's view: The right internal jugular vein. J Clin Monit 1:58-61, 1985.

198. Goldfarb G, Lebrec D: Percutaneous cannulation of the internal jugular vein in patients with coagulopathies: An experience based on 1,000 attempts. Anesthesiology 56:321-323, 1982.

199. Oliver WC Jr, Nuttall GA, Beynen FM, et al: The incidence of artery puncture with central venous cannulation using a modified technique for detection and prevention of arterial cannulation. J Cardiothorac Vasc Anesth 11:851-855, 1997.

200. Rosen M, Latto IP, Shang W: The internal jugular vein. *In* Handbook of Percutaneous Vein Catheterizations. London, WB Saunders, 1981.

201. Metz S, Horrow JC, Balcar I: A controlled comparison of techniques for locating the internal jugular vein using ultrasonography. Anesth Analg 63:673-679, 1984.

202. Willeford KL, Reitan JA: Neutral head position for placement of internal jugular vein catheters. Anaesthesia 49:202-204, 1994.

203. Jobes DR, Schwartz AJ, Greenhow DE, et al: Safer jugular vein cannulation: Recognition of arterial puncture and preferential use of the external jugular route. Anesthesiology 59:353-355, 1983.

204. Fabian JA, Jesudian MC: A simple method of improving the safety of percutaneous cannulation of the internal jugular vein. Anesth Analg 64:1032-1033, 1985.

205. Alexander R: Using continuous pressure monitoring to aid central vein cannulation. Can J Anaesth 44:99-100, 1997.

206. Seldinger SI: Catheter replacement of the needle in percutaneous arteriography. Acta Radiol 39:368, 1953.

207. Conahan TJI, Schwartz AJ, Geer RT: Percutaneous catheter introduction: The Seldinger technique. JAMA 237:446-447, 1977.

208. Oishi AJ, Zietlow SP, Sarr MG: Erroneous arterial placement of a central venous catheter. Mayo Clin Proc 69:287-288, 1994.

209. Gravenstein N, Blackshear RH: In vitro evaluation of relative perforating potential of central venous catheters: Comparison of materials, selected models, number of lumens, and angles of incidence to simulated membrane. J Clin Monit 7:1-6, 1991.

210. Fisher KL, Leung AN: Radiographic appearance of central venous catheters. AJR Am J Roentgenol 166:329-337, 1996.

211. Reeves ST, Roy RC, Dorman BH, et al: The incidence of complications after the double-catheter technique for cannulation of the right internal jugular vein in a university teaching hospital. Anesth Analg 81:1073-1076, 1995.

212. Reeves ST, Baliga P, Conroy JM, Cleaver TL: Avulsion of the right facial vein during double cannulation of the internal jugular vein. J Cardiothorac Vasc Anesth 9:429-430, 1995.

213. Inoue S, Ohnishi Y, Kuro M: Accidental penetration of an indwelling retrograde introducer sheath by an introducer needle during right internal jugular vein cannulation. J Cardiothorac Vasc Anesth 12:67-68, 1998.

214. Peres PW: Positioning central venous catheters—a prospective study. Anaesth Intensive Care 18:536-539, 1990.

215. Denys BG, Uretsky BF, Reddy PS, et al: An ultrasound method for safe and rapid central venous access. N Engl J Med 324:566-567, 1991.

216. Denys BG, Uretsky BF, Reddy PS: Ultrasound-assisted cannulation of the internal jugular vein: A prospective comparison to the external Landmark-guided technique. Circulation 87:1557-1562, 1993.

217. Gratz I, Afshar M, Kidwell P, et al: Doppler-guided cannulation of the internal jugular vein: A prospective, randomized trial. J Clin Monit 10:185-188, 1994.

218. Troianos CA, Jobes DR, Ellison N: Ultrasound-guided cannulation of the internal jugular vein. A prospective, randomized study. Anesth Analg 72:823-826, 1991.

219. Gualtieri E, Deppe S, Sipperly ME, Thompson DR: Subclavian venous catheterization: Greater success rate for less experienced operators using ultrasound guidance. Crit Care Med 23:692-697, 1995.

220. Lane P, Waldron RJ: Real-time ultrasound-guided central venous access via the subclavian approach. Anaesth Intensive Care 23:728-730, 1995.

221. Lefrant J-Y, Cuvillon P, Benezet J-F, et al: Pulsed Doppler ultrasonography guidance for catheterization of the subclavian vein. Anesthesiology 88:1195-1201, 1998.

222. Mansfield PF, Hohn DC, Fornage BD, et al: Complications and failures of subclavian-vein catheterization. N Engl J Med 331:1735-1738, 1994.

223. Sato S, Ueno E, Toyooka H: Central venous access via the distal femoral vein using ultrasound guidance. Anesthesiology 88:838-839, 1998.

224. Andropoulos DB, Stayer SA, Bent ST, et al: A controlled study of transesophageal echocardiography to guide central venous catheter placement in congenital heart surgery patients. Anesth Analg 89:65-70, 1999.

225. Randolph AG, Cook DJ, Gonzales CA, Pribble CG: Ultrasound guidance for placement of central venous catheters: A meta-analysis of the literature. Crit Care Med 24:2053-2058, 1996.

226. Rothschild JM: Ultrasound guidance of central vein catheterization. Evidence Report/Technology Assessment, N. 43. Making Health Care Safer. A Critical Analysis of Patient Safety Practices. Agency for Healthcare Research and Quality 2001, pp 245-253.

227. Denys BG, Uretsky BF: Anatomical variations of internal jugular vein location: Impact on central venous access. Crit Care Med 19:1516-1519, 1991.

228. Troianos CA, Kuwik RJ, Pasqual JR, et al: Internal jugular vein and carotid artery anatomic relation as determined by ultrasonography. Anesthesiology 85:43-48, 1996.

229. Khalil KG, Parker FB, Mukherjee N, Webb WR: Thoracic duct injury. A complication of jugular vein catheterization. JAMA 221:908-909, 1972.

230. Lobato EB, Myers JA, Sulek CA, Blas ML: A randomized study of right versus left internal jugular venous cannulation in adults. Anesthesiology 89:A1189, 1998.

231. Haire WD, Lieberman RP: Defining the risks of subclavian-vein catheterization. N Engl J Med 331:1769-1770, 1994.

232. Hoyt DB: Internal jugular vein cannulation versus subclavian vein cannulation. A surgeon's view: The subclavian vein. J Clin Monit 1:61-63, 1985.

233. Merrer J, De Jonghe B, Golliot R, et al: Complications of femoral and subclavian venous catheterization in critically ill patients. A randomized controlled trial. JAMA 286:700-707, 2001.

234. McGee DC, Gould MK: Preventing complications of central venous catheterization. N Engl J Med 348:1123-1133, 2003.

235. Blitt CD, Wright WA, Petty WC, Webster TA: Central venous catheterization via the external jugular vein: A technique employing the J-wire. JAMA 229:817-818, 1974.

236. Blitt CD, Carlson GL, Wright WA: J-wire versus straight wire for central venous system cannulation via the external jugular vein. Anesth Analg 61:536-537, 1982.

237. Schwartz AJ, Jobes DR, Levy WJ, et al: Intrathoracic vascular catheterization via the external jugular vein. Anesthesiology 56:400-402, 1982.

238. Joynt GM, Comersall CD, Buckley TA, et al: Comparison of intrathoracic and intra-abdominal measurements of central venous pressure. Lancet 347:1155-1157, 1996.

239. Ho KM, Joynt GM, Tan P: A comparison of central venous pressure and common iliac venous pressure in critically ill mechanically ventilated patients. Crit Care Med 26:461-464, 1998.

240. Andel H, Koller R, Andel D, et al: Central venous approach via vena axillaris in critically burned patients. Anesthesiology 89:B26, 1998.

241. Amar D, Melendez JA, Zhang H, et al: Correlation of peripheral venous pressure and central venous pressure in surgical patients. J Cardiothorac Vasc Anesth 15:40-43, 2001.

242. Philip JH, Philip BK: Hydrostatic and central venous pressure measurement by the IVAC 560 Infusion Pump. Med Instrum 19:232-235, 1985.

243. Ng PK, Ault MJ, Ellrodt AG, Maldonado L: Peripherally inserted central catheters in general medicine. Mayo Clin Proc 72:225-233, 1997.

244. Kellner GA, Smart JF: Percutaneous placement of catheters to monitor "central venous pressure." Anesthesiology 36:515-516, 1972.

245. Nichols PKT, Major E: Central venous cannulation. Curr Anaesth Crit Care 1:54-60, 1989.

246. Webre DR, Arens JF: Use of cephalic and basilic veins for introduction of central venous catheters. Anesthesiology 38:389-392, 1973.

247. Kuiper DH: Cardiac tamponade and death in a patient receiving total parenteral nutrition. JAMA 230:877, 1974.

248. Kasten GW, Owens E, Kennedy D: Ventricular tachycardia resulting from central venous catheter tip migration due to arm position changes: Report of two cases. Anesthesiology 62:185-187, 1985.

249. Shah KB, Rao TLK, Laughlin S, El-Etr AA: A review of pulmonary artery catheterization in 6,245 patients. Anesthesiology 61:271-275, 1984.

250. Heath KJ, Woulfe J, Lownie S, et al: A devastating complication of inadvertent carotid artery puncture. Anesthesiology 89:1273-1275, 1998.

251. Brown CQ: Inadvertent prolonged cannulation of the carotid artery. Anesth Analg 61:150-152, 1982.

252. Beilin Y, Bronheim D, Mandelbaum C: Hemothorax and subclavian artery laceration during "J" wire change of a right internal jugular vein catheter. Anesthesiology 88:1399-1400, 1998.

253. Bernard RW, Stahl WM: Mediastinal hematoma: Complication of subclavian vein catheterization. N Y State J Med 74:83-86, 1974.

254. Naguib M, Farag H, Joshi RN: Bilateral hydrothorax and hydromediastinum after a subclavian line insertion. Can Anaesth Soc J 32:412-414, 1985.

255. Rudge CJ, Bewick M, McColl I: Hydrothorax after central venous catheterization. BMJ 3:23-25, 1973.

256. Fangio P, Mourgeon E, Romelaer A, et al: Aortic injury and cardiac tamponade as a complication of subclavian venous catheterization. Anesthesiology 96:1520-1522, 2002.

257. Ezri T, Szmuk P, Cohen Y, et al: Carotid artery–internal jugular vein fistula: A complication of internal jugular vein catheterization. J Cardiothorac Vasc Anesth 15:231-232, 2001.

258. Brennan MF, Sugarbaker PH, Moore FD: Venobronchial fistula: A rare complication of central venous catheterization for parenteral hyperalimentation. Arch Surg 106:871-872, 1973.

259. Caron NR, Demmy TL, Curtis JJ: Bronchial erosion by an indwelling central venous catheter. Chest 106:1917-1918, 1994.

260. Danenberg HD, Hasin Y, Milgalter E, et al: Aorto-atrial fistula following internal jugular vein catheterization. Eur Heart J 16:279-281, 1995.

261. Collier PE, Ryan JJ, Diamond DL: Cardiac tamponade from central venous catheters. Report of a case and review of the English literature. Angiology 35:595-600, 1984.

262. Maschke SP, Rogove HJ: Cardiac tamponade associated with a multilumen central venous catheter. Crit Care Med 12:611-613, 1984.

263. Bowdle TA: Central line complications from the ASA Closed Claims Project. Am Soc Anesthesiol Newsl 60:22-26, 1996.

264. Mitchell MR, Wood DG, Naraghi M, Riopelle JM: Fatal cardiac perforation caused by the dilator of a central venous catheterization kit. J Clin Monit 9:288-292, 1993.

265. Bowdle TA: Central line complications from the ASA Closed Claims Project: An update. Am Soc Anesthesiol Newsl 66:11-25, 2002.

266. Tocino IM, Watanabe A: Impending catheter perforation of superior vena cava: Radiographic recognition. AJR Am J Roentgenol 146:487-490, 1986.

267. Bone DK, Maddrey WC, Eagan J, Cameron JL: Cardiac tamponade: A fatal complication of central venous catheterization. Arch Surg 106:868-870, 1973.

268. Eissa NT, Kvetan V: Guide wire as a cause of complete heart block in patients with preexisting left bundle branch block. Anesthesiology 73:772-774, 1990.

269. Oakes DD, Wilson RE: Malposition of a subclavian line. Resultant pleural effusions, interstitial pulmonary edema, and chest wall abscess during total parenteral nutrition. JAMA 233:532-533, 1975.

270. Klipper WS, Waite HD, Tomlinson CO: Endotracheal cuff perforation complicating subclavian venipuncture. JAMA 228:693, 1974.

271. Drachler DH, Koepke GH, Weg JG: Phrenic nerve injury from subclavian vein catheterization. JAMA 236:2880-2882, 1976.

272. Butsch JL, Butsch WL, Da Rosa JFT: Bilateral vocal cord paralysis. Arch Surg 111:828, 1976.

273. Burton AW, Controy BP, Sims S, et al: Complex regional pain syndrome type II as a complication of subclavian catheter insertion. Anesthesiology 89:804, 1998.

274. Qureshi GD, Lilly EL: Complications of CVP catheter insertion in cubital vein. JAMA 209:1906, 1969.

275. Reynen K: 14-year follow-up of central embolization by a guide wire. N Engl J Med 329:970-971, 1993.

276. Grace DM: Air embolism with neurologic complications: A potential hazard of central venous catheters. Can J Surg 20:51-53, 1977.

277. Levinsky WJ: Fatal air embolism during insertion of CVP monitoring apparatus. JAMA 209:1721-1722, 1969.

278. Tahir AH: Prevention of air embolism during subclavian venipuncture. JAMA 223:79-80, 1973.

279. Cohen MB, Mark JB, Morris RW, Frank E: Introducer sheath malfunction producing insidious air embolism. Anesthesiology 67:573-575, 1987.

280. Darouiche RO, Raad II, Heard SO, et al: A comparison of two antimicrobial-impregnated central venous catheters. N Engl J Med 340:1-348, 1999.

281. Wenzel RP, Edmond MB: The evolving technology of venous access. N Engl J Med 340:48-50, 1999.

282. Corona ML, Peters SG, Narr BJ, Thompson RL: Infections related to central venous catheters. Mayo Clin Proc 65:979-986, 1990.

283. Tebbs SE, Sawyer A, Elliott TS: Influence of surface morphology on in vitro bacterial adherence to central venous catheters. Br J Anaesth 72:587-591, 1994.

284. Cyna AM, Hovenden JL, Lehmann A, et al: Routine replacement of central venous catheters: Telephone survey of intensive care units in mainland Britain. BMJ 316:1944-1945, 1998.

285. Badley AD, Steckelberg JM, Wollan PC, Thompson RL: Infectious rates of central venous pressure catheters: Comparison between newly placed catheters and those that have been changed. Mayo Clin Proc 71:838-846, 1996.

286. Cook D, Randolph A, Kernerman P, et al: Central venous catheter replacement strategies: A systematic review of the literature. Crit Care Med 25:1417-1424, 1997.

287. Gilron I, Magder S: Monitoring complication due to a pulsatile femoral vein from tricuspid regurgitation. Can J Anaesth 42:141-143, 1995.

288. Oropello JM, Leibowitz AB, Manasia A, et al: Dilator-associated complications of central vein catheter insertion: Possible mechanisms of injury and suggestions for prevention. J Cardiothorac Vasc Anesth 10:634-637, 1996.

289. Kessler LG: FDA alert: Hypersensitivity reactions to central venous catheters. Am Soc Anesthesiol Newsl 62:24-25, 1998.

290. Terazawa E, Shimonaka H, Nagase K, et al: Severe anaphylactic reaction due to a chlorhexidine-impregnated central venous catheter. Anesthesiology 89:1296-1298, 1998.

291. Pomfret EA, Blackburn GL: Central venous access risk factors. Crit Care Med 22:196, 1994.

292. Nishimura RA, Housmans PR, Hatle LK, Tajik AJ: Assessment of diastolic function of the heart: Background and current applications of Doppler echocardiography. Part I. Physiologic and pathophysiologic features. Mayo Clin Proc 64:71-81, 1989.

293. Pagel PS, Grossman W, Haering JM, Warltier DC: Left ventricular diastolic function in the normal and diseased heart. Perspectives for the anesthesiologist (first of two parts). Anesthesiology 79:836-854, 1993.

294. Mark JB: Pressure-volume relations, transmural pressure, and preload. In Mark JB (ed): Atlas of Cardiovascular Monitoring. New York, Churchill Livingstone, 1998, pp 247-259.

295. Dwyer EM: Left ventricular pressure-volume alterations and regional disorders of contraction during myocardial ischemia induced by atrial pacing. Circulation 42:1111-1122, 1970.

296. Alderman EL, Glantz SA: Acute hemodynamic interventions shift the diastolic pressure-volume curve in man. Circulation 54:662-671, 1976.

297. Grossman W, McLaurin LP: Diastolic properties of the left ventricle. Ann Intern Med 84:316-326, 1976.

298. Gaasch WH, Levine HJ, Quinones MA, Alexander JK: Left ventricular compliance: Mechanisms and clinical implications. Am J Cardiol 38:645-653, 1976.

299. Brutsaert DL, Sys SU: Relaxation and diastole of the heart. Physiol Rev 69:1228-1315, 1989.

300. Labovitz AJ, Pearson AC: Evaluation of left ventricular diastolic function: Clinical relevance and recent Doppler echocardiographic insights. Am Heart J 114:836-851, 1987.

301. Pagel PS, Grossman W, Haering JM, Warltier DC: Left ventricular diastolic function in the normal and diseased heart. Perspectives for the anesthesiologist (second of two parts). Anesthesiology 79:1104-1120, 1993.

302. Shah PM, Pai RG: Diastolic heart failure. Curr Probl Cardiol 17:781-868, 1992.

303. Mark JB: Respiratory-circulatory interactions. In Mark JB (ed): Atlas of Cardiovascular Monitoring. New York, Churchill Livingstone, 1998, pp 261-285.

304. Kelman GR: Interpretation of CVP measurements. Anaesthesia 26:209-215, 1971.

305. Cohn JN: Central venous pressure as a guide to volume expansion. Ann Intern Med 66:1283-1287, 1967.

306. Mark JB: Getting the most from your central venous pressure catheter. In Barash PG (ed): ASA Refresher Courses in Anesthesiology. Philadelphia, Lippincott-Raven, 1995, pp 157-175.

307. Mark JB: Central venous pressure monitoring: Clinical insights beyond the numbers. J Cardiothorac Vasc Anesth 5:163-173, 1991.

308. Mark JB: Central venous pressure, left atrial pressure. In Mark JB (ed): Atlas of Cardiovascular Monitoring. New York, Churchill Livingstone, 1998, pp 15-25.

309. O'Rourke RA, Silverman ME, Schlant RC: General examination of the patient. In Schlant RC, Alexander RW (eds): The Heart Arteries and Veins. New York, McGraw-Hill, 1994, pp 238-241.

310. Mackay IFS, Walker RL: An experimental examination of factors responsible for the 'h' (d") wave of the jugular phlebogram in human beings. Am Heart J 71:228-239, 1966.

311. Mark JB: Arrhythmias. An integrated ECG and hemodynamic approach. In Mark JB (ed): Atlas of Cardiovascular Monitoring. New York, Churchill Livingstone, 1998, pp 219-245.

312. Mark JB: Patterns of valvular heart disease. In Mark JB (ed): Atlas of Cardiovascular Monitoring. New York, Churchill Livingstone, 1998, pp 287-312.

313. Swan HJC, Ganz W, Forrester J, et al: Catheterization of the heart in man with use of a flow-directed balloon-tipped catheter. N Engl J Med 283:447-451, 1970.

314. Crexells C, Chatterjee K, Forrester JS, et al: Optimal level of filling pressure in the left side of the heart in acute myocardial infarction. N Engl J Med 289:1263-1266, 1973.

315. Forrester JS, Diamond G, McHugh TJ, Swan HJC: Filling pressures in the right and left sides of the heart in acute myocardial infarction. A reappraisal of central-venous-pressure monitoring. N Engl J Med 235:190-193, 1971.

316. Forrester JS, Diamond G, Chatterjee K, Swan HJC: Medical therapy of acute myocardial infarction by application of hemodynamic subsets (first of two parts). N Engl J Med 295:1356-1362, 1976.

317. Forrester JS, Diamond G, Chatterjee K, Swan HJC: Medical therapy of acute myocardial infarction by application of hemodynamic subsets (second of two parts). N Engl J Med 295:1404-1413, 1976.

318. Roizen MF, Berger DL, Gabel RA, et al: Practice guidelines for pulmonary artery catheterization. An updated report by the American Society of Anesthesiologists Task Force on Pulmonary Artery Catheterization. Anesthesiology 99:988-1014, 2003.

319. Connors AF, McCaffree DR, Gray BA: Evaluation of right-heart catheterization in the critically ill patient without acute myocardial infarction. N Engl J Med 308:263-279, 1983.

320. Eisenberg PR, Jaffe AS, Schuster DP: Clinical evaluation compared to pulmonary artery catheterization in the hemodynamic assessment of critically ill patients. Crit Care Med 12:549-553, 1984.

321. Bernard GR, Sopko G, Cerra F, et al: Pulmonary artery catheterization and clinical outcomes. National Heart, Lung, and Blood Institute and Food and Drug Administration Workshop Project. JAMA 283:2568-2572, 2000.

322. Connors AF, Speroff T, Dawson NV, et al: The effectiveness of right heart catheterization in the initial care of critically ill patients. JAMA 276:889-897, 1996.

323. Polanczyk CA, Rohde LE, Goldman L, et al: Right heart catheterization and cardiac complications in patients undergoing noncardiac surgery. JAMA 286:309-314, 2001.

324. Sandham JD, Hull RD, Brant RF, et al: A randomized, controlled trial of the use of pulmonary-artery catheters in high-risk surgical patients. N Engl J Med 348:5-14, 2003.

325. Tuman KJ, Roizen MF: Outcome assessment and pulmonary artery catheterization: Why does the debate continue? Anesth Analg 84:1-4, 1997.

326. Erb J, Ramsay JG: Is your pulmonary artery catheter shedding? Anesthesiology 89:543, 1998.

327. Mark JB, Spillane R: Interluminal communication in a pulmonary artery catheter causing artifactual pressure measurement. Anesth Analg 78:1184-1186, 1994.

328. Baraka A, Nawfal M, Dahdah S: Difficult pulmonary artery catheterization in the patient with tricuspid regurgitation. Anesthesiology 74:393, 1991.

329. Swan HJC, Ganz W: Guidelines for use of balloon-tipped catheter. Am J Cardiol 34:119-120, 1974.

330. Donahue PJ, Satwicz PR: A method for ensuring proper function of multiorifice catheters. Anesthesiology 76:148-149, 1992.

331. Mark JB: Pulmonary artery pressure. In Mark JB (ed): Atlas of Cardiovascular Monitoring. New York, Churchill Livingstone, 1998, pp 27-37.

332. Johnston WE, Royster RL, Choplin RH: Pulmonary artery catheter migration during cardiac surgery. Anesthesiology 64:258, 1986.

333. Heard SO, Davis R, Sheretz RJ: Influence of sterile protective sleeves on the sterility of pulmonary artery catheters. Crit Care Med 15:499, 1987.

334. Bennett D, Boldt J, Brochard L, et al: Expert panel: The use of the pulmonary artery catheter. Intensive Care Med 17:I-VIII, 1991.

335. Noel TA: Pulmonary artery catheter sheath malfunction with sternotomy. Anesthesiology 61:633-634, 1984.

336. Bromley JL, Moorthy SS: Acute angulation of a pulmonary artery catheter. Anesthesiology 59:367-368, 1983.

337. Campbell FW, Schwartz AJ: Pulmonary artery catheter malfunction? Anesthesiology 60:513-514, 1984.

338. Azocar RJ, Narang P, Talmor D, et al: Persistent left superior vena cava identified after cannulation of the right subclavian vein. Anesth Analg 95:305-307, 2002.

339. Dhar P, Kaufman B, Doerfler M, Dadic P: Unusual course of a pulmonary artery catheter. J Cardiothorac Vasc Anesth 12:487-489, 1998.

340. Hanson EW, Hannan RL, Baum VC: Pulmonary artery catheter in the coronary sinus: Implications of a persistent left superior vena cava for retrograde cardioplegia. J Cardiothorac Vasc Anesth 12:448-449, 1998.

341. Hara Y Ota K, Fujita M, Suzuki H: Absence of right superior vena cava that was not detected by insertion of a pulmonary arterial catheter via the right internal jugular vein. J Clin Monit 10:210-212, 1994.

342. Schelling G, Briegel J, Eichinger K, et al: Pulmonary artery catheter placement and temporary cardiac pacing in a patient with a persistent left superior vena cava. Intensive Care Med 17:507-508, 1991.

343. Sweitzer BJ, Hoffman WJ, Allyn JW, Daggett WJ: Diagnosis of a left-sided superior vena cava during placement of a pulmonary artery catheter. J Clin Anesth 5:500-504, 1993.

344. Keusch DJ, Winters S, Thys DM: The patient's position influences the incidence of dysrhythmias during pulmonary artery catheterization. Anesthesiology 70:582-584, 1989.

345. Benumof JL, Saidman LJ, Arkin DB, Diamant M: Where pulmonary arterial catheters go: Intrathoracic distribution. Anesthesiology 46:336-338, 1977.

346. Kronberg GM, Quan SF, Schlobohm RM, et al: Anatomic locations of the tips of pulmonary-artery catheters in supine patients. Anesthesiology 51:467-469, 1979.

347. Parlow JL, Milne B, Cervenko FW: Balloon flotation is more important than flow direction in determining the position of flow-directed pulmonary artery catheters. J Cardiothorac Vasc Anesth 6:20-23, 1992.

348. Kelso LA: Complications associated with pulmonary artery catheterization. New Horizons 5:259-263, 1997.

349. Weil MH: The assault on the Swan-Ganz catheter. A case history of constrained technology, constrained bedside clinicians, and constrained monetary expenditures. Chest 113:1379-1386, 1998.

350. Damen J, Bolton D: A prospective analysis of 1400 pulmonary artery catheterizations in patients undergoing cardiac surgery. Acta Anesthesiol Scand 30:386-392, 1986.

351. Procaccini B, Clementi G, Miletti E, Lattanzi W: A review of pulmonary artery catheterization in 5,306 consecutive patients undergoing cardiac surgery. Br J Anaesth 80:A26, 1998.

352. Voukydis PC, Cohen SI: Catheter-induced arrhythmias. Am Heart J 88:588-592, 1974.

353. Sise CJ, Hollingsworth P, Brimm JE, et al: Complications of the flow-directed pulmonary-artery catheter: A prospective analysis in 219 patients. Crit Care Med 9:315-318, 1981.

354. Lopez-Sendon J, Lopez de Sa E, Maqueda IG, et al: Right ventricular infarction as a risk factor for ventricular fibrillation during pulmonary artery catheterization using Swan-Ganz catheters. Am Heart J 119:207-209, 1990.

355. Salmenperä M, Peltola K, Rosenberg P: Does prophylactic lidocaine control cardiac arrhythmias associated with pulmonary artery catheterization? Anesthesiology 56:210-212, 1982.

356. Shaw TJI: The Swan-Ganz pulmonary artery catheter. Anaesthesia 34:651-656, 1979.

357. Morris D, Mulvihill D, Lew WYW: Risk of developing complete heart block during bedside pulmonary artery catheterization in patients with left bundle-branch block. Arch Intern Med 147:2005-2010, 1987.

358. Sprung CL, Elser B, Schein RMH, et al: Risk of right bundle-branch block and complete heart block during pulmonary artery catheterization. Crit Care Med 17:1-3, 1989.

359. Thompson IR, Dalton BC, Lappas DG, Lowenstein E: Right bundle-branch block and complete heart block caused by the Swan-Ganz catheter. Anesthesiology 51:359-362, 1979.

360. Ezeugwu CO, Graham S: Evaluation of a hemodynamic tracing. J Cardiothorac Vasc Anesth 12:365-366, 1998.

361. Cooper SC, Desai M, Alpern JB: Beware the pulsating Swan. J Cardiothorac Anesth 4:474-475, 1990.

362. Daccache G, Depoix J-P, Provenchere S, et al: Pulmonary artery catheter during cardiac surgery: A rare but severe adverse effect. J Cardiothorac Vasc Anesth 12:125-130, 1998.

363. Eguaras MG, Luch M, Valdivia J, Chacon-Quevedo A: An unusual complication of Swan-Ganz catheter use. Tex Heart Inst J 19:149-150, 1992.

364. Klockgether-Radke A, Rathgeber J, Lange H: Inadvertant intracardiac entrapment of a Swan-Ganz catheter. Anaesthesist 44:116-118, 1995.

365. Troianos CA, Stypula RW: Transesophageal echocardiographic diagnosis of pulmonary artery catheter entrapment and coiling. Anesthesiology 79:602-604, 1993.

366. Huang G-S, Wang H-J, Chen C-H, et al: Pulmonary artery rupture after attempted removal of a pulmonary artery catheter. Anesth Analg 95:299-301, 2002.

367. Manecke JRJ, Brown JC, Landau AA, et al: An unusual case of pulmonary artery catheter malfunction. Anesth Analg 95:302-304, 2002.

368. Fitch JCK, Fang X-E, Dewar ML: Preinsertion pulmonary artery catheter flushing. Anesthesiology 88:1690-1691, 1998.

369. Paulsen AW: Artifactually low cardiac outputs resulting from a communication between the proximal and distal lumens of an Edwards pacing thermodilution Swan-Ganz catheter. Anesthesiology 68:308-309, 1988.

370. Arnaout S, Diab K, Al-Kutoubi A, Jamaleddine G: Rupture of the chordae of the tricuspid valve after knotting of the pulmonary artery catheter. Chest 120:1742-1744, 2001.

371. Fibuch EE, Tuohy GF: Intracardiac knotting of a flow-directed balloon-tipped catheter. Anesth Analg 59:217-222, 1980.

372. Lipp H: Intra-cardiac knotting of a flow-directed balloon catheter. N Engl J Med 284:220, 1971.

373. Dumensil JG, Proulx G: A new nonsurgical technique for untying tight knots in flow-directed balloon catheters. Am J Cardiol 53:395-396, 1984.

374. Michel L, Installe E, Joucken K: Knotting of intracardiac flow-directed balloon catheter. Chest 83:147-148, 1983.

375. Vincent J-L, Dhainaut J-F, Perret C, Suter P: Is the pulmonary artery catheter misused? A European view. Crit Care Med 26:1283-1287, 1998.

376. Chastre J, Cornud F, Bouchama A, et al: Thrombosis as a complication of pulmonary-artery catheterization via the internal jugular vein. N Engl J Med 306:278-281, 1982.

377. Hoar PF, Stone JG, Wicks AE, et al: Thrombogenesis associated with Swan-Ganz catheters. Anesthesiology 48:445-447, 1978.

378. Hoar PF, Wilson RM, Mangano DT, et al: Heparin bonding reduces thrombogenicity of pulmonary-artery catheters. N Engl J Med 305:993-995, 1981.

379. Böhrer H, Fleischer F, Lang J, Vahl C: Early formation of thrombi on pulmonary artery catheters in cardiac surgical patients receiving high-dose aprotinin. J Cardiothorac Anesth 4:222-225, 1990.

380. Dentz ME, Slaughter TF, Mark JB: Early thrombus formation on heparin bonded pulmonary artery catheters in patients receiving epsilon aminocaproic acid. Anesthesiology 82:583-586, 1995.

381. Randolph AG, Cook DJ, Gonzales CA, Andrew M: Benefit of heparin in central venous and pulmonary artery catheters. Chest 113:165-171, 1998.

382. Connors AF, Castele RJ, Farhat NZ, Tomashefski JF: Complications of right heart catheterization. A prospective autopsy study. Chest 88:567-572, 1985.

383. Foote GA, Schabel SI, Hodges M: Pulmonary complications of the flow-directed balloon-tipped catheter. N Engl J Med 290:927-931, 1974.

384. Yorra FH, Oblath R, Jaffe H, et al: Massive thrombosis associated with use of the Swan-Ganz catheter. Chest 65:682-684, 1974.

385. Applefield JJ, Caruthers TE, Reno DJ: Assessment of the sterility of long-term cardiac catheterization using the thermodilution Swan-Ganz catheter. Chest 74:377-380, 1978.

386. Mermel LA, McCormick RD, Springman SR, Maki DG: The pathogenesis and epidemiology of catheter-related infection with pulmonary artery Swan-Ganz catheters: A prospective study utilizing molecular subtyping. Am J Med 91:197S-205S, 1991.

387. Cobb DK, High KP, Sawyer R, et al: A controlled trial of scheduled replacement of central venous and pulmonary-artery catheters. N Engl J Med 327:1062-1068, 1992.

388. Bernardin G, Milhaud D, Roger PM, et al: Swan-Ganz catheter–related pulmonary valve infective endocarditis: A case report. Intensive Care Med 20:142-144, 1994.

389. Rowley KM, Clubb KS, Smith GJW, Cabin HS: Right-sided infective endocarditis as a consequence of flow-directed pulmonary-artery catheterization. N Engl J Med 311:1152-1156, 1984.

390. O'Toole JD, Wurtzbacher JJ, Wearner NE, Jain AC: Pulmonary-valve injury and insufficiency during pulmonary-artery catheterization. N Engl J Med 301:1167-1168, 1979.

391. Ali MJ, Omran AS, Rakowski HR, William WG: Pulmonary valve injury: Swan-Ganz or surgery. Can J Cardiol 17:467-470, 2001.

392. Sherman SV, Wall MH, Kennedy DJ, et al: Do pulmonary artery catheters cause or increase tricuspid or pulmonic valvular regurgitation? Anesth Analg 92:1117-1122, 2001.

393. Carlson TA, Goldenberg IF, Murray PD, et al: Catheter-induced delayed recurrent pulmonary artery hemorrhage. JAMA 261:1943-1945, 1989.

394. Kelly TF, Morris GC, Crawford ES, et al: Perforation of the pulmonary artery with Swan-Ganz catheters. Diagnosis and surgical management. Ann Surg 193:686-691, 1981.

395. McDaniel DD, Stone JG, Faltas AN, et al: Catheter-induced pulmonary artery hemorrhage. Diagnosis and management in cardiac operations. J Thorac Cardiovasc Surg 82:1-4, 1981.

396. Sirivella S, Gielchinsky I, Parsonnet V: Management of catheter-induced pulmonary artery perforation: A rare complication in cardiovascular operations. Ann Thorac Surg 72:2056-2059, 2001.

397. Mangar D, Connell GR, Lessin JL, Räsänen J: Catheter-induced pulmonary artery haemorrhage resulting from a pneumothorax. Can J Anaesth 40:1069-1072, 1993.

398. Urschel JD, Myerowitz PD: Catheter-induced pulmonary artery rupture in the setting of cardiopulmonary bypass. Ann Thorac Surg 56:585-589, 1993.

399. Barash PG, Nardi D, Hammond G, et al: Catheter-induced pulmonary artery perforation. J Thorac Cardiovasc Surg 82:5-12, 1981.

400. Hardy J-F, Morissette M, Taillefer J, Vauclair R: Pathophysiology of rupture of the pulmonary artery by pulmonary artery balloon-tipped catheters. Anesth Analg 62:925-930, 1983.

401. Lemen R, Jones JG, Cowan G: A mechanism of pulmonary-artery perforation by Swan-Ganz catheters. N Engl J Med 292:211-212, 1975.

402. Roberts LC, Ramsay MAE, Alivizatos PA, et al: Successfully treated pulmonary artery rupture complicated by aneurysm formation. J Cardiothorac Vasc Anesth 6:70-72, 1992.

403. Shin B, Ayella RJ, McAslan TC: Pitfalls of Swan-Ganz catheterization. Crit Care Med 5:125-127, 1977.

404. Klafta JM, Olson JP: Emergent lung separation for management of pulmonary artery rupture. Anesthesiology 87:1248-1250, 1997.

405. Bartter T, Irwin RS, Phillips DA, et al: Pulmonary artery pseudoaneurysm. Arch Intern Med 148:471-473, 1988.

406. Sprung J, Schoenwald PK, Hayden J, Kukreja N: Contained pulmonary artery perforation by pulmonary artery catheter. J Clin Monit 14:195-198, 1998.

407. Karak P, Dimick R, Hamrick KM, et al: Immediate transcatheter embolization of Swan-Ganz catheter–induced pulmonary artery pseudoaneurysm. Chest 111:1450-1452, 1997.

408. Ginosar Y, Thijs LG, Sprung CL: Raising the standard of hemodynamic monitoring: Targeting the practice or the practitioner? Crit Care Med 25:209-211, 1997.

409. De Backer D: Hemodynamic assessment: The technique or the physician at fault? Intensive Care Med 29:1865-1867, 2003.

410. Jain M, Canham M, Upadhyay D, Corbridge T: Variability in interventions with pulmonary artery catheter data. Intensive Care Med 29:2059-2062, 2003.

411. Squara P, Bennett D, Perret C: Pulmonary artery catheter. Does the problem lie in the users? Chest 121:2009-2015, 2002.

412. Iberti TJ, Fischer EP, Leibowitz AB, et al: A multicenter study of physicians' knowledge of the pulmonary artery catheter. JAMA 264:2928-2932, 1990.

413. Iberti TJ, Daily EK, Leibowitz AB, et al: Assessment of critical care nurses' knowledge of the pulmonary artery catheter. Crit Care Med 22:1674-1678, 1994.

414. Gnaegi A, Feihl F, Perret C: Intensive care physicians' insufficient knowledge of right-heart catheterization at the bedside: Time to act? Crit Care Med 25:213-220, 1997.

415. Trottier SJ, Taylor RW: Physicians' attitudes toward and knowledge of the pulmonary artery catheter: Society of Critical Care Medicine Membership Survey. New Horizons 5:201-206, 1997.

416. Komadina KH, Schenk DA, LaVeau P, et al: Interobserver variability in the interpretation of pulmonary artery catheter pressure tracings. Chest 100:1647-1654, 1991.

417. Jacka MJ, Cohen MM, To T, et al: Pulmonary artery occlusion pressure estimation: How confident are anesthesiologists? Crit Care Med 30:1197-1203, 2002.

418. Zarich S, Pust-Marcone J, Amoateng-Adjepong Y, Manthous CA: Failure of a brief educational program to improve interpretation of pulmonary artery occlusion pressure tracings. Intensive Care Med 26:698-703, 2000.

419. Feihl F, Gnaegi A, Perret C: Interpretation of the pulmonary artery occlusion (wedge) pressure: Physicians' knowledge versus the experts' knowledge. Crit Care Med 26:1763, 1998.

420. Marik P, Heard SO, Varon J: Interpretation of the pulmonary artery occlusion (wedge) pressure: Physicians' knowledge versus the experts' knowledge. Crit Care Med 26:1761-1764, 1998.

421. Trottier SJ, Taylor RW: Interpretation of the pulmonary artery occlusion (wedge) pressure: Physicians' knowledge versus the experts' knowledge. Crit Care Med 26:1763-1764, 1998.

422. Zidulka A, Hakim TS: Wedge pressure in large vs. small pulmonary arteries to detect pulmonary venoconstriction. J Appl Physiol 59:1329-1332, 1985.

423. Mark JB: Pulmonary artery wedge pressure. In Mark JB (ed): Atlas of Cardiovascular Monitoring. New York, Churchill Livingstone, 1998, pp 39-48.

424. Bouchard RJ, Gault JH, Ross J: Evaluation of pulmonary arterial end-diastolic pressure as an estimate of left ventricular end-diastolic pressure in patients with normal and abnormal left ventricular performance. Circulation 44:1072-1079, 1971.

425. Falicov RE, Resnekov L: Relationship of the pulmonary artery end-diastolic pressure to the left ventricular end-diastolic and mean filling pressures in patients with and without left ventricular dysfunction. Circulation 42:65-73, 1970.

426. Lappas D, Lell WA, Gabel JC, et al: Indirect measurement of left-atrial pressure in surgical patients—pulmonary-capillary wedge and pulmonary-artery diastolic pressures compared with left-atrial pressure. Anesthesiology 38:394-397, 1973.

427. Scheinman M, Evans GT, Weiss A, Rapaport E: Relationship between pulmonary artery end-diastolic pressure and left ventricular filling pressure in patients in shock. Circulation 47:317-324, 1973.

428. West JE, Dollery CT, Naimark A: Distribution of blood flow in isolated lung: Relation to vascular and alveolar pressures. J Appl Physiol 19:713-724, 1964.

429. Moore RA, Neary MJ, Gallagher JD, Clark DL: Determination of the pulmonary capillary wedge position in patients with giant left atrial V waves. J Cardiothorac Anesth 1:108-113, 1987.

430. Kern MJ, Deligonul U: The left-sided V wave. In Kern MJ (ed): Hemodynamic Rounds. Interpretation of Cardiac Pathophysiology from Pressure Waveform Analysis. New York, Wiley-Liss, 1993, pp 49-56.

431. Mark JB, Chetham PM: Ventricular pacing can induce hemodynamically significant mitral valve regurgitation. Anesthesiology 74:375-377, 1991.

432. Rao PS, Sathyanarayana PV: Transseptal insertion of left atrial line: A simple and safe technique. Ann Thorac Surg 55:785-786, 1993.

433. Zahorec R, Holoman M: Transatrial access for left atrial pressure monitoring in cardiac surgery patients. Eur J Cardiothorac Surg 11:379-380, 1997.

434. Leach JK, Friedlich AL, Myers GS, et al: Usefulness and limitations on left heart catheterization in mitral disease. Am J Cardiol 6:57-61, 1962.

435. Entress JJ, Dhamee S, Olund T, et al: Pulmonary artery occlusion pressure is not accurate immediately after cardiopulmonary bypass. J Cardiothorac Anesth 4:558-563, 1990.

436. Humphrey CB, Oury JH, Virgilio RW, et al: An analysis of direct and indirect measurements of left atrial filling pressure. J Thorac Cardiovasc Surg 71:643-647, 1976.

437. Gold JP, Jonas RA, Lang P, et al: Transthoracic intracardiac monitoring lines in pediatric surgical patients: A ten-year experience. Ann Thorac Surg 42:185-191, 1986.

438. Porter EJ, Norfleet EA, Boone FD, et al: Entrapment of a mitral valve prosthesis with a left atrial catheter. Anesthesiology 60:246-248, 1984.

439. Donahue PJ, Hansen DD, Mayer JE: A new complication of left atrial catheters. J Cardiothorac Anesth 3:757-759, 1989.

440. Yeo TC, Miller FA, Oh JK, Freeman WK: Retained left atrial catheter: An unusual cardiac source of embolism identified by transesophageal echocardiography. J Am Soc Echocardiogr 11:66-70, 1998.

441. Wiedemann HP: Wedge pressure in pulmonary veno-occlusive disease. N Engl J Med 315:1233, 1986.

442. Levy MM: Pulmonary capillary pressure. Clinical implications. Crit Care Clin 12:819-839, 1996.

443. Fang K, Krahmer RL, Rypins EB, Law WR: Starling resistor effects on pulmonary artery occlusion pressure in endotoxin shock provide inaccuracies in left ventricular compliance assessments. Crit Care Med 24:1618-1625, 1996.

444. Collee GG, Lynch KE, Hill RD, Zapol WM: Bedside measurement of pulmonary capillary pressure in patients with acute respiratory failure. Anesthesiology 66:614-620, 1987.

445. Cope DK, Allison RC, Parmentier JL, et al: Measurement of effective pulmonary capillary pressure using the pressure profile after pulmonary artery occlusion. Crit Care Med 14:16-22, 1986.

446. Gilbert E, Hakim TS: Derivation of pulmonary capillary pressure from arterial occlusion in intact conditions. Crit Care Med 22:986-993, 1994.

447. Hakim TS, Maarek JI, Chang HK: Estimation of pulmonary capillary pressure in intact dog lungs using the arterial occlusion technique. Am Rev Respir Dis 140:217-224, 1989.

448. Holloway H, Perry M, Downey J, et al: Estimation of effective pulmonary capillary pressure in intact lungs. J Appl Physiol 54:846-851, 1983.

449. Yamada Y, Komatsu K, Suzukawa M, et al: Pulmonary capillary pressure measured with a pulmonary arterial double port catheter in surgical patients. Anesth Analg 77:1130-1134, 1993.

450. Mark JB: Pulmonary artery and wedge pressure artifacts. In Mark JB (ed): Atlas of Cardiovascular Monitoring. New York, Churchill Livingstone, 1998, pp 49-58.

451. Morris AH, Chapman RH, Gardner RM: Frequency of technical problems encountered in the measurement of pulmonary artery wedge pressure. Crit Care Med 12:164-170, 1984.

452. Schmitt EA, Brantigan CO: Common artifacts of pulmonary artery and pulmonary artery wedge pressures: Recognition and interpretation. J Clin Monit 2:44-52, 1986.

453. Bashein G: Another source of artifact in the pulmonary artery pressure waveform. Anesthesiology 68:310, 1988.

454. Sharkey SW: Beyond the wedge: Clinical physiology and the Swan-Ganz catheter. Am J Med 83:111-122, 1987.

455. Dobson GM, Horan BF, Bradburn NT: Significance of diastolic pulmonary artery pressure peaks. J Clin Monit 8:62-65, 1992.

456. Bethea CF, Peter RH, Behar VS, et al: The hemodynamic simulation of mitral regurgitation in ventricular septal defect after myocardial infarction. Cathet Cardiovasc Diagn 2:97-104, 1976.

457. Fuchs RM, Heuser RR, Yin FCP, Brinker JA: Limitations of pulmonary wedge V waves in diagnosing mitral regurgitation. Am J Cardiol 49:849-854, 1982.

458. Grossman W: Profiles in valvular heart disease. *In* Grossman W, Baim DS (eds): Cardiac Catheterization, Angiography, and Intervention. Philadelphia, Lea & Febiger, 1991, pp 557-581.

459. Pichard AD, Kay R, Smith H, et al: Large V waves in the pulmonary wedge pressure tracing in the absence of mitral regurgitation. Am J Cardiol 50:1044-1050, 1982.

460. Snyder RW, Glamann DB, Lange RA, et al: Predictive value of prominent pulmonary arterial wedge V waves in assessing the presence and severity of mitral regurgitation. Am J Cardiol 73:568-570, 1994.

461. Royster RL, Johnson JC, Prough DS, et al: Differences in pulmonary artery wedge pressures obtained by balloon inflation versus impaction techniques. Anesthesiology 61:339-341, 1984.

462. Braunwald E, Awe WC: The syndrome of severe mitral regurgitation with normal left atrial pressure. Circulation 27:29-35, 1963.

463. Velky PJ, Harte FA: The appearance of large "V" waves in association with sternal retraction during coronary artery surgery. J Cardiothorac Vasc Anesth 6:453-455, 1992.

464. Bourdillon PD, Lorell BH, Mirsky I, et al: Increased regional myocardial stiffness of the left ventricle during pacing-induced angina in man. Circulation 67:316-323, 1983.

465. Dodek A, Kassebaum DG, Bristow JD: Pulmonary edema in coronary-artery disease without cardiomegaly. Paradox of the stiff heart. N Engl J Med 286:1347-1350, 1972.

466. Grossman W: Diastolic dysfunction in congestive heart failure. N Engl J Med 325:1557-1564, 1991.

467. Mark JB: Myocardial ischemia. Hemodynamic detection. *In* Mark JB (ed): Atlas of Cardiovascular Monitoring. New York, Churchill Livingstone, 1998, pp 181-204.

468. McLaurin LP, Rolett EL, Grossman W: Impaired left ventricular relaxation during pacing-induced ischemia. Am J Cardiol 32:751-757, 1973.

469. Waters DD, da Luz P, Wyatt HL, et al: Early changes in regional and global left ventricular function induced by graded reductions in regional coronary perfusion. Am J Cardiol 39:537-543, 1977.

470. Attia RR, Murphy JD, Snider M, et al: Myocardial ischemia due to infrarenal aortic cross-clamping during aortic surgery in patients with severe coronary artery disease. Circulation 53:961-965, 1976.

471. Haggmark S, Hohner P, Ostman M, et al: Comparison of hemodynamic, electrocardiographic, mechanical, and metabolic indicators of intraoperative myocardial ischemia in vascular surgical patients with coronary artery disease. Anesthesiology 70:19-25, 1989.

472. Kaplan JA, Wells PH: Early diagnosis of myocardial ischemia using the pulmonary arterial catheter. Anesth Analg 60:789-793, 1981.

473. Kaplan JA: Indications for pulmonary arterial catheterization. Anesth Analg 61:477-479, 1982.

474. Rahimtoola SH, Loeb HS, Ehsani A, et al: Relationship of pulmonary artery to left ventricular diastolic pressures in acute myocardial infarction. Circulation 46:283-290, 1972.

475. Sanchez R, Wee M: Perioperative myocardial ischemia: Early diagnosis using the pulmonary artery catheter. J Cardiothorac Vasc Anesth 5:604-607, 1991.

476. van Daele MERM, Sutherland GR, Mitchell MM, et al: Do changes in pulmonary capillary wedge pressure adequately reflect myocardial ischemia during anesthesia: A correlative preoperative hemodynamic, electrocardiographic, and transesophageal echocardiographic study. Circulation 81:865-871, 1990.

477. Stott DK, Marpole DGF, Bristow JD, et al: The role of left atrial transport in aortic and mitral stenosis. Circulation 41:1031-1041, 1970.

478. Wohlgelernter D, Jaffe CC, Cabin HS, et al: Silent ischemia during coronary occlusion produced by balloon inflation: Relation to regional myocardial dysfunction. J Am Coll Cardiol 10:491-498, 1978.

479. Leung JM, O'Kelly BF, Mangano DT: Relationship of regional wall motion abnormalities to hemodynamic indices of myocardial oxygen supply and demand in patients undergoing CABG surgery. Anesthesiology 73:802-814, 1990.

480. Slogoff S, Keats AS: Does perioperative myocardial ischemia lead to postoperative myocardial infarction? Anesthesiology 62:107-114, 1985.

481. Slogoff S, Keats AS: Further observations on perioperative myocardial ischemia. Anesthesiology 65:539-542, 1986.

482. Sabbah HN, Rosman H, Kono T, et al: On the mechanism of functional mitral regurgitation. Am J Cardiol 72:1074-1076, 1993.

483. Longabaugh JP, Sheikh KH, Bengtson JR, et al: Diagnosis and management of ischemic mitral regurgitation with the use of transesophageal echocardiography. Coronary Artery Dis 3:377-381, 1992.

484. Bashein G, Ivey TD: Con: A pulmonary artery catheter is not indicated for all coronary artery surgery. J Cardiothorac Anesth 1:362-365, 1987.

485. Keats AS: Adventures in perioperative myocardial ischemia. Tex Heart Inst J 20:5-11, 1993.

486. Lieberman RW, Orkin FK, Jobes DR, Schwartz AJ: Hemodynamic predictors of myocardial ischemia during halothane anesthesia for coronary-artery revascularization. Anesthesiology 59:36-41, 1983.

487. Weintraub AC, Barash PG: A pulmonary artery catheter is indicated in all patients for coronary artery surgery. J Cardiothorac Anesth 1:358-361, 1987.

488. Wickey GS, Larach DR, Keifer JC, et al: Combined interpretation of transesophageal echocardiography, electrocardiography, and pulmonary artery wedge waveform to detect myocardial ischemia. J Cardiothorac Anesth 4:102-104, 1990.

489. Lorell B, Leinbach RC, Pohost GM, et al: Right ventricular infarction. Clinical diagnosis and differentiation from cardiac tamponade and pericardial constriction. Am J Cardiol 43:465-471, 1979.

490. Goldstein JA, Barzilai B, Rosamond TL, et al: Determinants of hemodynamic compromise with severe right ventricular infarction. Circulation 82:359-368, 1990.

491. Kushwaha SS, Fallon JT, Fuster V: Restrictive cardiomyopathy. N Engl J Med 336:267-276, 1997.

492. Kern MJ, Aguirre F: Interpretation of cardiac pathophysiology from pressure waveform analysis: Pericardial compressive hemodynamics, part I. Cathet Cardiovasc Diagn 25:336-342, 1992.

493. Kern MJ, Aguirre F: Interpretation of cardiac pathophysiology from pressure waveform analysis: Pericardial compressive hemodynamics, part II. Cathet Cardiovasc Diagn 26:34-40, 1992.

494. Kern MJ, Aguirre F: Interpretation of cardiac pathophysiology from pressure waveform analysis: Pericardial compressive hemodynamics, part III. Cathet Cardiovasc Diagn 26:152-158, 1992.

495. Hirschmann JV: Pericardial constriction. Am Heart J 96:110-122, 1978.
496. Beloucif S, Takata M, Shimada M, Robotham JL: Influence of pericardial constraint on atrioventricular interactions. Am J Physiol 263:H125-H134, 1992.
497. Greenberg MA, Gitler B: Left ventricular rupture in a patient with coexisting right ventricular infarction. N Engl J Med 309:539-542, 1983.
498. Lorell BH, Braunwald E: Pericardial disease. In Braunwald E (ed): Heart Disease. A Textbook of Cardiovascular Medicine, 4th ed. Philadelphia, WB Saunders, 1992, pp 1465-1516.
499. Fowler NO: Cardiac tamponade. A clinical or an echocardiographic diagnosis? Circulation 87:1738-1741, 1993.
500. Hancock EW: Subacute effusive-constrictive pericarditis. Circulation 43:183-192, 1971.
501. Ellis DM: Interpretation of beat-to-beat blood pressure values in the presence of ventilatory changes. J Clin Monit 1:65-70, 1985.
502. Hoeksel SAAP, Blom JA, Jansen JRC, Schreuder JJ: Correction for respiration artifact in pulmonary blood pressure signals of ventilated patients. J Clin Monit 12:397-403, 1996.
503. Mitchell MM, Meathe EA, Jones BR, et al: Accurate, automated, continuously displayed pulmonary artery pressure measurement. Anesthesiology 67:294-300, 1987.
504. Teplick RS: Measuring central vascular pressures: A surprisingly complex problem. Anesthesiology 67:289-291, 1987.
505. Cengiz M, Crapo RO, Gardner RM: The effect of ventilation on the accuracy of pulmonary artery and wedge pressure measurements. Crit Care Med 11:502-507, 1983.
506. Bell H, Stubbs D, Pugh D: Reliability of central venous pressure as an indicator of left atrial pressure. A study in patients with mitral valve disease. Chest 59:169-173, 1971.
507. Buchbinder N, Ganz W: Hemodynamic monitoring: Invasive techniques. Anesthesiology 45:146-155, 1976.
508. Cohn JN, Tristani FE, Khatri IM: Relationship between left and right ventricular function. J Clin Invest 48:2008-2018, 1969.
509. Toussaint GPM, Burgess JH, Hampson LG: Central venous pressure and pulmonary wedge pressure in critical surgical illness. A comparison. Arch Surg 109:265-269, 1974.
510. Mangano DT: Monitoring pulmonary arterial pressure in coronary-artery disease. Anesthesiology 53:364-370, 1980.
511. Lowenstein E, Teplick R: To (PA) catheterize or not to (PA) catheterize—that is the question. Anesthesiology 53:361-363, 1980.
512. Tuman KJ, Carroll GC, Ivankovich AD: Pitfalls in interpretation of pulmonary artery catheter data. J Cardiothorac Anesth 3:625-641, 1989.
513. Mark JB: Predicting left ventricular end-diastolic pressure. In Mark JB (ed): Atlas of Cardiovascular Monitoring. New York, Churchill Livingstone, 1998, pp 59-79.
514. Mitchell JH, Gilmore JP, Sarnoff SJ: The transport function of the atrium. Factors influencing the relation between mean left atrial pressure and left ventricular end diastolic pressure. Am J Cardiol 9:237-247, 1962.
515. Herbert WH: Left ventricular compliance and pulmonary artery end-diastolic pressure. N Y State J Med 77:344-348, 1977.
516. Herbert WH: Pulmonary artery and left heart end-diastolic pressure relations. Br Heart J 32:774-778, 1970.
517. Berry AJ, Geer RT, Marshall BE: Alteration of pulmonary blood flow by pulmonary-artery occluded pressure measurement. Anesthesiology 51:164-166, 1979.
518. Wittnich C, Trudel J, Zidulka A, Chiu RC: Misleading "pulmonary wedge pressure" after pneumonectomy: Its importance in postoperative fluid therapy. Ann Thorac Surg 42:192-196, 1986.
519. Berryhill RE, Benumof JL: PEEP-induced discrepancy between pulmonary arterial wedge pressure and left atrial pressure: The effects of controlled vs. spontaneous ventilation and compliant vs. noncompliant lungs in the dog. Anesthesiology 51:303-308, 1979.

520. Guyton RA, Chiavarelli M, Padgett CA, et al: The influence of positive end-expiratory pressure on intrapericardial pressure and cardiac function after coronary artery bypass surgery. J Cardiothorac Anesth 1:98-107, 1987.
521. Nadeau S, Noble WH: Misinterpretation of pressure measurements from the pulmonary artery catheter. Can Anaesth Soc J 33:352-363, 1986.
522. Pinsky M, Vincent J-L, De Smet J-M: Estimating left ventricular filling pressure during positive end-expiratory pressure in humans. Am Rev Respir Dis 143:25-31, 1991.
523. Teboul JL, Zapol WM, Brun-Buisson C, et al: A comparison of pulmonary artery occlusion pressure and left ventricular end-diastolic pressure during mechanical ventilation with PEEP in patients with severe ARDS. Anesthesiology 70:261-266, 1989.
524. Cozzi PJ, Hall JB, Schmidt GA: Pulmonary artery diastolic-occlusion pressure gradient is increased in acute pulmonary embolism. Crit Care Med 23:1481-1484, 1995.
525. Case Records of the Massachusetts General Hospital (Case 21-1986). N Engl J Med 314:1435-1445, 1986.
526. Case records of the Massachusetts General Hospital (Case 48-1993). N Engl J Med 329:1720-1728, 1993.
527. Kern MJ, Aguirre FV: Mitral valve gradients: Part I. In Kern MJ (ed): Hemodynamic Rounds. Interpretation of Cardiac Pathophysiology from Pressure Waveform Analysis. New York, Wiley-Liss, 1993, pp 35-42.
528. Enson Y, Wood JA, Mantaras NB, Harvey RM: The influence of heart rate on pulmonary arterial–left ventricular pressure relationships at end-diastole. Circulation 56:533-539, 1977.
529. Dalen JE, Bone RC: Is it time to pull the pulmonary artery catheter? JAMA 276:916-918, 1996.
530. Soni N: Swan song for the Swan-Ganz catheter? The use of pulmonary artery catheters probably needs re-evaluation—but they should not be banned. BMJ 313:763-764, 1996.
531. Prielipp RC, Morell R: Con: Swan song for the Swan-Ganz? J Clin Monit 313:339-340, 1997.
532. Tuman KJ: Pro: A moratorium on PAC is unjustified. J Clin Monit 13:337-338, 1997.
533. Robin ED: The cult of the Swan-Ganz catheter. Intensive Crit Care Dig 5:18-21, 1986.
534. Robin ED: Death by pulmonary artery flow-directed catheter [editorial]. Time for a moratorium? Chest 92:727-731, 1987.
535. Shoemaker WC: Use and abuse of the balloon tip pulmonary artery (Swan-Ganz) catheter: Are patients getting their money's worth? Crit Care Med 18:1294-1296, 1990.
536. MacDonald D: Cerebral palsy and intrapartum fetal monitoring. N Engl J Med 334:659-660, 1996.
537. Nelson KB, Dambrosia JM, Ting TY, Grether JK: Uncertain value of electronic fetal monitoring in predicting cerebral palsy. N Engl J Med 334:613-618, 1996.
538. Shy KK, Luthy DA, Bennett FC, et al: Effects of electronic fetal-heart-rate monitoring, as compared with periodic auscultation, on the neurologic development of premature infants. N Engl J Med 322:588-593, 1990.
539. Cooper AB, Doig GS, Sibbald WJ: Pulmonary artery catheters in the critically ill. An overview using the methodology of evidence-based medicine. Crit Care Clin 12:777-794, 1996.
540. Berlauk J, Abrams JH, Gilmour IJ, et al: Preoperative optimization of cardiovascular hemodynamics improves outcome in peripheral vascular surgery. A prospective, randomized clinical trial. Ann Surg 214:289-299, 1991.
541. Del Guercio LRM, Cohn JD: Monitoring operative risk in the elderly. JAMA 243:1350-1355, 1980.
542. Flancbaum L, Ziegler DW, Choban PS: Preoperative intensive care unit admission and hemodynamic monitoring in patients scheduled for major elective noncardiac surgery: A retrospective review of 95 patients. J Cardiothorac Vasc Anesth 12:3-9, 1998.
543. Moore CH, Lombardo R, Allums JA, Gordon FT: Left main coronary artery stenosis: Hemodynamic monitoring to reduce mortality. Ann Thorac Surg 26:445-451, 1978.

544. Scalea TM, Simon HM, Duncan AO, et al: Geriatric blunt multiple trauma: Improved survival with early invasive monitoring. J Trauma 30:129-136, 1990.

545. Tuchschmidt J, Fried J, Astiz M, Rackow E: Elevation of cardiac output and oxygen delivery improves outcome in septic shock. Chest 102:216-220, 1992.

546. Bender JS, Smith-Meek MA, Jones CE: Routine pulmonary artery catheterization does not reduce morbidity and mortality of elective vascular surgery. Ann Surg 226:229-237, 1997.

547. Afessa B, Tefferi A, Hoagland HC, et al: Outcome of recipients of bone marrow transplants who require intensive-care unit support. Mayo Clin Proc 67:117-122, 1992.

548. Isaacson IJ, Lowdon JD, Berry AJ, et al: The value of pulmonary artery and central venous monitoring in patients undergoing abdominal aortic reconstructive surgery: A comparative study of two selected, randomized groups. J Vasc Surg 12:754-760, 1991.

549. Pearson KS, Gomez MN, Moyers JR, et al: A cost/benefit analysis of randomized invasive monitoring for patients undergoing cardiac surgery. Anesth Analg 69:336-341, 1989.

550. Rhodes A, Cusack RJ, Newman PJ, et al: A randomised, controlled trial of the pulmonary artery catheter in critically ill patients. Intensive Care Med 28:256-264, 2002.

551. Richard C, Warszawski J, Anguel N, et al: Early use of the pulmonary artery catheter and outcomes in patients with shock and acute respiratory distress syndrome. A randomized controlled trial. JAMA 290:2713-2720, 2003.

552. Dalen JE: The pulmonary artery catheter—friend, foe, or accomplice? JAMA 286:348-350, 2001.

553. Rao TLK, Jacobs KH, El-Etr AA: Reinfarction following anesthesia in patients with myocardial infarction. Anesthesiology 59:499-505, 1983.

554. Gore JM, Goldberg RJ, Spodick DH, et al: A community-wide assessment of the use of pulmonary artery catheters in patients with acute myocardial infarction. Chest 92:721-727, 1987.

555. Zion MM, Balkin J, Rosenmann D, et al: Use of pulmonary artery catheters in patients with acute myocardial infarction: Analysis of experience in 5,841 patients in the SPRINT Registry. Chest 98:1331-1335, 1990.

556. Bashein G, Johnson PW, Davis KB, Ivey TD: Elective coronary bypass surgery without pulmonary artery catheter monitoring. Anesthesiology 63:451-454, 1985.

557. Tuman KJ, McCarthy RJ, Spiess BD, et al: Effect of pulmonary artery catheterization on outcome in patients undergoing coronary artery surgery. Anesthesiology 70:199-206, 1989.

558. Saarela E, Kari A, Nikki P, et al: Current practice regarding invasive monitoring in intensive care units in Finland. Intensive Care Med 17:264-271, 1991.

559. Pulmonary Artery Catheter Consensus Conference Participants: Pulmonary artery catheter consensus conference: Consensus statement. Crit Care Med 25:910-925, 1997.

560. Sibbald WJ, Keenan SP: Show me the evidence: A critical appraisal of the Pulmonary Artery Catheter Consensus Conference and other musings on how critical care practitioners need to improve the way we conduct business. Crit Care Med 25:2060-2063, 1997.

561. Knaus WA, Harrell FEJ, Lynn J, et al: The SUPPORT prognostic model. Objective estimates of survival for seriously ill hospitalized adults. Ann Intern Med 122:191-203, 1995.

562. Lo B: Improving care near the end of life: Why is it so hard? JAMA 274:1634-1635, 1995.

563. Mark JB: Pulmonary artery catheterization wither. Cardiovasc Thorac Anesth J Club J 2:8-9, 1997.

564. SUPPORT Principal Investigators: A controlled trial to improve care for seriously ill hospitalized patients. JAMA 274:1591-1598, 1995.

565. Chernow B: Pulmonary artery flotation catheters. Chest 111:261-262, 1997.

566. Fowler RA, Cook DJ: The arc of the pulmonary artery catheter. JAMA 290:2732-2734, 2003.

567. Rapoport J, Teres D, Steingrub J, et al: Patient characteristics and ICU organizational factors that influence frequency of pulmonary artery catheterization. JAMA 283:2559-2567, 2000.

568. Ramsey SD, Saint S, Sullivan SD, et al: Clinical and economic effects of pulmonary artery catheterization in nonemergent coronary artery bypass graft surgery. J Cardiothorac Vasc Anesth 14:113-118, 2000.

569. Shoemaker WC, Kram HB, Appel PL, Fleming AW: The efficacy of central venous and pulmonary artery catheters and therapy based upon them in reducing mortality and morbidity. Arch Surg 125:1332-1338, 1990.

570. Shoemaker WC, Belzberg H: Pulmonary Artery Catheter Consensus Conference. Crit Care Med 26:1760-1761, 1998.

571. Pölönen P, Ruokonen E, Hippeläinen M, et al: A prospective, randomized study of goal-oriented hemodynamic therapy in cardiac surgical patients. Anesth Analg 90:1052-1059, 2000.

572. Rivers E, Nguyen B, Havstad S, et al: Early goal-directed therapy in the treatment of severe sepsis and septic shock. N Engl J Med 345:1368-1377, 2001.

573. Evans TW: Hemodynamic and metabolic therapy in critically ill patients. N Engl J Med 345:1417-1418, 2001.

574. Shoemaker WC, Thangathurai D, Wo CCJ, et al: Intraoperative evaluation of tissue perfusion in high-risk patients by invasive and noninvasive hemodynamic monitoring. Crit Care Med 27:2147-2152, 1999.

575. Boyd O, Grounds RM, Bennett ED: A randomized clinical trial of the effect of deliberate perioperative increase of oxygen delivery on mortality in high-risk surgical patients. JAMA 270:2699-2707, 1993.

576. Boyd O, Bennett ED: Achieving the goal. Crit Care Med 27:2298-2299, 1999.

577. Treasure T, Bennett D: Reducing the risk of major elective surgery. BMJ 318:1087-1088, 1999.

578. Wilson J, Woods I, Fawcett J, et al: Reducing the risk of major elective surgery: Randomised controlled trial of preoperative optimisation of oxygen delivery. BMJ 318:1099-1103, 1999.

579. Gattinoni L, Brazzi L, Pelosi P, et al: A trial of goal-oriented hemodynamic therapy in critically ill patients. N Engl J Med 333:1025-1032, 1995.

580. Hayes MA, Timmins AC, Yau EHS, et al: Elevation of systemic oxygen delivery in the treatment of critically ill patients. N Engl J Med 330:1717-1722, 1994.

581. Gasman JD, Ruoss SJ, Fishman RS, et al: Hazards with both determining and utilizing oxygen consumption measurements in the management of critically ill patients. Crit Care Med 24:6-9, 1996.

582. Heyland DK, Cook DJ, King D, et al: Maximizing oxygen delivery in critically ill patients: A methodologic appraisal of the evidence. Crit Care Med 24:517-524, 1996.

583. Hinds C, Watson D: Manipulating hemodynamics and oxygen transport in critically ill patients. N Engl J Med 333:1074-1075, 1995.

584. American College of Physicians/American College of Cardiology/American Heart Association Task Force on Clinical Privileges in Cardiology: Clinical competence in hemodynamic monitoring. J Am Coll Cardiol 15:1460-1464, 1990.

585. Naylor CD, Sibbald WJ, Sprung CL, et al: Pulmonary artery catheterization: Can there be an integrated strategy for guideline development and research promotion? JAMA 269:2407-2411, 1993.

586. Hemodynamic monitoring: A technology assessment. Technology Subcommittee of the Working Group on Critical Care, Ontario Ministry of Health. Can Med Assoc J 145:114-121, 1991.

587. Keats AS: The Rovenstine lecture, 1983: Cardiovascular anesthesia: Perceptions and perspectives. Anesthesiology 60:467-474, 1984.

588. Sandham JD, Hull RD, Brant RF: Ethics of technology assessment: Pulmonary artery flow directed catheter revisited. Am J Respir Crit Care Med 153:A422, 1996.

589. Sandham JD, Hull RD, Brant RF: Effect of the pulmonary artery catheter on morbidity and mortality, a multicenter trial. Am J Respir Crit Care Med 153:A601, 1996.

590. Sandham JD, Hull RD, Brant RF: Pulmonary artery flow directed catheter: The evidence. Lancet 348:1324, 1996.

591. Sandham JD, Hull RD, Brant RF: The pulmonary artery catheter takes a great fall. Crit Care Med 26:1288-1289, 1998.

592. Spodick DH: Analysis of flow-directed pulmonary artery catheterization. JAMA 261:1946-1947, 1989.

593. Spodick DH: Effectiveness of right heart catheterization: Time for a randomized trial. JAMA 277:113, 1997.

594. Guyatt G: A randomized control trial of right-heart catheterization in critically ill patients. Ontario Intensive Care Study Group. J Intensive Care Med 6:91-95, 1991.

595. Hall JB: Use of the pulmonary artery catheter in critically ill patients. Was invention the mother of necessity? JAMA 283:2577-2578, 2000.

596. Parsons PE: Progress in research on pulmonary-artery catheters. N Engl J Med 348:66-68, 2003.

597. Zaidan JR, Freniere S: Use of a pacing pulmonary artery catheter during cardiac surgery. Ann Thorac Surg 35:633-636, 1983.

598. Mora CT, Seltzer JL, McNulty SE: Evaluation of a new design pulmonary artery catheter for intraoperative ventricular pacing. J Cardiothorac Anesth 2:303-308, 1988.

599. Trankina MF, White RD: Perioperative cardiac pacing using an atrioventricular pacing pulmonary artery catheter. J Cardiothorac Anesth 3:154-162, 1989.

600. Teboul J-L: Dynamic concepts of volume responsiveness. Int J Intensive Care 10:XX-YY, 2003.

601. Perel A, Pizov R: Cardiovascular effects of mechanical ventilation. In Perel A, Stock MC (eds): Handbook of Mechanical Ventilatory Support. Baltimore, Williams & Wilkins, 1992, pp 51-65.

602. Robotham JL, Lixfeld W, Holland L, et al: Effects of respiration on cardiac performance. J Appl Physiol 44:703-709, 1978.

603. Robotham JL, Scharf SM: Effects of positive and negative pressure ventilation on cardiac performance. Clin Chest Med 4:161-187, 1983.

604. Robotham JL, Cherry D, Mitzner W, et al: A re-evaluation of the hemodynamic consequences of intermittent positive pressure ventilation. Crit Care Med 11:783-793, 1983.

605. Perel A: Assessing fluid responsiveness by the systolic pressure variation in mechanically ventilated patients. Anesthesiology 89:1309-1310, 1998.

606. Coriat P, Vrillon M, Perel A, et al: A comparison of systolic blood pressure variations and echocardiographic estimates of end-diastolic left ventricular size in patients after aortic surgery. Anesth Analg 78:46-53, 1994.

607. Pizov R, Segal E, Kaplan L, et al: The use of systolic pressure variation in hemodynamic monitoring during deliberate hypotension in spine surgery. J Clin Anesth 2:96-100, 1990.

608. Rooke GA: Systolic pressure variation as an indicator of hypovolemia. Curr Opin Anaesthesiol 8:511-515, 1995.

609. Parry-Jones AJD, Pittman JAL: Arterial pressure and stroke volume variability as measurements for cardiovascular optimisation. Int J Intensive Care 10:67-72, 2003.

610. Marik PE: The systolic blood pressure variation as an indicator of pulmonary capillary wedge pressure in ventilated patients. Anaesth Intensive Care 21:405-408, 1993.

611. Rasanen J, Howie MB: Mitral regurgitation during withdrawal of mechanical ventilatory support. J Cardiothorac Anesth 2:60-63, 1988.

612. Tavernier B, Makhotine O, Lebuffe G, et al: Systolic pressure variation as a guide to fluid therapy in patients with sepsis-induced hypotension. Anesthesiology 89:1313-1321, 1998.

613. Perel A: The value of ΔDown during hemorrhage. Br J Anaesth 83:967-968, 1999.

614. Gunn SR, Pinsky MR: Implications of arterial pressure variation in patients in the intensive care unit. Curr Opin Crit Care 7:212-217, 2001.

615. Michard F, Chemla D, Richard C, et al: Clinical use of respiratory changes in arterial pulse pressure to monitor the hemodynamic effects of PEEP. Am J Respir Crit Care Med 159:935-939, 1999.

616. Berkenstadt H, Margalit N, Hadani M, et al: Stroke volume variation as a predictor of fluid responsiveness in patients undergoing brain surgery. Anesth Analg 92:984-989, 2001.

617. Schwid HA, Rooke AG: Systolic blood pressure at end-expiration measured by the automated systolic pressure variation monitor is equivalent to systolic blood pressure during apnea. J Clin Monit 16:115-120, 2000.

618. Soncini M, Manfredi G, Redaelli A, et al: A computerized method to measure systolic pressure variation (SPV) in mechanically ventilated patients. J Clin Monit 17:141-146, 2002.

619. Stoneham MD: Less is more . . . using systolic pressure variation to assess hypovolemia. Br J Anaesth 83:550-551, 1999.

620. Denault AY, Gasior TA, Gorcsan J, et al: Determinants of aortic pressure variation during positive-pressure ventilation in man. Chest 116:176-186, 1999.

621. Dalibon N, Schlumberger S, Saada M, et al: Haemodynamic assessment of hypovolaemia under general anaesthesia in pigs submitted to graded haemorrhage and retransfusion. Br J Anaesth 82:97-103, 1999.

622. Dietzman RH, Ersek RA, Lillehei CW, et al: Low output syndrome. J Thorac Cardiovasc Surg 57:138-150, 1969.

623. Dupont H, Squara P: Cardiac output monitoring. Curr Opin Anaesthesiol 9:490-494, 1996.

624. Linton RAF, Linton NWF, Kelly F: Is clinical assessment of the circulation reliable in postoperative cardiac surgical patients? J Cardiothorac Vasc Anesth 16:4-7, 2002.

625. Sakka SG, Reinhart K, Wegscheider K, Meier-Hellmann A: Is the placement of a pulmonary artery catheter still justified solely for the measurement of cardiac output? J Cardiothorac Vasc Anesth 14:119-124, 2000.

626. Singer M: Cardiac output in 1998. Heart 79:425-428, 1998.

627. Ramsay J: How much cardiac output is enough? J Cardiothorac Vasc Anesth 16:1-3, 2002.

628. Stewart GN: Researches on the circulation time and on the influences which affect it. IV. The output of the heart. J Physiol 22:159, 1897.

629. Hamilton WF, Moore JW, Kinsman JM: Studies on the circulation. IV. Further analysis of the injection method, and changes in hemodynamics under physiologic and pathological conditions. Am J Physiol 99:534, 1932.

630. Bousvaros GA, Palmer WH, Sekelj P, McGregor M: Comparison of central and peripheral injection sites in the estimation of cardiac output by dye dilution curves. Circ Res 13:317-321, 1962.

631. Crane MG, Holloway JE, Sears C, et al: The effect of recirculation on the shape of the arterial concentration curve after an instantaneous injection of indicator. Int J Appl Radiat Isotopes 7:97-110, 1959.

632. Gunnells JC, Gorten R: Effect of varying indicator injection sites on values for cardiac output. J Appl Physiol 16:261-265, 1961.

633. Hetzel PS, Swan HJC, Wood EH: Influence of injection site on arterial dilution curves of T-1824. J Appl Physiol 7:66-72, 1954.

634. Fegler G: Measurement of cardiac output in anesthetized animals by a thermodilution method. Q J Exp Physiol 39:153-164, 1954.

635. Berger RL, Weisel RD, Vito L, et al: Cardiac output measurement by thermodilution during cardiac operations. Ann Thorac Surg 21:43-47, 1976.

636. Ganz W, Donoso R, Marcus HS, et al: A new technique for measurement of cardiac output by thermodilution in man. Am J Cardiol 27:392-396, 1971.

637. Weisel RD, Berger RL, Hechtman HB: Measurement of cardiac output by thermodilution. N Engl J Med 292:682-684, 1975.

638. Wong M, Skulsky A, Moon E: Loss of indicator in the thermodilution technique. Cathet Cardiovasc Diag 4:103-109, 1978.

639. Jansen JRC: The thermodilution method for the clinical assessment of cardiac output. Intensive Care Med 21:691-697, 1995.

640. Levett JM, Replogle RL: Thermodilution cardiac output: A critical analysis and review of the literature. J Surg Res 27:392-404, 1979.

641. Nishikawa T, Dohi S: Errors in the measurement of cardiac output by thermodilution. Can J Anaesth 40:142-153, 1993.

642. Conway J, Lund-Johansen P: Thermodilution method for measuring cardiac output. Eur Heart J 11:17-20, 1990.

643. Sharkey SW: A Guide to Interpretation of Hemodynamic Data in the Coronary Care Unit. Philadelphia, Lippincott-Raven, 1997.

644. Stetz CW, Miller RG, Kelly GE, Raffin TA: Reliability of the thermodilution method in the determination of cardiac output in clinical practice. Am Rev Respir Dis 126:1001-1004, 1982.

645. Bilfinger TV, Lin CY, Anagnostopoulos CE: In vitro determination of accuracy of cardiac output measurements by thermal dilution. J Surg Res 33:409-414, 1982.

646. Powner DJ, Snyder JV: In vitro comparison of six commercially available thermodilution cardiac output systems. Med Instrum 12:122-127, 1978.

647. Nishikawa T, Dohi S: Slowing of the heart during cardiac output measurement by thermodilution. Anesthesiology 57:538-539, 1982.

648. Boerboom LE, Kinney TE, Olinger GN, Hoffmann RG: Validity of cardiac output measurement by the thermodilution method in the presence of acute tricuspid regurgitation. J Thorac Cardiovasc Surg 106:636-642, 1993.

649. Cigarroa RG, Lange RA, Williams RH, et al: Underestimation of cardiac output by thermodilution in patients with tricuspid regurgitation. Am J Med 86:417-420, 1989.

650. Heerdt PM, Pleimann BE, Hogue CW: Flow-dependency of error in thermodilution cardiac output during tricuspid regurgitation in dogs. Anesthesiology 83:A614, 1995.

651. Boyd O, Mackay CJ, Newman P, et al: Effects of insertion depth and use of the sidearm of the introducer sheath of pulmonary artery catheters in cardiac output measurement. Crit Care Med 22:1132-1135, 1994.

652. Bearss MG, Yonutas DN, Allen WT: A complication with thermodilution cardiac outputs in centrally-placed pulmonary artery catheters. Chest 81:527, 1982.

653. Stoller JK, Herbst TJ, Hurford W, Rie MA: Spuriously high cardiac output from injecting thermal indicator through an ensheathed port. Crit Care Med 14:1064-1065, 1986.

654. Bazaral MG, Petre J, Novoa R: Errors in thermodilution cardiac output measurements caused by rapid pulmonary artery temperature decreases after cardiopulmonary bypass. Anesthesiology 77:31-37, 1992.

655. Griffin K, Benjamin E, DelGiudice R, et al: Thermodilution cardiac output measurement during simultaneous volume infusion through the venous infusion port of the pulmonary artery catheter. J Cardiothorac Vasc Anesth 11:437-439, 1997.

656. Wetzel RC, Latson TW: Major errors in thermodilution cardiac output measurement during rapid volume infusion. Anesthesiology 62:684-687, 1985.

657. Nelson LD, Anderson HB: Patient selection for iced versus room temperature injectate for thermodilution cardiac output determinations. Crit Care Med 13:182-184, 1985.

658. Pearl RG, Rosenthal MH, Nielson L, et al: Effect of injectate volume and temperature on thermodilution cardiac output determination. Anesthesiology 64:798-801, 1986.

659. Okamoto K, Komatsu T, Kumar V, et al: Effects of intermittent positive-pressure ventilation on cardiac output measurements by thermodilution. Crit Care Med 14:977-980, 1986.

660. Snyder JV, Powner DJ: Effects of mechanical ventilation on the measurement of cardiac output by thermodilution. Crit Care Med 10:677-682, 1982.

661. Woods M, Scott RN, Harken AH: Practical considerations for the use of a pulmonary artery thermistor catheter. Surgery 79:469-475, 1976.

662. Stevens JH, Raffin TA, Mihm FG, et al: Thermodilution cardiac output measurement. JAMA 253:2240-2242, 1985.

663. Groeneveld ABJ, Berendsen RR, Schneider AJ, et al: Effect of the mechanical ventilatory cycle on thermodilution right ventricular volumes and cardiac output. J Appl Physiol 89:89-96, 2000.

664. Lazor MA, Pierce ET, Stanley GD, et al: Evaluation of the accuracy and response time of STAT-Mode continuous cardiac output. J Cardiothorac Vasc Anesth 11:432-436, 1997.

665. Mihm FG, Gettinger A, Hanson CW, et al: A multicenter evaluation of a new continuous cardiac output pulmonary artery catheter system. Crit Care Med 26:1346-1350, 1998.

666. Philip JH, Long MC, Quinn MD, Newbower RS: Continuous thermal measurement of cardiac output. IEEE Trans Biomed Eng BME-31:393-400, 1984.

667. Yelderman M: Continuous measurement of cardiac output with the use of stochastic system identification techniques. J Clin Monit 6:322-332, 1990.

668. Yelderman ML, Ramsay MA, Quinn MD, et al: Continuous thermodilution cardiac output measurement in ICU patients. J Cardiothorac Vasc Anesth 6:270-275, 1992.

669. Yelderman M, Quinn MD, McKown RC: Continuous thermodilution cardiac output measurement in sheep. J Thorac Cardiovasc Surg 104:315-320, 1992.

670. Bottinger BW: Continuous cardiac output monitoring—further applications of the thermodilution principle. Intensive Care Med 25:131-133, 1999.

671. Cariou A, Monchi M, Dhainaut J-F: Continuous cardiac output and mixed venous oxygen saturation monitoring. J Crit Care 13:198-213, 1998.

672. Jansen JRC, Johnson RW, Yan JY, Verdouw PD: Near continuous cardiac output by thermodilution. J Clin Monit 13:233-239, 1997.

673. Aranda M, Mihm F, Garrett S, et al: Continuous cardiac output catheters. Anesthesiology 89:1592-1595, 1998.

674. Siegel LC, Hennessy MM, Pearl RG: Delayed time response of the continuous cardiac output pulmonary artery catheter. Anesth Analg 83:1173-1177, 1996.

675. Nelson LD: The new pulmonary artery catheters: Continuous venous oximetry, right ventricular ejection fraction, and continuous cardiac output. New Horizons 5:251-258, 1997.

676. Hogue CW, Rosenbloom M, McCawley C, Lappas DG: Comparison of cardiac output measurement by continuous thermodilution with electro magnetometry in adult cardiac surgical patients. J Cardiothorac Vasc Anesth 8:631-635, 1994.

677. Le Tulzo Y, Belghith M, Seguin P, et al: Reproducibility of thermodilution cardiac output determination in critically ill patients: Comparison between bolus and continuous method. J Clin Monit 12:379-385, 1996.

678. Gardner RM: Continuous cardiac output: How accurate and how timely? Crit Care Med 26:1302-1303, 1998.

679. Lichtenthal PR, Wade LD: Continuous cardiac output measurements. J Cardiothorac Vasc Anesth 8:668-670, 1994.

680. Hoff HE, Scott HJ: Physiology. N Engl J Med 239:120, 1948.

681. Fick A: Über die Messung des Blutquantums in den Herzventrikeln. Verh Phys Med Ges Wurzburg 2:16, 1870.

682. Carpenter JP, Nair S, Staw I: Cardiac output determination: Thermodilution versus a new computerized Fick method. Crit Care Med 13:576-579, 1985.

683. Davies GG, Jebson PJR, Glasgow BM, Hess DR: Continuous Fick cardiac output compared to thermodilution cardiac output. Crit Care Med 14:881-885, 1986.

684. Doi M, Morita K, Ikeda K: Frequently repeated Fick cardiac output measurements during anesthesia. J Clin Monit 6:107-112, 1990.

685. Norfleet EA, Watson CB: Continuous mixed venous oxygen saturation measurement: A significant advance in hemodynamic monitoring? J Clin Monit 1:245-258, 1985.

686. London MJ, Moritz TE, Henderson WG, et al: Standard versus fiberoptic pulmonary artery catheterization for cardiac surgery in the Department of Veterans Affairs. Anesthesiology 96:860-870, 2002.

687. Prewitt RM, Ghignone M: Treatment of right ventricular dysfunction in acute respiratory failure. Crit Care Med 11:346-352, 1983.
688. Sibbald WJ, Driedger AA: Right ventricular function in acute disease states: Pathophysiologic considerations. Crit Care Med 5:339-345, 1983.
689. Vlahakes GJ, Turley K, Hoffman JIE: The pathophysiology of failure in acute right ventricular hypertension: Hemodynamic and biochemical correlations. Circulation 63:87-95, 1981.
690. Weber KT, Janicki JS, Shroff SG, et al: The right ventricle: Physiologic and pathophysiologic considerations. Crit Care Med 11:323-328, 1983.
691. Cohn JN, Guiha NH, Broder M, Limas CJ: Right ventricular infarction. Clinical and hemodynamic features. Am J Cardiol 33:209-214, 1974.
692. Kinch JW, Ryan TJ: Right ventricular infarction. N Engl J Med 330:1211-1217, 1994.
693. Klein HO, Tordjman T, Ninio R, et al: The early recognition of right ventricular infarction: Diagnostic accuracy of the electrocardiographic V$_4$R lead. Circulation 67:558-565, 1983.
694. Zehender M, Kasper W, Kauder E, et al: Right ventricular infarction as an independent predictor of prognosis after acute inferior myocardial infarction. N Engl J Med 328:981-988, 1993.
695. Isner JM: Right ventricular myocardial infarction. JAMA 259:712-718, 1988.
696. Biondi JW, Schulman DS, Soufer R, et al: The effect of incremental positive end-expiratory pressure on right ventricular hemodynamics and ejection fraction. Anesth Analg 67:144-151, 1988.
697. Her C, Lees DE: Accurate assessment of right ventricular function in acute respiratory failure. Crit Care Med 21:1665-1672, 1993.
698. Nelson LD: Hemodynamic monitoring—a new day dawning. Crit Care Med 21:1626-1627, 1993.
699. Reuse C, Vincent J-L, Pinsky MR: Measurements of right ventricular volumes during fluid challenge. Chest 98:1450-1454, 1990.
700. Kay H, Afshan M, Barash PG: Measurement of ejection fraction by thermal dilution techniques. J Surg Res 34:337-346, 1983.
701. Dhainaut J-F, Brunet F, Monsallier JF, et al: Bedside evaluation of right ventricular performance using a rapid computerized thermodilution method. Crit Care Med 15:148-152, 1987.
702. Morrison DA, Stovall R, Sensecqua J: Thermodilution measurement of the right ventricular ejection fraction. Cathet Cardiovasc Diagn 13:167-173, 1987.
703. Urban P, Scheidegger D, Gabathuler J: Thermodilution determination of right ventricular volume and ejection fraction. Crit Care Med 15:652-655, 1987.
704. Stein KL, Breisblatt W, Wolfe C, et al: Depression and recovery of right ventricular function after cardiopulmonary bypass. Crit Care Med 18:1197-1200, 1990.
705. Boldt J, Kling D, Thiel A, et al: Revascularization of the right coronary artery: Influence on thermodilution right ventricular ejection fraction. J Cardiothorac Anesth 2:140-146, 1988.
706. Boldt J, Kling D, Moosdorf R, Hempelmann G: Influence of acute volume loading on right ventricular function after cardiopulmonary bypass. Crit Care Med 17:518-522, 1989.
707. Hines R, Barash PG: Intraoperative right ventricular dysfunction detected with a right ventricular ejection fraction catheter. J Clin Monit 2:206-208, 1986.
708. Chang MC, Mondy JS, Meredith JW, et al: Clinical application of ventricular end-systolic elastance and the ventricular pressure-volume diagram. Shock 7:413-419, 1997.
709. Harvey RM, Enson Y: Pulmonary vascular resistance. Adv Intern Med 15:73-93, 1969.
710. McGregor M, Sniderman A: On pulmonary vascular resistance: The need for more precise definition. Am J Cardiol 55:217-221, 1985.
711. Permutt S, Riley RL: Hemodynamics of collapsible vessels with tone: The vascular waterfall. J Appl Physiol 34:924-932, 1963.
712. Rouby J-J, Andreev A, Léger P, et al: Peripheral vascular effects of thiopental and propofol in humans with artificial hearts. Anesthesiology 75:32-42, 1991.
713. Gorback MS: Problems associated with the determination of pulmonary vascular resistance. J Clin Monit 6:118-127, 1990.
714. Hilgenberg JC: Pulmonary vascular impedance: Resistance versus pulmonary artery diastolic–pulmonary artery occluded pressure gradient. Anesthesiology 58:484-485, 1983.
715. Schulte-Sasse U, Hess W, Tarnow J: Pulmonary vascular impedance: Resistance versus pulmonary artery diastolic–pulmonary artery occluded pressure gradient. Anesthesiology 58:485-486, 1983.
716. Reeves JT, Grover RF, Filley GF: Cardiac output in normal resting man. J Appl Physiol 16:276, 1961.
717. Segal J, Pearl RG, Ford AJ, et al: Instantaneous and continuous cardiac output obtained with a Doppler pulmonary artery catheter. J Am Coll Cardiol 13:1382-1392, 1989.
718. Segal J, Nassi M, Ford AJ, Schuenemeyer TD: Instantaneous and continuous cardiac output in humans obtained with a Doppler pulmonary artery catheter. J Am Coll Cardiol 16:1398-1407, 1990.
719. Segal J, Gaudiani V, Nishimura T: Continuous determination of cardiac output using a flow-directed Doppler pulmonary artery catheter. J Cardiothorac Vasc Anesth 5:309-315, 1991.
720. Reich DL: Has continuous perioperative cardiac output monitoring finally arrived? J Cardiothorac Vasc Anesth 5:307-308, 1991.
721. Waxman K, Police AM, Cheung CK, et al: Laser Doppler velocimetry as a monitor of cardiac output changes in dogs. Crit Care Med 13:194-196, 1985.
722. Abrams JH, Weber RE, Holmen KD: Continuous cardiac output determination using transtracheal Doppler: Initial results in humans. Anesthesiology 71:11-15, 1989.
723. Abrams JH, Weber RE, Holmen KD: Transtracheal Doppler: A new procedure for continuous cardiac output measurement. Anesthesiology 70:134-138, 1989.
724. Hausen B, Schafers H-J, Rohde R, Haverich A: Clinical evaluation of transtracheal Doppler for continuous cardiac output estimation. Anesth Analg 74:800-804, 1992.
725. Perrino AC, O'Connor T, Luther M: Transtracheal Doppler cardiac output monitoring: Comparison to thermodilution during noncardiac surgery. Anesth Analg 78:1060-1066, 1994.
726. Huntsman LL, Gams E, Johnson CC, Fairbanks E: Transcutaneous determination of aortic blood-flow velocities in man. Am Heart J 89:605-612, 1975.
727. Colocousis JS, Huntsman LL, Curreri PW: Estimation of stroke volume changes by ultrasonic Doppler. Circulation 56:914-917, 1977.
728. Huntsman LL, Stewart DK, Barnes SR, et al: Noninvasive Doppler determination of cardiac output in man. Clinical validation. Circulation 67:593-602, 1983.
729. Mark JB, Steinbrook RA, Gugino LD, et al: Continuous noninvasive monitoring of cardiac output with esophageal Doppler ultrasound during cardiac surgery. Anesth Analg 65:1013-1020, 1986.
730. Nishimura RA, Callahan MJ, Schaff HV, et al: Noninvasive measurement of cardiac output by continuous-wave Doppler echocardiography: Initial experience and review of the literature. Mayo Clin Proc 59:484-489, 1984.
731. Chandraratna PA, Nanna M, McKay C, et al: Determination of cardiac output by transcutaneous continuous-wave ultrasonic Doppler computer. Am J Cardiol 53:234-237, 1984.
732. Cariou A, Monchi M, Joly L-M, et al: Noninvasive cardiac output monitoring by aortic blood flow determination: Evaluation of the Sometec Dynemo-3000 system. Crit Care Med 26:2066-2072, 1998.

733. Boulnois J-LG, Pechoux T: Non-invasive cardiac output monitoring by aortic blood flow measurement with the Dynemo 3000. J Clin Monit Comput 16:127-140, 2000.

734. Laupland KB, Bands CJ: Utility of esophageal Doppler as a minimally invasive hemodynamic monitor: A review. Can J Anaesth 49:393-401, 2002.

735. Freund PR: Transesophageal Doppler scanning versus thermodilution during general anesthesia. Am J Surg 153:490-494, 1987.

736. Perrino AC, Fleming J, LaMantia KR: Transesophageal Doppler ultrasonography: Evidence for improved cardiac output monitoring. Anesth Analg 71:651-657, 1990.

737. Perrino AC, Fleming J, LaMantia KR: Transesophageal Doppler cardiac output monitoring: Performance during aortic reconstructive surgery. Anesth Analg 73:705-710, 1991.

738. Schmid ER, Spahn DR, Tornic M: Reliability of a new generation transesophageal Doppler device for cardiac output monitoring. Anesth Analg 77:971-979, 1993.

739. Siegel LC, Shafer SL, Martinez GM, et al: Simultaneous measurements of cardiac output by thermodilution, esophageal Doppler, and electrical impedance in anesthetized patients. J Cardiothorac Anesth 2:590-595, 1988.

740. Wong DH, Tremper KK, Stemmer EA, et al: Noninvasive cardiac output: Simultaneous comparison of two different methods with thermodilution. Anesthesiology 72:784-792, 1990.

741. Wong DH, Watson T, Gordon I, et al: Comparison of changes in transit time ultrasound, esophageal Doppler, and thermodilution cardiac output after changes in preload, afterload, and contractility in pigs. Anesth Analg 72:584-588, 1991.

742. Kamal GD, Symreng T, Starr J: Inconsistent esophageal Doppler cardiac output during acute blood loss. Anesthesiology 72:95-99, 1990.

743. Marik PE: Pulmonary artery catheterization and esophageal Doppler monitoring in the ICU. Chest 116:1085-1091, 1999.

744. Singer M, Bennett D: Pitfalls of pulmonary artery catheterization highlighted by Doppler ultrasound. Crit Care Med 17:1060-1061, 1989.

745. Singer M, Clarke J, Bennett ED: Continuous hemodynamic monitoring by esophageal Doppler. Crit Care Med 17:447-452, 1989.

746. Singer M, Allen MJ, Webb AR, Bennett ED: Effects of alterations in left ventricular filling, contractility, and systemic vascular resistance on the ascending aortic blood velocity waveform of normal subjects. Crit Care Med 19:1138-1145, 1991.

747. Singer M, Bennett ED: Noninvasive optimization of left ventricular filling using esophageal Doppler. Crit Care Med 19:1132-1137, 1991.

748. Thys DM, Hillel Z: Left ventricular performance indices by transesophageal Doppler. Anesthesiology 69:728-737, 1988.

749. DiCorte CJ, Latham P, Greilich PE, et al: Esophageal Doppler monitor determinations of cardiac output and preload during cardiac operations. Ann Thorac Surg 69:1782-1786, 2000.

750. Poeze M, Ramsay G, Greve JWM, Singer M: Prediction of postoperative cardiac surgical morbidity and organ failure within 4 hours of intensive care unit admission using esophageal Doppler ultrasonography. Crit Care Med 27:1288-1294, 1999.

751. Guzzetta NA, Ramsay JG, Bailey JM, Palmer-Steele C: Clinical evaluation of the esophageal Doppler monitor for continuous cardiac output monitoring. Anesth Analg 86:SCA82, 1998.

752. Kuck K, Fine PG, Westenskow DR: Evaluation of a new esophageal Doppler cardiac output monitor. J Clin Monit 13:424, 1997.

753. Bengur AR, Meliones JN: Continuous monitoring of cardiac output: How many assumptions are valid? Crit Care Med 28:2168-2169, 2000.

754. Eachempati SR, Young C, Alexander J, et al: The clinical use of an esophageal Doppler monitor for hemodynamic monitoring in sepsis. J Clin Monit 15:223-225, 1999.

755. Gan TJ, Arrowsmith JE: The oesophageal Doppler monitor. BMJ 315:893-894, 1997.

756. Gan TJ, Wakeling H, Hardman D, et al: Intraoperative volume expansion guided by esophageal Doppler reduces the incidence of gastric mucosal hypoperfusion and may be associated with improved outcome following major surgery. Anesthesiology 87:A391, 1997.

757. Sinclair S, James S, Singer M: Intraoperative intravascular volume optimisation and length of hospital stay after repair of proximal femoral fracture: Randomised controlled trial. BMJ 315:909-912, 1997.

758. Kubicek WG, Karnegis JN, Patterson RP: Development and evaluation of an impedance cardiac output system. Aviat Space Environ Med 37:1208-1212, 1966.

759. Bernstein DP: A new stroke volume equation for thoracic electrical bioimpedance: Theory and rationale. Crit Care Med 14:904-909, 1986.

760. Mattar JA: Noninvasive cardiac output determination by thoracic electrical bioimpedance. Intensive Crit Care Dig 7:14-18, 1988.

761. Appel PL, Kram HB, MacKabee J: Comparison of measurements of cardiac output by bioimpedance and thermodilution in severely ill surgical patients. Crit Care Med 14:933-935, 1986.

762. Bernstein DP: Continuous noninvasive real-time monitoring of stroke volume and cardiac output by thoracic electrical bioimpedance. Crit Care Med 14:898-901, 1986.

763. Donovan KD, Dobb GJ, Woods WPD, Hockings BE: Comparison of transthoracic electrical impedance and thermodilution methods for measuring cardiac output. Crit Care Med 14:1038-1044, 1986.

764. Thomas AN, Ryan J, Doran BR, Pollard BJ: Bioimpedance versus thermodilution cardiac output measurement: The Bomed NCCOM3 after coronary bypass surgery. Intensive Care Med 17:383-386, 1991.

765. Tremper KK, Hufstedler SM, Barker SJ, et al: Continuous noninvasive estimation of cardiac output by electrical bioimpedance: An experimental study in dogs. Crit Care Med 14:231-233, 1986.

766. Young JD, McQuillan P: Comparison of thoracic electrical bioimpedance and thermodilution for the measurement of cardiac index in patients with severe sepsis. Br J Anaesth 70:58-62, 1993.

767. Shoemaker WC, Wo CCJ, Bishop MH, et al: Multicenter trial of a new thoracic electrical bioimpedance device for cardiac output estimation. Crit Care Med 22:1907-1912, 1994.

768. Thangathurai D, Charbonnet C, Roessler P, et al: Continuous intraoperative noninvasive cardiac output monitoring using a new thoracic bioimpedance device. J Cardiothorac Vasc Anesth 11:440-444, 1997.

769. Sageman WS, Riffenburgh RH, Spiess BD: Equivalence of bioimpedance and thermodilution in measuring cardiac index after cardiac surgery. J Cardiothorac Vasc Anesth 16:8-14, 2002.

770. Haryadi DG, Westenskow DR, Critchley LAH, et al: Evaluation of a new advanced thoracic bioimpedance device for estimation of cardiac output. J Clin Monit Comput 15:131-138, 1999.

771. Wallace AW, Salahieh A, Lawrence A, et al: Endotracheal cardiac output monitor. Anesthesiology 92:178-189, 2000.

772. Orr J, Westenskow D, Kofoed S, Turner R: A non-invasive cardiac output system using the partial re breathing Fick method. J Clin Monit 12:464-465, 1996.

773. Botero M, Lobato EB: Advances in noninvasive cardiac output monitoring: An update. J Cardiothorac Vasc Anesth 15:631-640, 2001.

774. Jaffe MB: Partial CO_2 rebreathing cardiac output—operating principles of the NICO system. J Clin Monit 15:387-401, 1999.

775. Capek JM, Roy RJ: Noninvasive measurement of cardiac output using partial CO_2 rebreathing. IEEE Trans Biomed Eng 35:653-661, 1988.

776. Gedeon A, Forslund L, Hedenstierna G, Romano E: A new method for noninvasive bedside determination of pulmonary blood flow. Med Biol Eng Comput 18:411-418, 1980.

777. Band DM, Linton RAF, O'Brien TK, et al: The shape of indicator dilution curves used for cardiac output measurement in man. J Physiol 498:225-229, 1997.

778. Linton RAF, Band DM, Hare KM: A new method of measuring cardiac output in man using lithium dilution. Br J Anaesth 71:262-266, 1993.

779. Linton RAF, Linton NWF, Band DM: A new method of analysing indicator dilution curves. Cardiovasc Res 30:930-938, 1995.

780. Kurita T, Morita K, Kato S, et al: Comparison of the accuracy of the lithium dilution technique with the thermodilution technique for measurement of cardiac output. Br J Anaesth 79:770-775, 1997.

781. Linton R, Band D, O'Brien T, et al: Lithium dilution cardiac output measurement: A comparison with thermodilution. Crit Care Med 25:1796-1800, 1997.

782. Garcia-Rodriguez C, Pittman J, Cassell CH, et al: Lithium dilution cardiac output measurement: A clinical assessment of central venous and peripheral venous indicator injection. Crit Care Med 30:2199-2204, 2002.

783. Jonas MM, Kelly FE, Linton RAF, et al: A comparison of lithium dilution cardiac output measurements made using central and antecubital venous injection of lithium chloride. J Clin Monit 15:525-528, 1999.

784. Kurita T, Morita K, Kato S, et al: Lithium dilution cardiac output measurements using a peripheral injection site: Comparison with central injection technique and thermodilution. J Clin Monit 15:279-285, 1999.

785. English JB, Hodges MR, Sentker C, et al: Comparison of aortic pulse-wave contour analysis and thermodilution methods of measuring cardiac output during anesthesia in the dog. Anesthesiology 52:56-61, 1980.

786. Tannenbaum GA, Mathews D, Weissman C: Pulse contour cardiac output in surgical intensive care unit patients. J Clin Anesth 5:471-478, 1993.

787. Gratz I, Kraidin J, Jacobi AG, et al: Continuous noninvasive cardiac output as estimated from the pulse contour curve. J Clin Monit 8:20-27, 1992.

788. Hirschl MM, Binder M, Gwechenberger M, et al: Noninvasive assessment of cardiac output in critically ill patients by analysis of the finger blood pressure waveform. Crit Care Med 25:1909-1914, 1997.

789. Lieshout JJ, Wesseling KH: Continuous cardiac output by pulse contour analysis? Br J Anaesth 86:467-469, 2001.

790. Zollner C, Haller M, Weis M, et al: Beat-to beat measurement of cardiac output by intravascular pulse contour analysis: A prospective criterion standard study in patients after cardiac surgery. J Cardiothorac Vasc Anesth 14:125-129, 2000.

791. Buhre W, Weyland A, Kazmaier S, et al: Comparison of cardiac output assessed by pulse-contour analysis and thermodilution in patients undergoing minimally invasive direct coronary artery bypass grafting. J Cardiothorac Vasc Anesth 13:437-440, 1999.

792. Godje O, Thiel C, Lamm P, et al: Less invasive, continuous hemodynamic monitoring during minimally invasive coronary surgery. Ann Thorac Surg 68:1532-1536, 1999.

793. Goedje O, Hoeke K, Lichtwarck-Aschoff M, et al: Continuous cardiac output by femoral arterial thermodilution calibrated pulse contour analysis: Comparison with pulmonary arterial thermodilution. Crit Care Med 27:2407-2412, 1999.

794. Rödig G, Prasser C, Keyl C, et al: Continuous cardiac output measurement: Pulse contour analysis vs thermodilution technique in cardiac surgical patients. Br J Anaesth 82:525-530, 1999.

795. Linton NWF, Linton RAF: Estimation of changes in cardiac output from the arterial blood pressure waveform in the upper limb. Br J Anaesth 86:486-496, 2001.

796. Sakka SG, Reinhart K, Meier-Hellmann A: Comparison of pulmonary artery and arterial thermodilution cardiac output in critically ill patients. Intensive Care Med 25:843-846, 1999.

797. Pittman JA, Sum Ping J, Sherwood M, et al: Continuous cardiac output measurement by arterial pressure waveform analysis: A 24-hour comparison with the lithium dilution indicator method. Anesth Analg 93:SCA71, 2002.

798. Lichtwarck-Aschoff M, Zeravik J, Pfeiffer UJ: Intrathoracic blood volume accurately reflects circulatory volume status in critically ill patients with mechanical ventilation. Intensive Care Med 18:142-147, 1992.

799. Preisman S, Pfeiffer U, Lieberman N, Perel A: New monitors of intravascular volume: A comparison of arterial pressure waveform analysis and the intrathoracic blood volume. Intensive Care Med 23:651-657, 1997.

800. Sakka SG, Bredle DL, Reinhart K, Meier-Hellmann A: Comparison between intrathoracic blood volume and cardiac filling pressures in the early phase of hemodynamic instability of patients with sepsis or septic shock. J Crit Care 14:78-83, 1999.

801. Lichtwarck-Aschoff M, Beale R, Pfeiffer UJ: Central venous pressure, pulmonary artery occlusion pressure, intrathoracic blood volume, and right ventricular end-diastolic volume as indicators of cardiac preload. J Crit Care 11:180-188, 1996.

802. Godje O, Peyerl M, Seebauer T, et al: Central venous pressure, pulmonary capillary wedge pressure and intrathoracic blood volumes as preload indicators in cardiac surgery patients. Eur J Cardiothorac Surg 13:533-539, 1998.

803. Hoeft A, Schorn B, Weyland A, et al: Bedside assessment of intravascular volume status in patients undergoing coronary bypass surgery. Anesthesiology 81:76-86, 1994.

804. Barker SJ: Blood volume measurement. The next intraoperative monitor? Anesthesiology 89:1310-1312, 1998.

805. Haruna M, Kumon K, Yahagi N, et al: Blood volume measurement at the bedside using ICG pulse spectrophotometry. Anesthesiology 89:1322-1328, 1998.

806. Iijima T, Aoyagi T, Iwao Y, et al: Cardiac output and circulating blood volume analysis by pulse dye-densitometry. J Clin Monit 13:81-89, 1997.

807. Iijima T, Iwao Y, Sankawa H: Circulating blood volume measured by pulse dye-densitometry. Anesthesiology 89:1329-1335, 1998.

808. Knichwitz G, Van Aken H, Brüssel T: Gastrointestinal monitoring using measurement of intramucosal P_{CO_2}. Anesth Analg 87:134-142, 1998.

809. Kolkman JJ, Zwaarekant LJ, Boshuizen K, et al: In vitro evaluation of intragastric P_{CO_2} measurement by air tonometry. J Clin Monit 13:115-119, 1997.

810. Welsby I, Mythen MG: Gut perfusion during cardiac surgery. Curr Opin Anaesthesiol 10:34-39, 1997.

811. Marik PE: Gastric intramucosal pH. A better predictor of multiorgan dysfunction syndrome and death than oxygen-derived variables in patients with sepsis. Chest 104:225-229, 1993.

812. Marshall JC: An intensivist's dilemma: Support of the splanchnic circulation in critical illness. Crit Care Med 26:1637-1638, 1998.

813. Silva E, DeBacker D, Créteur J, Vincent J-L: Effects of vasoactive drugs on gastric intramucosal pH. Crit Care Med 26:1749-1758, 1998.

814. Hirsh J: Heparin. N Engl J Med 324:1565-1574, 1991.

815. Bull BS, Korpman RA, Huse WM, Briggs BD: Heparin therapy during extracorporeal circulation. I. Problems inherent in existing protocols. J Thorac Cardiovasc Surg 69:674-684, 1975.

816. Metz S: Administration of protamine rather than heparin in a patient undergoing normothermic cardiopulmonary bypass. Anesthesiology 80:691-694, 1994.

817. Hattersley PG: Activated coagulation time of whole blood. JAMA 196:150-154, 1966.

818. Dietrich W, Jochum M: Effect of celite and kaolin on activated clotting time in the presence of aprotinin: Activated clotting time is reduced by binding of aprotinin to kaolin. J Thorac Cardiovasc Surg 109:177, 1995.

819. Gravlee GP, Whitaker CL, Mark LJ, et al: Baseline activated coagulation time should be measured after surgical incision. Anesth Analg 71:549-653, 1990.

820. Ammar T, Fisher CF, Sarier K, Coller BS: The effects of thrombocytopenia on the activated coagulation time. Anesth Analg 83:1185-1188, 1996.

821. Moliterno DJ, Califf RM, Aguirre FV, et al: Effect of platelet glycoprotein IIb/IIIa integrin blockade on activated clotting time during percutaneous transluminal coronary angioplasty or directional atherectomy (The EPIC Trial). Am J Cardiol 75:559-562, 1995.

822. Moorehead MT, Westengard JC, Bull BS: Platelet involvement in the activated clotting time of heparinized blood. Anesth Analg 63:394-398, 1984.

823. Gravlee GP, Case LD, Angert KC, et al: Variability of the activated coagulation time. Anesth Analg 67:469-472, 1988.

824. Bode AP, Eick L: Lysed platelets shorten the activated coagulation time (ACT) of heparinized blood. Am J Clin Pathol 91:430-434, 1989.

825. Bennett JA, Horrow JC: Activated coagulation time: One tube or two? J Cardiothorac Vasc Anesth 10:471-473, 1996.

826. Baugh RF, Deemar KA, Zimmermann JJ: Heparinase in the activated clotting time assay: Monitoring heparin-independent alteration in coagulation function. Anesth Analg 74:201-205, 1992.

827. Oberhardt BJ, Dermott SC, Taylor M, et al: Dry reagent technology for rapid, convenient measurements of blood coagulation and fibrinolysis. Clin Chem 37:520-526, 1991.

828. Mertzlufft F, Koster A, Hansen R, et al: Reliability of the heparin management test for monitoring high levels of unfractionated heparin. In vitro findings in volunteers versus in vivo findings during cardiopulmonary bypass. Anesthesiology 92:1594-1602, 2000.

829. Watke CM, Kern FH, Schulman SR, et al: The heparin management test (HMT): An improved method for monitoring anticoagulation during pediatric cardiac surgery. Anesthesiology 89:A910, 1998.

830. Koster A, Chew D, Grundel M, et al: Bivalrudin monitored with the ecarin clotting time for anticoagulation during cardiopulmonary bypass. Anesth Analg 96:383-386, 2003.

831. Huyzen RJ, van Oeveren W, Wei F, et al: In vitro effect of hemodilution on activated clotting time and high-dose thrombin time during cardiopulmonary bypass. Ann Thorac Surg 62:533-537, 1996.

832. Wang JS, Lin CY, Karp RB: Comparison of high-dose thrombin time with activated clotting time for monitoring of anticoagulant effects of heparin in cardiac surgical patients. Anesth Analg 79:9-13, 1994.

833. Macik GB: Designing a point-of-care program for coagulation testing. Arch Pathol Lab Med 119:929-938, 1995.

834. Despotis GJ, Summerfield AL, Joist JH: Comparison of activated coagulation time and whole blood heparin measurements with laboratory plasma anti-Xa heparin concentration in patients having cardiac operations. J Thorac Cardiovasc Surg 108:1076-1082, 1994.

835. Despotis GJ, Joist HJ, Hogue CW Jr, et al: More effective suppression of hemostatic system activation in patients undergoing cardiac surgery by heparin dosing based on heparin blood concentrations rather than ACT. Thromb Haemost 76:902-908, 1996.

836. Koster A, Fischer T, Praus M, et al: Hemostatic activation and inflammatory response during cardiopulmonary bypass: Impact of heparin management. Anesthesiology 97:837-841, 2002.

837. Despotis GJ, Joist JH, Hogue CW, et al: The impact of heparin concentration and activated clotting time monitoring on blood conservation. J Thorac Cardiovasc Surg 110:46-54, 1995.

838. Wahr JA, Yun J-H, Yang VC, et al: A new method of measuring heparin levels in whole blood by protamine titration using a heparin-responsive electrochemical sensor. J Cardiothorac Vasc Anesth 10:447-450, 1996.

839. Yang VC, Ma SC, Liu D, et al: A novel electrochemical heparin sensor. ASAIO J 39:M195-M201, 1993.

840. Hartert H: Blutgerinnungsstudien mit der Thrombelastographic, einen neuen Untersuchungsverfahren. Klin Wochenschr 16:257, 1948.

841. Mallett SV, Cox DJA: Thromboelastography. Br J Anaesth 69:307-313, 1992.

842. Shenaq SA, Saleem A: Viscoelastic measurement of clot formation: The Sonoclot. *In* Ellison N, Jobes DR (eds): Effective Hemostasis in Cardiac Surgery. Philadelphia, WB Saunders, 1988, pp 183-193.

843. Tuman KJ, Spiess BD, McCarthy RJ, Ivankovich AD: Comparison of viscoelastic measures of coagulation after cardiopulmonary bypass. Anesth Analg 69:69-75, 1989.

844. Saleem A, Blifeld C, Saleh SA, et al: Viscoelastic measurement of clot formation: A new test of platelet function. Ann Clin Lab Sci 13:115-124, 1983.

845. Zuckerman L, Cohen E, Vagher JP, et al: Comparison of thromboelastography with common coagulation tests. Thromb Haemost 46:752-756, 1981.

846. Cammerer U, Dietrich W, Rampf T, et al: The predictive value of modified computerized thromboelastography and platelet function analysis for postoperative blood loss in routine cardiac surgery. Anesth Analg 96:51-67, 2003.

847. Spiess BD, Tuman KJ, McCarthy RJ, et al: Thrombo-elastography as an indicator of post–cardiopulmonary bypass coagulopathies. J Clin Monit 3:25-30, 1987.

848. Royston D, von Kier S: Reduced haemostatic factor transfusion using heparinase-modified thromboelastography during cardiopulmonary bypass. Br J Anaesth 86:575-578, 2001.

849. Nicholson NS, Panzer-Knodle SG, Haas NF, et al: Assessment of platelet function assays. Am Heart J 135(5 Pt 2 Suppl):S170-S178, 1998.

850. Despotis GJ, Levine V, Filos KS, et al: Evaluation of a new point-of-care test that measures PAF-mediated acceleration of coagulation in cardiac surgical patients. Anesthesiology 85:1311-1323, 1996.

851. Ereth MH, Nuttall GA, Klindworth JT, et al: Does the platelet-activated clotting test (HemoSTATUS) predict blood loss and platelet dysfunction associated with cardiopulmonary bypass? Anesth Analg 85:259-264, 1997.

852. Ereth MH, Nuttall GA, Santrach PJ, et al: The relation between the platelet-activated clotting test (HemoSTATUS) and blood loss after cardiopulmonary bypass. Anesthesiology 88:962-969, 1998.

853. Coller BS, Lang D, Scudder LE: Rapid and simple platelet function assay to assess GPIIb/IIIa receptor blockade. Circulation 95:860-867, 1997.

854. Despotis GJ, Saleem R, Bigham M, Barnes P: Clinical evaluation of a new, point-of-care hemocytometer. Crit Care Med 28:1185-1190, 2000.

855. Lakkis NM, George S, Thomas E, et al: Use of ICHOR-platelet works to assess platelet function in patients treated with GP IIb/IIIA inhibitors. Cathet Cardiovasc Interv 53:346-351, 2001.

856. Carville DGM, Schleckser PA, Guyer KE, et al: Whole blood platelet function assay on the ICHOR point-of-care hematology analyzer. J Extracorpor Technol 30:171-177, 1998.

857. Kundu SK, Heilmann EJ, Sio R, et al: Description of an in vitro platelet function analyzer—PFA-100. Semin Thromb Hemost 21:106-112, 1995.

858. Fressinaud E, Veyradier A, Truchaud F, et al: Screening for von Willebrand disease with a new analyzer using high shear stress: A study of 60 cases. Blood 91:1325-1331, 1998.

859. Mammen EF, Koets MH, Washington BC, et al: Hemostasis changes during cardiopulmonary bypass surgery. Semin Thromb Hemost 11:281-292, 1985.

860. Slaughter TF, Sreeram G, Sharma AD, et al: Reversible shear-mediated platelet dysfunction during cardiac surgery as assessed by the PFA-100 platelet function analyzer. Blood Coagul Fibrinolysis 12:85-93, 2001.

861. Carr MEJ: Development of platelet contractile force as a research and clinical measure of platelet function. Cell Biochem Biophys 38:55-78, 2003.

862. Greilich PE, Brouse CF, Beckam J, et al: Reductions in platelet contractile force correlate with duration of cardiopulmonary bypass and blood loss in patients undergoing cardiac surgery. Thromb Res 105:523-529, 2002.

CHAPTER
33 Transesophageal Echocardiography

Daniel P. Vezina and Michael K. Cahalan

History   1363

Guidelines and Indications   1364

Ultrasound Principles and
   Echocardiographic Modalities   1364
   Ultrasound Principles   1364
   M-Mode and Two-Dimensional
      Echocardiography   1365
   Pulsed-Wave Doppler Echocardiography   1367
   Continuous-Wave Doppler
      Echocardiography   1369
   Color Doppler Echocardiography   1369

Equipment Design and Operation   1370

Transesophageal Echocardiographic
   Examinations   1370
   Precautions and Complications   1370
   Probe Placement   1371
   Abbreviated Examination   1372
   Comprehensive Examination   1374

Assessment of Hemodynamics   1376
   Preload   1376
   Left Ventricular Filling Pressure   1376
   Cardiac Output   1376

Global Left Ventricular Contractile
   Function   1376
Global Right Ventricular Contractile
   Function   1378
Hemodynamic Instability   1378

Myocardial Ischemia: Detection
   and Limitations   1378

Evaluation of Cardiovascular
   Pathologies   1379
   Aortic Diseases   1379
   Valvular Dysfunction   1379
   Other Pathologies   1381

Alterations of Surgical Plans and
   Assessment of Results   1383
   Atheromatous Disease of the Aorta   1383
   Valvular Heart Disease   1384
   Assessment of Surgical Results   1384

Data Storage, Documentation,
   and Quality Assurance   1384
   Data Storage and Documentation   1384
   Quality Assurance   1384

Conclusion   1385

Transesophageal echocardiography (TEE) is the most powerful cardiovascular diagnostic technique available in the practice of perioperative medicine today. Thousands of published reports document its vital role in the determination of hemodynamics, detection of myocardial ischemia, evaluation of cardiovascular pathology, and assessment of cardiac surgical plans and results. This chapter will review the literature after presenting a brief summary of TEE's history, its underlying physical principles, and the techniques required to perform it.

HISTORY

In 1976, Dr. Leon Frazin and colleagues published the results of studies using an esophageal M-mode transducer and thereby introduced the technique of TEE.[1] Subsequently, Matsumoto and coworkers used M-mode TEE to study left ventricular (LV) function during cardiovascular surgery.[2,3] However, M-mode echocardiography provides too limited a view of spatial relationships to be practical for intraoperative monitoring. In the early 1980s, Hanrath and associates introduced a two-dimensional, phased-array transducer mounted on the tip of a flexible gastroscope, and the intraoperative potential of TEE became apparent.[4] In the mid-1980s, TEE transducer design was refined,[5] and color flow Doppler technology became commercially available, thus making it possible for TEE to provide not only high-resolution, real-time images of cardiac structure and function but also simultaneous, superimposed maps of intracardiac blood flow. With these technical advances, TEE's role was ensured in the perioperative assessment of patients with a wide variety of cardiovascular diseases. With TEE as the catalyst, anesthesiologists, cardiovascular surgeons, and cardiologists began an unprecedented collaboration that has saved the lives and reduced the suffering of countless patients. No other perioperative diagnostic technique has had so great a beneficial impact on patient outcome.

GUIDELINES AND INDICATIONS

In 1996, a joint task force of the American Society of Anesthesiologists (ASA) and the Society of Cardiovascular Anesthesiologists (SCA) published guidelines for perioperative TEE in which two levels of practice (basic and advanced) were defined.[6] Anesthesiologists with basic training in perioperative TEE "should be able to use TEE for indications that lie within the customary practice of anesthesiology" and "must be able to recognize their limitations in this setting and request assistance, in a timely manner, from a physician with advanced training." Anesthesiologists with advanced training in perioperative TEE "should, in addition to the above, be able to exploit the full diagnostic potential of TEE in the perioperative period." These guidelines defined the general principles for training in perioperative TEE, including cognitive and technical objectives. In addition, the guidelines delineate three categories of evidence-based indications for TEE, including category I indications, for which TEE was judged to be frequently useful in improving clinical outcomes in the setting of hemodynamic instability, valvular pathology, cardiac source of emboli, and aortic pathology (Table 33-1). These indications were based on available data in 1995 when the task force wrote the guidelines. With the additional studies published on TEE since then, the number of category I indications would almost certainly increase should the task force revise the guidelines.

In 1999, a joint task force of the ASE and SCA published guidelines for a comprehensive TEE examination.[7] This examination will be presented in detail in a subsequent section of this chapter.

In 2002, a joint task force of the ASE and SCA published guidelines for training in perioperative TEE, including the prerequisite medical knowledge and training, echocardiographic knowledge and skills (Table 33-2), training components and duration, training environment and supervision, and equivalence requirements for postgraduate physicians already in practice.[8,9] Minimum numbers of cases are delineated (Table 33-3); however, these numbers are less important than the depth and diversity of the clinical experience and the quality of training. Like previous published guidelines, these guidelines provide training recommendations for a basic level and an advanced level of perioperative echocardiography. Unlike previous guidelines, these guidelines do not specify the duration of training. Instead, they emphasize the goals of training and the number and diversity of cases required to meet these goals. The time required for perioperative training will vary markedly and depends on the volume and diversity of the affiliated cardiac surgical program.

ULTRASOUND PRINCIPLES AND ECHOCARDIOGRAPHIC MODALITIES

Ultrasound Principles

Sound waves are mechanical vibrations that create refraction and compression of the medium through which they travel. Humans can hear sound waves with frequencies ranging from 20 cycles/sec (Hz) to 20 kHz. Beyond this range is ultrasound. Echocardiography uses ultrasound waves with frequencies of 2.5 to 7.5 million cycles/sec (MHz). Frequencies greater than 7.5 MHz are not routinely used in echocardiography because they produce wavelengths too short for adequate penetration into tissues (penetration is limited to about 200 to 400 times the wavelength). Frequencies less than 2.5 MHz are not routinely used because they produce wavelengths too long for resolution of small objects (resolution is limited to about twice the wavelength). The interrelationship of wavelength and frequency is described by the following equation:

$$C = \lambda \cdot F$$

where C = velocity of sound in tissue (1540 m/sec), F = frequency (Hz), and λ = wavelength (m). Because the velocity of sound is assumed to be constant, the wavelength of any frequency can be calculated as

$$\lambda \text{ (m)} = 1540 \text{ (m/sec)}/F \text{ (Hz), or}$$

$$\lambda \text{ (mm)} = 1,540,000 \text{ (mm/sec)}/F \text{ (Hz) or}$$

$$\lambda \text{ (mm)} = 1.54/F \text{ (MHz)}$$

Thus, ultrasound waves in the range of 2.5 to 7.5 MHz produce wavelengths of 0.2 to 0.6 mm, resolve objects 0.4 to 1.2 mm in size, and penetrate tissues up to 24 cm.

Ultrasound waves are generated by piezoelectric crystals that emit ultrasound when electricity is applied to them and emit electricity when struck by ultrasound. Thus, the same crystals can serve as emitters and receivers of ultrasound. Typically in echocardiography, the crystals emit very short pulses of ultrasound (approximately 1 μsec) and receive or "listen" for the reflected ultrasound for 250 to 500 μsec. When the emitted waves strike an interface of tissues of differing density, such as the pericardium and the heart, a portion of the ultrasound is reflected. The portion reflected depends on the difference in tissue density; that is, the greater the difference, the greater the portion reflected. For example, air in the left ventricle reflects a much greater portion of the transmitted ultrasound than blood does and is translated as a brighter signal on the display screen. Tissue is localized according to the time that it takes a sound wave to bounce back to the transducer; that is, the longer a sound wave takes to bounce back, the greater its distance from the transducer. For example, if it takes 26 μsec for the wave to return to the transducer, the ultrasonograph (often called an "echo machine") displays a structure that is 1 cm from the transducer. No ionizing radiation of any type is used in echocardiography, and no adverse effects of ultrasound have been demonstrated in humans.

Table 33–1   Indications for perioperative transesophageal echocardiography

Category I indications: Supported by the strongest evidence or expert opinion; TEE is frequently useful in improving clinical outcomes in the following settings and is often indicated, depending on individual circumstances:

Intraoperative evaluation of acute, persistent, and life-threatening hemodynamic disturbances in which ventricular function and its determinants are uncertain and have not responded to treatment

Intraoperative use in valve repair

Intraoperative use in congenital heart surgery for most lesions requiring cardiopulmonary bypass

Intraoperative use in repair of hypertrophic obstructive cardiomyopathy

Intraoperative use for endocarditis when preoperative testing was inadequate or extension of infection to perivalvular tissue is suspected

Preoperative use in unstable patients with suspected thoracic aortic aneurysms, dissection, or disruption who need to be evaluated quickly

Intraoperative assessment of aortic valve function in repair of aortic dissections with possible aortic valve involvement

Intraoperative evaluation of pericardial window procedures

Use in the intensive care unit for unstable patients with unexplained hemodynamic disturbances, suspected valve disease, or thromboembolic problems (if other tests or monitoring techniques have not confirmed the diagnosis or patients are too unstable to undergo other tests)

Category II indications: Supported by weaker evidence and expert consensus; TEE may be useful in improving clinical outcomes in the following settings, depending on individual circumstances, but appropriate indications are less certain:

Perioperative use in patients with an increased risk of myocardial ischemia or infarction

Perioperative use in patients with an increased risk of hemodynamic disturbances

Intraoperative assessment of valve replacement

Intraoperative assessment of repair of cardiac aneurysms

Intraoperative evaluation of removal of cardiac tumors

Intraoperative detection of foreign bodies

Intraoperative detection of air emboli during cardiotomy, heart transplant operations, and upright neurosurgical procedures

Intraoperative use during intracardiac thrombectomy

Intraoperative use during pulmonary embolectomy

Intraoperative use for suspected cardiac trauma

Preoperative assessment of patients with suspected acute thoracic aortic dissections, aneurysms, or disruption

Intraoperative use during repair of thoracic aortic dissections without suspected aortic valve involvement

Intraoperative detection of aortic atheromatous disease or other sources of aortic emboli

Intraoperative evaluation of pericardiectomy, pericardial effusions, or pericardial surgery

Intraoperative evaluation of anastomotic sites during heart and/or lung transplantation

Monitoring placement and function of assist devices

Category III indications: Little current scientific or expert support; TEE is infrequently useful in improving clinical outcomes in the following settings, and appropriate indications are uncertain:

Intraoperative evaluation of myocardial perfusion, coronary artery anatomy, or graft patency

Intraoperative use during repair of cardiomyopathies other than hypertrophic obstructive cardiomyopathy

Intraoperative use for uncomplicated endocarditis during noncardiac surgery

Intraoperative monitoring for emboli during orthopedic procedures

Intraoperative assessment of repair of thoracic aortic injuries

Intraoperative use for uncomplicated pericarditis

Intraoperative evaluation of pleuropulmonary diseases

Monitoring placement of intra-aortic balloon pumps, automatic implantable cardiac defibrillators, or pulmonary artery catheters

Intraoperative monitoring of cardioplegia administration

Adapted from Practice guidelines for perioperative transesophageal echocardiography. A report by the American Society of Anesthesiologists and the Society of Cardiovascular Anesthesiologists Task Force on Transesophageal Echocardiography. Anesthesiology 84:986-1006, 1996.

M-mode and Two-Dimensional Echocardiography

Because the propagation velocity of ultrasound in tissue is constant, the distance between the transducer and the reflective structure will be determined by the time that it takes the initial signal to go and come back.

This information can be displayed different ways. The first echocardiograms, "motion" or "M-mode" studies, were one-dimensional views of cardiac structures produced by single-crystal transducers with the results traced on moving photosensitive paper. Today, M-mode echocardiography is used principally to view rapidly moving structures,

Table 33–2   Recommended training objectives for basic and advanced perioperative echocardiography

Basic Training

Cognitive Skills

1. Knowledge of the physical principles of echocardiographic image formation and blood velocity measurement
2. Knowledge of the operation of ultrasonographs, including all controls that affect the quality of data displayed
3. Knowledge of equipment handling, infection control, and electrical safety associated with the techniques of perioperative echocardiography
4. Knowledge of the indications, contraindications, and potential complications of perioperative echocardiography
5. Knowledge of the appropriate alternative diagnostic techniques
6. Knowledge of the normal tomographic anatomy as revealed by perioperative echocardiographic techniques
7. Knowledge of commonly encountered blood flow velocity profiles as measured by Doppler echocardiography
8. Knowledge of the echocardiographic manifestations of native valvular lesions and dysfunction
9. Knowledge of the echocardiographic manifestations of cardiac masses, thrombi, cardiomyopathies, pericardial effusions, and lesions of the great vessels
10. Detailed knowledge of the echocardiographic manifestations of myocardial ischemia and infarction
11. Detailed knowledge of the echocardiographic manifestations of normal and abnormal ventricular function
12. Detailed knowledge of the echocardiographic manifestations of air embolization

Technical Skills

1. Ability to operate ultrasonographs, including the primary controls affecting the quality of the displayed data
2. Ability to insert a TEE probe safely in an anesthetized, tracheally intubated patient
3. Ability to perform a comprehensive TEE examination and differentiate normal from markedly abnormal cardiac structures and function
4. Ability to recognize marked changes in segmental ventricular contraction indicative of myocardial ischemia or infarction
5. Ability to recognize marked changes in global ventricular filling and ejection
6. Ability to recognize air embolization
7. Ability to recognize gross valvular lesions and dysfunction
8. Ability to recognize large intracardiac masses and thrombi
9. Ability to detect large pericardial effusions
10. Ability to recognize common echocardiographic artifacts
11. Ability to communicate echocardiographic results effectively to health care professionals, the medical record, and patients
12. Ability to recognize complications of perioperative echocardiography

Advanced Training

Cognitive Skills

1. All the cognitive skills defined under Basic Training
2. Detailed knowledge of the principles and methodologies of qualitative and quantitative echocardiography
3. Detailed knowledge of native and prosthetic valvular function, including valvular lesions and dysfunction
4. Knowledge of congenital heart disease (if congenital heart disease practice is planned, this knowledge must be detailed)
5. Detailed knowledge of all other diseases of the heart and great vessels that is relevant in the perioperative period (if pediatric practice is planned, this knowledge may be more general than detailed)
6. Detailed knowledge of the techniques, advantages, disadvantages, and potential complications of commonly used cardiac surgical procedures for the treatment of acquired and congenital heart disease
7. Detailed knowledge of other diagnostic methods appropriate for correlation with perioperative echocardiography

Technical Skills

1. All the technical skills defined under Basic Training
2. Ability to acquire or direct the acquisition of all necessary echocardiographic data, including epicardial and epiaortic imaging
3. Ability to recognize subtle changes in segmental ventricular contraction indicative of myocardial ischemia or infarction
4. Ability to quantify systolic and diastolic ventricular function and to estimate other relevant hemodynamic parameters
5. Ability to quantify normal and abnormal native and prosthetic valvular function
6. Ability to assess the appropriateness of cardiac surgical plans
7. Ability to identify inadequacies in cardiac surgical interventions and the underlying reasons for the inadequacies
8. Ability to aid in clinical decision making in the operating room

From Cahalan MK, Abel M, Goldman M, et al: American Society of Echocardiography and Society of Cardiovascular Anesthesiologists task force guidelines for training in perioperative echocardiography. Anesth Analg 94:1384-1388, 2002.

Table 33–3   Numbers of examinations and other key training recommendations for basic and advanced perioperative echocardiography

	Basic*	Advanced*
Minimum number of examinations†	150	300
Minimum number personally performed‡	50	150
Program director qualifications	Advanced perioperative echocardiography training	Advanced perioperative echocardiography training plus at least 150 additional perioperative TEE examinations
Program qualifications	Wide variety of perioperative applications of echocardiography	Full spectrum of perioperative applications of echocardiography

*Totals for basic training may be counted toward advanced training provided that the basic training was completed in an advanced training environment. See the text for additional details and explanation of training environments and program director qualifications.
†Complete echocardiographic examinations interpreted and reported by the trainee under appropriate supervision. Transthoracic studies recorded by qualified individuals other than the trainee may be included.
‡Comprehensive intraoperative TEE examinations personally performed, interpreted, and reported by the trainee under appropriate supervision.
From Cahalan MK, Abel M, Goldman M, et al: American Society of Echocardiography and Society of Cardiovascular Anesthesiologists task force guidelines for training in perioperative echocardiography. Anesth Analg 94:1384-1388, 2002.

such as valve leaflets, because M-mode transducers can produce up to 1800 images per second (Fig. 33-1). However, M-mode images reveal only a small portion of the heart at one time, thus making orientation and interpretation of spatial relationships difficult.

By using multiple crystals (linear or phased-array transducers) or rapidly moving a single crystal (mechanical transducer), multiple views can be obtained and collated into a two-dimensional image. Although two-dimensional techniques produce only about 30 images per second, definition in two dimensions provides an enormous advantage in recognizing anatomic and pathologic landmarks (Fig. 33-2). Images are displayed in "real time" on a monitor screen and recorded on videotape or digital format for later review. By altering the position or angle of the ultrasound beam, the operator produces multiple cross-sectional (tomographic) images revealing the external and internal anatomy and function of the heart and great vessels.

Pulsed-Wave Doppler Echocardiography

By measuring Doppler shift, modern ultrasonographs quantify blood flow velocities. Doppler shift is the shift in frequency of a wave when the source of the wave is moving (in this case, the wave reflected by moving red blood cells). When pulses of sound are used (pulsed-wave [PW] Doppler), the operator defines a small area (termed "sample volume") anywhere in the two-dimensional sector scan, and the ultrasonograph automatically converts the Doppler data in that sample volume to a display of the real-time blood flow velocities (Fig. 33-3). Thus, PW Doppler defines blood flow velocities and their location within the heart and great vessels.

However, two important limitations apply. First, Doppler shift is proportional to the cosine of the angle

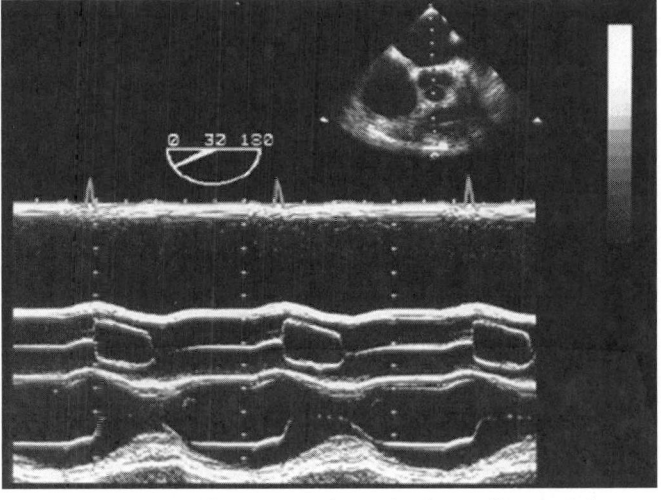

Figure 33–1 M-mode transesophageal echocardiogram of a normal aortic valve. For reference, a single frame (stop action) of the two-dimensional cross section is shown at the top right of the figure. The *dotted vertical line* through the two-dimensional echocardiogram depicts the single line of sampling provided by the M-mode echocardiogram over time (the horizontal axis for the lower two thirds of the figure). The electrocardiogram defines systole and diastole. Note in the middle of the M-mode image the three *tilted rectangles* connected by the *slightly undulating line*. These rectangles and lines are formed by the motion of the leaflets of the aortic valve as they open and close during the cardiac cycles shown. From top to bottom in this M-mode echocardiogram, the structures indicated by the *white lines* are the posterior wall of the left atrium (just under the electrocardiogram), the posterior wall of the aortic annulus, the aortic valve (as described above), the anterior wall of the aortic annulus, a pulmonary artery catheter, and the myocardium of the right ventricular outflow tract. (From Cahalan MK: Intraoperative Transesophageal Echocardiography. An Interactive Text and Atlas. New York, Churchill Livingstone, 1997.)

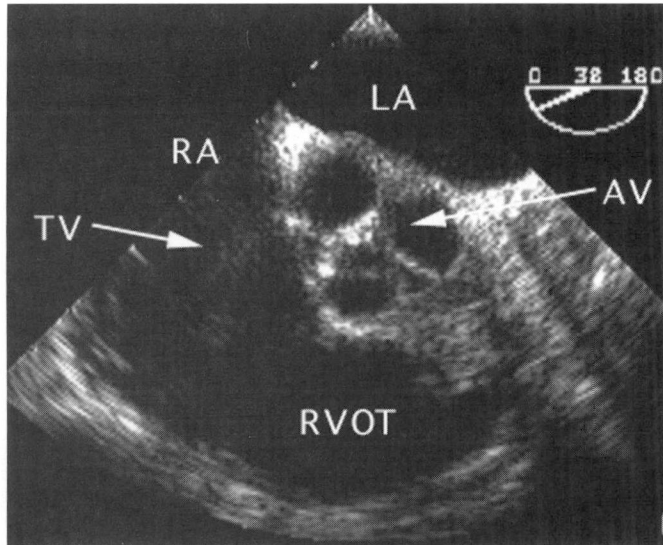

Figure 33–2 Short-axis two-dimensional cross section of a normal aortic valve (AV). This midesophageal short-axis view of the AV reveals the morphology of the three cusps of this normal valve. LA, left atrium; RA, right atrium; RVOT, right ventricular outflow tract; TV, tricuspid valve. (From Cahalan MK: Intraoperative Transesophageal Echocardiography. An Interactive Text and Atlas. New York, Churchill Livingstone, 1997.)

between the ultrasound beam and the direction of the blood cells. If the cells are moving directly parallel to the ultrasound beam, the angle is zero, and the cosine of zero is one. Thus, at an angle of zero, Doppler echocardiography provides a true estimate of blood flow velocity.

At all other angles the cosine is less than one, which results in less Doppler shift and an underestimation of flow velocity. Clinically, angles less than 15 degrees (the cosine is almost one) are insignificant in the estimation of velocity, whereas angles exceeding 20 degrees markedly attenuate the Doppler shift and thus necessitate caution in interpreting such data. This relationship is best stated in the following Doppler equation:

$$V = C \cdot (F_d)/(2F_0 \cdot \cos \theta)$$

where V is the velocity to be measured, C is the speed of sound in tissue (a constant), F_d is the Doppler shift in ultrasound frequency measured by the ultrasound machine, F_0 is the frequency of the transducer, and $\cos \theta$ is the cosine of the angle between the direction of the blood flow and the ultrasound waves. Second, the maximum velocity of blood flow that can be unambiguously measured is defined by the Nyquist limit. The Nyquist limit is directly related to the ultrasound frequency and the pulse repetition frequency. The pulse repetition frequency is the number of pulses of ultrasound emitted per second. Because an emitted pulse must return before the next pulse is emitted in PW Doppler, an increase in depth of the ultrasound scan decreases the pulse repetition frequency and the Nyquist limit. Thus, the depth of the ultrasound scan is the principal determinant of the Nyquist limit under the control of the operator. If the velocity of blood flow exceeds the Nyquist limit, sudden apparent flow reversal ("aliasing") will be depicted (Fig. 33-4). Aliasing is analogous to the sudden apparent reversal of direction in stagecoach wheels visible in old Westerns when the velocity of the wheel spokes exceeds the frame

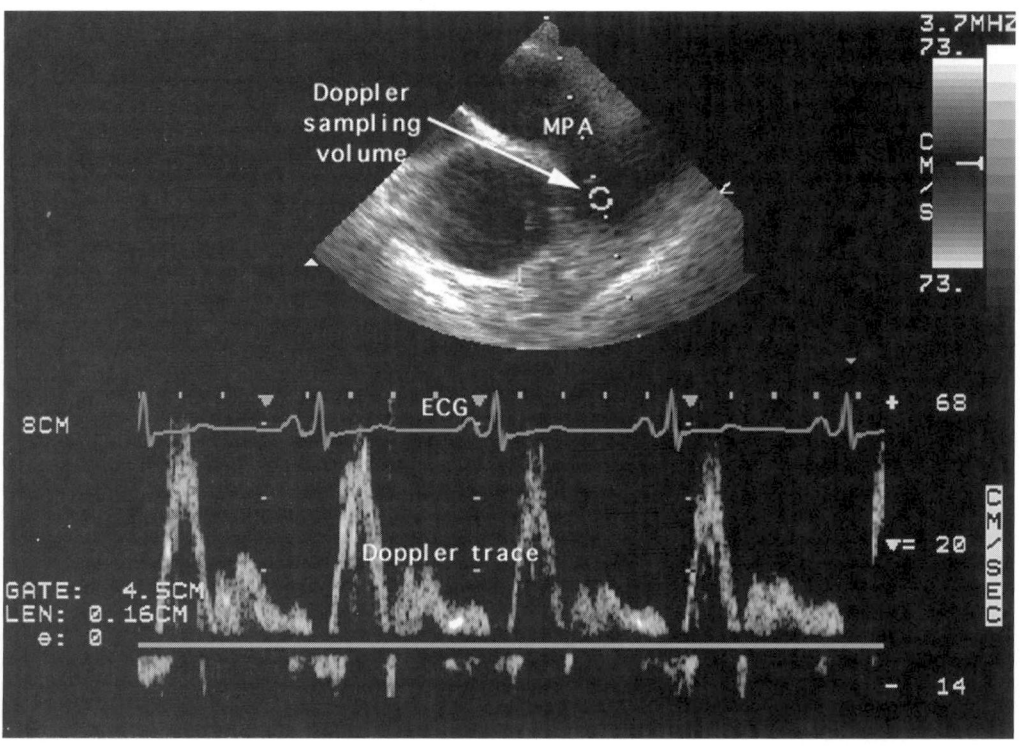

Figure 33–3 Pulsed-wave Doppler echocardiogram of the main pulmonary artery (MPA). At the top of the echocardiogram is a still-frame image of the two-dimensional cross section used to position the Doppler sample volume (the *round white sphere*). On the bottom two thirds of the echocardiogram is the display in white of the instantaneous blood flow velocities (vertical axis) versus time (horizontal axis) occurring in that sample volume. The electrocardiogram provides timing, and the *bold horizontal line* is the baseline (zero flow) for the flow velocities. Flow velocities above this line are positive (i.e., toward the transducer) to a maximum of 68 cm/sec. Flow below this line is negative (i.e., away from the transducer) to a maximum of −14 cm/sec. (From Cahalan MK: Intraoperative Transesophageal Echocardiography. An Interactive Text and Atlas. New York, Churchill Livingstone, 1997.)

Figure 33–4 Pulsed-wave Doppler with aliasing at high velocities. Pulsed-wave Doppler measurement of blood flow velocities in a mitral valve (MV) orifice during four cardiac cycles is shown. At the top of the figure is a still-frame image of the two-dimensional cross section used to position the Doppler sample volume (the *round white sphere*). On the bottom two thirds of the figure is the display in white of the instantaneous blood flow velocities (vertical axis) versus time (horizontal axis) occurring in that sample volume. The electrocardiogram provides timing, and the *bold horizontal line* is the baseline (zero flow) for the flow velocities. Flow velocities above this line are positive (i.e., toward the transducer) to a maximum of 183 cm/sec. Flow velocities below this line are negative (i.e., away from the transducer)

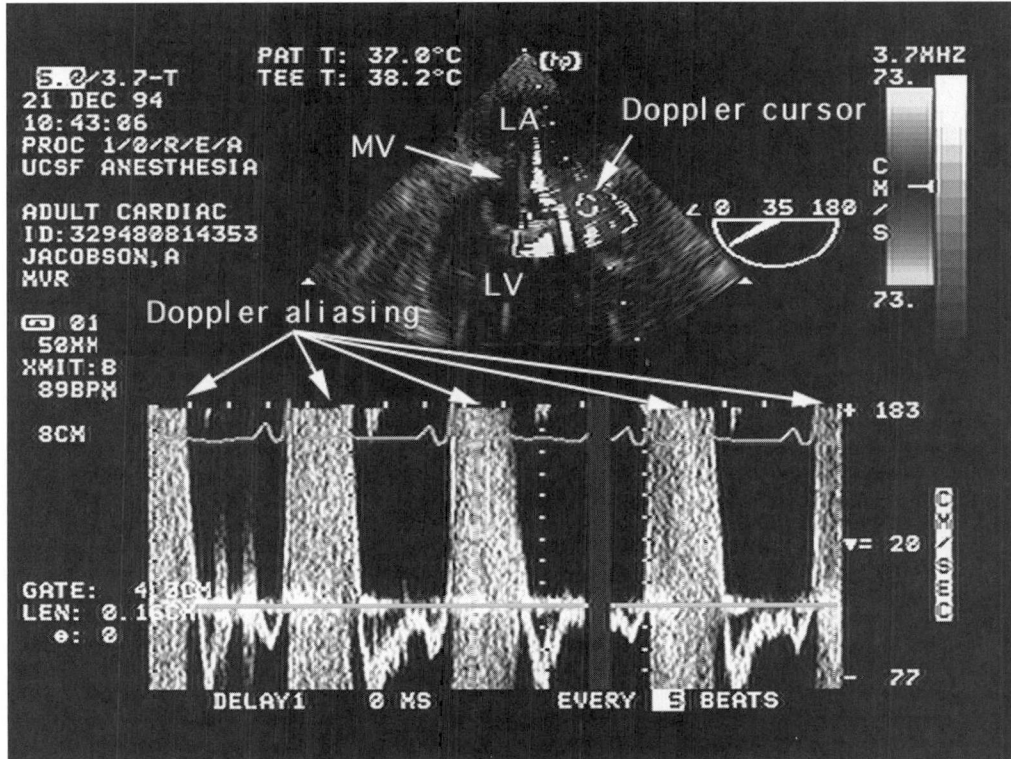

to a maximum of –77 cm/sec. This tracing documents significant mitral regurgitation (the positive systolic velocities) but does not measure the peak velocity of regurgitant flow because it is beyond the Nyquist limit—the systolic velocities off the top of the scale are said to alias, that is, they go off scale and wrap around into the domain of negative velocities. LA, left atrium; LV, left ventricle. (From Cahalan MK: Intraoperative Transesophageal Echocardiography. An Interactive Text and Atlas. New York, Churchill Livingstone, 1997.)

rate of the movie camera. Typically, aliasing of PW Doppler occurs at blood flow velocities of 0.8 to 1.0 m/sec. Normal flow within the heart may reach 1.4 m/sec, and pathologic flow, up to 6 m/sec. To measure these velocities, continuous-wave (CW) Doppler is needed.

Continuous-Wave Doppler Echocardiography

CW Doppler uses two separate crystals: one to continuously emit ultrasound and one to continuously receive it. CW Doppler is basically PW Doppler with an infinite pulse repetition frequency that eliminates the problem of aliasing (Fig. 33-5). However, this infinite pulse repetition rate allows insufficient time for the first pulse to return to the transducer before the next is emitted. Consequently, the ultrasonograph cannot determine which pulse of sound was frequency shifted and therefore cannot precisely define the location of the moving target. Nonetheless, the maximum velocity can prove to be vital information: by simplification of the Bernoulli equation, Holen and colleagues and Hatle and coworkers have proven that

$$\Delta P = 4V^2$$

where ΔP is the peak gradient across a stenosis and V is the maximum velocity determined by CW Doppler in meters per second.[10,11] Thus, CW Doppler defines higher blood flow velocities than PW does, but unlike the latter,

CW Doppler cannot precisely define the location of the velocities.

Color Doppler Echocardiography

Point-by-point determination of blood flow velocities by PW Doppler is too time consuming and does not reveal the instantaneous distribution of flow velocities within the cross-sectional image that is required for many diagnostic decisions. Color Doppler imaging was developed for this purpose. In color Doppler, which is a form of PW Doppler, a color code is used to depict flow toward (red) and away (blue) from the transducer; lighter and darker shades of red and blue respectively denote relatively faster and slower velocities. Continuous color maps of flow are superimposed on gray-scale cross-sectional echocardiograms. However, color Doppler is generally a semiquantitative technique and, like PW Doppler, will alias (color reversal) when the Nyquist limit is exceeded. Two aliasing patterns are easily recognized. The first is "normal" aliasing in which the area of apparent flow reversal forms one or more broad, relatively homogeneous color surfaces (Plate 33-1). Blood flow velocities within a normal heart often produce this type of aliasing because they exceed the Nyquist limit for color Doppler (0.6 to 0.8 m/sec). The second type of aliasing results from disturbed or turbulent flow within the heart (e.g., mitral regurgitation) and is never normal (Plate 33-2). When the ultrasonograph detects two different velocities

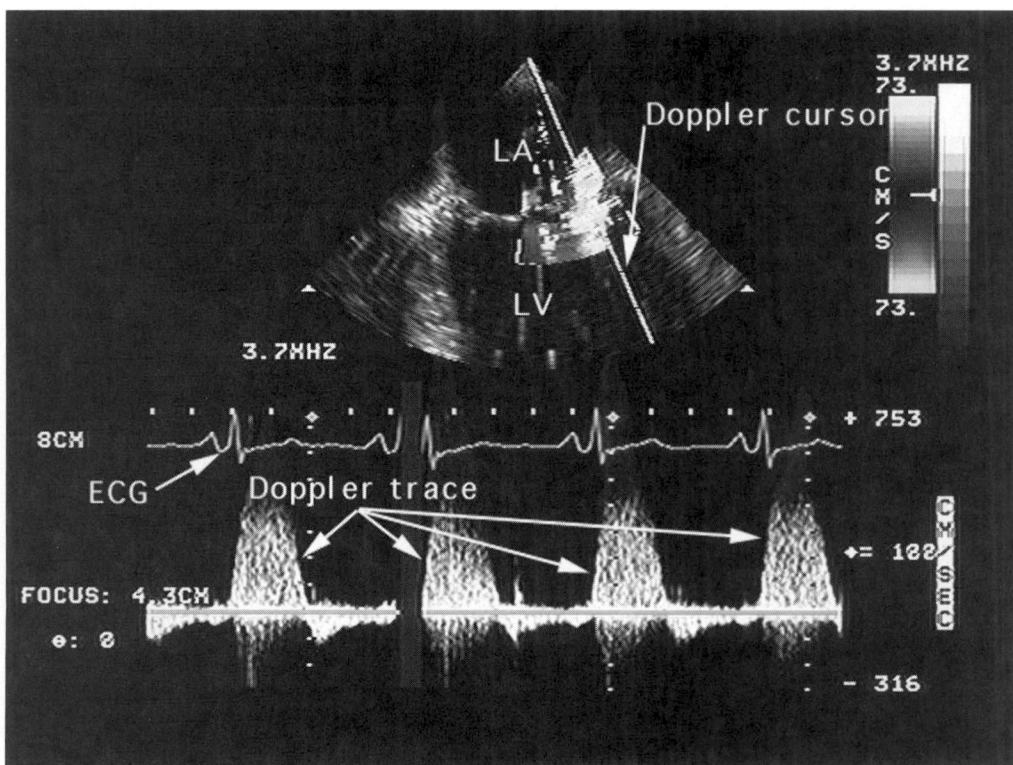

Figure 33–5 Continuous-wave Doppler measures high-velocity flow without aliasing. Continuous-wave Doppler measurement of blood flow velocities in a mitral valve orifice during four cardiac cycles is shown. At the top of the figure is a still-frame image of the two-dimensional cross section used to position the Doppler sample cursor (the *diagonal white line*). On the bottom two thirds of the figure is the display in white of all the instantaneous blood flow velocities (vertical axis) versus time (horizontal axis) occurring anywhere along that cursor. The electrocardiogram provides timing, and the *bold horizontal line* is the baseline (zero flow) for the flow velocities. Flow velocities above this line are positive (i.e., toward the transducer) to a maximum of 753 cm/sec. Flow velocities below this line are negative (i.e., away from the transducer) to a maximum of −316 cm/sec. This tracing documents significant mitral regurgitation (the positive systolic velocities) with a peak blood flow velocity of approximately 5 m/sec (each *white dot* on the vertical axis equals 100 cm/sec or 1 m/sec). LA, left atrium; LV, left ventricle. (From Cahalan MK: Intraoperative Transesophageal Echocardiography. An Interactive Text and Atlas. New York, Churchill Livingstone, 1997.)

within the same small sample volume (because of disturbed flow), it displays a mixture or mosaic of colors. These mosaics form jetlike configurations and are called "color jets." Because color Doppler presents the spatial relationships between structure and blood flow, it enhances the recognition of valvular abnormalities and intracardiac shunts.

EQUIPMENT DESIGN AND OPERATION

TEE probes are a marvel of engineering: a miniaturized echocardiographic transducer (about 40 mm long, 13 mm wide, and 11 mm thick) mounted on the tip of a gastroscope. Typically, the transducer is a phased-array configuration with 64 piezoelectric elements operating at 3.7 to 7.5 MHz. By means of sequential firing of the elements and an acoustic lens in the transducer housing, the ultrasound waves are formed into a 90-degree beam approximately 1 mm in thickness that emanates at right angles to the transducer. Like standard gastroscopes, two rotary knobs ("wheels") control movement of the tip of the scope. One of the wheels anteflexes and retroflexes the transducer (i.e., moves the transducer toward and away from the heart). The other wheel flexes the transducer rightward and leftward (Fig. 33-6).

Multiplane transducers use the same transducer technology, but mount the transducer on a rotating device that allows it to spin on its axis from 0 to 180 degrees within the tip of the gastroscope (transducer housing) (Fig. 33-6).

Because cardiac structures and blood flow are not precisely aligned relative to the transducer, this design has significantly refined imaging capability. By reducing the number of crystals and further miniaturizing transducers, manufacturers have produced transducers small enough for use in infants and neonates (Fig. 33-7).

Ultrasonographs contain high-powered computers capable of initiating the ultrasound beam and processing the returning data. A series of electronic transforms (some guarded commercial secrets) produce the real-time images displayed on the video screen. All ultrasonographs share common technical aspects, including gain, depth, and Doppler controls. However, the differences in technical aspects between manufacturers and even between models from the same manufacturer are sufficiently great that they prevent the formulation of any universal operating instructions. Fortunately, detailed instructions for each model are available in the operator's manual supplied with each ultrasonograph. Alternatively, cardiac sonographers are often excellent sources of instruction in the operation of these machines.

TRANSESOPHAGEAL ECHOCARDIOGRAPHIC EXAMINATIONS

Precautions and Complications

Before performing TEE, the operator must determine that the benefits of TEE outweigh the risks. Except in

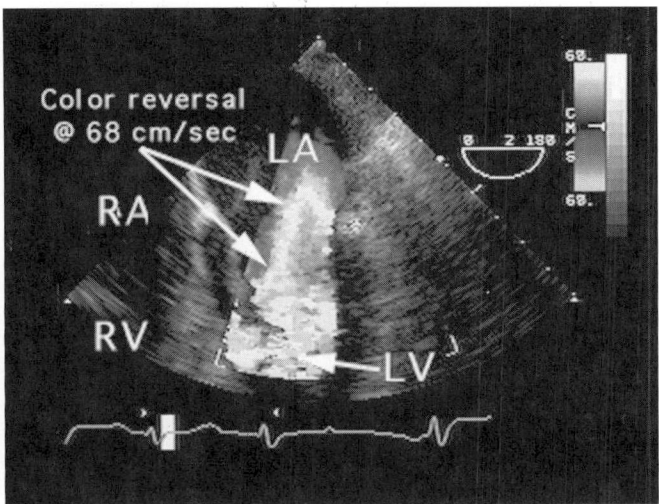

Plate 33–1 "Normal" color Doppler aliasing. In this echocardiogram, "normal" color Doppler aliasing is seen because laminar flow of blood through the mitral valve and into the left ventricle exceeds the Nyquist limit (68 cm/sec in this example—see the color reference icon at the upper right of the figure), thereby resulting in reversal of the color coding of flow direction. Notice that this color reversal occurs across fairly broad, regular areas and not in a random or point-by-point fashion as occurs with turbulent flow (always abnormal). In this example, follow the blue flow from high in the left atrium as it accelerates into the mitral orifice, and notice how color Doppler depicts the increasing flow velocities: the blue color becomes lighter and lighter until the Nyquist limit is reached. Then, color reversal occurs, with light blue becoming yellow. Just at that reversal point, the velocity equals the Nyquist limit, in this example 68 cm/sec. Subsequent reversals may occur at that limit or at multiples of that limit. LA, left atrium; LV, left ventricle; RA, right atrium; RV, right ventricle. (From Cahalan MK: Intraoperative Transesophageal Echocardiography. An Interactive Text and Atlas. New York, Churchill Livingstone, 1997.)

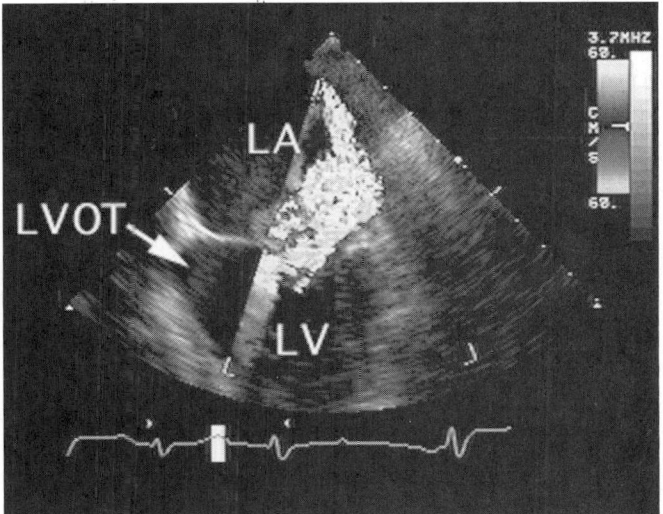

Plate 33–2 Color Doppler aliasing depicting turbulent flow. In this echocardiogram, color Doppler reveals aliasing caused by severe mitral regurgitation: a broad-based systolic color jet emanating from the mitral valve and extending far into the left atrium. This jet is composed of a mosaic of colors mixed in a seemingly random, point-by-point fashion because the jet results from the turbulent flow of mitral regurgitation. Turbulence is never normal in the heart, and thus mosaic jets such as the one shown here are highly valuable diagnostic signs of underlying pathology. LA, left atrium; LV, left ventricle; LVOT, left ventricular outflow tract. (From Cahalan MK: Intraoperative Transesophageal Echocardiography. An Interactive Text and Atlas. New York, Churchill Livingstone, 1997.)

the presence of esophageal disease or injury, the risk is quite low. Absolute contraindications include previous esophagectomy, severe esophageal obstruction, esophageal perforation, and ongoing esophageal hemorrhage. Relative contraindications include esophageal diverticula, varices, and fistulas; previous esophageal surgery; and a history of previous gastric surgery, mediastinal irradiation, unexplained swallowing difficulties, and other conditions that might be worsened by placement and manipulation of the TEE probe.

In some studies, TEE has been associated with an infrequent incidence of oral and pharyngeal injuries (0.1% to 0.3%), but in other studies the incidence of postoperative gastrointestinal complaints did not differ significantly from that in comparable patients who had not undergone TEE.[12-15] Uncontrolled studies have reported a 0.1% to 12% incidence of transient hoarseness after TEE. Serious pharyngeal or esophageal injury after TEE has been reported but is rare.[16-24] Two case report indicate the possibility of TEE-associated splenic injury.[25,26] Among 10,218 patients (European multicenter study) undergoing TEE (primarily outpatients), esophageal perforation occurred in 1, who subsequently died; autopsy revealed a malignant tumor invading the esophagus.[27]

Although bacteremia during TEE is uncommon, endocarditis has been reported in outpatients.[28-30] Endocarditis from intraoperative TEE has not been reported, and the risk is probably near zero because antibiotics are usually administered for prevention of surgical wound infection. In infants, TEE has a low complication rate, but even an appropriately sized TEE probe may obstruct the airway distal to the endotracheal tube or compress the descending aorta.[31-33]

Probe Placement

Once the patient is anesthetized and the trachea securely intubated, the contents of the stomach are suctioned. Gentle massage of the left upper quadrant of the abdomen during suctioning may help remove air, which can otherwise degrade imaging. The patient's neck is then extended, and a well-lubricated TEE probe is introduced into the midline of the hypopharynx with the transducer side facing anteriorly. Usually, with minimal force, the probe will pass blindly into the esophagus, especially if the neck is extended. If the probe does not pass blindly, a laryngoscope is used to lift the larynx anteriorly and the probe is placed into the esophagus under direct vision. During transducer insertion or withdrawal, the controls of the gastroscope must be in the neutral or relaxed position to allow the transducer to follow the natural course of the esophagus, thereby potentially minimizing the risk of injury.

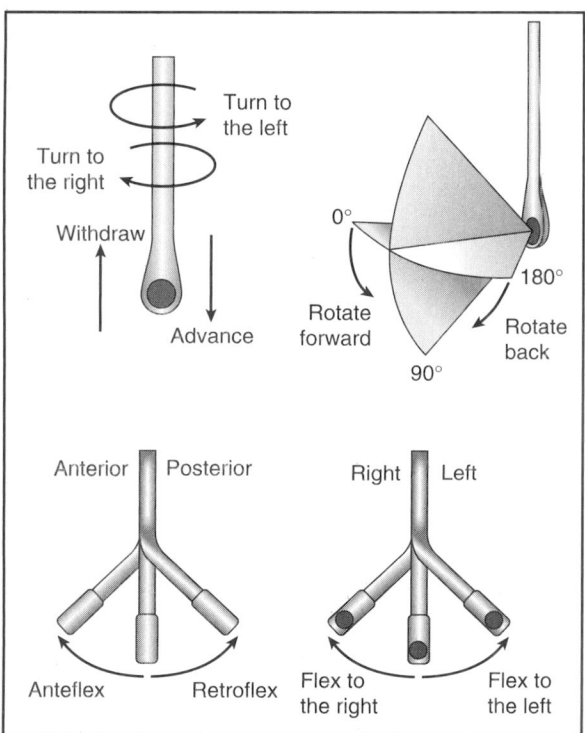

Figure 33–6 The terminology used to describe TEE probe movements is illustrated. (From Shanewise JS, Cheung AT, Aronson S, et al: ASE/SCA guidelines for performing a comprehensive intraoperative multiplane transesophageal echocardiography examination: Recommendations of the American Society of Echocardiography Council for Intraoperative Echocardiography and the Society of Cardiovascular Anesthesiologists Task Force for Certification in Perioperative Transesophageal Echocardiography. Anesth Analg 89:870-884, 1999.)

Abbreviated Examination

Because of time constraints and relatively narrow diagnostic goals, anesthesiologists often perform a more limited intraoperative examination than described in the ASE/SCA's task force recommendation for a comprehensive TEE examination (see the subsequent section).[7,34] However, even when time is critical, the examination performed should allow at least the basic applications of TEE as outlined in the 1996 guidelines for perioperative TEE: detection of markedly abnormal ventricular filling or function, extensive myocardial ischemia or infarction, large air embolism, severe valvular dysfunction, large cardiac masses or thrombi, large pericardial effusions, and major lesions of the great vessels.[6] A minimum of eight different cross sections drawn from the 20 cross sections delineated in the comprehensive examination are required to meet these diagnostic goals. Four of the cross sections are imaged in both two-dimensional and color Doppler to assess valvular function. The next paragraph describes the probe manipulations required to achieve these cross sections. The reader should review Figure 33-8 to understand the terms used in this description.

After the TEE probe is introduced safely into the esophagus, it is advanced to the midesophageal (ME) level (28 to 32 cm measured at the upper incisors), and the

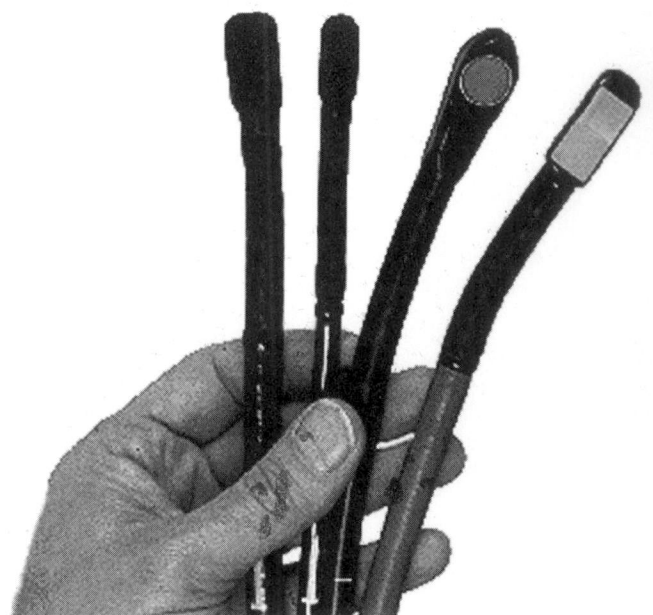

Figure 33–7 Four TEE probes compared. From left to right the probes are single plane, pediatric single plane, multiplane, and biplane. The probe tips are viewed in their maximum dimension. (From Cahalan MK: Intraoperative Transesophageal Echocardiography. An Interactive Text and Atlas. New York, Churchill Livingstone, 1997.)

aortic valve (AV) is imaged in the short axis (SAX) by turning the probe, adjusting its depth in the esophagus, and rotating the multiplane transducer to 25 to 45 degrees until the three cusps of the valve are seen as approximately equal in size and shape (Fig. 33-8H). Image depth is set at 10 to 12 cm as required to position the AV in the center of the video screen. This cross section is ideal for detection of aortic stenosis. The videotape is activated at this point and kept running throughout the rest of the examination. Videotape is very inexpensive relative to the cost of a missed diagnosis. Next, the probe is turned slightly to position the AV in the center of the video screen, and the multiplane angle is then rotated forward to 110 to 130 degrees to bring the long axis (LAX) of the AV in view (Fig. 33-8I). This cross section is best for detection of ascending aortic abnormalities, including type I aortic dissection. Color Doppler is used for assessment of AV competence. For detection of valvular stenosis and regurgitation, the maximum possible Nyquist limit is used (ideally, above 50 cm/sec). Next, Doppler is discontinued and the probe is turned rightward until the ME bicaval cross section comes into view (Fig. 33-8L). This cross section is usually seen best at a multiplane angle between 90 and 110 degrees and is ideal for assessing caval abnormalities, compression of the right atrium from anteriorly located masses or effusions, and compression of the left atrium from posteriorly located masses or effusions. In addition, the bicaval cross section may reveal collections of air located anteriorly in the left or right atrium, as well as the structure of the interatrial septum, including the foramen ovale. Next, the multiplane angle is rotated back to 60 to 80 degrees and the probe is turned leftward just past the AV to bring the ME right ventricular (RV) inflow

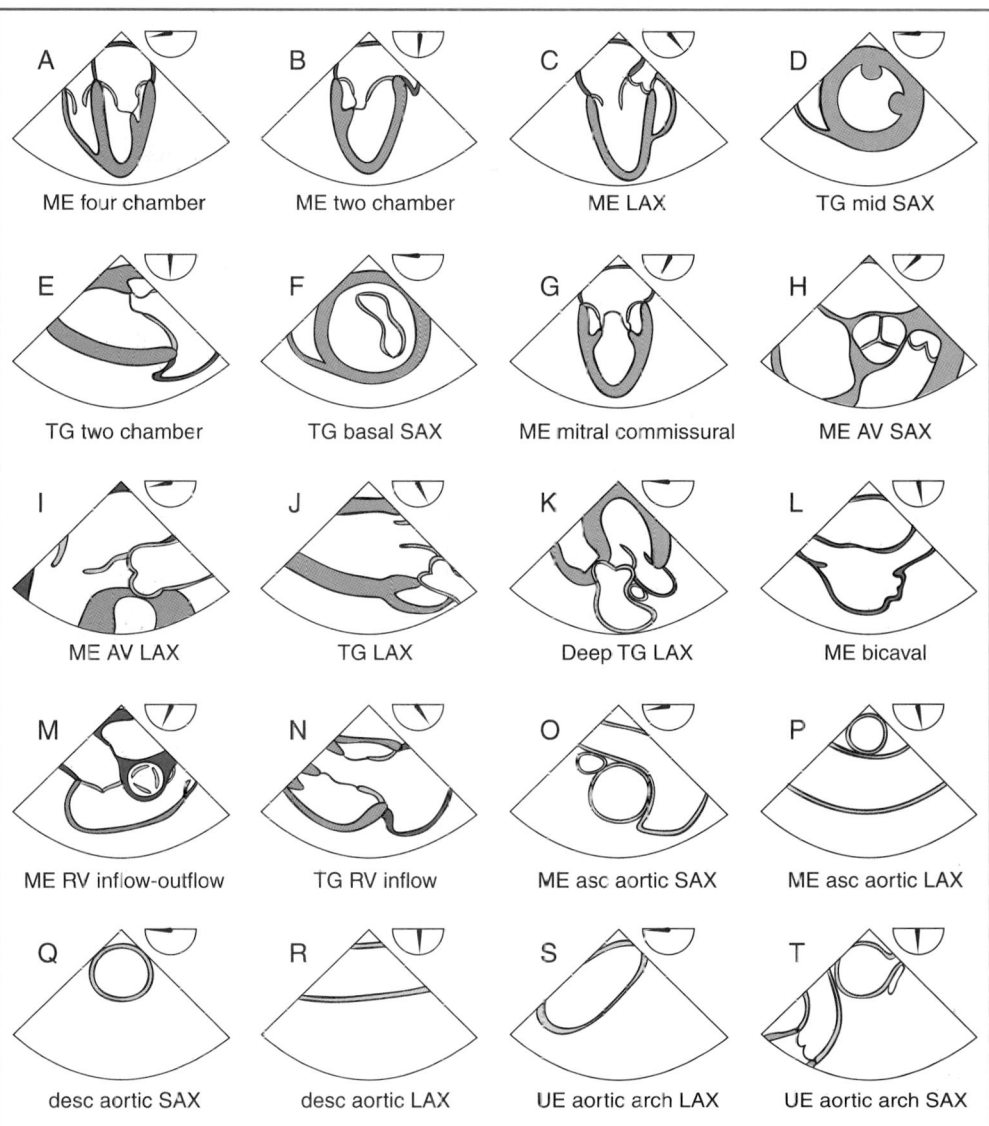

Figure 33-8 TEE cross sections in a comprehensive examination. Twenty standard cross sections and their abbreviated names are depicted by the line drawings. The text describes the probe manipulations required to produce each of the cross sections. (Redrawn from Shanewise JS, Cheung AT, Aronson S, et al: ASE/SCA guidelines for performing a comprehensive intraoperative multiplane transesophageal echocardiography examination: Recommendations of the American Society of Echocardiography Council for Intraoperative Echocardiography and the Society of Cardiovascular Anesthesiologists Task Force for Certification in Perioperative Transesophageal Echocardiography. Anesth Analg 89:870-884, 1999.)

A ME four chamber
B ME two chamber
C ME LAX
D TG mid SAX
E TG two chamber
F TG basal SAX
G ME mitral commissural
H ME AV SAX
I ME AV LAX
J TG LAX
K Deep TG LAX
L ME bicaval
M ME RV inflow-outflow
N TG RV inflow
O ME asc aortic SAX
P ME asc aortic LAX
Q desc aortic SAX
R desc aortic LAX
S UE aortic arch LAX
T UE aortic arch SAX

and outflow cross section into view (Fig. 33-8M). Usually, an image depth of 12 to 14 cm is required to position the RV outflow track in the center of the video screen. This cross section reveals the contractile function of the right ventricle, the outflow tract, and pulmonary valve function with the application of color Doppler. Next, the transducer is rotated back to 0 degrees and the probe is advanced 4 to 6 mm into the esophagus and gently retroflexed until all four cardiac chambers are visualized (ME four-chamber cross section) (Fig. 33-8A). Often, rotating the transducer 10 to 15 degrees will enhance the view of the tricuspid annulus. Generally, an image depth of 14 to 16 cm is required to include the LV apex in the sector scan. In two-dimensional imaging, the free wall of the right ventricle and the lateral and septal LV wall segments are evaluated for contractile function. With color Doppler, both the mitral and tricuspid valves are assessed. Stenotic and regurgitant lesions can be diagnosed accurately. During this assessment, image depth is decreased to 10 to 12 cm to afford a magnified view of the valves and maximization of the Nyquist limit (above 50 cm/sec).

Next, color Doppler is discontinued, the left ventricle is positioned in the center of the screen, and the multiplane angle is rotated forward to 90 degrees to bring into view the ME two-chamber cross section (Fig. 33-8B). Image depth is returned to 14 to 16 cm. This cross section is best for revealing the function of the basal and apical segments of the anterior and inferior LV walls, as well as anterior and inferior pericardial collections. When air emboli collect in the left ventricle, they can usually best be seen in this view as very echogenic areas located along the anterior apical endocardial surface. The transducer is then rotated forward to 135 degrees to reveal the ME LAX cross section that is best for assessment of the anteroseptal and posterior wall segments for contractile LV function (Fig. 33-8C). Together, the ME four-chamber, two-chamber, and LAX cross sections reveal all 16 segments of the left ventricle (Fig. 33-9). However, the next and last of the basic cross sections provides a second look at the midventricular segments, as well as other benefits. To achieve this cross section, the transducer is rotated back to 0 degrees, the left ventricle is centered in the screen, and the probe

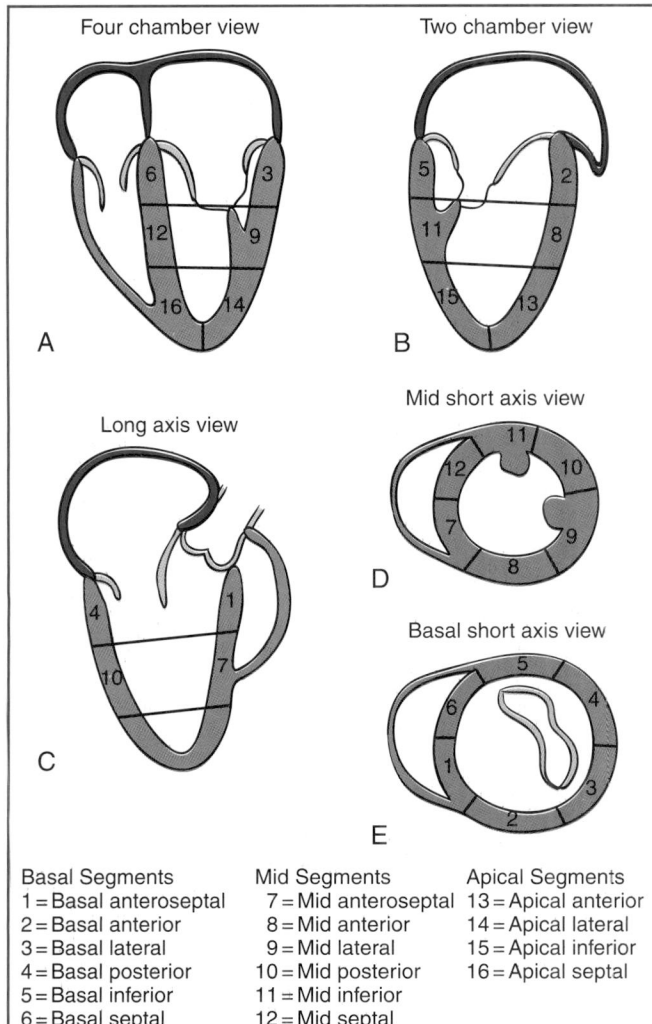

Four chamber view

Two chamber view

Long axis view

Mid short axis view

Basal short axis view

Basal Segments	Mid Segments	Apical Segments
1 = Basal anteroseptal	7 = Mid anteroseptal	13 = Apical anterior
2 = Basal anterior	8 = Mid anterior	14 = Apical lateral
3 = Basal lateral	9 = Mid lateral	15 = Apical inferior
4 = Basal posterior	10 = Mid posterior	16 = Apical septal
5 = Basal inferior	11 = Mid inferior	
6 = Basal septal	12 = Mid septal	

Figure 33–9 Five TEE cross sections with myocardial segments identified. A total of 16 myocardial segments are identified and named according to standards adopted by the American Society of Echocardiography and the Society of Cardiovascular Anesthesiologists. (Redrawn from Shanewise JS, Cheung AT, Aronson S. et al: ASE/SCA guidelines for performing a comprehensive intraoperative multiplane transesophageal echocardiography examination: Recommendations of the American Society of Echocardiography Council for Intraoperative Echocardiography and the Society of Cardiovascular Anesthesiologists Task Force for Certification in Perioperative Transesophageal Echocardiography. Anesth Analg 89: 870-884, 1999.)

is advanced 4 to 6 cm into the stomach. The probe is then flexed gently anteriorly to reveal the transgastric (TG) SAX cross section (Fig. 33-8D). This cross section is ideal for monitoring LV filling and contractile function. All major coronary arteries supplying the myocardium are viewed in this cross section. Moreover, changes in preload cause greater changes in the LV SAX dimension than the LV LAX dimension, and movement of the probe from this cross section is readily apparent because the papillary muscles provide prominent landmarks. Since this cross section is used to judge filling and ejection, image depth is consistently set to 12 cm so that the size and function

of the heart are judged easily relative to previously examined hearts.

Comprehensive Examination

In addition to the 8 cross sections described in the previous section, 12 other cross sections are required to complete the comprehensive perioperative TEE examination delineated in the 1999 ASE/SCA task force recommendations.[7] When time permits or the diagnostic question or questions require, the comprehensive examination can be completed in any order deemed most appropriate by the operator. Shanewise and associates described an examination sequence based on anatomic structures, and the reader is referred to this very detailed reference for one excellent approach.[7] However, when a single individual is responsible for anesthetic care and TEE, the comprehensive examination is completed as time permits after the basic examination has been recorded. When such is the case, the operator can use 3 of the 8 basic cross sections as takeoff points for the other 12 cross sections to make completion of the comprehensive examination a relatively easy sequence to remember and quick to perform.

With the probe positioned for the AV SAX cross section, the other six cross sections of the aorta are easily achieved. First, the probe is withdrawn slowly 1 to 3 cm while keeping the aorta in the center of the video screen to view the ascending aorta in SAX (Fig. 33-8O). As the probe is withdrawn, the operator views progressively more superior SAX cross sections of the aorta, beginning with the sinotubular junction, until the image is lost because of interposition of the trachea between the esophagus and aorta. Next, the multiplane angle is rotated forward to 100 to 120 degrees and advanced slowly 1 to 3 cm while keeping the aorta in the center of the video screen to view the ascending aorta in LAX (Fig. 33-8P). These two cross sections are ideal for assessment of pathology of the ascending aorta, such as type I aortic dissection and aortic atheromas. However, the most superior aspect of the aorta is rarely seen, including the takeoff of the innominate artery, because of the aforementioned tracheal interposition. Next, the transducer is returned to 0 degrees, the image depth decreased to 6 cm, and the probe turned leftward past the cardiac structures to reveal the descending aorta in SAX (Fig. 33-8Q). The probe is withdrawn and advanced with the aorta maintained in the center of the screen until the entire descending aorta has been examined in SAX. This maneuver is repeated with the transducer at 90 degrees to examine the descending aorta in LAX (Fig. 33-8R). Next, the transducer is returned to 0 degrees and the probe withdrawn until the distal aortic arch in LAX comes into view (Fig. 33-8S). Rotating the transducer to 90 degrees reveals the distal arch in SAX (Fig. 33-8T). The probe is turned leftward until the aorta just disappears from view and then turned slowly rightward to identify the takeoff of the left subclavian artery (well seen in most patients) and the left carotid artery (well seen in a minority of patients). These cross sections of the descending aorta and distal aortic arch reliably reveal dissections and atheromatous disease.

With the probe positioned for the ME four-chamber cross section, the ME mitral commissural cross section is achieved easily by centering the coaptation point of the mitral valve in the center of the video screen and rotating the multiplane angle forward to about 60 degrees (Fig. 33-8G). This maneuver positions the ultrasound beam parallel to the closure line of the mitral leaflets and completes the LAX examination of the mitral valve. Although a detailed discussion of mitral leaflet structure and function is beyond the scope of this chapter, Figure 33-10 summarizes an excellent approach to this challenging task.[35]

With the probe positioned for the TG mid SAX cross section, the remaining five cross sections of the comprehensive examination are easily achieved in most patients. First, the left ventricle is centered in the video screen and the multiplane angle is rotated forward to 90 degrees to reveal the TG two-chamber cross section (Fig. 33-8E). Although this cross section reveals the same structures as the ME two-chamber cross section, the viewing angle is orthogonal to the former viewing angle, and as a result, subvalvular structures are seen better. Next, the transducer is rotated to 100 to 120 degrees to reveal the TG LAX cross section (Fig. 33-8J). Again, this cross section reveals the same structures as the ME LAX, but the TG LAX view permits more parallel alignment of the ultrasound beam with blood flow through the LV outflow

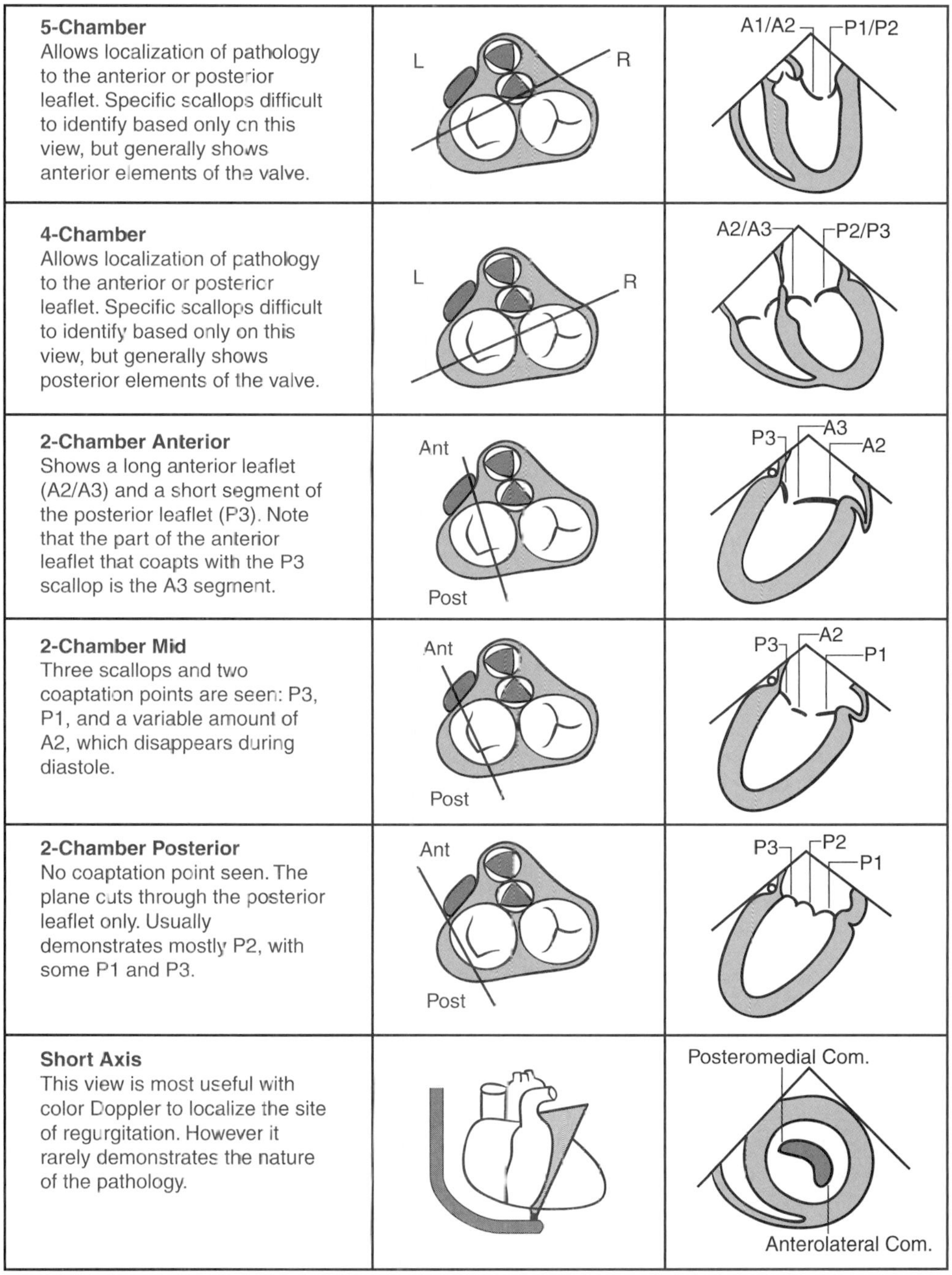

Figure 33–10 Systematic examination of the mitral valve. In this examination, the mitral valve is viewed in multiple cross sections to delineate leaflet anatomy. The "5-chamber" cross section is accomplished by withdrawing the probe slightly from the standard 4-chamber cross section until the left ventricular outflow track is in view. The *center column* shows the planes of the different cross sections as viewed from directly above the base of the heart. The 2-chamber "anterior," "mid," and "posterior" cross sections are variations of the standard 2-chamber cross section and are accomplished by turning the probe from the patient's right to left. "P1, P2, and P3" refer to the three scallops of the posterior mitral leaflet, and "A1, A2, and A3" refer to the juxtaposed segments of the anterior mitral leaflet. The *right column* shows the leaflet segments seen in the corresponding cross section. (Redrawn from Lambert AS, Miller JP, Foster E, et al: Improved evaluation of the location and mechanism of mitral valve regurgitation with a systematic transesophageal echocardiography examination. Anesth Analg 88:1205-1212, 1999.)

5-Chamber Allows localization of pathology to the anterior or posterior leaflet. Specific scallops difficult to identify based only on this view, but generally shows anterior elements of the valve.	A1/A2, P1/P2
4-Chamber Allows localization of pathology to the anterior or posterior leaflet. Specific scallops difficult to identify based only on this view, but generally shows posterior elements of the valve.	A2/A3, P2/P3
2-Chamber Anterior Shows a long anterior leaflet (A2/A3) and a short segment of the posterior leaflet (P3). Note that the part of the anterior leaflet that coapts with the P3 scallop is the A3 segment.	P3, A3, A2
2-Chamber Mid Three scallops and two coaptation points are seen: P3, P1, and a variable amount of A2, which disappears during diastole.	P3, A2, P1
2-Chamber Posterior No coaptation point seen. The plane cuts through the posterior leaflet only. Usually demonstrates mostly P2, with some P1 and P3.	P3, P2, P1
Short Axis This view is most useful with color Doppler to localize the site of regurgitation. However it rarely demonstrates the nature of the pathology.	Posteromedial Com. / Anterolateral Com.

track and AV. Next, the TG RV inflow cross section is achieved by returning the probe to the TG mid SAX position, turning it rightward until the right ventricle is in the centered in the video screen, and then rotating the multiplane angle to 100 to 120 degrees to bring the RV apex into view (Fig. 33-8N). This cross section is ideal for viewing the RV inferior free wall. Next, the TG basal SAX is achieved by returning the probe to the TG mid SAX, releasing the flexion of the probe, withdrawing 1 to 2 cm, and then flexing it gently until the orifice of the mitral valve is seen in SAX (Fig. 33-8F). This cross section can prove vital in determining the precise location of mitral regurgitation.[35] Finally, the deep TG LAX cross section is achieved by returning the probe to the TG mid SAX position, releasing the flexion of the probe, advancing it 6 to 8 cm into the stomach, fully flexing it once in the stomach, gently withdrawing it until minimal resistance is met at the gastroesophageal junction, and then slightly turning it leftward or rightward to reveal the LV outflow track and AV (Fig. 33-8K). Usually, this cross section does not resolve structures as well as the ME LAX does, but it does provide optimal beam alignment for Doppler interrogation of the LV outflow track and AV. Often, this cross section is the most difficult of the cross sections to achieve. If a few gentle attempts fail to accomplish it, it should be abandoned.

ASSESSMENT OF HEMODYNAMICS (see also Chapters 18 and 32)

Preload

Quantitative TEE measurements of ventricular preload reflect changes in ventricular diastolic volume more accurately than do data obtained from the pulmonary artery catheter.[36-39] For instance, in 30 patients scheduled for cardiac surgery, Cheung and colleagues removed 15% of each patient's blood volume (in six equal aliquots) before cardiopulmonary bypass while monitoring their TG mid SAX cross section with TEE.[40] A significant decrease in LV end-diastolic area was detected after removal of the first aliquot (2.5% of the estimated blood volume or about 200 mL). With subsequent aliquots, end-diastolic area decreased linearly ($0.3 \ cm^2/1.0\%$ of blood volume removed) such that after removal of all six aliquots, the end-diastolic area had decreased by 27% in patients with normal LV function and by 21% in patients with depressed LV function. Although pulmonary artery occlusion pressure and central venous pressure also declined during the study, their correlation with end-diastolic area and blood removal was very weak or nonexistent. In a different study, TEE Doppler estimates of transmitral flow provided a better method to predict cardiac output response to rapid intravenous fluid administration than did pulmonary artery occlusion pressure or LV end-diastolic area.[41]

Left Ventricular Filling Pressure

Surprisingly, TEE provides practical ways to estimate LV filling pressure. By placing the Doppler cursor at the junction of the left atrium and left superior pulmonary vein,

Kuecherer and coworkers demonstrated that a systolic fraction of flow of less than 55% was a specific and sensitive sign of left atrial pressure greater than 15 mm Hg. This sign is easily detected as predominance of flow during diastole (Figs. 33-11 and 33-12).[42] Significant mitral regurgitation, the presence of non-sinus rhythm, and extremes of cardiac output affect pulmonary venous flow and therefore limit this application of TEE. Alternative methods have been described that obviate these limitations.[43-46] Accordingly, TEE cannot estimate left atrial pressure precisely, but it can reliably identify clinically significant elevations.

Cardiac Output

Real-time images of LV filling and ejection permit qualitative, immediate assessment of marked changes in cardiac output. However, with PW and CW Doppler, TEE can quantify cardiac output. A Doppler measurement of blood flow velocity is combined with a two-dimensional measurement of cross-sectional area:

$$Cardiac \ output = VTI \cdot CSA \cdot cos \ \theta \cdot Heart \ rate$$

where VTI is the velocity time integral (the area under the Doppler-derived velocity-versus-time curve per systole), CSA is the cross-sectional area through which the velocity passes, and cos θ is the cosine of the angle between the ultrasound beam and blood flow (usually, the angle is assumed to be zero degrees so that this factor equals unity and can be disregarded). An initial study of flow in the main pulmonary artery and across the mitral valve versus thermodilution yielded somewhat disappointing results.[47] Subsequent studies excluding patients with tricuspid regurgitation and using other TEE cross sections demonstrated that TEE can estimate cardiac output reliably.[48-55]

Global Left Ventricular Contractile Function

Measuring LV contractility is much more difficult. The fractional area change (FAC) of the left ventricle can be measured by using the TG mid SAX or any of the LAX cross sections (provided that the LAX cross sections include the apex of the left ventricle) with the following formula:

$$(EDA - ESA)/EDA$$

where EDA is the cross-sectional area at end-diastole and ESA is the cross-sectional area at end-systole. EDA and ESA are easily measured with the standard software supplied with all ultrasonographs. In the absence of segmental dysfunction, FAC is a reasonable approximation of LV ejection fraction, but the ejection fraction is clearly load dependent and should be viewed cautiously as an index of ventricular function. However, the LV ejection fraction is an excellent predictor of survival in patients with coronary artery disease and is widely used in the perioperative assessment of high-risk patients. Load-independent measures of LV contractility are possible with TEE but are too complex for clinical practice.[56]

Figure 33–11 Normal pulmonary venous flow pattern. Pulsed-wave Doppler measurement of normal blood flow velocities in the left upper pulmonary vein (LUPV) is shown. At the top of the figure is a still-frame image of the two-dimensional cross section used to position the Doppler sample volume (the *round white sphere*). On the bottom two thirds of the figure is the display in white of the instantaneous blood flow velocities (vertical axis) versus time (horizontal axis) occurring in that sample volume. The electrocardiogram provides timing, and the *bold horizontal line* is the baseline (zero flow) for the flow velocities. Flow velocities above the *red line* are positive (i.e., toward the transducer) to a maximum of 69 cm/sec. Flow below the *red line* is negative (i.e., away from the transducer) to a maximum of –32 cm/sec. In this patient with normal left atrial pressure, systolic predominance of flow is evident; that is, more flow enters the atrium during the period of ventricular systole than during ventricular diastole as evidenced by the greater peak and average flow velocities during systole than during diastole. LA, left atrium. (From Cahalan MK: Intraoperative Transesophageal Echocardiography. An Interactive Text and Atlas. New York, Churchill Livingstone, 1997.)

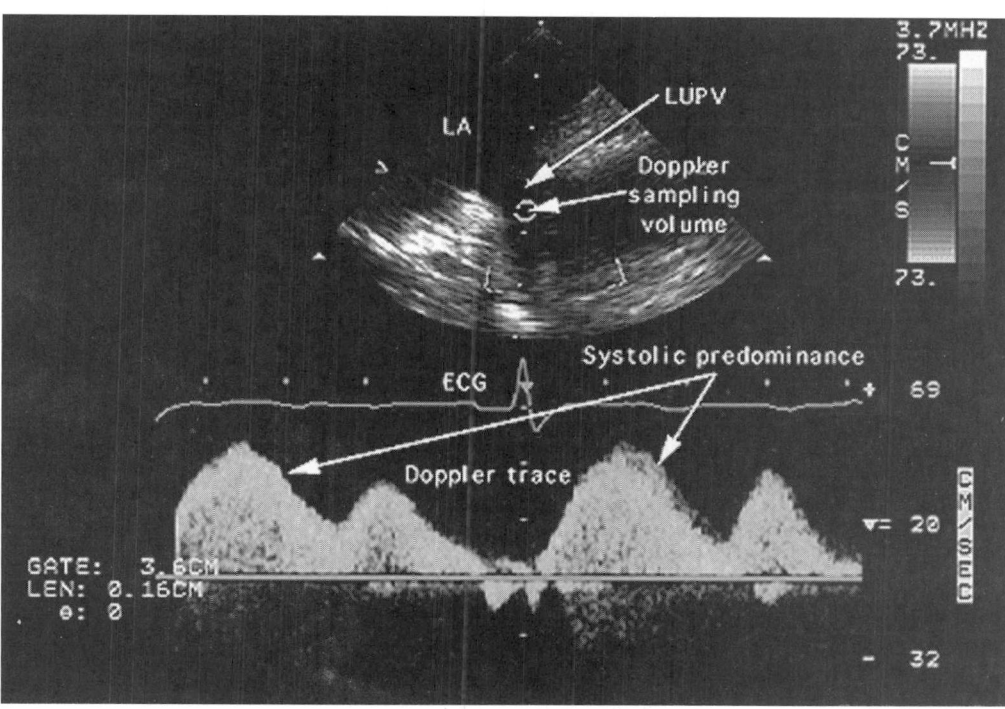

Figure 33–12 High left atrial pressure produces diastolic predominance in the pulmonary venous flow pattern. Pulsed-wave Doppler measurement of blood flow velocities in the left upper pulmonary vein (LUPV) in a patient with abnormally high left atrial pressure is shown. At the top of the figure is a still-frame image of the two-dimensional cross section used to position the Doppler sample volume (the *round white sphere*). On the bottom two thirds of the figure is the display in white of the instantaneous blood flow velocities (vertical axis) versus time (horizontal axis) occurring in that sample volume. The electrocardiogram provides timing, and the *bold horizontal line* is the baseline (zero flow) for the flow velocities. Flow velocities above the *red line* are positive (i.e., toward the transducer) to a maximum of 80 cm/sec. Flow below the *red line* is negative (i.e., away from the transducer) to a maximum of –44 cm/sec. In this patient with abnormally high left atrial pressure, diastolic predominance of flow is evident; that is, more flow enters the atrium during the period of ventricular diastole than during ventricular systole as evidenced by the greater peak and average flow velocities during diastole than during systole. The negative flow velocities are due to atrial contraction pushing blood back into the pulmonary vein. LA, left atrium. (From Cahalan MK: Intraoperative Transesophageal Echocardiography. An Interactive Text and Atlas. New York, Churchill Livingstone, 1997.)

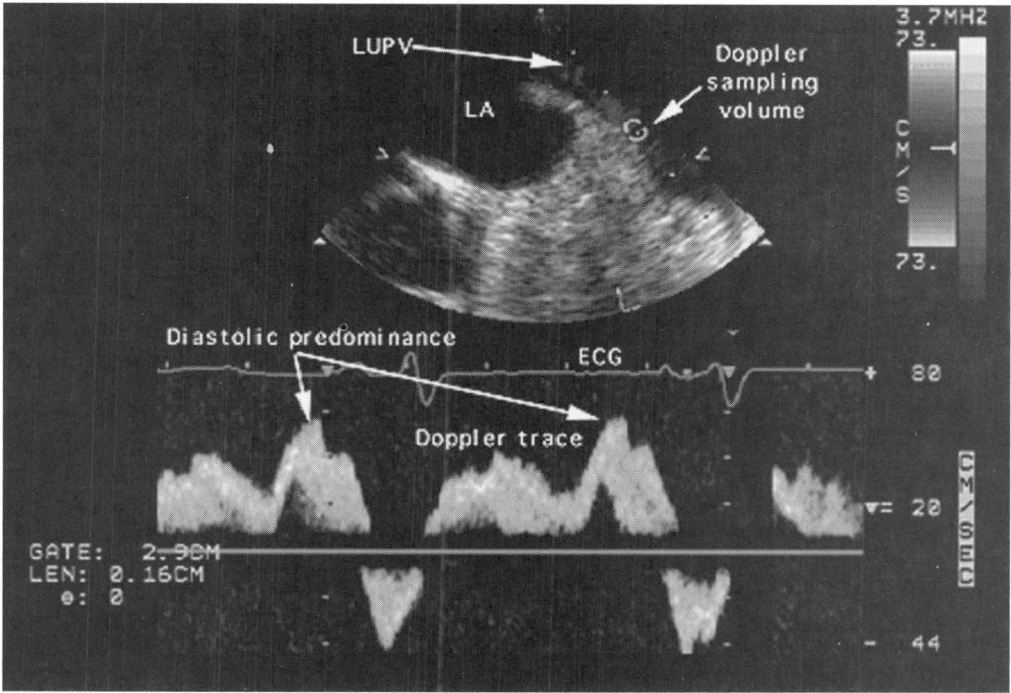

Global Right Ventricular Contractile Function

Measurement of RV function is more difficult than LV function because of the complex shape of the right ventricle, its large surface area relative to its volume, and its tendency to change shape with changes in loading. Normally, inward motion of the free wall of the right ventricle contributes most to RV ejection; however, some ejection is contributed by contraction of the RV outflow tract and by descent of the base of the heart. Thus, the four-chamber and ME RV inflow-outflow cross sections are the most useful for assessing RV function because they reveal the free wall best. In the four-chamber cross section, a normal right ventricle will appear smaller than a normal left ventricle (intracavitary area roughly two thirds of the LV cavity area) because it is crescent shaped and partially wrapped around the left ventricle. In the ME RV inflow-outflow cross section, the crescent shape of the right ventricle should be most apparent.

Although subtle RV dysfunction is hard to diagnose with TEE, severe dysfunction is not. The hallmarks are severe hypokinesis or akinesis of the RV free wall, enlargement of the right ventricle to exceed that of the apparent size of the left ventricle, a change in the shape of the right ventricle from crescent to round, and a flattening or bulging of the intraventricular septum to the left. These signs may be accompanied by tricuspid regurgitation secondary to tricuspid annular dilation. With very severe RV failure caused by RV pressure overload, RV dilation can be so great that it "tamponades" the left ventricle.

Hemodynamic Instability

When a sudden, severe change in hemodynamics occurs, qualitative estimates of LV filling and ejection serve as a practical guide for the administration of fluids and inotropes. With some ultrasonographs, computer technology converts the echocardiographic images from one cardiac cycle into digital code and then plays this cycle repetitively to allow side-by-side comparison with other cardiac cycles captured at other times during surgery. With this technology, an experienced observer can consistently detect decreases in preload before they result in greater than a 10% decrease in blood pressure.[57] This technology also facilitates qualitative assessment of changes in LV ejection and prompt differential diagnosis of the etiology of hypotension. For example, severe hypovolemia is easily recognized as a marked decrease in LV end-diastolic area with a marked increase in LV FAC, and LV failure is easily recognized as a marked increase in LV end-diastolic area with a marked decrease in LV FAC. During hypotension, arterial vasodilatation, aortic regurgitation, mitral regurgitation, and ventricular septal defects can manifest the same LV filling and ejection pattern at the TG mid SAX cross section: adequate LV end-diastolic filling area with an increased LV ejection fraction. Fortunately, distinguishing these etiologies of hypotension is not difficult with the use of other cross sections and color. Table 33-4 summarizes the most common causes of hypotension and their echocardiographic characteristics at the TG mid SAX cross section.

Table 33-4 Origin of hypotension*

EDA	EF	Cause
↓↓	>0.8	Hypovolemia
↑↑	<0.2	LV failure
Normal	>0.5	Low SVR or severe MR, AR, or VSD

*Obviously, other problems can cause hypotension, but the ones listed here include the most common occurring in the operating room. Two important caveats need to be mentioned. First, low systemic vascular resistance and hypovolemia sometimes occur simultaneously (for instance, in sepsis), and until hypovolemia is treated, low systemic vascular resistance will not be apparent. Second, one cannot assume that just because the papillary muscles meet during systole (i.e., LV cavity obliteration), the patient is hypovolemic. This finding can occur in the setting of either low systemic vascular resistance or hypovolemia. To make this differential diagnosis correctly, one must determine whether diastolic filling is adequate.

AR, aortic regurgitation; EDA, end-diastolic cross-sectional area; EF, ejection fraction; LV, left ventricular; MR, mitral regurgitation; SVR, systemic vascular resistance; VSD, ventricular septal defect.

From Cahalan MK: Intraoperative Transesophageal Echocardiography: An Interactive Text and Atlas. New York, Churchill Livingstone, 1996.

Prospective studies have established the value of this TEE application, sometimes called "rescue TEE."[58-64] For example, in 60 consecutive patients with severe, persistent hypotension after cardiac surgery, TEE corrected the presumed diagnosis in almost half of these patients.[59] In two patients, TEE prompted emergency surgery, and in five others it prevented unnecessary reoperations. In another study, unstable cardiac surgical patients in the operating room ($n = 57$) or intensive care unit ($n = 83$) underwent emergency TEE.[59] Based on the TEE findings alone, 22 of these patients had urgent surgical interventions. The average time to diagnosis was 11 minutes. In critically ill surgical patients, TEE is more cost-effective than transthoracic echocardiography because the latter so often fails to reveal diagnostic images.[60] Even in the setting of prolonged cardiopulmonary resuscitation, TEE may reveal crucial diagnostic information.[61]

MYOCARDIAL ISCHEMIA: DETECTION AND LIMITATIONS

Within seconds of the onset of myocardial ischemia, affected segments of the heart cease contracting normally.[65] This fact is the basis for the use of TEE for the detection of myocardial ischemia. For example, in 50 patients undergoing cardiovascular surgery, new severe segmental wall motion abnormalities (SWMAs) occurred in 24 patients and ischemic ST-segment changes in only 6.[66] In three patients who sustained intraoperative myocardial infarctions, severe SWMAs developed in the corresponding area of myocardium and persisted until the end of surgery, but only one of these three patients had ischemic ST-segment changes intraoperatively. Subsequent studies in comparable patients confirmed these advantages of TEE over electrocardiographic monitoring.[67-69] Moreover, when multiple TEE cross sections are monitored (not just the one cross section as was done in the aforementioned studies), the detection rate of SWMAs more than doubles.[70,71]

Limitations of TEE in the detection of ischemia should be recognized. When an area of myocardium is clearly in view, segmental contraction can be difficult to evaluate if the heart rotates or translates markedly during systole or if discoordinated contraction occurs because of bundle branch block or ventricular pacing. Consequently, a valid system for assessment of SWMAs must first compensate for global motion of the heart and then evaluate both regional endocardial motion and myocardial thickening. Marked worsening of segmental wall motion and wall thickening (in the absence of similar global changes) is required to make the diagnosis of ischemia (Table 33-5); less pronounced changes are not consistently interpreted even by experts. Interpretation of septal motion is the most problematic because it is often confounded by discoordinated contraction patterns. However, a simple rule applies: when the septum is viable and nonischemic, it thickens appreciably during systole, although its inward motion may begin slightly before or after the inward motion of the other ventricular segments. Thus, new SWMAs can be detected during bundle branch block, ventricular pacing, and marked global movements of the heart, but not by assessment of endocardial motion alone—wall thickening must also be assessed. Because not all hearts contract normally and not all parts of a normal heart contract to the same degree, not all SWMAs are indicative of myocardial ischemia.

Table 33–5 Classes of segmental wall motion and thickening*

Class of Wall Motion	Wall Thickening	Change in Radius
1. Normal or hyperkinesis	Marked	>30% ↓
2. Mild hypokinesis	Moderate	10%-30% ↓
3. Severe hypokinesis	Minimal	<10%, >0% ↓
4. Akinesis	None	No change
5. Dyskinesis	Thinning	↑

*Assessment of segmental wall motion is subjective, but this grading system helps limit the variability among readers by defining categories of inward endocardial motion and myocardial thickening. "Change in radius" refers to the percentage of change during systole in the radius from the endocardium to the imaginary center of the left ventricle. Because normal myocardial thickening is 2 to 5 mm and inward endocardial motion is 5 to 10 mm, thickening is more difficult to assess than endocardial motion. Nevertheless, thickening is the more reliable guide to myocardial function because it is unaffected by variables that confound assessment of endocardial motion: translational motion of the heart, conduction abnormalities, and ventricular pacing. In the absence of these variables, endocardial motion is usually an adequate indicator of function of the underlying myocardium.
From Cahalan MK: Intraoperative Transesophageal Echocardiography: An Interactive Text and Atlas. New York, Churchill Livingstone, 1996.

For instance, myocardial infarction, myocardial stunning, and myocarditis can cause SWMAs. However, a sudden, severe decrease or cessation of segmental contraction is almost certainly due to myocardial ischemia. One exception to this rule occurs when LV preload is severely reduced.[72]

Echocardiographic contrast agents can delineate myocardial blood flow, but to date, they have not proved to be a practical method to differentiate infarcted from acutely stunned myocardium.[73] Fortunately, dobutamine may facilitate this differential diagnosis because it can improve segmental function in stunned, but not infarcted myocardium.[74-76] For clinical purposes, when stunned myocardium is suspected after cardiopulmonary bypass, graft status should be re-evaluated and segmental myocardial function closely monitored for signs of improvement. A trial of low- to moderate-dose dobutamine may improve the function of stunned myocardium. If worsening occurs, if graft status is questionable, or if the patient's hemodynamics is tenuous, additional revascularization should be considered. Intraoperative stress testing has been evaluated and appears to be safe in the setting of cardiac surgery.[77,78]

EVALUATION OF CARDIOVASCULAR PATHOLOGIES (see also Chapter 50)

Aortic Diseases

TEE has a proven role in the assessment of aortic injury and aortic dissection when prompt and accurate diagnosis is vital to patient survival. In one study of 160 consecutive victims of blunt chest trauma, TEE was diagnostically superior to and faster than aortography for detection of aortic injury.[79] Unlike aortography, TEE reliably distinguishes between subadventitial disruptions that require emergency surgery and intimal tears that do not.[80,81] For the detection of aortic dissection, TEE has proved superior to aortography and computed tomography.[82] It is associated with a shorter time to diagnosis, less morbidity (renal dysfunction and neurologic events), and shorter hospital stays than aortography is.[83] Though marginally less sensitive and specific than magnetic resonance imaging (MRI) for some dissections (those originating in the aortic arch, where TEE imaging is partially obstructed by the trachea), TEE requires less time and expense than MRI or any other comparably reliable alternative does.[84] Moreover, TEE can delineate the mechanisms and severity of associated aortic regurgitation, thereby identifying patients in whom valve repair is likely to be successful.[85] Thus, TEE is the test of choice in unstable patients with suspected aortic injury or aortic dissection because a delay in surgery could prove fatal to these patients.

Valvular Dysfunction

TEE provides a highly reliable means for the assessment of valvular structure and function. Although a comprehensive review of this topic is beyond the scope of this chapter, a brief overview of the most commonly used techniques should prepare the reader to fulfill at least the requirements for basic TEE practice: to recognize gross valvular dysfunction. When performing color Doppler in the following assessments, the operator should use the minimum scan depth and maximum Nyquist limit possible.

The degree of aortic stenosis is easily appreciated in the ME AV SAX cross section, where the extent of leaflet opening can be estimated visually or measured directly with planimetry.[86] Severe stenosis is characterized by marked thickening of the leaflets and severely reduced leaflet motion (valve opening area <1 cm^2). In the deep TG LAX cross section, CW Doppler allows reliable estimation of the gradient across the AV (Fig. 33-13).[87] In severe stenosis, the peak instantaneous gradient will exceed 64 mm Hg (CW velocity exceeding 4 m/sec), provided that cardiac output has not been markedly compromised. Noteworthy is the fact that the echocardiographically derived AV gradient may be higher than the peak-to-peak gradient reported from a catheterization study because the latter does not measure the instantaneous gradient as Doppler echocardiography does. Additional information on the morphology of the AV, including the dimensions of the annulus, sinotubular junction, and ascending aorta, can be garnered from the ME AV LAX cross section. The degree of aortic regurgitation is appreciated best in this cross section. With color Doppler positioned over the leaflets and outflow track, aortic regurgitation is recognized as a color jet emanating from the valve during diastole.

Even modest degrees of aortic regurgitation can be clinically significant during cardiac surgery and produce LV distention during cardiopulmonary bypass, as well as diminish the effectiveness of antegrade cardioplegia.[88] Mild regurgitation is characterized by a narrow-based, diastolic color jet (<2 mm at its origin in the valve) that occupies less than a third of the cross-sectional area of the LV outflow tract and extends minimally into the left ventricle (1 to 2 cm). Moderate regurgitation is a broader-based, diastolic color jet (3 to 5 mm) that occupies less than two thirds of the cross-sectional area of the LV outflow tract and extends moderately into the left ventricle (3 to 5 cm). Severe regurgitation is a broad-based, diastolic color jet (>5 mm) occupying the entire LV outflow tract and extending well into the left ventricle (Table 33-6).

The presence and severity of mitral stenosis are easily determined with TEE by using the ME four-chamber, two-chamber, commissural, and/or LAX cross section, as well as the basal TG SAX cross section. Two-dimensional imaging reveals thickened leaflets that dome toward the left ventricle and open poorly. Color Doppler reveals laminar flow acceleration into the stenotic orifice and a turbulent jet emerging into the ventricle (Plate 33-3). PW and CW Doppler traces display a characteristic flow pattern with increased peak and mean velocities (Fig. 33-14). Mathematical calculations from these traces, such as the pressure half-time, are the most precise methods to assess the severity of mitral stenosis, and formulas for these

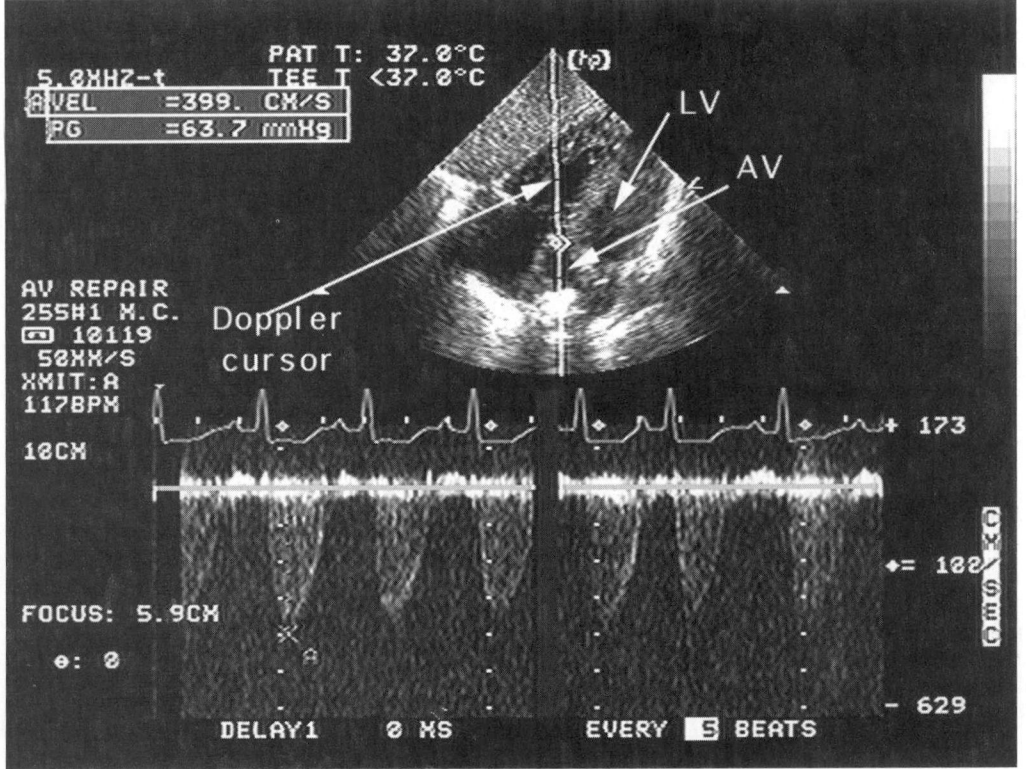

Figure 33–13 Continuous-wave Doppler estimation of the aortic valve (AV) gradient. Continuous-wave Doppler measurement of blood flow velocities immediately above the AV during seven cardiac cycles is shown. At the top of the figure is a still-frame image of the two-dimensional cross section used to position the Doppler sample cursor (the *diagonal white line*). On the bottom two thirds of the figure is the display in white of the instantaneous blood flow velocities (vertical axis) versus time (horizontal axis) occurring anywhere along that cursor. The electrocardiogram provides timing, and the *bold horizontal line* is the baseline (zero flow) for the flow velocities. With this Doppler alignment, all flow velocities are negative (i.e., away from the transducer). The Doppler scale has been set to a maximum of −629 cm/sec, and this tracing documents significant aortic stenosis: a peak blood flow velocity of approximately 4 m/sec (each *white dot* on the vertical axis equals 100 cm/sec or 1 m/sec) corresponding to a peak gradient across the aortic valve of 64 mm Hg. (From Cahalan MK: Intraoperative Transesophageal Echocardiography. An Interactive Text and Atlas. New York, Churchill Livingstone, 1997.)

Table 33–6 Simplified grading for aortic insufficiency*

	Jet Width at Origin (mm)	Jet Area (% of LVOT)	Jet Depth into LV (cm)
Mild	<2	<50	1-2
Moderate	3-5	50-75	3-5
Severe	>5	>75	>5

*Diastolic jet width is assessed with color Doppler in the five-chamber view at the closure point of the aortic valve (the origin of the regurgitant jet). The transducer should be repositioned until the origin of the jet is clearly imaged. Failure to image the origin of the jet may lead to overestimation of its severity. Diastolic jet area is assessed with color Doppler in the five-chamber view. % of LVOT is the percentage of the LVOT occupied by the plume of the color jet (the area of turbulent flow depicted by the mosaic of color pixels). This parameter is markedly affected by aortic diastolic pressure. Failure to adjust color or two-dimensional gains correctly may lead to underestimation or overestimation of the severity of the regurgitation. Color gain should be set just below the level that results in random color sparkle, and two-dimensional gains should be set at the minimum levels allowing adequate visualization of cardiac structures. Diastolic jet depth is assessed with color Doppler in the five-chamber view. The length of penetration of the jet from the LVOT into the LV is estimated in centimeters. This parameter is also markedly affected by aortic diastolic pressure and gain settings. LV, left ventricle; LVOT, LV outflow tract.
From Cahalan MK: Intraoperative Transesophageal Echocardiography: An Interactive Text and Atlas. New York, Churchill Livingstone, 1996.

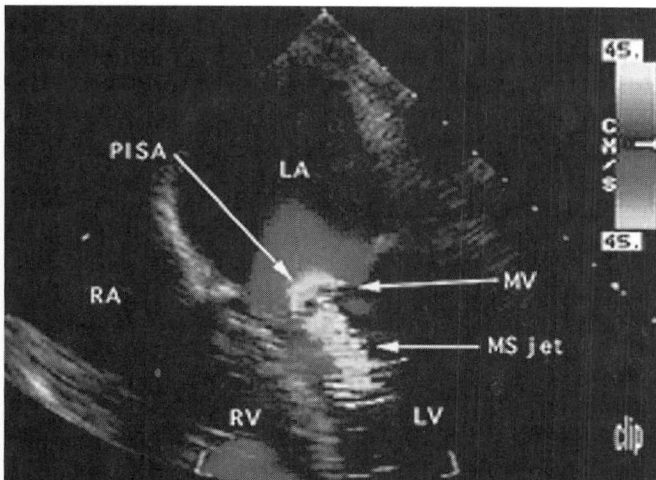

Plate 33–3 Color Doppler imaging of severe mitral stenosis. This four-chamber echocardiogram reveals a thickened and narrowed mitral valve (MV) indicative of mitral stenosis (MS). Color Doppler demonstrates (1) acceleration of blood flow into the stenotic valve (a light blue semicircular area immediately above the valve called "PISA"—proximal isovelocity surface area), (2) a narrow color jet across the valve itself, and (3) a 1 by 4-cm color jet extending from the undersurface of the valve into the left ventricle. LA, left atrium; LV, left ventricle; RA, right atrium; RV, right ventricle. (From Cahalan MK: Intraoperative Transesophageal Echocardiography. An Interactive Text and Atlas. New York, Churchill Livingstone, 1997.)

evaluations are built into the software of virtually every ultrasonograph.[89] In addition to the signs noted earlier, severe mitral stenosis always causes marked left atrial enlargement and left atrial spontaneous contrast. Spontaneous contrast is a swirling, smokelike appearance of 1- to 2-mm densities not caused by exogenously administered contrast agents but by aggregation of red cells in areas of low flow. Whenever left atrial enlargement and spontaneous contrast are noted, thrombus in the left atrium and, in particular, the left atrial appendage should be suspected and examined for carefully.

The presence and severity of mitral regurgitation are evaluated from the same cross sections used for evaluation of mitral stenosis and with the same grading strategy used for aortic regurgitation (Table 33-7). Mild regurgitation is characterized by a narrow-based, systolic color jet (<2 mm at its origin in the valve) that occupies less than 25% of the left atrial cross-sectional area and extends less than half the distance to the posterior wall of the left atrium. Moderate regurgitation is a broader-based, systolic color jet (3 to 5 mm at its origin in the valve) occupying less than 50% of the left atrial cross-sectional area and extending 50% to 90% of the distance to the posterior wall of the left atrium. Severe regurgitation is a broad-based, systolic color jet (>5 mm) that occupies most of the left atrium and extends into the pulmonary veins and left atrial appendage (Fig. 33-15). Eccentrically directed jets of mitral regurgitation that hug the wall of the atrium are generally associated with more severe valvular regurgitation than their cross-sectional area might suggest (Plate 33-4). Moreover, eccentrically directed jets usually point away from the defective leaflet (i.e., laterally directed jets are generally associated with anterior leaflet defects and medially directed jets with posterior leaflet defects), provided that the mechanism of regurgitation is leaflet prolapse or flail.[90] Severe mitral regurgitation is invariably associated with systolic reversal of pulmonary venous inflow.[91] The general guidelines listed earlier are widely used, but many more criteria have been described for assessment of mitral regurgitation.[92] Most importantly, the degree of regurgitation is exquisitely dependent on LV loading conditions. For practical purposes, quantitative measures of regurgitation, for example, the regurgitant orifice area based on the theory of proximal isovelocity surface area, are less often used in the operating room because of time restriction.[49]

Pulmonary and tricuspid valve pathology is assessed in a fashion analogous to that described for the aortic and mitral valves.

Other Pathologies

Thousands of published reports have documented that TEE can reveal virtually any significant morphologic or functional pathology of the heart. TEE is particularly sensitive for abnormalities involving the left atrium and mitral valve, including masses, thrombi, and emboli, because of the proximity of the left atrium and mitral valve to the TEE transducer. In contrast, pathologies of the RV and LV apex are less reliably detected. TEE is exquisitely sensitive to air embolism, and as a result, even insignificant amounts of air in the circulation give rise to

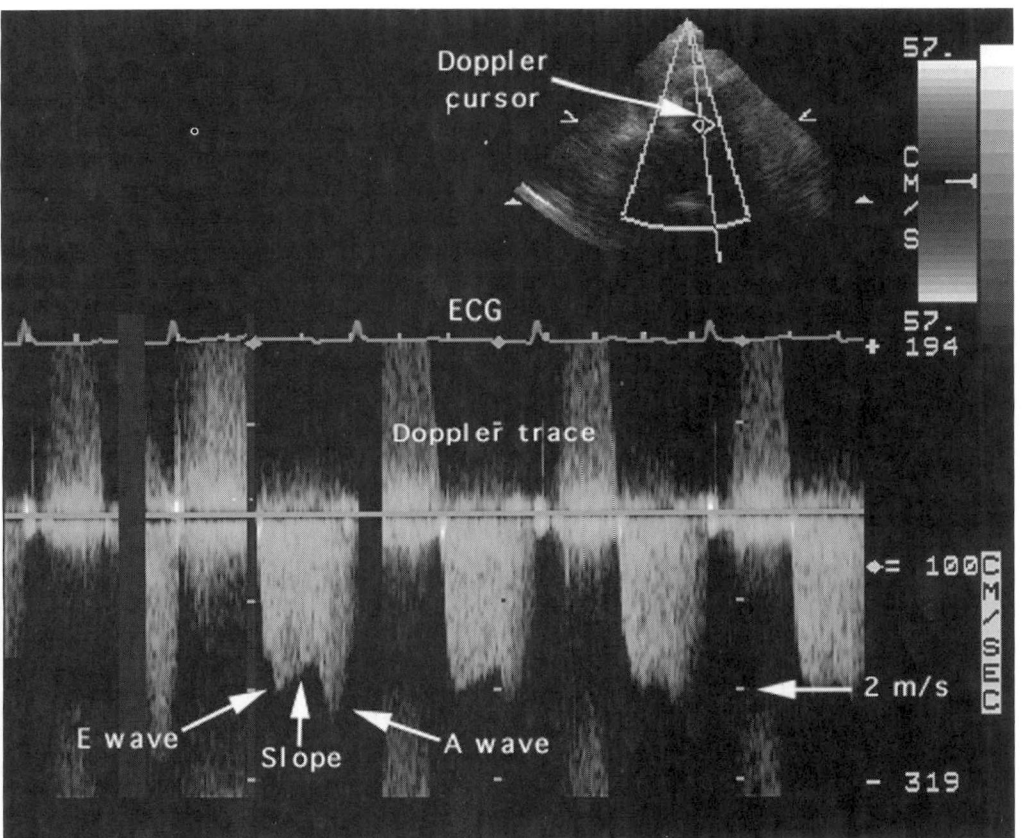

Figure 33–14 Continuous-wave Doppler evaluation of mitral stenosis. Continuous-wave Doppler measurement of blood flow velocities through a stenotic mitral valve is shown. At the top of the figure is a still-frame image of the four-chamber cross section used to position the Doppler cursor. On the bottom two thirds of the figure is the display in white of the instantaneous blood flow velocities (vertical axis) versus time (horizontal axis) occurring anywhere along that cursor. The electrocardiogram is shown for timing purposes, and the *red horizontal line* running through the Doppler tracing is the baseline (zero flow) for the flow velocities. Velocities displayed above the baseline are positive and represent flow toward the transducer. These velocities are due to mitral regurgitation and are so high that they exceed the scale used in this example. Velocities displayed below the baseline are negative and represent flow away from the transducer. These velocities are due to severe mitral stenosis and average about 2 m/sec, which is indicative of a gradient across the mitral valve of 16 mm Hg. Also note how slowly the flow velocity decreases after the peak of the E wave (indicated in the figure by "Slope"). The pressure half-time can be calculated from this slope and is markedly increased in the presence of severe mitral stenosis. (From Cahalan MK: Intraoperative Transesophageal Echocardiography. An Interactive Text and Atlas. New York, Churchill Livingstone, 1997.)

Table 33–7 Simplified grading for mitral regurgitation*

	Jet Width at Origin (mm)	Jet Area (%LA$_a$)	Jet Depth (%LA$_d$)
Mild	>2	<25	<50
Moderate	3-5	25-50	50-90
Severe	>5	>50	>100

*Systolic jet width is assessed with color Doppler in the five- or four-chamber view at the closure point of the mitral valve (the origin of the regurgitant jet). The transducer should be repositioned until the origin of the jet is clearly imaged. Failure to image the origin of the jet may lead to overestimation of its severity. Systolic jet area is assessed with color Doppler in the five- or four-chamber view. %LA$_a$ is the percentage of the LA$_a$ occupied by the plume of the color jet (the area of turbulent flow depicted by the mosaic of color pixels). This parameter is markedly affected by left ventricular systolic pressure. Failure to adjust color or two-dimensional gains correctly may lead to underestimation or overestimation of the severity of the regurgitation. Color gain should be set just below the level that results in random color sparkle, and two-dimensional gains should be set at the minimum levels allowing adequate visualization of cardiac structures. Systolic jet depth is assessed with color Doppler in the five- or four-chamber view. %LA$_d$ is the depth of penetration of the jet into the left atrium expressed as a percentage of the distance from the mitral annulus to the posterior wall of the left atrium. This parameter is also markedly affected by left ventricular systolic pressure. In severe mitral regurgitation, the regurgitant jet may extend into one or more pulmonary veins and may cause transient reversal of pulmonary venous blood flow.
LA$_a$, left atrial area; LA$_d$, LA depth.
From Cahalan MK: Intraoperative Transesophageal Echocardiography: An Interactive Text and Atlas. New York, Churchill Livingstone, 1996.

Figure 33–15 Pulmonary vein flow reversal and severe mitral regurgitation. Pulsed-wave Doppler measurement of blood flow velocities in the left upper pulmonary vein (LUPV) is shown. At the top of the figure is a still-frame image of the two-dimensional cross section used to position the Doppler sampling volume (the *white circle*). On the bottom two thirds of the figure is the display of the instantaneous blood flow velocities (vertical axis) versus time (horizontal axis) occurring in the left upper pulmonary vein. The electrocardiogram is shown for timing purposes, and the *gray horizontal line* running through the Doppler tracing is the baseline (zero flow) for the flow velocities. Velocities displayed above the baseline are positive and represent flow toward the transducer (in this case, into the left atrium). Velocities displayed below the baseline are negative and

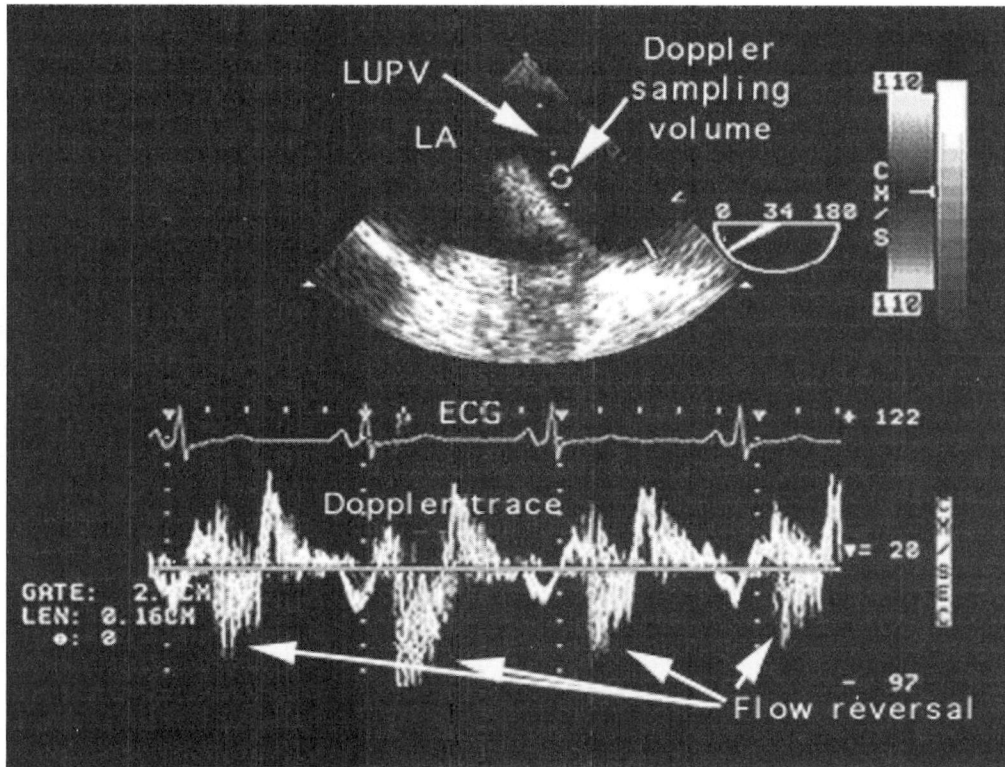

represent flow away from the transducer (in this case, into the left upper pulmonary vein). This Doppler tracing documents systolic flow reversal (normally it is positive, that is, toward the left atrium [LA] in systole) and confirms the presence of severe mitral regurgitation. (From Cahalan MK: Intraoperative Transesophageal Echocardiography. An Interactive Text and Atlas. New York, Churchill Livingstone, 1997.)

impressive densities on the video display. Currently, accurate estimation of the amount of air in the circulation is impossible with TEE. However, large amounts typically opacify the involved chambers until they form collections (very bright densities) in the most superiorly positioned parts of the chambers (i.e., the anterior endocardial surface of the left ventricle in a supine patient). Pulmonary emboli may be seen with TEE if they lodge proximal to the bifurcation of the main pulmonary artery. TEE is an exceedingly valuable tool for the evaluation of congenital heart defects. The reader is directed to an excellent review article on this topic by Miller-Hance and Silverman.[93]

ALTERATIONS OF SURGICAL PLANS AND ASSESSMENT OF RESULTS

Atheromatous Disease of the Aorta

TEE has had a positive influence on intraoperative management and outcome in patients with atheromatous disease of the aorta. In 130 patients older than 65 years undergoing coronary artery bypass grafting, TEE detection of protruding atheroma of the ascending aorta proved to be the most important independent predictor of stroke.[94] When a protruding atheroma or aortic arch intimal thickening of greater than 5 mm is detected by TEE, appropriate alteration of the aortic cannulation technique or avoidance of cannulation altogether will lower the chance of stroke.[95,96]

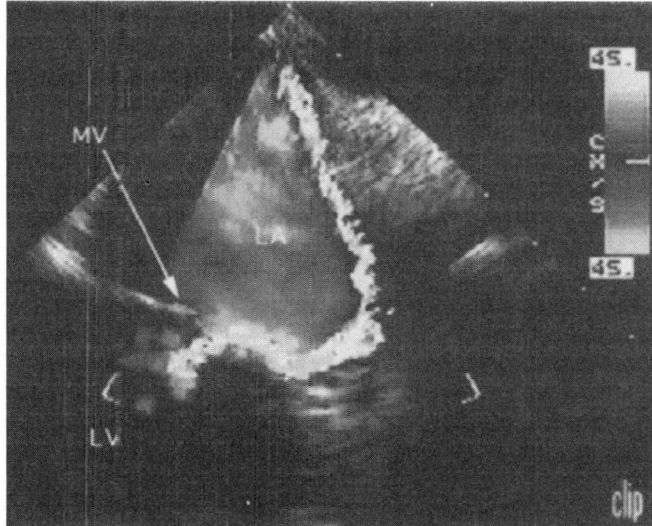

Plate 33–4 Severe mitral regurgitation with a wall-hugging jet. This honed-down five-chamber echocardiogram reveals severe mitral regurgitation. The long color jet has a fairly broad base and an eccentric direction indicative of severe mitral regurgitation. Wall-hugging jets such as this one have a small cross-sectional area because much of their energy is absorbed by the wall of the atrium. The mechanism of the regurgitation is apparent: the anterior leaflet (on the left side of the video screen) is prolapsing and allowing blood to escape beneath it and jet over the surface of the posterior leaflet into the left atrium (LA) LV, left ventricle; MV, mitral valve. (From Cahalan MK: Intraoperative Transesophageal Echocardiography. An Interactive Text and Atlas. New York, Churchill Livingstone, 1997.)

Valvular Heart Disease

Valvular abnormalities detected with TEE have important implications. In one study, intraoperative TEE detected mitral regurgitation so severe in 5 of 182 patients scheduled for coronary artery surgery that unscheduled mitral valve repair was performed.[97] Conversely, in 22 of 51 patients scheduled for combined coronary artery and mitral valve surgery, TEE revealed so little mitral valve dysfunction that the mitral repair was omitted. In another study, 6 of 383 patients undergoing aortic valve replacement had unscheduled mitral valve surgery based on the intraoperative diagnosis of severe mitral regurgitation by TEE.[98] In this same patient group, 25 scheduled mitral valve surgeries were omitted because of findings on intraoperative TEE. In a third study that prospectively evaluated 5016 patients, pre-bypass information from TEE led to modification of the surgical procedure in 12% of the patients undergoing valve procedures and 27% of the patients undergoing coronary surgery.[99] TEE is essential when mitral valve repair is anticipated. It provides a highly accurate anatomic assessment of the mitral valve and is strongly and independently predictive of valve reparability and postoperative outcome.[35,100,101]

Assessment of Surgical Results

After the planned surgical intervention, TEE can identify residual defects that need to be addressed to limit morbidity, mortality, and hospitalization costs. In a study of 50 patients, TEE identified 2 patients in whom new SWMAs provided the only sign of unsuspected graft occlusion and prompted graft thrombectomy.[102] In another study of 82 high-risk patients, Savage and coworkers used staged blinding of the cardiac surgeons and anesthesiologists at critical points during surgery.[103] After these clinicians documented their planned management at each stage, TEE results were revealed and led to at least one significant change in anesthetic management in 51% of patients and surgical management in 33% of patients, including additional unplanned or revised grafts (15%) and unplanned valve procedures (20%). Similarly, TEE has profoundly affected valvular heart surgery. In a study of 154 patients undergoing valve surgery, intraoperative TEE documented unsatisfactory repairs in 10 patients (6%) requiring immediate further surgery.[104] Although 6 of these 10 patients had abnormal V waves or elevated pulmonary capillary wedge pressure, hemodynamics was normal in the other 4 patients and only TEE indicated defective repair. At the conclusion of surgery, TEE revealed adequate valvular function in 123 of 154 patients (80%); 18 of these patients (15%) suffered a major postoperative complication, with 6 dying (5%). In contrast, TEE revealed moderate valve dysfunction in seven patients (5%), six of whom suffered major complications (86%), with three dying (50%). Subsequent studies have confirmed that intraoperative TEE assessment of mitral valve function is predictive of postoperative function and outcome.[105] However, during this assessment, the patient's hemodynamics must be restored to normal values; otherwise, the prognostic value of TEE can be lost. Even with the maturation of valve repair techniques, a significant number of repairs must be immediately revised.[106] During valve replacement surgery, TEE reliably detects periprosthetic leaks (surprisingly common).[107] Although moderate or severe periprosthetic leaks should almost always undergo immediate repair, almost half of small leaks resolve with the administration of protamine.[108] Even though immediate prosthetic valve malfunction is rare, it can occur and go undetected if TEE is not performed.[109,110]

TEE can be performed safely in infants as small as 3 kg (see also Chapter 51). Ungerleider and associates found that even with extensive experience as congenital heart surgeons, they were unable to predict without intraoperative echocardiography which of their repairs needed immediate revision.[111] Moreover, when immediate revision was performed, hospital costs were much less than when a second operation was needed to repair the residual defect ($34,000 versus $94,000). Stevenson and coauthors reported that intraoperative TEE reliably detected residual cardiac defects in 17 (7%) of 230 consecutive patients undergoing congenital heart surgery.[112] However, a subsequent publication from the same center reported that the number of residual defects missed by intraoperative TEE increased from 2% to 13% when TEE was performed by the attending anesthesiologist and not a separate echocardiographer.[33] Although this study does not resolve the issue of whether a separate echocardiographer is required to adequately perform TEE in patients undergoing congenital heart repairs, it does amply demonstrate that patients can suffer when intraoperative TEE is not expertly performed, interpreted, and acted on. In this study, the deaths of seven patients may have been related to delayed recognition of residual defects.

DATA STORAGE, DOCUMENTATION, AND QUALITY ASSURANCE

Data Storage and Documentation

Traditionally, echocardiograms are stored on videotape and written reports of the results are placed in the patient's medical record. The SCA has recommended a written report form for this purpose (*http://www.scahq.org/sca3/teereport.shtml*). Digital recording and storage of echocardiograms are growing more common, but because of the size of digital video files, some compression of the data is required. Preliminary studies indicate that compression need not result in loss of clinically important information, but definitive studies are lacking.[113] Regardless of the recording modality used, representative TEE images from all studies must be readily available for comparison with previous or subsequent studies or with both.

Quality Assurance

The ASE has published guidelines for continuous quality improvement (CQI) in echocardiography, but these guidelines were not designed specifically for perioperative TEE.[114] However, even relatively simple CQI interventions may produce dramatic results in the consistency of image acquisition and storage.[34] Periodic expert review of TEE interpretations is essential if practitioners are to reach and maintain their diagnostic potential. Collaboration between the departments of anesthesiology and cardiology is one approach to this review process that minimizes the duplication inherent in the formation of independent CQI programs.

CONCLUSION

TEE is the most powerful cardiovascular diagnostic technique available in the practice of perioperative medicine today. Thousands of published reports document its vital role in the determination of hemodynamics, detection of myocardial ischemia, evaluation of cardiovascular pathology, and assessment of cardiac surgical plans and results. TEE has become a vital part of cardiac anesthesia and surgery because it can provide information necessary for optimizing management and reducing morbidity and mortality. In addition, TEE is vital in the assessment of patients with severe, persistent hypotension because it often reveals the true cause of the hypotension not apparent from other diagnostic techniques available at the bedside. TEE interpretation is inherently subjective, so considerable training and ongoing quality assurance are essential.

KEY POINTS

1. One of the category I indications for TEE is evaluation of a hemodynamically unstable patient.
2. The speed of sound in the heart is assumed to be constant at 1540 m/sec.
3. The higher the transducer frequency, the better the image quality, but the more limited the depth of penetration.
4. Echocardiography relies on the time that it takes for the sound wave to travel between the probe and the imaged structure.
5. Doppler echocardiography is used to measure the velocity of blood in the cardiac chambers and across the valves.
6. The modified Bernoulli equation will transform the velocities into pressure units. $\Delta Pressure = 4V^2$, where V = velocity in m/sec.
7. Continuous-wave Doppler measures high velocities but does not precisely identify the location of the velocities.
8. Pulsed-wave Doppler permits measurement of velocities at an exact location but is limited in its ability to measure high velocities.
9. Color Doppler codes for flows: Blue Away from the probe, Red Toward the probe (BART).
10. The abbreviated TEE examination will be adequate for the practice of basic TEE as defined by the 1996 SCA/ASA TEE guidelines.
11. The differential diagnosis of severe hypotension includes hypovolemia, ventricular failure, severe valvular regurgitation, cardiac tamponade, and low systemic vascular resistance.
12. TEE has been shown to be more sensitive than electrocardiography for the intraoperative detection of myocardial ischemia.

REFERENCES

1. Frazin L, Talano JV, Stephanides L, et al: Esophageal echocardiography. Circulation 54:102-108, 1976.
2. Matsumoto M, Oka Y, Strom J, et al: Application of transesophageal echocardiography to continuous intraoperative monitoring of left ventricular performance. Am J Cardiol 46:95-105, 1980.
3. Matsumoto M, Oka Y, Lin YT, et al: Transesophageal echocardiography; for assessing ventricular performance. N Y State J Med 79:19-21, 1979.
4. Schluter M, Langenstein BA, Polster J, et al: Transesophageal cross-sectional echocardiography with a phased array transducer system. Technique and initial clinical results. Br Heart J 48:67-72, 1982.
5. Lancee CT, de Jong N, Bom N: Design and construction of an esophageal phased array probe. Med Prog Technol 13:139-148, 1988.
6. Practice guidelines for perioperative transesophageal echocardiography. A report by the American Society of Anesthesiologists and the Society of Cardiovascular Anesthesiologists Task Force on Transesophageal Echocardiography. Anesthesiology 84:986-1006, 1996.
7. Shanewise JS, Cheung AT, Aronson S, et al: ASE/SCA guidelines for performing a comprehensive intraoperative multiplane transesophageal echocardiography examination: Recommendations of the American Society of Echocardiography Council for Intraoperative Echocardiography and the Society of Cardiovascular Anesthesiologists Task Force for Certification in Perioperative Transesophageal Echocardiography. Anesth Analg 89:870-884, 1999.
8. Cahalan MK, Stewart W, Pearlman A, et al: American Society of Echocardiography and Society of Cardiovascular Anesthesiologists task force guidelines for training in perioperative echocardiography. J Am Soc Echocardiogr 15:647-652, 2002.
9. Cahalan MK, Abel M, Goldman M, et al: American Society of Echocardiography and Society of Cardiovascular Anesthesiologists task force guidelines for training in perioperative echocardiography. Anesth Analg 94:1384-1388, 2002.
10. Hatle L, Brubakk A, Tromsdal A, et al: Noninvasive assessment of pressure drop in mitral stenosis by Doppler ultrasound. Br Heart J 40:131-140, 1978.
11. Holen J, Simonsen S: Determination of pressure gradient in mitral stenosis with Doppler echocardiography. Br Heart J 41:529-535, 1979.
12. Messina AG, Paranicas M, Fiamengo S, et al: Risk of dysphagia after transesophageal echocardiography. Am J Cardiol 67:313-314, 1991.
13. Hulyalkar AR, Ayd JD: Low risk of gastroesophageal injury associated with transesophageal echocardiography during cardiac surgery. J Cardiothorac Vasc Anesth 7:175-177, 1993.
14. Owall A, Stahl L, Settergren G: Incidence of sore throat and patient complaints after intraoperative transesophageal echocardiography during cardiac surgery. J Cardiothorac Vasc Anesth 6:15-16, 1992.
15. Rousou JA, Tighe DA, Garb JL, et al: Risk of dysphagia after transesophageal echocardiography during cardiac operations. Ann Thorac Surg 69:486-489, 2000.
16. Dewhirst WE, Stragand JJ, Fleming BM: Mallory-Weiss tear complicating intraoperative transesophageal echocardiography in a patient undergoing aortic valve replacement. Anesthesiology 73:777-778, 1990.
17. Polhamus CD, Werth TE, Clement DJ, et al: Gastrointestinal bleeding complicating transesophageal echocardiography. Endoscopy 25:198-199, 1993.
18. Savino JS, Hanson CR, Bigelow DC, et al: Oropharyngeal injury after transesophageal echocardiography. J Cardiothorac Vasc Anesth 8:76-78, 1994.
19. Spahn DR, Schmid S, Carrel T, et al: Hypopharynx perforation by a transesophageal echocardiography probe. Anesthesiology 82:581-583, 1995.
20. Badacui R, Choufane S, Riboulot M, et al: Esophageal perforation after transesophageal echocardiography [in French]. Ann Fr Anesth Reanim 13:850-852, 1994.

21. Latham P, Hodgins LR: A gastric laceration after transesophageal echocardiography in a patient undergoing aortic valve replacement. Anesth Analg 81:641-642, 1995.

22. Kharasch ED, Sivarajan M: Gastroesophageal perforation after intraoperative transesophageal echocardiography. Anesthesiology 85:426-428, 1996.

23. Tam JW, Burwash IG, Ascah KJ, et al: Feasibility and complications of single-plane and biplane versus multiplane transesophageal imaging: A review of 2947 consecutive studies. Can J Cardiol 13:81-84, 1997.

24. Kallmeyer IJ, Collard CD, Fox JA, et al: The safety of intraoperative transesophageal echocardiography: A case series of 7200 cardiac surgical patients. Anesth Analg 92:1126-1130, 2001.

25. Olenchock SA Jr, Lukaszczyk JJ, Reed J 3rd, et al: Splenic injury after intraoperative transesophageal echocardiography. Ann Thorac Surg 72:2141-2143, 2001.

26. Chow MS, Taylor MA, Hanson CW 3rd: Splenic laceration associated with transesophageal echocardiography. J Cardiothorac Vasc Anesth 12:314-316, 1998.

27. Daniel WG, Erbel R, Kasper W, et al: Safety of transesophageal echocardiography. A multicenter survey of 10,419 examinations. Circulation 83:817-821, 1991.

28. Nikutta P, Mantey SF, Becht I, et al: Risk of bacteremia induced by transesophageal echocardiography: Analysis of 100 consecutive procedures. J Am Soc Echocardiogr 5:168-172, 1992.

29. Mentec H, Vignon P, Terre S, et al: Frequency of bacteremia associated with transesophageal echocardiography in intensive care unit patients: A prospective study of 139 patients. Crit Care Med 23:1194-1199, 1995.

30. Read RC, Finch RG, Donald FE, et al: Infective endocarditis after transesophageal echocardiography. Circulation 87:1426, 1993.

31. Gilbert TB, Panico FG, McGill WA, et al: Bronchial obstruction by transesophageal echocardiography probe in a pediatric cardiac patient. Anesth Analg 74:156-158, 1992.

32. Lunn RJ, Oliver WJ, Hagler DJ, et al: Aortic compression by transesophageal echocardiographic probe in infants and children undergoing cardiac surgery. Anesthesiology 77: 587-590, 1992.

33. Stevenson JG: Incidence of complications in pediatric transesophageal echocardiography: Experience in 1650 cases. J Am Soc Echocardiogr 12:527-532, 1999.

34. Miller JP, Lambert AS, Shapiro WA, et al: The adequacy of basic intraoperative transesophageal echocardiography performed by experienced anesthesiologists. Anesth Analg 92:1103-1110, 2001.

35. Lambert AS, Miller JP, Merrick SH, et al: Improved evaluation of the location and mechanism of mitral valve regurgitation with a systematic transesophageal echocardiography examination. Anesth Analg 88:1205-1212, 1996.

36. Swenson JD, Harkin C, Pace NL, et al: Transesophageal echocardiography: An objective tool in defining maximum ventricular response to intravenous fluid therapy. Anesth Analg 83:1149-1153, 1996.

37. Swenson JD, Bull D, Stringham J: Subjective assessment of left ventricular preload using transesophageal echocardiography: Corresponding pulmonary artery occlusion pressures. J Cardiothorac Vasc Anesth 15:580-583, 2001.

38. Tousignant CP, Walsh F, Mazer CD: The use of transesophageal echocardiography for preload assessment in critically ill patients. Anesth Analg 90:351-355, 2000.

39. Harpole DH, Clements FM, Quill T, et al: Right and left ventricular performance during and after abdominal aortic aneurysm repair. Ann Surg 209:356-362, 1989.

40. Cheung AT, Savino JS, Weiss SJ, et al: Echocardiographic and hemodynamic indexes of left ventricular preload in patients with normal and abnormal ventricular function. Anesthesiology 81:376-387, 1994.

41. Lattik R, Couture P, Denault AY, et al: Mitral Doppler indices are superior to two-dimensional echocardiographic and hemodynamic variables in predicting responsiveness of cardiac output to a rapid intravenous infusion of colloid. Anesth Analg 94:1092-1099, 2002.

42. Kuecherer HF, Muhiudeen IA, Kusumoto FM, et al: Estimation of mean left atrial pressure from transesophageal pulsed Doppler echocardiography of pulmonary venous flow. Circulation 82:1127-1139, 1990.

43. Hofmann T, Keck A, van Ingen G, et al: Simultaneous measurement of pulmonary venous flow by intravascular catheter Doppler velocimetry and transesophageal Doppler echocardiography: Relation to left atrial pressure and left atrial and left ventricular function. J Am Coll Cardiol 26:239-249, 1995.

44. Kusumoto FM, Muhiudeen IA, Kuecherer HF, et al: Response of the interatrial septum to transatrial pressure gradients and its potential for predicting pulmonary capillary wedge pressure: An intraoperative study using transesophageal echocardiography in patients during mechanical ventilation. J Am Coll Cardiol 21:721-728, 1993.

45. Castello R, Vaughn M, Dressler FA, et al: Relation between pulmonary venous flow and pulmonary wedge pressure: Influence of cardiac output. Am Heart J 130:127-134, 1995.

46. Nomura M, Hillel Z, Shih H, et al: The association between Doppler transmitral flow variables measured by transesophageal echocardiography and pulmonary capillary wedge pressure. Anesth Analg 84:491-496, 1997.

47. Muhiudeen IA, Kuecherer HF, Lee E, et al: Intraoperative estimation of cardiac output by transesophageal pulsed Doppler echocardiography. Anesthesiology 74:9-14, 1991.

48. Savino JS, Troianos CA, Aukburg S, et al: Measurement of pulmonary blood flow with transesophageal two-dimensional and Doppler echocardiography. Anesthesiology 75:445-451, 1991.

49. Pu M, Griffin BP, Vandervoort PM, et al: Intraoperative validation of mitral inflow determination by transesophageal echocardiography: Comparison of single-plane, biplane and thermodilution techniques. J Am Coll Cardiol 26:1047-1053, 1995.

50. Pu M, Griffin BP, Vandervoort PM, et al: The value of assessing pulmonary venous flow velocity for predicting severity of mitral regurgitation: A quantitative assessment integrating left ventricular function. J Am Soc Echocardiogr 12:736-743, 1999.

51. Darmon PL, Hillel Z, Mogtader A, et al: Cardiac output by transesophageal echocardiography using continuous-wave Doppler across the aortic valve. Anesthesiology 80:796-805, 1994.

52. Martin B, Jan P, Jan H: Effect of the degree of tricuspid regurgitation on cardiac output measurements by thermodilution. Intensive Care Med 28:1117-1121, 2002.

53. Feinberg MS, Hopkins WE, Davila RV, et al: Multiplane transesophageal echocardiographic Doppler imaging accurately determines cardiac output measurements in critically ill patients. Chest 107:769-773, 1995.

54. Perrino AC Jr, Harris SN, Luther MA: Intraoperative determination of cardiac output using multiplane transesophageal echocardiography: A comparison to thermodilution. Anesthesiology 89:350-357, 1998.

55. Gray PE, Perrino AC: Hemodynamic-induced changes in aortic valve area: Implications for Doppler cardiac output determinations. Anesth Analg 92:584-589, 2001.

56. Gorcsan J 3rd, Denault A, Gasior TA, et al: Rapid estimation of left ventricular contractility from end-systolic relations by echocardiographic automated border detection and femoral arterial pressure. Anesthesiology 81:553-562, discussion 27A, 1994.

57. Reich DL, Konstadt SN, Nejat M, et al: Intraoperative transesophageal echocardiography for the detection of cardiac preload changes induced by transfusion and phlebotomy in pediatric patients. Anesthesiology 79:10-15, 1993.

58. Reichert CL, Visser CA, Koolen JJ, et al: Transesophageal echocardiography in hypotensive patients after cardiac operations. Comparison with hemodynamic parameters. J Thorac Cardiovasc Surg 104:321-326, 1992.

59. Cicek S, Demirilic U, Kuralay E, et al: Transesophageal echocardiography in cardiac surgical emergencies. J Card Surg 10:236-244, 1995.

60. Cook CH, Praba AC, Beery PR, et al: Transthoracic echocardiography is not cost-effective in critically ill surgical patients. J Trauma 52:280-284, 2002.

61. van der Wouw PA, Koster RW, Delemarre BJ, et al: Diagnostic accuracy of transesophageal echocardiography during cardiopulmonary resuscitation. J Am Coll Cardiol 30:780-783, 1997.

62. Heidenreich PA, Stainback RF, Redberg RF, et al: Transesophageal echocardiography predicts mortality in critically ill patients with unexplained hypotension. J Am Coll Cardiol 26:152-158, 1995.

63. Costachescu T, Denault A, Guimond JG, et al: The hemo-dynamically unstable patient in the intensive care unit: Hemodynamic vs. transesophageal echocardiographic monitoring. Crit Care Med 30:1214-1223, 2002.

64. Colreavy FB, Donovan K, Lee KY, et al: Transesophageal echocardiography in critically ill patients. Crit Care Med 30:989-996, 2002.

65. Tennant R, Wiggers C: The effect of coronary occlusion on myocardial contraction. Am J Physiol 112:351-361, 1935.

66. Smith JS, Cahalan MK, Benefiel DJ, et al: Intraoperative detection of myocardial ischemia in high-risk patients: Electrocardiography versus two-dimensional transesophageal echocardiography. Circulation 72:1015-1021, 1985.

67. Leung JM, O'Kelly B, Browner WS, et al: Prognostic importance of postbypass regional wall-motion abnormalities in patients undergoing coronary artery bypass graft surgery. Anesthesiology 71:16-25, 1989.

68. van Daele ME, Sutherland GR, Mitchell MM, et al: Do changes in pulmonary capillary wedge pressure adequately reflect myocardial ischemia during anesthesia? A correlative preoperative hemodynamic, electrocardiographic, and transesophageal echocardiographic study. Circulation 81:865-871, 1990.

69. Comunale M, Body S, Ley C, et al: The concordance of intraoperative left ventricular wall-motion abnormalities and electrocardiographic S-T changes. Association with outcome after coronary revascularization. Anesthesiology 88:945-954, 1998.

70. Shah PM, Kyo S, Matsumura M, et al: Utility of biplane transesophageal echocardiography in left ventricular wall motion analysis. J Cardiothorac Vasc Anesth 5:316-319, 1991.

71. Rouine-Rapp K, Ionescu P, Balea M, et al: Detection of intraoperative segmental wall-motion abnormalities by transesophageal echocardiography: The incremental value of additional cross sections in the transverse and longitudinal planes. Anesth Analg 83:1141-1148, 1996.

72. Seeberger MD, Cahalan MK, Chu E, et al: Acute hypovolemia may cause segmental wall motion abnormalities in the absence of myocardial ischemia. Anesth Analg 85:1252-1257, 1997.

73. Aronson S, Lee BK, Wiencek JG, et al: Assessment of myocardial perfusion during CABG surgery with two-dimensional transesophageal contrast echocardiography. Anesthesiology 75:433-440, 1991.

74. Voci P, Bilotta F, Caretta Q, et al: Low-dose dobutamine echocardiography predicts the early response of dysfunctioning myocardial segments to coronary artery bypass grafting. Am Heart J 129:521-526, 1995.

75. Panza JA, Laurienzo JM, Curiel RV, et al: Transesophageal dobutamine stress echocardiography for evaluation of patients with coronary artery disease. J Am Coll Cardiol 24:1260-1267, 1994.

76. Baer FM, Voth E, Deutsch HJ, et al: Predictive value of low dose dobutamine transesophageal echocardiography and fluorine-18 fluorodeoxyglucose positron emission tomography for recovery of regional left ventricular function after successful revascularization. J Am Coll Cardiol 28:60-69, 1996.

77. Seeberger MD, Skarvan K, Buser P, et al: Dobutamine stress echocardiography to detect inducible demand ischemia in anesthetized patients with coronary artery disease. Anesthesiology 88:1233-1239, 1998.

78. Seeberger MD, Cahalan MK, Chu E, et al: Rapid atrial pacing for detecting provokable demand ischemia in anesthetized patients. Anesth Analg 84:1180-1185, 1997.

79. Buckmaster MJ, Kearney PA, Johnson SB, et al: Further experience with transesophageal echocardiography in the evaluation of thoracic aortic injury. J Trauma 37:989-995, 1994.

80. Vignon P, Lagrange P, Boncoeur MP, et al: Routine trans-esophageal echocardiography for the diagnosis of aortic disruption in trauma patients without enlarged mediastinum. J Trauma 40:422-427, 1996.

81. Goarin JP, Cluzel P, Gosgnach M, et al: Evaluation of transesophageal echocardiography for diagnosis of traumatic aortic injury. Anesthesiology 93:1373-1377, 2000.

82. Erbel R, Engberding R, Daniel W, et al: Echocardiography in diagnosis of aortic dissection. Lancet 1:457-461, 1989.

83. Torossov M, Singh A, Fein SA: Clinical presentation, diagnosis, and hospital outcome of patients with documented aortic dissection: The Albany Medical Center experience, 1986 to 1996. Am Heart J 137:154-156, 1999.

84. Nienaber CA, von Kodolitsch Y, Nicolas V, et al: The diagnosis of thoracic aortic dissection by noninvasive imaging procedures. N Engl J Med 328:1-9, 1993.

85. Movsowitz HD, Levine RA, Hilgenberg AD, et al: Transesophageal echocardiographic description of the mechanisms of aortic regurgitation in acute type A aortic dissection: Implications for aortic valve repair. J Am Coll Cardiol 36:884-890, 2000.

86. Hoffmann R, Flachskampf FA, Hanrath P: Planimetry of orifice area in aortic stenosis using multiplane trans-esophageal echocardiography. J Am Coll Cardiol 22:529-534, 1993.

87. Blumberg FC, Pfeifer M, Holmer SR, et al: Transgastric Doppler echocardiographic assessment of the severity of aortic stenosis using multiplane transesophageal echocardiography. Am J Cardiol 79:1273-1275, 1997.

88. Moisa RB, Zeldis SM, Alper SA, et al: Aortic regurgitation in coronary artery bypass grafting: Implications for cardioplegia administration. Ann Thorac Surg 60:665-668, 1995.

89. Stoddard MF, Prince CR, Tuman WL, et al: Angle of incidence does not affect accuracy of mitral stenosis area calculation by pressure half-time: Application to Doppler transesophageal echocardiography. Am Heart J 127:1562-1572, 1994.

90. Himelman RB, Kusumoto F, Oken K, et al: The flail mitral valve: Echocardiographic findings by precordial and transesophageal imaging and Doppler color flow mapping. J Am Coll Cardiol 17:272-279, 1991.

91. Klein AL, Obarski TP, Stewart WJ, et al: Transesophageal Doppler echocardiography of pulmonary venous flow: A new marker of mitral regurgitation severity. J Am Coll Cardiol 18:518-526, 1991.

92. Schiller NB, Foster E, Redberg RF: Transesophageal echocardiography in the evaluation of mitral regurgitation. Cardiol Clin 11:339-408, 1993.

93. Miller-Hance WC, Silverman NH: Transesophageal echocardiography (TEE) in congenital heart disease with focus on the adult. Cardiol Clin 18:861-892, 2000.

94. Katz ES, Tunick PA, Rusinek H, et al: Protruding aortic athero-mas predict stroke in elderly patients undergoing cardio-pulmonary bypass: Experience with intraoperative transesophageal echocardiography. J Am Coll Cardiol 20:70-77, 1992.

95. Mizuno T, Toyama M, Tabuchi N, et al: Thickened intima of the aortic arch is a risk factor for stroke with coronary artery bypass grafting. Ann Thorac Surg 70:1565-1570, 2000.

96. Trehan N, Mishra M, Kasliwal RR, et al: Surgical strategies in patients at high risk for stroke undergoing coronary artery bypass grafting. Ann Thorac Surg 70:1037-1045, 2000.

97. Sheikh KH, Bengtson JR, Rankin JS, et al: Intraoperative transesophageal Doppler color flow imaging used to guide patient selection and operative treatment of ischemic mitral regurgitation. Circulation 84:594-604, 1991.

98. Nowrangi SK, Connolly HM, Freeman WK, et al: Impact of intraoperative transesophageal echocardiography among patients undergoing aortic valve replacement for aortic stenosis. J Am Soc Echocardiogr 14:863-866, 2001.

99. Mishra M, Chauhan R, Sharma KK, et al: Real-time intraoperative transesophageal echocardiography—how useful? Experience of 5,016 cases. J Cardiothorac Vasc Anesth 12:625-632, 1998.

100. Enriquez-Sarano M, Freeman WK, Tribouilloy CM, et al: Functional anatomy of mitral regurgitation: Accuracy and outcome implications of transesophageal echocardiography. J Am Coll Cardiol 34:1129-1136, 1999.

101. Omran AS, Woo A, David TE, et al: Intraoperative transesophageal echocardiography accurately predicts mitral valve anatomy and suitability for repair. J Am Soc Echocardiogr 15:950-957, 2002.

102. Deutsch HJ, Curtius JM, Leischik R, et al: Diagnostic value of transesophageal echocardiography in cardiac surgery. Thorac Cardiovasc Surg 39:199-204, 1991.

103. Savage RM, Lytle BW, Aronson S, et al: Intraoperative echocardiography is indicated in high-risk coronary artery bypass grafting. Ann Thorac Surg 64:368-373, 1997.

104. Sheikh KH, de Bruijn NP, Rankin JS, et al: The utility of transesophageal echocardiography and Doppler color flow imaging in patients undergoing cardiac valve surgery. J Am Coll Cardiol 15:363-372, 1990.

105. Saiki Y, Kasegawa H, Kawase M, et al: Intraoperative TEE during mitral valve repair: Does it predict early and late postoperative mitral valve dysfunction? Ann Thorac Surg 66:1277-1281, 1998.

106. Click RL, Abel MD, Schaff HV: Intraoperative transesophageal echocardiography: 5-year prospective review of impact on surgical management. Mayo Clin Proc 75:241-247, 2000.

107. O'Rourke DJ, Palac RT, Malenka DJ, et al: Outcome of mild periprosthetic regurgitation detected by intraoperative transesophageal echocardiography. J Am Coll Cardiol 38:163-166, 2001.

108. Morehead AJ, Firstenberg MS, Shiota T, et al: Intraoperative echocardiographic detection of regurgitant jets after valve replacement. Ann Thorac Surg 69:135-139, 2000.

109. Kumano H, Suehiro S, Shibata T, et al: Stuck valve leaflet detected by intraoperative transesophageal echocardiography. Ann Thorac Surg 67:1484-1485, 1991.

110. Ionescu AA, West RR, Proudman C, et al: Prospective study of routine perioperative transesophageal echocardiography for elective valve replacement: Clinical impact and cost-saving implications. J Am Soc Echocardiogr 14:659-667, 2001.

111. Ungerleider RM, Kisslo JA, Greeley WJ, et al: Intraoperative echocardiography during congenital heart operations: Experience from 1,000 cases. Ann Thorac Surg 60:S539-S542, 1995.

112. Stevenson JG, Sorensen GK, Gartman DM, et al: Transesophageal echocardiography during repair of congenital cardiac defects: Identification of residual problems necessitating reoperation. J Am Soc Echocardiogr 6:356-365, 1993.

113. Lambert AS, Miller JP, Foster E, et al: The diagnostic validity of digitally captured intraoperative transesophageal echocardiography examinations compared with analog recordings: A pilot study. J Am Soc Echocardiogr 12:974-980, 1999.

114. Recommendations for continuous quality improvement in echocardiography. American Society of Echocardiography. J Am Soc Echocardiogr 8(Suppl):S1-28, 1995.

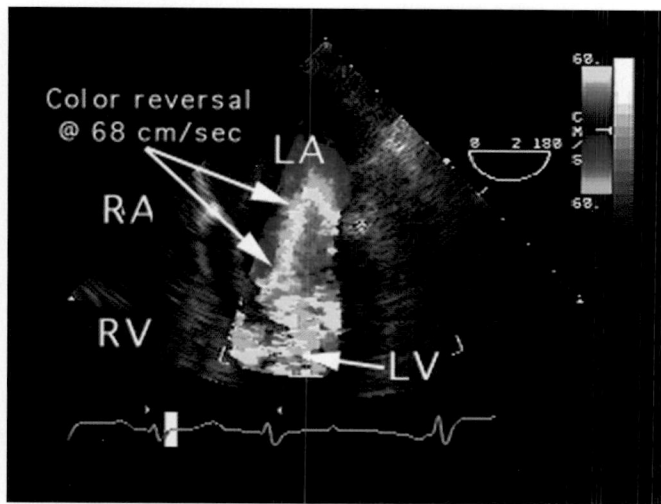

Plate 33–1 "Normal" color Doppler aliasing. In this echocardiogram, "normal" color Doppler aliasing is seen because laminar flow of blood through the mitral valve and into the left ventricle exceeds the Nyquist limit (68 cm/sec in this example—see the color reference icon at the upper right of the figure), thereby resulting in reversal of the color coding of flow direction. Notice that this color reversal occurs across fairly broad, regular areas and not in a random or point-by-point fashion as occurs with turbulent flow (always abnormal). In this example, follow the blue flow from high in the left atrium as it accelerates into the mitral orifice, and notice how color Doppler depicts the increasing flow velocities: the blue color becomes lighter and lighter until the Nyquist limit is reached. Then, color reversal occurs, with light blue becoming yellow. Just at that reversal point, the velocity equals the Nyquist limit, in this example 68 cm/sec. Subsequent reversals may occur at that limit or at multiples of that limit. LA, left atrium; LV, left ventricle; RA, right atrium; RV, right ventricle. (From Cahalan MK: Intraoperative Transesophageal Echocardiography. An Interactive Text and Atlas. New York, Churchill Livingstone, 1997.)

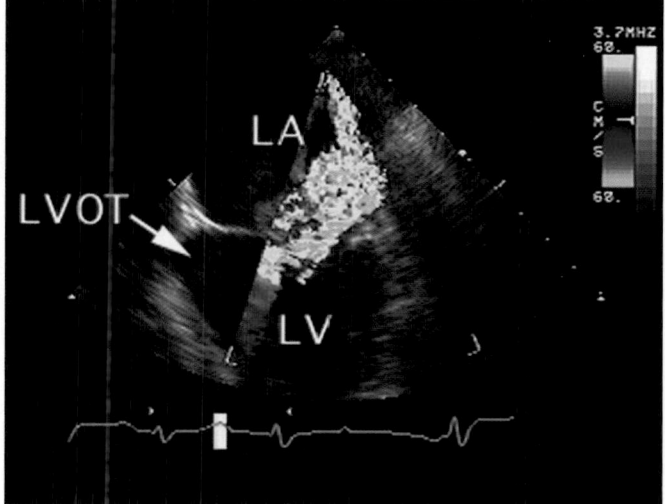

Plate 33–2 Color Doppler aliasing depicting turbulent flow. In this echocardiogram, color Doppler reveals aliasing caused by severe mitral regurgitation: a broad-based systolic color jet emanating from the mitral valve and extending far into the left atrium. This jet is composed of a mosaic of colors mixed in a seemingly random, point-by-point fashion because the jet results from the turbulent flow of mitral regurgitation. Turbulence is never normal in the heart, and thus mosaic jets such as the one shown here are highly valuable diagnostic signs of underlying pathology. LA, left atrium; LV, left ventricle; LVOT, left ventricular outflow tract. (From Cahalan MK: Intraoperative Transesophageal Echocardiography. An Interactive Text and Atlas. New York, Churchill Livingstone, 1997.)

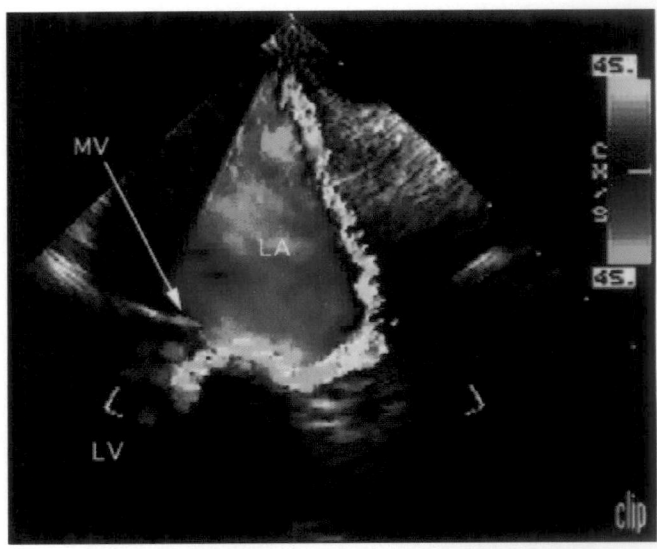

Plate 33–4 Severe mitral regurgitation with a wall-hugging jet. This honed-down five-chamber echocardiogram reveals severe mitral regurgitation. The long color jet has a fairly broad base and an eccentric direction indicative of severe mitral regurgitation. Wall-hugging jets such as this one have a small cross-sectional area because much of their energy is absorbed by the wall of the atrium. The mechanism of the regurgitation is apparent: the anterior leaflet (on the left side of the video screen) is prolapsing and allowing blood to escape beneath it and jet over the surface of the posterior leaflet into the left atrium (LA). LV, left ventricle; MV, mitral valve. (From Cahalan MK: Intraoperative Transesophageal Echocardiography. An Interactive Text and Atlas. New York, Churchill Livingstone, 1997.)

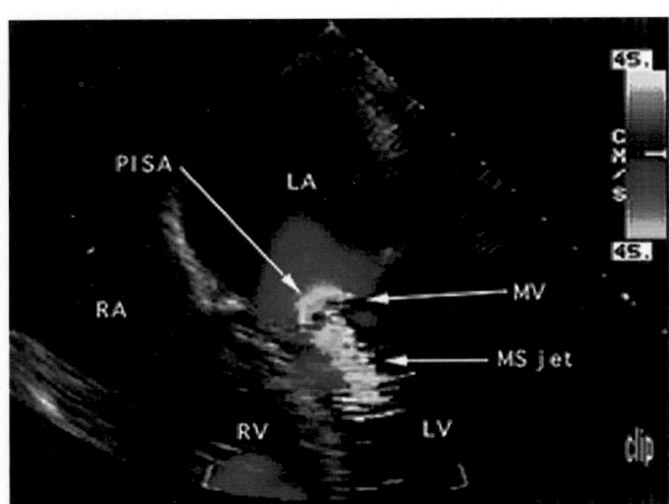

Plate 33–3 Color Doppler imaging of severe mitral stenosis. This four-chamber echocardiogram reveals a thickened and narrowed mitral valve (MV) indicative of mitral stenosis (MS). Color Doppler demonstrates (1) acceleration of blood flow into the stenotic valve (a light blue semicircular area immediately above the valve called "PISA"—proximal isovelocity surface area), (2) a narrow color jet across the valve itself, and (3) a 1 by 4-cm color jet extending from the undersurface of the valve into the left ventricle. LA, left atrium; LV, left ventricle; RA, right atrium; RV, right ventricle. (From Cahalan MK: Intraoperative Transesophageal Echocardiography. An Interactive Text and Atlas. New York, Churchill Livingstone, 1997.)

CHAPTER
34 Electrocardiography

Zaharia Hillel and Daniel M. Thys

Normal Electrical Activity   1389
P Wave   1389
PR Interval   1389
QRS Complex   1389
ST Segment and T Wave   1389

Lead Systems   1390
Standard Limb and Precordial Leads   1390
Electrocardiographic Monitoring Systems   1391

Display, Recording, and Interpretation   1395
Basic Requirements   1395
Artifacts   1396

Indications   1397
Diagnosis of Arrhythmias   1397

Treatment of Arrhythmias   1398
Diagnosis of Ischemia   1404
Diagnosis of Conduction
    Defects   1406

Automatic Recording   1409

Computer-Assisted Interpretation   1410
Arrhythmias   1411
Myocardial Ischemia   1411

Summary   1412

The intraoperative use of the electrocardiogram (ECG) has markedly developed over the past several decades.[1] Originally, this monitor was used during anesthesia for the detection of arrhythmias in high-risk patients.[2] At that time, standard limb lead II was displayed, because its electrical axis parallels the electrical axis of the heart and the P wave is usually easily observed. Since then, the importance of ECG as a standard monitor has been recognized, and its use while conducting any anesthetic regimen is now recommended.[3] Beyond the usefulness of the ECG for the recognition of intraoperative arrhythmias, one of the major indications for electrocardiographic monitoring is the intraoperative diagnosis of myocardial ischemia.[4] Despite widespread attempts at prevention, coronary artery disease continues to be a major health problem in the United States. Some patients undergoing different types of surgical procedures have significant coronary artery disease, and the ECG should be used to identify myocardial ischemia and to recognize arrhythmias. With many patients coming to surgery with pacemakers in place, the ECG also enables the physician to follow the function of the device during the surgical procedure. Since the first use of the ECG during anesthesia, the technology available to the anesthesiologist has become considerably more sophisticated. This chapter describes some of the newer developments in the use and interpretation of the ECG.

NORMAL ELECTRICAL ACTIVITY

P Wave

A complete electrocardiographic cycle, intervals, and segments are shown in Figure 34-1. Under normal circumstances, the sinoatrial node has the most rapid spontaneous depolarization rate and is therefore the dominant cardiac pacemaker (Table 34-1). From the sinoatrial node, the impulse spreads through the right and left atria. Specialized tracts conduct the impulse to the atrioventricular node, but they are not essential. The three selective inputs to the atrioventricular node are the right superior "fast" pathway, the right superior "slow" pathway, and a left-sided pathway that is less well characterized. On the ECG, depolarization of the atria is represented by the P wave. The initial depolarization involves primarily the right atrium and occurs predominantly in an anterior, inferior, and leftward direction. Subsequently, it proceeds to the left atrium, located in a more posterior position.

PR Interval

After the depolarization has reached the atrioventricular node, a delay is observed. The delay permits contraction

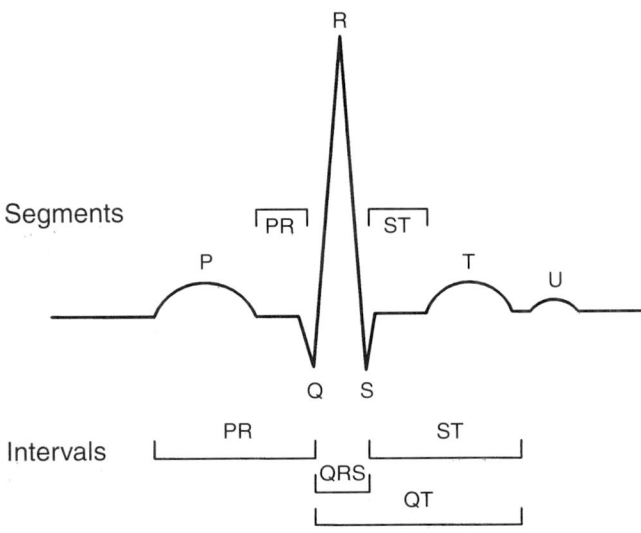

Figure 34–1 A single, normal electrocardiographic cycle with waves, segments, and intervals identified.

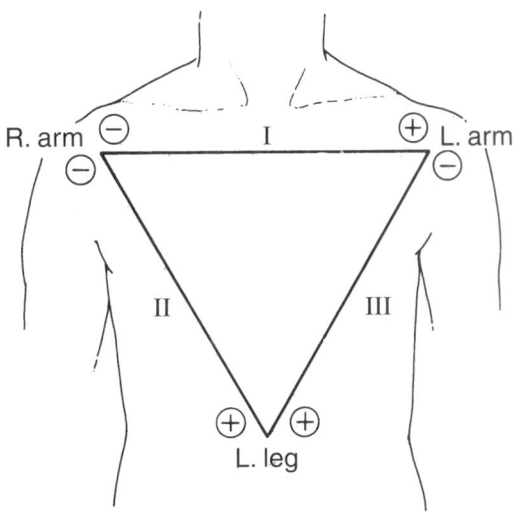

Figure 34–2 Einthoven triangle. (From Thys DM, Kaplan JA: The ECG in Anesthesia and Critical Care. New York, Churchill Livingstone, 1987.)

of the atria and supplemental filling of the ventricular chambers. On the ECG, it is represented by the PR interval.

QRS Complex

After passage through the atrioventricular node, the electrical impulse is conducted along the ventricular conduction pathways consisting of the common bundle of His, the left and right bundle branches, the distal bundle branches, and the Purkinje fibers. The QRS complex represents the progress of the depolarization wave through this conduction system. After terminal depolarization, the electrocardiographic pattern should normally return to baseline.

ST Segment and T Wave

Repolarization of the ventricles begins at the end of the QRS complex and consists of the ST segment and T wave. Whereas ventricular depolarization occurs along established conduction pathways, ventricular repolarization is a prolonged process that occurs independently in every cell. The T wave represents the uncancelled potential differences of ventricular repolarization. The junction of the QRS and the ST segment is the J junction. The T wave is sometimes followed by a small U wave, the origin of which is unclear. An inverted U wave has been associated with several clinically significant conditions, such as hypertension, coronary artery disease, valvular heart disease, and certain metabolic disorders. There may be an association between exercise- or rest-related U-wave

inversion and significant stenosis of the left anterior descending artery or the left main coronary artery.

LEAD SYSTEMS

Standard Limb and Precordial Leads

The small electric currents produced by the electrical activity of the heart spread throughout the body, which behaves as a volume conductor, allowing the surface ECG to be recorded at any site. The standard leads are bipolar leads, because they measure differences in potential between pairs of electrodes. The electrodes are placed on the right arm, the left arm, and the left leg. The leads are formed by the imaginary lines connecting the electrodes, and the polarities correspond to the conventions of the Einthoven triangle (Fig. 34-2). They are labeled leads I, II,

Table 34–1	Spontaneous electrical activity of cardiac tissues
Tissue	**Intrinsic Depolarization Rate (Beats/Min)**
Sinoatrial node	>60
Atrioventricular node	40–60
Purkinje fibers	<40

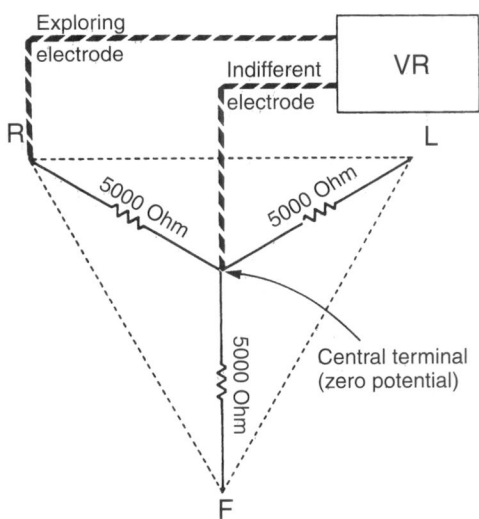

Figure 34–3 Unipolar limb lead circuit (VR). (From Thys DM, Kaplan JA: The ECG in Anesthesia and Critical Care. New York, Churchill Livingstone, 1987.)

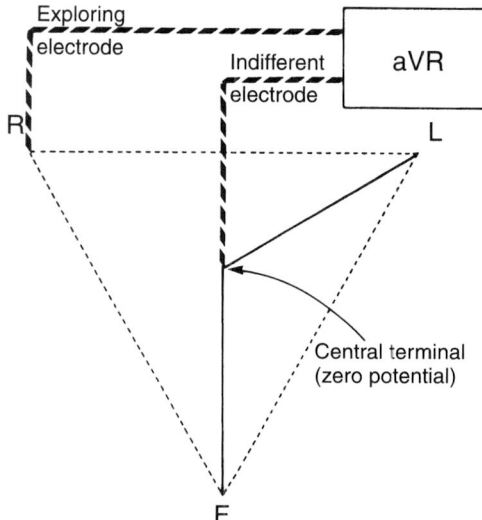

Figure 34–4 Goldberger modification to the unipolar lead aVR. (From Thys DM, Kaplan JA: The ECG in Anesthesia and Critical Care. New York, Churchill Livingstone, 1987.)

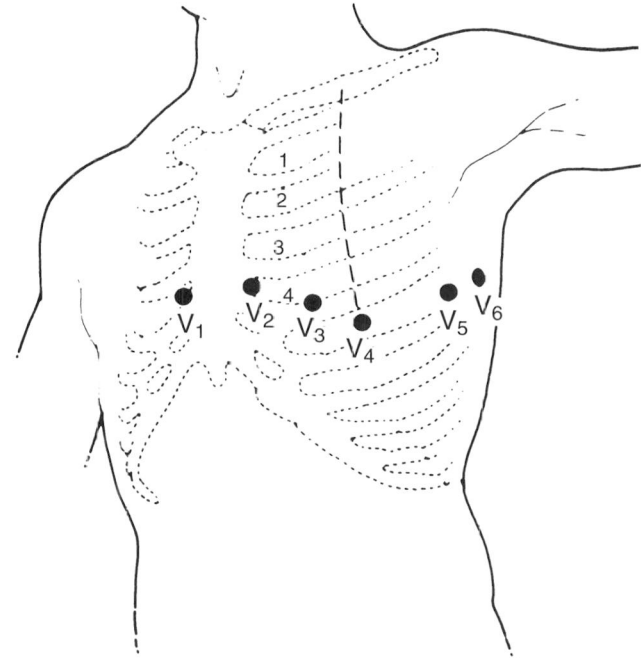

Figure 34–5 Anatomic location of the precordial unipolar leads V_1 through V_6. (From Thys DM, Kaplan JA: The ECG in Anesthesia and Critical Care. New York, Churchill Livingstone, 1987.)

and III. If the three electrodes of the standard leads are connected through resistances of 5000 ohms each, a common central terminal with zero potential is obtained. When this common electrode is used with another exploring electrode, the potential difference between them represents the actual potential (Fig. 34-3). On a standard 12-lead ECG, three unipolar limb leads are usually recorded: aVR, aVL, and aVF. The letter *a* indicates that they are augmented limb leads and were obtained using the Goldberger modification (Fig. 34-4). In this modification, the resistors are removed from the circuit, and the exploring electrode is disconnected from the central terminal. This modification produces larger electrocardiographic deflections.

Additional information on the heart's electrical activity is obtained by placing electrodes closer to the heart or around the thorax. In the precordial lead system, the neutral electrode is formed by the standard leads, and an exploring electrode is placed on the chest wall. The ECG is normally recorded with the exploring electrode in one or more of six precordial positions. They are indicated by the letter *V*, followed by a numeral from 1 to 6 indicating the location of the electrode on the chest wall (Fig. 34-5).

Electrocardiographic Monitoring Systems

Three-Electrode System

The three-electrode system uses only three electrodes to record the ECG. In such a system, the ECG is observed along one bipolar lead between two of the electrodes while the third electrode serves as a ground. A selector switch allows the user to alter the designation of the electrodes. Three electrocardiographic leads can be examined in sequence without changing the location of the electrodes. Although the three-electrode system has the advantage of simplicity, its use is limited in myocardial ischemia because it provides a narrow picture of myocardial electrical activity.

Modified Three-Electrode System

Numerous modifications of the standard bipolar limb lead system have been developed. Some of these are displayed

in Figure 34-6. They are used in an attempt to maximize P-wave height for the diagnosis of atrial arrhythmias or to increase the sensitivity of the ECG for the detection of anterior myocardial ischemia. In clinical studies, these modified three-electrode systems have been shown to be as sensitive as or more sensitive than the standard V_5 lead system for the intraoperative diagnosis of ischemia.[5]

Central Subclavicular Lead

The central subclavicular (CS_5) lead is particularly well suited for the detection of anterior myocardial wall ischemia. The right arm (RA) electrode is placed under the right clavicle, the left arm (LA) electrode is placed in the V_5 position, and the left leg electrode is in its usual position to serve as a ground. Lead I is selected for detection of anterior wall ischemia, and lead II can be selected for monitoring inferior wall ischemia or for the detection of arrhythmias. If a unipolar precordial electrode is unavailable, the CS_5 bipolar lead is the best and easiest alternative to a true V_5 lead for monitoring myocardial ischemia.

Central Back Lead

The central back (CB_5) lead is good for the detection of ischemia and supraventricular arrhythmias as demonstrated in a study comparing CB_5 and V_5 in patients with closed and open chests.[6] The P wave was 90% larger than in lead V_5, whereas a good correlation between ventricular deflections of CB_5 and V_5 leads was observed. CB_5 is obtained by placing the RA electrode over the center of the right scapula and the LA electrode in the V_5 position. The lead selector switch should be on lead I. The CB_5 lead may be useful in patients with ischemic heart disease who are susceptible to the development of arrhythmias during the perioperative period.

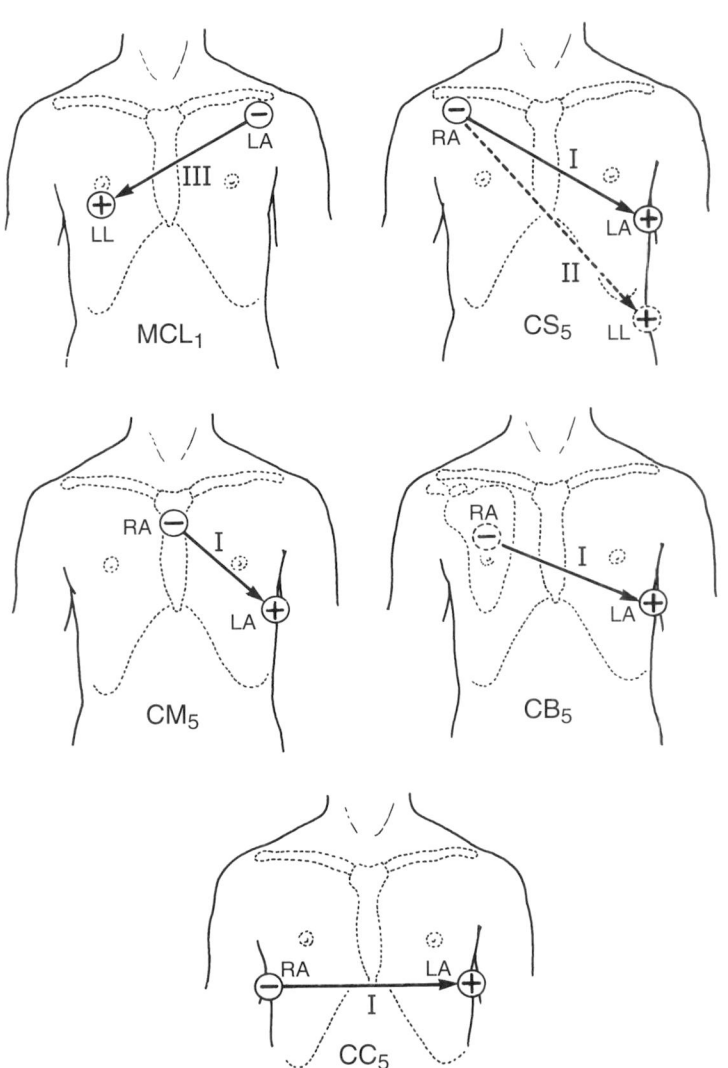

Figure 34–6 Modified bipolar standard limb lead system: MCL$_1$, CS$_5$, CM$_5$, CB$_5$, CC$_5$. (From Thys DM, Kaplan JA: The ECG in Anesthesia and Critical Care. New York, Churchill Livingstone, 1987.)

When modified bipolar limb leads are used, monitoring personnel should be aware that in certain aspects these leads differ significantly from true unipolar precordial leads. The modified precordial leads usually show greater R-wave amplitude than standard precordial leads, and this feature can result in amplification of the ST-segment response.

The criteria for diagnosing myocardial ischemia (discussed later) may need to be adjusted when modified bipolar leads are used. It has been shown during exercise stress testing that normalization of the degree of ST-segment depression to the height of the R wave increases the sensitivity and specificity of ECG for the recognition of myocardial ischemia.[7] In an intraoperative study, Mark and coworkers[8] observed that placement of a Canadian sternal retractor during cardiac surgery was associated with a reduction in V$_5$ R-wave amplitude from 15 ± 1 to 10 ± 1 mm. Simultaneously, V$_5$ S-wave amplitude and absolute ST-segment deviation were reduced from 3.5 ± 0.4 to 1.7 ± 0.3 mm and from 0.50 ± 0.04 to 0.39 ± 0.05 mm, respectively (Table 34-2). The researchers concluded that their results support the proposal that inclusion of an R-wave gain factor may improve perioperative electrocardiographic monitoring.

Five-Electrode System

The use of five electrodes allows the recording of the six standard limb leads (I, II, III, aVR, aVL, aVF), as well as one precordial unipolar lead. Generally, the unipolar lead is placed in the V$_5$ position, which is along the anterior axillary line in the fifth intercostal space (Fig. 34-7). With the addition of only two electrodes to the electrocardiographic system, up to seven different leads can be monitored simultaneously. This allows monitoring of several areas of the myocardium for ischemia or establishing a differential diagnosis between atrial and ventricular arrhythmias.

In 1976, Kaplan and King[9] suggested monitoring lead V$_5$ as the best choice for the detection of intraoperative ischemia. Using a single lead in high-risk patients undergoing noncardiac surgery, London and colleagues[10] demonstrated that the greatest sensitivity was obtained with lead V$_5$ (75%), followed by lead V$_4$ (61%). Combining leads V$_4$ and V$_5$ increased the sensitivity to 90%, whereas with the standard lead II and V$_5$ combination, the sensitivity was only 80%. London and colleagues also suggested that if three leads (II, V$_4$, and V$_5$) could be examined simultaneously, the sensitivity would rise to 98%. Most modern electrocardiographic monitors, however, do not readily allow the simultaneous display of more than one precordial lead. Some investigators

Table 34–2 Electrocardiographic changes during sternal retractor placement in 83 patients

Variable	Period	Mean ± SEM	n Increase	n Decrease	X^2	P
V_5 RWA	Baseline	15.1 ± 0.8	—	—	—	—
	Retractor	9.9 ± 0.7	9	69	44.6	0.001
V_5 SWA	Baseline	3.5 ± 0.4	—	—	—	—
	Retractor	1.7 ± 0.3	3	59	48.8	0.001
V_5 ST-ABS	Baseline	0.50 ± 0.04	—	—	—	—
	Retractor	0.40 ± 0.05	20	51	12.68	0.001

n, number of patients showing the indicated change; RWA, R-wave amplitude; ST-ABS, absolute value of ST displacement; SWA, S-wave amplitude; X^2, comparison between n increase and n decrease.
Adapted from Mark JB, Chien GL, Steinbrook RA, et al: Electrocardiographic R-wave changes during cardiac surgery. Anesth Analg 74:26, 1992.

have also suggested that the monitoring of a right-sided precordial lead (V_{4R}) may be of benefit in patients with occlusive disease of the right coronary artery.[11]

Great individual variability in the placement of precordial leads is a problem that has been recognized. In an attempt to reduce the error, Herman and coworkers[12] studied a device that facilitates precordial lead placement. The ECG obtained after device-guided electrode placement showed variations from those obtained without it in 60% of patients. Significant Q-wave appearance and disappearance or significant ST-segment elevation and depression, or both, occurred in 19% of patients.

Invasive Electrocardiographic Monitoring

The electrical potentials of the heart can be measured from a surface ECG and from body cavities adjacent to the heart (i.e., esophagus or trachea) or from within the heart itself.

Esophageal Electrocardiogram

The concept of esophageal ECG is not new; numerous studies have demonstrated the usefulness of this approach in the diagnosis of complicated arrhythmias. The esophageal electrodes are incorporated into an esophageal stethoscope and are welded to conventional electrocardiographic wires (Fig. 34-8). A prominent P wave is usually displayed in the presence of atrial depolarization, and its relation to the ventricular electrical activity can be examined (Fig. 34-9).

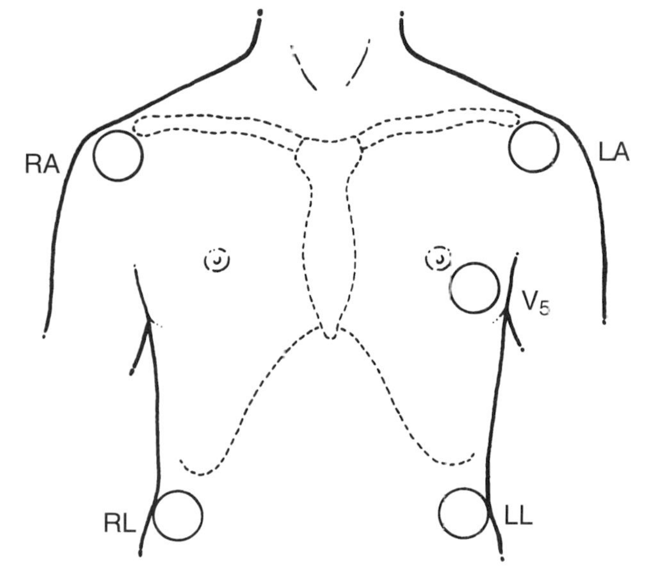

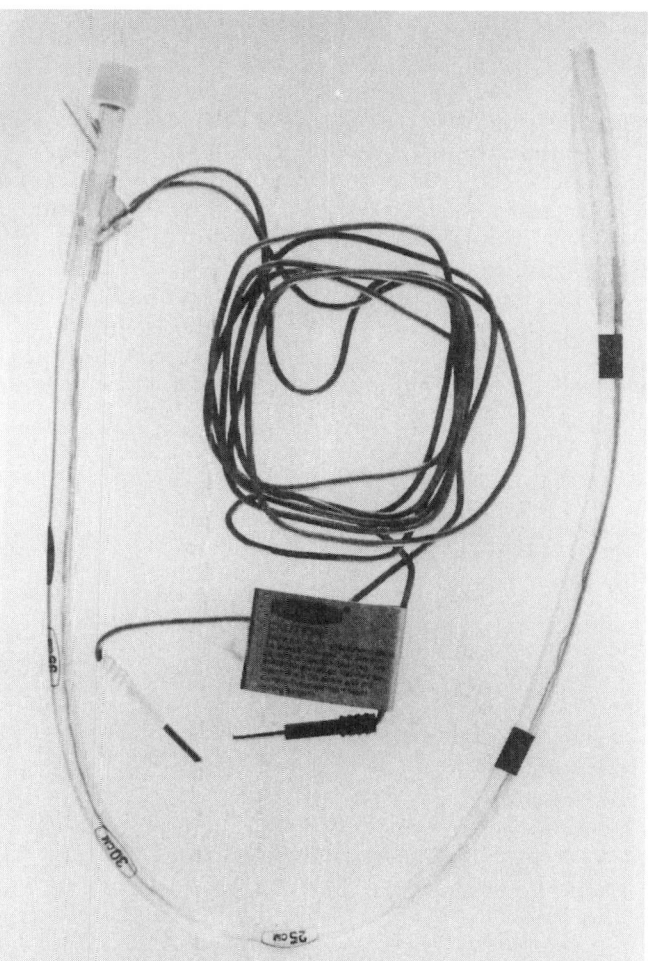

Figure 34–8 In the cardioesophagoscope, the esophageal leads are made of plastic. The electrocardiographic (ECG) wires are connected to the right and left arms, with lead I selected on the electrocardiographic monitor. (Adapted from Narang J, Thys DM: Electrocardiographic monitoring. In Ehrenwerth J, Eisenkraft JB [eds]: Anesthesia Equipment: Principles and Applications. St. Louis, Mosby–Year Book, 1992, p 284.)

Figure 34–7 Multiple-lead electrocardiographic system, consisting of four extremity electrodes and the V_5 lead. LA, left arm; LL, left leg ; RA, right arm; RL, right leg. (From Narang J, Thys DM: Electrocardiographic monitoring. In Ehrenwerth J. Eisenkraft JB [eds]: Anesthesia Equipment: Principles and Applications. St. Louis, Mosby–Year Book, 1992, p 284.)

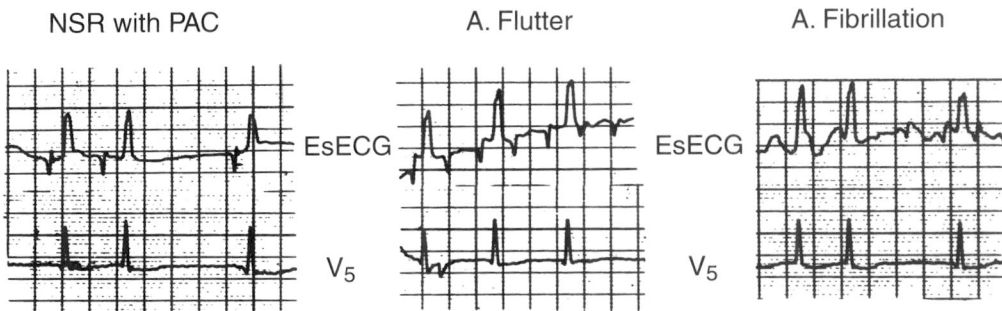

Figure 34–9 Enhanced detection of atrial electrical activity using an esophageal electrocardiogram (EsECG). The EsECG demonstrates arrhythmia progression from normal sinus rhythm (NSR), with one premature contraction (PAC), to atrial flutter (A flutter) and atrial fibrillation (A fibrillation). Lack of information about atrial activity from lead V_5 made definitive diagnosis impossible. (Adapted from Thys DM, Kaplan JA: The ECG in Anesthesia and Critical Care. New York, Churchill Livingstone, 1987.)

To observe a bipolar esophageal ECG, the electrodes are connected to the right and left arm terminals, and lead I is selected on the monitor. In a study of 20 cardiac patients, 100% of atrial arrhythmias were correctly diagnosed with the esophageal lead (using intracavitary ECG as the standard), whereas lead II led to a correct diagnosis in 54% of the cases and V_5 in 42% of cases (Table 34-3).[13] The esophageal ECG may be helpful in the detection of posterior wall ischemia because of its proximity to the posterior aspect of the left ventricle (Fig. 34-10). To minimize the risk of esophageal burn injury, an electrocautery protection filter capable of filtering radiofrequencies greater than 20 kHz should be inserted between the electrocardiographic cable and the esophageal lead.

Several investigators have described devices that allow electrocardiographic recording from the esophagus and pacing of the heart using the same device.[14] Esophageal electrodes have been found particularly useful in patients with emphysema and in critically ill patients for whom a satisfactory surface ECG cannot be obtained.[15,16]

Intracardiac Electrocardiogram

For many years, long saline-filled central venous catheters have been used to record an intracardiac ECG. More recently, Chatterjee and colleagues[17] described the use of a modified balloon-tipped flotation catheter for recording an intracavitary ECG (Fig. 34-11). The multipurpose pulmonary artery catheter that is available has all the features of a standard pulmonary artery catheter. Three atrial and two ventricular electrodes have been incorporated into the catheter. These electrodes permit recording of an intracavitary ECG and the establishment of atrial or atrioventricular pacing. The diagnostic capabilities with this catheter are great because atrial, ventricular, or atrioventricular nodal arrhythmias and conduction blocks can be demonstrated. The large voltages obtained from the intracardiac electrodes are relatively insensitive to electrocautery

Table 34–3 Comparison of esophageal and standard electrocardiography for correct arrhythmia diagnosis in 20 patients

Arrhythmia	No.	Correct Diagnosis from Single Leads		
		V_5	II	Esophageal
Sinus bradycardia	4	4	4	4
Sinus tachycardia	1	1	1	1
First-degree heart block	1	0	0	1
Second-degree heart block	2	0	0	2
Third-degree heart block	4	0	1	4
Frequent premature ventricular contractions	2	2	2	2
Frequent premature atrial contractions	5	2	3	5
Atrial flutter	2	0	0	2
Atrial fibrillation	3	2	2	3
Paroxysmal atrial tachycardia	1	0	0	1
Nodal rhythm	1	0	0	1
Percent correct		42.3%	53.8%	100%

Adapted from Kates RA, Zaidan JR, Kaplan JA: Esophageal lead for intraoperative electrocardiographic monitoring. Anesth Analg 61:781, 1982.

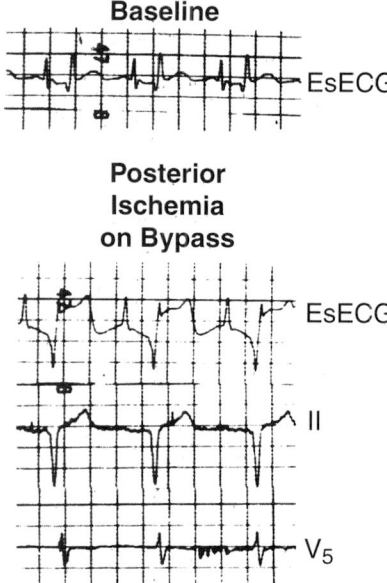

Baseline

EsECG

Posterior Ischemia on Bypass

EsECG

II

V₅

Figure 34–10 Tracings of the esophageal electrocardiogram (EsECG) and of leads II and V$_5$ indicate posterior ischemia. (Adapted from Kates RA, Zaidan JR, Kaplan JA: Esophageal lead for intraoperative electrocardiographic monitoring. Anesth Analg 61:781, 1982.)

interference, making them useful for intra-aortic balloon pump triggering.[18] Other pulmonary artery catheters have ventricular and atrial ports that allow passage of pacing wires. These catheters can also be used for diagnostic purposes and for therapeutic interventions (e.g., pacing).

Endotracheal Electrocardiogram
The endotracheal ECG allows monitoring of the ECG when it is impractical or impossible to monitor the surface ECG. The endotracheal ECG consists of a standard endotracheal tube in which two electrodes have been embedded (Fig. 34-12). This device may be most useful in pediatric patients for the diagnosis of atrial arrhythmias.[19] The same safety precautions as for esophageal ECG (discussed earlier) should be followed.

Intracoronary Electrocardiogram
The clinical use during angioplasty of a coronary guide wire for the recording of intracoronary ECG was first reported in 1985.[20] The major advantage was perceived to be a greater detection of acute ischemia than with surface ECG. In a study of 300 consecutive patients, intracoronary ECG detected ST-segment changes in 83% of lesions, compared with 67% on surface ECG.[21] Maeda and coworkers[22] observed a more rapid shortening of the QT interval with intracoronary ECG than with surface ECG after angioplasty balloon inflation.

DISPLAY, RECORDING, AND INTERPRETATION

The American Heart Association (AHA)[23] has published instrumentation and practice standards for electrocardiographic monitoring in special care units. They consist of performance standards, performance requirements, and disclosure requirements. They include recommendations that monitors be able to simultaneously display and analyze multiple leads and that users be informed of minimally acceptable accuracy in a standardized manner. Many of the principles detailed in these standards are also applicable to intraoperative monitoring.

Basic Requirements

The function of the electrocardiographic monitor is to detect, amplify, display, and record the electrocardiographic

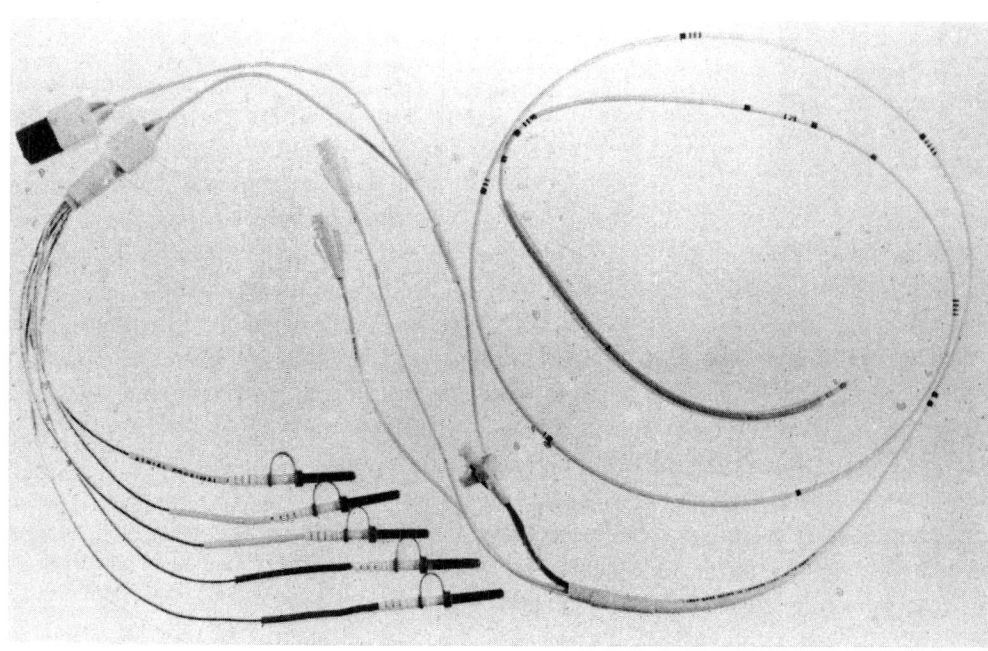

Figure 34–11 The multipurpose pacing pulmonary artery catheter. Three atrial and two ventricular electrodes can be seen. (From Narang J, Thys DM: Electrocardiographic monitoring. *In* Ehrenwerth J, Eisenkraft JB [eds]: Anesthesia Equipment: Principles and Applications. St. Louis, Mosby–Year Book, 1992, p 284.)

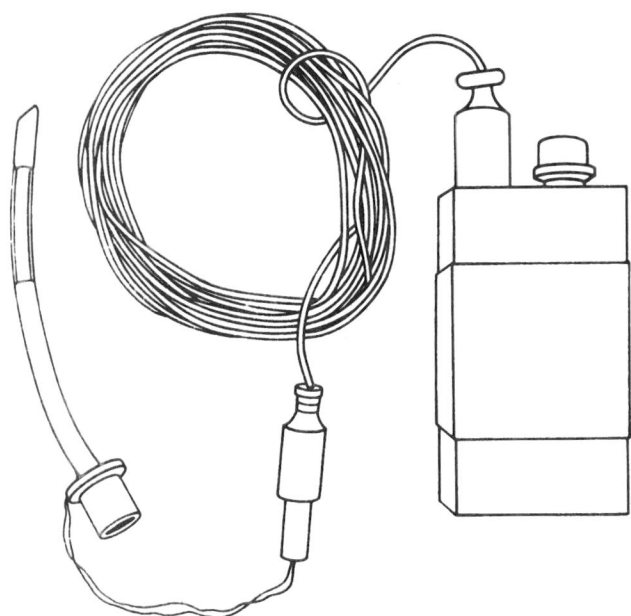

Figure 34–12 Diagram of tracheal tube electrocardiograph system. (From Narang J, Thys DM: Electrocardiographic monitoring. *In* Ehrenwerth J, Eisenkraft JB [eds]: Anesthesia Equipment: Principles and Applications. St. Louis, Mosby–Year Book, 1992, p 284.)

signal. The ECG is usually displayed on an oscilloscope. Several monitors offer nonfade storage oscilloscopes to facilitate wave recognition. All electrocardiographic monitors for use in patients with cardiac disease should also have paper recording capabilities. The recorder is needed to make accurate diagnoses of complex arrhythmias and to allow careful analysis of all the electrocardiographic waveforms. The recorder allows the examiner to differentiate real electrocardiographic changes from artifacts.

Oscilloscope Displays

Most modern oscilloscopes are high-resolution monochrome or color monitors, similar to those used in computer technology. They frequently allow considerable flexibility in screen configuration, including waveform positions, colors, and sweep speeds. The norm in modern technology is to display three electrocardiographic channels simultaneously. These usually consist of two limb leads and one unipolar precordial lead. In addition to the waveforms, average heart rates and optional arrhythmia and ST-segment information are displayed in alphanumeric format (discussed later).

Standard Electrocardiographic Recordings

The ECG is normally recorded on special paper consisting of grids of horizontal and vertical lines. Distances between vertical lines represent time intervals, whereas distances between horizontal lines represent voltages. The lines are 1 mm apart, with every fifth line intensified. The speed of the paper is standardized to 25 mm/second. On the horizontal axis, 1 mm represents 0.04 second, and 0.5 cm represents 0.20 second. On the vertical axis, 10 mm represents 1 mV. On every recording, a 1-cm (1-mV) calibration mark

should indicate that the ECG is appropriately calibrated. The user should follow the manufacturer's recommended calibration procedure for each monitoring episode. Strip chart recorders that are part of an electrocardiographic monitoring system should meet all the standards of time-based accuracy, frequency response, linearity, and so forth, proposed for conventional electrocardiographic recording systems.[24,25]

Artifacts

Patients

The electrical signal generated by the heart and monitored by the ECG is very weak, amounting to only 0.5 to 2 mV at the skin surface. It is therefore imperative that the skin be prepared optimally to avoid signal loss at the skin-electrode interface. Hair should be removed from the electrode sites with scissors and shavers. The skin should be cleaned with alcohol and should be free of any dirt. It is best to abrade the skin lightly to remove part of the stratum corneum, which can be a source of high resistance to the measured voltages. To avoid the problem of muscle artifact, electrodes should be placed over bony prominences, whenever possible. Muscle movement, in the form of shivering, can produce significant electrocardiographic artifact.

Electrodes and Leads

Loose electrodes and broken leads may produce a variety of artifacts that may simulate arrhythmias, Q waves, or inverted T waves. Pregelled, disposable silver/silver chloride electrodes are generally used in the operating room. The technical standards for such electrodes have been published by the American Association for the Advancement of Medical Instrumentation.[26] It is important that all the electrodes be moist, uniform, and not out of date. Needle electrodes should be avoided because of the risk of thermal injury. Some electrocardiographic monitors have built-in cable testers that enable a lead to be tested by connecting the cable's distal end into the monitor. A high resistance causes a large voltage drop, indicating that the lead is faulty. The main source of artifact from electrocardiographic leads is loss of the integrity of the lead insulation. This subsequently leads to pickup of other electric fields in the operating room, such as the 60-Hz alternating current (AC) from lights and currents from the electrocautery device. Any damaged electrocardiographic lead should be discarded for this reason. Lead movement can also lead to artifact.

Operating Room Environment

Many pieces of equipment found in the operating room emit electric fields that can interfere with the ECG: 60-Hz power lines for lights, electrosurgical equipment, cardiopulmonary equipment, and defibrillator discharges. Most of this interference can be minimized by proper shielding of the cables and leads of the ECG, although the interference created by the electrosurgical equipment cannot be reliably filtered without distortion of the ECG. Electrocautery is the most important source of interference on the ECG in the operating room; it usually completely obliterates the electrocardiographic tracing. Analysis of the electrocautery has identified three component frequencies.

The radiofrequency between 800 and 2000 kHz accounts for most of the interference, coupled with 60-Hz AC frequency and 0.1- to 10-Hz low-frequency noise from intermittent contact of the electrosurgical unit with the patient's tissues. Preamplifiers may be modified to suppress radiofrequency interference, but these filter circuits are still not widely available in the operating room.

Other causes of electrocardiographic artifacts in the operating room environment have been reported. Intraoperative monitoring of somatosensory-evoked potentials has been known to simulate pacemaker spikes.[27] They are caused by incorporation in certain monitors of a "pacer enhancement circuit." This problem can be eliminated by disabling the circuit. Artifactual spikes have been found to coincide with the drip rate in the drip chamber of a warming unit.[28] The spikes were probably related to the generation of static electricity from water droplets. The use of an automated percutaneous lumbar diskectomy nucleotome has been reported to simulate supraventricular tachycardia (SVT), related to a mechanical interference.[29]

Monitoring System

All electrocardiographic monitors use filters to narrow the bandwidth in an attempt to reduce environmental artifacts. The high-frequency filters reduce distortions from muscle movement, 60-Hz electrical current, and electromagnetic interference from other electrical equipment.[30] The low-frequency filters ensure a more stable baseline by reducing respiratory and body movement artifacts and those resulting from poor electrode contact. The AHA recommends that a flat frequency response be obtained at a bandwidth of 0.05 to 100 Hz.[25] The 100-Hz high-frequency limit ensures that tracings are of sufficient fidelity to assess QRS morphology and to evaluate rapid rhythms such as atrial flutter accurately. The low-frequency limit of 0.05 Hz allows accurate representation of slower events such as P-wave and T-wave morphology and ST-segment excursion.

Most modern electrocardiographic monitors allow the operator a choice among several bandwidths. The actual filter frequencies tend to vary among manufacturers. One manufacturer (Hewlett Packard, Andover, MA) allows a choice among a *diagnostic mode* with a bandwidth of 0.05 to 130 Hz for adults and 0.5 to 130 Hz for neonates, a *monitoring mode* with a bandwidth of 0.5 to 40 Hz for adults and 0.5 to 60 Hz for neonates, and a *filter mode* with a bandwidth of 0.5 to 20 Hz. The importance of bandwidth selection on the detection of perioperative myocardial ischemia was evaluated by Slogoff and coworkers.[31] These investigators simultaneously used five electrocardiographic systems: a Spacelabs (Redmond, WA) Alpha 14 model series 3200 Cardule with bandwidths of 0.05 to 125 Hz or 0.5 to 30 Hz, a Marquette Electronics (Milwaukee, WI) MAC II ECG with 0.05 to 40 Hz or 0.05 to 100 Hz, and a Del Mar (Cincinatti, OH) Holter recorder at 0.1 to 100 Hz. The ST-segment positions with the three systems using the lower filter limit (0.05 Hz) recommended by the AHA were similar, whereas on the Spacelabs device (0.5 to 30 Hz), they were consistently more negative. The ST-segment displacement on the Holter recorder was consistently less negative and less positive. In at least one automatic ST-segment analysis system

(Hewlett Packard), the lower frequency filter (0.05 Hz) is automatically activated when the ST analyzer is in use.

INDICATIONS

Diagnosis of Arrhythmias

Arrhythmias are common during surgery, and their causes are numerous (see Chapter 78). They can be classified by heart rate (HR) or by anatomic origin within the heart. Using heart rate criteria, arrhythmias can be broken down into three categories: bradyarrhythmias (HR < 60 beats/min), tachyarrhythmias (HR > 100 beats/min), and conduction blocks (at any heart rate). The anatomic origin of an arrhythmia can be ventricular, supraventricular, junctional, or elsewhere. Using continuous electromagnetic tape recordings, Bertrand and colleagues[32] reported an 84% incidence of supraventricular and ventricular arrhythmias in 100 patients during surgery. These arrhythmias were most common during endotracheal intubation or extubation and occurred more frequently in patients with pre-existing cardiac disease (60% versus 37%). Angelini and coworkers[33] reported that significant postoperative arrhythmias developed in 29 (58%) of 50 patients having valve surgery and in 35 (45%) of 78 patients undergoing coronary revascularization. There are several major factors contributing to the development of perioperative arrhythmias:

1. *General anesthetics:* Volatile anesthetics, such as halothane or enflurane, produce arrhythmias, probably by a reentrant mechanism.[34] Halothane also sensitizes the myocardium to endogenous and exogenous catecholamines. Drugs that block the reuptake of norepinephrine, such as cocaine and ketamine, can facilitate the development of epinephrine-induced arrhythmias (see Chapter 7).

2. *Local anesthetics:* Regional anesthesia by central neuraxial blockade, the goal of spinal or epidural anesthesia, may be associated with a profound albeit transient pharmacologic sympathectomy. This phenomenon may cause parasympathetic nervous system dominance leading to bradyarrhythmias from mild to very severe. This is especially true when the blockade extends to very high thoracic levels (see Chapter 43).

3. *Abnormal arterial blood gases or electrolytes:* Edwards and colleagues[35] showed that hyperventilation to a $PaCO_2$ of 30 or 20 mm Hg lowered a normal serum potassium to 3.64 or 3.12 mEq/L, respectively. If serum potassium and total-body potassium concentrations start at low levels, it is possible to decrease the serum potassium to the 2-mEq/L range by hyperventilation and precipitate severe cardiac arrhythmias. Alterations of blood gases or electrolytes may lead to arrhythmias by producing reentrant mechanisms or by altering phase 4 depolarization of conduction fibers. Electrolyte disturbances associated with cardiopulmonary bypass can also lead to intraoperative arrhythmias (see Chapters 46 and 50).

4. *Endotracheal intubation:* This maneuver may be the most common cause of arrhythmias during surgery and is often associated with hemodynamic disturbances (see Chapter 42).

5. *Reflexes:* Vagal stimulation may produce sinus brady-cardia and may allow ventricular escape mechanisms to occur. It may also produce atrioventricular block or even asystole. In vascular surgery, these reflexes may be related to traction on the peritoneum or to direct pressure on the vagus nerve during carotid surgery (see Chapter 52). During jugular vein cannulation, stimulation of the carotid sinus may occur because of pressure from fingers and can lead to bradyarrhythmias. Specific reflexes, such as the oculocardiac reflex, can produce severe bradycardia or asystole.

6. *Central nervous system stimulation and dysfunction of the autonomic nervous system:* Many electrocardiographic abnormalities can occur in patients with intracranial disease, especially subarachnoid hemorrhage. These abnormalities include changes in QT intervals, development of Q waves, ST-segment changes, and the occurrence of U waves[36] (see Chapter 53). The mechanism of these arrhythmias appears to be related to changes in autonomic nervous system tone.

7. *Preexisting cardiac disease:* Angelini and coworkers[33] showed that patients with known cardiac disease have a much higher incidence of arrhythmias during anesthesia than patients without known disease.

8. *Central venous cannulation:* The insertion of catheters or wires into the central circulation often leads to arrhythmias (see Chapter 32).

9. *Surgical manipulation of the cardiac structures:* Arrhythmias are often observed during insertion of atrial sutures or placement of venous bypass cannulas (see Chapters 50 and 51).

10. Location of surgery: Dental surgery is often associated with arrhythmias, because profound stimulation of sympathetic and parasympathetic nervous systems often occurs.[37] Junctional rhythms are often seen and may be caused by stimulation of the autonomic nervous system by the fifth cranial nerve.

After an arrhythmia is recognized, it is important to determine whether it produces a hemodynamic disturbance, what type of treatment is required, and how urgently therapy should be instituted. Treatment should be initiated promptly if the arrhythmia results in marked hemodynamic impairment. Treatment should be instituted if the arrhythmia is a precursor of a more severe arrhythmia (e.g., frequent multifocal ventricular premature beats [VPBs] with R-on-T phenomenon can lead to ventricular fibrillation) or the arrhythmia may be detrimental to the patient's underlying cardiac disease (e.g., tachycardia in a patient with mitral stenosis). For the detection of rhythm disturbances, the standard limb lead II is preferred because it usually displays large P waves.

Treatment of Arrhythmias

The diagnosis and treatment of arrhythmias can be simplified by using the following six questions as a checklist when looking at an electrocardiographic display and attempting to decide whether treatment is necessary:

1. What is the heart rate?
2. Is the rhythm regular?
3. Is there one P wave for each QRS complex?
4. Is the QRS complex normal?

5. Is the rhythm dangerous?
6. Does the rhythm require treatment?

Following are some common intraoperative arrhythmias to which the six questions should be applied.

Sinus Bradycardia

The pacemaker site is in the sinus node, but the rate is slower than normal. Etiologic factors include drug effects, acute inferior myocardial infarction, hypoxia, vagal stimulation, and high sympathetic blockade. Sinus bradycardia accounts for 11% of intraoperative arrhythmias:

1. *Heart rate:* The heart rate is slower than 60 beats/min. In patients on chronic β-blocker therapy, it is defined as a heart rate of less than 50 beats/min.

2. *Rhythm:* The rhythm is regular, except for occasional escape beats from other pacemaker sites.

3. *P:QRS:* There is a 1:1 relationship between the P waves and the QRS complexes.

4. *QRS complex:* Normal.

5. *Significance:* Heart rates lower than 40 beats/min are poorly tolerated even in healthy patients and should be evaluated on the basis of their effect on cardiac output. Treatment is recommended if hypotension, ventricular arrhythmias, or signs of poor peripheral perfusion are observed. Sinus bradycardia may be part of the sick sinus syndrome in which sinus node dysfunction can precipitate bradycardias, heart block, tachyarrhythmias, or alternating bradyarrhythmias and tachyarrhythmias (Fig. 34-13).[38]

6. *Treatment:* Usually, none is necessary. A progression from atropine (0.5 to 1.0 mg by intravenous bolus, repeated every 3 to 5 minutes, up to 0.04 mg/kg or approximately a 3.0-mg total dose for the average 75-kg male patient), to ephedrine (5 to 25 mg by intravenous bolus), dopamine (5 to 20 μg/kg/min by intravenous infusion), epinephrine (2 to 10 μg/min by intravenous infusion), or isoproterenol (2 to 10 μg/min by intravenous infusion) to temporary transcutaneous pacing or transvenous pacemaker insertion may be necessary for severe or refractory sinus bradycardia. Immediate institution of transcutaneous pacing is especially important if the patient is symptomatic.

Sinus Tachycardia

The pacemaker site is in the sinus node, but the rate is faster than normal. Sinus tachycardia is the most commonly occurring arrhythmia in the perioperative period. It occurs with such frequency that it is not included in most incidence studies. Common causes include pain, inadequate anesthesia, hypovolemia, fever, hypoxia, hypercarbia, heart failure, and drug effects.[4]

1. *Heart rate:* The rate is faster than 100 beats/min in the adult patient and can go up to 170 beats/min, which may be seen during a severe episode of hyperpyrexia.

2. *Rhythm:* Regular.

3. *P:QRS:* 1:1.

4. *QRS complex:* Normal. There may be associated ST-segment depression with severe increases in heart rate and resulting myocardial ischemia.

5. *Significance:* Prolonged tachycardias in patients with underlying heart disease can precipitate congestive heart failure because of the increased myocardial

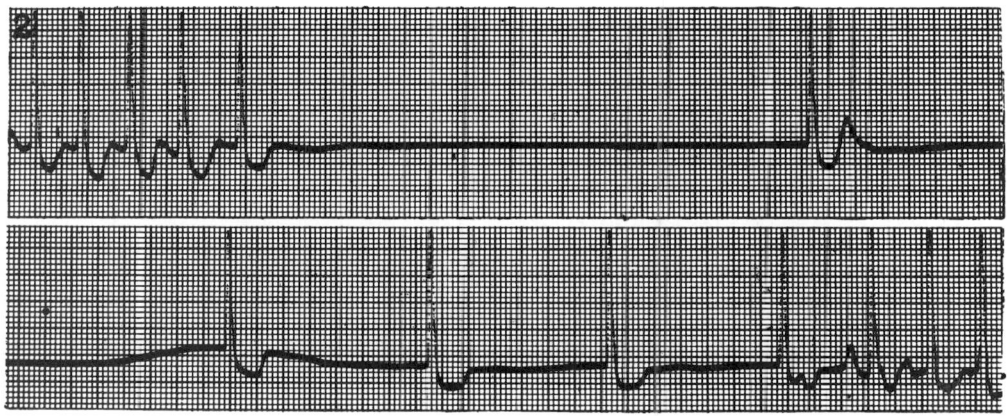

Figure 34–13 Sick sinus syndrome. (From Marriott HJL: Practical Electrocardiography, 7th ed. Baltimore, Williams & Wilkins, 1983.)

work required. The tachycardia decreases coronary perfusion time, which can cause secondary ST-T wave changes and can precipitate angina pectoris in patients with coronary artery disease. A major diagnostic problem is encountered when the heart rate is 150 beats/min, because this is a common rate for sinus tachycardia, paroxysmal atrial tachycardia (PAT), or atrial flutter with a 2:1 block. These three arrhythmias can sometimes be separated by the use of carotid sinus massage, intravenous administration of edrophonium, or atrial or esophageal electrocardiographic leads to identify the P waves on the ECG more accurately.

6. *Treatment:* The underlying disorder should be treated. Hypovolemia and light anesthesia are most common causes. If necessary, in patients with ischemic heart disease who develop tachycardia and ST-segment changes, after excluding hypovolemia and while determining the cause, esmolol should be used to prevent further myocardial ischemia.

Sinus Arrhythmia

The pacemaker impulse arises from the sinoatrial node, but the arrhythmia is manifested by alternating periods of slower and faster heart rates. The PR interval is normal, as is the QRS complex. Most commonly, but not invariably, the rate increases with inspiration and decreases with expiration. This arrhythmia occurs more often in children than in adults.[4]

1. *Heart rate:* 60 to 100 beats/min.
2. *Rhythm:* Irregular.
3. *P:QRS:* 1:1.
4. *QRS complex:* Normal.
5. *Significance:* Normal finding.
6. *Treatment:* None.

Atrial Premature Beats

An ectopic pacemaker site in the left or the right atrium initiates the atrial premature beat (APB). The shape of the P wave is different from the usual sinoatrial node P wave and may be inverted. The PR interval may be shorter or longer than normal, depending on the site of the ectopic focus and on the refractoriness of the atrioventricular nodal pathway. The APB spreads through the atrioventricular node and ventricular conduction system and, in retrograde fashion, reaches the sinoatrial node, resetting the sinus pacemaker. The interval from the APB to the next sinus beat is therefore a normal sinus cycle (i.e., no compensatory pause). The absence of a compensatory pause is an important distinguishing feature between APBs and VPBs. Occasionally, APBs may find part of the ventricular conduction system refractory. In that case, they travel down an aberrant pathway and create an abnormal QRS complex. They are then called APBs with aberrant ventricular conduction and can easily be confused with VPBs. Because the recovery period of the right ventricular conduction system outlasts that of the left, the most common form of aberration appears as a right bundle branch block (RBBB). Helpful points in separating APBs with aberrant ventricular conduction from VPBs include (1) the presence of a preceding P wave, usually abnormally shaped; (2) an RBBB configuration of the QRS complex; (3) the presence of an rsR′ ventricular complex in V_1; and (4) the finding that the initial vector forces are identical to the preceding beat but are usually the opposite with a VPB. Other characteristics of APBs are as follows:

1. *Heart rate:* Variable, depending on the frequency of APBs.
2. *Rhythm:* Irregular.
3. *P:QRS:* Usually 1:1. The P waves have various shapes and may even be lost in the QRS or T waves. Occasionally, the P wave is so early as to find the ventricle refractory, and a nonconducted beat occurs.
4. *QRS complex:* Usually normal unless there is ventricular aberration.
5. *Significance:* In one study, APBs represented 10% of all intraoperative arrhythmias. They have little clinical significance, but frequent APBs may lead to other more serious supraventricular arrhythmias or may be a sign of digitalis intoxication.
6. *Treatment:* Rarely necessary, but digitalis, β-blockers, or verapamil may be considered if hemodynamic function is impaired.

Paroxysmal Supraventricular Tachycardia

Paroxysmal SVT (PSVT) is characterized by a rapid regular rhythm, usually with a narrow QRS complex and lacking

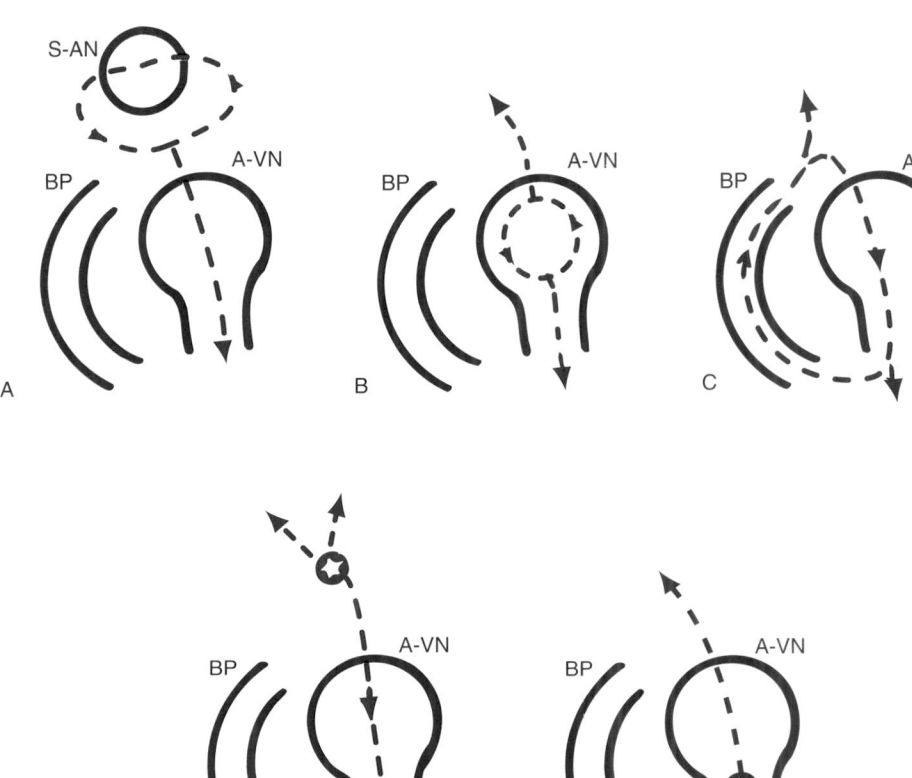

Figure 34–14 Diagrammatic representation of various mechanisms of supraventricular tachycardia. A-VN, A-V node; BP, bypass tract; S-AN, sinus node. (Adapted from Marriott HJL: Practical Electrocardiography, 7th ed. Baltimore, Williams & Wilkins, 1983.)

the normal sinoatrial node P wave. The inclusion of tachycardias involving the atrioventricular node (Fig. 34-14) allows their useful classification as caused by reentry in the atrioventricular node, apparent or concealed accessory atrioventricular pathways, or less often, sinoatrial node reentry (Table 34-4). Ectopic atrial or ectopic nodal tachycardias are also among the less frequent SVTs. Inappropriate or persistent sinus tachycardia is another variant. PSVT rhythms are usually abrupt in onset and termination. PSVT is easily distinguished from rapid atrial fibrillation, which is an irregular rhythm, or from rapid atrial flutter, which has flutter waves.

Table 34–4 Classification of supraventricular tachycardia
Reentry
Sinoatrial node (see Fig. 34–14A)
Atrial
Atrioventricular junction (see Fig. 34–14B)
Atrioventricular junction bypass (see Fig. 34–14C)
Kent bundle (Wolff-Parkinson-White syndrome)
Ectopic
Atrial (see Fig. 34–14D)
Atrioventricular junction (see Fig. 34–14E)

From Marriott HJL: Practical Electrocardiography, 7th ed. Baltimore, Williams & Wilkins, 1983.

1. *Heart rate:* 130 to 270 beats/min.
2. *Rhythm:* Usually regular unless the impulse originates from multiple atrial foci.
3. *P:QRS:* There is a 1:1 relationship, although the P wave may often be hidden in the QRS complex or T wave.
4. *QRS complex:* Generally normal, but ST-T changes indicative of ischemia may be observed. Aberration of ventricular conduction may occur, complicating the differential diagnosis with ventricular tachycardia. SVT may also be confused with sinus tachycardia, atrial flutter, and atrial fibrillation. In differentiating these rhythms, carotid sinus massage or edrophonium (5 to 10 mg given intravenously) traditionally was used. More recently, adenosine (6 to 12 mg by intravenous bolus) has been used to slow the rate by transiently enhancing the normal degree of atrioventricular block or terminate the arrhythmia.[39] Esophageal electrocardiographic leads may also be helpful to better define atrial activity.[40]
5. *Significance:* PSVT can be seen in 5% of normal young adults and in patients with Wolff-Parkinson-White syndrome or other preexcitation syndromes. During anesthesia, PSVT accounts for up to 2.5% of all arrhythmias, and the arrhythmia has been associated with intrinsic heart disease, systemic illness, thyrotoxicosis, digitalis toxicity, pulmonary embolism, and pregnancy. When a patient is under anesthesia, PSVT can be precipitated by changes in the autonomic nervous system tone, by drug effects, or by intravascular

volume shifts and can produce severe hemodynamic deterioration. Sometimes, the PSVT may be associated with atrioventricular block because of the fast atrial rate and slow atrioventricular conduction. PSVT with 2:1 block represents digitalis intoxication in many patients.

6. *Treatment:* This arrhythmia often must be treated because of its rapid rate and associated poor hemodynamic function. One or several of the following can be undertaken to treat this arrhythmia:

a. Vagal maneuvers such as carotid sinus massage should only be applied to one side.[41-43]

b. Adenosine, which is the drug of choice, is given by 6-mg rapid intravenous bolus, preferably through an antecubital or more central vein. If no response is elicited, second and third doses of 12 to 18 mg of adenosine may be administered by rapid intravenous bolus.[44]

c. Verapamil (2.5 to 10 mg given intravenously) terminates atrioventricular nodal reentry successfully in about 90% of cases. This was the drug of choice and is now the second choice.[45]

d. Amiodarone (150 mg infusion over 10 minutes for the loading dose) is a recent addition.[46]

e. Esmolol (1 mg/kg by bolus and 50 to 200 mg/kg/min by infusion) has been shown effective.[47]

f. Edrophonium (5 to 10 mg by intravenous bolus) can be given.[48]

g. Phenylephrine (100 μg by intravenous bolus) is administered if the patient is hypotensive.[48]

h. Intravenous digitalization is performed with one of the short-acting digitalis preparations: ouabain (0.25 to 0.5 mg given intravenously) or digoxin (0.5 to 1.0 mg given intravenously).[49]

i. Rapid overdrive pacing may be done in an effort to capture the ectopic focus.[50]

j. Synchronized cardioversion may be performed with incremental doses of energy of 100, 200, 300, and 360 J, preferably after light sedative premedication with a benzodiazepine.[51]

k. Procainamide is used in addition to cardioversion or antitachycardia pacing. Procainamide may be useful to treat SVT when antegrade conduction across an accessory atrioventricular path is the suspected mechanism.

Electrode catheter ablation using radiofrequency energy has evolved as the definitive, long-term treatment for most persistent atrioventricular reentrant or focal atrial SVT.[52]

Atrial Flutter

Atrial flutter most commonly represents a macro-reentrant arrhythmia that circulates in a specific manner in the right atrium (i.e., counterclockwise rotation as viewed in the angiographic left anterior oblique view). Because it is associated with very fast heart rates, it is usually accompanied by atrioventricular block. Classic sawtooth flutter waves (F waves) are usually present. The characteristics of atrial flutter are as follows:

1. *Heart rate:* The atrial heart rate is 250 to 350 beats/min with a ventricular rate of about 150 beats/min (2:1 or 3:1 atrioventricular conduction block).

2. *Rhythm:* The atrial rhythm is regular. The ventricular rhythm may be regular if a fixed atrioventricular block is present or irregular if a variable block exists.

3. *P:QRS:* Usually, there is a 2:1 block with an atrial rate of 300 beats/min and a ventricular rate of 150 beats/min, but it may vary between 2:1 and 8:1. F waves are best seen in leads V_1, II, and the esophageal lead.

4. *QRS complex:* Normal. T waves are lost in the f waves.

5. *Significance:* It usually indicates the presence of severe heart disease. It is seen with increased incidence in patients with coronary artery disease, mitral valve disease, pulmonary embolism, hyperthyroidism, cardiac trauma, cancers of the heart, and myocarditis.

6. *Treatment:* Pharmacologic or synchronized DC cardioversion, when indicated, should be performed only after careful consideration or evaluation of a possible thromboembolic event.

The initial treatment should be control of the ventricular response rate with agents that slow atrioventricular node conduction:

1. β-Blockers such as intravenous esmolol (1-mg/kg by intravenous bolus) or propranolol.

2. Calcium channel blockers such as verapamil (5 to 10 mg given intravenously) or diltiazem.[53]

If the ventricular response is excessively rapid or secondary hemodynamic instability is present, or both, use the following guidelines:

3. Synchronized direct current (DC) cardioversion starting with a relatively high energy of 100 J and gradually increasing to 360 J is indicated.[54]

4. The class III antiarrhythmic agent ibutilide (Corvert, 1 mg in 10 mL saline, or D_5W, infused intravenously slowly over 10 minutes) has been documented to convert atrial flutter to sinus rhythm in most patients with relatively new-onset atrial flutter.[55] This may be repeated once,[56] and although it is highly effective, life-threatening torsade de pointes (discussed later) may occur hours after ibutilide administration, making 4- to 8-hour monitoring after treatment highly desirable.

5. Procainamide (5 to 10 mg/kg for the intravenous loading dose, infused no faster than 0.5 mg/kg/min) may rarely be used in an attempt to restore sinus rhythm after the ventricular response has been adequately controlled.[57]

6. *Treatment:* Rapid atrial pacing from within the atrium enhanced by ibutilide or procainamide also effectively terminates atrial flutter.[58]

Atrial Fibrillation

Atrial fibrillation is an excessively rapid and irregular atrial focus with no P waves appearing on the ECG; instead, a fine fibrillatory activity (f waves) is seen. This is the most irregular rhythm; it is called *irregularly irregular* and may be associated with a pulse deficit. The characteristics are as follows:

1. *Heart rate:* The atrial rate is 350 to 500 beats/min, and the ventricular rate is 60 to 170 beats/min.

2. *Rhythm:* Irregularly irregular.

3. *P:QRS:* The P wave is absent and is replaced by f waves or no obvious atrial activity at all.

4. *QRS complex:* Normal.

5. *Significance:* The causes of atrial fibrillation are similar to those of atrial flutter. This rhythm is often associated

with significant cardiac disease; however, idiopathic, lone paroxysmal atrial fibrillation has become increasingly recognized. The clinical significance and treatment of atrial fibrillation are also similar to those of atrial flutter, except for two important considerations. The loss of an atrial "kick" from inefficient contraction of the atria may reduce ventricular filling and may significantly compromise cardiac output. After 24 hours, atrial fibrillation may be associated with the development of atrial thrombi, with resultant pulmonary and systemic embolization.

6. *Treatment:*

   a. *Acute atrial fibrillation:* The treatment of acute atrial fibrillation is very similar to that for atrial flutter. More attention should be focused on ventricular response, especially with the administration of intravenous diltiazem or esmolol. Ibutilide may restore sinus rhythm, but it is less effective than in the treatment of flutter.[55,56] Synchronized DC cardioversion should be relied on in patients with pronounced hemodynamic instability. However, if fibrillation is present for longer than 48 hours, attempts to restore sinus rhythm may be associated with a heightened risk of thromboembolism. In this setting for a patient with normal coagulation function, adequate anticoagulation for 3 to 4 weeks should be considered before attempting to restore sinus rhythm. New developments in electrophysiologic techniques for ventricular defibrillation with biphasic current shocks have shown superiority to the conventional monophasic current techniques (discussed later). However, data regarding biphasic shocks for conversion of AF are still emerging. A randomized, double-blind, multicenter trial by the BiCard Investigators[59] demonstrated that for the cardioversion of atrial fibrillation, a biphasic shock waveform has greater efficacy, requires fewer shocks and lower delivered energy, and results in less dermal injury than a monophasic shock waveform. These results mirror those seen in the ventricular fibrillation trials.

   b. *Long-term therapy:* Long-term therapy of atrial fibrillation varies and depends on factors such as whether the arrhythmia is constant or paroxysmal, the nature of the underlying heart disease, and the state of ventricular function or hemodynamic stability or reserve. In the older individual or in the setting of specific risk factors (e.g., hypertension, diabetes mellitus, severe left ventricular systolic dysfunction), anticoagulation with warfarin should be strongly considered. When control of ventricular response is difficult with standard agents (e.g., β-blockers, calcium channel blockers, digitalis), electrode catheter ablation of the atrioventricular junction and permanent pacemaker insertion have seen increased use. This is definitive, curative, and not merely a rate-control procedure. For patients who are in and out of atrial fibrillation, implanted atrial defibrillators have been introduced (see Chapter 35). They function automatically, much like the implanted ventricular defibrillators. A detailed discussion is beyond the scope here, but a review of their indications is available elsewhere.[60] These devices bypass the limitations and eliminate the side effects of current drug therapies, which may be life threatening. In the absence of coronary artery disease or significant left ventricular systolic dysfunction, class Ic antiarrhythmic agents (i.e., flecainide or propafenone) have become the agents of choice.[61] Use of class Ia drugs (i.e., quinidine, procainamide, and disopyramide) has sharply diminished because of concerns about their significant proarrhythmic function and their systemic and organ side effects. The use of antiarrhythmic drugs that block repolarizing potassium currents (i.e., sotalol[62] and amiodarone[63,64]) has gained popularity for the suppression of atrial fibrillation in individuals with significant structural heart disease. Sotalol, however, has a much lower efficiency of converting atrial fibrillation than class Ic agents.[65] New class III agents show good efficacy in converting atrial fibrillation. Ibutilide converts rapidly, can be effective in up to 50% of cases,[66] and is more effective than sotalol or procainamide.[67,68] Dofetilide, another class III agent, exhibits a 32% conversion rate over 72 hours.[69] All these drugs exhibit significant proarrhythmic properties, which are summarized in Table 34-5.[70] Their efficacy in maintaining sinus rhythm in patients with atrial fibrillation is summarized in Table 34-6.

Table 34–5 Proarrhythmia with medications used to prevent the recurrence of atrial fibrillation

Drugs	Cardiac Side Effects	Comments
Quinidine	Worsening of CHF, torsades de pointes	Most useful as a second-line agent
Flecainide, propafenone	Worsening of CHF, bradycardia, atrial and ventricular arrhythmias	Agents of choice in lone AF; contraindicated in those with a history of ischemia
Sotalol	Worsening of CHF, bradycardia, and torsades de pointes	Pronounced β-blocking effects useful in those with CAD but may exacerbate CHF
Amiodarone	Bradycardia, torsades de pointes (rare), and conduction abnormalities	Useful in those with CHF or as a second-line agent
Dofetilide	Torsades de pointes	Newer agent, useful in those with CHF

AF, atrial fibrillation; CAD, coronary artery disease; CHF, congestive heart failure.
From Donahue TP, Conti JB: Atrial fibrillation: Rate control versus maintenance of sinus rhythm. Curr Opin Cardiol 16:46–53, 2001.

Table 34–6 Efficacy of antiarrhythmic medications in maintaining sinus rhythm

Drug	Patients in Sinus Rhythm (%)	Duration of Treatment (Months)	Design of Trial
Quinidine	50	12	Meta-analysis
Flecainide	34	12	Meta-analysis
Amiodarone	60	12	Meta-analysis
Sotalol	36	10	Prospective
Dofetilide	65	12	Prospective

From Donahue TP, Conti JB: Atrial fibrillation: Rate control versus maintenance of sinus rhythm. Curr Opin Cardiol 16:46–53, 2001.

Junctional Rhythms

The atrioventricular node itself shows no intrinsic phase 4 depolarization. Cells in the node cannot act as pacemakers. Ectopic activity, however, may be initiated from sites just above and below the atrioventricular node. It makes sense to consider these arrhythmias as atrioventricular junctional in nature. The resultant P wave is abnormal and, depending on the position of the ectopic pacemaker, may be very close to, buried in, or after the QRS complex. Depending on the rate of fire of the ectopic pacemaker, the resultant rhythm is nodal premature, nodal quadrigeminy, trigeminy, or bigeminy, nodal rhythm, or nodal tachycardia.

1. *Heart rate:* Variable, 40 to 180 beats/min (i.e., nodal bradycardia to junctional tachycardia).
2. *Rhythm:* Regular.
3. *P:QRS:* 1:1 but, there are three varieties:
   a. *High-nodal rhythm:* The impulse reaches the atrium before the ventricle; the P wave therefore precedes the QRS but has a shortened PR interval (0.1 second).
   b. *Mid-nodal rhythm:* The impulse reaches the atrium and the ventricle at the same time. The P wave is lost in the QRS.
   c. *Low-nodal rhythm:* The impulse reaches the ventricle first and then the atrium, so that the P wave follows the QRS complex.
4. *QRS complex:* Normal, unless altered by the P wave.
5. *Significance:* Junctional rhythms are common in patients under anesthesia (about 20%) especially with halogenated anesthetic agents. The junctional rhythms frequently decrease blood pressure and cardiac output by about 15%, but they can decrease it up to 30% in patients with heart disease.[71]
6. *Treatment:* Usually, no treatment is required, and the rhythm reverts spontaneously. If hypotension and poor perfusion are associated with the rhythm, treatment is indicated. Atropine, ephedrine, or isoproterenol can be used in an effort to increase the activity of the sinoatrial node so it will take over as the pacemaker. Amiodarone is again the drug of choice in pharmacologic therapy. A small dose of succinylcholine (10 mg given intravenously) may revert a nodal rhythm to a sinus rhythm during anesthesia with halothane or enflurane. This probably works as a result of the effect of succinylcholine as a sympathetic ganglionic stimulator.

In some cases, propranolol may correct the rhythm disturbance if it is caused by sympathetic stimulation. Dual-chamber electrical pacing at a rate faster than a slow nodal rhythm is another option.

Ventricular Premature Beats

VPBs result from ectopic pacemaker activity arising below the atrioventricular junction. The VPB originates in and spreads through the myocardium or ventricular conducting system, resulting in a wide (>0.12-second), bizarre QRS complex. The ST segment usually slopes in the direction opposite to that of the main deflection of the QRS complex. There is no P wave associated with a VPB, but retrograde depolarization of the atria or blocked sinus beats may obscure the diagnosis.

The most important entity in the differential diagnosis is APB with aberrant ventricular conduction. The distinction should be made whenever possible.

Although an APB normally reaches the sinoatrial node and resets the sinus rhythm, such an occurrence is rare when the ectopic pacemaker is in the ventricle. A VPB often blocks the next depolarization from the sinoatrial node, but the following sinus beat occurs on time. The result is a compensatory pause, consisting of the interval from the VPB to the expected normal QRS, which is blocked at the atrioventricular node, plus a normal sinus interval.

VPBs are common during anesthesia, accounting for 15% of observed arrhythmias. They are much more common in anesthetized patients with preexisting cardiac disease. Other than heart disease, known etiologic factors include electrolyte and blood gas abnormalities, drug interactions, brainstem stimulation, and trauma to the heart.

1. *Heart rate:* Depends on the underlying sinus rate and frequency of the VPBs.
2. *Rhythm:* Irregular.
3. *P:QRS:* No P wave with the VPB.
4. *QRS complex:* Wide and bizarre, with a width of more than 0.12 second. If it is of an RBBB nature, prominent R forces are present in V_1. If it is a left bundle branch block (LBBB) in appearance, notching of the S wave and less acute downslopes are common.
5. *Significance:* The new onset of VPBs must be considered a life-threatening event because, in certain clinical situations, the arrhythmia may progress to ventricular tachycardia or fibrillation. These situations include coronary artery insufficiency, myocardial infarction, digitalis toxicity with hypokalemia, and hypoxemia. VPBs are more likely to lead to fibrillation if they are multiple, multifocal, or bigeminal; occur near the vulnerable period of the preceding ventricular repolarization (i.e., R-on-T phenomenon)[72]; or appear in short-long-short coupling sequences.
6. *Treatment:* The first step in treatment is to correct any underlying abnormalities such as decreased serum potassium or low arterial oxygen tension. If the arrhythmia is of hemodynamic significance or if it is believed to be a harbinger of worse arrhythmias, lidocaine is usually the treatment of choice, with an initial bolus dose of 1.5 mg/kg. Recurrent VPBs can be treated with a lidocaine infusion of 1 to 4 mg/min; additional therapy can be supplied with esmolol, propranolol,

procainamide, quinidine, disopyramide, atropine, verapamil, or overdrive pacing.

Ventricular Tachycardia

The presence of three or more sequential VPBs defines ventricular tachycardia. Diagnostic criteria include the presence of fusion beats, capture beats, and atrioventricular dissociation. The specific morphologic appearance of the QRS complex may also be helpful in distinguishing ventricular tachycardia from other arrhythmias. The characteristics of ventricular tachycardia are as follows:

1. *Heart rate:* 100 to 200 beats/min.
2. *Rhythm:* Usually regular, but may be irregular if the ventricular tachycardia is paroxysmal.
3. *P:QRS:* No fixed relationship because ventricular tachycardia is a form of atrioventricular dissociation in which the P waves can be seen marching through the QRS complex.
4. *QRS complex:* Wide, more than 0.12 second in width, with similar morphologic criteria in lead V_1 as for VPB.
5. *Significance:* Acute onset is life threatening and requires immediate treatment.
6. *Treatment:* Amiodarone administered as one or more doses of 150 mg given intravenously in 100 mL saline or D_5W over 10 minutes, followed by an intravenous infusion of 1 mg/min for 6 hours and 0.5 mg/min thereafter, is the recommended current treatment (maximum intravenous dose 2.2 g/24 hours). Intravenous amiodarone has been as effective as bretylium.[73] Although amiodarone is associated with substantially less hypotension compared with bretylium, hypotension and bradycardia are its main side effects. Amiodarone's pharmacologic effects persist for more than 45 days. Lidocaine and procainamide have been used in the past with various degrees of success to treat ventricular tachycardia. Synchronized cardioversion is the indicated nonpharmacologic intervention in any wide complex tachycardia, whether monomorphic ventricular tachycardia or a wide complex supraventricular tachycardia. Polymorphic ventricular tachycardia with a normal QT interval is treated with amiodarone and cardioversion. Metabolic abnormalities and drug toxicity must be considered and treated. Polymorphic ventricular tachycardia with prolonged QT interval is a more serious rhythm disturbance and the recommended current treatment is intravenous infusion of 1 g of magnesium over 2 to 3 minutes. Precipitating metabolic or toxic causes should be treated. Overdrive pacing may also be helpful in this setting.

Ventricular Fibrillation

Ventricular fibrillation is an irregular rhythm that results from a rapid discharge of impulses from one or more ventricular foci or from multiple wandering reentrant circuits in the ventricles. The ventricular contractions are erratic and are represented on the ECG by bizarre patterns of various sizes and configurations. P waves are not seen. Important causes of the arrhythmia include myocardial ischemia, hypoxia, hypothermia, electric shock, electrolyte imbalance, and drug effects. The characteristics are as follows:

1. *Heart rate:* Rapid and grossly disorganized.

2. *Rhythm:* Totally irregular.
3. *P:QRS:* None seen.
4. *QRS complex:* Not present.
5. *Significance:* There is no effective cardiac output, and life must be sustained by artificial means, such as external cardiac massage.
6. *Treatment:* Cardiopulmonary resuscitation must be initiated immediately, and then defibrillation must be performed as rapidly as possible. Asynchronous external defibrillation should be performed with a DC defibrillator, using incremental energies in the range of 200 to 360 J. In extreme situations, the use of two defibrillators in tandem across the chest, with one applied in the anteroposterior direction and the second applied in the left midaxillary to right midaxillary direction, has been suggested. The two devices are discharged simultaneously to increase the likelihood of successful defibrillation. Animal studies have failed to demonstrate the superiority of dual-pathway simultaneous shocks over single-pathway shock.[74] In contrast, introduction of the biphasic (and rectilinear) transthoracic shocks has reduced the energy levels required and increased the efficacy of ventricular defibrillation. In a prospective, randomized, multicenter trial conducted by the ZOLL Investigators,[75] 120 joules of biphasic current were superior to 200 joules of monophasic current, especially in patients with increased chest wall impedance.

Early administration of 1g of magnesium sulfate may facilitate defibrillation. In some instances, epinephrine has been used to coarsen the fibrillation just before and to facilitate defibrillation. Vasopressin has been added as a drug for the treatment of ventricular fibrillation. The vasopressin dose is a single 40-unit intravenous bolus. If elected, subsequent administration of epinephrine should be not earlier than 5 minutes after vasopressin. Supportive pharmacologic therapy may include lidocaine, amiodarone, bretylium, procainamide, phenytoin, or esmolol.

Torsade de pointes, which may mimic ventricular fibrillation or ventricular tachycardia, is a life-threatening arrhythmia that occurs in the presence of disturbed repolarization (hence its association with prolonged QT interval).[76] Discontinuation of drugs that predispose to QT-interval prolongation and correction of electrolyte abnormalities are essential in the treatment of torsades de pointes. Acute therapy may include defibrillation, 1 to 2 g of intravenous magnesium sulfate, intravenous amiodarone, intravenous isoproterenol, and overdrive pacing.[77]

Diagnosis of Ischemia

Perioperative myocardial ischemia is predictive of adverse cardiac outcomes[78] (see Chapters 32 and 50). Factors that predispose to the development of perioperative ischemia include the presence of preexisting coronary artery disease and perioperative events that affect the myocardial oxygen balance. Perioperative clinical studies have found a high incidence of electrocardiographic evidence of ischemia (20% to 80%) in patients with coronary artery disease who are undergoing cardiac or noncardiac surgery.[79,80] The incidence of perioperative myocardial infarction in patients with coronary artery disease with or without previous coronary artery bypass grafting (CABG) has been studied.[81] Most patients without prior CABG in whom perioperative infarction developed had three-vessel disease. The infarction rate in the CABG group was very low, supporting the protective effect of prior CABG before noncardiac surgery. In the anesthetized patient, the detection of ischemia by ECG becomes even more important because the hallmark symptom, angina, is not available. Prolonged ischemia lasting longer than 10 minutes after vascular surgery was associated significantly with myocardial infarction as demonstrated by serum troponin elevation.[82] Short-term ischemic events lasting less than 10 minutes were not correlated with postoperative infarction or cardiac complications. Prolonged ischemia was the major cause of cardiac morbidity after major vascular surgery.

It has also become evident that a significant number of patients suffer from asymptomatic or "silent" ischemia.[83] Silent ischemia is manifested by characteristic electrocardiographic signs of ischemia in the absence of angina and is not necessarily associated with changes in hemodynamics or heart rate. Among patients with chronic stable angina who have ST-segment depression during exercise, ambulatory electrocardiographic monitoring during daily life identifies transient ambulant ischemic episodes in approximately 40% to 50% of patients. In these patients, silent ischemic episodes account for about 75% of all ambulant ischemic episodes.[84]

The electrocardiographic changes occurring during myocardial ischemia are often characteristic and are detected with careful electrocardiographic monitoring. Although the electrocardiographic criteria for ischemia were established in patients undergoing exercise stress testing, they may also be applied to anesthetized patients (Table 34-7). These criteria are (1) horizontal or downsloping ST-segment depression of 0.1 mV, (2) ST-segment elevation of 0.1 mV in a non-Q wave lead, and (3) slowly upsloping ST-segment depression of 0.2 mV (all measured from 60 to 80 msec after the J point) (Fig. 34-15).[85] Okin and coworkers[86] studied the relation of the time after the J point at which ST depression is measured to the magnitude of ST-segment depression during peak exercise. These investigators found that a positive exercise ECG (0.1 mV or more of additional horizontal or downsloping ST depression at the end-exercise point) had a specificity of 96% for coronary artery disease when ST-segment depression was measured at the J point or J + 60 msec. There was no difference in sensitivity of electrocardiographic criteria at the J point or at J + 60 msec. However, at J + 60 msec,

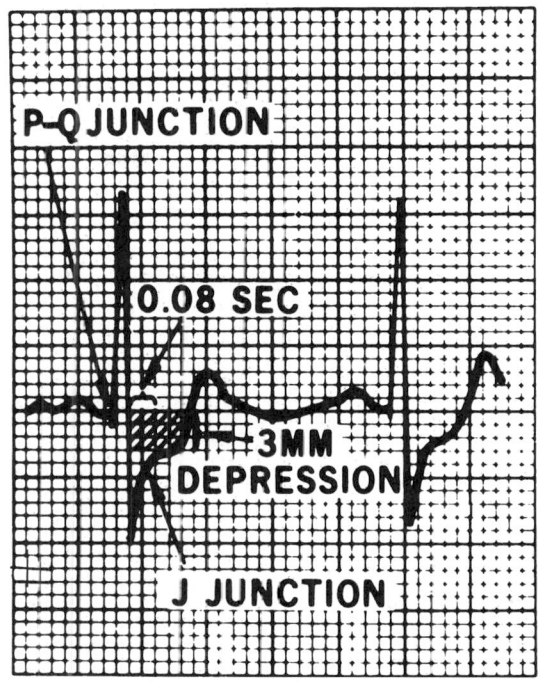

Figure 34–15 Assessment of ST-segment abnormality in the diagnosis of ischemia. (From Ellestad MH: Stress Testing: Principles and Practice. Philadelphia, FA Davis, 1975.)

there were significant differences in ST-segment depression at peak exercise among healthy persons, patients with clinical angina, and patients with documented coronary artery disease. Investigations focused on diagnosis and monitoring for myocardial ischemia have identified the minimum number and localization of electrocardiographic leads for detection. V_4 and V_5 were identified as the most sensitive (90% to 100% sensitivity) based on exercise stress testing[87,88] and intraoperative stress ischemia monitoring.[89]

In a perioperative study, investigators monitored 12 lead electrocardiographic changes larger than 0.2 mV from baseline in a single lead or more than 0.1 mV in two contiguous leads 60 msec after the J point to identify perioperative myocardial ischemia. These changes also had to last longer than 10 minutes.[90] Troponins were used as markers for myocardial infarction. In this study, leads V_3 and V_4 were identified as most sensitive for myocardial ischemia detection, with lead V_5 trailing close behind.[90] The sensitivity for detecting postoperative infarction was 100% for either combination of leads $V_3 + V_5$ or $V_4 + V_5$. When only a single precordial lead is available for perioperative ischemia monitoring, as is frequently encountered, the most isoelectric lead of V_3, V_4, or V_5 should be selected. Lead V_4 rather than V_5 detects ischemia earlier, is more sensitive, and shows a greater ST-segment deviation.[90] Lead V_4 appears to be more sensitive and appropriate for detection of prolonged postoperative ischemia and infarction. For patients with acute coronary syndromes (e.g., those with atherosclerotic plaque disruption), the recommendation is to monitor limb lead III and leads V_3 and V_5 as the most sensitive combination for ischemia detection.[91] Given the debate, the combination of an inferior limb lead along with lead V_4 or V_5 is prudent for ischemia detection along with good clinical care such as

Table 34–7 Electrocardiographic criteria for ischemia in anesthetized patients
Upsloping ST segment: 2-mm depression, 80 msec after J point
Horizontal ST segment: 1-mm depression, 60–80 msec after J point
Downsloping ST segment: >1 mm from top of curve to PQ junction
ST elevation
T-wave inversion

adequate control of stress, heart rate, and pain for the prevention of myocardial ischemia and infarction.[92]

It is commonly believed that monitoring for intraoperative myocardial ischemia is unnecessary in neonates. Whereas electrocardiographic lead systems for adults are concerned with the detection of ischemia and arrhythmias, neonatal electrocardiographic monitoring has focused on arrhythmia recognition alone. Results of some studies, however, suggest that the neonatal heart is more susceptible to ischemia than the adult heart.[93] These studies have demonstrated the importance of calibrated electrocardiographic monitoring in neonates with congenital heart disease (see Chapter 51).

Although ST-segment analysis provides sensitive information about myocardial ischemia, it should be remembered that underlying electrocardiographic abnormalities hinder the analysis in about 10% of patients. These abnormalities include hypokalemia, digitalis administration, LBBB, Wolff-Parkinson-White syndrome, left ventricular hypertrophy with strain, and acute pericarditis (Fig. 34-16). In these patients, other diagnostic modalities, such as transesophageal echocardiography, should be considered.

Diagnosis of Conduction Defects

Conduction defects can be observed during surgery. They can result from the passage of the pulmonary artery catheter through the right ventricle, or they can be a manifestation of myocardial ischemia. Because high-grade (second- and third-degree atrioventricular blocks) conduction defects often have deleterious effects on hemodynamic performance, their intraoperative recognition is important.

Three types of conduction system blocks are possible: sinoatrial block, atrioventricular heart block, and intraventricular conduction block (Table 34-8). The His bundle ECG has greatly improved the understanding of conduction through the heart.[94] In sinoatrial block, the block occurs at the sinus node. Because atrial excitation is not

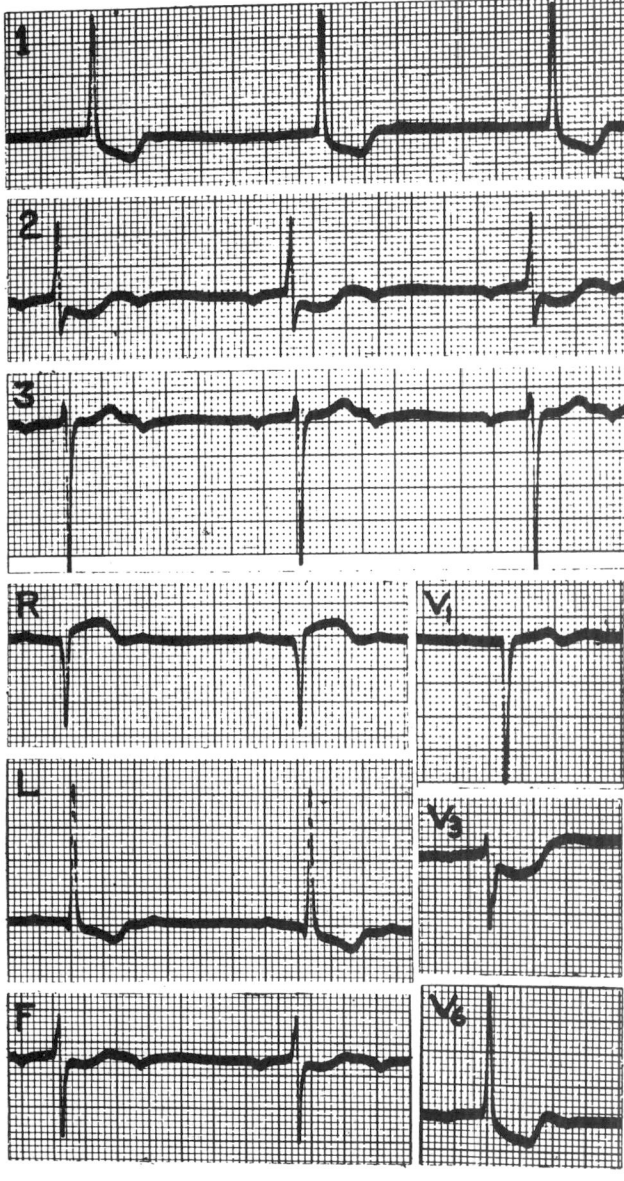

Figure 34–16 Digitalis effect on ST segments and T waves (i.e., ectopic atrial rhythm, 2:1 atrioventricular [AV] block, type 1 second-degree AV block, left ventricular hypertrophy with strain). (Adapted from Marriott HJL: Practical Electrocardiography, 7th ed. Baltimore, Williams & Wilkins, 1983.)

Table 34–8 Conduction defects

Sinus node block
AV conduction defects
  First-degree AV block
  Second-degree AV block
    Mobitz type I
    Mobitz type II
  Third-degree (complete) heart block
Intraventricular conduction defects
  RBBB
    Incomplete
    Complete
  LBBB
    Incomplete
    Complete
  Left fascicular block
    LAHB
    LPHB
  Bifascicular block
    RBBB + LAHB
    RBBB + LPHB
    Alternating LBBB/RBBB
    AV conduction defect + LBBB or RBBB
  Trifascicular block (bilateral bundle branch block + AV conduction defect)
  Indeterminate (bizarre defect, not included in any of the foregoing categories)

AV, atrioventricular; LAHB, left anterior hemiblock; LBBB, left bundle branch block; LPHB, left posterior hemiblock; RBBB, right bundle branch block.
From Thys DM, Kaplan JA: The ECG in Anesthesia and Critical Care. New York, Churchill Livingstone, 1987.

initiated, P waves are not found on the ECG. The next beat can be a normal sinus beat, a nodal escape beat, or a ventricular escape beat.

The second type of heart block is an atrioventricular heart block, or atrioventricular block, which may be incomplete or complete.[95] First- and second-degree atrioventricular blocks are usually considered incomplete, whereas a third-degree atrioventricular block is considered to be complete heart block. First-degree atrioventricular block is often found in healthy hearts, but it is also associated with coronary artery disease or digitalis administration. It is characterized by a PR interval longer than 0.21 second. All atrial impulses progress through the atrioventricular node to the Purkinje system. This form of heart block ordinarily requires no treatment (Fig. 34-17). Second-degree atrioventricular block is associated with the conduction of some of the atrial impulses to the atrioventricular node and into the Purkinje system. It is further subdivided into two specific types.[96] Mobitz type 1 block, or Wenckebach block, is characterized by progressive lengthening of the PR interval until an impulse is not conducted and the beat is dropped (Fig. 34-18). This form of block is relatively benign and often reversible, and it does not require a pacemaker. It may be caused by digitalis toxicity or myocardial infarction and is usually transient. Mobitz type 1 block reflects disease of the atrioventricular node.

The other form of second-degree heart block is Mobitz type 2 block, which may reflect disease of the bundle of His and Purkinje tissues, especially when the QRS complex is broad. In this, the less common and more serious form of second-degree heart block, dropped beats occur without any progressive lengthening of the PR interval (Fig. 34-19). This type of block has a serious prognosis, because it frequently progresses to complete heart block and may require pacemaker insertion before major surgical procedures. Third-degree atrioventricular block, also called complete heart block, occurs when all electrical activity from the atria fails to progress into the Purkinje system. The atrial and ventricular contractions have no relationship with each other, although each chamber contracts regularly. The ventricular rate is approximately 40 beats/min. The QRS complex may be normal if the pacemaker site is in the atrioventricular node, but it is usually widened to longer than 0.12 second when the pacemaker site is located in the ventricle (Fig. 34-20). The heart rate is usually too slow to maintain adequate cardiac

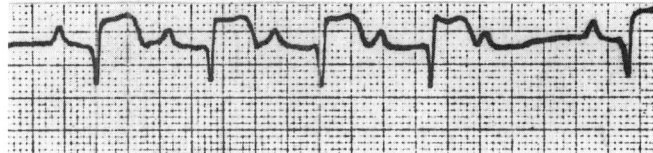

Figure 34–18 Mobitz type 1, or Wenckebach, block is diagnosed by the progressive lengthening of the PR interval until an impulse is not conducted and a dropped beat occurs. (Adapted from Thys DM, Kaplan JA: The ECG in Anesthesia and Critical Care. New York, Churchill Livingstone, 1987.)

output, and syncope or Adams-Stokes syndrome may occur, as well as heart failure. These patients usually require insertion of a transvenous endocardial or epicardial pacemaker to increase their heart rate and cardiac output.

The third type of block is an intraventricular conduction disturbance, which is usually classified as LBBB, RBBB, or hemiblock. LBBB is the most serious of these conduction disturbances. Impulses reach the ventricles exclusively through the right bundle branch—hence the wide QRS complex of more than 0.12 second and a wide-notched R wave in leads I, aVL, and V_6 (Fig. 34-21). The most important leads to study in bundle branch blocks are I, V_1, and V_6. The pattern of LBBB in V_6 is similar to that of left ventricular hypertrophy but exaggerated. An LBBB pattern is always associated with significant cardiac disease. In an RBBB, the QRS complex exceeds 0.11 second, and leads V_1 to V_3 have broad rSR' complexes, whereas leads I and V_6 have wide S waves (Fig. 34-22). RBBB may be of no clinical significance, as opposed to LBBB. However, it is frequently associated with chronic lung disease or atrial septal defects.

Hemiblock is a term used when one of two divisions of the left bundle is blocked, because if both divisions are blocked, complete LBBB exists. Even though hemiblocks are a form of intraventricular block, the QRS complex is not prolonged. Marriott's[97] criteria for left anterior hemiblock are as follows (Fig. 34-23): (1) left axis deviation (usually –60 degrees); (2) small Q in leads I and aVL and small R in leads II, III, and aVF; (3) a normal QRS duration; (4) a late intrinsicoid deflection in lead aVL (0.045 s); and (5) an increased QRS voltage in limb leads. In contrast, the criteria for a left posterior hemiblock are as follows (Fig. 34-24): (1) right axis deviation (usually +120 degrees);

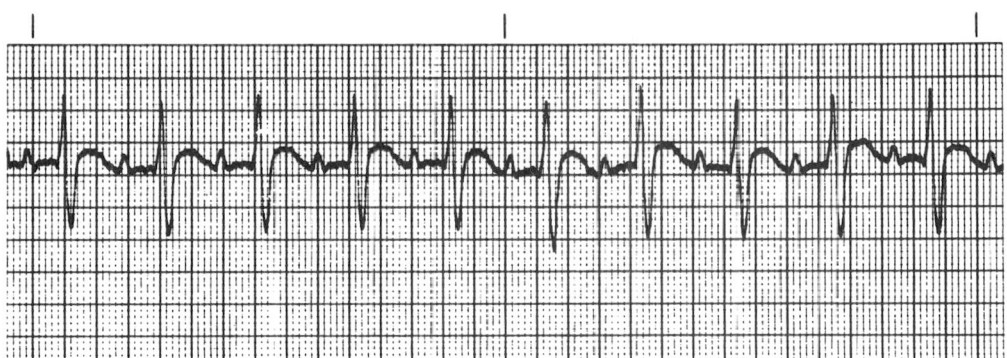

Figure 34–17 First-degree atrioventricular block is diagnosed by the presence of a PR interval longer than 0.21 second. (Adapted from Thys DM, Kaplan JA: The ECG in Anesthesia and Critical Care. New York, Churchill Livingstone, 1987.)

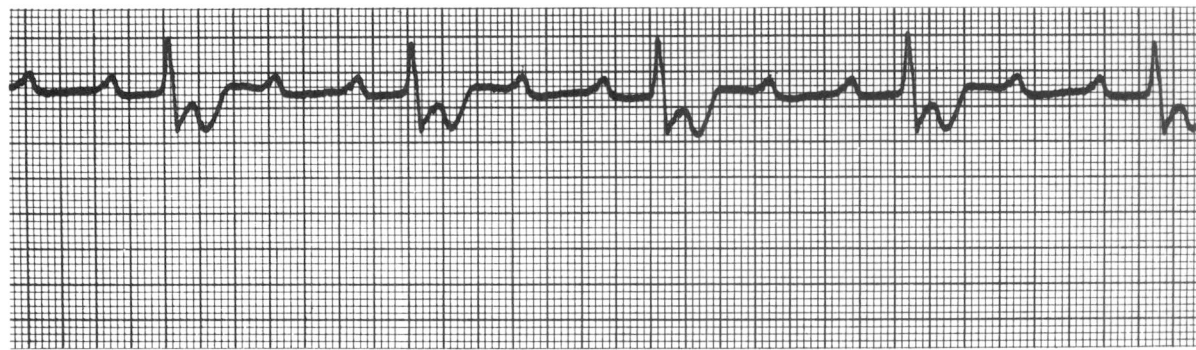

Figure 34–19 Mobitz type 2 second-degree heart block is demonstrated when dropped beats occur without progressive lengthening of the PR interval. (Adapted from Thys DM, Kaplan JA: The ECG in Anesthesia and Critical Care. New York, Churchill Livingstone, 1987.)

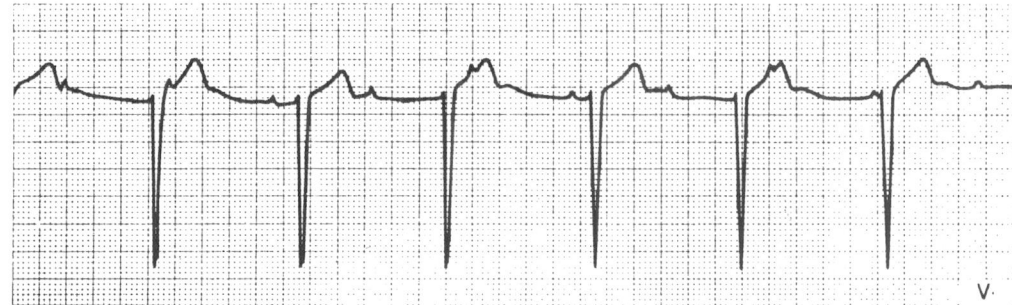

Figure 34–20 Complete, or third-degree, heart block is demonstrated by the total dissociation between atrial and ventricular complexes with a ventricular rate about 40 beats per minute. (Adapted from Thys DM, Kaplan JA: The ECG in Anesthesia and Critical Care. New York, Churchill Livingstone, 1987.)

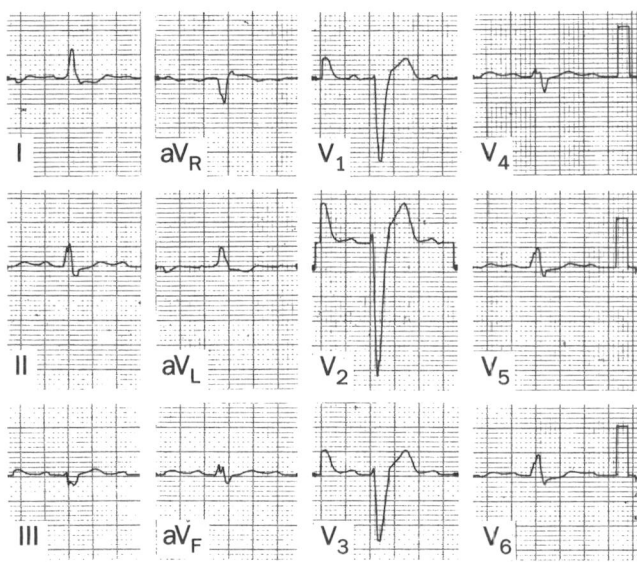

Figure 34–21 Left bundle branch block. Notice the rS pattern in V_1 and the notched rR′ pattern in V_6. In V_5 and V_6, a moderate depression of the ST segment is seen. (Adapted from Thys DM, Kaplan JA: The ECG in Anesthesia and Critical Care. New York, Churchill Livingstone, 1987.)

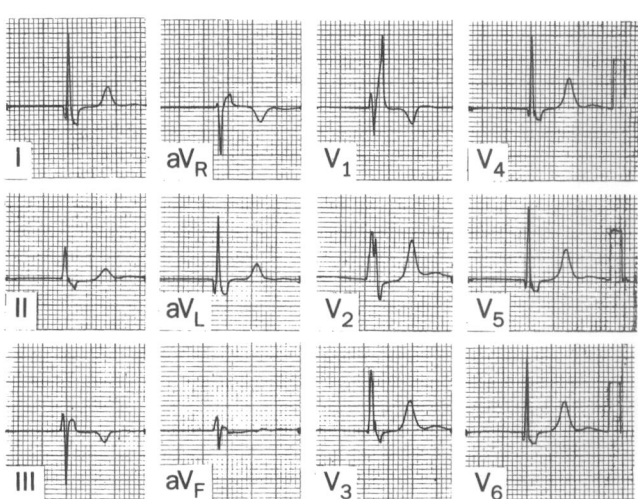

Figure 34–22 Right bundle branch block. Notice the rSR′ pattern in lead V_1, with slurring of R′ reflecting late right ventricular depolarization. (From Thys DM, Kaplan JA: The ECG in Anesthesia and Critical Care. New York, Churchill Livingstone, 1987.)

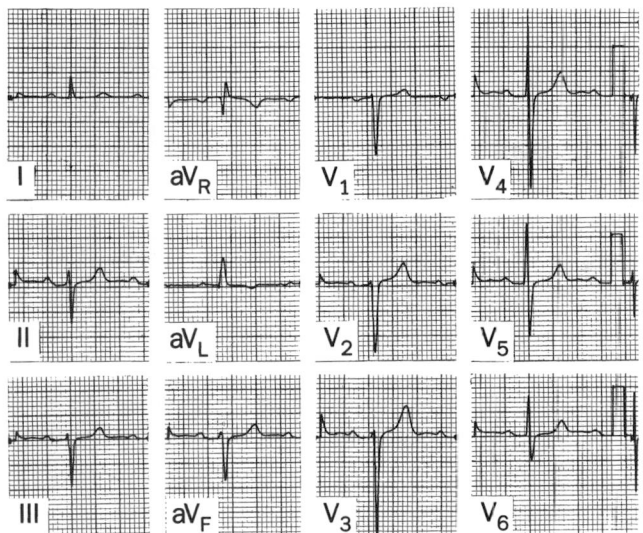

Figure 34–23 Left anterior hemiblock. Notice the left axis deviation and the terminal S in the inferior leads. (From Thys DM, Kaplan JA: The ECG in Anesthesia and Critical Care. New York, Churchill Livingstone, 1987.)

(2) small R in leads I and aVL and small Q in leads II, III, and aVF; (3) a normal QRS duration; (4) a late intrinsicoid deflection in lead aVF (>0.045 second); (5) an increased QRS voltage in limb leads; and (6) no evidence of right ventricular hypertrophy. The hemiblocks can occur by themselves but are often associated with an RBBB to form a bilateral bundle branch block. Only 10% of patients with an RBBB and a left anterior hemiblock (Fig. 34-25) progress to complete heart block, whereas patients with RBBB and a left posterior hemiblock (Fig. 34-26) often do proceed to complete heart block.

Trifascicular blocks usually consist of one of the foregoing bilateral bundle branch blocks (i.e., RBBB plus a left fascicular block) in addition to a prolonged PR interval (Fig. 34-27). Bundle of His ECGs are necessary to determine whether the atrioventricular conduction disturbance is localized in the atrioventricular node or whether it is distal, possibly representing an incomplete fascicular block in the last remaining fascicle.

AUTOMATIC RECORDING

Holter monitoring has been used by a number of anesthesiologists to document the perioperative incidence of arrhythmias and ischemia. In Holter monitoring, electrocardiographic information from one or two bipolar leads

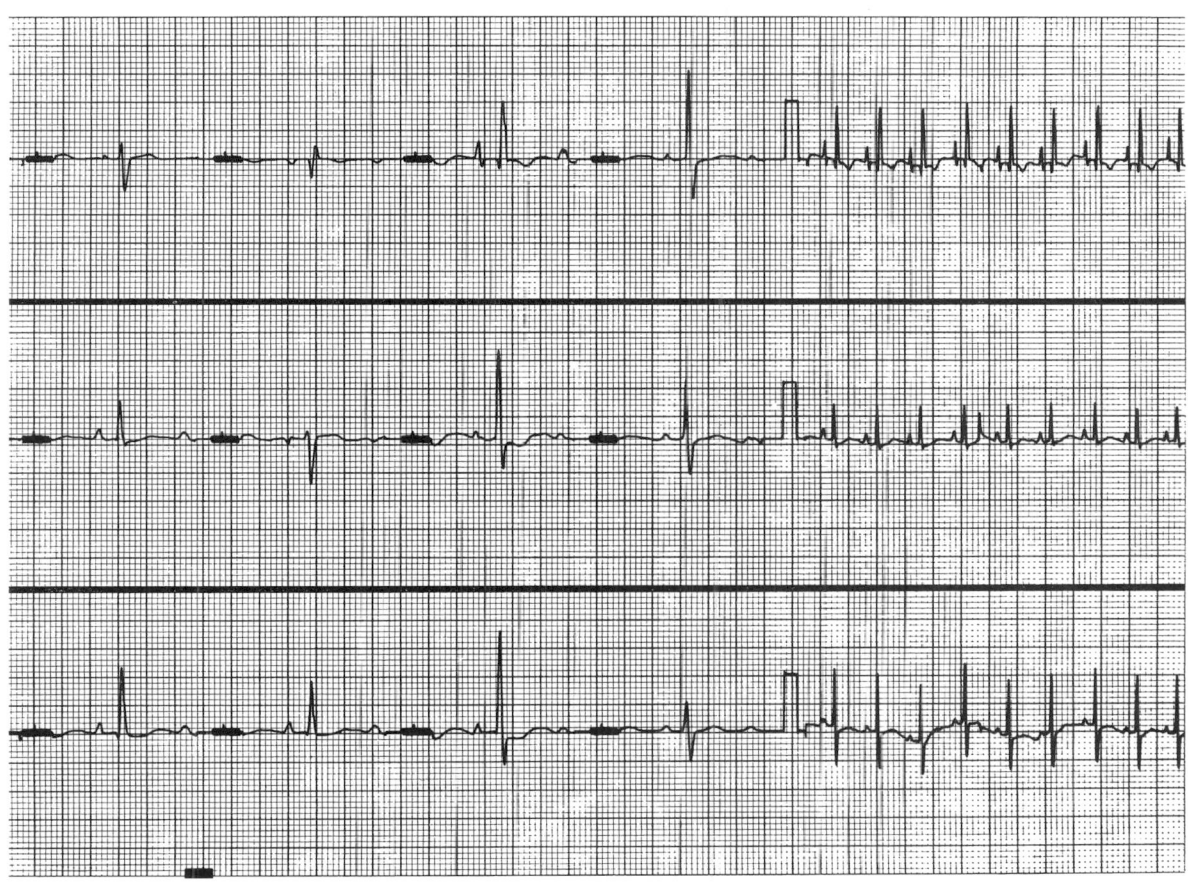

Figure 34–24 Left posterior hemiblock in association with biatrial enlargement and nonspecific ST- and T-wave abnormalities. (From Thys DM, Kaplan JA: The ECG in Anesthesia and Critical Care. New York, Churchill Livingstone, 1987.)

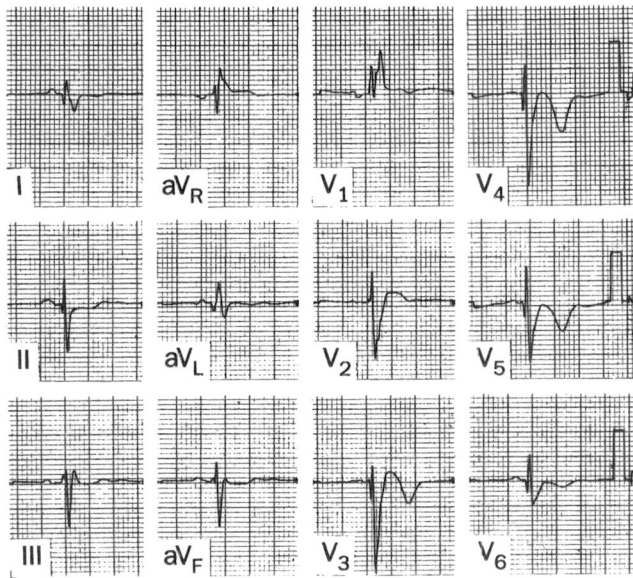

Figure 34–25 Right bundle branch block in association with left anterior hemiblock. Notice the RsR' pattern in V₁ and the wide S in the lateral leads. The axis of the initial QRS vector is –88 degrees. (From Thys DM, Kaplan JA: The ECG in Anesthesia and Critical Care. New York, Churchill Livingstone, 1987.)

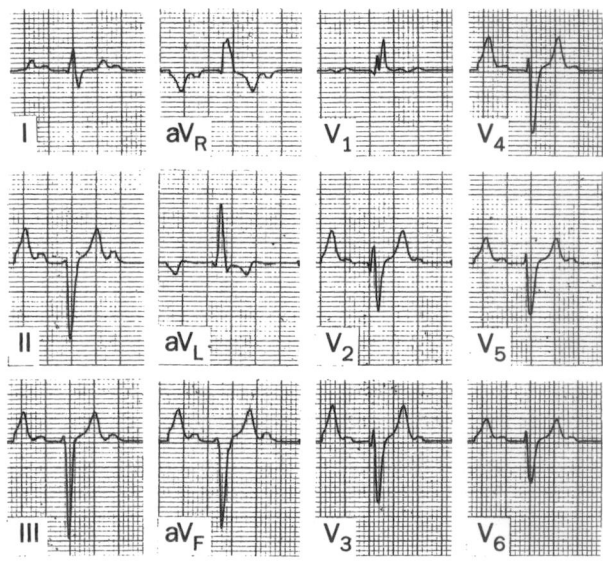

Figure 34–27 Trifascicular block. The PR interval is 232 msec, and a right bundle branch block is identified. The axis of the QRS vector is –85 degrees, indicating a left anterior hemiblock. (Adapted from Thys DM, Kaplan JA: The ECG in Anesthesia and Critical Care. New York, Churchill Livingstone, 1987.)

is recorded by a miniature magnetic tape recorder. Up to 48 hours of electrocardiographic signals can be collected. Subsequently, the tape is processed by a playback system, and the electrocardiographic signals are analyzed. On most modern systems, the playback unit includes a dedicated computer for rapid analysis of the data and automatic recognition of arrhythmias.

A significant early obstacle to the widespread use of conventional Holter monitoring in the perioperative period was the delayed, retrospective analysis and interpretation. This limitation was overcome by real-time Holter monitors. They record specific electrocardiographic segments for later playback, analyze the rhythm and ST segment in

real time, and alert the user to acute perturbations.[98] A report on validation testing of the SEER real-time digital Holter device (Marquette Electronics) found it highly accurate in detecting ST-segment deviations.[99] These results were obtained with digitally simulated electrocardiographic data, and accuracy in the clinical setting remains to be validated. A different device, the Q-Med (Q-Med, Inc., Clark, NJ), is a small, continuous electrocardiographic recording device that has been used in patients undergoing cardiac and noncardiac surgery.[100,101] The device records the electrocardiographic signals, performs an automatic analysis of the electrocardiographic tracing, and sounds an alarm when ischemic changes are recognized. Abnormal events are selectively stored and are subsequently retrievable. Despite significant technical progress, Holter monitoring continues to be limited primarily to clinical investigations.

COMPUTER-ASSISTED INTERPRETATION

Computer programs for the interpretation of ECG are widely used. In a large study, the ECGs of 1200 adult patients with known clinical conditions were interpreted by cardiologists and by nine computer programs.[102] The results demonstrated that, in some cases, computer interpretations of ECG were correct and cardiologists were incorrect when their diagnoses were tested against the clinical evidence. The opposite was twice as likely when the average computer program and the average cardiologist were compared. The computer programs with the best performance were almost as accurate as the best cardiologists in classifying the ECGs of patients in seven common diagnostic groups. The study did not test the computers' abilities, however, in two critical areas: acute myocardial ischemia and arrhythmia recognition. Modern monitoring

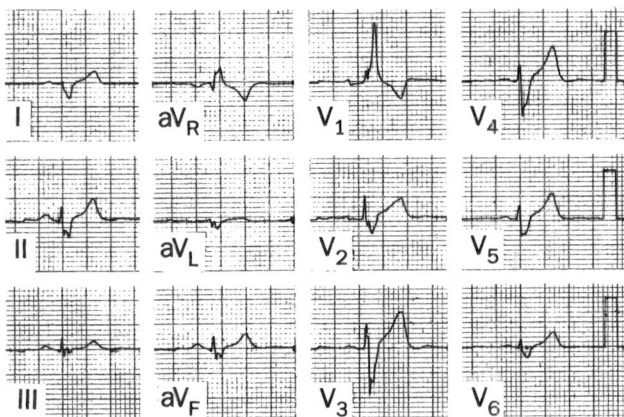

Figure 34–26 Right bundle branch block with left posterior hemiblock. Notice the wide S in the lateral leads and the rR' pattern in V₁. The axis of the initial QRS vector is +166 degrees. (From Thys DM, Kaplan JA: The ECG in Anesthesia and Critical Care. New York, Churchill Livingstone, 1987.)

equipment is highly computerized, and most of the physiologic information is manipulated, analyzed, and stored in the digital format. An early step in data collection therefore involves the conversion of analog signals (i.e., time-variable voltages or amplitudes) into digital format with an analog-to-digital converter. Once in the digital format, the physiologic information can readily be subjected to a variety of analyses. For ECGs, the most common analyses, besides rate calculations, are related to arrhythmia recognition and the detection of myocardial ischemia.

Arrhythmias

There is little doubt that during prolonged visual observation of the ECG on the oscilloscope, certain arrhythmias go undetected. This was clearly demonstrated by Romhilt and colleagues,[103] who showed that coronary care unit nurses failed to detect serious ventricular arrhythmias in 84% of their patients. Computers have therefore been designed for the automatic detection of arrhythmias in an attempt to increase the detection of abnormal rhythms. Using an early preprocessing algorithm called AZTEC, a computer accurately detected 78% of ventricular ectopic beats. It measured QRS width, offset, amplitude, and area to classify complexes into morphologic families.[104] In a prospective evaluation of such a system, it was found that the computer accurately detected 95.4% of VPBs but only 82.4% of supraventricular premature beats.

Other systems have depended on QRS recognition and cross-correlation with stored QRS complexes.[105] In cross-correlation, each detected QRS complex is compared with a list of previously detected complexes. If a complex does not correlate better than 0.9 with a previously stored complex, it is considered to have a new configuration and is added to the list (Fig. 34-28). Certain points of the complex, such as the PR interval and ST segment, are stored as a template for future comparison. Whenever a new complex matches an existing template, it is averaged into that template, so that each template represents a running average of all complexes of a particular configuration.[106] Each template is defined as normal, abnormal, or questionable according to previously defined criteria. The AHA has published several parameters that need to be tested to permit a meaningful understanding of a system's values and limitations and to permit reasonable comparison among systems.[25]

Myocardial Ischemia

One method of detecting intraoperative myocardial ischemia is automated ST-segment monitoring.[107] Several computer programs for online detection of ischemia and analysis of ST segments are available commercially. Each manufacturer uses different analysis techniques, and not all the algorithms are in the public domain. In one system (Marquette Electronics), an ST learning phase begins by looking at the first 16 beats in all leads for the dominant normal or paced shape. The shapes are correlated using a selected number of points on each of the active valid lead waveforms. An algorithm looks for leads in the fail or artifact mode to determine the number of valid leads used in the analysis. The algorithm also makes all leads positive to enable totaling the sum of the points on

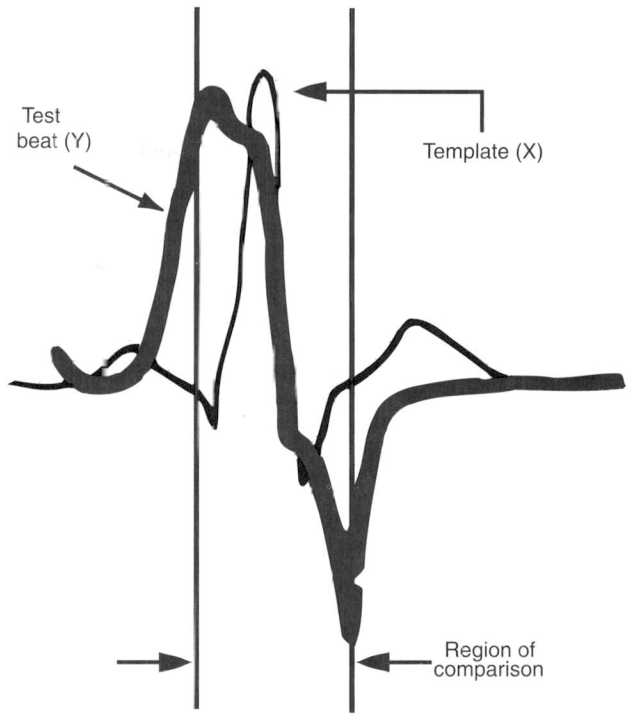

Figure 34-28 Computerized template of the underlying normal QRS complex (X) and an ectopic complex called a test beat (Y). Beat Y is matched to beat X by the computer during the region of comparison by cross-correlation algorithms. (Adapted from Morganroth J: Ambulatory Holter electrocardiography: Choice of technique and clinical uses. Ann Intern Med 102:73, 1985.)

the valid leads. This sum is used in determining a peak or fiducial point. The fiducial point is used as a point of reference on the QRS. A template is formed from selected points around the fiducial point for each electrocardiographic lead. As each beat is analyzed, its template is compared with templates of previous beats. If the templates correlate within 75% of a previously stored shape, it is deemed a match and is classified as an existing shape. If there is no match, it becomes a new shape. On the 17th beat, the dominant normal QRS shape or paced shape is determined. The algorithm then searches for an additional 16 beats that correlate with the dominant template. With the 18th beat, a process called *incremental averaging* is initiated. The incremental averaging is a method of tracking positive or negative changes occurring on the waveform. These changes are tracked for each of the valid leads. The changes may be physiologic, such as ST-segment changes resulting from ischemia or related to artifact caused by high-frequency noise. The tracking of the changes is achieved by only allowing a 0.1-mm adjustment, positive or negative, from the prior shape of each beat. On the 32nd beat, the product of the incrementally averaged templates becomes the learned ST templates. Until ST is relearned, all changes in the QRS shape are tracked against this learned template. The isoelectric point and ST points are determined during the learning phase and are based on the width of the QRS shape. The isoelectric point is placed 40 msec before the onset of the QRS, and the ST point is placed 60 msec past the offset of the QRS measurement. The isoelectric point provides the point of reference for determining the ST-segment measurement. The technique of incremental averaging is well suited to a continuous input with slow changes. However, it links the speed at which changes occur in the template to the heart rate.[108]

This system was evaluated in the intraoperative setting in patients undergoing cardiac surgery.[109] The device monitored three selected leads and displayed the absolute values of the ST segment as a line. Upward deflection of the trend line indicated worsening ischemia, whereas a downward trend reflected a return of the ST segment toward the isoelectric line. It was concluded that once the device was clinically accepted, the awareness for ischemic changes was heightened among the participating anesthesiologists and therapeutic interventions were more rapidly instituted, possibly leading to improved outcome.

A second ST-segment analysis system (Hewlett Packard) differs from the foregoing in several ways. A period of 15 seconds is analyzed first, and the ST displacement is determined on the basis of five "good" beats. These displacements are ranked, and the median value is determined. This technique eliminates the influence of occasional VPBs and ensures that a representative beat is selected. The objective of this procedure is to obtain a representative beat, rather than an average template. The measurement point for the ST segment can be selected as the R wave + 108 msec (default) or the J point + 60 or 80 msec. ST values and representative complexes are stored at 1-minute resolution for the most recent 30-minute trend and at 5-minute resolution for the preceding 7.5-hour trend.

In a third system (Spacelabs), a composite ST-segment waveform is developed every 30 seconds and is compared with a reference tracing acquired during an initial learning period. The isoelectric and ST-segment points can be manually adjusted to any location on the electrocardiographic tracing, or they may be automatically set to predetermined values. Using selective ST-segment displacement on seven different types of digitally simulated ECGs, London and Ahlstrom[110] bench-tested a version of a Spacelabs automated ST-analysis device, the PC2 Bedside Monitor. The device performed very well with five of the simulated ECGs, but it had some difficulty with two because of improper placement of the isoelectric point. Visual confirmation of ST-segment analyzer results was therefore advised.

The relative merits and shortcomings of the different ST-segment analysis systems in the clinical setting have not been fully elucidated. The ability of two automated ST-segment analysis systems to detect myocardial ischemia during noncardiac surgery was compared with 8-lead printed ECG and transesophageal echocardiography as reference standards.[111] In this study of 44 patients, the automated ST-analysis systems showed only fair agreement with transesophageal echocardiography or ECG in detecting ischemia. A different, brief, cautionary report mentions a case in which automated ST-segment monitoring falsely signaled the presence of intraoperative ischemia.[112]

SUMMARY

The ECG should be monitored in all patients undergoing anesthesia. Although it does not provide information on the mechanical function of the heart, it permits detection of electrical disturbances that can profoundly affect this function. With the judicious use of selected lead combinations, most arrhythmias and ischemic events can be precisely diagnosed in the intraoperative setting. This diagnostic activity is time consuming, however, and there is considerable evidence that many intraoperative electrocardiographic changes go undetected. There is little doubt that future technologic developments will facilitate the intraoperative recognition of electrocardiographic disturbances and lead to better patient outcomes.

REFERENCES

1. Thys DM, Kaplan JA: The ECG in Anesthesia and Critical Care. New York, Churchill Livingstone, 1987.
2. Cannard TH, Dripps RD, Helwig J, et al: The ECG during anesthesia and surgery. Anesthesiology 21:194, 1960.
3. Narang J, Thys DM: Electrocardiographic monitoring. In Ehrenwerth J, Eisenkraft JB (eds): Anesthesia Equipment: Principles and Applications. St. Louis, Mosby–Year Book, 1992, p 284.
4. Skeehan TM, Thys DM: Monitoring the cardiac surgical patient. In Hensley FA, Martin DE (eds): The Practice of Cardiac Anesthesia. Boston, Little, Brown, 1990, p 123.
5. Griffin RM, Kaplan JA: Comparison of ECG V, CS, CB, and II by computerized ST segment analysis [abstract]. Anesth Analg 65(Suppl 2):S1, 1986.
6. Bazaral MG, Norfleet EA: Comparison of CB and V leads for intraoperative electrocardiographic monitoring. Anesth Analg 60:849, 1981.
7. Hollenberg M, Mateo G, Massie BM, et al: Influence of the R-wave amplitude on exercise-induced ST depression: Need for a "gain factor" correction when interpreting a stress electrocardiogram. Am J Cardiol 56:13, 1985.
8. Mark JB, Chien GL, Steinbrook RA, et al: Electrocardiographic R-wave changes during cardiac surgery. Anesth Analg 74:26, 1992.
9. Kaplan JA, King SB: The precordial electrocardiographic lead (V) in patients who have coronary artery disease. Anesthesiology 45:570, 1976.
10. London MJ, Hollenberg M, Wong MG, et al: Intraoperative myocardial ischemia: Localization by continuous 12 lead electrocardiography. Anesthesiology 69:232, 1988.
11. De Hert SG, De Jongh RF, Van den Bossche AO, et al: The detection of intraoperative myocardial ischaemia: Preliminary experience with the right-sided precordial lead. Anaesthesia 44:881, 1989.
12. Herman MV, Ingram DA, Levy JA, et al: Variability of electrocardiographic precordial lead placement: A method to improve accuracy and reliability. Clin Cardiol 14:469, 1991.
13. Kates RA, Zaidan JR, Kaplan JA: Esophageal lead for intraoperative electrocardiographic monitoring. Anesth Analg 61:781, 1982.
14. Heinke M, Volkmann H: Balloon electrode catheter for transesophageal atrial pacing and transesophageal ECG recording. Pacing Clin Electrophysiol 15:1953, 1992.
15. Srivastava P, Mittal SR, Srivastava N: Role of oesophageal electrocardiograms in differentiation of old anteroseptal myocardial infarction from emphysema in cases with poor R wave progression in precordial leads. J Assoc Physicians India 39:249, 1991.
16. Katz A, Guetta V, Ovsyshcher IA: Transesophageal electrocardiography using a temporary pacing balloon-tipped electrode in acute cardiac care. Ann Emerg Med 20:961, 1991.
17. Chatterjee K, Swan HJC, Ganz W, et al: Use of a balloon-tipped flotation electrode catheter for cardiac monitoring. Am J Cardiol 36:56, 1975.
18. Lichtenthal PR: Multipurpose pulmonary artery catheter. Ann Thorac Surg 36:493, 1983.
19. Mylrea KC, Calkins JM, Carlson J, et al: ECG lead with the endotracheal tube. Crit Care Med 11:199, 1983.

20. Meier B, Killisch JP, Adatte JJ, et al: Intrakoronares Elektrokardiogramm wahrend transluminaler Koronarangioplasty. Schweiz Med Wochenschr 115:1590, 1985.
21. Pande AK, Meier B, Urban P, et al: Intracoronary electrocardiogram during coronary angioplasty. Am Heart J 124:337, 1992.
22. Maeda T, Saikawa T, Niwa H, et al: QT interval shortening and ST elevation in intracoronary ECG during PTCA. Clin Cardiol 15:525, 1992.
23. Mirvis DM, Berson AS, Goldberger AL, et al: Instrumentation and practice standards for electrocardiographic monitoring in special care units. Circulation 79:464, 1989.
24. Pipberger HV, Arzbaecher RC, Berson AS, et al: Report of the Committee on Electrocardiography, American Heart Association: Recommendations for standardization of leads and of specifications for instruments in electrocardiography and vectorcardiography. Circulation 52:11, 1975.
25. Sheffield LT, Berson AS, Bragg-Remschel D, et al: Recommendations for standards of instrumentation and practice in the use of ambulatory electrocardiography: The Task Force of the Committee on Electrocardiography and Cardiac Electrophysiology of the Council on Clinical Cardiology. Circulation 71:626A, 1985.
26. Association for the Advancement of Medical Instrumentation (AAMI): American National Standards for Pregelled Disposable Electrodes (EC12-1983). Arlington, VA, American National Standards Institute/AAMI, 1984.
27. Legatt AD, Frost EAM: ECG artifacts during intraoperative evoked potential monitoring. Anesthesiology 70:559, 1989.
28. Paulsen AW, Pritchard DG: ECG artifact produced by crystalloid administration through blood/fluid warmer sets. Anesthesiology 69:803, 1988.
29. Lampert BA, Sundstrom FD: ECG artifacts simulating supraventricular tachycardia during automated percutaneous lumbar discectomy. Anesth Analg 67:1096, 1988.
30. Arbeit SR, Rubin IL, Gross H: Dangers in interpreting the electrocardiogram from the oscilloscope monitor. JAMA 211:453, 1970.
31. Slogoff S, Keats A, David Y, et al: Incidence of perioperative myocardial ischemia detected by different electrocardiographic systems. Anesthesiology 73:1074, 1990.
32. Bertrand CA, Steiner NV, Jameson AG, et al: Disturbances of cardiac rhythm during anesthesia and surgery. JAMA 216:1615, 1971.
33. Angelini L, Feldman MI, Lufschonowski R, et al: Cardiac arrhythmias during and after heart surgery: Diagnosis and management. Prog Cardiovasc Dis 16:469, 1974.
34. Atlee JL, Rusy BF: Ventricular conduction times and AV nodal conductivity during enflurane anesthesia in dogs. Anesthesiology 47:498, 1977.
35. Edwards R, Winnie AP, Ramamurthy S: Acute hypocapnic hypokalemia: An iatrogenic anesthetic complication. Anesth Analg 56:786, 1977.
36. Smith M, Ray CT: Cardiac arrhythmias, increased intracranial pressure, and the autonomic nervous system. Chest 61:125, 1972.
37. Alexander JP: Dysrhythmia and oral surgery. Br J Anaesth 43:773, 1971.
38. Slapa WJ: The sick sinus syndrome. Am Heart J 92:648, 1976.
39. DiMarco JP, Sellers TD, Lerman BB, et al: Diagnostic and therapeutic use of adenosine in patients with supraventricular tachyarrhythmias. J Am Coll Cardiol 6:417, 1985.
40. Bushman GA: Clinical correlates of dysrhythmias requiring an esophageal ECG for accurate diagnosis in patients with congenital heart disease. J Cardiothorac Anesth 3:290, 1989.
41. Lim SH, Anantharaman V, Teo WS, et al: Comparison of treatment of supraventricular tachycardia by Valsalva maneuver and carotid sinus massage. Ann Emerg Med 31:30, 1998.
42. Hess DS, Hanlon T, Scheinman M, et al: Termination of ventricular tachycardia by carotid sinus massage. Circulation 65:627, 1982.
43. Aydin M, Baysal K, Kucukoduk S, et al: Application of ice water to the face in initial treatment of supraventricular tachycardia. Turk J Pediatr 37:15, 1995.
44. Camm AJ, Garratt CJ: Adenosine and supraventricular tachycardia. N Engl J Med 325:1621, 1991.
45. Di Marco JP, Miles W, Akhtar M, et al: Adenosine for paroxysmal supraventricular tachycardia: Dose ranging and comparison with verapamil. Assessment in placebo-controlled, multicenter trials: The Adenosine for PSVT Study Group. Ann Intern Med 113:104, 1990.
46. Balser JR. The rational use of intravenous amiodarone in the perioperative period. Anesthesiology 86:974-87, 1997.
47. The Esmolol Research Group: Intravenous esmolol for the treatment of supraventricular tachyarrhythmia: Results of a multicenter, baseline-controlled safety and efficacy study in 160 patients. Am Heart J 112:498, 1986.
48. Waxman MB, Wald RW, Sharma AD, et al: Vagal techniques for termination of paroxysmal supraventricular tachycardia. Am J Cardiol 46:655, 1980.
49. Basta M, Klein GJ, Yee R, et al: Current role of pharmacologic therapy for patients with paroxysmal supraventricular tachycardia. Cardiol Clin 15:587, 1997.
50. Altamura G, Bianconi L, Toscano S, et al: Transcutaneous cardiac pacing for termination of tachyarrhythmias. Pacing Clin Electrophysiol 13:2026, 1990.
51. Kerber RE: Electrical treatment of cardiac arrhythmias: Defibrillation and cardioversion. Ann Emerg Med 22:296, 1993.
52. Kay GN, Epstein AE, Daily SM, et al: Role of radiofrequency ablation in the management of supraventricular arrhythmias: Experience in 760 consecutive patients. J Cardiovasc Electrophysiol 4:371, 1993.
53. Ellenbogen KA, Dias VC, Cardello FP, et al: Safety and efficacy of intravenous diltiazem in atrial fibrillation or atrial flutter. Am J Cardiol 75:45, 1995.
54. Cummins RO (ed): Advanced Cardiac Life Support. Dallas, American Heart Association, 1997.
55. Ellenbogen KA, Stambler BS, Wood MA, et al: Efficacy of intravenous ibutilide for rapid termination of atrial fibrillation and atrial flutter: A dose-response study. J Am Coll Cardiol 28:130, 1996.
56. Stambler BS, Wood MA, Ellenbogen KA, et al: Efficacy and safety of repeated doses of ibutilide for rapid conversion of atrial flutter or fibrillation. Ibutilide Repeat Dose Study Investigators. Circulation 94:1613, 1996.
57. Chapman MJ, Moran JL, O'Fathartaigh MS, et al: Management of atrial tachyarrhythmias in the critically ill: A comparison of intravenous procainamide and amiodarone. Intensive Care Med 19:48, 1993.
58. Stambler BS, Wood MA. Ellenbogen KA: Comparative efficacy of intravenous ibutilide versus procainamide for enhancing termination of atrial flutter by atrial overdrive pacing. Am J Cardiol 77:960, 1996.
59. Page RL, Kerber RE, Russell JK, Trouton T: Biphasic versus monophasic shock waveform for conversion of atrial fibrillation: The results of an international randomized, double-blind multicenter trial. J Am Coll Cardiol 39:1956, 2002.
60. Griffin JC: Indications for atrial defibrillator. J Cardiovascular Electrophysiology 9(Suppl 8):S187, 1998.
61. Naccarelli GV, Dorian P, Hohnloser SH, et al: Prospective comparison of flecainide versus quinidine for the treatment of paroxysmal atrial fibrillation/flutter: The Flecainide Multicenter Atrial Fibrillation Study Group. Am J Cardiol 77:53A, 1996.
62. Gallik DM, Kim SG, Ferrick KJ, et al: Efficacy and safety of sotalol in patients with refractory atrial fibrillation or flutter. Am Heart J 134:155, 1997.
63. Opolski G, Stanislawska J, Gorecki A, et al: Amiodarone in restoration and maintenance of sinus rhythm in patients with chronic atrial fibrillation after unsuccessful direct-current cardioversion. Clin Cardiol 20:337, 1997.
64. Daoud EG, Strickberger SA. Man KC, et al: Preoperative amiodarone as prophylaxis against atrial fibrillation after heart surgery. N Engl J Med 337:1785, 1997.
65. Reisinger J, Gatterer E, Heinze G, et al: Prospective comparison of flecainide versus sotalol for immediate conversion of atrial fibrillation. Am J Cardiol 81:1450, 1998.
66. Stambler BS, Wood MA, Ellenbogen KA, et al: Efficacy and safety of repeated intravenous doses of ibutilide for rapid

conversion of atrial flutter or fibrillation. Ibutilide Repeat Dose Study Investigators. Circulation 94:1613, 1996.

67. Vos MA, Golitsyn SR, Stangl K, et al: Superiority of ibutilide (a new class III agent) over D,L-sotalol in converting atrial flutter and atrial fibrillation. Ibutilide/Sotalol Comparator Study Group. Heart 79:568, 1998.

68. Volgman AS, Carberry PA, Stambler B, et al: Conversion efficacy and safety of intravenous ibutilide compared with intravenous procainamide in patients with atrial flutter or fibrillation. J Am Coll Cardiol 31:1414, 1998.

69. Singh SN, Berk MR, Yellen LG, et al: Oral dofetilide for conversion of patients with chronic atrial fibrillation or atrial flutter to normal sinus rhythm: A multicenter study [abstract]. J Am Coll Cardiol 31:369A, 1998.

70. Donahue TP, Conti JB: Atrial fibrillation: Rate control versus maintenance of sinus rhythm. Curr Opin Cardiol 6:46, 2001.

71. Haldemann G, Sehaer H: Haemodynamic effects of transient atrioventricular dissociation in general anesthesia. Br J Anaesth 44:159, 1972.

72. Cranefeld PF: Ventricular fibrillation. N Engl J Med 289:732, 1973.

73. Kowey PR, Levine JH, Herre JM, et al: Randomized double blind comparison of intravenous amiodarone and bretylium in the treatment of patients with recurrent ventricular tachycardia or fibrillation. The Intravenous Amiodarone Multicenter Investigators Group. Circulation 92:3255, 1995.

74. Kerber RE, Bourland JD, Kallok MJ, et al: Transthoracic defibrillation using sequential and simultaneous dual shock pathways: Experimental studies. Pacing Clin Electrophysiol 13:207, 1990.

75. Mittal S, Ayati S, Stein KM, Knight BP: Comparison of a novel rectilinear biphasic waveform with a damped sine wave monophasic waveform for transthoracic ventricular defibrillation. ZOLL Investigators. J Am Coll Cardiol 34:1595, 1999.

76. Roden DM: Torsade de pointes. Clin Cardiol 16:683, 1993.

77. Roden DM: A practical approach to torsade de pointes. Clin Cardiol 20:285, 1997.

78. Slogoff S, Keats A: Does perioperative myocardial ischemia lead to postoperative myocardial infarction? Anesthesiology 62:107, 1985.

79. Sonntag H, Larsen R, Hilfiker O, et al: Myocardial blood flow and oxygen consumption during high-dose fentanyl anesthesia in patients with coronary artery disease. Anesthesiology 56:416, 1982.

80. Coriat P, Harari A, Daloz M, et al: Clinical predictors of intraoperative myocardial ischemia in patients with coronary artery disease undergoing non-cardiac surgery. Acta Anaesthesiol Scand 26:287, 1982.

81. Crutchley P, Kaplan JA, Hug CC, et al: Non-cardiac surgery in patients with prior myocardial revascularization. Can Anaesth Soc J 30:629, 1983.

82. Landesberg G, Mosseri M, Zahger D, et al: Myocardial infarction following vascular surgery: The role of prolonged stress-induced, ST-depression-type stress ischemia. J Am Coll Cardiol 37:1839, 2001.

83. Coy KM, Imperi GA, Lambert CR, et al: Silent myocardial ischemia during daily activities in asymptomatic men with positive exercise response. Am J Cardiol 59:45, 1987.

84. Pepine CJ: Is silent ischemia a treatable risk factor in patients with angina pectoris? Circulation 82(Suppl 2):135, 1990.

85. Chaitman BR, Hanson JS: Comparative sensitivity and specificity of exercise electrocardiographic lead systems. Am J Cardiol 47:1335, 1981.

86. Okin PM, Bergman G, Kligfield P: Effect of ST segment measurement point on performance of standard heart rate-adjusted ST segment criteria for the identification of coronary artery disease. Circulation 84:57, 1991.

87. Gianrossi R, Dotrano R, Mulvohill D, et al: Exercise-induced ST depression in the diagnosis of coronary artery disease: A meta analysis. Circulation 80:87, 1989.

88. Miller TD, Desser KB, Lawson M: How many ECG leads are required for exercise treadmill tests? J Electrocardiology 20:131, 1987.

89. London MJ, Hollenberg M, Wong MG, et al: Intraoperative myocardial ischemia: Localization by continuous 12-lead electrocardiography. Anesthesiology 69:232, 1988.

90. Landesberg G, Mosseri M, Wolf Y, et al: Perioperative myocardial ischemia and infarction. Anesthesiology 96:264, 2002.

91. Drew BJ, Krucoff MW: Multilead ST-segment monitoring in patients with acute coronary syndromes: A consensus statement for healthcare professionals. ST-Segment Monitoring Practice Guideline International Working Group. Am J Crit Care 8:372, 1999.

92. London MJ: Multilead precordial ST-segment monitoring [editorial]. Anesthesiology 96:261, 2002.

93. Bell C, Rimar S, Barash P: Intraoperative ST segment changes consistent with myocardial ischemia in the neonate: A report of three cases. Anesthesiology 71:601, 1989.

94. Hecht HH, Kossman EC, Childers RW, et al: Atrioventricular and intraventricular conduction: Revised nomenclature and concepts. Am J Cardiol 31:232, 1973.

95. Kastor JA: Atrioventricular block. N Engl J Med 292:462, 1976.

96. Wynands JE: Anesthesia for patients with heart block and artificial cardiac pacemakers. Anesth Analg 55:626, 1976.

97. Marriott HJL: Practical Electrocardiography, 7th ed. Baltimore, Williams & Wilkins, 1983.

98. Dodds TM, Delphin E, Stone G, et al: Detection of perioperative myocardial ischemia using Holter with real-time ST segment analysis. Anesth Analg 67:890, 1988.

99. London MJ: Validation testing of the SEER real-time digital Holter monitor. J Cardiothorac Vasc Anesth 10:497, 1996.

100. Levin RI, Cohen D, Frisbie W, et al: Potential for real-time processing of the continuously monitored electrocardiogram in the detection, quantitation, and intervention of silent myocardial ischemia. Cardiol Clin 4:735, 1986.

101. Clements FM, McCann RL, Levin RI: Continuous ST-segment analysis for the detection of perioperative myocardial ischemia. Crit Care Med 16:710, 1988.

102. Willems JL, Abreu-Lima C, Arnaud P, et al: The diagnostic performance of computer programs for the interpretation of electrocardiograms. N Engl J Med 325:1767, 1991.

103. Romhilt DW, Bloomfield SS, Chai TC, et al: Unreliability of conventional electrocardiographic monitoring of arrhythmia detection in coronary care units. Am J Cardiol 31:457, 1973.

104. Oliver GE, Nolle FM, Wolff GA, et al: Detection of premature ventricular contractions with a clinical system for monitoring electrocardiographic rhythms. Comput Biomed Res 4:523, 1971.

105. Shah PM, Arnold JM, Haberen NA, et al: Automatic real-time arrhythmia monitoring in the intensive coronary care unit. Am J Cardiol 39:701, 1977.

106. Morganroth J: Ambulatory Holter electrocardiography: Choice of technique and clinical uses. Ann Intern Med 102:73, 1985.

107. Kortly K, Kotter G, Mortara D, et al: Intraoperative detection of myocardial ischemia with an ST segment trend monitoring system. Anesth Analg 63:343, 1984.

108. London MJ: Monitoring for myocardial ischemia. In Kaplan JA (ed): Vascular Anesthesia. New York, Churchill Livingstone, 1991, p 249.

109. Kotter GS, Kotrly KJ, Kalbfleisch JH, et al: Myocardial ischemia during cardiovascular surgery as detected by an ST segment trend monitoring system. J Cardiothorac Anesth 1:190, 1987.

110. London MJ, Ahlstrom LD: Validation testing of the Spacelabs PC2 ST-segment analyzer. J Cardiothorac Vasc Anesth 9:684, 1995.

111. Ellis JE, Shah MN, Briller JE, et al: A comparison of methods for the detection of myocardial ischemia during noncardiac surgery: Automated ST-segment analysis systems, electrocardiography and transesophageal echocardiography. Anesth Analg 75:764, 1992.

112. Brooker S, Lowenstein E: Spurious ST segment depression by automated ST segment analysis. J Clin Monit 11:186, 1995.

113. Ellestad MH: Stress Testing: Principles and Practice. Philadelphia, FA Davis, 1975.

35 Implantable Cardiac Pulse Generators: Pacemakers and Cardioverter-Defibrillators

Marc A. Rozner

Pacemakers 1416
Overview 1416
Pacemaker Codes 1416
Pacemaker Indications 1418
Pacemaker Magnets 1419
Preanesthesia Evaluation and Pacemaker
    Reprogramming 1421
Intraoperative or Procedural Management of
    Pacemakers 1422
Pacemaker Failure 1426
Postanesthesia Pacemaker Evaluation 1427

**Implantable Cardioverter-
    Defibrillators 1427**
Overview 1427
Implantable Cardioverter-Defibrillator
    Indications 1428

Implantable Cardioverter-Defibrillator
    Magnets 1428
Preanesthesia Evaluation and
    Implantable Cardioverter-Defibrillator
    Reprogramming 1429
Intraoperative or Procedural Management of
    Implantable Cardioverter-
    Defibrillators 1429
Postanesthesia Implantable
    Cardioverter-Defibrillator
    Evaluation 1431

Summary 1431

Glossary 1431

Appendicies 1435

Battery operated pacing devices were introduced by CW Lillehei (a cardiothoracic surgeon) and Earl Bakken (an electrical technician) in 1958, just four years after the invention of the transistor. A few years later, Wilson Greatbatch, a cardiologist in Buffalo, NY, created the first implantable battery powered device in his barn.[1] Advances in electronic miniaturization as well as improvements in battery technology have led to the development of very small (10-mL volume), but electronically complicated, programmable pacing devices.

The natural progression of pacemaker developments led to the invention of the implanted cardioverter-defibrillator* (ICD) around 1980 by Michael Mirowski (Baltimore, MD). First approved by the U.S. Food and

Drug Administration (FDA) in 1985, implantation of these devices required a thoracotomy, a significant operation for the patient with poor heart function. However, four technologic advances (transvenous lead placement,

---

*The terms antibradycardia and antitachycardia will be used throughout this chapter. Antibradycardia refers to pacing to maintain a minimum rate. Conventional pacemakers are antibradycardia devices. Antitachycardia refers to therapy delivered in the setting of a tachycardia, and it is designed to reduce the underlying heart rate.

antitachycardia* pacing capability, miniaturization permitting pectoral pocket placement, and dual chamber, rate responsive antibradycardia pacing) have led to increases in implantations.

These changes in ICD implantation and indication have two important results for health care providers. First, a pectoral (rather than abdominal) pocket ICD with pacing capability might be mistaken, by virtue of pacing "spikes" on the surface electrocardiogram, for a (non-ICD) pacemaker. At many centers, electrocardiograms are collected from patients with "pacemakers" using a magnet. Since some ICDs from Guidant Medical and Cardiac Pacemakers, Inc. (CPI) can undergo permanent deactivation of antitachycardia therapy with magnet placement, this mistake could leave a patient unprotected.[2] Second, pacing functions in an ICD often respond to external stimuli (magnet placement, electromagnetic interference) differently than a pacemaker. These issues will be addressed in the text below.

The complexity of pacemakers and ICDs, as well as the multitude of programmable parameters, limits the number of generalizations that can be made about the perioperative care of the patient with an implanted pulse generator. Population aging, continued enhancements in implantable technology, and new indications for implantation of cardiac devices will lead to growing numbers of patients with these devices in the new millennium. The American College of Cardiology (ACC) has taken note of these issues, and guidelines (hereafter the ACC Guidelines) have been published regarding the care of the perioperative patient with a device.[3] The ACC is not alone in this endeavor; recently, Pinski and Trohman also reviewed this subject and published similar recommendations.[4,5] Because ICDs now also perform permanent cardiac pacing, some ICD issues related primarily to pacing will be discussed further on.

Patients with an implanted cardiac pulse generator (PG) often have significant comorbid diseases in addition to their cardiac rhythm disturbances. Our ability to care for these patients requires attention to their medical and psychological problems. We also need an understanding of the pulse generator, its functions, and its probable idiosyncrasies in the operating or procedure room.

Not all electronic generators implanted in the chest are cardiac devices, and devices resembling cardiac pulse generators are being implanted at increasing rates for indications unrelated to cardiac issues. When implanted in the pectoral position (the usual place for current cardiac generators), these devices can be mistakenly identified as cardiac generators.[6] Pulse generator implantation has been approved by the FDA for pain control, thalamic stimulation to control Parkinson's disease, phrenic nerve stimulation to stimulate the diaphragm in paralyzed patients, and vagus nerve stimulation to control epilepsy. When evaluating a patient with any pulse generator, one must now determine whether the PG will be pacing the heart, stimulating the central nervous system, stimulating the spinal cord, or stimulating the vagus nerve. Adding to this confusion, Cyberonics Corporation (Houston, TX) has a patent on a vagus nerve stimulator for heart failure, although, at this time, there have been no clinical trials

to evaluate vagus nerve stimulation in the setting of heart failure.

PACEMAKERS

Overview

Pacemaker manufacturers report that 26 companies have produced more than 1,500 models to date. Currently, more than 200,000 adults and children in the United States undergo new pacemaker placement each year, and nearly 2 million patients have pacemakers today. Many factors lead to confusion regarding the behavior of a device and the perioperative care of a patient with a device, especially since case reports, textbooks, and literature reviews have not kept pace with technologic developments.

A pacemaking system consists of an impulse generator and leads to carry the electrical impulse to the patient's heart. Leads are connected to the heart's chambers through the vena cava (transvenous leads) or are directly sewn onto the surface of the heart (epicardial leads). Leads can be unipolar (one electrode per lead), bipolar (two electrodes per lead), or multipolar (multiple electrodes and wires contained within one lead with connections in multiple chambers) (Fig. 35-1). Because two electrodes are required to complete a circuit, the second electrode in a unipolar configuration will be the metal generator case. Use of the case as an electrode requires that the generator pocket be devoid of gas, and electrical continuity has reportedly been disrupted by the use of nitrous oxide.[7]

Pacemakers with unipolar leads seem to be more sensitive to the effects of electromagnetic interference (EMI), and these systems produce larger "spikes" on an analogue-recorded electrocardiogram. Most pacemaking systems (except Autocapture devices from St. Jude Cardiac Rhythm Management, Sylmar, CA) use a bipolar pacing configuration, since bipolar pacing usually requires less energy. Also, bipolar sensing is more resistant to interference from muscle artifacts or stray electromagnetic fields. Often, bipolar electrodes can be identified on the chest film since they will have a ring electrode 1 to 3 cm proximal to the lead tip (see Fig. 35-1). However, generators with bipolar leads can be programmed to the unipolar mode for pacing, sensing, or both.

Pacemaker Codes

No discussion of pacemakers can take place without an understanding of the generic pacemaker code, which has been published by the North American Society of Pacing and Electrophysiology (NASPE) and British Pacing and Electrophysiology Group (BPEG). This code (NBG[†]) was

---

*Although many authors and references identify this device as an "automatic implantable cardioverter-defibrillator or AICD," the term "AICD" is a brand name and belongs to Cardiac Pacemakers Inc (CPI), which has been acquired by Guidant Medical Corporation, St. Paul, MN. The term "PCD" (for "Programmable Cardioverter-Defibrillator") belongs to the Medtronic Corporation.
†The NBG code is a joint project from NASPE (the "N") and BPEG (the "B"). The "G" stands for generic.

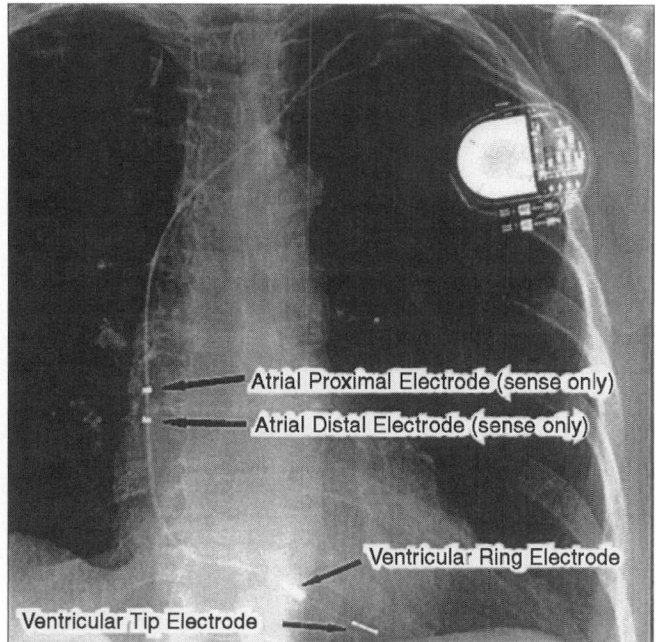

Atrial Proximal Electrode (sense only)
Atrial Distal Electrode (sense only)
Ventricular Ring Electrode
Ventricular Tip Electrode

Figure 35–1 Pacemaker with one quadripolar lead that provides atrial and ventricular sensing and ventricular pacing. This chest x-ray film shows a number of features of a modern pacing system. The generator is located in the left pectoral region. The single lead enters the subclavian vein under the clavicle but superficial to the first rib (a common site for lead problems, although no problem is demonstrated here). In this device, there are two electrodes in the right atrium that can provide sensing to detect intrinsic atrial activity. The ventricular portion of the lead shows the classic bipolar pattern, with a ring electrode just proximal to the tip electrode, and these electrodes can be used for sensing intrinsic ventricular activity and for depolarizing the ventricle. This is a ventricular pacing system with pacing in the triggered and inhibited mode (VDD), and this configuration is placed into patients with a functioning sinus node but a nonfunctioning atrioventricular node. This system cannot be used to depolarize the atrium. Because the surface electrocardiogram often demonstrates ventricular pacing that tracks the atrial activity, inspection of the surface electrocardiogram typically produces an erroneous diagnosis of a dual chamber (DDD) pacemaker.

initially published in 1983 and was last revised in 2002.[8] It describes the basic behavior of the pacing device (Table 35-1). Pacemakers also come with a variety of terms generally unfamiliar to the anesthesiologist, many of which are shown in the glossary at the end of this chapter.

The first two positions of this code (i.e., chamber paced and chamber sensed) seem relatively straightforward. Although early pacemakers provided only ventricular support, current models can provide pacing in the atria and ventricles, and these devices can also be programmed to determine intrinsic activity in these chambers as well. The code does not describe the array of diagnostic data that can be accumulated by these devices.

Probably the most confusing aspect of the NBG code is the third position (i.e., response to sensed event). Most pacemakers are programmed either to the DDD (dual chamber pacing and sensing, both triggered and inhibited mode) or VVI mode (for single chamber, ventricular pacing in the inhibited mode). Two other modes frequently found are VDD (ventricular pacing with atrial tracking) and DDI (dual chamber pacing and sensing, but inhibited mode only). In the United States, it is uncommon to find an atrial-only pacemaker (AAI), but these devices are indeed implanted in patients with sinus node disease in other countries. The third position describes the following behavior:

D (dual): For DDD pacemakers, atrial pacing will take place in the "inhibited" mode; i.e., the pacing device will emit an atrial pulse if no sensed atrial event (or intervening ventricular event, since any ventricular event will reset atrial timing) takes place within the appropriate timeframe. In DDD or VDD devices, once an atrial event has occurred (whether native or paced), the pacing device will ensure that a ventricular event follows (up to the Upper Tracking Rate [see glossary]). Dual response pacemakers are used to provide atrioventricular (AV) synchrony.

I (inhibited): The pacer will emit a pulse to the appropriate chamber unless it detects intrinsic electrical activity. In DDI mode, AV synchrony is provided only when the pacemaker paces the atrial chamber. If intrinsic atrial activity is present, then no AV synchrony is provided by the pacemaker.

Table 35–1   NASPE/BPEG revised (2002) NBG pacemaker code*

Position I	Position II	Position III	Position IV	Position V
(Chamber Paced)	(Chamber Sensed)	(Response to Sensed Event)	(Programmability, Rate Modulation)	(Multisite Pacing)
O = none	O = none	O = none	O = none	O = none
A = atrium	A = atrium	I = inhibited	R = rate modulation	A = atrium
V = ventricle	V = ventricle	T = triggered		V = ventricle
D = dual (A + V)	D = dual (A + V)	D = dual (T + I)		D = dual (A + V)

*The generic pacemaker code,[8] initially published in 1983, was last revised in 2002 in an effort to keep current with technologic developments in the pacing field. The NBG code is a joint project of the North American Society of Pacing and Electrophysiology (NASPE) and the British Pacing and Electrophysiology Group (BPEG).
NBG: North American Society of Pacing and Electrophysiology (N) and British Pacing and Electrophysiology Group (B) generic (G) pacemaker code.

T (triggered): The pacing device will emit a pulse only in response to a sensed event. Triggered mode is used when the device is being tested.

The VDD and DDI modes deserve further comment. VDD pacing is used for the patient with AV nodal dysfunction but intact and appropriate sinus node behavior. VDD pacing is accomplished with a single lead that incorporates atrial sensing electrodes and ventricular conductors that can pace and sense (see Fig. 35-1). A VDD device has no atrial pacing capability. As a result, in a patient who depends on atrial contraction to augment cardiac output, events that produce VVI pacing (e.g., sinus rate below the programmed rate, battery depletion) or asynchronous ventricular pacing (e.g., magnet placement in many devices, electromagnetic interference) can lead to deteriorating hemodynamics.[9,10]

DDI is rarely used as a primary mode of pacing. DDI pacing is indicated for the patient who has a dual-chamber pacemaker and has episodes of paroxysmal atrial dysrhythmia (e.g., paroxysmal atrial fibrillation). DDI pacing prevents high ventricular rates (i.e.; pacing at the upper tracking rate) that could result from attempted tracking of the atrial arrhythmia, and it provides AV synchrony only when the atrium is paced. Some DDD pacemakers are programmed to enter the DDI mode on the detection of high (programmable) atrial rates (called Mode Switch, Automatic Mode Switch, or Atrial Tachy Response, depending on manufacturer). For the DDD pacemaker that has switched to DDI, perturbations (e.g., such as atrial rates greater than 400/min), electromagnetic interference from the ESU or magnet placement and removal) can cause the pacemaker to transiently revert back to the DDD mode, with resultant appearance of AV pacing or ventricular pacing at the upper tracking rate (see "Pacemaker Magnets").

Rate modulation (the fourth position) also remains a poorly understood concept. Because some patients cannot increase their heart rate in response to increased oxygen demand (chronotropic incompetence), pacemaker manufacturers have devised a number of mechanisms to detect "patient exercise," such as sensors that detect vibration, respiration, and pressure (Table 35-2). As the sensor detects "exercise," it increases the pacing rate (termed "sensor indicated rate"). As the exercise tapers, this sensor indicated rate returns to the programmed LRL. The sensitivity of these sensors to their exercise signals and the rates of change in pacing are programmable features in current generators.

With the 2002 revision of the NBG, the fifth column now describes multisite pacing functionality (it had been used to describe antitachycardia function, but this scheme has been abandoned and a generic defibrillator code has been established). Atrial multisite pacing is being investigated as a means to prevent atrial fibrillation,[11] and ventricular multisite pacing is an acceptable treatment for pacing the patient with a dilated cardiomyopathy.[12-14]

Pacemaker Indications

Indications for permanent pacing are shown in Table 35-3 and are reviewed in detail elsewhere.[15] Classically, pacemakers are used to treat patients with diseases of the sinus node (improper impulse formation) and diseases of the AV node (improper impulse conduction).

Table 35–2 Rate modulation (activity) sensors

Approved in the United States*	Under Investigation*
Vibration sensor	Right ventricular stroke volume
Motion sensor	Blood pH
Minute ventilation (bio-impedance sensor)	Blood temperature
QT interval (Vitatron only)	Mixed venous oxygen sensor
Right ventricular pressure (Biotronik only)	Systolic time intervals
	Evoked response
	Intracardiac impedance

*Of the sensors used to detect exercise in a patient with a cardiac pacemaker, five types are approved in the United States, and many others are under investigation. Some devices have two sensors and can be programmed for cross-checking to prevent increases in heart rate from spurious causes. Minute ventilation sensors are very sensitive to stray electromagnetic interference, and patients have been inappropriately treated for pacemaker-driven tachycardias as a result. There is little perioperative experience with right ventricular pressure sensors. Most pacemaker experts[90] recommend programming rate modulation to the Off position in the perioperative period to prevent confusion between an intrinsic tachycardia and a pacemaker-induced tachycardia.

Pacing can be used to reduce the outflow tract obstruction in hypertrophic obstructive cardiomyopathy (HOCM) in both adults and children, since paced ventricular conduction takes place in a left bundle branch pattern (left ventricular septum depolarizes after the other segments, rather than as the early systolic event).[16,17] Finally, in August, 2001, devices were approved by the U.S. FDA for three-chamber pacing (right atrium, both ventricles) to treat dilated cardiomyopathy (DCM).[18] To accomplish left ventricular pacing, a wire is placed through the right atrium and into the coronary sinus (CS) (Fig. 35-2). Most of the current devices connect the electrodes from the CS lead in parallel with the electrodes on the RV lead. In the setting of ventricular noncapture, this parallel connection can lead to ventricular overcounting with resultant inappropriate antitachycardia therapy for the patient with a DCM pacing defibrillator.[19,20] Devices in clinical trial (as well as the Reveal Defibrillator from

Table 35–3 Indications for pacemaker placement

Symptomatic diseases of impulse formation
  (i.e., sinus node disease)*
Symptomatic diseases of impulse conduction
  (i.e., atrioventricular nodal disease)
Long QT syndrome
Hypertrophic obstructive cardiomyopathy[†]
Dilated cardiomyopathy (also called cardiac resynchronization therapy)[†]

*Indications for permanent pacing are shown. Most patients with pacemakers fall into the first two categories listed.
[†]Requires 100% ventricular pacing to be effective. Short atrioventricular delays (120 to 150 msec) are programmed.

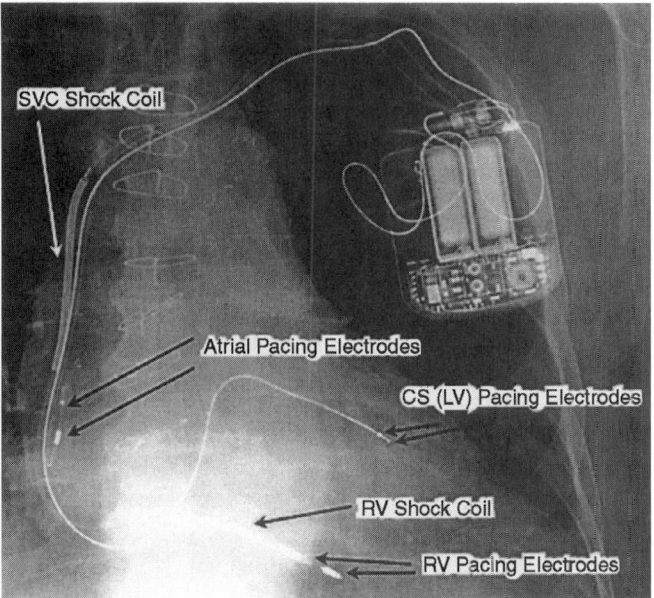

Figure 35–2 A defibrillator system with biventricular (BiV) pacemaker capability. Three leads are placed: a conventional, bipolar lead to the right atrium; a quadripolar lead to the right ventricle (RV); and a lead to the coronary sinus (CS). This system is designed to provide "resynchronization therapy" in the setting of a dilated cardiomyopathy with a prolonged QRS (and frequently with a prolonged PR interval). The bipolar lead in the right atrium performs sensing and pacing functions. Likewise, the bipolar tip in the RV performs pacing and sensing functions. The lead in the CS depolarizes the left ventricle (LV). In most BiV devices, both ventricles are depolarized simultaneously, because the electrode on the RV lead are connected in parallel with the electrode on the CS lead. This parallel connection can cause ventricular oversensing (and inappropriate antitachycardia therapy) in an implantable cardioverter-defibrillator (ICD) if the pacemaker fails to depolarize one or both of the ventricular chambers. The presence of "shock" conductors on the RV lead, called *coils*, in the RV and the superior vena cava (SVC) distinguish a defibrillation system from a conventional pacemaking system. Typically, the SVC shock coil is electrically identical to the defibrillator case, called the *can*. When the defibrillation circuitry includes the ICD case, it is called an *active can configuration*.

Guidant Medical and InSynch III from Medtronic) have separate sensing and output controls for the ventricular wires.

Pacing for HOCM and DCM requires careful attention to pacer programming. In order to be effective in these patients, the pacemaker must provide the stimulus for ventricular depolarization, and AV synchrony must be preserved.[21] Pacemaker inhibition or loss of pacing (i.e., from native conduction, atrial irregularity, ventricular irregularity, development of junctional rhythm, or electromagnetic interference) can lead to deteriorating hemodynamics in these patients.

Biventricular pacing might cause inappropriate lengthening of the Q-T interval in susceptible patients, and this lengthening has been reported to be associated with torsades de pointes.[22] As a result of this report, the prudent anesthesiologist should ensure adequate access to rapid defibrillation for the patient with biventricular pacing accomplished without an ICD.

Pacemaker Magnets

Despite the often-repeated folklore, most pacemaker manufacturers warn that magnets were never intended to treat pacemaker emergencies or prevent electromagnetic interference effects. Rather, magnet-activated reed switches were incorporated to produce pacing behavior that demonstrates remaining battery life and, sometimes, pacing threshold safety factors.

Placement of a magnet over a generator might produce no change in pacing since not all pacemakers switch to a continuous asynchronous mode when a magnet is placed. Also, not all models from a given company behave the same way. Only about 60% of pacemakers have high-rate (80 to 100 beats/min) asynchronous pacing with magnet application. About 25% switch to asynchronous pacing at program rate, and 15% respond with a brief (60 to 100 beats) asynchronous pacing event. Possible effects of magnet placement are shown in Table 35-4.[23-25] In some devices, magnet behavior can be altered by programming, and magnet behavior can be completely eliminated by programming in some devices.

For all generators, calling the manufacturer remains the most reliable method for determining magnet response and using this response to predict remaining battery life (phone numbers for the device manufacturers are shown in Appendix II). As battery voltage falls, the magnet response can be used to detect the following:

IFI (Intensified follow-up required)—the device must be checked frequently (approximately every 4 weeks for most models);

ERI (Elective replacement indicator)—the device is nearing the end of its useful life and should be electively replaced;

EOL (End of life)—the device has insufficient battery power remaining and should be replaced immediately.

On application of a magnet, some devices perform a threshold margin test (TMT). In this test, one or more of the pacemaker pulses is reduced in amplitude, pulse width, or both, in an attempt to gauge the safety margin for pacing voltage. Loss of capture on these TMT pulses indicates an inadequate safety margin for pacing (Fig. 35-3). Some devices from St. Jude Medical (formerly Pacesetter) with the Siemens "vario" engine reduce the ventricular pacing energy over 16 cycles to demonstrate the pacing threshold. As a result, many pacing cycles can take place at insufficient energy for ventricular capture, which can produce periods of asystole while the magnet is applied.[26]

Occasionally, a pacemaker mediated tachycardia (PMT) can ensue upon removal of the magnet from a dual chamber pacemaker (Fig. 35-4). These PMTs result from retrograde-conducted P waves during asynchronous ventricular pacing, most commonly when the magnet rate is lower than the patient's intrinsic rate. These retrograde P waves are then "tracked" after magnet removal by a dual chamber device (DDD, VDD modes only), resulting in pacing at the upper tracking rate. Each paced ventricular cycle results in another retrograde P wave, producing an endless loop tachycardia. Should this behavior be observed, it can be subverted by reapplication, then removal of the magnet. Some devices can be programmed to recognize these

Table 35–4 Pacemaker magnet behavior

No apparent rhythm or rate change*
    No magnet sensor (some pre-1985 Cordis, Telectronics models)
    Magnet mode disabled (possible with Cardiac Pacemakers, Inc. [CPI], Guidant, Pacesetter, Telectronics, and Biotronik models)
    Electrogram storage mode (EGM) enabled (CPI, Guidant, and other models)
    Program rate pacing in already paced patient (many CPI, Guidant, Intermedics, Telectronics, Vitatron, and other models)
    Improper monitor settings (pace filter on)
Brief (10-100 beats) asynchronous pacing; then a return to programmed values (most Intermedics and Biotronik models when
    programmed to their default state)
Continuous or transient loss of pacing
    Discharged battery (some pre-1990 devices)
    Pacer enters diagnostic threshold test mode (Siemans)
Asynchronous "high-rate" pacing
    Medtronic (most models) set at 85 beats/min; 65 beats/min if the battery is depleted
    Guidant Medical and CPI (models since 1990, magnet mode enabled) at more than 85 beats/min
      (maximum, 100 beats/min); 85 beats/min if the battery is depleted
    Pacesetter/St. Jude Medical (current models since 1990, magnet mode enabled) at more than 87 beats/min
      (maximum, 98.6 beats/min); 86.3 beats/min if the battery is depleted
    ELA Medical (models since 1989) at more than 80 beats/min (maximum, 96 beats/min); 80 beats/min if the battery
      is depleted. ELA Medical devices take eight additional asynchronous cycles (six at magnet rate, then two at
      programmed rate) on magnet removal. Placement of a magnet on an ELA device increases the pacing voltage to 5 V.
    Biotronik (only if programmed to asynchronous mode, which is not the default state) at 90 beats/min; 80 beats/min if
      the battery is depleted
Asynchronous pacing without rate responsiveness using parameters possibly not in patient's best interest

*Many pacemakers revert to some predetermined mode on placement of a magnet to indicate the remaining battery life. This table shows behaviors that can be observed on application of a magnet to an implanted cardiac pacemaker. Some devices perform a *threshold margin test* in which the pacing amplitude and/or pulse width is reduced briefly to test the pacing safety margin (see Fig. 35-3).

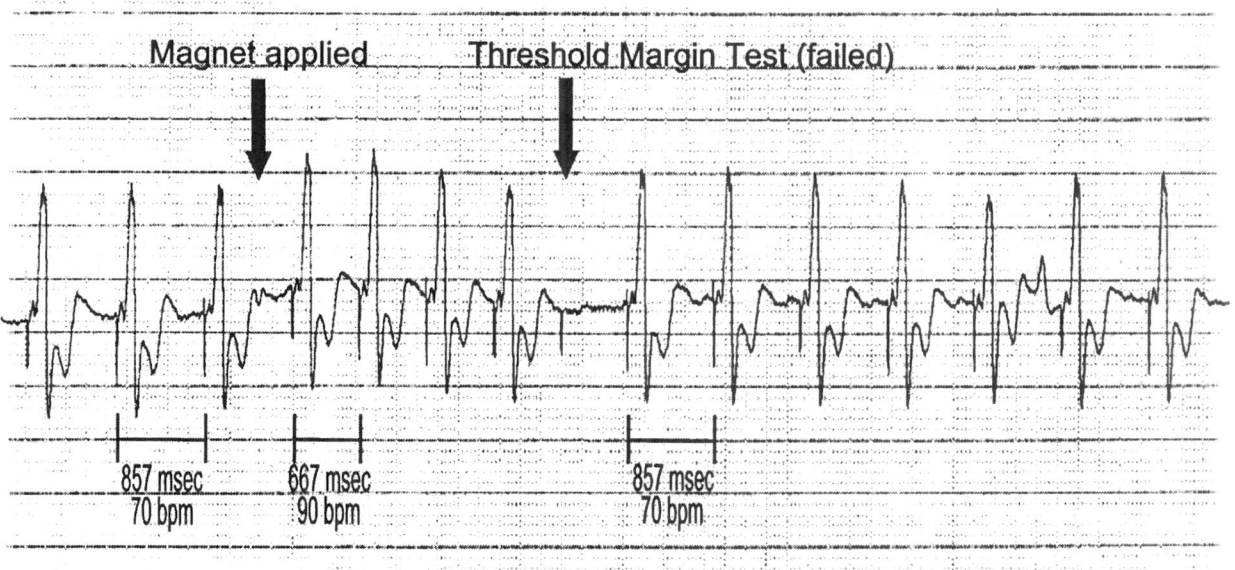

Figure 35–3 A threshold margin test (TMT), demonstrating inadequate safety margin for pacing. Application of a magnet to some pacemakers produces asynchronous pacing in which one or more pacing stimuli are emitted with a reduced ventricular pacing voltage, pulse width, or both. This sequence of the TMT is used to determine, without a formal pacemaker interrogation, the adequacy of the pacing energy settings. In this electrocardiographic strip from an Intermedics device, the patient was being paced in the VVI mode (ventricular pacing in the inhibited mode for a single chamber) at a rate of 70 beats/min, which is equal to 857-msec intervals. On application of the magnet, this pacemaker produced four intervals (i.e., five pacing stimuli) of asynchronous pacing at a rate of 90 beats/min (667-msec intervals), demonstrating adequate battery voltage for this device. At the fifth pacing stimulus after magnet application, the pacemaker performs a TMT by reducing the stimulus pulse width to 50% of the programmed value (equal to 50% of programmed pacing energy). The failure of this stimulus to produce a ventricular systole (i.e., failure to capture) demonstrates a dangerously low safety margin for ventricular pacing, because pacing pulse width should be at least three and usually four times the threshold for capture. After five initial stimuli, Intermedics pacemakers then pace asynchronously at the programmed lower rate (70 beats/min in this case) for 60 additional cycles. On completion of these 64 cycles (65 stimuli), Intermedics pacemakers return to programmed values and ignore the magnet.

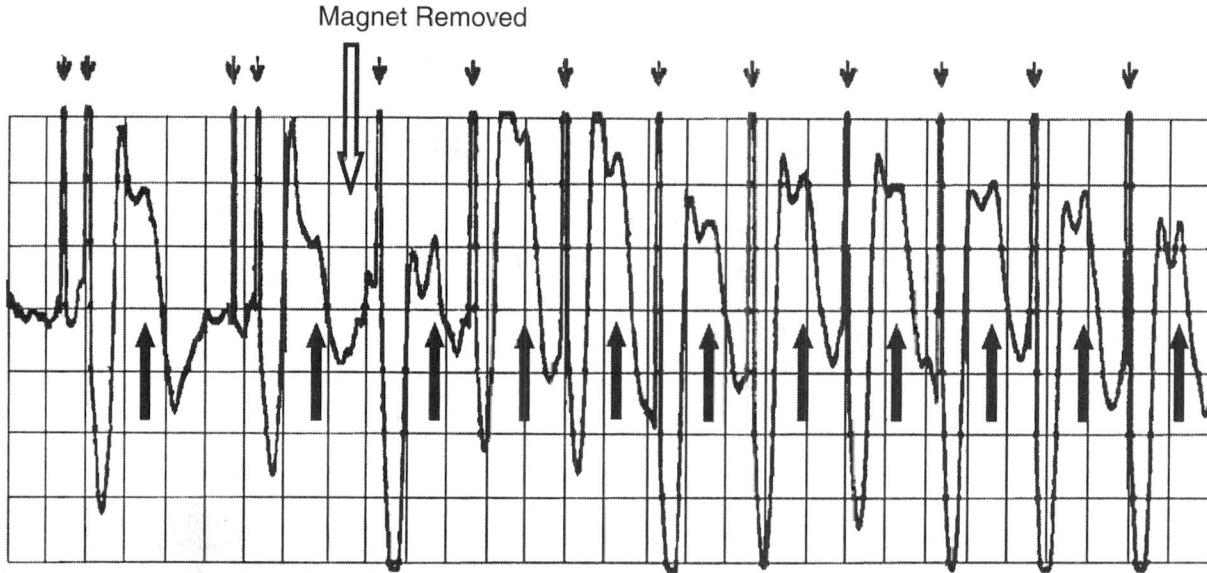

Figure 35–4 A pacemaker-mediated tachycardia (PMT) follows magnet removal from a pacemaker. This patient had a dual chamber pacemaker implanted for atrioventricular (AV) nodal disease, and she was pacemaker dependent for ventricular activity. She had a sinus rate of 75 beats/min before the magnet application with appropriate ventricular pacing (strip not shown). Her programmed AV delay is 200 msec. With magnet application, her pacemaker produced asynchronous AV sequential pacing (DOO mode) at a rate of 60 beats/min. This strip is from an electrocardiographic recorder that enhances the pacemaker artifact with *small, downward arrows*. Because the asynchronous magnet rate of this device is lower than her intrinsic atrial rate, many of the atrial pacing stimuli were applied during an atrial refractory period (i.e., functional noncapture). A consequence of atrial noncapture can be retrograde AV nodal conduction, with depolarization of the atria after the depolarization of the ventricles. The retrograde P waves are shown with the *upward arrows*. While the magnet is applied, this retrograde depolarization of the atria is ignored. Shortly after the magnet was removed *(open arrow)*, there was a paced ventricular event, followed by retrograde AV nodal conduction. With the ensuing depolarization of the atria from this retrograde conduction, the pacemaker sensed an atrial event and responded by pacing the ventricle 200 msec later. Another retrograde P wave appears, and each pace in response to a retrograde P wave created yet another ventricular pace. The result is a PMT at the upper tracking rate (programmed here to 130 beats/min) of the pacemaker. PMT from retrograde AV nodal conduction can occur in any DDD or VDD device with magnet removal, with a premature ventricular contraction, or with a noncaptured atrial pace. Treatment of this PMT entails reapplication of the magnet. Some pacemakers can be programmed to eventually break PMT by delaying one AV cycle when pacing at the upper tracking limit.

PMTs and will periodically omit one ventricular pacing pulse, or lengthen the AV delay, during UTR pacing.

The patient with a dual-chamber device that has detected a high atrial rate and "mode-switched" to prevent UTR pacing could have the mode-switch reset upon application and removal of the magnet. These patients will then undergo pacing at the upper tracking rate until criteria are met to return to the mode-switch mode. Distinguishing the PMT from retrograde P waves from the UTR pacing due to high atrial rates (prior to mode-switch entry) can be very difficult. In general, though, mode-switch due to high atrial rates will take place within 10-15 seconds, and PMT from retrograde P waves is quite persistent.

For generators with programmable magnet behavior [Guidant Medical, CPI, Pacesetter, St Jude Medical, Telectronics, Biotronik, others], only an interrogation with a programmer can reveal current settings. Many manufacturers publish a generator reference guide, although not all of these guides list all magnet idiosyncrasies.

Preanesthesia Evaluation and Pacemaker Reprogramming

Preoperative management of the patient with a pacemaker includes evaluation and optimization of coexisting diseases.

ACC guidelines suggest that cardiac testing (stress tests, echocardiograms) should be dictated by the patient's underlying diseases, medications, symptomatology, interval from the last testing, and planned intervention.[3]

No special laboratory tests or radiographs are needed for the patient with a conventional pacemaker. Chest films rarely depict lead problems, not all devices have radiographic markings, and a standard chest x-ray can exclude the generator or its markings. However, a patient with a BiV pacer (or defibrillator) might need a chest film to document the position of the coronary sinus (CS) lead, especially if central line placement is planned. Currently, there are no data or guidelines regarding the placement of a central line in the setting of a coronary sinus lead, and, since these leads have no fixation, they might be more easily dislodged than a standard pacemaker (or defibrillator) lead. In fact, in early studies, spontaneous CS lead dislodgement was found in more than 11% of patients.[27,28]

Important features of the preanesthetic device evaluation are shown in Appendix I. Current NASPE and Medicare guidelines include telephonic evaluation every 4-12 weeks (depending upon device type and age) and at least one direct evaluation (i.e., a device interrogation with a programmer) at least once per year.[29] In a recent abstract, Rozner et al reported significant noncompliance with these guidelines in 161 consecutive patients, as well as the need to replace 5% of pacemakers preoperatively for battery depletion.[30] Telephonic evaluation provides some assurance of battery longevity, but it does not provide rigorous evaluation of the pacemaking system. ACC guidelines now suggest a timely, preoperative interrogation of every pacemaker.[3]

For current pacemakers, interrogation with a programmer remains the most reliable method for evaluating battery voltage, battery impedance, lead performance, and adequacy of current settings. Special attention should be paid to patients from countries where pacemakers might be reused,[31,32] since battery life (typically 5-7 years, perhaps longer in some new devices) might not be related to length of implantation in the current patient. For any device with a battery voltage less than 2.6 volts or battery impedance (where available) greater than 3000 ohms, the device manufacturer should be consulted about the possible need for elective replacement of the device prior to the delivery of an anesthetic or surgery.

Appropriate reprogramming (Table 35-5) is the safest way to avoid intraoperative problems, especially if monopolar "Bovie" electrosurgery will be used. The pacemaker manufacturers stand ready to assist with this task (see Appendix II for company telephone numbers), however, any industry-employed allied professional must be supervised by an appropriately trained physician.[33] Hospital guidelines and policy should reflect the need for a physician with privileges to implant pacing devices to review and validate any pacing changes that are made to a pacemaker by a company representative.

Reprogramming a pacemaker to asynchronous pacing at a rate greater than the patient's underlying rate usually ensures that no over- or undersensing during EMI will take place, protecting the patient. However, there is one case report involving a Telectronics device which would open its output circuitry (i.e., no pacing stimuli would be delivered) in the presence of high voltage EMI.[34] At our institution, we have observed a Medtronic Kappa 400 dual chamber device in the DOO mode drop its rate during use of ESU, presumably due to high battery current drain.

Reprogramming a device will not protect the device from internal damage or reset caused by electromagnetic interference. Additionally, setting a device to asynchronous mode causes the pacemaker to ignore premature atrial or ventricular systoles, which could have the potential to create a malignant rhythm in the patient with significant structural compromise of the myocardium.[35]

In general, rate responsiveness and other "enhancements" (dynamic atrial overdrive, hysteresis, sleep rate, AV search, etc.) should be disabled by programming.[3,36,37] Note that for many Guidant and/or CPI devices, Guidant Medical recommends increasing the pacing voltage to "5 volts or higher" in any case where the monopolar electrosurgical unit will be used. Few cardiologists follow this recommendation, but there are reports of threshold changes during both intrathoracic[38] and non-chest surgery.[39] Recently, Levine and colleagues reported that significant noncardiac disease states could increase pacing threshold.[40]

Special attention must be given to any device with a minute ventilation (bioimpedance) sensor (Table 35-6), because inappropriate tachycardia has been observed secondary to mechanical ventilation,[41,42] monopolar "Bovie" electrosurgery,[41,43,44] and connection to an electrocardiographic monitor with respiratory rate monitoring.[45-50] Sometimes, this pacemaker driven tachycardia has led to inappropriate, unsuccessful pharmacologic treatment of the tachycardia.[42]

Intraoperative or Procedural Management of Pacemakers

Although no special monitoring or anesthetic technique is required for the patient with a pacemaker, attention must be given to a number of concerns. First, electrocardiographic monitoring of the patient must include the ability to detect pacemaker discharges. Currently, most electrocardiographic monitors in both the operating room and the intensive care unit perform digital acquisition and analysis of electrocardiographic signals. As a result, in their default settings, these monitors will filter the pacemaker artifacts, and no pacemaker "spikes" will

---

Table 35–5   Situations probably requiring pacemaker reprogramming

Any rate-responsive device* (Some problems are well known,[90,91] some problems have been misinterpreted with potential for patient injury,[37,41,46,50] and the U.S. FDA has issued an alert regarding devices with minute ventilation sensors[48] [see Table 35-6].)

Special pacing indication (e.g., hypertrophic obstructive cardiomyopathy, dilated cardiomyopathy, pediatric patients)

Pacemaker-dependent patient

Major procedure in the chest or abdomen

Rate enhancements that should be disabled

Special procedures

    Lithotripsy

    Transurethral resection

    Hysteroscopy

    Electroconvulsive therapy

    Succinylcholine use

    Magnetic resonance imaging (usually contraindicated by device manufacturers); might be possible in some pacemaker patients[92]

*In some situations and for certain patients, a pacemaker should be reprogrammed to avoid potential patient injury or to prevent a pacemaker rhythm that could be confused with pacemaker malfunction.

Table 35–6 Makers and models of pacemakers with minute ventilation sensors*

ELA Medical
    Brio (212, 220, 222)
    Chorus RM (7034, 7134)
    Opus RM (4534)
    Talent (130, 213, 223)
Guidant Medical and CPI Cardiac Pacemakers, Inc.
    Pulsar (1172, 1272)
    Pulsar Max (1170, 1171, 1270)
    Pulsar Max II (1180, 1181, 1280)
    Insignia Plus (1194, 1297, 1298)
Medtronic
    Kappa 400 series (KDR4C1, KDR403, KSR401, KSR403)
Telectronics/St. Jude
    Meta (1202, 1204, 1206, 1230, 1250, 1254, 1256)
    Tempo (1102, 1902, 2102, 2902)

*Pacemakers with minute ventilation (bioimpedance) sensors frequently respond to electromagnetic interference with pacing at the upper sensor rate.[46,50] These tachycardias also can be produced by connection to an operating room electrocardiographic monitor because many of these devices inject electrical signals through the electrocardiographic leads to determine respiratory rate or a lead disconnection.[45,47] In 1998, the U.S. Center for Devices and Radiologic Health issued a safety alert calling for the deactivation of any minute ventilation sensor before exposing a patient to a potential source of electromagnetic interference or connection to medical devices.[48]

be shown. This filtering must be disabled so that the monitor will "paint" pacemaker spikes onto the display. Even with the filtering disabled, though, pacemaker artifacts do not always appear. Atrial signals are weak, and current monitors do a poor job detecting them. Also, since the digital monitors generally analyze only one lead for these signals (and then "paint" on artifacts on every lead), placement of the electrocardiographic leads can markedly affect the detection axis. In practice, when a patient with known pacing is monitored, sometimes changing the "analysis" lead on the monitor will result in the appearance of pacing signals. Unfortunately, when the ESU artifact filter is disabled, any use of the monopolar ESU unit can lead to inappropriate "painting" of pacemaker artifacts on the monitor (Fig. 35-5).

Second, patient monitoring must include the ability to ensure that paced electrical activity is converted to mechanical systoles. Mechanical systoles are best evaluated by pulse oximetry plethysmography or arterial pressure waveform display.

Third, there is limited experience with intraoperative BiV pacing at this time. These patients often have ejection fractions less than 30%, and they depend on pacing in both ventricles to improve their cardiac output. Loss of ventricular pacing from any cause (AV dyssynchrony [atrial fibrillation, atrial flutter, appearance of junctional rhythm], myocardial ischemia, acid-base disturbance, change in pacing threshold, ESU interference, and so on) can cause an immediate decrease in cardiac output. Monitoring of these patients probably should include

beat-to-beat monitoring of cardiac output. The patient with HOCM pacing is also dependent upon forced ventricular pacing to limit left ventricular outflow tract obstruction.

Fourth, some patients might need an increased pacing rate during the perioperative period to meet an increased oxygen demand. This subject is often not addressed. Pacemaker patients reportedly have high postoperative morbidity and mortality,[51] and failure to address tissue oxygen demands and cardiac output needs might contribute to this problem.

Fifth, appropriate equipment must be on hand to provide backup pacing and/or defibrillation to the patient who might need it. The literature and anecdotal experience suggest that cardiac generators, while hardy, occasionally perform some untoward maneuver or fail, even in the absence of EMI.[52] Acceptable, but inappropriate behavior of a pacemaker or ICD can create an inhospitable situation. Even a properly working, dual chamber pacemaker can produce R-on-T pacing, especially in the setting of a junctional rhythm or PVCs (Fig. 35-6).

The medical team caring for the patient with an implanted cardiac pulse generator must understand that the patient has been deemed needy of this device by a physician who is an expert in the diagnosis and management of cardiac rhythm issues. Few anesthesiologists are qualified to contradict this diagnosis, yet some persist in providing an anesthetic without appropriate backup pacing and defibrillation equipment on hand.

Monopolar "Bovie" electrosurgery (ESU) use remains the principal intraoperative issue for the patient with a pacemaker. Between 1984 and 1997, the U.S. FDA was notified of 456 adverse events with pulse generators, 255 from electrosurgery, and a "significant number" of device failures.[53] Monopolar ESU is more likely to cause problems than bipolar ESU, and patients with unipolar electrode configuration are more sensitive to electromagnetic interference than those with bipolar configurations.[54] The most common effect of ESU on pacemakers is ventricular oversensing which causes pacemaker inhibition (see Fig. 35-5B). Sometimes, the pacemaker determines that significant EMI is present and begins pacing asynchronously at the programmed lower rate.[55] This behavior is called "noise reversion mode pacing," even though the pacemaker does not actually change "modes."

Magnet placement during electrosurgery might prevent aberrant pacemaker behavior, and it might allow reprogramming of an older (pre-1990) generator. Note that not all generators "open" their programming window during placement of a magnet (for example, devices from Guidant and/or CPI cannot be programmed in the presence of a magnet). Newer generators are believed to be relatively immune to spurious reprogramming from EMI.

If monopolar electrosurgery is to be used, then the electrosurgical current-return pad (often misidentified as the "grounding pad") must be placed to ensure that the electrosurgical current path does not cross the pacemaking system. Some authors recommend placement of this pad on the shoulder for head and neck procedures or the distal arm (with sterile draping of the wire) for breast and

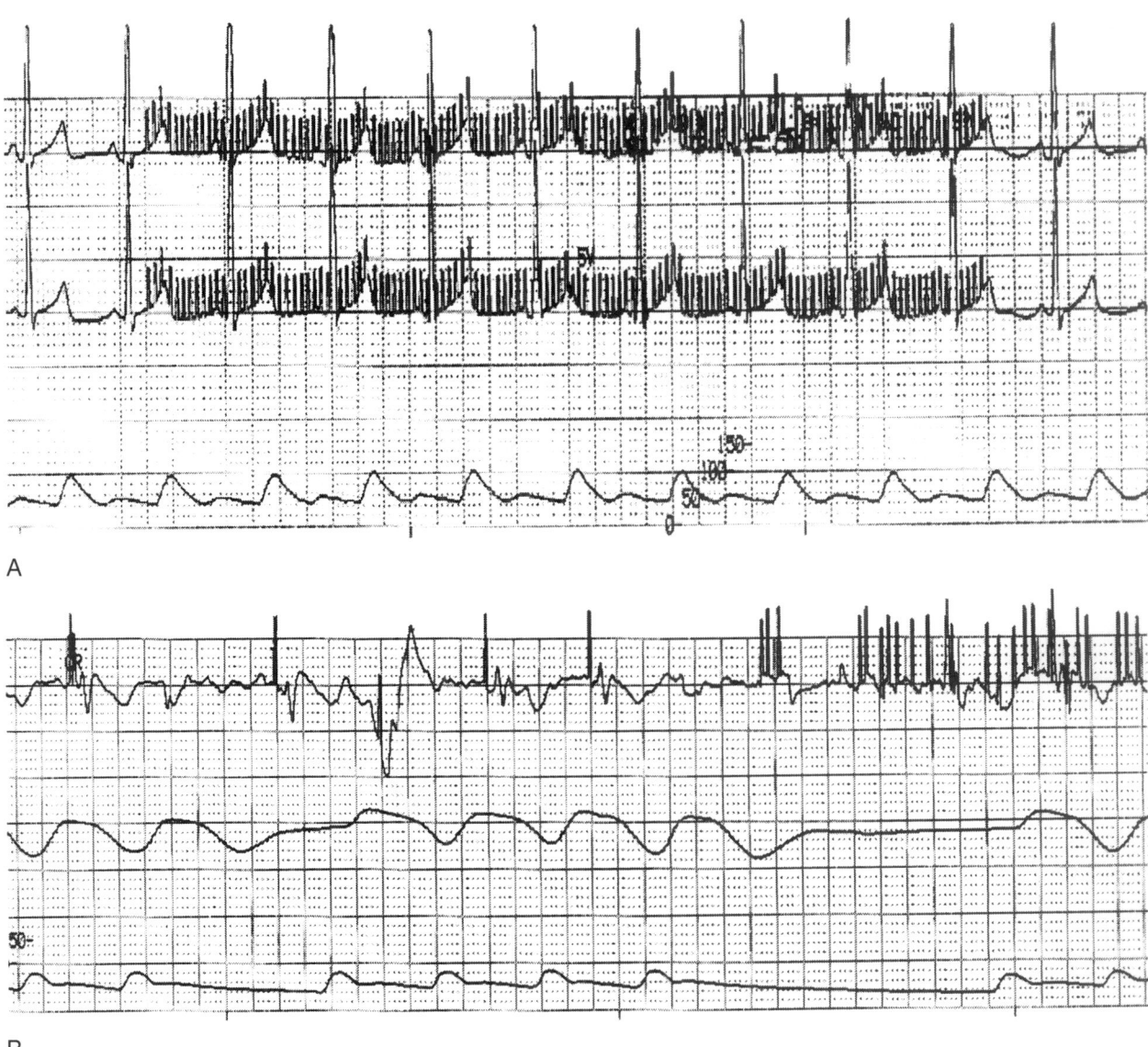

A

B

Figure 35–5 Disabling the pacemaker artifact filter on a digitally processed electrocardiographic (ECG) monitor results in the "painting" of environmental interference (EMI) as pacemaker artifacts. **A,** The patient's underlying rate exceeded the pacemaker's programmed lower rate limit, and no pacing took place. However, activation of the monopolar electrosurgical unit (ESU) in the "cut" mode produced sufficient electromagnetic noise that the monitor began painting pacemaker artifacts at a rate of about 20 Hz. The *top tracing* is ECG lead II, the *middle tracing* is ECG lead V5, and the *bottom tracing* is the invasive arterial pressure waveform. **B,** "Coagulation" ESU produced ventricular oversensing with pacemaker inhibition and left this patient with a compromised cardiac output. There is also evidence of inappropriate monitor painting of pacemaker artifacts from the EMI. The *top tracing* is ECG lead II, the *middle tracing* is the pulse oximeter plethysmogram, and the *bottom tracing* is the invasive arterial pressure waveform. (Adapted from Rozner MA: [untitled letter]. Pacing Clin Electrophysiol 26:923-925, 2003.)

Figure 35–6 Normal dual chamber pacemaker timing can produce R-on-T pacing. **A,** This strip demonstrates functional ventricular undersensing of a premature ventricular contraction (PVC) with a resultant R-on-T pace leading to torsades de pointes. This patient had a dual chamber pacemaker in the DDD mode with a programmed lower rate of 70 beats/min (R-R interval is 857 msec) and an atrioventricular delay of 200 msec. With these parameters, the pacemaker paces the atrium at 657 msec after any previous ventricular event. Atrial pacing (A) and ventricular pacing (V) are indicated. The *top tracing* is electrocardiographic (ECG) lead II, the *middle tracing* is ECG lead V5, and the *bottom tracing* is the invasive arterial blood pressure. Approximately 660 msec after the first QRS (1) on the strip (which was adequately sensed by the pacemaker), an atrial stimulus is emitted. At 200 msec after this atrial pace, a ventricular stimulus is emitted, appearing to depolarize the ventricle (2). About 660 msec later (3), the patient had a PVC. Because the pacemaker was preparing to emit the atrial stimulus, it had disabled its ventricular sensing element and failed to sense this PVC (i.e., functional undersensing). At 200 msec after the atrial stimulus, no ventricular event had been sensed, and the pacemaker emitted a ventricular stimulus on the T wave. Because the ventricle was in a refractory period from the PVC, there was no depolarization of the

Continued on facing page

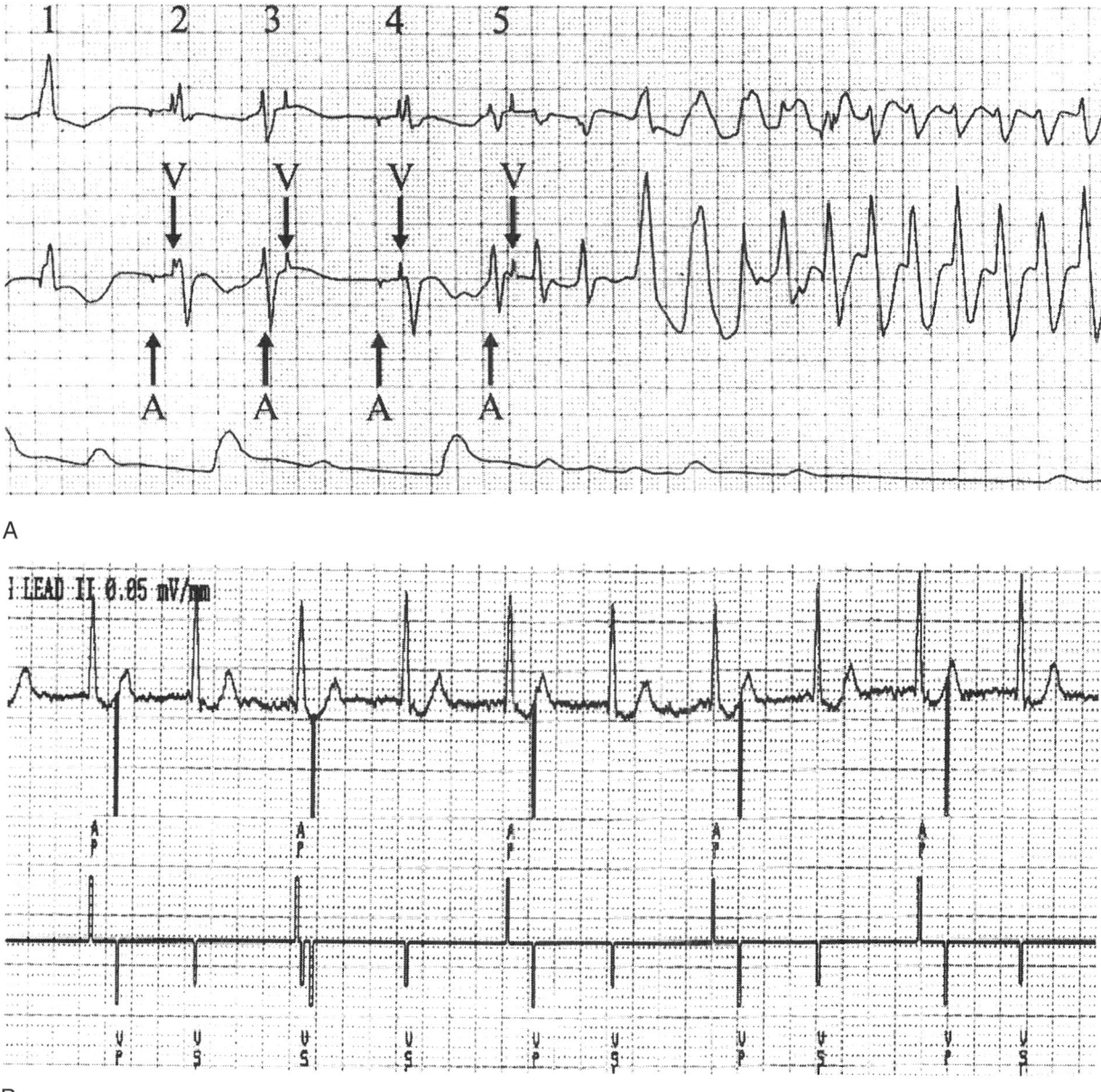

A

B

Figure 35–6—Cont'd ventricle (i.e., functional noncapture). At 660 msec from this attempted ventricular pacing, the pacemaker again paces the atrium (4), and it appears that the next ventricular pacing impulse captures the ventricle. At (5), there is a repeat of the events at (3); the pacemaker disabled its sensing elements in preparation to pace the atrium and failed to detect the PVC. This time, however, the ventricular pace on the T wave produced torsades de pointes. **B,** This strip was obtained from a Medtronic programmer during interrogation of a Kappa 700 dual-chamber pacemaker. The *top tracing* is ECG lead II, and the *bottom tracing* is the marker channel, which shows the pacemaker's interpretation of events. This pacemaker was programmed to the DDD mode with a lower rate of 60 beats/min. The atrioventricular (AV) delay was 200 msec. As a result, after any ventricular event, the pacemaker will emit an atrial pulse at 800 msec if no intervening atrial or ventricular event takes place. This patient had a junctional rhythm at 75 beats/min (corresponding to an R-R interval of 800 msec), and the pacemaker emitted an atrial pulse just as the junctional event occurred. Because the pacemaker disables its ventricular sensing element when emitting the atrial pulse, it failed to detect the ventricular event and emitted the ventricular pulse 200 msec later, falling on the T wave. This inappropriate pacing takes place every other cycle, because every other junctional event is sensed about 600 msec after the previous ventricular pace. Decreasing the AV delay decreases the likelihood of pacing during the vulnerable period of the ventricle. Atrial pace (AP), ventricular pace (VP), and ventricular sensed event (VS) are indicated. The third complex deserves comment. The pacemaker sensed this ventricular event as it re-enabled its sensing element, and the pacemaker could not tell whether the sensed event was a true ventricular depolarization or an echo of the atrial pace (called far-field oversensing). When a signal from the ventricle is sensed within 30 to 90 msec after an atrial pace, many pacemakers immediately emit a ventricular pacing stimulus. Called a *ventricular safety pace*, this pacing stimulus is designed to protect the patient from inappropriate sensing of the atrial signal by the ventricular channel, which would then inhibit the ventricular output. The safety pace is emitted at 110 msec to prevent R-on-T pacing. This feature is also called *nonphysiologic AV delay* by some manufacturers. R-on-T pacing can be appropriate (but not ideal) behavior of a DDD or DDI pacemaker in the setting of PVCs or a junctional rhythm. It can also be seen with atrial or ventricular undersensing.

axillary procedures.[54,56] Procedures using only monopolar ESU or with special pacing ramifications include the following:

Lithotripsy: The cardiac generator must be excluded from the lithotripter field. Since some lithotripters trigger their output on the sensed electrocardiographic "R" wave, atrial pacing should be disabled to prevent the lithotripter from inappropriately firing on the atrial pacing artifact;

Transurethral Resection and Uterine Hysteroscopy: TUR of the bladder or prostate and hysteroscopic procedures generally use monopolar ESU, and device reprogramming might be needed to prevent pacemaker oversensing with resultant pacemaker inhibition. A new resectoscope is in clinical trial that includes the current-return electrode on the shaft (the irrigation medium will be normal saline) which might limit EMI to the generator;

Magnetic Resonance Imaging (MRI)—Absolutely contraindicated by most device manufacturers, and deaths have been reported.* According to physicians' manuals from most manufacturers, MRI can lead to reed switch closure (magnet mode activation), reprogramming, inappropriate high rate pacing, generator damage, myocardial injury, or generator movement within the pocket, causing pain or lead failure. Nevertheless, safe performance of MRI with pacemakers has been reported[57];

Electroconvulsive Therapy—ECT requires non-sensing (asynchronous) mode to prevent myopotential-induced oversensing with resultant pacemaker inhibition[58];

Nerve Stimulator Testing/Therapy—Nerve stimulators can cause pacemaker oversensing with resultant pacemaker inhibition and cardiac arrest.[59] Nerve stimulators have been used intraoperatively to inhibit undesired cardiac pacing.[10] For the patient with an ICD, inappropriate detection of neuromuscular stimulators, TENS, and chiropractic electrical muscle stimulation as VT or VF has been reported[60,61];

Succinylcholine Use—There is one report of a problem in a pacemaker-dependent patient upon administration of succinylcholine.[62] In this case, muscle fasciculations might have caused ventricular oversensing with resultant pacemaker inhibition, but the case is difficult to interpret. No electrocardiographic tracings were published, and the pacemaker was damaged during a subsequent defibrillation. Using programmers, I have witnessed succinylcholine administration to over 50 patients with pacemakers or defibrillators, and I have not observed any myopotential oversensing. However, myopotential oversensing (in the absence of succinylcholine) has been observed to interfere with pacemaker function[63] or cause inappropriate ICD therapy.[64]

---

*Gimbel JR: Implantable pacemaker and defibrillator safety in the MR environment: New thoughts for the new millenium. In 2001 Syllabus, Special Cross-Specialty Categorical Course in Diagnostic Radiology: Practical MR Safety Considerations for Physicians, Physicists, and Technologists. Oak Lawn, IL, Radiological Society of North America, pp. 69-76, 2001.

Pacemaker Failure

Pacemaker failure has three causes: generator failure, lead failure, or failure of capture. Generator failure is rare in a device that has been previously evaluated and not near the end of useful battery life, unless the generator (or leads) is struck directly by ESU. Lead failure, also unusual, but reported during patient repositioning,[55] can result in undersensing (intrinsic activity is not detected); oversensing ("detection" of events unrelated to intrinsic activity); or failure to deliver sufficient energy to the myocardium to produce a depolarization (i.e., loss of capture). Myocardial changes that lengthen the refractory period or increase the energy requirement for depolarization (failure to capture) can result from myocardial ischemia/infarction, acid-base disturbance, electrolyte abnormalities, or abnormal antiarrhythmic drug levels.

The response to a pacemaker failure depends on the clinical situation: the patient with a perfusing rhythm and stable vital signs can be observed while a plan is made to correct the problem. For the patient with inadequate perfusion, the following steps can be tried (while cardiopulmonary resuscitation is in progress where appropriate):

1. A magnet can be applied if the pacemaker is known to revert to an asynchronous mode, which will also eliminate sensing behavior in these devices. For many of the Autocapture devices with magnet mode enabled, magnet application might increase pacing amplitude and restore capture. Devices from ELA medical typically increase their pacing amplitude when a magnet is applied. Some pacemakers perform threshold margin testing upon magnet placement, which can further reduce pacing.[24]

2. Temporary pacing can be initiated, and it can be transthoracic (transcutaneous), transvenous, or transesophageal. Transesophageal (atrial) pacing generally requires a functional atrium and AV node for ventricular activation, and it will likely be unsuccessful in the presence of atrial fibrillation or AV nodal disease. In the setting of external pacing, the electrocardiogram is often misinterpreted, since the pacemaker artifacts are large compared to the QRS complexes (Fig. 35-7). Successful ventricular pacing has been reported with transesophageal pacemakers, but it is not reliable at this time.[65] Note that any external pacing might further inhibit pacemaker output at energies that will not produce myocardial capture.[66,67]

3. Sympathomimetic drugs can be administered to decrease depolarization threshold and/or increase chronotropicity. Epinephrine (0.5 to 1 µg/min) or dopamine (5 to 20 µg/kg/min) should be considered. Isoproterenol (0.5 µg/min) is often recommended, but this drug is not widely available and its use is complicated by hypotension. Antimuscarinic drugs (atropine, glycopyrrolate) might be helpful.

4. Causes of myocardial ischemia should be sought and corrected. Myocardial ischemia can substantially increase the energy required for ventricular capture.[68]

5. Disturbances of electrolyte balance, antiarrhythmic drug levels, and acid-base equilibrium should be investigated and corrected. Potassium, calcium, and

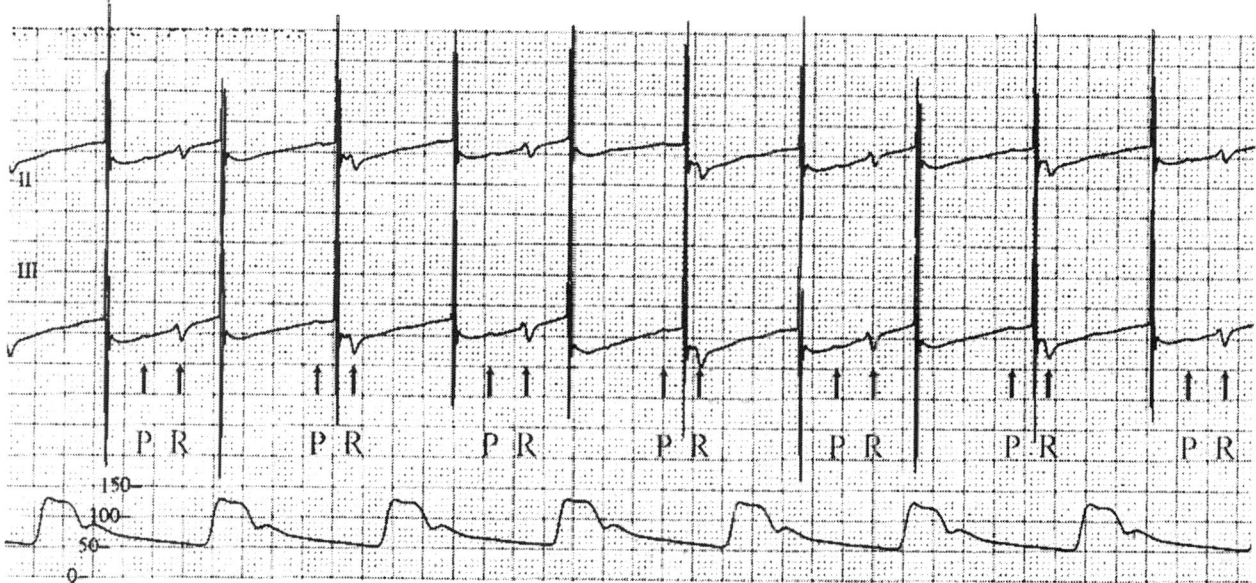

Figure 35–7 Improper placement of a transesophageal pacemaker. The *top recording* is electrocardiographic (ECG) lead II, the *middle recording* is ECG lead III, and the *bottom recording* is the invasive arterial pressure waveform. This 72-year-old man developed a sinus bradycardia with evidence of tissue underperfusion. A transesophageal pacemaker was placed, and the large electrocardiographic artifacts at 75 beats/min were misinterpreted as ventricular systoles (i.e., capture). They were the pacing stimuli as represented on the ECG monitor. This patient has a sinus rate of 50 beats/min with a first-degree atrioventricular block (PR interval of 280 msec). The patient's native atrial (P) and ventricular (R) depolarizations are identified. The arterial pressure waveform confirms pacing noncapture.

magnesium abnormalities can raise depolarization thresholds. Potassium flux, ionized calcium level, and acid-base equilibrium can be affected by hyperventilation and hypoventilation.

6. If none of the above measures succeeds, consideration should be given to placement of epicardial leads by the surgical staff.

Postanesthesia Pacemaker Evaluation

A pacemaker that was reprogrammed for the perioperative period should be reset appropriately. For non-reprogrammed devices, most manufacturers recommend interrogation to ensure proper functioning and remaining battery life if any electrosurgery was used. ACC Guidelines now recommend a post-procedure interrogation.[3]

IMPLANTABLE CARDIOVERTER-DEFIBRILLATORS

Overview

The development of an implantable, battery-powered device able to deliver sufficient energy to terminate ventricular tachycardia (VT) or fibrillation (VF) has represented a major medical breakthrough for patients with a history of ventricular tachydysrhythmias. These devices reduce deaths in the setting of malignant ventricular tachydysrhythmias,[69,70] and they clearly remain superior to antiarrhythmic drug therapy.[71] Initially approved by the U.S. FDA in 1985, industry sources report that more than 290,000 patients have these devices today.

Further, results from the Multicenter Automatic Defibrillator Implantation Trial-II (MADIT-II)—suggesting that prophylactic placement of an ICD is warranted in any patient with an ischemic cardiomyopathy and ejection fraction less than 0.30 *without* evidence of arrhythmic inducibility)—have significantly increased the number of patients for whom ICD therapy is indicated.[72] Currently, the Centers for Medicare and Medicaid Services (CMS) recognize some MADIT-II criteria for indication of an ICD.

A significant number of technologic advances have been applied since the first ICD was placed, including considerable miniaturization (pectoral pocket placement with transvenous leads is the norm) as well as battery improvements that now permit permanent pacing with these devices. An examiner could easily confuse a pectoral ICD with a pacemaker.

Like pacemakers, ICDs have a four-place generic code (NBD*) to indicate lead placement and function, which is shown in Table 35-7.[73] The most robust form of identification, called the "label form," expands the fourth character into its component generic pacemaker code (NBG).

Newer ICDs (since 1993) have many programmable features, but essentially they measure each cardiac R-R interval and categorize the rate as normal, too fast (short R-R interval), or too slow (long R-R interval). When the device detects a sufficient number of short R-R intervals within a period of time (all programmable), it will begin an antitachycardia event. The internal computer will

---

*The NBD code is a joint project from NASPE (the "N") and BPEG (the "B"). The "D" stands for defibrillator.

Table 35–7 NASPE/BPEG generic NBD defibrillator code*

Position I	Position II	Position III	Position IV†
(Shock Chamber)	(Antitachycardia Pacing Chamber)	(Tachycardia Detection)	(Antibradycardia Pacing Chamber)
O = none A = atrium V = ventricle D = dual (A + V)	O = none A = atrium V = ventricle D = dual (A + V)	E = electrogram H = hemodynamic	O = none A = atrium V = ventricle D = dual (A + V)

*The generic defibrillator code[73] is a joint project of the North American Society of Pacing and Electrophysiology (NASPE) and the British Pacing and Electrophysiology Group (BPEG).
†For robust identification, position IV is expanded into its complete NBG code. For example, a biventricular pacing-defibrillator with ventricular shock and antitachycardia pacing functionality would be identified as VVE-DDDRV, assuming that the pacing section was programmed DDDRV. No hemodynamic sensors have been approved for tachycardia detection (position III).
NBD: North American Society of Pacing and Electrophysiology (N) and British Pacing and Electrophysiology Group (B) generic defibrillator (D) code.

choose antitachycardia pacing (less energy use, better tolerated by patient) or shock, depending upon the presentation and device programming. If shock is chosen, an internal capacitor is charged. Charging time is dependent upon the desired output, and it can be 6 to 15 seconds for a maximum shock. Charging time is lengthened by lower battery voltage, time from last charge,* and lower temperature.

Most ICDs can be programmed to "reconfirm" VT or VF after charging in order to prevent inappropriate shock therapy. Typically, ICDs deliver 6-18 shocks per event. Once a shock is delivered, no further antitachycardia pacing can take place. Despite considerable improvement in detection of ventricular dysrhythmias, more than 10% of shocks are for rhythm other than VT or VF.[74,75] Supraventricular tachycardia remains the most common etiology of inappropriate shock therapy,[76,77] and causes of inappropriate shock have been reviewed elsewhere.[78] Programmable features in current ICDs to differentiate VT from a tachycardia of supraventricular origin (SVT) include the following[79]:
1. Onset criteria—in general, onset of VT is abrupt, whereas onset of SVT has sequentially shortening R-R intervals;
2. Stability criteria—in general, the R-R interval of VT is relatively constant, whereas the R-R interval of atrial fibrillation with rapid ventricular response is quite variable;
3. QRS width criteria—in general, the QRS width in SVT is narrow (<110 msec), whereas the QRS width in VT is wide (>120 msec);
4. "Intelligence" in dual chamber devices attempting to associate atrial activity to ventricular activity; and
5. Morphology waveform analysis with comparison to stored historical templates.
After the R-R interval becomes sufficiently short for VF detection, the ICD begins a shock sequence. After an ICD delivers any shock therapy, no further antitachycardia pacing will take place.

An ICD with antibradycardia pacing capability will begin pacing when the R-R interval is too long. In July, 1997, the U.S. FDA approved devices with sophisticated dual chamber pacing modes and rate responsive behavior for ICD patients who need permanent pacing (about 20% of ICD patients). Recently, though, a report has suggested that placement of a dual chamber device into a patient without a clear need for dual chamber pacing decreased survival when compared to single chamber device placement.[80] As a result of this study, many electrophysiologists are programming long (>250 msec) AV delays in these patients to limit ventricular pacing. As noted above, though (see Fig. 35-6A), long AV delays can lead to R-on-T pacing.

Implantable Cardioverter-Defibrillator Indications

Initially, ICDs were placed for hemodynamically significant VT or VF (Table 35-8). Newer indications associated with sudden death include: awaiting heart transplant,[81] long Q-T syndrome,[82] Brugada syndrome (right bundle branch block, S-T segment elevation in leads V1-V3), and arrhythmogenic right ventricular dysplasia.[83,84] Studies suggest that ICDs can be placed prophylactically (i.e., used for primary prevention) to prevent sudden death in young patients with hypertrophic cardiomyopathy,[85] as well as post-MI patients with ejection fraction less than 30%,[72] but are of no benefit post coronary artery bypass grafting. Three-chamber ICDs have been FDA approved for patients with dilated cardiomyopathy, and ICDs are in clinical trial for patients with HOCM who have experienced VT or VF.

Implantable Cardioverter-Defibrillator Magnets

Like pacemakers, magnet behavior in ICDs can be altered by programming. Most devices will suspend tachydysrhythmia detection (and therefore therapy) when a magnet is appropriately placed to activate the reed switch. Some devices from Angeion, CPI, Pacesetter (St. Jude Medical) or Ventritex can be programmed to ignore magnet placement. Depending on programming, antitachycardia therapy in some Guidant and/or CPI devices can be permanently

*The capacitor in an ICD "deforms" during inactivity, leading to increased time needed to charge the capacitor. To mitigate the effects of deformation, all ICDs perform a nontherapeutic charging of their capacitor (called "reforming") at a programmable periodic interval (usually one to six months).

Table 35–8 Indications for implantable cardioverter-defibrillator placement

Ventricular tachycardia

Ventricular fibrillation

Brugada syndrome (i.e., right bundle branch block, ST-segment elevation in V_1-V_3)

Arrhythmogenic right ventricular dysplasia

Long QT syndrome

Hypertrophic cardiomyopathy

Prophylactic use in the post–myocardial infarction patient who has an ejection fraction less than 30% (i.e., no electrophysiologic testing is needed to justify placement)[72]

Prophylactic use in any patient with a cardiomyopathy from any cause who has an ejection fraction less than 35%*

*Sudden cardiac death—heart failure trial. Presented at the American College of Cardiology Meeting, March 2004.

disabled by magnet placement for 30 seconds, and, as noted above, some patients have been discovered with their ICD antitachycardia therapy unintentionally disabled.[2] In Guidant and CPI devices, if magnet mode is enabled and the ICD is enabled for antitachycardia therapy, the ICD will emit beeps synchronized to R-waves, signifying adequate placement of magnet and suspension of tachyarrhythmia detection (thereby disabling therapy). If the ICD emits a constant tone, then antitachycardia therapy has been programmed to "off." Depending upon programming, ICDs from Guidant and CPI can toggle between activated and inactivated states with 30 seconds of magnet application. To re-enable therapy, the magnet must be removed, then replaced until the constant tone reverts to beeps synchronized to R-waves. Subsequent removal of the magnet then returns the antitachycardia therapy to the enabled state. Any Guidant or CPI device that emits either beeps or constant tones while a magnet is placed will have its antitachycardia therapy disabled during the magnet session.

To ensure correct magnet placement on their devices, Medtronic markets a device called the "Smart Magnet." This battery-powered instrument contains a magnet and a radio-frequency (RF) receiver. All Medtronic generators broadcast RF destined for the programmer upon magnet placement, and the Smart Magnet detects this radiofrequency transmission and illuminates a light to indicate that RF is being received. Medtronic recommends that the Smart Magnet be taped onto the patient. During the occurrence of EMI, the transmission from the ICD to the Smart Magnet is interrupted, and the ICD "found" light often turns off. In this setting, however, the ICD remains disabled, since it is the physical presence of the magnet, rather than the radiofrequency communication, that disables the antitachycardia therapy.

In general, magnets will not affect antibradycardia pacing mode or rate (except ELA [rate change] and Telectronics Guardian 4202/4203 [disabled]). Intermedics devices transiently change pacing rate (VVI mode) to reflect battery voltage. Interrogating the device and calling the manufacturer remain the most reliable method for determining magnet response.

Preanesthesia Evaluation and Implantable Cardioverter-Defibrillator Reprogramming

In addition to evaluating and optimizing any comorbid diseases in the ICD patient, every ICD should undergo preoperative interrogation. These devices store considerable data regarding the occurrence of dysrhythmias. Because antitachycardia pacing is well tolerated, many patients are not aware of this intervention. For any patient scheduled to undergo an elective procedure, the onset of new dysrhythmias warrants delay of the case and investigation of the problem (Fig. 35-8).

Determination of the need for elective replacement for battery depletion in ICDs is more complicated than in pacemakers. Since some ICDs have two batteries, predicting battery depletion based upon battery voltage is difficult. In general, the manufacturer should be consulted for any device with a "charging time" in excess of 12 seconds.

ALL ICDs should have their antitachycardia therapy disabled prior to the induction of anesthetic and commencement of the procedure (see ACC Guidelines[3]). The use of monopolar ESU can cause inappropriate shocks. Casavant and co-workers found a stored electrogram sequence in an ICD (similar to Fig. 35-8) suggesting that it had misinterpreted monopolar ESU during dermatologic facial surgery as VF,[86] and Figure 35-9 shows one of the 73 VT detections that occurred during an orthopedic procedure.

The comments in the pacing section (including Appendix I and Table 35-5) apply here for any ICD with antibradycardia pacing. Many ICDs have no noise reversion behavior, so ESU-induced ventricular oversensing might lead to nonpacing in the patients who are dependent upon their ICDs for pacing.

Intraoperative or Procedural Management of Implantable Cardioverter-Defibrillators

No special monitoring is required for the patient with an ICD. Electrocardiographic monitoring and the ability to deliver external cardioversion or defibrillation must be present during the time of ICD disablement. Should external cardioversion or defibrillation be needed, the defibrillator pads should be placed to avoid the pulse generator and lead system to the extent possible. Nevertheless, one should remember that the patient, not the ICD, is being treated. The recommendations in the section "Intraoperative or Procedural Management of Pacemakers" apply here as well.

No special anesthetic techniques have been championed for the patient with an ICD. Most of these patients will have severely depressed systolic function, dilated ventricular cavities, and significant valvular regurgitation. The choice of anesthetic technique should be dictated by the underlying physiologic derangements that are present. Conflicting data have been published regarding the choice of anesthetic agents and changes to defibrillation threshold (DFT). In 1992, Gill and colleagues examined DFT in dogs and concluded that neither halothane nor isoflurane changed DFT in open chest defibrillation compared to a pentobarbital infusion.[87] However, Weinbroum and associates recently evaluated defibrillation thresholds in humans during ICD implant

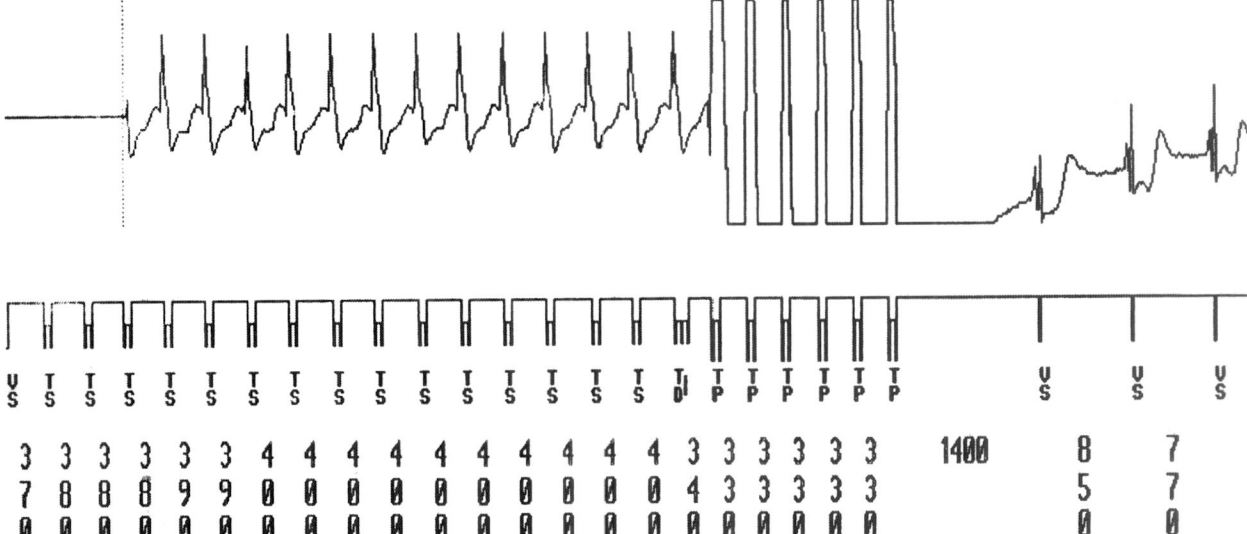

Figure 35–8 Unexpected ventricular tachycardia with antitachycardia pacing (ATP) was found in this patient during her preoperative visit. A 65-year-old woman with a history of ventricular tachycardia (VT) had undergone implantation of a Medtronic single-chamber defibrillator about 8 months earlier. She had no dizziness or syncopal episodes since the implantable cardioverter-defibrillator (ICD) placement. Interrogation of her device in the preoperative center revealed VVE-VVI programming, along with an episode of tachycardia at 150 to 162 beats/min that was detected by the ICD as VT. The ICD delivered a 6-beat burst of antitachycardia pacing at 182 beats/min, which converted the tachycardia back to sinus rhythm. No backup antibradycardia pacing was needed after the VT was terminated. The *upper tracing* is a digitized ventricular electrogram that was stored in the ICD during the tachycardic event. The *lower tracing* is the marker channel that reports the interpretation of the ICD for each event. The numbers below the marker channel represent the interval (in milliseconds). The heart rate is calculated by dividing the interval into 60,000 msec/min. TS represents an interval in the VT zone, TD marks the final event that starts therapy, TP is an ATP event, and VS is an intrinsic ventricular depolarization with a rate that is neither too fast (short interval) nor too slow (long interval). This device was set to detect VT as 16 consecutive ventricular events with a rate between 146 and 200 beats/min and to deliver ATP at 84% of the last R-R interval. The last interval was 400 msec, so ATP was delivered at a rate of 182 beats/min (330-msec intervals).

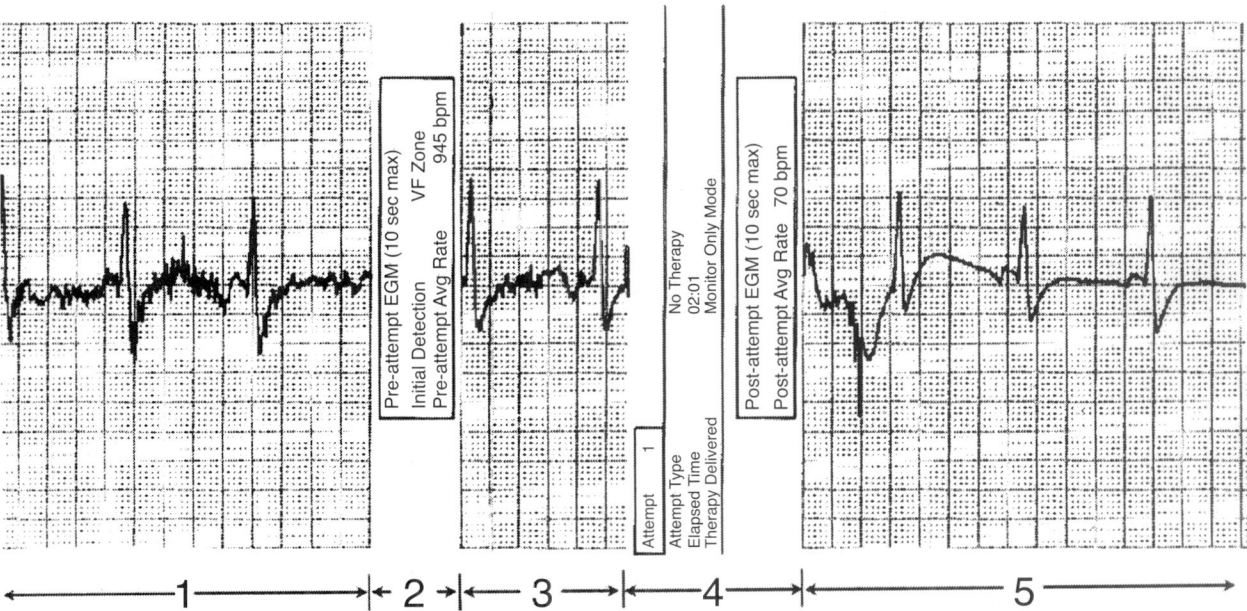

Figure 35–9 Electromagnetic interference from the monopolar electrosurgery (i.e., Bovie) caused an implantable cardioverter-defibrillator (ICD) to detect ventricular fibrillation (VF). This stored electrogram was one of 73 found at the end of a 4-hour surgical procedure in which considerable monopolar electrosurgery (ESU) was used. This patient had a Guidant Medical ICD in the VOE-VVI mode. This patient's ICD had been placed in a "monitor only" mode before surgery. As a result, the ICD recorded any instance of ventricular dysrhythmia that would have triggered therapy, but it could not deliver therapy. The electrogram demonstrates a ventricular rate of 70 beats/min but with considerable noise on the baseline (1); a ventricular fibrillation (VF) event was declared for the detected heart rate of 345 beats/min, and the ICD charged its capacitor (2); the ICD was programmed to "reconfirm before shock," and the ventricular rate remains 70 beats/min with noise on the baseline (3); the noise caused the ICD to believe that the patient remained in VF, and the ICD would have delivered a shock, except it was programmed to monitor only (4); and because the noise is gone (i.e., the ESU had stopped), the ICD declares the event over after a "successful" defibrillation (5).

and found that halothane, isoflurane, and fentanyl increased DFT.[88] Even with these increases, the increased DFTs found were still substantially lower than the maximum energy generally available in ICDs, and these increases would not have been noted under usual testing conditions.

Postanesthesia Implantable Cardioverter-Defibrillator Evaluation

The ICD must be reinterrogated and re-enabled. All events should be reviewed and counters should be cleared. The pacing parameters must be checked and reprogrammed as necessary.

SUMMARY

Electronic miniaturization has permitted the design and use of sophisticated electronics in patients who have need for artificial pacing and/or automated cardioversion/defibrillation of their heart. These devices are no longer confined to merely keeping the heart beating between a minimum rate (pacing function) and a maximum rate (ICD functions), as they are now being used as therapy to improve the failing heart.

The aging of the population and our ability to care for a patient with increasingly complex disease suggest that we will be caring for many more patients with these devices, and we must be prepared for this situation. Safe and efficient clinical management of these patients depends upon our understanding of implantable systems, indications for their use, and the perioperative needs that they create.

KEY POINTS

1. Have the pacemaker or defibrillator interrogated by a competent authority shortly before the anesthetic is delivered.
2. Obtain a copy of this interrogation, and ensure that the device will pace the heart.
3. Consider replacing any device near its elective replacement period in a patient scheduled to undergo major surgery or surgery within 15 cm (6 in.) of the generator.
4. Preoperatively determine the patient's underlying rate and rhythm, which then determines the need for backup (external) pacing support.
5. Identify the magnet rate and rhythm, if present.
6. Program minute ventilation rate responsiveness off, if present.
7. Program all rate enhancements off.
8. Consider increasing the lower rate limit rate to optimize oxygen delivery to tissues for major cases.
9. Disable antitachycardia therapy if using a defibrillator.
10. Intraoperatively, monitor cardiac rhythm with pulse oximeter (plethysmography) or arterial waveform.
11. Ask the surgeon to operate without the monopolar electrosurgical unit (ESU).
12. Use bipolar ESU if possible; if not possible, pure cut is better than "blend" or "coag."
13. Place the ESU return pad in such a way to prevent electricity from crossing the generator-heart circuit, even if the pad must be placed on the distal forearm and the wire covered with sterile drape.
14. If the ESU causes ventricular oversensing and pacer quiescence, limit the periods of asystole.
15. Have the device interrogated by a competent authority immediately postoperatively. Some rate enhancements can be reinitiated, and a determination of optimal heart rate and pacing parameters should be made. Any patient with a disabled antitachycardia therapy must be monitored until the antitachycardia therapy is restored.

GLOSSARY

Atrioventricular Delay - The time that a dual chamber system waits after detecting (or initiating) an atrial event before pacing the ventricle. Some generators shorten this time as heart rate increases (termed "rate adaptive AV delay" or "dynamic AV delay"). Some generators can be programmed to extend the AV delay to search for intrinsic conduction ("search AV delay"). Some generators will prolong an AV delay after any atrial event where the last ventricular event was intrinsic ("AV delay hysteresis"). In a patient with a conducting AV node, the sensed AV delay will be slightly longer than the PR interval on the surface electrocardiogram (see "Fusion Beat" and "Pseudofusion Beat"), since the ventricular sensing element is attached to the apex of the right ventricle and detects the depolarization only after right ventricular activation (typically greater than 60 msec after activation of the AV node).

Automatic Rate - See Lower Rate Limit.

Bipolar Lead - An electrode with two conductors. Bipolar pacing typically uses less energy than unipolar pacing, and it will produce smaller artifacts on analogue monitors. Bipolar sensing is more resistant to oversensing from muscle artifact or stray electromagnetic fields. Most pacing generators can be programmed to unipolar mode (separate settings for pacing and sensing) even in the presence of bipolar electrodes.

Dynamic Atrial Overdrive (DAO) - A programmable rate enhancement for pacemakers that increases the pacing rate in response to the presence of intrinsic atrial activity. DAO is designed to pace the atrium at a rate just above the intrinsic rate in order to prevent atrial fibrillation.[89] It should be disabled prior to an anesthetic to prevent high pacing rates. It is also called AF (for atrial fibrillation) suppression.

Electrogram Storage Mode (EGM Mode) - Passive acquisition and internal storage of electrocardiographic data for diagnostic purposes while pacing (or monitoring) with programmed parameters. A pacemaker programmed to enter the EGM mode upon application of a magnet will not demonstrate asynchronous pacing behavior.

Fusion Beat (FB) - A pacemaker impulse delivered shortly before a native depolarization of the ventricle which alters the morphology of the QRS, often misdiagnosed as undersensing. In a FB, the pacing stimulus is delivered after the activation of the AV node, but before the sensing element detects the pacemaker-induced depolarization. It is similar to a pre-excitation of the ventricle seen in Lown-Ganong-Levine syndrome or Wolff-Parkinson-White syndrome. Confirmation of appropriate sensing behavior can be made by lengthening the sensing interval (i.e., lengthening the AV delay). Fusion beats suggest, but should not be used to confirm, ventricular capture. See also Pseudofusion Beat.

Generator - The device with a power source and circuitry to produce an electrical impulse designed to be conducted to the heart. Typically, pacing generators are placed in a pectoral pocket, and leads are inserted into the right atrium, right ventricle, or both. Since 1995, implantable cardioverter-defibrillators (ICDs) have also been approved for pectoral pocket placement.

Hysteresis - If present, the amount by which the patient's intrinsic rate must fall below the programmed rate before the generator begins pacing. Some pacers periodically decrease the pacing rate in order to search for resumption of intrinsic activity (called "Search Hysteresis"). These functions, when present, can mimic pacemaker malfunction.

Implantable Cardioverter-Defibrillator (ICD) Mode - The designation of chambers shocked, chambers paced for antitachycardia pacing, method of tachycardia detection, and chambers paced for antibradycardia therapy. Table 35-7 shows the NASPE/BPEG generic ICD code.

Lower Rate Limit (LRL, also Automatic Rate or Programmed Rate) - The lowest sustained regular rate at which the generator will pace. Typically, the device begins pacing when the patient's intrinsic rate falls below this value. Hysteresis settings can permit an intrinsic heart rate lower than the LRL.

Oversensing - Detection of undesired signals that are interpreted as cardiac activity. Oversensing can lead to pacemaker driven tachycardia (pacing device, DDD mode with atrial oversensing and ventricular tracking); ventricular pause (pacing device with electrosurgically induced ventricular oversensing, leading the pacer to "detect" ventricular activity), or inappropriate shock (defibrillator, event oversensing).

Pacing Mode - The designation of chambers paced, chambers sensed, sensing response, rate responsiveness, and multisite function for a pacemaker system. Table 35-1 shows the NASPE/BPEG generic pacemaker code.

Programmed Rate - See Lower Rate Limit.

Pseudofusion Beat (PFB) - A pacemaker impulse delivered shortly after a native depolarization without alteration of the QRS morphology. PFBs are often misdiagnosed as undersensing, and they result from the position of the sensing electrode relative to the depolarizing wavefront (see Fusion Beat). Confirmation of appropriate sensing behavior can be made by lengthening the sensing interval (i.e., decreasing the program rate [atrial FB] or lengthening the AV delay

[ventricular PFB]). PFB cannot be used to confirm electronic capture.

Rate Enhancements - The features such as rate adaptive AV delay (shortens the AV delay with increasing heart rate); AV search hysteresis (lengthens/shortens the AV delay to produce intrinsic AV conduction); AF suppression (also called Dynamic Atrial Overdrive—increases the lower rate upon appearance of native atrial depolarization so as to create nearly constant atrial pacing but at a rate only slightly higher than the patient's intrinsic rate); rate smoothing (limits changes in paced rates due to changes in intrinsic activity, rising and falling rate limits can be programmed); Sleep Rate (see below); ventricular rate regulation (similar to rate smoothing but used to prevent atrial fibrillation); and hysteresis (see above). Each of these enhancements can produce pacing/nonpacing that can mimic pacemaker dysfunction, and these enhancements should be programmed "OFF" prior to any anesthetic.

Rate Modulation - The ability of the generator to sense the need to increase heart rate in response to patient activity. Mechanisms include a mechanical sensor in the generator to detect motion or vibration; electronic detection of QT interval (shortens during exercise); transthoracic impedance to measure changes in respiration; and sensors for central venous blood temperature or oxygen saturation (see Table 35-2). Some generators now incorporate multiple sensors. The pacing rate determined by the rate modulation algorithm is called "Sensor Indicated Rate."

Sensor Indicated Rate - The pacing rate determined by the sensor in a pacemaker programmed to a rate-responsive mode (fourth character of NBG = "R").

Sleep Rate (also Circadian Rate) - The rate (lower than the Programmed Rate) at which the pacing generator will pace during programmed "nighttime" hours.

Undersensing - Failure to detect a desired event.

Unipolar Lead - An electrode with only one conductor. Some devices with bipolar leads are programmed to the unipolar lead mode. Systems with unipolar leads produce larger spikes on the electrocardiogram than bipolar leads. Systems with unipolar leads utilize the generator case as the second conductor.

Upper Sensor Rate (USR, also called Upper Activity Rate [UAR]) - The maximum rate to which a rate modulated pacemaker can drive the heart. USR in a dual chamber mode is not affected by UTR, since, when USR becomes active, the pacemaker is pacing the atrium.

Upper Tracking Rate (UTR, also called Upper Rate Limit [URL]) - Pacemakers programmed to VDD or DDD mode cause the ventricles to track atrial activity. Should a patient develop an atrial tachyarrhythmia, such as a supraventricular tachycardia, atrial fibrillation, or atrial flutter, the generator acts to limit ventricular pacing. When the atrial rate exceeds the UTR, the generator can change mode (i.e., switch to DDI) or introduce second degree A-V block. Second degree blocks can be Mobitz type I (Wenckebach) or Mobitz type II, depending on a variety of programmed settings within the pacemaker.

REFERENCES

1. Chardick W, Gage A, Greatbatch W: A transistorized, self contained, implantable pacemaker for the long-term correction of complete heart block. Surgery 48:643-654, 1960.
2. Rasmussen MJ, Friedman PA, Hammill SC, Rea RF: Unintentional deactivation of implantable cardioverter-defibrillators in health care settings. Mayo Clin Proc 77:855-859, 2002.
3. Eagle KA, Berger PB, Caulkins H, et al: ACC/AHA guideline update for perioperative cardiovascular evaluation for non-cardiac surgery. Published January, 2002. Available at http://www.acc.org/clinical/guidelines/perio/update/pdf/perio_update.pdf./Accessed April 25, 2004.
4. Pinski SL, Trohman RG: Interference in implanted cardiac devices. Part I. Pacing Clin Electrophysiol 25:1367-1381, 2002.
5. Pinski SL, Trohman RG: Interference in implanted cardiac devices. Part II. Pacing Clin Electrophysiol 25:1496-1509, 2002.
6. Kazatsker M, Kusniek J, Hasdai D, et al: Two pacemakers in one patient: A stimulating case. J Cardiovasc Electrophysiol 13:522, 2002.
7. Lamas GA, Rebecca GS, Braunwald NS, Antman EM: Pacemaker malfunction after nitrous oxide anesthesia. Am J Cardiol 56:995, 1985.
8. Bernstein AD, Daubert JC, Fletcher RD, et al: The revised NASPE/BPEG generic code for antibradycardia, adaptive-rate, and multisite pacing. North American Society of Pacing and Electrophysiology/British Pacing and Electrophysiology Group. Pacing Clin Electrophysiol 25:260-264, 2002.
9. Forand JM, Schweiss JF: Pacemaker syndrome during anesthesia. Anesthesiology 60:588-590, 1984.
10. Ducey J, Fincher D, Baysinger C: Therapeutic suppression of a permanent ventricular pacemaker using a peripheral nerve stimulator. Anesthesiology 75:533-536, 1991.
11. Delfaut P, Saksena S: Electrophysiologic assessment in selecting patients for multisite atrial pacing. J Interv Card Electrophysiol 4(Suppl 1):81-85, 2000.
12. Peters RW, Gold MR: Pacing for patients with congestive heart failure and dilated cardiomyopathy. Cardiol Clin 18:55-66, 2000.
13. Abraham WT, Fisher WG, Smith AL, et al: Cardiac resynchronization in chronic heart failure. N Engl J Med 346:1845-1853, 2002.
14. Hare JM: Cardiac resynchronization therapy for heart failure. N Engl J Med 346:1902-1905, 2002.
15. Atlee J, Bernstein A: Cardiac rhythm management devices. Part I. Anesthesiology 95:1265-1280, 2001.
16. Hayes DL: Evolving indications for permanent pacing. Am J Cardiol 83:161D-165D, 1999.
17. Bevilacqua L, Hordof A: Cardiac pacing in children. Curr Opin Cardiol 13:48-55, 1998.
18. Auricchio A, Stellbrink C, Sack S, et al: The pacing therapies for congestive heart failure (PATH-CHF) study: Rationale, design, and endpoints of a prospective randomized multi-center study. Am J Cardiol 83:130D-135D, 1999.
19. Garcia-Moran E, Mont L, Brugada J: Inappropriate tachycardia detection by a biventricular implantable cardioverter defibrillator. Pacing Clin Electrophysiol 25:123-124, 2002.
20. Schreieck J, Zrenner B, Kolb C, et al: Inappropriate shock delivery due to ventricular double detection with a biventricular pacing implantable cardioverter defibrillator. Pacing Clin Electrophysiol 24:1154-1157, 2001.
21. Gras D, Mabo P, Tang T, et al: Multisite pacing as a supplemental treatment of congestive heart failure: Preliminary results of the Medtronic Inc. InSync Study. Pacing Clin Electrophysiol 21:2249-2255, 1998.
22. Medina-Ravell VA, Lankipalli RS, Yan GX, et al: Effect of epicardial or biventricular pacing to prolong QT interval and increase transmural dispersion of repolarization: Does resynchronization therapy pose a risk for patients predisposed to long QT or torsade de pointes? Circulation 107:740-746, 2003.
23. Rozner MA, Gursoy S, Monir G: Perioperative care of the patient with a pacemaker. In Stone DJ, Bogdanoff DL, Leisure GS, Spiekermann BF, Mathis DD (eds): Perioperative Care: Anesthesia, Surgery and Medicine. Philadelphia, Mosby, 1997, pp 53-67.
24. Purday JP, Towey RM: Apparent pacemaker failure caused by activation of ventricular threshold test by a magnetic instrument mat during general anaesthesia. Br J Anaesth 69:645-646, 1992.
25. Bourke ME: The patient with a pacemaker or related device. Can J Anaesth 43:24-41, 1996.
26. Shapiro WA, Roizen MF, Singleton MA, et al: Intraoperative pacemaker complications. Anesthesiology 63:319-322, 1985.
27. Valls-Bertault V, Mansourati J, Gilard M, et al: Adverse events with transvenous left ventricular pacing in patients with severe heart failure: Early experience from a single centre. Europace 3:60-63, 2001.
28. Alonso C, Leclercq C, d'Allonnes FR, et al: Six year experience of transvenous left ventricular lead implantation for permanent biventricular pacing in patients with advanced heart failure: Technical aspects. Heart 86:405-410, 2001.
29. Bernstein A, Irwin M, Parsonnet V, et al: Report of the NASPE policy conference on antibradycardia pacemaker follow-up: Effectiveness, needs and resources. Pacing Clin Electrophysiol 17:1714-1729, 1994.
30. Rozner MA, Nguyen AD, Roberson JC: Inadequate pacemaker follow-up detected at the preanesthetic visit [abstract]. Anesthesiology 96:A1071, 2002.
31. Sethi KK, Bhargava M, Pandit N, et al: Experience with recycled cardiac pacemakers. Indian Heart J 44:91-93, 1992.
32. Panja M, Sarkar CN, Kumar S, et al: Reuse of pacemaker. Indian Heart J 48:677-680, 1996.
33. Hayes JJ, Juknavorian R, Maloney JD: The role(s) of the industry employed allied professional. Pacing Clin Electrophysiol 24:398-399, 2001.
34. Kleinman B, Hamilton J, Hariman R, et al: Apparent failure of a precordial magnet and pacemaker programmer to convert a DDD pacemaker to VOO mode during the use of the electrosurgical unit. Anesthesiology 86:247-250, 1997.
35. Preisman S, Cheng DC: Life-threatening ventricular dysrhythmias with inadvertent asynchronous temporary pacing after cardiac surgery. Anesthesiology 91:880-883, 1999.
36. Andersen C, Madsen GM: Rate-responsive pacemakers and anaesthesia. A consideration of possible implications. Anaesthesia 45:472-476, 1990.
37. Levine PA: Response to "Rate-adaptive cardiac pacing: Implications of environmental noise during craniotomy" [letter] Anesthesiology 87:1261, 1997.
38. Levine PA, Balady GJ, Lazar HL, et al: Electrocautery and pacemakers: Management of the paced patient subject to electrocautery. Ann Thorac Surg 41:313-317, 1986.
39. Rozner MA, Nguyen AD: Unexpected pacing threshold changes during non-implant surgery [abstract]. Anesthesiology 96:A1070, 2002.
40. Levine PA, Gauch PRA: Utilizacão clinica da autocaptura. Reblampa 16:31-41, 2003 (translation [Portuguese] provided by author).
41. Madsen GM, Andersen C: Pacemaker-induced tachycardia during general anaesthesia: A case report. Br J Anaesth 63:360-361, 1989.
42. von Knobelsdorff G, Goerig M, Nagele H, Scholz J: Interaction of frequency-adaptive pacemakers and anesthetic management. Discussion of current literature and two case reports. Anaesthesist 45:856-860, 1996.
43. Van Hemel NM, Hamerlijnck RP, Pronk KJ, Van der Veen EP: Upper limit ventricular stimulation in respiratory rate responsive pacing due to electrocautery. Pacing Clin Electrophysiol 12:1720-1723, 1989.
44. Wong DT, Middleton W: Electrocautery-induced tachycardia in a rate-responsive pacemaker. Anesthesiology 94:710-711, 2001.
45. Chew EW, Troughear RH, Kuchar DL, Thorburn CW: Inappropriate rate change in minute ventilation rate responsive pacemakers due to interference by cardiac monitors. Pacing Clin Electrophysiol 20:276-282, 1997.
46. Rozner MA, Nishman RJ: Pacemaker-driven tachycardia revisited. Anesth Analg 88:965, 1999.

47. Wallden J, Gupta A, Carlsen HO: Supraventricular tachycardia induced by Datex patient monitoring system. Anesth Analg 86:1339, 1998.

48. Center for Devices and Radiologic Health. Interaction between minute ventilation rate-adaptive pacemakers and cardiac monitoring and diagnostic equipment. Published October 14, 1998. Available at http://www.accessdata.fda.gov/scripts/cdrh/cfdocs/cfTopic/topicinde/topindx.cfm/Accessed September 1, 2003.

49. Southorn PA, Kamath GS, Vasdev GM, Hayes DL: Monitoring equipment induced tachycardia in patients with minute ventilation rate-responsive pacemakers. Br J Anaesth 84:508-509, 2000.

50. Rozner MA, Nishman RJ: Electrocautery-induced pacemaker tachycardia: Why does this error continue? Anesthesiology 96:773-774, 2002.

51. Samain E, Schauveliege F, Henry C, Marty J: Outcome in patients with a cardiac pacemaker undergoing noncardiac surgery [abstract]. Anesthesiology 95:A142, 2001.

52. Samain E, Marty J, Souron V, et al: Intraoperative pacemaker malfunction during a shoulder arthroscopy. Anesthesiology 93:306-307, 2000.

53. Pressly N: Review of MDR Reports reinforces concern about EMI. FDA User Facility Reporting #20. Published 1997. Available at http://www.fda.gov/cdrh/fuse20.pdf/Accessed September 1, 2003.

54. Rozner MA: [Untitled letter]. Pacing Clin Electrophysiol 26:923-925, 2003.

55. Rozner MA, Trankina MF: Intrathoracic gadgets: Update on pacemakers and implantable cardioverter defibrillators. *In* Schwartz AJ (ed): ASA Refresher Courses in Anesthesiology. Philadelphia, Lippincott Williams & Wilkins, 2000, pp 183-199.

56. Trankina M.F., Black S, Gibby G: Pacemakers: Perioperative evaluation, management and complications. Anesthesiology 93:A1193, 2000.

57. Gimbel JR, Johnson D, Levine PA, Wilkoff BL: Safe performance of magnetic resonance imaging on five patients with permanent cardiac pacemakers. Pacing Clin Electrophysiol 19:913-919, 1996.

58. Alexopoulos GS, Frances RJ: ECT and cardiac patients with pacemakers. Am J Psychiatry 137:1111-1112, 1980.

59. O'Flaherty D, Wardill M, Adams AP: Inadvertent suppression of a fixed rate ventricular pacemaker using a peripheral nerve stimulator. Anaesthesia 48:687-689, 1993.

60. Philbin DM, Marieb MA, Aithal KH, Schoenfeld MH: Inappropriate shocks delivered by an ICD as a result of sensed potentials from a transcutaneous electronic nerve stimulation unit. Pacing Clin Electrophysiol 21:2010-2011, 1998.

61. Vlay SC: Electromagnetic interference and ICD discharge related to chiropractic treatment. Pacing Clin Electrophysiol 21:2009, 1998.

62. Finfer SR: Pacemaker failure on induction of anaesthesia. Br J Anaesth 66:509-512, 1991.

63. Bohm A, Kayser S, Pinter A, Preda I: Intermittent output failure of a VVI device due to the disintegration of the generator. Pacing Clin Electrophysiol 24:127-128, 2001.

64. Grimm W, Menz V, Hoffmann J, et al: Complications of third-generation implantable cardioverter defibrillator therapy. Pacing Clin Electrophysiol 22:206-211, 1999.

65. Roth JV, Brody JD, Denham EJ: Positioning the pacing esophageal stethoscope for transesophageal atrial pacing without P-wave recording: Implications for transesophageal ventricular pacing. Anesth Analg 83:48-54, 1996.

66. Mychaskiw G, Eichhorn JH: Interaction of an implanted pacemaker with a transesophageal atrial pacemaker: Report of a case. J Clin Anesth 11:669-671, 1999.

67. Moskowitz DM, Kahn RA, Camunas J, et al: External chest wall stimulation to suppress a permanent transvenous pacemaker in a patient during endovascular stent graft placement. Anesthesiology 89:531-533, 1998.

68. Snow N: Acute myocardial ischemia during pacemaker implantation: Implication for threshold determinations and potential complications. Pacing Clin Electrophysiol 6:35-37, 1983.

69. Moss AJ, Hall WJ, Cannom DS, et al: Improved survival with an implanted defibrillator in patients with coronary disease at high risk for ventricular arrhythmia. Multicenter Automatic Defibrillator Implantation Trial Investigators. N Engl J Med 335:1933-1940, 1996.

70. No authors listed: A comparison of antiarrhythmic-drug therapy with implantable defibrillators in patients resuscitated from near-fatal ventricular arrhythmias. The Antiarrhythmics versus Implantable Defibrillators (AVID) Investigators: N Engl J Med 337:1576-1583, 1997.

71. Buxton AE, Lee KL, Fisher JD, et al: A randomized study of the prevention of sudden death in patients with coronary artery disease. Multicenter Unsustained Tachycardia Trial Investigators. N Engl J Med 341:1882-1890, 1999.

72. Moss AJ, Zareba W, Hall WJ, et al: Prophylactic implantation of a defibrillator in patients with myocardial infarction and reduced ejection fraction. N Engl J Med 346:877-883, 2002.

73. Bernstein AD, Camm AJ, Fisher JD, et al: North American Society of Pacing and Electrophysiology policy statement. The NASPE/BPEG defibrillator code. Pacing Clin Electrophysiol 16:1776-1780, 1993.

74. Grimm W, Flores BF, Marchlinski FE: Electrocardiographically documented unnecessary, spontaneous shocks in 241 patients with implantable cardioverter defibrillators. Pacing Clin Electrophysiol 15:1667-1673, 1992.

75. Hurst TM, Krieglstein H, Tillmanns H, Waldecker B: Inappropriate management of self-terminating ventricular arrhythmias by implantable cardioverter defibrillators despite a specific reconfirmation algorithm: A report of two cases. Pacing Clin Electrophysiol 20:1328-1331, 1997.

76. Prasad K, Kishore AG, Anderson MH, et al: Inappropriate shocks in patients receiving internal cardioverter-defibrillators for malignant ventricular arrhythmias. Indian Heart J 49:403-407, 1997.

77. Schumacher B, Tebbenjohanns J, Jung W, et al: B: Radio-frequency catheter ablation of atrial flutter that elicits inappropriate implantable cardioverter defibrillator discharge. Pacing Clin Electrophysiol 20:125-127, 1997.

78. Rozner MA: The patient with an implantable cardioverter-defibrillator. Prog Anesthesiol 13:43-52, 1999.

79. Swerdlow CD: Supraventricular tachycardia-ventricular tachycardia discrimination algorithms in implantable cardioverter defibrillators: State-of-the-art review. J Cardiovasc Electrophysiol 12:606-612, 2001.

80. Wilkoff BL, Cook JR, Epstein AE, et al: Dual-chamber pacing or ventricular backup pacing in patients with an implantable defibrillator. The Dual Chamber and VVI Implantable Defibrillator (DAVID) Trial. JAMA 288:3115-3123, 2002.

81. Sandner SE, Wieselthaler G, Zuckermann A, et al: Survival benefit of the implantable cardioverter-defibrillator in patients on the waiting list for cardiac transplantation. Circulation 104(Suppl I):I171-I176, 2001.

82. Khan IA: Long QT syndrome: Diagnosis and management. Am Heart J 143:7-14, 2002.

83. McKenna WJ, Thiene G, Nava A, et al: Diagnosis of arrhythmogenic right ventricular dysplasia/cardiomyopathy. Task Force of the Working Group Myocardial and Pericardial Disease of the European Society of Cardiology and of the Scientific Council on Cardiomyopathies of the International Society and Federation of Cardiology. Br Heart J 71:215-218, 1994.

84. Brugada P, Geelen P: Some electrocardiographic patterns predicting sudden cardiac death that every doctor should recognize. Acta Cardiol 52:473-484, 1997.

85. Maron BJ, Shen WK, Link MS, et al: Efficacy of implantable cardioverter-defibrillators for the prevention of sudden death in patients with hypertrophic cardiomyopathy. N Engl J Med 342:365-373, 2000.

86. Casavant D, Haffajee C, Stevens S, Pacetti P: Aborted implantable cardioverter-defibrillator shock during facial electrosurgery. Pacing Clin Electrophysiol 21:1325-1326, 1998.

87. Gill RM, Sweeney RJ, Reid PR: The defibrillation threshold: A comparison of anesthetics and measurement methods. Pacing Clin Electrophysiol 16:708-714, 1993.

88. Weinbroum AA, Glick A, Copperman Y, et al: Halothane, isoflurane, and fentanyl increase the minimally effective defibrillation threshold of an implantable cardioverter defibrillator: First report in humans. Anesth Analg 95:1147-1153, 2002.

89. Carlson MD, Ip J, Messenger J, et al: A new pacemaker algorithm for the treatment of atrial fibrillation: Results of the Atrial Dynamic Overdrive Pacing Trial (ADOPT). J Am Coll Cardiol 42:627-633, 2003.
90. Schwartzenburg CF, Wass CT, Strickland RA, Hayes DL: Rate-adaptive cardiac pacing: Implications of environmental noise during craniotomy. Anesthesiology 87:1252-1254, 1997.
91. Aldrete JA, Brown C, Daily J, Buerke V: Pacemaker malfunction due to microcurrent injection from a bioimpedance noninvasive cardiac output monitor. J Clin Monit 11:131-133, 1995.
92. Martin ET, Coman JA, Shellock FG, et al: Magnetic resonance imaging and cardiac pacemaker safety at 105 Tesla. J Am Coll Cardiol 43:1315-1324, 2004.

APPENDIX I

Preanesthesia Pulse Generator Evaluation

Determining the indication for and date of initial device placement

Determining the patient's underlying rhythm and rate (if any)

Identifying the number and types of leads

Determining the last generator test date and battery status

Obtaining a history of generator events (if any)

Obtaining the current program information (device interrogation), including mode, rate, and rate enhancements

Ensuring that generator discharges become mechanical systoles with adequate pacing safety margins

Ensuring adequate safety margin for sensing events (if intrinsic events are present)

Ensuring that magnet detection is enabled (magnet behavior and rate should be recorded) if magnet use is indicated

Determining whether the pacemaker should be reprogrammed, which depends upon pacemaker dependency, surgery type and location, need for increased heart rate, etc.

The preanesthetic pacemaker evaluation should consist of a device interrogation. The statements, above, can be fashioned into a request to the cardiologist or pacemaker service. Note that for ICDs, the term "generator events" includes a history of antitachycardia therapy

APPENDIX II

Pulse Generator Company Phone Numbers

When calling for assistance, ask for "Brady tech support" for pacemaker assistance or "Tachy tech support" for ICD assistance.

Companies listed in boldface text market implanted cardioverter-defibrillators (ICDs):

AM Pacemaker Corporation (Guidant Medical): 800-227-3422

Angeion: 800-264-2466

Arco Medical (Guidant Medical): 800-227-3422

Biotronik: 800-547-0394

Cardiac Control Systems: unavailable

Cardio Pace Medical, Inc. (Novacon): unavailable

Cardiac Pacemakers, Inc. (CPI) (Guidant Medical): 800-227-3422

Cook Pacemaker Corporation: 800-245-4715

Coratomic (Biocontrol Technology): unavailable

Cordis Corporation (St. Jude Medical): 800-722-3774

Diag/Medcor (St. Jude Medical): 800-722-3774

Edwards Pacemaker Systems (Medtronic): 800-325-2518

ELA Medical: 800-352-6466

Guidant Medical: 800-227-3422

Intermedics (Guidant Medical): 800-227-3422

Medtronic: 800-505-4636

Pacesetter (St. Jude Medical): 800-722-3774

Siemans-Elema (St. Jude Medical): 800-722-3774

Telectronics Pacing (St. Jude Medical): 800-722-3774

Ventritex (St. Jude Medical): 800-722-3774

Vitatron (Medtronic): 800-328-2518

CHAPTER
36 Respiratory Monitoring

Richard E. Moon and Enrico M. Camporesi

Gas Exchange   1438
Alveolar Gases   1439
Arterial Gases   1439

**Measurement of Blood Gas
Tensions   1444**
Temperature Correction of Blood Gases   1445
Artifactual Effects on Gas Tension
Measurement   1446
Bedside Clinical Interpretation of Arterial
Po_2 and Pco_2 Measurements   1446

**Transcutaneous Gas Tension
Measurement   1447**

**Measurement of Oxygen
Saturation   1447**
Carbon Monoxide Oximetry   1447
Transcutaneous Oximetry   1448
Pulse Oximetry   1448

**Mixed Venous Oxygen
Monitoring   1453**

Tissue Oxygenation   1453

Expired Gas Analysis   1454
Mass Spectrometry and Raman
Gas Analysis   1454
Infrared Absorption   1454
Colorimetric Carbon Dioxide Analysis   1454
Polarographic Analysis   1454
Paramagnetic Analysis   1454
Nitric Oxide Analysis   1454

**Waveform Analysis of Expired
Respiratory Gases   1455**
Sidestream Capnographs   1455

Mainstream Capnometers   1456
Time Delays   1457
Capnographic Waveform   1458
Errors in Capnography   1462

**Oxygen and Carbon Dioxide
Exchange Monitoring   1462**

Respiratory Center Drive   1463

**Pulmonary and Chest Wall
Mechanical Function   1463**
Principles of Gas Flow
Measurement   1463
Respiratory Output   1463
Measurement of Respiratory
Mechanics   1465
Practical Measurement of Passive
Respiratory Mechanical Properties   1465

Apnea Monitoring   1467

Lung Water   1468

**Monitoring of High-Frequency
Ventilation   1468**

**Discontinuation of Mechanical
Ventilation and Tracheal
Extubation   1469**

**Tracheal Extubation after
Compromise of the Airway   1472**

**Transportation of the
Patient   1472**

**Epidural and Intrathecal
Opiates   1472**

A *monitor* has been variously defined as "something that reminds or gives warning"[1] and "an instrument used to measure continuously or at intervals a condition that must be kept within prescribed limits."[2] Although the former definition is applicable to self-contained instruments (e.g., pulse oximeters), we have used the wider view incorporated in the latter definition, including, for example, intermittent measurements and the relevant respiratory physiology as applied to assessment of patient well-being.

Although outcome data are sparse, there is general agreement that patient safety has been enhanced by the development of technologies that permit accurate physiologic monitoring; basic studies to elucidate the causes of mishaps, including incident monitoring; educational efforts by national patient safety organizations such as the Anesthesia Patient Safety Foundation and the Australian Patient Safety Foundation; and the promulgation of monitoring standards that have become widely accepted. Eichhorn and colleagues[3] outlined minimal recommended standards for patient monitoring during anesthesia at hospitals within the Harvard Medical School system, commonly referred to as the *Harvard Standards*.

In addition to monitors of cardiovascular function and patient temperature, these investigators suggested that mandatory respiratory monitors include methods of continuous monitoring of the patient's ventilation (including a breathing system disconnection monitor) and a monitor of oxygen (O_2) concentration within the patient's breathing system. A strong recommendation was made for monitoring end-tidal carbon dioxide (CO_2) concentrations. Since then, the American Society of Anesthesiologists (ASA) has also promulgated basic monitoring standards.[4] Included in the ASA Standards (www.asahq.org/publicationsServices.htm) are a requirement for measurement of inspired O_2 concentration and quantitative assessment of blood oxygenation, such as pulse oximetry. Adequate illumination and exposure of the patient are necessary to assess color. Adequacy of ventilation must be continually evaluated, and quantitative monitoring of CO_2 or volume of expired gas, or both, is strongly encouraged. When an endotracheal tube is inserted, correct placement of the tube must be verified by clinical assessment and by identification of CO_2 in the expired gas. Continual end-tidal CO_2 analysis using a quantitative method such as capnography should be performed from the time of endotracheal tube placement until extubation or initiation of transport to a postoperative care location. During mechanical ventilation, a device capable of detecting airway disconnects must be in continuous use. *Continual* is defined as repeated regularly and frequently in steady, rapid succession; *continuous* is defined as prolonged without any interruption at any time.

The limited ability of human organ systems to function anaerobically dictates a transport system that can maintain O_2 delivery to peripheral tissues. The monitoring of one component of this system, the cardiovascular system, is discussed in Chapter 32. This chapter discusses the other component, the respiratory system, and the appropriate monitoring necessary to detect malfunction in its gas exchange function.

GAS EXCHANGE

The major function of the lung is gas exchange: the addition of O_2 to blood and the elimination of CO_2 from blood. Because of the close relationship between the partial pressure of CO_2 in blood (Pco_2) and arterial (and hence tissue) pH, the goal is maintenance of arterial CO_2 within an appropriate physiologic range. Adequate O_2 delivery must also be maintained. Figure 36-1 shows the O_2 cascade from atmospheric gas to the intracellular site of use. Assessment of the adequacy of this delivery system may be made at any step of the cascade. For example, common clinical practice dictates that arterial O_2 content (Pao_2) should be sufficient. It is common practice to attempt to maintain arterial hemoglobin (Hb) O_2 saturation (Sao_2) level above 90%, a reasonable and practical goal for two reasons. First, clinical experience supports the notion that maintenance of hemoglobin at 90% saturation with O_2 in the presence of adequate cardiac output can provide sufficient O_2 delivery to the tissues. Second, because the Hb-O_2 dissociation curve becomes abruptly steeper at O_2 saturation levels below 90% (typical Po_2 of 55 to 60 mm Hg), further decreases in Pao_2 may result in sharp diminution of arterial O_2 content.

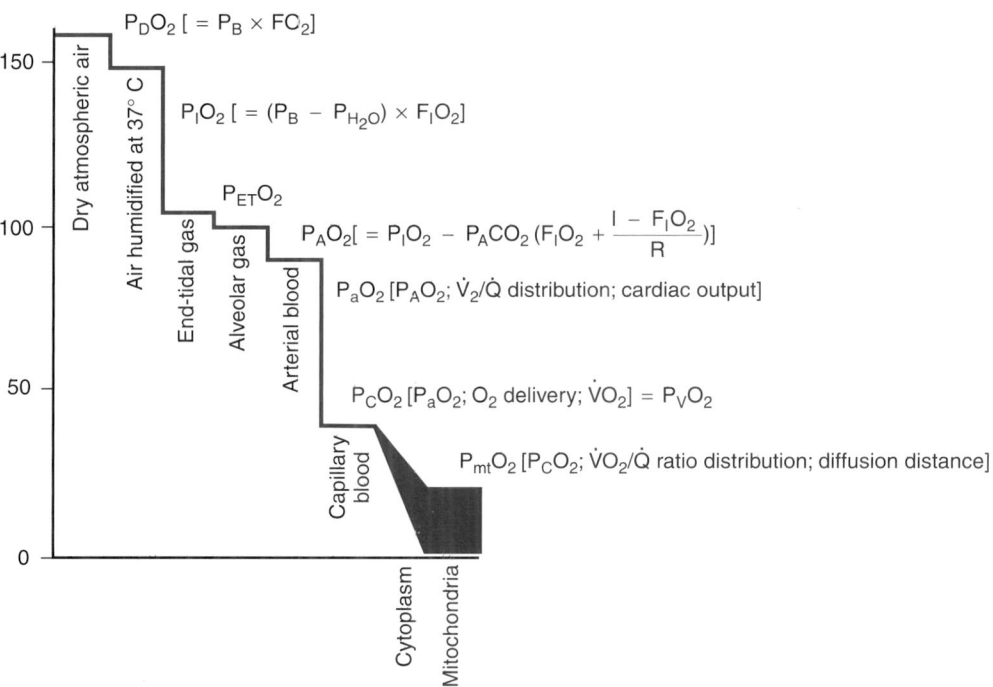

Figure 36–1 Oxygen transport cascade. A schematic view of the steps in oxygen transport from the atmosphere to the site of utilization in the mitochondrion is shown here. Approximate Po_2 values are shown for each step in the cascade, and factors determining those partial pressures are shown within the square brackets. There is a distribution of tissue Po_2 values depending on local capillary blood flow, tissue oxygen consumption, and diffusion distances. Mitochondrial Po_2 values are depicted as a range because reported levels vary widely. (Adapted from Nunn JF: Nunn's Applied Respiratory Physiology, 4th ed. Boston, Butterworth-Heinemann, 1993.)

In addition to Sa_{O_2}, O_2 delivery is a function of blood flow and hemoglobin concentration. A target value for Sa_{O_2} of 90% or greater should therefore not become a sacrosanct standard for all conditions. Acute altitude hypoxia with Sa_{O_2} values between 50% and 70% is well tolerated by normal individuals,[5,6] even during exercise, for periods of several hours or days, with no loss of consciousness, preservation of cardiac function, and minimal or no evidence of permanent sequelae.[7-11] Individuals with acute anemia may tolerate hypoxia less well because of the enhanced reduction in arterial O_2 content.

Alveolar Gases

The lung consists of a heterogeneous collection of gas exchange units (alveoli), with a range of O_2 and CO_2 gas tensions. It is therefore erroneous to speak of "the" alveolar P_{O_2} or P_{CO_2}. However, the concept of a homogeneous lung, in which all alveoli have the same gas tensions, is a useful one. The alveolar partial pressures calculated by using such a model may be thought of as averages for the O_2 and CO_2 partial pressures in the real (nonhomogeneous) lung. Equations for alveolar P_{O_2} and P_{CO_2} ($P_{A_{O_2}}$ and $P_{A_{CO_2}}$), or alveolar gas equations, are as follows:

$$P_{A_{CO_2}} = k\frac{\dot{V}_{CO_2}}{\dot{V}_A} \qquad (1)$$

$$P_{A_{O_2}} = P_{I_{O_2}} - P_{A_{CO_2}} \cdot \left(F_{I_{O_2}} + \frac{1 - F_{I_{O_2}}}{R}\right) \qquad (2)$$

In these equations, $\dot{V}_{CO_2}$ is the CO_2 production rate, $\dot{V}_{O_2}$ is the O_2 consumption rate, $\dot{V}_A$ is the alveolar ventilation rate, k is a constant, $F_{I_{O_2}}$ is the fractional inspired O_2 concentration, $P_{I_{O_2}}$ is the inspired P_{O_2} after humidification or $(P_{barometric} - P_{H_2O}) \cdot F_{I_{O_2}}$, and R is the respiratory exchange ratio or $\dot{V}_{CO_2}/\dot{V}_{O_2}$ (typically about 0.8).

An approximation to the O_2 alveolar gas equation follows:

$$P_{A_{O_2}} \cong P_{I_{O_2}} - 1.2 \times P_{CO_2} \qquad (3)$$

Unlike the alveolar equation for O_2, the equation for $P_{A_{CO_2}}$ is a function of only two variables. Because in clinical medicine $\dot{V}_{CO_2}$ is relatively constant, $P_{A_{CO_2}}$ is therefore mainly a function of alveolar ventilation $\dot{V}_A$, to which it is inversely proportional.

$$\dot{V}_A = \dot{V}_E - \dot{V}_D \qquad (4)$$

In Equation 4, $\dot{V}_E$ is the respiratory minute ventilation, and $\dot{V}_D$ is dead space ventilation. Because alveolar ventilation is usually a constant fraction of minute ventilation, the following relationship applies:

$$\dot{V}_A = k' \cdot \dot{V}_E \qquad (5)$$

The alveolar gas equation for CO_2 may be rewritten as follows:

$$P_{A_{CO_2}} = c \cdot \left(\frac{1}{\dot{V}_E}\right) \qquad (6)$$

In this form of the equation, c is a constant derived from constants k and k'.

This approximation may not hold if CO_2 production is substantially elevated, such as during a major motor seizure, shivering, or fever. CO_2 production may decrease as a result of general anesthesia or hypothermia. It is altered by approximately 7% for each 1°C change in body temperature. In young individuals, it has been observed to increase by 100% to 300% during violent shivering,[12] although in elderly patients (>60 years), the observed increase is only about 38%.[13]

The alveolar gas equation for O_2 (Equation 2) can be used to delineate the factors that result in low $P_{A_{O_2}}$. Several major factors apply:
1. Low $P_{I_{O_2}}$ caused by decreased barometric pressure (altitude) or breathing a gas mixture with inspired O_2 fraction ($F_{I_{O_2}}$) less than 0.21
2. Elevated $P_{A_{CO_2}}$ caused by hypoventilation or increased CO_2 production
3. Reduced respiratory exchange ratio (R), which is usually a minor effect because the physiologic range of R is on the order of 0.7 to 1.2, with the latter value seen during acute metabolic acidosis or excessive feeding.

Arterial Gases

The variables that determine alveolar gas tension have been described. The following additional factors also determine the gas tensions in arterial blood:
1. Ventilation-perfusion ($\dot{V}_A/\dot{Q}$) mismatching
2. Right-to-left shunt
3. Diffusion nonequilibrium

To understand fully the role of $\dot{V}_A/\dot{Q}$ in determining arterial gas tensions, it is necessary to discard the homogeneous lung model and consider a model with multiple parallel units of gas exchange and blood flow in which the resulting arterial gas tension is determined by the mixing of different proportions of blood from each gas exchange unit. The gas tensions in each unit depend on the regional ventilation, perfusion, and diffusion.

Gas exchange units with low or zero $\dot{V}_A/\dot{Q}$ ratios have low end-capillary P_{O_2}. The O_2-blood dissociation curve has a plateau at the point at which hemoglobin is fully saturated (see Fig. 36-9), and there is a maximum to which gas exchange units with normal ventilation and perfusion can raise the end-capillary O_2 content. Arterial O_2 content (and therefore P_{O_2}) is a flow weighted average of all gas exchange units. Under usual conditions, $\dot{V}_A/\dot{Q}$ mismatching always results in arterial hypoxemia. The only circumstance in which $\dot{V}_A/\dot{Q}$ mismatch results in increased arterial F_{O_2} is during the uptake of nitrous oxide.

The effect of $\dot{V}_A/\dot{Q}$ mismatching on Pa_{CO_2} is often erroneously assumed to be negligible because Pa_{CO_2} can usually be maintained within the normal range, even in the face of severe pulmonary pathology. This is true because the CO_2-blood dissociation curve (Fig. 36-2) is a monotonically increasing one. Moreover, the degree to which end-capillary P_{CO_2} (Pc'_{CO_2}) can be increased by gas exchange units with abnormal $\dot{V}_A/\dot{Q}$ is relatively small. The venoarterial P_{CO_2} difference is usually only 5 mm Hg under resting conditions and rarely exceeds 10 mm Hg. It is therefore usually possible for lung units with low Pa_{CO_2} (and therefore

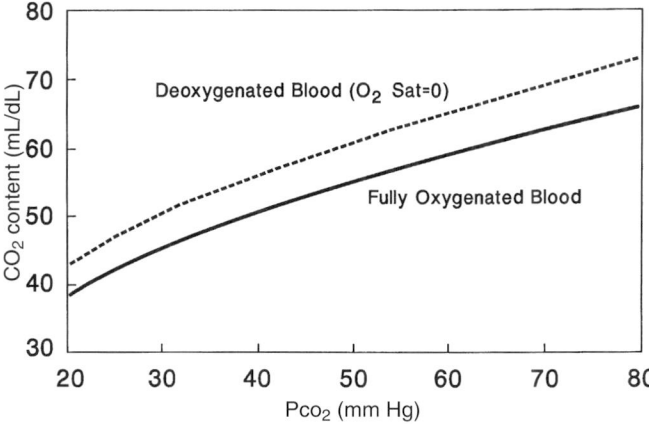

Figure 36–2 Carbon dioxide (CO_2) content of arterial blood as a function of Pco_2. For a given Pco_2 deoxygenated blood has a higher CO_2 content than oxygenated blood (i.e., Haldane effect). Unlike the HbO_2 saturation curve, the CO_2 content curve has no plateau and can be approximated by a straight line in the clinically useful range. (Data from Christiansen J, Douglas CG, Haldane JS: The absorption and dissociation of carbon dioxide by human blood. J Physiol [Lond] 48:244, 1914.)

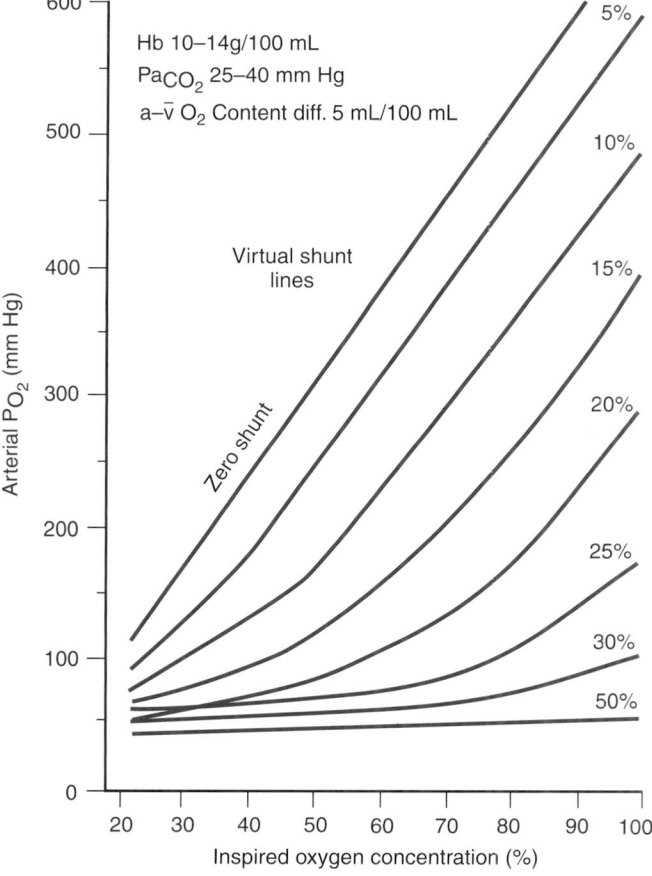

Figure 36–3 Arterial Po_2 as a function of FIo_2 and shunt fraction ($\dot{Q}s/\dot{Q}T$). Assumptions are shown on the upper left of the graph. The presence of a shunt decreases arterial Po_2 for a given FIo_2. As $\dot{Q}s/\dot{Q}T$ increases, supplemental O_2 has progressively less effect on arterial Po_2. (Adapted from Benumof JL: Anesthesia for Thoracic Surgery, 2nd ed. Philadelphia, WB Saunders, 1995, and Lawler PGP, Nunn JF: A reassessment of the validity of the iso-shunt graph. Br J Anaesth 56:1325, 1984.)

$Pc'co_2$) to "compensate" for alveoli with high Pco_2, producing a normal $Paco_2$, even in the face of a significant $\dot{V}A/\dot{Q}$ abnormality. Although $\dot{V}A/\dot{Q}$ mismatching affects CO_2 exchange to the same degree as it does O_2 exchange, this is often not reflected in the blood gases because compensatory hyperventilation can maintain $Paco_2$ within the normal range. The effect of $\dot{V}A/\dot{Q}$ mismatching on CO_2 exchange can be detected by an increase in $\dot{V}E$.

Right-to-left shunting is a special case of $\dot{V}A/\dot{Q}$ mismatch, with a $\dot{V}A/\dot{Q}$ ratio of zero. Blood flowing through a right-to-left shunt, whether intrapulmonary or intracardiac, has gas tensions equal to mixed venous values. The net effect on arterial Po_2 and Pco_2 depends on the magnitude of the shunt (Fig. 36-3) and the mixed venous and pulmonary capillary gas tensions. Because major determinant of mixed venous Po_2 (and to a lesser extent mixed venous Pco_2) is cardiac output ($\dot{Q}$), changes in $\dot{Q}$ may modify the degree to which arterial Po_2 is determined by pulmonary gas exchange (Fig. 36-4).

Diffusion nonequilibrium can exist when the gas tensions in the pulmonary capillary erythrocyte ($Pc'o_2$, $Pc'co_2$) are not equal to the alveolar gas tensions. This can occur under two physiologic conditions: increased pulmonary blood flow such that the erythrocyte does not have sufficient time in the alveoli to enable gas tensions to reach equilibrium or a thickening of the alveolar-capillary membrane such that the rate of diffusion of gas from alveolus to capillary (O_2) or vice versa (CO_2) is slowed. For CO_2 diffusion, nonequilibrium would result in an arterial Pco_2 ($Paco_2$) value higher than that of $PAco_2$. For O_2, nonequilibrium means that Pao_2 is less than PAo_2. In practice, there has never been any evidence for failure of diffusion equilibrium of CO_2. Despite much discussion of O_2 diffusion nonequilibrium, it probably rarely exists in clinical medicine. There is evidence for its existence during moderate exercise in patients with interstitial fibrosis and during severe exercise in normal individuals, particularly at higher altitudes.[7] In anesthesia or critical care, O_2 diffusion nonequilibrium would probably occur only under very unusual circumstances, such as a septic patient with high cardiac output breathing air at the top of Pike's Peak (i.e., altitude of 4301m and barometric pressure of 444 mm Hg).

The following are the most likely causes of low Pao_2:

1. Low PIo_2
2. Hypoventilation
3. $\dot{V}A/\dot{Q}$ mismatching, including right-to-left shunt (effect modified by mixed venous Po_2)

A common measurement used to assess the adequacy of pulmonary gas exchange is the alveolar-arterial (A-a) gradient:

$$\text{A-a gradient} = PAo_2 - Pao_2 \qquad (7)$$

Calculation of the A-a gradient takes into account any degree of hypoventilation or low inspired Po_2 such that an abnormally high A-a gradient reflects a $\dot{V}A/\dot{Q}$ mismatch (more specifically, low $\dot{V}A/\dot{Q}$ in gas exchange units) or shunt. The normal value of A-a gradient for a child or young adult is less than 10 mm Hg, with an increase due to aging[14] according to the following formula:

$$\text{A-a gradient} = 0.21 \times (\text{age in years} + 2.5) \qquad (8)$$

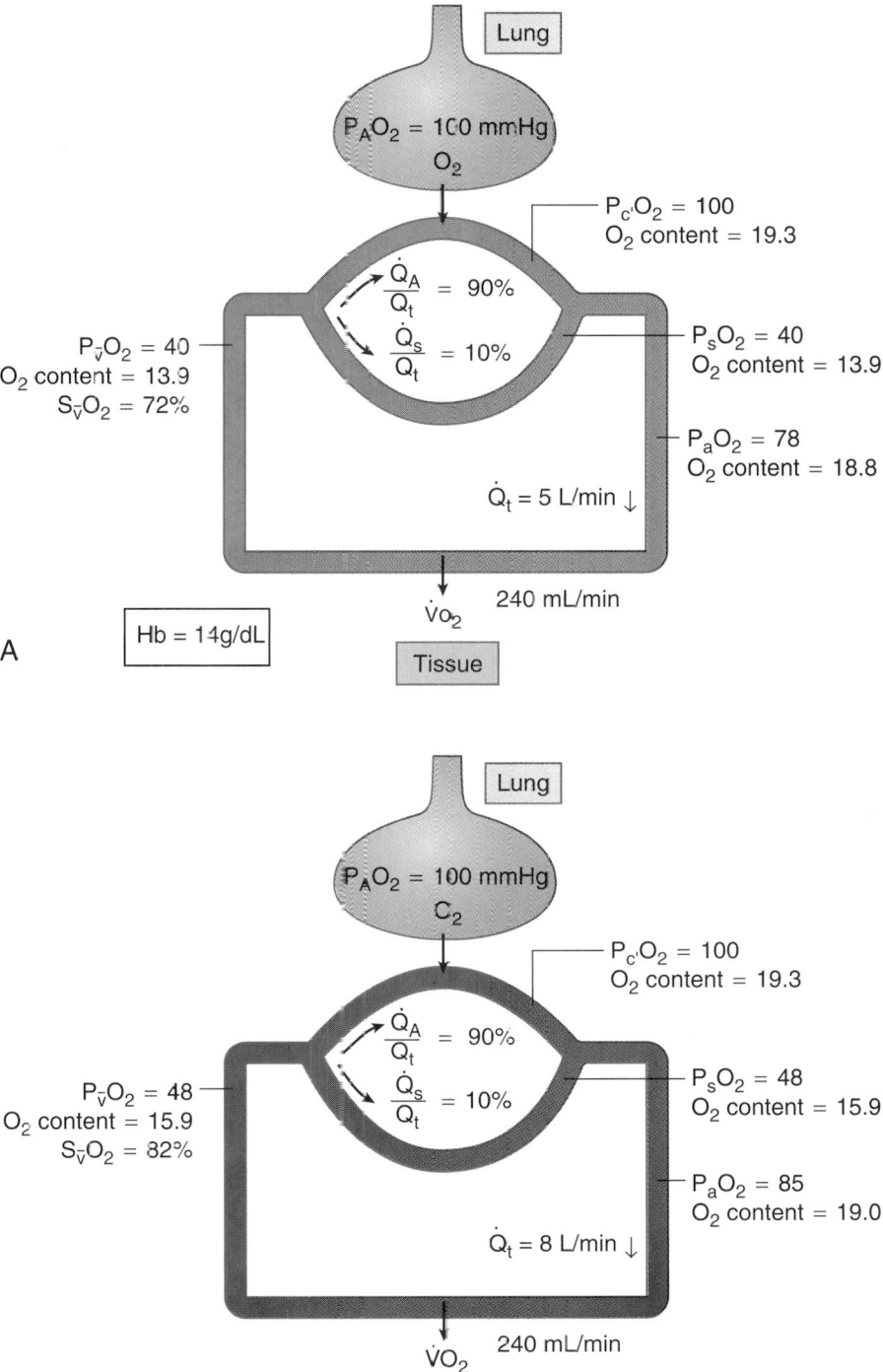

Figure 36–4 Effect of cardiac output on Po_2. **A,** Arterial and mixed venous O_2 tension and content are shown at a cardiac output of 5 L/min. **B,** Assuming a constant $\dot{V}o_2$, an increase in cardiac output to 8 L/min increases the Pao_2 from 78 to 85 mm Hg. This occurs because $S\bar{v}o_2$ increases at higher cardiac output. The resulting increase in O_2 content of the shunted blood (here assumed to be 10% of cardiac output) then raises arterial O_2 content and Pao_2. Po_2 values are in mm Hg, and O_2 content is in mL/dL.

There is considerable scatter of the data around the mean values predicted by the relationship in Equation 8, with individual values for the A-a gradient exceeding 30 mm Hg. The A-a gradient also increases with abnormalities of pulmonary gas exchange. The usefulness of the A-a gradient may be demonstrated by an example. Interpretation of the following arterial blood gases in an unconscious individual in an emergency room (breathing room air) may be aided by calculating the A-a gradient: $Pao_2 = 50$ mm Hg,

$Paco_2 = 76$ mm Hg, and pH = 7.17. Assuming that barometric pressure = 760 mm Hg, body temperature = 37°C (therefore $PH_2O = 47$ mm Hg), and R = 0.8 (in this case using Equation 2), $PAo_2 = 59$ mm Hg. The A-a gradient therefore equals $59 - 50 = 9$ mm Hg, a normal value. Because the impairment of arterial oxygenation is associated with a normal A-a gradient, there is no intrinsic abnormality of pulmonary gas exchange. The diagnosis is most likely central respiratory depression.

A problem with the clinical use of the a-a gradient is that its normal value is highly dependent on inspired O_2 concentration. As FIO_2 increases, the a-a gradient becomes larger. In a normal individual breathing 100% O_2, the a-a gradient can exceed 70 mm Hg. A more useful parameter that obviates this problem is the a/A ratio (i.e., PaO_2/PAO_2). Empirically, the a/A ratio has been shown to be relatively constant with varying FIO_2,[15] even in a hyperbaric chamber up to an ambient pressure of 3 atm absolute (see Chapter 70). The normal a/A ratio is 0.85; lower values indicate impaired pulmonary gas exchange.

If mixed venous blood is available for analysis, a solution can be found for a simplified but clinically useful compartmental model of the lung. This three-compartment model assumes the following division of gas exchange units within the lung:

A compartment with $\dot{V}A/\dot{Q} = 1$ (optimal matching of ventilation and perfusion)

A compartment with $\dot{V}A/\dot{Q} = 0$ (shunt compartment)

A compartment with $\dot{V}A/\dot{Q} = \infty$ (dead space compartment)

Shunt fraction (venous admixture) is the proportion of total blood flow perfusing the shunt compartment and can be calculated from the following equation:

$$\frac{\dot{Q}s}{\dot{Q}T} = \frac{Cc'O_2 - CaO_2}{Cc'O_2 - C\bar{v}O_2} \qquad (9)$$

In Equation 9, $\dot{Q}s$ is shunt blood flow, and $\dot{Q}T$ is cardiac output. $Cc'O_2$, CaO_2, and $C\bar{v}O_2$ are the O_2 contents of end-capillary, arterial, and mixed venous blood, respectively. CaO_2 and $C\bar{v}O_2$ can be calculated directly. $Cc'O_2$ must be calculated from PAO_2 and the Hb-O_2 dissociation curve.

$$O_2 \text{ content of blood} = \text{dissolved } O_2 + \text{Hb-bound } O_2$$
$$= 0.003 \times PO_2 + 1.39 \times \text{Hb}$$
$$\text{concentration} \qquad (10)$$

In Equation 10, the O_2 content is given in mL/dL; PO_2 is in mm Hg; and the hemoglobin concentration is in g/dL.

If PAO_2 is high enough that end-capillary blood has a hemoglobin O_2 saturation close to 100%, by dividing numerator and denominator by the O_2 capacity (i.e. O_2 content at 100% saturation) Equation 8 can be rewritten as the following approximation:

$$\frac{\dot{Q}s}{\dot{Q}T} \cong \frac{1 - SaO_2}{1 - S\bar{v}O_2} \qquad (11)$$

$\dot{Q}s/\dot{Q}T$ calculated using either equation (i.e., using O_2 as the "marker gas") includes gas exchange units of low $\dot{V}A/\dot{Q}$ in addition to pure shunt. Breathing 100% O_2, however, eliminates the contribution of low $\dot{V}A/\dot{Q}$ gas exchange units to $\dot{Q}s/\dot{Q}T$ because any lung unit with nonzero $\dot{V}A/\dot{Q}$ fully saturates with O_2 the capillary blood perfusing it. Use of this technique to assess shunt is complicated by the fact that breathing 100% O_2 results in the progressive development of resorption atelectasis and a parallel increase in shunt.[16]

Whereas pathology that affects pulmonary O_2 exchange (typically low $\dot{V}A/\dot{Q}$ or shunt) can be detected by inspection of the arterial blood gases and FIO_2 (or formal calculation of the a/A ratio), lung abnormalities that

affect pulmonary CO_2 exchange (typically high $\dot{V}A/\dot{Q}$ gas exchange units or dead space) require additional information. To measure physiologic dead space (VDS), the Bohr equation can be used:

$$V_{D\,PHYS} = V_T\left(1 - \frac{PECO_2}{PACO_2}\right) \qquad (12)$$

In Equation 12, $PECO_2$ is the mixed expired PCO_2 and VT is the tidal volume. $PACO_2$ can be assumed equal to $PaCO_2$ (i.e., Enghoff modification). To measure $PECO_2$, expired gas must be analyzed in a mixing box, or a bag must be used to collect several expired breaths. Alternatively, $PECO_2$ can be measured by placing a CO_2 sensor in a bypass flow-mixing chamber (i.e., bymixer) in the expiration limb of an anesthesia or ventilator circuit (Fig. 36-5).[17] The dead space calculated using this equation includes anatomic and physiologic dead space, as well as external dead space such as in the breathing circuit. Dead space can also be measured on a breath-by-breath basis if a volume capnogram is used (see Fig. 36-17). Dead space measured using this formula (i.e., total physiologic dead space) includes airway dead space (i.e., anatomic or series dead space) and alveolar dead space (i.e., intrapulmonary or parallel dead space). Dead space is usually expressed as a fraction of the tidal volume (VD/VT ratio).

Mixed expired gas analysis is often not clinically available, but an assessment of dead space ventilation may be made by examining the relationship between minute ventilation ($\dot{V}E$) and $PaCO_2$. $\dot{V}E$ is continuously displayed by modern ventilators, including anesthesia ventilators, and can be measured in spontaneously breathing individuals by using a spirometer. Assuming normal $\dot{V}CO_2$, the following equation[18] describes an empirical relationship:

$$\dot{V}E \times PaCO_2 \leq 8\ W \qquad (13)$$

In Equation 13, W is the body weight. If $\dot{V}E$ (L/min) times $PaCO_2$ (mm Hg) exceeds eight times the body weight (kg), an increase in dead space exists, indicating that to maintain a normal $PaCO_2$, higher than usual ventilation is required. $\dot{V}E \times PaCO_2$ can also be elevated by increased CO_2 production (e.g., shivering, fever, metabolic acidosis).

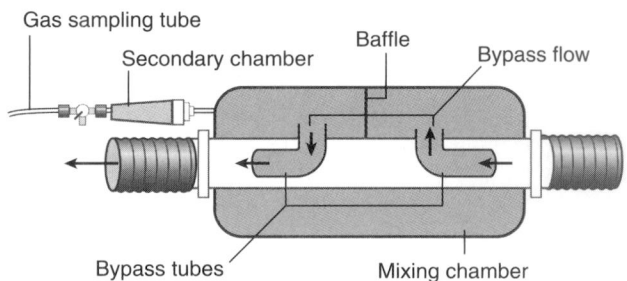

Figure 36–5 Bymixer. This compartment, placed in the expiratory limb of a circle system, provides a mixing chamber through which a portion of the exhaled gas flows. Mixing of gas within this chamber provides constant mixed expired O_2 and CO_2 concentrations, from which $\dot{V}O_2$, $\dot{V}CO_2$, and dead space can be calculated. (Adapted from Breen PH, Serina ER: Bymixer provides on-line calibration of measurement of CO_2 volume exhaled per breath. Ann Biomed Eng 25:164, 1997.)

Using the respiratory gases to assess pulmonary gas exchange has some drawbacks. First, the relationship between partial pressure and gas content is nonlinear for both O_2 and CO_2. Alterations in cardiac output, hemoglobin concentration (resulting in altered venous blood gas tensions), or inspired gas composition may lead to different calculated values of $\dot{Q}s/\dot{Q}T$ or Vd/Vt even if actual $\dot{V}A/\dot{Q}$ ratios in the lung are unchanged.[19] Second, changes in O_2 or CO_2 exchange can provide information only on a limited portion of the spectrum of $\dot{V}A/\dot{Q}$ ratios. An increase in calculated $\dot{Q}s/\dot{Q}T$ (Equation 9) cannot distinguish between a shift to lower $\dot{V}A/\dot{Q}$ ratios and an increase in true shunt.

In a more sophisticated technique described by Wagner and coworkers,[16,20] a dilute mixture of several inert (i.e., not metabolically active) tracer gases is infused intravenously. The ratio of partial pressures $Pc'/P\bar{v}$ or $PA/P\bar{v}$ at a gas exchange unit is described by the following equation:

$$\frac{Pc'}{P\bar{v}} = \frac{PA}{P\bar{v}} = \frac{\lambda}{\lambda + \dot{V}A/\dot{Q}} \qquad (14)$$

In Equation 14, Pc', P$\bar{v}$, and PA are the partial pressures of the gas in end-capillary blood, venous blood, and alveolar gas, respectively. The λ term is the blood-gas partition coefficient of the gas, and $\dot{V}A/\dot{Q}$ is the ventilation-perfusion ratio of the gas exchange unit.

In this technique of multiple inert gas (MIG) elimination, the six gases typically used are sulfur hexafluoride, ethane, cyclopropane, enflurane, diethyl ether, and acetone, spanning a partition coefficient of about 70,000. Each gas provides information about a particular region in the spectrum of $\dot{V}A/\dot{Q}$, permitting a multiple-compartment model to be calculated. The MIG method has been used to demonstrate the development of $\dot{V}A/\dot{Q}$ mismatching and shunt during general anesthesia.[21] Figure 36-6 demonstrates the use of MIG to calculate a 50-compartment model of $\dot{V}A/\dot{Q}$. Using this model, shunt fraction assessed by using the MIG method has been correlated with atelectatic areas in dependent lung regions visible on chest computed tomography (CT) (see Fig. 36-5).[22,23] The MIG method has been used to demonstrate improved $\dot{V}A/\dot{Q}$ matching

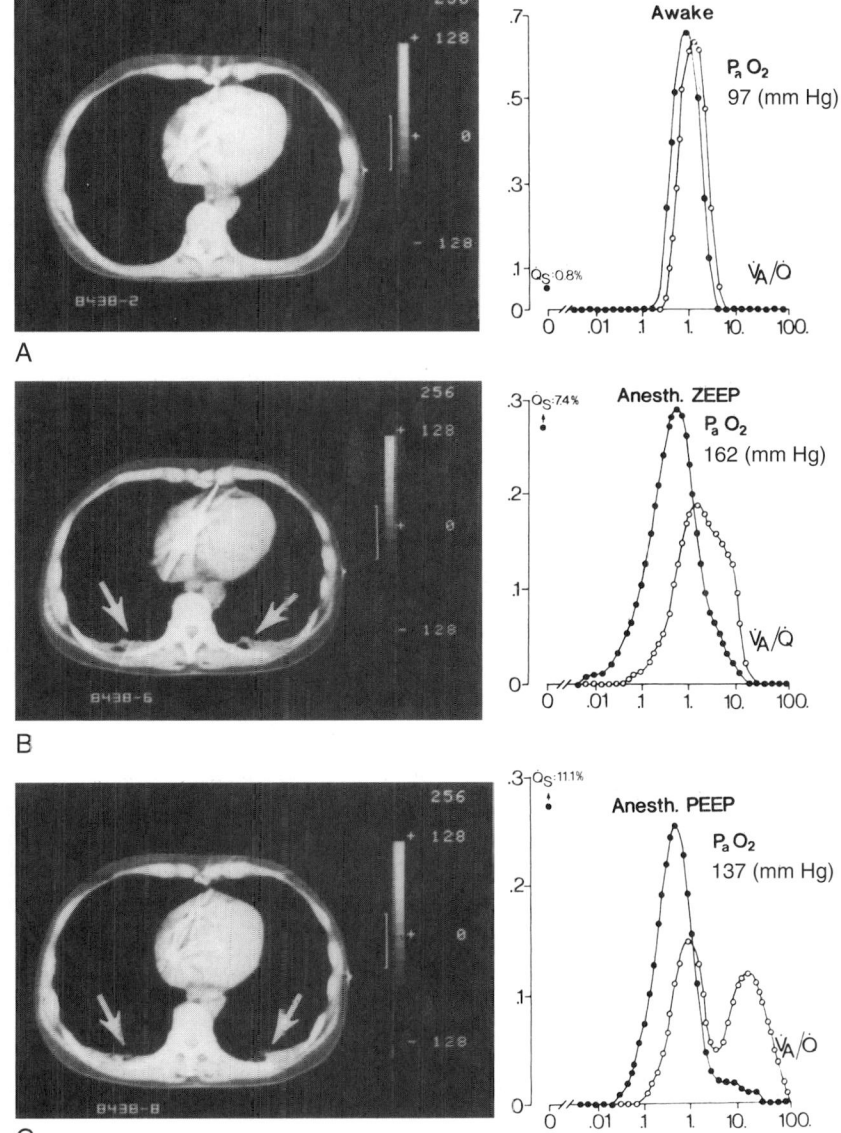

Figure 36–6 Effect of anesthesia on pulmonary atelectasis and gas exchange. **A,** Computed tomography of the chest of an awake patient. Adjacent to the scan is the distribution of ventilation (*open circles*) and perfusion (*solid circles*) in a 50-compartment lung model, determined by using the multiple inert gas method. A unimodal distribution is shown for the awake individual with a shunt fraction ($\dot{Q}s/\dot{Q}T$) of 0.8%. **B,** After a period of general anesthesia with positive-pressure ventilation, crescent-shaped areas of increased tissue density (*arrows*) appear in posterior lung regions. Corresponding to these changes are a widening of both $\dot{V}A$ and $\dot{Q}$ distributions and an increase in $\dot{Q}s/\dot{Q}T$ to 7.4%. **C,** The scan and data are shown for the same individual after application of 10 cm H_2O of PEEP. Very little change is observed in the areas of atelectasis, and $\dot{V}A/\dot{Q}$ matching is further worsened, with the development of a bimodal ventilation distribution and a further increase in $\dot{Q}s/\dot{Q}T$ to 11.1%. These changes are accompanied by a drop in Pao_2 from 162 to 137 mm Hg. (Adapted from Tokics L, Hedenstierna G, Strandberg A, et al: Lung collapse and gas exchange during general anesthesia: Effects of spontaneous breathing, muscle paralysis and positive end-expiratory pressure. Anesthesiology 66:157, 1987.)

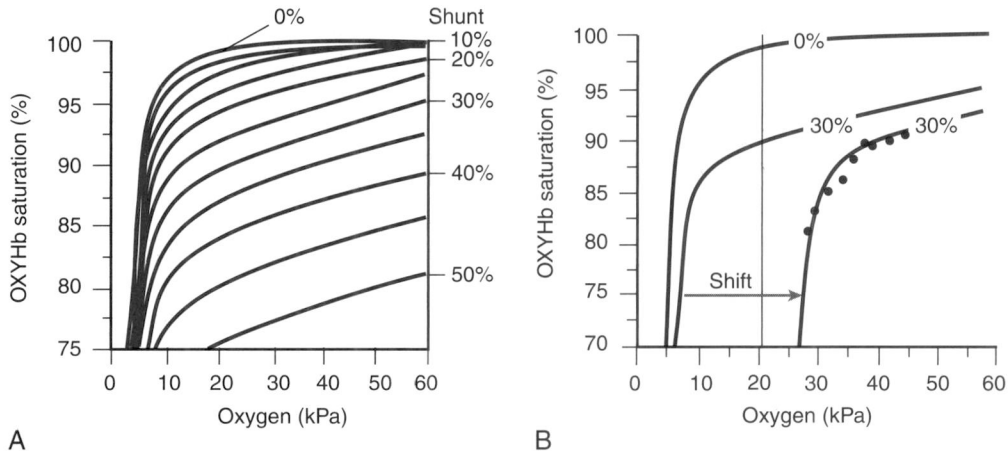

Figure 36–7 Hemoglobin-oxygen (OXYHb) saturation versus inspired partial pressure of oxygen (P_{O_2}). The curves are plotted by changing inspired P_{O_2} in a stepwise fashion. **A,** A series of theoretical curves obtained by calculating the effect of different degrees of right-to-left shunt. Increasing shunt displaces the curves downward. **B,** The curve on the left of the graph (0%) is from a normal subject. The middle curve (30%) represented a 30% right-to-left shunt from the 30% curve seen in **A**. The curve on the right of this graph is from a patient undergoing thoracotomy for esophageal surgery. The points cannot be fitted by any of the shunt curve, but the fit is quite good when the 30% curve is shifted to the right. This implies a combination of shunt and $\dot{V}_A/\dot{Q}$ mismatch. (Adapted from Jones JG, Jones SE: Discriminating between the effect of shunt and reduced V_A/Q on arterial oxygen saturation is particularly useful in clinical practice. J Clin Monit Comput 16:337, 2000.)

during continuous axial rotation in patients with acute lung injury[24] and to examine the effects on pulmonary gas exchange of cardiac surgery,[25] general anesthesia,[26] thoracic epidural block,[27] permissive hypercapnia,[28] and pneumoperitoneum.[29] Although this technique cannot yet be used as an on-line monitor, future development of rapid, inexpensive gas analyzers may allow continuous monitoring of $\dot{V}_A/\dot{Q}$ using this principle.

A noninvasive method of assessing the independent effects of shunt and $\dot{V}_A/\dot{Q}$ mismatching on arterial P_{O_2} is to plot simultaneously arterial O_2 saturation versus inspired P_{O_2} (Fig. 36-7).[30]

MEASUREMENT OF BLOOD GAS TENSIONS

The most straightforward method of ascertaining Pa_{O_2} is to measure it directly from a blood sample, usually by using a Clark electrode, which incorporates platinum and reference electrodes in an electrolyte bath (see Chapter 41). When a negative polarizing voltage is applied to the platinum electrode, O_2 molecules in solution are reduced by electrons from the electrode. The electrons from the cathode react as follows:

$$O_2 + 2H_2O + 2e^- \rightarrow H_2O_2 + 2OH^-$$
$$H_2O_2 + 2e^- \rightarrow 2OH^- \qquad (15)$$

Each molecule of O_2 is therefore reduced to two hydroxyl ions by four electrons. In the Clark electrode, the electrolyte solution is separated from the fluid being measured (e.g., blood) by a thin O_2-permeable membrane. The current generated is proportional to P_{O_2} within the sample.

When CO_2 is equilibrated with an aqueous solution, the concentration of carbonic acid is proportional to the P_{CO_2}.

$$H_2CO_3 = \alpha \, P_{CO_2} \qquad (16)$$

$$H_2CO_3 \leftrightarrow H^+ + HCO_3^- \qquad (17)$$

$$[H^+] = k \frac{P_{CO_2}}{[HCO_3^-]} \qquad (18)$$

In these equations, α is a constant, and k is a constant that equals 24 if the units are nanomoles/L for $[H^+]$, mm Hg for P_{CO_2}, and mmol/L for $[HCO_3^-]$. P_{CO_2} electrodes work by measuring the change in pH induced when blood equilibrates with a potassium chloride–sodium bicarbonate solution.[31]

The history of the development of blood gas analysis has been described by Severinghaus and Astrup[32] and that of O_2 monitoring in general by Severinghaus.[33] To obviate the need to withdraw blood samples for P_{O_2} analysis, intra-arterial P_{O_2} monitors have been developed. Initial attempts to use a Clark-type electrode were confounded by problems of drift and blood coagulation. This has been largely replaced by a fiberoptic technique, based on the property of O_2 to absorb energy from excited electrons in a fluorescent dye. Incident light is used to elevate electrons in the dye to a higher energy state. These excited electrons may then return to a lower energy level, emitting a photon in the process. Molecular O_2, by absorbing the energy, inhibits the photon emission. This process, called *fluorescence quenching*, is related to the P_{O_2}.[34]

A system using this technique (Diametrics Medical, St. Paul, MN), which has a ruthenium indicator to measure P_{O_2}, also incorporates an optical absorbance technique to measure P_{CO_2} and pH. Blood pH is measured by continuous monitoring of the absorbance of a pH-sensitive dye (i.e., phenol red) in polyacrylamide gel. At low pH, the color of the dye is yellow-orange; at high pH, it is dark red. Pulses of a green monochromatic light beam (wavelength of 555 nm) are transmitted along an optical fiber through the dye and reflected by a microscopic mirror. Pulses of red light (660 nm) are synchronized between the green pulses. The red light, the absorption of which is unaffected by pH changes, serves as a reference. Blood pH is related to the ratio of the intensities of the green and red light returned through the fiberoptic beam to the analyzer. Pco_2 measurement uses the same principle, in which the pH indicator with a fixed concentration of bicarbonate is sealed within a gas-permeable membrane that is impermeable to H^+ ions. CO_2 molecules diffusing into the cell liberate H^+ ions from water. Pco_2 can then be calculated from the measured pH (see Equation 18).

The fiberoptic probes of commercially available systems are somewhat fragile, and the probes can be subject to movement artifact. However, *bias*, the mean difference between instrument measurements and traditional blood gas analysis, is typically 5%, and *imprecision*,[35] the standard deviation of these differences, is about 10%, which are quite acceptable for clinical purposes. The 90% response time for pH is 70 to 80 seconds and 140 seconds for Po_2 and Pco_2; there is minimal drift over several days.[36] Use of continuous arterial blood gas monitoring systems has been described in several clinical settings[36-39] and its use reviewed.[40] Umbilical artery insertion of a probe

has been successfully used to monitor blood gas parameters in neonates.

When arterial puncture cannot be achieved or may be technically difficult (e.g., in neonates), capillary Po_2 may approximate the arterial value, particularly if the sampling site (e.g., heel) is prewarmed, causing an abundance of local blood flow relative to local tissue O_2 consumption. Although capillary Po_2 tends to be lower than the arterial value because of the shallow slope of the upper part of the Hb-O_2 dissociation curve, capillary O_2 saturation approximates arterial O_2 saturation (Sao_2) (capillary value is usually slightly lower).

Temperature Correction of Blood Gases

Conventionally, the temperature of the electrodes in blood gas analyzers is maintained at 37°C, but rarely is a patient's body temperature exactly this temperature (see Chapter 41). A blood gas sample from a patient is warmed or cooled to 37°C before analysis. Temperature changes cause alterations in gas solubility in plasma and O_2 affinity for hemoglobin. Because solubility and Hb-O_2 affinity decrease as temperature rises (and vice versa), if a syringe of blood is gas tight and no bubbles are present, heating the sample will elevate blood gas tensions and reduce the pH; cooling the sample will cause the reverse. Several algorithms exist for temperature correction, allowing the true partial pressure, predictive of physical and chemical activity at the tissue, to be calculated (Table 36-1).

Table 36–1   Algorithms for correction to body temperature of blood gas tensions measured at 37°C

pH

$$\Delta pH / \Delta T = -0.0146 + 0.0065 (7.4 - pH_m)$$

$$\Delta pH / \Delta T = -0.015$$

$$\Delta pH / \Delta T = -0.0147 + 0.0065 (7.4 - pH_m)^*$$

$$\Delta pH / \Delta T = -0.0146$$

Pco_2

$$\Delta \log_{10} Pco_2 / \Delta T = 0.019^*$$

$$\Delta \log_{10} Pco_2 / \Delta T = 0.021$$

Po_2

$$\Delta \log_{10} Po_2 / \Delta T = \left(\frac{0.0252}{0.243(Po_2 / 100)^{3.88} + 1} \right) + 0.00564$$

$$\Delta \log_{10} Po_2 / \Delta T = 0.0052 + 0.27 \left[1 - 10^{-0.13(100 - Sao_2)} \right]$$

$$\Delta \log_{10} Po_2 / \Delta T = \frac{5.49 \times 10^{-11} Po_2^{3.88} + 0.071^*}{9.72 \times 10^{-9} Po_2^{3.88} + 2.3}$$

$$\Delta \log_e Po_2 / \Delta T = \frac{0.012(Po_{2m}/714) + (So_2/100)(1 - So_2/100)(Hb/0.6) - 0.073}{Po_{2m}/714 + So_2/100(1 - So_2/100)(Hb/0.6)} \cdot (T - 37)$$

$So_2 \leq 95\%$: $\Delta \log_{10} Pco_2 / \Delta T = 0.31$

$So_2 > 95\%$: $\Delta \log_{10} Pco_2 / \Delta T = 0.032 - 0.0268 e^{(0.3So_2 - 30)}$

*National Committee for Clinical Laboratory Standards (NCCLS) approved standard.[41]
Hb, blood hemoglobin concentration in g/dL; pH_m and Po_{2m}, pH and Po_2 values measured at an electrode temperature of 37°C; Po_2, partial pressure of oxygen in mm Hg; So_2, hemoglobin-oxygen (Hb-O_2) saturation in percent; T, temperature in degrees centigrade (°C). Data from Ashwood ER, Kost G, Kenny M: Temperature correction of blood-gas and pH measurements. Clin Chem 29:1877, 1983, and Siggaard-Andersen O, Wimberley PD, Gothgen I, Siggaard-Andersen M: A mathematical model of the hemoglobin-oxygen dissociation curve of human blood and of the oxygen partial pressure as a function of temperature. Clin Chem 30:1646, 1984.)

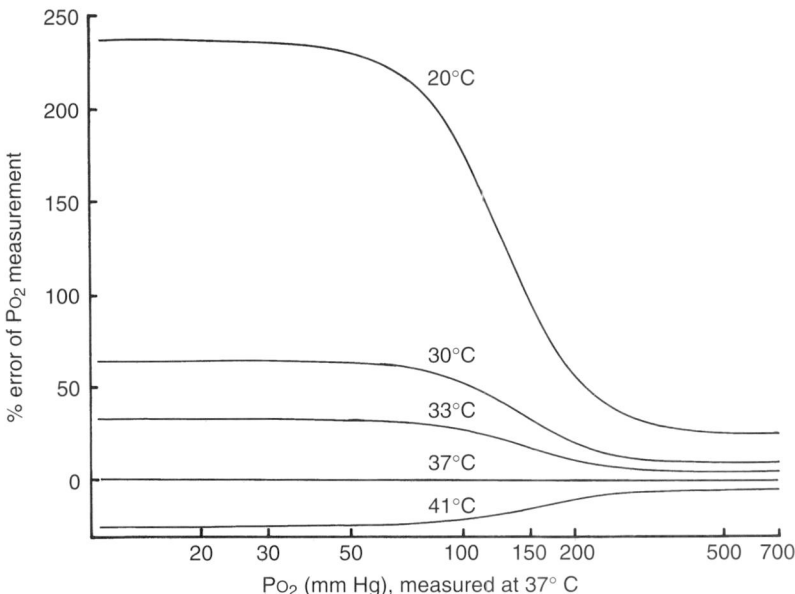

Figure 36–8 Temperature correction of blood P_{O_2}: percentage error of P_{O_2} measurement at various body temperatures with the blood gas electrode at 37°C. If the patient's temperature is 20°C, a P_{O_2} measurement performed at 37°C would overestimate the true value by more than 200%. The curves demonstrate that the percentage of error is greater for venous values ($P_{O_2} < 100$ mm Hg) than for arterial measurements ($P_{O_2} > 300$ mm Hg). (Adapted from Camporesi EM, Moon RE: Arterial blood gas values should be corrected for body temperature during hypothermia. *In* Fyman PN, Gotta AW [eds]: Controversies in Cardiovascular Anesthesia. Boston, Kluwer Academic Publishers, 1988, p 35.)

The algorithms approved by the National Committee for Clinical Laboratory Standards[41] and most commonly used in clinical instruments sold in the United States are provided in Table 36-1.

Application of the equation for P_{O_2} is shown in Figure 36-6. The P_{O_2} derived from a 37°C electrode is overestimated if the patient is hypothermic and underestimated if the patient is febrile. At high P_{O_2} values (>400 mm Hg) the effect is small, because hemoglobin is fully saturated in this region. At P_{O_2} values below 100 mm Hg, however, the degree of overestimation may be significant. For example, at a patient temperature of 30°C and a P_{O_2} below 80 mm Hg, the true P_{O_2} is overestimated by about 60% unless temperature correction is applied (Fig. 36-8).

Available evidence indicates that, during hypothermia, corrected arterial pH should be maintained in the alkalotic range (i.e., maintain uncorrected pH close to 7.4) (see Chapter 41). In contrast, the analysis previously presented suggests that P_{O_2} values should be corrected for temperature.[42]

Artifactual Effects on Gas Tension Measurement

Handling of arterial blood samples for measurement in a laboratory removed from the patient is important to maintain stability of gas tensions. Gas bubbles in the syringe allow diffusion of O_2 and CO_2 between the blood sample and the bubbles, usually lowering the values in the blood. This is particularly true for high P_{O_2} values, because in this region, O_2 is less soluble in blood. Small bubbles in the syringe tend to have less influence on P_{CO_2}. Removal of all air bubbles before capping the syringe and placing it in ice water can maintain stability of blood gas samples for several hours. Erythrocytes do not contain mitochondria and therefore do not consume O_2, but leukocytes and platelets do, and in the presence of extreme leukocytosis or thrombocytosis, significant O_2 consumption by the blood sample may occur.[43] This may be suspected when P_{O_2} values are inexplicably low in the presence of high leukocyte or platelet counts. Inhibition of cellular O_2 consumption may be accomplished by adding to the sample sodium fluoride[44] (available in evacuated tubes used for collection of blood for glucose measurement) or cyanide. Dilution of blood samples with saline (as may occur when drawing an insufficient volume of *dead space* from an indwelling arterial catheter before obtaining a sample) tends to lower P_{CO_2}, with less effect on P_{O_2}.

Bedside Clinical Interpretation of Arterial P_{O_2} and P_{CO_2} Measurements

Adequacy of O_2 exchange can be assessed at the bedside by examining the relationship between P_{O_2} and inspired O_2 fraction (F_{IO_2}). Although the A-a gradient (see Equation 6) varies with F_{IO_2}, the a/A ratio does not. A low a/A ratio (<0.8) implies abnormal gas exchange. A simpler alternative is to calculate P_{aO_2}/F_{IO_2} (i.e., P/F ratio). Although this varies with F_{IO_2}, it depends less on F_{IO_2} than the A-a gradient (Table 36-2). P_{aO_2}/F_{IO_2} normally exceeds 400 mm Hg. As gas exchange worsens, this ratio declines.

Table 36–2 A-a gradient and P_{aO_2}/F_{IO_2} in a person with normal pulmonary gas exchange*

F_{IO_2}	P_{AO_2}	a/A Ratio	P_{aO_2}	P_{aO_2}/F_{IO_2}	A-a Gradient
0.21	102	0.85	87	412	15
0.50	312	0.85	265	530	47
1.00	673	0.85	572	572	101
0.21	102	0.50	51	242	51
0.50	312	0.50	156	312	156
1.00	673	0.50	337	337	337

*Assuming $P_{aCO_2} = 40$ mm Hg, barometric pressure = 760 mm Hg, body temperature = 37°C, and respiratory exchange ratio (R) = 0.8.
A-a gradient, alveolar-arterial gradient; P_{aO_2}/F_{IO_2} (P/F ratio), arterial oxygen tension/fractional inspired oxygen concentration.

Table 36–3   Calculation of the VD/VT ratio*

$\dot{V}_E$	$\dot{V}_E \times Paco_2$	VD/VT
5	200	0.4
6	240	0.5
8	300	0.6
10	400	0.7
15	600	0.8
30	1200	0.9

*Calculated from measured $\dot{V}_E$ at $Paco_2 = 40$ mm Hg.
Interpretation of the adequacy of carbon dioxide exchange can
be inferred from the VD/VT ratio. Although this measurement is
usually not readily available, it can be estimated indirectly by
examining $Paco_2$ in the context of the minute ventilation using
the simple equation of $\dot{V}_E \times Paco_2$.
$Paco_2$, partial pressure of arterial carbon dioxide; $\dot{V}_E$, minute
ventilation; VD/VT, dead space expressed as a fraction of the
tidal volume.

CO_2 exchange can be assessed from the VD/VT ratio
(Equation 12). Although the VD/VT ratio is usually not
readily available, it can be estimated indirectly by examining $Paco_2$ in the context of the minute ventilation ($\dot{V}_E$)
by the simple calculation of $\dot{V}_E \times Paco_2$ (normally about
200 L/min/mm Hg during spontaneous breathing and
400 to 500 L/min/mm Hg during mechanical ventilation). As VD/VT increases (worsening CO_2 exchange), the
minute ventilation required to maintain a normal Pco_2
rises, as does the $\dot{V}_E \times Paco_2$ product (Table 36-3).

TRANSCUTANEOUS GAS TENSION MEASUREMENT

In areas of the skin where local blood flow exceeds the
amount required for local O_2 consumption, capillary Po_2
may approximate Pao_2. This may be particularly true if
the local area is warmed. This principle has been
exploited by manufacturers of transcutaneous Po_2 measuring instruments. These devices usually consist of a
small electrode that is attached with adhesive to the skin.
The skin is locally warmed to 40°C or 41°C. O_2 from capillaries diffuses through the intact skin into a Clark-type
electrode that measures Po_2 directly. This value usually
correlates well with Pao_2.[45] However, in the presence of
peripheral vasoconstriction[46] or with thick (adult) skin,
the measurement may be erroneous. A reduction in cardiac output tends to result in an artifactual decrease in
transcutaneous Po_2 because of the ensuing cutaneous
hypoxia. Peripheral vascular disease also reduces the
transcutaneous Po_2 value.[47,48]

Transcutaneous gas monitoring is particularly useful in
infants, in whom local skin blood flow tends to be high
and in whom repeated withdrawals of arterial blood may
cause anemia. These instruments require frequent calibration. The time constant of measurement is relatively
long, and a sudden decrease in Pao_2 may not be detectable
quickly enough to allow a timely therapeutic response.
Skin burns have sometimes resulted from prolonged
application of these devices.

Transcutaneous Pco_2 monitoring devices are also available.[49] Because changes in transcutaneous Pco_2 are slow
to detect apnea or airway disconnects, measurement of
these values by monitors is less widely used than monitoring of end-tidal CO_2 (see "Expired Gas Analysis").

MEASUREMENT OF OXYGEN SATURATION

Several species of hemoglobin may exist in blood, such as
oxyhemoglobin (HbO_2), deoxygenated hemoglobin
(HHb), carboxyhemoglobin (HbCO), and methemoglobin (HbMet). To avoid ambiguity, the following definitions have been proposed.[50]

$$So_2 = HbO_2/(HbO_2 + HHb) \qquad (19)$$

$$HbO_2 \text{ fraction} = HbO_2/\text{Total Hb} \qquad (20)$$

So_2 is most commonly reported as a percentage, obtained by
multiplying the value obtained from Equation 19 by 100.

Measurement of Sao_2 is an alternative method to Po_2 for
assessing arterial blood oxygenation. The fact that absorption and reflectance spectra of hemoglobin are affected by
its oxygenation allows for convenient optical methods of
measurement. The traditional method for monitoring Sao_2
is to observe the skin and mucous membranes for cyanosis.
In 1947, a systematic comparison of the clinical detection
of a cyanosis by medical staff and blood O_2 saturation
measurement with an ear oximeter in normal volunteers
demonstrated the poor accuracy of cyanosis as an indicator of hypoxemia.[51] In this study, a total of 7204 observations of skin and mucous membrane color were made in
normal volunteers breathing air or hypoxic gas over a
measured Sao_2 range of 71% to 100%. False-positive diagnosis of cyanosis was common; cyanosis was diagnosed
in 37% of 4587 observations despite a measured Sao_2 of
91% to 100%. However, in 1723 observations of hypoxic
volunteers with a measured Sao_2 between 71% and 80%,
normal color was observed in 12% of cases.

Cyanosis seems to be correlated best with the quantity
of deoxygenated arterial blood. It has been suggested that
for cyanosis to be detectable, 5 g/dL of deoxygenated
hemoglobin must be present in the arterial blood,[52]
although published evidence is consistent with a lower
detection threshold[53] (Fig. 36-9). Nevertheless, the
threshold for visual detection of cyanosis depends on
total hemoglobin concentration. If 3 g/dL of desaturated
blood is required to detect cyanosis by visual observation,
at a total hemoglobin concentration of 15 g/dL, cyanosis
occurs when Sao_2 is below 80%, compared with 66% for
a hemoglobin level of 9 g/dL. The evident inaccuracy and
uncertainty inherent in attempts to assess oxygenation
by visual inspection have led to its replacement with
highly successful quantitative methods.

Carbon Monoxide Oximetry

Simultaneous measurement of several hemoglobin
species with different absorption spectra can be accomplished by using multiple-wavelength absorption with at

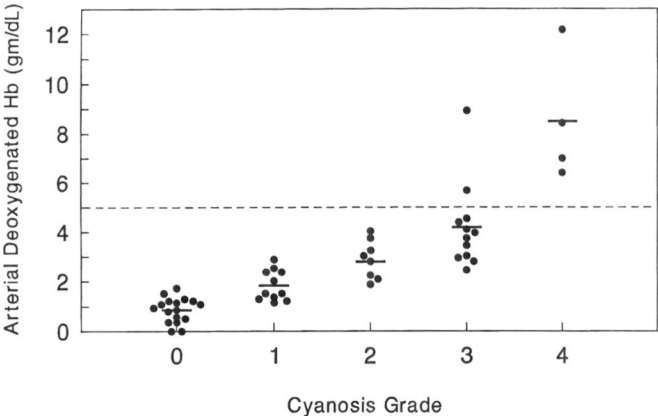

Figure 36–9 Quantity of deoxygenated hemoglobin (Hb) in arterial blood as a function of the degree of cyanosis. Traditionally, it has been assumed that 5 g/dL of deoxygenated hemoglobin is required for the detection of cyanosis, but mild cyanosis can be observed at lower values. (Data from Stadie WC: The oxygen of the arterial and venous blood in pneumonia and its relation to sepsis. J Exp Med 30:215, 1919.)

least one wavelength for each component hemoglobin.[54] This principle has been incorporated into clinical instruments capable of measurement of a blood sample in a cuvette within 1 to 2 minutes. Commonly available devices measure hemoglobin HHb, HbO_2, HbCO, and HbMet, and except when the patient has been administered a dye (e.g., methylene blue[55,56]) or there is a fifth hemoglobin species (e.g. fetal hemoglobin [HbF], cyanmethemoglobin), they are susceptible to few artifacts. The presence of HbF tends to produce an artifactual increase in the measured HbCO.[57]

Transcutaneous Oximetry

The fact that different hemoglobin species, particularly reduced hemoglobin and oxyhemoglobin (HbO_2) have different absorption spectra suggests the possibility of using absorption of light in vivo to calculate arterial hemoglobin O_2 saturation (SaO_2). A dual-wavelength system can be used to estimate SaO_2 if the following conditions are met:
1. The light is transilluminating arterial blood.
2. There are no significant quantities of other hemoglobin species, such as HbMet and HbCO.
3. The absorption of light by tissue is negligible.

The first condition may be met, for example, by transilluminating the earlobe, provided the tissue is kept warm. Under these circumstances, the ratio of blood flow to tissue O_2 consumption is relatively high, and the capillary blood is therefore predominantly arterial. The second condition is met under most clinical circumstances, in which the total of other hemoglobin species is usually less than 5% of the total. The third condition can be ensured by appropriate choice of wavelength.

Dual-wavelength oximeters became available in the 1940s. An eight-wavelength ear oximeter was produced by Hewlett-Packard,[58] in which active heating of the ear lobe by the sensor maintained a high proportion of arterial blood in the capillary bed. However, its cumbersome size prevented widespread use.

Pulse Oximetry

One of the major objections to the use of ear oximeters is the required assumption that the earlobe contains predominantly arterial blood, because these instruments had no means of differentiating between arterial and venous hemoglobin. The pulse oximeter is able to make this differentiation by assuming that the pulsatile portion of the signal is entirely arterial blood. This is almost always true except under unusual clinical circumstances, such as when there are prominent venous pulsations as in tricuspid regurgitation.[59]

The principle of pulse oximetry is shown schematically in Figure 36-10. The light passing through tissue is absorbed by tissue and by venous and arterial blood. The ratio S is calculated at two wavelengths of light, usually around 660 nm (red) and 940 nm (infrared), for which the following relationships apply:

$$S = \frac{AC_{660}/DC_{660}}{AC_{940}/DC_{940}} \qquad (21)$$

In Equation 21, AC_{660} and AC_{940} are pulsatile components of absorbance at wavelengths of 660 and 940 nm, respectively. DC_{660} and DC_{940} are the corresponding steady-state components. S is empirically related to O_2 saturation and incorporated into the design of the instrument. It has been proposed that the assessment of SaO_2 by pulse oximetry be designated as SpO_2.[50]

In practice, pulse oximeters use two light-emitting diodes (LEDs) and one photo diode as transmitting and sensing transducers, usually placed on opposite sides of a digit. The two LEDs are activated alternatively. The ratio S is calculated electronically; from the value of S, SpO_2 is derived by an internally stored algorithm.

One drawback of oximetry is that it is rather insensitive to large changes in arterial PO_2 at the high end of the Hb-O_2 dissociation curve, where large changes in PO_2 are associated with small changes in SpO_2. Another problem is that because only two wavelengths are used, only two species of hemoglobin can be resolved (assumed to be

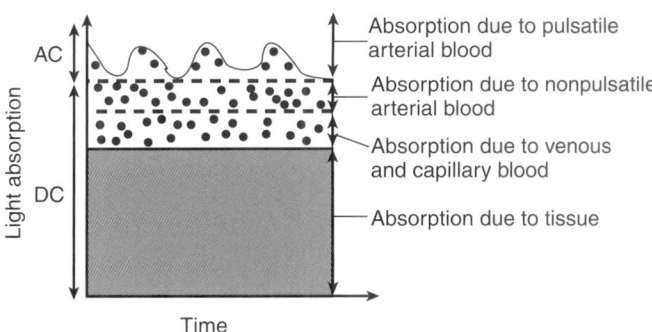

Figure 36–10 Principle of pulse oximetry. Light passing through tissue containing blood is absorbed by tissue and by arterial, capillary, and venous blood. Usually, only the arterial blood is pulsatile. Light absorption may therefore be split into a pulsatile component (AC) and a constant or nonpulsatile component (DC). Hemoglobin O_2 saturation may be obtained by application of Equation 19 in the text. (Data from Tremper KK, Barker SJ: Pulse oximetry. Anesthesiology 70:98, 1989.)

oxyhemoglobin and reduced hemoglobin). Depending on their absorption spectrum, significant quantities of other hemoglobin species may not be readily detected. Other disadvantages of pulse oximetry include inability to obtain a signal of sufficient amplitude during hypothermia or low cardiac output, interference by electrocautery and a variety of artifacts described subsequently. As a monitor of the adequacy of ventilation, because Sp_{O_2} is only minimally affected by P_{CO_2} (by the Bohr effect), pulse oximetry may fail to warn of inadequate ventilation, particularly when circumstances permit apneic oxygenation.[60] Pulse oximetry has been well reviewed by numerous investigators.[61-55]

Newer Pulse Oximeters

Although the inherently reliability of pulse oximetry has led to its wide use in anesthesia and critical care, remaining problems include motion sensitivity, causing false alarms and erroneous measurements, and hypoperfusion, causing loss of signal (see Chapter 30). Several manufacturers have developed proprietary methods to address these problems based on analysis of frequency, waveform morphology, or saturation.[66,67]

Published evidence supports the ability of new generation pulse oximeters to detect hypoxemic episodes more reliably than conventional devices under conditions of patient motion[68] and hypothermic hypoperfusion,[69] although they often falsely indicate hypoxemia, particularly when intra-aortic balloon pumps are used.[70]

Reflectance Oximeters

To assess arterial oxygenation when it is impossible to provide a transmission path, reflectance oximetry has been exploited. Reflectance oximetry has been used to monitor fetal scalp during labor.[71] An esophageal probe has been developed to monitor Sp_{O_2} when extremities are unavailable or have a pulse of insufficient amplitude.[72] Monitors using forehead skin probes are also commercially available.[73,74] Forehead sensors appear less susceptible to motion artifact during exercise, and during

hypothermia, they respond more quickly to changes in blood O_2 saturation than finger sensors (Fig. 36-11). However, forehead sensors can produce falsely low Sp_{O_2} values, particularly in the supine or head-down position. Measurement of gastric mucosal Sp_{O_2} has the potential to provide a monitor of splanchnic perfusion.[75]

Multiple-Wavelength Pulse Oximeters

Current pulse oximeters use only two wavelengths and can resolve only two hemoglobin species. Use of additional wavelengths provides the possibility of measuring additional hemoglobins. There are no commercially available devices, although research in this area is ongoing.

Use of Pulse Oximetry

Although oximetry has been available since the 1940s, the development of pulse oximetry triggered its wide acceptance because of the latter's reliability and convenience. The reliability and ease of use of such monitors has led to incorporation of their use within standards of care. Pulse oximetry has become a standard component of anesthesia monitoring, and it has gained acceptance in postanesthesia care units (PACUs) and intensive care units (ICUs) and for patients undergoing a variety of diagnostic procedures such as gastrointestinal endoscopy. The wide application of pulse oximetry attests to the clinical utility of this major advance in monitoring.

Intraoperative Monitoring

In a trial in which 20,802 patients scheduled for surgery were randomly assigned to receive monitoring with pulse oximetry or not, hypoxemia was detected during anesthesia 20 times and hypoventilation three times as frequently in the pulse oximetry group.[76,77] These differences persisted in the PACU, and bronchospasm, atelectasis, and bradycardia also were detected more frequently in the group monitored with oximetry. On the basis of favorable clinical experience with this technology, pulse oximetry is now a standard monitoring technique during anesthesia and monitored sedation.

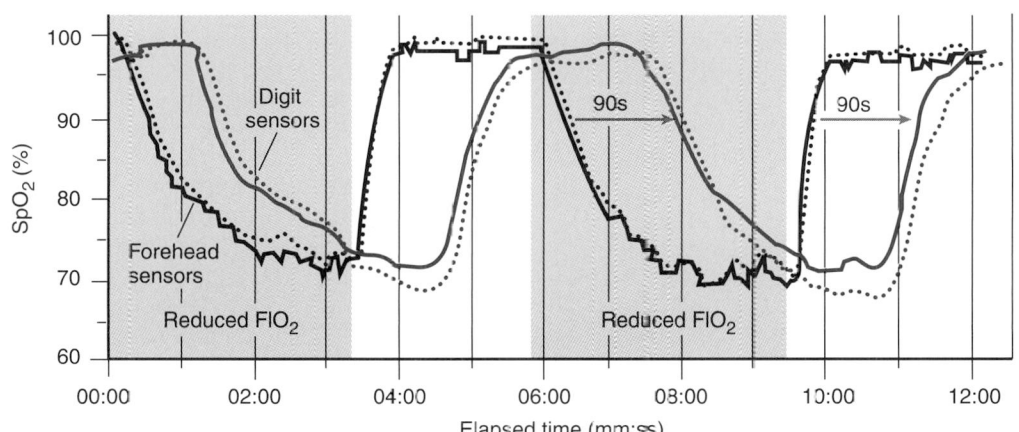

Figure 36–11 Effect of pulse oximeter probe replacement on delay from onset of hypoxemia to a drop in the measured Sp_{O_2}. During cold-induced peripheral vasoconstriction in normal volunteers, the onset of hypoxemia was detected more quickly using an oximeter probe on the forehead compared with the finger. Other studies have shown a similar advantage for pulse oximeter probes placed on the ear. (From Bebout DE, Mannheimer PD, Wun C-C: Site-dependent differences in the time to detect changes in saturation during low perfusion. Crit Care Med 29:A115, 2002.)

Postoperative Monitoring

In patients admitted to an ICU after elective cardiac surgery, the use of pulse oximetry has been reported to reduce the number of arterial blood gas analyses and to increase the probability of detecting hypoxemic episodes.[78] Continuous monitoring of patients for up to several days after surgery has been reported to detect hypoxemic episodes.[79-94] In this setting, some of the low readings can be caused by motion artifact, the elimination of which requires appropriate methods.[95]

These studies indicate that significant desaturation (SpO_2 of 80% to 85%) is relatively common. Desaturation also occurs in some patients before surgery,[86,87,89,90] and there is evidence that the existence of preoperative hypoxemic episodes may predict desaturation postoperatively. Hypoxemia is often correlated with peak effects of analgesia.[84,91] Detection or prevention of such episodes may be beneficial, because arterial desaturation can be correlated with an increase in heart rate[83,85] and electrocardiographic evidence of myocardial ischemia.[85,88]

Errors in Pulse Oximetry

Because pulse oximeters are dual-wavelength devices, the presence of hemoglobin species other than HHb and HbO_2 must therefore result in erroneous readings (Table 36-4).

Carboxyhemoglobin

The effect of HbCO may be discerned by examining its absorption spectrum. At 920 nm, HbCO has an extremely low absorbance and therefore does not contribute to total absorbance. At 660 nm, however, HbCO has an absorbance very similar to that of HbO_2, and SpO_2 will therefore be falsely high. This effect has been measured in a canine study in which the pulse oximeter reading of Nellcor and Ohmeda pulse oximeters was approximated[96] by the following formula:

$$SpO_2^* = \frac{[HbO_2] + 0.9 \cdot [HbCO]}{[Hb]} \quad (22)$$

In Equation 22, SpO_2^* is the pulse oximeter reading.

Using a pulse oximeter in the presence of HbCO provides a falsely high estimate of arterial SO_2. In that study, when HbCO was 50%, SpO_2 was approximately 95%. In human cases of carbon monoxide poisoning, a similar error has been observed.[97-101] In 30 patients with HbCO levels ranging from 25.2% to 54% (mean, 36.9%), Hampson[101] observed that each 8% increase in HbCO resulted in only a 1% decrease in SpO_2 reading.

Methemoglobin

HbMet has a larger absorbance than either of the two major species of hemoglobin at 940 nm but simulates hemoglobin at 660 nm. At high SaO_2 levels (>85%) the reading underestimates the true value; at a low SaO_2 (<85%), the value is falsely high.[102,103] In the presence of high HbMet concentrations, the measured SpO_2 approaches 85%, independently of the actual arterial oxygenation.

Other Toxic Alterations in Hemoglobin

Sulfhemoglobin, which can form after exposure to certain drugs and chemicals, and cyanmethemoglobin, a product of the pharmacologic induction of methemoglobinemia for treatment of cyanide poisoning, are nonfunctional hemoglobins. Although sulfhemoglobinemia is known to produce errors in CO oximetry,[104-106] usually with a false reading of methemoglobin, the effects of these species on pulse oximetry have not been reported.

Structural Hemoglobinopathies

In neonates, there is a large proportion of HbF. Because HbF has almost the same absorption spectrum as hemoglobin A, it has almost no measurable effect on SpO_2.[63]

SpO_2 has been reported to be accurate in patients with hemoglobin S (HbS) disease when SaO_2 determined by this method was compared with SaO_2 obtained by using in vitro oximetry,[107-109] although it is possible that the presence of HbS produces a similar artifact in both types of instrument. During sickle cell crisis, it has been reported that SpO_2 overestimates SaO_2 measured by CO oximetry[110] by an average of 6.9%. Patients with sickle cell disease have a rightward shift of the Hb-O_2 dissociation curve (i.e., increased P_{50}), and at any given PaO_2 value, the SpO_2 is lower than the normal Hb-O_2 dissociation curve would predict.

Pulse oximetry evaluation has been reported in a patient with hemoglobin H anemia. Two different pulse oximeters read 93% and 95% (artifactually high), respectively, in a patient who had a hematocrit of 9%.[111] Independent measurements of SaO_2 with which to compare the pulse oximeter readings were not reported.

Hemoglobin Köln, an unstable hemoglobin, has been associated with an artifactual reduction of 8% to 10% in SpO_2 reading.[112,113]

Hemoglobin Substitutes

Because of changes in their optical absorption spectra, hemoglobin substitutes could affect the readings of pulse oximeters or CO oximeters (see Chapter 47). Appropriate testing would have to incorporate independent measurement of O_2 content; however, little information exists on the effects of hemoglobin substitutes on CO oximetry or pulse oximetry. Artificial hemoglobin solutions such as diaspirin–cross-linked hemoglobin[114] and bovine polymerized hemoglobin (oxygen carrier-201)[115,116] have no apparent effect on SpO_2, at least after infusion of relatively low doses and under normoxic conditions. Whether administration of these solutions may artifactually increase SpO_2 readings has not been firmly established. Some errors are likely. An in vitro study of five hemoglobin substitutes suggested that CO oximeters could provide clinically acceptable measurements of total hemoglobin concentration, although measurement of components (e.g., methemoglobin) might be inaccurate.[117] In dogs, hemoglobin glutamer-200 administration (Oxyglobin, Biopure, Cambridge, MA) does not appear to affect significantly the readings of one commercially available CO oximeter (Nova Biomedical, Waltham MA).[118] The availability of a 128-nm-wavelength CO oximeter offers the potential for resolving HbF, sulfhemoglobin, and artificial blood substitutes.[119]

Hemoglobin Concentration

At normal oxygenation levels in humans, over a range of hemoglobin levels from 2.3 to 8.7 g/dL, SpO_2 accurately

Table 36–4 Artifacts in pulse oximetry

Factor	Effect	References
Toxic Alterations in Hemoglobin		
Carboxyhemoglobin (COHb)	Slight reduction of the assessment of Sao_2 by pulse oximetry (Spo_2) (i.e., overestimates fraction of Hb available for O_2 transport)	97-101
Cyanmethemoglobin	Not reported	
Methemoglobin (MetHb)	At high levels of MetHb, Spo_2 approaches 85%, independent of actual oxygen saturation (Sao_2)	102,103
Sulfhemoglobin	Not reported (affects CO oximetry by producing a falsely high reading of MetHb)	104-106
Structural Hemoglobinopathies		
Hemoglobin F	No significant effect	63
Hemoglobin H	No significant effect (i.e., overestimates fraction of Hb available for O_2 transport)	111
Hemoglobin Köln	Artifactual reduction in Spo_2 of 8-10%	112,113
Hemoglobin S	No significant effect	
Hemoglobin Replacement Solutions		
Diaspirin cross-linked hemoglobin	No significant effect	114
Bovine polymerized hemoglobin (oxygen carrier-201)	No significant effect	115,116
Dyes		
Fluorescein	No significant effect	62,125
Indigo carmine	Transient decrease	
Indocyanine green	Transient decrease	62,125
Isosulfan blue (patent blue V)	No significant effect at low dose; prolonged reduction in Spo_2 at high dose	130-132
Methylene blue	Transient, marked decrease in Spo_2, lasting up to several minutes; possible secondary effects due to effects on hemodynamics	124-128
Hemoglobin Concentration		
Anemia	If Sao_2 normal: no effect; during hypoxemia, at Hb values less than 14.5 g/dL: progressive underestimation of actual Sao_2	120,121
Polycythemia	No significant effect	122,123
Other Factors		
Acrylic fingernails	No significant effect	
Ambient light interference	Bright light, particularly if flicker frequency is close to a harmonic of light-emitting diode switching frequency, can falsely elevate Spo_2 reading.	64,142
Arterial O_2 saturation	Depends on manufacturer. During hypoxemia, Spo_2 tends to be artifactually low.	5,73,141,303
Blood flow	Reduced amplitude of pulsations can hinder obtaining a reading or cause a falsely low reading.	146,147
Henna	Red henna: no effect; black henna: may block light sufficiently to preclude measurement	134
Jaundice	No effect. Multi-wavelength laboratory oximeters may register a falsely low Sao_2 and a falsely high COHb and MetHb.	135-138
Motion	Movement, especially shivering, may depress Spo_2 reading.	64
Nail polish	Slight decrease in Spo_2 reading, with greatest effect using blue nail polish, or no change	133,304
Sensor contact	"Optical shunting" of light from source to detector directly or by reflection from skin results in falsely low Spo_2 reading.	145
Skin pigmentation	Small errors or no significant effect reported. Deep pigmentation can result in reduced signal.	62
Tape	Transparent tape between sensor and skin has little effect. Falsely low Spo_2 has been reported when smeared adhesive is in the optical path.	139,140
Vasodilatation	Slight decrease	148
Venous pulsation (e.g., tricuspid insufficiency)	Artifactual decrease in Spo_2	59

reflects SaO_2.[120] However, during hypoxia, SpO_2 tends to underestimate SaO_2 to a degree that increases linearly as the hemoglobin concentration falls. In a study by Severinghaus and Koh,[121] at a SaO_2 of 53% and a hemoglobin concentration of 8.2 g/dL, the average measured SpO_2 was approximately 15% low, of which 8% was attributed to anemia (the remaining error was caused by oximeter measurement errors unrelated to hemoglobin concentration).

Polycythemia has no apparent effect on pulse oximeter reading. In children with cyanotic congenital heart disease, many of whom were polycythemic, there was no systematic error in the SaO_2 reading that could be attributed to high hemoglobin concentration.[122,123]

Dyes
Clinically used dyes may also have an effect on pulse oximetry. Methylene blue results in a severe decrease in measured SaO_2.[124-128] Its administration can also cause alterations in cardiac output (i.e., an increase and then a decrease). In the presence of $\dot{V}A/\dot{Q}$ mismatch, this may result in a transient increase and then a decrease in actual SaO_2. The presence of high concentrations of methylene blue in blood can also alter CO oximeter readings such that an artifactual decrease in measured O_2 saturation may result. Quantitative information, however, is lacking.

Indocyanine green causes less artifactual decrease than methylene blue,[125] and a still smaller decrease occurs with indigo carmine.[62,125] Fluorescein injection has no measurable effect.[62,125]

Isosulfan blue (i.e., sulfan blue or patent blue V), a synthetic coal tar dye used to visualize lymphatic vessels for surgical procedures, has a peak absorption[129] at 640 nm and increased absorbance at 660 nm. Its administration has been associated with prolonged artifactual reduction in SpO_2.[130-132] It tends to affect CO oximetry by producing an artifactual increase in methemoglobin and a negative carboxyhemoglobin reading. This phenomenon is not observed with subcutaneous injection of up to 100 mg into an adult.

Nail Polish and Other Nail Pigments
Effects of nail polish have also been measured. Blue nail polish, with absorbance near 660 nm, has the greatest effect, an artifactual decrease, on the SaO_2 reading. Other colors have smaller effects.[133] Red henna, a pigment used for hand and nail decoration in some tropical countries, has no significant effect on SpO_2, although black henna can block enough light to prevent a satisfactory reading.[134]

Bilirubin
High levels of bilirubin have no significant effect on pulse oximeter readings,[135,136] although older types of ear oximeters may measure a falsely low value.[58] In the presence of jaundice, multiple-wavelength laboratory oximeters may also register falsely low SaO_2 and falsely high HbCO and HbMet values.[137,138]

Skin Pigment
Deeply pigmented skin can result in inability to pick up arterial pulsations by a pulse oximeter. Small errors in SaO_2 readings from black individuals have been reported

by some investigators, with others finding no significant effect.[62]

Tape
Four varieties of transparent tape have been shown not to alter SpO_2 measurements between 85% and 100%.[139] However, smeared adhesive caused by reusing a disposable oximeter probe has been reported to cause falsely low SpO_2 readings.[140]

Low Oxygen Saturation
Practical difficulties are associated with in vivo calibration of pulse oximeters in humans at low SaO_2 values. Using normal volunteers and direct measurement of SaO_2 in arterial blood, Severinghaus and associates[141] compared SpO_2 obtained from a variety of pulse oximeters during brief periods of profound hypoxemia. The mean nadir of arterial hemoglobin O_2 saturation was 56%. Within the pulse oximeters tested at that time, there was considerable variation. At 75% SaO_2, the bias (i.e., systematic error) was scattered uniformly around zero, with individual units either overestimating or underestimating the true SaO_2 by as much as 7%. Below 60% SaO_2, most units underestimated the actual SaO_2 (i.e., false low measurement).

Other Factors
Ambient light, particularly fluorescent light, can falsely increase the SpO_2 reading,[64,142] This occurs especially if the flicker frequency of the light is close to a harmonic of the diode switching frequency. Ambient light does not seem to affect readings when oxygenation is normal.[143] An artifact due to an optical interaction between a pulse oximeter probe and the plasma touch screen of an automated data recording system has been reported to cause an artifactual reading of 100%, even with the probe disconnected from the patient.[144] Poor contact of the sensor with the skin can result in direct "optical shunting" of light from source to detector, directly or by reflection from the skin, resulting in a falsely low SpO_2 reading.[145] Reduced blood flow to the extremity results in a diminished signal and can cause inability to obtain an SpO_2 reading[146] or a falsely low reading,[146,147] possibly caused in part by greater fractional tissue consumption of arterial O_2, resulting in a lower saturation in the pulsatile blood component that is measured. There may be a slight reduction (approximately 1%) in measured SpO_2 during the reactive hyperemia that occurs after ischemia in the arms,[148] perhaps due to venous pulsations. Pulse oximetry while using an intra-aortic balloon pump can produce false indication of hypoxemia.[70]

Vasoconstriction or hypotension can result in loss of SpO_2 signal. Successful countermeasures have included topical application of nitroglycerin ointment and digital nerve block is often successful. Topical application of EMLA cream (2.5% lidocaine and 2.5% prilocaine) (Astra Pharmaceuticals, Westborough, MA) to the earlobe, covered by an occlusive plastic dressing for 30 minutes, has been reported to facilitate a reliable signal.[149]

In a cold environment, studies in normal volunteers have shown delayed detection of hypoxemia and re-oxygenation when the probe is on a finger or ear compared with a reflectance forehead sensor[150,151] (see Fig. 36-11).

This suggests that when there is peripheral vasoconstriction, and arterial O_2 saturation may be changing rapidly (e.g., during difficult airway situations), forehead or ear oximetry may provide a more rapid indicator of desaturation.

MIXED VENOUS OXYGEN MONITORING

Mixed venous O_2 saturation ($S\bar{v}O_2$) is related to a number of factors:

$$S\bar{v}O_2 = SaO_2 - \frac{\dot{V}O_2}{13.9 \cdot \dot{Q} \cdot [Hb]} \quad (23)$$

In Equation 23, [Hb] is the hemoglobin concentration (g/dL), 13.9 is a constant (i.e., O_2 combining power of Hb [mL/10 g]), and $\dot{Q}$ is cardiac output. It can be seen that low SaO_2, low $\dot{Q}$, low [Hb], or an elevated O_2 level may decrease SO_2. All these conditions could produce impairment of O_2 delivery to the tissues. This single measurement ($S\bar{v}O_2$) may be uniquely helpful in detecting any condition that may result in impaired tissue oxygenation. $S\bar{v}O_2$ can be monitored by intermittent measurement of blood withdrawn through a pulmonary artery catheter or may be continuously monitored by using a pulmonary artery catheter equipped with fiberoptic bundles. These catheters have two fiberoptic bundles carrying an incident light beam and a reflected light beam. Using the fact that the reflected spectrum of hemoglobin depends on the degree of oxygenation, the appropriate calculations can be performed by the instrument and a continuous display of $S\bar{v}O_2$ provided. Low $S\bar{v}O_2$ (usually less than 60%) may sensitively reflect an abnormality of one or more of the factors on the right-hand side of Equation 23. However, several factors may artifactually elevate $S\bar{v}O_2$, including wedging of the catheter and mitral regurgitation (which tend to bring the catheter tip into contact with arterialized blood), sepsis, and intracardiac or peripheral left-to-right shunts.

Monitoring of $P\bar{v}O_2$ instead of $S\bar{v}O_2$ requires additional considerations. Although $S\bar{v}O_2$ is a function of four variables (Equation 23), other factors acting on the Hb-O_2 binding curve may alter $P\bar{v}O_2$ independently. In Figure 36-12, a normal curve is shown adjacent to curves depicting increased and decreased Hb-O_2 affinity. For the same SaO_2 and $S\bar{v}O_2$ (and the arteriovenous O_2 content difference), substantially different values for $P\bar{v}O_2$ occur under the three conditions. Correct interpretation of $P\bar{v}O_2$ values must therefore depend on the position of the Hb-O_2 dissociation curve, as dictated by pH, PCO_2, body temperature, and erythrocyte 2,3-diphosphoglycerate (DPG) concentration.

$S\bar{v}O_2$ measurement has been carried one step further by Räsänen and coworkers,[152] who have used this instrument (to measure $S\bar{v}O_2$) and a pulse oximeter (to measure SaO_2) to calculate shunt fraction continuously according to Equation 11. Räsänen and colleagues[152] demonstrated that continuous reading of $\dot{Q}s/\dot{Q}_T$ using this principle could be used as a guide to providing an optimal level of continuous positive airway pressure (CPAP) in a group of patients whose tracheas were intubated and in whom lowest $\dot{Q}s/\dot{Q}_T$ was desired. The investigators found that

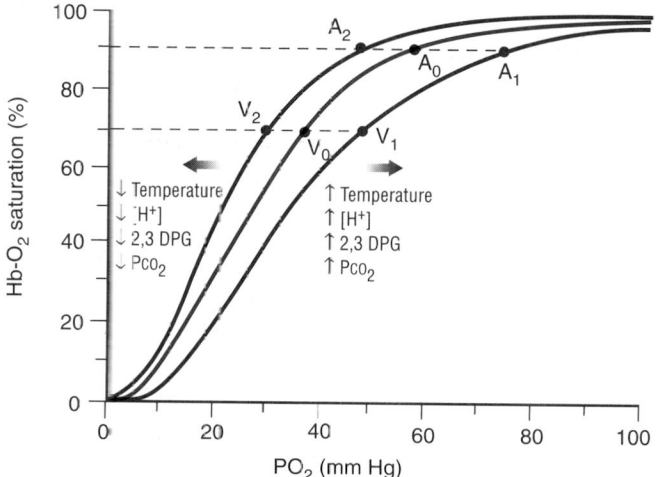

Figure 36–12 Hemoglobin-oxygen (Hb-O_2) saturation curves. *Dotted lines* indicate common arterial and venous values: $SaO_2 = 90\%$ and $S\bar{v}O_2 = 70\%$. The middle curve (A_0, V_0) represents the relationship with a pH of 7.40 and body temperature (T) of 37°C. The right-hand curve (A_1, V_1) would occur if pH = 7.20 or T = 41°C. The left-hand curve (A_2, V_2) represents the relationship when T = 33°C. Increased levels of any of the four factors shown (i.e., temperature, pH [H^+], erythrocyte 2,3-diphosphoglycerate [2,3 DPG], and partial pressure of carbon dioxide [PCO_2]) decreases Hb-O_2 affinity (i.e., rightward shift); decreased levels raise Hb-O_2 affinity (i.e. leftward shift). The same arterial and venous Hb-O_2 saturation under different conditions can therefore result in a wide range of arterial and venous gas tension values.

the on-line method was cost effective and concluded that CPAP therapy could be accurately titrated in the majority of patients with acute respiratory failure by using this noninvasive method to calculate shunt fraction.

TISSUE OXYGENATION

Arterial oxygenation as an indicator of respiratory function may be controversial, because an acceptable arterial O_2 content may not necessarily be associated with adequate tissue oxygenation because of abnormalities of blood flow. A more appropriate monitor of O_2 delivery would measure tissue oxygenation. Tissue PO_2 electrodes have been designed and implemented but have associated problems of sampling bias and tissue destruction. Because of heterogeneity of local tissue blood flow and O_2 consumption, there exists a distribution of tissue PO_2 values rather than a single value as in blood PO_2. Nevertheless, changes in tissue oxygenation have been demonstrated under various clinical conditions.[153]

Another approach is the noninvasive monitoring of O_2 saturation of blood within the tissue. This can be accomplished by transilluminating the tissue with at least two appropriately chosen wavelengths of light.[154] Light within the near-infrared band (650 to 1100 nm) can penetrate tissue reasonably well. Incident light is applied to the scalp, where it enters the tissue; a small proportion is scattered by the tissue and returned to the analyzer through a fiberoptic bundle. Instruments capable of monitoring blood O_2 saturation in vivo within brain tissue have been commercially available for some years. Measured saturation within the illuminated volume includes arterial, capillary, and venous blood but is heavily weighted toward venous values,[155] which reflect the adequacy of tissue oxygenation under normal circumstances.[156]

Reduction of O_2 to water occurs at the terminal end of the cytochrome chain, and monitoring of the cytochrome redox state is therefore more likely to provide a better estimate of O_2 availability at the cellular level than current clinical monitoring parameters. By using a similar technique with four wavelengths, it is possible to obtain information about the state of oxygenation of intracellular chromophores, including myoglobin and cytochrome a, a_3.[157,158] This technology has been used to monitor intracellular changes in muscle and brain due to respiratory acidosis in anesthetized cats,[155] in canine hearts during and after coronary occlusion,[159] in human forearm ischemia,[160] and in human brain during hypoxia[161] or cardiopulmonary bypass.[162]

EXPIRED GAS ANALYSIS

Mass Spectrometry and Raman Gas Analysis

Mass spectrometers are devices that measure concentrations of gases largely on the basis of their molecular weight. Gas samples are passed through an ionizer, typically an electron beam, which strips the individual molecules of one or more electrons, giving them a positive charge. The ionizing beam also splits some molecules, creating molecular fragments. After ionization, the gas mixture to be measured is accelerated through a magnetic field and then onto detectors according to charge-mass ratio. The rate at which ions hit the target is proportional to the concentration of that particular gas in the original mixture. These instruments are reliable and relatively rugged, with a delay time typically on the order of 100 to 200 msec.

When a photon from a light source (usually an argon laser) collides with a molecule of gas, it may be re-emitted (i.e., scattered light) with no loss of energy (i.e., Rayleigh scattering). Alternatively, there may be absorption of some of the kinetic energy from the photon, resulting in the scattered photon's having a lower energy level and longer wavelength (i.e., Raman scattering). Spectral analysis of the scattered light can be used to measure simultaneously the individual concentrations of a mixture of gases. Mass spectrometers and Raman gas analyzers in the operating room have been largely supplanted by infrared analyzers.

Infrared Absorption

In the infrared absorption method, an infrared light beam is projected through the gas sample, and the intensity of the transmitted light is measured. CO_2 absorbs light with a characteristic peak at a wavelength close to 4300 nm. Several other molecules, such as anesthetic gases (especially nitrous oxide), water vapor, CO, and O_2 also absorb light in this area of the spectrum, interfering with CO_2 measurement, especially if the incident light composition includes wavelengths other than those in a very narrow region around the CO_2 absorption peak. In practical use, the fixed geometry of the gas-sampling cell, a narrow-band infrared light source, and compensating electronic circuits can often automatically correct for interference by other gases. Most expired gas analyzers use infrared absorption.

Colorimetric Carbon Dioxide Analysis

Colorimetric detectors make use of the fact that CO_2 forms acidic solutions in water. Paper impregnated with an aqueous solution of a pH sensitive dye (e.g., metacresol purple) can be maintained inside a hydrophobic filter. When CO_2-containing gas comes into contact with the test paper, the pH drops and the indicator changes color. Disposable devices (e.g., Easy Cap, Nellcor Puritan Bennett, Pleasanton, CA) can analyze CO_2 semi-quantitatively and can be used to confirm tracheal intubation in the field.[163]

Polarographic Analysis

Because in the Clark electrode the electrolyte solution is contained within a gas-permeable membrane, the electrode can be used for Po_2 measurement in gaseous-O_2 mixtures. Polarographic O_2 analyzers have a slow response time and are not useful for rapid-response expired gas analysis. However, their low cost and mechanical sturdiness make them suitable for on-line inspired gas analysis in anesthesia or intensive care ventilator circuits.

Paramagnetic Analysis

O_2 has the property of paramagnetism, which results in its being attracted toward a magnetic field. Several types of instruments have been designed to use this property of O_2 to measure the Po_2 in a mixture of gases (Fig. 36-13). Paramagnetic sensors are commonly used for exhaled O_2 analysis in clinical monitors.

Nitric Oxide Analysis

Nitric oxide (NO) has been administered therapeutically in concentrations of 1 to 100 parts per million (ppm) as a pulmonary vasodilator. Continuous monitoring of the inhaled concentration can be accomplished using relatively inexpensive but specific and stable electrochemical detectors.[164,165] There has been interest in monitoring endogenously produced NO in exhaled gas.[166] Analysis of exhaled NO waveforms, in which end-tidal NO concentrations are typically on the order of 1 to 100 parts per billion (ppb), can be satisfactorily performed only by using mass spectrometry or rapid-response chemiluminescence analyzers,[167] which typically have a resolution of 0.1 ppb or less. Gaseous chemiluminescence analyzers usually rely on the chemical reaction of NO with ozone (O_3) to produce nitrogen dioxide (NO_2). Some NO_2 molecules are produced in an excited state (NO_2^*).[168] When NO_2^* then spontaneously reverts to its ground state, a photon is emitted. This emitted chemiluminescence signal, which has a wavelength at maximum intensity at approximately 1200 nm, can be detected using a photomultiplier.

Figure 36–13 Paramagnetic oxygen analyzer. Two sealed spheres filled with nitrogen are suspended in a magnetic field. Nitrogen (N_2) is slightly diamagnetic, and the resting position of the beam is such that the spheres are displaced away from the strongest portion of the field. If the surrounding gas contains oxygen, the spheres are pushed further out of the field by the relatively paramagnetic oxygen. The magnitude of the torque is related to the paramagnetism of the gas mixture and is proportional to the partial pressure of oxygen (Po_2). Movement of the dumbbell is detected by photocells, and a feedback current is applied to the coil encircling the spheres, returning the dumbbell to the zero position. The restoring current and output voltage are proportional to the Po_2. (Courtesy of Servomex Co., Norwood, MA.)

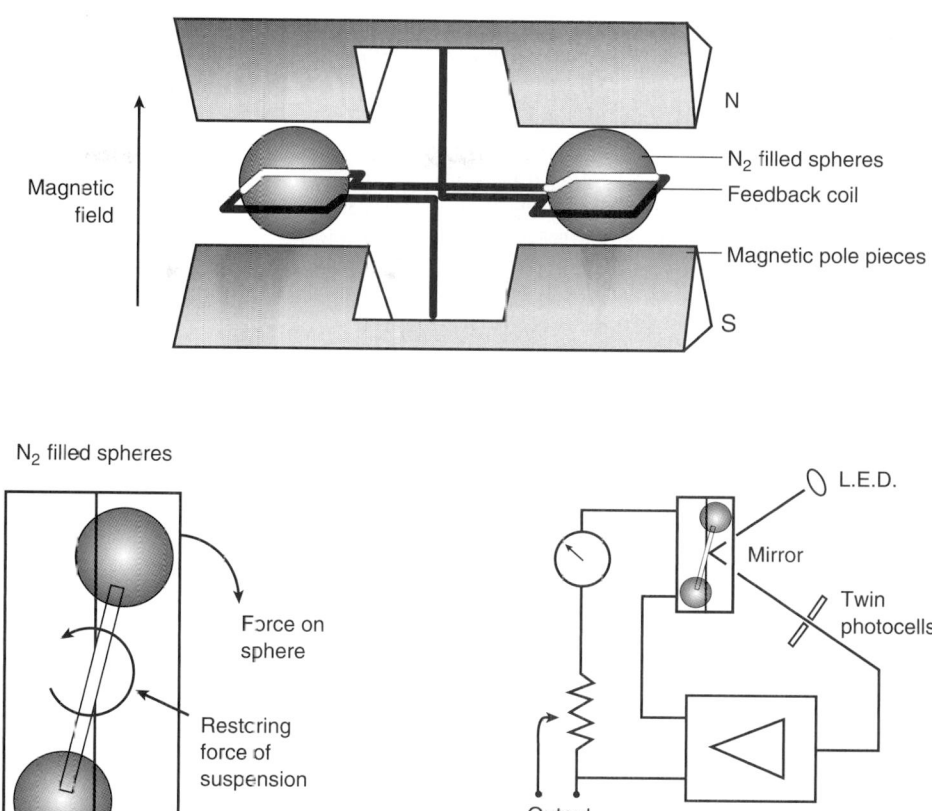

NO_2 in the original gas sample reacts slowly with O_3, even if it is present in high concentration. Chemiluminescence analyzers measure NO_2 concentration by first converting it to NO in a high-temperature reactor chamber.

WAVEFORM ANALYSIS OF EXPIRED RESPIRATORY GASES

Capnography, the measurement of CO_2 in expired gases, has evolved in the last few years into a commonly used procedure. Whereas a variety of techniques can be used for CO_2 measurement (e.g., mass spectrometry, Raman analysis), most capnographs rely on infrared absorption.[169] Use of this technique can reliably and quantitatively provide vital respiratory monitoring information in the operating room and in all critical care areas.

End-tidal Po_2 ($Peto_2$) may be used as an estimate of alveolar Po_2 and therefore Pao_2. Whereas end-tidal CO_2 ($Petco_2$) analysis has achieved a high degree of popularity, this has not occurred for Po_2 monitoring because of the variable A-a gradient. In normal individuals, this gradient may be less than 10 mm Hg, but in patients with severe $\dot{V}a/\dot{Q}$ mismatching, the gradient may be substantially increased. The A-a gradient is increased at high inspired O_2 concentrations, even with normal lungs. $Peto_2$ therefore almost always overestimates Pao_2. For example, the $Peto_2$ of a cadaver being ventilated with 100% O_2 would be approximately 700 mm Hg ($P_{barometric} - Ph_2o$)!

Nevertheless, exhaled O_2 analysis can be useful in monitoring the adequacy of nitrogen washout in preparation for induction of general anesthesia, particularly when a period of apnea is expected. Clinicians often select the time of induction of anesthesia at a point when the inspired-expired percentage of O_2 has decreased to a plateau (typically less than 10%). An example of a continuous tracing of expired Po_2, demonstrating nitrogen washout, is shown in Figure 36-14.

According to the gas sampling technique, infrared CO_2 monitors are in one of two categories: sidestream monitors, which draw a continuous sample of the gas from the respiratory circuit into the measuring cell, and mainstream monitors, which directly straddle the airway with a reading cell placed at the attachment between respiratory circuit and endotracheal tube or breathing mask. The key difference in use between the two types of capnographs depends on details of practical importance and on the type and duration of the monitoring environment.

Sidestream Capnographs

Sidestream capnographs depend crucially on a sampling flow that continuously aspirates from the side of the main respiratory gas flow a fixed amount of gas. The rate of gas sampling can usually be adjusted from 50 to 500 mL/min and sometimes up to 2 L/min. This continuous bias flow can be the source of significant methodologic error. If the sampling flow ever exceeds the expired gas flow,

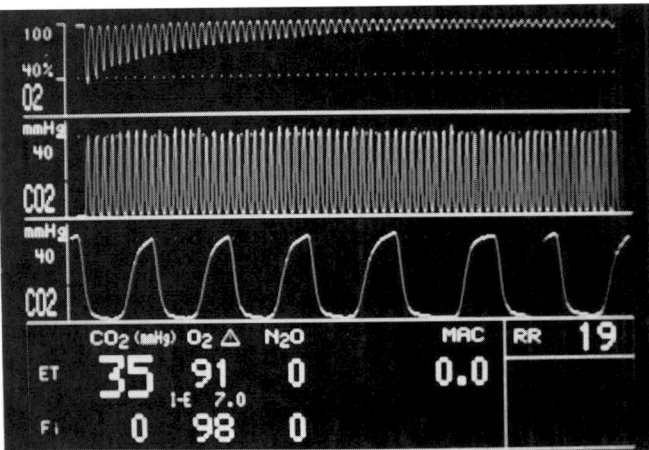

Figure 36–14 Monitoring of expired oxygen (O_2) to monitor lung nitrogen (N_2) washout. If preoxygenation is desired, its progress can be assessed by monitoring expired O_2. The top panel shows exhaled O_2 concentration on a compressed time scale while breathing 100% O_2 through an anesthesia mask. The next panel shows exhaled CO_2 on the same time scale. Exhaled O_2 steadily rises, and the difference between the inhaled and exhaled O_2 (I-e on the display) falls.

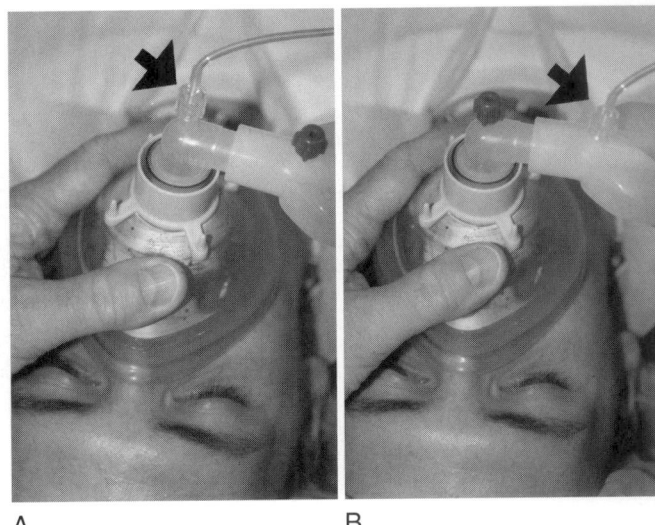

A   B

Figure 36–15 Sidestream sampling port placement. **A,** To minimize the effects of breathing circuit dead space, attachment of the sampling port should be as close to the patient as possible (*arrow*). **B,** Placement of the port as shown (*arrow*) can cause artifactual lowering of the end-tidal measurement.

contamination from the fresh gas flow source will occur. The sampling gas pump, flow regulator, sampling system (including the connector to the sampling port), and water trap or water separator constitute multiple sites for gas leak or breakage. Depending on the size and length of the sampling tube and the rate of gas flow, a certain delay in gas detection is introduced (i.e., CO_2 flight time), which can amount to several seconds when the sampling rate is low and the sampling dead space is high (e.g., long tubes). After measurement in the gas cell, the sampled gas may be exhausted into the atmosphere or retrieved and reinjected through a second tube into the breathing circuit to restore breathing circuit volume. This variable may be of great importance in closed-circuit and precise measurements of metabolic gas volumes. The analytic core of the instrument, the infrared measuring cell, must be carefully protected so that liquids and particulate matter do not enter it and cause erroneous readings of CO_2 because of their high infrared absorbance. The major problem is caused by water vapor, which is invariably present in expired air (at 37°C) with a saturated vapor pressure of 47 mm Hg. This condenses at lower (room) temperature on sampling tube walls. In critical care settings and often in the operating room, the inspired gas is kept warm and humid during long cases. This increases the load on water separation systems applied to capnographs. Water traps and filters have been designed to protect the measuring chamber.

The most faithful rendition of the capnograph waveform occurs when the sidestream sampling tubing is connected as close to the patient as possible (Fig. 36-15). Monitoring of end-tidal CO_2 in the spontaneously breathing patient whose trachea is not intubated requires some improvisation. Nasotracheal cannulae connected to a sidestream monitor usually provide a usable waveform but frequently become obstructed with saliva or mucus

and are uncomfortable. Taping a piece of intravenous tubing close to the nostril can provide an estimate of arterial P_{CO_2} that is adequate for clinical purposes. Alternatively, an intravenous catheter can be threaded into the common lumen of a pair of nasal O_2 cannulas such that the tip lies midway between the two nasal prongs. The extension tube normally connected to the O_2 source is tied off, and the intravenous catheter is then connected to a sidestream capnometer.[170] A commercially available version allows O_2 administration while end-tidal CO_2 is continuously monitored (Divided Canula, Salter Labs, Arvin, CA). Another device (Oridion, Needham, MA) samples exhalation from the mouth and nose (Fig. 36-16). Sampling CO_2 from a facemask, although adequate for monitoring respiratory rate, produces measured P_{ETCO_2} values that are significantly lower than Pa_{CO_2}.

Mainstream Capnometers

In a mainstream capnometer, with the measuring head placed close to the endotracheal tube, the measuring chamber is usually heated to about 40°C to prevent water condensation on the chamber window. The heating sensing head must be kept away from direct contact with the patient's skin; it is relatively heavy and must be supported to prevent endotracheal tube kinking. The sensor's window must be kept clean of mucus and particles to prevent false readings; calibration may be problematic. Despite all these problems, the response time is faster because no gas is subtracted from the breathing circuit, no sampling pumps or other suction devices add complexities to the mechanical system, and there is no uncertainty caused by the rate of gas sampling.

Capnographs must be calibrated periodically, at different intervals in various models, but usually at least daily. Equipment drift is most often caused by accumulation of

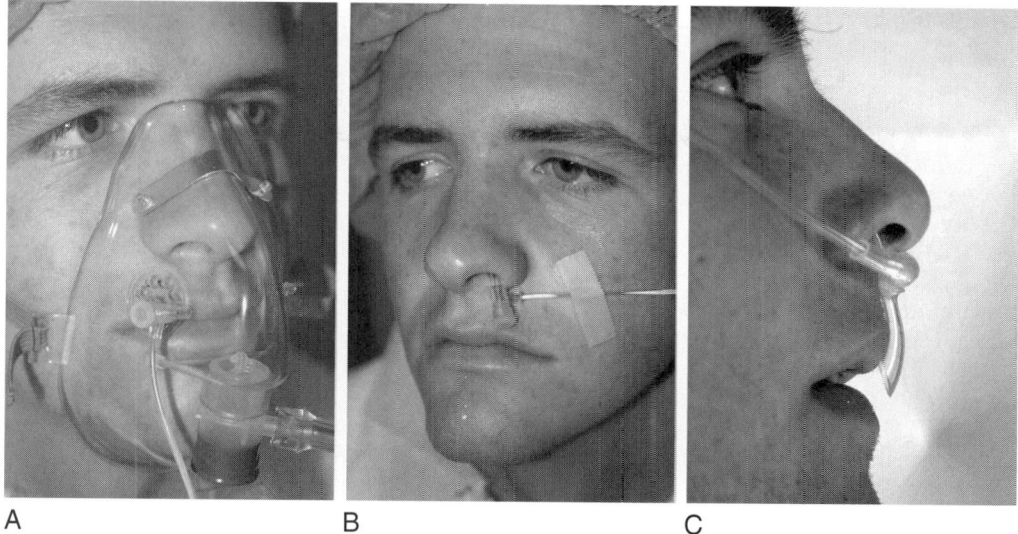

Figure 36–16 Monitoring a spontaneously breathing patient with a sidestream capnograph. **A,** Attachment of the sampling line to a non-rebreathing mask usually provides waveforms adequate for monitoring the respiratory rate, but end-tidal CO_2 tension is low because of mixing within the mask. **B,** Placement of a sample probe close to a nostril increases the accuracy of the P_{ETCO_2} measurement. **C,** A specially designed probe (Oridion, Needham, MA) samples exhaled gas from the nose and mouth for assessing exhaled gas from mouth-breathers. A second port in the same device can be used to administer supplemental oxygen.

saliva or other extraneous materials in the light path of the analyzer. Calibration can usually be performed by periodic use of calibrated gases. Mainstream capnometers are often equipped with calibration sample cells sealed with mixtures of CO_2 and N_2. In some instruments, room air is sampled in the mainstream cuvette to "zero" the CO_2 level automatically.

A useful analysis range varies from 0% to 10% (76 mm Hg) for end-tidal CO_2 to an extended range up to 100 mm Hg, which may be useful in rare cases of hypoventilation or malignant hyperthermia. The inspired CO_2 range must include 0 and extend up to 15 mm Hg for cases in which rebreathing must be detected and peak values determined.

Time Delays

A capnogram is produced by the sequential analysis of inspired and expired gas flowing by the mainstream window, which is usually positioned just proximal to the endotracheal tube or breathing mask, or sampled from a sidestream sampling site connected to the breathing circuit. In the case of sidestream sampling, a definite time delay is introduced by the length and volume of the tubing carrying the sampled gas to the detector. This delay caused by the transfer of the sampled gas into the reading cell can be minimized by using high flow rates for the sampling flow and narrow, short tubing assemblies compatible with the position of the equipment with respect to the patient breathing circuit. After the sampled gas reaches the sensing cell, an additional delay is introduced by the rise time of each instrument. The rise time is a characteristic delay induced by the exponential response to a square front of changing gas concentration, in which CO_2 concentration changes instantaneously from zero to

a new steady-state level (CO_{2ss}). This can be described by the following exponential equation:

$$S = CO_{2ss} \cdot (1 - e^{-t/\tau}) \tag{24}$$

In Equation 24, S is the signal at time t, e is the base of natural logarithms (≈ 2.718), and τ (tau) is the time constant. When $t = \tau$ (i.e., one time constant), it is possible to calculate that $S = 0.63 \cdot CO_{2ss}$ (or 63%). This approach is used to measure the speed of response of the circuitry. It is often presented in clinical instruments as a different fraction of the response, such as the 10% to 90% response time ($\approx 2.2\ \tau$).

If we assume a square-wave capnogram for argument's sake as the most difficult for an instrument to follow and assume a time constant of 100 msec (a frequent value for a clinical instrument), it is theoretically possible to follow respiratory profiles of CO_2 within 5% of the real value (accuracy better than 5%) up to respiratory rates of 100 breaths/min. In practice, most clinical capnographs display this accuracy up to 60 breaths/min.[169] A shared mass spectrometer, with the usually longer sampling line used in the share configuration, may display significant inaccuracy at respiratory rates of about 40 breaths/min.[171] The relative duration of inspiration and expiration (I/E ratio) can also affect the accuracy of the recording instrument. Standardized respiratory cycle profiles have been used to compare the most commonly employed clinical instruments.[172]

Sidestream capnographs are susceptible to errors related to gas diffusion. Radial diffusion of CO_2 out of the tubing can cause artificially low values.[173] This error is related to the tubing material and the length of exposure of the sample inside the tubing (i.e., related to the sample flow rate and tubing length). Polyethylene and Teflon tubing are much more permeable to CO_2 than nylon. Axial diffusion across the fronts of CO_2-rich boluses traveling along sampling lines can also smear the upstrokes and the downstrokes of waveforms. This type of diffusion has a significant effect on the interpretation of end-tidal CO_2 at higher respiratory frequencies.

Capnographic Waveform

Time Capnogram

The most commonly used display mode is P_{CO_2} versus time. Traditionally, several phases are distinguished in the capnograph trace. During inspiration and the first portion of expiration during which dead space gas is exhaled, there is no CO_2 (phase I). As expiration continues, a short phase of the capnogram is recognized (phase II), with a rapid upstroke toward the alveolar plateau, representing the rising front of CO_2 (Fig. 36-17A). The boundary of this front can be smeared by a variety of causes, but most notably by uneven mixing of the alveolar CO_2 bolus in the airways. Phase III, also called the alveolar plateau, represents the constant or slowly upsloping part of the capnogram.

In the time capnogram, the alveolar plateau lasts for the greater part of the trace (see Fig. 36-17), although the expiratory flow is highest at the beginning of the expiration and tapers off in exponential fashion during the last third of expiratory time. Most of the exhaled volume of a passive expiration therefore exits the trachea (and the

tracheal tube or the anesthetic mask) during the first half of exhalation time. Phase III reaches a peak, usually attained only during the final phase of exhalation and therefore called the end-tidal partial pressure of CO_2 (P_{ETCO_2}). P_{ETCO_2} in the normal individual is usually 2 to 3 mm Hg lower than Pa_{CO_2}. Chronic pulmonary disease and acute disturbances in $\dot{V}_A/\dot{Q}$ usually widen this difference to several millimeters of mercury. Slow exhalation, as during an acute asthmatic attack or in patients with chronic obstructive pulmonary disease, with reduced lung recoil usually induces a steeper alveolar plateau (Fig. 36-18D).

Why is the alveolar plateau upsloping in patients with diffuse airways obstruction? Several effects are responsible. A perfect lung would have perfect matching of ventilation and perfusion ($\dot{V}_A/\dot{Q} = 1$). However, diffuse airways obstruction is a nonuniform process in which there are gas exchange units with a spectrum of $\dot{V}_A/\dot{Q}$ ratios. Units with high $\dot{V}_A/\dot{Q}$ ratios are overventilated in relation to perfusion; alveolar P_{CO_2} in such units is low. Gas exchange units with low $\dot{V}_A/\dot{Q}$ ratios are underventilated in relation to perfusion and have high local alveolar P_{CO_2}. During exhalation, these gas exchange units empty at different rates; units that are unobstructed (normal or high $\dot{V}_A/\dot{Q}$) empty quickly, followed by obstructed units. Gas exhaled early in the breath tends to have a lower P_{CO_2} than gas exhaled later.

Another reason for the progressive rise in CO_2 concentration is that during the exhalation, CO_2 excretion from pulmonary capillaries into the alveoli continues at a nearly constant molar rate. CO_2 molecules entering a lung volume

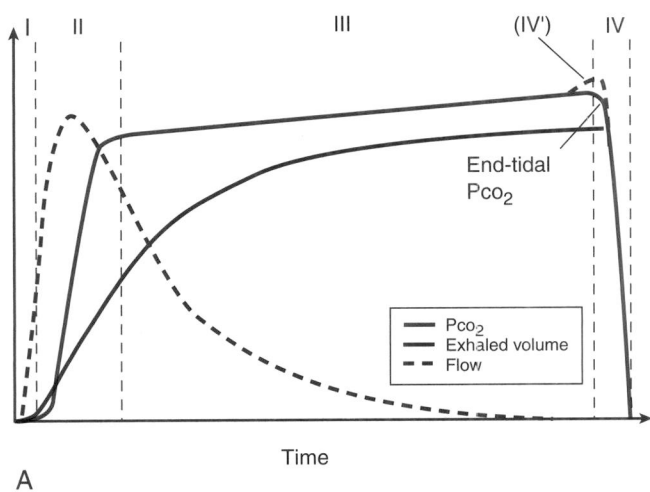

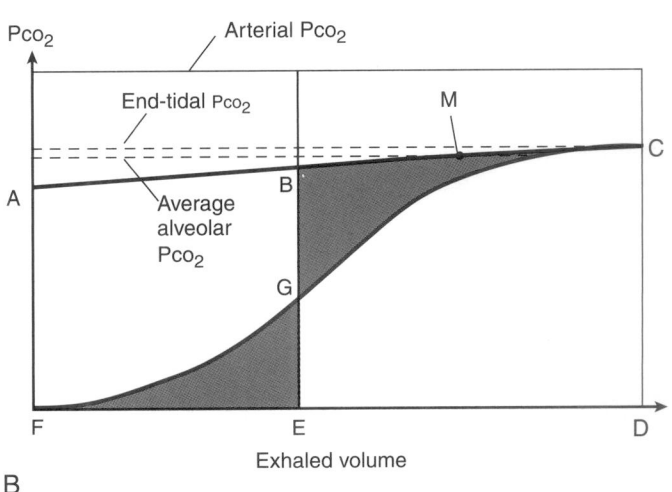

Figure 36–17 Time and volume capnographs. **A,** Expired P_{CO_2} versus time (i.e., standard time capnogram). The waveform is conventionally subdivided into phases. During phase I, exhaled gas from the large airways has a $P_{CO_2} = 0$. Phase II is the transition between airway and alveolar gas. Phase III (i.e., alveolar plateau) is normally flat, but in the presence of $\dot{V}_A/\dot{Q}$ mismatching, it has a positive slope. The down slope of the capnogram at the onset of inspiration is usually referred to as phase IV, but there is sometimes a terminal increase in the slope associated with the onset of airway closure (*dashed line* labeled IV'). This corresponds to the terminal upstroke seen in single inert gas washout curves, referred to in that setting as phase IV.[322] The P_{CO_2} value at the end of exhalation is referred to as the end-tidal P_{CO_2} (P_{ETCO_2}). Also shown are the exhaled gas flow rate and volume. **B,** Volume capnogram. In this form of the capnogram, exhaled P_{CO_2} is plotted against exhaled volume. Mixed expired P_{CO_2} can be measured for each breath as the area under the capnogram. Total physiologic dead space ($V_{DS PHYS}$) can there fore be measured using arterial P_{CO_2} and Equation 12 (Bohr equation, assuming $Pa_{CO_2} = Pa_{CO_2}$). Line AC is drawn tangent to the terminal portion of the alveolar plateau. Vertical line BE is constructed such that the two shaded areas (EDG and BCG) are equal in area. FE therefore represents anatomic dead space ($V_{DS ANAT}$),[323] which includes the volume in the trachea and large airways and any volume within a breathing circuit in which exhaled gas is rebreathed, such as the endotracheal tube, passive humidification device, or Y-piece. Alveolar dead space ($V_{DS ALV}$)[323] can therefore be calculated as the difference between $V_{DS PHYS}$ and $V_{DS ANAT}$.[324] Because the area of trapezoid BCDE is equal to the volume of CO_2 exhaled per breath, the mean (or average) alveolar P_{CO_2} is the value at the midpoint of segment BC (point P).[324]

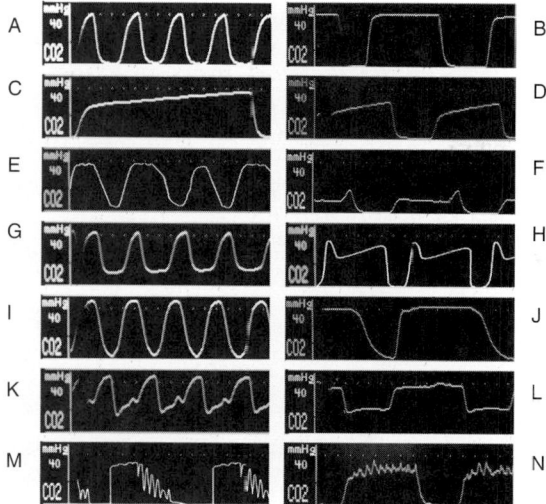

Figure 36–18 Examples of capnograph waves. **A,** Normal spontaneous breathing. **B,** Normal mechanical ventilation. **C,** Prolonged exhalation during spontaneous breathing. As CO_2 diffuses from the mixed venous blood into the alveoli, its concentration progressively rises (see Fig. 36-19). **D,** Increased slope of phase III in a mechanically ventilated patient with emphysema. **E,** Added dead space during spontaneous ventilation. **F,** Dual plateau (i.e. tails-up pattern) caused by a leak in the sample line.[325] The alveolar plateau is artifactually low because of dilution of exhaled gas with air leaking inward. During each mechanical breath, the leak is reduced because of higher pressure within the airway and tubing, explaining the rise in the CO_2 concentration at the end of the alveolar plateau. This pattern is not seen during spontaneous ventilation because the required increase in airway pressure is absent. **G,** Exhausted CO_2 absorbent produces an inhaled CO_2 concentration greater than zero. **H,** Double peak for a patient with a single lung transplant. The first peak represents CO_2 from the transplanted (normal) lung. CO_2 exhalation from the remaining (obstructed) lung is delayed, producing the second peak. **I,** Inspiratory valve stuck open during spontaneous breathing. Some backflow into the inspired limb of the circuit causes a rise in the level of inspired CO_2. **J,** Inspiratory valve stuck open during mechanical ventilation. The "slurred" downslope during inspiration represents a small amount of inspired CO_2 in the inspired limb of the circuit. **K and L,** Expiratory valve stuck open during spontaneous breathing or mechanical ventilation. Inhalation of exhaled gas causes an increase in inspired CO_2. **M,** Cardiogenic oscillations, when seen, usually occur with sidestream capnographs for spontaneously breathing patients at the end of each exhalation. Cardiac action causes to-and-fro movement of the interface between exhaled and fresh gas. The CO_2 concentration in gas entering the sampling line therefore alternates between high and low values. **N,** Electrical noise resulting from a malfunctioning component. The seemingly random nature of the signal perturbations (about three per second) implies a nonbiologic cause.

made progressively smaller by the exhalation process causes the CO_2 concentration to rise. For this reason, a prolonged exhalation, even in a person with normal lungs, can have an upsloping plateau (see Fig. 36-18C). Both factors are illustrated in Figure 36-19.

$PETCO_2$ can exceed arterial PCO_2.[174-177] Other than calibration error, the most common cause is slow respiratory rate or high mixed venous PCO_2. In these situations the cyclic variations in alveolar PCO_2 (which oscillates between

arterial and mixed venous values) may be relatively large, causing the $PETCO_2$ value to rise above the arterial value.

When patients are anesthetized in the lateral position, uneven ventilation of the dependent lung and lesser perfusion of the nondependent lung increase the range of alveolar gas disparity and the upslope of the alveolar plateau. This can be verified by alternating sampling sites between the two lungs when ventilating a patient in the lateral position with separate endobronchial tubes.

Sometimes, when expiration is prolonged and progresses to a lung volume below closing capacity, expired CO_2 concentration may rise sharply at the end of the alveolar plateau, in a fashion analogous to that of N_2 concentration after washout with 100% O_2.[178] One possible reason for this is that lung units subtended by airways predisposed to closure, at least in the spontaneously breathing patient, may contain alveolar gas with lower $PaCO_2$. Closure of these airways would therefore allow a greater proportion of CO_2-rich gas to reach the upper airway, producing the sharp upswing in CO_2 concentration. An alternative hypothesis is that during the course of expiration, well-ventilated lung units have a progressive, nonlinear, upsloping increase in PCO_2, whereas that of poorly ventilated (closure-prone) units increases in a linear fashion. When airway closure occurs, the rate of rise in well-ventilated units predominates, and the slope of the capnogram abruptly increases.[179] Using the terminology of the single-breath washout curve, this portion of the capnogram is occasionally referred to as phase IV.

The last segment of a capnograph is represented by the beginning of inspiration, when the CO_2 concentration rapidly decreases toward the inspired value. The capnogram value during inspiration represents the concentration of CO_2 in the inspirate and depends mostly on the breathing circuit used and inspiratory flow and fresh gas flow values. Rebreathing of dead space volume is often the cause of an inspired level above baseline (see Fig. 36-18E); this can be promptly corrected by removing the dead space. Exhaustion of the CO_2 absorber may also result in an elevated value of inspired PCO_2 (see Fig. 36-18G). The sampling flow rate of sidestream monitors must be taken into account when interpreting many features of the capnogram profile. Usually, sampling flow rates vary, and they can be set between 50 and 400 mL/min, with an average optimal value for an adult patient of about 200 mL/min. As soon as the respiratory gas flows decrease below the sidestream gas sampling rate, the characteristics of the sampling vary; instead of sampling a portion of the mainstream flow, the equipment contributes significantly to bulk flow in and out of the respiratory circuit. This is of great importance in the pediatric setting, during low-flow anesthesia, and when interpreting capnograms obtained during very low respiratory rates. For example, during a prolonged expiration or an end-expiratory pause, while the gas flow exiting the trachea approaches zero, the sampling of the monitor may aspirate gas alternately from the trachea and the inspiratory limb.

A profile that illustrates this effect is shown in Figure 36-18M; it is called *cardiogenic oscillation*, referring to the cause of the alteration. Synchronous changes in pulmonary blood flow during slow expiration and mechanical agitation of different lung regions induced by cardiac activity and

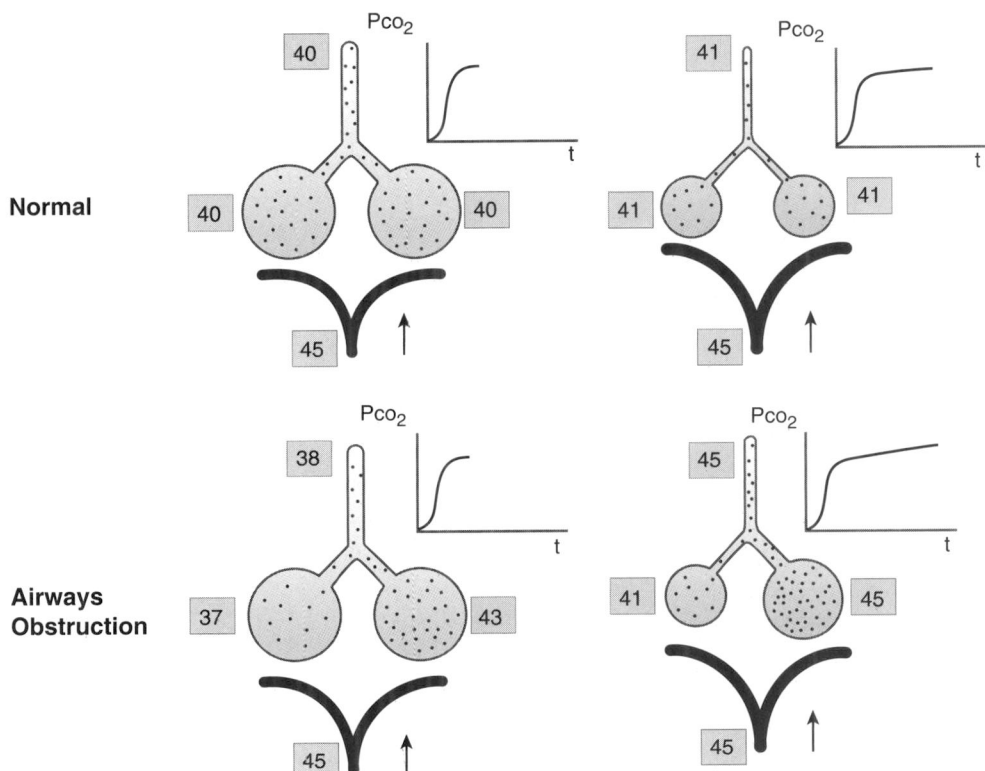

Figure 36–19 Mechanisms of airways obstruction producing an upsloping phase III capnogram. In a normal, healthy person (upper panel), there is a narrow range of $\dot{V}_A/\dot{Q}$ ratios with values close to 1. Gas exchange units therefore have similar P_{CO_2} and tend to empty synchronously, and the expired P_{CO_2} remains relatively constant. During the course of exhalation, the alveolar P_{CO_2} slowly rises as CO_2 continuously diffuses from the blood. This causes a slight increase in P_{CO_2} toward the end of expiration, and this increase can be pronounced if the exhalation is prolonged (see Fig. 36-18C). In a patient with diffuse airways obstruction (lower panel), the airway pathology is heterogeneous, with gas exchange units having a wide range of $\dot{V}_A/\dot{Q}$ ratios. Well-ventilated gas exchange units, with gas containing a lower P_{CO_2}, empty first; poorly ventilated units, with a higher P_{CO_2}, empty last. In addition to the continuous rise in P_{CO_2} mentioned previously, there is a progressive increase caused by asynchronous exhalation.

pulmonary blood flow contribute to the creation of ripples, often observed in a repetitive pattern during the alveolar plateau in synchrony with the heartbeat. The usual interpretation of cardiogenic oscillatory ripples is mechanical agitation of deep lung regions that expel CO_2-rich gas in synchrony with the heartbeat. Waveforms due to cardiogenic oscillation are more pronounced when sampling of gas is obtained from deeper tracheal and bronchial areas. Such fluctuations are often smoothed over when the sampling port is more distal to the airways or when lung volume is increased by application of positive end-expiratory pressure (PEEP).

Inspection of the whole curve rather than measurement only of peak expired and peak inhalation values, which may be reported digitally, improves the scope and interpretation of the trace. When a capnographic trace is displayed such that all characteristics of the various stages of the waveform are visible on a rapidly scrolling oscilloscope or on fast-moving paper, it is possible to recognize several features that may be of diagnostic value. When capnograms are plotted on slow-moving paper or trends of only inspired and P_{ETCO_2} values are produced, it is still possible to recognize important clinical information regarding rising or falling concentrations of inspired and expired CO_2. Examples of capnographic waveforms

are shown in Figure 36-18, and additional waveforms and didactic material on capnography can be found on the Internet (www.capnography.com).

Normal end-expiratory CO_2 partial pressure ranges between 35 and 45 mm Hg. An increase above this level (i.e., hypercapnia) must be interpreted in the light of additional information, because it depends on a variety of factors:

1. Increased CO_2 production, as during fever or malignant hyperpyrexia.
2. Depression of the respiratory center, with concomitant reduction of total ventilation and elevation of end-tidal CO_2
3. Reduction of ventilation induced by partial paralysis, neurologic disease, high spinal anesthesia, weakened respiratory muscle, or acute respiratory distress

If ventilation is controlled, inadequate mechanical ventilation must be the first interpretation of increased end-tidal CO_2. If an increasing trend in end-tidal CO_2 is observed while total ventilation remains constant, it is essential to verify the patient's temperature to exclude the diagnosis of hyperpyrexia. Other frequently observed causes of transient increases in end-tidal CO_2 are release of tourniquets with reperfusion of ischemic areas, release of aortic clamps, intravenous administration of bicarbonate

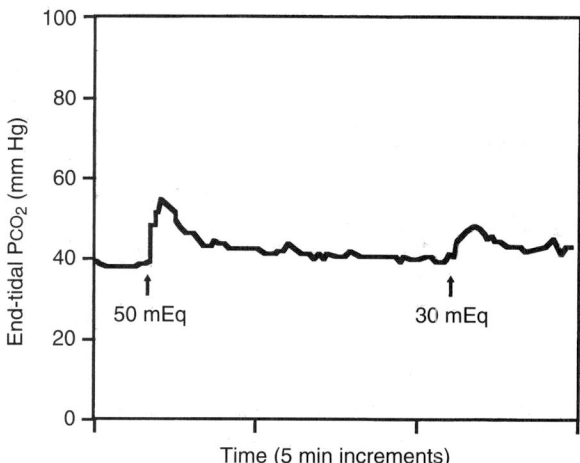

Figure 36–20 The effect of sodium bicarbonate administration on end-tidal P_{CO_2}. A continuous tracing of end-tidal P_{CO_2} is shown as a function of time. Intravenous administration of 50 mEq followed by 30 mEq of $NaHCO_3$ results in an abrupt increase in expired CO_2 because of neutralization of bicarbonate by hydrogen ions.

(Fig. 36-20), insufflation of CO_2 into the peritoneal cavity as during laparoscopy, and acute defects in mechanical ventilation systems.

Abnormally low end-tidal values (<35 mm Hg) most often reflect hyperventilation but may also be caused by increased dead space with normal Pa_{CO_2}. For example, alveolar gas emanating from a lung region with no blood flow (and therefore no local CO_2 transfer) dilutes exhaled gas and decreases PET_{CO_2} relative to Pa_{CO_2}. Hypocapnia may also be artifactually induced by high sampling rate of the sidestream monitor in the face of an elevated fresh gas flow rate. Low PET_{CO_2} may reflect decreased CO_2 (PET_{CO_2} during cardiac arrest may equal zero). The most common causes of an acute drop in PET_{CO_2} are a decrease in cardiac output, regional hypoperfusion of the lung due to pulmonary embolism, and airway disconnection or occlusion.

Similarly, areas of lung that are perfused but unventilated (e.g., in atelectasis) because of shunting of mixed venous blood have high regional Pa_{CO_2} and high arterial minus end-tidal CO_2 (Pa_{CO_2} – PET_{CO_2}), which has been used as a criterion for optimizing PEEP in ventilated patients.[180] Increasing levels of PEEP would be expected to resolve atelectasis and decrease Pa_{CO_2} – PET_{CO_2} in these areas. In normal areas, overdistension impairs perfusion and therefore increases regional Pa_{CO_2} – PET_{CO_2}. Optimal PEEP can be defined as when a balance is reached.

Irregularities in the alveolar plateau are often observed when mechanical factors acutely alter the pattern of alveolar emptying, such as when the arm of a surgeon compresses the chest in the middle of expiration. A cleft or a dip on the capnogram may indicate a spontaneous breath of small tidal volume, able to move just a small bolus of inspired gas past the sampling site. This often has been interpreted as indicating activation of respiratory centers by a patient recovering from anesthesia or activation of respiration induced by sudden increasing stimulation in the surgical field. It may also indicate inadequate inspiratory power during the switch from mechanical to spontaneous ventilation and can be the first sign of the need for reversal of neuromuscular blockade. However, it may indicate just the opposite, the need for increased total ventilation to induce apnea in the patient. The dip in the plateau of the capnogram must be interpreted with care, depending on the surgical stage, the drug exposure history of the patient, and the anesthetic plan.

The main use of the capnographic signal in anesthesia is the immediate verification of tracheal intubation beyond doubt by the immediate and continuous presence of metabolic CO_2 in the expired gas. Esophageal intubation may produce one or a few breaths containing CO_2 during expiration, but the concentration of this gas in exhalations from the stomach cavity rapidly decreases to zero. In this fashion, the continuous appearance of expired CO_2 is rapidly being adopted as a criterion for correct tracheal intubation. Another major use of this signal has been to determine the correct ventilatory needs (e.g., minute ventilation) during controlled ventilation. This use is easily extended to continuous monitoring of spontaneous ventilation and to monitoring of appropriate ventilation during titration of anesthetic agents that depress ventilation. In partial rebreathing circuits and in low-flow anesthesia, capnometry facilitates the adjustment of fresh gas flow, which is a major determinant of CO_2 levels insofar as it may increase minute ventilation. The shape of a partial rebreathing capnogram may vary greatly, depending on the ventilatory frequency and tidal volume. In all of these modes of use, the sensing head of the capnograph or the site of gas sampling is best kept close to the tracheal tube, connected with the minimal dead space assembly. In this mode, for instance, it is easy to reveal disconnection of the breathing system or inappropriate functioning of mechanical ventilators. Partial rebreathing circuit systems include a CO_2 absorber, whose exhaustion is manifested by hypercarbia.

Clinical signs of hypercarbia may be only slowly recognized, whereas an increase in inspired CO_2 is immediately observable with a capnograph. Rapid alterations in end-tidal CO_2 can be recognized within a single exhalation. In a different setting, capnography has been used on the exhaust side of a cardiopulmonary bypass oxygenator to track CO_2 excretion at different body temperatures.

Volume Capnogram

If exhaled volume and P_{CO_2} are measured simultaneously, exhaled P_{CO_2} can be plotted against exhaled gas volume (see Fig. 36-17). Volume capnography has several advantages over time capnography. First, the CO_2 signal can be integrated to obtain the volume of CO_2 exhaled per breath, obtaining an on-line, breath-by-breath measurement of CO_2. Second, significant changes in the morphology of the expired waveform can be detected in the volume capnogram (e.g., resulting from PEEP) but not in the traditional time capnogram.[181] Third, dead space can be partitioned into components of interest. Total physiologic dead space (V_D PHYS) can therefore be measured using arterial P_{CO_2} and Equation 12 (Bohr equation, assuming Pa_{CO_2} = Pa_{CO_2}). Anatomic dead space (V_D ANAT), including gas volume within a breathing circuit in which exhaled gas is rebreathed, such as the endotracheal tube, passive humidification device, or Y-piece, can be calculated directly from the volume capnogram (see Fig. 36-17B). Alveolar dead space (V_D ALV) is therefore the difference between V_D PHYS and V_D ANAT and is related to the difference between alveolar and arterial P_{CO_2} according to Equation 25:

$$V_D\ _{ALV} = (V_T - V_D\ _{ANAT})\left(1 - \frac{P_{A_{CO_2}}}{P_{a_{CO_2}}}\right) \quad (25)$$

Normally, alveolar P_{CO_2} can be estimated using $P_{ET_{CO_2}}$ obtained from the time capnogram as a measure of $P_{A_{CO_2}}$. However, when the alveolar plateau has a significant slope, $P_{ET_{CO_2}}$ can exceed $P_{a_{CO_2}}$,[174-177] and the average alveolar P_{CO_2} (see Fig. 36-17) obtained from the volume capnogram may be a more appropriate measure.[181] Commercial monitors incorporating volume capnometry are available.

Errors in Capnography

Because water vapor is often the major source of error, several "water trap" devices or heated suction tubes are used to deliver moisture-free gas to the reading cell. The effect of gas temperature can be calculated. Assume body temperature is 37°C and $P_{a_{CO_2}} = P_{ET_{CO_2}} = 40$ mm Hg. If the sampling tube and detector are maintained at a temperature above 37°C, there will be no condensation or "rain out" of water, and the measured P_{CO_2} will be 40 mm Hg. However, if the expired gas is allowed to cool to room temperature (e.g., 20°C), water will condense in the tubing, and the new water vapor pressure (P_{H_2O}) will decrease to the saturated P_{H_2O} at room temperature (typically 20 mm Hg). If a drying agent is used in the sample line, P_{H_2O} will drop to zero. In either case, the measured P_{CO_2} will increase slightly.

OXYGEN AND CARBON DIOXIDE EXCHANGE MONITORING

The most direct method of measuring O_2 uptake ($\dot{V}_{O_2}$) and CO_2 elimination ($\dot{V}_{CO_2}$) is by analysis of inspired (I) and expired (E) gas concentrations. If the minute volume is measured along with inspired and expired O_2 and CO_2 concentrations, $\dot{V}_{CO_2}$ can be calculated by the following equation:

$$\dot{V}_{CO_2} = \dot{V}_E \cdot F_{E_{CO_2}} - \dot{V}_I \cdot F_{I_{CO_2}} \quad (26)$$

In Equation 26, $\dot{V}_E$ and $\dot{V}_I$ are the expired and inspired respiratory minute volumes, respectively. $F_{E_{CO_2}}$ and $F_{I_{CO_2}}$ are the mixed expired and inspired CO_2 concentrations, respectively. Because the quantities of O_2 consumed and CO_2 eliminated are rarely exactly equal, $\dot{V}_E$ and $\dot{V}_I$ differ slightly. Because $F_{I_{CO_2}}$ is usually zero, Equation 26 can be simplified to the following form:

$$\dot{V}_{CO_2} = \dot{V}_E \cdot F_{E_{CO_2}} \quad (27)$$

Similarly, an equation can be written for the calculation of O_2 consumption:

$$\dot{V}_{O_2} = \dot{V}_I \cdot F_{I_{CO_2}} - \dot{V}_E \cdot F_{E_{CO_2}} \quad (28)$$

In practice, it is difficult to measure minute ventilation with the necessary degree of accuracy to be able to distinguish small differences between $\dot{V}_I$ and $\dot{V}_E$. Because the exchange of inert gas (i.e., gas in the breathing mixture that is neither CO_2 nor O_2) generally equals zero, $\dot{V}_I$ can be calculated as follows:

$$\dot{V}_I = \dot{V}_E \cdot \frac{F_E\ inert}{F_I\ inert} \quad (29)$$

$$F_I\ inert = 1 - F_{I_{O_2}} \quad (30)$$

$$F_E\ inert = 1 - (F_{E_{O_2}} + F_{E_{CO_2}}) \quad (31)$$

Equation 28 can be rewritten as follows:

$$\dot{V}_{O_2} = \dot{V}_E\left(F_{I_{O_2}}\frac{F_E\ inert}{F_I\ inert} - F_{E_{O_2}}\right) \quad (32)$$

$\dot{V}_{O_2}$ measurement using this equation becomes progressively less accurate as the inspired O_2 fraction is increased above 50%. At high $F_{I_{O_2}}$ values, because F_I inert becomes small, errors in the measurement of F_I inert result in correspondingly large errors in O_2. At $F_{I_{O_2}} = 1$, this equation breaks down completely.

Open-circuit measurement of $\dot{V}_{O_2}$ and $\dot{V}_{CO_2}$ under anesthesia using this method has been described by Viale and coworkers.[182] Self-contained analyzers have been designed.[183,184] These instruments have proved to be extremely satisfactory for gas exchange monitoring in patients in the critical care environment. One practical problem with systems incorporating zirconium oxide O_2 sensor is extremely sensitive to small concentrations of fluorinated anesthetic gases, which may cause severe malfunction. $\dot{V}_{O_2}$ and $\dot{V}_{CO_2}$ can be measured on a breath-by-breath basis by integrating $F_{I_{O_2}} - F_{E_{O_2}}$ with respect to exhaled volume.[185] A method of measurement of $\dot{V}_{O_2}$ by using rapid response temperature and humidity analyzers to make appropriate corrections may allow breath-by-breath monitoring even with high $F_{I_{O_2}}$ values.[186]

An alternative technique (i.e., reversed Fick) is to calculate the O_2 consumption as the product of the arteriovenous O_2 content difference and the cardiac output derived by thermodilution:

$$\dot{V}_{O_2} = (Ca_{O_2} - C\bar{v}_{O_2}) \cdot \dot{Q}_T \quad (33)$$

In Equation 33, Ca_{O_2} and $C\bar{v}_{O_2}$ are the arterial and mixed venous O_2 contents (mL/L), respectively. $\dot{Q}_T$ is cardiac output. Blood O_2 content may be calculated using Equation 10; when using Equation 31, the O_2 content values calculated using Equation 10 must be multiplied by 10 to obtain the O_2 in the correct units.

The reversed Fick technique is reasonably satisfactory for clinical purposes, although it becomes less accurate in the setting of high cardiac output and low arteriovenous O_2 content differences. It tends to underestimate the $\dot{V}_{O_2}$ measured directly by 30 to 60 mL/min.[187-189] This difference has been attributed to pulmonary O_2 consumption, which is not measured by the reversed Fick method. Use of continuous thermodilution cardiac output versus intermittent bolus injection may reduce the error.[190]

RESPIRATORY CENTER DRIVE

Classic techniques for assessment of respiratory drive have measured ventilatory output (i.e., minute ventilation [$\dot{V}E$]) as a function of varying levels of elevated $Paco_2$ (i.e., hypercapnic ventilatory response) or decreased levels of Pao_2 (i.e., hypoxic ventilatory response). However, these techniques are difficult to implement in clinical situations. Nevertheless, assessment of the respiratory drive is particularly important in clinical evaluation of the effects of anesthetic agents on the respiratory system and particularly in the process of weaning patients from mechanical ventilation. Of the various causes of respiratory failure, including pulmonary mechanical abnormalities and impairment of respiratory gas exchange, depressed ventilatory drive is probably the most common cause of failure to wean after general anesthesia.

Partitioning the respiratory waveform into inspiratory and expiratory components can provide further information. Mean inspiratory flow (i.e., tidal volume/inspiratory time) is an index of respiratory drive.[191] However, it is possible for a patient to have a high respiratory drive but not be able to translate that drive into respiratory output because of impaired ventilatory mechanics.

A low ventilation rate is conventionally considered to be a reasonable indicator of respiratory depression caused by anesthetic agents, particularly narcotics. Although parenteral narcotics usually slow the ventilation rate, several investigators have demonstrated in patients and normal volunteers that narcotic-induced ventilatory depression can manifest as a reduction in tidal volume, with little change in respiratory rate.[192-195] In a clinical series, one patient with a $Paco_2$ of 95 mm Hg had a respiratory rate of 12 breaths/min.[195] The published evidence indicates that apnea is not reliably predicted by bradypnea, and severe respiratory depression can exist in patients with acceptable respiratory rates.

A more sophisticated measure of respiratory drive is the maximum negative inspiratory airway pressure obtained 100 msec after a temporary occlusion of the airway (P_{100} or $P_{0.1}$) in a spontaneously breathing patient. Periodic transient airway occlusion that occurs in this way is not appreciably noticed by the patient. Chemosensitivity, determined in volunteers by CO_2 responsiveness, is not significantly affected by intermittent (every 30 seconds) P_{100} maneuvers.[196] The normal value for P_{100} during resting ventilation is 1 to 2 cm H_2O. P_{100} is a useful index of respiratory drive, requiring no voluntary effort on the part of the subject and being minimally affected by changes in respiratory mechanics. The technique is well described by Milic-Emili and associates.[197]

Under anesthesia, P_{100} is depressed,[198] but the effect of anesthesia depends highly on $Paco_2$, such that P_{100} at high $Paco_2$ values is increased, even under anesthesia. In acute respiratory failure due to other causes, P_{100} is generally elevated. Herrera and colleagues[199] and Sassoon and coworkers[200] observed values of P_{100} above 6 cm H_2O and 4.2 cm H_2O, respectively, during T-tube trials to be correlated to lack of success in weaning. Using similar threshold values, P_{100} can be used as a guide to the discontinuation of mechanical ventilation after general anesthesia.[201]

Montgomery and associates[202] found a similar relationship but reported a better prediction of weaning successes using the P_{100} response after breathing of 3% CO_2 ($P_{100}H$). The mean $P_{100}H/P_{100}$ ratio was 2.04 in seven successful weaning attempts and 1.17 in seven failures.

PULMONARY AND CHEST WALL MECHANICAL FUNCTION

Principles of Gas Flow Measurement

Monitoring of inspiratory and expiratory flow can be useful for a variety of reasons (see Chapter 26). First, measures of resistance (discussed later) require pressure and flow measurements. Second, flow may be integrated to provide a monitor of inspired or expired volume. Several types of flow meter exist. The most commonly used flow meter in anesthesia probably is the rotameter, in which gas flow imparts movement to a series of vanes connected to a wheel. The Wright spirometer integrates this movement, providing the user with a measure of volume. The Fleisch pneumotachograph consists of a bundle of small-diameter tubes in parallel. Flow within these capillary tubes is laminar, and pressure drop is therefore linearly related to gas flow.[203] Screen-type pneumotachographs work by measurement of the pressure drop across a mesh screen. These devices are usually smaller and lighter than Fleisch-type pneumotachographs, but they are inherently nonlinear. Moreover, their practical implementation is often limited by their tendency to collect moisture and debris, which changes their operating characteristics. Modern mechanical ventilators often incorporate vortex-type pneumotachographs, which work by measurement of interruptions in an ultrasonic beam placed across a tube in which struts disrupt the laminar flow, resulting in vortices.[203] Ultrasonic flow meters measure the speed of ultrasonic waves propagated parallel to the direction of flow.[204] Hot-wire anemometers consist of electrically heated wires placed in the gas stream, which tend to cool the wire and change the electrical conductivity. Flow is measured by the amount of additional electrical current generated by a feedback circuit that is necessary to maintain the wire at constant temperature. These devices characteristically have an extremely high-frequency response, but their behavior depends highly on gas temperature and contamination of the gas stream with mucus and water droplets.[203]

Respiratory Output

The mechanical output of the respiratory system may be assessed by measuring respiratory muscle activity and resulting gas flow. The electrical activity of the diaphragm, the most important inspiratory muscle, has been measured in adults with needle electrodes inserted into the eighth or ninth intercostal spaces in the midaxillary line[205] and in neonates with surface electrodes applied subcostally at the nipple line.[206] Diaphragmatic electromyograms can be obtained in this manner in neonates, but in adults, they are frequently contaminated by the simultaneous electrical activity of the overlying intercostals.

A cleaner diaphragmatic electromyographic signal may be obtained by using an esophageal electrode.[207] Electrical gating of the much larger electrocardiographic signal may allow relatively pure diaphragmatic electromyographic signals to be recorded.[208] Fatiguing muscle tends to produce electromyographic potentials at lower frequencies, allowing diaphragmatic fatigue in a variety of situations to be diagnosed by frequency analysis of the signal obtained in this way.[207] Mechanical activity of the diaphragm cannot be assessed directly. However, because of its approximately hemi-ellipsoidal shape, contraction of the diaphragm must result in a transdiaphragmatic pressure.

Esophageal and gastric pressure simultaneously measured may be used to calculate transdiaphragmatic pressure. A nasogastric tube with esophageal and gastric balloons is commercially available (Viasys Healthcare, Palm Springs, CA). Transdiaphragmatic pressure measurement has been used to assess diaphragmatic function[209] and loss of diaphragmatic contraction demonstrated in the early postoperative period after upper abdominal surgery.[210] Loss of transdiaphragmatic pressure generation implies lack of diaphragmatic contraction[211] (Fig. 36-21).

Diaphragm function can also be assessed by measuring either the compound action potential or transdiaphragmatic twitch pressure after phrenic nerve stimulation.[212-214] Diaphragm motion can be assessed somewhat more indirectly by observing or monitoring thoracic and abdominal movements during inspiration. The normal outward movement of the chest and abdomen during inspiration is replaced by paradoxical inward movement of the abdomen in the presence of diaphragmatic inaction,[215] which may be caused by phrenic nerve paresis or diaphragmatic fatigue.[216,217] External movement of the thorax and abdomen can be monitored in this way by using magnetometers, which can monitor anteroposterior and lateral thoracic and abdominal dimensions,[215,218] or by strain gauge displacement transducers.[219] Another method uses two coils of wire that encircle the torso at the thorax and abdomen. The self-inductances of the coils change in proportion to the encircled areas and can be calibrated to provide continuous monitoring of ventilation.[220] Unfortunately, these methods are rather sensitive to changes in posture or body position[221] and cannot be used during surgery on the thorax or abdomen. The final mechanical output of the respiratory system (i.e., gas flow) can be assessed by monitoring minute ventilation directly or monitoring its components, ventilation rate, and tidal volume.

Monitoring of breath sounds provides a low-cost, highly reliable, semi-quantitative measure of gas flow into and out of the lung. Continuous monitoring of breath sounds using an earpiece connected to a precordial or esophageal stethoscope allows immediate detection of breathing circuit disconnection in mechanically ventilated patients. It facilitates early detection of decreased tidal volume, changes in respiration rate, and endotracheal tube cuff leaks. It also provides qualitative data that may indicate changes in pulmonary mechanics. Wheezes (i.e., rhonchi) are produced when gas flow and airways interact such that airway walls become apposed. Oscillation of the airways between open and nearly closed causes airway vibration, which results in sound production detected as wheezing. Wheezes may occur when airway diameter is narrowed as a result of smooth muscle contraction (i.e., bronchospasm), mucosal thickening or edema, buildup of secretions, extrinsic compression, or an endobronchial mass such as a tumor or foreign body. Although severe generalized obstruction of airways may occur without wheezing, such as in emphysema, the presence of wheezes correlates with reversibility of airways obstruction.[222] Crackles (i.e., rales) are discontinuous sounds produced by the sudden opening of small airways during inspiration. They indicate airway closure and subsequent reopening, which may occur in interstitial fibrosis or in any situation resulting in premature closure of small airways, such as pneumonia, pulmonary edema, or low lung volumes. In patients with large amounts of airway secretions, particularly in the large airways, coarse crackles may also

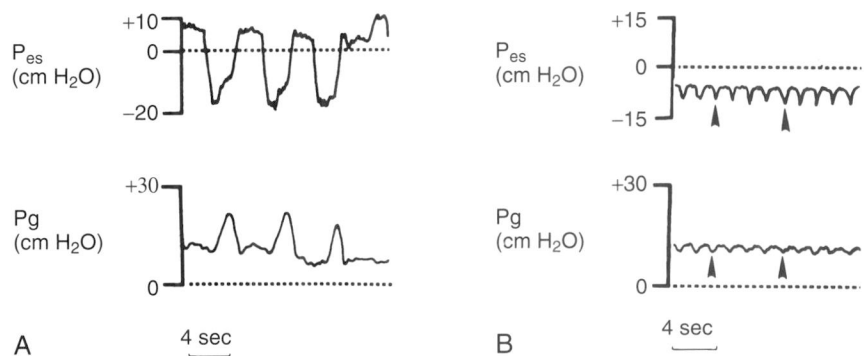

Figure 36–21 Examples of transdiaphragmatic pressure monitoring. **A,** Simultaneous esophageal and gastric pressure waveforms during tidal breathing in a normal individual. Negative esophageal (and therefore pleural) pressure swings are accompanied by positive gastric pressure waves, indicating the development of transdiaphragmatic pressure during inspiration. **B,** The same waveforms in a patient with phrenic nerve palsy (and therefore absent diaphragmatic contraction). Negative intrathoracic pressure swings (*arrowheads*) are accompanied by gastric pressure swings in the same direction. Intrathoracic pressure changes are directly transmitted through a passive diaphragm. These changes can also be observed in the early postoperative period in patients who have had upper abdominal surgery. (From Brown KA, Hoffstein V, Byrick RJ: Bedside diagnosis of bilateral diaphragmatic paralysis in a ventilator-dependent patient after open-heart surgery. Anesth Analg 64:1208, 1985.)

be caused by gas bubbling through airway secretions. The origin of lung sounds has been reviewed elsewhere.[223-225]

Minute ventilation and tidal volume are easy to measure directly in patients whose tracheas are intubated, and these parameters are routinely measured by modern mechanical ventilators. However, in the patient whose trachea is not intubated, these parameters can be obtained only somewhat inaccurately by monitoring external dimensions of the thorax and abdomen by direct observation or by using one of the techniques described. Subjective assessment is extremely inaccurate,[226] commonly done with overestimation of tidal volume by up to 60%. Alternatively, $\dot{V}_E$ can be monitored directly by using a head tent.[227] These methods are difficult to apply for routine clinical use. Measurement of the ventilation rate remains the mainstay of respiratory output monitoring. Mechanical measures of gas flow such as these provide combined assessments of respiratory drive and mechanical function of the respiratory system. However, in the presence of relatively normal thoracic mechanics, respiratory gas movement is considered to be a reasonable monitor of respiratory output.

Measurement of Respiratory Mechanics

Principles

Mechanical properties of the respiratory system include the passive mechanical properties of resistance, elastance, and inertance, in addition to the motor properties of the muscles of respiration. Resistance (R), in pulmonary mechanical terms, is the increment in pressure (ΔP) applied to the system divided by the increment in flow or rate of change of volume (ΔV):

$$R = \frac{P}{\dot{V}} = \frac{P}{dv/dt} \qquad (34)$$

Normal resistance is 1.5 cm $H_2O \cdot L^{-1} \cdot$ sec, but under anesthesia it may be as high as 9 cm H_2O/L/sec. Most of the resistance of the respiratory system results from the flow resistance of the major conducting airways. A small portion of the resistance is caused by the tissue viscosity.

Conductance (G) is the reciprocal of resistance:

$$G = \frac{1}{R} \qquad (35)$$

Elastance (E) is the applied pressure divided by the resulting static change in volume:

$$E = \frac{\Delta P}{\Delta V} \qquad (36)$$

A more commonly used variable is compliance (C), the reciprocal of elastance:

$$C = \frac{1}{E} \qquad (37)$$

A commonly used unit for compliance is mL/cm H_2O. Because the lung and chest wall are mechanically in series, the following relationships apply:

$$\frac{1}{C_{TH}} = \frac{1}{C_L} + \frac{1}{C_{CW}} \qquad (38)$$

In Equation 38, C_{TH}, C_L, and C_{CW} are the thoracic, lung, and chest wall compliances, respectively.

Inertance (I) is the applied pressure divided by the gas acceleration or the second derivative of volume with respect to time:

$$I = \frac{P}{\ddot{V}} = \frac{\Delta P}{d^2V/dt^2} \qquad (39)$$

Inertance is analogous to the mass of tissue and gas within the lung. Normal thoracic inertance is 0.02 to 0.04 cm $H_2O \cdot L \cdot sec^{-2}$. Ordinarily, because acceleration of gas flow and mass of gas and tissue are low, inertance plays a minor part in the mechanical behavior of the respiratory system. However, under conditions of high-frequency ventilation or high inspired gas density (e.g., in deep diving), inertance may play a major role in determining gas flow.

Practical Measurement of Passive Respiratory Mechanical Properties

Estimates of compliance and resistance in the respiratory system may be obtained by inspection of the airway pressure-volume (or time) relationships. Thoracic compliance may be obtained by inflating the lungs with known increments of volume and measuring the static pressure at each point. Under normal circumstances, the lung and chest wall have approximately equal compliance of approximately 200 mL/cm H_2O, resulting in a total thoracic compliance of 100 mL/cm H_2O. Individual measurements of chest wall and lung components of the total respiratory compliance cannot be made without some estimate of pleural pressure. Conventionally, pleural pressure is measured by inserting a pressure-monitoring balloon within the esophagus. Unfortunately, in the supine patient, the weight of the mediastinum results in a falsely high estimate of pleural pressure when using this technique. Direct pleural pressure measurement must therefore be obtained to measure lung and chest wall compliance accurately in this position. A noninvasive method of pleural pressure measurement, using a flat loop of Teflon-insulated wire attached to the skin of the suprasternal fossa, has been described.[228] The skin movement that accompanies changes in intrapleural pressure is transduced by the coil of wire by continuous measurement of its self-inductance. Measurements of pulmonary compliance using this technique correlated well with similar measurements using an esophageal balloon to estimate intrapleural pressure. However, the technique is time consuming, and measurements cannot be obtained in some individuals.

Thoracic compliance can be estimated on a breath-by-breath basis by monitoring the inspiratory pressure-time curve. If a constant tidal volume is being used to ventilate a patient, the thoracic compliance will be inversely related to the inspiratory pressure. It is important that the pressure used to calculate thoracic compliance be at end inspiration (i.e., plateau pressure), because during the period of inspiratory gas flow there is an additional component of pressure due to airways resistance. The changes in peak airway pressure (related to airways resistance and

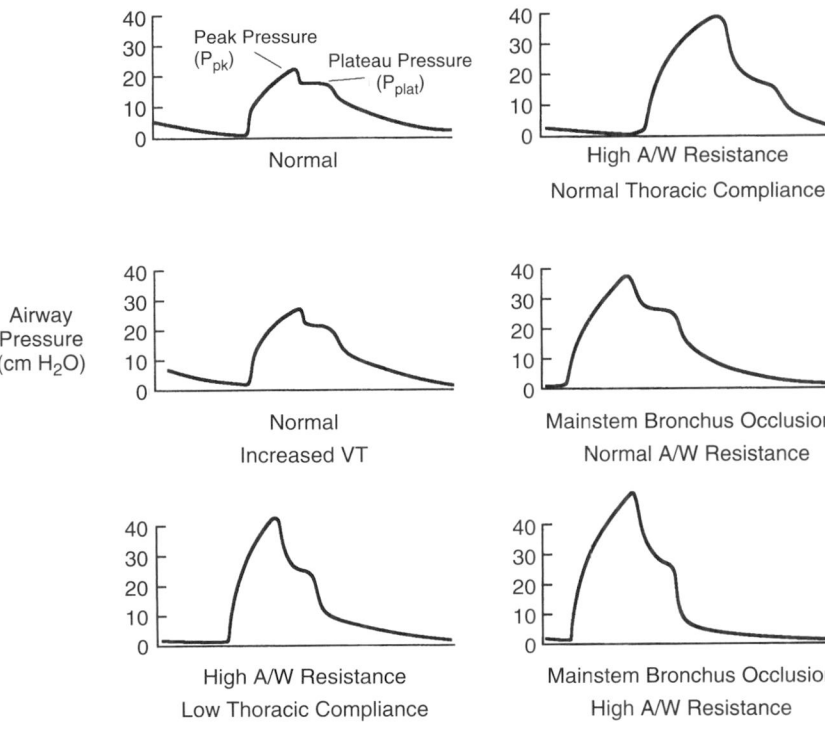

Figure 36–22 Examples of airway pressure waveforms. Airway pressure is plotted versus time. Decreased static thoracic compliance results in an increase in plateau pressure; increases in airway resistance cause increased peak airway pressure and decreased dynamic compliance.

thoracic compliance) and the plateau pressure (related only to compliance) may quickly identify pulmonary mechanical abnormalities in ventilated patients (Fig. 36-22). An empirically defined measurement, tidal volume divided by peak inspiratory pressure change, is defined as dynamic compliance (Cdyn):

$$Cdyn = \frac{V_T}{P_{pk} - PEEP} \qquad (40)$$

In Equation 40, V_T is the tidal volume, P_{pk} is the peak airway pressure, and PEEP is the positive end-expiratory pressure. The normal value is 40 to 80 mL/cm H_2O.

Static compliance (Cstat) can be calculated by measuring the plateau pressure and using the following equation:

$$Cstat = \frac{V_T}{P_{plat} - PEEP} \qquad (41)$$

The normal value for static compliance is 50 to 100 mL/cm H_2O.

To make these compliance calculations, any end-expiratory pressure must be subtracted from the peak pressure or plateau pressure. The PEEP value can usually be read directly from the airway pressure monitor at end expiration. However, when insufficient expiratory time prevents complete emptying of the lungs, significant end-expiratory elevation of alveolar pressure that is not detected at the airway pressure monitor (i.e., auto-PEEP) may occur.[229,230] Auto-PEEP is most likely to exist when elevation of airway resistance or compliance cause prolongation of expiratory time or when high ventilation rates are required.[229] Auto-PEEP can result in decreased cardiac output, hypotension, and electromechanical dissociation in mechanically ventilated patients. It also affects

compliance measurements. Detection of auto-PEEP can be accomplished by occluding the exhalation port of the ventilator while delaying the onset of the next ventilator breath. Alveolar pressure then equilibrates with the ventilator circuit, and auto-PEEP can be read on the airway pressure monitor (Fig. 36-23). During this temporary occlusion maneuver, it is important to prevent supplementary gas flow (e.g., fresh gas flow) from entering the circuit and falsely elevating the auto-PEEP value.

A decrease in static compliance may be caused by atelectasis, pulmonary edema, pneumothorax, external compression of the chest (i.e., intra-abdominal hemorrhage or, in the operating room, abdominal packing or the surgeon's leaning on the torso), or accumulation of pleural fluid. Decreased dynamic compliance may be caused by elevated airways resistance (e.g., bronchospasm, mucus accumulation) or obstruction or kinking of the endotracheal tube.

In parallel with the patient's thoracic compliance are the internal compliances of the breathing circuit and any associated humidification or gas warming systems. Circuit compliance may be as high as 10 mL/cm H_2O and must be accounted for if an accurate measurement of thoracic compliance is required. Decreased thoracic compliance places an additional load on the patient's respiratory muscles. Thoracic compliance less than 25 mL/cm H_2O is unlikely to result in successful weaning from mechanical ventilation.[231]

Thoracic resistance can be measured in the intubated patient by oscillating the airway with a sinusoidal or randomly varying flow with simultaneous measurements of flow and pressure. Significant increases in thoracic resistance have been observed in anesthetized patients after reversal of neuromuscular blockade with edrophonium (0.43 mg/kg).[232] An indirect estimate of airways resistance may also be obtained by monitoring the flow-time

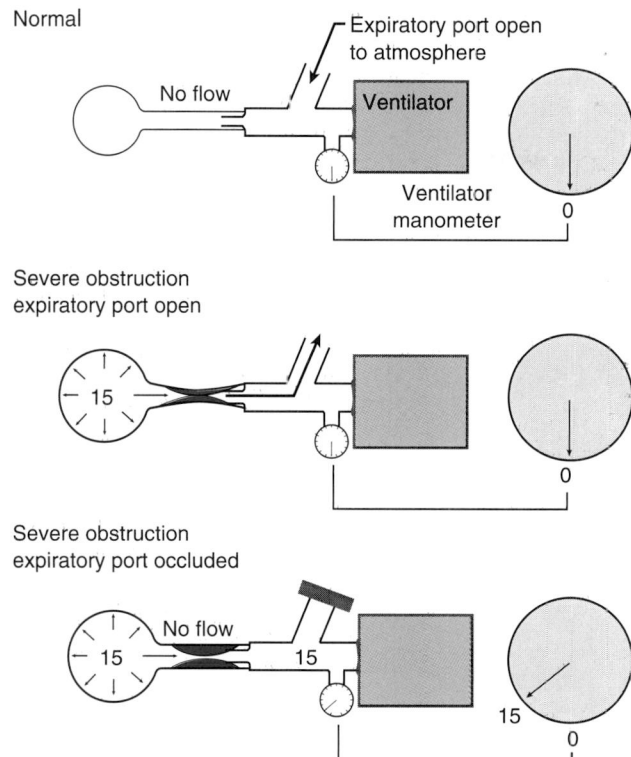

Normal

Expiratory port open to atmosphere

No flow

Ventilator

Ventilator manometer

Severe obstruction expiratory port open

Severe obstruction expiratory port occluded

No flow

Figure 36–23 Auto–positive end-expiratory pressure (auto-PEEP). Severe airway obstruction may result in high alveolar gas pressure at end expiration, which can exert the same effect on hemodynamics as externally applied PEEP. This is not usually detectable unless the expiratory port of the ventilator circuit is occluded. Auto-PEEP may then be read directly from the airway pressure monitor. (Adapted from Pepe PE, Marini JJ: Occult positive end-expiratory pressure in mechanically ventilated patients with airflow obstruction: The auto-PEEP effect. Am Rev Respir Dis 126:166, 1982.)

or volume-time relationship of a passive exhalation after manual inflation of a lung.[233] If a constant thoracic compliance is assumed, the time constant of exhalation is related to airways resistance.

Commercially available monitors can provide continuous displays of inspired volume versus airways pressure and flow versus inspired volume[234,235] (Fig. 36-24). These techniques can been used to monitor changes in pulmonary compliance caused by intraoperative pulmonary edema[234] or during laparoscopic instillation of gas into the peritoneal cavity,[236] to detect malpositioning of double-lumen endotracheal tubes,[237] and to assess pulmonary mechanics after lung volume–reduction surgery.[235]

APNEA MONITORING

Most of the principles of apnea monitoring have already been discussed. In practice, the appropriateness of a particular apnea monitor depends on the situation in which it is to be used. For example, a head canopy monitor of ventilation[227] may be appropriate in an ICU but entirely inappropriate for use at home in a young child. Apnea monitors are usually based on one of three general principles—detection of gas flow, chest wall movement, and gas exchange (i.e., monitors of $Paco_2$ or Sao_2). Guyatt and colleagues[238] described a method in which a pressure transducer was connected to a nasal O_2 cannula. Periodic fluctuations of about 1 cm H_2O due to cyclical respiratory flow were observed during nose breathing. Respiratory rates could easily be obtained with this technique, even when O_2 was flowing through the canula. Direct monitoring of ventilation can be obtained easily in a patient whose trachea is intubated. Use of a rigid, airtight canopy that encases the subject's head with a neck seal has been described by Sorkin and coworkers.[227] The canopy is continuously flushed with fresh gas. The subject's respiration produces a net flow in and out of the canopy,

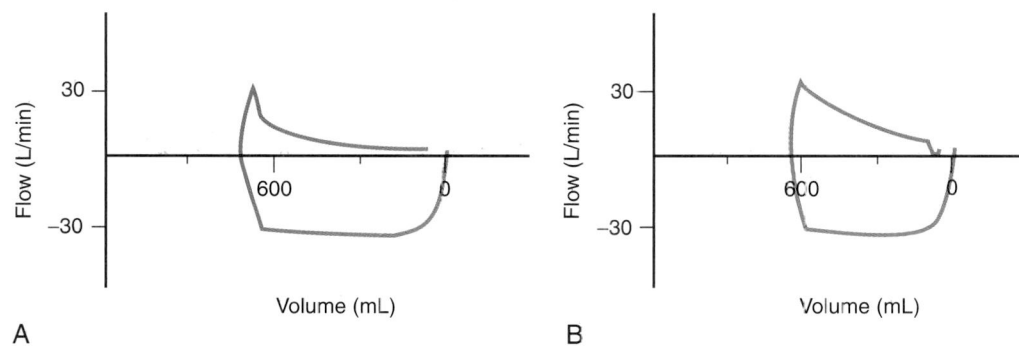

A   B

Figure 36–24 Flow (ordinate) versus volume (abscissa). **A,** Closed-chest positive-pressure ventilation under general anesthesia in a patient with severe airways obstruction and hyperinflation before surgery to reduce lung volume. The flow-volume curve shows inspiratory (negative) and expiratory (positive) flow on the ordinate, plotted clockwise from zero volume on the abscissa. Expiratory flow started with a sharp upward peak and then fell immediately to a low flow rate with convexity toward the volume axis, suggesting expiratory flow limitation. expiratory flow rate was so low that inflation of the next positive-pressure breath was initiated before expiratory flow reached zero. Because expiratory flow continued up to this point, there must have been intrinsic positive end-expiratory pressure (PEEPi). **B,** A similar closed-check flow-volume curve after lung resection shows that the characteristic pattern of expiratory flow limitation has disappeared and that expiratory flow rate fell to zero before inflation started for the next breath (i.e., no suggestion of PEEPi). (Adapted from Dueck R: Assessment and monitoring of flow limitation and other parameters from flow/volume loops. J Clin Monit Comput 16:425, 2000.)

which is unaffected by the fresh gas flow. The system can be worn comfortably while awake or asleep.

Another method of airflow detection was described by Werthammer and associates.[239] An acoustic monitor encapsulated in silicone rubber was taped 0.25 cm inside a nostril. Eight premature infants were continuously monitored for 1 to 2 hours; 26 episodes of apnea lasting 15 seconds or longer were detected and confirmed by direct observation. An impedance monitor detected only seven of these episodes. Hok and colleagues[240] described an acoustic method, which was demonstrated to detect hypoventilation and apnea with greater sensitivity than pulse oximetry. An extremely unobtrusive method is to use a tiny, rapid-response hygrometer taped close to a nostril. This type of sensor can monitor respiratory rates at least up to 60 breaths/min as effectively as capnometry in infants or adults.[241]

Chest wall movement may be detected in several ways. One method is inductive plethysmography,[220] in which the abdomen and thorax are each encircled by a coil, and respiratory movements are detected as changes in the self-inductance. A more commonly used approach is transthoracic impedance, a technique that is commonly implemented in commercially available electrocardiographic monitors. In this method, a small alternating current (typically 100 microamps) at about 100 kHz is passed through a pair of electrocardiographic leads, allowing transthoracic electrical impedance to be continuously measured by a change in the induced 100-kHz voltage. Low-frequency changes in respiratory impedance can easily be demodulated from the signal.[95,239] Electromyography of the respiratory muscles can also been used to monitor respiration,[206] although it is more difficult because of contamination of the electromyographic signal with a much higher voltage electrocardiographic potential. Photoplethysmography is the monitoring of changes induced by respiration in the light absorption of skin and blood vessels. Photoplethysmographic (PPG) sensors can detect cyclic changes in peripheral blood flow caused by breathing. PPG sensors, consisting of an infrared source and a photocell to measure back-scattered light, were applied near a forearm vein and could detect respiratory movements in patients after general anesthesia.[242] The main disadvantage of these monitors of patient movement is that they may fail to detect obstructive apnea, in which ventilatory effort or movement can occur without gas flow.

Because apnea may not result in any physiologic abnormality, a measure of its possible adverse effects (i.e., hypoxia or hypercapnia) may be preferable. Continuous measurement of end-tidal CO_2, although easy in an intubated patient, is more difficult in a patient whose trachea is not intubated because of discomfort from the catheter placement and clogging with mucus and saliva. This problem frequently accompanies direct placement of a cannula into the nasopharynx. Some improvements may be obtained if a catheter is placed inside a nasal airway. A more satisfactory solution is to use specially designed nasal cannulas in which one prong is used to sample exhaled gas while the other is used to deliver O_2.

Another approach is to use O_2 saturation. George and coworkers[243] compared arterial desaturation with manually detected events using a variety of monitors, including chin electromyography, airflow measurement, and respiratory movement measured by inductance plethysmography. Apnea was defined as cessation of respiration for more than 10 seconds. Nine overnight records from six patients with sleep apnea were analyzed and compared with Sao_2 measurement using an ear oximeter. Decreases in Sao_2 of more than 3% from baseline were considered significant. Using this criterion, only 1.32% of 4008 apneic episodes were undetected. Catley and associates[79] used ear oximetry and respiratory inductive plethysmography to monitor patients postoperatively, and they demonstrated that morphine analgesia, compared with regional analgesia with local anesthetic, was associated with a high incidence of hypoxemia and associated obstructive apnea, central apnea, paradoxic breathing, and slow respiratory rate.

Given the proven reliability of pulse oximetry, it seems that this method, perhaps in association with capnography, may provide an excellent method of apnea monitoring. Principles of apnea monitoring have been reviewed elsewhere in detail.[244]

LUNG WATER

The need to detect pulmonary edema has led to a variety of techniques for the early detection of increased lung water. Chest radiography, although it has a relatively low sensitivity (a 35% increase in extravascular lung water is required for the diagnosis of definite pulmonary edema), remains the gold standard. Techniques such as Compton scattering,[245,246] magnetic resonance imaing,[247,248] positron emission tomography,[249] double-indicator dilution using indocyanine green and a thermal marker[250,251] or heavy water (i.e., deuterium oxide [D_2O]),[252,253] multiple inert gases,[254,255] and impedance plethysmography[256] have been useful research tools but have not entered routine clinical use.

MONITORING OF HIGH-FREQUENCY VENTILATION

High-frequency ventilation has been variously defined but in general represents mechanical ventilation at high rates (usually 160 breaths/min). Several means of ventilating in this manner have been used experimentally and clinically. The use of conventional positive-pressure ventilators at high rates and small tidal volumes is called *high-frequency positive-pressure ventilation* (HFPV). Tidal volumes are usually on the order of 3 to 4 mL/kg of body weight, with a frequency of 60 to 100 breaths/min. The use of an oscillator providing positive and negative pressure fluctuations (e.g., a loudspeaker) is called *high-frequency oscillatory ventilation* (HFOV). Higher frequencies, upward of 3000 cycles/min, have been used with this modality. A *bias flow* of fresh gas at the level of the oscillator provides the source of the respiratory gas and washes out CO_2. Injection of a high-velocity pulse of gas into the airway through a narrow cannula, entraining with it fresh gas, is called *high-frequency jet ventilation* (HFJV).

In all these forms of high-frequency ventilation, instantaneous gas flows and pressure fluctuations cannot usually be monitored with conventional transducers. Moreover, because the system is basically open, a portion of the gas flow directed into the airway may leak out and not participate in intrapulmonary gas exchange. High-frequency ventilatory fluctuations generated by these ventilators may also in part do nothing more than compress and decompress the compliance of the ventilatory circuit and large conducting airways. Conventional mechanical monitoring is therefore difficult. Capnography is difficult to apply, because dilution of expired gas may render end-tidal measurements artificially low, even assuming a high-fidelity, high-frequency capnograph.

Monitoring of patients receiving high-frequency ventilation requires the ability to monitor O_2 and CO_2 exchange, as well as mechanical safety, including airway disconnection and obstruction. Hoskyns and colleagues[257] measured tidal volumes in 0.8- to 1.9-kg infants ventilated at 2 to 25 Hz using an external respiratory jacket. A side port of the jacket was used to monitor pressure changes, which correlated linearly with tidal volume.

Whereas patient oxygenation can readily be monitored with pulse oximetry, there is no reliable noninvasive monitor of CO_2 exchange. One way of monitoring CO_2 is to measure the mean waste gas CO_2 concentration by placing a capnograph in the expired circuit. If any condition that interferes with CO_2 exchange develops, the mean expired CO_2 decreases. Although this method provides a fairly gross measure of adequacy of CO_2 exchange, the expired CO_2 concentration highly depends on fresh gas flow rate. A more satisfactory monitor would multiply fresh gas flow by expired CO_2 fraction to obtain $\dot{V}_{CO_2}$. Changes in CO_2 could then reflect a mechanical problem with the ventilator. Unfortunately, other factors such as anesthesia or hypothermia may alter $\dot{V}_{CO_2}$. The clinician cannot obtain a measure of P_{ACO_2} or Pa_{CO_2} by this method. The most commonly used method is to interject a conventional breath periodically to measure end-tidal CO_2.[258] Capnometry can be used to measure end-tidal CO_2 during HFJV without such a maneuver, provided that gas is sampled from a port situated at the tip of the endotracheal tube.[259]

Monitoring of airway pressure is extremely important in high-frequency ventilation. In particular, HFJV uses high pressures and gas flows. Expiratory port occlusion can therefore result in extremely high airway pressures. Gas pressures commonly are measured on both sides of the jet valve (i.e., drive pressure and jet pressure), along with an independent pressure measurement in the airway (Fig. 36-25). An automated feedback loop is required to interrupt the jet ventilation by closing the solenoid valve in the event of excessively high pressures in the airway or on the jet side of the valve. Low pressures can be used as indications of airway disconnection or ventilator malfunction.

In addition to safety concerns, airway pressure has been shown in several studies to correlate with gas exchange efficiency during HFJV.[260] Increasing peak airway pressures result in lower Pa_{CO_2}. A superior indicator of Pa_{CO_2} is the difference between peak airway pressure and end-expiratory airway pressure.[261] However, there is no unique relationship, and the Pa_{CO_2} obtained for a given patient depends on properties of the lung. Position of the

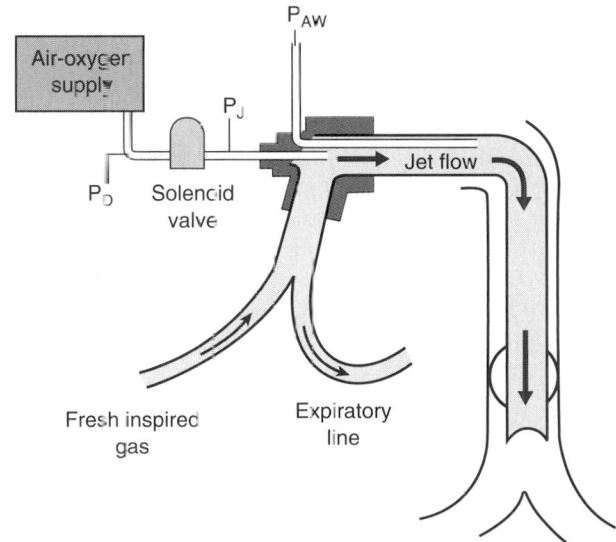

Figure 36–25 High-frequency jet ventilation. The jet is created when a high-pressure air-O_2 supply is rapidly modulated by the solenoid valve. Fresh inspired gas is from a low-pressure source, typically an anesthesia circuit. Drive pressure (PD) and jet pressure (PJ) are customarily monitored to detect solenoid or jet malfunction. An independent monitor of airway pressure (Paw), which can reliably detect overpressurization of the airway, circuit disconnection, or ventilator malfunction, should also be available.

monitoring transducer may be critical because proximal airway pressures may be artifactually low.[261]

Jet ventilation for prolonged periods should ideally be performed on patients with the ability to monitor arterial blood gases directly. Periodic measurement of Pa_{CO_2} may provide greater assurance of adequate pulmonary gas exchange than simple reliance on noninvasive measures.

DISCONTINUATION OF MECHANICAL VENTILATION AND TRACHEAL EXTUBATION

Mechanical ventilation may be instituted for a variety of reasons, including impaired respiratory drive, increased mechanical load, impaired respiratory motor function, and impaired pulmonary gas exchange (see Chapter 75). Endotracheal intubation is usually performed to facilitate mechanical ventilation but may also be instituted for maintenance of a patent upper airway, to enable suctioning of secretions, for bronchoscopy, and to provide airway protection. Development of criteria for the successful liberation of a patient from mechanical ventilation and extubation may be highly specific to the clinical situation.

The most common reason for mechanical ventilation during and after anesthesia is impaired respiratory drive. However, components of increased mechanical load and impaired neuromuscular function may contribute to an abnormally low ventilatory function. Patients with severe chronic obstructive pulmonary disease usually are mechanically ventilated because of transient increases in mechanical load superimposed on a chronic increase in airways resistance. However, impaired respiratory drive and abnormal respiratory muscle mechanics may also play a role. Abnormal arterial oxygenation may exist despite what appears to be adequate ventilatory effort. Ventilatory support may be required mainly to aid arterial oxygenation or CO_2 elimination. Assessment of the patient with regard to possible discontinuation of mechanical ventilation may therefore vary considerably, depending on the reason for mechanical ventilatory support.

Discontinuation of ventilatory support (i.e., weaning) from a patient whose only reason for mechanical ventilation is residual anesthesia is generally straightforward. A different approach is often required for a patient who has had prolonged ventilatory support for chronic respiratory disease.[262] Screening criteria are listed in Table 36-5. Commonly used discontinuation criteria include hemodynamic stability, a vital capacity not less than 10 mL/kg, maximum inspiratory pressure less than (i.e., more negative) –25 cm H_2O, respiratory rate not above 20 breaths/min, and $\dot{V}E$ not more than 10 to 20 L/min in the face of normal $PaCO_2$, and adequate arterial oxygenation (e.g., PaO_2/FIO_2 ratio > 150 to 200) maintained with an inspired O_2 concentration not above 40% to 50%, with less than 5 to 8 cm H_2O of PEEP. An extremely useful, easily measured variable is the ratio of ventilatory frequency to tidal volume (f/VT) during a 1- to 2-minute trial of spontaneous ventilation.[263,264] An f/VT ratio greater than 100 predicts unsuccessful weaning. A partial list of published weaning criteria is shown in Table 36-6.

Criteria used for patients being weaned from mechanical ventilation in the postoperative period are not applicable to patients who have been ventilator dependent for several days or weeks, in whom respiratory muscle atrophy, malnutrition, and peripheral neuropathy have often supervened. In the latter situation, any single criterion for discontinuation of ventilation has been shown to have poor predictive value.[262]

Extensive reviews and comments on weaning criteria and techniques have been published.[262,263,265-268] A task force of the American College of Chest Physicians, the American Association for Respiratory Care, and the American College of Critical Care Medicine has published a set of evidence-based guidelines for discontinuation of mechanical ventilation.[266] The first seven of these recommendations pertain to monitoring and weaning individual patients:

Recommendation 1: In patients requiring mechanical ventilation for more than 24 hours, a search for all the causes that may be contributing to ventilator dependence should be undertaken. This is particularly true for the patient who has failed attempts at withdrawing the mechanical ventilator. Reversing all possible ventilatory and nonventilatory issues should be an integral part of the ventilator-discontinuation process.

Recommendation 2: Patients receiving mechanical ventilation for respiratory failure should undergo a formal assessment of discontinuation potential if the following criteria are satisfied:
  A. Evidence for some reversal of the underlying cause for respiratory failure
  B. Adequate oxygenation (e.g., PaO_2/FIO_2 ratio > 150 to 200, requiring positive end-expiratory pressure [PEEP] = 5 to 8 cm H_2O and FIO_2 = 0.4 to 0.5) and pH (e.g., pH = 7.25)
  C. Hemodynamic stability, as defined by the absence of active myocardial ischemia and the absence of clinically significant hypotension (i.e., a condition requiring no vasopressor therapy or therapy with only low-dose vasopressors such as dopamine or dobutamine [<5 $\mu g \cdot kg^{-1} \cdot min$])
  D. The capability to initiate an inspiratory effort
  The decision to use these criteria must be individualized. Some patients not satisfying all of the above criteria (e.g., patients with chronic hypoxemia values below the thresholds cited) may be ready for attempts at the discontinuation of mechanical ventilation.

Recommendation 3: Formal discontinuation assessments for patients receiving mechanical ventilation for respiratory failure should be performed during spontaneous breathing rather than while the patient is still receiving substantial ventilatory support. An initial brief period of spontaneous breathing can be used to assess the capability of continuing onto a formal spontaneous breathing trial (SBT). The criteria with which to assess patient tolerance during SBTs are the respiratory pattern, the adequacy of gas exchange, hemodynamic stability, and subjective comfort. The tolerance of SBTs

---

Table 36–5 Screening criteria used in weaning trials to determine whether patients receiving high levels of ventilatory support can be considered for discontinuation

Criteria	Description
Objective	Adequate oxygenation (e.g., $PO_2 \geq 60$ mm Hg on $FIO_2 \leq 4$; PEEP ≤ 5-10 cm H_2O; $PaO_2/FIO_2 \geq 150$-300 mm Hg)
	Stable cardiovascular system (e.g., HR ≤ 140 beats/min, stable BP; no [or minimal] pressors)
	Afebrile (temperature < 38°C)
	No significant respiratory acidosis
	Adequate hemoglobin (e.g., Hb ≥ 8-10 g/dL)
	Adequate mentation (e.g., arousable, GCS ≥ 13, no continuous sedative infusions)
	Stable metabolic status (e.g., acceptable electrolytes)
Subjective clinical assessments	Resolution of disease acute phase; physician believes discontinuation possible; adequate cough

BP, blood pressure; GCS, Glasgow Coma Scale; Hb, hemoglobin; HR, heart rate; PaO_2/FIO_2 (P/F ratio), arterial oxygen tension/fractional inspired oxygen concentration; PEEP, positive end-expiratory pressure; PO_2, partial pressure of oxygen.
From MacIntyre NR, Cook DJ, Ely EW Jr, et al: Evidence-based guidelines for weaning and discontinuing ventilatory support: A collective task force facilitated by the American College of Chest Physicians, the American Association for Respiratory Care, and the American College of Critical Care Medicine. Chest 120:375S, 2001.

Table 36–6 Possible criteria for ventilator discontinuation

Test	Criterion for Weaning
Mechanical Function	
Forced vital capacity (FVC)	>10-15 mL/kg
Forced expiratory volume in 1 second (FEV$_1$)	>10 mL/kg
Tidal volume during spontaneous breathing (V$_T$)*	≥325-408 mL (4-6 mL/kg)
Maximum inspiratory pressure (P$_{Imax}$)*	≤ –15 - –30 cm H$_2$O
Negative inspiratory force (NIF)*	≤ –20 - –30 cm H$_2$O
Maximum voluntary ventilation (MVV)	>2 × resting V̇$_E$
Respiratory rate during spontaneous breathing (V$_F$)*	<30-38/min
Respiratory minute volume (V̇$_E$)	<10-15 L/min
V$_F$/V$_T$ (i.e., f/V$_T$ or rapid shallow breathing index [RSBI]) during spontaneous breathing*	≤60-105 breaths/min per 1 L
V$_F$/(V$_T$/kg) during spontaneous breathing†	<11 breaths/min per 1 mL/kg
Thoracic compliance	
Static	≥33 mL/cm H$_2$O
Dynamic	≥22 mL/cm H$_2$O
Work of breathing	
Per minute	≤1.6 kg · m/min
Per L/min V̇$_E$	≤0.14 kg · m/min
(0.75 V$_T$/C$_{dyn}$) · (T$_I$/T$_{tot}$)/(MIP)‡	<0.15
Functional residual capacity (FRC)	>50% of predicted
Gas Exchange Function	
A-a gradient (F$_{IO_2}$ = 1.0)	<350 mm Hg
Pao$_2$/Pao$_2$ ratio	≥0.35
Shunt fraction (Q̇s/Q̇T)	<0.2
Dead space/tidal volume ratio (V$_D$/V$_T$)	<0.6
Minute ventilation (V̇$_E$) with normal Paco$_2$	<180 mL/kg/min
Respiratory quotient (R)	<0.9
Pao$_2$/F$_{IO_2}$	>200
Respiratory Drive	
Pressure obtained 100 msec after temporary airway occlusion (P$_{100}$)	<6 cm H$_2$O
P$_{100}$/P$_{Imax}$*	<0.3
Other Tests	
Urine output	500 mL/6 hr
Arterial pH	>7.30
Gastric intramural pHi during pressure support trial	>7.30 or a change of <0.09
[C$_{dyn}$ · MIP · (Pao$_2$/Pao$_2$)] /V$_F$§	≥13 mL per 1 breath/min
[(C$_{dyn}$/kg) · MIP · (Pao$_2$/Pao$_2$)]/V$_F$†	≥0.1 mL/kg per 1 breath/min

*Measurements shown to have statistically significant likelihood ratios to predict the outcome of a ventilator discontinuation effort in more than one study.[266]

†Pediatric use.[305]

‡Inspiratory effort quotient (IEQ). If intrinsic positive end-expiratory pressure (PEEPi) is present,
IEQ = (PEEPi + 0.75 V$_T$/C$_{dyn}$) · (T$_I$/T$_{tot}$)/(MIP · PEEPi)[306]

§CROP index (i.e., compliance, rate, oxygenation, and pressure).[263]

C$_{dyn}$, dynamic thoracic compliance; P$_{Imax}$, maximum inspiratory pressure measured in an occluded airway after 20 seconds starting from residual volume; MIP, maximum inspiratory pressure; NIF, negative pressure measured after at least 1 second of inspiratory effort against an occluded airway, with the most negative value of three attempts recorded; T$_I$ inspiratory time; T$_{tot}$, total respiratory cycle length.

Data from references 18, 200, 202, 262, 263, and 306-317.

lasting 30 to 120 minutes should prompt consideration for permanent ventilator discontinuation.

Recommendation 4: The removal of the artificial airway from a patient who has successfully been discontinued from ventilatory support should be based on assessments of airway patency and the ability of the patient to protect the airway.

Recommendation 5: Patients receiving mechanical ventilation for respiratory failure who fail an SBT should have the cause for the failed SBT determined.

After reversible causes for failure are corrected and if the patient still meets the criteria listed in Table 36-5, subsequent SBTs should be performed every 24 hours.

Recommendation 6: Patients receiving mechanical ventilation for respiratory failure who fail an SBT should receive a stable, nonfatiguing, and comfortable form of ventilatory support.

Recommendation 7: Anesthesia or sedation strategies and ventilator management aimed at early extubation should be used in postsurgical patients.

TRACHEAL EXTUBATION AFTER COMPROMISE OF THE AIRWAY

Protection of the airway with potential encroachment by hemorrhage, edema, infection, or tumor using an endotracheal tube often engenders uncertainty at the time of extubation (see Chapters 74 and 75). Airway patency after extubation may not be ensured, and sudden loss of airway may occur. Reintubation may then be difficult or impossible.

Useful measures that can be taken at the time of extubation include inspection of the upper airway, directly or with a fiberoptic instrument to detect residual swelling of the oropharynx or nasopharynx, and occlusion of the endotracheal tube with cuff deflated. If the patient is able to breathe around the tube in this way, it is less likely that critical airway compromise will occur after extubation. If the endotracheal tube is large with respect to the patient's airway, the patient may not be able to breathe around it, even in the setting of a normal airway. Replacement of the tube with a smaller one may be accomplished over a rigid introducer. Extubation over a rigid introducer allows abrupt loss of the airway to be treated immediately with reinsertion. A nasogastric tube with the bulbous end cut off may be used, but a more rigid plastic introducer is preferable. Alternatively, a fiberoptic bronchoscope may be introduced into the endotracheal tube. If the patient is able to breathe after removal of the tube from the larynx and lower pharynx, direct inspection of the airway may be accomplished during removal of the fiberoptic instrument.

These measures should be undertaken while someone with the necessary skills to perform an emergency tracheotomy is available. Before removal of the endotracheal tube, the patient should be oxygenated with 100% O_2, providing a margin of safety in the event of loss of airway patency.

TRANSPORTATION OF THE PATIENT

Movement of the patient between various critical care units (i.e., operating room, ICU, or PACU) or between the ICU and diagnostic radiology presents special problems (see Chapter 69). Planning for such a move should include preparing for a worst-case scenario. Movement of the patient from the operating room to the PACU may engender problems of hypoxemia, loss of airway, hemodynamic instability or vomiting, and aspiration. After uncomplicated anesthesia, the most likely untoward event is arterial hypoxemia and loss of the airway. Because the patient is at risk for hypoxemia because of a variety of causes, including hypoventilation, atelectasis, impaired $\dot{V}_A/\dot{Q}$ matching, residual second gas effect (N_2O), shivering, and resulting decrease in mixed venous P_{O_2} and airway obstruction, it appears safest to transport the patient with supplemental O_2 unless the distance between operating room and PACU is short. Respiration can be continuously monitored using a tightly fitting mask and observing movements of a bag, a hand held under the chin to feel exhalations, a precordial stethoscope, or if the patient is still intubated, an esophageal stethoscope.

Patients at higher risk of hypoxemia during transport include children, patients with baseline gas exchange abnormality, and obese individuals. In these types of patients, relatively rapid desaturation may occur, even if the patient has been ventilated with 100% O_2 immediately before transport.[269,270] Continuous monitoring of Sp_{O_2} is an additional option.

A worst-case scenario for a patient undergoing transportation over a long distance, particularly in an elevator, includes accidental extubation or an inability to ventilate. In addition to the monitoring techniques described, long-distance transportation within the hospital should always occur with the ability to provide emergency positive-pressure ventilation and emergency endotracheal intubation. Several manufacturers produce portable pulse oximeters, which can be extremely useful in this setting.

EPIDURAL AND INTRATHECAL OPIATES

Many clinical reports suggest that spinal (epidural or intrathecal) opiate administration may result in prolonged superior analgesia after surgery compared with parenteral administration in the traditional fashion (see Chapter 72). Moreover, clinical investigation has suggested that respiratory function, particularly after upper abdominal surgery,[271] may be improved with epidural administration of morphine compared with intravenous administration. However, early reports of delayed respiratory depression after epidural and intrathecal morphine administration have led to scrutiny of the respiratory depressant effect of narcotics given by this route.[272]

Several detailed clinical investigations of blood gases, ventilation, and respiratory drive have shown acceptable degrees of depression after spinal narcotic administration. However, assessment of the mean response in small numbers of individuals may not predict the likelihood of an extreme response, which may occur infrequently. Few large-scale surveys are available. Rawal and coworkers[273] reported a survey of 93 departments of anesthesia in Sweden, in which during 1984 approximately 12,000 patients received epidural narcotics perioperatively, and 1000 patients received intrathecal narcotics. Most patients received morphine; 0.04% of patients showed clinical signs of ventilatory depression within 1 hour of epidural morphine injection, and 0.09% demonstrated delayed ventilatory depression. Delayed ventilatory depression occurred in 0.36% of patients who received intrathecal morphine. This occurred within 7 to 9 hours after injection. Stuart-Taylor and associates[274] reported that 7 of 800 patients receiving epidural diamorphine experienced respiratory depression to less than 10 breaths/min. Ready and colleagues[275] reported that 2 of 1106 consecutive patients treated with epidural morphine after surgery required medication for respiratory depression. Scherer and coworkers[276] reported that 1 of 1071 patients receiving thoracic epidural buprenorphine experienced respiratory depression. Lubenow[277] reported six incidents of respiratory depression in 5172 patients receiving epidural narcotics. The incidence of respiratory depression after epidural analgesia is acceptably low for routine clinical use[278-285] and, with appropriate monitoring procedures, can be detected and treated satisfactorily.

Although clinicians have tended to focus on the respiratory effects of epidural narcotics, respiratory depression and consequent hypoxemia can also occur after administration of narcotics by other routes. Periodic desaturation has also been reported after intravenous or intramuscular opiate administration.[79,80,85,86,89,90,92,93,286-291] One patient reported by Reeder[89] after abdominal vascular surgery experienced 229 episodes of desaturation to Spo_2 less than 70%, representing 43% of the third postoperative night. Etches and associates[292] reported eight cases of serious respiratory depression out of approximately 1600 patients who had received intravenous opioids by means of patient-controlled infusion pumps. A comparative study demonstrated a higher incidence of respiratory depression among patients receiving narcotics by means of a patient-controlled infusion pump than with the epidural route.[284] Subsets of patients who appear to be at higher risk for respiratory depression include the elderly[293] and patients with a history of sleep apnea.[294]

These observations suggest that narcotic administration through the epidural or intravenous routes carry a similar risk of mild or moderate episodic hypoxemia, although they have unknown clinical significance in most patients. Temporal association of transient hypoxemia with clinical events such as myocardial ischemia and confusion does not prove causation. Normal volunteers can be safely exposed to repetitive periods of hypoxemia (Sao_2 as low as 40%) for 30 to 45 seconds.[5,141] Although there is evidence that exposure to extreme hypoxia (mean lowest Sao_2 of 68%) for prolonged periods, along with hypocapnia, can cause minor psychomotor deficits,[295] there is little evidence that exposure to moderate-altitude hypoxia for hours (e.g., for astronomers commuting daily from sea level to the Mauna Kea observatories at barometric pressure = 468 mm Hg, mean arterial Po_2 = 39.7 mm Hg and Pco_2 = 27.7 mm Hg)[9] or even days results in permanent sequelae.[9,296,297] In terms of assessing the risks of various forms of postoperative analgesia, mild postoperative reduction in Spo_2 is only a surrogate end point, which may not reflect the risk of the most feared complication: major respiratory depression resulting in respiratory arrest or death.

Earlier reports recommended the routine use of apnea monitoring on patients given spinal narcotics, but apnea monitors are often associated with false alarms and are frequently ignored. Significant respiratory depression can occur with a normal respiratory rate.[192,193,195] However, significant respiratory depression is almost invariably associated with sedation. A periodic check of mental status may be more sensitive than mechanical monitors in detecting clinical respiratory depression and is an essential component of monitoring patients who have received epidural narcotics.

Several years of clinical experience with epidural opiates have suggested that monitoring beyond clinical assessment is not necessary, particularly in low-risk patients,[195 274-277,298,299] and have led to the implementation of less stringent policies in most institutions.[300] Standards of care after epidural opioid administration in the United States were illustrated by a survey of 197 institutions, including teaching and community hospitals, published by Muir and colleagues.[299] Patients were monitored in a general care ward after opioid administration through a thoracic epidural catheter in 88.6% of institutions and after lumbar administration in 96.8%. Pulse oximetry and electronic apnea monitoring were each routinely used in 28% of institutions after thoracic opioid administration, and in 27% and 5%, respectively, after lumbar administration. The frequency with which respiration rate and sedation are monitored is shown in Table 36-7.

There is a fairly widespread consensus that monitoring equipment and resuscitative drugs should be readily available in addition to regular monitoring of respiration rate and level of sedation. Naloxone and a syringe with which to administer it should be available. Dosage adjustment or more intensive monitoring may be suitable for individuals with cardiorespiratory disease or other risk factors for respiratory depression (Table 36-8). Because delayed respiratory depression can occur particularly after morphine administration, it is prudent to

Table 36–7 Frequency of respiratory rate and sedation monitoring following epidural analgesia in a survey of 197 institutions.

Frequency	Thoracic (N)		Lumbar (N)	
	Continuous	Bolus	Continuous	Bolus
q1h	28	17	31	19
q1h × 24 hours, then q2h	25	14	27	17
q1h × 12 hours, then q2h	19	9	19	9
q1h × 4 hours, then q2h	12	3	13	5
q1h × 4 hours, then q4h	25	13	31	16
q2h	2	1	3	1
q2h × 24 hours, then q4h	9	1	9	1
q2h × 12 hours, then q4h	6	2	4	1
q4h	7	3	7	3
Totals	133	63	144	72

Data from Muir MR, Sullivan FL, Dear G, Ginsberg B: Monitoring practices following epidural analgesics for pain management: A follow-up survey. J Pain Symptom Manage 14:36, 1997.

Table 36–8   Factors predisposing to the development of respiratory depression after administration of epidural opioids

Drug Factors
Hydrophilic drug (e.g., morphine)
Large doses
Repeated doses
Concomitant administration of parenteral opioids or other central nervous system depressants

Patient Factors
Elderly or debilitated patients
Coexisting respiratory disease
Thoracic epidural
High sensitivity to opioids (i.e., no previous exposure to opioids)
Intrathecal administration
Raised intrathoracic pressure (e.g., controlled ventilation, coughing, vomiting)

From Etches RC, Sandler AN, Daley MD: Respiratory depression and spinal opioids. Can J Anaesth 36:165, 1989.

continue the monitoring algorithm for several hours after the final dose has been administered.

The widespread clinical use of epidural narcotics, particularly morphine, suggests that this technique is safe for most patients without the need for monitoring beyond simple clinical observation.

7. In the presence of high carboxyhemoglobin levels, each 8% increase in carboxyhemoglobin causes only a 1% decrease in the Spo_2 value. With a high methemoglobin concentration, the measured Spo_2 approaches 85%, independent of the actual arterial oxygenation.

8. When the pulse oximeter reading is difficult to obtain because of hypothermic vasoconstriction, the anesthesiologist should consider using a digital nerve block or topical application of a local anesthetic cream (e.g., EMLA). When the patient is cold, rapid changes in Spo_2 are more quickly detected using an ear or forehead probe than a finger probe.

9. A sudden drop in $Petco_2$ most likely results from a decrease in cardiac output, regional hypoperfusion of the lung due to pulmonary embolism, or an airway problem. A rise in the $Petco_2$ value can occur only because of increased CO_2 production (e.g., fever, seizure, bicarbonate–hydrogen ion buffering) or hypoventilation.

10. When arterial blood is fully saturated, the shunt fraction can be approximated from the arterial and mixed venous saturation according to the following equation: $(\dot{Q}s/\dot{Q}T) \approx [(1 - Sao_2)/1 - S\bar{v}o_2)]$.

11. Although narcotic administration usually slows the respiratory rate, severe respiratory depression can occur in the face of a normal respiratory rate. However, narcotic overdosage is always associated with somnolence.

KEY POINTS

1. The causes of hypoxemia are low Pio_2, elevated $Paco_2$, ventilation-perfusion ($\dot{V}a/\dot{Q}$) mismatching, right-to-left shunt, and diffusion nonequilibrium.

2. The clinical approximation to the alveolar gas equation for O_2 is given by $Pao_2 \cong (P_{barometric} - 47) \times Fio_2 - 1.2 \times Pco_2$.

3. The A-a gradient = $Pao_2 - Pao_2 = 0.21 \times$ (age in years + 2.5); this gradient increases when supplemental O_2 is administered. The a/A ratio = Pao_2/Pao_2 (normal value of 0.8 to 0.85); this ratio does not significantly change when supplemental O_2 is given.

4. To assess the adequacy of O_2 exchange, use the a/A ratio or Pao_2/Fio_2 ratio (i.e., P/F ratio). An a/A ratio that is less than 0.8 or a P/F ratio that is less than 350 mm Hg implies abnormal gas exchange.

5. To assess the adequacy of CO_2 exchange, multiply minute ventilation ($\dot{V}e$) by the arterial Pco_2. Normal $\dot{V}e \times Pco_2$ is typically about 200 L/min/mm Hg during spontaneous breathing and 300 to 400 L/min/mm Hg during mechanical ventilation.

6. When Po_2 values are inexplicably low in the presence of high leukocyte or platelet counts, the clinician should consider an artifact caused by O_2 consumption by cells within the sample. Inhibition of cellular O_2 consumption may be accomplished by adding sodium fluoride to the sample.

Acknowledgments

The authors are grateful to Ms. Barbara Blank for her help in preparing the manuscript and to Andrew Moon and Peter Moon for their assistance in preparing the illustrations.

REFERENCES

1. The Shorter Oxford Dictionary. Oxford, Oxford University Press, 1987.
2. McGraw-Hill Dictionary of Scientific and Technical Terms. New York, McGraw-Hill, 1989.
3. Eichhorn JH, Cooper JB, Cullen DJ, et al: Standards for patient monitoring during anesthesia at Harvard Medical School. JAMA 256:1017, 1986.
4. American Society of Anesthesiologists: Standards for Basic Anesthetic Monitoring, 1998 Directory of Members. Park Ridge, IL, ASA, 1998, p 438.
5. Severinghaus JW, Naifeh KH, Koh SO: Errors in 14 pulse oximeters during profound hypoxia. J Clin Monit 5:72, 1989.
6. Barker SJ: Standardization of the testing of pulse oximeter performance. Anesth Analg 94(Suppl):S17, 2002.
7. Wagner PD, Gale GE, Moon RE, et al: Pulmonary gas exchange in humans exercising at sea level and simulated altitude. J Appl Physiol 61:260, 1986.
8. Rock PB, Johnson TS, Cymerman A, et al: Effect of dexamethasone on symptoms of acute mountain sickness at Pikes Peak, Colorado (4,300 m). Aviat Space Environ Med 58:668, 1987.
9. Heath D, Williams DR: High-Altitude Medicine and Pathology. Oxford, Oxford University Press, 1995.

10. Simon RP: Hypoxia versus ischemia. Neurology 52:7, 1999.
11. Hornbein TF: The high-altitude brain. J Exp Biol 204:3129, 2001.
12. Ciofolo MJ, Clergue F, Devilliers C, et al: Changes in ventilation, oxygen uptake, and carbon dioxide output during recovery from isoflurane anesthesia. Anesthesiology 70:737, 1989.
13. Frank SM, Fleisher LA, Olson KF, et al: Multivariate determinants of early postoperative oxygen consumption in elderly patients: Effects of shivering, body temperature, and gender. Anesthesiology 83:241, 1995.
14. Mellemgaard K: The alveolar-arterial oxygen difference: Its size and components in normal man. Acta Physiol Scand 67:10, 1966.
15. Gilbert R, Keighley JF: The arterial-alveolar oxygen tension ratio. An index of gas exchange applicable to varying inspired oxygen concentrations. Am Rev Respir Dis 109:142, 1974.
16. Wagner PD, Laravuso RB, Uhl R, West JB: Continuous distributions of ventilation-perfusion ratios in normal subjects breathing air and 100 per cent O_2. J Clin Invest 54:54, 1974.
17. Breen PH, Serina ER: Bymixer provides on-line calibration of measurement of CO_2 volume exhaled per breath. Ann Biomed Eng 25:164, 1997.
18. Sahn SA, Lakshminarayan S, Petty TL: Weaning from mechanical ventilation. JAMA 235:2208, 1976.
19. West JB: Ventilation-perfusion inequality and overall gas exchange in computer models of the lung. Respir Physiol 7:88, 1969.
20. Wagner PD, Saltzman HA, West JB: Measurement of continuous distributions of ventilation-perfusion ratios: Theory. J Appl Physiol 36:588, 1974.
21. Dueck R, Young I, Clausen J, Wagner PD: Altered distribution of pulmonary ventilation and blood flow following induction of inhalation anesthesia. Anesthesiology 52:113, 1980.
22. Tokics L, Hedenstierna G, Strandberg A, et al: Lung collapse and gas exchange during general anesthesia: Effects of spontaneous breathing, muscle paralysis and positive end-expiratory pressure. Anesthesiology 66:157, 1987.
23. Tokics L, Hedenstierna G, Svensson L, et al: V/Q distribution and correlation to atelectasis in anesthetized paralyzed humans. J Appl Physiol 81:1822, 1996.
24. Bein T, Reber A, Metz C, et al: Acute effects of continuous rotational therapy on ventilation-perfusion inequality in lung injury. Intensive Care Med 24:132, 1998.
25. Hachenberg T, Tenling A, Nystrom SO, et al: Ventilation-perfusion inequality in patients undergoing cardiac surgery. Anesthesiology 80:509, 1994.
26. Rothen HU, Sporre B, Engberg G, et al: Airway closure, atelectasis and gas exchange during general anaesthesia. Br J Anaesth 81:681, 1998.
27. Tenling A, Joachimsson PO, Tyden H, et al: Thoracic epidural anesthesia as an adjunct to general anesthesia for cardiac surgery: Effects on ventilation-perfusion relationships. J Cardiothorac Vasc Anesth 13:258, 1999.
28. Feihl F, Eckert P, Brimioulle S, et al: Permissive hypercapnia impairs pulmonary gas exchange in the acute respiratory distress syndrome. Am J Respir Crit Care Med 162:209, 2000.
29. Andersson L, Lagerstrand L, Thorne A, et al: Effect of CO_2 pneumoperitoneum on ventilation-perfusion relationships during laparoscopic cholecystectomy. Acta Anaesth Scand 46:552, 2002.
30. Jones JG, Jones SE: Discriminating between the effect of shunt and reduced VA/Q on arterial oxygen saturation is particularly useful in clinical practice. J Clin Monit Comput 16:337, 2000.
31. Severinghaus JW: Blood gas concentrations. In Fenn WO, Rahn H (eds): Handbook of Physiology. Section 3: Respiration. Washington, DC, American Physiological Society, 1965, p 1475.
32. Severinghaus JW, Astrup PB: History of blood gas analysis. Int Anesthesiol Clin 25:1, 1987.
33. Severinghaus JW: Historical development of oxygenation monitoring. In Payne JP, Severinghaus JW (eds): Pulse Oximetry. New York, Springer-Verlag, 1986, pp 1.
34. Barker SJ, Tremper KK, Hyatt J, et al: Continuous fiberoptic arterial oxygen tension measurements in dogs. J Clin Monit 3:48, 1987.
35. Barker SJ: Blood volume measurement: The next intraoperative monitor? Anesthesiology 89:1310, 1998.
36. Menzel M, Soukup J, Henze D, et al: Experiences with continuous intra-arterial blood gas monitoring: Precision and drift of a pure optode-system. Intensive Care Med 29:2180, 2003.
37. Vretzakis G, Papaziogas B, Matsaridou E, et al: Continuous monitoring of arterial blood gases and pH during intraoperative rapid blood administration using a Paratrend sensor. Vox Sang 78:158, 2000.
38. Coule LW, Truemper EJ, Steinhart CM, Lutin WA: Accuracy and utility of a continuous intra-arterial blood gas monitoring system in pediatric patients. Crit Care Med 29:420, 2001.
39. Ishikawa S, Nakazawa K, Makita K: Progressive changes in arterial oxygenation during one-lung anaesthesia are related to the response to compression of the non-dependent lung. Br J Anaesth 90:21, 2003.
40. Ganter M, Zollinger A: Continuous intravascular blood gas monitoring: Development, current techniques, and clinical use of a commercial device. Br J Anaesth 91:397, 2003.
41. National Committee for Clinical Laboratory Standards: Definitions of Quantities and Conventions Related to Blood pH and Gas Analysis; Approved Standard. NCCLS Document C12-A Villanova, PA, National Committee for Clinical Laboratory Standards, 1994.
42. Camporesi EM, Moon RE: Arterial blood gas values should be corrected for body temperature during hypothermia. In Fyman PN, Gotta AW (eds): Controversies in Cardiovascular Anesthesia. Boston, Kluwers Academic Publishers, 1988, p 35.
43. Hess CE, Nichols AB, Hunt WB, Suratt PM: Pseudohypoxemia secondary to leukemia and thrombocytosis. N Engl J Med 301:361, 1979.
44. Schmaier AH: Pseudohypoxemia due to leukemia and thrombocytosis. N Engl J Med 302:584, 1980.
45. Robertson PW, Hart BB: Assessment of tissue oxygenation. Respir Care Clin N Am 5:221, 1999.
46. Barker S, Hyatt J, Clarke C, Tremper KK: Hyperventilation reduces transcutaneous oxygen tension and skin blood flow. Anesthesiology 75:619, 1991.
47. Mathieu D, Neviere R, Pellerin P, et al: Pedicle musculocutaneous flap transplantation: Prediction of final outcome by transcutaneous oxygen measurements in hyperbaric oxygen. Plast Reconstr Surg 91:329, 1993.
48. Fife CE, Buyukcakir C, Otto GH, et al: The predictive value of transcutaneous oxygen tension measurement in diabetic lower extremity ulcers treated with hyperbaric oxygen therapy: A retrospective analysis of 1,144 patients. Wound Repair Regen 10:198, 2002.
49. Janssens JP, Howarth-Frey C, Chevrolet JC, et al: Transcutaneous P_{CO_2} to monitor noninvasive mechanical ventilation in adults: Assessment of a new transcutaneous P_{CO_2} device. Chest 113:768, 1998.
50. Severinghaus JW: Nomenclature of oxygen saturation. Adv Exp Med Biol 345:921, 1994.
51. Comroe JH Jr, Botelho S: The unreliability of cyanosis in the recognition of arterial hypoxemia. Am J Med Sci 214:1, 1947.
52. Lunsgaard C, Van Slyke DD: Cyanosis. Medicine (Baltimore) 2:1, 1923.
53. Stadie WC: The oxygen of the arterial and venous blood in pneumonia and its relation to sepsis. J Exp Med 30:215, 1919.
54. Severinghaus JW, Astrup PB: History of blood gas analysis. VI. Oximetry. J Clin Monit 2:270, 1986.
55. Kirlangitis JJ, Middaugh RE, Zablocki A, Rodriquez F: False indication of arterial oxygen desaturation and methemoglobinemia following injection of methylene blue in urological surgery. Mil Med 155:260, 1990.
56. Gourlain H, Buneaux F, Borron SW, et al: Interference of methylene blue with CO-oximetry of hemoglobin derivatives. Clin Chem 43:1078, 1997.
57. Shepherd Ali G, Ashoka Ali A, Steinke JM, Shepherd AP: A simple method for measuring fetal hemoglobin by CO-oximetry. Clin Chim Acta 307:249, 2001.
58. Chaudhary BA, Burki NK: Ear oximetry in clinical practice. Am Rev Respir Dis 117:173, 1978.

59. Skacel M, O'Hare E, Harrison D: Invalid information from the ear probe of a pulse oximeter in tricuspid incompetence. Anaesth Intensive Care 18:270, 1990.

60. Ayas N, Bergstrom LR, Schwab TR, Narr BJ: Unrecognized severe postoperative hypercapnia—A case of apneic oxygenation. Mayo Clin Proc 73:51, 1998.

61. Alexander CM, Teller LE, Gross JB: Principles of pulse oximetry: Theoretical and practical considerations. Anesth Analg 68:368, 1989.

62. Kelleher JF: Pulse oximetry. J Clin Monit 5:37, 1989.

63. Tremper KK, Barker SJ: Pulse oximetry. Anesthesiology 70:98, 1989.

64. Severinghaus JW, Kelleher JF: Recent developments in pulse oximetry. Anesthesiology 76:1018, 1992.

65. Wahr JA, Tremper KK, Diab M: Pulse oximetry. Respir Care Clin N Am 1:77, 1995.

66. Goldman JM, Petterson MT, Kopotic RJ, Barker SJ: Masimo signal extraction pulse oximetry. J Clin Monit Comput 16:475, 2000.

67. Jopling MW, Mannheimer PD, Bebout DE: Issues in the laboratory evaluation of pulse oximeter performance. Anesth Analg 94(Suppl):S62, 2002.

68. Bohnhorst B, Poets CF: Major reduction in alarm frequency with a new pulse oximeter. Intensive Care Med 24:277, 1998.

69. Irita K, Kai Y, Akiyoshi K, et al: Performance evaluation of a new pulse oximeter during mild hypothermic cardiopulmonary bypass. Anesth Analg 96:11, 2003.

70. Lutter NO, Urankar S, Kroeber S: False alarm rates of three third-generation pulse oximeters in PACU, ICU and IABP patients. Anesth Analg 94(Suppl):S69, 2002.

71. Kuhnert M, Seelbach-Goebel B, Butterwegge M: Predictive agreement between the fetal arterial oxygen saturation and fetal scalp pH: Results of the German multicenter study. Am J Obstet Gynecol 178:330, 1998.

72. Kyriacou PA, Powell SL, Jones DP, Langford RM: Evaluation of oesophageal pulse oximetry in patients undergoing cardiothoracic surgery. Anaesthesia 58:422, 2003.

73. Trivedi NS, Ghouri AF, Lai E, et al: Pulse oximeter performance during desaturation and resaturation: A comparison of seven models. J Clin Anesth 9:184, 1997.

74. Yamaya Y, Bogaard HJ, Wagner PD, et al: Validity of pulse oximetry during maximal exercise in normoxia, hypoxia, and hyperoxia. J Appl Physiol 92:162, 2002.

75. Fournell A, Schwarte LA, Kindgen-Milles D, et al: Assessment of microvascular oxygen saturation in gastric mucosa in volunteers breathing continuous positive airway pressure. Crit Care Med 31:1705, 2003.

76. Moller JT, Pedersen T, Rasmussen LS, et al: Randomized evaluation of pulse oximetry in 20,802 patients. I. Design, demography, pulse oximetry failure rate, and overall complication rate. Anesthesiology 78:436, 1993.

77. Moller JT, Johannessen NW, Espersen K, et al: Randomized evaluation of pulse oximetry in 20,802 patients. II. Perioperative events and postoperative complications. Anesthesiology 78:445, 1993.

78. Bierman MI, Stein KL, Snyder JV: Pulse oximetry in the postoperative care of cardiac surgical patients: A randomized controlled trial. Chest 102:1367, 1992.

79. Catley DM, Thornton C, Jordan C, et al: Pronounced, episodic oxygen desaturation in the postoperative period: Its association with ventilatory pattern and analgesic regimen. Anesthesiology 63:20, 1985.

80. Morris RW, Buschman A, Warren DL, et al: The prevalence of hypoxemia detected by pulse oximetry during recovery from anesthesia. J Clin Monit 4:16, 1988.

81. Brose WG, Cohen SE: Oxyhemoglobin saturation following cesarean section in patients receiving epidural morphine, PCA, or IM meperidine analgesia. Anesthesiology 70:948, 1989.

82. Choi HJ, Little MS, Garber SZ, Tremper KK: Pulse oximetry for monitoring during ward analgesia: Epidural morphine versus parenteral narcotics. J Clin Monit 5:87, 1989.

83. Rosenberg J, Dirkes WE, Kehlet H: Episodic arterial oxygen desaturation and heart rate variations following major abdominal surgery. Br J Anaesth 63:651, 1989.

84. Rosenberg J, Ullstad T, Larsen PN, et al: Continuous assessment of oxygen saturation and subcutaneous oxygen tension after abdominal operations. Acta Chir Scand 156:585, 1990.

85. Rosenberg J, Rasmussen V, von Jessen F, et al: Late postoperative episodic and constant hypoxaemia and associated ECG abnormalities. Br J Anaesth 65:684, 1990.

86. Wheatley RG, Somerville ID, Sapsford DJ, Jones JG: Postoperative hypoxaemia: Comparison of extradural, i.m. and patient-controlled opioid analgesia. Br J Anaesth 64:267, 1990.

87. Entwistle MD, Roe PG, Sapsford DJ, et al: Patterns of oxygenation after thoracotomy. Br J Anaesth 67:704, 1991.

88. Gill NP, Wright B, Reilly CS: Relationship between hypoxaemic and cardiac ischaemic events in the perioperative period. Br J Anaesth 68:471, 1992.

89. Reeder MK, Goldman MD, Loh L, et al: Late postoperative nocturnal dips in oxygen saturation in patients undergoing major abdominal vascular surgery: Predictive value of pre-operative overnight pulse oximetry. Anaesthesia 47:110, 1992.

90. Reeder MK, Goldman MD, Loh L, et al: Postoperative hypoxaemia after major abdominal vascular surgery. Br J Anaesth 68:23, 1992.

91. Rosenberg J, Pedersen MH, Gebuhr P, Kehlet H: Effect of oxygen therapy on late postoperative episodic and constant hypoxaemia. Br J Anaesth 68:18, 1992.

92. Wheatley RG, Shepherd D, Jackson IJ, et al: Hypoxaemia and pain relief after upper abdominal surgery: Comparison of i.m. and patient-controlled analgesia. Br J Anaesth 69:558, 1992.

93. Rosenberg J, Kehlet H: Postoperative mental confusion—Association with postoperative hypoxemia. Surgery 114:76, 1993.

94. Rosenberg J, Oturai P, Erichsen CJ, et al: Effect of general anesthesia and major versus minor surgery on late postoperative episodic and constant hypoxemia. J Clin Anesth 6:212, 1994.

95. Lewer BMF, Larsen PD, Torrance JM, Galletly DC: Artifactual episodic hypoxaemia during postoperative respiratory monitoring. Can J Anaesth 45:182, 1998.

96. Barker SJ, Tremper KK: The effect of carbon monoxide inhalation on pulse oximetry and transcutaneous Po_2. Anesthesiology 66:677, 1987.

97. Gonzalez A, Gomez-Arnau J, Pensado A: Carboxyhemoglobin and pulse oximetry. Anesthesiology 73:573, 1990.

98. Buckley RG, Aks SE, Eshom JL, et al: The pulse oximetry gap in carbon monoxide intoxication. Ann Emerg Med 24:252, 1994.

99. Nijland R, Jongsma HW, Nijhuis JG, et al: Notes on the apparent discordance of pulse oximetry and multi-wavelength haemoglobin photometry. Acta Anaesthesiol Scand Suppl 107:49, 1995.

100. Bozeman WP, Myers RAM, Barish RA: Confirmation of the pulse oximetry gap in carbon monoxide poisoning. Ann Emerg Med 30:608, 1997.

101. Hampson NB: Pulse oximetry in severe carbon monoxide poisoning. Chest 114:1036, 1998.

102. Eisenkraft JB: Pulse oximeter desaturation due to methemoglobinemia. Anesthesiology 68:279, 1988.

103. Barker SJ, Tremper KK, Hyatt J: Effects of methemoglobinemia on pulse oximetry and mixed venous oximetry. Anesthesiology 70:112, 1989.

104. Kouides PA, Abboud CN, Fairbanks VF: Flutamide-induced cyanosis refractory to methylene blue therapy. Br J Haematol 94:73, 1996.

105. Zijlstra WG, Maas AH, Moran RF: Definition, significance and measurement of quantities pertaining to the oxygen carrying properties of human blood. Scand J Clin Lab Invest Suppl 224:27, 1996.

106. Wu C, Kenny MA: A case of sulfhemoglobinemia and emergency measurement of sulfhemoglobin with an OSM3 CO-oximeter. Clin Chem 43:162, 1997.

107. Weston Smith SG, Glass UH, Acharya J, Pearson TC: Pulse oximetry in sickle cell disease. Clin Lab Haematol 11:185, 1989.

108. Pianosi P, Charge TD, Esseltine DW, Coates AL: Pulse oximetry in sickle cell disease. Arch Dis Child 68:735, 1993.
109. Rackoff WR, Kunkel N, Silber JH, et al: Pulse oximetry and factors associated with hemoglobin oxygen desaturation in children with sickle cell disease. Blood 81:3422, 1993.
110. Craft JA, Alessandrini E, Kenney LB, et al: Comparison of oxygenation measurements in pediatric patients during sickle cell crises. J Pediatr 124:93, 1994.
111. Jay GD, Renzi FP: Evaluation of pulse oximetry in anemia from hemoglobin-H disease. Ann Emerg Med 21:572, 1992.
112. Katoh R, Miyake T, Arai T: Unexpectedly low pulse oximeter readings in a boy with unstable hemoglobin Koln. Anesthesiology 80:472, 1994.
113. Gottschalk A, Silverberg M: An unexpected finding with pulse oximetry in a patient with hemoglobin Koln. Anesthesiology 80:474, 1994.
114. Przybelski RJ, Daily EK, Kisicki JC, et al: Phase I study of the safety and pharmacologic effects of diaspirin cross-linked hemoglobin solution. Crit Care Med 24:1993, 1996.
115. Hughes GS Jr, Francome SF, Antal EJ, et al: Hematologic effects of a novel hemoglobin-based oxygen carrier in normal male and female subjects. J Lab Clin Med 126:444, 1995.
116. Hughes GS, Francom SF, Antal EJ, et al: Effects of a novel hemoglobin-based oxygen carrier on percent oxygen saturation as determined with arterial blood gas analysis and pulse oximetry. Ann Emerg Med 27:164, 1996.
117. Ali AA, Ali GS, Steinke JM, Shepherd AP: CO-oximetry interference by hemoglobin-based blood substitutes. Anesth Analg 92:863, 2001.
118. Jahr JS, Driessen B, Lurie F, et al: Oxygen saturation measurements in canine blood containing hemoglobin glutamer-200 (bovine): In vitro validation of the NOVA CO-oximeter. Vet Clin Pathol 30:39, 2001.
119. Holbek CC: New developments in the measurement of CO-oximetry. Anesth Analg 94(Suppl):S89, 2002.
120. Jay GD, Hughes L, Renzi FP: Pulse oximetry is accurate in acute anemia from hemorrhage. Ann Emerg Med 24:32, 1994.
121. Severinghaus JW, Koh SO: Effect of anemia on pulse oximeter accuracy at low saturation. J Clin Monit 6:85, 1990.
122. Boxer RA, Gottesfeld I, Singh S, et al: Noninvasive pulse oximetry in children with cyanotic congenital heart disease. Crit Care Med 15:1062, 1987.
123. Schmitt HJ, Schuetz WH, Proeschel PA, Jaklin C: Accuracy of pulse oximetry in children with cyanotic congenital heart disease. J Cardiothorac Vasc Anesth 7:61, 1993.
124. Kessler MR, Eide T, Humayun B, Poppers PJ: Spurious pulse oximeter desaturation with methylene blue injection. Anesthesiology 65:435, 1986.
125. Sidi A, Paulus DA, Rush W, et al: Methylene blue and indocyanine green artifactually lower pulse oximetry readings of oxygen saturation: Studies in dogs. J Clin Monit 3:249, 1987.
126. Barker SJ, Tremper KK: Pulse oximetry: Applications and limitations. Int Anesthesiol Clin 25:155, 1987.
127. Gorman ES, Shnider MR: Effect of methylene blue on the absorbance of solutions of haemoglobin. Br J Anaesth 60:439, 1988.
128. Scott DM, Cooper MG: Spurious pulse oximetry with intrauterine methylene blue injection. Anaesth Intensive Care 19:267, 1991.
129. Larsen VH, Freudendal-Pedersen A, Fogh-Andersen N: The influence of patent blue V on pulse oximetry and haemoximetry. Acta Anaesthesiol Scand Suppl 107:53, 1995.
130. Morell RC, Heyneker T, Kashtan HI, Ruppe C: False desaturation due to intradermal patent blue dye. Anesthesiology 78:363, 1993.
131. Saito S, Fukura H, Shimada H, Fujita T: Prolonged interference of blue dye "patent blue" with pulse oximetry readings. Acta Anaesth Scand 39:268, 1995.
132. McEwan D, Lam K: Oximetry and patent blue five dye. Anaesth Intensive Care 25:587, 1997.
133. Coté CJ, Goldstein EA, Fuchsman WH, Hoaglin DC: The effect of nail polish on pulse oximetry. Anesth Analg 67:683, 1988.
134. al-Majed SA, Harakati MS: The effect of henna paste on oxygen saturation reading obtained by pulse oximetry. Trop Geogr Med 46:38, 1994.
135. Veyckemans F, Baele P, Guillaume JE, et al: Hyperbilirubinemia does not interfere with hemoglobin saturation measured by pulse oximetry. Anesthesiology 70:118, 1989.
136. Lebecque P, Shango P, Stijns M, et al: Pulse oximetry versus measured arterial oxygen saturation: A comparison of the Nellcor N100 and the Biox III. Pediatr Pulmonol 10:132, 1991.
137. Beall SN, Moorthy SS: Jaundice, oximetry, and spurious hemoglobin desaturation. Anesth Analg 68:806, 1989.
138. Veyckemans F, Baele PL: More about jaundice and oximetry. Anesth Analg 70:335, 1990.
139. Read MS: Effect of transparent adhesive tape on pulse oximetry. Anesth Analg 68:701, 1989.
140. Racys V, Nahrwold ML: Reusing the Nellcor pulse oximeter probe: Is it worth the savings? Anesthesiology 66:713, 1987.
141. Severinghaus JW, Naifeh KH: Accuracy of response of six pulse oximeters to profound hypoxia. Anesthesiology 67:551, 1987.
142. Costarino AT, Davis DA, Keon TP: Falsely normal saturation reading with the pulse oximeter. Anesthesiology 67:830, 1987.
143. Fluck RR Jr, Schroeder C, Frani G, et al: Does ambient light affect the accuracy of pulse oximetry? Respir Care 48:677, 2003.
144. Lindsay DR: False comfort from a pulse oximeter [letter]. Anesth Analg 88:1428, 1999.
145. Gardosi JO, Damianou D, Schram CM: Inappropriate sensor application in pulse oximetry. Lancet 340:920, 1992.
146. Severinghaus JW, Spellman MJ Jr: Pulse oximeter failure thresholds in hypotension and vasoconstriction. Anesthesiology 73:532, 1990.
147. Vegfors M, Lindberg LG, Lennmarken C: The influence of changes in blood flow on the accuracy of pulse oximetry in humans. Acta Anaesth Scand 36:346, 1992.
148. Broome IJ, Mills GH, Spiers P, Reilly CS: An evaluation of the effect of vasodilatation on oxygen saturations measured by pulse oximetry and venous blood gas analysis. Anaesthesia 48:415, 1993.
149. Bhargava M, Pothula SNM: Improvement of pulse oximetry signal by EMLA® cream. Anesth Analg 86:915, 1998.
150. Bebout DE, Mannheimer FD, Jopling MW: Site-dependent lag times for detecting changes in saturation during low perfusion. Anesth Analg 94(Suppl):S101, 2002.
151. Bebout DE, Mannheimer PD, Wun C-C: Site-dependent differences in the time to detect changes in saturation during low perfusion. Crit Care Med 29:A115, 2002.
152. Räsänen J, Downs JB, DeHaven B: Titration of continuous positive airway pressure by real-time dual oximetry. Chest 92:853, 1987.
153. Kersting T, Reinhart K, Fleckenstein W, et al: Tissue Po2 measurements in critical care: The effects of dopamine on muscular oxygen pressure fields. In Ehrly AM, Hauss J, Hach R (eds): Clinical Oxygen Pressure Measurement. New York, Springer-Verlag, 1985, p 109.
154. McCormick PW, Stewart M, Goetting MG, et al: Noninvasive cerebral optical spectroscopy for monitoring cerebral oxygen delivery and hemodynamics. Crit Care Med 19:89, 1991.
155. Hampson NB, Piantadosi CA: Near-infrared optical responses in feline brain and skeletal muscle tissues during respiratory acid-base imbalance. Brain Res 519:249, 1990.
156. Tenney SM: A theoretical analysis of the relationship between venous blood and mean tissue oxygen pressures. Respir Physiol 20:283, 1974.
157. Jöbsis FF: Noninvasive, infrared monitoring of cerebral and myocardial oxygen sufficiency and circulatory parameters. Science 198:1264, 1977.
158. Piantadosi CA, Comfort BJ: Development and validation of multiwavelength algorithms for in vivo near infrared spectroscopy. In Chance B, Blumberg WE (eds): Photon Migration in Tissue. New York, Plenum, 1989, p 69.
159. Parsons WJ, Rembert JC, Bauman RP, et al: Myocardial oxygenation in dogs during reactive hyperemia. J Biomed Opt 3:191, 1998.

160. Hampson NB, Piantadosi CA: Near-infrared monitoring of human skeletal muscle oxygenation during forearm ischemia. J Appl Physiol 64:2449, 1988.

161. Hampson NB, Camporesi EM, Stolp BW, et al: Cerebral oxygen availability by NIR spectroscopy during transient hypoxia in humans. J Appl Physiol 69:907, 1990.

162. Greeley WJ, Kern FH, Ungerleider RM, et al: The effect of hypothermic cardiopulmonary bypass and total circulatory arrest on cerebral metabolism in neonates, infants, and children. J Thorac Cardiovasc Surg 101:783, 1991.

163. Ornato JP, Shipley JB, Racht EM, et al: Multicenter study of a portable, hand-size, colorimetric end-tidal carbon dioxide detection device. Ann Emerg Med 21:55, 1992.

164. Malinski T, Czuchajowski L: Nitric oxide measurement by electrochemical methods. In Feelisch M, Stamler JS (eds): Methods in Nitric Oxide Research. New York, John Wiley & Sons, 1996, p 319.

165. Purtz EP, Hess D, Kacmarek RM: Evaluation of electrochemical nitric oxide and nitrogen dioxide analyzers suitable for use during mechanical ventilation. J Clin Monit 13:25, 1997.

166. Brett SJ, Evans TW: Measurement of endogenous nitric oxide in the lungs of patients with the acute respiratory distress syndrome. Am J Respir Crit Care Med 157:993, 1998.

167. Nishimura M, Imanaka H, Uchiyama A, et al: Nitric oxide (NO) measurement accuracy. J Clin Monit 13:241, 1997.

168. Hampl V, Walters CL, Archer SL: Determination of nitric oxide by the chemiluminescence reaction with ozone. In Feelisch M, Stamler JS (eds): Methods in Nitric Oxide Research. New York, John Wiley & Sons, 1996, p 309.

169. Gravenstein JS, Paulus DA, Hayes TJ: Gas Monitoring in Clinical Practice, 2nd ed. Boston, Butterworth-Heinemann, 1995.

170. Turner KE, Sandler AN, Vosu HA: End-tidal CO_2 monitoring in spontaneously breathing adults. Can J Anaesth 36:248, 1989.

171. Meny RG, Bhat AM, Aranas E: Mass spectrometer monitoring of expired carbon dioxide in critically ill neonates. Crit Care Med 13:1064, 1985.

172. Brunner JX, Westenskow DR: How the rise time of carbon dioxide analysers influences the accuracy of carbon dioxide measurements. Br J Anaesth 61:628, 1988.

173. Scamman FL, Fishbaugh JK: Frequency response of long mass-spectrometer sampling catheters. Anesthesiology 65:422, 1986.

174. Fletcher R, Veintemilla F: Changes in the arterial to end-tidal P_{CO_2} differences during coronary artery bypass grafting. Acta Anaesth Scand 33:656, 1989.

175. Russell GB, Graybeal JM, Strout JC: Stability of arterial to end-tidal carbon dioxide gradients during postoperative cardiorespiratory support. Can J Anaesth 37:560, 1990.

176. Russell GB, Graybeal JM: Reliability of the arterial to end-tidal carbon dioxide gradient in mechanically ventilated patients with multisystem trauma. J Trauma 36:317, 1994.

177. Russell GB, Graybeal JM: The arterial to end-tidal carbon dioxide difference in neurosurgical patients during craniotomy. Anesth Analg 81:806, 1995.

178. Bindslev L, Hedenstierna G, Santesson J, et al: Airway closure during anaesthesia, and its prevention by positive end expiratory pressure. Acta Anaesth Scand 24:199, 1980.

179. Bhavani-Shankar K, Kumar AY, Moseley HSL, Ahyee-Hallsworth R: Terminology and the current limitations of time capnography: A brief review. J Clin Monit 11:175, 1995.

180. Murray IP, Modell JH, Gallagher TJ, Banner MJ: Titration of PEEP by the arterial minus end-tidal carbon dioxide gradient. Chest 85:100, 1984.

181. Breen PH, Mazumdar B, Skinner SC: Comparison of end-tidal P_{CO_2} and average alveolar expired P_{CO_2} during positive end-expiratory pressure. Anesth Analg 82:368, 1996.

182. Viale JP, Annat G, Bertrand O, et al: Continuous measurement of pulmonary gas exchange during general anaesthesia in man. Acta Anaesth Scand 32:691, 1988.

183. Westenskow DR, Cutler CA, Wallace WD: Instrumentation for monitoring gas exchange and metabolic rate in critically ill patients. Crit Care Med 12:183, 1984.

184. Lewis WD, Chwals W, Benotti PN, et al: Bedside assessment of the work of breathing. Crit Care Med 16:117, 1988.

185. Zar HA, Noe FE, Szalados JE, et al: Monitoring pulmonary function with superimposed pulmonary gas exchange curves from standard analyzers. J Clin Monit Comput 17:241, 2002.

186. Breen PH, Isserles SA, Taitelman UZ: Non-steady state monitoring by respiratory gas exchange. J Clin Monit Comput 16:351, 2000.

187. Smithies MN, Royston B, Makita K, et al: Comparison of oxygen consumption measurements: Indirect calorimetry versus the reversed Fick method. Crit Care Med 19:1401, 1991.

188. Bizouarn P, Soulard D, Blanloeil Y, et al: Oxygen consumption after cardiac surgery—A comparison between calculation by Fick's principle and measurement by indirect calorimetry. Intensive Care Med 18:206, 1992.

189. Oudemans-van Straaten HM, Scheffer GJ, Eysman L, Wildevuur CR: Oxygen consumption after cardiopulmonary bypass—Implications of different measuring methods. Intensive Care Med 19:105, 1993.

190. Bizouarn P, Blanloeil Y, Pinaud M: Comparison between oxygen consumption calculated by Fick's principle using a continuous thermodilution technique and measured by indirect calorimetry. Br J Anaesth 75:719, 1995.

191. Schoene RB: The control of ventilation in clinical medicine: To breathe or not to breathe. Respir Care 34:500, 1989.

192. Camporesi EM, Nielsen CH, Bromage PR, Durant PA: Ventilatory CO_2 sensitivity after intravenous and epidural morphine in volunteers. Anesth Analg 62:633, 1983.

193. Rawal N, Wattwil M: Respiratory depression after epidural morphine—An experimental and clinical study. Anesth Analg 63:8, 1984.

194. Sandler AN, Chovaz P, Whiting W: Respiratory depression following epidural morphine: A clinical study. Can Anaesth Soc J 33:542, 1986.

195. Ready LB, Oden R, Chadwick HS, et al: Development of an anesthesiology-based postoperative pain management service. Anesthesiology 68:100, 1988.

196. Camporesi EM, Feezor M, Fortune J, Salzano J: An electro-magnetic valve for inspiratory occlusion pressures. J Appl Physiol 45:481, 1978.

197. Milic-Emili J, Whitelaw WA, Grassino AE: Measurement and testing of respiratory drive. In Hornbein TF (ed): Regulation of Breathing: Part II. New York, Marcel Dekker, 1981, p 675.

198. Derenne JP, Couture J, Iscoe S, et al: Occlusion pressures in men rebreathing CO_2 under methoxyflurane anesthesia. J Appl Physiol 40:805, 1976.

199. Herrera M, Blasco J, Venegas J, et al: Mouth occlusion pressure ($P_{0.1}$) in acute respiratory failure. Intensive Care Med 11:134, 1985.

200. Sassoon CS, Te TT, Mahutte CK, Light RW: Airway occlusion pressure: An important indicator for successful weaning in patients with chronic obstructive pulmonary disease. Am Rev Respir Dis 135:107, 1987.

201. Rivera L, Weissman C: Dynamic ventilatory characteristics during weaning in postoperative critically ill patients. Anesth Analg 84:1250, 1997.

202. Montgomery AB, Holle RH, Neagley SR, et al: Prediction of successful ventilator weaning using airway occlusion pressure and hypercapnic challenge. Chest 91:496, 1987.

203. Sullivan WJ, Peters GM, Enright PL: Pneumotachographs: Theory and clinical application. Respir Care 29:736, 1984.

204. Blumenfeld W, Turney SZ, Denman RJ: A coaxial ultrasonic pneumotachometer. Med Biol Eng 13:855, 1975.

205. de Troyer A, Bastenier J, Delhez L: Function of respiratory muscles during partial curarization in humans. J Appl Physiol 49:1049, 1980.

206. O'Brien MJ, Van Eykern LA, Oetomo SB, Van Vught HA: Transcutaneous respiratory electromyographic monitoring. Crit Care Med 15:294, 1987.

207. Schweitzer TW, Fitzgerald JW, Bowden JA, Lynne-Davies P: Spectral analysis of human inspiratory diaphragmatic electromyograms. J Appl Physiol 46:152, 1979.

208. Bloch R: Subtraction of electrocardiographic signal from respiratory electromyogram. J Appl Physiol 55:619, 1983.

209. Rochester DF: Tests of respiratory muscle function. Clin Chest Med 9:249, 1988.
210. Ford GT, Whitelaw WA, Rosenal TW, et al: Diaphragm function after upper abdominal surgery in humans. Am Rev Respir Dis 127:431, 1983.
211. Brown KA, Hoffstein V, Byrick RJ: Bedside diagnosis of bilateral diaphragmatic paralysis in a ventilator-dependent patient after open-heart surgery. Anesth Analg 64:1208, 1985.
212. Laghi F, Harrison MJ, Tobin MJ: Comparison of magnetic and electrical phrenic nerve stimulation in assessment of diaphragmatic contractility. J Appl Physiol 80:1731, 1996.
213. Laghi F, Cattapan SE, Jubran A, et al: Is weaning failure caused by low-frequency fatigue of the diaphragm? Am J Respir Crit Care Med 167:120, 2003.
214. Cattapan SE, Laghi F, Tobin MJ: Can diaphragmatic contractility be assessed by airway twitch pressure in mechanically ventilated patients? Thorax 58:58, 2003.
215. Stagg D, Goldman M, Newsom-Davis JN: Computer-aided measurement of breath volume and time components using magnetometers. J Appl Physiol 44:623, 1978.
216. Roussos C, Fixley M, Gross D, Macklem PT: Fatigue of inspiratory muscles and their synergic behavior. J Appl Physiol 46:897, 1979.
217. Roussos C, Zakynthinos S: Fatigue of the respiratory muscles. Intensive Care Med 22:134, 1996.
218. Mead J, Peterson N, Grimby G, Mead J: Pulmonary ventilation measured from body surface movements. Science 156:1383, 1967.
219. Faithfull D, Jones JG, Jordan C: Measurement of the relative contributions of rib cage and abdomen/diaphragm to tidal breathing in man. Br J Anaesth 51:391, 1979.
220. Cohn MA, Rao AS, Broudy M, et al: The respiratory inductive plethysmograph: A new non-invasive monitor of respiration. Bull Eur Physiopathol Respir 18:643, 1982.
221. Stradling JR, Chadwick GA, Quirk C, Phillips T: Respiratory inductance plethysmography: Calibration techniques, their validation and the effects of posture. Bull Eur Physiopathol Respir 21:317, 1985.
222. Marini JJ, Pierson DJ, Hudson LD, Lakshminarayan S: The significance of wheezing in chronic airflow obstruction. Am Rev Respir Dis 120:1069, 1979.
223. Forgacs P: The functional basis of pulmonary sounds. Chest 73:399, 1979.
224. Forgacs P: Lung Sounds. London, Baillière Tindall, 1978.
225. Loudon R, Murphy RL Jr: Lung sounds. Am Rev Respir Dis 130:663, 1984.
226. Semmes BJ, Tobin MJ, Snyder JV, Grenvik A: Subjective and objective measurement of tidal volume in critically ill patients. Chest 87:577, 1985.
227. Sorkin B, Rapoport DM, Falk DB, Goldring RM: Canopy ventilation monitor for quantitative measurement of ventilation during sleep. J Appl Physiol 48:724, 1980.
228. Tobin MJ, Jenouri GA, Watson H, Sackner MA: Noninvasive measurement of pleural pressure by surface inductive plethysmography. J Appl Physiol 55:267, 1983.
229. Pepe PE, Marini JJ: Occult positive end-expiratory pressure in mechanically ventilated patients with airflow obstruction: The auto-PEEP effect. Am Rev Respir Dis 126:166, 1982.
230. Bardoczky GI, Yernault JC, Engelman EE, et al: Intrinsic positive end-expiratory pressure during one-lung ventilation for thoracic surgery. The influence of preoperative pulmonary function. Chest 110:180, 1996.
231. Tobin MJ: Respiratory monitoring in the intensive care unit. Am Rev Respir Dis 138:1625, 1988.
232. Carle KA, Camporesi EM, Moon RE: Edrophonium-induced bronchoconstriction during reversal of muscle relaxants. Anesthesiology 65(Suppl):A495, 1986.
233. Wakakuri H, Camporesi EM: Peak expiratory flow during a passive exhalation: An index of expiratory resistance during anesthesia. Acta Anaesth Scand 23:207, 1979.
234. Bardoczky GI, deFrancquen P, Engelman E, Capello M: Continuous monitoring of pulmonary mechanics with the sidestream spirometer during lung transplantation. J Cardiothorac Vasc Anesth 6:731, 1992.

235. Dueck R: Assessment and monitoring of flow limitation and other parameters from flow/volume loops. J Clin Monit Comput 16:425, 2000.
236. Bardoczky GI, Engelman E, Levarlet M, Simon P: Ventilatory effects of pneumoperitoneum monitored with continuous spirometry. Anaesthesia 48:309, 1993.
237. Bardoczky GI, Levarlet M, Engelman E, deFrancquen P: Continuous spirometry for detection of double-lumen endobronchial tube displacement. Br J Anaesth 70:499, 1993.
238. Guyatt AR, Parker SP, McBride MJ: Measurement of human nasal ventilation using an oxygen cannula as a pilot tube. Am Rev Respir Dis 126:434, 1982.
239. Werthammer J, Krasner J, DiBenedetto J, Stark AR: Apnea monitoring by acoustic detection of airflow. Pediatrics 71:53, 1983.
240. Hok B, Wiklund L, Henneberg S: A new respiratory rate monitor: Development and initial clinical experience. Int J Clin Monit Comput 10:101, 1993.
241. Tatara T, Tsuzaki K: An apnea monitor using a rapid-response hygrometer. J Clin Monit 13:5, 1997.
242. Nilsson L, Johansson A, Kalman S: Monitoring of respiratory rate in postoperative care using a new photoplethysmographic technique. J Clin Monit Comput 16:309, 2000.
243. George CF, Millar TW, Kryger MH: Identification and quantification of apneas by computer-based analysis of oxygen saturation. Am Rev Respir Dis 137:1238, 1988.
244. Sackner MA, Krieger BP: Noninvasive respiratory monitoring. In Scharf SM, Cassidy SS (eds): Heart-Lung Interactions in Health and Disease. New York, Marcel Dekker, 1989, p 663.
245. Webber CE, Coates G: A clinical system for the in vivo measurement of lung density. Med Phys 9:473, 1982.
246. Coates G, Powles AC, Morrison SC, et al: The effects of intravenous infusion of saline on lung density, lung volumes, nitrogen washout, computed tomographic scans, and chest radiographs in humans. Am Rev Respir Dis 127:91, 1983.
247. Cutillo AG, Morris AH, Ailion DC, et al: Determination of lung water content and distribution by nuclear magnetic resonance imaging. J Thorac Imaging 1:39, 1986.
248. Mayo JR, MacKay AL, Whittall KP, et al: Measurement of lung water content and pleural pressure gradient with magnetic resonance imaging. J Thorac Imaging 10:73, 1995.
249. Serizawa S, Suzuki T, Niino H, et al: Using $H_2^{15}O$ and $C^{15}O$ in noninvasive pulmonary measurements. Chest 106:1145, 1994.
250. Sivak ED, Wiedemann HP: Clinical measurement of extravascular lung water. Crit Care Clin 2:511, 1986.
251. Mihm FG, Feeley TW, Jamieson SW: Thermal dye double indicator dilution measurement of lung water in man: Comparison with gravimetric measurements. Thorax 42:72, 1987.
252. Leksell LG, Schreiner MS, Sylvestro A, Neufeld GR: Commercial double-indicator-dilution densitometer using heavy water: Evaluation in oleic-acid pulmonary edema. J Clin Monit 6:99, 1990.
253. Wallin CJ, Leksell LG: Estimation of extravascular lung water in humans with use of ^2H_2O: Effect of blood flow and central blood volume. J Appl Physiol 76:1868, 1994.
254. Overland ES, Gupta RN, Huchon GJ, Murray JF: Measurement of pulmonary tissue volume and blood flow in persons with normal and edematous lungs. J Appl Physiol 51:1375, 1981.
255. Petrini MF, Norman JR: Soluble gas uptake from alveolar gas. Respir Care 34:470, 1989.
256. Van de Water JM, Mount BE, Barela JR, et al: Monitoring the chest with impedance. Chest 64:597, 1973.
257. Hoskyns EW, Milner AD, Hopkin IE: Measurement of tidal lung volumes in neonates during high-frequency oscillation. J Biomed Eng 14:16, 1992.
258. Fritsch T, Krafft P, Becker HD, et al: Intermittent capnography during high-frequency jet ventilation for prolonged rigid bronchoscopy. Acta Anaesth Scand 44:391, 2000.
259. Nishimura M, Imanaka H, Tashiro C, et al: Capnometry during high-frequency oscillatory ventilation. Chest 101:1681, 1992.

260. Waterson CK, Quan SF: Delivery equipment and monitoring techniques for high frequency ventilation. *In* Hamilton LH, Neu J, Calkins JM (eds): High Frequency Ventilation. Boca Raton, FL, CRC Press, 1986, p 90.

261. Waterson CK, Militzer HW, Quan SF, Calkins JM: Airway pressure as a measure of gas exchange during high-frequency jet ventilation. Crit Care Med 12:742, 1984.

262. Meade M, Guyatt G, Cook D, et al: Predicting success in weaning from mechanical ventilation. Chest 120:400S, 2001.

263. Yang KL, Tobin MJ: A prospective study of indexes predicting the outcome of trials of weaning from mechanical ventilation. N Engl J Med 324:1445, 1991.

264. Ely EW, Baker AM, Dunagan DP, et al: Effect on the duration of mechanical ventilation of identifying patients capable of breathing spontaneously. N Engl J Med 335:1864, 1996.

265. Weavind L, Shaw AD, Feeley TW: Monitoring ventilator weaning—Predictors of success. J Clin Monit Comput 16:409, 2000.

266. MacIntyre NR, Cook DJ, Ely EW Jr, et al: Evidence-based guidelines for weaning and discontinuing ventilatory support: A collective task force facilitated by the American College of Chest Physicians, the American Association for Respiratory Care, and the American College of Critical Care Medicine. Chest 120:375S, 2001.

267. Goldstone J: The pulmonary physician in critical care. 10. Difficult weaning. Thorax 57:986, 2002.

268. Manthous CA: The anarchy of weaning techniques. Chest 121:1738, 2002.

269. Chripko D, Bevan JC, Archer DP, Bherer N: Decreases in arterial oxygen saturation in paediatric outpatients during transfer to the postanaesthetic recovery room. Can J Anaesth 36:128, 1989.

270. Tait AR, Kyff JV, Crider B, et al: Changes in arterial oxygen saturation in cigarette smokers following general anaesthesia. Can J Anaesth 37:423, 1990.

271. Bromage PR, Camporesi E, Chestnut D: Epidural narcotics for postoperative analgesia. Anesth Analg 59:473, 1980.

272. Etches RC, Sandler AN, Daley MD: Respiratory depression and spinal opioids. Can J Anaesth 36:165, 1989.

273. Rawal N, Arner S, Gustafsson LL, Allvin R: Present state of extradural and intrathecal opioid analgesia in Sweden: A nationwide follow-up survey. Br J Anaesth 59:791, 1987.

274. Stuart-Taylor ME, Billingham IS, Barrett RF, Church JJ: Extradural diamorphine for postoperative analgesia: Audit of a nurse-administered service to 800 patients in a district general hospital. Br J Anaesth 68:429, 1992.

275. Ready LB, Loper KA, Nessly M, Wild L: Postoperative epidural morphine is safe on surgical wards. Anesthesiology 75:452, 1991.

276. Scherer R, Schmutzler M, Giebler R, et al: Complications related to thoracic epidural analgesia: A prospective study in 1071 surgical patients. Acta Anaesth Scand 37:370, 1993.

277. Lubenow TR: Epidural analgesia: Considerations and delivery methods. *In* Sinatra RS, Hord AH, Ginsberg B, Preble LM (eds): Acute Pain. Mechanisms and Management. St. Louis, CV Mosby, 1992, p 233.

278. Bozkurt P, Kaya G, Yeker Y: Single-injection lumbar epidural morphine for postoperative analgesia in children: A report of 175 cases. Reg Anesth 22:112, 1997.

279. Burstal R, Wegener F, Hayes C, Lantry G: Epidural analgesia: Prospective audit of 1062 patients. Anaesth Intensive Care 26:165, 1998.

280. Liu SS, Allen HW, Olsson GL: Patient-controlled epidural analgesia with bupivacaine and fentanyl on hospital wards: Prospective experience with 1,030 surgical patients. Anesthesiology 88:688, 1998.

281. Wigfull J, Welchew E: Survey of 1057 patients receiving postoperative patient-controlled epidural analgesia. Anaesthesia 56:70, 2001.

282. Rigg JR, Jamrozik K, Myles PS, et al: Epidural anaesthesia and analgesia and outcome of major surgery: A randomised trial. Lancet 359:1276, 2002.

283. Steinberg RB, Liu SS, Wu CL, et al: Comparison of ropivacaine-fentanyl patient-controlled epidural analgesia with morphine intravenous patient-controlled analgesia for perioperative analgesia and recovery after open colon surgery. J Clin Anesth 14:571, 2002.

284. Flisberg P, Rudin A, Linner R, Lundberg CJ: Pain relief and safety after major surgery: A prospective study of epidural and intravenous analgesia in 2696 patients. Acta Anaesth Scand 47:457, 2003.

285. Peyton PJ, Myles PS, Silbert BS, et al: Perioperative epidural analgesia and outcome after major abdominal surgery in high-risk patients. Anesth Analg 96:548, 2003.

286. Russell GB, Graybeal JM: Hypoxemic episodes of patients in a postanesthesia care unit. Chest 104:899, 1993.

287. Russell AW, Owen H, Ilsley AH, et al: Background infusion with patient-controlled analgesia: Effect on postoperative oxyhaemoglobin saturation and pain control. Anaesth Intensive Care 21:174, 1993.

288. Moller JT: Anesthesia related hypoxemia. The effect of pulse oximetry monitoring on perioperative events and postoperative complications. Dan Med Bull 41:489, 1994.

289. Rosenberg J, Wildschiodtz G, Pedersen MH, et al: Late postoperative nocturnal episodic hypoxaemia and associated sleep pattern. Br J Anaesth 72:145, 1994.

290. Rosenberg J, Ullstad T, Rasmussen J, et al: Time course of postoperative hypoxaemia. Eur J Surg 160:137, 1994.

291. Stone JG, Cozine KA, Wald A: Nocturnal oxygenation during patient-controlled analgesia. Anesth Analg 89:104, 1999.

292. Etches RC: Respiratory depression associated with patient-controlled analgesia: A review of eight cases. Can J Anaesth 41:125, 1994.

293. Flisberg P, Jakobsson J, Lundberg J: Apnea and bradypnea in patients receiving epidural bupivacaine-morphine for postoperative pain relief as assessed by a new monitoring method. J Clin Anesth 14:129, 2002.

294. Ostermeier AM, Roizen MF, Hautkappe M, et al: Three sudden postoperative respiratory arrests associated with epidural opioids in patients with sleep apnea. Anesth Analg 85:452, 1997.

295. Hornbein TF, Townes BD, Schoene RB, et al: The cost to the central nervous system of climbing to extremely high altitude. N Engl J Med 321:1714, 1989.

296. Clark CF, Heaton RK, Wiens AN: Neuropsychological functioning after prolonged high altitude exposure in mountaineering. Aviat Space Environ Med 54:202, 1983.

297. Jason GW, Pajurkova EM, Lee RG: High-altitude mountaineering and brain function: Neuropsychological testing of members of a Mount Everest expedition. Aviat Space Environ Med 60:170, 1989.

298. Brodsky JB, Brose WG, Vivenzo K: A postoperative pain management service. Anesthesiology 70:719, 1989.

299. Muir MR, Sullivan FL, Dear G, Ginsberg B: Monitoring practices following epidural analgesics for pain management: A follow-up survey. J Pain Symptom Manage 14:36, 1997.

300. Grichnik K, Ginsberg B: Epidural analgesia for patients recovering from surgery. *In* Sinatra RS, Hord AH, Ginsberg B, Preble LM (eds): Acute Pain. Mechanisms and Management. St. Louis, CV Mosby, 1992, p 243.

301. Ashwood ER, Kost G, Kenny M: Temperature correction of blood-gas and pH measurements. Clin Chem 29:1877, 1983.

302. Siggaard-Andersen O, Wimberley PD, Gothgen I, Siggaard-Andersen M: A mathematical model of the hemoglobin-oxygen dissociation curve of human blood and of the oxygen partial pressure as a function of temperature. Clin Chem 30:1646, 1984.

303. Carter BG, Carlin JB, Tibballs J, et al: Accuracy of two pulse oximeters at low arterial hemoglobin-oxygen-saturation. Crit Care Med 26:1128, 1998.

304. Brand TM, Brand ME, Jay GD: Enamel nail polish does not interfere with pulse oximetry among normoxic volunteers. J Clin Monit Comput 17:93, 2002.

305. Baumeister BL, el-Khatib M, Smith PG, Blumer JL: Evaluation of predictors of weaning from mechanical ventilation in pediatric patients. Pediatr Pulmonol 24:344, 1997.

306. Milic-Emili J: Is weaning an art or a science? Am Rev Respir Dis 134:1107, 1986.

307. Hall JB, Wood LD: Liberation of the patient from mechanical ventilation. JAMA 257:1621, 1987.

308. Hodgkin JE, Bowser MA, Burton GG: Respirator weaning. Crit Care Med 2:96, 1974.

309. Tahvanainen J, Salmenpera M, Nikki P: Extubation criteria after weaning from intermittent mandatory ventilation and continuous positive airway pressure. Crit Care Med 11:702, 1983.

310. Karpel JP, Aldrich TK: Respiratory failure and mechanical ventilation: Pathophysiology and methods of promoting weaning. Lung 164:309, 1986.

311. Tobin MJ, Perez W, Guenther SM, et al: The pattern of breathing during successful and unsuccessful trials of weaning from mechanical ventilation. Am Rev Respir Dis 134:1111, 1986.

312. Sporn PH, Morganroth ML: Discontinuation of mechanical ventilation. Clin Chest Med 9:113, 1988.

313. Gorback MS, Kantor K: Extubation without a trial of spontaneous ventilation in the general surgical population. Respir Care 32:178, 1987.

314. Tobin MJ, Yang K: Weaning from mechanical ventilation. Crit Care Clin 6:725, 1990.

315. Mohsenifar Z, Hay A, Hay J, et al: Gastric intramural pH as a predictor of success or failure in weaning patients from mechanical ventilation. Ann Intern Med 119:794, 1993.

316. Capdevila XJ, Perrigault PF, Perey PJ, et al: Occlusion pressure and its ratio to maximum inspiratory pressure are useful predictors for successful extubation following T-piece weaning trial. Chest 108:482, 1995.

317. Esteban A, Frutos F, Tobin MJ, et al: A comparison of four methods of weaning patients from mechanical ventilation. Spanish Lung Failure Collaborative Group. N Engl J Med 332:345, 1995.

318. Nunn JF: Nunn's Applied Respiratory Physiology, 4th ed. Boston, Butterworth-Heinemann, 1993.

319. Christiansen J, Douglas CG, Haldane JS: The absorption and dissociation of carbon dioxide by human blood. J Physiol (Lond) 48:244, 1914.

320. Benumof JL: Anesthesia for Thoracic Surgery, 2nd ed. Philadelphia, WB Saunders, 1995.

321. Lawler PGP, Nunn JF: A reassessment of the validity of the iso-shunt graph. Br J Anaesth 56:1325, 1984.

322. Gilmour I, Burnham M, Craig DB: Closing capacity measurement during general anesthesia. Anesthesiology 45:477, 1976.

323. Fowler WS: Lung function studies. II. The respiratory dead space Am J Physiol 154:405, 1948.

324. Fletcher R, Jonson B, Cumming G, Brew J: The concept of dead space with special reference to the single breath test for carbon dioxide. Br J Anaesth 53:77, 1981.

325. Zupan J, Martin M, Benumof JL: End-tidal CO_2 excretion waveform and error with gas sampling line leak. Anesth Analg 67:579, 1988.

CHAPTER
37 Renal Function Monitoring

Solomon Aronson

**The Basis of Renal Function
Monitoring   1484**
    Physiology of Urine Formation   1486
    Monitoring of Glomerular Filtration Rate   1488

**Understanding Changes in
Perioperative Renal Function   1489**
    Effects of Regional Anesthesia   1489
    Effects of Inhaled Anesthetics   1489
    Effects of Hemodynamic Changes   1491

**Preoperative Evaluation of
Renal Function   1492**

**Direct and Indirect Monitors of
Renal Function   1493**
    Intravascular Volume   1494
    Cardiopulmonary Function   1494
    Distribution of Cardiac Output
        to the Kidneys   1495
    Biochemical Markers of
        Renal Function   1499
    Renal Blood Flow   1501
    Use of Renal Blood Flow   1505

Summary   1506

Renal dysfunction remains a serious complication during the perioperative period in critically ill patients undergoing major surgery.[1-7] The onset of acute perioperative renal failure portends a poor prognosis from the loss of renal function with consequent volume and solute overload and from associated life-threatening complications, including sepsis, respiratory failure, gastrointestinal hemorrhage, and central nervous system dysfunction. Acute renal failure (ARF) requiring dialysis develops in 1% to 7% of patients after cardiac or major vascular surgery and is strongly associated with morbidity and mortality[8-11] (see Chapters 50 and 52). The mortality rate of ARF was 91% during World War II, 68% in Korea, and 67% in Vietnam. Today, depending on associated comorbidities, postoperative renal failure is responsible for up to 60% mortality in the postoperative period. ARF in the presence of no other comorbidities has about a 10% to 40% mortality rate, whereas ARF in the intensive care unit setting carries a 50% to 80% mortality rate.[12] Perioperative renal failure accounts for one half of all patients requiring acute dialysis.[12] Perhaps one reason for the persistently frequent incidence of perioperative renal failure is a shift in medical populations to older and more critically ill patients undergoing increasingly higher-risk procedures. The persistently frequent incidence of perioperative renal failure observed may also result from our inability to adequately monitor renal function changes and to predict the onset of ARF in the operative and critical care setting.

An understanding of how to interpret information derived from monitoring presumes an understanding of terms used to describe the observations made. In the case of renal function monitoring, these assumptions may not always be warranted. *Perioperative renal failure*, for example, has been defined clinically as the need for postoperative dialysis or, in some cases, as a postoperative serum creatinine level exceeding a predetermined preoperative value (e.g., an increase of 0.5 mg/dL or of 50% or more). In one review,[13] no two studies of 26 defined ARF the same way. The overall reported frequency of ARF among all patients admitted to the hospital is 1%[14] and may increase to 2% to 5%[4,15] during hospitalization; however, there is no universally accepted standard for detecting renal insufficiency or failure. Reporting on the cause, incidence, and management of renal dysfunction also varies greatly because of wide variations in the definition of terms used to describe degrees of renal dysfunction in the literature. It is not surprising therefore that an estimated 5% of the general population has renal disease (however defined) that is severe enough to adversely affect surgical outcome.[16]

Several mechanisms involving a renal tubule, a tubulointerstitial process, and a reduction in filtering capacity of the glomerulus have been implicated in renal dysfunction. Prerenal causes are responsible for most cases of perioperative ARF. Since World War II, it has become clear that ARF can result from decreased renal blood flow from myriad causes (Table 37-1). Prerenal azotemia accounts for 70% of general community-acquired ARF[14,15] and for

Table 37–1 Causes of renal hypoperfusion associated with acute renal failure

Intravascular Volume Depletion
Major trauma, burns, crush syndrome
Fever
Hemorrhage
Diuretic use
Pancreatitis, vomiting, diarrhea, peritonitis, dehydration, NPO status, bowel preparations

Decreased Cardiac Output
Congestive heart failure or low output syndrome
Pulmonary hypertension, massive pulmonary embolism
Positive pressure mechanical ventilation

Increased Renal/Systemic Vascular Resistance Ratio
Renal vasoconstriction
  α-Adrenergic agonists
  Hypercalcemia, amphotericin
  Cyclosporine
System vasodilation
  Afterload reduction
  Antihypertensive medications
  Anaphylactic shock
  Anesthesia sepsis

Renovascular Obstruction
Renal artery: atherosclerosis, embolism, thrombosis, dissecting aneurysm, vasculitis
Renal vein: thrombosis, compression

Glomerular and Small-Vessel Obstruction
Glomerulonephritis
Vasculitis
Toxemia of pregnancy
Hemolytic uremic syndrome
Disseminated intravascular coagulation
Malignant hypertension
Radiation injury

Increased Blood Viscosity
Macroglobulinemia
Polycythemia

Interference with Renal Autoregulation
Prostaglandin inhibitors in presence of congestive heart failure (CHF), nephritic syndrome, cirrhosis, hypovolemia
Angiotensin-converting enzyme inhibition in presence of renal artery stenosis or CHF

When describing prerenal azotemia progressing to renal failure, the terms *acute tubular necrosis*, *vasomotor nephropathy*, and *ischemic tubular injury* are often used interchangeably in the literature.

Although most causes of ischemic renal failure are reversible, after a critical point of prolonged severe ischemia, necrosis may be irreversible.[19] In patients with inadequate renal blood flow, this irreversible injury is commonly caused by the added risk of drugs that alter the intrarenal distribution of blood flow by abnormal hemodynamics or by preexisting disease[20] (see Chapters 52, 54, and 56). These predisposing variables, as well as the onset and pathogenesis of perioperative renal failure, are often difficult to determine because direct assessment of renal hemodynamics and renal tubular function is typically not possible. Renal function must often be indirectly assessed. An understanding of normal renal physiology and of the pathophysiology of ARF is critical. Because perioperative treatment strategies depend on differentiating normal from abnormal renal function, understanding the limitations of commonly used renal function monitoring techniques is also important.

THE BASIS OF RENAL FUNCTION MONITORING

In general, the renal response to any specific condition or insult is primarily determined by associated physiologic and hemodynamic conditions prevailing at the time (see Chapter 20). In patients with renal disease, the challenge of optimal perioperative management is demanding because recognition of subtle change is difficult. Renal failure symptoms typically are not detected until less than 40% of normal functioning nephrons remain, and uremic symptoms occur when less than 5% of normal functioning nephrons remain.[18]

The three general functions of the kidneys are to excrete potentially toxic metabolic end products, to regulate water and tonicity, and to produce hormones. The kidney excretes most of the waste products metabolized from dietary intake, chiefly urea formed from ammonia released in protein metabolism, creatinine from muscle metabolism, and uric acid from purine metabolism. Serum creatinine levels and blood urea nitrogen (BUN) levels are used to measure the efficiency of metabolic waste removal. The levels of these end products rise slightly with increased dietary intake or increased catabolism. With normal renal function, an increase in concentration of waste products in blood results in rapid excretion of the increased load. The waste products are filtered in the glomeruli and tend to remain in the tubular fluid because they cannot permeate the nephron wall. In contrast, more than 98% of the filtered water and solute is reabsorbed into the body. Some degradation products, such as uric acid, are reabsorbed in the proximal tubule, secreted back into the tubule fluid, and then eliminated in urine. Cells and proteins with molecular masses greater than 70,000 daltons do not cross the glomerular capillary wall. However, smaller proteins, peptides, amino acids, and glucose are filtered to a variable degree. The proximal

more than 90% of perioperative ARF.[13,17] Typically, an early compensatory phase of normal renal adaptation (e.g., pre-prerenal failure) progresses to become decompensatory as prerenal failure ensues.[18] ARF may be characterized as an abrupt decline in renal function at this transitional stage. Depending on preexisting reserve capacity, this stage may persist for hours to days. At this point, the key decline in renal function is sufficient to result in retention of nitrogenous end products of metabolism and cessation of fluid and electrolyte homeostasis. These events are not reversible by modifying nonrenal factors and are difficult to predict. Prerenal azotemia and tubular ischemic injury represent extreme examples of the same problem (i.e., insufficient renal blood flow).

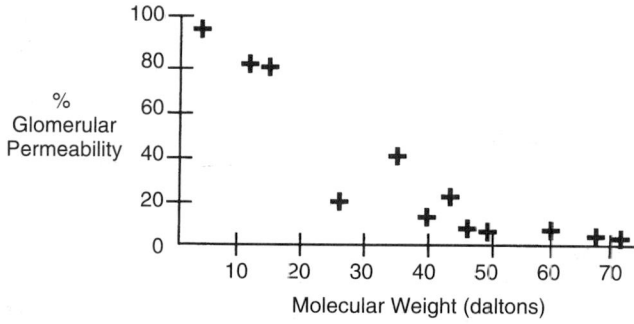

Figure 37–1 The glomerular permeability (i.e., filtration-to-plasma ratio) is represented on the *y* axis and compared with the molecular weight of the filtered substance represented on the *x* axis. (Data from Renkin EM, Robinson RR: Glomerular filtration. N Engl J Med 290:785, 1974.)

Figure 37–2 Renin released into the circulation interacts with angiotensinogen to cleave off the decapeptide angiotensin I; through converting enzymatic activity, this becomes the active octapeptide angiotensin II. Angiotensin II is a potent vasopressor and has a direct effect on the adrenals to stimulate aldosterone. By its vasoconstrictive action, angiotensin II increases salt retention.

tubule reabsorbs these substances, minimizing their loss in urine. Other substances that cannot be filtered are excreted primarily by active secretion into the tubular fluid (Fig. 37-1). The kidney is able to clear metabolic waste from the blood efficiently while conserving cells, proteins, and nutrients. When the glomerular membrane is damaged, red blood cells and large amounts of protein may enter the filtrate and later appear in urine.

The kidney regulates extracellular volume (approximately one third of total body water) primarily by manipulating sodium to maintain normal tonicity. The body senses intravascular volume losses through receptors in the left atrium, the afferent arteriole of the kidney, and the carotid sinus. Increased sympathetic neural tone to the kidney, decreased sodium delivery to the macula densa of the distal convoluted tubule, or reduced perfusion pressure stimulates renin release. The renin-angiotensin-aldosterone system acts to conserve sodium and water (Figs. 37-2 and 37-3). Normally, daily sodium intake (150 mEq/day) is excreted in the urine. With changes in water intake, sodium excretion in urine changes to maintain normal extracellular volume. The homeostatic range

Figure 37–3 Mechanism for renal sodium and volume regulation. ANF, atrial natriuretic factor; B.P., blood pressure; C.O., cardiac output; GFR, glomerular filtration rate; NaCl, sodium chloride.

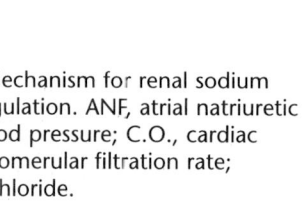

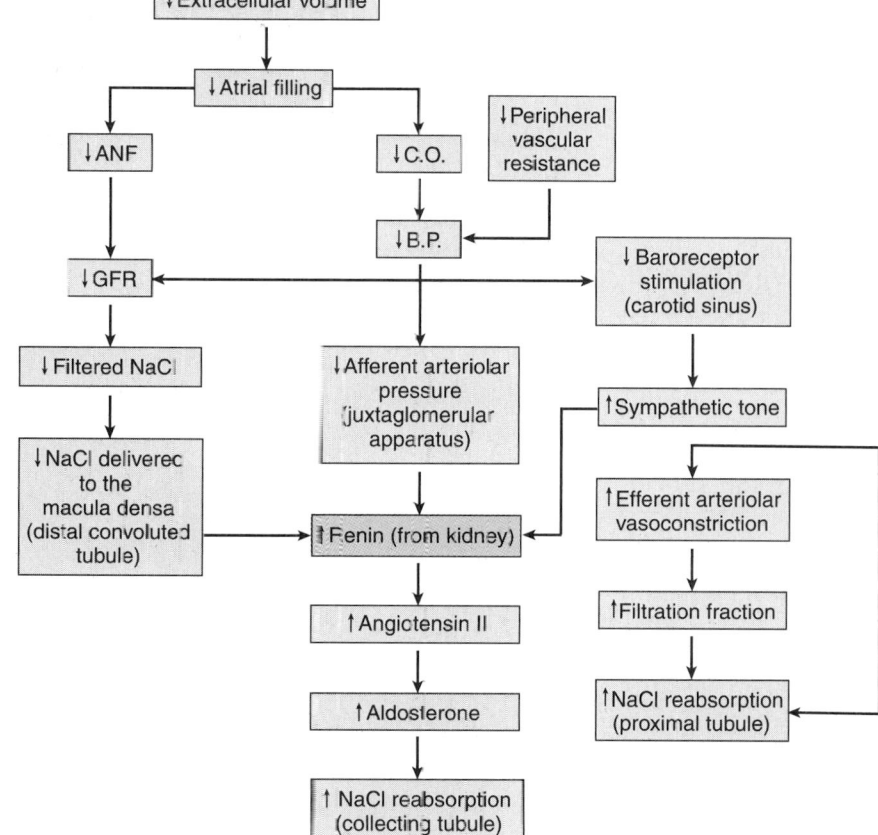

for the sodium intake and urinary excretion balance is great: less than 1 to more than 1000 mEq/day. Urinary excretion of sodium begins with filtration. The tubules then reabsorb 99% or more of the filtered sodium. Seventy percent is reabsorbed in the proximal tubule, 20% in the thick ascending limb of the loop of Henle and distal convoluted tubule, and 9% in the collecting ducts. The mechanisms regulating the urine excretion of sodium include systemic changes in circulating volume, causing decreased filtration and consequently decreased filtered sodium load. Less circulating volume also decreases levels of atrial natriuretic factor and increases aldosterone levels.

The second part of the tonicity function that the kidney serves is maintaining osmolarity within normal limits through regulation of water excretion. Reduced water intake with continued urinary water excretion leads to a rise in plasma osmolarity and vice versa. The major effector in the regulation of water excretion is the antidiuretic hormone (ADH) vasopressin. Vasopressin is secreted into the peripheral plasma by the posterior pituitary gland. The kidney is capable of wide variations in water excretion (i.e., urine flow) in response to changing levels of vasopressin in the peripheral plasma. Water excretion can be 100-fold lower in extreme antidiuresis (i.e., high vasopressin) than in extreme diuresis. These changes are achieved without substantial changes in steady-state rate of total solute excretion (i.e., osmolar excretion). This capability depends on the kidneys' ability to concentrate or dilute the urine. Water output from the kidneys of a 70-kg person normally ranges from 500 mL to 12 L/day. The kidney maintains a normal range of urinary concentrations and volumes first by producing a large amount of dilute fluid in the loop of Henle and the distal convoluted tubule. When the fluid passes through the highly concentrated solutes in the medulla in the presence of ADH, most of the water is reabsorbed. In the absence of ADH, only about one half of the water is reabsorbed. An acute (transient) effect of altered levels of circulating vasopressin (or ADH) is different from a steady-state response. Such transient behavior is observed in response to altered levels of circulating vasopressin and after induction of anesthesia.

The medullary concentration of solutes is high (1400 mOsm/L) because the ascending limb of the loop of Henle actively reabsorbs sodium and chloride without water into the medullary interstitium and because large amounts of urea enter the inner medulla from the collecting tubule. The cortical and outer medullary collecting tubules are sites of passive water reabsorption that are impermeable to urea. Urea becomes concentrated in the collecting ducts of the inner medulla, which are permeable to urea moving passively down its concentration gradient. The high concentrations of sodium, chloride, and urea are not washed out of the medulla because medullary blood flow is low and the configuration of the capillaries of the vasa recta permits a countercurrent exchange. Of the 140 to 180 L/day of fluid filtered at glomeruli, approximately 70% (100 L/day) is reabsorbed isosmotically in the proximal tubule, and 15% (20 L/day) is reabsorbed passively in the medulla in the descending loop of Henle. The remaining 15% (20 L/day) of highly concentrated tubular fluid reaches the papillary tip of the loop of Henle. As the fluid ascends the loop of Henle, sodium is reabsorbed (passively in the medulla and actively in the thick ascending limb in the outer medulla and cortex). Tubular fluid becomes hypotonic to plasma. Sodium reabsorption without water continues in the distal tubule. The collecting ducts may receive tubular fluid with concentrations below 100 mOsm/L. Tubular permeability to water increases or decreases, depending on the amount of ADH present, and may vary from 8 to 20 L, with subsequent urine volumes varying from 0.5 to 12 L/day in the normal 70-kg person.

The kidney functions as an endocrine gland in the renin-angiotensin system. Renin is secreted into the body by the granular cells of the juxtaglomerular apparatus of the kidney. Once in the bloodstream, renin catalyzes the splitting of angiotensin I from angiotensinogen, which is secreted from the liver and is always present in the plasma in high concentrations. The kidneys also secrete renal erythropoietic factor, which is involved in the control of erythrocyte production by the bone marrow. In response to decreased oxygen delivery to the kidney, renal erythropoietic factor is secreted and acts enzymatically in the plasma on a globulin secreted by the liver to form erythropoietin, which then acts to stimulate the bone marrow to increase its production of erythrocytes. The kidneys produce the active form of vitamin D and are linked to calcium metabolism; during times of prolonged fasting, the kidneys synthesize glucose from amino acids and other precursors and have the potential to be gluconeogenic organs.

Physiology of Urine Formation

Urine formation depends on hydraulic and oncotic pressures within the glomerular capillary, local and systemic neurohumoral influences, and an intact kidney-ureter-bladder feedback loop (see Chapter 20). The formation of urine begins with glomerular ultrafiltration and progresses to selective tubular reabsorption and tubular secretion. General anesthesia and surgery influence renal function primarily by affecting filtration and reabsorption.[21-25] All anesthetic agents, whether volatile or intravenous, have the potential to alter renal function by altering blood pressure and cardiac output so that renal blood flow is redistributed. This redistribution is accompanied by sodium and water conservation and decreased urine formation. Commonly used premedications can also influence urine output.[26] Narcotics and barbiturates, for example, can produce a small decrease in glomerular filtration rate (GFR) and, consequently, urine volume.

Regional anesthesia above level T4 reduces sympathetic tone to the kidney and makes renal blood flow and filtration directly dependent on perfusion pressure during sympathectomy.[27] Renal function and urine formation during regional anesthesia depend on the overall sum of the different homeostatic responses evoked, not just the sympathectomy. The combined effect of multiple factors, such as level of the block, preservation of autoregulatory mechanisms to preserve renal blood flow, circulating catecholamines, renin-angiotensin, ADH, steroids, and prostaglandins, determine the degree of urine formation.

Anesthetic drugs may increase or decrease catecholamines, alter renal vascular resistance, depress myocardium, and decrease renal blood flow, or they may have a direct nephrotoxic effect on renal tubular function. Surgery in general, aortic cross-clamping and declamping in particular, trauma, and stress also may indirectly influence urine formation by changing myocardial function, sympathetic activity, neuronal or hormonal activity (e.g., renin and angiotensin production), intravascular volume, or systemic vascular resistance.[28,29]

Starling Forces

Glomerular filtration is governed by the following equation:

$$GFR = K_f \times (P_{GC} - P_{BC} - P_{PO})$$

GFR is the glomerular filtration rate or the rate at which fluid is filtered through the glomerular capillaries into the Bowman capsule, K_f is the glomerular filtration coefficient or the factor that considers the permeability and surface area of the glomerular basement membrane, P_{GC} is the glomerular capillary pressure, P_{BC} is the pressure in the Bowman capsule, and P_{PO} is the plasma oncotic pressure.

The last three factors represent the Starling forces that govern the hydrostatic forces through the glomerular membrane. Acute changes in GFR, and consequently in urine formation, are commonly caused by changes in glomerular capillary pressure. For example, events that reduce plasma flow rates reduce the hydraulic pressure of glomerular capillaries and favor decreased ultrafiltration, whereas events that increase plasma flow rate have the opposite effect. Theoretically, varying concentrations of plasma proteins may influence urine formation and the GFR. As the concentration of proteins in plasma decreases, the oncotic pressure and the oncotic force opposing ultrafiltration also decrease. Conversely, a rise in oncotic pressure reduces the rate of glomerular filtration. This effect is most likely offset by the oncotic force of plasma proteins (e.g., albumin), which enables adequate intravascular volume to be maintained. The precise role in preserving renal function of oncotic pressure versus maintenance of adequate renal blood flow or other variables influencing glomerular filtration has never been studied. However, in one series,[30] patients resuscitated with albumin after massive transfusion had more renal dysfunction than those resuscitated with saline.

When the impact of normal saline–based intravenous fluid replacement was evaluated and compared with lactated Ringer's solution (i.e., albumin 5% in normal saline, hetastarch in normal saline, or lactated Ringer's solution), renal function indices (i.e., creatinine clearance, serum creatinine, and urine output) were all inferior in the normal saline–based vehicle groups.[31] The patients receiving lactated Ringer's solution were more likely to exhibit a hypercoagulable state.[31] Outcome data, however, did not enable a distinction between albumin and normal saline as a fluid replacement option.

Neurohumoral Influences

Because the tubules and the collecting ducts of the kidney reabsorb about 99% of the filtered solute, the daily filtration volume (approximately 180 L) greatly exceeds the typical daily urinary volume of 1 to 2 L. To clear nitrogenous wastes daily, 400 to 500 mL of urine is required. The countercurrent multiplier system in the loop of Henle is a critical component of the kidney's ability to excrete or conserve salt and water. Sodium and water reabsorption depend on the hypertonicity of the medullary interstitium, which depends on the maintenance of normal renal blood flow. The major hormonal influences determining conservation or loss of filtered sodium and water are aldosterone, ADH, atrial natriuretic factor, and the renal prostaglandins.

High concentrations of aldosterone stimulate reabsorption of sodium and water, primarily in the distal tubule and the collecting ducts. Aldosterone is produced by the adrenal cortex in response to the feedback from the renin-angiotensin-aldosterone system, simplified as follows. Reduced delivery of sodium to the macula densa causes release of renin from the granular cells of the juxtaglomerular apparatus. Renin catalyzes the release of angiotensin I from angiotensinogen. Angiotensin I is then transformed to angiotensin II in the lungs, catalyzed by angiotensin-converting enzyme. Angiotensin II stimulates the production of aldosterone.

ADH acts primarily on the collecting ducts to increase water reabsorption. ADH is released from the posterior pituitary gland in response to increased blood osmolarity, which stimulates osmoreceptors in the hypothalamus. ADH is inhibited by stimulation of atrial baroreceptors or increased atrial volume.[32] ADH release is also influenced by stress and increased partial pressure of arterial carbon dioxide.[33] A high level of ADH results in the excretion of small volumes of concentrated urine.

Atrial natriuretic peptide causes systemic vasodilation and promotes renal excretion of sodium and water by increasing glomerular filtration.[34] Atrial natriuretic peptide is secreted by the cardiac atria and other organs in response to increased intravascular volume. It decreases systemic blood pressure by relaxing vascular smooth muscle, reducing sympathetic stimulation, and inhibiting the renin-angiotensin-aldosterone system.

The kidney also synthesizes prostaglandins, which regulate the influence of other hormones. During hemodynamic instability and increased adrenergic stimulation, for example, prostaglandin E_2 decreases the vasoconstrictive effect of angiotensin II on the afferent arterioles and preserves renal blood flow. Inhibition of prostaglandin synthesis during normal states of hydration, renal perfusion, and sodium balance does not affect renal function. When the kidney is confronted with a vasoconstricted state, such as hypotension and hypovolemia, however, the presence of renal prostaglandins is essential for preserving adequate renal blood flow. Patients taking nonsteroidal anti-inflammatory drugs are at risk during conditions of impaired circulatory status because these agents inhibit cyclooxygenase activity, an important enzyme in the prostaglandin synthesis pathway, thereby rendering the kidney (afferent arteriole) susceptible to the systemic vasoconstrictive effect of angiotensin II and other catecholamines normally secreted to preserve intravascular volume and perfusion pressure.

Ureteral Peristalsis

Ureteral peristalsis influences urine formation. Interaction between the urinary bladder, the kidney, and the ureters regulates urine production by the kidney and urine transport to the bladder by the ureter.[35] General anesthesia decreases the rate of ureteral contractility (Fig. 37-4).[36] Normally, ureteral peristalsis originates with electrical activity at pacemaker sites located in the proximal portion of the urinary collecting system. The electrical activity is then propagated, giving rise to the mechanical event peristalsis and ureteral contraction, which propels the bolus of urine distally. Basal peristalsis within the ureter is influenced by pressures within the renal pelvis, the ureter, and the ureteral-vesical junction. The autonomic nervous system also plays an important role in ureteral function and consequently in urine formation.[37] Cholinergic agonists generally increase the frequency and the force of ureteral contraction. Drugs that act primarily on adrenergic receptors tend to stimulate ureteral activity, whereas agents that primarily activate adrenergic receptors tend to inhibit ureteral activity. Histamine stimulates ureteral activity. In a variety of preparations, morphine increases ureteral tone. Infections within the urinary tract may impair urine transport. In humans, irregular peristaltic contractions occur with retroperitoneal inflammation resulting from appendicitis, regional enteritis, ulcerative colitis, and peritonitis.[38] Clinically, the response of the ureter to pathologic conditions seems to vary with age. More marked degrees of ureteral dilation are observed in neonates and young children than in adults.[39] Aging brings a decrease in the effectiveness of β-adrenergic agonists to relax the ureter and a progressive increase in smooth muscle cell mass, producing the overall effect of no apparent change in the ureteral contractile process in the geriatric patient.

Monitoring of Glomerular Filtration Rate

Structure of the Glomerulus

In general, the GFR is determined by the rate of glomerular plasma flow (as it influences ultrafiltration pressure), systemic oncotic pressure, glomerular hydraulic pressure differences, and an ultrafiltration coefficient. The ultrafiltration coefficient is the product of glomerular capillary hydraulic permeability and total surface area available for filtration. The filtration rate across a capillary bed is therefore the product of surface area, pressure gradients, and permeability. In the glomerulus, the capillaries are configured in tufts, which increases their surface area. Hydrostatic pressures are normally maintained higher in glomerular capillaries than in other capillary beds by a delicate balance of preglomerular and postglomerular vascular tone in arterioles. The permeability of the glomerular capillary wall is equal for substances with molecular masses up to 5000 to 6000 daltons and decreases to almost zero at 60,000 to 70,000 daltons.[40] Metabolic wastes and essential nutrients are filtered freely, and larger proteins, such as albumin and immunoglobulin G, are filtered in trace amounts or not at all. The glomerulopathic process in diabetes,[41] for example, results from all of the factors that cause sustained increase in glomerular pressure and flow. Hyperglycemia induces a state of extracellular fluid volume expansion, structural hypertrophy of the kidney, and altered glucoregulatory and vasoregulatory hormone action. These hemodynamic consequences of hyperglycemia lead to renal vasodilation and increased plasma flow rate. The increase of plasma flow causes increased glomerular transcapillary flux of plasma proteins. The elevation in glomerular flow (i.e., pressure) also alters the permeability and selectivity of the glomerular basement membrane, resulting in increased protein filtration. The increased transglomerular flux of plasma proteins leads to their accumulation in the mesangium, which further propagates glomerulosclerosis.

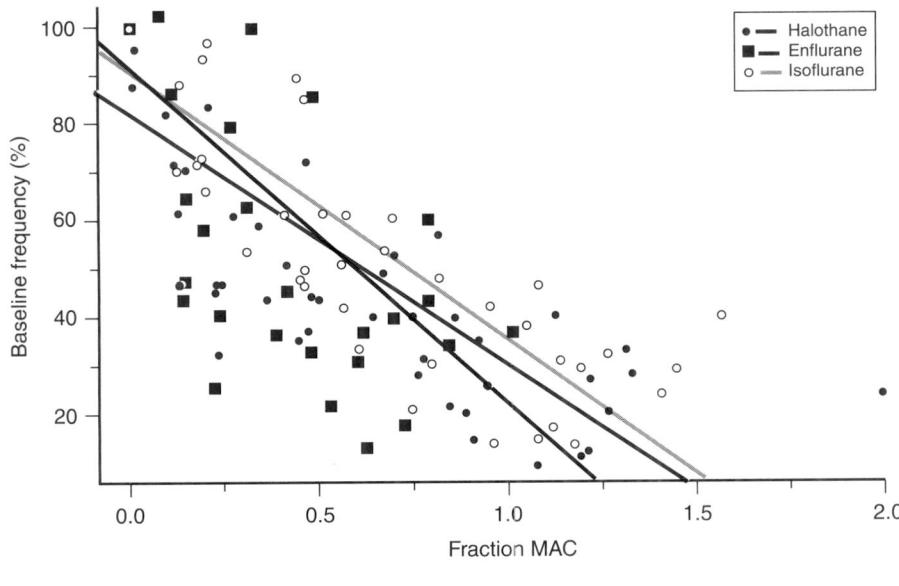

Figure 37–4 Effect of general anesthesia on the rate of ureteral contractility. (Adapted from Young CJ, Attele A, Toledano A, et al: Volatile anesthetics decrease peristalsis in the guinea pig ureter. Anesthesiology 81:452-458, 1994.)

Inulin Clearance

GFR, the rate at which plasma water is filtered across the glomerulus, is an important index of renal function. Because the tubule reabsorbs most of the water filtered through the glomerulus, urine volume cannot be used to measure GFR. For measurement, a substance is required that is filtered through the glomerulus at the same rate as water and is excreted in the urine (i.e., neither reabsorbed nor secreted). The amount of such a substance filtered is then equal to the amount eliminated in the urine and can be determined from the product of the substance's concentration in plasma and the amount of plasma water filtered.

Inulin, an exogenous polysaccharide with a molecular mass of 5200 daltons, has been used to measure GFR because it is filtered freely in the glomerulus, not reabsorbed or secreted, and is excreted in the urine. Since its introduction into clinical practice in 1934, inulin clearance had been considered the standard for measurement of GFR.[42] Its production is now limited, and it no longer remains a practical option in most clinical or experimental settings. To assess inulin clearance, the clinician administers a priming dose of inulin intravenously, followed by a continuous infusion calculated to maintain constant blood concentrations. After an equilibration period (usually 1 hour), clearance measurements are obtained. Urine is collected (typically with a Foley catheter), and venous blood samples are obtained at the midpoint of each clearance period. The longer the clearance period, the less likely is the introduction of error from incomplete voiding. The standard formula for calculation of clearance is as follows:

$$C_I = (U_I V)/P_I$$

U_I and P_I are the urine and plasma concentrations of inulin, C_I is the rate of insulin clearance, and V is the urine flow rate.

Creatinine Clearance

In clinical practice, the endogenous substance creatinine is used to measure clearance. Creatinine (molecular mass of 133 daltons) is a smaller substance than inulin and is produced from muscle metabolism. Creatinine is not an ideal substance for measuring clearance, because a small amount is secreted under normal conditions. Although creatinine clearance may exceed inulin clearance, the clearance of endogenous creatinine approximates that of inulin and has proved to be a reasonable measure of GFR.[43] The creatinine-to-inulin clearance ratio is almost identical in normal infants, children, and adults. In subjects with moderate to severe renal insufficiency, however, the creatinine-to-inulin clearance ratio is increased.[44] Increased secretion and clearance of creatinine in patients with renal insufficiency may therefore result in overestimates of true GFR.

Urea (molecular mass of 60 daltons) cannot be used to estimate GFR because, under normal conditions, it is filtered and reabsorbed. More importantly, urea clearance changes with the state of hydration; for example, under conditions of dehydration, urea clearance is significantly less than inulin clearance.

UNDERSTANDING CHANGES IN PERIOPERATIVE RENAL FUNCTION

The precise mechanisms heralding the transition from compensated preserved renal function to uncompensated renal failure during the perioperative period remain poorly understood, in part because the methods used to assess renal function changes are insensitive and nonspecific. All anesthetic techniques and perioperative events that decrease blood pressure and cardiac output have the potential to alter renal function because of blood flow redistribution within the kidney and decreased glomerular filtration.

Effects of Regional Anesthesia

Regional anesthetics and the kidneys interact in a complex manner that varies according to the underlying cardiovascular, renal, fluid, and electrolyte status of the patient[45] (see Chapters 43, 44, and 45). The combined effect of multiple factors (e.g., catecholamines, renin-angiotensin, ADH, steroids, prostaglandin) determines the consequences for renal function. The effect of sympathetic blockade depends on the level of the block and the presence of underlying disease. In a patient with global systolic ventricular dysfunction or dilated cardiomyopathy, regional anesthesia may exert the beneficial effects of an afterload-reducing and preload-reducing agent. However, the same anesthesia in a patient with hypovolemia may exacerbate hypotension and decrease renal perfusion. The interactions between regional anesthesia and renal function are different in patients with different underlying disease. In patients with ischemic heart disease, regional anesthesia may exacerbate regional myocardial dysfunction through vasodilation, hypotension, and decreased coronary perfusion pressure[46] and may thereby decrease renal perfusion.

Spinal cord segments T4 through L1 contribute to the sympathetic innervation of the renal vasculature, which is innervated through sympathetic fibers from the celiac and renal plexus.[27,47] As long as flow is maintained and perfusion pressure does not fall below the autoregulatory range during spinal and epidural anesthesia, there is little change in GFR or renal vascular resistance. Sulerman and colleagues[48] demonstrated in healthy volunteers that renal blood flow is unchanged during epidural anesthesia with a T6 sensory block. In their study, mean arterial pressure remained above 70 mm Hg and never decreased below 6% of the baseline level. The sympathetic innervation of the kidney affects multiple aspects of renal function, including hemodynamics, electrolyte and water reabsorption, and renin secretion.[45] Urine volume and free water clearance may decrease during spinal anesthesia as a result of increased ADH secretion. Increased renal sympathomimetic activity decreases renal blood flow through α-adrenergic mediation and increases renin release through β-adrenergic innervation directly or by interaction with the renal tubular macula densa and the baroreceptor reflex mechanism.[49]

Effects of Inhaled Anesthetics

There is a well-recognized renal nephrotoxic effect of the older volatile inhaled anesthetics that is attributed to the serum concentration of inorganic fluoride (F^-) (see Chapters 4 and 8). Increased serum levels of inorganic fluoride caused polyuric renal insufficiency.[50] Methoxyflurane, which is no longer used clinically, and enflurane, when used for prolonged periods (9.6 minimum alveolar concentration [MAC] hours), cause an increase in the serum level of inorganic fluoride.[50-52] After enflurane anesthesia, maximal urinary osmolality decreases in response to vasopressin for 5 days. These changes are of little consequence in patients with normal renal function. However, in patients with preexisting renal dysfunction, enflurane may cause further renal deterioration.

Sevoflurane appears to act as enflurane does in regard to the generation of inorganic fluoride as a result of metabolism.[53-56] Sevoflurane undergoes approximately 5% metabolism, and the primary metabolites are fluoride and hexafluoroisopropanol. Once formed, hexafluoroisopropanol is conjugated in the liver with glucuronic acid and excreted. The oxidative defluorination of sevoflurane in the liver causes liberation of free fluoride ions. Concerns have been raised that sevoflurane might impair the ability of the kidneys to concentrate urine (as methoxyflurane does).[54] Earlier research indicated that renal dysfunction from methoxyflurane was likely to occur when dose or duration of administration resulted in serum fluoride concentrations that exceeded 50 μM/L.[51] This presumed threshold for toxicity has been extrapolated for other halogenated anesthetic agents, including enflurane and sevoflurane. However, because sevoflurane is defluorinated by the cytochrome P450 enzyme system, renal defluorination of sevoflurane is not clinically significant. In American Society of Anesthesiologists (ASA) class I and II patients, it was shown that serum fluoride levels averaged 36.6 $\pm$ 4.3 μM/L after 9 MAC hours of sevoflurane anesthesia.[53,57] These fluoride levels peaked 2 hours after the end of anesthesia and decreased by 50% within 8 hours. The rapid decline of plasma fluoride was attributed to the insolubility and rapid pulmonary elimination of sevoflurane. Desmopressin was used to test urine-concentrating ability before anesthesia and on days 1 and 5 after 9.5 MAC hours of sevoflurane and enflurane anesthesia.[57] Mean plasma fluoride levels were approximately twice as high in volunteers receiving sevoflurane as in those receiving enflurane, and 43% of volunteers receiving sevoflurane had plasma fluoride levels that exceeded 50 μM/L. Despite these results, the kidneys of the volunteers receiving sevoflurane were not impaired in their ability to concentrate urine, whereas 20% of volunteers receiving enflurane had transient concentrating deficits on day 1. The investigators postulated that intrarenal production of fluoride ion was a more important factor in the pathogenesis of nephrotoxicity than the association between plasma fluoride levels and nephrotoxicity.[56] The intrarenal metabolism of methoxyflurane is fourfold greater than the intrarenal metabolism of sevoflurane.

All inhaled anesthetic agents interact with carbon dioxide absorbents to produce toxic compounds. A controversy has arisen concerning the relationships among sevoflurane, nephrotoxicity, and compound A. In circuit systems under conditions of high temperature and low flow rates, carbon dioxide absorbents degrade sevoflurane, resulting in detectable concentrations of fluoromethyl-2,2-difluoro-1-(trifluoroethyl) vinyl ether (i.e., compound A). These degradation products are conjugated in the liver with glutathione. Cysteine conjugates formed in the bile ducts and kidney by the conjugates are metabolized in the kidney by an enzyme (cysteine-conjugate β-lyase) to form end products that result in renal injury, which is characterized by diuresis, glycosuria, proteinuria, and elevated serum BUN and creatinine levels. This renal injury in experimental models was a function of the concentration and the duration of exposure of compound A.[58] The threshold for injury was exposure to compound A at 50 to 114 parts per million (ppm) for 3 hours, and the lethal dose of compound A was 331 ppm over 3 hours, 203 ppm over 6 hours, or 127 ppm over 12 hours.[59] The disparity between the results in humans and those in experimental rats may be caused by differences in the metabolic pathway of compound A in the species. Of the four recognized metabolic pathways for compound A, three do not involve renal β-lyase and do not result in organ toxicity. Humans have a 10-fold to 30-fold relative absence of the renal β-lyase enzyme pathway compared with rats, which may account for the apparent absence of renal injury from sevoflurane in humans. One study[60] evaluated the safety of low-flow sevoflurane anesthesia compared with low-flow isoflurane anesthesia in patients scheduled to have prolonged surgery (>6 hours). The average MAC hours in the sevoflurane group and in the isoflurane group were similar, and the average compound A concentration in the sevoflurane group was 20 $\pm$ 7 ppm. Markers of renal injury, including BUN, creatinine, N-acetyl-β-D-glucosaminidase (NAG), and alanine aminopeptidase, were increased similarly in all groups during the prolonged exposure to the volatile anesthetics.

The highest concentrations of compound A possible during anesthesia (mean arterial pressure, 56 mm Hg) was evaluated with sevoflurane in human volunteers.[61] Fresh carbon dioxide absorbent was used, and sevoflurane was given (without nitrous oxide) at 1.25 MAC while the esophageal temperature was maintained at 37°C. Volunteers were exposed to the anesthetic gas for 8 hours. In that study, compound A levels approached 50 ppm in the inspired limb of the breathing circuit, and the volunteers were asked to bring in 24-hour urine collections for 3 consecutive days after the anesthetic exposure. In most subjects, there were transient elevations of urinary protein, albumin, glucose, α-glutathione S-transferase (α-GST), and π-glutathione S-transferase (π-GST). No such increases were observed after a similar exposure to desflurane. The glutathione S-transferase (GST) protein protects cells by using reduced glutathione to inactivate reactive compounds before their excretion into the urine (or bile). The isolated forms (α-GST or π-GST) are specific to cells of the proximal and distal renal tubules and are released into the urine after renal damage. Urinary α-GST is a sensitive marker of tubular damage after nephrotoxic and ischemic insults.[62]

Another study[63] evaluated the safety and efficacy of sevoflurane versus isoflurane in patients during conditions of flow of less than 2 L/min. Patients from multiple institutions undergoing elective surgery lasting 2 to 8 hours were evaluated. Fresh Baralyme was used for all cases, and nitrous oxide was not permitted. The use of sevoflurane averaged 1 MAC hour. No differences were found in urine albumin, glucose, protein, or osmolality between treatment groups. Moreover, within the sevoflurane group, there were no significant correlations between compound A levels and BUN, creatinine or urinary excretion of protein, glucose, NAG, proximal tubule α-GST, or distal tubule π-GST.[63]

Effects of Hemodynamic Changes

Prerenal and renal factors can generate ischemic renal dysfunction. There appears to be an early phase of renal adaptation, or pre-prerenal failure, to the decreased delivery of blood to the glomerulus.[18] When these compensatory mechanisms become decompensatory, prerenal failure ensues. Renal clearance is determined by the delivery of waste products to the kidney (i.e., renal blood flow) and by the kidney's ability to extract them (i.e., the GFR).

A variety of experimental models have been devised to simulate hemodynamically mediated human ARF.[64-66] In these models, renal blood flow is commonly interrupted mechanically or pharmacologically. A reduction of flow by more than 50% is the rule during the initial phase of the experiment. After transient but total renal ischemia for 40 to 60 minutes, a lesion appears with clinical manifestations, laboratory features, and pathologic features of ARF. During the established phase, GFR is disproportionately depressed, compared with a moderate decline in renal blood flow. The maintenance of adequate blood supply to the kidneys therefore is critical; however, determining what constitutes adequate blood supply (i.e., oxygen) is difficult. The exact role and the timing of changes in renal blood flow in the initiation and the maintenance of ARF continue to be studied.

A number of theories have been proposed to explain the pathogenesis of hemodynamically mediated ARF.

Although a reduction in renal blood blow is clearly the initiating cause (Fig. 37-5),[67,68] the occurrence of ARF after hypotension is unpredictable. The precise circumstances precipitating a change from an underperfused healthy kidney to a damaged organ are difficult to define. Even with decreased delivery of blood to the glomerulus, a series of compensatory mechanisms may still preserve renal filtration function[18] (Fig. 37-6). Salt and water are retained to restore intravascular volume and fractional tubular reabsorption. The distribution of cardiac output to the kidneys is also regulated. At a given level of cardiac output, intrarenal factors affect the ratio of renal-to-systemic vascular resistance, thereby influencing the percentage of cardiac output received by the kidneys. Another critical component in the intrinsic modulation of renal filtration function is the regulation of filtration fraction. At the glomerular capillary, plasma is separated into a protein-free ultrafiltrate and a nonfiltered portion. Normally, the filtration fraction (i.e., relationship of GFR to renal plasma flow) is about 0.2. Initially, the filtration fraction is maintained by efferent arteriolar constriction. Unabated, the mechanisms that influence efferent arteriolar vasoconstriction ultimately may influence afferent arteriolar vasoconstriction. The resulting decrease in filtration fraction is the hallmark of postischemic ARF.[18] Ischemic tubular damage may be exacerbated further by an imbalance between oxygen supply and demand. Most vulnerable to the imbalance are the thick ascending tubular cells of the loop of Henle in the medulla.[68-71]

Intrarenal distribution of blood flow and total renal blood flow can be assessed with radioactive gases or

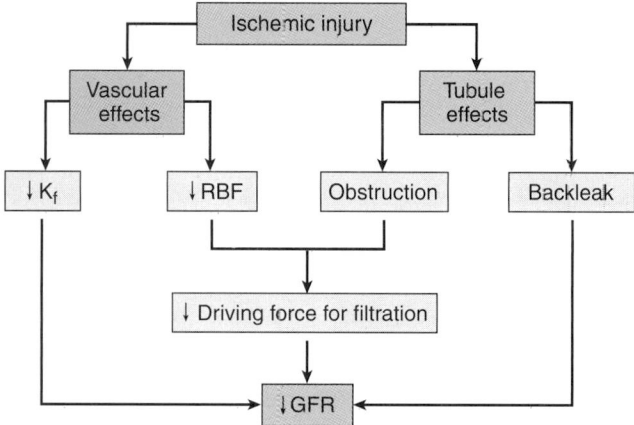

Figure 37–5 Schematic representation of the mechanisms that initiate and maintain decreased glomerular filtration seen in experimentally induced acute renal failure. GFR, glomerular filtration rate; K$_f$, glomerular capillary ultrafiltration coefficient; RBF, renal blood flow. (Adapted from Hostetter TH, Wilkes BM, Brenner BM: Mechanisms of impaired glomerular filtration in acute renal failure. *In* Brenner BM, Stein JH [eds]: Acute Renal Failure. New York, Churchill Livingstone, 1980, p 52.)

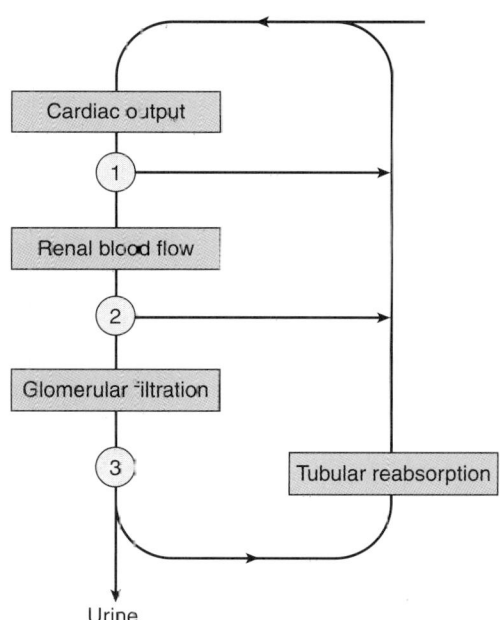

Figure 37–6 The regulatory mechanisms through which glomerular filtration is modulated include (1) fractional regional blood flow (renal blood flow/cardiac output); (2) filtration fraction (glomerular filtration rate/glomerular plasma flow rate); and (3) fractional tubular fluid reabsorption (tubular reabsorption/glomerular filtration rate). (Adapted from Badr KF, Ichikawa I: Prerenal failure: A deleterious shift from renal compensation to decompensation. N Engl J Med 319:623, 1988.)

radiolabeled microspheres. Microsphere, xenon washout, and angiographic techniques have shown that outer cortical blood flow decreases in ischemic models of ARF.[72-74] Because 85% to 90% of renal blood flow is distributed to cortical glomeruli, the finding of cortical pallor and redistribution of renal blood flow away from the cortex means that redistribution may be responsible for the functional lesions of ARF. In some cases, the return of perfusion to the cortex has correlated with a return of renal function.[73] The theory that intrarenal distribution of blood flow away from the outer cortex to the inner medulla decreases oxygen supply while increased tubular reabsorption of solute increases oxygen demand is further supported by studies of renal energetics during ARF.[75-77] It has been postulated that a decrease in the GFR and consequently in the energy requirement for tubular reabsorption may be a mechanism by which the kidney reduces energy demands before energy supply is critically limited. Increased demand and decreased supply are precipitated during states of inadequate perfusion, such as those resulting from depleted intravascular volume, maldistribution of systemic flow away from the renal vascular bed, cardiogenic shock, and destructive vascular conditions.

PREOPERATIVE EVALUATION OF RENAL FUNCTION

The greater the magnitude and duration of the surgical insult and the number of acute and chronic risk factors, the greater is the likelihood of perioperative renal compromise and the need for preoperative identification of renal function (see Chapters 25 and 27). In patients with inadequate blood flow, injury is commonly caused by the added risk of drugs, by abnormal hemodynamics, or by preexisting disease.[20] Studies have shown that 12% to 14% of patients who develop acute renal insufficiency disease during hospitalization do so after radiographic procedures with contrast. If preexisting renal insufficiency exists, progressive deterioration in renal function occurs 42% of cases, with a poor prognosis if dialysis is required.[78] Acute risk factors, such as volume depletion, aminoglycoside use, radiocontrast dye exposure, use of nonsteroidal anti-inflammatory drugs, septic shock, and pigmenturia, augment the risk of ARF rather than induce it. It appears that the combined interaction of these multiple acute risk factors is central in the pathogenesis of ARF (Table 37-2).[15] Patients with preexisting renal insufficiency, for example, are especially prone to develop ARF as a result of cardiovascular surgery. Patients with diabetes mellitus and renal insufficiency are especially vulnerable to radiocontrast agents. A review of the literature suggests that the most critical determinants of postoperative renal function are preoperative renal function, maintenance of appropriate intravascular volume, and normal myocardial function.[13] Although variables have been identified that increase the likelihood of renal dysfunction outcomes, there remains unexplained variability in prediction accuracy. Genetic polymorphism may predispose patients to acute perioperative renal dysfunction, similar to the situation that has been identified in chronic

Table 37-2   Risk factors associated with the development of acute renal failure

Acute Factors
Volume depletion
Use of aminoglycosides
Radiocontrast dye exposure
Use of nonsteroidal anti-inflammatory drugs
Septic shock
Pigmenturia
Chronic Factors
Preexisting renal disease
Hypertension
Congestive heart failure
Diabetes mellitus
Advanced age
Cirrhosis of the liver

renal disease. The apolipoprotein E4 was reported to be more associated with reduced postoperative increases in serum creatinine after cardiac surgery compared with the apolipoprotein E3 or E2 polymorphisms.[79]

Despite substantially reduced renal function, impaired functional reserve capacity may only become evident when stress imposes severe demands on renal function; therefore, a comprehensive evaluation of renal function reserve should be sought before surgery. In addition to intrinsic renal disease, several extrinsic variables influence the outcome of renal function tests: intracellular and extracellular volume, cardiovascular function, and neuroendocrine factors.[80,81] Advanced age also markedly decreases renal function reserve. GFR, normally about 125 mL/min in a young adult, decreases to about 80 mL/min at 60 years of age and to 60 mL/min at 80 years. Although not necessarily the primary cause for end-stage renal disease, hypertension in up to 85% of patients with renal failure is a major risk factor for the high cardiovascular morbidity that occurs.[82]

In addition to its contribution to renal failure in hypertensive nephrosclerosis, resulting from essential hypertension and hyperfiltration in diabetic nephropathy, hypertension also contributes to the loss of renal function associated with aging. Preoperative isolated systolic blood pressure (SBP) hypertension and wide pulse pressure (i.e., the difference between SBP and diastolic blood pressure [DBP]) are strong independent predictors of postoperative renal dysfunction.[10,11] It appears that an increase in conduit vessel stiffness with inadequate flow during low-pressure states contributes to increased preoperative renal dysfunction and hemodialysis-dependent renal failure. Four groups of preoperative hypertensive patients were identified in an analysis of 5065 patients undergoing coronary artery bypass surgery. Isolated SBP (SBP>160 mm Hg, DBP<90 mm Hg), isolated DBP (SBP<160 mm Hg, DBP>90 mm Hg), combined SBP and DBP, and wide pulse pressure (>80 mm Hg). In that analysis, the rate of wide pulse pressure was 8%, and that of isolated SBP was 2.3%. Mild hypertensive disease that is associated with renal disease therefore implies that renal disease may be primary.

Reliable evaluation requires knowledge of various renal function tests and their diagnostic limitations. For appropriate management, ischemic causes (e.g., prerenal azotemia) should ideally be distinguished from factors that maintain the intrinsic state of renal failure (e.g., acute tubular necrosis). Prerenal azotemia and acute tubular necrosis, however, may not be mutually exclusive. Unfortunately, there is no simple, inexpensive test that adequately quantifies renal function. The readily available tests fail to accurately reflect the status of the kidneys in a large percentage of patients, especially those who are elderly, malnourished, or dehydrated. Commonly obtained tests of renal function are urinalysis, BUN determination, serum creatinine determination, and creatinine clearance.

Urinalysis provides qualitative information that must be interpreted cautiously. Hematuria (i.e., more than one or two red blood cells per high-power field in a concentrated sediment) suggests glomerular disease or, in a trauma patient, injury to the kidneys or the lower urinary tract. A urine test result that is positive for blood in the absence of red blood cells suggests the presence of free hemoglobin or myoglobin in the urine. Pyuria (i.e., more than four white blood cells per high-power field) suggests urinary tract infection. Although urine may normally contain hyaline and granular casts, cellular casts represent a pathologic condition. Red blood cell casts suggest interstitial nephritis, including pyelonephritis. Urinary pH, although difficult to interpret on a spot urine sample, may assist in the diagnosis of some acid-base disturbances. The pH of urine tends to be more acidic when factors that initiate failure are prerenal rather than postrenal. The presence of proteinuria on a routine dipstick examination may be normal, or it may suggest severe renal disease. In a concentrated urine sample, trace or 1+ proteinuria is a nonspecific finding, whereas 3+ or 4+ proteinuria suggests glomerular disease. The existence of glucosuria without hyperglycemia indicates proximal tubular damage. Lysozymuria, an increase of the enzymatic protein lysozyme in urine, occurs if the serum level is elevated above the normal renal threshold (45 mg/mL) or when renal tubular function is impaired.[83] The normal urinary lysozyme level is less than 1.9 mg/mL, and a level greater than 5 mg/mL is regarded as evidence for significant renal tubular damage. Elevated serum levels of lysozyme may be a consequence of renal failure as well as a marker for it. Because white blood cells have a high concentration of lysozyme, urinary tract infections may also lead to elevated serum levels.

The BUN and serum creatinine levels offer rapid but inexact estimates of creatinine clearance. Acute elevations of BUN and serum creatinine levels occur in approximately 5% of all hospital admissions and in up to 20% of intensive care patients.[16] The incidence increases directly with the severity of trauma and the degree of injury or disease. The incidence and severity of ARF usually is greater when preoperative serum creatinine level is greater than 2 mg/dL[4]; however, an isolated serum creatinine measurement is an unreliable indicator of GFR when renal function is changing. There is an inverse logarithmic relationship between GFR and serum creatinine concentration (Fig. 37-7). Decreasing the rate by one half results in twice the serum creatinine level. For example,

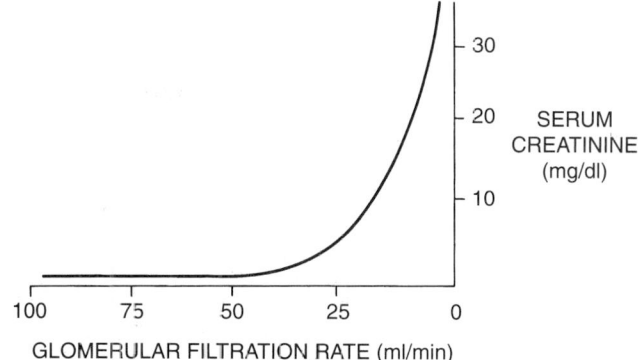

Figure 37–7 The inverse logarithmic relationship between serum creatinine concentration (*y* axis) and glomerular filtration rate (*x* axis). Notice that the serum creatinine level is not markedly increased until there is a reduction in glomerular filtration rate to about one fourth of normal (120 to 30 mL/min).

a patient with a preoperative serum creatinine level of 0.6 mg/dL whose filtration rate was reduced by one half (e.g., after a large preoperative contrast dye load) would have a serum creatinine level of 1.2 mg/dL, still in the normal range. A single serum creatinine measurement is not a very sensitive test for preoperative renal function reserve. However, it is relatively specific and useful in considering significant renal disease; it would be rare for someone who is not emaciated to have a creatinine level of 1.5 mg/dL and to have a creatinine clearance rate of less than 40 mL/min. The measurement of creatinine clearance may constitute the best overall indicator of GFR, although this index also has limitations. In one study, more than one half of 131 critically ill patients had normal values for urine output, BUN, and serum creatinine but had reduced creatinine clearance. Creatinine clearance was the best predictor of mortality among these patients compared with the other measures of renal function.[84] Although the serum creatinine level may be a more reliable measure of glomerular function than the BUN level, the simultaneous determination of BUN and serum creatinine levels offers a more complete evaluation of renal function than either determination alone. Ordinarily, the BUN-to-creatinine ratio is approximately 10, and if the BUN level is approximately 10 times as great as the serum creatinine level, the clinician may conclude that the measurements are probably correct. Conversely, if the ratio deviates significantly from 10, the clinician should consider the nonrenal factors influencing the BUN level or serum creatinine level, or both. All three measurements (i.e., BUN, serum creatinine level, and creatinine clearance) require careful interpretation.

DIRECT AND INDIRECT MONITORS OF RENAL FUNCTION

Means for direct, on-line evaluation of renal function are limited. We can monitor indirectly, however, the several factors that may contribute to the failure of compensatory mechanisms supporting renal function perioperatively. Among obstructive causes that may initiate ARF, an occluded or kinked urinary catheter can cause perioperative oliguria and must be eliminated as a source of obstruction. Toxic causes precipitated by antibiotics (e.g., aminoglycosides, amphotericin B) and radiocontrast agents also may be responsible for the development of ARF. For example, with aminoglycosides, nephrotoxicity is poorly correlated with kidney tissue or plasma levels of the drug but is markedly augmented by concomitant volume depletion or liver cirrhosis.[15] Similarly, ARF loosely correlates with the amount of radiocontrast material injected unless the patient has preexisting diabetic nephropathy or low cardiac output syndrome. The vigilance of the anesthesiologist is the first monitor required for preserving renal function.

Unlike the nephrologist, who can evaluate a patient's renal function under stable conditions over long periods, an anesthesiologist caring for hemodynamically unstable patients in the operating room is unable to use standard tests of renal function, such as creatinine clearance. To maintain the normal excretory functions of the kidney (i.e., filtration, reabsorption, and secretion), adequate perfusion is essential. The anesthesiologist often relies on indirect variables, such as urine volume, to assess renal perfusion. Unfortunately, urine output may not reliably reflect glomerular filtration and renal function under intraoperative conditions. Although not practical, monitoring renal perfusion directly would be ideal. Instead, we use monitors to ensure adequate intravascular volume (i.e., preload) and adequate cardiac performance or systemic perfusion as an indirect means to maintain normal renal function conditions. Serum chemistries and urinary indices may enable the assessment of adequate distribution of cardiac output to the kidneys themselves. Ultimately, however, only direct assessment of renal blood flow (and its regional distribution) can tell us whether a kidney is adequately perfused. Evidence of local renal tissue metabolism ensures that oxygen use is adequate. The combination of blood flow (i.e., oxygen delivery) and oxygen use should reflect normal function (Table 37-3).

Intravascular Volume

Central Venous Pressure versus Pulmonary Capillary Wedge Pressure

Monitoring techniques to ensure adequate intravascular volume should be selected after consideration of the physiologic condition of the patient in each situation

Table 37-3 Direct and indirect monitors of renal function

Preload
Ventricular function
Distribution of cardiac output to the kidneys
Intrarenal blood flow distribution
Regional renal utilization of substrate and oxygen delivery

(see Chapter 32). Epidemiologic studies have shown that renal failure commonly develops when dehydration acts in synergy with other chronic conditions. Diabetes mellitus and volume depletion together, for example, increase the chance of developing ARF by 100-fold.[15] Monitoring central venous pressure to assess adequate preload is contingent on normal left and right ventricular function, normal pulmonary vascular resistance, and normal mitral, pulmonary, and tricuspid valve function. Monitoring pulmonary artery pressure or pulmonary capillary wedge pressure to assess preload assumes normal left ventricular compliance, normal mitral valve function, and normal airway pressure.

Left Atrial Pressure

Directly measuring left atrial pressure may offer insights into the kidney pressure-flow relationship because left atrial hypotension has been shown to be a powerful stimulus for renal vasoconstriction.[85] Despite similar reductions in cardiac output and arterial blood pressure, renal blood flow appears to decrease much less during experimental conditions of cardiogenic shock, in which left atrial pressures are increased, compared with conditions of hemorrhagic shock, in which left atrial pressures are decreased.[85] It is postulated that when a decrease in cardiac output is accompanied by left atrial hypotension, reduction in systemic arterial pressure is followed by the normal response of renal vasoconstriction. The left atrial receptors are connected to the renal circulation by atrial natriuretic peptide, a hormone secreted by the cardiac atria in response to intravascular volume expansion.[86] Atrial natriuretic hormone acts on the arterial and venous systems, the adrenals, and the kidneys to reduce intravascular volume and decrease blood pressure.[34] Within the kidney, the hormone increases hydraulic pressure in the glomerular capillaries through afferent arteriolar dilation and efferent arteriolar vasoconstriction. Atrial natriuretic peptide reduces blood pressure by relaxing smooth muscle and reducing sympathetic vascular stimulation. It also inhibits renin and aldosterone secretion, producing renal vasodilation, natriuresis, and diuresis.[34]

Left Ventricular End-Diastolic Area

Although the most direct way to clinically monitor for adequate intravascular volume or preload may be during surgery by assessment of the left ventricular end-diastolic area with echocardiography,[87,88] the most practical method is by obtaining preoperative history and physical examination and by maintaining changes in systemic blood pressure to changing conditions. An awake patient may be observed for orthostatic changes in blood pressure, whereas an anesthetized patient may be observed for paradoxical arterial pulse changes with positive-pressure inspiration.[89] The clinician must decide which modality can most accurately reflect intravascular volume for a patient in a particular situation.

Cardiopulmonary Function

The next logical step in the algorithm of renal function monitoring is the assessment of adequate cardiac function through determination of systemic perfusion, pulse oximetry, acid-base assessment, cardiac output monitoring, or left ventricular fractional area of change as a surrogate for ejection fraction[90] (see Chapters 18 and 32).

Systemic Perfusion and Acid-Base Balance

Severe arterial hypoxemia to a partial pressure of arterial oxygen (PaO_2) value of less than 40 mm Hg is associated with decreased renal blood flow and renal vasoconstriction.[91,92] There is no consensus on the mechanism that underlies the antidiuresis response to hypoxia. It appears that systemic hypoxia can produce antidiuresis and antinatriuresis independent of renal nerve innervation.[93] Capnometry may be a useful monitor because hypercarbia has been associated with decreased renal blood flow in patients requiring mechanical ventilation.[94]

Cardiac Output

The electrocardiogram is essential to detect the depolarization-repolarization changes consistent with the electrolyte abnormalities of renal dysfunction and to monitor for normal rate and rhythm. The synchronized atrial kick preceding ventricular contraction may contribute significantly to cardiac output in the patient with a noncompliant left ventricle. The clinician can assess cardiac function by using the thermodilution technique for measuring cardiac output with the pulmonary artery catheter and can assess global and regional myocardial function with echocardiography.

Perfusion Pressure

Stone and Stahl[95] studied the effect of renal hemorrhage in otherwise healthy patients and concluded that a decrease in mean perfusion pressure from 80 to 60 mm Hg reduced renal blood flow about 30% without an autoregulatory response of the renal vasculature. It has been suggested that renal blood flow decreases precipitously when mean blood pressure drops below 80 mm Hg. In a study by Yao and associates,[96] mean arterial pressure during cardiopulmonary bypass was maintained with vasoactive drugs at 80 to 100 mm Hg in one group of patients and at 50 to 60 mm Hg in another group during moderate hypothermic conditions. It was found that renal circulation was maintained as long as mean arterial pressure was maintained above 50 mm Hg. Other studies challenge evidence that demonstrates decreased perfusion pressure as a cause of renal failure.[97-99]

We evaluated the relationship between preoperative isolated systolic hypertension[10] and wide pulse pressure hypertension[11] (both markers of abnormal central aortic compliance) and postoperative renal failure. In these two separate, large, multicenter epidemiologic studies, it was determined that preexisting central aortic disease manifesting as systolic wide pulse pressure hypertension is associated with significant increase risk of postoperative renal dysfunction outcomes. In the first case, preexisting systolic hypertension predicted a 40% greater risk of renal dysfunction outcome, and in the latter case, wide pulse pressure predicted postoperative renal dysfunction as well (odds ratio = 2:37, 1.69-3.33, $P < .005$). Mean arterial pressure less than 40 mm Hg during cardiopulmonary bypass in patients with preoperative isolated systolic hypertension (>160 mm Hg) predisposed them to renal insufficiency or failure postoperatively. These observations underscore the importance of renal physiology during surgery and perhaps pressure management during cardiopulmonary bypass. The systolic component of blood pressure is determined by stroke volume and the rate of ventricular ejection, whereas the pulsatile component of blood pressure is governed by the relationships among stroke volume, ventricular ejection, viscoelastic properties of large arteries, and peripheral vascular resistance. The latter factors contribute to the effect of arterial wave reflection from the periphery back to the central conduit arteries. Pulse pressure is an index of the effects of large artery stiffness and the rate of pressure on propagation and reflection within the arterial tree. Early return of reflected arterial waves during late systolic rather than early diastolic (from increased propagation velocity in stiff vessels) increases systolic blood pressure (i.e., afterload) and decreases diastolic blood pressure (i.e., perfusion pressure). It is likely that perfusion pressure and risk of perioperative renal dysfunction are linked by the preexisting capacity of the vasculature to compensate for low pressure as it determines flow. Future studies need to stratify the risk of pressure management according to specific diseases (i.e., systolic hypertension and wide pulse pressure hypertension groups). We might not have assigned risk and renal dysfunction to perfusion pressure appropriately. Those with a predisposition to low flow due to abnormal central aortic compliance may represent patients who require higher pressure to maintain adequate flow compared with normotensive patients.

The decision to use any monitor should depend on the patient's functional cardiac reserve status, the extent of the proposed surgical insult, and the capabilities of the anesthesiologist, the perioperative team, and the hospital. Differentiation between hypovolemic hypotension and cardiogenic hypotension, for example, is critical to properly tailor management and prevent exacerbation of renal ischemia. The best way to prevent intraoperative renal ischemia is to maintain renal blood flow. Although maintaining adequate cardiac output is necessary for maintaining adequate renal blood flow, it may not guarantee adequate flow. Monitoring with invasive devices, such as pulmonary artery catheters, arterial cannulas, and transesophageal echocardiography, has never been demonstrated to reduce the incidence of ARF.

Distribution of Cardiac Output to the Kidneys

Although the kidneys constitute less than 0.5% of body mass, they receive 20% to 25% of the total cardiac output in the normal adult. The distribution of cardiac output to the kidneys may be influenced by a number of factors, including hypovolemia, activation of the sympathetic nervous system or the renin-angiotensin system, extrinsically administered vasopressors and vasodilators, and local neurohumoral factors.

The fraction of cardiac output perfusing the kidneys depends on the ratio of renal vascular resistance to systemic vascular resistance.[18] In general, the response to renal hypoperfusion involves three major regulatory mechanisms that support renal function: afferent arteriolar dilation increases the proportion of cardiac output that perfuses the kidney; efferent arteriolar resistance increases the filtration fraction; and hormonal and neural responses improve renal perfusion by increasing intravascular volume, thereby indirectly increasing cardiac output. The afferent arterioles react to reductions in perfusion pressure by relaxing their smooth muscle elements to decrease renal vascular resistance. This property represents a relaxation response or myogenic reflex to reduced transmural pressure across the arteriolar wall. The kidney also possesses a tubuloglomerular feedback system, which is designed to maintain the homeostasis of salt and water excretion. Decreased solute delivery to the macula densa in the cortical portion of the thick ascending loop of Henle results in relaxation of the juxtaposed afferent arteriolar smooth muscle cells, improving glomerular perfusion and filtration.

The kidney produces vasodilator prostaglandins to counteract the effects of systemic vasoconstrictor hormones such as angiotensin II.[100] In a state of low cardiac output when systemic blood pressure is preserved by the action of systemic vasopressors, renal blood flow is not depressed because the effect of the vasopressors is blunted within the kidney.

A selective increase in efferent arteriolar resistance decreases glomerular plasma flow, thereby preserving GFR. Glomerular filtration is augmented because capillary pressure upstream from the site of vasoconstriction tends to rise. This mechanism enables the kidney to offer high organ vascular resistance to contribute to the maintenance of systemic blood pressure without compromising its function of filtration. Studies using specific inhibitors of angiotensin II have shown that efferent arteriolar resistance largely results from the action of angiotensin II.[101] At low concentrations, norepinephrine has a vasoconstricting effect on efferent arterioles, indicating that the adrenergic system may also be important for maintaining the renal compensatory response.[102]

There is abundant evidence to support the notion that reductions in cardiac output are accompanied by the release of vasopressin and by increased activity of the sympathetic nervous system and the renin-angiotensin-aldosterone system. These regulatory mechanisms to preserve renal blood flow conserve salt and water. The control of blood delivery to the kidney, the fraction of plasma filtered, and the amount of volume returned to the systemic circulation are determined by regulatory mechanisms within the kidney that attempt to preserve filtration function during compromised circulation. These compensatory mechanisms, however, have limits. Excessive vasoconstrictive forces may eventually induce a decrease in filtration function. This shift from compensation to decompensation may be exacerbated by pharmacologic interventions. Oliguria is both a symptom of ARF and a consequence of the normal compensatory mechanisms to prevent it. Differentiating between the two is critical for outcome and therapeutic strategies.

Clinical investigators have expended considerable effort to evaluate laboratory tests of serum and urinary indices that attempt to differentiate the cause of oliguric states, to predict outcome, and to direct therapy for the prevention of ARF. Unfortunately, none of the tests is sensitive or specific enough to predict which patients will or will not respond to therapy. Among the tests commonly obtained are urine volume, urine specific gravity, urine osmolality, serum creatinine level, serum GFR level, urine-to-plasma creatinine ratio, urine-to-plasma urea ratio, urine sodium level, fractional excretion of sodium, free rate clearance, and creatinine clearance.

Urine Volume

Monitoring urinary output as a sign of the adequacy of renal perfusion is easy and is based on the assumption that patients with diminished renal perfusion excrete a low volume of concentrated urine. Urinary flow rate is, however, an indirect parameter of renal function because many nonrenal factors may directly and profoundly affect urine output. Oliguria (anuria) during hypotensive anesthesia on one hand and polyuria on the other demonstrate that low urine output does not specifically reflect inadequate renal perfusion and that normal urine output does not guarantee a normally functioning kidney. The presence of urine flow (regardless of the amount) indicates that there is blood flow to the kidney, because without perfusion, glomerular filtration and generation of urine cease. The level of nitrogenous wastes in the blood depends on systemic production and renal clearance. Renal clearance depends on renal blood flow and glomerular filtration. The kidney concentrates the ultrafiltrate so that at maximal concentration, 400 to 500 mL of urine is required to clear the daily obligatory nitrogenous wastes.[103] Traditionally, inadequate urinary volume, or oliguria, is defined as urinary output of less than 0.5 mL/kg/hr. Multiple studies, however, have shown no correlation between urine volume and histologic evidence of acute tubular necrosis, GFR, creatinine clearance, or changes from preoperative to postoperative levels of BUN and creatinine levels in patients with burn injury,[104] trauma,[105,106] or shock status or in those undergoing cardiovascular surgery.[107-109] Moreover, measurement of mean and lowest hourly urinary output during aortic vascular surgery has not been predictive of postoperative renal insufficiency.[107]

Oliguria may reflect a variety of factors independent of GFR, and a normal hourly urine output does not rule out renal failure. Among these factors is tubular excretion of solute and water, which is determined by local and systemic levels of renin, aldosterone, and ADH. In the operating room, patients are often hemodynamically unstable; decreased blood volume or cardiac output, fluctuating hormone levels (e.g., aldosterone, renin, ADH), nervous system reflexes, and increased catecholamine concentrations, added to the effects of general anesthesia, can alter GFR. The data do not support oliguria as a reliable sign of pending renal dysfunction.[103-109]

Urine Indices and Serum Chemistries

Urine Specific Gravity

The specific gravity of urine is also easy to measure. In this test, the mass of 1 mL of urine is compared with the mass of 1 mL of distilled water to reflect renal concentrating ability. With poor perfusion or prerenal azotemia, urine specific gravity is 1.030, reflecting the kidney's conservation of sodium and water. With acute tubular necrosis, the loss of concentrating ability moves urine specific gravity toward 1.010. Because urine specific gravity is a measure of mass and the renal concentrating system responds to osmolality,[110,111] many substances and conditions can change the specific gravity of urine. The factors that make the test nonspecific appear in Table 37-4. For example, in patients of advanced age, distal renal tubular function is often impaired, whereas proximal tubular function is spared. The ability of the kidneys to concentrate urine after water deprivation is impaired in these patients, making urine specific gravity an unreliable test. Because the pathophysiology of acute tubular necrosis often reveals significant heterogeneity of tubular damage and the value of urine specific gravity depends on the extent of that damage, the test is unreliable unless the significance of the tubular damage has previously been assessed.

Urine Osmolality

Osmolality is a measure of the number of osmotically active particles in solution in the solvent phase. It is one of the major forces that move fluid throughout the body, especially in the kidney. Theoretically, urine osmolality is physiologically superior to urine specific gravity as a test of renal function; however, the same substances and conditions that render urine specific gravity a nonspecific test can also affect the reliability of urine osmolality (see Table 37-4). Since the late 1940s, physicians have recognized the inability of the kidneys to produce concentrated urine during acute tubular necrosis and have used as a guideline urine osmolality of greater than 500 mOsm/kg H_2O to identify prerenal azotemia and urine osmolality of less than 350 mOsm/kg H_2O to indicate acute tubular necrosis. A defective urinary concentrating mechanism tends to be one of the most consistent and lasting tubular defects of ARF.

The sensitivity and specificity of urine osmolality as a test for predicting or distinguishing acute tubular necrosis from prerenal azotemia are clinically inadequate.[109,112-117] With values greater than 500 mOsm, the positive predictive value for diagnosing prerenal azotemia ranges from 60% to 100%. With a value less than 350 mOsm, the positive predictive value for diagnosing acute tubular necrosis ranges from 69% to 95%. The measure of urine osmolality appears to be helpful at extreme values but is unfortunately a nonspecific test in most cases.

Serum Creatinine and Blood Urea Nitrogen

The relationship between serum creatinine or BUN levels and GFR seems to make the determination of either one an ideal indicator of filtration rate. However, elevations of serum creatinine and BUN levels are late signs of renal dysfunction because the GFR must often be reduced as much as 75% before elevations reach abnormal levels,[118] and many nonrenal variables affect serum creatinine and BUN levels (Table 37-5). A product of protein metabolism, BUN level is increased by high protein intake, blood in the gastrointestinal tract, and accelerated catabolism (e.g., in traumatized or septic patients). The normal range is 8 to 20 mg/dL. Because urea is synthesized in the liver, hepatic dysfunction decreases urea production and therefore BUN concentration. BUN concentration fails a key criterion as a reliable estimate of the GFR. Although urea is freely filtered at the glomerulus, it is reabsorbed to a large and variable extent. The reabsorption of urea is greater, approximately 60% of the filtered load, when urinary flow is low; only about 40% is reabsorbed when flow is high.

Creatinine, a product of skeletal muscle protein catabolism, is produced at a lower rate in elderly than in young adults and in women than in men. Consequently, serum creatinine levels may fail to accurately reflect the magnitude of nephron loss. Because creatinine production is proportional to muscle mass, many chronically ill, wasted, elderly patients have serum creatinine values in the normal range, despite reduced renal concentrating ability and GFR. Conversely, many critically ill patients at risk for developing ARF may have high metabolic rates because of hyperalimentation, sepsis, or post-traumatic states. Higher metabolic rates mean higher nitrogenous waste production requiring greater than average renal blood flow and urine flow rates to maintain normal serum creatinine concentration. In patients with ARF, edema may dilute serum creatinine concentrations. Because creatinine is excreted by glomerular filtration and tubular secretion, as the GFR decreases, the tubular secretion becomes a progressively more important fraction of creatinine excretion, such that creatinine clearance overestimates the GFR by 50% to 100% if the true GFR is less than 15 mL/min.[118,119] Postoperative serial serum creatinine

Table 37–4 Substances and conditions affecting urine specific gravity and urine osmolality
Proteins
Glucose
Mannitol
Dextran
Diuretics
Advanced age
Extremes of age
X-ray contrast media
Antibiotics (e.g., carbenicillin)
Hydrometer calibration
Detergents
Temperature
Hormonal imbalances

Table 37–5 Nonrenal variables affecting serum creatinine and blood urea nitrogen levels
Increased nitrogen absorption
Tissue breakdown
Body mass
Diet
Activity
Hepatic disease
Diabetic ketoacidosis
Large hematoma
Gastrointestinal bleeding
Drugs or steroids

measurements are predictive of renal dysfunction in only 33% of cases after noncardiac surgery[16] and are equally unreliable after cardiovascular surgery.[120] It was believed that combining BUN and serum creatinine levels would provide more reliable information than either alone. If ratios of BUN to serum creatinine exceeded 20:1, for example, dehydration was suspected. However, the same factors that render the individual tests nonspecific and insensitive remain true when their ratios are considered.

Urine and Plasma Creatinine Levels

The urine-to-plasma creatinine index was first introduced in 1950 by Bull and colleagues[121] as a method of evaluating patients with acute tubular necrosis. It was determined retrospectively that patients whose urine-to-plasma creatinine levels rose above 10 after having been below 10 were no longer at serious risk for "uncontrolled mineral and water loss." This index was introduced primarily as a prognostic aid and not as a diagnostic test.

The sensitivity and specificity of the urine-to-plasma creatinine index are unfortunately clinically unreliable for diagnosing acute tubular necrosis and prerenal azotemia.[122] Miller and coworkers[113] concluded that the index was not useful, except in extreme situations, because of significant overlap between groups. Espinel and Gregory[114] prospectively studied 87 patients (61 with acute tubular necrosis or prerenal azotemia) and concluded that the urine-to-plasma creatinine ratio might be a useful indicator of acute tubular necrosis if the ratio was less than 10 and that it might be an indicator of prerenal azotemia if the ratio was less than 40. However, a significant overlap in values was found for 33% of patients.

Urine and Plasma Urea Levels

In 1959, Perlmutter and colleagues[123] proposed that the ratio between urine and serum urea nitrogen levels could differentiate prerenal azotemia from acute tubular necrosis. These investigators thought that a ratio of greater than 14 was associated with transient oliguria and that a ratio of less than 10 was associated with acute tubular necrosis. In 1965, Eliahou and Bata[112] reported that the urine-to-blood urea ratio might not be useful for diagnosis in all cases. Subsequently, Chisholm and associatates[124] confirmed that the urine-to-plasma urea ratio was often misleading in the diagnosis of uremia.

Urea production is not constant and is affected by many nonrenal variables[125] (see Table 37-5). Variables include sudden increases or decreases in protein intake, states of increased protein catabolism (i.e., trauma, infections, hyperthermia, or steroid therapy), gastrointestinal bleeding, and liver dysfunction. Because urea levels can vary tremendously independent of renal function, it is not surprising that knowing the urine-to-plasma urea ratio does not make it possible to differentiate between prerenal azotemia and acute tubular necrosis.

Urinary Sodium

With decreasing perfusion, the normally functioning kidney conserves sodium and water. The factors affecting this phenomenon are numerous and include heterogenicity of nephrons, secretion of aldosterone, secretion of ADH, diuretic therapy, saline content of intravenous infusion solutions, sympathetic neural tone, and sodium-avid states (e.g., congestive heart failure, cirrhosis). It is traditionally accepted that a urinary sodium level of less than 20 mEq suggests prerenal azotemia and that a level of greater than 40 mEq indicates acute tubular necrosis.

The reported sensitivity and specificity of urinary sodium levels for diagnosis of acute tubular necrosis and prerenal azotemia suggest that the levels can be used for diagnosis of approximately one half of the patients with acute tubular necrosis.[109,113-115,121,126,127] Considering the complex physiology of sodium homeostasis, it is not surprising that levels of urinary sodium are unreliable indicators of prerenal azotemia or acute tubular necrosis. The test is nonspecific because a significant overlap exists between the diagnostic categories and because urinary sodium measurement tends to correlate more with volume and type of resuscitation fluid than with renal function.[106]

Fractional Excretion of Sodium

The fractional excretion of sodium was first described by Espinel.[126] It represents the fraction of sodium excreted of that filtered by the kidneys. Handa and Morrin[122] had previously described the renal failure ratio, which is also derived from the excreted fraction of filtered sodium. The only difference between the two is that in determining renal failure ratio, it is assumed that plasma sodium level is controlled within fairly narrow limits and is constant. The fractional excretion of sodium (FeNa) is calculated as follows:

$$FeNa = \frac{Excreted\ Na}{Filtered\ Na \times 100} = \frac{U_{Na}P_{Cr}}{(U_{Cr}P_{Na} \times 100)}$$

P_{Cr} is the plasma creatinine level, P_{Na} is the plasma sodium level, U_{Cr} is the urinary creatinine level, and U_{Na} is the urinary sodium level. All variables are easy to obtain.

At first investigators had reported that the fractional excretion of sodium clearly differentiated prerenal azotemia from acute tubular necrosis.[113-115,126] Subsequently, case reports demonstrated that the fractional excretion of sodium was a nonspecific indicator and was not as sensitive as initially believed.[126-130] Brown[128] suggested that the fractional excretion of sodium was diagnostic of acute tubular necrosis but was of little or no value for the early prediction of renal failure. Brosius and Lau[129] showed that early determinations of the fractional excretion of sodium were more likely to be misleading than later determinations, indicating that the measurement was unlikely to be helpful in the early diagnosis of acute tubular necrosis. Shin and colleagues[105] concluded that knowing the fractional excretion of sodium was useful only when oliguria was already present. A sodium excretion value of less than 1% compared with greater than 1% enables differentiation between prerenal azotemia and acute tubular necrosis in most cases. However, because this indicator is usually observed later in the course of renal disease than the changes in creatinine or free water clearance, the fractional excretion of sodium is less beneficial for predicting imminent renal failure.[131,132]

Free Water Clearance

Free water clearance is a measure of the kidney's ability to dilute or concentrate urine as necessary to maintain homeostasis. It is determined by the following equation:

$$C_{H_2O} = UV - (U_{Osm} \times UV / P_{Osm})$$

UV is urine volume, U_{Osm} is urinary osmolality, and P_{Osm} is plasma osmolality.

After an initial retrospective analysis, Jones and Weil[133] prospectively assessed the sensitivity of free water clearance and concluded that serial measurements predicted the patients who would experience progressive renal dysfunction.[109] In a prospective study, however, Rosenberg and coworkers[106] found no significant correlation between renal function and free water clearance in 69 patients with trauma or sepsis. After studying 38 patients in an intensive care unit, Baek and associates[134] concluded that the diagnosis of ARF was evident 1 to 3 days sooner with free water clearance than with other clinical and laboratory diagnostic criteria (creatinine clearance was not measured). These investigators recommended that sequential measurements of free water clearance could be used as an early indicator of pending ARF. A free water clearance rate of −15 to +15 mL/hr is a sign of incipient renal dysfunction. The normal range for free water clearance is −25 to −20 mL/hr.

After retrospectively reviewing the records of 675 trauma victims, Shin and colleagues[135] concluded that free water clearance alone was not sufficient for the early detection of renal dysfunction. They suggested that the combination of free water clearance greater than 20 mL/hr and creatinine clearance less than 25 mL/min predicted a high-risk group. When they prospectively monitored free water clearance in patients after surgery,[105] they concluded that this measure was not as sensitive as creatinine clearance for predicting ARF in trauma patients. The same substances and conditions that decrease the usefulness of urine osmolality for indicating renal failure can similarly decrease the usefulness of free water clearance (see Table 37-4).[136]

Creatinine Clearance

Creatinine clearance measures the ability of the glomeruli to filter creatinine from the plasma and approximates the rate of glomerular filtration. Measurements of creatinine clearance are most useful to quantify renal reserve. Creatinine clearance often is estimated in the stable patient by use of the following equation:

$$GFR = (140 - Age) \, wt/72 \times Serum \, creatinine \, level$$

The weight (wt) is weight in kilograms. However, this estimate is subject to the same limitations as the measurement of serum creatinine. Precise measurements of creatinine clearance require collection of timed urine samples using the following formula:

$$GFR = UV/P$$

U is the urinary concentration of creatinine (mg/dL), V is the volume of urine (mL/min), and P is the plasma concentration (mg/dL).

When Shin and associates[135] retrospectively reviewed the records of 26 patients who had acute tubular necrosis, they concluded that the diagnosis was likely to be made in patients who had a creatinine clearance of less than 25 mL/min and a free water clearance of greater than 15 mL/hr. In a follow-up study of 40 trauma patients who underwent surgery, Shin and colleagues[105] concluded that creatinine clearance of less than 25 mL/min alone permitted the early detection of renal dysfunction in patients with the potential for development of renal failure and that free water clearance was not as sensitive.

The major limitation in the determination of creatinine clearance is the necessity of collecting urine accurately. Although reasonable correlation between 2-hour and 24-hour creatinine clearance (R = 0.85) has been reported for intensive care patients[137,138] (Fig. 37-8), it remains true that the longer the urine collection period, the more accurate is the calculation of creatinine clearance. Changing hydration of the patient invalidates short-term determinations of the GFR, as does failure to record urine volume accurately. The error in calculation of creatinine clearance can vary from 10% to 27%, depending on the accuracy of urine collection,[139] body weight, surface area, and normal day-to-day variations. Another significant drawback is that for the patient with ARF, a test that requires 24-hour urine collection is often impractical. Nevertheless, it appears that creatinine clearance is the most efficient test available to assess glomerular filtration.

Biochemical Markers of Renal Function

The kidney contains many different cell types, and the primary roles are glomerular filtration, tubular reabsorption and secretion, and concentration of metabolites. Although complex, the kidney may be able to respond to

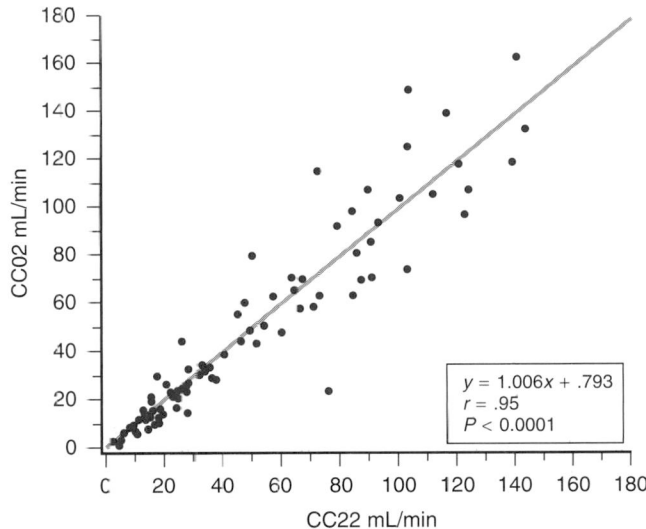

Figure 37–8 Correlation between the 2-hour creatinine clearance (CC02) and the 22-hour creatinine clearance (CC22). (Adapted from Sladen RN, Endo E, Harrison T: Two-hour versus 22-hour creatinine clearance in critically ill patients. Anesthesiology 67:1013, 1987.)

disease in only a limited number of ways at the cellular level. Noninvasive tests have been developed that reflect the morphologic, functional, and biochemical regional specialization.

NAG is a widely used urinary enzyme assay for the assessment of renal disease and the detection of nephrotoxicity. Unlike a number of unstable enzymes excreted into the urine, NAG remains suitable for clinical diagnosis of renal disease. Increased NAG activity detected in urine is a sensitive test for renal tubular damage.[140] Its molecular mass precludes filtration by the glomerulus, and it is neither absorbed nor secreted by the tubules. It is also the most active glycosidase found in the proximal tubule lysosomes. Any increase in urinary concentration of NAG may be considered a marker for tubular damage. The value of NAG as a diagnostic test is further enhanced by its presence in a number of isoenzyme forms. The relative amount of each isoenzyme varies at different stages of renal disease.

A number of analytical methods are available for the determination of urinary NAG, including fluorometric, colorimetric, spectrophotometric, and dipstick tests. Each of these methods is tedious and is associated with limitations that prevent widespread clinical adaptation. Low levels of NAG are excreted by normal individuals, and assay procedures must be sensitive enough to overcome the endogenous inhibitor urea.[141] Another factor to overcome is variation from urine collection that occurs over time. Factoring the enzyme activity with creatinine concentration over the same urine flow collection period is a reasonable approach for this problem.[142] In general, the sensitivity and reproducibility of the fluorometric method, when it is performed correctly, is excellent, but the equipment necessary is not commonly available in laboratories.

The colorimetric technique overcomes the limitations of the fluorometric technique by the incorporation of a calibrant for easy interlaboratory comparison and access in most clinical chemistry laboratories, with modification for use with spectrophotometric analysis.[143] The latest development is a dipstick method for detection of NAG in the urine.[144] The NAG strip incorporates a biochemical derivative that releases a blue-violet color on hydrolysis, and the test requires up to 30 minutes after the addition of reagents. However, problems can arise if the sample is contaminated with blood or bilirubin. Besides pigmented material in urine, a concentrated urine specimen that is high in urea also renders the test inaccurate.

Perhaps the most interesting discovery regarding urinary NAG for detection of renal disease is that there appears to be isoenzyme specificity for various types of pathology.[145] NAG is the most active lysosomal hydrolase and is normally found in tissues as two major forms: A and B. These major forms differ in their subunit composition. Traditionally, the main clinical interest in these isoenzymes had been their use in the detection of two autosomal recessive disorders, Tay-Sachs disease and Sandhoff disease. In 1970, Price and coworkers[146] reported that the B form increased in a urinary pattern of NAG after surgical trauma. Since that time, it has been appreciated that the relative amount of the B form

increased (i.e., the ratio of A to B forms decreased) compared with urine in the normal population. Automated methods for separation of NAG isoenzymes allow the pattern of excretion to be compared in various disease states (Table 37-6). Of interest to the anesthesiologist is that evidence suggests that after major surgery, the percentage of an intermediate form (I) increases in the urine.[147] Smaller increases in the I form were also observed in rejection of renal transplants. Rejection was more strongly associated with a decrease in the A/B ratio in a cohort of renal transplant patients. No change in the isoenzyme profile was found in stable transplant patients, whereas reversible rejection was characterized by an increase in the I form and a decrease in the relative amount of the A form present. When a patient did not respond to treatment, the I and the B forms were elevated, but levels of the A form decreased.[148]

Different nephrotoxic drugs or conditions appear to produce characteristic urinary isoenzyme profiles. For example, the B and I forms are elevated after administration of aminoglycosides. Total urinary and serum NAG activity also has been reported to increase in diabetic patients. Overall, NAG activity in the urine reflects the activity of the disease or severity of the damage. Serial monitoring is therefore most useful because trending is the most appropriate method to interpret the results. The NAG-to-creatinine ratio is a more sensitive and specific marker for renal tubular dysfunction. It is useful to express NAG as a ratio of urinary creatinine to minimize dilutional or concentration effects. The lack of sensitive, simple, inexpensive, and efficient methods is the limiting factor for widespread clinical use of NAG monitoring. Another urinary enzyme, clusterin, may prove to be more specific than NAG[149] for evaluating nephrotoxicity caused by aminoglycoside use while remaining equally sensitive.

Several other urinary constituents have been identified to detect cytotoxic and abnormal processes in specific regions of the kidney (Table 37-7). α-Glutathione S-transferase is found principally in the proximal convoluted tubules, and π-glutathione S-transferase is found principally in the distal convoluted tubule. β_2-Microglobulin is a subunit of the class I antigen of the

Table 37–6 Variation of urinary *N*-Acetyl-β-D-Glucosaminidase

Condition	Concentration of Isoenzyme Form		
	A	I	B
Severe renal damage	↓	↑	↑
Major surgery	↓	—	↑
Reversible renal transplant rejection	↓	↑	—
Nonreversible renal transplant rejection	↓	↑	↑
Aminoglycoside administration	—	↑	↑

↑, increased; ↓, decreased; —, no change.
From Campbell JAH, Conigall AV, Guy A, et al: Immunohistologic localization of alpha, mu, and pi class glutathione S-transferases in human tissue. Cancer 67:1608-1613, 1991.

Table 37–7 Urinary constituents used to measure renal function

Glomerular permeability and selectivity	Albumin
	Transferrin
	Aspartate aminotransferase
	Immunoglobulin G
Tubular protein uptake	β_2-Microglobulin
	Retinol binding protein
	Ribonuclease
Proximal tubular brush border	Alanine aminopeptidase
	γ-Glutamyl transpeptidase
Proximal tubule	N-Acetyl-β-D-glucosaminidase
	α-Glutathione S-transferase
Thick ascending limb	Tamm-Horsfall protein
Distal tubule	π-Glutathione S-transferase

From Baines AD: Strategies and criteria for developing new urinalysis tests. Kidney Int Suppl 47:S137-S141, 1994.

major histocompatibility complex and is structurally homologous to immunoglobulins.[150] Its mass is 11,600 daltons, it is freely filtered from plasma by the renal glomerulus, and more than 99.9% is reabsorbed in the proximal tubule. β_2-Microglobulin is measured by radioimmunoassay and immunodiffusion techniques.[151] Its secretion in urine is a sensitive indicator of tubular damage or disease. Limitations to its use include its unstable nature in urine of pH 5.5 or below, thereby precluding its use for patients with concomitant urinary tract infection or pyuria. Its degradation by proteolysis is affected by temperature, and its measurement requires a sophisticated laboratory that precludes widespread clinical use. α_1-Microglobulin is filtered at the glomerulus and is 95% reabsorbed at the proximal tubule, thereby indicating proximal tubular dysfunction when present in the urine.[152-154] Alanine aminopeptidase excretion has been identified as a specific marker for proximal tubular brush border dysfunction, as has γ-glutamyl transpeptidase excretion. Plasma and urinary cytokines, such as interleukin-8, interleukin-10, interleukin-1 receptor antagonist, and tissue necrosis factor soluble receptor-2, have been shown to correlate with proximal tubular dysfunction.[152] In general, enhanced excretion of biochemical markers, tubular enzymes, or antigens may be the consequence of an exfoliated damaged tubular cell, an increased turnover of tubular cells, or some other metabolic disturbance. The biologic variability of the sensitive analytes in response to physiologic stress is large compared with anticipated changes observed in early disease. The signals of early, irreversible disease may not always be distinguished from the noise of biologic variability, and use of these markers should be applied with appropriate caution.

Renal Blood Flow

Normally, the kidneys receive 1000 to 1250 mL/min of blood in the average adult. This amount far exceeds that needed to provide the kidney's intrinsic oxygen requirement but ensures optimal clearance of all wastes and drugs.

Essentially, all blood passes through glomeruli, and about 10% of renal blood flow is filtered (i.e., GFR of 125 mL/min in the normal adult). The basal normal blood flow is 3 to 5 mL/min/g of tissue, greater than in most other organs (i.e., seven to eight times as much as basal coronary blood flow and 400 times as much as skeletal muscle blood flow). This average primarily reflects blood flow in the cortical glomeruli because perfusion to the inner medulla and papilla is only about one tenth of total flow.

The vascular structure of the renal cortex is complex, and intracortical blood flow may not be evenly distributed[155] (Fig. 37-9). The renal artery enters the kidney at the hilum, where it divides into five interlobar arteries, each an end artery. At the junction of the renal medulla and cortex, the interlobar branches divide into arcuate arteries, which course at right angles to the interlobar arteries. The interlobular arteries arise at right angles to the arcuate arteries and penetrate through the renal cortex. The afferent arterioles, which arise from the interlobular arteries, divide within the cortical tissue to form the glomerular capillary network. The capillaries then reunite to form the efferent arterioles. The subsequent course of the efferent arterioles depends on whether they are located superficially in the cortex or are situated in the juxtamedullary cortex. Superficial efferent arterioles feed a plexus of peritubular venous capillary vessels. These vessels supply the proximal and distal tubules and portions of the loops of Henle and the collecting ducts before joining the interlobular veins and returning to the inferior vena cava through the arcuate, interlobar, and renal veins. Juxtamedullary efferent arterioles also supply the venous capillary network and give rise to the vasa recta, small-diameter vessels that penetrate deep into the medulla. These vessels provide most of the oxygen supply to the loop of Henle and join together to form the arcuate veins. The juxtaglomerular apparatus is between the afferent and efferent arterioles and the macula densa, a specialized group of cells in the distal convoluted tubule.

Because the renal cortex contains most of the glomeruli and depends on oxidative metabolism for energy, ischemic hypoxia injures the renal cortical structures, particularly the pars recta of the proximal tubules. As ischemia persists, the supply of glucose and substrates continues to decrease; glycogen is consumed, and the medulla, which depends to a greater extent on glycolysis for its energy sources, becomes more adversely affected. Interruption of blood flow to kidneys for more than 30 to 60 minutes results in ARF and irreversible cell damage. Early cell changes are reversible, such as the swelling of cell organelles, especially the mitochondria. As ischemia progresses, lack of adenosine triphosphate interferes with the sodium pump mechanism, water and sodium accumulate in the endoplasmic reticulum of tubular cells, and the cells begin to swell. In irreversible ARF, the several pathologic changes occur. Swelling of tubular epithelial cells leads to formation of bullae, which protrude into the tubular lumen distal to the cell; necrosis of tubular cells results in abnormal membrane permeability; structural changes in the glomerular epithelium may decrease glomerular filtration; and constriction of intrarenal arteries and arterioles may further reduce glomerular blood flow.

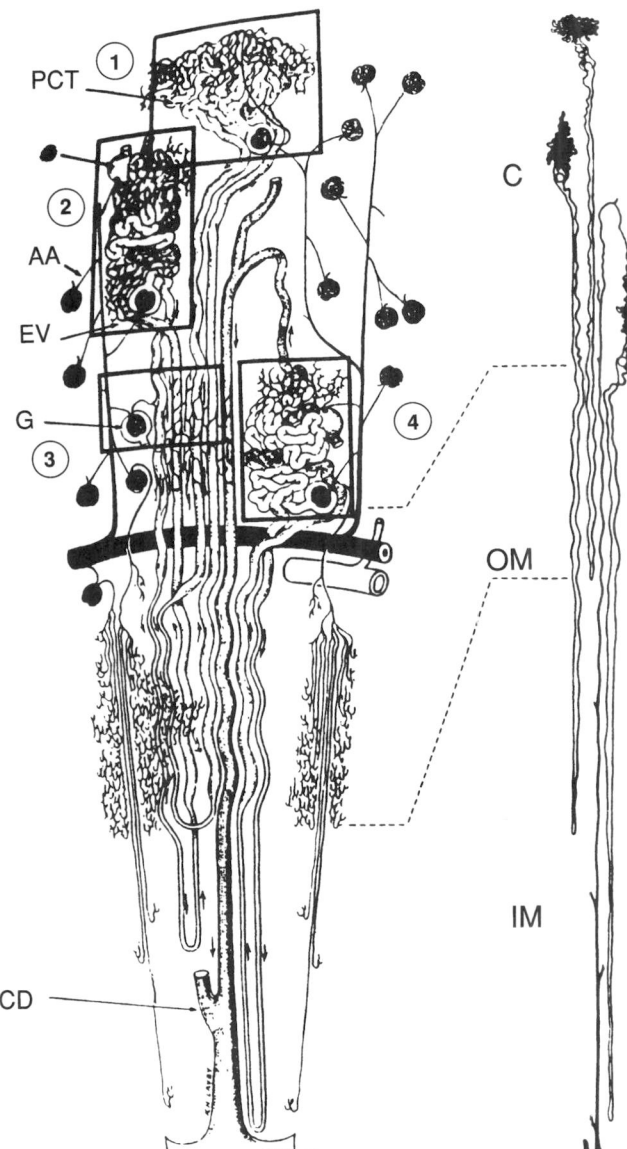

Figure 37–9 Diagram demonstrating the complex vascular and tubular organization of the kidney. The pattern of glomeruli (G) arising from afferent arterioles (AA) is demonstrated in the left-hand portion of the figure. Proximal convoluted tubules (PCT) are perfused by a peritubular capillary network derived from efferent vessels (EV). Loops of Henle are grouped with collecting ducts (CD). Only thin limbs of Henle extend with collecting ducts to the papillary tip. These are accompanied by vasa recta extending from the cores of the vascular bundles. C, cortex; OM, outer medulla; IM, inner medulla. (From Beeuwkes R, Bonventre JV: Tubular organization and vascular tubular relations in the dog kidney. Am J Physiol 229:695-713, 1975.)

Onset of tubular damage usually occurs within 25 minutes of ischemia as the microvilli of the proximal tubular cell brush borders begin to change. Within an hour, they slough off into the tubular lumen, and membrane bullae protrude into the straight portion of the proximal tubule. After a few hours, intratubular pressure rises, and tubular fluid backflows passively. Within 24 hours, obstructing casts appear in the distal tubular lumen. Even if renal blood flow is completely restored after 60 to 120 minutes of ischemia, the GFR may not immediately improve.[64]

In ischemia-induced ARF, lesions are unevenly distributed among nephrons, probably reflecting variability in blood flow. In nephrotoxin-induced failure, the necrosis of proximal tubular cells obstructs the tubular lumen with castlike material, and lesions are more evenly distributed among all nephrons.[156] After restoration of blood flow, intrarenal vascular resistance is high because of cell swelling and ischemic damage, and flow is as much as 50% below control values.[64] Renal hypoperfusion in the setting of a toxic insult may act in synergy to increase the risk of ARF. As blood flow becomes inadequate to support glomerular filtration, urine flow ceases, and toxic substances accumulate in the urine and renal parenchyma. Other factors contributing to increase the risk of renal failure include the interference of certain drugs (e.g., nonsteroidal anti-inflammatory drugs) with autoregulation and preservation of blood flow to strategic regions of the kidney, drug-induced membrane damage, or mitochondrial uncoupling, causing an insufficient use of oxygen. Toxic substances (e.g., aminoglycosides) and oxygen deprivation because of low blood flow produce depletion of adenosine triphosphate.

Distribution

Renal function reflects and is reflected by regional nephron heterogenicity and changes in regional renal blood flow. The vascular pattern of the kidney is complex, and the distribution of renal blood flow is nonhomogeneous (see Fig. 37-9). In the clinical setting of hypotension, the kidney appears to have a distinct susceptibility to injury. The reason for this susceptibility is not readily apparent, because renal blood flow is normally high and oxygen supply exceeds by far the requirements for oxygen use. This overall balance, however, may conceal regional hypoxia, predominantly in the outer medulla.

The interest in renal blood flow as a predictor of renal function was first stimulated in 1947, when Trueta and associates[157] introduced the concept of cortical ischemia and attributed the pathogenesis of ARF to increased blood flow through the medulla. Supporting evidence for this view has since been offered by many investigators who measured renal blood flow distribution with various methods.[158-161] Monitoring regional renal blood flow patterns may help us understand the physiology of renal salt and water excretion and the comparative pharmacologic effects on the so-called redistribution of blood flow within the cortex. Perhaps nephrons in the outer cortex are "salt losers," and those in the inner cortex are "salt retainers." If this is true, salt-retaining states should occur with the selective reduction of renal blood flow to the superficial cortex, and these states may or may not be accompanied by a rise in renal blood flow to the deep cortex.[30,161]

Because oliguria most commonly results from reduced cardiac output caused by hypovolemia, it is essential to understand how hypovolemia affects distribution of renal blood flow. Activation of the sympathetic nervous system and possibly the renin-angiotensin system reduces renal blood flow and the GFR. Despite well-maintained arterial blood pressure, blood flow may decrease to one third of its normal level. Constriction of afferent arterioles becomes sufficient to reduce the hydrostatic pressure in glomerular capillaries to levels inadequate for maintenance of normal filtration. Oliguria is initially caused by a decrease in filtration rate from reduced renal blood flow. This condition occurs before the metabolic function of the kidney itself becomes inadequate. As renal blood flow continues to decrease, arteriolar vasoconstriction leads to ischemia and morphologic damage.

Renal arteriographic and xenon washout studies in patients with ARF have shown selected, profound reduction in renal blood flow.[160] Arteriography revealed severe attenuation of the intrarenal arterial tree, inability to visualize cortical vessels, absence of a normal cortical nephrogram, and striking reduction in the velocity of contrast dye as it passed through the kidney. These same patients had no bleeding from the cortex during open renal biopsy. The xenon washout studies also show that the usual rapid transit of xenon through the cortex (indicating cortical perfusion) in the normal kidney is absent in acute oliguria. Renal cortical perfusion at one third of its normal level, involving constriction of the afferent arterioles, is a condition that is more than sufficient to stop renal functioning.

Assessment

The understanding that distribution of renal blood flow is nonhomogeneous, the recognition of nephron structure and functional heterogenicity, and the suggestion that changes in the zonal distribution of renal blood flow affect renal salt and water homeostasis have led investigators to focus on developing new techniques to measure intrarenal blood flow.[161] Methods to measure distribution of renal blood flow in humans include the clearance of para-aminohippurate, indicator dilution, renocortical tissue Po_2, radiolabeled tracers, Doppler ultrasonography, and external gas-washout techniques. The risks and limitations associated with these techniques limit their usefulness.

Any nontoxic substance cleared by the kidney and not metabolized may be used to measure renal blood flow by application of the Fick principle, whereby renal plasma flow is calculated as follows:

$$RPF = UV/(A - RV)$$

U is urinary concentration, V is urine flow rate, A is arterial plasma concentration, and RV is renal venous plasma concentration. Renal blood flow (RBF) is then calculated from the following formula:

$$RBF = RPF/(1 - Hematocrit)$$

The volume of plasma from which the kidney can extract and excrete a specific substance in a given time is the renal clearance of the substance. If a substance is completely eliminated from the plasma in one pass through the renal circulation, is filtered at the glomerulus, is not synthesized or destroyed, and is physiologically inert, it would be ideal for measuring renal plasma flow. Para-aminohippurate is a substance that almost meets these criteria.

The practical advantage of measuring the extraction of para-aminohippurate is that its renal extraction is approximately 90% in humans after one passage. Measurement of renal blood flow is based on the assumption that cortical extraction is 100% and that extraction in the medulla is 0%; therefore, it has been assumed that the nonextracted fraction (10%) should reflect the fraction of blood flowing through the medulla. However, experimental evidence shows that cortical extraction is not 100%,[162] casting doubt on the accuracy of intrarenal blood flow assessment with extraction techniques. Other limitations of the extraction technique include the requirement for a high rate of urine flow, a steady state for 15 to 30 minutes, and the sampling of systemic arterial and renal venous blood.

Indocyanine green, which is bound to albumin in plasma, has been used in the indicator dilution method with densitometry. The indicator dilution method necessitates catheterization of a renal artery and vein. Although attempts have been made to measure renocortical (fast) and medullar (slow) blood flows separately from dye dilution curves, no convincing results have been produced.[163] Measurement of renal blood flow by a continuous thermodilution technique, which requires renal venous cannulation and continuous injection of normal saline, has been proposed.[164] Measurements have correlated with calculated renal blood flows derived from clearance techniques in patients after cardiac catheterization; however, only total renal blood flow is measured with the thermodilution technique.

Tissue oxygen pressure is measured with a multiwire surface Po_2 electrode and temperature probe. This polarographic Clark-type electrode has multiple platinum microelectrodes arranged in an array in the center of the tissue contact area, with a polarographic silver anode positioned at its circumference. The probe is placed directly on the renal cortex and measures changes in local tissue Po_2, which is an indirect indicator of renal surface perfusion.[165-167] However, this device measures only outer cortical renal blood flow changes. Because ischemic insults to the kidney are associated with a marked decrease in blood flow to the outer cortex, a redistribution of blood flow to the juxtamedullary glomeruli in the inner cortex and medulla is presumed.

External krypton 85 and xenon 133 clearance techniques estimate local blood flow per gram of tissue from local gas clearance.[168] The gas-washout technique requires selective catheterization of the renal artery and is usually performed in conjunction with arteriography. The renal artery also may be punctured intraoperatively for injection. After intra-arterial injection, the gas diffuses rapidly into the renal tissue, theoretically equilibrating in tissue and blood. The renal washout curve is then assessed by external counting (Fig. 37-10). The reliability of washout methods has been questioned, and absolute flow rates cannot be determined with this method. In anuric subjects, various causes for unreliability of the method may be suspected. For example, the disappearance rate of the gas decreases when kidney volume increases, and kidney volume typically increases during ARF. The partition coefficient of 133 Xe may be less than 1.0 when the water content of the kidney is

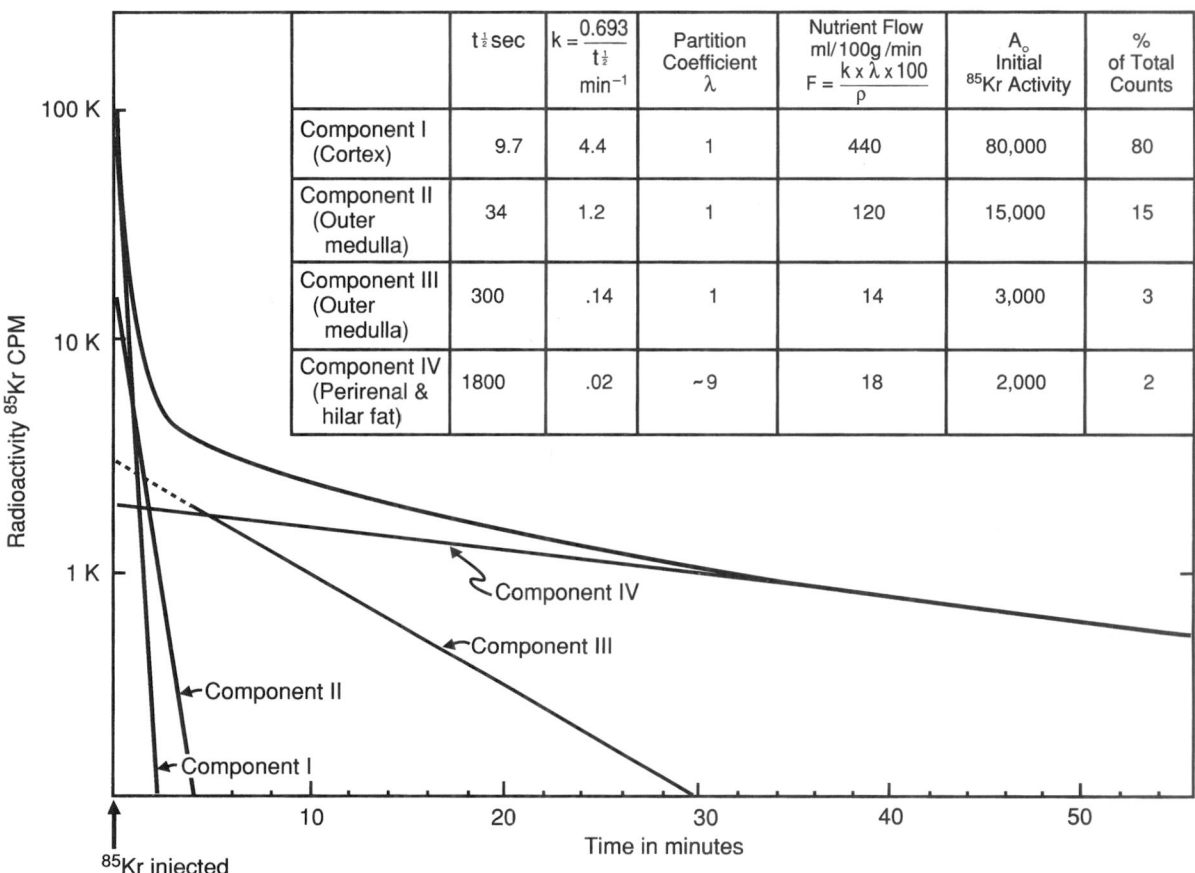

	$t\frac{1}{2}$ sec	$k = \dfrac{0.693}{t\frac{1}{2}}$ min^{-1}	Partition Coefficient λ	Nutrient Flow ml/100g /min $F = \dfrac{k \times \lambda \times 100}{\rho}$	A_o Initial ^{85}Kr Activity	% of Total Counts
Component I (Cortex)	9.7	4.4	1	440	80,000	80
Component II (Outer medulla)	34	1.2	1	120	15,000	15
Component III (Outer medulla)	300	.14	1	14	3,000	3
Component IV (Perirenal & hilar fat)	1800	.02	~9	18	2,000	2

Figure 37–10 Analysis of an externally monitored radioactive krypton washout curve for the kidney in a dog. Notice the logarithmic vertical scale. The rapid component (I) represents cortical blood flow. Half-times for each component together with estimated flow rates and compartment sizes are shown in the table above the plotted curves. (From Thorburn GD, Kopald HH, Herd A, et al: Intrarenal distribution of nutrient blood flow determined by krypton 85 in the unanesthetized dog. Circ Res 13:290, 1963.)

increased, as in ARF. If equilibrium of gas between tissue and capillaries is not achieved, actual flow rates may be underestimated. Hemodynamics must remain constant during washout curve recordings. The analysis is further complicated by the problem of resolving "external" summation curves into appropriate components representing flow through anatomic regions of the kidney. Theoretically, the desaturation curve after rapid injection of the radioactive isotope (recorded with a gamma counter placed over the kidney) is a summation of different desaturation curves. Each of the component curves represents a different region of the kidney, allowing flow rate per gram of tissue and relative volume of each region to be calculated.[169] What remains to be shown, however, is whether these calculated components really correspond to well-defined anatomic regions in the kidney. Little evidence supports such a conclusion beyond agreement that the first rapid washout component curve corresponds to flow in the renal cortex. The limitations of the gas-washout method should be kept in mind when clinical measurements are made. Another limitation of the gas-washout technique occurs because areas without perfusion cannot be demonstrated. The component representing an ischemic area is fused with components corresponding to regions that are normally perfused at

a slow rate. This procedure results in lack of detection of renal infarctions or segmental ischemic zones if the surrounding unaffected tissue is perfused normally.

Qualitative and semi-quantitative evaluation of renal perfusion can be obtained with a gamma camera recording of the transit of a radiopharmaceutical tracer through the kidney. Qualitative evaluation of renal perfusion consists of the visual assessment of the serial images and comparative assessment of the first transit of tracer from the aorta (or iliac-renal artery) to the kidney. Among the limitations associated with the renogram is movement of the radiopharmaceutical (injected intravenously as a bolus) before it reaches the kidney, necessitating that the pharmacokinetic model contain all the possible exchange compartments between the kidney and the plasma for accurate analysis of the tissue radioactivity curve. The presence of low urine flow rates, dilated pelvic caliceal cavities, or severely reduced renal function may also cause difficulties for test interpretation. In general, the information that can be derived from the renogram includes renal clearance (as a fraction of the radioisotope to blood volume) and blood flow of the two kidneys relative to each other.[170] Because the results obtained are comparative, lesions are revealed only when they have asymmetric distribution.

Duplex ultrasound has enabled evaluation of changes in renovascular resistance and intrarenal blood flow in patients. The technique is noninvasive and may be repeated as often as required. Typically, an interlobar artery is selected for evaluation for several reasons. The anatomic course and relationships of the vessel allow easy recognition on subsequent serial scans in the same patient; the vessel is large enough to assume laminar flow throughout its length; and the angle of the ultrasound beam can generally be minimized to assume maximum Doppler frequency shift. Renal vascular resistance can be assessed by the pulsatility index.[171] The lower the pulsatile index, the less resistance there is to flow. The value is derived by dividing the difference between systolic maximum height and diastolic minimum height of the waveform by its mean height (Fig. 37-11). Change in flow velocity can be assessed from a change in the mean frequency shift. The frequency shift is proportional to the mean velocity of blood flow within the vessel multiplied by the cosine of the angle between the ultrasound beam and the direction of flow. The angle is assumed to be close to zero. With this method, only blood flow velocity in large interlobar arteries and resistance can be assessed. The duplex Doppler ultrasound technique may provide a unique opportunity to demonstrate the effects of drugs on the renal vasculature and to predict the onset of pending renal failure or transplanted kidney rejection. Overall, this technique should provide an opportunity for measuring relative changes in large vessel flow velocity but not in absolute renal blood flow.

Contrast ultrasonography has been used to image renal blood flow.[172-175] The microbubbles produced by ultrasonic cavitation (i.e., sonication) are smaller than red blood cells and, in passing with them through the microcapillary vascular bed, reflect an echo beam to permit direct ultrasonic imaging of tissue volume and flow. Sonicated microbubbles have been shown to exhibit intracavitary velocities comparable to those of red blood cells, as observed by Doppler ultrasound techniques. Modest correlations have been found between calculated renal blood flow assessed by contrast ultrasonography and direct flow assessment.[175]

Use of Renal Blood Flow

Although the kidneys receive almost one fourth of the cardiac output and extract relatively little oxygen, there is a marked discrepancy between cortical and medullary blood flow and oxygen delivery and consumption. The apparent overabundance of blood flow to the cortex is designed to maximize flow-dependent functions, such as glomerular filtration and tubular reabsorption. In the medulla, blood flow and oxygen supply are restricted by a tubulovascular anatomy specifically designed for urinary concentration. There appears to be a physiologically important reason for the paucity of blood flow and, consequently, the oxygenation in the medulla.[176] The tubules carrying blood to the medulla are arranged in a hairpin-loop pattern to allow a countercurrent exchange of solute between the ascending and the descending limbs of the hairpin loop. In this way, urine in the tubule becomes highly concentrated. The osmotic gradient in the deeper portions of the medulla requires active transport of sodium in the thick ascending loop of Henle and limited blood flow through the medullary vessels to prevent washout of the solutes in those deeper tubules. To maintain this concentration gradient in the thick ascending limb, high energy demand (i.e., active sodium transport)

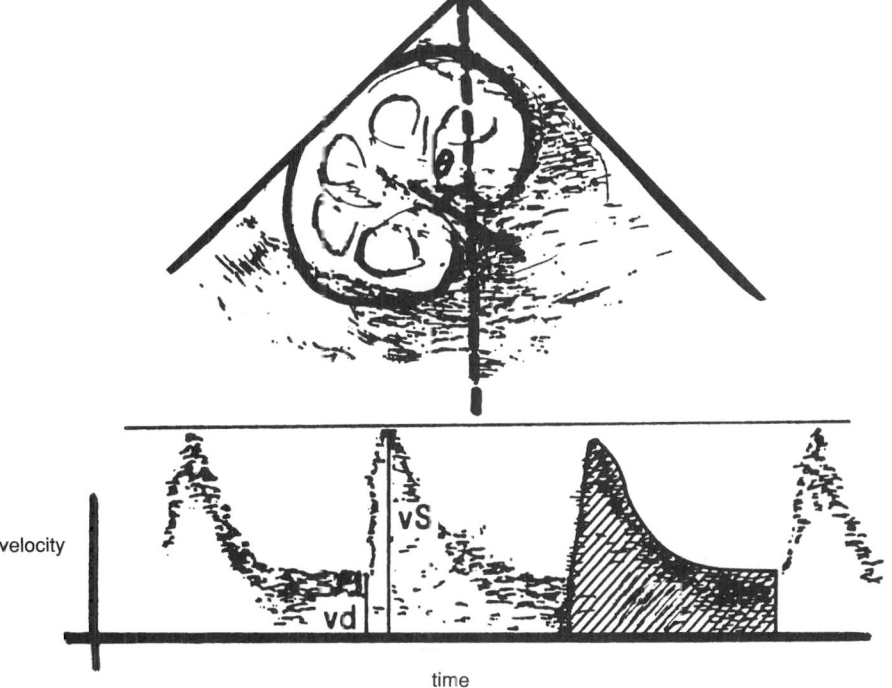

Figure 37–11 Renal duplex scan shows a sample volume superimposed over a B-scan image for a typical normal velocity flow pattern from the main renal artery at the hilum. θ, angle of incidence between transmitted ultrasound signal and received ultrasound signal; vd, diastolic velocity; vS, systolic velocity.

must be coupled with low oxygen delivery. The ambient partial pressure of oxygen in the medulla ranges from 10 to 15 mm Hg. The high metabolic requirement of the thick ascending loop of Henle in a hypoxic environment makes it especially vulnerable to injury associated with an imbalance in oxygen supply and demand.[177-178] Hypoxic perfusion of an isolated kidney preparation has demonstrated that the cells of the thick ascending limb of the loop of Henle in the medulla are extremely vulnerable to hypoxic damage.[69] This damage is patchy and is most evident in tubules farthest from a vessel. The selective vulnerability of the cells in the thick ascending loop of Henle is thought to result from their high oxygen consumption. Blood flow is approximately 90% to 95% to the cortex, compared with 5% to 10% to the medulla. Average blood flow is 5.0 mL/g/min and 0.03 mL/g/min for the cortex and medulla, respectively, and the oxygen extraction ratio (i.e., oxygen consumption over oxygen delivery) is 0.18 and 0.79 for the cortex and medulla, respectively. Normally, the partial pressure of oxygen is about 50 mm Hg in the cortex and 8 to 15 mm Hg in the medulla, making the thick ascending loop of Henle most vulnerable to tissue hypoxia. Severe hypoxia may therefore easily develop in the medulla if total renal blood flow is inadequate.

The initial response to decreased renal blood flow is an increase in sodium absorption in the ascending loop of Henle, which increases oxygen demand in the regions most vulnerable to decreased oxygen delivery. Ischemic renal damage may reflect hypoxic injury deep in the medulla to the metabolically active cells of the ascending loop of Henle. The normal response to systemic hypoperfusion is active sodium and water reabsorption, a metabolic response that demands oxygen at the time of greatest hypoxic vulnerability. To compensate, sympathoadrenal mechanisms cause cortical vasoconstriction and oliguria, which redistributes blood flow away from the outer cortex to the inner cortex and medulla. Determination of total RBF does not provide a reliable predictive index of organ function after an ischemic insult or surgery. Another compensatory mechanism, increased sodium delivery to the macula densa, results in afferent arteriolar constriction. With afferent arteriolar vasoconstriction, glomerular filtration decreases, after which solute reabsorption in the loop of Henle and oxygen consumption are reduced. In a hypoperfused kidney preparation, oxygen-enriched perfusion reduced cellular damage, hypoxic perfusion increased it, and complete cessation of perfusion (i.e., glomerular filtration equal to zero, preventing ultrafiltration) was associated with less cellular injury than hypoxic perfusion.[68] The severity of cellular injury appears related to the degree of imbalance between cellular oxygen supply and demand. Afferent arteriolar vasoconstriction may be a normal protective response to acute tubular injury. By reducing ultrafiltration, further energy expenditure by already ischemic medullary tubular cells is prevented, even at the cost of retaining nitrogenous waste.

Theoretically, therapeutic intervention designed to prevent renal insufficiency should be focused on preserving renal blood flow and oxygen delivery. Continuous monitoring of urinary oxygen tension has been examined as a method for assessing renal function during the perioperative period.[179-186] Urinary oxygen tension (Pu_{O_2}) decreases with clinical shock and dehydration. It has been demonstrated that Pu_{O_2} decreased when renal blood flow decreased or Pa_{O_2} decreased and that Pu_{O_2} increased when Pa_{O_2} increased. Changes in Pu_{O_2}, however, are relatively insensitive to oxygen content compared with changes in Pa_{O_2}. Because urinary oxygen tension depends on renal perfusion and renal oxygenation, it may be a useful tool for predicting renal cell injury, but it is not yet clinically practical to measure Pu_{O_2}. Urine samples obtained from bladder catheters provide artificially high Pu_{O_2} values because samples are easily contaminated with the oxygen in room air. Another problem with measuring urinary oxygen tension or saturation is that bladder measurements may be different from ureteral measurements. Ureteral measurements also may not reflect accurately the regional use of oxygen in the renal cortex versus the renal medulla or the renal pelvis. Interpreting the physiologic significance of changes in urine oxygen tension or saturation requires knowledge of where the oxygen comes from and its relationship to other physiologic variables.

SUMMARY

In patients with real or potential renal dysfunction, the perioperative management continues to be challenging. The causes of perioperative ARF vary but typically have a common mechanism of insufficient renal blood flow delivery or acute tubular necrosis, or both.

As our understanding of renal function continues to evolve, traditional answers turn into new questions. The introduction of new agents and the re-exploration of old techniques and their respective influence and reliance on renal function should become clearer with advances in renal function monitoring. Whether this information will modify the prognosis of renal dysfunction is unknown. Meanwhile, we are limited to relying on indirect variables of renal function that may or may not bear a reliable relationship to the GFR and renal blood flow—and therefore renal function—during the perioperative period. In the near future, we may be able to understand susceptibility to renal dysfunction on the basis of genetic screening and understand how to launch effective preventive management strategies by using this monitoring approach.

KEY POINTS

1. Perioperative ARF, although uncommon, is associated with extremely high morbidity and mortality rates.
2. The mechanism for perioperative ARF is complex and multifactorial but essentially can be characterized as hemodynamically mediated renal failure.
3. Direct assessment of renal hemodynamics, tubular function, or pathogenesis of perioperative renal dysfunction is difficult and not practical; therefore, indirect assessments must be used.

4. Intraoperative urine formation depends on a number of factors and is an insensitive and unreliable method for assessing postoperative risk of renal dysfunction outcome.
5. Serum chemistries and urine indices such as BUN, creatinine, fractional excretion of sodium, and free water clearance are generally late indicators of renal function deterioration and do not enable the clinician to clearly delineate the cause of renal failure.
6. Creatinine clearance is the most sensitive and specific method for determining renal risk, but it is limited by time and measurement restrictions.
7. Biochemical markers for renal function hold promise for differentiating glomerular from tubular causes but remain primarily limited to research settings.
8. Promising new technologies such as urine oximetry, ultrasound techniques, and radiopharmaceutical methods are being explored and may provide assessment of renal function in the operating room or critical care environment in the near future.

REFERENCES

1. McCarty JT: Prognosis of patients with acute renal failure in the intensive care unit: A tale of two eras. Mayo Clin Proc 71:117-126, 1996.
2. Drumk RN, Lax F, Grimn G, et al: Acute renal failure in the elderly 1975-1990. Clin Nephrol 41:342-349, 1994.
3. Butkus DE: Persistent high mortality in acute renal failure: Are we asking the right questions? Arch Intern Med 143:209-212, 1983.
4. Hou SH, Bushinsky DA, Wish JB, et al: Hospital-acquired renal insufficiency: A prospective study. Am J Med 74:243, 1983.
5. Maher ER, Robinson KN, Scoble JE, et al: Prognosis of critically ill patients with acute renal failure: Apache II score and other predictive factors. Q J Med 72:857-866, 1989.
6. Abreo K, Moorthy AV, Osborne M: Changing patterns and outcome of acute renal failure requiring hemodialysis. Arch Intern Med 146:1338-1341, 1986.
7. Kasiske BL, Kjellstrand CM: Perioperative management of patients with chronic renal failure and postoperative acute renal failure. Urol Clin North Am 10:35-50, 1983.
8. Chertow GM, Lazarus JM, Christianson CL, et al: Preoperative renal risk stratification. Circulation 95:878-884, 1997.
9. Mangano CM, Diamondstone LS, Ramsey JG, et al: Renal dysfunction after myocardial revascularization: Risk factors, adverse outcomes and hospital resource utilization. Ann Intern Med 128:194-203, 1998.
10. Aronson S, Fontes M, Mangano D: Wide pulse pressure confers a blow to the kidneys [abstract]. Anesthesiology, 2002.
11. Aronson S, Boisvert D, Lapp W: Isolated systolic hypertension is associated with adverse outcomes from coronary artery bypass grafting surgery. Anesth Analg 94:1079-1084, 2002.
12. Starr RA: Treatment of acute renal failure. Kidney Int 54:1817-1831, 1998.
13. Novis BK, Roizen MF, Aronson S, et al: Association of perioperative risk factors with postoperative acute renal failure. Anesth Analg 78:143-149, 1994.
14. Kaufman J, Dhakal M, Patel B, et al: Community-acquired acute renal failure. Am J Kidney Dis 17:191-198, 1991.
15. Shusterman N, Strom BL, Murray TG, et al: Risk factors and outcome of hospital acquired acute renal failure: Clinical epidemiology study. Am J Med 83:65-71, 1987.
16. Charlscn ME, MacKenzie CR, Gold JP, et al: Postoperative changes in serum creatinine: When do they occur and how much is important? Ann Surg 209:328-333, 1989.
17. Thadhani R, Pascual M, Bonventre JV: Acute renal failure. N Engl J Med 334:1448-1460, 1996.
18. Badr KF, Ichikawa I: Prerenal failure: A deleterious shift from renal compensation to decompensation. N Engl J Med 319:623, 1988.
19. Kellen M, Aronson S, Roizen MF, et al: Predictive and diagnostic tests of acute renal failure: A review. Anesth Analg 78:134-142, 1994.
20. Davidman M, Olson P, Kohen J, et al: Iatrogenic renal disease. Arch Intern Med 151:1809-1812, 1991.
21. Mazze RI, Cousins MJ, Barr GA: Renal effects and metabolism of isoflurane in man. Anesthesiology 40:536-542, 1974.
22. Mazze RI, Calverley RK, Smith NT: Inorganic fluoride nephrotoxicity: Prolonged enflurane and halothane anesthesia in volunteers. Anesthesiology 46:265-271, 1977.
23. Bastron RD, Pyne JL, Inagaki M: Halothane-induced renal vasodilation. Anesthesiology 50:126-131, 1979.
24. Seyde WC, Ellis JE, Longnecker DE: The addition of nitrous oxide to halothane decreases renal and splanchnic flow and increases cerebral blood flow in rats. Br J Anaesth 58:63-68, 1986.
25. Davidkova TI, Fujii K, Kikuchi H, et al: Urinary excretion of inorganic and organic fluoride after inhalation of sevoflurane. Hiroshima J Med Sci 36:99-104, 1987.
26. Papper S, Papper EM: The effects of preanesthetic, anesthetic and postoperative drugs on renal function. Clin Pharmacol Ther 5 205-215, 1964.
27. Kennedy WF, Sawyer TK, Gerbershagen HU, et al: Systemic cardiovascular and renal hemodynamic alterations during peridural anesthesia in normal men. Anesthesiology 31:414-421, 1969.
28. Gamulin Z, Forster A, Morel D, et al: Effects of infrarenal aortic cross-clamping on renal hemodynamics in humans. Anesthesiology 61:394, 1984.
29. Gamulin Z, Forster A, Simonet F, et al: Effects of renal sympathetic blockade on renal hemodynamics in patients undergoing major aortic abdominal surgery. Anesthesiology 65:688-692, 1986.
30. Lucas CE, Weaver D, Higgins RF, et al: Effects of albumin versus non-albumin resuscitation on plasma volume and renal excretory function. J Trauma 18:564-570, 1978.
31. Bennett-Guerrero E, et al: Impact of normal saline based versus balanced-salt intravenous fluid replacement on clinical outcomes: A randomized blinded clinical trial. Anesthesiology 94:A147, 2001.
32. Brennan LA Jr, Malvin RL, Jochim KE, et al: Influence of right and left atrial receptors on plasma concentrations of ADH and renin. Am J Physiol 221:273-278, 1971.
33. Philbin DM, Baratz RA, Patterson RW: The effect of carbon dioxide on plasma antidiuretic hormone levels during intermittent positive-pressure breathing. Anesthesiology 33:345-349, 1970.
34. Cogan MG: Renal effects of atrial natriuretic factor. Annu Rev Physiol 52:699-708, 1990.
35. Weiss RM: Ureteral function. Urology 12:114-133, 1978.
36. Young CJ, Attele A, Toledano A, et al: Volatile anesthetics decrease peristalsis in the guinea pig ureter. Anesthesiology 81:452-458, 1994.
37. Morita T, Wada I, Saeki H, et al: Ureteral urine transport changes in bolus volume, peristaltic frequency, intraluminal pressure and volume of flow resulting from autonomic drugs J Urol 137:132-135, 1987.
38. Makker SP, Tucker AS, Izant RJ Jr, et al: Nonobstructive hydronephrosis and hydroureter associated with peritonitis. N Engl J Med 287:535-537, 1972.
39. Wheeler MA, Cho YH, Hong KW, et al: Age-dependent alterations in beta-adrenergic receptor function in guinea pig ureter. Prog Clin Biol Res 327:711-715, 1990.
40. Renkin EM, Robinson RR: Glomerular filtration. N Engl J Med 290:785-792, 1974.
41. Mauer MS, Steffes MW, Ellis EN, et al: Structural-functional relationships in diabetic nephropathy. J Clin Invest 74:1143-1155, 1984.

42. Richards AN, Westfall BB, Bott PA: Renal excretion of inulin, creatinine, and xylose in normal dogs. Proc Soc Exp Biol 32:73, 1934.

43. Miller BF, Winkler AW: The renal excretion of endogenous creatinine in man, comparison with exogenous creatinine and inulin. J Clin Invest 17:31, 1938.

44. Skov PE: Glomerular filtration rate in patients with severe and very severe renal insufficiency. Acta Med Scand 187:419-428, 1970.

45. Mark JB, Steel SM: Cardiovascular effects of spinal anesthesia. Int Anesthesiol Clin 27:31-39, 1989.

46. Saada M, Duval AM, Bounet F, et al: Abnormalities in myocardial segmented wall motion during lumbar epidural anesthesia. Anesthesiology 71:26-32, 1989.

47. Kennedy WF, Sawyer TK, Gerbershagen HV: Simultaneous systemic cardiovascular and renal hemodynamic measurements during high spinal anesthesia in normal man. Acta Anaesthesiol Scand 37:163-171, 1970.

48. Sulerman MY, Passannante AN, Onder RL, et al: Alterations of renal blood flow during epidural anesthesia in normal subjects. Anesth Analg 84:1076-1080, 1997.

49. Halperin BD, Feeley TW: The effect of anesthesia and surgery on renal function. Int Anesthesiol Clin 22:157-168, 1984.

50. Mazze RI, Calverley RK, Smith NT: Inorganic fluoride nephrotoxicity: Prolonged enflurane and halothane anesthesia in volunteers. Anesthesiology 46:265-271, 1977.

51. Cousins MJ, Mazze RI: Methoxyflurane nephrotoxicity: A study of dose response in man. JAMA 225:1611-1616, 1973.

52. Mazze RI, Cousins MJ, Kosek JC: Dose-related methoxyflurane nephrotoxicity in rats: A biochemical and pathologic correlation. Anesthesiology 36:571-587, 1972.

53. Manday IT, Stoddart PA, Jones RM, et al: Serum fluoride concentration and urine osmolality after enflurane and sevoflurane anesthesia in male volunteers. Anesth Analg 81:353-359, 1995.

54. Kharasch ED, Armstrong AS, Gunn, et al: Clinical sevoflurane metabolism and disposition II. The role of cytochrome P450 2E1 in fluoride and hexafluoroisopropanol formation. Anesthesiology 82:1379-1388, 1995.

55. Conzen PF, Nuscheler M, Melotte A, et al: Renal function and serum fluoride concentration in patients with stable renal insufficiency after anesthesia with sevoflurane or enflurane. Anesth Analg 81:569-575, 1995.

56. Kharasch ED, Hawkins DC, Thummel KE: Human kidney methoxyflurane and sevoflurane metabolism: Intrarenal fluoride production as a possible mechanism of methoxyflurane nephrotoxicity. Anesthesiology 82:689-699, 1995.

57. Frink E, Malan T, Isner RJ, et al: Renal concentrating function with prolonged sevoflurane or enflurane anesthesia in volunteers. Anesthesiology 80:1019-1025, 1994.

58. Morio M, Fujii K, Satoh N, et al: Reaction of sevoflurane and its degradation products with soda lime: Toxicity of the byproducts. Anesthesiology 77:1155-1164, 1992.

59. Gonsowski CT, Laster MJ, Eger EI, et al: Toxicity of compound A in rats: Effects of increasing duration of administration. Anesthesiology 80:566-573, 1994.

60. Bito H, Ikewchi Y, Ikeda K: Effects of low-flow sevoflurane anesthesia on renal function. Anesthesiology 86:1231-1237, 1997.

61. Eger EI, Koblin DD, Bowland T, et al: Nephrotoxicity of sevoflurane versus desflurane anesthesia in volunteers. Anesth Analg 84:160-168, 1997.

62. Cressey G, Roberts DR, Snowden CP: Renal tubular injury after infrarenal aortic aneurysm repair. J Cardiothorac Vasc Anesth 16:290-293, 2002.

63. Kharasch ED, Frink EJ, Zager R, et al: Assessment of low-flow sevoflurane and isoflurane effects on renal function using sensitive markers of tubular function. Anesthesiology 86:1238-1253, 1997.

64. Schrier RW: Acute renal failure JAMA 247:2518-2522, 2524, 1982.

65. Donohoe JF, Venkatachalam MA, Bernard DB, et al: Tubular leakage and obstruction after renal ischemia: Structural-functional correlations. Kidney Int 13:208-222, 1978.

66. Cronin RE, Erickson AM, De Torrente A, et al: Norepinephrine-induced acute renal failure: A reversible ischemic model of acute renal failure. Kidney Int 14:187-190, 1978.

67. Myers BD, Moran SM: Hemodynamically mediated acute renal failure. N Engl J Med 314:97-105, 1986.

68. Brezis M, Rosen S, Silva P, et al: Renal ischemia: A new perspective. Kidney Int 26:375-383, 1984.

69. Brezis M, Rosen S, Silva P, et al: Selective vulnerability of the medullary thick ascending limb to anoxia in the isolated perfused rat kidney. J Clin Invest 73:182-190, 1984.

70. Byrick RJ, Rose DK: Pathophysiology and prevention of acute renal failure: The role of the anaesthetist. Can J Anaesth 37:457-467, 1990.

71. Zimmerhackl B, Robertson CR, Jamison RL: The microcirculation of the renal medulla. Circ Res 57:657-667, 1985.

72. Flamenbaum W: Pathophysiology of acute renal failure. Arch Intern Med 131:911-928, 1973.

73. Chedru M-F, Baethke R, Oken DE: Renal cortical blood flow and glomerular filtration in myohemoglobinuric acute renal failure. Kidney Int 1:232, 1972.

74. Knapp R, Hollenberg NK, Busch GJ, et al: Prolonged unilateral acute renal failure induced by intra-arterial norepinephrine infusion in the dog. Invest Radiol 7:164-173, 1972.

75. Ross B, Freeman D, Chan L: Contributions of nuclear magnetic resonance to renal biochemistry. Kidney Int 29:131-141, 1986.

76. Ratcliffe PJ, Moonen CT, Halloway PA, et al: Acute renal failure in hemorrhagic hypotension: Cellular energetics and renal function. Kidney Int 30:355-360, 1986.

77. Ratcliffe PJ, Moonen CTW, Ledingham JGG, et al: Timing of the onset of changes in renal energetics in relation to blood pressure and glomerular filtration in hemorrhagic hypotension in the rat. Nephron 51:225-232, 1989.

78. McCullough PA, Wolun R, Rocher LL, et al: ARF after coronary intervention incidence, risk factors, and relationship to mortality. Am J Med 103:368-375, 1997.

79. Chew ST, Newman MF, Whiter WD, et al: Preliminary report on the association of apolipoprotein E polymorphisms with postoperative peak serum creatinine concentrations in cardiac surgical patients. Anesthesiology 93:325-331, 2000.

80. Diehl JT, Cali RF, Hertzer NR, et al: Complications of abdominal aortic reconstruction: An analysis of perioperative risk factors in 557 patients. Ann Surg 197:49-56, 1983.

81. Crawford ES, Crawford JL, Safi HJ, et al: Thoracoabdominal aortic aneurysms: Preoperative and intraoperative factors determining immediate and long-term results of operations in 605 patients. J Vasc Surg 3:389-404, 1986.

82. Luke RG: Can renal function due to hypertension be prevented? Hypertension 3:139-142, 1991.

83. Harrison JF, Parker RW, De Silva KL: Lysozymuria and acute disorders of renal function. J Clin Pathol 26:278-284, 1973.

84. Wilson RF, Soullier G, Antonenko D: Creatinine clearance in critically ill surgical patients. Arch Surg 114:461-467, 1979.

85. Gorfinkel HJ, Szidon JP, Hirsch LJ, et al: Renal performance in experimental cardiogenic shock. Am J Physiol 222:1260-1268, 1972.

86. Kahl FR, Flint JF, Szidon JP: Influence of left atrial distension on renal vasomotor tone. Am J Physiol 226:240-246, 1974.

87. Smith MD, MacPhail B, Harrison MR, et al: Value and limitations of transesophageal echocardiography in determination of left ventricular volumes and ejection fraction. J Am Coll Cardiol 19:1213-1222, 1992.

88. Helak JW, Reichek N: Quantitation of human left ventricular mass and volume by two-dimensional echocardiography: In vitro anatomic validation. Circulation 63:1398-1407, 1981.

89. Perel A, Pizov R, Cotev S: Systolic blood pressure variation is a sensitive indicator of hypovolemia in ventilated dogs subjected to graded hemorrhage. Anesthesiology 67:498-502, 1987.

90. Folland ED, Parisi AF, Moynihan PF, et al: Assessment of left ventricular ejection fraction and volumes by real-time, two-dimensional echocardiography: A comparison of cineangiographic and radionuclide techniques. Circulation 60:760-766, 1979.

91. Kilburn KH, Dowell AR: Renal function in respiratory failure: Effects of hypoxia, hyperoxia and hypercapnia. Arch Intern Med 127:754-762, 1971.
92. Pelletier CL, Shepherd JT: Effect of hypoxia on vascular responses to the carotid baroreflex. Am J Physiol 228:331-336, 1975.
93. Neylon M, Johns EJ, Marshall JM: The renal response to systemic hypoxia in the anesthetized rat. J Physiol (Lond) 452:88P, 1992.
94. Sladen A, Laver MB, Pontoppidan H: Pulmonary complications and water retention in prolonged mechanical ventilation. N Engl J Med 279:448-453, 1968.
95. Stone AM, Stahl WM: Renal effects of hemorrhage in normal man. Ann Surg 172:825-836, 1970.
96. Yao FS, Hartman GS, Thomas SI, et al: Does arterial pressure during cardiopulmonary bypass effect renal and pulmonary complications following coronary artery surgery? Anesth Analg 80:113, 1995.
97. Hilberman M, Derby GC, Spencer RJ, et al: Sequential pathophysiological changes characterizing the progression from renal dysfunction to acute renal failure following cardiac operations. J Thorac Cardiovasc Surg 79:838-844, 1990.
98. Slogoff S, Reul GJ, Keats AS, et al: Role of perfusion pressure and flow in major organ dysfunction after cardiopulmonary bypass. Ann Thorac Surg 50:911-918, 1990.
99. Urzua J, Troncoso S, Bugedo G, et al: Renal function and cardiopulmonary bypass: Effects of perfusion pressure. J Cardiothorac Vasc Anesth 6:299-303, 1992.
100. Makhoul RG, Gewertz BL: Renal prostaglandins. J Surg Res 40:181-192, 1986.
101. Packer M, Lee WH, Kessler PD: Preservation of glomerular filtration rate in human heart failure by activation of the renin-angiotensin system. Circulation 74:766-774, 1986.
102. Edwards RM: Segmental effects of norepinephrine and angiotensin II on isolated renal microvessels. Am J Physiol 244:F526-F534, 1983.
103. Goldstein MB: Acute renal failure. Med Clin North Am 67:1325-1341, 1983.
104. Vertel RM, Knochel JP: Nonoliguric acute renal failure. JAMA 200:598-602, 1967.
105. Shin B, Mackenzie CF, Helrich M: Creatinine clearance for early detection of posttraumatic renal dysfunction. Anesthesiology 64:605-609, 1986.
106. Rosenberg IK, Gupta SL, Lucas CE, et al: Renal insufficiency after trauma and sepsis. Arch Surg 103:175-183, 1971.
107. Alpert RA, Roizen MF, Hamilton WK, et al: Intraoperative urinary output does not predict postoperative renal function in patients undergoing abdominal aortic revascularization. Surgery 95:707-711, 1984.
108. Knos GB, Berry AJ, Isaacson IJ, et al: Intraoperative urinary output and postoperative blood urea nitrogen and creatinine levels in patients undergoing aortic reconstructive surgery. J Clin Anesth 1:181-185, 1989.
109. Jones LW, Weil MH: Water, creatinine, and sodium excretion following circulatory shock with renal failure. Am J Med 51:314-318, 1971.
110. Pru C, Kjellstrand C: Urinary indices and chemistries in the differential diagnosis of prerenal failure and acute tubular necrosis. Semin Nephrol 5:224-233, 1985.
111. Haskell JP, Tannenberg AM: Elevated urinary specific gravity in acute oliguric renal failure due to hetastarch administration. N Y State J Med 88:387, 1988.
112. Eliahou HE, Bata A: The diagnosis of acute renal failure. Nephron 2:287, 1965.
113. Miller TR, Anderson RJ, Linas SL, et al: Urinary diagnostic indices in acute renal failure: A prospective study. Ann Intern Med 89:47-50, 1978.
114. Espinel CH, Gregory AW: Differential diagnosis of acute renal failure. Clin Nephrol 13:73-77, 1980.
115. Zager RA, Rubin NT, Ebert T, et al: Rapid radioimmunoassay for diagnosing acute tubular necrosis. Nephron 26:7-12, 1980.
116. Miller PD, Krebs RA, Neal BJ, et al: Polyuric prerenal failure. Arch Intern Med 140:907-909, 1980.
117. Heimann T, Brau S, Sakurai H, et al: Urinary osmolal changes in renal dysfunction following open-heart operations. Ann Thorac Surg 22:44-49, 1976.
118. Shemesh O, Golbetz H, Kriss JP, Myer BD: Limitations of creatinine as a filtration marker in glomerulopathic patients. Kidney Int 28:830-838, 1985.
119. Moran SM, Myers BD: Course of acute renal failure studied by a model of creatinine kinetics. Kidney Int 27:928-937, 1985.
120. Doolan PD, Alpen EL, Theil GB: A clinical appraisal of the plasma concentration and endogenous clearance of creatinine. Am J Med 32:65-79, 1962.
121. Bull GM, Joekes AM, Lowe KG: Renal function studies in acute tubular necrosis. Clin Sci 9:379, 1950.
122. Handa SP, Morrin PAF: Diagnostic indices in acute renal failure. Can Med Assoc J 96:78, 1967.
123. Perlmutter M, Grossman SL, Rothenberg S, et al: Urine-serum urea nitrogen ratio: Simple test of renal function in acute azotemia and oliguria. JAMA 170:1533-1537, 1959.
124. Chisholm GD, Charlton CAC, Orr WM: Urine-urea/blood-urea ratios in renal failure. Lancet 1:20, 1966.
125. Luke RG, Briggs JD, Allison MEM, et al: Factors determining response to mannitol in acute renal failure. Am J Med Sci 259:168-174, 1970.
126. Espinel CH: The FENa test: Use in the differential diagnosis of acute renal failure. JAMA 236:579-581, 1976.
127. Diamond JR, Yoburn DC: Nonoliguric acute renal failure associated with a low fractional excretion of sodium. Ann Intern Med 96:597-600, 1982.
128. Brown RS: Renal dysfunction in the surgical patient: Maintenance of the high output state with furosemide. Crit Care Med 7:63-68, 1979.
129. Brosius FC, Lau K: Low fractional excretion of sodium in acute renal failure: Role of timing of the test and ischemia. Am J Nephrol 6:450-457, 1986.
130. Saha H, Mustonen J, Helin H, et al: Limited value of the fractional excretion of sodium test in the diagnosis of acute renal failure. Nephrol Dial Transplant 2:79-82, 1987.
131. Steiner RW: Interpreting the fractional excretion of sodium. Am J Med 77:699-702, 1984.
132. Zarich S, Fang LS, Diamond JR: Fractional excretion of sodium: Exceptions to its diagnostic value. Arch Intern Med 145:108-112, 1985.
133. Jones LW, Weil MH: Changes in urinary output and free water clearance in patients with acute circulatory failure (shock). J Urol 102:121-125, 1969.
134. Baek SM, Brown RS, Shoemaker WC: Early prediction of acute renal failure and recovery. I. Sequential measurements of free water clearance. Ann Surg 177:253-258, 1973.
135. Shin B, Isenhower NN, McAslan TC, et al: Early recognition of renal insufficiency in post-anesthetic trauma victims. Anesthesiology 50:262-265, 1979.
136. Kosinski JP, Lucas CE, Ledgerwood AM: Meaning and value of free water clearance in injured patients. J Surg Res 33:184-188, 1982.
137. Sladen RN, Endo E, Harrison T: Two-hour versus 22-hour creatinine clearance in critically ill patients. Anesthesiology 67:1013-1016, 1987.
138. Wheeler LA, Sheiner LB: Clinical estimation of creatinine clearance. Am J Clin Pathol 72:27-32, 1979.
139. Greenblatt DJ, Ransil BJ, Harmatz JS, et al: Variability of 24-hour urinary creatinine excretion by normal subjects. J Clin Pharmacol 16:321-328, 1976.
140. Price RG: Urinary enzymes: Nephrotoxicity and renal disease. Toxicology 23:99-134, 1982.
141. Mueller PW, MacNeal ML, Steinberg KK: N-acetyl-β-D-glucosaminidase assay in urine urea inhibition. J Anal Toxicol 13:188-190, 1989.
142. Stolarek I, Howey JE, Frazer CG: Biological variation of urinary NAG: Practical and clinical implications. Clin Chem 35:550-563, 1989.
143. Yuen CT, Price RG, Chattagoon L, et al: Colorimetric assays for N-acetyl-β-D-glucosaminidase and beta-D-galactosidase in human urine using newly developed omega-nitrostyryl substrates. Clin Chim Acta 124:195-204, 1982.

144. Hofmann W, Guder WG: A diagnostic program for quantitative analysis of proteinuria. J Clin Chem Clin Biochem 27:589-600, 1989.

145. Robinson D, Sterling S: N-acetyl-β-glucosaminidases in human spleen. Biochem J 107:321-327, 1968.

146. Price RG, Dance N, Richards B, et al: The excretion of N-acetyl-beta-glucosaminidase and β-galactosidase following surgery to the kidney. Clin Chim Acta 27:65-72, 1970.

147. Tucker SM, Pierce RJ, Price RG, et al: Characteristics of human NAG isoenzymes as an indicator of tissue damage and disease. Clin Chim Acta 102:29-40, 1980.

148. Whiting PH, Peterson J, Power DA, et al: Diagnostic value of urinary N-acetyl-beta-D-glucosaminidase, its isoenzymes and the fractional excretion of sodium following renal transplantation. Clin Chim Acta 130:369-376, 1983.

149. Eti S, Cheng CY, Marshall A, et al: Urinary clusterin in chronic nephrotoxicity in the rat. Proc Soc Exp Biol Med 202:487-490, 1992.

150. Karlsson FA, Wibell L, Evrin PE: Beta-2-microglobulin in clinical medicine. Scan J Clin Lab Invest 154:27-37, 1980.

151. Norden AGW, Flynn FV: Degradation of β_2-microglobulin in infected urine by leukocyte elastase activity. Clin Chim Acta 134:167-176, 1983.

152. Flynn FV: Assessment of renal function: Selective developments. Clin Biochem 23:49-50, 1990.

153. Dehne MG, Boldt J, Heise D, et al: Tamm-Horsfall protein, alpha-1 and beta 2 microglobulin as kidney function markers in heart surgery. Anesthetist 44:545-551, 1995.

154. Gormley SM, McBride WT, Armstrong MA, et al: Plasma and urinary cytokine homostasis and renal dysfunction during cardiac surgery. Anesthesiology 93:1210-1216, 2000.

155. Barger AC, Herd JA: Renal vascular anatomy and distribution of blood flow. In Orlaff J, Berliner RW (eds): Handbook of Physiology, section 8. Baltimore, Williams & Wilkins, 1973, p 249.

156. Kreisberg JI, Venkatachalam MA: Morphologic factors in acute renal failure. In Brenner BM, Lazarus JM (eds): Acute Renal Failure, 2nd ed. New York, Churchill Livingstone, 1988, p 45.

157. Trueta J, Barclay AE, Daniel PM, et al: Studies on the Renal Circulation. Oxford, Blackwell Scientific Publications, 1947.

158. Carriere S, Thorburn GD, O'Morchoe CCC, et al: Intrarenal distribution of blood flow in dogs during hemorrhagic hypotension. Circ Res 19:167, 1966.

159. Barger AC, Herd JA: The renal circulation. N Engl J Med 284:482-490, 1971.

160. Rector JB, Stein JH, Bay WH, et al: Effect of hemorrhage and vasopressor agents on distribution of renal blood flow. Am J Physiol 222:1125-1131, 1972.

161. Auckland K: Intrarenal distribution of blood flow: Are reliable methods available for measurements in man? Scand J Clin Lab Invest 34:481, 1975.

162. Aukland K, Loyning EW: Intrarenal blood flow and para-aminohippurate (PAH) extraction. Acta Physiol Scand 79:95-108, 1970.

163. Reubi FC, Gossweiler N, Gurtler R: Renal circulation in man studied by means of a dye-dilution method. Circulation 33:426, 1966.

164. Haywood GA, Stewart JT, Counihan PJ, et al: Validation of bedside measurements of absolute human renal blood flow by a continuous thermodilution technique. Crit Care Med 20:659-664, 1992.

165. Muller M. Padberg W, Schindler E, et al: Renocortical tissue oxygen pressure measurement in patients undergoing living donor kidney transplantation. Anesth Analg 87:474-476, 1998.

166. Keam HB, Appel PL, Flemming AW, Shoemaker AC: Assessment of intestinal and renal perfusion using surface oxymetry Crit Care Med 14:707-713, 1986.

167. Schott G, Prom T: Intraoperative cortical P_{O_2} measurement in kidney transplantation: The effect of the calcium antagonist diltiazem. Urologe A 33:415-421, 1994.

168. Hollenberg NK, Epstein M, Rosen SM, et al: Acute oliguric renal failure in man: Evidence for preferential renal cortical ischemia. Medicine (Baltimore) 47:455-474, 1968.

169. Grunfeld J-P, Sabto J, Bankir L, et al: Methods for measurement of renal blood flow in man. Semin Nucl Med 4:39, 1974.

170. Farmelaut MH, Burrows BA: The renogram: Physiologic basis and current clinical use. Semin Nucl Med 4:61, 1974.

171. Stevens PE, Gwyther SJ, Hanson ME, et al: Noninvasive monitoring of renal blood flow characteristics during acute renal failure in man. Intensive Care Med 16:153-158, 1990.

172. Aronson S, Feinstein SB, Wiencek JG, et al: Assessment of renal blood flow with contrast ultrasonography. Anesth Analg 76:964-970, 1993.

173. Aronson S, Thisthelwaite R, Walker R, et al: Determination of renal blood flow during surgery with perfusion ultrasonography. Anesth Analg 80:353-359, 1995.

174. Wei K, Le E, Bin JP, et al: Quantification of renal blood flow with contrast-enhanced ultrasound. J Am Coll Cardiol 37:1135-1140, 2001.

175. Aronson S, Bilotta F, Wiencek JG, et al: Assessment of renal blood flow distribution in dogs with contrast ultrasound following dopamine infusion. Anesth Analg 74:S11, 1992.

176. Brezis M, Rosen SN, Epstein FH: The pathophysiological implications of medullary hypoxia. Am J Kidney Dis 13:253-258, 1989.

177. Brezis M, Rosen S, Spokes K, et al: Transport-dependent anoxic cell injury in the isolated perfused rat kidney. Am J Pathol 116:327-341, 1984.

178. Berzis M, Rosen S, Silva P, et al: Polyene toxicity in renal medulla: injury mediated by transport activity. Science 224:66-68, 1984.

179. Kainuma M, Kimura N, Shimada Y: Effect of acute changes in renal arterial blood flow on urine oxygen tension in dogs. Crit Care Med 18:309-312, 1990.

180. Rennie DW, Reeves RB, Pappenheimer JR: Oxygen pressure in urine and its relation to intrarenal blood flow. Am J Physiol 195:120-132, 1958.

181. Hong SK, Boylan JW, Tannenberg AM, et al: Total and partial gas tensions of human bladder urine. J Appl Physiol 15:115-120, 1960.

182. Thorburn GD, Kopald HH, Herd A, et al: Intrarenal distribution of nutrient blood flow determined by krypton 85 in the unanesthetized dog. Circ Res 13:290-307, 1963.

183. Hostetter TH, Wilkes BM, Brenner BM: Mechanisms of impaired glomerular filtration in acute renal failure. In Brenner BM, Stein JH (eds): Acute Renal Failure. New York, Churchill Livingstone, 1980, p 52.

184. Baines AD: Strategies and criteria for developing new urinalysis tests. Kidney Int Suppl 47:S137-S141, 1994.

185. Campbell JAH, Conigall AV, Guy A, et al: Immunohistologic localization of alpha, mu, and pi class glutathione S-transferases in human tissue. Cancer 67:1608-1613, 1991.

186. Beeuwkes R, Bonventre JV: Tubular organization and vascular tubular relations in the dog kidney. Am J Physiol 229:695-713, 1975.

38 Neurologic Monitoring

Michael E. Mahla, Susan Black, and Roy F. Cucchiara

Monitoring Modalities   1511

**The Standard
Electroencephalogram   1513**
Signal   1513
Normal Electroencephalogram   1514
Abnormal Electroencephalogram   1514

**The Processed
Electroencephalogram   1515**
Devices   1515
Data Acquisition Period   1516

**Anesthesia and the
Electroencephalogram   1516**
Intravenous Anesthetics   1517
Inhaled Anesthetics   1518

**Electroencephalographic Monitoring
for Surgical Procedures   1521**
Cardiopulmonary Bypass   1521
Carotid Endarterectomy   1521
Surgery for Epileptic Foci   1523

**Pathophysiologic Effects on the
Electroencephalogram   1523**
Hypoxia   1523
Hypotension   1524

Hypothermia   1524
Hypercarbia and Hypocarbia   1524
Untoward Events   1524
Brain Death   1525

**Intraoperative Monitoring of Sensory
Evoked Responses   1525**
Somatosensory Evoked Potentials   1527
Brainstem Auditory Evoked Potentials   1530
Visual Evoked Potentials   1532
Pharmacologic Factors Influencing Sensory
Evoked Responses   1532
Physiologic Factors Influencing Sensory Evoked
Responses   1537

**Monitoring of Motor Tracts
and Nerves   1537**
Electromyography   1537
Peripheral Nerve Monitoring   1539
Motor Evoked Potentials   1539

Monitors of Cerebral Blood Flow   1540
Transcranial Doppler Monitoring   1540
Jugular Bulb Venous Oxygen Saturation   1542
Cerebral Oximetry   1542

Summary   1542

In the 21st century, surgeons are attempting progressively more complex procedures involving the substance, supporting structures, and blood supply of the central and peripheral nervous systems. Direct, timely feedback about the effects of surgery on nervous system function and the adequacy of its blood supply can be extremely valuable to the surgeon. The best monitor of neurologic function remains the awake patient. In the awake patient, function of individual parts of the nervous system and the complex, often poorly understood interactions of different portions of the nervous system can be readily assessed. However, most surgical procedures involving the nervous system or its blood supply require general anesthesia. Current technology limits us to assessments of adequacy of blood flow to portions of the nervous system and the electrical function of groups of neurons and nervous system pathways that are not excessively depressed by the presence of anesthetic drugs.

This chapter focuses on monitoring nervous system electrical function and the adequacy of its blood supply using instruments also commonly used in the diagnostic laboratory. Types of operations in which neurologic monitoring has been used effectively are reviewed, and some of the changes that occur acutely in the operating room are described. How these signals are altered by commonly used anesthetics is reviewed in detail, and evidence for the utility and efficacy of neurologic monitoring is examined.

MONITORING MODALITIES

Multiple types of neurologic monitoring are used in the operating room (Table 38-1). To better understand the uses and limitations of each monitoring technique, neurologic monitors can be divided into monitors of electrical function and monitors of blood flow. Monitors of electrical function also indirectly monitor blood flow, because electrical function fails after a critical reduction in blood flow but before the onset of permanent cellular damage.

Table 38–1   The spectrum of neurologic monitoring

Monitor	Blood Flow	Electrical Function	Anesthetic Effect
Electroencephalogram	X (i)	X	X
Sensory evoked potentials	X (i)	X	X
Electromyogram	NU	X	NU
Motor evoked potentials	X (i)	X	NU
Transcranial Doppler ultrasound	X	NU	NU
Jugular venous oxygen saturation	X	NU	NU
Cerebral oximetry	X	NU	NU

(i), indirect measurement only; NU, not useful; X, used for neurologic monitoring.

Monitors of blood flow do not necessarily monitor electrical function, however, and only limited inferences about electroencephalograms (EEGs) and sensory evoked potentials (SEPs) can be made from measurements of blood flow. For example, surgically induced structural damage to the nervous system may not produce any change in blood flow or oxygen delivery to tissues, but function may permanently fail.

The most commonly used monitoring modalities are the EEG, sensory evoked responses (SERs), and the electromyogram (EMG). The EEG is a surface recording of the summation of excitatory and inhibitory postsynaptic potentials spontaneously generated by the pyramidal cells in the cerebral cortex. The signals are very small, and each electrode records only information generated directly beneath the electrode. Monitoring with the EEG is usually directed toward three perioperative uses. First, the EEG is used to help identify inadequate blood flow to the cerebral cortex caused by a surgical or anesthetic-induced reduction in blood flow or by retraction on cerebral tissue. Second, the EEG may be used to guide reduction of cerebral metabolism in anticipation of a loss of cerebral blood flow (CBF) or when a reduction in CBF and blood volume is desired in the patient with high intracranial pressure. Third, the EEG may be used to predict neurologic outcome after a brain insult.

More than one-half century of experience in monitoring with the EEG has led to many known correlations of electroencephalographic patterns with normal and pathologic clinical states of the cerebral cortex. The electroencephalographer can accurately identify consciousness, unconsciousness, seizure activity, stages of sleep, and coma. In the absence of changes in drug level, the electroencephalographer can also accurately identify inadequate oxygen delivery to the brain (from hypoxemia or ischemia). In the past decade, using high-speed, computerized analysis and statistical methods, the electroencephalographic patterns in the continuum from awake to deeply anesthetized are becoming, with few exceptions, much better understood. Although still far from perfect, correlations between electroencephalographic or evoked potential patterns and depth of hypnotic state have significantly improved,[1-6] and the likelihood of consciousness or amnesia can be assessed with most anesthetic techniques. These computer advances have made possible high-speed mathematic manipulation of the electroencephalographic signal to present the data in a manner more suitable to continuous, trended monitoring for surgical purposes.

Monitoring of the EEG in the operating room for surgical purposes requires significant training and experience. In contrast, electroencephalographic monitoring directed at assessing the depth of hypnosis can be readily mastered by most practicing clinicians in a short period.

Evoked potentials are electrical activity generated in response to a sensory or motor stimulus. Measurements of evoked responses may be made at multiple points along an involved nervous system pathway. The evoked responses are generally smaller than other electrical activity generated in nearby tissue (i.e., muscle or brain) and are readily obscured by these other biologic signals. Repeated sampling and sophisticated electronic summation and averaging techniques are needed to extract the desired evoked potential signal from background biologic signals.

SERs are by far the most common type of evoked potentials monitored intraoperatively. During the past 2 decades, much research has been carried out regarding the use of intraoperative motor evoked potentials (MEPs); however, routine use of MEP monitoring is not widespread. There are three basic types of SERs: somatosensory (SSEP), auditory (BAEP), and visual (VEP) potentials. The SSEP is produced by electrically stimulating a peripheral or cranial nerve. In the case of peripheral nerve stimulation, responses may be recorded proximally over the stimulated peripheral nerve, the spinal cord, and the cerebral cortex with assessment of the function of the peripheral nerve, the posterior and lateral aspects of the spinal cord, a small portion of the brainstem, the ventral posterolateral nucleus of the thalamus, the thalamocortical radiation, and a portion of the sensory cortex. The BAEP is usually produced by a series of rapid, loud clicks applied directly to the external auditory canal. Responses are most commonly recorded from scalp-applied electrodes, although more invasive direct recordings from auditory structures and nerves may be made. BAEPs assess function of the auditory apparatus itself, cranial nerve VIII, the cochlear nucleus, and a relatively small area of the rostral brainstem, the inferior colliculus, and the auditory cortex. After significant clinical research, cortically generated auditory responses (i.e., middle latency auditory responses) are being used to determine the depth of anesthetic induced hypnosis, similar to the bispectral index (BIS) monitor. The VEP is produced by flash stimulation of the retina. Recordings are made from cortically placed electrodes and assess visual pathways from the optic nerve to the occipital cortex.

THE STANDARD ELECTROENCEPHALOGRAM

Signal

The EEG is produced by a summation of excitatory and inhibitory postsynaptic potentials produced in cortical gray matter. Because the electroencephalographic signal is generated only by postsynaptic potentials and is much smaller than action potentials recorded over nerves or from the heart, extreme care must be taken when placing electrodes. The recording electrode impedances should be less than 5 kΩ and matched to each other to permit clear electroencephalographic signals, which may range from 5 to 500 mV. As electrode impedance increases above that value or becomes mismatched, significant signal loss occurs, and background electrical "noise" begins to obscure the electroencephalographic signal. Electrode impedance is kept low by using gold cup electrodes with silver–silver chloride electrolyte gel placed between the scalp and the electrode. The electrode is held tightly to the scalp with collodion, a biologic glue. Alternatively, subdermal needle electrodes may be used, particularly when sterile application of an electrode close to a surgical field is necessary. When electrodes are applied directly to the surface of the brain, impedance is minimized by close electrode contact and saturation of the area with an electrolyte solution.

Electroencephalographic electrodes usually are placed according to a mapping system that relates surface head anatomy to underlying brain cortical regions. The placement pattern of recording electrodes is called a *montage*. Use of a standard recording montage permits anatomic localization of signals produced by the brain and allows development of normative electroencephalographic patterns and comparison of recordings made at different times. The standard electroencephalographic map is called the International 10-20 System for electroencephalographic electrode placement (Fig. 38-1). This system is a symmetric array of scalp electrodes placed systematically based on the distance from the nasion to the inion and from the pretragal bony indentations associated with both temporomandibular joints. Based on 10% or 20% of these distances, recording electrodes are placed systematically over the frontal (F), parietal (P), temporal (T), and occipital (O) regions at increasing distances from the midline.

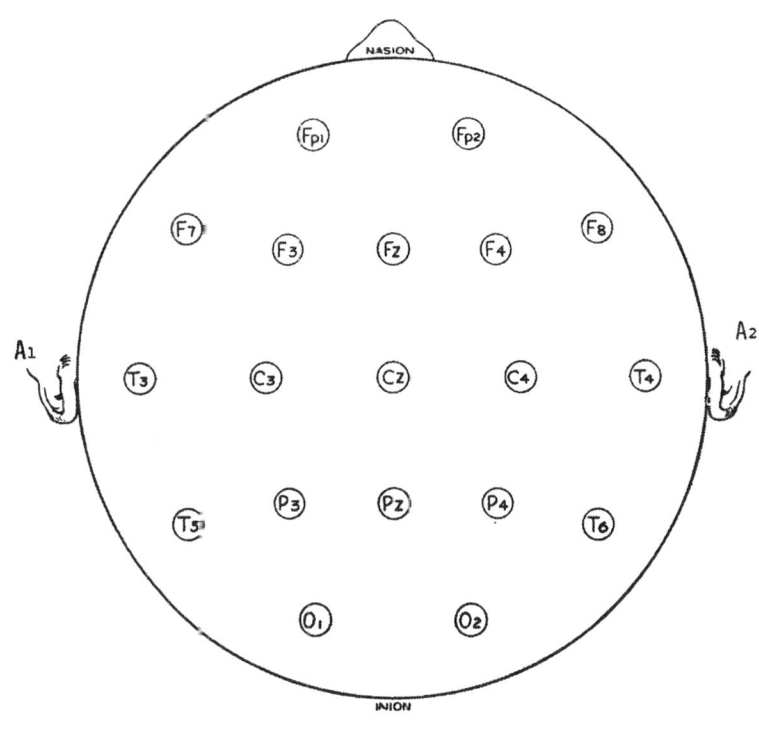

Figure 38–1 International 10-20 system of electrode placement for recording electroencephalograms and sensory evoked responses. (From Hughes JR: EEG in Clinical Practice, 2nd ed. Newton, ME, Butterworth-Heinemann, 1994.)

P3,4 = parietal
O1,2 = occipital
F7,8 = anterior temporal— records rhythms from that general region but placed on frontal bone

Fz = frontal midline
Cz = central vertex
Pz = parietal midline
(note: z = zero)

Left-sided electrodes are assigned odd numbers, and right-sided electrodes are assigned even numbers. Increasing numbers indicate an increasing distance from the midline. Midline electrodes are designated with a lower-case z. Recording electrodes may be referenced to other cephalic electrodes (i.e., bipolar recordings) or to electrodes placed away from cortical areas (i.e., referential recordings). The standard diagnostic EEG uses at least 16 channels of information,[7] but intraoperative recordings have been reported using 1 to 32 discrete channels.

The intraoperative EEG is most commonly recorded from electrodes placed on the scalp. Recordings may also be made from electrodes placed on the surface of the brain (i.e., electrocorticography) or from microelectrodes placed transcortically to record from individual neurons (e.g., during surgery for Parkinson's disease).[8,9] The electroencephalographic signal is described using three basic parameters: amplitude, frequency, and time. *Amplitude* is the size, or voltage of the recorded signal and ranges commonly from 5 µV to 500 mV (compared with 1 to 2 mV for the electrocardiographic signal). As neurons are irreversibly lost during the normal aging process, electroencephalographic amplitude decreases with age. *Frequency* can be thought of as the number of times per second the signal oscillates or crosses the zero voltage line. *Time* is the duration of the sampling of the signal; this is continuous and real time for the standard EEG but is a sampling epoch (i.e., data over a given period) for the processed EEG.

Normal Electroencephalogram

Normal patterns seen on the EEG vary somewhat among individuals but are consistent enough to allow for accurate recognition of normal and pathologic patterns. The usual base frequency in the awake patient is the β range (>13 Hz). This high-frequency and usually low-amplitude signal is common from the alert attentive brain and may be recorded from all regions. With eye closure, higher amplitude signals in the α frequency range (8 to 13 Hz) appear and are seen best in the occipital region (Fig. 38-2).

This eyes-closed resting pattern is the baseline awake pattern used when anesthetic effects on the EEG are described. When events that lead the brain to produce higher frequencies and larger amplitudes occur, the EEG is described as *activated*, and when slower frequencies are produced (θ = 4 to 7 Hz and δ < 4 Hz), the EEG is said to be *depressed*. The EEG for the sleeping patient may contain all of these frequencies at various times. The slower frequencies occur during deep natural sleep with sleep spindles (Fig. 38-3), but during light sleep or rapid eye movement (REM) sleep, the EEG becomes activated, and the eye muscle EMG appears on the EEG.

On normal EEGs for awake and asleep patients, patterns recorded from corresponding electrodes on each hemisphere are symmetric in terms of frequency and amplitude, the patterns are predictable if clinical states are known, and spike (epileptic) waveforms are absent. In most cases, normal electroencephalographic patterns are associated with normal underlying brain function.

Abnormal Electroencephalogram

General characteristics of the abnormal EEG include asymmetry with respect to frequency or amplitude, or both, recorded from corresponding electrodes on each hemisphere, and patterns of amplitude and frequency that are not predictable or expected in the normal recording. These abnormal patterns reflect anatomic or metabolic alterations in the underlying brain. Regional asymmetry can be seen with tumors, epilepsy, and cerebral ischemia or infarction. Epilepsy may be recognized by high-voltage spike and slow waves, whereas cerebral ischemia manifests with electroencephalographic slowing with preservation of voltage (mild or moderate) or loss of voltage (severe). Factors affecting the entire brain may produce symmetric abnormalities of the signal. Identifying pathologic abnormal patterns in the global electroencephalographic signal is very important, although sometimes quite difficult, in the clinical situation. Many of the normal global pattern changes produced by anesthetic

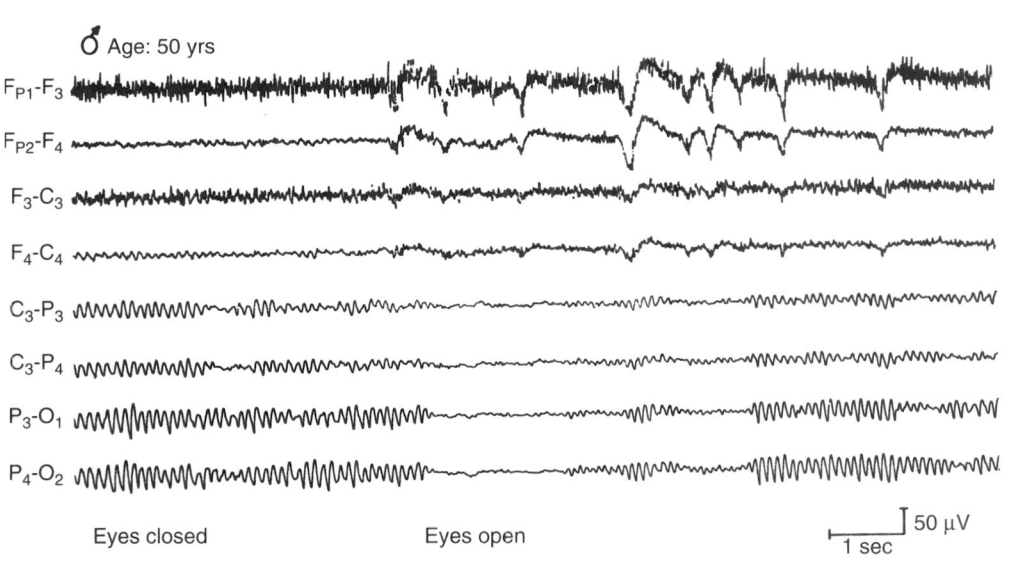

Figure 38–2 The loss and return of α activity can be seen as the eyes open and close. The large spikes are muscle artifact. (Courtesy of the Mayo Foundation, Rochester, MN.)

♂ Age: 50 yrs

F_{P1}-F_3

F_{P2}-F_4

F_3-C_3

F_4-C_4

C_3-P_3

C_3-P_4

P_3-O_1

P_4-O_2

Eyes closed   Eyes open   50 µV / 1 sec

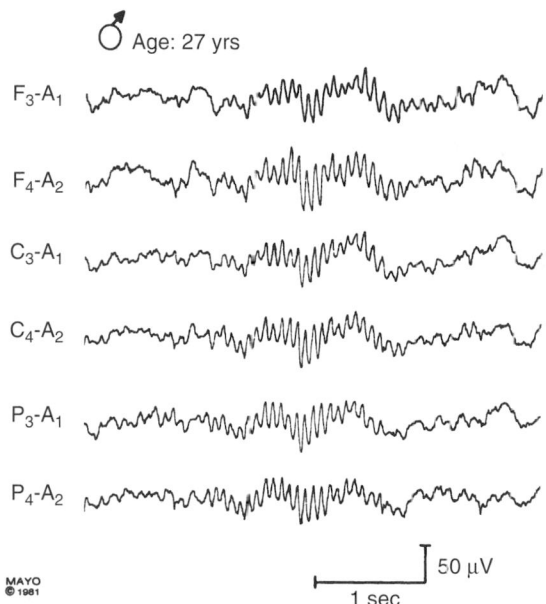

♂ Age: 27 yrs

F$_3$-A$_1$

F$_4$-A$_2$

C$_3$-A$_1$

C$_4$-A$_2$

P$_3$-A$_1$

P$_4$-A$_2$

MAYO
© 1981

50 μV

1 sec

Figure 38–3 Characteristic sleep spindles in normal sleep are shown in the center. (Courtesy of the Mayo Foundation, Rochester, MN.)

drugs are similar to pathologic patterns produced by ischemia or hypoxemia. Control of the anesthetic technique is important when the EEG is being used for clinical monitoring of the nervous system.

THE PROCESSED ELECTROENCEPHALOGRAM

Interpretation of the standard paper electroencephalographic tracing is a science and an art. All monitored waveforms during the case are compared with baseline signals. The interpreter has learned from experience the wide variety of normal changes that may occur in the perioperative period and promptly recognizes when changes occur that are not normal or expected. The baseline recordings and the qualitative overall impression of the record are important in interpreting the intraoperative EEG. Until recently, this qualitative approach was used because the waveforms could not be described mathematically in a timeframe that would make such information of any practical use. Analog-to-digital conversion technology associated with mainframe computers was used to convert the analog signal of the EEG to digital data and to mathematically manipulate the data. The process was complex, expensive, and still had little relevance to the clinician. Early techniques took 1 hour to digitize and analyze a 1-second epoch of electroencephalographic data. Computer hardware has dramatically improved in speed and size, and real-time signal processing is now possible and commonly used.

Several limitations are introduced when moving from the raw electroencephalographic domain to the processed electroencephalographic domain. First, as the processed electroencephalographic signal becomes more electronically remote (i.e., more processed), there is a point at

which it becomes increasingly difficult or impossible to relate what we know about the raw electroencephalographic data to the processed signal. An example of this problem was found in an early prototype electroencephalographic monitor used in the operating room. When the dominant electroencephalographic frequency and amplitude were kept in an acceptable reference range, a green light was visible. When values fell outside this range, a red light appeared. Most of the valuable information contained in the EEG was not visible to the clinician, and the displayed lights were of little value in many cases. Today, some clinicians with no experience in interpreting raw electroencephalographic data are using a processed EEG with little ability to understand how it relates to the original raw data and how artifacts may contaminate the signal and appear as perfectly believable processed electroencephalographic data. Second, the standard 16-channel electroencephalographic montage provides more information than can be practically analyzed or displayed in most processed electroencephalographic monitors and perhaps more than is needed for routine intraoperative use. Studies have not elucidated the optimal number of electroencephalographic channels for intraoperative monitoring, but most available processed electroencephalographic devices use four or fewer channels of information—translating to at most two channels per hemisphere. Processed electroencephalographic devices generally monitor less cerebral territory than a standard 16-channel EEG. Third, some intraoperative changes are unilateral, and some are bilateral. Display of the activity of both hemispheres is necessary to differentiate unilateral (i.e., not caused by global factors such as anesthesia) from bilateral changes. An appropriate number of leads over both hemispheres is needed. The gold standard for intraoperative electroencephalographic monitoring is the continuous visual inspection of a 16- to 32-channel analog EEG by an experienced electroencephalographer.[10,11] Adequate studies comparing processed EEG with fewer channels to this gold standard across multiple uses and operations have not been done, although limited data using processed electroencephalographic monitoring during carotid surgery suggest that two- or four-channel instruments can detect most significant changes.[12,13]

Devices

Two basic forms of electroencephalographic processing are used: power analysis and bispectral analysis. Power analysis uses Fourier transformation to convert the digitized raw electroencephalographic signal into component sine waves of identifiable frequency and amplitude. The raw electroencephalographic data, which are plots of voltage versus time, are converted to plots of frequency and amplitude versus time. Many commercially available processed electroencephalographic machines display power (i.e., voltage or amplitude squared) as a function of frequency and time. These monitors display the data in two general forms: compressed spectral array (CSA) or density spectral array (DSA). In CSA, frequency is displayed along the x axis, and power is displayed along the y axis, with the height of the waveform equal to the power at that frequency. Time is displayed along the z axis. Tracings overlap each other, with the most recent information in front (Fig. 38-4). DSA also displays frequency along the x axis and time along the y axis, and power is reflected by the density of the dots at each frequency. Each display format provides the same data, and the choice depends on the preference of the user.

Many changes that occur during anesthesia and surgery are reflected as changes in amplitude or frequency, or both. These changes can be clearly seen in the displays if adequate and appropriate channels are monitored. Power analysis has been used clinically for many years as a diagnostic tool during procedures with a risk for intraoperative cerebral ischemia such as carotid endarterectomy and cardiopulmonary bypass (CPB). Power analysis has proved to be a sensitive and reliable monitor in the hands of experienced operators using an adequate number of channels. Parameters obtained from power analysis have been investigated as monitors for depth of anesthesia.[14-17] Although earlier attempts to use parameters derived from power analysis for assessment of anesthetic depth were largely unsuccessful, these same parameters are now used to various degrees with much more success as a part of different algorithms (including BIS) to measure hypnotic states.

Bispectral analysis takes into account the phase relationships between the individual components of the raw electroencephalographic signal. These phase relationships

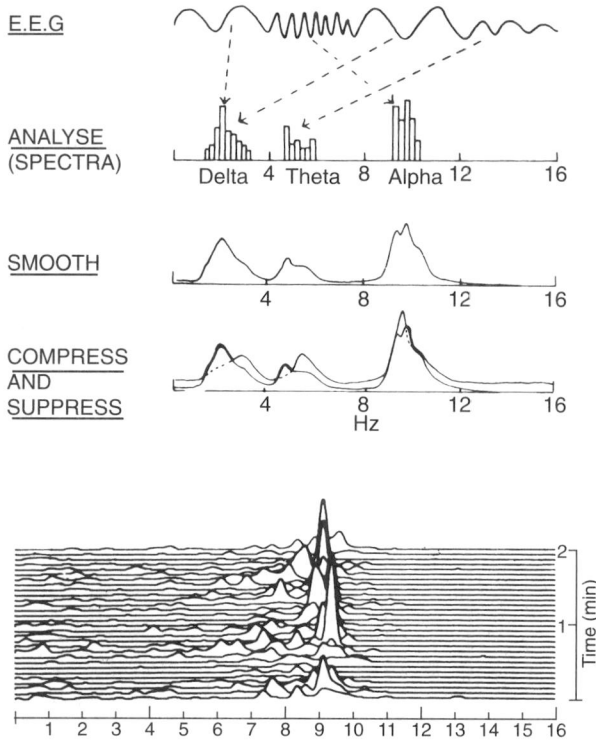

Figure 38–4 Diagram of the technique used to generate a compressed spectral array. Below the traces, the example shows compressed spectra of the α rhythm from a normal subject. (From Stockard JJ, Bickford RG: The neurophysiology of anesthesia. *In* Gordon E [ed]: A Basis and Practice of Neuroanesthesia. New York, Elsevier, 1981, p 3.)

are not included in power analysis. Bispectral analysis has seen extensive use in the past decade, and the primary use of this analysis technique is as a monitor of depth of hypnosis. Although the bispectral analysis may also yield information suggestive of cerebral pathologic states developing intraoperatively, such as cerebral ischemia, it is not recommended by the manufacturer for this use.[18-20]

Data Acquisition Period

An important consideration in the processed EEG is the element of time. The standard EEG is continuous in real time. The processed EEG samples data over a given period (i.e., epoch), processes the data, and then displays information in various formats. There is a relationship between epoch length and spectral resolution. If a long epoch length is chosen, the waveform can be described precisely, but the time required for data processing is long. If a short length of data is sampled, analysis may be done almost in real time, but the epoch chosen for analysis may not be representative of the overall waveform. There may also be insufficient data points for meaningful Fourier transformation. This issue, as related to the use of intraoperative EEG for analysis of anesthetic depth, has been studied by Levy.[21] A longer epoch may produce less epoch-to-epoch variability and allow more precise description of frequency and power; however, the longer epoch increases the delay before new information is processed and displayed, thereby reducing the amount and timeliness of information available for clinical decision-making. In studying epochs of 2 to 32 seconds, Levy concluded that 2-second epochs are appropriate during general anesthesia. Many of the commercially available devices have used 2-second epoch lengths, which are updated at various user-selected intervals. With better and faster computers, continuous monitoring of 2-second epochs is possible.

ANESTHESIA AND THE ELECTROENCEPHALOGRAM

With the advent of the then high-tech EEG in 1950, Courtin and colleagues[22] sought to monitor the brain and devise a servocontrolled system that could adjust the anesthetic concentration administered on the basis of the electroencephalographic pattern. It was an ingenious idea, but despite available descriptions of the EEG during anesthesia, knowledge and technology were not adequate at that time. Even using more modern devices with much higher degrees of computer power, servocontrolled administration of anesthetics remain imperfect at best.[23,24] Because all anesthetic drugs do not produce exactly the same changes in electroencephalographic pattern as anesthesia deepens, generic correlation of the EEG with depth of anesthesia across all anesthetic techniques remains an elusive goal. One of the major reasons that the EEG has been difficult to use for assessing anesthetic depth is that most modern anesthetics use many different classes of drugs, all of which have significant electroencephalographic effects, for premedication, induction, and

Table 38-2 Nonanesthetic factors affecting the electroencephalogram during anesthesia

Surgical Factors	Pathophysiologic Factors
Cardiopulmonary bypass	Hypoxemia
Occlusion of major cerebral vessel (carotid cross-clamping, aneurysm clipping)	Hypotension
Retraction on cerebral cortex	Hypothermia
Surgically induced emboli to the brain	Hypercarbia and hypocarbia
	Metabolic factors

maintenance of anesthesia. Other intraoperative factors may affect the EEG (Table 38-2), adding to the difficulty of its interpretation.

Much research has been directed at developing a processed electroencephalographic parameter that is indicative of depth of anesthesia. These processed parameters fall into two broad categories: parameters derived from power analysis of the raw electroencephalographic data and parameters derived from bispectral analysis of the EEG. Power analysis processes data from the raw EEG related to frequency and amplitude of the waveforms over time but does not consider phase relationships between the component waves. Bispectral analysis is a somewhat more complex process that includes phase relationship data. Several processed electroencephalographic parameters from Fourier analysis have been investigated as indicators of anesthetic depth. These parameters include *spectral edge frequency 95%* (SEF95), which is the frequency below which 95% of the electroencephalographic activity falls; *median frequency* (i.e., frequency at the midpoint of the power spectrum); *peak power frequency* (i.e., frequency with the highest electroencephalographic power), and *relative delta power* (i.e., percent of the EEG power in the delta band). Some investigators have had success in using one or more of these parameters to predict the depth of anesthesia.[14] Others have found that although these parameters change during anesthesia, they were not consistently predictive of depth of anesthesia as assessed by response to stimuli, movement, or return of consciousness during emergence from anesthesia.[25,26] In particular, these parameters depend on the type of anesthetic agent or combination of agents used. Whereas one parameter may correlate well with a primarily volatile anesthetic technique, it may perform less consistently during narcotic-based anesthesia.

Encouraging results have been obtained using the BIS to monitor anesthetic depth (see Chapter 31). The BIS is a processed parameter derived from multiple features generated by bispectral analysis of the EEG. Through clinical trials, features of the bispectral analysis that were predictive of response to stimuli under the effects of a variety of anesthetic agents were identified. These features were combined to a multivariate index using discriminant analysis.[18,27] After the BIS was developed, it was further tested and empirically refined to improve predictive ability.[27]

The BIS is displayed as a numeric value from 0 to 100 and can be trended over time. Many clinical trials have investigated the ability of the BIS to monitor anesthetic depth and predict response to stimuli. Trials have been directed at determining BIS values predictive of loss of consciousness, loss of recall, and prevention of movement in response to surgical stimulation. The BIS value indicative of a certain level of consciousness varies somewhat between different anesthetic techniques[27]; however, the ability of the BIS to predict loss of consciousness and lack of recall during sedation has been consistently demonstrated by a number of investigators using a variety of drugs and drug combinations.[14,27] However, the ability of BIS to predict hemodynamic response to surgical stimulation or movement in response to surgical stimulation has been less consistently demonstrated and may depend more on the anesthetic technique.[28,29] These results have suggested to some that the anesthetic state involves at least two different components. One is a reflection of hypnosis and consists of loss of consciousness and recall; the BIS value is indicative of this state. However, the obtundation of hemodynamic and movement responses to noxious stimuli is less well predicted by the BIS and probably is mainly mediated at the spinal cord level.[27] BIS monitoring of the level of sedation during an awake craniotomy with cortical mapping is shown in Figure 38-5.

Anesthetic drugs affect the frequency and amplitude of electroencephalographic waveforms. Although each drug class and each specific drug has some explicit, dose-related electroencephalographic effects (Table 38-3), some basic anesthesia-related electroencephalographic patterns may be described. Subanesthetic doses of intravenous and inhaled anesthetics usually produce an increase in frontal β activity and abolish the α activity normally seen in the occipital leads in the awake, relaxed patient with the eyes closed. As the patient goes to sleep with general anesthesia, the brain waves become larger in amplitude and slower in frequency. In the frontal areas, small β activity seen in the awake patient slows to the α range and increases in size. In combination with the loss of the occipital α activity, this phenomenon produces the appearance of a shift of the α activity from the posterior cortex to the anterior cortex. Further increases in the dose of the inhalation or intravenous agent produce further slowing of the EEG, and some agents have the capability to totally suppress electroencephalographic activity (see Table 38-3). Other agents (e.g., opioids, benzodiazepines) never produce burst suppression or an isoelectric EEG despite increasing dose because they are incapable of completely suppressing the EEG or because cardiovascular toxicity of the drug (e.g., halothane) prevents administration of a large enough dose.

Intravenous Anesthetics

Barbiturates, Propofol, and Etomidate

Despite widely varying potencies and durations of action, all of the intravenous anesthetics produce similar electroencephalographic patterns. Figure 38-6 shows the electroencephalographic effects of thiopental (see Chapter 10). These drugs all follow the basic anesthesia-related electroencephalographic pattern described previously, with

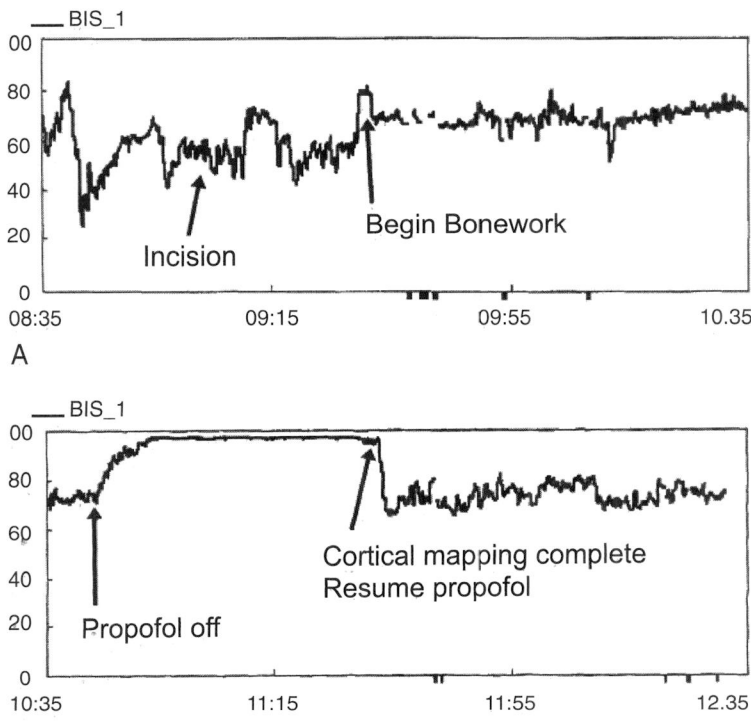

Figure 38–5 Bispectral index (BIS) tracings from an awake craniotomy with intraoperative cortical mapping. Propofol infusion was titrated against the BIS value to provide adequate sedation during the operative procedure. Termination of the propofol infusion during the cortical mapping is followed by a prompt increase in the BIS value and recovery of the patient to a fully alert state.

initial activation (see Fig. 38-6A) followed by dose-related depression. As the patient loses consciousness, characteristic frontal spindles are seen (see Fig. 38-6B), which are replaced by polymorphic 1- to 3-Hz activity (see Fig. 38-6C) as the drug dose is increased. Further increases in dose result in lengthening periods of suppression interspersed with periods of activity (i.e., burst suppression). With a very high dose, electroencephalographic silence results. All these drugs have been reported to cause epileptiform activity in humans, but epileptiform activity is clinically significant only after methohexital and etomidate when given in subhypnotic doses.

Ketamine

Ketamine does not follow the basic anesthesia-related electroencephalographic pattern. Anesthesia with ketamine is characterized by frontally dominant rhythmic, high-amplitude θ activity. Increasing doses produce intermittent polymorphic δ activity of very large amplitude interspersed with low-amplitude β activity.[30] Electrocortical silence cannot be produced with ketamine. Electroencephalographic activity may be very disorganized and variable at all doses. Recovery of normal electroencephalographic activity, even after a single bolus dose of ketamine, is relatively slow compared with barbiturates. There is no information available about the relationship between emergence reactions after ketamine and the EEG. Ketamine has also been associated with increased epileptiform activity.[30]

Benzodiazepines

Despite different potencies and durations of actions, benzodiazepines also follow the basic anesthesia-related electroencephalographic pattern. As a class, however, these drugs are incapable of producing burst suppression or an isoelectric EEG.

Opioids

As a class, opioids do not follow the basic anesthesia-related electroencephalographic pattern. In general, opioids produce a dose-related decrease in frequency and increase in amplitude of the EEG. If no further doses of opiates are given, α and β activity will return as drug redistribution occurs. The rapidity of return depends on the initial dose and on the drug. Remifentanil is associated with the most rapid return to normal.[31] Complete suppression of the EEG cannot be obtained with the opioids. Epileptiform activity occurs in humans and in animals receiving large to supramaximal clinical doses of opioids. For example, sharp wave activity is relatively common after induction of anesthesia with fentanyl, with 20% of patients showing this phenomenon after 30 μg/kg, 60% at 50 μg/kg, 58% at 60 μg/kg, and 80% at 70 μg/kg. This epileptiform activity is mainly observed in the frontotemporal region.[32]

Inhaled Anesthetics

Nitrous Oxide

Used alone, nitrous oxide causes a decrease in amplitude and frequency of the dominant occipital α rhythm (see Chapters 5 to 8). With the onset of analgesia and depressed consciousness, frontally dominant fast oscillatory activity (>30 Hz) is frequently seen.[33] This activity may persist to some extent for up to 50 minutes after discontinuation of nitrous oxide. When nitrous oxide is

Table 38–3 Anesthetic drugs and the electroencephalogram

Drug	Effect on EEG Frequency	Effect on EEG Amplitude of Dominant Frequency	Burst Suppression
Isoflurane			Yes, >1.5 MAC
Subanesthetic	Loss of α, ↑ frontal β	↑	
Anesthetic	Frontal 4-13 Hz activity	↑↑	
Increasing dose >1.5 MAC	Diffuse θ and δ → burst suppression → silence	↑ → 0	
Desflurane	Similar to equi-MAC dose of isoflurane	Similar to equi-MAC dose of isoflurane	Yes, >1.5 MAC
Sevoflurane	Similar to equi-MAC dose of isoflurane	Similar to equi-MAC dose of isoflurane	Yes, >1.5 MAC
Nitrous oxide (alone)	Frontal fast oscillatory activity (>30 Hz)	↑, especially with inspired concentration >50%	No
Enflurane			Yes, >1.5 MAC
Subanesthetic	Loss of α, ↑ frontal β	↑	
Anesthetic	↑ Frontal 7-12 Hz activity	↑	
Increasing dose >1.5 MAC	Spikes/spike and slow waves → burst suppression; hypocapnia → seizures	↑↑ → 0	
Halothane			Not seen in clinically useful dosage range
Subanesthetic	↑ Frontal 10-20 Hz activity	↑	
Anesthetic	↑ Frontal 10-15 Hz activity	↑	
Increasing dose >1.5 MAC	Diffuse θ, slowing with increasing dose	↑	
Barbiturates			Yes, with high doses
Low dose	Fast frontal β activity	Slight ↑	
Moderate dose	Frontal α-frequency spindles	↑	
Increasing high dose	Diffuse δ → burst suppression → silence	↑↑↑ → 0	
Etomidate			Yes, with high doses
Low dose	Fast frontal β activity	↑	
Moderate dose	Frontal α-frequency spindles	↑	
Increasing high dose	Diffuse δ → burst suppression → silence	↑↑ → 0	
Propofol			Yes, with high doses
Low dose	Loss of α, ↑ frontal β	↑	
Moderate dose	Frontal δ, waxing or waning α	↑	
Increasing high dose	Diffuse δ → burst suppression → silence	↑↑ → 0	
Ketamine			No
Low dose	Loss of α, ↑ variability	↑↓	
Moderate dose	Frontal rhythmic δ	↑	
High dose	Polymorphic δ, some β	↑↑ (β is low amplitude)	
Benzodiazepines			No
Low dose	Loss of α, increased frontal β activity	↑	
High dose	Frontally dominant δ and θ	↑	
Opiates			No
Low dose	Loss of β, α slows	↔↑	
Moderate dose	Diffuse θ, some δ	↑	
High dose	δ, often synchronized	↑↑	

EEG, electroencephalographic; MAC, minimum alveolar concentration; α, 8-13 Hz frequency; β, >13 Hz frequency; δ, <4 Hz frequency; θ, 4-7 Hz frequency.

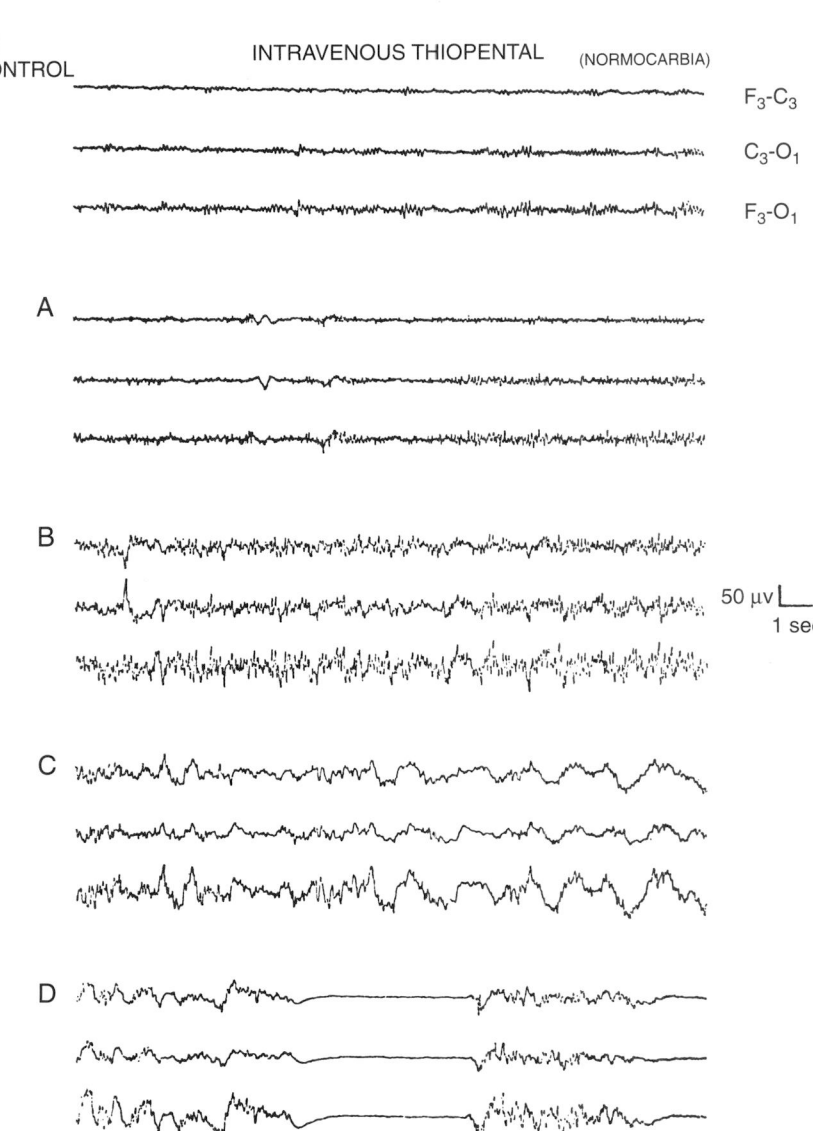

1-1
CONTROL   INTRAVENOUS THIOPENTAL (NORMOCARBIA)

F_3-C_3

C_3-O_1

F_3-O_1

A

B

50 μv
1 sec

C

D

Figure 38–6 Electroencephalographic effects of intravenous administration of thiopental in humans. **A,** Rapid activity. **B,** Barbiturate spindles. **C,** Slow waves. **D,** Burst suppression. (From Clark DL, Rosner BS: Neurophysiologic effects of general anesthetics. Anesthesiology 38:564, 1973.)

used in combination with other agents, it increases the clinical and electroencephalographic effects that are associated with the agent alone.

Isoflurane, Sevoflurane, Enflurane, Halothane, and Desflurane

Potent inhaled anesthetics follow the basic anesthesia-related electroencephalographic pattern. For example, isoflurane initially causes an activation of the EEG, followed by a slowing of the electroencephalographic activity that escalates with increasing dose. Isoflurane begins to produce periods of electroencephalographic suppression at 1.5 minimum alveolar concentration (MAC), which become longer with increasing dose until electrical silence is produced at 2 to 2.5 MAC. Sometimes, isolated epileptiform patterns can be seen during inter-suppression activity at 1.5 to 2.0 MAC of isoflurane.[34] Sevoflurane causes similar dose-dependent electroencephalographic effects. Equi-MAC concentrations of sevoflurane and isoflurane cause similar electroencephalographic changes.[35] Epileptiform activity has been

induced by administration of sevoflurane in patients without epilepsy, and seizure activity on EEG, but not clinical seizure activity, has been reported in pediatric patients with a history of epilepsy during induction of anesthesia with sevoflurane.[36,37] Despite these observations, sevoflurane, like other inhalation agents, is not suitable for use during electrocorticography for localization of seizure foci.[38] The electroencephalographic patterns seen with enflurane are similar to those seen with isoflurane, except that epileptiform activity is considerably more prominent. At 2 to 3 MAC, burst suppression is seen, but virtually all intersuppression activity consists of large spike and wave pattern discharges. Hyperventilation with high concentrations of enflurane increases the length of suppression, decreases the duration of bursts, but increases the amplitude and main frequency component of the intersuppression epileptiform activity. Frank seizures seen on the EEG may also occur with enflurane, which produces the same cerebral metabolic effects as pentylenetetrazol, a known convulsant. Halothane also produces electroencephalographic patterns similar to those of isoflurane, but dosages of halothane that would produce burst suppression on the EEG (3 to 4 MAC) are associated with profound cardiovascular toxicity. Desflurane produces electroencephalographic changes similar in nature to equi-MAC concentrations of isoflurane. In limited clinical studies, there has been no evidence of epileptiform activity with desflurane, despite hyperventilation and 1.6 MAC dosage,[39] and desflurane has been used as a treatment of refractory status epilepticus.[40]

Clinical studies have demonstrated that the EEG of inhalational anesthetic agents is influenced by age and baseline electroencephalographic characteristics. Older patients and those with electroencephalographic slowing at baseline were more sensitive to the electroencephalographic effects of isoflurane and desflurane. As anesthesia was deepened, similar electroencephalographic pattern changes were observed, but these changes occurred at lower end-tidal anesthetic concentrations.[41]

ELECTROENCEPHALOGRAPHIC MONITORING FOR SURGICAL PROCEDURES

Although the EEG has only recently achieved widespread use as a measure of the depth of anesthesia, its use as a monitor of the adequacy of CBF, especially during carotid endarterectomy, has been established for many years. Because anesthetic drugs do affect the EEG (see Table 38-3) and many of these electroencephalographic changes may mimic those associated with inadequate CBF, some guidelines about anesthetic management during electroencephalographic monitoring for cerebral ischemia may be helpful (Table 38-4).

Cardiopulmonary Bypass

In humans, changes that occur with the institution of CPB may alter the EEG by multiple different mechanisms (see Chapters 50 and 51). For example, plasma and brain levels of anesthetic drugs may be altered by CPB or by anesthetic drugs commonly given at the institution of bypass; alterations in arterial carbon dioxide tension and blood pressure may occur; and hemodilution with

Table 38–4	Anesthetic guidelines for intraoperative monitoring for ischemia

No changes in anesthetic technique should be made during critical periods of monitoring (e.g., induced hypotension, carotid clamping, aneurysm clipping).

Avoid major changes in anesthetic gas levels or boluses of opiates, barbiturates, or benzodiazepines near times of increased ischemic risk.

If drugs must be given that create extreme electroencephalographic slowing or an isoelectric pattern (e.g., barbiturates), it is sometimes possible to monitor somatosensory evoked potentials, which may remain relatively unaffected.

hypothermic perfusate usually occurs. These effects, all of which may produce electroencephalographic changes similar to the pathologic changes seen with ischemia, make it difficult to interpret the changes occurring around the time of institution of CPB.

Levy and colleagues[42,43] tried to differentiate the normal effects of hypothermia from other events occurring at the institution of and conclusion of CPB. Initially, they concluded that only a qualitative relationship could be determined, but later, with the use of a much more sophisticated analysis technique (i.e., approximate entropy), electroencephalographic changes associated with changes in temperature could be quantified.

Gugino and colleagues[44] in Boston and Edmonds and colleagues[45] in Louisville attempted to use quantitative (i.e., processed, multiple channel) EEG during CPB to detect cerebral hypoperfusion and relate these changes to postoperative neurologic function. Some minimal work has been done with intervention after detection of cerebral hypoperfusion using quantitative EEG. Such monitoring techniques have not been widely adopted, because although the data appear promising, only a small number of patients have been studied, and there are very few corroborating studies. This type of monitoring is extremely costly in time, personnel, and equipment, and given the lack of convincing outcome data, the cost-benefit ratio is unclear at best. Other investigators have failed to demonstrate any convincing relationship between intraoperative electroencephalographic parameters and postoperative neurologic function, especially in small infants and children.[46] Much work remains to be done studying the use of the processed, quantitative EEG to provide information for clinical management of patients during CPB. None of the currently available studies and recommendations would stand up to a close examination using evidence-based medicine.

Carotid Endarterectomy

Using the EEG during carotid vascular surgery to monitor the balance between oxygen supply and demand in the cerebral cortex is an example of the most accepted intraoperative use for the EEG (see Chapter 52). In a large series of patients undergoing carotid endarterectomy at the Mayo Clinic,[11] the EEG was compared with regional CBF using the ^{133}Xe-washout method. This study validated the EEG as an indicator of the adequacy of regional CBF.

Normal CBF in gray and white matter averages 50 mL/100 g/min. With most anesthetic techniques, the EEG begins to become abnormal when CBF decreases to 20 mL/100 g/min. However, the threshold for electroencephalographic changes appears to be much lower (8 to 10 mL/100 g/min) when isoflurane is used.[47] Cellular survival is not threatened until CBF decreases to 12 mL/100 g/min (lower with isoflurane). The difference in blood flow between when the EEG becomes abnormal and the blood flow at which cellular damage begins to occur provides a rational basis for monitoring with the EEG during carotid surgery. In many cases, prompt detection of electroencephalographic changes may allow intervention (e.g., shunting, increasing cerebral perfusion pressure) to restore CBF before onset of permanent neurologic damage. Standard hemodynamic monitoring provides no direct information about the adequacy of CBF. Blood pressure is not a specific indicator of the adequacy of CBF. Significant hypotension is not predictably associated with electroencephalographic evidence of cerebral ischemia. One study demonstrated that treatment of decreased blood pressure during carotid vascular surgery with phenylephrine resulted in a significant incidence of left ventricular wall motion abnormalities.[48] This finding suggests that treatment of hypotension with phenylephrine should be undertaken only when there is evidence of hypoperfusion on the ECG or EEG.

Severe anemia and decreases in oxygen saturation also decrease oxygen delivery. Electroencephalographic activity becomes abnormal after increased blood flow cannot compensate for decreased arterial oxygen content.

Serious intraoperative reduction in cerebral oxygen supply may result from surgical factors (e.g., carotid cross-clamping) that are usually beyond the anesthesiologist's control and from factors that the anesthesiologist can correct. Reduced CBF produced by hyperventilation, hypotension, or temporary occlusion of major blood vessels sometimes is corrected by reducing ventilation, by restoring normal blood pressure, or in the case of temporary vessel occlusion, by increasing blood pressure above normal. Because the cerebral ischemia may be readily detected by the EEG, electroencephalographic monitoring may be used to evaluate the effectiveness of therapy instituted to correct ischemia.

Ideally, electroencephalographic use is continuous; however, it has been described most frequently as a spot check to determine the need for shunt placement after carotid cross-clamping in anesthetized patients. This short-term use detects only a small portion of the neurologic injuries that can occur during and after carotid surgery. Critical carotid luminal narrowing risks cerebral hypoperfusion during hypotension or positioning. These problems are missed if the EEG is not monitored continuously.

If monitoring of the EEG could be proved scientifically to reduce the incidence of stroke, electroencephalographic monitoring during carotid surgery would be a clear standard of care. Data demonstrating this, however, do not yet exist. What information is available does not provide a basis to recommend universal use of electroencephalographic monitoring during carotid surgery. In a large series of patients undergoing carotid endarterectomy with selective shunting who were monitored with 16-channel unprocessed EEG, no patient awakened with a new neurologic deficit that was not predicted by the EEG.[49] Transient, correctable electroencephalographic changes were not associated with stroke. Persistent changes were associated with stroke. This study, however, had no comparison group analyzing stroke rate when electroencephalographic monitoring was not used during surgery. Because the EEG detects reductions in CBF that would not otherwise be apparent in unmonitored patients and permits intervention that may correct the problem (usually placement of a shunt), electroencephalographic monitoring should be useful in reducing the incidence of stroke when selective shunting is used.

More difficult to prove is that electroencephalographic monitoring is useful when all patients are shunted during carotid clamping. Such monitoring has detected correctable shunt malfunction, and investigators have described hypotension-related electroencephalographic changes in patients with critical stenoses and poor collateral circulation.[50] Advocates of selective shunting based on electroencephalographic (or other monitoring) criteria claim that inserting a shunt unnecessarily through a region of diseased vessel will surely increase embolization. A multicenter study of 1495 carotid endarterectomies provides some evidence that shunting of patients without evidence of decreased cerebral perfusion increases the incidence of stroke more than sixfold.[51] Although this study effectively advocates that selective shunting using some form of monitoring of the adequacy of CBF should improve perioperative stroke rate, an analysis by the Cochrane Stroke Group[52] failed to demonstrate sufficient evidence to advocate for routine shunting, selective shunting, or even no shunting at all. Until adequate studies addressing this issue are performed, it is unlikely that electroencephalographic monitoring during carotid vascular surgery will be proved useful.

Processed EEG has also been used during carotid vascular surgery. Two issues influence the efficacy and reliability of processed EEG as a monitor for cerebral ischemia. First, what is the minimum number of channels (i.e., areas of the brain) to be monitored? The 16-channel unprocessed EEG is a reliable and sensitive monitor for intraoperative cerebral ischemia during carotid endarterectomy. In a series of more than 2000 patients monitored with 16-channel EEG at the Mayo Clinic, there were no false-negative results[49]; no patient had undetected intraoperative cerebral injury. However, 16-channel EEG monitored by a dedicated technician is not available in most operating rooms where carotid surgery is performed. Processed EEGs using fewer than 16 channels are therefore used much more commonly. Clinical experience and clinical investigations suggest that the minimum number of channels for adequate sensitivity and specificity is four channels (i.e., two per side).[12] When a limited number of channels was compared with monitoring with a 16-channel EEG, 100% sensitivity and specificity were obtained using two channels per hemisphere, provided the channels monitored the middle cerebral artery territory. These results were obtained with the combination of a frontoparietal channel with a frontotemporal channel.[12]

The second issue is the experience level of the observer monitoring the processed EEG. Is a dedicated, experienced technician or electroencephalographer needed? In a study addressing this question, the 16-channel unprocessed EEG monitored by a dedicated technician was compared with a processed EEG reviewed by three anesthesiologists of different levels of experience with processed EEG. Fifty patients undergoing carotid endarterectomy were studied to compare the processed EEG with the full 16-channel EEG and regional CBF measurements as indicators of cerebral ischemia.[13] The three anesthesiologists interpreted the tracings without knowledge of the case. They were presented only with the written trace with an indication of the point at which

Figure 38–7 This Lifescan printout was obtained approximately 3 minutes after occlusion (XC) of the left carotid artery. It shows attenuation of activity on the left with occlusion. The electroencephalogram showed a similar change. The regional cerebral blood flow with occlusion was 9 mL/100 g/min. (From Spackman TN, Faust RJ, Cucchiara RF, et al: A comparison of a periodic analysis of the EEG with standard EEG and cerebral blood flow for detection of ischemia. Anesthesiology 66:229, 1987.)

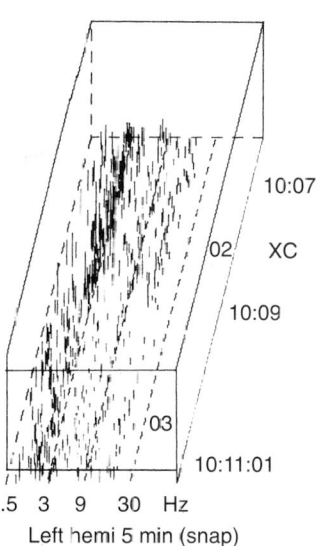

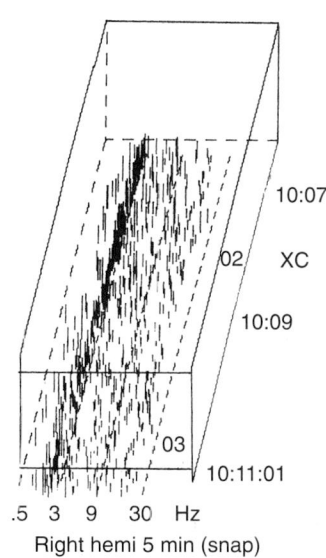

the carotid was clamped (Fig. 38-7). In these cases, the most important interpretation pitfall to avoid is the false-negative pattern. If the clinician interprets the EEG as demonstrating adequate CBF when it does not, the surgeon may fail to shunt an ischemic patient. A false-positive result may be less of a problem because the patient is not ischemic but is given a shunt anyway. In this case, only the risk of emboli from the possibly unnecessary shunt is incurred. The positive predictive value of the anesthesiologist correctly interpreting the trace as unchanged after clamping was 91% to 98%, which indicates that the device can be used by relatively novice interpreters with fair accuracy to determine the presence of cerebral ischemia at the time of carotid occlusion. In this study, the review by the anesthesiologist was not carried out during the course of the procedure but rather "off line." As such, it does not address the issue of whether an anesthesiologist providing the intraoperative anesthetic management of the patient can provide adequate monitoring of the processed EEG simultaneously.

Electroencephalographic monitoring does have limitations. Despite the data available from the Mayo Clinic, immediately evident postoperative strokes have been reported in patients without any evidence of electroencephalographic changes intraoperatively. In my (M.E.M.) experience, such strokes result from emboli through the lenticulostriate arteries to subcortical structures that do not generate or affect the EEG but are critically involved in the descending motor pathway. Overall, however, such events are rare.

Surgery for Epileptic Foci

It has long been recognized that seizures can begin with an anatomic focus of electrical synchrony that spreads to include the remainder of the cortex. Precise intraoperative localization of such a focus is an important part of surgery for drug-resistant seizures. This localization is performed by electrocorticography in the awake patient or by provocative techniques (discussed later), if necessary, during general anesthesia. Alternatively, a grid of subdural electrodes or depth electrodes may be placed in the anesthetized patient, with their locations based on preoperative surface electroencephalographic recordings and imaging studies. Subsequent detailed mapping is done in the awake patient in the electroencephalography laboratory over a period of several days to a week. The patient then returns to the operating room for resection of the excitable focus under local or general anesthesia. When intraoperative localization is desired, the anesthetic level is minimized, and a provocative technique such as hyperventilation or small-dose barbiturate (most commonly methohexital) administration can be employed to trigger the focus, aiding in its localization. If the cortex is excessively depressed pharmacologically, seizure activity cannot be provoked. Intraoperative seizure mapping requires the involvement of an electroencephalographer familiar with this technique. Rarely would an anesthesiologist possess the expertise required for intraoperative seizure focus localization.

PATHOPHYSIOLOGIC EFFECTS ON THE ELECTROENCEPHALOGRAM

Hypoxia

Hypoxia may produce inadequate delivery of oxygen to the cerebral cortex generating the EEG, and changes similar to those occurring with ischemia result. Initially, hypoxemia may not result in any electroencephalographic changes because the brain can increase blood flow to compensate. After the hypoxemia becomes severe enough, further increases in flow are impossible, and electroencephalographic changes occur. Slowing of the EEG during hypoxia is a nonspecific global effect.

Fast frequencies are lost, and low frequencies dominate. Eventually, the EEG is abolished as the brain shuts down electrical activity and diverts all oxygen delivered to the maintenance of cellular integrity.

Hypotension

In the normal, awake patient, significant levels of hypotension seem to be needed to cause the earliest of central nervous system (CNS) signs, as measured by discrimination tests such as the flicker-fusion test. This test examines the flicker rate at which the observer perceives the light to be continuous. In the early days of deliberate hypotension, this test was part of the preoperative evaluation to judge how far the pressure could be reduced for surgery. Clear signs of confusion and an inability to concentrate or respond properly to simple commands generally represent very low levels of cerebral perfusion when caused by hypotension because the normal cerebral circulation has a large capacity to vasodilate and maintain normal flow in the face of significant hypotension. The electroencephalographic changes associated with even this level of hypotension are not dramatic, although they are clear by comparison with a previously active recording. Herein lies the problem with using intraoperative EEG to determine whether a given level of hypotension has resulted in brain ischemia. Electroencephalographic changes are not very pronounced and are bilateral. These changes are also nearly identical to those caused by increasing doses of many anesthetic drugs. Electroencephalographic changes associated with hypotension can be detected, but when the hypotension is induced slowly and associated with changes in anesthetic drugs (e.g., use of isoflurane to reduce blood pressure), the changes are very difficult to interpret. Electroencephalographic changes associated with acute, severe hypotension, such as may be caused by sudden arrhythmias, are easier to read. A tracing of the effect of hypotension on the compressed spectral array is shown in Figure 38-8.[53]

Many patients undergoing surgery do not have a normal cerebral circulation. In these individuals, even mild hypotension may result in significant cerebral ischemia, and monitoring the EEG during planned hypotension may be very helpful, provided other causes of similar electroencephalographic changes can be carefully controlled. Little literature supports the use of electroencephalographic monitoring during hypotension, but in our opinion, when the EEG is being monitored (e.g., during carotid surgery), the changes caused by hypotension do represent cerebral ischemia of a significant degree and should be considered an important finding.

Hypothermia

During cooling for CPB, the total power and peak power frequency of the high-frequency band are highly correlated with temperature using Fourier analysis and spectral edge data; however, there is significant variability between subjects, especially during cooling.[53] Complete electroencephalographic suppression[43] usually develops at 15°C to 18°C. Levy and colleagues[43] demonstrated an improved ability to quantify the effects of hypothermia

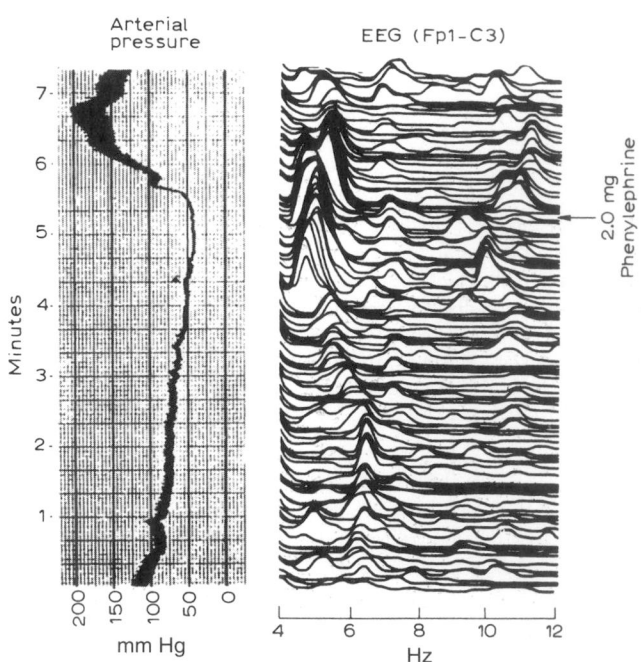

Figure 38–8 Changes in the compressed spectral array during hypotension. (From Stockard JJ, Bickford RG: The neurophysiology of anesthesia. *In* Gordon E [ed]: A Basis and Practice of Neuroanesthesia. New York, Elsevier, 1981, p 3.)

on the EEG using a processing technique known as *approximate entropy.*

Hypercarbia and Hypocarbia

Hyperventilation activates excitable seizure foci, and in rare cases, it may produce electroencephalographic evidence of cerebral ischemia even in awake subjects.[54] Hypoventilation, unless severe and associated with hypoxemia, has only indirect effects resulting from increased CBF. In the anesthetized patient, hypoventilation-associated increases in CBF may have effects similar to those seen with increasing end-tidal tension of volatile anesthetics.[55]

Untoward Events

One of the suggested reasons for monitoring the brain of the anesthetized patient is to enable detection of injuries to the nervous system that would not be otherwise apparent. Although there are hundreds of such case reports in the literature and many in our experience, the cost-effectiveness of such monitoring is not clear. In a case being prepared for publication, severe electroencephalographic changes occurred at the beginning of a carotid endarterectomy, before surgical incision, and were not associated with any other vital sign changes or hypotension. Immediate angiography revealed acute carotid occlusion and completely changed the operation performed, and the patient recovered completely. Some intraoperative events may lead to a CNS insult that, if detected early, can be rapidly reversed or treated to prevent permanent injury. However, given the rarity of such

Table 38–5   Criteria for determination of brain death

Absent cerebral and brainstem functions
Well-defined, irreversible cause
Persistent absence of all brain function after observation or treatment
Hypothermia, drug intoxication, metabolic encephalopathy, and shock excluded

Adapted from Darby JM, Stein K, Grenvik A, et al: Approach to management of the heart beating "brain dead" organ donor. JAMA 261:2222, 1989.

events, it is extremely unlikely that such monitoring could be shown to be beneficial in any foreseeable randomized trial. If the at-risk patient can be identified preoperatively, electroencephalographic monitoring may be useful in detecting untoward CNS events during anesthesia, such as a new stroke after elective general surgery.

Brain Death

The clinical diagnosis of brain death (see Chapter 79) is made when there is demonstration of the absence of all cerebral and brain stem function (Table 38-5). Various clinical tests have been devised to diagnose brain death (Table 38-6). Apnea testing is accepted as an essential component of the evaluation; however, electrocerebral silence on the EEG, when not confounded by the presence of high-dose barbiturates, metabolic encephalopathy, or very young age, supports the diagnosis of brain death.[51,56]

INTRAOPERATIVE MONITORING OF SENSORY EVOKED RESPONSES

Electroencephalographic signals provide information about cortical function but little or no information about neural pathways important to the daily function of

Table 38–6   Clinical tests of brain death

Cerebral unresponsiveness
No spontaneous motor activity
Absent pupillary, corneal, and oculocephalic or oculovestibular reflexes
Absent cough reflex with deep tracheal suctioning
No increase in heart rate in response to intravenous administration of atropine (2 mg)
No respiratory efforts on apnea testing ($Paco_2 > 60$ mm Hg)
Electrocerebral silence documented by electroencephalography in the absence of drug effect (desirable)

From Darby JM, Stein K, Crenvik A, et al: Approach to management of the heart beating "brain dead" organ donor. JAMA 261:2222, 1989.

the patient Intraoperative monitoring of SERs has gained increasing popularity over the past several decades because it provides the ability to monitor the functional integrity of sensory pathways in the anesthetized patient undergoing surgical procedures placing these pathways at risk. Because motor pathways are often adjacent anatomically to these sensory pathways or supplied by the same blood vessels, function of motor pathways may be, albeit imperfectly, inferred from the function of these sensory pathways.

SERs are electrical CNS responses to electrical, auditory, or visual stimuli. SERs are produced by stimulating a sensory system and recording the resulting electrical responses at various sites along the sensory pathway up to and including the cerebral cortex. Because of the very-low-amplitude of SERs (0.1 to 10 µV), it is often not possible to distinguish SERs from other background biologic signals such as those on the EEG or EMG that may be considered in this case undesirable noise. To extract the SER from the background noise, the recorded signal is digitized, and signal averaging is applied. With this technique, signal recording is time-locked to the application of the sensory stimulus. For example, during intraoperative SER monitoring of the median nerve, only signal information occurring less than 50 msec after the stimulus is recorded after nerve stimulation at the wrist. The SER occurs at a constant time after the stimulus application; other electrical activity such as spontaneous electroencephalographic activity occurs at random intervals after the sensory stimulus. The averaging technique improves the SER signal-to-noise ratio by eliminating random elements and enhancing the SER. This enhancing effect increases directly with the square root of the number of responses added into the averaged response.

SER recordings are of two general types determined by the distance of the recording electrode from the neural generator of the evoked response. SERs recorded from electrodes close to the neural generators (within approximately 3 to 4 cm in the average adult) are called *near-field potentials*.[57] Near-field potentials are transmitted to the recording electrode by propagated conduction along a discrete neural pathway,[58] and the morphology is directly affected by electrode location.[57] *Far-field potentials* are recorded from electrodes located a greater distance from the neural generator and are conducted to the recording electrode through a volume conductor (i.e., brain, cerebrospinal fluid, and membranes). It is more difficult to locate the source of the recorded signal because the current spreads diffusely throughout the conducting medium, and the electrode position has little effect on the morphology of the recorded evoked potential.[57,58] As the distance between the recording electrode and the neural generator increases, the recorded SER becomes smaller. More responses have to be averaged to record far-field potentials (up to several thousand) than near-field potentials (as few as 50 to 100).[57,58]

SERs may also be described as cortical or subcortical in origin. *Cortical responses* are generated by a summation of excitatory and inhibitory postsynaptic potentials produced by neurons in the gray matter. *Subcortical responses* may arise from many different structures, depending on the type of response, including peripheral nerves, spinal cord,

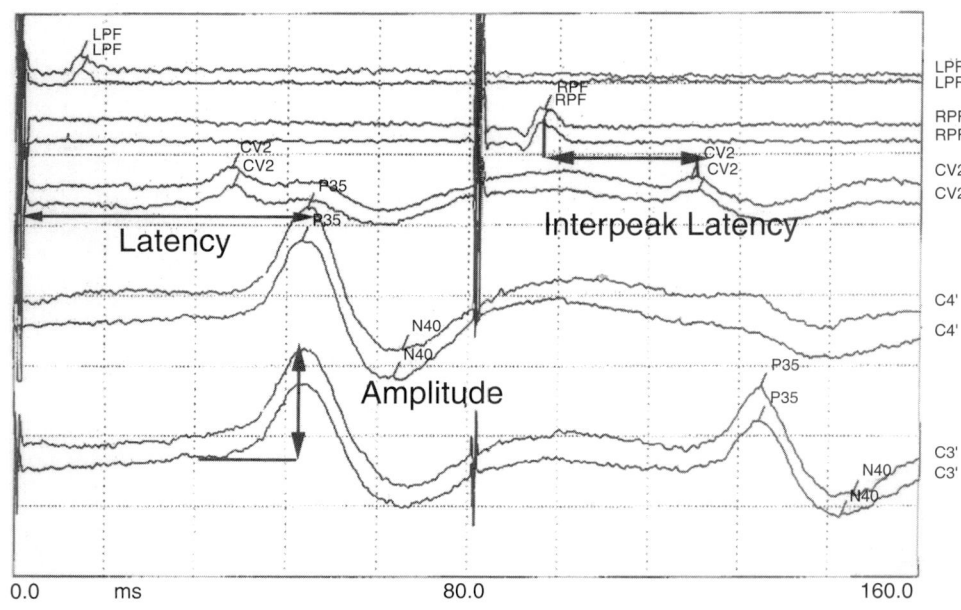

Figure 38–9 Sensory evoked responses are described in terms of latency (*upper left*) and amplitude (*lower left*). Interpeak latency is the measured time between two peaks. Interpeak latency may be measured between two peaks in the same channel or between peaks in different channels (*upper right*).

brainstem, thalamus, cranial nerves, and others. Cortical SERs are usually recorded from scalp electrodes placed according to the standard 10-20 system for electroencephalographic recordings (see Fig. 38-1). Subcortical evoked responses may also be recorded far-field from scalp electrodes or, as appropriate, from electrodes placed over the spinal column or peripheral nerve.

SERs are described in terms of latency and amplitude (Fig. 38-9). *Latency* is defined as the time measured from the application of the stimulus to the onset or peak (depending on convention used) of the SER. The *amplitude* is the voltage of the recorded response. According to convention, deflections below the baseline are labeled positive (P), and those above the baseline are negative (N). Standard identification of waveforms is by letter designating the direction of the deflection followed by a number representing the latency of that waveform (e.g., N14). Because amplitude and latency change with recording circumstances, normal values must be established for each neurologic monitoring laboratory and may differ somewhat from values recorded in other laboratories. SERs used for intraoperative monitoring include SSEPs, BAEPs, and rarely, VEPs. For all these techniques, recording electrodes are placed on the scalp, using the same standard 10-20 system as for recording the EEG and in various standardized subcortical locations. The surgical incision and the need for sterility may necessitate nonstandard electrode placements. Such deviations must be considered when interpreting baseline and subsequent SERs (Fig. 38-10).

NORMAL   ANESTHETIZED

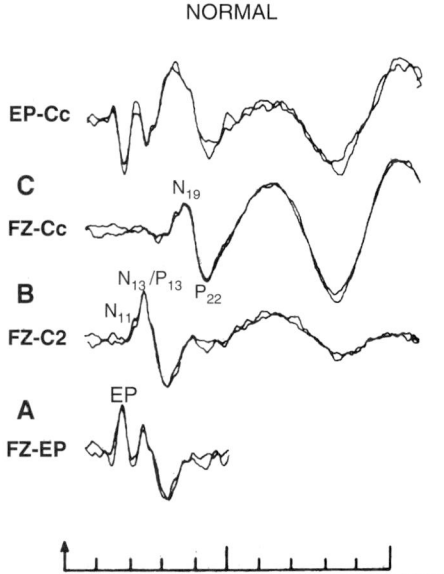

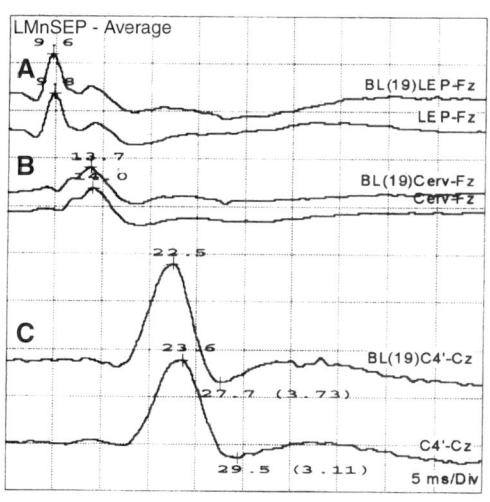

Figure 38–10 Short-latency somatosensory evoked potentials are produced by stimulation of the median nerve at the wrist. The ability to identify each of the labeled peaks shown in the tracing from the awake patient is compromised by the anesthetic state and use of different recording electrode locations. Corresponding tracings are labeled with the same letter. (Adapted from Chiappa KH, Ropper AH: Evoked potentials in clinical medicine. N Engl J Med 306:1205, 1982.)

Intraoperative changes in SERs, such as decreased amplitude, increased latency, or complete loss of the waveform, may result from surgical trespass or ischemia, or they may reflect systemic changes such as changes in anesthetic drug administration, temperature changes, or hypoperfusion. When these changes are detected and considered to be significant, the anesthesiologist or surgeon can make changes to relieve or lessen the insult to the monitored pathway. Interventions by the anesthesiologist are directed at improving perfusion to the nervous tissue at risk and include increasing arterial blood pressure, especially if induced hypotension is used or if the patient's pressure has fallen to below the preoperative level; transfusion if significant anemia is present; volume expansion; augmentation of cardiac output; and normalization of arterial blood gas tensions if indicated. Alterations in SERs may warn the surgeon of direct injury to nervous tissue in the operative field. For example, changes in SERs after retractor placement during a craniotomy or after compression of the blood supply to the spinal cord from spinal column distraction promptly allow the surgeon and the anesthesiologist to make appropriate changes to the operative procedure and anesthetic management that may prevent or minimize any postoperative neurologic deficit.

The degree and duration of SER changes that can be tolerated by patients during surgery is not well known or studied. Tolerance limits for the degree of change in SER signals or duration of complete loss of waveform before permanent neurologic dysfunction occurs are not clearly defined. Such ambiguity, unfortunately, is all too common among intraoperative monitors. For example, although we do know that increased frequency and duration of ST-depression during coronary bypass surgery is associated with an increased risk of perioperative infarction, exact limits for the degree and duration of ST-segment depression for surgery do not exist and probably vary significantly from patient to patient. Many centers using intraoperative SER monitoring define decreases in amplitude of 50% or more from baseline associated with a more than 10% prolongation in latency as clinically significant SER changes. Uncorrected, such changes are associated in clinical series and in case reports with onset of new postoperative neurologic deficits. As a result, such changes are immediately investigated. In practice, however, any SER changes directly associated with a surgical event are considered clinically significant, even if the magnitude of change is less than described earlier. Changes in SER that do not progress to complete loss of the waveform are less likely to be associated with a major new postoperative neurologic deficit. Complete loss of the SER waveform intraoperatively without recovery is highly likely to be associated with a major new deficit. If the SER recovers spontaneously or after intraoperative interventions, the likelihood of neurologic injury depends on the procedure and the duration of the SER loss. For example, in one study of aortic vascular surgery where SSEPs were monitored, loss of the SSEP waveform for less than 15 minutes was not associated with a new permanent neurologic deficit, whereas complete loss of the SSEP for longer periods was increasingly likely to

reflect permanent neurologic injury, even if the response recovered completely to normal during surgery.[59]

The operating room is a hostile environment for recording SERs. Because these potentials have very small amplitudes, the electrical noise that is quite common in most operating rooms often interferes with recording of good-quality SERs. Biologic noise, such as the cardiac electrical activity (i.e., electrocardiographic activity) and muscle movement or increased tone (i.e., electromyographic activity), may obscure the desired evoked response. To successfully record SERs in the operating room environment, these sources of noise must be recognized and the appropriate action taken to allow recording of the desired evoked response (e.g., unnecessary electrical equipment unplugged, small doses of muscle relaxant given to minimize electromyographic activity). Several physiologic changes and drugs administered intraoperatively can result in changes in the SERs unrelated to potential injury to nervous tissue. These factors must be recognized, minimized if possible, and included in the differential diagnosis as changes in SERs are detected intraoperatively. One of the most important principles of recording SERs intraoperatively is that reproducible, reliable tracings must be obtained at baseline before any intervention likely to cause changes in the evoked response. If good-quality tracings with identifiable waveforms cannot be recorded and reproduced at baseline, SER monitoring will be of little use in monitoring the integrity of the CNS intraoperatively. If significant variability exists or waveforms are difficult to identify, it will not be possible intraoperatively to distinguish SER changes that are clinically significant from a preexisting baseline variability of waveforms. When good, reproducible responses cannot be recorded at baseline, monitoring should not be used for clinical decision-making.

Somatosensory Evoked Potentials

SSEPs are recorded after electrical stimulation of a peripheral mixed nerve. Stimulation is provided most commonly with surface electrodes (e.g., electroencephalographic electrodes) placed on the skin above the nerve or with fine-needle electrodes. A square wave stimulus of 50 to 250 μsec duration is delivered to the peripheral nerve, and the intensity is adjusted to produce a minimal muscle contraction. Increasing the stimulus intensity beyond the sum of the motor and sensory threshold does not influence the amplitude or latency of the recorded evoked potential.[55] On a practical basis, however, many laboratories do not establish SSEP monitoring until after the patient is already anesthetized and paralyzed. In these cases, stimulus intensity is increased until no further increase in response size occurs at any recording site, and constant current stimulation of 20 to 50 mA is quite commonly used. For comparison, consider supramaximal stimulation used for neuromuscular blockade monitoring, commonly 80 mA. The rate of stimulation varies from 1 to 6 Hz. The common sites of stimulation include median nerve at the wrist, common peroneal nerve at the knee, and posterior tibial nerve at the ankle.[60] The tongue, trigeminal nerve, pudendal nerve, and ulnar nerve have also been studied,[60] but intraoperative experience with monitoring these nerves is limited.

SSEP responses consist of short- and long-latency waveforms. Short-latency SSEPs are most commonly recorded intraoperatively, because they are less influenced by changes in anesthetic drug levels. The pathways involved in the generation of upper extremity short-latency SSEPs include large-fiber sensory nerves with their cell bodies in the dorsal root ganglia and central processes traveling rostrally in the ipsilateral posterior column of the spinal cord and synapsing in the dorsal column nuclei at the cervicomedullary junction (i.e., first-order fibers), second-order fibers crossing and traveling to the contralateral thalamus through the medial lemniscus, and third-order fibers from the thalamus to the frontoparietal sensorimotor cortex.[55] These primary cortical evoked responses, which are recordable with most anesthetic techniques, result from the earliest electrical activity generated by the cortical neurons and are thought to arise from the postcentral sulcus parietal neurons. The longer-latency secondary cortical responses are thought to arise in the association cortex. These responses have much greater variability in the awake patient,[58] habituate rapidly on repetitive stimulation,[57] and are not reproducible during general anesthesia. Cortical SSEPs other than the primary cortical response are not monitored or interpreted intraoperatively because they are severely altered by general anesthesia.[57]

Whereas most evidence indicates that upper extremity evoked potentials are conducted rostrally in the spinal cord through dorsal column pathways, many data suggest that lower extremity SSEPs are conducted substantially by the lateral funiculus.[61] Stimulation of the posterior tibial nerve or common peroneal nerve at or above motor threshold activates group I fibers that synapse and travel rostrally through the dorsal spinocerebellar tract. After synapsing in nucleus Z at the spinomedullary junction, the pathway crosses and projects onto the ventral posterolateral thalamic nucleus.[62] Studies with dogs, cats, and monkeys support the concept that lower extremity SERs are conducted in all quadrants of the spinal cord but primarily in the dorsal lateral funiculus.[63,64] This pathway difference is important because the dorsal lateral funiculus is supplied primarily by the anterior spinal artery, the artery that also supplies the descending motor pathway and neurons in the spinal cord. Manipulations such as distraction of the spinal column to correct scoliosis, which may secondarily compress or distort radicular blood supply to the anterior spinal cord, should cause changes in the SSEP in the event blood supply is reduced to critical levels. This hypothesis is verified by the very low, but not zero, incidence of postoperative paraplegia on awakening without any intraoperative changes in SSEP.

For SSEP recordings with median nerve stimulation, recording electrodes (i.e., usually electrocardiographic pads) are first placed at Erb's point, just above the midpoint of the clavicle. This point overlies the brachial plexus, and signals recorded here assure the clinician that the stimulus is being delivered properly to the patient. The next electrode (i.e., an electrocardiographic pad or a gold cup electrode) is placed midline posteriorly over the neck at level of the second cervical vertebra, relatively

near the dorsal column nuclei. Signals recorded here ensure proper transmission of the response from the peripheral nervous system into the spinal cord and rostral along the spinal cord to the lower medulla. The final electrodes (i.e., gold cup electrodes or needle electrodes) are placed on the scalp overlying the sensory (parietal) cortex contralateral to the stimulated limb. Signals recorded here ensure the integrity of the pathway through the brainstem, thalamus, and internal capsule and may also assess adequacy of CBF in this area of the cortex.[65-69] For recording SSEPs after posterior tibial nerve stimulation, electrodes (i.e., electrocardiographic pads) are placed first over the popliteal fossa to ensure proper stimulus delivery to the nervous system. Electrodes may also be placed over the lower lumbar spine to ensure proper transmission of the signal into the spinal cord itself, but this site is not commonly used because of the proximity of sterile surgical incisions. Cervical spine and scalp recording electrodes are placed in a fashion similar to that described earlier, although different locations may be used as required by the placement of the surgical incision.

More invasive recording methods may also be used intraoperatively. These methods, although introducing an element of risk to the patient, have the advantage of producing much larger signals. For example, cortical SSEPs may be recorded from electrodes placed directly on the cerebral cortex, and subcortical potentials may be recorded using electrodes placed invasively into bone, ligament, or the epidural space in or near the operative site.[57]

Purported neural generators for short-latency SSEPs are listed in Table 38-7 and Figure 38-10.[57,60] Induction of anesthesia and use of different recording electrode locations (i.e., montage), necessitated by the surgical incision, may significantly alter the appearance of the SSEP. In these cases, attribution of a particular generator to a given wave on the tracing may be quite difficult. During neurologic monitoring, such precision is not needed, and recorded waveforms are compared with tracings obtained at baseline and during earlier portions of the surgical procedure. After lower limb stimulation, absolute latencies are increased because of the greater distance the response to stimulation must travel along the peripheral sensory nerve and spinal cord. Interpeak latencies (see Fig. 38-9)

Table 38–7 Generators of somatosensory evoked potentials after median nerve stimulation

Peak Waveforms	Neural Generators
N9 (EP)	Brachial plexus*
N11	Posterior columns or spinal roots
N13/P13	Dorsal column nuclei*
N14,15	Brainstem or thalamus
N19/P22	Parietal sensory cortex*

*Indicates sites commonly recorded during surgery. Other waveforms indicated are not commonly monitored.
EP, Erb point; N, indicates negative for the number of milliseconds between the stimulus and response; P, indicates positive for the number of milliseconds between the stimulus and response.

are also evaluated to assess specific conduction times such as N9 to N14 conduction time, reflecting transmission time from the brachial plexus to brainstem, or the N14 to N19 conduction time, reflecting transmission time between the dorsal column nuclei and the primary sensory cortex.[70]

Surgical Procedures Monitored with Somatosensory Evoked Potentials

For SSEP monitoring to benefit a patient, the neurologic pathway monitored must be potentially at risk during the procedure, and if SSEP changes occur, an option for intervention must exist. If both criteria are not true, monitoring is likely to offer little benefit to the patient. To optimize conditions for SSEP monitoring, the anesthesiologist should choose an anesthetic technique that does not markedly depress the SSEP, and the anesthetic depth and physiologic state of the patient should remain as constant as possible during periods of potential surgical injury to the monitored pathway. Reliable baseline tracings should be obtained before any intervention.

Intraoperative recording of SSEPs has been used to assess the functional integrity of the sensory pathways during operative procedures that place these pathways at risk as a result of surgical trespass along the course of the peripheral nerve, within the spinal canal, or in the brain or when there is potential for damage to the sensory pathway or compromise of its vascular supply. SSEP monitoring has also been used to assess the integrity of anatomically adjacent structures that are more difficult to monitor directly, such as the motor tracts. Intraoperative SSEP monitoring has been described for a wide variety of procedures, including correction of scoliosis with instrumentation[71,72]; spinal cord decompression and stabilization after acute spinal cord injury[73,74]; spinal fusion[75]; brachial plexus exploration after injury to the plexus[76]; resection of spinal cord tumor, cyst, or vascular lesion[77]; correction of cervical spondylosis[77]; resection of fourth ventricular cyst[77]; release of a tethered cord[77]; resection of intracranial vascular lesions involving the sensory cortex[77]; clipping of intracranial aneurysms[59]; carotid endarterectomy[78]; resection of thalamic tumor[79]; surgical correction after thoracic spine fracture[80]; abdominal and thoracic aortic aneurysm repair[55]; and repair of coarctation of the aorta.[81]

Two intraoperative uses of SSEPs have been most successful and deserve special mention. Intraoperative monitoring of SSEPs has been used most often in patients undergoing surgical procedures involving the spinal column or spinal cord, or both. Extensive experience has been gained in patients who have decompressive laminectomies or who have undergone corrective procedures for scoliosis. Intraoperative changes in SSEPs have been observed in 2.5% to 65% of patients undergoing surgical procedures on the spine or spinal cord.[72,75,80,82] When these changes are promptly reversed spontaneously or with interventions by the surgeon or anesthesiologist (e.g., lessening the degree of spine straightening in scoliosis surgery, increasing arterial blood pressure), the patients most often have preserved neurologic function postoperatively. When these changes persisted, however, the patients most often awakened with worsened neurologic function.

False-negative (rare) and false-positive (common) results have been reported with SSEP monitoring during spinal surgery. Patients with intact SSEPs throughout the procedure have awakened with a new significant neurologic deficit, but the total reported incidence of this finding is far less than 1% of all cases monitored. However, patients with no postoperative neurologic deficit commonly experience significant (as defined earlier) changes in intraoperative SSEPs.[82] This monitoring pattern is most commonly caused by failure to control for other, nonpathologic factors that may alter the SSEP. Overall, the reliability of properly performed SSEP monitoring to predict the postoperative sensory and motor function has been excellent.[57,77,80] However, motor tracts are not directly monitored by SSEPs. The blood supply to the dorsal columns of the spinal cord that carry all of the upper extremity SSEP, and at least a portion of the lower extremity SSEP, is derived primarily from the posterior spinal arteries. The blood supply to motor tracts and neurons is derived primarily from the anterior spinal artery. It is therefore possible for a significant motor deficit to develop postoperatively in patients with intact SSEPs throughout the operative course. Such events have been reported.[73,83]

In operations on the spinal column and after acute spinal cord injury, the sensory and motor changes generally correlate well[57]; however, in patients suffering neurologic dysfunction after thoracic aortic vascular surgery, posterior spinal cord function (e.g., proprioception, vibration, light touch) may be left intact when motor and other sensory functions (e.g., pain, temperature) are impaired. This result occurred in 32% of patients with neurologic injury after aortic aneurysm repair in one series,[84] with similar results in many other series. Intraoperative SSEP monitoring in these patients carries a significant risk for false-negative results, and as a result, use of such monitoring has not gained significant popularity.

SSEP monitoring has also been used to gauge the adequacy of CBF to the cerebral cortex and subcortical pathways during carotid vascular surgery[69,85,86] (see Chapter 52) and during intracranial aneurysm surgery[68,87-92] (see Chapter 53). SSEPs have been found in the laboratory to have a similar but slightly lower threshold for failure when compared with the EEG. SSEPs are generally intact until the cortical blood flow drops below 15 mL per 100 g of tissue per minute.[67] In a few studies comparing SSEP monitoring with the EEG, a similar sensitivity and specificity for postoperative neurologic function was found. These studies, however, involved few patients and are inadequate to support the hypothesis that SSEP monitoring may substitute for electroencephalographic monitoring of the adequacy of CBF.[85,93] Logic also suggests that changes in SSEP are unlikely, such as for ischemia involving the anterior portions of the frontal or temporal lobe, which could readily be detected by an appropriately placed electroencephalographic electrode. A meta-analysis does not support the use of SSEPs during carotid vascular surgery as a sole monitor of neurologic function.[94]

The SSEP has been much more extensively studied during cerebral aneurysm surgery. During these procedures, the surgical incision precludes placement of scalp electrodes that could detect cerebral ischemia in at-risk cortex.

Recording electrodes placed on the surface of the brain have been used successfully, but they are commonly considered "in the way" by neurosurgeons. Scalp electrodes may easily be placed for SSEP monitoring, although the recording montage is frequently not the same as that used in the awake patient. For aneurysms involving the anterior cerebral circulation, SSEP monitoring has an excellent, but not perfect, record for predicting postoperative neurologic function. Most patients without surgically induced SSEP changes during surgery awaken with an unchanged neurologic examination result. Those with significant SSEP changes that do not revert to normal awaken with a new neurologic deficit. Those with SSEP changes that return to normal after a significant intraoperative change may show at least a transient postoperative deficit, with the severity and duration increasing as the duration of the SSEP change increases. Many investigators have reported significant utility of SSEP monitoring in detecting improper aneurysm clip placement and in guiding intraoperative blood pressure management, particularly in patients already demonstrating or at significant risk for vasospasm after subarachnoid hemorrhage.[68,87-92] The same success, however, cannot be reported for posterior circulation aneurysms. In these cases, many areas of the cortex and subcortical structures are at risk for damage that cannot be monitored at all by somatosensory pathway function. A significant false-negative monitoring pattern exists for these patients, but changes can still be detected when a surgical insult is sufficiently severe to involve large portions of the brain.[95-98]

Coma Evaluation

SSEPs have been used diagnostically in the intensive care unit setting to evaluate comatose patients and assess prognosis. Prolongation of central conduction in comatose patients has been associated with a worse long-term prognosis.[99] Prolongation of central conduction time in patients after subarachnoid hemorrhage is associated with transient neurologic deficits and precedes the development of these deficits. The changes in central conduction time are probably related to cerebral ischemia.[100] If SSEPs have been irreversibly severely damaged or lost after head injury or global hypoxic or hypotensive cerebral injury, the best outcome that can be expected is a chronic vegetative state. In contrast, several reports suggest that patients with intact SSEPs after similar injury may have an excellent prognosis despite initially grave clinical presentations, and a meta-analysis suggests great utility for SSEPs in predicting which patients have the potential to awaken when performed early after the onset of coma.[101-104]

Brainstem Auditory Evoked Potentials

BAEPs are produced in the diagnostic laboratory by delivering repetitive clicks or tones through headphones. Headphones are not practical for surgical monitoring of neurosurgical procedures, and click stimuli are delivered using foam ear inserts attached to stimulus transducers. Stimulus intensity is usually set at 60 to 70 dB above the patient's click-hearing threshold, although practically, many intraoperative laboratories establish monitoring

after induction of anesthesia and instead begin with a stimulus intensity of 90 dB nHL. The duration of the click is approximately 100 μsec, and the stimulus is given usually between 10 and 15 times per second. Clicks are delivered using different polarities; the click may cause initial movement of the tympanic membrane away from the transducer (i.e., rarefaction) or toward the transducer (i.e., condensation). Use of these two different methods commonly produces very different waveforms, amplitudes, and latencies in individual patients, and the method is chosen that produces the largest reproducible response. If stimulus artifact is a serious problem, clicks of alternating polarity may be used to decrease stimulus artifact, but the waveforms produced are an average of those produced by either stimulating technique alone and may be more difficult to monitor. The rate and intensity of stimulus delivery affect the BAEP.[57,105] Unilateral stimulation is used because responses from the other ear, which may remain normal during surgery, may obscure any abnormal responses from the monitored ear. Recording electrodes (usually gold cup electrodes) are placed on the lobe of the stimulated ear and on the top (vertex) of the head.[105] White noise is delivered to the contralateral ear to prevent bone conduction from stimulation of the monitored ear from producing an evoked response from the contralateral ear. Five hundred to 2000 repetitions are required on average, because BAEPs recorded from the scalp are far-field potentials and extremely small (often less than 0.3 μV).[57,105]

Peaks in recordings of BAEP are labeled I through VII, and the purported neural generators for these peaks are shown in Figure 38-11. As with other SERs, amplitude, absolute latencies, and interpeak latencies are evaluated to assess integrity of the auditory system, localize the functional defect when it occurs, and assess peripheral and central conduction times. Because waves VI and VII are inconsistent and variable, they are not routinely monitored,[105] and most papers reporting use of BAEP for surgical monitoring in the operating room monitor waves only up to wave V.[106-108]

Surgical Procedures Monitored with Brainstem Auditory Evoked Potentials

BAEPs have been monitored intraoperatively during procedures involving or near the auditory pathway and during posterior fossa procedures when global brainstem function might be compromised. Cases in which BAEPs are commonly monitored include microvascular decompression of cranial nerves (especially V and VII), resection of acoustic neuroma, posterior fossa exploration for vascular or neoplastic lesions, clipping of basilar artery aneurysms, and sectioning of cranial nerve VIII for intractable tinnitus.[77,106,107]

Several of these procedures deserve special mention because monitoring appears to have significantly improved surgical results based on reported series (not controlled, randomized studies, however). During microvascular decompression of the facial nerve in patients with hemifacial spasm, hearing loss has been reported in up to 15% of cases, and this incidence can be greatly decreased with BAEP monitoring.[109,110] During this procedure, the cerebellum must be retracted to gain

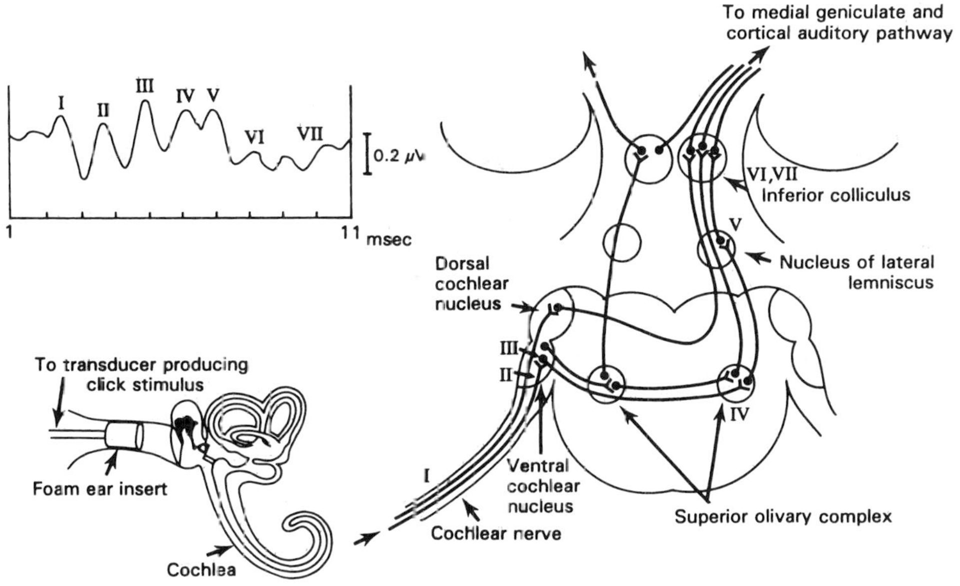

Figure 38–11 Schematic of auditory neural pathway. The brainstem auditory evoked potential (BAEP) is initiated by stimulation of the cochlea with a broadband click stimulus given through an ear insert in the external auditory canal. Neural generators of the BAEP peaks are shown.

exposure to the nerve root entry zone of the facial nerve. An insulating sponge is placed between the nerve root and an aberrant artery or, rarely, a vein that compresses and pulsates against the facial nerve root. Hearing loss may occur because the cerebellar retraction needed for operative exposure stretches cranial nerve VIII between its attachments at the brainstem and the internal auditory meatus. Hearing loss after the more common microvascular decompression of the trigeminal nerve for trigeminal neuralgia, although less common, has also been reduced with BAEP monitoring.[111-114] BAEP monitoring has been used during resection of small acoustic neuromas that have not yet caused severe, irreversible hearing loss.[113,115-118] This monitoring has helped surgeons determine the safety of tumor removal and has helped preserve hearing, particularly in younger patients in whom preservation of longer-term hearing may be more important. Changes in the BAEP can alert the surgeon that further resection of tumor will permanently damage hearing. The surgeon can then decide whether it is better to leave a small amount of residual tumor or to sacrifice hearing and achieve curative resection.

The most common BAEP change observed during monitoring of these operations is an increase in I-V interpeak latency and loss of amplitude of wave V. Other intraoperative BAEP changes include permanent or transient obliteration or severe distortion of waveforms distal to the operative site and, rarely, obliteration of BAEP contralateral to the operative side.[79,80,106,107] The most common BAEP change is usually caused by intraoperative stretch of cranial nerve VIII because of cerebellar retraction. Such changes may be reversed with repositioning or removal of the retractor. More significant changes may be caused by deliberate or unintentional sectioning of cranial nerve VIII, loss of blood supply to the nerve, brainstem compression or compromise to its blood supply, operative manipulation of cranial nerve VIII, severe cerebellar edema, and positioning of the head for retromastoid craniotomy[79,106,107,119] (Table 38-8). Technical and physiologic factors that may significantly alter the BAEP include drilling around the internal auditory canal (i.e., interferes with stimulus delivery), irrigation of cranial nerve VIII with cold saline, and hypotension and hypocarbia.

Patients with transient or persistent mild increases in latency or decreases in amplitude can be expected to have unchanged or only slightly worsened hearing postoperatively. Patients with complete but reversible loss of BAEP also have unchanged or mild worsening of hearing postoperatively. Patients with complete irreversible loss of BAEP have complete or near-complete loss of hearing in the ipsilateral ear postoperatively unless the change was caused by a technical problem or a neuropraxic type injury.[77,79,80,107]

Table 38–8 Correlation between brainstem auditory evoked potential changes and associated clinical events

Brainstem Auditory Evoked Potential Change	Associated Events
Transient latency increase, amplitude decrease	Drilling, irrigation, retraction, surgical irritation, hypocarbia and hypotension, positioning
Persistent latency increase, amplitude decrease	Retraction and stretching of the auditory nerve
Transient loss of evoked potential	Retraction, pressure, surgical dissection
Permanent loss of ipsilateral evoked potential	Surgical interruption of auditory pathway or interruption of cochlear blood supply
Loss of contralateral evoked potential	Cerebellar edema, damage to the brainstem or its blood supply

One series had a single false-positive result with a complete loss of BAEP with intact hearing postoperatively.[79] False-negative results are rare. In one series, BAEPs were monitored in a patient undergoing resection of a meningioma in the lateral ventricle and were unchanged intraoperatively and postoperatively; however, this patient did not regain consciousness postoperatively.[80] This case illustrates the fact that BAEP monitoring assesses only the health of the auditory pathway and involved structures. Function of the ascending reticular system and cortical functions are not monitored directly by the BAEP.

BAEPs are considered the easiest of the SERs to monitor intraoperatively and are least sensitive to changes in perioperative variables. Ability to record technically adequate BAEP has been reported in 90% to 100% of cases in which monitoring was attempted.[77,79,106,107] Unlike SSEPs, BAEPs are resistant to the effects of inhalation and intravenous anesthetics. Although latency and amplitude are altered, especially by inhalation anesthetics, the degree of change is small enough that changes in latency and amplitude associated with anesthetic agents used in clinically relevant doses would not be confused with significant surgically induced changes. Preservation of BAEP intraoperatively indicates preserved hearing postoperatively, and persistent changes indicate significant risk of injury.

Visual Evoked Potentials

VEPs are recorded after monocular stimulation with recording electrodes over the occipital, parietal, and central scalp.[107] Pattern reversal of a checkerboard pattern with constant luminance is the preferred stimulus because the generated evoked potentials have a narrower range of normal variation and are more sensitive to conduction defects. However, it is not possible to deliver this type of stimulation intraoperatively to the anesthetized patient. Instead, flash stimulation of the retina through closed eyelids is provided using light-emitting diodes embedded in soft plastic goggles. The flash rate is 1 to 3 Hz, with a duration of 3 to 5 msec. The major evoked response peak latencies are between 90 and 200 msec (Fig. 38-12), and signals are large enough that prolonged averaging is not needed, and frequently, as few as 20 responses may be averaged.[57,79,80,105] For some procedures, such as operations on the anterior cranial fossa, the goggles interfere with approach to the operative field. Light-emitting diodes embedded within a plastic contact lens have been used in these situations.[77] VEPs are cortical SERs that vary with the type of stimulus, part of the retina stimulated, degree of pupil dilation, and patient's attention level.[57] Because some of these factors change commonly and even constantly during the course of every anesthetic, VEPs would be expected to be highly variable during surgery even when no surgical trespass on the visual system occurs.

Surgical Procedures Monitored with Visual Evoked Potentials

Intraoperative VEP monitoring has been advocated for procedures placing the visual system at risk, especially for those in the area of the optic chiasm. Procedures in which

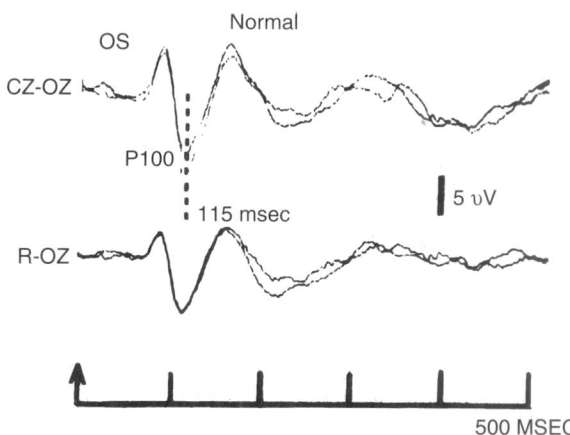

Figure 38–12 Pattern shift of visual evoked potentials. (Adapted from Chiappa KH, Ropper AH: Evoked potentials in clinical medicine. N Engl J Med 306:1140, 1982.)

VEP monitoring has been used include resection of pituitary tumors, craniopharyngioma, optic glioma, orbital pseudotumor, occipital arteriovenous malformation, meningioma impinging on the optic chiasm, and chondrosarcoma of the sphenoid wing; drainage of pituitary abscess; clipping of internal carotid artery and basilar artery aneurysms; surgical correction of cerebrospinal fluid rhinorrhea; and treatment of orbital fracture.[77,79,80] Changes in evoked potential latency and amplitude were used to guide operative manipulations or to indicate adequate systemic blood pressure in patients in whom induced hypotension was being used.[57,80] Intraoperative recordings can be recorded in 88% to 100% of patients.[77,79,80] However, intraoperative variability unrelated to changes in neurologic function may be as high as 68% to 81%.[79,80] In one large series, there was a relatively high incidence of false-positive and false-negative results. Thirteen percent of patients with intraoperative loss of VEPs had unchanged vision postoperatively, and 7% had intact VEPs with significant visual defects.[80]

VEPs are sensitive to a number of factors that cannot be controlled intraoperatively. Stimulus delivered to the retina is difficult to control because the flash must pass through the closed eyelid, and intraoperative changes in pupillary size and direction are common. Improved systems to deliver the stimulus intraoperatively need to be developed.[80] In the opinion of the investigator of one of the largest series of patients studied with intraoperative VEP monitoring using current techniques, VEPs cannot be reliably interpreted.[80] VEP responses, because they are entirely cortical in origin, suffer from the greatest sensitivity to changes in anesthetic drug levels or techniques. VEPs have enjoyed the least popularity of all forms of intraoperative evoked potential monitoring and at this point should be considered at best an experimental monitoring modality.

Pharmacologic Factors Influencing Sensory Evoked Responses

There are multiple drugs used in the perioperative period that can influence the ability to accurately monitor SERs (Table 38-9). An excellent review[120] provides a detailed

Table 38–9 Ability of an anesthetic drug to produce a change in sensory and motor evoked potentials that could be mistaken for a surgically induced change

Drug	SSEPs Lat	SSEPs Amp	BAEPs Lat	BAEPs Amp	VEPs Lat	VEPs Amp	Transcranial MEPs Lat	Transcranial MEPs Amp
Isoflurane	Yes*	Yes	No	No	Yes	Yes	Yes	Yes
Enflurane	Yes	Yes	No	No	Yes	Yes	Yes	Yes
Halothane	Yes	Yes	No	No	Yes	Yes	Yes	Yes
Nitrous oxide†	Yes	Yes	No	No	Yes	Yes	Yes	Yes
Barbiturates	Yes	Yes	No	No	Yes	Yes	Yes (p)	Yes (p)
Etomidate	No	No	No	No	Yes	Yes	No	No
Propofol	Yes	Yes	No	No	Yes	Yes	Yes	Yes
Droperidol	No	No	No	No	—	—	Yes	Yes
Diazepam	Yes	Yes	No	No	Yes	Yes	Yes (p)	Yes (p)
Midazolam	Yes	Yes	No	No	Yes	Yes	Yes (p)	Yes (p)
Ketamine	No	No	No	No	Yes	Yes	No	No
Opiates	No	No	No	No	No	No	No	No

*This table is not quantitative. Yes or no values indicate whether an individual drug is capable of producing an effect on any portion of the evoked response that could be mistaken for a surgically induced change.
†Increases the effect of the agents with which it is used.
Amp, amplitude; BAEPs, brainstem auditory evoked potentials; lat, latency; MEPs, motor evoked potentials; p, prohibitive in clinically useful doses because use of this drug at any dose may render this type of monitoring impossible for a significant period; SSEPs, somatosensory evoked potentials; VEPs, visual evoked potentials.

analysis of all drug effects on SERs that is beyond the scope of this chapter. Table 38-9 does not quantify drug effects, but rather lists whether an individual drug is capable of producing a change in any part of an evoked response that could be mistaken for a surgically induced change. A *No* designation in this table does not indicate a total lack of effects for a given drug on SERs. The *No* designation indicates that any effects that do occur would not be called clinically significant by *clinicians experienced in intraoperative monitoring*. Several general concepts (Table 38-10) can help the clinician who is trying to determine the best choice of drugs for use during monitored cases.

The volatile anesthetics isoflurane, sevoflurane, desflurane, enflurane, and halothane have similar effects in different degrees on all types of SERs. VEPs are the most sensitive to the effects of volatile anesthetics, and BAEPs are the most resistant to anesthetic-induced changes.

Table 38–10 Guidelines for choosing anesthetic techniques for procedures when sensory evoked potentials are monitored

Intravenous agents have significantly less effect than equipotent doses of inhaled anesthetics.
Combinations of drugs generally produce additive effects.
Subcortical (spinal or brainstem) sensory evoked potentials are very resistant to the effects of anesthetic drugs.
    If subcortical responses provide sufficient information for the surgical procedure, anesthetic technique is not important, and effects on cortically recorded responses may be ignored.

Spinal and subcortical SSEP responses are significantly less affected than the cortical potentials.[121-123]

SSEPs, because they are the most widely used intraoperative SER technique, are the most completely studied with respect to the effects of anesthetic drugs. The effects of the volatile agents on cortical SSEPs are dose-dependent increases in latency and conduction times and a decrease in amplitude of cortically but not subcortically recorded signals.[121-125] When comparing the different volatile agents, studies have reported conflicting results.[121,123] For example, one study[123] suggests that halothane has a greater impact on cortical SSEPs than isoflurane or enflurane, whereas another published report[121] supports a greater effect produced by enflurane and isoflurane than halothane. None of these differences is clinically important, and they may be ignored by the practicing clinician. Among the newer agents, desflurane and sevoflurane appear to have qualitatively and quantitatively similar effects on SERs as isoflurane.[126-130] Up to 0.5 to 1 MAC of any of the potent inhaled agents in the presence of nitrous oxide is compatible with monitoring of cortical SSEPs (Figs. 38-13 to 38-15) in neurologically normal patients.[121,125] Neurologically impaired patients may show a significantly greater sensitivity to inhaled agents, even to the point of not tolerating any recordable level of inhaled agent (see Fig. 38-19). In general, however, better monitoring conditions are obtained with narcotic-based anesthetics with less than 1 MAC total (nitrous oxide plus potent agent) end-tidal inhaled anesthetic concentration.

The volatile anesthetics result in increases in latency of BAEPs without significantly affecting the amplitude.[125,131-133] However, volatile anesthetics cause increases in latency and decreases in amplitude in the early (middle latency) cortical responses after auditory

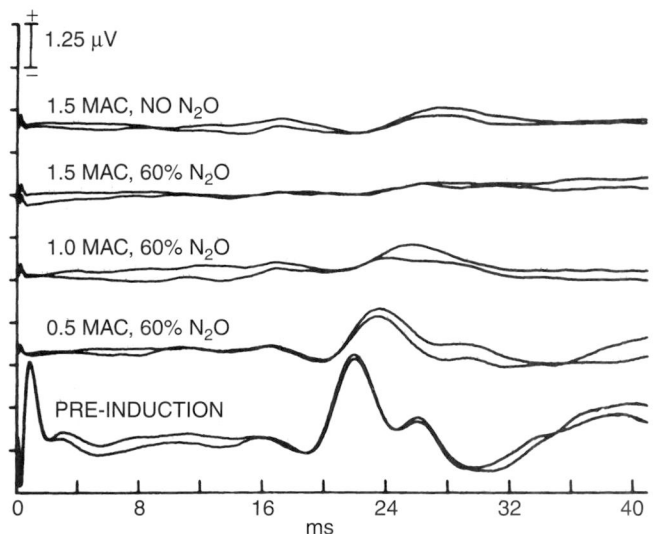

Figure 38–13 Representative somatosensory evoked potentials for cortical responses (C3, C4-FPz) at various minimum alveolar concentrations of isoflurane. (Adapted from Peterson DO, Drummond JC, Todd MM: Effects of halothane, enflurane, isoflurane, and nitrous oxide on somatosensory evoked potentials in humans. Anesthesiology 65:35, 1986.)

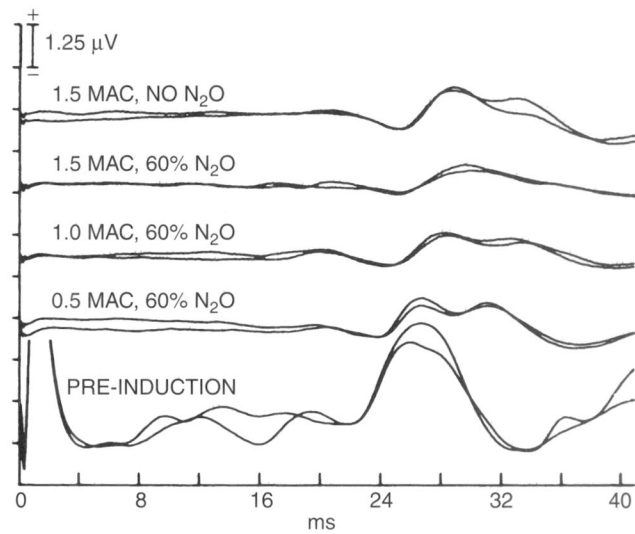

Figure 38–15 Representative somatosensory evoked potentials for cortical responses (C3, C4-FPz) at various minimum alveolar concentrations of halothane. (Adapted from Peterson DO, Drummond JC, Todd MM: Effects of halothane, enflurane, isoflurane, and nitrous oxide on somatosensory evoked potentials in humans. Anesthesiology 65:35, 1986.)

stimulation,[132] and these middle latency responses are being used to monitor the hypnotic component of general anesthetics.[7] Adequate monitoring of BAEPs is possible with any clinically useful concentrations of inhaled agents, with or without nitrous oxide (Figs. 38-16 and 38-17).[125,131-134]

Use of the volatile anesthetics during monitoring of VEPs results in dose-dependent increases in latency with or without changes in amplitude.[125,135-138] Isoflurane results

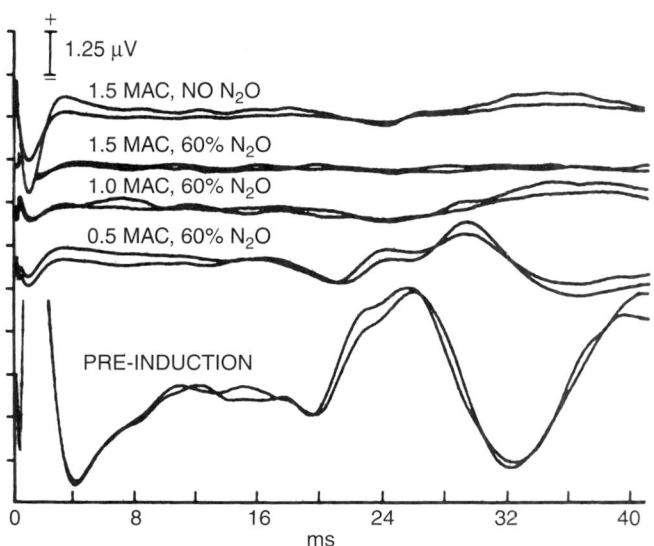

Figure 38–14 Representative somatosensory evoked potentials for cortical responses (C3 or C4-FPz) at various minimum alveolar concentrations of enflurane. (Adapted from Peterson DO, Drummond JC, Todd MM: Effects of halothane, enflurane, isoflurane, and nitrous oxide on somatosensory evoked potentials in humans. Anesthesiology 65:35, 1986.)

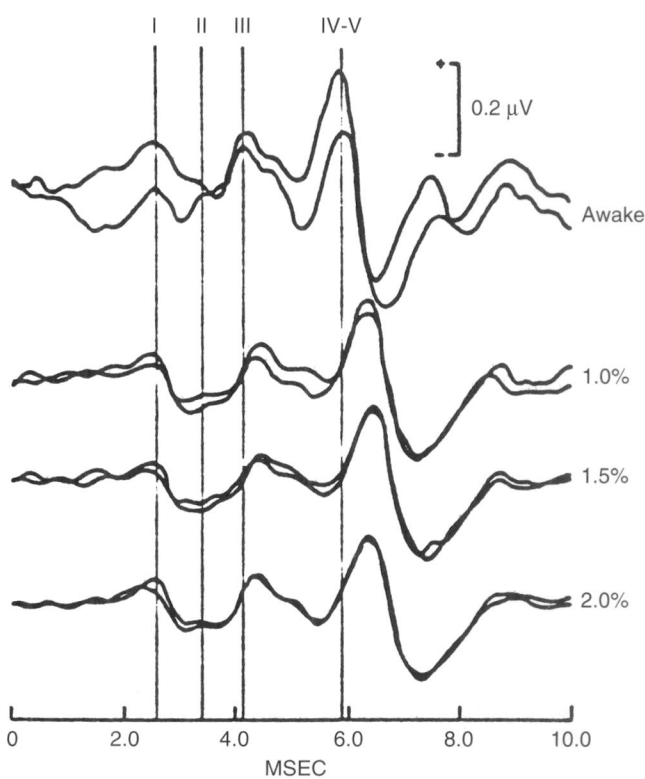

Figure 38–16 Influence of isoflurane alone on brainstem auditory evoked potentials in a typical subject. Latency of peaks III and IV to V increased at 1.0% but stabilized with increasing anesthetic depth. (Adapted from Manninen PH, Lam AM, Nicholas JF: The effects of isoflurane–nitrous oxide anesthesia on brainstem auditory evoked potentials in humans. Anesth Analg 64:43, 1985.)

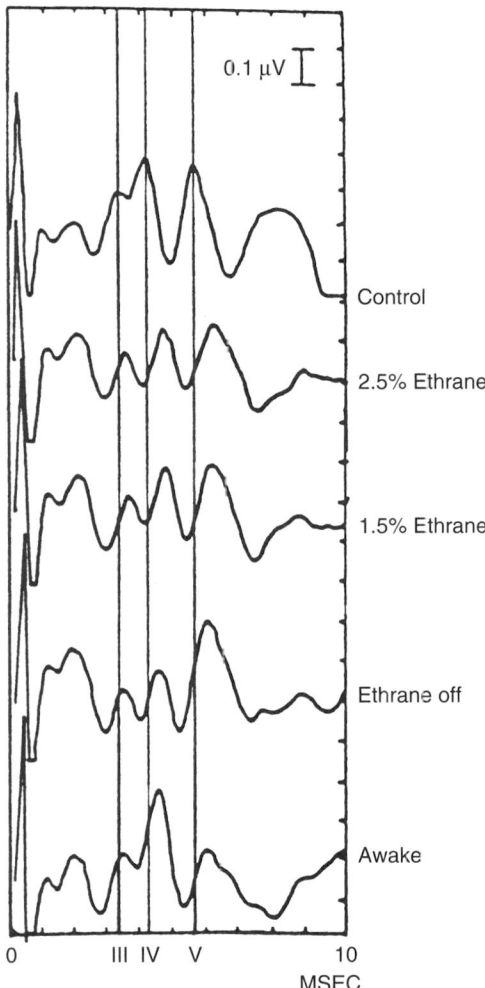

Figure 38–17 Brainstem auditory evoked potential recording obtained in one patient at different concentrations of inspired enflurane. (Adapted from Dubois MY, Sato S, Chassy J, et al: Effects of enflurane on brainstem auditory evoked responses in humans. Anesth Analg 61:898, 1982.)

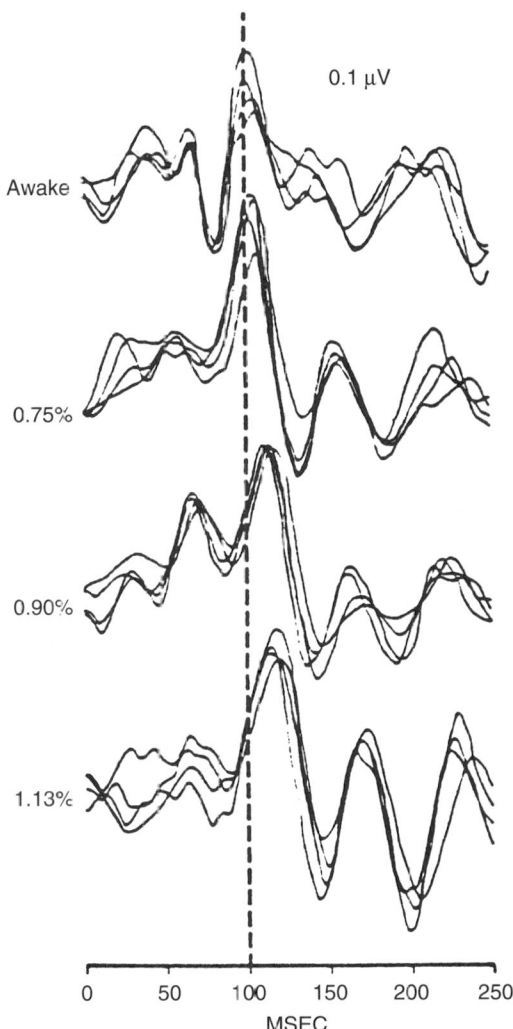

Figure 38–18 Waveforms of visual evoked responses from one patient were elicited when awake and anesthetized at three end-expired levels of halothane. Four separate tracings obtained during each condition have been superimposed. (From Uhl RR, Squires KC, Bruce DL, et al: Effect of halothane anesthesia on the human cortical visual evoked response. Anesthesiology 53:273, 1980.)

in dose-dependent increases in latency and decreases in amplitude up to 1.8% in 100% oxygen, at which time the waveform is lost.[125,135] Enflurane in the absence of hypocarbia also leads to decrease in amplitude.[135] Halothane causes increases in latency without changes in amplitude (Fig. 38-18).[136,137] Although the data from these studies appear valid, the results are really not clinically relevant, because the variability of VEPs in the anesthetized patient is so great that satisfactory monitoring, in the opinion of many experts, is not possible using any anesthetic technique.

Although volatile anesthetics cause significant changes in the SER waveforms, it is possible to provide adequate monitoring intraoperatively in the presence of anesthetic doses of volatile anesthetics. Doses of agents causing significant depression of the response to be monitored must be prevented. In our experience, end-tidal concentrations of inhaled agents totaling more than 1.3 MAC have a dose-related, increasing probability of obliterating cortical SSEPs, even in neurologically normal patients. Equally important, anesthetic concentration should not be

changed during the critical periods of intraoperative monitoring. Critical periods are defined as those in which surgical interventions are most likely to result in damage to neurologic tissue and changes in the SERs. Because the volatile anesthetic-induced changes in SERs are dose-dependent, increasing anesthetic dosage at a crucial point in the operative procedure can result in confusing changes in the SERs that potentially may be caused by the anesthetic or surgical procedure, or both. The appropriate intervention is then difficult to determine.

As with the volatile anesthetics, nitrous oxide causes different effects on the SERs, depending on the sensory system monitored. It causes decreases in amplitude without significant changes in latency in SSEPs when used alone or when added to a narcotic-based or volatile anesthetic.[121,122,139] The addition of nitrous oxide to a maintenance volatile anesthetic during the monitoring of BAEPs causes no further change.[131] Likewise, use of nitrous oxide alone causes no change in BAEPs unless gas accumulates in the middle ear.[139] Use of nitrous oxide alone results in an increase in latency and a decrease in amplitude in VEPs, but when it is added to a volatile anesthetic technique, it causes no further changes in VEPs.[135,139]

The effects of barbiturates on SERs have been studied in animal models and in humans. Increasing doses of thiopental in patients result in progressive dose-dependent increases in latency and decreases in amplitude of SSEPs and in progressive increases in the latency of wave V in BAEPs. The changes in SSEPs are more pronounced than are the changes in BAEPs, and waveforms beyond the initial primary cortical response are quickly obliterated. This finding is consistent with the theories that barbiturates affect synaptic transmission more than axonal conduction. Early waveforms in SERs result primarily from axonal transmission, and later waves depend on multisynaptic pathways in addition to axonal transmission. At doses of thiopental far in excess of those producing an isoelectric EEG, adequate monitoring of early cortical and subcortical SSEPs and BAEPs was preserved.[140] Other barbiturate compounds show similar effects. Somatosensory and auditory SERs were never obliterated, even at doses above those causing complete suppression of spontaneous electroencephalographic activity.[141] This observation is important, especially when attempting to monitor the adequacy of CBF during cerebrovascular surgery when the patient has been given large, "protective" doses of barbiturates. The EEG is isoelectric and not helpful for monitoring. The early cortical SSEP waveforms are, however, still preserved and may be very helpful in determining adequacy of CBF. Preserved ability to monitor SSEPs in head-injured patients receiving therapeutic thiopental infusions has been demonstrated.[142] VEPs are much more sensitive to barbiturates. Small barbiturate doses obliterate all except the earliest waveforms. The early potentials persisted with increases in latency, even in response to very high pentobarbital doses.[143] Except for VEPs, adequate perioperative monitoring of SERs is possible, even in the presence of high-dose barbiturate therapy, as long as the effects of the drug (i.e., increased latency with moderately decreased amplitude) are considered.

After bolus administration and intravenous infusions, etomidate causes increases in latency of all waves and prolongation of central conduction time in SSEPs. Unlike virtually all other commonly used anesthetics, etomidate causes increases in amplitude of the cortical SSEPs.[144,145] This effect may be caused by an alteration in the balance of inhibitory and excitatory influences or an increase in the irritability of the CNS. This effect seems to be present in the cortex but not in the spinal cord.[145] Etomidate infusions have been used to enhance SSEP recording in patients when it was not possible to obtain reproducible responses at the beginning of intraoperative monitoring because of the patients' pathologic findings (Fig. 38-19). After baseline responses that could not be monitored, etomidate augmentation of the SSEP allowed adequate monitoring and detection of intraoperative events leading to compromise of the spinal cord.[145] The effects of etomidate on BAEPs are dose-dependent increases in latency and decreases in amplitude that are not clinically significant.[146]

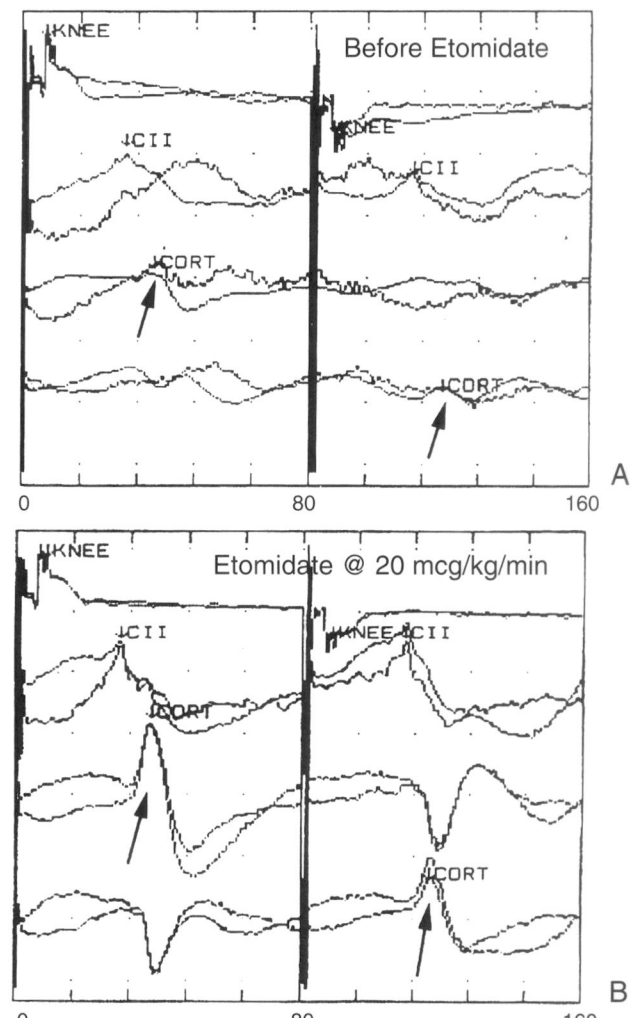

Figure 38–19 Effects of etomidate on somatosensory evoked potentials. **A,** The tracings were obtained from a mildly mentally impaired patient with severe kyphoscoliosis during the early maintenance phase of anesthesia using isoflurane and fentanyl. **B,** The tracings were obtained after discontinuing isoflurane and institution of an etomidate infusion at 20 μg/kg/min. Notice the dramatically increased amplitude and clarity of the signal in the cortical channels (*arrows*), which are both recorded with the same amplification scale.

Droperidol in premedicant doses has various effects on SSEPs. In most patients, decreases in amplitude and loss of late waves were observed, but in a few patients, increases in amplitude were seen. In all patients, conduction time was prolonged,[147] but effects were not clinically significant. Benzodiazepines also can cause changes in SERs.[148,149] Diazepam causes increases in latency and decreases in amplitude of SSEPs, increases in latency in the cortical response after auditory stimulation, and no change in BAEPs.[148,149] Midazolam causes decreases in amplitude without changes in the latency of SSEPs.[144]

In general, opioids cause small, dose-dependent increases in latency and decreases in the amplitude of SSEPs. These changes are not clinically significant. Effects on amplitude are more variable than the latency increases.[150,151] Even at large doses of fentanyl (≤60 μg/kg), reproducible

SSEPs can be recorded.[151] Other opiates cause similar dose-dependent changes in SSEPs.[150,152] Even in relatively large doses, opioids can be used in patients requiring intraoperative SSEP monitoring without impairment of ability to monitor neurologic function adequately. However, opioid-induced changes must be taken into account when evaluating the recordings. Large intravenous bolus administration of opioids should be avoided at times of potential surgical compromise to neurologic function to prevent confusing the interpretation of SEP changes if they develop. BAEPs were resistant to doses of fentanyl up to 50 µg/kg, with no changes observed in absolute latency, interpeak latency, or amplitude.[153]

Physiologic Factors Influencing Sensory Evoked Responses

A number of physiologic variables, including systemic blood pressure, temperature (local and systemic), and blood gas tensions, can influence SEP recordings. With decreases in mean arterial blood pressure to below levels of cerebral autoregulation due to blood loss or vasoactive agents, progressive changes in SERs have been observed. The SSEP changes observed are progressive decreases in amplitude until loss of the waveform with no changes in latency.[154,155] BAEPs are relatively resistant to even profound levels of hypotension (i.e., mean arterial pressure of 20 mm Hg in dogs).[154] Cortical (synaptic) function necessary to produce cortical SERs appears to be more sensitive to hypoperfusion than spinal cord or brainstem nonsynaptic transmission.[155] Rapid decreases in blood pressure to levels above the lower limit of autoregulation have also been associated with transient SSEP changes of decreased amplitude that resolve after several minutes of continued hypotension at the same level.[156] Reversible SSEP changes at systemic pressures within the normal range have been observed in patients undergoing spinal distraction during scoliosis surgery. These changes resolved with increases of systemic blood pressure to slightly above the patient's normal pressure, suggesting that the combination of surgical manipulation with levels of hypotension generally considered "safe" could result in spinal cord ischemia.[157]

Changes in temperature also affect SERs. Hypothermia causes increases in latency and decreases in amplitude of cortical and subcortical SERs after all types of stimulation.[158-160] Hyperthermia also alters SERs, with increases in temperature leading to decreases in the amplitude of SSEPs and loss of SSEPs at 42°C during induced hyperthermia.[161]

Changes in arterial blood gas tensions can alter SERs, probably in relation to changes in blood flow or oxygen delivery to neural structures.[162,163] Hypoxia produces SSEP changes (i.e., decreased amplitude) similar to those seen with ischemia.[163] Decreased oxygen delivery associated with anemia during isovolemic hemodilution results in progressive increases in the latencies of SSEPs and VEPs, which become significant at hematocrits below 15%. Changes in amplitude were variable until very low hematocrits (≈7%) were reached, at which point the amplitude of all waveforms decreased.[164]

MONITORING OF MOTOR TRACTS AND NERVES

Electromyography

Intraoperative monitoring of electromyographic responses generated by cranial and peripheral motor nerves allows early detection of surgically induced nerve damage and assessment of level of nerve function intraoperatively. In these cases, the ability of a nerve to produce a response in the innervated muscle is used to assess the health of a cranial or peripheral nerve at risk during surgery. Recordings are made from surface electrodes (i.e., electroencephalographic or gold cup) or needle electrodes placed directly in the muscle of interest.

Electromyographic monitoring may be active or passive. During active monitoring, a cranial or peripheral nerve is stimulated electrically, and the evoked electromyographic (i.e., compound muscle action potential [CMAP]) response from the muscle is recorded. Stimulation of the nerve proximal to the operative area or tumor can be used to assess functional integrity of the nerve.[165] Nerve function may also be assessed by observing the intensity of nerve stimulus needed to evoke a muscle response and by the morphology of the CMAP. Nerve function may be monitored passively during surgery with continuous recording of all generated responses from innervated muscle groups. "Popcorn" electromyographic discharges are produced by simple, benign contact with the monitored nerve. Response trains are produced with more significant nerve irritation. Neurotonic discharges are produced by significant nerve irritation or nerve damage (Fig. 38-20).[165] When these electromyographic responses reach a certain voltage threshold, they are usually converted into audible signals that provide immediate feedback to the surgeon and warn of impending nerve damage in real time. Real-time feedback is key, because the density and frequency of neurotonic discharges may correlate with the degree of postoperative nerve dysfunction, as demonstrated by data obtained from patients undergoing resection of acoustic tumors.[166]

Intraoperative monitoring of facial nerve function has been used in patients undergoing surgical procedures placing the facial nerve at risk, such as acoustic neuroma resection, microvascular decompression of the facial nerve for hemifacial spasm, resection of cerebellopontine angle meningiomas, removal of temporal bone neoplasms, resection of cerebellar hemangioblastomas, surgical treatment of glomus tympanicum, repair of traumatic facial nerve paralysis, and surgery risking the more peripheral facial nerve such as parotid tumor resection.[165,167] Much of the experience with intraoperative facial nerve monitoring has been obtained from patients undergoing acoustic neuroma resection. Improved preservation of facial nerve function after acoustic neuroma resection by intraoperative facial nerve electromyographic monitoring has been demonstrated, especially in patients with medium- to large-size tumors.[166] The National Institutes of Health Consensus Conference on Acoustic Neuroma[168] recommended that facial nerve monitoring should be used in all patients undergoing surgical resection of an acoustic neuroma.

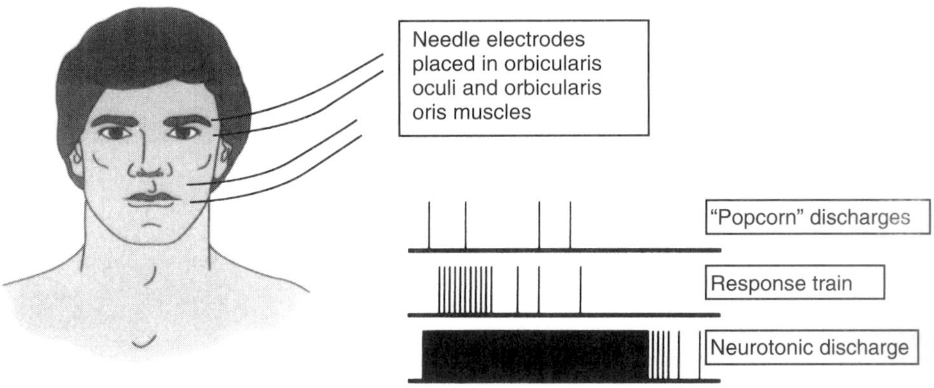

Figure 38–20 Schematic of facial nerve monitoring and typical responses seen during surgery.

The conference based its recommendations on clinical experience and research indicating that use of facial nerve monitoring results in improved neurologic outcome.

In patients undergoing microvascular decompression procedures for hemifacial spasm, two abnormal responses may be seen during electromyographic monitoring: autoexcitation and lateral spread response. *Autoexcitation* refers to late responses lasting 50 to 100 msec that follow the normal motor response to facial nerve stimulation. *Lateral spread* results when electrical stimulation of one branch of the facial nerve results in muscle response in the muscle innervated by that branch and in those innervated by other branches of the facial nerve. Both responses are abnormal and disappear intraoperatively when the facial nerve is adequately decompressed. During microvascular decompression for hemifacial spasm, intraoperative monitoring of the facial nerve provides warning of surgical damage to the nerve and information on the adequacy of the operative procedure to relieve the patient's symptoms intraoperatively.[169]

Intraoperative monitoring of the motor component of other cranial nerves has also been successfully performed. Electromyographic monitoring of the trigeminal nerve can be accomplished with electrodes placed over or in the temporalis or masseter muscles. Trigeminal nerve motor monitoring has been used during nerve section for tic douloureux to ensure preservation of the motor branch of the trigeminal nerve and in combination with facial nerve monitoring during resection of large posterior fossa lesions.[165] Using recording electrodes placed in or over the trapezius or sternocleidomastoid muscles, the spinal accessory nerve has been successfully monitored during resection of large meningiomas, glomus jugular tumors, and neck carcinomas.[165] Electromyographic monitoring of the hypoglossal nerve with needle electrodes placed in the tongue has been infrequently used for large posterior fossa lesions and clivus tumors.[165] Although electromyographic monitoring of the eye muscles can be performed using tiny hook wires for recording, it is rarely used.

Monitoring of peripheral motor nerves has been performed by placing needle electrodes in or over the muscles innervated by nerves that traverse the operative area and are at risk from the planned surgical procedure. Auditory feedback from electromyographic monitoring can warn the surgeon of unexpected surgical trespass of the nerve, help locate a nerve within the field (e.g., during untethering of the spinal cord), and localize the level of any conduction block or delay. Because radiculopathies have been reported to occur after spinal surgery, electromyographic monitoring of peripheral nerves has been used in patients undergoing spinal surgery to decrease the risk of nerve root injury during the procedure.[165]

In patients undergoing electromyographic monitoring of cranial or peripheral motor nerves, the choice of anesthetic technique is not important, but muscle relaxants should be avoided or limited during the period of monitoring. Although most clinicians avoid neuromuscular blocking agents completely during periods of electromyographic monitoring, adequate active monitoring of the facial nerve, which is relatively resistant to the effects of neuromuscular blocking agents, is possible during partial neuromuscular blockade (i.e., decrease of the CMAP by 50%). This level of blockade is associated with clinical weakness[170]; however, the most commonly used monitors of neuromuscular paralysis are not adequate to accurately quantify this level of relaxation. The trials in which partial neuromuscular paralysis was used during facial nerve monitoring are small, and large-scale trials evaluating outcome have not been performed. Effects of partial neuromuscular blockade on passive facial nerve monitoring have not been studied. As a result, most neuro-anesthesiologists continue to recommend complete avoidance of neuromuscular blocking agents after intubation until monitoring is completed.

Electromyographic monitoring has also been helpful during selective dorsal rhizotomy, usually performed in children with cerebral palsy for relief of spasticity. In this operation, sensory nerve roots are sectioned to reduce sensory input to the nervous system. The resultant pathologic spastic response is subsequently reduced. Sensory nerve rootlets are individually stimulated. In the normal patient, motor responses would be recorded only from muscle innervated by the corresponding motor nerve root. In patients with spasticity, the motor response produced by stimulation of a single sensory rootlet may generalize to other levels and muscle groups ipsilaterally and, in severe cases, to the opposite side. The most pathologic rootlets as indicated by electromyographic testing are sectioned. In some cases, volatile anesthetics and nitrous oxide may impair the ability to monitor adequately, and greater success may be obtained with narcotic-based techniques.[171,172]

Peripheral Nerve Monitoring

Monitoring of peripheral nerves has also been performed in patients undergoing nerve plexus or single-nerve explorations to locate areas of injury and assess axonal continuity. Patients with prolonged weakness and sensory loss after nerve injury may undergo nerve exploration to determine whether nerve reconstruction may improve outcome. The area of the lesion is determined by preoperative nerve conduction studies. Intraoperatively, the nerve is first stimulated proximal to the lesion, and a recording of the nerve action potential is made directly from the nerve distal to the lesion. If there is nerve conduction across the lesion, lysis of scar is performed, and the incision is closed. Natural recovery by means of axonal regrowth produces the best outcome. If, however, conduction does not occur across the lesion, resection of the damaged nerve and nerve cable grafting is performed.[165,173,174]

Motor Evoked Potentials

Monitoring of the integrity of the motor tracts within the spinal cord is a technique with great potential benefit, and even during the relative short history of MEP monitoring, there are reported cases of loss of MEPs with preservation of the SSEP.[175-180] This technique has potential applications in spinal surgery, in which transmission across the operative field can be assessed, and in aortic surgery with the potential for impairment of the blood supply to the vulnerable anterior spinal cord. Relative to SER monitoring, MEP monitoring is quite invasive, and until recently, some equipment associated with MEP testing was not approved by the U.S. Food and Drug Administration (FDA) for use in MEP monitoring in human subjects. These aspects of MEP monitoring have, until recently, substantially limited the applications of MEP monitoring.

MEP monitoring was developed specifically to assess the function of motor pathways and overcome one of the limitations of SEP monitoring. The first of several variants of MEP monitoring involves electrical or magnetic transcranial stimulation. During transcranial electrical MEP monitoring, stimulating electrodes are placed on the scalp overlying the motor cortex. During magnetic stimulation, a powerful magnetic stimulator is placed on the scalp over the motor cortex. Brief repetitive applications of electrical current or a strong magnetic field induce current in the motor cortex and produce an MEP. These transcranial stimulating methods may also activate surrounding cortical structures and subcortical white matter pathways (i.e., sensory and motor). Distal antidromic propagation of the transcranially applied stimulus is blocked by synapses in all of the ascending sensory pathways. The stimulus is propagated easily orthodromically through descending motor pathways. The evoked responses may be recorded over the spinal cord, the peripheral nerve, and the muscle itself. To enhance the MEP, these responses may be averaged in the same manner as

SERs, but averaging is often unnecessary. A third method of producing the MEP involves electrical stimulation of the spinal cord itself above the area of the cord at risk during surgery. Responses may be recorded over the distal spinal cord, peripheral nerve, and muscle.

MEP monitoring, although promising in some aspects, has some problems associated with it that still need to be resolved. The exact anatomic pathways and generators involved with MEP production have not been completely determined, and intraoperative experience with MEPs remains relatively limited. Multiple anecdotal reports suggest that MEP monitoring during surgery on the spine or its blood supply may be very useful, but whether this monitor can be used to guide management and predict postoperative neurologic function in a large series of patients is unclear.[181-184] For example, it was hoped that MEPs would be able to better predict postoperative motor function than SERs after occlusion of the blood supply to the spinal cord during operations on the thoracic aorta. Two studies suggest that MEPs may not be as effective as hoped. The first study[182] recorded MEPs from the lumbar spinal cord in dogs produced by transcranial electrical stimulation. Elmore and coworkers[185] found that these spinally recorded potentials did not accurately predict postoperative motor function. A second study[186] recorded MEPs at the spinal cord and peripheral nerve level in dogs produced by transcranial electrical stimulation. Reuter and associates[186] also found that the spinally recorded responses were inaccurate in predicting motor function postoperatively. The peripheral nerve responses disappeared in all animals and were not present 24 hours later, regardless of whether the animal could move its lower extremities. These studies suggest that the spinally recorded MEP probably represents a response generated by the descending corticospinal tract. This white matter pathway is relatively resistant to ischemia compared with the more metabolically active anterior horn cells (i.e., gray matter). Recovery of this white matter–generated MEP response may occur after reperfusion of the cord, but the gray matter may not recover. Responses recorded from the peripheral nerve can reflect postsynaptic anterior horn cell function, but lower extremity ischemia occurring after aortic cross-clamping often precludes recording this or the response from muscles during surgery.

Limited clinical work has shown much greater success with MEP monitoring during aortic vascular surgery in correctly detecting inadequate spinal cord blood flow and in improving operative outcome. The technique has proved useful, particularly when using operative strategies such as reimplantation of critical intercostal vessels based on results of MEP monitoring.[187-192] Although there is promise for this monitoring technique in aortic surgery, much more experimental and clinical work is needed before MEP monitoring during aortic surgery becomes widely accepted and used.

The greatest experience with MEP responses has been obtained using electrical stimulation of the spinal cord above the area at risk surgically.[193-195] Responses are recorded distally, usually over the peripheral nerve, and profound surgical muscle relaxation is used to prevent gross movement during surgery. This type of MEP is called a *neurogenic motor evoked potential* (NMEP). Initially, investigators thought that this response, recorded over a peripheral nerve in the lower extremity (typically the tibial nerve in the popliteal fossa), was generated by stimulation of the descending motor tracts, activation of the anterior horn cells, and propagation of the nerve action potential through the peripheral nerve. Multiple clinical trials using this technique and comparing results of MEP monitoring with those of SSEP reported good results.[193-195] Subsequent studies in animals and humans[196] have shown that NMEPs are, at best, mixed responses with a significant component of antidromically conducted responses along the sensory pathway. Stimulation of the dorsal column results in an antidromically conducted, recordable signal peripherally because the somesthetic system does not synapse in the dorsal root ganglion and fibers pass directly from the peripheral nerve through the cell body in the ganglion into the dorsal column. Because of this problem, use of NMEP monitoring has decreased significantly and has been replaced by the more invasive transcranial stimulation techniques that produce responses that are clearly produced by activation of the motor system alone. NMEP monitoring is very resistant to the effects of anesthetics and may be recorded with any commonly used anesthetic technique.

Except in the case of the NMEP, effects of anesthetics are surprisingly profound, particularly on MEP recordings from muscle produced by single-pulse transcranial electrical or by magnetic stimulation (see Table 38-9).[171,197-201] Anesthetic techniques typically used by most anesthesiologists for spinal surgery produce prohibitive depression of the MEP.[202,203] Investigators demonstrated in several studies that intravenous agents produce significantly less depression, and techniques using any combination of ketamine, opiates, etomidate, and propofol have been described.[204-210] Anesthetic effects on MEP responses recorded at spinal levels appear to be less serious. When responses are recorded from muscle, neuromuscular blocking agents should be monitored quantitatively, maintaining T1 twitch height at about 30% of control values to prevent excessive movement during the operation.[183,197] When responses are not recorded from muscle, profound relaxation is desirable because gross muscle movement produced by MEP stimulation is thereby eliminated, facilitating the surgical procedure. Fortunately for the practicing anesthesiologist, studies of transcranial electrical and magnetic stimulus techniques using rapid trains of stimuli have produced responses that are more resistant to the effects of anesthetic agents, and more traditional techniques using inhaled agents and narcotics may be used.[211-213] Precise control of the anesthetic and avoidance of boluses during critical monitoring periods appears to be even more important than for SSEPs. Although some centers have had consistent success using transcranial MEP monitoring, its use is not widespread. Early data are promising, and the clinician should expect to see increased use over the next decade. FDA approval of transcranial electrical stimulation should increase the intraoperative use of this monitoring modality, especially in spinal column surgery, during which modest movement would not be problematic, and provide considerably more data on the efficacy of its use.

MONITORS OF CEREBRAL BLOOD FLOW

Transcranial Doppler Monitoring

Transcranial Doppler (TCD) ultrasound is an easily applied, direct, noninvasive measurement of CBF. TCD is a diagnostic tool that has found application as a monitor in the operating room relatively recently.[201] TCD uses sound waves to measure the velocity of blood flowing in the basal arteries of the brain. Sound waves are transmitted through the relatively thin temporal bone (Fig. 38-21). When these sound waves come in contact with blood, they are reflected off the red blood cells through the brain and skull to a detector. The velocity of the sound waves reflected to the surface is changed because the blood cells themselves are in motion toward or away from the sound wave detector. This phenomenon is known as the *Doppler shift* and is directly related to the velocity and flow direction of the blood cells. The velocity of the blood cells is faster during systole and slower during diastole. The blood in the center of the lumen moves faster than the blood near the vessel wall. A spectrum of flow velocities is produced. This spectrum resembles the shape of the waveform produced by the pulse oximeter or an arterial pressure transducer (Fig. 38-22A). TCD measurements of flow velocity are most commonly and easily made in the middle cerebral artery but may also be measured in other arteries, including the anterior cerebral, anterior communicating, posterior cerebral, posterior communicating, and basilar arteries.

Two assumptions must be made for TCD-measured blood flow velocity to have a direct relationship to CBF. First, blood flow velocity is directly related to blood flow only if the diameter of the artery where the flow velocity is measured and the measurement angle of the Doppler probe remain constant. Second, CBF in the basal arteries of the

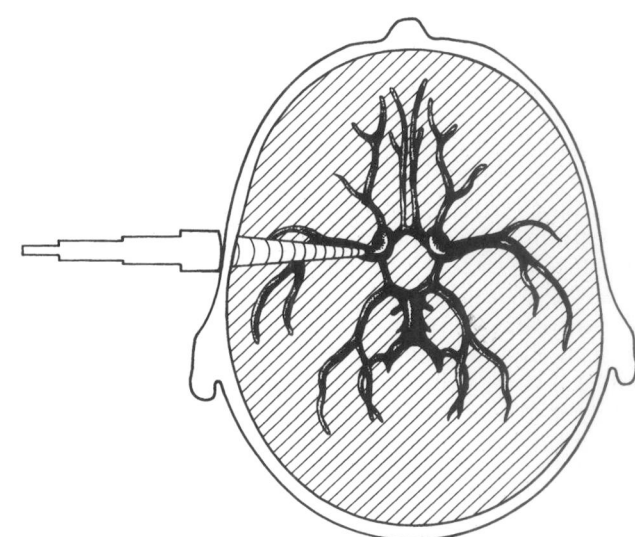

Figure 38–21 Schematic of transcranial Doppler ultrasonography. Sound waves are transmitted through the relatively thin temporal bone and reflected from red blood cells moving in the basal arteries of the brain.

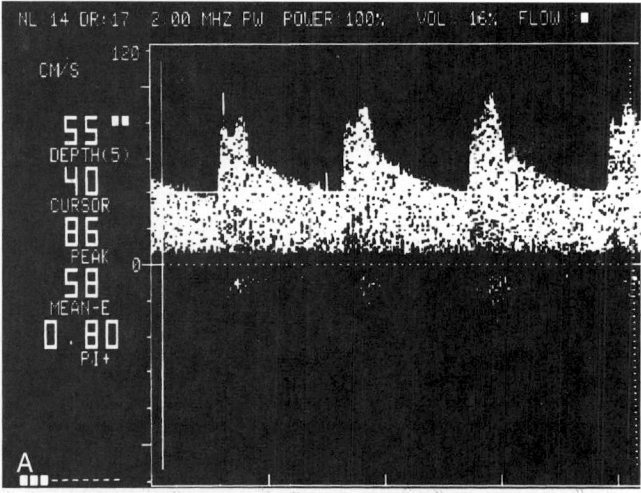

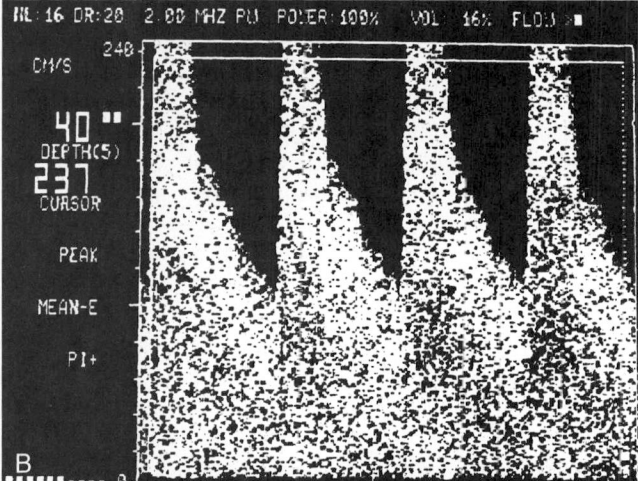

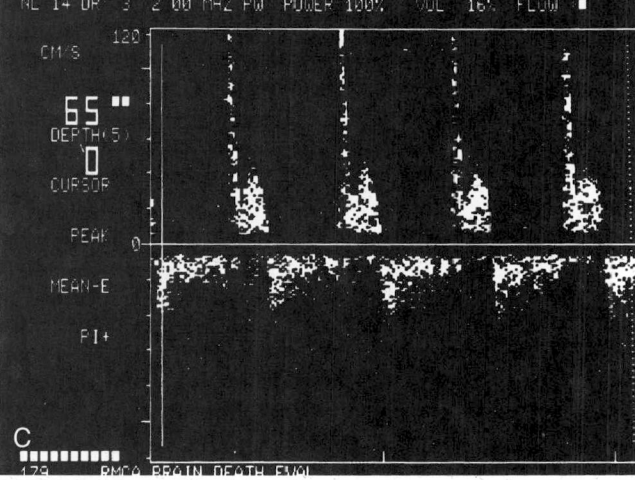

Figure 38–22 A, Normal transcranial Doppler (TCD) tracing from the middle cerebral artery at a depth of 55 mm. **B,** TCD tracing from a patient with cerebral vasospasm. Notice the very high flow velocities beyond the ability of the machine to quantify. **C,** TCD pattern from the middle cerebral artery in a case of brain death. Notice the brief systolic inflow of blood followed by flow reversal in diastole.

brain must be directly related to cortical CBF. Neither of these assumptions has been proved scientifically. The TCD has not been validated in a large series of intraoperative cases against established monitors of cerebral flow such as the EEG or against direct cortical CBF measurements.

The major reported intraoperative use of the TCD involves testing adequacy of CBF while the carotid artery is cross-clamped during carotid endarterectomy. Studies comparing measured CBF with the velocity in the middle cerebral artery have not shown a good correlation between the two measurements.[214] The period of carotid cross-clamping is only a relatively small portion of the time that the patient with carotid disease is at risk for ischemia, and most strokes occur at other times during or especially after surgery. Few data are available about the nature and degree of acceptable TCD changes during the remainder of the operation. Normal variations in blood flow velocities during surgery in patients without cerebrovascular disease appear to be large (Pashayan AG, Mahla ME: unpublished data). With increasing clinical experience with TCD during carotid endarterectomy, it has become one of the accepted monitors of CBF during carotid surgery, especially with respect to the detection of emboli. Preoperative TCD screening may be useful in defining which asymptomatic patients are at higher risk for stroke and may benefit from prophylactic surgery.[215] Surgeons using TCD monitoring have been able to alter their technique and reduce intraoperative microembolization.[216] TCD is becoming increasingly accepted as useful for the detection of emboli after completion of arterial repair, and studies are appearing that demonstrate the utility of TCD in detecting an abnormally high rate of postoperative embolization after carotid surgery.[217-221] These patients have been shown to be at higher risk for postoperative cerebral ischemia, and the implication is that excessive postoperative emboli counts merit urgent re-exploration of the arterial repair.

TCD is also used during CPB to detect air or particulate emboli during cannulation, during bypass, when weaning from bypass, and during decannulation.[222] Several small clinical studies have suggested that TCD monitoring is useful in identifying portions of the procedure with the highest risk for microemboli, potentially allowing alterations in the procedure to decrease microembolic events. The number of microemboli has been suggested to be predictive of postoperative neurologic dysfunction; however, most studies are relatively small, and the clinical utility of TCD emboli counts is still undefined.[223-227] Ease of application and interpretation of the characteristic spectra produced by emboli make this a very attractive monitor for cardiac surgery, but outcome data proving utility are still lacking.

TCD has been used in the intensive care unit to document the presence and severity of cerebral vasospasm after subarachnoid hemorrhage. As the major cerebral arteries narrow, flow velocity within the lumen must increase if blood flow is to be maintained (see Fig. 38-22B). Mean flow velocities of more than 120 cm per second seem to correlate well with angiographic vasospasm,[228,229] and the TCD is increasingly used for noninvasive, early detection of vasospasm, allowing therapy to be initiated before the onset of clinical symptoms.[230-234]

The TCD has also been used in the intensive care unit as an aid to the diagnosis of brain death. Studies have demonstrated a characteristic blood flow velocity pattern in patients who are clinically brain dead (see Fig. 38-22C).[235] TCD studies are easily performed at the bedside and can be used to determine whether definitive studies documenting brain death (which may require transporting the patient) need to be performed. Further studies documenting the sensitivity and specificity of this test in the diagnosis of brain death are needed before this test can be used as a sole criterion for brain death.

Jugular Bulb Venous Oxygen Saturation

Jugular bulb venous oxygen saturation (Sjvo$_2$) is thought to be a measure of the degree of oxygen extraction by the brain and represents the balance between cerebral oxygen supply and demand. As CBF decreases or demand increases without a flow increase, oxygen extraction increases, and Sjvo$_2$ falls. Conversely, when flow increases or metabolic demand decreases without a fall in flow, extraction decreases, and Sjvo$_2$ increases. Interpretation of the absolute value of Sjvo$_2$ is difficult if clinical circumstances are not clearly defined. For example, an increase in Sjvo$_2$ may be an ominous sign if the increase is caused by a fall in metabolism associated with cellular death.

Sjvo$_2$ can be measured by placing a sampling catheter or a fiberoptic catheter (for continuous monitoring) into the jugular bulb through the internal jugular vein or through a peripheral arm vein. In most clinical studies, Sjvo$_2$ measurements of below 50% are thought to indicate cerebral ischemia. Because venous blood in the jugular vein drains from a large portion of the brain, Sjvo$_2$ must be considered a monitor of global cerebral oxygenation. There is also significant variability from patient to patient about which areas of the brain are drained by which jugular vein. Focal areas of cerebral ischemia may therefore go undetected.

Sjvo$_2$ monitoring has been used most extensively in the intensive care unit to monitor patients with severe head injury and has been used to guide blood pressure and ventilatory management to optimize blood flow. This monitoring technology has had a major effect on ventilatory management of the head injured patient and has significantly reduced the routine use of hyperventilation in neurosurgical patients.[236-239] Its use to guide intraoperative management that may affect CBF has been described during carotid endarterectomy, craniotomy for neoplasms and vascular anomalies, and CPB procedures.[240-245] Although it is used routinely in some neurosurgical centers, it has not yet gained widespread clinical acceptance as a routine monitor of neurologic well-being intraoperatively during procedures placing the CNS at risk.

Cerebral Oximetry

Adaptation of the technology used for pulse oximetry and intravascular oximetry has been used to develop a monitor that can measure the oxygen saturation in the vascular bed (primarily venous component) of the cerebral cortex.[246] The rationale for monitoring this information is that as CBF falls, oxygen saturation decreases because of increased extraction by tissue. Proponents of this device, supported by some laboratory data, claim that cerebral oximetry can detect inadequate CBF before the more established and accepted EEG.[247] This finding is expected, because brain is able to increase oxygen extraction in the face of decreased flow and maintain function until the flow falls below a level at which increased extraction cannot compensate. Cerebral oximetry should therefore be a sensitive and specific indicator of the adequacy of regional blood flow in the tissue beneath the sensor.

Cerebral oximetry has been used with various degrees of success to monitor the adequacy of cerebral perfusion in head trauma patients,[248-252] during carotid vascular surgery,[253-255] and during CPB.[256-260] The monitoring device is easy to use and requires only the application of a probe similar to a pulse oximetry probe to the forehead (two for bilateral monitoring). This simplicity also gives rise to one of the limitations of this device. Frontal application of sensors allows monitoring only of a small portion of the cortex, and the well-being of the remainder of the cortex is inferred by the information derived from the frontopolar cerebral cortex. This assumption is frequently inaccurate. Vascular insufficiency in the distribution of the middle cerebral or posterior cerebral arteries cannot be detected with frontal sensors.

Samra and colleagues evaluated cerebral oximetry during 94 carotid endarterectomies in awake patients.[253] They found that the cerebral oximetry was able to identify 97.4% of patients with adequate CBF as indicated by the absence of clinical symptoms. However, the investigators found that there was a false-positive rate of 66.7%. The monitor frequently indicated inadequate CBF although the patient had no symptoms of inadequate CBF. This finding should not be surprising because oxygen extraction increases before any loss of function. The real problem is that the lower limit for acceptable regional oxygen saturation is not known in a large population of patients. This value may be different from patient to patient, and addition of anesthetic drugs that influence cerebral metabolism may further confuse the picture.

There has been much concern regarding the exact source of the signal monitored by cerebral oximetry.[261,262] Contamination of the oximetry signal by extracranial blood sources may be a source of serious error for this device. Adjustment of the algorithm is reported to have largely eliminated this problem,[263] but other serious concerns remain. No normative data exist across a large patient population for normal values or for expected changes during surgery. Trend patterns are emerging from various clinical reports and trials, but large-population data do not exist. The meaning of isolated values is even less clear. Technology associated with this monitoring is developing very fast, and cerebral oximetry will probably find a place in the clinical care of patients after more data become available and further technologic advances occur.

SUMMARY

Regardless of the type of intraoperative neurologic monitor, several principles must be followed for the use of neurologic monitoring to provide potential benefit to the patient. First, the pathway at risk during the surgical procedure must be amenable to monitoring. Second, if evidence of injury to the pathway is detected, some intervention must be possible. If changes in the neurologic monitor are detected and no intervention is possible, although the monitor may be of prognostic value, it does not have the potential to provide direct benefit to the patient by means of early detection of impending neurologic injury. Third, the monitor must provide reliable and reproducible data. If the data have a high degree of variability in the absence of clinical interventions, their utility for detecting clinically significant events is limited.

We have reviewed the most common clinically used intraoperative neurologic monitors. Ideally, clinical studies can provide outcome data on the efficacy of a neurologic monitor in a given procedure to improve neurologic outcome. Unfortunately, although there is a wealth of clinical experience with many of these monitoring modalities, there is little in the way of randomized, prospective studies evaluating the efficacy of neurologic monitoring. Based on clinical experience with neurologic monitoring and on nonrandomized clinical studies in which neurologic monitoring is used and typically compared with historical controls, practice patterns for use of neurologic monitoring have developed. For certain procedures, neurologic monitoring is recommended and used by most centers. For other procedures, monitoring is used almost routinely in some centers but not in others, and for some procedures, there is no clear clinical experience or evidence indicating that monitoring is useful at all (e.g., experimental use). For some procedures, monitoring is used selectively for patients believed to be at higher risk for intraoperative neurologic injury. Table 38-11 provides a summary of current clinical practice.

Table 38–11   Current practice in neurologic monitoring

Procedure	Monitors	Current Practice
Carotid endarterectomy	Neurologic examination of awake patient	Most available literature supports use of at least one of EEG, SSEP, TCD, awake patient
	EEG	
	SSEP	
	TCD	
	CO	Limited data available; inadequate normative population data
Scoliosis surgery	SSEP	Monitoring recommended and may substitute for wake-up testing
	Wake-up test	Largely abandoned in centers using electrophysiologic monitoring. Monitoring is not continuous, and false-negative monitoring patterns have been reported
	MEP	Increased clinical use since transcranial electrical stimulation was FDA approved; overall utility to be determined but probably useful
Acoustic neuroma	Facial nerve monitor	Facial nerve monitoring recommended
	BAEP	Shows some clinical evidence of improved outcome in some procedures
Intracranial aneurysm clipping	SSEP	Used routinely in some centers; limited clinical data on outcome but
	EEG	appears clinically useful during anterior circulation procedures
Cranial nerve V decompression	BAEP	Used in some centers; reduces hearing loss
Cranial nerve VII decompression	BAEP	Data from small series show improved hearing preservation
Supratentorial mass lesions	SSEP	Used in some centers in selected high-risk procedures
Infratentorial mass lesions	BAEP or SSEP	BAEP to detect retractor-related VIII nerve injury; SSEP for rare, high-risk lesions adjacent to ascending sensory pathways
Decompression of spinal stenosis	SSEP	Used in some centers in high-risk procedures (more often cervical)
Spinal cord trauma	SSEP	Used in some centers in high-risk procedures
Cardiopulmonary bypass	EEG	Used routinely in some centers; actively studied but no outcome data yet
	TCD	
	$Sjvo_2$	
	CO	
Aortic coarctation	SSEP	Used routinely in a few centers; no widespread acceptance
Aortic aneurysm repair	SSEP	Used routinely in a few centers; no widespread acceptance
	MEP	Used routinely in a few centers; no widespread acceptance

BAEP, brainstem auditory evoked potential; CO, cerebral oximetry; EEG, electroencephalogram; FDA, U.S. Food and Drug Administration; MEP, motor evoked potential; NIH, National Institutes of Health; $Sjvo_2$, jugular bulb venous oxygen saturation; SSEP, somatosensory evoked potential; TCD, transcranial Doppler ultrasound.

KEY POINTS

1. Monitors of the nervous system can monitor function or adequacy of blood flow, or both.

2. Most anesthetic drugs have a typical triphasic effect on the EEG: small doses produce activation, moderate doses produce slowing with maintenance or increase in amplitude, and large doses produce burst suppression.

3. The EEG is well established for monitoring the nervous system during carotid vascular surgery, during epilepsy surgery, and for depth of the hypnotic state. Other uses remain controversial and largely experimental.

4. Monitoring 16 or 32 channels of an analog EEG requires extensive resources, particularly with respect to personnel. Processed electroencephalographic monitors, by simplifying the display and using usually two or four channels of information, require fewer resources to use and may detect inadequate CBF during surgery nearly as well.

5. Electroencephalographic changes associated with inadequate CBF are similar to those observed with increasing doses of most anesthetic drugs.

6. Anesthetic effects on cortical SERs are significant and render monitoring of VEPs extremely difficult. Subcortical responses (i.e., auditory and somatosensory) are resistant to the effects of anesthetics. In general, the effects of intravenous drugs are less significant than those of inhaled anesthetics.

7. Electromyographic monitoring during neurologic or spinal surgery may allow the surgeon to identify nervous tissue and to detect impending damage to cranial and peripheral nerves. Use of muscle relaxant drugs is best avoided when such monitoring is used.

8. Monitoring of the motor pathways is feasible and will probably increase in coming years. Anesthetic effects may be quite significant, depending on the type of stimulation used, and precise control of the degree of muscle relaxation is necessary. Whether motor pathway monitoring with its accompanying anesthetic requirements will significantly improve our ability to monitor spinal cord or brain function remains to be seen.

9. TCD may provide information about the adequacy of CBF. More importantly, TCD readily detects emboli, and this information may help the surgeon improve technique and detect significant risk of stroke at any time during the perioperative period.

10. Measurement of $Sjvo_2$ may help determine the balance between cerebral oxygen supply and demand. This technology has helped us better understand the effects of hyperventilation on the neurosurgical patient and contributed to the ongoing reduction in the use of hyperventilation in the neurosurgical patient. Whether this technology will gain more widespread use, particularly intraoperatively, remains unclear.

11. Cerebral oximetry is a new technology designed to measure the adequacy of CBF. Use of this device remains controversial, particularly because there is no universal agreement about normal perioperative changes and the permissible degree of intraoperative change. Much more research is required before the roles of cerebral oximetry as a neurologic monitor can be determined.

REFERENCES

1. Drummond JC: Monitoring depth of anesthesia: With emphasis on the application of the bispectral index and the middle latency auditory evoked response to the prevention of recall. Anesthesiology 93:876, 2000.
2. Rosow C, Manberg PJ: Bispectral index monitoring. Anesthesiol Clin North Am 19:947, 2001.
3. Ge SJ, Zhuang XL, Wang YT, et al: Changes in the rapidly extracted auditory evoked potentials index and the bispectral index during sedation induced by propofol or midazolam under epidural block. Br J Anaesth 89:260, 2002.
4. Muncaster AR, Sleigh JW, Williams M: Changes in consciousness, conceptual memory, and quantitative electroencephalographical measures during recovery from sevoflurane- and remifentanil-based anesthesia. Anesth Analg 96:720, 2003.
5. Bruhn J, Bouillon TW, Radulescu L, et al: Correlation of approximate entropy, bispectral index, and spectral edge frequency 95 (SEF95) with clinical signs of "anesthetic depth" during coadministration of propofol and remifentanil. Anesthesiology 98:621, 2003.
6. Johansen JW, Sebel PS: Development and clinical application of electroencephalographic bispectrum monitoring. Anesthesiology 93:1336, 2000.
7. Hughes JR: EEG in Clinical Practice, 2nd ed. Newton, ME, Butterworth-Heinemann, 1994.
8. Vitek JL, Bakay RAE, Hashimoto T, et al: Microelectrode-guided pallidotomy: Technical approach and its application in medically intractable Parkinson's disease. J Neurosurg 88:1027, 1998.
9. Garonzik IM, Hua SE, Ohara S, et al: Intraoperative microelectrode and semi-microelectrode recording during the physiological localization of the thalamic nucleus ventral intermediate. Mov Disord 17:S135, 2002.
10. Martin JT, Faulconer A Jr, Bickford RG: Electroencephalography in anesthesiology. Anesthesiology 20:359, 1959.
11. Sharbrough FW, Messick JM Jr, Sundt TM: Correlation of continuous electroencephalograms with cerebral blood flow measurements during carotid endarterectomy. Stroke 4:674, 1973.
12. Craft RM, Losasso TJ, Perkins WJ, et al: EEG monitoring for cerebral ischemia during carotid endarterectomy (CEA): How much is enough? J Neurosurg Anesthesiol 6:301, 1994.
13. Spackman TN, Faust RJ, Cucchiara RF, et al: A comparison of a periodic analysis of the EEG with standard EEG and cerebral blood flow for detection of ischemia. Anesthesiology 66:229, 1987.
14. Billard V, Gambus PL, Chamoun N, et al: A comparison of spectral edge, delta power, and bispectral index as EEG measures of alfentanil, propofol, and midazolam drug effect. Clin Pharmacol Ther 61:45, 1997.
15. Schmidt GN, Bischoff P, Standl T, et al: Narcotrend and bispectral index monitor are superior to classic electroencephalographic parameters for the assessment of anesthetic states during propofol-remifentanil anesthesia. Anesthesiology 99:1072, 2003.
16. Willmann K, Springman S, Rusy D, et al: A preliminary evaluation of a new derived EEG index monitor in anesthetized patients. J Clin Monit Comput 17:345, 2002.

17. Drover DR, Lemmens HJ, Pierce ET, et al: Patient State Index: Titration of delivery and recovery from propofol, alfentanil, and nitrous oxide anesthesia. Anesthesiology 97:82, 2002.
18. Sigl JC, Chamoun NG: An introduction to bispectral analysis for the electroencephalogram. J Clin Monit 10:392, 1994.
19. Umegaki N, Hirota K, Kitayama M, et al: A marked decrease in bispectral index with elevation of suppression ratio by cervical haematoma reducing cerebral perfusion pressure. J Clin Neurosci 10:694, 2003.
20. Hayashida M, Chinzei M, Komatsu K, et al: Detection of cerebral hypoperfusion with bispectral index during paediatric cardiac surgery. Br J Anaesth 90:694, 2003.
21. Levy WJ: Effect of epoch length on power spectrum analysis of the EEG. Anesthesiology 66:489, 1987.
22. Courtin RF, Bickford RG, Faulconer A Jr: The classification and significance of electroencephalographic patterns produced by NO/ether anesthesia during surgical operations. Proc Staff Meeting Mayo Clin 25:197, 1950.
23. Struys MM, De Smet T, Versichelen LF, et al: Comparison of closed-loop controlled administration of propofol using Bispectral Index as the controlled variable versus "standard practice" controlled administration. Anesthesiology 95:6, 2001.
24. Absalom AR, Kenny GN: Closed-loop control of propofol anaesthesia using bispectral index: Performance assessment in patients receiving computer-controlled propofol and manually controlled remifentanil infusions for minor surgery. Br J Anaesth 90:737, 2003.
25. Ghouri AF, Monk TG, White PF: Electroencephalogram spectral edge frequency, lower esophageal contractility, and autonomic responsiveness during general anesthesia. J Clin Monit 9:176, 1993.
26. Long CW, Shah NK, Loughlin C, et al: A comparison of EEG determinants of near-awakening from isoflurane and fentanyl anesthesia. Anesth Analg 69:169, 1989.
27. Glass PS, Bloom M, Kearse L, et al: Bispectral analysis measures sedation and memory effects of propofol, midazolam, isoflurane, and alfentanil in healthy volunteers. Anesthesiology 86:836, 1997.
28. Vernon JM, Lang E, Sebel PS, et al: Prediction of movement using bispectral electroencephalographic analysis during propofol/alfentanil or isoflurane/alfentanil anesthesia. Anesth Analg 80:780, 1995.
29. Kearse LA, Manberg P, DeBros F, et al: Bispectral analysis of the electroencephalogram during induction of anesthesia may predict hemodynamic responses to laryngoscopy and intubation. Electroencephogr Clin Neurophysiol 90:194, 1994.
30. Rosen I, Hagerdal M: Electroencephalographic study of children during ketamine anesthesia. Acta Anaesthesiol Scand 20:32, 1976.
31. La Marca S, Lozito RJ, Dunn RW: Cognitive and EEG recovery following bolus intravenous administration of anesthetic agents. Psychopharmacology (Berl) 120:426, 1995.
32. Sebel PS, Bovill JG, Wauquier A, et al: Effects of high dose fentanyl anesthesia on the electroencephalogram. Anesthesiology 55:203, 1981.
33. Yamamura T, Fukuda M, Takeya H, et al: Fast oscillatory EEG activity induced by analgesic concentrations of nitrous oxide in man. Anesth Analg 60:283, 1981.
34. Clark DL, Hosick EC, Neigh JL: Neurophysiologic effects of isoflurane in man. Anesthesiology 39:261, 1973.
35. Artru AA, Lam AM, Johnson JO, et al: Intracranial pressure, middle cerebral artery flow velocity, and plasma inorganic fluoride concentrations in neurosurgical patients receiving sevoflurane or isoflurane. Anesth Analg 85:587, 1997.
36. Komatsu H, Taie S, Endo S, et al: Electrical seizures during sevoflurane anesthesia in two pediatric patients with epilepsy. Anesthesiology 81:1535, 1994.
37. Jaaskelainen SK, Kaisti K, Suni L, et al: Sevoflurane is epileptogenic in healthy subjects at surgical levels of anesthesia. Neurology 61:1073, 2003.
38. Endo T, Sato K, Shamoto H, et al: Effects of sevoflurane on electrocorticography in patients with intractable temporal lobe epilepsy. J Neurosurg Anesthesiol 14:59, 2002.
39. Rampil IJ, Lockhart SH, Eger EI, et al: The electroencephalographic effects of desflurane in humans. Anesthesiology 74:434, 1991.
40. Sharpe MD, Young GB, Mirsattari S, et al: Prolonged desflurane administration for refractory status epilepticus. Anesthesiology 97:261, 2002.
41. Hoffman WE, Edelman G: Comparison of isoflurane and desflurane anesthetic depth using burst suppression of the electroencephalogram in neurosurgical patients. Anesth Analg 81:811, 1995.
42. Levy WJ: Quantitative analysis of EEG changes during hypothermia. Anesthesiology 60:291, 1984.
43. Levy WJ, Pantin E, Mehta S, et al: Hypothermia and the approximate entropy of the electroencephalogram. Anesthesiology 98:53, 2003.
44. Chabot RJ, Gugino LD, Aglio LS, et al: QEEG and neuropsychological profiles of patients after undergoing cardiopulmonary bypass surgical procedures. Clin Electroencephalogr 28:98, 1997.
45. Edmonds HL Jr, Griffiths LK, van der Laken J, et al: Quantitative electroencephalographic monitoring during myocardial revascularization predicts postoperative disorientation and improves outcome. J Thorac Cardiovasc Surg 103:555, 1992.
46. Miller G, Rodichok LD, Baylen BG: EEG changes during open heart surgery on infants aged 6 months or less: Relationship to early neurologic morbidity. Pediatr Neurol 10:124, 1994.
47. Michenfelder JD, Sundt TM, Fode N, et al: Isoflurane when compared to enflurane and halothane decreases the frequency of cerebral ischemia during carotid endarterectomy. Anesthesiology 67:336, 1987.
48. Smith JS, Roizen MF, Cahalan MK, et al: Does anesthetic technique make a difference? Augmentation of systolic blood pressure during carotid endarterectomy: Effects of phenylephrine versus light anesthesia and of isoflurane versus halothane on the incidence of myocardial ischemia. Anesthesiology 69:846, 1988.
49. Sundt TW Jr, Sharbrough FW, Piepgras DG, et al: Correlation of cerebral blood flow and electroencephalographic changes during carotid endarterectomy: With results of surgery and hemodynamics of cerebral ischemia. Mayo Clin Proc 56:533, 1981.
50. Plestis KA, Loubser P, Mizrahi EM, et al: Continuous electroencephalographic monitoring and selective shunting reduces neurologic morbidity rates in carotid endarterectomy. J Vasc Surg 25:620, 1997.
51. Darby JM, Stein K, Grenvik A, et al: Approach to management of the heart beating "brain dead" organ donor. JAMA 261:2222, 1989.
52. Bond R, Rerkasem K, Counsell C, et al: Routine or selective carotid artery shunting for carotid endarterectomy (and different methods of monitoring in selective shunting). Cochrane Database Syst Rev 2:CD000190, 2000.
53. Stockard JJ, Bickford RG: The neurophysiology of anesthesia. *In* Gordon E (ed): A Basis and Practice of Neuroanesthesia. New York, Elsevier, 1981, p 3.
54. Kraaier V, van Huffelen AC, Wieneke GH: Changes in quantitative EEG and blood flow velocity due to standardized hyperventilation; a model of transient ischaemia in young human subjects. Electroencephalogr Clin Neurophysiol 70:377, 1988.
55. Clowes GHA Jr, Kretchmer HE, McBurney RW, et al: The electroencephalogram in the evaluation of the effects of anesthetic agents and carbon dioxide accumulation during surgery. Ann Surg 138:558, 1953.
56. Report of the Medical Consultants on the Diagnosis of Death to the President's Commission for the Study of Ethical Problems in Medicine and Biomedical and Behavioral Research: Guidelines for the determination of death. JAMA 246:2184, 1981.
57. Grundy BL: Monitoring of sensory evoked potentials during neurosurgical operation: Methods and applications. Neurosurgery 11:556, 1982.

58. Greenberg RP, Ducker TB: Evoked potentials in the clinical neurosciences. J Neurosurg 56:1, 1982.
59. Freedman WA, Chadwick GM, Verhoeven JS, et al: Monitoring of somatosensory evoked potentials during surgery of middle cerebral artery aneurysms. Neurosurgery 29:98, 1991.
60. Chiappa KH, Ropper AH: Evoked potentials in clinical medicine. N Engl J Med 306:1205, 1982.
61. Cohen AR, Young W, Ransohoff J: Intraspinal localization of the somatosensory evoked potential. Neurosurgery 9:157, 1981.
62. York DH: Somatosensory evoked potentials in man: Differentiation of spinal pathways responsible for conduction from the forelimb vs. hindlimb. Prog Neurobiol 25:1, 1985.
63. Ealand-Snyder BG, Holliday TA: Pathways of ascending evoked spinal cord potentials of dogs. Electroencephalogr Clin Neurophysiol 58:140, 1984.
64. Gaines R, York DH, Watts C: Identification of spinal cord pathways responsible for the peroneal-evoked response in the dog. Spine 9:810, 1984.
65. Bundo M, Inao S, Nakamura A, et al: Changes of neural activity correlate with the severity of cortical ischemia in patients with unilateral major cerebral artery occlusion. Stroke 33:61, 2002.
66. Symon L: Flow thresholds in brain ischaemia and the effects of drugs. Br J Anaesth 57:34, 1985.
67. Brainston NM, Ladds A, Symon L, et al: Comparison of the effects of ischaemia on early components of the somatosensory evoked potential in brainstem, thalamus, and cerebral cortex. J Cereb Blood Flow Metab 4:68, 1984.
68. Lopez JR, Chang SD, Steinberg GK: The use of electrophysiological monitoring in the intraoperative management of intracranial aneurysms. J Neurol Neurosurg Psychiatry 66:189, 1999.
69. Guerit JM, Witdoeckt C, de Tourtchaninoff M, et al: Somatosensory evoked potential monitoring in carotid surgery. I. Relationships between qualitative SEP alterations and intraoperative events. Electroencephalogr Clin Neurophysiol 104:459, 1997.
70. Ganes T: A study of peripheral, cervical, and cortical evoked potentials and afferent conduction times in the somatosensory pathway. Electroencephalogr Clin Neurophysiol 49:446, 1980.
71. Engler GL, Spielholz NI, Bernhard WN, et al: Somatosensory evoked potentials during Harrington instrumentation for scoliosis. J Bone Joint Surg Am 60:528, 1978.
72. Maccabee PJ, Pinkhasov EI, Tsairis P, et al: Spinal and short latency scalp derived somatosensory evoked potentials during corrective spinal column surgery. Electroencephalogr Clin Neurophysiol 53:P32, 1982.
73. Spielholz NI, Benjamin MV, Engler GL, et al: Somatosensory evoked potentials during decompression and stabilization of the spine: Methods and findings. Spine 4:500, 1979.
74. Spielholz NI, Benjamin MV, Engler G, et al: Somatosensory evoked potentials and clinical outcome in spinal cord injury. *In* Popp AJ, Bourke RS, Nelson LR, et al (eds): Neural Trauma. New York, Raven Press, 1979, p 217.
75. Luederes H, Gurd A, Hahn J, et al: A new technique for intraoperative monitoring of spinal cord function: Multichannel recording of spinal cord and subcortical evoked potentials. Spine 7:110, 1982.
76. Landi A, Copeland SA, Wynn-Parry CB, et al: The role of somatosensory evoked potentials and nerve conduction studies in the surgical management of brachial plexus injuries. J Bone Joint Surg Br 62:492, 1980.
77. Grundy BL: Intraoperative monitoring of sensory evoked potentials. *In* Nodar RH, Barber C (eds): Evoked Potentials II. Boston, Butterworth, 1984, p 624.
78. Markand ON, Dilley RS, Moorthy SS, et al: Monitoring of somatosensory evoked responses during carotid endarterectomy. Arch Neurol 41:375, 1994.
79. Allen A, Starr A, Nudleman K: Assessment of sensory function in the operating room utilizing cerebral evoked potentials: A study of fifty-six surgically anesthetized patients. Clin Neurosurg 28:457, 1981.
80. Raudzens PA: Intraoperative monitoring of evoked potentials. Ann N Y Acad Sci 388:308, 1982.
81. Kaplan BJ, Friedman WA, Alexander JA, et al: Somatosensory evoked potential monitoring of spinal cord ischemia during aortic operations. Neurosurgery 19:82, 1986.
82. McCallum JE, Bennett MH: Electrophysiologic monitoring of spinal cord function during intraspinal surgery. Surg Forum 26:469, 1975.
83. Halliday AM, Wakefield GS: Cerebral evoked potentials in patients with dissociated sensory loss. J Neurol Neurosurg Psychiatry 26:211, 1963.
84. Szilagyi DE, Hageman JH, Smith RF, et al: Spinal cord damage in surgery of the abdominal aorta. Surgery 83:38, 1978.
85. Lam AM, Manninen PH, Ferguson GG, et al: Monitoring of electrophysiologic function during carotid endarterectomy: A comparison of somatosensory evoked potentials and conventional electroencephalogram. Anesthesiology 75:15, 1991.
86. Ackerstaff RG, van de Vlasakker CJ: Monitoring of brain function during carotid endarterectomy: An analysis of contemporary methods. J Cardiothorac Vasc Anesth 12:341, 1998.
87. Friedman WA, Chadwick GM, Verhoeven FJ, et al: Monitoring of somatosensory evoked potentials during surgery for middle cerebral artery aneurysms. Neurosurgery 29:83, 1991.
88. Mizoi K, Yoshimoto T: Intraoperative monitoring of the somatosensory evoked potentials and cerebral blood flow during aneurysm surgery-safety evaluation for temporary vascular occlusion. Neurol Med Chir (Tokyo) 31:318, 1991.
89. Misoi K, Yoshimoto T: Permissible temporary occlusion time in aneurysm surgery as evaluated by evoked potential monitoring. Neurosurgery 33:434, 1993.
90. Holland NR: Subcortical strokes from intracranial aneurysm surgery: Implications for intraoperative neuromonitoring. J Clin Neurophysiol 15:439, 1998.
91. Schramm J, Zentner J, Pechstein U: Intraoperative SEP monitoring in aneurysm surgery. Neurol Res 16:20, 1994.
92. Wiedemayer H, Fauser B, Sandalcioglu IE: The impact of neurophysiological intraoperative monitoring on surgical decisions: A critical analysis of 423 cases. J Neurosurg 96:255, 2002.
93. Kearse LA Jr, Brown EN, McPeck K: Somatosensory evoked potentials sensitivity relative to electroencephalography for cerebral ischemia during carotid endarterectomy. Stroke 23:498, 1992.
94. Wober C, Zeitlhofer J, Asenbaum S, et al: Monitoring of median nerve somatosensory evoked potentials in carotid surgery. J Clin Neurophysiol 15:429, 1998.
95. Manninen PH, Patterson S, Lam AM, et al: Evoked potential monitoring during posterior fossa aneurysm surgery: A comparison of two modalities. Can J Anaesth 41:92, 1994.
96. Manninen PH, Cuillerier DJ, Gelb AW, et al: Monitoring of brain stem function during posterior fossa surgery. Can J Anaesth 37(Pt 2):S23, 1990.
97. Friedman WA, Kaplan BL, Day AL: Evoked potential monitoring during aneurysm operation: Observations after fifty cases. Neurosurgery 20:678, 1987.
98. Little JR, Lesser RP, Luders H: Electrophysiological monitoring during basilar aneurysm operation. Neurosurgery 20:421, 1987.
99. Hume AL, Cant BR, Shaw NA: Central somatosensory conduction time in comatose patients. Ann Neurol 5:379, 1979.
100. Symon L, Hargadine J, Zawirshi M, et al: Central conduction time as an index of ischemia in subarachnoid hemorrhage. J Neurol Sci 44:95, 1979.
101. Goodwin SR, Toney KA, Mahla ME: Sensory evoked potentials accurately predict recovery from prolonged coma caused by strangulation. Crit Care Med 21:631, 1993.
102. Tomita Y, Fukuda C, Maegaki Y, et al: Re-evaluation of short latency somatosensory evoked potentials (P13, P14, and N18) for brainstem function in children who once suffered from deep coma. Brain Dev 25:352, 2003.

103. Logi F, Fischer C, Mukrri L, et al: The prognostic value of evoked responses from primary somatosensory and auditory cortex in comatose patients. Clin Neurophysiol 114:1615, 2003.

104. Robinson LR, Micklesen PJ, Tirschwell DL, et al: Predictive value of somatosensory evoked potentials for awakening from coma. Crit Care Med 31:960, 2003.

105. Chiappa KH, Ropper AH: Evoked potentials in clinical medicine. N Engl J Med 306:1140, 1982.

106. Grundy BL, Jannetta PJ, Procopio PT, et al: Intraoperative monitoring of brain-stem auditory evoked potentials. J Neurosurg 57:674, 1982.

107. Raudzens PA, Shetter AG: Intraoperative monitoring of brain-stem auditory evoked potentials. J Neurosurg 57:341, 1982.

108. Duncan PG, Sanders RA, McCollough DW: Preservation of auditory-evoked responses in anaesthetized children. Can Anaesth Soc J 26:492, 1979.

109. Auger RG, Piepgras DG, Laws ER: Hemifacial spasm: Results of microvascular decompression of the facial nerve in 54 patients. Mayo Clin Proc 61:640, 1986.

110. Miller AR, Jannetta PJ: Monitoring auditory functions during cranial nerve microvascular decompression operations by direct recording from the eighth nerve. J Neurosurg 59:493, 1983.

111. Rizvi SS, Goyal RN, Calder HB: Hearing preservation in microvascular decompression for trigeminal neuralgia. Laryngoscope 109:591, 1999.

112. Moller AR, Moller MB: Does intraoperative monitoring of auditory evoked potentials reduce incidence of hearing loss as a complication of microvascular decompression of cranial nerves? Neurosurgery 24:257, 1989.

113. Watanabe E, Schramm J, Strauss C, et al: Neurophysiologic monitoring in posterior fossa surgery. II. BAEP—Waves I and V and preservation of hearing. Acta Neurochir (Wien) 98:118, 1989.

114. Friedman WA, Kaplan BJ, Gravenstein D, et al: Intraoperative brain-stem auditory evoked potentials during posterior fossa microvascular decompression. J Neurosurg 62:552, 1985.

115. Browning S, Mohr G, Dufour JJ, et al: Hearing preservation in acoustic neuroma surgery. J Otolaryngol 30:307, 2001.

116. Neu M, Strauss C, Romstock J, et al: The prognostic value of intraoperative BAEP patterns in acoustic neurinoma surgery. Clin Neurophysiol 110:1935, 1999.

117. Holsinger FC, Coker NJ, Jenkins HA: Hearing preservation in conservation surgery for vestibular schwannoma. Am J Otol 21:695, 2000.

118. Battista RA, Wiet RJ, Paauwe L: Evaluation of three intraoperative auditory monitoring techniques in acoustic neuroma surgery. Am J Otol 21:244, 2000.

119. Glascock ME III, Hays JW, Minor LB, et al: Preservation of hearing in surgery for acoustic neuromas. J Neurosurg 78:864, 1993.

120. Banoub M, Tetzlaff JE, Schubert A: Pharmacologic and physiologic influences affecting sensory evoked potentials. Anesthesiology 99:716, 2003.

121. Peterson DO, Drummond JC, Todd MM: Effects of halothane, enflurane, isoflurane, and nitrous oxide on somatosensory evoked potentials in humans. Anesthesiology 65:35, 1986.

122. McPherson RW, Mahla M, Johnson R, et al: Effects of enflurane, isoflurane, and nitrous oxide on somatosensory evoked potentials during fentanyl anesthesia. Anesthesiology 62:626, 1985.

123. Pathak KS, Amaddio BS, Scoles PV, et al: Effects of halothane, enflurane, and isoflurane in nitrous oxide on multilevel somatosensory evoked potentials. Anesthesiology 70:207, 1989.

124. Samra SK, Vanderzant CW, Domer PA, et al: Differential effects of isoflurane on human median nerve somatosensory evoked potentials. Anesthesiology 66:29, 1987.

125. Sebel PS, Ingram DA, Flynn PJ: Evoked potentials during isoflurane anaesthesia. Br J Anaesth 58:580, 1986.

126. Scholz J, Bischoff P, Szafarczyk W, et al: Comparison of sevoflurane and isoflurane in ambulatory surgery: Results of a multicenter study. Anaesthesist 45:S63, 1996.

127. Haghighi SS, Sirintrapun SJ, Johnson JC, et al: Suppression of spinal and cortical somatosensory evoked potentials by desflurane anesthesia. J Neurosurg Anesthesiol 8:148, 1996.

128. Bernard JM, Pereon Y, Fayet G, et al: Effects of isoflurane and desflurane on neurogenic motor- and somatosensory-evoked potential monitoring for scoliosis surgery. Anesthesiology 85:1013, 1996.

129. Boisseau N, Madany M, Staccini P, et al: Comparison of the effects of sevoflurane and propofol on cortical somatosensory evoked potentials. Br J Anaesth 88:785, 2002.

130. Vaugha DJ, Thornton C, Wright DR, et al: Effects of different concentrations of sevoflurane and desflurane on subcortical somatosensory evoked responses in anaesthetized, non-stimulated patients. Br J Anaesth 86:59, 2001.

131. Manninen PH, Lam AM, Nicholas JF: The effects of isoflurane–nitrous oxide anesthesia on brainstem auditory evoked potentials in humans. Anesth Analg 64:43, 1985.

132. Thornton C, Catley DM, Jordan C, et al: Enflurane anaesthesia causes graded changes in the brainstem and early cortical auditory evoked response in man. Br J Anaesth 55:479, 1983.

133. Dubois MY, Sato S, Chassy J, et al: Effects of enflurane on brainstem auditory evoked responses in humans. Anesth Analg 61:898, 1982.

134. Cohen MS, Britt RH: Effects of sodium pentobarbital, ketamine, halothane, chloralose on brainstem auditory evoked responses. Anesth Analg 61:338, 1982.

135. Chi OZ, Field C: Effects of isoflurane on visual evoked potentials in humans. Anesthesiology 65:328, 1986.

136. Uhl RR, Squires KC, Bruce DL, et al: Effect of halothane anesthesia on the human cortical visual evoked response. Anesthesiology 53:273, 1980.

137. Domino EF, Corssen G, Sweet RB: Effects of various general anesthetics on the visually evoked response in man. Anesth Analg 42:735, 1963.

138. Burchiel KG, Stockard JJ, Myers RR, et al: Visual and auditory evoked responses during enflurane anesthesia in man and cats. Electroencephalogr Clin Neurophysiol 39:434P, 1973.

139. Sebel PS, Flynn PJ, Ingram DA: Effect of nitrous oxide on visual, auditory, and somatosensory evoked potentials. Br J Anaesth 56:1403, 1984.

140. Drummond JC, Todd MM, Sang H: The effect of high dose sodium thiopental on brain stem auditory and median nerve somatosensory evoked responses in humans. Anesthesiology 63:249, 1985.

141. Shimoji K, Kano T, Nakashima H, et al: The effects of thiamylal sodium on electrical activities of the central and peripheral nervous systems in man. Anesthesiology 40:234, 1974.

142. Ganes T, Lundar T: The effect of thiopentone on somatosensory evoked responses and EEGs in comatose patients. J Neurol Neurosurg Psychiatry 46:509, 1983.

143. Sutton LN, Frewen T, Marsh R, et al: The effects of deep barbiturate coma on multimodality evoked potentials. J Neurosurg 57:178, 1982.

144. Koht A, Schutz W, Schmidt G, et al: Effects of etomidate, midazolam, and thiopental on median nerve somatosensory evoked potentials and the additive effects of fentanyl and nitrous oxide. Anesth Analg 67:435, 1988.

145. Sloan TB, Ronai AK, Toleikis JR, et al: Improvement of intraoperative somatosensory evoked potentials by etomidate. Anesth Analg 67:582, 1988.

146. Navaratnarajah M, Thornton C, Heneghan CPH, et al: Effect of etomidate on the auditory evoked response in man Proc Anaesth Res Soc 55:1157P, 1983.

147. Grundy BL, Brown RH, Clifton PC: Effect of droperidol on somatosensory cortical evoked potentials. Electroencephalogr Clin Neurophysiol 50:158, 1980.

148. Doring WH, Daub D: Akustisch evozierte Hirstamm und Rindepotentiale bei sedierung mit diazepam. Arch Otorhinolaryngol 227:522, 1980.

149. Grundy BL, Brown RH, Greenbergh BA: Diazepam alters cortical potentials. Anesthesiology 51:538, 1979.

150. Pathak KS, Brown RH, Cascorbi HF, et al: Effects of fentanyl and morphine on intraoperative somatosensory cortical-evoked potentials. Anesth Analg 63:833, 1984.

151. Schubert A, Peterson DO, Drummond JC, et al: The effect of high-dose fentanyl on human median nerve somatosensory evoked responses. Anesth Analg 65:S136, 1986.

152. Grundy BL, Brown RH: Meperidine enhances somatosensory cortical evoked potentials. Electroencephalogr Clin Neurophysiol 50:177, 1980.

153. Samra SK, Lilly DJ, Rush NL, et al: Fentanyl anesthesia and human brain-stem auditory evoked potentials. Anesthesiology 61:261, 1984.

154. Eng DY, Dong WK, Bledsoe SW, et al: Electrical and pathological correlates of brain hypoxia during hypotension. Anesthesiology 53:S92, 1980.

155. Kobrine AI, Evans DE, Rizzoli HV: Relative vulnerability of the brain and spinal cord to ischemia. J Neurol Sci 45:65, 1980.

156. Bunegin L, Albin MS, Helsel P, et al: Evoked responses during trimethaphan hypotension. Anesthesiology 55:A232, 1981.

157. Grundy BL, Nash CL, Brown RH: Arterial pressure manipulation alters spinal cord function during correction of scoliosis. Anesthesiology 54:249, 1981.

158. Russ W, Kling D, Loesevitz A, et al: Effect of hypothermia on visual evoked potential (VEP) in humans. Anesthesiology 61:207, 1984.

159. Stockard JJ, Sharbrough FW, Tinker JA: Effects of hypothermia on the human brainstem auditory response. Ann Neurol 3:368, 1978.

160. Spetzler RF, Hadley MN, Rigamonti D, et al: Aneurysms of the basilar artery treated with circulatory arrest, hypothermia, and barbiturate cerebral protection. J Neurosurg 68:868, 1988.

161. Dubois M, Loppola R, Buchsbaum MS, et al: Somatosensory evoked potentials during whole body hyperthermia in humans. Electroencephalogr Clin Neurophysiol 52:157, 1981.

162. Nakagawa Y, Ohtsuka T, Tsura M, et al: Effects of mild hypercapnia on somatosensory evoked potentials in experimental cerebral ischemia. Stroke 25:275, 1984.

163. Grundy BL, Heros RC, Tung AS, et al: Intraoperative hypoxia detected by evoked potential monitoring. Anesth Analg 60:437, 1981.

164. Nagao S, Roccaforte P, Moody RA: The effects of isovolemic hemodilution and reinfusion of packed erythrocytes on somatosensory and visual evoked potentials. J Surg Res 25:S30, 1978.

165. Harper CM, Daube RJ: Surgical monitoring with evoked potentials: The Mayo Clinic experience. *In* Desmedt JE (ed): Neuromonitoring in Surgery. New York, Elsevier Science, 1989, p 275.

166. Harner SG, Daube JR, Beatty CW: Improved preservation of facial nerve function with use of electrical monitoring during removal of acoustic neuromas. Mayo Clin Proc 62:92, 1987.

167. Harner SG, Daube JR, Ebersold MJ: Electrophysiologic monitoring of facial nerve during temporal bone surgery. Laryngoscope 96:65, 1986.

168. Acoustic neuroma. Consens Statement 9:1, 1991.

169. Miller AR, Jannetta PJ: Microvascular decompression in hemifacial spasm: Intraoperative electrophysiological observations. Neurosurgery 16:612, 1985.

170. Lennon RL, Hosking MP, Daube JR, et al: Effect of partial neuromuscular blockade on intraoperative electromyography in patients undergoing resection of acoustic neuroma. Anesth Analg 75:729, 1992.

171. Zentner J, Kiss I, Ebner A: Influence of anesthetics—nitrous oxide in particular—on electromyographic response evoked by transcranial electrical stimulation of the cortex. Neurosurgery 24:253, 1989.

172. Zentner J, Abner A: Nitrous oxide suppresses the electromyographic response evoked by electrical stimulation of the motor cortex. Neurosurgery 24:60, 1989.

173. Kline DG, Kim D, Midha R, et al: Management and results of sciatic nerve injuries: A 24-year experience. J Neurosurg 89:13, 1998.

174. Kim DH, Cho YJ, Tiel RL, et al: Outcomes of surgery in 1019 brachial plexus lesions treated at Louisiana State University Health Sciences Center. J Neurosurg 98:1005, 2003.

175. Levy WJ, York DH, McCaffrey M, et al: Motor evoked potentials from transcranial stimulation of the motor cortex in humans. Neurosurgery 15:287, 1984.

176. Legatt AD: Current practice of motor evoked potential monitoring: Results of a survey. J Clin Neurophysiol 19:454, 2002.

177. MacDonald DB, Al Zayed Z, Khoudeir I, et al: Monitoring scoliosis surgery with combined multiple pulse transcranial electric motor and cortical somatosensory-evoked potentials from the lower and upper extremities. Spine 28:194, 2003.

178. Szelenyi A, Bueno de Camargo A, Flamm E, et al: Neurophysiological criteria for intraoperative prediction of pure motor hemiplegia during aneurysm surgery: Case report. J Neurosurg 99:575, 2003.

179. Meylaerts S, Jacobs MJ, van Iterson V, et al: Comparison of transcranial motor evoked potentials and somatosensory evoked potentials during thoracoabdominal aortic aneurysm repair. Ann Surg 230:742, 1999.

180. Pelosi L, Lamb J, Grevitt M, et al: Combined monitoring of motor and somatosensory evoked potentials in orthopaedic spinal surgery. Clin Neurophysiol 113:1082, 2002.

181. Zentner J: Motor evoked potential monitoring during neurosurgical operations on the spinal cord. Neurosurg Rev 14:29, 1991.

182. Owen JH, Laschinger J, Bridwell K, et al: Sensitivity and specificity of somatosensory and neurogenic-motor evoked potentials in animals and humans. Spine 13:1111, 1988.

183. Edmonds HL, Paloheimo MPJ, Backman MH, et al: Transcranial magnetic motor evoked potentials for functional monitoring of motor pathways during scoliosis surgery. Spine 14:683, 1989.

184. Boyd SG, Rothwell JC, Cowan JMA, et al: A method of monitoring function in corticospinal pathways during scoliosis surgery with a note on motor conduction velocities. J Neurol Neurosurg Psychiatry 49:251, 1986.

185. Elmore JR, Gloviczki P, Harper CM, et al: Failure of motor evoked potentials to predict neurologic outcome in experimental thoracic aortic occlusion. J Vasc Surg 14:131, 1991.

186. Reuter DG, Tacker WA, Badylak SF, et al: Correlation of motor-evoked potential response to ischemic spinal cord damage. J Thorac Cardiovasc Surg 104:262, 1992.

187. Dong CC, MacDonald DB, Janusz MT: Intraoperative spinal cord monitoring during descending thoracic and thoracoabdominal aneurysm surgery. Ann Thorac Surg 74:S1873, 2002.

188. Guerit JM, Dion RA: State-of-the-art of neuromonitoring for prevention of immediate and delayed paraplegia in thoracic and thoracoabdominal aorta surgery. Ann Thorac Surg 74:S1867, 2002.

189. Jacobs MJ, Elenbaas TW, Schurink GW, et al: Assessment of spinal cord integrity during thoracoabdominal aortic aneurysm repair. Ann Thorac Surg 74:S1864, 2002.

190. MacDonald DB, Janusz M: An approach to intraoperative neurophysiologic monitoring of thoracoabdominal aneurysm surgery. J Clin Neurophysiol 19:43, 2002.

191. Meylaerts SA, Jacobs MJ, van Iterson V, et al: Comparison of transcranial motor evoked potentials and somatosensory evoked potentials during thoracoabdominal aortic aneurysm repair. Ann Surg 230:742, 1999.

192. de Haan P, Kalkman CJ, Jacobs MJ: Spinal cord monitoring with myogenic motor evoked potentials: Early detection of spinal cord ischemia as an integral part of spinal cord protective strategies during thoracoabdominal aneurysm surgery. Semin Thorac Cardiovasc Surg 10:19, 1998.

193. Owen JH, Bridwell KH, Grubb R, et al: The clinical application of neurogenic motor evoked potentials to

monitor spinal cord function during surgery. Spine 16(Suppl):S385, 1991.

194. Darden BV 2nd, Hatley MK, Owen JH: Neurogenic motor evoked-potential monitoring in anterior cervical surgery. J Spinal Disord 9:485, 1996.

195. Pereon Y, Bernard JM, Fayet G, et al: Usefulness of neurogenic motor evoked potentials for spinal cord monitoring: Findings in 112 consecutive patients undergoing surgery for spinal deformity. Electroencephalogr Clin Neurophysiol 108:17, 1998.

196. Toleikis JR, Skelly JP, Carlvin AO, et al: Spinally elicited peripheral nerve responses are sensory rather than motor. Clin Neurophysiol 111:736, 2000.

197. Jellinek D, Jewkes D, Symon L: Noninvasive intraoperative monitoring of motor evoked potentials under propofol anesthesia: Effects of spinal surgery on the amplitude and latency of motor evoked potentials. Neurosurgery 29:551, 1991.

198. Taniguchi M, Nadstawek J, Langenbach U, et al: Effects of four intravenous anesthetic agents on motor evoked potentials elicited by magnetic transcranial stimulation. Neurosurgery 33:407, 1993.

199. Ubags LH, Kalkman CJ, Been HD, et al: The use of ketamine or etomidate to supplement sufentanil/N$_2$O anesthesia does not disrupt monitoring of myogenic transcranial motor evoked responses. J Neurosurg Anesthesiol 9:228, 1997.

200. Kalkman CJ, Drummond JC, Patel PM, et al: Effects of droperidol, pentobarbital and ketamine on myogenic motor evoked responses in humans. Neurosurgery 35:1066, 1994.

201. DeWitt LD, Wechsler LR: Transcranial Doppler. Stroke 19:915, 1988.

202. Sloan TB, Heyer EJ: Anesthesia for intraoperative neurophysiologic monitoring of the spinal cord. J Clin Neurophysiol 19:430, 2002.

203. Zentner J, Thees C, Pechstein U, et al: Influence of nitrous oxide on motor-evoked potentials. Spine 22:1002, 1997.

204. Nathan N, Tabaraud F, Lacroix F, et al: Influence of propofol concentrations on multipulse transcranial motor evoked potentials. Br J Anaesth 91:493, 2003.

205. Ghaly RF, Ham JH, Lee JJ: High-dose ketamine hydrochloride maintains somatosensory and magnetic motor evoked potentials in primates. Neurol Res 23:881, 2001.

206. Scheufler KM, Zentner J: Total intravenous anesthesia for intraoperative monitoring of the motor pathways: An integral view combining clinical and experimental data. J Neurosurg 96:571, 2002.

207. Taniguchi M, Nadstawek J, Langenbach U, et al: Effects of four intravenous anesthetic agents on motor evoked potentials elicited by magnetic transcranial stimulation. Neurosurgery 33:407, 1993.

208. Ubags LH, Kalkman CJ, Been HD, et al: The use of ketamine or etomidate to supplement sufentanil/N$_2$O anesthesia does not disrupt monitoring of myogenic transcranial motor evoked responses. J Neurosurg Anesthesiol 9:228, 1997.

209. Yang LH, Lin SM, Lee WY, et al: Intraoperative transcranial electrical motor evoked potential monitoring during spinal surgery under intravenous ketamine or etomidate anesthesia. Acta Neurochir (Wien) 127:191, 1994.

210. Ubags LH, Kalkman CJ, Been HD, et al: A comparison of myogenic motor evoked responses to electrical and magnetic transcranial stimulation during nitrous oxide/opioid anesthesia. Anesth Analg 88:568, 1999.

211. Pechstein U, Nadstawek J, Zentner J, et al: Isoflurane plus nitrous oxide versus propofol for recording of motor evoked potentials after high frequency repetitive electrical stimulation. Electroencephalogr Clin Neurophysiol 108:175, 1998.

212. Pelosi L, Stevenson M, Hobbs GJ, et al: Intraoperative motor evoked potentials to transcranial electrical stimulation during two anaesthetic regimens. Clin Neurophysiol 112:1076, 2001.

213. Ubaga LH, Kalkman CJ, Been HD: Influence of isoflurane on myogenic motor evoked potentials to single and multiple transcranial stimuli during nitrous oxide/opioid anesthesia. Neurosurgery 43:90, 1998.

214. Halsey JH, McDowell HA, Gelman S: Transcranial Doppler and rCBF compared in carotid endarterectomy. Stroke 17:1206, 1986.

215. Molloy J, Markus HS: Asymptomatic embolization predicts stroke and TIA risk in patients with carotid artery stenosis. Stroke 30:1440, 1999.

216. Ackerstaff RG, Moons KG, van de Vlasakker CJ, et al: Association of intraoperative transcranial Doppler monitoring variables with stroke from carotid endarterectomy. Stroke 31:1817, 2000.

217. Laman DM, Wieneke GH, van Duijn H, et al: High embolic rate early after carotid endarterectomy is associated with early cerebrovascular complications, especially in women. J Vasc Surg 36:278, 2002.

218. Munts AG, Mess WH, Bruggemans EF, et al: Feasibility and reliability of on-line automated microemboli detection after carotid endarterectomy: A transcranial Doppler study. Eur J Vasc Endovasc Surg 25:262, 2003.

219. Levi CR, O'Malley HM, Fell G, et al: Transcranial Doppler detected cerebral microembolism following carotid endarterectomy. High microembolic signal loads predict postoperative cerebral ischaemia. Brain 120(Pt 4):621, 1997.

220. Levi CR, Roberts AK, Fell G, et al: Transcranial Doppler microembolus detection in the identification of patients at high risk of perioperative stroke. Eur J Vasc Endovasc Surg 14:170, 1997.

221. Smith JL, Evans DH, Gaunt ME, et al: Experience with transcranial Doppler monitoring reduces the incidence of particulate embolization during carotid endarterectomy. Br J Surg 85:56, 1998.

222. van der Linden J, Casimir AH: When do cerebral emboli occur during open heart operations? A transcranial Doppler study. Ann Thorac Surg 51:237, 1991.

223. Pugsley W, Klinger L, Paschalis C, et al: The impact of microemboli during cardiopulmonary bypass on neuropsychological functioning. Stroke 25:1393, 1994.

224. Clark RE, Brillman J, Davis DA, et al: Microemboli during coronary artery bypass grafting. J Thorac Cardiovasc Surg 109:249, 1995.

225. Fearn SJ, Pole R, Burgess M, Ray SG, et al: Cerebral embolisation during modern cardiopulmonary bypass. Eur J Cardiothorac Surg 20:1163, 2001.

226. Borger MA, Djaiani G, Fedorko L, et al: Reduction of cerebral emboli during cardiac surgery: Influence of surgeon and perfusionist feedback. Heart Surg Forum 6:204, 2003.

227. Groom RC, Likosky DS, O'Connor GT, et al: Identification of techniques associated with changes in embolic count, hemodynamics and cerebral desaturation. II. Perfusion. Heart Surg Forum 6:205, 2003.

228. Sloan MA, Haley EC, Kassell NF, et al: Sensitivity and specificity of transcranial Doppler ultrasonography in the diagnosis of vasospasm following subarachnoid hemorrhage. Neurology 39:1514, 1989.

229. Sekhar LN, Wechsler LR, Yonas H, et al: Value of transcranial Doppler examination in the diagnosis of cerebral vasospasm after subarachnoid hemorrhage. Neurosurgery 22:813, 1988.

230. Suarez JI, Qureshi AI, Yahia AB, et al: Symptomatic vasospasm diagnosis after subarachnoid hemorrhage: Evaluation of transcranial Doppler ultrasound and cerebral angiography as related to compromised vascular distribution. Crit Care Med 30:1348, 2002.

231. Topcuoglu MA, Pryor JC, Ogilvy CS, et al: Cerebral vasospasm following subarachnoid hemorrhage. Curr Treat Options Cardiovasc Med 4:373, 2002.

232. Jarus-Dziedzic K, Juniewicz H, Wronski J, et al: The relation between cerebral blood flow velocities as measured by TCD and the incidence of delayed ischemic deficits: A prospective study after subarachnoid hemorrhage. Neurol Res 24:582, 2002.

233. Aaslid R: Transcranial Doppler assessment of cerebral vasospasm. Eur J Ultrasound 16:3, 2002.

234. Mascia L, Fedorko L, terBrugge K, et al: The accuracy of transcranial Doppler to detect vasospasm in patients with

aneurysmal subarachnoid hemorrhage. Intensive Care Med 29:1088, 2003.

235. Petty GW, Mohr JP, Pedley T, et al: The role of transcranial Doppler in confirming brain death. Neurology 40:300, 1990.

236. Fortune JB, Feustel PJ, Graca L, et al: Effect of hyperventilation, mannitol, and ventriculostomy drainage on cerebral blood flow after head injury. J Trauma 39:1091, 1995.

237. Skippen P, Seear M, Poskitt K, et al: Effect of hyperventilation on regional cerebral blood flow in head-injured children. Crit Care Med 25:1402, 1997.

238. Imberti R, Bellinzona G, Langer M: Cerebral tissue Po$_2$ and Sjvo$_2$ changes during moderate hyperventilation in patients with severe traumatic brain injury. J Neurosurg 96:97, 2002.

239. Coles JP, Minhas PS, Fryer TD, et al: Effect of hyperventilation on cerebral blood flow in traumatic head injury: Clinical relevance and monitoring correlates. Crit Care Med 30:1950, 2002.

240. Williams IM, Picton A, Farrell A, et al: Light-reflective cerebral oximetry and jugular bulb venous oxygen saturation during carotid endarterectomy. Br J Surg 81:1291, 1994.

241. Gopinath SP, Cormio M, Ziegler J, et al: Intraoperative jugular desaturation during surgery for traumatic intracranial hematomas. Anesth Analg 83:1014, 1996.

242. Unterberg AW, Kiening KL, Härtl R, et al: Multimodal monitoring in patients with head injury: Evaluation of the effects of treatment on cerebral oxygenation. J Trauma 42:S32, 1997.

243. Matta BF, Lam AM: The rate of blood withdrawal affects the accuracy of jugular venous bulb oxygen saturation measurements. Anesthesiology 86:806, 1997.

244. Moss E, Dearden NM, Berridge JC: Effects of changes in mean arterial pressure on Sjo$_2$ during cerebral aneurysm surgery. Br J Anaesth 75:527, 1995.

245. Croughwell ND, White WD, Smith LR, et al: Jugular bulb saturation and mixed venous saturation during cardiopulmonary bypass. J Card Surg 10:503, 1995.

246. Smythe PR, Samra SK: Monitors of cerebral oxygenation. Anesthesiol Clin North Am 20:293, 2002.

247. Rampil IJ, Litt L, Mayevsky A: Correlated, simultaneous, multiple-wavelength optical monitoring in vivo of localized cerebrocortical NADH and brain microvessel hemoglobin oxygen saturation. J Clin Monit 8:216, 1992.

248. Dunham CM, Sosnowski C, Porter JM, et al: Correlation of noninvasive cerebral oximetry with cerebral perfusion in the severe head injured patient: A pilot study. J Trauma 52:40, 2002.

249. Buchner K, Meixensberger J, Dings J, et al: Near-infrared spectroscopy—Not useful to monitor cerebral oxygenation after severe brain injury. Zentralbl Neurochir 61:69, 2000.

250. Macmillan CS, Andrews PJ: Cerebrovenous oxygen saturation monitoring: Practical considerations and clinical relevance. Intensive Care Med 26:1028, 2000.

251. McLeod AD, Igielman F, Elwell C, et al: Measuring cerebral oxygenation during normobaric hyperoxia: A comparison of tissue microprobes, near-infrared spectroscopy, and jugular venous oximetry in head injury. Anesth Analg 97:851, 2003.

252. Kirkpatric PJ, Smielewski P, Czosnyka M, et al: Near-infrared spectroscopy use in patients with head injury. J Neurosurg 83:963, 1995.

253. Samra SK, Dy EA, Welch K, et al: Evaluation of a cerebral oximeter as a monitor of cerebral ischemia during carotid endarterectomy. Anesthesiology 93:964, 2000.

254. Grubhofer G, Lassnigg A, Manlik F, et al: The contribution of extracranial blood oxygenation on near-infrared spectroscopy during carotid thromboendarterectomy. Anaesthesia 52:116, 1997.

255. Beese U, Langer H, Lang W, et al: Comparison of near-infrared spectroscopy and somatosensory evoked potentials for the detection of cerebral ischemia during carotid endarterectomy. Stroke 29:2032, 1998.

256. Reents W, Muellges W, Franke D, et al: Cerebral oxygen saturation assessed by near-infrared spectroscopy during coronary artery bypass grafting and early postoperative cognitive function. Ann Thorac Surg 74:109, 2002.

257. Janelle GM, Mnookin S, Gravenstein N, et al: Unilateral cerebral oxygen desaturation during emergent repair of a DeBakey type 1 aortic dissection: Potential aversion of a major catastrophe. Anesthesiology 96:1263, 2002.

258. Brown R, Wright G, Royston D: A comparison of two systems for assessing cerebral venous oxyhaemoglobin saturation during cardiopulmonary bypass in humans. Anaesthesia 48:697, 1993.

259. Daubeney PE, Smith DC, Pilkington SN, et al: Cerebral oxygenation during paediatric cardiac surgery: Identification of vulnerable periods using near-infrared spectroscopy. Eur J Cardiothorac Surg 13:370, 1998.

260. Kadoi Y, Kawahara F, Saito S, et al: Effects of hypothermic and normothermic cardiopulmonary bypass on brain oxygenation. Ann Thorac Surg 68:34, 1999.

261. Germon TJ, Young AE, Manara AR, et al: Extracerebral absorption of near-infrared light influences the detection of increased cerebral oxygenation monitored by near-infrared spectroscopy. J Neurol Neurosurg Psychiatry 58:477, 1995.

262. Fearn SJ, Picton AJ, Mortimer AJ, et al: The contribution of the external carotid artery to cerebral perfusion in carotid disease. J Vasc Surg 31:989, 2000.

263. Samra SK, Stanley JC, Zelenock GB, et al: An assessment of contributions made by extracranial tissues during cerebral oximetry. J Neurosurg Anesthesiol 11:1, 1999.

264. Clark DL, Rosner BS: Neurophysiologic effects of general anesthetics. Anesthesiology 38:564, 1973.

39 Neuromuscular Monitoring

Jørgen Viby-Mogensen

**Types of Peripheral Nerve
Stimulation   1552**

**Principles of Peripheral Nerve
Stimulation   1552**

Patterns of Nerve Stimulation   1552
Single-Twitch Stimulation   1552
Train-of-Four Stimulation   1552
Tetanic Stimulation   1553
Post-Tetanic Count Stimulation   1554
Double-Burst Stimulation   1555

The Nerve Stimulator   1555

The Stimulating Electrodes   1557

**Sites of Nerve Stimulation and
Different Muscle Responses   1557**

Recording of Evoked Responses   1558
Mechanomyography   1558
Electromyography   1558
Acceleromyography   1560

Piezoelectric Neuromuscular
Monitors   1561
Phonomyography   1561

**Evaluation of Recorded Evoked
Responses   1561**
Nondepolarizing Neuromuscular
Blockade   1561
Depolarizing Neuromuscular Blockade
(Phase I and II Blocks)   1563

**Use of Nerve Stimulators Without
Recording Equipment   1563**
Use of a Peripheral Nerve Stimulator During
Induction of Anesthesia   1564
Use of a Peripheral Nerve Stimulator
During Surgery   1564
Use of a Peripheral Nerve Stimulator During
Reversal of Neuromuscular Blockade   1565

**When to Use a Peripheral Nerve
Stimulator   1565**

Traditionally, the degree of neuromuscular block during and after anesthesia is evaluated with clinical criteria alone. However, many studies have documented that routine clinical evaluation of recovery of neuromuscular function does not exclude clinically significant residual curarization.[1-4] Therefore, there is a growing understanding that more attention should be paid to objective monitoring of the degree of neuromuscular block during and after anesthesia and to the problems of residual curarization.[5,6]

In awake patients, muscle power can be evaluated through tests of voluntary muscle strength, but during anesthesia and recovery from anesthesia this is not possible. Instead, the clinician uses clinical tests to assess muscle power directly and to estimate neuromuscular function indirectly (muscle tone, the feel of the anesthesia bag as an indirect measure of pulmonary compliance,

tidal volume, and inspiratory force). All of these tests, however, are influenced by factors other than the degree of neuromuscular blockade. Therefore, whenever more precise information regarding the status of neuromuscular functioning is desired, the response of muscle to nerve stimulation should be assessed. This procedure also takes into account the considerable variation in individual response to muscle relaxants.

This chapter reviews the basic principles of peripheral nerve stimulation and the requirements for effective use of nerve stimulators. It also describes the response to nerve stimulation during depolarizing (phase I and phase II) and nondepolarizing neuromuscular blocks. Finally, this chapter discusses methods of evaluating evoked neuromuscular responses both with and without the availability of recording equipment.

TYPES OF PERIPHERAL NERVE STIMULATION

Neuromuscular function is monitored by evaluating the muscular response to supramaximal stimulation of a peripheral motor nerve. Two types of stimulation can be used: electrical and magnetic. Electrical nerve stimulation is by far the most commonly used method in clinical practice and is described in detail in this chapter. In theory, magnetic nerve stimulation has several advantages over electrical nerve stimulation.[7,8] It is less painful and does not require physical contact with the body. However, the required equipment is bulky and heavy, it cannot be used for train-of-four stimulation and it is difficult to achieve supramaximal stimulation with this method. Therefore, it is very seldom used in clinical anesthesia.

PRINCIPLES OF PERIPHERAL NERVE STIMULATION

The reaction of a single muscle fiber to a stimulus follows an all-or-none pattern. In contrast, the response of the whole muscle depends on the number of muscle fibers activated. If a nerve is stimulated with sufficient intensity, all fibers supplied by the nerve will react, and the maximum response will be triggered. After administration of a neuromuscular blocking drug, the response of the muscle decreases in parallel with the number of fibers blocked. The reduction in response during constant stimulation, reflects the degree of neuromuscular blockade.

For the preceding principles to be in effect, the stimulus must be truly maximal throughout the period of monitoring; therefore, the electrical stimulus applied is usually at least 20% to 25% above that necessary for a maximal response. For this reason the stimulus is said to be supramaximal; however, supramaximal electrical stimulation hurts, which is not a concern during anesthesia, but during recovery the patient may be awake enough to experience the discomfort of nerve stimulation. Therefore, some researchers advocate stimulation with submaximal current during recovery. Although several investigations indicate that testing of neuromuscular function can be reliably performed postoperatively using submaximal stimulation,[9-11] the accuracy of the monitoring is unacceptable at low current.[12]

PATTERNS OF NERVE STIMULATION

For evaluation of neuromuscular function the most commonly used patterns of electrical nerve stimulation are single-twitch, train-of-four (TOF), tetanic, post-tetanic count (PTC), and double-burst stimulation (DBS).

Single-Twitch Stimulation

In the single-twitch mode of stimulation, single supramaximal electrical stimuli are applied to a peripheral motor nerve at frequencies ranging from 1.0 Hz (once every second) to 0.1 Hz (once every 10 seconds) (Fig. 39-1).

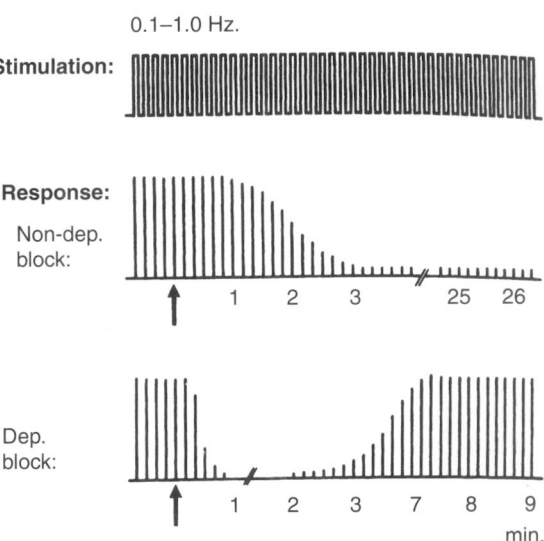

Figure 39–1 Pattern of electrical stimulation and evoked muscle responses to single-twitch nerve stimulation (at frequencies of 0.1 to 1.0 Hz) after injection of nondepolarizing (Non-dep) and depolarizing (Dep) neuromuscular blocking drugs (*arrows*). Note that except for the difference in time factors, no differences in the strength of the evoked responses exist between the two types of block.

The response to single-twitch stimulation depends on the frequency with which the individual stimuli are applied. If the rate of delivery is increased to more than 0.15 Hz, the evoked response will gradually decrease and settle at a lower level. As a result, a frequency of 0.1 Hz is generally used. Because 1-Hz stimulation shortens the time necessary to determine supramaximal stimulation, this frequency is sometimes employed during induction of anesthesia; however, the apparent time of onset and length of neuromuscular blockade depend on the pattern and duration of stimulation. Therefore, results obtained using 1-Hz single-twitch stimulation cannot be compared with results obtained by using, for instance, 0.1-Hz single-twitch stimulation or TOF stimulation.[13]

Train-of-Four Stimulation

In TOF nerve stimulation, introduced by Ali and associates[14,15] during the early 1970s, four supramaximal stimuli are given every 0.5 seconds (2 Hz) (Fig. 39-2). When used continuously, each set (train) of stimuli normally is repeated every 10th to 20th second. Each stimulus in the train causes the muscle to contract, and "fade" in the response provides the basis for evaluation. That is, dividing the amplitude of the fourth response by the amplitude of the first response provides the TOF ratio. In the control response (the response obtained before administration of muscle relaxant), all four responses are ideally the same: The TOF ratio is 1.0. During a partial nondepolarizing block, the ratio decreases (fades) and is inversely proportional to the degree of blockade. During a partial depolarizing block, no fade occurs in the TOF response; ideally, the TOF ratio is approximately 1.0. Fade in the TOF response after injection of succinylcholine signifies the development of a phase II block (discussed later in the section on Depolarizing Neuromuscular Blockade).

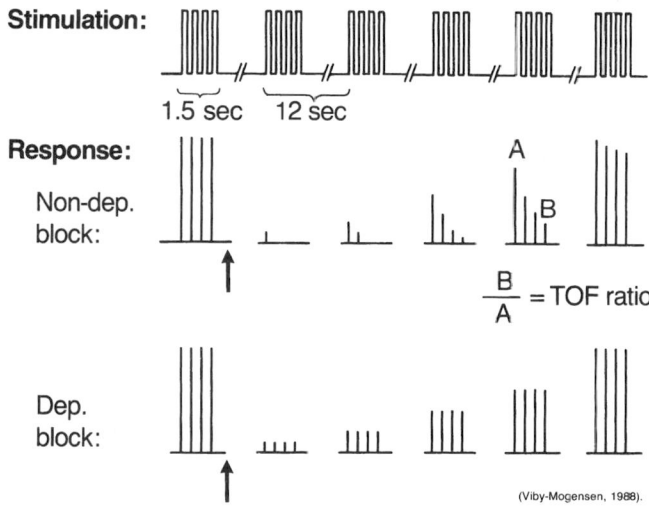

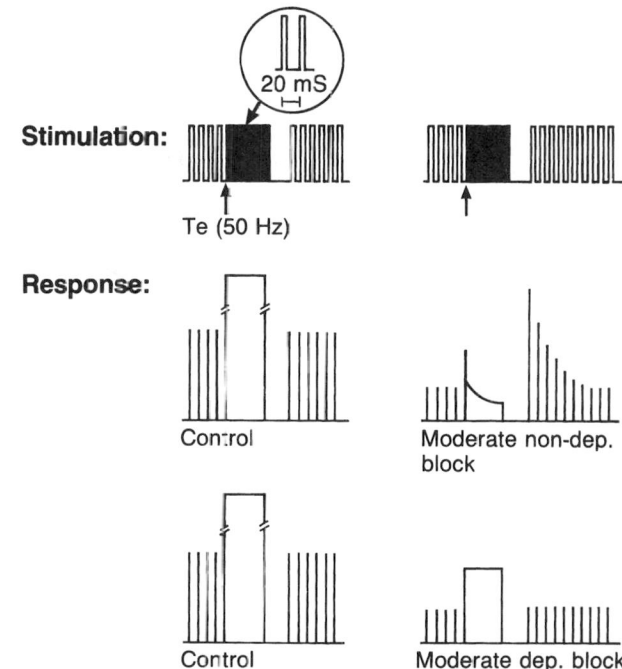

Figure 39–2 Pattern of electrical stimulation and evoked muscle responses to TOF nerve stimulation before and after injection of nondepolarizing (Non-dep) and depolarizing (Dep) neuromuscular blocking drugs (*arrows*).

Figure 39–3 Pattern of stimulation and evoked muscle responses to tetanic (50-Hz) nerve stimulation for 5 seconds (Te) and post-tetanic stimulation (1.0-Hz) twitch. Stimulation was applied before injection of neuromuscular blocking drugs and during moderate nondepolarizing and depolarizing blocks. Note fade in the response to tetanic stimulation, plus post-tetanic facilitation of transmission during nondepolarizing blockade. During depolarizing blockade, the tetanic response is well sustained and no post-tetanic facilitation of transmission occurs.

The advantages of TOF stimulation are greatest during nondepolarizing blockade, because the degree of block can be read directly from the TOF response even though a preoperative value is lacking. In addition, TOF stimulation has some advantages over tetanic stimulation: it is less painful and, unlike tetanic stimulation, generally does not affect the degree of neuromuscular blockade.

Tetanic Stimulation

Tetanic stimulation consists of very rapid (e.g., 30-, 50-, or 100-Hz) delivery of electrical stimuli. The most commonly used pattern in clinical practice is 50-Hz stimulation given for 5 seconds, although some investigators have advocated the use of 50-, 100-, and even 200-Hz stimulation for 1 second. During normal neuromuscular transmission and a pure depolarizing block, the muscle response to 50-Hz tetanic stimulation for 5 seconds is sustained. During a nondepolarizing block and a phase II block after injection of succinylcholine, the response will not be sustained (i.e., fade occurs) (Fig. 39-3).

Fade in response to tetanic stimulation is normally considered a presynaptic event; the traditional explanation is that at the start of tetanic stimulation, large amounts of acetylcholine are released from immediately available stores in the nerve terminal. As these stores become depleted, the rate of acetylcholine release decreases until equilibrium between mobilization and synthesis of acetylcholine is achieved. Despite this equilibrium, the muscle response caused by tetanic stimulation of the nerve at, for example, 50 Hz, is maintained (given normal neuromuscular transmission) simply because the release of acetylcholine is many times greater than the amount necessary to evoke a response. When the "margin of safety"[16] of the postsynaptic membrane (i.e., the number of free cholinergic receptors) is reduced by a nondepolarizing neuromuscular blocking agent, the decrease in release of acetylcholine during tetanic stimulation produces fade.

In addition to blocking the postsynaptic receptors, nondepolarizing neuromuscular blocking drugs may also impair the mobilization of acetylcholine within the nerve terminal. This effect may contribute to the fade in the response to tetanic (and TOF) stimulation. The degree of fade depends primarily on the degree of neuromuscular blockade. Fade also depends on the frequency (Hz) and the length (seconds) of stimulation and on how often tetanic stimuli are applied. Unless these variables are kept constant, results from different studies using tetanic stimulation cannot be compared.

During partial nondepolarizing blockade, tetanic nerve stimulation is followed by a post-tetanic increase in twitch tension (i.e., post-tetanic facilitation [PTF] of transmission) (see Fig. 39-3). This event occurs because the increase in mobilization and synthesis of acetylcholine caused by tetanic stimulation continues for some time after discontinuation of stimulation. The degree and duration of PTF depend on the degree of neuromuscular blockade, with PTF usually disappearing within 60 seconds of tetanic stimulation. PTF is evident in electromyographic, acceleromyographic, and mechanical recordings during a partial nondepolarizing neuromuscular blockade. In contrast, post-tetanic twitch potentiation, which sometimes occurs in mechanical recordings before any neuromuscular blocking drug has been given, is a muscular phenomenon that is not accompanied by an increase in the compound muscle action potential.

Tetanic stimulation has several disadvantages. It is very painful and therefore normally not acceptable to the unanesthetized patient. Furthermore, especially in the late phase of neuromuscular recovery, tetanic stimulations may produce a lasting antagonism of neuromuscular blockade in the stimulated muscle, such that the response of the tested site may no longer be representative of other muscle groups.[17,18]

Traditionally, tetanic stimulation has been used to evaluate residual neuromuscular blockade. However, except in connection with the technique of post-tetanic count (see later), tetanic stimulation has very little place in everyday clinical anesthesia. If the response to nerve stimulation is recorded, all the information required can be obtained from the response to TOF nerve stimulation. In contrast, if the response to nerve stimulation is evaluated only by feel[19] or by eye (Viby-Mogensen and colleagues, unpublished observation), even experienced observers are unable to judge the response of tetanic stimulation with sufficient certainty to exclude residual neuromuscular blockade.

Post-Tetanic Count Stimulation

Injection of a nondepolarizing neuromuscular blocking drug in a dose sufficient to ensure smooth tracheal intubation causes intense neuromuscular blockade of the peripheral muscles. Because no response to TOF and single-twitch stimulation occurs under these conditions, these modes of stimulation cannot be used to determine the degree of blockade. It is possible, however, to quantify intense neuromuscular blockade of the peripheral muscles by applying tetanic stimulation (50 Hz for 5 seconds) and observing the post-tetanic response to single-twitch stimulation given at 1 Hz starting 3 seconds after the end of tetanic stimulation.[20] During very intense blockade, there is no response to either tetanic or post-tetanic stimulation (Fig. 39-4). However, when the very intense neuromuscular blockade dissipates and before the first response to TOF stimulation reappears, the first response to post-tetanic twitch stimulation occurs. As the intense block dissipates, more and more responses to post-tetanic twitch stimulation appear. For a given neuromuscular blocking drug, the time until return of the first response to TOF stimulation is related to the number of post-tetanic twitch responses present at a given time (the post-tetanic count)[20-25] (Fig. 39-5).

The main application of the PTC method is in evaluating the degree of neuromuscular blockade when there is no reaction to single twitch or TOF nerve stimulation, as may be the case after injection of a large dose of a nondepolarizing neuromuscular blocking drug. However, PTC can also be used whenever sudden movements must be eliminated (e.g., during ophthalmic surgery). The necessary level of block of the adductor pollicis muscle to ensure paralysis of the diaphragm depends on the type of anesthesia and, in the intensive care unit, on the level of sedation.[23,26] To ensure elimination of any bucking or coughing in response to tracheobronchial stimulation, neuromuscular blockade of the peripheral muscles must be so intense that no response to post-tetanic twitch stimulation can be elicited (PTC-0)[20-22,24,25] (Fig. 39-6).

The response to PTC stimulation depends primarily on the degree of neuromuscular blockade. It also depends on the frequency and duration of tetanic stimulation, the length of time between the end of tetanic stimulation and the first post-tetanic stimulus, the frequency of the single-twitch stimulation, and also (probably) the length

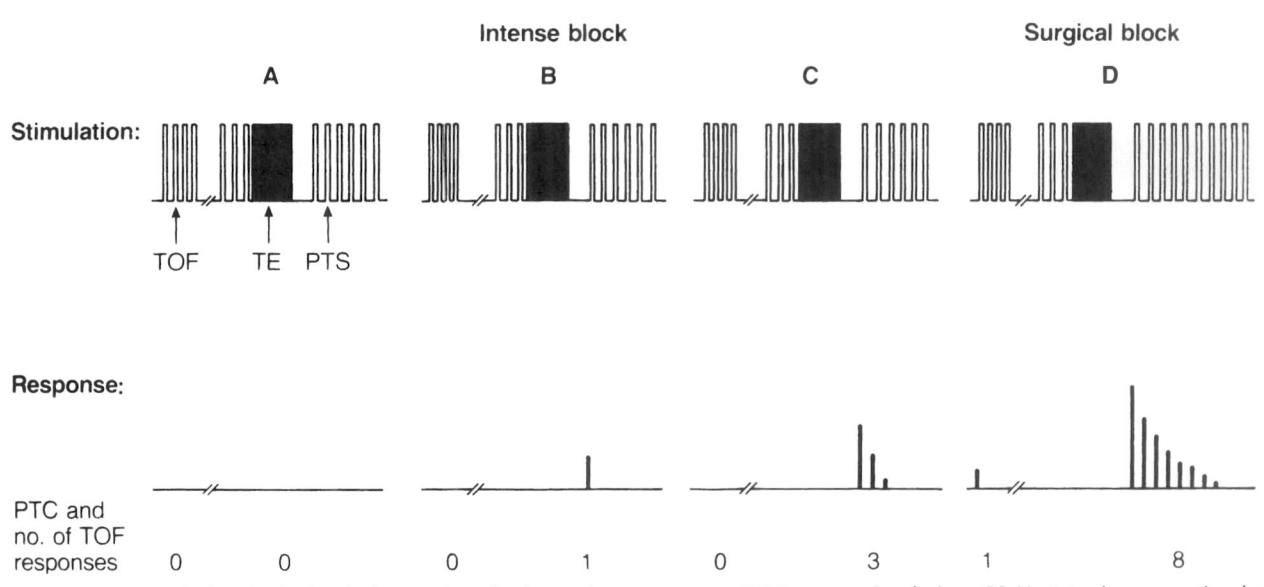

Figure 39-4 Pattern of electrical stimulation and evoked muscle responses to TOF nerve stimulation, 50-Hz tetanic nerve stimulation for 5 seconds (TE), and 1.0-Hz post-tetanic twitch stimulation (PTS) during four different levels of nondepolarizing neuromuscular blockade. During very intense blockade of the peripheral muscles (A), no response to any of the forms of stimulation occurs. During less pronounced blockade (B and C), there is still no response to stimulation, but post-tetanic facilitation of transmission is present. During surgical block (D), the first response to TOF appears and post-tetanic facilitation increases further. The post-tetanic count (see text) is 1 during intense block (B), 3 during less intense block (C), and 8 during surgical block (D).

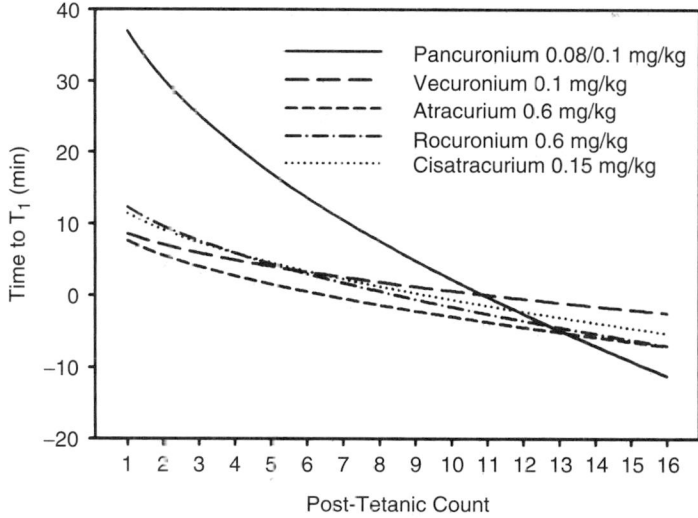

Figure 39–5 Relationship between the post-tetanic count (PTC) and time when onset of train-of-four (T_1) is likely to be elicited for various neuromuscular blocking agents. (From El-Orbany MI, Joseph JN, Salem MR: The relationship of posttetanic count and train-of-four responses during recovery from intense cisatracurium-induced neuromuscular blockade. Anesth Analg 97:80, 2003.)

of single-twitch stimulation before tetanic stimulation. When the PTC method is used, these variables should therefore be kept constant. Also, because of possible antagonism of neuromuscular blockade in the hand, tetanic stimulation should not be given more often than every 6 minutes.[20] If the hand muscles undergo antagonism of neuromuscular blockade while the rest of the body is still paralyzed, the hand muscles are no longer useful for monitoring.

Double-Burst Stimulation

DBS consists of two short bursts of 50-Hz tetanic stimulation separated by 750 msec. The duration of each square wave impulse in the burst is 0.2 msec (Fig. 39-7). Although the number of impulses in each burst can vary, most commonly used is DBS with three impulses in each of the two tetanic bursts ($DBS_{3,3}$).[27-30]

In nonparalyzed muscle, the response to $DBS_{3,3}$ is two short muscle contractions of equal strength. In the partly paralyzed muscle, the second response is weaker than the first (i.e., the response fades) (see Fig 39-7). Measured mechanically, the TOF ratio correlates closely with the $DBS_{3,3}$ ratio. DBS was developed with the specific aim of allowing manual (tactile) detection of small amounts of residual blockade under clinical conditions,[27] and during recovery and immediately after surgery, tactile evaluation of the response to $DBS_{3,3}$ is superior to tactile evaluation of the response to TOF stimulation.[29,31,32] However, as shown in Figure 39-8, absence of fade in the manually evaluated response to $DBS_{3,3}$ (and TOF) does not exclude residual neuromuscular blockade.[33]

THE NERVE STIMULATOR

Although many nerve stimulators are commercially available, not all meet the basic requirements for clinical use.

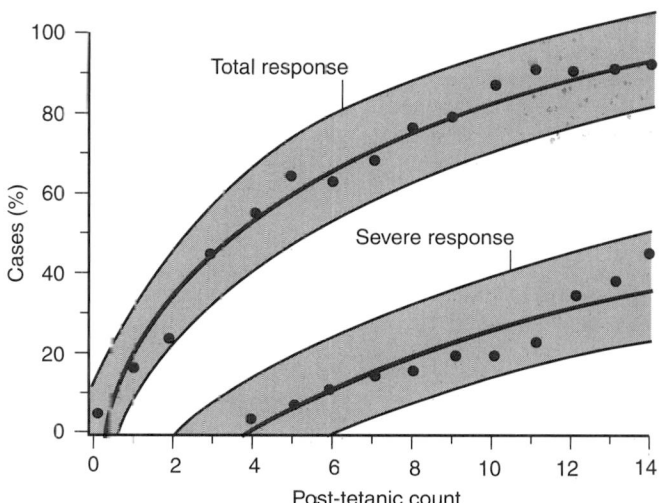

Figure 39–6 Relationship between the rate of muscle response to stimulation of the tracheal carina and the degree of neuromuscular blockade of peripheral muscles, as evaluated by using post-tetanic count. The subjects were 25 patients anesthetized with thiopental, nitrous oxide, and fentanyl who were given vecuronium (0.1 mg/kg) for tracheal intubation. For comparison, the first response to TOF stimulation usually occurs when PTC is approximately 10 (range, 6 to 16). The carina was stimulated with a soft sterile rubber suction catheter introduced via the endotracheal tube. The total response consisted of mild responses plus severe response. A mild response was said to occur if stimulation of the carina induced only slight bucking that did not interfere with surgery. A severe response was said to occur if stimulation elicited bucking that interfered with surgery and required intervention. Elimination of severe responses requires an intense neuromuscular blockade; PTC must be less than 2 to 3, and elimination of all reactions requires that PTC be 0. (From Fernando PUE, Viby-Mogensen J, Bonsu AK, et al: Relationship between post-tetanic count and response to carinal stimulation during vecuronium-induced neuromuscular blockade. Acta Anaesthesiol Scand 31:593, 1987. Copyright 1987, Munksgaard International Publishers, Ltd. Copenhagen, Denmark.)

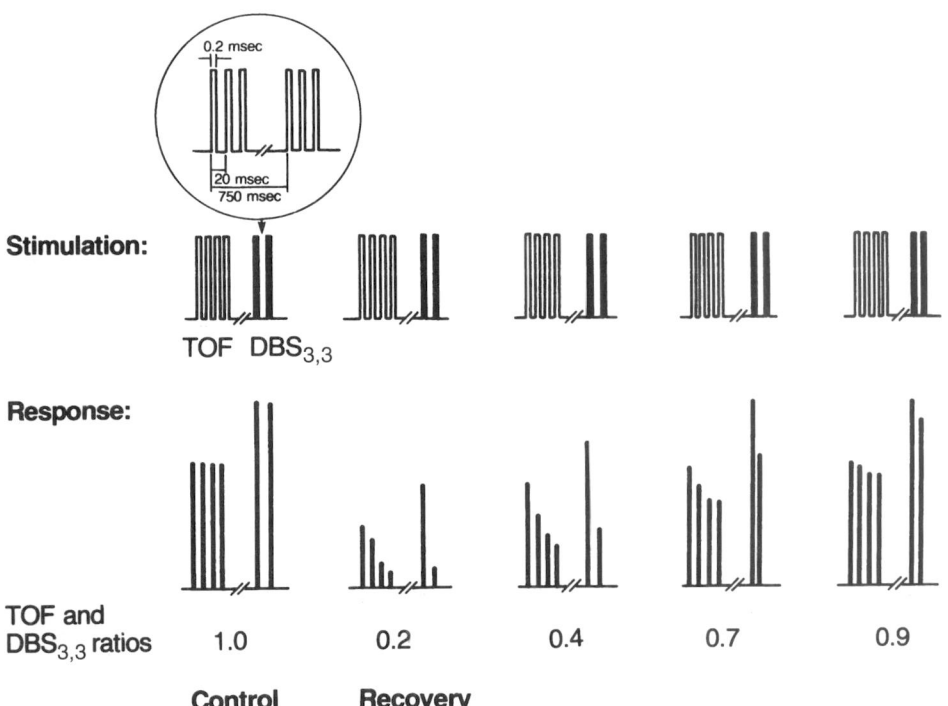

Figure 39–7 Pattern of electrical stimulation and evoked muscle responses to TOF nerve stimulation and double-burst nerve stimulation (i.e., three impulses in each of two tetanic bursts, DBS$_{3,3}$) before injection of muscle relaxants (control) and during recovery from nondepolarizing neuromuscular blockade. TOF ratio is the amplitude of the fourth response to TOF divided by the amplitude of the first response. DBS$_{3,3}$ ratio is the amplitude of the second response to DBS$_{3,3}$ divided by the amplitude of the first response. (See text for further explanation.)

The stimulus should produce a monophasic and rectangular waveform, and the length of the pulse should not exceed 0.2 to 0.3 msec. A pulse exceeding 0.5 msec may stimulate the muscle directly or cause repetitive firing. Stimulation at a constant current is preferable to stimulation at a constant voltage because current is the determinant of nerve stimulation. Also, for safety reasons, the nerve stimulator should be battery-operated, include a battery check, and be able to generate 60 to 70 mA, but not more than 80 mA. Many commercially available stimulators can deliver only 25 to 50 mA and provide a constant current only when skin resistance ranges from 0 Ω to 2.5 kΩ. This deficiency is a disadvantage; during cooling, skin resistance may increase to approximately 5 kΩ, which may cause the current delivered to the nerve to fall below the supramaximal level, leading to a decrease in the response to stimulation. As a result, the anesthesiologist may misjudge the degree of neuromuscular blockade. Ideally, the nerve stimulator should have a built-in warning system or a current level display that alerts the user when the current selected is not delivered to the nerve.

The ideal nerve stimulator should have other features as well. The polarity of the electrodes should be indicated. Also, the apparatus should be capable of delivering the following modes of stimulation: TOF (as both a single train and in a repetitive mode, with TOF stimulation being given every 10 to 20 seconds); single-twitch stimulations at 0.1 and 1.0 Hz; and tetanic stimulation at 50 Hz. In addition, the stimulator should have a built-in time constant system to facilitate post-tetanic count. Tetanic stimulus should last 5 seconds and be followed 3 seconds later by the first post-tetanic stimulus. If the nerve stimulator does not allow objective measurement of the response to TOF stimulation, at least one DBS mode should be available, preferably DBS$_{3,3}$. Single-twitch stimulation at 1 Hz is useful during initiation of monitoring because it shortens the time necessary to determine supramaximal stimulation. Most investigators agree that there is no need for tetanus at 100 or 200 Hz because 50-Hz tetanic stimulation stresses neuromuscular function to the same extent as does a maximal voluntary effort.

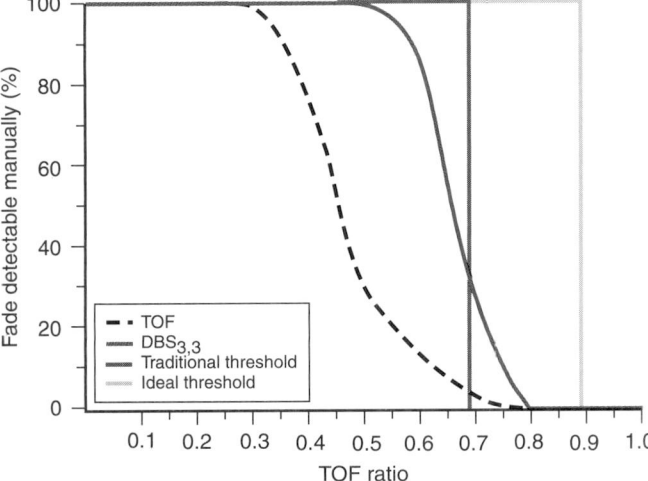

Figure 39–8 Fade detectable by feel in the response to TOF and double burst stimulation (DBS$_{3,3}$) in relation to the true TOF ratio, as measured mechanically. The axis indicates the percentage of instances in which fade can be felt at a given TOF ratio.[28,29] It appears that it is not possible to exclude residual neuromuscular block by any of the methods, whether a TOF ratio of 0.7 or 0.9 is taken to reflect adequate recovery of neuromuscular function. (See text for further explanation.)

Furthermore, in contrast to 100- and 200-Hz stimulation, 50-Hz tetanic stimulation does not cause fatigue (fade) in nonparalyzed muscle.

THE STIMULATING ELECTRODES

Electrical impulses are transmitted from stimulator to nerve by means of surface or needle electrodes, the former being the more commonly used in clinical anesthesia. Normally, disposal pregelled silver or silver chloride surface electrodes are used. The actual conducting area should be small, approximately 7 to 8 mm in diameter. Otherwise, the current produced in the underlying nerve may not be adequate. The skin should always be cleansed properly and preferably rubbed with an abrasive before application of the electrodes. When a supramaximal response cannot be obtained by using surface electrodes, needle electrodes should be used. Although specially coated needle electrodes are commercially available, ordinary steel injection needles can be used. The needles should be placed subcutaneously but never in a nerve.

SITES OF NERVE STIMULATION AND DIFFERENT MUSCLE RESPONSES

In principle, any superficially located peripheral motor nerve may be stimulated. In clinical anesthesia, the ulnar nerve is the most popular site; the median, the posterior tibial, common peroneal, and facial nerves are also sometimes used. For stimulation of the ulnar nerve, the electrodes are best applied at the volar side of the wrist (Fig. 39-9). The distal electrode should be placed about 1 cm proximal to the point at which the proximal flexion crease of the wrist crosses the radial side of the tendon to the flexor carpi ulnaris muscle. The proximal electrode preferably should be placed 2 to 5 cm proximal to the

distal electrode. With this placement of the electrodes, electrical stimulation normally elicits only finger flexion and thumb adduction. If the one electrode is placed over the ulnar groove at the elbow, thumb adduction is often pronounced because of stimulation of the flexor carpi ulnaris muscle. When this latter placement of electrodes (sometimes preferred in small children) is used, the active negative electrode should be at the wrist to ensure a maximal response. Polarity of the electrodes is less crucial when both electrodes are close to each other at the volar side of the wrist; however, placement of the negative electrode distally normally elicits the greatest neuromuscular response.[34] When the temporal branch of the facial nerve is stimulated, the negative electrode should be placed over the nerve, and the positive electrode should be placed somewhere else over the forehead.

Because different muscle groups have different sensitivities to neuromuscular blocking agents, results obtained for one muscle cannot be extrapolated automatically to other muscles. The diaphragm is among the most resistant of all muscles to both depolarizing[35] and nondepolarizing neuromuscular blocking drugs.[36] In general, the diaphragm requires 1.4 to 2.0 times as much muscle relaxant as the adductor pollicis muscle for an identical degree of blockade (Fig. 39-10).[36] Also of clinical significance are the facts that onset time is normally shorter for the diaphragm than for the adductor pollicis muscle and that the diaphragm recovers from paralysis more quickly than do the peripheral muscles (Fig. 39-11).[37] The other respiratory

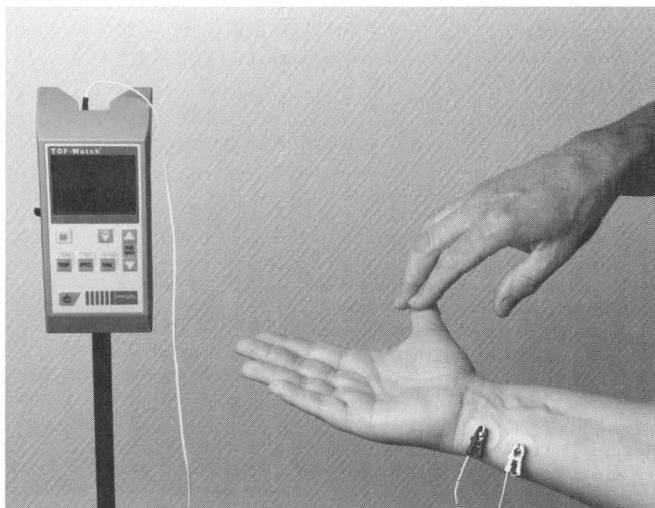

Figure 39–9 Evaluation of neuromuscular blockade by feeling the response of the thumb to stimulation of the ulnar nerve. (Courtesy of Organon Ltd., Dublin, Ireland.)

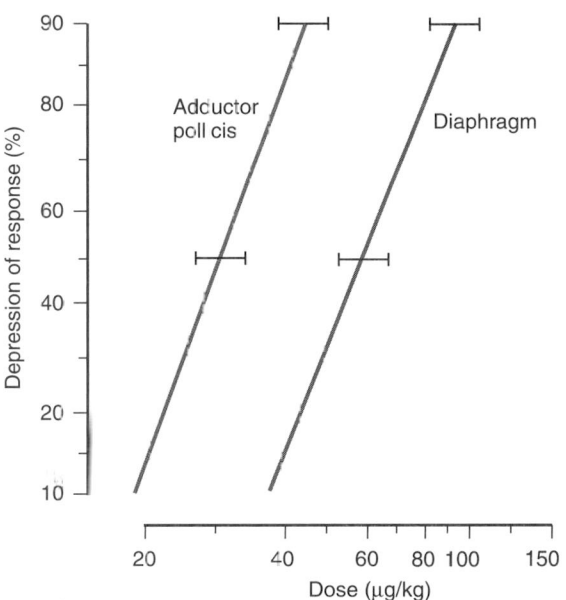

Figure 39–10 Mean cumulative dose-response curve for pancuronium in two muscles shows that the diaphragm requires approximately twice as much pancuronium as does the adductor pollicis muscle for the same amount of neuromuscular blockade. The depression in muscle response to the first stimulus in TOF nerve stimulation (probit scale) was plotted against dose (log scale). Force of contraction of the adductor pollicis was measured on a force-displacement transducer; response of the diaphragm was measured electromyographically. (From Donati F, Antzaka C, Bevan DR: Potency of pancuronium at the diaphragm and the adductor pollicis muscle in humans. Anesthesiology 65:1, 1986.)

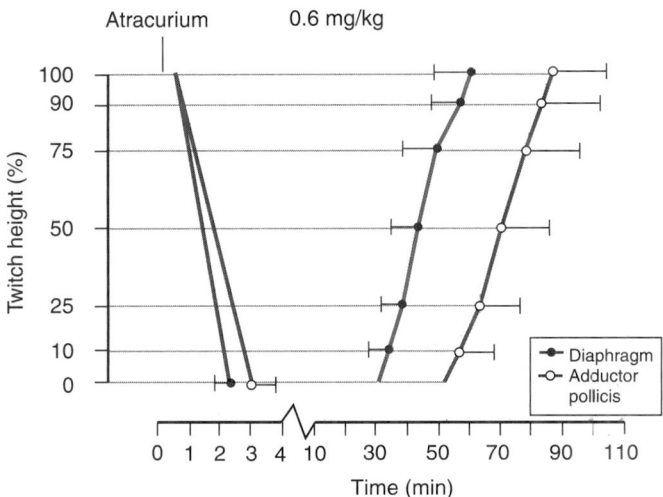

Figure 39–11 Evolution of twitch height (mean ± SD) of the diaphragm (*closed circles*) and of the adductor pollicis muscle (*open circles*) in 10 anesthetized patients after administration of atracurium 0.6 mg/kg. (From Pansard J-L, Chauvin M, Lebrault C, et al: Effect of an intubating dose of succinylcholine and atracurium on the diaphragm and the adductor pollicis muscle in humans. Anesthesiology 67:326, 1987.)

muscles are less resistant than the diaphragm, as are the larynx and the corrugater supercilii muscles.[38-43] Most sensitive are the abdominal muscles, the orbicularis oculi muscle, the peripheral muscles of the limbs, and the geniohyoid, masseter, and upper airway muscles.[44-48] From a practical clinical point of view, it is worth noting that (1) the corrugator supercilii response to facial nerve stimulation reflects the extent of neuromuscular blockade of the laryngeal adductor muscles (and the diaphragm?) better than does the response of the adductor pollicis to ulnar nerve stimulation[38,39] and (2) the upper airway muscles seem to be more sensitive than peripheral muscles.[45,46] Although three investigations using acceleromyography have indicated small differences in the response to TOF nerve stimulation in the arm (adductor pollicis muscle) and the leg (flexor hallucis brevis muscle), these differences are probably of little clinical significance.[49-52]

The precise source of these differences is unknown. Possible causes may be differences in acetylcholine receptor density, acetylcholine release, acetylcholinesterase activity, fiber composition, innervation ratio (number of neuromuscular junctions), blood flow, and muscle temperature.

In assessing neuromuscular function, the use of a relatively sensitive muscle such as the adductor pollicis of the hand has both disadvantages and advantages. Obviously, during surgery it is a disadvantage that even total elimination of the response to single-twitch and TOF stimulation does not exclude the possibility of movement of the diaphragm, such as hiccupping and coughing. PTC stimulation, however, allows for evaluation of the very intense blockade necessary to ensure total paralysis of the diaphragm. On the positive side, the risk of overdosing the patient decreases if the response of a relatively sensitive muscle is used as a guide to the administration of muscle relaxants during surgery. Also, during recovery,

when the adductor pollicis has recovered sufficiently, it can be assumed that no residual neuromuscular blockade exists in the diaphragm or in other resistant muscles.

RECORDING OF EVOKED RESPONSES

The choice of recording method is a practical decision. Five methods are available: measurement of evoked mechanical response of the muscle (mechanomyography [MMG]), measurement of evoked electrical response of the muscle (electromyography [EMG]), measurement of acceleration of the muscle response (acceleromyography [AMG]), measurement of evoked electrical response in a piezoelectric film sensor attached to the muscle (piezoelectric neuromuscular monitors [P$_Z$EMG], and phonomyography [PMG]).

Mechanomyography

A requirement for correct and reproducible measurements of evoked tension is that the muscle contraction be isometric. In clinical anesthesia, this condition is most easily achieved by measuring thumb movement after application of a resting tension of 200 to 300 g (a preload) to the thumb. When the ulnar nerve is stimulated, the thumb (the adductor pollicis muscle) acts on a force-displacement transducer. The force of contraction is then converted into an electrical signal, which is amplified, displayed, and recorded. The arm and hand should be fixed rigidly, and care should be taken to prevent overloading of the transducer. Also, the transducer should be placed in correct relationship to the thumb (i.e., the thumb should always apply tension precisely along the length of the transducer). It is important to remember that the response to nerve stimulation depends on the frequency with which the individual stimuli are applied and that the time used to achieve a stable control response may influence the subsequent determination of onset time and duration of block.[53] Generally, the reaction to supramaximal stimulation increases during the first 8 to 12 minutes after commencement of the stimulation. Therefore, in clinical studies, control measurements (before injection of muscle relaxant) should not be made before the response has stabilized for 8 to 12 minutes or a 2-second or 5-second 50-Hz tetanic stimulation has been given.[54] Even then, twitch response often recovers to 110% to 150% of the control response after paralysis with succinylcholine. This increase in response, thought to be caused by a change in the contractile response of the muscle, normally disappears within 15 to 25 minutes.

Although numerous methods for mechanical recording of evoked mechanical responses exist, not all meet the criteria outlined.

Electromyography

Evoked EMG records the compound action potentials produced by stimulation of a peripheral nerve. The compound action potential is a high-speed event that for many years could only be picked up by means of a preamplifier and a storage oscilloscope. Modern neuromuscular transmission analyzers are able to make on-line electronic analyses and graphic presentations of the EMG response.

The evoked EMG response is most often obtained from muscles innervated by the ulnar or the median nerves. Stimulating electrodes are applied as in force measurements. Although both surface and needle electrodes may be used for recording, no advantage is obtained by using the latter. Most often, the evoked EMG is obtained from the thenar or hypothenar eminence of the hand or from the first dorsal interosseous muscle of the hand, preferably with the active electrode over the motor point of the muscle (Fig. 39-12). The signal picked up by the analyzer is processed by an amplifier, a rectifier, and an electronic integrator. The results are displayed either as a percentage of control or as a TOF ratio.

Two new sites for recording the electromyography response have been introduced: the larynx and the diaphragm.[39,55-58] Using a non-invasive disposable laryngeal electrode attached to the tracheal tube and placed between the vocal cords, it is possible to monitor onset of neuromuscular block in the laryngeal muscles.[55,56] So far, however, the method is mainly of interest in clinical research when investigating onset times of the laryngeal muscles.[59] In paravertebral surface diaphragmal electromyography the recording electrodes are placed on the right of the vertebrae T12/L1 or L1/L2 for EMG monitoring of the response of the right diaphragmatic crux to transcutaneous stimulation of the right phrenic nerve at the neck.[53,57,58] As is the case with surface laryngeal EMG, surface diaphragmal EMG is mainly of interest in clinical research, because of the difficulties connected with the stimulation of the phrenic nerve transcutaneously at the neck.[59]

Evoked electrical and mechanical responses represent different physiologic events. Evoked EMG records changes in electrical activity of one or more muscles, whereas evoked MMG records changes associated with excitation-contraction coupling and the contraction of the muscle as well. For these reasons, the results obtained with these

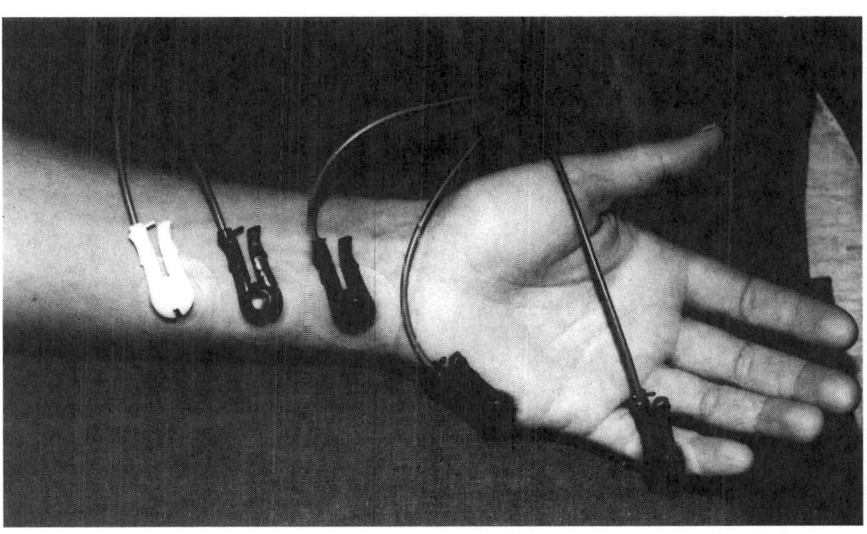

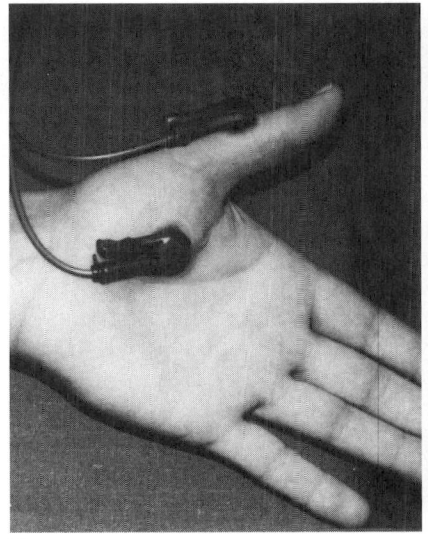

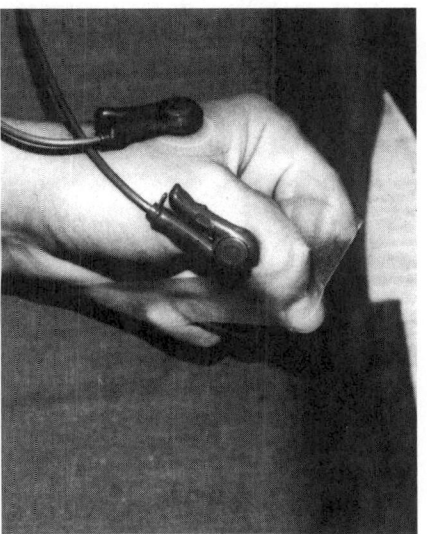

Figure 39–12 Electrode placement for stimulation of the ulnar nerve and for recording of the compound action potential from three sites of the hand. **A,** Abductor digiti minimi muscle (in the hypothenar eminence). **B,** Adductor pollicis muscle (in the thenar eminence). **C,** First dorsal interosseus muscle. (Courtesy of Datex-Ohmeda, Helsinki, Finland.)

methods may differ.[60,61] Although evoked EMG responses generally correlate well with evoked mechanical responses,[62] marked differences may occur, especially in the response to succinylcholine and in the TOF ratio during recovery from a nondepolarizing block.[60-62]

In theory, recording of evoked EMG responses has several advantages over recording of evoked mechanical responses. Equipment for measuring evoked EMG responses is easier to set up, the response reflects only those factors influencing neuromuscular transmission, and the response can be obtained from muscles not accessible to mechanical recording. However, evoked EMG does entail some difficulties. Although good recordings are possible in most patients, results are not always reliable. For one thing, improper placement of electrodes may result in inadequate pickup of the compound EMG signal. If the neuromuscular transmission analyzer does not allow observation of the actual waveform of the compound EMG, determining the optimal placement of the electrodes is difficult. Another source of unreliable results may be that fixation of the hand with a preload on the thumb may be more important than generally appreciated,[62,63] as changes in the position of the electrodes in relationship to the muscle may affect the EMG response. In addition, direct muscle stimulation sometimes occurs. If muscles close to the stimulating electrodes are stimulated directly, the recording electrodes may pick up an electrical signal even though neuromuscular transmission is completely blocked. Another difficulty is that the EMG response often does not return to control value. Whether this situation is the result of technical problems, inadequate fixation of the hand, or changes in temperature is unknown (Fig. 39-13). Finally, the

evoked EMG response is very sensitive to electrical interference, such as that caused by diathermy.

Acceleromyography

The technique of AMG is based on Newton's second law: force equals mass times acceleration.[64,65] If mass is constant, acceleration is directly proportional to force. Accordingly, after nerve stimulation, one can measure not only the evoked force but also the acceleration of the thumb.

AMG uses a piezoelectric ceramic wafer with electrodes on both sides. Exposure of the electrode to a force generates an electrical voltage proportional to the acceleration of the thumb in response to nerve stimulation. When the accelerometer is fixed to the thumb and the ulnar nerve is stimulated, an electrical signal is produced whenever the thumb moves. This signal is then analyzed in a specially designed analyzer[65] or perhaps displayed on a recording system. At least one detached monitor based on measurement of acceleration is commercially available: the TOF-Watch (Organon Teknika, Boxtel, Holland) (Fig. 39-14).

AMG is a simple method of analyzing neuromuscular function, both in the operating room and in the intensive care unit.[66,67] However, although a good correlation exists between the TOF ratio measured by this method and TOF ratio measured with a force-displacement transducer or using EMG,[64,65,68] measurements made with an AMG are not directly comparable with results obtained using the other two methods.[69,70-75] When an AMG is used, as originally suggested, with a free-moving thumb,[64] wide limits of agreements in twitch height (T1) and TOF ratio and differences in the onset and recovery course of blockade between AMG and MMG have been found. Also, the AMG control TOF ratio is consistently higher than when measured using a force-displacement transducer. In accordance with this, one study has indicated that when using AMG, the threshold TOF ratio for sufficient postoperative neuromuscular recovery is 1.0, rather than 0.9 as when measured with MMG or EMG.[76]

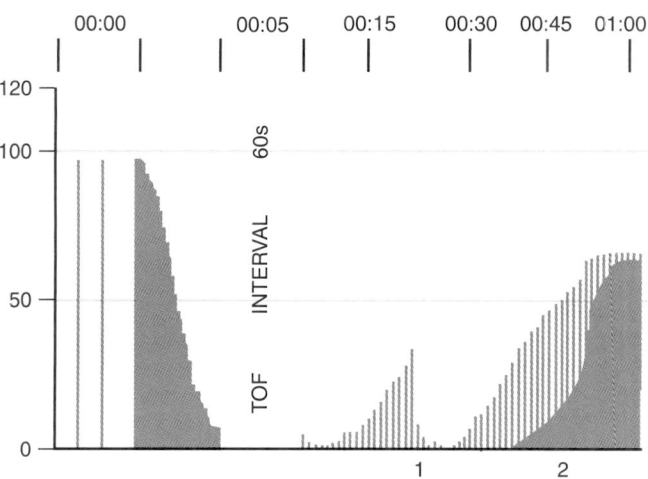

Figure 39–13 Evoked electromyographic printout from a Relaxograph. Initially, single-twitch stimulation was given at 0.1 Hz, and vecuronium (70 µg/kg) was given intravenously for tracheal intubation. After approximately 5 minutes, the mode of stimulation was changed to TOF stimulation every 60 seconds. At a twitch height (first twitch in TOF response) of approximately 30% of control (marker 1), 1 mg of vecuronium was given intravenously. At marker 2, 1 mg of neostigmine was given intravenously, preceded by 2 mg of glycopyrrolate. The printout also illustrates the common problem of failure of the electromyographic response to return to control level. (Courtesy of Datex-Ohmeda, Helsinki, Finland.)

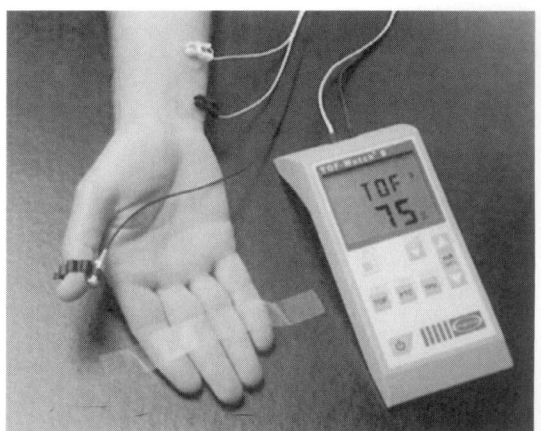

Figure 39–14 TOF-Watch (Organon Ltd., Dublin, Ireland). This neuromuscular transmission monitor is based on measurement of acceleration using a piezoelectric transducer.[64,65] Note the transducer fastened to the thumb and the stimulating electrodes. On the display of the TOF-Watch, the TOF ratio is given in percentage.

One reason for the wide limits of agreement between AMG and MMG is probably and paradoxically connected with one of the originally claimed advantages of the method, that fixation of the hand could be reduced to a minimum as long as the thumb could move freely.[64] However, in daily clinical practice it is often not possible to ensure that the thumb can move freely, and that the position of the hand does not change during a surgical procedure. The evoked response may therefore vary considerably. Several solutions have been proposed, and ongoing clinical research indicates that the use of an elastic preload to the thumb may improve the agreement between results obtained using AMG and MMG (Fig. 39-15). In spite of the above reservations, it is my opinion that AMG at the thumb is a valuable clinical tool that used with intelligence may eliminate the problem of postoperative residual neuromuscular block.[77,78]

When the thumb is not available for monitoring during surgery, some clinicians prefer to monitor the AMG response of the orbicularis oculi or the corrugator supercilii in response to facial nerve stimulation. However, it is important to realize that neuromuscular monitoring with AMG from both these sites are subject to a large uncertainty as a measure of paralysis, and it cannot therefore be recommended for routine monitoring. It only provides a rough estimate of the degree of block of the peripheral muscles.[39,79,80]

Piezoelectric Neuromuscular Monitors

The technique of the piezoelectric monitor is based on the principle that stretching or bending a flexible piezoelectric film, for example, attached to the thumb, in response to nerve stimulation generates a voltage that is proportional to the amount of stretching or bending.[81,82] At least two devices based on the this principle are available commercially: The ParaGraph Neuromuscular Blockade Monitor (Vital Signs, Totowa, NJ) and the M-NMT MechanoSensor, which is a part of the Datex AS/3 monitoring system (Datex-Ohmeda, Helsinki, Finland) (Fig. 39-16).

Few studies have evaluated the function of these monitors.[81-83] The scarce data indicate a good relationship between results obtained using P_ZEMG, AMG and MMG, but also wide limits of agreement between the methods.

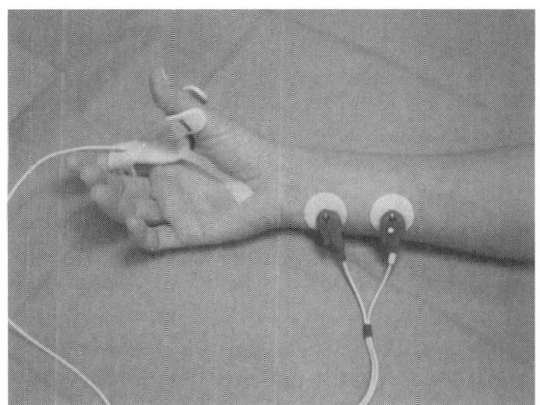

Figure 39–16 Datex-Engstrøm M-NMT MechanoSensor (a piezoelectric neuromuscular monitor).

Therefore, although P_ZEMG may be a valuable clinical tool, the values obtained in the individual patient using this method may vary from those obtained using MMG or AMG.

Phonomyography

PMG (acoustic myography) is a relatively new method of monitoring neuromuscular function.[84-89] The contraction of skeletal muscles generates intrinsic low-frequency sounds, which can be recorded using special microphones. This method has been evaluated for clinical and research purposes. Several reports indicate a good correlation between the evoked acoustic responses and responses obtained using more traditional methods of recording, such as MMG, EMG, and AMG. However, it is uncertain whether PMG will ever be used for monitoring neuromuscular block during routine anesthesia. What does make PMG interesting, however, is that in theory the method can be applied not only to the adductor pollicis muscle but also to other muscles of interest such as the diaphragm, the larynx, and the eye muscles. Also, the ease of application is attractive.

For further information on recording evoked responses, the reader is referred to guidelines for Good Clinical Research Practice in pharmacodynamic studies of neuromuscular blocking agents, published in Acta Anaesthesiologica Scandinavica.[53]

EVALUATION OF RECORDED EVOKED RESPONSES

Nerve stimulation in clinical anesthesia is usually synonymous with TOF nerve stimulation. Therefore, the recorded response to this form of stimulation is used to explain how to evaluate the degree of neuromuscular blockade during clinical anesthesia.

Nondepolarizing Neuromuscular Blockade

After injection of a nondepolarizing neuromuscular blocking drug in a dose sufficient for smooth tracheal

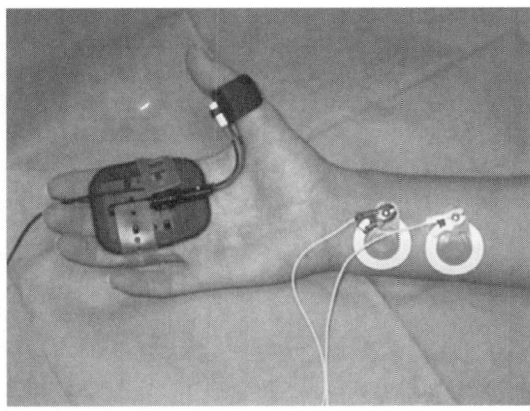

Figure 39–15 Hand adaptor (elastic preload) for the TOF-Watch transducer. (Accelleromyography, Organon Ltd., Dublin, Ireland.)

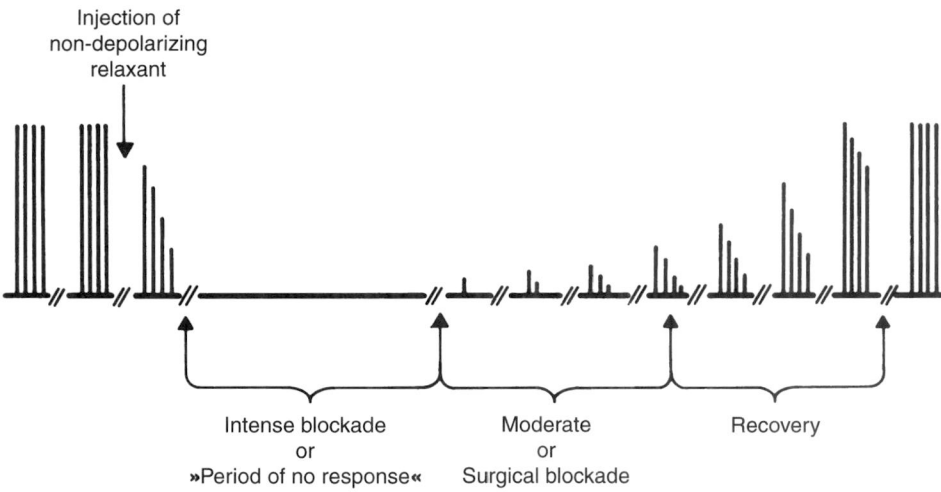

Figure 39–17 Diagram of the changes in response to TOF nerve stimulation during nondepolarizing neuromuscular blockade.

intubation, TOF recording demonstrates three phases or levels of neuromuscular blockade: intense blockade, moderate or surgical blockade, and recovery (Fig. 39-17).

Intense Neuromuscular Blockade

Intense neuromuscular blockade occurs within 3 to 6 minutes of injection of an intubating dose of a nondepolarizing muscle relaxant, depending on the drug and the dose given. This phase is also called the "period of no response" because no response to TOF or single-twitch stimulation occurs. The length of this period varies, again depending primarily on the duration of action of the muscle relaxant and the dose given. The sensitivity of the patient to the drug also affects the period of no response. Although during this phase it is not possible to determine exactly how long intense neuromuscular blockade will last, correlation does exist between PTC stimulation and the time to reappearance of the first response to TOF stimulation (see Fig. 39-5).

Moderate or Surgical Blockade

Moderate or surgical blockade begins when the first response to TOF stimulation appears. This phase is characterized by a gradual return of the four responses to TOF stimulation. Furthermore, good correlation exists between the degree of neuromuscular blockade and the number of responses to TOF stimulation. When only one response is detectable, the degree of neuromuscular blockade (the depression in twitch tension) is 90% to 95%. When the fourth response reappears, neuromuscular blockade is usually 60% to 85%.[90,91] The presence of one or two responses in the TOF pattern normally indicates sufficient relaxation for most surgical procedures. During light anesthesia, however, patients may move, buck, or cough. Therefore, when elimination of sudden movements is crucial, a more intense block (or a deeper level of anesthesia) may be necessary. The more intense block can then be evaluated by using the post-tetanic count (see Fig. 39-6).

Antagonism of neuromuscular blockade should normally not be attempted when blockade is intense because reversal will often be inadequate, regardless of the dose of antagonist administered.[92] Also, after the administration of large doses of muscle relaxants, reversal of the block to clinically normal activity is not always possible if only one response in the TOF is present. In general, antagonism should not be initiated before at least two, preferably three or four, responses are observed.

Recovery

The return of the fourth response in the TOF heralds the recovery phase. During neuromuscular recovery, a reasonably good correlation exists between the actual TOF ratio measured using MMG and clinical observations, but the relationship between TOF ratio and signs and symptoms of residual blockade varies greatly among patients.[92] When the TOF ratio is 0.4 or less, the patient is generally unable to lift the head or arm. Tidal volume may be normal, but vital capacity and inspiratory force will be reduced. When the ratio is 0.6, most patients are able to lift the head for 3 seconds, open the eyes widely, and stick out the tongue, but vital capacity and inspiratory force are often still reduced. At a TOF ratio of 0.7 to 0.75, the patient can normally cough sufficiently, and lift the head for at least 5 seconds, but the grip strength may still be as low as about 60% of control.[93] When the ratio is 0.8 and higher, vital capacity and inspiratory force are normal.[15,94-96] The patient may, however, still have diplopia and facial weakness (Table 39-1).[92]

In clinical anesthesia, a TOF ratio of 0.70 to 0.75, or even 0.50, has been thought to reflect adequate recovery of neuromuscular function.[96] However, studies have shown that the TOF ratio, whether recorded mechanically or by EMG, must exceed 0.80 or even 0.90 to exclude clinically important residual neuromuscular blockade.[5,6,48,62,76,97-102] Eriksson and colleagues have shown that moderate degrees of neuromuscular block decrease the chemoreceptor sensitivity to hypoxia, leading to insufficient response to a decrease in oxygen tension in blood.[97,98,100,102] They also showed that residual block (TOF < 0.90) is associated with functional impairment of the muscles of the pharynx and upper esophagus, most

Table 39–1   Clinical signs and symptoms of residual paralysis in awake volunteers after mivacurium-induced neuromuscular block

TOF ratio	Signs and Symptoms
0.70-0.75	Diplopia and visual disturbances Decreased hand-grip strength Inability to maintain incisor teeth apposition "Tongue depressor test" negative Inability to sit up without assistance Severe facial weakness Speaking a major effort Overall weakness and tiredness
0.85-0.90	Diplopia and visual disturbances Generalized fatigue

From Kopman AF, Yee PS, Neuman GG: Relationship of the train-of-four fade ratio to clinical signs and symptoms of residual paralysis in awake volunteers. Anesthesiology 86:765, 1997.

probably predisposing to regurgitation and aspiration.[48] In accordance with this, it has been documented that residual block (TOF < 0.70) caused by the long-acting muscle relaxant, pancuronium, is a significant risk factor for the development of postoperative pulmonary complications (Table 39-2 and Fig. 39-18).[99] Kopman et associates[93] have documented that even in volunteers without sedation or impaired consciousness a TOF ratio ≤ 0.9 may impair the ability to maintain the airway. Available evidence thus indicates that adequate recovery of neuromuscular function requires return of a MMG or EMG TOF ratio to ≥? 0.90, which cannot be guaranteed without objective neuromuscular monitoring.[77,78,103,104]

Depolarizing Neuromuscular Blockade (Phase I and II Blocks)

Patients with normal plasma cholinesterase activity who are given a moderate dose of succinylcholine (0.5 to 1.5 mg/kg) undergo a typical depolarizing neuromuscular block (phase I block) (i.e., the response to TOF or tetanic stimulation does not fade, and no post-tetanic facilitation

of transmission occurs). In contrast, some patients with genetically determined abnormal plasma cholinesterase activity who are given the same dose of succinylcholine undergo a non-depolarizing–like block characterized by fade in the response to TOF and tetanic stimulation and occurrence of post-tetanic facilitation of transmission (Fig. 39-19). This type of block is called a phase II block (dual, mixed, or desensitizing block). Also, phase II blocks sometimes occur in genetically normal patients after prolonged infusion of succinylcholine.

From a therapeutic point of view, a phase II block in normal patients must be differentiated from a phase II block in patients with abnormal cholinesterase activity. In normal patients, a phase II block can be antagonized by administering a cholinesterase inhibitor a few minutes after discontinuation of succinylcholine. In patients with abnormal genotypes, the effect of intravenous injection of an acetylcholinesterase inhibitor (e.g., neostigmine) is unpredictable. For example, neostigmine can potentiate the block dramatically, temporarily improve neuromuscular transmission, and then potentiate the block or partially reverse the block, all depending on the time elapsed since administration of succinylcholine and the dose of neostigmine given. Therefore, unless the cholinesterase genotype is known to be normal, antagonism of a phase II block with a cholinesterase inhibitor should be undertaken with extreme caution. Even if the neuromuscular function improves promptly, patient surveillance should continue for at least 1 hour.

USE OF NERVE STIMULATORS WITHOUT RECORDING EQUIPMENT

Although it is my opinion that neuromuscular function should be monitored objectively whenever a neuromuscular blocking drug is administered to a patient, tactile or visual evaluation of the evoked response is still the most common form of clinical neuromuscular monitoring. The following is a description of how this is best done.

First, for supramaximal stimulation, careful cleansing of the skin and proper placement and fixation of electrodes are essential. Second, every effort should be taken

Table 39–2   Relationship between train-of-four ratio at first postoperative recording and postoperative pulmonary complications (POPC)*

	Pancuronium (n = 226)			Atracurium or Vecuronium (n = 450)		
		Patients with POPC			Patients with POPC	
	No. of patients	n	%	No. of patients	n	%
TOF ≥ 0.70	167	8	4.8	426	23	5.4
TOF < 0.70	59	10	16.9†	24	1	4.2

*Results from a prospective, randomized, and blinded study of postoperative POPC in a total of 691 adult patients undergoing abdominal, gynecologic, or orthopedic surgery, receiving either pancuronium, atracurium, or vecuronium.[99] In 4 of the 46 patients with POPC (1 in the pancuronium group and 3 in the atracurium and vecuronium groups) the TOF ratio was not available. Because there were no significant differences in the two groups of patients given the intermediate-acting muscle relaxants, the data from these groups are pooled.
†P < 0.02 compared with patients in the same group with TOF ratio ≥0.70.

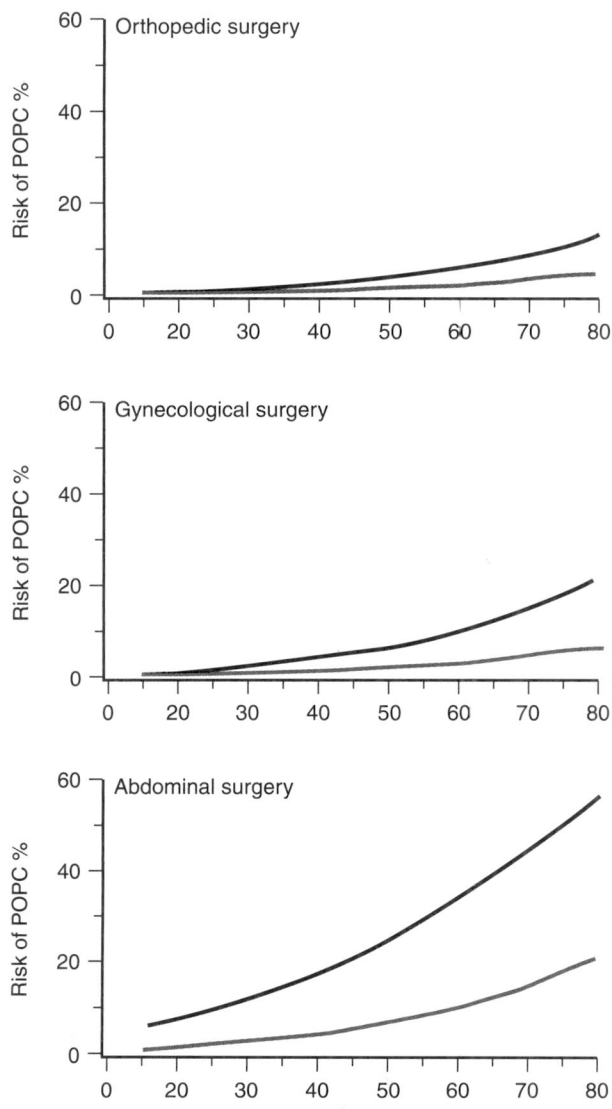

Figure 39–18 Predicted probabilities of postoperative pulmonary complications in different age groups in orthopedic, gynecologic, and major abdominal surgery with a duration of anesthesia of less than 200 minutes. The solid lines represent patients having residual neuromuscular block (TOF < 0.70) following the use of pancuronium; the broken lines represent patients with TOF ≥ 0.70 following the use of pancuronium as well as all patients following the use of atracurium and vecuronium, independent of the TOF ratio at the end of anesthesia.[99]

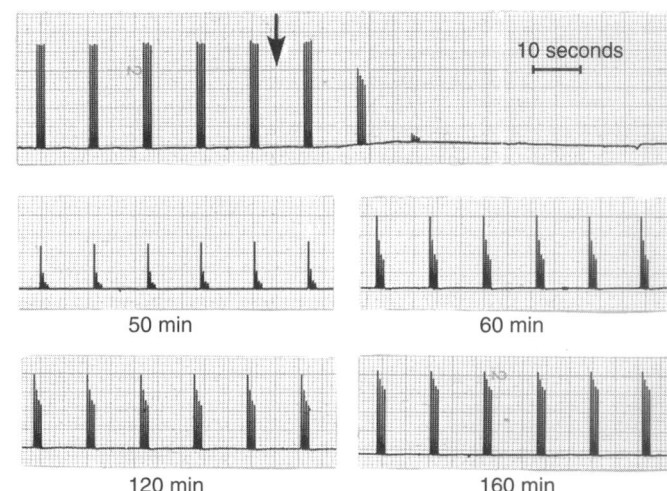

Figure 39–19 Typical recording of the mechanical response (Myograph 2000) to TOF nerve stimulation of the ulnar nerve after injection of 1 mg/kg of succinylcholine (arrow) in a patient with genetically determined abnormal plasma cholinesterase activity. The prolonged duration of action and the pronounced fade in the response indicate a phase II block.

to prevent central cooling as well as cooling of the extremity being evaluated. Both central and local surface cooling of the adductor pollicis muscle may reduce the twitch tension and the TOF ratio.[105,106] Peripheral cooling may affect nerve conduction, decrease the rate of release of acetylcholine and muscle contractility, increase skin impedance, and reduce blood flow to the muscles, thus decreasing the rate of removal of muscle relaxant from the neuromuscular junction. These factors may account for the occasional very pronounced difference in muscle response between a cold extremity and the contralateral warm extremity.[107] Third, when possible, the response to

nerve stimulation should be evaluated by feel and not by eye, and the response of the thumb (rather than that of the fifth finger) should be evaluated. Direct stimulation of the muscle often causes subtle movements of the fifth finger when no response is present at the thumb. Finally, the different sensitivities of various muscle groups to neuromuscular blocking agents should always be kept in mind.

Figure 39-20 shows which modes of nerve stimulation can be used at various perioperative times.

Use of a Peripheral Nerve Stimulator During Induction of Anesthesia

The nerve stimulator should be attached to the patient before induction of anesthesia but should not be turned on until after the patient is unconscious. Single-twitch stimulation at 1 Hz may be used initially when seeking supramaximal stimulation. However, after supramaximal stimulation has been ensured and before muscle relaxant is injected, the mode of stimulation should be changed to TOF (or 0.1-Hz twitch stimulation). Then, after the response to this stimulation has been observed (the control response), the neuromuscular blocking agent is injected. Although the trachea is often intubated when the response to TOF stimulation disappears, postponement of this procedure for 30 to 90 seconds, depending upon the muscle relaxant used, usually produces better conditions.

Use of a Peripheral Nerve Stimulator During Surgery

If tracheal intubation is facilitated by the administration of succinylcholine, no more muscle relaxant should be given until the response to nerve stimulation reappears or until the patient shows other signs of returning neuromuscular function. If the plasma cholinesterase

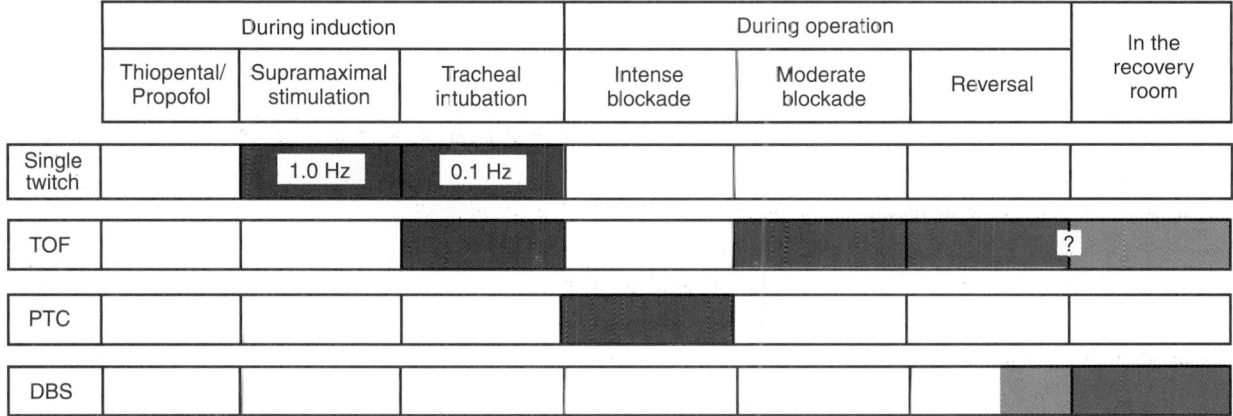

Figure 39–20 This diagram shows when the different modes of electrical nerve stimulation can be used during clinical anesthesia. Dark areas indicate appropriate use; light areas, less effective use. Modes of nerve stimulation: TOF, train-of-four stimulation; PTC, post-tetanic count; DBS, double-burst stimulation; and ?, indicating that TOF is less useful in the recovery room unless measured using mechano-, electro-, or acceleromyography. (See text for further explanation.)

activity is normal, the muscle response to TOF nerve stimulation reappears within 4 to 8 minutes.

When a nondepolarizing neuromuscular drug is used for tracheal intubation, a longer-lasting period of intense blockade usually follows. During this period of no response to TOF and single-twitch stimulation, the time until return of response to TOF stimulation may be evaluated by using post-tetanic count (see Fig. 39-5).

For most surgical procedures requiring muscle relaxation, a twitch depression of approximately 90% will be sufficient, provided the patient is properly anesthetized. If a nondepolarizing relaxant is used, one or two of the responses to TOF stimulation can be felt. However, because the respiratory muscles (including the diaphragm) are less sensitive to neuromuscular blocking agents than are the peripheral muscles, the patient may breathe, hiccup, or even cough at this depth of block. To ensure paralysis of the diaphragm, neuromuscular blockade of the peripheral muscles must be so intense that PTC stimulation is zero in the thumb.

An added advantage of keeping the neuromuscular blockade at a level of one or two responses to TOF stimulation is that antagonism of the block is facilitated at the end of surgery.

Use of a Peripheral Nerve Stimulator During Reversal of Neuromuscular Blockade

Antagonism of a nondepolarizing neuromuscular block should not be initiated before at least two responses to TOF stimulation can be felt or before obvious clinical signs of returning neuromuscular function are present. To achieve rapid reversal (within 10 minutes) to a TOF ratio of 0.7 in more than 90% of patients, three and preferably four responses should be present at the time of neostigmine injection.[108] It is not possible to achieve a TOF ratio of 0.9 in all patients using this method, but critical episodes of postoperative residual block should be an infrequent occurrence.[109]

During recovery of neuromuscular function, when all four responses to TOF stimulation can be felt, an estimation of the TOF ratio may be attempted. However, manual (tactile) evaluation of the response to TOF stimulation (see Fig. 39-8) is not sensitive enough to exclude the possibility of residual neuromuscular blockade.[29,104,110] Greater sensitivity is achieved with $DBS_{3,3}$, but even absence of manual fade in the $DBS_{3,3}$ response does not exclude clinically significant residual blockade.[33] Therefore, manual evaluation of responses to nerve stimulation should always be considered in relation to reliable clinical signs and symptoms of residual neuromuscular blockade (Table 39-3).

WHEN TO USE A PERIPHERAL NERVE STIMULATOR

At some institutions, nerve stimulators are used routinely whenever a neuromuscular blocking drug is given. In most cases, the response is evaluated by touch, and only in selected cases are the responses recorded. Many anesthesiologists do not agree with an extensive use of nerve stimulators and argue that they manage quite well without

Table 39–3   Clinical tests of postoperative neuromuscular recovery

Unreliable
Sustained eye opening
Protrusion of the tongue
Arm lift to opposite shoulder
Normal tidal volume
Normal or near normal vital capacity
Maximum inspiratory pressure <40-50 cm H_2O
Reliable
Sustained head-lift for 5 seconds
Sustained leg lift for 5 seconds
Sustained hand grip for 5 seconds
Sustained "tongue depressor test"
Maximum inspiratory pressure ≥40-50 cm H_2O
(Normal swallowing?)

these devices. However, the question is not how little an experienced anesthetist can manage with, but rather, how to ensure that all patients receive optimal treatment.

In daily clinical practice significant residual block can be excluded with certainty only if objective methods of neuromuscular monitoring are used.[77,78] In my opinion[5] and those of others,[6] good evidence-based practice dictates that clinicians should always quantitate the extent of neuromuscular recovery using objective monitoring. At a minimum, the TOF ratio should be measured during recovery whenever a non-depolarizing neuromuscular block is not antagonized.[5]

However, in many departments clinicians do not have access to equipment for measuring the degree of block. How then to evaluate and, as far as possible, exclude clinically significant postoperative block? First, long-acting neuromuscular blocking agents should not be used. Second, the tactile response to TOF nerve stimulation should be evaluated during surgery. Third, avoid if possible total twitch suppression. Keep the block so that there is always one or two tactile TOF responses. Fourth, the block should be antagonized at the end of the procedure, but reversal should not be initiated before at least two and preferably three or four responses to TOF stimulation are present. Fifth, during recovery, tactile evaluation of the response to DBS is preferable to tactile evaluation of the response to TOF stimulation, because it is easier to feel fade in the DBS than in the TOF response. Sixth, recognize that absence of tactile fade in both the TOF and the DBS responses does not exclude significant residual block.[33,103,104,110] Finally, reliable clinical signs and symptoms of residual block (see Table 39-3) should be considered in relation to the response to nerve stimulation.

Considering the uncertainty connected with both the use of clinical tests of postoperative neuromuscular recovery and tactile evaluation of the response to nerve stimulation, at a minimum every anesthesia department and every recovery room should have at least one apparatus for recording evoked responses. Whether the functioning of such a neuromuscular transmission analyzer is based on EMG, MMG, AMG, P_ZEMG or PMG is not crucial, as long as the physician knows how to use the apparatus in question.

KEY POINTS

1. Residual postoperative neuromuscular block causes decreased chemoreceptor sensitivity to hypoxia, functional impairment of the muscles of the pharynx and upper esophagus, impaired ability to maintain the airway, and an increased risk for the development of postoperative pulmonary complications.

2. It is difficult, and often impossible, by clinical evaluation of recovery of neuromuscular function, to exclude with certainty clinically significant residual curarization.

3. Absence of tactile fade in the response to TOF stimulation, tetanic stimulation and DBS does not exclude significant residual block.

4. Adequate recovery of postoperative neuromuscular function cannot be guaranteed without objective neuromuscular monitoring.

5. Good evidence-based practice dictates that clinicians should always quantitate the extent of neuromuscular blockade using objective monitoring.

6. To exclude clinically significant residual neuromuscular blockade the TOF ratio when measured mechanically or by electromyography must exceed 0.9.

7. Avoid total twitch depression during surgery. Keep, whenever possible one or two TOF responses.

8. Antagonism of the neuromuscular block should not be initiated before at least two, preferably three or four, responses to TOF stimulation are observed.

9. If sufficient recovery (TOF ≥ 0.9) has not been documented objectively at the end of the surgical procedure, the neuromuscular block should be antagonized.

REFERENCES

1. Viby-Mogensen J, Chraemmer-Jorgensen B, Ørding H: Residual curarization in the recovery room. Anesthesiology 50:539, 1979.
2. Baillard C, Gehan G, Reboul-Marty, et al: Residual curarization in the recovery room after vecuronium. Br J Anaesth 84:394, 2000.
3. Hayes AH, Mirakhur RK, Breslin DS, et al: Postoperative residual block after intermediate-acting neuromuscular blocking drugs. Anaesthesia 56:312, 2001.
4. Debaene B, Plaud B, Dilly M-P, et al: Residual paralysis in the PACU after a single intubating dose of nondepolarizing muscle relaxant with an intermediate duration of action. Anesthesiology 98:1042, 2003.
5. Viby-Mogensen J: Postoperative residual curarization and evidence-based anaesthesia. Br J Anaesth 84:301, 2000.
6. Eriksson LI: Evidence-based practice and neuromuscular monitoring. It's time for routine quantitative assessment. Anesthesiology 98:1037, 2003.
7. Iwasaki H, Igarashi M, Namiki A: A preliminary evaluation of magnetic stimulation of the ulnar nerve for monitoring neuromuscular transmission. Anaesthesia 49:814, 1994.
8. Moerer O, Baller C, Hinz J et al: Neuromuscular effects of rapacuronium on the diaphragm and skeletal muscles in anaesthetized patients using cervical magnetic stimulation for stimulating the phrenic nerves. Eur J Anaesth 19:883, 2002.
9. Brull SJ, Ehrenwerth J, Silverman DG: Stimulation with submaximal current for train-of-four monitoring. Anesthesiology 72:629, 1990.
10. Brull SJ, Ehrenwerth J, Connelly NR, et al: Assessment of residual curarization using low-current stimulation. Can J Anaesth 38:164, 1991.
11. Silverman DG, Brull SJ: Assessment of double-burst monitoring at 10 mA above threshold current. Can J Anaesth 40:502, 1993.
12. Helbo-Hansen HS, Bang U, Nielsen HK, et al: The accuracy of train-of-four monitoring at varying stimulating currents. Anesthesiology 76:199, 1992.
13. Curran MJ, Donati F, Bevan DR: Onset and recovery of atracurium and suxamethonium-induced neuromuscular blockade with simultaneous train-of-four and single twitch stimulation. Br J Anaesth 59:989, 1987.
14. Ali HH, Utting JE, Gray C: Stimulus frequency in the detection of neuromuscular blocks in humans. Br J Anaesth 42:967, 1970.

15. Ali HH, Utting JE, Gray C: Quantitative assessment of residual antidepolarizing block (part II). Br J Anaesth 43:478, 1971.
16. Paton WDM, Waud DR: The margin of safety of neuromuscular transmission. J Physiol 191:59, 1967.
17. Brull SJ, Silverman DG: Tetanus-induced changes in apparent recovery after bolus doses of atracurium or vecuronium. Anesthesiology 77:642, 1992.
18. Saitoh Y, Masuda A, Toyooka H, et al: Effect of tetanic stimulation on subsequent train-of-four responses at various levels of vecuronium-induced neuromuscular block. Br J Anaesth 73:416, 1994.
19. Dupuis JY, Martin R, Tessonnier JM, et al: Clinical assessment of the muscular response to tetanic nerve stimulation. Can J Anaesth 37:397, 1990.
20. Viby-Mogensen J, Howardy-Hansen P, Chraemmer-Jorgensen B, et al: Post-tetanic count (PTC). A new method of evaluating an intense nondepolarizing neuromuscular blockade. Anesthesiology 55:458, 1981.
21. Bonsu AK, Viby-Mogensen J, Fernando PUE, et al: Relationship of post-tetanic count and train-of-four response during intense neuromuscular blockade caused by atracurium. Br J Anaesth 59:1089, 1987.
22. Muchhal KK, Viby-Mogensen J, Fernando PUE, et al: Evaluation of intense neuromuscular blockade caused by vecuronium using post-tetanic count (PTC). Anesthesiology 66:846, 1987.
23. Fernando PUE, Viby-Mogensen J, Bonsu AK, et al: Relationship between post-tetanic count and response to carinal stimulation during vecuronium-induced neuromuscular blockade. Acta Anaesthesiol Scand 31:593, 1987.
24. Schultz P, Ibsen D, Østergaard D, et al: Onset and duration of action of rocuronium: from tracheal intubation, through intense block to complete recovery. Acta Anaesthesiol Scand 45:612, 2001.
25. El-Orbany MI, Joseph JN, Salem MR: The relationship of posttetanic count and train-of-four responses during recovery from intense cisatracurium-induced neuromuscular blockade. Anesth Analg 97:80, 2003.
26. Werba A, Klezl M, Schramm W, et al: The level of neuromuscular block needed to suppress diaphragmatic movement during tracheal suction in patients with raised intracranial pressure: A study with vecuronium and atracurium. Anaesthesia 48:301, 1993.
27. Engbæk J, Østergaard D, Viby-Mogensen J: Double burst stimulation (DBS). A new pattern of nerve stimulation to identify residual curarization. Br J Anaesth 62:274, 1989.
28. Viby-Mogensen J, Jensen NH, Engbæk J, et al: Tactile and visual evaluation of the response to train-of-four nerve stimulation. Anesthesiology 63:440, 1985.
29. Drenck NE, Olsen NV, Ueda N, et al: Clinical assessment of residual curarization. A comparison of train-of-four stimulation and double burst stimulation. Anesthesiology 70:578, 1989.
30. Ueda N, Muteki T, Tsuda H, et al: Is the diagnosis of significant residual neuromuscular blockade improved by using double-burst nerve stimulation? Eur J Anaesth 8:213, 1991.
31. Saddler JM, Bevan JC, Donati F, et al: Comparison of double-burst and train-of-four stimulation to assess neuromuscular blockade in children. Anesthesiology 73:401, 1990.
32. Gill SS, Donati F, Bevan DR: Clinical evaluation of double-burst stimulation. Its relationship to train-of-four stimulation. Anaesthesia 45:543, 1990.
33. Fruergaard K, Viby-Mogensen J, Berg H, et al: Tactile evaluation of the response to double burst stimulation decreases, but does not eliminate the problem of postoperative residual paralysis. Acta Anaesthesiol Scand, 42:1168, 1998.
34. Brull SJ, Silverman DG: Pulse width, stimulus intensity, electrode placement, and polarity during assessment of neuromuscular block. Anesthesiology 83:702, 1995.
35. Smith CE, Donati F, Bevan DR: Potency of succinylcholine at the diaphragm and the adductor pollicis muscle. Anesth Analg 67:625, 1988.
36. Donati F, Antzaka C, Bevan DR: Potency of pancuronium at the diaphragm and the adductor pollicis muscle in humans. Anesthesiology 65:1, 1986.
37. Pansard J-L, Chauvin M, Lebrault C, et al: Effect of an intubating dose of succinylcholine and atracurium on the diaphragm and the adductor pollicis muscle in humans. Anesthesiology 67:326, 1987.
38. Plaud B, Debaene B, Donati F: The corrugator supercilii, not orbicularis oculi, reflects rocuronium neuromuscular blockade at the laryngeal adductor muscles. Anesthesiology 95:96, 2001.
39. Hemmerling TM, Donati F: Neuromuscular blockade at the larynx, the diaphragm and the corrugator supercilii muscle: a review. Can J Anesth 50:779, 2003.
40. Donati F, Meistelman C, Plaud B: Vecuronium neuromuscular blockade at the diaphragm, the orbicularis oculi, and adductor pollicis muscles. Anesthesiology 73:870, 1990.
41. Donati F, Meistelman C, Plaud B: Vecuronium neuromuscular blockade at the adductor muscles of the larynx and adductor pollicis. Anesthesiology 74:833, 1991.
42. Ungureanu D, Meistelman C, Frossard J, et al: The orbicularis oculi and the adductor pollicis muscles as monitors of atracurium block of laryngeal muscles. Anesth Analg 77:775, 1993.
43. Rimaniol JM, Dhonneur G, Sperry L, et al: A comparison of the neuromuscular blocking effects of atracurium, mivacurium, and vecuronium on the adductor pollicis and the orbicularis oculi muscle in humans. Anesth Analg 83:808, 1996.
44. Smith CE, Donati F, Bevan DR: Differential effects of pancuronium on masseter and adductor pollicis muscles in humans. Anesthesiology 71:57, 1989.
45. Isono S, Ide T, Kochi T, et al: Effects of partial paralysis on the swallowing reflex in conscious humans. Anesthesiology 75:980, 1991.
46. Pavlin EG, Holle R, Schone R: Recovery of airway protection compared with ventilation in humans after paralysis with curare. Anesthesiology 70:381, 1989.
47. D'Honneur G, Guignard B, Slavov V, et al: Comparison of the neuromuscular blocking effect of atracurium and vecuronium on the adductor pollicis and the geniohyoid muscle in humans. Anesthesiology 82:649, 1995.
48. Eriksson LI, Sundman E, Olsson R, et al: Functional assessment of the pharynx at rest and during swallowing in partially paralyzed humans. Anesthesiology 87:1035, 1997.
49. Sopher MJ, Sears DH, Walts LF: Neuromuscular function monitoring comparing the flexor hallucis brevis and adductor pollicis muscles. Anesthesiology 69:129, 1988.
50. Suzuki T, Suzuki H, Katsumata N, et al: Evaluation of twitch responses obtained from abductor hallucis muscle as a monitor of neuromuscular blockade: Comparison with the results from adductor pollicis muscle. J Anesth 8:44, 1994.
51. Kern SE, Johnson JO, Orr JA, et al: Clinical analysis of the flexor hallucis brevis as an alternative site for monitoring neuromuscular block from mivacurium. J Clin Anesth 9:383, 1997.
52. Saitoh Y, Fujii Y, Takahashi K, et al: Recovery of post-tetanic count and train-of-four responses at the great toe and thumb. Anaesthesia 53:244, 1998.
53. Viby-Mogensen J, Engbæk J, Gramstad L, et al: Good Clinical Research Practice (GCRP) in pharmacodynamic studies of neuromuscular blocking agents. Acta Anaesthesiol Scand 40:59, 1996.
54. Lee GC, Iyengar S, Szenohradszky J, et al: Improving the design of muscle relaxant studies. Anesthesiology 86:48, 1997.
55. Hemmerling TM, Schmidt J, Hanusa C, et al: Simultaneous determination of neuromuscular block at the larynx, diaphragm, adductor pollicis, orbicularis oculi and corrugator supercilii muscles. Br J Anaesth 856:860, 2000.
56. Hemmerling TM, Schurr C, Walter S, et al: A new method of monitoring the effect of muscle relaxants on laryngeal muscle using surface laryngeal electromyography. Anesth Analg 90:494, 2000.
57. Hemmerling TM, Schmidt J, Wolf T, et al: Intramuscular versus surface electromyography of the diaphragm for determining neuromuscular blockade. Anesth Analg 92:106, 2001.

58. Hemmerling TM, Schmidt J, Hanusa C, et al: The lumbar paravertebral region provides a novel site to assess neuromuscular block at the diaphragm. Can J Anesth 48:356, 2001.

59. Viby-Mogensen J: Neuromuscular monitoring. Curr Opin Anaesthesiol 14:655, 2001.

60. Engbæk J, Skovgaard LT, Fries B, et al: Monitoring of neuromuscular transmission by electromyography (II). Evoked compound EMG area, amplitude and duration compared to mechanical twitch recording during onset and recovery of pancuronium-induced blockade in the cat. Acta Anaesthesiol Scand 37:788, 1993.

61. Kopman AF: The relationship of evoked electromyographic and mechanical responses following atracurium in humans. Anesthesiology 63:208, 1985.

62. Engbæk J, Østergaard D, Viby-Mogensen J: Clinical recovery and train-of-four ratio measured mechanically and electromyographically following atracurium. Anesthesiology 71:391, 1989.

63. Kosek PS, Sears DHJ, Rubinstein EH: Minimizing movement-induced changes in twitch response during integrated electromyography [letter]. Anesthesiology 69:142, 1988.

64. Viby-Mogensen J, Jensen E, Werner M, et al: Measurement of acceleration: A new method of monitoring neuromuscular function. Acta Anaesthesiol Scand 32:45, 1988.

65. Jensen E, Viby-Mogensen J, Bang U: The Accelograph: A new neuromuscular transmission monitor. Acta Anaesthesiol Scand 32:49, 1988.

66. Viby-Mogensen J: Monitoring neuromuscular function in the Intensive Care Unit. Intensive Care Med 19:S74, 1993.

67. Hodges UM: Vecuronium infusion requirements in paediatric patients in intensive care units: The use of acceleromyography. Br J Anaesth 76:23, 1996.

68. Werner MU, Kirkegaard Nielsen H, et al: Assessment of neuromuscular transmission by the evoked acceleration response. An evaluation of the accuracy of the acceleration transducer in comparison with a force displacement transducer. Acta Anaesthesiol Scand 32:395, 1988.

69. Ansermino JM, Sanderson PM, Bevan DR: Acceleromyography improves detection of residual neuromuscular blockade in children. Can J Anaesth 43:589, 1996.

70. May O, Kirkegaard Nielsen H, Werner MU: The acceleration transducer—an assessment of its precision in comparison with a force displacement transducer. Acta Anaesthesiol Scand 32:239, 1988.

71. Harper NJN, Martlew R, Strang T, et al: Monitoring neuromuscular block by acceleromyography: Comparison of the Mini-Accelograph with the Myograph 2000. Br J Anaesth 72:411, 1994.

72. McCluskey A, Meakin G, Hopkinson JM, et al: A comparison of acceleromyography and mechanomyography for determination of the dose-response curve of rocuronium in children. Anaesthesia 52:345, 1997.

73. Kirkegaard-Nielsen H, Helbo-Hansen HS, Pedersen SH, et al: New equipment for neuromuscular transmission monitoring: A comparison of the TOF-Guard with the Myograph 2000. J Clin Monitor Comput 14:19, 1998.

74. Kopman AF, Klewicka MM, Neuman GG: The relationship between acceleromyographic train-of-four fade and single twitch depression. Anesthesiology 96:583, 2002.

75. Kopman AF: Measurement and monitoring of neuromuscular blockade. Curr Opin Anaesthesiol 15:415, 2002.

76. Eikermann M, Groeben H, Hüsing J, et al: Accelerometry of adductor pollicis muscle predicts recovery of respiratory function from neuromuscular blockade. Anesthesiology 98:1133, 2003.

77. Mortensen CR, Berg H, El-Mahdy A, et al: Perioperative monitoring of neuromuscular transmission using acceleromyography prevents residual neuromuscular block following pancuronium. Acta Anaesthesiol Scand 39:797, 1995.

78. Gätke MR, Viby-Mogensen J, Rosenstock C, et al: Postoperative muscle paralysis after rocuronium: Less residual block when acceleromyography is used. Acta Anaesthesiol Scand 46:207, 2002.

79. Gätke MR, Larsen PB, Engbæk J, et al: Acceleromyography of the orbicularis oculi muscle I: significance of the electrode position. Acta Anaesthesiol Scand 46:1124, 2002.

80. Larsen PB, Gätke MR, Fredensborg BB, et al: Acceleromyography of the orbicularis oculi muscle. II: Comparing the orbicularis oculi and adductor pollicis muscles. Acta Anaesthesiol Scand 46:1131, 2002.

81. Kern SE, Johnson JO, Westenkow DR, et al: An effectiveness study of a new piezoelectric sensor for train-of-four measurement. Anesth Analg 78:978, 1994.

82. Pelgrims K, Vanacker B: Comparative study of the TOF-ratio measured by the ParaGraph versus the TOF-Guard, with and without thumb repositioning. Acta Anaesthesiol Belg 52:297, 2001.

83. Dahaba AA, von Klobucar F, Rehak PH, et al: The neuromuscular transmission module versus the relaxometer mechanomyograph for neuromuscular block monitoring. Anesth Analg 94:591, 2002.

84. Barry DT: Muscle sounds from evoked twitches in the hand. Arch Phys Med Rehabil 72:573, 1991.

85. Dascalu A, Geller E, Moalem Y, et al: Acoustic monitoring of intraoperative neuromuscular block. Br J Anaesth 83:405, 1999.

86. Hemmerling TM, Donati F, Beaulieu P, et al: Phonomyography of the corrugator supercilii muscle: Signal characteristics, best recording site and comparison with acceleromyography. Br J Anaesth 88:389, 2002.

87. Hemmerling TM, Donati F, Babin D, et al: Duration of control stimulation does not affect onset and offset of neuromuscular blockade at the corrugator supercilii muscle measured with phonomyography or acceleromyography. Can J Anesth 49:913, 2002.

88. Hemmerling TM, Babin D, Donati F: Phonomyography as a novel method to determine neuromuscular blockade at the laryngeal adductor muscles. Anesthesiology 98:359, 2003.

89. Hemmerling TM, Michaud G, Trager G, et al: Phonomyography and mechanomyography can be used interchangeably to measure neuromuscular block at the adductor pollicis muscle. Anesth Analg 98:377, 2004.

90. Gibson FM, Mirakhur RK, Clarke RSJ, et al: Quantification of train-of-four responses during recovery of block from non-depolarizing muscle relaxants. Acta Anaesthesiol Scand 31:655, 1987.

91. O'Hara DA, Fragen RJ, Shanks CA: Comparison of visual and measured train-of-four recovery after vecuronium-induced neuromuscular blockade using two anaesthetic techniques. Br J Anaesth 58:1300, 1986.

92. Engbæk J, Østergaard D, Theil Skovgaard L, et al: Reversal of intense neuromuscular blockade following infusion of atracurium. Anesthesiology 72:803, 1990.

93. Kopman AF, Yee PS, Neuman GG: Relationship of the train-of-four fade ratio to clinical signs and symptoms of residual paralysis in awake volunteers. Anesthesiology 86:765, 1997.

94. Ali HH, Wilson RS, Savarese JJ, et al: The effect of tubocurarine on indirectly elicited train-of-four muscle response and respiratory measurements in humans. Br J Anaesth 47:570, 1975.

95. Ali HH, Utting JE, Gray C: Quantitative assessment of residual antidepolarizing block (part I). Br J Anaesth 43:473, 1971.

96. Brand JB, Cullen DJ, Wilson NE, et al: Spontaneous recovery from non-depolarizing neuromuscular blockade: Correlation between clinical and evoked responses. Anesth Analg 56:55, 1977.

97. Eriksson LI, Lennmarken C, Wyon N, et al: Attenuated ventilatory response to hypoxaemia at vecuronium-induced partial neuromuscular block. Acta Anaesthesiol Scand 36:710, 1992.

98. Eriksson LI, Sato M, Severinghaus JW: Effect of a vecuronium-induced partial neuromuscular block on hypoxic ventilatory response. Anesthesiology 78:693, 1993.

99. Berg H, Viby-Mogensen J, Roed J, et al: Residual neuromuscular block is a risk factor for postoperative pulmonary complications. Acta Anaesthesiol Scand 41:1095, 1997.

100. Wyon N, Joensen H, Yamamoto Y, et al: Carotid body chemoreceptor function is impaired by vecuronium during hypoxia. Anesthesiology 89:1471, 1999.
101. Sundman E, Witt H, Olsson R, et al: The incidence and mechanism of pharyngeal and upper esophagus dysfunction in partially paralyzed humans. Anesthesiology 92:997, 2000.
102. Jonsson M, Kim C, Yamamoto Y, et al: Atracurium and vecuronium block nicotine-induced carotid body responses. Acta Anaesthesiol Scand 94:117, 2002.
103. Shorten GD, Merk H: Perioperative train-of-four monitoring and residual curarization. Can J Anaesth 42:711, 1995.
104. Kopman AF, Ng J, Zank LM, et al: Residual postoperative paralysis. Pancuronium versus mivacurium, does it matter? Anesthesiology 85:1253, 1996.
105. Heier T, Caldwell JE, Sessler DI, et al: The effect of local surface and central cooling on adductor pollicis twitch tension during nitrous oxide/isoflurane and nitrous oxide/fentanyl anesthesia in humans. Anesthesiology 72:807, 1990.
106. Eriksson LI, Lennmarken C, Jensen E, et al: Twitch tension and train-of-four ratio during prolonged neuromuscular monitoring at different peripheral temperatures. Acta Anaesthesiol Scand 35:247, 1991.
107. Thornberry EA, Mazumdar B: The effect of changes in arm temperature on neuromuscular monitoring in the presence of atracurium blockade. Anaesthesia 43:447, 1988.
108. Kirkegaard H, Heier T, Caldwell JE: Efficacy of tactile-guided reversal from cisatracurium-induced neuromuscular block. Anesthesiology 96:45, 2002.
109. Kopman AF, Zank LM, Ng J, et al: Antagonism of cisatracurium and rocuronium block at a tactile train-of-four count of 2: Should quantitative assessment of neuromuscular function be mandatory? Anesth Analg 98:102, 2004.
110. Pedersen T, Viby-Mogensen J, Bang U, et al: Does perioperative tactile evaluation of the train-of-four response influence the frequency of postoperative residual neuromuscular blockade? Anesthesiology 73:835, 1990.

40 Temperature Monitoring

Daniel I. Sessler

Introduction   1571

Normal Thermoregulation   1572
Afferent Input   1572
Central Control   1572
Efferent Responses   1573

Thermoregulation during General Anesthesia   1574
Response Thresholds   1574
Responses in Infants and the Elderly   1575
Gain and Maximum Response Intensity   1575

Development of Hypothermia during General Anesthesia   1576
Heat Transfer   1576
Patterns of Intraoperative Hypothermia   1576

Neuraxial Anesthesia   1577
Thermoregulation   1578
Heat Balance   1580
Shivering   1580

Consequences of Mild Intraoperative Hypothermia   1581
Benefits   1581
Complications   1581
Postanesthetic Shivering   1582

Perioperative Thermal Manipulations   1583

Effects of Vasomotor Tone on Heat Transfer   1584
Preventing Redistribution Hypothermia   1584
Airway Heating and Humidification   1585
Intravenous Fluids   1585
Cutaneous Warming   1585
Induction of Mild Therapeutic Hypothermia   1587

Deliberate Severe Intraoperative Hypothermia   1588
Organ Function   1588
Acid-Base Changes   1588

Hyperthermia and Fever   1589
Passive Hyperthermia and Malignant Hyperthermia   1589
Fever   1589
Hyperthermia during Epidural Analgesia   1590

Temperature Monitoring   1590
Thermometers   1590
When Temperature Monitoring Is Required   1590
Temperature-Monitoring Sites   1591
Temperature-Monitoring and Thermal Management Guidelines   1591

Summary   1592

INTRODUCTION

Mammals and birds are homeothermic; that is, they require a nearly constant internal body temperature. When internal temperature deviates significantly from normal, metabolic functions usually deteriorate, and death may result. The thermoregulatory system usually maintains core body temperature within 0.2°C of "normal," which is about 37°C in humans. Anesthetic-induced inhibition of thermoregulation combines with exposure to a cold operating room environment to make most unwarmed patients hypothermic.

In recent years, major outcome studies have shown that mild hypothermia (≈1°C to 2°C) (1) triples the incidence of morbid cardiac outcomes, (2) triples the incidence of surgical wound infections and prolongs hospitalization by 20%, and (3) significantly increases surgical blood loss and the need for allogeneic transfusion. An understanding of normal and anesthetic-influenced thermoregulation will facilitate prevention and management of these and numerous other temperature-related complications.

NORMAL THERMOREGULATION

Thermoregulation is similar to many other physiologic control systems in that the brain uses negative and positive feedback to minimize perturbations from preset, "normal" values. Since 1912, animals have been known to regulate body temperature poorly when the hypothalamus is destroyed. The importance of thermal input from the skin surface was recognized in the late 1950s, when it was observed that mice placed in a cold environment shivered *before* decreasing their hypothalamic temperature.

In the early 1960s, physiologists reported active thermoregulation in response to isolated warming and cooling at sites other than the hypothalamus or skin surface, including extrahypothalamic portions of the brain, deep abdominal tissues, and the spinal cord.[1] Thus, thermoregulation is based on multiple, redundant signals from nearly every type of tissue. The processing of thermoregulatory information occurs in three phases: *afferent thermal sensing, central regulation,* and *efferent responses.*

Afferent Input

Temperature information is obtained from thermally sensitive cells throughout the body. Cold-sensitive cells are anatomically and physiologically distinct from those that detect warmth. Warm receptors increase their firing rates when temperature increases, whereas cold receptors do so when temperature decreases. Cutaneous warm receptors rarely depolarize at normal skin temperatures and are probably important only during heat stress. Cold signals travel primarily by means of Aδ nerve fibers and warm information by unmyelinated C fibers, although some overlap occurs.[2] C fibers also detect and convey pain sensation, which is why intense heat cannot be distinguished from sharp pain. Most ascending thermal information traverses the spinothalamic tracts in the anterior spinal cord, but no single spinal tract is critical for conveying thermal information. Consequently, the entire anterior cord must be destroyed to ablate thermoregulatory responses. The hypothalamus, other parts of the brain, the spinal cord, deep abdominal and thoracic tissues, and the skin surface each contribute roughly 20% of the total thermal input to the central regulatory system.[3,4]

Central Control

Temperature is regulated by central structures (primarily the hypothalamus) that compare integrated thermal inputs from the skin surface, neuraxis, and deep tissues with *threshold* temperatures for each thermoregulatory response. Though integrated by the hypothalamus, most thermal information is "preprocessed" in the spinal cord and other parts of the central nervous system. This hierarchic arrangement presumably developed when the evolving thermoregulatory control system co-opted previously existing mechanisms (e.g., shivering from muscles previously used for posture and locomotion).[1] It is likely that

some thermoregulatory responses can be mounted by the spinal cord alone.[4] For example, animals and patients with high spinal cord transections regulate temperature better than might be expected.

The slope of response intensity versus core temperature defines the *gain* of a thermoregulatory response. A response intensity no longer increasing with further deviation in core temperature identifies the *maximum intensity.* This system of thresholds and gains is a model for a thermoregulatory system that is further complicated by interactions between other regulatory responses (i.e., vascular volume control) and time-dependent effects.

How the body determines absolute threshold temperatures is unknown, but the mechanism appears to be mediated by norepinephrine, dopamine, 5-hydroxytryptamine, acetylcholine, prostaglandin E_1, and neuropeptides. Thresholds vary daily in both sexes (circadian rhythm) and monthly in women by approximately 0.5°C. Exercise, food intake, infection, hypothyroidism and hyperthyroidism, anesthetic and other drugs (including alcohol, sedatives, and nicotine), and cold and warm adaptation alter threshold temperatures.

Control of autonomic responses is approximately 80% determined by thermal input from core structures (Fig. 40–1).[5,6] In contrast, a large fraction of the input controlling behavioral responses is derived from the skin surface. The *interthreshold range* (core temperatures *not* triggering autonomic thermoregulatory responses) is only 0.2°C.[7] This range is bounded by the sweating threshold at its upper end and by vasoconstriction at the lower end. Because energy cost and nutrients are conserved without excessive autonomic control within this range, some animals such as camels and desert rats use this strategy extensively to allow core temperature changes of up to 10°C each day.

Both sweating and vasoconstriction thresholds are 0.3°C to 0.5°C higher in women than men, even during the follicular phase of the monthly cycle (first 10 days).[8] Differences are even greater during the luteal phase.[9] Central thermoregulatory control is apparently intact even in somewhat premature infants.[10] In contrast, thermoregulatory control is sometimes impaired in the elderly.[11]

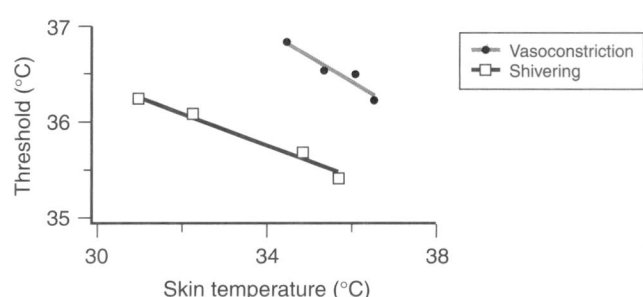

Figure 40–1 There is a linear relationship between mean skin temperature and the core temperature triggering vasoconstriction and shivering. Skin temperature contributes about 20% to control of each thermoregulatory defense. (Redrawn from Cheng C, Matsukawa T, Sessler DI, et al: Increasing mean skin temperature linearly reduces the core-temperature thresholds for vasoconstriction and shivering in humans. Anesthesiology 82:1160–1168, 1995.)

Efferent Responses

The body responds to thermal perturbations (body temperatures differing from the appropriate threshold) by activating effector mechanisms that increase metabolic heat production or alter environmental heat loss. Each thermoregulatory effector has its own threshold and gain, so there is an orderly progression of responses and response intensities in proportion to need. In general, energy-efficient effectors such as vasoconstriction are maximized before metabolically costly responses such as shivering are initiated. The interaction between thermal input, central control, and effector responses is shown in Figure 40–2; this figure also shows normal values for the major autonomic response thresholds.

Effectors determine the ambient temperature range that the body will tolerate while maintaining a normal core temperature. When specific effector mechanisms are inhibited (e.g., shivering prevented by the administration of muscle relaxants), the tolerable range is decreased. Still, temperature will remain normal unless other effectors cannot compensate for the imposed stress. Quantitatively, *behavioral regulation* (e.g., dressing appropriately, modifying the environmental temperature, assuming positions that oppose skin surfaces, and voluntary movement) is the most important effector mechanism.

Infants regulate their temperatures remarkably well. In contrast, advanced age, infirmity, or medications can diminish the efficacy of thermoregulatory responses and increase the risk of hypothermia. For example, decreased

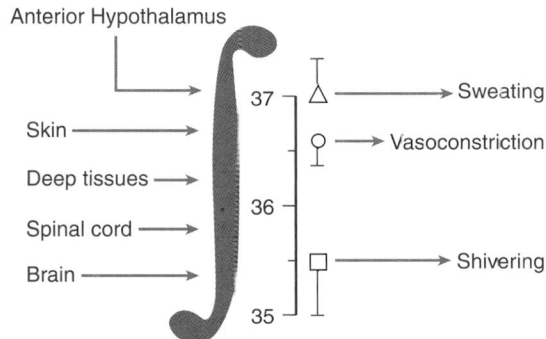

Figure 40–2 Schematic illustrating thermoregulatory control mechanisms. Mean body temperature is the integrated thermal input from a variety of tissues, including the brain, skin surface, spinal cord, and deep core structures. This input is shown entering the hypothalamus from the *left*. However, thresholds are usually expressed in terms of core temperature. A core temperature below the thresholds for response to cold provokes vasoconstriction, nonshivering thermogenesis, and shivering. Core temperature exceeding the hyperthermic thresholds produces active vasodilation and sweating. No thermoregulatory responses are initiated when the core temperature is between these thresholds; these temperatures identify the interthreshold range, which in humans is usually only about 0.2°C. (Threshold data from Lopez M, Sessler DI, Walter K, et al: Rate and gender dependence of the sweating, vasoconstriction, and shivering thresholds in humans. Anesthesiology 80:780–788, 1994. Figure redrawn from Sessler DI: Perioperative hypothermia. N Engl J Med 336:1730–1737, 1997.)

muscle mass, neuromuscular diseases, and muscle relaxants all inhibit shivering, which increases the minimum tolerable ambient temperature. Similarly, anticholinergic drugs inhibit sweating, which decreases the maximum tolerable temperature.

Cutaneous vasoconstriction is the most consistently used autonomic effector mechanism. Metabolic heat is lost primarily through convection and radiation from the skin surface, and vasoconstriction reduces this loss. Total digital skin blood flow is divided into nutritional (mostly capillary) and thermoregulatory (mostly arteriovenous shunt) components.[12] The arteriovenous shunts are anatomically and functionally distinct from the capillaries supplying nutritional blood to the skin (thus vasoconstriction does not compromise the needs of peripheral tissues). Shunts are typically 100 μm in diameter, which means that one shunt can convey 10,000-fold as much blood as a comparable length of capillary 10 μm in diameter.

Control of blood flow through arteriovenous shunts tends to be "on" or "off." In other words, the gain of this response is high. Local α-adrenergic sympathetic nerves mediate constriction in the thermoregulatory arteriovenous shunts, and flow is minimally affected by *circulating* catecholamines. Roughly 10% of cardiac output traverses arteriovenous shunts; consequently, shunt vasoconstriction increases mean arterial pressure approximately 15 mm Hg.

Nonshivering thermogenesis increases metabolic heat production (measured as whole-body oxygen consumption) without producing mechanical work. It doubles heat production in infants[13] but increases it only slightly in adults.[14] The intensity of nonshivering thermogenesis increases in linear proportion to the difference between mean body temperature and its threshold. Skeletal muscle and brown fat tissue are the major sources of nonshivering heat in adults. The metabolic rate in both tissues is controlled primarily by norepinephrine release from adrenergic nerve terminals and is further mediated locally by an uncoupling protein.[15]

Sustained shivering augments metabolic heat production 50% to 100% in adults. This increase is small in comparison to that produced by exercise (which can, at least briefly, increase metabolism 500%) and is thus surprisingly ineffective. Shivering does not occur in newborn infants and is probably not fully effective until children are several years old. The rapid tremor (up to 250 Hz) and unsynchronized muscular activity of thermogenic shivering suggest no central oscillator. However, superimposed on the fast activity is usually a slow (4 to 8 cycle/min), synchronous "waxing-and-waning" pattern that presumably is centrally mediated.[16]

Sweating is mediated by postganglionic cholinergic nerves.[17] It is thus an active process that is prevented by nerve block or atropine administration.[18] Even untrained individuals can sweat up to 1 L/hr, and athletes can sweat at twice that rate. Sweating is the only mechanism by which the body can dissipate heat in an environment exceeding core temperature. Fortunately, the process is remarkably effective, with 0.58 kcal of heat dissipated per gram of evaporated sweat.

Active vasodilation is mediated by a yet-to-be-identified factor released from sweat glands; the mediator may be a protein because it is not blocked by any standard drugs.[19]

Active vasodilation requires intact sweat gland function, so it is also largely inhibited by nerve blocks. During extreme heat stress, blood flow through the top millimeter of skin can reach 7.5 L/min—equal to the entire resting cardiac output.[20] The threshold for active vasodilation is usually similar to the sweating threshold, but the gain may be less. Consequently, maximum cutaneous vasodilation is generally delayed until core temperature is well above that provoking the maximum sweating intensity.

THERMOREGULATION DURING GENERAL ANESTHESIA

Behavioral regulation is not relevant during general anesthesia because patients are unconscious and frequently paralyzed. All general anesthetics tested thus far markedly impair normal autonomic thermoregulatory control. Anesthetic-induced impairment has a specific form: warm-response thresholds are elevated slightly whereas cold-response thresholds are markedly reduced. Consequently, the interthreshold range is increased from its normal

values near 0.2°C to approximately 2°C to 4°C.[21–25] The gain and maximum intensity of some responses remain normal,[8] whereas others are reduced by general anesthesia.[26,27]

Response Thresholds

Propofol,[21] alfentanil,[22] and dexmedetomidine[23] all produce a slight linear increase in the sweating threshold combined with a marked linear decrease in the vasoconstriction and shivering thresholds. Isoflurane[25] and desflurane[24] also slightly increase the sweating threshold; however, they decrease the cold-response thresholds nonlinearly. Consequently, the volatile anesthetics inhibit vasoconstriction and shivering less than propofol does at low concentrations, but more than propofol does at typical anesthetic doses. In all cases (except during meperidine administration[28]), vasoconstriction and shivering decrease synchronously, thereby maintaining their normal approximately 1°C difference.

The dose-dependent response thresholds for four anesthetic drugs are shown in Figure 40–3. The combination

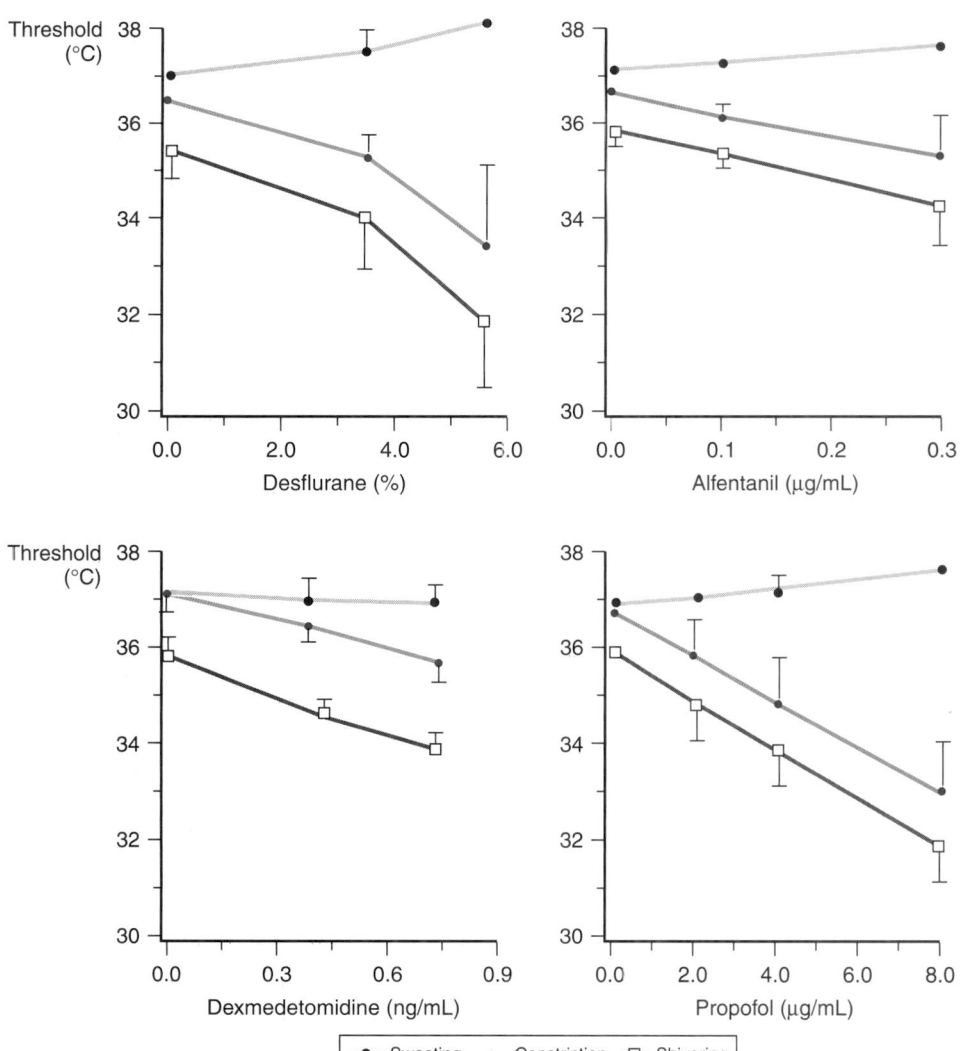

Figure 40–3 Major autonomic thermoregulatory response thresholds in volunteers given desflurane, alfentanil, dexmedetomidine, or propofol. All the anesthetics slightly increase the sweating threshold (triggering core temperature) while markedly and synchronously decreasing the vasoconstriction and shivering thresholds. Standard deviation bars smaller than the data markers have been deleted. (Data from references 21–24.)

of increased sweating thresholds and reduced vasoconstriction thresholds increases the interthreshold range about 20-fold, from its normal value near 0.2°C to around 2°C to 4°C. Temperatures within this range do *not* trigger thermoregulatory defenses; by definition, patients are thus poikilothermic within this temperature range.

Halothane,[29] enflurane,[30] and the combination of nitrous oxide and fentanyl[31] decrease the vasoconstriction threshold 2°C to 4°C from its normal value near approximately 37°C. However, the effect of these drugs on sweating or shivering remains unknown. Clonidine synchronously decreases cold-response thresholds[32] while slightly increasing the sweating threshold.[33] Nitrous oxide decreases the vasoconstriction[34] and shivering[35] thresholds less than equipotent concentrations of volatile anesthetics do. The only sedative or anesthetic drug tested that minimally influences thermoregulatory control is midazolam.[36] Painful stimulation slightly increases vasoconstriction thresholds[30]; consequently, thresholds will be somewhat lower when surgical pain is prevented by simultaneous local or regional anesthesia.

Responses in Infants and the Elderly (also see Chapters 59, 60, and 62)

Thermoregulatory vasoconstriction is comparably impaired in infants, children, and adults given isoflurane[37] or halothane (Fig. 40–4).[38] In contrast, the vasoconstriction threshold is about 1°C less in patients aged 60 to 80 years than in those between 30 and 50 years old (Fig. 40–5).[39,40]

Nonshivering thermogenesis does not occur in anesthetized adults,[41] which is unsurprising because this

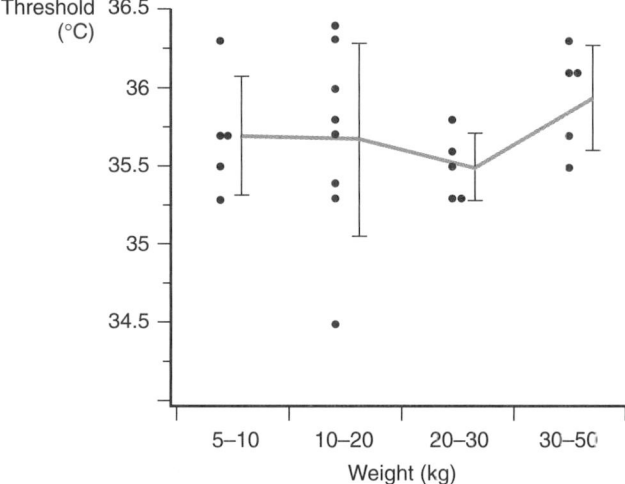

Figure 40–4 The core thermoregulatory threshold in 23 healthy children and infants undergoing abdominal surgery with halothane anesthesia. Differences among the groups are not statistically significant. Results are presented as means ± SD. (Redrawn from Bissonnette B, Sessler DI: Thermoregulatory thresholds for vasoconstriction in pediatric patients anesthetized with halothane or halothane and caudal bupivacaine. Anesthesiology 76:387–392, 1992.)

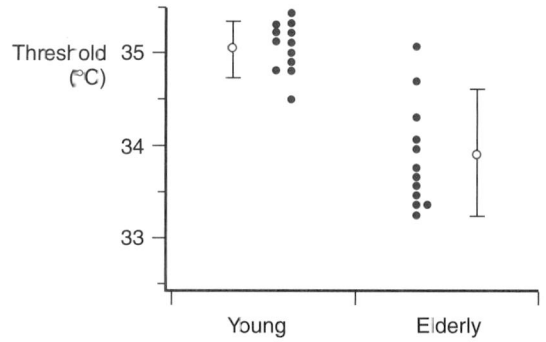

Figure 40–5 The vasoconstriction threshold was significantly less in the elderly (33.9 ± 0.6°C) than in younger patients (35.1 ± 0.3°C) during 60% nitrous oxide and isoflurane (0.75% end-tidal concentration). *Filled circles* indicate the vasoconstriction threshold in each patient; *open circles* show the mean and standard deviation in each group. (Redrawn from Kurz A, Plattner O, Sessler DI, et al: The threshold for thermoregulatory vasoconstriction during nitrous oxide/isoflurane anesthesia is lower in elderly than young patients. Anesthesiology 79:465–469, 1993.)

response is not particularly important in unanesthetized adults.[14] In contrast to adult humans, nonshivering thermogenesis is an important thermoregulatory response in animals and human infants. However, nonshivering thermogenesis in animals is inhibited by volatile anesthetics,[42] and it fails to increase the metabolic rate in infants anesthetized with propofol.[43]

Gain and Maximum Response Intensity

Both the gain and maximum intensity of sweating remain normal during isoflurane[8] and enflurane anesthesia.[44] However, the gain of arteriovenous shunt vasoconstriction is reduced threefold during desflurane anesthesia (Fig. 40–6),[26] even though the maximum vasoconstriction intensity remains normal.[45]

Shivering is rare during surgical doses of general anesthesia, which is consistent with its threshold being roughly 1°C less than the vasoconstriction threshold.[21–25] (Vasoconstriction usually prevents additional hypothermia,[46] so even unwarmed patients rarely become cold enough to shiver.) Nonetheless, shivering can be induced by sufficient active cooling.

Gain and maximum shivering intensity remain normal during both meperidine and alfentanil administration.[47] Gain also remains nearly intact during nitrous oxide administration, although maximum intensity is reduced.[48] Isoflurane changes the macroscopic pattern of shivering to such an extent that it is no longer possible to easily determine gain. The drug does, however, reduce maximum shivering intensity.[27]

Taken together, sweating appears to be the thermoregulatory defense that is best preserved during anesthesia. Not only is the threshold only slightly increased, but the gain and maximum intensity are also well preserved. In contrast, the thresholds for vasoconstriction and shivering are markedly reduced, and furthermore, these responses are less effective than normal even after being activated.

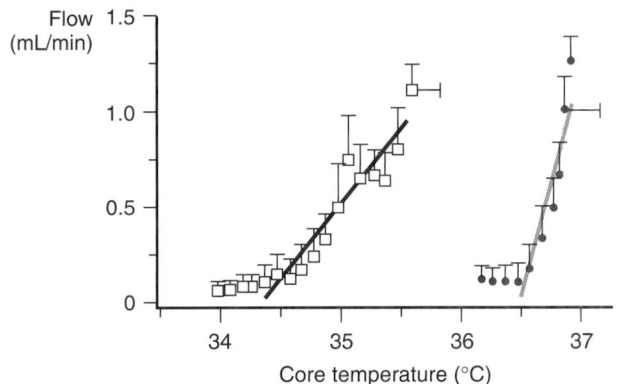

Figure 40–6 Finger blood flow without *(open squares)* and with *(filled circles)* desflurane administration. Values were computed relative to the thresholds (finger flow = 1.0 mL/min) in each subject. Flows of exactly 1.0 mL/min are not shown because flows in each individual were averaged over 0.1°C or 0.05°C increments; each data point thus includes both higher and lower flows. The horizontal standard deviation bars indicate variability in the thresholds among the volunteers; although errors bars are shown only at a flow near 1.0 mL/min, the same temperature variability applies to each data point. The slopes of the flow–versus–core temperature relationships (1.0 to approximately 0.15 mL/min) were determined by linear regression. These slopes defined the gain of vasoconstriction with and without desflurane anesthesia. Gain was reduced by a factor of 3, from 2.4 to 0.8 mL/min/°C (*P* < .01). (Redrawn from Kurz A, Xiong J, Sessler DI, et al: Desflurane reduces the gain of thermoregulatory arteriovenous shunt vasoconstriction in humans. Anesthesiology 83:1212–1219, 1995.)

DEVELOPMENT OF HYPOTHERMIA DURING GENERAL ANESTHESIA

Inadvertent hypothermia during anesthesia is by far the most common perioperative thermal disturbance. Hypothermia results from a combination of anesthetic-impaired thermoregulation and exposure to a cold operating room environment.

Heat Transfer

Heat can be transferred from a patient to the environment in four ways: (1) radiation, (2) conduction, (3) convection, and (4) evaporation. Among these mechanisms, radiation and convection contribute most to perioperative heat loss. All surfaces with a temperature above absolute zero radiate heat; similarly, all surfaces absorb radiant heat from surrounding surfaces. Heat transfer by this mechanism is proportional to the fourth power of the absolute temperature difference between the surfaces. It is likely that radiation is the major type of heat loss in most surgical patients.[49]

Conductive heat loss is proportional to the temperature difference between two adjacent surfaces and the strength of the thermal insulation separating them. In general, conductive losses are negligible during surgery because patients usually only directly contact the foam pad (an excellent thermal insulator) covering most operating room tables.

Conductive loss of heat directly to air molecules is limited by the development of a layer of still air adjacent to the skin that serves as an insulator. When this layer is disturbed by air currents, the insulative properties diminish substantially, and heat loss therefore increases. This increase is termed *convection* and is proportional to the square root of air speed; it is the basis of the familiar "wind chill" factor. Air speed in operating rooms—even those with high rates of air turnover—is typically just about 20 cm/sec, which only slightly increases loss in comparison to that in still air. Nonetheless, convective loss is usually the second most important mechanism by which heat is transferred from patients to the environment. Presumably, convective loss increases substantially in operating rooms equipped to provide laminar flow. However, the actual augmentation has not been quantified and may be less than expected from the increase in air speed because surgical draping provides considerable thermal insulation.

Sweating increases cutaneous evaporative loss enormously but is rare during anesthesia. In the absence of sweating, evaporative loss from the skin surface is limited to less than 10% of metabolic heat production in adults. In contrast, infants lose a higher fraction of their metabolic heat from transpiration of water through thin skin. The problem becomes especially acute in premature infants, who may lose a fifth of their metabolic heat production through transcutaneous evaporation.[50,51] Simple thermodynamic calculations and clinical measurements indicate that only trivial amounts of heat are lost from the respiratory system.[52] However, evaporation inside a surgical wound can contribute substantially to total heat loss.[53]

Patterns of Intraoperative Hypothermia

Hypothermia during general anesthesia develops with a characteristic pattern. An initial rapid decrease in core temperature is followed by a slow, linear reduction in core temperature. Finally, core temperature stabilizes and subsequently remains virtually unchanged (Fig. 40–7). Each portion of this typical pattern has a different etiology.

Volatile anesthetics cause vasodilation through a direct peripheral action.[54] More importantly, they also inhibit tonic thermoregulatory vasoconstriction, which results in arteriovenous shunt dilation.[21-25] Nonetheless, anesthetic-induced vasodilation increases cutaneous heat loss only slightly.[55] Anesthetics reduce the metabolic rate 20% to 30%.[56] However, even the combination of increased heat loss and reduced heat production is insufficient to explain the 0.5°C to 1.5°C decrease in core temperature usually observed during the first hour of anesthesia.

The key to understanding the initial decrease in core temperature is to appreciate that body heat is not normally evenly distributed. Core temperature represents only about half the body mass (mostly the trunk and head); the remaining mass is typically 2°C to 4°C cooler than the core. This core-to-peripheral tissue temperature gradient is normally maintained by tonic thermoregulatory vasoconstriction. Anesthetic-induced vasodilation, however, allows core heat to flow peripherally. This heat redistribution warms the arms and legs, but does so at the expense of the core (Figs. 40–8 and 40–9).[57]

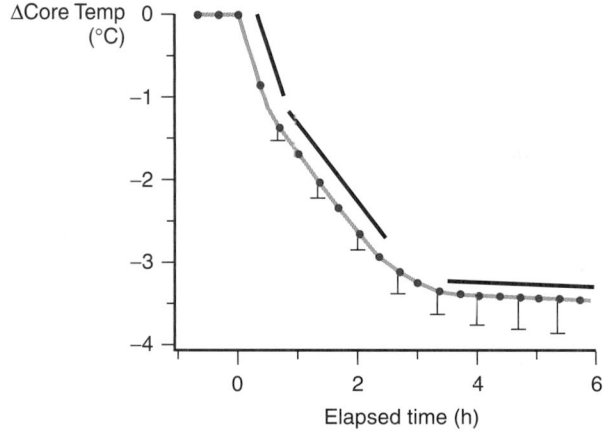

Figure 40–7 Hypothermia during general anesthesia develops with a characteristic pattern. An initial rapid decrease in core temperature results from a core-to-peripheral redistribution of body heat. This redistribution is followed by a slow, linear reduction in core temperature that results simply from heat loss exceeding heat production. Finally, core temperature stabilizes and subsequently remains virtually unchanged. This plateau phase may be a passive thermal steady state or might result when sufficient hypothermia triggers thermoregulatory vasoconstriction. Results are presented as means ± SD.

After the initial redistribution hypothermia, core temperature usually decreases in a slow, linear fashion for 2 to 4 hours. This reduction results simply from heat loss exceeding metabolic heat production.[58] After 3 to 4 hours of anesthesia, core temperature generally reaches a plateau and remains virtually constant for the duration of surgery.[31] The core temperature plateau may simply represent a thermal steady state (heat production equaling heat loss) in patients remaining relatively warm.[59] In others, however, the plateau phase is associated with peripheral thermoregulatory vasoconstriction triggered by core temperatures of 33°C to 35°C.[60]

Thermoregulatory vasoconstriction during anesthesia significantly decreases cutaneous heat loss,[45] but this decrease alone is usually insufficient to produce a thermal steady state. Furthermore, neither adults[41] nor infants[43]

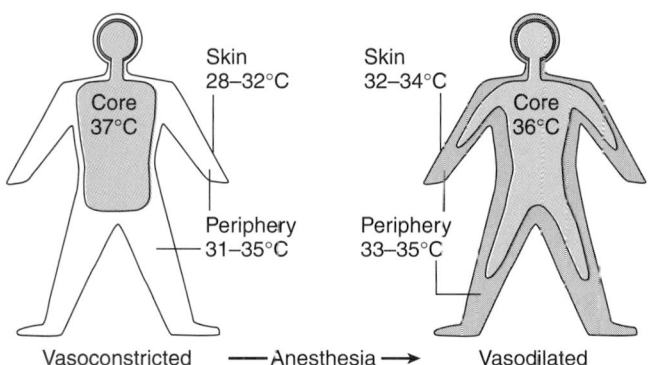

Figure 40–8 Cartoon illustrating internal redistribution of body heat after induction of general anesthesia. Hypothermia after induction of spinal or epidural anesthesia results similarly, but redistribution is restricted to the legs.

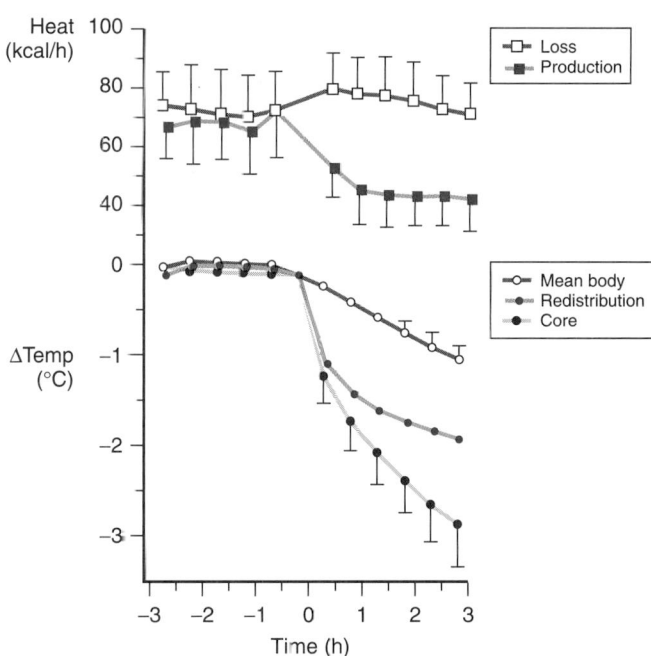

Figure 40–9 Changes in body heat content and distribution of heat within the body during induction of general anesthesia (at elapsed time zero). Subtraction of the change in mean body temperature from the change in core (tympanic membrane) temperature results in the core hypothermia specifically attributable to redistribution. Redistribution hypothermia was thus not a measured value; instead, it is defined by the decrease in core temperature not explained by the relatively small decrease in systemic heat content. After 1 hour of anesthesia, core temperature had decreased 1.6°C ± 0.3°C, with redistribution contributing 81% to the decrease. Even after 3 hours of anesthesia, redistribution contributed 65% to the entire 2.8°C ± 0.5°C decrease in core temperature. Results are presented as means ± SD. (Redrawn with modification from Matsukawa T, Sessler DI, Sessler AM, et al: Heat flow and distribution during induction of general anesthesia. Anesthesiology 82:662–673, 1995.)

appear to be able to increase intraoperative heat production in response to hypothermia. An additional mechanism must therefore contribute to the core temperature plateau. Evidence suggests that a primary factor is constraint of metabolic heat to the core thermal compartment. In this scenario, the distribution of metabolic heat (which is largely produced centrally) is restricted to the core compartment to maintain its temperature. Peripheral tissue temperature, in contrast, continues to decrease because it is no longer being supplied with sufficient heat from the core (Fig. 40–10).[46] A core temperature plateau resulting from thermoregulatory vasoconstriction is thus not a thermal steady state, and body heat content continues to decrease even though core temperature remains nearly constant.

NEURAXIAL ANESTHESIA (also see Chapters 43 to 45)

Autonomic thermoregulation is impaired during regional anesthesia, and the result is typically intraoperative core hypothermia. Interestingly, this hypothermia is often not

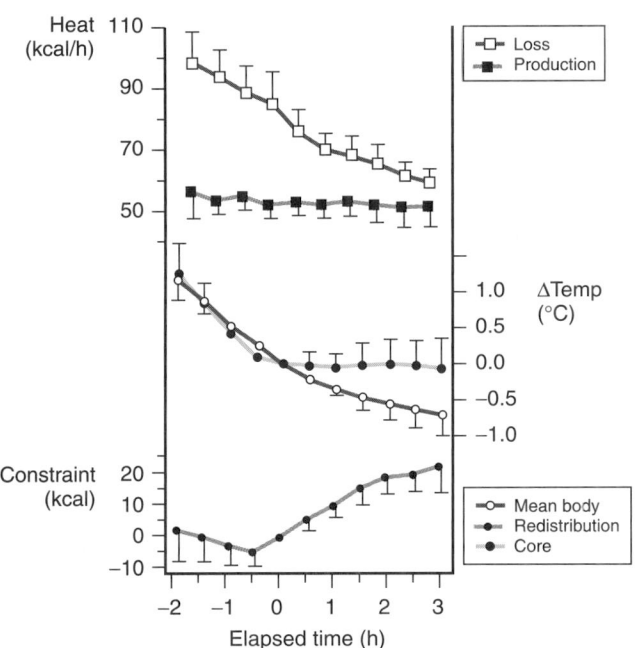

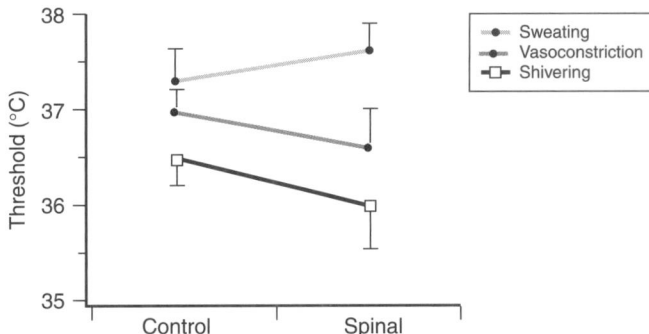

Figure 40–11 Spinal anesthesia increased the sweating threshold but reduced the thresholds for vasoconstriction and shivering. Consequently, the interthreshold range increased substantially. The vasoconstriction-to-shivering range, however, remained normal during spinal anesthesia. Results are presented as means ± SD. (Redrawn from Kurz A, Sessler DI, Schroeder M, Kurz M: Thermoregulatory response thresholds during spinal anesthesia. Anesth Analg 77:721–726, 1993.)

Figure 40–10 Changes in body heat content and distribution of heat within the body during the core temperature plateau. Elapsed time zero indicates the onset of arteriovenous shunt vasoconstriction, which causes the plateau. Core temperature decreased 1.3°C in 2 hours before constriction and then remained constant. The difference between core temperature and mean body temperature (which continued to decrease) indicates how much heat was retained in the core thermal compartment by thermoregulatory vasoconstriction. In this case, 22 ± 8 kcal was constrained to the core. Results are presented as means ± SD. (Redrawn with modification from Kurz A, Sessler DI, Christensen R, Dechert M: Heat balance and distribution during the core-temperature plateau in anesthetized humans. Anesthesiology 83:491–499, 1995.)

consciously perceived by patients, but it nonetheless triggers shivering. The result is frequently a potentially dangerous clinical paradox: a shivering patient who denies feeling cold.

Thermoregulation

Epidural anesthesia[61,62] and spinal anesthesia[62,63] each decrease the thresholds triggering vasoconstriction and shivering (above the level of the block) about 0.6°C (Fig. 40–11). Presumably, this decrease does not result from recirculation of neuraxially administered local anesthetic because the impairment is similar during epidural and spinal anesthesia,[61-63] even though the amount and location of administered local anesthetic differ substantially. Furthermore, lidocaine administered intravenously in doses producing plasma concentrations similar to those occurring during epidural anesthesia has no thermoregulatory effect.[64] Finally, neuraxial administration of 2-chloroprocaine, a local anesthetic that has a plasma half-life near 20 seconds, also impairs thermoregulatory control.[65]

The vasoconstriction and shivering thresholds are comparably decreased during regional anesthesia,[63] thus suggesting an alteration in central rather than peripheral control. The mechanism by which peripheral administration of a local anesthetic impairs centrally mediated thermoregulation may involve an alteration in afferent thermal input from the legs. The key factor here is that tonic cold signals dominate thermal input at leg skin temperatures in typical operating room environments.[2,66] Regional anesthesia blocks all thermal input from blocked regions, which in the typical case is primarily cold information. The brain may then interpret decreased cold information as relative leg warming. This appears to be an unconscious process because perceived temperature does not increase.[67] Because skin temperature is an important input to the thermoregulatory control system, leg warming proportionately reduces the vasoconstriction and shivering thresholds. Consistent with this theory, a leg skin temperature near 38°C is required to produce the same reduction in cold-response thresholds in an unanesthetized subject as is produced by regional anesthesia.[68] Furthermore, the reduction in thresholds is proportional to the number of spinal segments blocked (Fig. 40–12).[69] Major conduction anesthesia may thus reduce the vasoconstriction and shivering thresholds by producing an abnormal elevation in *apparent* (as opposed to actual) leg temperature.

Because neuraxial anesthesia prevents vasoconstriction and shivering in blocked regions, it is not surprising that epidural anesthesia decreases the maximum intensity of shivering. However, epidural anesthesia also reduces the gain of shivering, which suggests that the regulatory system is unable to compensate for lower body paralysis (Fig. 40–13).[27] Thermoregulatory defenses, once triggered, are thus less effective than usual during regional anesthesia.

Neuraxial anesthesia is frequently supplemented with sedative and analgesic medications. With the exception of midazolam,[36] all significantly impair thermoregulatory control.[22,28,70] Such inhibition may be severe when combined with the intrinsic impairment produced by regional anesthesia and other factors, including advanced age and preexisting illness (Fig. 40–14).[11]

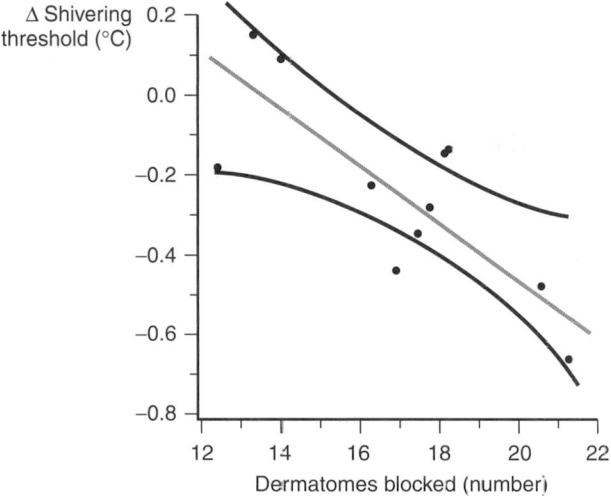

Figure 40–12 The number of dermatomes blocked (sacral segments, 5; lumbar segments, 5; thoracic segments, 12) versus reduction in the shivering threshold (difference between the control shivering threshold and the spinal shivering threshold). The shivering threshold was reduced more by extensive spinal blocks than by less extensive ones (Δ threshold = 0.74 − 0.06 [dermatomes blocked]; r^2 = .58, P < .006). The curved lines indicate the 95% confidence intervals for the slope. (Redrawn from Leslie K, Sessler DI: Reduction in the shivering threshold is proportional to spinal block height. Anesthesiology 84:1327–1331, 1996.)

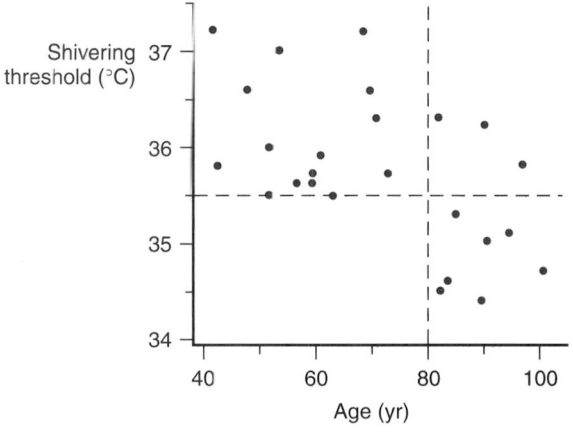

Figure 40–14 Fifteen patients younger than 80 years (58 ± 10 years [mean ± SD]) shivered at 36.1°C ± 0.6°C during spinal anesthesia; in contrast, 8 patients 80 years or older (89 ± 7 years) shivered at a significantly lower mean temperature, 35.2°C ± 0.8°C. The shivering thresholds in seven of the ten patients older than 80 years was less than 35.5°C, whereas the threshold equaled or exceeded this value in all the younger patients. (Redrawn from Vassilieff N, Rosencher N, Sessler DI, Conseiller C: The shivering threshold during spinal anesthesia is reduced in the elderly. Anesthesiology 83:1162–1166, 1995.)

Interestingly, core hypothermia during regional anesthesia may not trigger a perception of cold.[61,71] The reason is that thermal perception (behavioral regulation) is largely determined by skin rather than core temperature. During regional anesthesia, core hypothermia is accompanied by a real increase in skin temperature. The result is typically a perception of continued or increased warmth accompanied by autonomic thermoregulatory responses, including shivering (Fig. 40–15).[61,71]

Taken together, these data indicate that neuraxial anesthesia inhibits numerous aspects of thermoregulatory control. The vasoconstriction and shivering thresholds

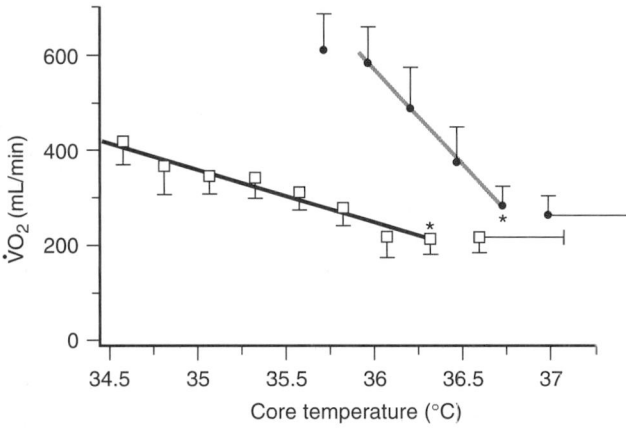

Figure 40–13 Systemic oxygen consumption without (circles) and with (squares) epidural anesthesia. The horizontal standard deviation bars indicate variability in the thresholds among the volunteers; although errors bars are shown only once in each series, the same temperature variability applies to each data point. The slopes of the oxygen consumption–versus–core temperature relationships (solid lines) were determined by linear regression. These slopes defined the gain of shivering with and without epidural anesthesia. Gain was reduced 3.7-fold, from −412 mL/min/°C (r^2 = .99) to −112 mL/min/°C (r^2 = .96). (Redrawn from Kim J-S, Ikeda T, Sessler D, et al: Epidural anesthesia reduces the gain and maximum intensity of shivering. Anesthesiology 88:851–857, 1998.)

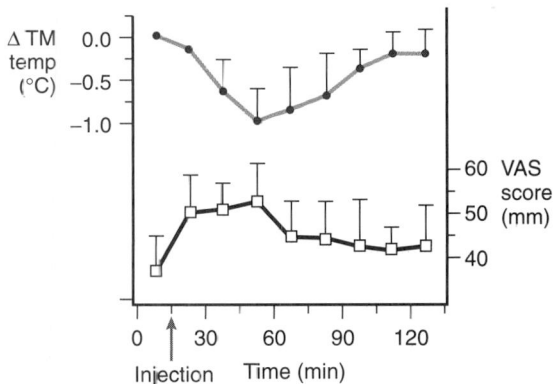

Figure 40–15 Induction of epidural anesthesia at an elapsed time of 15 minutes decreased core temperature and increased thermal comfort as determined by a 100-mm visual analog scale (VAS). Interestingly, however, maximal thermal comfort coincided with the minimum core temperature. Results are presented as means ± SD. TM, tympanic membrane. (Redrawn with modification from Sessler DI, Ponte J: Shivering during epidural anesthesia. Anesthesiology 72:816–821, 1990.)

are reduced by regional anesthesia[61-63,68,69] and further reduced by adjuvant drugs[22,36] and advanced age.[11] Even once triggered, the gain and maximum response intensity of shivering are about half normal.[72] Finally, behavioral thermoregulation is impaired.[71] The result is that cold defenses are triggered at a lower temperature than normal during regional anesthesia, defenses are less effective once triggered, and patients frequently do not recognize that they are hypothermic. Because core temperature monitoring remains rare during regional anesthesia, substantial hypothermia often goes undetected in these patients.[73]

Heat Balance

Hypothermia is common during regional anesthesia and may be nearly as severe as during general anesthesia.[74-76] Core temperature typically decreases 0.5°C to 1.0°C shortly after induction of anesthesia. However, the vasodilation induced by regional anesthesia only slightly increases cutaneous heat loss. Furthermore, metabolic heat production remains constant or increases because of shivering thermogenesis. This rapid decrease in core temperature, similar to that noted after induction of general anesthesia, also results from an internal core-to-peripheral redistribution of body heat (Fig. 40–16).[77] As during general anesthesia, redistribution hypothermia during regional anesthesia can be minimized by cutaneous warming before induction.[78]

Subsequent hypothermia results simply from heat loss exceeding metabolic heat production. Unlike patients given general anesthesia, however, core temperature does not necessarily plateau after several hours of surgery. Not only is the vasoconstriction threshold centrally impaired by regional anesthesia,[62,63] but more importantly, vasoconstriction in the legs is also directly prevented by nerve block.[79,80] Because the legs constitute the bulk of the thermal compartment, an effective plateau cannot develop without vasoconstriction in the legs and the resulting decrease in cutaneous heat loss and constraint of metabolic heat to the core.

The importance of intraoperative leg vasoconstriction is illustrated during combined regional/general anesthesia. Consistent with the impairment in thermoregulatory responses with regional anesthesia alone,[62,63] vasoconstriction during combined regional/general anesthesia is triggered at a core temperature approximately 1°C less than during general anesthesia alone. Furthermore, once triggered, vasoconstriction produces a core temperature plateau during general anesthesia alone but not during combined regional/general anesthesia. The result is that core temperature during combined regional/general anesthesia continues to decrease throughout surgery.[81] Consequently, core temperature monitoring and thermal management are particularly important in patients given simultaneous regional and general anesthesia.

Shivering

Shivering-like tremor in volunteers given neuraxial anesthesia is always preceded by core hypothermia and vasoconstriction (above the level of the block).[61] Furthermore, electromyographic analysis indicates that

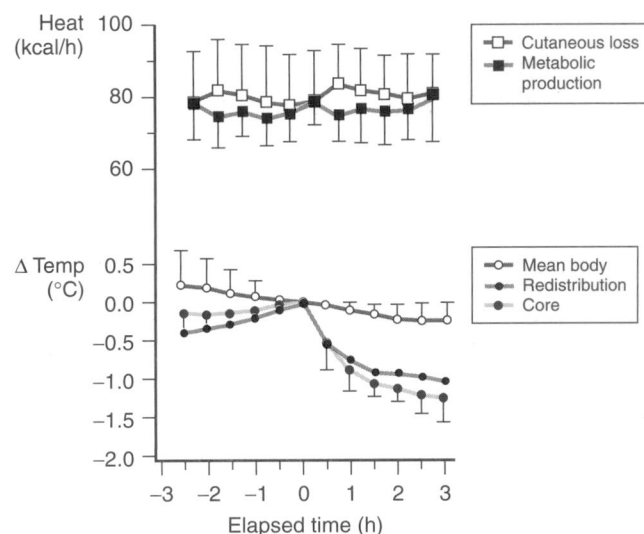

Figure 40–16 Overall, heat balance was only slightly negative (loss exceeding production) before induction of anesthesia and subsequently changed little. To separate the contributions of decreased overall heat balance and internal redistribution of body heat to the decrease in core temperature, the change in overall heat balance was divided by body weight and the specific heat of humans. The resulting change in mean body temperature ("mean body") was subtracted from the change in core temperature ("core"), thus leaving the core hypothermia specifically resulting from redistribution ("redistribution"). After 1 hour of anesthesia, core temperature had decreased 0.8°C ± 0.3°C, with redistribution contributing 89% to the decrease. During the subsequent 2 hours of anesthesia, core temperature decreased an additional 0.4°C ± 0.3°C, with redistribution contributing 62%. Redistribution thus contributed 80% to the entire 1.2°C ± 0.3°C decrease in core temperature during the 3 hours of anesthesia. The increase in the "redistribution" curve before induction of anesthesia indicates that thermoregulatory vasoconstriction was constraining metabolic heat to the core thermal compartment. Such constraint is, of course, the only way in which core temperature could increase while body heat content decreased. Induction of epidural anesthesia is identified as elapsed time zero. Results are presented as means ± SD. (Redrawn with modification from Matsukawa T, Sessler DI, Christensen R, et al: Heat flow and distribution during epidural anesthesia. Anesthesiology 83:961–967, 1995.)

the tremor has the 4- to 8-cycle/min waxing-and-waning pattern that characterizes normal shivering.[65] The tremor is thus apparently normal thermoregulatory shivering that is triggered when redistribution hypothermia decreases core temperature.

It remains probable, though, that tremor during regional anesthesia in pregnant women has a different etiology. Similarly, the shivering-like tremor so often observed during labor without neuraxial anesthesia has yet to be adequately characterized. In both cases, there appears to be a significant incidence of shivering-like tremor in normothermic and vasodilated patients. This observation suggests that some tremor is nonthermoregulatory because shivering should always be preceded by hypothermia and arteriovenous shunt vasoconstriction.

Spinal thermal receptors have been detected in every mammal and bird tested. Experimental stimulation of these receptors reliably produces shivering in animals. Stimulation of these putative receptors by injection of an epidural anesthetic in humans could theoretically initiate thermoregulatory responses, including shivering. Consistent with this possibility, the incidence of shivering in pregnant women is greater when they are given a refrigerated epidural anesthetic than when the anesthetic is warmed before injection.[82] However, epidural administration of large amounts of ice-cold saline does not trigger shivering in nonpregnant volunteers.[83] Furthermore, the incidence of shivering is comparable in volunteers[61] and nonpregnant patients[84] given warm or cold epidural anesthetic injections. These data indicate—at least in nonpregnant individuals—that the temperature of injected local anesthetic does not influence the incidence of shivering during major conduction anesthesia.

The risk of shivering during neuraxial anesthesia is markedly diminished by maintaining strict normothermia.[61] However, there is a distinct incidence of low-intensity, shivering-like tremor that occurs in normothermic patients and is not thermoregulatory.[85] The cause of this muscular activity remains unknown, but it is associated with pain and may thus result from activation of the sympathetic nervous system.

Shivering during neuraxial anesthesia can sometimes be treated by warming sentient skin. Such warming increases cutaneous thermal input to the central regulatory system, thus increasing the degree of core hypothermia tolerated.[86] Because the entire skin surface contributes 20% to thermoregulatory control[5] and the lower part of the body contributes about 10%,[68] sentient skin warming is likely to compensate for only small reductions in core temperature. The same drugs that are effective for postanesthetic tremor are also useful for shivering during regional anesthesia; these drugs include meperidine (25 mg intravenously [IV] or epidurally),[87] clonidine (75 μg IV),[88] ketanserin (10 mg IV),[88] and magnesium sulfate (30 mg/kg IV).[89]

CONSEQUENCES OF MILD INTRAOPERATIVE HYPOTHERMIA

Perianesthetic hypothermia produces potentially severe complications as well as distinct benefits. Thermal management thus deserves the same thoughtful analysis of potential risks and benefits as other therapeutic decisions do.

Benefits

Substantial protection against cerebral ischemia and hypoxia is provided by just 1°C to 3°C hypothermia in animals.[90–92] Similar benefits have been demonstrated for acute myocardial infarction in human-sized pigs.[93] Mild hypothermia reduces intracranial pressure, but randomized studies have yet to demonstrate that therapeutic hypothermia improves outcomes in patients with brain trauma, stroke, or subarachnoid hemorrhage.

Hypothermia for brain trauma was initially claimed to be therapeutic based on a post hoc subgroup analysis of a study that overall showed no benefit.[94] A subsequent large randomized trial was unable to demonstrate any benefit overall or in subgroups—although the study was somewhat limited by serious protocol violations in some patients.[95] Most recently, hypothermia was shown to be beneficial in a nonrandomized but nonetheless fairly convincing study: brain trauma patients with elevated intracranial pressure refractory to conventional treatment were assigned to therapeutic hypothermia. Despite being sicker than the comparison patients (who had low intracranial pressure), the hypothermic patients demonstrated improved outcomes.[95] The only situation in which therapeutic hypothermia has been unequivocally shown in randomized trials to improve outcome is during recovery from cardiac arrest.[97,98]

Protection was initially thought to result from the approximately 8%/°C linear reduction in tissue metabolic rate. However, the efficacy of mild hypothermia far exceeds that of treatments such as high-dose isoflurane or barbiturate coma, which comparably reduce the metabolic rate.[99] These data suggest that other factors (e.g., decreased release of excitatory amino acids) explain the protective action of hypothermia. As such, there is no reason to expect protection to decrease linearly with temperature, and in animals it appears that much of the total benefit from moderate hypothermia occurs within the first couple of degrees.

The potential protection afforded by mild hypothermia is so great that reduced core temperature (i.e., ≈34°C) is increasingly being used during neurosurgery and other procedures in which tissue ischemia can be anticipated. Mild hypothermia may also be useful for the treatment of acute myocardial infarction.[93] The difficulty is that currently, few outcome data in humans have substantiated this extrapolation from animal data. Furthermore, the appropriate target temperature for therapeutic hypothermia has yet to be established in humans, and there are currently little data on which to base such decisions.

Acute malignant hyperthermia is more difficult to trigger in mildly hypothermic swine than in those kept normothermic. Moreover, once triggered, the syndrome is less severe.[100,101] These data suggest that active warming should be avoided in patients known to be susceptible to malignant hyperthermia; instead, they should be allowed to become slightly hypothermic during surgery.

Complications

Coagulation is impaired by mild hypothermia. The most important factor appears to be a cold-induced defect in platelet function.[102] Interestingly, the defect in platelet function is related to local temperature, not core temperature.[103] Wound temperature, however, is largely determined by core temperature and will be distinctly higher in normothermic patients. Perhaps as important, hypothermia directly impairs enzymes of the coagulation cascade. This impairment will not be apparent during routine coagulation screening because the tests are performed at 37°C. When these tests are performed at hypothermic temperatures, however, the defect becomes apparent.[104,105] Consistent with these in vitro defects, prospective, randomized clinical trials indicate that mild hypothermia significantly increases blood loss during hip arthroplasty and increases allogeneic transfusion requirements.[106,107] In contrast, a similar study failed to identify any benefit.[108] It nonetheless seems likely that hypothermia impairs coagulation at least to some extent.

Wound infections are among the most common serious complication of anesthesia and surgery in that they probably cause more morbidity than all other anesthetic complications combined do.[109,110] Hypothermia can contribute to wound infections both by directly impairing immune function[111] and by triggering thermoregulatory vasoconstriction, which in turn decreases wound oxygen delivery.[112] It is well established that fever is protective and that infections are aggravated when naturally occurring fever is prevented.[113,114] Similarly, mild hypothermia, maintained only during anesthesia, impairs subsequent resistance to both *Escherichia coli* and *Staphylococcus aureus* dermal infections in guinea pigs.[115,116] As might be expected from these in vitro and animal data, a prospective, randomized clinical trial has indicated that mild intraoperative hypothermia triples the incidence of surgical wound infection in patients undergoing colon surgery. Furthermore, hypothermia delayed wound healing and prolonged the duration of hospitalization 20%, even in patients without infection.[117] Consistent with poor wound healing, urinary nitrogen excretion remains elevated for several postoperative days in patients allowed to become hypothermic during surgery.[118]

Thermal comfort is markedly impaired by postoperative hypothermia.[119] Patients, asked years after surgery, often identify feeling cold in the immediate postoperative period as the worst part of their hospitalization—sometimes rating it worse than surgical pain. Postoperative thermal discomfort is also physiologically stressful because it elevates blood pressure, heart rate, and plasma catecholamine concentrations.[120,121] These factors presumably contribute to what may be the most important consequence of mild perioperative hypothermia: morbid myocardial outcomes.[122] Given that myocardial ischemia is among the leading causes of unanticipated perioperative death, the results of this prospective, randomized trial must be taken extremely seriously.

Drug metabolism is markedly decreased by perioperative hypothermia. The duration of action of vecuronium is more than doubled by a 2°C reduction in core temperature, and the prolongation is a pharmacokinetic effect, not a pharmacodynamic one.[123] Atracurium's duration of action is less dependent on core temperature: a 3°C reduction in core temperature increases the duration of muscle relaxation by only 60%.[124] With each drug, the recovery index (time for 25% to 75% twitch recovery) remains normal during hypothermia. Interestingly, core hypothermia per se decreases twitch strength 10% to 15%, even without muscle relaxants.[125] The efficacy of neostigmine as an antagonist of vecuronium-induced neuromuscular blockade is not altered by mild hypothermia, although onset time is about 20% longer.[126]

During a constant infusion of propofol, the plasma concentration is approximately 30% greater than normal when individuals are 3°C hypothermic.[124] The effects of mild hypothermia on the metabolism and pharmacodynamics of most other drugs have yet to be reported. However, the results for muscle relaxants and propofol suggest that the effects are substantial. Hypothermia also alters the pharmacodynamics of the volatile anesthetics, with the minimum alveolar concentration being reduced about 5%/°C.[127,128] Consequently, no anesthesia whatsoever is required to prevent movement in response to skin incision at core temperatures below 20°C.[129] As might be expected from the pharmacokinetic and pharmacodynamic effects of hypothermia, the duration of postanesthetic recovery is significantly prolonged—even when temperature is not a discharge criterion. When "fitness for discharge" and a core temperature exceeding 36°C are required (as in many postanesthesia care units), the duration of recovery is prolonged several hours.[130] Table 40–1 lists the proven consequences of mild perioperative hypothermia.

Postanesthetic Shivering

The incidence of postoperative shivering-like tremor is reportedly approximately 40%, but it now appears to be less as more patients are kept normothermic and opioids are administered more frequently and in larger doses than in the past. It is a potentially serious complication, with oxygen consumption increased roughly 100% in proportion to intraoperative heat loss.[132] Interestingly, though, myocardial ischemia is poorly correlated with shivering, thus suggesting that an increased metabolic rate is not the primary etiology of this complication.[122] In addition to increasing intraocular and intracranial pressure, postoperative shivering probably aggravates wound pain by stretching incisions.

Over the years, postanesthetic tremor has been attributed to uninhibited spinal reflexes, pain, decreased sympathetic activity, pyrogen release, adrenal suppression, respiratory alkalosis, and most commonly, simple thermoregulatory shivering in response to intraoperative hypothermia. Unfortunately, the etiology of postanesthetic shivering-like tremor remains unclear. Certainly, much postoperative tremor is simply normal shivering. As early as 1972, however, investigators recognized the existence of at least two distinct tremor patterns.[133] That perceptive observation was subsequently confirmed in a study that used electromyography to demonstrate that postoperative tremor has (1) a tonic pattern resembling normal shivering, typically with a 4- to 8-cycle/min waxing-and-waning component, and (2) a phasic, 5- to 7-Hz bursting pattern resembling pathologic clonus.[134] The clonic pattern was consistent with the previous observation that pathologic spinal cord responses, including clonus, nystagmus, and exaggerated deep tendon reflexes, were common during recovery from general anesthesia.[135]

It was not until 1991 that a triple crossover study in volunteers established that the tonic and clonic patterns were both thermoregulatory, that is, always preceded by core hypothermia and arteriovenous shunt vasoconstriction.[136] The tonic pattern consistently demonstrated the 4- to 8-cycle/min waxing-and-waning pattern of normal shivering[16] and is apparently a simple thermoregulatory response to intraoperative hypothermia. In contrast, the clonic pattern is not a normal component of thermoregulatory shivering and appears to be specific to recovery

Table 40–1 Major in vivo consequences of mild perioperative hypothermia in humans

Consequence	Author	N	ΔT_{core} (°C)	Normothermic	Hypothermic	P
Surgical wound infection	Kurz et al.[117]	200	1.9	6%	19%	<.01
Duration of hospitalization	Kurz et al.[117]	200	1.9	12.1 ± 4.4 days	14.7 ± 6.5 days	<.01
Intraoperative blood loss	Schmied et al.[106]	60	1.6	1.7 ± 0.3 L	2.2 ± 0.5 L	<.001
Allogeneic transfusion requirement	Schmied et al.[106]	60	1.6	1 U	8 U	<.05
Morbid cardiac events	Frank et al.[122]	300	1.3	1%	6%	<.05
Postoperative ventricular tachycardia	Frank et al.[122]	300	1.3	2%	8%	<.05
Urinary excretion of nitrogen	Carli et al.[118]	12	1.5	982 mmol/day	1798 mmol/day	<.05
Duration of vecuronium	Heier et al.[123]	20	2.0	28 ± 4 min	62 ± 8 min	<.001
Duration of atracurium	Leslie et al.[124]	6	3.0	44 ± 4 min	68 ± 7 min	<.05
Postoperative shivering	Just et al.[131]	14	2.3	141 ± 9 mL/min/m²	269 ± 60 mL/min/m²	<.001
Duration of postanesthetic recovery	Lenhardt et al.[130]	150	1.9	53 ± 36 min	94 ± 65 min	<.001
Adrenergic activation	Frank et al.[121]	74	1.5	330 ± 30 pg/mL	480 ± 70 pg/mL	<.05
Thermal discomfort	Kurz et al.[119]	74	2.6	50 ± 10 mm VAS	18 ± 9 mm VAS	<.001

Only prospective, randomized human trials are included; subjective responses were evaluated by observers blinded to the treatment group and core temperature. Different outcomes of the first three studies are shown on separate lines.

N, total number of subjects; ΔT_{core}, difference in core temperature between the treatment groups; VAS, 100-mm-long visual analog scale (0 mm = intense cold, 100 mm = intense heat).

Reprinted, by permission, from Sessler DI: Perioperative hypothermia. N Engl J Med 336:1730–1737, 1997.

from volatile anesthetics. Although the precise etiology of this tremor pattern remains unknown, it may result from anesthetic-induced disinhibition of normal descending control over spinal reflexes. Recent data in surgical patients, however, belie the simple conclusion from the volunteer study[136] that all postanesthetic tremor is thermoregulatory. Instead, there appears to be a distinct incidence of nonthermoregulatory tremor in normothermic postoperative patients;[137] similar nonthermoregulatory tremor has been observed in women during labor.[85] The etiology of this tremor and why volunteers and patients should respond differently remain unknown, but surgical pain appears to be a key factor.[138]

Postanesthetic shivering can be treated by skin surface warming[86] because the regulatory system tolerates more core hypothermia when cutaneous warm input is augmented.[5] However, the skin surface contributes only 20% to control of shivering,[5] and the available skin surface warmers increase mean skin temperature just a few degrees centigrade.[139] Consequently, cutaneous warming compensates for only small amounts of core hypothermia and will not usually prove effective in most patients with core temperatures much below 35°C.[140] Postanesthetic shivering can also be treated with a variety of drugs, including clonidine (75 μg IV),[88,141] ketanserin (10 mg IV),[88] tramadol,[142,143] physostigmine (0.04 mg/kg IV),[144] and magnesium sulfate (30 mg/kg IV).[89] The specific mechanisms by which ketanserin, tramadol, physostigmine, and magnesium sulfate stop shivering remain unknown. Similarly, how clonidine arrests shivering also remains unknown, but clonidine[32] and dexmedetomidine[23] comparably reduce the vasoconstriction and shivering

thresholds, thus suggesting that they act on the central thermoregulatory system rather than preventing shivering peripherally. Postoperative shivering has recently been reviewed in detail.[145]

Alfentanil, a pure μ-receptor agonist, significantly impairs thermoregulatory control.[22] However, meperidine is reportedly considerably more effective in treating shivering than equianalgesic doses of other μ-agonists are.[146] Clinically, this efficacy is manifested as a shivering threshold that is reduced twice as much as the vasoconstriction threshold[28] without a decrease in the gain or maximum intensity of shivering.[47] The efficacy of meperidine is, at least partially, preserved during the administration of moderate doses of naloxone (0.5 μg/kg/min) but virtually obliterated by enormous doses (5.0 μg/kg/min).[147] These data suggest that the action of this drug is, in part, mediated by non–μ-opioid receptors. Meperidine possesses considerable κ activity[148] and also has central anticholinergic activity. However, neither mechanism appears to mediate meperidine's special antishivering activity.[149] Instead, it may result from agonist activity at central α-adrenoceptors.[150] Whatever the mechanism, meperidine appears to be considerably more effective in the treatment of postoperative shivering than other opioids are.

PERIOPERATIVE THERMAL MANIPULATIONS

Intraoperative thermoregulatory vasoconstriction, once triggered, is remarkably effective in preventing further core hypothermia.[38,46] Nonetheless, most patients are poikilothermic during surgery because they do not become sufficiently hypothermic to trigger thermoregulatory responses.[21,22,24,25] Therefore, intraoperative hypothermia can be minimized by any technique that limits cutaneous heat loss to the environment as a result of cold operating rooms, evaporation from surgical incisions, and conductive cooling produced by the administration of cold intravenous fluids.

Mean body temperature will decrease when heat loss to the environment exceeds metabolic heat production. Heat production during anesthesia is approximately 0.8 kcal/kg/hr. Because the specific heat of the human body is about 0.83 kcal/kg,[151] body temperature decreases approximately 1°C/hr when heat lost to the environment exceeds metabolic production by a factor of 2. Normally, about 90% of metabolic heat is lost through the skin surface. During anesthesia, additional heat is lost directly from surgical incisions and by the administration of cold intravenous fluids.

Effects of Vasomotor Tone on Heat Transfer

Thermoregulatory vasodilation causes the initial core-to-peripheral redistribution of body heat[57]; similarly, re-emergence of vasoconstriction in patients becoming sufficiently hypothermic produces a core temperature plateau.[46] It is thus evident that vasomotor tone alters intercompartmental heat transfer. In addition to thermoregulatory arteriovenous shunt status, arteriolar tone is directly modulated by anesthetics per se.[54] Both factors potentially influence the speed with which peripherally applied heat reaches the core thermal compartment.

Thermoregulatory vasoconstriction slightly impairs induction of therapeutic hypothermia during neurosurgery.[152] However, arteriovenous shunt tone has little effect on intraoperative cooling[153] or heating.[154] Intraoperative vasoconstriction thus only slightly impedes peripheral-to-core transfer of cutaneous heating and cooling. Little clinical effect presumably results because intraoperative thermoregulatory vasoconstriction is opposed by direct anesthetic-induced peripheral vasodilation.

During postanesthetic recovery, however, the situation differs markedly. Here, anesthetic-induced peripheral dilation[54,155] dissipates, with thermoregulatory vasoconstriction left unopposed. As might be expected, this vasoconstriction then becomes an important factor and significantly impairs transfer of peripherally applied heat to the core thermal compartment. Patients with a residual spinal anesthetic block thus warm considerably faster than those recovering from general anesthesia alone (Fig. 40–17).[156] Heat balance studies indicate that core warming is slowed because vasoconstriction constrains up to 30 kcal in peripheral tissues.[157]

Because postoperative thermoregulatory vasoconstriction decreases peripheral-to-core transfer of heat, applied warming is most effective during surgery when patients are vasodilated. From a practical point of view, this means that it is easier to maintain intraoperative normothermia (when most patients are vasodilated) than to rewarm them postoperatively (when virtually all hypothermic patients

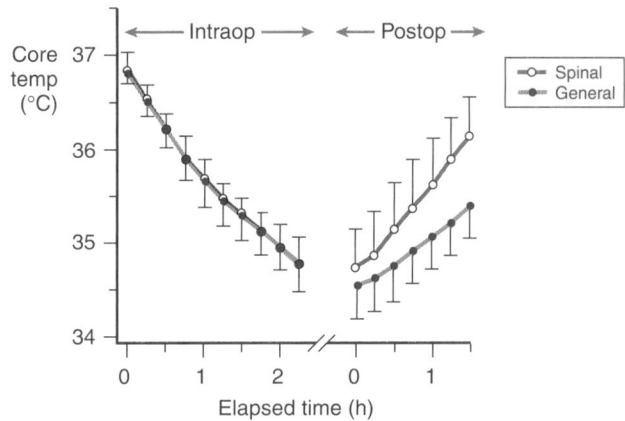

Figure 40–17 Intraoperative and postoperative core temperatures in patients assigned to general anesthesia (*n* = 20) and spinal anesthesia (*n* = 20). All patients were warmed with forced air during the postoperative period. Core temperature did not differ significantly during surgery, but it increased significantly faster postoperatively in patients given spinal anesthesia (1.2 ± 0.1°C/hr versus 0.7 ± 0.2°C/hr, means ± SD). (Redrawn from Szmuk P, Ezri T, Sessler DI, et al: Spinal anesthesia only minimally increases the efficacy of postoperative forced-air rewarming. Anesthesiology 87:1050–1054, 1997.)

are vasoconstricted). In addition to being more effective, intraoperative warming is more appropriate than postoperative treatment of hypothermia because it prevents the complications resulting from hypothermia.[106,117,122] Patients unavoidably becoming hypothermic during surgery should nonetheless be actively heated postoperatively to increase thermal comfort, decrease shivering, and hasten rewarming.

Preventing Redistribution Hypothermia

The initial 0.5°C to 1.5°C reduction in core temperature is difficult to prevent because it results from redistribution of heat from the central thermal compartment to cooler peripheral tissues.[57] Consequently, surface warming usually fails to prevent hypothermia during the first hour of anesthesia.[58,117] Lack of efficacy during this period results because the central-to-peripheral flow of heat is massive and because transfer of applied cutaneous heat to the core requires nearly an hour, even in vasodilated patients.

Although redistribution cannot be treated effectively,[58,117] it can be prevented. Redistribution results when anesthetic-induced vasodilation allows heat to flow peripherally down the normal temperature gradient. Skin surface warming before induction of anesthesia does not significantly alter core temperature (which remains well regulated), but it does increase body heat content. Most of the increase is in the legs, the most important component of the peripheral thermal compartment. When peripheral tissue temperature is sufficiently increased, subsequent inhibition of normal tonic thermoregulatory vasoconstriction produces little redistribution hypothermia because heat can flow only down a temperature gradient (Fig. 40–18).[158,159] Although substantial amounts of heat must be transferred across the skin surface, active

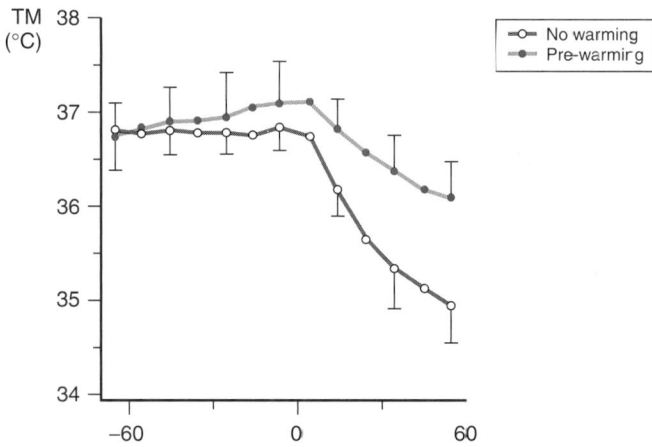

Figure 40–18 During the preinduction period (−120 to 0 minutes), volunteers were either actively warmed or passively cooled (no warming). At induction of anesthesia (time = 0 minutes), active warming was discontinued and volunteers were exposed to the ambient environment. Initial tympanic membrane temperatures were similar before each preinduction treatment. During the 60 minutes after induction of anesthesia, core temperature decreased less when volunteers were prewarmed. (ΔT = −1.1°C ± 0.3°C) than when the same volunteers were not warmed (ΔT = −1.9°C ± 0.3°C). Data are presented as means ± SD. (Redrawn from Hynson JM, Sessler DI, Moayeri A, et al: The effects of pre-induction warming on temperature and blood pressure during propofol/nitrous oxide anesthesia. Anesthesiology 79:219–228, 1993.)

prewarming for as little as 30 minutes probably prevents considerable redistribution.[160]

The "afterdrop" associated with discontinuation of cardiopulmonary bypass is a type of redistribution hypothermia that results from a substantial core-to-peripheral tissue temperature gradient. As might be expected, it is more impressive after bypass at 17°C[161] than at 27°C to 31°C.[162] Cutaneous warming during and after bypass reduces core temperature afterdrop by 60%. However, heat balance data indicate that this reduction results primarily because cutaneous warming prevents the typical decrease in body heat content after discontinuation of bypass rather than by reducing redistribution.[163]

Airway Heating and Humidification

Simple thermodynamic calculations indicate that less than 10% of metabolic heat production is lost through the respiratory tract. The loss results from both heating and humidifying inspiratory gases, but humidification requires two thirds of the heat.[52] Because little heat is lost through respiration, even active airway heating and humidification minimally influence core temperature.[58,164] The *apparent* clinical efficacy of these devices probably results from artifactual warming of proximally positioned esophageal stethoscopes.[165]

Because respiratory heat loss remains virtually constant during anesthesia, the fraction of total heat lost through the respiratory tract decreases dramatically during large operations in which substantial heat is lost from evaporation within surgical incisions.[53] Consequently, airway heating and humidification are even less effective

than usual in patients most in need of effective warming. Cutaneous warming maintains normothermia so much better than respiratory gas conditioning does that intraoperative active airway heating and humidification are rarely if ever indicated. Airway heating and humidification are more effective in infants and children than adults,[166] but cutaneous warming is also more effective in these patients and transfers more than 10 times as much heat. Hygroscopic condenser humidifiers and heat- and moisture-exchanging filters ("artificial noses") retain substantial amounts of moisture and heat within the respiratory system. In terms of preventing heat loss, these passive devices are about half as good as active systems[166]; however, they cost only a fraction as much. Heat retention is comparable in all clinically available heat and moisture exchangers.[52]

Intravenous Fluids

It is not possible to warm patients by administering heated fluids because the fluids cannot (much) exceed body temperature. On the other hand, heat loss from cold intravenous fluids becomes significant when large amounts of crystalloid solution or blood are administered. One unit of refrigerated blood or 1 L of crystalloid solution administered at room temperature decreases mean body temperature approximately 0.25°C. Fluid warmers minimize these losses and should be used when large amounts of intravenous fluid or blood are administered.

For routine cases, there are no clinically important differences among the available warmers. Although most warmers allow fluid to cool in the tubing between the heater and the patient, this cooling is of little consequence in adults: at high flows, little cooling occurs, and at low flows, the amount of fluid given is trivial.[167] Special high-volume systems with powerful heaters and little resistance to flow facilitate the care of trauma victims and are useful in other cases in which large amount of fluid must be administered quickly.

Cutaneous Warming

Operating room temperature is the most critical factor influencing heat loss because it determines the rate at which metabolic heat is lost by radiation and convection from the skin and by evaporation from within surgical incisions. Consequently, increasing room temperature is one way to minimize heat loss. However, room temperatures exceeding 23°C are generally required to maintain normothermia in patients undergoing all but the smallest procedures[168]; most operating room personnel find such temperatures uncomfortably warm. Infants may require ambient temperatures exceeding 26°C to maintain normothermia. Such temperatures are sufficiently high to impair the performance of operating room personnel and decrease their vigilance.

The easiest method of decreasing cutaneous heat loss is to apply passive insulation to the skin surface. Insulators readily available in most operating rooms include cotton blankets, surgical drapes, plastic sheeting, and reflective composites ("space blankets"). A single layer of each reduces heat loss approximately 30%, with no clinically

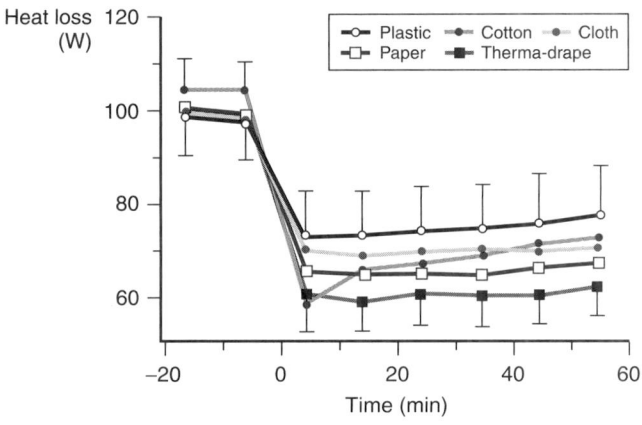

Figure 40–19 Insulators readily available in most operating rooms include cotton blankets, surgical drapes, plastic sheeting, and reflective composites ("space blankets"). A single layer of each reduces total cutaneous heat loss approximately 30%, without any clinically important differences among the insulation types. Data are presented as means ± SD. (Redrawn from Sessler DI, McGuire J, Sessler AM: Perioperative thermal insulation. Anesthesiology 74:875–879, 1991.)

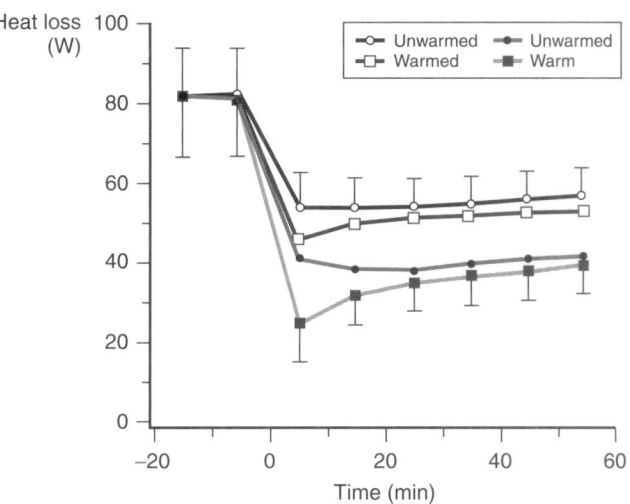

Figure 40–20 Total cutaneous heat loss when the volunteers were covered with a single warmed *(open circles)* or unwarmed blanket *(open squares)* or three warmed *(filled circles)* or unwarmed *(filled squares)* blankets. These data indicate that warming cotton blankets is of little benefit and that adding additional blankets only slightly decreases cutaneous heat loss. Data are presented as means ± SD. (Redrawn from Sessler DI, Schroeder M: Heat loss in humans covered with cotton hospital blankets. Anesth Analg 77:73–77, 1993.)

important differences noted among the insulation types (Fig. 40–19).[169] Insulators should therefore be chosen strictly based on cost; paying a premium to purchase reflective composites, for example, is not justified.

The reduction in heat loss from all the commonly used passive insulators is similar because most of the insulation is provided by the layer of still air trapped beneath the covering. Consequently, adding additional layers of insulation further reduces heat loss only slightly. For example, one cotton blanket reduces heat loss by about 30%, but three cotton blankets reduce heat loss by only 50%. Furthermore, warming the cotton blankets provides little benefit, and the benefit is short-lived (Fig. 40–20).[170] These data indicate that simply adding additional layers of passive insulation or warming the insulation before application will usually be insufficient in patients becoming hypothermic while covered with a single layer of insulation.

Cutaneous heat loss is roughly proportional to surface area throughout the body.[171] (The popular perception that a large fraction of metabolic heat is lost from the head is false in adults. Loss from the head can be substantial in small infants,[172,173] but the loss is high mostly because the head represents a large fraction of the total surface area.) Consequently, the amount of skin covered is more important than which surfaces are insulated. It does not make sense, for example, to cover the head and leave the arms exposed; the arms have more surface area than the head does and account for more heat loss.

Passive insulation alone is rarely sufficient to maintain normothermia in patients undergoing large operations; active warming will be required in these cases. Because about 90% of metabolic heat is lost through the skin surface, only cutaneous warming will transfer sufficient heat to prevent hypothermia. Most infrared systems are little more effective than passive insulation.[139,169] Consequently, for intraoperative use, circulating water

and forced air are the two major systems requiring consideration.

Studies consistently report that circulating-water mattresses are nearly ineffective.[174] Presumably, they are unable to maintain normothermia because little heat is lost from the back into the 5 cm of foam insulation covering most operating room tables. Furthermore, the combination of heat and decreased local perfusion (resulting when the patient's weight reduces capillary blood flow) increases the propensity for pressure/heat necrosis ("burns").[175] Such tissue injury can occur even when water temperature does not exceed 40°C.[176] Circulating water is more effective—and safer—when placed *over* patients rather than *under* them and, in that position, can almost completely eliminate metabolic heat loss.[139] Metabolic heat production will increase mean body temperature approximately 1°C/hr when cutaneous heat loss is eliminated. Recently developed circulating-water garments transfer large amounts of heat by increasing the warmed surface area or using materials that facilitate conduction.[177,178]

The most common perianesthetic warming system is forced air. The best forced-air systems transfer more than 30 W across the skin surface, which rapidly increases mean body temperature.[139,179] Forced air usually maintains normothermia even during the largest operations[58,117,180] and is superior to circulating-water mattresses.[181] Resistive heating (electric blankets) is as effective as forced air but is much less expensive because it does not require a disposable product (Fig. 40–21).[182] Nonetheless, carbon-fiber resistive heaters should be avoided because they frequently cause burns. Figure 40–22 shows the relative effect of common patient warming methods and the

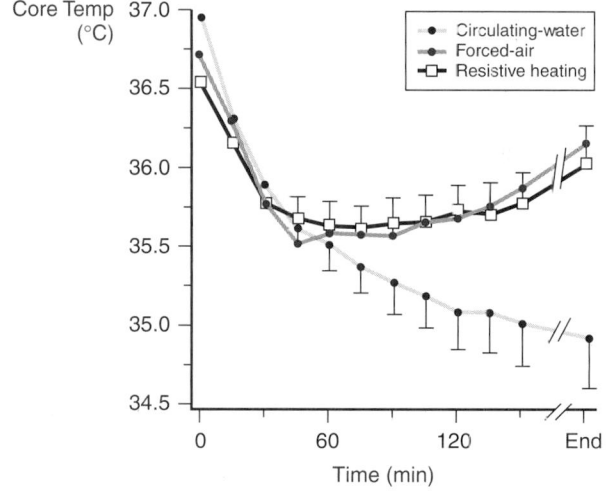

Figure 40–21 Core temperature as a function of time in patients assigned to the circulating-water, forced-air, and carbon-fiber (resistive heating) groups. Temperature changes in the control group differed significantly from changes in the other groups after 150 elapsed minutes. Temperatures in the circulating-water and carbon-fiber groups never differed significantly. Results are presented as means ± SEM. Despite similar efficacy, carbon-fiber heating is associated with patient burns and should be avoided. (Redrawn from Negishi C, Hasegawa K, Mukai S, et al: Resistive-heating and forced-air warming are comparably effective. Anesth Analg 96:1683–1687, 2003.)

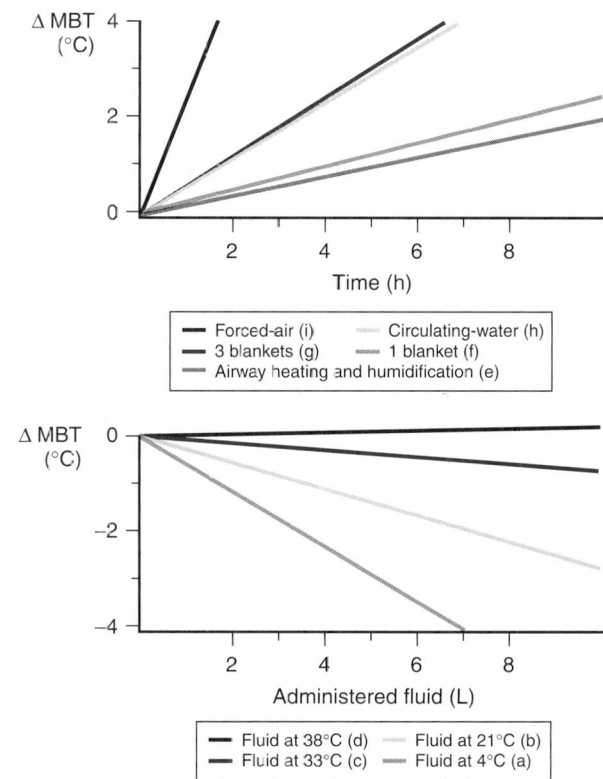

Figure 40–22 Relative effects of warming methods on mean body temperature (ΔMBT) as a function of time *(upper portion)* or administered fluid *(lower portion)*. Mean body temperature is the average temperature of body tissues and is usually somewhat less than core temperature. The calculations assume an undressed 70-kg patient with a metabolic rate of 80 kcal/hr, in thermal steady state, and with a typical 21°C operating room environment. Only the changes resulting from specific treatments are shown; changes from combined interventions will be additive. a to d, Changes in MBT per liter of administered blood or crystalloid at various fluid temperatures; e, inspiring warmed, humidified gas; f and g, warmed or unwarmed blankets, with all skin below the neck covered; savings are similar with a single layer of other passive insulators; h, full-length circulating water mattress; i, full-length forced-air warmer. (Redrawn from Sessler AM, Sessler DI: Consequences and treatment of perioperative hypothermia. Anesthiol Clin North Am 12:425–456, 1994. See the original figure legend for equations and citations justifying the assumptions.)

changes in mean body temperature resulting from infusion of unwarmed crystalloid or blood.

Induction of Mild Therapeutic Hypothermia

Rapid core cooling may be required when the target core temperature is low (e.g., 32°C or 33°C) or for stroke or acute myocardial infarction when cooling must be induced expeditiously. In such cases, passive cooling is not practical. Immersion in cold water is by far the quickest noninvasive method of actively cooling patients. However, immersion is difficult under clinical conditions and poses a substantial electrical safety risk. Administration of refrigerated intravenous fluids is also effective and reduces mean body temperature 0.5°C/L.[183] However, this method is usually impractical in neurosurgical patients, in whom fluids must be restricted.

Forced-air cooling is easy to implement, but relatively slow, with approximately 2.5 hours needed to cool neurosurgical patients to 33°C.[152] Conventional circulating-water mattresses are unlikely to be efficient because relatively little skin surface contacts the mattress and the patient's own body weight reduces blood-borne convection of heat to the back. That is, circulating water probably does not cool well for the same reason that it heats poorly.[139] Newer circulating-water systems include garment-like covers that cover far more skin surface and transfer large amounts of heat, and they are fairly effective.[177,184]

The best way to rapidly induce therapeutic hypothermia is probably endovascular cooling. These systems consist of a heat-exchanging catheter, usually inserted

into the inferior vena cava through the femoral artery, and a servocontroller. They can decrease core temperatures at rates approaching 4°C/hr (Fig. 40–23).[185]

Inducing therapeutic hypothermia during surgery is relatively easy because anesthetics profoundly impair thermoregulatory responses. In contrast, unanesthetized patients—even those who have suffered a stroke—vigorously defend core temperature by vasoconstricting and shivering.[186] It is thus necessary to pharmacologically induce tolerance to hypothermia. The best method thus far identified is the combination of buspirone and meperidine, drugs that synergistically reduce the shivering threshold to approximately 34°C without provoking excessive sedation or respiratory toxicity.[187] The combination of dexmedetomidine and meperidine may also be helpful, although the interaction is simply additive in this case.

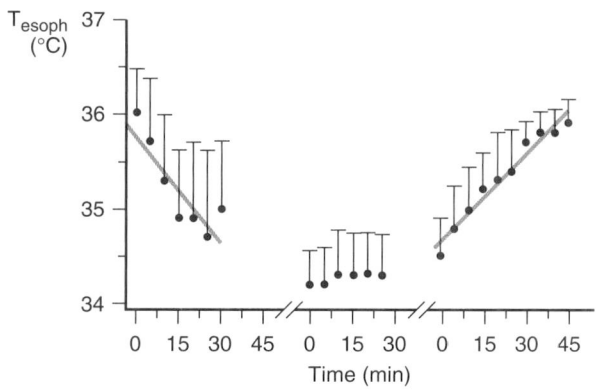

Figure 40–23 Average (± SD) intraoperative esophageal temperatures (T_{esoph}) during the cooling, temperature maintenance, and rewarming periods in eight neurosurgical patients who were cooled with endovascular heat-exchanging catheters in the vena cava. Time zero identified the beginning of each thermal management period; the duration of these periods differed in individual patients, depending on the length of surgery and other factors. The regression lines (gray lines) are shown for the cooling and rewarming periods. (Redrawn from Doufas AG, Akça O, Barry A, et al: Initial experience with a novel heat-exchanging catheter in neurosurgical patients. Anesth Analg 95:1752–1756, 2002.)

DELIBERATE SEVERE INTRAOPERATIVE HYPOTHERMIA

Severe hypothermia may be induced deliberately to confer protection against tissue ischemia, specifically during cardiac surgery and occasionally during neurosurgery. Drugs such as barbiturates and volatile anesthetics provide considerably less protection than even mild hypothermia does.[99] Because many organs compensate poorly for hypothermia, temperatures as low as those deliberately induced are usually lethal when unintentional. Deliberate hypothermia is safe only because anesthesiologists understand and treat the physiologic changes caused by core temperatures 10°C to 15°C below normal.

Although deep hypothermia (i.e., 28°C) has been used to facilitate cardiopulmonary bypass for decades, recent evidence suggests that hypothermia is either unhelpful or simply harmful. For example, hypothermia may be associated with prolonged ventricular dysfunction[188] and does not limit cognitive impairment after bypass.[189] Furthermore, normothermia appears to improve major outcomes after bypass surgery.[190] Consequently, cardiac surgery is increasingly performed at either "tepid" temperatures (i.e., 33°C) or normothermia.

Organ Function

Ischemia damages tissues because oxygen deprivation forces cells to obtain energy anaerobically. Because this mechanism is inefficient, it may not provide adequate energy. Anaerobic metabolism also produces more toxic metabolic waste products (e.g., lactate and superoxide radicals) than the Krebs cycle does, which is particularly serious when these waste products are not removed by circulating blood.

Hypothermia decreases the whole-body metabolic rate by approximately 8%/°C to approximately half the normal rate at 28°C. Whole-body oxygen demand diminishes, and oxygen consumption in tissues that have higher than normal metabolic rates, such as the brain, is especially reduced. Low metabolic rates allow aerobic metabolism to continue during periods of compromised oxygen supply; toxic waste production declines in proportion to the metabolic rate. Although a decreased metabolic rate certainly contributes to the observed protection against tissue ischemia, other specific actions of hypothermia (including "membrane stabilization" and decreased release of toxic metabolites and excitatory amino acids) may be most important.

Cerebral blood flow also decreases in proportion to the metabolic rate during hypothermia because of an autoregulatory increase in cerebrovascular resistance. The arteriovenous Po_2 difference thus remains constant, and the venous lactate concentration does not increase. Cerebral function is well maintained until core temperatures reach around 33°C, but consciousness is lost at temperatures below 28°C. Primitive reflexes such as the gag, pupillary constriction, and monosynaptic spinal reflexes remain intact until approximately 25°C. Nerve conduction decreases, but peripheral muscle tone increases, and rigidity and myoclonus ensue at temperatures near 26°C. Somatosensory and audio evoked potentials are temperature dependent, but not significantly modified at core temperatures of 33°C or higher.

Hypothermic effects on the heart include a decrease in the heart rate, increased contractility, and well-maintained stroke volume.[191] Cardiac output and blood pressure both decrease. At temperatures below 28°C, sinoatrial pacing becomes erratic and ventricular irritability increases. Fibrillation usually occurs between 25°C and 30°C, and electrical defibrillation is generally ineffective at these temperatures. Because coronary artery blood flow decreases in proportion to cardiac work, hypothermia per se does not cause myocardial ischemia. However, even mild hypothermia decreases tissue damage in response to experimental cardiac ischemia.[93]

Hypothermia decreases blood flow to the kidneys by increasing renal vascular resistance. Inhibition of tubular absorption maintains normal urinary volume. As temperature decreases, reabsorption of sodium and potassium is progressively inhibited, and an antidiuretic hormone–mediated "cold diuresis" results. Despite increased excretion of these ions, plasma electrolyte concentrations usually remain normal. Kidney function returns to normal when patients are rewarmed. Respiratory strength is diminished at core temperatures less than 33°C, but the ventilatory CO_2 response is minimally affected. Hepatic blood flow and function also decrease, which significantly inhibits the metabolism of some drugs.

Acid-Base Changes (also see Chapter 41)

The pH of neutral water ($[OH^-] = [H^+]$) increases 0.017 U for each 1°C reduction in temperature; the pH of blood in a closed system (e.g., test tube or artery) changes similarly. Cold-blooded animals allow the pH to vary with body temperature as it would in vitro (i.e., blood becomes more alkalotic as the temperature decreases), whereas homeotherms, which decrease body temperature during hibernation, maintain an arterial pH near 7.4. Interpretation of arterial pH in hypothermic humans is difficult because it is unclear which strategy is optimal.[192] To mimic the compensatory mechanisms used by hibernating homeotherms, blood pH (which is measured by electrodes at 37°C) has traditionally been "corrected" to the patient's actual body temperature. Without correction, tissue oxygen availability decreases because hemoglobin's affinity for oxygen increases approximately 1.7%/°C. This effect is small when compared with the 5.7%/°C increase in oxyhemoglobin affinity caused by hypothermia itself. Fortunately, the combined increases in affinity are offset by the 8%/°C reduction in metabolic rate caused by hypothermia. Tissue hypoxia is thus unlikely, with or without correction, and has not been demonstrated experimentally.

The ectothermic strategy is also known as "alphastat" because the dissociation constant of the α-imidazole group in histidine changes in parallel with that of water. Maintaining constant imidazole ionization results in optimal enzyme function as temperature changes. In contrast, homeothermic dynamics significantly decreases metabolic function, and animals are essentially anesthetized by cold. Constant relative alkalinity also maintains a stable intracellular-to-extracellular gradient that promotes the removal of acidic products of intracellular metabolism.

No studies have convincingly indicated that an ectothermic strategy is better than that adopted by hibernating homeotherms. However, most anesthesiologists now use "uncorrected" values. This technique facilitates comparison between serial blood gas values because "normal" arterial pH remains approximately 7.4 and "normal" $Paco_2$ remains about 40 mm Hg at any temperature. However, both techniques work well, and physiologic differences between them appear to be subtle and have minimal if any effect on patient outcome.

HYPERTHERMIA AND FEVER

Hypothermia is by far the most common perianesthetic thermal perturbation. However, hyperthermia is more dangerous than a comparable degree of hypothermia. Hyperthermia is a generic term simply indicating a core body temperature exceeding normal values. In contrast, fever is a regulated increase in the core temperature targeted by the thermoregulatory system. Hyperthermia can result from a variety of causes and usually indicates a problem of sufficient severity that physician intervention is required.

Passive Hyperthermia and Malignant Hyperthermia

Passive intraoperative hyperthermia results from excessive patient heating and is most common in infants and children. It is especially frequent when effective active warming is used without adequate core temperature monitoring. Passive hyperthermia, by definition, does not result from thermoregulatory intervention.

Consequently, it can easily be treated by discontinuing active warming and removing excessive insulation.

The increase in body temperature during malignant hyperthermia results from an enormous increase in metabolic heat produced by both internal organs and skeletal muscle. Central thermoregulation presumably remains intact during acute crises, but efferent heat loss mechanisms may be compromised by the intense peripheral vasoconstriction resulting from circulating catecholamine concentrations 20 times normal.[193]

Fever

Normal body temperature is neither set nor maintained by circulating factors. In contrast, fever results when endogenous pyrogens increase the thermoregulatory target temperature ("set point"). Identified endogenous pyrogens include interleukin-1, tumor necrosis factor, interferon-α, and macrophage inflammatory protein-1.[194] Although it was initially believed that these factors acted directly on hypothalamic thermoregulatory centers,[195] there is increasing evidence for a more complicated system involving vagal afferents.[196] Most endogenous pyrogens have peripheral actions (e.g., immune system activation) in addition to their central generating capabilities.

Fever is relatively rare during general anesthesia when one considers how often febrile stimuli are likely to be present. It is rare because volatile anesthetics per se inhibit the expression of fever (Fig. 40–24),[197] as do opioids.[198] Infection is by far the most common cause of fever. Such fever may reflect preexisting infection or result, for

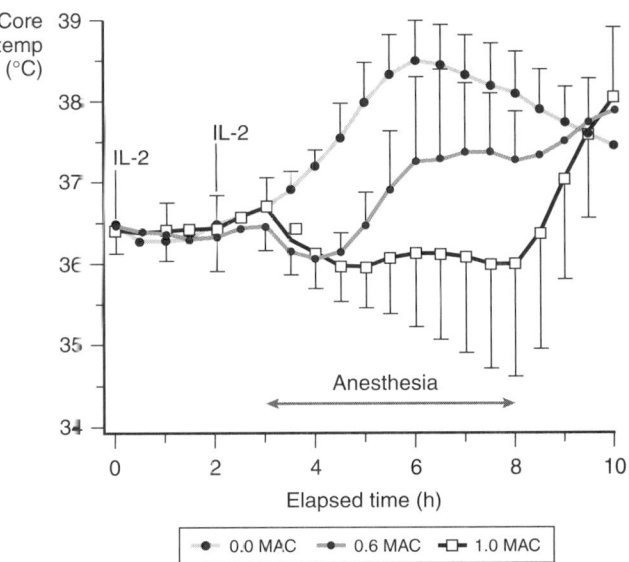

Figure 40–24 Change in core temperature after the administration of 50,000 IU/kg of interleukin-2 (IL-2) followed by a second dose of 100,000 IU/kg 2 hours later. The first dose of IL-2 defined elapsed time zero; anesthesia was started after 3 elapsed hours and continued for 5 hours. Data are presented as means ± SD. MAC, minimum alveolar concentration. (Redrawn from Negishi C, Lenhardt R, Sessler DI, et al: Desflurane reduces the febrile response to interleukin-2 administration. Anesthesiology 88:1162–1169, 1998.)

example, from urologic manipulations. However, perioperative fever also occurs in response to mismatched blood transfusions, blood in the fourth cerebral ventricle, and allergic reactions.[199] In addition, some degree of fever is typical after surgery.[200] The causes of fever are sufficiently diverse—and potentially serious—that a search for a specific etiology is usually warranted.

Treatment of hyperthermia depends on the etiology, with the critical distinction being between fever and the other causes of hyperthermia. (In general, patients with fever and increasing core temperature will have constricted fingertips, whereas those with other types of hyperthermia will be vasodilated.) It is always appropriate to treat the underlying causes, but nonfebrile hyperthermia will also improve with cooling. The first- and second-line treatments of fever are amelioration of the underlying cause and administration of antipyretic medications. The first treatment strategy often fails because the etiology of fever remains unknown; alternatively, the source may be known but unresponsive. The second strategy also often fails or is only partially effective, perhaps because some fever is mediated by mechanisms that bypass conventional antipyretics.[194] It is in these patients that third-line treatment is most likely to be implemented: active cooling. Active cooling of febrile patients is intuitive. However, it often fails to reduce core temperature—while simultaneously worsening the situation by triggering thermoregulatory defenses, including intense discomfort, shivering, and activation of the autonomic nervous system.[201]

Hyperthermia during Epidural Analgesia

Hyperthermia frequently complicates epidural analgesia in patients undergoing labor and delivery[202–205] and in nonpregnant postoperative patients.[206] A clinical consequence of this hyperthermia is that women given epidural analgesia are more often administered antibiotics than those treated conventionally, and their offspring are more commonly treated for sepsis.[203,207,208]

Because passive hyperthermia and excessive heat production are unlikely etiologies, elevated body temperature in laboring and postoperative patients is presumably true fever resulting from infection, tissue damage atelectasis, and other causes. This theory is consistent with reports demonstrating a correlation between hyperthermia during epidural analgesia and clinical signs of infection.[209] Some evidence also indicates that hyperthermia during epidural analgesia is highly associated with placental inflammation.[210] These authors concluded that "Epidural analgesia is associated with intrapartum fever, but only in the presence of placental inflammation. This suggests that the fever reported with epidural analgesia is due to infection rather than the analgesia itself."

The conventional assumption is that hyperthermia is *caused* by the technique, although no convincing mechanism has been proposed. However, it is worth remembering that pain in "control" patients is usually treated with opioids—which themselves attenuate fever. Fever associated with infection or tissue injury might then be suppressed by the low doses of opioids usually given to "control" patients while being expressed normally in patients given epidural analgesia. The extent to which this mechanism contributes remains to be determined, but no convincing alternative explanation has been advanced.

TEMPERATURE MONITORING

Core temperature measurements (e.g., tympanic membrane, pulmonary artery, distal portion of the esophagus, and nasopharynx) are used to monitor intraoperative hypothermia, prevent overheating, and facilitate detection of malignant hyperthermia. Muscle or skin surface temperatures may be used to evaluate vasomotion[211] and ensure the validity of peripheral neuromuscular monitoring.[212] Both core and skin surface temperature measurements are required to determine the thermoregulatory effects of different anesthetic drugs. Temperatures are not uniform within the body; consequently, temperatures measured at each site have different physiologic and practical significance.

Thermometers

Traditionally, the medical community has used mercury-in-glass thermometers. These slow and cumbersome thermometers have largely been replaced by electronic systems. The most common electronic thermometers are thermistors and thermocouples. Both devices are sufficiently accurate for clinical use and inexpensive enough to be disposable. Also sufficiently accurate for clinical use are "deep tissue" thermometers based on actively reducing cutaneous heat flux to zero[213,214]; unfortunately, these monitors are not currently available in Europe or the United States. True infrared tympanic membrane thermometers are another alternative.[215,216] However, the more common infrared monitors that extrapolate tympanic membrane temperature from outer ear temperature are often unreliable,[217] as are infrared systems that scan forehead skin.[218]

When Temperature Monitoring Is Required

The local anesthetics (including amides) used to produce regional blocks and the sedatives used during monitored anesthesia care do not trigger malignant hyperthermia.[219] Nonetheless, core hypothermia is as common during epidural and spinal anesthesia as during general anesthesia and can be nearly as severe.[73] Therefore, core temperature should be measured during regional anesthesia in patients likely to become hypothermic (e.g., those undergoing body cavity surgery).

Core temperature monitoring is appropriate during the administration of most general anesthetics both to facilitate detection of malignant hyperthermia and to quantify hyperthermia and hypothermia. Malignant hyperthermia is best detected by tachycardia and an increase in end-tidal P_{CO_2} out of proportion to minute ventilation.[220] Although an increasing core temperature is not the first sign of acute malignant hyperthermia, it certainly helps confirm the diagnosis. More common than malignant hyperthermia is intraoperative hyperthermia of other etiologies, including excessive warming, infectious fever, blood in the fourth cerebral ventricle, and mismatched blood transfusions.

By far the most common perioperative thermal disturbance is inadvertent hypothermia. Core temperature usually decreases 0.5°C to 1.5°C in the first 30 minutes after induction of anesthesia. Hypothermia results from internal redistribution of heat and a variety of other factors whose importance in individual patients is hard to predict.[57,77] Core temperature perturbations during the first 30 minutes of anesthesia are thus difficult to interpret, and measurements are not usually required. Body temperature should, however, be monitored in patients undergoing general anesthesia exceeding 30 minutes in duration and in all patients whose surgery lasts longer than 1 hour.

Temperature-Monitoring Sites

The core thermal compartment is composed of highly perfused tissues whose temperature is uniform and high in comparison to the rest of the body. Temperature in this compartment can be evaluated in the pulmonary artery, distal part of the esophagus, tympanic membrane, or nasopharynx.[221,222] Temperature probes incorporated into esophageal stethoscopes must be positioned at the point of maximal heart sounds, or even more distally, to provide accurate readings.[165] Even during rapid thermal perturbations (e.g., cardiopulmonary bypass), these temperature-monitoring sites remain reliable. Core temperature can be estimated with reasonable accuracy by using oral, axillary, rectal, and bladder temperatures, except during extreme thermal perturbations.[221,222]

Skin surface temperatures are considerably lower than core temperature.[223] Skin surface temperatures—when adjusted with an appropriate offset—nonetheless reflect core temperature reasonably well.[224] However, skin temperatures fail to reliably confirm the clinical signs of malignant hyperthermia (tachycardia and hypercarbia) in swine[225] and have not been evaluated for this purpose in humans (Fig. 40–25).[225] Rectal temperature also normally correlates well with core temperature,[221,222] but it fails to increase appropriately during malignant hyperthermia crises[225] and in other documented situations.[226,227] Consequently, rectal and skin surface temperatures must be used with some caution.

Even during cardiopulmonary bypass, the core temperature–monitoring sites (e.g., tympanic membrane, nasopharynx, pulmonary artery, and esophagus) remain useful. In contrast, rectal temperatures lag behind those measured in core sites. Consequently, rectal temperature is considered an "intermediate" temperature in deliberately cooled patients. During cardiac surgery, bladder temperature is equal to rectal temperature (and therefore intermediate temperature) when urine flow is low, but equal to pulmonary artery temperature (and thus core temperature) when flow is high.[228] Because bladder temperature is strongly influenced by urine flow, it may be difficult to interpret in these patients. The adequacy of

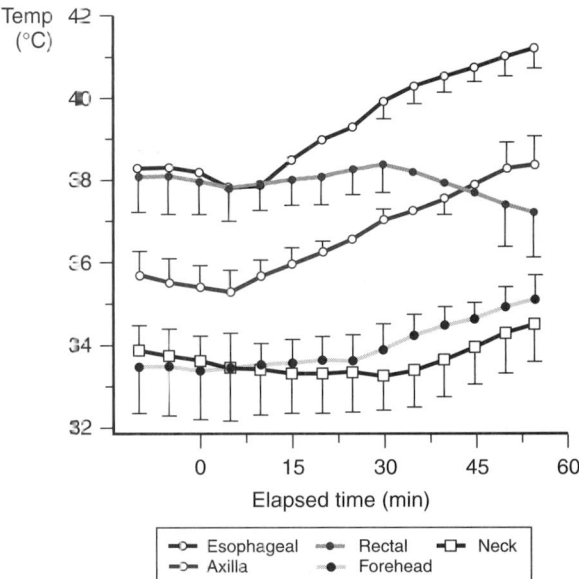

Figure 40–25 Axillary and esophageal temperatures correlated well during acute malignant hyperthermia in swine, but forehead and neck skin temperatures did not. Rectal temperature also failed to promptly identify the onset of malignant hyperthermia. Elapsed time zero indicates an end-tidal Pco_2 of 70 mm Hg. These data indicate that forehead and neck skin surface temperatures will not adequately confirm other clinical signs of malignant hyperthermia. Valid core temperature monitoring sites include the distal part of the esophagus, pulmonary artery, nasopharynx, and tympanic membrane. Except during cardiopulmonary bypass, body temperature can also be measured in the mouth, axilla, and bladder. Data are presented as means ± SD. (Redrawn with modification from Iaizzo PA, Zink RS, Kehler CH, et al: Skin and central temperature during malignant hyperthermia in swine [abstract]. Anesthesiology 77:A569, 1992.)

rewarming is best evaluated by considering both "core" and "intermediate" temperatures.

Temperature-Monitoring and Thermal Management Guidelines

The objective of temperature monitoring and perioperative thermal management is to detect thermal disturbances and maintain appropriate body temperature during anesthesia. The available data suggest the following guidelines:

1. Core body temperature should be measured in most patients given general anesthesia for longer than 30 minutes.
2. Temperature should also be measured during regional anesthesia when changes in body temperature are intended, anticipated, or suspected.
3. Unless hypothermia is specifically indicated (e.g., for protection against ischemia), effort should be made to maintain an intraoperative core temperature higher than 36°C.*

---

*Opinions are the author's and are not necessarily shared by the American Society of Anesthesiologists, but they should be.

SUMMARY

Body temperature is normally controlled by a negative feedback system in the hypothalamus, which integrates thermal information from most tissues. Approximately 80% of this thermal input is derived from core body temperature, which can be measured with distal esophageal, nasopharyngeal, or tympanic membrane thermometer probes. The hypothalamus coordinates increases in heat production (nonshivering thermogenesis and shivering), increases in environmental heat loss (sweating), and decreases in heat loss (vasoconstriction) as needed to maintain normothermia.

Thermal steady state requires that heat loss to the environment equal metabolic heat production; hypothermia occurs when heat loss exceeds production. Mild core hypothermia is common during surgery and anesthesia and results initially from redistribution of body heat from the core to peripheral tissues and subsequently from heat loss exceeding metabolic heat production. Clinical doses of all tested general anesthetics decrease the threshold for response to hypothermia from approximately 37°C (normal) to 33°C to 35°C. Thus, anesthetized patients with core temperatures exceeding these temperatures are usually poikilothermic and do not actively respond to thermal perturbations. Patients becoming sufficiently hypothermic do trigger thermoregulatory vasoconstriction, and the vasoconstriction is remarkably effective in minimizing further core hypothermia.

Mild intraoperative hypothermia provides significant protection against tissue ischemia and hypoxia. It also decreases triggering of malignant hyperthermia and reduces the severity of the syndrome once triggered. However, most consequences of inadvertent hypothermia are harmful. Major adverse effects include morbid myocardial outcomes, reduced resistance to surgical wound infections, impaired coagulation, prolonged duration of drug action, shivering, and decreased postoperative thermal comfort.

Little metabolic heat is lost through the respiratory tract. Consequently, even active airway heating and humidification are of little benefit and virtually never indicated. Administration of sufficient volumes of cold intravenous fluid can produce substantial hypothermia. Fluids should therefore be warmed for patients requiring intravenous administration of more than several liters per hour. Among the clinically available active systems, forced-air heating and resistive heating (electric blankets) are the most effective and can usually maintain normothermia even during the largest operations.

Regional anesthesia produces both peripheral and central inhibition of thermoregulatory control. Peripheral inhibition results when local anesthetics block nerves that are required for thermoregulatory defense. Hypothermia during neuraxial anesthesia results initially from core-to-peripheral redistribution of body heat and subsequently from heat loss exceeding heat production. Hypothermia during major conduction anesthesia may be as severe as that during general anesthesia.

Increased core temperature can result from augmented thermogenesis (malignant hyperthermia), excessive heating (passive hyperthermia), or a specific increase in the thermoregulatory target temperature (fever). Because the causes of hyperthermia are varied and often serious, the etiology of observed increases in core temperature should be sought and appropriate treatments instituted.

A reasonable strategy for detecting and preventing thermal disturbances is to monitor core temperature in patients subjected to general anesthesia lasting longer than 30 minutes and in those undergoing major surgery with regional anesthesia. Unless hypothermia is specifically indicated (i.e., for protection against cerebral ischemia), core temperature should be maintained above 36°C.

Acknowledgments

Many of the studies described in this chapter were supported by the National Institutes of Health, the Commonwealth of Kentucky Research Challenge Trust Fund (Louisville, KY), and the Joseph Drown Foundation (Los Angeles). Mallinckrodt Anesthesiology Products, Inc. (St. Louis), donated the thermocouples used in many of the studies described. Dr. Sessler has a personal financial interest in Radiant Medical, Inc. (Redwood City, CA).

KEY POINTS

1. The normal interthreshold range is only a few tenths of a degree centigrade.
2. General anesthetics slightly increase the sweating threshold, but profoundly and synchronously reduce the vasoconstriction and shivering thresholds.
3. Hypothermia during anesthesia develops in three phases: (1) a rapid decrease in core temperature during the first hour resulting from redistribution of body heat from the core to peripheral thermal compartments; (2) a slower, linear decrease in core temperature from heat loss exceeding heat production; and (3) a core temperature plateau that results from thermal equilibrium or re-emergence of thermoregulatory vasoconstriction.
4. Neuraxial anesthesia inhibits behavioral and autonomic thermoregulatory control; consequently, hypothermia is nearly as common and severe during spinal or epidural anesthesia as during general anesthesia.
5. The three most important complications associated with mild hypothermia are a threefold increase in morbid myocardial events, a threefold increase in the risk of surgical wound infection and prolonged hospitalization, and increased blood loss and transfusion requirements.
6. Airway heating and humidification and circulating-water mattresses are nearly ineffective. Intravenous fluid warming should be used when large volumes of fluid are being given. However, fluid warming alone will not prevent hypothermia. Forced-air heating is the most effective, commonly available, inexpensive, noninvasive warming method.
7. Any increase in body temperature is hyperthermia; fever is a *regulated* hyperthermia that is mediated by endogenous pyrogens. Anesthetics and opioids inhibit fever.

8. Core temperature–monitoring sites include the pulmonary artery, tympanic membrane (with a thermocouple), distal end of the esophagus, and nasopharynx. "Intermediate" sites that can be used in most patients include the axilla, mouth, and bladder. Rectal and skin temperatures may fail to track core temperature during malignant hyperthermia crises. Infrared aural canal thermometers are insufficiently accurate for clinical use.

REFERENCES

1. Satinoff E: Neural organization and evolution of thermal regulation in mammals—several hierarchically arranged integrating systems may have evolved to achieve precise thermoregulation. Science 201:16–22, 1978.
2. Poulos DA: Central processing of cutaneous temperature information. Fed Proc 40:2825–2829, 1981.
3. Jessen C, Feistkorn G: Some characteristics of core temperature signals in the conscious goat. Am J Physiol 247:R456–R464, 1984.
4. Simon E: Temperature regulation: The spinal cord as a site of extrahypothalamic thermoregulatory functions. Rev Physiol Biochem Pharmacol 71:1–76, 1974.
5. Cheng C, Matsukawa T, Sessler DI, et al: Increasing mean skin temperature linearly reduces the core-temperature thresholds for vasoconstriction and shivering in humans. Anesthesiology 82:1160–1168, 1995.
6. Wyss CR, Brengelmann GL, Johnson JM, et al: Altered control of skin blood flow at high skin and core temperatures. J Appl Physiol 38:839–845, 1975.
7. Lopez M, Sessler DI, Walter K, et al: Rate and gender dependence of the sweating, vasoconstriction, and shivering thresholds in humans. Anesthesiology 80:780–788, 1994.
8. Washington D, Sessler DI, Moayeri A, et al: Thermoregulatory responses to hyperthermia during isoflurane anesthesia in humans. J Appl Physiol 74:82–87, 1993.
9. Hessemer V, Brück K: Influence of menstrual cycle on thermoregulatory, metabolic, and heart rate responses to exercise at night. J Appl Physiol 59:1911–1917, 1985.
10. Mestyan J, Jarai I, Bata G, Fekete M: The significance of facial skin temperature in the chemical heat regulation of premature infants. Biol Neonate 7:243–254, 1964.
11. Vassilieff N, Rosencher N, Sessler DI, Conseiller C: The shivering threshold during spinal anesthesia is reduced in the elderly. Anesthesiology 83:1162–1166, 1995.
12. Hales JRS: Skin arteriovenous anastomoses, their control and role in thermoregulation. In Burggren W, Johansen K (eds): Cardiovascular Shunts: Phylogenetic, Ontogenetic and Clinical Aspects. Copenhagen, Munksgaard, 1985, pp 433–451.
13. Dawkins MJR, Scopes JW: Non-shivering thermogenesis and brown adipose tissue in the human new-born infant. Nature 206:201–202, 1965.
14. Jessen K: An assessment of human regulatory nonshivering thermogenesis. Acta Anaesthesiol Scand 24:138–143, 1980.
15. Nedergaard J, Cannon B: The uncoupling protein thermogenin and mitochondrial thermogenesis. New Comp Biochem 23:385–420, 1992.
16. Israel DJ, Pozos RS: Synchronized slow-amplitude modulations in the electromyograms of shivering muscles. J Appl Physiol 66:2358–2363, 1989.
17. Hemingway A, Price WM: The autonomic nervous system and regulation of body temperature. Anesthesiology 29:693–701, 1968.
18. Boudet J, Qing W, Boyer-Chammard A, et al: Dose-response effects of atropine in human volunteers. Fundam Clin Pharmacol 5:635–640, 1991.
19. Rowell LB: Active neurogenic vasodilation in man. In Vanhoutte P, Leusen I (eds): Vasodilatation. New York, Raven, 1981, pp 1–17.
20. Detry JM, Brengelmann GL, Rowell LB, Wyss C: Skin and muscle components of forearm blood flow in directly heated resting man. J Appl Physiol 32:506–511, 1972.
21. Matsukawa T, Kurz A, Sessler DI, et al: Propofol linearly reduces the vasoconstriction and shivering thresholds. Anesthesiology 82:1169–1180, 1995.
22. Kurz A, Go JC, Sessler DI, et al: Alfentanil slightly increases the sweating threshold and markedly reduces the vasoconstriction and shivering thresholds. Anesthesiology 83:293–299, 1995.
23. Talke P, Tayefeh F, Sessler DI, et al: Dexmedetomidine does not alter the sweating threshold, but comparably and linearly reduces the vasoconstriction and shivering thresholds. Anesthesiology 87:835–841, 1997.
24. Annadata RS, Sessler DI, Tayefeh F, et al: Desflurane slightly increases the sweating threshold, but produces marked, non-linear decreases in the vasoconstriction and shivering thresholds. Anesthesiology 83:1205–1211, 1995.
25. Xiong J, Kurz A, Sessler DI, et al: Isoflurane produces marked and non-linear decreases in the vasoconstriction and shivering thresholds. Anesthesiology 85:240–245, 1996.
26. Kurz A, Xiong J, Sessler DI, et al: Desflurane reduces the gain of thermoregulatory arteriovenous shunt vasoconstriction in humans. Anesthesiology 83:1212–1219, 1995.
27. Ikeda T, Kim J-S, Sessler DI, et al: Isoflurane alters shivering patterns and reduces maximum shivering intensity. Anesthesiology 88:866–873, 1998.
28. Kurz A, Ikeda T, Sessler DI, et al: Meperidine decreases the shivering threshold twice as much as the vasoconstriction threshold. Anesthesiology 86:1046–1054, 1997.
29. Sessler DI, Olofsson CI, Rubinstein EH, Beebe JJ: The thermoregulatory threshold in humans during halothane anesthesia. Anesthesiology 68:836–842, 1988.
30. Washington DE, Sessler DI, McGuire J, et al: Painful stimulation minimally increases the thermoregulatory threshold for vasoconstriction during enflurane anesthesia in humans. Anesthesiology 77:286–290, 1992.
31. Sessler DI, Olofsson CI, Rubinstein EH: The thermoregulatory threshold in humans during nitrous oxide–fentanyl anesthesia. Anesthesiology 69:357–364, 1988.
32. Delaunay L, Bonnet F, Liu N, et al: Clonidine comparably decreases the thermoregulatory thresholds for vasoconstriction and shivering in humans. Anesthesiology 79:470–474, 1993.
33. Delaunay L, Herail T, Sessler DI, et al: Clonidine increases the sweating threshold, but does not reduce the gain of sweating. Anesth Analg 83:844–848, 1996.
34. Ozaki M, Sessler DI, Suzuki H, et al: Nitrous oxide decreases the threshold for vasoconstriction less than sevoflurane or isoflurane. Anesth Analg 80:1212–1216, 1995.
35. Imamura M, Matsukawa T, Ozaki M, et al: Nitrous oxide decreases shivering threshold in rabbits less than isoflurane. Br J Anaesth 90:88–90, 2003.
36. Kurz A, Sessler DI, Annadata R, et al: Midazolam minimally impairs thermoregulatory control. Anesth Analg 81:393–398, 1995.
37. Bissonnette B, Sessler DI: The thermoregulatory threshold in infants and children anesthetized with isoflurane and caudal bupivacaine. Anesthesiology 73:1114–1118, 1990.
38. Bissonnette B, Sessler DI: Thermoregulatory thresholds for vasoconstriction in pediatric patients anesthetized with halothane or halothane and caudal bupivacaine. Anesthesiology 76:387–392, 1992.
39. Kurz A, Plattner O, Sessler DI, et al: The threshold for thermoregulatory vasoconstriction during nitrous oxide/isoflurane anesthesia is lower in elderly than young patients. Anesthesiology 79:465–469, 1993.
40. Ozaki M, Sessler DI, Suzuki H, et al: The threshold for thermoregulatory vasoconstriction during nitrous oxide/sevoflurane anesthesia is reduced in elderly patients. Anesth Analg 84:1029–1033, 1997.
41. Hynson JM, Sessler DI, Moayeri A, McGuire J: Absence of nonshivering thermogenesis in anesthetized humans. Anesthesiology 79:695–703, 1993.
42. Dicker A, Ohlson KB, Johnson L, et al: Halothane selectively inhibits nonshivering thermogenesis. Anesthesiology 82:491–501, 1995.

43. Plattner O, Semsroth M, Sessler DI, et al: Lack of nonshivering thermogenesis in infants anesthetized with fentanyl and propofol. Anesthesiology 86:772–777, 1997.

44. Lopez M, Ozaki M, Sessler DI, Valdes M: Physiological responses to hyperthermia during epidural anesthesia and combined epidural/enflurane anesthesia in women. Anesthesiology 78:1046–1054, 1993.

45. Sessler DI, Hynson J, McGuire J, et al: Thermoregulatory vasoconstriction during isoflurane anesthesia minimally decreases heat loss. Anesthesiology 76:670–675, 1992.

46. Kurz A, Sessler DI, Christensen R, Dechert M: Heat balance and distribution during the core-temperature plateau in anesthetized humans. Anesthesiology 83:491–499, 1995.

47. Ikeda T, Sessler DI, Tayefeh F, et al: Meperidine and alfentanil do not reduce the gain or maximum intensity of shivering. Anesthesiology 88:858–865, 1998.

48. Passias TC, Mekjavic IB, Eiken O: The effect of 30% nitrous oxide on thermoregulatory responses in humans during hypothermia. Anesthesiology 76:550–559, 1992.

49. Hardy JD, Milhorat AT, DuBois EF: Basal metabolism and heat loss of young women at temperatures from 22 degrees C to 35 degrees C. J Nutr 21:383–403, 1941.

50. Hammarlund K, Sedin G: Transepidermal water loss in newborn infants III. Relation to gestational age. Acta Paediatr Scand 68:795–801, 1979.

51. Maurer A, Micheli JL, Schutz Y, et al: Transepidermal water loss and resting energy expenditure in preterm infants. Helv Paediatr Acta 39:405–418, 1984.

52. Bickler P, Sessler DI: Efficiency of airway heat and moisture exchangers in anesthetized humans. Anesth Analg 71:415–418, 1990.

53. Roe CF: Effect of bowel exposure on body temperature during surgical operations. Am J Surg 122:13–15, 1971.

54. Robinson BJ, Ebert TJ, O'Brien TJ, et al: Mechanisms whereby propofol mediates peripheral vasodilation in humans. Anesthesiology 86:64–72, 1997.

55. Sessler DI, McGuire J, Moayeri A, Hynson J: Isoflurane-induced vasodilation minimally increases cutaneous heat loss. Anesthesiology 74:226–232, 1991.

56. Stevens WC, Cromwell TH, Halsey MJ, et al: The cardiovascular effects of a new inhalation anesthetic, Forane, in human volunteers at constant arterial carbon dioxide tension. Anesthesiology 35:8–16, 1971.

57. Matsukawa T, Sessler DI, Sessler AM, et al: Heat flow and distribution during induction of general anesthesia. Anesthesiology 82:662–673, 1995.

58. Hynson J, Sessler DI: Intraoperative warming therapies: A comparison of three devices. J Clin Anesth 4:194–199, 1992.

59. Sessler DI, Rubinstein EH, Eger EI II: Core temperature changes during N₂O/fentanyl and halothane/O₂ anesthesia. Anesthesiology 67:137–139, 1987.

60. Belani K, Sessler DI, Sessler AM, et al: Leg heat content continues to decrease during the core temperature plateau in humans. Anesthesiology 78:856–863, 1993.

61. Sessler DI, Ponte J: Shivering during epidural anesthesia. Anesthesiology 72:816–821, 1990.

62. Ozaki M, Kurz A, Sessler DI, et al: Thermoregulatory thresholds during spinal and epidural anesthesia. Anesthesiology 81:282–288, 1994.

63. Kurz A, Sessler DI, Schroeder M, Kurz M: Thermoregulatory response thresholds during spinal anesthesia. Anesth Analg 77:721–726, 1993.

64. Glosten B, Sessler DI, Ostman LG, et al: Intravenous lidocaine does not cause tremor or alter thermoregulation. Reg Anesth 16:218–222, 1991.

65. Hynson J, Sessler DI, Glosten B, McGuire J: Thermal balance and tremor patterns during epidural anesthesia. Anesthesiology 74:680–690, 1991.

66. Pierau F-K, Wurster RD: Primary afferent input from cutaneous thermoreceptors. Fed Proc 40:2819–2824, 1981.

67. Rajek A, Greif R, Sessler DI: Effects of epidural anesthesia on thermal sensation. Reg Anesth Pain Med 26:527–531, 2001.

68. Emerick TH, Ozaki M, Sessler DI, et al: Epidural anesthesia increases apparent leg temperature and decreases the shivering threshold. Anesthesiology 81:289–298, 1994.

69. Leslie K, Sessler DI: Reduction in the shivering threshold is proportional to spinal block height. Anesthesiology 84:1327–1331, 1996.

70. Leslie K, Sessler DI, Bjorksten A, et al: Propofol causes a dose-dependent decrease in the thermoregulatory threshold for vasoconstriction, but has little effect on sweating. Anesthesiology 81:353–360, 1994.

71. Glosten B, Sessler DI, Faure EAM, et al: Central temperature changes are not perceived during epidural anesthesia. Anesthesiology 77:10–16, 1992.

72. Kim J-S, Ikeda T, Sessler D, et al: Epidural anesthesia reduces the gain and maximum intensity of shivering. Anesthesiology 88:851–857, 1998.

73. Arkilic CF, Akça O, Taguchi A, et al: Temperature monitoring and management during neuraxial anesthesia: An observational study. Anesth Analg 91:662–666, 2000.

74. Frank SM, Beattie C, Christopherson R, et al: Epidural versus general anesthesia, ambient operating room temperature, and patient age as predictors of inadvertent hypothermia. Anesthesiology 77:252–257, 1992.

75. Jenkins J, Fox J, Sharwood-Smith G: Changes in body heat during transvesical prostatectomy: A comparison of general and epidural anesthesia. Anaesthesia 38:748–753, 1983.

76. Hendolin H, Lansimies E: Skin and central temperatures during continuous epidural analgesia and general anaesthesia in patients subjected to open prostatectomy. Ann Clin Res 14:181–186, 1982.

77. Matsukawa T, Sessler DI, Christensen R, et al: Heat flow and distribution during epidural anesthesia. Anesthesiology 83:961–967, 1995.

78. Glosten B, Hynson J, Sessler DI, McGuire J: Preanesthetic skin-surface warming reduces redistribution hypothermia caused by epidural block. Anesth Analg 77:488–493, 1993.

79. Valley MA, Bourke DL, Hamill MP, Srinivasa NR: Time course of sympathetic blockade during epidural anesthesia: Laser Doppler flowmetry studies of regional skin perfusion. Anesth Analg 76:289–294, 1993.

80. Modig J, Malmberg P, Karlstrom G: Effect of epidural versus general anesthesia on calf blood flow. Acta Anaesthesiol Scand 24:305–309, 1980.

81. Joris H, Ozaki M, Sessler DI, et al: Epidural anesthesia impairs both central and peripheral thermoregulatory control during general anesthesia. Anesthesiology 80:268–277, 1994.

82. Ponte J, Collett BJ, Walmsley A: Anaesthetic temperature and shivering in epidural anaesthesia. Acta Anaesthesiol Scand 30:584–587, 1986.

83. Ponte J, Sessler DI: Extradurals and shivering: Effects of cold and warm extradural saline injections in volunteers. Br J Anaesth 64:731–733, 1990.

84. Harris MM, Lawson D, Cooper CM, Ellis J: Treatment of shivering after epidural lidocaine. Reg Anesth 14:13–18, 1989.

85. Panzer O, Ghazanfari N, Sessler DI, et al: Shivering and shivering-like tremor during labor with and without epidural analgesia. Anesthesiology 90:1609–1616, 1999.

86. Sharkey A, Lipton JM, Murphy MT, Giesecke AH: Inhibition of postanesthetic shivering with radiant heat. Anesthesiology 66:249–252, 1987.

87. Brownbridge P: Shivering related to epidural blockade with bupivacaine in labour, and the influence of epidural pethidine. Anaesth Intensive Care 14:412–417, 1986.

88. Joris J, Banache M, Bonnet F, et al: Clonidine and ketanserin both are effective treatments for postanesthetic shivering. Anesthesiology 79:532–539, 1993.

89. Kizilirmak S, Karakas SE, Akça O, et al: Magnesium sulphate stops postanesthetic shivering. Proc N Y Acad Sci 813:799–806, 1997.

90. Busto R, Globus MY-T, Dietrich WD, et al: Effect of mild hypothermia on ischemia-induced release of neurotransmitters and free fatty acids in rat brain. Stroke 20:904–910, 1989.

91. Minamisawa H, Smith M-L, Siesjo BK: The effect of mild hyperthermia and hypothermia on brain damage following 5, 10, and 15 minutes of forebrain ischemia. Ann Neurol 28:26–33, 1990.

92. Wass CT, Lanier WL, Hofer RE, et al: Temperature changes of ≥1°C alter functional neurologic outcome and histopathology in a canine model of a complete cerebral ischemia. Anesthesiology 83:325–335, 1995.

93. Dae MW, Gao DW, Sessler DI, et al: Effect of endovascular cooling on myocardial temperature, infarct size, and cardiac output in human-sized pigs. Am J Physiol Heart Circ Physiol 282:H1584–H1591, 2002.

94. Marion DW, Penrod LE, Kelsey SF, et al: Treatment of traumatic brain injury with moderate hypothermia. N Engl J Med 336:540–546, 1997.

95. Clifton GL, Miller ER, Choi SC, et al: Lack of effect of induction of hypothermia after acute brain injury. N Engl J Med 344:556–563, 2001.

96. Polderman KH, Joe RTT, Peerdeman SM, et al: Effects of therapeutic hypothermia on intracranial pressure and outcome in patients with severe head injury. Intensive Care Med 28:1563–1573, 2002.

97. Bernard SA, Gray TW, Buist MD, et al: Treatment of comatose survivors of out-of-hospital cardiac arrest with induced hypothermia. N Engl J Med 346:557–563, 2002.

98. Hypothermia after Cardiac Arrest Study Group: Mild therapeutic hypothermia to improve the neurologic outcome after cardiac arrest. N Engl J Med 346:549–556, 2002.

99. Todd MM, Warner DS: A comfortable hypothesis reevaluated: Cerebral metabolic depression and brain protection during ischemia [editorial]. Anesthesiology 76:161–164, 1992.

100. Nelson TE: Porcine malignant hyperthermia: Critical temperatures for in vivo and in vitro responses. Anesthesiology 73:449–454, 1990.

101. Iaizzo PA, Kehler CH, Carr RJ, et al: Prior hypothermia attenuates malignant hyperthermia in susceptible swine. Anesth Analg 82:782–789, 1996.

102. Michelson AD, MacGregor H, Barnard MR, et al: Reversible inhibition of human platelet activation by hypothermia in vivo and in vitro. Thromb Haemost 71:633–640, 1994.

103. Valeri CR, Khabbaz K, Khuri SF, et al: Effect of skin temperature on platelet function in patients undergoing extracorporeal bypass. J Thorac Cardiovasc Surg 104:108–116, 1992.

104. Reed L, Johnston TD, Hudson JD, Fischer RP: The disparity between hypothermic coagulopathy and clotting studies. J Trauma 33:465–470, 1992.

105. Staab DB, Sorensen VJ, Fath JJ, et al: Coagulation defects resulting from ambient temperature–induced hypothermia. J Trauma 36:634–638, 1994.

106. Schmied H, Kurz A, Sessler DI, et al: Mild intraoperative hypothermia increases blood loss and allogeneic transfusion requirements during total hip arthroplasty. Lancet 347:289–292, 1996.

107. Winkler M, Akça O, Birkenberg B, et al: Aggressive warming reduces blood loss during hip arthroplasty. Anesth Analg 91:978–984, 2000.

108. Johansson T, Lisander B, Ivarsson I: Mild hypothermia does not increase blood loss during total hip arthroplasty. Acta Anaesthesiol Scand 43:1005–1010, 1999.

109. Bremmelgaard A, Raahave D, Beir-Holgersen R, et al: Computer-aided surveillance of surgical infections and identification of risk factors. J Hosp Infect 13:1–18, 1989.

110. Polk HC, Simpson CJ, Simmons BP, Alexander JW: Guidelines for prevention of surgical wound infection. Arch Surg 118(Suppl):S1213–S1217, 1983.

111. Van Oss CJ, Absolam DR, Moore LL, et al: Effect of temperature on the chemotaxis, phagocytic engulfment, digestion and O_2 consumption of human polymorphonuclear leukocytes. J Reticuloendothel Soc 27:561–565, 1980.

112. Sheffield CW, Sessler DI, Hopf HW, et al: Centrally and locally mediated thermoregulatory responses alter subcutaneous oxygen tension. Wound Rep Reg 4:339–345, 1997.

113. Kluger MJ: Is fever beneficial? Yale J Biol Med 59:89–95, 1986.

114. Kluger MJ, Ringler DH, Anver MR: Fever and survival. Science 188:166–168, 1975.

115. Sheffield CW, Sessler DI, Hunt TK: Mild hypothermia during isoflurane anesthesia decreases resistance to E. coli dermal infection in guinea pigs. Acta Anaesthesiol Scand 38:201–205, 1994.

116. Sheffield CW, Sessler DI, Hunt TK, Scheuenstuhl H: Mild hypothermia during halothane anesthesia decreases resistance to S. aureus dermal infection in guinea pigs. Wound Rep Reg 2:48–56, 1994.

117. Kurz A, Sessler DI, Lenhardt RA: Perioperative normothermia to reduce the incidence of surgical-wound infection and shorten hospitalization. Study of Wound Infections and Temperature Group. N Engl J Med 334:1209–1215, 1996.

118. Carli F, Emery PW, Freemantle CAJ: Effect of perioperative normothermia on postoperative protein metabolism in elderly patients undergoing hip arthroplasty. Br J Anaesth 63:276–282, 1989.

119. Kurz A, Sessler DI, Narzt E, et al: Postoperative hemodynamic and thermoregulatory consequences of intraoperative core hypothermia. J Clin Anesth 7:359–366, 1995.

120. Frank SM, Fleisher LA, Olson KF, et al: Multivariate determinants of early postoperative oxygen consumption in elderly patients. Anesthesiology 83:241–249, 1995.

121. Frank SM, Higgins MS, Breslow MJ, et al: The catecholamine, cortisol, and hemodynamic responses to mild perioperative hypothermia. Anesthesiology 82:83–93, 1995.

122. Frank SM, Fleisher LA, Breslow MJ, et al: Perioperative maintenance of normothermia reduces the incidence of morbid cardiac events: A randomized clinical trial. JAMA 277:1127–1134, 1997.

123. Heier T, Caldwell JE, Sessler DI, Miller RD: Mild intraoperative hypothermia increases duration of action and spontaneous recovery of vecuronium blockade during nitrous oxide–isoflurane anesthesia in humans. Anesthesiology 74:815–819, 1991.

124. Leslie K, Sessler DI, Bjorksten AR, Moayeri A: Mild hypothermia alters propofol pharmacokinetics and increases the duration of action of atracurium. Anesth Analg 80:1007–1014, 1995.

125. Heier T, Caldwell JE, Eriksson LI, et al: The effect of hypothermia on adductor pollicis twitch tension during continuous infusion of vecuronium in isoflurane-anesthetized humans. Anesth Analg 788:312–317, 1994.

126. Heier T, Clough D, Wright PM, et al: The influence of mild hypothermia on the pharmacokinetics and time course of action of neostigmine in anesthetized volunteers. Anesthesiology 97:90–95, 2002.

127. Eger EI II, Johnson BH: MAC of I-653 in rats, including a test of the effect of body temperature and anesthetic duration. Anesth Analg 66:974–976, 1987.

128. Vitez TS, White PF, Eger EI II: Effects of hypothermia on halothane MAC and isoflurane MAC in the rat. Anesthesiology 41:80–81, 1974.

129. Antognini JF: Hypothermia eliminates isoflurane requirements at 20°C. Anesthesiology 78:1152–1156, 1993.

130. Lenhardt R, Marker E, Goll V, et al: Mild intraoperative hypothermia prolongs postoperative recovery. Anesthesiology 87:1318–1323, 1997.

131. Just B, Delva E, Camus Y, Lienhart A: Oxygen uptake during recovery following naloxone. Anesthesiology 76:60–64, 1992.

132. Lienhart A, Fiez N, Deriaz H: Frisson postopératoire: Analyse des principaux facteurs associés. Ann Fr Anesth Reanim 11:488–495, 1992.

133. Soliman MG, Gillies DMM: Muscular hyperactivity after general anaesthesia. Can Anaesth Soc J 19:529–535, 1972.

134. Sessler DI, Israel D, Pozos RS, et al: Spontaneous postanesthetic tremor does not resemble thermoregulatory shivering. Anesthesiology 68:843–850, 1988.

135. Rosenberg H, Clofine R, Bialik O: Neurologic changes during awakening from anesthesia. Anesthesiology 54:125–130, 1981.

136. Sessler DI, Rubinstein EH, Moayeri A: Physiological responses to mild perianesthetic hypothermia in humans. Anesthesiology 75:594–610, 1991.

137. Horn E-P, Sessler DI, Standl T, et al: Non-thermoregulatory shivering in patients recovering from isoflurane or desflurane anesthesia. Anesthesiology 89:878–886, 1998.

138. Horn E-P, Schroeder F, Wilhelm S, et al: Postoperative pain facilitates non-thermoregulatory tremor. Anesthesiology 91:979–984, 1999.

139. Sessler DI, Moayeri A: Skin-surface warming: Heat flux and central temperature. Anesthesiology 73:218–224, 1990.

140. Alfonsi P, Nouredine K, Chauvin M, Sessler DI: Contribution of skin and core temperatures to postoperative shivering threshold [abstract]. Anesthesiology 93:A387, 2000.

141. Delaunay L, Bonnet F, Duvaldestin P: Clonidine decreases postoperative oxygen consumption in patients recovering from general anaesthesia. Br J Anaesth 67:397–401, 1991.

142. De Witte J, Rietman GW, Vandenbroucke G, Deloof T: Post-operative effects of tramadol administered at wound closure. Eur J Anaesthesiol 15:190–195, 1998.

143. De Witte JL, Kim J-S, Sessler DI, et al: Tramadol reduces the sweating, vasoconstriction, and shivering thresholds. Anesth Analg 87:173–179, 1998.

144. Horn E-P, Standl T, Sessler DI, et al: Physostigmine prevents postanesthetic shivering as does meperidine or clonidine. Anesthesiology 88:108–113, 1998.

145. De Witte J, Sessler DI: Perioperative shivering: Physiology and pharmacology. Anesthesiology 96:467–484, 2002.

146. Guffin A, Girard D, Kaplan JA: Shivering following cardiac surgery: Hemodynamic changes and reversal. J Cardiothorac Vasc Anesth 1:24–28, 1987.

147. Kurz M, Belani K, Sessler DI, et al: Naloxone, meperidine, and shivering. Anesthesiology 79:1193–1201, 1993.

148. Magnan J, Paterson SJ, Tavani A, Kosterlitz HW: The binding spectrum of narcotic analgesic drugs with different agonist and antagonist properties. Naunyn Schmiedebergs Arch Pharmacol 319:197–205, 1982.

149. Greif R, Laciny S, Rajek AM, et al: Neither nalbuphine nor atropine possesses special antishivering activity. Anesth Analg 93:620–627, 2001.

150. Takada K, Clark DJ, Davies MF, et al: Meperidine exerts agonist activity at the alpha(2B)-adrenoceptor subtype. Anesthesiology 96:1420–1426, 2002.

151. Burton AC: Human calorimetry: The average temperature of the tissues of the body. J Nutr 9:261–280, 1935.

152. Kurz A, Sessler DI, Birnbauer F, et al: Thermoregulatory vasoconstriction impairs active core cooling. Anesthesiology 82:870–876, 1995.

153. Plattner O, Xiong J, Sessler DI, et al: Rapid core-to-peripheral tissue heat transfer during cutaneous cooling. Anesth Analg 82:925–930, 1996.

154. Clough D, Kurz A, Sessler DI, et al: Thermoregulatory vasoconstriction does not impede core warming during cutaneous heating. Anesthesiology 85:281–288, 1996.

155. Weiskopf RB: Cardiovascular effects of desflurane in experimental animals and volunteers. Anaesthesia 50(Suppl):S14–S27, 1995.

156. Szmuk P, Ezri T, Sessler DI, et al: Spinal anesthesia only minimally increases the efficacy of postoperative forced-air rewarming. Anesthesiology 87:1050–1054, 1997.

157. Plattner O, Ikeda T, Sessler DI, et al: Postanesthetic vasoconstriction slows postanesthetic peripheral-to-core transfer of cutaneous heat, thereby isolating the core thermal compartment. Anesth Analg 85:899–906, 1997.

158. Hynson JM, Sessler DI, Moayeri A, et al: The effects of pre-induction warming on temperature and blood pressure during propofol/nitrous oxide anesthesia. Anesthesiology 79:219–228, 1993.

159. Just B, Trévien V, Delva E, Lienhart A: Prevention of intraoperative hypothermia by preoperative skin-surface warming. Anesthesiology 79:214–218, 1993.

160. Sessler DI, Schroeder M, Merrifield B, et al: Optimal duration and temperature of pre-warming. Anesthesiology 82:674–681, 1995.

161. Rajek A, Lenhardt R, Sessler DI, et al: Tissue heat content and distribution during and after cardiopulmonary bypass at 17°C. Anesth Analg 88:1220–1225, 1999.

162. Rajek A, Lenhardt R, Sessler DI, et al: Tissue heat content and distribution during and after cardiopulmonary bypass at 31°C and 27°C. Anesthesiology 88:1511–1518, 1998.

163. Rajek A, Lenhardt R, Sessler DI, et al: Efficacy of two methods for reducing post-bypass afterdrop. Anesthesiology 92:447–456, 2000.

164. Deriaz H, Fiez N, Lienhart A: Influence d'un filtre hygrophobe ou d'un humidificateur-réchauffeur sur l'hypothermie peropératoire. Ann Fr Anesth Reanim 11:145–149, 1992.

165. Kaufman RD: Relationship between esophageal temperature gradient and heart and lung sounds heard by esophageal stethoscope. Anesth Analg 66:1046–1048, 1987.

166. Bissonnette B, Sessler DI: Passive or active inspired gas humidification increases thermal steady-state temperatures in anesthetized infants. Anesth Analg 69:783–787, 1989.

167. Faries G, Johnston C, Pruitt KM, Plouff RT: Temperature relationship to distance and flow rate of warmed IV fluids. Ann Emerg Med 20:1198–1200, 1991.

168. Morris RH: Operating room temperature and the anesthetized, paralyzed patient. Surgery 102:95–97, 1971.

169. Sessler DI, McGuire J, Sessler AM: Perioperative thermal insulation. Anesthesiology 74:875–879, 1991.

170. Sessler DI, Schroeder M: Heat loss in humans covered with cotton hospital blankets. Anesth Analg 77:73–77, 1993.

171. Sessler DI, Moayeri A, Støen R, et al: Thermoregulatory vasoconstriction decreases cutaneous heat loss. Anesthesiology 73:656–660, 1990.

172. Simbruner G, Weninge RM, Popow C, Herholdt WJ: Regional heat loss in newborn infants: Part I. Heat loss in healthy newborns at various environmental temperatures. S Afr Med J 68:940–944, 1985.

173. Simbruner G, Weninger W, Popow C, Herholdt WJ: Regional heat loss in newborn infants: Part II. Heat loss in newborns with various diseases—a method of assessing local metabolism and perfusion. S Afr Med J 68:945–948, 1985.

174. Morris RH, Kumar A: The effect of warming blankets on maintenance of body temperature of the anesthetized, paralyzed adult patient. Anesthesiology 36:408–411, 1972.

175. Kokate JY, Leland KJ, Held AM, et al: Temperature-modulated pressure ulcers: A porcine model. Arch Phys Med Rehabil 76:666–673, 1995.

176. Crino MH, Nagel EL: Thermal burns caused by warming blankets in the operating room. Anesthesiology 29:149–151, 1968.

177. Nesher N, Wolf T, Kushnir I, et al: Novel thermoregulation system for enhancing cardiac function and hemodynamics during coronary artery bypass graft surgery. Ann Thorac Surg 72(Suppl):S1069–S1076, 2001.

178. Stanley TO, Grocott HP, Phillips-Bute B, et al: Preliminary evaluation of the Arctic Sun temperature-controlling system during off-pump coronary artery bypass surgery. Ann Thorac Surg 75:1140–1144, 2003.

179. Giesbrecht GG, Ducharme MB, McGuire JP: Comparison of forced-air patient warming systems for perioperative use. Anesthesiology 80:671–679, 1994.

180. Camus Y, Delva E, Just B, Lienhart A: Leg warming minimizes core hypothermia during abdominal surgery. Anesth Analg 77:995–999, 1993.

181. Kurz A, Kurz M, Poeschl G, et al: Forced-air warming maintains intraoperative normothermia better than circulating-water mattresses. Anesth Analg 77:89–95, 1993.

182. Negishi C, Hasegawa K, Mukai S, et al: Resistive heating and forced-air warming are comparably effective. Anesth Analg 96:1683–1687, 2003.

183. Rajek A, Greif R, Sessler DI, et al: Core cooling by central-venous infusion of 4°C and 20°C fluid: Isolation of core and peripheral thermal compartments. Anesthesiology 93:629–637, 2000.

184. Nesher N, Wolf T, Uretzky G, et al: A novel thermoregulatory system maintains perioperative normothermia in children undergoing elective surgery. Paediatr Anaesth 11:555–560, 2001.

185. Doufas AG, Akça O, Barry A, et al: Initial experience with a novel heat-exchanging catheter in neurosurgical patients. Anesth Analg 95:1752–1756, 2002.

186. Zweifler RM, Sessler DI, Zivin JA: Thermoregulatory vasoconstriction and shivering impede therapeutic hypothermia in acute ischemic stroke victims. J Stroke Cerebrovasc Dis 6:100–104, 1997.

187. Mokhtarani M, Mahgob AN, Morioka N, et al: Buspirone and meperidine synergistically reduce the shivering threshold. Anesth Analg 93:1233–1239, 2001.
188. Tveita T, Ytrehus K, Myhre ES, Hevroy O: Left ventricular dysfunction following rewarming from experimental hypothermia. J Appl Physiol 85:2135–2139, 1998.
189. Grigore AM, Mathew J, Grocott HP, et al: Prospective randomized trial of normothermic versus hypothermic cardiopulmonary bypass on cognitive function after coronary artery bypass graft surgery. Anesthesiology 95:1110–1119, 2001.
190. Randomised trial of normothermic versus hypothermic coronary bypass surgery. The Warm Heart Investigators. Lancet 343:559–563, 1994.
191. Weisser J, Martin J, Bisping E, et al: Influence of mild hypothermia on myocardial contractility and circulatory function. Basic Res Cardiol 96:198–205, 2001.
192. White FN: A comparative physiological approach to hypothermia. J Thorac Cardiovasc Surg 82:821–831, 1981.
193. Gronert GA, Theye RA, Milde JH, Tinker JH: Catecholamine stimulation of myocardial oxygen consumption in porcine malignant hyperthermia. Anesthesiology 49:330–337, 1978.
194. Davatelis G, Wolpe SD, Sherry B, et al: Macrophage inflammatory protein-1: A prostaglandin-independent endogenous pyrogen. Science 243:1066–1068, 1989.
195. Blatteis C: Role of the OVLT in the febrile response to circulating pyrogens. Prog Brain Res 91:409–412, 1992.
196. Blatteis C, Sehic E: Fever: How may circulating pyrogens signal the brain? News Physiol Sci 12:1–9, 1997.
197. Negishi C, Lenhardt R, Sessler DI, et al: Desflurane reduces the febrile response to interleukin-2 administration. Anesthesiology 88:1162–1169, 1998.
198. Negishi C, Kim J-S, Lenhardt R, et al: Alfentanil reduces the febrile response to interleukin-2 in men. Crit Care Med 28:1295–1300, 1999.
199. Kotani N, Kushikata T, Matsukawa T, et al: A rapid increase in foot tissue temperature predicts cardiovascular collapse during anaphylactic and anaphylactoid reactions. Anesthesiology 87:559–568, 1997.
200. Frank SM, Kluger MJ, Kunkel SL: Elevated thermostatic setpoint in postoperative patients. Anesthesiology 93:1426–1431, 2000.
201. Lenhardt R, Negishi C, Sessler DI, et al: The effects of physical treatment on induced fever in humans. Am J Med 106:550–555, 1999.
202. Fusi L, Maresh MJA, Steer PJ, Beard RW: Maternal pyrexia associated with the use of epidural analgesia in labour. Lancet 1:1250–1252, 1989.
203. Philip J, Alexander JM, Sharma SK, et al: Epidural analgesia during labor and maternal fever. Anesthesiology 90:1271–1275, 1999.
204. Vinson DC, Thomas R, Kiser T: Association between epidural analgesia during labor and fever. J Fam Pract 36:617–622, 1993.
205. Macaulay JH, Mrcog KB, Steer PJ: Epidural analgesia in labor and fetal hyperthermia. Obstet Gynecol 80:665–669, 1992.
206. Bredtmann RD, Herden HN, Teichmann W, et al: Epidural analgesia in colonic surgery: Results of a randomized prospective study. Br J Surg 77:638–642, 1990.
207. Lieberman E, Lang JM, Frigoletto F, et al: Epidural analgesia, intrapartum fever, and neonatal sepsis evaluation. Pediatrics 99:415–419, 1997.
208. Lieberman E, Cohen A, Lang J, et al: Maternal intrapartum temperature elevation as a risk factor for cesarean delivery and assisted vaginal delivery. Am J Public Health 89:506–510, 1999.
209. Churgay CA, Smith MA, Blok B: Maternal fever during labor—what does it mean? J Am Board Fam Pract 7:14–24, 1994.
210. Dashe JS, Rogers BB, McIntire DD, Leveno KJ: Epidural analgesia and intrapartum fever: Placental findings. Obstet Gynecol 93:341–344, 1999.
211. Rubinstein EH, Sessler DI: Skin-surface temperature gradients correlate with fingertip blood flow in humans. Anesthesiology 73:541–545, 1990.
212. Heier T, Caldwell JE, Sessler DI, et al: The relationship between adductor pollicis twitch tension and core, skin and muscle temperature during nitrous oxide–isoflurane anesthesia in humans. Anesthesiology 71:381–384, 1989.
213. Togawa T, Nemoto T, Yamazaki T, Kobayashi T: A modified internal temperature measurement device. Med Biol Eng 14:361–364, 1976.
214. Matsukawa T, Sessler DI, Ozaki M, Kumazawa T: Comparison of distal esophageal temperature to "deep sternal," "deep forehead," and tracheal temperatures. Can J Anaesth 44:433–438, 1997.
215. Lopez M, Ozaki M, Sessler DI, Valdes M: Mild core hyperthermia does not alter electroencephalographic responses during epidural/enflurane anesthesia in humans. J Clin Anesth 5:425–430, 1993.
216. Matsukawa T, Kashimoto S, Miyaji T, et al: A new infrared tympanic thermometer in surgery and anesthesia. J Anesth 7:33–39, 1993.
217. Imamura M, Matsukawa T, Ozaki M, et al: The accuracy and precision of four infrared aural canal thermometers during cardiac surgery. Acta Anaesthiol Scand 42:1222–1226, 1998.
218. Suleman MI, Doufas AG, Akca O, et al: Insufficiency in a new temporal-artery thermometer for adult and pediatric patients. Anesth Analg 95:67–71, 2002.
219. Wingard DW, Bobko S: Failure of lidocaine to trigger porcine malignant hyperthermia. Anesth Analg 58:99–103, 1979.
220. Baudendistel L, Goudsouzian N, Coté C, Strafford M: End-tidal CO_2 monitoring. Its use in the diagnosis and management of malignant hyperthermia. Anaesthesia 39:1000–1003, 1984.
221. Bissonnette B, Sessler DI, LaFlamme P: Intraoperative temperature monitoring sites in infants and children and the effect of inspired gas warming on esophageal temperature. Anesth Analg 69:192–196, 1989.
222. Cork RC, Vaughan RW, Humphrey LS: Precision and accuracy of intraoperative temperature monitoring. Anesth Analg 62:211–214, 1983.
223. Burgess GE III, Cooper JR, Marino RJ, Peuler MJ: Continuous monitoring of skin temperature using a liquid-crystal thermometer during anesthesia. South Med J 71:516–518, 1978.
224. Ikeda T, Sessler DI, Marder D, Xiong J: The influence of thermoregulatory vasomotion and ambient temperature variation on the accuracy of core-temperature estimates by cutaneous liquid-crystal thermometers. Anesthesiology 86:603–612, 1997.
225. Iaizzo PA, Kehler CH, Zink RS, et al: Thermal response in acute porcine malignant hyperthermia. Anesth Analg 82:803–809, 1996.
226. Ash CJ, Cook JR, McMurry TA, Auner CR: The use of rectal temperature to monitor heat stroke. Mo Med 89:283–288, 1992.
227. Iaizzo PA, Zaritsky AL: Occult core hyperthermia complicating cardiogenic shock. Pediatrics 83:782–784, 1989.
228. Horrow JC, Rosenberg H: Does urinary catheter temperature reflect core temperature during cardiac surgery? Anesthesiology 69:986–989, 1988.

Patrick J. Neligan and Clifford S. Deutschman

Physical Chemistry of Water   1599

Acids and Bases   1600

Stewart Approach to Acid-Base Balance   1601
What Determines the Acidity or Alkalinity of a Solution?   1601
Strong Ions   1601
Weak Acid Buffer Solutions   1601
Carbon Dioxide   1602
Factors Independently Influencing Water Dissociation   1602

Acid-Base Abnormalities   1602
Respiratory Acid-Base Abnormalities   1603
Metabolic Acid-Base Disturbances   1603

Regulation of Acid-Base Balance   1604

Analytic Tools Used in Acid-Base Chemistry   1605
Carbon Dioxide–Bicarbonate (Boston) Approach   1606
Base Deficit or Excess (Copenhagen) Approach   1606
Anion Gap Approach   1607
Stewart-Fencl Approach   1608

Acid-Base Problems in Different Clinical Settings   1609
Acid-Base Disturbances in Emergency Settings   1609
Perioperative Acid-Base Disturbances   1611
Acid-Base Disturbances in Critical Illness   1613

Summary   1614

The chemical composition of the extracellular and intracellular spaces is tightly controlled to facilitate homeostatic function. This includes, but is not limited to, hydrogen and hydroxyl ion concentrations. Alterations in the relative concentrations of these ions are associated with significant clinical problems. Consequently, the detection, interpretation, and treatment of acid-base abnormalities have become core elements of clinical care. Traditional educational approaches to acid-base balance have tended to focus on methods of interpretation of laboratory data, rather than on understanding the underlying biophysical chemistry. The field has been confusing for students and clinicians alike, and several commonly recognized acid-base problems have escaped explanation. The modern physical-chemical approach to acid-base balance has significantly enhanced our understanding of these problems and simplified the clinical approach.[1-4]

Acid-base abnormalities should be seen as resulting from other biochemical changes in the extracellular environment.[5] Alterations in the relative concentrations of hydronium (hydrogen) and hydroxyl ions are less important than the chemical abnormalities causing them.

Hydronium and hydroxyl ions are the dissociation products of water, whose concentrations are modulated to maintain electrical neutrality depending on the local concentration of strong ions, weak acids, and carbon dioxide. In this chapter, we explore the physical chemistry of water, examine the evolution of acid-base medicine, and apply clinical approaches to acid-base conundrums.

PHYSICAL CHEMISTRY OF WATER

The human body is made up principally of water. Consequently, the physical properties of water have enormous implication for maintenance of homeostasis. Water is a simple triatomic molecule. Its chemical formula is H_2O, and its structural formula is H-O-H. Because the charge distribution of each covalent bond is unequal, the molecule has a polar conformation, and the H-O-H bond angle is 105 degrees. Water molecules attract and form hydrogen bonds with one another. These bonds are fundamental to the existence of life on this planet. Water has a high surface tension, low vapor pressure, high specific heat capacity, high heat of vaporization, and a high boiling point.

Water molecules are in continuous motion. Occasionally, when molecules collide, enough energy is produced to transfer a proton from one water molecule to another. Water slightly dissociates into a negatively charged hydroxyl ion (OH^-) and positively charged hydronium ion (H_3O^+). Conventionally, this self-ionization of water is written as follows:

$$H_2O \rightleftharpoons H^+ + OH^-$$

The symbol H^+ is convenient because, although protons dissociating from water have many aliases (e.g., H_3O^+, $H_9O_4^+$), most physicians and chemists refer to them as hydrogen ions.

The self-ionization of water is miniscule. In pure water at 25°C, the $[H^+]$ and $[OH^-]$ are 1.0×10^{-7} mmol/L. The tendency for water to dissociate into its component parts is represented by the following expression:

$$K_{eq} H_2O = [H^+][OH^-]$$

The molarity of water is extremely high—55.5 M ("there is a lot of water in water"). Because the concentration of water and the K_{eq} are constants, the ion-product dissociation constant for water (Kw) can be expressed as follows:

$$K_{eq} H_2O = K_{eq}(55.5) = Kw = [H^+][OH^-]$$

The implication is that the relative concentrations of hydroxyl and hydrogen are constant, and when there is an increase in the concentration of hydrogen ions, there is a concomitant decrease in the concentration of hydroxyl ions and vice versa.

Pure water is considered neutral because the relative concentrations of hydrogen and hydroxyl are equal at 1.0×10^{-7} mmol/L. A solution is considered *acidic* if the concentration of hydrogen ions exceeds that of hydroxyl ions ($[H^+] > 1.0 \times 10^{-7}$ mmol/L, $[OH^-] < 1.0 \times 10^{-7}$ mmol/L). A solution is considered *alkaline* if the hydroxyl ion concentration exceeds the hydrogen ion concentration.

ACIDS AND BASES

The concept of acids and bases is relatively new. In the early part of the 20th century, it was known that the carbon dioxide (CO_2) content of the blood decreased in cases of critical illness. As early as 1831, O'Shaughnessy identified loss of "carbonate of soda" from the blood as a fundamental disturbance in patients dying of cholera.[2] We now know that the loss of bicarbonate was related to hyperventilation and buffering of free hydrogen ions in dysoxic or dysmetabolic states. In 1909, L.J. Henderson coined the term *acid-base balance*.[6] He was able to define this process in terms of carbonic acid equilibrium, work that was later refined by Hasselbalch (1916).[7] Essentially, their method described acid-base balance in terms of the hydration equation for carbon dioxide.[4] The latter was the only clinical chemistry test available at that time.

$$CO_2 + H_2O \rightarrow H_2CO_3 \rightarrow H^+ + HCO_3^-$$
$$pH = pK_a + \log [HCO_3^-] / [H_2CO_3]$$
$$\text{Total } CO_2 = [HCO_3^-] + [\text{Dissolved } CO_2]$$
$$+ [\text{Carbamino } CO_2] + [H_2CO_3]$$
$$\approx P_{CO_2} \times 0.03 \text{ mmol of } CO_2/L/\text{mm Hg}$$

Substituting into the first previous equation provides the Henderson-Hasselbalch equation:

$$pH = 6.1 + \log [HCO_3^-] / P_{CO_2} \times 0.03$$

The revolutionary theory of Svante Arrhenius (1859-1927) in 1903 established the foundations of acid-base chemistry. In an aqueous solution, an Arrhenius acid is any substance that delivers a hydrogen ion into the solution.[2] A base is any substance that delivers a hydroxyl ion into the solution. Water is a highly ionizing solution because of its high dielectric constant, and substances with polar bonds dissociate into their component parts (i.e., dissolve) in it. Hydrogen chloride (HCl) is an acid, and potassium hydroxide (KOH) is a base.

The degree of dissociation of substances in water determines whether they are strong acids or strong bases. Lactic acid, which has an ion dissociation constant (pK_a) of 3.4, is completely dissociated at physiologic pH and is a strong acid. Carbonic acid, which has a pK_a of 6.4, is incompletely dissociated and is a weak acid. Similarly, ions such as sodium, potassium, and chloride, which do not easily bind other molecules, are considered strong ions; they exist free in solution. In any solution, the ion dissociation constant for water (Kw) dictates that the relative ratio of $[H^+]$ to $[OH^-]$ must always be constant, and electrical neutrality must always hold. Consequently, strong cations (Na^+, K^+, Ca^{2+}, Mg^{2+}) act as Arrhenius bases because they drive hydroxyl out of and hydrogen into solution to maintain electrical neutrality, and strong anions (Cl^-, LA^- [lactate], ketones, sulfate, formate) act as Arrhenius acids.

One problem with the Arrhenius theory is that it is not comprehensive enough. Aqueous solutions such as ammonia (NH_3), sodium carbonate (Na_2CO_3), and sodium bicarbonate ($NaHCO_3$) are bases, but none is a hydroxide. In 1923, Brønsted and Lowry proposed an expanded theory of acids and bases. They defined acids as proton donors and bases as proton acceptors. All Arrhenius acids and bases were therefore also Brønsted-Lowry acids and bases, and the peculiar behavior of carbon dioxide and ammonia could be accounted for.

$$NH_3 + H_2O \rightleftharpoons NH_4^+ + OH^-$$

In this situation, water is the proton donor, the Brønsted-Lowry acid, and ammonia the proton acceptor, the Brønsted-Lowry base. Conversely, consider the following reaction:

$$HCl + H_2O \rightarrow H_3O^+ + Cl^-$$

In the previous reaction, hydrogen chloride acts as a Brønsted-Lowry acid and water as a Brønsted-Lowry base.

$$CO_2 + H_2O \rightleftharpoons H_2CO_3 \rightleftharpoons H^+ + HCO_3^-$$

In this reaction, carbon dioxide is hydrated to carbonic acid, a Brønsted-Lowry acid, which subsequently dissociates to hydrogen (H^+) and bicarbonate (HCO_3^-) ions.

STEWART APPROACH TO ACID-BASE BALANCE

What Determines the Acidity or Alkalinity of a Solution?

The extracellular fluid (ECF) is a solution containing a number of different molecules that directly influence the dissociation of water. It is inconvenient to use the molar concentration of hydrogen and hydroxide to reflect the relative acidity and alkalinity of a solution. The pH scale, developed by Sorenson in the 1920s, is a simple device for acid-base quantification. By using the negative logarithm (p) of the hydrogen ion concentration (H), the pH scale was developed. Neutral pH for pure water is 7.0 (1.0×10^{-7} mmol/L). Physiologic pH for the ECF is 7.4, which is alkaline. Conventionally, we refer to relative acidity and alkalinity from this starting point. If the pH is more than 7.4, the ECF is alkaline (relative to normal), and if the pH is less than 7.4, the ECF is acidic (relative to normal). The pH of the intracellular space is 6.8 to 7.0, and remains constant despite dramatic changes in extracellular pH. The reason for the difference in acidity between the spaces is unclear.[8,9]

To determine the hydrogen ion concentration of ECF, the investigator must look at the dissociation equilibria for all fully dissociated and partially dissociated ionic compounds and apply three simple rules:

1. *Electrical neutrality.* In aqueous solutions in any compartment, the sum of all of the positive charged ions must equal the sum of all of the negative charged ions.
2. *Dissociation equilibria.* The dissociation equilibria of all incompletely dissociated substances, as derived from the law of mass action, must be satisfied at all times.
3. *Mass conservation.* The amount of a substance remains constant unless it is added, removed, generated, or destroyed. The total concentration of an incompletely dissociated substance is the sum of concentrations of its dissociated and undissociated forms.

To determine the acid-base status of a fluid, all substances to which these rules may be applied must be accounted for. A discussion of key groups follows.

Strong Ions

The strong ions, the first group of ions, are relatively simple to incorporate because they dissociate completely. The most abundant strong ions in the extracellular space are Na^+ and Cl^-. Other important strong ions include K^+, SO_4^{2-}, Mg^{2+}, and Ca^{2+}. In a solution containing strong ions created, for example, using specified concentrations of NaOH and HCl, the hydrogen ion concentration can be calculated by solving for electric neutrality:

$$([Na^+] - [Cl^-]) + ([H^+] - [OH^-]) = 0$$

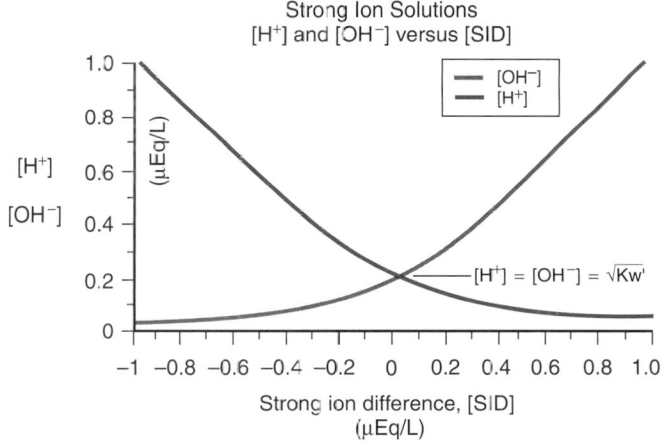

Strong Ion Solutions
$[H^+]$ and $[OH^-]$ versus [SID]

Figure 41–1 Effect of changes in the strong ion gap (SID) on hydrogen and hydroxyl ion concentration. (Adapted from Stewart PA: Modern quantitative acid-base chemistry. Can J Physiol Pharmacol 61:1444-1461, 1983.)

This creates two simultaneous equations:

$$[H^+] = \sqrt{K_w + ([Na^+] - [Cl^-])^2 / 4} - ([Na^-] - [Cl^-])/2$$
$$[OH^-] = \sqrt{K_w + ([Na^+] - [Cl^-])^2 / 4} + ([Na^+] - [Cl^-])/2$$

These equations tell us that hydrogen and hydroxyl concentrations are determined by the Kw and the difference in charge between sodium and chloride. Because the former is constant, in this system, ($[Na^+] - [Cl^-]$) must determine $[H^+]$ and $[OH^-]$. Because the concentration of sodium and chloride are known, the net positive charge minus net negative charge can be quantified. It is the strong ion difference (SID). In any solution, the sum total of the charges imparted by strong cations minus the charges from strong anions represents the SID. The SID independently influences hydrogen ion concentration (Fig. 41-1). In human ECF, the SID is positive.

$$SID = ([Na^+] + [K^+] + [Ca^{2+}] + [Mg^{2+}]) - ([Cl^-] + [A^-])$$
$$= 40 \text{ to } 44 \text{ mEq/L}$$

The pioneering work of Peter Stewart revealed several facts regarding $[H^+]$ that had not previously been understood. SID is always positive in human ECF, and hydroxyl ions almost always exceed hydrogen ions quantitatively in solution. The relationship between the SID and $[H^+]$ is nonlinear in these conditions. Any change in the SID changes the $[H^+]$ and $[OH^-]$ concentrations. Because of the water dissociation constant, this relationship is inverse: as $[H^+]$ increases, $[OH^-]$ decreases. SID is an independent variable, and $[H^+]$ and $[OH^-]$ are dependent, meaning that the addition of hydrogen ions alone (without strong corresponding anions) cannot influence the pH of the solution.

Weak Acid Buffer Solutions

The degree of water dissociation, and therefore the hydrogen ion concentration, is also influenced by charges derived from weak acids. These are partially dissociated compounds whose degree of dissociation is determined by the prevailing temperature and pH. The predominant molecules in this group are albumin and phosphate. Stewart used the term A_{TOT} to represent the total concentration of weak ions that influenced acid-base balance.[10]

The acid, HA, only partly dissociates, represented by the following equilibrium:

$$[HA] = K_A [H^+][A^-]$$

K_A is the weak acid (A^-) dissociation constant. If we assume that HA and A^- play no further part in this reaction (because of the law of mass conservation), the amount of A^- present in the solution must equal the amount initially present:

$$[HA][A^-] = [A_{TOT}]$$

In this equation, $[A_{TOT}]$ is the total weak acid concentration.

To calculate the effect of weak acid dissociation on $[H^+]$, we must take into account water dissociation and electrical neutrality:

$$[H^+] \times [OH^-] = Kw \text{ (water dissociation)}$$
$$[SID] + [H^+] - [A^-] - [OH^-] = 0 \text{ (electrical neutrality)}$$

The four previous simultaneous equations determine the $[H^+]$ in this solution containing strong ions and weak acids. SID and A_{TOT} are independent variables, whose concentration was determined during the production of the system. Kw and K_A are constants. Consequently, the other variables [HA], [H+], $[OH^-]$, and $[A^-]$ must adjust to satisfy the previous equations. They are dependent variables.

Carbon Dioxide

Along with strong ions and weak bases, ECF contains carbon dioxide. The concentration of carbon dioxide in ECF is determined by tissue production and alveolar ventilation. Carbon dioxide, when in solution, exists in four forms: carbon dioxide, denoted $CO_2(d)$; carbonic acid (H_2CO_3); bicarbonate ions (HCO_3^-); and carbonate ions (CO_3^{2-}).

The concentration of $CO_2(d)$ is determined by the solubility coefficient of carbon dioxide (S_{CO_2}), which depends on body temperature, P_{CO_2}, and other factors. Several equilibria equations can be derived from the hydration of CO_2.

$$[CO_2(d)] = [S_{CO_2}] \times P_{CO_2}.$$

The tendency for CO_2 to hydrate to H_2CO_3 and subsequently dissociate to H^+ and HCO_3^- is reflected in the following equation:

$$[CO_2(d)] \times [OH^-] = K_1 \times [HCO_3^-]$$

These equations can be combined together and with water equilibrium to produce the following formula:

$$[H^+] \times [HCO_3^-] = K_c \times P_{CO_2}.$$

Bicarbonate also dissociates to release hydrogen ions and carbonate, the equilibrium reaction for which follows:

$$[H^+] \times [CO_3^{2-}] = K_3 \times [HCO_3^-]$$

Factors Independently Influencing Water Dissociation

After considering the factors that can influence the concentration of hydrogen ions in a solution—strong ions, weak acids, and CO_2—we can combine the derived equations to solve for $[H^+]$:

Water dissociation equilibrium:	$[H^+] \times [OH^-] = K_W$
Weak acid dissociation equilibrium:	$[H^+] \times [A^-] = K_A \times [HA]$
Conservation of mass for weak acids:	$[HA] + [A^-] = [A_{TOT}]$
Bicarbonate ion formation equilibrium:	$[H^+] \times [HCO_3^-] = K_C \times P_{CO_2}$
Carbonate ion formation equilibrium:	$[H^+] \times [CO_3^{2-}] = K_3 \times [HCO_3^-]$
Electrical neutrality:	$[SID] + [H^+] - [HCO_3^-] - [A^-] - [CO_3^{2-}] - [OH^-] = 0$

There are six independent simultaneous equations and just six unknown, dependent variables determined by them: [HA], $[A^-]$, $[HCO_3^-]$, $[CO_3^{2-}]$, $[OH^-]$, and $[H^+]$. There are three known independent variables: [SID], $[A_{TOT}]$, and P_{CO_2}.

Although these equations look relatively simple, they require fourth-order polynomials for solution. This is not possible without computer technology. Solving the equations for $[H^+]$:

$$[H^+]^4 + ([SID] + K_A) \times [H^+]^3 + (K_A \times ([SID] - [A_{TOT}]) - K_w - K_c \times P_{CO_2}) \times [H^+]^2 - (K_A \times (K_w + K_c \times P_{CO_2}) - K_3 \times K_c \times P_{CO_2}) \times [H^+] - K_A \times K_3 \times K_c \times P_{CO_2} = 0$$

In other words, $[H^+]$ is a function of SID, A_{TOT}, P_{CO_2}, and several constants. All other variables, most notably $[H^+]$, $[OH^-]$, and $[HCO_3^-]$, are dependent and cannot independently influence the acid-base balance.

ACID-BASE ABNORMALITIES

The value of the Stewart approach is that it allows us to use a simple model for explaining acid-base disturbances, because all abnormalities can be explained in terms of SID, A_{TOT}, or P_{CO_2}. Traditionally, acid-base disturbances have been classified as caused by alterations in arterial carbon dioxide (Pa_{CO_2}) tension (e.g., respiratory acidosis or alkalosis), and alterations in blood chemistry metabolic acidosis, or alkalosis. This remains a useful classification, although respiratory and metabolic abnormalities rarely occur independently of one another.

Respiratory Acid-Base Abnormalities

Respiratory acidosis occurs when there is an acute rise in $Paco_2$, principally because of respiratory failure (see Chapters 74 and 75). Clinically, there are signs of CO_2 retention: cyanosis, vasodilatation, and narcosis. Respiratory alkalosis occurs when there is an acute decrease in $Paco_2$ caused by hyperventilation. The patient presents with symptoms and signs of vasoconstriction: lightheadedness, visual disturbances, dizziness, and perhaps hypocalcemia because of increased binding of calcium to albumin. The latter condition is caused by an increase in the available negative charge on albumin in alkaline states. Acute hypocalcemia is associated with paresthesia and tetany.

Respiratory acidosis causes a rapid increase in $[H^+]$. Compensation for hypercarbia is slow, requiring increased urinary excretion of chloride.[8] There is a concomitant increase in the serum bicarbonate, reflecting a higher total CO_2 load, rather than compensation. The acuity of respiratory failure can be deduced by looking at the relative ratio of CO_2 to HCO_3^- (Table 41-1). Many investigators have suggested that respiratory acidosis may not necessarily be harmful. There has been extensive clinical experience with "permissive hypercapnia" for acute respiratory failure, which appears to be well tolerated.[9,11,12]

Metabolic Acid-Base Disturbances

Metabolic acid-base abnormalities are caused by alterations in the SID or A_{TOT}, or both. An increase in the SID causes alkalemia; a decrease in the SID causes acidemia. The alternation may be caused by a change in the total or relative concentration of strong ions. For example, a decrease in the SID (i.e., more anions relative to cations) causes acidosis; this may occur because of a net increase in anions (e.g., hyperchloremia, lacticemia) or an increase in the volume of distribution of the same quantity of ions (e.g., dilutional acidosis) (see Table 41-1).

Metabolic acidosis is of clinical significance for two reasons: pathologies arising from the acidosis itself and pathologies arising from the cause of the acidosis. Acidosis is associated with alterations in transcellular ion pumps and increased ionized calcium. The result is vasodilation,

diminished muscular performance (particularly myocardial), and arrhythmias. The oxyhemoglobin dissociation curve shifts rightward to increase oxygen offload into the tissues. Rapid-onset metabolic acidosis may be associated with profound hypotension, cardiac arrhythmias, and death. The malignancy of the acidosis is strongly related to the underlying disease process; lactic acidosis caused by circulatory shock is more malevolent than hyperchloremic acidosis due to excessive administration of normal saline.[13] The body is hyperresponsive to acidosis. Increasing the hydrogen ion content in cerebrospinal fluid activates the respiratory center to stimulate respiration. Alveolar ventilation increases, reducing arterial CO_2 content and reducing the total body $[H^+]$. Bicarbonate concentration simultaneously decreases because of buffering activity and the reduction in total CO_2. This prevents abrupt reductions in plasma pH in acute metabolic acidosis.

Metabolic alkalosis rarely occurs as a result of acute illness. Symptoms and signs of metabolic alkalosis include widespread vasoconstriction, lightheadedness, tetany, and paresthesia. The main compensatory mechanism is hypoventilation, which may delay weaning from mechanical ventilation in critically ill patients (see Chapters 74 and 75).

An understanding of the mechanisms by which alterations in the SID affect acid-base balance clarifies many of the abnormalities that have remained unexplained by traditional teaching. Of key importance is the ability to differentiate the change in the SID that results from altered free water balance from that arising from altered concentrations of measured and unmeasured electrolytes.

An average man of 70 kg has a total-body water content of approximately 45 L, two thirds of which are in the intracellular space. Approximately 15 L are extracellular. The $[Na^+]$ in this compartment is 140 mEq/L, $[Cl^-]$ is 100 mEq/L, and $[K^+]$ is 4 mEq/L. For simplicity, we ignore magnesium, calcium, other strong ions, and CO_2. In this system, the SID is 44 mEq/L, with this positive charge being balanced principally by weak acids. Anything that increases the SID increases the relative concentration of strong cations to strong anions and alkalinizes the solution. Anything that decreases the SID decreases the relative concentration of cations to anions and acidifies the solution.

When the volume of this compartment is expanded by 2 L, as occurs with rapid infusion of 5% dextrose, the $[Na^+]$ falls to 123 mEq/L, the $[K^+]$ falls to 3.5 mEq/L, and the $[Cl^-]$ falls to 88 mEq/L. The relative ratio of cations to anions also falls, and the SID decreases to 38.5 mEq/L. The system becomes more acidic. This is the basis of *dilutional acidosis*.

Conversely, if 2 L of free water are removed from the system and the total concentration of ions remains unchanged (as would occur with profuse sweating or dehydration), the opposite would occur. $[Na^+]$ rises to 161 mEq/L, $[K^+]$ increases to 4.6 mEq/L, and $[Cl^-]$ increases to 115 mEq/L. The relative ratio of cations to anions actually rises, and SID increases to 50.6 mEq/L. The system becomes more alkaline. This is the basis of *contraction alkalosis*.

In perioperative medicine, normal saline (0.9% NaCl), containing 154 mEq/L of sodium and 154 mEq/L of

Table 41–1 Changes in $Paco_2$ and $[HCO_3^-]$ in response to acute and chronic acid-base disturbances

Disturbances	$[HCO_3^-]$ vs. $Paco_2$
Acute respiratory acidosis	$\Delta HCO_3^- = 0.2 \, \Delta Paco_2$
Acute respiratory alkalosis	$\Delta HCO_3^- = 0.2 \, \Delta Paco_2$
Chronic respiratory acidosis	$\Delta HCO_3^- = 0.5 \, \Delta Paco_2$
Metabolic acidosis	$\Delta Paco_2 = 1.3 \, \Delta HCO_3^-$
Metabolic alkalosis	$\Delta Paco_2 = 0.75 \, \Delta HCO_3^-$

Δ, change in value; $[HCO_3^-]$, concentration of bicarbonate ion; $Paco_2$, partial pressure of arterial carbon dioxide.
Modified from Narins RB, Emmett M: Simple and mixed acid-base disorders: A practical approach. Medicine (Baltimore) 59:161-187, 1980.

chloride, is commonly used. The SID of this solution is 0. For example, a patient who loses 5 L of ECF and is given 5 L of NaCl as replacement would be expected to have a net gain in sodium and chloride. In this scenario, [Na$^+$] increases to 144 mEq/L, [K$^+$] decreases to 2.6 mEq/L, and [Cl$^-$] increases to 118 mEq/L. The SID decreases to 29 mEq/L. This is the basis of *hyperchloremic acidosis.*[14]

Any process that leads to dilution of the total number of ions (i.e., charged particles) in the solution can be expected to cause acidosis. As examples, consider the use of mannitol therapeutically (before the diuresis) or hyperglycemia or ethylene glycol or the pathology of methanol poisoning. This process increases the volume of water without changing the net charge and results in a dilutional acidosis. Any process that removes chloride without sodium, such as aggressive nasogastric suctioning that removes HCl, causes metabolic alkalosis (i.e., hypochloremic alkalosis) because of an increase in the SID. The alkalosis is caused by chloride loss, which obeys the law of conservation of mass (i.e., there is a finite quantity available in the ECF), not hydrogen ions, whose source, water, is unlimited. Severe diarrhea, which is associated with loss of potassium and sodium, reduces the SID, and is associated with metabolic acidosis. Aggressive use of diuretics causes a net loss of free water over sodium and chloride and causes contraction alkalosis.

The most malignant form of metabolic acidosis is associated with a net gain of *unmeasured* anions (i.e., electrolytes not conventionally measured on serum chemistry analysis) and, consequently, a decreased SID.

1. In dysoxia, lactate is produced, reducing the SID and causing acidosis.
2. In out-of-control diabetes (i.e., ketoacidosis), β-hydroxybutyrate and acetoacetate are produced, reducing the SID and causing acidosis.
3. In severe renal failure, SO$_4^{2-}$ and PO$_4^{3-}$ (i.e., fixed renal acids) are not excreted, causing acidosis.

The mechanism of acidosis is similar to previous examples. If, in our patient with [Na$^+$] = 140 mEq/L, [Cl$^-$] = 100 mEq/L, and [K$^+$] = 4 mEq/L, an additional anion (i.e., lactate) is added at a concentration of 10 mEq/L, the SID decreases to 34 mEq/L, and the system becomes more acidemic.

The total weak acid pool, principally serum albumin and phosphate, is also an important determinant of acid-base status. Hyperphosphatemia has long been associated with the acidosis of renal failure, and hypoalbuminemia is common in clinical practice. There is a strong association between hypoalbuminemia and the severity of critical illness. This occurs because of hepatic reprioritization of visceral protein production toward acute-phase reactants, capillary leak, breakdown of preexisting albumin (so that its constituent amino acids can be used for protein synthesis), and hemodilution with isotonic fluids. Hypoalbuminemia decreases A$_{TOT}$ and is associated with metabolic alkalosis.[15]

The impact of hypoalbuminemia on acid-base balance has been grossly underestimated. Stewart's original theory was modified by Fencl and Figge.[16] The serum albumin concentration is the core negative charge offsetting the net positive charge of the SID.[17] Consequently, the presence of hypoalbuminemia may mask the detection of acidosis,[18] such as by unmeasured anions (UMAs), when using the conventional tools of acid-base chemistry, pH, base deficit, and the anion gap.[19] The presence of hypoalbuminemia has significant implications, not least for its association with adverse outcomes,[18,20] unlike abnormalities of the SID, which have not been shown to have prognostic significance. Hyperalbuminemia is very unusual; nonetheless, in cholera, when associated with hemoconcentration, it is associated with acidosis.[21]

Fencl neatly categorized acid-base disturbances along respiratory and metabolic lines (Table 41-2). This elegantly explains all known acid-base disturbances.

Table 41–2 Classification of primary acid-base abnormalities

Abnormalities	Acidosis	Alkalosis
Respiratory	Increased Pco$_2$	Decreased Pco$_2$
Metabolic		
Abnormal SID		
Caused by water excess or deficit	Water excess = dilutional ↓ SID + ↓ [Na$^+$]	Water deficit = contraction ↑ SID ↑ [Na$^+$]
Caused by electrolytes	Chloride excess	Chloride deficit
Chloride (measured)	↓ SID ↑ [Cl$^-$]	↑ SID + ↓ [Cl$^-$]
Other (unmeasured) anions, such as lactate and keto acids	↓ SID ↑ [UMA$^-$]	—
Abnormal A$_{TOT}$		
Albumin [Alb]	↑ [Alb] (rare)	↓ [Alb]
Phosphate [Pi]	↑ [Pi]	

[Alb], concentration of serum albumin; A$_{TOT}$, to represent the total concentration of weak ions; [Cl$^-$], concentration of chloride ions; [Na$^+$], concentration of sodium ions; Pco$_2$, partial pressure of carbon dioxide; [Pi], concentration of inorganic phosphate; SID, strong ion difference; [UMA$^-$], unmeasured anions; ↑, increased; ↓, decreased.
Adapted from Fencl V, Jabor A, Kazda A, Figge J: Diagnosis of metabolic acid-base disturbances in critically ill patients. Am J Respir Crit Care Med 162:2246-2251, 2000.

There are significant differences between the mechanisms causing acid-base imbalances. It would be reasonable to predict significantly different outcomes for patients developing acidosis from dilution, poisoning, hyperchloremia, excessive use of normal saline infusions, or dysoxia due to increased production of lactate. The acid-base abnormalities, in themselves, may be of less clinical significance than previously thought.[9]

REGULATION OF ACID-BASE BALANCE

Extracellular hydrogen ion concentration appears to be tightly controlled by the body. This should be viewed in terms of volatile and metabolic acids. A variety of intracellular and extracellular weak acid buffering systems have developed to prevent rapid changes in the electrochemical balance in the extracellular space from interfering with transcellular ion pumps. A *buffer* is a solution of two or more chemicals that minimizes changes in pH in response to the addition of an acid or base. Most buffers are weak acids. Ideally, a buffer has a pK_a that is equal to the pH, and an ideal body buffer has a pK_a between 6.8 and 7.2.

The major source of acid in the body is CO_2, from which is produced 12,500 mEq of H^+ each day. This is excreted by the lungs. In contrast, only 20 to 70 mEq of H^+-promoting anions are excreted through the kidney each day. Volatile acid is principally buffered by hemoglobin. Deoxygenated hemoglobin is a strong base, and there would be a huge rise in the pH of venous blood if hemoglobin did not bind hydrogen ions (derived from oxidative metabolism). Venous blood contains 1.68 mmol/L of extra CO_2 over arterial blood: 65% as HCO_3^- and H^+ bound to hemoglobin, 27% as carbaminohemoglobin (i.e., CO_2 bound to hemoglobin), and 8% dissolved.

CO_2 easily passes through cell membranes. Within the erythrocyte, CO_2 combines with H_2O under the influence of carbonic anhydrase to form H_2CO_3, which ionizes to hydrogen and bicarbonate. Hydrogen ions bind to histidine residues on deoxyhemoglobin, and bicarbonate is actively pumped out of the cell. Chloride moves inward to maintain electroneutrality (i.e., chloride shift). Large increases in Pco_2 (i.e., respiratory acidosis) overwhelm this system, leading to a rapid, dramatic drop in pH. The *metabolic compensation*[3] for respiratory acidosis is increased SID by removal of chloride from the extracellular space, initially transcellularly and subsequently through urinary loss. There is a concomitant increase in $[HCO_3^-]$, often misrepresented as compensation for the increase in $Paco_2$. $[HCO_3^-]$ is a dependent variable, which increases or decreases with Pco_2. The rate of conversion of CO_2 to HCO_3^- depends on carbonic anhydrase activity and occurs slowly. It is possible to mathematically determine whether a rise in $Paco_2$ is acute or long-standing (see Table 4-2).

Metabolic acid is buffered principally by increased alveolar ventilation, producing respiratory alkalosis and extracellular weak acids. These weak acids include plasma proteins, phosphate, and bicarbonate. The bicarbonate buffering system (92% of plasma buffering and 13% overall) is probably the most important extracellular buffer.

The pK_a of bicarbonate is relatively low (6.1), but the system derives its importance because of the enormous quantity of CO_2 in the body. The coupling of bicarbonate and H_2O produces CO_2, which is then excreted through the lungs. There is an increase in alveolar ventilation. Physicians must be aware of the importance of this compensatory mechanism. For example, anesthetized or critically ill patients on controlled mechanical ventilation lose the capacity to regulate their own Pco_2. Consequently, the combination of acute metabolic and respiratory acidosis can cause a devastating reduction in pH.

The major effect of the kidney on acid-base balance is related to renal handling of sodium and chloride ions. Because dietary intake of sodium and chloride is roughly equal, the kidney excretes a net chloride load, using NH_4^+, a weak cation, to accompany chloride (electrochemically) in the urine.

In metabolic acidosis, chloride is preferentially excreted by the kidney. In metabolic alkalosis, chloride is retained, and sodium and potassium are excreted. The presence of bicarbonate in the urine reflects the needs to maintain electrical neutrality. In renal tubular acidosis, there is an inability to excrete Cl^- in proportion to Na^+. The diagnosis can be made by observing a hyperchloremic metabolic acidosis with inappropriately low levels of Cl^- in the urine; the urinary SID is positive. If the urinary SID is negative, the process is not renal. The other causes of hyperchloremic metabolic acidosis are gastrointestinal losses (e.g., diarrhea, small bowel or pancreatic drainage), parenteral nutrition, excessive administration of saline; and the use of carbonic anhydrase inhibitors.

ANALYTIC TOOLS USED IN ACID-BASE CHEMISTRY

Textbooks and clinical practice have tended to overestimate the importance of isolated changes in hydrogen or bicarbonate ion concentration. An emerging body of evidence suggests that the clinical significance of acid-base perturbations is determined by the underlying cause rather than the serum concentration of hydrogen and hydroxyl ions. Nevertheless, acid-base chemistry remains a mainstay of clinical data interpretation because of ubiquitous availability, low cost, and universal acceptance. The accuracy of acid-base measurements, however, is not determined by the blood gas value alone, which measures volatile acid and pH. Rather, measurement of each of the strong and weak ions that influence water dissociation, although cumbersome, is essential.

Acid-base abnormalities are best described by alterations in Pco_2, SID, and A_{TOT}. Unfortunately, many approaches used to teach and describe the acid-base status of a patient fail to adequately explain many commonly seen perioperative acid-base abnormalities (e.g., dilutional or hyperchloremic acidosis) and mislead us about the cause of the problem (i.e., dilutional acidosis is caused by reduced SID, not dilution of bicarbonate). Although it is important to consider historically used approaches, modern approaches to acid-base interrogation focus on physical chemistry to calculate the magnitude of the disturbance in the SID or recalculate the base deficit or excess (BDE) using the SID and A_{TOT}. We next consider some of the tools that have evolved over the past 50 years to assist in interpretation of acid-base conundrums. None is entirely accurate, and each has a dedicated group of followers.[23] We deal with each of these approaches chronologically and discuss the merits and demerits.

Carbon Dioxide–Bicarbonate (Boston) Approach

Schwartz, Brackett, and others,[21a,21b] at Tufts University in Boston, developed an approach to acid-base chemistry using acid-base maps and the mathematical relationship between carbon dioxide tension and serum bicarbonate (or total CO_2), derived from the Henderson-Hasselbalch equation, to predict the nature of acid-base disturbances (see Table 41-2). A number of patients with known acid-base disturbances at steady states of compensation were evaluated. The degree of compensation from what was considered normal was measured for each disease state. The investigators were able to describe six primary states of acid-base imbalance using linear equations or maps relating hydrogen ion concentration to Pco_2 for respiratory disturbances and Pco_2 to HCO_3^- concentration for metabolic disturbances (Fig. 41-2). For any given acid-base disturbance, an expected HCO_3^- concentration was determined. For most simple disturbances, this is a reasonable approach.

Using these maps and equations, physicians have been able to determine the nature of most respiratory and metabolic acid-base disturbances. Although there is a mathematical relationship in place, alterations in H^+ and HCO_3^- do not reflect cause and effect. For example, chronic hypoventilation is associated with an increase in Pco_2 and HCO_3^-. Many physicians have incorrectly assigned the increase in HCO_3^- as compensation for raised Pco_2. It is not. The increased HCO_3^- concentration reflects increased total CO_2 in the body. Alterations in HCO_3^- reflect its role as a buffer, CO_2 by-product, and weak acid.

Although the Pco_2-HCO_3^- approach is relatively accurate for most disturbances, there are several inherent pitfalls, particularly in relation to the metabolic component. First, the approach is not as simple as it seems, requiring the clinician to refer to confusing maps or to learn formulas and perform mental arithmetic. Second, the system neither explains nor accounts for many of the complex acid-base abnormalities seen in perioperative and critically ill patients, such as those with acute acidosis in the setting of hypoalbuminemia, hyperchloremic acidosis, or dilutional acidosis or with lactic acidosis in the setting of chronic respiratory acidosis.

Base Deficit or Excess (Copenhagen) Approach

Singer and Hastings[24] pioneered an alternative approach to acid-base chemistry in 1948, by moving away from the Henderson-Hasselbalch description toward quantifying the metabolic component. They proposed that the whole blood buffer base (BB) could be used for this purpose. The buffer base represented the sum of the bicarbonate and the nonvolatile buffer ions (essentially the serum albumin, phosphate, and hemoglobin). Applying the law of electrical neutrality, the buffer base was forced to equal the electrical charge difference between strong (fully dissociated) ions. Normally, $BB = [Na^+] + [K^+] - [Cl^-]$. Alterations in buffer base essentially represented changes in strong ion concentrations (which could not be easily measured in 1948), buffer base increases in metabolic alkalosis, and decreases in metabolic acidosis. The major drawback of the use of buffer base measurements is the potential for changes in buffering capacity associated with alterations in hemoglobin concentration.

In 1958, Siggard-Anderson and colleagues[24a] developed a simpler measure of metabolic acid-base activity, the BDE (base deficit or excess). They defined the BDE as the amount of strong acid or base required to return pH to 7.4, assuming a Pco_2 of 40 mm Hg and temperature of 38°C. The initial use of whole blood base excess was criticized because of the dynamic activity of red blood cells within the acid-base paradigm of gas and electrolyte exchange. This approach was modified in the 1960s to use only serum base excess (BE), and the calculation became the *standardized* base excess (SBE). Like the Boston group, their data were based on observations of a large population of patients, leading to the development of nomograms (Fig. 41-3 and see Table 41-3). Current algorithms for computing the SBE are derived from the Van Slyke equation (1977).[25] The BDE approach to acid-base chemistry has been successfully validated by Schlitig[26] and Morgan.[27]

The SBE is computed by blood gas analyzers by using the following equation:

$$SBE = 0.9287 \times [HCO_3^- - 24.4 + (pH - 7.4)].$$

Simple mathematical rules can be applied using the BDE in each of the common acid-base disturbances. For example,

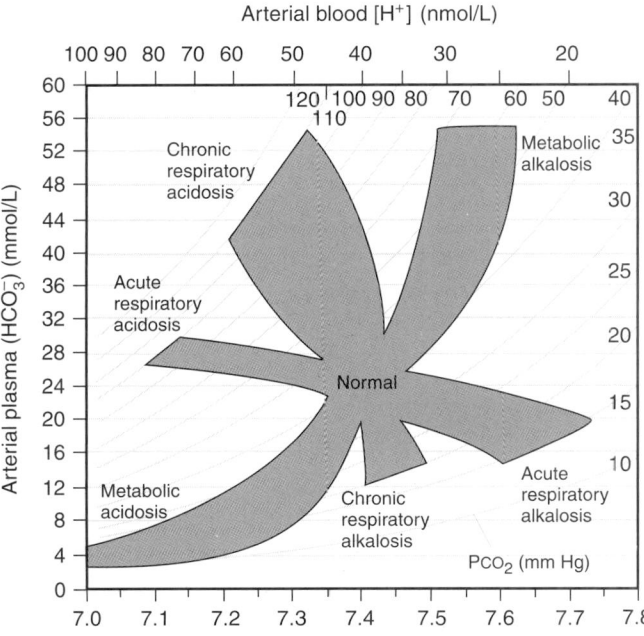

Arterial blood [H⁺] (nmol/L)

Figure 41–2 Acid-base nomogram using the Boston approach. Different acid-base disturbances can be distinguished based on the relative values of Pco_2 and HCO_3^-. (Adapted from Brenner BM, Rector FC: The Kidney, 3rd ed. Philadelphia, WB Saunders, 1986, p 473.)

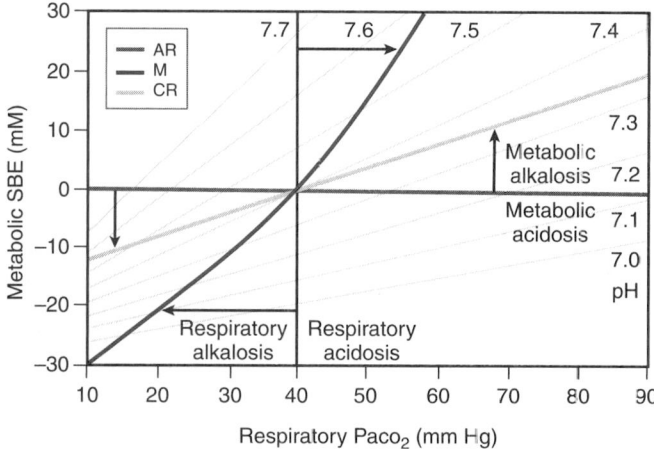

Figure 41–3 Acid-base nomogram using the Copenhagen approach as revised by Schlichtig. The various acid-base disturbances can be distinguished based on P_{CO_2} and base deficit or excess, here referred to as standard base excess (SBE). *Arrows* represent changes as the body compensates for acute acidosis or alkalosis. AR, acute respiratory acidosis or alkalosis; CR, chronic respiratory acidosis or alkalosis; M, metabolic acidosis or alkalosis. (From Schlichtig R, Grogono AW, Severinghaus JW: Human Pa_{CO_2} and standard base excess compensation for acid-base imbalance. Crit Care Med 26: 1173-1179, 1998.)

in acute respiratory acidosis or alkalosis, BDE does not change. Conversely, in acute metabolic acidosis, the magnitude of change of the P_{CO_2} (in millimeters of mercury) is the same as that of the BDE (in milliequivalents per liter) (Table 41-3).

There has been considerable discussion over the past 30 years about the merits and demerits of the BDE compared with the CO_2-HCO_3^- system. In reality, there is little difference between the two; both equations and nomograms were derived from in vivo patient data and abstracted backward. Consequently, for most patients, either approach is relatively accurate but misleading. Using measures of buffer base as a means of quantifying acid-base disturbances, these techniques do not allow the clinician to distinguish between, for example, acidosis

Table 41–3   Changes in standardized base deficit or excess in response to acute and chronic acid-base disturbances

Disturbance	BDE vs. Pa_{CO_2}
Acute respiratory acidosis	$\Delta BDE = 0$
Acute respiratory alkalosis	$\Delta BDE = 0$
Chronic respiratory acidosis	$\Delta BDE = 0.4\ \Delta Pa_{CO_2}$
Metabolic acidosis	$\Delta Pa_{CO_2} = \Delta BDE$
Metabolic alkalosis	$\Delta Pa_{CO_2} = 0.6\ \Delta BDE$

BDE, base deficit or excess; Δ, change in value; Pa_{CO_2}, partial pressure of arterial oxygen.
Modified from Narins RB, Emmett M: Simple and mixed acid-base disorders: A practical approach. Medicine (Baltimore) 59:161-187, 1980.

due to lactate or chloride, or alkalosis due to dehydration or hypoalbuminemia. These measures may miss the presence of an acid-base disturbance entirely; for example a hypoalbuminemic (metabolic alkalosis), critically ill patient with a lactic acidosis may have a normal range pH, bicarbonate, and BE. This may lead to inappropriate therapy.

Anion Gap Approach

The first and most widely used tool for investigating metabolic acidosis is the anion gap (AG), developed by Emmit and Narins in 1975.[28] This is based on the law of electrical neutrality and is entirely consistent with the work of Stewart and Fencl. The system is based on data that were not easily available or known at the time of publication: the contribution to electrical neutrality ascribed to weak acids (phosphate and albumin) and UMAs. The sum of the difference in charge of the common extracellular ions reveals an unaccounted for a gap of -10 to -12 mEq/L, because the AG is equal to $Na^+ + K^+ - (Cl^- + HCO_3^-)$ (Fig. 41-4). If the patient develops a metabolic acidosis, and the gap "widens" to, for example, -16 mEq/L, the acidosis is caused by UMAs (lactate or ketones). If the gap does not widen, the anions are being measured, and the acidosis has been caused by hyperchloremia (bicarbonate cannot independently influence acid-base status). Although this is a useful tool, it is weakened by the assumption of what is or is not a normal gap.[29] Most critically ill patients are hypoalbuminemic, and many are also hypophosphatemic.[30] Consequently, the gap may be normal in the presence of UMAs. This has been extensively studied by Fencl and Figge,[19] who provided a variant known as the *corrected anion gap*:

Anion gap corrected = calculated anion gap + 2.5
(for albumin)   × (normal albumin [in g/dL]
                         – observed albumin [in g/dL])

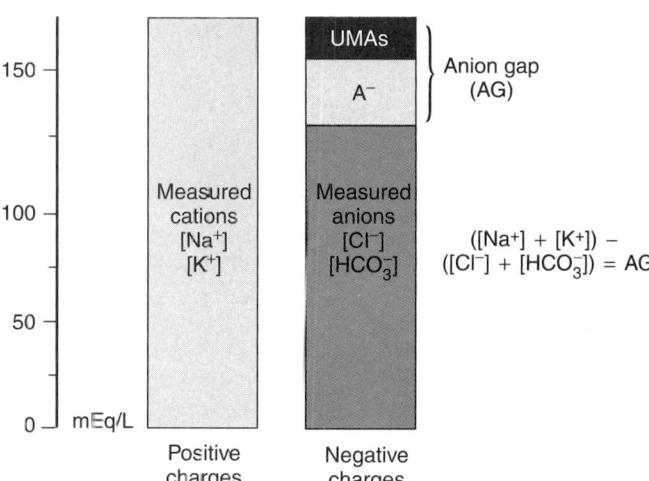

Figure 41–4 The anion gap represents the difference in charge between measured cations and measured anions. The missing negative charge is made up of weak acids (A^-), such as albumin and phosphate, and strong unmeasured anions (UMAs), such as lactate.

The second weakness with this approach is the use of bicarbonate in the equation. An alteration in $[HCO_3^-]$ concentration can occur for reasons independent of metabolic disturbance, such as hyperventilation. The base deficit (BD) and AG frequently underestimate the extent of the metabolic disturbance.[18] Nonetheless, the AG is useful in differentiating acidosis from UMAs from hyperchloremic acidosis in a previously healthy patient (e.g., in acute trauma).

Stewart-Fencl Approach

A more accurate reflection of true acid-base status can be derived using the Stewart-Fencl approach.[1,2] This is based on the concept of electrical neutrality, a small advance from using the AG. There exists in plasma a SID of $[(Na^+ + Mg^{2+} + Ca^{2+} = K^+) - (Cl^- + A^-)]$ of 40 to 44m Eq/L, balanced by the negative charge on bicarbonate and A_{TOT} (the buffer base). There is a small difference between SIDa (apparent SID) and buffer base (effective SID [SIDe]). This represents a strong ion gap (SIG), which quantifies the amount of unmeasured anions present (Fig. 41-5).

$$SIDa = ([Na^+] + [K^+] + [Mg^{2+}] + [Ca^{2-}]) - [Cl^-]$$
$$SIDe = [HCO_3^-] + (\text{charge on albumin}) + (\text{charge on inorganic phosphate [Pi]}) \text{ (in mmol/L)}$$

Weak acids' degree of ionization is pH dependent, and calculations must include this:

$$[alb] = [alb] \text{ (in g/L)} \times (0.123 \times pH - 0.631)$$
$$[Pi] \text{ (in mg/dL)} = [Pi] / 10 \times pH - 0.47.$$
$$SIG = SIDa - SIDe$$

The weakness of this system is that the SIG does not necessarily represent unmeasured strong anions but merely all anions that are unmeasured. SID changes quantitatively in absolute and relative terms when there are changes in plasma water concentration. Fencl addressed this problem by correcting the chloride concentration for free water, [Cl⁻]corrected with the following equation:

$$[Cl^-]\text{corrected} = [Cl^-]\text{observed} \times ([Na^+]\text{normal}/ [Na^+]\text{observed})$$

This corrected chloride concentration may be then inserted into the previous SIDa equation. Likewise, the derived value for UMAs should also be corrected for free water using UMAs instead of Cl^- in the previous equation.[18] In a series of nine normal subjects, Fencl estimated the normal SIG as 8 ± 2 mEq/L.[18]

Although accurate, the SIG is cumbersome and expensive, requiring measurement of multiple ions and albumin. An alternative approach, used by Gilfix and colleagues[31] and subsequently by Balasubramanyan and coworkers,[32] is to calculate the BD or base excess gap (BEG). This allows recalculation of BDE using strong ions, free water, and albumin. The resulting BEG (i.e., BE caused by UMAs) should mirror the SIG and AG, and these terms may be manipulated to provide the following equations and definitions:

BEG = BDE – CBE
BDE = Standard BDE
CBE = Calculated BDE
    BEfw = Changes in free water = 0.3 × (Na – 140)
    BECl = Changes in chloride = 102 – (Cl – 140/Na)
    BEalb = Changes in albumin = 3.4 × (4.5 – albumin)
CBE = BEfw + BECl + BEalb

It is probable that no single number will ever allow us to make sense of complex acid-base disturbances. Fencl[18] has suggested that, rather than focusing on AG or BDE, physicians should address each blood gas in terms of all alkalinizing and acidifying effects: respiratory acidosis or alkalosis, the presence or absence of abnormal SID (due to water excess or deficit, measured electrolytes or unmeasured electrolytes), and abnormal A_{TOT}. This does not necessarily mean that when examining a blood gas result and serum chemistry profile, the physician is required to perform a series of calculations. Many acid-base abnormalities can be inferred by "eyeballing" the laboratory values[18]:

1. Hyperchloremic acidemia is usually present if the corrected serum chloride level is more than 112 mEq/L.
2. Hypochloremic alkalemia is usually present when the corrected serum chloride level is less than 100 mEq/L.
3. Dilutional acidemia is usually present when the serum sodium level is less than 136 mEq/L.
4. Contraction alkalemia is usually present when the serum sodium level is more than 148 mEq/L.
5. Hyperphosphatemic acidemia is usually present when the serum phosphate level is more than 2.0 mmol/L.
6. Hypoalbuminemic alkalosis is usually present when the serum albumin level is less than 3.5 g/dL.

Although this approach may appear inelegant, it has the advantage of being comprehensive. Consider the following data for a patient described by Fencl[18] (in mEq/L unless

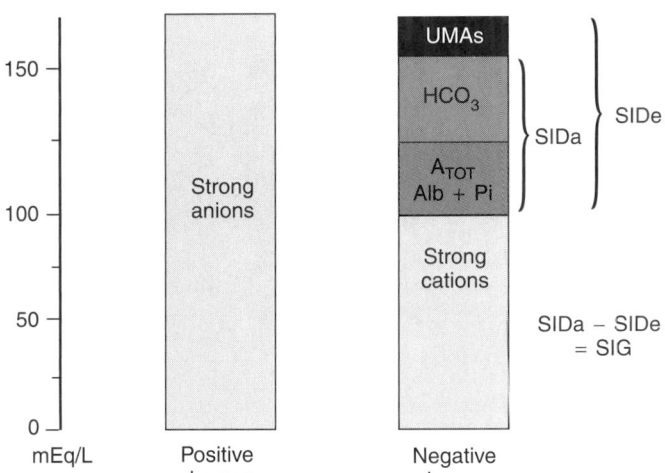

Figure 41–5 The strong ion gap apparent (SIDa) is the sum of the total concentration of weak ions (A_{TOT}), such as albumin (Alb) and inorganic phosphate (Pi), plus the concentration of bicarbonate ions $[HCO_3^-]$. SID effective (SIDe) is the real SID. The difference between the two is made up of unmeasured anions (UMAs).

otherwise stated): Na = 117, K = 3.9, Ca = 3.0, Mg = 1.4, Cl = 92, Pi = 0.6 mmol/L, albumin = 6.0 g/L, pH = 7.33, P_{CO_2} = 30 mm Hg, HCO_3 = 15, AG = 13, $AG_{corrected}$ = 23, BE = −10, SID = 18, $Cl_{corrected}$ = 112, and $UMA_{corrected}$ = 18. Using traditional methodology, this would be described as a non-AG metabolic acidosis, and the physician would look for causes of bicarbonate wasting, such as renal tubular acidosis or gastrointestinal losses. The degree of respiratory alkalosis is appropriate for the degree of acidosis ($\Delta BD = \Delta P_{CO_2}$). However, the Fencl-Stewart method reveals a much more complex situation. SID is reduced to 18 mEq/L, caused by free water excess, UMAs, and surprisingly, hyperchloremia (see the corrected chloride value). However, the degree of acidosis does not mirror this metabolic disturbance because of the alkalizing force at play: hypoalbuminemia. The corrected AG mirrors the change in SID, but this is grossly underestimated by the BD. This patient has a dilutional acidosis, a hyperchloremic acidosis, and a lactic acidosis!

For most patients presenting to the emergency room or operating suite who have been previously healthy, the use of tools such as the BD or AG to assess metabolic disturbances remains reasonable. However, for critically ill patients, the most effective method of interpreting acid-base conundrums involves unraveling synchronous acidifying and alkalinizing processes and using calculations or rules of thumb to distinguish between the various forces at play. Unfortunately, a clinician's ability to interpret such information depends on the amount of available data. A simple blood gas determination alone may camouflage a significant acid-base disturbance.

ACID-BASE PROBLEMS IN DIFFERENT CLINICAL SETTINGS

Simple acid-base disturbances can be evaluated using the following strategy.

Step 1. Look at the pH.

    <7.35 = acidosis

    7.35 to 7.5 = normal or compensated acidosis

    >7.5 = alkalosis

Step 2. Look for respiratory component (volatile acid = CO_2).

    P_{CO_2} < 35 mm Hg = respiratory alkalosis or compensation for metabolic (if so, BD > −5) acidosis.

    P_{CO_2} = 35 to 45 (normal range)

    P_{CO_2} >45 = respiratory acidosis (acute if pH < 7.35; chronic if pH in normal range and BE > 5).

Step 3. Look for a metabolic component (i.e., buffer base use). BD is the amount of strong cation required to bring pH back to 7.4, with P_{CO_2} corrected at 40 mm Hg. BE is the amount of strong anion required to bring pH back to 7.4, with P_{CO_2} corrected at 40 mm Hg.

    BD > −5 = metabolic acidosis

    BE −5 to +5 = normal range

    BE >5 = alkalosis

Combining this information, the following options are possible:

1. Acidosis, CO_2 < 35 mm Hg, ± BD > −5 = acute metabolic acidosis

2. Normal-range pH, CO_2 < 35, BD > −5 = acute metabolic acidosis plus compensation

3. Acidosis, P_{CO_2} > 45, normal-range BDE = acute respiratory acidosis

4. Normal-range pH, P_{CO_2} >45, BE >+5 = prolonged respiratory acidosis

5. Alkalosis, P_{CO_2} > 45, BE > +5 = metabolic alkalosis

6. Alkalosis, P_{CO_2} < 35, normal-range BDE = acute respiratory alkalosis

7. If the acid-base picture does not conform to any of these options, a mixed pattern exists.

Acid-Base Disturbances in Emergency Settings

Acid-base disturbances are an important part of laboratory investigation of acutely ill patients. The common disturbances are acute respiratory acidosis or alkalosis and acute metabolic acidosis. Acute metabolic alkalosis is unusual. Mixed respiratory acidosis and metabolic acidosis is seen in the severely injured or infected patient.

Acute respiratory acidosis results from hypoventilation due to loss of respiratory drive, neuromuscular or chest wall disorders, or rapid, shallow breathing, which increases the fraction of dead-space ventilation. Acute respiratory alkalosis is caused by hyperventilation due to anxiety, central respiratory stimulation (e.g., in salicylate poisoning), or excessive artificial ventilation. Acute respiratory alkalosis usually accompanies acute metabolic acidosis, in which case the reduction in P_{CO_2} from baseline (usually 40 mm Hg) is equal to the magnitude of the BD. For example, in a patient with lactic acidosis with a lactate concentration of 10 mEq/L, the BD should be −10, and the P_{CO_2} should be 30 mm Hg. If the P_{CO_2} is higher than expected, there is a problem with the respiratory apparatus. This is seen, for example, in a multitrauma patient who has massive blood loss, causing lactic acidosis, and a flail chest, causing respiratory acidosis.

Acute metabolic acidosis is caused by an alteration in the SID or A_{TOT}. The SID is changed by an alteration in the relative quantity of strong anions to strong cations. This can be caused by anion gain, as occurs with lactic acidosis, renal acidosis, ketoacidosis, and hyperchloremic acidosis, or by cation loss, as occurs with severe diarrhea or renal tubular acidosis. Acidosis also results from increased free water relative to strong ions; dilutional acidosis, which occurs with excessive hypotonic fluid intake; certain poisonings, such as methanol, ethylene glycol, or isopropyl alcohol; hyperglycemia; or after mannitol administration.

To investigate acute metabolic acidosis in previously healthy patients, simple observational and mathematical tools such as the AG and BD are useful (Table 41-4). The BD merely demonstrates the presence of an acid-base anomaly; the AG (= $[Na^+ + K^+] - [Cl^- + HCO_3^-]$) separates acidosis due to hyperchloremia (e.g., renal tubular acidosis, excessive administration of normal saline) from that caused by UMAs and dilution. Many UMAs, such as lactate and ketones, are measurable. When a patient presents with acute metabolic upset caused by trauma, exsanguination, loss of consciousness, or tachypnea, a blood gas determination, electrolyte panel, serum osmolality level, and urinalysis should be obtained.

Table 41–4 Evaluation of a patient with metabolic acidosis

1. Is the acidosis caused by measured or unmeasured anions (e.g., chloride)?

Look at the blood chemistry:
  Calculate the anion gap: Na + K – Cl = 10 to 12.
  If the gap is normal, there is too much chloride present from excessive administration, excess loss of sodium (e.g., diarrhea, ileostomy), or renal tubular acidosis.
  If the gap is wide (>16), other unmeasured anions are present, causing the acidosis.

Check the serum lactate level; if > 2, lactic acidosis is probably the cause:
  If the high lactate level is explained by circulatory insufficiency (e.g., shock, hypovolemia, oliguria, under-resuscitation, anemia, carbon monoxide poisoning, seizures), this is type A lactic acidosis.
  If not explained by circulatory insufficiency, consider the type B lactic acidosis (rare) causes, such as biguanides, fructose, sorbitol, nitroprusside, ethylene glycol, cancer, and liver disease.

Look at the creatinine and urine output:
  If the patient is in acute renal failure, the identified molecules may be renal acids.
  Assess the blood glucose and urinary ketone levels.
  If the patient is hyperglycemic and ketotic, this condition is diabetic ketoacidosis.
  If the patient is ketotic (unmeasured anion) and normoglycemic, this condition is alcoholic (check blood alcohol) or starvation ketosis.
  Check for chronic alcohol abuse (e.g., high mean corpuscular volume, raised γ-glutamyl-transferase level on the liver panel).

2. If all of the previous tests are negative, consider intoxication as a cause.
  The toxicology laboratory can assess samples (particularly salicylates) and serum osmolality. Osmolality is calculated with the following formula: 2 (Na + K) + Glucose/18 + BUN/2.8.
  Look for an unmeasured source of osmoles. If the gap between the measured and calculated serum osmolality is more than 12, consider an alcohol, particularly ethylene glycol, isopropyl alcohol, and methanol, as the cause.

In cases of acute metabolic acidosis, three diagnoses should be immediately investigated: lactic acidemia (the serum lactate level should mirror the magnitude of the BD), ketoacidosis due to diabetes (the patient should be hyperglycemic and have positive urinary ketones), and acute renal failure, demonstrated by high serum urea and creatinine levels and a low total CO_2 level. The latter condition is a diagnosis of exclusion. A low serum sodium concentration (>135 mEq/L) should alert the clinician to the possibility of a dilutional acidosis caused by alcohol poisoning. Alcohols such as ethanol, methanol, isopropyl alcohol, and ethylene glycol are osmotically active molecules that expand extracellular water; glucose and mannitol have the same effect but also promote diuresis because the molecules are small enough to be filtered by the kidney. Alcohol poisoning is suspected by the presence of an *osmolar gap*; a difference between the measured and calculated serum osmolality of greater than 12 mOsm demonstrates the presence of unmeasured osmoles. Toxicology laboratories can investigate for the presence of various toxic alcohols.

Acid-base disturbances are indicative of significant underlying pathology. Acute respiratory failure may be caused by a variety of pathologies, including neurologic injury (e.g., stroke, spinal cord injury, botulism, tetanus), toxic suppression of the respiratory center (e.g., opioids, barbiturates, benzodiazepines), neuromuscular disorders (e.g., Guillain-Barré syndrome, myasthenia gravis), abdominal hypertension, flail chest, hydro-hemo-pneumo-thorax, pulmonary edema, and pneumonia. Frequently, mechanical ventilation is required to reverse the acidosis.

Lactic acidosis is caused by increased glycolytic production of lactate. When hypoxemia or hypoperfusion is present, it is called *type A lactic acidosis*. When hypoxemia or hypoperfusion is absent, it is called *type B lactic acidosis*, which is associated with inborn errors of metabolism, some drugs such as biguanides, and toxins. Lactate is metabolized to carbon dioxide and water in the liver by means of the Cori cycle.

Diabetic ketoacidosis is characterized by ketosis and hyperglycemia. Ketone bodies are produced from β-hydroxylated fatty acids in states of starvation or insulin deficiency. They include acetate, acetoacetate, and β-hydroxybutyrate. The ketone bodies act as strong ions, causing metabolic acidosis. Patients with diabetic ketoacidosis have acidosis caused by ketones and lactate, as well as hypoperfusion. They are characteristically dehydrated because of hyperglycemia-induced diuresis.

CASE 1

A 45-year-old man is admitted after a motor vehicle crash. He is bleeding, and his pulse is thready. His blood pressure is 90/50 mm Hg, heart rate is 120 beats/min, respiratory rate is 36, and temperature is 35°C. A serum chemistry panel and blood gas determinations are obtained. Consider the resulting data for the patient (in mEq/L unless otherwise stated): Na^+ = 144, K^+ = 4, Cl^- = 110, total CO_2 = 8, urea = 10, creatinine = 2.0, albumin = 4.0, lactate = 16.0, pH = 7.28, Pco_2 = 24, HCO_3 = 8, BE = –16, AG = 26, and corrected AG = 27.25. Does he have any acid-base disturbances?

Using traditional tools, the patient has a widened AG acidosis. This is a lactic acidosis, with appropriate respiratory compensation. The BDE and AG approach accurately detects the "unmeasured" anion, lactate.

The patient is aggressively volume resuscitated and brought to the operating room. Twelve hours later, blood gas determinations and a serum chemistry panel are obtained for the patient, who is now mechanically ventilated in the intensive care unit. Consider the data obtained for the patient (in mEq/L unless otherwise stated): Na^+ = 148, K^+ = 3, Cl^- = 120, total CO_2 = 22, urea = 10, creatinine = 2.0, albumin = 2.0, lactate = 5.0, pH = 7.33, P_{CO_2} = 35, HCO_3 = 18, and BE = −11. Is the patient still under-resuscitated, and what intravenous fluid was used?

In this situation, traditional tools are unreliable. Using the Fencl-Gilfix[31,32] approach, correcting the base deficit or excess for acidifying and alkalinizing processes, reveals a complex situation. Base deficit corrected (BDC) – base excess corrected (BEC) = −10.1.

Acidifying Processes	Magnitude	BDC	Alkalinizing Processes	Magnitude	BEC
Hyperchloremia	120 mEq/L	−17	Hypernatremia	148 mEq/L	+2.4
Lacticemia	5 mEq/L	−5	Hypoalbuminemia	2.0 g/dL	+8.5
Total		−22	Total		+11.9

Using simple measures such as BDE to follow the resuscitation, the clinician might assume, based on the BD, that serum lactate was significantly higher that it was and that the patient is under-resuscitated. This is not so. The patient was resuscitated with normal saline.

Renal acidosis is caused by accumulation of strong ion products of metabolism excreted exclusively by the kidney. These include sulfate and formate. There also is accumulation of a weak acid, phosphate, which is caused by relative deficiency of vitamin D. Lactic acidosis is treated by volume resuscitation and source control. Diabetic ketoacidosis is treated with volume resuscitation and insulin. Renal acidosis is treated with dialysis.

The use of sodium bicarbonate boluses or infusions is controversial in treating metabolic acidosis. There is little evidence of benefit using this agent in lactic acidosis or ketoacidosis.[9] This situation is related not to the ability of sodium bicarbonate to reverse the acidosis, which it does by increasing the SID, but to the perception that the acidosis is the problem. Nevertheless, sodium bicarbonate (8.4%) is a hypertonic solution, which should have a plasma-expanding effect similar to that of hypertonic saline, albeit at the cost of increasing P_{aCO_2}. This probably explains the perceived hemodynamic benefit in shock.[9] Sodium bicarbonate infusions, with the purpose of increasing the SID, have been used in patients awaiting dialysis to reduce symptoms and prevent hyperkalemia.

Methanol is metabolized to formaldehyde and formate by alcohol dehydrogenase. These are highly toxic compounds, causing blindness, cardiovascular instability, and death. Treatment strategies include the use of ethanol, which competes for binding to alcohol dehydrogenase, and fomepizole, which inhibits the enzyme. Ethylene glycol poisoning causes central nervous system depression, lactic acidosis, formation of calcium oxalate urinary crystals leading to hypocalcemia and renal failure, cardiovascular depression, and death. Treatment is with fomepizole, with or without hemodialysis.

Perioperative Acid-Base Disturbances

In addition to the acid-base disturbances seen in emergency situations, a number of acid-base conundrums are peculiar to the perioperative and critically ill patient.

These include respiratory acidosis and alkalosis associated with mechanical ventilation, acidosis due to hyperchloremia or dilution, and alkalosis due to sodium gain, chloride loss or volume contraction.

Perioperatively, respiratory acidosis is caused by poor mechanical ventilation strategy, narcosis, or incomplete reversal of neuromuscular blockade. Respiratory alkalosis is caused by hyperventilation in response to pain or anxiety.

Metabolic acid-base disturbances are relatively common perioperatively. Pathologic causes involve lactic acidosis, ketoacidosis, and renal acidosis as described in the previous section. Iatrogenic causes include manipulation of the SID by administration of electrolyte- or osmolite-imbalanced solutions.

Hyperchloremic acidosis is frequently seen in the operating suite. It usually follows large-volume administration of 0.9% saline solution. This solution contains 154 mEq of both Na^+ and Cl^+, with an SID of 0. Each liter of normal saline is associated with a decline in the SID value. Hyperchloremic acidosis is also associated with acute normovolemic hemodilution with 5% albumin solution or 6% hetastarch (both formulated in normal saline).[33] Kellum,[34] in an experimental model of sepsis, showed that dogs treated with lactated Ringer's solution and 5% hydroxyethyl starch diluted in lactated Ringer's solution (Hextend) (both with an SID of 20) had less acidosis and longer survival than those treated with normal saline.

There has been an unfortunate tendency to confuse hyperchloremic and dilutional acidosis.[35] Hyperchloremic acidosis is caused by chloride gain, such as by NaCl administration; serum sodium may stay the same or even increase. Dilutional acidosis refers to a condition in which there is an alteration in the relative quantity of sodium and chloride in free water; serum sodium decreases. This can occur perioperatively from administration of sodium-poor fluids. The perioperative stress response is associated with reduced ability to excrete free water because of increased secretion of antidiuretic hormone. Excessive administration of hypotonic fluids, such as 5% dextrose or 0.45% NaCl, leads to an expansion in free water, hyponatremia, and acidosis.

Traditional teaching explains dilutional acidosis in terms of dilution of bicarbonate by the added volume.[35] However, acids and bases alike should be diluted in this fashion. Moreover, no study has been able to quantitatively explain dilutional acidosis on the basis of reduced serum bicarbonate.[35,36] Bicarbonate concentration is determined by carbon dioxide equilibrium.[37] Alterations in pH associated with changes in the relative ratio of sodium and chloride have been elegantly demonstrated by Morgan and colleagues.[38] With in vitro hemodilution, there was a simple linear relationship between diluent crystalloid SID and the rate and direction of change of plasma SID and whole blood BE.

What is the relevance of hyperchloremic acidosis? Waters and colleagues[39] demonstrated a significant difference in perioperative acidosis in patients undergoing aneurysm surgery who were treated with normal saline rather than lactated Ringer's solution. There were, however, no significant differences in outcomes. Brill and colleagues[13] found that acidosis due to hyperchloremia was associated with better outcomes than those associated with lactic acidosis or ketoacidosis. This supports the contention that it is the underlying problem that increases the patient's risk, not the acidosis itself.

Hyperchloremic acidosis is treated by increasing the SID of infused fluids, such as by infusing sodium without chloride. Although no such fluid is available commercially, one can be easily made up by diluting 3 ampules of 7.5% sodium bicarbonate in 1 L of 5% dextrose. This is run as maintenance fluid (the SID is 144) until the BD returns to zero.

Perioperative metabolic alkalosis is usually of iatrogenic origin. Hyperventilation of patients with chronic respiratory failure results in acute metabolic alkalosis because of the chronic compensatory alkalosis associated with chloride loss in urine[8] (Fig. 41-6 and Table 41-5). More frequently, metabolic alkalosis is associated with increased SID due to sodium gain. This is caused by administration of fluids in which sodium is "buffered" by weak ions, citrate (in blood products), acetate (in parenteral nutrition), and bicarbonate. Buffer ions such as citrate, acetate, gluconate, and lactate are, under normal conditions, rapidly cleared by the liver and do not contribute to acid-base balance. Sodium and chloride obey the law of conservation of mass. Sodium gain is chloride-sensitive alkalosis, treated by administration of net loads of chloride in the form of 0.9% NaCl, potassium chloride, calcium chloride, and occasionally, hydrogen chloride. It is important to correct chloride-sensitive alkalosis, because the normal compensatory measure is hypoventilation, which increases $Paco_2$ and may lead to CO_2 narcosis or failure to liberate the patient from mechanical ventilation.

Another cause of metabolic alkalosis in perioperative patients is chloride loss caused by removal of chloride from the gastrointestinal tract by continuous suctioning or vomiting. Gastric juice contains hydrochloric acid, and loss of chloride leads to alkalosis. Loss of hydrogen ions does not.

Anesthesiologists should understand the effects of fluids on acid-base disturbances (see Chapter 46). Hypotonic and

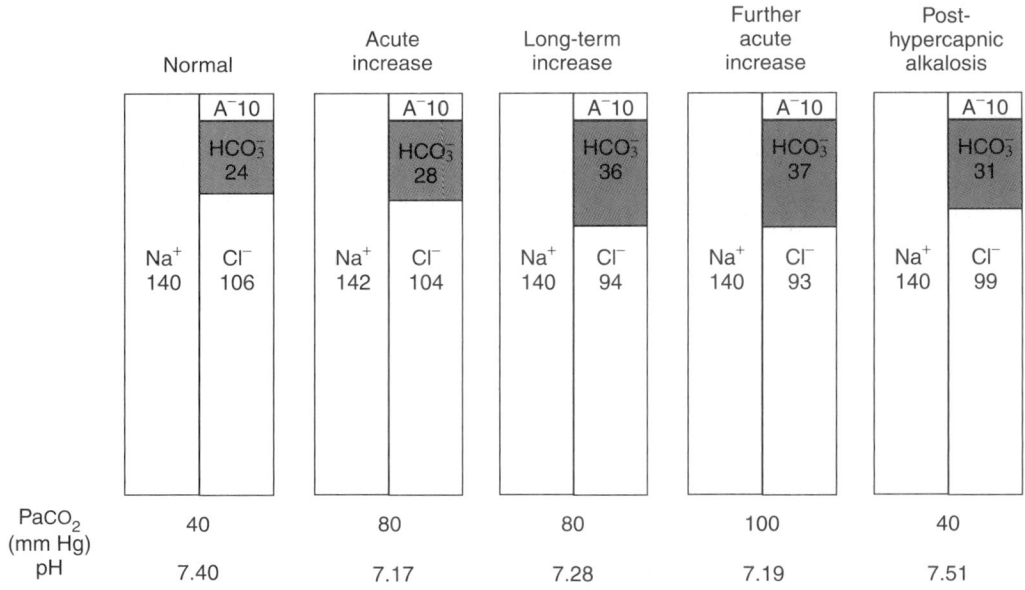

Figure 41–6 Changes in acid-base and electrolyte composition in patients with respiratory acidosis. *Left to right*, the panels depict normal acid-base status; adaptation to an acute rise in the partial pressure of arterial carbon dioxide ($Paco_2$) to 80 mm Hg; adaptation to a long-term rise in $Paco_2$ to 80 mm Hg; superimposition of an acute further increment in $Paco_2$ (to a level of 100 mm Hg) in the same patient; and post-hypercapnic alkalosis resulting from an abrupt reduction in $Paco_2$ to the level of 40 mm Hg in the same patient. A^- denotes unmeasured plasma anions, and the numbers within the bars give ion concentrations in millimoles per liter. (Adapted from Androgue H, Madias N: Management of life-threatening acid-base disorders. First of two parts. N Engl J Med 338:26-34, 1998.)

Table 41-5 Acid-base disturbances commonly occurring perioperatively

Disorder	Cause
Respiratory acidosis	Hypoventilation; narcosis, incomplete reversal of neuromuscular blockade
Respiratory alkalosis	Hyperventilation; anxiety, pain
Metabolic acidosis due to unmeasured anions (e.g., widened gap acidosis)	Hypoperfusion (e.g., lactic acidosis; diabetic ketoacidosis); renal failure
Metabolic acidosis due to measured anions (non–anion gap hyperchloremic acidosis)	Hyperchloremia (e.g., "normal" saline, hetastarch, albumin infusions); renal tubular acidosis; bladder reconstructions
Metabolic acidosis due to free water excess (e.g., hyponatremia, dilution acidosis)	Hypotonic fluid administration; sodium loss (e.g., diarrhea); administration of hyperosmolar fluids (e.g., mannitol, alcohol); hyperproteinemia
Metabolic alkalosis	Hyperventilation of patient with history of carbon dioxide retention (e.g., chronic obstructive pulmonary disease); sodium gain (e.g., sodium bicarbonate, massive blood transfusion); chloride loss (e.g., nasogastric suctioning)

dextrose-containing fluids should be avoided. For patients receiving 1 or 2 L of fluid perioperatively, there is little difference between the choices of fluids. If larger-volume crystalloid resuscitation is expected, balanced buffered solutions that mirror the electrolyte content of the ECF, such as lactated Ringer's solution, Normosol, or Plasmalyte, are recommended. If the patient has been on continuous nasogastric suctioning, normal saline should be administered until the BD returns to zero; then balanced buffered solutions should be used. Likewise, if large volumes of blood or frozen plasma are administered, normal saline should be given. Care must be taken to avoid hypokalemia, hypocalcemia, hypomagnesemia, and hypophosphatemia. Patients who have received purgatives for bowel surgery should be treated with balanced buffer solutions. The same rules apply to colloid solutions. Human albumin solution, some hetastarches, and gelatins (available in Europe) are formulated in NaCl, and large volumes cause hyperchloremic acidosis.

Acid-Base Disturbances in Critical Illness

The emergence of the Stewart approach to acid-base balance in recent years owes much to the dissatisfaction of intensivists with the traditional approach. Critically ill patients may have many confounding acid-base disturbances that may not be revealed with a single quantitative measure such as BD. Patients frequently have perturbations of PCO_2, SID, and A_{TOT}, and significant pathology may be overlooked because of apparently normal blood gas results.

The most important single disturbance in acid-base chemistry in critically ill patients is hypoalbuminemia.[15] This condition is ubiquitous and causes an unpredictable metabolic alkalosis. It may mask significant alterations in the SID, such as lactic acidemia. Although Figge and colleagues[19] presented a mechanism for adjusting the AG for albumin, this implies that the physician is aware of an acid-base abnormality. Likewise, the use of BD to predict lactate levels is unreliable in critical illness, particularly in

patients undergoing secondary deterioration.[18] Prolonged respiratory failure with associated hypercarbia leads to additional metabolic alkalosis because of chloride loss in urine.[8] Mechanical ventilation increases the circulating volume of atrial natriuretic peptide and antidiuretic hormone. The result is increased total body water, leading to dilutional acidosis. This may be further complicated by renal insufficiency or renal failure, with concomitant accumulation of metabolic by products, renal anions, and other UMAs. Polyuric renal failure may be associated with significant contraction alkalosis due to the loss of sodium, potassium, and free water.

Critically ill patients are vulnerable to significant changes in the SID and free water. Nasogastric suctioning causes chloride loss. Diarrhea causes loss of sodium and potassium. Surgical drains placed in tissue beds may remove fluids with various electrolyte concentrations (e.g., the pancreatic bed secretes fluid rich in sodium). Fever, sweating, oozing tissues, and inadequately humidified ventilator circuits lead to large-volume insensible loss and contraction alkalosis.

Infusions administered to patients may be responsible for stealth alterations in serum chemistry. Many antibiotics, such as piperacillin-tazobactam, are diluted in sodium-rich solutions. Others, such as vancomycin, are administered in large volumes of free water (5% dextrose). Lorazepam is diluted in propylene glycol, large volumes of which cause metabolic acidosis similar to that seen with ethylene glycol.[41]

Continuous renal replacement therapy (CRRT) is used in critical illness for hemofiltration and hemodialysis of patients who are hemodynamically unstable. Rocktaschel and colleagues[42] demonstrated that CRRT resolved the acidosis of acute renal failure by removing strong ions and phosphate. However, metabolic alkalosis ensued because of the unmasking of metabolic alkalosis due to hypoalbuminemia.

Other, seemingly innocuous therapies may cause significant disturbances in the acid-base balance. Loop diuretics are often administered to critically ill patients in

CASE 2

A 56-year-old man is chronically critically ill. A serum chemistry panel and blood gas determinations are obtained. Consider the resulting data for the patient (in mEq/L unless otherwise stated): Na^+ = 130, K^+ = 4, Cl^- = 100, total CO_2 = 24, urea = 10, creatinine = 1.0, albumin = 1.0, lactate = 6.0, pH = 7.42, Pco_2 = 40, HCO_3 = 24, and BE = +1. Does he have any acid-base disturbances?

Using the Fencl-Gilfix[31,32] approach, correcting the base deficit or excess for acidifying and alkalinizing processes reveals a complex situation. Base deficit corrected (BDC) – base excess corrected (BEC) = 0.9.

Acidifying Processes	Magnitude	BDC	Alkalinizing Processes	Magnitude	BEC
Hyponatremia	130 mEq/L	−3	Hypoalbuminemia	1.0 g/dL	+11.9
Hyperchloremia	100 mEq/L	−3			
Lacticemia	5 mEq/L	−5			
Total		−11	Total		+11.9

In this example, the patient has three significant acidifying processes going on, and the presence of lactic acidosis is sinister. However, using traditional approaches would not reveal the abnormalities.

the mistaken view that they can liberate sequestered fluids. These agents cause hypochloremic and contraction alkalosis. Similarly, the use of carbonic anhydrase inhibitors to treat patients with metabolic alkalosis is misguided. These agents increase tissue CO_2 levels, causing respiratory acidosis, and they cause diuresis, worsening contraction alkalosis. There is no treatment for hypoalbuminemic metabolic alkalosis except recovery. Contraction alkalosis is treated by correcting the free water deficit using the following formula:

$$\text{Free water deficit} = 0.6 \times \text{patient's weight (in kg)} \times ([\text{patient's sodium level}/140] - 1)$$

Hypochloremic alkalosis should be treated by correcting the chloride deficit, using normal saline.

Neurosurgical patients are vulnerable to a variety of acid-base disturbances related to osmotherapy and brain injury (see Chapter 53). Mannitol, which is administered to reduce intracranial pressure, initially causes dilutional acidosis. A contraction alkalosis follows because of diuresis. Moreover, these patients are routinely treated with normal saline solution and frequently treated with hypertonic saline, both of which cause acidosis.[43] Diabetes insipidus frequently occurs as a complication of severe head injury, usually in the terminal stages. It is caused by damage to or destruction of the pituitary gland or hypothalamus. In the absence of antidiuretic hormone, the kidney is unable to concentrate the urine, and a massive diuresis follows. The disorder is characterized by an increase in plasma osmolality in the presence of a low urinary osmolality. It typically manifests as a contraction alkalosis. The treatment is hormonal replacement with vasopressin or desmopressin.

SUMMARY

Much of the confusion regarding acid-base chemistry reflects the attempt to apply observational approaches, such as that of Henderson and Hasselbalch as well as

Schwartz and Brackett, to the entire spectrum of pathophysiologic processes. The use of physical chemistry principles has provided improved explanations of acid-base balance and superior tools to apply in a wide variety of clinical situations. This does not suggest that the traditional approach is incorrect, merely that it looks at a mirror image of that proposed by Stewart, Fencl, and others. All acid-base disorders can be explained in terms of the SID, A_{TOT}, and Pco_2. This is important to anesthesiologists, who may significantly affect the acid-base balance by their choice of fluids and strategy for mechanical ventilation.

KEY POINTS

1. A significant acid-base abnormality often signals a sinister underlying problem.
2. All acid-base abnormalities result from alterations in the dissociation of water.
3. Only three factors independently affect acid-base balance: $Paco_2$, SID, and A_{TOT}.
4. Respiratory acidosis and alkalosis are caused by hypercarbia and hypocarbia, respectively.
5. Metabolic acidosis is caused by decreased SID or increased A_{TOT}. Decreased SID results from accumulation of metabolic anions (i.e., shock, ketoacidosis, and renal failure), hyperchloremia, and free water excess. Increased A_{TOT} results from hyperphosphatemia.
6. Metabolic alkalosis is caused by increased SID or decreased A_{TOT}. The SID increases because of sodium gain, chloride loss, or free water deficit. A_{TOT} decreases in hypoalbuminemia and hypophosphatemia. This condition is particularly common in critical illness.
7. Most acid-base disorders are treated by reversal of the cause.

REFERENCES

1. Stewart PA: Modern quantitative acid-base chemistry. Can J Physiol Pharmacol 61:1444-1461, 1983.
2. Fencl V, Leith DE: Stewart's quantitative acid-base chemistry: Applications in biology and medicine. Respir Physiol 91:1-16, 1993.
3. Kellum JA: Diagnosis and treatment of acid-base disorders. *In* Grenvik A, Ayres S, Holbrook P, Shoemaker W (eds): Textbook of Critical Care, 4th ed. Philadelphia, WB Saunders, 2000, pp 839-853.
4. Sirker AA, Rhodes A, Grounds RM, Bennett ED: Acid-base physiology: The "traditional" and the "modern" approaches. Anaesthesia 57:348-356, 2002.
5. Wooten EW: Analytic calculation of physiological acid-base parameters in plasma. J Appl Physiol 86:326-334, 1999.
6. Henderson LJ: Das Gleichgewicht zwischen Sauren und Bases im tierischen Organismus. Ergebn Physiol 8:254-325, 1909.
7. Hasselbalch KA: Die Berechnung der Wasserstoffzahl des Blutes aus der freien und gebundenen Kohlensaure desselben, und die Sauerstoffbindung des Blutes als Funktion der Wasserstoffzahl. Biochem Z 78:112-144, 1916.
8. Alfaro V, Torras R, Ibanez J, Palacios L: A physical-chemical analysis of the acid-base response to chronic obstructive pulmonary disease. Can J Physiol Pharmacol 11:1229-1235, 1996.
9. Forsythe SM, Schmidt GA: Sodium bicarbonate for the treatment of lactic acidosis. Chest 117:260-267, 2000.
10. Stewart PA: Independent and dependent variables of acid-base control. Respir Physiol 33:9-26, 1978.
11. Laffey JG, Kavanagh BP: Carbon dioxide and the critically ill—Too little of a good thing? Lancet 354:1283-1286, 1999.
12. Hickling KG: Permissive hypercapnia. Respir Care Clin N Am 8:155-169, v, 2002.
13. Brill SA, Stewart TR, Brundage SI, Schreiber MA: Base deficit does not predict mortality when secondary to hyperchloremic acidosis. Shock 17:459-462, 2002.
14. Scheingraber S, Rehm M, Sehmisch C, Finsterer U: Rapid saline infusion produces hyperchloremic acidosis in patients undergoing gynecologic surgery. Anesthesiology 90:1265-1270, 1999.
15. Story DA, Poustie S, Bellomo R: Quantitative physical chemistry analysis of acid-base disorders in critically ill patients. Anaesthesia 56:530-533, 2001.
16. Figge J, Rossing TH, Fencl V: The role of serum proteins in acid-base equilibria. J Lab Clin Med 117:453-467, 1991.
17. Figge J, Mydosh T, Fencl V: Serum proteins and acid-base equilibria: a follow-up. J Lab Clin Med 120:713-719, 1992.
18. Fencl V, Jabor A, Kazda A, Figge J: Diagnosis of metabolic acid-base disturbances in critically ill patients. Am J Respir Crit Care Med 162:2246-2251, 2000.
19. Figge J, Jabor A, Kazda A, Fencl V: Anion gap and hypoalbuminemia. Crit Care Med 26:1807-1810, 1998.
20. Goldwasser P, Feldman J: Association of serum albumin and mortality risk. J Clin Epidemiol 50:693-703, 1997.
21. Wang F, Butler T, Rabbani GH, Jones PK: The acidosis of cholera. Contributions of hyperproteinemia, lactic acidemia, and hyperphosphatemia to an increased serum anion gap. N Engl J Med 315:1591-1595, 1986.
21a. Brackett NC Jr, Cohen JJ, Schwartz WB: Carbon dioxide titration curve of normal man. Effect of increasing degrees of acute hypercapnia on acid-base equilibrium. N Engl J Med 272:6-12, 1965.
21b. Schwartz WB, Brackett NC Jr, Cohen JJ: The response of extracellular hydrogen ion concentration to graded degrees of chronic hypercapnia: The physiologic limits of the defense of pH. J Clin Invest 44:291-301, 1965.
22. Narins R, Emmett M: Simple and mixed acid-base disorders: A practical approach. Medicine (Baltimore) 59:161-187, 1980.
23. Severinghaus JW: Acid-base balance nomogram—A Boston-Copenhagen detente. Anesthesiology 45:539-541, 1976.
24. Singer RB, Hastings AB: An improved clinical method for the estimation of disturbances of the acid-base balance of human blood. Medicine (Baltimore) 10:242, 1948.
24a. Astrup P, Siggard-Andersen O: Micromethods for measuring acid-base values of blood. Adv Clin Chem 69:1-28, 1963.
25. Siggaard-Andersen O: The van Slyke equation. Scand J Clin Lab Invest Suppl 37:15-20, 1977.
26. Schlichtig R, Grogono AW, Severinghaus JW: Human $Paco_2$ and standard base excess compensation for acid-base imbalance. Crit Care Med 26:1173-1179, 1998.
27. Morgan TJ, Clark C, Endre ZH: Accuracy of base excess—An in vitro evaluation of the Van Slyke equation. Crit Care Med 28:2932-2936, 2003.
28. Emmett M, Narins RG: Clinical use of the anion gap. Medicine (Baltimore) 56:38-54, 1977.
29. Salem MM, Mujais SK: Gaps in the anion gap. Arch Intern Med 152:1625-1629, 1992.
30. Wilkes P: Hypoproteinemia, strong-ion difference, and acid-base status in critically ill patients. J Appl Physiol 84:1740-1748, 1998.
31. Gilfix BM, Bique M, Magder S: A physical chemical approach to the analysis of acid-base balance in the clinical setting. J Crit Care 8:187-197, 1993.
32. Balasubramanyan N, Havens PL, Hoffman GM: Unmeasured anions identified by the Fencl-Stewart method predict mortality better than base excess, anion gap, and lactate in patients in the pediatric intensive care unit. Crit Care Med 27:1577-1581, 1999.
33. Rehm M, Orth V, Scheingraber S, et al: Acid-base changes caused by 5% albumin versus 6% hydroxyethyl starch solution in patients undergoing acute normovolemic hemodilution: A randomized prospective study. Anesthesiology 93:1174-1183, 2000.
34. Kellum JA: Fluid resuscitation and hyperchloremic acidosis in experimental sepsis: improved short-term survival and acid-base balance with Hextend compared with saline. Crit Care Med 30:300-305, 2002.
35. Prough D, White R: Acidosis associated with perioperative saline administration: Dilution or delusion? Anesthesiology 93:1167-1169, 2000.
36. Garella S, Chang BS, Kahn SI: Dilution acidosis and contraction alkalosis: Review of a concept. Kidney Int 8:279-283, 1975.
37. Kellum JA: Saline-induced hyperchloremic metabolic acidosis. Crit Care Med 30:259-261, 2002.
38. Morgan TJ, Venkatesh B, Hall J: Crystalloid strong ion difference determines metabolic acid-base change during in vitro hemodilution. Crit Care Med 30:157-160, 2002.
39. Waters J, Gottlieb A, Schoenwald P, Popovich M: Normal saline versus lactated Ringer's solution for intraoperative fluid management in patients undergoing abdominal aortic aneurysm repair: An outcome study. Anesth Analg 93:817-822, 2001.
40. Androgue H, Madias N: Management of life-threatening acid-base disorders. First of two parts. N Engl J Med 338:26-34, 1998.
41. Tayar J, Jabbour G, Saggi SJ: Severe hyperosmolar metabolic acidosis due to a large dose of intravenous lorazepam. N Engl J Med 346:1253-1254, 2002.
42. Rocktaschel J, Morimatsu H, Uchino S, et al: Impact of continuous veno-venous hemofiltration on acid-base balance. Int J Artif Organs 26:19-25, 2003.
43. Moon P, Kramer GC: Hypertonic saline-dextran resuscitation from hemorrhagic shock induces transient mixed acidosis. Crit Care Med 23:323-331, 1995.

Index

Note: Page number followed by f refer to figures; page numbers followed by t refer to tables.

A

A-a (alveolar-arterial) gradient, 1010, 1440–1442, 1446–1447, 1446t, 1455
ABCDDEF, in toxic releases, 2521–2522, 2522t
Abciximab, in coronary angiography, 2649
Abdomen, trauma to, 2481–2482
Abdominal aorta
  aneurysm of, 2070–2071
    mortality with, 2071
    natural history of, 2071
    risk factors for, 2070–2071
    rupture of, 2071
  reconstruction of
    anesthesia for, 2079–2081
    aortic cross-clamping in, 2072–2076, 2073t, 2074f, 2074t, 2075f
    blood transfusion during, 2079
    care after, 2080–2081
    endovascular, 2089–2092
    extubation after, 2081
    monitoring during, 2077–2079
    normothermia for, 2081
    normovolemic hemodilution during, 2079
Abel, John J., 8
Abiomed BVS 5000 system, 1992, 1992t
ABO blood typing, 1802, 1802t, 1804
Abortion, in minor, 3182
Abscess
  lung, 1926
  peritonsillar, 2544
Acceleration, 1192, 1218
Acceleromyography, 1560–1561, 1560f
Accessory nerve block, 1707–1708
Accommodation reflex, 2996, 2997t
Acebutolol, 653–654, 655
Acetaminophen
  hepatotoxicity of, 2221t
  in chronic pain, 2769
  postoperative, 2735t, 2736f
Acetazolamide
  metabolic acidosis with, 1783
  neuromuscular blocking agent interaction with, 517–518
N-Acetyl-β-D-glucosaminidase, in renal function monitoring, 1500, 1500t
Acetyl-CoA, in lipid metabolism, 748
Acetylcholine. See also Acetylcholine receptor.
  bronchial response to, 156
  enteric, 624
  formation of, 862, 863f
  function of, 625t, 627–630, 629f, 860
  in cardiac function, 735–737, 736f, 737f
  inactivation of, 642
  inhaled anesthetic effects on, 112
  ocular preparations of, 2537
  secretion of, 641–642, 863–864, 863f, 864f
  synthesis of, 640–641, 640f
  vascular tone and, 629–630, 629f
  vasoactive intestinal polypeptide and, 620–621, 621f
  vesicle storage of, 641–642, 641f
Acetylcholine receptor, 642–644, 643f, 860, 861, 865–866, 865f, 866f
  α-bungarotoxin binding of, 874
  desensitization of, 869–870, 870t
  fetal, 871
  immature (extrajunctional), 871–873
    in burn patient, 530
    in muscular dystrophy, 536
    in myasthenia syndromes, 541
    in myopathy of critical illness, 873
  mature (junctional), 871–873, 872f

Acetylcholine receptor (Continued)
  muscarinic, 513–514, 513f, 644
    in cardiac function, 735, 736f
  nicotinic, 482–483, 483f, 642–644, 643f, 874–875
    fetal, 483
    in spinal cord injury, 102
    inhaled anesthetic effects on, 120–121, 121f
  prejunctional, 873–875
  subunits of, 871, 874
Acetylcholinesterase, 642
  abnormal, 1563, 1564f
  deficiency of, 540t, 865
  in neuromuscular transmission, 860, 864–865
  inhibitors of. See Anticholinesterases.
N-Acetylcysteine
  aerosol, 2816–2817
  in phosgene exposure, 2512
  renal effects of, 804
Acid, 1600–1601
  weak, 1601–1602
Acid-base balance, 1599–1614
  abnormalities of, 1602–1604, 1603t, 1782–1783
    anion gap approach to, 1607–1608, 1607f, 1781–1782
    base deficit/excess (Copenhagen) approach to, 1606–1607, 1607f, 1607t
    carbon dioxide-bicarbonate (Boston) approach to, 1606, 1606f
    evaluation of, 1609–1614, 1610f, 1613t
    hypoalbuminemia and, 1604, 1608, 1613
    in critical illness, 1613–1614
    in emergency setting, 1609–1611, 1610t
    neuromuscular blockade and, 522–523
    oxygen-hemoglobin dissociation curve and, 701
    perioperative, 1611–1613, 1612f, 1613t
    Stewart-Fencl approach to, 1608–1609, 1608f
  carbon dioxide and, 1602
  equations for, 1602
  hypothermia and, 1588–1589, 1980–1981
  in blood transfusion, 1814–1815, 1814f
  in cardiopulmonary bypass, 1980–1981, 1981f
  in renal function monitoring, 1495
  opioids and, 409
  regulation of, 1604–1605, 1605t
  Stewart approach to, 1601–1602, 1601f
  strong ion difference and, 1601, 1601f, 1603–1604, 1603t
  weak acid buffer solutions and, 1601–1602
α₁-Acid glycoprotein, drug binding to, 74–76, 75f, 1722–1723
  age-related changes in, 100–101
Acidosis
  dilutional, 1604, 1608, 1611–1612
  hyperchloremic, 1604, 1608, 1611, 1612, 1775
  lactic, 1610–1611
  local anesthetics and, 593, 596
  metabolic, 1603–1604, 1603t, 1605t
    anion gap, 1781–1782
    blood transfusion and, 1814–1815, 1814f
    compensatory response to, 1605
    diuretic administration and, 1782
    high-altitude acclimation and, 1783
    hyperventilation and, 1783
    hypoventilation and, 1783
    in alcohol poisoning, 1610
    in emergency setting, 1609–1611, 1610t
    in kidney failure, 2181–2182, 2181t, 2182t
    in neonatal respiratory failure, 1782–1783
    liver transplantation and, 1782
    low cardiac output and, 1782
    perioperative, 1613t
    succinylcholine-related hyperkalemia and, 489
    treatment of, 1781

Acidosis (Continued)
  neonatal, 1782–1783, 2357–2358, 2357f, 2358f
  renal, 1611
  respiratory, 1603, 1603t, 1605t
    compensatory response to, 1605
    in emergency setting, 1609
    perioperative, 1611, 1613t
Acivicin, 253–254, 255f
Acoustic apnea monitor, 1468
Acoustic neuroma, 1531, 1537–1538, 1538f
Acquired immunodeficiency syndrome (AIDS)
  hotline for, 3156
  in children, 2871, 2872–2873
  in health care worker, 919, 3155–3156, 3156t
  testing for, 942, 956, 959
  transfusion-transmitted, 1818t, 1819
Acromegaly, 1051–1052
Actin, 733, 733f, 734, 734f
Action potential
  cardiac, 730–731, 731f
  neural, 577–579, 579f
Activated clotting time, 1339–1340
  in heparin monitoring, 1973–1974, 1973f
Activated partial thromboplastin time, 1340
Active compression-decompression, in basic life support, 2926
Acupressure, 2599
Acupuncture, 612–613, 613f, 2599
  in chronic pain, 2777
  postoperative, 2744
Acute intermittent porphyria, 749
Acute normovolemic hemodilution, 1834–1836
  clinical trials of, 1835–1836, 1836t
  cost-effectiveness of, 1836
  hematocrit level with, 1834–1835, 1835f
  hemostasis with, 1835
  oxygenation with, 1835
  patient selection for, 1836t
Acute-phase proteins, in sepsis, 2901–2903, 2902f, 2902t
Acute respiratory distress syndrome, 2848, 2848t
  in critical care patient, 2790–2791, 2792f–2793f
Acute tubular necrosis
  after infrarenal aortic reconstruction, 2076
  free water clearance in, 789
  in hepatic disease, 761
Adaptive pressure ventilation, 2824–2825, 2824f, 2824t
Addiction, 3164–3170
  causes of, 3166–3167, 3167f
  management of, 3167–3169, 3167t, 3168t
  prevalence of, 3165–3166
  prognosis for, 3169–3170
  suicide and, 3167
  work reentry after, 3169
Addisonian crisis, 1039
Addison's disease, 1038–1039, 1048
Adenoma
  adrenal, 1038
  pituitary, 1037, 1041, 1052
Adenosine
  in pediatric life support, 2947t
  in renal regulation, 798, 798t
  in supraventricular tachyarrhythmias, 2930–2932, 2932f, 2932t
  inhaled anesthetic effects on, 113
  pulmonary vascular resistance and, 688, 688t
Adenosine monophosphate, cyclic (cAMP), inhaled anesthetic effects on, 113–114
Adenosine receptors, in renal regulation, 798, 798t
Adenosine triphosphate
  as cotransmitter, 619, 619f
  in cerebral ischemia, 834–836, 835f

Adenylyl cyclase, 92, 92f
Adhesive tape, pulse oximetry errors and, 1451t, 1452
Adrenal cortex
  adenoma of, 1038
  age-related function of, 1041
  disorders of, 1035–1042, 1037t
  etomidate effects on, 1041
  hormones of, 1035–1037
  incidentaloma of, 1038, 1041–1042
  resection of, 1037–1038
Adrenal gland. See also Adrenal cortex; Adrenal medulla.
  catecholamine synthesis in, 633
  congenital hyperplasia of, 2861
  in hemorrhagic shock, 2459–2460
  opioid effects on, 396
Adrenal insufficiency, in children, 2861
Adrenal medulla, pheochromocytoma of, 1042–1044, 1042t, 1043t, 2861
Adrenalectomy, 1037–1038
α-Adrenergic receptor(s), 635f, 636, 636t
  bronchial, 156
  desensitization of, 101–102
  G protein interaction with, 637–639, 638f
  in cardiac function, 735–737, 736f, 737f
β-Adrenergic receptor(s), 89–90, 89f, 90f, 635f, 636–637, 636t, 637f
  bronchial, 156
  desensitization of, 639–640
  downregulation of, 639–640
  G protein interaction with, 637–639, 638f
  genetic variability in, 99–100, 100f
  in cardiac function, 735–737, 736f, 737f
  subtypes of, 637
α₁-Adrenergic receptor agonists, 650. See also Phenylephrine.
α₂-Adrenergic receptor agonists, 355–359, 650–651, 650t, 1121. See also Clonidine; Dexmedetomidine.
β-Adrenergic receptor agonists, 651–652. See also Dobutamine; Isoproterenol.
  halothane MAC and, 113, 113f
α-Adrenergic receptor antagonists, 652–653
β-Adrenergic receptor antagonists, 653–657, 654f, 654t, 1120–1121
  adverse effects of, 656–657
  cerebral blood flow and, 819
  contraindications to, 656–657
  drug interactions with, 656
  in arrhythmias, 656
  in congestive heart failure, 655
  in glaucoma, 656
  in hypertension, 655–656
  in myocardial ischemia, 655, 1946–1947
  in tachycardia, 656
  in thyrotoxicosis, 656
  indications for, 655–656
  overdose of, 656–657
  perioperative, 655, 2068, 2069f
  pharmacology of, 653–655, 654f, 654t
Adrenocorticotropic hormone, 1036
  deficiency of, 1038
Adrenomedullin, in cardiac function, 737, 737t
Adult respiratory distress syndrome. See Respiratory distress syndrome.
Advanced cardiac life support, 2929–2941
  arrhythmia monitoring and recognition in, 2929–2935, 2930f–2937f
  cardiac arrest management in, 2935, 2937–2941, 2938f, 2939f
  do-not-resuscitate orders and, 2940–2941
  in children, 2942–2947, 2943f–2946f, 2947t
Advanced trauma life support protocol, 2452, 2453f
Aerosols, 2815–2817, 2815f, 2816t, 2817t
  anti-inflammatory, 2816, 2817t
  antimicrobial, 2816
  bronchodilating, 2816, 2817, 2817t
Afterload, 725–726, 725f
  inhaled anesthetic effects on, 197–198, 198f
Age. See also Children; Elderly patient.
  cerebral blood flow and, 820
  creatinine clearance and, 74
  drug response and, 100–101
  minimum alveolar concentration and, 108
  opioid effects and, 406, 406f
Aging, 2435–2439, 2436t. See also Elderly patient.
  drug metabolism and, 2438–2439, 2439t
  of cardiovascular system, 2436–2437, 2436f, 2436t
  of central nervous system, 2435–2436
  of kidneys, 2438

Aging (Continued)
  of liver, 2438
  of respiratory system, 2437–2438
Agonist, 86, 86f
  dose-response relationship of, 95f, 96
  full, 86, 86f, 87f, 95f, 96
  inverse, 86f, 87, 87f
  partial, 86, 86f, 87f
Agrin, 866, 866f, 872
Ahlquist, R., 9
Air
  cranial retention of, 2138, 2138f
  intramyocardial, in pediatric cardiopulmonary bypass, 2030, 2030f
  transpulmonary passage of, 2142
Air bubbles, in blood gas measurement, 1446
Air cysts, 1916–1917
Air embolism, 2672–2673
  after orthopedic surgery, 2411
  arterial blood pressure monitoring and, 1277
  experimental, 141, 142f
  in head and neck surgery, 2539
  in pediatric anesthesia, 2394
  left atrial pressure monitoring and, 1311
  mediastinoscopy and, 1911
  paradoxical, 2141–2142
  transesophageal echocardiography in, 1381, 1383
  venous, 2138–2142, 2139f, 2140f, 2140t, 2141f, 2672
Air travel, 2691, 2693
Airflow absence testing, in double-lumen endotracheal tube placement, 1882, 1883f
Airway
  closing capacity of, 694–697
    in abnormal lungs, 695, 695f
    in normal lungs, 694–695, 695f
    tracer gas test of, 695–697, 696f, 697f
  difficult, 2545–2548. See also Airway management.
    algorithm for, 1636–1637, 1638f, 1639f
    BURP maneuver in, 1637
    cart for, 1640, 1641t, 2386t
    Combitube in, 1637, 2458
    cricothyroidotomy in, 1639–1640
      for children, 2386–2387
    disease-specific, 1621t
    fiberoptic bronchoscopy in, 1645–1646
    gum elastic bougie in, 1637, 2458, 2458f
    in children, 2385–2387, 2386t, 2387f
    in trauma patient, 2458–2459, 2458f
    laryngeal block in, 2545–2546
    laryngeal mask airway in, 1637, 1640f, 2458
      for children, 2386, 2386t
    predictability of, 1623
    tracheostomy in, 2539–2540, 2546–2547
    transtracheal jet ventilation in, 1637–1639, 1640f, 2458–2459
      for children, 2386–2387, 2387f
  evaluation of, in airway management, 1620–1623, 1620t, 1621t, 1622f
  foreign body in, 2545
  functions of, 1619–1620
  in basic life support, 2923–2925
  in pediatric life support, 2942
  intraoperative heating and humidification of, 1585
  ketamine effects on, 348
  laser surgery on, 2542–2543
  nerve blocks for, 1708–1709, 1708f
  normal, 1624f
  preoperative rehabilitation of, 1014
  secretions of, preoperative removal of, 1014
  structure of, 1617–1619, 1618f
    in children, 2840, 2841t, 2842
    in infant, 2369–2370, 2370f
Airway (artificial). See also Endotracheal intubation; Tracheostomy.
  nasopharyngeal, 1619, 1624–1625, 1625f
  oropharyngeal, 1619, 1624–1625, 1625f
Airway conductance, in pulmonary function testing, 1003, 1003f
Airway management, 1617–1651
  airway evaluation in, 1620–1623, 1620t, 1621t, 1622f
  chest radiography in, 1623
  Combitube in, 1627–1628, 1628f, 1637
  computed tomography in, 1623
  consultation on, 1650–1651
  cricothyroidotomy in, 1639–1640
    for children, 2386–2387
    in basic life support, 2924
    in emergency, 2547

Airway management (Continued)
  disease-specific difficulties in, 1621t
  endotracheal intubation in, 1628–1646. See also Endotracheal intubation.
  general recommendations for, 1651
  head position in, 1622–1623, 1622f
  historical perspective on, 36–40, 36f
  hoarseness and, 1623
  hyomental distance in, 1621
  in brain injury, 2470–2471
  in children, 1646–1647
  in congenital syndromes, 1620, 1620t
  in edentulous patients, 1620
  in goiter, 1046–1047
  in laryngeal trauma, 2540–2541
  in spinal cord injury, 2475–2476
  in trauma, 2452–2453, 2452t, 2454–2459, 2455f
    aspiration and, 2456
    cervical spine in, 2456
    cricoid pressure in, 2456
    endotracheal intubation in, 2455–2459, 2456t, 2457f, 2458f
    extubation for, 2483, 2483t
    in facial trauma, 2459
    in pharyngeal trauma, 2459
    indications for, 2454–2455
    induction anesthetics for, 2457
    mechanical ventilation for, 2485–2487, 2485t, 2486f, 2486t
    neuromuscular blocking drugs for, 2457–2458
    oral vs. nasal intubation in, 2459
    personnel for, 2456–2457
  laryngeal mask airway in, 1625–1628, 1626f, 1627f, 1637, 1640f
  Mallampati score in, 1621
  mandibular hypoplasia and, 1621–1622
  mask ventilation in, 1623–1624, 1623f, 1624f
  mouth opening size in, 1620
  nasopharyngeal airway in, 1624–1625, 1625f
  neck examination in, 1622–1623, 1622f
  oral cavity examination in, 1620–1621, 1622f
  oropharyngeal airway in, 1624–1625, 1625f
  patient history in, 1620, 1621t
  physical examination in, 1620–1623
  soft nasal airway in, 1625
  thyromental distance in, 1621
  transtracheal jet ventilation in, 1637–1639, 1640f, 2458–2459, 2545, 2546
Airway obstruction, 1618–1619, 1624f. See also Airway management.
  airway resistance measurement in, 1005–1006, 1006f
  alveolar-arterial oxygen tension difference in, 1010
  diffusing capacity in, 1010–1011
  expiratory air flow in, 1004–1005, 1005t
  flow-volume loops in, 1007–1009, 1008f, 1009f
  forced expiration measurements in, 1006–1007, 1007f, 1008f
  gas exchange function in, 1010–1011, 1010f
  in children, 2387–2388, 2387f, 2388f, 2844–2845, 2848–2849, 2854, 2870. See also Respiratory failure, pediatric.
  in rheumatoid arthritis, 2410
  mechanisms of, 1004–1005, 1005t
  mediastinal mass and, 2870
  multiple-breath nitrogen washout test in, 1010, 1010f
  postoperative, 2711–2712, 2711f, 2712f
  pulmonary function testing in, 1005–1010, 1007f–1009f, 1009t
  treatment of, 1618–1619
Airway pressure
  during laparoscopy, 2288, 2288f
  in high-frequency ventilation, 1469, 1469f
  inspiratory (P₁₀₀), 1463
  monitoring of, 1463–1467, 1464f, 1466f, 1467f
Airway receptors, 171–174, 174f
  inhaled anesthetic effects on, 172–173
Airway resistance, 690–691
  endotracheal intubation and, 1649
  hypoxemia and, 709–710, 710f
  in children, 2842
  in pulmonary function testing, 1002–1003, 1003f, 1005–1006, 1006f
  inhaled anesthetic-related changes in, 155–161, 157f–160f
  lung volumes and, 709–710, 710f
Alanine aminopeptidase, in renal function monitoring, 1501

Alanine aminotransferase, 753–754, 753t
  preoperative, 2214–2215, 2215f
Albumin
  drug binding to, 74–76, 75f, 120, 1722–1723
    age-related changes in, 100–101, 2438
  five percent, 1787
  hepatic metabolism of, 747
  serum, 753t, 754
    preoperative, 962
  transfusion of, 1825
  twenty-five percent, 1787
Albuterol, 652, 2817t
  halothane with, 161
  preoperative, 1859
Alcohol dehydrogenase, 760
Alcohol use, 1096–1097. See also Substance abuse.
  alfentanil use and, 1248
  hepatotoxicity of, 759–760, 2221t
  hypophosphatemia in, 1774
  in elderly patient, 2443
Alcuronium, 493t, 497, 497t
  autonomic effects of, 511, 511t, 512t
  dosage for, 501t
  elimination of, 506t
  metabolism of, 506t, 509
  pharmacodynamics of, 502t
Aldehyde dehydrogenase, 760
Aldosterone, 1036–1037
  excess of, 1038
  in cardiac function, 737–738, 737t
  in renal function, 793, 793f, 1487
Alertness, 3055. See also Sleep deprivation.
Alfentanil, 380t. See also Intravenous anesthetics.
  age-related pharmacokinetics of, 406, 406f, 2439, 2439t
  arterial concentration of, 84, 84f
  automated delivery system for, 472
  C_{50} of, 446–448, 447t
  cardiovascular effects of, 394, 395
  cerebral blood flow effects of, 389, 390, 823
  context-sensitive decrement time of, 455–456, 456f
  context-sensitive half-time of, 404, 404f
  depth of anesthesia and, 1245
  electroencephalographic effects of, 388–389, 388f, 389f
  endocrine effects of, 396–397
  epileptogenic properties of, 833
  for children, 2377
  hepatic effects of, 398
  hepatic metabolism of, 2213
  high-dose, 414
  in alcohol-consuming patient, 1248
  in awake craniotomy, 2160
  in balanced anesthesia, 411, 412f
  in endotracheal intubation, 1647
  in kidney transplantation, 2241
  in outpatient anesthesia, 2606
  in outpatient monitored anesthesia care, 2610
  in pediatric cardiac surgery, 2022
  in single-agent anesthesia, 414
  in total intravenous anesthesia, 413, 413t
  infusion rate of, 459t
  intracranial pressure effects and, 390, 823
  isoflurane interaction with, 449–450
  manual infusion of, 460, 460t
  midazolam interaction with, 450, 453f
  myocardial ischemia and, 395
  patient-controlled, 2733–2734, 2733t
  peak effect of, 404, 405f
  pharmacodynamics of, 1249
  pharmacokinetics of, 400, 400f, 401t, 402–403
    age and, 406, 406f, 2439, 2439t
    liver failure and, 408
    target-controlled infusion and, 466–468, 468t
  plasma concentration ranges for, 453t
  propofol with, 90, 97f, 398, 413, 422, 449, 449f, 450, 453t
  respiratory effects of, 392–393
  seizures and, 833
  single-bolus, 410
  single-dose, 2737, 2738t
  structure of, 381f
  thermoregulatory response thresholds with, 1574–1575, 1574f
  volume of distribution of, 454t
Aliflurane, oil-gas partition coefficient of, 115t
Alkali therapy, in neonatal acidosis, 2357–2358, 2358f
Alkaline phosphatase, 753t, 754–755
  parenteral nutrition and, 2911
  preoperative, 2214–2215, 2215f

Alkaline solution, 1600
Alkalosis
  contraction, 1604, 1608, 1614
  hypocapnic, hypoxemia and, 708
  hypochloremic, 1608
  metabolic, 1603–1604, 1603t, 1605t
    hypercapnia and, 718
    perioperative, 1512–1513, 1612f, 1613t
  respiratory, 1603, 1603t, 1605t
    fentanyl effects and, 409
    perioperative, 1611
n-Alkanes, 116
Alkylating agents, 1118
Allele frequency, 98
Allen test, 1272, 2069
Allergic reaction
  anaphylactic, 514, 1092–1093, 1093t
  barbiturates and, 333
  blood transfusion and, 1817
  chymopapain, 1092, 1093t
  latex and, 919, 1092, 1093, 3161–3162
  local anesthetics and, 596–597
  nondepolarizing muscle relaxants and, 514
  opioids and, 399
Allopurinol, hepatotoxicity of, 2221t
Alpha bungarotoxin, 2515t
Alpha-fetoprotein, 756
  hepatic metabolism of, 747
Alpha value, in statistics, 885
Alphaprodine, 417
Althesin, intraocular pressure effects of, 2552
Altitude, 2656, 2667t
  decompression illness and, 2672–2673, 2678, 2691, 2693
  gas density and, 2691
  high, 2687–2693
    anesthesia at, 2691–2693, 2692t, 2693t
    birth at, 2689
    bleeding at, 2691
    cardiovascular response to, 2667–2669, 2668f, 2669f, 2670t
    cerebral edema at, 2690–2691
    decompression illness and, 2691
    hypoxia and, 687, 2688–2689, 2688f, 2689f
    metabolic acidosis at, 1783
    mountain sickness at, 2690, 2691
    oxygen therapy at, 2692–2693
    pulmonary artery pressure at, 687
    pulmonary edema at, 2690
Altitude illness, 2690–2691
Alveolar-arterial (A-a) gradient, 1010, 1440–1442, 1455
  interpretation of, 1446–1447, 1446t
Alveolar dead space, 680, 697–698, 697f, 698f
  hypercapnia and, 714, 714f
  measurement of, 1442, 1442f
Alveolar gases, 1439. See also Carbon dioxide (CO_2); Oxygen (O_2).
Alveolar/inspired pressure ratio (FA-FI), 131–136, 132f, 132t, 133t, 134f–136f
  anesthetic metabolism and, 136
  anesthetic solubility and, 132, 132t, 134, 134f, 139–140
  cardiac output and, 138–139, 138f, 139f
  intertissue anesthetic diffusion and, 135
  second gas effect and, 135, 136f
  ventilation-to-perfusion ratio and, 139–140, 140f, 141f
  ventilatory changes and, 136–137, 137t, 139, 139f, 140f
Alveolar pressure
  blood flow and, 679–681, 680f
  pulmonary artery catheter monitoring and, 1308–1309, 1308f
Alveoli, 703–705, 704f
  pediatric, 2840, 2841t
Alzheimer's disease, 1096
Ambu bag, in neonatal resuscitation, 2350
Ambulation, after spinal anesthesia, 1679
Ambulatory (outpatient) anesthesia, 58–59, 58f, 2589–2623
  α_2-adrenergic agonists for, 2596–2597, 2596t
  acupressure with, 2599
  acupuncture with, 2599
  analgesics for, 2597
  antacids with, 2600
  anticholinergics with, 2599
  antihistamines with, 2599
  aspiration pneumonitis prevention and, 2599–2601, 2600t
  benzodiazepines for, 2596, 2596t

Ambulatory (outpatient) anesthesia (Continued)
  cerebral monitoring for, 2611–2612
  complications of, 2621–2622
  contraindications to, 2593
  cost effectiveness of, 2612–2613
  dexamethasone with, 2599
  discharge after, 2612–2613, 2613t, 2619–2621, 2620t
  domperidone with, 2598
  droperidol with, 2598
  facilities for, 2590–2591, 2591f
  fast-tracking, 2613–2614, 2613t, 2614t, 2615t
  for electroconvulsive therapy, 2618–2619, 2619t
  for gastroenterology suite, 2618
  for magnetic resonance imaging, 2618
  future trends in, 2622
  gastrokinetic agents with, 2598, 2600
  general, 2602–2608, 2602t
  H_2 receptor antagonists with, 2599–2600, 2600t
  hospital admission after, 2621–2622
  hydration guidelines for, 2601, 2601f
  in elderly patient, 2593
  in infant, 2593
  local, 2609, 2616
  malignant hyperthermia and, 2593
  metoclopramide with, 2598, 2600
  monitored anesthesia care in, 2609–2611
  monitoring for, 2609–2612
  nausea with, 2597–2599, 2597t, 2598f
  neurokinin-1 antagonists with, 2599
  nonopioid analgesics for, 2597
  nonpharmacologic preparation for, 2595, 2595f
  NPO guidelines for, 2600–2601, 2601f
  office-based, 2616–2617
  opioid analgesics for, 2597
  optimal, 2612–2613, 2613t
  outcomes of, 2621–2622
  patient age and, 2593
  patient physical status and, 2592–2593, 2592t
  patient selection for, 2591–2593, 2592t
  phenothiazines with, 2598
  premedication for, 2595–2601, 2596t, 2597t, 2598f
  preoperative assessment for, 2593–2594, 2594t
  preoperative preparation for, 2595–2601, 2595f, 2596t, 2597t, 2598f
  procedure duration and, 2592
  proton pump inhibitors with, 2599–2600, 2600t
  psychological preparation for, 2595, 2595f
  rationale for, 2590, 2590t
  recovery after, 2612, 2614–2616, 2615t, 2616t, 2619–2620, 2620t
  regional, 2608–2609, 2620
  remote-location, 2617–2619. See also Remote locations.
  screening tests for, 2593–2594, 2594t
  serotonin antagonists with, 2599
  side effects of, 2614–2616, 2615t, 2616t
  vomiting with, 2597–2599, 2597t, 2598f
Amenorrhea, 1052
American Society of Anesthesiologists, 41
  physical status classification of, 902, 902f, 906, 907t
American Society of Anesthesiologists Standards, for monitoring, 1438
Ames Salmonella assay, 261
Amikacin, renal effects of, 803
Amino acids
  branched-chain, in sepsis, 2901
  excitatory, inhaled anesthetic effects on, 113
  in hepatic failure, 2916
  in parenteral nutrition, 2912t
  metabolism of, in sepsis, 2897–2899, 2898f
  muscle release of, 2890–2891
p-Aminobenzoic acid, allergic reactions to, 596–597
γ-Aminobutyric acid (GABA)
  inhaled anesthetic effects on, 111–112, 112f, 113, 121, 122f, 174–175, 175f
  kava effects on, 610–611
  valerian effects on, 612
γ-Aminobutyric acid (GABA$_A$) receptor, 89f, 90–92, 91f
  benzodiazepine binding to, 337–339, 337f, 338f
  in barbiturate-induced anesthesia, 330
ε-Aminocaproic acid, 1811
Aminoglycosides
  neuromuscular blockade with, 516
  renal effects of, 803, 805
Aminooxyacetic acid (AOAA), 253–254, 255f
Aminophylline, 1124, 1859
4-Aminopyridine, 516

Aminotransferases, 753–754, 753t
  preoperative, 2214–2215, 2215f
Amiodarone, 1125
  hepatotoxicity of, 2221t
  in atrial fibrillation, 1402, 1402t, 1403t
  in cardiac arrest, 2938
  in ventricular tachycardia, 1404
  preoperative, 1860–1861
  thyroid dysfunction and, 1047
Amitriptyline, in chronic pain, 2771
Ammonia, toxicity of, transurethral resection of
  prostate and, 2192–2193
Amoxicillin/clavulanic acid, hepatotoxicity of, 2221t
Ampere, 1208
Amphetamines, 1124, 3061
Amphotericin B, 2816
Amplification artifact, 1220–1221
Amputation, 2479
Amrinone, with aortic cross-clamping, 2077
Amyl nitrite, in cyanide poisoning, 2513t
Amyloidosis, 1047
Amyotrophic lateral sclerosis, neuromuscular
  blockade in, 534
Anabolic steroids, 2221t
Analgesia
  epidural, 2720, 2737–2743, 2737t, 2738t. See also
    Epidural analgesia.
  for vaginal delivery, 2319–2322. See also Vaginal
    delivery, regional analgesia for.
  inter/intrapleural, 587–588, 1909, 2744
    for children, 1753
  patient-controlled, 30, 410, 2733–2734, 2733t,
    2741–2742, 2741t, 2748
  postoperative, 2729–2751. See also Pain,
    postoperative.
  preemptive, 2731–2732
Analgesia, 56
Anaphylactoid reaction, 514, 1092–1093
Anaphylaxis, 1092–1093
  barbiturates and, 333
  blood transfusion-induced, 1817
  neuromuscular blocking agents and, 514
Anaritide, renal protection with, 800
Andrews, Edmund, 17
Androgens, adrenal, 1035–1036
Anemia, 1111–1114
  drug-induced, 1114
  enzyme-deficient, 1113–1114
  hemolytic, autoimmune, 1114
  hyperbaric oxygen therapy in, 2674
  in critically ill patient, 2803
  in hepatic disease, 761
  in kidney failure, 2181t, 2182, 2239
  pernicious, 1097
  sickle cell, 1112–1113
  uremia and, 1101
Anemometry, 1463
Anencephalic infant, organ donation from, 2962
Anesoft patient simulators, 3077t, 3078–3079,
  3079f
Anesthesia
  definition of, 1230–1231
  depth of, 1227–1259. See also Depth of anesthesia.
  education for, 64, 64f, 3105–3113, 3106f. See also
    Anesthesia education.
  historical perspective on, 12–19
  machines for. See Anesthesia machines.
  practice of, 55–65
  risk of. See Anesthesia-related risk.
  value-based, 62–64, 62f, 63f, 63t
  workforce for, 60–62, 61f. See also
    Anesthesiologist.
Anesthesia, 56
Anesthesia crisis resource management, 3082–3084,
  3083t
Anesthesia education, 64, 64f, 3105–3113, 3106f,
  3113f
  affective learning and, 3111
  audiovisual aids in, 3113
  Board certification in, 3107–3108
  curriculum for, 3111, 3116–3117
  for continued demonstration of qualifications,
    3109
  for nurses, 3108
  goals of, 3107–3109
  methods of, 3112–3113
  question type in, 3112
  simulation in, 3091–3092, 3095–3096, 3112. See
    also Patient simulators.
  students of, 3106–3107
  teachers of, 3109–3111, 3110t

Anesthesia machines, 273–311
  barotrauma and, 301
  carbon dioxide absorption systems of, 296–298,
    297f
  check valve of, 275, 276
  checkout procedure for, 307–310, 308f, 308t, 309f,
    310f, 315–316
  circle breathing system of, 295–296, 295f
    problems in, 300–301, 300f
    test of, 310
  circuits of, 293–296, 294f, 295f
  cylinder supply source of, 274–275, 275f, 276
  Datex-Ohmeda Aladin cassette, 292–293
  Datex-Ohmeda S/5 ADU, 301–302, 307–308, 308t
  Datex-Ohmeda Tec 6, 281t, 289–292, 290f
  defects in, 283
  Diameter Index Safety System of, 276
  Drager Narkomed 6000, 302–303, 303f
  electronic alarm of, 276
  Fabius GS, 302–303, 307–308, 308t
  fail-safe valves of, 275, 277, 277f
  flow meter assembly of, 277–281, 278f–281f. See
    also Flow meter assembly.
  hazards of, 276, 282–283, 288–289, 300–301
  high-pressure circuit of, 274
  historical perspective on, 33–35
  intermediate-pressure circuit of, 274
  leak test of, 283, 307–309, 308f, 308t, 309f
  Link-25 proportioning system for, 281, 281f, 283
  low-pressure circuit of, 274
  malfunction of
    hypercapnia and, 715
    hypoxemia and, 707–708
    tests for, 307–310, 308t, 309f, 310f, 315–316
  negative-pressure leak test of, 309–310, 310f
  oxygen analyzer calibration for, 307
  oxygen failure protection device of, 277, 278f
  oxygen flush valve of, 283–284
  oxygen ratio monitor controller for, 281–282,
    282f, 283
  oxygen regulator of, 275, 277
  Pin INdex Safety System of, 276
  pipeline crossover hazard of, 276
  pipeline supply source of, 274–275, 275f, 276
  pneumatic alarm of, 276
  positive-pressure leak test of, 309, 309f
  pressure regulator of, 276
  proportioning systems of, 281–283, 281f, 282f
    errors with, 283
  safety devices of, 276–277, 277f
  scavenging systems of, 303–307, 304f, 304t, 305f,
    306f, 3151–3152
  second-stage pressure regulator of, 277
  self-tests of, 310
  shut-off valve of, 277, 277f
  two-gas machine of, 274–275, 275f
  vaporizers of, 284–296. See also Vaporizer(s).
  ventilators of, 298–301, 299f. See also
    Ventilator(s).
  workstations for, 273–274, 274f, 301–303, 303f
Anesthesia Patient Safety Foundation, 41
Anesthesia preoperative evaluation clinic, 980–991,
  981t, 982t, 983f, 983t, 984f–987f
Anesthesia-related risk, 893–920, 895f, 919t
  ACCS study of, 904–905, 905t, 906f
  anesthesiologist factors in, 917–918, 918f
  anesthetic agent in, 914–915
  ASA physical status classification and, 902, 902f,
    906, 907t
  cardiovascular disease and, 908–909, 910t, 915,
    916t
  hospital-specific, 915–916
  in geriatrics, 914
  in obstetrics, 909–912, 911t, 912f
  in ophthalmologic surgery, 915
  in outpatient surgery, 902–903, 903f, 916–917
  in pediatrics, 912–914, 913t, 914f
  intraoperative cardiac arrest and, 903–904, 904t
  long-term, 905–906
  outcome measures and, 893–894, 894t
  patient factors in, 906–909, 907f, 907t, 910t
  reduction of, 919–920, 919t
  studies of, 894–902
    after 1980, 899–902, 899t, 900t, 901t, 902f,
      902t
    before 1980, 897–899, 897t
    computer analysis for, 904
    design of, 894–897
  surgical factors in, 906t, 915
  surrogate end points and, 894
  vs. surgery without anesthesia, 897

Anesthesiologist, 60–62, 61f
  ability requirements for, 3041–3042, 3042t
  abstract reasoning by, 3026t, 3027–3028
  accident response by, 3033–3035, 3034f,
    3043–3047, 3044f, 3045f
  action by, 3026t, 3028, 3030–3031
  action density and, 3036–3037, 3036f–3038f,
    3036t
  anesthesia-related risk and, 917–918, 918f
  anesthetic plan of, 3032–3033, 3033f
  attention management by, 3029–3031
  automation and, 3037–3038
  chemical dependence in, 3164–3170. See also
    Substance abuse.
  cognitive demands on, 3023–3031, 3025f, 3025t,
    3026t, 3028t, 3029t, 3030t
  decision-making by, 3024–3026, 3025f, 3025t,
    3026t, 3027–3028, 3043–3047, 3044f,
    3045t
  direct observations of, 3046
  education for, 64, 64f, 3105–3113, 3106f. See also
    Anesthesia education.
  empirical studies of, 3035–3038, 3036f–3038f
  equipment preparation by, 3032
  errors by, 3028, 3029, 3029t, 3044–3045, 3046
  event response by, 3033–3035, 3034f, 3043–3047,
    3044f, 3045t
  FIT-System analysis of, 3036–3037, 3036f–3038f,
    3036t
  fixation errors of, 3029, 3029t
  hazardous attitudes of, 3029, 3030t
  heuristics use by, 3027
  idle time of, 3035
  indirect observations of, 3046
  infection in, 918–919, 3155–3161, 3157t, 3158t
  job stress and, 3163–3164
  latex allergy in, 3161–3162
  mental simulations by, 3031
  mental workload of, 3038–3040, 3039f
  noise effects on, 3054–3055, 3162
  novice, 3035–3036, 3039–3040, 3039f
  observations by, 3026, 3026t
  occupational risks of, 918–919, 3155–3162, 3157t,
    3158t
  overwork and, 3162
  performance of, 3021–3064
    aging and, 3062–3063
    cognitive demands in, 3023–3031, 3025f,
      3025t, 3026t, 3028t, 3029t, 3030t
    drug use and, 3063. See also Substance abuse.
    environmental demands in, 3023–3024
    illness and, 3063
    investigation of, 3022–3024
    noise and, 3054–3055
    operating room safety and, 3047–3054,
      3047f–3049f, 3049t, 3050t, 3051t, 3052t,
      3053f. See also Operating room, safety of.
    reading and, 3055
    sleep deprivation and, 3055–3062
    tasks analysis in, 3031–3042, 3033f, 3034f,
      3036f–3039f, 3041f
    work hour regulation and, 3062
  predictions by, 3026t, 3027
  preoperative evaluation by, 3031–3032
  problem recognition by, 3027
  prospective memory of, 3028–3029
  radiation hazards to, 3153–3155, 3154f
  reevaluation by, 3028, 3028t
  resource management by, 3031
  situation awareness of, 3028
  sleep deprivation effects on, 3162–3163
  stress effects on, 3163–3164
  task patterns and, 3035–3036, 3036f
  verification by, 3026–3027, 3026t
  video analysis of, 3046–3047
  vigilance of, 3038–3040, 3039f, 3042–3043, 3042t
    during transesophageal echocardiography,
      3040–3041, 3041f
  visual attention by, 3035
  waste gas effects on, 3151–3153
  workload management by, 3030
Anesthetic analyzer, 1213, 1213f
Anesthetic circuits, 293–296. See also Anesthesia
  machines.
  Bain, 293–295, 294f
  circle, 295–296, 295f
  Mapleson, 293–295, 294f
Aneurysm
  aortic, 1963–1964, 1964f, 1964t
    abdominal, 2070–2071. See also Abdominal
      aorta, reconstruction of.

Aneurysm (Continued)
   intracranial, 2146–2151. See also Intracranial
      aneurysm.
Angina, 1074, 1075t. See also Myocardial ischemia.
   Ludwig's, 2544
Angiography
   coronary, 2648–2649
      before peripheral vascular surgery, 2062, 2063t,
         2064t
      cortical blindness after, 3011–3012
   in brain death, 2965t, 2966
   intraoperative, in intracranial aneurysm
      treatment, 2151
   spinal cord, before thoracoabdominal aortic
      reconstruction, 2088, 2088f
Angiotensin
   in carcinoid-related hypotension, 1109
   in cardiac function, 737, 737t
Angiotensin-converting enzyme (ACE) inhibitors,
   659, 793, 1120
Angiotensin I, 659
   in sodium homeostasis, 1765
Angiotensin II, 659
   in hepatic blood flow, 747
   in renal regulation, 792–793, 792f
   in sodium homeostasis, 1765
Anion gap, 1607–1608, 1607f, 1781–1782
Ankle
   nerve blocks at, 1703–1704, 1703f, 1704f, Plate 15
   surgery on, 2422
Ankle-brachial index, 2093
Ankylosing spondylitis, 2411
Anorexia nervosa, 1034
Antacids
   for outpatient premedication, 2600, 2600t
   preoperative, 1860
Antagonist, 86–87, 86f, 87f
   competitive, 86, 95f, 96
   discontinuation of, 102
   dose-response relationship of, 95f, 96
   noncompetitive, 86–87
Anterior interosseous nerve, position-related injury
   to, 1156t
Anthrax, 2503, 2515t, 2516–2517, 2518t. See also
   Chemical and biological warfare agents.
Antiarrhythmic drugs, 1124–1125
Antibiotics, 1125
   aerosol, 2816
   neuromuscular blockade and, 516, 523
   preoperative, 1859
      for endocarditis, 1079, 1080t–1081t
Anticholinesterases, 662, 875–876
   in kidney failure, 2186, 2186t
   in phase II block, 1563
   neuromuscular blockade recovery with, 519,
      521–522, 521f, 523–524, 524t, 875–876
      acid-base state and, 522–523
      antibiotic interactions with, 523
      anticholinesterase dose and, 521, 522
      anticholinesterase potency and, 521, 521f
      atropine with, 523
      depth of block and, 520, 520f
      electrolyte imbalance and, 523
      exogenous butyrylcholinesterase in, 522
      hypothermia interactions with, 523
      nausea with, 523
      pharmacokinetics of, 523–524, 524t
      plasma drug concentration and, 521–522, 521f
      verapamil interactions with, 523
      vomiting with, 523
   organophosphate effects on, 2504, 2505f, 2506t
Anticoagulation
   epidural analgesia and, 2742–2743
   epidural anesthesia and, 1677
   in cardiopulmonary bypass, 1972–1974, 1973f,
      1974f
   in orthopedic surgery, 2426
   in pediatric cardiac surgery, 2034–2035
   prophylactic, 1079, 1082–1083, 1082t
Anticonvulsants, 517, 2134
Antidepressants, 1122–1124
   electroconvulsive therapy and, 2654
   in chronic pain, 2771–2772
   tricyclic, 1121, 1123
Antidiuretic hormone
   deficiency of, 1053
   in renal function, 1487
   secretion of, 1766
   syndrome of inappropriate secretion of,
      1052–1053
Antidotes, for toxic ingestions, 2875

Antiepileptic agents
   age-related effects of, 101
   in chronic pain, 2771
Antifibrinolytics
   in cardiopulmonary bypass, 1974–1975
   in intracranial aneurysm, 2148
Antihypertensive drugs, 1119–1122, 1119f, 1120f
Antimitochondrial antibodies, 755
Antipsychotic agents, neuroleptic malignant
   syndrome with, 1183
Antithymocyte globulin, in organ transplantation,
   2271–2273, 2272t
α_1-Antitrypsin
   deficiency of, 755–756
   in sepsis, 2902, 2902f
AOAA (aminooxyacetic acid), 253–254, 255t
Aorta
   abdominal. See Abdominal aorta.
   aneurysm of, 1963–1964, 1964f, 1964t
   atheroma of, 1383
   coarctation of, 2010–2011, 2039–2040
   cross-clamping of. See Aortic cross-clamping.
   dissection of, 1964, 1965f, 1965t
   endovascular surgery on, 2089–2092
      anesthesia for, 2090–2091
      complications of, 2091–2092
      endoleak with, 2091
      monitoring during, 2091
      outcomes of, 2091–2092
      technique of, 2089–2090
      vs. open repair, 2092
   infrarenal, occlusive disease of, 2071–2072,
      2075–2076
   normal pressures of, 1297t
   thoracoabdominal. See Thoracoabdominal aorta.
   transesophageal echocardiography of, 1379, 1383
   trauma to, 2480
Aortic arch
   aneurysm of, 2086
   interruption of, 2010–2011
Aortic cannula, 1995
Aortic cross-clamping. See also Cardiopulmonary
   bypass.
   afterload reduction in, 2077
   arterial hypertension and, 2072–2073
   blood volume redistribution with, 2073–2074,
      2075f
   cardiac output and, 2073, 2074f, 2075
   in abdominal aortic reconstruction, 2072–2076,
      2073t, 2074f, 2074t, 2075f
   in thoracoabdominal aortic reconstruction, 2085
   infrarenal, 2075–2076
   metabolic effects of, 2073t, 2075
   preload effects of, 2074–2075
   preload normalization in, 2077
   pulmonary capillary wedge pressure and,
      2073–2074, 2074t
   unclamping for, 2077, 2078f
Aortic regurgitation, 1958–1959, 1959f, 1960f
   arterial blood pressure monitoring in, 1285
   left ventricular end-diastolic pressure in, 1321,
      1321t
   transesophageal echocardiography in, 1380, 1381t
Aortic stenosis, 1954–1957
   arterial blood pressure monitoring in, 1284–1285
   congenital, 2010–2011
   ejection fraction reduction in, 1956
   pathophysiology of, 1954–1955, 1955t
   pseudo-, 1956, 1956t
   sudden death in, 1955–1956
   symptomatic, 1955
   transesophageal echocardiography in, 1380,
      1380f
   ventricular response to, 726, 726f
Aortic valve, sclerosis of, 2437
Aortoiliac occlusive disease, 2071–2072
Aoyagi, Takuo, 6
Apgar, Virginia, 42–43, 43f
Apgar score, 2348–2349, 2349t, 2352–2353
Apnea. See also Respiratory failure.
   benzodiazepine-induced, 340
   in infant, 2397–2398, 2397f, 2723
   monitoring for, 1467–1468, 1473
   sleep, 1096
      obesity and, 1030–1031
      postoperative pain management and,
         2748–2749
      pulmonary complications and, 1038
Apnea test, for brain death, 2961
Apneic insufflation, 1901
Apneic threshold, 178, 178f

Apoptosis
   hepatic, 757
   neuronal, 834–837, 835f, 838f
Aprotinin, 1811
   in cardiopulmonary bypass, 1974–1975
   in pediatric cardiac surgery, 2035–2036
Arachidonic acid, in prostaglandin synthesis, 795,
   795f
Arachnoid mater, 1655, 1655f
Area under the curve, 80
L-Arginine, nitrate tolerance and, 1950–1951
Arginine vasopressin
   in renal regulation, 793–794, 794f
   in septic shock, 806–807, 807f
Argon, oil-gas partition coefficient of, 115t
Argon beam coagulator, 3147
Aristotle, 4
Arm. See also Elbow.
   surgery on, 2421
Arndt bronchial blockers, 1887–1888, 1888f, 1888t
Arnold-Chiari malformation, 2164t
Arrhythmias, 1083–1085, 2929–2935. See also specific
   arrhythmias.
   β-adrenergic receptor antagonists in, 656
   before peripheral vascular surgery, 2059
   catheter ablation in, 2653
   cimetidine and, 1053
   drug treatment of, 1124–1125
   during laparoscopy, 2293
   electrocardiography in. See Electrocardiography.
   epinephrine-induced, inhaled anesthetic effects
      on, 203
   extracorporeal shock wave lithotripsy and, 2196
   halothane-related, 203, 649
      in children, 2374
   hypercapnia and, 717
   hypoxemia and, 716
   in head and neck surgery, 2539
   in hypokalemia, 1107
   inhaled anesthetics and, 203
   magnesium effects on, 1773
   nitrous oxide and, 214
   pacemakers for, 1084–1085, 1084t. See also
      Pacemaker.
   pediatric, 1732, 1732t, 2374, 2378, 2839
   percutaneous transluminal coronary angioplasty
      and, 2649
   postoperative, 2717
   pulmonary artery catheter-related, 1304–1305
   risk factors for, 1397–1398
   succinylcholine-related, 489, 873
      in children, 2378
   tonsillectomy and, 2544
   vasopressin and, 1053
Arterial blood gases, 1439–1447. See Carbon dioxide
   (CO_2), arterial; Oxygen (O_2), arterial.
Arterial blood pressure, 1268–1286
   aortic cross-clamping and, 2072–2073, 2073t,
      2074t
   automated measurement of
      continuous, 1271–1272
      intermittent, 1269–1271, 1270f, 1271t
   cerebral blood flow and, 816f, 817, 829
   dexmedetomidine effects on, 357, 357f
   direct measurement of, 1272–1286, 1284t
      air bubble dampening in, 1277, 1278f
      anacrotic notch on, 1284
      axillary artery cannulation for, 1274
      brachial artery cannulation for, 1274
      calibration procedure in, 1280
      complications of, 1274–1275, 1275t
      damping coefficient in, 1276, 1277f,
         1278–1279, 1278f
      dicrotic notch on, 1282, 1282f
      distal pulse amplification in, 1282–1283, 1282f
      drug effects on, 1283
      dynamic (frequency) response in, 1275–1279,
         1275f–1278f
      equipment for, 1279
      fast-flush test in, 1277–1278, 1279
      femoral artery cannulation for, 1274
      guidelines for, 1279
      in aortic regurgitation, 1285
      in aortic stenosis, 1284–1285
      in cardiopulmonary bypass, 1283–1284, 1284f,
         1286
      in children, 2393
      in hypertrophic cardiomyopathy, 1285
      in intra-aortic balloon counterpulsation, 1286,
         1287f
      in pulsus alternans, 1285, 1286f

Arterial blood pressure (Continued)
  direct measurement of (Continued)
    in pulsus paradoxus, 1285–1286, 1286f
    in sepsis, 1283
    inaccuracy in, 1279
    indications for, 1272, 1272f
    interpretation of, 1280–1281, 1281f
    leveling procedure in, 1280–1281, 1281f
    monitor for, 1282
    natural frequency in, 1275–1279, 1275f–1278f
    normal waveform characteristics in, 1281–1282, 1282f
    overdamped waveform in, 1276, 1276f
    patient position and, 1280–1281, 1281f, 1283
    pressure wave reflection in, 1283, 1283f
    radial artery cannulation for, 1272–1274, 1273f
    shock and, 1283
    surgical procedure and, 1283
    system frequency in, 1275–1277, 1276f, 1277f
    technical aspects of, 1275–1281, 1275f–1278f
    transducer setup for, 1279–1281, 1281f
    ulnar artery cannulation for, 1274
    underdamped waveform in, 1276, 1276f
    waveform characteristics in, 1275–1279, 1275f–1278f, 1281–1282, 1282f
    zeroing procedure in, 1279–1280
  during pregnancy, 2312
  epidural anesthesia and, 1660
  historical studies on, 6–8
  in aortic reconstruction, 2077
  in aortic regurgitation, 1285
  in aortic stenosis, 1284–1285
  in autonomic function assessment, 663t
  in basic life support, 2927
  in cardiopulmonary bypass, 1283–1284, 1284f, 1286, 1979
  in cholestasis, 764–765
  in diabetes mellitus, 665
  in head injury, 2154–2155, 2154t
  in hypertrophic cardiomyopathy, 1285
  in intra-aortic balloon counterpulsation, 1286, 1287f
  in neonate, 2358, 2359t
  in neurosurgery, 2133, 2136–2137
  in pediatric cardiac surgery, 2016–2017
  in peripheral vascular surgery, 2069–2070
  in pulsus alternans, 1285, 1286f
  in pulsus paradoxus, 1285–1286, 1286f
  in renal function monitoring, 1495
  in sepsis, 1283
  in spinal transection, 666
  indirect measurement of, 1269–1272, 1269f, 1270f, 1271t
  inhaled anesthetic effects on, 202, 211–212, 212f, 213f
  intermittent measurement of
    automated, 1269–1271, 1270f
    manual, 1269, 1269f
  measurement principles for, 1199–1201, 1199f–1201f
  neuraxial anesthesia effects on, 1658–1660
  nitrous oxide effects on, 214
  noninvasive measurement of, 1201, 1202f
  normal, 2834t
  oscillometry for, 1270, 1270f
  regulation of, 627, 628f
  somatosensory evoked potential monitoring and, 1537
  sphygmomanometry for, 1269, 1269f
  spinal anesthesia and, 1660
Arteriovenous malformation, intracranial, 2151–2152, 2647
Arteriovenous shunts, in thermoregulation, 1573
Arthroplasty
  deep venous thrombosis with, 2425–2426
  hip, 2413–2417, 2414t
  knee, 2414t, 2417–2418
  robotic, 2568
Aryepiglottic folds, 1618
ASA (American Society of Anesthesiologists), 41
  monitoring standards of, 1438
  physical status classification of, 902, 902f, 906, 907t
Ascites
  fluid therapy in, 1789, 1791
  in liver disease, 762–763, 763f
  in portal hypertension, 2222–2223
Aspartate aminotransferase, 753–754, 753t
  preoperative, 2214–2215, 2215f
Asphyxia, neonatal, 2347–2348, 2348f, 2876–2877

Aspiration
  endotracheal intubation and, 1635, 1635t, 1647, 2456
  enteral nutrition and, 2913
  heart transplantation and, 2259
  in children with full stomach, 2384–2385
  in obese patient, 1029–1030, 1030f
  kidney transplantation and, 2241
  laparoscopy and, 2290
Aspiration pneumonitis, prevention of, in outpatient, 2599–2601, 2600t
Aspirin
  bleeding and, 956
  epidural anesthesia and, 1676
  hepatotoxicity of, 2221t
  in cardiopulmonary bypass, 1985
  platelet function and, 1116
  postoperative, 1944, 2735t, 2736f
  preoperative, 1944
  renal effects of, 803
Asthma, 1091
  airway closure in, 695
  anaphylactic reaction in, 1092–1093
  Ascaris antigen-induced, 157
  halothane treatment of, 159–160
  inhaled anesthetic effects on, 155
  opioids in, 392
  preoperative bronchodilation in, 1859
  status, 348, 2852–2853
Astronauts, 2693–2694
Astrup, Paul B., 6
Asymmetric mixed-onium chlorofumarates (430A), 493t, 495, 496f, 497t, 506t, 509
  metabolism of, 506t, 509
Asystole, 2939
  in children, 2944–2946, 2945f, 2947t
Atelectasis
  absorption, 711
  hypoxia and, 687, 2713
  in children, 2844–2845
  PETCO$_2$ and, 1461
  postoperative, 2713
Atenolol, 653–655, 654t, 1120
Atherosclerosis, 1027–1028, 2052. See also Vascular surgery.
  coexisting disease with, 2053
  coronary, 1943–1944, 1944f–1946f. See also Myocardial infarction; Myocardial ischemia.
  kidney failure and, 2238
  sites of, 2051, 2052f
Atlantoaxial instability, 2410, 2410f, 2410t
ATP-binding cassette transport proteins, 751
Atracurium, 493–494, 493t, 494f, 497t
  allergic reaction to, 514
  autonomic effects of, 511, 511t, 512t
  bradycardia with, 513
  calcium interaction with, 517
  cerebral physiology and, 831
  dosage for, 501t
  elimination of, 506t, 509, 511
  hepatobiliary disease and, 529–530, 529t
  histamine release with, 512
  Hofmann degradation of, 74
  hypothermia effect on, 516
  in children, 525, 2379
  in elderly patients, 527
  in ICU patient, 532–533
  in kidney transplantation, 2241
  in myasthenia gravis, 541–542, 542f
  in renal failure, 2184–2186, 2185t
  metabolism of, 506t, 509, 510f
  mivacurium maintenance dose after, 515
  pharmacodynamics of, 500t, 502f
  renal failure and, 527, 528t
  succinylcholine interaction with, 515
Atrial fibrillation, 2930, 2931f, 2932, 2932f, 2936f
  after cardiac surgery, 1993
  after thoracic surgery, 1860–1861
  central venous pressure monitoring in, 1298–1299, 1299f
  electrocardiography in, 1401–1402, 1402t, 1403t
  treatment of, 1402, 1402t, 1403t
Atrial flutter, 2932, 2932f, 2936f
  after thoracic surgery, 1860–1861
  electrocardiography in, 1401
Atrial natriuretic peptide
  in cardiac function, 737, 737t
  in renal function, 795–796, 796f, 797f, 1487
  infusion of, 800
Atrial premature beats, 1399

Atrial pressure, 1297–1298, 1297t, 1298f
  left, 1297t, 1310–1311, 1311f
  right, 1297t
Atrial rupture, 2481
Atrial septal defect, 2009–2010, 2009t
  pulmonary artery catheter monitoring and, 1303
  robotic surgery for, 2564
Atrial tachycardia, multifocal, 2933, 2933f
Atrial-to-femoral bypass, during thoracoabdominal aorta reconstruction, 2085–2086, 2085f
Atrioventricular canal, 2009–2010, 2009t
Atrioventricular dissociation
  central venous pressure monitoring in, 1299, 1299f
  nitrous oxide and, 214
Atrioventricular heart block, 1406t, 1407, 1407f, 1408f
Atropine, 660–662, 660t, 661f
  anticholinesterases with, 523
  for children, 2381
  in electroconvulsive therapy, 2655
  in neonatal resuscitation, 2361t
  in oculocardiac reflex, 2530
  in organophosphate poisoning, 2507, 2507f
  in outpatient premedication, 2599
  in pediatric shock, 2836
  toxicity of, 662
Auditory evoked potentials. See Brainstem auditory evoked potentials.
Auditory input recall, depth of anesthesia and, 1238
Auer, John, 33
Auerbach plexus, 624
Auricular nerve block, 2548
Auriculotemporal nerve block, 2548
Autonomic hyperreflexia syndrome, 1044
Autonomic nervous system, 617–666
  adrenergic function of, 625t, 626–627, 626t, 627t, 628f
  aging-related changes in, 665
  assessment of, 663–666, 663t
  chemical coding of, 619
  cholinergic function of, 625t, 627–630, 629f
  drug effects on, 645–662, 646t, 1119. See also at specific drugs.
  dysfunction of, 663–666, 663t
  enteric, 624–625
  function of, 625–630, 625t, 626t, 627t, 628f, 629f
  functional anatomy of, 621–625, 622f, 623f
  ganglia of, 644–645, 645t
  historical studies on, 8–9, 617–618
  in diabetes mellitus, 664–665
  in spinal cord transection, 665–666
  in surgical stress response, 664
  parasympathetic, 617, 618, 618f, 622–623
  sympathetic, 617, 618, 618f, 621–622, 622f, 623f
  transmitters of, 618–622, 618f–621f. See also Acetylcholine; Epinephrine; Norepinephrine.
Autonomic neuropathy, in diabetes mellitus, 1025, 1026f
Autoreceptor, 636
Aviation simulators, 3074
Awareness, depth of anesthesia and, 1236–1239, 1256
Axillary artery
  cannulation of, 1274. See also Arterial blood pressure.
  in axillary nerve block, 1691, 1692
Axillary nerve, position-related injury to, 1156t
Axillary nerve block, 1690–1692, 1691f, Plate 5
  needle localization for, 1692
  pediatric, 1738–1739, 1739f, 1740t
  side effects of, 1692
Axillary vein, cannulation of, 1293. See also Central venous pressure monitoring.
Axon, 576–577, 576f, 577f
  inhaled anesthetic effects on, 111
Ayres system, in neonatal resuscitation, 2350
Azathioprine
  hepatotoxicity of, 2221t
  in organ transplantation, 2271–2273, 2272t
  muscle blockade and, 2273
  nondepolarizing muscle relaxant interaction with, 518

B

B-type natriuretic peptide, in cardiac function, 737, 737t
Bacillus anthracis, 2515t, 2516–2517, 2518t

Back pain, 1096. *See also* Pain, chronic.
 after spinal anesthesia, 1670
 postpartum, 2329
Baclofen, in complex regional pain syndrome, 2775
Bacteremia, transurethral resection of prostate and, 2193
Bain anesthetic circuit, 293–295, 294f
Bainbridge reflex, 739
Balanced salt solutions, 1785
Balloon valvuloplasty, 2652
Balloon valvulotomy, in children, 2042
Baralyme, 296. *See also* Carbon dioxide (CO₂) absorbents.
Barbiturate(s), 326–334. *See also specific barbiturates.*
 after cardiac arrest, 838–839
 allergic reaction to, 333
 awakening from, 331–332, 332f
 brainstem auditory evoked potential effects of, 1533t, 1536
 cardiovascular system effects of, 333–334
 central nervous system effects of, 331
 cerebral blood flow and, 821, 821f
 cerebral metabolism and, 330, 815, 821, 821f, 839
 complications of, 333–334
 contraindications to, 334
 cyclosporine interaction with, 2273
 dosing for, 333, 333t
 during labor, 2318
 electroencephalographic effects of, 330, 1517–1518, 1519t
 formulation of, 328
 historical perspective on, 326–327, 327f
 in ambulatory anesthesia, 2602–2603, 2602t
 in heart disease patient, 334
 in pediatric ICP increase, 2857
 induction with, 332–333
 intra-arterial injection of, 333
 intraocular pressure effects of, 2532
 lipid solubility of, 331
 mechanism of action of, 330
 metabolism of, 329, 336, 336t
 neuroprotection with, 839, 2087
 pharmacodynamics of, 330–331
 pharmacokinetics of, 329–330, 332
 physiochemical characteristics of, 328–329, 328f, 328t, 329t
 plasma concentration of, 331
 protein binding of, 331
 redistribution of, 331–332, 332f
 respiratory system effects of, 334
 sensory evoked potential effects of, 1533t, 1536
 side effects of, 333–334
 somatosensory evoked potential effects of, 1533t, 1536
 stereoisomerism of, 328–329
 structure-activity relationships of, 328, 329t
 structure of, 328, 328f
 visual evoked potential effects of, 1533t, 1536
Barbiturate coma, in traumatic brain injury, 2472
Bariatric surgery, 1028–1034. *See also* Obesity.
Barker, Arthur E., 26
Barlow's syndrome, 1962
Barometric pressure, 2667t. *See also* Altitude, high; Hyperbaric oxygen therapy.
 increase in, 2667, 2668f, 2668t
  anesthesia reversal and, 2669
  drug disposition and, 2669, 2671
  high-pressure nervous syndrome and, 2669
Baroreceptors, 738–739, 738f
 opioid effects on, 395
 pediatric, 2833
Barotrauma, 2487, 2679. *See also* Hyperbaric oxygen therapy.
Bartling v Superior Court, 3183
Basal energy expenditure, 2905
Base, 1600–1601
Basic life support, 2923–2929
 airway control and ventilation in, 2923–2925
 automated external defibrillator for, 2928–2929
 chest compression in, 2925–2926, 2925f, 2926f
 in children, 2941–2942, 2941f
 monitoring for, 2927–2928, 2928t
Basiliximab, in organ transplantation, 2271–2273, 2272t
Batrachotoxin, 2515t
Battelli, F., 40
Battered child syndrome, 2874
Bayesian statistics, 888–889. *See also* Statistics.
Beck, Claude, 40
Becker's muscular dystrophy, 535, 535t, 536–537, 536f

Beclomethasone, 2817t
Beddoes, Thomas, 13
Beecher, Henry, 10, 33
Beer-Lambert law, 1212–1213, 1212f
Bell, Benjamin, 22
Bell, Charles, 9
Benign prostatic hypertrophy, saw palmetto in, 611
Bennett, Abram E., 32
Benzocaine, 575t, 589–590, 590t
Benzodiazepines, 334–343. *See also specific benzodiazepines.*
 age-related pharmacokinetics of, 2439, 2439t
 awakening from, 341
 cardiovascular system effects of, 340, 340t
 central nervous system effects of, 339
 contraindications to, 342
 during labor, 2318–2319
 electroencephalographic effects of, 339, 1518, 1519t
 for children, 2375–2376
 half-life of, 337–338
 historical perspective on, 334–335
 in ambulatory anesthesia, 2603
 in organophosphate poisoning, 2508–2509
 in outpatient premedication, 2596, 2596t
 in renal failure, 2184
 in trauma, 2485
 induction with, 340t, 341–342, 341f, 342f
 ketamine with, 347
 lipid solubility of, 337–338
 maintenance with, 340t, 341–342
 metabolism of, 335–336
 opioid interactions with, 422
 pharmacokinetics of, 336–337, 336f, 337f
 pharmacology of, 337–340, 337f–339f
 physiochemical characteristics of, 335, 335t
 receptor for, 337–339, 337f, 338f
 respiratory system effects of, 339–340, 339f, 341
 sedation with, 340–341, 340t
 side effects of, 342
 somatosensory evoked potential effects of, 1533t
 structure of, 335, 335f
 tolerance to, 337
 visual evoked potential effects of, 1533t
 with neuraxial anesthesia, 1678
Benzylisoquinolinium compounds, 492–494, 493f, 493t, 494f, 508–509, 508f, 510f. *See also specific benzylisoquinolinium compounds.*
Berger, Johannes Hans, 42
Bernard, Claude, 8, 20, 30, 31f, 85
Bernoulli equation, 1202
Bernoulli's principle, 1221–1222
Bert, Paul, 17
Beta-blockers. *See* β-Adrenergic receptor antagonists.
Beta error, in statistics, 885
Betamethasone, neuromuscular blocking agent interaction with, 518
Betaxolol, 653, 656
Bethanecol, 660
Bevantolol, 653
Bezold-Jarisch reflex, 739, 1688
Bias, in statistics, 886
Bicarbonate
 coagulation and, 1815
 in metabolic acidosis, 1781
 with epidural anesthesia, 1675
Bier, August, 24, 25f, 26
Bier block, 1695, 2608–2609
Bigelow, Henry J., 14–15, 15f
Bile acids, 748–749
Bile salts, cardiac effects of, 764
Biliary tract, 529–530, 530t. *See also* Liver.
 atresia of, 2854
 opioid effects on, 398
Bilirubin, 753t, 755
 conjugated, 750, 753t, 755
 in cholestasis, 764
 postoperative, 2219–2220, 2219t
 preoperative, 2215
 production of, 750
 pulse oximetry errors and, 1451t, 1452
 renal effects of, 805
Bioimpedance cardiac output monitoring, 1336–1337
Biological warfare agents. *See* Chemical and biological warfare agents.
Birth. *See also* Fetus; Neonate.
 catecholamines at, 2345–2346
 neonatal assessment at, 2348–2349
 resuscitation at, 2345–2363. *See also* Neonate, resuscitation of.

Bischoff, Johann J., 21
Bisferiens pulse, 1285
Bispectral index, 42, 1251–1256, 1251f–1254f. *See also* Electroencephalography, bispectral.
Bisquaternary tropinyl diester derivatives, 493t, 495, 496f
Bitolterol, 2817t
Blacher, R. S., 42
Black, Joseph, 13
Black cohosh, hepatotoxicity of, 2222t
Bladder
 innervation of, 2176, 2177f
 pain in, 2200
 perforation of, 2191, 2193
 transitional cell carcinoma of, 2200
Blalock-Taussig shunt, 2040
Blankets, 1585–1587, 1586f, 1587f
Bleeding. *See also* Hemorrhage.
 after cardiopulmonary bypass, 1982–1985, 1983f, 1986f
 after heart transplantation, 2262
 after pediatric cardiopulmonary bypass, 2035–2036, 2036f
 after tonsillectomy, 2544
 after transurethral resection of prostate, 2193
 aspirin and, 956
 gastrointestinal, in children, 2863–2864
 kidney failure and, 2239
 mediastinal, 2262
 saw palmetto-related, 611
 variceal, 761
Bleomycin, 1118
 hepatotoxicity of, 2221t
 oxygen toxicity and, 2677–2678
Blinded study, 886. *See also* Statistics.
Blindness. *See also* Vision, postoperative loss of.
 cortical, 1158, 3011–3012
  computed tomography in, 2997–2998
  eye examination in, 2996, 2997t
  magnetic resonance imaging in, 2997–2998
Blood
 synthetic, 1826–1827
 transfusion of. *See* Blood transfusion.
 warming of, 2391–2392
Blood-brain barrier, 832–833
 in ischemic optic neuropathy, 3007
Blood chemistry, 955–956, 957t–958t
Blood flow
 cerebral, 813–830. *See also* Cerebral blood flow.
 hepatic, 743–744, 745f, 746f. *See also* Liver, blood flow in.
 pulmonary, 679–681, 680f, 683–689. *See also* Lung(s), blood flow in.
 renal, 783, 783t, 2177–2178, 2178f. *See also* Kidney(s), blood flow in.
 shunt fraction of, 1442
 uterine, 2312
Blood-gas partition coefficient, of inhaled anesthetics, 132, 132t
Blood gases. *See* Carbon dioxide (CO₂), arterial; Oxygen (O₂), arterial.
Blood pressure. *See* Arterial blood pressure; Central venous pressure monitoring.
Blood transfusion, 1799–1821. *See also* Transfusion therapy.
 ABO-Rh typing for, 1802, 1802t, 1804
 acid-base abnormalities in, 1814–1815, 1814f
 acute lung injury in, 1820
 alternatives to, 1839–1840, 1840t
 antibody screening for, 1803
 autologous, 1801, 1831–1841
  acute normovolemic hemodilution for, 1834–1836
   clinical trials of, 1835–1836, 1836t
   cost-effectiveness of, 1836
   hematocrit level with, 1834–1835, 1835f
   hemostasis with, 1835
   oxygenation with, 1835
   patient selection for, 1836t
  historical perspective on, 1832, 1832t
  intraoperative blood collection for, 1836–1837, 1838t
  postoperative blood collection for, 1837–1838
  preoperative, 1832–1834
   cost-effectiveness of, 1834
   erythropoietin in, 1833–1834, 1833t
   hematocrit trigger for, 1834, 1834t
   patient selection for, 1832–1833, 1833t
   phlebotomy in, 1833–1834, 1833t
 blood storage for, 1804–1805, 1805t
 citrate intoxication in, 1812–1813

Blood transfusion *(Continued)*
  clotting deficiency with, 1117
  coagulopathy in, 1807–1812, 1808f, 1811f–1813f
  compatibility testing for, 1801–1803, 1802f, 1802t
  complications of, 1806–1815, 1806f, 1808f, 1809f, 1811f–1814f
  crossmatch-to-transfusion ratio in, 1803
  crossmatching for, 1802–1803, 1802f
  cytomegalovirus transmission with, 1818t, 1819
  delayed hemolytic reaction to, 1817
  dilutional thrombocytopenia in, 1807–1809, 1808t, 1809f
  disseminated intravascular coagulation-like syndrome in, 1809–1810
  during orthopedic surgery, 2413
  emergency, 1804
  factor V deficiency in, 1809
  factor VII deficiency in, 1809
  fever with, 1817
  frozen blood for, 1805
  graft-versus-host disease in, 1820
  hematocrit value for, 1799–1801
  hemoglobin value for, 1799–1801
  hemolytic reaction to, 1810, 1815–1817, 1815t, 1816f, 1816t
  hepatitis transmission with, 1818–1819, 1818t
  historical studies on, 21–22
  human immunodeficiency virus transmission with, 1818t, 1819
  human T-cell lymphotropic virus type 1 transmission with, 1818t, 1819
  hyperkalemia in, 1813
  immune extravascular reaction to, 1817
  immunomodulatory effects of, 1820–1821
  in abdominal aorta reconstruction, 2079
  in children, 2869
  in critically ill patient, 2803–2804
  in hemorrhagic shock, 2465, 2466
  in neonatal hypovolemia, 2359
  in sepsis, 2795
  in sickle cell anemia, 1113
  in transfusion-induced coagulopathy, 1811
  indications for, 1799–1801, 1800t
  infection transmission with, 1817–1820, 1818t, 1820t
  informed consent for, 1827
  leukoreduction for, 1821
  malaria transmission with, 1820
  nonhemolytic reactions to, 1817
  ocular reaction to, 1820
  order schedule for, 1803
  oxygen transport in, 1806–1807, 1806f
  particulate matter infusion in, 1815
  pediatric, 2389–2390
    refusal of, 3181–3182
  refusal of, 1839–1840, 1840t, 3181–3182
  syphilis transmission with, 1820
  temperature effects on, 1803–1804
  type and hold for, 1803
  type and screen for, 1803
  type-specific, 1804
  uncrossmatched blood for, 1804
  universal donor for, 1804
  urticaria with, 1817
  vs. packed red blood cells, 1821–1822, 1822t
  warmed blood for, 1814, 1814t
  West Nile virus transmission with, 1818t, 1819
  Yersinia enterocolitica transmission with, 1820
Blood typing, 1802, 1802t, 1804
Blood urea nitrogen, 753t, 2179, 2179f
  in compound A exposure, 252–253
  in renal function monitoring, 1497–1498, 1497t
  preoperative, 956, 969f, 1493
Blood warmer, for children, 2391–2392
Blundell, James, 21
BODY patient simulators, 3078
Body temperature. *See* Temperature, body.
Bohr effect, 703
Bohr equation, 1442
Bone(s). *See also* Orthopedic surgery.
  trauma to, 2476–2479, 2477t, 2478t
Bone graft, 2420–2421, 2420f
Bone marrow transplantation, in sickle cell anemia, 1113
Bonica, John, 24, 28
Bosentan, hepatotoxicity of, 2221t
Botulinum toxin, 2515–2516, 2515t
Bourdon tube, 1205, 1205f
Bowel obstruction, postoperative, 1790–1791
Bowman's capsule, 777
Boyle, H. Edmund G., 34

Boyle, Robert, 12
Brachial artery, cannulation of, 1274. *See also* Arterial blood pressure.
Brachial plexus
  anatomy of, 1686, 1687f
  injury to
    position-related, 1152t, 1154, 1159–1160
    with orthopedic surgery, 2411–2412, 2412t
Brachial plexus block, 1686–1692
  anesthetics for, 588, 588t
  axillary approach to, 1690–1692, 1691f, Plate 5
  contraindications to, 1692
  epinephrine in, 588
  in outpatient procedures, 2609
  infraclavicular approach to, 1690
  interscalene approach to, 1686, 1688–1689, 1688f
  pediatric, 1738–1742
    anatomy for, 1738
    axillary approaches in, 1738–1739, 1739f, 1740t
    contraindications to, 1738
    coracoid approaches in, 1739–1740, 1740f
    indications for, 1738
    interscalene approach in, 1741–1742, 1742f
    parascalene approach in, 1740–1741, 1740t, 1741f
    peri-subclavian artery approaches in, 1742
  sufentanil with, 387
  supraclavicular approach to, 1689–1690, 1689f, 1690f, Plate 3
Bradley, A. F., 6
Bradyarrhythmia, 1083
  supraventricular, 2929–2930
    in children, 2942, 2943f
  ventricular, 2933f
    in children, 2944
Bradycardia
  after cardiopulmonary bypass, 1982
  atropine-induced, 661–662
  fetal, 2833
  interscalene block and, 1688
  muscle relaxants and, 513
  oculocardiac reflex and, 2530
  opioid-related, 394–395
  spinal transection and, 666
Brain. *See also at* Cerebral.
  acetylcholine of, inhaled anesthetic effects on, 112
  γ-aminobutyric acid of, inhaled anesthetic effects on, 113
  arteriovenous malformation of, 2151–2152, 2647
  blood flow of. *See* Cerebral blood flow.
  death of. *See* Brain death.
  dopamine of, inhaled anesthetic effects on, 113
  epinephrine of, inhaled anesthetic effects on, 112–113
  glycine of, inhaled anesthetic effects on, 113
  highly sensitive neurons of, inhaled anesthetic effects on, 110–111, 111f
  inhaled anesthetic effects on, 109, 110–113, 111f
  inhaled anesthetic uptake by, 133–134, 133t
  injury to. *See* Brain injury.
  norepinephrine of, inhaled anesthetic effects on, 112–113
  oxygen consumption by, 813. *See also* Cerebral metabolic rate of oxygen (CMRO$_2$).
  serotonin of, inhaled anesthetic effects on, 113
  tumor of
    cerebral blood flow and, 842–843
    in children, 2856
  weight of, 813
Brain death, 2232, 2232t, 2955–2968
  angiography in, 2965t, 2966
  apnea test in, 2961
  blood flow measurement in, 2965–2966
  brainstem auditory evoked potentials in, 2965
  brainstem reflexes in, 2961
  cardiovascular function and, 2958–2959, 2959f
  clinical diagnosis of, 2962
  computed tomography in, 2966
  concept of, 2957
  confirmatory tests for, 2964–2967, 2965t
  consciousness and, 2958
  diagnostic criteria for, 2956t, 2961–2962
  Doppler ultrasonography in, 2966
  edema in, 2957
  electrocerebral inactivity in, 2965
  electroencephalography for, 2964–2965, 2965t
  evoked responses in, 2965
  historical perspective on, 2955–2956
  hypotension in, 2962

Brain death *(Continued)*
  hypothalamic-pituitary function and, 2960
  immune system function and, 2960
  in children, 2858, 2877, 2963–2964, 2964t
  loss of consciousness in, 2958
  magnetic resonance imaging in, 2966
  mechanism of, 2957
  neurophysiologic basis of, 2958–2961, 2959f
  organ donation and, 2967
  poikilothermia in, 2959–2960, 2961–2962
  positron emission tomography in, 2967
  pupils in, 2961
  respiration and, 2958
  somatosensory evoked potentials in, 2965
  spinal cord reflexes and, 2962–2963, 2963f
  thermoregulation and, 2959–2960
  tonsillar herniation and, 2959
  transcranial Doppler ultrasonography for, 1541f, 1542
Brain injury, 2469–2476
  airway management in, 2470–2471
  analgesics in, 2472
  barbiturate coma in, 2472
  cerebral perfusion pressure in, 2154–2155, 2154f, 2471–2473, 2472f
  classification of, 2470
  decompressive craniectomy in, 2472–2473
  hemorrhagic shock in, 2471
  hypothermia in, 1581, 2473
  in children, 2856
  intracranial pressure in, 2471, 2473
  mannitol in, 2472
  mild, 2470
  moderate, 2470
  positional therapy in, 2471–2472
  severe, 2470
  total parenteral nutrition in, 2915
  ventilation in, 2470–2471
Brain tumor
  cerebral blood flow and, 842–843
  in children, 2856
Brainstem, surgical stimulation of, 2157–2158, 2157t
Brainstem anesthesia, retrobulbar block and, 2530–2531
Brainstem auditory evoked potentials, 1512, 1530–1532, 1531f, 1531t
  anesthetic effects on, 1532–1537, 1533t, 1534f, 1535f
  barbiturate effects on, 1533t, 1536
  enflurane effects on, 1533t, 1534, 1535, 1535f
  etomidate effects on, 352
  in acoustic neuroma resection, 1531
  in anesthetic depth monitoring, 1258
  in brain death, 2965
  in facial nerve decompression, 1530–1531
  in outpatient procedures, 2611
  in trigeminal nerve decompression, 1531
  indications for, 1530–1532
  inhaled anesthetic effects on, 1533–1534, 1533t, 1534f, 1535f
  isoflurane effects on, 1533–1534, 1533t, 1534f
  physiologic factors and, 1537
Brainstem death, 2958. *See also* Brain death.
Brainstem reflexes, in brain death, 2961
Branch retinal artery occlusion, 2998–3005
  amniotic fluid emboli and, 3004
  cardiopulmonary bypass surgery and, 3003
  etiology of, 3003–3004
  eye examination in, 2996–2997, 2997t
  head and neck injection and, 3003
  head position and, 3004–3005
  local anesthesia injection and, 3004
  mechanisms of, 2998, 3000
  nasal septal surgery and, 3004
  pathogenesis of, 3000, 3002
  patient characteristics in, 3000, 3001t–3002t
  prevention of, 3004–3005
  prognosis for, 3004
  pterygopalatine fissure injection and, 3003–3004
  treatment of, 3004
Branched-chain amino acids, in sepsis, 2901
Braun, Heinrich, 23, 27
Breasts
  mammography of, 942–943, 944
  outpatient removal of, 916–917
  positioning of, 1162–1163
Breath nitrogen washout test, 1010, 1010f
Breath sounds
  in neonate, 2354
  monitoring of, 1464–1465

Breathing. *See also* Respiration; Ventilation.
deep, for bronchial hygiene, 2818
neonatal, 2349, 2349t
rescue, 2924
shallow, rapid, 711
work of, 177, 692–693, 692f, 693f
Brettauer, Josef, 23
Bretylium, 658
Brocklesby, Richard, 30
Brodie, Benjamin, 30, 31f
Bromage, Philip, 28
Bromochlorotrifluoroethane, nephrotoxicity of, 254
Bromocriptine, 1052
Bromsulphalein test, 753t, 756
Bronchial blockers (single-lumen endotracheal
        tubes), 1883–1885, 1884f, 1885f, 1885t
    Arndt type, 1887–1888, 1888f, 1888t
    Fogarty catheter with, 1887–1888, 1887f
    independent, 1887–1889, 1887f, 1888f, 1888t
    indications for, 1887
    just-seal volume and, 1886–1887
    limitations of, 1885–1886, 1886t
    technique of, 1889–1890
Bronchial hygiene therapy, 2818–2820, 2818f, 2818t
Bronchiolitis, 2852
Bronchitis, 707, 707f
Broncho-Cath continuous positive airway pressure
        system, in one-lung ventilation, 1895f,
        1897–1900, 1898f
Bronchodilation
    inhaled anesthetic-induced, 156–159, 157f–159f
    preoperative, 1859
Bronchodilators, 1124, 2816, 2817, 2817t
Bronchopleural fistula, 1900, 1902, 1925–1926
Bronchopulmonary dysplasia, 2853
Bronchopulmonary lavage, 1918–1920, 1918f, 1919t
Bronchoscope, in laser surgery, 2543
Bronchoscopy
    in bronchial hygiene, 2820
    in double-lumen endotracheal tube positioning,
        1879–1882, 1880f, 1881f
    in endotracheal intubation, 1645–1646
    in hemoptysis, 1923, 1924f
    in lung cancer, 1852
    in nosocomial infection, 2796
Bronchospasm
    anesthetic-related, 155
    carcinoid tumor-related, 1110
    endotracheal intubation and, 1648
    inhaled anesthetic effects on, 156–157
    ketamine effects on, 348
    neuromuscular blocking agents and, 514
    surgical risk of, 161
Bronchus (bronchi). *See also* Lung(s).
    inhaled anesthetic effects on, 156–161, 157f–160f
    intubation of, 708, 1648–1649
    mucociliary function of, 161–162
        inhaled anesthetic effects on, 161–165, 163f, 164f
        nasal nitric oxide and, 162
        postoperative, 162
        tantalum clearance study of, 163
        videomicroscopy of, 162
    pharmacology of, 155–156
    trauma to, 2480
Brucella spp., in biological warfare, 2518t
Bubonic plague, 2517
Budesemide, in experimental chlorine exposure,
        2512
Budesonide, 2817t
Buffer, 1605
Bulimia, 1034
Bullectomy, 1916–1917
Bullous emphysema, 1916–1917
Bundle branch block
    left, 1406t, 1407–1408, 1408f
    right, 1406t, 1407, 1407f, 1409, 1410f
        left ventricular end-diastolic pressure in,
            1321–1322, 1321t
        pulmonary artery catheter-related, 1305
Bupivacaine, 24, 575t
    biotransformation of, 592
    cardiovascular effects of, 593–596, 594t
    chloroprocaine and, 585–586
    differential sensory/motor blockade with, 584
    duration of action of, 584
    during labor, 2321, 2321t, 2322
    in cesarean section, 2324, 2324f
    in continuous epidural analgesia, 2321, 2321t
    in elderly patient, 2439
    in epidural anesthesia, 588–589, 588t, 1674t, 1675
    in nerve block, 587–588, 587t, 588t

Bupivacaine *(Continued)*
    in pediatric regional anesthesia, 1723, 1723f,
        1723t, 1724, 1728, 1728t
    in pregnancy, 595
    in spinal anesthesia, 589, 589t, 1661t, 1666–1667
    infiltration of, 586–587, 586t
    intravenous, 587
    onset of action of, 584
    pKa of, 574, 574f
    potency of, 576t
    structure of, 575f
    tissue distribution of, 592, 592t
    ventricular arrhythmias with, 594–595
    vs. ropivacaine, 595–596
Buprenorphine, 380t, 418t, 419
    for patient-controlled intravenous analgesia,
        2733–2734, 2733t
    respiratory depression with, 1472
    structure of, 382t
    transmucosal, 416
Burkholderia mallei, in biological warfare, 2518t, 2519
Burn(s). *See also* Electrical safety.
    fluid management in, 1793–1794
    neuromuscular blockade and, 530
    nondepolarizing muscle relaxants in, 530, 530t
    with pulse oximetry, 3144
Burney, Fanny, 11–12
BURP maneuver, in endotracheal intubation,
        1634–1635
Butorphanol, 380t, 418t, 419
    during labor, 2318
    in outpatient anesthesia, 2606
    structure of, 382t
Butyrophenones, 1123
Butyrylcholinesterase, 486–488, 488f, 488t, 642
    exogenous, in neuromuscular blockade
        recovery, 522
    genetic variability in, 99
    in elderly patients, 527
    in liver disease, 530
Bymixer, 1442, 1442f
BZ, 2516

C

C-Kit ligand, 1114t
C-reactive protein, in sepsis, 2902, 2902f
Cabergoline, 1052
Caenorhabditis elegans, inhaled anesthetic study in,
        123–124
Caffeine, 3061
    in post-dural puncture headache, 2328
Caffeine clearance test, 756
Caglieri, Guido, 26
Calcitonin
    in calcium physiology, 1771
    in hyperparathyroidism, 1050
Calcium, 1770–1772. *See also* Hypercalcemia;
        Hypocalcemia.
    antibiotic interaction with, 516
    citrate binding of, 1812–1813
    in cardiac function, 731–734, 732f, 734f
    in cerebral ischemia, 835–836, 835f
    in children, 2838
    in malignant hyperthermia, 1176–1177,
        1178–1179
    in parenteral nutrition, 2912t
    in pediatric left ventricular dysfunction, 2032
    inhaled anesthetic effects on, 114, 156, 157–158,
        158f, 159f, 167, 168f, 207
        myocardial depression and, 194–195
    minimum alveolar concentration and, 109
    nitrous oxide effects on, 214
    nondepolarizing muscle relaxants and, 517
    serum, 1770–1771
Calcium channel
    in neurotransmission, 862–863, 863f
    opioid effects on, 423–424
Calcium channel blockers, 1121–1122, 1122f
    after cardiac arrest, 838–839
    for neuroprotection, 840, 2087
    for renal protection, 799–800, 804
    hepatotoxicity of, 2221t
    in intracranial aneurysm, 2148
    malignant hyperthermia and, 1179
Calcium chloride
    in citrate intoxication, 1812
    in pediatric life support, 2947t
Calcium gluconate, in neonatal resuscitation, 2361t

Calculi
    renal, 2195–2197
    ureteral, 2194, 2195–2197
Calmodulin, 732
    ryanodine receptor interaction with, 1173
Calorimetry, indirect, 2906
Calreticulin, 732
Calsequestrin, 732, 1173
Cancer, 1117–1118
    inhaled anesthetic-related, 261–262
    lung. *See* Lung cancer.
    pain in, 2770. *See also* Pain, chronic.
Cannon, Walter B., 8, 20
Caordean-Cobra aortic cannula, 1995
Capacitance, 1209, 1209f, 1210, 1210f
Capacitor, 1209–1210
Capacity limited drugs, 72
Capnography, 1213, 1213f, 1455–1462
    alveolar plateau in, 1458–1459, 1459f, 1461
    cardiogenic oscillation in, 1459–1460, 1459f
    during laparoscopy, 2286, 2288, 2288f
    errors in, 1457–1458, 1462
    for children, 2392
    in awake craniotomy, 2160
    in basic life support, 2927
    in double-lumen endotracheal tube positioning,
        1882
    in endotracheal intubation, 1461
    in mechanical ventilation, 1460–1461
    in pediatric cardiac surgery, 2017
    in renal function monitoring, 1495
    interpretation of, 1458–1462, 1458f–1461f
    mainstream, 1456–1457
    sidestream, 1455–1456, 1456f, 1457f
        errors in, 1457–1458
    time, 1458–1461, 1458f–1461f
        time delays in, 1457–1458
    volume, 1458f, 1461–1462
Captopril, 659, 2221t
Carbachol, 660
Carbamazepine, 517, 2221t
Carbohydrates, hepatic metabolism of, 747–748
Carbon dioxide (CO_2)
    alveolar, partial pressure of (P_{ACO_2}), 698–699, 698f,
        1439
    arterial, 177
        minute ventilation and, 178–179
        organ function and, 179
        partial pressure of (P_{aCO_2}), 1438
            artifactual effects on, 1446
            diffusion nonequilibrium and, 1440
            during laparoscopy, 2286–2288, 2287f, 2287t
            during neurosurgery, 2131–2133, 2133f
            gas bubbles and, 1446
            in brain death, 2961
            in children, 2843
            in hemorrhagic shock, 2468–2469
            in one-lung ventilation, 1890–1891, 1890f
            limitations of, 1443
            minute ventilation and, 1442, 1447, 1447t
            multiple inert gas elimination technique for,
                1443–1444
            P_{ETCO_2} and, 1459
            temperature correction of, 1445–1446, 1445f
            ventilation-perfusion mismatch and,
                1439–1440, 1440f
    ventilatory response to, 177–179, 178f
    capillary, partial pressure of, 1440
    colorimetric analysis of, 1454
    end-tidal, 1442, 1442f
        in apnea monitoring, 2927–2928, 2928t
        in basic life support, 2927–2928, 2928t
        partial pressure of (P_{ETCO_2}), 1458–1461, 1459f,
            1460f. *See also* Capnography.
            interpretation of, 1460–1461, 1461f
    expired, 1454–1462. *See also* Capnography.
    hypercapnia and, 714f, 715
    in acid-base balance, 1602, 1605
    in hyperbaric oxygen therapy, 2679, 2682, 2684
    infrared absorption analysis of, 1454
    intraocular pressure and, 2532
    open-circuit measurement of, 1462
    transport of, 703
Carbon dioxide (CO_2) absorbents, 296–298, 297f
    anesthetic interactions with, 142–143, 251–256,
        251f, 254f, 297–298, 1490
    carbon monoxide production and, 255–256,
        255f, 256f
    chemistry of, 296
    inadvertent switching off of, 715
    indicators for, 296–297, 297f

Carbon dioxide-blood dissociation curve, 703, 1439–1440, 1440f
Carbon dioxide embolism, during laparoscopy, 2289–2290
Carbon dioxide tension, cerebral ischemia and, 840–841
Carbon monoxide
  diffusing capacity of, 1011, 1089
  production of, 297–298
  pulmonary vascular resistance and, 165
  toxicity of, 255–256, 256f
Carbon monoxide oximetry, 1447–1448
Carbon monoxide poisoning, 2671–2672, 2671t
Carbon octofluorine, intravitreal injection of, 2533
Carbon tetrafluoride, oil-gas partition coefficient of, 115t
Carbonation
  for epidural anesthesia, 1675
  of local anesthetics, 585
Carbonyl chloride (phosgene), 297, 2510–2513, 2511t, 2512f
Carboxyhemoglobin
  production of, 297–298
  pulse oximetry errors and, 1450, 1451t
Carcinoid tumors, 1108–1110
Cardiac. See also at Heart; Myocardial.
Cardiac arrest, 2935, 2937–2941, 2940t
  after spinal anesthesia, 1670
  cerebral blood flow and, 837–839
  cerebral injury after, 2800, 2803
  hypothermia after, 2800, 2803
  organ donation and, 2233–2234
  pediatric, 2392–2393, 2944–2947, 2944f
    in malignant hyperthermia, 1181
Cardiac catheterization, 2650–2653. See also Angiography.
  complications of, 2652
  in children, 2015–2016, 2651–2652
  interventions during, 2652–2653
Cardiac cycle, 723–724, 724f, 731–732, 732f, 734f
  inhaled anesthetic effects on, 202–203
Cardiac efficiency, 727
Cardiac index, 2834t. See also Cardiac risk index.
Cardiac massage, in neonate, 2360, 2360f
Cardiac output, 683–684, 684f, 728–729, 728f, 729f
  age-related changes in, 100
  alveolar/inspired pressure ratio and, 138–139, 138f, 139f
  aortic cross-clamping effects on, 2075
  barbiturate effects on, 333–334
  continuous thermodilution monitoring of, 1330–1331
  dexmedetomidine effects on, 357–358, 357f
  drug effects on, 101
  during laparoscopy, 2290–2292, 2291f
  during pregnancy, 2308, 2308t
  fetal, 2312, 2312f
  Fick method monitoring of, 1331
  hypoxic pulmonary vasoconstriction and, 168–169
  in hepatic disease, 762
  in neonatal asphyxia, 2348
  in obese patient, 1033
  in renal function monitoring, 1495–1496
  inhaled anesthetic uptake and, 133, 138–139, 138f, 139f
  metabolic acidosis and, 1782
  monitoring of, 1222–1223, 1327–1331, 1327t, 1329t
    bioimpedance methods of, 1336–1337
    double indicator dilution method of, 1338
    equations for, 1333–1334
    gastric tonometry for, 1338
    iced injectate for, 1330
    lithium dilution method of, 1337–1338
    partial CO$_2$ rebreathing Fick method of, 1337
    pulmonary artery catheter for, 1327–1331, 1327t, 1329t
    pulse contour method of, 1338
    pulse dye densitometry for, 1338
    respiratory cycle and, 1330
    thermodilution methods of, 1328–1330, 1329t
    ultrasound methods of, 1334–1336
  neonatal, 2358
  nitrous oxide effects on, 214
  oxygen consumption and, 712, 712f
  Pao$_2$ and, 1440, 1440f, 1441f
  postoperative hypoxemia and, 2714, 2714f
  pulmonary artery catheter monitoring of, 1327–1331, 1327t, 1329t
  shunt blood flow and, 1442

Cardiac output (Continued)
  thermodilution monitoring of, 1328–1330, 1329t
    errors in, 1329–1330, 1330t
  transesophageal echocardiography for, 1376
Cardiac pump mechanism, in basic life support, 2925–2926, 2925f
Cardiac resuscitation. See also Cardiopulmonary resuscitation.
  after local anesthetic administration, 595
Cardiac risk index, 1067–1072, 1068t, 1069f, 1069t, 1070t, 1071f–1072f, 1071t
Cardiac tamponade, 1966–1967, 1966t, 1967f
  central venous catheterization and, 1294
  central venous pressure monitoring in, 1316–1317, 1318f
Cardiac work, 727
Cardio-West Total Artificial Heart, 1992, 1992t
Cardiogenic oscillation, in capnography, 1459–1460, 1459f
Cardiogenic reflex, opioid effects on, 395
Cardiomyocytes, 729–735
  contractile system of, 732–735, 733f, 734f
  excitation-contraction coupling of, 731–732, 732f
  excitation system of, 730–731, 731f
  structure of, 729–730, 730f
Cardiomyopathy
  after radiofrequency ablation, 2043
  dilated
    familial, 734–735
    kidney failure and, 2238
  hypertrophic, 1956–1957, 1957f, 1958f
    familial, 733
    kidney failure and, 2238
  inhaled anesthetic effects on, 193–194, 193f, 196, 196f, 198, 199f, 202
  restrictive, central venous pressure monitoring in, 1316
Cardioplegia, 1977–1978, 1977t
Cardiopulmonary bypass, 1971–1982
  acid-base management in, 1980–1981, 1981f
  anticoagulation for, 1972–1974, 1973f, 1974f
  antifibrinolytics for, 1974–1975
  arterial blood pressure monitoring in, 1283–1284, 1284f, 1286
  at remote locations, 2650
  bleeding after, 1982–1985, 1983f, 1986f
  blood temperature in, 1329
  branch retinal artery occlusion and, 3003
  cardiac output measurement in, 1329
  cerebral blood flow for, 1979
  circuitry of, 1971–1972, 1972f
  coagulation after, 1982–1985, 1983f
  discontinuation of, 2260–2262, 2260t
    hypothermia after, 1585
  electrocardiography after, 1985–1986, 1987f
  electroencephalography during, 1521, 1521t
  glycemic control for, 1981
  hematocrit for, 1979–1980, 1979f, 1980f
  hemodilution in, 1983
  heparin rebound after, 1984
  heparin reversal for, 1982
  hepatic dysfunction and, 2219
  in aortic arch aneurysm, 2086
  in lung transplantation, 2266–2267
  in tracheal resection, 1915
  inflammatory response to, 1975–1976, 1975f, 1975t, 1976f
  mean arterial pressure for, 1979
  myocardial dysfunction after, 1986–1991, 1987f, 1988f, 1988t, 1989f, 1990f
  myocardial ischemia after, 1985–1986, 1987t
  myocardial protection for, 1976–1978, 1977t, 1978f
  opioid pharmacokinetics in, 408–409, 409f
  pathobiology of, 1975–1976, 1975f, 1975t, 1976f
  pediatric, 2022–2034
    cannulation for, 2024–2025
    cerebral blood flow during, 2019, 2019f
    coagulation profile in, 2034–2036, 2035f
    discontinuation of, 2029–2030, 2032–2034
    echocardiography in, 2017–2018, 2017f, 2018f
    flow rate for, 2025–2026
    glucose regulation and, 2027–2028
    hematocrit formula for, 2024
    hemodilution in, 2024, 2030–2032, 2031f
    hyperglycemia in, 2028
    hypoglycemia in, 2028
    hypothermia for, 2024, 2025, 2026–2027, 2026f
    initiation of, 2024–2026
    intramyocardial air and, 2030, 2030f
    left ventricular dysfunction after, 2032

Cardiopulmonary bypass (Continued)
  pediatric (Continued)
    low-flow, 2027
    management after, 2036–2037
    modified ultrafiltration in, 2030–2032, 2031f
    pain control after, 2036–2037
    priming solutions for, 2023
    pulmonary effects of, 2028f, 2029
    pulmonary hypertension after, 2033–2034
    renal effects of, 2028–2029, 2028t
    right ventricular dysfunction after, 2032–2033
    stress response during, 2028t, 2029
    ultrafiltration in, 2030–2032, 2031f
    vs. adult, 2022–2023, 2023t
    xenon clearance study in, 2019, 2019f
  platelet dysfunction after, 1984–1985, 1984f
  preoperative platelet collection in, 1834
  renal effects of, 802–803
  renal protection during, 802–803
  separation from, 1981–1982, 1981t
  temperature for, 1978–1979, 2087
  transcranial Doppler ultrasonography during, 1541
  ventricular dysfunction after, 1990–1991, 1991t
Cardiopulmonary resuscitation, 2923–2948
  advanced cardiac life support for, 2929–2941
    arrhythmia monitoring and recognition in, 2929–2935, 2930f–2937f
    cardiac arrest management in, 2935, 2937–2941, 2938f, 2939f
    do-not-resuscitate orders and, 2940–2941
  basic life support for, 2923–2929
    airway control and ventilation in, 2923–2925
    automated external defibrillator for, 2928–2929
    chest compression in, 2925–2926, 2925f, 2926f
    monitoring for, 2927–2928, 2928t
  in ventricular fibrillation, 1404
  neonatal, 2345–2363
    Apgar score in, 2352–2353
    cardiac massage in, 2360, 2360f
    case study of, 2361–2363
    discontinuation of, 2361
    drugs for, 2360–2361, 2361t
    equipment for, 2349–2351, 2350f, 2351f
    evaluation for, 2351–2353, 2352f, 2352t
    pulmonary, 2353–2356, 2353f
    tracheal intubation in, 2353–2354, 2353f
    tracheal suctioning in, 2354–2355
    vascular, 2356–2359, 2357f, 2358f, 2358t
    ventilation monitoring in, 2354
  outcomes of, 2939–2940
  pediatric, 2877–2878, 2941–2947, 2941t
    advanced cardiac life support in, 2942–2947, 2943f–2946f, 2947t
    basic life support in, 2941–2942, 2941t
    vascular access for, 2944–2945, 2946f
  refusal of, 3183–3186, 3185t
Cardiovascular disease, 1941–1996. See also specific diseases.
  aging and, 1941–1942, 1942f, 1943t
  anesthesia for, 1970–1971. See also at specific procedures.
  anesthesia-related risk and, 908–909, 915, 916t
  fast-tract anesthesia for, 1970–1971
  intraoperative monitoring in, 1968–1970, 1970f, 1970t
  kidney failure and, 2238, 2239–2240
  preoperative evaluation of, 1968, 1969t
  robotic surgery in, 2562–2566, 2563t, 2563t, 2564t, 2565f, 2565t, 2566f, 2566t
Cardiovascular monitoring, 1265–1344
  arterial blood pressure in, 1268–1286. See also Arterial blood pressure.
  cardiac output in, 1327–1331, 1327t, 1329t
  central venous pressure for, 1286–1327. See also Central venous pressure monitoring.
  clinical observation in, 1266
  coagulation measures in, 1338–1343, 1339t, 1342f
  continuous mixed venous oximetry for, 1331–1332
  electrocardiography in, 1267–1268, 1268f
  heart rate in, 1267–1268, 1268f
  palpation in, 1266
  pulmonary artery catheter for, 1301–1327. See also Pulmonary artery catheter monitoring.
  pulse rate in, 1268
  pulses in, 1266
  right ventricular ejection fraction pulmonary artery for, 1332–1333
  stethoscopy in, 1266–1267
  stroke volume variation in, 1327
  systolic pressure variation in, 1326–1327, 1326f

Cardiovascular system. *See also* Heart.
  age-related changes in, 2436–2437, 2436f, 2436t
  barbiturate effects on, 333–334
  benzodiazepine effects on, 340, 340t
  brainstem stimulation effects on, 2157–2158, 2157t
  development of, 2368–2369
  dexmedetomidine effects on, 357–358, 357f
  droperidol effects on, 360
  etomidate effects on, 353
  in brain death, 2958–2959, 2959f
  in preeclampsia, 2331, 2331f
  ketamine effects on, 348
  pediatric, 2832–2833
  pregnancy-related changes in, 2308–2309, 2308t
  sitting position effects on, 2136–2137
Cardioversion, elective, 2653–2654
Cardioverter-defibrillator, implantable. *See* Implantable cardioverter-defibrillator.
Carlens tube, 1875, 1875f. *See also* Endotracheal tubes, double-lumen.
Carnitine:acyl transferase-1, 2904
Carotid artery
  compression of, with mediastinoscopy, 1911
  stenosis of, 2098–2106. *See also* Carotid endarterectomy.
    endovascular surgery for, 2105–2106, 2162
Carotid artery stump pressure, 2103
Carotid body, denervation of, after carotid endarterectomy, 2105
Carotid bruits, 1060–1061, 1061t
Carotid endarterectomy, 2098–2106. *See also* Vascular surgery.
  anesthesia for, 2100–2103
  bradycardia with, 2102
  care after, 2104–2105
  carotid body denervation with, 2105
  cerebral blood flow monitoring during, 2103
  cerebral hyperperfusion syndrome after, 2105
  cerebral oximetry in, 1542
  cervical nerve injury with, 2105
  cranial nerve injury with, 2105
  electroencephalography during, 1521–1523, 1521t, 1523f, 2103–2104
  general anesthesia for, 2101–2103
  hematoma after, 2105
  hemodynamic changes with, 2101–2102
  hyperglycemia during, 2103
  hypertension after, 2105
  hypocapnia during, 2103
  hypotension and, 2102, 2105
  indications for, 2099–2100
  local anesthesia for, 2102
  monitoring during, 2101, 2103–2104
  morbidity of, 2100
  mortality with, 2100
  neurologic complications of, 2102, 2103, 2104–2105
  neurologic monitoring during, 2103–2104
  outcomes of, 2099–2100
  preoperative evaluation in, 2100
  regional anesthesia for, 2102–2103
  somatosensory evoked potentials during, 2104
  transcranial Doppler ultrasonography during, 1541, 2104
Carotid sinus reflex, 738–739, 738f
Carteolol, 653–654
Carvedilol, 653–655, 654t, 657
Case-control study, 887. *See also* Statistics.
CASE patient simulators, 3079
Castor beans, 2516
Cataract surgery, 1709
Catecholamines, 646. *See also* Dopamine; Epinephrine; Norepinephrine.
  at birth, 2345–2346
  in carcinoid tumor, 1109
  inhaled anesthetic effects on, 112–113
  MAC effects of, 102
  opioid effects on, 395–396
  pulmonary vascular resistance and, 688, 688t
Cathelin, Fernand, 27
Catheter ablation, 2653
Cauda equina syndrome, microcatheter-related, 2320
Caudal anesthesia, 1673–1674, 1674f. *See also* Neuraxial anesthesia.
  anatomy for, 1657–1658, 1658f, 1659f
  in transurethral resection of prostate, 2190
  pediatric, 1732–1734, 1733f, 1734f, 2609
    anatomy in, 1732–1733
    anesthetic volume for, 1734
    catheter for, 1733

Caudal anesthesia *(Continued)*
  pediatric *(Continued)*
    complications of, 1734
    contraindications to, 1733
    equipment for, 1729t, 1733
    failure of, 1734
    indications for, 1733
    technique of, 1733–1734, 1733f, 1734f
Celandine, hepatotoxicity of, 2222t
Celiac artery stenosis, 2072
Celiac plexus blockade, 1711–1712, 1712f
  in complex regional pain syndrome, 2775
Celiotomy, 2482
Celiprolol, 653–654
Central core disease, 538t
Central nervous system. *See also* Brain; Spinal cord.
  aging-related changes in, 2435–2436
  functional development of, 2854–2855, 2854t
Central pontine myelinolysis, 1767
Central retinal artery, 2992–2994, 2993f
Central retinal artery occlusion, 2998–3005
  electroretinography in, 2998, 2999f
  etiology of, 3002–3003
  eye examination in, 2996–2997, 2997t, 2998f
  head position and, 3003, 3004–3005
  mechanisms of, 2998, 3000
  nasal/sinus surgery and, 3003, 3005
  ocular compression and, 3003
  pathogenesis of, 3000, 3002
  patient characteristics in, 3000, 3001t–3002t
  prevention of, 3004–3005
  prognosis for, 3004
  surgical factors and, 3003
  treatment of, 3004
Central retinal vein, 2994
Central tendency, measures of, 883, 883t
Central venous catheter, 1290. *See also* Central venous pressure monitoring.
  antibiotic-coated, 2797, 2798t
  as intravascular ECG electrode, 2141, 2141f
  for children, 2393
  infection of, 1293t, 1295, 2797–2798, 2798t
  insertion of, 2797–2798
Central venous pressure monitoring, 1201, 1286–1327
  abnormal waveform characteristics on, 1298–1301, 1299f, 1299t, 1300f, 1316
  aortic cross-clamping and, 2073
  axillary vein for, 1293
  cannulation for, 1286–1293, 1287t, 1288f, 1291f
    axillary vein for, 1293
    complications of, 1293–1296, 1293t
    double, 1290
    external jugular vein in, 1292
    femoral vein in, 1292–1293
    left internal jugular vein in, 1291–1292
    peripheral veins in, 1293
    radiographic confirmation of, 1289
    right internal jugular vein in, 1287–1291, 1288f, 1291f
    site for, 1290–1291
    subclavian vein in, 1292
    techniques of, 1289–1291
    ultrasound-guided, 1291, 1291f
  cardiac filling pressure in, 1297, 1297t
  catheters for, 1290
    complications of, 1293t, 1295–1296, 2797–2798, 2798t
    for children, 2393
  complications of, 1293–1296, 1293t
    prevention of, 2797–2798, 2798t
  diastolic pressure-volume relationship and, 1296–1297, 1296f
  external jugular vein for, 1292
  femoral vein for, 1292–1293
  for renal function, 1494
  in aortic reconstruction, 2077
  in atrial fibrillation, 1298–1299, 1299f
  in atrioventricular dissociation, 1299, 1299f
  in cardiac tamponade, 1316–1317, 1318f
  in kidney transplantation, 2241
  in living liver donation, 2236
  in neonatal hypovolemia, 2359
  in pediatric shock, 2836
  in pericardial constriction, 1316, 1317f
  in peripheral vascular surgery, 2070
  in preeclampsia, 2332, 2332f
  in pulmonary artery hypertension, 1316
  in restrictive cardiomyopathy, 1316
  in right ventricular ischemia, 1316
  in tricuspid regurgitation, 1299, 1300f

Central venous pressure monitoring *(Continued)*
  in tricuspid stenosis, 1299–1300, 1300f
  in ventricular pacing, 1299, 1299f
  infectious complications of, 1293t, 1295
    prevention of, 2797–2798, 2798t
  left internal jugular vein for, 1291–1292
  left ventricular preload estimation in, 1319–1320, 1319f
  mechanical complications of, 1293–1294, 1293t
  misinterpretation of, 1295–1296
  nerve injury with, 1295
  nitrous oxide effects on, 214
  normal waveform characteristics on, 1297–1298, 1297t, 1298f
  operator errors in, 1295–1296
  peripheral veins for, 1293
  physiologic considerations in, 1296–1297, 1296f
  pneumothorax with, 1294
  respiratory influences on, 1300–1301, 1300f
  right internal jugular vein for, 1287–1291, 1288f, 1291f
  subclavian vein for, 1292
  thromboembolic complications of, 1293t, 1295
  transmural pressure in, 1296–1297
  vascular complications of, 1294
  waveform characteristics of
    abnormal, 1298–1301, 1299f, 1299t, 1300f, 1316
    normal, 1297–1298, 1297t, 1298f
Central volume of distribution, 68, 69f
Cephalosporins, neuromuscular blockade and, 516
Cerebral aneurysm. *See* Intracranial aneurysm.
Cerebral arteries. *See also* Cerebral blood flow; Cerebral ischemia.
  innervation of, 817
  posterior, 2994
Cerebral atrophy, age-related, 2435–2436
Cerebral blood flow, 813–830
  age-related effects on, 820
  alfentanil and, 823
  arterial pressure and, 829
  barbiturates and, 330, 821, 821f
  benzodiazepines and, 824
  brain tumor and, 842–843
  cardiac arrest and, 837–839
  cerebral blood volume and, 820, 829, 829f
  cerebral metabolic rate and, 814–817, 814t, 815f, 816f
  chemical regulation of, 814–817, 814t, 815f, 816f
  clonidine and, 820
  critical thresholds of, 833–834, 834f
  dexmedetomidine and, 356, 820, 821f
  diazepam and, 821f, 824
  dopamine and, 819–820, 819t
  droperidol and, 360, 824
  during carotid endarterectomy, 2103
  epinephrine and, 819, 819t
  esmolol and, 819
  etomidate and, 352, 821f, 822
  fentanyl and, 821f, 823
  flumazenil and, 824
  hematocrit and, 817–818
  hemorrhagic shock and, 817
  hypocapnia-induced reduction in, 2132–2133, 2133f
  hypothermia and, 1588
  in brain death, 2965–2966
  in cardiopulmonary bypass, 1979
  in coma, 843
  in epilepsy, 843
  in head injury, 2154–2155, 2154t
  in pediatric cardiac surgery, 2019, 2019t
  inhaled anesthetics and, 825–831, 826f–830f, 2130–2131
  intravenous anesthetics and, 821–825, 821f, 2130
  ketamine and, 347, 821f, 824–825
  labetalol and, 819
  lidocaine and, 825
  local anesthetics and, 593
  lorazepam and, 824
  midazolam and, 821f
  morphine and, 821f, 822–823
  muscle relaxants and, 831–832, 2131
  myogenic regulation of, 817
  neurogenic regulation of, 817
  nitrous oxide and, 830–831, 830f, 2130–2131
  norepinephrine and, 818–819, 819t
  normal values for, 813–814, 814t
  opioid effects on, 389–390
  $Paco_2$ and, 816–817, 816f
  Pao_2 and, 816f, 817

Cerebral blood flow (Continued)
  pH and, 816–817
  phenylephrine and, 818–819
  propofol and, 821–822, 821f, 827f
  propranolol and, 819
  regulation of, 814–818, 814t, 815f, 816f
  remifentanil and, 821f, 823–824
  seizures and, 843
  somatosensory evoked potential monitoring of, 1529
  succinylcholine and, 831–832
  sufentanil and, 821f, 823
  thiopental and, 821f
  transcranial Doppler ultrasound monitoring of, 1540–1542, 1540f, 1541f
  vasodilators and, 818
  viscosity and, 817–818
Cerebral blood volume, 820
  cerebral blood flow and, 829, 829f
Cerebral death, 2962. See also Brain death.
Cerebral edema, 2957
  at high altitude, 2690–2691
  fluid management in, 1792–1793
  post-TURP visual changes and, 3014
Cerebral hyperperfusion syndrome, after carotid endarterectomy, 2105
Cerebral ischemia, 833–837
  after coronary artery bypass surgery, 1061
  blindness with, 1158, 2996, 2997–2998, 2997t, 3011–3012
  carbon dioxide tension and, 840–841
  cerebral blood flow thresholds in, 833–834, 834f
  cerebral perfusion pressure and, 840
  diabetes mellitus and, 1022
  elective surgery and, 842
  energy failure in, 834–836, 836f
  glucose and, 841–842
  hemodilution in, 818, 842
  hypocapnia-induced, 2132–2133, 2133f
  hypotension and, 840
  hypothermia and, 841, 841t, 1581, 2144
  models of, 834, 834f
  neuronal death in, 836–837, 837f
  neuroprotection and, 837–842, 838t. See also Neuroprotection.
  nitrous oxide and, 836
  postoperative, 2718
  prevention of. See Carotid endarterectomy.
  thrombolytic therapy for, 2647
Cerebral metabolic rate, 815–816, 815f
  barbiturates and, 330, 821, 821f, 839
  benzodiazepines and, 821f, 824
  BIS index and, 1254
  cerebral blood flow and, 814–817, 814t, 819, 819t
  dexmedetomidine and, 821f
  diazepam and, 821f
  droperidol and, 824
  etomidate and, 821f, 822
  fentanyl and, 821f, 823
  flumazenil and, 824
  functional state and, 815
  inhaled anesthetics and, 825–831, 826f
  ketamine and, 821f, 824–825
  midazolam and, 821f
  morphine and, 821f, 822–823
  nitrous oxide and, 831
  normal values for, 813–814, 814t
  propofol effects on, 821–822, 821f
  remifentanil and, 821f
  seizures and, 843
  sufentanil and, 821f, 823
  temperature and, 816, 816f
  thiopental and, 821f
Cerebral metabolic rate of oxygen ($CMRO_2$), 814t, 815, 815f
  age and, 820
  barbiturates and, 330, 821, 821f
  benzodiazepines and, 821f, 824
  dexmedetomidine and, 821f
  diazepam and, 821f, 824
  etomidate and, 352, 821f
  fentanyl and, 821f, 823
  hyperthermia and, 816
  hypothermia and, 816, 816f
  inhaled anesthetics and, 826f, 827–828
  ketamine and, 347, 821f
  lidocaine and, 825
  midazolam and, 821f
  morphine and, 821f, 822–823
  opioids and, 389, 390, 821f, 822–823
  propofol and, 821–822, 821f

Cerebral metabolic rate of oxygen (Continued)
  remifentanil and, 821f
  sufentanil and, 821f, 823
  temperature and, 816, 816f
  thiopental and, 821f
Cerebral palsy, orthopedic surgery in, 2427
Cerebral perfusion pressure, 817, 2127, 2133, 2133f
  etomidate effects on, 822
  in brain injury, 2154–2155, 2154t, 2471–2473, 2472f
  in cerebral ischemia, 840
Cerebrospinal fluid, 822t, 832
  accumulation of, 2162–2163, 2856
  drainage of
    for spinal cord protection, 2087
    in intracranial aneurysm treatment, 2149–2150
  leak of, after transsphenoidal hypophysectomy, 2159
  lumbosacral volume of, 1655
Ceruloplasmin, in sepsis, 2902, 2902f
Cervical nerves, dysfunction of, after carotid endarterectomy, 2105
Cervical plexus block, 1706–1707, 1706f, 1707f, Plate 4
  in outpatient procedures, 2609
  pediatric, 1753
Cervical spine
  injury to, 2152–2153, 2153f
  instability of, 2410, 2410f, 2410t
  subluxation of, 2410, 2411f
  surgery on, 2418
Cervicothoracic ganglion block, pediatric, 1753–1754
Cesarean section, 2323–2326
  anesthesia-related risk in, 909–912, 911t
  continuous spinal anesthesia for, 2325
  epidural anesthesia for, 2324–2325
  failed endotracheal intubation in, 2325–2326, 2327f
  general anesthesia for, 2325–2326, 2326t
  regional anesthesia for, 2323–2324
    complications of, 2326, 2328–2329
  spinal anesthesia for, 2324, 2324f
  spinal-epidural anesthesia for, 2325
Channelopathies, 537–538, 538t, 539f, 543–546
  myotonic, 543–546, 544t
Channels of Martin, 692
Chaparral, hepatotoxicity of, 2222t
Charcot-Marie-Tooth disease, 534–535, 538t
Charles, Jacques, 12
Chemical and biological warfare agents, 2497–2524
  accidental release of, 2503, 2503t
  biological agents as, 2516–2519, 2518t
  cellular toxins as, 2513, 2513t–2514t
  classified information on, 2498
  definitions of, 2498–2500
  detection of, 2520–2521
  evidence-based studies of, 2498
  hazard spectrum of, 2499, 2499f
  historical perspective on, 2501, 2502t
  incident management of, 2519–2523, 2520f, 2520t
    anesthesia-related effects in, 2523
    early medical response in, 2521–2522, 2521f, 2522f
    personal protection in, 2520, 2520f, 2520t
    problems in, 2523
  latency properties of, 2499
  LD_{50} of, 2499
  Lemmler plates for, 2500, 2500f
  lethality coefficient of, 2499
  literature sources on, 2498
  lung-damaging agents as, 2510–2513, 2511t, 2512f
  military release of, 2502–2503, 2503t
  NBC classification of, 2499–2500
  nerve agents as, 2504–2509, 2504f, 2505t, 2506t, 2507f
  persistency properties of, 2499
  personal protection against, 2520, 2520f, 2520t
  terrorist release of, 2503
  threat and, 2501–2502
  toxicity properties of, 2499
  toxins as, 2513, 2515–2516, 2515t
  transmissibility properties of, 2499
  United Nations HAZMAT classification of, 2500, 2500t
  vesicant agents as, 2509–2510, 2509f, 2510f
  viral diseases as, 2519
Chemoreceptors, 739
  in respiration, 177
  pediatric, 2833

Chemotherapy, 1118
  oxygen toxicity and, 2677–2678
Cherry-red spot, 2997, 2998f
Chest. See also Thoracic surgery.
  trauma to, 2479–2481
Chest compressions, in basic life support, 2925–2926, 2925f
Chest massage, in neonate, 2360, 2360f
Chest pain, 1074, 1075t. See also Myocardial ischemia.
  in lung cancer, 1850
Chest physiotherapy, 2818–2819, 2818f
  preoperative, 1859–1860
Chest radiography
  in airway management, 1623
  in double-lumen endotracheal tube positioning, 1882
  in lung cancer, 1851–1852, 1852f, 1852t
  in pregnancy, 2309, 2309t
  preoperative, 947–949, 948t–949t, 951, 968f
Chest wall. See also Thoracic surgery.
  inhaled anesthetic effects on, 174–177, 174f–176f
  neonatal, 2842
  pediatric, 2842
Child-Pugh score, 2217–2218, 2217t
Children. See also Infant; Neonate; Pediatric intensive care unit.
  abuse of, 2874
  acute respiratory distress syndrome in, 2848, 2848t
  adrenal hyperplasia in, 2861
  adrenal insufficiency in, 2861
  airway management in, 1646–1647, 2382t, 2384–2388, 2385f
    difficult airway in, 2385–2387, 2386t, 2387f
    endotracheal intubation for, 1630, 1630t, 2384, 2384t
    laryngoscope blades for, 2384, 2384t
  airway obstruction in, 2387–2388, 2387f, 2388f, 2844–2845, 2854. See also Respiratory failure, pediatric.
  ambulatory anesthesia for, 2607–2608
  anesthesia circuits for, 2393, 2394f
  anesthesia for, 2379–2398
    airway management for, 2384–2388, 2384t, 2385f, 2386t, 2387f, 2388f
    equipment for, 2393
    induction of, 2375, 2382–2384
    intramuscular induction of, 2384
    intravenous induction of, 2384
    principles of, 2393–2395, 2394f
    rectal induction of, 2383–2384
  anesthesia-related risk in, 912–914, 913t, 914f
  anomalous origin of coronary arteries in, 2840
  apnea in, 2723
  arrhythmias in, 2839
  arterial catheter for, 2393
  asphyxiation of, 2876–2877
  asystole in, 2944–2946, 2945f, 2947t
  at high altitude, 2689
  biliary atresia in, 2864
  blood transfusion in, 2869
  blood warmers for, 2391–2392
  brain death in, 2858, 2877, 2963–2964, 2964t
  bronchiolitis in, 2852
  bronchopulmonary dysplasia in, 2853
  cardiac arrest in, 2392–2393
  cardiac catheterization in, 2015–2016, 2651–2652
  cardiac surgery in, 2005–2043, 2006t. See also Congenital heart disease.
  cardiopulmonary bypass in, 2022–2034. See also Cardiopulmonary bypass, pediatric.
  cardiopulmonary resuscitation in, 2941–2947, 2941t
    advanced cardiac life support in, 2942–2947, 2943f–2946f, 2947t
    basic life support in, 2941–2942, 2941t
    vascular access for, 2944–2945, 2946f
  cardiovascular system of, 2006–2008, 2007f, 2832–2833
  caudal anesthesia for, 1732–1734, 1733f, 1734f, 2609
    anatomy in, 1732–1733
    anesthetic volume for, 1734
    catheter for, 1733
    complications of, 1734
    contraindications to, 1733
    equipment for, 1729t, 1733
    failure of, 1734
    indications for, 1733
    technique of, 1733–1734, 1733f, 1734f

Children (*Continued*)
  central venous catheter for, 2393
  cerebral palsy in, 2427
  coagulation system of, 2867, 2867f
  congenital heart disease in, 2005–2043, 2006t, 2009t, 2010t. *See also* Congenital heart disease.
  cystic fibrosis in, 2853
  diabetes insipidus in, 2861
  diabetic ketoacidosis in, 2862–2863
  disseminated intravascular coagulation in, 2868
  droperidol for, 360
  emergence delirium in, 2723
  epidural analgesia in, 2748
  epiglottitis in, 2852
  epilepsy in, 2858
  equipment cart for, 2393
  external beam radiotherapy for, 2657–2658
  extracorporeal membrane oxygenation in, 2851
  extrahepatic biliary atresia in, 2864
  eye injury in, 2534
  factor VIII deficiency in, 2867–2868
  fasting by, 2381, 2381t
  fearfulness in, 2380–2381
  fluid therapy in, 1790
  foreign body aspiration in, 2853–2854
  fresh frozen plasma for, 2390, 2391f
  gastrointestinal disorders of, 2863–2867
  Glasgow Coma Scale for, 2855, 2855t
  heart of, 2832–2833
  heart transplantation in, 2037–2039, 2037f, 2038f
  hemochromatosis in, 2869
  hemolytic-uremic syndrome in, 2859–2860
  hepatic failure in, 2864
  hereditary thrombocytopenia in, 2868
  Hirschsprung's disease in, 2863
  human immunodeficiency virus infection in, 2871, 2872–2873
  hyperbaric oxygen therapy in, 2673
  hypertension in, 2839–2840, 2839t, 2840t
  hypoglycemia in, 2862
  immunosuppression in, 2871–2873, 2872t–2873t
  infection in, 2870–2873, 2870t, 2872t–2873t
  inflammatory bowel disease in, 2864
  informed consent for, 3180–3182, 3180t, 3181t
  inotropic drugs for, 2836–2839, 2837t
  intensive care for, 2831–2879. *See also* Pediatric intensive care unit.
  intestine of, 2863
  intracranial pressure increase in, 2856–2857
  intravenous fluids for, 2388–2389, 2388t
  intussusception in, 2864
  Kawasaki's disease in, 2840
  ketamine in, 348, 349
  laparoscopy in, 2295
  laryngotracheobronchitis in, 2851–2852
  larynx in, 2540
  left atrial pressure monitoring in, 1311
  leukemia in, 2869–2870
  leukostasis in, 2869
  liquid ventilation in, 2851
  liver development in, 2863
  liver transplantation in, 2865
  malignant hyperthermia in, 1181
  malrotation in, 2863
  maximal allowable blood loss from, 2389–2390
  mechanical ventilation in, 2846–2851, 2848t
  Meckel's diverticulum in, 2863
  mediastinal mass in, 2870
  meningomyelocele in, 2854
  methohexital for, 333
  monitoring for, 2392–2393
  necrotizing enterocolitis in, 2864
  neurologic function in, 2855–2856, 2855t
  neurosurgery for, 2163, 2164t
  neutropenia in, 2870
  nondepolarizing muscle relaxants in, 525–526, 525f
  nutritional support for, 2865–2867
  opioid effects in, 406, 406f
  orthopedic surgery in, 2426–2427
  outpatient procedures for, 2607–2608
  packed red blood cells for, 2389–2390
  pain control for, 2398, 2747–2748
  pain perception in, 1720–1721
  parenteral nutrition in, 2865–2867, 2866f
  parents with, 2382, 2384, 2607–2608, 2722
  patient-controlled analgesia for, 2748
  pharmacodynamics/pharmacokinetics in, 2371–2379, 2371f
    alfentanil and, 2377

Children (*Continued*)
  pharmacodynamics/pharmacokinetics in (*Continued*)
    desflurane and, 2374–2375
    diazepam and, 2375–2376
    fentanyl and, 2376–2377, 2377f
    halothane and, 2373–2374, 2373t
    inhaled anesthetics and, 2372–2375, 2372f, 2372t, 2373t
    isoflurane and, 2374
    meperidine and, 2376
    methohexital and, 2375
    midazolam and, 2376
    morphine and, 2376
    muscle relaxants and, 2378–2379, 2380t
    propofol and, 2375
    remifentanil and, 2377–2378, 2378f
    sevoflurane and, 2372–2373, 2373t
    succinylcholine and, 2378–2379
    sufentanil and, 2377
    thiopental and, 2375
  pheochromocytoma in, 2861
  platelet disorders in, 2868
  platelets for, 2390–2391, 2391f
  Pneumocystis carinii pneumonia in, 2871, 2872
  poisoning in, 2875
  postanesthesia care unit for, 2722–2723
  postanesthetic apnea in, 2723
  postintubation croup in, 2723
  postoperative pain control for, 2398, 2747–2748
  premedication for, 2381
  pulmonary function testing in, 2841t, 2843
  red cell abnormalities in, 2868–2869
  regional anesthesia for, 1719–1756, 2398, 2427
    anesthetic selection for, 1728–1729, 1728t
    assessment of, 1730
    cardiac complications of, 1732, 1732t
    catheter-related infection with, 1731
    caudal block in, 1732–1734, 1733f, 1734f
    cervical plexus blocks for, 1753
    cervicothoracic ganglion block for, 1753–1754
    clonidine for, 1725–1726, 1725t
    complications of, 1730–1732
      epidemiology of, 1730–1731
    conduction blocks for, 1738–1749
      anesthetic absorption with, 1722
    contraindications to, 1727
    developmental considerations in, 1720, 1721t
    epidural, 1734–1737, 1735f, 1736t
    epidural space location for, 1729
    epinephrine for, 1725, 1728
    equipment for, 1729, 1729t
    flip-flop effect in, 1722
    iliohypogastric nerve block for, 1749, 1749f
    ilioinguinal nerve block for, 1749, 1749f
    indications for, 1726–1727, 1727t
    infraorbital nerve block for, 1754
    injection technique for, 1730
    intercostal nerve block for, 1752–1753, 1752f
    interpleural block for, 1753
    intracapsular injections for, 1756
    intradermal wheals for, 1755
    intraperitoneal injections for, 1756
    intrapleural block for, 1753
    intravenous, 1755
    ketamine for, 1725t, 1726
    laryngeal nerve block for, 1753, 1753f
    local anesthetics for, 1722–1724
      absorption of, 1722
      clearance of, 1724
      clinical characteristics of, 1724
      distribution phase of, 1723, 1723f, 1723t
      metabolism of, 1723–1724
      plasma protein binding of, 1722–1723
      red blood cell storage of, 1722
      toxicity of, 1724
    local complications of, 1731
    local infiltrations for, 1755–1756
    lower extremity conduction blocks for, 1742–1749
      anatomy for, 1742–1743
      contraindications to, 1743–1744
      fascia iliaca compartment block in, 1745
      femoral nerve, 1744–1745, 1744f
      indications for, 1743–1744
      lateral cutaneous nerve, 1746
      lumbar plexus, 1743–1746, 1744f–1745f
      psoas compartment, 1745, 1745f
      sacral plexus, 1743, 1744, 1746–1748, 1747f, 1748f
      saphenous nerve, 1745–1746, 1746f

Children (*Continued*)
  regional anesthesia for (*Continued*)
    lower extremity conduction blocks for (*Continued*)
      sciatic nerve, 1746–1748, 1747f, 1748f
      three-in-one block in, 1744–1745, 1744f
      umbilical block in, 1751
      vastus medialis nerve block in, 1746, 1746f
    mental nerve block for, 1754–1755
    metatarsal block for, 1748–1749
    monitoring procedures for, 1730
    nerve injury with, 1731
    nerve trunk location for, 1729
    neuraxial blocks for, 1720, 1732–1738, 1733f–1735f, 1736t, 1737t
    opioids for, 1724–1725, 1725t, 1728–1729
    penile block for, 1750–1751, 1750f
    physiologic considerations in, 1726
    procedure section for, 1727–1728
    psychological considerations in, 1726
    pudendal nerve block for, 1749–1750, 1750f
    rectus sheath block for, 1751, 1751f
    regional complications of, 1731
    safety procedures for, 1730, 1731t
    scalp blocks for, 1755
    sedation for, 1730
    spinal, 1737–1738, 1737t
    stellate ganglion block for, 1753–1754
    subarachnoid space location for, 1729
    supraorbital nerve block for, 1754, 1754f
    supratrochlear nerve block for, 1754, 1754f
    systemic complications of, 1731–1732, 1732t
    techniques for, 1729–1730, 1729t
    thoracic paravertebral space block for, 1751–1752, 1752f
    topical, 1755
    transthecal block for, 1748–1749
    transtracheal injections for, 1756
    trigeminal nerve block for, 1754
    truncal blocks for, 1749–1753, 1749f–1752f
    upper extremity conduction blocks for, 1738–1742
      anatomy for, 1738
      axillary approaches in, 1738–1739, 1739f, 1740t
      contraindications to, 1738
      coracoid approaches in, 1739–1740, 1740f
      distal, 1742
      indications for, 1738
      interscalene approach in, 1741–1742, 1742f
      metacarpal, 1742, 1742f
      parascalene approach in, 1720–1741, 1740t, 1741f
      peri-subclavian artery approaches in, 1742
      transthecal, 1742, 1742f
  renal failure in, 2859–2861
  renal system of, 2858–2859, 2859t
  respiratory failure in, 2843–2851. *See also* Respiratory failure, pediatric.
  respiratory system of, 2840–2842, 2841t
  rheumatoid arthritis in, 2427
  seizures in, 2858
  sevoflurane in, 253, 830
  shock in, 2834–2836, 2835f, 2835t
  sick sinus syndrome in, 2839
  sickle cell disease in, 2869
  sinus bradycardia in, 2839
  sleep apnea in, 2853
  status epilepticus in, 2858
  strabismus surgery in, 2535–2536
  stress response in, 2394–2395
  stridor in, 2387–2388, 2387f, 2388f
  supraventricular tachycardia in, 2839
  syndrome of inappropriate secretion of antidiuretic hormone in, 2861–2862
  tonsillectomy in, 2543–2544
  topical anesthesia for, 1755
  total parenteral nutrition in, 2865–2867, 2866t
  transesophageal echocardiography in, 1384
  transport of, 2875
  trauma in, 2873–2874
  tumor lysis syndrome in, 2869–2870
  upper respiratory tract infection in, 2381–2382
  ventilation in, 2842–2843
  ventricular fibrillation in, 1732, 1732t, 2946–2947
  ventriculoperitoneal shunt in, 2163
  vocal cord paralysis in, 2854
  volvulus in, 2863
  von Willebrand disease in, 2868
  with full stomach, 2384–2385
  with stridor, 2387–2388, 2387f, 2388f

Chiropractic, in chronic pain, 2777
Chirurgia, 11f
Chloride
    depletion of, 1775
    physiology of, 1775
Chlorine
    experimental inhalation study of, 2512
    warfare use of, 2510, 2511t
1-Chloro-1,2,2,2-tetrafluoroethyl
            chlorodifluoromethyl ether, 116–117,
            116f
Chlorobutanol, 350
Chloroform
    historical studies on, 16–17
    oil-gas partition coefficient of, 115t
    structure of, 106f
Chloroprocaine, 24, 575t
    biotransformation of, 592
    bupivacaine and, 585–586
    cardiovascular toxicity of, 594–595, 594t
    during labor, 2323
    half-life of, 74
    in epidural anesthesia, 588–589, 588t, 1674–1675,
            1674t
    in nerve block, 587–588, 587t
    in pediatric regional anesthesia, 1728t
    infiltration of, 586–587, 586t
    intravenous, 587
    neurotoxicity of, 597
    onset of action of, 584
    pK_a of, 574, 574f
    potency of, 576t
    structure of, 575t
Chlorpromazine
    hepatotoxicity of, 2221t
    in outpatient premedication, 2598
Choanal atresia, 2352
Cholecystectomy, robotic, 2561–2562, 2562f
Cholera, 2515t, 2517, 2519
Cholestasis, 763–765, 764t, 805
    cardiovascular dysfunction in, 764–765
    coagulopathy in, 764
    renal dysfunction in, 764
Cholinergic agonists, 618, 659–660
Cholinergic antagonists, 618
Chondocurine, 493t
Choroid, blood flow to, 2995, 2995f
Christmas disease, 1824
Chromaffin cells, 633
Chronic obstructive pulmonary disease, 1090–1091,
            2264–2265. *See also* Lung
            transplantation.
    diffusing capacity of carbon monoxide in, 1089
    hypoventilation in, 177, 177f
    in lung cancer patient, 1854–1856, 1855f, 1855t
    metered-dose inhaler in, 1090, 1090t
    postoperative respiratory function in, 164
    preoperative bronchodilation in, 1859
    Shapiro score in, 1089
Chvostek's sign, 1051, 2540
Chymopapain allergy, 1092, 1093t
Cigarette smoking
    cessation of, 1014, 1086, 1858–1859, 1859t
    postoperative mucociliary function and, 164
Cimetidine, 1125
    in outpatient premedication, 2599–2600, 2600t
    vasopressin with, 1053
Ciprofloxacin, in anthrax infection, 2517
Circadian rhythms, 3055, 3062
Circle breathing system, 295–296, 295f
    problems in, 300–301, 300f
    test of, 310
Circle of Zinn-Haller, 2994
Circulation. *See also* Heart.
    development of, 2368–2369
    fetal, 2347, 2347f
Circumcision, 2609
Cirrhosis, 760–763, 763f
    ascites with, 762–763
    cardiovascular dysfunction with, 762
    central nervous system dysfunction with, 761–762
    Child-Pugh score in, 2217–2218, 2217t
    circulatory volume in, 762
    endocrinopathy with, 761
    fluid therapy in, 1791–1792
    gastrointestinal complications of, 761
    hematologic dysfunction with, 761
    intravenous anesthetic metabolism in, 2213
    morphine metabolism in, 2212–2213
    neuromuscular blocking drug metabolism in,
            2213–2214, 2214f

Cirrhosis *(Continued)*
    opioid metabolism in, 2212–2213
    portal hypertension and, 762
    preoperative, 2217–2218, 2217f, 2218f
    pulmonary dysfunction with, 760–761
    renal dysfunction with, 761
Cisatracurium, 493t, 494, 494f, 497t
    autonomic effects of, 511, 511t, 512t
    bradycardia with, 513
    dosage for, 501t
    elimination of, 506t, 509, 511
    for children, 2379, 2380t
    hepatobiliary disease and, 529–530, 529t
    Hofmann degradation of, 74
    in elderly patients, 527
    in kidney transplantation, 2241
    in outpatient anesthesia, 2607
    in renal failure, 2184–2186, 2185t
    metabolism of, 506t, 509
    pharmacodynamics of, 500t, 502t
    renal failure and, 527, 528t
    skin testing with, 514
Cisplatin, 1118
    hepatotoxicity of, 2221t
Citrate intoxication, 1812–1813, 2466
Citrate phosphate dextrose adenine, for blood
            storage, 1804–1805, 1805t
Clarck, Timothy, 28–29
Clark, Leland C., 6, 6f
Clearance, 69–74
    definition of, 69–70, 70f
    distribution, 74
    hepatic, 70–74, 71f–74f
    intercompartmental, 68–69
    intrinsic, 72–73, 74f
    protein binding and, 76
    renal, 73–74, 784–789, 787f
    tissue, 74
Clement, F. W., 17
Clinical trial, 886, 887. *See also* Statistics.
Clonidine, 650–651, 650t, 1121
    cerebral blood flow and, 820
    epidural, 651
    in outpatient monitored anesthesia care, 2611
    in outpatient premedication, 2596–2597, 2596t
    in pain treatment, 651
    in pediatric regional anesthesia, 1725–1726, 1725t
    in postoperative shivering, 1583
    nonanesthetic uses of, 651
    thermoregulatory response thresholds with, 1575
Closing capacity, 695–697
    in abnormal lungs, 695, 695f
    in normal lungs, 694–695, 695f
    measurement of, 695–696, 696f
    residual capacity and, 696–697, 696f, 697f
    tracer gas test of, 695–697, 696f, 697f
Clostridium infection, 2673
Clover, Joseph T., 33
Cluster headache, 1096
Coagulation, 1983–1983, 1983f
    during pregnancy, 2310, 2310t
    during thoracoabdominal aorta reconstruction,
            2089
    epidural analgesia and, 2742
    fluid therapy and, 1786–1787
    hypothermia-related impairment of, 1581
    in children, 2867–2868, 2867f
    in cholestasis, 764
    monitoring of, 1338–1343, 1339f, 1342f
    postoperative pain and, 2730
    preoperative evaluation of, 955–956, 960t, 961f
    transfusion-induced disorders of, 1807–1812,
            1808f, 1808t, 1809f, 1811f, 1812f
    viscoelastic monitoring of, 1341–1342, 1342f
Coagulation factors
    disorders of, 1116–1117
    during pregnancy, 2310, 2310t
    hepatic synthesis of, 749
    in cardiopulmonary bypass, 1983
    vitamin K-dependent, 749
Cobo, Bernabe, 22
Cobratoxin, 2515t
Cocaine, 20f, 575t. *See also* Substance abuse.
    cardiovascular toxicity of, 594–595, 594t
    channel blockade by, 870
    historical perspective on, 22–23
    in awake intubation, 1641–1642
    intranasal, 2547
    laryngeal, 2548
    ocular, 2537
    organ response to, 633, 634t

Cocaine *(Continued)*
    structure of, 575t
    topical, 589–590, 590t, 2537, 2547
Codeine, 380t, 417
    postoperative, 2735t, 2736f
    structure of, 382t
Codman, A. E., 41
Cognition
    in anesthesiologist, 3023–3031, 3025f, 3025t,
            3026f, 3028t, 3029t, 3030t
    in elderly patient, 2441
    sleep deprivation and, 3162–3163
Cohort study, 887. *See also* Statistics.
Cold. *See* Hypothermia.
Coleman, Alfred, 34
Colistin, 2816
Colitis, ulcerative, 1108
Collagen, of cardiac ventricles, 725
Colloids, 1787–1788
    in hemorrhagic shock, 2464
    vs. crystalloids, 1786–1787
Colony-stimulating factor-1, 1114t
Colt, Samuel, 13
Colton, Gardner Q., 13, 14f, 17
Coma, 1094
    barbiturate, 2472
    cerebral blood flow in, 843
    deep, 2958, 2961. *See also* Brain death.
    somatosensory evoked potentials in, 1530
Combitube, 1627–1628, 1628f, 1637
    in basic life support, 2924
    in trauma patient, 2458
Comfrey, hepatotoxicity of, 2222t
Common peroneal nerve, position-related injury to,
            1155, 1156f, 1157f
Common rule, in research, 3190, 3190t
Compartment syndrome, 2478–2479
    lithotomy position and, 1159
    supine position and, 1158
    trauma-related, 2478–2479
Complementary and alternative medicine,
            605–613, 606t
    acupuncture for, 612–613, 613f
    dietary supplement for, 612
    herbal, 605–612. *See also specific plants.*
    music for, 613
Complex regional pain syndrome, 2774–2775
Compound 485
    convulsions with, 116
    oil-gas partition coefficient of, 115t
    structure of, 106f
Compound A, 251–256, 251f, 254f, 1490
    in pediatric cardiac surgery, 2021
Computed tomography
    anesthesia for, 2642–2643
    in airway management, 1623
    in brain death, 2966
    in cortical blindness, 2997–2998
    in ischemic optic neuropathy, 2998
    in lung cancer, 1851
    in pediatric neurologic impairment, 2855
Concentration
    drug, vs. response, 95, 95f
    minimum alveolar, 107–109, 107f, 108f,
            108t, 2438
        catecholamine effects on, 102
        depth of anesthesia and, 1239–1241,
            1240f, 1241f
        lipid solubility and, 115, 115f
        movement response and, 1239–1241, 1240f,
            1241t, 1243f
Concentration over time curve, 79–80
Conduction, heat loss with, 1576
Confidentiality, informed consent and,
            3179–3180, 3181
Conflicts of interest, 3190–3191
Confounding bias, in statistics, 886
Confusion assessment method (CAM) score, 2442
Congenital adrenal hyperplasia, 2861
Congenital heart disease, 2008–2012, 2009t, 2010t,
            2834, 2834t
    angioplasty in, 2042, 2042f
    chronic effects of, 2011–2012
    halothane effects on, 2374
    heart failure in, 2011–2012, 2012f
    nonoperative approaches to, 2040–2043, 2041f
    surgery for, 2012–2014, 2013t. *See also*
            Cardiopulmonary bypass, pediatric.
        anesthesia in, 2020–2022, 2020f, 2022f, 2022t
        anticoagulation in, 2034–2035
        aprotinin for, 2035–2036

Congenital heart disease (Continued)
  surgery for (Continued)
    body temperature monitoring in, 2017
    capnography in, 2017
    cardiac catheterization before, 2015–2016
    closed heart, 2039–2040
    Doppler echocardiography before, 2015
    echocardiography during, 2017–2018,
        2017f, 2018f
    electroencephalography in, 2018–2019
    heparin in, 2035
    management after, 2036–2037
    monitoring in, 2016–2017, 2016t
    neurologic monitoring in, 2018–2019, 2019f
    operating room preparation for, 2016
    pain control after, 2036–2037
    premedication in, 2016
    preoperative evaluation in, 2014–2016
    pulmonary artery catheter in, 2017
    pulse oximetry in, 2017
  ventricular remodeling in, 2011–2012, 2012f
Congenital myasthenic syndrome, 540–541, 540t
Conjunctival erythema, transfusion-associated, 1820
Conn's syndrome, 1038
Consciousness, loss of, 2961. See also Brain death.
Consensual light reflex, 2996, 2997t
Consultation, 989, 1018–1019, 1019t
  form for, 970f
Continuous mandatory (assist/control) ventilation,
    2822–2823, 2823t
Continuous positive airway pressure (CPAP), 2824.
        See also Mechanical ventilation,
        positive-pressure.
  in bronchial hygiene, 2819
  in children, 2847–2848
  in obese patient, 1032–1033
  in one-lung ventilation, 1895f, 1897–1900, 1898f,
      1899f
  in postoperative hypoxemia, 2714–2715
  in premature infant, 2356
  physiology of, 2820–2821
Continuous renal replacement therapy, 1102–1103,
    1103t
  acid-base balance and, 1613
Contrast media, 2640–2641, 2641t
  anaphylaxis with, 1092–1093
  renal effects of, 804, 2180
Conus medullaris, 1654
Convection, heat loss with, 1576
Cor pulmonale, 1089–1090
Cordus, Valerius, 11
Corneal abrasion, 2537
  position-related, 1157, 1158f
Corning, James Leonard, 24–25
Coronary arteries
  angiography of, 2648–2649
    before peripheral vascular surgery, 2062, 2063t,
        2064t
    cortical blindness after, 3011–3012
  anomalous origin of, 2840
  disease of. See Coronary artery disease.
  inhaled anesthetic effects on, 203–211
    blood flow and, 210–211
    in vitro, 203
    in vivo, 203–204
    ischemia and, 205–206, 206f
    protective effects and, 206–210, 206f, 208f,
        209f, 211
    vasodilation and, 205
    vasodilator reserve and, 204–205, 204f
  nitrous oxide effects on, 214–215
  opioid effects on, 395
Coronary artery bypass graft surgery, 2650
  cardiopulmonary bypass for, 1971–1982. See also
      Cardiopulmonary bypass.
  cerebral ischemia after, 1061
  cortical blindness after, 3011–3012
  diabetes mellitus and, 1022
  history of, 1073–1074, 1074f
  in lung cancer patient, 1856
  minimally invasive, 1994–1995, 1994f
  off-pump, 1994
  peripheral vascular surgery and, 1073–1074,
      1074f, 2062–2063
  port-access, 1995
  robotic, 1995, 2565–2566, 2565f, 2565t, 2566f,
      2566t
Coronary artery disease, 1027–1028, 2053. See also
      Myocardial infarction; Myocardial
      ischemia.
  angiography in, 2648–2649

Coronary artery disease (Continued)
  carotid artery stenosis and, 2100
  cortical blindness and, 3011–3012
  drug treatment of, 1027–1028, 1028t
  electrocardiography in, 1060–1061
  hypothyroidism and, 1048
  in lung cancer patient, 1856
  intraoperative monitoring in, 1968–1970, 1970f,
      1970t
  ischemic optic neuropathy and, 3010
  management of, 1946–1951, 1948f–1951f
    β-adrenergic blockers in, 1946–1947
    myocardial oxygen supply and demand in,
        1946, 1948f
    nitrates in, 1947–1951, 1949f–1951f
    pathophysiology of, 1943–1944, 1944f–1946f
    percutaneous transluminal angioplasty in,
        2649–2650
  peripheral vascular disease and, 2055, 2058t
  peripheral vascular surgery and, 2059–2062,
      2060t, 2061f
  premedications in, 1968, 1969t
  preoperative antihypertensive therapy and,
      1057–1058, 1058t
  preoperative evaluation of, 1064–1073, 1064t,
      1065f, 1069f, 1969t
    algorithms for, 1068–1072, 1070t, 1071f–1072f,
        1071t
    cardiac risk index for, 1067–1072, 1068t, 1069f,
        1069t, 1070t, 1071f–1072f, 1071t
    dipyridamole-thallium scanning for, 1064t,
        1065f, 1066–1067
    dobutamine stress echocardiography for, 1064t,
        1065f, 1067
    electrocardiography for, 1064, 1065f
    Holter monitoring for, 1064t, 1065f, 1067
    summary of, 1074–1075, 1076f, 1077f
    treadmill exercise testing for, 1064, 1066, 1066t
  preoperative therapy in, 1075–1077
  radiation therapy in, 2650
  stent placement in, 2650
  transvascular procedures in, 2649–2650
Coronary sinus, unroofed, pulmonary artery catheter
    monitoring and, 1303
Cortical blindness, 1158, 3011–3012
  computed tomography in, 2997–2998
  eye examination in, 2996, 2997t
  magnetic resonance imaging in, 2997–2998
Cortical somatosensory evoked responses,
    815, 815f
Corticosteroids
  adrenal insufficiency with, 2861
  aerosol, 2816, 2817t
  in carcinoid tumor, 1109
  in neuroprotection, 2087
  in neurosurgery, 2133–2134, 2146
  in pediatric ICP increase, 2857
  in sepsis, 2795–2796
  neuromuscular blockade and, 518
  perioperative, 1039–1041, 1040t
    complications of, 1040–1041
    infection and, 1041
    wound healing and, 1040–1041
Cortisol, 1036
  age-related secretion of, 1041
  etomidate effects on, 353–354, 354f
  in sepsis, 2899–2900
  stress-related secretion of, 1040
Cotransmitters, 619, 619f
Cotugno, Domenico, 26
Coughing, 1619–1620
  preoperative, 1859–1860
Coulomb, 1208
Courville, C. B., 17
Cousins, Michael, 28
COX-II inhibitors, in chronic pain, 2769
Cox maze procedure, 1993
Coxiella burnetii, in biological warfare, 2518t
Crackles, 1464–1465
Cranial nerves
  dysfunction of, after carotid endarterectomy, 2105
  electromyographic monitoring of, 1537–1539
  injury to, 2157
Craniectomy, decompressive, 2472–2473
Craniofacial abnormalities, 2164t
  ocular pathology in, 2536
Craniopharyngioma, 2146
Craniosynostosis, 2164t
Craniotomy, 2145–2146
  awake, 2159–2161
Cranium, air retention in, 2138, 2138f

Creatine kinase, in malignant hyperthermia,
    1182, 1185
Creatinine, 2179
  during pregnancy, 2311, 2311t
  in children, 2859t
  in compound A exposure, 252–253
  in renal function monitoring, 1497–1498, 1497t
  preoperative, 969f, 1493, 1493f
  serum, 788–789, 788f
  urinary, 1498
Creatinine clearance, 73–74, 786–788, 787f,
    1101–1102, 1489, 2179, 2179f
  after pediatric cardiopulmonary bypass, 2028t,
      2029
  during pregnancy, 2311, 2311t
  in compound A exposure, 252–253
  in renal function monitoring, 1499, 1499f
  normal variation in, 787
  preoperative, 1493
  serial, 788
Creutzfeldt-Jakob disease, in health care worker,
    3159–3160
Cricoid pressure, in endotracheal intubation, 1635,
    2456
Cricothyrotomy, 1639–1640
  emergency, 2547
  for children, 2386–2387
  in basic life support, 2924
Crile, George W., 21, 35
Crisis resource management, 3082–3084, 3083t
Critical care medicine, 59–60, 2787–2804, 2788t.
        See also Pediatric intensive care unit.
  evidence-based management in, 2789–2790,
      2790f, 2790t
    for acute lung injury, 2790–2791, 2792f–2793f
    for acute respiratory distress syndrome,
        2790–2791, 2792f–2793f
    for cerebral injury prevention, 2800, 2803
    for glycemic control, 2799–2800, 2801f–2802f
    for nosocomial infection, 2796–2798, 2797t
    for pain control, 2798–2799, 2799t
    for sedation, 2798–2799, 2799t
    for sepsis, 2794–2796
    for transfusion, 2803–2804
    for venous catheter infection, 2797–2798, 2798t
    for ventilator-associated pneumonia,
        2796–2797, 2797t
    for ventilator weaning, 2791, 2793–2794, 2794f
Critical illness myopathy, 531–532
Critical illness polyneuropathy, 532
Critical volume hypothesis, of inhaled anesthetics,
    117, 119
Crossmatch-to-transfusion ratio, 1803
Crossmatching, for blood transfusion, 1802–1803,
    1802f
Croup, 2851–2852
  postintubation, 2723
Crush syndrome, 2478–2479
Cruzan v Director, Missouri Department of Health,
    3183
Cryoanalgesia, 1906–1907, 2744
Cryoprecipitate, 1824
  during thoracoabdominal aorta reconstruction,
      2089
Cryoshock syndrome, 2224
Cryotherapy, hepatic, 2224
Cryptorchidism, 2200
Crystalloids, 1785
  body temperature changes with, 1585
  for packed red blood cells, 1822
  historical studies on, 20–21
  in hemorrhagic shock, 2463
  vs. colloids, 1786–1787
  with neuraxial anesthesia, 1659–1660
Cullen, Stuart, 32
Curare, 20f, 30–32, 32f
  in kidney transplantation, 2241
Curbelo, Manuel Martinez, 27–28
Curry, James, 39
Cushing, Harvey, 35–36, 35f, 41
Cushing's disease, 1041
Cushing's reflex, 739
Cushing's syndrome, 1037–1038, 1037t
Cyanide, 2513, 2513t–2514t
Cyanmethemoglobin, pulse oximetry errors and,
    1450, 1451t
Cyanosis, detection threshold of, 1447, 1448f
Cyclic AMP diesterase inhibitors, in phosgene
    exposure, 2512
γ-Cyclodextrin (ORG 25969), 524–525, 524f, 876
Cyclonine, topical, 589–590, 590t

Cyclooxygenase-1, in prostaglandin synthesis, 795, 795f
Cyclooxygenase-2, in prostaglandin synthesis, 795, 795f
Cyclooxygenase-2 inhibitors, in outpatient premedication, 2597
Cyclopentolate, 2537
Cyclophosphamide, 1118
Cycloplegics, 1126t
Cyclopropane, 17–18
   minimum alveolar concentration of, 107–109, 107f, 108t
   oil-gas partition coefficient of, 115t
   structure of, 106f
Cyclosporine
   hepatotoxicity of, 2221t
   in organ transplantation, 2271–2273, 2272t
   renal effects of, 803–804
Cyst, air, 1916–1917
Cystic fibrosis, 1091, 2264–2265, 2853. *See also* Lung transplantation.
Cystitis, interstitial, 2200
Cytochrome P450
   in drug metabolism, 750–751, 758–759
   St. John's wort effects on, 611
Cytochrome P450 3A4, 99, 101
Cytochrome P450 2C19, 99
Cytochrome P450 2D6, 99, 101
Cytokines, 1114t–1115t
Cytomegalovirus, transfusion-transmitted, 1818t, 1819

D

Daclizumab, in organ transplantation, 2271–2273, 2272t
Dale, Henry H., 8
Dalton, John, 12
Damping coefficient, in arterial blood pressure monitoring, 1276, 1277f, 1278–1279, 1278f
Danazol, hepatotoxicity of, 2221t
Dantrolene
   hepatotoxicity of, 2221t
   in malignant hyperthermia, 1177–1178, 1179, 1184
   muscle relaxant interaction with, 518
Dapsone, hepatotoxicity of, 2221t
Data, 882, 882t
   for anesthesia-related risk studies, 896–897
Data dredging, 887
Datex-Ohmeda S/5 ADU anesthesia machine, 301–302
Datex-Ohmeda S/5 ADU cassette vaporizer, 292–293, 292f
Datex-Ohmeda Tec 6 vaporizer, 281t, 289–292, 290f
   at altitude, 291
   carrier gas composition for, 291
   operating principles of, 289–291, 290f, 291t
   safety features of, 291–292
Datex Ultima monitor, 1204
Davy, Humphry, 5, 5f, 13
De la Condamine, Charles-Marie, 30
De Petit, Ponfour, 8
Dead space, 680, 697–698, 697f, 698f
   hypercapnia and, 714, 714f
   measurement of, 1442, 1442f
1-Deamino-8-D-arginine vasopressin, 1811
Death
   brain, 2955–2968. *See also* Brain death.
   brainstem, 2958
   cerebral, 2962
Debrisoquine hydroxylase, 99
Decamethonium, channel blockade by, 870
n-Decane, cutoff effect with, 116
Decastello, A. V., 21
Decerebration, isoflurane MAC and, 109, 110f
Decision-making, 3024–3026, 3025f, 3025t, 3026t, 3027–3028, 3043–3047, 3044f, 3045t
Decision-making capacity, informed consent and, 3176
Declaration of Helsinki, 3189
Decompression sickness, 2672–2673, 2691, 2693
   heliox in, 2678
Decompressive craniectomy, in traumatic brain injury, 2472–2473
Deep breathing, for bronchial hygiene, 2818
Deep hypothermic circulatory arrest
   in aortic arch aneurysm, 2086

Deep hypothermic circulatory arrest *(Continued)*
   in pediatric cardiopulmonary bypass, 2026–2027, 2026f, 2027f
Deep venous thrombosis
   orthopedic surgery and, 2425–2426, 2425f, 2426f
   prophylaxis for, 1079, 1082–1083, 1082t
   transurethral resection of prostate and, 2190–2191
Dehydration. *See also* Fluid therapy.
   in elderly patient, 2443
   neuromuscular blockade and, 523
   sodium clearance in, 790
Delirium
   in children, 2723
   in elderly patient, 2441–2442, 2442t, 2746
Delirium tremens, 1097, 2485
Delta sleep-inducing peptide, 2516
Dementia, 1095–1096, 2441
Demyelinating disease, 1096
15-Deoxyspergualin, in organ transplantation, 2271–2273, 2272t
Depression, 1100
   in elderly patient, 2442
   St. John's wort in, 611
   treatment of, 1122–1123
Depth of anesthesia, 1227–1259
   awareness and, 1236–1239
   definition(s) of, 1227–1236
      components of, 1230–1231, 1230t
      historical, 1227–1230, 1228f, 1229f
      modern, 1230–1236, 1230t, 1231f–1234f, 1236f
   electrophysiologic monitoring of, 1249–1258
      bispectral electroencephalography for, 1250–1257, 1251f–1254f, 1257f. *See also* Electroencephalography, bispectral.
      evoked responses for, 1257–1258
      spontaneous electroencephalography for, 1249–1250
   experimental characterization of, 1233–1235, 1233f, 1234f
   historical definitions of, 1227–1230, 1228f, 1229f
   inhaled anesthetics and, 1235–1236, 1236f, 1239–1243, 1240f, 1241t, 1242f, 1242t
   intravenous nonopioid anesthetics and, 1243–1245, 1243f, 1244f, 1245t
   isolated arm movement monitoring of, 1237
   memory and, 1236–1239
   minute ventilation and, 706, 706f
   modern definitions of, 1230–1236, 1230t, 1231f–1234f, 1236f
   nonresponsiveness and, 1230–1231, 1231f, 1232f, 1233f, 1234–1235, 1234f
   opioid anesthetics and, 1231–1233, 1231f, 1246–1249, 1246f, 1247f, 1247t, 1248f, 1248t
   pharmacologic model of, 1231–1233, 1231f, 1232f
   respiratory pattern and, 706, 706f
   response surfaces for, 1235–1236, 1236f
Dermatomyositis, 1098
Desensitization, 101–102
Desflurane, 18, 284–285, 284f
   airway resistance and, 160, 160f
   arterial pressure and, 202
   BIS index and, 1254, 1255–1256
   bronchodilation and, 157
   central ventilatory effects of, 171, 172f
   cerebral blood flow and, 825–827, 826f
   cerebral metabolic rate and, 826f, 827–828
   cerebrospinal fluid dynamics and, 832, 832t
   Datex-Ohmeda Tec 6 vaporizer for, 281t, 289–292, 290f
   diastolic function and, 195–196, 195f
   during labor, 2319
   electroencephalographic effects of, 1519t, 1520–1521
   fluoride-associated nephrotoxicity of, 251
   for children, 2372, 2372f, 2372t, 2374–2375
   heart rate and, 202
   hepatic function and, 2209–2212, 2211f
   hepatotoxicity of, 244f, 245
   hypoxic pulmonary vasoconstriction and, 166, 167–168, 167f, 168f
   in ambulatory anesthesia, 2604–2605, 2604t, 2605f
   in kidney transplantation, 2241
   in pediatric cardiac surgery, 2021
   in renal failure, 2183
   left atrial function and, 199–200, 201f
   left ventricular-arterial coupling and, 196–197
   metabolism of, 135, 238, 239f
   minimum alveolar concentration of, 107–109, 107f, 108t

Desflurane *(Continued)*
   myocardial contractility and, 192, 193f
   neuromuscular blockade and, 515–516, 516f
   partition coefficients of, 132, 132t
   pulmonary blood flow and, 169
   recovery from, 147–151, 148f, 149f, 150f, 2707–2708, 2707t, 2708t
   structure of, 106f
   thermoregulatory response thresholds with, 1574–1575, 1574f, 1576f
   toxicity of, 244f, 245. *See also* Malignant hyperthermia.
   tubing uptake of, 142, 143t
   vasodilating effect of, 829
Desmopressin
   in diabetes insipidus, 1053
   in von Willebrand's disease, 1117
Desmosomes, 730, 730f
Detsky Modified Risk Index, 908
Dexamethasone
   in experimental chlorine exposure, 2512
   in neurosurgery, 2146
   in outpatient premedication, 2599, 2614
   neuromuscular blocking agent interaction with, 518
Dexmedetomidine, 355–359, 651
   cardiovascular system effects of, 357–358, 357f
   central nervous system effects of, 356
   cerebral blood flow and, 820, 821f
   cerebral metabolic rate and, 821f
   dosing for, 358–359
   halothane MAC and, 113, 113f
   hepatic metabolism of, 2213
   historical perspective on, 355–356
   in awake craniotomy, 2160
   in neurosurgery, 2145
   in outpatient monitored anesthesia care, 2611
   in outpatient premedication, 2596–2597, 2596t
   maintenance with, 358–359
   metabolism of, 356, 2213
   pharmacokinetics of, 319t, 356
   pharmacology of, 356–358
   physiochemical characteristics of, 356
   respiratory system effects of, 357
   sedation with, 358
   structure of, 356, 356f
   thermoregulatory response thresholds with, 1574–1575, 1574f
Dextran 40, 1787, 1826
   allergy to, 1093t
Dextran 70, 1787, 1826
Dextropropoxyphene, postoperative, 2735t, 2736f
Dextrorphan, for neuroprotection, 2088
Dextrose
   five percent, 1786
   in diabetes mellitus, 1779
   in pediatric cardiopulmonary resuscitation, 2946
Dezocine, 420
   in outpatient anesthesia, 2606
Diabetes insipidus, 1053
   acid-base balance and, 1614
   after transsphenoidal hypophysectomy, 2159
   central, 1767–1768
   in brain death, 2960
   in children, 2861
   nephrogenic, 1767–1768, 1768t
Diabetes mellitus, 1019–1025, 1776–1781
   acute hyperglycemia in, 1780
   age-induced physiologic changes in, 1025
   anesthetic considerations in, 1778–1780
   autonomic dysfunction in, 664–665, 1778
   autonomic neuropathy in, 1025, 1026f
   blood glucose in, 1778–1780
      cerebral ischemia and, 1022
      control of, 1021, 1022t, 1023–1024, 1024f
   cardiovascular effects of, 1778
   cerebral ischemia in, 1022
   classification of, 1776, 1776t
   complications of, 1021, 1022t
   coronary artery bypass graft surgery and, 1022
   diagnosis of, 1020
   dysautonomia in, 1044–1045
   end-organ effects of, 1025
   gastrointestinal effects of, 1025, 1026f, 1778, 1779
   hemoglobin A_{1c} in, 1779
   hypoglycemia in, 1781
   infection and, 1021
   insulin requirements in, 1021
   ischemic optic neuropathy and, 3010
   ketoacidosis in, 1022–1023, 1780
      in children, 2862–2863

Diabetes mellitus (Continued)
  kidney failure and, 2238
  kidney transplantation in, 2240
  microangiopathy and, 1025
  myocardial ischemia and, 1026, 1027t
  obesity and, 1025
  pancreas transplantation in, 2242–2245, 2244f
  pathology of, 1776–1777, 1777t
  treatment of, 1021, 1025–1026, 1777–1778, 1777t, 1778t
  type 1 vs. type 2, 1020–1021
Diabetic ketoacidosis, 1022–1023, 1780
  in children, 2862–2863
Diallyl derivative of toxiferine, 493t, 497, 497f, 509. See also Alcuronium.
Dialysis, 1102–1103, 1103t
  in pediatric hemolytic-uremic syndrome, 2860
  in renal failure, 2188–2189
3,4-Diaminopyridine, in Lambert-Eaton myasthenic syndrome, 540
Diamorphine
  respiratory depression with, 1472
  single-dose, 2737, 2738t
Diaphragm
  cephalad displacement of, 708–709, 709f
  electromyographic monitoring of, 1463–1464
  inhaled anesthetic effects on, 174–177, 174f–176f
  neuromuscular blockade of, 1557–1558 4731f, 1558f
  paralysis effect on, 709, 712–713
  pressure monitoring of, 1464, 1464f
Diaphragmatic hernia, 2355–2356, 2396–2397
Diastole, 724, 724f, 728
Diazepam
  cardiovascular system effects of, 323t, 340, 340t
  central nervous system effects of, 339
  cerebral blood flow and, 821f, 824
  cerebral metabolic rate and, 821f, 824
  during labor, 2318–2319
  for children, 2375–2376
  half-life of, 337–338
  in awake intubation, 1641
  in outpatient premedication, 2596, 2596t
  in renal failure, 2184
  induction with, 340t
  maintenance with, 340t
  metabolism of, 335–336
  metabolites of, 336
  pharmacokinetics of, 319t, 336–337, 336f
  physiochemical characteristics of, 335, 335t
  respiratory system effects of, 339–340, 339f
  sedation with, 340–341, 340t
  side effects of, 342
  somatosensory evoked potential effects of, 1533t
  structure of, 335, 335f
  visual evoked potential effects of, 1533t
Dibucaine, 575t
  in spinal anesthesia, 589, 589t
  structure of, 575t
  topical, 589–590, 590t
Dibucaine number, 487–489, 488t
1,2-Dichlorohexafluorocyclobutane, 116–117, 116f
2,3-Dichlorooctafluorobutane, 116–117, 116f
Diclofenac, postoperative, 2735t, 2736f
Dicobalt edetate, in cyanide poisoning, 2514t
Dietary supplements, 612
Diethyl ether
  oil-gas partition coefficient of, 115t
  partition coefficients of, 132, 132t
  structure of, 106f
Difficult airway. See Airway, difficult; Airway management.
Diffusing capacity, 1010–1011
Diffusion hypoxia
  nitrous oxide and, 150, 150f
  postoperative, 2713, 2714f
DiGeorge's syndrome, 2838
DiGiovanni, Anthony J., 27
Digitalis, 1125
  in children, 2837–2838
  in kidney failure, 2186
Digoxin, age-related effects of, 101
Dihydrocodeine, postoperative, 2735t, 2736f
Dihydromorphone, 380t
Dilevalol, 653–654
Diltiazem, 1121–1122, 1122f
  for renal protection, 799–800, 804
  in kidney failure, 2186–2187
  in supraventricular arrhythmias, 2933
  neuromuscular blocking agent interaction with, 517

Dimenhydrinate, in outpatient premedication, 2599
Dioxychlorane
  oil-gas partition coefficient of, 115t
  structure of, 106f
Dip-and-plateau pattern, in pericardial constriction, 1316, 1317f
Diphenhydramine, opioid interaction with, 424
Diphenoxylate, 381f
2,3-Diphosphoglycerate, 1806–1807, 1806f
Diplopia, anesthetic-related, 2531
Dipyridamole-thallium imaging
  before peripheral vascular surgery, 2059–2061, 2060t, 2061f
  in anesthesia-related risk evaluation, 909
  in coronary artery disease evaluation, 1064t, 1065f, 1066–1067
Disclosure, informed consent and, 3176–3177
Disopyramide, 1125
Disseminated intravascular coagulation
  in children, 2868
  in malignant hyperthermia, 1180
  transfusion-related, 1809–1810, 1811
Dissociation constant (PK_a), 1600
Distribution clearance, 74
Disulfiram, hepatotoxicity of, 2221t
Diuretics, 1121
  in neurosurgery, 2134
  metabolic acidosis with, 1782
  neuromuscular blocking agent interaction with, 517–518
  nondepolarizing muscle relaxant interaction with, 517–518
Dixon, Walter E., 8
4-DMAP, in cyanide poisoning, 2514t
DNase, recombinant, 2816
Do-not-resuscitate order, 2940–2941, 3183–3186, 3185f
  documentation of, 3185–3186
  perioperative, 3185
Dobutamine, 651–652
  in children, 2032, 2837
  structure of, 647f
Dobutamine stress echocardiography
  before peripheral vascular surgery, 2060t, 2061–2062
  in anesthesia-related risk evaluation, 909
  in coronary artery disease evaluation, 1064t, 1065f, 1067
Dofetilide, in atrial fibrillation, 1402, 1402t, 1403t
Dogliotti, Achille M., 25f, 27
Dolasetron, 2721
Domperidone, in outpatient premedication, 2598–2599
Dopamine
  cerebral blood flow and, 819–820, 819t
  during cardiopulmonary bypass, 803
  for renal protection, 798–799, 802
  in children, 2837, 2837t
  in infrarenal aortic reconstruction, 2075
  in kidney transplantation, 2242
  in neonatal resuscitation, 2361t
  in pediatric left ventricular dysfunction, 2032
  in pediatric life support, 2947t
  in renal regulation, 796–797, 796t
  in septic shock, 806
  inhaled anesthetic effects on, 113
  intravenous administration of, 649
  metabolism of, 631
  receptors for, 637, 638f
  renal effects of, 798–799
  structure of, 647f
Dopaminergic receptors, in renal regulation, 796–797, 796t
Dopexamine
  for renal protection, 799
  in septic shock, 806
  intravenous administration of, 649
  renal effects of, 799
Doppler effect, 1206, 1206f, 1208
Doppler ultrasonography
  during carotid endarterectomy, 2104
  in brain death, 2966
  in cardiac output monitoring, 1334–1336
  in pediatric cardiopulmonary bypass, 2017–2018, 2018f
  in pediatric neurologic impairment, 2855
  transcranial, 1512t, 1540–1542, 1540f, 1541f
    in pediatric cardiac surgery, 2019
Dorsal rhizotomy, electromyographic monitoring in, 1538–1539

Dorsalis pedis artery, cannulation of, 1274. See also Arterial blood pressure.
Dose
  effective, 95–96, 96f
  lethal, 95–96, 96f
Double-blind study, 886. See also Statistics.
Double indicator dilution method, for cardiac output monitoring, 1338
Down syndrome, 1099, 2536
Doxacurium, 493t, 494, 494f, 497t
  autonomic effects of, 511, 511t, 512t
  dosage for, 501t
  elimination of, 506t, 509
  hepatobiliary disease and, 529–530, 529t
  in elderly patients, 527
  in renal failure, 2186
  metabolism of, 506t, 509
  opioid interactions with, 423
  pharmacodynamics of, 502t
  renal failure and, 528t
Doxepin, in chronic pain, 2771
Drager, Bernhard, 34
Drager, Heinrich, 34
Drager Narkomed 6000 anesthesia machine, 302–303, 303f
Dressler's syndrome, 1967
Dripps, Robert, 27
Droperidol, 359–360, 412–413, 1123, 2720
  antiemetic effects of, 360
  cardiovascular system effects of, 323t, 360
  central nervous system effects of, 360
  cerebral blood flow and, 824
  cerebral metabolic rate and, 824
  electroencephalographic effects of, 360
  for children, 360
  historical perspective on, 359
  in awake craniotomy, 2160
  in awake intubation, 1641
  in outpatient premedication, 2598, 2598f, 2615
  metabolism of, 360
  pharmacokinetics of, 319t, 360
  pharmacology of, 360
  physicochemical characteristics of, 359–360, 359f, 360f
  respiratory system effects of, 360
  somatosensory evoked potential effects of, 1533t, 1536
  structure of, 359, 359f
  visual evoked potential effects of, 1533t
Drosophila, inhaled anesthetic study in, 124
Drowsiness, 3057. See also Sleep deprivation.
Drug discontinuation, 1125–1127, 1127t
Duchenne's muscular dystrophy, 535, 535t, 536f, 1099
  anesthesia in, 536–537
  malignant hyperthermia and, 1183
Ductus arteriosus, 2347
Dunbar, Burdett S., 27
Dura mater, 1655, 1655f
  puncture of, 2326, 2328
Dural sac, 1655f, 1657–1658
Dying. See also End-of-life care.
  good death and, 3186–3187, 3187t
  physician aid in, 3187–3188, 3188t
Dynorphin, 382
Dysautonomia, 1044–1045
Dysfibrinogenemia, 761
Dysmenorrhea, 2201
Dyspareunia, 2201
Dyspnea
  in lung cancer, 1851
  preoperative evaluation of, 1086–1087, 1087t
  spinal anesthesia and, 1670
Dyspnea differentiation index, 1010
Dysrhythmias. See also Arrhythmias.
  anticholinesterase effects on, 523
  laryngoscopy and, 1647
  nondepolarizing muscle relaxants and, 513
  postoperative, 1993
  succinylcholine and, 489
Dystroglycan, 872

E

Ear
  pressure equilibration in, 2679–2680
  surgery on, 2548–2549
Eating disorders, 1034. See also Obesity.
Eaton-Lambert myasthenic syndrome, 863

Ebullism, 2694
Echinacea *(Echinacea purpurea)*, 606, 607t, 608, 2222t
Echocardiography, 1363–1385. *See also*
        Transesophageal echocardiography.
  before peripheral vascular surgery, 2060t,
    2061–2062
  for monitoring, 1208
  in anesthesia-related risk evaluation, 909
  in coronary artery disease evaluation, 1064t,
    1065f, 1067
  in pediatric cardiopulmonary bypass, 2017–2018,
    2017f, 2018f
  in pediatric shock, 2836
  in pregnancy, 2309, 2309t
Echothiophate, 1125, 1126t, 2536–2537
Eclampsia, 1125. *See also* Preeclampsia.
ED$_{50}$ (effective dose), 95–96, 96f
Edema
  cerebral, 2957
    at high altitude, 2690–2691
    fluid management in, 1792–1793
    post-TURP visual changes and, 3014
  fluid management in, 1789–1790, 1790t
  laryngeal, after endotracheal intubation, 1650
  pulmonary, 680–681m 704–705, 704f, 705t
    after thoracic surgery, 1903
    at high altitude, 2690
    detection of, 1468
    in kidney failure, 2181t, 2182
    in preeclampsia, 2330–2331
    postoperative hypoxemia and, 2713, 2713f
Edentulous patients, 1620
Edrophonium, 519, 521–522, 521f, 662, 875–876.
        See also Anticholinesterases.
  for children, 526, 2380t
  in kidney failure, 2186, 2186t
  in outpatient anesthesia, 2607
  neuromuscular blocking agent interaction
    with, 517
  pharmacokinetics of, 523–524, 524t
Effective dose, 95–96, 96f
Efficacy, drug, 95, 96f
Eger II, Edmund I., 18
Eicosanoids. *See also* Prostaglandin(s).
  pulmonary vascular resistance and, 685t, 686,
    688, 688t
Einhorn, Alfred, 24
Einthoven, Willem, 40
Eisberg, C. A., 33
Eisenmenger complex, 2009–2010, 2009f, 2259,
    2263
Elam, James O., 40
Elastin, 2840
Elbow
  median nerve block at, 1693, 1693f
  musculocutaneous nerve block at, 1694
  radial nerve block at, 1693, 1693f
  surgery on, 2421
  ulnar nerve block at, 1694
Elderly patient
  alcoholism in, 2443
  anesthesia for, 2443, 2444
    pharmacokinetics of, 2438–2439, 2439t
    risk of, 914
  bispectral index in, 2612
  chronic pain in, 2443
  cognitive status in, 2441
  dehydration in, 2443
  delirium in, 2441–2442, 2442t, 2746
  dementia in, 2441
  depression in, 2442
  disease manifestations in, 2441
  edentulous, 1620
  emergency surgery in, 2440
  general anesthesia in, 2443
  hypotensive resuscitation in, 2463
  hypothermia in, 2443
  immobility in, 2443
  informed consent from, 2441
  intraoperative care for, 2443
  malnutrition in, 2442, 2443t
  opioid effects in, 406, 406f
  pain management in, 2444–2445, 2745–2746
  postoperative care for, 2444, 2444t
  preoperative evaluation of, 2440–2443
  preoperative testing for, 2443
  risk assessment in, 914, 2440
  surgical mortality in, 2440
  trauma in, 2482
Electric blankets, 1586–1587, 1587f
Electric shock injury, 3144–3146, 3145f, 3145t

Electric shock therapy. *See* Electroconvulsive therapy.
Electrical energy, 1208–1210, 1209f
Electrical resistance, 1209, 1209f, 1210, 1210f
Electrical safety, 3139–3148
  capacitive coupling and, 3143–3144, 3143f
  electrical ground for, 3139–3140
  failures of, 3144–3146, 3145f, 3145t
  for argon beam coagulator, 3147
  for electrocardiology monitor, 3141, 3141f
  for electrosurgery, 3146–3147, 3146f
  ground fault current interruption outlets for, 3140
  isolation transformer for, 3141–3143, 3141f, 3142f
  line isolation monitor for, 3142–3143, 3142f
  resistive coupling and, 3143
  vigilant approach to, 3147–3148
Electricity, 1208–1212
  alternating current, 1210, 1210f
  direct current, 1208–1210, 1209f
  static, 1208
Electrocardiography, 723, 724f, 1210–1211, 1211f,
    1389–1412
  after cardiopulmonary bypass, 1985–1986, 1987t
  ambulatory, 2060t, 2061
  artifacts with, 1396–1397
  at remote locations, 2653
  automatic, 1409–1410
  before peripheral vascular surgery, 2059, 2060t,
    2061
  central back lead for, 1391–1393, 1392t
  central subclavicular lead for, 1391
  computer-assisted interpretation of, 1410–1412,
    1411f
  display monitor for, 1395–1396
  during electroconvulsive therapy, 2654
  electrical interference with, 1268
  electrode preparation for, 1396
  endotracheal, 1395, 1396f
  esophageal, 1393–1394, 1393f, 1394f, 1394t,
    1395f
  five-electrode system for, 1393, 1393f
  in angina, 1856
  in atrial fibrillation, 1401–1402, 1402t, 1403t
  in atrial flutter, 1401
  in atrial premature beats, 1399
  in conduction defects, 1406–1409, 1406t,
    1407f–1410f
  in coronary artery disease evaluation, 1064, 1065f
  in hypercalcemia, 1049–1050, 1049f
  in hyperkalemia, 1106
  in hypermagnesemia, 1773
  in hypocalcemia, 1050
  in hypokalemia, 1106
  in intracranial aneurysm, 2148–2149, 2148f
  in junctional rhythms, 1403
  in myocardial ischemia, 1404–1406, 1405f, 1405t,
    1406f, 1411–1412, 1411f
  in obesity, 1031
  in paroxysmal supraventricular tachycardia,
    1399–1401, 1400t
  in pregnancy, 2309, 2309t
  in renal evaluation, 2180
  in sick sinus syndrome, 1398, 1399f
  in sinus arrhythmia, 1399
  in sinus bradycardia, 1398, 1399f
  in sinus tachycardia, 1398–1399
  in ventricular fibrillation, 1404
  in ventricular premature beats, 1403–1404
  in ventricular tachycardia, 1404
  indications for, 1397–1398
  intracardiac, 1394–1395, 1395f
  intracoronary, 1395
  intraoperative, 1267–1268, 1268f
  invasive, 1393–1395, 1393f–1396f
  lead systems for, 1390–1395, 1390f–1395f
  microshocks with, 3145–3146
  monitoring system for, 1397
  normal, 1389–1390, 1390f
  oscilloscope display for, 1396
  P wave on, 1389, 1390f
  paper for, 1396
  perioperative, 2067–2068, 2067f
  PR interval on, 1389, 1390f
  precordial leads for, 1391, 1391f
  preoperative, 951–954, 951t–952t, 953t
  QRS complex on, 1389, 1390f
  room environment for, 1396–1397
  skin preparation for, 1396
  ST segment on, 1390, 1390f
  standard limb leads for, 1390–1391, 1390f, 1391f
  T wave on, 1390, 1390f
  three-electrode system for, 1391, 1392f

Electrocerebral inactivity (silence), 2965. *See also*
    Brain death.
Electroconvulsive therapy, 2618–2619, 2619t,
    2654–2656
  anesthesia for, 2655–2656
  in pacemaker patient, 1426
  side effects of, 2655
Electroencephalography, 1211, 1512, 1512t,
    1513–1525
  abnormal, 1514–1515
  anesthesia-related changes in, 1516–1521, 1519t
  barbiturate effects on, 330, 1517–1518, 1519t
  benzodiazepine effects on, 339, 1518, 1519t
  bispectral, 1250–1257, 1517, 1518f
    clinical application of, 1256–1257, 1257f
    conceptual basis of, 1251
    development of, 1251–1252, 1251f, 1252f
    interpretation of, 1253–1255, 1253f, 1254f
    signal processing in, 1251, 1252f
    utility of, 1255–1256
    validation of, 1252–1253
  compressed spectral array for, 1515–1516, 1516f
  cost-effectiveness of, 1524–1525
  data processing for, 1515–1516, 1516f
  density spectral array for, 1515–1516
  desflurane effects on, 1519t, 1520–1521
  droperidol effects on, 360
  during cardiopulmonary bypass, 1521, 1521t
  during carotid endarterectomy, 1521–1523, 1521t,
    1523f, 2103–2104
  during sleep, 1514, 1515f
  electrode placement for, 1513–1514, 1513f
  enflurane effects on, 1519t, 1520–1521
  epoch length for, 1516
  etomidate effects on, 352, 1517–1518, 1519t
  fentanyl effects on, 1518
  for brain death, 1525, 1525t, 2964–2965, 2965t
  for depth of anesthesia, 1516–1521, 1517t
  halothane effects on, 1519t, 1520–1521
  hypercarbia effects on, 1524
  hypocarbia effects on, 1524
  hypotension effects on, 1524, 1524f
  hypothermia effects on, 1524
  hypoxia effects on, 1523–1524
  in children, 2855
  in coma, 2958
  in elderly patient, 2612
  in epilepsy, 1094, 1514, 1523
  in intracranial aneurysm, 2151
  in outpatient procedures, 2611, 2612
  in pediatric brain death, 2964, 2964t
  in pediatric cardiac surgery, 2018–2019
  inhaled anesthetic effects on, 1518–1521, 1519t
  interpretation of, 1515–1516
  intravenous anesthetic effects on, 1517–1518,
    1519t
  isoflurane effects on, 1519t, 1520–1521
  ketamine effects on, 1518, 1519t
  nitrous oxide effects on, 1518, 1519t, 1520
  normal, 1514, 1514f, 1515f
  on awakening from anesthesia, 1250
  opioid effects on, 388–389, 388f, 389f, 405–406,
    1518, 1519t
  propofol effects on, 1517–1518, 1518f, 1519t
  sevoflurane effects on, 1519t, 1520–1521
  signal generation in, 1513–1514, 1513f
  spontaneous, in depth of anesthesia monitoring,
    1249–1250
  thiopental effects on, 1517–1518, 1520f
  vs. somatosensory evoked potential monitoring,
    1529
Electrolytes, 1764, 1764t. *See also specific electrolytes.*
  disorders of, 1104–1107
  urinary, 2180
Electromagnetic flow probe study, in renal blood
    flow measurement, 790
Electromotive force, 1208–1209
Electromyography, 1512, 1512t, 1558–1560, 1559f,
    1560f
  after spinal anesthesia, 1670
  for monitoring, 1537–1539, 1538f
  in spinal surgery, 2418–2419
Electroretinography, 2535, 2998, 2999f
Electrosurgery
  bipolar, 3147
  in implantable cardioverter-defibrillator patient,
    1429, 1430f
  in pacemaker patient, 1423, 1426
  safety for, 3146–3147, 3146f
  unipolar, 3146–3147
Elliott, Thomas R., 8

Elliptocytosis, hereditary, 1113–1114
Emancipated minor, informed consent by, 3182
Emboli-X device, 1995
Embolism
    air. *See* Air embolism.
    carbon dioxide, 2289–2290
    during hip replacement, 2415, 2416f
    during knee replacement, 2417
    fat, 2425, 2478
    gas, 2672–2673. *See also* Air embolism.
        laparoscopy-related, 2289–2290
        laser-induced, 2579–2580
    nitrous oxide, 141, 142f
    pulmonary, 1089–1090
        after bariatric surgery, 1033, 1034
        hypoxemia in, 713, 713f
        postoperative hypoxemia and, 2713
        prophylaxis for, 1079, 1082–1083, 1082t
        pulmonary artery catheter-related, 1305–1306
        with orthopedic surgery, 2425–2426, 2425f, 2426f
Emergence
    in children, 2723
    ketamine-related reactions with, 347
Emery-Dreifuss muscular dystrophy, 535t, 536, 536f
EMLA (eutectic mixture of lidocaine and prilocaine), 589–590, 590t, 596
Emphysema, 1091
    bullous, 1916–1917
        lung volume reduction surgery for, 1917–1918
        respiration in, 707, 707f, 709
    subcutaneous, during laparoscopy, 2288
Empyema, 1926
Enalapril, 659, 2221t
Enantiomers, 76
Encephalitis, viral, in biological warfare, 2518t
Encephalocele, 2164t
Encephalopathy
    hepatic, 761–762, 2222, 2247
        total parenteral nutrition in, 2915–2916
    hypoxic-ischemic, in children, 2856
End-of-life care, 3182–3189, 3187t
    DNR orders and, 3183–3186, 3185t
    futile therapy and, 3186
    legal decisions about, 3182–3183
    pain treatment in, 3186–3187
    physician aid in dying and, 3187–3188, 3188t
Endobronchial intubation
    endotracheal intubation and, 708, 1648–1649
    laparoscopy and, 2289
Endocarditis
    antibiotic prophylaxis for, 1079, 1080t–1081t
    pulmonary artery catheter-related, 1306
    transesophageal echocardiography and, 1371
Endoleak, with aortic endovascular reconstruction, 2091
Endomorphins, 383
β-Endorphin, 382
    knockout mouse study of, 386
Endoscopic retrograde cholangiopancreatography, 2618
Endothelial cells, acetylcholine effects on, 629–630, 629f
Endothelin, 629–630
    in cardiac function, 737t
    in liver disease, 762
    pulmonary vascular resistance and, 685–686, 685t
Endotoxin
    hepatic effects of, 758
    renal effects of, 805
Endotracheal intubation, 1628–1646. *See also* Airway management.
    airway resistance and, 1649
    apnea monitoring and, 1467–1468
    aspiration with, 1635, 1635t, 1647
    awake extubation after, 1649–1650
    BIS index and, 1254
    bronchial intubation with, 708, 1648–1649
    bronchoscopy in, 1645–1646
    bronchospasm with, 1648
    BURP maneuver in, 1634–1635
    capnography in, 1461
    cardiovascular complications of, 1647
    cloth tape for, 1632
    complications of, 1647–1649, 2547
    conscious (awake), 1640–1645, 1643f, 1644f
        anticholinergics for, 1641–1642
        blind, 1643–1644
        in obese patient, 1029–1030
        nasal route for, 1644
        nerve blocks for, 1642, 1643f
        oral route for, 1642–1644

Endotracheal intubation (Continued)
    conscious (Continued)
        retrograde, 1644–1645, 1644f
        sedation for, 1641
        topical anesthesia for, 1641–1642
    cricoid pressure in, 1635, 2456
    cuff for, 1629–1630
    cuff pressures in, 1630
    curved blade for, 1631, 1631f
    dental injury with, 1647
    difficult, 2546–2547. *See also* Airway, difficult.
    discontinuation of, 1472
    epistaxis with, 1649
    equipment for, 1629–1632, 1629f, 1630t, 1631f
        in children, 2384, 2384t, 2847
    Eschmann introducer for, 1632
    esmolol in, 1647–1648
    esophageal intubation with, 1461, 1648
    extubation after, 1649–1650
    failure of, 708, 1636–1640, 1637f–1639f, 1640f.
        See also Airway, difficult.
    fiberoptic bronchoscopy in, 1645–1646
    for cesarean section, 2325–2326, 2327f
    for microlaryngoscopy, 2542
    high-dose neuromuscular blocker for, 505
    hypercarbia with, 1647
    hypoxemia with, 1647
    in basic life support, 2924
    in cervical spine injury, 2153, 2153f
    in children, 2384–2388, 2384t, 2385f, 2386t, 2842, 2846–2847, 2850
        in status asthmaticus, 2853
    in head injury, 2152, 2152t, 2153, 2153f
    in hemoptysis, 1924–1925
    in infant, 2382, 2384–2388, 2384t, 2385f, 2386t
    in neonate, 2350, 2353–2354, 2353f
    in orthopedic patients, 2410, 2410f
    in spinal cord injury, 2476
    in status asthmaticus, 2853
    in trauma, 2455–2456, 2456f, 2457f, 2458–2459, 2458f
    indications for, 1628–1629, 1629f
    infection with, 1649
    intracranial pressure elevation with, 1648
    intraocular pressure effects of, 2533
    laryngeal edema after, 1650
    laryngoscope for, 1631, 1631f, 1634, 1634f
    laryngospasm with, 1647
    laser-related fire in, 2580–2584, 2580f, 2582f
    lidocaine in, 1647
    lubrication for, 1632
    mechanical injury with, 1648
    mucociliary clearance and, 711–712
    mucosal tear with, 2541
    neuromuscular blockers for, 491–492, 503–505, 503f, 504t, 505f
        low-dose, 505
    monitoring of, 1560, 1560f, 1561–1562, 1562f
    opioids in, 392, 411, 412f
    Parker Flex-Tip tube for, 1632
    pneumothorax with, 1649
    priming technique for, 504
    RAE tube for, 1630, 1631f
    rapid, 504–505
    reinforced tubes for, 1630
    soft tissue injury with, 1647
    sore throat after, 1650
    straight blade for, 1631, 1631f
    stylet for, 1631–1632
    techniques of, 1632–1636
        anesthesia for, 1632–1633
        conscious (awake), 1640–1645, 1643f, 1644f
        nasal route for, 1633, 1636
        oral route for, 1633–1636, 1633f–1635f, 1635t
        succinylcholine for, 1633
        tube position and, 1635, 1635f
    tubes for, 1629–1630, 1630t. *See also* Endotracheal tubes.
    vocal cord paralysis after, 1650
Endotracheal tubes, 1629–1630, 1630t
    aluminum tape protection of, 2581–2582
    colored signaling cuff of, 2583
    composition of, 2581
    copper tape protection of, 2581–2582
    double-lumen
        in bronchopleural fistula, 1925–1926
        one-lung ventilation with, 1874–1889, 1874f–1876f
        airflow absence testing of, 1882, 1883f
        chest radiography with, 1882
        complications of, 1882–1883, 1883t

Endotracheal tubes (Continued)
    double-lumen (Continued)
        contraindications to, 1883
        conventional intubation procedure for, 1877–1879, 1878f, 1879f
        cuff seal pressure hold with, 1882, 1883f
        fiberoptic bronchoscopy with, 1879–1882, 1880f, 1881f, 1882t
        malposition of, 1879, 1879f
        selection of, 1876–1877
        tracheobronchial tree disruption and, 1883, 1883t
    size of, 1877
    for children, 2384, 2384t, 2847
    historical perspective on, 37–38
    laser-related fire in, 2580–2584, 2580f, 2582f
    laser-resistant coating of, 2582–2583, 2582f
    metal, 2583
    metal foil tape protection of, 2581–2582, 2582f
    mucociliary flow and, 711–712
    nonflammable, 2583
    position of, 1635, 1635f
    single-lumen
        in hemoptysis, 1889–1890
        one-lung ventilation with, 1883–1885, 1884f, 1885f, 1885t
        independent, 1887–1889, 1887f, 1888f, 1888t
        indications for, 1887
        just-seal volume and, 1886–1887
        limitations of, 1885–1886, 1886t
        technique of, 1889–1890
    tape protection of, 2581–2583, 2582f
    uncuffed, 1630
Energy, 1197–1198, 1198f, 1199t
    requirements for, 2905–2907, 2906t, 2907f, 2908
Enflurane, 18, 284–285, 284f
    airway receptor effects of, 173
    arrhythmias and, 203
    brainstem auditory evoked potential effects of, 1533t, 1534, 1535, 1535f
    calcium channel effects of, 194–195
    cardiac conduction and, 202–203
    central ventilatory effects of, 171, 172f
    cerebral blood flow and, 825–827, 826f
    cerebrospinal fluid dynamics and, 832, 832t
    coronary artery effects of, 203–211
        blood flow and, 210–211
        in vitro, 203
        in vivo, 203–204
        protective effects and, 206–210
        vasodilation and, 205
        vasodilator reserve and, 204–205, 204f
    coronary blood flow and, 210–211
    depth of anesthesia and, 1246–1247, 1246f, 1247f
    during labor, 2319
    electroencephalographic effects of, 1519t, 1520–1521
    epileptogenic properties of, 829–830
    fluoride-associated nephrotoxicity of, 248–249, 249f
    heart rate and, 201–202
    hepatic effects of, 243–244, 244f, 2209–2212, 2210f
    hypoxic pulmonary vasoconstriction and, 166, 167–168
    in ambulatory anesthesia, 2604–2605, 2604t
    in obese patient, 1033
    in renal failure, 2184t
    metabolism of, 238, 239f
    minimum alveolar concentration of, 107–109, 107f, 108t
    myocardial contractility and, 191–194
    neuromuscular blockade reversal and, 522
    ocular blood flow and, 2995
    oil-gas partition coefficient of, 115t, 116
    partition coefficients of, 132, 132t
    renal effects of, 800–801, 1490
    somatosensory evoked potential effects of, 1533, 1533t
    structure of, 106f
    synaptic effects of, 111–112, 112f
    thermoregulatory response thresholds with, 1575
    toxicity of, 243–244, 244f. *See also* Malignant hyperthermia.
    tubing uptake of, 142, 143t
    visual evoked potential effects of, 1533t, 2535
Enkephalin, 382
Enlimomab, in organ transplantation, 2271–2273, 2272t
Enteral nutrition, 2913–2914, 2914f
    aspiration in, 2913
    vs. parenteral nutrition, 2907–2908

Enteric nervous system, 624–625
Enterocolitis, necrotizing, in children, 2864
Enterotoxin, 2515t
Entonox, during labor, 2319
Environmental safety. *See* Operating room, safety of.
Ephedra (*Ephedra sinica,* ma huang), 607t, 608–609, 609t
Ephedrine
  autonomic nervous system effects of, 650
  during pregnancy, 2312
  with neuraxial anesthesia, 1659
Epidural analgesia. *See also* Epidural anesthesia.
  after thoracic surgery, 1907–1909, 1908t
  anticoagulation with, 2742–2743
  catheter for, 1868, 2739, 2739t, 2742, 2743
  coagulation and, 2742
  continuous, 2738–2743, 2738t, 2739t, 2741t
    adjuvant drugs for, 2739
    catheter location for, 2739, 2739t, 2743
    during labor, 2321, 2321t
    local anesthetics for, 2738, 2739
    opioids for, 2738–2739, 2738t
    side effects of, 2739–2741
  during labor, 2319–2320
  gastrointestinal function and, 2742
  historical studies of, 27–28
  hyperthermia and, 1590
  hypotension and, 2740
  in children, 2037, 2748
  infection and, 2743
  ketamine in, 2375
  motor block and, 2740
  myocardial infarction risk and, 2742
  nausea and vomiting with, 2740
  patient-controlled, 2741–2742, 2741t
    during labor, 2322, 2322t
  postoperative, 2720, 2737–2743, 2737t
    after orthopedic surgery, 2422–2423
    benefits of, 2742
    continuous infusion for, 2738–2743, 2738t, 2739t, 2741t
    risks of, 2742–2743
    side effects of, 2739–2741
    single-dose opioids for, 2737, 2737t, 2738t
  pruritus with, 2740
  pulmonary function and, 2742
  respiratory depression with, 1472–1474, 1473t, 1474t, 2740
  risks of, 2742–2743
  side effects of, 2739–2741
  single-dose, 2737, 2737t, 2738t
    side effects of, 2739–2741
  urinary retention with, 2740–2741
Epidural anesthesia, 1670–1673. *See also* Neuraxial anesthesia.
  ambulatory, 2608
  anesthetics for, 588–589, 588t, 589t
  anticoagulant use and, 1677
  arterial blood pressure with, 1660
  aspirin use and, 1676
  benzodiazepine use and, 1678
  bicarbonate with, 1675
  BIS index and, 1255
  bupivacaine for, 1674t, 1675
  carbonation for, 1675
  2-chloroprocaine for, 1674–1675, 1674t
  clinical outcomes and, 1678
  complications of, 1675–1677
  drugs for, 1674–1675, 1674t
  dural puncture with, 2326, 2328
  epinephrine-containing test dose for, 1677–1678
  epinephrine with, 1675
  equipment for, 1670–1671, 1671f–1672f
  etidocaine for, 1674t, 1675
  hanging-drop technique of, 1673
  height of, 1677
  heparin and, 2426
  in cesarean section, 2324–2325
  in elderly patient, 2439
  in obstetric patient, 1677–1678
  intravascular injection of, 1675–1676
  levobupivacaine for, 1674t, 1675
  lidocaine for, 1674t, 1675
  loss-of-resistance technique of, 1673
  low molecular weight heparin use and, 1677
  lumbar approach to, 1672–1673, 1673f
  mepivacaine for, 1674t, 1675
  needle insertion for, 1672–1673, 1673f
  neurologic injury with, 1676–1677
  patient position for, 1671–1672, 1672f

Epidural anesthesia *(Continued)*
  pediatric, 1734–1737, 1735f, 1736t
    anatomy for, 1734
    anesthetic dosage for, 1735, 1736t
    complications of, 1736–1737
    contraindications to, 1735
    equipment for, 1729t
    indications for, 1735
    lumbar, 1735, 1735f
    sacral, 1735–1736
    techniques of, 1735–1736, 1735f, 1736t
    thoracic, 1736
  physiologic effects of, 1660–1661
  ropivacaine for, 1674t, 1675
  seizures with, 1676
  soak time for, 1677
  spinal anesthesia with, 1678, 1678t
  subarachnoid injection of, 1676
  thoracic approach to, 1672–1673, 1673f
Epidural blood patch, 1669–1670, 2328
Epidural space, 1656, 1656f
  drug spread in, 1656–1657
  septa in, 1656–1657
Epidural steroid injections, in chronic pain, 2773–2774
Epiglottitis, 2544
  in children, 2852
Epilepsy. *See* Seizures.
Epinephrine, 1124
  aerosol, 2816, 2817t
  arrhythmias with, 203, 649
  cerebral blood flow and, 819, 819t
  drug interactions with, 648–649
  during labor, 2321, 2321t
  effects of, 625t, 626–627, 626t, 627t
  endotracheal administration of, 647
  epidural anesthesia with, 1675
  in anaphylactic reaction, 514
  in cardiac arrest, 2937–2938
  in hepatic blood flow, 747
  in hip replacement–related hypotension, 2415
  in malignant hyperthermia, 1180
  in neonatal resuscitation, 2361t
  in pediatric cardiac arrest, 2837, 2837t
  in pediatric left ventricular dysfunction, 2032
  in pediatric life support, 2947t
  in pediatric regional anesthesia, 1725, 1728
  in pediatric right ventricular dysfunction, 2032
  in pediatric supraventricular bradyarrhythmia, 2942, 2943f
  in renal regulation, 791–792, 791f
  in sepsis, 2897, 2900
  in vivo kinetics of, 664
  inhalation of, 648
  inhaled anesthetic effects on, 112–113
  intraosseous administration of, 647
  intravenous, 514, 646–649, 648t
  local anesthetics with, 585, 591
  metabolism of, 635f
  mucosal application of, 648
  ocular preparations of, 2536
  plasma, 663
  pulmonary vascular resistance and, 688, 688t
  reversal of, 648
  spinal anesthesia with, 1667
  structure of, 647f
  subcutaneous administration of, 648
  synthesis of, 630f
Epistaxis, endotracheal intubation and, 1649
Epoprostenol, pulmonary vascular resistance and, 686
Equal pressure point, in pulmonary function testing, 1004, 1005f
Erhlich, Paul, 85
Errors. *See also* Safety.
  anesthesia machine, 283, 307–310, 308t, 309f, 310f, 315–316
  anesthesiologist, 3028, 3029, 3029t, 3044–3045, 3046
  in capnography, 1457–1458, 1462
  in central venous pressure monitoring, 1295–1296
  in flow meter assembly, 280
  in laboratory test orders, 971–972
  in measurement, 1192t, 1193
  in pulmonary artery wedge pressure, 1307
  in pulse oximetry, 1450–1453, 1451t
  in thermodilution monitoring, 1329–1330, 1330t
  operating room, 3047–3048, 3047f–3049f
  statistical, 883–884, 885
Erythromycin
  hepatotoxicity of, 2221t
  opioid interaction with, 424

Erythropoiesis, hepatic, 749–750
Erythropoiesis-stimulating factor, 2180
Erythropoietin, 1112, 1114t
  in critically ill patient, 2803–2804
  in kidney failure, 2182
  recombinant, 1826
Erythroxylon coca, 20f, 22–23
Escherichia coli O157 infection, in children, 2859–2860
Escherichia coli O157.H2, in biological warfare, 2518t
Eschmann introducer, for endotracheal intubation, 1632
Esmarch, Johann F., 25
Esmarch bandage, 2412t
Esmolol, 653, 657
  BIS index and, 1255
  butyrylcholinesterase interaction with, 488
  cerebral blood flow and, 819
  in endotracheal intubation, 1647–1648
  in neurosurgery, 2145
  pharmacology of, 653–655, 654t
Esophageal varices, 761, 1053
Esophagectomy, robotic, 2567
Esophagogastroscopy, 756
Esophagus
  atresia of, 2355
  Doppler ultrasonography of, for cardiac output monitoring, 1335–1336
  intubation of, 1648
    capnography in, 1461
  stethoscope for, 1267
  varices of, 761, 1053
Estrogen, 1125
Ethanol. *See* Alcohol use.
Ether, 11, 11f, 13–16
Ethics
  conflicts of interest and, 3190–3191
  consultation on, 3192
  end-of-life care and, 3182–3189, 3187t. *See also* End-of-life care.
  health insurance and, 3191–3192
  in aid in dying, 3187–3188, 3188t
  in organ procurement, 3189
  informed consent and, 3176–3179. *See also* Informed consent.
  research, 3189–3190
Ethyl violet, for carbon dioxide absorption indicator, 296–297, 297f
Ethylene, 17
  oil-gas partition coefficient of, 115t
Ethylene glycol poisoning, 1611
Ethyleneglycoltetraacetic acid, 597
Etidocaine
  cardiovascular toxicity of, 594–595, 594t
  differential sensory/motor blockade with, 584
  duration of action of, 584
  in epidural anesthesia, 588–589, 588t, 1674t, 1675
  in nerve block, 587–588, 587t, 588t
  infiltration of, 586–587, 586t
  intravenous, 587
  potency of, 576t
  tissue distribution of, 592, 592t
  ventricular arrhythmias with, 594–595
Etomidate, 29, 350–355
  adrenal effects of, 1041
  cardiovascular system effects of, 323t, 353
  central nervous system effects of, 352–353
  cerebral blood flow and, 821f, 822
  cerebral metabolic rate and, 821f, 822
  cerebrospinal fluid dynamics and, 832, 832t
  dosing for, 351, 351t
  electroencephalographic effects of, 352, 1517–1518
  endocrine effects of, 353–354, 354f
  epileptogenic properties of, 833
  hepatic metabolism of, 2213
  historical perspective on, 350–351
  in ambulatory anesthesia, 2602t, 2603
  in cardiovascular surgery, 353, 355
  in heart disease patient, 353, 355
  induction with, 351, 351t, 355
  injection pain with, 354–355
  intraocular pressure effects of, 2532
  maintenance with, 351, 351t
  manual infusion of, 462
  metabolism of, 351
  myoclonus with, 355
  nausea and vomiting with, 354
  neuroprotection with, 840
  opioids with, 422
  pharmacokinetics of, 319t, 351–352, 352f

Etomidate (Continued)
  pharmacology of, 352–355
  physicochemical characteristics of, 351
  plasma concentration ranges for, 453t
  propylene glycol carrier for, 355
  respiratory system effects of, 353
  sedation with, 355
  seizures and, 833
  somatosensory evoked potential effects of, 1533t, 1536, 1536f
  structure of, 351, 351f
  thrombophlebitis with, 354
  visual evoked potential effects of, 1533t
Etorphine, 380t
Euthanasia, voluntary, 3187–3188, 3188t
Evaporation, heat loss with, 1576
Evidence-based medicine, 889, 2789–2790, 2790f, 2790t
  for acute lung injury, 2790–2791, 2792f–2793f
  for acute respiratory distress syndrome, 2790–2791, 2792f–2793f
  for cerebral injury prevention, 2800, 2803
  for glycemic control, 2799–2800, 2801f–2802f
  for nosocomial infection, 2796–2798, 2797t
  for pain control, 2798–2799, 2799t
  for sedation, 2798–2799, 2799t
  for sepsis, 2794–2796
  for transfusion, 2803–2804
  for venous catheter infection, 2797–2798, 2798t
  for ventilator-associated pneumonia, 2796–2797, 2797t
  for ventilator weaning, 2791, 2793–2794, 2794f
Evoked responses. See Peripheral nerve stimulation.
Exchange transfusion, in sickle cell anemia, 1113
Excitation-contraction coupling, in muscle, 1170–1174, 1171f, 1172f
Exercise, malignant hyperthermia with, 1182–1183
Exercise testing
  before peripheral vascular surgery, 2059
  in coronary artery disease evaluation, 1064, 1066, 1066t
  in pulmonectomy patient, 1013–1014
Expiratory reserve volume, 694, 694f
External beam radiotherapy, 2657–2658
External cephalic version, 2338
Extracellular fluid, 1764, 1764t
Extracorporeal life support, in trauma, 2488
Extracorporeal membrane oxygenation, in children, 2033, 2851
Extracorporeal shock wave lithotripsy, 2195–2197, 2196t, 2609, 2617–2619
  anesthesia for, 2196–2197
  biomechanical effects of, 2195–2196
  cardiac injury with, 2196
  contraindications to, 2197
  lung injury with, 2196
  physiologic changes with, 2196, 2196t
Extraction ratio, 72–73, 73f, 74f
Extraocular muscles
  examination of, 2996, 2997t
  innervation of, 860–861
  succinylcholine effects on, 869
Extubation, 1649–1650
  in trauma, 2483, 2483t
Eye(s), 2991–2995. See also Eye surgery; Vision.
  blood supply to, 2992–2994, 2993f, 2994f
  choroid of, 2995, 2995f
  drops for, 2531, 2536–2537
  drugs for, 1125, 1126t
  examination of, 2996–2997, 2997t
  glaucoma of, 1125, 1126t
  laser injury to, 2580, 3154
  optic nerve of, 2992, 2994–2995
  oxygen toxicity to, 2678
  position-related injury to, 1155, 1157–1158, 1158f
  protection of, 2580
  retina of, 2992, 2992f, 2995, 2995f
  trauma to, 2530
Eye surgery, 2527–2537
  complications of, 2536
  drug effects during, 2536–2537
  in children, 2534
  in congenital syndromes, 2536
  in ocular trauma, 2533–2534
  in strabismus, 2535–2536
  intraocular pressure during, 2531–2533
  intravitreal gas injection in, 2533
  pain after, 2537
  regional anesthesia in, 2527–2531
    blocks for, 2528–2531
    brainstem anesthesia with, 2530–2531

Eye surgery (Continued)
  regional anesthesia in (Continued)
    care after, 2528
    diplopia with, 2531
    intra-arterial injection of, 2531
    monitoring of, 2528
    ocular trauma with, 2530
    oculocardiac reflex with, 2529–2530
    peribulbar block for, 2529
    preoperative preparation for, 2527–2528
    ptosis and, 2531
    retrobulbar hemorrhage with, 2530
    shivering with, 2530
    sub-Tenon block for, 2529
  robotic, 2568–2569
  topical anesthesia in, 2531
Eyedrops
  acetylcholine, 2537
  anesthetic, 2531
  cocaine, 2537
  cyclopentolate, 2537
  echothiophate, 2536–2537
  epinephrine, 2535
  phenylephrine, 2536
  scopolamine, 2537
  timolol, 2536
Ez-PAP, for bronchial hygiene, 2819

F

F-wave, inhaled anesthetic effects on, 109
Fabius GS anesthesia machine, 302–303
Face
  fractures of, 2541–2542, 2541f
  trauma to, airway management in, 2459
Facet blocks, in chronic back pain, 2774
Facial nerve
  decompression of
    brainstem auditory evoked potentials in, 1530–1531
    electromyography in, 1538
  intraoperative monitoring of, 1537–1538, 1538f
  preservation of, 2548
Facioscapulohumeral muscular dystrophy, 535t, 536, 536f
Factor V, transfusion-related decrease in, 1809
Factor VII, recombinant, 1811
Factor VIIa, recombinant, 1838–1839
Factor VIII
  deficiency of, 2867–2868
  transfusion-related decrease in, 1809
Factor IX, 1824
Fail-safe valves, of anesthesia machines, 275, 277, 277f
Falconer, Jr., Albert, 42
False vocal cords, 1618
Famotidine, preoperative, 1860
Fascia iliaca compartment block, in children, 1745
Fasciculations, succinylcholine-induced, 874
Fasciitis, perinephritic, 2200
Fast-flush test, in arterial blood pressure monitoring, 1277–1278
Fast-track ambulatory (outpatient) anesthesia, 2613–2614, 2613t, 2614t, 2615t
Fasting, 2888–2892, 2889f–2891f, 2891t, 2892f
  by children, 2381, 2381t
  for outpatient procedures, 2600–2601
Fat, inhaled anesthetic uptake by, 134
Fat-blood coefficient, of inhaled anesthetics, 132t, 133
Fat embolism
  orthopedic surgery and, 2425
  orthopedic trauma and, 2478
Fatigue, 3162. See also Sleep deprivation.
  countermeasures for, 3060–3063
Fatty acids, metabolism of, 748
  in sepsis, 2903, 2903t
Fearfulness, in children, 2380–2381
Federal Aviation Administration, Age 60 Rule of, 3062–3063
Fell-O-Dwyer apparatus, 35
Femoral artery, cannulation of, 1274. See also Arterial blood pressure.
Femoral nerve
  anatomy of, 1743
  in orthopedic surgery, 2411–2412, 2412t
  position-related injury to, 1155, 1156t

Femoral nerve block, 1697–1699, 1698f, Plates 12 and 20
  in outpatient procedures, 2609
  pediatric, 1743, 1744–1745, 1744f
Femoral vein
  cannulation of, 1292–1293. See also Central venous pressure monitoring.
  catheterization of, in hemorrhagic shock, 2466
Femur
  fracture of
    fat embolism and, 2425
    patient positioning for, 1163, 1163f
  neck of, fracture of, 2417
Fenoldopam
  for renal protection, 799
  in infrarenal aortic reconstruction, 2076
  in kidney transplantation, 2242
  intravenous administration of, 649–650
  renal effects of, 799, 804
Fentanyl, 380t. See also Intravenous anesthetics.
  abuse of, 3166. See also Substance abuse.
  age-related pharmacokinetics of, 2439, 2439t
  allergic reactions to, 397
  arterial concentration of, 84, 84f
  BIS index and, 1255–1256
  bolus dose calculations for, 450–451, 454f
  C_{50} of, 446–448, 447t
  cardiovascular effects of, 394
  cerebral blood flow and, 389, 821f, 823
  cerebral metabolic rate and, 821f, 823
  cerebrospinal fluid dynamics and, 832, 832t
  context-sensitive decrement time of, 455–456, 456f
  context-sensitive half-time of, 404, 404f
  cyclosporine interaction with, 2273
  depth of anesthesia and, 1245, 1245t, 1246–1247, 1246f, 1247f
  during labor, 2317–2318, 2321, 2321t
  during pregnancy, 399
  electroencephalographic effects of, 388–389, 388f, 389f, 1518
  endocrinologic effects of, 396–397
  epileptogenic properties of, 833
  for children, 2376–2377, 2377f
  for continuous epidural analgesia, 2321, 2321t
  for patient-controlled intravenous analgesia, 2733–2734, 2733t
  hepatic effects of, 398
  hepatic metabolism of, 2213
  high-dose, 414, 414f
  in anesthetic induction, 411
  in asthma, 392
  in awake intubation, 1641
  in balanced anesthesia, 411
  in endotracheal intubation, 1647
  in hemorrhagic shock, 409, 409f
  in kidney transplantation, 2241
  in oocyte retrieval, 399
  in outpatient anesthesia, 2606, 2606f
  in pediatric cardiac surgery, 2021
  in pediatric regional anesthesia, 1725, 1725t
  in pediatric respiratory failure, 2849
  in renal failure, 2183, 2184t
  in single-agent anesthesia, 414, 414f
  in thoracic surgery, 1867, 1868
  in total intravenous anesthesia, 413, 413t
  in trauma, 2484
  infusion rate of, 459t
  intracranial pressure effects of, 390
  intranasal, 417
  isoflurane interaction with, 96, 97f, 387–388, 388f, 449, 450f
  manual infusion of, 460–461, 460t
  memory effects of, 1238
  myocardial ischemia and, 395
  neuroexcitation with, 391
  neuroprotective effects of, 390
  peak effect of, 404, 405f
  pharmacokinetics of, 401t, 402
    acid-base changes and, 409
    age and, 406, 406f
    cardiopulmonary bypass and, 409
    hydraulic model of, 82, 82f
    renal failure and, 407–408
    target-controlled infusion and, 466–468, 468t, 470f
  plasma concentration ranges for, 453t
  postoperative, 2737, 2737t, 2738t
  propofol interaction with, 413, 422, 449, 449f, 457, 458f
  respiratory effects of, 392–393

Fentanyl (Continued)
  seizures and, 833
  single-bolus, 410
  somatosensory evoked potential effects of, 1536–1537
  structure of, 381f
  target-controlled infusion and, 466–468, 468t, 470f
  terrorist use of, 2516
  thermoregulatory response thresholds with, 1575
  transdermal, 415–416, 416f
  transmucosal, 416
  volume of distribution of, 454t
Ferromagnetic objects, magnetic resonance imaging and, 2644
Ferrous sulfate, hepatotoxicity of, 2221t
Fetal heart rate, 2313–2314
  maternal trauma and, 2337–2338
Fetus, 2311–2312, 2311f, 2312f. See also Neonate; Pregnancy.
  acetylcholine receptor of, 871
  cardiovascular system of, 2006–2008, 2007f, 2833
  circulation of, 2347, 2347f
  evaluation of, 2313–2314
  external cephalic version of, 2338
  heart rate of, 2313–2314, 2337–2338
  hemoglobin of, 2843
  informed consent for, 3182
  intestine of, 2863
  intrauterine resuscitation of, 2314
  liver of, 2863
  lungs of, 2346–2347, 2347f
  respiratory system of, 2840, 2841–2842, 2841t
  surgery on, 2338
  trauma to, 2873
FEV$_1$. See Forced expiratory volume in 1 second.
Fever, 1589–1590, 1589f
  blood transfusion and, 1817
Fibrin glue, 1838
Fibrinogen
  deficiency of, 1117
  in sepsis, 2902, 2902f
Fibrinolysis, 1983–1984
  after transurethral resection of prostate, 2193
  secondary, 1809–1810
Fibromyalgia, vs. myofascial pain, 2772
Fibula, autograft from, 2420, 2420f
Fick principle, 702–703, 728–729, 728f, 2313
  in cardiac output measurement, 1331
  renal clearance and, 784–785
Fight or flight response, 617
Filtration fraction, glomerular, 786
Fingers, operating table injury to, 1159, 1159f
Fire
  airway, 2580–2584, 2580f, 2582f
  hyperbaric oxygen therapy and, 2680, 2684–2685
  laser surgery and, 2543
Fischer, Emil, 29
Fistula
  bronchopleural, 1900, 1902, 1925–1926
  tracheoesophageal, 2355, 2396
Fixation reflex, 2996, 2997t
FKBP12, ryanodine receptor interaction with, 1174
Flagg, Paluel J., 17
Flecainide, in atrial fibrillation, 1402, 1402t, 1403t
Flip-flop effect, in pediatric regional anesthesia, 1722
Flourens, Maire Jean, 16
Flow, 1202–1205
  principles of, 1202–1203, 1202t, 1203f
Flow limited drugs, 72
Flow meter, 1221–1222, 1463. See also Pulmonary function testing; Spirometry.
Flow meter assembly, 277–281, 278f, 1463
  ambiguous scales in, 280–281
  annular space and, 278, 279f
  components of, 278–280, 278f
  constant-pressure, 278
  electronic, 281
  float stops of, 279
  flow tubes of, 278f, 279
  inaccuracy errors in, 280
  indicator floats of, 279
  leaks in, 280, 280f, 281f
  physical principles of, 278
  safety features of, 279, 280
  scale of, 279–281
  variable orifice and, 278
Flow test, 310
Flow-volume relationships, in pulmonary function testing, 1003–1004, 1003f, 1004f, 1007–1009, 1008f, 1009f

Floxuridine, hepatotoxicity of, 2221t
Fluid therapy, 1783–1795, 1784t
  balanced salt solutions in, 1785
  body temperature changes with, 1585
  coagulation and, 1786–1787
  colloids in, 1786–1788
  compensatory, 1788–1789
  composition of, 1784t
  crystalloids in, 1785, 1786–1787
  during liposuction, 1794–1795
  five percent albumin in, 1787
  five percent dextrose in, 1786
  hetastarch in, 1784t, 1787
  historical studies on, 20–22
  hyperbaric oxygen therapy and, 2680–2681
  hypertonic salt solutions in, 1785–1786
  in adult respiratory distress syndrome, 1793
  in burn patient, 1793–1794
  in cerebral edema, 1792–1793
  in decompression sickness, 2672
  in diabetes insipidus, 2159
  in diabetic ketoacidosis, 1780
  in fluid deficits, 1789
  in fluid losses, 1789–1795, 1790t
  in gas embolism, 2672
  in head injury, 2155
  in heart failure, 1792
  in hemorrhagic shock, 2460–2466, 2461t, 2462f, 2462t, 2463t, 2464f, 2467–2469, 2467t, 2468f
  in intracranial aneurysm, 2147
  in ketoacidosis, 1023
  in liver failure, 1791–1792
  in neonate, 2358–2359, 2358t, 2359t, 2360f, 2388t, 2389
  in neurosurgery, 2143–2144
  in organ donation, 2233
  in pancreas transplantation, 2245
  in pediatric diabetic ketoacidosis, 2862
  in pediatric ICP increase, 2857
  in pediatric patient, 1790, 2388–2389, 2388t
  in pediatric shock, 2835–2836, 2835f
  in postoperative bowel obstruction, 1790–1791
  in postoperative shock, 2716–2717
  in preeclampsia, 1794
  in renal failure, 1793
  in sepsis, 2480
  in shock, 1784–1785, 2716–2717, 2835–2836, 2835f
  in spinal cord injury, 2475
  in third-space losses, 1789–1790
  intraoperative, 1788
  ischemic optic neuropathy and, 3009
  maintenance, 1788, 1788t
  normal saline in, 1785
  pentastarch in, 1787
  perfluorochemical emulsions in, 1787–1788
  preoperative
    for children, 2381, 2381t
    for outpatient, 2600–2601, 2601f
  renal effects of, 1487
  routine, 1788, 1788t
  six percent Dextran 70 in, 1787
  stroma-free hemoglobin in, 1787–1788
  twenty-five percent albumin in, 1787
Flumazenil, 343–345
  cerebral blood flow and, 824
  cerebral metabolic rate and, 824
  contraindications to, 345
  diagnostic use of, 344, 345t
  dosing for, 344, 345, 345t
  for benzodiazepine reversal, 344–345, 345t
  in outpatient anesthesia, 2607
  metabolism of, 343–344
  pharmacokinetics of, 319t, 344
  pharmacology of, 344
  physicochemical characteristics of, 343
  receptor binding of, 337f
  respiratory effects of, 344
  side effects of, 345
  structure of, 335, 335f
Flunisolide, 2817t
Fluorescein angiography, in ischemic optic neuropathy, 2997, 3000f
Fluoride, renal effects of, 1489–1490
Fluorouracil, 1118
Fluosol-DA, 1826
Flurothyl, convulsions with, 116
Fluroxene
  oil-gas partition coefficient of, 115t
  structure of, 106f

Fluticasone, 2817t
Fogarty catheter, in one-lung ventilation, 1887–1888, 1887f
Folate, serum, parenteral nutrition and, 2911
Fontana, Felix, 30
Foods
  drug interactions with, 101
  monoamine oxidase inhibitors interaction with, 658
Foot, surgery on, 2421–2422
Foramen, intervertebral, 1656
Foramen ovale, right-to-left shunt across, 689, 713, 1903
Force
  electromotive, 1208–1209
  electrostatic, 1208, 1208f
  unit of, 1192
Forced-air cooling, 1587
Forced air heating, 1586–1587, 1587f
Forced expiration technique, preoperative, 1859–1860
Forced expiratory flow between 200 and 1200 mL of FVC, 1000f, 1001
Forced expiratory volume in 1 second, 1000–1001, 1000t, 1001t
  clinical significance of, 1012, 1013
  in pulmonectomy patient, 1013, 1852–1854, 1853t
Forced midexpiratory flow, 1001, 1007, 1007f
Forced vital capacity, 1000–1001, 1000f, 1001t, 1007, 1007f, 1008f
Forearm, surgery on, 2421
Foreign body, airway, 2545
  in children, 2853–2854
Formoterol, 2817t
Forssman, Werner, 7
Fourier series, 1194, 1196f
Fracture
  fat embolism and, 2425
  femoral, 1163, 1163f
  femoral neck, 2417
  Le Fort, 2541f, 2542
  mandibular, 2459, 2541
  maxillary, 2459, 2541f, 2542
  osteoporotic, 1051
  pelvic, 2476–2477
  rib, 2480–2481
Francisella tularensis infection, 2518t
Frank-Starling relationship, 725f, 726–727, 727f, 733–734
Fraser, T. R., 9
Free radicals, in cerebral ischemia, 835f, 836
Free water clearance, 789, 1102, 1499
Free water deficit, 1614
Freeman, Walter, 32
Fresh frozen plasma, 1809, 1823–1824
  for children, 2390
  indications for, 1824
Freud, Sigmund, 22, 23
Functional residual capacity, 693–694, 693f, 694f
  during pregnancy, 2310
  hypoxemia and, 708–712, 709f, 710f
  inhaled anesthetic effect on, 161, 174–177, 174f, 175f
  patient positioning and, 708, 711
Furosemide
  in hyperparathyroidism, 1050
  in neurosurgery, 2134
  metabolic acidosis with, 1782
  neuromuscular blocking agent interaction with, 517
Futile therapy, 3186

G

G protein(s)
  halothane interaction with, 639
  in signal transduction, 637–639, 638f
  inhaled anesthetic effects on, 122–123
  muscarinic cholinergic receptor interaction with, 644
G protein-coupled receptors, in cardiac function, 735–737, 736f, 737f
Gabapentin
  in chronic pain, 2771
  opioid interactions with, 422–423
Gainesville patient simulators, 3080, 3081f
Galactorrhea, 1052

Galen, 4, 9
  vein of, aneurysm of, 2151f
Gallamine, 33, 493t, 495, 497f, 497t
  autonomic effects of, 511, 511t, 512t
  dosage for, 501t
  dysrhythmia and, 513
  elimination of, 506t, 509
  hepatobiliary disease and, 529–530, 529t
  in kidney transplantation, 2241
  renal failure and, 527, 528t
  tachycardia and, 512, 513
Ganglion (ganglia), 644–645, 645t, 662
Ganglionic agonists, 645, 662
Ganglionic antagonists, 645, 662
Ganglioplegia, 412
Garlic (ajo, Allium sativum), 607t, 609–610
Garments, circulating-water, 1586
Gas, intravitreal injection of, 2533
Gas embolism, 2672–2673. See also Air embolism.
  during laparoscopy, 2289–2290
  laser-induced, 2579–2580
Gas exchange, 697–703, 1438–1439, 1438–1444, 1438f
  alveolar gas tensions in, 697–698, 697f, 698f
  evaluation of, 1010–1011, 1010f
  monitoring of, 1439–1444
  oxygen transport in, 699–703, 699t, 700f–702f
  parenteral nutrition and, 2906–2907, 2907f
Gas tracer study
  in renal blood flow measurement, 790–791
  of closing capacity, 695–697, 696f, 697f
Gaskell, Walter H., 8
Gastric emptying
  during pregnancy, 2310–2311
  in kidney failure, 2238
  opioid effects on, 398
Gastric tonometry, for cardiac output monitoring, 1338
Gastric ulcers, in children, 2864
Gastroesophageal reflux disease, preoperative therapy in, 1860
Gastrointestinal tract
  carcinoid tumors of, 1108–1110
  disorders of, 1107–1110
    in children, 2863–2867
    5-hydroxytryptophan effects on, 1109
  in hemorrhagic shock, 2460
  maturation of, 2371
  opioid effects on, 398–399, 399f
  preoperative identification of, 1107–1108
Gastroparesis, in diabetes mellitus, 665, 1025, 1026f
Gastropathy, hypertensive, 761
Gastroschisis, 2395–2396, 2395t
Genetic polymorphism, 97
Genetic testing, informed consent for, 3180
Genioglossus muscle, inhaled anesthetic effects on, 173–174
Gentamicin, renal effects of, 803
Germander, hepatotoxicity of, 2222t
Giant bullous emphysema, 1916–1917
Gill, Richard C., 31–32
Gill's familial dysautonomia, 1044–1045
Ginkgo biloba, 607t, 610, 1095–1096
Ginseng (Panax ginseng, Panax quinquefolius), 607t, 610
Glanders, in biological warfare, 2518t, 2519
Glasgow Coma Scale, 2453–2454, 2454t
  in children, 2855, 2855t
  in head injury, 2152, 2152t
Glaucoma, 1125, 1126f, 2537
  acute, 3012–3014
  β-adrenergic receptor antagonists in, 656
  angle-closure, 3012
Glioma, 2145–2146
Glomerular filtration pressure, 779, 780f
Glomerular filtration rate, 778, 779, 780f, 1101–1102, 1487, 1488–1489, 2178–2179, 2180–2181
  after pediatric cardiopulmonary bypass, 2028t, 2029
  creatinine clearance for, 1489
  during pregnancy, 2311
  in children, 2859t
  in hepatic disease, 761
  inulin clearance for, 1489
  preoperative, 1493, 1493f
  radioisotopic markers for, 790
Glomerulus, 777–780, 779f, 780f. See also Glomerular filtration rate.
  filtration fraction of, 786

Glossopharyngeal nerve block, 1709
  in awake intubation, 1642
  in endotracheal intubation, 1647
Gloves, latex, 919, 1092, 1093, 3161–3162
Glucagon
  in hepatic blood flow, 747
  in sepsis, 2897
Glucocorticoids
  adrenal, 1036
    deficiency of, 1038–1039
    excess of, 1037–1038, 1037t
  before peripheral vascular surgery, 2063
  synthetic, 1036, 1036t, 1037
    calcium levels and, 1049
Gluconeogenesis, 748
Glucose, 1775–1781
  catecholamine effects on, 627
  cerebral ischemia and, 841–842
  in diabetes mellitus, 1021, 1022, 1022t, 1023–1024, 1024f
  in neonatal hyperglycemia, 2361
  in parenteral nutrition, 2892–2894, 2894t, 2908, 2912t
  in pediatric cardiopulmonary bypass, 2027–2028
  in pediatric cardiopulmonary resuscitation, 2946
  in pediatric head injury, 2857
  in pediatric hypoglycemia, 2862
  in sepsis, 2895–2897, 2895f, 2896f
  monitoring of, 1775–1776
  preoperative evaluation of, 969f
  renal tubule reabsorption of, 781
  requirement for, 2888–2890, 2889f
  urinary, 2180
Glucose-6-phosphate dehydrogenase deficiency, 1114
Glucose transporters, 2896
Glutamic oxaloacetate, serum, parenteral nutrition and, 2911
Glutamic pyruvate transaminase, serum, parenteral nutrition and, 2911
Glutamine, in sepsis, 2898
γ-Glutamyl-transpeptidase, 753t, 755
γ-Glutamyltransferase, 2215
Glutathione, 757–758
Glutathione peroxidase, 757
Glutathione S-transferase, 754, 757
α-Glutathione S-transferase, in renal function monitoring, 1500
Glycine
  inhaled anesthetic effects on, 113, 121, 122f
  toxicity of, transurethral resection of prostate and, 2192, 3013–3014
Glycogen phosphorylase, 748
Glycogen synthase, 748
Glycoprotein IIb/IIIa inhibitors, in cardiopulmonary bypass, 1985
Glycopyrrolate, 660t, 661, 661f
  in awake intubation, 1641
  in outpatient premedication, 2599
  with anticholinesterases, 523
  with electroconvulsive therapy, 2655
Goggles, 3154
Goiter, 1046–1047
Gold, hepatotoxicity of, 2221t
Goldan, S. Ormond, 26
Goldman Cardiac Risk Index, 908
Goldstein, A., 10
Gordh, Torsten, 24
Gormley, James F., 27
Gould, August A., 15f
Graft-versus-host disease, transfusion-associated, 1820
Granisetron, 2721
Granulocyte colony-stimulating factor, 1114t
Granulocyte-macrophage colony-stimulating factor, 1114t
Granulocytopenia, 1114, 1116
Grapefruit, cytochrome P450 3A4 interactions with, 101
Graves' disease, 1046–1047
Gravitational force, 1196
Gravity, space travel and, 2693–2694, 2694f
Gray E. Cecil, 32
Gregory, George, 43
Griffith, Harold, 32, 32f
Gross, Samuel, 22
Growth factors, 1114t–1115t
Growth hormone
  anabolic effects of, 2891
  deficiency of, 1052
  dexmedetomidine effects on, 356

Growth hormone (Continued)
  excess of, 1051–1052
  in brain death, 2960
  in sepsis, 2900
Guanabenz, 1121
Guanethidine, 658
Guanfacine, 1121
Guanosine monophosphate, cyclic (cGMP), inhaled anesthetic effects on, 113–114, 156
Guedel, Arthur, 39, 40, 43–44, 43f
Guidelines, 919–920
Guillain-Barré syndrome, 534, 1096
Guillotine, Joseph, 11
Gum elastic bougie, in difficult airway, 2458, 2458f
Guthrie, Samuel, 16
Gutierrez, A., 27
Gwathmey, James T., 17, 38f, 42

H

H₂ receptor antagonists, in outpatient premedication, 2599–2600, 2600t
Haldane, John S., 5
Haldane effect, 703
Hales, Stephen, 6, 7f
Hall, Alfred, 23
Haloperidol, 1123
Halothane, 18, 284–285, 284f
  airway receptor effects of, 173
  airway resistance and, 160, 160f
  albuterol with, 161
  aminophylline interaction with, 1124
  arrhythmias with, 203, 649
    in children, 2374
  arterial pressure and, 211–212, 212f, 213f
  bronchial effects of, 158, 159f
  calcium channel effects of, 194–195
  calcium effects of, 158, 159f, 167, 168f
  cardiac conduction and, 202–203
  central ventilatory effects of, 171, 172f
  cerebral blood flow and, 825–827, 826f
  cerebral metabolic rate and, 826f, 827–828
  cerebrospinal fluid dynamics and, 832, 832t
  choroidal blood flow and, 2995, 2995f
  congenital heart disease and, 2374
  coronary artery effects of, 203–211
    blood flow and, 210–211
    in vitro, 203
    in vivo, 203–204
    ischemia and, 205–206, 206f
    protective effects and, 206–210, 206f
    vasodilation and, 205
    vasodilator reserve and, 204–205, 204f
  coronary blood flow and, 210–211
  diaphragm effects of, 174–177, 174f–176f
  diastolic function and, 195–196, 195f, 196f
  electroencephalographic effects of, 1519t, 1520–1521
  ephedra interaction with, 609
  epinephrine interaction with, 1124
  fluoride-associated nephrotoxicity of, 251
  for children, 2372, 2372f, 2372t, 2373–2374, 2373f
  G protein interaction with, 639
  heart rate and, 201–202
  hepatic function and, 2209–2212, 2210f, 2211f
    in children, 2373–2374
  hepatotoxicity of, 18, 240–243, 242t, 243f, 244f, 245t, 759
    assays for, 247–248, 247t
    in children, 243, 2373–2374
    risk factors for, 246–247
  hippocampal effects of, 109, 110f
  hyperbaric oxygen therapy and, 2685, 2686–2687
  hypoxic pulmonary vasoconstriction and, 166, 167–168, 167f
  in ambulatory anesthesia, 2604–2605, 2604t
  in children, 161
  in pediatric cardiac surgery, 2020, 2020f
  in renal failure, 2184t
  in status asthmaticus, 159–160
  left atrial function and, 199–200
  left ventricular afterload and, 197–198, 198f
  left ventricular-arterial coupling and, 196–197
  metabolism of, 135, 237–238, 237f, 239f
  minimum alveolar concentration of, 107–109, 107f, 108t
    adenosine effects on, 113
    bronchodilation and, 156, 157, 157f

Halothane *(Continued)*
   minimum alveolar concentration of *(Continued)*
      clonidine effects on, 651
      dexmedetomidine effects on, 113, 113f
      hypernatremia and, 108
      hyponatremia and, 108
   mucociliary clearance and, 712
   myocardial contractility and, 191–194, 193f
   neuromuscular blockade and, 515–516
   occupational health risks of, 3151–3153
   oil-gas partition coefficient of, 115
   partition coefficients of, 132, 132t
   phrenic nerve effects of, 175, 176f
   pulmonary blood flow and, 169, 169f
   renal effects of, 800–801
   retinal blood flow and, 2995, 2995f
   serotonin with, 161
   somatosensory evoked potential effects of, 1533,
      1533t
   structure of, 106f
   surfactant effects of, 162, 164f
   synaptic effects of, 111–112, 112f
   thermoregulatory response thresholds with, 1575
   tubing uptake of, 142, 143t
   vasodilating effect of, 829
   visual evoked potential effects of, 1533t, 1535,
      1535f, 2535
Halsted, William, 23, 3164
Hamburger, Hartog J., 20
Hand
   operating table injury to, 1159, 1159f
   surgery on, 2421
Harcourt, Augustus Vernon, 33
Harger, John R., 27
Harris-Benedict equation, 2905
Harroun, Phyllis, 32
Harvard Standards, for monitoring, 1437–1438
Harvey, William, 28, 439
Hayward, George, 15f, 40, 41
Hazardous materials, 2500. *See also* Chemical and
      biological warfare agents.
Head and neck. *See also* Head injury.
   dermatomes of, Plate 2
   position of, in airway management, 1622–1623,
      1622f
   surgery on
      air embolism with, 2539
      arrhythmias with, 2539
Head and neck nerve block, 1704–1710
   accessory nerve, 1707–1708
   cervical plexus, 1706–1707, 1706f, 1707f, Plate 4
   glossopharyngeal nerve, 1709
   peribulbar, 1709
   retrobulbar, 1709
   stellate ganglion, 1709–1710, 1709f
   superior laryngeal nerve, 1708, 1708f
   translaryngeal, 1708–1709, 1709f
   trigeminal nerve, 1704–1706, 1705f, 1706f,
      Plates 1 and 2
Head injury, 2152–2159, 2479. *See also* Brain injury.
   anesthesia in, 2153–2155, 2154f
   blood pressure management in, 2154–2155, 2154t
   brain tissue Po_2 monitoring in, 2156
   cervical spine injury and, 2152–2153, 2153f
   corticosteroids in, 2133–2134
   fluid management in, 2143, 2155
   hyperventilation in, 2155
   hypothermia in, 841, 2144, 2156
   in children, 2856, 2857
   intracranial pressure monitoring in, 2156–2157
   intubation in, 2152, 2152t, 2153, 2153f
   jugular venous oxygen saturation in, 2155–2156
   succinylcholine-related hyperkalemia and, 490
Head tilt–chin maneuver, in basic life support, 2924
Headache
   dural puncture and, 2328
   pediatric epidural anesthesia and, 1736–1737
   spinal anesthesia and, 1669–1670, 1669t
Health care proxy, 3183
Health insurance, 3191–3192
Hearing loss, brainstem auditory evoked potentials
      for, 1530–1532
Heart. *See also at* Cardiac; Cardiovascular;
      Myocardial.
   acetylcholine effects on, 628
   action potential of, 730–731, 731f
   adrenergic receptor stimulation in, 639
   age-related changes in, 2436–2437, 2436f, 2436t
   barbiturate effects on, 333–334
   cardiomyocytes of, 729–735, 729f. *See also*
      Cardiomyocytes.

Heart *(Continued)*
   cellular anatomy of, 729, 729f
   cessation of, 2957. *See also* Brain death.
   contractility of, 726–727, 727f, 728–729, 728f
      inhaled anesthetics effects on, 191–194,
         192f–194f
      nitrous oxide effects on, 212–214
   cycle of, 723–724, 724f
   development of, 2369
   efficiency of, 727
   electrical events of, 723, 724f
   ephedra effect on, 607t, 608–609, 609t
   excitation-contraction coupling in, 731–732,
      732f
   force-frequency relationship in, 727–728
   halothane effects on, 203, 649
      in children, 2374
   herniation of, 1901–1902
   hormonal regulation of, 737–738, 737t
   hypothermia effect on, 1588
   in cholestasis, 764–765
   in hemorrhagic shock, 2460
   in hepatic disease, 762
   in malignant hyperthermia, 1179
   inhaled anesthetic effects on, 191–211. *See also at*
      specific cardiac parameters.
   inhaled anesthetic uptake by, 133–134, 133t
   ketamine effects on, 348
   local anesthetic effects on, 593–594
   magnesium effects on, 1773
   maximal velocity of contraction (Vmax) of, 727
   mechanical events of, 724
   neural regulation of, 735–737, 735f, 736f
   opioid effects on, 394–396, 395f
   organophosphate effects on, 2507
   output of, 728–729, 728f, 729f. *See also* Cardiac
      output.
   pediatric, 2832–2833
   pressure-volume loop of, 727, 727f
   reflex regulation of, 738–739, 738f
   rupture of, 2481
   stroke work of, 727
   transplantation of, 1964–1966, 1966t, 2253–2263,
      2262t. *See also* Heart transplantation.
   trauma to, 2481
   treppe phenomenon of, 727–728
   tumors in, 1967–1968
   ultrasonography of. *See* Transesophageal
      echocardiography.
   ventricles of, 724–728, 725f–727f. *See also* Left
      ventricle; Right ventricle.
   work of, 727
Heart block, 1083
   electrocardiography of, 1406–1409, 1406t,
      1407f–1410f
   pulmonary artery catheter-related, 1305
Heart failure
   β-adrenergic receptor antagonists in, 655
   β-adrenergic receptor downregulation in, 640
   after cardiopulmonary bypass, 1986–1991, 1987f,
      1988f, 1988t, 1989f, 1990f
   autonomic nervous system in, 633–634
   fluid therapy in, 1792
   in congenital heart disease, 2011–2012, 2012f
   neonatal, 2358
   right-sided, after thoracic surgery, 1903
   uremia and, 1101
Heart murmurs, 1078t
Heart rate, 727–728
   dexmedetomidine effects on, 357–358, 357f
   during pregnancy, 2308, 2308t
   fetal, 2313–2314
      maternal trauma and, 2337–2338
   in autonomic function assessment, 663t
   in heart transplantation, 2259
   in hyperthyroidism, 1046
   in neonatal asphyxia, 2348–2349
   in spinal transection, 666
   inhaled anesthetic effects on, 201–202
   intraoperative monitoring of, 1267–1268, 1268f
   neuraxial anesthesia effects on, 1658
   nitrous oxide effects on, 214, 215
   normal, 2834t
Heart transplantation, 1964–1966, 1966t,
      2253–2263, 2262t
   ABO typing in, 2255
   anesthesia after, 2262–2263
   anesthetics in, 2259
   anticoagulants in, 2259–2260
   antifibrinolytics in, 2259
   aspiration and, 2259

Heart transplantation *(Continued)*
   cardiopulmonary bypass in, 2255, 2258,
      2260–2261, 2260t. *See also*
      Cardiopulmonary bypass.
   care after, 2261–2262
   contraindications to, 2254–2255, 2255t
   heart rate in, 2259
   hemodynamic factors in, 2259
   inotropic medications in, 2259
   intraoperative management in, 2258–2260
   mediastinal bleeding after, 2262
   nitrous oxide after, 2261
   organ harvest for, 2233
   organ matching in, 2254–2255
   organ preservation for, 2234
   pediatric, 2037–2039, 2037f, 2038f
   recipient evaluation for, 2254–2255, 2255t, 2258
   recipient selection for, 2254, 2255t
   rejection of, 2261–2262
   renal function after, 2261
   right ventricular failure and, 2260–2261, 2260t
   technique of, 2255–2258, 2256f, 2257f
Heartmate mechanical circulatory support system,
      1992, 1992t
Heat, 1193. *See also* Hyperthermia; Hypothermia.
   latent, of vaporization, 285
   transfer of, 1576
Heat stroke, malignant hyperthermia with,
      1182–1183
Heidbrink, Jay Albion, 34
Heliox, 2539, 2815
   in decompression sickness, 2678
   in status asthmaticus, 2852
HELLP syndrome, 2331
Hematocrit
   cerebral blood flow and, 817–818
   in acute normovolemic hemodilution, 1834–1835,
      1835f
   in blood transfusion, 1799–1801
   in cardiopulmonary bypass, 1979–1980, 1979f,
      1980f
   in peripheral vascular surgery, 2066
   neuroprotection and, 842
   preoperative, 954, 969f
   retinal blood flow and, 2995
Hematoma
   carotid endarterectomy and, 2105
   central venous catheterization and, 1294
   postpartum, 2329
Hematuria, preoperative, 1493
Heme, hepatic production of, 749
Hemiblock, 1407, 1410, 1410f
Hemifacial spasm, facial nerve decompression for,
      1530–1531, 1538
Hemochromatosis, in children, 2869
Hemodialysis, 1102–1103, 1103t, 2188–2189
Hemodyne Hemostasis Analyzer, 1343
Hemofiltration, in pediatric hemolytic-uremic
      syndrome, 2860
Hemoglobin
   absorption spectra of, 1447
   acid-base balance and, 1605
   anesthetic binding sites of, 120
   artificial, pulse oximetry errors and, 1450,
      1451t
   concentration of, pulse oximetry errors and, 1450,
      1451t, 1452
   fetal, 2843
   in blood transfusion, 1799–1801
   in peripheral vascular surgery, 2066
   metabolism of, 750
   normal, 2834t
   oxygen saturation of, 1438, 1439, 1447–1453. *See
      also* Oximetry; Pulse oximetry.
   preoperative, 954, 955t, 969f
   pulse oximetry errors and, 1450, 1451t, 1452
   recombinant, 1826
   renal effects of, 805
   species of, 1447
   stroma-free, 1787–1788
Hemoglobin-based oxygen carriers, in hemorrhagic
      shock, 2466
Hemoglobin F, pulse oximetry errors and, 1450,
      1451t
Hemoglobin H, pulse oximetry errors and, 1450,
      1451t
Hemoglobin Köln, pulse oximetry errors and, 1450,
      1451t
Hemoglobin-oxygen dissociation curve, 699–701,
      700f, 1438
   blood transfusion and, 1806–1807, 1806f

Hemoglobin-oxygen dissociation curve (Continued)
  Pv̄o₂ and, 1453, 1453f
  vs. inspired Po₂ and, 1444, 1444f
Hemoglobin S, pulse oximetry errors and, 1450, 1451t
Hemoglobinemia, renal effects of, 805
Hemolysis, renal effects of, 805
Hemolytic transfusion reaction, 1815–1817, 1815t
  clinical manifestations of, 1815–1816, 1816f, 1816t
  delayed, 1817
  treatment of, 1816–1817, 1816t
Hemolytic-uremic syndrome, in children, 2859–2860
Hemophilia, 1116–1117, 1824
  in children, 2867–2868
Hemoptysis
  bronchoscopy in, 1923, 1924f
  endobronchial intubation in, 1889–1890, 1925
  in catheter-related pulmonary artery rupture, 1306–1307
  massive, 1923–1925, 1924f
Hemopure, 1826–1827
Hemorrhage
  after thoracic surgery, 1902
  dilutional thrombocytopenia and, 1807–1809, 1808f, 1808t, 1809f
  during mediastinoscopy, 1911
  in hepatic dysfunction, 2222
  ischemic optic neuropathy and, 3007, 3008–3009, 3010
  obstetric, 2333–2336, 2334f, 2335f
  postpartum, 2335–2336
  retrobulbar, 2530, 3010
  subarachnoid, 2146–2151, 2146t, 2147t
    transcranial Doppler ultrasonography after, 1541
  transfusion-related, 1807–1812, 1808f, 1808t, 1809f, 1811f, 1812f
  with endotracheal intubation, 1649
Hemorrhagic fever, 2518t
Hemorrhagic shock. See Shock, hemorrhagic.
Hemostasis, acute normovolemic hemodilution and, 1835
HemoSTATUS monitor, 1342–1343
Henderson-Hasselbalch equation, 1600, 2313
Henna, pulse oximetry errors and, 1451t, 1452
Henry, William, 12
Henry's law, 703
Heparin
  contraindications to, 1974
  electrochemical monitoring of, 1341
  epidural catheter risk and, 2422
  in cardiopulmonary bypass, 1972–1974, 1973f, 1974f, 1984
  in coronary angiography, 2649
  in interventional neuroradiology, 2648
  in orthopedic surgery, 2426
  in pediatric cardiac surgery, 2035
  measurement of, 1340–1341
  monitoring of, 1338–1341, 1339t
  physiologic effects of, 1973
  protamine reversal of, 1982
  spinal hematoma and, 2329
  thrombocytopenia with, 1116
  with epidural analgesia, 2742–2743
  with epidural anesthesia, 1677
Heparin management test, 1340
Heparinase, 1982
HepatAmine, 2916
Hepatectomy, for liver donation, 2235–2237, 2236f
Hepatic arterial buffer response, 2211
Hepatitis, 755
  acute, 2216
  chronic, 2217
  disopyramide and, 1125
  halothane, 18, 240–243, 242t, 243f, 244f, 245t, 759, 1111
    assays for, 247–248, 247t
    in children, 243, 2373–2374
    risk factors for, 246–247
  transfusion-related, 1818–1819, 1818t
  vaccines against, 1111
Hepatitis A, 755
Hepatitis B, 755
  in health care worker, 919, 3157–3158, 3158t
  transfusion-related, 1818–1819, 1818t
Hepatitis C, 755
  in health care worker, 919, 3158–3159
  transfusion-related, 1818–1819, 1818t
Hepatobiliary disease. See Liver, disease/injury of.
Hepatopulmonary syndrome, 2223, 2247–2248

Hepatorenal syndrome, 761, 2223
Herbal medicine, 605–612, 607t, 608t, 609t
Hereditary angioneurotic edema, 1093
Herniation
  cardiac, 1901–1902
  diaphragmatic, 2355–2356, 2396–2397
  intervertebral, 1095
Heroin, 380t, 382t, 417. See also Addiction.
Herrick, James B., 40
Hetastarch, 1039t, 1787, 1825–1826
Heteroreceptor, 636
Hewer, Christopher L., 18
Hewitt, Frederick, 37
Hexafluorodiethyl ether, synaptic effects of, 111–112, 112f
Hexafluoroisopropanol, 253
Hexamethonium, 662
HI-6, in organophosphate poisoning, 2508
Hiccups, etomidate-related, 355
Hickman, Henry Hill, 13
High altitude. See Altitude, high.
High-dose thrombin time, 1340
High-frequency jet ventilation
  in thoracic surgery, 1900–1901
  in tracheal resection, 1915
  monitoring of, 1468–1469, 1469f
High-frequency oscillatory ventilation
  in children, 2851
  monitoring of, 1468–1469
High-frequency positive-pressure ventilation
  for microlaryngoscopy, 2542
  in thoracic surgery, 1900–1901
  in tracheal resection, 1915
  monitoring of, 1468–1469
High-frequency ventilation
  in children, 2851
  in thoracic surgery, 1900–1901
  monitoring of, 1468–1469
High-pressure nervous syndrome, 2669
High reliability organization theory, 3050–3052, 3050f, 3051t
Hildebrandt, August, 26
Hill coefficient, 95
Hill equation, 95
Hip
  dislocation of, 2476
  replacement of, 2413–2417, 2414t
    blood loss during, 2413
    cement fixation in, 2413–2414
    deep venous thrombosis and, 2425–2426
    hypotension during, 2414–2417, 2414t, 2415f
    monitoring during, 2413, 2414t
    pain management after, 2417
    patient positioning for, 2413
    pulmonary artery catheter monitoring during, 2415–2417, 2416f
    robotic, 2568
Hippocampus, inhaled anesthetic effects on, 109, 110f
Hippocrates, 10
Hirschel, G., 23, 24f
Hirschsprung's disease, 2863
Histamine
  bronchial response to, 156
  in carcinoid tumor, 1109
  intracranial pressure and, 831
  neuromuscular blocker-induced release of, 511–512, 514
  opioid effects on, 395–396
  pulmonary vascular resistance and, 688, 688t
Hoarseness, 1623
Hofmann degradation, 74
Holmes, Oliver Wendell, 15
Holter monitoring, 1064t, 1065f, 1067, 1409–1410
Homer proteins, ryanodine receptor interaction with, 1174
Homocystinuria, ocular pathology in, 2536
Hook, Robert, 4
Horner's syndrome, 1590
Horsepower, 1193
Hughes, J., 10
Human immunodeficiency virus (HIV) infection
  hotline for, 3156
  in children, 2871, 2872–2873
  in health care worker, 919, 3155–3156
  postexposure prophylaxis for, 3156, 3156t
  testing for, 942, 956, 959
  transfusion-transmitted, 1818t, 1819
Human performance, 3021–3064. See also
    Anesthesiologist, performance of.

Human T-cell lymphotropic virus type 1, transfusion-transmitted, 1818t, 1819
Humidification, for bronchial hygiene, 2818, 2818t
Hunter, Charles, 19
Hustin, Albert, 21
Hydralazine
  in children, 2838
  in kidney failure, 2187
  in preeclampsia, 2331, 2332t
Hydration. See also Fluid therapy.
  before outpatient procedures, 2600–2601, 2601f
  preoperative, 1859
Hydrocephalus
  in children, 2856
  shunt for, 2162–2163
Hydrochloric acid, minimum alveolar concentration and, 109
Hydrochlorofluorocarbons, hepatotoxicity of, 245–246, 245f
Hydrocodone, structure of, 382t
Hydrocortisone, 1039
Hydrogen, 106f
Hydrogen cyanide, 2513, 2513t–2514t
Hydromorphone, 417
  for patient-controlled intravenous analgesia, 2733–2734, 2733t
  in outpatient anesthesia, 2606
  in trauma, 2484
  single-dose, 2737, 2737t, 2738t
  structure of, 382t
Hydrophobicity, of local anesthetics, 574, 579, 583
Hydrostatic pressure, 1219–1220
Hydroxocobalamin, in cyanide poisoning, 2514t
Hydroxyethyl starch (hetastarch), 1787, 1825–1826
  allergy to, 1093t
11β-Hydroxylase, etomidate effects on, 353–354, 354f
5-Hydroxytryptophan, 1108–1109
Hydroxyzine, in outpatient premedication, 2599
Hyomental distance, in airway management, 1621
Hyperaldosteronism, 1038
Hyperalgesia, opioid-induced, 397
Hyperalimentation. See Nutrition, parenteral.
Hyperbaric oxygen therapy
  anesthesia and, 2685–2687, 2686f, 2687f
  atmosphere control in, 2684
  barotrauma in, 2679
  battery use in, 2684
  blood gas assessment in, 2681–2684, 2682f, 2682t, 2683f
  carbon dioxide control in, 2684
  cardiovascular response to, 2669, 2670t
  chambers for, 2674–2675, 2674f, 2675f
  fire hazards in, 2684–2685
  fluid administration with, 2680–2681
  halothane anesthesia and, 2685, 2686–2687, 2686f, 2687f
  history of, 2665–2667, 2666f, 2666t
  in anemia, 2674
  in carbon monoxide poisoning, 2671–2672
  in children, 2673
  in Clostridium infection, 2673
  in cyanotic heart disease, 2673
  in decompression sickness, 2672
  in gas embolism, 2672
  in one-lung ventilation, 2673, 2674f
  intravenous anesthesia and, 2687
  mechanical ventilation in, 2682–2684, 2683f
  middle ear pressure equilibration in, 2679–2680
  nitrogen narcosis in, 2678–2679
  nitrous oxide anesthesia and, 2686, 2686f
  ocular toxicity of, 2678
  patient monitoring in, 2680
  pulmonary pressure equilibration in, 2680
  pulmonary toxicity with, 2677–2678
  regional anesthesia and, 2687
  safety of, 2685
  seizures with, 2678
  side effects of, 2676–2679, 2677f
  toxicity of, 2676–2678
  trace gases in, 2679, 2684
  treatment schedules for, 2675–2676, 2676f
Hyperbilirubinemia, 755, 2215
Hypercalcemia, 1771, 1771t
  hyperparathyroidism and, 1048–1050
  hypertension and, 1049
Hypercapnia, 714–715, 714f, 717–718, 717t
  arrhythmias and, 717
  carbon dioxide production and, 714f, 715
  cerebral blood flow and, 816–817, 816f
  cerebral ischemia and, 840–841

Hypercapnia (Continued)
    dead space ventilation and, 714, 714f
    electroencephalographic effects of, 1524
    hypoventilation and, 714, 714f
    in lung transplantation, 2268
    local anesthetics and, 593, 596
    with endotracheal intubation, 1647
Hyperglycemia, 1776. See also Diabetes mellitus.
    during carotid endarterectomy, 2103
    glomerular filtration rate in, 1488
    in cardiopulmonary bypass, 1981
    in critically ill patient, 2893
    in neonate, 2361
    in pediatric cardiopulmonary bypass, 2028
    in pediatric head injury, 2857
    in sepsis, 2799-2800
    infection and, 2800
Hyperkalemia, 1106-1107, 1769-1770, 1770t
    acute, 1770
    chronic, 1770
    hypercapnia and, 718
    in burn patient, 530
    in citrate intoxication, 1813
    in kidney failure, 2181t, 2182
    minimum alveolar concentration and, 108-109
    succinylcholine-induced, 489-490, 873
    treatment of, 1770
Hyperkalemic periodic paralysis, 538t, 543, 544t, 545
Hyperlipidemia, 1027-1028
Hyperlipoproteinemia, 1027-1028
Hypermagnesemia, 1772-1774
    in neonate, 2359
Hypernatremia, 1104-1105, 1767-1768, 1768t
    minimum alveolar concentration and, 108
Hypernephroma (renal cell carcinoma), 2198, 2198t,
        2199
Hyperoxia, 716-717, 2676-2678, 2677f
Hyperparathyroidism, 1048-1050
    neuromuscular blockade in, 517
Hyperphosphatemia, 1774, 1775t
    acid-base balance and, 1604, 1608
Hyperreninemia, 2238
Hypertension
    β-adrenergic receptor antagonists in, 655-656
    after carotid endarterectomy, 2105
    aortic cross-clamping and, 2072-2073, 2073t
    blood pressure reduction in, 842
    fenoldopam in, 649-650
    hypercalcemia and, 1049
    in anesthesia-related risk evaluation, 909, 910t
    in hyperaldosteronism, 1038
    in kidney failure, 2181t, 2182
    in kidney transplantation, 2241
    in neurosurgery, 2145
    in pheochromocytoma, 1044
    intraoperative blood pressure values in, 1058,
        1058f
    ischemic optic neuropathy and, 3010
    isoflurane-related, in children, 2374
    ketamine-induced, 348
    opioid effects on, 395
    pediatric, 2839-2840, 2839f, 2840t
    peripheral vascular surgery and, 2056
    portal, 760-763, 763f, 1110-1111. See also
        Cirrhosis.
      in end-stage liver disease, 2247
      pathogenesis of, 762
    postoperative, 2717, 2717f
    preoperative evaluation of, 1492-1493, 1492t,
        1495
    preoperative treatment of, 1053-1058, 1054t,
        1055f, 1056t, 1057t, 1058t
      β-blocking drugs in, 1057, 1057t
      coronary artery disease and, 1057-1058, 1058t
      criteria for, 1054-1055
      drug administration for, 1059-1060
      end-organ assessment and, 1059
      perioperative morbidity and, 1055-1057, 1056t,
        1058
      recommendations for, 1058-1059
      surgical timing and, 1054-1055
    pulmonary, 684, 1089-1090
      after pediatric cardiopulmonary bypass,
        2033-2034
      central venous pressure monitoring in, 1316
      diaphragmatic hernia and, 2356
      high-altitude, 687
      in lung cancer patient, 1854-1856, 1855f, 1855t
      left ventricular end-diastolic pressure in,
        1322-1323, 1322t
      nitric oxide therapy for, 2815

Hypertension (Continued)
    pulmonary vascular resistance in, 684
    with laryngoscopy, 1647
Hyperthermia
    cerebral metabolic rate and, 816
    during epidural analgesia, 1590
    intraoperative, 1589-1590, 1589f
    malignant, 538t, 539f, 1169-1186. See also
        Malignant hyperthermia.
    somatosensory evoked potential monitoring and,
        1537
Hyperthyroidism, 1046-1047
    adrenergic receptor function in, 640
Hypertonic saline, 1785-1786, 1826
    in hemorrhagic shock, 2463-2464
    in pediatric ICP increase, 2857
    in traumatic brain injury, 2472
Hyperventilation
    hypocapnia and, 718
    hypoxemia and, 708
    in neurosurgery, 2132-2133, 2133f
    in traumatic brain injury, 2155, 2470-2471
    metabolic acidosis with, 1783
    opioid prevention of, 392
    $PETCO_2$ and, 1461
Hypervolemia
    neonatal, 2348
    renal response to, 784
Hypoalbuminemia
    acid-base balance and, 1604, 1608, 1613
    hypocalcemia and, 1050-1051
Hypoaldosteronism, 1039
Hypocalcemia, 1050-1051, 1771-1772, 1772t
    after thyroid surgery, 2540
    hyperphosphatemia and, 1774
    in citrate intoxication, 1812
    in liver transplantation, 1813
    in neonate, 2359
Hypocapnia, 715, 718
    cerebral blood flow and, 816-817, 816f
    during carotid endarterectomy, 2103
    during neurosurgery, 2131-2133, 2133f
    electroencephalographic effects of, 1524
    in one-lung ventilation, 1893
    in transsphenoidal hypophysectomy, 2159
Hypogastric plexus block, in pelvic pain, 2201
Hypoglycemia, 1026-1027, 1781. See also Diabetes
        mellitus.
    in children, 2862
    in critically ill patient, 2800
    in neonate, 2359
    in parenteral nutrition, 2913
    in pediatric cardiopulmonary bypass, 2028
    in pediatric head injury, 2857
    postoperative, 2718
Hypokalemia, 1105-1106, 1769, 1769t
    in ketoacidosis, 1023
    neuromuscular blockade and, 523
Hypokalemic periodic paralysis, 538t, 544t, 545-546
Hypolipidemia, 1028
Hypomagnesemia, 1772, 1773, 1773t
    hypocalcemia and, 1050-1051, 1771-1772
    testing for, 959, 962, 962t
Hyponatremia, 1104-1105, 1765-1767, 1766t, 1767t
    after thoracolumbar surgery, 2419
    in post-TURP visual changes, 3014
    minimum alveolar concentration and, 108
    neurologic sequelae of, 1766
    transurethral resection of prostate and, 2192
    treatment of, 1766-1767
Hypoparathyroidism, 2540
    hyperphosphatemia in, 1774
    hypocalcemia and, 1050-1051
Hypophosphatemia, 1774-1775, 1775t
    total parenteral nutrition and, 1035
Hypotension
    after carotid endarterectomy, 2105
    aortic unclamping and, 2077
    arginine vasopressin response to, 794, 794f
    brain death and, 2962
    carcinoid tumor and, 1109
    cerebral ischemia and, 840
    during labor, 2326
    during pregnancy, 2312
    electroencephalographic effects of, 1524, 1524f
    epidural analgesia and, 2740
    hip replacement and, 2414-2417, 2414t, 2415f,
        2416f
    in cholestasis, 764-765
    in kidney transplantation, 2240-2242
    in pheochromocytoma, 1044

Hypotension (Continued)
    interscalene block and, 1688
    ischemic optic neuropathy and, 3008
    neuromuscular blocking agents and, 512, 513f
    nondepolarizing muscle relaxants and, 512
    postoperative, 2716-2717
    renal effects of, 802
    sitting position and, 2136
    somatosensory evoked potential monitoring
        and, 1537
    transesophageal echocardiography in, 1378,
        1378t
Hypothalamus
    in brain death, 2960
    in thermoregulation, 1572, 1572f
Hypothermia
    acid-base balance and, 1980-1981
    after cardiac arrest, 839
    cerebral metabolic rate and, 816, 816f
    electroencephalographic effects of, 1524
    in brain injury, 2156, 2473
    in cardiopulmonary bypass, 1977, 1977t,
        1978-1979
    in elderly patient, 2443
    in infant, 2371
    in intracranial aneurysm treatment, 2150-2151
    in neuroprotection, 841, 841t, 2087
    in neurosurgery, 2144
    in pediatric cardiopulmonary bypass, 2024, 2025,
        2026-2027, 2026f, 2027f
    in pediatric ICP increase, 2857
    in spinal cord protection, 2087
    in spinal transection, 666
    intraoperative
      benefits of, 1581
      complications of, 1581-1582, 1583t
      core temperature plateau and, 1577, 1578f
      inadvertent, 1576-1577, 1577f, 1578f
      induction of, 1587-1589, 1588f
      neuraxial anesthesia and, 1577-1581,
        1578f-1580f
      prevention of, 1583-1587, 1584f-1587f
      vasodilation and, 1576-1577, 1577f
    neuromuscular blockade and, 516, 523, 524
    postoperative, 1582, 1583t, 2718, 2721
    somatosensory evoked potential monitoring and,
        1537
    transurethral resection of prostate and, 2193
Hypothyroidism, 1047-1048
Hypoventilation
    hypercapnia and, 714, 714f
    hypoxia and, 687, 687f, 708
    in strabismus surgery, 2530
    metabolic acidosis with, 1783
    obesity and, 1031-1033
    pediatric, 2844
    postoperative, 2715, 2715f
Hypovolemia
    in kidney failure, 2181, 2181t
    neonatal, 2348, 2358-2359, 2358t, 2359f, 2359t
    pediatric, 2835, 2835t
    renal response to, 784
    sodium clearance in, 790
    succinylcholine-related hyperkalemia and, 489
    systolic pressure variation in, 1326-1327, 1326f
Hypoxemia, 707-714, 715-716, 2812, 2812t
    absorption atelectasis and, 711
    airway resistance increase and, 709-710, 710f
    arrhythmias and, 716
    cardiac output decrease and, 712, 712f
    cardiovascular response to, 715-716, 715t
    endotracheal intubation and, 1647
    endotracheal tube failure and, 708
    equipment failure and, 707-708
    expiratory muscle tone and, 709
    functional residual capacity decrease and,
        708-712, 709f, 710f
    hyperventilation and, 708
    hypoventilation and, 708
    immobility and, 710-711
    in adult respiratory distress syndrome, 713-714,
        713f
    in one-lung ventilation, 1891-1894, 1891f,
        1892f
    in pulmonary embolism, 713, 713f, 2713
    mucociliary flow decrease and, 711-712
    muscle tone and, 708-709
    obesity and, 1030, 1031-1032
    oxygen consumption increase and, 712
    paralysis and, 709, 712-713
    posthyperventilation, 2713, 2714f

Hypoxemia (Continued)
  postoperative, 2712–2715, 2713f, 2714f
    atelectasis and, 2713
    cardiac output and, 2714, 2714f
    iatrogenic, 2712
    pneumothorax and, 2713
    pulmonary edema and, 2713, 2713f
    pulmonary embolism and, 2713
    right-to-left pulmonary shunt and, 2713
    treatment of, 2714–2715, 2714f
  pulmonary vasoconstriction and, 712
  rapid shallow breathing and, 711
  right-to-left interatrial shunting and, 713
  right-to-left pulmonary shunt and, 701, 701f,
      2713
  supine position and, 708, 709f, 710–711, 710f
  ventilation pattern and, 711
Hypoxia, 715–716, 715t, 716t, 2811, 2812, 2812t.
    See also Hypoxemia.
  at high altitude, 2688–2689, 2688f, 2689f
  biphasic response to, 180
  diffusion
    nitrous oxide and, 150, 150f
    postoperative, 2713, 2714f
  during hip replacement, 2415, 2417
  electroencephalographic effects of, 1523–1524
  fetal, 2314, 2689, 2833
  hepatic injury with, 760
  hypothermia protection against, 1581
  in one-lung ventilation, 1891–1894, 1891f, 1892f
  local anesthetics and, 596
  maternal, 2689
  neonatal, 2842
  pulmonary vasoconstriction and, 166–168, 167f,
      168f, 686–687, 687f
    in one-lung ventilation, 1891–1893, 1891f,
        1892f
    inhaled anesthetics and, 166–170, 167f–169f,
        1864–1865, 1865f
  somatosensory evoked potential monitoring and,
      1537
  ventilatory response to, 179–181, 180f
Hysteresis, 84, 84f, 85f, 444
Hysteroscopy, in pacemaker patient, 1426

I

Ibsen, Bjørn, 35
Ibuprofen, postoperative, 2735t, 2736f
Ibutilide, in supraventricular tachyarrhythmias,
    2932–2933
Ikeda, S., 39
Ileus, postoperative, 624
Iliac artery, occlusive disease of, 2071–2072
Iliohypogastric nerve block, pediatric, 1749, 1749f
Ilioinguinal nerve block, pediatric, 1749, 1749f
Iloprost, pulmonary vascular resistance and, 686
Immobility, in elderly patient, 2443
Immune extravascular reaction, 1817
Immune system
  echinacea effects on, 606, 608
  hepatic, 750
  in brain death, 2960
  in hepatic injury, 759
  in trauma, 2488
  opioid effects on, 399–400
Immunization, 1104
Immunodeficiency disease, 1093
Immunoglobulin, intravenous, in Lambert-Eaton
    myasthenic syndrome, 540
Immunoglobulin A, selective deficiency of, 1093
Immunoglobulin E, in anaphylaxis, 1092
Immunoglobulin G, in hepatitis, 755
Immunomodulation, transfusion-associated,
    1820–1821, 1820t
Immunonutrition, 2908, 2910
Immunosuppressive drugs, 2271–2273, 2272t
  anesthesia interaction with, 2273
Implantable cardioverter-defibrillator, 1415–1416,
    1427–1431
  at remote locations, 2653
  code for, 1427, 1428t
  company phone numbers for, 1435
  indications for, 1428, 1429t
  intraoperative management of, 1429, 1431
  magnet application to, 1428–1429
  monopolar electrosurgery and, 1429, 1430f
  postanesthesia evaluation of, 1431
  preanesthesia evaluation of, 1429, 1430f

Implantable cardioverter-defibrillator (Continued)
  programming for, 1427–1428
  reprogramming for, 1429
  terminology for, 1431–1432
Implicit memory, depth of anesthesia and, 1239
Incentive spirometry
  for bronchial hygiene, 2818
  preoperative, 1085
Incidentaloma, 1038, 1041–1042
Indicator dilution technique, for cardiac output,
    729, 729f
Indigo carmine, pulse oximetry errors and, 1451t,
    1452
Indocyanine green, pulse oximetry errors and,
    1451t, 1452
Indocyanine green test, 753t, 756
Indomethacin, renal effects of, 803
Inductor, 1210, 1210f
Inert gas dilution, for lung volumes, 694
Infant. See also Children; Neonate.
  airway management in, 2382t, 2384–2388, 2385f,
      2386t, 2387f, 2388f
    endotracheal tube for, 2384, 2384t
    laryngoscope blades for, 2384, 2384t
  airway of, 2369–2370, 2370f
  anesthesia circuits for, 2393, 2394f
  anesthesia for, 2379–2398
    air embolism with, 2394
    complications of, 2394–2395
    induction of, 2375, 2382, 2383–2384
    prematurity and, 2397–2398, 2397f
    preoperative evaluation for, 2379–2380
    principals of, 2393–2395
    pulse oximetry with, 2394
  arterial catheter for, 2393
  asphyxiation of, 2347–2348, 2348f, 2875–2877
  at high altitude, 2689
  blood warmers for, 2391–2392
  body composition of, 2371, 2371f
  cardiac arrest in, 2392–2393
  central venous catheter for, 2393
  croup in, 2851–2852
  development of, 2367–2371, 2368f
    cardiovascular, 2368–2369
    gastrointestinal, 2371
    hepatic, 2370
    pulmonary, 2369–2370, 2369f, 2370f
    renal, 2370, 2370f
    thermoregulatory, 2371
  diaphragmatic hernia in, 2396–2397
  emergence delirium in, 2723
  equipment cart for, 2393
  fasting by, 2381, 2381t
  fluid requirements in, 2389
  fresh frozen plasma for, 2390, 2391f
  gastroschisis in, 2395–2396, 2395t
  Glasgow Coma Scale for, 2855, 2855t
  heat loss in, 2371
  hypothermia in, 2371
  infection in, 2870–2871, 2870t, 2872t–2873t
  intensive care unit for. See Pediatric intensive care
      unit.
  intravenous fluids for, 2388–2389, 2388t
  laryngotracheobronchitis in, 2851–2852
  maximal allowable blood loss from, 2389–2390
  mechanical ventilation in. See Mechanical
      ventilation, pediatric.
  meningomyelocele in, 2395
  monitoring for, 2392–2393
  omphalocele in, 2395–2396, 2395t
  packed red blood cells for, 2389–2390
  parents with, 2382, 2384, 2722
  pharmacodynamics/pharmacokinetics in,
      2371–2379, 2371f
    alfentanil and, 2377
    desflurane and, 2374–2375
    diazepam and, 2375–2376
    fentanyl and, 2376–2377, 2377f
    halothane and, 2373–2374, 2373t
    inhaled anesthetics and, 2372–2375, 2372f,
        2372t, 2373t
    isoflurane and, 2374
    meperidine and, 2376
    methohexital and, 2375
    midazolam and, 2376
    morphine and, 2376
    muscle relaxants and, 2378–2379, 2380t
    propofol and, 2375
    remifentanil and, 2377–2378, 2378f
    sevoflurane and, 2372–2373, 2373t
    succinylcholine and, 2378–2379

Infant (Continued)
  pharmacodynamics/pharmacokinetics in (Continued)
    sufentanil and, 2377
    thiopental and, 2375
  platelets for, 2390–2391
  postanesthesia apnea in, 2397–2398, 2397f,
      2723
  postintubation croup in, 2723
  premedication for, 2381
  preoperative evaluation of, 2379–2380
  pyloric stenosis in, 2395
  respiration in, 2369–2370, 2369f, 2370f
  retinopathy of prematurity in, 2534–2535
  stress response in, 2394–2395
  sudden death in, 2875–2876
  tracheoesophageal fistula anomaly in, 2396
  trauma to, 2873
  water loss from, 2389
  with stridor, 2387–2388, 2387f, 2388f
Infarction
  cerebral. See Cerebral ischemia.
  myocardial. See Myocardial infarction.
  pulmonary artery catheter-related, 1306
Infection, 1103–1104. See also specific infections.
  abdominal, succinylcholine-related hyperkalemia
      and, 490
  central venous pressure monitoring and, 1293t,
      1295
  endotracheal intubation and, 1649
  epidural analgesia and, 2743
  gastrointestinal tract disease and, 1108
  in children, 2870–2873, 2870t, 2872t–2873t
  in trauma patient, 2487–2488
  isolation precautions for, 3160–3161
  nosocomial, 2796–2798, 2797t
  occupational health risk of, 3155–3162, 3157t,
      3158t
  postpartum, 2329
  pulmonary artery catheter-related, 1306
  respiratory
    in children, 2381–2382
    preoperative, 1088, 1090
  transfusion-related, 1817–1820, 1818t, 1820t
  wound, hypothermia effects on, 1582
Inflammation
  in atherosclerosis, 2052
  in hemorrhagic shock, 2459, 2460f
  with cardiopulmonary bypass, 1975–1976, 1975f,
      1975t, 1976f
Inflammatory bowel disease, in children, 2864
Information management, 972–980
  data collation in, 976–977
  data integration in, 977–979, 979f
  date collection in, 972–975, 973f–978f
  information dissemination in, 979–980
Informed consent, 3176–3179
  by emancipated minor, 3182
  confidentiality and, 3179–3180, 3181
  controversies in, 3179–3182
  decision-making capacity and, 3176
  disclosure and, 3176–3177
  for genetic testing, 3180
  for transfusion, 1827
  from Jehovah's Witnesses, 3179, 3181–3182
  in elderly patient, 2441
  in emergencies, 3179
  legal issues in, 3177–3178
  maternal-fetal conflicts and, 3182
  patient authorization and, 3179
  patient decision and, 3178–3179
  patient understanding and, 3178
  pediatric, 3180–3182, 3180t, 3181t
    abortion and, 3182
    parent-physician disagreements and, 3181
    transfusion refusal and, 3181–3182
  physician recommendation and, 3178
  reasonable person preferences and, 3177
  refusal to provide care and, 3179
  voluntariness and, 3176
Infraclavicular nerve block, 1690
Infraorbital nerve block, 1706, 1706f
  pediatric, 1754
Infrared absorption, for gas analysis, 1454
Inhaled anesthetics. See also specific agents.
  abuse of. See Substance abuse.
  acetylcholine levels and, 112
  additive effects of, 116
  adenosine levels and, 113
  age-related MAC for, 108, 2438
  airway hyperreactivity with, 174
  alveolar-to-venous gradient of, 133

Inhaled anesthetics *(Continued)*
γ-aminobutyric acid effects of, 111–112, 112f, 113, 121, 122f
anesthetic depth and, 1239–1243, 1240f, 1241t, 1242f, 1242t
  hemodynamic response and, 1241–1243, 1242f, 1242t
  movement response and, 1239–1241, 1240f, 1241t
animal models of, 123–125, 124f
  dietary studies with, 123
  genetic studies with, 123–125, 124f
  tolerance studies with, 123
arrhythmias and, 203
axonal transmission and, 111
blood-gas partition coefficient of, 132, 132t
brain effects of, 109, 110f, 825–831, 826f–830f, 2130–2131
brainstem auditory evoked potential effects of, 1532–1536, 1533t, 1534f, 1535f
bronchodilation with, 156–157, 157f
bronchomotor tone and, 155–161, 157f–160f
Caenorhabditis elegans model of, 123–124
calcium channel effects of, 194–195
calcium effects of, 109, 114, 156, 157–158, 158f, 159f, 167, 168f
carbon dioxide absorbent interactions of, 297–298
carcinogenicity of, 261–262
cardiac conduction and, 202–203
cardioprotective effects of, 203
catecholamine levels and, 112–113, 113f
cerebral blood flow and, 825–831, 826f–830f, 2130–2131
cerebral blood volume and, 829, 829f
cerebral vasodilation and, 828–829, 828f
circulatory effects of, 211–212, 212f
convulsions with, 116
coronary vascular effects of, 203–204, 205, 210–211
coronary vasodilator reserve and, 204–205, 204f
critical volume hypothesis of, 117, 119
cutoff effect with, 116
cyclic nucleotide levels and, 113–114
cytoplasmic activity of, 118
decerebration effects and, 109, 110f
delivery systems for, 142–143, 273–311. *See also* Anesthesia machines.
  anesthetic loss in, 142–143, 143t
  breathing system of, 295–296, 295f
    test of, 316
  carbon dioxide absorption systems of, 296–298, 297f
  checkout procedure for, 307–310, 308f, 308t, 309f, 310f, 315–316
  circle breathing system of, 295–296, 295f, 300–301, 300f, 310
  closed-circuit, 143–146, 144f, 145f
  cylinder supply source of, 275f, 276
  electronic alarm of, 276
  fail-safe valves of, 277, 277f
  flow meter assembly of, 277–281, 278f–281f. *See also* Flow meter assembly.
  leak test of, 307–309, 308f, 308t, 309f
  low-flow, 146–147, 147t
  negative-pressure leak test of, 309–310, 310f
  oxygen analyzer calibration for, 307
  oxygen failure protection device of, 277, 278f
  oxygen flush valve of, 283–284
  pediatric, 2393
  pipeline supply source of, 275f, 276
  pneumatic alarm of, 276
  positive-pressure leak test of, 309, 309f
  proportioning systems of, 281–283, 281f, 282f
  rebreathing effects and, 143
  safety devices of, 276–277, 277f
  scavenging systems of, 303–307, 304f, 304t, 305f, 306f
  second-stage pressure regulator of, 277
  self-tests of, 310
  two-gas machine of, 274–275, 275f
  vaporizers of, 284–296. *See also* Vaporizer(s).
  ventilators of, 298–301, 299f
  washin of, 142, 142f
  workstations of, 273–274, 274f, 301–303, 303f
depth of anesthesia and, 1235–1236, 1236f, 1239–1243, 1240, 1241f, 1242f, 1242t
diaphragm effects of, 174, 174f
diastolic function and, 195–196, 195f, 196f
Drosophila model of, 124
during labor, 2319
ED$_{50}$ of, 107, 107f, 108t

Inhaled anesthetics *(Continued)*
electroencephalographic effects of, 1518–1521, 1519f
endogenous opiate levels and, 114
epinephrine-induced arrhythmias and, 203
excitatory amino acid levels and, 113
fluidization theory of, 120
for children, 2372–2375, 2372f, 2372t, 2373t
genotoxicity of, 260–261
glycine effects of, 113, 121, 122f
hepatic function and. 2209–2212, 2210f, 2211f
historical perspective on, 12–13, 16–19
hydrate theory of, 117
hydrogen bond disruption by, 117
hydrophilic sites for, 117
hydrophobic sites for, 115–117, 115f, 115t, 116f
hyperbaric oxygen therapy and, 2686–2687, 2686f, 2687f
hyperkalemia and, 108–109
hypernatremia and, 108
hyponatremia and, 108
hypoxic pulmonary vasoconstriction and, 166–168, 167f, 168f, 1864–1865, 1865f
in ambulatory anesthesia, 2604–2605, 2604t, 2605f
in obese patient, 1033
in renal failure, 2183, 2184t
in thoracic surgery, 1867, 1868
inflammatory response and, 181
intertissue diffusion of, 136
isomers of, 116
left atrial function and, 199–200, 200f, 201f
left ventricular afterload and, 197–198, 198f, 199f
left ventricular-arterial coupling and, 196–197, 197f
lipid solubility of, 115–117, 115f, 115t, 116f
magnesium effects on, 109
mechanism of action of, 869
membrane site of action of, 117–123, 118f, 119f, 121f, 122f. *See also* at Plasma membrane.
metabolism of, 135, 231–264, 232f. *See also* specific *inhaled anesthetics.*
  hepatic, 231–234, 232f, 233f
  in children, 234
  pharmacogenetics of. 234–235, 235f
  pharmacogenomics of, 236
  recovery and, 150
  stereoselective, 240, 240f, 241f
Meyer-Overton rule and, 115–116, 115f, 115t
minimum alveolar concentration of, 107–109, 107f, 108t
  catecholamine effects on, 102
  depth of anesthesia and, 1239–1241, 1240f, 1241t
  lipid solubility and, 115, 115f
  movement response and, 1239–1241, 1240f, 1241t, 1243f
mouse models of, 123, 124–125, 124f
mucociliary function and, 161–165, 163f, 164f
myocardial effects of, 191–195, 192f–194f, 205–206, 206f
myocardial protection with, 206–210, 206f, 208f, 209f, 211
neuromuscular blockade and, 515–516, 516f, 522
neuronal sensitivity to, 110–111, 111f
nicotinic acetylcholine receptor effects of, 120–121, 121f
nitric oxide levels and, 114
occupational health risks of, 3151–3153
opioid interactions with, 96–97, 97f, 423
percutaneous loss of, 135
peripheral receptors and, 109–110
physiochemistry of, 114–117, 115f, 115t, 116f, 125t
postsynaptic action of, 111–112, 112f
potency of, 107, 107f, 108t
pressure effects on, 108
presynaptic action of, 111
protein interaction with, 120–123, 121f, 122f
pulmonary blood flow and, 168–170, 169f, 1865–1866, 1866f
pulmonary vascular resistance and, 165–170, 167f–169f, 1864–1865, 1865f
recovery from, 147–151
  anesthetic circuit and, 151
  diffusion hypoxia and, 150, 150f
  metabolic effects in, 150
  principles of, 147, 148f
  rapid, 149–150, 150f
  routine, 2707–2708, 2707t, 2708t, 2709t
  vs. induction, 147–149, 148f, 149f

Inhaled anesthetics *(Continued)*
renal effects of, 800–801, 1489–1491
right ventricular function and, 199
scavenging systems for, 303–307, 304f, 304t, 305f
sensory evoked potential effects of, 1532–1536, 1533t, 1534f
serotonin effects of, 113, 121
solubility of
  recovery and, 148, 148f, 149f
  uptake and, 132, 132t, 134, 134f
somatosensory evoked potential effects of, 1532–1536, 1533f, 1534f
spinal cord effects of, 109
stereoisomers of, 116
structure of, 106f
surfactant effects of, 162, 164f
synaptic transmission and, 111–112, 112f
systemic hemodynamics and, 201–202
temperature effects on, 108, 108f
tissue-blood partition coefficients of, 132t, 133
toxicity of, 240–262, 242f. *See also* specific *inhaled anesthetics.*
  Ames *Salmonella* assay for, 261
  carbon dioxide absorbent-related, 251–256, 251f, 254f
  carbon monoxide in, 255–256, 255f, 256f
  carcinogenesis and, 261–262
  developmental defects and, 259–260
  during pregnancy, 257–260, 258f
  fluoride-associated, 248–251, 248f
  gene mutation and, 260–261
  hepatic, 231–248. *See also* specific *inhaled anesthetics.*
    assays for, 247–248, 247t
    risk factors for, 246–247, 247t
  nephrotoxicity of, 248–251, 248f
  occupational exposures and, 256–257, 260, 262
    to dentists, 262
    to nurse anesthetists, 262
    to sperm, 258
unitary theory of, 114–117, 115f, 115t
uptake of, 131–150
  alveolar-to-venous gradient and, 133
  anesthetic concentration and, 134f, 135, 135f
  anesthetic metabolism and, 136
  anesthetic solubility and, 132, 132t, 134, 134f, 139–140
  blood-gas partition coefficient and, 132, 132t
  cardiac output and, 133, 138–139, 138f, 139f
  concentration effects in, 134f, 135, 135f
  FA-FI relationship in, 131–136, 132f, 132t, 133t, 134f–136f
    cardiac output and, 138–139, 138f, 139f
    ventilation-to-perfusion ratio and, 139–140, 140f, 141f
    ventilatory changes and, 136–137, 137f, 139, 139f, 140f
  in closed circuit, 143–146, 144f, 145f
  in low-flow circuit, 146–147, 147t
  intertissue diffusion and, 136
  percutaneous anesthetic loss and, 135
  second gas effect in, 135, 136f
  tissue-specific, 133–134, 133t
  ventilation and, 131–132, 132f, 135, 136–137, 137f, 139, 139f, 140f
  ventilation-to-perfusion ratio and, 139–140, 140f, 141f
  washin and, 142, 142f
ventilation and, 170–171, 179–181, 180f. *See also* Ventilation, inhaled anesthetic effects on.
visceral loss of, 135
visual evoked potential effects of, 1532–1536, 1533t, 1535f
volume expansion by, 117
waste, 3151–3153
Inolimomab, in organ transplantation, 2271–2273, 2272t
Insomnia
  chronic pain and, 2772
  valerian in, 611–612
Inspiratory airway pressure (P$_{100}$), 1463
Inspiratory capacity, 694, 694f, 1007
Inspiratory reserve volume, 694, 694f
Insulin, 1020
  hepatic metabolism of, 750
  in critically ill patient, 2800, 2801f–2802f, 2893
  in diabetes mellitus, 1023–1024, 1024f, 1777–1778, 1777t, 1778t, 1779, 1780
  in ketoacidosis, 1023
  in pediatric diabetic ketoacidosis, 2862
  in sepsis, 2900

Insulin analogs, in diabetes mellitus, 1777–1778, 1778t
Insulin-like growth factor-1
  in hepatic disease, 761
  in sepsis, 2900
Insulin resistance
  acetylcholine receptors in, 871
  in hepatic disease, 761
  in sepsis, 2904–2905
Insulinoma, 1026–1027
β-Integrin, in muscle development, 856
Intensive care unit. See also Critical care medicine; Pediatric intensive care unit.
  director of, 2789
  staffing of, 2788–2789, 2789t
Inter/intrapleural analgesia, 587–588, 1909, 2744
  for children, 1753
Intercalated discs, 730, 730f
Intercostal nerve block, 1710–1711, 1710f
  catheter placement for, 1711
  cryoprobe for (cryoanalgesia), 1906–1907
  in thoracoscopy, 1912
  pediatric, 1752–1753, 1752f
Interleukin-1, 1114t
  in sepsis, 2901
Interleukin-2, 1114t
Interleukin-3, 1114t
Interleukin-4, 1114t
Interleukin-5, 1114t
Interleukin-6, 1114t
  in brain death, 2960
  in sepsis, 2900
Interleukin-7, 1114t
Interleukin-8, 1114t
Interleukin-9, 1114t
Interleukin-10, 1114t
Interleukin-11, 1114t
Intermediate filaments, 734
Intermittent mandatory ventilation, 2823, 2823f
  after thoracic surgery, 1904–1906, 1904t, 1905t
  in children, 2848
Intermittent positive-pressure breathing
  efficacy of, 696–697
  for bronchial hygiene, 2819
  preoperative, 1086
Internet, 2973–2978, 2974f
  clinician-oriented information on, 2974–2975
  department sites on, 2977
  discussion groups on, 2977
  journals on, 2975, 2975t
  research-related information on, 2975–2977, 2976f
Interosseous nerve, anterior, injury to, 2411–2412, 2412t
Interpleural analgesia
  for children, 1753
  for postoperative pain, 2744
Interposed abdominal counterpulsation, in basic life support, 2926
Interscalene block, 1686, 1688–1689, 1688f
  pediatric, 1741–1742, 1742f
  postoperative, 1688
  side effects of, 1688–1689
Interventional study, 886. See also Statistics.
Intervertebral disk herniation, 1096
Intestine
  malrotation of, 2863
  opioid effects on, 398
  transplantation of, 2253
Intocostrin, 32
Intra-aortic balloon pump counterpulsation, 1991
  arterial blood pressure monitoring in, 1286, 1287f
Intra-articular analgesia, 2744
Intra-/interpleural analgesia, 587–588, 1909, 2744
  for children, 1753
Intracapsular anesthetic injection, in children, 1756
Intracellular fluid, 1764, 1764t
Intracranial aneurysm, 2146–2151, 2146t, 2147t, 2647
  antifibrinolytics in, 2148
  calcium channel blockers in, 2148
  electrocardiography in, 2148–2149, 2148f
  evaluation of, 2147–2149, 2148f
  fluid management in, 2147
  intervention for, 2162
    anesthesia in, 2149–2151
    angiography in, 2151
    brain protection during, 2150
    CSF drainage in, 2149–2150
    early, 2147
    electroencephalography in, 2151

Intracranial aneurysm (Continued)
  intervention for (Continued)
    hypocapnia in, 2149
    hypothermia in, 2150–2151
    induced hypertension in, 2149
    induced hypotension in, 2149
    mannitol in, 2150
    monitoring in, 2149, 2151
    trapping, 2150
  of ophthalmic artery, 2151
  of vein of Galen, 2151
  of vertebrobasilar artery, 2151
  somatosensory evoked potential monitoring in, 1529–1530
  vasospasm in, 2147–2148
Intracranial pressure (ICP), 2127–2131, 2128f
  alfentanil effects on, 823
  dexmedetomidine effects on, 356
  endotracheal intubation and, 1648
  etomidate effects on, 352, 822
  histamine and, 831
  in children, 2855–2856, 2864
  in end-stage liver disease, 2247
  in head injury, 2156–2157
  in pediatric liver failure, 2864
  in traumatic brain injury, 2471–2473
  increased, 1099–1100, 2128–2131, 2128f, 2131t
    anesthetic selection and, 2130–2131
    hyperventilation in, 2132–2133, 2133f
    in children, 2856–2857
    pathophysiology of, 2128, 2129f
    treatment of, 2129–2130, 2129t, 2130f, 2130t, 2131, 2131t
  inhaled anesthetic effects on, 829, 829f
  ketamine effects on, 347, 825
  lidocaine effects on, 825
  opioid effects on, 390
  pancuronium, 831
  pressure-volume relationship in, 2128, 2128f
  remifentanil effects on, 823–824
  succinylcholine effects on, 491, 831–832
  sufentanil effects on, 823
Intradermal wheal anesthesia, in children, 1755
Intradiscal electrothermal annuloplasty, 2774
Intragastric pressure, succinylcholine effect on, 490–491
Intraocular pressure, 2531–2533
  anesthesia effects on, 2532–2533
  ischemic optic neuropathy and, 3009
  opioid effects on, 399
  physiology of, 2531–2532
  post-TURP, 3014
  retinal blood flow and, 2995
  succinylcholine effect on, 490
Intraperitoneal anesthetic injection, for children, 1756
Intrathecal drug therapy, in chronic pain, 2774
Intravascular coils, in children, 2042
Intravenous anesthetics. See also specific intravenous anesthetics.
  α-adrenergic agonists as, 355–359. See also Dexmedetomidine.
  automated delivery systems for, 463–475, 463f–467f, 468t, 469f–471f. See also Intravenous anesthetics, target-controlled delivery systems for.
  barbiturates as 326–334. See also Barbiturate(s).
  benzodiazepines as, 334–343. See also Benzodiazepines.
  bolus dose calculations for, 450–451, 454f
  C_{50} of, 446–448, 447t, 450, 452t, 453f
  cerebral blood flow and, 821–825, 821f
  cerebral metabolic rate and, 821–825, 821f
  closed-loop delivery systems for, 473–475, 475f
  context-sensitive decrement time of, 455–456, 455f, 456f
  delivery systems for, 439–476
    automated, 463–475, 463f–467f, 468t, 469f–471f. See also Intravenous anesthetics, target-controlled delivery systems for.
    bolus dose calculations for, 450–451, 454f, 454f
    closed-loop, 473–475, 475f
    dosing regimens and, 450–458, 454f–457f
    historical perspective on, 439–440, 440f
    infusion devices for, 463–475, 463f–467f, 468t, 469f–471f
    maintenance infusion rate for, 451–455, 454f, 455f
    manual infusion for, 458–462, 460t

Intravenous anesthetics (Continued)
  delivery systems for (Continued)
    pharmacodynamics and, 444–450, 445t, 446f, 447t, 449f–453f
    pharmacokinetics and, 440–444, 441f–443f
    pumps for, 463
    target-controlled, 464–473, 464f–467f, 468t, 469f–471f. See also Intravenous anesthetics, target-controlled delivery systems for.
  depth of anesthesia and, 1243–1245, 1244f, 1245t
    during induction, 1243–1244
    during maintenance, 1244–1245, 1244f, 1245t
  droperidol as, 359–360, 360f
  drug interactions with, 448–450, 449f–453f, 456–457, 457f–459f
  effect-site concentration of, 447–448
  electroencephalographic effects of, 1517–1518, 1519t
  etomidate as, 350–355. See also Etomidate.
  flumazenil as, 343–345, 343f, 345t
  for electroconvulsive therapy, 2655–2656
  hepatic function and, 2212, 2213
  historical studies on, 28–30
  hyperbaric oxygen therapy and, 2687
  in renal failure, 2183–2184, 2184t
  in thoracic surgery, 1867
  maintenance infusion rate of, 451–455, 454f, 455f
  manual infusion of, 458–462, 460t
  minimum alveolar concentration of, 448–450, 450f
  nonopioid, 317–362. See also specific anesthetics.
    depth of anesthesia and, 1243–1245, 1244f, 1245t
  opioid, 379–424. See also Opioids.
  pharmacodynamics of, 444–450
    biophase of, 444–445, 446
    direct effect models of, 445, 445t
    drug interactions and, 448–450, 449f–453f
    EEG assessment of, 444–445
    indirect effect models of, 445–446
    patient variability and, 448, 450, 453t
    potency and, 446–450, 447t, 449f–453f
  pharmacokinetics of, 440–444, 441f–443f
    mathematical model of, 442–444, 442f, 443f
    target-controlled infusion and, 466–468, 468t
  phencyclidines as, 345–350. See also Ketamine.
  plasma concentration ranges for, 450, 453t
  propofol as, 318–326. See also Propofol.
  pseudo-steady state of, 448
  recovery from, 455–458, 455f–459f, 459t
  target-controlled delivery systems for, 464–473
    age-associated variability and, 469
    Bayesian forecasting for, 471
    BET scheme of, 464
    components of, 463–464, 463f
    effect-site concentration in, 471–472, 471f
    evaluation of, 465–466, 465f
    gender-associated variability and, 469
    intraindividual variability and, 470–471
    median absolute performance error in, 466–468, 468t
    microcomputer of, 464, 464f
    optimization of, 466–472, 466f, 467f, 468t, 469f–471f
    outcome of, 472–473
    patient-associated variability and, 469–471
    pharmacokinetic model for, 464–465, 465f, 467, 468t, 469f–471f, 471–472
    set point for, 463
    shock-associated variability and, 469–470
Intrinsic clearance, 72–73, 74f
Intubating laryngeal mask airway, 1627, 1627f
Intubation
  bronchial, 708, 1648–1649
    during laparoscopy, 2289
  endotracheal. See Endotracheal intubation.
  esophageal, 1461, 1648
Intussusception, 2864
Inulin clearance, 786, 1489
Inverse agonist, 86f, 87, 87f
Ion channels, 89f, 90–92, 91f, 538
  disorders of, 537–538, 538t
  inhaled anesthetic effects on, 120–122, 121f
Ion pumps, 92
Ipratropium, 2817t
Iron lung, 35, 2850–2851
Isaacs' syndrome (neuromyotonia), 543
Ischemia
  cerebral. See Cerebral ischemia.
  hepatic, 758

Ischemia (Continued)
  myocardial. See Myocardial ischemia.
  optic. See Optic neuropathy, ischemic.
  pulmonary artery catheter-related, 1306
  renal, 1491–1492, 1491f
  spinal cord, in thoracoabdominal aortic
      reconstruction, 2086–2088, 2086f
Iso-indoklon, oil-gas partition coefficient of, 115t
Isocyanates, accidental release of, 2510
Isoflurane, 18, 284–285, 284f
  abuse of. See Substance abuse.
  airway hyperreactivity with, 174
  airway receptor effects of, 173
  airway resistance and, 160, 160f
  arrhythmias and, 203
  arterial pressure and, 202
  brainstem auditory evoked potential effects of,
      1533–1534, 1533t, 1534f
  bronchial effects of, 158, 158f
  bronchodilation and, 157
  calcium channel effects of, 194–195
  calcium effects of, 158, 158f, 167, 168f
  cardiac conduction and, 202–203
  central ventilatory effects of, 171, 172f
  cerebral blood flow and, 825–827, 826f, 828–829,
      828f
  cerebral metabolic rate and, 826f, 827–828
  cerebral metabolism and, 815, 815f
  cerebrospinal fluid dynamics and, 832, 832t
  coronary artery effects of, 203–211
      blood flow and, 210–211
      in vitro, 203
      in vivo, 203–204
      ischemia and, 205–206, 206f
      protective effects and, 206–210, 206f, 208f,
          209f, 211
      vasodilation and, 205
      vasodilator reserve and, 204–205, 204f
  coronary blood flow and, 211
  cortical somatosensory evoked responses with,
      815, 815f
  cyclosporine interaction with, 2273
  depth of anesthesia and, 1235–1236, 1236f,
      1241–1243, 1242f, 1242t, 1243f
  diastolic function and, 195–196, 195f, 196f
  during labor, 2319
  electroencephalographic effects of, 1519t,
      1520–1521
  fentanyl interaction with, 96, 97f
  fluoride-associated nephrotoxicity of, 249
  for children, 2372, 2372f, 2372t, 2374
  heart rate and, 201–202
  hepatic effects of, 244–245, 244f, 2209–2212,
      2210f, 2211f
  hippocampal effects of, 109, 110f
  hypoxic pulmonary vasoconstriction and, 166,
      167–168
  in ambulatory anesthesia, 2604–2605, 2604t
  in kidney transplantation, 2241
  in renal failure, 2184t
  left atrial function and, 199–200, 201f
  left ventricular afterload and, 197–198, 198f, 199f
  left ventricular-arterial coupling and, 196–197
  memory effects of, 1238
  metabolism of, 135, 238, 239f
  minimum alveolar concentration of, 107–109,
      107f, 108t
      alfentanil effects on, 411
      decerebration and, 109, 110f
      esmolol effects on, 388
      fentanyl effects on, 387–388, 388f, 411
      ondansetron and, 113
      opioid effects on, 449–450, 450f, 451f
  myocardial contractility and, 191–194, 192f–194f
  myocardial preconditioning and, 1954
  neuromuscular blockade and, 515–516, 516f
  neuromuscular blockade reversal and, 522
  neuroprotection with, 839–840
  oil-gas partition coefficient of, 115t, 116
  partition coefficients of, 132, 132t
  peripheral effects of, 109–110
  plasma membrane effects of, 117, 118f
  pulmonary blood flow and, 169, 169f, 1866, 1866f
  recovery from, 147–151, 148f, 149f, 150f,
      2707–2708, 2708t
  remifentanil interaction with, 449–450, 451f
  renal effects of, 800–801, 1490–1491
  seizures and, 829–830
  serotonin with, 161
  somatosensory evoked potential effects of, 1533,
      1533t

Isoflurane (Continued)
  structure of, 106f
  tubing uptake of, 142, 143t
  vasodilating effect of, 828–829, 828f
  visual evoked potential effects of, 1533t, 2535
Isoflurophate, 1125, 1126t
Isolation, 1104, 3160–3161
Isoniazid, hepatotoxicity of, 2221t
Isoproterenol, 652, 1120, 2817t
  calcium levels and, 1812
  in children, 2837, 2837t
  in neonatal resuscitation, 2361, 2361t
  structure of, 647f, 654f
Isosulfan blue, pulse oximetry errors and, 1451t,
      1452

J

Jackson, Charles T., 16
Jackson, Chevier, 39
Jackson, Dennis, 34
Jarvik 2000 system, 1993
Jaundice
  in cholestasis, 764
  postoperative, 2219–2220, 2219t
  renal effects of, 805
Jaw spasm
  in malignant hyperthermia, 1180–1181, 1181f
  succinylcholine-induced, 491, 2378–2379
Jehovah's Witnesses, 1839–1840, 1840t
  informed consent from, 3179, 3181–3182
  transfusion and, 3181–3182
  trauma in, 2482–2483
Jet ventilation system. See also High-frequency jet
      ventilation.
  in basic life support, 2924–2925
  in laser surgery, 2583–2584
  transtracheal, 1637–1639, 1640t, 2458–2459,
      2545, 2546, 2924–2925
Jin bu huan, hepatotoxicity of, 2222t
Journals, 2975, 2975t
Jugular vein
  external, cannulation of, 1292. See also Central
      venous pressure monitoring.
  internal
      left, cannulation of, 1291–1292, 1303. See also
          Central venous pressure monitoring.
      puncture of, 1293–1294
      right, cannulation of, 1287–1291, 1288f, 1291f,
          1301–1304, 1302f. See also Central
          venous pressure monitoring; Pulmonary
          artery catheter monitoring.
          anatomy for, 1287, 1288f
          asepsis for, 1288
          needle insertion for, 1288–1289, 1288f
  oxygen saturation of, 1512t, 1542
      in head injury, 2155–2156
Junctional rhythms
  electrocardiography in, 1403
  succinylcholine-induced, 489
Junker, Ferdinand, 33
Juvenile rheumatoid arthritis, 2427
Juxtaglomerular apparatus, 778–779, 780f

K

Kappis, M., 23
Kava (Piper methysticum), 607t, 610–611
Kavain bu huan, hepatotoxicity of, 2222t
Kawasaki's disease, 2840
Kearns-Sayre syndrome, 537
Ketamine, 29, 345–350
  abuse of. See Substance abuse.
  administrative routes for, 350
  analgesic effects of, 347, 349
  applications of, 348–350, 349t
  awakening from, 347
  benzodiazepine with, 347
  BIS index and, 1255
  cardiovascular system effects of, 323t, 348
  central nervous system effects of, 346–347
  cerebral blood flow and, 821f, 824–825
  cerebral metabolic rate and, 821f, 824–825
  chlorobutanol preservative for, 350
  contraindications to, 350
  dosing for, 349t, 350
  during labor, 2318

Ketamine (Continued)
  electroencephalographic effects of, 1518, 1519t
  emergence reactions with, 347
  epileptogenic properties of, 833
  for children, 348, 349, 350, 1725t, 1726, 2375,
      2381
  half-life of, 346, 346f
  historical perspective on, 345
  in ambulatory anesthesia, 2602t, 2603
  in depressive patient, 349
  in heart disease patient, 349
  in outpatient monitored anesthesia care, 2610,
      2611
  in pediatric cardiac surgery, 2020, 2020f
  in pediatric regional anesthesia, 1725t, 1726
  in thoracic surgery, 1867
  in trauma patient, 349, 2457
  induction with, 349, 349t
  intracranial pressure effects of, 825
  intraocular pressure effects of, 2532
  maintenance with, 349, 349t
  manual infusion of, 460t, 462
  mechanism of action of, 869
  metabolism of, 346, 2213
  neuroprotective effects of, 347
  opioids with, 422
  pain treatment with, 2735–2736
  pharmacokinetics of, 319t, 346, 346f
  pharmacology of, 346–348
  physiochemical characteristics of, 345–346, 345f
  plasma concentration ranges for, 453t
  receptor binding of, 347
  respiratory system effects of, 347–348
  sedation with, 349–350, 349t
  seizures and, 833
  side effects of, 350
  somatosensory evoked potential effects of, 1533t
  stereoisomers of, 345, 345f, 346
  visual evoked potential effects of, 1533t, 2535
  with regional anesthesia, 350
Ketanserin, in postoperative shivering, 1583
Ketoacidosis, 1022–1023
  diabetic, 1610, 1780
      in children, 2862–2863
Ketoconazole, hepatotoxicity of, 2221t
Ketone bodies, 748, 2891, 2891t, 2892f, 2904
Ketorolac
  in outpatient monitored anesthesia care,
      2610–2611
  postoperative, 2719–2720, 2735t, 2736f
  renal effects of, 803
Kety, Seymore S., 18
Kidney(s), 777–807
  age-related changes in, 2438
  aminoglycoside-induced injury to, 803
  anesthetic drug effects on, 800–801
  antihypertensive drug effects on, 2186–2187
  aortic cross-clamping effects on, 802
  atrial natriuretic peptide infusion effects on, 800
  autoregulation of, 779, 779f
  benign neoplasms of, 2199
  bilirubin-induced injury to, 805
  blood flow in, 783, 783t, 2177–2178, 2178f
      assessment of, 1503–1506, 1504f, 1505f
      calculation of, 1503
      cortical vs. medullary, 1505–1506
      electromagnetic probes for, 790
      gamma camera measurement of, 1504
      gas-washout measurement of, 1503–1504, 1504f
      hypothermia effect on, 1588
      indocyanine green measurement of, 1503
      monitoring of, 790–791, 1501–1505, 1502f,
          1504f
      para-aminohippurate measurement of, 1503
      postischemic, 1491–1492, 1491f
      tissue oxygen pressure measurement of, 1503
      ultrasound measurement of, 1505, 1505f
  bromochlorotrifluoroethane effects on, 254
  calcium channel blocker effects on, 799–800
  calculi of, 2195–2197
  cancer of, 2198, 2198t, 2199
  cardiopulmonary bypass effects on, 802–803
  compound A toxicity to, 251–256, 251f, 254f,
      1490
  contrast-induced injury to, 804, 2180
  cyclosporine-induced injury to, 803–804
  digitalis effects on, 2186
  disease of, 1100–1103, 1103t
      hypocalcemia and, 1050–1051
      in cholestasis, 764
      in liver disease, 761, 2247–2248

Kidney(s) (Continued)
  donation of, 3189
  dopamine effects on, 798–799
  dopexamine effects on, 799
  drug clearance by, 73–74
  drug effects on, 803–805, 2182–2187, 2183t,
      2184t, 2185t, 2186t
  effective blood flow of, 786
  evaluation of, 2178–2181, 2178t, 2179f
      before peripheral vascular surgery, 2065
  excretory function of, 1484–1485, 1485f
  failure of. See Kidney failure.
  fenoldopam effects on, 799, 804
  function of, 784, 785f, 1484–1489, 1485f. See also
      Kidney function.
  glomerulus of, 777–780, 779f, 780f
  hemoglobin-induced injury to, 805
  hypotension effects on, 802
  idiopathic pain in, 2200
  imaging of, 2180–2181
  in hemorrhagic shock, 2459–2460
  in hypervolemia, 784
  in hypovolemia, 784
  in pediatric cardiopulmonary bypass, 2028–2029,
      2028f
  inflammatory disease of, 2199–2200
  inhaled anesthetic effects on, 248–251, 248f, 801,
      2183, 2184t
  inhaled anesthetic uptake by, 133–134, 133t
  innervation of, 2175–2176, 2176f
  intravenous anesthetic effects on, 2183–2184,
      2184t
  ischemia of, 1491–1492, 1491f, 1501–1502
  mannitol effects on, 802
  maturation of, 2370, 2370f
  muscle relaxant effects on, 2184–2186, 2185t,
      2186t
  myoglobin-induced injury to, 804–805
  N-acetylcysteine-induced injury to, 804
  neuraxial anesthesia effects on, 1660
  neurohumoral influences on, 1487–1488
  NSAID-induced injury to, 803
  opioid effects on, 2183
  pediatric, 2858–2859, 2859t
  pharmacologic protection of, 798–800, 802
      in sepsis, 805–807
  pigment-induced injury to, 804–805
  positive-pressure ventilation effects on, 801–802
  prostaglandin infusion effects on, 799
  radionuclide imaging of, 2180–2181
  sepsis-related failure of, 805–807
  sodium regulation by, 1485–1486, 1485f, 1506
      in liver disease, 762
  Starling forces in, 1487
  stones in, 1101
  sympathetic innervation of, 1489
  toxic injury to, 783, 800–807
  transplantation of, 1103, 2235, 2237–2242, 2239f.
      See also Kidney transplantation.
  tubules of, 781–784, 781f, 782f, 783t. See also
      Renal tubules.
  tubuloglomerular feedback in, 779
  urine formation by, 1486–1488, 1765
      tests of, 789
  vascular structure of, 1501, 1502f
  vasopressor effects on, 2186–2187
  volume regulation by, 1485–1486, 1485f
Kidney failure. See also Kidney function.
  acidemia in, 2181–2182, 2181t, 2182t
  acute, 2187–2188
  after thoracoabdominal aortic reconstruction,
      2088–2089
  anemia in, 2181t, 2182
  antihypertensive drugs in, 2186–2187
  blood flow evaluation of, 1503–1506, 1504f, 1505f
  cardiac manifestations of, 2181t, 2182
  cardiovascular disease and, 2238, 2239–2240
  classification of, 2187–2188, 2187t
  clinical manifestations of, 2181–2182, 2181t
  diabetes mellitus and, 2238
  dialysis in, 1102–1103, 1103t, 2188–2189
  digitalis in, 2186
  drug effects in, 1103, 2182–2187, 2183t, 2184t,
      2185t, 2186t
  etiology of, 1483–1484, 1484t
  filtration fraction in, 1491, 1491f
  fluid management in, 1793
  glomerular filtration rate in, 2180–2181
  hematologic manifestations of, 2181t, 2182
  hyperkalemia in, 2181t, 2182
  hyperreninemia and, 2238

Kidney failure (Continued)
  hypovolemia in, 2181, 2181t
  in children, 2859–2861
  in hepatic disease, 761
  infrarenal aortic cross-clamping and, 2075
  inhaled anesthetics in, 2183, 2184t
  intravenous anesthetics in, 2183–2184, 2184t
  muscle relaxants in, 2184–2186, 2185t, 2186t
  neuromuscular blockade and, 527–529, 528t
  nondepolarizing muscle relaxants in, 527–529,
      528t
  opioid effects in, 406–408, 407f, 2183
  pathophysiology of, 2238–2239
  perioperative, 1483–1484, 1484t
  postischemic, 1491–1492, 1491f, 1501–1502
  postoperative, 1102
  preoperative risk for, 1492–1493, 1492t
  pulmonary manifestations of, 2181t, 2182
  total parenteral nutrition in, 2915
  vasopressors in, 2186–2187
Kidney function, 784, 785f, 1484–1489, 1485f
  adenosine system and, 798, 798t
  after heart transplantation, 2261
  arginine vasopressin and, 793–794, 794f
  atrial natriuretic peptide and, 795–796, 796f, 797f
  compound A effects on, 1490
  dopaminergic system and, 796–797, 796t
  inhaled anesthetic effects on, 1489–1491
  investigational tests of, 790–791
  ischemia effects on, 1491–1492, 1491f
  kinins and, 795
  monitoring of, 1493–1506, 1494t
      α-glutathione Z-transferase in, 1500, 1501t
      alanine aminopeptidase in, 1501, 1501t
      β2-macroglobulin in, 1500–1501, 1501t
      biochemical markers in, 1499–1501, 1500t
      blood urea nitrogen in, 1497–1498, 1497t
      capnometry in, 1495
      cardiac output in, 1495
      central venous pressure in, 1494
      creatinine clearance in, 1499, 1499f
      creatinine levels in, 1498
      fractional excretion of sodium in, 1498
      free water clearance in, 1499
      glomerular filtration rate for, 1488–1489
      left atrial pressure in, 1494
      left ventricular end-diastolic area in, 1494
      N-acetyl-β-D-glucosaminidase in, 1500, 1500t
      perfusion pressure in, 1495
      pulmonary capillary wedge pressure in, 1494
      renal blood flow in, 1495–1496, 1501–1506,
          1502f, 1504f, 1505f
      serum creatinine in, 1497–1498, 1497t
      urea levels in, 1498
      urinary sodium in, 1498
      urine osmolality in, 1497, 1497t
      urine specific gravity in, 1496–1497
      urine volume in, 1496
  neurohormonal regulation of, 791–798, 791f–797f
  nitric oxide and, 797–798
  pharmacologic protection of, 798–800, 802
  preoperative evaluation of, 1492–1493, 1492t,
      1493f
  preservation of, 1102
  prostaglandins and, 794–795, 795f
  regional anesthesia effect on, 1489
  renin-angiotensin-aldosterone system and,
      792–793, 792f, 793f
  sympathoadrenal axis and, 791–792
  tests of, 784–791, 787f. See also Renal clearance.
Kidney transplantation, 2235, 2237–2242, 2239f
  anesthesia after, 2241
  anesthetic in, 2241
  aspiration with, 2241
  cardiovascular evaluation for, 2239–2240
  care after, 2241
  central venous pressure monitoring, 2241
  coagulation evaluation in, 2240
  donor organ for, 2235, 2237–2238
  hypotension and, 2240–2242
  in diabetes mellitus, 2240
  intraoperative management in, 2240–2242
  living donor for, 2235
  organ harvest for, 2233
  organ preservation for, 2234
  pain control in, 2241
  preoperative evaluation for, 2239–2240
  urine output after, 2242
  vascular anastomoses for, 2239, 2239f
Killian, Gustav, 39
Kilopascal, 1196

Kinetic energy, 1197, 1198f, 1219
King-Denborough syndrome, 1183
Kinins
  in carcinoid tumor, 1109
  in renal regulation, 795
Kirstein, Alfred, 39
Kitagawa, Otojiro, 26
Klebanoff, G., 21
Kleihauer-Betke blood test, 2482
Knee replacement, 2414t, 2417–2418
  blood loss in, 2417–2418
  cement in, 2417
  deep venous thrombosis and, 2425–2426
  emboli in, 2417
  pain management after, 2418
  robotic, 2568
Koenig, Franz, 40
Koenigstein, Leopold, 23
Kohn, pores of, 692
Koller, Carl, 22–23
Konyne, 1824
Korotkoff sounds, 1269, 1270f
Korotkov, Nikolai, 7
Kouwenhoven, William B., 40
Krantz, Jr., John C., 18
Krypton, oil-gas partition coefficient of, 115t
Kuhn, Franz, 34, 37
Kuhne, Willy, 30
Kulenkampff, D., 23, 24f
Kupffer cells, 750

L

Labat, Gaston L., 9, 24
Labetalol, 657
  cerebral blood flow and, 819
  in neurosurgery, 2145
  in preeclampsia, 2331, 2332t
  pharmacology of, 653–655, 654t
Labor, 2314–2315, 2314f, 2314t. See also Vaginal
      delivery.
Laboratory testing, 939–946. See also specific imaging
      modalities and tests.
  abnormal results in, 947–949, 948t–949t
  ASA Advisory on, 940, 942–944, 942t
  benefit-risk analysis of, 949–950, 949f, 950t
  cardiovascular, 967f
  effectiveness of, 441f, 940, 962–972, 964t–965t,
      966t, 967f–969f
  hematologic, 969f
  hepatic, 968f
  in asymptomatic patient, 962–972, 964t–965t,
      966t, 967f–969f
  in children, 943
  in elderly, 943
  lead-time bias and, 950
  length-time bias and, 950
  medicolegal liability and, 944–946, 945t, 946f,
      946t
  operating room schedules and, 946
  ordering errors and, 971–972
  patient risk with, 944, 945t
  predictive value of, 947–949, 948t–949t
  procedure-related, 942t, 950–951
  pulmonary, 968f
  recommendations for, 962–972, 964t–965t, 966t,
      967f–969f
  renal, 969f
  underordering of, 971
Lactate dehydrogenase, 754
Laennec, Rene T., 41
Lambert, E. H., 7
Lambert-Eaton syndrome, 540, 540t, 1098
  neuromuscular blockade in, 542–543
Laminar flow, 1202, 1203f, 1221–1222
Lamm, H., 39
Landsteiner, Karl, 21
Langley, John N., 8, 85
Laparoscopy, 2285–2299
  anesthesia for, 2296–2299, 2296t, 2297t
      general, 2297–2298
      local, 2298
      monitoring after, 2298–2299
      recovery after, 2298–2299
      regional, 2298
  arrhythmias during, 2293
  aspiration during, 2290
  carbon dioxide subcutaneous emphysema in,
      2288

Laparoscopy (Continued)
  cardiac output during, 2290–2292, 2291f
  cerebral blood flow during, 2292
  complications of, 2295–2296, 2299
  during pregnancy, 2295, 2338
  endobronchial intubation during, 2289
  endocrine response after, 2294
  gas embolism during, 2289–2290
  gasless, 2295
  head-down position for, 2293
  head-up position for, 2293
  hemodynamic changes during, 2290–2293, 2291f
  in cardiac patient, 2292, 2296, 2296t
  in children, 2295
  inert gases for, 2295
  metabolic response after, 2294
  monitoring during, 2297
  mortality with, 2299
  nausea after, 2294
  nerve injury with, 2293
  PaCO2 during, 2286–2288, 2287f, 2287t
  pain after, 2293, 2294
  patient evaluation for, 2296, 2296t
  patient positioning for, 2293, 2297
  pneumomediastinum during, 2288–2289
  pneumopericardium during, 2288–2289
  pneumoperitoneum during, 2290–2292, 2291f,
      2294–2295
  pneumothorax during, 2288–2289
  postoperative benefits of, 2293–2294
  premedication for, 2296
  pulmonary function after, 2294
  respiratory changes with, 2293
  respiratory complications of, 2288–2290, 2288f
  splanchnic blood flow during, 2292
  stress response after, 2293, 2294
  systemic vascular resistance during, 2291–2292,
      2291f
  thromboembolism during, 2292
  urologic, 2194–2195
  venous stasis during, 2293
  ventilatory changes during, 2286–2288, 2286f,
      2287f
  vomiting after, 2294
  vs. laparotomy, 2297
Laparotomy, decompressive, in traumatic brain
      injury, 2473
Laplace equation, 690, 726
Larrey, Dominique J., 11–12, 22
Laryngeal block, 2545–2546
Laryngeal edema, after endotracheal intubation,
      1650
Laryngeal mask airway, 1625–1628, 1626f, 1627f,
      1637, 1640f
  design of, 1625–1627, 1626f, 1627f
  for children, 2386, 2386t
  in basic life support, 2924
  in postoperative airway obstruction, 2711–2712
  in trauma patient, 2458
  insertion of, 1625–1627, 1626f
  intubating, 1627, 1627f
  problems with, 1627
  ProSeal, 1627, 1627f
Laryngeal nerve(s), 2537, 2538f
  injury to, 2538, 2547
Laryngeal nerve block, 1708, 1708f
  pediatric, 1753, 1753f
Laryngeal receptors, inhaled anesthetic effects on,
      173
Laryngoscope, 1631, 1631f
  historical perspective on, 39
  in awake intubation, 1642–1643
  intraocular pressure effects of, 2533
  positioning of, 1634, 1634f
Laryngospasm, 2538–2539
  after tonsillectomy, 2543
  sounds of, 1619
  treatment of, 1619
  with endotracheal intubation, 1647
Laryngotracheobronchitis, 2851–2852
Larynx
  anatomy of, 1618, 1618t, 2537–2539, 2538f
  innervation of, 1618, 1618t
  laser surgery on, 2542–2543
  microlaryngoscopy of, 2542
  pediatric, 2540
  trauma to, 2540–2542
Laser lithotripsy, 2194
Laser prostatectomy, 2194
Laser surgery, 2573–2585, 2574t
  biologic effects of, 2578, 2578f

Laser surgery (Continued)
  clinical applications of, 2577–2578
  embolism with, 2579–2580
  endotracheal tube fires with, 2580–2584, 2580f,
      2582f
  eye protection for, 2580
  FDA regulation of, 2578–2579
  hardware for, 2576–2577, 2576f, 2577f, 2577t
  hazards of, 2543, 2579–2584, 2579f, 2584f
  inappropriate energy transfer with, 2580
  jet ventilation system in, 2583–2584
  occupational health risks of, 3154–3155
  physics of, 2573, 2575–2576, 2575f
  pneumothorax with, 2579
  risks of, 2578–2579
  smoke plume with, 2579, 3154–3155
  smoke production with, 2579
  tissue perforation with, 2579
  upper airway, 2542–2543
Latent heat of vaporization, 285
Lateral cutaneous nerve block, pediatric, 1743, 1746
Lateral femoral cutaneous nerve, injury to
  position-related, 1155, 1156t
  with orthopedic surgery, 2411–2412, 2412t
Lateral femoral cutaneous nerve block, 1698f, 1699,
      Plate 12
Lateral oblique position, nerve injury with,
      1160–1162, 1161f, 1162f
Lateral position
  for neurosurgery, 2135
  nerve injury with, 1159–1160
Latex allergy, 919, 1092, 1093, 3161–3162
Laudanosine, 509, 510f
  cerebral physiology and, 831
Laurie, R., 21
Lavage, bronchopulmonary, 1918–1920, 1918f,
      1919t
Lavoisier, Antoine-Laurent, 4–5, 5f
Läwen, Arthur, 27
LD50 (lethal dose), 95–96, 96f
Leak tests
  low-pressure, 307–309, 308f, 308t, 309f, 315
  negative-pressure, 309–310, 310f
  oxygen flushing in, 309, 309f
Leake, Chauncey, 17
Lee-White whole blood clotting time, 1973, 1973f
Left atrial function, inhaled anesthetic effects on,
      199–200, 200f, 201f
Left atrial pressure
  in renal function monitoring, 1494
  paradoxical air embolism and, 2141
Left bundle branch block, 1406t, 1407–1408, 1408f
Left ventricle
  afterload of, 725–726, 725f
    inhaled anesthetic effects on, 197–198, 198f
  compliance of, 728
  contractility of, transesophageal echocardiography
      for, 1376
  diastolic function of
    inhaled anesthetic effects on, 195–196, 195f,
        196f
    left ventricular end-diastolic pressure and, 1321,
        1321t
    nitrous oxide effects on, 212–214, 213f
  diastolic pressure-volume relationship of,
      1296–1297, 1296f
  dysfunction of
    after cardiopulmonary bypass, 1990–1991
    in lung disease, 1856
    inhaled anesthetic effects on, 193–194, 193f,
        194f, 202
    left ventricular end-diastolic pressure and, 1321,
        1321t
    xenon and, 215, 216f
  filling of, 1320–1323, 1320f, 1321f, 1322t, 1376,
      1377f
  fractional area change of, 1376
  function of, 725–728, 725f–727f
  in congenital heart disease, 2011–2012, 2012f
  normal pressures of, 1297t
  peak instantaneous pressure decline in, 728
  preload of, 1318–1320, 1318f, 1319f, 1326–1327,
      1376
  structure of, 724–725, 725f
  thickness of, 726
  wall motion abnormalities of, intraoperative
      monitoring of, 2079
Left ventricular-arterial coupling, inhaled anesthetic
      effects on, 196–197, 197f
Left ventricular end-diastolic area, in renal function
      monitoring, 1494

Left ventricular end-diastolic pressure
  overestimation of, 1322–1323, 1322t
  pulmonary artery wedge pressure and, 1320–1323,
      1320f, 1321f, 1321t, 1322t, 1323t
  underestimation of, 1321–1322, 1321t
Left ventricular filling pressure, 1376, 1377f
Leg, surgery on, 2421–2422
Legal aspects, 3175–3194. See also End-of-life care;
      Ethics; Informed consent.
Length, 1192
Leroy, J., 39
Lesch-Nyhan syndrome, 1044–1045
LET (lidocaine-epinephrine-tetracaine), 589–590, 590t
Lethal dose, 95–96, 96f
Leukemia, in children, 2869–2870
Leukocytosis, oxygen consumption in, 1446
Leukopenia, mustard gas and, 2510
Leukoreduction, 1821
Leukostasis, in children, 2869
Leukotrienes, pulmonary vascular resistance and,
      685t, 686
Levalbuterol, 2817t
Levallorphan, structure of, 382t
Levobupivacaine
  during labor, 2323
  for epidural anesthesia, 1674t, 1675
  for pediatric regional anesthesia, 1728, 1728t
  for spinal anesthesia, 1661t, 1667
Levorphanol, 380t, 382t, 417
Levothyroxine, 1048
Lidocaine, 24, 575t
  biotransformation of, 592
  cardiovascular toxicity of, 594–595, 594t
  cerebral metabolic rate and, 825
  duration of action of, 584
  during labor, 2323
  electrophysiologic effect of, 580–581, 580f
  in awake intubation, 1642
  in cardiac arrest, 2938
  in chronic pain, 2770
  in endotracheal intubation, 1647
  in epidural anesthesia, 588–589, 588t, 1674t, 1675
  in liposuction, 591
  in nerve block, 587–588, 587t, 588t
  in neuropathic pain, 591
  in pediatric ICP increase, 2857
  in pediatric life support, 2947t
  in pediatric regional anesthesia, 1723, 1723t,
      1724, 1728t
  in spinal anesthesia, 589, 589t, 1661t, 1665–1666
  infiltration of, 586–587, 586t
  intracranial pressure effects of, 825
  intravenous, 587
    postoperative meperidine requirements and,
        1661, 1661f
  neural toxicity of, 597
  peripheral vascular effects of, 594
  pKa of, 574, 574f
  potency of, 576t
  structure of, 573–574, 574f, 575t
  tissue distribution of, 592, 592t
  topical, 589–590, 590t
Life support, basic, 2923–2929. See also
      Cardiopulmonary resuscitation.
  airway control and ventilation in, 2923–2925
  automated external defibrillator for, 2928–2929
  chest compression in, 2925–2926, 2925f, 2926f
  in children, 2941–2942, 2941t
  monitoring for, 2927–2928, 2928t
Ligamentum flavum, 1656, 1656f, 1657f, 1657t
Light, 1212–1215
  Beer-Lambert law of, 1212–1213, 1212f
  principles of, 1212
  Raman scattering of, 1215
Light reflex, 2996, 2997t
Light therapy, 3062
Limb-girdle muscular dystrophy, 535, 535t, 536f,
      1099
  anesthesia in, 536–537
Link-25 proportioning system, for anesthesia
      machines, 281, 281f, 283
Lipid(s)
  hepatic metabolism of, 748
  in intravenous alimentation, 2866, 2867t
  in parenteral nutrition, 2908, 2912t, 2913
  membrane, inhaled anesthetic action at,
      118–120, 119f
Lipogenesis, in sepsis, 2903–2904
Lipophilicity
  of inhaled anesthetics, 115–117, 115f, 115t
  of local anesthetics, 574, 579

Liposuction
  fluid management in, 1794–1795
  lidocaine in, 591
Liquid crystals, for temperature monitoring, 1217
Liquid ventilation, in children, 2851
Liston, Robert, 15
Lithium
  electroconvulsive therapy and, 2654
  in syndrome of inappropriate secretion of
    antidiuretic hormone, 1053
  neuromuscular blockade and, 517
Lithium dilution technique, for cardiac output
    monitoring, 1337–1338
Lithotomy position, 1155, 1157f
  nerve injury with, 597, 1157f, 1158–1159, 1159f
Lithotripsy, 2609, 2617
  extracorporeal, 2195–2197, 2196f. See also
    Extracorporeal shock wave lithotripsy.
  in pacemaker patient, 1426
  laser, 2194
Liver, 743–766
  acinus of, 744–745, 747f
  age-related changes in, 100, 2438
  anatomy of, 743, 744f
  anesthetic effects on, 2209–2212, 2210f, 2211f
  ATP-binding cassette transport proteins of, 751
  bile metabolism by, 748–749
  bilirubin metabolism in, 749–750
  blood flow in, 743–744, 745f, 746f
    angiotensin II effect on, 747
    autoregulation of, 745
    buffer response regulation of, 745–746
    direct measurement of, 756
    drug effects on, 752, 752t, 753t
    epinephrine effect on, 747
    extrinsic regulation of, 746
    glucagon effect on, 747
    humoral regulation of, 746f, 747
    indicator dilution measurement of, 756
    intrinsic regulation of, 745–746
    local anesthetics and, 592
    metabolic regulation of, 745
    neural regulation of, 746
    tests of, 756
  carbohydrate metabolism by, 747–748
  cirrhosis of, 760–763, 763f, 2217–2218, 2217f,
    2218f. See also Cirrhosis.
  coagulation factor synthesis by, 749
  cryotherapy for, 2224
  cytochrome P-450 of, 750–751
  development of, 2863
  disease/injury of, 757–765, 1110–1111
    anesthetic drugs effects and, 2212–2214, 2214f
    antibodies in, 759
    apoptosis in, 757, 759
    cholestatic, 763–765, 764t
    cirrhotic, 760–763, 763f. See also Cirrhosis.
    drug-induced, 758–759, 2221t
    during transplantation, 758
    ethanol-induced, 759–760
    glutathione system in, 757–758
    halothane-induced, 18, 240–243, 242t, 243f,
      244f, 245t, 759, 1111
      assays for, 247–248, 247t
      in children, 243, 2373–2374
      risk factors for, 246–247
    herb-induced, 2222t
    hypoxia and, 760
    in alcoholism, 759–760
    infectious, 758
    ischemia in, 758
    necrosis in, 757
    neuromuscular blockade and, 529–530, 529t
    oxidative stress in, 757–758
    postoperative, 2214–2219, 2217f, 2218f
    preoperative laboratory screening for, 2213f,
      2214–2215, 2220, 2222–2223
    xanthine dehydrogenase in, 758
    xanthine oxidase in, 758
  drug clearance in, 70–74, 71f–74f
  drug metabolism in, 70–71, 71f, 72f, 750–752
    determinants of, 751–752
    pharmacokinetics of, 752, 752t, 753t
    phase 1 reactions in, 750–751
    phase 2 reactions in, 751
    phase 3 reactions in, 751
  endocrine function of, 750
  endotoxin injury to, 758
  erythropoiesis in, 749–750
  evaluation of, 752–757
    biochemical, 753–756, 753t

Liver (Continued)
  evaluation of (Continued)
    blood flow measurement in, 756
    clinical, 752–753
    quantitative, 756
    radiologic, 756–757
  failure of. See Liver failure.
  fatty, 2216–2217
  function of, 1110
  halothane-induced injury to, 240–243, 242t, 243f,
    244f, 245t, 759, 1111
    assays for, 247–248, 247t
    in children, 243, 2373–2374
    risk factors for, 246–247
  hemoglobin metabolism in, 750
  hormone metabolism in, 750
  immune function of, 750
  in hemorrhagic shock, 2460
  in malignant hyperthermia, 1180
  inhaled anesthetic effects on, 2209–2212, 2210f,
    2211f
  inhaled anesthetic toxicity to, 231–248. See also
    specific inhaled anesthetics.
    assays for, 247–248, 247t
    risk factors for, 246–247, 247t
  inhaled anesthetic uptake by, 133–134, 133t
  intravenous anesthetic effects on, 2212
  Kupffer cells of, 750
  lactate metabolism by, 2890
  lipid metabolism by, 748
  maturation of, 2370
  microcirculation of, 744–745, 747f
  necrosis of, 757
  neuraxial anesthetic effects on, 2212
  opioid effects on, 398
  protein metabolism in, 747
    in sepsis, 2901–2903, 2902f, 2902t, 2903f
  radiology of, 756–757
  reactive oxygen species in, 757–758
  reperfusion injury of, 758
  resection of, 2224
    anesthesia in, 2224
    for liver donation, 2235–2237, 2236f
  stellate cells of, 750
  transplantation of, 2235–2237, 2236f, 2245–2253,
    2251f. See also Liver transplantation.
Liver failure, 2246
  fluid therapy in, 1791–1792
  hemostatic abnormalities in, 2248
  in children, 2864
  opioid effects and, 408, 408f
  pathophysiology of, 2247–2248
  postoperative, 2218–2219
    acute hepatitis and, 2216
    cardiothoracic surgery and, 2219
    obstructive jaundice and, 2220
    prevention of, 2220, 2222–2223
    surgical procedure and, 2218–2219
  total parenteral nutrition in, 2915–2916
Liver transplantation, 2235–2237, 2236f, 2245–2253,
    2251f
  ABO matching in, 2246
  anastomoses in, 2251f, 2252
  anesthesia after, 2253
  anesthetics in, 2249, 2250
  blood products in, 2249, 2250
  care after, 2252–2253
  coagulation monitoring in, 2250
  contraindications to, 2246
  exploratory laparotomy after, 2253
  glucose monitoring in, 2250
  hepatic injury during, 758
  hypocalcemia with, 1813
  immunosuppression for, 2249–2250
  in children, 2865
  indications for, 2246
  infracaval interposition technique in, 2251–2252,
    2251f
  intraoperative management in, 2249–2252, 2251f
  living donor for, 2235–2237, 2236f
  MELD risk score in, 2246
  metabolic acidosis with, 1782
  organ for, 2245, 2246
    harvest of, 2233
    preservation of, 2234
  orogastric/nasogastric tube in, 2249
  pain control after, 2253
  piggyback technique in, 2251
  preoperative evaluation in, 2248
  reperfusion phase of, 2251
  stages of, 2250–2252, 2251f

Liver transplantation (Continued)
  venous-venous bypass in, 2250–2251
Living will, 3183
Livingstone, David, 10
Local anesthetics, 573–599. See also specific
    anesthetics.
  absorption of, 591–592
  acidosis and, 593, 596
  active form of, 579–580
  age-related factors and, 592
  allergic-type reaction with, 596–597
  binding site for, 581, 582f
  biotransformation of, 592
  blood levels of, 591
  carbonation of, 585
  cardiovascular system toxicity of, 593–596, 594t
  CC(cardiovascular collapse)/CNS ratio of, 594
  central nervous system toxicity of, 593
  chemistry of, 573–574, 574f, 575t, 576t
  clinical pharmacology of, 583–586
  concentration of, 574, 576
  continuous infusion of, 598
  differential sensory/motor blockade by, 584
  distribution of, 592, 592t
  dosage of, 584–585
  duration of action of, 584
  during labor, 2322–2323
  during pregnancy, 586, 595
  electrophysiologic effects of, 580–581, 580f
  epidural infusion of, 2738
  epinephrine with, 585, 591
  excretion of, 592
  hepatic dysfunction and, 592
  hydrophobicity of, 574, 579, 583
  hypercapnia and, 593, 596
  hypoxia and, 596
  in children, 1755–1756
  in laparoscopy, 2298
  in neuropathic pain, 591
  in newborns, 592
  in spinal anesthesia, 589, 589t
  infiltration, 586–587, 586t
    in children, 1755–1756
    in outpatient, 2609, 2616
  injection site for, 585
  intrapleural administration of, 587–588
  intravenous, 587. See also Regional anesthesia.
  lipophilicity of, 574, 579
  mechanisms of action of, 582–583
  methemoglobinemia with, 596
  mixtures of, 585–586
  muscle effects of, 597–598
  neuromuscular blockade with, 517
  neurotoxicity of, 597
  onset of action of, 584
  peripheral vascular effects of, 594
  pH and, 574, 585
  pharmacodynamics of, 579–583
  pharmacokinetics of, 591–592, 592t
  phasic inhibition by, 581–582, 583f, 584
  pKₐ of, 574, 574f, 576
  potency of, 583
  prolonged-duration, 598
  sodium bicarbonate with, 585
  sodium channel binding of, 580–581, 580f, 582f
  sodium channel susceptibility to, 581–582, 583f
  structure-activity relationships of, 574, 576
  structure of, 573–574, 574t
  systemic administration of, 591
  tachyphylaxis with, 598
  tissue distribution of, 592, 592t
  tissue toxicity of, 597–598
  tolerance to, 598
  topical, 589–591, 590t
  toxicity of, 592–598
    cardiac resuscitation for, 595–596
    systemic, 592–596
  tumescent, 591
  vasoconstrictors with, 585
  ventricular arrhythmias with, 594–595
LocaNerve block, postoperative, 2743–2744
Loewi, Otto, 8
Long, Crawford, 16
Long QT syndrome, 203
Loperamide, 381f
Lorazepam
  cardiovascular system effects of, 323t, 340, 340t
  central nervous system effects of, 339
  cerebral blood flow and, 824
  cerebral metabolic rate and, 824
  during labor, 2318–2319

Lorazepam *(Continued)*
　half-life of, 337–338
　in awake intubation, 1641
　in outpatient premedication, 2596, 2596t
　in pediatric respiratory failure, 2849
　in pediatric seizures, 2858
　induction with, 340t
　maintenance with, 340t
　metabolism of, 335–336
　pharmacokinetics of, 319t, 336–337, 337f
　physiochemical characteristics of, 335, 335t
　respiratory system effects of, 339–340
　sedation with, 340–341, 340t
　side effects of, 342
　structure of, 335, 335f
Lou Gehrig's disease, 534
Low-flow apneic ventilation, 1901
Low-molecular-weight heparin
　epidural catheter risk and, 2422
　in orthopedic surgery, 2426
　spinal hematoma and, 2329
　with epidural analgesia, 2742–2743
　with epidural anesthesia, 1677
Low-pressure leak test, 307–309, 308f, 308t, 309f, 315
Lowenstein, Edward, 36
Lower extremity nerve block, 1695–1704
　anatomy for, 1695–1696, 1696f, 1697f, Plate 11
　femoral nerve, 1697–1699, 1698f, Plates 12 and 20
　lateral femoral cutaneous nerve, 1698f, 1699, Plate 12
　obturator nerve, 1698f, 1699, Plate 12
　peroneal nerve, 1703–1704, 1704f, 1705f, Plate 16
　popliteal fossa, 1701–1703, 1702f, Plate 14
　posterior tibial nerve, 1703, 1703f, Plate 15
　psoas compartment, 1696–1697, Plate 11
　saphenous nerve, 1703–1704, 1704f, 1705f, Plate 16
　sciatic nerve, 1699–1701, 1700f, 1701f, Plate 13
　sural nerve, 1703, 1703f, Plate 15
Luciferase, anesthetic inhibition of, 120
Ludwig's angina, 2544
Lumbar plexus, anatomy of, 1695–1696, 1696f, 1697f, Plate 11
Lumbar plexus block, pediatric, 1743–1746, 1744f–1745f
Lumbar spine
　anatomy of, 8, 9, Plate 6
　surgery on, 2420
Lundy, John S., 21
Lung(s). *See also at* Airway; Pulmonary; Respiratory system; Ventilation.
　abscess of, 1926
　acute injury of, in critical care patient, 2790–2791, 2792f–2793f
　age-related changes in, 2437–2438
　barotrauma to, in hyperbaric oxygen therapy, 2680
　blood flow in, 679–689, 680f, 682f, 683f. *See also* Pulmonary vascular resistance.
　　cardiac output and, 683–685, 684f
　　during one-lung ventilation, 1891–1892, 1891f, 1892f, 1893–1894
　　during thoracic surgery, 1865–1866, 1866f
　　eicosanoids and, 685t, 686
　　endothelin-1 and, 685–686, 685t
　　hormones and, 688, 688t
　　hypoxia and, 686, 687f
　　inhaled anesthetics and, 168–170, 169f
　　lung volume and, 684–685, 684f
　　neural systems in, 687–688
　　nitric oxide and, 685, 685t
　　nonalveolar, 688–689
　　oxygen content and, 701–702, 701f, 702f
　bullae of, 1916–1917
　cancer of. *See* Lung cancer.
　closing capacity of, 694–697, 695f, 696f
　　in children, 2842
　collateral ventilation of, 692
　compliance of, 689–690, 690f, 1465
　　in children, 2842
　cysts of, 1916–1917
　dead space of, 680, 697–698, 697f, 698f
　　hypercapnia and, 714, 714f
　　measurement of, 1442, 1442f
　development of, 2369–2370, 2369f, 2370f
　diffusing capacity of, 1010–1011
　edema of. *See* Pulmonary edema.
　end-stage disease of, 2264–2265
　fetal, 2346–2347, 2347f, 2841

Lung(s) *(Continued)*
　functional residual capacity of, 693–694, 693f, 694f
　　during pregnancy, 2310
　　hypoxemia and, 708–712, 709f, 710f
　　inhaled anesthetic effect on, 161, 174–177, 174f, 175f
　　patient positioning and, 708, 711
　gas exchange in, 697–703, 697f–699f, 1438–1439, 1438f. *See also* Carbon dioxide (CO_2); Oxygen (O_2).
　　carbon dioxide transport and, 703
　　oxygen transport and, 699–703, 699t, 700f–702f, 702t
　gravity effects on, 681–682, 681f
　hygiene therapy for, 2818–2820, 2818f, 2818t, 2817
　immune-mediated disease of, 1091
　in hemorrhagic shock, 2460
　in hepatic disease, 760–761
　in malignant hyperthermia, 1180
　infection of, 1090
　injury to
　　extracorporeal shock wave lithotripsy and, 2196
　　in pediatric cardiopulmonary bypass, 2028t, 2029
　interstitial disease of, 1091
　　in children, 2844
　interstitial fluid of, 680–681, 704–705, 704f, 705t. *See also* Pulmonary edema.
　interstitial pressure of, 680f, 681
　intubation of, 708
　laser plume deposition in, 2579
　lavage of, 1918–1920, 1919f
　microcirculation of, 703–705, 704f, 705t
　mustard gas effect on, 2509, 2510, 2510f, 2522t
　neonatal, 2840, 2841–2842, 2841t
　nitrogen washout of, 1455, 1456f
　norepinephrine inactivation by, 633
　opioid uptake by, 401
　oxygen toxicity to, 2677–2678
　pediatric, 2840, 2841, 2841t
　phosgene damage to, 2510–2513, 2511t, 2512f, 2522t
　pleural pressure of, 681–682, 681f
　preoperative rehabilitation of, 1014
　regional time constants of, 691–692, 691f
　resection of. *See* Thoracic surgery.
　resistance of, 690–691, 1465
　separation of, 1873–1900. *See also* One-lung ventilation.
　stretch receptors of, inhaled anesthetic effects on, 173
　surface-active material of, 2346
　testing of, 999–1025. *See also* Pulmonary function testing.
　three-compartment model of, 1442
　transfusion-related injury to, 1815, 1820
　transplantation of. *See* Lung transplantation.
　trauma to, 2479–2480
　vascular pressures of, 679–681, 680f
　ventilation-perfusion ratio of, 682–683, 682f, 683f
　volumes of
　　airway resistance and, 709–710, 710f
　　functional residual capacity and, 693–694, 693f, 694f
　　pulmonary vascular resistance and, 684–685, 684f
　　respiratory dysfunction and, 707, 707f
　　work of breathing and, 692–693, 692f
Lung cancer, 1091–1092. *See also* Thoracic surgery.
　bronchopulmonary symptoms in, 1850–1851
　bronchoscopic examination in, 1852
　cardiovascular evaluation in, 1854–1856, 1855f, 1855t
　chest pain in, 1850
　chest radiography in, 1851–1852, 1852f, 1852t
　chronic obstructive pulmonary disease in, 1854–1856, 1855f, 1855t
　computed tomography in, 1851
　coronary artery disease and, 1856
　dyspnea in, 1851
　extrapulmonary intrathoracic symptoms in, 1850–1851
　extrathoracic symptoms in, 1851
　histology of, 1848, 1849t
　laboratory tests in, 1851–1854, 1852f, 1852t, 1853t
　left ventricular function in, 1856
　metastatic, 1851

Lung cancer *(Continued)*
　non-small cell, 1091, 1848, 1849t
　paraneoplastic syndromes in, 1851
　preoperative evaluation of, 1849–1856, 1852f, 1852t, 1853t, 1855f, 1855t
　pulmonary function tests in, 1852–1854, 1853t
　pulmonary history in, 1849–1851
　pulmonary physical examination in, 1851
　risk for, 1849–1850
　small cell, 1091–1092, 1848, 1849t
　sputum formation in, 1850
　staging of, 1848–1849, 1850t
　wheezing in, 1851
Lung transplantation, 2237, 2263–2271, 2263t, 2264t, 2266f, 2267f
　anesthesia after, 2271
　cardiopulmonary bypass in, 2266–2267, 2269
　care after, 2270–2271
　hypercapnia during, 2268
　immunosuppression in, 2269
　indications for, 2263
　intraoperative management in, 2267–2270
　intubation for, 2268
　living donor for, 2237
　monitoring during, 2267–2268
　nitrous oxide in, 2269, 2270
　organ harvest for, 2233
　organ matching for, 2263
　organ preservation for, 2234
　pain control after, 2270–2271
　patient position for, 2268
　positive end-expiratory pressure in, 2268–2269
　postoperative mucociliary function and, 164–165
　preoperative evaluation for, 2265–2267
　pulmonary reimplantation response after, 2269–2270
　recipient selection for, 2263–2264, 2264t
　rejection of, 2270
　reperfusion after, 2269–2270
　respiratory failure after, 2270
　technique of, 2266f–2267f
　ventilation after, 2270
　ventilation during, 2268–2269
Lymphatic capillaries, pulmonary, 705
Lysine acetylsalicylate, in succinylcholine-induced pain prevention, 491
Lysozymuria, preoperative, 1493

M

M current, 645
Macewen, Sir William, 37
Macintosh, Sir Robert R., 38f, 39
Macroglossia
　in neonate, 2355
　neurosurgery and, 2137
Macroshock, 3144–3145, 3145f, 3145t
MacWilliam, John, 40
Magendie, François, 9
Magill, Sir Ivan Whiteside, 37, 38, 38f
Magnesium, 1125, 1772–1774
　deficiency of, 1772, 1773, 1773t
　　hypocalcemia and, 1050–1051, 1771–1772
　　testing for, 959, 962t
　for neuroprotection, 2088
　in malignant hyperthermia, 1184
　minimum alveolar concentration and, 109
　nondepolarizing muscle relaxant interaction with, 516–517
　opioid interaction with, 424
　succinylcholine interaction with, 517
Magnesium sulfate
　in postoperative shivering, 1583
　in preeclampsia, 2331–2332
　in status asthmaticus, 2852
　neuromuscular blocking agent interaction with, 516–517
Magnetic objects, magnetic resonance imaging and, 2644
Magnetic resonance imaging, 2618, 2643–2646, 2645f
　anesthesia for, 2645–2646, 2645f
　contraindications to, 1426, 2644
　cranial, 2161–2162
　hazards of, 2644–2645
　in brain death, 2966
　in cortical blindness, 2997–2998
　in ischemic optic neuropathy, 2998
　in pediatric neurologic impairment, 2855

Magnetic resonance imaging *(Continued)*
  limitations of, 2643–2644
  patient monitoring during, 2645–2646
  principles of, 2643
  safety for, 2644–2645
Malaria, transfusion-transmitted, 1818t, 1820
Malignant hyperthermia, 1099, 1169–1186
  anesthesia guidelines and, 1184–1185
  anesthetic triggering of, 1182
  cardiac abnormalities in, 1179–1180
  cardiac arrest in, 1181
  central nervous system in, 1179–1180
  clinical manifestations of, 1180–1182, 1181f,
      1181t
  coagulation abnormalities in, 1180
  creatine kinase and, 1183–1184
  dantrolene for, 1177–1178, 1184
  diagnosis of, 1183
  exercise triggering of, 1182–1183
  genetics of, 1170, 1174–1177, 1175f, 1175t
  heat stroke triggering of, 1182–1183
  hepatic abnormalities in, 1180
  historical perspective on, 1170
  hotline for, 1170
  hyperkalemic periodic paralysis and, 545
  in Charcot-Marie-Tooth disease, 535
  in outpatient setting, 2593
  mimics of, 1181t
  molecular events in, 1171–1173, 1172f
  muscle abnormalities in, 1178–1179
  myotonia and, 543
  nerve system abnormalities in, 1180
  pathophysiology of, 1170–1171, 1171f
  resources on, 1169–1170
  rhabdomyolysis in, 1181–1182
  ryanodine receptor in, 1173–1174, 1176–1177
  RYR1 gene and, 100
  screening for, 1176, 1185–1186
  syndromic associations of, 1183–1184
  temperature monitoring in, 1591, 1591f
  testing for, 959, 961f
  tissue abnormalities in, 1178–1180
  treatment of, 1184
  trismus-masseter spasm in, 1180–1181, 1181f
Mallampati score, 1621
Malnutrition. *See also* Nutrition.
  in elderly patient, 2442, 2443t
Malonyl CoA, 2904
Malrotation, intestinal, 2863
Mammary artery, internal, robotic harvest of, 2564
Mammillary model, 69, 81–82, 82f, 83f
Mammography, 942–943, 944
Managed care organizations, 3192
Mandible
  fracture of, 2459, 2541
  hypoplasia of, 1621–1622
Mandibular nerve block, 1704–1705, 1705f
Mannitol
  acid-base balance and, 1614
  for renal protection, 802
  in infrarenal aortic reconstruction, 2076
  in intracranial aneurysm, 2150
  in kidney transplantation, 2242
  in neurosurgery, 2134
  in pediatric ICP increase, 2857
  in thoracoabdominal aortic reconstruction,
      2088–2089
  in traumatic brain injury, 2472
  neuromuscular blockade and, 518
  renal effects of, 802
Manometry, 1198–1199, 1199f
Mapleson anesthetic circuits, 293–295, 294f
Marfan's syndrome, 2536
Margosa oil, hepatotoxicity of, 2222t
Marijuana, 1118
Martin, channels of, 692
Mask ventilation, 1623–1624, 1623f, 1624f
  historical perspective on, 36–37
  one-handed grip for, 1623, 1623f
  two-handed grip for, 1623, 1624f
Mass (m), 1192
Mass reflex, in spinal transection, 666
Mass spectrometry, 1454
Masseter spasm
  in malignant hyperthermia, 1180–1181, 1181f
  succinylcholine-induced, 491
    in children, 2378–2379
Mastectomy, outpatient, 916–917
Matas, Rudolph, 25f, 26
Mattresses, circulating-water, 1586
Mature minor doctrine, 3182

Maxilla, fracture of, 2541f, 2542
  airway management in, 2459
Maxillary nerve block, 1704–1705, 1705f
Maximal velocity of contraction (Vmax), 727
Maximum expiratory flow rate, 1000f, 1001
Maximum static expiratory pressure, 1002, 1002f
Maximum static inspiratory pressure, 1002, 1002f
Maximum voluntary ventilation, 1002
McDowell, Ephraim, 35
McGill, Ivan W., 37
McGill pain questionnaire, 2315, 2315f
McIntyre, A. R., 32
McKesson, Elmer I., 17
McMechan, Francis Hoffer, 41
Mean, 883, 883t
  standard error of, 883–884
Measurement, 1192–1193, 1192f
Measurement bias, in statistics, 886
Mechanical assist devices, 1991–1993, 1992t. *See also*
      Cardiopulmonary bypass.
Mechanical circulatory support, 1991–1993, 1992t
Mechanical ventilation. *See also* Oxygen therapy.
  acid-base balance and, 1613
  after bullectomy, 1917
  after thoracic surgery, 1904–1906, 1904t, 1905t
  discontinuation of, 1469–1471, 1470t, 1471t
  guidelines for, 1470–1471, 1471t
  high-frequency. *See* High-frequency ventilation.
  hyperbaric oxygen therapy and, 2682–2684, 2683f
  in acute lung injury, 2790–2791, 2792f–2793f
  in acute respiratory distress syndrome, 2790–2791,
      2792f–2793f
  in critical care patient, 2790–2791, 2792f–2793f
  in microlaryngoscopy, 2542
  in obese patient, 1032–1033
  in phosgene exposure, 2511–2512, 2512f
  in spinal cord injury, 2475
  in status asthmaticus, 2853
  infection with, 2796–2797, 2797t
  left ventricular end-diastolic pressure in, 1322,
      1322t
  metered-dose inhalers with, 2817
  monitoring of, 1468–1469, 1469f
  pediatric, 2846–2851, 2848t
    adjunctive pharmacologic therapy in, 2849
    after cardiopulmonary bypass, 2033
    extubation after, 2850
    negative-pressure, 2850–2851
    positive-pressure, 2848–2849, 2848t
    surfactant and, 2851
    weaning from, 2849–2850
  PETCO₂ and, 1460–1461
  positive-pressure, 2820–2828. *See also* Continuous
      positive airway pressure (CPAP); Positive
      end-expiratory pressure (PEEP).
    assist/control (continuous mandatory),
        2822–2823, 2823f
    cardiovascular effects of, 2820–2821
    dual-control modes of, 2824–2825, 2824f,
        2824f, 2825f
    in children, 2848–2849
    intermittent mandatory, 2823, 2823f
      after thoracic surgery, 1904–1906, 1904t, 1905t
      in children, 2848
    modes of, 2821–2825, 2821f–2824f
    noninvasive, 2825–2828, 2826f, 2827f
    physiology of, 2820–2821
    pressure-support, 2823–2824
    pressure-targeted, 2821, 2822f, 2822t
    pulmonary effects of, 2820
    renal effects of, 801–802
    volume-targeted, 2821–2822, 2822t, 2823f
  pulmonary artery catheter monitoring in,
      1317–1318, 1318f
  quality improvement for, 2986
  renal effects of, 801–802
  weaning from, protocol-driven, 2791, 2793–2794,
      2794f
Mechanomyography, 1558
Mechanoreceptors, in ventilation, 171, 174–177,
      174f–177f
Mechlorethamine, 1118
Meckel's diverticulum, 2863
Meclofenamate, renal effects of, 803
Meconium aspiration, 2354–2355
Median, statistical, 883, 883t
Median nerve
  for somatosensory evoked potential monitoring,
      1528
  position-related injury to, 1152t, 1155, 1156f

Median nerve block, 1693, 1693f, 1694f
Mediastinal masses, 1920–1923, 1921f, 1921t
  cardiac compression with, 1922
  in children, 2870
  pulmonary artery compression with, 1922
  superior vena cava syndrome with, 1922–1923
  tracheobronchial tree compression with,
      1921–1922
Mediastinal shift, 1868–1869, 1869f
Mediastinoscopy, 1909–1911, 1910f
  complications of, 1911
Medical necessity, 3192
MedicAlert System, 1620
MEDLINE, 2974–2977, 2975f
  search strategies for, 2976–2977
MedSim patient simulators, 3077t, 3079–3080,
      3080f, 3081f
Mein, A., 9
Meissner plexus, 624
MELAS syndrome, 537
Meltzer, Samuel, 33
Melzack, R., 10
Memory
  age-related declines in, 3062
  depth of anesthesia and, 1236–1239
Mendelssohn, Curtis L., 40
Meningioma, 2139, 2139f, 2145–2146
Meningocele, 2164t
Meningomyelocele, 2395, 2854
Menstruation, painful, 2201
Mental disorders, 1100. *See also* Depression.
Mental nerve block, 1706, 1706f
  pediatric, 1754–1755
Meperidine, 380t
  allergic reactions to, 399
  biliary effects of, 398
  during labor, 2317, 2317f
  during pregnancy, 399
  for children, 2376
  for patient-controlled intravenous analgesia,
      2733–2734, 2733t
  in outpatient anesthesia, 2606
  in shivering, 391, 1583
  neuroexcitation with, 391
  pharmacokinetics of, 401t, 402
  postoperative, 2735t, 2736f, 2737, 2738t
  renal metabolism of, 407
  single-bolus, 410
  single-dose, 2737, 2738t
  sodium channel effects of, 386, 386f
  structure of, 381f
Mephentermine, autonomic nervous system effects
      of, 650
Mepivacaine, 24, 575t
  biotransformation of, 592
  cardiovascular toxicity of, 594–595, 594t
  duration of action of, 584
  in epidural anesthesia, 588–589, 588t, 1674t, 1675
  in nerve block, 587–588, 587t, 588t
  in pediatric regional anesthesia, 1723, 1723t,
      1724, 1728t
  in spinal anesthesia, 1666
  infiltration of, 586–587, 586t
  intravenous, 587
  potency of, 576t
  structure of, 575t
  tissue distribution of, 592, 592t
Meptazinol, 420
Mercaptopurine, 1118
MERRF syndrome, 537
Merrill, Sayre, 32
Mesenteric artery stenosis, 2072
Mesmer, Franz Anton, 11
Meta-analysis, 889. *See also* Statistics.
Metabolic rate. *See also* Cerebral metabolic rate.
  hypothermia effect on, 1588
Metacarpal block, pediatric, 1742, 1742f
Metachromism, 161
Metaproterenol, 652, 2817t
Metaraminol, autonomic nervous system effects
      of, 650
Metatarsal block, pediatric, 1748–1749
Metered-dose inhaler, 2815–2817, 2815f, 2816f, 2817t
  in chronic obstructive pulmonary disease, 1090,
      1090t
Metformin, in diabetes mellitus, 1779
Methacholine, 660
Methadone, 380t, 417
  for patient-controlled intravenous analgesia,
      2733–2734, 2733t
  single-dose, 2737, 2738t

Methamphetamines, 1124
Methanol, toxicity of, 1611
Methemoglobin, pulse oximetry errors and, 1450, 1451t
Methemoglobinemia, local anesthetics and, 596
Methimazole, 1046, 2221t
Methohexital
    cardiovascular system effects of, 333–334
    contraindications to, 334
    distribution of, 332
    dosing for, 333, 333t
    duration of action of, 328t
    epileptogenic properties of, 833
    for children, 333, 2375
    for electroconvulsive therapy, 2655
    hepatic metabolism of, 2213
    in ambulatory anesthesia, 2602t
    in heart disease patient, 334
    in outpatient monitored anesthesia care, 2610
    induction with, 332–333
    lipid solubility of, 331
    manual infusion of, 460t, 462
    metabolism of, 329
    neuroprotection with, 839
    pharmacokinetics of, 319t
    plasma concentration ranges for, 453t
    respiratory system effects of, 334
    seizures and, 833
    side effects of, 333–334
    structure of, 328, 328f
Methotrexate, 1118, 2221t
Methoxamine, 650
Methoxyflurane
    fluoride-associated nephrotoxicity of, 248
    hepatotoxicity of, 246
    left atrial function and, 199–200
    metabolism of, 135
    minimum alveolar concentration of, 107–109, 107f, 108t
    oil-gas partition coefficient of, 115t
    partition coefficients of, 132, 132t
    renal effects of, 801
    structure of, 106f
    tubing uptake of, 142, 143t
N-Methyl-D-aspartate (NMDA) receptors
    antagonists of, for neuroprotection, 2087–2088
    ketamine effects on, 348
Methyldopa, 657–658
    hepatotoxicity of, 2221t
    in kidney failure, 2187
Methylene blue, pulse oximetry errors and, 1451t, 1452
Methylisocyanate, accidental release of, 2510
Methylnaltrexone, 421
Methylparathyrosine, 658
Methylprednisolone
    in septic shock, 806
    in spinal cord injury, 2475
Methylxanthines, preoperative, 1859
METI patient simulator, 3077t, 3081, 3082f
Metoclopramide, 2720
    in outpatient premedication, 2598–2599, 2600
    preoperative, 1860
Metocurine, 493f, 493t, 497t
    autonomic effects of, 511, 511t, 512t
    dosage for, 501t
    elimination of, 506t, 509
    histamine release with, 512
    in elderly patients, 526, 526f
    in kidney transplantation, 2241
    in renal failure, 527, 528t, 2184–2186, 2185t
    metabolism of, 506t, 509
    opioid interactions with, 423
    pharmacodynamics of, 502t
Metoprolol, 653–655, 654t, 657, 1120
Mexiletine, in neuropathic pain, 591
Meyer-Overton rule, 115–117, 115f, 115t, 116f
    exceptions to, 116–117, 116f
Michaelis constant, 71
β_2-Microglobulin, in renal function monitoring, 1500–1501
Micrognathia, 2355
Microlaryngoscopy, 2542
Microshock, 3145–3146
Microsleep, 3057
Microtubules, 734
Micturition, opioid effects on, 398
Midazolam. See also Intravenous anesthetics.
    age-related pharmacokinetics of, 2439, 2439t
    alfentanil interaction with, 450, 453f
    awakening from, 341

Midazolam (Continued)
    C_{50} of, 446–448, 447t
    cardiovascular system effects of, 323t, 340, 340t
    central nervous system effects of, 339
    cerebral blood flow and, 821f
    cerebral metabolic rate and, 821f
    during labor, 2318–2319
    for children, 2376, 2381
    half-life of, 337–338
    hepatic metabolism of, 2213
    in ambulatory anesthesia, 2602t, 2603
    in awake intubation, 1641
    in outpatient monitored anesthesia care, 2610
    in outpatient premedication, 2596, 2596t
    in pediatric respiratory failure, 2849
    in renal failure, 2183–2184, 2184t
    induction with, 340t, 341–342, 341f, 342f
    inhaled anesthetics with, 342
    maintenance with, 340t
    manual infusion of, 460t, 462
    memory effects of, 1238
    metabolism of, 335–336
    metabolites of, 336, 336t
    opioids with, 342, 413, 422
    pharmacokinetics of, 319t, 336–337, 336f
        target-controlled infusion and, 466–468, 468t
    physiochemical characteristics of, 335, 335t
    plasma concentration ranges for, 453t
    propofol with, 341, 342f, 450, 453f
    receptor binding of, 337–339, 337f, 338f
    respiratory system effects of, 339–340, 339f
    sedation with, 340–341, 340t
    side effects of, 342
    somatosensory evoked potential effects of, 1533t
    structure of, 335, 335f
    visual evoked potential effects of, 1533t
    volume of distribution of, 454t
Middle ear, pressure equilibration in, 2679–2680
Midgut volvulus, 2863
Midhumeral block, 1693
Midlatency auditory evoked potentials, in anesthetic depth monitoring, 1258
Migraine headache, 1096
Milrinone
    in children, 2837, 2837t
    in pediatric left ventricular dysfunction, 2032
    in pediatric shock, 2836
Mineralocorticoids, 1036–1037
    deficiency of, 1039
    excess of, 1038
Miniature end-plate potentials, 862
Minimum alveolar concentration, 107–109, 107f, 108f, 108t, 2438
    catecholamine effects on, 102
    depth of anesthesia and, 1239–1241, 1240f, 1241t
    lipid solubility and, 115, 115f
    movement response and, 1239–1241, 1240f, 1241t, 1243f
Minor, informed consent by, 3182
Minute ventilation, 1465
    anesthetic depth and, 706, 706f
    $Paco_2$ and, 1442, 1447, 1447t
Miotics, 1126v
Mitochondrial myopathy, 537
Mitomycin C, oxygen toxicity and, 2677–2678
Mitral regurgitation, 1962–1963, 1962t, 1963f
    ejection fraction in, 1963
    left ventricular end-diastolic pressure in, 1322t, 1323
    pulmonary artery catheter monitoring in, 1312–1314, 1313f, 1313t
    transesophageal echocardiography in, 1381, 1382t, 1383, 1383f, 1384, Plate 33–4
Mitral stenosis, 1959–1961, 1961f
    left ventricular end-diastolic pressure in, 1322t, 1323
    mitral valve area in, 1960–1961, 1961f
    pulmonary artery catheter monitoring in, 1314, 1315f
    thromboembolism in, 1961
    transesophageal echocardiography in, 1380–1381, 1381f, 1382f, 1384, Plate 33–3
Mitral valve, 1960–1961
    calcification of, 2437
    robotic surgery on, 2563–2564, 2563f, 2563t
Mitral valve prolapse, 1079, 1962–1963, 1963f
Mivacurium, 493t, 494, 494f, 497t
    autonomic effects of, 511, 511t, 512t
    dosage for, 501t
    elimination of, 506t, 508–509, 511
    for children, 526, 2379, 2380t

Mivacurium (Continued)
    for tracheal intubation, 503–505, 503f, 504t
    half-life of, 74
    hepatic metabolism of, 2214
    hepatobiliary disease and, 529–530, 529t
    histamine release with, 512
    hypotension with, 512, 513f
    in outpatient anesthesia, 2607
    in renal failure, 2184–2186, 2185t
    maintenance dose of, 515
    metabolism of, 506t, 508–509, 508f
    opioid interactions with, 423
    pharmacodynamics of, 500t, 502t
    recovery from, 521–522, 521f
    renal failure and, 528–529, 528t
Mixed expired gas analysis, 1442, 1442f
Mixed venous oximetry, 1331–1332
Mixed venous oxygen monitoring, 1453, 1453f
Mode, 883, 883t
Moerch, E. Trier, 35
Molecular adsorbents recirculating system, in end-stage liver disease, 2247
Molecular pharmacology, 93–95, 94t
Monitored anesthesia care, in outpatient procedures, 2609–2611
Monitoring, 1191–1217
    acid-base balance, 1599–1614. See also Acid-base balance.
    anesthetic analyzer for, 1213, 1213f
    arterial blood pressure, 1201, 1202f, 1268–1286. See also Arterial blood pressure.
    balance-of-pressure flow meter for, 1204–1205, 1204f, 1205f
    capnography in, 1213, 1213f, 1455–1462. See also Capnography.
    cardiac output, 1327–1331, 1327t, 1329t. See also Cardiac output, monitoring of.
    cardiovascular, 1265–1344. See also Cardiovascular monitoring.
    central venous pressure, 1201, 1286–1327. See also Central venous pressure monitoring.
    definition of, 1192
    dynamic pressure measurement for, 1199–1201, 1199f–1201f
    echocardiography for, 1208
    electric measurement for, 1208–1212, 1208f–1211f
    electrocardiography for, 1210–1211, 1211f
    electroencephalography for, 1211, 1513–1525. See also Electroencephalography.
    flow measurement for, 1202–1205, 1203f–1205f, 1203t
    in hyperbaric oxygen therapy, 2680
    in postanesthesia care unit, 2706–2707
    in thoracic surgery, 1861–1864, 1862t
    light measurement for, 1212–1215, 1212f–1214f
    liquid crystals for, 1217
    manometry for, 1198–1199, 1199f
    measurement for, 1192–1193, 1192f
        accuracy of, 1193, 1194f
    neurologic, 1511–1544, 2142. See also Neurologic monitoring.
    neuromuscular, 1551–1566. See also Peripheral nerve stimulation.
    pediatric, 2392–2393
    percussion for, 1206–1207
    Pitot tube for, 1204, 1204f
    postoperative, anesthesia-related mortality and, 916
    pressure measurements for, 1196–1201, 1198f–1202f
    pulmonary artery pressure, 1301–1327. See also Pulmonary artery catheter monitoring.
    pulse oximetry in, 1213–1215, 1214f. See also Pulse oximetry.
    renal, 1493–1506, 1494t. See also Kidney function, monitoring of.
    respiratory, 1437–1474. See also Respiratory monitoring.
    sensory evoked potentials for, 1525–1537. See also Brainstem auditory evoked potentials; Motor evoked potentials; Somatosensory evoked potentials; Visual evoked potentials.
    signal-processed pressure measurement for, 1201, 1202f
    signal processing for, 1193–1196, 1195f–1197f
    sound measurement for, 1205–1208, 1205f–1207f
    static pressure measurement for, 1198–1199, 1199f
    stethoscope for, 1206
    temperature, 1216–1217, 1216f, 1590–1591, 1591f
    thermistors for, 1216–1217

Monitoring *(Continued)*
thermodilution for, 1203, 1222–1223
thermometers for, 1216
ultrasound for, 1207–1208, 1207f
vane spirometer for, 1205, 1205f
venous pressure for, 1286–1327. *See also* Central venous pressure monitoring.
Venturi tube for, 1203, 1204f
Monoamine oxidase inhibitors, 634, 658, 1122–1123
drug/food interactions with, 658
electroconvulsive therapy and, 2654
ephedra interaction with, 609
opioid interactions with, 423
Monoethylglycinexylidide test, 756
Monosialotetrahexosylganglioside, in spinal cord injury, 2475
Mood, sleep deprivation and, 3057
Mood-altering drugs, 1122–1124
Moore, Francis D., 21
Morgagni, Giovanni Battista, 12
Morphine, 19, 380t. *See also* Addiction.
age-related pharmacokinetics of, 2439, 2439t
allergic reactions to, 399
cardiac myocyte effects of, 386
cerebral blood flow and, 821f, 822–823
cerebral metabolic rate and, 821f, 822–823
during pregnancy, 399
endocrine effects of, 396–397
for children, 2376
for patient-controlled intravenous analgesia, 2733–2734, 2733t
hepatic metabolism of, 401–402, 402f
in cirrhosis, 2212–2213
high-dose, 414f
hormonal effects of, 395–396
in outpatient anesthesia, 2606
in pediatric regional anesthesia, 1724–1725, 1725t, 1728–1729
in renal failure, 2183
in trauma, 2484
inotropic effects of, 394
intranasal, 417
myocardial ischemia and, 395, 395f
nalbuphine after, 420, 420f
pharmacokinetics of, 401–402, 401t, 402f
cardiopulmonary bypass and, 408–409
liver failure and, 408
renal failure and, 407, 407f
postoperative, 2735t, 2736f, 2737, 2737t, 2738t
rectal, 417
respiratory effects of, 392–393, 394f, 1472
sex-related response to, 387
single-dose, 2737, 2737t, 2738t
structure of, 382f
tolerance to, 397
transmucosal, 416, 416f
Morphine-6-glucouronide, 418
Morphinone, 380t
Morris, Lucien, 34–35
Mortality
anesthesia-related, 914–915, 919t. *See also* Anesthesia-related risk.
ASA physical status classification and, 902, 902f, 906, 907t
BIS index and, 1256
cardiovascular disease and, 908–909
in geriatrics, 914
in obstetrics, 909–912, 911t, 912f
in outpatient surgery, 902–903, 903f, 916–917
in pediatrics, 912–914, 913t, 914f
indices for, 907–908, 907f
intraoperative, 903–904, 904t
long-term, 905–906
patient factors in, 906–909, 907f, 907t
postoperative monitoring and, 916
studies of, 893–902, 894t, 895f
ACCS, 904–905, 905t, 906f
after 1980, 899–902, 899t, 900t, 901t, 902f, 902t
before 1980, 897–899, 897t
CEPOD, 901–902, 901t, 902t
computer analysis for, 904
data for, 896–897
design of, 894–897
intraoperative, 903–904, 904t
problems in, 896–897
surgical factors in, 915
risk for, 928, 928t, 929f
without anesthesia, 897
Morton, A. W., 26
Morton, William T. G., 4, 14, 14f, 15f, 16

Morvan's syndrome, 543
Motor block, with epidural analgesia, 2740
Motor evoked potentials, 1512, 1512t, 1539–1540
anesthetic effects on, 1533t, 1540
in spinal surgery, 2418–2419
Motor neuron disease, 534
Motor unit, 860, 861f
Mountain sickness, 687, 2690–2691
Mouse, inhaled anesthetic study in, 123–125, 124f
Moya, Frank, 43
Moyer, Carl, 21
Mu huang, hepatotoxicity of, 2222t
Mucus, 161–162
decreased flow of, 711–712
endotracheal cuff effect on, 711–712
postoperative bronchial transport of, 162–165, 163f, 164f
Müller, Johannes, 9
Multifocal atrial tachycardia, 2933, 2933f
Multiple-breath nitrogen washout test, 1010, 1010f
Multiple gestation, 2336
Multiple inert gas (MIG) elimination technique, for ventilation-perfusion mismatch, 1443–1444, 1443f
Multiple sclerosis, 533–534, 1096
Murad, Ferid, 9
Murmurs, 1078t
Murrell, William, 9
Muscarinic antagonists, 660–661, 660t. *See also* Atropine; Glycopyrrolate; Scopolamine.
Muscarinic drugs, 618
Muscle(s)
acetylcholine effects on, 628
anesthetic toxicity to. *See* Malignant hyperthermia.
biopsy of, in malignant hyperthermia, 1185
catabolism of, in sepsis, 2897–2901, 2898f, 2899f
contracture testing of, in malignant hyperthermia, 1185–1186
excitation-contraction coupling in, 1170–1174, 1171f, 1172f
illness-related weakness of, 873
in hemorrhagic shock, 2460
in malignant hyperthermia, 1178–1179
inhaled anesthetic uptake by, 134
local anesthetic effects on, 597–598
neonatal, 2349, 2349t
nerve contact of, 860–861, 861f
opioid-induced rigidity of, 390–391, 391t
succinylcholine-induced fasciculations of, 874
succinylcholine-induced pain in, 491
Muscle-blood coefficient, of inhaled anesthetics, 132t, 133
Muscle relaxant(s), 481–547
cerebral blood flow and, 831–832, 2131
depolarizing, 486–492. *See also* Succinylcholine.
drug interactions with, 514–518, 516f
economics of, 546–547
hepatic metabolism of, 2213–2214
historical perspective on, 30–33, 482
in brain injury, 2472
in Charcot-Marie-Tooth disease, 534–535
in children, 525–526, 525f, 2378–2380, 2380t
in critically ill patient, 530–533, 531t, 532t, 533t
in elderly patient, 526–527, 526f, 2439
in electroconvulsive therapy, 2655–2656
in Guillain-Barré syndrome, 534
in hepatobiliary disease, 529–530, 529t
in ICU patient, 530–533, 531t, 532t, 533t
in motor neuron diseases, 534
in multiple sclerosis, 533–534
in myasthenia gravis, 101
in obese patient, 527, 1033
in outpatient anesthesia, 2607
in pediatric ICP increase, 2857
in pediatric respiratory failure, 2849–2850
in renal failure, 527–529, 528t, 2184–2186, 2185t
in trauma patient, 2457–2458, 2472
intraocular pressure effects of, 2532
mechanism of action of, 482–484, 483f, 867–868, 867f
monitoring of, 484–486, 484f, 485f, 487t, 1551–1556. *See also* Peripheral nerve stimulation.
nondepolarizing, 492–514, 493t
additive interactions of, 514–515
adverse effects of, 511–514, 511t, 512t, 513f, 546–547
allergic reactions with, 514
antagonists of. *See* Anticholinesterases.
antibiotic interaction with, 516

Muscle relaxant(s) *(Continued)*
nondepolarizing *(Continued)*
anticonvulsant interaction with, 517
asymmetric mixed-onium chlorofumarates as, 493t, 495, 496f, 509
autonomic effects of, 511, 511t, 512t
azathioprine interaction with, 518
benzylisoquinolinium compounds as, 492–494, 493f, 493t, 494f, 508–509, 508f, 510f. *See also specific benzylisoquinolinium compounds.*
bisquaternary tropinyl diester derivatives as, 493t, 495, 496f
bradycardia with, 513
calcium effects on, 517
cerebral blood flow and, 831
clinical use of, 501
combinations of, 514–515
costs of, 546–547
critical illness myopathy and, 531–532
critical illness polyneuropathy and, 532
dantrolene interaction with, 518
diuretic interaction with, 517–518
dosage guidelines for, 501–503, 501t, 502t
drug interactions with, 514–518, 516f
dysrhythmias with, 513
economic considerations and, 546–547
elimination of, 505–511, 506f, 507f, 508f, 510t
histamine release with, 511–512
hypotension with, 512
in burn injury, 530, 530t
in Charcot-Marie-Tooth disease, 534–535
in critically ill (ICU) patient, 530–533, 531t, 532t, 533t
in elderly patients, 526–527, 526f
in Guillain-Barré syndrome, 534
in hepatobiliary disease, 529–530, 529t
in ICU patient, 532–533, 533t
in motor neuron diseases, 534
in multiple sclerosis, 533–534
in obese patients, 527
in pediatric patients, 525–526, 525f, 2379–2380, 2380t
in renal failure, 527–529, 528t
inhaled anesthetic interaction with, 515–516, 516f
lithium effects on, 517
local anesthetic interaction with, 517
magnesium effects on, 516–517
mannitol interaction with, 518
mechanism of action of, 867–868, 867f
metabolism of, 505–511, 506f, 507f, 508f, 510t
monitoring of, 484–486, 484f, 485f, 1561–1563, 1562f, 1563f, 1564f
pharmacodynamics of, 498–500, 498f, 499f, 500t
pharmacokinetics of, 498–500, 498f, 499f
phenolic ether derivative as, 493t, 495, 497f, 509
potency of, 497–498, 497t, 498f
quinidine interaction with, 517
recovery from, 518–525, 519f, 875–876
5-second head lift monitoring of, 486, 487t
acid-base status and, 522–523
anticholinesterases for, 519, 521–522, 521f, 523–524, 524t, 875–876. *See also* Anticholinesterases.
antidote drugs for, 876
atropine in, 523
depth of block and, 520, 520f
electrolyte imbalance and, 523
evoked responses in, 1562–1563, 1564f, 1565, 1565t, 1581t
handgrip monitoring of, 486, 487t
in children, 2380, 2380t
magnesium and, 516–517
nausea and, 523
ORG 25969 (γ-cyclodextrin) for, 524–525, 524f, 876
plasma concentration and, 499–500, 499f
rate of, 519–522, 520f, 521f
recommendations for, 522
respiratory function and, 486, 487t
sustained bite monitoring of, 486, 487t
train-of-four stimulation monitoring of, 485–486, 487t
verapamil effects and, 523
volatile anesthetic concentration and, 522
vomiting and, 523
residual, 546–547
respiratory effects of, 513–514, 513f

Muscle relaxant(s) (Continued)
  nondepolarizing (Continued)
    sequences of, 515
    steroid interaction with, 518
    steroidal compounds as, 493t, 494–495, 495f,
        507–508, 507f
    succinylcholine interaction with, 515
    tachycardia with, 512–513
    tamoxifen interaction with, 518
    temperature effects on, 516
    toxiferine diallyl derivative as, 493t, 497,
        497f, 509
    tracheal intubation and, 503–505, 503f,
        504t, 505f
  opioid interactions with, 423
  postjunctional effects of, 482–483, 483f
  prejunctional effects of, 483–484
  succinylcholine as, 486–492. See also
      Succinylcholine.
  train-of-four stimulation monitoring of, 484–486,
      484f, 487t
Muscular dystrophy, 535–537, 535t, 536f, 1099
  anesthesia in, 536–537
Musculocutaneous nerve, position-related injury to,
    1156t
Musculocutaneous nerve block, 1694
Music, 613
Mustard gas, 2509–2510, 2509f, 2510f, 2512–2513
Myalgia, succinylcholine-induced, 491
Myasthenia gravis, 539–540, 540t, 1098
  anesthesia in, 541–543, 541f, 542f
  drug effects in, 101
  neuromuscular blockade in, 541–542, 542f
Myasthenic syndromes, 538–543, 538t, 539f, 540t,
    1098
  anesthesia in, 541–543, 541f, 542f
  congenital, 540–541, 540t
  succinylcholine resistance in, 541–542, 541f, 542f
Mycophenolate mofetil, in organ transplantation,
    2271–2273, 2272t
Mydriatics, 1126t
Myelin, 576, 577t
Myelinization, in children, 1720
Myelomeningocele, 2164t
Myocardial hibernation, 1947t, 1952
Myocardial infarction, 2650
  classification of, 1944, 1949f
  epidural analgesia and, 2742
  history of, 1061–1064, 1062t, 1063t
  in anesthesia-related risk evaluation, 909, 910t
  mechanisms of, 1943–1944, 1944f–1946f
  oxygen supply and demand in, 1944, 1948f
  peripheral vascular surgery and, 2053–2054,
      2054t, 2058–2059, 2059t
  pulmonary artery catheterization in, 1304–1305
  rupture-type, 1944, 1948f
  serum markers after, 1948f
  stress-type, 1944, 1948f
  transient ischemic attack and, 1061
Myocardial ischemia, 1942–1954, 1947t. See also
    Coronary artery disease.
  acute, 1944, 1946–1951, 1948f–1951f
  β-adrenergic receptor antagonists in, 655
  angina with, 1944, 1946–1951, 1948f–1951f
  electrocardiography in, 1404–1406, 1405f, 1405t,
      1406f, 1411–1412, 1411f
  in diabetes mellitus, 1026, 1027f
  inhaled anesthetic effects on, 193, 205–206, 206f,
      207, 208f
  intraoperative, inhaled anesthetics and, 211
  management of, 1946–1951, 1948f–1951f
    β-adrenergic blockers in, 1946–1947
    myocardial oxygen supply and demand in,
        1946, 1948f
    nitrates in, 1947–1951, 1949f–1951f
  mortality with, 1942–1943, 1943f
  opioid effects in, 395, 395f
  perioperative, 1060–1077, 2065–2068, 2065f,
      2066f, 2066t, 2067f
    etiology of, 2065, 2065t
    identification of, 1060–1061
    incidence of, 2065, 2066t
    management of, 2106–2107, 2106f
    monitoring for, 2066–2068
    pathophysiology of, 2066, 2066f, 2067f
  pulmonary artery catheter monitoring in,
      1314–1316, 1315f
  right ventricular, central venous pressure
      monitoring in, 1316
  silent, 1060–1061, 1405, 1951
  ST segment in, 1406, 1411–1412

Myocardial ischemia (Continued)
  sufentanil and, 397
  transesophageal echocardiography in, 1378–1379,
      1379t, 1384
Myocardial perfusion imaging, before peripheral
    vascular surgery, 2059–2061, 2060t,
    2061f
Myocardial preconditioning, 1947t, 1952–1954,
    1953f, 1953t, 1954f
Myocardial protection, 1976–1978, 1977t, 1978f
  inhaled anesthetic-induced, 206–210, 206f, 208f,
      209f
Myocardial stunning, 1947t, 1951–1952, 1977
  inhaled anesthetic effects on, 206–207, 206f
  transesophageal echocardiography of, 1379
Myocardium. See also at Heart; Myocardial.
  air in, in pediatric cardiopulmonary bypass, 2030,
      2030f
  fetal, 2833
  hibernating, 1947t, 1952
  in growth hormone deficiency, 1052
  stunned, 1947t, 1951–1952, 1977
    inhaled anesthetic effects on, 206–207, 206f
    transesophageal echocardiography of, 1379
  trauma to, 2481
Myoclonus, etomidate-related, 355
Myofascial pain, 2772. See also Pain, chronic.
Myofibril, 730
Myoglobin
  anesthetic binding sites of, 120
  renal effects of, 804–805
Myoglobinemia, renal effects of, 804–805
Myonecrosis, clostridial, 2673
Myopathy
  anesthesia-induced. See Malignant hyperthermia.
  of critical illness, 873
Myosin, 733, 733f, 734f
Myotonia
  ion-channel, 543–546, 544t
  potassium-aggravated, 538t, 543, 544t, 545
Myotonia congenita, 538t, 543, 544t
Myotonic muscular dystrophy, 535t, 536, 1099
  anesthesia in, 536–537
Myringotomy, 2549

N

Nadolol, 653, 654–655
Nafcillin, hepatotoxicity of, 2221t
Nail polish, pulse oximetry errors and, 1451t, 1452
Nalbuphine, 418t, 419–420, 420f
  during labor, 2318
  in outpatient anesthesia, 2606
  in patient-controlled intravenous analgesia,
      2733–2734, 2733t
  structure of, 382t
Nalmefene, 382t, 421
Nalorphine, 382t, 418
Naloxone, 36, 420–421
  channel blockade by, 870
  in opioid-addicted patient, 397
  in outpatient anesthesia, 2607
  inhaled anesthetic effects and, 114
  postoperative, 2718
  structure of, 382t
Naltrexone, 421
  channel blockade by, 870
  in opioid-addicted patient, 397
  structure of, 382t
Napping, 3061
Narcosis
  nitrogen, 2669, 2678–2679
  unitary theory of, 114–117, 115f, 115t
Narcotics. See Opioids.
NARP syndrome, 537
Nasal airway, soft, in airway management, 1625
National Guideline Clearinghouse, 2974
National Library of Medicine, 2974–2977, 2975f
National Research Act, 3190
Nausea, 2720–2721
  acupuncture for, 612–613
  after laparoscopy, 2294
  after outpatient anesthesia, 2597–2599, 2597t,
      2614–2615, 2621
  anticholinesterase effects on, 523
  droperidol for, 360
  epidural analgesia and, 2740
  etomidate-related, 354
  middle ear surgery and, 2549

Nausea (Continued)
  neuraxial anesthesia and, 1660
  opioid-related, 398, 399f
NBC agents, 2499–2500. See also Chemical and
    biological warfare agents.
Neck. See also Head and neck; Nose and throat
    surgery.
  examination of, in airway management,
      1622–1623, 1622f
  flexion of, in neurosurgery, 2136, 2137
  pain in, 1096
  trauma to, 2479
Necrosis
  hepatic, 757
  renal
    after infrarenal aortic reconstruction, 2076
    free water clearance in, 789
    in hepatic disease, 761
Necrotizing enterocolitis, in children, 2864
Needles
  for axillary nerve block, 1692
  for epidural anesthesia, 1672–1673, 1673f
  for nerve blocks, 1685–1686, Plates 6 and 7
  for right internal jugular vein cannulation,
      1288–1289, 1288f
  for spinal anesthesia, 1663–1665, 1663f–1666f,
      1669
  historical perspective on, 19–20
  injury with, 919, 3155–3156, 3161
Needlestick injury, 919, 3155–3156, 3161
Neff, William, 32
Negative-pressure leak test, 309–310, 310f
Negative-pressure ventilation, 35, 2850–2851
Neimann, Albert, 22
Neonate. See also Fetus; Infant; Pregnancy.
  acidosis in, 2357–2358, 2357f, 2358f
  acoustic apnea monitor for, 1468
  asphyxia in, 2347–2348, 2348f
  blood gases in, 2354
  breathing by, 2346
  cardiac output in, 2358
  cardiorespiratory physiology of, 2346–2347, 2346f
  cardiovascular system of, 2006–2008, 2007f
  choanal atresia in, 2352
  color of, 2349, 2349t
  congenital anomalies in, 2355. See also Congenital
      heart disease.
  diaphragmatic hernia in, 2355–2356
  ductus arteriosus of, 2347
  esophageal atresia in, 2355
  heart failure in, 2358
  heart rate in, 2348–2349, 2349t
  hypermagnesemia in, 2359
  hypervolemia in, 2348
  hypocalcemia in, 2359
  hypoglycemia in, 2359
  hypovolemia in, 2348, 2358–2359, 2358t, 2359f,
      2359t
  local anesthetics in, 592
  meconium aspiration in, 2354–2355
  micrognathia in, 2355
  muscle tone of, 2349, 2349t
  persistent fetal circulation syndrome in, 2355
  pneumothorax in, 2355
  polycythemia in, 2359–2360
  pulmonary vascular resistance in, 2347
  reflex irritability of, 2349, 2349t
  respiratory effort of, 2349, 2349t
  resuscitation of, 2353–2361
    Apgar score in, 2352–2353
    cardiac massage in, 2360, 2360f
    case study of, 2361–2363
    discontinuation of, 2361
    drugs for, 2360–2361, 2361t
    equipment for, 2349–2351, 2350f, 2351f
    evaluation for, 2351–2353, 2352f, 2352t
    pulmonary, 2353–2356
    tracheal intubation in, 2353–2354, 2353f
    tracheal suctioning in, 2354–2355
    vascular, 2356–2359, 2357f, 2358f, 2358t
    ventilation monitoring in, 2354
  surfactant administration to, 2356
  tracheoesophageal fistula in, 2355
  transient tachypnea of, 2346
  umbilical artery catheterization in, 2356
  umbilical venous catheterization in, 2356–2357
Neostigmine, 519, 520f, 521–522, 521f, 662,
    875–876. See also Anticholinesterases.
  for children, 526, 2380t
  in kidney failure, 2186, 2186t
  in outpatient anesthesia, 2607

Neostigmine (Continued)
  pharmacokinetics of, 523–524, 524t
  succinylcholine interaction with, 492
  temperature and, 516
Nephrectomy, 2197, 2198, 2198t
Nephrolithiasis, in hyperparathyroidism, 1049
Nephron, 777, 778f. See also Kidney(s).
Nephrotic syndrome, 1100
Nernst equation, 578
Nerve(s), 576–579. See also Nerve block(s).
  action potential of, 862–863, 863f
  cholinergic, 618, 618f
  classification of, 618
  conductive physiology of, 577–579, 577t, 579f
  injury to, 1151–1166
    by age, 1151, 1152t
    by gender, 1151, 1152t
    cardiovascular considerations in, 1152
    central venous pressure monitoring and, 1295
    classification of, 1153
    lateral oblique position and, 1160–1162, 1161f,
        1162f
    lateral position and, 1159–1160, 1160f
    lithotomy position and, 1158–1159, 1159f
    neurologic considerations in, 1153–1158, 1154f,
        1156t, 1157f
    orthopedic surgery and, 1163, 1163f, 1164f
    pathophysiologic considerations in, 1152–1158,
        1154f, 1156t, 1157f
    practice advisory on, 1151, 1153t
    prevention of, 1151, 1153t
    prone position and, 1162–1163
    pulmonary considerations in, 1152–1153
    shoulder surgery and, 1163–1164, 1164f
    sitting position and, 1164–1166, 1165f
    somatosensory evoked potentials in, 1154
    supine position and, 1158
    Trendelenburg position and, 1162
    upper extremity, 1154–1155, 1154f
  muscle contact of, 860–861, 861f
  stimulation of. See Peripheral nerve stimulation.
  structure of, 576–577, 576f–578f
Nerve agents, 2504–2509, 2504f, 2505t, 2506t,
    2507f. See also Organophosphates.
Nerve block(s), 1685–1715
  anesthetics for, 587–588, 587t, 588t
  auricular, 2548
  auriculotemporal, 2548
  continuous catheter techniques for, 1713, 1714f
  head and neck, 1704–1710
    accessory nerve, 1707–1708
    cervical plexus, 1706–1707, 1706f, 1707f,
        Plate 4
    glossopharyngeal nerve, 1709
    peribulbar, 1709
    retrobulbar, 1709
    stellate ganglion, 1709–1710, 1709f
    superior laryngeal nerve, 1708, 1708f
    translaryngeal, 1708–1709, 1709f
    trigeminal nerve, 1704–1706, 1705f, 1706f,
        Plates 1 and 2
  historical perspective on, 22–24, 24f
  in ambulatory surgery, 2609
  in chronic pain, 2772–2776
  laryngeal, 2545–2546
  local anesthetic selection for, 1714
  lower extremity, 1695–1704
    anatomy for, 1695–1696, 1696f, 1697f,
        Plate 11
    femoral nerve, 1697–1699, 1698f, Plates 12
        and 20
    lateral femoral cutaneous nerve, 1698f, 1699,
        Plate 12
    obturator nerve, 1698f, 1699, Plate 12
    peroneal nerve, 1703–1704, 1704f, 1705f,
        Plate 16
    popliteal fossa, 1701–1703, 1702f, Plate 14
    posterior tibial nerve, 1703, 1703f, Plate 15
    psoas compartment, 1696–1697, Plate 11
    saphenous nerve, 1703–1704, 1704f, 1705f,
        Plate 16
    sciatic nerve, 1699–1701, 1700f, 1701f,
        Plate 13
    sural nerve, 1703, 1703f, Plate 15
  needle localization for, 1685–1686, Plates 6 and 7
  neurologic complications of, 1714–1715
  ocular, 2529–2531
    complications of, 2529–2531
    peribulbar, 2529
    sub-Tenon, 2529
  postoperative, 2720, 2743–2744

Nerve block(s) (Continued)
  thorax and abdomen, 1710–1712
    celiac plexus, 1711–1712, 1712f
    intercostal nerve, 1710–1711, 1710f
    paravertebral, 1712, 1713f, Plate 10
    tympanic, 2548
  upper extremity, 1686–1695
    anatomy for, 1686, 1687f
    axillary, 1690–1692, 1691f, Plate 5
    infraclavicular, 1690
    interscalene, 1686, 1688–1689, 1688f
    intravenous, 1695
    median nerve, 1693, 1693f, 1694f
    midhumeral, 1693
    musculocutaneous, 1694
    supraclavicular, 1689–1690, 1689f, 1690f,
        Plate 3
    ulnar nerve, 1693–1694
Nerve stimulator testing/therapy, in pacemaker
    patient, 1426
Nesiritide, for renal protection, 800
Neuraxial anesthesia, 1653–1679. See also Caudal
    anesthesia; Epidural anesthesia; Spinal
    anesthesia.
  anatomy for, 1654–1658, 1655f–1659f
  arterial blood pressure with, 1658–1660
  cardiovascular effects of, 1658–1660, 1971
    treatment of, 1659–1660
  contraindications to, 1654
  for obstetric patient, 1677–1678
  gastrointestinal effects of, 1660
  heart rate with, 1658
  heat balance during, 1580, 1580f
  hepatic function and, 2212
  historical perspective on, 24–28, 1653–1654
  indications for, 1654
  nausea with, 1660
  physiologic effects of, 1658–1661, 1661f
  redistribution hypothermia during, 1580, 1580f
  renal effects of, 1660
  respiratory effects of, 1660
  shivering during, 1580–1581
  skin warming during, 1581
  thermoregulation during, 1578–1580, 1578f,
      1579f
    perceived warmth and, 1579, 1579f
  urinary retention with, 1660
  vomiting with, 1660
Neuregulins, 866, 866f
Neurexin, 862
Neuroendocrine stress response, 2730–2731
Neurogenic motor evoked potential, 1539–1540
Neurokinin-1 antagonists, in outpatient
    premedication, 2599
Neuroleptanalgesia, 412–413
Neuroleptanesthesia, 412
Neuroleptic malignant syndrome, 1183
Neurologic disorders. See also Neurologic
    monitoring.
  after nerve blocks, 1714–1715
  postpartum, 2329
  with hyponatremia, 1767
Neurologic examination, in trauma, 2453–2454,
    2454t
Neurologic monitoring, 1511–1544, 1512t, 2142
  cerebral oximetry for, 1542
  electroencephalography in, 1513–1525. See also
      Electroencephalography.
  electromyography for, 1537–1539, 1538f
  in children, 2855, 2855t
  in outpatient procedures, 2611–2612
  in pediatric cardiac surgery, 2018–2019, 2019f
  jugular bulb venous oxygen saturation for, 1542
  motor evoked potentials for, 1533t, 1539–1540
  neurogenic motor evoked potential for,
      1539–1540
  sensory evoked potentials for, 1512–1513, 1512t,
      1525–1537. See also Brainstem auditory
      evoked potentials; Motor evoked
      potentials; Somatosensory evoked
      potentials; Visual evoked potentials.
  transcranial Doppler ultrasonography for,
      1540–1542, 1540f, 1541f
Neurolytic blocks, in chronic pain, 2775–2776
Neuroma, acoustic, 1531, 1537–1538, 1538f
Neuromodulators, 619–620
Neuromuscular blocking agents. See Muscle
    relaxant(s).
Neuromuscular junction, 862–867
  acetylcholine release at, 863–864, 863f, 864f
  action potential at, 862–863, 863f

Neuromuscular junction (Continued)
  electrophysiology of, 866–867, 867f
  morphology of, 860–861, 861f
  neurotransmitter formation at, 862, 863f
  perijunctional zone of, 861, 861f
  storage vesicles of, 863–864, 863f
Neuromuscular transmission, 860–862
  morphology of, 860–861, 861f
  quantal theory of, 861–862
Neuromyotonia, acquired (Isaacs' syndrome), 543
Neurons. See also Nerve(s).
  apoptosis of, in cerebral ischemia, 834–837,
      835f, 838f
  enteric, 624
Neuropathic pain, 2763–2778. See also Pain, chronic.
Neuropathy. See Nerve(s), injury to.
Neuropeptide, in cardiac function, 737t
Neuropeptide Y, 620, 620f
Neuroplegia, 412
Neuroprotection, 837–842, 838t
  barbiturates in, 839, 2087
  calcium channel blockers in, 840, 2087
  carbon dioxide tension and, 840–841
  cerebral perfusion pressure and, 840
  cerebrospinal fluid drainage in, 2087
  corticosteroids in, 2087
  etomidate in, 840
  glucose levels and, 841–842
  hemodilution in, 818, 842
  hypothermia in, 841, 841t, 2087
  isoflurane in, 839–840
  N-methyl-D-aspartate receptor antagonists in,
      2087–2088
  pH and, 842
  propofol in, 840
Neuroradiology, 2161–2162
  interventional, 2646–2648
    anesthesia for, 2647–2648
Neurosurgery, 2127–2165
  anticonvulsants in, 2134
  blood pressure in, 2133, 2133f
  corticosteroids in, 2146
  diuretics in, 2134
  emergence after, 2144–2145
  fluid management during, 2143–2144
  hypertension during, 2145
  hyperventilation in, 2132–2133, 2133f
  hypocapnia-induced cerebral blood flow reduction
      in, 2132–2133, 2133f
  hypothermia during, 2144
  in arteriovenous malformations, 2151–2152
  in head injury, 2152–2159, 2152t, 2153f, 2154f.
      See also Head injury.
  in intracranial aneurysm, 2146–2152, 2146t,
      2147t, 2148f
  in pituitary tumors, 2158–2159, 2158t
  in posterior fossa disease, 2157–2158, 2157t
  in seizures, 2159–2161
  in shunt insertion, 2162–2163
  in supratentorial tumors, 2145–2146
  intra-arterial pressure monitoring during, 2142,
      2143t
  intracranial pressure in, 2127–2131, 2128f, 2129f,
      2129t, 2130f, 2130t, 2131t
  lateral positioning for, 2135
  macroglossia after, 2137
  mannitol in, 2134
  monitoring during, 2142, 2143t
  nitrous oxide elimination in, 2142
  Paco2 in, 2131–2133, 2133f
  paradoxical air embolism during, 2141–2142
  patient positioning for, 2134–2138, 2135t
  pediatric, 2163, 2164t
  pneumocephalus with, 2138, 2138f
  positive end-expiratory pressure in, 2141, 2142
  prone positioning for, 2135–2136
  quadriplegia after, 2137–2138
  rebound swelling in, 2134
  right heart catheter in, 2140–2141, 2141f
  robotic, 2567
  semilateral positioning for, 2135
  sitting positioning for, 2136–2138, 2137f
  stereotactic, 2161
  steroids in, 2133–2134
  supine positioning for, 2135
  transpulmonary air passage in, 2142
  venous air embolism with, 2138–2142, 2139f,
      2140f, 2140t
Neurotransmission, 618–622, 618f–621f
  cerebral blood flow and, 814–815
  channel-blocking drug effects on, 870

Neurotransmission *(Continued)*
  depolarizing muscle relaxant action at, 868–869, 868f, 870–871
  electrophysiology of, 866–867, 867f
  inhaled anesthetic effects on, 111–112, 112f, 869
  ketamine effects on, 869
  nondepolarizing muscle relaxant action at, 867–868, 867f
  procaine effects on, 869
Neutropenia, in children, 2870
Nevirapine, hepatotoxicity of, 2221t
Newborn. *See* Neonate.
Newton (N), 1192
Niacin, hepatotoxicity of, 2221t
Nicardipine, neuromuscular blocking agent interaction with, 517
Nicotine, 618, 645, 662
Nifedipine, 1121–1122, 1122f
  in kidney failure, 2186–2187
Nimodipine, after cardiac arrest, 839
Nissen fundoplication, robotic, 2561–2562, 2562f
Nitrates
  in myocardial ischemia, 1947–1951, 1948f–1951f
  tolerance to, 1949–1951, 1950f, 1951f
Nitric oxide, 629, 630
  in cerebral ischemia, 836
  in hypoxia, 178
  in renal injury, 798
  in renal regulation, 797–798
  inhaled anesthetic effect and, 114
  monitoring of, 1454–1455
  pulmonary vascular resistance and, 165, 685, 685t
  therapeutic, 1454, 2815
    after pediatric cardiopulmonary bypass, 2034
    in children, 2839
Nitric oxide synthase, 685
  in renal regulation, 797–798
  uncoupling of, 1949–1950, 1950f
Nitric oxide synthase inhibitors, inhaled anesthetic effect and, 114
Nitrofurantoin, hepatotoxicity of, 2221t
Nitrogen
  elevated partial pressure of, 2669
  oil-gas partition coefficient of, 115t
  structure of, 106f
  urinary, 2906, 2906t
Nitrogen balance, in sepsis, 2897–2898, 2898f
Nitrogen narcosis, 2669, 2678–2679
Nitrogen washout, 694, 1010, 1010f, 1455, 1456f
Nitroglycerin
  in children, 2837t, 2838
  in kidney failure, 2187
  with aortic cross-clamping, 2077
Nitrous oxide. *See also* Inhaled anesthetics.
  abuse of. *See* Substance abuse.
  after heart transplantation, 2261
  airway resistance and, 161
  BIS index and, 1254–1256
  cardiac electrophysiology and, 214
  central ventilatory effects of, 171, 172f
  cerebral blood flow and, 830–831, 830f, 2130–2131
  cerebral metabolic rate and, 831
  coronary circulation and, 214–215
  depth of anesthesia and, 1244–1245, 1245t
  desflurane with, for children, 2374–2375
  diffusion hypoxia and, 150, 150f
  electroencephalographic effects of, 1518, 1519t, 1520
  embolus of, 141, 142f
  hematologic toxicity of, 256–257, 257f
  hemodynamic effects of, 214
  historical studies on, 17
  hyperbaric oxygen therapy and, 2686
  hypoxic pulmonary vasoconstriction and, 166
  in ambulatory anesthesia, 2604–2605, 2604t
  in closed gas spaces, 140–141, 141f, 143f
  in lung transplantation, 2269, 2270
  in malignant hyperthermia, 1182
  in poorly compliant spaces, 142
  intravitreal injection of, 2533
  left ventricular diastolic function and, 212–214
  memory effects of, 1238
  metabolism of, 236–237, 236f
  middle ear pressure and, 2548–2549
  minimum alveolar concentration of, 107–109, 107f, 108t
  myocardial contractility and, 212–214, 213f
  N-methyl-D-aspartate glutamate inhibition by, 121
  neuromuscular blockade and, 515–516

Nitrous oxide *(Continued)*
  neurotoxicity of, 256–257
  occupational exposure to, 256–257, 3151–3153
  oil-gas partition coefficient of, 115t
  opioids with, 423
  partition coefficients of, 115t, 132, 132t
  recovery from, 147–151, 149f, 150f
  second gas effect and, 135, 136f
  somatosensory evoked potential effects of, 1533t
  structure of, 106f
  systemic circulation and, 215
  teratogenicity of, 259–260
  thermoregulatory response thresholds with, 1575
  tolerance to, 123
  tubing uptake of, 142, 143t
  vasodilating effect of, 831
  venous air embolism and, 2142
  visual evoked potential effects of, 1533t
Nitrous oxide challenge, 141
Nobel, Alfred, 9
Nociceptin (orphanin FQ), 382–383, 387
Nociception. *See* Pain.
Nociceptors, 2729–2730
  inhaled anesthetic effects on, 109–110
Noise, 3054–3055, 3162
Non-operating room anesthesia. *See* Ambulatory (outpatient) anesthesia; Remote locations.
Nonimmobilizers, 116–117, 116f, 122
Noninvasive positive-pressure ventilation, 2486–2487, 2826t, 2827f
Nonresponsiveness, definition of, 1230
Nonsteroidal anti-inflammatory drugs
  hepatotoxicity of, 2221t
  in chronic pain, 2768–2769
  in outpatient premedication, 2597
  in trauma, 2484
  opioid interaction with, 424
  postoperative, 2719–2720, 2734–2735, 2735t
  renal effects of, 803
Norepinephrine
  as cotransmitter, 619, 619f
  cerebral blood flow and, 818–819, 819t
  enteric, 624
  extravasation of, 649
  in cardiac function, 735–737, 736f, 737f
  in children, 2836, 2837, 2837t
  in hepatic failure, 2916
  in malignant hyperthermia, 1180
  in pediatric shock, 2836
  in renal regulation, 791–792, 791f
  in sepsis, 2897
  in septic shock, 806
  in vivo kinetics of, 664
  inactivation of, 633–634
  inhaled anesthetic effects on, 112–113
  inhibitors of, 657–658
  intravenous administration of, 649
  ketamine effects on, 348
  kiss and run release of, 633
  metabolism of, 634, 635f
  nitrous oxide interaction with, 214
  plasma, 663–664
  pulmonary vascular resistance and, 688, 688t
  receptors for, 634–637, 635f, 636t
  release of, 631–633, 632f
  structure of, 647f
  synthesis of, 630–631, 630f
  tissue effects of, 93, 93f
  vesicle storage of, 631
Normal accident theory, 3049–3050, 3050t
Normal distribution, in statistics, 882–884, 883t
Normeperidine, hepatic metabolism of, 2212–2213
Nose, 1617, 2540
  apnea monitor for, 1468
Nose and throat surgery, 2537–2548
  cocaine in, 2547–2548
  in epiglottitis, 2544
  in foreign body removal, 2545
  in Ludwig's angina, 2544
  in peritonsillar abscess, 2544
  in sinus disease, 2540
  in thyroid disease, 2540
  in tonsillitis, 2543–2544
  in trauma, 2540–2542, 2541f
  laryngeal anatomy in, 2537–2539, 2538f
  laryngospasm and, 2538–2539
  laser, 2542–2543
  microlaryngoscopic, 2542
  phenylephrine in, 2548
  stridor and, 2539
  vasoconstrictors in, 2547–2548

Novocor mechanical circulatory support system, 1992, 1992t
5'-Nucleotidase, 753t, 755
Nucleotides, cyclic, inhaled anesthetic effects on, 113–114, 156
Nutrition, 2887–2917
  drug metabolism and, 2914–2915, 2914f
  enteral, 2913–2914, 2914f
    vs. parenteral nutrition, 2907–2908
  in critically ill child, 2865–2867
  in trauma, 2488
  parenteral, 1034–1035, 2905–2907, 2914f
    albumin levels with, 1035, 1035f
    amino acids in, 2908, 2910
    assessment for, 2905
    central catheter for, 2910–2911, 2911t
    complications of, 1035, 2911–2914, 2912t
    drug metabolism and, 2914–2915, 2914f
    energy estimation for, 2905–2907, 2906t, 2907f
    for children, 2389, 2865–2867, 2866f
    gas exchange and, 2906–2907, 2907f
    glucose homeostasis during, 2892–2894, 2894t
    hepatotoxicity of, 2221t
    hypoglycemia and, 2913
    in hepatic encephalopathy, 2915–2916
    in hepatic failure, 2915, 2916
    in neurosurgical patient, 2915
    in renal failure, 2915
    in trauma, 2488
    intraoperative, 2916–2917
    lipids in, 2913
    omega-3 fatty acids in, 2908, 2910
    preoperative check for, 2916–2917
    prescription for, 2907–2914, 2909f–2910f
    requirements for, 2887–2892, 2888f, 2888t
    respiratory complications of, 2913
    serum folate and, 2911
    substrate requirements for, 2908
    vs. enteral nutrition, 2907–2908
    water retention and, 2913

O

Obesity, 1028–1034
  airway obstruction and, 1029
  cardiovascular disease and, 1033–1034
  definition of, 1028, 1029t
  hypoventilation and, 1031–1033
  neuromuscular blockade and, 527
  pain management and, 2748–2749
  positioning in, 1034
  psychological evaluation in, 1034
  pulmonary complications and, 1088
  respiration in, 707, 707f
  sleep apnea and, 1030–1031
  supine position in, 1032
  thromboembolism and, 1033
  venous stasis and, 1033
Obesity-hypoventilation syndrome, 1031–1033
Obidoxime, in organophosphate poisoning, 2508
Observational study, 886. *See also* Statistics.
Obstetric procedures, 2307–2339. *See also* Cesarean section; Pregnancy; Vaginal delivery.
  anesthesia-related risk in, 909–912, 911t, 912f
  hemorrhage with, 2333–2336, 2334f, 2335f
  robotic, 2568
Obstructive sleep apnea
  pain management and, 2748–2749
  pulmonary complications and, 1088
Obturator nerve, position-related injury to, 1155, 1156f
Obturator nerve block, 1698f, 1699, Plate 12
Occult hypoperfusion syndrome, in trauma patient, 2467
Octreotide, in insulinoma resection, 1027
Oculocardiac reflex, 739, 2530
  strabismus surgery and, 2535–2536
Oculopharyngeal muscular dystrophy, 536f
Odom, Charles B., 27
O'Dwyer, Joseph, 37
Office-based anesthesia, 59, 2616–2617. *See also* Ambulatory (outpatient) anesthesia.
Ohm's law, 1209
Oliguria, 1496, 1502–1503, 2187–2188, 2187t, 2188t. *See also* Kidney failure.
Omphalocele, 2395–2396, 2395t
Ondansetron, 2721
  in outpatient premedication, 2598f, 2599, 2615
  isoflurane MAC and, 113

One-lung ventilation, 1873–1900
arterial oxygenation with, 1865–1866, 1866f, 1890–1891, 1890f
blood flow distribution with, 1891–1894
conventional management of, 1894–1895, 1894t
dependent lung positive end-expiratory pressure in, 1894
differential lung positive end-expiratory pressure/continuous positive airway pressure in, 1895f, 1897–1899, 1898f
differential management of, 1895–1899, 1895f, 1897f, 1898f
double-lumen endotracheal tubes for, 1874–1889, 1874f–1876f
chest radiography with, 1882
complications of, 1882–1883, 1883t
contraindications to, 1883
conventional intubation procedure for, 1877–1879, 1878f, 1879f
cuff seal pressure hold with, 1882, 1883f
fiberoptic bronchoscopy with, 1879–1882, 1880f, 1881f, 1882t
selection of, 1876–1877
indications for, 1873–1874, 1873t
inspired oxygen concentration in, 1894
intermittent collapsed lung ventilation in, 1895, 1895f
management of
conventional, 1894–1895, 1894t
differential, 1895–1899, 1895f, 1897f, 1898f
recommendation for, 1899–1900, 1899f
physiology of, 1890–1894, 1890f–1892f
respiratory rate in, 1894–1895
selective dependent lung positive end-expiratory pressure in, 1895–1896, 1895f
selective nondependent lung CPAP in, 1895f, 1896–1897, 1897f
single-lumen endotracheal tube for (bronchial blocker), 1883–1885, 1884f, 1885f, 1885t
independent, 1887–1889, 1887f, 1888f, 1888t
indications for, 1887
just-seal volume and, 1886–1887
limitations of, 1885–1886, 1886t
technique of, 1889–1890
tidal volume in, 1894
Operating room, 57–58
errors in, 3047–3048, 3047f–3049f
management of, 3119–3134
anesthesia service in, 3130–3131
between-case turnover in, 3125–3126, 3126t
conflict resolution in, 3130, 3131t
cost accounting in, 3132–3134, 3133t
daily schedule completion in, 3128–3130, 3129t, 3130f
historical perspective on, 3119–3120
human performance and, 3021–3064. See also Human performance.
information systems for, 3131–3132
medical director for, 3120–3122, 3121f, 3121t
noise levels and, 3162
on-time starts in, 3123, 3125, 3125t
postoperative activities and, 3131
preoperative activities and, 3131
regulatory issues in, 3134, 3134t
scheduling system in, 3122–3123, 3123f, 3124t, 3125t
utilization tracking in, 3126–3128, 3127f, 3127t, 3128t
safety of, 3047–3054, 3151–3164
chemical dependence and, 3164–3170. See also Substance abuse.
communication and, 3052–3054, 3053f
culture of, 3050–3052, 3051t
electrical, 3139–3148, 3141f–3143f. See also Electrical safety.
error causation and, 3047–3048, 3047f–3049f
goals of, 3049, 3049t
high reliability organization theory of, 3050–3052, 3050t, 3051t
incident reporting system for, 3052, 3052t
infection and, 3155–3161, 3157t, 3158
job stress and, 3163–3164
latex allergy and, 3161–3162
noise and, 3054–3055, 3162
normal accident theory of, 3049–3050, 3050t
overwork and, 3162
radiation and, 3153–3155, 3154f
reading and, 3055
risk factor assessment and, 3052
sleep deprivation and, 3055–3059, 3162–3163

Operating room (Continued)
safety of (Continued)
stress and, 3163–3164
team structure and, 3052–3054, 3053f
vs. production, 3051–3052, 3054, 3054t
waste gases and, 3151–3153
Ophthalmic artery, 2992–2994, 2993f
aneurysm of, 2151
Ophthalmic vein, 2994
Ophthalmoscopy, 2996–2997
Opioids. See also Addiction; Intravenous anesthetics and specific opioids.
addiction to, 397, 2746
agonist-antagonist, 418–420, 418t
allergic reactions to, 399
analgesic mechanisms of, 385, 387
anesthetic mechanisms of, 387–388, 388f
antagonists of, 420–421
antishivering effects of, 391–392
baroreception and, 395
benzodiazepine interactions with, 422
biliary effects of, 398
BIS index and, 1254
calcium channel effects of, 423–424
cardiac conduction effects of, 395
cardiac myocyte effects of, 386
cardiogenic reflex and, 395
cardiovascular effects of, 394–396, 395f
cerebral blood flow effects of, 389–390
cerebral metabolic rate effects of, 390
classification of, 380, 380t
computer-controlled infusion of, 405
concentration-effect relationship of, 404–405
context-sensitive half-time of, 404, 404f
controlled-release, 417
coronary circulation and, 395
δ-receptor for, 381, 383t
knockout mouse study of, 386
dependence on, 397
depth of anesthesia and, 1231–1233, 1231f, 1246–1249, 1246f, 1247f, 1247t, 1248f, 1248t
diphenhydramine interaction with, 424
doxacurium interactions with, 423
drug interactions with, 421–424
during labor, 2317–2318, 2317f
during pregnancy, 399
effect site of, 404
electroencephalographic effects of, 388–389, 388f, 389f, 405–406, 1518, 1519t
endocrine effects of, 396–397
endogenous, 382–383
inhaled anesthetic effects on, 114
epidural, 2738–2739. See also Epidural analgesia.
respiratory depression with, 1472–1474, 1473t, 1474t
κ-receptor for, 381, 383t, 385
equianalgesic dosing conversion for, 2747, 2747t
erythromycin interaction with, 424
etomidate and, 422
for analgesia, 410–413, 410t
for children, 2376–2378, 2377f, 2378f
for sedation, 410–413, 410t
gabapentin interactions with, 422–423
gastrointestinal effects of, 398–399, 399f
half-life of, 403–404, 404f
hepatic effects of, 398, 2212–2213
high-dose, 414–415, 414f
hormonal effects of, 395–396
hydrophilicity of, 2737, 2737t
hyperalgesia with, 397
immune effects of, 399–400
in asthma, 392
in balanced anesthesia, 410–411
in chronic pain, 2769–2771, 2769t, 2770t, 2781–2784
in endotracheal intubation, 392
in myocardial ischemia, 395, 395f
in obstetrics, 399
in outpatient anesthesia, 2605–2606, 2606f
in outpatient premedication, 2597
in pediatric cardiac surgery, 2022
in pediatric regional anesthesia, 1724–1725, 1725t, 1728–1729
in renal failure, 2183
in single-agent anesthesia, 414–415, 414f
in total intravenous anesthesia, 413, 413t
in trauma, 2484
inadequate anesthesia with, 1247–1249, 1247t, 1248f, 1248t

Opioids (Continued)
inhaled anesthetic interactions with, 96–97, 97f, 423
inotropic effects of, 394
intracranial pressure effects of, 390
intranasal, 416–417
intraocular pressure effects of, 399
intravenous, 410–415, 410t
agent selection for, 411–412, 412f
postoperative, 2733–2734, 2733t
respiratory depression with, 1473
ketamine and, 422
knockout mouse study of, 385–386
lipid solubility of, 400, 401f
lipophilicity of, 2737, 2737t
magnesium interaction with, 424
MAOI interactions with, 423
metocurine interactions with, 423
midazolam interactions with, 422
mivacurium interactions with, 423
mood altering mechanisms of, 385
μ-receptor for, 381, 383t, 384f, 385
knockout mouse study of, 385–386
muscle relaxant interactions with, 423
muscle rigidity with, 390–391, 391t
nausea with, 398, 399f
neuroexcitation with, 391
neurophysiologic effects of, 387–392, 388f, 389f, 391t
neuroprotective effects of, 390
nitrous oxide with, 423
nonsteroidal anti-inflammatory drug interaction with, 424
pancuronium interactions with, 423
peak effect of, 404, 405f
pharmacokinetics of, 400–406, 400f–406f
acid-base changes and, 409
age and, 406, 406f, 2439, 2439t
body weight and, 406, 407f
cardiopulmonary bypass and, 408–409, 409f
hemorrhagic shock and, 409, 409f, 410f
hepatic failure and, 408, 408f
renal failure and, 406–408, 407f
physical dependence on, 2746
physicochemical properties of, 400, 401f, 401t
postoperative, 2719, 2732–2734, 2733t
intravenous, 2733–2734, 2733t
transdermal, 415–416, 416f
transmucosal, 416–417, 416f
potency of, 405–406, 406f
propofol and, 422
protein binding of, 400
pruritus with, 392, 2740
pulmonary uptake of, 401
pupillary effects of, 391
receptors for, 380–382, 383t, 384f
distribution of, 385
gastrointestinal, 398
signal transduction of, 383–385, 384f
renal effects of, 397–398
respiratory effects of, 392–394, 393f, 393t, 1463, 1472–1474, 1473t, 1474t, 2740
drug-related factors in, 393
hyperventilation and, 393–394
patient-related factors in, 393
renal factors in, 393
sensory evoked potential effects of, 389
sex-related response to, 387
shivering attenuation with, 391–392
single-bolus, 410
skin-incision potency test of, 405, 406f
sodium channel effects of, 386–387, 386f
somatosensory evoked potential effects of, 1533t
sphincter of Oddi spasm and, 2220
structure of, 380, 381f, 382t
teratogenicity of, 399
thermoregulatory effects of, 391–392
thiopental and, 422
tissue distribution of, 400–401, 401f, 401t
tolerance to, 384–385, 397, 2746–2747, 2747t
transdermal, 415–416, 416f
transmucosal, 416–417, 416f
urodynamic effects of, 397–398
vascular mechanisms of, 396
vecuronium interactions with, 423
ventilatory effects of, 392–394, 393f, 393t
visual evoked potential effects of, 1533t
vomiting with, 398, 399f
Opium, 20f
Optic nerve, 2992
blood supply to, 2992–2995, 2993f
microvasculature of, 2994

Optic nerve sheath, anesthetic injection into, 2531
Optic neuropathy, ischemic, 3005–3011
  after thoracolumbar surgery, 2420
  anterior, 3001t–3002t, 3005
  arteritic, 3005
  blood-brain barrier in, 3007
  case reports on, 3001t–3002t
  coronary artery disease and, 3010
  cup-to-disk ratio and, 3006
  diabetes and, 3010
  emboli and, 3010
  eye examination in, 2996–2997, 2997t
  fluid therapy and, 3009
  fluorescein angiography in, 2997, 3000f
  funduscopy in, 2997, 2999f
  hypertension and, 3010
  hypotension and, 3008
  imaging in, 2998
  intraocular pressure and, 3009
  mechanisms of, 3006–3007
  nonarteritic, 3005
  nonsurgical bleeding and, 3007
  ophthalmoscopic examination in, 3007
  optic nerve anatomy and, 3009–3010
  optic nerve blood supply and, 3006
  pathophysiology of, 3007–3010
  patient characteristics in, 3005–3006
  position-related, 1157–1158, 1158f
  posterior, 3001t–3002t, 3005
  posterior ciliary artery anatomy and, 2993–2994
  prevention of, 3010–3011
  previous stroke and, 3010
  prognosis for, 3010
  retrobulbar hemorrhage and, 3010
  sleep apnea syndrome and, 3007
  spinal surgery and, 3006, 3008
  spontaneous occurrence of, 3007–3008
  surgical blood loss and, 3008–3009
  symptoms of, 2996
  treatment of, 3010
  ultrasonography in, 2997
  vasopressors and, 3010
Oral cavity, in airway management, 1620–1621,
    1622f
Oral contraceptives, 1125, 2221t
Ore, Pierre-Cyprien, 29
Oregon Death with Dignity Act, 3188
Organ donation, 3189
  brain death and, 2232, 2232t, 2967
  cadaveric, 2232–2233, 2232t
  fluid therapy for, 2233
  from anencephalic infant, 2962
  from non-heart-beating donor, 2233–2234
  intraoperative management for, 2232–2233
  living, 2234–2237
  physiologic guidelines for, 2233
  preservation for, 2234
Organ transplantation, 2231–2273
  contraindications to, 2237
  heart, 2253–2263, 2255t, 2256f–2257f, 2260t,
    2262t
  immunosuppression for, 2271–2273, 2272t
  intestine, 2253
  kidney, 2235, 2237–2242, 2239f
  liver, 2235–2237, 2236f, 2245–2253, 2251f. See
    also Liver transplantation.
  lung, 2237, 2263–2271, 2263t, 2264t, 2266f,
    2267f. See also Lung transplantation.
  pancreas, 2242–2245, 2244f
  team approach in, 2231–2232
Organophosphates, 2504–2509
  chemical formulas of, 2504, 2504f
  enzyme inhibition by, 2504, 2505f
  physical properties of, 2504, 2505t
  poisoning by, 2504–2507, 2506t
    atropine in, 2507
    benzodiazepine in, 2508–2509
    oxime in, 2507–2508
    pyridostigmine in, 2508–2509
    treatment of, 2507–2509, 2507f
Orphanin FQ (nociceptin), 382–383, 387
Orr, Malcolm D., 21
Orthoclone (OKT3), in organ transplantation,
    2271–2273, 2272t
Orthodeoxia, 2247
Orthopedic surgery, 2409–2427
  air embolism after, 2411
  allograft/autograft, 2414t, 2420–2421, 2420f
  analgesia after, 2422–2423
  anesthetic technique in, 2412
  blood loss during, 2413

Orthopedic surgery (Continued)
  complications of, 2423–2426, 2423t, 2424f–2426f
    patient position and, 2411–2412, 2412t
  deep venous thrombosis after, 2425–2426, 2425f,
    2426f
  epidural analgesia after, 2422–2423
  fat embolism after, 2425
  in ankylosing spondylitis, 2411, 2411t, 2412t
  in cerebral palsy patient, 2427
  in juvenile rheumatoid arthritis, 2427
  in rheumatoid arthritis, 2409–2410, 2410f, 2410t,
    2411f
  monitoring in, 2413, 2414t
    on cervical spine, 2414t, 2418
    on femur, 2417
    on hip, 2413–2417, 2414t, 2415f, 2416f
    on knee, 2414t, 2417–2418
    on lower extremity, 2421–2422
    on lumbar spine, 2420
    on pelvis, 2414t, 2421
    on sacrum, 2421
    on thoracolumbar spine, 2418–2420
    on upper extremity, 2421
  patient positioning for, 1163, 1163f, 1164f
  pediatric, 2426–2427
  peripheral nerve injury in, 2411–2412, 2412t
  positioning for, 2411–2412, 2411t, 2412t
  tourniquet problems after, 2423–2425, 2423t,
    2424f
O'Shaughnessy, William B., 21
Osler, William, 4
Osmolality, urine
  in diabetes insipidus, 1768
  in renal function monitoring, 1497, 1497t
Osteitis fibrosa cystica, 1049
Osteopenia, in hyperparathyroidism, 1049
Osteoporosis, 1051
Outpatient surgery. See also Ambulatory (outpatient)
    anesthesia; Remote locations.
  anesthesia-related risk with, 902–903, 903f,
    916–917
  pain management after, 2745
  postanesthesia care unit for, 2721–2722, 2722f,
    2722t
Overwork, 3162–3163
Oximes, in organophosphate poisoning, 2507–2508
Oximetry
  carbon monoxide, 1447–1448
  cerebral, 1512t, 1542
  pulse, 1213–1215, 1214f, 1448–1453, 1448f,
    1449f. See also Pulse oximetry.
  reflectance, 1449, 1449f
  transcutaneous, 1448
  venous, mixed, 1331–1332
Oxprenolol, 653–654
Oxycodone
  controlled-release, 417
  in chronic pain, 2770
  postoperative, 2735t, 2736f
  structure of, 382t
Oxygen (O$_2$). See also Hypoxemia; Hypoxia; Oxygen
    therapy.
  alveolar, partial pressure of (Pao$_2$), 1439
    increase in, 2667–2669, 2669f, 2670t
    measurement of, 1010
    ventilation and, 698, 698f, 699f
  alveolar-arterial (A-a) gradient of, 1010,
    1440–1442, 1455
    interpretation of, 1446–1447, 1446t
  arterial, 729
    hemoglobin saturation with (Sao$_2$), 699–701,
      700f, 1438, 1439, 1447–1453. See also
      Oximetry; Pulse oximetry.
      blood transfusion and, 1806–1807, 1806f
      in apnea monitoring, 1468
    partial pressure of (Pao$_2$), 1438, 1438f,
      1439–1444, 1440f–1445f
      artifactual effects on, 1446
      carbon dioxide-blood dissociation curve and,
        1439–1440, 1440f
      cardiac output and, 1440, 1441f
      cerebral blood flow and, 816f, 817
      Clark electrode for, 1444
      continuous monitoring of, 1444–1445
      diffusion nonequilibrium and, 1440
      fiberoptic technique for, 1444–1445
      Fio$_2$ and, 701, 701f, 1440, 1440f
      gas bubbles and, 1446
      in children, 2843
      in hyperbaric oxygen therapy, 2681–2684,
        2682f, 2682t

Oxygen (O$_2$) (Continued)
  arterial (Continued)
    partial pressure of (Pao$_2$) (Continued)
      in hypothermia, 1446
      in kidneys, 1505–1506
      in one-lung ventilation, 1890–1891, 1890f
      in thoracic surgery, 1863
      interpretation of, 1446–1447, 1446t
      limitations of, 1443
      measurement of, 1010, 1444–1447, 1445f,
        1446f, 1446t
      multiple inert gas elimination technique for,
        1443–1444, 1443f
      right-to-left shunt and, 701–702, 701f, 702f,
        702t, 1440, 1440f, 1441f
      temperature correction of, 1445–1446, 1445f,
        1446f
      transcutaneous measurement of, 1447
      ventilation-perfusion mismatch and, 1439
  brain, 813, 1453–1454. See also Cerebral metabolic
    rate of oxygen (CMRO$_2$).
    partial pressure of (Ptio$_2$), in head injury, 2156
  capillary, 701–702, 701f
    cardiac output and, 712, 712f
    partial pressure of, 1440, 1445
    transcutaneous measurement of, 1447
  cardiac delivery of, 728–729, 728f, 729f
  chromophore measurement of, 1454
  consumption of, 702–703, 1462
    neonatal, 2833, 2843
    pediatric, 2834t
  end-tidal, 1455
  exercise-related uptake of, in pulmonectomy
    patient, 1013
  expired, 1454–1455, 1455f, 1456f, 1462
  in cyanide poisoning, 2513t
  inspired (Fio$_2$), 1439, 1462
    alveolar-arterial gradient and, 1442
    Pao$_2$ and, 701, 701f, 1440, 1440f
    vs. hemoglobin-oxygen saturation, 1444, 1444f
  inspired-expired percentage of, 1455, 1456f
  jugular vein saturation of, 1512t, 1542
    in head injury, 2155–2156
  mixed venous saturation of, 1453, 1453f
  muscle, 1454
  ocular toxicity of, 2678
  open-circuit measurement of, 1462
  paramagnetic analysis of, 1454, 1454f
  polarographic analysis of, 1454
  renal distribution of, 783, 783t, 798
  saturation of, vs. inspired Po$_2$, 1444, 1444f
  synthetic carriers of, 1826–1827
  therapeutic. See Oxygen therapy.
  tissue, 1453–1454
    acute normovolemic hemodilution and, 1835
  toxicity of, 716–717, 2676–2678, 2677f
  transport of, 699–703, 699t, 700f–702f, 702t,
    1438–1439, 1438f
    Cao$_2$ and, 701–702, 701f, 702f
    Fick principle and, 702–703
    hemoglobin and, 699–701, 699f, 700f
    Qs/Qt and, 701, 701f, 702t
  urinary, 1506
  venous, mixed, 1453, 1453f
Oxygen failure protection device, 277, 278f
Oxygen flush valve, 283–284
Oxygen-hemoglobin dissociation curve, 699–701,
    700f, 1438
  blood transfusion and, 1806–1807, 1806f
  Pv̄o$_2$ and, 1453, 1453f
  vs. inspired Po$_2$ and, 1444, 1444f
Oxygen ratio monitor controller, 281–282, 282f, 283
Oxygen regulator, 275, 277
Oxygen-sensing catheter, in neonatal resuscitation,
    2350–2351, 2351f
Oxygen therapy, 2812–2815
  atelectasis and, 711
  delivery systems for, 2812–2813, 2813t, 2814f
  face mask for, 2813, 2813t, 2814f
  high-concentration, 717
  high-flow system for, 2813, 2814f
  hyperbaric. See Hyperbaric oxygen therapy.
  in neonatal resuscitation, 2349, 2350–2351, 2351f
  in obese patient, 1032
  in pediatric respiratory failure, 2845
  in postoperative hypoxemia, 2712–2715, 2714f
  in septic shock, 806
  low-flow system for, 2813, 2813t
  nonrebreathing face mask for, 2813, 2814f
  rebreathing face mask for, 2813, 2814f
  reservoir system for, 2813, 2813t, 2814f

Oxygen therapy (Continued)
　retinal effects of, 2535
　toxicity of, 716–717, 2535
　Venturi mask for, 2813
Oxymorphone, 417
　in outpatient anesthesia, 2606
　in patient-controlled intravenous analgesia,
　　2733–2734, 2733t
　structure of, 382t

P

P value, 885
P wave, 1389, 1390f
Pacemaker, 1084–1085, 1084t, 1416–1427. See also
　　Implantable cardioverter-defibrillator.
　at remote locations, 2653
　backup equipment for, 1423
　biventricular, 1418–1419, 1419f, 1423
　codes for, 1416–1418, 1417t, 1418t
　company phone numbers for, 1435
　electrocardiographic monitoring of, 1422–1423,
　　1424f–1425f
　electrosurgery and, 3147
　failure of, 1425–1427, 1426f
　indications for, 1418–1419, 1418t
　intraoperative management of, 1422–1426,
　　1424f–1425f
　magnet application to, 1419–1421, 1420f, 1420t,
　　1421f
　minute ventilation sensor in, 1422, 1423t
　monopolar electrosurgery and, 1423, 1426
　postanesthesia evaluation of, 1427
　preanesthesia evaluation of, 1421–1422, 1435
　reprogramming of, 1422, 1422t
　structure of, 1416, 1417f
　terminology for, 1431–1432
　threshold margin test of, 1419, 1420f
Packed red blood cells, 1812, 1812f, 1821–1822,
　　1822f
　for children, 2389–2390
　in hemorrhagic shock, 2465
Pagés, Fidel, 27
Pain, 60, 60f
　after laparoscopy, 2293, 2294
　at end of life, 3186–3187
　back, 1096, 2772, 2773–2774
　　after spinal anesthesia, 1670
　　postpartum, 2329
　chronic, 2763–2778
　　evaluation of, 2765–2767
　　in cancer, 2770
　　in elderly patient, 2443
　　insomnia with, 2772
　　laboratory studies in, 2766–2767
　　low back, 2772, 2773–2774
　　multispecialty treatment of, 2767–2768
　　outpatient treatment of, 2768
　　patient history in, 2765–2766
　　physical examination in, 2766
　　postoperative, 2731
　　psychosocial assessment in, 2767
　　systemic local anesthetics for, 591
　　treatment of, 2767, 2768–2777
　　　acetaminophen in, 2769
　　　acupuncture in, 2777
　　　antidepressant drugs in, 2771–2772
　　　antiepileptic drugs in, 2771
　　　chiropractic in, 2777
　　　COX-II inhibitors in, 2769
　　　epidural steroid injections in, 2773–2774
　　　facet blocks in, 2774
　　　guidelines for, 2781–2784
　　　intradiscal electrothermal annuloplasty in,
　　　　2774
　　　intrathecal drugs in, 2774
　　　nerve blocks in, 2772–2776
　　　neurolytic blocks in, 2775–2776
　　　nonsteroidal anti-inflammatory drugs in,
　　　　2768–2769
　　　opioids in, 2769–2771, 2769t, 2770t,
　　　　2781–2784
　　　oxycodone in, 2770
　　　psychological therapy in, 2776
　　　rehabilitation in, 2776–2777
　　　spinal cord stimulation in, 2774
　　　sympathetic nerve blocks in, 2774–2775
　　　topical creams for, 2771
　　　tramadol in, 2769

Pain (Continued)
　chronic (Continued)
　　treatment of (Continued)
　　　transcutaneous electrical nerve stimulation
　　　　in, 2776–2777
　　　transdermal, 2770–2771
　　　trigger point injections in, 2772
　　Waddell signs in, 2766
　clonidine for, 651
　CNS response in, 2764
　dorsal root ganglion in, 2764
　etomidate-related, 354–355
　gate control theory in, 2764
　genitourinary, 2200–2202
　historical studies on, 9–10
　inflammatory, 2763–2764
　myofascial, 2772
　N-methyl-D-aspartate receptors in, 2764, 2765
　neurobiology of, 2729–2730, 2764–2765
　neuropathic, 2763–2778. See also Pain, chronic.
　　in trauma, 2484
　perception of, 2718, 2718t, 2744
　　in children, 1720–1721
　post-traumatic, 2483–2485
　　in brain injury, 2472
　　in orthopedic injury, 2477
　postoperative, 2718–2720, 2729–2751
　　acute effects of, 2730–2731
　　after pediatric cardiac surgery, 2036–2037
　　after thoracic surgery, 1906–1909
　　chronic effects of, 2731
　　coagulation and, 2730
　　in elderly patient, 2444–2445
　　neuroendocrine stress response and, 2730–2731
　　ocular, 2537
　　preemptive analgesia for, 2731–2732
　　risk factors for, 2719, 2719f
　　treatment of, 2732–2744, 2732t
　　　epidural analgesia in, 2720, 2738–2743,
　　　　2739t, 2741t
　　　in ambulatory patient, 2615–2616, 2616t,
　　　　2745
　　　in children, 2398, 2747–2748
　　　in elderly patient, 2745–2746
　　　in obese patient, 2748–2749
　　　in obstructive sleep apnea patient, 2749
　　　in opioid-tolerant patients, 2746–2747
　　　intra-articular analgesia in, 2744
　　　ketamine in, 2735–2736
　　　multimodal strategy in, 2732
　　　nerve block in, 2720
　　　nonsteroidal anti-inflammatory agents in,
　　　　2719–2720, 2734–2735, 2735t
　　　opioids in, 2719, 2732–2734, 2733t
　　　pain service for, 2749–2750, 2750t
　　　peripheral regional analgesia in, 2743–2744
　　　preemptive, 2731–2732
　　　regional analgesia in, 2737–2744, 2737t,
　　　　2738t
　　　respiration and, 2731
　　　sleep disruption and, 2749
　　　thoracic analgesia in, 2744
　　　tramadol in, 2736–2737
　　　transcutaneous electrical nerve stimulation
　　　　in, 2744
　　undertreatment of, 2718–2719
Pain services, 2749–2750, 2750t
Pal, Jacob, 9
Pancreas
　adrenergic receptors in, 627
　cells of, 1020
　disease of, 1019–1027. See also Diabetes mellitus.
　transplantation of, 2242–2245, 2244f
　　anesthesia after, 2245
　　autonomic neuropathy and, 2245
　　care after, 2245
　　fluid therapy in, 2245
　　glucose monitoring in, 2245
　　immunosuppression for, 2244
　　intraoperative management in, 2244–2245
　　organ matching for, 2243
　　organ preservation for, 2244
　　preoperative evaluation for, 2243–2244
Pancuronium, 493t, 494, 495f, 497t
　autonomic effects of, 511, 511t, 512t
　calcium interaction with, 517
　cerebral physiology and, 831
　dosage for, 501t
　dysrhythmias with, 513
　elimination of, 506t, 507
　for children, 2379, 2380t

Pancuronium (Continued)
　hepatobiliary disease and, 529–530, 529t
　in elderly patients, 526
　in kidney transplantation, 2241
　in pediatric cardiac surgery, 2021
　in pediatric respiratory failure, 2849
　in renal failure, 2184–2186, 2185t
　intracranial pressure and, 831
　metabolism of, 506t, 507
　opioid interactions with, 423
　pharmacodynamics of, 500t, 502t
　recovery from, 1562–1563, 1562t, 1563f
　renal failure and, 527, 528t
　succinylcholine interaction with, 515
　tachycardia with, 512–513
　vecuronium maintenance dose after, 515
Pantoprazole, in outpatient premedication,
　　2599–2600, 2600t
Papaver somniferum, 20f
Papaverine, 380t
Para-aminohippurate clearance, 785–786
Paracelsus, 11
Paracervical block, during labor, 2322
Paradoxical respiration, 1869, 1869f
Paraldehyde, in pediatric seizures, 2858
Paralysis
　after thoracic surgery, 1903–1904
　hypoxemia and, 709, 712–713
　periodic, 1098–1099
　　hyperkalemic, 538t, 543, 544t, 545
　　hypokalemic, 538t, 544t, 545–546
　vocal cord, 1650
Paramyotonia congenita, 538t, 543, 544t, 545
Paranasal sinuses, surgery on, 2540
Paraneoplastic syndromes, in lung cancer, 1851
Paraplegia, after thoracic surgery, 1903–1904
Parascalene block, pediatric, 1740–1741, 1740t,
　　1741f
Parathyroid gland, in calcium physiology, 1771
Paravertebral block, 1712, 1713f, Plate 10
　in outpatient procedures, 2609
　lumbar, 1712, 1713f, Plate 10
　　during labor, 2322
　thoracic, 1712
Paré, Ambroise, 22
Parecoxib, in outpatient premedication, 2597
Parenteral nutrition, 2905–2907. See also Nutrition,
　　parenteral.
Parents
　of pediatric ICU patient, 2878–2879
　with children, 2382, 2384, 2607–2608, 2722
Park bench position, 1162
Parker Flex-Tip tube, 1632
Parkinson's disease, 1095
Parkman, Samuel, 15f
Paroxysmal supraventricular tachycardia,
　　2930–2931, 2930f
　electrocardiography in, 1399–1401, 1400t
Partial CO₂ rebreathing Fick technique, for cardiac
　　output monitoring, 1337
Partial liquid ventilation, in children, 2851
Partial thromboplastin time
　in children, 2390
　in heparin monitoring, 1973, 1973f
　preoperative, 956, 960t, 961f
Pascal (Pa), 1196
Patent ductus arteriosus, 2009–2010, 2009t
　ligation of, 2039
Patent foramen ovale
　air passage through, 2141–2142
　right-to-left shunt across, 689, 713, 1903
Patient-controlled analgesia, 30, 410, 2719,
　　2741–2742, 2741t
　epidural, 2741–2742, 2741t
　in trauma, 2484
　intravenous, 2733–2734, 2733t
　　in children, 2748
　　side effects of, 2734
　target-controlled infusion in, 473
Patient history, 933–938, 934t, 936f–937f
　airway disorders in, 934–935
　bleeding problems in, 937
　cardiovascular disease in, 933–934, 934t
　endocrine disturbances in, 937–938
　gastrointestinal disease in, 935
　hepatic disorders in, 935
　musculoskeletal disease in, 938
　neurologic disease in, 938
　renal disease in, 937
　sensitive areas in, 938
　three aspects of, 933

Patient-physician relationship, 3175–3182. *See also* Informed consent.
Patient positioning, 1151–1166
    atelectasis and, 711
    blood pooling in, 1152
    hypoxemia and, 708, 709f, 710–711, 710f
    in awake craniotomy, 2161
    in neurosurgery, 2134–2138, 2135t, 2137f
    in obesity, 1034
    in orthopedic surgery, 1163, 1163f, 1164f, 2411–2412, 2411t, 2412t
    in pediatric respiratory failure, 2845
    in shoulder surgery, 1163–1164, 1164f
    lateral
        in neurosurgery, 2135
        nerve injury with, 1159–1160
    lateral decubitus, 1869–1873, 1872f
        anesthetized
            closed-chest, 1870–1871, 1871f
            open-chest, 1871–1872, 1871f
                paralyzed, 1871f, 1872
        awake, closed-chest, 1869–1870, 1870f
        hypoxemia and, 710–711, 710f
        pulmonary vascular monitoring and, 1863–1864, 1864f
    lateral oblique, nerve injury with, 1160–1162, 1161f, 1162f
    lithotomy, 1155, 1157f
        nerve injury with, 597, 1157f, 1158–1159, 1159f
    park bench, nerve injury with, 1162
    prone
        chest rolls for, 1163
        hypotension and, 1163
        in neurosurgery, 2135–2136
        lumbar flexion for, 1163
        nerve injury with, 1162–1163
    semilateral, in neurosurgery, 2135
    semirecumbent, 1163–1164, 1164f
    sitting
        in neurosurgery, 2136–2138, 2137f
        nerve injury with, 1164–1166, 1165f
    supine
        hypoxemia and, 709, 709f, 710, 711
        in neurosurgery, 2135
        nerve injury with, 1158
    Trendelenburg
        functional residual capacity and, 711
        nerve injury with, 1162
Patient simulators, 3073–3099
    Anesoft, 3077t, 3078–3079, 3079f
    applications of, 3074, 3074t
    BODY, 3078
    CASE, 3079
    centers for, 3096–3098, 3097f, 3098f
    classification of, 3074
    components of, 3074–3075, 3075f, 3076t, 3077t
    cost-effectiveness of, 3093–3094, 3096
    development of, 3078
    ecologic validity of, 3095, 3095f
    for biomedical industry, 3093
    for continuing medical education, 3091–3092
    for medicolegal proceedings, 3093
    for nonanesthesia health care personnel, 3092–3093, 3092f, 3093f
    for research, 3093, 3094t
    for resident training, 3090–3091, 3095–3096
    Gainesville, 3080, 3081f
    in crisis resource management training, 3045–3046, 3082–3084, 3083t, 3085t
    mannequin-based, 3074–3075, 3075f, 3076t, 3077t, 3079–3082, 3080f–3082f
    MedSim, 3077t, 3079–3080, 3080f, 3081f
    METI, 3077t, 3081, 3082f
    performance evaluation with, 3084–3090
        nontechnical skills in, 3086–3088, 3087t, 3088t, 3089t
        pitfalls of, 3089–3090
    screen-based, 3078–3079
    SimMan, 3077t, 3080, 3082, 3082f
    SLEEPER, 3078
    team-oriented, 3084
    virtual reality, 3075–3078
    websites on, 3098t
Patient transport
    in trauma, 2487
    risks of, 1472
    to pediatric intensive care unit, 2875
    to postanesthesia care unit, 2708, 2710
Peak flow, 1001, 1001f

Pediatric intensive care unit, 2831–2879
    asphyxial injury care in, 2876–2877
    cardiopulmonary resuscitation in, 2877–2878. *See also* Cardiopulmonary resuscitation, pediatric.
    cardiovascular care in, 2832–2840, 2834t, 2835f, 2835t, 2837t, 2839t, 2840t
    endocrine care in, 2861–2863
    gastrointestinal care in, 2863–2867, 2866t
    hematologic care in, 2867–2869, 2867f
    infectious disease care in, 2870–2873, 2870t, 2872t–2873t
    neurologic care in, 2854–2858, 2854t, 2855t
    oncologic care in, 2869–2870
    organization of, 2832
    parent/family support in, 2878–2879
    patient transport to, 2875
    renal care in, 2858–2861, 2859t
    respiratory care in, 2840–2854, 2841t, 2845t, 2846t, 2848t
    staff of, 2832
    trauma care in, 2873–2875
Pelvic pain, 2201
Pelvis
    fracture of, 2476–2477
    resection of, 2414t
    surgery on, 2421
Pemoline, hepatotoxicity of, 2221t
Penbutolol, 653–654
Penicillins
    allergy to, 1093t
    hepatotoxicity of, 2221t
    neuromuscular blockade with, 516
Penile block, pediatric, 1750–1751, 1750f
Penis
    innervation of, 2177
    prolonged erection of, 2201
Pentamorphone, 417
n-Pentane, 106f
Pentastarch, 1787
Pentazocine, 380t, 418t, 419
    for patient-controlled intravenous analgesia, 2733–2734, 2733t
Pentobarbital
    duration of action of, 328t
    in pediatric ICP increase, 2857
    lipid solubility of, 331
    neuroprotection with, 839
Pentolamine, in children, 2838
Percentile, 883
Percutaneous transluminal coronary artery angioplasty, 2649–2650
    peripheral vascular surgery and, 1073–1074, 1074f, 2063
Perfluoroalkanes, cutoff effect with, 116
Perfluorochemical emulsions, 1787–1788
Perfluorochemical liquid ventilation, in children, 2851
Perfluorooctylbromide, 1826
Perfringens toxin, 2515t
Perfusion pressure, 680
    in renal function monitoring, 1495
Peribulbar block, 1709, 2529
Pericardial tamponade, 2649, 2652
Pericarditis
    constrictive, 1967, 1968f
        central venous pressure monitoring in, 1316, 1317f
    in kidney failure, 2181t, 2182
Perimetry, 2997, 2997t
Periodic paralysis, 1098–1099
    hyperkalemia, 538t, 543, 544t, 545
    hypokalemic, 538t, 544t, 545–546
Peripheral arterial disease, 2092–2098. *See also* Vascular surgery.
    acute, 2092–2093
    ankle-brachial index in, 2093
    chronic, 2093
    operative treatment of, 2093–2098. *See also* Vascular surgery.
        anesthesia for, 2094–2098
        cardiac morbidity with, 2095–2096, 2096t
        general anesthesia for, 2094, 2098
        monitoring for, 2094
        pain control after, 2097–2098
        regional anesthesia for, 2095, 2096–2097, 2096f, 2097f, 2098
    percutaneous transluminal coronary artery angioplasty and, 1073–1074, 1074f, 2063

Peripheral nerve stimulation, 1539, 1551–1566
    acceleromyography for, 1560–1561, 1560f, 1561f
    double-burst, 1555, 1556f
    during induction, 1564
    during neuromuscular blockade reversal, 1565, 1565t
    during surgery, 1564–1565
    electrical, 1552
    electrodes for, 1557
    electromyography for, 1558–1560, 1558f, 1560f
    in anesthetic depth monitoring, 1257–1258
    in brain death, 2965
    in depolarizing neuromuscular blockade, 1563, 1564f
    in nondepolarizing neuromuscular blockade, 1561–1563, 1562f, 1563t, 1564f
    indications for, 1565–1566
    magnetic, 1552
    mechanomyography for, 1558
    muscle sites for, 1557–1558, 1557f, 1558f
    of diaphragm, 1557–1558, 1558f
    of ulnar nerve, 1559–1560, 1559f
    patterns of, 1552–1555, 1552f–1555f
    phonomyography for, 1561
    piezoelectric monitors for, 1561, 1561f
    post-tetanic single-twitch, 1554–1555, 1554f, 1555f
    principles of, 1552
    recording methods for, 1558–1561, 1559f–1561f
    single-twitch, 1552, 1552f
    stimulator for, 1555–1557
    tetanic, 1553–1554, 1553f
    train-of-four, 1552–1553, 1553f
    types of, 1552
    without recording equipment, 1563–1565, 1565f
Peripheral volume of distribution, 68–69
Peripherally inserted central venous catheters, 1293
Peritoneal dialysis, 1102–1103, 1103t
    in pediatric hemolytic-uremic syndrome, 2860
    in renal failure, 2188–2189
Peritonitis, in cirrhosis, 2248
Pernicious anemia, 1097
Peroneal nerve
    atrophy of, in Charcot-Marie-Tooth disease, 535
    common, with orthopedic surgery, 2411–2412, 2412t
    position-related injury to, 1155, 1156t, 1158
Peroneal nerve block, 1703–1704, 1704f, 1705f, Plate 16
Persistence of left superior vena cava, 1303
Persistent fetal circulation syndrome, 2355
Persistent vegetative state, 2962
Pesticides. *See* Organophosphates.
Peyronie's disease, 2201
PFA-100 platelet monitor, 1343
Pflüger, Wilhelm, 5
pH, 1601
    cerebral blood flow and, 816–817
    hypothermia effect on, 1588–1589
    local anesthetics and, 574, 585
    urinary, 1493, 2180
Pharmacodynamics, 84–97. *See also* Pharmacokinetics.
    genetic variability in, 99–100
    molecular, 93–95, 94t
    receptors in, 85–93. *See also* Receptor(s).
Pharmacokinetics, 68–84
    area under the curve for, 80
    bolus, 77–80, 79f, 80f, 81–84, 82f, 83f
    central volume of distribution and, 68, 69f
    clearance and, 69–74, 70f–74f
    concentration over time curve for, 79–80
    distribution clearance and, 74
    elimination phase in, 82, 82f
    first-order, 76–77
    genetic variability in, 99
    hepatic clearance and, 70–74, 71f–74f
    hepatic dysfunction effects on, 2212–2214, 2214f
    hysteresis and, 84, 84f, 85f
    infusion, 80–81
    models of, 76–84, 77f
        compartmental, 77–84, 79f, 80f, 82f, 83f
        hydraulic, 82–83, 82f
        mammillary, 81–82, 82f, 83f
        multicompartmental, 79f, 81–84, 82f, 83f
        one-compartment, 77–81, 79f, 80f
        physiologic, 77, 78f
    peripheral volume of distribution and, 68–69
    protein binding and, 74–76, 75f
    rapid-distribution phase in, 81–82, 82f
    rate of absorption and, 81

Pharmacokinetics *(Continued)*
  renal clearance and, 73–74
  slow-distribution phase in, 82, 82f
  stereochemistry and, 76
  terminal phase in, 82, 82f
  time and, 76–77, 77f
  tissue clearance and, 74
  volume of distribution and, 68–69, 68f, 69f
  zero-order, 76–77
Pharmacophore, 90
Pharyngitis, after tracheal intubation, 2547
Pharynx, 1617
  trauma to, 2459
Phencyclidines, 345–350. *See also* Ketamine.
Phenobarbital
  in pediatric seizures, 2858
  metabolism of, 329
Phenolic ether derivative, 493t, 495, 497f, 509.
    See also Gallamine.
Phenoperidine, 417
Phenothiazines, 1123–1124
  drug interactions of, 1123–1124
  in outpatient premedication, 2598
Phenoxybenzamine, 652–653
  in pheochromocytoma, 1042, 1043
Phentolamine, 653
  in pediatric shock, 2836
Phenylalanine, in hepatic failure, 2916
Phenylephrine, 650
  cerebral blood flow and, 818–819, 819t
  during pregnancy, 2312
  guidelines for, 2548
  in awake intubation, 1642
  in pediatric shock, 2836
  ocular preparations of, 2536
  with spinal anesthesia, 1667
Phenytoin
  hepatotoxicity of, 2221t
  in pediatric seizures, 2858
Pheochromocytoma, 1042–1044, 1042t, 1043t
Phonomyography, 1561
Phosgene, 297, 2510–2513, 2511t, 2512f
Phosphate, 1774–1775, 1775t
  in hyperparathyroidism, 1050
Phosphatidylinositol, 92
Phospholipase A$_2$, in prostaglandin synthesis,
    795, 795f
Phosphorus
  deficiency of, in ketoacidosis, 1023
  in parenteral nutrition, 2912t
Photoplethysmography, in apnea monitoring, 1468
Photoreceptors, 2992, 2992f
Phrenic nerve
  halothane effects on, 175, 176f
  injury to, with thoracic surgery, 1903
Phrenic nerve block
  with interscalene block, 1688
  with supraclavicular block, 1690
Physical examination, 938–939. *See also* Preoperative
    evaluation.
  three aspects of, 933
Physician. *See also* Anesthesiologist; Ethics.
  aid in dying by, 3187–3188, 3188t
  conflicts of interest of, 3190–3191
  informed consent and, 3175–3182. *See also*
    Informed consent.
  parent disagreements with, 3181
  primary care, 1018–1019
  professionalism of, 3192–3193, 3193t–3194t
Physics, 1192–1193
Physostigmine, 662
  postoperative, 662, 1583
Pia mater, 1655, 1655f
Pierre Robin syndrome, 2355
Piezoelectric neuromuscular monitors, 1561, 1561f
Pilots, Age 60 Rule for, 3062–3063
Pindolol, 653–654
Pipecuronium, 493t, 494, 495f, 497t
  autonomic effects of, 511, 511t, 512t
  cerebral physiology and, 831
  dosage for, 501t
  elimination of, 506t, 507
  hepatobiliary disease and, 529–530, 529t
  in elderly patients, 527
  lithium interaction with, 517
  metabolism of, 506t, 507
  pharmacodynamics of, 502t
  renal failure and, 527, 528t
  vecuronium maintenance dose after, 515
Piperocaine, channel blockade by, 870
Pirbuterol, 2817t

Piritramide, 417
Pirogoff, Nikolai Ivanovitch, 15
Pitot tube, 1204, 1204f
Pituitary gland
  adenoma of, 1037, 1041, 1052
  anterior
    hypersecretion disorders of, 1051–1052
    hypofunction of, 1052
  in brain death, 2960
  posterior, disorders of, 1052–1053
  transsphenoidal resection of, 2158–2159, 2158t
  tumors of, 2146, 2158–2159, 2158t
PK$_a$, 1600
Placenta, 2311, 2311f
  anesthetic drug transfer by, 2312–2313
Placenta accreta, 2334–2335, 2335f
Placenta previa, 2334, 2334f
Placental abruption, 2334, 2334f
Plague, 2503, 2517
Plants, 605–612, 607t, 608t, 609t
Plasma, 1825
  in hemorrhagic shock, 2465
Plasma membrane, inhaled anesthetic action at,
    117–123
  electrophysiologic studies of, 117, 118f
  G proteins and, 122–123
  ligand-gated ion channels and, 120–122, 121f
  lipid bilayer fluidization and, 120
  lipid bilayer site of, 118–120, 119f
  metabotropic receptors and, 122–123
  permeability and, 119
  potassium channels and, 122
  protein kinase C and, 123
  protein site of, 119f, 120–123, 121f, 122f
  voltage-gated ion channels and, 122
Plasmapheresis, in Lambert-Eaton myasthenic
    syndrome, 540
Plastic surgery, local anesthetics in, 591
Plastic tubing, anesthetic loss to, 142, 143t
Platelet(s)
  activation of, cardiopulmonary bypass and,
    1984–1985, 1984f
  assays for, 1342–1343
  disorders of, 1116
    end-stage liver disease and, 2248
    in children, 2868
    kidney failure and, 2239
    transfusion-related, 1807–1809, 1808f, 1808t,
      1809f, 1810–1811
  during pregnancy, 2310
  garlic effects on, 609–610
  heparin-induced inhibition of, 1984
  in preeclampsia, 2331
  preoperative collection of, 1834
  transfusion of, 1822–1823
    for children, 2390–2391, 2391f
    in dilutional thrombocytopenia, 1810–1811
    in hemorrhagic shock, 2465–2466
    indications for, 1823
  transfusion-related decrease in, 1807–1809, 1808f,
    1808t, 1809f, 1810–1811
Platelet inhibitors, in coronary angiography, 2649
Plateletworks, 1343
Plethysmography, 694, 1468
Pleura, anesthetic loss from, 135
Pleural analgesia, 587–588, 1909, 2744
  for children, 1753
Pleural effusion, fluid therapy in, 1789
Pleural pressure, 681–682, 681f, 1465
Pleuroscopy, 1912
Pneumatic vest, in basic life support, 2926, 2927f
Pneumocephalus, 2138, 2138f
Pneumocystis carinii pneumonia, in children, 2871,
    2872
Pneumomediastinum, during laparoscopy,
    2288–2289
Pneumonectomy
  in trauma, 2480
  left ventricular end-diastolic pressure after, 1321t,
    1322
Pneumonia
  postoperative, 1087, 1088t
  ventilator-associated, 2796–2797, 2797t
Pneumonic plague, 2517
Pneumopericardium, during laparoscopy, 2288–2289
Pneumotachography, 1463
Pneumothorax
  after mediastinoscopy, 1911
  after supraclavicular block, 1690
  central venous catheterization and, 1294
  during laparoscopy, 2288–2289

Pneumothorax *(Continued)*
  in hyperbaric oxygen therapy, 2680
  in neonate, 2355
  laser-induced, 2579
  postoperative hypoxemia and, 2713
  spontaneous, 1925
  tension, 1902
  with endotracheal intubation, 1649
Poikilothermia, in brain death, 2959–2960,
    2961–2962
Poiseuille, Jean L., 6
Poisoning, in children, 2875
Polycythemia, 1111–1114
  in neonate, 2359–2360
Polymorphic ventricular tachycardia, 2934, 2935f
Polymyositis, 1098
Polysomnography, 1030–1031
Polystyrene beads, radiolabeled, in renal blood flow
    measurement, 791
Popliteal fossa block, 1701–1703, 1702f, Plate 14
Pores of Kohn, 692
Porphyria, 749, 1097–1098, 1097f
Portal hypertension, 760–763, 763f, 1110–1111.
    See also Cirrhosis.
  ascites and, 2222–2223
  pathogenesis of, 762
Porter, W., 8
Portopulmonary syndrome, 2247
Positioning. *See* Patient positioning.
Positive end-expiratory pressure (PEEP). *See also*
    Mechanical ventilation, positive-
    pressure.
  after thoracic surgery, 1904–1906, 1904t, 1905t
  after trauma, 2485–2486, 2486t
  auto-, 1466, 1467f
  in children, 2847–2848
  in lung transplantation, 2268–2269
  in neurosurgery, 2141, 2142
  in one-lung ventilation, 1893, 1894, 1895f,
    1897–1900, 1898f, 1899f
  physiology of, 2820–2821
Positive expiratory pressure, for bronchial hygiene,
    2819
Positive-pressure ventilation, 2820–2828, 2848–2849.
    See also Mechanical ventilation, positive-
    pressure.
Positron emission tomography, in brain death, 2967
Post-traumatic stress disorder, intraoperative recall
    and, 1238–1239
Postanesthesia care unit, 59, 2703–2723
  airway obstruction in, 2711–2712, 2711f, 2712f
  complications in, 2710–2721
    circulatory, 2715–2717, 2717f
    rate of, 2710–2711, 2711f
    respiratory, 2711–2715, 2711f–2715f
  design of, 2705–2706, 2706f
  discharge from, 2708, 2709t, 2710
  dysrhythmias in, 2717
  economics of, 2704–2705, 2704t
  equipment for, 2706–2707
  for outpatient surgery, 2721–2722, 2722f, 2722t
  historical perspective on, 2703–2704
  hypertension in, 2717, 2717f
  hypotension in, 2716–2717, 2717f
  hypothermia in, 2721
  hypoventilation in, 2715, 2715f
  hypoxemia in, 2712–2715, 2713f, 2714f
  location of, 2705
  nausea in, 2720–2721
  pain management in, 2718–2720, 2718t, 2719f
    epidural analgesia for, 2720
    nerve blocks for, 2720
    nonsteroidal anti-inflammatory drugs for,
      2719–2720
    opioids for, 2719
  patient stay in, 2708–2709
  pediatric, 2722–2723
    emergence delirium in, 2723
    parents in, 2722
    postanesthetic apnea in, 2723
    postintubation croup in, 2723
  persistent somnolence in, 2717–2718
  prolonged patient stay in, 2709
  quality improvement for, 2710
  report for, 2708, 2710
  routine recovery in, 2707–2709, 2707t, 2708t,
    2709t
  shivering in, 2721
  size of, 2705
  staffing for, 2705
  standards for, 2709–2710

Postanesthesia care unit *(Continued)*
  transport to, 2708, 2710
  unconsciousness in, 2717–2718
  vomiting in, 2720–2721
Posterior ciliary arteries, 2992–2994, 2993f, 2994f
Posterior fossa surgery, 2157–2158, 2157f
Posterior tibial nerve block, 1703, 1703f, Plate 15
Postmature infant, 2367, 2368f, 2368t. *See also* Infant.
Postpartum hemorrhage, 2335–2336
Potassium, 1768–1770. *See also* Hyperkalemia; Hypokalemia.
  epinephrine effects on, 627
  in hypokalemia, 1107
  in ketoacidosis, 1023
  physiology of, 1768–1769
  requirements for, 1769
Potassium-aggravated myotonia, 543, 544t, 545
Potassium channel
  in nerve conduction, 577–578, 579f
  inhaled anesthetic effects on, 207–210, 209f
  reactive oxygen species generation and, 210
Potassium chloride, supplemental, 1769
Potency, drug, 95, 96f
Potential energy, 1197, 1198f
Power, statistical, 885
Power spectrum, 1194, 1197f
PR interval, 1389, 1390f
Pralidoxime, in organophosphate poisoning, 2508
Prazosin, 653
  in pheochromocytoma, 1042
Pre-excitation syndrome, 1084
Prednisolone
  in organ transplantation, 2271–2273, 2272t
  neuromuscular blocking agent interaction with, 518
Prednisone. *See also* Corticosteroids.
  before peripheral vascular surgery, 2063
Preeclampsia, 2329–2333
  anesthetic management in, 2332–2333, 2333t
  antihypertensive agents in, 2331, 2332t
  central venous pressure in, 2332, 2332f
  classification of, 2330, 2330t
  clinical features of, 2330–2331, 2331f
  fluid management in, 1794
  HELLP syndrome in, 2331
  magnesium effects in, 1773
  pathophysiology of, 2330
  treatment of, 2331–2332, 2332t
Pregnancy. *See also* Fetus.
  anesthesia-related risk in, 909–912, 911t, 912f
  anesthesia sensitivity in, 2311
  anesthetic toxicity during, 257–260, 258t
  blood volume during, 2309–2310
  bupivacaine toxicity in, 595
  cardiovascular changes of, 2308–2309, 2308t, 2309f
  chest radiography during, 2309, 2309t
  coagulation during, 2310, 2310t
  echocardiography during, 2309, 2309t
  electrocardiography during, 2309, 2309t
  ephedrine during, 2312
  functional residual capacity during, 2310
  gastric emptying during, 2310–2311
  gastrointestinal changes of, 2310–2311
  glomerular filtration rate during, 2311
  hematologic changes of, 2309–2310, 2310t
  hypotension during, 2312
  intubation during, 2310
  laparoscopy during, 2295, 2338
  local anesthetics during, 586, 595
  multiple-gestation, 2336
  nervous system changes of, 2311
  nonobstetric surgery during, 2337–2338, 2337t
  opioids during, 399
  phenylephrine during, 2312
  physiologic changes of, 2308–2311, 2308t, 2309f, 2309t, 2310t, 2311t
  platelet count during, 2310
  renal changes of, 2311, 2311t
  respiratory changes of, 2310
  supine hypotension syndrome in, 2308–2309
  testing for, 956, 959
  trauma during, 2337–2338, 2482
  uterine blood flow during, 2312
  venography in, 2308, 2309f
Preload, 725–726, 725f
  aortic cross-clamping effects on, 2074–2075
  transesophageal echocardiography for, 1376
Premature atrial contractions, 1084

Premature infant, 2367, 2368f, 2368t. *See also* Infant.
  postanesthesia apnea and, 2397–2398, 2397f, 2723
  retinopathy in, 2354, 2534–2535
  retrolental fibroplasia in, 717
  surfactant for, 2851
Premature ventricular contractions, 1083–1084
Preoperative and preprocedure assessment clinic, 57, 980–991, 981t, 982t, 983f, 983t, 984f–987f
  cancellations and, 990–991, 991t
  cost-effectiveness of, 989–991
  cost reductions in, 991
  daily operations of, 988–989
  delays and, 990–991
  economics of, 984–985, 987t
  facilities renovation for, 988, 988t
  goals for, 981, 983f, 984, 987f
  marketing of, 985–988
  patient statements for, 981, 984f, 985f
  policy statement for, 981, 983f
  quality assurance in, 989, 990f
  teamwork for, 981, 984
  testing guidelines for, 986f, 989–990
Preoperative evaluation, 57, 927–992, 3031–3032
  clinic for, 980–991, 981t, 982t, 983f, 983t, 984f–987f
  in children, 2379–2380
  in elderly patient, 2440–2443
  information management in, 972–980. *See also* Information management.
  laboratory tests in, 939–962. *See also* Laboratory testing.
  of herbal medicine use, 606
  patient history in, 933–938, 934t, 936f–937f. *See also* Patient history.
  patient satisfaction with, 980
  physical examination in, 938–939
  rationale for, 927–932, 928t, 929f, 930t, 931t
  reform in, 932
Preproenkephalin, knockout mouse study of, 386
Pressure, 1196–1198, 1198f. *See also specific pressures.*
  dynamic, 1199–1201, 1199f–1201f
  hydrostatic, 1219–1220
  static, 1198–1199, 1199f
Pressure reversal of anesthesia, 108
Pressure sores, with epidural analgesia, 2740
Pressure-support ventilation, 2823–2824
Pressure-targeted ventilation, 2821, 2822f, 2823f
Pressure-volume loop, in myocardial contraction, 727, 727f
Prevost, J. L., 40
Priapism, 2201
Priestly, Joseph, 4, 5f, 12, 42
Prilocaine, 575t
  cardiovascular toxicity of, 594–595, 594t
  duration of action of, 584
  in epidural anesthesia, 588–589, 588t
  in nerve block, 587–588, 587t, 588t
  in pediatric regional anesthesia, 1728t
  infiltration of, 586–587, 586t
  intravenous, 587
  methemoglobinemia and, 596
  potency of, 576t
  structure of, 575f
  tissue distribution of, 592, 592t
Primary care physician, 1018–1019
Priming, for tracheal intubation, 504
Prion diseases, in health care worker, 3159–3160
Probability, 888–889. *See also* Statistics.
Procaine, 24, 575t
  cardiovascular toxicity of, 594–595, 594t
  in pediatric regional anesthesia, 1728t
  in spinal anesthesia, 589, 589t, 1665
  infiltration of, 586–587, 586t
  intravenous, 587
  mechanism of action of, 869
  neuromuscular blocking agent interaction with, 517
  structure of, 573–574, 574f, 575t
Professionalism, 3192–3193, 3193t–3194t
Prolactin, excess of, 1052
Promethazine
  during labor, 2318
  in outpatient premedication, 2598f
Prone position
  chest rolls for, 1163
  hypotension and, 1163
  in neurosurgery, 2135–2136
  lumbar flexion for, 1163
  nerve injury with, 1162–1163

Propafenone
  hepatotoxicity of, 2221t
  in atrial fibrillation, 1402, 1402t
Proplex, 1824
Propofol, 29, 318–326
  abuse of. *See* Substance abuse.
  alfentanil interaction with, 97, 97f, 398, 449, 449f, 450, 453f
  antiemetic activity of, 324
  automated delivery system for, 472–473
  BIS index and, 1254, 1255
  cardiovascular system effects of, 323–324, 323t
  central nervous system effects of, 320–322, 321f
  cerebral blood flow and, 821–822, 821f, 827f
  cerebral metabolic rate and, 821–822, 821f
  chemotactic activity of, 324–325
  contraindications to, 326
  depth of anesthesia and, 1245, 1245t
  electroencephalographic effects of, 1517–1518, 1518f, 1519t
  fentanyl interaction with, 449, 449f, 457, 458f
  hepatic metabolism of, 2213
  historical perspective on, 318
  hypothermia effects on, 1582
  in ambulatory anesthesia, 2602t, 2603–2604, 2603f
  in awake craniotomy, 2160
  in children, 173–174, 2375
  in eye surgery, 2528
  in kidney transplantation, 2241
  in malignant hyperthermia-like reaction, 1182
  in microlaryngoscopy, 2542
  in myotonic muscular dystrophy, 537
  in outpatient monitored anesthesia care, 2610
  in renal failure, 2184
  induction with, 325–326, 325t
  intraocular pressure effects of, 2532
  maintenance with, 325–326, 325t
  manual infusion of, 460t, 461–462
  memory effects of, 1238
  metabolism of, 318
  midazolam interaction with, 341, 342f, 450, 453f
  neuromuscular blockade and, 515–516
  neuroprotection with, 840
  opioid interaction with, 388, 413, 422
  pharmacokinetics of, 318–320, 319f, 319t
    target-controlled infusion and, 466–468, 468t, 469f
  pharmacology of, 320–325, 321f, 323t
  physiochemical characteristics of, 318, 318f
  plasma concentration ranges for, 453t
  recovery from, 2707–2708, 2707f
  remifentanil interaction with, 457–458, 459f
  respiratory system effects of, 322–323
  sedation with, 326
  side effects of, 326
  somatosensory evoked potential effects of, 1533t
  thermoregulatory response thresholds with, 1574–1575, 1574f
  visual evoked potential effects of, 1533t
  volume of distribution of, 454t
Proportioning systems, of anesthesia machines, 281–283, 281f, 282f
Propranolol, 653, 657, 1120–1121
  cerebral blood flow and, 819
  in kidney failure, 2186
  in pheochromocytoma, 1043
  pharmacology of, 653–655, 654f, 654t
  structure of, 654f
Propylthiouracil, 1046, 2221t
ProSeal laryngeal mask airway, 1627, 1627f
Prostacyclin, 629, 630
Prostaglandin(s)
  in renal function, 794–795, 795f, 1487–1488
  in renal protection, 799
  pulmonary vascular resistance and, 685t, 686
  synthesis of, 795, 795f
Prostaglandin E_1, in children, 2838–2839
Prostate gland
  cancer of, 2201
  cryosurgery for, 2194
  hypertrophy of, 2189
  innervation of, 2176
  laparoscopic surgery on, 2194–2195
  laser resection of, 2194
  microwave ablation of, 2194
  pain in, 2200–2201
  removal of, 2198–2199, 2198t. *See also* Transurethral resection of prostate (TURP).
  robotic, 2567–2568

Prostatitis, 2200–2201
Prosthetic cardiac valves, 1079, 1082–1083, 1082t, 1083f
Protamine
    for heparin monitoring, 1340–1341
    heparin reversal with, 1982
Protein(s)
    acute-phase, in sepsis, 2901–2903, 2902f, 2902t
    drug binding to, 74–76, 75f
        age-related changes in, 100–101
    metabolism of, 747
        by infant, 2370
        in sepsis, 2897–2899, 2898f
    plasma, 1825
Protein C, activated, in sepsis, 2796
Protein kinase C
    in myocardial protection, 209–210
    inhaled anesthetic effects on, 123
Proteinuria, 1493, 2179
Prothrombin complex, 1824
Prothrombin time, 753t, 754, 1340
    in children, 2390
    preoperative, 956, 960t, 961f, 2215
    prolongation of, 749
Proton pump inhibitors, in outpatient premedication, 2599–2600, 2600t
Pruritus
    droperidol for, 360
    epidural analgesia and, 2740
    in cholestasis, 764
    opioid-related, 392
Pseudo-aortic stenosis, 1956, 1956t
Pseudoaneurysm, catheter-related pulmonary artery rupture and, 1307
Pseudocholinesterase deficiency, cocaine hazard in, 2548
Pseudohypoparathyroidism, 1050
Pseudopseudohypoparathyroidism, 1050
Pseudorenal pain syndromes, 2200
Psoas compartment block, 1696–1697, Plate 11
    pediatric, 1743, 1745, 1745f
Ptosis, postoperative, 2531
Pudendal block
    during labor, 2322
    pediatric, 1749–1750, 1750f
Pulmonary arteriointerstitial pressure difference, 681
Pulmonary arteriovenous pressure difference, 680
Pulmonary artery
    catheter-related rupture of, 1306–1307
    congenital stenosis of, 2042, 2042f
    hypoxia-induced vasoconstriction of, 686–687, 687f, 712
        in one-lung ventilation, 1891–1893, 1891f, 1892f
        inhaled anesthetics and, 166–168, 167f, 168f, 1864–1865, 1865f
    mediastinal mass compression of, 1921f, 1922
    pediatric, 2841
Pulmonary artery banding, 2040
Pulmonary artery catheter monitoring, 1301–1327, 1333–1334
    after pneumonectomy, 1321t, 1322
    alveolar pressure effects on, 1308–1309, 1308f
    arrhythmias with, 1304–1305
    artifacts in, 1311–1312, 1311f
    artifactual pressure peaks in, 1312, 1312f
    atrial septal defect and, 1303
    body surface area in, 1334
    capillary pressure in, 1311
    cardiac output on, 1327–1331, 1327t, 1329t
    catheter flotation for, 1304
    catheter for, 1325–1326
        defects in, 1305
        placement of, 1301–1304, 1302f, 1308–1309, 1308f
        overwedging with, 1312, 1312f
    catheter knots with, 1305
    complications of, 1304–1307, 1304t
        incidence of, 1304
        knowledge deficit and, 1307
    controversial outcome studies of, 1323–1325
    during hip replacement, 2415–2417, 2416f
    endocarditis with, 1306
    goal-directed, 1325
    heart block with, 1305
    hemodynamic calculations for, 1333–1334
    hemoptysis with, 1306–1307
    in aortic reconstruction, 2077–2078
    in aortic regurgitation, 1321, 1321t
    in children, 2393
    in hyperbaric oxygen therapy, 2680

Pulmonary artery catheter monitoring (Continued)
    in left ventricular diastolic dysfunction, 1321, 1321t
    in mitral regurgitation, 1312–1314, 1313f–1315f, 1313t, 1322t, 1323
    in mitral stenosis, 1314, 1315f, 1322t, 1323
    in myocardial ischemia, 1314–1316, 1315f, 2068
    in pediatric cardiac surgery, 2017
    in pediatric shock, 2836
    in pericardial constriction, 1316, 1317f
    in positive end-expiratory pressure ventilation, 1322, 1322t
    in positive-pressure mechanical ventilation, 1317–1318, 1318f
    in preeclampsia, 2332
    in pulmonary hypertension, 1322–1323, 1322t, 1323f
    in pulmonary veno-occlusive disease, 1322t, 1323
    in pulmonic regurgitation, 1321, 1321t
    in right bundle branch block, 1321–1322, 1321t
    in sepsis, 2795
    in tachycardia, 1322t, 1323
    in thoracic surgery, 1863–1864, 1864f
    in ventricular septal defect, 1314, 1322t, 1323
    indications for, 1325
    infectious complications of, 1306
    knowledge deficit in, 1324
    left atrial pressure in, 1310–1311, 1310f, 1311f
    left ventricular end-diastolic pressure estimate with, 1320–1323, 1320f, 1321f, 1321t, 1322t, 1323f
    left ventricular filling pressure in, 1307–1309, 1308f
    left ventricular preload estimation in, 1318–1320, 1318f, 1319f
    lung zone effects on, 1308–1309, 1308f
    mechanical complications of, 1305
    misinterpretation of, 1307
    mixed venous oximetry with, 1331–1332
    outcome studies of, 1323–1325
    overwedging artifact in, 1312, 1312f
    persistence of left superior vena cava and, 1303
    physiologic considerations in, 1307–1309, 1308f
    practice variability in, 1324
    pressure waveform characteristics in
        artifactual, 1311–1312, 1311f
        normal, 1309–1310, 1309f, 1310f
    pseudoaneurysm with, 1307
    pulmonary artery rupture with, 1306–1307
    right bundle branch block with, 1305
    right ventricular ejection fraction in, 1332–1333
    thromboembolic complications of, 1305–1306
    valvular regurgitation with, 1306
    wedge pressure waveform in. See Pulmonary artery wedge pressure.
Pulmonary artery occlusion pressure. See Pulmonary artery wedge pressure.
Pulmonary artery pressure, 1308, 1309, 1309f. See also Pulmonary artery catheter monitoring.
    aortic cross-clamping and, 2073
    at high altitude, 687
    distribution of, 679–681, 680f
    during catheterization, 1302–1303, 1302f
    hypoxic pulmonary vasoconstriction and, 169, 687, 687f, 712
    measurement of, 1201
    normal, 679–681, 680f, 1297t
    pulmonary vascular resistance and, 684, 684f
Pulmonary artery wedge pressure, 1307–1308, 1308f, 1309–1310, 1310f, 1311
    abnormal, 1312–1316, 1313f–1315f
    during catheterization, 1302–1303, 1302f
    errors in, 1307
    fluid challenge test for, 1319
    in mitral regurgitation, 1312–1314, 1313f, 1313t, 1314f
    in mitral stenosis, 1314, 1315f
    in myocardial ischemia, 1314–1316, 1315f
    in ventricular septal defects, 1314
    interpretation of, 1318–1320, 1318f, 1319f
    left ventricular end-diastolic pressure estimate with, 1320–1323, 1320f, 1321f, 1321t, 1322t, 1323t
    left ventricular filling and, 1320–1323, 1320f, 1321f, 1322f
    left ventricular preload and, 1318–1320, 1318f, 1319f
Pulmonary capillary, 703–704, 704f
    fluid movement across, 704–705, 705t
Pulmonary capillary pressure, 1311

Pulmonary capillary wedge pressure
    aortic cross-clamping and, 2073, 2074t
    in renal function monitoring, 1494
Pulmonary compliance, 689–690, 690f
Pulmonary edema, 680–681, 704–705, 704f, 705t
    after thoracic surgery, 1903
    at high altitude, 2690
    detection of, 1468
    in kidney failure, 2181t, 2182
    in preeclampsia, 2330–2331
    postoperative hypoxemia and, 2713, 2713f
    with phosgene, 2511–2512
Pulmonary embolism, 1089–1090
    after bariatric surgery, 1033, 1034
    hypoxemia and, 2713
    hypoxemia in, 713, 713f
    prophylaxis for, 1079, 1082–1083, 1082t
Pulmonary fibrosis, idiopathic, 2264–2265
Pulmonary function testing, 999–1010
    after laparoscopy, 2294
    airway conductance and, 1003, 1003f
    airway resistance in, 1002–1003, 1003f, 1005–1006, 1006f
    before peripheral vascular surgery, 2063
    dynamic airway compression and, 1004, 1005f
    equal pressure point and, 1004, 1005f
    expiratory flow limitation on, 1004–1005, 1005f, 1005t
    flow-volume relationships in, 1003–1004, 1003f, 1004f, 1007–1009, 1008f, 1009f
    forced expiratory flow between 200 and 1200 mL of FVC in, 1000f, 1001
    forced expiratory volume in 1 second in, 1000–1001, 1000t, 1001t, 1006–1007, 1012, 1013
    forced midexpiratory flow in, 1001, 1007, 1007f
    forced vital capacity in, 1000–1001, 1000f, 1001t, 1007, 1007f, 1008f
    guidelines for, 1011–1012, 1011t, 1012t
    in airway obstruction, 1005–1010, 1007f–1009f, 1009t
    in asthma, 1005, 1005t
    in emphysema, 1005, 1005t
    in lung cancer, 1852–1854, 1853t
    in lung resection patient, 1012–1014
    in neuromuscular disease, 1005, 1005t
    in obesity, 1031–1032
    in surgical patient, 1011–1012, 1011t, 1012t
    in variable airway obstruction, 1009, 1009f, 1009t
    indications for, 1011–1012, 1011t, 1012t
    inspiratory capacity in, 1007
    maximum expiratory flow rate in, 1000f, 1001
    maximum static expiratory pressure in, 1002, 1002f
    maximum static inspiratory pressure in, 1002, 1002f
    maximum voluntary ventilation in, 1002
    normal values on, 1009–1010
    peak flow in, 1001, 1001f
    pediatric, 2841t, 2843
    recoil pressures in, 1002, 1003f
    total lung capacity in, 1000f, 1007, 1007f, 1008f
    vital capacity in, 999–1000
Pulmonary hypertension, 684, 1089–1090
    after pediatric cardiopulmonary bypass, 2033–2034
    central venous pressure monitoring in, 1316
    diaphragmatic hernia and, 2356
    high-altitude, 687
    in lung cancer patient, 1854–1856, 1855f, 1855t
    left ventricular end-diastolic pressure in, 1322–1323, 1322t
    nitric oxide therapy for, 2815
Pulmonary infarction, pulmonary artery catheter-related, 1306
Pulmonary interstitial pressure, 681
Pulmonary perfusion. See Lung(s), blood flow in.
Pulmonary reimplantation response, 2269–2270
Pulmonary stretch receptors, inhaled anesthetic effects on, 173
Pulmonary torsion, 1902
Pulmonary vascular resistance, 679–681, 680f
    after pediatric cardiopulmonary bypass, 2033–2034
    calculation of, 1333–1334
    carbon monoxide effect on, 165
    cardiac output and, 683–685, 684f
    determinants of, 165–166
    during one-lung ventilation, 1864–1865, 1865f, 1891–1893, 1891f, 1892f
    endothelin-1 and, 685–686, 685t

Pulmonary vascular resistance (Continued)
  hormonal effects on, 688, 688t
  hypoxia and, 686–687, 687f
  in hypertension, 684
  in lung cancer patient, 1854–1856, 1855f, 1855t
  inhaled anesthetic effects on, 165–170, 167f–169f
  lung volume and, 684–685, 684f
  neonatal, 2008, 2347, 2833, 2834
  neural systems in, 687–688
  nitric oxide and, 165, 685, 685t
  nitrous oxide effects on, 214
  nonalveolar blood flow and, 688–689
  normal, 1327t
  prostaglandins and, 685t, 686
  regional blood flow and, 166
  therapeutic reduction of, 686
Pulmonary veno-occlusive disease, left ventricular
      end-diastolic pressure in, 1322t, 1323
Pulmonary venous pressure, 679–681, 680f
Pulmonectomy. See Thoracic surgery.
Pulmonic regurgitation
  cardiac output measurement in, 1329
  left ventricular end-diastolic pressure in, 1321,
      1321t
  pulmonary artery catheter-related, 1306
Pulmonic stenosis, 2010–2011
Pulse
  in basic life support, 2927
  intraoperative monitoring of, 1268
Pulse contour technique, for cardiac output
      monitoring, 1338
Pulse dye densitometry, for cardiac output
      monitoring, 1338
Pulse oximetry, 1213–1215, 1214f
  accuracy of, 1193, 1194f
  artificial hemoglobin effects on, 1450, 1451t
  bilirubin effects on, 1451t, 1452
  burns with, 3143
  carboxyhemoglobin effects on, 1450, 1451t
  cyanmethemoglobin effects on, 1450, 1451t
  during laparoscopy, 2286, 2288, 2288f
  dye effects on, 1451t, 1452
  environmental temperature effects on, 1452–1453
  errors in, 1450–1453, 1451t
  fetal, 2313–2314
  hemoglobin concentration effects on, 1450,
      1451t, 1452
  hemoglobinopathy effects on, 1450, 1451t
  henna effects on, 1451t, 1452
  hypotension effects on, 1452
  in children, 2392, 2844
  in infant, 2394
  in pediatric cardiac surgery, 2017
  instrument design for, 1214, 1214f
  intraoperative, 1449
  light effects on, 1452
  limitations of, 1448–1449
  low oxygen saturation on, 1451t, 1452
  methemoglobin effects on, 1450, 1451t
  motion artifact with, 1215
  multi-wavelength, 1449
  nail polish effects on, 1451t, 1452
  polycythemia effects on, 1452
  postoperative, 1450
  principle of, 1448, 1448f
  reflectance, 1449, 1449f
  signal artifact with, 1214–1215
  skin pigmentation effects on, 1451t, 1452
  sulfhemoglobin effects on, 1450, 1451t
  tape effects on, 1451t, 1452
  vasoconstriction effects on, 1452
  vasodilation effects on, 1451t, 1452
  venous noise reference signal in, 1215
  venous pulsation effects on, 1451t
Pulseless electrical activity, 2939, 2940t
  in children, 2944–2946, 2945f
Pulseless ventricular tachycardia, 2935, 2937–2939
  in children, 2946–2947
Pulsus alternans, arterial blood pressure monitoring
      in, 1285, 1286f
Pulsus paradoxus, arterial blood pressure monitoring
      in, 1285–1286, 1286f
Pumping effect, variable-bypass vaporizer and, 286f,
      287, 287f
Pupil(s). See also Eye(s).
  examination of, 2996
    in brain death, 2961
  in basic life support, 2927
  light reflex of, 2996, 2997t
  opioid effects on, 391
Pupillary light reflex, 2996, 2997t

Purkinje cells, 730–731. See also Cardiomyocytes.
Pyloric stenosis, 2395
Pyridostigmine, 519, 521–522, 521f, 662, 875–876.
      See also Anticholinesterases.
  in kidney failure, 2186, 2186t
  in organophosphate poisoning, 2508–2509
  pharmacokinetics of, 523–524, 524t
  succinylcholine interaction with, 492
Pyruvate dehydrogenase, 2890–2891, 2890f, 2891f,
      2896–2897, 2897f
Pyuria, preoperative, 1493

Q

QRS complex, 1389, 1390f, 1411, 1411f
Quadriplegia, neurosurgery and, 2137–2138
Quality improvement, 2979–2988
  approaches to, 2982–2983, 2982f, 2986–2987
  care bundle concept in, 2987
  data analysis for, 2985–2986
  evidence-based medicine in, 2982t, 2983
  for mechanical ventilation, 2986
  incident report and review for, 2980–2982, 2981t
  performance measurements for, 2983–2986,
      2984f
  process measurements for, 2984
  public demand for, 2987
  quality of care definition and, 2980
  quantitative measurements for, 2984–2985
Quincke, Heinrich I., 25–26
Quinidine, 1125
  channel blockade by, 870
  hepatotoxicity of, 2221t
  in atrial fibrillation, 1402, 1402t, 1403t
  neuromuscular blocking agent interaction
      with, 517
Quinlan, Karen Ann, 3183

R

Radial artery, cannulation of, 1272–1274, 1273f.
      See also Arterial blood pressure.
Radial nerve block, 1693, 1693f, 1694f
Radial nerve injury
  position-related, 1152t, 1155, 1156f
  with orthopedic surgery, 2411–2412, 2412t
Radiation, occupational health risks of, 3153–3155,
      3154f
Radiation therapy, 1118, 2656–2658, 2657f
  in coronary artery disease, 2650
  intraoperative, 2656, 2657f
  safety for, 2640
Radioactive microspheres, in renal blood flow
      measurement, 791
Radiofrequency ablation, in children, 2042–2043
Radioisotopes, in glomerular filtration rate
      measurement, 790
Radiology suite, 2639–2643, 2641t
  anesthesia in, 2641–2642
  contrast media use in, 2640–2641, 2641t
Radiosurgery, 2658
RAE tube, 1630, 1631f
Raleigh, Sir Walter, 30
Raman gas analysis, 1454
Raman scattering, 1215
Ranitidine
  in outpatient premedication, 2599–2600, 2600t
  preoperative, 1860
Rapacuronium, 493t, 495, 495f, 497t
  autonomic effects of, 511, 511t, 512t
  bronchospasm with, 514
  elimination of, 506t, 508
  metabolism of, 506t, 508
Raper, Howard R., 16
Rapid Platelet Function Analyzer, 1343
Rapsyn, 866, 866f, 872
Rash, barbiturate-induced, 333
Raventos, James, 18
Reactive oxygen species
  hepatic, 757–758
  in myocardial reperfusion, 210
Reading, by anesthesiologist, 3055
Rebreathing, of inspired gas, 143
Recall, intraoperative
  depth of anesthesia and, 1237–1239
  postoperative consequences of, 1238–1239
Receptive substance, 85

Receptor(s), 85–93
  agonists at, 86, 86f
  antagonists at, 86–87, 86f
  classic theory of, 85–89, 86f–89f
  cold, 1572
  definition of, 85
  desensitization of, 101–102
  drug interactions at, 95f, 96–97, 97f
  G protein-coupled, 89–90, 90f
  $GABA_A$, 89f, 90–92, 91f
  historical studies of, 85
  in mice models, 93–95, 94t
  increased sensitivity of, 102
  ion channel, 89f, 90–92, 91f
  ion pump, 92
  ligand interaction with, 87–89, 88f, 89f
  molecular approaches to, 93–95, 94t
  R/R^* state of, 87–89, 88f, 89f
  second messenger, 92–93, 92f, 93f
  sensitivity of, 101–102
  states of, 87–89, 88f, 89f
  structure of, 89–93, 89f–93f
  warm, 1572
Recovery, 2707–2709, 2707t, 2708t, 2709t
  after ambulatory (outpatient) anesthesia, 2612,
      2614–2616, 2615t, 2616t, 2619–2620,
      2620t
  after inhaled anesthetics, 147–151. See also
      Inhaled anesthetics, recovery from.
  after intravenous anesthetics, 455–458, 455f–459f,
      459t
  after neuromuscular blockade, 519, 521–522, 521f,
      523–524, 524t, 875–876. See also
      Anticholinesterases.
  at remote locations, 2639
Rectus sheath block, pediatric, 1751, 1751f
Recurrent laryngeal nerve, 2537, 2538f
  injury to, 1047, 2538, 2547
  with mediastinoscopy, 1911
Red blood cells
  abnormalities of, in children, 2868–2869
  packed, 1812, 1812f, 1821–1822, 1822t
    for children, 2389–2390
    in hemorrhagic shock, 2465
Red henna, pulse oximetry errors and, 1451t, 1452
Reflectance oximetry, 1449, 1449f
Reflex(es)
  accommodation, 2996, 2997t
  Bainbridge, 739
  baroreceptor, 738–739, 738f
  Bezold-Jarisch, 739
  cardiac, 738–739, 738f
  carotid sinus, 738–739, 738f
  chemoreceptor, 739
  Cushing's, 739
  ocular, 2996, 2997t
  oculocardiac, 739
Reflex sympathetic dystrophy, 2774–2775
Refusal to provide care, 3179
Regional analgesia
  for vaginal delivery, 2319–2322. See also Vaginal
      delivery, regional analgesia for.
  in trauma, 2484–2485
  inter/intrapleural, 587–588, 1753, 1909, 2744
Regional anesthesia. See also Caudal anesthesia;
      Epidural anesthesia; Nerve block(s);
      Neuraxial anesthesia; Spinal anesthesia.
  ambulatory, 2608–2609
  historical studies on, 22–28
  hyperbaric oxygen therapy and, 2687
  in children, 1719–1756. See also Children, regional
      anesthesia for.
  in elderly patient, 2443
  in laparoscopy, 2298
  in orthopedic trauma, 2477–2478, 2477t, 2478t
  intravenous, 587
  ketamine with, 350
  renal effects of, 1489
  thermoregulation during, 1578–1580, 1578f,
      1579f
Regression analysis, 884–885
Rehabilitation, after trauma, 2479
Remifentanil, 380t. See also Intravenous anesthetics.
  age-related pharmacokinetics of, 2439, 2439f
  C_{50} of, 446–448, 447t
  cerebral blood flow and, 390, 821f, 823–824
  cerebral metabolic rate and, 821f
  context-sensitive decrement time of, 455–456,
      456f
  context-sensitive half-time of, 404, 404f
  during labor, 2318

Remifentanil (Continued)
electroencephalographic effects of, 388–389, 389f
for children, 2377–2378, 2378f
hepatic metabolism of, 2213
high-dose, 415, 415f
in balanced anesthesia, 411–412
in eye surgery, 2528
in head and neck surgery, 2539
in hemorrhagic shock, 409, 410f
in kidney transplantation, 2241
in outpatient anesthesia, 2606, 2606f
in outpatient monitored anesthesia care, 2610
in pediatric cardiac surgery, 2022
in single-agent anesthesia, 415, 415f
in total intravenous anesthesia, 413, 413t
infusion rate of, 459t
intracranial pressure effects of, 823–824
isoflurane interaction with, 449–450, 451f
manual infusion of, 460t, 461
metabolism of, 1248–1249
pharmacodynamics of, 1248–1249
pharmacokinetics of, 401t, 403, 403f
liver failure and, 408, 408f
target-controlled infusion and, 466–468, 468t
plasma concentration ranges for, 453t
propofol interaction with, 388, 413, 457–458, 459f
skin-incision potency test of, 405, 406f
sphincter of Oddi effects of, 2220, 2222
structure of, 381f
tolerance to, 397
volume of distribution of, 454t
Remote locations, 2637–2658
anesthesia at, 2617–2619. See also Ambulatory (outpatient) anesthesia.
cardiac catheterization at, 2650–2653
cardioverter-defibrillator implantation at, 2653
catheter ablation at, 2653
computed tomography at, 2642–2643
contrast media use at, 2640–2641, 2641t
coronary angiography at, 2648–2649
elective cardioversion at, 2653–2654
electroconvulsive therapy at, 2654–2656
electrophysiologic studies at, 2653
equipment for, 2638
external beam radiotherapy at, 2657–2658
interventional cardiology at, 2648–2654
interventional neuroradiology at, 2646–2648
anesthesia for, 2647–2648
methods for, 2647
magnetic resonance imaging at, 2643–2646, 2645f
anesthesia for, 2645–2646
medications for, 2639
pacemaker implantation at, 2653
patient monitoring at, 2638
personnel for, 2638–2639
radiation safety at, 2640
radiology suite for, 2639–2643, 2641t
anesthesia in, 2641–2642
recovery care at, 2639
stereotactic radiosurgery at, 2658
therapeutic radiation at, 2656–2658, 2657f
transvascular coronary arterial procedures at, 2649–2650
Renal. See also Kidney(s).
Renal artery
fibromuscular dysplasia of, 2072
stenosis of, 2072
Renal cell carcinoma, 2198, 2198t, 2199
Renal clearance, 73–74, 784–789
creatinine, 786–788, 787f
definition of, 785
Fick principle and, 784–785
free water, 789
inulin, 786
para-aminohippurate, 785–786
Renal erythropoietic factor, 1486
Renal insufficiency, after pediatric cardiopulmonary bypass, 2028t, 2029
Renal tubules, 781–784, 781f, 782f, 783t. See also Kidney(s).
acute necrosis of
after infrarenal aortic reconstruction, 2076
free water clearance in, 789
in hepatic disease, 761
collecting duct of, 781f, 784
distal, 781f, 784
evaluation of, 2179–2180
function of, 784, 785f, 1484–1486, 1485f
neurohumoral influences on, 1487–1488
oxygen balance in, 783, 783t

Renal tubules (Continued)
proximal, 781f, 782–783
reabsorption by, 781–782, 782f, 784
secretion by, 781–782, 782f
structure of, 781, 781f
tests of, 789–790
thick ascending loop of Henle of, 781f, 782f, 783
urine concentration by, 784, 785f
Renal vein, thermodilution measurements of, 790
Renin, 792–793, 792f, 1486
Renin-angiotensin-aldosterone system
drug effects on, 659
in blood pressure regulation, 627, 628f
in renal regulation, 792–793, 792f, 796, 796f
in spinal transection, 666
Renin-angiotensin system, 1486
in cardiac function, 737
in sodium homeostasis, 1765
Reperfusion injury, in liver transplantation 758, 2251
Rescue breathing, 2924
Research, internet use for, 2975–2977, 2975f
Reserpine, 658
organ response to, 633, 634t
Residual volume, 694, 694f
Respiration, 679–718. See also at Airway; Lung(s); Pulmonary.
after laparoscopy, 2294
airway resistance and, 690–691
alveolar filling with, 691–692, 691f
anesthetic depth and, 706, 706f
anesthetic effects on, 705–707, 706f, 707f. See also Hypoxemia.
intraoperative events and, 707
preexisting disease and, 707, 707f
barbiturate effects on, 334
benzodiazepine effects on, 339–340, 339f, 341
bronchitis and, 707, 707f
cardiac output monitoring and, 1330
cessation of, 2957, 2958. See also Brain death.
with pediatric spinal anesthesia, 1738
collateral ventilation with, 692
dexmedetomidine effects on, 357
droperidol effects on, 360
during central venous pressure monitoring, 1300–1301, 1300f
emphysema and, 707, 707f
epidural analgesia and, 2740
etomidate effects on, 353
evaluation of. See Pulmonary function testing.
flumazenil effects on, 344
historical studies on, 4–6
in emphysema, 709
in infant, 2369–2370, 2369f, 2370f
in malnourished patient, 2892, 2897f
in one-lung ventilation, 1894–1895
inhaled anesthetic effects on, 171, 172f
ketamine effects on, 347–348
light or inadequate general anesthesia and, 709
lung volumes and, 693–697, 693f
naloxone effects on, 420–421
neonatal, 2346, 2347, 2349, 2349t
neuraxial anesthesia and, 1660
obesity and, 707, 707f
opioid effects on, 392–394, 393f, 393t, 1463, 1472–1474, 1473t, 1474t
paradoxical, 1869, 1869f
post-traumatic, 2892, 2892f
postoperative depression of, 2715, 2715f
pressure-volume characteristics of, 692–693, 692f
pulmonary compliance and, 689–690, 690f
starvation and, 2913
toxic agent effects on, 2521–2522, 2522t
work of breathing and, 692–693, 692f, 693f
Respiratory centers, injury to, 2157–2158
Respiratory distress syndrome
evidence-based management in, 2790–2791, 2792f–2793f
fluid therapy in, 1793
hypoxemia in, 713–714, 713f
in children, 2848, 2848t
in critical care patient, 2790–2791, 2792f–2793f
Respiratory drive, 1463
Respiratory exchange ratio, 1010
Respiratory failure, 2811–2812
aerosol therapy for, 2815–2817, 2815f, 2816t, 2817t
after lung transplantation, 2270
bronchial hygiene therapy and, 2818–2820, 2818f, 2818t
bronchoscopic suctioning in, 2820

Respiratory failure (Continued)
classification of, 2811–2812
continuous positive airway pressure for, 2819
helium therapy for, 2815
in critical care patient, 2790–2791, 2792f–2793f
in mitochondrial myopathy, 537
intermittent positive-pressure breathing for, 2819
nasotracheal suctioning in, 2819–2820
nitric oxide therapy for, 2815
oxygen therapy for, 2812–2814, 2813t, 2814f. See also Oxygen therapy.
pathogenesis of, 2811–2812, 2812f, 2812t
pediatric, 2843–2851
alveolar disorders and, 2844, 2845t
arterial blood gases in, 2843–2844
causes of, 2844–2845, 2845t, 2846t
evaluation of, 2843–2844
hypoventilation and, 2844, 2845t
in bronchiolitis, 2852
in bronchopulmonary dysplasia, 2853
in cystic fibrosis, 2853
in epiglottitis, 2852
in foreign body aspiration, 2853–2854
in laryngotracheobronchitis, 2851–2852
in meningomyelocele, 2854
in sleep apnea, 2853
in status asthmaticus, 2852–2853
interstitial disorders and, 2844
metabolic acidosis with, 1782–1783
obstructive airway disease and, 2844–2845, 2845t
pulse oximetry in, 2844
treatment of, 2845–2851
analgesics in, 2849
continuous positive airway pressure in, 2847–2848
endotracheal intubation in, 2846–2847
extracorporeal membrane oxygenation in, 2851
extubation in, 2850
high-frequency ventilation in, 2851
liquid ventilation in, 2851
negative-pressure ventilation in, 2850–2851
partial liquid ventilation in, 2851
patient position in, 2845
perfluorochemical ventilation in, 2851
positive end-expiratory pressure in, 2847–2848
positive-pressure ventilation in, 2848–2849
sedatives in, 2849
surfactant in, 2851
ventilatory therapy in, 2846–2851, 2848t
positive expiratory pressure for, 2819
positive-pressure ventilation for, 2820–2828. See also Mechanical ventilation, positive-pressure.
risk index for, 1087, 1087t
Respiratory insufficiency, after thoracic surgery, 1902–1903
Respiratory monitoring, 1437–1474
alveolar gases in, 1439. See also Carbon dioxide (CO_2), alveolar; Oxygen (O_2), alveolar.
apnea monitor in, 1467–1468
arterial gases in, 1439–1447, 1440f–1444f, 1445t, 1446f, 1446t, 1447t. See also Carbon dioxide (CO_2), arterial; Oxygen (O_2), arterial.
capnography in, 1455–1462. See also Capnography.
continual vs. continuous, 1438
during patient transportation, 1472
expired gas analysis in, 1454–1455, 1455f
gas concentration measurement in, 1462
gas flow measurement in, 1463
high-frequency ventilation monitor in, 1468–1469, 1469f
in narcotic-related respiratory depression, 1472–1474, 1473t, 1474t
lung water in, 1468
mixed venous oxygen in, 1453, 1453f
oxygen saturation in, 1447–1453, 1448f, 1449f. See also Oximetry; Pulse oximetry.
respiratory drive measurement in, 1463
respiratory mechanics in, 1465–1467, 1466f, 1467f
respiratory output in, 1463–1465, 1464f
tissue oxygenation in, 1453–1454
transcutaneous gas tensions in, 1447
Respiratory muscles, 1463–1465, 1464f
Respiratory quotient, 703, 2906–2907, 2907f

Respiratory system. *See also* Lung(s); Respiration; Respiratory failure.
    age-related changes in, 2437–2438
    auto-positive end-expiratory pressure of, 1466, 1467f
    complicance of, 1465
    conductance of, 1465
    elastance of, 1465
    inertance of, 1465
    mechanical properties of, 1465–1467, 1466f, 1467f
    pediatric, 2840–2842, 2841t
    preoperative evaluation of, 1085–1089, 1087t, 1088t
    resistance of, 1465
    static compliance of, 1466
Respiratory tract infection
    in children, 2381–2382
    preoperative, 1088, 1090
Response, drug
    age and, 100–101
    disease state and, 101
    drug-drug interactions and, 102
    genetic variability in, 99–100
    pharmacodynamic interactions and, 101–102
    pharmacokinetic interactions and, 101
    receptor sensitivity and, 102
    variability in, 97–102, 98f
    vs. concentration, 95, 95f
Response surfaces, in pharmacodynamics, 97, 98f
Rest breaks, 3060–3061
Resting energy expenditure, 2906, 2906t
Reticular formation, inhaled anesthetic effects on, 109
Retina, 2992, 2992f
    blood supply to, 2995, 2995f
    venous hemorrhage of, 3003
Retinopathy of prematurity, 2354, 2534–2535
Retrobulbar block, 1709
Retrobulbar hemorrhage, 2530
Retrolental fibroplasia, 717, 2354
Rh blood typing, 1802, 1802t, 1804
Rhabdomyolysis, 1160
    exercise-induced, 1182–1183
    in malignant hyperthermia, 1181–1182
    in muscular dystrophy, 537
    renal effects of, 804–805
Rheumatic fever, 1959–1962
Rheumatoid arthritis, 2409–2410
    juvenile, orthopedic surgery in, 2427
    patient positioning in, 2412
Rib fracture, 2480–2481
Ribavirin
    aerosol, 2816
    in bronchiolitis, 2852
Richardson, Benjamin Ward, 22, 44, 44f
Richet, Charles R., 42
Ricin, 2515t, 2516
Rifampin, 2221t
Right atrial pressure, paradoxical air embolism and, 2141
Right bundle branch block, 1406t, 1407, 1407f, 1409, 1410f
    left ventricular end-diastolic pressure in, 1321–1322, 1321t
    pulmonary artery catheter-related, 1305
Right heart catheter, in neurosurgery, 2140–2141, 2141f
Right ventricle
    contractility of, transesophageal echocardiography for, 1378
    failure of
        after cardiopulmonary bypass, 1990–1991, 1991t
        after pneumonectomy, 2480
        in cardiac injury, 2481
        in heart transplantation, 2260–2261, 2260t
        in congenital heart disease, 2011–2012, 2012f
    inhaled anesthetic effects on, 199
    ischemia of, central venous pressure monitoring in, 1316
    normal pressures of, 1297t
    structure of, 724–725, 725f
Right ventricular ejection fraction, pulmonary artery catheter monitoring of, 1332–1333
Riley-Day syndrome, 1044–1045
Riluzole, hepatotoxicity of, 2221t
Ringer, Sydney, 21
Risk, anesthesia. *See* Anesthesia-related risk.
Ritodrine, 652

Robertshaw tube, 1875–1876, 1875f, 1877–1878, 1878f. *See also* Endotracheal tubes, double-lumen.
Robinson, James, 15
Robotic surgery, 2557–2569, 2694
    cardiac, 1995, 2562–2566, 2563f, 2563t, 2564t, 2565f, 2565t, 2566f, 2566t
    gastrointestinal, 2561–2562, 2562f
    gynecologic, 2568
    historical perspective on, 2557–2558
    neurologic, 2567
    ophthalmologic, 2568–2569
    orthopedic, 2568
    systems for, 2558–2561, 2559f–2561f
    thoracic, 2566–2567
    urologic, 2567–2568
Rocci, Scipione Riva, 6–7
Rocuronium, 493t, 494–495, 495f, 497t
    allergic reaction to, 514
    autonomic effects of, 511, 511t, 512t
    cerebral physiology and, 831
    dosage for, 501t
    elimination of, 506t, 508, 511
    for tracheal intubation, 503–505, 503f, 504t, 505f
    hepatic metabolism of, 2214
    hepatobiliary disease and, 529–530, 529t, 2214
    hypothermia effect on, 516
    in children, 525–526, 2379, 2380t
    in elderly patients, 526
    in renal failure, 2184–2186, 2185t
    in trauma patient, 2458
    metabolism of, 506t, 508
    pharmacodynamics of, 500t, 502t
    renal failure and, 528, 528t
    skin testing with, 514
Roe, Cecil, 26
Rofecoxib
    in outpatient premedication, 2597
    postoperative, 2735t, 2736f
Roizen, Michael, 36
Ropivacaine, 575t
    during labor, 2321, 2321t, 2323
    for epidural anesthesia, 1674t, 1675
    for spinal anesthesia, 1661t, 1667
    in pediatric regional anesthesia, 1723, 1723f, 1723t, 1724, 1728, 1728t
    structure of, 575t
    vs. bupivacaine, 595–596
Rose bengal test, 756
Rotameter, 1463
Rous, P., 21
Rovenstine, Emery A., 24
Rowbotham, Edgar S., 37
Ryanodine receptors, 1172–1174, 1172f
    genes for, 1173, 1174–1176, 1175f, 1175t
    in malignant hyperthermia, 1176–1177
Rynd, Francis, 19
RYR1 gene, 100

S

Sacral hiatus, 1657, 1658f, 1659f
    in children, 1720
Sacral plexus block, pediatric, 1743, 1744, 1746–1748, 1747f, 1748f
Sacrum
    in children, 1720
    surgery on, 2421
Sadove, Max S., 18
Safar, Peter, 40
Safety
    electrical, 3139–3148. *See also* Electrical safety.
    for machines, 276–277, 277f, 279, 280, 288, 291–292
    for magnetic resonance imaging, 2644–2645
    for radiation therapy, 2640
    of anesthesia, 893–920, 895f, 919t. *See also* Anesthesia-related safety.
    of hyperbaric oxygen therapy, 2685
    operating room, 3047–3054, 3151–3164. *See also* Operating room, safety of.
St. John's wort (*Hypericum perforatum*), 607t, 611
Saline
    hypertonic, 1785–1786, 1826
        in hemorrhagic shock, 2463–2464
        in pediatric ICP increase, 2857
        in traumatic brain injury, 2472
    normal, 1785
Salmeterol, 2817t

Salmonella assay, for mutagenicity, 261
Salt intolerance, postoperative, 21
Salt solutions
    balanced, 1785
    hypertonic, 1785–1786
Sameridine, 418
Saphenous nerve, position-related injury to, 1156t
Saphenous nerve block, 1703–1704, 1704f, 1705f, Plate 16
    pediatric, 1743, 1745–1746, 1746f
Sarcolemma, 730, 730f
    in cardiac excitation-contraction coupling, 731–732, 732f
Sarcomere, 732–733, 733f
    Frank-Starling relationship and, 725f, 726–727, 727f
    length of, 726
Sarin, 2504–2509, 2505t, 2506t, 2507f
Sassafras, hepatotoxicity of, 2222t
Sauerbruch, Ernst Ferdinand, 37
Saw palmetto (*Serenoa repens*), 607t, 611
Saxitoxin, 2515t, 2516
Scalp blocks, pediatric, 1755
Scavenging systems, 303–307
    checkout for, 315
    closed interface of, 305f, 306–307
    components of, 304–307, 304f
    gas-collecting assembly of, 304–305, 304f
    gas-disposal assembly of, 307
    hazards of, 307
    NIOSH recommendations for, 304, 304t
    open interface of, 305–306, 305f
    scavenging interface of, 305–307, 305f, 306f
    transfer means of, 305
    tubing of, 307
Scheele, Carl W., 4, 12–13
Schiff, Moritz, S., 9
Schimmelbusch, Curt, 37
Schizophrenia, 1123
Schleich, Carl, 23
Schwarz, Emil, 21
Schwilden, Helmut, 439
Sciatic nerve
    anatomy of, 1743
    position-related injury to, 1155, 1156t
Sciatic nerve block, 1699–1701, 1700f, 1701f, Plate 13
    anterior approach to, 1701, 1701f
    classic (posterior) approach to, 1700, 1700f, Plate 13
    pediatric, 1744, 1746–1748, 1747f, 1748f
        lateral, 1748, 1748f
        popliteal, 1746–1747, 1747f
        proximal, 1747–1748, 1747f, 1748f
Scopolamine, 660t, 661, 661f, 2720–2721
    in outpatient premedication, 2599
    toxicity of, 662, 2537
Scrotum, innervation of, 2177
SDZ-RAD, in organ transplantation, 2271–2273, 2272t
Second gas effect, 135, 136f
Second messengers, 92–93, 92f, 93f
Sedation. *See also* Barbiturate(s).
    benzodiazepines for, 340–341, 340t
    dexmedetomidine for, 358
    etomidate for, 355
    for children, 1730, 2381
    for conscious (awake) endotracheal intubation, 1641
    for critically ill patient, 2798–2799, 2799t
    in pediatric ICP increase, 2857
    in pediatric respiratory failure, 2849
    ketamine for, 349–450, 349t
    opioids for, 410–413, 410t
    propofol for, 326
    scoring scales for, 2798, 2799t
Segmental wall motion, transesophageal echocardiography of, 1378–1379, 1379t, 1384
Seizures, 833, 1094–1095
    awake craniotomy in, 2159–2161
    cerebral blood flow and, 843
    cerebral ischemia and, 842
    compound 485 and, 116
    electroencephalography in, 1514, 1523
    enflurane and, 829
    epidural anesthesia and, 1676
    flurothyl and, 116
    in alcohol withdrawal, 1097
    in children, 2857, 2858
    in hypocalcemia, 1050

Seizures (Continued)
    in preeclampsia, 2331–2332
    intracranial pressure and, 2857
    isoflurane and, 829–830
    laudanosine and, 831
    opioids and, 391
    oxygen toxicity and, 2678
    sevoflurane and, 830
Selection bias, in statistics, 886
Selective serotonin reuptake inhibitors, 1123
    in chronic pain, 2771–2772
Sellick, B., 40–41
Sellick maneuver, 2456
Semilateral position, for neurosurgery, 2135
Semirecumbent position, 1163–1164, 1164f
Sensitivity, test, 889
Sensory evoked potentials, 1512–1513, 1512t.
                  See also Brainstem auditory evoked
                  potentials; Motor evoked potentials;
                  Somatosensory evoked potentials; Visual
                  evoked potentials.
    abnormal changes in, 1527
    amplitude of, 1526, 1526f
    anesthetic effects on, 1532–1537, 1533t
    cortical, 1525
    latency of, 1526, 1526f
    near-field, 1525
    noise interference with, 1527
    opioid effects on, 389
    physiologic factors and, 1537
    short-latency, 1526, 1526f
    subcortical, 1525–1526
Sensory receptors, inhaled anesthetic effects on,
                  109–110
Sepsis, 1104, 2894–2905
    amino acid metabolism in, 2898–2899, 2899f
    arterial blood pressure monitoring in, 1283
    branched-chain amino acid metabolism in,
                  2901
    cardiovascular response to, 2894–2895, 2894f
    cortisol in, 2899–2900
    cytokines in, 2900–2901
    epinephrine in, 2900
    fatty acid metabolism in, 2903, 2903f
    glucose metabolism in, 2895–2897, 2895f, 2896f
    growth hormone in, 2900
    hepatic protein metabolism in, 2901–2903, 2902f,
                  2902t
    hormonal response to, 2897, 2899–2900
    hyperglycemia in, 2799–2800
    insulin in, 2900
    insulin-like growth factor-1 in, 2900
    insulin resistance in, 2904–2905
    interleukin-1 in, 2901
    interleukin-6 in, 2900
    ketone bodies in, 2904
    lipogenesis in, 2903–2904
    metabolic response to, 2894–2897, 2894f–2897f
    neonatal, 2870–2871, 2870t
    nitrogen balance in, 2897–2898, 2898f
    pediatric, 2871
    protein metabolism in, 2897–2898, 2898f
    renal protection in, 805–807
    transurethral resection of prostate and, 2193
    treatment of, 2794–2796
    tumor necrosis factor in, 2900–2901
Sepsis syndrome, 806
Septicemic plague, 2517
Serotonin
    bronchial response to, 156
    halothane with, 161
    inhaled anesthetic effects on, 113, 121
    isoflurane with, 161
    pulmonary vascular resistance and, 688, 688t
Sertuerner, Friedrich W., 19
Severinghaus, John W., 6, 6f
Sevoflurane, 19, 284–285, 284f
    age-related interactions with, 1255
    airway hyperreactivity with, 174
    airway resistance and, 160, 160f
    arterial pressure and, 202
    BIS index and, 1255–1256
    bronchial effects of, 157, 158, 158f
    calcium effects of, 158, 158f, 167
    carbon dioxide absorbent interaction with,
                  251–256, 251f, 254f, 297–298
    central ventilatory effects of, 171, 172f
    cerebral blood flow and, 825–827, 826f, 827f
    cerebral metabolic rate and, 826f, 827–828
    diaphragm effects of, 174–177, 175f, 177f
    diastolic function and, 195–196

Sevoflurane (Continued)
    electroencephalographic effects of, 1519t,
                  1520–1521
    emergence from, in children, 2373
    fluoride-associated nephrotoxicity of, 249–250
    hepatic function and, 246, 2209–2212, 2211f
    hypoxic pulmonary vasoconstriction and, 166,
                  167–168, 168f
    in ambulatory anesthesia, 2604–2605, 2604t
    in children, 253, 2372–2373, 2372f, 2372t, 2373t
    in kidney transplantation, 2241
    in outpatient monitored anesthesia care, 2611
    in pediatric cardiac surgery, 2020, 2021
    in renal failure, 2183
    left atrial function and, 199–200, 201f
    left ventricular-arterial coupling and, 196–197,
                  197f
    metabolism of, 135, 238–240, 239f
    minimum alveolar concentration of, 107–109,
                  107f, 108t
    myocardial contractility and, 192
    myocardial preconditioning and, 1954
    nephrotoxicity of, 251–256, 251f, 254f, 1490
    neuromuscular blockade and, 515–516, 516t
    neuromuscular blockade reversal and, 522
    oil-gas partition coefficient of, 115t
    partition coefficients of, 132, 132t
    pulmonary blood flow and, 169
    recovery from, 147–151, 148f, 149f, 2707–2708,
                  2708t
    renal effects of, 801, 1490–1491
    seizures and, 830
    structure of, 106f
    toxicity of, 914. See also Malignant hyperthermia.
    tubing uptake of, 142, 143t
    vasodilating effect of, 829
Sheehan's syndrome, 1052
Shellfish poisoning, 2516
Shift work, 3057–3058. See also Sleep deprivation.
Shipway, Francis E., 33
Shires, G., 21
Shivering, 1575
    during eye surgery, 2530
    opioid effects on, 391–392
    postoperative, 1582–1583, 2714, 2721
    threshold for, 1575
        during neuraxial anesthesia, 1578, 1578f, 1579f,
                  1580–1581
Shnider, Sol M., 43
Shock
    cardiogenic
        pediatric, 2835
        postoperative, 2716
    fluid therapy in, 1784–1785
    hemorrhagic
        cerebral blood flow and, 817
        opioid effects in, 409, 409f, 410f
        trauma-related, 2459–2469
            pathophysiology of, 2459–2460, 2460f
            Pco2 in, 2468–2469
            resuscitation for, 2453, 2453t, 2454t
                early, 2460–2463, 2461t, 2462t, 2462t,
                  2463t, 2464f
                equipment for, 2466–2467, 2466t, 2467t
                fluids for, 2463–2466
                in vulnerable patient populations, 2463
                late, 2467–2469, 2467t, 2468f
    hypovolemic, postoperative, 2716
    pediatric, 2834–2836, 2835f, 2835t, 2871
    postoperative, 2716–2717
    septic
        in children, 2871
        postoperative, 2716–2717
        treatment of, 2794–2796
Shock lung, blood transfusion and, 1815
Shock therapy. See Electroconvulsive therapy.
Shoulder surgery, 2421
    patient positioning for, 1163–1164, 1164f
Shunt
    arteriovenous, 1573
    Blalock-Taussig, 2040
    congenital, 2009–2010, 2009t
    CSF, 2162–2163
    portal-systemic, 2223–2224, 2223f
    right-to-left
        arterial gas tensions and, 77, 701–702, 701f,
                  702f, 1440, 1440f, 1441f
        hypoxemia and, 701, 701f, 713, 2713
        in patent foramen ovale, 689, 713, 1903
        thoracic surgery and, 1903
    ventriculoperitoneal, 2163

Shunt fraction, 1442
Shy-Drager syndrome, 1044–1045
Sibson, Francis, 37
Sicard, Jean Enthuse, 27
Sick sinus syndrome
    electrocardiography in, 1398, 1399f
    pediatric, 2839
Sickle cell disease, 1112–1113
    in children, 2869
    ocular pathology in, 2536
    tonsillectomy and, 2544
Sigmoid-E$_{max}$ relationship, 95
Signal processing, for monitoring, 1193–1196,
                  1195f–1197f
Significance, statistical, 885
SimMan patient simulators, 3080, 3082, 3082f
Simpson, James Young, 16
Simulators. See Patient simulators.
Single nucleotide polymorphism, 97–98
Sinoatrial block, 1406–1407, 1406f
Sinoatrial node, inhaled anesthetic effects on, 202
Sinus arrest/pause, dexmedetomidine-induced, 358
Sinus arrhythmia, electrocardiography in, 1399
Sinus bradycardia
    electrocardiography in, 1398, 1399f
    pediatric, 2839
    succinylcholine-induced, 489
Sinus tachycardia, electrocardiography in,
                  1398–1399
Sinuses, surgery on, 2540
Sirolimus, in organ transplantation, 2271–2273, 2272t
Sitting position
    in neurosurgery, 2136–2138, 2137f
    nerve injury with, 1164–1166, 1165f
Six-minute walk test, in pulmonectomy patient,
                  1013
Skin
    anesthetic loss by, 135
    inhaled anesthetic uptake by, 134
    kava effects on, 611
    mustard gas effect on, 2509, 2509f
    of neonate, 2349, 2349f
    pigmentation of, pulse oximetry errors and,
                  1451t, 1452
    warming of, 1585–1587, 1586f, 1587f
        during neuraxial anesthesia, 1581
        postoperative, 1583
Skullcap, hepatotoxicity of, 2222t
Sleep
    assessment of, 3058
    determinants of, 3056–3057
    electroencephalography during, 1514, 1515f
    medications for, 3061–3062
    micro-, 3057
    nonresponsiveness of, 1230
    normal, 3055
    postoperative disruptions in, 2749
    recommendations for, 3060
Sleep aids, 3061–3062
Sleep apnea, 1096
    in children, 2853
    obesity and, 1030–1031
    postoperative pain management and, 2748–2749
    pulmonary complications and, 1088
Sleep debt, 3055
Sleep deprivation, 3055–3059, 3162–3163
    aging and, 3062
    assessment of, 3058
    consequences of, 3058–3059
    countermeasures for, 3060–3063
    perception of, 3059
    work hours regulation and, 3062
SLEEPER patient simulators, 3078
Sleepiness, 3058
Smallpox, in biological warfare, 2519
Smith, G., 8
Smith, W. D. A., 17
SNARE (soluble N-ethylmaleimide-sensitive
                  attachment protein receptor), 864, 864f
Snow, John, 33, 44, 44f
Snyder, S. H., 10
Sobrero, Ascanio, 9
Soda lime, 296. See also Carbon dioxide (CO2)
                  absorbents.
Sodium, 1764–1768. See also Hypernatremia;
                  Hyponatremia.
    fractional excretion of, 790, 1498
    physiology of, 1764–1765
    renal regulation of, 1485–1486, 1485f, 1506
    requirements for, 1764–1765
    urinary, 789–790, 1498

Sodium (Na⁺)-calcium (Ca²⁺) exchanger, in cardiac function, 731, 731f, 732f
Sodium bicarbonate
   in cardiac arrest, 2938–2939
   in children, 2838
   in metabolic acidosis, 1611
   in neonatal acidosis, 2357–2358, 2357f, 2358f
   in pediatric cardiac arrest, 2946
   in pediatric life support, 2947t
   local anesthetics with, 585
   minimum alveolar concentration and, 109
   PETCO₂ and, 1460–1461, 1461f
Sodium bisulfite, 597
Sodium channel
   in nerve conduction, 578, 579f
   isoforms of, 581–582
   local anesthetic binding to, 580–581, 580f, 582f
   neurotoxin effects on, 583f
   opioid effects on, 386–387, 386f
   selective sensitivity of, 581–582, 583f
Sodium channel-blocking factor, in Guillain-Barré syndrome, 534
Sodium citrate, in outpatient premedication, 2600, 2600t
Sodium nitrite, in cyanide poisoning, 2514t
Sodium nitroprusside
   in children, 2837t, 2838
   in kidney failure, 2187
   in pediatric shock, 2836
   with aortic cross-clamping, 2077
Sodium-potassium-ATPase pump, digitalis inhibition of, 92
Sodium thiosulfate, in cyanide poisoning, 2514t
Soft tissue injury, 2479
   with endotracheal intubation, 1647
Solubility, drug, 69
Soluble N-ethyl maleimide sensitive factor (NSF), 632
Soman, 2504–2509, 2505t, 2506t, 2507f
Somatosensory evoked potentials, 1211–1212, 1512, 1527–1530
   abnormal changes in, 1527
   anesthetic effects on, 1532–1537, 1533t, 1534f, 1536f
   barbiturate effects on, 1533t, 1536
   blood gas effects on, 1537
   droperidol effects on, 1533t, 1536
   during carotid endarterectomy, 2104
   etomidate effects on, 352–353, 1533t, 1536, 1536f
   false-positive results with, 1529
   fentanyl effects on, 1536–1537
   for cerebral blood flow, 1529
   in aortic aneurysm repair, 1529
   in brain death, 2965
   in cerebral aneurysm surgery, 1529–1530
   in coma, 1530
   in spinal cord procedures, 1529
   in spinal surgery, 2418–2419
   indications for, 1529
   long-latency, 1528
   median nerve stimulation for, 1528
   opioid effects on, 1533t, 1536–1537
   physiologic factors and, 1537
   short-latency, 1526, 1526f, 1528–1529, 1528t
   temperature effects on, 1537
   vs. electroencephalography, 1529
Somatostatin, in carcinoid-related hypotension, 1109
Sonoclot system, 1341–1342
Soporific sponge, 10–11
Soranus, 8
Sore throat, after intubation, 1650, 2547
Sotalol, 653, 654–655
   in atrial fibrillation, 1402, 1402t, 1403t
Soubeiran, Eugene, 16
Sound, 1205–1208
   principles of, 1205–1206, 1205f, 1206f
Space, medical care in, 2693–2694, 2694f
Sparteine oxygenase, 99
Spasm
   in malignant hyperthermia, 1180–1181, 1181f
   succinylcholine-related, 491, 2378–2379
Specific gravity, urine, in renal function monitoring, 1496–1497
Specific heat, 285
Specificity, test, 889
Spectrometry, mass, 1454
Spherocytosis, hereditary, 1113–1114
Sphincter of Oddi, drug effects on, 2220, 2222
Sphygmomanometry, 1269, 1269f

Spinal analgesia. See also Epidural analgesia; Spinal-epidural analgesia.
   during labor, 2320–2321
   historical studies of, 25–27
Spinal anesthesia, 1661–1670. See also Neuraxial anesthesia.
   ambulation after, 1670
   ambulatory, 2608
   arterial blood pressure with, 1660
   backache after, 1670
   benzodiazepine use and, 1678
   bupivacaine for, 589, 589t, 1661t, 1666–1667
   cardiac arrest after, 1670
   CNS depressants with, 1670
   complications of, 597, 1668–1670, 1669t
   continuous, 1665, 1666f
      for cesarean section, 2325
   drug selection for, 589, 589t, 1661, 1661t, 1665–1667
   dyspnea with, 1670
   electromyography after, 1670
   epidural anesthesia with, 1678, 1678t
   epidural blood patch after, 1669–1670
   epinephrine with, 1667
   equipment for, 1661, 1662f
   failure of, 1668
   for cesarean section, 2324, 2324f
   headache after, 1669–1670, 1669t
   height of, 1668, 1668t
   hypobaric, 1667–1668
   in transurethral resection of prostate, 2190
   isobaric, 1667–1668
   lateral decubitus position for, 1662, 1662f
   levobupivacaine for, 1661t, 1667
   lidocaine for, 589, 589t, 1661t, 1665–1666
   lumbosacral approach to, 1665, 1665f
   mepivacaine for, 1666
   midline approach to, 1663–1664, 1664f
   needle insertion for, 1663–1665, 1663f–1666f, 1669
   neurologic injury with, 1669, 1670
   paramedian approach to, 1664–1665, 1664f
   patient position for, 1662–1663, 1662f, 1663f
   pediatric, 1737–1738, 1737t
      anatomy for, 1737
      anesthetic dosage for, 1737, 1737t
      complications of, 1738
      contraindications to, 1737
      equipment for, 1729t
      indications for, 1737
      limitations of, 1738
      technique for, 1737–1738, 1737t
   phenylephrine with, 1667
   physiologic effects of, 1658–1660
   preparation for, 1661, 1661t, 1662f
   procaine for, 1665
   prone position for, 1663
   respiratory arrest with, 1660
   ropivacaine for, 1661t, 1667
   sitting position for, 1662, 1663f
   tetracaine for, 589, 589t, 1661t, 1666, 1666t
   transient neurologic symptoms with, 1666
Spinal block, total, 2328–2329
Spinal cord, 1654–1658, 1655f
   angiography of, before thoracoabdominal aortic reconstruction, 2088, 2088f
   development of, 1720
   inhaled anesthetic effects on, 109
   ischemia of, in thoracoabdominal aortic reconstruction, 2086–2088, 2086f
   nitrous oxide-induced subacute combined degeneration of, 256–257
   surgery on, 2164, 2165t
Spinal cord injury, 2473–2476, 2474f
   autonomic changes with, 665–666
   autonomic hyperreflexia syndrome in, 1044
   cervical, 2456, 2474–2475
   dysautonomia with, 1044–1045
   early supportive care in, 2475–2476
   intraoperative management of, 2476
   ischemic, 2086–2088, 2086f
   neuraxial blocks and, 1151
   nicotinic receptor upregulation in, 102
   with thoracic surgery, 1903–1904
Spinal cord reflexes, brain death and, 2962–2963, 2963f
Spinal cord stimulation
   in chronic pain, 2774
   in complex regional pain syndrome, 2775
Spinal-epidural analgesia, during labor, 2320–2321, 2321f

Spinal-epidural anesthesia, for cesarean section, 2325
Spinal nerve roots, 1654–1655, 1655f
Spinal shock, 666
Spinal surgery, 2164, 2165t, 2414t
   cervical, 2418
   thoracolumbar, 2418–2420
Spine
   ossification of, 1720
   radiosurgery on, 2567
Spirometer, 1205, 1205f
Spirometry, 694, 694f, 999–1002, 1463. See also Pulmonary function testing.
   for preoperative rehabilitation, 1014
   in double-lumen endotracheal tube positioning, 1882
   in pulmonectomy patient, 1013–1014
   incentive
      for bronchial hygiene, 2818
      preoperative, 1086
   time-expired, 1000–1001, 1000f, 1000t, 1001t, 1006–1007, 1007f
Spironolactone, in hyperaldosteronism, 1038
Spiropulsator, 35
Splenic sequestration, in sickle cell disease, 2869
Splenoportography, 757
Spondylosis, 1096
Sputum, preoperative removal of, 1859–1860
Square root sign, in pericardial constriction, 1316, 1317f
ST segment, 1390, 1390f
   computer-assisted interpretation of, 1411–1412
   in ischemia monitoring, 2068
   in myocardial ischemia, 1406, 1411–1412
Stahl, Georg Ernst, 4
Standard deviation, 883
Standard error of the mean, 883–884
Standard precautions, 3161
Standards, 919
Starling, Ernest H., 20
Starling forces, in renal function, 1487
Starvation, 1034, 2888–2892, 2889f–2891f, 2891t, 2892f. See also Nutrition.
   respiration and, 2892, 2897f, 2913
   ventilation and, 2892, 2893f
Statins, 1027–1028, 1028t
Statistics, 881–889
   alpha value in, 885
   beta error in, 885
   bias in, 886
   central tendency measure in, 883, 883t
   confidence intervals in, 885–886
   contingency tables in, 888
   data dredging and, 887
   data for, 882, 882t
   dispersion measures in, 883–884
   evidence-based medicine and, 889
   for hypothesis testing, 885–886
   graphic format for, 884
   level of significance in, 885
   meta-analysis and, 889
   multiple comparisons and, 887
   multiple-group analysis in, 888t
   multivariate analysis in, 884–885
   nonparametric, 882, 887–888, 888t
   normal distribution in, 882–884, 883t
   P value in, 885
   paired data in, 888
   parametric, 882, 888t
   power in, 885
   probability in, 888–889
   regression analysis in, 884–885
   standard deviation in, 883
   standard error of the mean in, 883–884
   study design and, 886–887
   two-group analysis in, 888t
   univariate analysis in, 884
   unpaired data in, 888
   variables in, 884–885
Status asthmaticus, 2852–2853
   ketamine in, 348
Status epilepticus, 1094
   in children, 2858
Steatohepatitis, postoperative, 2216–2217
Steatosis, postoperative, 2216–2217
Stellate cells, hepatic, 750
Stellate ganglion block, 1709–1710, 1709f
   pediatric, 1753–1754
Stereochemistry, 76
Stereotactic neurosurgery, 2161
Stereotactic radiosurgery, 2658

Steroidal compounds, 493t, 494–495, 495f, 507–508, 507f. *See also specific steroidal compounds.*
Steroids. *See* Corticosteroids.
Stethoscope, 1206
Stethoscopy, intraoperative, 1266–1267
Stool, in cholestasis, 764
Strabismus, 2530, 2535–2536
Streptokinase, bleeding with, 1117
Stress
  post-traumatic, 1238–1239
  work-related, 3162–3164
    substance abuse and, 3166
Stress-free anesthesia, historical studies on, 35–36, 35f
Stress response, 2730–2731, 2892, 2892f. *See also* Sepsis.
  in neonate, 2345–2346, 2394–2395
  in pediatric cardiopulmonary bypass, 2028t, 2029
  opioid effects on, 396–397
  renal effects of, 783
Stridor, 2387–2388, 2387f, 2388f, 2539
  after tonsillectomy, 2543
Stroke. *See* Cerebral ischemia.
Stroke volume
  inhaled anesthetic effects on, 196–197, 197f
  nitrous oxide effects on, 214
  normal, 2834t
  variation in, 1327
Stroke work, of heart, 727
Strong ion difference, 1601, 1601f, 1603–1604, 1603t
Strychnine, 19, 20f
Strychnos toxifera, 20f
Study design, 886–887, 894–897
Sturge-Weber syndrome, 2536
Stylet, for endotracheal intubation, 1631–1632, 2458, 2458f
Sub-Tenon block, 2529
Subarachnoid hemorrhage, 2146–2151, 2146t, 2147t. *See also* Intracranial aneurysm.
  transcranial Doppler ultrasonography after, 1541
Subclavian artery, mediastinoscopy-related compression of, 1911
Subclavian vein
  cannulation of, 1292, 1303. *See also* Central venous pressure monitoring.
  catheterization of
    in hemorrhagic shock, 2466
    in parenteral nutrition, 2910–2911
Subdural space, 1655–1656, 1655f
Substance abuse, 3063, 3164–3170
  causes of, 3166–3167, 3167f
  consequences of, 3167
  identification of, 3167–3168, 3167t, 3168t
  management of, 3167–3169, 3167t, 3168t
  mortality rates and, 3167
  prevalence of, 3165–3166
  prognosis for, 3169–3170
  workplace reentry after, 3169
Succinylcholine, 486–492
  acetylcholine receptor effects of, 483
  allergic reaction to, 514
  anticholinesterase interaction with, 492
  anticonvulsant interaction with, 517
  autonomic effects of, 512t
  butyrylcholinesterase effect on, 487–489, 488f, 488t
  cardiovascular effects of, 489
  cerebral blood pressure and, 831–832
  channel blockade by, 870
  clinical uses of, 491–492, 492t
  contraindications to, in children, 525
  diltiazem interaction with, 517
  diuretic interaction with, 517–518
  dysrhythmia and, 513
  economic considerations and, 546–547
  ED$_{95}$ of, 486
  elimination of, 506t
  extraocular muscle effects of, 869
  for children, 2378–2379
  for children with full stomach, 2385
  furosemide interaction with, 517
  half-life of, 74
  hyperkalemia with, 489–490, 873
  in burn patient, 530
  in electroconvulsive therapy, 2655–2656
  in endotracheal intubation, 491–492, 503–505, 503f, 504t, 1633
  in head injury, 2153
  in ICU patient, 532
  in kidney transplantation, 2241

Succinylcholine (*Continued*)
  in microlaryngoscopy, 2542
  in motor neuron diseases, 534
  in myasthenic syndromes, 541, 541f, 542f
  in outpatient anesthesia, 2607
  in pacemaker patient, 1426
  in renal failure, 2184–2185
  in spinal cord injury, 102
  in trauma patient, 2457–2458
  intracranial pressure and, 491, 831–832
  intragastric pressure and, 490–491
  intraocular pressure and, 490, 2532–2533
  lithium interaction with, 517
  magnesium interaction with, 517
  masseter spasm with, 491, 2378–2379
  mechanism of action of, 868–869, 868f, 870–871
  metabolism of, 506t
  monitoring of, 484–485, 484f
  myalgia with, 491
  nodal rhythms with, 489
  nondepolarizing neuromuscular blocking agent interaction with, 515
  pediatric contraindications to, 525
  pharmacodynamics of, 486–487, 502t
  pharmacokinetics of, 486–487
  phase II block with, 1563, 1564f
  side effects on, 489–491
  sinus bradycardia with, 489
  structure of, 488, 488f
  toxicity of, 1180, 1182. *See also* Malignant hyperthermia.
  ventricular dysrhythmias with, 489
  verapamil interaction with, 517
Suckling, Charles, 18
Sudden death
  in aortic stenosis, 1955–1956
  in hypertrophic cardiomyopathy, 1957
Sudden infant death syndrome, 2875–2876
Sufentanil, 380t. *See also* Intravenous anesthetics.
  abuse of, 3166. *See also* Substance abuse.
  adrenal effects of, 396
  age-related pharmacokinetics of, 2439, 2439t
  allergic reactions to, 399
  C$_{50}$ of, 446–448, 447t
  cardiovascular effects of, 395
  cerebral blood flow and, 389, 821f, 823
  cerebral metabolic rate and, 821f, 823
  context-sensitive half-time of, 404, 404f
  during labor, 2321, 2321t
  endocrine effects of, 396–397
  epileptogenic properties of, 833
  for children, 2377
  for patient-controlled intravenous analgesia, 2733–2734, 2733t
  hepatic metabolism of, 2213
  high-dose, 414f, 415
  in balanced anesthesia, 411
  in kidney transplantation, 2241
  in outpatient anesthesia, 2606, 2606f
  in pediatric cardiac surgery, 2021, 2022, 2022t, 4230f
  in pediatric regional anesthesia, 1725, 1725t
  in single-agent anesthesia, 414f, 415
  in total intravenous anesthesia, 413, 413t
  infusion rate of, 459t
  intracranial pressure effects of, 390, 823
  intranasal, 416–417
  isoflurane interaction with, 449–450
  manual infusion of, 460t, 461
  myocardial ischemia and, 395, 397
  peak effect of, 404, 405f
  pharmacokinetics of, 401t, 403
    cardiopulmonary bypass and, 409, 409f
    liver failure and, 408
    target-controlled infusion and, 465–468, 468t
  plasma concentration ranges for, 455t
  postoperative, 2737, 2737t, 2738t
  propofol with, 413
  seizures and, 833
  single-bolus, 410
  structure of, 381f
  volume of distribution of, 454t
Suicide, 3167
  addiction and, 3167
  physician-assisted, 3187–3188, 3188t
Sulfhemoglobin, pulse oximetry errors and, 1450, 1451t
Sulfonamides, hepatotoxicity of, 2221t
Sulfur hexafluoride
  intravitreal injection of, 2533
  oil-gas partition coefficient of, 115t

Sulfur mustard, 2509–2510, 2509f, 2510f, 2512–2513
Superior hypogastric plexus blockade, in complex regional pain syndrome, 2775
Superior laryngeal nerve block, 1708, 1708f
  in awake intubation, 1642, 1643f
  in endotracheal intubation, 1647
Superior vena cava, left, persistence of, 1303
Superior vena cava syndrome, 1921f, 1922–1923
Supine position
  in neurosurgery, 2135
  nerve injury with, 1158
Supraclavicular nerve block, 1689–1690, 1689f, 1690f, Plate 3
Supraorbital nerve block, 1706, 1706f, Plates 1 and 2
  pediatric, 1754, 1754f
Supraorbital nerve injury, with orthopedic surgery, 2411–2412, 2412t
Supratentorial tumor, 2145–2146
Supratrochlear nerve block, 1706, 1706f, Plates 1 and 2
  pediatric, 1754, 1754f
Supraventricular bradyarrhythmia, 2929–2930
  in children, 2942, 2943f
Supraventricular tachyarrhythmias, 2930–2933, 2930f–2933f, 2936f
  in children, 2942–2943
Supraventricular tachycardia, 2930, 2931f, 2936f
  after cardiac surgery, 1993
  in children, 2839
Sural nerve, position-related injury to, 1156t
Sural nerve block, 1703, 1703f, Plate 15
Surfactant, 690
  for neonate, 2356
  in premature infant, 2851
  inhaled anesthetic effects on, 162, 164f
Surgical stress response, 664
Sweating, threshold for, 1572, 1572f, 1573, 1573f, 1575
  during neuraxial anesthesia, 1578, 1578f
Sympathetic nerve block, in chronic pain, 2774–2775
Synapse, 860, 861f
  inhaled anesthetic effects on, 111–112, 112f
Synaptosome-associated protein 25, in acetylcholine release, 864, 864f
Syntaxin, in acetylcholine release, 864, 864f
Syndrome of inappropriate antidiuretic hormone secretion, 1052–1053, 1766
Syndrome of inappropriate secretion of antidiuretic hormone
  after subarachnoid hemorrhage, 2147
  in children, 2861–2862
Syndrome X, 1777, 1951
Synthane, oil-gas partition coefficient of, 115t
Syphilis, transfusion-transmitted, 1820
Syringe, historical perspective on, 19–20, 19f
Systeme International d' Unites, 1192–1193
Systemic vascular resistance, 1327t, 1333–1334
  during laparoscopy, 2291–2292, 2291f
  sitting position effects on, 2136
Systole
  atrial, 724, 724f
  ventricular, 724, 724f, 725–728, 725f–727f
Systolic pressure variation, 1326–1327, 1326f

T

T wave, 1390, 1390f
TAAC3, 493t, 495, 496f
Tabun, 2504–2509, 2505f, 2506t, 2507f
TAC (tetracaine-epinephrine-cocaine), 589–590, 590t
Tachycardia
  β-adrenergic receptor antagonists in, 656
  ketamine-induced, 348
  laryngoscopy and, 1647
  left ventricular end-diastolic pressure in, 1322t, 1323
  neonatal, 2836–2837
  neuromuscular blocking agents and, 512–513
  pancuronium and, 513
Tacrine, hepatotoxicity of, 2221t
Tacrolimus, in organ transplantation, 2271–2273, 2272t
Tait, Frederick Dudley, 26
Tamoxifen
  hepatotoxicity of, 2221t
  neuromuscular blocking agent interaction with, 518
Tape (adhesive), pulse oximetry errors and, 1451t, 1452

Target-controlled anesthetic infusion, 464–473
  age-associated variability and, 469
  Bayesian forecasting for, 471
  BET scheme of, 464
  components of, 463–464, 463f
  effect-site concentration in, 471–472, 471f
  evaluation of, 465–466, 465f
  gender-associated variability and, 469
  intraindividual variability and, 470–471
  median absolute performance error in, 466–468, 468t
  microcomputer of, 464, 464f
  optimization of, 466–472, 466f, 467f, 468t, 469f–471f
  outcome of, 472–473
  patient-associated variability and, 469–471
  pharmacokinetic model for, 464–465, 465f, 467, 468t, 469f–471f, 471–472
  set point for, 463
  shock-associated variability and, 469–470
Teeth
  absence of, 1620
  intubation-related injury to, 1647
Temazepam, in outpatient premedication, 2596, 2596t
Temperature, 1193
  body. See also Hyperthermia; Hypothermia.
    behavioral regulation of, 1573
    BIS index and, 1255
    cerebral metabolic rate and, 816, 816f
    distribution of, 1576–1577, 1584–1585
    in blood transfusion, 1814, 1814t
    in cardiopulmonary bypass, 1977, 1977t, 1978–1979
    interthreshold range of, 1572
    minimum alveolar concentration and, 108, 108f
    monitoring of, 1216–1217, 1216f, 1590–1591, 1591f
    neuromuscular blockade and, 516
    perception of, 1579, 1579f
    regulation of. See Thermoregulation.
    somatosensory evoked potential monitoring and, 1537
    threshold, 1572
Temperature scale, 1193
Temporal artery, cannulation of, 1274. See alsoArterial blood pressure.
Tension headache, 1096
Tension pneumocephalus, 2138, 2138f
Tension pneumothorax, 1902
Terbutaline, 652, 1120
  in status asthmaticus, 2852
Terrell, Ross C., 18
Testis (testes)
  innervation of, 2177
  pain in, 2200
  tumor of, 2200
Tetanus toxin, 2515t
Tetracaine, 575t
  cardiovascular toxicity of, 594–595, 594t
  duration of action of, 584
  in nerve block, 587–588, 588t
  in spinal anesthesia, 589, 589t, 1661t, 1666, 1666t
  pKa of, 574, 574f
  potency of, 576t
  structure of, 575t
  topical, 589–590, 590t
Tetracycline
  hepatotoxicity of, 2221t
  neuromuscular blockade and, 516
Tetrahydrocannabinol, 1118
Tetralogy of Fallot, 2009–2010, 2009t
Tetrodotoxin, 2515t
Thalassemia, 1113
THAM (trishydroxymethylaminomethane), in neonatal acidosis, 2357
Theodoric of Cervia, 11
Theophylline, 1124
  in post-dural puncture headache, 2328
  preoperative, 1859
Thermal conductivity, 285
Thermistors, 1216–1217
Thermodilution
  in cardiac output monitoring, 1203, 1222–1223
  in renal vein evaluation, 790
Thermogenesis
  in spinal transection, 666
  nonshivering, 1573, 1575
Thermometers, 1216, 1590

Thermoregulation, 1572–1574. See also Hyperthermia; Hypothermia; Temperature, body.
  afferent input in, 1572
  central control in, 1572, 1572f
  during anesthesia, 1574–1576, 1574f–1576f
  efferent responses in, 1573–1574, 1573f
  heat transfer and, 1576
  in brain death, 2959–2960, 2961–2962
  in elderly, 1575, 1575f
  in infants, 1575, 1575f
  opioid effects on, 391–392
  shivering response in, 1575
  sweating thresholds in, 1574–1575, 1574f
Thiamylal
  duration of action of, 328
  neuroprotection with, 839
  side effects of, 333–334
  structure of, 328, 328f
Thigh, surgery on, 2422
Thioguanine, 1118
Thiomethoxyflurane
  oil-gas partition coefficient of, 115t
  structure of, 106f
Thiopental. See also Intravenous anesthetics.
  airway resistance and, 160, 160f
  C50 of, 446–448, 447t
  cardiovascular system effects of, 333–334
  cerebral blood flow and, 821, 821f
  cerebral metabolic rate and, 821, 821f
  cerebral metabolism and, 815, 815f
  contraindications to, 334
  cortical somatosensory evoked responses with, 815, 815f
  depth of anesthesia and, 1244–1245, 1244f
  distribution of, 332
  dosing for, 333, 333t
  duration of action of, 328t
  electroencephalographic effects of, 1517–1518, 1520f
  for children, 2375
  hepatic metabolism of, 2213
  in ambulatory anesthesia, 2602–2603, 2602t
  in heart disease patient, 334
  in myotonic muscular dystrophy, 537
  in pediatric ICP increase, 2857
  in renal failure, 2183–2184, 2184t
  induction with, 332
  intraocular pressure effects of, 2532
  lipid solubility of, 331
  manual infusion of, 462
  memory effects of, 1238
  metabolism of, 329
  neuroprotection with, 839
  opioids with, 422
  pharmacokinetics of, 319t, 330
    in elderly patient, 2438–2439, 2439t
    target-controlled infusion and, 466–468, 468t
  physiologic model of, 77, 78f
  plasma concentration ranges for, 453t
  respiratory system effects of, 334
  side effects of, 333–334
  structure of, 328, 328f
  volume of distribution of, 454t
Third spacing, in postoperative bowel obstruction, 1790
Thoracic analgesia, postoperative, 2744
Thoracic paravertebral block
  pediatric, 1751–1752, 1752f
  postoperative, 2744
Thoracic pump mechanism, in basic life support, 2925f, 2926
Thoracic surgery, 1847–1926
  anesthesia for, 1864–1868, 1909–1926
    arterial oxygenation and, 1865–1866, 1866f
    in bronchopleural fistula, 1925–1926
    in bronchopulmonary lavage, 1918–1920, 1918f, 1919t
    in bullectomy, 1916–1917
    in empyema, 1926
    in lung abscess, 1926
    in lung volume reduction, 1917–1918
    in massive hemoptysis, 1923–1925, 1924f
    in mediastinal mass resection, 1920–1923, 1921f, 1921t
    in mediastinoscopy, 1909–1911, 1910f
    in thoracoscopy, 1912
    in tracheal resection, 1912–1916, 1913f–1915f
    inhaled anesthetics for, 1867
    intravenous anesthetics for, 1867

Thoracic surgery (Continued)
  anesthesia for (Continued)
    pulmonary vasoconstriction and, 1864–1865, 1865f, 1891–1893, 1891f, 1892f
    techniques for, 1867–1868
  bronchial disruption with, 1902
  cardiac herniation with, 1901–1902
  complications of, 1901–1904
  epidural catheter for, 1868
  extubation after, 1868
  fentanyl in, 1867, 1868
  hemorrhage with, 1902
  high-frequency ventilation in, 1900–1901
  inhaled anesthetics in, 1867, 1868
  ketamine in, 1867
  lateral decubitus position for, 1869–1873, 1872f
    anesthetized
      closed-chest, 1870–1871, 1871f
      open-chest, 1871–1872, 1871f
      paralyzed, 1871f, 1872
    awake, closed-chest, 1869–1870, 1870f
    pulmonary vascular monitoring and, 1863–1864, 1864f
  liver failure and, 2219
  low-flow apneic ventilation in, 1901
  mechanical ventilation after, 1904–1906, 1904t, 1905f
  monitoring during, 1861–1864, 1862t, 1864f
  neural injury with, 1903–1904
  one-lung ventilation for, 1873–1900
    arterial oxygenation with, 1890–1891, 1890f
    blood flow distribution with, 1891–1894
    conventional management of, 1894–1895, 1894t
    dependent lung positive end-expiratory pressure in, 1894
    differential lung positive end-expiratory pressure/continuous positive airway pressure in, 1895f, 1897–1899, 1898f
    differential management of, 1895–1899, 1895f, 1897f, 1898f
    double-lumen endotracheal tubes for, 1874–1889, 1874f–1876f
      chest radiography with, 1882
      complications of, 1882–1883, 1883t
      contraindications to, 1883
      conventional intubation procedure for, 1877–1879, 1878f, 1879f
      cuff seal pressure hold with, 1882, 1883f
      fiberoptic bronchoscopy with, 1879–1882, 1880f, 1881f, 1882t
      selection of, 1876–1877
    indications for, 1873–1874, 1873t
    inspired oxygen concentration in, 1894
    intermittent collapsed lung ventilation in, 1895, 1895f
    management of
      conventional, 1894–1895, 1894t
      differential, 1895–1899, 1895f, 1897f, 1898f
      recommendation for, 1899–1900, 1899f
    physiology of, 1890–1894, 1890f–1892f
    respiratory rate in, 1894–1895
    selective dependent lung positive end-expiratory pressure in, 1895–1896, 1895f
    selective nondependent lung CPAP in, 1895f, 1896–1897, 1897f
    single-lumen endotracheal tube for (bronchial blocker), 1883–1885, 1884f, 1885f, 1885t
      independent, 1887–1889, 1887f, 1888f, 1888t
      indications for, 1887
      just-seal volume and, 1886–1887
      limitations of, 1885–1886, 1886f
      technique of, 1889–1890
    tidal volume in, 1894
  pain management after, 1906–1909
    cryoanalgesia in, 1906–1907
    epidural analgesia in, 1907–1909, 1908t
    interpleural analgesia in, 1909
  paradoxical respiration and, 1869
  preoperative evaluation for, 1849–1856
    cardiovascular evaluation in, 1854–1856, 1855f, 1855t
    chest radiography in, 1851–1852, 1852f, 1852t
    laboratory tests in, 1851–1854, 1852f, 1852t, 1853t
    pathology review in, 1848, 1849t
    pulmonary function tests in, 1012–1014, 1852–1854, 1853t
    staging in, 1848–1849, 1850t

Thoracic surgery (Continued)
  preoperative preparation for, 1856–1861, 1857f, 1858f, 1858t
    airway dilation in, 1859
    atrial fibrillation/flutter prophylaxis in, 1860–1861
    chest physiotherapy in, 1859–1860
    gastroesophageal reflux prophylaxis in, 1860
    secretion loosening in, 1859
    secretion removal in, 1859–1860
    smoking discontinuation in, 1858–1859, 1859t
  pulmonary complications of, 1856–1857, 1857f, 1902, 1903
    pulmonary edema with, 1903
    pulmonary torsion with, 1902
    respiratory insufficiency after, 1902–1903
    right heart failure with, 1903
    right-to-left shunt with, 1903
    spontaneous ventilation and, 1868–1869, 1869f
    unilateral pulmonary edema with, 1903
Thoracic vest system, in basic life support, 2926, 2927f
Thoracoabdominal aorta
  aneurysm of, 2081–2089
    classification of, 2082–2083, 2082f, 2083f
    etiology of, 2081–2083
    morbidity of, 2083
    mortality with, 2083
  dissection of, 2082–2083, 2083f
  reconstruction of, 2083–2089
    anesthesia for, 2085–2086
    aortic cross-clamping in, 2085
    atrial-to-femoral bypass during, 2085–2086, 2085f
    blood transfusion in, 2083
    coagulopathy and, 2089
    endovascular, 2089–2092
    extracorporeal support during, 2085–2086, 2085f
    intravenous access for, 2083
    metabolic management in, 2089
    monitoring during, 2083–2084
    motor evoked potential monitoring during, 2083
    neuromuscular blockade during, 2083
    one-lung ventilation in, 2083–2084
    paraplegia and, 2086–2088, 2086f
    renal failure after, 2088–2089
    somatosensory evoked potential monitoring during, 2083
    spinal cord ischemia and, 2086–2088, 2086f
    temperature monitoring during, 2083
Thoracolumbar spine surgery, 2418–2420
  blood conservation in, 2419
  complications of, 2419–2420
  pulmonary complications of, 2419
  visual loss after, 2419–2420
  wake-up test in, 2419
Thoracoscopy, 1912
Thoratec mechanical circulatory support system, 1992, 1992t
Thorax
  compliance of, 1465–1466, 1466f
  muscle tone of, 708–709, 709f
  resistance of, 1466–1467
Thorax and abdomen nerve block, 1710–1712
  celiac plexus, 1711–1712, 1712f
  intercostal nerve, 1710–1711, 1710f
  paravertebral, 1712, 1713f, Plate 10
Thorpe, P. H., 277, 1204, 1204f
Three-in-one block, pediatric, 1744–1745, 1744f
Throat. See also Nose and throat surgery.
  sore, 1650, 2547
Thrombin, in coagulation, 1983, 1983f
Thrombin time, 1340
Thrombocytopenia, 1116
  dilutional, 1807–1809, 1808f, 1808t, 1809f, 1810–1811
  hereditary, 2868
  in end-stage liver disease, 2248
  in hepatic disease, 761
Thrombocytosis, oxygen consumption in, 1446
Thromboelastography, 1341–1342, 1342f
Thromboembolism
  central venous catheter-related, 1293t, 1295
  in mitral stenosis, 1961
  in obese patient, 1033, 1034
  pulmonary artery catheter-related, 1305–1306
Thrombolytic agents
  bleeding with, 1117
  for stroke, 2647

Thrombophlebitis, etomidate-related, 354
Thrombosis
  recombinant factor VIIa and, 1838–1839
  risk factors for, 1116
  venous, with orthopedic surgery, 2425–2426, 2425f, 2426f
  with percutaneous transluminal coronary angioplasty, 2649–2650
Thrombotic thrombocytopenic purpura, 1116
Thromboxane, pulmonary vascular resistance and, 685t, 686
Thromboxane A$_2$, 795, 795f
Thyroid gland
  amiodarone-induced dysfunction of, 1047
  carcinoma of, 1048
  dysfunction of, 1045–1048, 1045t
  in brain death, 2960
  nodules of, 1048
  surgery on, 2540
Thyroid storm, 1047
Thyromental distance, in airway management, 1621
Thyrotoxicosis, β-adrenergic receptor antagonists in, 656
Thyroxine (T$_4$), 1045–1046, 1045t
  hepatic metabolism of, 750
  in brain death, 2960
Tibial artery, cannulation of, 1274. See also Arterial blood pressure.
Tibial fracture, fat embolism and, 2425
Tibial nerve, position-related injury to, 1156t
Tibial nerve block, 1703, 1703f, Plate 15
Ticlopidine, hepatotoxicity of, 2221t
Tidal volume, 694, 694f, 1465
  assessment of, 1463
  in one-lung ventilation, 1894
  reduction of. See Hypoventilation.
Time, 1192
Timolol, 653, 656, 2536
Tiotropium, 2817t
Tissue-blood partition coefficient, of inhaled anesthetics, 132t, 133
Tissue clearance, 74
Tissue plasminogen activator, bleeding with, 1117
Titin, 733, 733f
Tobramycin
  aerosol, 2816
  renal effects of, 803
Todd, D. P., 33
Tolazoline, in children, 2836, 2838
Tolcapone, hepatotoxicity of, 2221t
Tomlinson, Herbert, 7
Tongue, in neurosurgery, 2136, 2137
Tonsillar herniation, brain death and, 2959
Tonsillectomy, 2543–2544
Topical anesthesia
  anesthetics for, 589–591, 590t
  ocular, 2531
  pediatric, 1755
Torsades de pointes, 1404, 2934, 2934f
  droperidol-related, 360
Total energy expenditure, 2905
Total intravenous anesthesia, 29
Total lung capacity, 694, 694f, 1007, 1007f, 1008f
Total parenteral nutrition. See Nutrition, parenteral.
Tourniquet, 2423–2425, 2423t, 2424f
  deflation of, 2423–2424, 2424f
  inflation of, 2423, 2424, 2424f
  neurologic consequences of, 2424–2425
  pain with, 2424
Toxiferine diallyl derivative, 493t, 497, 497f, 509. See also Alcuronium.
Toxins
  biological, 2513, 2515–2516, 2515t
  pediatric ingestion of, 2875
Trachea
  anatomy of, 1618
  mediastinal mass compression of, 1921–1922, 1921f, 1921t
  receptors of, 1618
  resection of, 1912–1916, 1913f–1915f
    for carinal lesion, 1914–1915, 1915f
    for high lesion, 1913–1914, 1913f
    for low lesion, 1914, 1914f
    high-frequency jet ventilation in, 1915
    high-frequency positive-pressure ventilation in, 1915
  suctioning of
    for bronchial hygiene, 2819–2820
    in neonate, 2354–2355
  trauma to, 2480

Tracheobronchial tree, mediastinal mass compression of, 1921–1922, 1921f, 1921t
Tracheoesophageal fistula, 2355, 2396
Tracheostomy
  emergency, 2546–2547
  tube change for, 2539–2540
Train-of-four stimulation, in muscle relaxant monitoring, 484–486, 484f
Tramadol, 417–418
  in chronic pain, 2769
  in outpatient anesthesia, 2606
  in postoperative pain, 2735t, 2736–2737, 2736f
  in postoperative shivering, 1583
  shivering attenuation with, 391–392
Tranexamic acid, 1812
Transcranial Doppler ultrasonography, 1512t, 1540–1542, 1540f, 1541f
  for cerebral blood flow monitoring, 1540–1542, 1540f, 1541f
  in pediatric cardiac surgery, 2019
Transcutaneous electrical nerve stimulation
  during labor, 2317
  in chronic pain, 2776–2777
  postoperative, 2744
Transdiaphragmatic pressure monitoring, 1464, 1464f
Transducer
  for dynamic pressure measurement, 1199–1201, 1199f–1201f
  for signal processing, 1194, 1195f
Transesophageal echocardiography, 1363–1385
  abbreviated examination in, 1372–1374, 1373f, 1374f
  anesthesiologist performance during, 3040–3041, 3041f
  cardiac output on, 1376
  complications of, 1371
  comprehensive examination in, 1373f, 1374–1376, 1375f
  contraindications to, 1371
  data storage in, 1384
  Doppler
    color, 1369–1370, 1371f, Plates 33–1 and 33–2
    continuous-wave, 1369, 1370f
    pulsed-wave, 1367–1369, 1368f, 1369f
  endocarditis and, 1371
  equipment for, 1370, 1372f
  global left ventricular contractile function on, 1376
  global right ventricular contractile function on, 1378
  guidelines for, 1364
  historical perspective on, 7–8, 1363–1364
  hypotension on, 1378, 1378t
  in air embolism, 1381, 1383
  in aortic disease, 1379, 1383
  in children, 1384
  in congenital heart disease, 1384
  in myocardial ischemia, 1378–1379, 1379f, 2068
  in patent foramen ovale, 689
  in surgical decision-making, 1383–1384
  in valvular disease, 1379–1381, 1380f, 1381t, 1382f, 1383f, 1384, Plates 33–3 and 33–4
  indications for, 1364, 1365f
  intraoperative, 1969–1970
    in aortic reconstruction, 2078–2079
  left ventricular filling pressure on, 1376, 1377f
  M-mode, 1365, 1367, 1367f
  precautions for, 1370–1371
  preload on, 1376
  principles of, 1364
  probes for, 1371, 1372f
  quality assurance for, 1384–1385
  rescue, 1378, 1378t
  surgical implications of, 1383–1384
  training for, 1364, 1366t, 1367t
  two-dimensional, 1365, 1367, 1368f
Transfusion therapy, 1799–1827
  albumin preparations for, 1825
  blood components for, 1821–1825, 1821f, 1822t
  blood for, 1799–1821. See also Blood transfusion.
  cryoprecipitate for, 1824
  dextrans for, 1826
  frequent-donor plasma for, 1825
  fresh frozen plasma for, 1809, 1823–1824
  hydroxyethyl starch for, 1825–1826
  informed consent for, 1827
  oxygen-carrying substances for, 1826–1827
  packed red blood cells for, 1821–1822, 1822t

Transfusion therapy (Continued)
plasma protein preparations for, 1825
platelet concentrates for, 1822–1823
prothrombin complex for, 1824
single-donor plasma for, 1825
synthetic colloids for, 1825–1828
synthetic oxygen-carrying substances for, 1826–1827
Transient ischemic attack, myocardial infarction and, 1061
Transient neurologic symptoms, with lithotomy position, 1155
Transjugular intrahepatic portal-systemic shunt procedure, 2223–2224, 2223f
Translaryngeal nerve block, 1708–1709, 1709f
Transmural pressure, in central venous pressure monitoring, 1296–1297
Transmyocardial revascularization, 1995
Transparent tape, pulse oximetry errors and, 1451t, 1452
Transphenoidal hypophysectomy, 2158–2159, 2158t
Transplantation, 2231–2273
contraindications to, 2237
heart, 2253–2263, 2255t, 2256f–2257f, 2260t, 2262t. See also Heart transplantation.
immunosuppression for, 2271–2273, 2272t
intestine, 2253
kidney, 2235, 2237–2242, 2239f
liver, 2235–2237, 2236f, 2245–2253, 2251f. See also Liver transplantation.
lung, 2237, 2263–2271, 2263t, 2264t, 2266f, 2267f. See also Lung transplantation.
pancreas, 2242–2245, 2244f
team approach to, 2231–2232
Transport. See Patient transport.
Transthecal block
distal, 1742
pediatric, 1742, 1742f, 1748–1749
Transthoracic impedance, in apnea monitoring, 1468
Transtracheal anesthetic injection, in children, 1756
Transtracheal jet ventilation, 1637–1639, 1640f, 2458–2459, 2545, 2546
in basic life support, 2924–2925
Transurethral resection of prostate (TURP), 2189–2194
ammonia toxicity and, 2192–2193
anesthesia for, 2190–2191
bacteremia and, 2193
bladder perforation and, 2193
bleeding and, 2193
circulatory overload and, 2192
coagulopathy and, 2193
complications of, 2191–2194
glycine toxicity and, 2192
hypo-osmolality and, 2192
hyponatremia and, 2192
hypothermia and, 2193
in pacemaker patient, 1426
irrigation solutions for, 2189–2190, 2190t, 2191–2192
morbidity of, 2191
mortality and, 2191
robotic, 2567–2568
septicemia and, 2193
TURP syndrome after, 1766–1767, 2193–2194, 2194t
visual changes after, 3012–3014
cerebral edema and, 3014
glycine toxicity and, 3013–3014
hyponatremia and, 3014
intraocular pressure and, 3014
irrigating fluid and, 3013
spinal anesthesia and, 3014
symptoms of, 3013
Transurethral resection of prostate (TURP) syndrome, 1766–1767, 2193–2194, 2194t
Transverse (T) tubules, 730
Trauma, 2451–2489
abdominal, 2481–2482
airway management in, 2452–2453, 2452t, 2454–2459, 2455f
aspiration and, 2456
cervical spine in, 2456
cricoid pressure in, 2456
endotracheal intubation in, 2455–2456, 2456t, 2457f, 2458–2459, 2458f
extubation for, 2483, 2483t
in facial trauma, 2459
in pharyngeal trauma, 2459
indications for, 2454–2455

Trauma (Continued)
airway management in (Continued)
induction anesthetics for, 2457
mechanical ventilation for, 2485–2487, 2485t, 2486f, 2486t
neuromuscular blocking drugs for, 2457–2458
oral vs. nasal intubation in, 2459
personnel for, 2456–2457
analgesia in, 2483–2485
aortic, 2480
ATLS protocol for, 2452–2454, 2453f
cardiac, 2481
central nervous system, 2469–2476. See also Brain injury; Spinal cord injury.
chest, 2479–2481
compartment syndrome with, 2478–2479
crush syndrome with, 2478–2479
during pregnancy, 2337–2338, 2482
epidemiology of, 2451
extracorporeal life support in, 2488
Glasgow coma score in, 2453–2454, 2454t
hemorrhagic shock in, 2459–2469
pathophysiology of, 2459–2460, 2460f
resuscitation for, 2453, 2453t, 2454t
early, 2460–2463, 2461t, 2462f, 2462t, 2463t, 2464f
equipment for, 2466–2467, 2466t, 2467t
fluids for, 2463–2466
in vulnerable patient populations, 2463
late, 2467–2469, 2467t, 2468f
in elderly patients, 2482
in Jehovah's Witness patient, 2482–2483
infection and, 2487–2488
intrahospital transport in, 2487
mechanical ventilation after, 2485–2487, 2485t, 2486f, 2486t
neck, 2479
neurologic assessment in, 2453–2454, 2454t
nutritional support in, 2488
orthopedic, 2476–2479, 2477t, 2478t
pain management in, 2483–2485
pulmonary, 2479–2480
rib, 2480–2481
sepsis in, 2454
soft tissue, 2479
stress response to, 2892, 2892f
surgical management in, 2454, 2455f
training for, 2452
Trazodone, hepatotoxicity of, 2221t
Treadmill exercise testing, in coronary artery disease evaluation, 1064, 1066, 1066t
Tremor, shivering-like, 1580–1581
Trendelenburg, Friedrich, 37
Trendelenburg position, nerve injury with, 1162
Treppe phenomenon, 727–728
Triamcinolone, 2817t
neuromuscular blocking agent interaction with, 518
Triazolam, in outpatient premedication, 2596, 2596t
Trichloroethylene, 18
structure of, 106f
Trichothecenes, 2515t
Tricuspid insufficiency, pulse oximetry errors and, 1451t
Tricuspid regurgitation
cardiac output measurement in, 1329
central venous pressure monitoring in, 1299, 1300f
pulmonary artery catheter-related, 1306
Tricuspid stenosis, central venous pressure monitoring in, 1299–1300, 1300f
Tricuspid valve, Ebstein's malformation of, 2011
Tricyclic antidepressants, 1121, 1123
channel blockade by, 870
electroconvulsive therapy and, 2654
in chronic pain, 2771–2772
Trifascicular block, 1409, 1410f
Trifluoroacylated adducts, antibodies to, 759
Trigeminal nerve block, 1704–1706, 1705f, 1706f, Plates 1 and 2
pediatric, 1754
Trigeminal nerve injury
brainstem auditory evoked potentials in, 1531
diagnostic nerve blocks in, 1705–1706, 1706f
electromyography in, 1538
Trigger point injections, in chronic pain, 2772
Triglycerides, in sepsis, 2904
Triiodothyronine (T_3), 1045–1046, 1045t
in brain death, 2960
in sepsis, 2897
Trimethaphan, in kidney failure, 2187

Trishydroxymethylaminomethane (THAM), in neonatal acidosis, 2357
Trismus-masseter spasm, in malignant hyperthermia, 1180–1181, 1181f
Trisomy 21, 1099
Tropomyosin, 733, 734f
Troponins, 733, 734f
Trousseau, Armand, 37
Trousseau's sign, 1051, 2540
Tuberculosis, in health care worker, 3159
Tubing, anesthetic loss to, 142, 143t
d-Tubocurarine, 492–494, 493f, 493t, 494f, 497t, 508–509, 508f, 510f
autonomic effects of, 511, 511t, 512t
calcium interaction with, 517
dosage for, 501t
dysrhythmias and, 513
elimination of, 506t, 509
furosemide interaction with, 517–518
histamine release in, 512
hypotension with, 512
in elderly patients, 526
in malignant hyperthermia, 1182
in renal failure, 2184–2186, 2185t
metabolism of, 506t, 509
neuromuscular junction effects of, 867–868, 867f
pharmacodynamics of, 500t, 502t
renal failure and, 527, 528t
succinylcholine interaction with, 515
Tuffier, Theodore, 8, 25f, 26
Tularemia, 2503
Tumor lysis syndrome, in children, 2869–2870
Tumor necrosis factor
in brain death, 2960
in sepsis, 2900–2901
Turbulent flow, 1202–1203, 1203f, 1221–1222
Turner, J. R., 21
TURP syndrome, 1766–1767, 2193–2194, 2194t. See also Transurethral resection of prostate (TURP).
Tympanic nerve block, 2548
Tympanoplasty, 2549
Tyndall, John, 39
Tyramine
metabolism of, 634
monoamine oxidase inhibitors interaction with, 658
Tyrosine, in hepatic failure, 2916

U

Ulcerative colitis, 1108
Ulcers, in children, 2864
Ulnar artery, cannulation of, 1274
Ulnar nerve
electrical stimulation of, 1559, 1559f
in muscle relaxant monitoring, 484, 485, 485f
injury to
position-related, 1152t, 1154–1155, 1154f, 1156t
with orthopedic surgery, 2411–2412, 2412t
Ulnar nerve block, 1693–1694
Ultrafiltration, in pediatric hemolytic-uremic syndrome, 2860
Ultrasonography
cardiac, 1363–1385. See also Transesophageal echocardiography.
during carotid endarterectomy, 2104
in cardiac output monitoring, 1334–1336
in central venous catheter insertion, 1291, 1291f
in ischemic optic neuropathy, 2997
in pediatric neurologic impairment, 2855
in renal blood flow measurement, 790, 1505, 1505f
M-mode, 1365, 1367
Ultrasound, 1207–1208, 1207f, 1223–1225, 1364. See also Ultrasonography.
Umbilical artery catheter, 2356, 2843–2844
Umbilical block, 1751, 1751f
Umbilical cord, prolapse of, 2336
Umbilical vein, catheterization of, 2356–2357
Unconsciousness, postoperative, 2717–2718
Univent bronchial blocker system, 1883–1885, 1884f, 1885f, 1885t
independent, 1887–1889, 1887f, 1888f, 1888t
indications for, 1887
just-seal volume and, 1886–1887
limitations of, 1885–1886, 1886t
technique of, 1889–1890

Unroofed coronary sinus, pulmonary artery catheter monitoring and, 1303
Upper extremity nerve block, 1686–1695
    anatomy for, 1686, 1687f
    axillary, 1690–1692, 1691f, Plate 5
    infraclavicular, 1690
    interscalene, 1686, 1688–1689, 1688f
    intravenous, 1695
    median nerve, 1693, 1693f, 1694f
    midhumeral, 1693
    musculocutaneous, 1694
    supraclavicular, 1689–1690, 1689f, 1690f, Plate 3
    ulnar nerve, 1693–1694
Urea
    during pregnancy, 2311, 2311t
    in renal function monitoring, 1498
Uremia, 1100–1101
Uremic polyneuropathy, 1097
Ureter
    calculi of
        extracorporeal shock wave lithotripsy for, 2195–2197
        laser lithotripsy for, 2194
    innervation of, 2175–2176, 2176f
    peristalsis of, 1488, 1488f
Urethra, innervation of, 2176, 2177f
Uric acid, during pregnancy, 2311, 2311t
Urinalysis, 955–956, 959t, 1493, 2180
Urinary tract. See Bladder; Kidney(s); Ureter; Urethra.
Urine
    blood in, 1493
    concentration of, 2179
        in children, 2859t
    creatinine in, in renal function monitoring, 1498
    electrolytes of, 2180
    formation of, 789, 1486–1488, 1765
    glucose in, 2180
    lysozyme in, 1493
    nitrogen in, 2906, 2906t
    osmolality of
        in diabetes insipidus, 1768
        in renal function monitoring, 1497, 1497t
    output of
        after kidney transplantation, 2242
        in pediatric shock, 2836
        in renal function monitoring, 1496
    oxygen tension of, 1506
    pH of, 1493, 2180
    protein in, 1493, 2179
    renal concentration of, 784, 785f
    retention of
        epidural analgesia and, 2740–2741
        neuraxial anesthesia and, 1660
    sodium in, 789–790, 1498
    specific gravity of, 1496–1497
    tubular concentration of, 789
    urea in, 1498
Urine-to-plasma creatinine ratio, 789
Urine-to-plasma osmolar ratio, 789
URL (uniform resource locator), 2974, 2974f
Urokinase, bleeding with, 1117
Urticaria, blood transfusion and, 1817
USENET, 2977
Uterus, disorders of, 2336
Utrophin, 872

V

Vaccination, 1104
    anthrax, 2517
Vacco v Quill, 3188
VACTERL association, 2396
Vaginal delivery, 2315–2323
    bupivacaine for, 2322
    butorphanol for, 2318
    2-chloroprocaine for, 2323
    external cephalic version during, 2338
    fentanyl for, 2317–2318
    hemorrhage with, 2333–2336, 2334f, 2335f
    inhalational analgesia for, 2319
    levobupivacaine for, 2323
    lidocaine for, 2323
    local anesthetics for, 2322–2323
    meperidine for, 2317, 2317f
    opioids for, 2317–2318, 2317f
    pain during, 2315, 2315f, 2316f
    psychoprophylaxis for, 2315, 2317
    regional analgesia for, 2319–2322
        backache after, 2329

Vaginal delivery (Continued)
    regional analgesia for (Continued)
        complications of, 2326, 2328–2329
        continuous, 2321, 2321t
        dural puncture with, 2326, 2328
        epidural, 2319–2320
        hematoma with, 2329
        hypotension with, 2326
        infectious complications of, 2329
        neurologic complications of, 2329
        paracervical, 2322
        paravertebral, 2322
        patient-controlled, 2322, 2322t
        patient evaluation for, 2319
        post-dural puncture headache with, 2328
        pudendal, 2322
        spinal, 2320
        spinal-epidural, 2320–2321, 2321f
        total spinal block with, 2328–2329
    remifentanil for, 2318
    ropivacaine for, 2323
    sedative-tranquilizers for, 2318–2319
    transcutaneous electrical nerve stimulation for, 2317
    umbilical cord prolapse during, 2336
    uterine rupture during, 2336
Vaginismus, 2201
Vagus nerve, 623
Valdecoxib, in outpatient premedication, 2597
Valerian (Valerian officinalis), 607t, 611–612
Valproic acid, hepatotoxicity of, 2221t
Valsalva hemorrhagic retinopathy, 3003
Valsalva maneuver, 739
    visual impairment with, 3014
Valvular heart disease, 1077–1083, 1078f, 1078t, 1080t–1081t, 1082t, 1083f. See also specific disorders.
Valvuloplasty, balloon, 2652
Van Haller, Albrecht, 9
Van Helmont, Jean Baptiste, 12
Van Slyke, Donald D., 6
Vandam, Leroy, 27
Vanillylmandelic acid, 634
Vapor pressure, 284–285, 284f
Vaporization, latent heat of, 285
Vaporizer(s), 284–296
    add-on, 310
    Datex-Ohmeda S/5 ADU cassette, 292–293, 292f
    Datex-Ohmeda Tec 6, 281t, 289–292, 290f
    for desflurane, 289–292, 290f
    latent heat of vaporization and, 285
    physics of, 284–285, 284f
    specific heat and, 285
    thermal conductivity and, 285
    vapor pressure and, 284–285, 284f
    variable-bypass, 285–289, 285f–288f
Variable-bypass vaporizer, 285–289
    carrier gas composition and, 287–288, 288f
    contamination of, 288
    flow rate of, 286
    hazards of, 288–289
    intermittent back pressure and, 286f, 287, 287f
    leaks in, 289
    misfilling of, 288
    operating principles of, 285–286, 285f, 286f
    overfilling of, 288
    pumping effect and, 286f, 287, 287f
    safety features of, 288
    temperature of, 286–287, 286f, 287f
    tipping of, 288
    underfilling of, 288
    vapor interlock (vapor exclusion) system of, 289
Varices, esophageal, 761, 1053
Variola, in biological warfare, 2518t
Vasa previa, 2335
Vascular surgery
    β-blockers before, 2068, 2069f
    cardiac assessment for, 2054–2063, 2056f–2057f
        ambulatory electrocardiography in, 2060t, 2061
        angiography in, 2062, 2063t, 2064t
        cardiac catheterization in, 2062, 2063t, 2064t
        dipyridamole thallium imaging in, 2060t
        dobutamine stress echocardiography in, 2060t, 2061–2062
        echocardiography in, 2061
        electrocardiography in, 2059
        hypertension in, 2056
        myocardial perfusion imaging in, 2059–2061, 2061f
        previous myocardial infarction in, 2058–2059, 2059t

Vascular surgery (Continued)
    cardiac assessment for (Continued)
        prior coronary artery bypass in, 2062–2063
        prior percutaneous transluminal coronary angioplasty in, 2063
        radionuclide ventriculography in, 2062
        risk indices for, 2054–2055, 2058t
    cardiac morbidity and, 2053–2054, 2054t, 2106–2107, 2106f
    endovascular, 2089–2092, 2105–2106
    for abdominal aortic reconstruction, 2070–2081. See also Abdominal aorta, reconstruction of.
    for carotid disease, 2098–2106. See also Carotid endarterectomy.
    for lower extremity arterial insufficiency, 2092–2098, 2096f, 2096t, 2097f
    for thoracoabdominal aortic reconstruction, 2081–2089. See also Thoracoabdominal aorta, reconstruction of.
    hemodynamic monitoring in, 2068–2070
    mortality and, 2053–2054, 2054t
    myocardial infarction and, 2053–2054, 2054t. See also Coronary artery bypass graft surgery.
    myocardial ischemia and, 2065–2068, 2065t, 2066t, 2106–2107, 2106f
        monitoring for, 2066–2068
        prevention of, 2065–2066, 2066f, 2067f, 2068
    prophylactic coronary artery revascularization and, 2054, 2055f
    pulmonary assessment for, 2063
    renal assessment for, 2065
Vasoactive intestinal polypeptide
    acetylcholine coexistence with, 620–621, 621f
    in cardiac function, 737t
Vasoconstriction
    intraoperative, 1584
    postoperative, 1584
    pulmonary
        hypoxic, 166–168, 167f, 168f, 684, 686–687, 687f
        in one-lung ventilation, 1891–1893, 1891f, 1892f
        inhaled anesthetics and, 166–170, 167f–169f, 1864–1865, 1865f
        inhibition of, 712
        threshold for, 1572, 1572f, 1573, 1573f, 1575
        during neuraxial anesthesia, 1578, 1578f, 1580
Vasodilation
    anesthesia-induced, 1584–1585, 1585f
    cerebral, 818, 828–829, 828f
    droperidol-related, 360
    in thermoregulation, 1573–1574
    pulse oximetry errors and, 1451t, 1452
Vasodilators
    after pediatric cardiopulmonary bypass, 2034
    hypoxia-induced vasoconstriction and, 687, 1892
    in children, 2837t, 2838–2839
Vasopressin
    in brain death, 2960
    in cardiac arrest, 2938
    in cardiac function, 737, 737t
    in diabetes insipidus, 1053
    in esophageal varices, 1053
    in water excretion, 1486
Vasospasm, in intracranial aneurysm, 2147–2148
Vastus medialis nerve block, pediatric, 1746, 1746f
VATER association, 2396
Vecuronium, 493t, 494, 495f, 497t
    autonomic effects of, 511, 511t, 512t
    bradycardia with, 513
    bronchospasm with, 514
    carbamazepine interaction with, 517
    cerebral physiology and, 831
    dosage for, 501t
    elimination of, 506t, 508, 511
    for tracheal intubation, 503–505, 503f, 504t
    hepatic metabolism of, 2213–2214, 2214f
    hepatobiliary disease and, 529–530, 529t
    hypothermia effects on, 516, 1582
    in children, 525, 2379, 2380t
    in elderly patients, 526
    in ICU patient, 533
    in kidney transplantation, 2241
    in myasthenia gravis, 541–542, 542f
    in obese patient, 1033
    in pediatric respiratory failure, 2849
    in renal failure, 2184–2186, 2185t
    in trauma patient, 2458
    magnesium sulfate interaction with, 516–517

Vecuronium (Continued)
  maintenance dose of, 515
  metabolism of, 506t, 507–508, 507t
  opioid interactions with, 423
  pharmacodynamics of, 500t, 502t
  recovery from, 1562–1563, 1562t, 1563f
  renal failure and, 527–528, 528t
  succinylcholine interaction with, 515
Vein of Galen, aneurysm of, 2151
Velocity, 1192, 1218–1219
Vena cava, superior, 1303, 1921f, 1922–1923
Venipuncture, for right internal jugular vein,
    1288–1289, 1288f
Venous air embolism, 2138–2142, 2139f, 2140f,
    2140t, 2141f
  detection of, 2139, 2139f, 2140f, 2140t
Venous oxygen, 1453, 1453f
Venous stasis, in obese patient, 1033, 1034
Venous thrombosis
  orthopedic surgery and, 2425–2426, 2425f, 2426f
  prophylaxis for, 1079, 1082–1083, 1082t
  transurethral resection of prostate and, 2190–2191
Venous-venous bypass, in liver transplantation,
    2250–2251
Ventilation, 681–682, 681f–683f. See also Respiration.
  alveolar, 681–682, 681f–683f, 691–692, 691f,
    697–698, 697f, 698f
  carbon dioxide effects on, 178–179
  collateral, 692
  failure of, 2811–2812, 2812f
  historical perspective on, 36–40, 36f
  in basic life support, 2923–2925
  in chronic obstructive pulmonary disease,
    177, 177f
  in pediatric life support, 2942
  inhaled anesthetic effects on, 170–181
    airway receptors and, 171–174, 174f
    apneic threshold and, 178, 178f
    carbon dioxide and, 177–179, 178f
    chemical stimuli and, 177
    hypoxia and, 179–181, 180f
    inflammation and, 181
    mechanoreceptors and, 171, 174–177,
      174f–177f
    pulmonary stretch receptors and, 173
    respiratory rate and, 171, 172f
  inhaled anesthetic uptake and, 131–132, 132f,
    136–137, 137f
  mask, 36–37, 1623–1624, 1623f, 1624f
  mechanical. See Mechanical ventilation.
  minute, 706, 706f, 1442, 1447, 1447t, 1465
  motor system in, 170f, 171
  one-lung, 1873–1900. See also One-lung
    ventilation.
  opioid effects on, 392–394, 393f, 393t
  pediatric, 2842–2843
  reflex control of, 170–171, 170f
  respiratory control system in, 170, 170f
  sensory system in, 170, 170f
  spontaneous, in open chest, 1868–1869, 1869f
  starvation effects on, 2892, 2893f
  voluntary, maximum, 1002
Ventilation-perfusion mismatch
  arterial gas tensions and, 1439–1440, 1440f,
    1441f
  arterial O_2 saturation vs. inspired Po_2 for, 1444,
    1444f
  in end-stage lung disease, 2264
  multiple inert gas (MIG) elimination technique
    for, 1443–1444, 1443f
Ventilation-perfusion ratio, 682–683, 682f, 683f
Ventilator(s)
  anesthesia, 298–301
    ascending bellows, 298–300, 299f
    bellows classification of, 298, 299f
    circuit designation of, 298
    cycling mechanism of, 298
    drive mechanism of, 298
    electrical problems in, 301
    leaks in, 301
    mechanical problems in, 301
    power source of, 298
    problems with, 300–301
    relief valve problems in, 301
    test of, 316
  historical perspective on, 35
  mechanical. See Mechanical ventilation.
Ventricles
  cardiac, 724–728. See also Left ventricle; Right
    ventricle.
  cerebral, surgery on, 2157–2158

Ventricular arrhythmias
  bupivacine-induced, 594–595
  etidocaine-induced, 594–595
  PTCA-related, 2649
  pulmonary artery catheter-related, 1304–1305
  succinylcholine-induced, 489
Ventricular bradyarrhythmia, 2933, 2933f
  in children, 2944
Ventricular fibrillation, 2935, 2937–2939
  after cardiac surgery, 1993
  automated external defibrillator for, 2928–2929
  electrocardiography in, 1404
  in children, 1732, 1732t, 2946–2947
  pulmonary artery catheter-related, 1304–1305
Ventricular pacing, central venous pressure
    monitoring in, 1299, 1299f
Ventricular premature beats, 1403–1404
Ventricular septal defect, 2009–2010, 2009t,
    2017–2018, 2017f, 2018f
  left ventricular end-diastolic pressure in, 1322t,
    1323
  pulmonary artery catheter monitoring in, 1314
Ventricular tachyarrhythmias, 2933–2935,
    2934f–2937f
  in children, 2944
Ventricular tachycardia, 2937f
  after cardiac surgery, 1993
  electrocardiography in, 1404
  hyperkalemia, 2938f
  pulseless, 2935, 2937–2939
    in children, 2946–2947
  with pediatric regional anesthesia, 1732, 1732t
Ventriculography, before peripheral vascular surgery,
    2062
Ventriculoperitoneal shunt, 2163
Venturi jet ventilation, for microlaryngoscopy, 2542
Venturi tube, 1203, 1204f
Verapamil, 1121–1122, 1122f
  contraindications to, 2935, 2937f, 2943
  in kidney failure, 2186–2187
  in supraventricular arrhythmias, 2933
  neuromuscular blockade interaction with,
    517, 523
Vertebrobasilar artery, aneurysm of, 2151
Vesicant agents, 2509–2510, 2509f, 2510f
Vestibular folds, 1618
Vestibulitis, 2201
Video-assisted thoracoscopy, 2566–2567
Videotelemetry, in awake craniotomy, 2159–2160
Vierrordt, Karl, 6
Vigilance, 3038–3040, 3039f, 3042–3043, 3042t
  during transesophageal echocardiography,
    3040–3041, 3041f
  sleep deprivation and, 3057
Vinamar, 18
Vinethene, 17
Viral encephalitis, in biological warfare, 2518t
Viral hemorrhagic fever, 2518t
Virchow, Rudolph, 12
Virtual reality patient simulators, 3075–3078
Viscera, anesthetic loss by, 135
Vision
  disturbances of, transurethral resection of prostate
    and, 2191, 3012–3014
  postoperative loss of, 2996–3015
    after thoracolumbar surgery, 2419–2420
    computed tomography in, 2997–2998
    cortical, 1158, 2996, 2997–2998, 2997t,
      3011–3012
    electroretinography in, 2998, 2999f
    eye examination in, 2996–2997, 2997t
    fluorescein angiography in, 2998, 3000f
    ischemic optic neuropathy and, 3005–3011.
      See also Optic neuropathy, ischemic.
    literature review of, 2996
    magnetic resonance imaging in, 2998
    occipital infarction and, 3011–3012
    ophthalmoscopy in, 2996–2997, 2998f
    perimetry in, 2997
    pupil signs in, 2996
    retinal ischemia and, 2998–3005. See also
      Branch retinal artery occlusion; Central
      retinal artery occlusion.
    symptoms of, 2996
    ultrasonography in, 2998
    visual evoked potentials in, 2998
    visual fields in, 2997
Visual evoked potentials, 1512–1513, 1532, 1532f,
    2998
  anesthetic effects on, 1532–1537, 1533t, 1535f,
    2535

Visual evoked potentials (Continued)
  barbiturate effects on, 1533t, 1536
  halothane effects on, 1533t, 1535, 1535f
  indications for, 1532
  inhaled anesthetic effects on, 1533t, 1534–1535,
    1535f
  physiologic factors and, 1537
Vital capacity, 694, 694f, 999–1000, 2715
Vitamin A, hepatotoxicity of, 2221t
Vitamin B_{12}, deficiency of, 1097
Vitamin C, after etomidate, 353
Vitamin D, in calcium physiology, 1771
Vitamin K-dependent factors, 749, 1117
Vitrectomy, visual impairment with, 3014
Vitreous, gas injection into, 2533
Vocal cords, 1618
  microlaryngoscopy for, 2542
  paralysis of, 2538
    after endotracheal intubation, 1650, 2547
    in children, 2854
Volatile anesthetics. See Inhaled anesthetics.
Volume-assured pressure support ventilation, 2824t,
    2825, 2825f
Volume of distribution, 68–69, 68f, 69f
  protein binding and, 76
  steady state, 69
Volume-targeted ventilation, 2821–2822, 2822t,
    2823f
Volumeter, 1203, 1203f
Volutrauma, 2487
Volvulus, midgut, 2863
Vomiting, 2720–2721
  acupuncture for, 612–613
  after laparoscopy, 2294
  after outpatient anesthesia, 2597–2599, 2597t,
    2614–2615, 2621
  anticholinesterase effects on, 523
  droperidol for, 360
  etomidate-related, 354
  middle ear surgery and, 2549
  opioid-related, 398, 399f
  strabismus surgery and, 2535–2536
  with epidural analgesia, 2740
  with neuraxial anesthesia, 1660
Von Anrep, Vasili, 22
Von Baeyer, Adolf, 29
Von Esmarch, Friedrich, 36–37, 36f
Von Euler, Ulf Svante, 8
Von Haller, Albrecht, 7f
Von Hohenheim, Theophrastus Bombastus, 11
Von Hufner, Carl Gustav, 5–6
Von Liebig, Justus, 16
Von Mickulicz-Radecki, Johann, 37
Von Willebrand's disease, 1116–1117
  in children, 2868
Vulvodynia, 2201
VX, 2504–2509, 2505t, 2506t, 2507f

W

Waddell signs, in chronic pain, 2766
Wake-up test, in spinal surgery, 2419
Walk test, in pulmonectomy patient, 1013
Wall, P., 10
Waller, Augustus, 40
Wang, J., 28
Warfarin, in orthopedic surgery, 2426
Warming
  for infant, 2371
  in hemorrhagic shock, 2466
  postoperative, 2721
  skin, 1585–1587, 1586f, 1587f
    postoperative, 1583
Warren, John, 14, 15f, 37
Washington v Glucksberg, 3188
Waste gases, 3151–3153
Water, 1599–1600
  body, 1764, 1764t, 1765t
    renal regulation of, 1485–1486, 1485f
  free clearance of, 1102
  molarity of, 1600
  self-ionization of, 1600
Water clearance, in renal function monitoring,
    1499
Water overload, in parenteral nutrition, 2913
Waters, Ralph M., 17–18, 34, 38f, 39, 40
Waterton, Charles, 30, 31f
Weakness syndromes, neuromuscular blockade in,
    530–533, 531t, 532t

Weapons of mass destruction, 2499, 2500. *See also* Chemical and biological warfare agents.
Weese, Helmut, 29
Weight, body. *See also* Obesity.
opioid effects and, 406, 407f
Weighted mean, 883
Wells, Horace, 13–14, 16
West Nile virus, transfusion-transmitted, 1818t, 1819
Wheatstone bridge, 1216, 1216f, 1220
Wheezing, 1464
in lung cancer, 1851
preoperative, 1088
White blood cell count, preoperative, 955t
Whytt, Robert, 8
Willis, Thomas, 8
Winnie, Alon P., 24
Wölfler, Anton, 23
Wood, Alexander, 19
Wood, E. H., 7
Woolley, Albert, 26
Work, definition of, 1196
Workstations, 273–274, 274f, 301–303, 303f
standards for, 274
World Wide Web, 2973–2978, 2974f
clinician-oriented information on, 2974–2975
department sites on, 2977

World Wide Web *(Continued)*
discussion groups on, 2977
journals on, 2975, 2975t
research-related information on, 2975–2977, 2976f
Wound healing, hypothermia effects on, 1582
Wren, Christopher, 28–29, 439, 440f
Wright, Lewis H., 32
Wright spirometer, 1205, 1205f, 1463
Wrist
median nerve block at, 1693, 1694f
radial nerve block at, 1693, 1694f
ulnar nerve block at, 1694, 1694f
Wulfing, H., 19
Wynter, Walter, 26

X

Xanthine dehydrogenase, 758
Xanthine oxidase, 758
Xanthines, 1124
Xenon
airway resistance and, 160–161
cardiovascular effects of, 215, 216f

Xenon *(Continued)*
metabolism of, 236–237, 236t
N-methyl-D-aspartate glutamate inhibition by, 121
oil-gas partition coefficient of, 115t
Xenopus oocyte, opioid effects on, 386–387, 386f

Y

Yerba, hepatotoxicity of, 2222t
Yersinia enterocolitica, transfusion-transmitted, 1818t, 1820
Yersinia pestis, 2503, 2517, 2518t
Yohimbine, 653

Z

Zafirlukast, hepatotoxicity of, 2221t
Zinn-Haller, circle of, 2994
Zion, Libby, 3162, 3163